AVERY'S DISEASES OF THE NEWBORN

AVERY'S DISEASES OF THE NEWBORN

Seventh Edition

H. William Taeusch, M.D.

Professor and Vice Chair of Pediatrics
University of California–San Francisco

Chief of Pediatrics
San Francisco General Hospital
San Francisco, California

Roberta A. Ballard, M.D.

Professor of Pediatrics, Obstetrics and Gynecology
University of Pennsylvania School of Medicine

Director, Division of Neonatology
Children's Hospital of Philadelphia and
   Hospital of the University of Pennsylvania
Philadelphia, Pennsylvania

W.B. SAUNDERS COMPANY
A Division of Harcourt Brace & Company
Philadelphia   London   Toronto   Montreal   Sydney   Tokyo

W.B. SAUNDERS COMPANY
A Division of Harcourt Brace & Company

The Curtis Center
Independence Square West
Philadelphia, Pennsylvania 19106

Library of Congress Cataloging-in-Publication Data

Avery's diseases of the newborn / [edited by] H. William Taeusch,
Roberta A. Ballard.—7th ed.

p.   cm.

Rev. ed. of: Schaffer and Avery's diseases of the newborn. 6th ed. c 1991.

Includes bibliographical references and index.

ISBN 0–7216–5751–6

1. Infants (Newborn)—Diseases.   I. Taeusch, H. William.   II. Ballard, Roberta A.
III. Schaffer and Avery's diseases of the newborn.
    [DNLM: 1. Infant, Newborn, Diseases   WS 420 A955 1998]

RJ254.S3   1998   618.92′01—dc21

DNLM/DLC   97-42374

AVERY'S DISEASES OF THE NEWBORN   ISBN 0–7216–5751–6

Last digit is the print number: 9   8   7   6   5   4   3   2   1

To the newborns,
infants, and parents
who challenge us
to get it right.

CONTRIBUTORS

STEVEN A. ABRAMS, M.D.
Associate Professor of Pediatrics, Baylor College of Medicine, Houston, Texas.
Parenteral and Enteral Nutrition; Special Gastrointestinal Concerns

N. SCOTT ADZICK, M.D.
C. Everett Koop Professor of Pediatric Surgery, University of Pennsylvania School of Medicine; Surgeon-in-Chief, Children's Hospital of Philadelphia, Philadelphia, Pennsylvania.
Fetal Surgery

MARILEE C. ALLEN, M.D.
Associate Professor of Pediatrics, Johns Hopkins University School of Medicine; Associate Director of Neonatology, Johns Hopkins Hospital; Co-Director of the NICU Developmental Clinic, Kennedy Krieger Institute, Baltimore, Maryland.
Outcome and Follow-Up of High-Risk Infants

MAUREEN ANDREW, M.D., F.R.C.P.
Professor of Pediatrics, McMaster University and Hamilton Civic Hospitals Research Centre, Hamilton, Ontario; Professor of Pediatrics, The Hospital for Sick Children, Toronto, Ontario, Canada.
Hemostatic Disorders in Newborns

MARY ELLEN AVERY, M.D.
Thomas Morgan Rotch Distinguished Professor of Pediatrics, Harvard Medical School; Physician-in-Chief Emeritus, Children's Hospital, Boston, Massachusetts.
History and Epidemiology; Malformations of the Mediastinum and Lung Parenchyma

PHILIP L. BALLARD, M.D., Ph.D.
Professor of Pediatrics, University of Pennsylvania School of Medicine; Director of Neonatal Research, Children's Hospital of Philadelphia, Philadelphia, Pennsylvania.
General Strategies of Fetal Development; Hormonal Influences on Fetal Development

ROBERTA A. BALLARD, M.D.
Professor of Pediatrics, Obstetrics and Gynecology, University of Pennsylvania School of Medicine; Director, Division of Neonatology, Children's Hospital of Philadelphia and Hospital of the University of Pennsylvania, Philadelphia, Pennsylvania.
Nonimmune Hydrops; Resuscitation in the Delivery Room; Disorders of the Chest Wall and Diaphragm

STEPHEN BAUMGART, M.D.
Professor and Vice Chairman, Department of Pediatrics, Thomas Jefferson University, Jefferson Medical College, and Thomas Jefferson University Hospital, Philadelphia, Pennsylvania; Pediatrician, A.I. DuPont Children's Hospital, Wilmington, Delaware.
Temperature Regulation of the Premature Infant

XYLINA BEAN, M.D.
Associate Professor of Pediatrics, Charles R. Drew University and University of California–Los Angeles; Director of Neonatology, King/Drew Medical Center, Los Angeles, California.
Perinatal Substance Abuse

STEPHANIE A. BERMAN, M.S.W., L.C.S.W.
Supervisor, Maternal and Child Health Social Work Services, University of California–San Francisco, San Francisco, California.
Caring for Parents of Infants in Intensive Care

MERTON BERNFIELD, M.D.
Clement A. Smith Professor of Pediatrics and Professor of Cell Biology, Harvard Medical School; Director, Joint Program in Neonatology, Children's Hospital, Boston, Massachusetts.
General Strategies of Fetal Development

GERARD T. BERRY, M.D.
Professor, University of Pennsylvania School of Medicine; Senior Physician, Children's Hospital of Philadelphia, Philadelphia, Pennsylvania.
Introduction to the Metabolic or Biochemical Genetic Diseases; Inborn Errors of Carbohydrate, Ammonia, Amino Acid, and Organic Acid Metabolism

CAROL LYNN BERSETH, M.D.
Associate Professor of Pediatrics, Newborn Section and Pediatric Gastroenterology and Nutrition Section; Associate Professor, Center for Ethics, Baylor College of Medicine; Pediatrician, Texas Children's Hospital, Ben Taub General Hospital, Texas Women's Hospital, and Methodist Hospital, Houston, Texas.
Developmental Anatomy and Physiology of the Gastrointestinal Tract; Disorders of the Teeth, Mouth, and Neck; Disorders of the Esophagus; Disorders of the Stomach; Disorders of the Intestine and Pancreas; Disorders of the Liver; Disorders of the Umbilical Cord, Abdominal Wall, Urachus, and Omphalomesenteric Duct; Ascites and Peritonitis; Parenteral and Enteral Nutrition; Special Gastrointestinal Concerns

DIANA W. BIANCHI, M.D.

Associate Professor, Departments of Pediatrics, Obstetrics, and Gynecology, Tufts University School of Medicine; Chief, Division of Genetics, Department of Pediatrics, New England Medical Center, Boston, Massachusetts.

Prenatal Genetic Diagnosis; Genetic Examination of the Newborn Infant

MARY L. BRANDT, M.D.

Associate Professor of Surgery and Associate Professor of Pediatrics, Baylor College of Medicine, Houston, Texas.

Gastrointestinal Surgical Emergencies of the Newborn

LELA W. BRINK, M.D.

Assistant Professor, Department of Pediatrics–Pediatric Critical Care, University of North Carolina School of Medicine; Director, Pediatric Intensive Care Unit, North Carolina Children's Hospital, Chapel Hill, North Carolina.

Preoperative and Postoperative Care of the Newborn with Congenital Heart Disease

MICHAEL BROOK, M.D.

Pediatric Cardiologist, University of California–San Francisco, San Francisco, California.

Evaluation of Newborns with Possible Cardiac Problems

LU ANN BROOKER, R.T.

Research Assistant, Hamilton Civic Hospitals Research Centre, Hamilton, Ontario, Canada.

Hemostatic Disorders in Newborns

MITCHELL S. CAIRO, M.D.

Attending Physician, Director of Cancer Research, Pediatric Hematology-Oncology, Childrens Hospital of Orange County, Orange, California.

Leukocyte Disorders in the Newborn

VALERIE CHARLTON, M.D., M.P.H.

Professor of Pediatrics, University of California–San Francisco; Director, Extracorporeal Life Support, University of California Medical Center, San Francisco, California.

Fetal Growth: Nutritional Issues (Perinatal and Long-Term Consequences)

RONALD I. CLYMAN, M.D.

Professor of Pediatrics and Senior Staff Member, Cardiovascular Research Institute, University of California–San Francisco, San Francisco, California.

Patent Ductus Arteriosus in the Premature Infant

ROBERT M. COHN, M.D.

Associate Professor, Department of Pediatrics, University of Pennsylvania School of Medicine; Deputy Director, Clinical Laboratories, and Senior Physician, Division of Metabolism, Children's Hospital of Philadelphia, Philadelphia, Pennsylvania.

Lysosomal and Peroxisomal Disorders Presenting in the Newborn

F. SESSIONS COLE, M.D.

Professor of Pediatrics, Cell Biology and Physiology and Vice Chairman, Edward Mallinckrodt Department of Pediatrics, Washington University School of Medicine; Director Division of Newborn Medicine, Medical Director of the Pediatric Region, St. Louis Children's Hospital, St. Louis, Missouri.

Immunology; Fetal/Newborn Human Immunodeficiency Virus Infection; Viral Infections of the Fetus and Newborn; Bacterial Infections of the Newborn; Other Specific Bacterial Infections; Fungal Infections; Protozoal Infections: Congenital Toxoplasmosis and Malaria; Infections with Spirochetal and Parasitic Organisms

ANTHONY CORBET, M.B., B.S.

Clinical Professor of Pediatrics, University of Texas Health Science Center; Partner, South Texas Newborn Associates; Attending Neonatologist, Santa Rosa Children's Hospital, Southwest Texas Methodist Hospital, Methodist Women's and Children's Hospital, San Antonio, Texas.

Lung Development and Function; Control of Breathing; Pulmonary Physiology of the Newborn; Principles of Respiratory Monitoring and Therapy; Therapies for Intractable Respiratory Failure; Disorders of the Transition; Air Block Syndromes; Chronic Lung Disease; Neonatal Pneumonias; Diseases of the Airways; Malformations of the Mediastinum and Lung Parenchyma; Accumulation of Fluid in the Pleural Space; Disorders of the Chest Wall and Diaphragm

JOHN L. COTTON, M.D.

Assistant Professor of Pediatrics, Division of Pediatric Cardiology, School of Medicine, University of North Carolina at Chapel Hill; Attending Physician, University of North Carolina Hospitals, Chapel Hill, North Carolina.

Fetal Cardiology/Telemedicine

NANCY B. ESTERLY, M.D.

Professor of Pediatrics and Professor of Dermatology, Medical College of Wisconsin; Chief, Dermatology Service, Children's Hospital of Wisconsin, Milwaukee, Wisconsin.

Newborn Skin: Basic Concepts; Congenital and Hereditary Disorders of the Skin; Infections of the Skin; Common Newborn Dermatoses; Cutaneous Congenital Defects

JACQUELYN EVANS, M.D., F.R.C.P.

Clinical Associate Professor of Pediatrics, University of Pennsylvania School of Medicine; Director, Community Neonatology, Children's Hospital of Philadelphia, Philadelphia, Pennsylvania.

Acid-Base, Fluid, and Electrolyte Management; Clinical Evaluation of Renal and Urinary Tract Disease; Renal Insufficiency and Acute Renal Failure; Renal Vascular Disease in the Newborn

DELBERT A. FISHER, M.D.

Professor of Pediatrics and Internal Medicine Emeritus, University of California–Los Angeles School of Medicine, Los Angeles; Senior Scientist, Walter Martin Research Center, Harbor-UCLA Medical Center, Torrance; Senior Science Officer, Quest Diagnostics–Nichols Institute, San Juan, Capistrano, California.

Disorders of the Thyroid Gland

ELMAN G. FRANTZ, M.D.

Associate Professor, Pediatrics (Cardiology), University of North Carolina School of Medicine; Director, Pediatric Cardiac Catheterization Laboratory, University of North Carolina Hospitals and Clinics, Chapel Hill, North Carolina.

Evaluation of Newborns with Possible Cardiac Problems; Therapeutic Cardiac Catheterization

MICHAEL D. FREED, M.D.

Associate Professor of Pediatrics, Harvard Medical School; Senior Associate in Cardiology and Chief, Cardiology Inpatient Service, Children's Hospital, Boston, Massachusetts.

Evaluation of Newborns with Possible Cardiac Problems

ROBERT H. FRIESEN, M.D.

Clinical Professor of Anesthesia and Pediatrics, University of Colorado School of Medicine; Associate Director of Anesthesiology, The Children's Hospital, Denver, Colorado.

Anesthesia and Analgesia: Issues for the Fetus and Newborn

WILLIAM M. GILBERT, M.D.

Associate Professor of Obstetrics/Gynecology, University of California–Davis; Chief of Obstetrics, University of California–Davis Medical Center, Sacramento, California.

Placental Function and Diseases: The Placenta, Fetal Membranes, and Umbilical Cord

BERTIL E. GLADER, Ph.D., M.D.

Professor of Pediatrics, Stanford University School of Medicine; Director, Division of Hematology/Oncology, Lucille Packard Children's Hospital, Stanford, California.

Erythrocyte Disorders in Infancy

JAN GODDARD-FINEGOLD, M.D.

Associate Professor of Pediatrics and Pathology, Division of Pediatric Neurology, Baylor College of Medicine and Texas Children's Hospital, Houston, Texas.

Introduction and Overview of Antenatal Central Nervous System Insults; The Intrauterine Nervous System; The Nervous System During Birth; The Newborn Nervous System

MICHAEL GOMEZ, M.D.

Attending Neonatologist, Santa Rosa Children's Hospital, Southwest Texas Methodist Hospital, and Women's and Children's Hospital, San Antonio, Texas.

Principles of Respiratory Monitoring and Therapy; Therapies for Intractable Respiratory Failure

PEGGY GORDIN, M.S., R.N.

Director, Neonatal Nursing, Children's Hospital of Philadelphia, Philadelphia, Pennsylvania.

Issues in Nursing Care of the Newborn

PETER A. GORSKI, M.D., M.P.A.

Assistant Professor of Pediatrics, Harvard Medical School; Director of Education, The Brazelton Institute, Boston Children's Hospital; and Executive Director, Massachusetts Caring for Children Foundation, Boston, Massachusetts.

Behavioral Assessment of the Newborn

CAROL L. GREENE, M.D.

Associate Professor of Pediatrics, University of Colorado School of Medicine; Director, Inherited Metabolic Diseases Clinic, Children's Hospital and University of Colorado Health Sciences Center, Denver, Colorado.

Lysosomal Storage and Peroxisomal Disorders Presenting in the Newborn

JEAN-PIERRE GUIGNARD, PROF. DR. MED.

Professor of Pediatrics, University Children's Hospital; Director, Pediatric Nephrology Unit, Centre Hospitalier Universitaire, Lausanne, Switzerland.

Renal Morphogenesis and Development of Renal Function

G. WILLIAM HENRY, A.B., M.D.

Professor of Pediatrics and Chief, Pediatric Cardiology, University of North Carolina School of Medicine; Attending Physician, University of North Carolina Hospitals and North Carolina Children's Hospital, Chapel Hill, North Carolina.

Evaluation of Newborns with Possible Cardiac Problems

THOMAS HANSEN, M.D.

Professor of Pediatrics and Chairman, Department of Pediatrics, Ohio State University School of Medicine; Medical Director and Acting Chief Executive Officer, Children's Hospital, Columbus, Ohio.

Lung Development and Function; Control of Breathing; Pulmonary Physiology of the Newborn; Principles of Respiratory Monitoring and Therapy; Therapies for Intractable Respiratory Failure; Disorders of the Transition; Air Block Syndromes; Chronic Lung Disease; Neonatal Pneumonias; Diseases of the Airways; Malformations of the Mediastinum and Lung Parenchyma; Accumulation of Fluid in the Pleural Space; Disorders of the Chest Wall and Diaphragm

ANDREW HULL, B.Med.Sci., B.M.B.S., M.R.C.O.G.

Instructor, Reproductive Medicine, University of California–San Diego; Fellow, Maternal-Fetal Medicine, University of California–San Diego Medical Center, San Diego, California.

Antepartum Fetal Assessment; Preterm Labor and Birth

BERNARD S. KAPLAN, M.B., B.Ch.

Professor of Pediatrics and Professor of Medicine, University of Pennsylvania School of Medicine; Director of Nephrology, Children's Hospital of Philadelphia, Philadelphia, Pennsylvania.

Developmental Abnormalities of the Kidneys; Glomerulonephropathies and Disorders of Tubular Function

PAIGE KAPLAN, M.B., B.Ch.

Professor of Pediatrics, University of Pennsylvania School of Medicine; Senior Physician, Children's Hospital of Philadelphia and Hospital of the University of Pennsylvania, Philadelphia, Pennsylvania.

Connective Tissue Disorders and Skeletal Dysplasias

THOMAS KELLY, M.D.

Assistant Clinical Professor of Reproductive Medicine, University of California–San Diego School of Medicine, La Jolla; Perinatologist, University of California–San Diego Medical Center, San Diego; Consultant, Scripps Memorial Hospital, La Jolla; Consultant, Mercy Hospital, San Diego, California.

Maternal Medical Disorders of Fetal Significance: Seizure Disorders, Hypertension, and Isoimmunization

SOOK Z. KIM, M.D., Ph.D.

Fellow in Genetics, Harvard Medical School and Children's Hospital, Boston, Massachusetts.

Newborn Screening

KENNETH G. KUPKE, M.D.

Neonatologist and Clinical Geneticist, Neonatology Associates, Northside and Scottish Rite Hospitals, Atlanta, Georgia.

Genetics of Common Problems Presenting in the Newborn; Specific Genetic Disorders Presenting in the Newborn; Human Teratogens

RITA T. LEE, M.D.

Associate Professor of Pediatrics and Neurology, Division of Pediatric Neurology, Baylor College of Medicine and Texas Children's Hospital, Houston, Texas.

The Newborn Nervous System

ROBERT LEVIN, Pharm.D.

Professor, Department of Clinical Pharmacy, University of California–San Francisco School of Pharmacy; Clinical Professor, Department of Pediatrics, University of California–San Francisco School of Medicine; and Associate Director of Pharmaceutica, San Francisco General Hospital, San Francisco, California.

Appendix 1: Drugs

HARVEY L. LEVY, M.D.

Associate Professor of Pediatrics, Harvard Medical School; Senior Associate in Medicine/Genetics, Children's Hospital, Boston, Massachusetts.

Newborn Screening

HELEN LILEY, M.B., B.Ch.

Clinical Senior Lecturer, Christchurch School of Medicine, Otago University; Director, Neonatal Intensive Care Unit, Christchurch Women's Hospital, Christchurch, New Zealand.

General Strategies of Fetal Development

JAMES P. LOEHR, M.D.

Assistant Professor of Pediatrics, Division of Pediatric Cardiology, University of North Carolina at Chapel Hill; Attending Physician, North Carolina Memorial Hospital, Chapel Hill, North Carolina.

Fetal Cardiology/Telemedicine

WALKER A. LONG, M.D.

Associate Professor of Pediatrics and Director, Office of Telemedicine, University of North Carolina at Chapel Hill School of Medicine; Attending Physician, University of North Carolina Hospital, Chapel Hill; Attending Physician, New Hanover Regional Medical Center, Wilmington, North Carolina.

Evaluation of Newborns with Possible Cardiac Problems; Fetal Cardiology/Telemedicine

JAMES R. MacMAHON, M.D., C.M.

Assistant Professor of Pediatrics, Stanford University School of Medicine; Director of Well Baby Nursery, Stanford Health Services, Stanford, California.

Bilirubin Metabolism; Physiologic Jaundice; Bilirubin Toxicity, Encephalopathy, and Kernicterus; Unconjugated Hyperbilirubinemias; Obstructive Jaundice Due to Biliary Atresia and Neonatal Hepatitis; Other Conjugated Hyperbilirubinemias; Management of Neonatal Hyperbilirubinemia

ERIC B. MALLOW, M.D.
Assistant Professor of Pediatrics, Section of Newborn Medicine, Pennsylvania State University College of Medicine; Attending Neonatologist, Hershey Medical Center, Hershey, Pennsylvania.
Nonimmune Hydrops

ALMA MARTINEZ, M.D., M.P.H.
Assistant Professor of Pediatrics, University of California–San Francisco and San Francisco General Hospital, San Francisco, California.
Perinatal Substance Abuse

KATHERINE K. MATTHAY, M.D.
Professor of Pediatrics and Director, Pediatrics Oncology, University of California–San Francisco, San Francisco, California.
Congenital Malignant Disorders

MARIE C. McCORMICK, M.D., Sc.D.
Sumner and Esther Feldberg Professor of Maternal and Child Health, Harvard School of Public Health; Professor of Pediatrics, Joint Program in Neonatology, Harvard Medical School; Associate Pediatrician, Newborn Medicine, Brigham and Women's Hospital; Senior Associate in Medicine (Newborn) and Co-Director of the Infant Follow-up Program, Children's Hospital; and Senior Associate in Pediatrics, Beth Israel Deaconess Medical Center, Boston, Massachusetts.
Long-Term Costs of Perinatal Disabilities

WILLIAM C. MENTZER, M.D.
Professor of Pediatrics and Director, Division of Hematology/Oncology, Department of Pediatrics, University of California–San Francisco, San Francisco, California.
Erythrocyte Disorders in Infancy

ELI M. MIZRAHI, M.D.
Associate Professor of Neurology and Pediatrics, Neurophysiology Department and Division of Pediatric Neurology, Baylor College of Medicine and Texas Children's Hospital, Houston, Texas.
The Newborn Nervous System

THOMAS R. MOORE, M.D.
Professor and Chairman of Reproductive Medicine, University of California–San Diego School of Medicine; Chief of Obstetrics and Gynecology, University of California–San Diego Medical Center, San Diego, California.
Endocrine Disorders in Pregnancy; Maternal Medical Disorders of Fetal Significance: Seizure Disorders, Hypertension, and Isoimmunization; Abnormalities of Fetal Growth; Antepartum Fetal Assessment; Intrapartum Fetal Management

FRANK A. OSKI, M.D. (deceased)
Late Given Professor of Pediatrics and Chairman, Department of Pediatrics, Johns Hopkins University School of Medicine, Baltimore, Maryland; Late Pediatrician-in-Chief, Johns Hopkins Hospital Children's Center, Baltimore, Maryland.
Bilirubin Metabolism; Physiologic Jaundice; Bilirubin Toxicity, Encephalopathy, and Kernicterus; Unconjugated Hyperbilirubinemias; Obstructive Jaundice due to Biliary Atresia and Neonatal Hepatitis; Other Conjugated Hyperbilirubinemias; Management of Neonatal Hyperbilirubinemia

J. COLIN PARTRIDGE, M.D., M.P.H.
Associate Professor, Department of Pediatrics, University of California–San Francisco and San Francisco General Hospital, San Francisco, California.
Perinatal Substance Abuse

DANIEL H. POLK, M.D.
Professor, Division of Neonatology, Department of Pediatrics, Northwestern University Medical School; Acting Chief, Division of Neonatology, Northwestern University Medical School; Chief of Pediatric Services, Prentice Women's Hospital; and Director, Neonatal Services, Children's Memorial Hospital, Chicago, Illinois.
Disorders of the Adrenal Gland; Abnormalities of Sexual Differentiation; Disorders of the Thyroid Gland; Disorders of Carbohydrate Metabolism

GRAHAM E. QUINN, M.D.
Associate Professor of Ophthalmology, University of Pennsylvania School of Medicine; Pediatric Ophthalmologist, Children's Hospital of Philadelphia, Philadelphia, Pennsylvania.
Retinopathy of Prematurity

DOUGLAS RICHARDSON, M.D., M.B.A.
Associate Professor of Pediatrics, Harvard Medical School; Associate Professor of Maternal and Child Health, Harvard School of Public Health; Director of Newborn Research, Beth Israel Deaconess Medical Center; and Attending Neonatologist, Joint Program in Neonatology at BIDMC, Brigham and Women's, and Children's Hospitals, Boston, Massachusetts.
History and Epidemiology; Long-Term Costs of Perinatal Disabilities

DONALD ROBERTS, M.D.
Fellow, Maternal-Fetal Medicine, University of California–San Diego Medical Center, San Diego, California.
Intrapartum Fetal Management

JOSEPH ROSENTHAL, M.D.
Director, Pediatric Bone Marrow Transplant Program,
City of Hope National Medical Center, Duarte,
California.
Leukocyte Disorders in the Newborn

LEWIS P. RUBIN, M.D.
Associate Professor of Pediatrics, Brown University School
of Medicine; Attending Neonatologist, Women and
Infants Hospital, Providence, Rhode Island.
Disorders of Calcium and Phosphorus Metabolism

RICHARD J. SCHANLER, M.D.
Professor of Pediatrics, Baylor College of Medicine,
Houston, Texas.
Parenteral and Enteral Nutrition

ISTVAN SERI, M.D., Ph.D.
Assistant Professor of Pediatrics, University of
Pennsylvania School of Medicine; Clinical Director of
Newborn Services, Children's Hospital of Philadelphia,
Philadelphia, Pennsylvania.
*Acid-Base, Fluid, and Electrolyte Management; Clinical
Evaluation of Renal and Urinary Tract Disease; Renal
Insufficiency and Acute Renal Failure; Renal Vascular
Disease in the Newborn*

BARBARA SHEPHARD, M.D.
Assistant Professor of Pediatrics, Tufts University School
of Medicine, New England Medical Center, Boston,
Massachusetts.
*Genetics of Common Problems Presenting in the
Newborn; Specific Genetic Disorders Presenting in the
Newborn*

ELAINE C. SIEGFRIED, M.D.
Associate Professor of Pediatrics and Dermatology, St.
Louis University Health Sciences Center, St. Louis,
Missouri.
*Newborn Skin: Basic Concepts; Congenital and
Hereditary Disorders of the Skin; Infections of the Skin;
Common Newborn Dermatoses; Cutaneous Congenital
Defects*

JOHN C. SINCLAIR, M.D.
Professor, Departments of Pediatrics and of Clinical
Epidemiology and Biostatistics, McMaster University,
Hamilton, Ontario, Canada.
Evaluation of Therapeutic Recommendations

SUSAN SNIDERMAN, M.D.
Professor of Clinical Pediatrics, University of California
Medical Center; Chief, Newborn Services, San Francisco
General Hospital, San Francisco, California.
*Initial Evaluation: History and Physical Examination of
the Newborn*

BRYAN SOHL, M.D.
Fellow in Maternal-Fetal Medicine, University of
California–San Diego School of Medicine, San Diego,
California.
Abnormalities of Fetal Growth

DAVID K. STEVENSON, M.D.
Harold K. Faber Professor and Chief, Division of
Neonatal and Developmental Medicine, and Associate
Chair, Department of Pediatrics, Stanford University
School of Medicine, Stanford, California.
*Bilirubin Metabolism; Physiologic Jaundice; Bilirubin
Toxicity, Encephalopathy, and Kernicterus; Unconjugated
Hyperbilirubinemias; Obstructive Jaundice Due to Biliary
Atresia and Neonatal Hepatitis; Other Conjugated
Hyperbilirubinemias; Management of Neonatal
Hyperbilirubinemia*

ROBERT W. SWEETMAN, M.D.
Assistant Professor, Department of Pediatrics, University
of Louisville School of Medicine; Attending Physician,
Pediatric Hematology/Oncology, Kosair Children's
Hospital, Louisville, Kentucky.
Leukocyte Disorders in the Newborn

H. WILLIAM TAEUSCH, M.D.
Professor and Vice Chair of Pediatrics, University of
California–San Francisco; Chief of Pediatrics, San
Francisco General Hospital, San Francisco, California.
*Perinatal Substance Abuse; Initial Evaluation: History and
Physical Examination of the Newborn*

JANET A. THOMAS, M.D.
Assistant Professor of Pediatrics, University of Colorado
School of Medicine, Children's Hospital, and University of
Colorado Health Sciences Center, Denver, Colorado.
*Lysosomal Storage and Peroxisomal Disorders Presenting
in the Newborn*

TIVADAR TULASSAY, M.D., D.Sc.
Professor of Pediatrics and Physician-in-Chief,
Department of Pediatrics, Semmelweis University
Medical School, Budapest, Hungary.
*Renal Insufficiency and Acute Renal Failure; Renal
Vascular Disease in the Newborn*

ROBERT J. VOSATKA, M.D., Ph.D.
Assistant Professor, Columbia University, New York, New
York.
*Modes of Inheritance; Techniques of Molecular Diagnosis;
Other Resources for Genetic Diagnosis*

MARTIN WALKER, B.M., B.S., D.M.

Assistant Professor, University of California–San Diego
School of Medicine; Director of Maternity Services,
University of California–San Diego Medical Center, San
Diego, California.

Preterm Labor and Birth

ROBERT M. WARD, M.D.

Professor of Pediatrics, University of Utah, Salt Lake City,
Utah.

Pharmacologic Principles and Practicalities

STEPHEN A. ZDERIC, M.D.

Assistant Professor of Surgery, University of Pennsylvania
School of Medicine; Staff Physician, Division of Urology,
Children's Hospital of Philadelphia, Philadelphia,
Pennsylvania.

*Developmental Abnormalities of the Genitourinary
System; Infection of the Urinary Tract and Vesicoureteral
Reflux*

PREFACE

While mainstream pediatrics focused on diseases of infants and young children, specific interest in the diagnosis and treatment of the few recognized problems of the newborn and the premature infant (feeding, temperature regulation, inanition, icterus, hemorrhagic diseases, and "diatheses") was a smaller parallel rivulet until the 1960s, when the ability to quantify respiratory insufficiency with micro samples of blood from arterial catheters for gas tensions and the ability to treat the condition with ventilators led to the change from obstetrics-based nurseries to neonatal intensive care units. Thereafter, a small number of remarkably cooperative and creative clinical investigators and medical scientists from Europe, Asia, and North America, aided by continual contributions from basic science and technology, have helped develop the field to its present level of sophistication. The degree of medical progress in the diagnosis and care of newborn infants in just a few decades is unprecedented in nearly all other medical fields of endeavor.

This seventh edition of *Diseases of the Newborn* continues a legacy started by Alexander Schaffer in Baltimore nearly 40 years ago. These editions have tracked the exponential success of neonatology in the care of newborns. At the time, Schaffer, a former chief resident of Dr. Edwards Park, was a leading practitioner at the Hospital for Women of Maryland and Johns Hopkins Hospital. For years he accumulated case histories of newborns, the compilation of which led to the first edition of this text. Dr. Mary Ellen Avery joined Dr. Schaffer for the third edition. She emphasized the scientific contributions to the field particularly in the areas of fetal and neonatal physiology.

The sixth edition appeared in 1991 and summarized the standard of care in what now is known as the "presurfactant era" of neonatology. Since that time the infant mortality rate has dropped from about 10 to 7 deaths per 100 livebirths in the United States, a result largely due to the use of antenatal glucocorticoids to mature the fetus as well as the widespread advent of surfactant treatment for respiratory distress syndrome (hyaline membrane disease) over this period.

Many diagnostic and therapeutic problems are receding in the face of current investigations and changes in the state of the art since the last edition: to name a few advances—improved molecular biologic techniques for diagnosis, better imaging techniques, rapid solid-state microchemistries, inhaled nitric oxide, improved formulations and new uses for surfactant, new approaches to ventilation, clearer definition of the limits of viability, improved extracorporeal membrane gas exchange (ECMO), antivirals and anti-infection strategies, improved nutrition, ability to arrest the progression of retinopathy, indomethacin for closure of the ductus, improved pain control, better surgical and nonsurgical approaches to fetal and neonatal anomalies, and information access on the Internet.

Some problems remain intractable, such as the exposure of the fetus to tobacco, alcohol, and illicit drugs. The major problem in perinatology, that of premature birth, has not changed, nor at the time of this writing is any major new understanding of its cause or prevention foreseen.

Therefore, major long-term problems that are simply defined remain unsolved, while extraordinary discoveries both solve and create new problems. Lambs have been cloned in 1997, raising the specter of cloning of humans. Human genes have been inserted into fetal fibroblast donor nuclei to produce lambs that contain the gene for human clotting factor IX in the germline, allowing for easy animal production of human proteins for treatment of human diseases. In 1998, normal human somatic cells have been immortalized. The spectacular successes of science relevant to reproduction can be contrasted with the sluggish progress in ethical application of these discoveries and application of known solutions to the societal ills that ultimately produce many of our major medical problems in neonatology.

In this seventh edition, much of the book has been rewritten with many new section editors and a 30% increase in contributors. The art of writing a textbook lies in the choice of what is important and in choosing the right line of specificity versus generality. As in past editions, we have attempted to create a book that is primarily for those caring for newborns who may want to review areas unfamiliar to them or to screen for diagnostic or therapeutic approaches for an unusual condition, or refresh themselves on how our contributors have defined the state of the art for common problems. We have tried to present diagnosis and treatment options for the most important and/or the most frequent conditions, and we have emphasized areas that are currently advancing rapidly or that remain problematic. We have not included sections on aftercare of the infant who has required intensive care or who may leave the nursery with a chronic condition.

In this age of the Internet and rapid access to current medical information, the question may arise as to why create yet another textbook. Are current journal articles and reviews not sufficient? At least for the time being, we submit that a text can allow a second order of expertise to put medical information into context, and we thank our many contributors for their wisdom and success in carrying out this aim. In part this edition is the product of feedback that you readers have given us about prior editions. We look forward to knowing whether you find this edition useful, whether you like the format, what omissions you find, and God forbid, what errors of commission you may perceive. We would like to hear from you.

We are also grateful to our patient, wise, and persistent publishers (Janice Gaillard and Judy Fletcher of W.B. Saunders Company), our copy editor (Sue Reilly), our colleagues who have educated us, our academic institutions, and our families for their support of this effort.

H. William Taeusch
Roberta A. Ballard
Mary Ellen Avery

CONTENTS

PART I
INTRODUCTION

CHAPTER **1**

History and Epidemiology

Mary Ellen Avery and Douglas Richardson

EARLY HISTORY OF CARE OF INFANTS*

In the late nineteenth century and the early part of the twentieth century, deaths from infectious diseases in the first years of life were so common that it is not surprising to find so few students of premature birth and so few articles concerning the special needs of low-birth-weight infants. These small infants were not expected to live. In fact, in the 1940s, some authorities thought of birth weights under 3 pounds as incompatible with life, although rare exceptions have always been noted, as in the case of the Dionne quintuplets, each of whom weighed under 3 pounds. Dafoe, who delivered them on May 28, 1934, wrote, "There were no scales small enough to measure accurately the separate weights of the babies, but on May 29 [second day] their combined weight was 13 pounds 6 ounces." They were born about 2 months early. Marie, the smallest, weighed 1 1/2 pounds. Yvonne, the largest, weighed nearly 3 pounds. (Accurate scales arrived on the 6th day.)

As many infectious diseases came under control, physicians turned more attention to newborn infants. It is believed that Budin in Paris published one of the first articles on premature infants in 1888. At about the same time, German physicians, one of whom was Finkelstein in Berlin, became interested in the problems of premature infants and initiated special programs for their care. In Helsinki in 1912, Ylppo pioneered the research on prenatal and postnatal growth and the pathology of prematurity. Hess, an American physician who studied in Europe, was the founder of the first center in the United States that specialized in the care of premature infants; it was established at Michael Reese Hospital in Chicago in 1922. The criterion of 2500 g (5 1/2 pounds) birth weight was used to distinguish a premature from a term infant, and not until much later was the concept of gestational age widely accepted as being a more accurate measure of the stage of development of an infant than weight alone. Physicians who were first concerned with premature infants noted early that these children were unable to maintain their own body temperatures. Various devices, including double-walled metal tubs with the space between the walls filled with circulating hot water, were in use in Europe and Russia in the mid-nineteenth century. Other devices, such as hot-water bottles and electrically heated cribs, were the predecessors of

more modern incubators. Occasionally the whole room in which many infants were cared for was kept at high temperatures, paving the way for the modern requirements that constant year-round temperature and humidity be maintained in nurseries where premature infants are cared for.

It is not surprising that much attention was focused on ways to feed immature infants, particularly because some of them were too weak to suckle. Tarnier is credited with introducing the practice of tube feeding for premature infants at the Maternity Hospital in Paris in 1884. Many other devices for oral and nasal feeding of premature infants have been advocated, but it wasn't until the 1980s that research made total intravenous nutrition possible.

The first physicians to care for premature infants considered human milk indispensable for the infants' welfare. In fact, in 1828, Meissner in Leipzig, Germany, was so convinced of the benefits of human milk that he advised that the infant be fed mother's milk and be given enemas of milk and at least two milk baths daily.

A number of physicians, puzzled by the inability of many infants to tolerate cow's milk, proceeded to compare the chemical composition of human milk and cow's milk, with the expectation that they could modify cow's milk to make it a suitable substitute for mother's milk. In this regard, a number of extreme views were taken, including the idea that cow's milk contained an indigestible protein, casein, and that diluting it with 3 or 4 parts of water to keep the protein under 1% would improve the infant's tolerance to this formula. Later it was believed that a higher percentage of protein was necessary to support adequate growth. Over subsequent years, many pediatricians have continued the quest for optimal nutrition for infants of different gestational ages and birth weights, but no universal recommendations have emerged.

Some early students of the care of premature infants recognized that any epidemic of respiratory tract infection and diarrheal disease could be lethal among such infants. In fact, special units for the care of premature infants were established to avoid the dangers of acquired infection and epidemics within nurseries by providing separate facilities from other patients who might bring infection to the infants. In the early 1900s, guidelines for the care of premature infants specified that incubators that could be easily disinfected should be constructed, that rooms should not be crowded, that personnel should wear gowns and should wash their hands before handling an infant, and that infants with infections should be isolated from other infants.

---

*Portions of this chapter appeared in Avery ME, Litwack G: Born Early. Boston, Little, Brown, 1983.

It was not until after World War II that a new generation of pediatricians focused their attention on the medical needs of premature infants and, working with pathologists, began to study systematically the causes of death that occurs immediately after birth. Examination of the infants after death showed that not infrequently their lungs were airless, and when examined microscopically they revealed a material, hyaline membrane, in the terminal air spaces that should not have been there. From this discovery, the condition was named *hyaline membrane disease*; thereafter, the label *respiratory distress syndrome* was applied to describe the outstanding clinical feature of the disorder. The first obvious assumption was that the material in the lungs was aspirated from the amniotic fluid, but the absence of it in the lungs of infants who were stillborn made that an improbable explanation. Miller made this point in an article in 1949, suggesting that the affected infants acquired the membranes postnatally. Thereafter, many pathologists and pediatricians, through careful study of the infants during their first 2 or 3 days of life and examination of the infants' lungs after death, clarified this condition as a functional immaturity of the lung with respect to synthesis of pulmonary surfactants. Because of improved understanding, deaths from hyaline membrane disease have decreased from about 10,000 per year in the United States in the 1950s to about 2000 per year in 1994.

Meanwhile, the 1940s were marked by the construction of many new nurseries and the introduction of more modern incubators that increased the amount of oxygen in the infants' environment. At that time, it was evident that some of the infants had a newly recognized eye condition, called *retrolental fibroplasia*, which by the late 1940s became the leading cause of blindness in the United States. The epidemic of this new condition led to enormous speculation about its origin and to a number of studies that culminated in the work by Ashton in England and Patz in Washington. When they exposed kittens to environments containing high levels of oxygen, the kittens acquired the condition. Although oxygen undoubtedly plays a role in retrolental fibroplasia, more recent experience with very immature infants indicates that other as yet undefined circumstances contribute to its severity.

Increased attention to the needs of small infants resulted in a gradual reduction in their mortality. As more very small infants lived, new problems came into focus. Some could be defined for the first time because of the availability of chemical techniques that allowed measurements on small samples of blood. The application of these newer methods of measurement permitted study of the physiologic adaptations of the infant to extrauterine life. Parallel to increased attention to the infants themselves was the evolution of a field of perinatal physiology, stimulated largely through the work of Barcroft and colleagues in England in the 1930s and 1940s and subsequently by many of their students and colleagues in the 1950s and thereafter. *The Physiology of the Newborn Infant* by Smith brought many of these observations to the attention of pediatricians in 1945 and again in the three subsequent editions of his classic text.

The fetal lamb became the experimental model because the animal could be delivered from the uterus with umbilical cord intact and continue to receive oxygen and remove carbon dioxide across the placenta, since the uterus of the ewe does not contract under these circumstances. More recently, it has been possible to place catheters in vessels in the fetal lamb in the uterus for more physiologic studies of fetal life. The events surrounding delivery could then be witnessed in a carefully controlled manner with suitable measurements made to define qualitatively and quantitatively changes in the heart and lungs at birth. From these studies, many suggestions emerged for less direct measurements on the infants that were possible without jeopardizing their condition.

RAPID ADVANCES IN NEONATAL CARE: SCIENTIFIC AND TECHNICAL FOUNDATIONS (1955–1970)

The first edition of *Diseases of the Newborn*, which was published in 1960, presented the observations of Schaffer and a few colleagues in diagnosis and management of newborn infants and, in so doing, provided a description of the state of neonatology in the late 1950s and stimulated another generation to try to augment the scientific base of a new subspecialty that had long been relatively neglected in medical research and education. Consider for example that neonatal mortality was *20.5/1000* live births in 1950 compared with *7.5/1000* live births in the United States in 1985, *5.4/1000* live births in 1993, and *4.8/1000* live births in 1995.

The major diagnostic tools in the 1960s were cultures, blood counts, urinalyses, radiographs, and biopsies. Little was known of the pathophysiology of many major disorders of infancy. Pulmonary hyaline membrane syndrome of the newborn was diagnosed by chest film and follow-up of clinical course. Surfactant deficiency, described the year before (1959), was not sufficiently recognized to warrant much discussion in the early 1960s. Blood gases were not available, respirators were not used, and half the infants in whom the diagnosis was made died.

Mother's milk was recommended for term infants, but if the mother did not wish to nurse her infant, she was assured the baby would thrive on evaporated milk diluted with water (2 parts to 3), with 5% to 10% added carbohydrate. Premature infants had been observed to have fat intolerance and hence were given half-skimmed milk with added carbohydrate to achieve an average intake of 120 cal/kg per day. Little discussion related to infants smaller than 1300 g (3 pounds) because only 28% survived in 1954.

In the early 1960s, serial amino acid measurements in the blood of the infants receiving the accepted half-skimmed milk formula revealed transient elevations of phenylalanine and tyrosine that could be damaging to the developing brain. Banking of breast milk, which was common in the 1950s, was markedly decreased when formulas of modified cow's milk became available. Breast-milk banks have little chance of reappearing now that it is known that viruses can be transmitted by breast milk, and infants without maternal antibody protection can become infected.

This level of active research attracted a larger number of young clinicians into the special care units, where they began to apply their evolving knowledge of the fetus and newborn. This resulted in the use of intravenous glucose and bicarbonate, blood gas analysis, and improved incubators. Early attempts at mechanical ventilation had dismal outcomes, but any survivors were considered evidence of success.

EMERGENCE OF NEONATAL INTENSIVE CARE (1971–1989)

A clinical breakthrough in neonatal care was the introduction of continuous positive airway pressure (CPAP) by Gregory and associates (1971). This technique had a powerful and immediate effect on the survival of sick premature infants, but it required around-the-clock care by specialized physicians and nurses. This spurred development of neonatal intensive care units and the impetus to transfer sick newborns from community hospitals to such centers of newborn expertise. CPAP was soon successfully incorporated into strategies for mechanical ventilation that led to design of new ventilators specifically for newborns. The evolution of newborn intensive care required microchemical determinations that permitted controlled intravenous alimentation, devices to measure blood gases, and devices to monitor pulse, respiration, and blood pressure. The rapid influx of pediatricians specializing in newborn care led to the development of fellowships and subspecialty certification in neonatology. Nursing specialization developed concomitantly with a mission not only to provide care to the infants but also to be interactive with and supportive of the infants' families.

The advances in survival attributable to neonatal intensive care made it imperative to make intensive care unit services available to a wider population. Initially, this took the form of professionalizing the emergency transport of sick newborns from community hospitals to regional centers using skilled physician/nurse teams dispatched from neonatal centers. In a regionalized system, all hospitals are designated by level according to the intensity of obstetric and neonatal services they provide, including level I (normal birthing and newborn care); level II (common obstetric complications and intermediate newborn care); and level III (around-the-clock high-risk maternal care and intensive care for newborns, including subspecialty and surgical services). Regionalization also included the coordinated movement of patients between hospitals as their needs changed. Bed planning was undertaken on a regionwide basis to provide one level III bed and four to six level II beds per 1000 births. Other components of regionalization included outreach education to the community hospitals, uniform medical records, and standardized statistical reporting for the region. Although regionalization progressed differently in various areas of the United States, overall it had a major impact on reducing neonatal mortality (McCormick et al, 1985). Central to this success was the emerging practice of transferring high-risk mothers so that an increasing proportion of all very-low-birth-weight infants was born in perinatal centers. This concentration of patients and obstetric expertise, in turn, facilitated the development of the subspecialty of maternal-fetal medicine and of an array of new diagnostic and treatment technologies in obstetrics.

The field of neonatology became well established and emerged as the largest subspecialty within pediatrics. Neonatologists developed their own special areas of research interest, focusing on organ systems, epidemiology, and mobilization of the tools of cellular and molecular biology. This combination of basic science and clinical trials resulted in steady improvements in nutrition, ventilators, diagnostic technologies, catheters, and surgical techniques. In addition, changes in practice evolved from the relative isolation of sick infants to involvement of family members and primary nurses, and to consultations with other concerned members of society, including pediatricians and ethicists.

With the increasing survival of extremely premature infants came concern about a possible increase in numbers of handicapped survivors. Numerous studies were undertaken to document risk factors and outcomes. These have indicated that the *proportion* of handicapped infants has not changed, but the larger number of survivors has led to a larger total number of impaired survivors. Large trials have indicated the value of early educational intervention in optimizing longer-term outcomes (McCormick et al, 1993), and such developmentally appropriate care is being incorporated into nursery routines.

Innovations in neonatal anesthesia and surgical techniques have permitted earlier and more decisive intervention for a variety of major congenital anomalies. This has been most dramatic for congenital heart disease. Previously lethal conditions (such as transposition of the great vessels) can be definitively repaired in the newborn period, and others (such as hypoplastic left heart syndrome) can be successfully palliated. Long-term outcomes are improving steadily.

Extracorporeal membrane oxygenation (ECMO) was developed in the 1980s as a heroic treatment for total but reversible pulmonary failure. Early successes in treating persistent pulmonary hypertension of the newborn and diaphragmatic hernia led to widespread adoption of ECMO before its efficacy was established in randomized trials. Improving early medical treatments and ventilator strategies, and most recently, nitric oxide, have reduced the number of infants who require ECMO in the 1990s.

The emergence of a competitive health care environment in the 1980s significantly shaped neonatal intensive care in the United States. The ready availability of well-trained neonatologists and nurses and standardized neonatal technologies have facilitated the proliferation of level III centers, which are predominantly suburban and nonacademic. The traditional models of levels of care and regionalization are being replaced by entrepreneurial intensive care units and contract-based networks.

EXPANSION OF CLINICAL TRIALS TO ASSESS THERAPY: SURFACTANT ERA (1980–1996)

Administration of glucocorticoids to mothers 24 to 48 hours before delivery to accelerate fetal lung maturation was shown to be effective in the early 1970s. Numerous controlled trials confirmed efficacy and safety, but wide acceptance did not occur until the 1990s. Glucocorticoids are not appropriate in the event of precipitous labor or other maternal contraindications. Rapid acceptance of surfactant replacement therapy and the evidence that prenatal glucocorticoids act to "condition" the lung to enhance the efficacy of postnatal surfactant replacement have widened the use of both interventions.

Early successful clinical trials of surfactant replacement led to the globalization of neonatology in Europe, North America, and Japan. The evident clinical successes were followed by clear documentation of reduction of national neonatal mortality rates for respiratory distress syndrome, formerly the leading cause of death of liveborn preterm infants. Surfactant replacement therapy has had a profound impact on neonatal care as it has shifted the emphasis from acute survival to quality of survival. Increasing numbers of extremely premature survivors remain dependent on sophisticated nursing regimens. Nutritional issues are emerging to dominate neonatology along with optimizing developmental interventions, infection control, and environmental regulation.

The reduction in deaths from prematurity leaves congenital anomalies, asphyxia and meconium aspiration, and persistent pulmonary hypertension in term infants as major remaining challenges. Newer technologies or combinations of treatments indicate promise in early trials, including surfactant replacement, high-frequency oscillators, inhaled nitric oxide, and less invasive venovenous ECMO. The rapid expansion of prenatal diagnosis, made feasible by genetic probes and high-quality ultrasound, has permitted earlier identification, and counseling has facilitated multidisciplinary planning before birth for correctable anomalies and provided parental options for severe or lethal anomalies. The anticipated promise of fetal surgery remains largely unfulfilled. Neurologic morbidity among premature infants remains a significant problem, and it is the focus of extensive research aimed at preventing intracranial hemorrhage and white matter damage. The most effective strategy remains aggressive use of antenatal corticosteroids that reduce severity of respiratory distress and risk of intraventricular hemorrhage. An increase in retinopathy of prematurity has been related simply to the survival of larger numbers of extremely immature infants. Great variation in outcomes that has been described among centers may represent differences in the antecedent risks (birth weight, race, obstetric events, illness severity) or differences in the successful application of these neonatal intensive care unit technologies. Efforts to identify the most successful treatment strategies are emerging worldwide through the development of neonatal networks and standardized comparisons.

It has been customary in the conduct of prospective, controlled clinical trials to match the group receiving the intervention with those who receive a placebo. The matching has traditionally been on the basis of birth weight or gestational age (or both) and occasionally, where relevant, race. It has long been apparent that infants of given gestational age can have widely disparate birth weights, and similarly infants of like birth weights may be of different gestational ages. A more valid approach to constructing a comparable control group and in analyzing the results takes into consideration the severity of the illness to be treated. Both Tarnow-Mordi and colleagues (1990) in the United Kingdom and Richardson and coworkers (1993) in the United States have proposed similar scales for assessing the severity of illness as a predictor of neonatal mortality.

In an evaluation of the score, Richardson and coworkers (1993) showed that birth weight and severity of illness are each powerful independent predictors of neonatal mortality across a broad range of birth weights and that their effects are additive.

New questions focus on: How small is too small? When is a new treatment too expensive? What is the physician's responsibility with respect to starting or discontinuing life support systems in the face of major or irreversible medical problems? Attempts to involve the judicial system have not proven fruitful. Most neonatologists choose to individualize difficult decisions in consultation with the most concerned adults, chiefly parents, nurses, and primary care physicians. A consensus is almost always reached. The enormous costs of such infants at the borderline of viability and the increasing cost consciousness of society have led to substantial debate about whether a lower limit of gestational age (e.g., 23 to 24 weeks) can be defined as eligibility for neonatal intensive care. The tension between patient autonomy, the uncertainty of prognosis, and society's increasing unwillingness to bear the costs will continue over the coming decades.

DEFINITIONS OF TERMS USED IN CARE OF THE NEWBORN

In a clarification of definitions by the World Health Organization (WHO) in 1974, Dunn wrote,

> The perinatal period occupies less than 0.5% of the average life span, yet accounts in many countries for more deaths than the next 30 years. With the reduction in infant and childhood mortality, attention is increasingly being focused on the prevention of perinatal mortality.

The definitions agreed on by a WHO group in 1974 for reporting purposes remain appropriate in the 1990s. The perinatal period extends from the 28th completed week of pregnancy to the 7th day of life. Clearly, some infants survive after only 25 weeks' gestation, and, in the future, recording of these births and deaths will be appropriate in societies that are prepared to provide intensive care for newborns. Of course, infant deaths also occur after 7 days, and in the United States, neonatal deaths are often defined as deaths that occur within 28 days of birth, or, for local hospital purposes, deaths that occur before discharge from the hospital after preterm birth.

A reason to maintain the WHO nomenclature for worldwide comparisons relates to the incomplete records available in some societies for very immature infants. Although infants born before 28 weeks' gestation account for fewer than 1% of live births, careful recording of births and deaths and inclusion in national statistics penalize the countries that have the best reporting.

Preterm. Preterm is defined as less than 37 completed weeks', or 259 days', gestation. The definition is, of course, arbitrary, but it is based on the greater likelihood of conditions associated with immaturity, such as hyaline membrane disease, in the group of infants born before 259 days. For most developed countries, 37 completed weeks of gestation corresponds to a birth weight of 3000 g.

Stillbirth and Fetal Death. By definition, early fetal death occurs at less than 20 completed weeks of gestation, intermediate fetal death occurs at more than 20 and less than 28 completed weeks, and late fetal death occurs after 28 weeks. The term *stillbirth* is usually applied to late fetal deaths.

Live Birth. WHO defines live birth as

> The complete expulsion or extraction from its mother of a product of conception, irrespective of the duration of pregnancy, which after such separation, breathes or shows any other evidence of life, such as beating of the heart, pulsation of the umbilical cord, or definite movement of voluntary muscles, whether or not the umbilical cord has been cut or the placenta is attached; each product of such a birth is considered liveborn.

Term. Term defines births that occur from 37 to less than 42 completed weeks, measured from the day of onset of the last normal menstrual period (259 to 293 days, with an average of 280 days).

Post-Term. Post-term refers to births that occur at 42 or more completed weeks (294 days).

Early Neonatal Death. Early neonatal death describes the death of a liveborn infant during the first 7 completed days of life.

Late Neonatal Death. Late neonatal death refers to the death of a liveborn infant after 7 but before 28 completed days of life.

In-Hospital Death. Although this term is not included in the WHO system, the authors have found that it is useful to record as in-hospital neonatal mortality any death that occurs within a hospital period that is continuous from birth. Therefore, infants who die at 3 to 6 months or later and who have been hospitalized continuously from birth because of complications and chronic disease following respiratory distress syndrome, congenital anomalies, and other conditions are included in this category.

EPIDEMIOLOGY
Changing Social Scene in United States

Major changes in life-style and family composition affect the number of infants born and their morbidities. In 1900, children younger than 15 years of age were 34% of the population; in 1990, they were only 22%. Life expectancy at birth in 1920 was 54 years and in 1993 was 75.5 years. The number of children per family was only 1.8 in 1985. Births to unmarried mothers were 22.6% of white births and 68% of black births.

Marital status relates to unintended pregnancies, which,

in turn, is a marker for contraceptive failure (Forrest, 1994). An unintended pregnancy occurs if it had not been wanted at the time of conception, regardless of whether or not contraception was being used. Among unintended pregnancies there is a distinction between missed timing and unwanted conception. Missed-time conceptions are those that occur among women who at some time intended to be pregnant but not at the time they conceived. An unwanted conception occurs to a woman when she did not want to have any more pregnancies at all.

A woman can change her attitude with respect to a pregnancy as the pregnancy proceeds. Occasionally an unanticipated pregnancy can result in a much cherished newborn. These definitions are important because unintended pregnancies are far more likely to end in abortion than are intended pregnancies (Brown and Eisenberg, 1995). More than half of all unintended pregnancies end in abortion. These pregnancies are a major contribution to the 1.5 million abortions per year that have been performed for more than a decade. These data highlight the need for improved sex education and more safe and effective means of contraception.

Other less quantifiable social trends include frequent moves to other locations, often far from grandparents or other relatives. Immigration is increasing and with it considerable poverty and illnesses.

An increase in multiple-gestation pregnancies has occurred with assisted reproduction techniques (Luke and Keith, 1992). The number of mothers who delivered twins at Brigham and Women's Hospital, Boston, in 1991 was 221 compared with 146 in 1986. Higher-order multiple gestations increased by 19% per year, to 23 sets in 1990 from 8 sets in 1986 (Callahan et al, 1994). Many of the infants are preterm and require intensive care.

It is estimated that nearly one fifth of all children in the United States are poor, principally associated with adolescent pregnancies, single-parent households, and race. One third of black children live in a household with less than $14,335 annual income for a family of four, defined as the poverty level. Poverty is one of many risk factors associated with an increase in violence against individuals of all ages. Parenting practices are of crucial importance and provide the pediatrician with the possibility of early recognition and prevention (Rivara and Farrington, 1995).

A nationally representative survey of use of illicit drugs has revealed the wide use of stimulants and tranquilizers.* Among women in the 15- to 44-year-old age range, almost half have used illicit drugs once in their life, and 2 million have used cocaine, mostly in the form of crack. In the 1992 survey, it was estimated that 17 million women in that age range were smokers, and 2 million drank five or more alcoholic beverages on one or more occasions in the preceding month. An unexpected finding in the survey was that about 70% of women who reported using drugs also reported having been sexually abused before the age of 16. These women were characterized as having poor nutrition, low self-esteem, depression, and, if pregnant, an increased

---

*Data obtained from the National Institute on Drug Abuse, 5600 Fishers Lane, Rockville, MD 20857.

risk of preterm labor. In addition, they had a greater than expected incidence of sexually transmitted diseases.

From 1981 to 1997, the Centers for Disease Control and Prevention documented more than 488,300 cases of acquired immunodeficiency syndrome (AIDS) among women in the United States. Nearly 70% were related to either the woman's own injecting drug use or sexual contact with an injecting drug user.

Despite the wide publicity given to the adverse effects of cigarette smoking and alcohol use during pregnancy, it is estimated that approximately 19% of women used alcohol and 20% smoked cigarettes at some time during pregnancy. The national survey also found that illicit drug use was more prevalent in women who were not married and had had less than 16 years of formal education, were not working, and relied on some public source of funding to pay for their hospital stay.

These findings underscore the compelling need to consider the health of the mother and the adequacy of her support services whenever efforts are undertaken to reduce the morbidities and mortality of newborn infants.

Pregnancy Outcomes

The outlook for a successful outcome of pregnancy has improved dramatically (Fig. 1–1). A rough chronology of major advances is listed in Table 1–1. The impact of new knowledge and its application has resulted in an impressive reduction in deaths in the first year of life in the United States, with a 50% reduction in mortality rates from 1970 to 1985 and a 15% reduction in the rate of low-birthweight infants. Most of the reduction in infant mortality has been attributed to the decline in birth weight–specific mortality, presumably related to improvements in perinatal care. The number of deaths from respiratory distress syndrome and hyaline membrane disease in the United States in four different 5-year periods is shown in Table 1–2.

Race

Overall the mortality rate of nonwhite infants in the first year of life is twice as high as that of white infants. The higher rate of preterm births (12.8% in nonwhite compared with 7.4% for whites) was a large factor in the Massachusetts experience reported by Wise and coworkers (1985). The weight-specific mortality is actually lower in black infants weighing less than 2500 g (Table 1–3). Infant mortality rates by age and race from 1940 to 1992 are shown in Table 1–4.

The reasons for the relative advantage of blacks when they are born prematurely may relate to biologic factors, such as their accelerated lung maturation. The marked disadvantages in the first year of life of black infants born with weights greater than 2000 g are thought to be related to adverse socioeconomic factors (Miller and Jekel, 1987).

An interval of less than 9 months between pregnancies is associated with a greater prevalence of preterm birth and low birth weight among black women. This observation was seen among white women only with intervals of less than 3 months. An interpregnancy interval of less than 9 months was more than 10 times more common among black women in a study of 1922 women reported by Rawlings and colleagues (1995). This is surely a factor in understanding the continuing wide disparity in pregnancy outcome.

Maternal Age

In general, the best outcome of pregnancy takes place when the mother is over age 20 and under age 35. Extension of maternal age in either direction has generally been thought to result in an increase in infant mortality. Berkowitz and coworkers (1990) have reported that although pregnancy complications are increased, mortality need not be increased in pregnancies of healthy middle-class women. An association between the percentage of mothers under

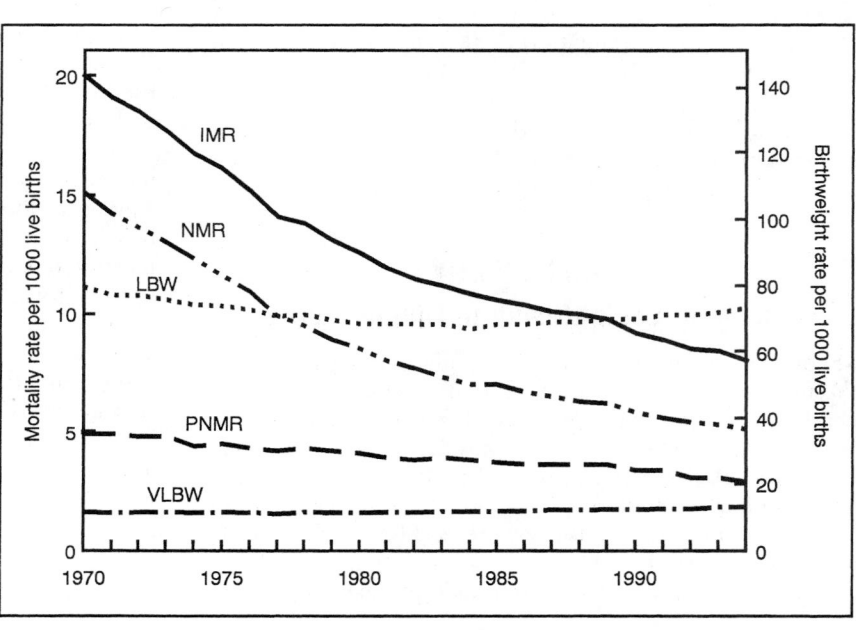

FIGURE 1–1. Infant, neonatal, and postneonatal mortality and low- and very-low birth weight, United States, 1970–1994. IMR, infant mortality rate; NMR, neonatal mortality rate; PNMR, postneonatal mortality rate; LBW, low birth weight (<2500 g); VLBW, very-low birth weight (<1500 g). (From Guyer B, Strobino DM, Ventura SJ, et al: Annual summary of vital statistics—1995. Pediatrics 98:1007–1019, 1996. Reproduced by Permission of PEDIATRICS, Vol 98 Pages 1007–1019 Copyright 1996.)

TABLE 1–1

Diagnostic and Therapeutic Advances in Perinatology

		Pediatrics	Obstetrics
1950–1960	Infections	Nursery infection control Widespread use of antibiotics	Control of endometritis Near elimination of maternal mortality in childbirth
	Rh disease	Exchange transfusions	Serum antibody testing Amniocentesis for bilirubin pigments
	Surgery	Patent ductus arteriosus, imperforate anus, tracheoesophageal fistula	Avoidance of midforceps delivery, improved maternal anesthesia
	Toxicology	Chloramphenicol, sulfonamides, oxygen	Thalidomide, diethylstilbestrol
1961–1970	Rh disease/jaundice	Phototherapy	Prevention of isoimmunization
	Regionalization	High-risk infants: neonatal intensive care units, intermediate care units	High-risk mothers: perinatal centers
	Monitoring	Intra-arterial blood gases, blood pressure Continuous heart and respiratory rate monitoring	Fetal heart rate monitoring, fetal scalp pH Maternal estrogen excretion
	Amniotic fluid testing	Improved genetic counseling	Detection of fetal genetic disorders
1971–1980	Infection	Cord blood serologies for detection of chronic fetal infections	Rubella immunization
	Respiratory disease	Ventilator support with continuous distending airway pressure Microtesting of blood samples Transcutaneous O_2 and CO_2 monitoring	Amniotic fluid testing for respiratory distress syndrome risk Prenatal glucocorticoids to accelerate fetal lung maturation Improved suctioning techniques for removal of meconium in the upper airway
	Genetics	Neonatal screening: phenylketonuria, hypothyroidism, and other metabolic diseases	Heterozygote definition (Tay-Sachs) Fetal diagnosis of hemoglobinopathies
	Imaging	Computed tomography scanning and ultrasonography	Fetal ultrasonography
	Prematurity	Intravenous hyperalimentation Psychological support of parents of intensive care unit infants	Suppression of premature labor
1981–1990	Respiratory disease	Surfactant replacement Selective use of extracorporeal membrane oxygenator for severe cardiopulmonary failure	
	Cardiac disorders	Indomethacin for closure of ductus Total correction of heart malformations in infancy O_2 saturation monitoring	
	Genetics		Expanded molecular diagnosis Percutaneous fetal blood sampling Expanded use of fetal ultrasonography
	Prematurity	Cryotherapy for retinopathy of prematurity	Improved access to prenatal care
1991–1998	Respiratory disease	High-frequency ventilation Permissive hypercapnia	
	Prematurity	Hearing screening Laser therapy for retinopathy	Fetal reduction after in vitro fertilization Molecular probe for diagnosis Rh isoimmunization
	Cardiac disorders	Transthoracic ligation of patent ductus Inhaled nitric oxide for pulmonary hypertension	
	Infection		Prenatal zidovudine for prevention of fetal infection with human immunodeficiency virus

age 20 years and infant mortality in four countries is shown in Table 1–5. Because pregnancy among adolescents occurs more commonly among mothers of lower socioeconomic status and more often among nonwhites than whites, assigning relative importance to these and other factors that coexist with young maternal age has been a challenge.

Several reasons are often cited for the rise in teenage pregnancies, principally the growing number of teenagers and the increase in sexual activity. In the United States, more than 900,000 teenage women between ages 15 and 19 become pregnant each year, and almost 25,000 are 15 years old or younger. Adolescent mothers contribute 19% of the births but have 26% of the low-birth-weight infants. These mothers have increased risks for death in childbirth, toxemia, anemia, and neurologic disorders in their offspring. On the average, infants born to adolescent mothers may be less well nurtured, have a greater risk of child abuse, and receive less health supervision as children. Similarly, adolescent mothers who have infants are more prone to marital dissolution and emotional disturbances. Obviously, causes and effects are difficult to unravel, but there is little doubt that for a young woman between 15 and 19 years of age, pregnancy may contribute to what Smith described in 1980 as "a dismal future of unemployment, poverty, dropping out of school, family breakdowns, emotional stress, dependency on public health agencies, and health problems for mother and child."

Pregnancy after age 40 years is associated with another set of hazards for the baby. For pregnant women over 40 years, a sharp increase in deaths around the time of birth (perinatal mortality) occurs with each subsequent year of age. After 40 years of age, the hazards are greater if it is the woman's first pregnancy rather than a subsequent pregnancy. One of the risks of pregnancy after age 40 years is the approximately 2.6% incidence of Down syndrome in the infant compared with an overall incidence of 0.15%. Another problem relates to diminished elasticity of the pelvic structures, which results in difficulties with delivery and a greater likelihood of preterm labor. Diagnostic amniocentesis for detection of chromosome abnormalities such as Down syndrome can alert the mother to that possibility and provide her with the option of abortion. Skillful obstetric management can reduce these hazards around the time of delivery.

TABLE 1–2

Annual Respiratory Distress Syndrome/Hyaline Membrane Disease Specific Mortality (U.S. Vital Statistics)

	1969–1973	1974–1978	1979–1983	1993*
White	7880	5945	3837	1490
Black	1989	1897	1345	740
Rates/1000 live births	2.89	2.47	1.46	
Change (%) in rates within 5-year period	+2.7	−9.4	−8.8	

*Provisional.

TABLE 1–3

Births, Neonatal Deaths, and Neonatal Mortality Rates by Race and Birth Weight: United States, 1987

		White	Black	Other	All Races
<500 g	no. live births	2778	2178	140	5096
	no. deaths	2476	1891	126	4493
	nmr	891.29	868.23	900.00	881.67
500–749 g	no. live births	4820	3579	272	8671
	no. deaths	3259	2118	168	5545
	nmr	676.14	591.79	617.65	639.49
750–999 g	no. live births	5752	3725	352	9829
	no. deaths	1772	763	87	2622
	nmr	308.07	204.83	247.16	266.76
1000–1249 g	no. live births	6690	3701	367	10,758
	no. deaths	957	307	48	1312
	nmr	143.05	82.95	130.79	121.96
1250–1499 g	no. live births	8087	4338	477	12,902
	no. deaths	583	174	33	790
	nmr	72.09	40.11	69.18	61.23
1500–1999 g	no. live births	32,274	15,668	1927	49,869
	no. deaths	1133	347	63	1543
	nmr	35.11	22.15	32.69	30.94
2000–2499 g	no. live births	109,505	48,282	7569	165,356
	no. deaths	1146	350	75	1571
	nmr	10.47	7.25	9.91	9.50
2500–2999 g	no. live births	424,055	150,628	33,706	608,389
	no. deaths	1223	417	73	1713
	nmr	2.88	2.77	2.17	2.82
3000–3499 g	no. live births	1,079,851	243,647	71,200	1,394,698
	no. deaths	1307	368	71	1746
	nmr	1.21	1.51	1.00	1.25
3500–3999 g	no. live births	945,180	130,569	45,214	1,120,963
	no. deaths	735	176	48	959
	nmr	0.78	1.35	1.06	0.86
4000–4499 g	no. live births	307,121	28,812	11,603	347,536
	no. deaths	236	54	13	303
	nmr	0.77	1.87	1.12	0.87
4500–4999 g	no. live births	56,051	4730	1993	62,774
	no. deaths	77	15	4	96
	nmr	1.37	3.17	2.01	1.53
5000+ g	no. live births	6869	740	271	7880
	no. deaths	57	27	3	87
	nmr	8.30	36.49	11.07	11.04
Total°	no. live births	2,992,659	641,661	175,350	3,809,670
	no. deaths	15,552	7397	861	23,810
	nmr	5.20	11.53	4.91	6.25

°Total includes cases with unknown birth weights.
nmr, neonatal mortality rate (per 1000 live births).
Adapted by the Harvard Institute for Reproductive and Child Health, Harvard Medical School, from the National Linked Birth/Infant Death Data Set: 1987 Birth Cohort. Atlanta, National Center for Health Statistics, Centers for Disease Control and Prevention, 1987.

Prenatal Care

Numerous studies have documented the higher incidence of prematurity and growth retardation in infants of mothers from a lower socioeconomic group, and among the findings is a specific association of these developmental problems with lack of prenatal care (Miller and Jekel, 1987; Wise et al, 1985). Many confounding factors complicate the interpretation of these and similar findings. It is not known what aspects of prenatal care have a significant bearing on the outcome of a pregnancy. It seems reasonable to give much credit to health education (Kogan et al, 1994). The mothers who want to do what is best for their babies are

TABLE 1–4

Infant Mortality Rates by Age and Race: Selected Years

	Year							% Decline, 1940–1991
	1992°	1991†	1990†	1990‡	1980‡	1960†	1940‡	
Total§	848.7	8.9	9.2	9.2	12.6	26.0	47.0	81.1
White		7.3	7.6	7.7	11.0	22.9	43.2	83.1
Black		17.6	18.0	17.0	21.4	44.3	72.9	75.9
B:W ratio		2.4	2.4	2.2	1.9	1.9	1.7	
<28 d	538.6	5.6	5.8	5.8	8.5	18.7	28.8	80.6
White		4.5	4.8	4.9	7.5	17.2	27.2	83.5
Black		11.2	11.6	10.9	14.1	27.8	39.9	71.9
B:W ratio		2.5	2.4	2.2	1.9	1.6	1.5	
Postneonatal	309.7	3.4	3.4	3.4	4.1	7.3	18.3	81.4
White		2.8	2.8	2.8	3.5	5.7	16.0	82.5
Black		6.3	6.4	6.1	7.3	16.5	33.0	80.9
B:W ratio		2.3	2.3	2.2	2.1	2.9	2.1	

°Provisional, estimated from a 10% sample of deaths; rates per 100,000 live births. 1940–1991 final; rates per 1000 live births.
†Race according to race of mother (introduced in 1989).
‡Race according to race of child.
§Includes races other than white and black.
  Data from National Center for Health Statistics. From Wegman ME: Annual summary of vital statistics, 1993. Pediatrics 94:792, 1994. Reproduced by Permission of PEDIATRICS, Vol 94 Page 792 Copyright 1994.

probably the ones who elect prenatal care. Early detection of risk factors, hypertension, and poor or excessive weight gain surely dictates appropriate interventions, which on the whole improve the outcome of pregnancy.

GLOBAL PERSPECTIVES IN THE FUTURE OF NEWBORN CARE

Currently, focus is on the national embarrassment of the relatively high infant mortality rate in the United States compared with other developed nations and the persistently high mortality among nonwhite infants. Goals set in 1979 for the year 1990 were not met and require a concerted federal and state effort to reduce the social and economic barriers to access to prenatal care in the 1990s (Table 1–6).

There is increasing worldwide attention to the disparities in infant mortality and the circumstances that are deemed responsible. The lowest rates ever recorded were set in the mid-1980s when Japan achieved an infant mortal-

ity rate of 5.5 per 1000 live births, followed closely by Finland and Sweden, with the United States well behind at 10.6. By 1993, Japan reported a rate of 4.4 per 1000 live births, Sweden 4.8, and the United States 8.3 (Wegman, 1994). These so-called developed countries have vastly lower infant mortality rates than most of the countries in the world. According to data collected by the United Nations Children's Fund in 1992, at least 32 countries reported infant mortality rates of greater than 100 per 1000 live births. These included many of the countries of sub-Saharan Africa, Southeast Asia, and Central and South America.

Maternal Perspectives

In some societies, the maternal mortality rate is also shockingly high. In the developed countries, the maternal mortality rate is approximately 1 per 10,000 births, whereas among the poorest countries it is more than 100 times as high.

Priorities must differ in the context of the existing situations in each country. In a careful examination of the problem in the Zaria area of northern Nigeria, Harrison (1985) commented that preventing stillbirths of term infants who died in utero before their mothers arrived at the hospital is the highest priority.

Although there is recognition that the prevention of low birth weight by preterm delivery is clearly important, the high mortality of normal-birth-weight infants remains the central concern. Among the factors that contribute to the problem are the observation that in a traditional sub-Saharan society, African women are accorded an inferior status. They take a limited part in the decision-making process, even when it involves child-bearing. The decision to transfer a desperately ill pregnant woman to a hospital is nearly always made by the husband, and in his absence

TABLE 1–5

Association of Infant Mortality in Four Countries and Percentage of Mothers Under Age 20 Years

Country	1985 Infant Mortality per 1000 Live Births	Percentage of Mothers <20 Years of Age
Japan	5.5	1.1
Finland	6.3	5.0
United Kingdom	9.3	8.9
United States	10.4	14.8

  Mortality data from Wegman ME: Annual summary of vital statistics, 1986. Pediatrics 80:817, 1987.

TABLE 1–6

1990 Federal Priority Objectives for Pregnancy and Infant Health

Improved Health Status
1. National IMR should be reduced to no more than 9 deaths per 1000 live births
2. The neonatal death rate should be reduced to no more than 6.5 deaths per 1000
3. The perinatal death rate should be reduced to no more than 5.5 deaths per 1000
4. No county, racial, or ethnic group should have an IMR in excess of 12 deaths per 1000
5. No county, racial, or ethnic group should have a maternal mortality rate of more than 5 deaths per 100,000 live births

Reduced Risk Factors
6. LBW infants (<2500 g) should constitute not more than 5% of live births
7. No county, racial, or ethnic group should have an LBW rate that exceeds 9%
8. The majority of infants should leave hospitals in car safety seats

Increased Public Awareness
9. 85% of women of child-bearing age should be able to choose foods wisely and should understand the hazards of smoking, alcohol, and drugs during pregnancy and lactation

Improved Services and Protection
10. All women and infants should be served at a level appropriate to their need by a regionalized system of perinatal care
11. The proportion of women in any county, racial, or ethnic group who obtain no prenatal care during the first trimester of pregnancy should not exceed 10%
12. All newborns should be screened for metabolic disorders for which effective tests and treatments are available
13. All infants should be able to participate in comprehensive primary health care

IMR, infant mortality rate; LBW, low birth weight.
From U.S. Public Health Service: Promoting Health/Preventing Disease: Objectives for the Nation. Washington, DC, Department of Health and Human Services, 1980. *In* Centers for Disease Control and Prevention, National Center for Health Statistics: Progress toward achieving the 1990 objectives for pregnancy and infant health. MMWR 37:406, 1988.

others may be unwilling to make the decision. There is a traditional dislike of operative deliveries, so that even when labor is obstructed, consent to relieve the obstruction by cesarean section may require prolonged discussion. Marriage soon after puberty is widely practiced among the illiterate traditional majority of individuals. Most of the girls of this age are underdeveloped and also nutritionally deprived so that pelvic contraction is common. A further problem is that young primigravidae are often shy about their pregnancies, strive to conceal the fact, and therefore have no prenatal care. Home delivery is nearly always preferred by that particular population.

Although the biosocial issues that have an impact on the outcome of pregnancy are complex, some of the solutions are straightforward. It is fair enough to say that major structural changes in the existing political, economic, and cultural milieu are necessary for major improvements to occur over the long-term. It is also clear that providing facilities for antenatal care and an educational program that promotes their use can make an immediate difference. The development of facilities for performing cesarean sec-

tion safely has to be a priority, as does the availability of safe blood transfusions.

Pediatric Perspectives

Experiences in developed and developing countries suggest that perinatal mortality may be reduced by 30% to 40% within a few years by the application of some straightforward, commonsense interventions. These include the recognition of risk factors and the identification of women who are likely to have difficulty during the perinatal period so that they may be delivered in safe settings. It also means applying current knowledge, such as ensuring the availability of appropriate resuscitation and thermal environment for an infant, the encouragement of timely breastfeeding, and the minimizing of the risk of infection by making hand-washing a consistent practice. It is extraordinary to realize that in some hospital-based intensive care nurseries or even routine care nurseries, the caretakers move from infant to infant without washing hands between examinations. In many nurseries, no sinks are readily available except those at a considerable distance, and even then they may not be equipped with soap or disposable towels. The high prevalence of nosocomial infection in such environments is not surprising. In fact, the leading cause of death in many such settings is acquired infection in the period after delivery. Encouraging mothers to care for their own infants is, of course, an important intervention to provide where possible and is widely practiced in some of the developing countries. If individuals other than the mother are to care for infants, they must be required to wash their hands; be taught not to insert their fingers into the infants' mouths; and be encouraged to make sure that sheets, blankets, and other objects with which the infant comes in contact have been washed and preferably sterilized. It is essential to realize that where the infant mortality rate is high, it can be reduced by at least one third, if not one half, through the application of the straightforward caretaking measures just cited.

Clearly major contributions to the reduction in the mortality of both term and low-birth-weight infants that has taken place in the developed countries have been the use of better incubators, temperature control devices, and respirators and the ability to monitor blood gases and to have microchemical determinations promptly available.

TABLE 1–7

Fertility Rates and Birth Rates Between 1790 and 1985 (U.S. Vital Statistics)

Year	Birth Rate (per 1000)	Births per Woman (Fertility Rate)
1790	55	8
1900	30	—
1940	20	2.3
1950	22	3.2
1957	22	3.7
1970	19	2.5
1985	15.5	1.8

TABLE 1–8

Live Births, Total Fertility Rates, and Birth Rates by Age of Mother

	Live Births	Total Fertility Rate	Birth Rate by Age of Mother			
			15–19 Yr	20–24 Yr	25–39 Yr	40–44 Yr
All races°						
1992	4,065,014	2,065.0	60.7	114.6	32.5	5.9
1990	4,158,212	2,081.0	59.9	116.5	31.7	5.5
1985	3,760,561	1,844.0	51.0	108.3	24.0	4.0
1980†	3,612,258	1,839.5	53.0	115.1	19.8	3.9
1970‡	3,731,386	2,480.0	68.3	167.8	31.7	8.1
Race—1992°						
White	3,201,678	1,993.5	51.8	108.2	32.2	5.7
Black	673,633	2,442.0	112.4	158.0	28.8	5.6
American Indian§	39,453	2,190.0	84.4	145.5	28.0	6.1
Asian/Pacific Islander	150,250	1,942.0	26.6	74.6	50.6	11.0
Hispanic origin—1992°						
All Hispanic	643,271	3,043.0	107.1	190.6	45.6	10.9
Mexican	432,047	3,196.5	108.8	202.3	47.7	11.8
Puerto Rican	59,569	2,644.5	110.4	204.9	30.0	6.5
Cuban	11,472	1,485.5	26.3	51.6	28.9	4.7
Other Hispanic	140,183	3,076.0	112.1	172.9	50.3	12.5
Non-Hispanic White	2,527,217	1,810.5	41.7	93.9	30.5	5.1
Non-Hispanic Black	657,450	2,514.0	116.0	163.0	29.4	5.7

°All races, U.S., selected years; by race, U.S., 1992; Hispanic and non-Hispanic origin, 49 states and District of Columbia (New Hampshire does not collect information on Hispanic origin), 1992.

†Based on 100% of births in selected states and on a 50% sample of births in all other states.

‡Based on a 50% sample of births.

§Includes births to Aleuts and Eskimos.

Data from National Center for Health Statistics, final natality rates, 1992. From Wegman ME: Annual summary of vital statistics, 1993. Pediatrics 94:792, 1994. Reproduced by Permission of PEDIATRICS, Vol 94 Page 792, Copyright 1994.

Because such advanced equipment and the highly trained personnel to work with it cannot be reproduced in all settings where babies are born, it is inappropriate to assign their availability the highest priority.

Each society must identify its own problems and ascertain the most appropriate, feasible interventions. In 1979, the U.S. Public Health Service defined a list of objectives for 1990, which were not achieved (see Table 1–6). Nothing will improve, however, without the advocacy of those who care about the health of mothers and infants in any social context. The remarkable success that has been achieved in the Scandinavian countries and Japan is encouraging. Maternal mortality is almost always preventable, and infant mortality should be less than 5/1000 live births. Fortunately, when infant mortality falls, fertility rates also fall because there is less need for a woman to have multiple pregnancies if there is reasonable assurance of the survival of each infant. This observation has been duplicated in every society in which there has been a reduction in infant mortality, including the United States (Tables 1–7 and 1–8). The coupling of efforts to reduce maternal and infant mortality with advice on family planning and child spacing would seem to be the most important goal for the next decades. Universal access to prenatal care is a high priority. Stimulated by the leadership shown by WHO, UNICEF, and the International Pediatric Association as well as local pediatric societies and religious groups, the goals for the year 2000 could be attainable. At least, clinicians should

not rest until progress in reaching the goals is seen being made in all parts of the world.

REFERENCES

AAP Special Report: Barriers to Care. Elk Grove Village, IL, American Academy of Pediatrics, 1989.

Behrman RE: Premature births among black women. N Engl J Med 317:763, 1987.

Berkowitz GS, Skouron ML, Lapinski RH, et al: Delayed child bearing and the outcome of pregnancy. N Engl J Med 322:659, 1990.

Braverman P, Oliva G, Miller MG, et al: Adverse outcomes and lack of health insurance among newborns in an eight-county area of California, 1982 to 1986. N Engl J Med 321:508, 1989.

Brown SS, Eisenberg L: The best intentions: The causes, consequences and prevention of unintended pregnancy. Washington, DC, Committee on Unintended Pregnancy, Institute of Medicine, National Academy of Sciences, 1995.

Callahan TL, Hall JE, Ettner SL, et al: The economic impact of multiple-gestation pregnancies and the contribution of assisted-reproduction techniques to their incidence. N Engl J Med 331:244, 1994.

Centers for Disease Control and Prevention: Update: Trends in AIDS incidence, deaths, and prevalence—United States, 1996. MMWR 46:162, 1997.

Cloherty JP, Stark AR (Eds): Manual of Neonatal Care. Boston, Little, Brown, 1980.

Editorial: Maternal health in sub-Saharan Africa. Lancet 1:255, 1987.

Forrest JD: Epidemiology of unintended pregnancy and contraceptive use. Am J Obstet Gynecol 170(part 2):1485, 1994.

Gould JB, Davey B, Stafford RS: Socioeconomic differences in rates of cesarean section. N Engl J Med 321:233, 1989.

Gregory GA, Kitterman JA, Phibbs RH, et al: Treatment of the idiopathic respiratory-distress syndrome with continuous positive airway pressure. N Engl J Med 284:1333, 1971.

Guyer B, Strobino DM, Ventura SJ, et al: Annual summary of vital statistics, 1995. Pediatrics 98:1007, 1996.

Harrison KA: Childbearing, health and social priorities: A survey of 2274 consecutive hospital births in Zaria, Northern Nigeria. Br J Obstet Gynaecol 92(Suppl 5):1, 1985.

Kiely JL, Paneth N, Susser M: An assessment of the effects of maternal age and parity in different components of perinatal mortality. Am J Epidemiol 123:444, 1986.

Kleinman JD, Kessel SS: Racial differences in low birth weight. N Engl J Med 317:749, 1987.

Kogan MD, Alexander GR, Kotelchuck M, Nagey DA: Relation of the content of prenatal care to the risk of low birth weight. JAMA 271:1340, 1994.

Lee KS, Corpuz M: Teenage pregnancy: Trend and impact on rates of low birth weight and fetal, maternal, and neonatal mortality in the United States. Clin Perinatol 15:929, 1988.

Luke B, Keith LG: The contribution of singletons, twins and triplets to low birth weight, infant mortality and handicap in the United States. J Reprod Med 37:661, 1992.

Mahler H: The safe motherhood initiative: A call to action. Lancet 1:668, 1987.

McCormick MC, McCarton C, Tonascia J, Brooks-Gunn J: Early educational intervention for very low birth weight infants: Results from the Infant Health and Development Program. J Pediatr 123:527, 1993.

McCormick MC, Shapiro S, Starfield BH: The regionalization of perinatal services: Summary of the evaluation of a national demonstration program. JAMA 253:799, 1985.

Miller HC, Jekel JF: The effect of race on the incidence of low birth weight: Persistence of effect after controlling for socioeconomic, educational, marital, and risk status. Yale J Biol Med 60:221, 1987.

Modanlou H, Dorchester W, Freeman R, Rommal C: Perinatal transport to a regional perinatal center in a metropolitan area: Maternal vs. neonatal transport. Am J Obstet Gynecol 138:1157, 1980.

Murray JL, Bernfield M: The differential effect of prenatal care on the incidence of low birth weight among blacks and whites in a prepaid health care plan. N Engl J Med 319:1385, 1988.

National Commission to Prevent Infant Mortality: Death Before Life: The Tragedy of Infant Mortality. August 1988.

Rawlings JS, Rawlings VB, Read JA: Prevalence of low birth weight and preterm delivery in relation to the interval between pregnancies among white and black women. N Engl J Med 332:69, 1995.

Richardson DK, Gray JE, McCormick MC, et al: Score for neonatal acute physiology: A physiologic severity index for neonatal intensive care. Pediatrics 91:617, 1993.

Richardson DK, Phibbs CS, Gray JE, et al: Birth weight and severity independent predictors of neonatal mortality. Pediatrics 91:969, 1993.

Rivara FP, Farrington DP: Prevention of violence. Arch Pediatr Adolesc Med 149:421, 1995.

Smith P, Mumford P (Eds): Adolescent Pregnancy. Boston, CK Hall, 1980, p 18.

Tarnow-Mordi W, Ogston S, Wilkinson AR, et al: Predicting death from initial disease severity in very low birthweight infants: A method for comparing the performance of neonatal units. BMJ 300:1611, 1990.

Wegman ME: Annual summary of vital statistics, 1993. Pediatrics 94:792, 1994.

Wise PH, Kotelchuck M, Mills M: Racial and socioeconomic disparities in childhood mortality in Boston. N Engl J Med 313:360, 1985.

CHAPTER 2

Evaluation of Therapeutic Recommendations

John C. Sinclair

That pediatricians can differ in their beliefs about effective treatment is not a new phenomenon. What *is* new is the accelerating pace of therapeutic innovation resulting from the explosion of new knowledge concerning the causes, natural history, diagnosis, treatment, and prevention of diseases of the newborn and older child. Today's pediatrician needs up-to-date information concerning ever more powerful therapies and, more importantly, the ability to "separate the wheat from the chaff" when it comes to evaluating the validity and applicability of therapeutic recommendations (Evidence-Based Medicine Working Group, 1992, 1993, 1994).

What standards of evidence should be met before new tests or treatments are widely applied in clinical practice? The history of the development of perinatal and neonatal medicine has included both triumphs and disasters. The fact that therapeutic innovations can be effective, useless, or even harmful has been amply demonstrated in this field. One need only cite, as examples of the last-mentioned, the unsuspected and initially undetected occurrence of retrolental fibroplasia following the uncritical introduction of unrestricted oxygen therapy, kernicterus resulting from the use of sulfisoxazole, and the gray baby syndrome owing to intoxication with chloramphenicol. These examples, taken from the 1940s and 1950s, serve as reminders that it may be not only unhelpful but also disastrous to apply untested new treatments on a wide scale.

In the present era, the problem persists. For example, concerning the supportive care of premature newborn infants, clinicians know on the basis of well-designed clinical research that keeping them warmer than was done previously reduces neonatal mortality, but an alarming report (Lucas et al, 1988) of an association between low but asymptomatic neonatal glucose levels in low-birth-weight infants and impaired later neurodevelopment exposes the fact that there has never been an experimental test of the effect of contrasting policies of neonatal glycemic control on neurodevelopmental outcome in such patients. Concerning the treatment of diseases of the newborn and infant, well-designed clinical research has shown the effects of surfactant replacement for the treatment or prevention of respiratory distress syndrome (RDS) and cryotherapy for the treatment of stage 3+ retinopathy of prematurity. Can one point to research of comparable caliber to justify the use of tolazoline in persistent pulmonary hypertension or (to choose a common, everyday problem in neonatal intensive care) phenobarbital as the preferred first drug in the treatment of neonatal seizures?

For many, if not most, therapies in use at present, valid evidence of their effectiveness is lacking. Based on past experience, one can predict that many of the therapies that are presently incorporated into clinical practice will fall into disuse in the future. In fact, seven stages in the typical career of an innovative treatment or technology have been described (McKinlay, 1981):

1. Promising report.
2. Professional and organizational adoption.
3. Public acceptance and state (third-party) endorsement.
4. Incorporation into standard practice, observational reports.
5. Rigorous evaluation using randomized, controlled trials.
6. Professional denunciation.
7. Abandonment and replacement by a newer technology.

This sequence of events demonstrates a failure to evaluate properly new therapies or diagnostic technologies at an early stage of their diffusion. The case of intrapartum electronic fetal heart rate monitoring is a much studied example of widespread diffusion of a new technology before rigorous evaluation (Shy et al, 1987). This chapter describes a scheme for the evaluation of new therapies and demonstrates the application of this scheme in the field of perinatology.

MEASUREMENT ITERATIVE LOOP

A framework, called the *measurement iterative loop*, which is useful for the type of evaluation just discussed, is shown in Figure 2–1 (Tugwell et al, 1985). This scheme identifies distinct research and evaluation questions that constitute a logical progression: What is the burden of disease? What are the causes of health problems contributing to the burden? What is the effectiveness of treatment (a function of treatment efficacy, screening and diagnostic accuracy, physician and patient compliance, and coverage)? What are the costs in relation to the effects of the treatment? What interventions or programs should be selected for widespread use? What are the effects on quality of care and patient outcomes? How has the disease burden been affected? This chapter focuses particularly on the efficacy and effectiveness of treatment.

Evaluating the Efficacy of Treatment

The clinical questions to be asked about any treatment are the following:

1. What is the magnitude of the baseline risk (i.e., without treatment, what proportion of patients will experience an adverse outcome)?
2. Is there an effect of treatment (i.e., is there an effect that is real and not due to chance)?
3. What are the direction and size of treatment effect?
4. What is the duration of treatment effect?

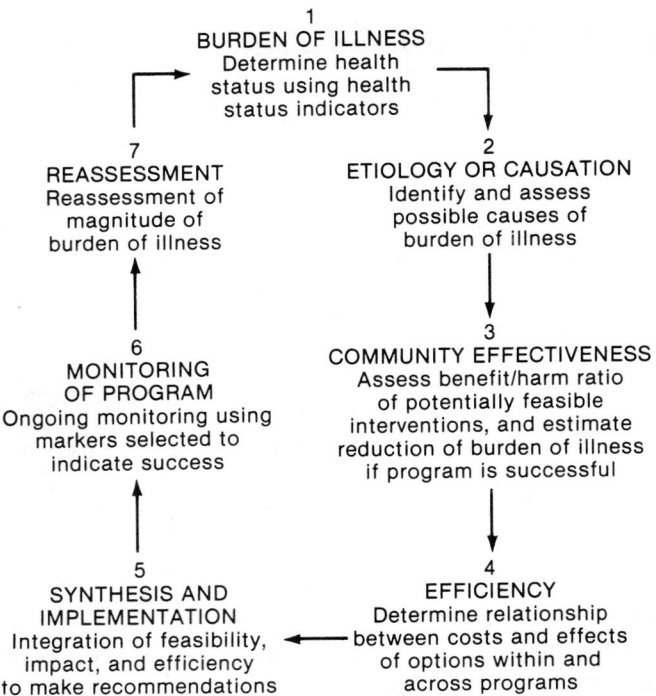

FIGURE 2–1. The measurement iterative loop.

5. Are there unwanted side effects that are attributable to the treatment?
6. What are the economic costs?
7. Do the clinical benefits of treatment outweigh the unwanted side effects or economic costs?
8. To whom are these results applicable?

Obtaining answers to these questions is not a simple matter. Research may sometimes result in a wrong answer because of systematic error (bias) or random error (imprecision). Even valid conclusions from research can be of limited generalizability to clinical practice. Thus, the physician needs to be concerned not only with the proclaimed results of clinical research concerning treatment but also with the methodologic issues of bias, precision, and applicability.

Expressing the Effect of Treatment

Table 2–1 displays the structure of a typical study that seeks to evaluate treatment. There are two exposure groups (labeled as *treated* or *control*) and two possible outcome categories (labeled as *event* or *no event*). An event may be

any outcome, such as occurrence of disease, complication of disease, or death. Such a study design permits answers to clinically relevant questions about the effect of treatment (Sinclair and Bracken, 1994), as explained in the following:

1. The magnitude of risk in the absence of treatment is given by the event rate in the control group, $c/c + d$.
2. The effect of treatment is given by comparing the event rate in the treated group with that in the control group. This comparison is expressed as either the *relative risk* (RR), $a/(a+b) \div c/(c+d)$, or the *risk difference* (RD), $a/(a+b) - c/(c+d)$. (Another measure of the association between treatment and outcome is given by the relative odds or odds ratio, $a/c \div b/d$. The odds ratio, an approximation of the relative risk at low prevalence, is used to estimate strength of association between outcome and exposure in case-control studies, in which relative risk cannot be calculated. In cohort studies including randomized clinical trials, however, strength of association is directly estimated as relative risk. Odds ratio is not considered further in this chapter.)

The relative risk and the risk difference convey different (and to some extent complementary) information. The relative risk indicates the *relative,* but not absolute, magnitude of reduction in the event rate. The complement of the relative risk $(1 - RR)$ gives the proportionate risk reduction. Thus, a relative risk of 0.75 represents a 25% reduction in the rate of events in the treated group relative to the rate of events in the controls.

The risk difference indicates the *absolute* magnitude of reduction of risk. For example, a risk difference of -0.10 represents an absolute 10 percentage point reduction of events in the treated group. The reciprocal of the risk difference (1/RD) indicates the number of patients who must be treated to expect to prevent the event in one patient. This latter measure is particularly relevant when considering whether to use a treatment that is effective but whose effect is bought at considerable cost (in the form of either clinical side effects or economic cost). In the example here, 1/0.10, 10 patients need to be treated to prevent one with an event. When outcome data are reported on a continuous scale (e.g., blood pressure measured in millimeters of mercury), a different measure of effect, the mean difference, is computed.

CONTROLLING BIAS

The fundamental goal of clinical research concerning the efficacy and safety of treatment is that it should obtain an unbiased answer to the question posed. Bias means a force that leads to an answer that is systematically different from the truth.

Most studies on treatment or prevention use designs that can be classified into one of four categories. These designs are listed in order of ascending methodologic rigor:

1. Single case reports or case series without controls.
2. Nonrandomized studies using historical controls (e.g., comparing current patients who receive the innovative treatment with previous patients, from the same institution or from the literature, who did not).

TABLE 2–1

Structure of a Study to Evaluate the Effect of a Treatment

		Outcome	
		Event	**No Event**
Exposure	*Treated*	a	b
	Control	c	d

3. Nonrandomized studies using concurrent controls (e.g., comparing contemporaneous patients who did or did not receive the experimental treatment).
4. Randomized, controlled trials.

The case report and case series (without controls) are the designs most prone to bias. The absence of a control group generally leads to an overestimate of the effect of treatment: Any improvement in the clinical course of patients in a case series is attributed to treatment, even when the improvement would have occurred in the absence of treatment.

Studies that use controls provide a much more valid basis for reaching conclusions about the effect of treatment. The performance of a controlled study, however, is not, in itself, a sufficient guarantee of a valid result. Biases can seriously impair studies using either historical or nonrandomized concurrent controls (Sackett, 1979). Sacks and colleagues (1982) surveyed reports of controlled studies of six different therapies and found that for each therapy, studies using historical controls were much more likely to find an apparent benefit than studies using randomized controls. The difference was due to the fact that the control group in the historical control studies had worse outcomes than the controls in the randomized control studies; the treated patients in the two types of studies generally had similar outcomes. Historical control groups tend to fare poorly in part because they typically include all patients who meet the diagnostic criteria, even poor-risk or noncompliant patients or patients who have other adverse characteristics that might exclude them from enrollment in prospective, randomized trials.

The randomized trial is based on principles originally developed for agricultural research by Fisher in the 1920s and subsequently applied to clinical research in the pioneering work of Hill, Silverman, and others in the 1940s and 1950s. The randomized trial is the strongest design for evaluating the effect of treatment. It offers maximum protection against selection biases that can invalidate comparisons between groups of patients because of *confounding*. A confounder is extraneous to the question being posed, is unequally distributed between the treatment groups being compared, and is itself a determinant of the outcome. In nonrandomized studies, the investigator tries to control confounding by strategies such as exclusion, stratification at the time of sampling, matching, stratification in the analysis, adjustment and standardization, and modeling. These techniques, however, require that the source of confounding be known. In clinical medicine, the confounders are often unknown; a presently unknown confounder may be discovered tomorrow. It is the unique property and strength of randomization that it has the capacity to allocate not only known but also unknown confounders in an unbiased manner.

Methodologic standards for the design, conduct, and analysis of randomized trials continue to be refined (Chalmers et al, 1981; Reisch et al, 1989; Tyson et al, 1983). Several features of the design deserve emphasis

1. There must be an a priori hypothesis, stated in quantitative terms, susceptible to disproof. This requires a predetermined sample size based on estimates of the hypothesized clinical effect of the new treatment

and the investigators' predetermined probabilities of missing a real treatment effect and of incorrectly identifying the treatment as being effective. (The reader of a report of a randomized trial that did not find a statistically significant effect of treatment may well wonder whether the trial was large enough to have found a clinically significant difference [e.g., relative risk reduction of 25% or 50%] if it had occurred. Such post facto consideration of the results of completed trials is aided by tables prepared by Detsky and Sackett [1985].)

2. The allocation process should be truly random and impervious to code-breaking or tampering. (Quasi-random allocation procedures such as alternation and day of week are not preferred.)
3. When feasible, blinding of both physician and patient to the treatment allocation should be accomplished. (Among other advantages, this defends against cointervention bias—the selective use of additional screening, diagnostic, or therapeutic procedures in one group more than in the other.)
4. Outcome measurements should be made by observers who are blinded to the treatment allocation.
5. All patients randomized must be accounted for in the primary analysis.

The methodologic criterion (item 5) that all patients randomized must be accounted for in the primary analysis has specific application in the case of *competing events*. For example, neonatal death and chronic lung disease are competing events: chronic lung disease cannot occur if the patient has died early. An intervention that is effective in reducing the incidence of neonatal death (e.g., mechanical ventilation) may also increase the incidence of chronic lung disease among survivors. An unbiased view of the effect of mechanical ventilation requires that outcomes be related to the number of patients exposed to the intervention—that is, the number of patients with the event as a proportion of the number randomized in each arm of the trial. In the case of competing events, outcomes expressed in this way can then be aggregated—that is, *either* neonatal death *or* chronic lung disease—to obtain a global view of the effect of the intervention. Note that the incidence of chronic lung disease among survivors of mechanical ventilation, taken alone, would give a biased impression of the treatment effect if mechanical ventilation also caused an important difference in the neonatal death rate.

Of the above-mentioned criteria, the avoidance of bias in treatment allocation is arguably the most fundamental requirement. Chalmers and associates (1983) obtained empiric evidence of the importance of unbiased allocation by surveying 145 reports of controlled studies of the treatment of myocardial infarction. This group of papers included 57 in which the randomization process was blinded (i.e., neither the investigator nor the patient knew the treatment assignment until after the patient had been enrolled in the study and informed consent had been obtained), 45 in which the randomization process may have been unblinded in that the patient could be selected or rejected for the study after the physician knew the treatment assignment, and 43 in which historical or nonrandomized concurrent controls were used. It was found that studies in which the assignment of controls was unblinded or nonrandom suffered from dissimilar distributions of prognostic variables (typically favoring the experimental group) and were also more likely to find a significant difference (again in favor of the experimental group). Treatment assignment in randomized trials should occur only after the patient has been accepted and formally enrolled in the study; then random assignment should be performed according to a prearranged scheme such as a telephone call to a statistical center or consecutively arranged blinded medications or treatment instructions contained in opaque envelopes.

Table 2–2 indicates the relative frequency of use of different study designs in a survey of the literature on treatment or prevention of diseases of the newborn (Schmidt et al, 1987). An increasing use of randomized, controlled trials is apparent in published reports of research. In neonatology, the use of randomized trials has increased to the point where they currently account for close to 25% of published studies concerning treatment and prevention of diseases of the newborn (Kirpalani et al, 1989). There are presently more than 3000 reports of randomized trials in neonatology, a number that is doubling every 6 years.

Example: Expressing the Effect of Treatment and Controlling Bias

The outcome data of the Auckland trial (Crowley, 1989, 1994; Liggins and Howie, 1972) of antepartum glucocorticoid therapy to prevent RDS in premature infants are shown in Table 2–3. This was a randomized, controlled trial of betamethasone therapy in mothers in whom premature delivery threatened or was planned before 37 weeks' gestation. The risk of RDS in the absence of betamethasone therapy is given by the RDS rate in the control group, 84/538 = 15.6%. The effect of treatment expressed as the relative risk is 49/532 ÷ 84/538 = 0.59. Risk of RDS after glucocorticoid treatment is reduced to 59% of the risk in the control group—that is, a relative risk reduction of 41%. Alternatively the effect of treatment can be expressed as the risk difference, 49/532 − 84/538 = − 0.064. The risk of RDS has been reduced, in absolute terms, by 6.4%; the reciprocal (1/0.064) indicates that approximately 16 patients need to be treated to prevent one case of RDS.

TABLE 2–2

Articles on Treatment or Prevention of Diseases of the Newborn, by Study Design

Study Design	No. of Articles	Percent
Randomized trials	57	24
Concurrent controls, nonrandomized	69	29
Historical controls, nonrandomized	24	10
No controls (case series or case reports)	84	36
Total	234	100

Data from Schmidt B, Kirpalani H, Sinclair JC: Unpublished observations, 1987.

TABLE 2–3

Effect of the Administration of Betamethasone Before Preterm Delivery on Respiratory Distress Syndrome and Stillbirth Without Lethal Malformation

Treatment Group	n	Respiratory Distress Syndrome	Stillbirth
Betamethasone	532	49 (9.2%)	31 (5.8%)
Control	538	84 (15.6%)	28 (5.2%)
Relative risk		0.59	1.12
95% CI		0.42, 0.82	0.68, 1.84
Risk difference		− 6.4	+ 0.6
95% CI		− 10.3, − 2.5	− 2.1, + 3.3

CI, confidence interval.

These estimates of treatment effect are likely to be unbiased because of the following:

1. The investigators employed the strongest design for the control of selection bias: the randomized trial.
2. The allocation process was truly random and probably impervious to code-breaking or tampering (a pharmacist at arm's length from the trial controlled the randomization).
3. The active and control injections appeared to be identical so that neither the patient nor the health-care professionals knew the identity of the treatment.
4. The diagnosis of RDS was made using objective clinical and radiologic criteria; however, it is not certain whether assessors were blind to treatment allocation.
5. Virtually all randomized patients were included in the analysis.

The issue of competing events would arise in this trial if glucocorticoid treatment also substantially affected the fetal death rates: RDS could not occur if the fetus were not born alive. This issue is resolved by computing both the fetal death rates and the RDS rates as a proportion of the number randomized in each arm of the trial. In this instance, there is no important difference in the incidence of stillbirth, and this competing event, therefore, does not explain the reduction in incidence of RDS.

ESTIMATING PRECISION

Randomized trials are concerned with *estimation* (estimating the size of effect of treatment) as well as with *hypothesis testing* (testing whether an effect is real or due to chance). Although a randomized trial offers the most powerful design for providing an unbiased estimate of the size of difference in outcomes of the treatment regimens being compared, the estimate can be imprecise.

The confidence interval (Bulpitt, 1987) displays the uncertainty in the study's estimate of the size of effect by presenting the upper and lower bounds for the anticipated true treatment difference. The 95% confidence interval indicates that if the study were to be repeated 100 times, the true value would be included within the calculated confidence interval on 95 occasions.

The confidence interval tends to widen when the data

are variable, the sample size is small, or both. Thus, imprecision in estimation is a particular problem in trials that enroll only small numbers of patients. As the number of patients increases, the confidence interval narrows.

The *clinical* significance of a true treatment effect depends on the size of treatment effect and on the complications and costs of treatment. Weighing these considerations is a matter of clinical judgment. The declaration of *statistical* significance is a determination that a treatment effect is real—i.e., unlikely to be due to chance. A clinically significant difference may be suggested in a study whose sample size is too small to achieve statistical significance. Alternatively a difference that is so small that it is of little or no clinical importance can be rendered statistically significant if the sample size is large. In evaluating treatment recommendations, therefore, the clinician is most impressed by the demonstration of treatment effects that are both clinically and statistically significant.

Example: Estimating Precision

Returning to the data shown in Table 2–3, one can ask, "How precise is the estimate of treatment effect in this study?" Precision can be expressed by calculating the 95% confidence interval around the *point estimate* for treatment effect. It was calculated previously that the relative risk of RDS was reduced by betamethasone treatment to 0.59. The 95% confidence interval attached to this estimate is 0.42 to 0.82. This interval would contain the true value for the effect of betamethasone treatment in 95 of 100 replications of this trial. Similarly, it was calculated previously that the risk of RDS, in absolute terms, was reduced by 6.4%; the confidence interval around this estimate is 2.5% to 10.3%.

JUDGING APPLICABILITY

The applicability of the results of a trial depends on the appropriateness of generalizing the trial's conclusion to a particular clinical practice. This, in turn, depends on the physician's answers to the following questions:

1. Were the study patients recognizably similar to his or her own?
2. Is the intervention feasible in practice?
3. Were all clinically relevant outcomes reported?

Underlying these specific questions is the more general issue of whether the trial is of the *management* or *explanatory* type (Sackett and Gent, 1987). The conceptual distinction is that a management trial determines the *effectiveness* of an intervention in actual clinical practice, whereas an explanatory trial determines the *efficacy* of an intervention under optimal or narrowly defined conditions. The primary analysis of a management trial, based on all patients randomized, takes into account real-life problems such as diagnostic errors that are appreciated only after treatment, patients with additional diseases or with outcomes not obviously caused by the treatment being studied, and patients who die early before treatment takes hold. The primary analysis of a management trial is sometimes described as an *intention-to-treat* analysis, thus reflecting the

clinical reality that a management decision to treat does not necessarily mean that the full course of treatment will be received as prescribed. Moreover, with some treatments, the patient may die before the treatment is given. For example, it may take several hours to prepare a granulocyte transfusion, leading to a significant delay in treatment. Such an important treatment effect can be identified only by counting all deaths in a study instead of only those occurring after treatment.

The limits of applicability of the results of a randomized trial are generally determined by the range of variation among entry characteristics and intervention policies as described in the index trial. The wider these limits, the wider the limits of applicability of the conclusions. It is not warranted, however, to extend the results beyond the limits tested in the trial. A famous example of inappropriate application in neonatal practice was the extrapolation of the restricted oxygen policy to all premature infants after the report in 1954 that oxygen restriction greatly reduced the incidence and severity of retrolental fibroplasia. The fact that all infants who entered the trial had to be at least 48 hours old was overlooked in making this recommendation. It was estimated subsequently (Cross, 1973) that 16 deaths (mainly from respiratory disorders in the first days of life) were caused for every case of retrolental fibroplasia prevented, even though the original trial demonstrated no mortality owing to oxygen restriction. The extension of a study's results to a different patient population, therefore, should be done first under the auspices of a new randomized trial.

Even when a randomized trial exists that appears to be applicable to one's patient, there remains the issue that the conclusions from clinical research based on groups of patients do not necessarily apply to each individual patient. Indeed, in virtually all randomized trials that prove a therapy to be effective, there are some treated patients who do not benefit or are even harmed; conversely, in trials that generate a negative result, there are nevertheless some treated patients that appear to have benefited. These considerations have prompted the development of the strategy of randomized trials in individual patients—so-called N-of-1 trials—in which a single patient undergoes a series of pairs of treatments (one active and one placebo or alternative treatment per pair) with the order determined by random allocation (Guyatt et al, 1986). The results of such a trial apply without reservation to the patient who was the participant in the trial; however, the N-of-1 design does not provide information on how to treat other patients with the same disorder.

Applicability also depends on the range of outcomes that are evaluated in a trial of a new treatment. Although the investigator may assess only a single outcome, many interventions have the capacity to affect more than one outcome of clinical importance. Before a new therapy is adopted for widespread use, evidence is needed concerning its effect on all the major outcomes it is likely to influence. This is an exceedingly difficult dictum to carry over into practice because neither investigators nor clinicians are wise enough to know all the places they should look. Moreover, some effects are not expressed until considerable time has elapsed. Nevertheless, a few suggestions can be made, as follows:

1. Concerning choice of outcome, the reader should beware of what has been called the *substitution game,* in which a risk factor (e.g., blood cholesterol level) is substituted for events of prime clinical importance (i.e., heart attack, stroke). This issue arises also when an intermediate outcome (e.g., arterial-to-alveolar oxygen ratio) is substituted for the more relevant clinical outcomes of death or major morbidity.

2. Although scientific rationale can provide a strong lead in determining where to look in assessing the effects of a new therapy, one should not easily dismiss apparent effects for which no scientific rationale presently exists. This is particularly true if the effect has been exposed in a well-designed and well-conducted randomized trial (e.g., the demonstration that sulfisoxazole causes an increase in the incidence of and death from kernicterus in premature infants) (Silverman et al, 1956).

3. Total mortality as well as mortality from the specific disease under investigation should be considered.

4. Long-term follow-up to determine late outcomes should be undertaken.

Example: Judging Applicability

Do the data shown in Table 2–3 entirely justify the widespread use of antenatal glucocorticoid treatment of mothers who threaten to deliver prematurely? Liggins and Howie (1972) from the outset pointed to the need for further trials that would refine treatment indications and that would assess multiple outcomes, including both early and late effects. Such trials have examined the effects of corticosteroids by gestational age at treatment, by status of the membranes (whether intact or ruptured), and by presence or absence of maternal hypertension. The effect of glucocorticoids has been assessed in male and female fetuses. Trials have examined the effects on major neonatal problems, such as infection, periventricular hemorrhage, and necrotizing enterocolitis. Effects on perinatal mortality (all causes) and on neurologic abnormality at follow-up have been assessed. Even length of stay in the hospital and cost savings have been estimated. Thus, the clinician is now armed with a wide range of clinically important information concerning the indications for, and likely clinical effects of, antepartum glucocorticoid treatment.

WHY RESULTS OF RANDOMIZED, CONTROLLED TRIALS MAY DIFFER

Does phenobarbital prevent intraventricular hemorrhage? Does vitamin E prevent bronchopulmonary dysplasia? The reader of clinical literature may well be perplexed at the apparently conflicting answers that have been obtained in randomized trials.

In considering this issue, it is first necessary to be satisfied that the trials are addressing the same question—that is, that they enroll comparable patients, test the same (or closely similar) intervention, and define and measure the same outcome. Having been satisfied that this is so, there are two commonly cited reasons why the results of randomized trials may differ (Horwitz, 1987):

1. There may be a failure to control bias in individual trials (systematic error).

2. There may be variation in the results of individual trials owing to chance, particularly in trials of small sample size (random error). If a theoretical population of identical trials of an efficacious drug is considered, having typically set power for avoiding the incorrect acceptance of the null hypothesis of no treatment effect at 80%, then one in five trials incorrectly reports the drug as having no benefit. In fact, many trials have power closer to only 50% (Freeman et al, 1978), and half of such trials miss a true treatment effect. Alternatively, in a population of trials of a drug that has no real efficacy, 1 in 20 ($\alpha = 0.05$) incorrectly finds a significant treatment effect. Thus, to place the result of an apparently unbiased but small trial in context, the physician needs access to all the relevant (and unbiased) trials that have tested the same intervention.

META-ANALYSIS

A formal overview of a series of comparable trials of an intervention (sometimes termed a *meta-analysis* [Sacks et al, 1987]) seeks to obtain a summary estimate of the effect of that intervention on each outcome of interest. A valid overview requires that all clinically relevant trials be identified by predefined inclusion and exclusion criteria. There is some evidence of a publication bias favoring trials claiming so-called positive results (as compared with those claiming no difference); to ensure that a meta-analysis represents all trials to date, the method requires a search for unpublished as well as published trials. Next, the trials are examined for their methodologic quality; those whose methods fail to meet predefined criteria for methodologic quality are excluded. Then, and only then, the results of the included trials are tabulated, and a summary estimate of treatment effect is calculated. This summary effect (sometimes termed a *typical effect*) is some form of weighted average across trials; the weights are inversely related to the variance in the estimate of treatment effect provided by each participating trial. The variance in any single trial is a function of the number of patients studied, the homogeneity of the patients on entry to the trial, the homogeneity of the response in untreated (control) patients, and the homogeneity of response in treated patients.

The results of a meta-analysis of randomized trials have several uses:

1. A meta-analysis provides increased statistical power, especially when individual trials are all relatively small; this increased power can resolve uncertainty arising from disagreement between individual trials as to whether a treatment effect is real or due to chance.

2. A meta-analysis provides increased precision in the estimate of effect size; this increased precision can be critical in weighing benefits of a treatment against clinical side effects, in choosing between alternative treatments when more than one has a true beneficial effect, and in quantitating the cost-effectiveness of the treatment.

TABLE 2–4

Effect of Corticosteroid Before Preterm Delivery on Incidence of Respiratory Distress Syndrome

| Study | Corticosteroid | | Control | | | | Risk Difference | |
	n	Percent	n	Percent	Relative Risk	(95% CI)	(%)	(95% CI)
Liggins and Howie, 1972	49/532	9.2	84/538	15.6	0.59	(0.42, 0.82)	−6.4	(−10.3, −2.5)
Block et al, 1977	5/69	7.3	12/61	19.7	0.37	(0.14, 0.99)	−12.4	(−24.1, −0.7)
Morrison et al, 1978	6/67	9.0	14/59	23.7	0.38	(0.16, 0.92)	−14.8	(−27.5, −2.1)
Papageorgiou et al, 1979	7/71	9.9	23/75	30.7	0.32	(0.15, 0.70)	−20.8	(−33.3, −8.3)
Schutte et al, 1979	11/64	17.2	17/58	29.3	0.59	(0.30, 1.15)	−12.1	(−27.0, +2.8)
Taeusch et al, 1979	7/56	12.5	14/71	19.7	0.63	(0.28, 1.46)	−7.2	(−19.9, +5.5)
Doran et al, 1980	4/81	4.9	10/63	15.9	0.31	(0.10, 0.95)	−10.9	(−21.1, −0.8)
Teramo et al, 1980	3/38	7.9	3/42	7.1	1.11	(0.24, 5.15)	+0.8	(−10.8, +12.3)
Collaborative Group, 1981	42/371	11.3	59/372	15.9	0.71	(0.49, 1.03)	−4.5	(−9.5, +0.4)
Schmidt et al, 1984	9/34	26.5	10/31	32.3	0.82	(0.39, 1.75)	−5.8	(−27.9, +16.4)
Morales et al, 1986	30/121	24.8	63/124	50.8	0.49	(0.34, 0.70)	−26.0	(−37.7, −14.3)
Gamsu et al, 1989	7/131	5.3	16/137	11.7	0.46	(0.20, 1.08)	−6.3	(−13.0, +0.3)
Carlen et al, 1991	1/11	9.1	4/13	30.8	0.30	(0.04, 2.27)	−21.7	(−52.1, +8.7)
Garite et al, 1992	21/40	52.5	28/42	66.7	0.79	(0.55, 1.14)	−14.2	(−35.2, +6.8)
Eronen et al, 1993	13/29	44.8	16/37	43.2	1.04	(0.60, 1.79)	+1.6	(−22.5, +25.7)
Typical effect°					0.59	(0.51, 0.68)	−7.9	(−10.2, −5.6)

°Typical effects calculated by MB Bracken, Perinatal Epidemiology Unit, Yale University. (Data are those used for meta-analysis by Crowley, 1994.)
CI, confidence interval.

3. A meta-analysis can also be useful in exploring the differences between studies in their results and in generating hypotheses (not posed at the start of individual trials) about the source of such differences.
4. A meta-analysis provides an existing structure for the incorporation of new evidence from comparable trials performed in the future.

Example: Meta-Analyses of All Trials of Glucocorticoid Treatment for Prevention of Respiratory Distress Syndrome

Between 1972 and 1993, at least 15 randomized trials were reported, enrolling almost 3500 cases of threatened preterm delivery (Table 2–4). The summary or *typical* estimate of treatment effect based on all trials confirms the original finding of Liggins and Howie (1972) that glucocorticoid treatment reduces the incidence of RDS. Note that there is considerable variation between trials, both in the *point estimate* of treatment effect (due to the play of chance and to variable success in control of bias) and in the width of the 95% confidence intervals (due to differences in sample size). Note also, however, that despite such differences between the individual trials, the confidence interval around the typical estimate of treatment effect is narrower than for that of any single trial.

Similar meta-analyses have been conducted to assess the effect, across trials, of the typical effect of glucocorticoid treatment with respect to a range of maternal, fetal, and neonatal outcomes (Crowley, 1989, 1994). These overviews indicate that glucocorticoid treatment is effective in reducing the incidence of RDS in both male and female fetuses. Such treatment reduces the incidence of both periventricular hemorrhage and necrotizing enterocolitis. Overall, there is no effect on the incidence of fetal or neonatal infection,

although there is a statistically nonsignificant trend of an increase in the rate of infection if a steroid is given after rupture of membranes. Most importantly, the overview shows that there is an important reduction in early neonatal deaths (all causes) and a trend (not quite significant) toward a decrease in the rate of neurologic abnormality at follow-up. These data were important determinants of the National Institutes of Health (NIH) Consensus Development Panel's recommendation that all fetuses between 24 and 34 weeks of gestation should be considered candidates for antenatal corticosteroid treatment (NIH Consensus Development Panel, 1995).

Overviews of randomized trials of perinatal interventions (such as that shown in Table 2–4) are included in the Cochrane Database of Systematic Reviews (Chalmers, 1993; Enkin, 1995) and in two related publications: *Effective Care in Pregnancy and Childbirth* (Chalmers et al, 1989) and *Effective Care of the Newborn Infant* (Sinclair and Bracken, 1992).

REFERENCES

Bulpitt CJ: Confidence intervals. Lancet 1:494, 1987.
Chalmers I: The Cochrane Collaboration: Preparing, maintaining and disseminating systematic reviews of the effects of health care. Ann NY Acad Sci 703:156, 1993.
Chalmers I, Enkin M, Keirse MJNC (Eds): Effective Care in Pregnancy and Childbirth. New York, Oxford University Press, 1989.
Chalmers TC, Celano P, Sacks HS, Smith H: Bias in treatment assignment in controlled clinical trials. N Engl J Med 309:1358, 1983.
Chalmers TC, Smith H, Blackburn B, et al: A method for assessing the quality of a randomized controlled trial. Contr Clin Trials 2:31, 1981.
Cross KW: Cost of preventing retrolental fibroplasia. Lancet 2:954, 1973.
Crowley P: Promoting pulmonary maturity. *In* Chalmers I, Enkin M, Keirse MJNC (Eds): Effective Care in Pregnancy and Childbirth. New York, Oxford University Press, 1989, pp 746–764.
Crowley P: Update of the antenatal steroid meta-analysis: Current knowledge and future research needs. Consensus Development Conference

on the Effect of Corticosteroids for Fetal Maturation on Perinatal Outcomes, Bethesda, MD, 1994.

Detsky AS, Sackett DL: When was a "negative" clinical trial big enough? How many patients you needed depends on what you found. Arch Intern Med 145:709, 1985.

Enkin MW: Systematic summaries and dissemination of evidence: The Cochrane Pregnancy and Childbirth Database. Semin Perinatol 19:155, 1995.

Evidence-Based Medicine Working Group: Evidence-based medicine: A new approach to teaching the practice of medicine. JAMA 268:2420, 1992.

Evidence-Based Medicine Working Group: Users' guide to the medical literature: II. How to use an article about therapy or prevention: A. Are the results of the study valid? JAMA 270:2598, 1993.

Evidence-Based Medicine Working Group: Users' guide to reading the medical literature: II. How to use an article about therapy or prevention: B. What are the results and will they help me in caring for my patients? JAMA 271:59, 1994.

Freeman JA, Chalmers TC, Smith H, Kuebler RR: The importance of beta, the type II error and sample size in the design and interpretation of the randomized control trial. N Engl J Med 299:690, 1978.

Guyatt G, Sackett DL, Taylor DW, et al: Determining optimal therapy—randomized trials in individual patients. N Engl J Med 314:889, 1986.

Horwitz RI: Complexity and contradiction in clinical trial research. Am J Med 82:498, 1987.

Kirpalani H, Schmidt B, McKibbon KA, et al: Searching MEDLINE for randomized clinical trials involving care of the newborn. Pediatrics 83:543, 1989.

Liggins GL, Howie RN: A controlled trial of antepartum glucocorticoid treatment for prevention of the respiratory distress syndrome in premature infants. Pediatrics 50:515, 1972.

Lucas A, Morley R, Cole TJ: Adverse neurodevelopmental outcome of moderate neonatal hypoglycemia. Br Med J 297:1304, 1988.

McKinlay JB: From "promising report" to "standard procedure": Seven stages in the career of a medical innovation. Milbank Q 59:374, 1981.

NIH Consensus Development Panel on the Effect of Corticosteroids for Fetal Maturation on Perinatal Outcomes: Effect of corticosteroids for fetal maturation on perinatal outcomes. JAMA 273:413, 1995.

Reisch JS, Tyson JE, Mize SG: Aid to the evaluation of therapeutic studies. Pediatrics 84:815, 1989.

Sackett DL: Bias in analytic research. J Chron Dis 32:51, 1979.

Sackett DL, Gent M: Controversy in counting and attributing events in clinical trials. N Engl J Med 316:450, 1987.

Sacks H, Chalmers TC, Smith H: Randomized versus historical controls for clinical trials. Am J Med 72:233, 1982.

Sacks HS, Berrier J, Reitman D, et al: Meta-analysis of randomized controlled trials. N Engl J Med 316:450, 1987.

Schmidt B, Kirpalani H, Sinclair JC: Unpublished observations, 1987.

Shy KK, Larson EB, Luthy DA: Evaluating a new technology: The effectiveness of electronic fetal heart rate monitoring. Annu Rev Public Health 8:165, 1987.

Silverman WA, Andersen DH, Blanc WA, Crozier DN: A difference in mortality rate and incidence of kernicterus among premature infants allotted to two prophylactic antibacterial regimens. Pediatrics 18:614, 1956.

Sinclair JC, Bracken MB (Eds): Effective Care of the Newborn Infant. Oxford, Oxford University Press, 1992.

Sinclair JC, Bracken MB: Clinically useful measures of effect in binary analyses of randomized trials. J Clin Epidemiol 47:881, 1994.

Tugwell P, Bennett KJ, Sackett DL, Haynes RB: The measurement iterative loop: A framework for the critical appraisal of needs, benefits and costs of health interventions. J Chron Dis 38:339, 1985.

Tyson JE, Furzan JA, Reisch JS, Mize SG: An evaluation of the quality of therapeutic studies in perinatal medicine. J Pediatr 102:10, 1983.

PART II

MAJOR INFLUENCES ON FETAL GROWTH AND DEVELOPMENT

CHAPTER 3

General Strategies of Fetal Development

Helen Liley, Merton Bernfield and Philip L. Ballard

The sequence of human development can be viewed as a progression of successive stages. These stages involve the generation of cells that organize and specialize, yielding tissues that show new functional properties and structural complexities. Development is a cellular process, in which various factors orchestrate the behavior of single cells so that they become the functional tissues that make up organs. The development from zygote to newborn is the change from independent cells to tissues and organs that are assemblies of cells that function in concert. As organs emerge, they become increasingly interdependent for normal function. This chapter shows how developmental biology, which addresses the control of cells, merges with classic embryology, which considers the assembly of cells into organs.

FIVE MILESTONES OF HUMAN EMBRYOGENESIS

Human development begins with the formation of the gametes and consists of five stages (Fig. 3–1): (1) fertilization, the formation of the fertilized zygote by union of the egg and sperm; (2) cleavage, the rapid set of cell divisions initiated by the fusion of egg and sperm; (3) implantation, the invasion of the embryo into maternal tissue; (4) gastru-

lation, the movement of cells that creates the basic body plan; and (5) organogenesis, the relatively lengthy process of formation of individual organs. This progression occurs early in human development. Organogenesis, the final stage, begins in the 3rd week after fertilization. Growth of the embryo ensues, achieved largely by increasing the number of cells and by deposition of extracellular materials.

Gametogenesis produces highly specialized male and female gametes that have undergone meiosis and thus contain a haploid number of chromosomes. The general schemes by which egg and sperm form are similar; the major differences are the duration of meiosis and the amount of cytoplasm. During meiosis, the genome of the gamete precursor cell undergoes extensive recombination as a result of crossing-over between homologous chromosomes in the first meiotic division. The genotype of each gamete is further varied because the chromosomal homologues sort independently of each other at the end of the first division. These processes cause the genetic complement of each human gamete to be unique. DNA present in the mitochondria of the egg, the source of mitochondria in the zygote, provides another source of genetic diversity because each zygote inherits mitochondrial DNA only from its mother.

The gametes are highly differentiated cells. The sperm head contains condensed DNA and is topped by the acrosome, a membrane-bound structure containing enzymes used to penetrate the ovum. The neck contains numerous mitochondria to provide energy for the motion generated by the flagellum tail. In contrast to the sperm, the egg is large; in fact, it is the largest human cell. Eggs contain stores of RNA and ribosomes that enable protein synthesis to start rapidly following fertilization. Egg differentiation includes the production of a covering layer, the zona pellucida, that protects the egg, if fertilized, during its passage through the fallopian tube.

Fertilization

Fertilization restores the diploid number of chromosomes, determines sex, and initiates the developmental sequence. Fertilization of the egg occurs in the fallopian tube near the ovary by fusion of a recently ovulated egg with a sperm that has undergone capacitation induced by uterine fluids. Capacitation involves changes in the membrane covering the acrosome, allowing release of hydrolytic enzymes that

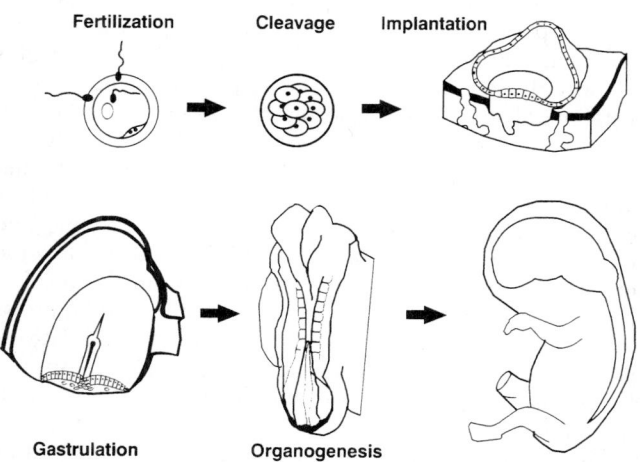

FIGURE 3–1. Human development begins with formation of the gametes and consists of five stages (see text).

enable the sperm to penetrate the zona pellucida. The sperm head attaches to the surface of the egg, and their plasma membranes fuse. The egg reacts to this contact with depolarization of its plasma membrane and polymerization of the zona pellucida, changes that prevent the entry of other sperm. The fertilized egg completes meiosis, a process that began during the fetal life of its mother. Once in the egg cytoplasm, the nucleus of the sperm enlarges. The male and female haploid nuclei fuse, and their chromosomes intermingle, forming the zygote or fertilized egg.

Cleavage

The zygote undergoes rapid cell divisions or cleavages to form a ball of cells, the morula, which then develops an internal cavity, the blastocyst. The first division of the zygote occurs about 30 hours after fertilization, and repeated cleavages produce smaller cells, called blastomeres. The absence of cell growth between these divisions distinguishes them from most cell divisions at later stages. The divisions occur as the zygote, still surrounded by the zona pellucida, is transported along the fallopian tube toward the uterus. About 3 days after fertilization, the morula, now a solid ball of 16 to 32 cells, enters the uterine cavity. On the 4th day, a fluid-filled cavity develops within the morula, creating the blastocyst. Meanwhile, the internal cells divide at a greater rate than the outer cells so that the blastocyst consists of two distinct cell populations, an outer trophoblast and an inner cell mass. The trophoblast cells form the extraembryonic structures, the amnion and the chorion. The cells of the inner cell mass produce the embryo and the yolk sac, which later contributes chorionic mesoderm to the trophoblast. Because of this contribution, chorionic villus sampling can allow the biopsy of cells derived both from the trophoblast shell and from the inner cell mass.

Development to this point can occur without maternal influence after in vitro fertilization, and results in the pre-embryo. The term *pre-embryo* was coined to refer to the multicellular organism before it implants.

Implantation

The blastocyst begins to implant into the endometrial lining of the uterus, thus initiating the formation of the placenta. On about the 5th day, the zona pellucida degenerates, exposing an adhesive region on the trophoblast cells overlying the inner cell mass. This region adheres to endometrial cells that have been prepared by steroid hormone stimulation of the ovarian cycle. At about the 7th day, implantation begins as the trophoblast cells invade between the uterine lining cells. Thus, by the end of the 1st week, the blastocyst is superficially implanted within the uterus, but it does not have functional connections with the mother. The trophoblast then differentiates into two layers—the syncytiotrophoblast, an outer layer lacking cell boundaries, and the cytotrophoblast, an inner, cellular layer. As the syncytiotrophoblast continues to invade, it produces chorionic gonadotropin that converts the corpus luteum in the ovary into the corpus luteum of pregnancy. Steroid hormones produced by the corpus luteum then maintain the lining of the uterus to support subsequent development of the embryo.

During the 2nd week of human development, the trophoblast cells further differentiate and begin to form the placenta and the extraembryonic membranes, including the amniotic sac. The embryo subsequently grows into the cavity formed by the amniotic sac. The amniotic sac enlarges and obliterates the chorionic cavity that is formed by the surrounding chorion, another derivative of the trophoblast. Implantation is normally completed by the end of the 2nd week.

Gastrulation

Gastrulation begins at about the 15th day, coincident with the first missed menstrual period. During the formation of the extraembryonic membranes, the inner cell mass flattens to form two epithelial sheets, the embryonic endoderm and ectoderm, that lie between the primary yolk sac and the amniotic cavity. The events of gastrulation convert these two flat circular layers of the embryonic disc into a three-dimensional organism and create a basic body plan. This plan has three axes, anterior-posterior, dorsal-ventral, and left-right. During gastrulation, the embryo forms three distinct germ layers: the ectoderm, the mesoderm, and the endoderm.

Gastrulation begins at a midline groove, the primitive streak. This groove forms in the embryonic ectoderm near the posterior end of the embryonic disc. A population of embryonic ectoderm cells migrates into this groove and begins to fill the potential space between the cell sheets of embryonic ectoderm and endoderm. These cells, which migrate anteriorly and laterally, form the embryonic mesoderm or mesenchyme. A cord of these cells coalesces anterior to the primitive streak to form the midline notochord that lengthens, causing the embryonic disc to become elongated. By the end of the 3rd week, when gastrulation is completed, the embryo has three layers and has each of the three body axes.

Organogenesis

Cells form specific tissues and organs by differentiation, the acquisition of specialized cell structure and function, and morphogenesis, change in shape and location. The ectoderm, the first layer to undergo organogenesis, begins to form the central nervous system on the 18th day of gestation. The ectoderm forms the brain, its accessory organs, the adrenal medulla, and the melanocytes. It also forms the epidermis and its derivatives, the sweat and mammary glands. Neurulation, the initial step in formation of the central nervous system, occurs by thickening and folding of the ectoderm in the dorsal midline to form the neural tube, a continuous canal running from the head to the tail end of the embryo. Because the neural tube grows at a greater rate than the rest of the embryo, the relatively flat embryonic disc takes on increasing convexity, so that the originally dorsal ectoderm ultimately almost surrounds the embryo.

The originally ventral endoderm becomes enveloped by the other two germ layers and folds to form a tube that later becomes the gut epithelium and its derivatives. These derivatives, which include the liver, pancreas, salivary glands, and lungs, form as outgrowths from the tube. By the 30th day, the embryo has become rounded and elongated, and the organ anlagen are nearly in their final positions relative to one another.

The mesoderm organizes into specialized regions, the major ones being in the center of the embryo between the base of the head and the tail. The mesoderm consists of loose connective tissue, the mesenchymal cells. In some places, these cells interact with epithelia of ectodermal and endodermal origin to form various organs. The somite (or paraxial) mesoderm is adjacent to the notochord. It condenses into segments or somites, each of which soon splits into three parts. These are the dermatome, which forms the dermis; the myotome, which forms the muscles of the limbs and trunk; and the sclerotome, which forms the skeleton of the vertebral column.

Lateral to the somites is the intermediate (or nephrogenic) mesoderm, which forms the urogenital system and its associated glands. Lateral to the intermediate mesoderm is the lateral plate mesoderm, which forms the serous linings, the lymphatic and blood vascular systems, and the bone marrow. In response to cues from surface ectoderm, this mesoderm forms the bones and cartilage of the limbs.

Although organogenesis begins during the 3rd week, it is a lengthy process, and the different organs develop at different rates. The earliest organ system to become functional is the cardiovascular system, which begins early in the 4th week of development to bring nutrients and oxygen from the uterine lining to the developing embryo. The last organ system to begin to develop is the urogenital system. The development of particular organs is described in standard textbooks of human embryology, a few of which are listed in the references.

By term, most organs have achieved their adult shape, but almost none have achieved their adult histoarchitecture. The growth and development of most organs is not complete until the end of adolescence. Maturation of several organs is accelerated around the time of birth, however, to enable the fetus to accommodate to extrauterine life. These developmental changes are induced at different times and rates and by a variety of stimuli. For example, before birth, various stimuli, including increased levels of cortisol, increase surfactant production in the lung. At birth, changes in afterload caused by absence of the placenta, dilation of the pulmonary vasculature, and closure of the ductus arteriosus induce changes in the molecular and cellular structure of the heart. After birth, as the infant is exposed to new antigens and as maternally derived immunoglobulins decline, B-cell production of immunoglobulins gradually increases.

DEVELOPMENTAL BIOLOGY AND THE PROCESSES INVOLVED IN EMBRYOGENESIS

To develop functioning tissues and organs, cells must control their own fate and direct the behavior of other cells. Developmental biology is the study of how cells accomplish these ends.

Genes Control Development

The blueprint for development is encoded in DNA, which is present in all nucleated cells in the body. With rare exceptions, such as in B cells where immunoglobulin genes undergo rearrangement, each diploid cell contains identical DNA sequences. Each cell type, however, expresses only about 1% of its genes. The programming of each cell type to acquire distinct patterns of gene expression is one of the processes needed for the formation of functioning tissues and organs.

Cells Commit to Distinct Developmental Fates

The zygote and its early daughter cells are capable of giving rise to any type of cell in the body. These totipotent cells give rise to lineages of progressively more specialized cells (Fig. 3–2). The cells that begin the formation of organs have a less extensive repertoire but can still develop into multiple different cell types. For example, as the lung starts to develop, epithelial cells bud from the foregut endoderm. They eventually form the wide range of specialized epithelial cells found in the airways and acini. The cells of the splanchnic mesoderm, into which the bud grows, become fibroblasts, smooth muscle cells, and chondrocytes. The processes by which cells become specialized are known as *determination* and *differentiation*.

Determination, or commitment, is the process of gradual reduction of developmental options that eventually renders the cells capable of becoming only a single cell type. The cells become committed to a particular type of differentiation. These changes in the developmental potential of cells are heritable by daughter cells and are irreversible. Although determination is induced by factors in the environment of cells, changes in the environment can induce new determination events but cannot reverse existing ones. Determination does not result from a loss of DNA but from stable changes in how and when genes are expressed. Importantly a cell becomes determined before one can recognize changes in phenotype. Thus, one cannot establish when a cell has become committed until after the commitment has occurred.

Cells Become Specialized in Form and Function

In contrast to determination, which narrows developmental options, differentiation is the acquisition of characteristics that enable cells to fulfill specialized functions. For example, neural crest cells eventually differentiate into cells with a wide variety of specialized functions, including conduction and transmission of signals, mechanical support, nutrition of other cells, and hormone production.

The expression of differentiated characteristics is influenced by a cell's hormonal milieu and physical environment. For example, if cells are dissociated and grown in culture dishes, they rarely perform their full range of specialized functions exactly as they did in vivo. These changes in environment, however, do not reverse a cell's commitment. A pancreatic islet cell cannot be made into a thyroid epithelial cell or vice versa.

Determination and differentiation occur in a series of overlapping steps. Cells frequently have some differentiated characteristics even though they have not yet undergone their final determination. For example, cells from embryonic bone have characteristics that distinguish them as osteogenic cells, yet they are able to develop into osteo-

ZYGOTE

PLURIPOTENTIAL
CELLS

COMMITTED
PRECURSOR CELLS

DIFFERENTIATED
CELLS

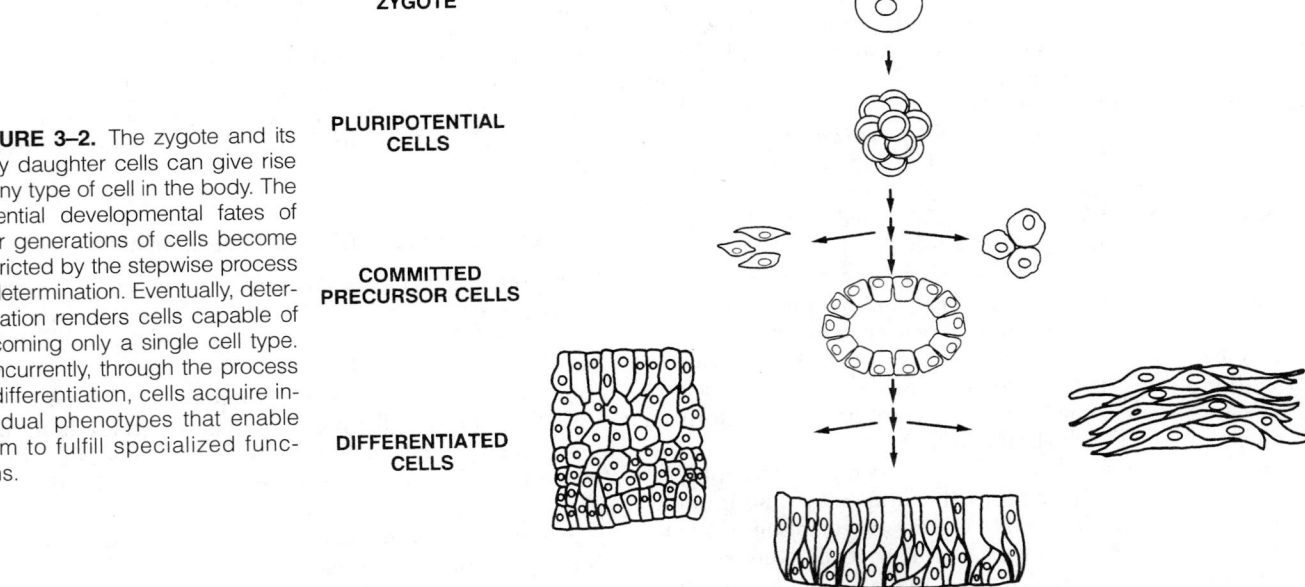

FIGURE 3–2. The zygote and its early daughter cells can give rise to any type of cell in the body. The potential developmental fates of later generations of cells become restricted by the stepwise process of determination. Eventually, determination renders cells capable of becoming only a single cell type. Concurrently, through the process of differentiation, cells acquire individual phenotypes that enable them to fulfill specialized functions.

blasts, osteoclasts, and osteocytes. They also give rise to a population of stem cells, the osteoprogenitor cells. Stem cells differ from embryonic cells in that they persist into adult life and have extensive capacity for self-renewal, but they give rise to at least one and often several types of differentiated progeny.

Acquisition of Specialized Function and the Generation of Unique Forms

The development of functioning organs requires not only that cells acquire specialized roles but also that they arrange themselves correctly. A type I pneumocyte cannot perform its most important function, gas exchange, unless it is organized properly with respect to its adjacent cells, including type II pneumocytes to provide surfactant, capillary endothelial cells to conduct blood, and fibroblasts to produce scaffolding. To form functioning organs, the behavior of populations of cells must be coordinated. Thus the genome of cells contains information needed not only for a variety of specialized functions, but also for the plan that will orchestrate the formation of organs and the whole organism. The origins of this plan may reside in a number of genes that act as switches (Blau, 1988).

When activated, these genes permit or inhibit the expression of other genes that alter the expression of yet more genes. Thus, these genes may form a regulatory hierarchy in which activation of *master* genes turns on entire developmental sequences. Such genes may also repress developmental sequences, but evidence for this is not as clear. The number of master genes required to regulate development is not known. A small number of genes, probably fewer than the number of differentiated cell types, likely act in various sequences and combinations to control the many steps of determination and differentiation.

Some of the genes regulating development in organisms with short life cycles, such as the fruit fly, *Drosophila melanogaster*, have been identified. Genes that may regulate some of the early processes of mammalian development have been identified because they share sequences with the *Drosophila melanogaster* genes (Dressler and Gruss, 1988; Gehring, 1987). The functions of most of these genes in mammals are still unknown, but their temporal and spatial patterns of expression suggest that, similar to their insect counterparts, they control formation of tissue patterns and organs. Examples of the genes that control development in *Drosophila melanogaster* include genes of the homeo box family that code for proteins controlling the identity of body segments, genes of the paired box family that code for proteins controlling segmentation, and genes for proteins with multiple *zinc-finger* DNA-binding motifs that may control cell determination. Putative genes involved in regulating development have also been identified and their roles explored in mammals by gene transfer (Gossler et al, 1989). For example, candidate genes from committed, although as yet undifferentiated, cells have been introduced into uncommitted recipient cells so that the effects of the genes on cell lineage could be explored.

Cell Specialization and Selective Gene Activation

Products of regulatory genes act at many levels to control the expression of many hundreds of other genes at precise times during development. Sites of regulation include the synthesis, processing, and degradation of numerous RNA and protein molecules. This large repertoire of mechanisms is used both to control where genes are transcribed and to diversify their products.

DNA Structure

RNA synthesis is regulated by factors that change the conformation (or shape) of DNA. These include nuclear proteins that control DNA-folding, specific chemical modifications of DNA, short DNA sequences in or near genes themselves (so-called *cis*-acting factors), and proteins that interact with DNA sequences to increase or decrease transcription (so-called *trans*-acting factors). The products of genes can also control protein synthesis by affecting RNA processing, messenger RNA stability and transport, and transfer RNA availability. In addition, various modifications of proteins can alter their location, activity, and rate of degradation. Each of these post-translational modifications can affect the cell's phenotype.

DNA Conformation. DNA is a linear polymer, but it exists in cells as a double helical strand that is highly and precisely contorted. Slight differences in its folding appear to affect gene expression profoundly. Some of the folding is controlled by histones, which are small, highly basic proteins that bind tightly to the negatively charged DNA. Histone-DNA complexes, in which DNA strands are looped at regular intervals around several histone molecules, form chromatin. Chromatin is contorted into higher-order filamentous structures, also by interactions with histone proteins. A third level of DNA conformation is heterochromatin, a highly condensed form of DNA. One of the X chromosomes in each mammalian female cell is almost entirely heterochromatin. Other chromosomes, although not entirely condensed, can also develop lengthy regions of heterochromatin.

These methods of progressively increasing the order of DNA-folding produce stable decreases in the likelihood of gene transcription. The folding must be undone to allow DNA replication, but the patterns of folding can be passed on to many generations of daughter cells. Little is known about how these patterns are maintained and inherited.

Chemical Modification of DNA. Physiologic methylation of certain DNA bases, the cytidines, also affects the local conformation of segments of DNA (Cedar, 1988). Methylation alters the binding of regulatory factors, histones, and other proteins. So-called housekeeping genes, which are expressed in nearly all cells, are predominantly unmethylated. In contrast, tissue-specific genes are typically almost fully methylated during early development in germ line and somatic cells, but they become unmethylated in those cells that can express them. Moreover, daughter cells inherit specific methylation patterns. The factors responsible for site-specific changes in methylation are unknown. Furthermore, because methylation of DNA does not occur in some eukaryotic organisms, there must be other mechanisms for selecting genes for transcription.

Protein Interactions with DNA: *Cis*-Acting and *Trans*-Acting Factors. So-called *trans*-acting factors are proteins that transiently interact with DNA to activate or suppress transcription. They appear to change the local conformation of DNA and thus alter the binding of RNA synthetic enzymes. *Trans*-acting proteins bind to specific DNA sequences, designated as *cis* elements. *Cis* elements are promoters, which by definition, include the site where transcription is initiated, and both enhancers and silencers, which are more distant from the gene and can act on more than one gene. DNA-folding may bring *cis* elements together to allow protein-binding, enabling distant elements to interact (Dynan, 1989; Schüle et al, 1988).

Some genes have multiple promoters, each used in different tissues or at different times (Schibler and Sierra, 1989). The alternative promoters can be affected distinctly by *trans*-acting factors to vary the rate of transcription, and their transcripts can have differing rates of degradation or translation, leading to diverse expression of the same gene. Less commonly, use of an alternative promoter changes the translation initiation codon and, therefore, the primary structure of the protein.

Other DNA sequences can also produce tissue-specific or development-specific variations of a protein. For example, short sequences determine where messenger RNA molecules can be spliced, thus determining which sections of the transcript are removed (Breitbart et al, 1987). Alternative splicing and alternative promoters are mechanisms whereby a wide variety of myosin and troponin isoforms are produced from a limited number of genes. These different isoforms are expressed in different sites and at different times in development to vary the functional properties of cardiac and skeletal muscles.

Certain other sequences in genes can render their transcripts susceptible, in certain circumstances, to degradation (Klausner and Harford, 1989). For example, a sequence in transferrin transcripts causes them to be less stable when the cells expressing them are exposed to iron.

Various proteins produced or activated in response to extracellular signals can serve as *trans*-acting factors. Examples of *trans*-acting factors include steroid hormone receptors. Hormone-binding causes these receptors to interact with regulatory elements common to many inducible genes.

There are probably only a limited number of *trans*-acting factors, and their effects are also regulated. For example, modifications of the DNA, *cis* elements, and cooperative binding of different *trans*-acting factors can permit, amplify, reduce, or negate the effects of transcriptional activation.

Generation of Tissue and Organ Forms

The generation of tissue and organ forms requires coordination of multiple gene products. Although genes control expression of specific proteins and can act as switches to begin formation of tissue patterns, such as segments and limbs, how they dictate these patterns is not known. Establishment of patterns requires interaction between cells. Morphogenesis, the process whereby cells organize into correct arrangements to form functional organs, involves the basic mechanisms whereby cells control and are controlled by the behavior of their neighbors. Although there is enormous diversity in the structure and function of organs, cells regulate multiple gene products to produce a limited repertoire of behaviors that control all of morphogenesis.

Cellular Behaviors of Morphogenesis

To form organs, cells must adhere, change in shape, and change in number. These behaviors are coordinated and propagated by the insoluble extracellular matrix and the diffusible peptide growth factors.

Cell Adhesion. Embryonic tissues can be dissociated into suspensions of single cells that, under certain circumstances, can reassemble and reform structures resembling the original tissue. This property depends on the ability of cells to adhere to and to recognize one another.

Cell adhesion and recognition behaviors are vital to the establishment of tissue boundaries, the migration of cells along specific pathways, and the relative placement of cells. Cell adhesion and cell recognition are accomplished by cell adhesion molecules. Subsequently, specialized cell junctions arise that maintain and stabilize the adhesions and allow intercellular communication.

Cell Adhesion Molecules. A variety of cell adhesion molecules have been identified and have been characterized to varying degrees (Edelman, 1986; Ekblom et al, 1986; Takeichi, 1988). All have extracellular domains that interact with other cell adhesion molecules and intracellular domains that interact with the cytoskeleton. The molecules can be grouped based on whether or not they require calcium ions to mediate adhesion and whether the molecule they bind to on adjacent cells is identical (homophilic) or nonidentical (heterophilic). Examples include E-cadherin (also known as uvomorulin or ECAM [epithelial cell adhesion molecule]), a calcium-dependent cell adhesion molecule that is found initially on blastomeric cells and cells of the inner cell mass. Its distribution changes during development, and ultimately it is confined to epithelial cells, where it forms part of the junctional complex between cells. Another example is N-cadherin (NCAM) (originally neural cell adhesion molecule). Binding with NCAM is calcium independent. It is found on endoderm, mesoderm, and ectoderm of the early embryo, but it is later confined to neural cells, smooth muscle, and motor endplates.

Each cell adhesion molecule has a specific tissue and developmental distribution. The expression of cell adhesion molecules is regulated in ways that are important in morphogenesis. For example, the density, distribution, and number relative to other cell adhesion molecules can all be regulated. In addition, in some cases the extracellular domains of cell adhesion molecules may be altered by post-translational modifications, and their cytoplasmic domains can be varied by differential splicing of messenger RNAs. These changes can lead to altered binding with other cell adhesion molecules and altered interactions with the cytoskeleton (Cunningham et al, 1987).

Cell Junctions. Once simple epithelial cells form a sheet or tube, they become connected at their lateral borders by a junctional complex that encircles the apex of each cell. It has several components. The tight junction, or zonula occludens, the most apical part of the complex, appears earliest in development and acts to polarize the epithelium. Tight junctions act as a fence to limit the diffusion of membrane constituents between the apical and lateral membranes and to regulate selectively the passage of ions between cells. The extent of this gating function varies widely between epithelia.

The intermediate junction (zonula adherens) also encircles the cell within the junctional complex and connects to the actin network in the cell (see the section, Change in Cell Shape).

Spot desmosomes (macula adherens) appear to act as rivets between lateral cell membranes. These junctions also consist of a membrane domain and a cytoplasmic plaque that is anchored to the structural cytokeratin network within the cell.

Gap junctions provide passageways connecting adjacent cells. They are assembled from subunits of hydrophobic proteins to form channels within the plasma membrane that admit various ions and molecules with a molecular mass of less than 500 daltons. The intercellular transfer of these small molecules may regulate and coordinate the differentiation of certain cell types.

Change in Cell Shape. When a cell differentiates, it acquires a specific shape that is one of its differentiated characteristics. Cell shape results, in part, from a cytoplasmic framework, the cytoskeleton. This framework is composed of polymers of fibril-forming proteins and various accessory proteins organized together into microfilaments, intermediate filaments, and microtubules (Table 3–1). The accessory proteins affect filament assembly or link the filaments to one another or to other cell components. The cytoskeleton is not a permanent structure but changes rapidly in response to cellular events. In addition to its role in cell shape, the cytoskeleton (1) interacts extensively with cell membranes and regulates the mobility of integral proteins within the membrane; (2) organizes the cytoplasm by binding various organelles; (3) forms specialized regions of cells, such as microvilli; and (4) contributes to secretory mechanisms.

The other influences on cell shape are various external factors, which include cell-cell and cell-matrix adhesion. These adhesions are transduced by a variety of transmembrane signaling systems. Changes in shape are generally initiated by changes in linkages between membrane proteins and the microfilament network and are maintained by microfilaments and microtubules.

Cell culture evidence suggests that specific cell shape is needed to maintain differentiated cell function. The details of how cell shape exerts these effects are not known but may include traction of cytoskeletal components on the nucleus and organelles and activation of various second messenger systems.

Cell shape has other important effects during morphogenesis. Cells can move when they change shape. If the cells are linked together, as in an epithelial sheet, a change in cell shape results in a change in the form of the entire sheet. If the cells are not linked, a change in their shape can begin a locomotory sequence, in which coordinated adhesion of the leading edge to the substratum and change in cell shape together result in cell migration.

Change in Cell Number. Localized differences in rates of proliferation change the shape of developing organs. Higher rates of mitosis of some groups of cells relative to others initiate the formation of many organs and lead to the development of specialized forms, such as branches and lobes. Both the rate of mitosis and the plane of cleavage, which determines the position of the daughter cells relative to one another, are important. Also, mitosis can yield two identical progeny or be asymmetric, yielding two different daughter cells (O'Farrell et al, 1989).

The local control of proliferation of cells is complex. It

TABLE 3–1

Major Classes of Cytoskeletal Components

Components	Composition	Functions
Microfilaments	Actin and diverse group of actin-binding proteins	Contractile systems necessary to generate tension and for cell extension movement and division Mechanical support for cell structures and extensions by lamellipodia, microvilli Interactions with cell adhesion molecules, extracellular matrix receptors
Microtubules	Alpha and beta tubulins	Strength and motility of cilia and flagella Anchorage of nucleus Formation of mitotic spindle
Intermediate filaments	Vimentin, desmin, cytokeratins, and others (characteristic of cell type)	Tension bearing

is mediated partly by peptide growth factors and growth inhibitory factors and partly by changes in the extracellular matrix. The molecular mechanisms whereby these local environmental influences affect cell proliferation are also not well understood. Two families of intracellular proteins, cyclins and cyclin-dependent kinases, interact to control transition of eukaryotic cells from the G1 phase of the cell cycle into DNA synthesis and cell division. Studies are elucidating the cell cycle checkpoints and regulatory pathways involved in cell cycle transitions in normal and malignant cells (Elledge, 1996; Sherr, 1996; Stillman, 1996).

Programmed cell death, termed apoptosis, at specific localized sites (see Table 3–1) is a normal event in morphogenesis, illustrated in the interdigital areas of the limb buds, where the death of cells allows separation of the digits. In the developing central and peripheral nervous system, cell death is a ubiquitous phenomenon. Survival or death of a neuron appears to be determined by events in its projection field. Another example of localized cell death is the death of the intimal cell layer of the ductus arteriosus when it closes after birth. Cell death in this case may be secondary to failure of nutrition because of cessation of blood flow through the vessel. Cell death had also been presumed to cause loss of epithelia at several sites during organogenesis. Loss of some of these epithelia, however, is now thought to result from the conversion of epithelium to mesenchymal cells (e.g., the medial palatine epithelium at the time of palatal fusion).

Extracellular Coordinating Molecules

Morphogenesis is wholly dependent on the molecules that organize the behavior of individual cells into morphologically and functionally defined groups. Two classes of molecules can serve this function—the extracellular matrix components and the peptide growth factors. These molecules are the predominant influences on the differentiation, proliferation, shape, and migration of cells. The extracellular matrix components are large, multidomain molecules that are extensively cross-linked to each other, predominantly by noncovalent bonds, to form an insoluble matrix that spans multiple cells. The growth factors are small, soluble peptides that can diffuse locally to affect groups of cells.

Thus, extracellular matrix composites and peptide growth factors differ in fundamental ways, yet they share biologic effects. They both act (1) locally, influencing a particular population of cells; (2) via autocrine or paracrine mechanisms, influencing their tissue of origin or adjacent tissues; and (3) at the cell surface, by binding receptors. The insoluble matrix can modulate the effect of the otherwise diffusible growth factors. The matrix binds some growth factor peptides and thus can partition their effects, protect them from degradation, or serve as a reservoir for growth factors.

Extracellular Matrix Components. All cells undergoing morphogenesis produce and deposit an insoluble mesh, the extracellular matrix, beyond their cell membranes. Each cell type produces a specific type of matrix. For example, parenchymal cells produce a basal lamina, and mesenchymal cells produce an interstitial matrix (Fig. 3–3). The major components of each matrix are the structural proteins, which include the collagens and elastin, the adhesive glycoproteins, and the proteoglycans. The exact composition and organization of matrices, however, vary from tissue to tissue and change during development (McDonald, 1988).

Collagens. The collagens provide resiliency to all matrices. There are at least 12 genetically distinct forms of collagen, each sharing a characteristic triple helix, and most are formed by assembly of nonidentical subunits transcribed from several genes. These heterotrimers are generally polymerized into macroscopic fibrils. Some collagen types (e.g., Type IV, the predominant collagen in basal laminae) do not form fibrils but produce a chicken wire–like mesh. Collagen fibrils have great tensile strength because of intermolecular cross-linking of the molecules.

Elastin. Elastin is a constituent of the matrix in organs such as the lung, skin, and aorta in which considerable elasticity is required. Elastin is composed of a single type of hydrophobic polypeptide that forms random coils. These are highly cross-linked to produce multimers that can both stretch and recoil. Elastin combines with a variety of microfibril proteins, which serve as a scaffolding, to form the elastic fiber of matrix.

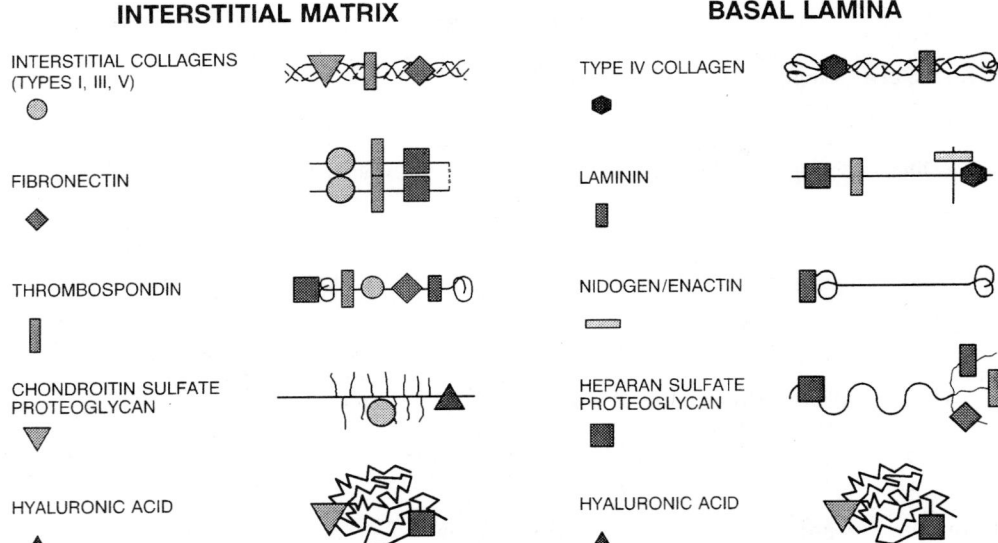

FIGURE 3–3. Mesenchymal cells produce an interstitial matrix, and parenchymal cells produce a basal lamina. Both of these extracellular matrix types contain collagens, adhesive glycoproteins (such as fibronectin, thrombospondin, laminin, and nidogen), and glycosaminoglycan–containing molecules (the proteoglycans and hyaluronic acid). The interstitial matrix and the basal lamina each contain characteristic molecular species of these large, extensively cross-linked, insoluble components. Major extracellular matrix components are shown. The symbols represent each component, and molecular interactions are indicated. For example, the interstitial collagens bind chondroitin sulfate proteoglycan, thrombospondin, and fibronectin.

Adhesive Glycoproteins. These large proteins contain multiple distinct polypeptide domains that bind tightly to various other matrix molecules and to specific cell surface receptors. The most abundant types, laminin, found predominantly in the basal lamina, and fibronectin, located in the interstitial matrix, typify matrix adhesive glycoproteins. Each contains specific amino acid sequences that are recognized by cell surface receptors, notably arg-gly-asp in fibronectin and tyr-ile-gly-ser-arg in laminin, and the heparin-binding regions of both fibronectin and laminin.

Proteoglycans. Surrounding and bound to the protein components of the matrix are proteoglycans and hyaluronate. Proteoglycans consist of glycosaminoglycan chains covalently linked to a core protein. Hyaluronate is a large linear glycosaminoglycan. These polysaccharides are composed of alternating hexuronate and N-acetyl hexosamine residues. The glycosaminoglycans can bind many large and small molecules, including water, and can occupy a huge volume for their mass, thus allowing diffusion of nutrients, metabolites, and hormones across the extracellular matrix. Variations in the core proteins and in the glycosaminoglycan chains permit considerable diversity of the proteoglycans. For example, the proteoglycans organize components of the basal lamina, lubricate joints, provide turgor to the dermis, stabilize collagen fibrils, and resist compressive forces in cartilage (Ruoslahti, 1988).

Peptide Growth Factors. These factors were originally identified by their ability to stimulate proliferation of cultured cells and, thus, are usually referred to as growth factors. They can have a much wider range of actions,

however, including altering responsiveness to other hormones or growth factors, inducing or repressing differentiation, and changing the composition of the extracellular matrix. Although usually autocrine or paracrine in action, some, such as the insulin-like growth factors, circulate in blood and may have endocrine functions. The actions of combinations of growth factor peptides are not necessarily predictable from an analysis of their actions when examined separately, and their effects can differ after changes in differentiation of the target cells (Mercola and Stiles, 1988; Slack, 1989).

There are several families of peptide growth factors. Examples are given in Table 3–2. Each family has several members that share at least one amino acid sequence and activity and may be recognized by the same receptor. Related forms are found in a wide variety of animal species. Some oncogenes also encode family members of growth factors or their receptors. Oncogenes are genes whose products confer on cells properties common to cells of many malignant tumors.

Any list of peptide growth factors is likely to be incomplete because this is a rapidly expanding field of research. Examples other than those in Table 3–2 include a group of neurotropic growth factors that promote growth and prevent programmed death of neurons in both the peripheral and the central nervous systems. The cytokines, which include the interferons, the interleukins, and tumor necrosis factor, are structurally unrelated but together control the determination and differentiation of bone marrow–derived cells.

Localization of growth factors and their messenger RNAs has provided valuable insights into the functions of

TABLE 3-2

Examples of Peptide Growth Factors

Family	Examples	Examples of Functions
Epidermal growth factors	EGF	Stimulate proliferation of many embryonic cells
	TGF-α	Promote expression of differentiation of many mature cells, especially epithelial cells
Platelet-derived growth factors	PDGF-A	Mitogenic for mesenchymal cells
	PDGF-B	Chemotactic for vascular endothelial cells
	PDGF-AB	
Transforming growth factor-beta	TGF-β 1	Induction of other growth factors
	TGF-β 2	Cause accumulation of matrix components
	Inhibins	Control development of the genital tract
	Activins	
	Müllerian growth factor	
	Inhibitory factor	
Heparin-binding growth factors (fibroblast growth factors)	Acidic FGF	Promotion of angiogenesis
	Basic FGF	Mitogens for mesodermal and neuroectodermal cells
	KFGF	
	FGF5	
Insulin-like growth factors	IGF-1	Mitogenic for some cells
	IGF-2	Promote differentiation of others, e.g., muscle, cartilage
	Relaxin	Maturation of female reproductive tract

these factors in development but requires cautious interpretation because their actions are complex. For example, the presence of the messenger RNA for a factor in a developing tissue does not prove that the message is translated, that the active form of the factor is secreted, that it encounters functional receptors, or what other influences might modify its actions.

Receptors for Peptide Growth Factors and Matrix Components. The actions of both growth factor peptides and matrix components in changing cell behavior are mediated through binding to receptors, which are proteins with extracellular, *trans*-membrane, and intracellular domains. In each case, binding can lead to altered production of various proteins. The steps between receptor-binding and the alteration of transcription, translation, and protein-processing, however, are not yet well understood. The receptors for peptide growth factors and matrix components have different properties.

Binding of the soluble peptide growth factors to their receptors is specific and of high affinity. It leads to activation of intracellular signaling mechanisms and, often, to internalization and degradation or recycling of the receptor. Members of the epidermal growth factor, insulin-like growth factor, and platelet-derived growth factor families have receptors that activate intracellular pathways by phosphorylating tyrosines in various enzymes. Availability of growth factors for binding to receptor, at least in the case of the insulin-like growth factors, is determined by the level of specific binding proteins.

Because the matrix is insoluble, its receptors act differently (Buck and Horowitz, 1987). Matrix receptors often interact with more than one type of matrix component and

can have small intracellular domains that interact with components of the cytoskeleton. Binding does not lead to internalization or degradation of the receptor. Although different matrix receptors, such as the syndecans or the members of the integrin superfamily, can bind cells to virtually identical matrix components, each may have distinct effects on cell behaviors.

Hyaluronic acid regulates the motility of various cell types through interaction with specific cell surface receptors. CD44 was the first receptor to be identified; however, evidence indicates a major role for RHAMM (receptor for HA-mediated motility) in cell locomotion related to processes such as lymphocyte homing to tissues, tumorigenesis, and responses to injury. Hyaluronic acid and RHAMM may also have an important role in cell movement during both embryogenesis and organogenesis (Yang et al, 1994).

Developmental Strategies

Nature Versus Nurture on a Cellular Level. The overall sequence of development involves the generation of precursor cells to produce progeny that become determined and differentiated and organize into functional tissues and organs. Multicellular organisms use two strategies to accomplish these processes—mosaic and regulative development.

In mosaic development, cells are instructed by events within themselves corresponding to their intrinsic nature. Information dictating cellular development is derived from cellular genes and is independent of the behavior or even the existence of neighboring cells. Cell diversity is achieved by genetically induced changes in lineages. Some invertebrates, such as nematodes, develop primarily in this manner.

In regulative development, cells in a developing organism influence or nurture the development of other cells or tissues. These cell–cell interactions have profound effects on the determination, differentiation, and morphogenetic behavior of cells. Regulative development allows for a great degree of developmental plasticity. As a cell matures, however, its responses to its neighbors are affected to an increasing degree by previous cell–cell interactions and, therefore, by its own intrinsic nature. Thus, the degree of plasticity diminishes with increasing maturity of the organism. This regulative strategy predominates in vertebrates.

Developmental Strategies Are Time Dependent and Sequential. Both cell lineage and cell interactions dictate development in mammals, but responses to these influences are not stereotyped; rather, they undergo changes during development. Changes in cell behavior induced by any interaction modify the cell's response to all subsequent interactions. Thus, the response to a developmental influence is critically dependent on the history of the target cell, specifically how and when it was previously influenced. Thus, the sequential changes in phenotype of cells in developing tissues occur in parallel with changes in their potential patterns of response. This concept underlies the familiar differential effect of various teratogens. For example, the distinct phenotypes caused by thalidomide exposure resulted from effects on different tissues. The tissues that were affected depended on when during gestation exposure occurred, and thalidomide had essentially no teratogenic effect if exposure was sufficiently late.

NORMAL ORGAN FORM AND FUNCTION

The generation of organ form and function is affected by other developing organs, just as the behaviors of cells are governed partly by adjacent cells. Normal growth of the lung, for example, depends on growth of the chest wall and the fetal breathing movements of the diaphragm. How physical factors such as distention, compression, and stretch regulate behaviors of cells to form and deform organs is not well understood but is likely to be mediated in part through the extracellular matrix and intercellular junctions.

Malformations

Earlier sections of this chapter have shown that the cell is the simplest functional unit of morphogenesis and that a limited number of cell behaviors form all organs. Conceptually, congenital anomalies have been divided into malformations, deformations, and disruptions. In all of these, however, the anomalies result partly because the spatial and temporal distributions of expression of the molecules that govern cell behavior, such as the growth factors, matrix molecules, and their receptors, are altered. In the case of the abnormal collagen gene in Type I osteogenesis imperfecta, the mechanism is known and directly affects expression of a matrix component; but most of the defects are unknown, and it is likely that many are indirect.

Mutations of the genes that regulate segmentation and other aspects of pattern formation may also account for some congenital anomalies. As discussed earlier, these genes may be near the top of a hierarchy of genes that regulate the patterns of expression of other genes, including those for growth factors, matrix molecules, and factors that control cell lineage. The pattern-forming genes of *Drosophila melanogaster* have been identified and characterized because mutant forms of them cause anomalies. To date, no human genes that determine body form have been identified or linked to congenital anomalies. Mutation or abnormal expression of these pattern-forming genes early in gestation, however, could account for malformations of single organs and for multiple malformation sequences.

Premature Birth and Abnormal Development

When birth occurs prematurely, developmental influences occur out of sequence. There is sufficient flexibility in development of many organs for them to attain full size, form, and function despite their incomplete development when an infant is born in the late second or early third trimester. The delivery and postnatal support of premature infants, however, frequently result in the superimposition of tissue damage on the events of development.

Tissue repair can modify developmental processes, and the results of repair may differ in mature and in developing tissue. For example, a variety of agents, including hyperoxia, affect the lung differently early in development than in a mature individual. In preterm infants, these agents can induce coarse emphysema and scarring and reduced alveolar number, whereas in adults hyperoxia induces diffuse interstitial fibrosis. The responses differ but are both mediated through the controls that cells exert over one another.

Developmental processes can also modify tissue repair, presumably because the same types of cell behaviors and molecular controls are operating. Additionally, developing tissues may contain cells that are less committed than those in adult tissues. The developing tissues may therefore have a greater capacity to restore normal architecture at a site of injury. Although the mechanism is unclear, the rapid and remarkably complete repair of some developing tissues such as skin, cartilage, and bone of the fetus and infant is well known.

REFERENCES

Alberts D, Bray D, Lewis J, et al: Molecular biology of the cell. New York, Garland, 1989.

Blau HM: Hierarchies of regulatory genes may specify mammalian development. Cell 53:673, 1988.

Breitbart RE, Andreadis A, Nadal-Ginard B: Alternative splicing: A ubiquitous mechanism for the generation of multiple protein isoforms from single genes. Annu Rev Cell Biol 56:467, 1987.

Buck CA, Horowitz AF: Cell surface receptors for extracellular matrix molecules. Annu Rev Cell Biol 3:179, 1987.

Carraway KL, Carraway CAC: Membrane–cytoskeleton interactions in animal cells. Biochim Biophys Acta 988:147, 1987.

Cedar H: DNA methylation and gene activity. Cell 53:3, 1988.

Chen S, Teicher LC, Kazim D, et al: Commitment of mouse fibroblasts to adipocyte differentiation by DNA transfection. Science 244:582, 1989.

Cunningham BA, Hemperly JJ, Murray BA, et al: Neural cell adhesion molecule: Structure, immunoglobulin-like domains, cell surface modulation and alternative RNA splicing. Science 236:799, 1987.

Dressler GR, Gruss P: Do multigene families regulate vertebrate development? Trends Genet 4:214, 1988.

Dynan WS: Modularity in promoters and enhancers. Cell 58:1, 1989.

Edelman GM: Cell adhesion molecules in the regulation of animal form and tissue pattern. Annu Rev Cell Biol 2:81, 1986.

Ekblom P, Vestweber D, Kemler R: Cell–matrix interactions and cell adhesion during development. Annu Rev Cell Biol 2:27, 1986.

Elledge SJ: Cell cycle checkpoints: Preventing an identity crisis. Science 274:1664, 1996.

Gaunt SJ, Sharpe PT, Duboule D: Spatially restricted domains of homeogene transcripts in mouse embryos: Relation to a segmented body plan. Development 104S:169, 1988.

Gehring WJ: Homeo boxes in the study of development. Science 236:1245, 1987.

Gossler A, Joyner AL, Rossant J, et al: Mouse embryonic stem cells and reporter constructs to detect developmentally regulated genes. Science 244:463, 1989.

Hall PA, Watt FM: Stem cells: The generation and maintenance of cellular diversity. Development 106:619, 1989.

Klausner RD, Harford JB: *Cis-trans* models for post-transcriptional gene regulation. Science 246:870, 1989.

Maniatis T, Goodbourn S, Fischer JA: Regulation of inducible and tissue-specific gene expression. Science 236:1237, 1987.

McDonald JA: Extracellular matrix assembly. Annu Rev Cell Biol 4:183, 1988.

Mercola M, Stiles CD: Growth factor superfamilies and mammalian embryogenesis. Development 102:451, 1988.

Metcalf D: The molecular control of cell division, differentiation, commitment and maturation in haemopoietic cells. Nature 339:27, 1989.

O'Farrell PH, Edgar BA, Lakich D, Lehner CF: Directing cell division during development. Science 246:635, 1989.

Pelton RW, Nomura S, Moses HL, Hogan BL: Expression of transforming growth factor beta-2 RNA during murine embryogenesis. Development 106:759, 1989.

Rizzino A: Transforming growth factor-β: Multiple effects on cell differentiation and extracellular matrices. Dev Biol 130:411, 1988.

Ross R: Platelet-derived growth factor. Lancet 1:1179, 1989.

Ruoslahti E: Structure and biology of proteoglycans. Annu Rev Cell Biol 4:229, 1988.

Sadler T: Langman's Medical Embryology, 6th ed. Baltimore, Williams & Wilkins, 1990.

Schibler U, Sierra F: Alternative promoters in developmental gene expression. Annu Rev Genet 21:237, 1989.

Schüle R, Muller M, Kaltschmidt C, Renkawitz R: Many transcription factors interact synergistically with steroid receptors. Science 242:1418, 1988.

Sherr CJ: Cancer cell cycles. Science 274:1672, 1996.

Slack JMW: Peptide regulatory factors in embryonic development. Lancet 1:1312, 1989.

Stillman B: Cell cycle control of DNA replication. Science 274:1659, 1996.

Takeichi M: The cadherins: Cell–cell adhesion molecules controlling animal morphogenesis. Development 102:639, 1988.

Yang B, Yang BL, Savani RC, Turley E: Identification of a common hyaluronan (HA) binding motif in the HA-binding proteins RHAMM, CD44 and link protein. EMBO J 13:286, 1994.

Yarden Y, Ullrich A: Growth factor receptor tyrosine kinases. Annu Rev Biochem 57:443, 1988.

CHAPTER 4

Hormonal Influences on Fetal Development

Philip L. Ballard

The physiology of the fetal endocrine system differs from that of the adult with regard to the hormonal milieu, production sites, plasma levels, rates and pathways of degradation, and biologic function. The unique endocrine environment of the fetus and placenta is important for both normal growth and differentiation of the fetus and timely parturition. Although there are major differences in endocrine physiology and regulated genes between the fetus and adult, the basic cellular mechanisms of hormone action do not change during development.

SITES OF PRODUCTION AND ACTION

Autocrine. Some hormones act primarily on the cells where they are synthesized. Hormones are synthesized within the cells, secreted at the cell surface into the extracellular domain, and then bind to specific cell surface receptors on the same cell. This interaction initiates a series of intracellular events, as described subsequently, which modify growth, differentiation, or function of the cell.

Paracrine. In this system, hormones are secreted by one cell type and act on adjacent neighboring cells of another type. This mechanism provides for cell-cell communication within a tissue and is involved in regulating both growth and differentiation. In the fetal lung and other tissues, for example, insulin-like growth factors (IGFs) are produced and secreted by mesenchymal cells and influence the growth of adjacent epithelial cells.

Endocrine. Most hormones are produced in a specific cell type of a tissue, are secreted into the circulation, and exert their regulatory effects on distant tissues. Included in this category are polypeptide hormones synthesized in the hypothalamus, pituitary, placenta, and other tissues as well as the steroid hormones (androgens, estrogens, progestins, mineralocorticoids, vitamin D, and glucocorticoids). The steroid hormones and many of the protein hormones are bound to specific binding proteins in the serum, providing a hormone reservoir that is less susceptible to degradation. For most hormones, the plasma concentration of free (unbound) hormones represents the physiologically active hormones available to target cells. After secretion, the activity of hormones may be modified by metabolism in the circulation or tissues. For example, inactive cortisone may be converted to active cortisol by target tissues (e.g., lung and liver), and thyroxine (T_4) can undergo deiodination to either active triiodothyronine (T_3) or inactive reverse T_3 (rT_3) in the adult and fetus, respectively.

Cellular Mechanisms

The signal inherent in a hormone is expressed through the binding of a hormone to its receptor, which initiates a series of biochemical events within the cell leading to altered replication or function. In general, the steps in this process of signal transduction are identical for adult and fetal cells, although different genes or proteins (or both) of a given cell type may be responsive during the developmental process. Furthermore, in the fetus, developmental immaturity or deficiency of specific components in the signal transduction system can alter hormone responsiveness.

Membrane Receptors

The protein and peptide hormones as well as biogenic amines exert their effects on cells by binding to specific receptor proteins located on the cell membrane. The receptors are membrane-spanning proteins with an extracellular domain containing the binding site for the hormone and a cytoplasmic domain that transmits the hormonal signal to intracellular molecules. For many hormonal systems, binding of hormone to receptor results in increased intracellular levels of a second messenger, such as cyclic adenosine monophosphate (cAMP). Membrane receptors are capable of moving within the cell membrane and may aggregate and be endocytosed after binding of the hormone. Receptors are also substrates for various protein kinases, and in some cases phosphorylation is dependent on the binding of hormones. These processes can produce a transient deficiency or inactivity of receptors (down regulation) and relative unresponsiveness of the cells to continued hormonal exposure. For example, down regulation and hormone refractoriness may be observed clinically with continued administration of a beta-agonist.

One of the best described membrane receptor systems is that for beta-adrenergic agonists. The receptor has been isolated, purified, and sequenced, and complementary DNAs have been cloned for studying receptor structure, function, and regulation (Lefkowitz and Caron, 1988). The cytoplasmic domain of the receptor is associated with G proteins, which either activate or inhibit the catalytic component of adenyl cyclase. In the case of activation, binding of the hormone results within minutes in increased production of cAMP from adenosine triphosphate (ATP); the response is transient, and levels rapidly return to near baseline values. cAMP, in turn, binds to the regulatory subunit of protein kinase A, releasing and activating the catalytic subunit. This enzyme phosphorylates specific cellular proteins resulting in either activation or inactivation with subsequent effects on enzyme activity (e.g., glycogen phosphorylase), intracellular structure (e.g., in the cytoskeleton), or gene expression in the nucleus. This sequence of events is summarized in Figure 4–1.

Intracellular Receptors

Thyroid hormones, steroid hormones, and certain polypeptide hormones enter target cells and bind to specific recep-

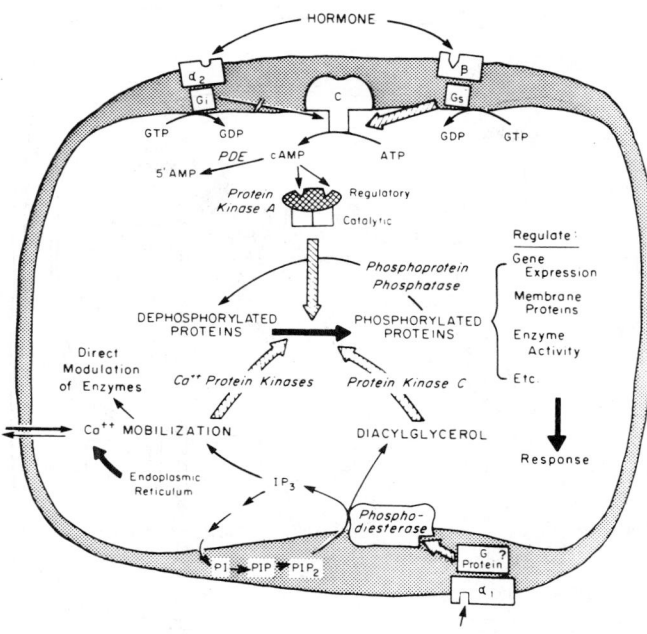

FIGURE 4–1. Molecular mechanism of catecholamine action. This model applies for a variety of hormones that act through either cAMP or IP3 as secondary messengers. ATP, adenosine-5′-triphosphate; cAMP, adenosine-3′,5′-cyclic monophosphate; 5′-AMP, adenosine-5′-monophosphate; C, catalytic subunit of adenylate cyclase; GTP, guanosine-5′-triphosphate; GDP, guanosine-5′-diphosphate; G, guanine nucleotide regulatory protein (stimulatory or inhibitory); PI, phosphatidylinositol; PIP, phosphatidylinositol-4-phosphate; PIP₂, phosphatidylinositol-4,5-diphosphate; IP₃, inositol triphosphate; PDE, phosphodiesterase. (From Ballard PL: Mechanism of hormone action. *In* Rudolph AM, Hoffman JIE [Eds]: Pediatrics. Norwalk, CT, Appleton & Lange, 1987.)

tors in the cytoplasm, on the nuclear membrane, or within the nucleus. In the case of steroid hormones, interaction with a receptor protein modifies receptor structure and increases its affinity for specific binding sites (response elements) on regulated genes. This alters the rate of gene transcription and subsequently the levels of the encoded protein. Hormones can also alter messenger RNA levels by influencing stability or efficiency of translation of the transcript. When the hormone is removed, steroid dissociates from the receptor through the law of mass action, and the response is reversed. Although binding of hormones to membrane receptors often produces responses within minutes (e.g., adrenocorticotropic hormone [ACTH] stimulation of cortisol production), steroid and other hormones that regulate gene expression require several hours to increase the content of specific messenger RNAs and the encoded proteins. The mechanism of steroid hormone action is depicted in Figure 4–2.

Evans (1988) has established that the receptors for steroid hormones and thyroid hormones have striking structural similarities. In particular, the region of the receptor involved in DNA binding is quite homologous among the various proteins. This finding suggests an evolutionary relationship between these receptors as well as similarities in their mechanism of action at target genes.

Postreceptor Events

Hormones have diverse effects on cells, but their mechanism of action is in general limited to one of three categories: (1) directly modifying an enzyme or a protein and altering function (e.g., phosphorylation), (2) activating specific genes that increase synthesis and content of the encoded protein, or (3) repressing the expression of a gene. All three processes occur during fetal life. One effect of beta-agonists in the fetal lung is secretion of surfactant from type II cells, and this response occurs within minutes on hormone exposure, presumably reflecting phosphorylation of specific proteins involved in the exocytic process (Walters, 1985). Catecholamines also stimulate production of pulmonary surfactant lipids and proteins, and this response involves de novo RNA and protein synthesis over a longer time scale (Ballard, 1989). Glucocorticoid treatment of fetal lung induces a number of proteins but also inhibits the synthesis of others (Odom et al, 1989); the stimulatory and inhibitory effects of glucocorticoids appear to be mediated through distinct nucleotide sequences (response elements) in the promoter region of the regulated genes.

Hormonal responsiveness of a cell is determined by both the levels of circulating hormone and the concentration and activity of cellular receptors and other mediating proteins. In the undisturbed adult organism, for example, responsiveness is determined primarily by the level of circulating hormone that normally fluctuates over a relatively limited range (e.g., diurnal variation). As hormone levels increase, the percentage of receptors occupied by hormone also increases, often in a nearly linear fashion, resulting in a highly responsive and tightly regulated stimulus-response system. In the fetus, particularly early in gestation, hormonal responsiveness is limited by developmental deficiencies in hormone levels, number of receptors, necessary cofactors, or mediating proteins. In the adrenergic system, for example, low receptor number and altered ratio of G protein subunits result in relative insensitivity of fetal tissues to adrenergic stimulation. Furthermore, cells may be hormonally unresponsive at certain points in development owing to alterations in chromatin structure that prevent receptor-hormone binding.

UNIQUE FEATURES OF THE FETAL ENDOCRINE SYSTEM

The endocrine environment of the fetus is unique with regard to the endocrine organs, the presence of certain hormones, changing and often high circulating concentrations of hormones, hormone metabolism, and specialized responses related to in utero development. Although the pattern of fetal growth and development is not generally dependent on hormones, with some important exceptions, the timing of these events is modulated by levels of endogenous hormones and exposure to hormone treatment.

Hormones and Sources

During the first trimester of gestation, the fetal testes produce an inhibitor of müllerian duct differentiation. Müllerian inhibiting factor (MIF) is a glycoprotein with a molecular weight of approximately 72,000, which acts locally

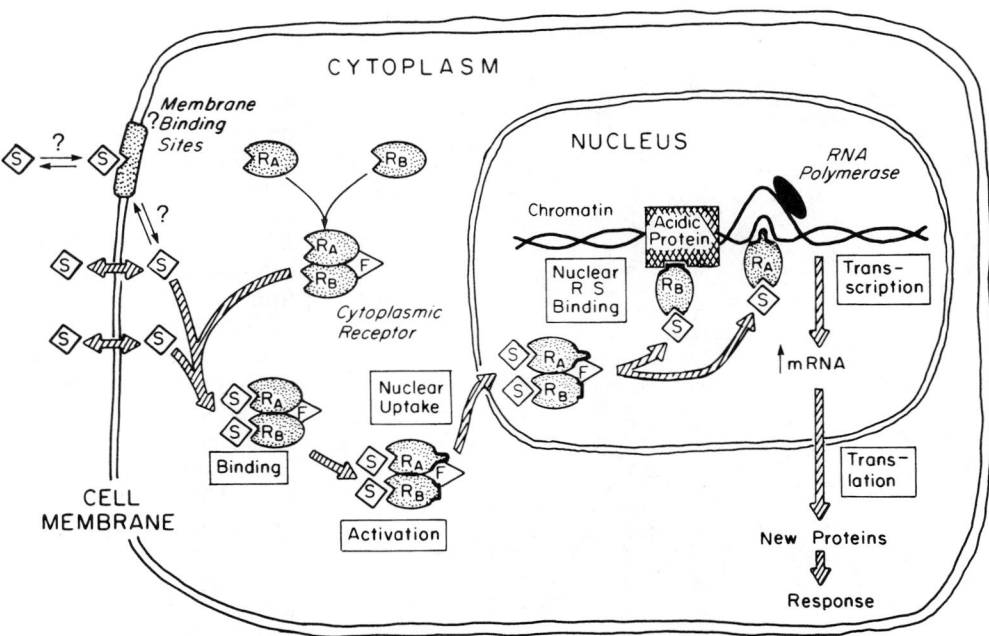

FIGURE 4–2. Molecular mechanism of action of steroid hormones in their target cells. This model applies in general to glucocorticoids, estrogens, androgens, progestins, mineralocorticoids, and vitamin D. S, steroid; R$_A$, subunit A of receptor; R$_B$, subunit B of receptor; RS, receptor-steroid complex; F, heat shock proteins. (From Ballard PL: Mechanism of hormone action. *In* Rudolph AM, Hoffman JIE, Rudolph CE [Eds]: Pediatrics, 20th ed. San Mateo, CA, Appleton & Lange, 1996, p 1678.)

through paracrine mechanisms to cause involution of the müllerian structures and may inhibit oocyte meiosis in the ovary (Ueno et al, 1988). The cellular mechanism of action of MIF is uncertain but may involve dephosphorylation of a membrane protein.

During pregnancy, steroid hormones are produced through complex interaction of mother, fetus, and placenta. Progesterone is initially synthesized by the maternal corpus luteum, whereas during the second and third trimester, the placenta is the major source. Progesterone is synthesized from maternal low-density lipoprotein and occurs independent of the fetus. The high levels of progesterone appear to serve at least two functions: suppressing uterine activity and decreasing maternal immune responses against fetal antigens.

The adult zone of the fetal adrenal produces cortisol (in increasing amounts during gestation), and the inner fetal zone acts in concert with the placenta to produce estrogens and their precursors. The fetal zone is deficient in delta-5,3-beta-OH dehydrogenase and delta-4,5,3-ketosteroid isomerase and has considerable steroid sulfokinase activity, resulting in production of dehydroepiandrosterone sulfate (DHAS) from pregnenolone supplied by the placenta. DHAS undergoes 16-hydroxylation in the fetal liver and then is transported to the placenta where it and DHAS (of both fetal and maternal origin) are the major substrates for estrogen synthesis. Much of the estrogen, predominantly estriol, enters the maternal circulation and subsequently is excreted in the urine. High levels of estrogen also accumulate in the fetus and amniotic fluid, but the function of estrogen in the fetus is uncertain. Estrogen biosynthesis is greatly reduced in infants with steroid sulfatase deficiency; development of the fetus under these circumstances, however, appears to be normal.

In addition to production of progesterone, the placenta synthesizes a number of polypeptide hormones throughout pregnancy. These include human chorionic somatomam-motropin (hCS), human chorionic gonadotropin (hCG), human chorionic corticotropin (hCC), human chorionic thyrotropin (hCT), beta endorphin, alpha-melanocyte–stimulating hormone (α-MSH), and both beta and alpha lipotropin. The placenta also produces most, if not all, of the releasing hormones synthesized by the hypothalamus. Thus, the placenta contributes to the circulating pool of pituitary and hypothalamic hormones in the fetus. In addition to the placenta, other fetal tissues, particularly the gut and pancreas, synthesize a number of the releasing hormones characteristic of the hypothalamus. The presence of extrahypothalamic peptides is established, but their role in fetal development is not certain.

Another unique source of hormone production in the fetus is the para-aortic chromaffin system. These extramedullary paraganglia, the largest of which are referred to as the organs of Zuckerkandl, are located along the abdominal and pelvic sympathetic plexuses during fetal life and disappear completely in the first years after birth. By the second trimester of gestation, this tissue actively produces norepinephrine but relatively little epinephrine because of low levels of phenylethanolamine-*N*-methyl transferase. The chromaffin cells of the para-aortic system as well as the sympathetic nerve cells are derived from a neuroectodermal stem cell and are responsive to nerve growth factor.

The catecholamine responses at birth are due in part to the para-aortic chromaffin system as well as increased postganglionic sympathetic neuronal and adrenal medullary catecholamine secretion. Circulating catecholamines (norepinephrine, epinephrine, and dopamine) increase exponentially after delivery and cord cutting. In the newborn sheep, which lacks para-aortic chromaffin tissue, the increased circulating norepinephrine is derived predominantly from the spillover of postganglionic sympathetic neurons, whereas the increased epinephrine derives solely from adrenal medullary secretion. Lacking complete organ sympathetic innervation and maturation of adrenergic receptor mechanisms, the fetus and newborn exhibit profound dependence on circulating catecholamines for maintenance of cardiovascular and metabolic homeostasis in response to physiologic stress such as the transition to extrauterine life (Padbury and Martinez, 1988). Adrenalectomized animals, deficient in the normally increased levels of circulating epinephrine in the newborn period, are impaired in their ability to increase cardiac output and myocardial contractility, secrete surfactant, and mobilize energy substrates for successful postnatal adaptation. It is not known precisely how long this dependence on circulating catecholamines persists postnatally, but basal myocardial function and the high resting cardiac output characteristic of the first weeks of life remain dependent on an intact sympathoadrenal system. Survival during hypoxic stress in newborn rats has been shown to be dependent on similar mechanisms (Slotkin and Seidler, 1988).

In addition to the anterior and posterior lobes of the pituitary, the fetus has an intermediate lobe that regresses after birth and is not found in adults. In animals, however, the intermediate lobe is maintained through adult life. The intermediate lobe secretes primarily α-MSH and beta-endorphin, which are derived from proopiomelanocortin (POMC). In the anterior lobe of the pituitary, POMC is cleaved primarily to beta-lipotropin and ACTH. By the second trimester of gestation, the fetal neurohypophysis contains arginine vasopressin (AVP), oxytocin, and arginine vasotocin (AVT). The pituitary gland contains AVT throughout fetal life, but this hormone disappears after birth. AVT is also present in the pineal glands of both fetuses and adults.

Ontogeny

The function of hormones in the fetus is determined primarily by the developmental pattern of the hormones or their receptor system. In general, most endocrine systems of the fetus are functional by the end of the first trimester, although circulating levels of many hormones increase substantially only during the third trimester. One exception to this pattern is illustrated by the hypothalamic-pituitary-gonad axis. Secretion of hypothalamic gonadotropin-releasing hormone (Gn-RH) becomes active in the first trimester, resulting in pulsatile release of luteinizing hormone (LH) and follicle-stimulating hormone (FSH), which stimulates production of testosterone or estradiol by the fetal gonads. Throughout the rest of fetal life and through childhood, until the onset of puberty, this hormonal axis remains quiescent. Control of this hormonal system is believed to reside in the central nervous system.

Hormones known to influence terminal differentiation (acquisition of specialized functions by cells) have developmental patterns consistent with this role. For example, cortisol is detected in fetal plasma at low levels during the second trimester and then increases exponentially during the third trimester (Murphy, 1982). Glucocorticoid receptors are detected relatively early in gestation in many fetal tissues and appear to be fully functional. The influence of endogenous cortisol on fetal development, therefore, is determined by the rate of adrenal production of cortisol and perhaps by postreceptor responsiveness in target tissues. Similarly, plasma levels of T_3 and T_4 increase only

during the third trimester, whereas thyroid hormone receptors are present throughout the second trimester (Fisher and Klein, 1981; Gonzales and Ballard, 1981). Prolactin levels in plasma and amniotic fluid increase throughout the third trimester to levels much greater than those found in the adult or in the mother. By contrast, levels of growth hormone increase during the first two thirds of pregnancy and then decline toward term.

The adrenergic response system appears to be constrained throughout most of gestation. The catecholamine response to the stress of delivery is greater at term than in preterm deliveries, and in the fetal lung and heart, for example, the number of beta-adrenergic receptors and the ability to provoke cAMP are low in the midgestation fetus as compared with the adult (Davis et al, 1987).

Metabolism

In the human fetus, the levels of circulating cortisol (an active glucocorticoid) and cortisone (inactive) are similar. Although most adult tissues, particularly the liver, readily convert cortisone to cortisol, fetal tissues generally lack this ability because of deficiency of the enzyme 17-beta-hydroxysteroid dehydrogenase or cofactors NADP and NADPH. The low enzymatic activity in most tissues reduces the possible contribution of cortisone to tissue glucocorticoid activity. In the fetal lung of animals, the ability to convert cortisone to cortisol increases markedly during the third trimester, coincident with lung maturation (Nicholas et al, 1978). Lung tissue from the second-trimester human fetus is similarly responsive to cortisone and cortisol during explant culture, reflecting rapid conversion of cortisone to cortisol (Gonzales et al, 1986; Liley et al, 1989). In this tissue, therefore, cortisone contributes to the pool of circulating glucocorticoids. Administered corticosteroids are rapidly cleared from the fetal circulation by metabolism in the maternal liver, whereas similar doses to the newborn infant are metabolized slowly because of liver immaturity.

Thyroid hormone metabolism also varies markedly in the fetus when compared to that of the adult (see Chapter 102). In the fetus, T_4 is deiodinated preferentially to inactive rT_3 rather than active T_3. This occurs in most fetal tissues but particularly the placenta. In fetal sheep, at least, the switch from production of rT_3 to T_3 is regulated by endogenous cortisol (levels increase markedly in late gestation) and is stimulated precociously by administered glucocorticoids (Thomas et al, 1978). The generalized inactivation of T_4 during most of fetal life appears to have at least two beneficial effects in the fetus: first, to protect most fetal tissues from the catabolic effects of thyroid hormone and, second, to provide a mechanism whereby selected tissues could increase their exposure to active T_3 by increasing local T_3 production. Moreover, several fetal tissues in animals are relatively unresponsive to administered T_3 with regard to thermogenesis, a function that is not needed by the fetus before birth.

HORMONES AND TISSUE DEVELOPMENT

The developmental processes of organogenesis and subsequent maturation of tissue structure and function are, for the most part, programmed and occur in the absence of hormonal influences. Chapter 3 reviews current understanding of the genetic control of tissue development, which involves coordination and interaction of multiple gene products. Maintenance of the differentiated state appears to be an active process requiring continued synthesis of specific regulatory proteins. Hormones and growth factors have three general roles in the process of differentiation. First, they modulate the rate of tissue development by virtue of increased concentrations or tissue responsiveness during normal gestation. Hormonal effects involve both enzyme induction, resulting in differentiated tissue function (e.g., pulmonary surfactant production), and repression of specific genes (e.g., hepatic alpha-fetoprotein) with loss of a fetal-specific protein. Within a given tissue, the response to a particular hormone typically involves a specific subset of cellular proteins (e.g., glucose-metabolizing enzymes of the intestine), providing a coordinated maturational response. Second, hormones can accelerate the normal timetable of development resulting in precocious organ maturation. This accelerating effect is observed with exogenous hormone treatment and at times of increased hormone production, such as during chronic in utero stress, during both premature and term labor and delivery, in the immediate postnatal period, and, in animals, around the time of weaning. The third area of hormonal influence relates to tumorigenesis, in which there is loss of growth control and dedifferentiation. A number of oncogenes have been described whose overexpression is associated with the genesis of cancer. The oncogenes of retroviruses represent slightly mutated cellular genes that have been obtained by the virus and that are constitutively expressed on viral infection. Many of the oncogenes encode growth factors, their receptors, other hormone receptors, or proteins involved in signal transduction (Drucker et al, 1989). For example, oncogenes encode for proteins related to epidermal growth factor receptor (erbB), platelet-derived growth factor (sis), fibroblast growth factor (int-2), the G proteins

of adenyl cyclase (ras), and thyroid hormone receptor (erbA). Thus, appropriate expression of hormones, growth factors, and receptors is important in both initial differentiation and maintenance of the differentiated state. Table 4–1 gives a partial listing of hormones that probably have a role in fetal development.

Intrinsic Timetable

Experiments of nature, such as anencephaly with panhypopituitarism, indicate that fetal growth and development proceed in a near-normal fashion in the absence of hypothalamic and pituitary input. Such fetuses are still exposed to hormones from the mother and placenta. Circulating levels of many hormones are much lower than in normal fetuses but apparently sufficient to ensure organ maturity at term. In experimental animals with a genetically engineered knock-out of corticotropin-releasing hormone, rendering homozygous fetuses deficient in both fetal-derived and maternal-derived corticosteroids, newborns died of respiratory failure because of inadequate surfactant and air space development (Muglia et al, 1995). Absence of corticosteroids, however, did not appear to interfere with organogenesis (e.g., airway branching in the lung). When fetal tissue is placed in explant culture in the absence of serum or added hormones, growth, structural development, and biochemical differentiation continue at a rate equal to or greater than that in in vivo. Fetal lung, for example, undergoes airway branching, formation of peripheral air spaces, and cytodifferentiation of epithelial cells into surfactant-producing type II cells (Fig. 4–3). These findings in vivo and in vitro suggest that tissue growth and differentiation proceed even in the absence of circulating hormones as a result of gene expression that is apparently determined by cell lineage and cell interactions. It is likely that tissue interactions, which are essential for normal development, are mediated in part through the production of growth

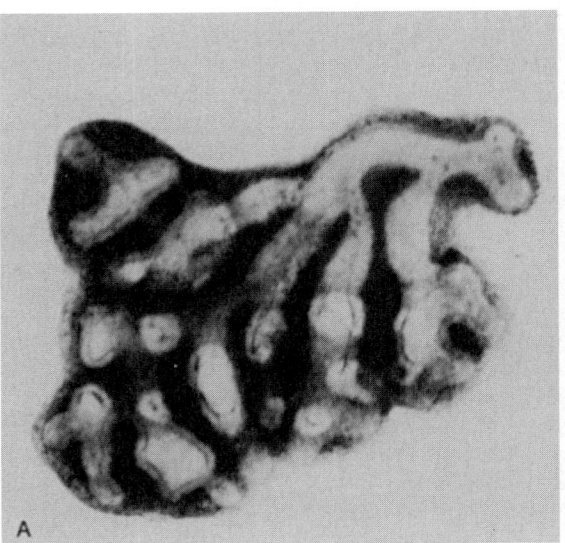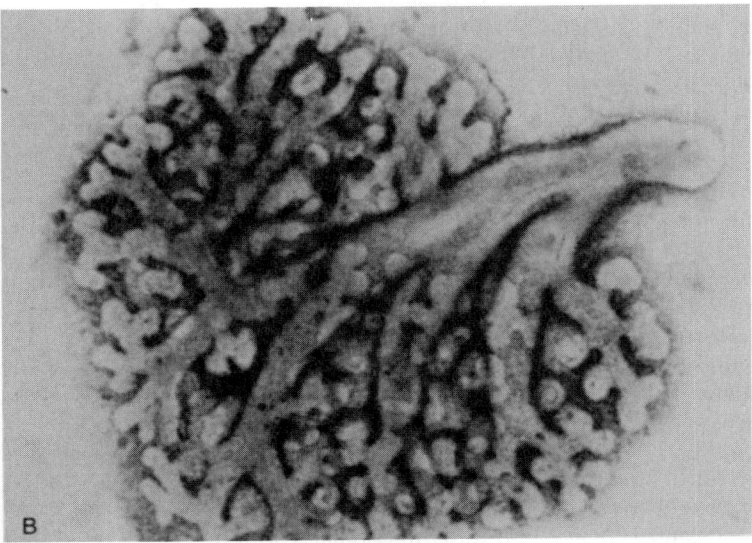

FIGURE 4–3. Development of the fetal lung in vitro. Intact lungs from 14-day rat fetuses were cultured as explants in medium without hormones for 1 day *(A)* and 4 days *(B)*. (From Gross I, Wilson CM: Fetal rat lung maturation: Initiation and modulation. J Appl Physiol 55:1725, 1731, 1983.)

TABLE 4–1

Hormones of the Fetus that Influence Growth or Differentiation (in vitro and/or in vivo)

Hormone or Growth Factor	Sources	Fetal Effects
Adrenocorticotropic hormone (ACTH)	Pituitary, placenta	Activates fetal adrenal gland
Androgens (testosterone)	Testes, adrenals, liver	Produces male sexual differentiation
		Delays lung maturation?
β-Endorphin	Pituitary, placenta	Maintains vasoregulation?
Calcitonin	Thyroid	Promotes bone mineralization and anabolism?
Catecholamines	Adrenal	Produces lung differentiation
		Increases cardiac output, thermogenesis, and glycogen and fat mobilization
Human chorionic corticotropin (hCC)	Placenta	Regulates fetal adrenal cortex
Human chorionic gonadotropin (hCG)	Placenta	Luteotropic; stimulates steroid production by the fetal testes and adrenals
Human chorionic somatomammotropin (hCS), human placental lactogen (hPL)	Placenta	Promotes secretion of insulin-like growth factors (IGFs)?
Cortisol	Adrenal adult zone	Needed for parturition and differentiation of numerous tissues
Eicosanoids (prostaglandins, leukotrienes, and thromboxanes)	Most tissues	Initiates uterus contraction; regulates vessel tone and lung maturation; activates fetal adrenals
Epidermal growth factor (EGF)	Multiple tissues	Regulates epithelial cell division
Estrogens (estrone, estradiol, and estriol)	Placenta	Regulates lung differentiation?
		Increases uteroplacental blood flow
Fibroblast growth factors (FGFs)	Fibroblasts	Regulate cell division
Insulin-like growth factors (IGFs)	Multiple tissues	Regulate cell division (and differentiation?)
Interferon-γ	White blood cells, other cell type	Differentiates lungs and other tissues?
α-Melanocyte-stimulating hormone (α-MSH)	Pituitary and placenta	Activates fetal adrenals
Müllerian-inhibiting factor (MIF)	Testes (Sertoli cells)	Activates involution müllerian ducts
Nerve growth factor (NGF)		Needed for development and maintenance of neurons and Sertoli cells?
Parathyroid hormone	Parathyroids	Produce 1,25-vitamin D
Platelet-derived growth factor (PDGF)	Platelets, other tissues	Needed for cell replication
Progesterone	Placenta	Precursor for fetal steroids, needed for pregnancy maintenance
Prolactin	Pituitary	Needed for water balance and lung development?
Releasing hormones (TRH, SRIF, CRF, gonadotropin-releasing hormone [Gn-RH])	Hypothalamus, placenta, gut	Augment output of fetal pituitary hormones and placental hormones?
Thyroid hormones (thyroxine [T₄], triiodothyronine [T₃])	Thyroid, liver	Activate lung and heart differentiation
Transforming growth factor (TGF)	Multiple tissues	Regulates cell division, deposition of extracellular matrix, and differentiation
Vasopressin, vasotocin	Neurohypophysis, pineal	Maintain placental and lung water transport
		Stimulate ACTH release from fetal pituitary?
Vitamin D	Maternal skin, liver, kidney	Placental calcium transport

TRH, thyroid-releasing hormone; SRIF, somatotropin-releasing inhibiting factor; CRF, coagulase-reacting factor.

factors and possibly other regulators acting in an autocrine or a paracrine fashion. The primary role of circulating hormones in the fetus, therefore, is to modulate the rate of differentiation, in part as a response to changes in the fetal environment.

Sexual Differentiation

The patterns of hormonal secretion and response vital to sexual differentiation are described in Chapter 101. Figure 4–4 summarizes the major events in sexual differentiation. Besides affecting sexual development, the patterns of sex steroid secretion may have important effects on other organ systems. In experimental animals, the surge of circulating

androgens near midgestation appears to influence the subsequent pattern of lung maturation. Male fetuses have a transient developmental delay in the production of pulmonary surfactant, which can be abolished by treatment with antiandrogen agents (Nielsen et al, 1982). These experimental observations may relate to the situation in human infants in which males have an increased risk for respiratory distress syndrome (RDS) and may be less responsive to prenatal betamethasone treatment.

Terminal Differentiation

In addition to modulating normal tissue development, circulating hormones accelerate the process in stressful condi-

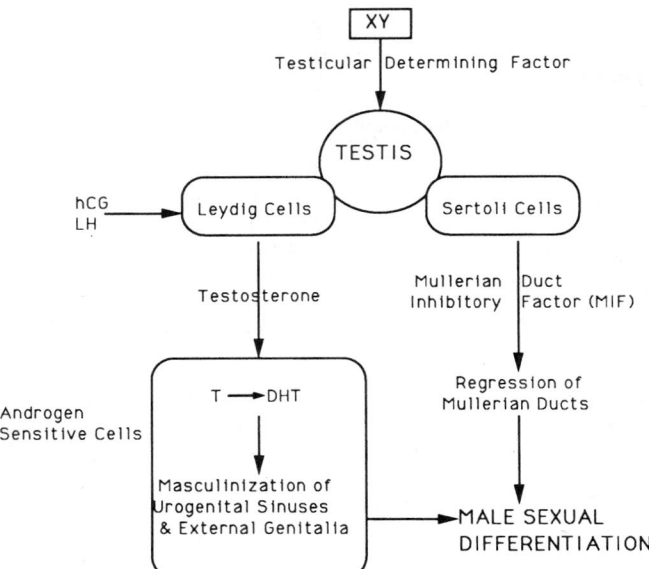

FIGURE 4–4. Outline of hormonal effects in fetal sexual differentiation. hCG, human chorionic gonadotropin; LH, luteinizing hormone; T, testosterone; DHT, dihydrotestosterone.

tions (e.g., placental insufficiency, prolonged rupture of membranes, premature labor), a process that has been described as preparation for birth. Several different hormones, as described subsequently, are involved in the stress response, and in several tissues there is an interaction between hormones to stimulate maturation. Many of the problems encountered by the premature infant may be thought of as developmental deficiencies or immaturity of critical functions in select tissues. Table 4–2 lists diseases that result from immature hormonally regulated systems.

Glucocorticoids

Endogenous cortisol, and in some tissues, cortisone, is the most important hormone regulating tissue maturation. Cortisol levels increase continually through the third trimester and are elevated in both acutely and chronically stressful situations. Glucocorticoids are known to have the following effects in fetal and newborn tissues of animals:

1. In the lung, glucocorticoids accelerate structural development and the appearance, accumulation, and secretion of surfactant (see Chapter 48).
2. In some species, they increase pulmonary receptors for insulin, epidermal growth factor (EGF), and beta-adrenergic agonists.
3. They induce the adrenal medullary enzyme phenyl-ethanolamine-N-methyl transferase, which catalyzes epinephrine synthesis from norepinephrine.
4. In animals, but probably not in the human fetus, they induce the hepatic enzyme that catalyzes production of T_3 from T_4.
5. They decrease the sensitivity of the ductus arteriosus (in fetal sheep) to dilating prostaglandins, facilitating closure of the ductus in response to increased oxygen concentration.

6. They accelerate secretory activity of the fetal pancreas.
7. In the liver, they stimulate glycogen deposition, induce gluconeogenic and other enzymes important in postnatal function, and repress hematopoietic cells and production of alpha-fetoprotein.
8. In the placenta of sheep, they promote estrogen biosynthesis, which in turn stimulates prostaglandin $F_{2\alpha}$ production and subsequently the initiation of parturition.
9. They influence the rate of myelination in the brain, accelerating or retarding this process depending on species, timing, and dose.
10. They induce glutamine synthetase activity in the embryonic neural retina.
11. In suckling or weaning animals, they induce brush border enzymes, such as peptidases, sucrase, maltase, and alkaline phosphatase, which are required for normal function of the adult intestine.
12. They inhibit cell division in some but not all tissues.

Experimentally these findings with glucocorticoids arise from studies with administered hormone, ablation procedures (e.g., hypophysectomy or adrenalectomy) that delay organ maturation, and temporal associations between circulating corticosteroids and inducible responses. A prepartum rise in circulating fetal corticosteroids occurs in all species that have been studied, and the experimental manipulations of steroid treatment or withdrawal provide consistent results in a variety of animal models.

In many tissues, the maturational effects of glucocorticoids require or are synergistic with effects of other hormones such as T_3 and catecholamines (cAMP). Although it is not possible to extrapolate all of the findings in animals to the human infant, a number of these regulatory events appear to occur in the human and have clinical implications (see Table 4–2).

The effects and physiologic role of glucocorticoids are well described with regard to maturation of the fetal lung. Studies with explant cultures of human tissue have established that glucocorticoids affect both lung structure and production of surfactant by type II cells (Gonzales et al, 1986). Treatment accelerates differentiation of the epithelial cells into type II cells (loss of glycogen and the appearance of apical microvilli and intracellular lamellar bodies), reduces mesenchymal volume, narrows the intra-alveolar septal distance, and increases maximal lung volume and compliance. Surfactant production and secretion are increased, and the response includes all of the known components of pulmonary surfactant (saturated phosphatidylcholine and the three surfactant-associated proteins). The response to glucocorticoids in fetal lung is mediated by glucocorticoid receptors and involves increased gene expression (i.e., increased content of messenger RNA) for the surfactant-associated proteins. Glucocorticoids increase the activity of cholinephosphate cytidylyltransferase (via increased levels of lipid cofactor), the rate-limiting enzyme of the choline incorporation pathway, and stimulate production of fatty acid synthetase, the rate-limiting enzyme for fatty acid production from malonyl coenzyme A. Prenatal treatment of rats with dexamethasone causes a precocious increase in antioxidant enzyme activities in the fetal

TABLE 4–2

Abnormalities of the Newborn that May Be Related to Hormonal Conditions

Abnormality	Hormone	Cause (Known or Postulated)
Male pseudohermaphroditism	Testosterone	Genetic defects in testosterone biosynthesis, metabolism (5α-reductase), or responsiveness (receptor deficiency or abnormality)
Testicular feminization	Dihydrotesterone	Decreased receptors in androgen target tissues yield female phenotype in genetic male
Female pseudohermaphroditism (congenital hyperplasia)	Cortisol, insulin	Enzymatic defects in cortisol biosynthesis with excess androgen
Infant diabetic mother	Insulin	Fetal hyperinsulinemia increases growth and fat deposition and delays lung development
Infant leprechaunism	Insulin	Decreased insulin receptors with intrauterine growth retardation
Congenital hypothyroidism	T_4, T_3	Hormone deficiency alters development of brain, heart, lung, and other tissues
Respiratory distress syndrome	Cortisol, T_3, catecholamines, prolactin?	Developmental deficiency in one or more hormones may delay lung development
Transient tachypnea of newborn	Cortisol, catecholamines, arginine vasopressin, and others?	Decreased hormone levels or responsiveness of lung epithelium for fluid clearance
Lung hypoplasia	Unknown growth factors	Presumed decreased production of lung factors
Persistent pulmonary hypertension of newborn	?	Stress-related hormones may delay pulmonary vascular development in utero
Patent ductus arteriosus	Cortisol, prostaglandins?	Possible imbalance in levels and/or responsiveness for dilating and constricting prostaglandins
Necrotizing enterocolitis	Cortisol, glucagon?	Developmental deficiency in hormones may delay gut development

T_4, Thyroxine; T_3, triiodothyronine.

lung, but at present there are no data in the human. It is likely that glucocorticoids have other maturational effects in the lung because a number of as yet unidentified proteins are induced by glucocorticoid treatment of cultured tissue. The clinical effects of prenatal corticosteroid therapy are discussed in Chapters 2 and 48. The improved survival rates in treated infants result from precocious maturation of the lung as well as other organs.

Thyroid Hormones

Levels of both T_3 and T_4 increase in the human fetus during the third trimester. Although thyroid hormones are important for normal postnatal growth, the athyroid human fetus grows normally and does not display signs or symptoms of hypothyroidism seen in children and adults (see Chapter 102). Thyroid hormones, however, may play an important role in the maturation of the fetal lung and perhaps other tissues. Surfactant production and structural pulmonary development are retarded in hypothyroid sheep fetuses. Treatment with thyroid hormone accelerates phospholipid synthesis in cultured lung (Ballard, 1989), and thyroid hormones are necessary for maximal response to cortisol treatment in fetal sheep (Schellenberg et al, 1988).

The in vitro effects of thyroid hormone on lipid synthesis are receptor-mediated, indicating that physiologic levels of hormones can be effective in vivo. At present, the enzymatic sites of thyroid hormone action are not known. Combined treatment with both glucocorticoid and thyroid hormone results in an additive or synergistic stimulation of phospholipid synthesis in cultured tissue (Fig. 4–5). In vivo, cortisol treatment of sheep fetuses also increases circulating T_3 concentrations via increased conversion from T_4. These and other observations on the interactions of glucocorticoids and thyroid hormones led to clinical trials of prenatal therapy with betamethasone plus thyrotropin-releasing hormone (TRH) for prevention of RDS. Initial results indicated benefit with regard to incidence of RDS and chronic lung disease for treated infants (Morales et al, 1989; Ballard et al, 1992); however, more recent trials have not found benefit (ACTOBAT Study Group, 1995; Maturana et al, 1997).

Thyroid hormones are also important for cardiac development. In the sheep fetus, thyroidectomy during late gestation blunts the increase in heart rate, cardiac output, and oxygen consumption normally seen after birth, and replacement T_3 therapy before birth is corrective. This T_3 effect appears to be mediated through beta-adrenergic

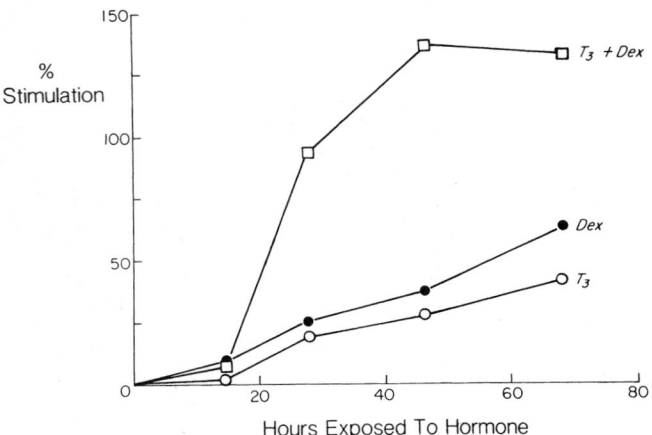

FIGURE 4–5. Synergistic interaction between glucocorticoids and thyroid hormones in phosphatidylcholine synthesis. Explant cultures of fetal rabbit lung were treated with dexamethasone (Dex) or triiodothyronine (T_3) (or both) for the times shown; data are expressed as percent stimulation over control. (From Ballard PL, Hovey ML, Gonzales LK: Thyroid hormone stimulation of phosphatidylcholine synthesis in cultured fetal rabbit lung. J Clin Invest 74:898, 1984.)

receptor concentration and responsiveness to endogenous catecholamines (Birk et al, 1988). The normal hypertrophic growth of the myocardium also depends on thyroid hormones but apparently does not involve the beta-adrenergic system.

Catecholamines

Circulating catecholamine concentrations increase dramatically with labor and delivery, and amniotic fluid levels, which probably reflect production by the fetus, are generally elevated in complicated pregnancies. A well-described effect of catecholamines on terminal differentiation is in the fetal lung. Treatment with beta-adrenergic agonists causes a prompt increase in surfactant secretion both in vivo and in isolated type II cells, and endogenous catecholamines contribute to release of surfactant at the time of birth. For example, the amount of surfactant in airways of fetal animals is decreased by blockade of the beta-adrenergic receptors with an irreversible antagonist, by treatment with an inhibitor of catecholamine biosynthesis, and by adrenalectomy.

A second effect of catecholamines is to stimulate the rate of surfactant synthesis. In cultured lung tissue, treatment with analogues of cAMP, beta-agonists, or other agents that induce cAMP increases synthesis of surfactant phospholipids and surfactant-associated proteins A and B. Alveolar structure in cultured lung explants is also modified by these treatments, probably resulting from altered ion and fluid transport.

A third effect of catecholamines is reduction of lung fluid. In fetal animals, beta-agonists decrease fluid accumulation in the air spaces by inhibiting the chloride pump and promoting fluid reabsorption through a sodium pump in epithelial cells. The physiologic relevance of these responses has been demonstrated in the fetal lamb, in which

there is a close correlation between fluid flux and endogenous levels of catecholamines during labor. Responsiveness to catecholamines normally increases during the third trimester; the response is markedly blunted in thyroidectomized fetuses but restored by combined treatment with T_3 and hydrocortisone but not by treatment with either hormone alone (Barker et al, 1988, 1989). These findings suggest that increasing concentrations of cortisol and T_3 during development enhance the sensitivity of epithelial cells for responding to catecholamines. This system illustrates the interaction of hormones in regulating a developmental process important for successful adaptation to extrauterine life. Clinical aspects of lung fluid are discussed in Chapters 34 and 50.

All three catecholamine effects in fetal lung are mediated by beta-adrenergic receptors and increased intracellular levels of cAMP. Protein kinase A is activated by cAMP, resulting in phosphorylation of specific cell proteins that affect the secretory process (surfactant) and ion channels or pumps (fluid flux) or regulate gene expression (synthesis of surfactant components and the sodium channel). Obviously this chain of intracellular events can be modified at various levels to affect the response. For example, glucocorticoid treatment increases adrenergic receptor concentration and accordingly the sensitivity to catecholamines (in animals) and may also affect the G protein of adenyl cyclase (Cheng et al, 1980; Bottari et al, 1988). In fetal sheep, chronic infusion of glucose delayed the developmental increase in lung beta-adrenergic receptor concentration (Warburton et al, 1988). Clinically it is conceivable that exposure of the fetus to xanthines or other inhibitors of cAMP phosphodiesterase would enhance cAMP responses and lung maturation.

Catecholamines are also involved in increasing myocardial contractility and systemic vascular resistance and in triggering the onset of thermogenesis through mobilization of energy substrates. Infants born prematurely are thus at increased risk with regard to cardiac function and thermal stability because of both decreased metabolic reserves and suboptimal catecholamine levels.

Insulin

The infant of a diabetic mother is at increased risk for a number of abnormalities, including macrosomia with organomegaly, placental hypertrophy, polyhydramnios, congenital anomalies, and intrauterine death (see Chapter 7). Based on animal models of diabetes, it is generally believed that fetal hyperinsulinemia also delays the appearance of pulmonary surfactant and may alter surfactant composition (and therefore its function) or alveolar structure (or both). One possible explanation for this effect relates to the mitogenic activity of insulin and the general biologic principle that cell differentiation (e.g., production of surfactant) is associated with decreased cell division. Thus, under the stimulation of increased circulating insulin, lung type II cells may remain in an active cell cycle, not entering the G_0 stage when specialized cell products are synthesized. Another possible explanation is an inhibitory effect of insulin on synthesis of surfactant per se. Experiments with cultured lung tissue found that insulin can inhibit synthesis of surfactant proteins A, B, and C, which are required for normal surfactant structure and function (Guttentag et al, 1992; Snyder and Mendelson, 1987). A third possible explanation suggested by in vitro studies is that insulin blocks cortisol stimulation of lung structure and type II cell function. Infants of diabetic mothers also have an increased incidence of respiratory distress because of delayed fluid clearance. The mechanism of this abnormality is not known but could relate to either increased cell division or antagonism of glucocorticoid effects in the lung.

The inhibitory effects of insulin on lung development are presumably mediated by plasma membrane receptors. High-affinity binding sites have been described for whole fetal lung tissue and on isolated adult type II cells of the rat. Receptor levels may be influenced by other hormones in the fetus, although down regulation of receptors by insulin appears not to occur. This latter observation could indicate that the fetus of a diabetic pregnancy is subject to both hyperinsulinemia and increased receptor concentration.

Eicosanoids

These compounds, which include prostaglandins, thromboxanes, and leukotrienes, are produced from arachidonic acid (released from phospholipids) in the placenta and various fetal tissues. Although many effects of prostaglandins are paracrine, these hormones are present in the circulation, and levels of some (e.g., prostaglandin E_2 [PGE_2]) are much higher in the fetus than the adult, reflecting in part decreased metabolic clearance by the poorly perfused fetal lung. Synthesis of prostaglandins is increased by a variety of stimuli, many of which involve perturbation of cell membrane integrity, and production is inhibited by glucocorticoids (induction of lipocortin, which blocks phospholipase A_2) and drugs such as xanthine derivatives that block synthetic enzymes. Effects of prostaglandins are mediated through membrane receptors (primarily on the cell surface) and, at least in part, by the generation of cAMP.

In addition to their important role in initiation of parturition, prostaglandins have several known effects in maturational events of the cardiopulmonary system. Prostaglandins, in particular PGE_2, maintain the patency of the ductus arteriosus in fetal life; in fetal sheep, sensitivity to PGE_2 decreases during late gestation and in response to glucocorticoid treatment, allowing increased responsiveness to the contracting influence of oxygen (Clyman et al, 1981).

The increased incidence of patent ductus arteriosus in premature infants (and closure with prenatal glucocorticoid and postnatal indomethacin treatment) probably results from changing prostaglandin levels and sensitivity. Prostaglandins also influence the tone of the pulmonary vessels in utero and after birth. Maintenance of pulmonary vasoconstriction in the fetus is due in part to leukotrienes produced within the lung. The rapid fall in pulmonary vascular resistance at the time of birth results in part from the vasodilating effects of prostacyclin as well as other agents (e.g., prostaglandin D_2, bradykinin, and histamine) that are released by stretching the lung. Thus, altered prostaglandin production or responsiveness could conceiv-

ably contribute to the development of persistent pulmonary hypertension in some newborn infants.

Prostaglandins may also have physiologic roles in other aspects of lung development. Treatment of fetal sheep with inhibitors of prostaglandin synthesis increases fetal breathing movements and in some studies decreases both the rate of lung fluid production and its surfactant content. In newborn lambs, treatment with PGE_2 produces hyperventilation and apnea (Guarra et al, 1988). In cultured lung tissue, PGE_2 and prostaglandin E_1, presumably acting through cAMP, stimulate syntheses of surfactant lipids and surfactant protein A and promote the release of surfactant from type II cells. Thus, endogenous prostaglandins may contribute to lung growth (via fluid production and breathing movements) and maturation of the surfactant system in utero. Conceivably the administration of inhibitors of prostaglandin synthesis such as tocolytics might adversely affect lung maturation in the human fetus.

Arginine Vasopressin and Arginine Vasotocin

Although AVP and AVT are present in the pituitary gland of the human fetus, it is not known whether they have a unique physiologic role in the fetus. In addition to conserving water for the fetus, vasopressin is increased in response to hypoxic stress to levels greater than those occurring with osmolar stimuli. As a stress response hormone, AVP may contribute to maintenance of fetal blood pressure during hemorrhage or hypoxia. Administration of AVP to fetal animals decreases production of fetal lung fluid without affecting fluid osmolarity (Hooper et al, 1989; Ross et al, 1984). This response was greater in older fetuses, indicating developmental changes in responsiveness. Plasma AVP is elevated in infants delivered vaginally compared with cesarean section deliveries, and exposure to labor reduces the incidence of respiratory distress after birth. It is possible, therefore, that increased levels of endogenous AVP or AVT associated with labor and delivery contribute to the clearance of lung water.

Atrial Natriuretic Peptide

Fluid production, and possibly other lung functions, may be influenced by atrial natriuretic peptide (ANP) which is synthesized and secreted from atrial myocytes under glucocorticoid regulation. ANP is also synthesized in pulmonary type II cells of newborn rats and high-affinity binding sites occur within lung tissue (Matsubara et al, 1988). In fetal sheep, infusion of ANP or saline decreases lung fluid production. In the human, plasma concentrations of ANP are higher in term newborns than in adults and are further elevated in infants with RDS (Shaffer et al, 1986). Thus, ANP, whose levels are regulated by cortisol, may have a developmental influence in fluid production by both the kidney and the lung. ANP also has vasorelaxant properties and thus could have an effect on pulmonary blood flow and the occurrence of patent ductus arteriosus in the newborn (Hargrave et al, 1990; Pesonen et al, 1990).

Studies indicate that ANP is also synthesized in a number of extra-atrial tissues such as adrenal, gut, pancreas, nerve, and endocrine cells of the adult animal. The presence of ANP receptors in many of these same tissues suggests possible autocrine or paracrine roles of ANP in addition to its regulation of water and salt homeostasis. Possible roles of ANP in developing tissues other than the lung have not yet been investigated.

Neuropeptides

A variety of regulatory peptides are synthesized and secreted by a diffuse endocrine system of small granule cells of the intestine, pancreas, thyroid, lung, and other organs. Products of these cells are the biogenic amines and neuropeptides such as bombesin (gastrin-releasing peptide), bombesin-related compounds, calcitonin, calcitonin gene–related peptides, leucine enkephalin, somatostatin, and cholecystokinin. The neuroendocrine cells and their products are present in the fetus from early gestation, increase during fetal life, and then generally decline during childhood. The developmental pattern and distribution of these endocrine and paracrine systems suggest that the neuropeptides may have a role in fetal growth and development. At present, specific biologic functions have not been defined, although there is evidence for stimulatory effects on lung development.

Activin and inhibin are protein hormones, isolated from the adult ovary, which regulate in opposite manner both secretion of FSH and gonadotropin-mediated steroidogenesis. These hormones may also influence early embryogenesis and cell differentiation in the fetus. For example, activin (also termed *erythroid differentiation factor*) and inhibin, acting antagonistically, modulate hemoglobin production in human bone marrow and an erythroid cell line, and expression of the inhibin gene occurs in several tissues other than the ovary (e.g., bone marrow, thymus, placenta, and adrenal cortex).

Other Hormones

Other hormones have less well-defined roles in tissue differentiation. Levels of prolactin are high in the fetus, increase throughout the third trimester, and correlate with lung maturity (and the occurrence of RDS). In fetal lambs, at least, treatment with prolactin increases the stimulatory effect of T_3 and cortisol on lung development, but prolactin alone has no effect (Schellenberg et al, 1988). Prolactin may also play a role in water regulation in the fetus and across the placenta. A role for α-MSH, derived from pro-opiomelanocortin of the intermediate lobe of the fetal pituitary, in activation of the fetal adrenal has been proposed; this effect may occur before adrenal activation by ACTH. Beta-endorphin, another cleavage product of POMC, is present in fetal serum, and levels increase during gestation. This hormone may contribute to the circulatory responses to stress, but its role is not well defined.

Fetal Growth

Growth of the fetus is determined primarily by genetic factors, the capacity of the mother to provide nutrients, and the ability of the placenta to transfer nutrients. Relatively little is known regarding the role of hormones and growth factors in the complex process of fetal growth.

Although growth hormone and thyroid hormones are important for postnatal growth, they appear to have no growth-promoting role in utero. In fact, growth retardation is not a feature of anencephaly, which often involves complete absence of hypothalamic and pituitary hormones.

A number of different and related growth-promoting factors have been identified and studied. The biologic responses to these proteins depend on the target cells and may involve differentiation, stimulation of replication, or growth inhibition. It is likely that tissue growth in the fetus is determined in large part by an interplay of locally produced growth factors. Studies in cell lines indicate that stimulation of cell division requires both competence factors (e.g., platelet-derived growth factor [PDGF] and fibroblast growth factor [FGF]), which render growth-arrested cells capable of entering the cell cycle (G_0 to G_1), and progression factors (e.g., IGFs), which promote entry into the DNA synthesis phase of the cell cycle.

Insulin

One fetal hormone known to influence fetal growth is insulin. It is present in the human fetal pancreas and circulation by 10 weeks of gestation, and its levels are influenced by the blood glucose concentration. The rare condition of congenital absence of the pancreas is associated with marked reduction in birth length and weight. The syndrome of leprechaunism, which involves a genetic deficiency of insulin receptors and therefore lack of responsiveness, is also characterized by severe growth retardation. In animals, experimental hypoinsulinism leads to fetal growth retardation, and infusion of insulin increases fetal weight and causes organomegaly. Infants of diabetic mothers with poorly controlled disease are often macrosomic; this overgrowth is not observed when the diabetes is well controlled. In severe diabetes, with vascular disease and decreased uterine blood flow, fetuses are growth retarded because of nutrient deprivation. Infants with the Beckwith-Wiedemann syndrome are macrosomic with generalized organomegaly and appear to be hypersensitive to circulating insulin. The mechanism of insulin action in fetal growth is not fully defined but probably includes a direct stimulation of cell division through insulin receptors (insulin promotes cell division in culture), enhanced glucose and amino acid uptake into cells, and possible interactions with IGFs.

Insulin-Like Growth Factors

IGFs (or somatomedins) are a family of proteins that are structurally related to insulin, have some insulin-like metabolic activities, and mediate the action of growth hormone on postnatal growth. They circulate bound to specific binding proteins and act via cell membrane receptors. IGFs and their receptors are present in most fetal tissues (except the brain) and undoubtedly have a role in both organ and somatic growth. There is a correlation between size at birth and levels of IGFs in cord blood consistent with a physiologic role. Production of IGFs by tissues is developmentally controlled and cell specific. For example, in the lung, messenger RNA for IGF-II is high in the fetus, decreases markedly by term, and is not detected in adult lung; by contrast, IGF-I messenger RNA is found in both fetal and adult tissue (Scott et al, 1985). IGF-II messenger RNA is found only in lung mesenchymal cells, indicating the cellular site of synthesis, whereas immunostaining occurs in epithelial cells but not mesenchymal fibroblasts. These and other findings suggest that IGFs are produced by certain cell types (e.g., fibroblasts), are secreted, and stimulate proliferation of neighboring cells after binding to cell surface receptors. Agents or hormones that influence either IGFs or their receptors could potentially influence the rate of fetal growth. For example, secretion of IGF by cultured lung tissue is inhibited by cortisol (Stiles and D'Ercole, 1990). This finding may reflect one aspect of the general reciprocal relationship between cellular proliferation and differentiation that is modulated by glucocorticoids (i.e., promotion of maturation at the expense of growth).

Epidermal Growth Factor

EGF was first identified as a protein from the mouse submaxillary gland, which accelerated eruption of the incisors and eyelid opening in the newborn animal. EGF has generalized effects on epithelial growth and keratinization in several species and in a variety of cell types (mammary epithelial cells, chondrocytes, corneal cells, vascular smooth muscle cells, prostatic cells, glial cells, fibroblasts, and epithelial cells of the female reproductive organs). In vitro, EGF stimulates DNA synthesis in cultured cells. In explant culture of fetal lung, EGF stimulates both cell division and phospholipid biosynthesis. Infusion of EGF into fetuses stimulates epithelial growth in many tissues, with major effects on the weight of the placenta, intestine, kidneys, and adrenals, but does not affect general somatic growth. These observations suggest that endogenous EGF may have a role in growth and maturation of the kidney, adrenal cortex, intestine, and lung.

Nerve Growth Factor

Nerve growth factor (NGF) was also first isolated from mouse salivary glands but has been detected in various tissues, including human placenta. Treatment of chick embryos with NGF increases the size of sensory and sympathetic ganglia owing to survival of neurons that normally degenerate. Sympathetic ganglia of newborn animals contain more NGF than adult ganglia and are more responsive in terms of transformation of sympathetic neuroblasts into differentiated neurons. It has been postulated that locally produced NGF is important in the maturation of adrenergic neurons, the sympathetic nervous system, and fetal brain development in general. Administration of T_4 to rats increases NGF in brain and other tissues, suggesting a possible mechanism for postnatal T_4 effects on brain development. NGF and its receptor are also present in the testes of rats, but the possible role of EGF in this tissue is not known (Persson et al, 1990).

Other Growth Factors

Basic FGF (B-FGF) and related proteins (A-FGF, K-FGF, int-2, and FGF-5) appear to play an important role in early embryonic induction, angiogenesis of myocardial and vascular disease, and wound healing. They are mitogenic for vascular endothelial cells through an autocrine mechanism and promote endothelial cell migration and invasion and production of plasminogen activator—all necessary features of angiogenesis in vivo. Acidic FGF appears to be essential for branching morphogenesis in embryonic lung based on observations in animals with FGF receptor knockout (Peters et al, 1994). PDGF, in combination with other growth factors, stimulates division of glial cells, muscle cells, ovarian granulosa cells, pancreatic beta cells, and certain cell types of the immune system.

The transforming growth factors, in particular transforming growth factor-beta (TGF-β), have multiple effects on a variety of tissues. For example, TGF-β stimulates growth and extracellular matrix production by fibroblasts, promotes a switch from chondrocytic to osteoblastic phenotype, and inhibits the synthesis of surfactant components in cultured lung. TGF-β messenger RNA appears to be localized to epithelial cells adjacent to the mesenchyme of cartilage, bone, teeth, and other tissues consistent with a paracrine mechanism of action on these connective tissue cells. These findings suggest that TGF-β may act in the fetus as both a growth stimulator (e.g., of bone) and differentiation inhibitor (e.g., in the lung). It is also conceivable that TGF-β (and other growth factors) plays a role in the disordered growth and repair process that is a part of bronchopulmonary dysplasia in infants.

REFERENCES

ACTOBAT Study Group: Australian Collaborative Trial of Antenatal Thyrotropin-Releasing Hormone (ACTOBAT) for Prevention of Neonatal Respiratory Disease. Lancet 345:877, 1995.

Ballard PL: Hormonal regulation of pulmonary surfactant. Endocr Rev 10:165, 1989.

Ballard PL, Hovey ML, Gonzales LK: Thyroid hormone stimulation of phosphatidylcholine synthesis in cultured fetal rabbit lung. J Clin Invest 74:898, 1984.

Ballard RA: Antenatal glucocorticoid therapy: Clinical effects. In Hormones and Lung Maturation, vol 28. Monographs on Endocrinology. Berlin, Springer-Verlag, 1986, pp 137–172.

Ballard RA, Ballard PL, Creasy R, et al: Respiratory disease in very-low-birthweight infants after prenatal thyrotropin-releasing hormone and glucocorticoid. Lancet 339:510, 1992.

Barker PM, Brown MJ, Ramsden CA, et al: The effect of thyroidectomy in the fetal sheep on lung liquid readsorption induced by adrenaline or cyclic AMP. J Physiol 407:373, 1988.

Barker PM, Markiewicz M, Parker KA, et al: Induction of the adrenaline-dependent reabsorption of lung liquid in the fetal sheep by synergistic action of triiodothyronine and hydrocortisone. Proc Physiol Soc 146P:137, 1989.

Birk E, Rudolph AM, Roberts JM: Fetal thyroidectomy reduces postnatal myocardial beta-adrenergic receptor responses in newborn lambs. Pediatr Res 23:431A, 1988.

Bottari SP, King IN, Liley HG, et al: Changes in G-proteins may determine development of adrenergic sensitivity in human lung. Clin Res 36:239A, 1988.

Cheng JB, Goldfien A, Ballard PL, et al: Glucocorticoids increase pulmonary β-adrenergic receptors in fetal rabbit. Endocrinology 107:1646, 1980.

Clyman RI, Mauray F, Roman C, et al: Glucocorticoids alter the sensitivity of the lamb ductus arteriosus to prostaglandin E₂. J Pediatr 98:126, 1981.

Davis DJ, Dattel BJ, Ballard PL, et al: β-Adrenergic receptors and cyclic adenosine monophosphate generation in human fetal lung. Pediatr Res 21:142, 1987.

Drucker BJ, Harvey J, Mamon BS, et al: Oncogenes, growth factors and signal transduction. N Engl J Med 321:1383, 1989.

Evans RM: The steroid and thyroid hormone receptor superfamily. Science 240:889, 1988.

Fisher DA, Klein AH: Thyroid development and disorders of thyroid function in the newborn. N Engl J Med 304:702, 1981.

Gonzales LW, Ballard PL: Identification and characterization of nuclear 3,5,3′-triiodothyronine-binding sites in fetal human lung. J Clin Endocrinol Metab 53:21, 1981.

Gonzales LW, Ballard PL, Ertsey R, et al: Glucocorticoids and thyroid hormones stimulate biochemical and morphological differentiation of human fetal lung in organ culture. J Clin Endocrinol Metab 62:678, 1986.

Gross I, Wilson CM: Fetal rat lung maturation: Initiation and modulation. J Appl Physiol 55:1725, 1983.

Guarra FA, Savich RD, Wallen RD, et al: Prostaglandin E$_2$ causes hyperventilation and apnea in newborn lambs. J Appl Physiol 64:2160, 1988.

Guttentag SH, Phelps DS, Warshaw JB, et al: Delayed hydrophobic surfactant protein (SP-B, SP-C) expression in fetuses of streptozotocin-treated rats. Am J Respir Cell Mol Biol 7:190, 1992.

Hargrave B, Roman C, Morville P, et al: Pulmonary vascular effects of exogenous atrial natriuretic peptide in sheep fetuses. Pediatr Res 27:140, 1990.

Hooper SB, Wallace MJ, Harding R: Development of the lung liquid secretory response to vasopressin in fetal sheep. Fetal Neonatal Physiol 118A:7, 1989.

Lefkowitz RJ, Caron MC: Adrenergic receptors: Models for the study of receptors coupled to guanine nucleotide regulatory proteins. J Biol Chem 263:4993, 1988.

Liley HG, White RT, Warr RG, et al: Regulation of messenger RNAs for the hydrophobic surfactant proteins in human lung. J Clin Invest 83:1191, 1989.

Matsubara H, Mori Y, Umeda Y, et al: Atrial natriuretic peptide gene expression and its secretion. Biochem Biophys Res Commun 156:619, 1988.

Maturana A, Torres J, Salinas R, et al: Controlled trial of prenatal thyrotropin-releasing hormone and betamethasone for prevention of respiratory distress syndrome. Pediatr Res 41:163A, 1997.

Morales WJ, O'Brien WF, Angel JF, et al: Fetal lung maturation: The combined use of corticosteroids and thyrotropin-releasing hormone. Obstet Gynecol 73:111, 1989.

Muglia L, Jacobson L, Dikkes P, Majzoub JA: Corticotropin-releasing hormone deficiency reveals major fetal but not adult glucocorticoid need. Nature 373:427, 1995.

Murphy BEP: Human fetal serum cortisol levels related to gestational age: Evidence of a midgestational fall and a steep late gestational rise independent of sex or mode of delivery. Am J Obstet Gynecol 144:276, 1982.

Nicholas TE, Johnson RG, Lugg MA, et al: Pulmonary phospholipid biosynthesis and the ability of the fetal rabbit lung to reduce cortisone to cortisol during the final ten days of gestation. Life Sci 22:1517, 1978.

Nielsen HC, Zinman HM, Torday JS: Dihydrotestosterone inhibits fetal rabbit pulmonary surfactant production. J Clin Invest 69:611, 1982.

Odom MW, Ertsey R, Ballard PL: Hormonal effects on protein synthesis in human fetal lung. Pediatr Res 26:321A, 1989.

Padbury JF, Martinez AM: Sympathoadrenal system activity at birth and integration of postnatal adaptation. Semin Perinatol 12:163, 1988.

Persson H, Lievre CA-L, Soder O, et al: Expression of β-nerve growth factor receptor mRNA in sertoli cells downregulated by testosterone. Science 247:704, 1990.

Pesonen E, Merritt AT, Heldt G, et al: Correlation of patent ductus arteriosus shunting with plasma atrial natriuretic factor concentration in preterm infants with respiratory distress syndrome. Pediatr Res 27:137, 1990.

Peters K, Werner S, Liao X, et al: Targeted expression of a dominant negative FGF receptor blocks branching morphogenesis and epithelial differentiation of the mouse lung. EMBO J 13:3296, 1994.

Ross MG, Ervin G, Leake RD, et al: Fetal lung liquid regulation by neuropeptides. Am J Obstet Gynecol 150:421, 1984.

Schellenberg JC, Liggins GC, Manzai MK, et al: Synergistic hormonal effects on lung maturation in fetal sheep. J Appl Physiol 65:94, 1988.

Scott J, Cowell J, Robertson ME, et al: Insulin-like growth factor-II gene expression in Wilms' tumour and embryonic tissues. Nature 317:260, 1985.

Shaffer SG, Geer PG, Goetz KL: Elevated atrial natriuretic factor in neonates with respiratory distress syndrome. J Pediatr 109:1028, 1986.

Slotkin TA, Seidler FJ: Adrenomedullary catecholamine release in the fetus and newborn: Secretory mechanisms and their role in stress and survival. J Dev Physiol 10:1, 1988.

Snyder JM, Mendelson CR: Insulin inhibits the accumulation of the major lung surfactant apoprotein in human fetal lung explants maintained in vitro. Endocrinology 120:1250, 1987.

Stiles A, D'Ercole J: Insulin-like growth factors and the lung. Am J Respir Cell Molec Biol 3:93, 1990.

Thomas AL, Krane EJ, Nathanielsz PW: Changes in the fetal thyroid axis after induction of premature parturition by low-dose continuous intravascular cortisol infusion to the fetal sheep at 130 days of gestation. Endocrinology 103:17, 1978.

Ueno S, Manganaro TF, Donahoe PK: Human recombinant müllerian-inhibiting substance inhibition of rat oocyte meiosis is reversed by epidermal growth factor in vitro. Endocrinology 123:1652, 1988.

Walters DV: The role of β-adrenergic agents in the control of surfactant secretion. Biochem Soc Trans 13:1089, 1985.

Warburton D, Parton L, Buckley S, et al: Combined effects of corticosteroid, thyroid hormones, and β-receptor binding in fetal lamb lung. Pediatr Res 24:166, 1988.

SUGGESTED READINGS

Albrecht ED, Pepe GJ: Placental steroid hormone biosynthesis in primate pregnancy. Endocr Rev 11:124, 1990.

Ballard PL: Hormones and Lung Maturation, vol 28. Monographs on Endocrinology. Berlin, Springer-Verlag, 1986.

Ballard PL: Mechanism of hormone action. *In* Hoffman JIE (Eds): Pediatrics. Norwalk, CT, Appleton & Lange, 1987, pp 1447–1453.

Ballard PL: Hormonal regulation of pulmonary surfactant. Endocr Rev 10:165, 1989.

Browne CA, Thorburn GD: Endocrine control of fetal growth. Biol Neonate 55:331, 1989.

Challis JRG, Brooks AN: Maturation and activation of hypothalamic-pituitary-adrenal function in fetal sheep. Endocr Rev 10:182, 1989.

Evans RM: The steroid and thyroid hormone receptor superfamily. Science 240:889, 1988.

Fisher DA: The unique endocrine milieu of the fetus. J Clin Invest 78:603, 1986.

Jones CT (Ed): The Biochemical Development of the Fetus and Neonate. Oxford, Elsevier Biomedical Press, 1982, pp 65–619.

Jones CT (Ed): Perinatal endocrinology. Baillière's Clin Endocrinol Metabol 3:579, 1989.

Lefkowitz RJ, Caron MC: Adrenergic receptors: Models for the study of receptors coupled to guanine nucleotide regulatory proteins. J Biol Chem 263:4993, 1988.

Pepe GJ, Albrecht ED: Regulation of the primate fetal adrenal cortex. Endocr Rev 11:151, 1990.

CHAPTER 5

Fetal Growth: Nutritional Issues
(Perinatal and Long-Term Consequences)

Valerie Charlton

PATTERN OF NORMAL FETAL GROWTH
Changes in Weight and Length

Fetal growth does not occur at a uniform rate but rather changes over gestation (Moore, 1988). The rate of increase in crown-rump length occurs most rapidly early in gestation and then continues at a steady, somewhat slower pace. Fetal weight gain, viewed as a percentage increase in fetal weight, is also greatest in the earliest stages of gestation when the fetus is actively increasing its mass. This represents only a small increase in absolute weight, however. Absolute weight increases most steeply during the last half of gestation. These changing growth patterns can be appreciated in Table 5–1. Fetal weight and crown-rump length are presented, beginning with fetuses of 9 weeks' conceptual age and extending up to near-term fetuses of 36 weeks. Early in gestation, the change in crown-rump length is approximately 50 mm per month. This later declines to 40 mm per month. Fetal weight increases 460% between 9 and 12 weeks, but this represents an absolute increase of only 37 g. In contrast, fetal weight increases 800 g between 32 and 36 weeks, yet this is an increase of only 38%.

The rapid increase in absolute fetal weight and the increases in total length and head circumference that occur in later gestation are seen in Figure 5–1. These graphs were constructed by Usher and McLean (1969) from information on size at birth at various gestations for infants in Montreal. Mean values ± 2 standard deviations are given. Over the majority of the intervals shown, fetal size increases linearly. During the last few weeks of gestation, however, size begins to level off.

TABLE 5–1

Average Fetal Weight and Length at Different Ages*

Conceptual Age (weeks)	Weight (g)	Crown-Rump Length (mm)
9	8	50
12	45	87
16	200	140
20	460	190
24	820	230
28	1300	270
32	2100	300
36	2900	340

*Weights are from fixed fetuses and are approximately 5% greater than fresh weights.

Adapted from Moore KL: The fetal period. *In* The Developing Human, 4th ed. Philadelphia, WB Saunders, 1988, pp 87–103.

Organ Growth

The rate of increase in total fetal size is not necessarily matched by the growth rate of individual organs. Organ growth varies so that body proportions change over gestation. The relative size of the fetal head decreases from almost 50% of fetal length at 9 conceptual weeks to 25% near term, whereas the contribution of limb length to overall length increases (Moore, 1988). Organ weights as a percentage of body weight also change. For example, between midgestation (20 to 24 weeks) and term, there is an increase in liver weight from 3.7% to 5.1% of total fetal weight, an increase in small intestinal weight from 0.5% to 1.0%, and a decrease in skeletal weight from 22% to 18% (Shah and Rajalakshmi, 1988; Widdowson, 1974).

Body Composition

As the fetus develops from midgestation to term, there is a change in body composition (Apte and Iyengar, 1972; Ziegler et al, 1976). The percentage of fetal weight that is water decreases from 89% to 74% and the absolute accretion rate of major body constituents changes markedly, as can be seen in Table 5–2. Along with the higher rates of accretion, there are increases in the percent both of body weight that is lipid (rising from <1% to 11%) and of protein (increasing from 9% to 12%). Tissue concentrations of calcium, magnesium, and phosphorus also increase by 17% to 40%, whereas sodium and chloride concentrations decrease slightly (Ziegler et al, 1976). Fetal iron stores triple (Apte and Iyengar, 1972). At the end of gestation, some slowing in the rates of fetal tissue accretion again occurs, coincident with the plateauing in overall growth.

ROLE OF NUTRIENTS IN FETAL GROWTH AND DEVELOPMENT

Throughout gestation, the quantity and balance of nutrients available to the fetus affect the patterns of fetal development and growth. Early in gestation, when the absolute increase in fetal weight is small, abnormalities in nutrient supply are associated with abnormal embryogenesis and organ development. Later in gestation, abnormalities in nutrient supply have a more pronounced effect on the growth rate, influencing both the total size and the growth of specific organs.

Early Gestation
Nutritional Deficiencies

Maternal deficiencies and excesses of vitamins and trace minerals during early pregnancy result in fetal dysgenesis

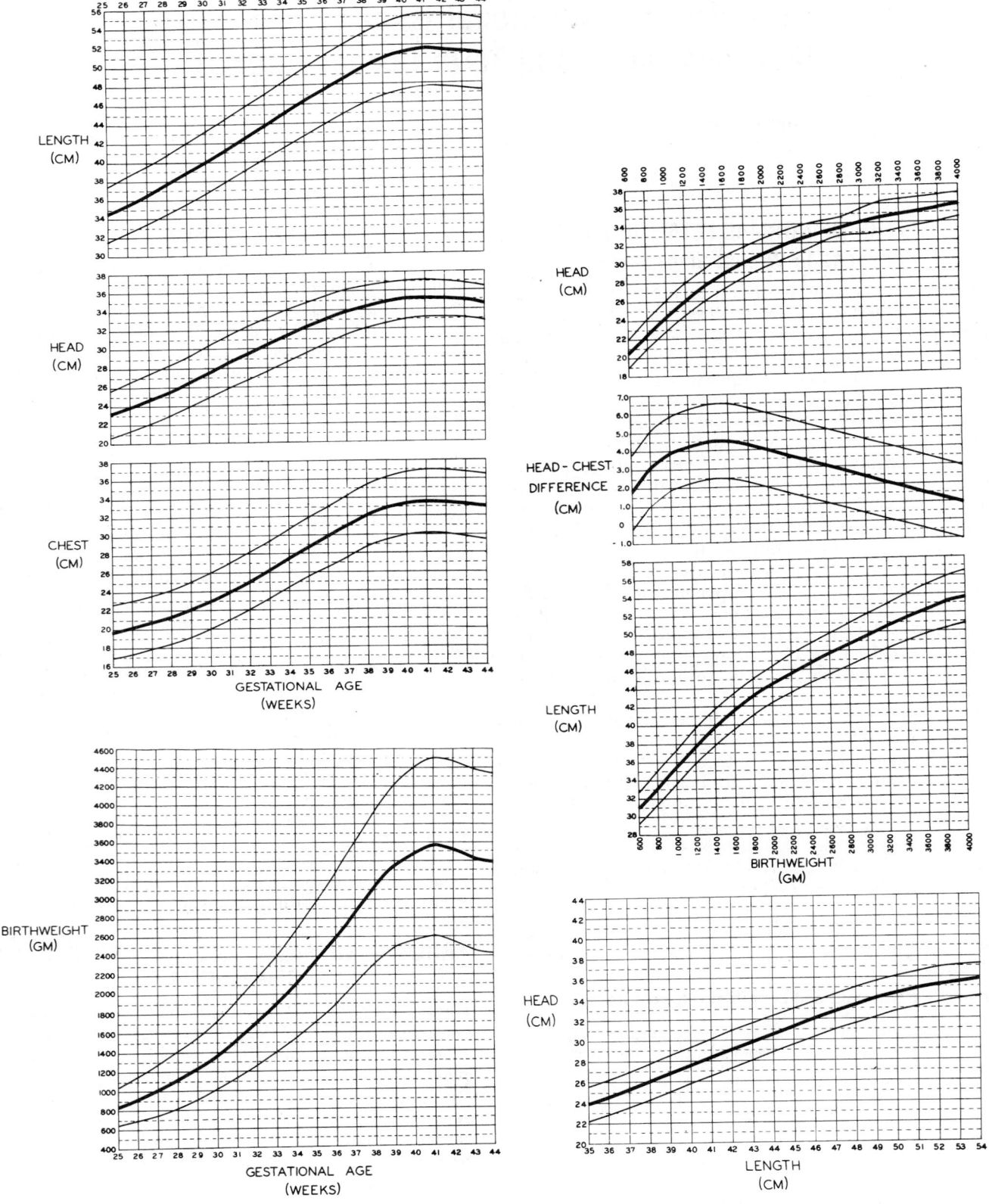

FIGURE 5–1. Size at birth versus gestational age. Smooth curve values of the mean ±2 standard deviations (3rd and 97th percentiles) for white infants at sea level (Montreal). (See also Appendix 3.) (From Usher R, McLean F: Intrauterine growth of live born Caucasian infants at sea level. J Pediatr 74:901, 1969.)

TABLE 5–2

Daily Increments in Body Weight and Constituents of the Reference Fetus

Gestation (weeks)	Weight (g)	Protein (g)	Lipid (g)	Ca (mg)	P (mg)	Mg (mg)	Na (mEq)	K (mEq)	Cl (mEq)
24–25	11.4	1.25	0.5	61	39	1.8	0.9	0.5	0.8
29–30	23.1	2.76	2.6	138	89	3.7	1.7	1.0	1.3
34–35	31.4	4.23	4.4	258	162	6.0	2.2	1.0	1.3
39–40	17.1	2.50	5.0	302	179	5.0	1.0	0.6	0.3

Adapted from Ziegler E, O'Donnell A, Nelson S, et al.: Body composition of the reference fetus. *Growth 40:*329, 1976.

(Hurley, 1980). Examples of such abnormalities in experimental animals are listed in Table 5–3. Besides fetal abnormalities, reduced maternal fertility and increased numbers of preterm offspring and stillbirths are observed in animals with deficiencies of specific vitamins and minerals (e.g., riboflavin, folate, thiamine, pantothenic acid, vitamin C, vitamin E, and zinc).

In the human, microcephaly and eye anomalies have been reported in the offspring of vitamin A–deficient mothers. Vitamin D deficiency leads to fetal rickets. Zinc deficiency has been linked to low birth weight and, when severe, malformations of the central nervous system (Hurley, 1980; Worthington-Roberts, 1985).

Mothers giving birth to infants with neural tube defects (NTDs) have been found to have low blood cell levels of folate, riboflavin, and vitamin C (Smithells et al, 1976). Further, prospective studies in Hungary and Britain have shown that prophylactic ingestion of multivitamin and mineral preparations, starting before and continuing after conception, prevent the first occurrence of NTDs and reduce the risk of recurrence after a prior NTD (Czeizel and Dudas, 1992; Smithells et al, 1989). Supplementation with folic acid alone reduces the risk of NTD recurrence threefold (Medical Research Council, 1991). On the basis of these studies, it has been recommended that all women capable of becoming pregnant ingest 400 μg of folic acid per day (Committee on Genetics, 1993). Periconceptual use of multivitamins containing folate has also been associated with decreased risk of fetal urinary tract anomalies, but the exact vitamin responsible for this effect is not clear (Li et al, 1995).

Nutritional Excesses

Increased maternal vitamin intake has also been associated with fetal abnormalities in the human. An example is vitamin A, which when taken in excess may cause fetal genitourinary, neural, and cardiac malformations and cleft lip and palate (Bernhardt and Dorsey, 1974; Gal et al, 1972; Rothman et al, 1995). Vitamin A analogues used to treat severe acne (e.g., isotretinoin) have also been associated with a constellation of defects, including central nervous system malformations, microtia, and cardiac defects (Lammer et al, 1985).

Excessive intake of vitamin D during pregnancy may cause hypercalcemia in the infant. The infant may have supravalvular aortic stenosis or peripheral pulmonic arterial stenoses and elfin faces (Worthington-Roberts, 1985). Hypotonia, irritability, vomiting, and dehydration may be present when the serum calcium is elevated and may resolve with low calcium and low vitamin D intake and appropriate hydration.

Derangements in macronutrient availability early in pregnancy can also lead to fetal dysgenesis. Hyperglycemia and related metabolic abnormalities in lipid and protein metabolism have been associated with an increased risk of multiple fetal anomalies in diabetics (Becerra et al, 1990; Cousins, 1983). These include fetal cardiac disease, anal atresia, vertebral abnormalities, microcolon, caudal regression syndrome, and NTDs. Hyperphenylalaninemia in mothers with phenylketonuria has been associated with a high incidence of central nervous system abnormalities and poor growth in utero in their nonphenylketonuric offspring (Lipson et al, 1984).

Mid to Late Gestation

Later in gestation, during the period when absolute growth and tissue accretion rates are high, wide variation in fetal size becomes apparent. In Figure 5–1, the range in weight encompassed between 2 standard deviations above and below the mean is approximately 2000 g at term.

FACTORS INFLUENCING VARIABILITY IN FETAL SIZE

The differences in fetal size are influenced both by inherent fetal genetic variation and by extrinsic maternal and environmental factors. Studies comparing weights of monozygotic twins, who share a genotype and womb environment, and dizygotic twins, who are genetically different but share the intrauterine environment, have suggested that the fetal genotype normally accounts for only 10% to 18% of the variation in birth weight (Yates, 1988). The majority of variation is usually due to extrinsic factors. These include environmental, maternal, and placental factors as well as insults that adversely alter the fetus (Table 5–4). Most of these factors affect the delivery of nutrients and oxygen to the fetus (Charlton, 1986; Gross, 1989). Their association with fetal growth suggests that availability of adequate substrates is a major determinant of intrauterine growth. The estimated variations in fetal size attributable to some of these extrinsic factors include maternal height and prepregnancy weight, 8%; total weight gain during pregnancy, 3% to 6%; weight gain from midpregnancy to term, 3%; and maternal age, education, and a prior low-birth-weight infant, 8% (Metcoff et al, 1981).

TABLE 5–3

Abnormalities of Fetal Development in Animals Associated with Maternal Deficiencies and Excesses of Trace Nutrients

Nutrient	Species Studied	Resulting Fetal Abnormality
Deficiency		
Vitamin A	Rat, pig	Defects in eyes, cardiovascular system, urogenital system, and lungs
Vitamin D	Rat, cow	Fetal rickets
Riboflavin	Rat, pig	Bone and rib anomalies, fused or missing digits, hydrocephaly, and cleft palate
Folate	Rat	Eye defects, hydrocephaly, cleft lip, and failure of closure of the thoracic and abdominal walls
Vitamin B$_{12}$	Rat	Hydrocephaly
Magnesium	Rat	Anemia, red cell abnormalities, and multiple malformations
Iron	Rat	Anemia, reduced tissue iron, and hyperlipidemia
Copper	Sheep	Spastic paralysis, blindness, central nervous system anomalies, anemia
Zinc	Guinea pig	Ataxia
	Rat	Stunted growth, short limbs, missing digits and tail, and hydrocephaly
Manganese	Rat	Severe ataxia
Excess		
Vitamin A	Rat, mouse, guinea pig, pig, rabbit, monkey	Severe anomalies of skull and brain, cleft lip, cleft palate, and eye defects
Vitamin C	Guinea pig	Increased fetal mortality
Vitamin D	Rat	Growth retardation, multiple fractures, and abnormal bone development
	Rabbit	Cranial, facial, and aortic lesions
Calcium	Rat	Low birth weight and neonatal hypocalcemia

Adapted from Hurley L: Developmental Nutrition. Englewood Cliffs, NJ, Prentice Hall, 1980.

Reductions in fetal weight of 3% to 8% are induced by varying degrees of alcohol consumption and cigarette smoking (Shu et al, 1995). Several earlier studies suggested an association between caffeine consumption and increased risk of low birth weight or fetal growth retardation, but this has not been found in subsequent studies that controlled for relevant confounders (Shu et al, 1995; Worthington-Roberts, 1985).

It should be noted that the growth curves presented in Figure 5–1 were collected at sea level using white infants. Because of variations in populations and environment, data collected in other locations differ. Lower mean birth weights at 40 weeks' gestation have been reported in Denver (3230 g) and in Baltimore (3280 g), presumably reflecting differences in altitude and population composition (Naeye and Dixon, 1978). The growth curve appropriate for each population should be used when assessing infant size.

CLASSIFICATION OF FETAL SIZE AT BIRTH
Appropriately Grown Fetus

Infants at the extremes of the range in growth, either too small or too large, are at increased risk of perinatal mortality versus infants of normal growth (Williams et al, 1982). Normal intrauterine growth, or appropriate size for gestational age, is commonly defined as a birth weight between 2 standard deviations below and 2 standard deviations above the mean for gestation on the birth weight curve (e.g., approximately between the 3rd and 97th percentiles). Some investigators, however, use a narrower definition of appropriate growth, such as between the 10th and 90th birth weight percentiles.

Undergrown Fetus

Inadequate growth in utero has commonly been defined as a birth weight less than 2 standard deviations below the

TABLE 5–4

Maternal, Placental, Environmental, and Fetal Factors Affecting Intrauterine Growth

Maternal Factors
Maternal nutrient levels and nutrient stores: *Reduced by* inadequate or poorly balanced nutrient intake, low prepregnancy weight, small maternal size, poor gestational weight gain, poor late-pregnancy weight gain, recent pregnancy, young maternal age, hypoglycemia, chronic illness, and alcoholism. *Increased by* good dietary intake, normal prepregnancy weight, and good gestational weight gain
Oxygen level: *Reduced by* cyanotic heart disease, hemoglobinopathies, respiratory failure, and smoking
Uteroplacental blood flow: *Reduced by* hypertension, renal disease, vascular disease, cocaine, smoking, and caffeine
Multiple gestation: Decreases substrates available for each fetus
Medications: Fetal growth reduced by antimetabolites, phenytoin, warfarin, and beta blockers
Previous low-birth-weight infant: Increases risk for low birth weight
Placental Factors
Placental size and surface area: Reduced substrate transfer with decreased size and surface area
Structural abnormalities: Reduced transfer area with infarcts, villous changes, and abnormal cord insertion
Transport: Alcohol reduces placental amino acid and zinc transport
Environmental Factors
Socioeconomic and educational status: Low socioeconomic and educational status associated with reduced birth weight
Altitude: High altitude reduces maternal oxygen levels
Fetal Factors
Infections: Intrauterine infections can adversely affect fetal growth
Chromosomal: Identifiable chromosomal abnormalities and dysmorphic syndromes can alter growth
Toxins: Can lead to abnormal fetal development, e.g., methyl mercury exposure

Adapted from Campbell, 1974; Charlton, 1986; Fisher et al, 1983; Gross, 1989; Metcoff et al, 1981; Mochizuki et al, 1984; Socol et al, 1982; Van den Berg, 1981; Woods et al, 1987.

mean for gestation (approximately the 3rd percentile) on fetal weight curves. Some authors use a less restrictive definition of a birth weight below the 10th percentile. Infants whose size falls below these levels are termed *intrauterine growth retarded, small for gestational age* (SGA), or *small for dates.* Unfortunately, these definitions, based on birth weight alone, do not differentiate infants who are also reduced in length or head circumference and completely overlook long, wasted infants whose birth weight is slightly above the defined cut off. A plea has been made for a fresh approach to categorizing normal and abnormal intrauterine growth, including some indicator of weight for length (Miller and Jekel, 1989).

Infants who are SGA are a heterogeneous group. Some appear symmetrically growth retarded, with proportionally reduced size in weight, length, and head circumference. These infants have a slow growth rate beginning early in gestation and are more likely to have marked genetic constraints on growth or underlying fetal abnormalities of the type listed in Table 5–4, such as congenital infections, chromosomal abnormalities, or dysmorphic syndromes (Campbell, 1974).

Most growth-retarded infants, however, are asymmetrically growth retarded. Their severest growth reductions are in weight and perhaps length. They often are low weight for their length and have a reduced ponderal index (weight/length³). There is relative sparing of head growth, but despite this relative sparing, absolute head size is usually decreased for gestation (Kramer et al, 1989). In fact, growth-retarded infants who have died in the newborn period have been found to have a 19% to 20% decrease in cerebral size and cellularity and a 35% to 37% reduction in size and cellularity of the cerebellum (Chase et al, 1972).

The asymmetric form of growth retardation is usually due to extrinsic influences on the fetus and becomes apparent later in gestation, when growth should be most rapid. Abnormalities of the maternal, placental, and environmental factors listed in Table 5–4 lead to this fetal phenotype. These infants have a malnourished, wasted appearance, and the individual organs most reduced in size are those compromised by postnatal malnutrition—the liver, spleen, thymus, and adrenals. This growth pattern again suggests a causative role for malnutrition in poor fetal growth (Naeye, 1965). Intestinal length is also reduced (Shanklin and Cooke, 1993). Animal studies indicate that key organs, such as the brain, maintain somewhat better growth because they are given a larger share of the available nutrients, through preferential blood distribution patterns and increased rates of blood flow (Charlton, 1986).

Growth-retarded infants also have undergrown placentas (Molteni et al, 1978). They are at increased risk for perinatal complications and long-term sequelae. These consequences of abnormal fetal growth are discussed later.

Large Fetus

Excessive growth in utero has been defined as a birth weight either greater than 2 standard deviations above the mean for gestation (the 97th percentile) or above the 90th percentile. Infants with weights above these levels are termed *large for gestational age* (LGA) or *large for dates.*

Infants who are LGA can be either normal large infants or infants whose growth has been stimulated by abnormal conditions in utero. These abnormal conditions usually involve exposure to increased levels of glucose or hyperinsulinism (or both), suggesting that a surplus of substrate and increased glucose metabolism promote fetal growth. Examples are infants of diabetic mothers (IDMs) (Willman et al, 1986) and infants with Beckwith-Wiedemann syndrome. The latter includes pancreatic hyperplasia and hyperinsulinism (Jones, 1988). High C-peptide levels, indicating high insulin secretory activity, have also been found in LGA infants of nondiabetic mothers, with no other recognized syndromes (Akinbi and Gerdes, 1995). Placental size tends to be increased in large infants (Molteni et al, 1978), but higher rates of substrate utilization raise the demand for oxygen (Milley et al, 1984; Phillips et al, 1985). These fetuses are at risk for birth asphyxia and birth trauma. The perinatal and long-term outcomes for the LGA fetus are discussed later.

FETAL NUTRITIONAL NEEDS DURING THE PERIOD OF RAPID GROWTH

To achieve normal growth, a balanced quantity of nutrients must reach the fetus during the latter part of gestation. Normal caloric entry into the human fetus near term has been estimated as approximately 90 to 100 kcal/kg/day. Of this, 40 kcal/kg/day are used for growth (Sparks et al, 1980). The major nutrients that provide these calories are glucose and amino acids.

Glucose

Glucose is the major source of energy for the fetus and a large source of carbon. It is also the major substrate used by the fetal brain (Jones, 1979). Glucose crosses the placenta by facilitated diffusion, and fetal uptake of glucose is proportional, over a wide range, to maternal glucose levels and the concentration gradient between mother and fetus (Aldoretta and Hay, 1995; Hauguel et al, 1986). Glucose levels in the human fetus at birth are 70% to 80% of maternal venous values, with fetal umbilical venous concentrations reported as 55 to 85 mg/dL (Morriss et al, 1975). Studies of cesarean sections indicate that if all the glucose entering the fetus were completely oxidized, glucose use could account for approximately 80% of fetal oxygen consumption (Morriss et al, 1975).

Availability of glucose appears to play a major role in fetal growth. Intrauterine blood glucose concentrations are reduced in the growth-retarded fetus, and cord blood glucose levels are low in growth-retarded newborns (Economides and Nicolaides, 1989; Haymond et al, 1974). Both low fasting maternal glucose levels and rapid maternal utilization of glucose have been found in women giving birth to small infants (Langer et al, 1986; Raman, 1981). The association between increased levels of glucose and insulin and increased fetal size has been mentioned. In women with diabetes, the chance of fetal macrosomia is increased twofold when mean maternal glucose levels exceed 130 mg/dL (Willman et al, 1986).

In third-trimester fetal sheep, the total quantity of glucose taken up across the umbilical circulation normally averages 27 g/day. In experimentally growth-retarded fetal lambs, total glucose uptake falls by up to 50%. The quantity of glucose taken up per kilogram of fetal weight declines by only 10% to 30%, however, suggesting that fetal growth adapts in response to the substrate supply (Charlton, 1986).

Amino Acids

Amino acids serve as the source of nitrogen for the fetus and as a major source of carbon. They are used during anabolism and are rapidly catabolized, as indicated by a high fetal urea production rate. They are actively transported into the fetus against a concentration gradient, resulting in higher amino acid levels in the fetus than in the mother (Aldoretta and Hay, 1995; Rosso, 1983). Total fetal amino acid concentrations average 2.3 mmol/L in the mid-trimester human, and with the decrease in maternal amino acids during pregnancy, fetal levels average 2.4 times maternal. Although fetal amino acid levels are higher than maternal, there is a direct correlation between fetal and maternal values for most amino acids in the human (Soltesz et al, 1985). Amino acid abnormalities in maternal blood, therefore, are magnified in the fetus. This undoubtedly relates to the previously mentioned high incidence of malformations in nonphenylketonuric infants born to mothers with phenylketonuria (Lipson et al, 1984).

Poor fetal growth has been associated with decreased total plasma amino acid levels in the mother and decreased maternal levels of specific amino acids (Metcoff et al, 1981). Further, growth-retarded human fetuses have been found to have decreased cord blood levels of total and specific amino acids (Cetin et al, 1988).

In third-trimester fetal sheep, approximately 20 g of amino acids are taken up across the umbilical circulation each day. With maternal malnutrition, fetal umbilical uptake of amino acids decreases, and amino acids are diverted from fetal protein synthesis to use as oxidative fuels (Aldoretta and Hay, 1995; Charlton, 1986).

Lactate

Under conditions of normal oxygenation, lactate has been identified as an additional major fetal nutrient in sheep (Charlton and Creasy, 1976a). It is produced by placental metabolism and excreted into the fetal and maternal circulations. Further, it is produced by fetal metabolism and used as a substrate by fetal organs such as the heart and gastrointestinal tract (Sparks et al, 1982). In sheep, fetal umbilical uptake of lactate averages 7 g/day (Charlton, 1986). Lactate is also produced by the human placenta, and cord blood measurements, made at elective repeat cesarean section, suggest that it is taken up across the umbilical circulation by the human fetus (Charlton and Creasy, 1976b).

Fats, Ketones, and Acetate

Fats are a major source of calories postnatally, but there is great species variation in the extent to which fatty acids are transferred across the placenta. In the human, there appears to be some placental lipid transport as well as lipid synthesis within the fetus (Rosso, 1983). Essential fatty acids and acetate, which can be used to synthesize lipids and cholesterol, cross the human placenta (Plotz et al, 1968). In the fetal lamb, acetate uptake across the umbilical circulation has been documented in quantities that could explain up to 10% of fetal oxygen consumption (Charlton and Creasy, 1976c). Ketone transfer in animals is usually low but increases slightly when maternal levels are elevated (Morriss et al, 1974). In the human, fetal cord blood levels of ketones correlate with maternal levels (Bencini and Symonds, 1972). Of concern are the findings that elevated ketone levels adversely affect brain metabolism in the fetal lamb and that beta-hydroxybutyrate levels in pregnant human diabetics correlate inversely with later developmental and intelligence scores in their offspring (Harding and Charlton, 1990; Rizzo et al, 1995).

Relation Between Macronutrient Supply and Growth-Promoting Hormones

The effects of macronutrients on fetal growth may in part be mediated by their effects on growth-promoting hormones. The increased insulin levels in macrosomic infants have been mentioned, but the somatomedins, or insulin-like growth factors (IGFs), appear to play a larger role in fetal growth (Sara, 1988). Cord blood levels of IGFs show a correlation with birth weight in the human, and growth-retarded infants have low IGF levels (Engstrom and Heath, 1988). In animals, malnutrition during pregnancy leads to decreased fetal levels of IGFs as well as decreased fetal growth (D'Ercole, 1987).

In the human fetus, the predominant IGFs are a variant form of IGF-1 and IGF-2. The IGFs are produced in all fetal tissues, and their production is independent of growth hormone regulation. Placental lactogen may regulate IGF production in some species, but in the human it has been suggested that IGF biosynthesis is regulated by availability of substrate to the cell. This would provide a local mechanism for controlling cellular growth (Sara, 1988).

Trace Minerals and Vitamins

Besides macronutrients, micronutrients are needed for normal late fetal growth. The high accretion rates of some minerals in late gestation are given in Table 5–2. Adequate fetal supply of key minerals, such as calcium, phosphorus, and iron, enters the fetus by active transport, and near term, fetal blood levels of these minerals exceed maternal. Nonetheless, fetal anemia and depleted iron stores can occur with maternal iron deficiency (Hurley, 1980). Ensuring adequate maternal intake of zinc, by supplementation of women with zinc levels below the median, increases birth weight by approximately 250 g and increases head circumference by 0.7 cm (Goldenberg et al, 1995).

Both fat-soluble and water-soluble vitamins are needed by the fetus. Fat-soluble vitamins (A, D, E, and K) cross the placenta by diffusion, and fetal levels are less than or equal to maternal levels. Because water-soluble vitamins (B and C) cross the placenta by active transport, fetal levels are greater than maternal (Rosso, 1983). Specific vitamin abnormalities can present as derangements in the newborn period. Fetal thiamine deficiency can lead to congenital beriberi with cardiac failure, aphonia, or a pseudomeningitis. Excess fetal vitamin C can lead to high rates of ascorbate metabolism and neonatal scurvy (Hurley, 1980).

Oxygen

To allow utilization of all the substrates discussed in this chapter, sufficient oxygen must also enter the fetus. In animal studies, it has been estimated that 20% of normal fetal oxidative metabolism is consumed by growth (Clapp et al, 1981). Because oxygen enters the fetus rapidly by simple diffusion, oxygen levels are usually adequate. In fetuses with abnormal growth, both small and large, however, there may be evidence of decreased oxygenation, indicated by low cord blood oxygen tensions, increased hemoglobin levels, and increased erythropoietin levels (Charlton, 1986; Georgieff et al, 1989).

Plateauing of Fetal Growth

Fetal growth usually plateaus near term. Even under normal intrauterine conditions, fetal requirements eventually outstrip substrate supply, so that high rates of growth cannot be maintained. After birth and adjustment to ex utero conditions, rapid growth resumes.

MATERNAL NUTRITION DURING PREGNANCY
Normal Weight Gain

To provide the fetus with the proper quantity and mix of substrates, the normal pregnant woman in a developed country gains an average of 27 pounds (range 25 to 35 pounds [12 to 16 kg]). Of this, approximately 33% is fetal and placental weight, 23% is increase in maternal blood volume and extracellular fluid, 7% is amniotic fluid, and the remainder is made up of new maternal tissue (e.g., uterus and breasts) plus fat stores for lactation (Chez, 1993). Maternal weight gain during the first and second trimesters goes mainly toward maternal components (blood, extracellular fluid, tissue, and fat stores) and the placenta, and weight gain during the third trimester goes mainly toward fetal tissue. This is why maternal weight gain during late pregnancy is a specific risk factor influencing fetal size (Van den Berg, 1981).

Caloric and Dietary Needs

The extra nutritional intake required by the mother to achieve this increase in weight and optimum fetal growth has been estimated at 80,000 kcal in developed countries. The National Research Council of the American Academy of Sciences (1989) has, therefore, recommended an intake of 300 kcal/day over nonpregnant needs, or an approximate total caloric intake of 2500 kcal/day. Whether pregnant women with adequate body reserves need caloric supplementation in the first trimester has been questioned, but supplementation in the second and third trimesters is clearly advocated. As Table 5–5 shows, the National Academy of Sciences also recommends that protein intake be

TABLE 5–5

Recommended Daily Dietary Allowances During Pregnancy

Nutrient, Unit	Amount
Energy, kcal	+300 (above usual)*
Protein, g	60
Fat-soluble vitamins	
Vitamin A, μg as retinol equivalents	800
Vitamin D, μg as cholecalciferol	10
Vitamin E, mg α-tocopherol equivalents	10
Vitamin K, μg	65
Water-soluble vitamins	
Vitamin C, mg	70
Thiamine, mg	1.5
Riboflavin, mg	1.6
Niacin, mg niacin equivalent	17
Vitamin B_6, mg	2.2
Folate, μg	400
Vitamin B_{12}, μg	2.2
Minerals	
Calcium, mg	1200
Phosphorus, mg	1200
Magnesium, mg	320
Iron, mg	30
Zinc, mg	15
Iodine, μg	175
Selenium, μg	65

*Most important in the second and third trimesters.

Reprinted with permission from the National Research Council, Food and Nutrition Board: Recommended Dietary Allowances, 10th rev ed. Copyright 1989 by the National Academy of Sciences. Courtesy of the National Academy Press, Washington, DC.

increased up to a total of about 60 g/day. Excessive protein intake, however, is undesirable and may lead to an increased incidence of preterm births (Susser, 1981). The recommended dietary intake for most vitamins is increased during pregnancy by 10% to 50% versus intakes recommended for nonpregnant women, and the recommended intake for calcium and iron is increased by 50% to 100%.

In some nations, apparently normal fetal growth is achieved with lower maternal caloric intakes than those recommended by the American National Research Council. Caloric needs during pregnancy have been investigated in a large seven-country study, which included developed and developing nations. The results of the study suggest that in some populations actual maternal caloric needs are lessened by maternal physiologic adaptations, including decreased basal metabolic rate, activity levels, body temperature, and fat stores (Durnin, 1987; Poppitt et al, 1994). Below maternal caloric intakes of around 1800 kcal/day, however, fetal growth can no longer be protected (Whitehead, 1988).

Attempts to Improve Fetal Growth
Maternal Dietary Supplementation

To try to improve fetal size and outcome, trials of dietary supplementation have been carried out in different parts of the world. Supplementation rates of up to 1000 kcal and

40 g of protein per day have been given. The benefits of supplementation have been variable, and where an effect has been seen, it has been only in the range of a 100 to 300 g increase in birth weight (Whitehead, 1988). Even these small increases, however, can have a marked effect in reducing the incidence of low birth weight in some populations (e.g., from 28% to 5% in Gambia) (Nutrition Reviews, 1984). A number of questions have also been raised about these studies with respect to the mother's ingestion of the supplement instead of her regular diet, rather than consuming it as additional intake, and the prior level of maternal physiologic adaptation to malnutrition (Whitehead, 1988).

Nondietary Approaches

In developed nations, in settings in which maternal oral nutrition is considered sufficient, fetal growth retardation continues to occur. Therefore, other approaches have been taken to help augment delivery of substrates to the fetus and even bypass a possibly poorly functioning placenta (Charlton, 1986; Harding and Charlton, 1989). Variable success has been achieved with nutritional therapies such as intravenous infusion of glucose and amino acids into the mother, infusion of amino acids into the amniotic fluid, and infusion of amino acids directly into the fetal peritoneal cavity. Non-nutritional therapies aimed at improving uterine blood flow (such as bed rest and maternal aspirin therapy) have been used as well as maternal oxygen therapy to improve fetoplacental oxygenation. To date, the advantages and risks of each of these therapies are still undefined.

PERINATAL AND LONG-TERM CONSEQUENCES OF ABNORMAL FETAL GROWTH AND NUTRITION
Small-for-Gestational-Age Infant
Perinatal Complications

Classification of size at birth, the neonatal phenotypes indicating poor growth in utero, and factors affecting fetal growth were discussed earlier in this chapter. Although poor growth in utero may be due to causes intrinsic to the fetus, most intrauterine growth retardation is caused by factors extrinsic to the fetus, that occur in the mother, placenta, or environment (see Table 5–4). Common to these extrinsic causes is that they decrease delivery of nutrients, oxygen, or both to the fetus (Charlton, 1986). It is, therefore, not surprising that infants born SGA are at increased risk of perinatal complications.

Compared with infants who are normally grown, SGA newborns are more likely to show signs of fetal distress, be acidotic at birth, and have low Apgar scores (Charlton, 1996). In California, fetal death rates of 1.5 to 2.4 per 1000 and neonatal death rates of 1.2 to 2.4 per 1000 have been reported for normally grown singletons, between 38 and 42 weeks' gestation and weights of 3000 to 4000 g. In contrast, fetal death rates of 18 to 46 per 1000 and neonatal death rates of 12 to 33 per 1000 were reported for SGA singletons of the same mature gestation but with weights of 2000 to 2500 g (Williams et al, 1982).

Because of chronic intrauterine hypoxia, SGA infants are likely to be polycythemic (i.e., have a venous hematocrit of 65% or greater). In term and near-term SGA infants, the incidence of polycythemia is 8% to 15%, compared to 1% to 2% in normally grown newborns (Wirth et al, 1979; Wiswell et al, 1986).

The reduced amount of subcutaneous tissue in SGA infants makes them susceptible to hypothermia and reduced nutrient stores, as well as large red blood cell mass and a high rate of cerebral glucose use in relation to liver size, makes them likely to develop hypoglycemia (Charlton, 1996). Before close monitoring of blood glucose and early feedings were instituted, 21% of term SGA infants had serum glucose levels less than 20 mg/dL before their first feeding at 3 to 6 hours of life versus 2% of normally grown term infants. Twenty-five percent of term SGA infants had glucose levels less than 30 mg/dL (Lubchenco and Bard, 1971).

To avoid these perinatal complications, there should be close fetal monitoring when delivery of an SGA infant is anticipated and personnel and facilities available for postnatal resuscitation. Postnatally, SGA infants should be kept warm. Blood glucose levels should be initially checked within an hour of birth and thereafter monitored closely, (e.g., rechecked at 2, 4, 6, 12, 24, and 48 hours). In moderately growth-retarded infants, early feedings (e.g., 5% dextrose in water) should be given by 2 hours of age, as tolerated, if feedings are not contraindicated by birth asphyxia, illness, or preterm gestation. In asphyxiated, sick, preterm, or severely SGA infants, intravenous glucose administration should be begun prophylactically and glucose levels monitored. Hypoglycemia should be treated if it occurs, and, in asphyxiated or preterm infants, hypocalcemia may also be seen (see Chapters 99 and 103 for treatment of hypoglycemia and hypocalcemia). The hematocrit should be checked by 2 hours of age, and a partial exchange transfusion may need to be carried out if there is polycythemia. If the hematocrit is between 60% and 65%, a follow-up hematocrit should be done at 4 hours for treatment of polycythemia). If the physical examination suggests possible intrinsic fetal abnormality, such as a chromosomal anomaly or intrauterine infection, pertinent tests should be done.

Long-Term Sequelae

Infants who are SGA have been followed through adolescence and as a group have been found to have reduced ultimate stature (Paz et al, 1993). The prognosis for postnatal growth, however, differs somewhat between the SGA phenotypes. The symmetrically growth-retarded fetus with inherent abnormalities is likely to continue to manifest growth failure. Asymmetrically growth-retarded infants, who are of normal or near-normal length at birth, usually catch up in weight and attain relatively normal stature, whereas infants who are stunted in length as well as weight often remain comparatively short (Fitzhardinge and Inwood, 1989; Henrichson et al, 1986; Villar et al, 1984). These short infants may exhibit some catch-up growth and end up in a height percentile that is within the normal range, but many remain more than 2 standard deviations below normal mean height; individuals who were of short stature at birth later account for approximately 22% of the short adult population (Karlberg and Albertsson-Wikland, 1995). The duration of the growth insult in utero may be causally related to the presence of poor later growth. Short stature and lower than average weight at 4 years are more likely to be found if there is slowing of fetal growth by 34 weeks' gestation than if growth failure occurs after 34 weeks (Fancourt et al, 1976).

SGA infants have an increased incidence of neurologic deficits. Twenty-five percent of term SGA infants, who were followed for up to 8 years, were found to have speech defects and minimal brain dysfunction, including hyperactivity, short attention span, poor fine coordination, and learning difficulties (Fitzhardinge and Steven, 1972). Possible relationships between a variety of perinatal complications and learning deficits at age 9 to 11 years have also been assessed, and only fetal growth retardation has been found to be related (Low et al, 1992). In studies of monozygous twins, reduced global and performance intelligence quotients (IQ) have been found at 9 to 17 years of age in the twin who was growth compromised at birth compared to the better grown sibling (Henrichson et al, 1986). As mentioned earlier, brain and head size are often reduced in SGA infants (Chase et al, 1972; Kramer et al, 1989). The timing of the insult to fetal head growth may be important in determining later performance, because early intrauterine slowing of head growth has been associated with subsequent developmental deficits (Harvey et al, 1982).

In addition to the association with growth and developmental outcomes, different SGA phenotypes have been linked in retrospective epidemiologic studies with health problems in adults. In general, individuals who were SGA at birth have a threefold to fourfold increased risk of hypertension in adolescence and early adulthood (Barker et al, 1989; Gennser et al, 1988). Individuals who are born thin, with a low ponderal index, have a 10-fold increased risk for developing syndrome X (non-insulin-dependent diabetes, hypertension, and hyperlipidemia) by age 65 versus individuals of higher birth weight (Barker et al, 1993a). Individuals born SGA, with a low ponderal index and a small head size, have an increased risk of death from cardiovascular disease by age 65 (Barker et al, 1993b). It has been hypothesized that abnormalities in the intrauterine metabolic environment affect organ development and lead to the long-term health effects.

Large-for-Gestational-Age Infant

Perinatal Complications

As was noted earlier in this chapter, LGA infants are often exposed in utero to increased levels of nutrients (particularly glucose) and may have hyperinsulinism and high rates of glucose and oxygen use (Akinbi and Gerdes, 1995; Jones, 1988; Milley et al, 1984; Phillips et al, 1985; Willman et al, 1986). Their metabolic and size abnormalities put them at increased risk for perinatal complications, such as asphyxia, birth trauma, polycythemia, and hypoglycemia. LGA infants, particularly IDMs, are also at increased risk of cardiac and other birth defects (Cousins, 1983).

Compared to normally grown infants, infants who are LGA have higher fetal and neonatal death rates. For singleton LGA gestations, between 38 and 42 weeks and weights of 4000 g or greater, the fetal death rate in California has been reported as 1.8 to 8.2 per 1000 and the neonatal death rate as 1.4 to 5.4 per 1000. In appropriately grown infants, of the same gestation with birth weights of 3000 to 4000 g, the maximal fetal and neonatal death rates are 2.4 per 1000 (Williams et al, 1982).

Increased nutrient availability and oxidative demands can serve as a stimulus to raise in utero hemoglobin (Charlton and Johengen, 1985). Term and near-term LGA infants have a 3% to 6% incidence of polycythemia (venous hematocrit of 65% or greater) versus the 1% to 2% incidence in normally grown infants (Wirth et al, 1979).

With termination of the placental supply line at birth and increased glucose consumption, LGA infants may become hypoglycemic. Before initiation of prophylactic early feedings, serum glucose levels of less than 30 mg/dL were found at 3 to 6 hours of age in 38% of preterm LGA infants less than 38 weeks' gestation versus 15% of normally grown infants of similar gestation (Lubchenco and Bard, 1971). Even with current approaches to management, plasma glucose levels less than 35 mg/dL have been found during the first day of life in 20% of a cohort of LGA neonates, weighing greater than 4000 g (Akinbi and Gerdes, 1995).

To avoid these perinatal complications, there must be close assessment of the LGA fetus during labor and personnel and facilities available to carry out obstetric intervention, or neonatal resuscitation, or both if needed. After birth, hematocrit and blood glucose should be monitored and early feedings or administration of glucose begun, as described previously for the SGA infant. Polycythemia and hypoglycemia should be treated, if they occur. IDMs and asphyxiated infants are also at risk of hypocalcemia, and levels should be checked and corrected. (See Chapter 7 for specific discussion of the IDM and Chapters 89, 99, and 103 on polycythemia, hypocalcemia, and hypoglycemia.)

Long-Term Sequelae

The extent to which LGA infants have later sequelae related to their perinatal environment is unclear. Most follow-up studies have focused on the IDM. Many of these infants are relatively obese, with increased weight-to-length ratios. These obese infants initially appear to normalize in weight over the first year of life but often become obese again later. In a follow-up study of 139 IDMs, by 8 years of age, half of the children had weights greater than the 90th percentile on normal growth charts (Rizzo et al, 1995). In another study of LGA IDMs, 42% were found to be obese (with increased weight-for-height indices) at 7 years of age versus 7% of the control population that was normally grown at birth. Weight-for-height indices were also higher in young adults between 12 to 17 years of age who had been LGA newborns (Vohr et al, 1980). Adult obesity has been reported as more frequent in individuals who were LGA IDMs (Verdy et al, 1974).

Intellectual development may also be compromised in IDMs exposed to ketones in utero. The presence of acetone in the urine of pregnant diabetics has been related to lower IQ scores in their offspring at 5 years of age (Stehbens et al, 1977). Maternal second-trimester and third-trimester beta-hydroxybutyrate levels have been found to correlate with the children's psychomotor scores at age 6 to 9 years. The more aberrant the mother's metabolism during gestation, the poorer the child's psychomotor development (Rizzo et al, 1995).

The risk for developing diabetes is increased in children of diabetic mothers. This risk, however, does not appear necessarily to be related to being LGA in size at birth and includes a genetic component (Farquhar, 1969; Persson et al, 1984).

SUMMARY

The substrates available to the fetus play an important role in fetal development and growth. To provide the best environment for the fetus, the mother should be optimally treated for any underlying medical conditions, should be in good nutritional status before pregnancy, and should consume an adequate balanced diet during pregnancy that results in a normal gestational weight gain. Abnormalities in maternal nutrition or metabolism that affect fetal size and development increase perinatal morbidity and mortality and have lifelong consequences.

REFERENCES

Aldoretta P, Hay W: Metabolic substrates for fetal energy metabolism and growth. Clin Perinatol 22:15, 1995.

Akinbi H, Gerdes J: Macrosomic infants of nondiabetic mothers and elevated C-peptide levels in cord blood. J Pediatr 127:481, 1995.

Apte S, Iyengar L: Composition of the human fetus. Br J Nutr 27:305, 1972.

Barker D, Osmond C, Golding J: Growth in utero, blood pressure in childhood and adult life, and mortality from cardiovascular disease. BMJ 298:564, 1989.

Barker D, Hales C, Fall C, et al: Type 2 (non-insulin-dependent) diabetes mellitus, hypertension and hyperlipidemia (syndrome X): Relation to reduced fetal growth. Diabetologia 36:62, 1993a.

Barker D, Osmond C, Simmonds S, et al: The relation of small head circumference and thinness at birth to death from cardiovascular disease in adult life. BMJ 306:422, 1993b.

Becerra J, Khoury M, Cordero J, et al: Diabetes mellitus during pregnancy and the risks for specific birth defects: A population based case-control study. Pediatrics 85:1, 1990.

Bencini F, Symonds E: Ketone bodies in fetal and maternal blood during parturition. Aust NZ Obstet Gynaecol 12:176, 1972.

Bernhardt I, Dorsey D: Hypervitaminosis A and congenital renal anomalies in a human infant. Obstet Gynecol 43:750, 1974.

Campbell S: The assessment of fetal development by diagnostic ultrasound. Clin Perinatol 2:507, 1974.

Cetin I, Marconi A, Bozzetti P, et al: Umbilical amino acid concentrations in appropriate and small for gestational age infants: A biochemical difference present in utero. Am J Obstet Gynecol 158:120, 1988.

Charlton V: Nutritional supplementation of the growth retarded fetus: Rationale, theoretical considerations, and in vivo studies. *In* Milunsky, A, Friedman E, Gluck L (Eds): Advances in Perinatal Medicine, vol 5. New York, Plenum Press, 1986, pp 1–42.

Charlton V: The small-for-gestational age infant. *In* Rudolph A (Ed): Rudolph's Pediatrics, 20th ed. San Mateo, CA, Appleton & Lange, 1996, pp 245–248.

Charlton V, Creasy R. Lactate and pyruvate as fetal metabolic substrates. Pediatr Res 10:231, 1976a.

Charlton V, Creasy R: Unpublished observations, 1976b.

Charlton V, Creasy R: Acetate as metabolic substrate in the fetal lamb. Am J Physiol 230:357, 1976c.

Charlton V, Johengen M: Effects of intrauterine nutritional supplementation on fetal growth retardation. Biol Neonate 48:125, 1985.

Chase P, Welch N, Dabiere C, et al: Alterations in human brain biochemistry following IUGR. Pediatrics 50:403, 1972.

Chez R: Nutritional factors in pregnancy affecting fetal growth and subsequent infant development. *In* Suskind R, Lewinter-Suskind L (Eds): Textbook of Pediatric Nutrition, 2nd ed. New York, Raven Press, 1993, pp 9–15.

Clapp J, Szeto H, Larrow R, et al: Fetal metabolic response to experimental placental vascular damage. Am J Obstet Gynecol 140:446, 1981.

Committee on Genetics of the American Academy of Pediatrics: Folic acid for the prevention of neural tube defects. Pediatrics 92:493, 1993.

Cousins L: Congenital anomalies among infants of diabetic mothers. Am J Obstet Gynecol 147:333, 1983.

Czeizel A, Dudas I: Prevention of the first occurrence of neural tube defects by periconceptual vitamin supplementation. N Engl J Med 327:1832, 1992.

D'Ercole A: Somatomedins/insulin-like growth factors and fetal growth. J Dev Physiol 9:481, 1987.

Durnin J: Energy requirements of pregnancy. Lancet 2:895, 1987.

Economides D, Nicolaides K: Blood glucose and oxygen tension levels in small for gestational age fetuses. Am J Obstet Gynecol 160:385, 1989.

Engstrom W, Heath J: Growth factors in early embryonic development. *In* Cockburn F (Ed): Fetal and Neonatal Growth: Perinatal Practice, vol 5. New York, John Wiley & Sons, 1988, pp 11–32.

Fancourt R, Campbell S, Harvey D, et al: Follow-up study of small-for-date babies. BMJ 1:1435, 1976.

Farquhar J: Prognosis for babies born to diabetic mothers in Edinburgh. Arch Dis Child 44:36, 1969.

Fisher S, Atkinson M, Jacobsen S, et al: Selective fetal malnutrition: The effect of in vivo ethanol exposure upon in vitro placental uptake of amino acids in the non-human primate. Pediatr Res 17:704, 1983.

Fitzhardinge P, Inwood S: Long-term growth in small-for-date children. Acta Paediatr Scand 349(suppl):27, 1989.

Fitzhardinge P, Steven E: The small for date infant: II. Neurological and intellectual sequelae. Pediatrics 50:50, 1972.

Gal I, Sharman I, Pryse-Davies J: Vitamin A in relation to human congenital malformations. Adv Teratol 5:143, 1972.

Gennser G, Rymark P, Isberg P: Low birth weight and risk of high blood pressure in adulthood. BMJ 296:1498, 1988.

Georgieff M, Widness J, Mills M, et al: The effect of prolonged intrauterine hyperinsulinemia on iron utilization in fetal sheep. Pediatr Res 26:467, 1989.

Goldenberg R, Tamura T, Neggers Y, et al: The effect of zinc supplementation on pregnancy outcome. JAMA 274:463, 1995.

Gross T: Maternal and placental causes of intrauterine growth retardation. *In* Gross T, Sokol R (Eds): Intrauterine Growth Retardation: A Practical Approach. Chicago, Year Book Medical Publishers, 1989, pp 57–67.

Harding J, Charlton V: Treatment of the growth retarded fetus by augmentation of substrate supply. Semin Perinatol 14:211, 1989.

Harding J, Charlton V: Effect of lactate and β-hydroxybutyrate infusion on brain metabolism in the fetal sheep. J Dev Physiol 14:139, 1990.

Harvey D, Prince J, Bunton J, et al: The abilities of children who were small for gestational age babies. Pediatrics 69:296, 1982.

Hauguel S, Desmaizieres V, Challier J: Glucose uptake, utilization and transfer by the human placenta as a function of maternal glucose concentration. Pediatr Res 20:269, 1986.

Haymond M, Karl I, Pagliara A: Increased gluconeogenic substrates in the small for gestational age infant. N Engl J Med 291:322, 1974.

Henrichson L, Skinoj K, Andersen G: Delayed growth and reduced intelligence in 9–17 year old intrauterine growth retarded children compared with their monozygous co-twins. Acta Paediatr Scand 75:31, 1986.

Hurley L: Nutritional influences on embryonic and fetal development: Fat-soluble vitamins, water-soluble vitamins, major mineral elements, trace elements. *In* Hurley L: Developmental Nutrition. Englewood Cliffs, NJ, Prentice Hall, 1980, pp 125–227.

Jones D: Energy metabolism in developing brain. Semin Perinatol 3:121, 1979.

Jones K: Beckwith-Wiedemann syndrome. *In* Graham JM Jr (Ed): Smith's Recognizable Patterns of Human Malformation. Philadelphia, WB Saunders, 1988, pp 136–139.

Karlberg J, Albertsson-Wikland K: Growth in full term small for gestational age infants: From birth to final height. Pediatr Res 38:733, 1995.

Kramer M, McLean F, Olivier M, et al: Body proportionality and head and length "sparing" in growth retarded neonates: A critical reappraisal. Pediatrics 84:717, 1989.

Lammer E, Chen D, Holar R, et al: Retinoic acid embryopathy. N Engl J Med 313:837, 1985.

Langer O, Damus K, Maiman M, et al: A link between relative hypoglycemia-hypoinsulinemia during oral glucose tolerance tests and intrauterine growth retardation. Am J Obstet Gynecol 155:711, 1986.

Li D, Daling J, Mueller B, et al: Periconceptual multivitamin use in relation to the risk of congenital urinary tract anomalies. Epidemiology 6:212, 1995.

Lipson A, Beuhler B, Bartley J, et al: Maternal hyperphenylalaninemia fetal effects. J Pediatr 104:216, 1984.

Low J, Handley-Derry M, Burke S, et al: Association of intrauterine fetal growth retardation and learning deficits at age 9 to 11 years. Am J Obstet Gynecol 167:1499, 1992.

Lubchenco L, Bard H: Incidence of hypoglycemia in newborn infants classified by birth weight and gestational age. Pediatrics 47:831, 1971.

Medical Research Council Vitamin Study Group: Prevention of neural tube defects: Results of the Medical Research Council Vitamin Study. Lancet 338:131, 1991.

Metcoff J, Costiloe JP, Crosby W, et al: Maternal nutrition and fetal outcome. Am J Clin Nutr 34(suppl 4):708, 1981.

Miller H, Jekel J: Malnutrition and growth retardation in newborn infants. Pediatrics 83:443, 1989.

Milley R, Rosenberg A, Phillips A, et al: The effect of insulin on ovine fetal oxygen extraction. Am J Obstet Gynecol 149:673, 1984.

Mochizuki M, Maruo T, Masuko K, et al: Effect of smoking on fetoplacental-maternal system during pregnancy. Am J Obstet Gynecol 149:413, 1984.

Molteni R, Stys S, Battaglia F: Relationships of fetal and placental weight in human beings: Fetal/placental weight ratios at various gestational ages and birth weight distributions. J Reprod Med 21:327, 1978.

Moore K: The fetal period. *In* The Developing Human, 4th ed. Philadelphia, WB Saunders, 1988, pp 87–103.

Morriss F, Boyd R, Makowski E, et al: Umbilical V-A differences of acetoacetate and β-hydroxybutyrate in fed and starved ewes. Proc Soc Exp Biol Med 145:879, 1974.

Morriss F, Makowski E, Meschia G, et al: The glucose/oxygen quotient of the term human fetus. Biol Neonate 25:44, 1975.

Naeye R: Malnutrition—probable cause of fetal growth retardation. Arch Pathol 79:284, 1965.

Naeye R, Dixon J: Distortions in fetal growth standards. Pediatr Res 12:987, 1978.

National Research Council, Food and Nutrition Board: Recommended Dietary Allowances, 10th rev ed. Washington, DC, National Academy of Science, 1989.

Nutrition Reviews Editorial: Nutrition intervention in pregnancy. Nutr Rev 42:42, 1984.

Paz I, Seidman D, Danon Y, et al: Are children born small for gestational age at increased risk of short stature? Am J Dis Child 147:337, 1993.

Persson B, Gentz J, Moller E: Follow-up of children of insulin dependent (Type 1) and gestational diabetic mothers. Acta Paediatr Scand 73:778, 1984.

Phillips A, Rosenkrantz T, Porte P, et al: The effects of chronic fetal hyperglycemia on substrate uptake by the ovine fetus and conceptus. Pediatr Res 19:659, 1985.

Plotz E, Kabara J, Davis M, et al: Studies on the synthesis of cholesterol in the brain of the human fetus. Am J Obstet Gynecol 4:534, 1968.

Poppitt S, Prentice A, Goldberg G, et al: Energy sparing strategies to protect human fetal growth. Am J Obstet Gynecol 171:118, 1994.

Raman L: Influence of maternal nutritional factors affecting birth weight. Am J Clin Nutr 34(suppl 4):775, 1981.

Rizzo T, Dooley S, Metzger B, et al: Prenatal and perinatal influences on long term psychomotor development in offspring of diabetic mothers. Am J Obstet Gynecol 173:1753, 1995.

Rosso P: Nutritional needs of the human fetus. Clin Nutr 2:4, 1983.

Rothman K, Moore L, Singer M, et al: Teratogenicity of high vitamin A intake. N Engl J Med 333:1369, 1995.

Sara V: The role of somatomedins in fetal growth. *In* Lindbland B (Ed): Perinatal Nutrition. New York, Academic Press, 1988, pp 63–74.

Shah R, Rajalakshmi R: Studies on human fetal tissues: I. Fetal weight and tissue weights in relation to gestational age, fetal size, and maternal status. Ind J Pediatr 55:261, 1988.

Shanklin D, Cooke R: Effects of intrauterine growth on intestinal length in the human fetus. Biol Neonate 64:76, 1993.

Shu X, Hatch M, Mills J, et al: Maternal smoking, alcohol drinking, caffeine consumption, and fetal growth: Results from a prospective study. Epidemiology 6:115, 1995.

Smithells R, Sheppard S, Schorah CJ: Vitamin deficiencies and neural tube defects. Arch Dis Child 51:944, 1976.

Smithells R, Sheppard S, Wild J, et al: Prevention of neural tube defect recurrences in Yorkshire: Final report. Lancet 2:498, 1989.

Socol M, Manning F, Murata Y, et al: Maternal smoking causes fetal hypoxia: Experimental evidence. Am J Obstet Gynecol 142:214, 1982.

Soltesz G, Harris D, MacKenzie I, et al: The metabolic and endocrine milieu of the human fetus and mother at 18–21 weeks of gestation: I. Plasma amino acid concentration. Pediatr Res 19:91, 1985.

Sparks J, Girard J, Battaglia F: An estimate of the caloric requirements of the human fetus. Biol Neonate 38:113, 1980.

Sparks J, Hay W, Bonds D, et al: Simultaneous measurements of lactate turnover rate and umbilical lactate uptake in the fetal lamb. J Clin Invest 70:179, 1982.

Stehbens J, Baker G, Mitchell M: Outcomes at ages 1, 3, and 5 years of children born to diabetic women. Am J Obstet Gynecol 127:408, 1977.

Susser M: Prenatal nutrition, birth weight and psychological development. Am J Clin Nutr 34(suppl 4):784, 1981.

Usher R, McLean F: Intrauterine growth of live born Caucasian infants at sea level. J Pediatr 74:901, 1969.

Van den Berg B: Maternal variables affecting fetal growth. Am J Clin Nutr 34(suppl 4):722, 1981.

Verdy M, Gagnon M, Caron D: Birth weight and adult obesity in children of diabetic mothers. N Engl J Med 290:576, 1974.

Villar J, Smerglio V, Martorell R, et al: Heterogeneous growth and mental development of intrauterine growth retarded infants during the first 3 years of life. Pediatrics 74:783, 1984.

Vohr B, Lipsitt L, Oh W: Somatic growth of children of diabetic mothers with reference to birth size. J Pediatr 97:196, 1980.

Whitehead R: Birth from the nutritional point of view. *In* Lindbland B (Ed): Perinatal Nutrition. New York, Academic Press, 1988, pp 197–206.

Widdowson E: Change in body proportion and composition during growth. *In* Davis J, Dobbing J (Eds): Scientific Foundation in Pediatrics. Philadelphia, WB Saunders, 1974, pp 153–163.

Williams R, Creasy R, Cunningham G, et al: Fetal growth and perinatal viability in California. Obstet Gynecol 59:624, 1982.

Willman S, Leveno K, Guzick D, et al: Glucose threshold for macrosomia in pregnancy complicated by diabetes. Am J Obstet Gynecol 154:470, 1986.

Wirth F, Goldberg K, Lubchenco L: Neonatal hyperviscosity: I. Incidence. Pediatrics 63:833, 1979.

Wiswell T, Cornish J, Northam R: Neonatal polycythemia: Frequency of clinical manifestations and other associated findings. Pediatrics 78:26, 1986.

Woods R, Plessinger M, Clark K: Effect of cocaine on uterine blood flow and fetal oxygenation. JAMA 257:957, 1987.

Worthington-Roberts B: Nutrition deficiencies and excesses: Impact on pregnancy, Part 2. J Perinatol 5:12, 1985.

Yates J: The genetics of fetal and postnatal growth. *In* Cockburn F (Ed): Fetal and Neonatal Growth. New York, John Wiley & Sons, 1988, pp 1–10.

Ziegler E, O'Donnell A, Nelson S, et al: Body composition of the reference fetus. Growth 40:329, 1976.

CHAPTER **6**

Placental Function and Diseases: The Placenta, Fetal Membranes, and Umbilical Cord

William M. Gilbert

In most normal pregnancies, the newborn is healthy and goes home in a day or two with the mother. If unexpected complications should develop in the newborn period, quite often the placenta has been discarded and is unavailable for examination for clues to help determine possible causes of these problems. Physicians involved in the delivery of high-risk pregnant patients usually send the placenta to the pathology department for a pathologic examination. A detailed examination often provides clues helpful in the management of these high-risk pregnancies. The same is not true of the normal pregnancy. Thorough examination of the placenta at the time of birth may identify some abnormality that would be of assistance in explaining complications in the newborn. For this reason, anyone involved in the care of pregnant women or their newborns should be able to examine a placenta and know the basics about normal and abnormal architecture. This chapter examines the normal development of the placenta and the development of particular disease states relating to it. In addition, placental hormones, the immunology of the placenta, and abnormalities of amniotic fluid volume are summarized.

EMBRYOLOGIC DEVELOPMENT

Shortly after fertilization takes place in the ampullary portion of the fallopian tube, the fertilized ovum or zygote begins dividing into a ball of cells called a morula. As the morula enters the uterus (by the 4th day after fertilization), it forms a central cystic area and is called a blastocyst. The blastocyst implants within the endometrium by day 7 (Moore, 1988).

The blastocyst contains two components: an inner cell mass, which becomes the developing embryo, and the outer cell layer, which becomes the placenta and fetal membranes (Hertig, 1968). The cells of the developing blastocyst, which eventually become the placenta, are differentiated quite early in gestation (within 7 days after fertilization). The outer cell layer, the trophoblast, invades the endometrium to the level of the decidual basalis. Maternal blood vessels are also invaded en route (Fig. 6–1). Once entered and controlled by trophoblast, these maternal blood vessels form lacunae, which provide nutrition and substrates for the developing products of conception. The trophoblast differentiates into two cell types: the inner cytotrophoblast and the outer syncytiotrophoblast (see Fig.

6–1). The former has distinct cell walls and is thought to represent the more immature form of trophoblast. The syncytiotrophoblast is essentially acellular and the site of most placental hormone and metabolic activity. Once the trophoblast has invaded the endometrium, it begins to form outpouchings called villi, which extend into the blood-

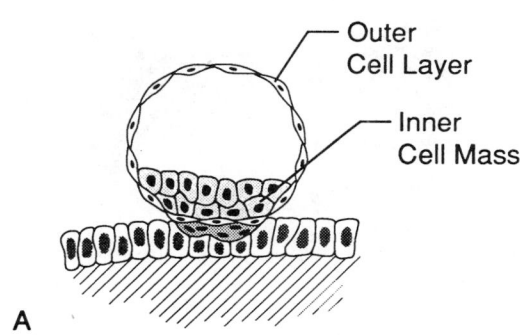

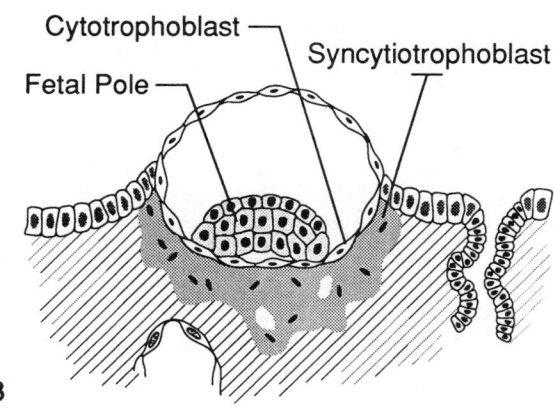

FIGURE 6–1. *A,* The human blastocyst contains two portions: an inner cell mass, which develops into the embryo, and an outer cell layer, which develops into the placenta and membranes. *B,* The outer acellular layer is the syncytiotrophoblast, and the inner cellular layer is the cytotrophoblast. (From Gilbert WM: Anatomy and physiology of the placenta, fetal membranes, and amniotic fluid. *In* Moore TR, Reiter RC, Rebar RW, Baker VV [Eds]: Gynecology and Obstetrics: A Longitudinal Approach. New York, Churchill Livingstone, 1993, pp 209–222.)

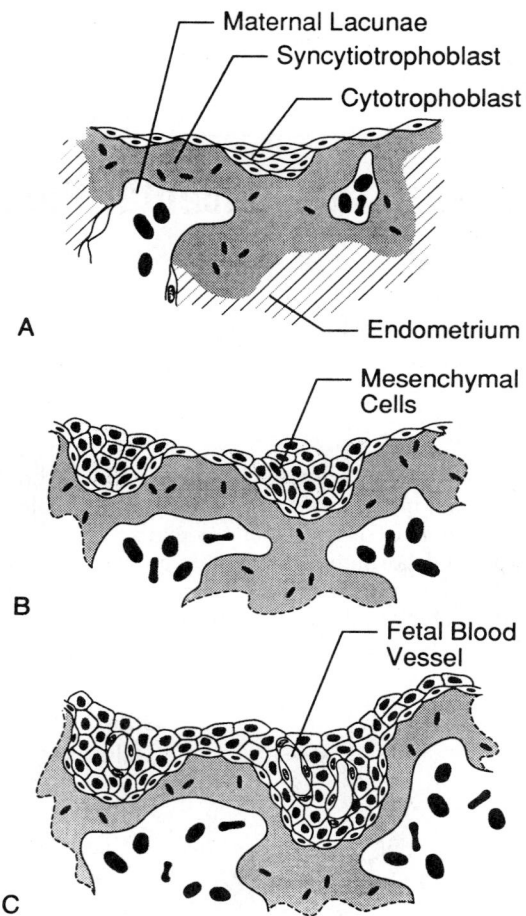

FIGURE 6–2. *A,* The cytotrophoblast indents the syncytiotrophoblast to form primary villi. *B,* Mesenchymal cells invade the cytotrophoblast 2 days after formation of the primary villi to form secondary villi. *C,* Blood vessels arise de novo and eventually connect with blood vessels from the embryo, forming tertiary villi. (From Gilbert WM: Anatomy and physiology of the placenta, fetal membranes, and amniotic fluid. *In* Moore TR, Reiter RC, Rebar RW, Baker VV [Eds]: Gynecology and Obstetrics: A Longitudinal Approach. New York, Churchill Livingstone, 1993, pp 209–222.)

filled maternal lacunae or further invade the endometrium to attach more solidly with the decidua, forming anchoring villi.

There are three types of villi, depending on the location and stage of development. Figure 6–2 demonstrates the three types of villi: primary, secondary, or tertiary, depending on whether cytotrophoblastic tissue with or without fetal blood vessels is present.

PLACENTAL CIRCULATION

With the formation of the tertiary villi (19 days after fertilization), a direct vascular connection is made between the developing embryo and placenta (Moore, 1988). Umbilical circulation between the placenta and embryo is evident by 5½ weeks of gestation. Figure 6–3 demonstrates aspects of the maternal and fetal circulation in the mature placenta.

The umbilical arteries from the fetus reach the placenta and then divide repetitively and branch to cover the fetal surface of the placenta. Terminal arteries then penetrate the individual cotyledons, forming capillary beds for substrate exchange within the tertiary villi. These capillaries then reform into tributaries of the umbilical venous system, which carries oxygenated blood back to the fetus.

It is evident that the fetal circulatory system is a closed system with no direct connection with the maternal blood. Indeed, maternally delivered substrates must cross three tissue layers within the villus in order to reach the fetal blood. Despite this barrier, however, fetal cells have been identified within the maternal circulation and vice versa. Current research is underway in an attempt to use these cells of fetal origin within the maternal circulation for prenatal diagnosis (Steel et al, 1996).

Maternal blood enters the intervillous space in a pulsatile fashion, with each maternal heartbeat, bathing the fetal villi with blood and providing a site for exchange of nutrients and waste products. The maternal blood then collects in sinuses at the basilar layer of the intervillous space and flows into the uterine vein. This type of placenta, in which the maternal blood is in contact only with the fetal trophoblast, is called a hemochorial type of placentation.

PLACENTAL ANATOMY

At term, the normal placenta covers roughly one third of the interior portion of the uterus and weighs approximately 500 g. The appearance is of a flat circular disc about 2 to 3 cm thick and 15 to 20 cm across (Benirschke and Kaufmann, 1990). The umbilical cord normally inserts into the center of the placenta but may insert in other locations such as at the margin (marginal or battledore insertion) or onto the membranes (velamentous insertion) (Fig. 6–4) before they join the border of the placenta. In the case of a velamentous insertion, in which the umbilical cord inserts into the amnionic membrane and fetal blood vessels travel within the membranes for a distance, poor perinatal outcome may occur. If the fetal vessels cross the cervical os, a high-risk condition called a vasa praevia is present (Pent, 1979). Rupture of the amniotic membrane in labor may rupture fetal vessels near the cervical os, resulting in fatal hemorrhage. Although most vaginal bleeding before and during labor is of maternal origin, in the case of new-onset vaginal bleeding and simultaneous evidence of fetal distress, the diagnosis of vasa praevia must be considered if fetal death from exsanguination is to be prevented.

In early pregnancy the placenta covers the majority of the inside of the uterus. At 20 weeks of gestation, approximately 5% of placentas will cover the cervix and thus be classified as a placenta previa (Townsend et al, 1986). By 37 weeks, however, fewer than 1% will still be "previa" (Newton et al, 1984). The term applied to this apparent placental movement away from the cervical os is *placental migration.* The placenta does not actually migrate, but differential growth of the uterus compared with that of the placenta results in the placenta moving away from the cervix. When the placental tissue remains centrally placed over the cervix, a diagnosis of complete placenta previa is made. The complications of pregnancy associated with placenta previa derive from the risk of massive

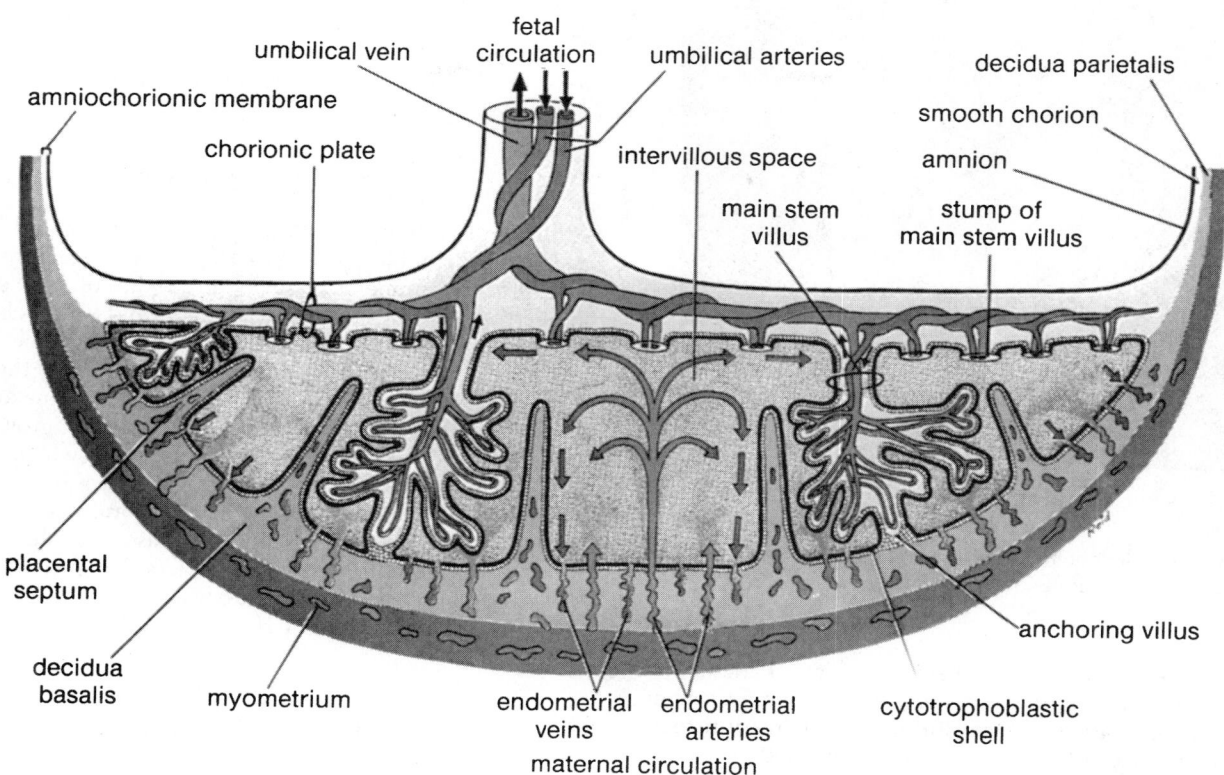

FIGURE 6–3. Schematic drawing of a section of a mature placenta showing (1) the relation of the villous chorion (fetal part of the placenta) to the decidua basalis (maternal part of the placenta), (2) the fetal placental circulation, and (3) the maternal placental circulation. Maternal blood flows into the intervillous spaces in funnel-shaped spurts, and exchanges occur with the fetal blood as the maternal blood flows around the villi. Note that the umbilical arteries carry deoxygenated fetal blood to the placenta, and the umbilical vein carries oxygenated blood to the fetus. Note that the cotyledons are separated from each other by decidual septa of the maternal portion of the placenta. Each cotyledon consists of two or more main stem villi and their main branches. In this drawing, only one main stem villus is shown in each cotyledon, but the stumps of those that have been removed are indicated. (From Moore KL: The Developing Human: Clinically Oriented Embryology, 5th ed. Philadelphia, WB Saunders, 1993, p 117.)

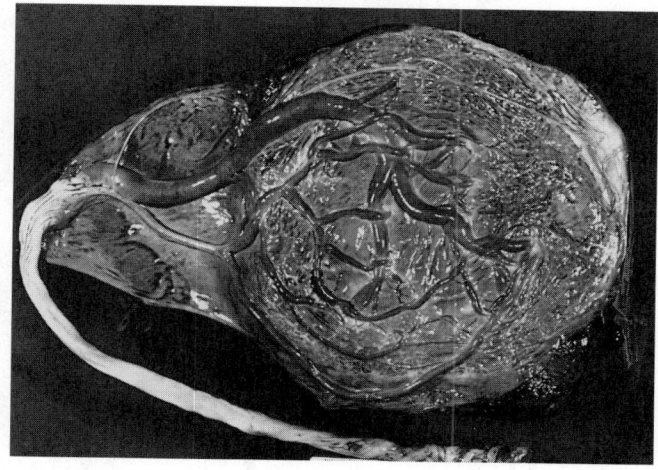

FIGURE 6–4. Velamentous insertion of the umbilical cord onto the membranes with fetal vessels running onto the placenta.

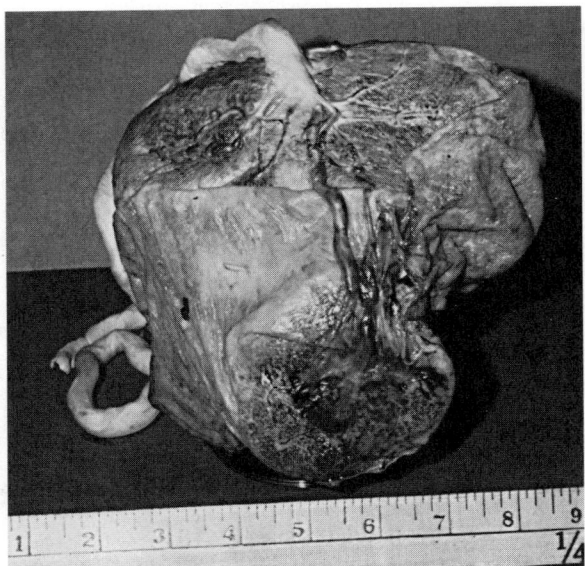

FIGURE 6–5. Succenturiate placental lobe. Note the membrane connecting the separate lobes of placental tissue.

hemorrhage when the cervix begins to dilate. Patients with placenta previa almost always require a cesarean section, although rare cases of successful vaginal delivery through a complete placenta previa have been reported.

Other abnormalities of placental development include the presence of an accessory lobe of placenta, which may be connected to the main portion of the placenta by only a strand of fetal blood vessels. This condition is called a succenturiate lobe (Fig. 6–5) and may be problematic if that lobe of placenta is inadvertently left within the uterus at the time of delivery. The retained placental tissue may cause postpartum hemorrhage or infection and require curettage for removal. For this reason, placental examination after delivery should include inspection of the placental edges to look for ragged portions suggestive of succenturiate lobe.

Another recognized placental abnormality is when the chorionic portion of the fetal membranes does not insert at the edge of the placenta but rather inserts some distance more centrally. This condition, called a circumvallate placenta, occurs in about 5% of pregnancies (Fig. 6–6) and is associated with antepartum bleeding, preterm labor, intrauterine growth restriction, and single umbilical artery (Naftolin et al, 1973). The cause of this condition is largely unknown.

FETAL MEMBRANES

After delivery the placenta and membranes should be inspected for completeness. What appears at delivery to be a single membrane is actually made up of two closely applied membranes: an inner amnion and outer chorion. The chorion is covered with villi early in pregnancy. Later, the majority of the villi degenerates, except in the area where the placenta is located. The inner membrane amnion is derived from the developing embryo and grows and expands to fill the extraembryonic coelom, which is the fluid-filled area surrounding the early embryo. By 14 weeks gestation, the amnion joins with the chorion. Before this time, the amnion may be seen on ultrasonographic examination as a thin inner membrane surrounding the embryo. The two membranes remain closely applied for the remainder of the pregnancy and can be manually separated after birth.

UMBILICAL CORD

The umbilical cord averages 50 cm in length, although a wide range of normal lengths is recognized. The cord should be measured only if it is at one or the other extremes of length (Benirschke and Kaufmann, 1990). The overall length of the umbilical cord is determined by fetal activity in utero, with longer cords in more active fetuses and shorter cords associated with decreased activity. The umbilical cord usually contains two umbilical arteries and one umbilical vein. An umbilical cord with only two vessels (one artery, one vein) occurs about 1% of the time and is associated with an increase in fetal structural malformations and chromosomal abnormalities (Leung and Robson, 1989). When the diagnosis of a single umbilical artery is made either before or after birth, a complete examination of the fetus or newborn should be made to look for other

FIGURE 6–6. Circumvalate placenta. Note the insertion of the membranes into the placenta halfway between the edge of the placenta and the center.

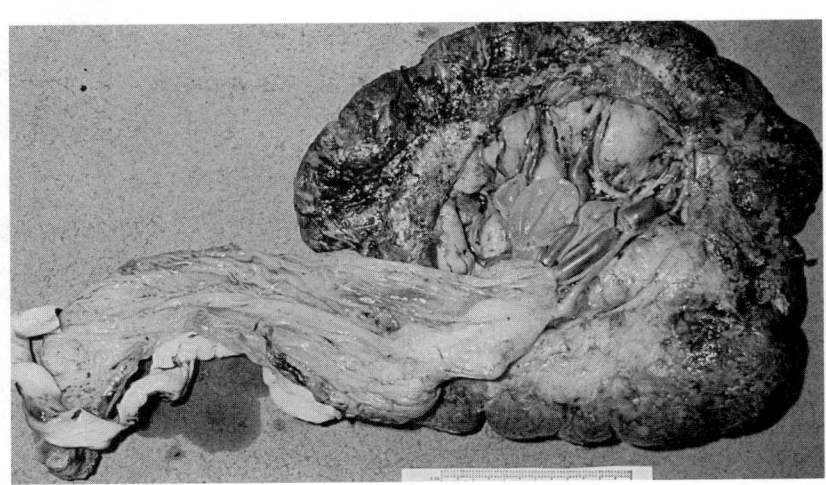

abnormalities, with particular attention to fetal kidneys and heart. In some cases, a two-vessel cord should be an indication for an amniocentesis for chromosomal analysis (Nicolaides et al, 1993).

EXAMINATION OF THE PLACENTA

All placentas should undergo an examination at the time of birth regardless of whether or not the newborn has any immediate problems. Most placentas will invert with traction at the time of delivery, and the fetal membranes will cover the maternal surface. It is important to reinvert the membranes and examine all surfaces of the placenta and membranes, looking for abnormalities. The edges of the placenta should be examined for completeness. The membranes and fetal surface should be shiny and translucent. An odor may suggest infection, and cultures of the placenta may be beneficial (Benirschke and Kaufmann, 1990). Greenish discoloration may represent meconium staining or old blood; such placentas should be sent to the pathologist for complete histologic examination. The finding of deep meconium staining of the membranes and umbilical cord suggests that the meconium was passed at least 2 hours before delivery. This fact may be helpful in cases of meconium aspiration syndrome when legal questions arise as to whether or not the aspiration occurred before or during labor. If the membranes are deeply stained, the meconium passage by the fetus may have predated labor onset; thus, the aspiration could have occurred before labor. The umbilical cord should also be examined for the number of vessels and insertion into the placenta. Vessels on the fetal surface of the placenta should be examined for evidence of clot or thrombosis. Normally, the fetal arteries cross superficially over the veins. Clots or thrombosis may be firm, whitish knots on the placental surface. Table 6–1 provides guidelines for when placentas should be sent to the pathologist for examination.

PLACENTAL PHYSIOLOGY
Placental Transport

The developing embryo obtains all of its nutrients from the mother during gestation. Initial nutrient transport to the conceptus is via simple diffusion from the maternal blood in the decidua. The early primitive vitelline circulation, which circulates blood from the yolk sac to the embryo at 5 to 6 weeks, is replaced by a true umbilical circulation by 7 weeks. This circulation functions as the

TABLE 6–1

Guidelines for Pathologic Examination of the Placenta

Fetal congenital anomaly
Maternal or fetal infection
Preterm delivery
Maternal disease states (e.g., hypertension, diabetes)
Multiple gestation
Intrauterine growth restriction
Newborn admission to the neonatal intensive care unit

TABLE 6–2

Mechanisms of Placental Transport

Mechanism	Substance
Simple diffusion	Oxygen, carbon dioxide, sodium, and chloride
Facilitated diffusion	Glucose
Active transport	Certain amino acids, calcium
Pinocytosis	Immunoglobulins

mature transport system throughout pregnancy until delivery.

The four main substrate transport mechanisms across the placenta are simple diffusion, facilitated diffusion, active transport, and pinocytosis. Examples of substances that are delivered to the fetus by each of these routes are shown in Table 6–2. The major osmotic ions of sodium, chloride, and free water move by simple diffusion. Fetal concentrations of amino acids may be 20 times that of the maternal levels as a result of active transport (Faber and Thornburg, 1985). Glucose moves by both simple and facilitated diffusion, resulting in fetal levels that are about 80% of maternal levels.

Water Transport

The fetus is capable of producing water as a by-product of the breakdown of glucose and the formation of energy. This, however, is insufficient for fetal requirements. Two additional forces driving water into the fetal compartment include pure hydrostatic forces and osmotic forces measured in milliosmole per kilogram (Schroder, 1989). Both forces are important for fluid movement, but the interplay of these mechanisms is poorly understood in the human placenta.

In the past, the fluid homeostasis of the mother and developing fetus were thought to be largely independent. However, mounting evidence indicates they are intricately intertwined. With maternal dehydration in the sheep, amniotic fluid volume is observed to decrease (oligohydramnios). With maternal rehydration, normal amniotic fluid volume returns. A study in humans demonstrated that maternal oral hydration in cases of decreased amniotic fluid volume resulted in an increase in amniotic fluid volume as measured ultrasonographically by the amniotic fluid index. These studies provide strong evidence of the interconnectiveness of maternal and fetal fluid spaces across the membranes and placenta (Kilpatrick et al, 1991).

HORMONE PRODUCTION

Shortly after fertilization, the blastocyst synthesizes and releases human chorionic gonadotropin (hCG) into the maternal circulation as it implants into the endometrium. This embryonic control of maternal hCG levels is vital to maintain the corpus luteum and prevent rejection of the conceptus. The hCG molecule is very similar in structure to luteinizing hormone released by the pituitary gland with a primary difference in the hCG beta chain. Placental production of hCG peaks at 8 to 10 weeks of gestation, after which its levels decrease markedly. hCG maintains the production of progesterone from the corpus luteum until the placenta takes over at about 9 weeks of gestation. Progesterone, produced in the syncytiotrophoblast, is the primary hormone of pregnancy involved in maintaining uterine and other smooth muscle relaxation. It also functions in immune suppression. Many of the vasodilatory and gastrointestinal symptoms of pregnancy noted by the mother are due to the action of progesterone.

Several estrogens are produced by the placenta, with the greatest proportion secreted into the maternal compartment. A primary role of estrogens is to increase uterine blood flow and help maintain the pregnancy (Resnik et al, 1974). The synthetic pathway of estriol involves both the fetal adrenal gland and the placenta. Measurement of this hormone in either maternal urine or plasma was historically believed to be an effective method of fetal surveillance in high-risk pregnancies because the estriol concentration reflected both fetal and placental well-being. With a significant decrease in maternal estriol levels, placental function was supposed to be declining as well. However, studies have shown that measurement of estriol is not predictive of fetal jeopardy. Interestingly, studies have shown that abrupt elevations of estriol in saliva may be predictive of preterm labor (Hedriana et al, 1996). In the future, a simple saliva test may predict the onset of labor either preterm or at term.

The final major hormone of pregnancy is human chorionic somatomammotropin (hCS), which is also termed human placental lactogen. This hormone is a growth factor primarily involved with mobilization of maternal stores of glucose, fatty acids, and ketones (Speroff et al, 1989). hCS increases with placental mass and is a major mediator of glucose intolerance in pregnancy. With the larger placental mass associated with multiple gestations, there is likewise a higher rate of glucose intolerance.

IMMUNOLOGY

Pregnancy is a unique state in which the mother has a functionally intact immune system, able to eliminate infection and suppress neoplasia while allowing a genetically different "tumor" (the fetus) to grow relatively unchecked within the uterus. The uterus itself does not prevent rejection because intra-abdominal pregnancies are not immunologically rejected. Although the exact mechanisms that prevent maternal rejection are not completely clear, several key facts are known. The invading trophoblast does not express HLA antigens, which leaves the embryo largely unrecognized by the maternal immune system (Colbern and Main, 1991). In addition, the trophoblast secretes a sialomucin coating over its outer surface, which shields the trophoblast from maternal recognition. Finally, the trophoblast produces extremely high levels of progesterone, which is known to effectively suppress mitogen activation, mixed lymphocyte reactions, and cytotoxic T-cell generation in human blood lymphocytes (Stites et al, 1985; Szekeres-Bartho et al, 1985).

Historically, one mechanism that was thought to prevent maternal rejection of the embryo was the development of "blocking antibodies" (Rocklin et al, 1976). These antibodies, produced by the mother in response to the antigenically foreign embryo, were thought to bind antigens that were found on the trophoblast. By blocking these fetal antigens, the mother would not reject the fetus. The follow-up studies examining these antibodies have not supported the initial studies, and further work in this area is needed (Neppert et al, 1989). It appears that the maternal-fetal immune interaction is largely a local one occurring at the placental interface and not related to systemic factors.

AMNIOTIC FLUID VOLUME

Amniotic fluid is an integral part of and closely connected with the fetus, placenta, and membranes. All of these tissues contribute at one time or another to amniotic fluid formation and removal. Structural or physiologic abnormalities of either the fetus or placenta may first present as too much (polyhydramnios) or too little (oligohydramnios) amniotic fluid. To understand the associations with abnormal amniotic fluid, the mechanisms involved in formation and removal of amniotic fluid must be conceptualized. In this there is a problem because the mechanisms that regulate amniotic fluid volume in the normal state are understood only rudimentarily.

It is known that the main contributor to amniotic fluid formation is fetal urination, and either absence or obstruction of the fetal urinary system will result in severe oligohydramnios and fetal or neonatal death. With uteroplacental insufficiency, which is often associated with maternal conditions such as chronic hypertension or preeclampsia, oligohydramnios may be the first presenting sign of fetal compromise (Wladimiroff and Campbell, 1974). The fetal lung is another major source of amniotic fluid. See also Chapter 49, Lung Development and Function.

Fetal swallowing is the main route of amniotic fluid removal, and any interruption in fetal swallowing, such as is found with duodenal atresia, may result in polyhydramnios. Whenever extremes of amniotic fluid volume are suspected, a detailed ultrasonogram should be performed. Particular attention should be given to identifying structural abnormalities in the gastrointestinal and genitourinary systems. Under normal conditions, the fetus is able to maintain its amniotic fluid volume in a relatively narrow range (800–1200 mL) of normal, as demonstrated in Figure 6–7 (Brace and Wolf, 1989).

MULTIPLE GESTATIONS

The frequency of multiple gestations is increasing largely because of the increase in assisted reproductive technologies. The most common multiple gestation is twins, with two thirds or more resulting from two separate zygotes. The major problems associated with dizygotic twins are the complications of prematurity and growth restriction resulting from overcrowding in the uterus. Monozygotic twins are the result of the splitting of a single zygote and most commonly have two amnions and one chorion (Benirschke, 1961). The perinatal morbidity and mortality associated with monozygotic twins are increased relative to those of dizygotic twins (with two chorions and two amnions) largely because of the twin transfusion syndrome. It is important antenatally to distinguish chorionicity of all

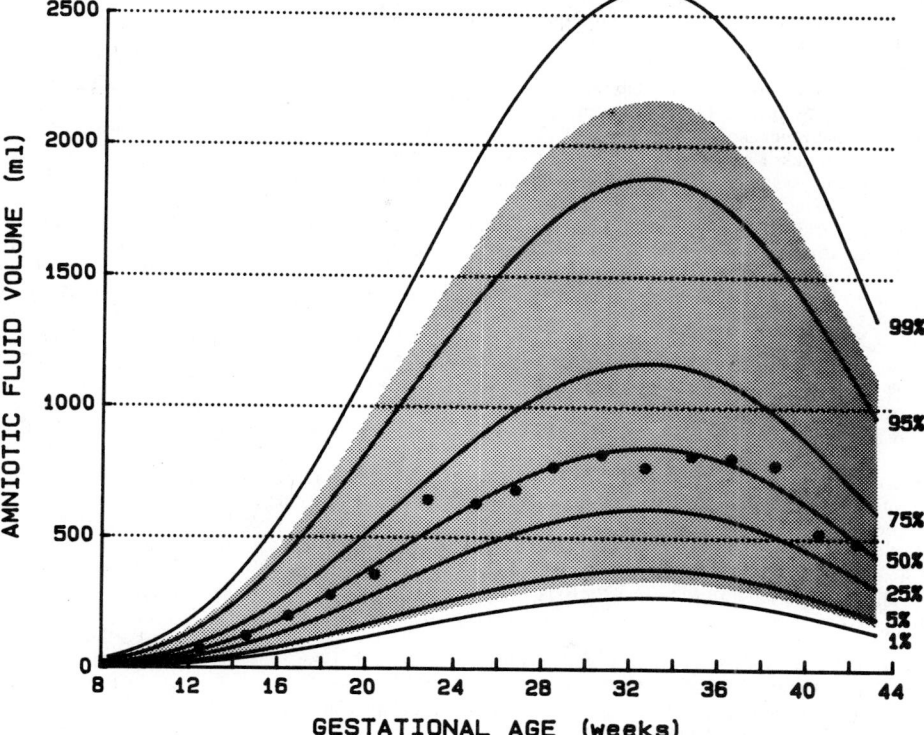

FIGURE 6–7. Nomogram shows amniotic fluid volumes as a function of gestational age. Dots are means for 2-week intervals. Percentiles are calculated from polynomial regression equation and standard deviation of residuals. Shaded area covers 95% confidence interval. (From Brace RA, Wolf EJ: Characterization of normal gestational changes in amniotic fluid volume. Am J Obstet Gynecol 161:382, 1989.)

twin gestations because of different risk factors for both. The easiest way to differentiate this is if the sex is different between twins (dichorionic). If the twins have the same sex, close examination early in pregnancy should demonstrate a "thick" dividing membrane in dichorionic twins and a "thin" membrane in monochorionic twins.

Twin-to-Twin Transfusion Syndrome

Virtually all monochorionic twins have a single placenta with vascular connections within the placenta between the two fetuses. The most common connection is arterial to arterial (Benirschke, 1961). The next most common vascular connection is venous to venous. Little morbidity is associated with these anastomoses. The final and most important is when an artery from one fetus connects with the vein of another fetus, resulting in a flow of blood and fluid from one fetus to the other. The typical clinical presentation is that of acute polyhydramnios in the sac of the fetus receiving the transfusion and severe oligohydramnios in the donor twin. The perinatal mortality rate is virtually 100% if diagnosed before 25 weeks of gestation and left untreated (Wier et al, 1979).

There are two main treatment options. The first is repetitive reduction amniocentesis, which is begun at the first sign of maternal or fetal compromise. An 18-gauge spinal needle is used, and the polyhydramniotic amniotic sac is entered, removing enough fluid (up to 5–6 L) to return the amniotic fluid volume to a normal range. This procedure may need to be repeated every week or two, usually increasing in frequency until a viable gestation is reached or there is either maternal or fetal compromise (Elliott,

1991; Saunders et al, 1992). With this modality, survival rates of 40% to 79% have been reported.

A second, more ingenious modality is the utilization of a laser by fetoscopy to photocoagulate the interconnecting arteriovenous connection (De Lia et al, 1990). A similar survival rate as previously mentioned has been reported. A final technique reported by Berry and associates in 1997 used an amniocentesis needle to puncture the two amniotic sacs between the twins, allowing amniotic fluid to flow from the polyhydramniotic sac to the oligohydramniotic sac. In nine cases the authors reported a survival rate of 83% compared with historic controls with a survival rate of approximately zero.

SUMMARY

It is common to underappreciate the importance of the placenta, membranes, and amniotic fluid when all attention is focused on the fetus during pregnancy and the newborn after birth. Abnormalities in amniotic fluid volume may suggest structural or developmental abnormalities in the growing fetus that require further examination. A simple but complete examination of the placenta and membranes at the time of delivery may provide important clues that may be helpful in the future care of the mother and newborn.

REFERENCES

Benirschke K: Twin placenta in perinatal mortality. NY State J Med 61:1499, 1961.
Benirschke K, Kaufmann P: Pathology of the Human Placenta, 2nd ed. New York, Springer-Verlag, 1990.

Berry D, Montgomery L, Johnson A, et al: Amniotic septostomy for the treatment of the stuck twin sequence. Am J Obstet Gynecol 176:S19, 1997.

Brace RA, Wolf EJ: Characterization of normal gestational changes in amniotic fluid volume. Am J Obstet Gynecol 161:382, 1989.

Colbern GT, Main EK: Immunology of the maternal-placental interface in normal pregnancy. Semin Perinatol 15:196, 1991.

De Lia JE, Cruikshank DP, Koye WR: Fetoscopic neodymium: YAG laser occlusion placental vessels in severe twin-twin transfusion syndrome. Obstet Gynecol 75:1046, 1990.

Elliott JP, Urig MA, Clewell WH: Aggressive therapeutic amniocentesis for treatment of twin-twin transfusion syndrome. Obstet Gynecol 77:537, 1991.

Faber II, Thornburg KL: Placental Physiology. New York, Raven Press, 1985, p 151.

Gilbert WM: Anatomy and physiology of the placenta, fetal membranes, and amniotic fluid. *In* Moore TR, Reiter RC, Rebar RW, Baker VV (Eds): Gynecology and Obstetrics: A Longitudinal Approach. New York, Churchill Livingstone, 1993, pp 209–222.

Gilbert WM, Moore TR, Brace RA: Amniotic fluid volume dynamics. Fetal Med Rev 3:89, 1991.

Hedriana HL, Monroe CJ, Eby-Wilkins EM, Lasley BL: Changes in rates of salivary estriol increase prior to parturition at term. J Soc Gynecol Invest 3:316A, 1996.

Hertig AT: Human Trophoblast. Springfield, IL, Charles C Thomas, 1968.

Kilpatrick SJ, Safford KL, Pomeroy T: Maternal hydration increases amniotic fluid index. Obstet Gynecol 78:1098, 1991.

Leung AKC, Robson WLM: Single umbilical artery: A report of 159 cases. Am J Dis Child 148:108, 1989.

Moore KI: The Developing Human. Philadelphia, WB Saunders, 1988.

Naftolin F, Khudr G, Benirschke K, Hutchinson D: The syndrome of chronic abruptio placentae, hydrorrhea, and circumvallate placenta. Am J Obstet Gynecol 116:347, 1973.

Neppert J, Mueller-Eckhardt G, Neumeyer H, et al: Pregnancy-maintaining antibodies: Workshop report (Giessen, 1988). J Reprod Immunol 15:159, 1989.

Newton ER, Barass V, Cetrulo CL: The epidemiology and clinical history of asymptomatic midtrimester placentae previa. Am J Obstet Gynecol 148:161, 1984.

Nicolaides K, Shawwa L, Brizot M, Snijders R: Ultrasonographically detectable markers of fetal chromosomal defects. Ultrasound Obstet Gynecol 2:56, 1993.

Pent D: Vasa previa. Am J Obstet Gynecol 134:151, 1979.

Resnik R, Killam AP, Battaglia FC, et al: The stimulation of uterine blood flow by various estrogens. Endocrinology 94:1192, 1974.

Rocklin RE, Kitzmiller JL, Carpenter CB, et al: Absence of an immunologic blocking factor from the serum of women with chronic abortions. N Engl J Med 295:1209, 1976.

Saunders NJ, Snijders RJM, Nicolaides KH: Therapeutic amniocentesis in twin-twin transfusion syndrome appearing in the second trimester of pregnancy. Am J Obstet Gynecol 166:820, 1992.

Schroder HJ: Basics of placental structures and transfer functions in fetal and neonatal body fluids. The scientific basis for clinical practice. *In* Brace RA, Ross MG, Robillard JE (Eds): Fetal and Neonatal Body Fluids: The Scientific Basis for Clinical Practice. Ithaca, NY, Perinatology Press, 1989, p 187.

Speroff L, Glass RH, Kase NG: Clinical Gynecologic Endocrinology and Infertility, 4th ed. Baltimore, MD, Williams & Wilkins, 1989.

Steel CD, Wapner RJ, Smith JB, et al: Prenatal diagnosis using fetal cells isolated from maternal peripheral blood: A review. Clin Obstet Gynecol 39:801, 1996.

Stites DP, Bugbee S, Siiteri PK: Differential action of progesterone and cortisol on lymphocyte and monocyte interaction during lymphocyte activation—Relevance to immunosuppression in pregnancy. J Reprod Immunol 5:215, 1985.

Szekeres-Bartho J, Hadnagy J, Pacsa AS: The suppressive effects of progesterone on lymphocytes. J Reprod Immunol 7:121, 1985.

Townsend RR, Lainge FC, Nyberg DA, et al: Technical factors responsible for "placental migration": Sonographic assessment. Radiology 160:105, 1986.

Wier PE, Raten G, Beisher N: Acute polyhydramnios—A complication of monozygous twin pregnancy. Br J Obstet Gynaecol 86:849, 1979.

Wladimiroff JW, Campbell S: Fetal urine-production rates in normal and complicated pregnancy. Lancet 2:151, 1974.

CHAPTER 7

Endocrine Disorders in Pregnancy

Thomas R. Moore

DIABETES IN PREGNANCY

Depending on the population surveyed, recognizable abnormalities in maternal glucose regulation occur in 3% to 8% of pregnancies. Although 80% or more of this glucose intolerance arises only during pregnancy (gestational diabetes) and involves relatively modest episodes of hyperglycemia, the attendant fetal and newborn morbidity is disproportionate. Compared to weight-matched controls, in infants of diabetic mothers (IDMs), the risk of serious birth injury is doubled, the likelihood of cesarean section is tripled, and the incidence of newborn intensive care unit admission is quadrupled. Studies indicate that the magnitude of risk of these maloccurrences is proportional to the degree of maternal hyperglycemia. Therefore, to some extent, the excessive fetal and neonatal morbidity of diabetes in pregnancy is preventable or at least reducible by meticulous prenatal and intrapartum care.

Maternal-Fetal Metabolism in Normal and Diabetic Pregnancy

Normal Maternal Glucose Regulation

With each meal, a complex combination of maternal hormonal actions—including the secretion of pancreatic insulin, glucagon, somatomedins, and adrenal catecholamines—ensures an ample but not excessive supply of glucose to mother and fetus during pregnancy. The key modifications in maternal metabolic regulation during pregnancy are as follows:

- Because the fetus continues to draw glucose from the maternal bloodstream across the placenta even during periods of fasting, the tendency toward maternal hypoglycemia between meals becomes increasingly marked as pregnancy progresses and fetal glucose demand grows.
- Placental steroid and peptide hormone production—estrogens, progesterone, and chorionic somatomammotropin—rises linearly throughout the second and third trimesters, resulting in a progressively increasing tissue resistance to maternal insulin action.
- Progressive maternal *insulin resistance* requires a significant augmentation (more than twice nonpregnant levels) in pancreatic insulin production during feeding to maintain euglycemia. Twenty-four-hour mean insulin levels are 30% higher in the third trimester than in the nonpregnant state.
- Failure to augment pancreatic insulin output adequately results in maternal, then fetal, hyperglycemia. The degree of hyperglycemia and its timing depend on the relative inadequacy of insulin production.

Fetal Effects of Maternal Hyperglycemia

Congenital Anomalies

A major threat to the IDM is the possibility of a life-threatening structural anomaly. Among the general population, the risk in pregnancy of a major birth defect is 1% to 2%. Among women with overt diabetes before conception, the risk of a structural anomaly in the fetus is increased fourfold to eightfold (Fig. 7–1). The typical defects and their frequency of occurrence noted in a prospective study of infants with major malformations are noted in Table 7–1. The majority of lesions involve the central nervous system and the cardiovascular system, although other series have reported an excess of genitourinary and limb defects as well (Cousins, 1991).

There is no increase in birth defects among offspring of diabetic fathers, prediabetic women, and women who develop gestational diabetes after the first trimester. This suggests that glycemic control during embryogenesis is a critical factor in the genesis of diabetes-associated birth defects. In a study by Miller and colleagues (1981), the

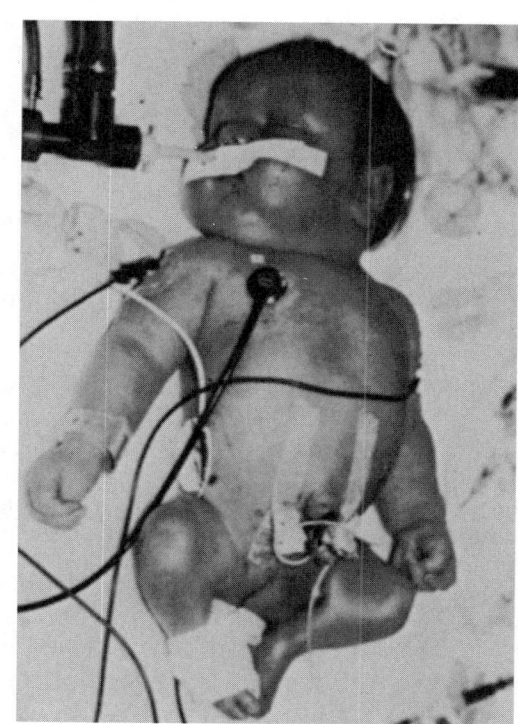

FIGURE 7–1. Newborn with caudal regression syndrome, macrosomia, and respiratory distress. The mother had Type I diabetes and and HbA$_{1c}$ concentration of 13.5% when first seen for prenatal care at 12 weeks' gestation. (From Creasy RK, Resnik R [Eds]: Maternal-Fetal Medicine: Principles and Practice, 2nd ed. Philadelphia, WB Saunders, 1989.)

TABLE 7–1

Congenital Malformations in Infants of Insulin-Dependent Diabetic Mothers

Anomaly	Approximate Risk Ratio	Percent Risk
All cardiac defects	18×	8.5
All central nervous system anomalies	16×	5.3
Anencephaly	13×	
Spina bifida	20×	
All congenital anomalies	8×	18.4

Adapted from Becerra JE, Khoury MJ, Cordero JF, Erickson JD: Diabetes mellitus during pregnancy and the risks for specific birth defects: A population based case-control study. Reproduced by Permission of PEDIATRICS Vol 85, Page 1–9, Copyright 1990.

frequency of congenital anomalies was proportional to the maternal glycohemoglobin in the first trimester (3.4% anomalies with HbA_{1c} <8.5%; 22.4% with HbA_{1c} >8.5%). Lucas and associates (1989) reported a similar experience with 105 diabetic patients with an overall malformation rate of 13.3%. The risk of delivering a malformed infant, however, was nil with HbA_{1c} less than 7.1%, 14% with HbA_{1c} 7.2% to 9.1%, 23% with HbA_{1c} 9.2% to 11.1%, and 25% with HbA_{1c} greater than 11.2%.

Pathogenesis. The mechanism by which hyperglycemia disturbs embryonic development is controversial, but reduced arachidonic acid and *myo*-inositol levels and accumulation of sorbitol and trace metals in the conceptus have been postulated. Maternal, then fetal hyperglycemia may promote excessive formation of oxygen radicals in the mitochondria of susceptible fetal tissues, leading to the formation of hydroperoxides, which are inhibitors of prostacyclin. The resulting overabundance of thromboxanes and other prostaglandins may then disrupt the vascularization of developing tissues. In support of this theory, addition of prostaglandin inhibitors to mouse embryos in culture medium prevented glucose-induced embryopathy (Pinter et al, 1986).

Prevention. Because the critical time for teratogenesis is during the period 3 to 6 weeks after conception, normal glycemic control must be instituted before pregnancy to minimize the risk of birth defects. Several clinical trials of preconception care and education of diabetic women have demonstrated that malformation rates equivalent to the general population can be achieved with meticulous preconceptional glycemic control (Fuhrmann et al, 1983). The safe level of glycemic control, as evidenced by the HbA_{1c} level, to normalize a patient's risk of congenital anomalies seems to be a near-normal value. Above normal, the risk of teratogenesis rises proportionately.

Macrosomia

Fetal overgrowth is a major problem in pregnancies complicated by diabetes. A study of birth weights in the past 20 years indicated that 21% of infants with birth weight 4540 g or greater were born to mothers who were glucose intolerant, a rate clearly disproportionate to the only 2% to 5% of gravidas with some form of diabetes (Shelley-Jones et al, 1992). Thus the problem of abnormal fetal growth in diabetic pregnancy remains an important challenge for the clinician.

Defined variously as birth weight above the 90th percentile for gestational age or birth weight greater than 4000 g, macrosomia occurs in 15% to 45% of diabetic pregnancies. Excessive fetal size contributes to increased frequency of intrapartum injury in diabetic pregnancy (shoulder dystocia, brachial plexus and facial nerve injuries, and asphyxia). Macrosomia is also a major factor in the increased rate of cesarean delivery among diabetic women. Because the risk of macrosomia is fairly constant across all classes of diabetes, it is likely that first-trimester metabolic control has less effect on fetal growth than glycemic regulation in the third trimester.

Growth Dynamics. The macrosomic IDM does not follow the growth patterns observed in euglycemic pregnancies. During the first and second trimesters, differentiation of diabetic from nondiabetic fetuses is extremely difficult using ultrasound measurements. After 24 weeks, however, the growth velocity of the abdominal circumference typically begins to rise above normal (Ogata et al, 1980). Reece and colleagues (1990) found that the IDM fetus has normal head growth, even when advanced degrees of hyperglycemia are present. Landon and coworkers (1989) noted that although IDM fetal head and femur growth were similar to normals, abdominal circumference growth exceeded that of controls beginning at 32 weeks (diabetic abdominal circumference growth = 1.36 cm/week versus 0.901 cm/week in normals).

Morphometric studies of the IDM newborn indicate that the increased growth of the abdominal circumference is due to deposition of fat in the abdominal and interscapular area. This central deposition of fat is a key characteristic of diabetic macrosomia and underlies the pathology associated with vaginal delivery in these pregnancies. Acker and colleagues (1986) showed that although the incidence of shoulder dystocia is 3% among infants weighing greater than 4000 g, 16% of infants weighing greater than 4000 g from diabetic pregnancies sustained shoulder dystocia.

Childhood Effects. Increased growth velocity, begun in fetal life during pregnancy complicated by diabetes, may extend into childhood and adult life. Silverman and coworkers (1995) reported follow-up of IDMs through age 8 years in which half the infants weighed greater than the 90th percentile for gestational age at birth. By age 8 years, approximately half of the IDMs weighed more than the heaviest 10% of the nondiabetic children. The asymmetry index was 30% higher in diabetic offspring than the controls by age 8 years. These investigators also found that the diabetic offspring have permanent derangement of glucose-insulin kinetics, resulting in increased incidence of impaired glucose tolerance.

Pathophysiology. The pathophysiology of excessive fetal growth is complex and reflects the delivery of an abnormal nutrient mixture to the fetoplacental unit, regulated by an abnormal confluence of growth factors. Pedersen (1952) hypothesized that maternal hyperglycemia stimulates fetal hyperinsulinemia, which, in turn, mediates accelerated fuel utilization and growth. The features of the abnormal growth in diabetic pregnancy include excessive adipose deposition, visceral organ hypertrophy, and acceleration of body mass accretion (Ogata et al, 1980). Freinkel and Metzger (1979) further postulated that abnormal fetal growth was related to altered delivery of lipids, amino acids, and ketones across the placenta.

Data from the Diabetes In Early Pregnancy (DIEP) project suggest that maternal metabolic control is a critical factor in fetal macrosomia (Jovanovic-Peterson et al, 1991). In this project, in which meticulous glycemic care was maintained in early pregnancy, fetal weight did not correlate significantly with fasting glucose levels. During the second and third trimesters, however, *postprandial* blood glucose levels were strongly predictive of both birth weight and the overall percentage of macrosomic infants. With postprandial glucose values averaging 120 mg/dL, approximately 20% of infants were macrosomic; a 30% rise in postprandial levels to 160 mg/dL resulted in a predicted percentage of macrosomia of 35%.

The Pedersen hypothesis presumes that abnormal fuel milieu in the maternal compartment is reflected contemporaneously in the fetal compartment. *Maternal hyperglycemia = fetal hyperglycemia.* Studies by Hollingsworth and Cousins (1981) have confirmed much of Pedersen's hypothesis and note that during normal pregnancy:

- Maternal fasting blood glucose levels decline from mid-80s mg/dL to mid-70s mg/dL. Mean blood glucose declines also.
- At night, maternal glucose levels drop markedly as the fetus continues to draw glucose stores from the maternal circulation.
- Postprandial peaks in maternal blood glucose rarely exceed 120 mg/dL at 2 hours or 130 mg/dL at 1 hour.
- Should maternal glucose levels surge excessively postprandially, the consequent fetal hyperglycemia is accompanied by episodic fetal hyperinsulinemia.
- Fetal hyperinsulinemia, lasting only episodically for 1 to 2 hours, has detrimental consequences to fetal growth and well-being in that it (1) promotes storage of excess nutrients, resulting in macrosomia, and (2) drives catabolism of the oversupply of fuel, using energy and depleting fetal oxygen stores.

Episodic fetal hypoxia stimulated by episodic maternal hyperglycemia leads to outpouring of adrenal catecholamines, which, in turn, causes:

- Hypertension, cardiac remodeling, and cardiac hypertrophy.
- Stimulation of erythropoietin, red cell hyperplasia, and increased hematocrit.
- High hematocrits, which lead to poor circulation and postnatal hyperbilirubinemia.

Diagnostic Classification of Diabetes

A classification scheme based on the pathophysiology of hyperglycemia was developed by the National Diabetes

TABLE 7–2

Classification of Diabetes Mellitus

Type	Old Nomenclature	Clinical Features
Type I diabetes	Juvenile-onset diabetes	Insulin deficient, ketosis prone. Virtually all Type I patients are insulin dependent
Type II diabetes	Adult-onset diabetes	Insulin resistant, not ketosis prone. Few Type II patients are truly insulin dependent
Gestational diabetes		Occurs in and resolves after pregnancy. Insulin resistant, not ketosis prone

Data Group (NDDG) of the National Institutes of Health (1979). The types are summarized in Table 7–2. This nomenclature is a useful guide because it categorizes patients by their underlying pathogenesis (insulin-deficient [Type I] and insulin-resistant [Type II and gestational]).

Another useful concept in classifying diabetes during pregnancy contrasts overt, pre-existing diabetes (Types I and II) from gestational diabetes because the teratogenic effects of hyperglycemia occur only in overt diabetic women, and the timing of onset (and therefore the severity of diabetic effects on fetal growth) of hyperglycemia is highly variable in gestational diabetes.

Overt Diabetes

Patients with Type I diabetes typically present with hyperglycemia, ketosis, and dehydration in childhood or adolescence, rarely during pregnancy. Often the diagnosis is made during a hospital admission for diabetic ketoacidosis and coma. It is not unusual for women tentatively diagnosed with gestational diabetes to be found to have overt diabetes after delivery. The diagnosis of Type II diabetes in nonpregnant subjects is made using the 75-g, 2-hour glucose tolerance test (GTT). Diagnostic criteria are listed in Table 7–3.

TABLE 7–3

Seventy-Five–g Glucose Tolerance Test for Type II Diabetes Mellitus (Venous Plasma Glucose)*

Diagnosis	Fasting (mg/dL)	2-Hour (mg/dL)
Normal	<140	<200
Impaired glucose tolerance	<140	>140 and <200
Diabetes	≥140	≥140

*Note: Diagnosis of non–insulin-dependent diabetes mellitus after pregnancy requires a 1-hour value >200 mg/dL in addition to abnormal fasting and 2-hour values.

TABLE 7–4

One Hundred-g 3-Hour Glucose Tolerance Test for Gestational Diabetes

Test Prerequisites

1-h 50-g glucose challenge result ≥135 mg/dL
Overnight fast of 8–14 h
Carbohydrate loading 3 d including ≥150 g carbohydrate
Seated, not smoking during the test
Two or more values must be met or exceeded

	Venous Plasma (mg/dL)	Capillary Whole Blood (mg/dL)
Fasting	105	114
1-h	190	211
2-h	165	183
3-h	145	157

Adapted from Metzger BE: Summary and recommendations of the Third International Workshop-Conference on Gestational Diabetes Mellitus. Diabetes 40 Suppl 2:197, 1991.

Gestational Diabetes

Gestational diabetes is diagnosed from a 3-hour GTT using 100 g of glucose. The diagnostic criteria, shown in Table 7–4, require an overnight fast and carbohydrate loading before the test. Although many experts believe that the capillary reflectance meters are not sufficiently accurate to be used to diagnose gestational diabetes, some clinics use the finger-stick system because of economy. The corresponding capillary glucose levels are also shown in Table 7–4.

The Third International Workshop-Conference on Gestational Diabetes Mellitus has continued to recommend the use of a two-stage screening/diagnosis system first proposed by O'Sullivan and Mahan in 1964. A 50-g oral glucose challenge test is the preferred initial screening test because it is better tolerated than the 3-hour oral GTT and reduces the number of 3-hour tests administered. Measurements of maternal glycosylated hemoglobin, although predictive of fetal anomalies in overt diabetic women, have not been shown to be sensitive diagnostic indicators for gestational diabetes.

Timing of glucose tolerance testing for gestational diabetes is critical. Because the insulin resistance that causes hyperglycemia becomes increasingly evident as the third trimester progresses, early testing may miss some patients who become glucose intolerant later. Performing the test later in the third trimester, however, limits the time in which metabolic intervention can take place. Thus, the need for glucose screening is assessed at the initial prenatal visit and again at 26 to 28 weeks. Clinical features that should lead to a first-trimester glucose challenge test are listed in Table 7–5.

Perinatal Complications of Diabetes During Pregnancy
Fetal Morbidity and Mortality
Perinatal Mortality

Perinatal mortality in diabetic pregnancy has decreased 30-fold since the discovery of insulin in 1922 and intensive obstetric and infant care in the 1970s (Fig. 7–2). Improved techniques of maintaining maternal euglycemia have led to later timing of delivery and reduced incidence of iatrogenic respiratory distress syndrome (RDS).

Nevertheless, the currently reported perinatal mortality rates among diabetic women remain approximately twice those observed in the nondiabetic population (Table 7–6). Congenital malformations, RDS, and extreme prematurity account for most perinatal deaths in contemporary diabetic pregnancy. Figure 7–3 demonstrates the differences in RDS in diabetic and euglycemic pregnancy. In the past decade, fewer intrauterine deaths have been reported, probably reflecting more careful fetal monitoring. Nevertheless, intrapartum asphyxia and fetal demise remain a persistent problem.

Birth Injury

Birth injury, including shoulder dystocia (Keller et al, 1991) and brachial plexus trauma, is more common among IDMs,

TABLE 7–5

Indications for First-Trimester 50-g Glucose Challenge

Maternal age >25 years
Previous infant >4 kg
Previous unexplained fetal demise
Previous pregnancy with gestational diabetes
Strong immediate family history of adult-onset or gestational diabetes
Obesity (>90 kg)
Fasting glucose >140 mg/dL (7.8 mM) or random glucose >200 mg/dL (11.1 mM)

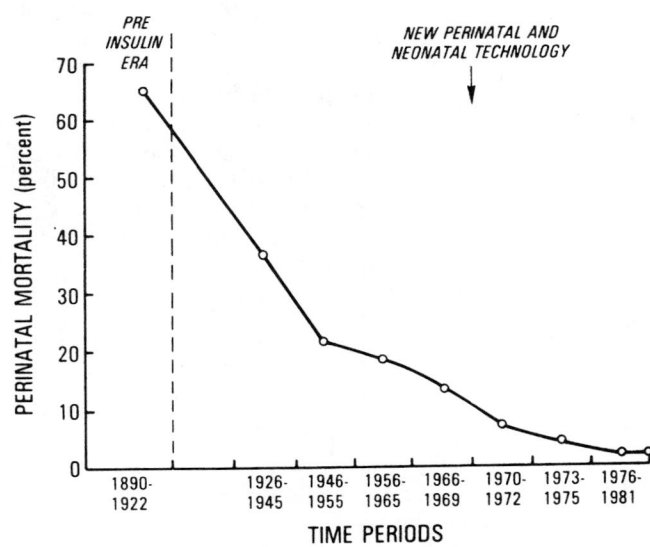

FIGURE 7–2. Perinatal mortality rate (percent) among infants of diabetic mothers from 1890 to 1981. Data plotted from reports of Craigin and Ryder (1916), DeLee (1920), Williams (1925), Pederson (1977), Gabbe and colleagues (1978), and Jorge and colleagues (1981). (From Creasy RK, Resnik R [Eds]: Maternal-Fetal Medicine: Principles and Practice, 2nd ed. Philadelphia, WB Saunders, 1989.)

TABLE 7-6

Perinatal Mortality Rates in Diabetic Pregnancy (Deaths per 1000 Births)

	Gestational Diabetes	Pre-Existing Diabetes	Normals*
Fetal mortality	4.7	10.4	5.7
Neonatal mortality	3.3	12.2	4.7
Perinatal mortality	8.0	22.6	10.4

*California data 1986, birth weight, sex, and race corrected.

and macrosomic fetuses are at the highest risk (Mimouni et al, 1992). Shoulder dystocia, defined as difficulty in delivering the fetal body after expulsion of the fetal head, is an obstetric emergency that places the fetus and mother at great risk. Shoulder dystocia occurs in 0.3% to 0.5% of vaginal deliveries among normal pregnant women, whereas the incidence is twofold to fourfold higher in women with diabetes, probably because the hyperglycemia of diabetic pregnancy causes the fetal shoulder and abdominal widths to become massive. Although half of shoulder dystocias occur in infants of normal birth weight (2500 to 4000 g), the incidence of shoulder dystocia rises 10-fold to 5% to 7% among infants weighing 4000 g or more and up to 31% if diabetes is involved (Acker et al, 1986).

The clinical signs associated with shoulder dystocia include (1) protracted labor progress, (2) pushing for more than 2 to 3 hours, (3) the use of midforceps, and (4) a known diabetic pregnancy. The presence of two or more of these factors multiplies the risk of shoulder dystocia significantly.

The major risks of shoulder dystocia are damage to the brachial plexus during forcible extraction of the fetus and asphyxiation because of the excessive time necessary to perform the extraction. The risk of permanent brachial plexus palsy associated with shoulder dystocia is approximately 1%. If delivery occurs within 8 minutes of recognition of the shoulder dystocia, significant asphyxial damage to the fetus' brain is unlikely.

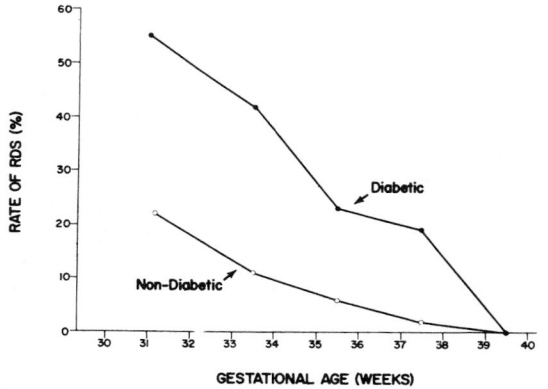

FIGURE 7-3. Rate of respiratory distress syndrome (RDS) versus gestational age. Improved management of maternal glycemic control permits delaying delivery until after 38 weeks when the risk of RDS approaches that of nondiabetic pregnancy.

Ideally, shoulder dystocia should be avoided by awareness of the aforementioned warning signs. Fewer than 30% of these events, however, can be predicted on the basis of clinical factors (Sandmire and OHalloin, 1988). Thus, a decision to perform cesarean section for suspected fetal macrosomia should be approached cautiously. Given the risk of shoulder dystocia of 30% for a fetus weighing greater than 4300 to 4500 g, some authorities consider it prudent to perform an outright cesarean section with coexisting diabetes. If the fetal weight is estimated to be less than 4300 g, a trial of labor (with avoidance of forceps assistance) is appropriate for most patients unless extreme fetal abdominal obesity is documented on ultrasound.

Neonatal Morbidity and Mortality

Polycythemia and Hyperviscosity

Polycythemia (central venous hemoglobin concentration >20 g/dL or hematocrit >65%) is not uncommon in IDMs and apparently related to glycemic control. Widness and associates (1990) demonstrated that hyperglycemia is a powerful stimulus to fetal erythropoietin production, probably mediated by decreased fetal oxygen tension. Untreated, neonatal polycythemia may promote vascular sludging, ischemia, and infarction of vital tissues, including the kidneys and central nervous system.

Neonatal Hypoglycemia

The hyperinsulinemic IDM is at increased risk for low plasma glucose levels after birth. This complication is usually much milder and less common in the infant whose insulin-dependent diabetic mother is well controlled throughout the *entire* pregnancy and euglycemic during labor and delivery. Unrecognized postnatal hypoglycemia may lead to neonatal seizures, coma, and brain damage. Thus, it is imperative that the nursery receiving the IDM have a protocol for frequent monitoring of the infant's blood glucose until metabolic stability is ensured.

Neonatal Hypocalcemia

Low levels of serum calcium (<7 mg/100 mL) have been reported in up to 50% of IDMs during the first 3 days of life. Tsang and coworkers (1979) reported normal levels of parathyroid hormone in cord blood of IDMs, indicating normal fetal parathyroid function. Decreased parathyroid function in such infants was associated with decreased serum calcium levels and increased serum phosphorus values. These changes in infants of insulin-dependent diabetics did not evoke an increase in serum parathyroid hormone. The resulting functional hypoparathyroidism was considered to be related to (1) prematurity, (2) birth asphyxia, or (3) suppressed parathyroid function secondary to hypercalcemia in utero.

Neonatal Hypomagnesemia

Tsang and coworkers (1976) followed 56 IDMs prospectively from birth and noted that 38% of the infants had a serum magnesium level of less than 1.5 mg/dL at some time during the first 3 days of life. Decreased levels of serum magnesium were related to low maternal age, severity of maternal diabetes, and prematurity. Neuromuscular irritability did not correlate with decreased serum magnesium or ionized calcium levels. Decreased serum magnesium levels observed in IDMs are associated with decreased maternal serum magnesium, decreased ionized and total calcium, increased serum phosphorus, and decreased parathyroid function. Neonatal parathyroid hormone and calcium responses to magnesium sulfate infusions are inversely related to neonatal serum magnesium concentrations.

Hyperbilirubinemia

The risk of hyperbilirubinemia is higher in IDMs than in normal infants. There are multiple causes of hyperbilirubinemia in IDMs, but prematurity and polycythemia are the primary contributing factors. Increased destruction of red blood cells contributes to the risk of jaundice and kernicterus. Treatment of this complication is usually by phototherapy, but exchange transfusions may be necessary if bilirubin levels are markedly elevated.

Hypertrophic and Congestive Cardiomyopathy

In some macrosomic infants of poorly controlled diabetic mothers, a thickened myocardium and significant septal hypertrophy have been described (Gutgesell et al, 1976). Although the prevalence of myocardial hypertrophy in IDMs may exceed 30% at birth, almost all cases have resolved by 1 year of age (Mace et al, 1979).

Hypertrophic cardiac dysfunction in a newborn IDM often leads to respiratory distress, which may be mistaken for hyaline membrane disease. IDMs with cardiomegaly may have either congestive or hypertrophic cardiomyopathy. Echocardiograms show a hypercontractile, thickened myocardium, often with septal hypertrophy disproportionate to the ventricular free walls. The ventricular chambers are often smaller than normal, and there may be anterior systolic motion of the mitral valve producing left ventricular outflow tract obstruction.

The pathogenesis of hypertrophic cardiomyopathy in IDMs is unclear, although it is recognized to be associated with poor maternal metabolic control. There is evidence that the fetal myocardium is particularly sensitive to insulin during gestation, and Susa and colleagues (1979) reported a doubling of cardiac mass in hyperinsulinemic fetal rhesus monkeys. The myocardium is known to be richly endowed with insulin receptors.

IDMs may also have *congestive* cardiomyopathy without hypertrophy. On echocardiogram, the myocardium is overstretched and poorly contractile. This condition is often rapidly reversible with correction of neonatal hypoglycemia, hypocalcemia, and polycythemia; it responds to digoxin or diuretics or both. In contrast, treatment of hypertrophic cardiomyopathy with an inotropic or diuretic agent tends to decrease further the size of the ventricular chambers and leads to obstruction of blood flow. Echocardiographic examination of IDMs with enlarged hearts is recommended to detect and treat clinically silent cardiomyopathy.

Respiratory Distress Syndrome

Since the 1970s, improved maternal management and better protocols for timing delivery have resulted in a dramatic decline in the incidence of RDS from 31% to 3% (Frantz et al, 1979). Nevertheless, respiratory dysfunction in the newborn IDM continues to be a frequent and all-too-common complication of diabetic pregnancy. This may be due to surfactant deficiency or some other form of pulmonary distress. Late timing of surfactant production occurs in diabetic pregnancy. Studies of fetal lung ion transport in the diabetic rat by Pinter and coworkers (1991) demonstrated decreased fluid clearance and lack of thinning of the lung's connective tissue in diabetics compared to controls. In humans, Kjos (1990) noted *respiratory distress* in 18 of 526 infants delivered of diabetic gestations (3.4%). Surfactant-deficient airway disease accounted for less than one third of cases, with transient tachypnea, hypertrophic cardiomyopathy, and pneumonia responsible for the majority.

Thus, the near-term infant of a poorly controlled diabetic mother is more likely to have neonatal RDS than the infant of a nondiabetic mother at the same gestational age. This circumstance further compounds the diabetic infant's metabolic and cardiovascular difficulties after birth. The nondiabetic fetus achieves pulmonary maturity at a mean gestational age of 34 to 35 weeks. By 37 weeks, more than 99% of normal newborn infants have mature lung profiles as assessed by phospholipid assays. In a diabetic pregnancy, however, it is unwise to assume that the risk of respiratory distress has passed until after 38.5 gestational weeks have been completed. Any delivery contemplated before 38.5 weeks for other than the most urgent fetal and maternal indications should be preceded by documentation of pulmonary maturity by amniocentesis.

Obstetric Complications

Pregnancy complicated by diabetes is subject to a number of obstetric disorders, including ketoacidosis, preeclampsia, polyhydramnios, and abnormal labor, in increased frequency over controls.

Preeclampsia

An unpredictable multisystem disorder, in which maternal neurologic, renal, and cardiovascular status can decline precipitously and which may threaten fetal health through placental ischemia and abruptio placentae, preeclampsia occurs in approximately 12% of insulin-requiring diabetics, as compared to 8% of nondiabetics (Moore et al, 1985). Diamond and colleagues (1985) encountered preeclampsia in 19% of diabetics, noting that the risk was related to maternal age and duration of pre-existing diabetes. Fetal deaths are increased in diabetics with preeclampsia. In the diabetic patient with chronic hypertension, preeclampsia may be difficult to distinguish from near-term blood pressure elevations. The onset is typically insidious and not confidently recognized until severe.

When a patient with diabetes develops preeclampsia, she should be evaluated for delivery. If severe signs are present (e.g., blood pressure >160/110 mm Hg, neurologic symptoms, or significant renal dysfunction), delivery should be performed promptly. In mild cases, the patient may be observed if the fetal lungs are immature. Preeclampsia after 38 weeks' gestation, however, is adequate grounds for initiating delivery.

Polyhydramnios

Polyhydramnios is defined as excessive amniotic fluid. The clinical definition varies, including greater than 2000 mL amniotic fluid recorded at delivery and various measures of amniotic fluid pocket depths as observed on ultrasound. In practice, polyhydramnios is usually diagnosed when any single vertical pocket of amniotic fluid is deeper than 8 cm (equivalent to the 97th percentile) or when the sum of four pockets from each quadrant of the uterus (amniotic fluid index) exceeds approximately 24 cm (95th percentile) (Moore and Cayle, 1990). The principal causes of hydramnios in diabetic pregnancy include fetal gastrointestinal anomalies (e.g., esophageal atresia) and poor glycemic control. A rapid increase in fundal height should prompt a thorough ultrasound examination by a skilled examiner. The main clinical problems associated with hydramnios are fetal malposition and preterm labor.

Management of the patient with hydramnios is predominantly symptomatic, focused on improving glycemic control and preventing premature labor. Enhanced patient awareness of contractions and the signs and subtle sensations of preterm labor is essential.

Management
Preconceptional Management

Preconceptional counseling and a detailed medical risk assessment are recommended for all women with overt diabetes and those with a history of gestational diabetes during a previous pregnancy. Significant impact on the maternal and neonatal complications of diabetic pregnancy cannot be realized until meticulous preconceptional metabolic control is achieved in all women contemplating pregnancy.

The important elements to be considered in preconceptional counseling of the diabetic patient include the patient's level of glycemic control; current status of the patient's retinal and renal health; and any medications being taken, especially antihypertensive or thyroid medications. A realistic assessment of the patient's risk of complications during pregnancy, including worsening of renal or ophthalmologic function, should be provided.

The preconceptional program should lead to a comprehensive program of glucose control. The major goals of the prepregnancy metabolic program include:

- Establishing a regimen of frequent, regular monitoring of capillary glucose levels.
- Adopting an insulin dosing regimen that results in smooth interprandial glucose profile (fasting glucose 80 to 100 mg/dL, 2-hour postprandial glucose < 120 mg/dL, no reactions between meals or at night).

- Bringing HbA$_{1c}$ level into the normal range.
- Developing family, financial, and personal resources to assist the patient should pregnancy complications necessitate lost time from job or bed rest.

Prenatal Metabolic Management

The goals of glycemic monitoring, dietary regulation, and insulin therapy in diabetic pregnancy are to prevent the postnatal sequelae of diabetes in the newborn: macrosomia, shoulder dystocia, and postnatal metabolic instability. These measures must be instituted early and aggressively if they are to be effective.

Principles of Dietary Therapy

Because women with diabetes have inadequate insulin action after feeding, the goal of dietary therapy is to avoid single, large meals and foods with a large percentage of simple carbohydrates. Three major meals and three snacks are prescribed. The use of *nonglycemic foods* that release calories into the gut slowly also improves metabolic control.

The American Diabetes Association (1979), British Diabetic Association (1980), and Canadian Diabetes Association (1981) recommended diet contains 50% to 60% carbohydrate, 12% to 20% protein, less than 10% saturated fatty acids, and up to 10% polyunsaturated fatty acids.

Principles of Glucose Monitoring: Home Glucose Monitoring

The availability of capillary glucose chemical test strips has revolutionized the management of diabetes and should now be considered the standard of care for pregnancy monitoring. The discipline of measuring and recording blood glucose levels before and after meals may have the effect of improving glycemic control (Goldberg et al, 1986).

The frequency and timing of home glucose monitoring should be individualized, but *postprandial* values must be assessed because they have the strongest correlation with fetal growth. Data from the DIEP (Jovanovic-Peterson et al, 1991) project found that the correlation of fasting glucose levels with fetal weight was nonsignificant, but *postprandial* levels were strongly predictive of both birth weight and the overall percentage of macrosomic infants. With postprandial glucose values averaging 120 mg/dL, approximately 20% of infants were macrosomic; a 30% rise in postprandial levels to 160 mg/dL resulted in a predicted percentage of macrosomia of 35%.

Similar results were reported by de Veciana and associates (1995). Women randomly assigned to have their diabetes managed according to 1-hour postprandial blood glucose concentrations had markedly better results than women using premeal glucose levels. In the postprandial group, the mean ($\pm$ SD) change in the glycosylated hemoglobin value was greater ($-3.0\% \pm 2.2\%$ versus $0.6\% \pm 1.6\%$, P <.001), the birth weights were lower (3469 ± 668 versus 3848 ± 434 g, P =.01), the rates of neonatal hypoglycemia were less (3% versus 21%, P =.05), and the rates of macrosomia were less (12% versus 42%, P =.01).

A typical schedule involves blood glucose checks on rising in the morning, 1 or 2 hours after breakfast, before and after lunch, before dinner, and before bedtime. The goal of *physiologic* glycemic control in pregnancy, however, is not met by simply avoiding hypoglycemia. The data summarized here regarding fetal macrosomia and postnatal morbidity emphasize the key role of excessive postprandial glucose excursions. Thus, close attention must be paid to both preprandial and postprandial glycemic profiles.

Principles of Insulin Therapy

No available insulin delivery method approaches the precise secretion of the hormone from the human pancreas. The therapeutic goal of exogenous insulin therapy during pregnancy is to achieve diurnal glucose excursions similar to those of nondiabetic pregnant women. Normal pregnant women maintain postprandial blood glucose excursions within a relatively narrow range (70 to 120 mg/dL). As pregnancy progresses, the fasting and between-meal blood glucose levels drop progressively lower, as a result of the continual uptake of glucose from the maternal circulation by the growing fetus. Any insulin regimen for pregnant women must be designed to avoid excessive unopposed insulin action during the fasting state.

Insulin type and dosing frequency should be individualized. Use of regular insulin before each major meal helps limit postprandial hyperglycemia. To provide basal insulin levels between feedings, a longer-acting preparation is necessary, such as NPH or Lente. Typical dose ratios are 2:3 of total insulin in the morning, with 2:3 intermediate-acting and 1:3 regular insulin.

Prenatal Obstetric Management

The overall strategy of management of diabetic pregnancy in the third trimester involves preventing stillbirth and asphyxia and monitoring growth of the fetus to select the proper time and route of delivery to minimize maternal and infant morbidity. The first is accomplished by testing fetal well-being at frequent intervals and the second through ultrasound trending of fetal size.

Periodic Fetal Biophysical Testing

A variety of fetal tests are available to the clinician, including fetal heart rate testing, fetal movement assessment, ultrasound biophysical scoring, and fetal umbilical Doppler studies. Most of these can be used with confidence to provide assurance of fetal well-being while awaiting fetal maturity if applied properly. These tests are summarized in Table 7–7.

Testing should be initiated early enough to avoid significant risk of stillbirth but not so early so that a high false-positive rate is encountered. In patients with poor glycemic control or significant hypertension, testing should begin as early as 28 weeks. In lower risk patients, most centers begin formal fetal testing by 34 weeks. Fetal movement counting is performed in all pregnancies from 28 weeks onward.

Assessing Fetal Growth

Monitoring fetal growth continues to be a challenging and highly inexact process. Although today's tools, serial plotting of fetal growth parameters, are superior to earlier clinical estimations, accuracy is still ±15%. Both single and multiple longitudinal assessments of fetal size have been attempted.

Calculation of Estimated Fetal Weight. Several polynomial formulas using combinations of head, abdominal, and limb measurements have been proposed to predict the weight of the macrosomic fetus from ultrasound parameters (Ferrero et al, 1994; Tongsong et al, 1994). Unfortunately, in such formulas small errors in individual measurements of the head, abdomen, and femur are typically multiplied together. In the obese fetus, the inaccuracies are further magnified. Bernstein and Catalano (1992) observed that significant correlation exists between the degree of error in the ultrasound estimated fetal weight and the percent body fat on the fetus (r = 0.28, $P < .05$). Perhaps this problem is why no single formula has proven to be adequate in identifying the macrosomic fetus (Tamura et al, 1985).

TABLE 7–7

Tests of Fetal Well-Being

Test	Frequency	Reassuring Result	Comment
Fetal movement counting	Every night from 28 weeks	Ten movements in <60 min	Performed in all patients
Nonstress test	Twice weekly	Two heart rate accelerations in 20 min	Begin at 28–34 weeks with insulin-dependent diabetes. Start at 36 weeks in diet-controlled gestational diabetes
Contraction stress test	Weekly	No heart rate decelerations in response to ≥3 contractions in 10 min	Same as for nonstress test
Ultrasound biophysical profile	Weekly	Score of 8 in 30 min	3 movements = 2 1 flexion = 2 30 sec breathing = 2 2 cm amniotic fluid = 2

The relative accuracy of the various available formulas has been reviewed. Approximately 75% of the fetal weight predictions were within 10% of actual birth weight, with sensitivity for detecting macrosomia varying greatly (11% to 76%) (Shamley and Landon, 1994). In another study (McLaren et al, 1995), 65% of weight estimates using a simple abdominal circumference and femur length formula were within 10%. A similar accuracy was achieved with more complex models (53% to 66%).

The formula by Shepard and colleagues (1982), which uses biparietal diameter and abdominal circumference, is readily available in textbooks and is used most commonly in current sonographic equipment software. It has accuracy levels similar to the statistics quoted.

Serial Estimated Fetal Weight Assessments. Because prediction of fetal weight from a single set of measurements is inaccurate, serial trending of ultrasonographic parameters (typically every 1.5 to 3 weeks) might theoretically offer a better estimate of actual weight percentile. A comparison of the efficacy of serial estimated fetal weight calculations to a single measurement, however, did not improve predictive accuracy (Larsen et al, 1995). Predictions based on the average of repeated weight estimates or linear extrapolation from two estimates or extrapolation by a second-order equation fitted to four estimates were no better than the prediction from the last estimate before delivery. Similar findings (that a single estimate is as accurate as multiple assessments) were reported by Hedriana and Moore (1994).

Choosing Timing and Route of Delivery

Timing of delivery should be selected to minimize maternal and neonatal morbidity and mortality. Delaying delivery as near as possible to the estimated date of confinement helps maximize cervical ripeness and improve the chances of spontaneous labor and vaginal delivery. Yet the risks of fetal macrosomia, birth injury, and fetal death increase as the due date approaches (Rasmussen et al, 1992). Although earlier delivery at 37 weeks might reduce the risk of shoulder dystocia, an increase in failed labor inductions and poor neonatal pulmonary status must be considered. Thus, an optimal time for delivery of most diabetic pregnancies is between 38.5 and 40 weeks.

Delivery of a diabetic patient before 38.5 weeks' gestation without documented fetal lung maturity should be performed only for compelling maternal or fetal reasons. Fetal lung maturity should be verified in such cases by the presence of greater than 3% phosphotidyl glycerol or the equivalent on an amniocentesis specimen. After 38.5 weeks, the obstetrician can await spontaneous labor if the fetus is not macrosomic and biophysical testing is reassuring. In patients with gestational diabetes and superb glycemic control, continued fetal testing and expectant management can be considered until 41 weeks (Lurie et al, 1992).

Kjos and associates (1993) compared the outcomes associated with labor induction in gestational diabetics at 38 weeks versus expectant management with fetal testing. Expectant management increased the gestational age at delivery by 1 week, but the cesarean delivery rate was not significantly different. The prevalence of macrosomic infants in the expectantly managed group (23%) was significantly greater than that in the active induction group (10%). This finding suggests that routine induction of diabetics on or before 39 weeks does not increase the risk of cesarean section and may reduce the risk of macrosomia.

Given the previous data, the decision to attempt vaginal delivery or perform a cesarean section is inevitably based on limited data. The patient's past obstetric history, the best estimation of fetal weight, fetal adipose profile (abdomen larger than head), and clinical pelvimetry should all be considered. Most large series of diabetic pregnancies report a cesarean section rate of 30% to 50%. The best means by which this rate can be lowered is by early and strict glycemic control in pregnancy. Conducting long labor inductions in patients with a large fetus and marginal pelvis may increase rather than lower morbidity and costs.

Intrapartum Glycemic Management

Maintenance of intrapartum metabolic homeostasis is essential to avoid fetal hypoxemia and promote a smooth postnatal infant transition. Strict maternal euglycemia during labor does not guarantee newborn euglycemia in infants with macrosomia and long-established islet cell hypertrophy. Nevertheless, the use of a combined insulin and glucose infusion during labor to maintain maternal blood glucose in a narrow (80 to 110 mg/dL) range during labor is common and reasonable practice (Caplan et al, 1982). Typical infusion rates are 5% dextrose in Ringer's lactate at 100 mL per hour and regular insulin at 0.5 to 1.0 units per hour. Capillary blood glucose levels are monitored hourly in such patients.

For patients with diet-controlled gestational diabetes in labor, avoiding dextrose in all intravenous fluids normally maintains excellent blood glucose control. After 1 to 2 hours, no further assessments of capillary blood glucose are typically necessary.

Neonatal Management

Neonatal Transitional Management

One of the metabolic problems common to IDMs is hypoglycemia, which is related to the degree of maternal control over the 6 to 12 weeks before birth. Neonatal hypoglycemia is most likely to occur between 1 and 5 hours after birth, as the rich supply of maternal glucose stops with ligation of the umbilical cord, and the infant's levels of circulating insulin remain elevated. These infants therefore require close monitoring for blood glucose concentration during the first hours after birth. IDMs also appear to have disorders of both catecholamine and glucagon metabolism and have diminished capability to mount normal compensatory responses to hypoglycemia.

In the past, IDMs were treated with glucagon; however, this treatment frequently results in high blood glucose levels that trigger insulin secretion and repeated cycles of hypoglycemia-hyperglycemia. Current recommendations, therefore, include early oral feeding when possible, along with infusion of intravenous glucose.

Ordinarily, blood glucose levels can be controlled satisfactorily with an infusion of 10% glucose. If greater amounts of glucose are required, bolus administration of 5 mL/kg of 10% glucose is recommended, with gradually increasing concentrations of glucose administered every 30 to 60 minutes, if necessary. Close monitoring to correct hypoglycemia while avoiding hyperglycemia and consequent stimulation of insulin secretion is important.

Breast-Feeding

Most authorities prefer to maintain strict monitoring of newborn IDM glucose levels for at least 4 to 6 hours, frequently necessitating admission to a newborn special care unit. IDMs delivered atraumatically and well oxygenated, however, can be kept with their mothers under close glycemic monitoring for the first 1 to 2 hours of life. This permits early breast-feeding, which may reduce the need for intravenous glucose therapy.

Summary

Intensive management of women with glucose intolerance during pregnancy has resulted in markedly improved outcomes. Despite these advances, care of the IDM continues to require vigilance and meticulous monitoring with a full understanding of the quality of the glycemic milieu in which it developed.

DISORDERS OF THE THYROID
Incidence

Thyroid disorders, in general, are more frequent in women than men and represent a common endocrine abnormality during pregnancy. Both hyperthyroidism and hypothyroidism in the mother put the infant at risk and require careful management by the perinatal-neonatal team. Table 7–8 presents an overview of the approach to infants who are thought to be at risk for abnormal thyroid function because of maternal thyroid abnormalities. The most frequently described problem is the syndrome of postpartum thyroiditis, which has been reported to complicate as many as 5% of all pregnancies. The diagnosis of thyroid disease in pregnancy is complicated by the natural changes that occur in immunologic status of the mother and fetus and that complicate assessment of any of the autoimmune thyroid disorders.

Hyperthyroidism

Hyperthyroidism occurs in approximately 0.2% of pregnancies and results in a significant increase in the prevalence of both low-birth-weight delivery and a trend toward increased neonatal mortality. The most common cause of thyrotoxicosis (85% of cases) in women of child-bearing age is Graves disease; other causes include acute (or subacute) thyroiditis (transient), Hashimoto disease, hydatidiform mole, choriocarcinoma, toxic nodular goiter, and toxic adenoma. Graves disease has a peak incidence during the reproductive years, but patients with Graves disease may actually have remissions during pregnancy and then postpartum exacerbations. The unique feature of these pregnancies is that the fetus may also be affected, regardless of the mother's concurrent medical condition. Thyroid function is difficult to evaluate in the fetus, and the status of the fetus may not correlate with that of the mother.

Diagnosis

The differential diagnosis of thyrotoxicosis becomes more difficult during pregnancy because normal pregnant women may have a variety of hyperdynamic signs and symptoms. These may include intolerance to heat, nervousness, irritability, emotional lability, and increased perspiration, along with tachycardia and anxiety. Laboratory data are also difficult to evaluate because total serum thyroxin values are normally elevated during pregnancy as a result of estrogen-induced increases in thyroxine-binding globulin. Thus, if thyroxine-binding globulin is increased, resin tri-iodothyronine uptake may be in the euthyroid to slightly increased range in a patient who has true hyperthyroidism.

Hollingsworth (1989) has reviewed the assessment of thyroid function tests in nonpregnant and pregnant women, along with the differential diagnosis of hyperthyroidism during pregnancy.

Pathogenesis of Graves Disease

The pathogenesis of Graves disease is not completely understood, but it probably represents an overlapping spectrum of disorders that are characterized by production of polyclonal antibodies. It has been appreciated since the 1960s (Sunshine et al, 1965) that abnormal thyroid-stimulating immunoglobulins, which appear to be immunoglobulin G (IgG), are present in pregnant women with Graves disease and cross the placenta easily to cause neonatal hyperthyroidism in some infants (McKenzie and Zakarija, 1978). The clinical spectrum of Graves disease in utero is quite broad and may result in stillbirth or preterm delivery. Some affected infants have widespread evidence of autoimmune disease, including thrombocytopenic purpura and generalized hypertrophy of the lymphatic tissues. Thyroid storm can occur shortly after birth, or infants may have disease that is transient in nature, lasting from 1 to 5 months. Infants born to mothers who have been treated with thioamides may appear normal at birth but subsequently develop signs of thyrotoxicosis at 7 to 10 days of age, when the effect of thioamide suppression of thyroxine synthesis is no longer present. The measurement of thyroid-stimulating antibodies (TSAbs) is useful in predicting whether the fetus will be affected.

Management of the Mother

Because radioactive iodine therapy is contraindicated during pregnancy, treatment of the pregnant woman with thyrotoxicosis involves a choice between antithyroid drugs and surgery. The therapeutic goal is to achieve a euthyroid, or perhaps slightly hyperthyroid, state in the mother while preventing fetal hypothyroidism or hyperthyroidism. Either propylthiouracil (PTU) or methimazole may be used to treat thyrotoxicosis during pregnancy. Because methimazole therapy may be associated with aplasia cutis in the

TABLE 7–8

Approach for Infants Judged to Be at Risk for Abnormal Thyroid Function

Possible Thyroid Abnormality	Cord Blood Analysis	Assessment at Birth	Assessment at 2–7 Days of Life
Congenital hyperthyroidism because mother has: Graves disease with hyperthyroidism; and may have been treated with PTU, methimazole, ^{131}I, or iodides, or surgery History of maternal Graves disease or Hashimoto disease	T$_4$, RSH, TSAb	Physical examination for IUGR, goiter, exophthalmos, tachycardia, bradycardia, size of anterior fontanel, synostosis, congenital anomalies Gestational age by dates, ultrasonography during pregnancy, or Dubovitz examination Plot intrauterine growth by gestational age Neurologic examination Bone age (knee) For selected cases: electrocardiogram, auditory and visual evoked potentials, motor conduction, velocity tests, skull x-rays	T$_4$, TSH, TSAb (if available) determinations: If normal, given no treatment; observe and repeat T$_4$, T$_3$, TSH at 7–10 d[*] If hypothyroid, repeat T$_4$, TSH; if abnormal, treatment at 7–10 d[†] If hyperthyroid, begin treatment with PTU (8 mg/kg) and propranolol
Congenital or early childhood hypothyroidism because mother has: Graves disease with excessive PTU therapy Hashimoto disease ?Acute (subacute) thyroiditis Familial genetic defect in thyroxine synthesis Treatment with iodides or lithium for nonthyroidal illness Exposure to ^{131}I while pregnant	T$_4$, RSH, ThyAb	Same as for suspected hyperthyroidism	T$_4$, TSH, ThyAb determinations: If hypothyroid, perform thyroid ultrasound scan to define presence, size, location of thyroid tissue If hypothyroidism confirmed, begin treatment with Synthroid (0.05 mg/d)

[*]The children of mothers who receive PTU may not develop neonatal Graves disease at age 7–10 d.

[†]Children who receive PTU in utero may have transient or longer lasting hypothyroidism.

PTU, propylthiouracil; IUGR, intrauterine growth retardation; T$_4$, thyroxine; T$_3$, triiodothyronine; TSH, thyroid-stimulating hormone; TSAb, thyroid-stimulating antibody.

From Creasy RK, Resnik R (Eds): Maternal-Fetal Medicine: Principles and Practice, 2nd ed. Philadelphia, WB Saunders, 1989.

offspring of treated women and because PTU crosses the placenta more slowly than methimazole, PTU has become the drug of choice during pregnancy. Ordinarily the disease can be controlled with doses of 300 mg per day. Once the disorder is under control, however, it is important to keep the dose as low as possible, preferably less than 100 mg daily, because these drugs do cross the placenta and block fetal thyroid function and may produce hypothyroidism in the fetus. In women with cardiovascular effects, the use of beta blockers may be appropriate to achieve rapid control of thyrotoxicosis. Because administration of propranolol to pregnant women has been associated with intrauterine growth retardation and impaired responses of the fetus to anoxic stress as well as postnatal bradycardia and hypoglycemia, the dosages must be closely controlled. Iodides have also been used, particularly in combination with beta-blocking agents, to control thyrotoxicosis. Long-term iodide therapy, however, presents a risk to the fetus. Because of the inhibition of the incorporation of iodide into thyroglobulin, the fetus can develop a large, obstructive goiter. Surgery during pregnancy is best reserved for cases in which a woman is hypersensitive to antithyroid drugs or there is poor compliance with medication or, in rare cases, when drugs are ineffective in controlling the disease.

Effects on the Newborn

Approximately 1% of infants born to mothers with some degree of thyrotoxicosis themselves have thyrotoxicosis (Fig. 7–4). Assessment of fetal risk in utero includes measurement of thyroid-stimulating immunoglobulins, with expectation that if the titers are high, there is increased risk of thyrotoxicosis. Additional assessment of the fetus should pay particular attention to elevated resting heart rate and poor fetal growth. Daneman and Howard (1980) reported on the outcome of nine infants with neonatal thyrotoxicosis and noted normal growth but a high incidence of craniosynostosis and intellectual impairment. It may, therefore, be necessary to treat the asymptomatic mother with thioamides and propranolol (and thyroid replacement) during

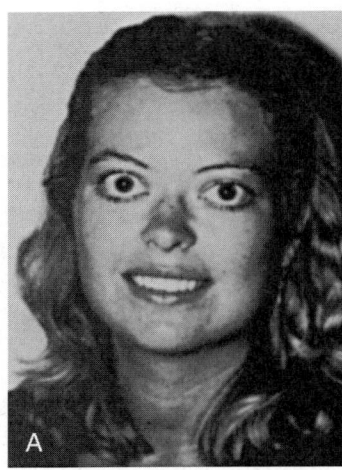
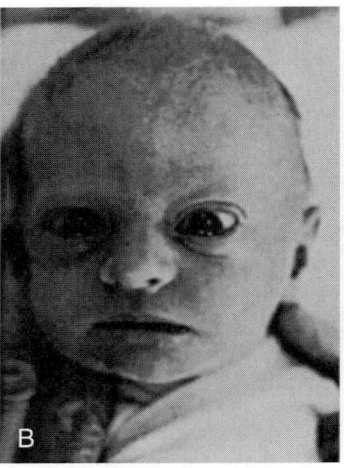
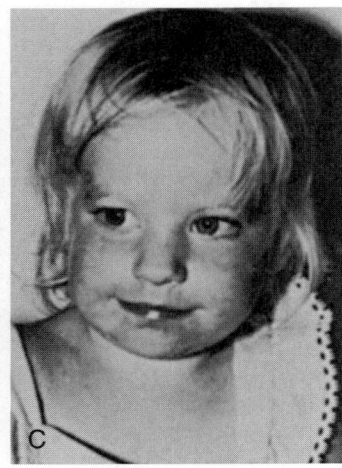

FIGURE 7–4. *A,* Hypothyroid 21-year-old mother who developed Graves disease at age 7 and was treated by subtotal thyroidectomy. She was given maintenance therapy with daily levothyroxine sodium (Synthroid), 0.15 mg, throughout pregnancy. *B,* Her infant girl was born at term with severe Graves disease, goiter, and exophthalmos that persisted for 6 months. *C,* Child was normal at age 20 months. (From Creasy RK, Resnik R [Eds]: Maternal-Fetal Medicine: Principles and Practice, 2nd ed. Philadelphia, WB Saunders, 1989.)

pregnancy to treat the infant and prevent serious neonatal morbidity and long-term problems.

Mothers with thyrotoxicosis who are taking normal doses of thioamides may safely breast-feed their infants, although thioamides do appear in breast milk in low amounts. Currently, there does not appear to be any long-term adverse outcome for infants whose mothers have received PTU during pregnancy.

Hypothyroidism

Maternal hypothyroidism ordinarily can be classified as primary in nature because secondary hypothyroidism owing to pituitary disease is rare in young women, accounting for fewer than 5% of the cases. The principal causes of hypothyroidism in pregnant women are chronic lymphocytic thyroiditis and previous treatment for Graves disease. Other causes include previous therapy with ^{131}I, subtotal thyroidectomy, or exposure to excessive doses of PTU. Ordinarily, maternal hypothyroidism occurring during pregnancy is relatively mild because severe hypothyroidism results in failure of ovulation. This makes diagnosis particularly difficult during pregnancy. Many women have an increased requirement for thyroxine replacement during pregnancy (Mandel et al, 1990). Pregnancies complicated by untreated hypothyroidism may be associated with increased fetal loss or prolongation of gestation.

Treatment with replacement doses of thyroid hormone is usually well tolerated and easily titrated. The clinician must be aware of the fact that the increased thyroid-binding globulin levels in maternal plasma may result in movement of thyroid hormone from the fetus to the mother with a decrease in severity of her disease during the pregnancy. Hypothyroidism has occurred in the fetus when the mother has received ^{131}I inadvertently during pregnancy. There is currently no reliable method for diagnosing hypothyroidism in utero.

REFERENCES

Acker DB, Sachs BP, Friedman EA: Risk factors for shoulder dystocia in the average weight infant. Obstet Gynecol 67:614, 1986.

Becerra JE, Khoury MJ, Cordero JF, Erickson JD: Diabetes mellitus during pregnancy and the risks for specific birth defects: A population based case-control study. Pediatrics 85:1, 1990.

Bernstein IM, Catalano PM: Influence of fetal fat on the ultrasound estimation of fetal weight in diabetic mothers. Obstet Gynecol 79:561, 1992.

Caplan RH, Pagliara AS, Beguin EA, et al: Constant intravenous insulin infusion during labor and delivery in diabetes mellitus. Diabetes Care 5:6, 1982.

Cousins L: The California Diabetes and Pregnancy Programme: A state-wide collaborative programme for the pre-conception and prenatal care of diabetic women. Balliere's Clin Obstet Gynecol 5:443, 1991.

Craigin EB, Ryder GH: Obstetrics: A Practical Textbook for Students and Practitioners. Philadelphia, Lea & Febiger, 1916.

Creasy RK, Resnik R (Eds): Maternal Fetal Medicine: Principles and Practice, 2nd ed. Philadelphia, WB Saunders, 1989.

Daneman D, Howard NJ: Neonatal thyrotoxicosis: Intellectual impairment and craniosynostosis in later years. J Pediatr 97:257, 1980.

DeLee JB: The Principles and Practice of Obstetrics, 3rd ed. Philadelphia, WB Saunders, 1920.

de Veciana M, Major CA, Morgan MA, et al: Postprandial versus preprandial blood glucose monitoring in women with gestational diabetes mellitus requiring insulin therapy [see comments]. N Engl J Med 333:1237, 1995.

Diamond MP, Shah DM, Hester RA, et al: Complication of insulin-dependent diabetic pregnancies by pre-eclampsia and/or chronic hypertension: Analysis of outcome. Am J Perinatol 2:263, 1985.

Ferrero A, Maggi E, Giancotti A, et al: Regression formula for estimation of fetal weight with use of abdominal circumference and femur length: A prospective study. J Ultrasound Med 13:823, 1994.

Frantz ID III, Epstein MF: Fetal lung development in pregnancies complicated by diabetes. *In* Merkatz IR, Adam PAJ (Eds): The Diabetic Pregnancy: A Perinatal Perspective. New York, Grune & Stratton, 1979.

Freinkel N, Metzger BE: Pregnancy as a tissue culture experience: The critical implications of maternal metabolism for fetal development. *In* Pregnancy Metabolism, Diabetes and the Fetus. CIBA Foundation Symposium 63 (new series). Amsterdam, Excerpta Medica, 1979.

Fuhrmann K, Reiher H, Semmler K, et al: Prevention of congenital malformations in infants of insulin-dependent diabetic mothers. Diabetes Care 6:219, 1983.

Gabbe SG, Lowensohn RI, Wu PYK, Guerra G: Current patterns of neonatal morbidity and mortality in infants of diabetic mothers. Diabetes Care 1:334, 1978.

Goldberg JD, Franklin B, Lasser D, et al: Gestational diabetes: Impact of home glucose monitoring on neonatal birth weight. Am J Obstet Gynecol 154:546, 1986.

Gutgesell HP, Mullins CE, Gillette PC, et al: Transient hypertrophic subaortic stenosis in infants of diabetic mothers. J Pediatr 89:120, 1976.

Hedriana H, Moore TR: Comparison of single vs multiple growth sonography in predicting birthweight. Am J Obstet Gynecol 170:1600, 1994.

Hollingsworth DR: Endocrine disorders in pregnancy. *In* Creasy RK, Resnik R (Eds): Maternal-Fetal Medicine: Principles and Practice, 2nd ed. Philadelphia, WB Saunders, 1989.

Hollingsworth DR, Cousins L: Diabetes in pregnancy: A new perspective. *In* Milunsky A, Friedman E, Gluck L (Eds): Advances in Perinatal Medicine, Vol 2. New York, Plenum Press, 1981.

Jorge CS, Artal R, Paul RH, et al: Antepartum fetal surveillance in diabetic pregnant patients. Am J Obstet Gynecol 141:641, 1981.

Jovanovic-Peterson L, Peterson CM, Reed GF, et al: Maternal postprandial glucose levels and infant birth weight: The Diabetes in Early Pregnancy Study. The National Institute of Child Health and Human Development—Diabetes in Early Pregnancy Study. Am J Obstet Gynecol 164:103, 1991.

Keller JD, Lopez-Zeno JA, Dooley SL, Socol ML: Shoulder dystocia and birth trauma in gestational diabetes: A five-year experience. Am J Obstet Gynecol 165(4 Pt 1):928, 1991.

Kjos SL, Henry OA, Montoro M, et al: Insulin-requiring diabetes in pregnancy: A randomized trial of active induction of labor and expectant management. Am J Obstet Gynecol 169:611, 1993.

Kjos SL, Walther FJ, Montoro M, et al: Prevalence and etiology of respiratory distress in infants of diabetic mothers: Predictive value of fetal lung maturation tests. Am J Obstet Gynecol 163:898, 1990.

Landon MB, Mintz MC, Gabbe SG: Sonographic evaluation of fetal abdominal growth: Predictor of the large for gestational age infant in pregnancies complicated by diabetes mellitus. Am J Obstet Gynecol 160:115, 1989.

Larsen T, Greisen G, Petersen S: Prediction of birth weight by ultrasound-estimated fetal weight: A comparison between single and repeated estimates. Eur J Obstet Gynecol Reprod Biol 60:37, 1995.

Lucas MJ, Leveno KJ, Williams ML, et al: Early pregnancy glycosylated hemoglobin, severity of diabetes, and fetal malformations. Am J Obstet Gynecol 161:426, 1989.

Lurie S, Matzkel A, Weissman A, et al: Outcome of pregnancy in class A1 and A2 gestational diabetic patients delivered beyond 40 weeks' gestation. Am J Perinatol 9:484, 1992

Mace S, Hirschfeld SS, Riggs T, et al: Echocardiographic abnormalities in infants of diabtic mothers. J Pediatr 95:1013, 1979.

Mandel SJ, Larsen PR, Seely EW, et al: Increased need for thyroxine during pregnancy in women with primary hypothyroidism. N Engl J Med 323:91, 1990.

McKenzie JM, Zakarija M: Pathogenesis of neonatal Graves' disease. J Endocrinol Invest 2:183, 1978.

McLaren RA, Puckett JL, Chauhan SP: Estimators of birth weight in pregnant women requiring insulin: A comparison of seven sonographic models. Obstet Gynecol 85:565, 1995

Miller E, Hare JW, Cloherty JP, et al: Elevated maternal HbA1c in early pregnancy and major congenital anomalies in infants of diabetic mothers. N Engl J Med 304:1331, 1981.

Mimouni F, Miodovnik M, Rosenn B, et al: Birth trauma in insulin-dependent diabetic pregnancies. Am J Perinatol 9:205, 1992.

Moore TR, Cayle JE: The amniotic fluid index in normal human pregnancy. Am J Obstet Gynecol 162:1168, 1990.

Moore TR, Key TC, Reisner LS, et al: Evaluation of the use of continuous lumbar epidural anesthesia for hypertensive pregnant women in labor. Am J Obstet Gynecol 152:85, 1985.

Ogata ES, Sabbagha R, Metzger BE, et al: Serial ultrasonography to assess evolving fetal macrosomia: Studies in 23 pregnant diabetic women. JAMA 243:2405, 1980.

Pedersen J: Diabetes and Pregnancy: Blood Sugar of Newborn Infants. Copenhagen, Danish Science, 1952.

Pederson J: The Pregnant Diabetic and Her Newborn, 2nd ed. Baltimore, Williams & Wilkins, 1977, p 9.

Pinter E, Peyman JA, Snow K, et al: Effects of maternal diabetes on fetal rat lung ion transport: Contribution of alveolar and bronchiolar epithelial cells. J Clin Invest 87:821, 1991.

Pinter E, Reece EA, Leranth CZ, et al: Arachidonic acid prevents hyperglycemia-associated yolk sac damage and embryopathy. Am J Obstet Gynecol 155:691, 1986.

Rasmussen MJ, Firth R, Foley M, Stronge JM: The timing of delivery in diabetic pregnancy: A 10-year review. Aust N Z J Obstet Gynaecol 32:313, 1992.

Reece EA, Winn HN, Smikle C, et al: Sonographic assessment of growth of the fetal head in diabetic pregnancies compared with normal gestations. Am J Perinatol 7:18, 1990.

Sandmire HF, OHalloin TJ: Shoulder dystocia: Its incidence and associated risk factors. Int J Gynaecol Obstet 26:65, 1988.

Shamley KT, Landon MB: Accuracy and modifying factors for ultrasonographic determination of fetal weight at term. Obstet Gynecol 84:926, 1994.

Shelley-Jones DC, Beischer NA, Sheedy MT, Walstab JE: Excessive birth weight and maternal glucose tolerance—a 19-year review. Aust N Z J Obstet Gynaecol 32:318, 1992.

Shepherd MJ, Richards VA, Berkowitz RL, et al: An evaluation of two equations for predicting fetal weight by ultrasound. Am J Obstet Gynecol 142:47, 1982.

Silverman BL, Metzger BE, Cho NH, Loeb CA: Impaired glucose tolerance in adolescent offspring of diabetic mothers: Relationship to fetal hyperinsulinism. Diabetes Care 18:611, 1995.

Sunshine P, Kusomoto H, Kriss JP: Survival time of long-acting thyroid stimulator in neonatal thyrotoxicosis: Implications of diagnosis and therapy of the disorder. Pediatrics 36:869, 1965.

Susa JB, McCormick KL, Widness JA, et al: Chronic hyperinsulinemia in the fetal rhesus monkey: Effects of fetal growth and composition. Diabetes 25:1058, 1979.

Tamura RK, Sabbagha RE, Dooley SL, et al: Real-time ultrasound estimations of weight in fetuses of diabetic gravid women. Am J Obstet Gynecol 153:57, 1985.

Tongsong T, Piyamongkol W, Sreshthaputra O: Accuracy of ultrasonic fetal weight estimation: A comparison of three equations employed for estimating fetal weight. J Med Assoc Thai 77:373, 1994.

Tsang RC, Brown DR, Steicher JJ: Diabetes and calcium: Calcium disturbances in infants of diabetic mothers. *In* Merkatz IR, Adam PAJ (Eds): The Diabetic Pregnancy: A Perinatal Perspective. New York, Grune & Stratton, 1979.

Tsang RC, Strub R, Brown DR, et al: Hypomagnesemia in infants of diabetic mothers: Perinatal studies. J Pediatr 89:115, 1976.

Widness JA, Teramo KA, Clemons GK, et al: Direct relationship of antepartum glucose control and fetal erythropoietin in human type 1 (insulin dependent) diabetic pregnancy. Diabetologia 33:378, 1990.

Williams JW: Obstetrics: A Textbook for the Use of Students and Practitioners. New York, D Appleton, 1925.

CHAPTER 8

Maternal Medical Disorders of Fetal Significance: Seizure Disorders, Hypertension, and Isoimmunization

Thomas Kelly and Thomas R. Moore

A significant spectrum of medical complications may complicate pregnancy. Some of these, very manageable in the nonpregnant patient, can be lethal to the gravid woman. Thus, two basic questions arise when dealing with the pregnant female who is experiencing a medical complication. First, is the condition affected by the patient's normal adaptations to pregnancy? Second, how does the medical problem affect the patient and her fetus? Although many medical conditions during pregnancy can be managed similarly to those in the nonpregnant woman, there are usually nuances to the care during gestation to which the obstetrician must be attuned.

During pregnancy, medical therapeutics should be carefully scrutinized so that fetal risks are minimized. In the past, thalidomide and diethylstilbestrol were prescribed for morning sickness and recurrent miscarriages but resulted in significant and tragic congenital anomalies in the offspring. Today the benefit expected of each medication prescribed to a pregnant woman should be weighed against potential risk, such as phenytoin in the patient with epilepsy. Also, because pharmacokinetics may be altered by changes in maternal physiology, dosage of familiar medications may have to be adjusted. Classic examples include thyroid hormone replacement (in which an increased thyroid-binding globulin increases total thyroxine [T_4] but leaves serum free T_4 unchanged) and aminoglycoside antibiotic therapy (increased glomerular filtration results in lower serum drug levels). This chapter focuses on three maternal conditions that may influence fetal growth, development, and outcome: seizure disorders, hypertensive states, and red blood cell isoimmunization. The basics of management, the potential effects of pregnancy on the condition, and the effects of the condition on the gravida and the fetus are discussed.

MATERNAL SEIZURE DISORDERS

Epilepsy is not uncommon, affecting more than 2 million people in the United States. The prevalence in pregnancy is approximately 0.5%. Seizures range from complex partial to generalized tonic-clonic and generalized absence (petit mal). Physiologically, they arise from paroxysmal episodes of abnormal brain electrical discharges, and when associated with motor activity they are termed *convulsive*.

The effect of pregnancy on the course of the seizure disorder is controversial, with significant variability from patient to patient. Although in a few patients the condition worsens (approximately 25% of cases) (Willhelm et al, 1990), some do improve, but most remain the same. Prepregnancy medical control may influence the patient's course during gestation; those who are poorly controlled

tend to have increased seizure frequency, whereas those who are seizure free for 2 years have only a 10% risk of convulsing during gestation (Schmidt et al, 1983).

Perinatal Risk

Women with seizures have more obstetric complications during pregnancy and an increased rate of poor perinatal outcomes. Preeclampsia, preterm delivery, small-for-gestational-age infants, congenital malformations, cerebral palsy, and perinatal mortality all are increased in women with an antecedent seizure disorder (Nelson and Ellenberg, 1982). Pregnancy outcome is also influenced greatly by the patient's socioeconomic status, prenatal care, and maternal age.

The well-documented increased frequency of congenital malformations among women with seizure disorders is curious because it is observed irrespective of fetal exposure to anticonvulsant medications (Bjerkedal, 1982). The malformation risk is, however, correlated with the severity of epilepsy and the number of medications used. Overall, the risk is increased over baseline by 3.5% to 4.4%. Specific malformations reported include a fivefold increase in orofacial clefts (Friis et al, 1986); an increase in congenital heart disease, particularly with trimethadione (Friis and Hauge, 1985); and a 1% to 2% incidence of neural tube defects in fetuses exposed to valproic acid (Lammer et al, 1987). Facial abnormalities (e.g., midface hypoplasia) are not specific to any particular antiepileptic drug and are seen with phenytoin, carbamazepine, and trimethadione.

The classic features of the hydantoin syndrome include facial clefting, broad nasal ridge, hypertelorism, epicanthal folds, distal phalangeal hypoplasia, and growth and mental deficiency; however, these features are shared with other antiseizure medications as well. The postulated cause for this common syndrome is a common epoxide intermediate of these medications acting on a teratogen. The hydantoin syndrome developed in those fetuses with inadequate epoxide hydrolase activity (Buehler et al, 1990). This enzymatic deficiency appears to be recessively inherited.

Management

Management of the patient with epilepsy is based on keeping the patient seizure free. Theoretically, this approach reduces maternal physical risk and lowers the incidence of fetal complications. Preconceptional counseling is preferable and should entail adjusting medication dosages into the therapeutic range, attempting to limit the patient to one drug if possible, and choosing an agent with the least risk of teratogenesis. Frank discussion of the various risks of each agent should be conducted, particularly regarding those associated with valproic acid and trimethadione. Usually if the patient is adequately controlled on one agent, it rarely needs to be changed, because the risks of increasing seizures are believed to outweigh the potential for reducing congenital malformations.

Patients taking antiepileptic medication should also have preconceptional folic acid supplements because inhibition of folate absorption has been proposed as a teratogenic mechanism, particularly with phenytoin. During gestation, the anticonvulsant levels should be checked monthly and the dose adjusted accordingly. Medications should not be changed unless they are proven ineffective at the optimal serum level. If a patient reports increased seizure activity, the serum level should be checked immediately. A common source of increased seizures is the patient not taking her medication, usually because of the fear of teratogenicity.

Mothers taking phenytoin, phenobarbital, or primidone may have an increased incidence of neonatal coagulopathy as a result of vitamin K–dependent clotting factor deficiency. Maternal vitamin K supplementation in the third trimester is reasonable; a single parenteral dose of 10 mg can be given.

HYPERTENSIVE DISORDERS

Hypertension is one the most common disorders complicating pregnancy, affecting approximately 1 in 10 gravidas. The majority of hypertensive disease is preeclampsia; only about 30% is chronic essential hypertension. Differentiating between the two is important because the significant fetal and maternal complications associated with preeclampsia are usually more common and more devastating. Additionally, management strategies are markedly different. Preeclampsia may lead to maternal convulsions, renal failure, and coagulopathy. However, the chronic hypertension, apart from threatening maternal well-being with stroke and fetal well-being with placental abruption, does not typically lead to multisystem dysfunction.

Chronic Hypertension

Classification

Four categories of hypertensive disorders have been classified by the American College of Obstetricians and Gynecologists (Table 8–1). *Chronic hypertension* is defined as (1) blood pressure of 140/90 mm Hg before pregnancy or before 20 weeks' gestation in cases in which the preconception blood pressures are unknown or (2) persistent hypertension more than 6 weeks' postpartum. In distinction, *preeclampsia* usually presents in the third trimester, only

TABLE 8–1

Hypertensive Disorders in Pregnancy

Preeclampsia/eclampsia
Chronic hypertension
Chronic hypertension with superimposed preeclampsia
Transient hypertension

TABLE 8–2

High-Risk Factors in the Hypertensive Patient

Maternal age >40 years
Duration of hypertension >15 years
Blood pressure >160/110 mm Hg early in pregnancy
Pregestational diabetes
Cardiomyopathy
Renal disease
Connective tissue disease

rarely is noted earlier than 26 weeks, and resolves within the first few weeks' postpartum. *Transient* or *gestational hypertension*, usually recognized in the near-term patient, commonly presents as increased blood pressure in labor without the classic stigmata of preeclampsia and resolves promptly after delivery. It may be difficult to differentiate among the various types of hypertension because the patient may not have blood pressure measurements recorded preconceptionally, and the midtrimester decreases in blood pressure may be due to exacerbation of chronic hypertension or the onset of superimposed preeclampsia.

Etiology

Most chronic hypertension does not have an identifiable cause such as renovascular stenosis, pheochromocytoma, or coarctation of the aorta, although these discrete diagnoses should be excluded. What remains is essential hypertension. High blood pressure is associated with increased maternal and perinatal morbidity and mortality (Page et al, 1975). These complications are more severe in those with underlying renal disease or other medical condition coexistent with the hypertension.

Perinatal Risk

Risks to the patient and fetus can be classified as either low or high depending on the presence of factors listed in Table 8–2. Preconceptional assessment of the patient allows exploration of these factors and permits counseling of the patient about the risks not only of hypertension but also of medications used to control blood pressure. Low-risk hypertensive patients tend to have outcomes similar to those of normotensive population. "High-risk" patients have an increased frequency of superimposed preeclampsia (52%), stillbirth, and neonatal death (Sibai and Anderson, 1986). The poor outcomes usually are the result of the development of superimposed preeclampsia early in the third trimester, necessitating preterm delivery.

Diagnosis and Treatment

The initial evaluation of the hypertensive patient includes a careful search for the physical clues for the cause of hypertension. This should include blood pressure in all extremities, antinuclear antibody, possibly urine metanephrines, as well as funduscopy, 24-hour urine for protein and creatinine clearance, and electrocardiogram. Careful dating of the pregnancy is important not only to establish reliable due dates but also to enable the obstetrician to assess the adequacy of fetal growth.

Patients should be seen twice monthly until 30 weeks and weekly thereafter. At each visit the blood pressure should be recorded, performed with the patient seated upright. Mean arterial pressure usually falls in the mid-trimester and then returns to the prepregnancy value as the patient approaches term. This trend is seen in both normotensive and most hypertensive patients but may not occur in individuals destined to become preeclamptic or in those with significant essential hypertension. Urine is checked for proteinuria, and weight is noted. Edema that is 3+ or 4+ or a 4-pound weight gain in 1 week is a signal of evolving preeclampsia. Lack of maternal weight gain may be a sign of fetal growth restriction. Serial sonograms are usually obtained monthly to assess fetal growth and amniotic fluid volume. Antenatal biophysical testing to assess fetal well-being is started by 34 to 36 weeks and sooner if there is a specific fetal or maternal indication such as growth retardation or the development of superimposed preeclampsia. Fetal movement counting is a helpful adjunct from 28 weeks onward. Delivery is usually at term or earlier if complications develop, such as superimposed preeclampsia or significant intrauterine growth retardation. Only in rare cases is a hypertensive patient allowed to go beyond 40½ weeks' gestation.

Antihypertensive therapy in the mildly hypertensive, pregnant patient is usually withheld because use of antihypertensives does not appear to decrease the incidence of superimposed preeclampsia (Sibai et al, 1990). However, most experts treat patients when blood pressure exceeds 160/110 mm Hg. The main role of antihypertensive medication is to reduce the patient's risk of stroke. In the short period of a 9-month gestation, mild hypertension (140/90 mm Hg) is well tolerated in the gravida without significant morbidity. However, medications used to lower systemic blood pressure pose two potential threats to the fetus: (1) direct pharmacologic effects such as teratogenesis, metabolic consequences such as hypoglycemia in the case of beta blockers, and renal effects (oligohydramnios) with angiotensin-converting enzyme inhibitors; and (2) reduction of uterine blood flow, which may result in poor fetal growth or hypoxia.

The antihypertensive agent used most commonly is methyldopa. It acts centrally by stimulating alpha$_2$-adrenergic receptors, and blood pressure effect is maximal by 4 hours. The drug is given orally in divided doses that usually range from 1 to 2 g/day. Because the safety of this drug is well documented (Cockburn et al, 1982), methyldopa is the first-line agent, and failure to control blood pressure necessitates adding or switching to medications that may pose more of a risk. Beta blockers such as atenolol and labetalol are typical second-line agents, but the side effects, such as ominous fetal heart patterns, poor fetal growth, and neonatal hypoglycemia, can be difficult to manage. Nifedipine, a calcium channel blocker used not only for hypertension but also for management of preterm labor, is a commonly used second- or third-line drug, but large-scale studies of its safety and efficacy in pregnancy are lacking at present.

TABLE 8–3

Diagnosis of Preeclampsia

Blood pressure >140/90 mm Hg, two measurements 6 or more hours apart or an increase of 30 mm Hg systolic/15 mm Hg diastolic from first-trimester values
Proteinuria >300 mg/24 hr *or* > 1+ on two consecutive specimens
Significant nondependent edema

Preeclampsia

Preeclampsia is a uniquely human pregnancy disorder characterized by unpredictable onset of *edema, hypertension,* and *proteinuria.* The criteria for diagnosis are listed in Tables 8–3 and 8–4. A defining characteristic of preeclampsia is its typically prompt and complete resolution with delivery of the fetus. Variously referred to as *toxemia, gestosis, hypertension with proteinuria,* and *pregnancy-induced hypertension,* preeclampsia usually results in successful vaginal delivery of a healthy neonate. However, some patients experience severe multisystem decompensation. In its full-blown form, severe preeclampsia may lead to pulmonary and cerebral edema; convulsions and intracerebral hemorrhage; oliguria and renal failure; cardiovascular collapse; and death of mother, fetus, or both. Despite advances in many areas of perinatal medicine, the incidence of preeclampsia has not changed, affecting 5% to 7% of pregnancies in the United States. It continues to be a major cause of maternal and perinatal morbidity and mortality (Chamberlain et al, 1978).

Etiology

Preeclampsia is a disease of theories, but no single etiologic thesis adequately explains the protean manifestations of

---

TABLE 8–4

Diagnosis of Severe Preeclampsia

Diagnostic Criterion	Finding
Blood pressure	Persistently >160/110 mm Hg
Proteinuria, oliguria	>5 g/24 hr
	<30 mL/hr, <400 mL/24 hr
RUQ or epigastric pain	Suggests liver-capsule distention
Central nervous system dysfunction	Blurry vision, scotomata, severe headaches, altered sensorium
Pulmonary edema, cyanosis	Rales, chest radiograph evidence of pulmonary edema, hypoxia on blood gas
Eclampsia	Seizures or postictal state
HELLP syndrome	Hemolysis, elevated transaminases (2 × normal), low platelets (<100,000 mm³)
Significant fetal growth retardation	Tapering or cessation of growth, growth at or below the 10th percentile

RUQ, right upper quadrant.

TABLE 8–5

Theories of Cause of Preeclampsia

Theory	Evidence
Excessive placental mass	Increased incidence in twins, molar gestation
Immunologic	Increased incidence in first pregnancy
Placental ischemia	Increased incidence of fetal growth retardation
Genetic	Autosomal recessive inheritance pattern
Imbalance of prostaglandins	Aspirin therapy somewhat protective
Endothelial injury	Renal hepatic dysfunction, coagulopathy

this disorder. Current etiologic candidates are listed in Table 8–5. Despite the paucity of knowledge of fundamental mechanisms underlying its multisystem effects, certain common themes are evident:

■ Hypertension is a central symptom, with affected patients having hyperresponsiveness to endogenous pressor mechanisms, suggesting deranged regulation of vascular tone.

■ Total body water is increased and maternal vascular volume is reduced compared with nonpreeclamptic pregnant control subjects, suggesting disordered vascular permeability mechanisms. Reduced circulating volume is associated with poor placental perfusion, fetal growth retardation, and fetal distress.

■ An imbalance of prostaglandin metabolites is found in affected patients, with thromboxanes (TXs) (and their vasospastic properties) exceeding prostacylin levels, leading to tissue ischemia, platelet consumption, and microvascular coagulation.

■ Histologically, the uterine spiral arteries that supply the placenta have atherotic deposits that compromise their caliber and reduce transplacental nutrient flow (Fig. 8–1). This suggests that endothelial damage is a primary mechanism underlying placental ischemia (Roberts et al, 1989).

Effects on the Fetus and Neonate

Perinatal Morbidity and Mortality

The fetal-neonatal mortality associated with preeclampsia is twofold to fivefold higher than in normotensive pregnancy, mostly because of iatrogenic prematurity, occasioned to preserve maternal health. However, with severe preeclampsia, a number of other complications may threaten fetal survival as well. The risk of placental abruption increases with advancing maternal hypertension. Once progressive placental separation begins to evolve, oxygen transfer capacity falls, uterine hypertonus is induced, and fetal asphyxia follows. Eclamptic seizures pose a particularly significant danger to the fetus. Typically starting with tonic-clonic spasms, eclampsia is rapidly followed by maternal apnea, which may last 3 to 10 minutes. During this time, with rapid maternal oxygen desaturation, the fetus quickly

becomes hypoxic and bradycardic. Although maternal respiration is typically restored during the postictal phase, the previous hypoxia may leave the fetus significantly compromised. Maternal pulmonary aspiration of gastric contents or abruptio placentae may further complicate maternal and fetal status. Severe fetal heart rate abnormalities are usual both during and for up to 30 minutes after the seizure. Long-term effects range from fetal death to other sequelae of hypoxic ischemic damage, such as long-term neurologic deficit, acute tubular necrosis, and necrotizing enterocolitis.

Intrauterine Growth Retardation

Elevated vascular resistance associated with preeclampsia is seen in the uterine vasculature as well. Studies by Hutter and associates (1993) indicate that uterine artery flow characteristics are abnormal (high resistance indicated by diastolic "notching") and can be detected in patients destined to become preeclamptic as early as the first trimester using Doppler velocimetry. Ultimately, this long-standing restriction in uterine perfusion leads to intrauterine growth retardation (IUGR). Depending on the degree of growth restriction and placental dysfunction, affected infants have a high rate of stillbirth and perinatal asphyxia, tolerate labor poorly, and are often delivered through meconium, which contributes further to their perinatal morbidity. Polycythemia, hyperviscosity, and hypoglycemia resulting from decreased glycogen stores are frequent complications in the newborn.

Respiratory Distress Syndrome

Gluck and Kulovich (1973) postulated that maternal hypertensive states provided a stimulative effect on fetal lung

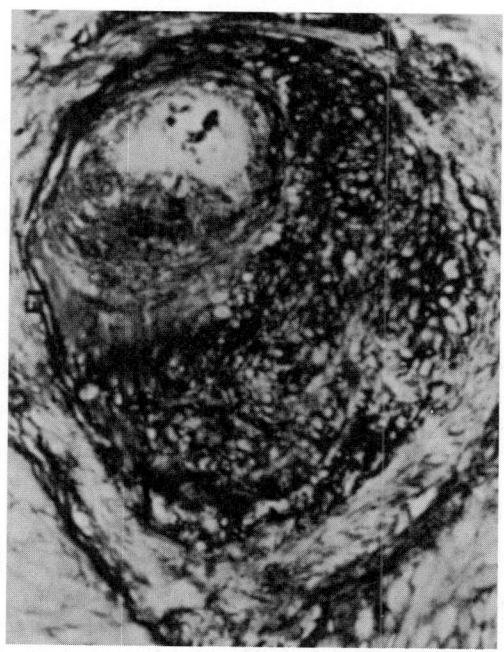

FIGURE 8–1. Atherosis: numerous lipid-laden cells and fibrin deposition are present in the media of this occluded decidual vessel. (From Sheppard BD, Bonnar J: Uteroplacental arteries and hypertensive pregnancy. *In* Bonnar J, MacGillivray I, Symonds G [Eds]: Pregnancy Hypertension. Baltimore, MD, University Park Press, 1980.)

maturation. Similarly, Yoon and coworkers (1980) observed that the incidence of respiratory distress syndrome (RDS) was less among infants of mothers with hypertensive disease, controlled for gestational age. In infants younger than 32 weeks' gestation, the incidence of RDS was reduced from 41% to 26%. Morbidity and mortality were similar among infants with RDS regardless of maternal hypertension, and mortality was actually increased in the hypertensive group *without* RDS, suggesting that although preeclampsia promotes advanced fetal pulmonary maturation, it also carries other risks related to chronic hypoxemia.

Effect of Maternal Pharmacotherapy

Because preeclamptic mothers typically receive magnesium sulfate infusions as seizure prophylaxis, their infants often exhibit hypermagnesemia, apnea, hypotension, and slow responsiveness postnatally. On balance, given the usual maternal magnesium levels of 4.5 to 6.0 mg/dL associated with infusion rates of 2 g/hour, newborn levels, usually roughly equivalent, are not high enough to cause significant newborn morbidity unless IUGR or extreme prematurity is present.

Thrombocytopenia and Neutropenia

Preeclampsia is frequently complicated by platelet dysfunction and thrombocytopenia (see later discussion of HELLP syndrome). Infants of preeclamptic mothers may share in these coagulation disorders; almost half of infants born to mothers with thrombocytopenia also have platelet counts less than 150,000/mm^3 at birth. Again, this rarely impacts the neonate long term unless extreme prematurity or intrapartum asphyxia are coexistent. Typically, affected newborns' platelet counts rise rapidly to normal levels within 1 to 3 days. Infants born to mothers with the HELLP syndrome may also have neutropenia, the cause of which is not clear. It may be related to agents that cause endothelial damage in the mother and cross the placenta (Weinstein, 1986).

Prevention of Preeclampsia

By the time preeclampsia becomes clinically manifest, the disease process is usually quite advanced, and the clinician's role is to minimize associated morbidity. Ideally, it is preferable to prevent, not treat, preeclampsia. However, a successful preventive strategy requires not only an effective intervention but a sensitive and specific screening test to identify those susceptible to the disease.

To date, a reliable and clinically useful preeclampsia screening test has not been developed. Although provocative tests that identify those with abnormal vascular responses to pressor stimuli have been proposed (e.g., angiotensin challenge test and the "rollover test") (Gant et al, 1973), these have proven to be expensive, time consuming, and difficult to apply to a large clinical population.

However, certain groups of patients at high risk for preeclampsia have been identified, namely

- Those who are nulliparous
- Adolescents

- Members of lower socioeconomic groups
- Those with preexisting vascular disease such as chronic hypertension, insulin-dependent diabetes, and collagen vascular disease
- Those with preeclampsia in a prior pregnancy
- Those who are pregnant with multifetal gestations

Typically, most of the currently favored preventive or ameliorative therapies for preeclampsia are applied to the high-risk groups just listed.

Pharmacologic Prevention of Preeclampsia

Currently, the principal pharmacologic agent used in prevention of preeclampsia is low-dose aspirin (40–81 mg/day). The theory behind this approach involves the ability of low-dose aspirin to inhibit platelet TX synthesis while minimally affecting prostacyclin (PGI) synthesis (Benigni et al, 1986; Schiff et al, 1986). Presumably, low-dose aspirin therapy favorably alters the PGI-TX ratio, protects the endothelial cell from damage, and prevents initiation of the cascade of intravascular events that leads to clinically evident preeclampsia.

Initially, multiple, small clinical trials successfully demonstrated that low-dose aspirin markedly reduces the incidence of preeclampsia. In a meta-analysis of 394 patients in six randomized trials, Imperiale and colleagues (1991) reported a 65% reduction in clinical disease. However, more recent larger trials have shown less dramatic results. A large European multicenter trial (CLASP) of 9364 women demonstrated a reduction of only 12% in the incidence of preeclampsia, which was not significant. Nor was there any significant effect on the incidence of IUGR or of stillbirth and neonatal death. Aspirin did, however, significantly reduce the likelihood of preterm delivery (19.7% aspirin vs. 22.2% control). Another study of 3135 women reported that the incidence of preeclampsia was lower in the aspirin group (4.6%) than in the placebo group (6.3%) with a relative risk of 0.7. There were no significant differences in the infants' birth weight or in the incidence of fetal growth retardation, postpartum hemorrhage, or neonatal bleeding problems between the two groups (Sibai et al, 1993). Thus, it now appears that although low-dose aspirin is safe and moderately efficacious, the major desired end points (prematurity and perinatal morbidity) are not sharply reduced. At present, the use of aspirin in pregnancy is controversial and probably useful only with patients at substantial risk for preeclampsia.

In informing the patient of the possible benefits of low-dose aspirin therapy, the potential risks should be mentioned. Although several early studies suggested that exposure to aspirin could have teratogenic effects (McNeil, 1973; Sloan et al, 1976)—specifically increased risk for various congenital cardiac anomalies—18-month follow-up of the CLASP infants demonstrated no differences in congenital malformations, motor deficit, developmental delay, respiratory problems or bleeding problems; height or weight below the third percentile; and delayed acquisition of certain developmental skills (CLASP Collaborative Group, 1995). Other concerns include fetal pulmonary hypertension, delay of onset of labor, coagulation disorders in the mother or fetus (or both), and reduced intelligence quotient scores. The large trials have also failed to confirm these complications (Hauth et al, 1995; Streissguth et al, 1987).

Until the issue regarding low-dose aspirin for the prevention of preeclampsia is clearer, such therapy should be undertaken only after informed consent and under the supervision of a knowledgeable physician. When indicated, aspirin therapy is usually begun at 18 to 20 weeks at a dose of 60 to 81 mg orally daily or every other day. Ideally, this therapy should be discontinued 2 weeks before delivery to permit restoration of normal platelet function.

Dietary Prevention of Preeclampsia

Over the past decades, a number of nonpharmacologic "cures" for preeclampsia have been proposed, but most have met with limited success. These include severe sodium restriction, increases and limitations in protein intake, and reduction of medium-chain triglycerides in the diet. Other nutritional approaches have included zinc, magnesium, and calcium supplementation. Although several reports suggested that relative zinc deficiency may be associated with an increased incidence of preeclampsia, zinc supplementation has not been clinically successful.

Dietary magnesium supplementation in early pregnancy was proposed based on its use intravenously in the treatment of overt preeclampsia. Although several early studies suggested that magnesium supplementation may effectively reduce the incidence of preeclampsia, (Conradt, 1984; Spatling and Spatling, 1988), a randomized clinical trial has failed to support that association (Sibai et al, 1989).

Calcium supplementation has also been proposed to reduce the incidence of preeclampsia (Repke and Villar, 1991). There is a well-described relationship between serum and urinary calcium balance and blood pressure. Increased dietary calcium has been associated with reduced blood pressure in both pregnant and nonpregnant populations. Hypertensive, nonpregnant subjects have higher calcium excretion and lower serum calcium levels than normotensive groups. In pregnant patients, several randomized clinical trials have demonstrated that calcium supplementation (1500–2000 g/day) may reduce vascular sensitivity to angiotensin II and thus lower the clinical incidence of preeclampsia (Repke and Villar, 1991). However, a preliminary report of a large multicenter clinical trial of calcium supplementation in patients at high risk for preeclampsia was disappointing. Clearly, dietary interventions, which appear to offer therapeutic promise with minimal downside, require further investigation to be used effectively.

Treatment of Preeclampsia

With effective primary prevention of preeclampsia an unrealized goal, clinical management that minimizes maternal and fetal morbidity is essential. This begins with precise diagnosis, ensuring that late-gestation hypertension and exacerbations of chronic hypertension are not confused with preeclampsia (see Table 8–4). Strictly defined, preeclampsia is the triad of hypertension with proteinuria or edema or both. Given that the diagnosis of preeclampsia is made with relative certainty, decisions regarding manage-

ment and timing of delivery should be made carefully, with due consideration for the age of the fetus, the severity of the preeclampsia, and the rate at which it appears to be worsening. If delivery is too early, maternal health will be maintained at the potential expense of newborn morbidity from prematurity. If delivery is too late, both maternal and fetal health may be seriously jeopardized.

Antepartum Management

Management should be governed by the severity of symptoms and the gestational age of the pregnancy. An algorithm for triage management of these patients is presented in Figure 8–2. In stable, compliant, preterm patients with mild disease, strict bed rest at home with close fetal and maternal surveillance is reasonable. For the motivated patient, this may include dipstick urinalysis for proteinuria and blood pressure measurements at home. Semiweekly fetal biophysical testing, either in the home or clinic, is also recommended. In general, once the patient with mild preeclampsia reaches 37 weeks' gestation, induction of labor should be considered. If the cervix is unfavorable, the patient may cautiously be managed expectantly for 7 to 14 days until spontaneous labor or a favorable Bishop cervical score occurs. However, any sign of worsening preeclampsia or fetal compromise should prompt immediate hospitalization and evaluation for delivery.

Once the patient is hospitalized, the goal is to minimize maternal morbidity, optimize perinatal outcome, and effect prompt delivery when indicated. This is accomplished by closely monitoring for signs of severe disease or fetal maturity. When severe preeclampsia is diagnosed at any time in pregnancy, delivery should be performed relatively promptly. Although the notion of continued observation of the preterm patient with severe preeclampsia may be attractive, in fact delay in delivery of such patients actually increases the fetal mortality rate. A possible exception to this rule is during 24 to 27 weeks' gestation in which neonatal mortality and morbidity are high. Cautious observation of such patients may yield a small percentage of

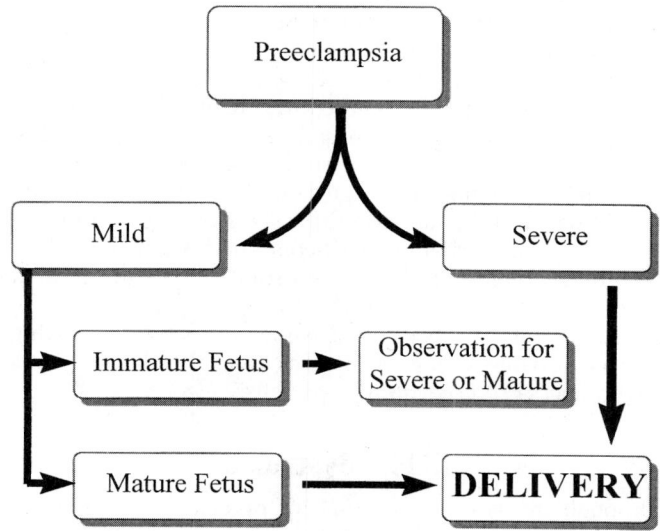

FIGURE 8–2. Management scheme for preeclampsia.

viable neonates, but the overall prognosis is dismal in either case.

Intrapartum Management

Once preeclampsia has progressed to the point at which delivery is required (see Fig. 8–2), the next priority is prevention of progression to eclamptic convulsions. Magnesium sulfate remains the drug used most commonly in the United States for prevention of eclampsia. Although it is not universally accepted that mild preeclampsia requires magnesium sulfate therapy during the intrapartum period, it is the most common practice to begin magnesium infusions during labor and to continue therapy for 24 to 48 hours postpartum. Until recently, there has been considerable controversy as to whether other agents could produce equivalent or superior results in preventing and treating eclamptic seizures. Because convincing animal data regarding magnesium's efficacy in preventing or ameliorating experimentally induced seizures are lacking, the use of other agents such as benzodiazepines and phenytoin has been advocated despite the considerable accumulated clinical experience suggesting its superiority over other single or polypharmaceutical regimens (Pritchard et al, 1984). However, definitive data are now available on this issue. A 1995 randomized trial of magnesium versus hydantoin in more than 2000 women demonstrated clear superiority of magnesium in preventing seizures (Lucas et al, 1995). When magnesium was compared with diazepam in the prevention of eclamptic seizure recurrence in another study, those patients treated with magnesium had 37% fewer adverse events (Collaborative Eclampsia Trial, 1995).

Treatment Protocols

Because the pathogenesis of the eclamptic seizure is incompletely understood, proper use of magnesium sulfate is somewhat empirical. It is known that magnesium competes with calcium for specific ion channels and may, therefore, minimize cellular excitability. Clinically, magnesium also exerts a peripheral effect at the neuromuscular junction, resulting in maternal and newborn flaccidity and respiratory depression if given in high doses. These complications can be avoided by monitoring magnesium levels during labor, with levels between 4 and 8 mEq/L generally accepted as therapeutic. These are achieved by use of a 4-g bolus of intravenous magnesium sulfate followed by 2 g/hour infusion. Because magnesium is primarily excreted by the kidney, patients with oliguria or altered renal function should be carefully monitored for signs of magnesium toxicity. Magnesium therapy is discontinued when the risk of eclampsia is considered to have abated. Although duration of therapy is typically until 24 to 36 hours postpartum, the infusion should be continued while the patient is having central nervous system symptoms (e.g., headache, visual disturbances) or is severely hypertensive.

HELLP Syndrome

Although the typical syndrome of preeclampsia has been recognized for several millennia, only recently has a constellation of hematologic findings been described as a unique subdiagnostic entity. Redman and colleagues in 1978 described a reduction in platelet count as an early manifestation of preeclampsia. The larger syndrome, named in 1982 by Weinstein, is characterized by *h*emolytic anemia, *e*levated *l*iver enzymes, and *l*ow *p*latelet counts (HELLP syndrome). Although usually considered a variant of severe preeclampsia, HELLP syndrome may appear before hypertensive complications and proteinuria become evident. Associated findings with the HELLP syndrome include jaundice; elevated blood urea and creatinine levels; severe right upper quadrant pain; and a firm, tense liver with evidence of subcapsular hematoma. Clotting factors other than platelets are usually normal. The management scheme for HELLP syndrome is the same as for preeclampsia (see Fig. 8–2). The primary objective is stabilization of the mother and the fetus and appropriate decisions regarding timing and route of delivery.

Eclampsia

Eclampsia was recognized by Hippocrates as a convulsive disorder in pregnant women with unusual premonitory visual symptoms (eclampsia is Greek for "lightning," descriptive of the flashing lights seen by many gravidas before their seizure) (Table 8–6). Eclampsia remains a leading cause of maternal death in the United States, England, and Wales (Kaunitz et al, 1985). Eclampsia in the United States currently occurs in approximately 1 per 2500 deliveries.

Initial Management

The best management of eclamptic seizures is to prevent them by infusing magnesium sulfate as soon as preeclampsia is recognized and initiating delivery procedures when it is severe. However, many eclamptic events do not occur in labor. In a study of 186 cases of eclampsia at the University of Tennessee (Sibai et al, 1980), researchers found that seizures occurred postpartum in 28%, and half of these occurred more than 48 hours after delivery. Indeed, only approximately one third of eclamptic events occur during labor, with almost half of all patients convulsing before admission to the delivery unit.

The initial management of the patient who experiences an eclamptic seizure includes prevention of maternal injury and protection of the airway. Most eclamptic seizures are

TABLE 8–6

Patient Symptoms Preceding Eclampsia

Symptom	Percentage of Patients
Headache	83
Hyper-reflexia	80
Clonus	46
Proteinuria	80
Visual signs	45
Epigastric pain	20

Adapted with permission from The American College of Obstetricians and Gynecologists (Obstetrics and Gynecology, 1981, Vol. 57, pp 199–203).

self-limited and, if appropriate maternal protection is afforded, resolve without significant sequelae. Recurrent eclamptic seizures may follow, however, resulting in maternal cardiovascular collapse, intracerebral hemorrhage, fetal asphyxia, or abruptio placentae.

As with most grand mal seizures, the seizure event is characterized by maternal apnea and transient hypoxia, accompanied almost routinely by transient fetal bradycardia. Patience and administration of oxygen usually result in eventual in utero resuscitation of the fetus. The initial resolution of the fetal bradycardia is followed by compensatory tachycardia, usually with some loss of baseline variability. The patient recovers usually within 20 to 30 minutes, and the fetal heart rate returns to its preseizure state unless maternal intracerebral hemorrhage or massive abruptio placentae has occurred.

Delivery

Once the eclamptic patient has been stabilized, timing and route of delivery must be planned. However, emergency delivery, especially "crash" cesarean section, places the mother and fetus at substantially increased risk for morbidity. When maternal status is stable, both vaginal and cesarean delivery routes should be considered. If fetal distress is present and not improving with maternal resuscitation or if the cervix is unfavorable, cesarean section affords the advantage of prompt delivery. Regardless of delivery mode, newborns of eclamptic patients are fragile, typically requiring close observation and hematologic monitoring, indicating the importance of having a skilled neonatal team available at delivery.

ISOIMMUNIZATION

Hydrops fetalis, a condition associated with abnormal fluid collections in various body cavities of the fetus, was first described in 1892. The causes are many but can be broken down into two basic categories: immune and nonimmune. In immune-mediated hydrops, circulating immunoglobulins lead to the destruction of fetal red blood cells and hemolytic anemia. Landsteiner and Weiner first elucidated the rhesus factor in 1940. The pathogenesis of erythroblastosis was shown to be due to maternal isoimmunization in 1941 (Levine et al, 1941). The development of Rh immunoglobulins occurred in the mid-1960s and significantly reduced the number of cases of D isoimmunization and increased the relative frequency of antibody formation against atypical red blood cell antigen. The pathophysiology of immune-mediated fetal hemolytic disease is similar irrespective of the blood group antigen; therefore, the bulk of the discussion is concerned with the Rh system.

Genetics

The Rh blood group actually represents a number of antigens, designated the *D, Cc,* and *Ee antigens.* The genes for these are located on the short arm of chromosome 1 and are inherited in a set of three from each parent. The presence of D determines whether the individual is Rh positive, and the absence of D (d has not been found as

an antigen) types as Rh negative. The combinations of these various antigens occur with different frequencies. For example, Cde prevalence (41%) is higher than CDE (0.08%) (Lewis et al, 1971). Although the Rh phenotype is the result of D status, the various genotype combinations help predict the zygosity of an individual.

There are no sex differences in the frequency of Rh negativity. However, racial variations are striking. It is common in the Basque population (30% to 35%) but rare (1% to 2%) among Chinese, Japanese, and North American Indians. The average incidence in white populations is about 15%. North American blacks have a higher incidence (8%) than African blacks (4%).

Pathogenesis

Before modern blood banking, the Rh-negative patient became immunized from transfusion of Rh-positive blood. In the case of atypical red blood cell antigen (e.g., Duffy, Kidd) isoimmunization, blood transfusion is still a significant cause. Fetal transplacental hemorrhage is currently the primary cause of Rh isoimmunization. Transplacental hemorrhage of fetal cells into the maternal circulation is surprisingly common: 75% of women have evidence of this at some time during gestation (Bowman et al, 1986). Usually, the amount of fetal blood is small, but approximately 1% of women have 5 mL and 0.25% have 30 mL or more. Historic events increase the chance of transplacental hemorrhage (Table 8–7), as does the incidence and amount of hemorrhage with advancing gestational age (from 12% in the first trimester to 45% in the third trimester). As little as 0.3 mL of Rh-positive blood produces immunization, and the risk is dose dependent. ABO blood group incompatibility between fetus and mother affords some protection, reducing the risk from 16% to 2%.

The primary maternal immune response is slow and may take as long as 6 months to develop. IgM class antibodies form first and do not cross the placenta; the IgG class antibodies are produced soon after the IgM class and do cross the placenta. Therefore, the initial event causing sensitization rarely results in fetal hemolysis. A second transplacental hemorrhage then results in the more rapid and abundant immunoglobulin G response, which, in the presence of fetal D-positive cells, may cause significant hemolysis and fetal anemia. The degree of hemolytic disease is related to the maternal antibody titer, the affinity

TABLE 8–7

Pregnancy Events Associated with Transplacental Hemorrhage

Abortion
Antepartum hemorrhage (abruptio placentae, placenta previa, marginal sinus separation)
Manual removal of the placenta
Cesarean section
External breech version
Amniocentesis
Placenta accreta/percreta
Preeclampsia

TABLE 8–8

Classification of the Severity of Hemolytic Disease

Degree of Severity	Description	Incidence (%)
Mild	Indirect bilirubin 16–20 mg/dL; no anemia; no treatment needed	45–50
Moderate	Fetal hydrops does not develop; moderate anemia; severe jaundice with risk of kernicterus unless treated after birth	25–30
Severe	Fetal hydrops develops in utero	20–25
	Before 34 weeks gestation	10–12
	After 34 weeks gestation	10–12

From Bowman JM: Maternal blood group immunization. *In* Creasy R, Resnik R (eds): Maternal-Fetal Medicine: Principles and Practice. Philadelphia, WB Saunders, 1984, pp 561–602.

for the red blood cell membrane, and the ability of the fetus to compensate for the red blood cell destruction. The degree of fetal and neonatal disease is listed in Table 8–8. Most cases are mild in nature and result in normal outcomes. The cord blood is strongly Coombs positive, but the infants do not become significantly anemic or hyperbilirubinemic. Moderate disease results from the red blood cell destruction and the increased production of indirect bilirubin, and although the mother is able to clear this product for the fetus in utero, the neonate is deficient in the liver glucuronyl transferase enzyme, leading to the build-up of this water-insoluble molecule. Albumin carries the indirect bilirubin, but if the binding capacity is exceeded, diffusion of the bilirubin into the fatty tissues occurs. Neural tissue is high in lipid content. Ultimate destruction of neurons can occur, resulting in kernicterus. Treatment is dependent on the recognition of the hyperbilirubinemia and usually entails phototherapy and exchange transfusion in the nursery.

Severe disease occurs when the fetal red blood cell production cannot compensate for the increased red blood cell destruction. Extramedullary hematopoiesis is prominent and ultimately portal hypertension develops and is associated with placental edema and ascites. Albumin production diminishes because of hepatocellular damage and results in anasarca, giving rise to the finding of hydrops fetalis. There is a variable relationship of the fetal anemia and hydrops, but most hydropic fetuses have hemoglobin levels less than 60 g/L.

Management

Management of the sensitized patient, for both Rh and atypical red blood cell antigens, requires the understanding of the mechanism of disease and the skill and experience to predict its severity. Although management schemes follow some basic guidelines, successful management requires access to a blood bank with expertise in antibody typing and with clinicians skilled in prenatal diagnostic procedures (e.g., cordocentesis). Referral to experienced high-risk centers for the management of this problem is common in the United States.

Monitoring

At their first visit, all pregnant patients should have a blood type and antibody screen. This will identify the Rh-negative woman as well as screen for the presence of anti-D or other atypical red blood cell antigen–associated immunoglobulins (Table 8–9) capable of causing fetal hemolytic disease. Any positive antibody screen should be evaluated aggressively and identified, and the amount should be quantified by titer. Consulting a blood bank pathologist may be necessary in cases of atypical antibodies.

Once the isoimmunized patient has been identified, the maternal history is important. All prior pregnancies and their outcomes must be documented to attempt to elucidate the timing and cause of the sensitization as well as to assess the degree of risk for the current pregnancy. In general, the condition is worse with each pregnancy. In a first-sensitized pregnancy, the risk of hydrops is approximately 10%. Ninety percent of patients delivering a hydropic infant will have another one subsequently.

Paternal blood typing and Rh genotyping should be done to calculate the fetal risk of Rh positivity. For atypical blood group immunization, history of outcomes plus transfusions (a significant cause for these antibodies) and determination of the paternal antigen status is of similar importance. For example, a woman with anti-Kell antibody titer of 1:128 would be at moderate risk for hydrops, unless the father of the infant is found to be Kell negative. No invasive procedures for isoimmunization should be performed until paternal antibody status is established.

Ultrasonographic screening for the affected fetus is notoriously unreliable in that significantly anemic fetuses may not be grossly hydropic. However, clues that have been proposed to suggest impending hydrops include polyhydramnios, skin thickening, early ascites (particularly around the fetal bladder), placental thickening, and low umbilical artery Doppler resistance.

Antibody titers are followed monthly to predict fetuses at risk (in the absence of a history of a prior hydropic infant). If the indirect antibody titer is less than 1:16, the development of hydrops is unlikely. Most centers consider the critical titer to be 1:16 because at and above this level

TABLE 8–9

Examples of Atypical Red Cell Antigens Associated with Fetal Hemolytic Disease

Blood Group System	Antigen	Severity of Hemolytic Disease
Kell	K	Mild to severe
Duffy	Fya	Mild to severe
Kidd	JKa	Mild to severe
	JKb	Mild to severe
MNSs	M	Mild to severe
	N	Mild
	S	Mild to severe
	s	Mild to severe
	U	Mild to severe
P	PP	Mild to severe
Public antigens	Yta	Moderate to severe

one cannot ensure the absence of hydrops. When the patient's titer is at or above this level, more invasive testing is necessary. This is usually accomplished by amniocentesis and less commonly by direct fetal blood sampling.

Amniocentesis is the primary screening technique because amniotic fluid contains breakdown products of hemolysis, including bilirubin. The supernatant is run in a spectrophotometer, and the bilirubin peak at 450-nm wavelength is quantified. The change from the baseline is calculated and results in a ΔOD_{450}. The amount of the increase in the optical density correlates reasonably well with severity of hemolysis. In 1961, Liley developed a graph that has been used to predict the severity of fetal hemolytic disease using the ΔOD_{450}. The graph is broken into three zones: Zone I represents the lowest risk and indicates an unaffected fetus, whereas Zone III strongly suggests a severely affected fetus in which fetal hydrops and death can ensue if untreated within the next 7 to 10 days (Fig. 8–3). The Liley curve is authoritative in the third trimester, but its reliability before 26 weeks has been questioned (Queenan et al, 1993). Furthermore, before 20 weeks' gestation, the ΔOD_{450} must be greater than 0.15 or less than 0.09 to be predictive of severe or mild disease, respectively, with a "gray zone" between the two values being unpredictable (Ananth and Queenan, 1989). Thus, the clinician must integrate clinical history and ultrasonogram clues for possible impending hydrops or consider fetal blood sampling in the 18- to 25-week fetus at risk.

Amniocytes can be obtained at the amniocentesis, and, using polymerase chain reaction, fetal D antigen typing can be obtained as early as 14 weeks (Dildy et al, 1996). This allows the identification of the fetus who is at no risk when the paternal status is heterozygous or unknown. It is hoped that in the future immunization with other red blood cell antigens can be detected similarly, reducing the amount of unnecessary invasive procedures on otherwise unaffected fetuses.

Direct ultrasonogram-guided fetal umbilical blood sampling provides valuable data for the fetus at risk, particularly after 18 weeks. Cordocentesis is used most often when the risk, determined by history, indirect antibody titer, or ultrasonogram clues, is significant. It also provides vascular access should fetal transfusion be necessary. Although most obstetricians are well skilled in amniocentesis, cordocentesis is usually performed in tertiary centers by perinatologists. It carries a higher risk of fetal loss and morbidity and is associated with a more significant risk of worsening maternal sensitization (Bowman and Pollock, 1994).

Therapy

Fetal transfusion therapy is the mainstay of treatment for the severely affected fetus. Intraperitoneal transfusions were the primary therapy in the past and are still useful. Tightly packed, irradiated O-negative blood is percutaneously infused into the fetal peritoneal cavity via an amnio-

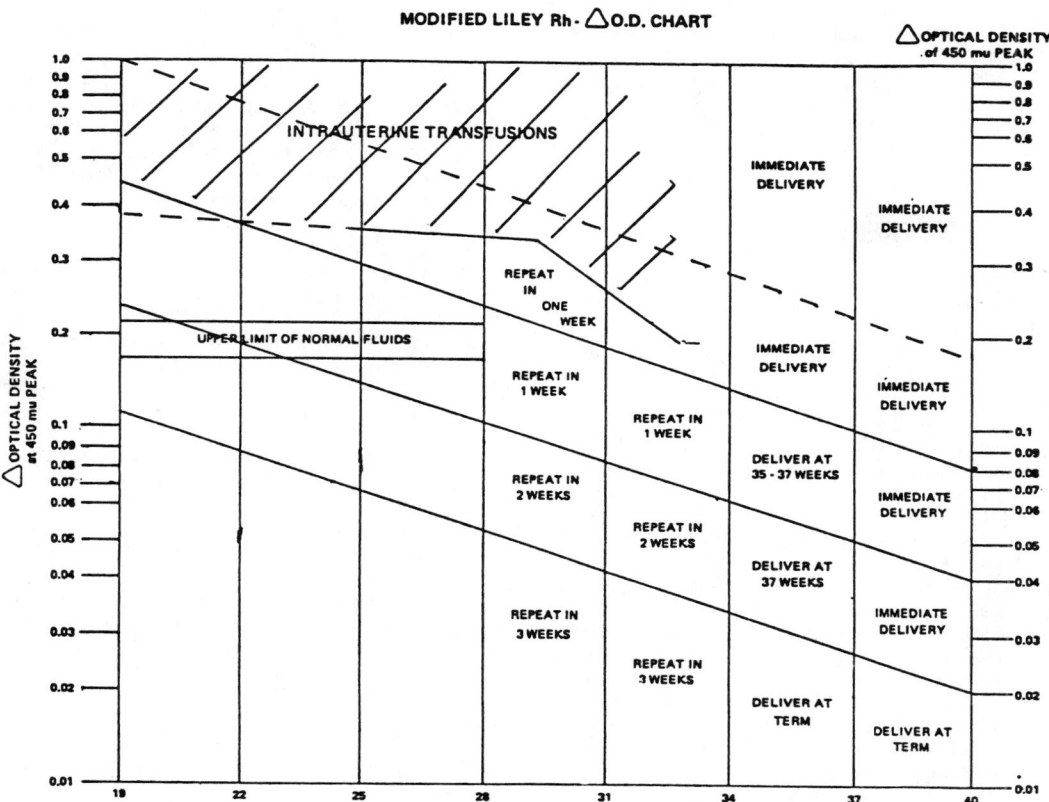

FIGURE 8–3. Liley graph used to assess severity of fetal hemolysis. (From Liley AW: Liquor amnii analysis in management of pregnancy complicated by rhesus immunization. Am J Obstet Gynecol 82:1359, 1961.)

centesis needle. Approximately 1 mL is transfused for each week of gestation greater than 20 weeks. Red blood cell absorption occurs through the lymphatics and may be erratic, particularly in the hydropic fetus. Success rates near 100% in the nonhydropic fetus and 75% in hydropic fetuses have been reported (Harman et al, 1983). Problems associated with this procedure include potential vascular or other intra-abdominal organ injury as well as the inability to obtain fetal blood type and blood count.

Direct intravascular transfusions are now the first-line treatment. The advantages of this procedure include gaining an assessment of the fetal anemia and determining fetal blood type. In addition, ultimate success does not appear to be affected by the presence of hydrops (Ney et al, 1991). Overall success is about 85%. Limitations are usually procedure related. The most accessible site usually requires an anterior placenta in which the cord root can be visualized and posterior placentation makes this technique more difficult. Also risks include bleeding from the cord puncture site, fetal exsanguination, cord hematoma, ruptured membranes, and chorioamnionitis. Because the transfusions are repeated every 2 to 3 weeks as a result of the finite transfused red blood cell life and ongoing hemolysis of fetal red blood cells, ultimately the entire fetal blood supply is replaced with Rh-negative blood. The major neonatal side effect is bone marrow depression, which typically peaks at 3 to 6 weeks of life.

As the pregnancy proceeds through the third trimester, vigorous fetal testing is carried out either with nonstress tests and amniotic fluid index or biophysical profiles. Delivery is carried out 3 to 6 weeks before term, usually after demonstration of a mature fetal lung profile. However, preterm delivery may be indicated in the severely affected fetus, regardless of lung profile, because the procedural risk of transfusions may exceed the risk of morbidity associated with delivery of a near-term, yet premature infant.

REFERENCES

Ananth U, Queenan JT: Does midtrimester ΔOD450 of amniotic fluid reflect severity of Rh disease? Am J Obstet Gynecol 161:47, 1989.

Benigni D, Gregorini G, Frusca T, et al: Effect of low-dose aspirin on fetal and maternal generation of thromboxane by platelets in women at risk for pregnancy-induced hypertension. N Engl J Med 321:357, 1986.

Bjerkedal T: Outcome of pregnancy in women with epilepsy, Norway, 1966 to 1978: Congenital malformations. *In* Janz D, Dam M, Richens A (Eds): Epilepsy, Pregnancy, and the Child. New York, Raven Press, 1982, p 289.

Bowman JM, Pollock JM: Fetomaternal hemorrhage following funipuncture: Increase in severity of maternal red-cell alloimmunization. Obstet Gynecol 84:839, 1994.

Bowman JM, Pollock JM, Penston LE: Fetomaternal transplacental hemorrhage during pregnancy and after delivery. Vox Sang 51:117, 1986.

Brazie JE, Grumm JK, Little VA: Neonatal manifestations of severe maternal hypertension occurring before the thirty-sixth week of pregnancy. J Pediatr 100:265, 1982.

Buehler BA, Delimont D, van Waes M, Finnell RH: Prenatal prediction of risk of the fetal hydantoin syndrome. N Engl J Med 322:1567, 1990.

Chamberlain F, Philipp E, Howlett B, et al: British Births 1970, vol. 2. London, Heinemann, 1978, pp 80–107.

CLASP: A randomised trial of low-dose aspirin for the prevention and treatment of preeclampsia among 9364 pregnant women. CLASP (Collaborative Low-dose Aspirin Study in Pregnancy) Collaborative Group [see comments]. Lancet 343:619, 1994.

CLASP Collaborative Group: Low dose aspirin in pregnancy and early

childhood development: Follow up of the collaborative low dose aspirin study in pregnancy. B J Obstet Gynaecol 102:861, 1995.

Cockburn J, Ounsted M, Moar VA, Redman CWG: Final report of the study on hypertension during pregnancy: The effects of specific treatment on the growth and development of the children. Lancet 1:647, 1982.

Collins R, Wallenburg HCS: Pharmacological prevention and treatment of hypertensive disorders in pregnancy. *In* Chalmers I, Enkin M, Keirse MJNC (Eds): Effective Care in Pregnancy, vol. 1. Oxford, Oxford University Press, 1989, pp 512–531.

Conradt A, Weidinger H, Algayer H: On the role of magnesium in fetal hypotrophy, pregnancy-induced hypertension, and preeclampsia. Magnesium Bull 6:68, 1984.

Crowther C: Magnesium sulfate versus diazepam in the management of eclampsia: A randomized controlled trial. Br J Obstet Gynaecol 97:110, 1990.

Cunningham FG, Fernandez CO, Hernandez C: Blindness associated with preeclampsia and eclampsia. Am J Obstet Gynecol 172:1291, 1995.

Cunningham FG, Gant NF: Prevention of preeclampsia—a reality? N Engl J Med 321:606, 1989.

Dildy GA, Jackson GM, Ward K: Determination of fetal RhD status from uncultured amniocytes. Obstet Gynecol 88:207, 1996.

Doll R, Hanington E: International survey of eclampsia and preeclampsia 1958–1959. Epidemiologic aspects. Pathol Microbiol 24:531, 1961.

Domisse J: Phenytoin, sodium and magnesium sulfate in the management of eclampsia. Br J Obstet Gynaecol 7:104, 1990.

Douglas KA, Redman CW: Eclampsia in the United Kingdom. BMJ 309:1395, 1994.

Easterling TR, Benedetti TH: Preeclampsia: A hyperdynamic disease model. Am J Obstet Gynecol 160:1447, 1989.

Eclampsia Trial Collaborative Group: Which anticonvulsant for women with eclampsia? Evidence from the Collaborative Eclampsia Trial. Lancet 345:1455, 1995.

Friis ML, Hauge M: Congenital heart defects in liveborn children of epileptic patients. Arch Neurol 42:374, 1985.

Friis ML, Holm NV, Sindrop EH: Facial clefts in sibs and children of epileptic patients. Neurology 30:346, 1986.

Gant NF, Donley GL, Chand S, et al: A study of angiotensin II pressor response throughout primagravida pregnancy. J Clin Invest 52:2682, 1973.

Gant NF, Worley RJ: Hypertension in Pregnancy: Concepts and Management. New York, Appleton-Century-Crofts, 1980.

Gluck L, Kulovich MV: Lecithin/sphingomyelin ratio in amniotic fluid in normal and abnormal pregnancy. Am J Obstet 115:539, 1973.

Harman CR, Manning JA, Bowman JM, Lange IR: Severe Rh disease—poor outcome is not inevitable. Am J Obstet Gynecol 145:823, 1983.

Hauth JC, Goldenberg RL, Parker CR Jr, et al: Low-dose aspirin: Lack of association with an increase in abruptio placentae or perinatal mortality. Obstet Gynecol 85:1055, 1995.

Hauth JC, Goldenberg RL, Parker CR, et al: Maternal serum thromboxane B₂ reduction versus pregnancy outcome in a low-dose aspirin trial. Am J Obstet Gynecol 173:578, 1995.

Hubel CA, Roberts JM, Taylor RN, et al: Lipid peroxidation in pregnancy: New perspectives on preeclampsia. Am J Obstet Gynecol 161:1025, 1989.

Hutter W, Grab D, Schneider D, et al: The value of continuous wave Doppler ultrasound in risk pregnancy-intrauterine growth retardation and pregnancy-induced hypertension. Zentralbl Gynakol 115:51, 1993.

Imperiale TF, Petrulis AS: A meta-analysis of low-dose aspirin for the prevention of pregnancy-induced hypertensive disease. JAMA 266:260, 1991.

Kaunitz AM, Hughes JB, Grimes DA, et al: Causes of maternal mortality in the United States. Obstet Gynecol 65:605, 1985.

Kleikner HB, Giles HR, Corrigan JJ: The association of maternal and neonatal thrombocytopenia in high-risk pregnancies. Am J Obstet Gynecol 128:235, 1977.

Knutzen VK, Davey DA: Hypertension in pregnancy: Perinatal mortality and causes of fetal death. S Afr Med J 51:675, 1977.

Lammer EJ, Sever LE, Oakley GP: Teratogen update: Valproic acid. Teratology 35:465, 1987.

Landsteiner K, Weiner AS: An agglutinable factor in human blood recognized by immune sera for rhesus blood. Proc Soc Exp Biol Med 43:223, 1940.

Levine P: Isoimmunization in pregnancy and the pathogenesis of erythroblastosis fetalis. *In* Karsner HT, Hooker SB (Eds): 1941 Yearbook of Pathology and Immunology. Chicago, Yearbook, 1941, p 505.

Lewis M, Kaita H, Chown B: The inheritance of the Rh blood groups: Frequencies in 1000 unrelated caucasian families consisting of 2000 parents and 2806 children. Vox Sang 20:502, 1971.

Liley AW: Liquor amnii analysis in management of pregnancy complicated by rhesus immunization. Am J Obstet Gynecol 82:1359, 1961.

Lucas MJ, Leveno KJ, Cunningham FG: A comparison of magnesium sulfate with phenytoin for the prevention of eclampsia [see comments]. N Engl J Med 333:201, 1995.

McNeil J: The possible teratogenic effects of salicylates on the developing fetus: Brief summaries of eight suggestive cases. Clin Pediatr 12:347, 1973.

Nelson KB, Ellenberg JH: Maternal seizure disorder, outcome of pregnancy, and neurologic abnormalities in the children. Neurology 32:1247, 1982.

Ney JA, Socol ML, Dooley SN, et al: Perinatal outcome following intravascular transfusion in severely isoimmunized fetuses. Int J Gynaecol Obstet 35:41, 1991.

Page EW, Christianson R: The impact of mean arterial pressure in the middle trimester upon the outcomes of pregnancy. Am J Obstet Gynecol 125:740, 1975.

Pritchard JA, Cunningham FG, Pritchard SA: The Parkland Memorial Hospital protocol for treatment of eclampsia: Evaluation of 245 cases. Am J Obstet Gynecol 148:951, 1984.

Queenan JT, Tomai TP, Ural SH, King JC: Deviation in amniotic fluid optical density at a wavelength of 450 nm in Rh isoimmunized pregnancies from 14 to 40 weeks gestation: A proposal for clinical management. Am J Obstet Gynecol 168:1370, 1993.

Redman CWG, Bonnar J, Berlin L: Early platelet consumption in preeclampsia. BMJ 1:467, 1978.

Repke JT, Villar J: Pregnancy-induced hypertension and low birth weight: The role of calcium. Am J Clin Nutr 54:237S, 1991.

Roberts JM, May WJ: Consumptive coagulopathy in severe preeclampsia. Obstet Gynecol 48:163, 1976.

Roberts JM, Taylor RN, Musci TJ: Preeclampsia: An endothelial cell disorder. Am J Obstet Gynecol 161:1200, 1989.

Schiff E, Peley E, Goldenberg M, et al: The use of aspirin to prevent pregnancy-induced hypertension and lower the ratio of thromboxane A$_2$ to prostacyclin in relatively high-risk pregnancies. N Engl J Med 321:351, 1986.

Schmidt D, Canger R, Avanzini G, et al: Change of seizure frequency in pregnant epileptic women. J Neurol Neurosurg Psychiatry 46:751, 1983.

Sibai BM, Anderson GD: Pregnancy outcome of intensive therapy in severe hypertension in the first trimester. Obstet Gynecol 67:517, 1986.

Sibai BM, Caritis SN, Thom E, et al: Prevention of preeclampsia with low-dose aspirin in healthy, nulliparous pregnant women. The National Institute of Child Health and Human Development Network of Maternal-Fetal Medicine Units [see comments]. N Engl J Med 329:1213, 1993.

Sibai BM, Lipsshitz J, Anderson GD, Dilts PV: Reassessment of intravenous MgSO$_4$ therapy in preeclampsia-eclampsia. Obstet Gynecol 57:199, 1981.

Sibai BM, Mabie WC, Shasma F, et al: A comparison of no medication versus methyldopa or labetolol in chronic hypertension during pregnancy. Am J Obstet Gynecol 162:960, 1990.

Sibai BM, Schneider JM, Morrison JC: The late postpartum eclampsia controversy. Obstet Gynecol 55:75, 1980.

Sibai BM, Villar MA, Bray E: Magnesium supplementation during pregnancy: A double blind randomized controlled clinical trial. Am J Obstet Gynecol 161:115, 1989.

Sloan D, Heinonen OP, Kaufman DW, et al: Aspirin and congenital malformations. Lancet 1:1373, 1976.

Spatling L, Spatling G: Magnesium supplementation in pregnancy: A double blind study. Br J Obstet Gynaecol 95:120, 1988.

Streissguth AP, Treder RP, Barr HM, et al: Aspirin and acetaminophen use by pregnant women and subsequent child IQ and attention deficits. Teratology 35:211, 1987.

Wallenburg HCS: Detecting hypertensive disorders of pregnancy. *In* Chalmers I, Enkin M, Keirse MJNC (Eds): Effective Care in Pregnancy, vol. 1. Oxford, England, Oxford University Press, 1989, pp 382–402.

Weinstein L: The HELLP syndrome: A severe consequence of hypertension in pregnancy. J Perinatol 6:316, 1986.

Wilhelm J, Morris D, Hotham N: Epilepsy and pregnancy—a review of 98 pregnancies. Aust N Z J Obstet Gynaecol 4:290, 1990.

Yoon JJ, Kohl S, Harpers RG: The relationship between maternal hypertensive disease of pregnancy and the incidence of idiopathic RDS. Pediatrics 65:735, 1980.

CHAPTER 9

Abnormalities of Fetal Growth

Bryan Sohl and Thomas R. Moore

INTRAUTERINE GROWTH RESTRICTION

When making diagnostic or therapeutic decisions regarding a fetus suspected to be small for dates, it is important to distinguish the fetus with intrauterine growth restriction (IUGR) from a fetus who is small on the basis of prematurity or constitutional factors. Although in 1935 the American Academy of Pediatrics defined prematurity as a live-born infant weighing 2500 g or less (Cone, 1985), clinical practice has taught us that many neonates weighing less than 2500 g are not in fact premature but are of term gestation in whom growth has been limited by intrinsic or extrinsic factors. In 1967 the World Health Organization recognized this and termed newborns weighing 2500 g or less as being of low birth weight. Low-birth-weight infants therefore consist of three populations

▌ Appropriately grown premature infants, delivered prior to 37 weeks' completed gestation, who weigh 2500 g or less
▌ Term infants, born at or after 37 completed weeks' gestation who weigh 2500 g or less; these infants are small for gestational age (SGA) or growth restricted
▌ Infants born both premature and SGA

Accurate Determination of Gestational Age

Confidence in the diagnosis of IUGR depends on an accurate assessment of the gestational age. The most precise clinical determinant of gestational age is the last menstrual period (LMP), especially if the patient has regular menstrual cycles and did not use oral contraceptives in the cycle preceding the LMP. The estimated day of confinement (EDC), which is 280 days after the first day of the LMP, can be calculated by subtracting 3 months and then adding 7 days to the first day of the LMP (Naegle rule).

Clinical milestones used to support or contradict the EDC based on the LMP include

▌ *First trimester uterine size*—assessed by bimanual pelvic examination
▌ *Quickening*—the first fetal movement perceived by the mother, usually felt by 18 weeks' gestation in a first pregnancy and often by 16 weeks' gestation in subsequent pregnancies
▌ *Fetal heart auscultation*—fetal heart tones are usually detected by 12 weeks with an electronic Doppler device and heard by 19 or 20 weeks with a DeLee fetoscope
▌ *Uterine fundal height measurements*—the uterine fundus has usually reached the maternal umbilicus by 20 weeks' gestation and between 20 and 31 weeks' gestation the symphysis pubis–to–fundus measurement in centimeters equals the estimated gestational age in weeks ±3 weeks (Jimenez et al, 1983).

However, because of uncertainties in maternal recall of the LMP and the frequent discrepancies between the LMP-determined gestational age and clinical milestones, the true age of the fetus is often in question. For many patients, ultrasonography is the best way to establish gestational age confidently.

In general, the earlier in pregnancy ultrasonography is performed, the more accurate are the results. Important rules for dating pregnancies by ultrasonography include the following:

▌ The gestational sac is seen by 5 menstrual weeks on transvaginal scanning and 6 menstrual weeks on transabdominal scanning.
▌ Fetal heart motion is seen by 6 menstrual weeks on transvaginal scanning and 7 menstrual weeks on transabdominal scanning.
▌ Measurement of the fetal crown-rump length between 7 and 13 menstrual weeks is accurate to within 3 to 5 days.
▌ In the second and third trimesters measurements of fetal biparietal diameter (BPD), head circumference (HC), abdominal circumference (AC), and femur length (FL) provide accuracies varying from ±1 to 1.5 weeks at 14 to 20 weeks' gestation, to ±2 weeks from 20 to 30 weeks' gestation, and ±3 weeks beyond 30 weeks' gestation.

Standards for Normal Fetal Growth

Obtaining enough birth-weight data from live births throughout gestation to make accurate standards for normal human fetal growth is difficult because of the inherent uncertainty about gestational age. Nevertheless, fetal growth standards have been published by a number of investigators, defining a normal range typically between the 10th and 90th percentile.

The standards used most commonly in the United States over the last 3 decades were developed in Denver and first published by Lubchenco and colleagues in 1963. However, since these curves were developed at high altitude (5280 feet), their applicability to the general population has been questioned, given that altitude is known to negatively affect birth weight. More widely applicable standards include the data collected from 31,102 deliveries and prostaglandin-induced abortions in Cleveland published by Brenner and associates in 1976, data of Williams and associates in 1982 from 2 million births in California between 1970 and 1976, and data from more than a million singleton and 10,000 twin gestations in Canada published by Arbuckle and co-workers in 1993. These standards are not in complete uniformity with each other and may vary by up to 100 to 200 g at any particular gestational age. In clinical practice, SGA is usually defined as birth weight below the 10th percentile; at term this may vary from 2500 to 2750 g. Large for gestational age (LGA) may be defined as birth weight greater than the 90th percentile but is often defined as birth weight greater than 4000 g. The birth-weight curves derived from the California data are shown in Figure 9–1.

The various influences on fetal birth weight are summarized in Table 9–1. At times the terms SGA and IUGR do not necessarily reflect identical clinical situations. Some perfectly normal, constitutionally small babies are below the 10th percentile for gestational age at birth, whereas some babies born above the 10th percentile exhibit growth restriction, having come from an in utero environment that prevented the fetus from reaching its full growth potential.

Perinatal and Long-Term Consequences of IUGR

Suboptimal weight at birth may have perinatal, childhood, and adult consequences. As shown in Figure 9–1, perinatal mortality is higher for growth-restricted fetuses than for normal-sized fetuses. Hobbins (1980) reported an eight times higher rate of perinatal death in growth-restricted fetuses. Infants weighing between 1500 and 2500 g at term have a perinatal mortality rate 5 to 30 times greater than infants born between the 10th and 50th percentiles, and infants born at less than 1500 g near term have a perinatal mortality rate that is 70 to 100 times greater (Williams et

TABLE 9–1

Factors Affecting Fetal Weight at Birth

Factor	Comment
Sex	Males weigh more than females
Race	White babies at term weigh more than black babies
Parity	Birth weight increases with parity through at least para 2
Constitutional factors	As a rough general rule, small parents make small babies and large parents make large babies; maternal constitutional factors have a greater influence on fetal growth than do paternal factors
Multiple gestation	Singletons are larger than twins, which are larger than triplets, and so forth
Maternal disease states and maternal placental infarction	Diseases include obesity, diabetes, hypertension, infections, and substance abuse, among others

al, 1982). Fetal mortality rates are approximately 50% higher than neonatal rates. Much of this increased mortality is because of the high association of anomalous development and chromosome abnormalities with IUGR, but anatomically and chromosomally normal fetuses with IUGR still have significantly increased mortality rates.

IUGR fetuses are more likely to experience fetal distress in labor and be acidotic at birth (Lin et al, 1976). Meconium staining and aspiration are more common in IUGR infants born after 34 weeks. Growth-restricted neonates are at risk for many neonatal complications, including hypoglycemia, hypocalcemia, hyponatremia, hypothermia, and polycythemia. On the other hand, when IUGR infants are born prematurely, they appear to be relatively protected against respiratory distress syndrome and intraventricular hemorrhage when compared with normally grown infants (Procianoy et al, 1980) (see Chapters 5 and 51).

The relative effects of IUGR on long-term development are related to the specific causes of IUGR and the timing and duration of the insult. It has been reported that between 36% and 50% of children born with IUGR suffer poor school performance (Fitzhardinge and Steven, 1972). Commey and Fitzhardinge (1979) found that 49% of SGA infants, most of whom weighed less than 1500 g, had developmental handicaps at 2 years of age. This group, however, contained only "outborn" neonates, a skewed group of infants transferred after birth to a regional medical center. Goldenberg and associates (1997) recently reported that the I.Q. of IUGR infants at 5 years of age averaged 3.3 points lower than term children who are appropriate for their gestational age. If both premature and IUGR, such children averaged 6.7 points lower on standard intelligence tests, suggesting that the IUGR fetus has less postnatal adaptability and greater susceptibility to injury in the perinatal period. Infants with early growth insults (such as those associated with congenital viral infections) fare much worse than do children with later restric-

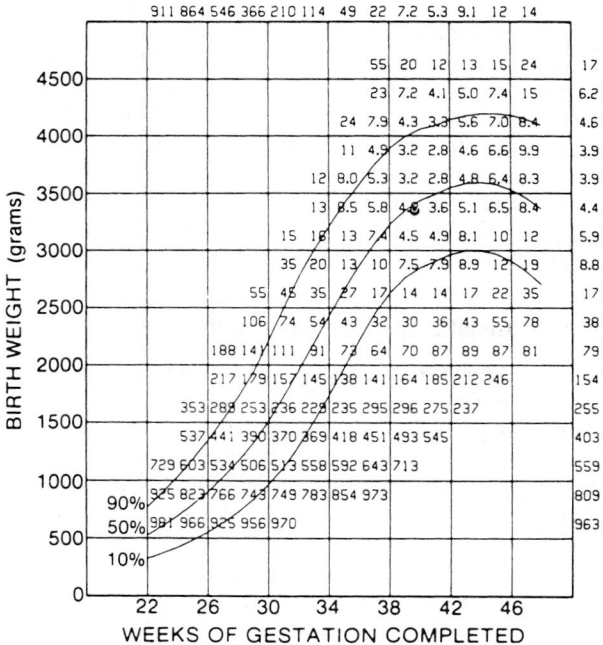

FIGURE 9–1. Growth and perinatal viability in California. The 10th, 50th, and 90th percentiles of birth weight in a large California birth cohort for various gestational ages are shown. The perinatal mortality risk for each combination of birth weight and gestational age is shown (per 1000 live births). (From Williams RL, Creasy RK, Cunningham GC, et al: Fetal growth and perinatal viability in California. Obstet Gynecol 59:624, 1982. Reprinted with permission from The American College of Obstetricians and Gynecologists.)

tion, typically from impaired uteroplacental perfusion. Lipper and colleagues (1981) demonstrated that neonatal HC percentile is a strong predictor of neurologic development. IUGR infants born with an HC less than the 10th percentile had two to three times the incidence of long-term neurologic sequelae as compared with normocephalic IUGR infants. Hack and coworkers (1991) similarly showed that infants born with a small HC who do not exhibit catch-up growth are at increased risk of suboptimal downstream neurologic function. However, the child unlikely to suffer significant neurologic sequelae is one whose IUGR does not result from anomalous development, chromosome abnormalities, or in utero infection and whose head size at birth is normocephalic or if small, exhibits catch-up growth. However, this child may still be at risk for language delay, behavioral problems, and potential school problems (Fanaroff et al, 1994).

Recently, a number of epidemiologic studies have suggested that IUGR offspring, especially those born with a relatively large placenta, may be at increased risk of developing hypertension as an adult (Stewart et al, 1995).

Etiologies of Intrauterine Growth Restriction

The causes of IUGR are myriad but can be grouped into intrinsic and extrinsic types. These are summarized in Table 9–2. An additional classification system is based on relative restriction in the growth of fetal head and abdomen. Those with symmetrically reduced intrauterine growth are believed to derive from an early in utero insult that globally resets the growth potential of most, if not all, organs. Histology of IUGR fetal organs demonstrates a decreased number of cells. The early insult leads to cellular

hypoplasia and subsequent limitation in overall organ and, thus, fetal growth. Examples of this process include chromosome abnormalities, congenital infections, and syndromes of anomalous development.

Asymmetric growth restriction, on the other hand, is believed to reflect a relatively late insult, after fetal organ development has for the most part already occurred, and usually reflects an abnormal delivery of substances necessary for fetal well-being and growth, such as nutrition, water, and oxygen. Individual organs may have a normal number of smaller, or hypotrophic, cells. This often results from uteroplacental insufficiency secondary to maternal disease states such as hypertension and diabetes complicated by vascular disease. In symmetric growth restriction, substrate delivery to vital organs such as the brain and heart are usually spared to some degree, at the expense of other parts of the fetus, such as the liver and subcutaneous tissue. This division of IUGR into symmetric and asymmetric patterns is an oversimplification, and often mixed patterns of abnormal growth are noted.

Constitutional Influences on Growth

There are definite genetic and constitutional influences on growth. It has been estimated that the genetic contribution to birth weight is approximately 40%, whereas environmental factors contribute 60% (Polani, 1974). Small mothers are more likely to make small babies. If a mother weighs less than 100 lb, her risk of delivering an SGA infant is at least doubled (Simpson et al, 1975). Maternal influences on fetal growth are greater than are paternal, whereas in childhood and young adulthood maternal and paternal influences are more even. In 1955, Morton showed that maternal half siblings and full siblings are closer in birth weight than are paternal half and full siblings. Emanuel and associates in 1992 published a longitudinal study of all births in 1 week that occurred in England, Scotland, and Wales in 1958 and found that there are intergenerational influences on birth weight that are passed on through the maternal side.

Genetic and Developmental Influences

There are known chromosome influences on fetal growth. The Y chromosome is a case in point. Males at term weigh 150 to 200 g more than do females. Fetuses born with trisomy 21 are slightly small, having a mean birth weight of 2900 g at term, which is 1 SD below the normal mean. Typically, the lag in growth in fetuses with trisomy 21 manifests itself after 34 weeks' gestation.

On the other hand, infants born with trisomy 13 or 18 are often severely and symmetrically growth restricted, having mean birth weights of 2600 and 2240 g, respectively (Grouchy and Turleau, 1984). Trisomy 18 fetuses in particular usually exhibit early symmetric IUGR, which is often detectable by 18 weeks' gestational age. Turner syndrome (45, X) is associated with mild growth lag, with an average birth weight of 85% of normal. Other chromosome abnormalities such as deletions, duplications, and translocations have variable effects on fetal growth, depending on the chromosomes affected and the amount of unbalanced genetic material. Often syndromes that cause multiple con-

---

TABLE 9–2

Fetal Growth Restriction

Intrinsic Causes

Constitutional (e.g., parents of small stature)
Genetic (especially trisomy 18, 13 syndromes)
Toxic: alcohol, nicotine, virus, hydantoin, coumarin
Infectious: TORCH,° syphilis, malaria
Teratogenic: radiation, drugs

Extrinsic Causes

Decreased Maternal Nutrient Delivery

   Maternal cardiac disease
   High altitude
   Maternal anemia (e.g., sickle cell)
   Maternal starvation/inanition

Placental Dysfunction

   Hypertensive disease
   Autoimmune disease (e.g., lupus)
   Placental infection (e.g., syphilis)
   Reduced placental area (chronic abruptio placentae, multifetal gestation, placental infarction)

In Utero Constraint

   Müllerian anomaly
   Extrinsic mass (e.g., fibroid)

°See text for complete term.

genital abnormalities are associated with IUGR, including Meckel-Gruber and Roberts syndromes. Likewise, single but massive congenital malformations such as anencephaly and gastroschisis are often associated with IUGR. Fetal cardiac anomalies, especially those associated with septal defects, can also be associated with IUGR (Richards et al, 1955).

Congenital Infection

A number of microorganisms are capable of crossing the placenta and causing fetal infection. If the infection occurs at a critical time in fetal development, some organisms can cause enough disruption of fetal cells to result in IUGR. In general, intrauterine infections have more severe consequences when they occur early in gestation. First-trimester infections may disrupt organogenesis directly or, indirectly, as a consequence of hyperthermia or placentitis.

Most of the agents associated with the TORCH syndrome (*t*oxoplasmosis, *o*ther infections, *r*ubella, *c*ytomegalovirus [CMV] infection, *h*erpes simplex) cause IUGR. CMV infection during early pregnancy has been associated with IUGR, occurring as a result of cellular lysis and a subnormal number of cells in fetal organs. First-trimester varicella infection has also been associated with a syndrome of congenital anomalies that includes IUGR. Although most women of child-bearing age are immune to rubella, as a result of infection or vaccination, nonimmunized women are at risk for infection, and this can lead to IUGR. It is not entirely clear if an HIV-caused embryopathy involving IUGR exists. Varner and Galask (1984) reviewed infectious causes of IUGR (see Chapters 43 and 47). Bacterial infections, with the exception of syphilis, have not been associated with IUGR.

Maternal Drug Exposure

Tobacco, the most common fetal drug exposure, is associated with a 200-g lower birth weight in infants of heavy smokers as compared with nonsmoking controls (ACOG, 1993). Fetal alcohol syndrome (FAS) is characterized by three major findings: abnormal facies, central nervous system dysfunction, and IUGR (Rosett, 1980). Occasional or rare alcohol use during pregnancy probably has no deleterious effect on fetal growth. Development of FAS is likely dose and timing-of-exposure related, with the greatest risk occurring with first-trimester exposure. Hanson and colleagues reported in 1978 that up to 10% of offspring of moderate drinkers (1 to 2 oz of absolute ethanol per day) will have some features of FAS.

Illicit drugs have also been associated with IUGR. Cocaine use, especially of the "crack" form, has been associated with IUGR. This may occur as a result of vasoconstriction of uterine vessels impeding substrate delivery to the fetus (Moore et al, 1986). Up to 25% to 30% of cocaine users during pregnancy may deliver a fetus with IUGR (MacGregor et al, 1987). Crystal methamphetamine use has also been associated with IUGR (Little et al, 1988). The use of "crank" has been rapidly escalating in recent years, particularly on the West Coast. Narcotics including heroin have been associated with IUGR, with rates three to seven times that of the general public (Fricker and

Segal, 1978), although it is not clear that opioids independently cause fetal growth restriction. Methadone use, in the absence of other drug usage, does not seem to be associated with IUGR (Newman et al, 1975). The use of marijuana and hallucinogens in pregnancy does not seem to be associated with IUGR. It is hard to isolate the effects of illicit drug use on growth because often there may be concomitant tobacco use and poor nutrition. Some prescription drugs indicated for specific maternal medical conditions have been associated with IUGR, most notably coumarin and phenytoin (ACOG, 1985).

Maternal Disease States

Several maternal disease states can lead to IUGR in the fetus. This can occur in conjunction with reductions in uteroplacental perfusion as is seen in patients with chronic hypertension. IUGR can also occur as the result of low availability of substrates needed for growth, such as oxygen in severe anemia or cyanotic heart disease, or protein and calories in poor nutritional states.

Maternal vascular disease including chronic hypertension, pregnancy-induced hypertension, severe diabetes with vasculopathy, chronic renal disease, systemic lupus erythematosus with vascular involvement, and antiphospholipid syndromes all have been associated with poor fetal growth (Aulman et al, 1980; Katz et al, 1980; Long et al, 1980). The common thread in all these diseases is vascular pathology that reduces uteroplacental perfusion. Campbell and coworkers in 1987 studied the uterine circulation in hypertensive pregnancies complicated by IUGR and found a high incidence of abnormal vascular resistance in the uterine artery. Easterling and coworkers (1991) have shown that high-uterine-artery-resistance hypertension is more likely to be associated with IUGR than is low-resistance hypertension. Clinically, maternal hypertension unaccompanied by underlying vascular or renal disease is unlikely to be associated with IUGR (Robertson et al, 1975).

Maternal medical complications that compromise delivery of oxygen to the fetus are associated with IUGR. Patton and associates in 1990 demonstrated that cyanotic maternal heart disease is associated with IUGR. Severe maternal anemia (hemoglobin <8 g/dL), such as associated with sickle cell disease, is also linked with IUGR, with up to 30% of infants born to women with hemoglobin sickle cell disease weighing less than 2500 g at birth (Fort et al, 1971). Similarly, living at high altitude is associated with decreased birth weight—at 10,000 feet altitude mean birth weight at term is decreased by 250 g, presumably from a decrease in available oxygen to the fetus (Lichty et al, 1957).

Maternal malnutrition has been known for many years to be a cause of IUGR, although the magnitude of this effect is moderate. Much of our knowledge of severe malnutrition in humans comes from studies of two populations (from Netherlands and Leningrad) subjected to starvation during World War II. The Leningrad studies examined a group of women subjected to prolonged famine throughout their pregnancy and who entered pregnancy in poor nutritional status (Antonov, 1947). In Holland, previously well-nourished women endured a 6-month famine that abruptly ended in 1945 (Stein and Susser, 1975). The two groups most affected were Leningrad women with very poor nutritional status entering pregnancy and Dutch women in whom calorie deprivation occurred in the third trimester. The Leningrad population had babies 400 to 600 g lighter in weight than those born during periods of normal feeding. In Dutch women starved in the third trimester, birth weight dropped by 250 g compared with weights of mothers with normal intake. No lowering of birth weight was noted if the famine occurred in the first or second trimester.

Obstetric Factors

Multiple pregnancy is associated with IUGR. Arbuckle and associates in 1993 published data from a large Canadian birth registry showing that up to 25% of twins are born with IUGR. Miller and Merritt in 1979 showed that up to two thirds of twins at birth showed some signs of growth restriction. Although twins have growth rates similar to singletons through the first two trimesters of pregnancy, fetal growth rates peak in singletons at 220 to 240 g per week at 34 weeks' gestation and in twins at 160 to 170 g per week at 30 weeks' gestation (Williams et al, 1982). Higher-order gestations experience even higher rates of IUGR, probably owing to placental crowding in some of the fetuses. At 38 weeks the average birth weight of a triplet is at the 10th percentile for singletons (Elster et al, 1991).

Placental and umbilical cord abnormalities are associated with IUGR, including chronic placental abruptio, placental infarcts, placental hemangiomas, two-vessel umbilical cords, and velamentous cord insertions. Confined placental mosaicism, a discrepancy between the fetal and placental chromosome complements, has been shown to be associated with IUGR by Kalousek and Dill (1983).

Diagnosis of Fetal Growth Restriction

Diagnosing fetal growth restriction in utero requires an awareness of risk factors, skills at physical examination, and an understanding of the abilities and limitations of ultrasonography in identifying the fetus at risk. Historically, clinical examination has been ineffective at identifying the growth-restricted fetus. In 1977, Tejani and Mann showed that only one third of babies born with IUGR had been detected prior to birth. Similar results were reported by Cetrulo and Freeman (1977), with only 37% of fetuses at-risk for IUGR diagnosed correctly before birth.

Fundal Height

Clinically, measurements of the distance from the maternal symphysis pubis to the top of the uterus are obtained at every prenatal visit from 16 weeks' gestation until delivery. This measurement is most valid if done in the same manner by the same practitioner at each visit. However, even careful fundal height measurements have a high false-negative rate, with normal measurements in 60% of fetuses with confirmed growth restriction (Jensen and Larsen, 1991). Fundal height measurements are, at best, a crude screening tool for the detection of IUGR.

Ultrasonography

Currently, ultrasonography is the most effective clinical tool for identification of the IUGR fetus. Measurements of BPD, HC, AC, and FL are compared with normal values obtained from published tables or as displayed in the ultrasound machine software package. Additional evaluation tools include assessment of amniotic fluid volume, maturation or grading of the placenta, and Doppler studies of blood flow in various maternal and fetal vascular beds.

The fetus who has suffered an early pregnancy insult, whether from genetic, developmental, or infectious causes, often is symmetrically growth restricted. All biometric indices are small. There is usually no sparing of the growth of the fetal head. In symmetric IUGR, fetal head size often is compromised early in gestation. An HC less than the third percentile is strongly suggestive of IUGR, provided dating criteria are firmly established. Although IUGR may be diagnosed with ultrasonography in the late first trimester (Benacerraf, 1988), diagnostic confidence is better in the second trimester.

In contrast, the fetus who is growth restricted from causes related to inadequate uteroplacental perfusion and substrate deprivation, such as the offspring of a woman with severe hypertension or diabetes with vascular disease, more typically has IUGR of late onset, characterized by an asymmetric growth pattern, with a small AC owing to glycogen depletion in the fetal liver and decreased subcutaneous fat deposition. Long bone growth is affected only by a prolonged and relatively early insult. Restriction of head growth is a late finding in cases of asymmetric IUGR because of the fetus's ability to shunt blood flow to the brain at the expense of the body. Thus, in a fetus with asymmetric growth restriction who has had numerous serial ultrasound biometric measurements, typically the AC falls off established growth curves first, followed by the FL, and lastly by the HC.

The best single biometric measurement for predicting IUGR is the AC. Hadlock and colleagues in 1983 and Brown and coworkers in 1987 found the sensitivity of the AC for detecting IUGR to be 100% and 96%, respectively. The FL is less predictive of IUGR. A decreased FL is a late finding in asymmetric IUGR but can be seen early in fetuses with symmetric IUGR caused by chromosome abnormalities. Hadlock and colleagues (1983) found the FL to be less than the third percentile in 20% of fetuses with IUGR, and Brown and coworkers (1987) reported the FL to be less than the 10th percentile in 45% of fetuses with IUGR in the third trimester.

Fetal weight is often used to predict IUGR. However, it must be kept in mind that fetal weight is a calculated value, usually the product of various combinations of head, abdominal, and femoral measurements. These calculations multiply the inherent errors of each single measurement, resulting in a 90% confidence interval of ±15%. Hadlock and colleagues (1983), using a calculated fetal weight devised from their population, identified 87% of fetuses with IUGR in the third trimester using a 10th percentile cutoff. Vintzileos and coworkers in 1987 reported similar results using a different formula for fetal weight.

Various ratios of fetal body measurements, particularly the HC-to-AC and AC-to-FL ratios, have been proposed as a means to identify the IUGR fetus. Campbell and Thoms first reported on the use of the HC-to-AC ratio in identifying IUGR in 1977. Hadlock and colleagues, again in 1983, found that the HC-to-AC ratio detected IUGR two thirds of the time. Hadlock and colleagues (1983) and Jeanty and coworkers (1984) independently proposed that the AC-to-FL ratio be used as an "in-utero ponderal index" for the prediction of IUGR. This ratio is relatively constant at 22 weeks' gestation and beyond. This ratio also detects about two thirds of fetuses with IUGR using a cut-off of 24%.

Amniotic Fluid Volume

Oligohydramnios is often associated with IUGR, particularly asymmetric IUGR. The theoretical basis for this is that IUGR associated with poor placental perfusion results in decreased transplacental water transfer and, thus, oligohydramnios. The clinical observation that IUGR neonates are frequently hemoconcentrated is consistent with this thesis. Manning and colleagues reported on the relationship of IUGR and oligohydramnios in 1981. For a definition of oligohydramnios, they used a sonographically measured maximal vertical pocket of amniotic fluid of less than 1 cm. However, this degree of near-absolute oligohydramnios is a rare and late finding with IUGR. More recently, Moore and Cayle in 1990 presented standard values for the four-quadrant Amniotic Fluid Index (AFI) for normal pregnancy. They included in their report values for the third percentile, which varies depending on gestational age. This has clinically been used as a cut-off for diagnosing oligohydramnios (AFI = 75 mm). Others use an absolute cut-off of 50 mm to diagnose oligohydramnios independent of gestational age. The presence of oligohydramnios in the absence of ruptured amniotic membranes should alert the practitioner to the potential presence of IUGR.

Placental Grade

Sonographically, the placenta can be graded (0 to 3) on the basis of increasing calcium deposits, believed to reflect the process of placental "aging." In normal gestations it is rare to have a Grade 3 placenta prior to 36 weeks' gestation. Kazzi and coworkers in 1983 showed a fourfold increase in IUGR in fetuses with an estimated fetal weight of less than 2700 g and a Grade 3 placenta, as compared with fetuses of the same size with less than a Grade 3 placenta. When oligohydramnios, an estimated fetal weight of less than 2700 g and a Grade 3 placenta, is identified, a high index of suspicion for IUGR should be raised.

Doppler Velocimetry

In recent years, there has been much interest in the use of Doppler velocity assessments of vascular flow to evaluate pregnancies at risk for IUGR. Various fetal vessels, along with the maternal uterine arteries, have been studied. Currently, the umbilical artery is the most commonly studied vessel. Most studies have evaluated the ratio of Doppler velocities during systolic and diastolic phases of the fetal cardiac cycle. Theoretically, as downstream resistance rises, the velocity of blood flow during diastole decreases, causing

the ratio of systolic-to-diastolic velocity (S/D ratio) to rise. These are illustrated in Figure 9–2. In cases of very high resistance, diastolic flow velocity may fall to zero or even reverse. In the third trimester, the S/D ratio is typically less than 3. A ratio of greater than 4 after 30 weeks is distinctly abnormal, and absence of end-diastolic flow has a high correlation with IUGR. Reversed diastolic flow is highly abnormal and almost universally associated with severe IUGR. Fetal death within 24 to 48 hours of observing reversed flow is not unusual. Use of Doppler velocimetry to identify and manage the fetus with IUGR is summarized in Table 9–3.

With the use of ultrasonographic evaluation of the fetus to detect IUGR, the role of serial sonography must be emphasized. A set of single measurements is helpful in identifying severe IUGR, but earlier growth disorders are better detected using serial measurements taken 2 to 4 weeks apart and looking for a fall-off in growth, particularly of the AC. A falling-off in growth from established growth curves and the detection of oligohydramnios are the most helpful clinical predictors of IUGR.

Management of Intrauterine Growth Restriction

The management of pregnancy complicated by IUGR depends on the gestation of the pregnancy, the degree and type of IUGR, and the suspected cause of the IUGR.

Genetic Analysis

When severe, symmetric IUGR is detected remote from term, a diagnostic regimen is necessary to determine the etiology of the growth restriction. Chromosome analysis, amniotic fluid viral culture, polymerase chain reaction studies directed against pathogenic genetic material, and acute IgM antibody titers can be performed by either amniocentesis or fetal umbilical cord blood sampling. A high-resolution ultrasound study should be performed in an effort to

---

TABLE 9–3

Use of Doppler Ultrasonography to Assess Fetal Growth

S/D or resistance indices (RI) should normally decrease as term nears

Rising RI is characteristic of increasing placental resistance and typically accompanies declining fetal growth. At the same time, RI in the cerebral circulation falls as flow increases to compensate for limitation in oxygen supply

Absent end-diastolic velocity is associated with IUGR and distress but can exist for 2 to 12 weeks before signs of fetal compromise become evident on FHR or BPP testing

Reversed diastolic velocity is an end-stage finding, associated with fetal death within 24–72 hours of its appearance. Delivery is mandatory when reversed diastolic flow is persistent. Intermittent flow reversal precedes persistent flow reversal; planned fetal intervention is possible at that stage

IUGR, intrauterine growth restriction; FHR, fetal heart rate; BPP, biophysical profile; S/D, systolic to diastolic.

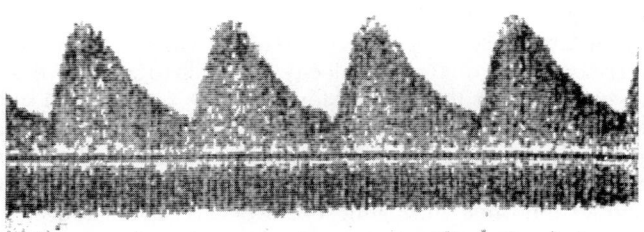

NORMAL SYSTOLIC-DIASTOLIC RATIO

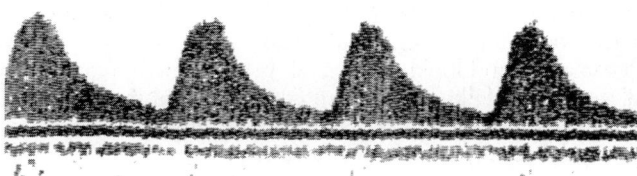

HIGH SYSTOLIC-DIASTOLIC RATIO

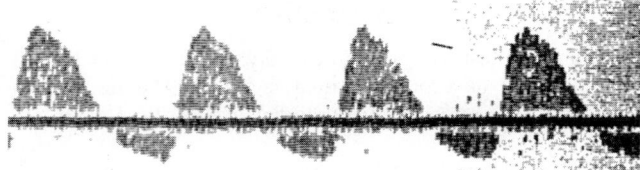

EXTREME SYSTOLIC-DIASTOLIC RATIO

FIGURE 9–2. Doppler velocity assessment in the fetal umbilical artery: flow velocity waveforms from the umbilical artery. Flow velocity is plotted vertically against time of the cardiac cycle. A normal waveform is shown in the upper panel. In the middle panel, absent diastolic blood flow is evident. In the lower panel, diastolic flow is reversed, a highly ominous sign.

uncover structural anomalies. Early detection of a severe chromosome or developmental abnormality allows parents maximal options regarding continuation or termination of the pregnancy. Knowledge of such an abnormality could also alter the management of the rest of the pregnancy, allowing antepartum consultations with subspecialists and delivery at a tertiary center; on the other hand, it may allow a couple to deliver a severely affected child in a noninvasive and private manner.

Maternal Intervention

When IUGR is identified, an effort should be made to improve the in utero environment. Life-style modifications, such as improved nutrition and cessation of tobacco, alcohol, or illicit drug use, should be made. The fetus may benefit by maternal bed rest or at least a restriction in maternal activity.

Fetal Surveillance

When the diagnosis of IUGR is made prior to term, careful surveillance of the pregnancy is mandatory. Immediate

institution of regular fetal testing should be begun. Currently, most centers use non-stress testing (NST) of the fetal heart rate or the biophysical profile (BPP). If the NST is used, amniotic fluid adequacy should be assessed (AFI >50 mm) at each test, and testing should be performed twice weekly. If the BPP is used, weekly testing is usually adequate. Details of these tests and their interpretation are given in Chapter 13. Testing is continued until delivery. Ultrasound measurements of fetal growth parameters are done every 10 to 21 days. The inherent errors in fetal measurements performed more frequently than every 10 days cause overlap and potentially misleading trends. Women with a suspected IUGR fetus should be instructed in fetal kick counting, which should be performed and recorded daily (Moore and Piacquadio, 1989).

When to Deliver

The ideal timing of delivery of the IUGR fetus may be difficult to determine, especially if the diagnosis is somewhat uncertain. If the pregnancy with IUGR reaches 36 weeks or more, delivery should be performed because further significant fetal growth is unlikely, the requirements for intensive fetal surveillance are high, and the risk of fetal demise or perinatal asphyxia is substantial. Although amniocentesis for fetal lung maturity should be performed if doubt about the gestational age exists, an IUGR pregnancy with well-documented dates of 36 weeks or longer should be delivered without further evaluation. As for delivery mode, a vaginal delivery is preferred unless clear contraindications to labor exist. However, in a pregnancy with severe IUGR and oligohydramnios, a primary cesarean section should be considered if the fetus has persistent late decelerations or a BPP of 2.

If the IUGR gestation is preterm, the risks of continuing the pregnancy and risking intrauterine fetal demise or asphyxia must be weighed against the risks of preterm delivery and the potential complications of prematurity. In general, if a preterm fetus with IUGR has reassuring fetal testing and adequate AFIs (≥5 cm) and demonstrates continuing fetal growth on serial ultrasound studies, the pregnancy may be safely followed until term.

If suspicious or nonreassuring fetal testing occurs in the preterm gestation, consideration should be given to hospital admission and intensive fetal surveillance and support (Table 9–4). These efforts are to optimize the in utero

---

TABLE 9–4

Indications for Intensive, In-Hospital Fetal Surveillance in IUGR Pregnancy

Fetal growth stops (especially arrest of growth in abdominal circumference)

Severe oligohydramnios (AFI <50) is noted

FHR testing is persistently nonreactive, has late decelerations or prolonged, spontaneous decelerations

Doppler studies demonstrate absent end-diastolic velocity or flow reversal

IUGR, intrauterine growth restriction; AFI, Amniotic Fluid Index; FHR, fetal heart rate.

environment with maternal blood volume expansion, oxygen administration, bed rest in a lateral decubitus position, and continuous fetal monitoring. Amniocentesis to document status of fetal lung maturity and administration of corticosteroids should be considered. If despite these efforts, fetal biophysical status deteriorates, delivery must be contemplated.

Intrapartum Management

During labor and delivery, the IUGR fetus must be closely monitored for evidence of distress. Although external Doppler fetal heart rate monitoring is adequate in most cases, a fetal scalp electrode, intrauterine pressure catheter, and fetal scalp pH analysis may be helpful in evaluating confusing fetal heart rate tracings.

It is imperative to provide early notification of both the pediatric and anesthesia services when a patient with suspected IUGR is present in the labor and delivery suite. Pediatric personnel should be present at the birth of a growth-restricted fetus because fetal distress and meconium staining are both increased. Early anesthesia notification assists in management of pain and fetal distress, especially if emergent cesarean section is needed.

The recognition of patients with risk factors for fetal IUGR, careful ultrasound surveillance of their fetus's growth combined with antenatal testing, well-timed delivery, and a multidisciplinary approach to the management of the labor and delivery of such fetuses help to maximize the chances of delivering a healthy fetus free from hypoxic insult. Fortunately, in many instances, the fetus diagnosed with IUGR has excellent prospects of normal postnatal development.

FETAL MACROSOMIA

Similar to fetal growth restriction, fetal macrosomia represents a tail end of the spectrum of fetal growth. As in IUGR, there is not a single definition of fetal macrosomia. It has been variously defined as birth weight above the 90th percentile, birth weight above 4500 g, and birth weight above 4000 g at term. The American College of Obstetricians and Gynecologists (ACOG) (1991) defines macrosomia as birth weight above 4500 g.

Using 4000 g and 4500 g as diagnostic cut-offs for macrosomia, the Obstetrical Statistical Cooperative found the incidence of macrosomia to be 5.3% and 0.4%, respectively, whereas at Parkland Hospital in Dallas in 1991, using similar diagnostic criteria, macrosomia was identified in 7.7% and 1.0% of deliveries (Cunningham et al, 1993). In contrast, at the University of California at San Diego, 13% of births are greater than 4000 g. Thus, it appears that 4000 g offers a reasonable working criterion for macrosomia in a typical U.S. population, with approximately 5% to 7% of term babies defined as "macrosomic."

Risk Factors for Fetal Macrosomia

There are many risk factors for the development of fetal macrosomia. These are often found in combination. Risk factors include gestational age, multiparity, male sex of the fetus, constitutional factors, a history of birthing a previous macrosomic infant, labor difficulties, maternal obesity, and, in particular, maternal diabetes. In addition, there are rare fetal syndromes associated with macrosomia.

Pollack and associates in 1992 reported that among pregnancies 41 weeks or longer, 23% of newborns weighed greater than 4000 g and 4% weighed more than 4500 g. Post-term infants account for approximately 10% to 20% of macrosomic infants. Infants born to parous women are two or three times more likely to be macrosomic than those born to nulliparous women (Mondanlou et al, 1980). Birth weight increases an average of 80 to 120 g in succeeding pregnancies through the fifth pregnancy (O'Leary and Leonetti, 1990). In the third trimester male fetuses weigh on average 150 g more than do females and hence account for 60% to 70% of macrosomic newborns (Spellacy et al, 1985). O'Leary and Leonetti (1990) reported that if a woman has given birth to an infant weighing greater than 4500 g, she is five to ten times more likely in a subsequent pregnancy to deliver a fetus weighing more than 4000 g.

Labor difficulties, such as arrest and protraction abnormalities, and operative vaginal deliveries (particularly mid-pelvic forceps and vacuum types) have been associated with macrosomic infants (Benedetti and Gabbe, 1978; McFarland et al, 1986). Maternal obesity has been associated with a 4- to 120-fold increased risk for fetal macrosomia (Johnson et al, 1987). Maternal diabetes, both pregestational insulin-dependent and gestational, predisposes to macrosomia and shoulder dystocia. Because these fetuses have greater shoulder-to-head and chest-to-head disproportion than do fetuses born to nondiabetic mothers (Mondanlou et al, 1982), they experience greater rates of shoulder dystocia for a similar birth weight (Acker et al, 1985).

Although genetic disorders are more commonly associated with IUGR, there are some rare syndromes associated with macrosomia. These include Beckwith-Wiedemann, Carpenter, Marshall, Nevo, Ruvalcaba-Myhre, Simpson-Golabi-Behmel, and Weaver syndromes.

Complications of Fetal Macrosomia

Maternal Morbidity

Most of the maternal complications of fetal macrosomia are related to an increased risk for cesarean section and its increased maternal morbidity as compared with vaginal delivery. Spellacy and associates (1985) found that infants weighing more than 4500 g were delivered by cesarean section 34% of the time compared with an approximate 20% cesarean section rate overall. With cesarean section there are increased risks for anesthetic complications, bleeding, and postoperative infection. Obstetric complications are also more frequent with macrosomia, including postpartum hemorrhage from uterine atony, uterine lacerations, and vaginal and perineal trauma associated with operative vaginal delivery (e.g., forceps).

Fetal and Neonatal Morbidity

Spellacy and colleagues in 1985 reported perinatal mortality more than doubled for infants with birth weights greater than 4500 g as compared with infants born weighing between 2500 and 3500 g. Most of the increase in mortality was due to birth trauma related to macrosomia. The most common birth injury was brachial plexus damage. This is highly correlated with shoulder dystocia, although Hardy in 1981 was able to document shoulder dystocia in only 50% of those infants displaying evidence of brachial plexus injury.

Lipscomb and associates (1995) reported that 18.5% of 157 infants weighing more than 4500 g experienced shoulder dystocia. Of the 29 fetuses with shoulder dystocia, seven developed Erb palsy. Fortunately, all were transient. In 1991 at Parkland Hospital in Dallas four (3%) of 118 infants weighing more than 4500 g at birth sustained a brachial plexus injury compared with only 4 (0.7%) of 737 infants weighing 4000 to 4500 g. The frequency of permanent nerve palsy was not documented by these authors (Ramin and Cunningham, 1995). Although brachial plexus injury occurs more commonly with vaginal delivery, it has been reported to occur even with cesarean section.

Other birth injuries associated with macrosomia include fractures of the clavicle and humerus. Fortunately, these usually heal well and cause no permanent sequelae. Although lower 1- and 5-minute Apgar scores are associated with macrosomia (Lazer et al, 1986), asphyxial injury is not (Boyd et al, 1983). Macrosomic neonates are also at risk for complications typical of infants of diabetic mothers, including hypoglycemia, hyperbilirubinemia, hyperviscosity, and disorders of calcium homeostasis.

Diagnosis of Fetal Macrosomia

The diagnosis of fetal macrosomia remains extremely difficult to make with confidence. In the macrosomic infant, clinical estimates of fetal weight by Leopold maneuvers (abdominal palpation of the fetus) are unreliable, even more so with an obese gravida. Typically, actual birth weight is underestimated by at least 500 g in more than half of fetuses weighing more than 4000 g and in up to 80% of fetuses larger than 4500 g (ACOG, 1991).

Advances in fetal imaging with ultrasonography have created the hope that ultrasound estimation of fetal weight and especially prediction of macrosomia would lessen the incidence of macrosomia-associated birth injury. Despite numerous published studies, different polynomial equations, and various biometric ratios, accurate prediction of fetal weight in the term infant remains highly imprecise. A study by Jennett and coworkers (1992) showed that, despite an increased cesarean section rate in the last 10 years, the incidence of shoulder dystocia and brachial plexus injury has not changed.

There are various reasons for the disappointing progress in management of this important problem, including the fact that most shoulder dystocias occur with nonmacrosomic infants. Nevertheless, the clinician must be aware of the best current methods for estimating fetal size and have a full understanding of their limitations. For the neonatologist attending births of suspected or unexpected macrosomic infants, an appreciation for the issues regarding fetal measurements and decisions based on them is helpful.

Various formulas have been proposed for predicting fetal weight using ultrasonography. These formulas, derived from a variety of fetal measurements through a multivariate regression model, typically use a combination of BPD, HC, AC, and FL. As might be expected from multiplying multiple coefficients together, the resultant product (estimated fetal weight) has an inherent inaccuracy of $\pm 15\%$. Watson and Seeds in 1991 found that fetuses predicted to weigh 4000 g and 4500 g by ultrasonography actually weighed that much only 50% of the time. Benacerraf and associates (1988), in a study involving more than 300 fetuses who weighed more than 4000 g at birth, found that ultrasonography had a sensitivity of only 65% in identifying macrosomic fetuses. Pollack and associates (1992) found that in post-term pregnancies the positive predictive value of ultrasonography in correctly predicting a fetus to be macrosomic at birth was only 64%.

More recently, O'Reilly-Green (1996) found that ultrasonography had a positive predictive value of 79% for weight greater than 4000 g but only 33% for 4500 g in 202 consecutive post-term pregnancies. Tamura and colleagues (1986) found in 147 diabetics that a single measurement of the fetal AC above the 90th percentile predicted macrosomia 78% of the time. However, a sensitivity of approximately 80% is typically associated with a specificity of 50% to 60%. This means a false-positive rate of 30% to 50% occurs even with the more predictive formula, possibly requiring an "unnecessary" cesarean section of more than 100 fetuses to prevent one permanent Erb palsy (see later).

Given the inaccuracy of a single ultrasound measurement in predicting macrosomia, some investigators have proposed "trending" fetal growth over two to four measurements. However, Hedriana and Moore (1994) suggested that for all weight classes, serial measurements provided no benefit over a single measurement between 32 to 36 weeks' gestation. In their study, serial measurements were averaged, and the fetal weight was within 10% of actual birth weight only 42% of the time. However, in a subgroup of 46 macrosomic fetuses, serial measurements of the AC as compared with a single AC measurement at 32 to 36 weeks improved the sensitivity of detection of LGA from 54% to 84% and the positive predictive value from 53% to 100% (Hedriana and Moore, 1994).

Watson and coworkers in 1988, and subsequently a number of studies by Chauhan and various associates (1992, 1994, 1995) have shown that when ultrasound prediction of fetal weight is directly compared with a clinical estimate of fetal weight, ultrasonography has no advantage. In fact, in two of Chauhan's studies it was shown that parous women with previous birth experience who were in early labor were as accurate in predicting their fetuses' birth weight as were their health care provider's clinical and ultrasound fetal weight predictions.

Management of Macrosomia

Once the diagnosis of macrosomia has been established, there is little that can be done to reverse the condition. This is surprising, since prenatal management of maternal diabetes has traditionally oriented to achieving excellent glucose control to reduce the incidence of macrosomia. However, the actual clinical results obtained have been mixed. Moore and coworkers in 1987 administered subcutaneous insulin to an obese type II diabetic mother whose fetus was believed to be macrosomic at 28 weeks' gestation. Despite achieving excellent glucose control, they were unable to prevent macrosomia or alter fetal growth. Coustan and colleagues in 1980 found that the risk of macrosomia did not correlate with maternal blood glucose values in diabetic women. On the other hand, Jovanovic-Peterson and coworkers (1991) found that while fasting glucose levels were not predictive of macrosomia, second- and third-trimester postprandial glucose levels were highly correlated with fetal birth weight. This suggests that at least in diabetic patients control of postprandial blood glucose excursions conceivably could help prevent macrosomia. Studies by O'Sullivan in 1975 and Coustan and Lewis in 1978 suggested that use of prophylactic insulin in gestational diabetics can reduce the incidence of macrosomia as compared with treatment with diet alone.

In an effort to minimize the incidence of shoulder dystocia and associated birth injury associated with suspected macrosomia, a number of management schemes have been proposed. In diabetic patients, it has historically been common to deliver an infant at 37 to 38 weeks' gestation after documentation of fetal lung maturity at least partly in an effort to avoid macrosomia associated with postdatism (gestation $\geq$42 weeks). This has led to high rates of induction of labor (>50%), failed induction, and cesarean section (approximately 50%) without appreciably decreasing attendant perinatal mortality and morbidity rates.

Combs and associates in 1993 showed that induction of labor versus awaiting spontaneous labor in patients with suspected macrosomia led to an increased cesarean section rate without an improvement in perinatal mortality or morbidity rates. The induced group had a cesarean section rate of 57% versus 31% in the spontaneous labor group. Weeks and colleagues in 1995 found a high bias toward cesarean section and "failed induction" in patients suspected of having a macrosomic fetus. They reviewed the records of more than 500 patients delivered of a fetus weighing more than 4200 g and compared those who were predicted before birth to have a macrosomic infant and those not predicted to deliver a macrosomic infant. Patients were induced more often (42.5% vs. 26.6%), failed to achieve active labor ($\geq$4 cm dilation) more frequently (49.0% vs. 16.5%), and underwent cesarean section more frequently (52% vs. 30%). Despite these changes in labor management, the incidence of shoulder dystocia in the predicted and nonpredicted groups was the same (11.8% and 11.7%, respectively).

Sandmire in 1993 editorialized that no reliable data are available to support a policy of cesarean section or early induction of labor in cases of suspected fetal macrosomia. He believed that there is not enough information to support an "evidence-based decision-making policy" of early induction of labor or "prophylactic" cesarean section in an effort to decrease fetal birth injury. On the other hand, Langer and associates (1991) have argued strenuously that all mothers with fetuses estimated to have weights greater than 4250 g should be offered cesarean section.

If one accepts that 8% to 20% of fetuses born weighing 4500 g or greater will experience shoulder dystocia, 15% to 30% of these will have recognizable brachial plexus injury, and 5% of these injuries will result in some perma-

nent damage, one can calculate that 333 to 1667 cesarean sections would have to be performed in women carrying a suspected macrosomic infant to prevent one case of permanent nerve injury due to shoulder dystocia. In fact, McFarland and associates (1986) found an incidence of brachial plexus injury in infants weighing greater than 4500 g delivered vaginally of 1:124. This translates into a persistent brachial plexus palsy incidence of 1:2480 for infants weighing greater than 4500 g delivered vaginally. Combined 1991 data from Los Angeles County Hospital and Parkland Hospital showed that of 275 infants delivered vaginally and weighing more than 4500 g, no perinatal deaths related to asphyxia or shoulder dystocia occurred (Lipscomb et al, 1995; Ramin and Cunningham, 1995).

In light of the inability to adequately predict fetal weight and macrosomia prior to delivery, ACOG has no specific recommendations regarding the management of macrosomia. Each case should be evaluated individually on its own merits. Special attention must be given to a patient whose labor is not progressing normally, because this has been shown by Acker and coworkers in 1985 to be a risk factor for shoulder dystocia, although McFarland and associates in 1995 found that labor abnormalities did not predict shoulder dystocia.

Despite the methodologic difficulties in predicting macrosomia, common sense and prudence are important attributes of well-managed pregnancy. Midpelvic operative deliveries should be avoided when macrosomia is suspected, and low pelvic or even outlet operative deliveries must be approached with extreme caution if labor is protracted. Many investigators have reported on the increased risk of shoulder dystocia with midforceps or vacuum deliveries (Benedetti and Gabbe, 1978; Levine et al, 1984; McFarland et al, 1986). The delivering practitioner must be well versed in the variety of maneuvers used to free an impacted fetus when shoulder dystocia presents. Finally, pediatric, anesthesia, and nursing staff should be notified in advance of delivery of a suspected macrosomic infant to maximize resuscitative efforts should the neonate need them.

In summary, fetal macrosomia occurs in association with a number of pathologic processes during pregnancy, including, notably, glucose intolerance and obesity in the mother. Contemporary management must be underpinned with caution and prudence. Although the risk of fetal injury is increased, with close consultation with pediatric and obstetric teams, successful management and excellent outcomes are achievable.

REFERENCES

Acker DB, Sachs BP, Friedman EA: Risk factors for shoulder dystocia. Obstet Gynecol 66:762, 1985.

American College of Obstetricians and Gynecologists: Teratology. ACOG Technical Bulletin #84. Washington, DC, ACOG, 1985.

American College of Obstetricians and Gynecologists: Fetal Macrosomia. Technical Bulletin #159. Washington, DC, ACOG, September 1991.

American College of Obstetricians and Gynecologists: Smoking and Reproductive Health. ACOG Technical Bulletin #180. Washington, DC, ACOG, 1993.

Antonov AN: Children born during the siege of Leningrad in 1942. J Pediatr 30:250, 1947.

Arbuckle TE, Wilkens R, Sherman GJ: Birth weight percentiles by gestational age in Canada. Obstet Gynecol 81:39, 1993.

Aulman JI, Talal N, Hoffman GS, Epstein WV: Problems associated with the management of pregnancies in patients with systemic lupus erythematosus. J Rheumatol 7:327, 1980.

Benacerraf BR: Intrauterine growth retardation in the first trimester associated with triploidy. J Ultrasound Med 7:153, 1988.

Benacerraf BR, Gelman R, Frigoletto RD: Sonographically estimated fetal weights: Accuracy and limitations. Am J Obstet Gynecol 159:1118, 1988.

Benedetti TJ, Gabbe SG: Shoulder dystocia: A complication of fetal macrosomia and prolonged second-stage labor with midpelvic delivery. Obstet Gynecol 52:526, 1978.

Boyd ME, Usher RH, McLean FH: Fetal macrosomia: Prediction, risks, proposed management. Obstet Gynecol 61:715, 1983.

Brenner WE, Edelman DA, Hendricks CH: A standard of fetal growth for the United States of America. Am J Obstet Gynecol 126:555, 1976.

Brown HL, Miller JM, Gabert, Kissling G: Ultrasonic recognition of the small-for-gestational-age fetus. Obstet Gynecol 69:693, 1987.

Campbell S, Bewley S, Cohen-Overbeek T: Investigation of the uteroplacental circulation by Doppler ultrasound. Semin Perinatol 11:362, 1987.

Campbell S, Thoms A: Ultrasound measurement of the fetal head-to-abdomen circumference ratio in the assessment of growth retardation. Br J Obstet Gynecol 84:165, 1977.

Cetrulo CL, Freeman RF: Bioelectric evaluation in intrauterine growth retardation. Clin Obstet Gynecol 20:979, 1977.

Chauhan SP, Lutton PM, Bailey KJ, et al: Intrapartum clinical, sonographic, and parous patients' estimates of newborn birth weight. Obstet Gynecol 79:956, 1992.

Chauhan SP, Sullivan CA, Lutton TC, et al: Parous patient's estimate of birth weight in postterm pregnancy. J Perinatol 15:192, 1995.

Chauhan SP, Sullivan CA, Magann EF, et al: Estimate of birthweight among post-term pregnancy: Clinical versus sonographic. J Matern Fetal Med 3:208, 1994.

Combs CA, Nackaran BS, Khoury JC: Elective induction versus spontaneous labor after sonographic diagnosis of fetal macrosomia. Obstet Gynecol 81:492, 1993.

Commey JOO, Fitzhardinge PM: Handicap in the preterm small-for-gestational-age infant. J Pediatr 94:779, 1979.

Cone JE: History of the Care and Feeding of the Premature Infant. Boston, Little, Brown, 1985, p 180.

Coustan DR, Berkowitz RL, Hobbins JC: Tight metabolic control of overt diabetes in pregnancy. Am J Med 68:845, 1980.

Coustan DR, Lewis SB: Insulin therapy for gestational diabetes. Obstet Gynecol 51:306, 1978.

Cunningham FG, MacDonald PC, Leveno KJ, et al (Eds): In Williams Obstetrics, 19th ed. Norwalk, CT, Appleton & Lange, 1993, p 508.

Easterling TR, Benedetti TJ, Carlson KC, et al: The effect of maternal hemodynamics on fetal growth in hypertensive pregnancies. Am J Obstet Gynecol 165:902, 1991.

Elster AD, Bleyl JL, Craven TE: Birth weight standards for triplets under modern obstetric care in the United States: 1984–1989. Obstet Gynecol 77:387, 1991.

Emanuel I, Alberman HFE, Evans SJ: Intergenerational studies of human birthweight from the 1958 birth cohort: I. Evidence for a multigenerational effect. Br J Obstet Gynaecol 99:67, 1992.

Fanaroff AA, Matin RJ, Miller MJ: Identification and management of high-risk problems in the neonate. In Creasy RK, Resnik R (Eds): Maternal-Fetal Medicine, 3rd ed. Philadelphia, WB Saunders, 1994, p 1151.

Fitzhardinge PM, Steven EM: The small-for-date infant: II. Neurological and intellectual sequellae. Pediatrics 50:50, 1972.

Fort AT, Morrison JC, Berreras L, et al: Counseling the patients with sickle cell disease about reproduction: Pregnancy outcome does not justify the maternal risk. Am J Obstet Gynecol 111:391, 1971.

Fricker HS, Segal S: Narcotic addiction, pregnancy, and the newborn. Am J Dis Child 132: 360. 1978.

Goldenberg RL, DuBard MB, Cliver SP, et al: Pregnancy outcome and intelligence at age five years. Am J Obstet Gynecol 175:1511, 1997.

Grouchy J, Turleau C: Clinical Atlas of Human Chromosomes, 2nd ed. New York, Wiley & Sons, 1984.

Hack M, Breslau N, Weissman B, et al: Effect of very low birth weight and subnormal head size on cognitive abilities at school age. N Engl J Med 325:231, 1991.

Hadlock FP, Deter RL, Harrist RB, et al: A date-independent predictor of intrauterine growth retardation: Femur length/abdominal circumference ratio. Am J Radiol 141:979, 1983.

Hanson JW, Streissguth AP, Smith DW: The effects of moderate alcohol consumption during pregnancy on fetal growth and morphogenesis. J Pediatr 92:457, 1978.

Hardy AE: Birth injuries of the brachial plexus: Incidence and prognosis. J Bone Joint Surg 63:98, 1981.

Hedriana HL, Moore TR: A comparison of single versus multiple growth ultrasonographic examinations in predicting birth weight. An J Obstet Gynecol 170:1600, 1994.

Hobbins J: Intrauterine growth retardation. In Quilligan E (Ed): Current Therapy in Obstetrics and Gynecology. Philadelphia, WB Saunders, 1980, p 50.

Jovanovic-Peterson L, Peterson CM, Reed GF, et al: Maternal postprandial glucose levels and infant birth weight: The National Institute of Child Health and Human Development—Diabetes in Early Pregnancy Study. Am J Obstet Gynecol 164:103, 1991.

Jeanty P, Cantraine F, Romero R, et al: A longitudinal study of fetal weight growth. J Ultrasound Med 3:321, 1984.

Jennett RJ, Tarby TJ, Kreinick CJ: Brachial plexus palsy: An old problem revisited. Am J Obstet Gynecol 166:431, 1992.

Jensen OH, Larsen S: Evaluation of symphysis fundus measurements and weighing during pregnancy. Acta Obstet Gynecol Scand 70:13, 1991.

Jimenez Jm, Tyson JE, Reisch JS: Clinical measures of gestational age in normal pregnancies. Obstet Gynecol 61:438, 1983.

Johnson SR, Kolberg BH, Varner MW: Maternal obesity and pregnancy. Surg Gynecol Obstet 164:431, 1987.

Kalousek DK, Dill FJ: Chromosomal mosaicism confined to the placenta in human conceptions. Science 221:665, 1983.

Katz AE, Davison JM, Hayslett JP, et al: Pregnancy in women with kidney disease. Kidney Int 18:192, 1980.

Kazzi GM, Gross TL, Sokol RJ, Kazzi NJ: Detection of intrauterine growth retardation: A new use for sonographic placental grading. J Obstet Gynecol 145:733, 1983.

Langer O, Berkus MD, Huff RW, Samueloff A: Shoulder dystocia: Should the fetus weighing greater than or equal to 4000 grams be delivered by cesarean section? Am J Obstet Gynecol 165:831, 1991.

Lazer S, Biale Y, Mazor M, et al: Complications associated with the macrosomic fetus. J Reprod Med 31:501, 1986.

Levine MG, Holroyde J, Woods JR, et al: Birth trauma: Incidence and predisposing factors. Obstet Gynecol 63:792, 1984.

Lichty JA, Ting RY, Burns PD, Dyar E: Studies of babies born at high altitude. Am J Dis Child 93:666, 1957.

Lin C-C, Moawad AH, Rosenow PJ, River P: Acid-base characteristics of fetuses with IUGR during labor and delivery. Am J Obstet Gynecol 126:712, 1976.

Lipper E, Lee K-S, Gartner LM, Brellong B: Determinants of neurobehavioral outcome in low-birthweight infants. Pediatrics 67:502, 1981.

Lipscomb KR, Gregory K, Show K: The outcome of macrosomic infants weighing at least 4500: Los Angeles County and University of Southern California experience. Obstet Gynecol 85:558, 1995.

Little BB, Snell LM, Gilstrap LC II: Methamphetamine abuse during pregnancy: Outcome and fetal effects. Obstet Gynecol 72:541, 1988.

Long PA, Abell DA, Beischer NA: Fetal growth retardation and preeclampsia. Br J Obstet Gynaecol 87:13, 1980.

Lubchenco LO, Hansman C, Dressler M, Boyd, E: Intrauterine growth as estimated form liveborn birth-weight data at 24 to 42 weeks of gestation. Pediatrics 32:793, 1963.

MacGregor SN, Keith LG, Chasnoff IJ, et al: Cocaine use during pregnancy: Adverse perinatal outcome. Am J Obstet Gynecol 157:686, 1987.

Manning FA, Hill LM, Platt LD: Qualitative amniotic fluid volume determination by ultrasound: Antepartum detection of intrauterine growth retardation. Am J Obstet Gynecol 139:254, 1981.

McFarland LV, Raskin M, Daling JR, Benedetti TJ: Erb/Duchenne's palsy: A consequence of fetal macrosomia and method of delivery. Obstet Gynecol 68:784, 1986.

McFarland M, Hod M, Piper JM, et al: Are labor abnormalities more common in shoulder dystocia? Am J Obstet Gynecol 173:1211, 1995.

Miller HC, Merritt TA: Fetal Growth in Humans. Chicago, Year Book, 1979.

Mondanlou HD, Dorchester WL, Thorosian A, Freeman RK: Macrosomia: Maternal, fetal, and neonatal implications. Obstet Gynecol 55:420, 1980.

Mondanlou HD, Komatsu G, Dorchester W, Freeman RK, Bosu SK: Large-for-gestational-age neonates: Anthropometric reasons for shoulder dystocia. Obstet Gynecol 60:417. 1982.

Moore TR, Cayle JE: The Amniotic Fluid Index in normal human pregnancy. Am J Obstet Gynecol 162:1168, 1990.

Moore TR, Hollingworth DR, Kolterman O, et al: Continuous subcutaneous insulin infusion in an obese insulin-resistant pregnant woman with type II diabetes: Accelerated fetal growth and neonatal complications. Obstet Gynecol 70:480, 1987.

Moore TR, Piacquadio K: A prospective assessment of fetal movement screening to reduce fetal mortality. Am J Obstet Gynecol 160:1075, 1989.

Moore TR, Sorg J, Miller L, et al: Hemodynamic effects of intravenous cocaine on the pregnant ewe and fetus. Am J Obstet Gynecol 155:883, 1986.

Morton NE: The inheritance of human birth weight. Ann Hum Genet 20:125, 1955.

Newman RG, Bashkow S, Calko D: Results of 313 consecutive live births of infants delivered to patients in the New York City Methadone Maintenance Treatment Program. Am J Obstet Gynecol 121: 233, 1975.

O'Leary JA, Leonetti HB: Shoulder dystocia: Prevention and treatment. Am J Obstet Gynecol 162:5, 1990.

O'Reilly-Green C: Positive and negative predictive value of estimated fetal weight for macrosomia in postdates patients. Am J Obstet Gynecol 174:350, 1996.

O'Sullivan JB: Prospective study of gestational diabetes and its treatment. *In* Sutherland HW, Stowers JM (Eds): Carbohydrate Metabolism in Pregnancy and the Newborn. Edinburgh, Churchill Livingstone, 1975.

Patton DE, Lee W, Cotton DB, et al: Cyanotic heart disease: I. Pregnancy. Obstet Gynecol Surv 45:594, 1990.

Polani PE: Chromosomal and other genetic influences on birth weight variation. *In* Elliot K, Knight J (Eds): Size at Birth. Amsterdam, Associated Scientific Publishers, 1974.

Pollack RN, Hauer-Pollack G, Divon MY: Macrosomia in postdates pregnancies: The accuracy of routine ultrasonographic screening. Am J Obstet Gynecol 167:7, 1992.

Procianoy RS, Garcia-Prats FA, Adams JM, et al: Hyaline membrane disease and intraventricular hemorrhage in small-for-gestational-age infants. Arch Dis Child 55:502, 1980.

Ramin SM, Cunningham FG: Obesity in pregnancy. *In* Cunningham FG, MacDonald PC (Eds): Williams Obstetrics, 19th ed. (suppl 13), Stamford, CO, Appleton & Lange, June/July 1995.

Richards MR, Merrit KK, Samuels JH, Langman A: Congenital malformations of the cardiovascular system in a series of 6053 infants. Pediatrics 15:12, 1955.

Robertson WB, Brosens I, Dixon G: Maternal uterine vascular lesions in the hypertensive complications of Pregnancy. *In* Lindheimer M, Katz A, Zuspan F (Eds): Hypertension in Pregnancy. New York, Wiley, 1975.

Rosett HL: A clinical perspective of the fetal alcohol syndrome. Alcohol Clin Exp Res 4:119, 1980.

Sandmire HF: Whither ultrasonic prediction of fetal macrosomia? Obstet Gynecol 82:260, 1993.

Simpson JW, Lawless RW, Mitchell AC: Responsibility of the obstetrician to the fetus: II. Influence of prepregnancy weight and pregnancy weight gain on birth weight. Obstet Gynecol 45:481, 1975.

Spellacy WN, Miller MS, Winegar A, Peterson PQ: Macrosomia: Maternal characteristics and infant complications. Obstet Gynecol 66:158, 1985.

Stein Z, Susser M: The Dutch famine, 1944–1945: I. Effects on six indices at birth. Pediatr Res 9:70, 1975.

Stewart PM, Rogerson FM, Mason JI: Type 2 11-beta-hydroxysteroid dehydrogenase messenger ribonucleic acid and activity in human placenta and fetal membranes: Its relationship to birth weight and putative role in fetal adrenal steroidogenesis. J Clin Endocrinol Metab 80(3):885, 1995.

Tamura RK, Sabbagha RE, Depp R, et al: Diabetic macrosomia: Accuracy of third trimester ultrasound. Obstet Gynecol 67:828, 1986.

Tejani N, Mann LL: Diagnosis and management of the small-for-gestational-age fetus. *In* Frigoletto FD (Ed): Clinical Obstetrics and Gynecology. Hagerstown, Harper & Row, 1977, p 943.

Varner MW, Galask RP: Infectious causes. *In* Lin CC, Evans MI (Eds): Intrauterine Growth Retardation. New York, McGraw-Hill, 1984.

Vintzileos AM, Campbell WA, Rodis JF, et al: Fetal weight estimation formulas with head, abdominal, femur, and thigh circumference measurements. Am J Obstet Gynecol 157:410, 1987.

Watson W, Seeds J: Sonographic diagnosis of macrosomia. *In* Divon MR (Ed): Abnormal Fetal Growth. New York, Elsevier, 1991, p 237.

Watson WJ, Soisson AP, Harlass FE: Estimated weight of the term fetus: Accuracy of ultrasound versus clinical examination. J Reprod Med 33:369, 1988.

Weeks JW, Pitman T, Spinnato JA II: Fetal macrosomia: Does antenatal prediction affect delivery route and birth outcome? Am J Obstet Gynecol 173:1215, 1995.

Williams RL, Creasy RK, Cunningham GC, et al: Fetal growth and perinatal viability in California. Obstet Gynecol 59:624, 1982.

World Health Organization: Prevention of perinatal morbidity and mortality. *In* Public Health Papers, Geneva, World Health Organization, 1972, p 8.

CHAPTER 10

Perinatal Substance Abuse

Alma Martinez, J. Colin Partridge, Xylina Bean and H. William Taeusch

Substance abuse during pregnancy, as defined by excessive use of alcohol and, to a lesser extent, narcotics, barbiturates, amphetamines, and marijuana, has been recognized for many decades. Since the 1950s, awareness has also grown regarding the adverse impact of tobacco on pregnancy. It is only in the past 15 years, however, that cocaine/crack use has assumed epidemic proportions in the United States.

Psychotropic substances both legal (such as alcohol, cigarettes, and prescription drugs) and illegal (such as heroin, amphetamine, cocaine, and phencyclidine [PCP]) may cause obstetric complications and fetal injury. These substances have short-term and long-term consequences for the newborn infant. Although chronic or sporadic abuse of a single substance can occur in a person who functions well in upper-class or middle-class society, more often several elements, such as life-style; health risks; poverty; and drug, tobacco, and alcohol abuse, are coexistent (Table 10–1). From this point of view, substance abuse, similar to many other health conditions, is a downstream consequence of multiple societal, governmental, familial, psychological, medical, educational, and personal ills. In turn, substance abuse often exacerbates the conditions associated with its use.

Why do women who are pregnant, who frequently are aware of potential adverse effects on the fetus, use drugs and smoke cigarettes? The reasons may vary depending on individuals and type of substance used and are summarized in Table 10–2.

The circumstances listed in Table 10–1 illustrate how difficult it has been to attribute effects on the fetus, newborn, infant, or child of a single drug. Nonetheless, the general effects of substances that may be abused during pregnancy are listed in Table 10–3. Consequences of exposure during pregnancy specifically attributed to drugs, alcohol, and smoking are poor intrauterine growth, prematurity, fetal distress, abortion, stillbirth, cerebral infarctions and other vascular accidents, malformations, and neurobehavioral dysfunction.

Nationally, women make up approximately 30% of drug treatment admissions and 25% of alcohol treatment admissions. Women, however, are underrepresented in treatment because many treatment programs do not admit pregnant women.

National Institute of Drug Abuse Surveys conducted in 1982 estimated that 90,000 women from 19 to 25 years of age used heroin, and 970,000 women in this same age group used cocaine or other stimulants, an increase of 250% from 1979 (NIDA, 1985). The present epidemic of drug abuse is attributable primarily to the marked increase in the use of cocaine. In 1982, 4.2 million women over age 12 years had used cocaine during the past year, and 1.4 million had used cocaine in the month before the survey. In 1991, Gomby and Shiono estimated that exposure rates during pregnancy for women in the United States are 4% to 5% for cocaine, 17% for marijuana, 38% for cigarettes, and 73% for alcohol.

Some of the most comprehensive, geographically based data on substance abuse by pregnant women have been obtained by the Perinatal Substance Exposure Study Group (Vega et al, 1993). This group collected urine from more than 30,000 women at delivery in California in 1992. (California has approximately 600,000 deliveries per year or about 15% of all deliveries in the United States.) Major

---

TABLE 10–1

Drug Use, Alcohol Use, Smoking, and Other Issues for Child-Bearing Women

Suboptimal parenting
Physical, sexual, domestic violence
Poverty
Poor schooling, illiteracy, school dropout
Limited job skills, training
Limited jobs
Poor self-image, poor coping skills
Peer pressure
Ineffectual birth control, STD protection
Unplanned, unwanted pregnancy; teenage pregnancy
Poor nutrition and preconception health care
Poor access, receipt, and quality of prenatal care
Little family/father support
Stress
Psychological disorders, depression
Limited access to support services in community
Dependence/addiction
Pregnancy wastage
Increased risk of premature birth
Increased risk of fetal malformations
Fetal growth retardation
Fetal/neonatal death
Newborn to foster care
Attempts at rehabilitation
Increased risk of HIV, syphilis, hepatitis B or C, STDs
Incarceration
Recapitulation in next generation

STD, sexually transmitted disease; HIV, human immunodeficiency virus.

TABLE 10–2

Common Reasons for Using Potentially Toxic Substances

Anxiety reduction	Escapism
Antidepressants	Fun, high, euphoria
Peer group pressure	Energy
Appetite suppression	Need, addiction

TABLE 10–3

Enhanced Risk for Various Events After Substance Use During Pregnancy*

	Ethanol	Cigarettes	Cannabis	Opiates	Cocaine	Amphetamines	Barbiturates	PCP
Malformation	+	−	?	−	+	−	−	+
Abortion	−	+	?	?	+	+	−	+
IUGR	+	+	?	+	+	+	−	?
Prematurity	−	+	?	±	+	+	−	?
Withdrawal	±	−	−	+	−	−	−	−
Central nervous system sequelae	+	?	?	?	+	?	−	?
SIDS risk	+	+	?	+	+	?	−	?
Foster care	+	−	−	+	+	+	±	+

*Although risk is increased, the risk ratio ranges for the most part from 1 to 2 for these associations.
IUGR, intrauterine growth retardation; SIDS, sudden infant death syndrome; PCP, phencyclidine.

results are shown in Table 10–4. These results (except for the higher rates of alcohol in California) are similar to earlier statewide surveys from South Carolina and Rhode Island. If results from this study can be extrapolated to the United States at large, an estimated 450,000 infants per year (of 4 million livebirths; 11%) are exposed to alcohol or drugs (or both) in the days before delivery.

Table 10–5 indicates substance exposure by ethnic group. Race/ethnic distributions of births in California are 44% Hispanic, 36% White non-Hispanic, 8% black, and 6% Asian/Pacific Islander. Prevalence of alcohol, smoking, and drugs are highest among blacks and lowest among Asian/Pacific Islanders. Despite lower risk, because they represent a larger segment of the population, the white, non-Hispanic group has roughly half the newborns exposed to drugs, smoking, and alcohol. Substance exposure was twofold higher in groups identified as *poor* on the basis of eligibility for Medicaid health insurance, indicating the

TABLE 10–4

California Prevalence Rates at Delivery of Substance Abuse, 1992

Substance	Percentage*
Amphetamines	0.7
Barbiturates	0.3
Benzodiazepines	0.1
Tetrahydrocannabinol/marijuana	1.9
Cocaine	1.1
Methadone	0.2
Opiates	1.5
PCP	0.0
Alcohol	6.7
Illicit drugs	3.5
Drugs and/or alcohol†	11.3
Tobacco‡	8.8

*Percentages represent the positive urine tests obtained from 29,494 women delivering infants from March through October 1992.
†Includes alcohol and/or any drug; excludes tobacco.
‡Tobacco was self-reported and not based on urine testing.
PCP, phencyclidine.
Data from Vega W, Kolody B, Hwang J, Noble A: Prevalence and magnitude of prenatal substance exposures in California. N Engl J Med 329:850, 1993.

expected association between substance abuse and poverty. Smoking was self-reported in this study and served as a major risk for illicit substance exposure (e.g., there was a 22-fold increased risk for cocaine use among those who smoked).

The emotional, medical, legal, familial, financial, and societal impact resulting from the fact that 10% to 15% of liveborn infants have been exposed during fetal life to substances with toxic effects is profound. Frustrated by this fact, some prosecutors have charged substance-abusing women with fetal/child abuse—for the most part unsuccessfully. Hospital costs average $5000 more for drug-exposed infants than for non–drug-exposed infants. A *positive toxicology screen* is associated with a 26% to 58% chance of referral to foster care placement compared with 1% to 2% in nonexposed infants (U.S. General Accounting Office, 1990). Costs of foster care are roughly $5000/year for normal infants and $20,000/year for infants with special needs.

In the California prevalence study, polydrug use was not common (0.5%). This figure may underestimate polydrug use because women may use drugs sequentially according to preference and availability rather than simultaneously. In the authors' experience, many use cigarettes and alcohol as primary drugs with either heroin or crack as the preferred substance when finances allow. Studies that attempt to learn over a long term true dose and duration exposures are not available.

OPIATES

Opium is obtained from the poppy *Papaver somniferum*, which is indigenous to the Middle East and Southeast Asia. Opium derivatives have been used as analgesics for centuries and remain the most effective analgesics available. Morphine is obtained from the seed capsules of the poppy plant and is the major alkaloid of opium. Other opioids of clinical interest include heroin, methadone, meperidine, and codeine.

Morphine's potential for abuse and addiction was documented in the mid-1800s, shortly after it began to be used extensively. Opium along with cocaine was a common additive to popular patent medicines. Perinatal problems associated with opium were reported in the late 1800s as a result of women using these preparations. In 1914, the

TABLE 10–5

Race/Ethnicity and Substance Exposure at Term in California, 1992*

Race/Ethnicity	Alcohol	Illicit Drugs	Nonillicit	Any Drug†	Total Positives‡	Tobacco§
Asian/Pacific Islander	5	0.4	1	2	7	2
Black	12	12	2	14	24	20
Hispanic	7	2	1	3	9	3
White, non-Hispanic	6	5	2	7	12	15
Other	4	2	1	3	7	5

°Numbers equal percentage of sample in which substance was identified at delivery.
†Excludes alcohol and tobacco. Indicates percentage of women in whom one or more drugs was identified in urine.
‡Includes alcohol and/or any drug; excludes tobacco.
§Tobacco was self-reported and not based on urine testing.

Harrison Act resulted in a marked decrease in the availability of opiate-containing medications. Since the 1950s, heroin has become endemic in most major American cities.

During the past decade, specific opiate receptors have been identified in the nervous system and the bowel that are activated by endogenous opiates, such as the naturally occurring endorphins and enkephalins (Olson et al, 1994). The endogenous opiates are believed to be modulators of the sympathoadrenal system and are important during periods of diverse forms of stress (Martinez et al, 1990, 1991). Activation of the different receptor types by the endogenous opiates produces different effects, including analgesia, drowsiness, respiratory depression, decreased gastrointestinal motility, nausea, and vomiting as well as alterations in the endocrine and autonomic nervous systems. These same endogenous opiate receptors are activated by exogenous opioid drugs and result in similar clinical effects.

Use of the opioid drugs can result in the development of tolerance, physiologic dependence, and addiction. With *tolerance*, there is a shortened duration of action of opioids and a decrease in the intensity of the drug action. There is a subsequent need for a higher dose of drug to obtain the same clinical effect. Tolerance is believed to result because of continued occupancy of the opioid receptor. Continuous administration of opioids, therefore, results in more rapid onset of tolerance (Anand and Arnold, 1994). With physiologic *dependence*, there is a need for further drug administration to prevent withdrawal symptoms (agitation, dysphoria, temperature instability). *Addiction* is a more severe form of dependence that includes a complex pattern of drug-seeking behavior.

Epidemiology

Prevalence of opiate use among pregnant women is reported to range from 1% to 2% (Vega et al, 1993; Yawn et al, 1994) to as high as 21% in a highly selected group of women (Behnke and Eyler, 1993; Ostrea et al, 1992b). Rates for heroin use are higher in metropolitan areas and cities and are more concentrated in Northeast and West Coast cities. Opiate abuse is more common in groups of lower socioeconomic status. Studies of the distribution of opiate abuse among ethnic groups in the United States have shown inconsistencies and apparent contradictions.

Reports showing blacks and Hispanics disproportionately represented (Hartnoll, 1994) can be contrasted with those showing a higher incidence among white women (Edelin et al, 1988; Gillogley et al, 1990). In a population-based study in California, the prevalence of opiate use during pregnancy was highest in blacks, followed by white women, and lowest in Asian and Hispanic women (Vega et al, 1993).

Women using opiates during pregnancy are more likely to use other drugs (Edelin et al, 1988; Gillogley et al, 1990; van Baar et al, 1994a, 1994b). Additionally, women who smoke during pregnancy are more likely to use opiates, alcohol, cocaine, amphetamines, and cannabis during pregnancy than nonsmoking women (Vega et al, 1993). In a study from Amsterdam, only 7% of heroin-using and methadone-using women did not smoke during pregnancy (Boer et al, 1994).

Of the opiate drugs known to be abused during pregnancy, heroin has been the most extensively studied. Heroin can be ingested by smoking or by the intranasal or intravenous routes. Intranasal use is common among women, especially in the western United States, whereas the intravenous route is more popular among users on the eastern seaboard. Reports from European countries suggest a trend away from intravenous injection of opiates (Hartnoll, 1994). The use of noninjectable heroin may reduce the risk of human immunodeficiency virus (HIV) transmission; however, its wider use ensures the emergence of new groups of heroin users for whom intravenous use and risk is a major deterrent.

Clinical Aspects

Maternal Aspects

Many heroin-addicted pregnant women have poor general health with multiple medical problems associated with the drug abuse life-styles (see Table 10–1). Intravenous use places the woman at risk for multiple infectious complications, including cellulitis, thrombophlebitis, hepatitis, endocarditis, syphilis, gonorrhea, and acquired immunodeficiency syndrome (AIDS). In an prospective study from New York City, close to 40% of women enrolled in a methadone maintenance program tested positive for HIV (Selwyn et al, 1989). Additionally, opiate abusers are less likely to receive prenatal care or obtain late prenatal care (Edelin et al, 1988; Lindenberg, 1993). Heroin-addicted mothers are often malnourished. Heroin is an appetite suppressant and appears to interfere directly with the absorption of nutrients (Raye et al, 1980). Iron-deficiency anemia appears to be more common in pregnant opiate users than nonusers.

Fetal and Neonatal Aspects

Obstetric complications reported in the literature include higher incidence of spontaneous abortions, premature delivery and preterm labor, abruptio placentae, chorioamnionitis, increased risk for cesarean section associated with breech presentation, and fetal distress. Chasnoff and colleagues (1985) reported a 46% incidence of spontaneous abortions in women using both methadone and cocaine and 16% in women using methadone alone. These rates were significantly greater than the control group. Similarly, higher incidence of fetal losses has been reported by others (Gillogley et al, 1990).

The incidence of preterm labor and premature delivery ranges between 25% and 33% for women using opiates (Chiriboga, 1993; Oro and Dixon, 1987). Investigators have found that infants exposed to opiates have higher risk for intrauterine growth retardation (Chasnoff et al, 1985; Oats et al, 1984) and smaller head circumference (Boer et al, 1994; Fulroth et al, 1989; Lifschitz et al, 1983). Investigators have also found that maternal opiate use is associated with increased rates of meconium staining, lower Apgar scores, and increased time of rupture of membranes (Edelin et al, 1988; Gillogley et al, 1990).

The increased risks for fetal loss, intrauterine growth retardation, prematurity, and low birth weight are thought to be multifactorial. Maternal life-style as well as frequent polydrug abuse is likely to result in poor perinatal outcomes. The increased incidence of maternal infections reported by some investigators is believed to contribute to intrauterine growth retardation and prematurity. Finally, because the drug supply is often uncertain, the pregnant woman addict is subject to episodes of withdrawal and overdose, thereby subjecting the fetus to intermittent episodes of hypoxia in utero, hindering growth and increasing the risk for spontaneous abortion, stillbirth, fetal distress, and prematurity. Infants born to these mothers are, therefore, more likely to be of low birth weight, to be premature, and to suffer from infection and perinatal asphyxia. The incidence of respiratory distress syndrome is reportedly decreased in heroin-exposed infants. This decrease may represent a direct effect of heroin on lung maturation or stress-induced accelerated lung maturation (or both) (Taeusch et al, 1973).

Neonatal Withdrawal Syndrome

The classic neonatal withdrawal or abstinence syndrome includes a wide variety of central nervous system signs of irritability, gastrointestinal and feeding problems (diarrhea, hyperphagia), autonomic signs of dysfunction, and respiratory symptoms (Table 10–6). The incidence of neonatal withdrawal syndrome in women using heroin or methadone is quite high, with wide ranges reported between 16% and 90% (Boer et al, 1994; Maas et al, 1990; van Baar et al, 1994a). One study suggests that the use of other drugs

---

TABLE 10–6

Clinical Signs of Neonatal Withdrawal Syndrome

Central Nervous System Dysfunction
Irritable, excessive crying
Jittery, tremulous
Hyperactive reflexes
Increased tone
Sleep disturbance
Seizures
Autonomic Dysfunction
Excessive sweating
Mottling
Hyperthermia
Hypertension
Respiratory Symptoms
Tachypnea
Nasal stuffiness
Gastrointestinal and Feeding Disturbances
Diarrhea
Excessive sucking
Hyperphagia

---

in addition to opiates during gestation may increase the newborn's risk for withdrawal symptoms (Fulroth et al, 1989).

The mortality rate in the past for withdrawing infants has been estimated as high as 10% during the years of 1969 through 1979 in Amsterdam (Boer et al, 1994). Current estimates show marked improvement, with perinatal mortality rates currently less than 1% (Boer et al, 1994). Mortality is rarely associated with withdrawal alone but occurs as a consequence of prematurity, infection, and severe perinatal asphyxia.

There are a number of evaluation tools that are frequently used to assess the severity of opiate withdrawal after birth. The Neonatal Abstinence Score is a scale based on nursing observations of the severity signs of withdrawal (Finnegan et al, 1975). Others have introduced the Neonatal Narcotic Withdrawal Index (Green and Suffet, 1981) as a rapid physician-based evaluation for neonatal signs of withdrawal. Using these scoring systems, the severity of the infant's withdrawal can thus be *quantified*. The score is used to guide the clinician's treatment of the withdrawing infant. These methods have shown good interobserver reliability and can increase clinicians' ability to treat the withdrawing infant appropriately (Anand and Arnold, 1994; Franck and Vilardi, 1995).

Treatment

Treatment includes soothing (swaddling, rocking, decreased environmental stimulation) as well as pharmacologic management. Medications most commonly used for opiate withdrawal include dilute tincture of opium, benzodiazepines, and phenobarbital (Levy and Sino, 1993). The mainstay of treatment, however, continues to be the opioids, used alone or in combination with other medications. The medication is titrated to the severity of the signs of withdrawal for each infant.

The authors use starting doses of tincture of opium (0.4

mg/mL of morphine equivalent) of 0.1 mL/kg given orally. This dose can be increased by 0.05- to 0.1-mL increments until the symptoms are controlled. The usual dose for infants withdrawing at birth can range from 0.2 to 0.5 mL every 3 to 4 hours (American Academy of Pediatrics, 1983; Anand and Arnold, 1994; Levy and Sino, 1993). Because of the occurrence of adverse effects with the use of paregoric in preterm infants, this medication should be avoided in the treatment of opiate withdrawal. Paregoric has been reported to be associated with acidosis, central nervous system depression, respiratory distress, hypotension, renal failure, seizures, and death (American Academy of Pediatrics, 1983; Anand and Arnold, 1994). Methadone has been used in the treatment of withdrawal in infants and older children as well (Tobias et al, 1990). Methadone has a longer duration of action and can be administered by either the oral or the parenteral route. The initial dose for methadone is 0.05 to 0.1 mg/kg given every 6 to 12 hours, with increases of 0.05 mg/kg until symptoms are controlled. Tobias and colleagues showed that the methadone could be given every 12 to 24 hours because of the longer half-life with this drug. The authors rarely use phenobarbital for withdrawal because it does not reduce diarrhea and because studies comparing phenobarbital and paregoric (morphine equivalent) showed that 11% of infants treated with phenobarbital had clinical seizures, whereas none of the infants treated with paregoric had this complication (Kandall et al, 1983). At higher doses, phenobarbital has also been shown to impair infant sucking. Diazepam may be used as an additional drug in withdrawing infants. The usual starting dose is 0.1 mg/kg every 6 to 8 hours and increasing to 0.3 mg/kg depending on the symptoms (Anand and Arnold, 1994; Levy and Sino, 1993).

Sudden Infant Death Syndrome and Opiates

Numerous small studies and reports have suggested a link between maternal opiate use during pregnancy and an increased risk for sudden infant death syndrome (SIDS). In a large 10-year study from New York, Kandall and associates (1993) showed that after controlling for known associated high-risk factors, the corrected risk ratio for SIDS among opiate exposed infants was two to four times greater than among infants not exposed to any perinatal drugs. These investigators found that differences in the rates of SIDS among ethnic groups disappear when women used drugs during their pregnancy. Whether the association between maternal opiate use and increased SIDS risk reflects pathology in the respiratory center of infants who eventually die from SIDS or whether this association is a reflection of other associated confounder(s) is still unclear. There are a number of maternal risk factors that may be associated with both opiate use and SIDS. Reports point to the strong association of maternal smoking in SIDS (Taylor and Sanderson, 1995).

Maternal Methadone Maintenance

Because maternal withdrawal is believed to be associated with subsequent fetal withdrawal, fetal asphyxia, and spontaneous abortions, detoxification of a pregnant heroin user is infrequently attempted (Barr and Jones, 1994; Zuspan et al, 1975). Most women are treated with daily methadone maintenance throughout pregnancy.

A retrospective comparison of opiate-using women enrolled in a maintenance program found that these women continued to use other illicit drugs at equally high rates and had infants of similar birth weight when compared to women not in enrolled in a program. The women in the methadone program received more prenatal care, however, and had a decreased incidence of anemia (Edelin et al, 1988). In a separate study, investigators showed that measures of adequacy of prenatal care, such as the number of visits and onset of care, were correlated with improved perinatal outcomes in women enrolled in a methadone program during pregnancy (Suffet and Brotman, 1984). In the Netherlands, women enrolled in a methadone program also had higher rates of prenatal care. In this study, higher prenatal care rates were associated with higher birth weights and less prematurity in the offspring the women (Soepatmi, 1994). When women in a methadone maintenance program were enrolled in an *enhanced* prenatal care program, their infants' birth weights were significantly larger than the control group of women receiving regular methadone maintenance during their pregnancy (Chang et al, 1992). These favorable outcomes are believed to be related to a stable intrauterine environment uncomplicated by periods of intoxication and withdrawal as well as less stress and better nutrition by the mother.

Controversy continues over the most appropriate dose of methadone maintenance during pregnancy. Several investigators have not found that neonatal withdrawal symptoms, birth weight, length of pregnancy, and number of days infants require treatment for abstinence correlate with maternal methadone dosage (Finnegan, 1991; Madden et al, 1977; Rosen and Pippenger, 1976). In contrast, others have reported significant correlation between the severity of neonatal withdrawal and maternal methadone dose (Harper et al, 1977; Kandall et al, 1983; Maas et al, 1990; Madden et al, 1977). Studying maternal and neonatal serum levels of methadone does not help to clarify this dilemma. Investigators have found no correlation between neonatal serum levels of methadone and the maternal methadone dose at delivery, the maternal serum levels, or the severity of withdrawal symptoms in the neonates (Harper et al, 1977; Mack, 1991). Doberczak and colleagues (1993) reported that the withdrawal signs were found to correlate with the *rate of decline* of the neonatal plasma level during the first few days of life.

These divergent findings have been used to argue either for weaning pregnant women to a low methadone maintenance dose or for attempting complete maternal detoxification during pregnancy. Others believe in maintaining high methadone doses to prevent the mother from "chipping" with additional street drugs that would put her at risk not only for enhanced drug-induced pregnancy complications, but also for increased risk of infections transmitted by intravenous use of drug (HIV, hepatitis) or of sexually transmitted disease wherein sex is traded for drugs. Some also believe that the fetus is placed at risk during maternal detoxification. The medical management of pregnant women addicted to opiates remains controversial.

Prognosis

A number of studies have shown that opiate exposure in utero can have a prolonged effect on infant growth. Chasnoff and colleagues (1980) showed that methadone-exposed infants remain small for the first 4 months of life and after that show accelerated growth. This growth spurt was found to coincide with improvement in the infants' neurobehavioral clinical findings. Others have also shown that growth-retarded infants exposed to opiates in utero experience an accelerated postnatal growth through early childhood (Soepatmi, 1994). A separate study of 18-month-old infants, however, found that infants exposed to methadone in utero showed a greater incidence of small head size, developmental delays, poor fine motor coordination, and lower Bayley mental and motor developmental scores when compared to a control group of infants (Rosen and Johnson, 1982). Various investigators have shown that behavioral characteristics of infants are affected by prenatal exposure to opiates. These infants showed significant differences in interactive behaviors, visual and auditory orientation, consolability, and state control.

Other significant developmental and learning deficits occur in both methadone-exposed and heroin-exposed children (Soepatmi, 1994; van Baar and de Graaf, 1994; van Baar et al, 1994; Wilson et al, 1979). Because opiate drug abusers use multiple drugs, including cigarettes, alcohol, cocaine, PCP, and amphetamines, it is impossible to ascribe all adverse developmental effects to opiates alone. Additionally, maternal intelligence and maternal behaviors have significant effects on their children's performance on intelligence measures and social adaptive behaviors. Using regression analysis, Lifschitz (1985) showed that the amount of prenatal care obtained by the mother and the postnatal home environment were most predictive of the infant's future intellectual performance. Conversely the amount of maternal opiate use during pregnancy was not found to be predictive. Others have pointed to the adverse environmental effects of poverty and poor learning environment on the development of methadone-exposed children. A multifactorial model, which includes both prenatal and postnatal influences on childhood development in drug-exposed infants, has been proposed by investigators that incorporates many of these diverse findings (Zuckerman and Bresnahan, 1991).

COCAINE

Cocaine is a highly psychoactive stimulant with a long history of abuse. Cocaine, a naturally occurring anesthetic of the tropane family of alkaloids, is obtained from the *Erythroxylon coca* plant, which is indigenous to the mountain slopes of Central and South America. The coca leaf has been chewed or made into a stimulant tea for centuries by the natives of these areas to decrease fatigue and hunger. Introduced to Europe in the sixteenth century, cocaine was isolated by Newman in 1860. Cocaine's euphoria-producing effect was exploited extensively in the United States in the late nineteenth and early twentieth centuries, when cocaine became an active ingredient in a number of elixirs and tonics. These over-the-counter preparations were widely used, and cocaine abuse became a major medical problem. The Harrison Narcotic Act of 1914 regulated the distribution of narcotics and cocaine, which at that time was erroneously classified as a narcotic. In 1970, the older federal drug laws were replaced by the Comprehensive Drug Abuse Prevention and Control Act, and cocaine was classified with the opiates, barbiturates, and amphetamines as a Schedule II drug (i.e., one of "high abuse potential with restricted medical use"). Cocaine use markedly decreased, and, until recently, cocaine held the status of an exotic drug used primarily by those in sports and entertainment to enhance performance. The limitation on its importation made cocaine a relatively expensive drug, available primarily to the affluent. Its reputation as a glamor drug, the widely held misconception that cocaine is nonaddictive, and the development and marketing of crack, a cheap version of cocaine, were the major factors in the resurgence of drug use (Abelson and Miller, 1985; Adams and Kozel, 1985).

Cocaine and other stimulants have become the drugs of choice for women in the United States (Berger et al, 1990), with estimates that up to 13% of women aged 18 to 25 use cocaine regularly. Women's use of cocaine as well as sexual activity to obtain drugs and maintain their habit has resulted in a marked increase nationwide in the birth of infants exposed to cocaine in utero. A survey of 18 metropolitan hospitals conducted by the U.S. House Select Committee on Children, Youth and Families found threefold to fourfold increases in deliveries of cocaine-exposed infants between 1985 and 1989 (Miller, 1989). Studies based on urine toxicology screening report a prevalence ranging from 5% of parturients (in urban New York City) to 1.1% (in a geographic sample in California) and to less than 0.5% (in private hospitals in Denver) (Burke and Roth, 1993). Prevalence increases to 18% when both self-report and urine testing are used, and the highest prevalence rates are reported from studies using meconium testing. In these studies, up to 31% of women delivering in a high-risk urban setting and 3.4% of women randomly tested in more representative urban samples tested positive for cocaine use (Ostrea et al, 1992a, 1992b; Zuckerman et al, 1989).

The pharmacologic actions of cocaine include inhibition of postsynaptic reuptake of norepinephrine, dopamine, and serotonin neurotransmitters by sympathetic nerve terminals. Cocaine allows higher concentrations of neurotransmitters to interact with receptors (Kurth et al, 1993). Higher levels of epinephrine and norepinephrine produce vasoconstriction, hypertension, and tachycardia. In adults, cocaine binds strongly to neuronal dopamine-reuptake transporters, thereby increasing postsynaptic dopamine at the mesolimbic and mesocortical levels and producing the addictive cycle of euphoria and dysphoria (Leshner, 1996). Tryptophan uptake is similarly inhibited, altering serotonin pathways with resultant effects on sleep. Sodium ion permeability is blocked, producing the anesthetic effect of cocaine. The metabolites of cocaine are pharmacologically active and may themselves produce neurotoxicity in the pregnant woman or her fetus. Two forms of cocaine are commonly used, cocaine hydrochloride and cocaine base (either extracted by organic solvents or precipitated as crack using ammonia and baking soda). Cocaine hydrochloride is a water-soluble white powder that is used orally, intranasally (snorting), or intravenously (running). Intravenous users are more likely to have a past history of heroin abuse and often use the drug in combination with heroin (speedballing). Cocaine hydrochloride decomposes on heating. Therefore, cocaine is converted to the freebase for inhalation. Freebasing involves extraction of cocaine from aqueous solution into an organic solvent such as ether. Crack, the most widely available form of freebase, is almost pure cocaine, and when it is smoked, it readily enters the bloodstream to produce levels similar to those occurring with intravenous use. Crack cocaine is popular in urban minority communities, where it may be smoked in combination with PCP (spacebasing). Crack smoking appears to be particularly reinforcing and is associated with compulsive use, binges, and acceleration of the addictive process.

Many of the adverse perinatal outcomes with cocaine abuse are thought to be related to the effects of cocaine on uterine blood supply (Woods et al, 1987). An increase in maternal mean arterial blood pressure, a decrease in uterine blood flow, and a transient rise in fetal systemic blood pressure after an intravenous cocaine infusion have been found in fetal sheep (Moore et al, 1986). Additional animal studies demonstrated significant fetal hypoxemia associated with changes in uterine blood flow with cocaine infusion (Woods et al, 1987). Maternal hypertension and intermittent fetal hypoxia contribute to the increased risks for abruptio placentae, intrauterine growth retardation, and potentially the congenital anomalies seen in cocaine-exposed infants.

Cocaine and some of its metabolites readily cross the placenta and achieve pharmacologic fetal levels (Schenker et al, 1993), although the exact mechanisms by which cocaine affects the fetus are not fully elucidated. Amniotic fluid may serve as a reservoir for cocaine and its metabolites, prolonging fetal exposure and potentially exacerbating the direct fetopathic effects of cocaine. Additionally the confounding effects of increased use of multiple drugs, tobacco, or alcohol and the less frequent use of prenatal care among cocaine-using women make interpretation of the causal relationships between gestational cocaine exposure and intrauterine growth and subsequent neurobehavioral development difficult (Chiriboga, 1993; Racine et al, 1993).

Maternal Effects of Cocaine

Cocaine use results in a sense of well-being, increased energy, increased sexual achievement, and an intense euphoria or high. The sympathomimetic action can have potentially devastating physiologic effects on the cardiovascular system. In adults, cocaine has been associated with cerebral hemorrhage, cardiac arrest, cardiac arrhythmias, myocardial infarction, intestinal ischemia, and seizures. Chronic use is associated with anorexia, nutritional problems, and paranoid psychosis. Chronic use ultimately results in neurotransmitter depletion and a crash characterized by lethargy, depression, anxiety, severe insomnia, hyperphagia, and cocaine craving (Kleber and Gawin, 1987).

Women who use cocaine during pregnancy are at high risk for stillbirths, spontaneous abortions, abruptio placentae, intrauterine growth deficiency, anemia and malnutrition, and maternal death from intracerebral hemorrhage

(Table 10–7). Cocaine directly stimulates uterine contractions because of its alpha-adrenergic, prostaglandin, or dopaminergic effects, with resulting increased risk for fetal distress and premature deliveries. Abruptio placentae appears related to cocaine only when use occurs shortly before delivery (Ostrea et al, 1992b). Other problems include evidence of fetal distress associated with abnormal fetal heart rate tracing and meconium staining (but not aspiration syndrome). These women are at high risk for premature labor, low-birth-weight infants, premature rupture of the membranes, and perinatal infections. The higher prevalence of sexually transmitted disease has been associated with the trading of sex for drugs. A fourfold increased odds of cocaine exposure among infants with congenital syphilis has been documented (Greenberg et al, 1991; Webber et al, 1993); both injection and noninjection use of cocaine increase risks for HIV acquisition, with a 3.5-increased risk among women who trade sex for crack (Lindsay et al, 1992).

TABLE 10–7

Associated Clinical Features in the Mother and Infant with Cocaine Use During Pregnancy

Pregnancy
Spontaneous abortions
Abruptio placentae
Stillbirths
Premature delivery
Growth
Low birth weight
Intrauterine growth retardation
Small head size
Infections
Perinatal HIV
Congenital syphilis
Malformations
Urogenital
Brain
   Midline defects (agenesis of the corpus callosum, septo-optic dysplasia)
   Skull defects, encephaloceles
   Ocular
   Vascular disruption (limb reduction, intestinal atresia)
   Cardiac
Neurodevelopmental Findings
Neonates
   Impaired organizational state
   Hypertonia, tremor
   Strokes, porencephaly
   Seizures
   Brain stem conduction delays
   SIDS
Infants and children
   Hypertonia in infancy
   Abnormal behaviors(?)

HIV, human immunodeficiency virus; SIDS, sudden infant death syndrome.

Reprinted with permission from Chiriboga CA: Cocaine and the fetus: Methodological issues and neurologic correlates. *In* Konkol RJ, Olsen GD: Prenatal Cocaine Exposure. Copyright CRC Press, Boca-Raton, Florida. © 1996.

Fetal Growth

Diminished intrauterine growth is the most common effect of gestational cocaine exposure (Chouteau et al, 1988; Zuckerman et al, 1989), with effects on weight, height, and head circumference at birth (see Table 10–7) (Frank et al, 1993). Head circumference among exposed infants is decreased, and it is postulated that fetal brain growth is impaired more than somatic growth. Abstinence after the first trimester appears to diminish the intrauterine growth-retarding process but may not prevent diminished head growth or neurobehavioral abnormalities (Chasnoff et al, 1985; Zuckerman et al, 1989). One large prospective study suggested direct cocaine effects on intrauterine growth as well as indirect effects of cocaine-associated undernutrition (Zuckerman et al, 1989). The effects of suboptimal intrauterine growth on subsequent neurodevelopmental outcome abnormalities have not been distinguished from the effects of cocaine or its metabolites.

Congenital Malformations

Cocaine has been reported in association with a variety of congenital anomalies in animals, although the teratogenicity of cocaine has yet to be established in humans. Some of the fetal malformations could be explained by norepinephrine-mediated vasoconstrictive effects during organogenesis (Mahalik and Hitner, 1994). Limb reduction deformities, intestinal atresia or infarction, and other vascular disruption sequences have been reported, although no increase was found in a population-based prevalence study (Martin et al, 1992). Central nervous system ischemic and hemorrhagic lesions have been reported inconsistently (Dusick et al, 1993; Konkol et al, 1994), both in term and in premature infants. The risk of genitourinary anomalies appears to be increased fourfold; these are the only anomalies well demonstrated in association with cocaine exposure (Martin et al, 1992). Cardiac malformations, such as cardiomegaly, atrial septal defects, and ventricular septal defects, have been inconsistently reported (Lipschultz et al, 1991), and this association may be confounded by higher rates of maternal tobacco, marijuana, or alcohol use among the cocaine-exposed groups. Ocular abnormalities attributed to cocaine have included retinopathy, persistent hyperplastic vitreous, dilated and tortuous iris blood vessels, delayed visual maturation, palpebral edema, and structural anomalies of the eye among cocaine-exposed infants (Dominguez et al, 1991). Overall, both animal studies and some human studies suggest a vasoconstrictive cause for cocaine-associated anomalies, particularly for limb reduction and urogenital anomalies (Hoyme et al, 1990). A teratogenic potential for cocaine remains controversial, and to date a well-identified cocaine-associated syndrome has not been identified. Multiple studies have not reported increased rates of congenital anomalies among cocaine-exposed infants.

Cocaine and Premature Delivery

Of all the problems attributed to cocaine use in the pregnant woman, the most common problem is that of premature delivery (Bateman et al, 1993). Accordingly, infants born to these women may develop sequelae of prematurity:

cerebral palsy, developmental delay, diminished intellectual capacity, and behavioral impairment. Four of five studies with sample sizes large enough to assess independent effects of cocaine on prematurity demonstrated this association (Chouteau et al, 1988; Gillogley et al, 1990; Handler et al, 1991; Petitti and Coleman, 1990); the fifth (Zuckerman et al, 1989) showed no such association but was done in woman receiving prenatal care, suggesting that in the absence of prenatal care, cocaine may bear an independent association with prematurity. Prematurity and intrauterine growth retardation also appear to be closely related to maternal life-style. In those populations studied in which the mother receives good prenatal care associated with drug treatment, the incidence of prematurity and intrauterine growth retardation is low (Chasnoff et al, 1985; Shiono et al, 1995). In the presence of poor prenatal care and no documented drug treatment, however, the rates of premature birth and intrauterine growth retardation are high (Burkett et al, 1990; Chouteau et al, 1988; Oro and Dixon, 1987). These findings have obvious implications for the development of effective treatment strategies to minimize adverse perinatal outcome in substance-abusing women, as has been suggested by cohort studies demonstrating improved rates of prematurity in women with adequate prenatal care. The risk of respiratory distress syndrome is not affected specifically by cocaine use; however, because of the increased risks of premature delivery, the frequency is greater in cocaine-exposed infants.

Neurobehavioral Abnormalities

Cocaine-exposed infants manifest a range of neurobehavioral abnormalities initially described as drug withdrawal, but these are more likely due to acute intoxication (Chasnoff et al, 1985; Dempsey et al, 1996). Signs are present at birth or a few days thereafter, waning as cocaine and benzoylecgonine are cleared from plasma. The infants are hypertonic, irritable, and tremulous (Chiriboga, 1993) and may have abnormal crying, sleep, and feeding patterns, although controlled, blinded studies have demonstrated cocaine withdrawal signs in a lower proportion of cocaine-exposed infants than have unblinded studies. Tachycardia, tachypnea, and apnea have been noted in two blinded, controlled studies, with significant elevations in cardiac output, stroke volume, mean arterial blood pressure, and cerebral artery flow velocity resolving by day 2, consistent with an intoxicant effect of cocaine (van de Bor et al, 1990a, 1990b). Other early and late patterns of neurobehavioral abnormalities include a depressed state occurring immediately after birth and lasting 3 to 4 days (resembling the adult cocaine crash) and a late-emerging (onset 3 to 30 days) hyperirritable phase, which may be a manifestation of fetopathic effects of cocaine (Mott et al, 1994). Cocaine-exposed infants may have abnormal electroencephalograms or clinical seizures, perhaps the result of toxicity from benzoylecgonine, a major metabolite of cocaine (Konkol et al, 1994). Although up to 50% of exposed infants in one series had seizures (Doberczak et al, 1989), this was not confirmed by another study (Legido et al, 1992), and in the authors' experience neonatal seizures stemming directly from maternal cocaine use are rare. Seizures may occur because of asphyxial complications associated with maternal cocaine use.

Persisting behavioral, neurologic, and rearing problems are reported in these children (Chasnoff et al, 1989a, 1992). Significant impairment of orientation, motor, and state regulation among infants with documented cocaine exposure during only the first trimester has been reported (Chasnoff et al, 1989a). In contrast, Chasnoff and colleagues (1992) noted no significant differences between a cocaine and polydrug group and a drug-negative group in mean developmental scores, although a significantly larger proportion of children scored in the abnormal cognitive range. Compromised motor performance in late infancy has been reported in exposed infants in a controlled longitudinal study (Fetters and Tronick, 1996). These motor abnormalities did not persist at 15 months, and both the exposed and the control group had motor scores significantly below norms for age. Variable outcomes of these studies may depend on the amounts and style of drug usage that vary with geographic area or on other covariates, such as nutritional status, poverty, and parental educational level.

The neurodevelopmental problems among children exposed to cocaine may occur either from direct encephalopathic drug effects during gestation or from indirect effects of the social environment in which the developing infant is reared. Chasnoff (1987) reported that opiate-exposed, cocaine-exposed, and stimulant-exposed infants demonstrated a downward trend in mean developmental scores by age 2 consistent with a deleterious effect of the environment, parental stimulation, socioeconomic status, or potentially other indirect effects of drugs on the developing central nervous system. At 3 years of age, the four- to five-point decrease on the Stanford-Binet intelligence quotient did not significantly differ from unexposed controls. Prospective studies have demonstrated increased rates of hypertonia, peaking at 6 months of age and resolving in most children over the next 2 to 3 years (Chiriboga et al, 1995; Hurt et al, 1995). To date, little is known about subsequent effects on adult behavior and learning.

Postnatal Growth

Growth-retarded infants exposed to cocaine generally exhibit catch-up growth. Their length does not differ from nonexposed controls at 18 months. At 2 years, mean length of cocaine-exposed infants was lower but did not differ from alcohol-exposed or marijuana-exposed infants. At all ages, drug-exposed infants (cocaine, ethanol, or marijuana) had lower mean head circumferences than unexposed infants.

Sudden Infant Death Syndrome and Cocaine

The incidence of SIDS may be greater in cocaine-exposed infants (Chasnoff et al, 1989b; Kandall et al, 1993), although this increase appears less significant than those for methadone-exposed or heroin-exposed infants (Bauchner and Zuckerman, 1990). Other studies demonstrate abnormal respiratory patterns and ventilatory control (Chasnoff et al, 1989b).

Management

Intrapartum Management

The pregnant woman with suspected or admitted gestational or intrapartum cocaine use should undergo urine toxicology screening after informed consent, recognizing that both self-report and urine screening are neither sensitive nor specific tools for identifying intrapartum complications, neonatal morbidity, long-term outcome, or families at risk of child neglect or abuse (Jessup, 1990; Ostrea and Welch, 1991). Identification offers the potential benefits of screening for sexually transmitted diseases, closer obstetric monitoring of maternal and fetal well-being, drug counseling, support and referrals for rehabilitation, and social service needs assessment. Use of prenatal care should be encouraged on the basis of the benefits to mother and fetus, rather than enforced by incarceration or prosecution (Chavkin, 1991). Obstetric care should be offered in a nonjudgmental manner and should avoid being codependent or punitive. Recommendations for intrapartum medications do not differ from recommendations for drug-free women; however, cocaine-using women may require treatment for hypertension or for agitation. The authors recommend using standardized criteria for perinatal toxicology screening to avoid risks of differential screening and reporting. Routine prenatal laboratory tests, including third-trimester (or intrapartum) syphilis serology, should be performed. The authors also encourage HIV antibody testing for cocaine-using women, in keeping with current obstetric recommendations. Postpartum education should stress general health, routine postpartum teaching, breast-feeding risks, neonatal care, parenting skills, and need for obstetric and neonatal follow-up. Referrals for drug treatment and counseling should be facilitated before discharge, recognizing the scarce resources available to substance-using women with children. Public health nurse follow-up is recommended.

Neonatal Care

The majority of infants, although at higher risk for medical complications, do not require intensive neonatal care; however, symptomatic infants often require more nursing care. Admission physical examination should document a maturational age examination, birth weight, head circumference, and length. Infants should be examined for any evidence of cocaine-associated malformations (or anomalies related to concurrent alcohol exposure) or of complications of prematurity. Hypertonic, tremulous infants usually respond to swaddling, being held, decreases in ambient environmental stimuli (light and noise), pacifiers, and more frequent feedings. Studies such as electroencephalography, brain imaging, or renal sonography may add diagnostic or prognostic information when physical or neurologic abnormalities are noted, but these are not indicated for all exposed infants. Neurologic or ophthalmologic evaluation may document tone and ocular abnormalities in some otherwise asymptomatic infants, but it is not clear that all exposed infants should be referred for examination. Feedings in premature infants with cocaine exposure should be started with diluted formula with lower than usual volume increments because premature infants exposed to cocaine have been found to be at increased risk for both early-onset and late-onset necrotizing enterocolitis. Maternal cocaine use exposes infants to higher than expected problems with postasphyxial syndrome, and organ malfunction on this basis should be sought and treated.

Toxicology testing should be performed on neonatal urine (or meconium, where possible) as soon as possible. Infants should undergo screening for anemia, polycythemia, hypoglycemia, congenital syphilis, and perinatal HIV exposure. Discharge planning should identify a continuity provider as well as support services for the mother and infant (e.g., nutritional, social/familial, parenting) and a plan for neurodevelopmental follow-up. Although there are reports of increased risks of SIDS among cocaine-exposed infants, neither polysomnography nor home apnea monitoring is indicated in the absence of other risk factors for SIDS.

Mother-Infant Care

Breast-feeding has benefits of improved bonding; however, the risks of hepatitis, HIV, and recurring drug exposure may outweigh these benefits. Women who wish to breast-feed despite these potential risks should undergo drug monitoring of their breast milk and sequential HIV antibody testing. Close observation of visiting patterns and of mother-infant interaction should be documented in the infant's chart. Parenting and child-care skills should be stressed as part of the discharge education for the mother. All physician interactions with the family should be documented in detail.

Disposition of Cocaine-Exposed Infants

Many states include maternal substance abuse among reasons for mandated reporting to child protective services for evaluation of potential foster care placement. Cocaine exposure increases the risk for foster care placement from a background rate of 1% to 2% among nonexposed infants to 26% to 58% in exposed infants (U.S. General Accounting Office, 1990). Cocaine use has become the dominant characteristic of child welfare caseloads in 22 states and the District of Columbia (Besharov, 1989). Variations in screening and reporting protocols lead to inconsistent reporting practices. Referrals to child protective services were more frequent for black women using crack cocaine in a Florida study (Chasnoff et al, 1990). In California, cases involving maternal cocaine use are more apt to reach court adjudication for foster care placement than are cases involving maternal use of amphetamines (Chasnoff et al, 1990; Sagatun-Edwards et al, 1995).

The number of children in foster care increased 81% in the first 4 years of the crack cocaine epidemic (County Welfare Directors Association of California, 1990). The increases are attributed to the cocaine epidemic, with the effects of lowering the age of children in foster care and of rapidly increasing the number of out-of-home placements (Halfon et al, 1990). Maltreatment of infants of cocaine-using women has been described in a controlled cohort study (Wasserman and Leventhal, 1993); however, the neurobehavioral abnormalities seen in foster children suggest

that separation of mother and infant should occur only in high-risk cases.

Costs of care for cocaine-exposed infants are significantly higher than for nonexposed infants and outweigh the costs of providing prenatal care. The added costs of gestational cocaine exposure include the costs of perinatal care for the substance-using woman, the costs of neonatal intensive care, and the costs of boarding infants awaiting release to foster care, in addition to the costs of later specialized services to infants with anatomic or neurodevelopmental sequelae of cocaine exposure (Phibbs et al, 1991).

AMPHETAMINES

The clinical effects of amphetamines are often indistinguishable from those of cocaine. Amphetamines also potentiate the action of norepinephrine, dopamine, and serotonin and are sympathomimetics similar to cocaine. Amphetamine (methylphenethylamine) was synthesized in 1887 and introduced into the United States in 1931 and the *d,l*-isomer marketed as Benzedrine. A number of other isomers soon followed, including dextroamphetamine (Dexedrine) and the *N*-methylated form, methamphetamine. Clinically the amphetamine isomers have the same effect and can be distinguished only in the laboratory. Amphetamines were initially marketed for the treatment of obesity and narcolepsy and continue to be used for treatment of attention deficit disorders in children. Amphetamines are classified as Schedule II drugs, similar to cocaine and the narcotics. Amphetamines may have some ability to block reuptake of released neurotransmitters. In contrast to cocaine, however, they appear to exert their central nervous system effects primarily by enhancing the release of neurotransmitters from presynaptic neurons. They may also exert a direct stimulatory action on postsynaptic catecholamine receptors.

Amphetamines are taken orally, inhaled, or injected. The clinical effects and toxicity of amphetamines are indistinguishable from those of cocaine. The primary difference is in the duration of action. The psychotropic effects of cocaine are of short duration, 5 to 45 minutes. The effects of amphetamines may last from 2 to 12 hours (Robbins et al, 1983). Methamphetamine (*crystal*) has been the primary form abused. Amphetamines have always been popular among adolescents, especially adolescent females. The drug's popularity has been increasing owing to the appearance of a new smokable form of methamphetamine, *ice*. Ice is currently the major drug abused in some parts of the United States, especially Hawaii and San Diego. Crystal and ice both can be produced locally and fairly cheaply. With increased restrictions on the importation of cocaine, a resurgence in amphetamine use has been noted. The popularity of amphetamines among women of child-bearing age places this group at high risk for perinatal abuse (Dixon, 1989). A California study of drug-exposed infants in the social welfare system documented a higherprevalence of amphetamine use among White pregnant women compared to women of other ethnicities (Sagatun-Edwards et al, 1995).

The medical and obstetric complications of amphetamines are similar to those described for cocaine. Amphetamine toxicity has been described as more intense and prolonged than that seen with cocaine. Visual, auditory, and tactile hallucinations are common (Schmidt, 1987), and microvascular damage has been seen in the brains of chronic users (Rothrock et al, 1988). Amphetamine withdrawal is characterized by prolonged periods of hypersomnia, depression, and intense, often violent paranoid psychosis (Smith et al, 1979). Obstetric complications include an increased incidence of stillbirth (Dearlove et al, 1992). As in cocaine-using women, the pregnancies of amphetamine users are characterized by poor prenatal care, sexually transmitted diseases, and cardiovascular problems including abruptio placentae and postpartum hemorrhage.

Neonatal problems include prematurity and intrauterine growth retardation (Dixon, 1989; Oro and Dixon, 1987). Cardiovascular malformations have been described (Fein et al, 1987), but other studies have failed to show an increased risk. Neurodevelopmental abnormalities have been described both during the neonatal period and in long-term follow-up studies as late as 14 years (Cernerud et al, 1996; Dixon, 1989). Intellectual capacity does not appear to be diminished among exposed infants. These children are described as exhibiting disturbed behavior, including hyperactivity, aggressiveness, and sleep disturbances. The neurobehavioral abnormalities appear to be associated with the extent and the duration of fetal exposure. Children with the most severe problems were those born to mothers who abused amphetamines throughout pregnancy and those being reared in homes with an addicted parent (Billings et al, 1985).

Children of amphetamine abusers appear to be at high risk for social problems, including abandonment, abuse, and neglect (Eriksson et al, 1986). In two Swedish studies, only 22% of amphetamine-exposed infants remained in the care of their biologic mothers, whereas 70% were in foster care at 10 years of age (Cernerud et al, 1996; Eriksson and Zetterstrom, 1994).

PHENCYCLIDINE

Phencyclidine hydrochloride (1-phenyl cyclohexyl piperidine) is an arylcyclohexamine developed in 1956 and marketed for the first time in 1963 as an anesthetic (Sernyl) and in the early 1970s as a veterinary drug (Sernylan). PCP was withdrawn following reports of delirium and hallucinations and following recognition of its potential for abuse. No longer legally manufactured, PCP remains included in the Comprehensive Drug Abuse Prevention and Control Act of 1970. The first reports of the illicit use of PCP occurred in 1967 from the Haight-Ashbury district of San Francisco. Epidemic use of PCP began in the mid-1970s and peaked in 1983, when it was the most frequently used hallucinogen among young adults in the United States. Since it developed a reputation as a dangerous drug, its popularity has been episodic and often geographically and demographically concentrated. Use is common among polysubstance users, particularly in combination with marijuana, heroin, and alcohol (Golden et al, 1987).

PCP, also known as angel dust, is a white crystalline powder soluble in water and alcohol. It can be inhaled, taken orally, or injected intravenously. Its popularity among young adults, especially women, however, relates to its low cost and its ability to be smoked. PCP is usually smoked sprinkled (dusted) on cigarettes (lovely) or marijuana (sherm). PCP increases epinephrine release, but its exact mechanism of action is not clearly understood. PCP receptors have been identified in the brain, but how they interact with PCP is unclear. The effects of the drug are dose-related and differ according to the duration of exposure. Low doses primarily cause euphoria associated with disturbances in body image. Moderate doses result in confusion, disorientation, and impaired sensory perception (analgesia and anesthetic effects). High doses are followed by hypertension, seizures, hyperpyrexia, an acute toxic paranoid psychosis, coma, and death. Chronic, continuing use results in violent behaviors; depressive anxiety; an organic brain syndrome; and, rarely, delayed, prolonged, or recurrent schizophrenia-like reactions. The toxic psychosis is treated by sensory isolation and diazepam, whereas the prolonged PCP psychosis requires antipsychotic medications.

There are limited data on the effects of PCP on pregnancy and the newborn. PCP readily crosses the placenta and has been documented in both the fetus and the newborn as well as in breast milk (Golden et al, 1984; Kaufman et al, 1983). Animal studies demonstrate alterations in septohippocampal cholinergic innervations with later behavioral consequences (Yanai et al, 1992). From 1981 to 1984, PCP was the primary drug of abuse among parturients in some urban areas; in 1985, crack cocaine replaced PCP as the drug of choice for substance-abusing women. Since the mid-1980s, use of PCP has decreased. Its use was more prevalent among pregnant Latinas in one study in California (Sagatun-Edwards et al, 1995).

The effects of PCP on the outcome of pregnancy appear to be dose related. In low doses, PCP has few side effects, although the anesthetic nature of the drug increases the frequency of precipitous deliveries at home, in ambulances, and in emergency departments. Other obstetric complications are not known to be increased. PCP is not associated with increased risks for prematurity, but 40% of PCP-exposed infants are small for gestational age.

A severe syndrome associated with PCP exposure in utero has been reported, with onset shortly after birth (Golden et al, 1980; Strauss et al, 1981). The timing and severity of the symptoms, however, often present at birth, raise the question of whether the neurologic findings represent drug intoxication rather than drug withdrawal effects (Rahbar et al, 1993) because PCP persists in the body, and especially in fetal brains, for prolonged periods (Ahmad et al, 1987). The neurologic findings in PCP-exposed infants were striking for the severity of the hypertonicity and hyperreflexia, often associated with spontaneous clonus and persisting for several weeks (Chasnoff et al, 1986; Golden et al, 1987). Sudden episodes of agitation and fluctuating levels of consciousness have been described. Gastrointestinal symptoms, including abdominal distention, vomiting, and diarrhea, were also present in about 20% of the infants. The morbidity of significant PCP withdrawal can be attributed to gastrointestinal complications and the prolonged duration of symptoms. The mean duration of hospitalization in the authors' population was 14 days (range 10 to 21 days). The withdrawal syndrome seen in infants exposed to PCP in combination with other drugs appears to be less intense, most likely related to a lower dose exposure or to inadvertent or erratic exposure when other drugs, such as cocaine, are "cut" with PCP.

Congenital anomalies have been reported (Chasnoff et al, 1983a; Golden et al, 1980; Strauss et al, 1981), but a clear causal association with PCP has not been verified. The authors found no increased risk of congenital anomalies, in contrast to the report of Golden and coworkers (1987). The reported somatic growth of PCP-exposed infants appears similar to that of polydrug-exposed infants. Isolated microcephaly, usually less severe than that seen in cocaine-exposed infants, has also been described and may be dose related (Rahbar et al, 1993).

Long-term outcome studies of chronically PCP-exposed infants show an increased prevalence of severe developmental and behavioral problems (Chasnoff et al, 1983a). Early alterations in state lability and consolability more severe than in all other drug-exposed groups have been documented, but these do not appear to persist later in infancy (Chasnoff et al, 1983a).

ALCOHOL

First described in Europe by Lemoine in 1968 and subsequently recorded in a number of studies in the United States, the fetal alcohol syndrome (FAS) is an extensively documented teratogenic syndrome. FAS occurs in 1 to 2 per 1000 live births in most industrialized countries (as high as 20% of live births in a few reported subgroups of Native Americans), making it a major cause of mental retardation. FAS is estimated to occur in the infants of 30% to 40% of pregnant women who consume 3 or more ounces of absolute alcohol per day. The prevalence and incidence of the syndrome may be on the rise in the United States (Update, 1995). The adverse effects of alcohol on the fetus are related to the gestational stage at which exposure occurs, the amount of liquor the mother consumes, the presence of binge drinking, and the individual susceptibility of the fetus. There is no documented safe level of alcohol ingestion, and women should be advised to abstain from alcohol during pregnancy. The high incidence of FAS led the U.S. government to add a warning label on beer, wine, hard liquor, and wine cooler containers.

FAS is diagnosed by history and physical examination (Olsen and Tuntiseranee, 1995). There are no laboratory tests as yet that summate alcohol exposure during fetal life (Robinson et al, 1995). The syndrome consists of prenatal and postnatal growth deficiency, microcephaly, and mental retardation associated with characteristic facies and diverse ocular defects. The microcephaly is a reflection of the damage to brain tissues that results from alcohol exposure. The facial features consist of short palpebral fissures, broad flat nasal bridge, short upturned nose, and long upper lip without distinct philtrum (Abel et al, 1983). Abnormal hand creases and cardiac anomalies have been described.

Women who are chronic alcoholics may also have a greater risk for abruptio placentae, spontaneous abortions, and stillbirths. Lesser degrees of alcohol consumption have been associated with fetal growth retardation, congenital anomalies, behavioral and neurologic abnormalities, and milder degrees of mental retardation—a condition termed by some *fetal alcohol effects* as compared with the more severe and clearly identifiable FAS. Because fetal effects

of alcohol are dose related and all part of a spectrum, Aase and colleagues (1995) have questioned the value of using the term *fetal alcohol effects*. A neonatal withdrawal syndrome with jitteriness and poor feeding has been reported in infants born to mothers who were intoxicated at the time of delivery.

The subsequent degree of mental retardation correlates with the degree of physical stigmata. The postnatal growth deficiency is prominent in infancy and persists into early childhood and may be associated with vomiting. Speech and language problems are common in older children. Behavioral problems, including severe hyperactivity and attention deficit disorders, contribute to the learning disabilities characteristically seen in these children (Wekselman et al, 1995; West et al, 1994).

The approach to a newborn with FAS is to establish the diagnosis by ruling out other causes of malformations, determining the extent of malformation, and establishing long-term care for both the mother and infant. A reasonable postnatal assessment includes cranial, renal, and cardiac ultrasonography; social service; and genetic, neurologic, and ophthalmologic consultation. Unfortunately the long-term prognosis for alcohol addiction may be particularly high among women who remain high users during pregnancy, so it is reasonable to encourage birth control in situations in which future newborns with FAS are likely.

Despite supportive intervention programs for FAS, moderate to severe mental retardation persists in two thirds of the children with the most clearly defined syndrome (Ernhart et al, 1995). The relative severity and timing of neurobehavioral symptoms that result from various prenatal exposures to drugs are shown in Table 10–8.

CIGARETTES

Cigarettes are the drug most often used during pregnancy. Cigarette smoking has been associated with an increased risk of spontaneous abortion, stillbirth, fetal growth retardation, prematurity, and SIDS (Abel, 1984). The degree of intrauterine growth retardation is related to the number of cigarettes smoked. One pack (20 cigarettes) per day correlates with a 280-g weight decrement in term newborn infants. Maternal cotinine excretion is used as a marker to quantitate the degree of smoking. Eskenazi and coworkers (Eskenazi et al, 1995; Eskenazi and Trupin, 1995) found a 1-g reduction in birth weight for every nanogram per milli-

| TABLE 10–8 |

Neonatal Neurobehavioral Symptoms After Fetal Drug Exposure

	Onset	Peak	Duration	Relative Severity
Alcohol	0–1 d	1–2 d	1–2 d	Mild
Cocaine	0–3 d	1–4 d	? mo	Mild–moderate
Amphetamine	0–3 d	3–7 d	2–8 wk	Mild–moderate
Phencyclidine	0–2 d	5–7 d	2–6 mo	Moderate–severe
Heroin	0–3 d	3–7 d	2–4 wk	Mild–moderate
Methadone	3–7 d	10–21 d	2–6 wk	Mild–severe

liter of cotinine increase in maternal urine. The exact mechanism of the adverse effect on pregnancy is unknown. Cigarettes contain a number of potentially toxic compounds. Most theories involve the induction of fetal hypoxia either from carbon monoxide production or from nicotine-induced vasospasm; however, a direct cytotoxic effect has not been ruled out. Slotkin and colleagues (1995) have shown loss of neonatal hypoxia tolerance after prenatal nicotine exposure and suggested this as a causative factor in the increased risk of SIDS among offspring of mothers who smoke. Mothers who smoke during pregnancy commonly smoke during their infants' childhoods. A 5-year follow-up study has identified neurobehavioral differences among children who have been exposed to passive smoking, but no differences were found in offspring of mothers who smoked during pregnancy (Eskenazi et al, 1995; Eskenazi and Trupin, 1995). Asthma as well as recurrent otitis media is increased for infants exposed to passive smoking (Ey et al, 1995; Martinez et al, 1995).

MARIJUANA

Marijuana is the illegal drug that is probably most frequently used during pregnancy. Marijuana is derived from the hemp plant Cannabis, with the most active ingredient being delta-9-tetrahydrocannabinol. Marijuana is associated with growth retardation (Abel, 1980). Neurologic abnormalities similar to a mild withdrawal syndrome with hypertonicity, irritability, and jitteriness have been seen in the newborn but without documented evidence of long-term sequelae. Marijuana is often used in combination with other drugs and potentiates the risk for prematurity and low birth weight (Abel, 1985). FAS may be more common among women who abuse alcohol with marijuana.

CAFFEINE

Caffeine exposure may occur in 75% of pregnancies in the United States (Eskenazi, 1993). Caffeine is contained in coffee, tea, colas, and chocolate (100 mg/cup of coffee). Most studies detect increased risk of intrauterine growth retardation with intake in excess of 300 mg/day. That is to say a detectable and significant increase of growth retardation occurs (relative risk about 1.5). Many studies also report increased risk of spontaneous abortion with caffeine exposure (e.g., risk of abortion increases by 1.017 for each cup of coffee/day in first trimester [Armstrong et al, 1992]). Most studies of caffeine, similar to those of other licit and illicit drugs, share problems of ascertainment; dose, duration, response, and confounding factors. For example, genetic differences may affect susceptibility to caffeine, caffeine may have fetotoxic additive effects with smoking, and drinks such as coffee may contain ingredients that have effects on pregnancy that are independent of caffeine. Granted these considerations, and to a greater degree than with other drugs discussed in this chapter, it is usually not possible to attribute growth retardation or spontaneous abortion in a specific case to caffeine. It is prudent to advise women to limit maximum caffeine intake to less than 100 mg/day both when pregnant and when anticipating pregnancy (Infante-Rinard et al, 1993).

BREAST-FEEDING

Psychotropic drugs are low molecular weight and lipophilic, which means that they are readily excreted in breast milk. Seizures and overdose symptoms have been reported in one infant whose mother used cocaine. Amphetamines appear in large quantities in breast milk. PCP has also been found to cross into breast milk readily. Because of the risk of toxicity, breast-feeding should be discouraged for known abusers of the above-named drugs with the exception of those mothers in drug treatment programs in which their drug use is monitored closely. Methadone is excreted in small quantities in breast milk and is considered safe if the mother is well controlled, that is to say on low doses of methadone with no evidence of additional licit or illicit drug intake. Breast-feeding longer than 3 to 6 months should be avoided because of the potential for increased exposure to methadone as the amount of milk consumption increases. Alcohol intake while breast-feeding is not listed as a contraindication by the American Academy of Pediatrics, but excessive maternal alcohol intake during breast-feeding may be as deleterious for the infant as fetal exposure (Lawrence, 1994) (see Appendix 1).

HUMAN IMMUNODEFICIENCY VIRUS INFECTION

Nationwide, intravenous drug abusers are the second largest risk group for HIV infection. Drug abusers also may be the primary source of infection for non–drug-using heterosexuals as well as for children (Chamberland and Dondero, 1987). Pediatric AIDS is a perinatally acquired infection in 75% of cases nationwide. The seropositivity rate among female intravenous drug users in New York City and northern New Jersey is estimated at 50% to 70% compared to 5% to 20% in California. Heroin and cocaine addicts often resort to prostitution to support their habit. Amphetamine and methamphetamine users often inject drug several times daily. Alcohol decreases sexual inhibition, impairs judgment, and increases the chance of unsafe sexual activity. Every infant born to a substance abuser should be evaluated for HIV infection, and universal precautions must be strictly observed.

IDENTIFICATION AND INTERVENTION

The abuse of a variety of drugs during pregnancy has adverse consequences for the mother, fetus, and newborn. Clearly, it is important to ascertain and distinguish the causes for fetal and neonatal consequences of suboptimal placentation, intrauterine growth retardation, vascular problems, and acute neurobehavioral symptoms. It is less clear why one should identify infants who have had fetal drug exposure if they are asymptomatic. Reasons commonly offered are that a positive toxicology screen (sometimes backed by the threat of loss of her newborn to foster care) may break through maternal denial about drug abuse and enable the mother to accept treatment. In addition, courts are more apt to accept hard evidence such as a positive toxicology test than historical data of drug abuse that may be denied by the mother.

Therefore, a drug and alcohol history should be routinely included as part of the initial contact with every pregnant patient. To be effective, such histories must be nonjudgmental and taken in the context of other life-style questions. When a positive history is obtained, intervention should begin immediately. The person taking the history should be prepared to offer preliminary counseling on risk reduction and concrete referrals for treatment programs.

A more controversial method of identification is routine drug screening of mothers and infants in cases in which drug abuse is suspected. Rapid reliable drug testing using urine or blood is readily available in most clinical laboratories. Drug screening should be combined with a history and should be a part of a well-delineated protocol that clearly defines which infants and mothers should be screened. Screening protocols should be based on well-defined, high-risk behavior documented to be associated with perinatal drug abuse. High-risk behavior during the prenatal period includes a history of drug abuse, physical evidence of drug use (track marks or altered mental status), noncompliance with medical treatment and appointments, history of child abuse or children removed from the home, and history of a partner using drugs or excessive alcohol. Homelessness and recent prostitution or incarceration are also risk factors. A large percentage of drug abusers have no prenatal care or inadequate prenatal care (onset in last trimester or only a few visits), and this group has the highest rate of complicated deliveries. In addition, screening should include patients entering labor and delivery with complications associated with drug abuse, such as hemorrhage, untreated sexually transmitted diseases, and prematurity. Infants born to mothers who received no prenatal care and those born precipitously or prematurely should also be included in a social/toxicology screening protocol. Screening should always be done in a manner to ensure as much as possible the right of privacy of the mother while allowing physicians to provide optimal medical care to both mother and infant.

In the absence of intervention, infants discharged to mothers who abuse alcohol or illegal drugs are at high risk for subsequent physical abuse and neglect, but the degree of risk is unknown. Most states require some form of reporting to a child protective service agency. States differ in the aggressiveness with which they deal with this issue. In some states, the child's drug exposure is prima facie evidence of abuse. In general, however, the mother's addiction is evaluated in the context of its impact on her ability to care for the child. The primary focus of physicians caring for the mother and infant should be to ensure that all interventions are therapeutic and designed to foster the health of both patients.

REFERENCES

Aase JM, Jones KL, Clarren SK: Do we need the term "FAE"? Pediatrics 95:428, 1995.

Abel EL: Prenatal exposure to cannabis: A critical review of effects on growth development and behavior. Behav Neurol Biol 29:137, 1980.

Abel EL: Smoking and pregnancy. J Psychoact Drugs 16:327, 1984.

Abel EL: Effects of prenatal exposure to cannabinoids. *In* Pinker MG (Ed): Current Research on the Consequences of Maternal Drug Abuse. Washington, DC, National Institute on Drug Abuse Research Monograph Series 59, 1985.

Abel EL, Jacobson S, Sherman BT: In utero alcohol exposure: Functional and structural brain damage. Neurobehav Toxicol Teratol 5:363, 1983.

Abelson HJ, Miller JD: A decade of trends in cocaine use in the household population. Natl Inst Drug Abuse Res Monogr Ser 61:35, 1985.

Adams EH, Kozel NJ: Cocaine use in America: Introduction and overview. Natl Inst Drug Abuse Res Monogr Ser 61:1, 1985.

Ahmad G, Halsall LC, Bondy SC: Persistence of phencyclidine in fetal brain. Brain Res 415:194, 1987.

American Academy of Pediatrics: Neonatal drug withdrawal statement. Pediatrics 72:895, 1983.

Anand K, Arnold J: Opioid tolerance and dependence in infants and children. Crit Care Med 22:334, 1994.

Armstrong BG, McDonald AD, Sloan M: Cigarettes, alcohol and coffee consumption and spontaneous abortion. Am J Pub Health 82:85, 1992.

Barr G, Jones K: Opiate withdrawal in the infant. Neurotoxicol Teratol 16:219, 1994.

Bateman DA, Ng SK, Hansen CA, Heagarty MC: The effects of intrauterine cocaine exposure in newborns. Am J Pub Health 83:190, 1993.

Bauchner H, Zuckerman BS: Cocaine, sudden infant death syndrome, and home monitoring. J Pediatr 117:904, 1990.

Behnke M, Eyler F: The consequences of prenatal substance use for the developing fetus, newborn and young child. Int J Addict 28:1341, 1993.

Berger CS, Sorenson L, Gendler B, Fitzsimmons J: Cocaine and pregnancy: A challenge for health care providers. Health Soc Work 15:310, 1990.

Besharov D: The children of crack: Will we protect them? Public Welfare 47:6, 1989.

Billings L, Eriksson M, Steneroth G, Zetterstrom R: Pre-school children of amphetamine-addicted mothers: 1. Somatic and psychomotor development. Acta Paediatr Scand 74:179, 1985.

Boer K, Smit B, van Huis A, Hogerzeil H: Substance use in pregnancy: Do we care? Acta Paediatr 404(suppl):65, 1994.

Burke MS, Roth D: Anonymous cocaine screening in a private obstetric population. Obstet Gynecol 81:354, 1993.

Cernerud L, Eriksson M, Jonsson B, et al: Amphetamine addiction during pregnancy: 14-year follow-up of growth and school performance. Acta Paediatr 85:204, 1996.

Chamberland ME, Dondero TJ: Heterosexually acquired infection with human immunodeficiency virus (HIV): A view from the III International Conference on AIDS. Ann Intern Med 107:763, 1987.

Chang G, Carroll K, Behr H, Kosten T: Improving treatment outcome in pregnant opiate-dependent women. J Subst Abuse Treat 9:327, 1992.

Chasnoff IJ, Burns WJ, Hatcher RP, Burns KA: Phencyclidine effects on the fetus and neonate. Dev Pharmacol Ther 6:404, 1983a.

Chasnoff IJ, Burns WJ, Schnoll SH: Prenatal drug exposure: Effect on neonatal and infant growth and development. Neurobehav Toxicol Teratol 8:357, 1986.

Chasnoff IJ, Burns WJ, Schnoll SH, Burns KA: Cocaine use in pregnancy. N Engl J Med 313:666, 1985.

Chasnoff IJ, Griffith DR, Freier C, Murray J: Cocaine/polydrug use in pregnancy: Two-year follow-up. Pediatrics 89:284, 1992.

Chasnoff IJ, Griffith DR, MacGregor S: Temporal patterns of cocaine use in pregnancy: Perinatal outcome. JAMA 261:1741, 1989a.

Chasnoff IJ, Hatcher R, Burns W: Early growth patterns of methadone-addicted infants. Am J Dis Child 134:1049, 1980.

Chasnoff IJ, Hatcher R, Burns W, Schnoll SH: Pentazocine and tripelennamine ("T's and Blue's"): Effects on the fetus and neonate. Dev Pharmacol Ther 6:162, 1983b.

Chasnoff IJ, Hunt CE, Kletter R, Kaplan D: Prenatal cocaine exposure is associated with respiratory pattern abnormalities. Am J Dis Child 143:583, 1989b.

Chasnoff IJ, Landress HJ, Barrett ME: The prevalence of illicit-drug or alcohol use during pregnancy and discrepancies in mandatory reporting in Pinellas County, Florida. N Engl J Med 332:1202, 1990.

Chavkin W: Mandatory treatment for drug use during pregnancy. JAMA 266:1556, 1991.

Chiriboga CA: Neurologic complications of drug and alcohol abuse: Fetal effects. Neurol Clin 11:707, 1993.

Chiriboga CA: Cocaine and the fetus: Methodological issues and neurologic correlates. *In* Konkol RJ, Olsen GD: Prenatal Cocaine Exposure. Boca Raton, FL, CRC Press, 1996.

Chiriboga CA, Vibbert M, Malouf R: Neurological correlates of fetal cocaine exposure: Transient hypertonia of infancy and early childhood. Pediatrics 96:1070, 1995.

Centers for Disease Control: Urogenital anomalies in the offspring of women using cocaine during early pregnancy—Atlanta, 1968–1980. MMWR 38:536, 1989.

County Welfare Directors Association of California, Chief Probation Officers Association of California, Mental Health Directors Association: Ten Reasons to Invest in the Families of California. Sacramento, 1990.

Dearlove JC, Betteridge TJ, Henry JA: Stillbirth due to intravenous amphetamine. BMJ 304:548, 1992.

Dempsey DA, Ferriero DM, Jacobson SN: Critical review of evidence for neonatal cocaine intoxication and withdrawal. *In* Konkol R, Olsen G (Eds): Effects of Cocaine Exposure: Mechanisms and Outcome. Boca Raton, FL, CRC Press, 1996.

Dixon SD: Effects of transplacental exposure to cocaine and methampethamine on the neonate. West J Med 150:436, 1989.

Doberczak T, Kandall S, Friedmann P: Relationships between maternal methadone dosage, maternal-neonatal methadone levels and neonatal withdrawal. Obstet Gynecol 81:936, 1993.

Doberczak TM, Shanzer S, Senie RT, Kandall SR: Neonatal neurologic and electroencephalographic effects of intrauterine cocaine exposure. J Pediatr 113:354, 1989.

Dominguez R, Aguirre V, Coro A, et al: Brain and ocular abnormalities in infants with in utero exposure to cocaine and other street drugs. Am J Dis Child 145:688, 1991.

Dusick AM, Covert RF, Schreiber MD: Risk of intracranial hemorrhage and other adverse outcomes after cocaine exposure in a cohort of 323 very low birth weight infants. J Pediatr 122:438, 1993.

Edelin K, Gurganious L, Golar K, et al: Methadone maintenance in pregnancy: Consequences to care and outcome. Obstet Gynecol 71:399, 1988.

Ernhart CB, Greene T, Sokol RJ, et al: Neonatal diagnosis of fetal alcohol syndrome: Not necessarily a hopeless prognosis. Alcohol Clin Exp Res 19:1550, 1995.

Eriksson M, Stenoroth G, Zetterstrom R: Influence of pregnancy and child-rearing on amphetamine-addicted women: Five-year follow-up after delivery. Acta Psychiatr Scand 73:634, 1986.

Eriksson M, Zetterstrom R: Amphetamine addiction during pregnancy: 10-year follow-up. Acta Paediatr 404(suppl):27, 1994.

Eskenazi B: Caffeine during pregnancy: Grounds for concern? JAMA 270(24):2973, 1993.

Eskenazi B, Prehn AW, Christianson RE: Passive and active maternal smoking as measured by serum cotinine: The effect on birthweight. Am J Public Health 85:395, 1995.

Eskenazi B, Trupin LS: Passive and active maternal smoking during pregnancy as measured by serum cotinine and postnatal smoke exposure: II. Effects on neurodevelopment at age 5 years. Am J Epidemiol (suppl 9)S19, 1995.

Ey JL, Holberg CJ, Aldous MB, et al: Passive smoke exposure and otitis media in the first year of life. Pediatrics 95:670, 1995.

Fein AF, Shviro Y, Manoach M, Nebel L: Teratogenic effect of d-amphetamine sulfate: Histodifferentiation and electrocardiogram pattern of mouse embryonic heart. Teratology 35:27, 1987.

Fetters L, Tronick EZ: Neuromotor development of cocaine-exposed and control infants from birth through 15 months: Poor and poorer performance. Pediatrics 98:938, 1996.

Finnegan L: Perinatal substance abuse: Comments and perspectives. Semin Perinatol 15:331, 1991.

Finnegan L, Connaughton J, Kron R: Neonatal abstinence syndrome: Assessment and management. Addict Dis 2:141, 1975.

Franck L, Vilardi J: Assessment and management of opioid withdrawal in ill neonates. Neonatal Network 14:39, 1995.

Frank DA, Bresnahan K, Zuckerman BS: Maternal cocaine use: Impact on child health and development. Adv Pediatr 40:65, 1993.

Fulroth R, Phillips B, Durand D: Perinatal outcome of infants exposed to cocaine and/or heroin in utero. Am J Dis Child 143:905, 1989.

Gillogley K, Evans A, Hansen R, et al: The perinatal impact of cocaine, amphetamine and opiate use detected by universal intrapartum screening. Am J Obstet Gynecol 163:1535, 1990.

Golden NL, Kuhnert BR, Sokol RJ: Neonatal manifestations of maternal phencyclidine exposure. J Perinat Med 15:185, 1987.

Golden NL, Kuhnert BR, Sokol RJ, et al: Phencyclidine use during pregnancy. Am J Obstet Gynecol 148:254, 1984.

Golden NL, Sokol RJ, Rubin IL: Angel dust: Possible effects on the fetus. Pediatrics 65:18, 1980.

Gomby DS, Shiono PH: Estimating the number of substance-exposed infants. *In* Behrman RE (Ed): Drug Exposed Infants. Los Altos, CA, The David and Lucile Packard Foundation, Center for the Future of Children, 1991.

Green M, Suffet F: The Neonatal Narcotic Withdrawal Index: A device

for the improvement of care in the abstinence syndrome. Am J Drug Alcohol Abuse 8:203, 1981.

Greenberg MS, Singh T, Htoo M, Schultz S: The association between congenital syphilis and cocaine/crack in New York City: A case control study. Am J Public Health 81:1316, 1991.

Halfon N, Berkowitz G, Klee L: Health and mental health utilization by children in foster care in California. Berkeley, California Policy Seminar Brief, University of California, 1990.

Handler A, Kistin N, Davis F, Ferre C: Cocaine use during pregnancy: Perinatal outcome. Am J Epidemiol 133:818, 1991.

Harper R, Solish G, Feingold E, et al: Maternal ingested methadone, body fluid methadone, and the neonatal withdrawal syndrome. Am J Obstet Gynecol 129:417, 1977.

Hartnoll R: Opiates: Prevalence and demographic factors. Addiction 89:1377, 1994.

Hoyme HE, Jones KL, Dixon SD: Prenatal cocaine exposure and fetal vascular dusruption. Pediatrics 85:743, 1990.

Hurt H, Brodsky NL, Betancourt L: Cocaine-exposed children: Follow-up through 30 months. J Dev Behav Pediatr 16:29, 1995.

Infante-Rinard C, Fernandez A, Gauthier R, et al: Fetal loss associated with caffeine intake before and during pregnancy. JAMA 270:2940, 1993.

Jessup M: The treatment of perinatal addiction—identification, intervention, and advocacy. West J Med 152(spec iss):553, 1990.

Kandall S, Doberczak T, Mauer K, et al: Opiate vs CNS depressant therapy in neonatal drug abstinence syndrome. Am J Dis Child 137:378, 1983.

Kandall S, Gaines J, Habel L, et al: Relationship of maternal substance abuse to subsequent sudden infant death syndrome in offspring. J Pediatr 123:120, 1993.

Kaufman KR, Petruchka RA, Pitts TN, Weekes ME: PCP in amniotic fluid and breast milk: Case report. J Clin Psychiatry 44:269, 1983.

Kleber HD, Gawin FH: Cocaine withdrawal. Arch Gen Psychiatry 44:298, 1987.

Konkol RJ, Murphey L, Ferriero DM, et al: Cocaine metabolites in the neonate: Potential for toxicity. J Child Neurol 9:242, 1994.

Kurth CD, Monitto C, Albuquerque ML: Cocaine and its metabolites constrict cerebral arterioles in newborn pigs. J Pharmacol Exp Ther 265:587, 1993.

Lawrence R: Breastfeeding, 4th ed. St. Louis, Mosby-Year Book, 1994.

Legido A, Clancy RR, Spitzer AR, Finnegan LP: Electroencephalographic and behavioral-state studies in infants of cocaine-addicted mothers. Am J Dis Child 146:748, 1992.

Leshner AI: Molecular mechanisms of cocaine addiction. N Engl J Med 335: 128, 1996.

Levy M, Sino M: Neonatal withdrawal syndrome: Associated drugs and pharmacologic management. Pharmacotherapy 13:202, 1993.

Lifschitz M, Wilson G, Smith EM, Desmond M: Fetal and postnatal growth of children born to narcotic-dependent women. J Pediatr 102:686, 1983.

Lifschitz M, Wilson G, Smith E, Desmond M: Factors affecting head growth and intellectual function in children of drug addicts. Pediatr 75:269, 1985.

Lindenberg C: Opiate abuse in pregnancy. Ann Rev Nursing Res 11:249, 1993.

Lindsay MK, Peterson HB, Boring J: Crack/cocaine: A risk factor for human immunodeficiency virus infection type I among inner-city parturiens. Obstet Gynecol 80:981, 1992.

Lipshultz SE, Frassica JJ, Orav EJ: Cardiovascular abnormalities in infants prenatally exposed to cocaine. J Pediatr 118:44, 1991.

Maas U, Kattner E, Weingart-Jesse B, et al: Infrequent neonatal opiate withdrawal following maternal methadone detoxification during pregnancy. J Perinat Med 18:111, 1990.

Mack G, Giles W, Thomas D, Buchanan N: Methadone levels and neonatal withdrawal. J Paediatr Child Health 27:96, 1991.

Madden J, Chappel J, Zuspan F, et al: Observation and treatment of neonatal narcotic withdrawal. Am J Obstet Gynecol 127:199, 1977.

Mahalik MP, Hitner HW: Antagonism of cocaine-induced fetal anomalies by prazosin and diltiazem in mice. Reprod Technol 6:161, 1994.

Martin ML, Khoury MJ, Cordero JF, Waters GD: Trends in rates of multiple vascular disruption defects, Atlanta 1968–1989: Is there evidence of a cocaine teratogenic epidemic? Teratology 45:647, 1992.

Martinez A, Kastner B, Taeusch HW: Hyperphagia in newborns withdrawing from methadone. Pediatr Res 39:315A, 1996.

Martinez A, Padbury J, Burnell E, et al: The effects of hypoxia on methionine enkephalin peptide and catecholamine release in fetal sheep. Pediatr Res 27:52, 1990.

Martinez A, Padbury J, Burnell E, Thio S: Plasma methionine enkephalin levels in the human newborn at birth. Biol Neonate 60:102, 1991.

Martinez FD, Wright AL, Taussig LM, et al: Asthma and wheezing in the first six years of life. N Engl J Med 332:133, 1995.

Miller G: Addicted infants and their mothers: A survey conducted for the House Select Committee on Children, Youth, and Families. National Center for Clinical Infant Programs, Zero to Three IX:20, 1989.

Moore TR, Sorg J, Thomas CK, et al: Hemodynamic effects of intravenous cocaine on the pregnant ewe and fetus. Am J Obstet Gynecol 155:883, 1986.

Mott SH, Packer RJ, Soldin SJ: Neurological manifestations of cocaine exposure in childhood. Pediatrics 93:557, 1994.

National Institute of Drug Abuse (NIDA): Drug Use Among American High School Students and Other Young Adults: National Trends through 1985. DHHS Pub. (ADM) 86-145. Washington DC, U.S. Government Printing Office, 1985.

Oats J, Beischer N, Breheny J, Pepperell R: The outcome of pregnancies complicated by narcotic drug addiction. Aust NZ J Obstet Gynaecol 24:14, 1984.

Olsen J, Tuntiseranee P: Is moderate alcohol intake in pregnancy associated with the craniofacial features related to the fetal alcohol syndrome? Scand J Soc Med 23:156, 1995.

Olson GA, Olson RD, Kastin AJ: Endogenous opiates: 1993 review. Peptides 15:1513, 1994.

Ostrea E, Brady M, Parks P, et al: Drug screening of meconium in infants of drug-dependent mothers: An alternative to urine testing. J Pediatr 115:474, 1992a.

Ostrea EM Jr, Brady MJ, Gause S, et al: Drug screening of newborns by meconium analysis: A large-scale, prospective, epidemiological study. Pediatrics 89:107, 1992b.

Ostrea EM Jr, Welch, RA: Detection of prenatal drug exposure in the pregnant woman and her newborn infant. Clin Perinatol 18:629, 1991.

Petitti DB, Coleman C: Cocaine and the risk of low birth weight. Am J Public Health 80:25, 1990.

Phibbs CS, Bateman DA, Schwartz RM: The neonatal costs of maternal cocaine use. JAMA 266:1521, 1991.

Racine A, Joyce T, Anderson R: The association between prenatal care and birth weight among women exposed to cocaine in New York City. JAMA 270:1581, 1993 [Erratum, 271:1161, 1994].

Rahbar F, Fomufod A, White D, Westney LS: Impact of intrauterine exposure to phencyclidine (PCP) and cocaine on neonates. J Natl Med Assoc 85:349, 1993.

Raye J, Dubin J, Blechner J: Alterations in fetal metabolism subsequent to maternal morphine administration. Am J Obstet Gynecol 137:505, 1980.

Robbins TW, Watson CA, Gastin M, Ennis C: Contrasting interactions of pipradrol, d-amphetamine, cocaine, cocaine analogues, apomorphine and other drugs with conditioned reinforcement. Psychopharmacology 80:113, 1983.

Robinson MK, Myrick JE, Henderson LO, et al: Two-dimensional protein electrophoresis and multiple hypothesis testing to detect potential serum protein biomarkers in children with fetal alcohol syndrome. Electrophoresis 16:1176, 1995.

Rosen T, Johnson H: Children of methadone-maintained mothers: Follow-up to 18 months of age. J Pediatr 101:192, 1982.

Rosen T, Pippenger C: Pharmacologic observations on the neonatal withdrawal syndrome. J Pediatr 88:1044, 1976.

Rothrock JF, Rubenstein B, Lyden PD: Ischemic stroke associated with methamphetamine inhalation. Neurology 38:589, 1988.

Sagatun-Edwards IJ, Saylor C, Shifflett B: Drug exposed infants in the social welfare system and juvenile court. Child Abuse Neglect 19:83, 1995.

Schenker S, Yang Y, Johnson RF: The transfer of cocaine and its metabolites across the term human placenta. Clin Pharmacol Ther 53:329, 1993.

Schmidt CJ: Neurotoxicity of the psychedelic amphetamine, methyenedioxymethamphetamine. J Pharmacol Exp Ther 240:1, 1987.

Selwyn P, Schoenbaum E, Davenny K, et al: Prospective study of human immunodeficiency virus infection and pregnancy outcomes in intravenous drug users. JAMA 261:1289, 1989.

Shiono PH, Klebanoff MA, Nugent RP: The impact of cocaine and marijuana use on low birth weight and preterm birth: A multicenter study. Am J Obstet Gynecol 172:19, 1995.

Slotkin TA, Lappi SE, McCook EC, et al: Loss of neonatal hypoxia tolerance after prenatal nicotine exposure: Implications for sudden infant death syndrome. Brain Res Bull 38:69, 1995.

Smith DE, Wesson DR, Buxson ME (Eds): Amphetamine Use, Misuse, and Abuse. Boston, G. K. Hall, 1979.

Soepatmi S: Developmental outcomes of children of mothers dependent on heroin or heroin/methadone during pregnancy. Act Paediatr 404(suppl):36, 1994.

Strauss AA, Modanlou HD, Bosu SK: Neonatal manifestations of maternal phencyclidine (PCP) abuse. Pediatrics 68:550, 1981.

Strauss M, Starr R, Ostrea E, et al: Behavioral concomitants of prenatal addiction to narcotics. J Pediatr 89:842, 1976.

Suffet F, Brotman R: A comprehensive care program for pregnancy addicts: Obstetrical, neonatal, and child development outcomes. Int J Addict 19:199, 1984.

Taeusch HW Jr, Carson S, Wang NS, et al: Heroin induction of lung maturation and growth retardation in fetal rabbits. J Pediatr 82:869, 1973.

Taylor J, Sanderson M: A reexamination of the risk factors for the sudden infant death syndrome. J Pediatr 126:887, 1995.

Tobias J, Schleien C, Haun S: Methadone as treatment for iatrogenic narcotic dependency in pediatric intensive care unit patients. Crit Care Med 18:1292, 1990.

Tsay CH, Partridge JC, Villarreal SF, et al: Neurologic and ophthalmologic findings in children with gestational cocaine exposure. J Child. Neuro 11:25, 1996.

United States General Accounting Office: Drug Exposed Infants: A Generation at Risk. Washington, DC, Human Resources Division 90-138, 1990.

Update: Trends in fetal alcohol syndrome—United States, 1979–1993. MMWR 44:249, 1995.

van Baar A, de Graaff B: Cognitive development at preschool-age of infants of drug-dependent mothers. Dev Med Child Neurol 36:1063, 1994.

van Baar A, Soepatmi S, Gunning W, Akkerhuis G: Development after prenatal exposure to cocaine, heroin and methadone. Acta Paediatr 404(suppl):40, 1994b.

van de Bor M, Walther FJ, Ebrahimi M: Decreased cardiac output in infants of mothers who abused cocaine. Pediatrics 85:30, 1990a.

van de Bor M, Walther FJ, Sims ME: Increased cerebral blood flow velocity in infants of mothers who abuse cocaine. Pediatrics 85:733, 1990b.

Vega W, Kolody B, Hwang J, Noble A: Prevalence and magnitude of prenatal substance exposures in California. N Engl J Med 329:850, 1993.

Wasserman DR, Leventhal JM: Maltreatment of children born to cocaine-dependent mothers. Am J Dis Child 147:1324, 1993.

Webber MP, Lambert G, Bateman DA, Hauser, WA: Maternal risk factors for congenital syphilis: A case-control study. Am J Epidemiol 137:415, 1993.

Wekselman K, Spiering K, Hetteberg C, et al: Fetal alcohol syndrome from infancy through childhood: A review of the literature. J Pediatr Nurs 10:296, 1995.

West JR, Chen WJ, Pantazis NJ: Fetal alcohol syndrome: The vulnerability of the developing brain and possible mechanisms of damage. Metab Brain Dis 9:291, 1994.

Wilson F, McCreary R, Kean J, Baster J: The development of preschool children of heroin-addicted mothers: A controlled study. Pediatrics 63:135, 1979.

Woods JR Jr, Plessinger MS, Clark KE: Effects of cocaine on uterine blood flow. JAMA. 257:957, 1987.

Yanai J, Avraham Y, Levy S: Alterations in septohippocampal cholinergic innervations and related behaviors after early exposure to heroin and phencyclidine. Brain Res 69:207, 1992.

Yawn B, Thompson L, Lupo V, et al: Prenatal drug use in Minneapolis–St. Paul, Minnesota: A 4 year trend. Arch Fam Med 3:520, 1994.

Zuckerman B, Bresnahan K: Developmental and behavioral consequences of prenatal drug and alcohol exposure. Pediatr Clin North Am 38:1387, 1991.

Zuckerman B, Frank DA, Hingson R: Effects of maternal marijuana and cocaine on fetal growth. N Engl J Med 320:762, 1989.

Zuspan F, Gumpel J, Mejia-Zelaya A, et al: Fetal stress from methadone withdrawal. Am J Obstet Gynecol 122:43, 1975.

CHAPTER 11

Nonimmune Hydrops

Eric B. Mallow and Roberta A. Ballard

Hydrops describes the infant who has generalized edema owing to accumulation of excess fluid. The condition varies from mild, generalized edema to massive edema, with ascites and pleural and pericardial effusions and with peripheral edema so severe that the extremities are fixed in extension. Severely hydropic fetuses die in utero if they cannot be delivered under controlled circumstances, and even if delivered alive, they may die in the neonatal period either from the severity of their underlying disease or from severe cardiorespiratory failure caused by the hydrops.

Hydrops fetalis is the term used to describe hydrops that occurs as a result of end-stage, severe erythroblastosis fetalis (alloimmune hemolytic anemia). In the past, the great majority of cases were due to maternal-fetal incompatibility for the D-antigen in the Rh system. Advances in the use of anti-D immune globulin to prevent maternal sensitization, however, have markedly decreased the incidence of hydrops due to Rh disease (Phibbs and Naiman, 1989). Alloimmune disease does occur occasionally from incompatibility of other important blood group antigens and can be severe enough to cause hydrops (Baker et al, 1988; Beal, 1979). (See Chapter 89 for further discussion of alloimmune hydrops.)

NONIMMUNE FETAL HYDROPS

Potter (1943) first distinguished between hydrops secondary to erythroblastosis fetalis and nonimmune hydrops in describing a group of infants with generalized body edema who did not have hepatosplenomegaly or abnormal erythropoiesis. With the decrease in incidence of alloimmune hydrops, it was estimated that by 1970 approximately 20% of the cases of hydrops in western countries would be of the nonimmune type. With the nearly universal use of anti-D globulin and refinement of the schedule and doses for administration, the occurrence of immune hydrops has decreased still further. The increasing use of ultrasound in pregnancy has permitted early diagnosis (and, therefore, cataloguing) of more infants with nonimmune hydrops. Current estimates of incidence vary from 1 in 2500 to 1 in 4000 (Norton, 1994). In patients undergoing prenatal ultrasound scans, half of the cases of hydrops reported were due to either cardiac lesions or chromosomal abnormalities.

PATHOPHYSIOLOGY
Normal Fluid Homeostasis

To understand the pathogenesis of hydrops, it is necessary to consider the forces underlying normal fluid homeostasis. Body water exists in two principal spaces: intracellular and extracellular. Intracellular volume is maintained largely by osmotic forces across the cell membrane and by the energy-dependent sodium transporter. In hydrops, the disorder is in the regulation of extracellular water such that fluid accumulates in the interstitium and body cavities.

Starling Equation

The Starling equation describes the movement of water across a semipermeable membrane both in terms of hydrostatic and osmotic pressures and in terms of the degree of permeability of the membrane to water and solutes. The mechanisms in the pathogenesis of hydrops can ultimately be integrated through the Starling relationship. The Starling equation as applied to the balance of fluid across a capillary is as follows:

$$\text{Filtration} = K\left[(P_c - P_t) - R(O_p - O_t)\right]$$

where K = capillary filtration coefficient, P_c = hydrostatic pressure—capillary, P_t = hydrostatic pressure—tissue, R = reflection coefficient for solute, O_p = osmotic pressure—plasma, and O_t = osmotic pressure—tissue fluid.

It is useful to consider each variable individually and then to consider the physiologic effects when the values of these parameters are altered.

Capillary Filtration Coefficient (K). The capillary filtration coefficient represents the degree of permeability of the capillary wall to water. A value of 1 implies complete permeability. This value is always less than 1 but may be increased by factors that reduce the integrity of the capillary endothelium, such as inflammatory mediators, endotoxins, and hypoxia. Clinical settings that predispose to increased permeability include sepsis and asphyxia. The net effect is an increase in filtration of water from the capillary into the extravascular space. This increase in tissue fluid is compensated for by lymphatic drainage and the intrinsic fluid buffering effect of the intercellular gel. These mechanisms are sufficiently effective that an increase in interstitial water may not result in a significant rise in tissue hydrostatic pressure, a force that would act to oppose filtration from the intravascular to the extravascular space.

Capillary Hydrostatic Pressure (Pc). An increase in capillary hydrostatic pressure results in an increase in water flux from the intravascular to the interstitial space. Forces opposing capillary hydrostatic pressure are the interstitial hydrostatic pressure and the oncotic pressure of intravascular plasma. Factors that may increase the capillary hydrostatic pressure include increased central venous pressure, increased arterial pressure, and postcapillary venous obstruction.

Tissue Hydrostatic Pressure (Pt). Tissue hydrostatic pressure is subject to less fluctuation than the other parameters because of lymphatic drainage and fluid buffering capacity of the interstitial gel. Tissue hydrostatic pressure can be increased if lymphatic drainage is impaired or if the rate of interstitial fluid formation exceeds the capacity of compensatory mechanisms. Opposing forces are capillary hydrostatic pressure and tissue oncotic pressure.

Reflection Coefficient (R). The reflection coefficient for a solute represents the degree of permeability of the capillary wall to that solute. The contribution by a given solute to osmotic pressure on either side of the capillary wall is determined by its reflection coefficient. A reflection coefficient of zero for a solute implies free permeability of the capillary to that solute; therefore, the solute exerts no osmotic force. A value of 1 implies total impermeability and thus a maximum osmotic force exerted by the solute.

Large molecules, such as albumin, have higher reflection coefficients and thus make greater contributions to total intravascular and extravascular osmotic forces. Clinically available preparations of salt-poor albumin have been treated in a way that results in smaller molecules with lower reflection coefficients. Reflection coefficients are also lowered when the capillary integrity is diminished. Conditions such as sepsis and hypoxia, which increase the capillary filtration coefficient, also decrease reflection coefficients, thereby enhancing edema formation.

Plasma Osmotic Pressure (Op). The osmotic pressures of all intravascular solutes contribute to the total plasma osmotic pressure, which acts to keep water in the intravascular space. Because of complex behaviors of molecules at the capillary membrane surface, the total osmotic pressure is not an absolute sum of the osmotic contributions of all molecules. The forces opposing plasma osmotic pressure are tissue osmotic pressure and capillary hydrostatic pressure.

Conditions that result in decreased plasma osmotic pressure may contribute to increased interstitial fluid accumulation. Clinical settings include reduced plasma protein synthesis in hepatic failure or malnutrition, plasma dilution owing to administration of excess free water, excess urinary excretion of protein, and loss of plasma proteins from the intravascular compartment owing to either increased capillary leak or hemorrhage.

Tissue Osmotic Pressure (Ot). Osmotic pressure of intercellular fluid acts to retain water in the interstitial space. Normally, tissue osmotic pressure is less than capillary osmotic pressure. Conditions that increase capillary permeability may result in a net loss of osmotically active molecules from the intravascular compartment to the interstitial space. This loss results in increased extracellular water accumulation as a result of a decrease in the osmotic difference between the intravascular and extravascular spaces. The forces opposing tissue osmotic pressure are plasma osmotic pressure and tissue hydrostatic pressure.

These factors must be considered in the fetus in the context of the fact that, in utero, 40% of fetal cardiac output goes through the placenta, allowing rapid transfer of water from the fetus to the mother. Because of this situation, it is unlikely that either low plasma colloid osmotic pressure or elevated capillary hydrostatic pressure could contribute to fluid retention in the fetus. Increased capillary permeability, allowing water and protein to leak from the fetal circulation, would lead to higher colloid osmotic pressures in the tissues, including the interstitial spaces of the fetoplacental villi. Therefore, factors leading to increased capillary permeability, whether from severe anemia and hypoxia or from congestive heart failure, are more likely to contribute to hydrops.

Clinical Manifestations

Diamond and coworkers (1932) suggested three possible mechanisms that might be operative in infants with hydrops. These mechanisms included anemia, low colloid osmotic pressure with hypoproteinemia, and congestive heart failure with hypervolemia. Others (Barnes et al, 1977; Phibbs, 1992) have reviewed these potential mechanisms, and they remain among central hypotheses addressed by investigators in this area.

Anemia

Infants with alloimmune hydrops (and several of the nonimmune hydrops conditions as well) have significant anemia. It has been proposed that anemia leads to congestive heart failure with increased hydrostatic pressure in the capillaries, causing vascular damage that results in edema. There is significant overlap in the hematocrit values of infants who do and who do not have hydrops, however, suggesting that anemia alone is not a satisfying explanation. It is clear that a rapidly lowered hemoglobin concentration results in a need for greater cardiac output to maintain adequate oxygen delivery. This results in higher oxygen demands by the myocardium, which may be difficult to meet because of the anemia itself. The hypoxic myocardium may become less contractile and less compliant, with ventricular stiffness causing an increased afterload to the atria. As in the case of supraventricular tachycardia (SVT) (see later), a right ventricle with reduced compliance may result in flow reversal in the inferior vena cava (IVC), which may, in turn, cause end-organ damage to the liver, with consequent hypoalbuminemia and portal hypertension enhancing edema and ascites formation. High-output congestive heart failure may then exist, resulting in elevated central venous pressure (CVP). In turn, elevated CVP leads to increased capillary filtration pressures and impairment of lymphatic return. Hydrops has been produced using experimentally induced anemia in fetal lambs (Blair et al, 1994). Hemoglobin content was lowered in 12 fetuses through exchange transfusion using cell-free plasma, and six became hydropic. The hydropic fetuses had a more rapid development of anemia and had an elevated CVP as compared to those without hydrops. In the most severely anemic fetuses, it is probable that decreased oxygen transport causes tissue hypoxia, which, in turn, causes increased capillary permeability to both water and protein. It is probable that the changes in capillary permeability also contribute to the development of hydrops.

Low Colloid Osmotic Pressure with Hypoproteinemia

Infants who have erythroblastosis and hydrops seem to demonstrate a correlation between serum albumin concentration and the degree of hydrops (Phibbs et al, 1974). Initial therapy after birth, however, tends to raise the serum albumin toward normal rapidly, and with diuresis, these infants appear to have normal albumin concentrations. This suggests that their hypoalbuminemia may have been the result of dilution rather than the cause of the hydrops.

Hypoproteinemia

To elucidate the role of isolated hypoproteinemia in the genesis of hydrops, hypoproteinemia has been induced in fetal lambs (Moise et al, 1991). Using sets of twin fetuses, one twin underwent serum protein reduction by repeated removal of plasma and replacement with normal saline. Over 3 days, an average of a 41% reduction of plasma protein was achieved, with a 44% reduction in colloid osmotic pressure. No fetuses became edematous, and total body water content was similar in experimental and control animals. Thus, hypoproteinemia alone was not sufficient to cause hydrops fetalis over the course of the study. Transcapillary filtration probably increased with hypoproteinemia but was compensated by lymphatic return. In agreement with this study, it has been observed that human fetuses with hypoproteinemia owing to nephrotic syndrome or analbuminemia rarely develop hydrops. Hypoproteinemia may, however, lower the threshold for edema formation in the presence of impaired lymphatic return or increased intravascular hydrostatic pressures.

Cardiac Mechanisms

The most commonly diagnosed causes of nonimmune hydrops are cardiac disorders (about 40%) (Norton, 1994). Any state in which cardiac output is less than the rate of venous return results in an elevated CVP. Increased CVP raises capillary filtration pressures and, if high enough, restricts lymphatic return. Both of these mechanisms may then contribute to interstitial fluid accumulation. Structural cardiac causes of elevated CVP include obstructive lesions and valvular regurgitation. Tachycardia (particularly supraventricular) and bradycardia may reduce cardiac output, resulting in an elevated CVP. Myocardial hypoxia (most often due to severe anemia) and myocarditis (usually infectious) reduce both contractility and compliance and can cause an increase in CVP.

The most common single cause of nonimmune hydrops is SVT. Fortunately, SVT is also the most easily reversible cause of nonimmune hydrops. In general, cardiac output increases with heart rate. At increasingly high rates, however, cardiac output plateaus and then diminishes as rate increases further. The rates observed with SVT are often associated with decreased cardiac output. Impaired cardiac output results in elevated CVP, which may give rise to edema through mechanisms discussed previously.

Hydrops has been induced experimentally in fetal lambs by rapid atrial pacing (Gest et al, 1990a). Twenty-eight fetal lambs were paced at 320 beats per minute. All fetuses developed peripheral edema and ascites, as early as 15 hours after the onset of pacing. CVP was found to increase to 8 torr from a baseline of 4 torr, whereas aortic pressures were unaffected. Edema in these fetuses probably arose because of increased capillary filtration pressures or im-

paired lymphatic return (or both). Hypoproteinemia was not observed, possibly because of the short study duration.

In a separate study (Gest et al, 1990b), the effect of rapid atrial pacing on central venous hemodynamics was investigated. Seven fetal lambs were paced at 320 beats per minute. Hydrops developed in four fetuses in 4 hours, and all were hydropic by 48 hours. An increase in CVP of 75% was seen during pacing. A reversal of IVC blood flow, constituting 21% of forward flow, was seen immediately with the onset of pacing and ceased immediately on restoration of a normal heart rate. The reversal occurred during ventricular diastole, coincident with atrial contraction. IVC flow reversal was due, therefore, to changes in atrioventricular coupling dynamics and not tricuspid regurgitation.

It is important to be aware, however, that most infants with hydrops owing to erythroblastosis do not appear to be hypervolemic but conversely may have a low circulating blood volume and require transfusion after their asphyxia has been corrected (Phibbs et al, 1974).

Impaired Lymphatic Return

A fourth factor that contributes to hydrops is decreased lymph flow (Brace, 1989; Gest et al, 1992). If the rate of fluid filtration from plasma to tissues exceeds the rate of lymph return to the central venous system, edema and effusions form. Impairment of lymph flow may be caused by either a structural impedance or an increased CVP opposing lymphatic return. To determine the effects of alterations in CVP on lymphatic return, an opposing hydrostatic pressure was applied to the thoracic duct in fetal lambs (Gest et al, 1992). In each of 10 fetuses, a catheter was inserted into the thoracic duct. By varying the height of the catheter, the thoracic duct outflow pressure was altered. Thoracic duct flow was nearly constant over the physiologic range of CVPs. Lymph flow decreased sharply at 5.1 torr, however, and ceased at 18 torr. Thus, lymphatic flow may be reduced or essentially blocked in pathologic states associated with elevated CVPs.

Thus, the cause of hydrops appears to be multifactorial, with mechanisms that produce elevated CVP, capillary leakage, and impaired lymphatic drainage contributing to its development.

ETIOLOGY

Alloimmune hydrops is discussed in Chapter 89 and is most commonly associated with anti-D Rh-isoimmunization. Nonimmune hydrops has been described in association with a wide range of conditions (Table 11–1). The majority of the conditions that have been associated with nonimmune hydrops would be expected to cause edema either through anemia with hypoxia and consequent capillary leak or through cardiovascular anomalies with heart failure. The latter may also result in tissue hypoxia with increased vascular permeability as well as decreased lymphatic flow. Other conditions associated with hydrops, such as arteriovenous malformations and pulmonary masses, may also act to increase the occurrence of capillary leak and may be associated with lymphatic abnormalities as well. The causal mechanism of hydrops in association with many other conditions is not clear.

TABLE 11–1

Conditions Associated with Hydrops Fetalis

Hemolytic anemias
    Alloimmune, Rh, Kell, c
    Alpha-chain hemoglobinopathies (homozygous alpha-thalassemia)
    Red blood cell enzyme deficiencies (glucose phosphate
        isomerase deficiency, glucose-6-phosphate dehydrogenase)
Other anemias
    Fetomaternal hemorrhage
    Twin–twin transfusion
Cardiac conditions
    Premature closure of foramen ovale
    Ebstein's anomaly
    Hypoplastic left or right heart
    Subaortic stenosis with fibroelastosis
    Cardiomyopathy, myocardial fibroelastosis
    Atrioventricular canal
    Myocarditis
    Right atrial hemangioma
    Intracardiac hamartoma or fibroma
    Tuberous sclerosis with cardiac rhabdomyoma
Cardiac arrhythmias
    Supraventricular tachycardia
    Atrial flutter
    Congenital heart block
Vascular malformations
    Hemangioma of liver
    Any large arteriovenous malformation
    Angiosteohypertrophy (Klippel-Trenaunay syndrome)
Vascular accidents
    Thrombosis of umbilical vein or inferior vena cava
    Recipient in twin–twin transfusion
Infections
    Cytomegalovirus, congenital hepatitis, human parvovirus, other
        viruses
    Toxoplasmosis, Chagas disease
    Coxsackie virus
    Syphilis
    Leptospirosis
Lymphatic abnormalities
    Lymphangiectasia
    Cystic hygroma
    Noonan syndrome
    Multiple pterygium syndrome
Nervous system lesions
    Absent corpus callosum
    Encephalocele
    Cerebral arteriovenous malformation
    Intracranial hemorrhage (massive)
    Holoprosencephaly
    Fetal akinesia sequence

Pulmonary conditions
    Cystic adenomatoid malformation of lung
    Mediastinal teratoma
    Diaphragmatic hernia
    Lung sequestration syndrome
    Lymphangiectasia
Renal conditions
    Urinary ascites
    Congenital nephrosis
    Renal vein thrombosis
Invasive and storage processes
    Tuberous sclerosis
    Gaucher disease
    Mucopolysaccharidosis
    Mucolipidosis
Chromosome abnormalities
    Trisomy 13, trisomy 18, trisomy 21
    Turner syndrome
    XX/XY
Bone diseases
    Osteogenesis imperfecta
    Achondroplasia
    Asphyxiating thoracic dystrophy
Gastrointestinal conditions
    Bowel obstruction with perforation and meconium peritonitis
    Small-bowel volvulus
    Other intestinal obstruction
    Prune-belly syndrome
Tumors
    Neuroblastoma
    Choriocarcinoma
    Sacrococcygeal teratoma
    Hemangioma of the liver
    Congenital leukemia
Maternal or placental conditions
    Maternal diabetes
    Maternal therapy with indomethacin
    Multiple gestation with parasitic fetus
    Chorioangioma of placenta, chorionic vessels, or umbilical vessels
    Toxemia
    Systemic lupus erythematosus
Miscellaneous
    Neu-Laxova syndrome
    Myotonic dystrophy
Idiopathic

ANTENATAL MANAGEMENT OF NONIMMUNE HYDROPS

The diagnosis of hydrops is now frequently made antenatally, as a result of evaluation of polyhydramnios, a pregnancy that is considered high risk for other reasons, or simply as part of a routine ultrasound screening.

Prenatal Diagnosis of Hydrops Fetalis

Prenatal ultrasound diagnosis of hydrops is made by observing generalized skin thickening of greater than 5 mm and two of the following: ascites, pleural effusions, pericardial effusion, or placental enlargement. Because the mortality and morbidity risk for hydrops is high, a rapid determination of the cause must be undertaken when the diagnosis is made so that appropriate intervention may preserve fetal well-being when possible. Ultrasound, in addition to revealing hydrops, may also yield information as to the cause. Cardiac defects and dysrhythmias are evident by fetal echocardiography and Doppler blood flow analysis. Fetal heart rate monitoring may be used to follow dysrhythmias. Other anomalies, including lesions such as teratomas and hemangiomas, which may create high-output failure states, may be visible as well.

The goals of antenatal evaluation are as follows:

1. *Identify conditions in which therapy is futile*, so that the mother is not subjected to unnecessary additional testing or unnecessary cesarean section for fetal distress.

2. *Identify those fetuses whose conditions can be corrected by intrauterine therapy.* SVT is the most common cause of nonimmune hydrops but is also the most amenable to treatment. Commonly the mother is given antiarrhythmic agents, and the fetus is monitored closely for resolution of the SVT. Digoxin is the drug most commonly administered, although quinidine, procainamide, or other drugs may be used. Transplacental transfer of digoxin may be impaired in the setting of hydrops.

If the cause of hydrops is determined to be anemia, transfusions of packed red blood cells may be administered to the fetus. Transfusions may be given under ultrasound guidance, into the intraperitoneal space or umbilical vein. Blood instilled into the abdominal cavity is taken up by lymphatics. This uptake may be impaired, however, in the setting of hydrops (Phibbs, 1992), probably because elevated CVP impedes lymphatic flow in the thoracic duct. If uptake of intraperitoneal blood is incomplete, degeneration of the remaining hemoglobin may create a substantial bilirubin load necessitating phototherapy or exchange transfusion after the infant is delivered.

Fetal surgery is now making possible the prenatal correction or palliation of several anomalies that cause hydrops. Defects that may be correctable include congenital cystic adenomatoid malformation of the lung, pulmonary sequestration, and sacrococcygeal teratomas. Several investigators are also attempting to treat congenital diaphragmatic hernia. Conditions resulting in fetal hydrothorax can be ameliorated using intrapleural catheters draining to the amniotic space. (See also Chapter 12.)

3. *Identify those conditions that can be corrected by appropriate care at the time of delivery*, such as elimination of a chorioangioma of the placenta or immediate neonatal surgical treatment. Obviously, these interventions need to be balanced against the degree of prematurity and the likelihood of the infant's surviving the problems of prematurity plus the treatment of the underlying cause of hydrops.

Carlton and associates (1989) outlined a multidisciplinary approach to the evaluation and management of the mother, fetus, and newborn infant. Table 11–2 provides recommendations for the investigation of fetal hydrops. It is important in evaluating these mothers that one person coordinate the fetal assessment and serve as the consultant with the family. The suggested steps in evaluation are as follows:

1. A complete review of the mother's health history as well as family and pregnancy history should be performed, including documentation of ethnic origin, possibility of consanguinity, and history of similarly affected infants within the family. Maternal disorders such as diabetes, systemic lupus erythematosus, myotonic dystrophy, or any type of liver disease should also be noted.

2. Maternal blood studies should be obtained, including complete blood count, blood group typing, assessment for

---

TABLE 11–2

Investigation of Fetal Hydrops

Maternal
  Complete blood count and indices
  Hemoglobin electrophoresis
  Kleihauer-Betke stain of peripheral blood
  VDRL, rapid plasma reagin, and TORCH titers
  Ant-Ro, systemic lupus erythematosus preparation, sedimentation rate
  Parvovirus IgM, IgG
  Glucose-6-phosphate dehydrogenase, pyruvate kinase deficiency screening
Fetal
  Serial ultrasound evaluation
  Limb length, fetal movement
  Echocardiography
Amniocentesis
  Karyotype
  Alpha-fetoprotein
  Viral cultures; polymerase chain reaction for toxoplasmosis, parvovirus 19
  Establish culture for appropriate metabolic or DNA testing
Fetal Blood Sampling
  Karyotype
  Complete blood count
  Hemoglobin analysis
  IgM; specific cultures
  Albumin and total protein
  Measurement of umbilical venous pressure

From McGillivray BC, Hall JC: Nonimmune hydrops. Pediatr Rev 9:197, 1987. Reproduced by permission of Pediatrics.

---

thalassemia, possible glucose-6-phosphate dehydrogenase deficiency, viral infection, or hemorrhage.

3. Serial ultrasound scans should be obtained during pregnancy, with attention to fluid accumulation, development of the fetus' cardiac structure and rhythm, assessment of limb shape (because of possible dwarfing), and fetal movement.

4. In addition, assessment of the fetus (via either amniocentesis or umbilical cord sampling) should include karyotyping, viral titers, metabolic testing, and determination of hemoglobin and protein levels. Measurement of umbilical venous pressure may provide a reflection of fetal CVP (Weiner, 1993).

5. It may be necessary to tap a fetal fluid cavity, such as the peritoneal or pleural cavity, for diagnosis or therapy.

6. Because of the possibility of fetal demise, preparations should be made for maximal evaluation at the time of delivery, including pathologic studies and radiographs.

7. Consideration should be given to possible therapeutic measures from nonspecific therapy, such as amniocentesis to remove excess fluid, increase maternal comfort, and decrease risk of premature labor as well as to specific therapy, such as treatment of fetal cardiac arrhythmia. In addition, plans should be made for delivery of the infant with a skilled resuscitation team present (see Chapter 30).

NEONATAL EVALUATION

Table 11–3 presents the diagnostic evaluation recommended for newborn infants with nonimmune hydrops of unknown cause.

TABLE 11-3

**Diagnostic Evaluation of Newborns
with Nonimmune Hydrops**

System	Type of Evaluation
Cardiovascular	Echocardiogram, electrocardiogram
Pulmonary	Chest radiograph, pleural fluid examination
Hematologic	Complete blood cell count, differential platelet count, blood type and Coombs test, blood smear for morphology
Gastrointestinal	Abdominal radiograph, abdominal ultrasound, liver function tests, peritoneal fluid examination, total protein, albumin
Renal	Urinalysis, BUN, creatinine
Genetic	Chromosomal analysis, skeletal radiographs, genetic consultation
Congenital infections	Viral cultures or serology (including TORCH agents and parvovirus)
Pathologic	Complete autopsy, placental examination

Adapted from Carlton DP, McGillivray BC, Schreiber MD: Nonimmune hydrops fetalis: A multidisciplinary approach. Clin Perinatol 16:844, 1989.

Intensive Care of the Infant with Hydrops Fetalis

After successful resuscitation, including the intubation and administration of surfactant and placement of umbilical catheters, the clinical management can address both the cause and the complications of the hydrops. Morbidity and mortality may be due to the hydropic state, the underlying conditions giving rise to hydrops, or both. A hydropic fetus delivered prematurely is subject to the additional complications of prematurity.

Respiratory Management

Virtually all infants with hydrops require mechanical ventilation because of effusions, pulmonary hypoplasia, surfactant deficiency, pulmonary edema, poor chest wall compliance from edema, or, in some cases, persistent pulmonary hypertension of the newborn. The presence of persistent pleural effusions may necessitate the placing of chest tubes. Ascites may also compress the diaphragm and make lung expansion difficult. Breath sounds, chest movement, blood gases, and radiograms must all be monitored frequently, so that ventilator support can be reduced in response to increasing lung compliance and water clearance. Pneumothorax and pulmonary interstitial emphysema remain potential complications as long as ventilator support is continued. Infants, particularly those born prematurely, who require prolonged or aggressive courses of ventilation may develop bronchopulmonary dysplasia. Chronic lung disease may result in a longer and more complicated hospital course and contributes to the late mortality of hydrops.

Fluid and Electrolyte Management

A primary goal of fluid management is resolution of the hydrops itself. Maintenance fluids should be restricted, with volume boluses given only in response to clear signs of inadequate intravascular volume. The hydropic newborn has not only an excess of free extracellular water, but also an excess of sodium. Volume given during resuscitation increases further the amount of water and sodium that must be removed. Initial maintenance fluids should not contain sodium. Serum and urine sodium levels, urine volume, and daily weights should be monitored carefully to guide fluid and electrolyte administration. Urinary sodium levels may help to differentiate between hyponatremia owing to hemodilution and urinary losses.

Cardiovascular Management

Shock may be a prominent feature in patients with hydrops. This may result from hypovolemia owing to capillary leakage, poor vascular tone and impaired myocardial contractility owing to hypoxia or infection, impaired venous return owing to shifting or compression of mediastinal structures, or pericardial effusion. Adequate intravascular volume must be maintained, and correctable causes of impaired venous return should be addressed. Peripheral perfusion, heart rate, blood pressure, and acid-base status should be monitored carefully.

CLINICAL COURSE AND OUTCOME

Despite major advances in the ability to diagnose hydrops in utero by ultrasound techniques, the overall prognosis of patients with nonimmune hydrops remains poor. In cases in which the diagnosis is made antenatally, reported survival has ranged from 20% to 33% (Holtzgreve et al, 1990; Tomic et al, 1985). Of those infants with hydrops who are born alive, approximately 40% to 50% survive; these figures are misleading, however, because many of the underlying conditions are lethal. Obviously the degree of prematurity has a major impact on the overall mortality rate. As a group, the idiopathic cases currently seem to have the best prognosis.

Carlton and coworkers (1989) reported on a group of 36 infants with nonimmune hydrops and noted that 90% of those who died within 24 hours had pleural effusions compared with only 50% of those who survived. They also noted that more than one third of the infants in their study required thoracentesis in the delivery room to aid in lung expansion. All of the infants who lived more than 24 hours were mechanically ventilated and received supplemental oxygen. They required ventilation for an average of 11 days (range 2 to 48 days). Most of these infants lose a minimum of 15% of their birth weight, and some lose as much as 30%. Ordinarily, diuresis begins on the 2nd or 3rd day after birth and continues for a period of 2 to 4 days. Once the edema has resolved, the infants have normal levels of circulating protein and eventually appear to recover from their apparent capillary leak syndrome. If the hydrops is treated successfully or if it is of the idiopathic variety, the long-term outcome is good in the absence of serious birth asphyxia.

REFERENCES

Anand A, Gray ES, Brown T, et al: Human parvovirus infection in pregnancy and hydrops fetalis. N Engl J Med 316:183, 1987.

Baker JW, Harrison KL, Harvey PJ: Anti-C haemolytic disease requiring intrauterine and exchange transfusion. Med J Aust 2:296, 1988.

Barnes SE, Bryan EM, Harris DA, et al: Oedema in the newborn. Mol Aspects Med 1:187, 1977.

Bawle EV, Black V: Nonimmune hydrops fetalis in Noonan's syndrome. Am J Dis Child 140:758, 1986.

Beal RW: Non-rhesus (D) blood group isoimmunization in obstetrics. Clin Obstet Gynecol 6:493, 1979.

Bierman FZ, Baxi L, Jaffe I, et al: Fetal hydrops and congenital complete heart block: Response to maternal steroid therapy. J Pediatr 112:646, 1988.

Blair DK, Vander Straten MC, Gest AL: Hydrops in fetal sheep from rapid induction of anemia. Pediatr Res 35:5, 1994.

Boyd PA, Keeling JW: Fetal hydrops. J Med Genet 29:91, 1992.

Brace RA: Effects of outflow pressure on fetal lymph flow. Am J Obstet Gynecol 160:494, 1989.

Carlton DP, McGillivray BC, Schreiber MD: Nonimmune hydrops fetalis: A multidisciplinary approach. Clin Perinatol 16:839, 1989.

Diamond LK, Blackfan KD, Baty JM: Erythroblastosis fetalis and its association with universal edema of the fetus, icterus gravis neonatorum and anemia of the newborn. J Pediatr 1:269, 1932.

Etches PC, Lemons JA: Nonimmune hydrops fetalis: Report of 22 cases including three siblings. Pediatrics 64:326, 1979.

Gest AL, Blair DK, Vander Straten MC: The effect of outflow pressure upon thoracic duct lymph flow rate in fetal sheep. Pediatr Res 32:5, 1992.

Gest AL, Hansen TN, Moise AA, Hartley CJ: Atrial tachycardia causes hydrops in fetal lambs. Am J Physiol 258:27, 1990a.

Gest AL, Martin CG, Moise AA, Hansen TN: Reversal of venous blood flow with atrial tachycardia and hydrops in fetal sheep. Pediatr Res 28:3, 1990b.

Hansmann M, Gembruch U, Bald R: New therapeutic aspects in nonimmune hydrops fetalis based on four hundred and two prenatally diagnosed cases. Fetal Ther 4:29, 1989.

Holtzgreve W, Hansmann M, Genbruch U, et al: The fetus with nonimmune hydrops. *In* Harrison MR, Golbus MS, Filly RA (Eds): The Unborn Patient: Prenatal Diagnosis and Treatment, 2nd ed. Philadelphia, WB Saunders, 1990.

Hutchinson AA, Drew JH, Yu VYH, et al: Nonimmunologic hydrops fetalis: A review of 61 cases. Obstet Gynecol 59:347, 1982.

Machin GA: Hydrops revisited: Literature review of 1414 cases published in the 1980s. Am J Med Genet 34:366, 1989.

McGillivray BC, Hall JG: Nonimmune hydrops. Pediatr Rev 9:197, 1987.

Moise AA, Gest AL, Weickmann PH, McMicken HW: Reduction in plasma protein does not affect body water content in fetal sheep. Pediatr Res 29:6, 1991.

Newburger JW, Keane JF: Intrauterine supraventricular tachycardia. J Pediatr 95:780, 1979.

Norton ME: Nonimmune hydrops fetalis. Semin Perinatol 18:321, 1994.

Phibbs RH: Hydrops fetalis and other causes of neonatal edema and ascites. *In* Polin RA, Fox WW (Eds): Fetal and Neonatal Physiology. Philadelphia, WB Saunders, 1992.

Phibbs RH, Johnson P, Kitterman JA, et al: Cardiorespiratory status of erythroblastotic infants: I. Relationship of gestational age, severity of hemolytic disease and birth asphyxia to idiopathic respiratory distress syndrome and survival. Pediatrics 49:5, 1972.

Phibbs RH, Johnson P, Tooley WH: Cardiorespiratory status of erythroblastotic newborn infants: II. Blood volume, hematocrit and serum albumin concentrations in relation to hydrops fetalis. Pediatrics 53:13, 1974.

Phibbs RH, Naiman JL: Hemolytic disease of the newborn. *In* Mentzer WC, Wagner GH (Eds): Congenital Hemolytic Anemias. New Edinburgh, Churchill-Livingstone, 1989, pp 319–390.

Potter EL: Universal edema of the fetus unassociated with erythroblastosis. Am J Obstet Gynecol 46:30, 1943.

Ravindranath U, Paglia DE, Warrier I, et al: Glucose phosphate isomerase deficiency as a cause of hydrops fetalis. N Engl J Med 316:258, 1987.

Santolaya J, Alley D, Jaffe R, et al: Antenatal classification of hydrops fetalis. Obstet Gynecol 79:256, 1992.

Tomic S, McGillivray BC: A protocol for fetal hydrops: Summer Research Study. Vancouver, BC, University of British Columbia, 1985.

Weiner CP: Umbilical pressure measurement in the evaluation of nonimmune hydrops fetalis. Am J Obstet Gynecol 168:817, 1993.

CHAPTER 12

Fetal Surgery

N. Scott Adzick

The womb once shielded the fetus from observation and treatment. Powerful new imaging and sampling techniques, as well as a better understanding of fetal pathophysiology derived from animal models, have successfully stripped the veil of mystery from the once secretive fetus. Fetal therapy is the logical culmination of progress in fetal diagnosis. Stated simply, the fetus is now a patient (Adzick and Harrison, 1994).

The accurate diagnosis of a fetal anomaly permits the physician and parents to decide knowledgeably among various management options for the pregnancy. Although most prenatally diagnosed malformations are best managed by maternal transport, planned delivery near term, and appropriate neonatal therapy, other choices include elective abortion, a change in the timing or mode of delivery, or consideration of in utero therapy. A few anomalies with predictable and life-threatening prenatal pathophysiologic consequences may benefit from surgical correction before birth.

In the 1960s, direct fetal exposure with catheterization of fetal vessels for exchange transfusion was unsuccessful, and the procedure was abandoned. In the 1970s, increasingly sophisticated sonographic experience led to the accurate diagnosis before birth of many anatomic defects. In the 1980s, the rationale and feasibility of in utero repair for a number of fetal anomalies were explored. The succession of steps leading from the laboratory to the bedside included the following: The pathophysiology of potentially treatable fetal abnormalities was delineated in fetal animal models, and experimental in utero correction was shown to be efficacious; serial sonographic study of human fetuses with anatomic lesions determined the features that affect clinical outcome and helped craft selection criteria for prenatal intervention; and the surgical, anesthetic, and tocolytic techniques for hysterotomy and fetal surgery were developed in nonhuman primates, shown to be safe for the mother and her future reproductive potential, and finally introduced clinically. In the 1990s, more widespread clinical implementation is under way, and critical evaluation of the efficacy, safety, and cost of this new therapeutic approach is anticipated. The unique experience with fetal surgery at the Children's Hospital of Philadelphia (CHOP) and the University of California, San Francisco (UCSF) is reviewed in this chapter.

FETAL THORACIC LESIONS

Congenital cystic adenomatoid malformation is a benign cystic lung mass. In a series of more than 100 prenatally diagnosed cases, the author has found that the overall prognosis depends on the size of the lung mass and the secondary physiologic derangement: A large mass causes mediastinal shift, hypoplasia of normal lung tissue, polyhy-

dramnios, and cardiovascular compromise leading to fetal hydrops and death (Adzick, 1993). Esophageal compression by the thoracic mass with consequent decreased fetal swallowing of amniotic fluid leads to polyhydramnios, which is a common obstetric indication for sonography. Some prenatally diagnosed fetal lung lesions can shrink during gestation (MacGillivray et al, 1993).

The finding that the fetus with a large lung mass and associated hydrops is at high risk for fetal or neonatal demise has led to successful fetal lobectomy (Adzick et al, 1993). Fetal thoracentesis alone is usually ineffective because cyst fluid rapidly reaccumulates. Placement of thoracoamniotic shunts in fetuses with a single large cyst has provided long-term decompression in some cases. Fetal surgical resection of the massively enlarged pulmonary lobe was performed at 21 to 27 weeks' gestation in 12 patients with 7 healthy survivors at 1 to 5 years' follow-up. Developmental and pulmonary function testing at yearly intervals has been normal in these patients. Initial experience suggests that in appropriately selected cases of fetal cystic adenomatoid malformation (Fig. 12–1), resection is reasonably safe, reverses hydrops, and allows sufficient lung growth to permit survival.

Congenital pleural effusions are often caused by fetal chylothorax. Small effusions may be harmless, whereas large effusions may result in pulmonary compression, pulmonary hypoplasia, and a tension hydrothorax leading to hydrops (Longaker et al, 1989). For large effusions causing hydrops, in utero decompression may offer the only hope for survival. Although success with repeated fetal thoracenteses has been reported, the author and others have placed thoracoamniotic shunts in many afflicted fetuses to decompress the chylothorax successfully after a single aspiration failed to drain the fetal chest permanently (Nicolaides and Azar, 1989; Rodeck et al, 1988).

CONGENITAL DIAPHRAGMATIC HERNIA

Many infants born with congenital diaphragmatic hernia die despite optimal postnatal care because their lungs are too hypoplastic to support extrauterine life (Adzick et al, 1989; Sharland et al, 1992). The pulmonary hypoplasia is caused by in utero compression of the developing lungs by herniated abdominal viscera (Harrison et al, 1980). Because retrospective reviews of mortality for congenital diaphragmatic hernia vary widely and are flawed by a *hidden mortality* of unknown magnitude, Harrison and colleagues prospectively studied the outcome of 83 fetuses with potentially correctable isolated diaphragmatic hernia diagnosed before 24 weeks' gestation and arranged optimal postnatal care, including extracorporeal membrane oxygenation. The mortality was 58%, reflecting a substantial number of infants who died in utero or soon after birth (Harrison et al, 1994).

The Fetus with Congenital Cystic Adenomatoid Malformation

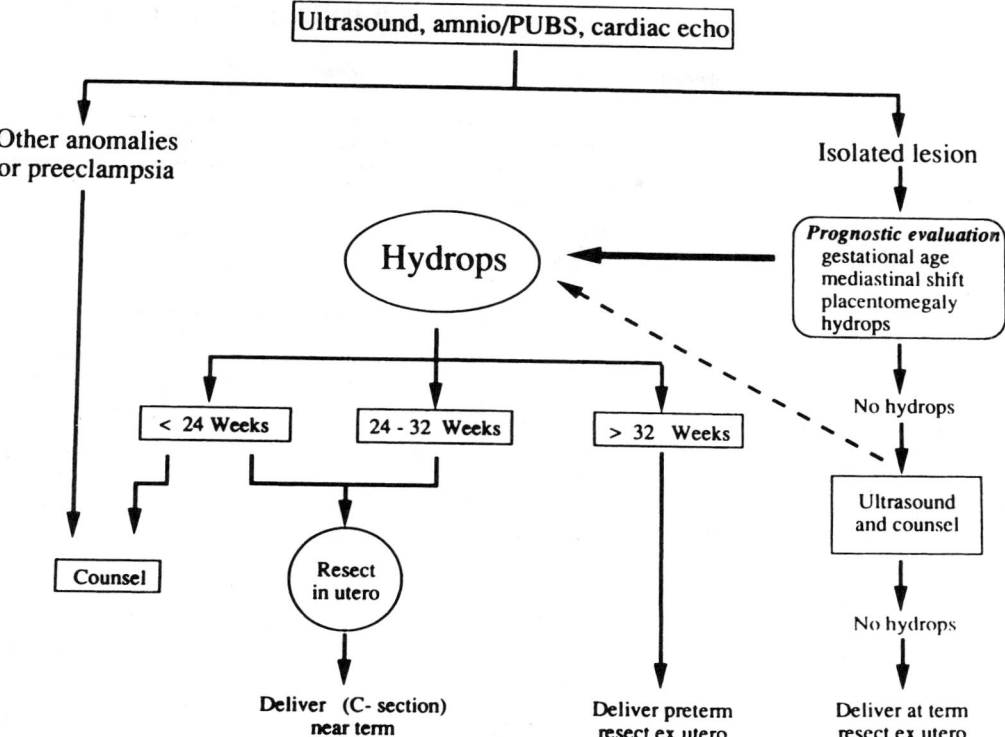

FIGURE 12–1. Management algorithm for the fetus with a cystic adenomatoid malformation. Amnio, amniocentesis; PUBS, percutaneous umbilical blood sampling; echo, echocardiography.

For fetuses with liver herniation, a less invasive approach to enhance fetal lung growth appears promising. Impeding the normal egress of fetal lung fluid by controlled tracheal obstruction in fetal lambs with surgically created diaphragmatic hernia dramatically enlarges the hypoplastic lungs, pushes the viscera back into the abdomen, and improves pulmonary function at birth (DiFiore et al, 1994; Hedrick et al, 1994a). The author has begun to apply this PLUG (*Plug the Lung Until It Grows*) procedure in human fetuses with large fetal diaphragmatic hernias containing fetal liver. In the future, prenatal tracheal occlusion using less invasive videofetoscopic techniques may simplify the fetal surgical approach to diaphragmatic hernia.

Sonographic studies have demonstrated that there is a broad range of clinical severity for fetal diaphragmatic hernia. An algorithm for management is shown in Figure 12–2. Some mildly affected fetuses are detected later in gestation, develop polyhydramnios later or not at all, and have a smaller volume of viscera in the chest. These fetuses should be delivered at an appropriate tertiary perinatal center after the lungs are mature. Unfortunately most fetuses are on the severe end of the clinical spectrum and do not survive even with optimal postnatal management. In general, these fetuses are detected earlier, develop polyhydramnios earlier, and have a larger volume of viscera in the chest (dilated stomach, impressive mediastinal shift, little lung visible in either thorax). Some of these fetuses may be salvaged by treatment in utero.

EX UTERO INTRAPARTUM TREATMENT PROCEDURE

In the course of treating 13 fetuses with predictable airway obstruction, a systematic approach to secure the airway during delivery was developed. Eight patients had their trachea clipped in utero for treatment of congenital diaphragmatic hernia, and five patients had prenatally diagnosed teratoma or lymphangioma of the neck and oropharynx. The author has found fast-image fetal magnetic resonance imaging (MRI) useful for the prenatal assessment of the fetal airway. The ex utero intrapartum treatment (EXIT) procedure was performed by using high doses of inhaled halogenated agents to facilitate uterine relaxation during cesarean section, securing the fetal airway while fetoplacental circulation remained intact (for up to 45 to 60 minutes), and then dividing the umbilical cord. A variety of procedures were performed during the EXIT procedure, including bronchoscopy, orotracheal intubation, tracheostomy, tracheoplasty, and installation of surfactant. This approach necessitates the coordinated efforts of pediatric surgeons, obstetricians, anesthesiologists, sonographers, and neonatologists. The combination of intensive maternal-fetal monitoring, cesarean section with maximal uterine relaxation, and maintenance of intact fetoplacental circulation provides a controlled environment for securing the airway in infants with prenatally diagnosed airway obstruction.

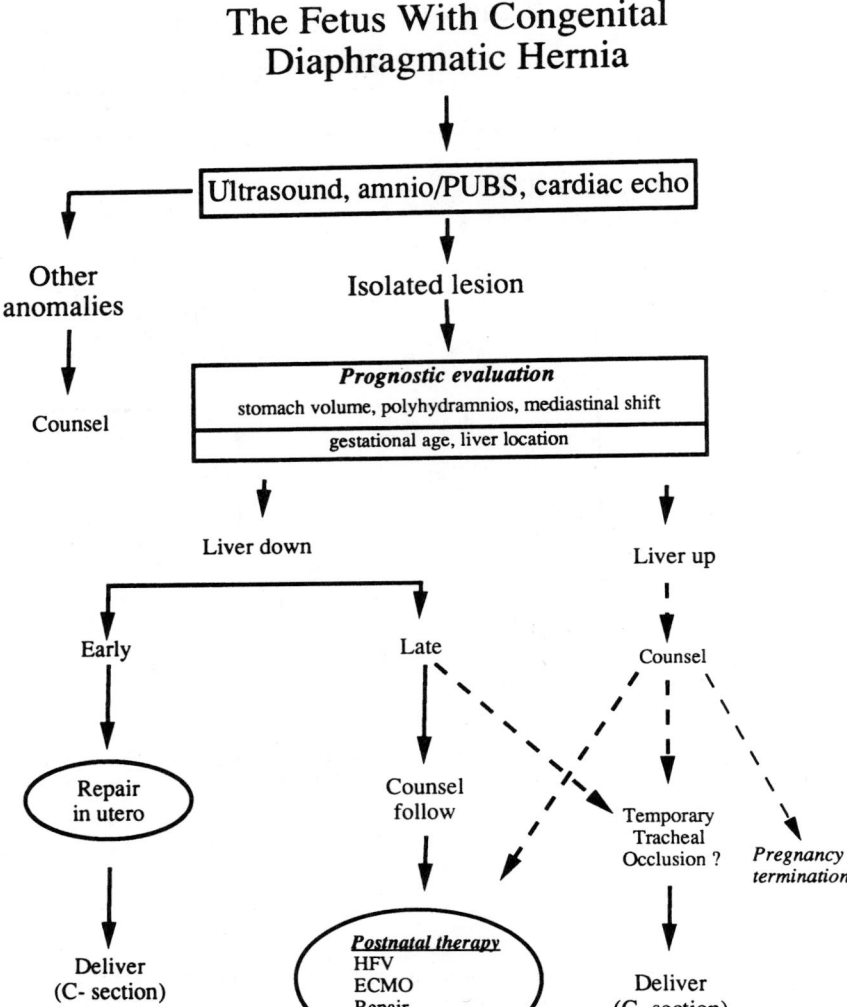

FIGURE 12–2. Management algorithm for the fetus with congenital diaphragmatic hernia. Amnio, amniocentesis; PUBS, percutaneous umbilical blood sampling; echo, echocardiography; HFV, high-frequency ventilation; ECMO, extracorporeal membrane oxygenation.

URINARY TRACT OBSTRUCTION

Unrelieved urinary tract obstruction interferes with fetal development. The severity of damage at birth depends on the type, degree, and duration of the obstruction. Although infants born with partial bilateral obstruction may have only mild hydronephrosis that is reversible with decompression after birth, male fetuses with high-grade urethral obstruction secondary to urethral valves develop renal dysplasia. In addition, oligohydramnios secondary to decreased fetal urine output produces fatal pulmonary hypoplasia.

Animal studies have demonstrated that these devastating renal and pulmonary consequences can be alleviated by urinary tract decompression before birth (Adzick et al, 1985). Sonographic study of hundreds of human fetuses with urinary tract obstruction has helped trace the natural history of this fetal condition, and selection criteria for in utero treatment have been developed. The sonographic detection of renal cortical cysts or increased renal echogenicity is predictive of renal dysplasia. High levels of sodium, chloride, calcium, and beta₂-microglobulin in fetal urine obtained by a percutaneous fetal bladder aspiration correlates with poor fetal renal function (Estes and Harrison, 1993).

Most fetuses with obstructive uropathy do not require intervention (Fig. 12–3). If bilateral hydronephrosis is an isolated condition and the amniotic fluid volume is adequate, the mother should be followed by serial ultrasonography, and the fetus should be evaluated and treated postnatally. If moderate to severe oligohydramnios develops, the fetus should undergo a complete prognostic evaluation to determine its potential for normal renal and pulmonary function at birth. For the fetus with predicted renal dysplasia, aggressive obstetric care or in utero decompression is not indicated. For the fetus with predicted preserved renal function, early delivery for postnatal decompression is indicated if the lungs are mature. If the lungs are immature, in utero decompression is recommended using either a double-pigtail catheter shunt placed percutaneously under sonographic guidance or creation of a vesicostomy using open fetal surgical techniques. Survival after catheter placement is approximately 70% in appropriately selected male fetuses with posterior urethral valves (Holzgreve and Evans, 1993). A newly developed fetoscopic technique for placement of an expandable mesh stent may solve some of the technical problems encountered with double-pigtail catheters (occlusion, dislodgment, abdominal wall disruption) and avoid the potential morbidity of open surgery (Estes et al, 1992a).

Important lessons have been gleaned from evaluating several hundred fetuses in many institutions over the past decade. Patient selection is accurate enough to avoid intervention in cases that do not need it. In utero decompression with restoration of amniotic fluid can prevent the development of fatal oligohydramnios-induced pulmonary hypoplasia. It is still unclear whether fetal treatment can arrest or reverse renal dysplastic changes initiated before birth that may compromise renal function as demand increases during postnatal growth.

SACROCOCCYGEAL TERATOMA

Sacrococcygeal teratoma is the most common neonatal tumor. Most sacrococcygeal teratomas are diagnosed in newborns when the malignant potential is low and the prognosis is good. Prenatal sonographic diagnosis, however, has identified fetuses with large teratomas and associated hydrops who die (Flake, 1993). Fetal demise occurs because of high-output cardiac failure associated with a *vascular steal* owing to the extremely high blood flow through the tumor (Fig. 12–4).

The development of fetal hydrops and placentomegaly may lead to the potentially devastating maternal mirror syndrome, in which the mother's condition begins to mirror that of the sick fetus. The affected mother develops progressive symptoms of preeclampsia, including vomiting, hypertension, proteinuria, peripheral edema, and pulmo-

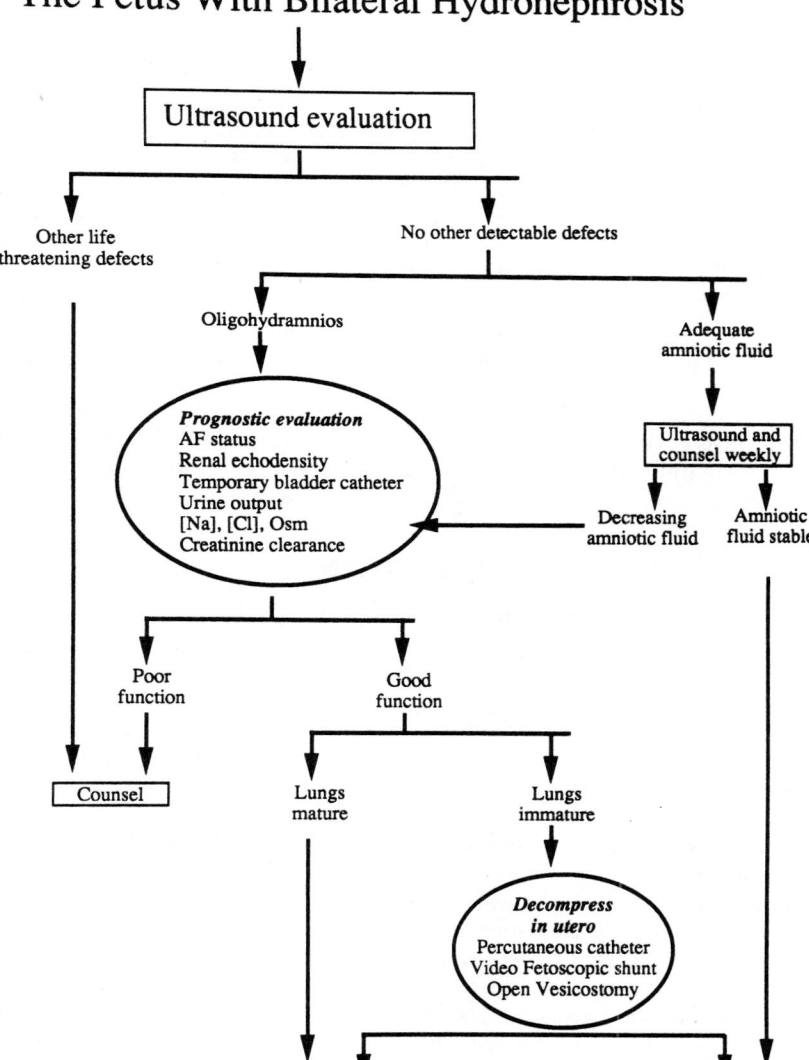

FIGURE 12–3. Management algorithm for the fetus with bilateral hydronephrosis. AF, amniotic fluid; Osm, osmolality.

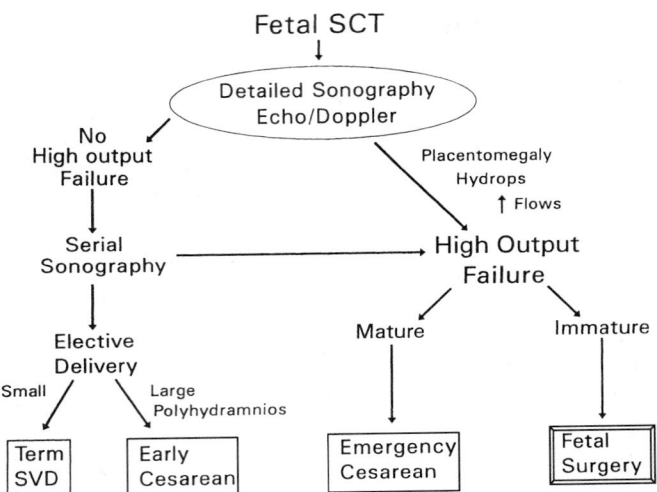

FIGURE 12–4. Management algorithm for the fetus with sacrococcygeal teratoma (SCT). SVD, spontaneous vaginal delivery.

nary edema, all of which may be a consequence of vasoactive factors or endothelial toxins released from the edematous placenta.

Clear documentation of high-output failure secondary to tumor vascular steal using color flow Doppler ultrasound combined with the uniformly fatal outcome of immature fetuses who develop placentomegaly and hydrops suggests that in utero tumor resection might reverse hydrops and prevent fetal demise. Initial experience with two cases indicated that fetal teratoma excision leads to resolution of hydrops, but resection must be done before initiation of placentomegaly and the associated mirror syndrome (Flake, 1993). More recently, a fetal sacrococcygeal teratoma resection was performed at CHOP with good outcome (Adzick, 1997). Less invasive sonographically guided or videofetoscopic techniques may soon be used selectively to occlude the tumor vessels and interrupt the vascular steal.

TWIN-TWIN TRANSFUSION

Abnormalities of twin pregnancies that may require in utero treatment occur when abnormal placental chorionic vessels connect the circulations of the twins, leading to an imbalance of blood flow. This parabiosis can put both twins in jeopardy because of marked changes in amniotic fluid volume, growth retardation, and hydrops. Both twin-twin transfusion syndrome and heart failure of the normal "pump" twin in an acardiac twin pregnancy are associated with high perinatal mortality secondary to premature birth or in utero death, especially when these conditions occur in previable pregnancies in which delivery is not an option. Therapy has focused on interrupting the abnormal placental vascular circulation by severing the abnormal placental vessels. For twin-twin transfusion syndrome, these vessels have been divided using a fetoscopically directed laser (Ville et al, 1995). For the acardiac twin pregnancy, the normal twin has been salvaged by occluding the umbilical circulation of the abnormal twin (Porreco et al, 1991), by removing the abnormal fetus via a hysterotomy at 26 weeks' gestation or less (four of five normal twins survived at the

author's center) (Fries et al, 1992), or by umbilical cord ligation under videofetoscopic guidance (Quintero et al, 1994). Future studies will determine the most effective approach.

THERAPY FOR OTHER ANATOMIC LESIONS

A few lesions may be treatable prenatally once their pathophysiology is deciphered and new methods of treatment are developed. For example, fetal aortic valvular stenosis often causes irreversible left ventricular damage, and percutaneous balloon catheter dilation of the stenotic fetal aortic valve has been performed (Maxwell et al, 1991). Fetal complete heart block in the setting of maternal collagen vascular disease can lead to cardiac failure, hydrops, and fetal demise (Schmidt et al, 1991). After establishing the efficacy of pacing for heart block in fetal lambs (Crombleholme et al, 1990), a pacemaker was successfully placed in a 22-week hydropic fetus, but the heart was already irreversibly damaged by more than 6 weeks of heart failure, so earlier intervention may be required.

Progressive ventriculomegaly as a result of obstruction of the aqueduct of Sylvius can compress and injure the developing brain. A large multicenter experience with in utero drainage procedures for fetal hydrocephalus has not clearly improved outcome, and a moratorium for fetal treatment of this condition has been observed because of current inadequacies in diagnosis, ineffective fetal shunting techniques, and improper selection criteria (Hudgins et al, 1988; Manning et al, 1986). If these shortcomings can be overcome, some hydrocephalic fetuses may benefit from ventricular decompression before birth.

Fetuses with laryngeal atresia develop large lungs distended with fetal lung fluid that can lead to cardiac compression and hydrops. These fetuses may be salvaged in utero by decompressing the obstructed trachea (fetal tracheostomy). If hydrops is not present, planned near-term cesarean delivery permits airway access by tracheostomy while the fetus remains connected to the placenta (Hedrick et al, 1994b).

Myelomeningocele is becoming less common because it can be detected early in gestation (when pregnancy termination is an option), and this lesion may be prevented by vitamin supplementation. There is evidence that neurologic impairment is secondary to exposure of the spinal cord in utero, so it may be possible to ameliorate the progressive disabling sequelae by repairing the anatomic defect in utero (Meuli et al, 1995).

MATERNAL-FETAL MANAGEMENT

Clinical fetal surgical principles are derived from more than 1600 operations in fetal lambs and more than 400 operations in fetal rhesus monkeys at the author's center during the past 15 years. Indomethacin and antibiotics are given preoperatively, and halogenated inhalation agents provide anesthesia for both mother and fetus. Perioperative maternal monitoring requires a radial arterial catheter, blood pressure cuff, intravenous and central venous pressure catheters, bladder catheter, electrocardiogram leads, and transcutaneous pulse oximeter.

The uterus is exposed through a low transverse abdominal incision. Fentanyl and pancuronium are injected into the fetus under sterile intraoperative ultrasound guidance to help ablate the fetal stress response. The fetal and placental positions are determined sonographically, some amniotic fluid is aspirated through a trocar, the hysterotomy is extended with a specially developed absorbable uterine stapler (Bond et al, 1989), and the appropriate fetal part is exposed. For fetal monitoring, a miniaturized pulse oximeter is wrapped around the fetal hand, and an implanted radiotelemetry device reliably measures the fetal electrocardiogram, temperature, and intrauterine pressure both intraoperatively and postoperatively (Jennings et al, 1993a). The fetus and uterus are continually bathed in warm saline. After repair of the defect, the fetus is returned to the uterus, the staples are removed from the uterine edge, a watertight two-layer uterine closure is performed that is supplemented with fibrin glue to help seal the membranes, and a transparent dressing is placed on the closed laparotomy wound to prevent interference with postoperative sonographic monitoring.

Optimal perioperative management of the maternal-fetal unit requires continuous monitoring of maternal hemodynamics, fetal condition, and uterine contractions in an intensive care setting, usually for 48 hours. Vigilant maternal-fetal monitoring continues on the obstetrics unit for 5 to 7 days postoperatively, followed by outpatient examinations, sonograms, and subcutaneous terbutaline tocolysis given via a portable pump. Cesarean section is performed when either the membranes rupture or labor cannot be controlled, which usually occurs before 36 weeks' gestation.

Appropriate surveillance and treatment of preterm labor remain the "Achilles heel" of fetal surgery, and the tocolytic regimen that was successful in nonhuman primate experiments is fraught with potential clinical difficulties. Indomethacin can cause fetal ductus arteriosus constriction, tricuspid regurgitation, and right-sided heart failure, so serial fetal echocardiographic monitoring is essential. Although deep halogenated anesthesia can provide satisfactory intraoperative uterine relaxation, this regimen can produce fetal and maternal myocardial depression and decrease placental perfusion. Maternal pulmonary edema is a known side effect of magnesium sulfate and beta-mimetics used for tocolysis, and fluid restriction to avoid this complication may compromise maternal-placental-fetal circulation and exacerbate preterm labor. Experimental studies suggest that endogenous nitric oxide mediates normal uterine relaxation during pregnancy (Natuzzi et al, 1993; Yallampalli et al, 1993). Nitric oxide donors have been shown to inhibit hysterotomy-induced uterine contractions in rhesus monkeys (Jennings et al, 1993b), and this approach appears promising for the future management of preterm labor during and after human fetal surgery.

Maternal safety is the cardinal issue (Longaker et al, 1991a). Clearly the healthy mother accepts some risk to help her unborn child. Only a handful of open fetal surgery cases have been performed at other institutions, so the 70 cases from CHOP and UCSF provide the best data on maternal outcome. Although there have been few maternal complications, all patients had uterine contractions after fetal surgery, which accounted for some misery and morbidity from the treatment regimen (e.g., one patient devel-

oped pulmonary edema from the tocolytic medications). Amniotic fluid leaks developed in five patients: Two patients had leaks through the hysterotomy site requiring reoperation and closure, and three other patients had vaginal amniotic fluid leaks that were presumably from fluid dissecting internally from the hysterotomy site to the cervix. There were two infections: one case of pseudomembranous colitis owing to parenteral antibiotic therapy that responded promptly to a course of oral vancomycin and one superficial wound infection. Seven patients required blood transfusion.

Because the midgestation hysterotomy is invariably in the upper segment of the uterine corpus and thus is comparable to a classic cesarean section, there is potential for uterine disruption during labor. Thus, delivery after the fetal surgery and for all future deliveries should be by cesarean section. Two disruptions occurred in subsequent pregnancies before a cesarean section could be done. Maternal and neonatal outcome were excellent in both cases. Finally, future reproductive potential does not appear to be jeopardized by fetal surgery. Although most fetal operations have taken place in the past 5 years, more long-term follow-up from earlier cases reveals that 26 patients have had 28 normal children in subsequent pregnancies.

SCIENTIFIC SPINOFFS

Investigative studies that were initially focused on prenatal treatment have led to other potential benefits that extend beyond the nascent field of fetal surgery. The natural history and pathophysiologic consequences of a growing list of fetal anatomic abnormalities have been clarified for perinatologists, neonatologists, and pediatric surgical specialists. A uterine stapling device containing absorbable staples that was developed to open the gravid uterus quickly and bloodlessly during fetal surgery has now been applied to routine cesarean sections (Bond et al, 1989). Continuous transmission of intrauterine pressure and fetal electrocardiogram by a fetal radiotelemeter may prove useful in the management of high-risk pregnancies threatened with preterm labor. Nitric oxide donors may provide a promising new approach to the broader problem of preterm labor (Lees et al, 1994).

Fetal endoscopic surgery (which the author calls "fetendo") may permit fetal surgery through small puncture sites in the uterus, thereby obviating the potential morbidity of a large hysterotomy. Videofetoscopic techniques have been developed in fetal lambs and monkeys for in utero bladder and pleural fluid decompression, temporary tracheal occlusion for pulmonary hypoplasia, umbilical cord ligation for acardiac twin pregnancies, and cleft lip and palate repair (Estes et al, 1992b). Using videofetoscopic visualization, extra-amniotic catheterization of chorionic vessels for long-term fetal vascular access may provide a portal for fetal blood sampling, transfusion, hematopoietic stem cell transplantation, and gene therapy (Hedrick et al, 1993).

The fetus has taught clinicians some important lessons about fetal biology. By serendipity, it was learned that the fetus heals surgical incisions without scar. This observation has fostered a multidisciplinary approach to unravel the biology of scarless fetal wound healing. This unique repair

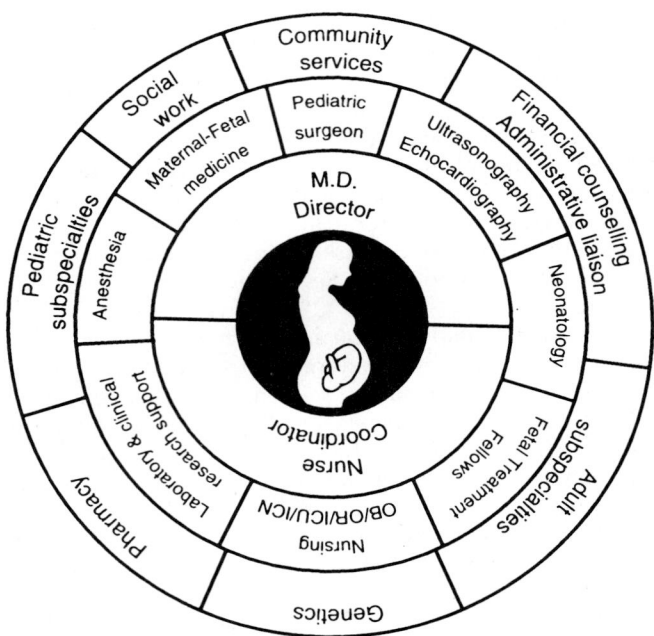

FIGURE 12–5. The fetal treatment center requires the expertise of many different specialists in an institutional setting that fosters high-level perinatal care, clinical investigation, and experimental work.

process is not dependent on the sterile, aqueous intrauterine environment. The differences between fetal and adult skin healing reflect processes intrinsic to fetal tissue, such as an extracellular wound matrix rich in hyaluronic acid and a markedly reduced inflammatory infiltrate and cytokine profile (Adzick and Longaker, 1992). By mimicking the scarless fetal wound healing blueprint, therapeutic strategies have emerged to ameliorate scar in children and adults (Shah et al, 1992).

The observation that fetal wounds heal without scar formation before midgestation has stimulated interest in the possibility of correcting cleft lip and palate in utero to avoid scarring, midfacial growth restriction, and secondary nasal deformity. The theoretical benefits of repair are unproven, however, and do not yet justify the risks of intervention (Longaker et al, 1991b).

Fetal immune tolerance permits stable, long-term chimerism after in utero transplantation of normal fetal hematopoietic stem cells without graft-versus-host disease or the need for immunosuppression (Flake et al, 1986; Harrison et al, 1989). This tactic to avoid transplant rejection may allow a wide variety of prenatally diagnosed inherited diseases such as thalassemia and Hurler disease to be cured by fetal hematopoietic stem cell transplantation (Touraine, 1992). Furthermore, fetuses diagnosed with impending organ failure may undergo the prenatal infusion of allogeneic or xenogeneic hematopoietic stem cells to render them tolerant for donor-specific organ transplantation after birth (West et al, 1994).

FUTURE OF FETAL INTERVENTION

The promise of fetal therapy is that the earliest possible intervention for a life-threatening fetal disorder may pro-

duce the best result. Because fetal surgery jeopardizes the pregnancy and entails potential risks to the mother as well as the fetus, fetal surgery should be pursued only in centers committed to ongoing research concomitant with cautious clinical application. A fetal treatment center requires the close collaboration of dedicated pediatric surgeons, perinatal obstetricians, sonographers, echocardiographers, neonatologists, intensivists, geneticists, ethicists, neonatal and obstetric nurses, and a compassionate nurse coordinator (Fig. 12–5). The fetal treatment team should make a commitment to have this innovative therapy reviewed by uninvolved professional colleagues (institutional review board), to publish all results (bad as well as good), to avoid media reports until cases are peer reviewed, and to test the validity and cost-effectiveness of this approach in properly controlled trials.

REFERENCES

Adzick NS: Fetal thoracic lesions. Semin Pediatr Surg 2:103, 1993.
Adzick NS, Crombleholme TM, Morgan MA, et al: A rapidly growing fetal teratoma. Lancet 349:538, 1997.
Adzick NS, Harrison MR: Fetal surgical therapy. Lancet 343:897, 1994.
Adzick NS, Harrison MR: The unborn surgical patient. *In* Current Problems in Surgery. Littleton, MA, Mosby-Year Book, 1994.
Adzick NS, Harrison MR, Flake AW, et al: Fetal urinary tract obstruction: Experimental pathophysiology. Semin Perinatol 9:79, 1985.
Adzick NS, Harrison MR, Flake AW, et al: Fetal surgery for cystic adenomatoid malformation of the lung. J Pediatr Surg 28:806, 1993.
Adzick NS, Longaker MT (Eds): Fetal Wound Healing. New York, Elsevier, 1992.
Adzick NS, Vacanti JP, Lillehei CW, et al: Fetal diaphragmatic hernia: Ultrasound diagnosis and clinical outcome in 38 cases from a single medical center. J Pediatr Surg 24:654, 1989.
Bond SJ, Harrison MR, Slotnick RN, et al: Cesarean delivery and hysterotomy using an absorbable stapling device. Obstet Gynecol 74:25, 1989.
Crombleholme TM, Harrison MR, Longaker MT, et al: Complete heart block in fetal lambs: I. Technique and acute physiologic response. J Pediatr Surg 25:587, 1990.
DiFiore JW, Fauzo DO, Slavin R, et al: Experimental fetal tracheal ligation reverses the structural and physiological effects of pulmonary hypoplasia in congenital diaphragmatic hernia. J Pediatr Surg 29:248, 1994.
Estes JM, Harrison MR: Fetal obstructive uropathy. Semin Pediatr Surg 2:932, 1993.
Estes JM, Macgillivray TE, Hedrick MH, et al: Fetoscopic surgery for the treatment of congenital anomalies. J Pediatr Surg 27:950, 1992a.
Estes JM, Whitby DJ, Lorenz HP, et al: Endoscopic creation and repair of fetal cleft lip. Plast Reconstr Surg 90:743, 1992b.
Flake AW: Fetal sacrococcygeal teratoma. Semin Pediatr Surg 2:113, 1993.
Flake AW, Harrison MR, Adzick NS, Zanjani E: Transplantation of fetal hematopoietic stem cells in utero: The creation of hematopoietic chimeras. Science 233:776, 1986.
Fries MH, Goldberg JD, Golbus MS: Treatment of acardiac-acephalus twin gestations by hysterotomy and selective delivery. Obstet Gynecol 79:601, 1992.
Harrison MR, Adzick NS, Estes JM, Howell LJ: A prospective study of the outcome for fetuses with diaphragmatic hernia. JAMA 271:382, 1994.
Harrison MR, Adzick NS, Flake AW, et al: Correction of congenital diaphragmatic hernia in utero: VI. Hard-earned lessons. J Pediatr Surg 28:1411, 1993.
Harrison MR, Adzick NS, Longaker MT, et al: Successful repair in utero of a fetal diaphragmatic hernia after removal of herniated viscera from the left thorax. N Engl J Med 322:1582, 1990.
Harrison MR, Bressack MA, Churg AM, et al: Correction of congenital diaphragmatic hernia in utero: II. Simulated correction permits fetal lung growth with survival at birth. Surgery 88:260, 1980.
Harrison MR, Slotnick RN, Crombleholme TM, et al: In utero transplantation of fetal liver hematopoietic stem cells in monkeys. Lancet 2:1425, 1989.

Hedrick MH, Estes JM, Sullivan KM, et al: Plug the lung until it grows (PLUG): A new method to treat congenital diaphragmatic hernia in utero. J Pediatr Surg 29:612, 1994a.

Hedrick MH, Jennings RW, MacGillivray TE, et al: Chronic fetal vascular access. Lancet 342:1086, 1993.

Hedrick MH, Martinez-Ferro M, Flake AW, et al: Prenatal diagnosis of congenital high airway obstruction (CHAOS): Potential for perinatal intervention. J Pediatr Surg 29:271, 1994b.

Holzgreve W, Evans MI: Nonvascular needles and shunt placements for fetal therapy. West J Med 159:333, 1993.

Hudgins KJ, Edwards MSB, Goldstein RB, et al: Natural history of fetal ventriculomegaly. Pediatrics 82:692, 1988.

Jennings RW, Adzick NS, Longaker MT, et al: Radio-telemetric fetal monitoring during and after open fetal surgery. Surg Gynecol Obstet 176:59, 1993a.

Jennings RW, MacGillivray TE, Harrison MR: Nitric oxide inhibits preterm labor in the rhesus monkey. J Maternal Fetal Med 2:170, 1993b.

Lees C, Campbell S, Jauniaux E, et al: Arrest of preterm labor and prolongation of gestation with glyceryl trinitrate, a nitric oxide donor. Lancet 343:1325, 1994.

Longaker MT, Golbus MS, Filly RA, et al: Maternal outcome after open fetal surgery: A review of the first 17 human cases. JAMA 265:737, 1991a.

Longaker MT, Laberge JM, Dansereau J, et al: Primary fetal hydrothorax: Natural history and management. J Pediatr Surg 24:573, 1989.

Longaker MT, Whitby DJ, Adzick NS, et al: Fetal surgery for cleft lip: A plea for caution. Plast Reconstr Surg 88:1087, 1991b.

MacGillivray TE, Harrison MR, Goldstein RB, Adzick NS: Disappearing fetal lung lesions. J Pediatr Surg 28:1321, 1993.

Manning FA, Harrison MR, Rodeck CH, et al: Special report: Catheter shunts for fetal hydronephrosis and hydrocephalus. N Engl J Med 315:336, 1986.

Maxwell D, Allan L, Tynan MJ: Balloon dilatation of the aortic valve in the fetus: A report of two cases. Br Heart J 65:256, 1991.

Meuli M, Meuli-Simmen C, Yingling CD, et al: Creation of myelomeningocele in utero: A model of functional damage from spinal cord exposure in fetal sheep. J Pediatr Surg 30:1028, 1995.

Natuzzi ES, Ursell PC, Harrison MR, et al: Uterine nitric oxide synthase activity in the gravid uterus decreases at parturition. Biochem Biophys Res Commun 179:1, 1993.

Nicolaides KH, Azar GB: Thoraco-amniotic shunting. Fetal Diagn Ther 5:153, 1989.

Porreco RP, Barton SM, Havercamp AD: Occlusion of umbilical artery in acardiac, acephalic twin. Lancet 337:326, 1991.

Quintero RA, Reich H, Puder KS, et al: Umbilical-cord ligation of an acardiac twin by fetoscopy at 19 weeks' gestation. N Engl J Med 330:469, 1994.

Rodeck CH, Fisk NM, Fraser DI, et al: Long-term in utero drainage of fetal hydrothrax. N Engl J Med 319:1135, 1988.

Schmidt KG, Ulmer HE, Silverman NH, et al: Perinatal outcome of fetal complete heart block: A multicenter experience. J Am Coll Cardiol 17:360, 1991.

Shah M, Foreman DM, Ferguson MWJ: Control of scarring in adult wounds by neutralising antibody to transforming growth factor beta. Lancet 339:213, 1992.

Sharland GK, Lockhart SM, Heward AJ, et al: Prognosis in fetal diaphragmatic hernia. Am J Obstet Gynecol 166:9, 1992.

Touraine JL: In utero transplantation of fetal liver stem cells into human fetuses. Hum Reprod 7:44, 1992.

Ville Y, Hyett J, Hecher K, Nicolaides K: Preliminary experience with endoscopic laser surgery for severe twin-twin transfusion syndrome. N Engl J Med 332:224, 1995.

West LJ, Morris PJ, Wood KJ: Fetal liver haematopoietic cells and tolerance to organ allografts. Lancet 343:148, 1994.

Yallampalli C, Izumi H, Bryan-Smith M, et al: An L-arginine-nitric oxide-cyclic guanosine monophosphate system exists in the uterus and inhibits contractility during pregnancy. Am J Obstet Gynecol 170:175, 1993.

CHAPTER 13

Antepartum Fetal Assessment

Andrew Hull and Thomas R. Moore

In an ideal world, astute clinicians would be able to correct any inadequacies of the intrauterine environment so as to optimize fetal growth, development, and well-being. With such corrections, fetal outcome would be uniformly excellent. Because this is, as yet, an unattainable goal, clinicians must carefully observe fetal status and effect delivery when extrauterine life seems safer or more desirable than continuing the pregnancy. To that end, obstetricians have developed a set of tests that can assist in determining the timing of delivery so as to minimize unexpected fetal morbidity.

Although the primary aim of antenatal fetal surveillance is the prevention of stillbirth, a secondary, although no less important, aim is minimizing fetal and neonatal morbidity. In comparing the efficacy of various surveillance methods, reduction in fetal mortality is a convenient outcome measure. The best tests, however, result in the birth of better newborns. The various methods of assessing fetal status currently are listed in Table 13–1, and the details of each are discussed subsequently.

GENERAL PRINCIPLES OF FETAL BIOPHYSICAL ASSESSMENT

The ideal test of fetal well-being would be simple to carry out, cheap, and accurate and generate clear, reproducible results not subject to variable interpretation. Equally, it should be easy to apply to an entire patient population and thus select all patients at significant risk of poor fetal outcome. Such a test does not yet exist. Given the problems with designing the perfect test, clinicians have, over time, begun testing more and more pregnancies to reduce to a minimum poor fetal outcome.

Platt and colleagues (1987) studied the impact of increasing use of antepartum fetal testing in the period 1971 through 1986. The results are shown in Table 13–2. Clearly, although the outcomes of the small minority tested population improved, the largest number of fetal deaths occurred in the larger untested population, despite a marked increase in the percentage of patients undergoing expensive antepartum testing.

The financial impact of this trend can be roughly calculated. Using estimated charges of approximately $125 per test, the cost of fetal testing in a cohort of 1000 pregnant patients would be $37,500, discounting the expense to the patient associated with child care or job absence to visit the testing center. If, as Platt and colleagues have shown, such testing reduces fetal mortality rate by 2 per 1000 births, the cost per fetal life saved equals $18,750.

In reviewing the data, Platt and colleagues have suggested that better means of identifying the at-risk fetus should be devised so that antepartum testing could be applied to the population most likely to experience benefit. Based on the accumulated experience with traditional bio-physical testing, further increasing the indications for non-stress or biophysical profile testing is not likely to be economical or effective in reducing the fetal mortality rate.

Indications for Fetal Testing

As noted previously, 30% or more of stillbirths occur in patients without identifiable risk factors (Hovatta et al, 1983). Thus, simply screening or testing high-risk patients is not enough. Nevertheless, conditions in which fetal surveillance is traditionally considered mandatory are listed in Table 13–3. This list can almost be expanded indefinitely. Optimally, fetal testing should involve use of an inexpensive, widely applied test, with further, specific testing for those pregnancies identified as *at risk*.

When to Begin Fetal Testing

Given that testing is indicated in an individual pregnancy, the next question is when to begin testing. Because there is little to be gained in identifying a fetus that is in distress before viability, testing typically begins after 24 to 26 weeks. Gestational age at entry into a surveillance program for specific groups may be arbitrarily chosen or based on risk assessment. For instance, routine testing is performed on most insulin-dependent diabetics from 32 to 34 weeks' gestation and in most uncomplicated patients after 41.5 weeks' gestation based on the relative risk of poor fetal outcome as a function of time.

Frequency of Fetal Testing

Fetal assessment clearly lends itself to the use of algorithms both for selecting patients and for designing a cascade of testing methods. Such a sequential approach is commonly used (Devoe et al, 1990) and potentially nullifies some of the subjective shortcomings of fetal testing.

Clearly, if clinicians are willing to use methods of fetal surveillance, they must be willing to act on the results. Given that for the most part this action is delivery, it is imperative that the testing method chosen yields few false-positive results and even fewer false-negative results. This topic is addressed following the accounts of each testing modality.

ULTRASOUND

Ultrasound has become an increasingly important tool in the evaluation of high-risk obstetric patients. In many obstetric practices, all pregnant women are offered an ultrasound evaluation of the fetus at some time. Although this practice is controversial, there are several well-recognized indications for sonography.

TABLE 13–1

Fetal Biophysical Assessment Modalities

Maternal assessment of fetal movement	Biophysical profile
Cardiotocography	Doppler flow studies
Nonstress testing	Amniocentesis
Contraction stress testing	Cordocentesis
Assessment of amniotic fluid volume	

TABLE 13–3

Indications for Fetal Surveillance

Threatened preterm delivery	Chronic maternal illness
Post-term pregnancy	Diabetes
Hypertensive disorders	Anemia
Intrauterine growth retardation	Hemoglobinopathies
Previous stillbirth	Cyanotic heart disease
Decreased fetal movement	Collagen vascular disease
Multiple gestation	Renal impairment

Determination of Gestational Age

Accurate determination of pregnancy duration is a central goal of prenatal care. Although precise pregnancy dating is valuable in even uncomplicated pregnancies, this information is of critical importance in situations of marginal fetal viability and salvageability. A typical scenario involves the problem of performing or avoiding cesarean delivery in a pregnancy with fetal distress at 23 (<5% survival) to 26 (30% survival) weeks' gestation. Typical dating criteria and their accuracy are listed in Table 13–4. Although a crown-rump length measurement obtained between 7 and 10 weeks' gestation provides the smallest error (± 3 days), a single sonographic study in the 16- to 22-week time period affords acceptable dating accuracy (± 10 days) while allowing visualization of most of the fetal organs.

Diagnosis of Fetal Anomalies

A major additional benefit of routine sonographic scanning of pregnancies is the diagnosis of unexpected fetal anomalies. Several secondary benefits are associated with antenatal identification of the anomalous fetus:

1. Selection of appropriate level of obstetric and neonatal care. *Antenatal counseling by pediatric and neonatal specialists provides smoother transition for both parents and newborn.* Typical anomalies in which antenatal counseling improves postnatal care include congenital diaphragmatic hernia and cyanotic heart disease.
2. *Identification of lethal anomalies, avoiding unnecessary cesarean delivery and futile neonatal intervention.* Examples include anencephaly, holoprosencephaly, thanatophoric dwarfism, and bilateral renal

agenesis, all of which have a high incidence of distress during labor often leading to emergent cesarean delivery. Antenatal recognition of these lethal conditions permits families to make rational choices regarding delivery route.

3. Identification of chromosome anomalies *in otherwise low-risk women.* Most major chromosome anomalies have typical sonographic features, which may suggest further diagnostic procedures, such as amniocentesis or umbilical cord blood sampling.
4. Identification of nonlethal but significantly debilitating fetal anomalies *before viability permits the option of pregnancy termination or in utero fetal therapy.* Examples include large meningomyelocele, multiple amputations associated with the amniotic band syndrome, and fetal hydrops arising from perinatal viral infections such as cytomegalovirus. Conditions that may be amenable to in utero therapy include congenital hydrothorax and posterior urethral valves.

Factors that may adversely affect the accuracy and sensitivity of ultrasound screening for fetal anomalies include

TABLE 13–2

Antepartum Fetal Deaths in Tested and Untested Pregnancies

	1971–1975	1976–1980	1981–1985
Pregnancies tested	1233	4163	11,263
Rate/1000	10.5	6.3	4.4
% all deaths	1.9	3.4	6.7
Pregnancies untested	51,254	61,963	69,677
Rate/1000	13.3	11.9	10.0
% all deaths	98	96	93

Adapted from Platt LD, Paul RH, Phelan J, et al: Fifteen years of experience with antepartum fetal testing. Am J Obstet Gynecol 156:1509, 1987.

TABLE 13–4

Accuracy of Gestational Age Estimation

Parameter	Accuracy	Comment
Clinical		
Last menstrual period	± 2 wk	Depends on cycle length and maternal recollection
First-trimester uterine size	± 2 wk	Depends on operator skill
Auscultation of fetal heart tones	± 2 wk	Typically at 20 wk (fetoscope), 12 wk with Doppler scope
Fundal height measurements	± 3 wk	Varies with maternal body habitus
Sonographic		
Gestational sac diameter	± 5 d	Variable shape distorts measurements Performed from 4.5–5.5 wk
Embryonic crown-rump length	± 3 d	Performed from 6.0–12 wk
Biparietal diameter, femur length, cerebellar transverse diameter	± 10 d ± 14–20 d	If obtained from 15–22 wk If obtained after 22 wk

fetal position, maternal obesity, and decreased amniotic fluid volume. Further, accurate evaluation of fetal anatomy requires a skilled team of experienced sonographers and perinatologists using equipment with optimal image resolution. Counseling of the affected family and formulation of the management plan should involve neonatologists, pediatric subspecialists, and geneticists. Even with optimal equipment and personnel, up to 25% of significant structural defects may be missed.

ASSESSMENT OF FETAL MOVEMENT

The use of maternally perceived fetal activity to identify fetuses at risk for distress or death has been proposed because of its relatively low cost, convenience, and applicability to a large population. The optimal technique, frequency, and duration of fetal movement monitoring have not been clarified. Factors such as fetal waking and quiet cycles, maternal attention span, compliance, and motivation must be considered. The role of maternal body habitus, placental position, and amniotic fluid volume may be important. An understanding of the biology of fetal movement may provide important clues helpful in devising an effective program of fetal testing.

Maturational and Circadian Influences

Patrick and colleagues (1982) monitored fetal body movements in third-trimester human pregnancy from 30 to 40 weeks using continuous 24-hour ultrasonographic observation. The results of their study are shown in Table 13–5. There was no statistically significant change in the number of movements per hour as gestational age advanced in this study. This finding was confirmed by Manning and colleagues (1979), Valentin and Marsal (1986), and Rayburn (1982). The Valentin and Marsal study documented a mean of 85 fetal movements in a 45-minute period, with a 95% confidence limit of 14 to 232 movements.

Effect of Fetal Oxygenation on Body Movements

The thesis that fetal movements decrease with hypoxia is central to understanding of the nonstress test (NST) and biophysical profile. Bekedam and Visser (1985) monitored fetal body movements in growth-retarded fetuses before, during, and after uterine contractions. During contractions associated with late decelerations, fetal body movement

frequency fell by 85% when compared with the frequency before such contractions. In contractions associated with normal fetal heart rate, no change in fetal body movements occurred. The exquisite sensitivity of fetal movement frequency to reductions in oxygenation is similar to that reported by Natale and associates (1981).

Valentin and Masal's study found that the 97.5th percentile for absence of fetal activity was 28 minutes, suggesting an ideal observation interval of approximately 1 hour. Moore and Piacquadio (1989) found that the mean time to perceive 10 fetal movements was 18 ± 12 (standard deviation) minutes. A 1-hour observation period lacking 10 movements represented 3.5 standard deviations (99th percentile).

Based on these observations, various methods of "kick counting" have been proposed. Perhaps the simplest of proven worth is that of Moore and Piacquadio (1989), in which the patient records the time taken for 10 fetal movements to occur between 7 and 11 P.M. (the period of peak fetal activity). If the requisite 10 movements are not obtained after 1 hour of recording, further fetal evaluation is performed. An example of the card used for self-recording of fetal movement times is shown in Figure 13–1.

Other investigators have confirmed the utility of fetal movement counting in normal and high-risk patients (Neldham, 1980). The results of general population screening are mixed, ranging from no benefit in a British multicenter randomized trial (Grant et al, 1989) to a significant reduction in stillbirth rate in a case-control study of patients in a military population (Moore and Piacquadio, 1989). Despite the varied results, it is difficult to formulate a good argument against maternal kick counting, and thus it should probably be widely used as an initial screen from 28 weeks of gestation onward.

Fetal movement assessment thus is a simple screening test that enables the pregnant patient to participate in her pregnancy care in a useful way. Although subjective and showing poor correlation with objective assessment of fetal movement, such maternal reportage is an important first step in monitoring fetal well-being.

CARDIOTOCOGRAPHY (CONTRACTION STRESS TEST, NONSTRESS TEST)

The most widely used method of assessing fetal well-being combines electronic fetal heart rate and uterine contraction monitoring. Antenatal fetal heart rate monitoring arose from the finding that certain intrapartum fetal heart rate patterns were associated with poor fetal outcomes, hypoxia, acidemia, and asphyxia.

Contraction Stress Test

The earliest fetal wellness test involving fetal heart rate monitoring was the contraction stress test (CST). This test assesses the response of the fetal heart rate to uterine contractions produced by administration of exogenous oxytocin or by nipple stimulation (Evertson et al, 1979). In an oxygen-compromised fetus, contractions typically lead to late decelerations in the fetal heart rate. Such a test is shown in Figure 13–2. Although the CST remains a useful

---

TABLE 13–5

Frequency of Fetal Body Movements (FBMs) in the Human Fetus

	30–31 Wk	34–35 Wk	38–39 Wk
No. FBM/h	33 ± 2	28 ± 2	32 ± 2
% time spent in FBM	9.3 ± 0.9	9.8 ± 0.7	11.2 ± 0.9

Mean ± SD.

Adapted from Patrick J, Campbell K, Carmichael L, et al: Patterns of gross fetal body movements over 24 hour observation intervals during the last 10 weeks of pregnancy. Am J Obstet Gynecol 142:363, 1982.

FETAL MOVEMENT RECORD

Name:_____

Due Date:_____

Start Date	Number of weeks pregnant

Date	Time First Movement Felt	Time 10th Movement Felt	Total Time
EXAMPLE 11/4/91	6:50 p.m.	7:28 p.m.	38 minutes

INSTRUCTIONS

1. Count the baby's movements **EVERY NIGHT**.

2. A movement may be a kick, swish or roll. Do not count hiccups or small flutters.

3. You can start counting any time in the evening when the baby is active. **BUT: COUNT EVERY NIGHT**.

4. Count baby's movements while lying down, preferably on your left side.

5. Mark down the **time** you feel the baby move for the first time.

6. Mark down the **time** you feel the 10th fetal movement.

7. You should feel at least 10 fetal movements within one hour. Call Labor and Delivery (543-6600) **immediately** if

   a) you do not feel 10 movements within 1 hour .
   b) it takes longer and longer for your baby to move 10 times.
   c) you have not felt the baby move all day.

DO NOT WAIT UNTIL TOMORROW.

FIGURE 13–1. Sample card for self-recording of fetal movement times. The patient records the starting time and the time at which the 10th fetal movement is felt. If 10 movements cannot be appreciated in less than 60 minutes, the patient is instructed to contact her physician.

test, its disadvantages include significant time investment (45 to 60 minutes), the high frequency of uterine contraction hyperstimulation, and the need for close supervision. Furthermore, the CST is contraindicated in several high-risk groups:

- Threatened preterm delivery.
- Premature ruptured membranes.
- Previous classic cesarean section.
- Placenta previa.

The criteria for a satisfactory test include a minimum of three contractions in 10 minutes and a continuous fetal heart rate signal. Tests are categorized as negative (reassuring), equivocal, positive, and unsatisfactory. A negative CST requires the absence of late decelerations after all contractions. The diagnostic categories of the CST are summarized in Table 13–6. If more than three contractions occur in 10 minutes and late decelerations are noted, the test is classified as hyperstimulatory or unsatisfactory, requiring further testing. Reassuring tests can be repeated weekly.

Nonstress Test

Several observers noted that CSTs were rarely abnormal when fetal heart rate accelerations were present in associa-

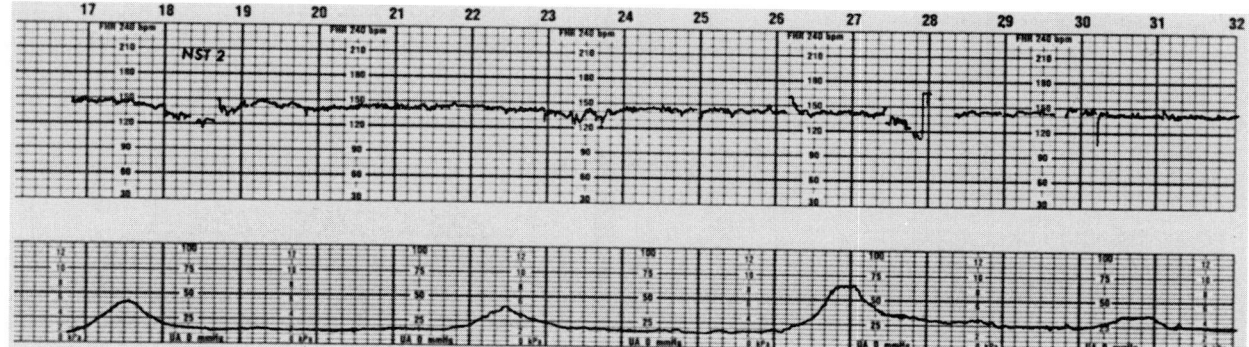

FIGURE 13–2. A contraction stress test. The fetal heart rate (FHR) is plotted above the uterine contraction signal. Note the *late* deceleration following a contraction. NST, nonstress test.

TABLE 13–6

Diagnostic Categories of the Contraction Stress Test

Result	Criteria	Comment
Negative (reassuring)	No late decelerations after a minimum of 3 contractions in 10 min	Retest weekly
Positive	Late decelerations after >50% of contractions	Further testing or delivery indicated
Equivocal	Late decelerations noted, but after <50% of contractions	Retest in <24 h
Unsatisfactory	Hyperstimulation noted (>3 contractions/10 min with decelerations or inadequate fetal heart rate tracing)	Retest immediately

tion with movement. This clinical observation led to omission of the contractions, with simple monitoring for fetal heart rate accelerations (Lee et al, 1976; Rochard et al, 1976). Because of its ease of use, universal applicability, and lack of contraindications, the NST has replaced the CST as a first-line surveillance tool.

The NST is carried out with the patient supine with a lateral tilt. The fetal heart rate and uterine activity are recorded using an external transducer for up to 40 minutes. Usually uterine activity is monitored simultaneously, and the patient records perceived fetal movement with an event marker. A normal (reactive) NST is shown in Figure 13–3.

Criteria for a reassuring test are as follows:

- Observation period of 20 minutes.
- Baseline fetal heart rate between 110 and 160 beats/min.
- Short-term variability of ±5 beats/min.
- Two or more fetal heart rate accelerations of at least 15 beats/min lasting at least 15 seconds.

- No nonreassuring features (decelerations, tachycardia, bradycardia).

Factors Influencing the Nonstress Test

Fetal heart rate is modified by autonomic activity and may show reduced or absent reactivity in conditions of hypoxia, neurologic depression, maternal drug ingestion, and acidosis. Fetal behavioral state influences the cardiac reactivity. The human fetus commonly exhibits periods of lowered activity referred to as sleep cycles. These may produce decreased or absent reactivity on an NST. These sleep cycles rarely last more than 20 minutes and may be discounted by observing the fetus for up to 40 minutes.

Adjustments must be made when monitoring the fetus remote from term (Lagrew, 1987). Between 24 and 32 weeks, the fetus may show accelerations of lesser amplitude that are of shorter duration, reduced reactivity (Druzin et al, 1985; Lavin et al, 1984), and spontaneous low-amplitude decelerations with movement (Sorokin et al, 1982), which do not carry the same ominous portent as in later gestations.

Indications for and Frequency of Nonstress Testing

The typical indications for the NST are as follows:

- Multiple gestation.
- Post-term pregnancy.
- Intrauterine growth retardation.
- History of previous stillbirth.
- Maternal chronic illness.
- Decreased fetal movement.
- Collagen vascular disorders.
- Diabetes mellitus.

Although originally performed weekly, studies suggest that the fetal death rate with weekly testing is excessive, especially compared with the CST (Freeman et al, 1982). Twice-weekly NST often coupled with simultaneous mea-

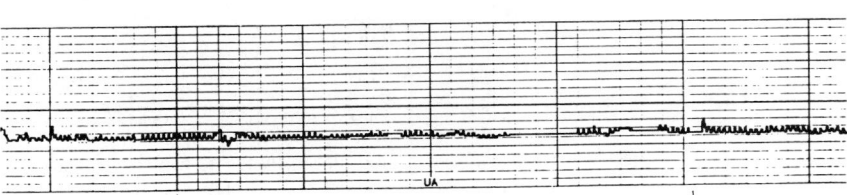

FIGURE 13–3. A reassuring nonstress test. Note two fetal heart rate (FHR) accelerations exceeding 15 beats/min and lasting at least 15 seconds during the monitoring period.

surement of amniotic fluid volume is the mainstay of fetal monitoring in most complicated pregnancies today.

It has been suggested that diabetes and post-term pregnancy presents increased risk of fetal mortality and morbidity and thus is ideally suited to the application of fetal monitoring (Slavensen et al, 1993). Several studies have convincingly shown that waiting for spontaneous labor to occur up to 42 weeks' gestation in the presence of reassuring fetal testing results in healthy newborns and lower cesarean section rates than when a more aggressive induction policy is followed. Nonetheless the increasing risk to the fetus with pregnancy extending beyond 42 completed weeks leads many obstetricians arbitrarily to terminate pregnancy by induction at that point.

Sequential NSTs performed in fetuses with intrauterine growth retardation provide an ideal way of following fetal well-being and aid significantly in timing delivery for optimal outcome, especially when combined with assessment of amniotic fluid volume.

ASSESSMENT OF AMNIOTIC FLUID VOLUME

Abnormalities of amniotic fluid volume are associated with suboptimal pregnancy outcome. *Oligohydramnios* (inadequate fluid volume) is associated with increased frequency of fetal urinary obstruction, placental insufficiency, umbilical cord compression, fetal distress, meconium passage, and fetal asphyxia (Hill et al, 1984). Prolonged oligohydramnios interferes with normal lung growth, resulting in potentially lethal pulmonary hypoplasia (Nimrod et al, 1984). *Hydramnios* (excessive amniotic fluid volume) is associated with maternal diabetes, fetal esophageal obstruction, and duodenal atresia. Pregnancies complicated by hydramnios have increased rates of abnormal fetal lie, cesarean delivery, and abruptio placentae (Hill et al, 1987). The major diagnostic entities associated with abnormal amniotic fluid volume are listed in Tables 13–7 through 13–9.

Normal Amniotic Fluid Volume

Twelve studies devoted to the direct quantitation of human amniotic fluid volume have been published since 1965. Brace and Wolf (1989) summarized the changes in amniotic fluid volume during gestation derived from 705 observational studies of normal pregnancies as follows:

TABLE 13–7

Diagnostic Categories of the Amniotic Fluid Index

Amniotic Fluid Volume	% Patients	Amniotic Fluid Index Value (cm)
Very low	8	5
Low	20	5.1–8.0
Normal	66	8.1–18.0
High	6	>18

Adapted from Phelan JP, Smith CV, Broussard P, Small M: Amniotic fluid volume assessment using the four-quadrant technique in the pregnancy between 36 and 42 weeks' gestation. J Reprod Med 32:540, 1987.

TABLE 13–8

Principal Diagnoses Associated with Oligohydramnios

Occult or overt premature rupture of membranes
Placental insufficiency
   Maternal hypertensive disease
   Autoimmune condition
   Chronic abruption
   Placental crowding in multifetal pregnancy
Urinary tract anomaly
   Renal agenesis
   Ureteral obstruction
   Urethral obstruction
   Polycystic or multicystic dysplastic kidneys

- Amniotic fluid volume rises progressively during gestation until approximately 32 weeks.
- From 22 to 39 weeks, the mean volume remains relatively constant, ranging from 630 to 817 mL.
- After 40 weeks, amniotic fluid volume declines at a rate of 8% per week, averaging only 400 mL at 42 weeks. Although amniotic fluid volume varies significantly during pregnancy, the lower 5th percentile in the third trimester (oligohydramnios) is approximately 300 mL. Hydramnios (>95th percentile) is greater than approximately 2000 mL.

Sonographic Assessment of Amniotic Fluid Volume

Although the increase in perinatal complications associated with abnormal amniotic fluid volume has been recognized for many decades, only recently with ultrasound has it been possible to estimate amniotic fluid volume. Because of the complex shape of the fetus within the uterus, however, direct calculation of the volume of amniotic fluid surrounding the fetus is not presently feasible. Current techniques to estimate with ultrasound the relative amount of fluid include subjective estimates (Moore et al, 1989), measurement of the largest pocket of amniotic fluid (Chamberlain et al, 1984), and sampling pocket depths in several areas of the uterus (Rutherford et al, 1987). The amniotic fluid index (AFI) appears to provide improved reproducibility and predictive value.

Measuring the AFI involves imaging the amniotic fluid pockets in each of four uterine quadrants and summing

TABLE 13–9

Principal Diagnoses Associated with Polyhydramnios

Gastrointestinal obstruction	Cardiac anomalies
Esophageal atresia	Fetal anemia
Thoracic mass, pleural effusion	Fetomaternal hemorrhage
Duodenal atresia	Blood group isoimmunization
Central nervous system	Parvovirus infection
abnormalities	Twin transfusion syndrome
Structural	Maternal diabetes
Chromosome	Constitutional macrosomia

the deepest measurements. Longitudinal measurements of the AFI in normal pregnancies have shown that the AFI varies significantly during gestation (Moore and Cayle, 1990). The normal and boundary values for the AFI are depicted in Figure 13–4.

Although the percentile lines of Figure 13–4 define the limits of normal AFI, the values of AFI that constitute *action* points are less clear. Currently accepted values are shown in Table 13–7, although they have not necessarily been rigorously established. Typically, AFIs greater than 80 mm are regarded as normal, values between 50 and 80 mm require further evaluation, and values less than 50 mm mandate further more complex testing or delivery.

BIOPHYSICAL PROFILE

Theoretically, identification of the compromised fetus could be improved by assessing several biophysical variables using real-time ultrasonography, rather than simply monitoring the fetal heart rate, as is done in cardiotocography. Manning and associates (1980) recognized the limitations of existing means of fetal heart rate monitoring and developed the biophysical profile (BPP), which encompasses observations of fetal behavioral activity on ultrasound in addition to fetal heart rate reactivity. Prospective clinical studies have demonsrated generally good but varying predictive accuracies for each individual variable, but a combination of these measures improves the predictive accuracy substantially (Manning et al, 1987). The components of this BPP are listed in Table 13–10.

A positive finding in each of the BPP parameters is awarded a value of 2 to give a total score of 10. Outcomes in Manning's initial study were collected prospectively, and scores of 8 to 10 were found to correlate with good outcome. Scores of 2 and 4 are associated with high perinatal

TABLE 13–10
Elements of the Biophysical Profile

Nonstress test
  Reactive test = 2 points
Fetal breathing movements
  At least one episode of fetal breathing of 60 sec duration = 2 points
Gross fetal body movements
  At least three discrete episodes of fetal movement = 2 points
Fetal tone
  At least one episode of extension and return to flexion of extremities or spine or hand open/close = 2 points
Amniotic fluid volume
  At least one amniotic fluid pocket of at least 1 cm in depth = 2 points
Total available
  10 points

mortality and warrant intervention. A summary of possible scores and recommended actions is given in Table 13–11.

Although a number of studies have demonstrated the worth of the BPP, it is time-consuming and somewhat more expensive in resources to perform. Many centers now use the so-called *modified BPP* score, in which the NST provides the estimate of short-term fetal acid-base status and the AFI assesses comparatively longer-term alterations in placental function and fetal well-being (Clark et al, 1989; Vintzileos and Knuppel, 1994).

DOPPLER FLOW STUDIES

Reports of the use of Doppler ultrasound for the evaluation of maternal and fetal condition have increased in frequency in the obstetric literature. Despite the increasing number of publications reporting a variety of applications of Doppler ultrasound in obstetrics, however, there is still considerable question as to the reliability of and the indications for its use.

It is possible to study flow in many fetal vessels using Doppler ultrasound. The umbilical artery has been widely studied, but considerable interest has been generated by studies of cerebral blood flow and other regional circulations. Despite the enthusiasm of the proponents of Doppler, it remains an investigational tool only and is never required in any given situation, although it may aid decision making.

Physiology of Doppler Velocimetry

In conditions of fetal hypoxia or other forms of stress, abnormalities of the fetal velocity waveforms develop. Although the systolic component reflects the vigor of fetal cardiac function, the *diastolic component* of the fetal velocity waveforms is of greatest value in assessing fetal status because it reflects the amount of peripheral resistance that the downstream vascular bed presents to the heart. As peripheral resistance increases, blood flow velocity decreases during cardiac diastole. Therefore, the fetus with an infarcted placenta and associated increase in intraplacental

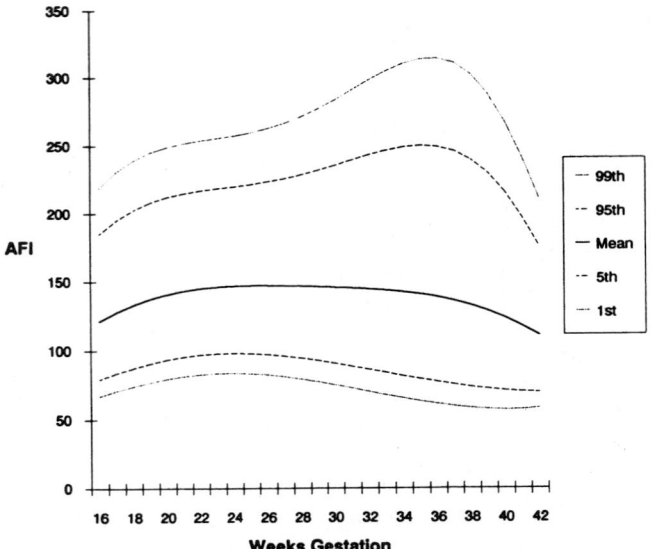

FIGURE 13–4. Amniotic fluid index (AFI) (in millimeters) plotted against gestational age. The darker line represents the 50th percentile, and the thinner lines represent the 10th and 90th percentiles.

TABLE 13–11

Interpretation and Management of Biophysical Profile Score

Score	Comment	Perinatal Mortality Within 1 Wk Without Intervention	Management
10 of 10	Risk of fetal asphyxia extremely rare	<1/1000	Intervention only for obstetric and maternal factors
8 of 10 (normal fluid)	No indication for intervention for fetal disease		
8 of 8 (NST not done)	Equivalent to BPP = 10 with NST		
8 of 10 (abnormal fluid)	Probable chronic fetal compromise	89/1000	Determine that there is functioning renal tissue and intact membranes; if so, deliver for fetal indications
6 of 10 (normal fluid)	Equivocal test, possible fetal asphyxia	Variable	If the fetus is mature, deliver. In the immature fetus, repeat test within 24 h; if <6/10 deliver
6 of 10 (abnormal fluid)	Probable fetal asphyxia	89/1000	Deliver for fetal indications
4 of 10	High probability of fetal asphyxia	91/1000	Deliver for fetal indications
2 of 10	Fetal asphyxia almost certain	125/1000	Deliver for fetal indications
0 of 10	Fetal asphyxia certain	600/1000	Deliver for fetal indications

NST, nonstress test; BPP, biophysical profile.

From Manning FA, Morrison I, Harman CR, et al: Fetal assessment based on fetal biophysical profile scoring: Experience in 19,221 referred high-risk pregnancies. Am J Obstet Gynecol 157:880, 1987.

resistance develops rising systolic-diastolic ratios over time. If resistance rises high enough, flow in diastole may cease completely. In extreme cases, reversed diastolic flow may be seen. The association of absent end-diastolic velocities in the umbilical artery with intrauterine growth retardation, meconium aspiration, intrauterine fetal death, and birth asphyxia has been reported by many investigators.

In pregnancies complicated by intrauterine growth retardation, between two thirds and three quarters of fetuses exhibit an excessively high index of placental resistance (systolic-diastolic ratio or resistance index) (Trudinger et al, 1991). Fetuses with abnormal flow-velocity waveforms have a higher incidence of neonatal morbidity than those with a normal study.

Histologically the high placental resistance evidenced by the abnormal umbilical Doppler flow velocity waveform is associated with reduced numbers of small (<90 μm diameter) arteries in the tertiary villi of the placenta (the resistance vessels) (Giles et al, 1985) and obliterative changes in the remaining vessels.

Abnormalities of blood flow velocity may occur in other vascular beds in the fetus experiencing hypoxemia. As oxygen level in the umbilical venous blood drops, the cerebral circulation compensates by increasing flow in the carotids. Accordingly, with progressive hypoxia, intracerebral vascular resistance typically falls, and diastolic velocity increases. Flow velocity in the descending aorta, supplying the majority of the fetus' visceral organs, may be adversely affected. The degree of intrauterine hypoxemia at any given time may be best expressed as the sum of effects on umbilical, cerebral, and aortic circulations.

Because the relationship of the fetal heart to the placental, cerebral, and visceral circulations is in a dynamic state of flux during pregnancy, the fetal velocity waveform indices must be corrected for gestational age. *Normative tables*

for the pulsatility index and systolic-diastolic ratio have been published by Schulman and coworkers (1984).

Abnormalities in the fetal velocity waveform (particularly the diastolic changes) generally become evident 1 to 3 weeks before the onset of abnormalities in other clinical parameters, such as fetal heart rate monitoring, amniotic fluid volume, and fetal BPP. During pregnancy, uterine blood flow is markedly increased with minimal resistance secondary to the effects of estrogen on the uterine circulation. From reasonably early in gestation, the fetal velocity waveforms of the uteroplacental circulation can be documented, and in certain cases of maternal disease such as chronic hypertension or pregnancy-induced hypertension, abnormalities in the uteroplacental fetal velocity waveforms can be documented. In fact, Campbell and associates (1986) noted abnormalities in uteroplacental circulation from approximately 20 weeks onward in pregnancies that developed either severe intrauterine growth retardation or pregnancy-induced hypertension.

Applications of Doppler Waveform Analysis in Fetal Management
Rule Out Chronic Fetal Hypoxia

Despite the flurry of papers concerning the use of Doppler ultrasound throughout pregnancy, its most frequent indication is as an advisory adjunct in the evaluation of fetal status. As an example, in pregnancies remote from term with no evidence of intrauterine growth retardation, decreased amniotic fluid volume, or abnormal fetal heart rate changes, it is unlikely that one would deliver on the basis of a grossly abnormal Doppler blood flow unless the BPP was less than 4 also. The controversy surrounding use of Doppler in fetal testing has been well characterized by Low (1991).

More recently, investigators have used pulsed Doppler to examine the carotid or descending aortic blood flow. They have found that under normal conditions there is decreased diastolic blood flow in the carotid arteries. With the development of intrauterine growth retardation or hypoxia, there is a dilation of the cerebral blood flow during diastole. These findings are consistent with the known increase in cerebral blood flow with hypoxia in laboratory animals.

Overall, the decision to intervene in a pregnancy at risk for intrauterine growth retardation is strengthened by knowing the trend in Doppler ratios. Most experts believe that Doppler alone is not adequate evidence of urgent fetal compromise unless diastolic flow is actually reversed. Doppler velocimetry should be used to guide the use of more traditional biophysical tests (e.g., NST, CST).

Investigate Discordance in Twins

Finding one large, possibly hydramniotic twin and another with oligohydramnios and growth failure can present a difficult diagnostic challenge if the genders are concordant (twin-twin transfusion versus placental abnormality and intrauterine growth retardation). Use of serial Doppler velocimetry can help differentiate twin-twin transfusion from intrauterine growth retardation: In twin-twin transfusion, the systolic-diastolic ratio in umbilical fetal velocity waveforms of the small twin is usually normal or decreased. Following with Doppler studies in a twin with intrauterine growth retardation can help identify the starting point for biophysical testing (when systolic-diastolic ratios rise or end-diastolic velocity disappears) and may provide an early signal of the need for urgent delivery.

Doppler ultrasound is a helpful tool to assist in the evaluation of fetal status. In some cases, it can be predictive of abnormal future fetal or maternal outcomes, but it is neither sensitive nor specific enough at this time to be completely reliable unless extremes of flow velocity are present.

AMNIOCENTESIS

Examination of amniotic fluid in late pregnancy for biochemical evidence of lung maturity may precede elective delivery or aid in timing of delivery in a compromised pregnancy. A variety of tests are available:

1. Lecithin-sphingomyelin ratio.
2. Phosphatidyl glycerol.
3. Phosphatidyl inositol.
4. Abbott TDx-FLM fluorescence polarization assay.

In certain cases of apparent fetal compromise, it may be necessary to exclude potentially lethal chromosome anomalies before intervention and delivery. Amniocentesis for karyotyping or the more rapid fluorescent in-situ hybridization for identification of trisomies 13, 18, and 21 may thus be indicated.

CORDOCENTESIS

Access to fetal blood provides the ultimate means of assessing fetal status—although not without significant proce-

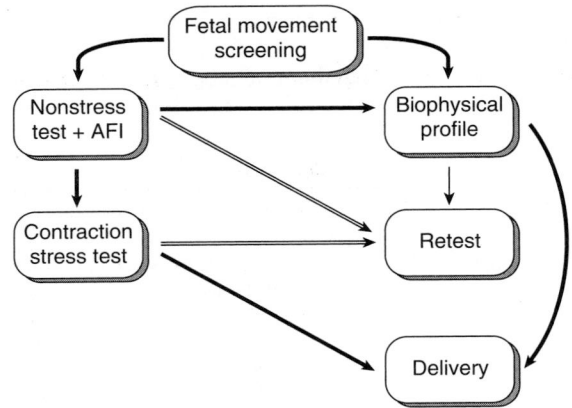

FIGURE 13–5. Fetal testing cascade. Filled lines indicate abnormal, or nonreassuring, test result. Open lines indicate normal, or reassuring, test result. AFI, amniotic fluid index.

dural risk, carrying a fetal loss rate of 1%. Acid-base status and blood gases may be measured (Soothill et al, 1992), although critical values for intervention have not been firmly established (Sonek and Nicolaides, 1994).

SUMMARY

Clearly fetal surveillance encompasses a wide range of modalities, each with advantages and disadvantages. A suggested cascade of complexity is shown in Figure 13–5. There is no agreement among authorities as to the ideal test(s) of fetal well-being. Because there are no large randomized, prospective studies comparing the various methods available, none may be considered superior to others. The key is to identify the fetus potentially at risk and then to ensure that a reassuring test result is obtained at each scheduled encounter. Avoidable mortality occurs most often when the practitioner does not act on concerning test results.

REFERENCES

Bekedam MD, Visser GHA: Effects of hypoxemic events on breathing, body movements, and heart rate variation: A study in growth-retarded human fetuses. Am J Obstet Gynecol 153:52, 1985.

Boehm FH, Salyer S, Shah DM, Vaughn WK: Improved outcome of twice weekly nonstress testing. Obstet Gynecol 67:566, 1986.

Brace RA, Wolf EJ. Normal amniotic fluid volume changes throughout pregnancy. Am J Obstet Gynecol 161:382, 1989.

Campbell S, Pearch JMF, Hackett G, et al: Qualitative assessment of uteroplacental bloodflow: Early screening test for high-risk pregnancies. Obstet Gynecol 68:649, 1986.

Chamberlain MB, Manning GA, Morrison I, et al: Ultrasound evaluation of amniotic fluid: I. The relationship of marginal and decreased amniotic fluid volume to perinatal outcome. Am J Obstet Gynecol 150:245, 1984.

Clark SL, Sabey P, Jolley K: Nonstress testing with acoustic stimulation and amniotic fluid volume assessment: 5973 tests without unexpected fetal death. Am J Obstet Gynecol 160:694, 1989.

Devoe LD, Gardner P, Dear C, et al: The diagnostic values of concurrent nonstress testing, amniotic fluid measurement, and Doppler velocimetry in screening a general high-risk population. Am J Obstet Gynecol 163:1040, 1990.

Druzin ML, Fox A, Kogut E, et al: The relationship of the nonstress test to gestational age. Am J Obstet Gynecol 153:386, 1985.

Evertson LR, Gauthier RJ, Schifrin BS, et al: Antepartum fetal heart rate testing: I. Evolution of the nonstress test. Am J Obstet Gynecol 133:29, 1979.

Freeman RK, Anderson G, Dorchester W: A prospective multi-institutional study of antepartum fetal heart rate monitoring: II. Contraction stress test versus nonstress test for primary surveillance. Am J Obstet Gynecol 143:778, 1982.

Giles WB, Trudinger BJ, Baird P: Fetal umbilical artery flow velocity waveforms and placental resistance: Pathological correlation. Br J Obstet Gynaecol 92:31, 1985.

Grant A, Valentin L, Elbourne D, Alexander S: Routine formal fetal movement counting and risk of antepartum late death in normally formed singletons. Lancet 2:345, 1989.

Hill LM, Breckle R, Thomas ML, et al: Polyhydramnios: Ultrasonically detected prevalence and neonatal outcome. Obstet Gynecol 69:21, 1987.

Hill LM, Breckle R, Wolfgram KR, O'Brien PC: Oligohydramnios: Ultrasonically detected incidence and subsequent fetal outcome. Am J Obstet Gynecol 147:407, 1984.

Hovatta O, Lipasti A, Rapola J, et al: Causes of stillbirth: A clinicopathological study of 243 patients. Br J Obstet Gynaecol 90:691, 1983.

Lagrew DC: Fetal evaluation in early gestational ages. Clin Obstet Gynecol 30:992, 1987.

Lagrew DC, Pircon RA, Nageotte M, et al: How frequently should the amniotic fluid index be repeated? Am J Obstet Gynecol 167:1129, 1992.

Lavin JP, Miodovnik M, Barden TP: Relationship of nonstress reactivity and gestational age. Obstet Gynecol 63:338, 1984.

Lee CY, DiLoreto PC, Logrand B: Fetal activity acceleration determination for the evaluation of fetal reserve. Obstet Gynecol 48:19, 1976.

Low JA: The current status of maternal and fetal blood flow velocimetry. Am J Obstet Gynecol 164:1049, 1991.

Manning FA, Morrison I, Harman CR, et al: Fetal assessment based on fetal biophysical profile scoring: Experience in 19,221 referred high-risk pregnancies. Am J Obstet Gynecol 157:880, 1987.

Manning FA, Platt LD, Sipos L: Fetal movements in human pregnancies in the third trimester. Obstet Gynecol 6:699, 1979.

Manning FA, Platt LD, Sipos L: Antepartum fetal evaluation: Development of a fetal biophysical profile. Am J Obstet Gynecol 136:787, 1980.

Moore TR, Cayle JE: The amniotic fluid index in normal human pregnancy. Am J Obstet Gynecol 162:1168, 1990.

Moore TR, Longo J, Leopold G, et al: The reliability and predictive value of an amniotic fluid scoring system in severe second trimester oligohydramnios. Obstet Gynecol 73:739, 1989.

Moore TR, Piacquadio K: A prospective evaluation of fetal movement screening to reduce the incidence of antepartum fetal death. Am J Obstet Gynecol 162:1168, 1989.

Natale R, Clelow F, Dawes GS: Measurement of fetal forelimb movements in lambs in utero. Am J Obstet Gynecol 140:545–551, 1981.

Neldham S: Fetal movements as an indicator of fetal well-being. Lancet 1:1222, 1980.

Nimrod C, Varela-Gittings F, Machin G, et al: The effect of very prolonged membrane rupture on fetal development. Am J Obstet Gynecol 148:540, 1984.

Patrick J, Campbell K, Carmichael L, et al: Patterns of gross fetal body movements over 24 hour observation intervals during the last 10 weeks of pregnancy. Am J Obstet Gynecol 142:363, 1982.

Phelan JP, Smith CV, Broussard P, Small M: Amniotic fluid volume assessment using the four-quadrant technique in the pregnancy between 36 and 42 weeks' gestation. J Reprod Med 32:540, 1987.

Platt LD, Paul RH, Phelan J, et al: Fifteen years of experience with antepartum fetal testing. Am J Obstet Gynecol 156:1509, 1987.

Rayburn WF: Clinical applications of monitoring fetal activity. Am J Obstet Gynecol 144:967, 1982.

Rochard F, Schifin BS, Goupil F, et al: Nonstressed fetal heart rate monitoring in the antepartum period. Am J Obstet Gynecol 126:699, 1976.

Rutherford SE, Phelan JP, Smith CV, Jacobs N: The four-quadrant assessment of amniotic fluid volume: An adjunct to antepartum fetal heart rate testing. Obstet Gynecol 70:353, 1987.

Schifrin BS: More Exercises in Fetal Monitoring. St. Louis, Mosby, 1993.

Schulman H, Fleischer A, Sterm W, et al: Umbilical velocity wave ratios in human pregnancy. Am J Obstet Gynecol 148:986, 1984.

Slavesen DR, Freeman J, Brudenell JM, et al: Prediction of fetal acidemia in pregnancies complicated by maternal diabetes mellitus by biophysical profile scoring and fetal heart rate monitoring. Br J Obstet Gynaecol 100:227, 1993.

Sonek J, Nicolaides K: The role of cordocentesis in the diagnosis of fetal well being. Clin Perinatol 21:743, 1994.

Soothill PW, Ajayi RA, Campbell EM, et al: Relationship between fetal acidemia at cordocentesis and subsequent neurodevelopment. Ultrasound Obstet Gynecol 2:80, 1992.

Sorokin Y, Dierker LJ, Pillay SK, et al: The association between fetal heart rate patterns and fetal movements in pregnancies between 20 and 30 weeks gestation. Am J Obstet Gynecol 143:243, 1982.

Trudinger BJ, Cook CM, Giles WB, et al: Fetal umbilical artery velocity waveforms and subsequent neonatal outcome. Br J Obstet Gynaecol 98:378, 1991.

Valentin L, Marsal K: Fetal movement in the third trimester of normal pregnancy. Early Hum Dev 14:295, 1986.

Vintzileos AM, Knuppel RA: Multiple parameter biophysical testing in the prediction of fetal acid-base status. Clin Perinatol 21:823, 1994.

CHAPTER 14

Preterm Labor and Birth

Martin Walker and Andrew Hull

Premature delivery is the unfortunate end of many pregnancies. Although most preterm infants do well, infants born before 26 to 27 weeks' gestation may have a turbulent, painful, and often short life. Along with the tragedy of the extremely preterm infant, the other family members suffer the often chronic illness and disability that result from this catastrophic perturbation of normal gestation. Premature birth afflicted 11% of all pregnancies, resulting in 431,613 deliveries in the United States in 1994 (Ventura et al, 1996). Fewer than 1% of the deliveries were of infants less than 27 weeks' gestation, however.

DEFINITIONS
Premature Labor

Premature labor is defined as the presence of regular uterine contractions resulting in dilation of the cervix and descent of the presenting part at a gestation of greater than 20 completed weeks and less than 37 completed weeks. This definition, although semantically correct, ignores the reality of clinical medicine in the 1990s. Because of the gravity of the consequences of preterm delivery, premature labor is liberally diagnosed in the presence of lesser signs and symptoms. Clinically significant premature labor is considered between the lower limit of viability (usually 23 or 24 weeks) and the upper limit of statistically significant morbidity (usually 34 weeks).

Premature Delivery

Premature delivery is the delivery of any infant, of whatever cause, between 20 and 37 completed weeks of gestation. As with premature labor, clinically significant premature delivery occurs between the limit of viability and the limits of statistically significant neonatal morbidity (usually 23 to 34 weeks).

Preterm Premature Rupture of the Membranes

Preterm premature rupture of the membranes (PPROM) (sometimes called *preterm spontaneous rupture of the membranes*) is spontaneous rupture of the amniotic sack before the onset of labor (premature) before 37 completed weeks of gestation (preterm). It is distinguished from term premature rupture of the membranes (PROM) only by the gestational age of the pregnancy.

HISTORICAL PERSPECTIVE
Prematurity

The definition of prematurity at less than 37 completed weeks of pregnancy is based on the definition of *term* as being between 37 and 42 completed weeks. This definition is neither precise nor clinically useful. A more utilitarian definition of prematurity is based on the expected outcome of a delivery at any particular gestation. This definition will clearly change over time as medical technology advances. Additionally, maternal conditions, such as gestational diabetes, alter the fetal maturity at a given gestation.

Before the 1960s, a gestational age of less than 37 weeks could be associated with both minor and major morbidities. With the introduction of fine feeding tubes and intravenous lines, it is now uncommon to experience significant morbidity beyond 34 completed weeks (Fig. 14–1). For practical purposes then, 34 to 35 weeks is used as the cutoff before which the patient is considered to be significantly premature (Lewis et al, 1996). If the mother is diabetic, different criteria are used because fetal lung maturity may be delayed. Under these circumstances, 35 to 36 weeks may be more appropriate gestational ages before which the patient may be considered truly premature.

Past Therapies

Therapies that have been employed in the past to suppress premature labor include intravenous ethanol (Spearing, 1979). These therapies fell out of favor because their side effects, combined with lack of efficacy, made their use impractical.

RISK FACTORS
Socioeconomic Factors

Premature delivery is strongly associated with social deprivation. Poverty, work away from home, teenage pregnancy, and single motherhood have all been identified as risk factors for preterm delivery (Main, 1988). In the United States, race continues to be a major risk factor for prematurity, with blacks having a preterm birth rate of 18.1% compared with 9.6% in whites in 1994 (Ventura et al, 1996). Despite increasing access to health care, blacks continue to have a higher preterm delivery rate than their white counterparts regardless of economic status (Ventura et al, 1996).

Smoking is strongly associated with premature delivery as well as other perinatal morbidities (Andres, 1996). Increased circulating carboxyhemoglobin, decreased oxygen delivery to the placenta and fetus, and nicotine have been postulated as reasons for the higher incidence of premature labor (Bureau et al, 1983).

The use of recreational drugs, such as cocaine and crystal metamphetamine, is strongly associated with premature labor and delivery. Although associated comorbidities, such as sexually transmitted diseases, are undoubtedly important, these drugs have direct effects on the uterus and placenta (Keith et al, 1989). Cocaine especially is well known to result in maternal hypertension and placental abruption (Slutsker, 1992). There is some evidence that

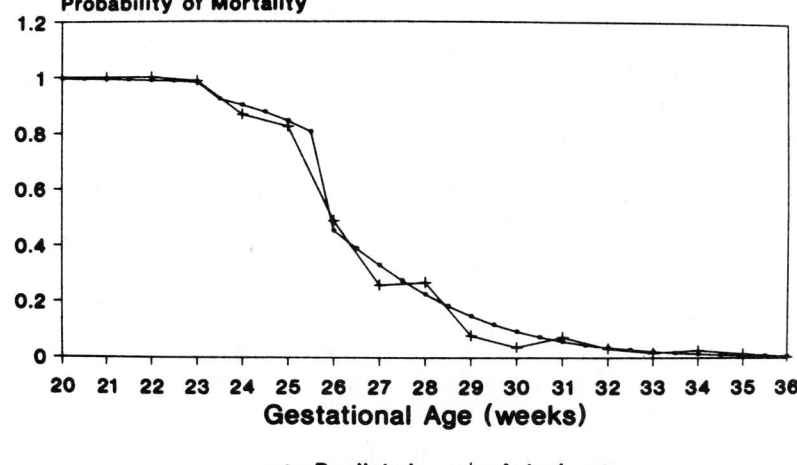

FIGURE 14–1. Perinatal mortality across gestational age.

cocaine may also have a direct stimulatory effect on the myometrium resulting in contractions (Nakahara et al, 1996).

Infections

The most important advance in medical science regarding prematurity has been the understanding of the role of infectious agents in the cause of the condition. It is now clear that many women who deliver prematurely after spontaneous premature labor have an intra-amniotic infection (Romero and Mazor, 1988) (Fig. 14–2).

Work by Romero and Mazor (1988) has demonstrated that up to 16% of women presenting with premature labor and intact membranes have microbiologic evidence of intra-amniotic infection on amniocentesis. Further work has demonstrated an even higher incidence of infection when markers such as intra-amniotic glucose and interleukin-6 are used (Mazor et al, 1995).

Such evidence of overt and subclinical infection has led to much work on the use of antibiotics in premature labor. Related research has demonstrated that vaginal infection with anaerobic organisms, such as bacterial vaginosis, is a major risk factor for premature delivery. Early diagnosis and treatment of such infections has been shown to reduce the incidence of premature delivery (Hauth et al, 1995). In addition, the presence of untreated urinary infections, including pyelonephritis, is associated with preterm labor and delivery (Whalley, 1967).

Multiple Gestation

As the number of fetuses per pregnancy increases, the mean gestational age at delivery decreases. Twins deliver at 35 weeks, on average; triplets, 33 weeks; quadruplets, 29 weeks; and so on (Caspi et al, 1976). The mechanism of prematurity includes an increased risk of iatrogenic delivery as well as spontaneous premature labor (Newman and Ellings, 1995). The increased incidence of premature labor may be related to the increase in volume of the uterus as well as the increased rate of volume change during the pregnancy (Neilson and Crowther, 1993). In

early gestation, the phenomenon of silent cervical dilation is well recognized in multiple gestations, and it is probable that the cervix remains more easily dilated throughout gestation. The mechanism for this relative increase in cervical compliance is unknown but is possibly related to increased levels of relaxin and progesterone.

Diethylstilbestrol Exposure

The use of diethylstilbestrol (DES) in an attempt to salvage pregnancies at risk for spontaneous miscarriage was popu-

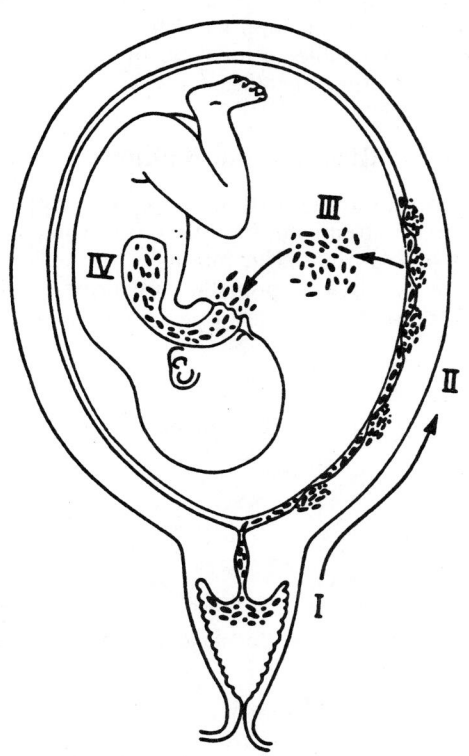

FIGURE 14–2. Amnionitis and intact membranes. I, Bacteria colonize the upper vagina and cervix; II, a bacteria deciduitis develops; III, amniotic fluid bacterial colonization occurs; and IV, the fetus ingests the infected amniotic fluid.

lar in the 1950s through the 1970s. It has become apparent that DES exposure in utero may result in genitourinary abnormalities in both male and female fetuses (Sandberg et al, 1981). Female congenital abnormalities include tubal, uterine, cervical, and vaginal conditions that result in infertility, spontaneous miscarriage, incompetent cervix, premature labor, and malpresentation. The abnormalities that result in premature delivery include cervical shortening and cervical matrix abnormalities that may result in painless cervical dilation or cervical incompetence (Cousins et al, 1980). Further abnormalities described after DES exposure include uterine cavity restrictions (the T-shaped uterus). These abnormalities behave similarly to other congenital uterine abnormalities described subsequently.

Uterine Abnormalities

As a result of the embryologic formation of the uterus by the uniting of bilaterally formed müllerian ducts, congenital abnormalities tend to be those of incomplete fusion. In general, the more incomplete the fusion, the greater the risk of premature delivery. The incidence of prematurity with bicornuate uterus is 16%, ranging to 8% in septate uterus (Ludmir et al, 1990).

Iatrogenic Risk Factors

It should not be forgotten that despite the importance of spontaneous preterm labor, the vast majority of preterm infants are delivered for reasons of maternal necessity, such as severe preeclampsia, or fetal necessity, such as growth restriction. In all, only approximately 5% of premature deliveries are amenable to tocolytic therapy and potential prolongation of pregnancy (Tucker et al, 1991) (Fig. 14–3).

Risk-Scoring Methods

A variety of risk-scoring methods have been employed over the years in an attempt to identify those women at risk of delivering prematurely. The rationale for such systems is to direct the women to prenatal care providers that may ameliorate these risks. The scoring systems currently in use

derive a score from the weighted answers to a number of questions designed to explore the factors discussed previously. From the final numerical score, the patient is placed in a risk category.

The major problem with all scoring systems is the fact that they are designed retrospectively from particular populations and often validated in these same populations (Chard, 1991). A further problem with risk scoring for prematurity is that the major risk factor for preterm delivery is a prior history of a preterm delivery (Keirse et al, 1978). In nulliparous patients, this historical risk factor is not available for analysis, and thus risk-scoring systems are less useful. Given that a large proportion of preterm deliveries occur in first pregnancies, the utility of risk-scoring systems is limited (Chard, 1991).

Summary

There are many risk factors for the delivery of a premature infant. Some of these are amenable to therapy, such as DES exposure, and some not, such as poverty. It appears that the integration of these factors by an experienced caregiver is at least as useful as a formal risk-scoring process. Despite the recognition of these risk factors, the majority of preterm deliveries are either indicated or unexpected.

PRESENTATION
At Home

The pregnant woman calling from home with concerns about premature labor may have a variety of signs and symptoms. As with normal labor, events proceed at a gradual pace under usual circumstances, and precipitous premature delivery at home is an unusual event. More commonly, symptoms have arisen over a number of days, even weeks, but have not been sufficiently worrying to precipitate a visit to the hospital.

Contractions are the most common complaint in premature labor (Katz et al, 1990). This complaint presents occasional difficulty because contractions are normally present during pregnancy from early in the third trimester (Moore,

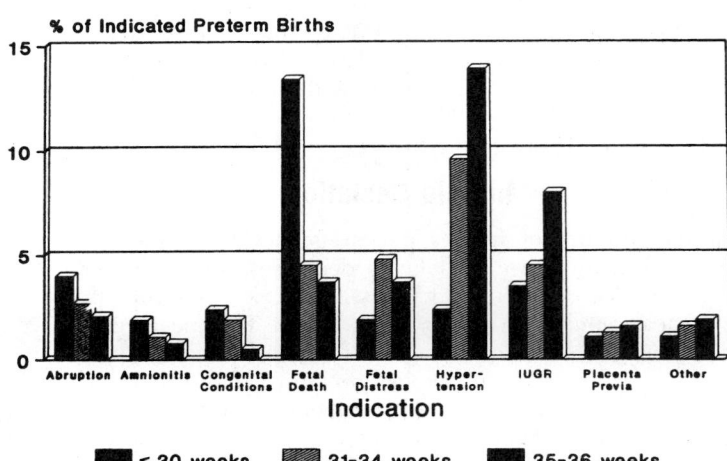

FIGURE 14–3. Causes of premature delivery.

1995). Contractions increase in both strength and frequency as pregnancy progresses, eventually turning into labor at term. Under normal circumstances, contraction frequency displays a diurnal rhythm, increasing during the hours of darkness (Moore, 1995). The innocent preterm contraction is usually called a *Braxton-Hicks* contraction and is characterized by a painless tightening, usually felt abdominally. These may occur up to 5 times per hour and occasionally more frequently.

More sinister contractions are associated with painful uterine tightening, more frequent tightening, and pain felt in the back as well as the abdomen. Needless to say, premature delivery is poorly predicted by uterine contractions. Associated symptoms that are of concern include vaginal bleeding, an increase in vaginal discharge, pelvic pressure, and any loss of fluid from the vagina (Katz et al, 1990).

The symptoms of premature labor can be summarized as follows:

- Uterine contractions
- Increased vaginal discharge
- Pelvic pressure
- Vaginal bleeding
- Leakage of fluid

In the Clinic

Atypically, premature labor is diagnosed at a clinic visit. Under these circumstances, the presenting signs are either asymptomatic cervical dilation, usually in multiple pregnancy, or asymptomatic uterine contractions found during nonstress testing.

At the Hospital

On arrival at the hospital, the patient in premature labor describes one or all of the aforementioned symptoms. In addition, cervical dilation may be found as well as a sensation of filling of the lower segment on pelvic examination. Cervical effacement is a worrisome finding in both multiparas and primiparas (Cooper et al, 1990).

Diagnosis

The definition of premature labor is that process which results in a premature delivery. Because of the gravity of the consequences of missing a diagnosis of premature labor, and the necessity to diagnose the process prospectively rather than retrospectively, the diagnosis is made liberally. This is witnessed by the fact that 70% of patients admitted to the labor unit with a diagnosis of premature labor are discharged undelivered (Keirse et al, 1989).

From a practical perspective, premature labor is diagnosed in the presence of regular uterine contractions associated with a cervical dilation of 2 cm or effacement of 50% or greater in a primipara and 3 cm or 80% in a multipara. These criteria provide maximum sensitivity for premature labor but little specificity.

Initial Investigations

After the diagnosis of premature labor is made, the patient is admitted to bed rest in labor and delivery. Initial investigations should include a complete blood count, including a white cell count, and a urinalysis. Should the urinalysis be suggestive, a urine culture should be ordered. Further tests that may be helpful under special circumstances include a urine toxicology screen, vaginal cultures, and an amniocentesis for lung maturity.

Once initial stabilization has occurred, an obstetric ultrasound is invaluable both to determine fetal lie and to confirm approximate dates. In addition, the discovery of significant fetal abnormalities is important in determining optimal management.

Initial investigations in preterm labor can be summarized as follows:

- Complete blood count
- Sterile speculum for amniotic fluid
- Cervical cultures
- Urinalysis
- Urine toxicology
- Urine culture and sensitivity
- Ultrasound for size, presentation, and gestational age

TREATMENT
Premature Labor
Bed Rest

Bed rest, with or without sedation, is the most commonly used therapy for premature labor. Although there is evidence that strenuous activity may increase uterine activity, and walking is a commonly used method of encouraging early labor, there is no evidence that bed rest alone has any effect on the course of premature labor (Goldenberg et al, 1994). Beyond its lack of proven efficacy, bed rest is difficult both to enforce and to comply with voluntarily.

Hydration

The use of hydration to suppress premature labor is based on the premise that the inhibition of pituitary vasopressin also suppresses pituitary oxytocin production. The theory further posits that maternal pituitary oxytocin is the causal agent in premature labor. Randomized, controlled trials have shown no benefit of maternal hydration in the treatment of premature labor (Keirse et al, 1995a).

Under conditions of maternal dehydration and ketosis, the patient may present with increased uterine activity. Although rehydration is the correct therapy, there is no evidence that contractions under these circumstances result in preterm delivery.

Sedation

The use of benzodiazepines, barbiturates, and narcotics for the suppression of premature labor is common. There is no evidence that true premature labor can be halted by such measures, although the time that the patient spends sleeping may allow natural resolution of uterine irritability. The downside to the use of these drugs for this condition lies in the subsequent inability for the patient to be assessed for continuing symptoms. Occasionally, this results in unexpected premature delivery of a significantly depressed infant. In addition, benzodiazepines are known to result in an increased risk of neonatal jaundice secondary to displacement of bilirubin from albumin (McElhatton, 1994).

Antibiotics

Because of the importance of infection as a cause of premature labor, the use of antibiotics has been proposed as therapy for premature labor. Antibiotics have been demonstrated to be useful under specific circumstances: maternal group B streptococcus colonization, antenatal bacterial vaginosis, and PPROM. The use of antibiotics to suppress premature labor has been proposed and tested but has not been shown to be of benefit (Romero et al, 1993).

Steroids

When premature delivery seems inevitable or even likely, the only medical intervention that has been demonstrated to be beneficial is the administration of glucocorticoids (National Institute of Child Health and Development, 1994). The glucocorticoid of choice is either betamethasone, 12 mg intramuscularly every 24 hours for two doses, or dexamethasone, 6 mg intramuscularly every 6 hours for four doses.

Antenatal glucocorticoids are maximally effective if delivery occurs between 48 hours and 7 days after first administration. Their use has been shown to result in a reduction in neonatal morbidity from respiratory distress, necrotizing enterocolitis, and intraventricular hemorrhage (National Institute of Child Health and Development, 1994).

There are no contraindications to the use of corticosteroids in preterm labor except for imminent delivery (minutes away). Their use in PPROM has been demonstrated to be beneficial, with no increase in infection rate. Repeated courses of steroids in undelivered patients is controversial.

Tocolytics

When a patient presents in active premature labor and there is no indication for delivery, tocolysis may be attempted. Tocolysis is the pharmacologic attempt to halt uterine contractions in an effort either to administer antenatal steroids or to improve maturity. All methods of tocolysis share common contraindications: cervical dilation greater than 4 cm, a contraindication to continued intrauterine existence for the fetus, and a contraindication to continued pregnancy for the mother (Table 14–1). Such contraindications include evidence of intrauterine infection, significant antepartum hemorrhage, and fetal distress.

Many different regimens are used to attempt to halt premature labor. Their variety testifies to their relative inefficacy.

Magnesium Sulfate

Proposed Mechanism of Action. Magnesium sulfate is the most commonly used tocolytic in the United States. Although its mechanism of action is not entirely determined, as a calcium antagonist it has a relaxant effect on

TABLE 14–1
Tocolytic Contraindications

Maternal
Severe preeclampsia
Severe maternal heart disease
Diabetic ketoacidosis (beta-mimetic agents)
Antepartum hemorrhage
Advanced labor

Fetal
Severe intrauterine growth retardation
Lethal fetal anomalies
Chorioamnionitis
Fetal distress

both vascular smooth muscle and uterine muscle (Popper, et al 1989).

Evidence of Efficacy. Magnesium sulfate clearly relaxes uterine smooth muscle. Tetanic uterine contractions are halted within 1 minute of institution of an intravenous infusion. There are two randomized, controlled studies examining the utility of magnesium sulfate as a tocolytic (Cotton et al, 1984; Cox et al, 1990). Both of these studies, although small, show no improvement over placebo in time to delivery or perinatal outcome.

Administration. Magnesium sulfate may be given intravenously or intramuscularly. For use as a tocolytic, it is usually administered intravenously as a bolus of 4 g over 15 minutes followed by 2 to 3 g per hour. While magnesium sulfate is being administered, the patient should be on fluid restriction to prevent overhydration and pulmonary edema. Blood levels may be followed every 6 hours and should remain under 8 mEq/L (Monga and Creasy, 1995). Levels are especially important if the patient has any degree of renal dysfunction.

Side Effects

Maternal. Minor maternal side effects include flushing, weakness, blurred vision, and shortness of breath. The drug gives some patients a metallic taste in their mouths. In overdose, the patient becomes progressively weaker and develops respiratory depression, coma, cardiac depression, and death. When magnesium sulfate is given for prolonged periods of time, pulmonary edema may develop. Calcium gluconate is the antidote for overdosage.

Fetal and Neonatal. Because magnesium sulfate freely crosses the placenta, short-term exposure results in similar muscular weakness in the newborn as the mother. This hypotonia may exacerbate respiratory difficulties in the nursery (Petrie, 1981). Long-term exposure has been associated with distinctive radiologic findings in neonatal long bones (Holcomb et al, 1991).

Beta-Mimetic Agents

Proposed Mechanism of Action. Terbutaline and ritodrine are the beta agonists used to suppress preterm uterine contractions. Their mechanism of action is the stimulation of beta-adrenergic receptors on smooth muscle cell walls, which results in smooth muscle relaxation (Monga and Creasy, 1995). Stimulation of these receptors results in activation of adenylate cyclase and thus increases in intracellular cyclic adenosine monophosphate (cAMP). cAMP then activates protein kinase and phosphorylates intracellular proteins, decreasing intracellular calcium. In addition, myosin light chain kinase is phosphorylated, reducing its affinity for calmodulin. These combined actions result in smooth muscle relaxation

Evidence of Efficacy. Ritodrine has been extensively investigated in randomized comparisons to other tocolytics and to placebo (Keirse et al, 1989). It has been demonstrated to result in up to a 48-hour delay in delivery in the gestational age group 26 to 28 weeks (The Canadian Preterm Labor Investigators Group, 1992). This delivery delay has not contributed to an improvement in perinatal outcome. Long-term use results in tachyphylaxis and diminished utility (Casper and Lye, 1986).

Administration. Ritodrine is commonly administered intravenously, titrated to contraction frequency. In addition, it may be given intramuscularly for acute relief of uterine hypertonus or orally for long-term prophylaxis. Terbutaline is commonly used subcutaneously for the immediate suppression of uterine contractions. For long-term use, it is administered by subcutaneous pump or orally (Monga and Creasy, 1995).

Side Effects

Maternal. Immediate maternal side effects of beta-mimetic use include tachycardia, hyperglycemia, and hypokalemia. More serious complications include pulmonary edema and diabetic ketoacidosis (Keirse et al, 1989). Ritodrine is the tocolytic most commonly associated with serious maternal side effects, including death.

Fetal and Neonatal. Fetal tachycardia is invariably seen with beta-mimetic use. Maternal hyperglycemia may result in neonatal hypoglycemia (Monga and Creasy, 1995).

Prostaglandin Synthesis Inhibitors

Proposed Mechanism of Action. The inhibition of oxytocic prostaglandins $PGF_{2\alpha}$ and PGE_2 by indomethacin, ibuprofen, and sulindac is achieved via the inhibition of cyclooxygenase in the decidua (Lundin-Schiller and Mitchell, 1990).

Evidence of Efficacy. Indomethacin is an effective tocolytic. It has been demonstrated in controlled trials to be effective in delaying delivery by 24 and 48 hours and 7 and 10 days (Keirse, 1995b). This delay has not, however, translated into an improvement in perinatal outcome in treated pregnancies. The size of the trials available to date has not been sufficiently large to exclude a beneficial effect.

Administration. Indomethacin is given as an initial oral or rectal dose of 50 mg. This dose is followed by 25 to 50 mg orally every 6 to 8 hours for 48 to 72 hours. Because of

neonatal side effects discussed subsequently, it should not be administered beyond 32 weeks or for longer than 72 hours at a time (Moise et al, 1988).

Side Effects

Maternal. Rectal administration of indomethacin may result in diarrhea. In addition, oral indomethacin may give rise to gastrointestinal discomfort in 1% to 5% of women. Rarely, indomethacin may result in idiosyncratic headache in some women.

Fetal and Neonatal. Indomethacin and other prostaglandin synthesis inhibitors result in a fall in fetal and neonatal urine output, probably by the enhancement of the renal action of arginine vasopressin (Walker et al, 1994). This condition is readily reversible within hours of drug discontinuation (Hickok et al, 1989).

Indomethacin results in a constriction of the ductus arteriosus both in utero (Moise et al, 1988) and ex utero (Douidar et al, 1988). The sensitivity of the ductus increases with both gestational age and arterial oxygen content (Eronen et al, 1991). Thus, the preterm fetus before 32 weeks exhibits mild partial constriction, if any at all. Prolonged use may result in permanent constriction and, hypothetically, primary pulmonary hypertension (Manchester et al, 1976). This complication has not been described in the controlled studies of indomethacin published to date.

Prolonged use of indomethacin has been associated with ileal perforation and meconium peritonitis as well as oligohydramnios (Iskovitz et al, 1980). There are anecdotal and uncontrolled reports of increased rates of necrotizing enterocolitis and intraventricular hemorrhage with prolonged high-dose indomethacin usage (Norton et al, 1993).

Calcium Channel Blockers

Proposed Mechanism of Action. By blocking the free flow of calcium into and within smooth muscle cells, nifedipine and other calcium channel blockers relax vascular and uterine smooth muscle (Jannis and Triggle, 1986).

Evidence of Efficacy. There is no evidence that nifedipine acts as a tocolytic or has any beneficial effect in premature labor.

Administration. Nifedipine is given orally at a dose of 10 to 30 mg every 4 to 6 hours.

Side Effects

Maternal. Maternal hypotension is a recognized effect of nifedipine. This effect is particularly exacerbated when magnesium sulfate is being concurrently administered.

Fetal and Neonatal. There are no serious fetal or neonatal side effects from the use of calcium channel blockers. Reduction in uteroplacental blood flow has been demonstrated in some animal models (Vielle et al, 1986).

Oxytocin Antagonists

Proposed Mechanism of Action. Oxytocin acts to cause uterine contractions through activation of a cell surface receptor on smooth muscles. Atosiban is a competitive inhibitor of the oxytocin receptor (Akerlund et al, 1987).

Evidence of Efficacy. Although still in the development phase, atosiban has been demonstrated to reduce uterine contraction frequency before term (Goodwin et al, 1994). Comparative and placebo controlled trials have demonstrated a short-term delay in delivery when another oxytocin antagonist, antocin, is administered (Sibai et al, 1997). This delay has not been demonstrated to result in an improvement in perinatal outcome.

Administration. Atosiban is administered as a dilute intravenous infusion titrated to uterine activity.

Side Effects
Maternal. There are no specific maternal side effects of atosiban.

Fetal and Neonatal. There are no specific fetal or neonatal side effects of atosiban.

Nitric Oxide Donors

Currently investigational, nitric oxide donors such as glyceryl trinitrate show promise as tocolytics (Lees et al, 1994). The use of glyceryl trinitrate as a short-term uterine relaxant for breech version and breech extraction is described and appears safe. Further research is currently under way in this area.

Preterm Premature Rupture of the Membranes

PPROM is the most common precursor of preterm labor and delivery (Meis et al, 1987). It appears that many episodes of PPROM are the result of subclinical membrane infections or chorioamnionitis (Romero and Mazor, 1988). Twenty-four percent of women suffering PPROM deliver within 24 hours, and of the remainder a proportion require induction within 24 hours for infection (Graham et al, 1982). The remaining pregnancies may remain undelivered for some time and are managed expectantly until the fetus is mature, the patient enters spontaneous labor, or chorioamnionitis ensues.

Bed Rest

The basis of management is close observation and bed rest. The patient is monitored for signs and symptoms of chorioamnionitis, and the fetus is monitored daily. No examining finger should be placed in the vagina of the PPROM patient until labor unequivocally occurs because digital examination is associated with early chorioamnionitis (Muldoon, 1968).

Antibiotics

The PPROM patient is placed on an intravenous or oral antibiotic at the time of admission to (1) obtain prophylaxis against group B streptococcus should the patient deliver; and (2) prolong the latency period between rupture and the onset of chorioamnionitis. For these reasons, the antibiotics of choice are either ampicillin or erythromycin, although there are many different regimens described. These prophylactic antibiotics have been shown to result in increased time to delivery, reduced neonatal infectious morbidity, and reduced maternal infectious morbidity (Crowley et al, 1995). Although concern has been raised regarding resistant organisms and fungal infections, this does not appear to be an important factor in clinical practice (Lewis et al, 1996).

Delivery Timing

If the patient enters spontaneous labor, infection is almost always the underlying cause, and delivery should be allowed to proceed unimpeded (Garite, 1985). Likewise, chorioamnionitis, once diagnosed, is an indication for immediate induction or cesarean section if appropriate. Absent either of these events, delivery timing becomes controversial. The practitioner must calculate the gestational age at which the risk of chorioamnionitis and in utero infection exceeds the risk of prematurity. The gestational age at which this occurs depends on the pregnancy (diabetic or not) and the underlying prevalence of infection in the population from which the patient comes. The gestational age at which this determination occurs usually varies between 33 and 36 weeks (Garite, 1985).

MONITORING
Electronic Fetal Heart Rate Monitoring

While in labor, the preterm infant should be monitored similar to its term counterpart. Electronic fetal monitoring is commonly employed, although intermittent auscultation is acceptable. The interpretation of fetal heart rate monitoring strips in the preterm infant is more problematic than in the term infant. Even in the term infant, there is little evidence that accurate and useful information can be gleaned from this method of surveillance (Thacker et al, 1995). The preterm infant has a generally higher heart rate baseline, fewer accelerations, and lower beat-to-beat variability (Natale et al, 1984). Fetal heart rate decelerations are generally considered to have the same prognostic importance as in the term infant.

There are few objective studies of electronic fetal heart rate monitoring in the preterm fetus, but the largest randomized trial of electronic fetal monitoring in premature labor suggested no benefit over intermittent auscultation and perhaps an adverse effect (Shy et al, 1990).

Uterine Activity Monitoring

Uterine activity monitoring in preterm labor can be accomplished by the external tocodynamometer, an intrauterine pressure catheter, or an examining hand on the gravid abdomen. All three methods are acceptable.

DELIVERY OPTIONS
Vaginal Delivery

Prematurity is not a contraindication to vaginal delivery. The delivery route should be chosen for obstetric indications only. When delivering a preterm infant vaginally, care should be taken not to cause unnecessary bruising or trauma. To that end, vacuum assistance is not generally recommended before 36 weeks (Vacca, 1990). There is no evidence that the use of a scalp clip is harmful. Although a common practice in the past, the prophylactic use of forceps and episiotomy is no longer recommended (Thacker and Banta, 1983).

Cesarean Section

The use of cesarean section for delivery of the preterm infant is reserved for obstetric indications. When performing a cesarean section for a premature infant, the obstetrician should be aware that the lower uterine segment may not be fully developed. This may lead to the need to make a classical incision in the uterus.

A cesarean section can be a physically traumatic event for the easily bruised preterm infant, and care should be taken to handle the infant with gentleness. A good rule is the smaller the infant, the larger the incision.

En Caul

One method of ensuring a bruise-free delivery is to attempt to deliver the infant without rupturing the membranes. Such a delivery is cushioned by the remaining amniotic fluid. These deliveries are difficult to achieve and are known as *en caul* deliveries.

Preterm Breech

The preterm breech is an area of continuing controversy. The issue of the optimal method of delivery remains disputed, although most are still delivered by cesarean section. The major consideration is the relative size of the presenting part and the after-coming head. If the breech is flexed (either complete or frank), the bitrochanteric diameter equals the biparietal diameter at approximately 34 weeks or 2500 g. At fetal weights of less than 750 g, there is no evidence of benefit to cesarean section, and vaginal delivery is often employed. Between 750 and 2500 g lays the area of controversy, and delivery choices are usually made on the basis of the experience and comfort levels of the attending obstetrician (Effer et al, 1983).

PREVENTION

Because the consequences of preterm delivery are so grave, much effort has been employed to prevent preterm labor. Risk scoring, discussed previously, is an attempt to identify women at whom these efforts should be directed. The pitfalls of risk scoring have limited the utility of such prevention efforts.

Home Uterine Activity Monitoring

Home uterine activity monitoring (HUAM) is the formal electronic monitoring of uterine activity using external tocodynamometry. The frequency of contractions is reviewed by nursing personnel at a central site, and advice is then given to the patient to take tocolytics or come to the hospital.

The theory behind HUAM is that preterm labor is preceded by a recognizable increase in uterine contraction frequency and that the recognition of this increase allows more successful treatment and thus prolongs gestation (Hill and Gookin, 1997). The first of these assumptions is correct, with recognizable increases in uterine activity appearing some days before the formal diagnosis of preterm labor (Bell, 1983). The second assumption, however, does not appear to be so clearly true (Utter et al, 1990).

Randomized trials of HUAM versus standard care show a decrease in the rate of preterm delivery in the HUAM group. Further trials, however, have shown that the intervention that accounts for the improvement in outcome in these patients is the daily nursing contact (Grimes and Schulz, 1992). Randomized trials of HUAM versus daily nursing contact have shown no improvement in outcome (Grimes and Schulz, 1992).

Education

At the basis of all attempts to reduce the preterm delivery rate is the education of women regarding the risk factors and symptoms of preterm labor. Clearly the early use of antenatal care reduces the preterm delivery rate by allowing early detection and treatment of bacterial vaginosis. In patients at known increased risk of preterm delivery, teaching of the signs and symptoms of preterm labor allows for earlier presentation to the hospital in the process. This earlier presentation allows use of antibiotics and steroids at critical time points in the labor.

CONCLUSION

Preterm labor and delivery accounts for the majority of the perinatal morbidity and mortality seen in the United States. The prevention, treatment, and amelioration of prematurity is of the utmost importance. To date, the interventions of proven utility are prenatal care, treatment of sexually transmitted diseases, antenatal steroids, the use of antibiotics in group B streptococcus colonized women and PPROM, and delivery in a tertiary care center. The search for an effective tocolytic continues.

REFERENCES

Akerlund M, Stromberg P, Hauksson A, et al: Inhibition of uterine contractions of premature labour with an oxytocin analogue: Results from a pilot study. Br J Obstet Gynaecol 94:1040, 1987.

Andres RL: The association of cigarette smoking with placenta previa and abruptio placentae. Semin Perinatol 20:2, 1996.

Bell R: The prediction of preterm labour by recording spontaneous antenatal uterine activity. Br J Obstet Gynaecol 90:884, 1983.

Bureau MA, Shapcott D, Bertiaume Y, et al: Maternal cigarette smoking and fetal oxygen transport: A study of P50, 2,3-diphosphoglycerate, total hemoglobin, hematocrit, and type F hemoglobin in fetal blood. Pediatrics 72:1, 1983.

Casper RF, Lye SJ: Myometrial desensitization to continuous but not to intermittent β-adrenergic agonist infusion in the sheep. Am J Obstet Gynecol 154:301, 1986.

Caspi E, Ronen J, Schreyer P, Goldberg MD: The outcome of pregnancy after gonadotrophin therapy. Br J Obstet Gynaecol 83:12, 1976.

Chard T: Obstetric risk scores. Fetal Med Rev 3:1, 1991.

Cooper RL, Goldenberg RL, Creasy RK, et al: A multicenter study of preterm birth weight and gestational age–specific neonatal mortality. Am J Obstet Gynecol 168:78, 1993.

Cooper RL, Goldenberg RL, Davis RO, et al: Warning symptoms, uterine contractions, and cervical examination findings in women at risk of preterm delivery. Am J Obstet Gynecol 162:3, 1990.

Cotton DB, Stassner HT, Hill LM, et al: Comparison of magnesium sulfate, terbutaline and a placebo for inhibition of preterm labor: A randomized study. J Reprod Med 29:2, 1984.

Cousins L, Karp W, Lacey C, Lucas WE: Reproductive outcome of women exposed to diethylstilbestrol in utero. Obstet Gynecol 56:1, 1980.

Cox SM, Sherman ML, Leveno KJ: Randomized investigation of magnesium sulfate for prevention of preterm birth. Am J Obstet Gynecol 163:767, 1990.

Crowley P, Enkin MW, Keirse MJNC, et al (Eds): Pregnancy and Childbirth Module of The Cochrane Database of Systematic Reviews. London, BMJ, 1995.

Douidar SM, Richardson J, Snodgrass WR: Role of indomethacin in ductus closure: An update evaluation. Dev Pharmacol Ther 11:196, 1988.

Effer S, Saigal S, Rand C, et al: Effect of delivery method on outcomes in the very low-birth weight breech infant: Is the improved survival related to cesarean section or other perinatal care maneuvers? Am J Obstet Gynecol 145:2, 1983.

Eronen M, Pesonen E, Kurki T, et al: The effects of indomethacin and a β-sympathomimetic agent on the fetal ductus arteriosus during treatment of premature labor: A randomized double-blind study. Am J Obstet Gynecol 164:141, 1991.

Garite TJ: Premature rupture of the membranes: The enigma of the obstetrician. Am J Obstet Gynecol 151:8, 1985.

Goldenberg RL, Cliver SP, Bronstein J, et al: Bed rest in pregnancy. Obstet Gynecol 84:1, 1994.

Goodwin TM, Paul R, Silver H, et al: The effect of the oxytocin antagonist atosiban on preterm uterine activity in the human. Am J Obstet Gynecol 170:2, 1994.

Graham RL, Gilstrap LC, Hauth JC, et al: Conservative management of patients with premature rupture of fetal membranes. Obstet Gynecol 59:5, 1982.

Grimes DA, Schulz KF: Randomized controlled trials of home uterine activity monitoring: A review and critique. Am J Obstet Gynecol 79:1, 1992.

Hauth JC, Goldenberg RL, Andrews WW, et al: Reduced incidence of preterm delivery with metronidazole and erythromycin in women with bacterial vaginosis. N Engl J Med 333:26, 1995.

Hickok DE, Hollenbach KA, Reilley SF, Nyberg DA: The association between decreased amniotic fluid volume and treatment with nonsteroidal anti-inflammatory agents for preterm labor. Am J Obstet Gynecol 160:1525, 1989.

Hill CW, Gookin KS: Home uterine activity monitoring. Clin Perinatol 19:2, 1997.

Holcomb WL, Shackelford GD, Petrie RH: Magnesium tocolysis and neonatal bone abnormalities: A controlled study. Obstet Gynecol 78:611, 1991.

Iskovitz J, Abramovici H, Brandes JM: Oligohydramnion, meconium and perinatal death concurrent with indomethacin treatment in human pregnancy. J Reprod Med 24:137, 1980.

Jannis RA, Triggle DJ, Huszar A (Eds): The Physiology and Biochemistry of the Uterus in Pregnancy and Labor. Boca Raton, FL, CRC Press, 1986.

Katz M, Goodyear K, Creasy RK: Early signs and symptoms of preterm labor. Am J Obstet Gynecol 162:1150, 1990.

Keirse MJNC, Enkin MW, Renfrew MJ, Neilson JP (Eds): Pregnancy and Childbirth Module of The Cochrane Database of Systematic Reviews. London, BMJ, 1995a.

Keirse MJNC, Enkin MW, Renfrew MJ, Neilson JP (Eds): Pregnancy and Childbirth Module of The Cochrane Database of Systematic Reviews. London, BMJ Publishing Group, 1995b.

Keirse MJNC, Grant A, King JF, et al (Eds): Effective Care in Pregnancy and Childbirth. Oxford, Oxford University Press, 1989.

Keirse MJNC, Rush RW, Anderson AB: Risk of preterm delivery in patients with previous preterm delivery or abortion. Br J Obstet Gynaecol 85:81, 1978.

Keith LG, MacGregor S, Friedell S, et al: Substance abuse in pregnant women: Recent experience at the Perinatal Center for Chemical Dependency of Northwestern Memorial Hospital. Obstet Gynecol 73:5, 1989.

Lees C, Campbell S, Jauniaux E, et al: Arrest of preterm labour and prolongation of gestation with glyceryl trinitrate, a nitric oxide donor. Lancet 343:8909, 1994.

Lewis DF, Brody K, Edwards MS, et al: Preterm premature ruptured membranes: A randomized trial of steroids after treatment with antibiotics. Obstet Gynecol 88:5, 1996.

Lewis DF, Futayyeh S, Towers CV, et al: Preterm delivery from 34 to 37 weeks of gestation: Is respiratory distress syndrome a problem? Am J Obstet Gynecol 174:2, 1996.

Ludmir J, Samuels P, Brooks S, Mennuti MT: Pregnancy outcome of patients with uncorrected uterine anomalies managed in a high-risk obstetric setting. Obstet Gynecol 75:6, 1990.

Lundin-Schiller S, Mitchell MD: The role of prostaglandins in human parturition. Prostaglandins Leukot Essent Fatty Acids 39:1, 1990.

Main DM: The epidemiology of preterm birth. Clin Obstet Gynecol 31:521, 1988.

Manchester D, Margolis HS, Sheldon RE: Possible association between maternal indomethacin therapy and primary pulmonary hypertension of the newborn. Am J Obstet Gynecol 126:467, 1976.

Mazor M, Cohen J, Romero R, et al: Cytokines and preterm labour. Fetal Med Rev 7:4, 1995.

McElhatton PR: The effects of benzodiazepine use during pregnancy and lactation. Reprod Toxicol 8:6, 1994.

Meis PJ, Ernest JM, Moore ML: Causes of low birth weight in public and private patients. Am J Obstet Gynecol 156:1165, 1987.

Moise KJ, Huhta JC, Sharif DS, et al: Indomethacin in the treatment of premature labor. N Engl J Med 319:327, 1988.

Monga M, Creasy RK: Pharmacologic management of preterm labor. Semin Perinatol 19:1, 1995.

Moore TRM: Patterns of human uterine contractions: Implications for clinical practice. Semin Perinatol 19:1, 1995.

Muldoon MJ: A prospective study of intrauterine infection following surgical induction of labour. J Obstet Gynaecol Br Commnwlth 75:1144, 1968.

Nakahara K, Iso A, Chao CR, et al: Pregnancy enhances cocaine-induced stimulation of uterine contractions in the chronically instrumented rat. Am J Obstet Gynecol 175:1, 1996.

Natale R, Nasello C, Turliuk R: The relationship between movements and accelerations in FHR at twenty-four to thirty-two weeks gestation. Am J Obstet Gynecol 148:5, 1984.

National Institute of Child Health and Development: Report of the Consensus Development Conference on the Effect of Corticosteroids for Fetal Maturation on Perinatal Outcomes. NIH Publication, Washington, DC, 1994.

Neilson JP, Crowther CA: Preterm labour in multiple pregnancies. Fetal Med Rev 5:2, 1993.

Newman RB, Ellings JM: Antepartum management of the multiple gestation: The case for specialized care. Semin Perinatol 19:5, 1995.

Norton ME, Merrill J, Cooper BAB, et al: Neonatal complications after the administration of indomethacin for preterm labor. N Engl J Med 329:1602, 1993.

Petrie RH: Tocolysis using magnesium sulfate. Semin Perinatol 5:266, 1981.

Popper LD, Batra SC, Akerlund M: The effect of magnesium on calcium uptake and contractility in the human myometrium. Gynecol Obstet Invest 28:78, 1989.

Romero R, Mazor M: Infection and preterm labor. Clin Obstet Gynecol 31:3, 1988.

Romero R, Sibai B, Caritis S, et al: Antibiotic treatment of preterm labor with intact membranes: A multicenter, randomized, double-blinded, placebo-controlled trial. Am J Obstet Gynecol 169:4, 1993.

Sandberg EC, Riffle NL, Higdon JV, Getman CE: Pregnancy outcome in women exposed to diethylstilbestrol in utero. Am J Obstet Gynecol 140:2, 1981.

Shy KK, Luthy DA, Bennett FC, et al: Effects of electronic fetal-heart-rate monitoring, as compared with periodic auscultation, on the neurologic development of premature infants. N Engl J Med 322:9, 1990.

Sibai BM, Romero R, Sanchez-Ramos L, et al: A double-blind placebo-controlled trial of an oxytocin-receptor antagonist (antocin) in the treatment of preterm labor (Abstract). Am J Obstet Gynecol 176(1 pt 2):S2, 1997.

Slutsker L: Risks associated with cocaine use during pregnancy. Obstet Gynecol 79:5, 1992.

Spearing G: Alcohol, indomethacin, and salbutamol: A comparative trial of their use in preterm labor. Am J Obstet Gynecol 53:2, 1979.

Thacker SB, Banta HD: Benefits and risks of episiotomy: An interpretive review of the English literature, 1860–1980. Obstet Gynecol Surv 38:322, 1983.

Thacker SB, Stroup DF, Peterson HB: Efficacy and safety of intrapartum electronic fetal montoring: An update. Obstet Gynecol 86:4, 1995.

The Canadian Preterm Labor Investigators Group: Treatment of preterm labor with the beta-adrenergic agonist ritodrine. N Engl J Med 327:308, 1992.

Tucker JM, Goldenberg RL, Davis RO, et al: Etiologies of preterm birth in an indigent population: Is prevention a logical expectation? Obstet Gynecol 77:3, 1991.

Utter GO, Dooley SL, Tamura RK, Socol ML: Awaiting cervical change for the diagnosis of preterm labor does not compromise the efficacy of ritodrine tocolysis. Am J Obstet Gynecol 163:3, 1990.

Vacca A: The place of the vacuum extractor in modern obstetric practice. Fetal Med Rev 2:103, 1990.

Ventura SJ, Martin JA, Mathews TJ, Clarke SC: Advance report of final natality statistics, 1994. Monthly Vital Statistics Report Vol 44: 1996.

Vielle JC, Bissonnette JM, Hohimer AR: The effect of a calcium channel blocker (nifedepine) on uterine blood flow in the pregnant goat. Am J Obstet Gynecol 154:1160, 1986.

Walker MPR, Moore TR, Brace RA: Indomethacin and AVP interaction in the fetal kidney: A mechanism of oliguria. Am J Obstet Gynecol 171:1234, 1994.

Whalley RJ: Bacteriuria of pregnancy. Obstet Gynecol 97:723, 1967.

CHAPTER 15

Intrapartum Fetal Management

Thomas R. Moore and Donald Roberts

INTRAPARTUM FETAL MONITORING

Because maternal safety during the parturitional process has improved so dramatically in the past five decades, monitoring of the fetus during labor has now become paramount in the United States. In other cultures, however, the prime goal of intrapartum monitoring is to ensure the survival of the mother, with fetal outcome considered secondary. This chapter focuses on key actions designed to ensure fetal well-being, including fetal heart rate (FHR) monitoring, performance of assisted vaginal delivery, management of shoulder dystocia, and management of meconium.

Fetal Heart Rate Monitoring

History

Until the technology (cesarean section) allowing intervention to rescue the fetus during labor became safe in the late 1960s, little attention was paid to the fetus during parturition. Auscultation of the fetal heart tones first became practical with the invention of the De Lee-Hillis fetoscope in 1917, and the fetoscope remained the state-of-the-art until the late 1950s, but it was used only to demonstrate the continuing life of the fetus at the start and end of labor, not to diagnose fetal distress. In 1958, Hon noted that clinical auscultation of FHR was inaccurate from observer to observer. In 1968, Benson and colleagues reported that auscultation was an unreliable indicator of fetal distress unless an extreme degree of compromise had already occurred.

In an attempt to provide more reproducible estimates of actual FHR, Hon (1963) developed the first reliable continuous recording of the FHR obtained from a clip on the fetal scalp. Subsequently, Kubli and associates (1969) described a number of patterns of change in the FHR that correlated with low Apgar scores and newborn acidemia.

Because of its convenience and technologic attraction, electronic FHR monitoring became the standard of care in most obstetric hospitals by the mid-1970s. The ability remotely to display continuously the FHR in a central location reduced the number of nurses necessary and thus was eagerly adopted by maternity hospitals. The technology was so rapidly integrated into the mainstream of obstetric therapy, however, that no clear documentation of its efficacy was demonstrated before its adoption. An entire industry developed to educate physicians and nurses in the nuances of FHR interpretation, and millions of dollars were won in lawsuits for negligence in the use of this new technology. As a result, physicians have become progressively reliant on electronic FHR monitoring to guide obstetric decision making.

The effectiveness of electronic FHR monitoring in prevention of perinatal morbidity has undergone a radical reassessment. Better understanding of the pathophysiology underlying intrapartum asphyxia and neurologic damage has demonstrated that not all causes of fetal neurologic damage can be identified by the use of FHR monitoring. In a meta-analysis of randomized trials of electronic FHR monitoring versus auscultation, Neilson (1994) noted that the cesarean section rate increased by 270%, the intervention rate for fetal distress rose fourfold, and the likelihood of cesarean section for dystocia doubled. These increases in medical cost and maternal morbidity were not accompanied by improvements in newborn outcome.

Despite concerns about the reliability of FHR monitoring to prevent perinatal morbidity, its use continues to be widespread. In contemporary use, electronic FHR monitoring should be viewed as a helpful adjunct in assessing fetal well-being. Overinterpretation of these tracings, however, is likely to increase unnecessary operative intervention without reducing significantly the incidence of long-term newborn morbidity.

Elements of the Fetal Heart Rate

There are few instances in modern medicine in which judgments about an individual's health are made on the basis of a single biologic signal; in the case of the fetus, obstetricians rely only on the FHR to ensure fetal health. Nevertheless, an amazingly rich amount of information can be gleaned from this simple tracing. In its essential form, the art of FHR monitoring is a form of pattern recognition. Thus, the clinician should be knowledgeable regarding the various elements of the FHR tracing (Table 15–1).

Physiology of the Fetal Heart Rate

Fetal oxygenation is maintained by continuous delivery of oxygenated maternal blood into the intervillous spaces of the placenta. A number of factors influence the availability of oxygen for transfer to the fetus across the placental interface (Table 15–2).

Maternal Blood Pressure

Maternal blood reaches the placenta from the uterine arteries by traversing the myometrium via the spiral arteries and ultimately bathing the fetal tissue. Any factor that decreases uterine blood flow or affects diffusibility affects the amount of oxygen delivered to the fetus. Decreased maternal cardiac output, whether from hypotension associated with epidural analgesia or by supine positioning, has a profound effect on fetal oxygenation, resulting in marked FHR changes with relatively small changes in maternal status. Maternal conditions such as hypertension, diabetes, and preeclampsia are associated with a decrease in the

TABLE 15–1

Elements of the Fetal Heart Rate Tracing

Element	Comment
Uterine contractions	Displays uterine contraction frequency. Note frequency and amplitude of contractions. Amplitude is on a relative scale unless an intrauterine pressure catheter is used
Fetal heart rate baseline rate	The average value of fetal heart rate between contractions. Normal limits are 120–160 beats/min
Short-term or beat-to-beat variability	The wiggle in the baseline. Amplitude varies with fetal sleep/wake state
Accelerations	Upward excursions in fetal heart rate. An acceleration must be ≥15 beats/min, lasting ≥15 sec
Decelerations	
Early	Uniform deceleration with a nadir coinciding with the contraction peak
Variable	Irregular-shaped deceleration of *variable* onset and duration
Late	Uniform deceleration with a nadir *later* than the contraction peak

caliber of vessels supplying the placenta, and decreased placental blood flow may result.

Uterine Contractions

The increases in myometrial pressure associated with uterine contractions inhibit venous outflow from the intervillous spaces, resulting in a *breath-holding* effect for the fetus. In a typical labor pattern with contractions lasting 45 seconds and occurring every 3 minutes, the episodic reduction in the fetal oxygenation is tolerable. With frequent contractions (e.g., every 1 to 2 minutes) or with prolonged systole (e.g., 2 minutes), however, even the most healthy fetus may decompensate, causing the venous outflow channels to collapse. During this time, the intervillous circulation is acutely depleted of oxygen. If the contractions are prolonged or tetanic, the uteroplacental reserve can be exceeded and fetal hypoxia produced. Exaggerated FHR

TABLE 15–2

Factors Affecting Fetal Oxygenation

Factor	Examples
Maternal blood pressure	Maternal hypotension due to hemorrhage, anesthesia, or supine positioning
Maternal blood oxygen-carrying capacity	Nutritional anemias, hemoglobinopathies
Maternal oxygen intake, circulation	High altitude, lung disease, cardiac disease
Placental circulation	Vascular disease (e.g., lupus, diabetes)
Placental surface area	Abruptio placentae, infarcts with antiphospholipid syndrome, placental crowding with multifetal gestation

accelerations and tachycardia are often early responses to hypoxia, and late decelerations are the hallmark of fetal hypoxia being present.

Neurologic Control of the Fetal Heart Rate

The baseline FHR is a continuously negotiated compromise between the tachycardic pressure of the sympathetic nervous supply to the heart and the deceleratory influence of vagal tone. Parasympathetic nerve impulses, generated in the brain stem and reaching the heart via the vagus nerve, respond to intracerebral signals and baroreceptor activation. Sympathetic stimuli, carried from the brain stem to the heart via cervical sympathetic nerve fibers, respond to neurologic activity in the fetal cortex (*waking*).

Thus, beat-to-beat variability is the product of vagal and sympathetic tone, which, in turn, are controlled by fetal behavioral state: more with *waking* activity, less with *sleeping* activity. Accelerations are evidence of sustained sympathetic discharge associated with fetal motor and cognitive activity.

Pathophysiology of Fetal Heart Rate Decelerations

Deciding whether a FHR pattern is reassuring or nonreassuring can be complex. Interpretation of the severity of decelerations requires assessment of the remainder of the fetal milieu, including the baseline FHR; the presence of accelerations; the frequency, type, and severity of decelerations; and the presence or absence of variability. Other factors, such as labor progress, contraction frequency, maternal condition, and obstetric complications, must be considered. Late decelerations occurring intermittently with a normal baseline and frequent accelerations are viewed differently than a single, prolonged late deceleration surrounded by a *flat line* baseline. Three distinct types of decelerations are recognized, each resulting from unique physiologic circumstances.

Early Decelerations

Early decelerations are uniform (smooth, concave) decelerations characterized by a nadir at the same time as the contraction peak, forming a mirror of the uterine activity. Early decelerations, associated with fetal head compression during a contraction, are most common in the early second stage of labor when the fetal head is descending into the pelvis. Early decelerations are self-limited and not associated with a loss of variability or chronic hypoxia and should not be considered an ominous pattern.

Variable Decelerations

Variable decelerations, commonly referred to as *v-shaped* or *w-shaped*, are characterized by an abrupt onset and sharp return to baseline (Fig. 15–1). The duration, intensity, and timing relative to the contraction are diverse, hence the name *variable*. Accelerations commonly precede and follow a variable deceleration.

Variable decelerations can be reproduced in the laboratory with intermittent umbilical cord compression. During early cord vessel compression, the umbilical vein is oc-

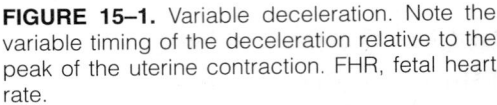

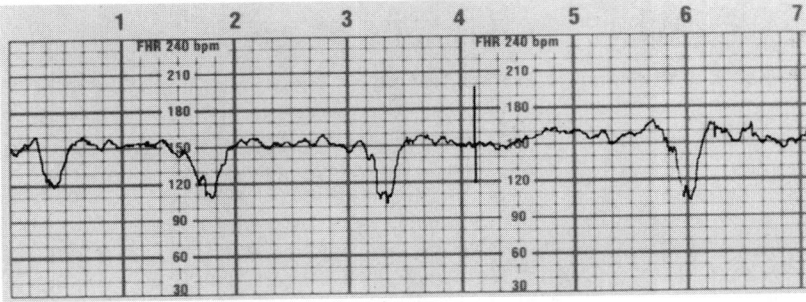

FIGURE 15–1. Variable deceleration. Note the variable timing of the deceleration relative to the peak of the uterine contraction. FHR, fetal heart rate.

cluded, resulting in reduced cardiac return and reflex fetal tachycardia. As compression continues, the umbilical artery is occluded, causing hypertension and activation of the baroreceptor-vagus circuit, resulting in abrupt and deep deceleration in the FHR. As the contraction remits, first the umbilical artery opens and a reflex tachycardia occurs. As the vein is finally opened, the FHR returns to normal. The jagged appearance of the variable is due to the intermittent and often intense vagal stimulation, which exerts powerful control over the FHR.

Variables are graded as mild and severe depending on the depth and duration of FHR deceleration and associated hypoxia. Mild variable decelerations last less than 30 seconds or have a level of deceleration not below 70 beats/min regardless of duration. Severe variable decelerations descend to fetal heart rates below 70 beats/min or drop more than 40 beats/min for greater than 60 seconds' duration (Kubli et al, 1969).

The finding of frequent variable decelerations does not constitute fetal distress. The fetus' ability to tolerate persistent variable decelerations depends on a number of factors, including reserve oxygen capacity, the frequency and depth of heart rate decelerations, and the presence or absence of infection. Loss of variability or baseline tachycardia suggests the possibility of hypoxia and acidosis. If the return to baseline is gradual rather than abrupt, the clinician should be suspicious of progressively worsening hypoxia. If variability and baseline are normal, the fetus can be assumed to be tolerating the intermittent stress.

Late Decelerations

Late decelerations are of uniform, concave shape, but the timing of the low point in the deceleration is *late* compared to the peak in the contraction amplitude (Fig. 15–2). Late decelerations usually return to baseline after the contraction has ended. Persistent late decelerations, especially those occurring in a setting of poor or absent variability, are ominous. Late decelerations may be shallow or deep, but depth does not correlate with the degree of hypoxia present.

Late decelerations can be reliably produced in the laboratory by restricting fetal oxygen supply, either by constricting the uterine artery or by reducing maternal inspired oxygen. With compromised oxygen content in the maternal blood bathing the intervillous space, uterine contractions further decrease oxygen delivery to the fetus for the duration of uterine systole. During this period, inflow of oxygenated blood slows or even stops, causing the equivalent of

breath holding during the contraction. Dropping intervillous oxygen content results in a decrease in FHR. As the contraction abates, circulation returns, restoring oxygen flow and returning FHR to normal.

Other Types of Abnormal Fetal Heart Rate Patterns

Prolonged Bradycardia. Prolonged bradycardias are defined as decelerations more than 30 beats/min below baseline and lasting longer than 60 to 90 seconds. They can occur with umbilical cord prolapse, tetanic uterine contractions, rapid descent of the fetal head, abruption, or profound maternal hypotension. Prognosis for the fetus depends on the length and repetition of prolonged deceleration as well as the underlying cause of fetal circulatory compromise.

Sinusoidal Pattern. A sinusoidal pattern is frequently seen with severe fetal anemia or after use of certain synthetic opioids. True sinusoidal pattern is characterized by a normal baseline with smooth, regular *sine-wave* oscillations above and below the baseline two to five times per minute and not exceeding 15 beats in amplitude. Ultrasound evaluation of the fetus with a sinusoidal FHR pattern is indicated.

Fetal and Newborn pH Assessment

Umbilical cord blood pH and blood gas values are a valuable tool in assessing the immediate condition of the newborn. The technique is simple, is inexpensive, and is widely used. Normal values for umbilical cord blood pH and blood gas values for term infants have been studied. The mean values reported for normal umbilical arterial blood pH in the term newborn range from 7.27 to 7.28. A value of 7.15 is 2 standard deviations below the mean.

The normal values for premature infants have also been studied. Although the Apgar scores for premature infants may be significantly lower than those for term infants, the pH and acid-base status are similar. The mean values reported for normal umbilical arterial blood pH in the preterm newborn range from 7.26 to 7.29. A value of 7.14 is 2 standard deviations from the mean.

Traditionally, newborn acidemia has been defined as an umbilical venous pH of less than 7.20. Most newborns with this pH, however, have normal Apgar scores and show normal development neurologically. Because of this finding, some authors have recommended that a pH concentra-

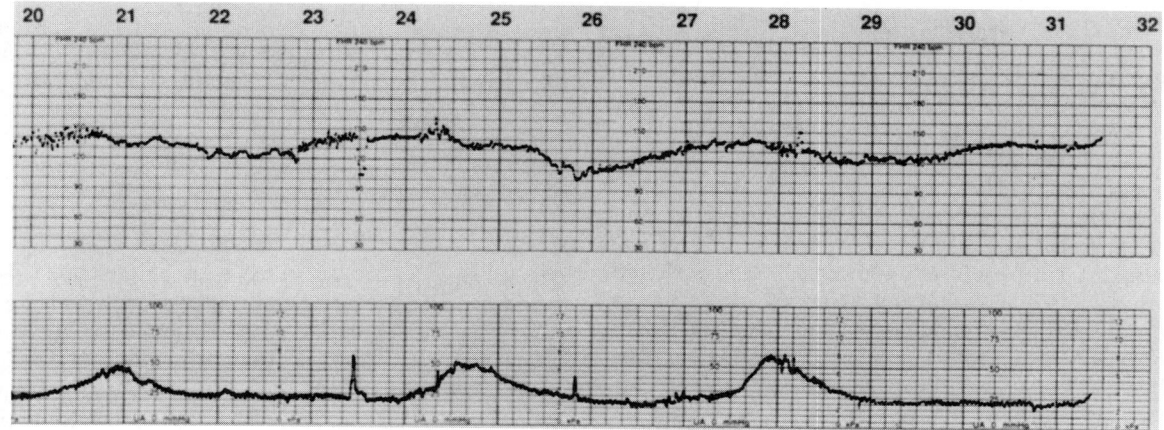

FIGURE 15–2. Late deceleration. Note the uniform shape, mirroring but peaking later than the contraction.

tion of 2 standard deviations below the mean (pH 7.10 to 7.18) be used to define significant fetal acidemia. However as Sykes and coworkers (1982) reported, this cutoff may not even be useful. In that study, greater than 85% of newborns with cord blood pH of less than 7.1 had normal 5-minute Apgar scores.

A pH of 7.00 was found by at least one study to be a more accurate assessment of longterm morbidity in the newborn. Winkler and associates in 1991 found that an umbilical artery blood pH of less than 7.00 with a metabolic component was an important indicator of birth asphyxia and subsequent neurologic dysfunction. Even at this low threshold, however, most newborns are neurologically normal.

OPERATIVE VAGINAL DELIVERY
Forceps

Although obstetric forceps have gained a popular reputation of brutality and lack of finesse, these instruments have undoubtedly spared countless gravidas and their offspring significant morbidity over the past three centuries. Modern obstetric forceps date back to the 1620s, when the Chamberlen family invented and refined a paired instrument that could be used to extract a living fetus. Earlier forceps were two-bladed instruments used for fetal destruction. Today's forceps are remarkably similar to those used by the Chamberlens, having evolved little over the past 300 years.

Obstetric forceps consist of a set of forged steel blades with a cephalic curve and, usually, a pelvic curve. The blades connect to branches and handles; the branches articulate or lock in some way to maintain stability during traction. Each pair is a unique set, and each is numbered; thus, blades are not interchangeable. Various forceps differ in construction of one or more of the components of blade, shank, lock, or handle. Each model was designed to assist in management of a specific set of clinical problems and for convenience of the operator.

The most successful and commonly used obstetric forceps are the designs by Simpson and Elliot. These forceps are most commonly used for elective outlet applications or lower pelvic rotations. Other forceps include the Hawkes-

Dennen (for occiput posterior outlet deliveries), Barton (deep transverse arrest), Kielland (midpelvic rotation), and Piper (delivery of the after-coming head of the breech). In a knowledgeable and skilled obstetrician's hands, forceps can be applied gently and assist in delivery without significant maternal or fetal trauma.

Indications

Indications for operative vaginal delivery are either fetal or maternal (Table 15–3). Fetal indications include fetal distress and failure to deliver spontaneously after an appropriately managed second stage. Maternal indications for operative vaginal delivery include the need to avoid Valsalva effort, as in a patient with severe cardiac or cerebrovascular disease. With certain pulmonary or neuromuscular diseases, pushing efforts may also be either inadequate or insufficient. Exhaustion, lack of cooperation, and excessive analgesia more often impair voluntary efforts and may indicate the need for instrumental delivery.

TABLE 15–3

Indications for Operative Vaginal Delivery

Indication	Criteria
Fetal distress	Nonspecific. Fetal heart rate, scalp pH, or other indicators should be recorded in the chart. Criteria for outlet or midforceps should be met
Maternal indications Shorten the second stage of labor Intervene with maternal exhaustion	Performed to avoid bearing down in patients with contraindications (e.g., cardiac disease) or exhaustion. Criteria for outlet forceps should be met
Prolonged second stage of labor	Nullipara: arrest of descent for >2 h (>3 h with epidural anesthetic) Multipara: arrest of descent for >1 h (>2 h with epidural)

Prerequisites

Careful attention to the prerequisites for forceps application minimizes the risk of trauma. The maternal bladder should be emptied for procedures other than outlet forceps. The cervix should be completely dilated and the membranes ruptured. The fetal head should be engaged, implying that the biparietal diameter is in the pelvic inlet (below zero station).

Positioning of the patient is important. The legs should be supported in stirrups but not strapped or taped in because the possibility of shoulder dystocia and the possible use of the McRoberts maneuver should be remembered. The operator should know as precisely as possible the station and position of the fetal head to permit an accurate application of the forceps blades. Additional prerequisites include adequate anesthesia, an experienced operator, and the capability of performing an emergency cesarean delivery if unexpected difficulty is encountered.

Forceps Classification

For more than 30 years, the definition of station has been the focus of the controversy regarding what actually constitutes a midforceps delivery. Under the older classification, any forceps rotation was considered a midforceps delivery as was any operation ranging from one with the fetal head barely engaged to one with the fetal head just above the perineum.

In 1988, forceps operations were redefined by the American College of Obstetricians and Gynecologists (Table 15–4). The new classification describes station as the level of the leading bony point of the fetal head in centimeters above or below the level of the maternal ischial spines. Zero station is at the ischial spines, and +5 coincides with the fetal scalp visible at the labia. Midforceps operations

are performed above +2 station, and low forceps operations are performed between +2 and the pelvic outlet. The American College of Obstetricians and Gynecologists classification scheme was validated in a series of 357 forceps deliveries defined under the old and the new systems. The classification does not recognize forceps procedures in which the fetal head is unengaged (*high forceps*).

Vacuum

The application of the vacuum as an obstetric instrument was first reported in the mid-nineteenth century by Simpson. A vaginal speculum was originally fitted with wetted leather, and suction was created by use of a piston. It was initially used in cases of dystocia or second-stage arrest. It was also used reportedly to remove retained placenta. Today's vacuum consists of a Silastic cup connected by a flexible tubing to a vacuum source. The vacuum extractor is intended to create traction on the fetal scalp to assist the normal forces of labor. Depending on the type of device and the length of application, a characteristic caput succedaneum of edema fluid accumulates in the subcutaneous tissues of the scalp. In most instances, the caput is of cosmetic concern only and quickly resolves postpartum. The vacuum extractor, however, is associated with an increased incidence of cephalohematoma.

Pressure changes both on and within the fetal head have been studied for forceps and vacuum, both in clinical settings and in the laboratory. Vacuum cup displacement depends on the strength of the vacuum, the height of the cup, and the angle of traction. Using a series of mathematic models, Rosa calculated that the maximal traction that the vacuum extractor can exert until it breaks loose amounts to 14.8 kg. Further, Rosa noted that oblique pulls reduced the net effective force obtainable with the extractor owing to lifting of the cup edge and loss of vacuum. Studies also indicate that the vacuum extractor can generate cranial pressures similar to forceps.

The same respect and clinical judgment should be given vacuum extraction that is given forceps. The larger the fetus, the more difficult the pull and the greater likelihood of scalp injury or shoulder dystocia. Regardless of the type, the vacuum cup should always be located in the midline toward the fetal occiput. This way the head is flexed and not extended when traction is applied. Failure to position the cup correctly to favor cranial flexion is likely the greatest factor in failure of extraction from the midpelvis.

Before any attempted extraction, careful attention is given to alternative management, including oxytocin administration, continued observation, forceps application, and cesarean section. Once the vacuum extractor has been chosen and the instrument applied, checks similar to those seen with forceps are performed by the operator. Delivery should usually be completed within two to four contractions. The direction of traction should be the same as for forceps delivery.

Neonatal Outcome

Outlet forceps, as defined previously, have no significant adverse effect on neonatal well-being. The IQ scores of children delivered by outlet forceps were no different than those of children with spontaneous vaginal delivery by age 4 (Friedman et al, 1977).

For *midforceps*, the risks are not as clear. In the ex-

TABLE 15–4

Criteria of Forceps Deliveries According to Station and Rotation

Types of Procedure	Criteria
Outlet forceps	Scalp is visible at the introitus without separating labia
	Fetal skull has reached pelvic floor
	Sagittal suture is in anteroposterior diameter or right or left occiput anterior or posterior position
	Fetal head is at or on perineum
	Rotation does not exceed 45 degrees
Low forceps	Leading point of fetal skull is at station ≥ +2 cm and not on the pelvic floor
	Rotation ≤45 degrees (left or right occiput anterior to occiput anterior, or left or right occiput posterior to occiput posterior)
	Rotation >45 degrees
Midforceps	Station above +2 cm but head engaged
High	Not included in classification

From American College of Obstetricians and Gynecologists. Operative Vaginal Delivery. (Technical Bulletin No. 196). Washington, DC, © ACOG, August 1994.

treme, Kielland forceps used in rotation of the fetal head have been associated with spinal cord transection and brain-stem injury (Gould and Smith, 1984). Friedman (1987), citing outcome data from the Collaborative Perinatal Project of the 1960s, noted that infants delivered with midforceps after a protracted active phase had markedly increased perinatal mortality. Hughey and McElin (1978) reported an "unfavorable neonatal outcome" in 31% of midforcep operations involving rotation and 13.5% of all midforceps procedures.

More recent reports, however, have failed to reproduce these dire findings. Dierker and colleagues (1986) noted that the neurologic status at 2 years of age and older of 110 infants delivered by midforceps was no different than a matched group delivered by cesarean section for similar indications. The differences in these more recent studies may be attributable to more restrictive selection of midforceps candidates and avoidance of mid-midforceps and high-midforceps by contemporary practitioners.

SHOULDER DYSTOCIA
Incidence and Risk Factors

Shoulder dystocia, defined as the failure of the shoulders to deliver following the head despite standard assisting maneuvers, is one of the true obstetric emergencies that causes terror for the obstetrician, the patient, and her family. Although it is encountered with an incidence varying from 0.15% to 0.5% of all deliveries, the frequency is directly related to fetal size and the presence of diabetes. Benedetti and Gabbe (1978) have identified a series of high-risk factors for shoulder dystocia (Table 15–5). These include a previous large infant, estimated fetal weight more than 4000 g in the present pregnancy, maternal diabetes, a prolonged second stage of labor, and use of forceps or vacuum with the fetal head in the midpelvis. The highest estimate of the risk of shoulder dystocia (estimated fetal weight >4500 g and the presence of diabetes) is approximately 35%. Notably, more than half of shoulder dystocias occur in infants weighing less than 4000 g.

TABLE 15–5

Risk Factors for Shoulder Dystocia

Risk Factor	Comment
Macrosomia	Weight >4000 g in present or prior pregnancy
Protracted active phase labor	Cervical dilation progress <1 cm/h after 4 cm
Prolonged second stage	Nulliparas: pushing >3 h Multiparas: pushing >2 h
Maternal diabetes	Pre-existing diabetes or gestational diabetes
Maternal obesity	Prepregnant weight >200 lb or body mass index >26
Use of midforceps or midpelvic vacuum	Application above +2 station
Previous shoulder dystocia	

Management
Philosophy

In the best possible scenario, shoulder dystocia is managed expertly, and both mother and newborn emerge unscathed from the experience. With increasing severity of the dystocia, some degree of fetal and maternal injury may be unavoidable. Therefore, the following priorities should be followed, in descending order:

1. Avoid infant death.
2. Avoid asphyxiation and permanent brain injury to the infant.
3. Avoid permanent peripheral nerve injury to the infant.
4. Avoid asphyxiation and perinatal depression of the infant.
5. Avoid skeletal bone fracture in the infant.
6. Avoid or minimize maternal soft tissue injury.

Time to complete delivery of the fetus after emergence of the head is the critical factor in achieving success in items 1, 2, and 4 because oxygen delivery to the fetal brain is severely reduced while the head is trapped against the maternal vulvar tissues. Animal studies indicate that permanent brain damage begins to occur 8 to 10 minutes after restriction of brain blood flow. The assisting nursing staff should keep the obstetrician and pediatric team informed of this critical time. Avoiding brachial nerve palsy requires the skilled application of maneuvers to help release the fetus (see later).

Preparedness

In most shoulder dystocia cases, the infant can be delivered uninjured if simple guidelines are followed. The first rule is to be prepared for possible shoulder dystocia in the high-risk patient. This preparation includes having at least one experienced obstetrician present at the delivery, an anesthesiologist present in case general anesthesia is necessary, and a neonatology team. The attending nursing staff should be familiar with the correct application of various maneuvers and when not to apply certain maneuvers. In some institutions, shoulder dystocia drills are conducted for this purpose.

Specific Maneuvers

Because it is impossible to predict every case of shoulder dystocia, all obstetricians should be familiar with procedures used to correct the condition (Lurie et al, 1994) (Table 15–6). Once shoulder dystocia is encountered, the McRoberts maneuver is used first because this alone may release the anterior shoulder. In this technique, the obstetric nursing staff assists the mother in flexing her hips, bringing her legs sharply against her abdomen. This movement results in a straightening of the sacrum relative to the lumbar spine, widening the pelvic inlet and thus freeing the impacted anterior shoulder (Gonik et al, 1989). This procedure reportedly has a 70% to 80% success rate.

If the dystocia persists, suprapubic pressure should be applied to the mother's lower abdomen. To apply adequate pressure, a step stool is helpful. The heel of the hand is

TABLE 15-6

Maneuvers to Resolve Shoulder Dystocia

Maneuver	Comment
McRoberts maneuver	Flex patient's hips, bringing knees up onto chest. Increases the pubosacral distance
Suprapubic pressure	Assistant attempts to push anterior shoulder beneath pubis. Usually not successful by itself
Wood's maneuver (corkscrew)	Displace shoulders from a vertical into an oblique alignment. Oblique diameters are larger than the direct pubosacral distance
Enlarge the episiotomy	Ensures minimal maternal soft tissue resistance
Deliver the posterior arm	Reduces shoulder width. Arm extraction may fracture humerus
Fracture the clavicle	Difficult to perform
Cephalic replacement (Zavanelli maneuver)	Requires cesarean delivery

applied to the suprapubic area (similar to a cardiopulmonary resuscitation chest compression maneuver) while the obstetrician applies gentle traction on the head. Excessive traction on the fetal head must be avoided.

If this simple maneuver fails, the operator should attempt to rotate the anterior fetal shoulder posteriorly away from the symphysis pubis toward an oblique corner of the pelvis. If the shoulder moves, continuing downward traction on the fetus coupled with continued rotation through 180 degrees frees the shoulders from the pubis allowing delivery to occur (*corkscrew maneuver*). If delivery is still not accomplished, an episiotomy should be performed or widely enlarged to provide maximal room for fetal shoulder movement.

Delivery of the posterior arm is usually successful in disimpacting the fetus in difficult cases. Preferably under adequate anesthesia, the operator slips a hand beneath the posterior fetal shoulder and follows the arm to the hand. The hand is grasped, and delivered over the fetal chest and face. Incidental to this technique, the humerus can be broken. After the posterior arm and shoulder have been delivered, the infant should be rotated and the anterior shoulder is delivered easily from the posterior position.

No more than a total of 8 minutes should be expended in the above-mentioned attempts to effect delivery. By 6 to 7 minutes, preparations should be made to replace the fetal head and perform a cesarean section (Zavanelli maneuver) (O'Leary, 1993; O'Leary and Cuva, 1992).

Administration of external pressure on the uterine fundus, without first releasing the fetal shoulders, worsens the impaction and increases risk of fetal injury and nerve damage. Thus, it is contraindicated until at least one fetal shoulder has been freed.

Outcome

Reliable information about the outcome of shoulder dystocia is difficult to obtain because of irregularities in charting of both mother and infant. Maternal risks are low to moderate: Many patients with shoulder dystocia have had long labors complicated by chorioamnionitis; thus, the incidence of postpartum fever and hemorrhage are increased. For the newborn, the major risks are humerus or clavicular fracture, brachial nerve palsy, and asphyxia. Most studies indicate the risk of fetal injury is approximately 30%. About one third of these injuries are bone fractures, which have no sequelae, leaving a 20% risk of nerve injury. Of these, at most 10% are unresolved at hospital discharge, and of those, 90% resolve over the next 6 months (Morrison et al, 1992). Thus, the prospective risk of permanent injury to the fetus at high risk of shoulder dystocia is 20% × 10% or 0.2%. In the case of the fetus with an estimated risk of shoulder dystocia of 33% before labor, the risk of permanent injury is 0.06%. Clearly, this risk is too low to make cesarean section before labor a realistic option because more than 300 cesarean sections would be performed to avoid this complication (Nocon et al, 1993). Avoiding high-risk circumstances is prudent, however, and that implies avoidance of midpelvic forceps or vacuum procedures in patients with slow labor progress and a macrosomic fetus (Keller et al, 1991).

NONVERTEX PRESENTATION
Clinical Issues

The frequency of cesarean section increased significantly from 11% in 1940 to greater than 75% in the 1980s. Several factors have contributed to the abrupt increase in cesarean sections for breech presentation. First, the breech delivery carries an increased risk of fetal injury and death in almost every situation. Morgan and Kane (1964) demonstrated a fivefold increase in perinatal mortality when all breech deliveries were compared with vertex deliveries. Subsequent reports by Brenner and colleagues (1974) and Kaupilla (1975) supported the contention that vaginal delivery of the breech produces fetal injuries that would be avoided with cesarean section.

A further stimulus to increased cesarean delivery of the breech has been popular demand. Well-informed patients have increasingly demanded that birth be as free as possible of trauma and asphyxia, forcing many experienced obstetricians to reconsider their former practices involving higher-risk vaginal deliveries. As cesarean birth has become more frequent, many patients and practitioners believe that the maternal risks accompanying cesarean section are of less long-term impact than the neonatal sequelae following suboptimal breech vaginal birth. Appropriately selected patients and fetuses, however, can achieve successful vaginal breech delivery if high-risk circumstances are recognized and avoided (Croughan-Minihane et al, 1990).

Incidence and Types

The incidence of breech presentation varies with the gestational age of the pregnancy. At term, breeches account for 3% to 4% of deliveries, but before 32 weeks 20% of fetuses are in a nonvertex presentation. Presumably the increasing prevalence of vertex presentation as term approaches is due to some form of fetal selection because an excess of anomalous and damaged fetuses is found among term breeches.

There are basically three types of breech presentation. In the frank breech, the legs are flexed at the hips and extended at the knee (*pike* position). This is the most common in the primigravida and accounts for 60% of breeches overall. The complete breech (10%) has both hips and knees flexed (*tailor fashion*). The remainder are single or double footling breech (30%), in which one or both feet are presenting.

Morbidity and Mortality

Piper (Piper and Bachman, 1929), after whom the specialized forceps designed for the breech was named, recognized three major factors contributing to increased breech perinatal morbidity when he introduced his breech forceps: umbilical cord prolapse, nuchal arms, and entrapment of the aftercoming head. The risk of these complications depends on the size of the fetus, its gestational age, and the type of breech presentation.

Umbilical Cord Prolapse

The frequency of umbilical cord prolapse is increased 5- to 20-fold in the breech presentation, most of which occurs when the breech is nonfrank. The risk of prolapse with footling breech is 8% to 25% and with complete breech 10%. The frank breech has cord prolapse in only 2%, however, a figure similar to that experienced with vertex presentation (Gimovsky and Paul, 1982).

Nonfrank Breech

Accumulated data suggest that vaginal delivery of the nonfrank breech invites excessive risk taking because of the cord prolapse risk. Gimovsky and Paul (1982) randomized nonfrank breech fetuses to vaginal versus cesarean section. On final analysis, there was no statistical difference between fully *evaluated* breech deliveries and vertex vaginal births. Among the breech infants delivered vaginally without complete fetal and maternal evaluation, however, 15% had 5-minute Apgar scores less than 7, and one fetus delivered vaginally died intrapartum.

Frank Breech

The outcome of the frank breech is less morbid than nonfrank breech because of the lesser risk of umbilical cord prolapse. Collea and associates (1980) randomized frank breeches to cesarean section and vaginal trial of labor and found the differences in outcome to be nonsignificant. From Collea's study, it can be concluded that of patients trying labor, only 44% eventually deliver vaginally, and most of the fetal morbidity (in Collea's study, three with nuchal arms resulting in two brachial palsies and acidotic umbilical cord pH) occurs in the vaginal group.

Entrapment of the Fetal Head

Entrapment of the fetal head is an obstetric emergency that can occur in association with fetal macrosomia, deflexion of the fetal head, and delivery of the fetal body through an incompletely dilated cervix. Macrosomic fetuses face additional hazards regardless of presentation, but a breech fetus weighing greater than 4000 g multiplies the risk of perinatal death by a factor of 10. This problem is compounded by the currently inaccurate methods for judging fetal weight. For these reasons, setting an upper limit of estimated fetal weight of 3800 g helps minimize the chance of head entrapment during delivery.

Hyperextension of the fetal neck in labor increases the risk of head entrapment. Ballas and Toaff (1976) reported more than 70% incidence of spinal cord transection during vaginal breech delivery if the attitude of the fetal head was extended beyond 90 degrees. The nondeflexed, or *military*, head position carries no increased risk during vaginal birth.

Head entrapment may also occur in the premature gestation if the fetal body (which has diameters some 20% smaller than the fetal head diameters) *prolapses* through an incompletely dilated cervix. Releasing the head of the entrapped fetus frequently results in permanent fetal injury or death. Because fetal head dimensions exceed those of the abdomen until approximately 35 weeks, many practitioners exclude preterm pregnancies from trial of labor.

Selective Vaginal Delivery of the Breech Presentation

Frank Breech

The National Institutes of Health Task Force on Cesarean Birth recommended that vaginal delivery at term should remain an acceptable obstetric choice, provided that the physician and patient meet certain criteria, as follows:

- Term pregnancy (>35 weeks).
- Frank breech.
- Fetal weight between 2500 and 3800 g.
- Nondeflexed fetal head.
- Adequate x-ray pelvimetry.
- Skilled operator.

Key points to be emphasized are:

1. Informed consent, which must be complete and frank.
2. Full fetal evaluation, including comprehensive estimation of fetal weight and exclusion of neck extension.
3. A skilled delivery team, including experienced obstetrician, immediately available anesthesia, and neonatal resuscitation team.

Management of Labor and Delivery

The use of oxytocin in a breech labor is controversial. In Collea's study, oxytocin was unsuccessful in resolving dystocia and led to two cases of brachial plexus injury (Collea et al, 1980). There should be no contraindications to giving oxytocin with prolonged rupture of the membranes or prolonged latent phase, but it may be unwise to augment the active phase of labor.

There are two types of vaginal breech deliveries: assisted and total breech extraction. In the first, the obstetrician assists and controls the birth of the infant while maternal pushing provides most of the motive power. The second type, typically applied to a second twin, involves grasping the fetal feet in the uterus, and delivering the fetus by external traction. With total breech extraction, there is a higher incidence of perinatal morbidity because the infant has less time to adapt to the process.

Of particular concern is head entrapment and nuchal arms. In the latter, one or more of the fetal arms are crossed above the fetal head, blocking delivery. In either case, gentle attempts to reduce the obstruction by a skilled operator should be successful within 5 minutes of recognition of the complication if fetal asphyxia is to be avoided. If such attempts are unsuccessful, general anesthesia is administered to relax the uterus, and one further attempt to deliver the fetus is undertaken while cesarean section preparations go forward simultaneously. In these instances, the pediatric resuscitation team should be prepared to receive a depressed newborn. When general anesthesia has been administered, a period of assisted ventilation helps clear the anesthetic from the newborn's bloodstream and hasten resuscitation.

Under certain strict criteria, vaginal delivery of the term breech should be an accepted procedure. If labor does not progress satisfactorily, a primary cesarean section should be performed.

MANAGEMENT OF MECONIUM
Clinical Issues

Considering all births, meconium staining of the amniotic fluid occurs in one of seven deliveries. Although the presence of meconium is considered by most clinicians to be a marker for fetal distress, the data are conflicting. Overall perinatal outcomes with meconium-stained fluid are suboptimal compared with those with clear fluid. Nathan and colleagues (1994) compared outcomes in 8136 meconium-stained versus 34,573 clear amniotic fluid deliveries and found the perinatal mortality increased fivefold with meconium ($P<.001$). Most of these deaths resulted from meconium aspiration. Umbilical artery blood pH less than 7.00 increased 2.5 times ($P<.001$), and cesarean delivery increased from 7% to 14% ($P<.001$). An association between the presence of meconium and fetal distress is suggested by the work of Garcia-Alix and coworkers (1992), who noted a fourfold increase in serum catecholamines in meconium-stained fetuses compared with controls.

Correlations are not perfect, however, as demonstrated by the findings of Richey and colleagues (1995) (Table 15-7). The significant differences in erythropoietin levels but not catecholamines suggests that chronic, not acute stress may be linked to meconium passage. During amniocentesis on 514 term patients not in labor, King and associates (1978) found meconium staining in only 10 (0.2%), a figure considerably less than the 15% prevalence of meconium noted after labor. These results, together with the recognition that most often meconium staining is accompanied by no signs of fetal hypoxia or distress, raise significant questions about how the discovery of meconium-stained amniotic fluid should be routinely managed by the obstetric team.

TABLE 15–7

Comparison of Perinatal Outcome in Deliveries with Meconium-Stained and Clear Amniotic Fluid

Factor	Meconium	Clear	P Value
Gestational age (wk)	39.7 ± 1.4	38.9 ± 1.6	NS
Weight (g)	3548 ± 416	3339 ± 368	NS
Cord pH	7.26 ± 0.06	7.25 ± 0.1	NS
Lactate (mg/dL)	30.5 ± 11.5	30.4 ± 14.2	NS
Hypoxanthine (μMol/L)	13.6 ± 7.1	14.5 ± 5.9	NS
Erythropoietin (mIU/mL)	39.5	26.8	.05

From Richey SD, Ramin SM, Bawdon RE, et al: Markers of acute and chronic asphyxia in infants with meconium-stained amniotic fluid. Am J Obstet Gynecol 172(4 Pt 1):1212, 1995.

Pathophysiology

The pathologic relationship between fetal hypoxia, intestinal hyperstalsis, and smooth muscle relaxation has been affirmed by many studies. Walker (1954) demonstrated that meconium was released more commonly when the oxygen saturation of the umbilical vein was below 30% and that heavy meconium was more often associated with a lower oxygen saturation than was light meconium.

The precise relationship of meconium passage to fetal distress, however, is not as well documented. In at least half of meconium deliveries, there is no demonstrable fetal distress. In the study by Low and colleagues (1995) of 20 newborns with severe acidemia at birth (base deficit >34 mmol/L), the meconium was not statistically associated. A study by Kariniemi and Harrela (1990), however, examined the problem from the other direction using multivariate analysis of all meconium-stained cases to associate various clinical variables. The predictors of meconium staining were older gestational age, fetal acidemia, a calcified placenta, late decelerations, and placental weight. Other variables having no effect on the frequency of meconium included maternal age, parity, fetal sex, duration of labor, entanglement of the umbilical cord, FHR variability, variable decelerations, oxytocin usage, type of anesthesia, and maternal smoking and alcohol consumption habits. Thus, the presence of meconium does not itself predict asphyxia well; however, the presence of acidemia at birth is correlated with meconium staining.

Composition

Meconium is the net product of swallowed squames, hair, vernix, sloughed gastrointestinal cells, gastrointestinal mucin, and bilirubin pigments. It accumulates during gestation and moves progressively from the upper intestinal tract into the large bowel, where it collects awaiting a stimulus for passage. Although meconium is sterile, it contains powerful stimulants for release of cytokines and other vasoactive substances, which may mediate strong cardiovascular responses in the fetus and newborn. Chemically, meconium can induce a marked inflammatory response in susceptible tissues (e.g., respiratory epithelium), and mechanically, it can obstruct small airways, particularly if it is thick in consistency.

Passage of Meconium

The stimuli initiating passage of meconium in the fetus and newborn are complex, probably involving interaction of meconium load in the bowel, gestational age, levels of catecholamines, motilin and other gastrointestinal hormones, and the presence of hypoxia. Although it is recognized that most newborns pass meconium within 24 hours, up to one third have passed meconium as fetuses at or before delivery. What proportion of these are due to physiologic mechanisms and how many are related to in utero hypoxemia is unclear. Several facts are known:

- Meconium is typically passed near the time of delivery or shortly postpartum.
- Ten percent to 15% of term deliveries have meconium-stained amniotic fluid, and most fetuses show no signs of distress.
- Meconium is virtually never released before 32 weeks.
- Physiologic release of meconium is regulated by motilin and dependent on parasympathetic tone.
- *Distressed* release of meconium can be mediated by strong vagal outflow associated with umbilical cord compression or by sympathetic overdrive during hypoxia.

Meconium Thickness and Outcome

The entire medical literature devoted to meconium lacks a precise definitional basis for thickness. Meconium is usually classified as thin, moderate, or thick, although the definitions vary according to the observer. Typically, thin meconium is translucent, and thick meconium, strictly defined, is sticky, tenacious, and "pea soup," whereas moderate meconium fits in between. However defined, thick meconium is unique because it is viscid enough to obstruct neonatal airways, concentrated enough to cause significant chemical injury to tissues, and, most importantly, occurs in the setting of oligohydramnios, which itself is associated with poor placental function.

In an effort to bring more exactness to this diagnosis, Trimmer and Gilstrap (1991) defined meconium thickness on the basis of centrifuged solids. They found that 58% of meconium was thin, 34% was moderate, and 8% was thick. In their study, there was no correlation between the type of meconium and newborn acidemia (umbilical artery pH <7.20)—13% for thin, 19% for moderate, and 11% for thick (Fig. 15–3). Starks (1980), however, found that thick meconium was associated with a higher percentage of low Apgar scores, and Mahomed and colleagues (1994) reported that patients with thin meconium had outcomes indistinguishable from those with clear fluid. In the latter study, those with thick meconium had higher frequencies of poor perinatal outcome in every parameter studied. The key role of amniotic fluid volume in meconium morbidity was highlighted in a study by Jeng and associates (1992), in which it was noted that pregnancies with an amniotic fluid index of 8 cm or less had higher incidences of meconium staining, cesarean delivery for fetal distress, abnormal FHR monitoring, and Apgar scores of 7 or less at 1 minute.

Thus, the importance of meconium thickness is probably derived from its clinical setting, whether or not placental insufficiency, oligohydramnios, intermittent umbilical cord compression, and intrauterine growth retardation are coexistent. With one or more of these clinical risk factors present with thick meconium, fetal jeopardy rises significantly.

Meconium Aspiration

Meconium aspiration may be defined as the presence of meconium below the vocal cords. Meconium is found below the vocal cords in 11% to 58% (mean 35%) of live births with meconium-stained amniotic fluid, approximately 4% of all live births.

Meconium aspiration syndrome comprises a significant range of respiratory compromise. In its mildest form, the disease may present with neonatal tachypnea, associated with normal pH and lower P_{CO_2}, which resolves within 2 to 3 days. Clinically, this mild respiratory morbidity may be indistinguishable from transient tachypnea of the newborn. In the more severe form, the syndrome can present as severe hypoxemia, acidosis, pneumothorax, and respiratory failure a few hours after birth. Pulmonary arterial vasospasm may lead to right-to-left shunting through the patent foramen ovale or ductus arteriosus. Hypoxia further stimulates pulmonary hypertension, and the downward spiral continues, ultimately leading to convulsions, renal failure, disseminated intravascular coagulation, and heart failure.

Mechanism of Meconium Aspiration

It appears that passage of meconium can occur in response to asphyxial stress or in conjunction with normal physio-

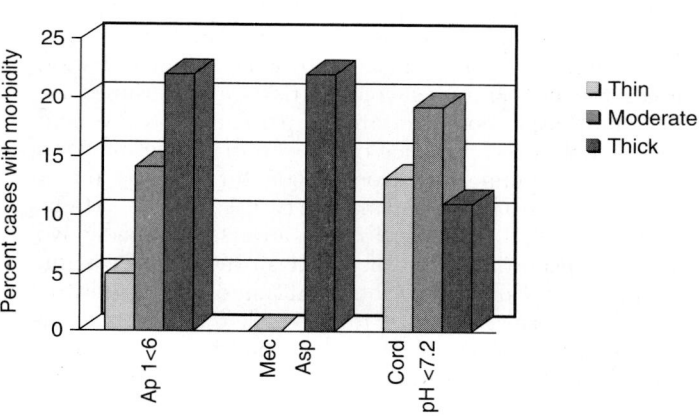

FIGURE 15–3. Frequency of perinatal morbidity with various levels of meconium thickness. Vertical axis plots percent of cases with morbidity. Ap, Apgar score, Mec Asp, meconium aspiration. (Adapted from Trimmer KJ, Gilstrep LC III: "Meconiumcrit" and birth asphyxia. Am J Obstet Gynecol 165:1010, 1991.)

logic processes. Regardless of the mechanism of passage, however, if meconium is released in utero, the fetus is then at risk for meconium aspiration. How and when does this occur?

Experiments in a wide variety of mammals have demonstrated a typical sequence of asphyxial meconium passage and in utero aspiration. A key event is the gasping reflex, which is stimulated by severe hypoxia and usually occurs after meconium release. Dawes and colleagues (1972) induced meconium aspiration in fetal lambs with umbilical cord occlusion, which caused the lambs to pass meconium, gasp, and aspirate the meconium into their lungs. Gasping has been similarly induced in rhesus monkeys and baboons (Block et al, 1987).

Human gasping has been described in high-risk fetuses 24 to 72 hours before intrauterine death. Amniotic fluid, cellular debris, and meconium may be found in the lungs of fetuses who have died in utero of asphyxia (Brown and Gleicher, 1981). Autopsies of severely asphyxiated preterm stillborn fetuses consistently demonstrate amniotic fluid and debris in the fetal lung parenchyma, but meconium is rarely found (Turbeville et al, 1979).

Therefore, in patients presenting with meconium-stained amniotic fluid, meconium aspiration could be potentially prevented by the following measures:

- During labor, ensuring that in utero gasping owing to hypoxic stress and vagal stimulation is avoided.
- During labor, diluting thick meconium via amnioinfusion of intravenous fluids so that if gasping or deep fetal breathing occurs, meconium aspiration is minimized.
- After delivery, ensuring that meconium is cleared from the airways before neonatal gasping or breathing occurs.

Pathologic Effects

The deleterious effects of meconium aspiration are mechanical, chemical, infectious, and neuroadaptive. First, simple plugging of the neonatal airways with particulate matter from the meconium reduces air-exchange area in the lung and may necessitate high ventilator pressures or even extracorporeal membrane oxygenation (ECMO) to achieve satisfactory oxygenation. Pneumothorax and pulmonary interstitial emphysema may ensue. Chemical inflammation of the lung initiated by meconium constituents, such as bilirubin metabolites, stimulates diffuse alveolitis characterized by vascular leak, neutrophil and macrophage invasion, and cytokine release (Lopez and Bildfell, 1992).

The inflammation stimulated by meconium aspiration places the newborn at increased risk for superinfection. Meconium aspiration syndrome is particularly severe and often lethal in the presence of infection because infection may lead to pulmonary hypertension through the direct action of toxins on the pulmonary vasculature (Hammerman et al, 1988). Finally, the adverse neuroadaptive effects of exposure of the neonatal airways to meconium are uncertain. Considering the significant olfactory sensitivities of the normal newborn, it is possible that the chemical and physical impact of meconium on the airways may inhibit normal maternal-infant bonding and feeding behaviors.

Intrapartum Management of Meconium
Combined Obstetric and Pediatric Airway Suctioning

Carson and associates (1976) reported that suction of the fetal nasopharynx immediately after delivery of the head but before delivery of the body combined with tracheal intubation and suction by the pediatrician was effective in reducing the incidence and severity of meconium aspiration. Retrospectively, they identified five neonatal deaths in 18 cases of meconium aspiration syndrome without combined suction and no deaths among seven cases of meconium aspiration syndrome after the institution of the combined suction protocol. A prospective study supported these findings (Gregory et al, 1974). As a result of these small studies, a De Lee suction catheter has traditionally been used to accomplish this. The procedure is outlined in Table 15–8.

Potential Downside of Aggressive Management of Cases of Meconium Staining

Although the protocol outlined in Table 15–8 has been applied almost universally in hospital delivery units since the late 1970s, concerns have arisen about its potential shortcomings. These include doubts about the efficacy of combined suctioning in preventing meconium aspiration syndrome and a perceived worsening of neonatal status in some newborns subjected to laryngoscopy who appear to be vigorous and breathing successfully before intervention. The traditional method assumes most, if not all, meconium aspiration occurs at first neonatal breath, whereas Suresh and Sarkar (1994) noted that despite careful De Lee suctioning and lack of neonatal breathing before intubation, 75% still had meconium in the trachea.

In response to these concerns, Yoder (1994) conducted a program of selective suctioning, in which suctioning of term infants was avoided if the infants were vigorous at

---

TABLE 15–8

Traditional Protocol for Combined Approach to Meconium

Used at both cesarean and vaginal delivery
Resuscitation unit readied
   Warmer on
   Suction apparatus connected, tested
   Bag, mask unit connected to oxygen supply, tested
   Laryngoscope available, light tested
At delivery of the head but before first breath using De Lee trap, obstetrician clears airway (mouth, hypopharynx, nasopharynx), then delivers body
Umbilical cord rapidly clamped and cut
Neonatal respirations suppressed or avoided during prompt neonatal transfer to pediatrician or trained resuscitation team
Newborn placed on resuscitation unit
Laryngoscopy performed to assess meconium volume, thickness, location
Flexible tracheal suctioning as necessary to visualize vocal cords
Intubate unless infant vigorous and vocal cords clear
Suction trachea via endotracheal tube until clear. Reintubate and suction as indicated until no further meconium is aspirated
When airway is clear, resuscitate newborn

birth—regardless of meconium thickness. Those with and without suctioning were compared with matched controls with clear amniotic fluid. Meconium aspiration syndrome was significantly more common in suctioned infants as compared with those selectively not suctioned, those with light meconium, and those with clear fluid (11% versus 3% versus 0% versus 0%; $P<.01$). The need for ventilator or oxygen support was similar among infants with clear fluid, lightly stained fluid, and moderate to thick fluid who were selectively not suctioned but was significantly greater among suctioned infants ($P<.01$).

A further reconsideration of *deep hypopharyngeal suctioning* with the De Lee catheter was conducted by Locus and coworkers (1990) in which meconium-stained deliveries were randomized between traditional De Lee catheter and the standard bulb suction device. Of the 107 infants studied, 4 developed meconium aspiration syndrome, 3 in the De Lee group and 1 in the bulb group. There was no difference in the amount of meconium found below the vocal cords, comparing pharyngeal De Lee suction with bulb suction (0.22 mL versus 0.24 mL; P = not significant).

The above-mentioned suggests that a cautious modification of the currently advocated protocol for meconium can be undertaken to include (1) use of the bulb syringe or De Lee catheter at delivery of the head and (2) laryngoscopy and intubation only for newborns with thick meconium and those who are depressed or had evidence of fetal distress just before delivery.

REFERENCES

Aladjem S, Vuolo K: Antepartum fetal testing: Evaluation and redefinition of criteria for clinical interpretation. Semin Perinatol 5:145, 1981.

Allen R: The significance of meconium in midtrimester genetic amniocenteses. Am J Obstet Gynecol 152:413, 1985.

Anate M: Instrumental (operative) vaginal deliveries: Vacuum extraction compared with forceps delivery at Ilorin University Teaching Hospital, Nigeria. West Afr J Med 10:127, 1991.

Ballas S, Toaff R: Hyperextension of the fetal head in breech presentation: Radiological evaluation and significance. Br J Obstet Gynaecol 83:201, 1976.

Benedetti TJ, Gabbe SG: Shoulder dystocia: Complication of fetal macrosomia and prolonged second stage of labor with midpelvic delivery. Obstet Gynecol 52:526, 1978.

Benson RC, Shubeck F, Deutschberger J, et al: Fetal heart rate as a predictor of fetal distress, a report from the Collaborative Project. Obstet Gynecol 35:529, 1968.

Block JC, Kallenberger DA, et al: In utero meconium aspiration by the baboon fetus. Obstet Gynecol 57:37, 1987.

Bocking AD, Harding R: Effects of reduced uterine blood flow on accelerations and decelerations in heart rate of fetal sheep. Am J Obstet Gynecol 154:329, 1986.

Boehm FH, Slayer SF: Improved outcome of twice weekly nonstress testing. Obstet Gynecol 67:566, 1986.

Brady JP, Goldman SL: Management of meconium aspiration syndrome. *In* Thibault DW, Gregory GA (Eds): Neonatal Pulmonary Care. Norwalk, CT, Appleton-Century-Crofts, 1986.

Brenner WE, Bruce RD, Hendricks CH: The characteristics and perils of breech presentation. Am J Obstet Gynecol 118:700, 1974.

Brown BL, Gleicher N: Intrauterine meconium aspiration. Obstet Gynecol 57:26, 1981.

Carson BJ, Cogney RW, et al: Combined obstetric and pediatric approach to prevent meconium aspiration syndrome. Am J Obstet Gynecol 126:712, 1976.

Cibils LA: Clinical significance of FHR patterns during labor. Am J Obstet Gynecol 123:473, 1975.

Collea JV, Rabin SC, Weghorst GR, Quilligan EJ: The randomized management of the frank breech presentation: Vaginal delivery vs. cesarean section. Trans Pacific Coast Obstet Gynecol Soc 45:88–97, 1978.

Collea JV, Chien C, Quilligan EJ: The randomized management of term frank breech presentation: A study of 208 cases. Am J Obstet Gynecol 137:235, 1980.

Committee on Obstetrics: Maternal and Fetal Medicine 59: Obstetric Forceps. Washington, DC, American College of Obstetricians and Gynecologists, 1988.

Croughan-Minihane MS, Petitti DB, Gordis L, Golditch I: Morbidity among breech infants according to method of delivery. Obstet Gynecol 75:821, 1990.

Dalton KJ, Dawes GS: The autonomic nervous system and FHR variability. Am J Obstet Gynecol 146:456, 1983.

Davis RO, Philips JB, et al: Fetal meconium aspiration syndrome occurring despite airway management considered appropriate. Am J Obstet Gynecol 151:731, 1985.

Dawe GS, Fox HE, Leduc BM, et al: Respiratory movements and rapid eye movement sleep in the foetal lamb. J Physiol 220:119, 1972.

Dierker LJ, Rosen MG, Thompson K, Lynn P: Midforceps deliveries: Long-term outcome of infants. Am J Obstet Gynecol 154:764, 1986.

Emmanouilides GC, Townsend DE: Effects of single umbilical artery ligation in the lamb fetus. Pediatrics 42:919, 1968.

Fee SC, Malee K, Deddish R, et al: Severe acidosis and subsequent neurologic status. Am J Obstet Gynecol 162:802, 1990.

Friedman EA: Midforceps delivery: No? Clin Obstet Gynecol 30:90, 1987.

Friedman EA, Sachtleben MR, Bresky PA: Dysfunctional labor: XII. Long term effects on infant. Am J Obstet Gynecol 127:779, 1977.

Garcia-Alix A, Perlman JM, Amon E: Catecholamine levels and associated cardiovascular responses in infants with meconium-stained amniotic fluid. Eur J Pediatr 151:855, 1992.

Gimovsky ML, Paul RH: Singleton breech presentation in labor: Experience in 1980. Am J Obstet Gynecol 143:733, 1982.

Golde SH, Montoro M: The role of nonstress tests, fetal biophysical profile and contraction stress test in the outpatient management of insulin requiring diabetic pregnancies. Am J Obstet Gynecol 148:269, 1984.

Gonik B, Allen R, Sorab J: Objective evaluation of the shoulder dystocia phenomenon: Effect of maternal pelvic orientation on force reduction. Obstet Gynecol 74:44, 1989.

Gonik B, Stringer CA, Held B: An alternate maneuver for management of shoulder dystocia. Am J Obstet Gynecol 145:882, 1983.

Gould SJ, Smith JF: Spinal cord transection, cerebral ischaemic and brain-stem injury in a baby following a Kielland's forceps rotation. Neuropathol Appl Neurobiol 10:151, 1984.

Gregory GA, Gooding CA, Phibbs RH, Tooley WH: Meconium aspiration in infants: A prospective study. J Pediatr 85:848, 1974.

Hagadorn-Freathy AS, Yeomans ER, Hankins GD: Validation of the 1988 ACOG forceps classification system. Obstet Gynecol 77:356, 1991.

Hammerman C, Komar K, Abu-Khudair H: Hypoxic vs septic pulmonary hypertension. Am J Dis Child 142:319, 1988.

Hon EH: The electronic evaluation of the FHR. Am J Obstet Gynecol 75:1215, 1958.

Hon EH: Instrumentation of FHR and electrocardiography: II. A vaginal electrode. Am J Obstet Gynecol 86:772, 1963.

Hughey MJ, McElin TW: Forceps operations in perspective: I. Midforceps rotation operations. J Reprod Med 20:253, 1978.

James LS, Morishima HO: Mechanism of late deceleration of the FHR. Am J Obstet Gynecol 113:578, 1972.

Jeng CJ, Lee JF, Wang KG, et al: Decreased amniotic fluid index in term pregnancy: Clinical significance. J Reprod Med 37:789, 1992.

Johnson JWC, Riley W: Cord blood gas studies: A survey. Clin Obstet Gynecol 36:99, 1993.

Kariniemi V, Harrela M: Significance of meconium staining of the amniotic fluid. J Perinat Med 18:345, 1990.

Kaupilla O: The perinatal mortality in breech deliveries and observations on affecting factors: A retrospective study of 2227 cases. Acta Obstet Gynecol Scand 39:1, 1975.

Keller JD, Lopez-Zeno JA, Dooley SL, Socol ML: Shoulder dystocia and birth trauma in gestational diabetes: A five-year experience. Am J Obstet Gynecol 165(4 Pt 1):928, 1991.

King CR, Prescott G, Pernoll M: Significance of meconium in midtrimester diagnostic amniocenteses. Am J Obstet Gynecol 132:667, 1978.

Krebs HB, Petres RE, Dunn LJ: Intrapartum FHR monitoring: Association of meconium with abnormal FHR patterns. Am J Obstet Gynecol 137:936, 1980.

Kubli F, Ruttgers H, Haller U, et al: Observations on heart rate and pH in the human fetus during labor. Am J Obstet Gynecol 104:1190, 1969.

Locus P, Yeomans E, Crosby U: Efficacy of bulb versus DeLee suction at deliveries complicated by meconium stained amniotic fluid [see comments]. Am J Perinatol 7:87, 1990.

Lopez A, Bildfell R: Pulmonary inflammation associated with aspirated meconium and epithelial cells in calves. Vet Pathol 29:104, 1992.

Low JA, Simpson LL, Tonni G, Chamberlain S: Limitations in the clinical prediction of intrapartum fetal asphyxia. Am J Obstet Gynecol 172:801, 1995.

Lurie S, Ben-Arie A, Hagay Z: The ABC of shoulder dystocia management. Asia Oceania J Obstet Gynaecol 20:195, 1994.

Luthy DA, Shy KK: A randomized trial of electronic fetal monitoring in preterm labor. Obstet Gynecol 69:687, 1987.

Mahomed K, Nyoni R, Masona D: Meconium staining of the liquor in a low-risk population. Paediatr Perinat Epidemiol 8:292, 1994.

Miller FC, Sacks DA, Yeh SY: Significance of meconium during labor. Am J Obstet Gynecol 122:573, 1975.

Morgan HS, Kane SH: An analysis of 16,327 breech births. JAMA 187:262, 1964.

Morrison JC, Sanders JR, Magann EF, Wiser WL: The diagnosis and management of dystocia of the shoulder. Surg Gynecol Obstet 175:515, 1992.

Murata Y, Martin CB: Fetal heart rate accelerations and late decelerations during the course of intrauterine death in chronically catheterized rhesus monkeys. Am J Obstet Gynecol 144:218, 1982.

Murphy JD, Vawter GF, Reid LM: Pulmonary vascular disease in fatal meconium aspiration. J Pediatr 104:758, 1984.

Myers RE, Mueller-Huebach E: Predictability of the state of fetal oxygenation from a quantitative analysis of the components of late deceleration. Am J Obstet Gynecol 115:1083, 1973.

Nathan L, Leveno KJ, Carmody TJ 3rd, et al: Meconium: A 1990s perspective on an old obstetric hazard. Obstet Gynecol 83:329, 1994.

Neilson JP: EFM alone vs intermittent auscultation in labour. *In* Enkin MW, Keirse MJNC, Renfrew MJ, Neilson JP (Eds): Pregnancy and Childbirth Module. Cochrane Database of Systematic Reviews: Review No. 03298, 4 May 1994. Oxford, Cochrane Updates on Disk, Update Software, 1994, Disk Issue 1.

Nocon JJ, McKenzie DK, Thomas LJ, Hansell RS: Shoulder dystocia: An analysis of risks and obstetric maneuvers. Am J Obstet Gynecol 168(6 Pt 1):1732, 1993.

O'Leary JA: Cephalic replacement for shoulder dystocia: Present status and future role of the Zavanelli maneuver. Obstet Gynecol 82:847, 1993.

O'Leary JA, Cuva A: Abdominal rescue after failed cephalic replacement. Obstet Gynecol 80(3 Pt 2):514, 1992.

Paul RH, Miller FC: Antenatal FHR monitoring. Clin Obstet Gynecol 21:375, 1978.

Piper EB, Bachman C: The prevention of fetal injuries in breech delivery. JAMA 92:217, 1929.

Ramin SM, Gilstrap LC III, Leveno KJ, et al: Umbilical artery acid-base status in the preterm infant. Obstet Gynecol 74:256, 1989.

Ray M, Freeman R: Clinical experience with the oxytocin challenge test. Am J Obstet Gynecol 114:1, 1972.

Richey SD, Ramin SM, Bawdon RE, et al: Markers of acute and chronic asphyxia in infants with meconium-stained amniotic fluid. Am J Obstet Gynecol 172(4 Pt 1):1212, 1995.

Rochard F, Schifrin BS: Nonstressed FHR monitoring in the antepartum period. Am J Obstet Gynecol 126:699, 1976.

Ruth VJ, Raivio KO: Perinatal brain damage: Predictive value of metabolic acidosis and the Apgar score. BMJ 297:24, 1988.

Saling E: Fetal and Neonatal Hypoxia in Relation to Clinical Obstetric Practice. London, Deward Arnold, 1968.

Saling E, Hartung M: Analyses of tractive forces during the application of vacuum extraction. J Perinat Med 1:245, 1973.

Schifrin BS: More Exercises in Fetal Monitoring. St Louis, Mosby-Year Book, 1993.

Starks GC: Correlation of meconium-stained amniotic fluid early intrapartum fetal pH and Apgar scores as predictors of perinatal outcome. Obstet Gynecol 56:604, 1980.

Suresh GK, Sarkar S: Delivery room management of infants born through thin meconium stained liquor. Indian J Pediatr 31:1177, 1994.

Sykes GS, Molloy PM, Johnson P, et al: Do Apgar scores indicate asphyxia? Lancet 1:494, 1982.

Tank ES, Davis R, Holt JF, et al: Mechanisms of trauma during breech delivery. Obstet Gynecol 38:761, 1971.

Thacker SB, Berkelman RL: Assessing the diagnostic accuracy and efficiency of selected antepartum fetal surveillance techniques. Obstet Gynecol Surv 41:121, 1986.

Thiery M: Obsteric vacuum extraction. Obstet Gynecol Annu 14:73, 1985.

Trimmer KJ, Gilstrap LC 3d: "Meconiumcrit" and birth asphyxia. Am J Obstet Gynecol 165(4 Pt 1):1010, 1991.

Turbeville DF, McCaffree MA, Block MF, Krous HF: In utero distal pulmonary meconium aspiration. South Med J 72:535, 1979.

Walker J: Fetal anoxia. Obstet Gynecol Br Emp 61:162, 1954.

Winkler CL, Hauth JC, Tucker JM, et al: Neonatal complications at term as related to the degree of umbilical artery acidemia. Am J Obstet Gynecol 164:637, 1991.

Yeomans ER, Hauth JC, Gilstrap LC III, et al: Umbilical cord pH, Pco$_2$ and bicarbonate following uncomplicated term vaginal deliveries. Am J Obstet Gynecol 151:798, 1985.

Yoder BA: Meconium-stained amniotic fluid and respiratory complications: Impact of selective tracheal suction. Obstet Gynecol 83:77, 1994.

CHAPTER 16

Anesthesia and Analgesia: Issues for the Fetus and Newborn

Robert H. Friesen

OBSTETRIC ANESTHESIA AND ANALGESIA

Obstetric anesthesia and analgesia is a unique and challenging field in which the goals of maternal safety and comfort during childbirth are shared with that of preserving the well-being of the fetus and newborn. Drugs and methods of administration in the mother may have direct or indirect effects on the baby. Current aspects of these issues are discussed in this chapter.

Intravenous Analgesia and Sedation

Most sedative and narcotic drugs cross the placenta readily, primarily by passive diffusion, and can cause dose-related neonatal depression. Barbiturates are rarely used for maternal sedation for this reason. Diazepam has minimal effects on the newborn when small doses are given to the mother. Although meperidine is associated with less neonatal respiratory depression than morphine (Way et al, 1965) and remains the most commonly used intravenous narcotic in obstetrics, observable effects on neonatal breathing patterns do occur with its use (Hamza et al, 1992). The timing of meperidine administration in relation to delivery of the newborn is important, with the greatest neonatal depression being observed 2 to 3 hours after maternal intravenous injection (Kuhnert et al, 1979). Preterm newborns are more easily depressed by maternal sedatives and narcotics than are term newborns.

Regional Analgesia and Anesthesia

Regional analgesia and anesthesia with local anesthetics are widely used during labor and delivery. Such techniques provide the mother with excellent pain relief without sedation and exert minimal effects on the fetus and newborn. Several regional blocks can be used, including lumbar epidural, subarachnoid (spinal), caudal epidural, pudendal, and paracervical. Recently, epidural narcotic analgesia was introduced for labor and delivery. When regional analgesia and anesthesia techniques are used, important issues that affect the status of the fetus and newborn must be considered.

Maternal Hypotension

Sympathetic blockade, with accompanying maternal hypotension and decreased uteroplacental blood flow, is the most common undesired side effect of lumbar epidural and subarachnoid anesthesia. Maternal hypotension can usually be prevented by prior intravenous administration of 15 to 20 mL/kg of dextrose-free balanced salt solution and, for epidural block, incremental injection of local anes-

thetic solutions at a rate not exceeding 5 mL/30 seconds (Shnider and Levinson, 1986). Aortocaval compression by the gravid uterus causes supine maternal hypotension and reduces uterine arterial and venous blood flow (Bieniarz et al, 1968; Kerr et al, 1964), so the mother should be kept in the lateral position, or left uterine displacement (usually by means of a wedge under the right hip) should be used. If hypotension develops, the mother should receive oxygen and be placed in a slight Trendelenburg position. Ephedrine, 5 to 15 mg intravenously, is the drug of choice for treatment of persistent maternal hypotension. Drugs that are direct alpha-adrenergic agonists, such as phenylephrine and epinephrine, should not be used to treat maternal hypotension because they cause uterine vasoconstriction and reduction in uteroplacental blood flow. Treatment of maternal hypotension is summarized in Table 16-1.

Epidural Local Anesthetics

When used for uncomplicated epidural anesthesia for labor and delivery, lidocaine, bupivacaine, and chloroprocaine do not exert adverse effects on neonatal Apgar scores or acid-base status (Abboud et al, 1982, 1983; Kangas-Saarela et al, 1989). Lidocaine has been associated with neurobehavioral impairment of the newborn (Kuhnert et al, 1984), but those effects were subtle and have not been consistently observed (Abboud et al, 1982, 1983; Loftus et al, 1991). Although baseline fetal heart rate and beat-to-beat variability of fetal heart rate are not affected, late deceleration patterns of fetal heart rate during labor appear to be more common during epidural anesthesia with bupivacaine (Abboud et al, 1982). In the absence of labor, epidural local anesthetics do not affect fetal heart rate or uteroplacental blood flow when administered for elective cesarean section (Alahuhta et al, 1991; Loftus et al, 1991).

If there is accidental maternal vascular injection, all local anesthetics can cause central nervous system depression and seizures. Amide local anesthetics cause myocardial depression, with bupivacaine being more cardiotoxic than

---

TABLE 16-1

Treatment of Maternal Hypotension

1. Administer 15 to 20 mL/kg balanced salt solution intravenously (IV)
2. Left uterine displacement for aortocaval decompression
3. Administer oxygen by face mask
4. Place patient in slight Trendelenburg position
5. Administer ephedrine 5–15 mg IV

lidocaine (Clarkson and Hondeghem, 1985). Fetal plasma levels of local anesthetics are directly related to maternal plasma levels.

Epidural and Intrathecal Narcotics

Narcotics can be added to lumbar epidural local anesthetic blocks for enhanced analgesia during labor and cesarean section. Studies of epidural morphine, fentanyl, and sufentanil have demonstrated an absence of deleterious effects on uteroplacental blood flow (Alahuhta et al, 1993), fetal heart rate (Viscomi et al, 1990), and neonatal condition (Benlabed et al, 1990; Cohen et al, 1987; Hughes et al, 1984). Similarly, intrathecal narcotics appear to enhance maternal analgesia without significant fetal or neonatal effects (Abouleish et al, 1988; Cohen et al, 1993; Hunt et al, 1989.).

Paracervical Block

The paracervical block, which provides analgesia during the first stage of labor, is associated with fetal anesthetic toxicity, manifested by a high incidence of bradycardia and acidosis. When fetal bradycardia occurs a few minutes after administration of the block, fetal blood levels of local anesthetic are high and are significantly greater than maternal levels (Asling et al, 1970). This implies rapid uptake of the local anesthetic by the uterine artery, located near the injection site. Duration of bradycardia is up to 15 minutes (Asling et al, 1970) and is probably limited by transfer of the local anesthetic across the placenta to the mother (Morishima and Adamsons, 1967). Neonatal depression can occur if the neonatal blood level is still elevated. If feasible, delay of delivery for 30 to 60 minutes following local anesthetic–related fetal bradycardia may reduce this risk (Morishima and Adamsons, 1967).

Similar fetal and neonatal depression can occur after accidental injection of local anesthetic into the fetal head, which can occur during attempted paracervical, pudendal, and caudal blocks.

General Anesthesia

General anesthesia is often preferred for emergency cesarean section for fetal distress because the risk of maternal hypotension is less than during regional anesthesia. To minimize the effects of anesthetic drugs on the fetus, anesthesia is not induced until the patient is prepped and draped and the surgeon is ready to make the incision.

Thiopental is the usual choice for induction of anesthesia. It crosses the placenta readily but has minimal effect on the newborn if the mother's dose is less than 4 mg/kg (Kosaka et al, 1969). Propofol, a newer anesthetic induction agent, does not adversely affect the fetus (Alon et al, 1993) but is associated with neonatal neurobehavioral depression (Celleno et al, 1989). Muscle relaxants, used to facilitate tracheal intubation and to relax abdominal muscles, have only poor placental transfer and, thus, do not generally affect the fetus. Narcotics are not administered until the umbilical cord is clamped.

Anesthetic concentrations of inhalation anesthetics can cause neonatal depression and uterine relaxation. However, subanesthetic concentrations of nitrous oxide and the potent inhalation anesthetics are not associated with such problems and can be safely administered to the mother during the few minutes after thiopental induction prior to delivery of the baby (Shnider and Levinson, 1986).

Controlled ventilation is necessary to maintain adequate maternal oxygenation during general anesthesia for cesarean section. However, it is imperative to avoid hyperventilation of the mother before delivery of the baby. Hypocapnia decreases uterine and umbilical blood flow, increases the affinity of maternal hemoglobin for oxygen, and may be associated with fetal hypoxemia and acidosis (Levinson et al, 1974).

NEONATAL ANESTHESIA AND ANALGESIA

Neonatal anesthesia has progressed remarkably during the past 20 years. Great strides have been made in the development of monitoring devices, the understanding of neonatal physiology, and the medical and surgical treatment of diseases of the newborn. The number of pediatric anesthesiologists has increased 10-fold, and anesthesia for the newborn has become notably safer.

Response to Pain

Provision of adequate anesthesia and analgesia to the newborn has been hampered by long-held misconceptions regarding the newborn's neurophysiologic maturity and by a paucity of studies documenting the newborn's response to pain. Although the newborn does display functional immaturity of several organ systems, including the neurologic system, there is no question that the newborn perceives and reacts appropriately to pain, even at 26 weeks of conceptual age (Dargassies, 1977). Acceptance of this fact and confidence in the ability to safely prevent pain have been slow to develop. However, the newborn's response to pain and the consequences of that response are better documented than they were during the early years of neonatal anesthesia (Anand and Hickey, 1987; Porter, 1989).

Major Surgery

It has become increasingly evident that the paralyzed, but inadequately anesthetized, newborn displays a marked stress response to major surgical procedures, measurable by cardiovascular, hormonal, and metabolic parameters. Yaster (1987) studied newborns undergoing major surgical operations. Those patients who were inadequately anesthetized (<10 μg/kg fentanyl) responded to surgical stimuli with significant increases in heart rate and systolic blood pressure.

Anand and colleagues (1987) followed the intraoperative and postoperative hormonal and metabolic responses of two groups of preterm newborns undergoing ligation of patent ductus arteriosus. One group was lightly anesthetized with 50% nitrous oxide and immobilized with a muscle relaxant. This group displayed a major stress response to surgery (Fig. 16-1), characterized by significant elevations of plasma levels of catecholamines, corticosteroids,

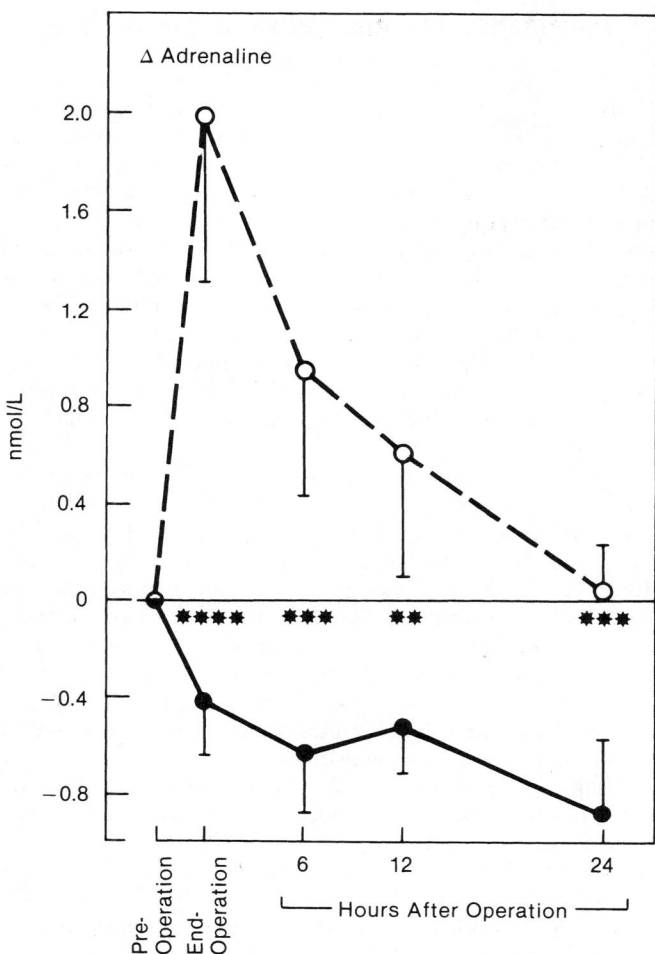

FIGURE 16–1. The stress response of the inadequately anesthetized preterm newborn during major surgery can be prevented by general anesthesia with fentanyl. (○, 50% N_2O; ●, 50% N_2O + 10 μg/kg fentanyl; all asterisks, statistically significant differences.) (Reprinted with permission from Anand KJS, Sippell WG, Aynsley-Green A: Randomised trial of fentanyl anaesthesia in preterm babies undergoing surgery: Effects on the stress response. Lancet 1:243–248, 1987.)

and glucagon. Metabolically, this group exhibited a marked and sustained hyperglycemia and an intraoperative increase and postoperative decrease in blood levels of gluconeogenic substrates. A catabolic response, as indicated by an increase in the urinary 3-methylhistidine/creatinine ratio, was evident on the 2nd and 3rd postoperative days. Administration of intravenous fentanyl, 10 μg/kg, to a second group of similar patients prevented these changes and reduced the number of postoperative clinical complications.

Circumcision and Minor Procedures

The stress response of newborns undergoing minor surgical procedures during inadequate anesthesia can also be deleterious. Williamson and Williamson (1983) and Maxwell and associates (1987) studied two groups of awake newborns undergoing circumcision. The patients who were not provided analgesia displayed prolonged crying, increased

heart rate and blood pressure, and decreased transcutaneous P_{O_2} or oxygen saturation. These changes were significantly less in similar groups of newborns who underwent dorsal penile nerve block with lidocaine before circumcision. Use of dorsal penile nerve block also attenuated the behavioral disruptions observed following circumcision without local anesthesia (Dixon et al, 1984). Acetaminophen alone provided inadequate analgesia for circumcision (Howard et al, 1994). Despite this evidence, most physicians who perform newborn circumcisions do not use appropriate analgesia (Wellington and Rieder, 1993), a situation that can be reversed by educational programs (Ryan and Finer, 1994).

Chest tube insertion, cutdown for vascular access, and other procedures performed in the neonatal intensive care unit (NICU), must be assumed to trigger responses similar to those of circumcision. Accordingly, adequate intravenous or local analgesia should be used for such procedures. For example, narcotic analgesia was shown to reduce distress and the duration of hypoxemia associated with tracheal suctioning and other routine care procedures in the NICU (Pokela, 1994). On the other hand, the unchecked use of analgesia or sedation for every noxious stimulus in the NICU is probably not warranted either; overdosage and oversedation are genuine hazards. There is some evidence that analgesic creams applied to the penis under an occlusive dressing 60 to 80 minutes before circumcision are safe and may be effective in reducing pain (Taddio et al, 1997).

Pulmonary Hypertension and Stress

Although the newborn's pulmonary vascular resistance decreases at birth, it does not decrease to normal childhood levels during the neonatal period. Pulmonary hypertension and fluctuations in pulmonary vascular resistance occur in several diseases of the newborn. In patients with these diseases, a variety of noxious stimuli can cause abrupt increases in pulmonary vascular resistance and clinical deterioration. Chest physiotherapy and tracheal suctioning of preterm newborns with respiratory distress syndrome was associated with increased plasma catecholamines, a hormonal stress response that was diminished by sedation with phenobarbital (Greisen et al, 1985). Fentanyl, 25 μg/kg, was shown to significantly attenuate the increases in pulmonary artery pressure and pulmonary vascular resistance as well as other circulatory stress responses that accompanied tracheal suctioning in infants after repair of congenital heart defects (Hickey et al, 1985). A similar stabilizing effect on the pulmonary vasculature was achieved by continuing fentanyl anesthesia during the postoperative period in critically ill newborns with congenital diaphragmatic hernia (Vacanti et al, 1984). Thus, anesthetic doses of fentanyl significantly blunt the pulmonary hemodynamic response to stressful stimuli and may be beneficial in diseases in which pulmonary hypertension is a problem.

Tracheal Intubation and Intracranial Pressure

Although the perianesthetic period does not appear to be one of greater risk for the development of intracranial hemorrhage in preterm newborns (Friesen et al, 1987a; Strange et al, 1985), specific procedures associated with fluctuations of cerebral blood flow and intracranial pressure may occur during that time. One such procedure is tracheal intubation. In a study of preterm newborns requiring anesthesia for surgical operations, anterior fontanel pressure was observed to increase markedly during laryngoscopy and intubation in awake patients (Friesen et al, 1987b). Those patients exhibited a vigorous motor response, in the form of coughing and sustained forced expiratory effort, to intubation. In contrast, newborns who were paralyzed with pancuronium and anesthetized before laryngoscopy and intubation did not have significant changes in anterior fontanel pressure (Fig. 16–2). This situation is analogous to that of a study by Perlman and colleagues (1985) of preterm newborns with respiratory distress syndrome who required mechanical ventilation. Wide fluctuations in the velocity of cerebral blood flow, presumably caused by fluctuations in intrathoracic pressure, were observed in newborns breathing out of synchrony with their ventilators. Muscle relaxation with pancuronium eliminated the fluctuations in the cerebral blood flow and reduced the incidence and severity of intracranial hemorrhage.

These observations have led the author to recommend that, during anesthetic management of preterm newborns, tracheal intubation should be performed only after paralysis and anesthesia have been induced, unless a specific indication for intubation with the patient awake (such as in the case of a moribund or unstable patient, a gastric or small bowel obstruction, or a difficult airway) exists. A similar recommendation regarding intubation in the NICU or delivery room is probably not warranted because patients in those settings usually require intubation during periods of clinical deterioration or resuscitation. However, neonatologists should be aware of the effects of tracheal intubation in the awake patient and should consider the use of pancuronium and mask ventilation before intubation in selected patients at greatest risk for intracranial hemorrhage.

Anesthetics and Analgesics in Current Use
General Anesthetics

Early in the development of pediatric anesthesia, anesthetizing a preterm newborn was considered to be an uncommon emergency procedure entailing high risk. Hypovolemia, sepsis, respiratory failure, and cardiovascular immaturity frequently resulted in hypotension during anesthesia. Such problems, combined with the misconception that newborns did not sense pain well, created a setting in which anesthesiologists provided cardiovascular stability and immobility by using muscle relaxants and minimal or no anesthetic. Clinical research has since established that adequate anesthesia can be provided to preterm and term newborns without causing significant cardiovascular depression.

Nitrous oxide was, because of its cardiovascular stability, the most commonly used anesthetic in newborns for many years. However, it is a weak inhalation anesthetic that fails to prevent the stress response to surgery (Anand et al, 1987). Furthermore, its use is contraindicated in many commonly encountered disease states of the newborn, including conditions requiring high amounts of oxygen, pneumothorax, pulmonary interstitial emphysema, necrotizing enterocolitis, and bowel obstruction or perforation. When use of nitrous oxide is not contraindicated, its role is limited to supplementing other anesthetics.

Fentanyl, an intravenously administered synthetic narcotic, has been extensively studied as a neonatal anesthetic. A dose of 10 µg/kg in preterm newborns prevents the hemodynamic response to surgical stimuli for 75 minutes (Yaster, 1987) and, when added to 50% nitrous oxide, blocks the hormonal and metabolic stress response to surgery (Anand et al, 1987). Even at high doses of 30 to 50 µg/kg, cardiovascular effects of fentanyl are minimal (Robinson and Gregory, 1981). At anesthetic doses, fentanyl is a profound ventilatory depressant, and postopera-

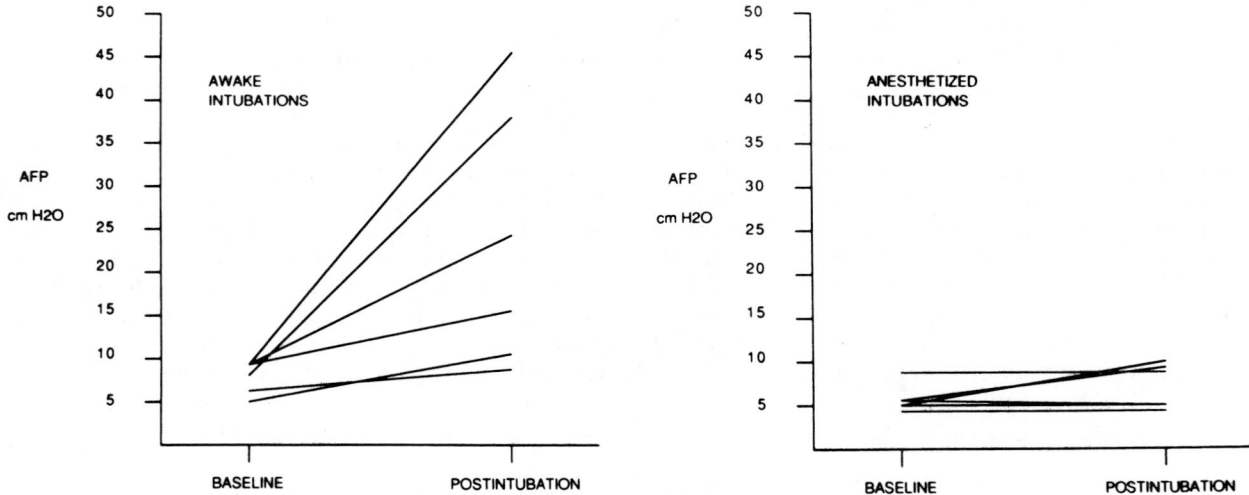

FIGURE 16–2. The marked increase in anterior fontanel pressure during tracheal intubation of the awake preterm neonate can be prevented by general anesthesia and muscle relaxation. (Reprinted with permission from the International Anesthesia Research Society from Friesen RH, Honda AT, Thieme RE: Changes in anterior fontanel pressure in preterm neonates during tracheal intubation. Anesth Analg 66:874–878, 1987.)

tive mechanical ventilation is required. Because it is slowly eliminated by the newborn (Collins et al, 1985; Koehntop et al, 1986), its effects are prolonged.

The concentration of an inhalation anesthetic required to prevent a motor response to painful stimulation in 50% of subjects is known as its minimum alveolar concentration. The minimum alveolar concentrations of the inhalational anesthetics for the newborn are somewhat lower than those of other pediatric age groups (Cameron et al, 1984; LeDez and Lerman, 1987; Lerman et al, 1983). Cardiovascular depression can be a problem in newborns receiving these anesthetics. Even at concentrations at or below the minimum alveolar concentration, systolic blood pressure decreases by 25% to 30% (Friesen and Henry, 1986; LeDez and Lerman, 1987; Lerman et al, 1983). This sensitivity to the cardiovascular depressant effects of inhalation anesthetics is age related (Fig. 16–3) (Cook et al, 1981; Krane and Su, 1987; Rao et al, 1986) and is probably due to the immaturity of the neonatal myocardium, which has fewer contractile elements, immature sympathetic innervation, lower norepinephrine stores, and poorer compliance than

the myocardium of the adult (Friedman, 1972). This cardiovascular depression can be minimized by the administration of atropine (Friesen and Lichtor, 1982) and intravenous fluids or by using lower doses of halothane or isoflurane combined with a low dose of fentanyl. Inhalation anesthetics are eliminated rapidly and their effects are short lived after administration ceases.

The newborn's requirement for the intravenous anesthetic ketamine has not been extensively studied. An induction dose of 2 mg/kg is associated with cardiovascular stability (Friesen and Henry, 1986) and does not appear to increase intracranial pressure in preterm newborns (Friesen et al, 1987c) as it does in adults. Transient ventilatory depression follows ketamine administration.

Local Anesthetics

Traditional dose limitations for local infiltration and nerve blocks in children and adults are 4 mg/kg of lidocaine solution or, because of delayed absorption and slower increase in plasma concentration, 7 mg/kg of lidocaine mixed with epinephrine. Although specific dose recommendations for newborns are not available, greater caution is indicated during administration of local anesthetics. Newborns have low serum concentrations of alpha$_1$ acid glycoprotein, the plasma protein that binds local anesthetics (LeDez et al, 1986). The resulting increased free fraction of local anesthetics and their prolonged elimination by the newborn (LeDez et al, 1987) may place newborn patients at greater risk of local anesthetic toxicity. Nevertheless, dorsal penile nerve block for neonatal circumcision results in safe lidocaine plasma levels (Maxwell et al, 1987), and even conservative dosage guidelines allow satisfactory local anesthesia for vascular cutdown and chest tube insertion. Such uses should be encouraged. Topical cutaneous application of a eutectic mixture of prilocaine and lidocaine provides effective analgesia for venous cannulation and similar procedures in children (Halperin et al, 1989; Soliman et al, 1988), but it has not been evaluated in newborns.

Parenteral Analgesics

Intravenous fentanyl, 1 to 2 μg/kg, or morphine, 0.05 to 0.1 mg/kg, is a useful analgesic for pain that does not require general or local anesthesia. These medications can enjoy wide application in the NICU. Narcotics have minimal direct cardiovascular effects, but they are potent ventilatory depressants and, like most drugs, have prolonged elimination phases in the newborn (Collins et al, 1985; Koehntop et al, 1986; Lynn and Slattery, 1987). Appropriate monitoring and vigilance for cumulative effects on ventilation and consciousness should be practiced. Usually, doses should not be repeated for several hours. When fentanyl is administered for continuous sedation over a prolonged period, as is done during extracorporeal membrane oxygenation, development of tolerance and dependence can be clinical problems (Arnold et al, 1990).

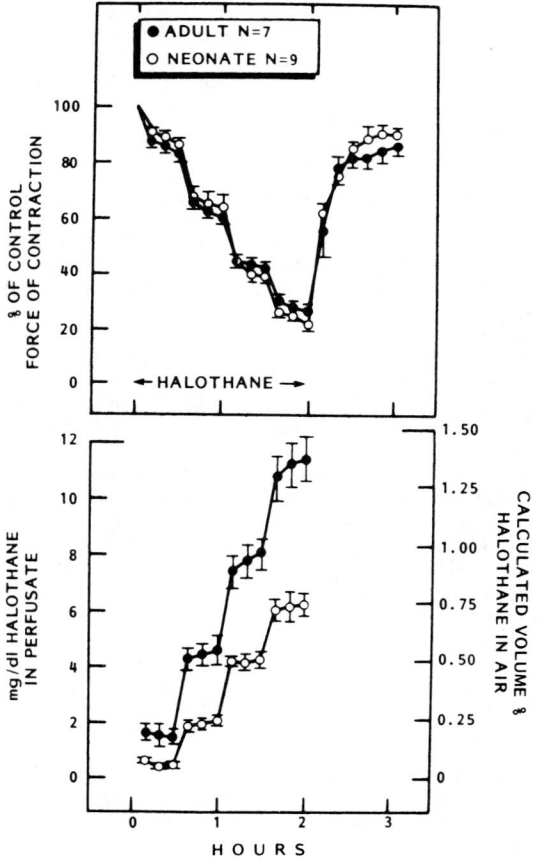

FIGURE 16–3. The newborn mammal is far more sensitive to the myocardial depressant effects of inhalation anesthetics than is the mature mammal. In this study, the concentration of halothane (lower graph) required to depress atrial contractility (upper graph) in the newborn rat was only half that required in the adult. (From Rao CC, Boyer MS, Krishna G, Paradise RR: Increased sensitivity of the isometric contraction of the neonatal isolated rat atria to halothane, isoflurane, and enflurane. Anesthesiology 64:13–18, 1986.)

REFERENCES

Abboud TK, Khoo SS, Miller F, et al: Maternal, fetal, and neonatal responses after epidural anesthesia with bupivacaine, 2-chloroprocaine, or lidocaine. Anesth Analg 61:638–644, 1982.

Abboud TK, Kim KC, Noueihed R, et al: Epidural bupivacaine, chloro-procaine, or lidocaine for cesarean section—maternal and neonatal effects. Anesth Analg 62:914–919, 1983.

Abouleish E, Rawal N, Fallon K, Hernandez D: Combined intrathecal morphine and bupivacaine for cesarean section. Anesth Analg 67:370–374, 1988.

Alahuhta S, Rasanen J, Jouppila R, et al: Effects of extradural bupivacaine with adrenaline for caesarean section on uteroplacental and fetal circulation. Br J Anaesth 67:678–682, 1991.

Alahuhta S, Rasanen J, Jouppila P, et al: Epidural sufentanil and bupiva-caine for labor analgesia and Doppler velocimetry of the umbilical and uterine arteries. Anesthesiology 78:231–236, 1993.

Alon E, Ball RH, Gillie MH, et al: Effects of propofol and thiopental on maternal and fetal cardiovascular and acid-base variables in the preg-nant ewe. Anesthesiology 78:562–576, 1993.

Anand KJS, Hickey PR: Pain and its effects in the human neonate and fetus. N Engl J Med 317:1321–1329, 1987.

Anand KJS, Sippell WG, Aynsley-Green A: Randomised trial of fentanyl anaesthesia in preterm babies undergoing surgery: Effects on the stress response. Lancet 1:243–248, 1987.

Arnold JH, Truog RD, Orav EJ, et al: Tolerance and dependence in neonates sedated with fentanyl during extracorporeal membrane oxy-genation. Anesthesiology 73:1136–1140, 1990.

Asling JH, Shnider SM, Margolis AJ, et al: Paracervical block anesthesia in obstetrics. II. Etiology of fetal bradycardia following paracervical block anesthesia. Am J Obstet Gynecol 107:626–634, 1970.

Benlabed M, Dreizzen E, Ecoffey C, et al: Neonatal patterns of breathing after cesarean section with or without epidural fentanyl. Anesthesiol-ogy 73:1110–1113, 1990.

Bieniarz J, Crottogini JJ, Curuchet E: Aortocaval compression by the uterus in the late human pregnancy. II. An arteriographic study. Am J Obstet Gynecol 100:203–217, 1968.

Cameron CB, Robinson S, Gregory GA: The minimum anesthetic concen-tration of isoflurane in children. Anesth Analg 63:418–420, 1984.

Celleno D, Capogna G, Tomassetti M, et al: Neurobehavioural effects of propofol on the neonate following elective caesarean section. Br J Anaesth 62:649–654, 1989.

Clarkson CW, Hondeghem LM: Mechanism for bupivacaine depression of cardiac conduction: Fast block of sodium channels during the action potential with slow recovery from block during diastole. Anesthesiol-ogy 62:396–405, 1985.

Cohen SE, Tan S, Albright GA, Halpern J: Epidural fentanyl/bupivacaine mixtures for obstetric analgesia. Anesthesiology 67:403–407, 1987.

Cohen SE, Cherry CM, Holbrook RH Jr, et al: Intrathecal sufentanil for labor analgesia—sensory changes, side effects, and fetal heart rate changes. Anesth Analg 77:1155–1160, 1993.

Collins C, Koren G, Crean P, et al: Fentanyl pharmacokinetics and hemodynamic effects in preterm infants during ligation of patent ductus arteriosus. Anesth Analg 64:1078–1080, 1985.

Cook DR, Brandom BW, Shiu G, Wolfson B: The inspired median effective dose, brain concentration at anesthesia, and cardiovascular index for halothane in young rats. Anesth Analg 60:182–185, 1981.

Dargassies SS: Neurological Development in the Full-Term and Prema-ture Neonate. Amsterdam, Excerpta Medica, 1977, pp 248–256.

Dixon S, Synder J, Holve R, Bromberger P: Behavioral effects of circum-cision with and without anesthesia. J Dev Behav Pediatr 5:246–250, 1984.

Friedman WF: The intrinsic physiologic properties of the developing heart. Prog Cardiovasc Dis 15:87–111, 1972.

Friesen RH, Henry DB: Cardiovascular changes in preterm neonates receiving isoflurane, halothane, fentanyl, and ketamine. Anesthesiology 64:238–242, 1986.

Friesen RH, Honda AT, Thieme RE: Perianesthetic intracranial hemor-rhage in preterm neonates. Anesthesiology 67:814–816, 1987a.

Friesen RH, Honda AT, Thieme RE: Changes in anterior fontanel pres-sure in preterm neonates during tracheal intubation. Anesth Analg 66:874–878, 1987b.

Friesen RH, Lichtor JL: Cardiovascular depression during halothane anesthesia in infants: A study of three induction techniques. Anesth Analg 61:42–45, 1982.

Friesen RH, Thieme RE, Honda AT, Morrison JE Jr: Changes in anterior fontanel pressure in preterm neonates receiving isoflurane, halothane, fentanyl, or ketamine. Anesth Analg 66:431–434, 1987c.

Greisen G, Frederiksen PS, Hertel J, Christensen NJ: Catecholamine

response to chest physiotherapy and endotracheal suctioning in pre-term infants. Acta Pediatr Scand 74:525–529, 1985.

Halperin DL, Koren G, Attias D, et al: Topical skin anesthesia for venous, subcutaneous drug reservoir and lumbar punctures in children. Pediat-rics 84:281–284, 1989.

Hamza J, Benlabed M, Orhant E, et al: Neonatal pattern of breathing during active and quiet sleep after maternal administration of meperi-dine. Pediatr Res 32:412–416, 1992.

Hickey PR, Hansen DD, Wessel DL, et al: Blunting of stress responses in the pulmonary circulation of infants by fentanyl. Anesth Analg 64:1137–1142, 1985.

Howard CR, Howard FM, Weitzman ML: Acetaminophen analgesia in neonatal circumcision: The effect on pain. Pediatrics 93:641–646, 1994.

Hughes SC, Rosen MA, Shnider SM, et al: Maternal and neonatal effects of epidural morphine for labor and delivery. Anesth Analg 63:319–324, 1984.

Hunt CO, Naulty JS, Bader AM, et al: Perioperative analgesia with subarachnoid fentanyl-bupivacaine for cesarean delivery. Anesthesiol-ogy 71:535–540, 1989.

Kangas-Saarela T, Jouppila R, Alahuhta S, et al: The effect of lumbar epidural analgesia on the neurobehavioural responses of newborn infants. Acta Anaesthesiol Scand 33:320–325, 1989.

Kerr MG, Scott DB, Samuel E: Studies of the inferior vena cava in late pregnancy. BMJ 1:532–533, 1964.

Koehntop DE, Rodman JH, Brundage DM, et al: Pharmacokinetics of fentanyl in neonates. Anesth Analg 65:227–232, 1986.

Kosaka Y, Takahashi T, Mark LC: Intravenous thiobarbiturate anesthesia for cesarean section. Anesthesiology 31:489–506, 1969.

Krane EJ, Su JY: Comparison of the effects of halothane on newborn and adult rabbit myocardium. Anesth Analg 66:1240–1244, 1987.

Kuhnert BR, Harrison MJ, Linn PL, Kuhnert PM: Effects of maternal epidural anesthesia on neonatal behavior. Anesth Analg 63:301–308, 1984.

Kuhnert BR, Kuhnert PM, Tu AL, Lin DCK: Meperidine and normeperi-dine levels following meperidine administration during labor. II. Fetus and neonate. Am J Obstet Gynecol 133:909–914, 1979.

LeDez KM, Lerman J: The minimum alveolar concentration (MAC) of isoflurane in preterm neonates. Anesthesiology 67:301–307, 1987.

LeDez KM, Strong A, Reider M, Burrows FA, Lerman J: Effect of age on the pharmacokinetics of intravenous lidocaine in pediatrics. Anesthesiology 67:A500, 1987.

LeDez KM, Swartz J, Strong A, Burrows FA, Lerman J: The effect of age on the serum concentration of alpha-1 acid glycoprotein in newborns, infants, and children. Anesthesiology 65:A421, 1986.

Lerman J, Robinson S, Willis MM, Gregory GA: Anesthetic requirements for halothane in young children 0–1 month and 1–6 months of age. Anesthesiology 59:421–424, 1983.

Levinson G, Shnider SM, deLorimier AA, Steffenson JL: Effects of maternal hyperventilation on uterine blood flow and fetal oxygenation and acid-base status. Anesthesiology 40:340–347, 1974.

Loftus JR, Holbrook RH, Cohen SE: Fetal heart rate after epidural lidocaine and bupivacaine for elective cesarean section. Anesthesiology 75:406–412, 1991.

Lynn AM, Slattery JT: Morphine pharmacokinetics in early infancy. Anes-thesiology 66:136–139, 1987.

Maxwell LG, Yaster M, Wetzel RC, Niebyl JR: Penile nerve block for newborn circumcision. Obstet Gynecol 70:415–418, 1987.

Morishima HO, Adamsons K: Placental clearance of mepivacaine follow-ing administration to the guinea pig fetus. Anesthesiology 28:343–348, 1967.

Perlman JM, Goodman S, Kreusser KL, Volpe JJ: Reduction in intraven-tricular hemorrhage by elimination of fluctuating cerebral blood-flow velocity in preterm infants with respiratory distress syndrome. N Engl J Med 312:1353–1357, 1985.

Pokela M: Pain relief can reduce hypoxemia in distressed neonates during routine treatment procedures. Pediatrics 93:379–383, 1994.

Porter F: Pain in the newborn. Clin Perinatol 16:549–564, 1989.

Rao CC, Boyer MS, Krishna G, Paradise RR: Increased sensitivity of the isometric contraction of the neonatal isolated rat atria to halothane, isoflurane, and enflurane. Anesthesiology 64:13–18, 1986.

Robinson S, Gregory GA: Fentanyl-air-oxygen anesthesia for ligation of patent ductus arteriosus in preterm infants. Anesth Analg 60:331–334, 1981.

Ryan CA, Finer NN: Changing attitudes and practices regarding local analgesia for newborn circumcision. Pediatrics 94:230–233, 1994.

Shnider SM, Levinson G: Obstetric anesthesia. *In* Miller RD (Ed): Anesthesia, 2nd ed. New York, Churchill Livingstone, 1986, pp 1681–1728.

Soliman IE, Broadman LM, Hannallah RS, McGill WA: Comparison of the analgesic effects of EMLA (eutectic mixture of local anesthetics) to intradermal lidocaine infiltration prior to venous cannulation in unpremedicated children. Anesthesiology 68:804–806, 1988.

Strange MJ, Myers G, Kirklin JK, et al: Surgical closure of patent ductus arteriosus does not increase the risk of intraventricular hemorrhage in the preterm infant. J Pediatr 107:602–604, 1985.

Taddio A, Stevens B, Craig K, et al: Efficacy and safety of lidocaine-prilocaine cream for pain during circumcision. N Engl J Med 336:1197–1201, 1997.

Vacanti JP, Crone RK, Murphy JD, et al: The pulmonary hemodynamic response to perioperative anesthesia in the treatment of high-risk infants with congenital diaphragmatic hernia. J Pediatr Surg 19:672–679, 1984.

Viscomi CM, Hood DD, Melone PJ, Eisenach JC: Fetal heart rate variability after epidural fentanyl during labor. Anesth Analg 71:679–683, 1990.

Way WL, Costley EC, Way EL: Respiratory sensitivity of the newborn infant to meperidine and morphine. Clin Pharmacol Ther 6:454–461, 1965.

Wellington N, Rieder MJ: Attitudes and practices regarding analgesia for newborn circumcision. Pediatrics 92:541–543, 1993.

Williamson PS, Williamson ML: Physiologic stress reduction by a local anesthetic during newborn circumcision. Pediatrics 71:36–40, 1983.

Yaster M: The dose response of fentanyl in neonatal anesthesia. Anesthesiology 66:433–435, 1987.

PART IV
GENETICS AND METABOLISM

CHAPTER 17

Modes of Inheritance

Robert J. Vosatka

FOUNDATIONS OF HUMAN GENETICS

Modern concepts of patterns of inheritance are derived from the work of Gregor Mendel in 1865 with pea plants. He proposed three laws of inheritance:

1. The law of segregation defined genetic traits as discrete categorical properties (as opposed to continuously variable properties).
2. The law of uniformity provided an operational definition for dominant and recessive inheritance.
3. The law of independence predicted the independent inheritance of traits.

INHERITANCE PATTERNS AND MENDEL'S LAWS

In a paper entitled *The Incidence of Alkaptonuria: A Study in Chemical Individuality*, Garrod noted that the occurrence of a human disorder was in accordance with the patterns of inheritance formulated by Mendel (Garrod, 1902). Garrod studied alkaptonuria, characterized by the excretion of homogentisic acid in the urine, and observed that the familial occurrence of this biochemical disorder was consistent with a recessive mode of inheritance. Additionally, he found that this disease occurred more commonly in consanguineous progeny. These observations form the basis of the mendelian approach to human genetic disease.

Therapies for Disease

In the year 1900, Landsteiner began to decipher the ABO blood group system and proved that these blood groups were an inherited trait (Landsteiner, 1900). The understanding of the pattern of inheritance of these major blood group antigens and the subsequent discovery of the Rh factor led to the development of Rho (D) immune globulin as a therapeutic approach to Rh hemolytic disease of the newborn in women at risk (Freda et al, 1967). This was the first instance in which knowledge of the genetics of a human disease led directly to a therapy for that disease.

Genetic Traits Connected in a Linear Array

Studies in plants have had further major contributions to the understanding of genetic principles in humans. Over the course of many years, Barbara McClintock described genetic control elements in corn plants that affected expression of genetic traits based on their physical location (McClintock, 1956). Thus, she was the first investigator to describe a linear arrangement of genes along structures that have come to be known as chromosomes. This concept that human genes could reside together in a locus suggested a physical nature of genetic elements. Understanding of the concept of the linear arrangement of genes is crucial to understanding the concept of linkage, one of the most important concepts in prenatal diagnosis.

DNA

The work of McClintock in the 1940s long preceded the work by James Watson and Francis Crick, who deduced the double stranded nature of DNA that gave a chemical basis for her physical model (Watson and Crick, 1953). The concept of the double helix gave information not only about the chemical nature of the gene and the physical relationship of one gene to another but also about a chemical basis for the ability of an organism to reproduce its genome by copying one strand of DNA against the other.

LINKAGE

Bernstein, referring to the ABO blood groups, wrote, "Accustomed as we now are to thousands of polymorphisms useful as human chromosome markers, it is hard to realize that in the first quarter century of Mendelism there was only one good marker. It is all the more remarkable that its simple mode of inheritance was not understood until the trait had been known for 25 years" (Crow, 1993). One major aspect of the identification of locations on the chromosome occurred from the concept of linkage that was developed primarily from work in the *Drosophila* (Morgan, 1910). The converse of Mendel's law of segregation explained the coinheritance of genes as studied by these early workers on *Drosophila*. Thus, physical linkage of the gene of one trait to another through an intervening strand of DNA produces the linkage or the association of the inheritance of one trait to the inheritance of others.

Physical linkage experiments on humans did not occur until the development of somatic cell genetics in which cells from humans could be fused to cells from other animals, such as mice. The resulting heterokaryons retained different human chromosomes; therefore, biochemical traits could be correlated with the inheritance of a particular chromosome. These types of experiments allowed the physical separation of different chromosomes from each other. Long before the identification of individual genes or individual mutations became feasible, it was possible to study mutations by their physical linkage or location on a chromosome. Mendel first chose a number of genetic traits in peas from which he developed his theory of independent segregation. In humans, linkage to gender or, later, cell surface antigen markers were the first types of linkage that were readily available. In 1980, the possibility of linking genes to markers throughout the genome became possible with the introduction of a technique called restriction fragment length polymorphism analysis.

Chromosomes

Chromosomes were first recognized as subcellular structures in the 1800s and named by Waldeyer in 1880 (Vogel and Motulsky, 1986). It was not until 1956 that the correct number of chromosomes in humans was identified as 46.

Proteins Encoded in DNA

In the early 1940s it had already been elucidated that genetic elements worked by producing proteins. The one-gene, one-enzyme hypothesis was developed from the work of Beadle and Tatum. This produced a model whereby genes could be expressed based on changes induced in the activity of enzymes (Beadle and Tatum, 1941). The first observation of a defective enzyme in humans that could cause disease was described by Gibson (1948), who identified the mutant enzyme in the autosomal recessive disease methemoglobinemia. This extension of the work of Beadle and Tatum led to the human correlate of their work: one gene, one disease.

Genetic Disease

The first observation that a physical change in the structure of a protein could be a cause of human disease was first identified by Ingram (1956). He showed that the autosomal recessive disease sickle cell anemia was caused by a structural abnormality of hemoglobin. The identification of the genetic triplet code in the 1960s led to the molecular basis of how changes in the DNA could be incorporated into RNA and affect the structure of proteins. These observations by a number of workers ultimately led to current understanding that abnormalities of the structure of proteins could result from an incorrect codon for an amino acid, a premature termination of protein synthesis, or a frame shift mutation that could alter the structure of a protein by changing the reading frame relative to the triplet amino acid code.

SINGLE GENE (MENDELIAN) TRAITS
Autosomal Dominant
Inheritance Patterns

The first pedigree that demonstrated autosomal dominant inheritance was published in 1866 by Broca. An early dominant pedigree is shown in Figure 17–1. Autosomal dominant transmission of traits is commonly observed in

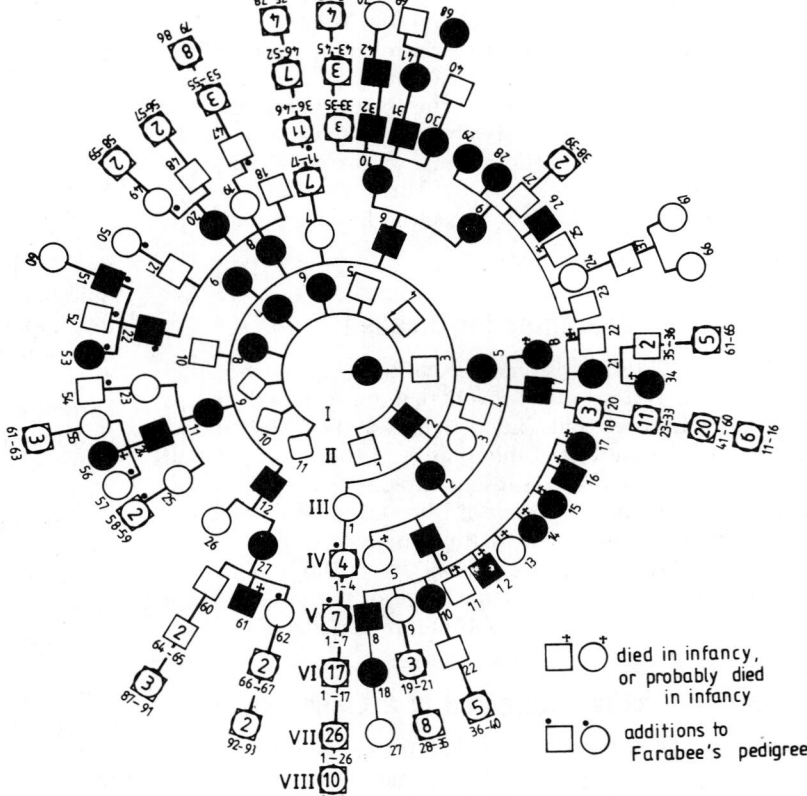

FIGURE 17–1. An early autosomal dominant pedigree showing vertical transmission with several affected members in each generation (Farabee's brachyphalangy pedigree). (From Haws DV, McKusick VA: Farabee's bradydactylous kindred revisited. Johns Hopkins Med J 113:20–30, 1963. © 1963, The Johns Hopkins University Press.)

the neonatal intensive care unit (NICU). The term *traits* is used here because all recognizable genetic characteristics, for example, hair color, are not necessarily causes of disease. Characteristics of autosomal dominant traits include the presence of vertical transmission from one generation to the next, with affected individuals in multiple generations. Because the genes for these traits are found on the autosomes and not on the sex chromosomes, there is an equal distribution of affected males and females. The transmission is independent of the sex of the transmitting parent, and the presence of male-to-male transmission is a key feature of autosomal dominant patterns of inheritance. The inheritance requires transmission of a gene from a single affected parent to an offspring. Because each trait is encoded on a single autosome, there is a 50% chance of transmission of the autosome carrying the trait in an affected individual for each offspring. The remaining 50% of the time, the other (unaffected) autosome is transmitted. Sporadic cases of autosomal dominant traits can be found consistent with new mutations. In subsequent generations, the pattern is identical to other cases of autosomal dominant inheritance. The mean age of fathers of individuals with newly occurring cases of autosomal dominant diseases is advanced (Jones et al, 1975).

Mechanisms

The known molecular mechanisms that can result in an autosomal dominant pattern of inheritance are considerably more complex than those known for autosomal recessive diseases (Wilkie, 1994). The following discussion defines some of those mechanisms.

Haploinsufficiency

In haploinsufficiency, the amount of gene product necessary for normal function is inadequate. The disease gene fails to produce a functional product and the second allele on the other chromosome is unable to generate enough of the product to replace that normally made by the disease allele.

Dominant Negative Model

In the dominant negative model, a defective product from the disease gene causes inactivation of the normal gene product. In this case, the abnormal gene product can interact with the normal product, resulting in an inactive dimer. Alternatively, the abnormal gene product can compete with the normal gene product for a substrate.

Structural Protein Abnormality

Abnormalities of structural proteins can result in a dominant phenotype. For example, in some forms of osteogenesis imperfecta, an abnormal collagen peptide becomes incorporated into the bony matrix, resulting in decreased bone strength.

Features

In addition to the patterns of inheritance, there are other features of autosomal dominant traits that can often be demonstrated. Autosomal dominant disorders often have associated malformations of physical features. There are often variations in the severity of expression from generation to generation. Some autosomal dominant disorders express *anticipation*, in which subsequent generations are more severely affected than earlier generations. The molecular basis of anticipation has recently been discerned (see Trinucleotide Repeats). Autosomal dominant disorders are often less clinically severe than recessive disorders, because dominant disorders must preserve survival to sexual maturity and fertility to be transmitted to subsequent generations. Some autosomal dominant disorders are transmitted homozygously to offspring. In these instances, two affected individuals produce an offspring who receives both copies of the affected allele. When this occurs in achondroplasia, the affected offspring is more severely affected and does not survive infancy (Aterman et al, 1983). In contrast, homozygous transmission of the gene for Huntington chorea, another autosomal dominant disorder, produces a clinical syndrome indistinguishable from heterozygous transmission (Wexler et al, 1987).

Some autosomal dominant traits exhibit codominance. This is most commonly observed in the neonatal period in the inheritance pattern of ABO blood group antigens (Table 17–1). Here, the A and B blood types are codominant. The O blood type is the result of the inheritance of the genes for neither the A nor the B blood group. The AB blood type is obtained when both the A and B blood group alleles are inherited, one from each parent.

Trinucleotide Repeats

The identification of the DNA sequence of a large number of genes has led to the understanding of novel pathogenetic mechanisms of disease that were hitherto inconceivable. The most unexpected mutations involve amplification of trinucleotide repeats. A number of diseases have been identified that are related to the amplification of what are termed trinucleotide repeats, which are identical three-base-pair segments of DNA repeated along a stretch of DNA. The number of repeat sequences is inherited as an autosomal dominant trait from parent to child.

A new vocabulary has been developed to describe the events associated with expansion of these repeats and their relationship to disease. Normal individuals can have a small number of repeats that are transmitted from generation to generation (and from cell to cell within an individual) without a change in size. Some individuals can have what

TABLE 17–1

Relationship Between Genetics and Immunology of the Codominant Inheritance of the ABO Antigens

Blood Type	Red Cell Antigen	Natural Antibodies	Relevant Gene
A	A	B	A transferase
B	B	A	B transferase
AB	A, B	—	A transferase, B transferase
O	H	A, B	Mutated transferases

is termed a *premutation*, wherein they are clinically unaffected but have an increased number of a particular repeat, as compared with normal individuals. This premutation is an unstable, heritable segment of DNA. Progeny of an individual with a premutation can inherit an expansion of the repeat, which results in clinical disease. Trinucleotide repeats are common and occur every 300 to 500 kilobases of genomic DNA. Pathologic expansions of these repeats several-fold have been found in at least six different disorders: fragile X syndrome, spinal and bulbar muscular atrophy, myotonic dystrophy, Huntington disease, spinocerebellar ataxia type I, and dentato-rubra-pallidoluysian atrophy. These disorders have some clinical features in common, including variable age of onset and severity, and a decrease in age of onset of symptoms in each successive generation. Amplifications of the trinucleotide repeat sequences occur during both meiosis and mitosis. How the expansion of these trinucleotide repeats results in disease is poorly understood. Some of these trinucleotide expansions occur in the coding region on proteins, resulting in variable repeats of a specific amino acid.

Myotonic Dystrophy—An Example of Anticipation

Myotonic dystrophy is an autosomal dominant disorder characterized by progressive myotonia, cataracts, and frontal baldness. Myotonic dystrophy is the most common form of muscular dystrophy in adults with an incidence of approximately 1 in 8000. A congenital form exists in which the child of an affected mother transmits the disorder to her fetus. The fetus may have polyhydramnios caused by decreased fetal swallowing and profound hypotonia. Newborns with the disorder often have respiratory failure. Although myotonic dystrophy is an autosomal dominant disorder caused by a mutation on chromosome 19, the congenital form exhibits genomic imprinting, commonly presenting when the gene is transmitted from an affected mother. Paternal transmission is rare but has been reported (Nakagawa et al, 1994). The gene for this disorder has been referred to as DM1, the myotonin protein kinase (Brook et al, 1992; Fu et al, 1992; Mahadevan et al, 1992).

Trinucleotide expansions in the myotonic dystrophy gene region occur downstream from the coding region. It is presently unclear how these expansions result in disease (Richards and Sutherland, 1992) (Fig. 17–2).

Normal individuals have from 5 to 27 copies of a CTG trinucleotide repeat sequence, whereas affected persons have greater than 50 copies of this repeat. In individuals with greater than 50 copies, each subsequent meiosis results in expansion of the number of these repeats. A correlation exists between number of copies of repeats and the clinical severity of myotonic dystrophy. Changes in the number of trinucleotide repeats can occur in somatic as well as germ line tissues. These changes offer a molecular explanation for the clinically observed inheritance pattern known as anticipation (Harley et al, 1992). The number of trinucleotide repeats correlates with muscular disability and inversely with age at diagnosis. Mental dysfunction is more common in patients with a larger number of repeats. Other symptoms, however, including cataracts, gastrointestinal dysfunction, and cardiac abnormalities, have not been shown to be correlated with amplification of the repeat (Jaspert et al, 1995). The pathogenesis of variation in number of these repeats is not clearly understood but may involve slipping of the DNA polymerase during DNA replication (Schlotterer and Tautz, 1992). It is unclear what distinguishes a stable repeat from a premutation to a slightly longer repeat that can undergo amplification. How these repeats ultimately result in disease is not clearly understood. Tissue mRNA levels of DM1 are decreased in late onset cases and profoundly decreased in congenital cases (Fu et al, 1993; Gennarelli et al, 1996). These reduced mRNA levels are associated with only modestly reduced levels of the encoded DM1 protein, however. Why a modest reduction in this protein or a decrease in the amount of RNA from this region might result in an autosomal dominant mode of inheritance is unclear.

Charcot-Marie-Tooth Disease

One newly observed mode of inheritance highlights the complexity of the changes in the genome that can result in disease. Charcot-Marie-Tooth disease represents a group of chronic demyelinating polyneuropathies for which at least three disease genes exist. The most common form of this disease, referred to as CMT1A, has been mapped to a small region on human chromosome 17. Most patients with this disorder appear to have a tandem duplication of a small 1.5-megabase region, resulting in a duplication of the peripheral myelin protein 22, also known as the PMP 22 gene. Occasionally, CMT1A is caused by a point mutation in the same protein. In contrast, other point mutations in PMP 22 or another gene P0 (myelin protein 0) result in Dejerine-Sottas disease. This is a severe polyneuropathy

FIGURE 17–2. Molecular basis of anticipation: unstable amplification of a trinucleotide repeat (AGC)ₙ in the myotonic dystrophy gene (DM-1). (From Richards RI, Sutherland GR: Dynamic mutations: A new class of mutations causing human disease. Cell 70:709–712, 1992. © Cell Press.)

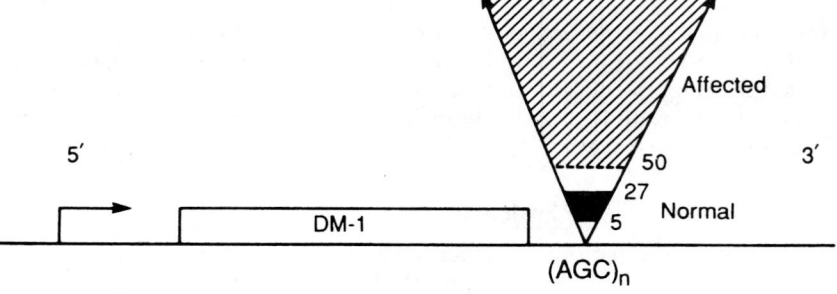

DM-1 - Myotonic Dystrophy

with an infantile onset that is distinct from Charcot-Marie-Tooth disease. A third disorder, hereditary neuropathy with liability to pressure palsies, is another inherited disorder, which results in recurrent demyelinating neuropathy, again distinct from Charcot-Marie-Tooth type 1A and Dejerine-Sottas disease. This disorder results from a deletion of the PMP 22 gene. Thus, duplication, deletion, or point mutation in a single protein can lead to three distinct genetic disorders of man (Roa and Lupski, 1993).

Autosomal Recessive

Inheritance Patterns

Autosomal recessive pattern of inheritance is also a common pattern observed in infants. Pedigrees of autosomal recessive traits feature a horizontal pattern of inheritance, with affected members in a single generation, and, in general, no affected members in prior or subsequent generations. To be affected with an autosomal recessive disease, an individual must inherit two disease genes, one from each parent. The parents of an affected individual are heterozygotes, or *carriers*, of the recessive allele and are generally clinically normal. Because the genes for autosomal recessive traits are not on the sex chromosomes, males and females are equally affected. Each offspring of two carriers of a particular autosomal recessive trait has a 25% chance of inheriting the two copies of the affected gene and thus expressing the disease. Each offspring has a 50% chance of inheriting a single copy of the affected gene and being a clinically unaffected carrier of the trait. Alternatively, an offspring has a 25% chance of inheriting neither affected allele from the parents and thus being unaffected. Consanguinity increases the likelihood that the two parents will share a recessive gene and thus increase the likelihood of bearing affected offspring. Subsequent nonconsanguineous generations are not at increased risk of expressing an autosomal recessive trait.

Autosomal recessive disease genes often encode enzymes and are thus termed *inborn errors of metabolism*.

Clinical Features

Many autosomal recessive diseases have severe clinical manifestations, often leading to death in the newborn period or before sexual maturity. Unlike autosomal dominant traits, which often exhibit great variability of expression, autosomal recessive diseases often exhibit less clinical variability. In contrast, alternative alleles of a gene can produce distinct phenotypes.

Alternative Alleles and Clinical Variability

Although inheritance of an autosomal recessive disease requires the inheritance of an affected gene from each parent, the genes from each parent can have a different specific mutation within the affected gene. Affected individuals with an autosomal recessive trait but with two different alleles are called *genetic compounds* or *compound heterozygotes*. Specific genetic compounds can have distinguishable phenotypes. For example, inheritance of two copies of the autosomal recessive allele for cystic fibrosis gene CFTR called delta F508 (deletion of the 508th codon encoding phenylalanine) results in the classic phenotype of cystic fibrosis with progressive, severe lung disease and pancreatic insufficiency. In contrast, inheritance of another mutation of the CFTR gene called 5T from one parent along with delta F508 (Chillon et al, 1995) results in agenesis of the vas deferens in males, with no respiratory disease and pancreatic dysfunction. Inheritance of the delta F508 mutation with a "pancreatic sufficiency" mutation from the other parent produces a third phenotype of progressive, severe lung disease but without pancreatic insufficiency.

Frequency of Carriers

Because the inheritance of an autosomal recessive disease requires the inheritance of a defective gene from each of both parents, the frequency of carriers of a recessive allele in a population greatly influences the frequency of affected individuals in that population. The frequency of defective genes varies greatly among various ethnic groups. For example, the gene for Tay-Sachs disease is commonly carried among Ashkenazi Jews but is less common among other ethnic groups.

X-Linked

A large number of single gene defects have been mapped to the X chromosome based on their relationship to the sex of affected and carrier individuals. An example of an X-linked pedigree is shown in Figure 17–3. Specifically, the X chromosome cannot be transmitted from father to son, so that no traits carried on the X chromosome can be carried from father to son. Unaffected males cannot transmit an X-linked trait, but all daughters of an affected father are carriers of the trait. Because females carry two X chromosomes, they often have a milder phenotype than males, who do not have the potential benefit of a second, normal X chromosome. Because females can have a milder phenotype than males, it is possible for an unaffected (but carrier) female to have a severely affected son. The concept of "dominant" or "recessive" modes of X-linked inheritance depends both on the particular disease gene and on how sensitive an assay is used to detect the presence of the disease phenotype. For example, female carriers of ornithine transcarbamylase deficiency are, generally, unaffected. However, some carriers are vegetarian or otherwise avoid protein-rich food, presumably to avoid the symptoms of hyperammonemia, which is potentially lethal in an affected male (Gilchrist and Coleman, 1987). As in sporadic cases of an autosomal dominant trait, advanced paternal age is often found in the father of the first heterozygous female in a pedigree.

Y-Linked

Although single gene traits such as tooth size or height have been mapped to the Y chromosome, none are clinically relevant in the newborn period. Some genes present on the Y chromosome map to a region referred to as the pseudoautosomal region. Y-linked traits are passed exclusively from father to son and are never transmitted to genetic females.

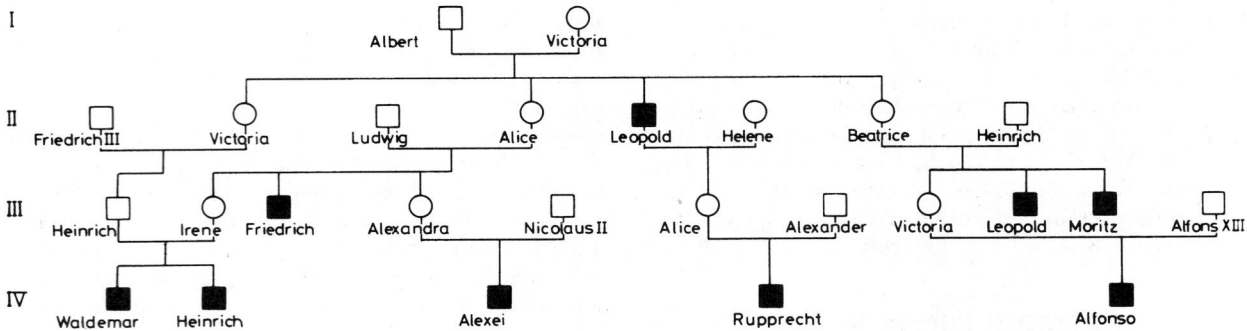

FIGURE 17–3. X-linked pedigree: X-linked recessive hemophilia A in the European royal houses. (From Vogel F, Motulsky AG: Human Genetics, 3rd ed. New York, Springer-Verlag, 1996.)

NON-MENDELIAN INHERITANCE

Clear concepts of mendelian inheritance have led to the recognition of non-mendelian patterns of inheritance as well.

Mitochondrial Mode

Mitochondrial disorders do not have a typical mendelian inheritance pattern. Mitochondrial DNA is transmitted within the mitochondria. Although mitochondria are present in spermatozoa, they are not inherited by the fertilized egg. Thus, genetic material is passed matrilineally, that is, strictly from mothers to their offspring of either sex. Normal cells contain hundreds of copies of the small mitochondrial chromosome present in multiple copies within each mitochondrion. This small chromosome encodes only 13 known genes. A variety of different mutations in these genes have produced a number of distinct clinical phenotypes in humans. Most mitochondrial disorders manifest well beyond the newborn period and affect organs that use large amounts of adenosine triphosphate such as muscle and brain (Wallace, 1992).

Genomic Imprinting

Genomic imprinting is a novel mode of inheritance that affects the expression of inherited genes. Genomic imprinting is an epigenetic phenomenon, resulting in modification of the expression of independently inherited genes. This mode of inheritance is an active research area and the details of its importance to human inheritance patterns, health, and disease are emerging. Imprinted genes have a novel inheritance pattern as shown in the hypothetical pedigrees in Figure 17–4 (Hall, 1990). These pedigrees demonstrate expression of a trait based on the sex of the transmitting parent. The best understood examples of human genomic imprinting have been derived from studies of the inheritance of Prader-Willi and Angelman syndromes. These two disorders illustrate how genomic imprinting affects clinical syndromes and contributes to understanding the link of classic mendelian single-gene modes of inheritance to non-mendelian chromosomal modes of inheritance.

A number of models to explain the modification of gene expression by the presence of a second inherited gene have been proposed. One mechanism whereby genome imprinting most likely occurs is through the inheritance of specific patterns of DNA methylation of either the maternal or paternal chromosome genes (Li et al, 1983).

Uniparental Disomy

The concept that an individual could inherit two copies of a chromosome from one parent and none of the same chromosome from the other parent was first proposed in 1980 (Engel, 1980). The first demonstration that uniparental disomy could occur at all came primarily from work in mouse models (Cattanach and Kirk, 1985).

In 1988, Spence and colleagues were the first to confirm the speculation of Engel that uniparental disomy could be a novel mode of inheritance in humans. These workers described a case in which cystic fibrosis was inherited through transmission of two copies of a single chromosome 7 from the child's mother who had been a carrier of a cystic fibrosis gene (maternal uniparental isodisomy). This observation raised the specter that other usually autosomal recessive diseases could be transmitted in a mode that mimicked an autosomal dominant pattern of inheritance. This mode of inheritance is rare and may not be possible for all chromosomes.

Specific Diseases

Prader-Willi Syndrome

Prader-Willi syndrome is characterized by obesity, mental retardation, characteristic facies, and hypogonadism. The hypogonadism is readily identified in males and often alerts the clinician to the diagnosis. In the neonate, the usual clinical presentation is hypotonia and prolonged need for gavage feeding. High-resolution karyotypes identify a characteristic chromosomal anomaly, a deletion of the proximal long arm of chromosome 15, termed the *Prader-Willi syndrome critical region* (PWSCR), in approximately half of patients. Molecular analysis with probes within the deleted region can confirm the deletion of this material from one of the number 15 chromosomes. The other half of patients have a cytogenetically and molecularly normal chromosome by the same analysis. However, careful molecular analysis

PATERNAL

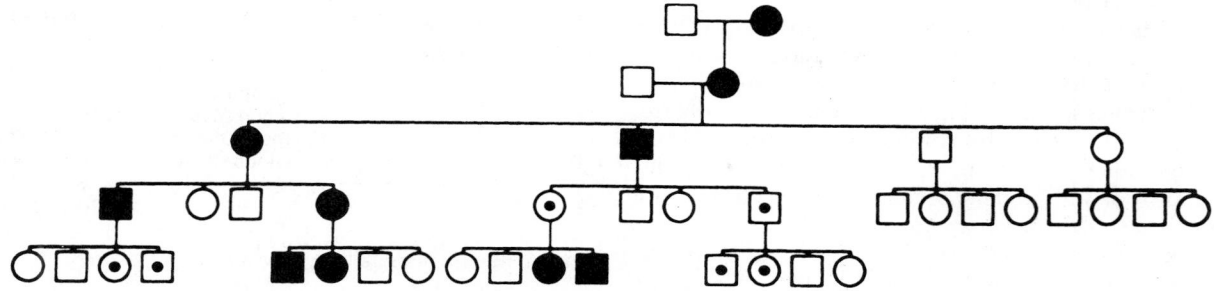

FIGURE 17–4. Genomic imprinting. Hypothetical pedigree demonstrates paternal imprinting effects on expression of the imprinted phenotype. Expression of the phenotype requires inheritance of the imprinted gene from the mother (solid filled). Females who inherit the imprinted gene from their father are unaffected but can transmit the phenotype to their offspring (dot filled, female). Males who inherit the imprinted gene from their father do not express the phenotype, nor will their children who inherit the gene (dot filled, male). (From Hall JG: How imprinting is relevant to disease. Development Suppl 141:148, 1990; with permission of Company of Biologists Ltd.)

of the inheritance of the chromosome 15 in patients from their parents gives an unusual result. Most of these patients with cytogenetically normal chromosomes 15 are found to have inherited both of their chromosomes 15 from their mother, known as maternal uniparental disomy for chromosome 15. Examples of both maternal uniparental isodisomy 15 (two identical chromosomes from the mother) and maternal uniparental heterodisomy 15 (one of each chromosome 15, both from the mother) have been observed in Prader-Willi syndrome patients (Nichols et al, 1989). In all cases of uniparental disomy, there is no contribution of genetic material derived from a paternal copy of chromosome 15. Differing expression of genetic material from one parent or the other is called a *parent of origin effect*. When the deleted chromosome 15 from the other patients with Prader-Willi syndrome was studied, the parent of origin of the deleted chromosome was found to be paternal. Thus, patients who express the Prader-Willi syndrome phenotype also fail to inherit the PWSCR of chromosome 15 from their father.

In 1993, Chan and colleagues reported that the reciprocal uniparental disomy, that is, the inheritance of two chromosomes 15 from the mother and none from the father (termed uniparental maternal disomy), resulted in a different disorder called Angelman syndrome.

In addition to sharing uniparental disomy as a cause of both Prader-Willi syndrome and Angelman syndrome, it had previously been noted that the regions of chromosome 15 involved in both syndromes were overlapping (Magenis et al, 1990). Together, the observations that both deletions of chromosome 15 and parent of origin–specific inheritance result in two different disorders suggest that there is unequal transmission of genetic information from the maternal and paternal genomes. The molecular basis of these changes has yet to be fully elucidated but it is likely to involve methylation of the DNA.

It is likely that uniparental disomy results from "rescue" of a lethal trisomy of the affected chromosome. If an embryo inherits three chromosomes 15, for example, the embryo cannot survive. If, however, a line of cells loses the extra chromosome 15, resulting in a correction to a "normal" karyotype, the situation is no longer lethal. If the remaining two chromosomes have arisen from only one parent, uniparental disomy results (Fig. 17–5).

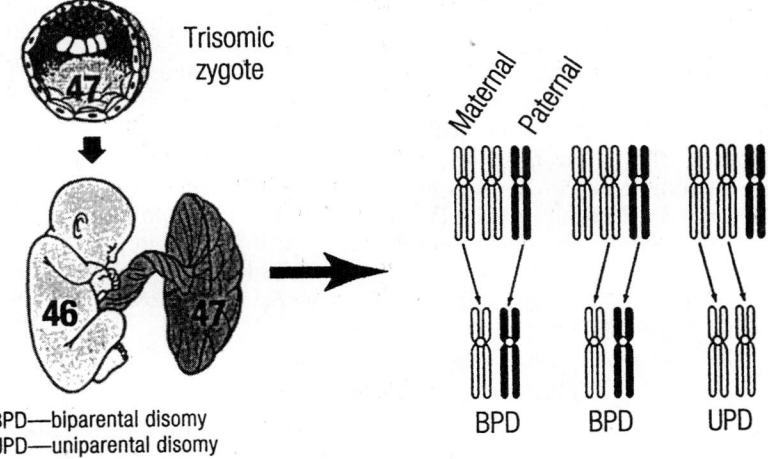

FIGURE 17–5. Mechanism whereby uniparental disomy can result from a trisomic zygote. (From Kalousek DK, Harrison K: Uniparental disomy and unexplained intrauterine growth retardation. CONTEMPORARY OB/GYN 9:41–48, 1995; with permission of Medical Economics Publishing.)

Intrauterine Growth Retardation

Since the initial observations were made, more than 100 other patients have been identified with uniparental disomy of a number of different chromosomes (Kalousek and Barrett, 1994). Uniparental disomy is most frequently associated with chromosomes 7, 11, 14, 15, and 16 (Ledbetter and Engel, 1995). The observation that abnormal karyotypes in chorionic villi can be resolved as uniparental disomy has provided an understanding of the mechanism for the occurrence of uniparental disomy, confirming the work of Eric Engel (Engel, 1980) (see Fig. 17–5). The introduction of chorionic villus sampling (CVS) has allowed the simultaneous ability to discern the karyotypes of fetuses and placentas prenatally. Approximately 1% of CVS cases reveal the presence of two or more cell lines identified by different karyotypes. When the mosaicism is not expressed in the fetus, this is termed *confined placental mosaicism.* Kalousek and coworkers (1991) have observed a high incidence of intrauterine growth retardation (IUGR) in patients with confined placental mosaicism. It is unclear whether the IUGR results from residual trisomic cells in the placenta or from uniparental disomy (Ledbetter and Engel, 1995).

MULTIFACTORIAL INHERITANCE

Not all inherited syndromes are transmitted as single genetic traits. A large number of disorders that afflict humanity are transmitted as multifactorial traits. Multifactorial syndromes that are manifest in the neonatal period include cleft lip and palate, congenital heart disease, neural tube defects, and pyloric stenosis. In these disorders contributions of both genetic and environmental factors allow for predisposition to a particular phenotype. As such, monozygotic twins who share the identical genetic makeup can be discordant for multifactorial traits. Because the genetic component of a multifactorial trait represents only a portion of the genetic basis, linkage studies elucidating the underlying genetic basis for multifactorial traits are considerably hampered compared with studies of single gene (mendelian) traits (Patterson and Todd, 1995). Genes that contribute to the multifactorial inheritance patterns, however, have already been identified (Frogul et al, 1992; Paul et al, 1990).

Pyloric Stenosis

Pyloric stenosis is much more common among males than females. However, its incidence is increased in families in which there is a previously diagnosed relative. The first model for its inheritance pattern was proposed in 1976 (Carter, 1976). Carter hypothesized that there was a threshold of genetic influence that was lower in the male relatives compared with females such that male children were more likely to express the phenotype. Females with pyloric stenosis, therefore, have a greater genetic burden and are more likely to have offspring who also have pyloric stenosis (see Chapter 73).

Neural Tube Defects

Neural tube defects, including anencephaly and spina bifida, commonly present in the perinatal period. Epidemio-

---

TABLE 17–2

Empiric Risk Estimates for Various Forms of Congenital Heart Disease*

Defect	Empiric Recurrence Risk (One Previous Child)	Empiric Recurrence Risk (Other Risk Factors)
Overall	2%	10% (2 affected children)
Aortic valvular atresia	4%	
Coarctation of the aorta	7%	
Complex congenital heart disease	10%	
Truncus arteriosus	10%	
Atrioventricular septal defects	2% to 9%	15% (affected parent)

*Empiric recurrence risk estimations should be used only when more specific modes of inheritance have been excluded.

logic studies have identified folic acid and perhaps vitamin B_{12} as important nongenetic factors that can influence the rate of neural tube defects occurring in a population (Czeizel and Dudas, 1992; Mills et al, 1995). The ability to prenatally screen mothers for risk of having a fetus with these neural tube defects has lowered the incidence of live born babies with these defects (see Chapter 67).

Congenital Heart Disease

Many forms of congenital heart disease are thought to involve a multifactorial mode of inheritance. Recent advances have identified a number of chromosomal, subchromosomal, or single gene defects as causes of congenital heart disease. The recurrence risks for various forms of congenital heart disease are related either to the recurrence risk of the specific underlying genetic disorder (e.g., Down syndrome and atrioventricular canal, Williams syndrome and supravalvular aortic stenosis) or can be estimated based on empiric (population based) risks, when an underlying syndromic diagnosis cannot be discerned. Empiric recurrence risk estimates based on cardiac diagnosis are listed in Table 17–2 (Allan et al, 1986; Sanchez-Cascos, 1978). In the newborn, consideration should be given to the exclusion of newly described genetic disorders with prominent cardiac manifestations, such as microdeletions of chromosome 22, before considering recurrence risk estimation based on empiric data (reviewed in Payne et al, 1995).

REFERENCES

Allan LD, Crawford DC, Chita SK, et al: Familial recurrence of congenital heart disease in a prospective series of mothers referred for fetal echocardiography. Am J Cardiol 58:334–337, 1986.

Aterman K, Welch JP, Taylor PG: Presumed homozygous achondroplasia: A review and report of a further case. Path Res Pract 178:27–39, 1983.

Beadle GW, Tatum EL: Genetic control of biochemical reactions in neurospora. Proc Nat Acad Sci U S A 27:499–506, 1941.

Broca PP: Traite des Tumeurs. Vol 1. Paris, P Asselin, 1866, 1:80.

Brook JD, McCurrach ME, Harley HG, et al: Molecular basis of myotonic dystrophy: Expansion of a trinucleotide (CTG) repeat at the 3′ end of a transcript encoding a protein kinase family member [Erratum published in Cell 69:385, 1992]. Cell 68:799–808, 1992.

Carter CO: Genetics of common single malformations. Br Med Bull 32:21–26, 1976.

Cattanach B, Kirk M: Differential activity of maternally and paternally derived chromosomes regions in mice. Nature 315:496–498, 1985.

Chan CT, Clayton-Smith J, Cheng XJ, et al: Molecular mechanisms in Angelman syndrome: A survey of 93 patients. J Med Genet 30:895–902, 1993.

Chillon M, Casals T, Mercier B, et al: Mutations in the cystic fibrosis gene in patients with congenital absence of the vas deferens. N Engl J Med 332:1475–1480, 1995.

Crow JF: Felix Bernstein and the first human marker locus. Genetics 133:4–7, 1993.

Czeizel AE, Dudas I: Prevention of the first occurrence of neural tube defects by periconceptional vitamin supplementation. N Engl J Med 327:1832–1835, 1992.

Engel E: A new concept: Uniparental disomy and its potential effect. Am J Med Genet 6:137–143, 1980.

Freda VJ, Gorman JG, Pollack W: Suppression of the primary Rh immune response with passive Rh IgG immunoglobulin. N Engl J Med 277:1022–1023, 1967.

Frogul P, Daxillaire M, Sun S, et al: Close linkage of glucose kinase locus on chromosome 7P to early onset non-insulin dependent diabetes mellitus. Nature 356:162, 1992.

Fu Y-H, Friedman DL, Richards S, et al: Decreased expression of myotonin protein kinase in adult form of myotonic dystrophy. Science 260:235–238, 1993.

Fu Y-H, Pizzuti A, Fenwick RG, et al: An unstable triplet repeat in a gene related to myotonic dystrophy. Science 255:1256–1258, 1992.

Garrod AE: The incidence of alkaptonuria: A study in chemical individuality. Lancet 2:1616–1620, 1902.

Gennarelli M, Novelli G, Andreasi Bassi F, et al: Prediction of myotonic dystrophy clinical severity based on the number of intragenic [CTG]n trinucleotide repeats. Am J Med Genet 65:342–427, 1996.

Gibson QH: The reduction of methemoglobin in red blood cells and stays on the cause of etiopathy methemoglobinemia. Biochem J 42:13–23, 1948.

Gilchrist JM, Coleman RA: Ornithine transcarbamylase deficiency: Adult onset of severe symptoms. Ann Intern Med 106:556–558, 1987.

Hall JG: How imprinting is relevant to disease. Development Suppl 141:148, 1990.

Harley HG, Brooks JD, Rundle SA, et al: Expansion of an unstable DNA region and phenotypic variation in myotonic dystrophy. Nature 355:545–548, 1992.

Ingram VM: A specific chemical difference between the globins of normal human and sickle cell anemia hemoglobin. Nature 178:792, 1956.

Jaspert A, Fahsold R, Grehl H, Claus D: Myotonic dystrophy: Correlation of clinical symptoms with the size of the CTG trinucleotide repeat. J Neurol 242:99–104, 1995.

Jones KL, Smith DW, Harvey MA, et al: Older paternal age and fresh gene mutation: Data on additional disorders. J Pediatr 86:84–88, 1975.

Kalousek DK, Barrett I: Genome imprinting related to prenatal diagnosis. Prenat Diagn 14:1191–1201, 1994.

Kalousek DK, Howard-Peebeles PN, Olson SB, et al: Confirmation of CVS mosaicism in term placentae and high frequency of intrauterine growth retardation associated with confined placental mosaicism. Prenat Diagn 11:743–750, 1991.

Landsteiner K: Zur Kenntnis der antifermentativen, lytischen und agglutinierenden Wirkungen des Blutserums und der Lymphe. Zentralbl Bakteriol 27:357–362, 1900.

Ledbetter DH, Engel E: Uniparental disomy in humans: Development of an imprinting map and its implications for prenatal diagnosis. Hum Mol Genet 4:1757–1764, 1995.

Li E, Beard C, Jaenich R: Role for DNA methylation in genome imprinting. Nature 356:362, 1983.

Magenis RE, Toth-Fejal S, Allen LJ, et al: Comparison of the 15q deletions in Prader-Willi and Angelman's syndromes: Specific regions, extent of deletions, parental origins and clinical consequences. Am J Med Genet 35:333–349, 1990.

Mahadevan M, Tsilfidis C, Sabourin L, et al: Myotonic dystrophy mutation: An unstable CTG repeat in the 3′ untranslated region of the gene. Science 255:1253–1255, 1992.

McClintock B: Controlling elements in the gene. Cold Spring Harbor Symposium in Quantitative Biology 21:197–216, 1956.

Mills JL, McPartlin JM, Kirke PN, et al: Homocysteine metabolism in pregnancies complicated by neural tube defects. Lancet 343:149–151, 1995.

Morgan TH: Sex-limited inheritance in drosophila. Science 32:120–122, 1910.

Nakagawa M, Yamada H, Higuchi I, et al: A case of paternally inherited congenital myotonic dystrophy. J Med Genet 31:397–400, 1994.

Nichols RD, Knoll JHM, Butler MG, et al: Genetic imprinting suggested by maternal heterodisomy in non-deletion Prader-Willi syndrome. Nature 342:381–385, 1989.

Patterson M, Todd JA: A complex issue. Trends in genetics 11:463, 1995.

Paul JM, Lee MK, Newman B, et al: Linkage of the early onset familial breast cancer to chromosome 17Q21. Science 250:64, 1990.

Payne RM, Johnson MC, Grant JW, et al: Toward a molecular understanding of congenital heart disease. Circulation 91:494–504, 1995.

Richards RI, Sutherland GR: Dynamic mutations: A new class of mutations causing human disease. Cell 70:709–712, 1992.

Roa BB, Lupski JR: Molecular basis of Charcot-Marie-Tooth disease type IA: Gene dosage as a novel mechanism for a common autosomal dominant condition. Am J Med Sci 306:177–184, 1993.

Sanchez-Cascos A: The recurrence risk in congenital heart disease. Eur J Cardiol 7:197–210, 1978.

Schlotterer C, Tautz D: Slippage synthesis of single sequence DNA. Nucleic Acids Res 20:211–215, 1992.

Spence JE, Perciccante RG, Greig GM, et al: Uniparental disomy as a mechanism for human disease. Am J Hum Genet 42:217–226, 1988.

Vogel F, Motulsky AG: Human Genetics, 2nd ed. New York, Springer-Verlag, 1986, pp 9–19.

Wallace DC: Mitochondrial genetics: A paradigm for aging in degenerative diseases? Science 256:628–632, 1992.

Watson J, Crick F: The Structure of DNA, Cold Spring Harbor Symposium in Quantitative Biology 18:123–132, 1953.

Wexler NS, Young AB, Tanzi RE, et al: Homozygotes for Huntington's disease. Nature 326:194–197, 1987.

Wilkie AOM: The molecular basis of genetic dominance. J Med Genet 31:89–98, 1994.

CHAPTER 18

Techniques of Molecular Diagnosis

Robert J. Vosatka

The focus of this chapter is on clinically relevant techniques useful for the diagnosis of genetic or infectious disease by DNA analysis.

CONVENTIONAL CYTOGENETICS

Conventional cytogenetic techniques are suitable for the detection of most clinically important abnormalities of chromosome number and structure.

Detection of Aneuploidy

Despite advances in prenatal diagnosis and prenatal screening, the most common disorder of chromosome number diagnosed in the newborn nursery is Down syndrome (Fig. 18–1). The overall birth incidence of Down syndrome (trisomy 21) is approximately 1 in 700 live births. However, the incidence at conception is significantly higher. Many chromosomally abnormal fetuses spontaneously miscarry.

The incidence of trisomy 21 is related to the age of the mother. Ninety-five percent of cases of Down syndrome are due to trisomy 21 (47 chromosomes present). Of these, 80% are due to nondisjunction occurring during the first meiotic division. As may be predicted from the association of advanced maternal age with increased risk for Down syndrome, in 85% of the cases, the extra chromosome 21 is of maternal origin (Boue et al, 1985). Table 18–1 summarizes the relative live birth incidences of commonly observed aneuploidies.

Detection of Abnormal Chromosome Structure

A number of techniques have led to considerable advancement in the ability to detect subtle alterations in chromosome structure. A variety of banding techniques allow cytogeneticists to distinguish individual chromosomes based on their size, location of the centromere, and the specific pattern of bands unique to each chromosome. High-resolution techniques allow the visualization of 700 to 1000 bands

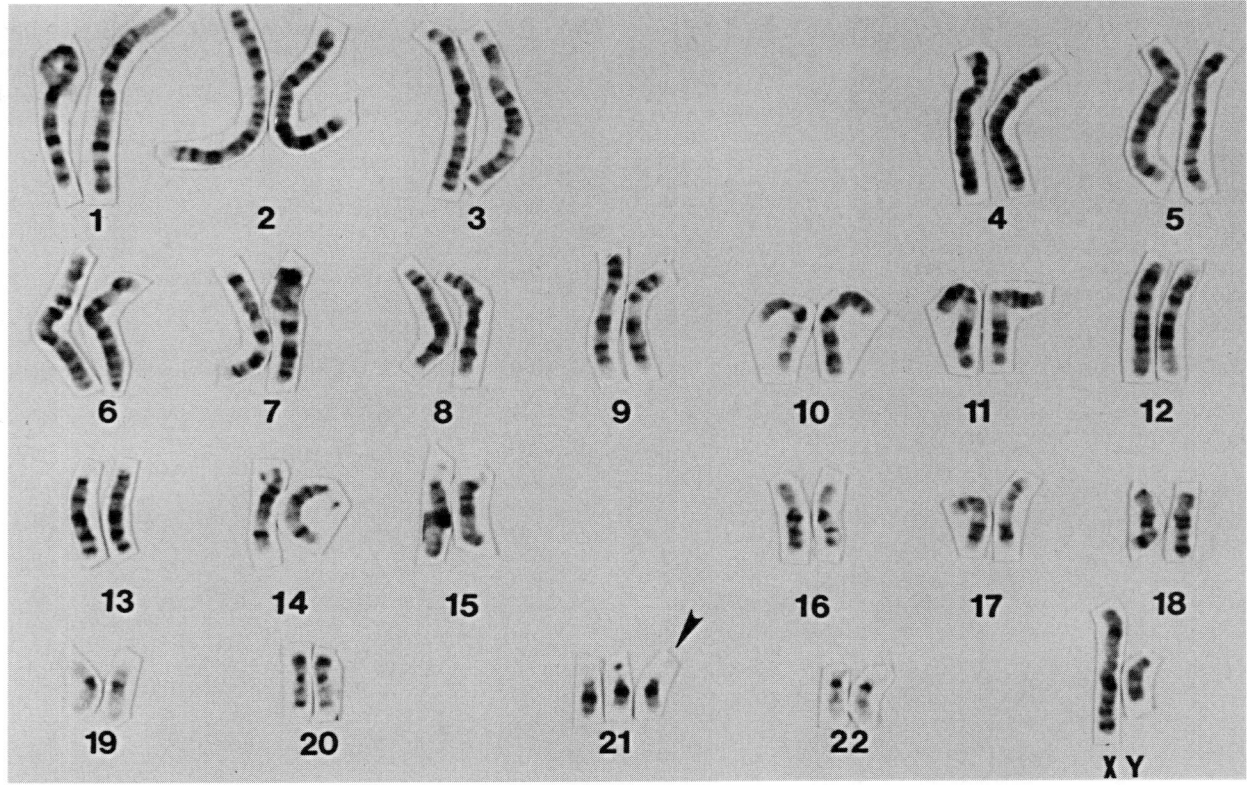

FIGURE 18–1. G-banded karyotype of a male with Down syndrome (trisomy 21) at 575 band resolution. The arrowhead indicates an additional copy of chromosome 21. The different satellite regions on the three copies of chromosome 21 suggest that the trisomy is a result of meiosis I error. (Courtesy of Janet M. Cowan, PhD, New England Medical Center, Boston, MA.)

TABLE 18-1

Birth Incidence of Common Aneuploids

Syndrome	Abnormality	Birth Incidence
Down	Trisomy 21	1 in 700
Edward	Trisomy 18	1 in 3000
Patau	Trisomy 13	1 in 5000
Turner	X	1 in 5000
Triple X female	XXX	1 in 1000
Klinefelter	XXY	1 in 1000

across the 46 human chromosomes. The smallest segment of a chromosome that can be distinguished using these high-resolution techniques contains approximately 1 million base pairs of DNA. The most commonly used technique in the United States for the routine karyotype uses G, or giemsa, banding (see Fig. 18–1). R, or reverse banding, and C banding specific for the centromere are additional techniques that can enhance the ability of a skilled cytogeneticist to detect specific abnormalities. Once a structural abnormality is suspected, specific techniques such as fluorescence in situ hybridization (FISH) (Fig. 18–2) or chromosome painting can be used to further define the abnormality.

Chromosome Analysis: Blood Sampling

It is important to understand the technique for obtaining appropriate samples for chromosome analysis. The cells in a blood sample that are studied in the standard preparation of a metaphase karyotype are lymphocytes. Packed red blood cell transfusions generally deliver small numbers of lymphocytes to a patient. Additionally, leukocyte filtration can physically remove these cells. Irradiation of blood products produces cells that do not divide in culture and thus do not interfere with the production of a karyotype. Thus, an accurate karyotype can be generated even in the infant who has received multiple transfusions. Generally, 2 to 10 mL of blood are obtained for a karyotype in a sodium heparin (green top) tube and kept at room temperature. Samples should be transported to the cytogenetics laboratory within a short period of time (hours) because living cells are needed to place into cell culture. Colchicine is later added to these cells to arrest the cells in metaphase to produce the standard banded karyotype.

MOLECULAR TECHNIQUES
Hybridization Techniques

Many types of DNA and RNA analysis techniques make use of the property of DNA (or RNA) to bind to its complementary sequence. Each of the four bases—cytosine (C), guanosine (G), adenosine (A), and thymidine (T)—binds to a specific second base (RNA uses uracil, U, in place of thymidine). C binds to G, and T binds to A. Linear sequences of nucleotides bind to their complementary sequences. Although very short sequences of DNA (three to six bases) can bind at many different places throughout a genome-sized collection of DNA, slightly longer sequences (18 to 20 bases) are unique within the genome.

Restriction Endonucleases

Restriction endonucleases are enzymes that can recognize short (3 to 8 bases) DNA sequences and digest the DNA at these recognition sequences. These enzymes are obtained from bacteria that use them as a form of immunity, identifying and destroying foreign DNA. Hundreds of these enzymes have been identified, and many are purified and sold commercially as reagents for molecular biologic uses. These enzymes are useful for cutting specific pieces of DNA so that they may be used for construction of specific DNA structures. They are also useful in analytic techniques such as Southern blots (Southern, 1975).

Southern Blots

Southern blots allow the identification of specific fragments of DNA based on their length and ability to hybridize to a DNA probe. DNA from a patient or other source is often cut with one or more restriction enzymes before analysis. The DNA is physically separated into different sized fragments by a technique known as agarose gel electrophoresis. Agarose gel electrophoresis separates fragments of DNA by causing them to move in an electric field. The negatively charged DNA moves toward the positive electric pole. Agarose, a three-dimensional sugar matrix, impedes the rate of movement of the DNA within the electric fields. Larger pieces of DNA containing greater numbers of bases have greater difficulty moving through this agarose matrix. The smaller DNA pieces thus travel relatively farther. After a suitable length of time to allow separation of the DNA pieces, the size-fractionated DNA contained within the agarose is transferred to a piece of filter paper or membrane by another electric field, or capillary action. This paper, or "blot," then holds a size-fractionated collection of the DNA of interest. The test probe DNA of interest is then made radioactive, through labeling techniques. This radioactive probe DNA is dissolved in a solution of water and salt, and the blot of size-fractionated DNA molecules is soaked in it. After several hours, the radioactive DNA hybridizes to its specific complementary DNA on the blot. The nonhybridized radioactive DNA is removed by extensive washing. This radioactive blot is exposed to x-ray film. The radioactive DNA exposes the film, which is then developed normally. The exposed film identifies the piece of DNA based on its ability to hybridize to the radioactive probe and its length. This information is sufficient for sophisticated analysis of DNA structure and analysis of unique patterns known as restriction fragment length polymorphisms (RFLPs), which are transmitted from parent to child.

Restriction Fragment Length Polymorphisms

RFLPs are unique, polymorphic-sized DNA fragments from a region of interest in the human genome. The DNA fragments are generated by digestion of the DNA with a restriction enzyme that recognizes a specific site within or near the DNA sequence. The DNA fragments are separated by size by electrophoresis followed by detection of the gene segment of interest by Southern blotting. RFLPs are found throughout the genome and do not necessarily consist of genes themselves but frequently reside in regions of DNA not known to contain any specific genetic information (introns). Minor variations in the DNA sequence, such as point deletions or small amplifications, alter the region recognized by the DNA restriction enzymes. These polymorphisms are transmitted from parent to child, and the inheritance follows a strictly dominant mendelian pattern. Because each RFLP is present at a unique position within the genome, the introduction of this technique allowed the possibility of correlating disease or absence of disease with the inheritance of an RFLP (Botstein et al, 1980). This powerful technique also facilitated the ability to begin to map genes based solely on their position within the genome. Linkage analysis, therefore, allows tracking of the inheritance of gene segments that are physically connected to a disease-causing mutation. The closer that a disease gene resides on a chromosome relative to an RFLP, the more likely it is that the two will be transmitted together as a unit. In this way, the RFLP can serve as an indirect marker of the inheritance of a disease gene.

Fluorescence in Situ Hybridization

The ability to physically locate genes along specific chromosomes once a DNA probe became available is not new (Gall and Pardue, 1969). The original technique used radioactive probes to detect hybridization to white blood cell chromosomes during mitosis. Because of the great complexity of this approach, the technique remained a purely research tool until 1985 (Landegent et al, 1985, 1987). The introduction of highly fluorescent probes allowed detection of genetic elements within human chromosomes without the use of radioactivity (Fig. 18–2). This technique for the first time allowed visualization of DNA segments within the human genome to look for small deletions of chromosomes, smaller than the bands that could be detected by visual inspection of a karyotype.

One of the most clinically important uses of this technique in the newborn is to assist in the detection and diagnosis of small deletions associated with the DiGeorge syndrome (Driscoll et al, 1993). These small deletions can be found in the DiGeorge syndrome critical region (DGSCR) on chromosome 22. Patients with features suggestive of the DiGeorge syndrome should have a banded karyotype and FISH studies using the DGSCR probe to identify a deletion in the DGSCR.

Polymerase Chain Reaction

The introduction of the technique known as polymerase chain reaction (PCR) has revolutionized the analysis of DNA. In PCR, short pieces of DNA known as *primers* are used to result in the specific amplification of short pieces of DNA (Fig. 18–3). Quantities of DNA that were previously too small to be studied by any other technique can be rapidly reproduced over and over until they represent

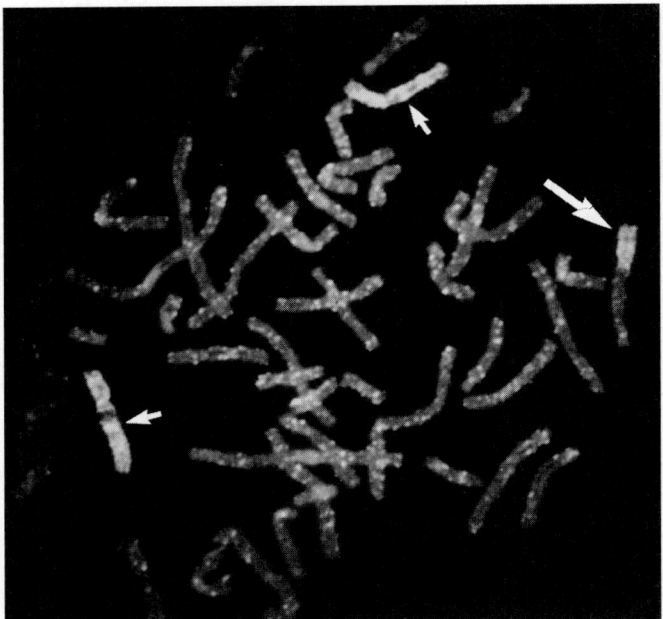

FIGURE 18–2. Fluorescence in situ hybridization is useful in confirming structural rearrangements of chromosomes. Here, a chromosome 10–specific painting probe identifies two normal chromosomes 10 (small arrowheads) and a rearranged chromosome containing genetic material from chromosome 10 (large arrowhead). (From Fallet S, Babu A, Ely S, Wilner JP: Prenatal diagnosis of partial trisomy 10q using fluorescence in situ hybridization. Children's Hospital Quarterly 6:75–80, 1994.)

large amounts of DNA, suitable for analysis by other simple, low-sensitivity techniques. The PCR primers are designed based on their ability to hybridize to a specific piece of target DNA that is desired to be amplified. Pairs of primers, each 15 to 25 bases in length, uniquely flank the area of interest. These short primer sequences can be synthesized chemically using commercially available devices. The target DNA of interest is hybridized to the primers at a low temperature. A thermostable enzyme, Taq polymerase—which can copy DNA when present with the primer, or starting piece—is added. In a short time, the Taq polymerase copies the target DNA, including the region complementary to the second primer. The mixture is then heated, and the newly synthesized DNA and the target DNA separate. Upon cooling, the primers, which are in vast excess, hybridize to the target DNA as well as the DNA synthesized during the first round of amplification. Again, the Taq polymerase copies the target DNA (and newly synthesized DNA), once again doubling the quantities of each. Repetition of these heating and cooling cycles results in a doubling of DNA quantity with each cycle. After 20 to 30 cycles, relatively huge quantities of DNA are available for further analysis.

Uses of Polymerase Chain Reaction

The products of a PCR reaction are useful for a number of clinically important investigations. The presence or absence of a PCR product can be used to measure the presence or absence of a piece of DNA. PCR, especially

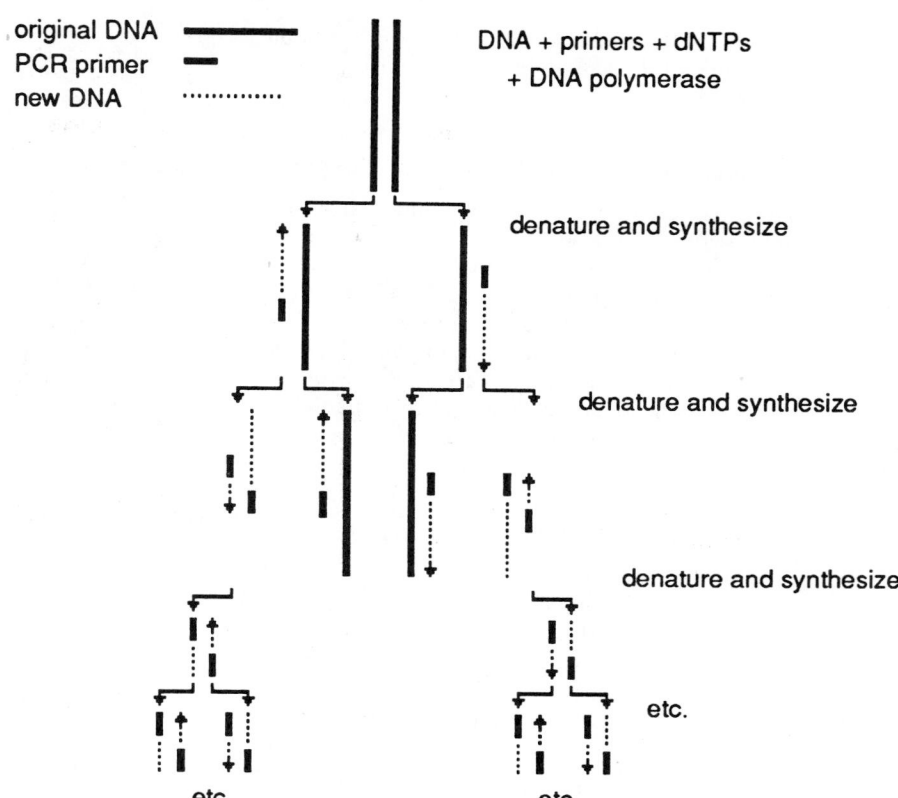

original DNA ———
PCR primer —
new DNA ············

DNA + primers + dNTPs
+ DNA polymerase

denature and synthesize

denature and synthesize

denature and synthesize

etc.

etc.

etc.

FIGURE 18–3. Polymerase chain reaction. The figure shows cycles of heating (denature) and cooling (synthesis) that result in denaturation and in hybridization and polymerization, respectively. The key ingredients are listed at the top. The DNA polymerase used is heat stable, allowing multiple cycles of heating and cooling without loss of activity. After typically 20 to 30 cycles of heating and cooling, the original DNA sequence is amplified several million times. (From Ausubel FM, Brent R, Kingston RE: Current Protocols in Molecular Biology. Copyright 1994 John Wiley & Sons. Reprinted by permission of John Wiley & Sons, Inc., New York.)

when extended by some subtle variations, may be helpful at quantifying small quantities of DNA. Additionally, the amplified pieces of DNA can be subjected to RFLP analysis for further linkage studies.

Diagnosis of Infectious Disease

PCR is a useful test to supplement current microbiologic techniques, relying on the ability to amplify small quantities of infectious material. In particular, it is possible to identify the presence of organisms that are either impossible or difficult to culture.

Whipple Disease. One organism that is impossible to culture is the Whipple disease–associated bacillus (Fleming, 1989). Whipple disease is a multisystem disorder with gastrointestinal, heart, and central nervous system involvement. Previously the diagnosis was entirely made by pathologic studies. PCR has allowed the uncultured detection of the Whipple disease–associated bacillus using a PCR technique (Relman et al, 1982).

Toxoplasma gondii. Other potential clinical indications for PCR diagnosis of infectious disease include tests for toxoplasmosis. *Toxoplasma gondii* can be cultured in fibroblasts from cerebrospinal fluid (CSF) or after inoculation of postmortem clinical specimens. These techniques, however, are of limited sensitivity and often take weeks before a result is obtained (Hitt and Filice, 1992). PCR offers an increased sensitivity to the presence of toxoplasma relative to fibroblast culture and can be performed not only on CSF but also on amniotic fluid, thus allowing rapid prenatal

diagnosis (Grover et al, 1990). This technique also permits diagnosis in those few individuals who do not mount an immune response to the organism.

Tuberculosis. Another disease that has become amenable to PCR diagnostics is *Mycobacterium tuberculosis*. Currently, cultivation of tuberculosis can take 2 to 3 months until final identification of an organism. Using the PCR technique, it is possible to identify the DNA from fewer than 10 organisms in a clinical specimen and to detect antibiotic resistance genes in such specimens (deWit et al, 1993). The molecular cloning of the mycobacterial gene inhA confers a missense mutation in that gene, resulting in resistance to both isonicotinic acid hydrazide (INH) and ethionamide. Molecular cloning of this gene and the mutation within it allows the possibility not only to detect the presence of mycobacterial tuberculosis but also to detect sensitivity or resistance to INH. Thus, PCR amplification can potentially allow the identification of tuberculosis and its antibiotic sensitivity without culturing the organism. This can be done rapidly so that the information is available to the physician before the initiation of chemotherapy.

Rapid Identification of Bacterial Antibiotic Resistance

PCR has been useful in rapidly distinguishing methicillin-resistant *Staphylococcus aureus* specimens from non–methicillin-resistant *Staphylococcus aureus* specimens. This technique uses PCR to identify the small MECA gene that encodes a low-affinity penicillin-binding protein. This type of PCR analysis is very sensitive to the presence of the MECA gene and is more sensitive than conventional methods of identification of methicillin-resistant organisms (Tokue et al, 1992).

Rapid Detection of Common Bacterial Pathogens

A recent paper has identified a PCR technique that specifically amplifies the 16-S ribosomal RNA from a variety of clinically important bacteria from blood samples to accurately identify bacteremic patients (McCabe et al, 1995). This technique can detect in blood the presence of *Haemophilus influenzae* type B, *Klebsiella pneumoniae, Proteus mirabilis, Pseudomonas aeruginosa, Salmonella, Shigella,* group A beta hemolytic streptococcus, group B hemolytic streptococcus, and *Staphylococcus aureus,* all in a single rapid reaction.

Human Immunodeficiency Virus

PCR is also helpful in cases of neonatal acquired immunodeficiency virus in distinguishing infants who acquire maternal antibodies at birth and in whom human immunodeficiency virus (HIV) infection will develop. Maternal antibodies to HIV can persist in infants for 6 to up to 15 months after birth. The PCR technique is more sensitive than either culture or antigen detection, offering more than 97% sensitivity to infection in children who will go on to have neonatal HIV infection (Comeau et al, 1993; Petru et al, 1992).

REFERENCES

Botstein D, White RL, Skolnick M, Davis RW: Construction of a genetic linkage map in man using restriction fragment length polymorphisms. Am J Hum Genet 32:314–331, 1980.

Boue A, Gropp A, Boue J: Cytogenetics of pregnancy wastage. Adv Hum Genet 14:1–58, 1985.

Comeau AN, Hsu H-W, Schwezler M, et al: Identifying human immunodeficiency virus infection at birth: Application of preliminary chain reaction to Guthrie cards. J Pediatr 123:252–258, 1993.

deWit D, Wootton M, Allan B, Steyn L: Simple method for production of internal control DNA for *Mycobacterium tuberculosis* polymerase chain reaction assays. J Clin Microbiol 31:2204–2207, 1993.

Driscoll DA, Salvin J, Sellinger B, et al: Prevalence of 22q11 microdeletions in DiGeorge and velocardiofacial syndromes: Implications for genetic counselling and prenatal diagnosis. J Med Genet 30:813–817, 1993.

Fleming JL: Whipple's disease: Clinical biochemical and histopathology and assessment of treatment in 29 patients. Mayo Clin Proc 63:539–551, 1989.

Gall JG, Pardue NL: Formation and detection of RNA–DNA hybrid molecules in preparations. Proc Nat Acad Sci USA 63:378, 1969.

Grover CM, Thulliez P, Remington JS, et al: Rapid prenatal diagnosis of congenital toxoplasma infection by using polymerase chain reaction and amniotic fluid. J Clin Microbiol 28:2297–2301, 1990.

Hitt JA, Filice GA: Detection of *Toxoplasma gondii* parasitemia by gene amplifications and cell culture in mouse inoculation. J Clin Microbiol 30:3181–3184, 1992.

Landegent JE, Jansen IN, Dewal N, et al: Chromosomal localization of a unique gene by non-autoradiography in situ hybridization. Nature 317:175, 1985.

Landegent JE, Jansen IN, Dewal N, et al: Use of whole cosmid clone genome sequences for chromosomal localization by non-radioactive in situ hybridization. Hum Genet 77:366, 1987.

McCabe KM, Khan G, Zhang YH, et al: Amplification of bacterial DNA using highly conserved sequences: Automated analysis and potential for molecular triage of sepsis. Pediatrics 95:165–169, 1995.

Petru A, Dunphy MG, Azimi P, et al: Reliability of polymerase chain reaction detection of human immunodeficiency virus in children. Pediatr Infect Dis J 11:30–33, 1992.

Relman DA, et al: Identification of the uncultured bacillus of Whipple's disease. N Engl J Med 327:293–301, 1982.

Southern EM: Detection of specific sequences among DNA fragments separated by gel electrophoresis. J Molec Biol 98(3):503–517, 1975.

Tokue Y, Shoji S, Satoh K, et al: Comparison of a polymerase chain reaction assay and a conventional microbiologic method for detection of methicillin-resistant *Staphylococcus aureus* [see comments]. Antimicrob Agents Chemother 36:6–9, 1992.

Tokue Y, et al: Comparison of a polymerase chain reaction assay and a conventional microbiology method for the detection of methicillin resistant *Staphylococcus aureus* [comment]. Antimicrob Agents Chemother 36:1585–1586, 1992.

CHAPTER 19

Prenatal Genetic Diagnosis

Diana W. Bianchi

As a result of the ever-expanding number of prenatal diagnostic tests that are performed on pregnant women, clinicians know a lot about their patients long before they even touch them. This chapter discusses the common methods of prenatal genetic diagnosis, the information they convey, and the implications for the newborn.

MATERNAL SERUM SCREENING

Maternal serum screening has been incorporated into routine obstetric care. It is used to identify a high-risk pregnancy in a low-risk population of pregnant women. Currently, maternal serum screening consists of measurement of alpha-fetoprotein (AFP), human chorionic gonadotropin (hCG), and unconjugated estriol (uE3), proteins that are made by the fetus or placenta. The most clinical experience has been achieved with assay of AFP.

AFP is one of the major proteins in fetal serum. Its precise physiologic role is unknown. It can be detected as early as 4 weeks' gestation, when it is synthesized by the yolk sac (Bergstrand, 1986). Subsequently, it is produced in the fetal liver and peaks in the fetal serum between 10 and 13 weeks' gestation. AFP is then excreted into the fetal urine or leaks into the amniotic fluid through the skin before keratinization at 20 weeks' gestation. It is also present in cerebrospinal fluid. AFP in maternal serum is exclusively fetal in origin (Crandall, 1981). Maternal serum AFP peaks at 32 weeks' gestation owing to increased placental permeability for the protein (Ferguson-Smith, 1983). Most clinical assays are performed at 16 weeks' gestation. Accurate gestational dating, maternal race, weight, and presence of diabetes are critical to the interpretation of results.

In 1972, Brock and Sutcliffe observed that there were markedly increased levels of AFP in the amniotic fluid of fetuses with anencephaly and open neural tube defects. Subsequently, it was shown that elevated amniotic fluid AFP levels were associated with increased maternal serum AFP (Ferguson-Smith, 1983). The possibility of a screening test for open neural tube defects became apparent. In the initial collaborative efforts aimed at studying maternal serum AFP, results were expressed as multiples of the median (MoM) to allow comparison between laboratories. It has become a convention to describe results of greater than 2.5 MoM as abnormally high and less than 0.6 MoM as abnormally low. Both require further investigation.

If the AFP is elevated, the patient is offered an ultrasonographic examination to verify gestational age, determine fetal viability, and diagnose many of the structural abnormalities that can be associated with an elevated AFP. Although the AFP test was developed to screen for neural tube defects, abnormally high results are not specific for this condition (Table 19–1). If the ultrasonographic examination is unrevealing, the patient undergoes amniocentesis

to assay the amniotic fluid for the presence of AFP and acetylcholinesterase, which are elevated in open spina bifida (Crandall et al, 1983). Even though an elevated AFP is compatible with a normal diagnosis, a study of 277 infants with elevated maternal serum AFP and normal amniotic fluid AFP revealed an increased incidence of intrauterine growth restriction and non-neural tube anomalies (Burton and Dillard, 1986).

Maternal serum AFP screening has also been used to detect chromosomally abnormal fetuses since the observation was made that a low AFP value was more likely in a trisomy 18 or 21 fetus than in a normal fetus (Merkatz et al, 1984). Several prospective studies have demonstrated that, by expressing risk for Down syndrome as a combined function of maternal age and AFP value and by offering amniocentesis to all women with a risk of 1:270 or greater (the equivalent risk in a 35-year-old woman based on age alone), it is possible to detect approximately one third of otherwise unexpected Down syndrome fetuses (Dimaio et al, 1987; Palomaki and Haddow, 1987). Low AFP values are probably caused by decreased hepatic production in the affected fetus. Although it would make sense to ascribe this phenomenon to the small size of the liver, one study found no association between fetal weight and low AFP values in chromosomally abnormal fetuses (Librach et al, 1988). The differential diagnosis of a decreased AFP level is shown in Table 19–2. Because a low AFP value detects only one third of Down syndrome fetuses, a normal AFP value does not rule out trisomy 21.

Experience with using low maternal AFP levels as a screen for fetal chromosome abnormalities has led to the

---

TABLE 19–1

Differential Diagnosis of Abnormally High Maternal Serum Alpha-Fetoprotein

Incorrect gestational dating
Multiple pregnancy
Threatened pregnancy loss
Fetomaternal hemorrhage
Anencephaly
Open spina bifida
Anterior abdominal wall defects
Congenital nephrosis
Acardia
Lesions of the placenta and umbilical cord
Turner syndrome
Cystic hygroma
Renal agenesis
Polycystic kidney disease
Epidermolysis bullosa
Hereditary persistence (autosomal dominant trait)

TABLE 19–2

TABLE 19–2

Differential Diagnosis of Abnormally Low Maternal Serum Alpha-Fetoprotein

Incorrect gestational dating	Trisomy 18
Trisomy 21	Intrauterine growth restriction

evaluation of many other proteins produced by both the fetus and placenta. Two of these, uE3 and hCG, have been incorporated into maternal serum screening panels. AFP, uE3, and hCG are only weakly correlated with each other and their values are all independent of maternal age (Norton, 1994). Measurement of all three can be combined to improve sensitivity and specificity of Down syndrome detection. Elevated hCG values are the most specific markers for fetal trisomy 21 (Bogart et al, 1987; Rose and Mennuti, 1993), whereas estriol levels are approximately 25% less than normal. Pregnancies affected by fetal trisomy 18 also have reduced levels of uE3 and hCG. Women whose serum screens indicate a fetal Down syndrome risk of greater than 1:270 should be offered gestational dating by sonography, because all biochemical measurements are interpreted in relation to gestational age.

Future trends in maternal serum screening include measurements during the first trimester of pregnancy. Particularly promising are pregnancy-associated plasma protein A (PAPP-A) and the free beta subunit of hCG (Brambati et al, 1994), both of which are abnormal in cases of fetal trisomy 21. Research is also ongoing to correlate higher levels of excretion of the beta-core fragment of hCG in maternal urine in cases complicated by fetal aneuploidy (Hayashi and Kozu, 1995).

ULTRASONOGRAPHY

The routine use of ultrasound imaging in pregnancy has been controversial in the United States (Bakketeig et al, 1984; Eik-Neis et al, 1984; Ewigman et al, 1993). Nevertheless, it remains the best noninvasive method for gestational dating, definition of fetal anatomy, serial measurements of fetal growth, and evaluation of dynamic parameters such as cardiac contractility, fetal urine production, and fetal movement. Additionally, it has been suggested that antenatal visualization of the fetus promotes maternal-infant bonding (Fletcher and Evans, 1983). Despite controversies, it has been estimated that 40% of obstetric patients undergo at least one ultrasonographic examination during pregnancy (Hill et al, 1983). The advent of antenatal ultrasonography has had a large impact on the types of patients who present to the neonatal intensive care unit.

Within the context of prenatal genetic diagnosis, ultrasonography may be used to detect congenital anomalies. In 2% to 3% of live births, a malformation is present (Nelson and Holmes, 1989). Fetal structures that are normally filled with fluid are especially well visualized. In approximately 10% of infants with anomalies, the central nervous system is involved (Hill et al, 1983). Ultrasonography is particularly useful in the diagnosis of anencephaly, microcephaly, en-

cephalocele, and hydrocephalus. By 20 weeks' gestation, the fetal facial structures may be examined for cyclopia, cleft lip, or micrognathia. Nuchal membrane thickening is suggestive of Down syndrome, familial pterygium coli, or other chromosome abnormalities (Benacerraf et al, 1987; Chervenak et al, 1983). Fetal cardiovascular structures may be reliably examined at 20 weeks' gestation. The presence of four cardiac chambers, the dynamic relationships between the cardiac valves, and the location of the vessels allow such diagnoses as hypoplastic left heart, double outlet right ventricle, tricuspid atresia, tetralogy of Fallot, and Ebstein anomaly to be made. Pericardial effusion and arrhythmias may be similarly observed.

Gastrointestinal anomalies occur in approximately 0.6% of live births, and one third of them are associated with chromosome abnormalities (Barss et al, 1985). The decrease in fetal swallowing seen in some cases of bowel obstruction (from atresia, stenosis, annular pancreas, or diaphragmatic hernia) may lead to polyhydramnios that results in a uterine size greater than expected for gestational dates. Although gastroschisis and omphalocele are readily diagnosed, they may be confused with each other, and their differing prognoses may cause considerable parental anxiety (Griffiths and Gough, 1985). Gastroschisis usually occurs as an isolated anomaly; infants generally do well after surgical repair. The kidneys are identifiable by 14 weeks' gestation, but the presence of perirenal fat and large adrenals may obscure the diagnosis of renal agenesis (Hill et al, 1983). Renal cysts, hydronephrosis, and obstructive uropathy are easily visualized. Oligohydramnios is indicative of poor renal function. Multiple standard curves exist for fetal anthropometric measurements (Elejalde and Elejalde, 1986; Saul et al, 1988). These are particularly helpful in the diagnosis of skeletal dysplasias and evaluation of growth retardation. Fetal genitalia may be reliably determined by 24 weeks' gestation (Birnholz, 1983). Additionally, ultrasonographic examination is of benefit in the diagnosis and management of multiple pregnancies (Fig. 19–1).

Although there have been no documented adverse outcomes related to ultrasound exposure during human pregnancy, the reported experimental biologic effects of altered immune response, cell death, change in cell membrane functions, free radical formation, and reduced cell reproductive potential necessitate judicious use of this technology. Another concern is the appropriate pediatric follow-up for prenatally observed conditions with unclear clinical significance, such as minimal hydronephrosis and echogenic bowel.

The accuracy of ultrasonographic diagnosis has been addressed in several papers. In one study of 1737 referrals, 244 malformations were correctly diagnosed. Six results were falsely called abnormal (0.3%), and 16 were incorrectly called normal (0.9%) (Campbell and Pearce, 1983). In 596 women referred for ultrasonography, 81 had fetal anomalies diagnosed, with a falsely abnormal rate of 0.6% and a falsely normal rate of 0.5% (Sabbagha et al, 1985). The limitations of ultrasonography were delineated in a study correlating anatomic pathologic findings at autopsy with prenatal diagnosis (Rutledge et al, 1986). Fifty-two malformations in 45 fetuses were correctly diagnosed antenatally, but 90 additional malformations were missed.

Recently, a randomized trial was conducted involving

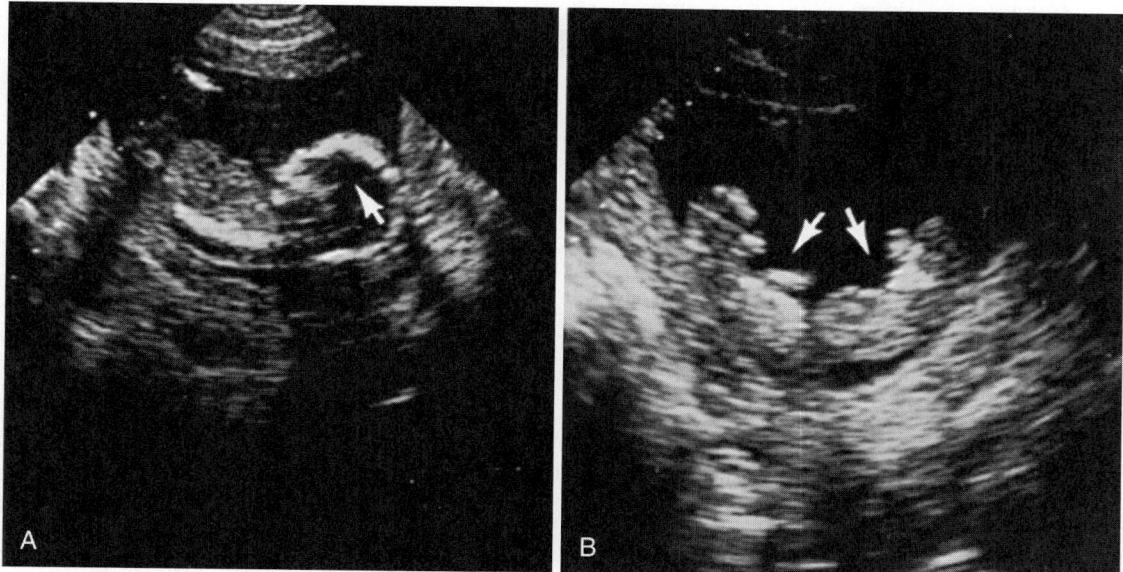

FIGURE 19–1. Appearance on ultrasonographic examination (B-mode scan, 5.0 MHz) of a singleton pregnancy, *A*, at approximately 4 months' gestation, and a twin pregnancy, *B*, at approximately 12 weeks' gestation. The arrow in *A* points to the fetal cranium; the arrows in *B* indicate the fetuses. (Courtesy of Dr. Jason Birnholz.)

15,151 pregnant women to determine whether the routine use of sonographic screening decreased the occurrence of adverse perinatal outcomes (Ewigman et al, 1993). This study, which received considerable attention, did not show improved rates of preterm delivery or birth weight. Approximately 35% of the fetuses with anomalies were detected by antenatal sonography in the screened population versus only 11% in the control group (Crane et al, 1994). Despite this difference, neither clinical management nor outcome of the pregnancy was significantly improved in the screened population.

Continuous ultrasonographic fetal imaging is important in improvement of the safety and efficacy of the more invasive diagnostic procedures such as amniocentesis, chorionic villus sampling, and cordocentesis, which are discussed in the following sections.

AMNIOCENTESIS

Amniocentesis refers to the removal of up to 20 mL of amniotic fluid from the pregnant uterus. Contained within this fluid are cellular components (desquamated fetal epithelial and bladder cells), which serve as a source of chromosomes, DNA, or enzymes. Most of these cellular elements are nonviable. Hence, amniocytes generally require tissue culture under specific conditions to provide enough material for diagnosis (Gosden, 1983). Herein lies one of the major disadvantages of the procedure—results are received late in the second trimester after fetal movement has been perceived by the pregnant woman. In contrast, the amniotic fluid itself may be assayed immediately after removal for the biochemical presence of alpha-fetoprotein, acetylcholinesterase, bilirubin, lecithin, sphingomyelin, or phosphatidylcholine.

The indications for genetic amniocentesis are (1) mater-

nal age of 35 years or older at the time of delivery because there is an increased risk for fetal chromosome abnormalities, (2) a previous pregnancy that resulted in an infant with chromosome abnormalities, (3) either parent with a balanced chromosome translocation, (4) an abnormal maternal serum screen, (5) a family history of a child with a neural tube defect, (6) a family history of a metabolic disorder for which the enzyme defect is known, (7) a maternal history of X-linked disorder, or (8) a family history of a disorder for which DNA diagnosis is available.

Extensive clinical experience with amniocentesis has accrued since the results of the first large-scale randomized trials were published in the 1970s (National Institute of Child Health and Human Development National Registry, 1976; Simpson et al, 1976). Most institutions in the United States currently quote a 1% to 2% incidence of minor complications, such as amniotic fluid leakage, uterine cramping, or vaginal spotting, following the procedure; a 0.25% to 0.5% incidence of more serious complications, such as chorioamnionitis and miscarriage, also exists (Centers for Disease Control and Prevention, 1995). There is a significant inverse relationship between procedural experience and risk of miscarriage (Verjaal and Leschot, 1981).

In a series of 3000 amniocenteses performed at a single institution over 8 years, there was a diagnostic accuracy rate of more than 99%. Chromosome abnormalities were detected in 2.4% of 2404 women with advanced maternal age, 1.2% of 240 women who had previously had an infant with trisomy 21, and 9.1% of 55 women with other cytogenetic indications (Golbus et al, 1979).

Because results of amniocentesis are received relatively late in the pregnancy, research efforts have focused on evaluation of the procedure if performed between 12 and 15 weeks' gestation. No significant increased risks associated with early amniocentesis are known (Nevin et al, 1990). This area is under study with regard to safety and accuracy. Even though a smaller amount of amniotic fluid is withdrawn, there does not appear to be any increased difficulty in obtaining enough cells to make a diagnosis (Hanson et al, 1987). In some medical centers, early amniocentesis is offered as an alternative to chorionic villus sampling.

CHORIONIC VILLUS SAMPLING

Despite the wealth of experience with amniocentesis, its usefulness has been somewhat limited by the timing of the procedure. Since the publication of the first English language report on sampling of the chorion (Kazy et al, 1982), there has been enormous medical and scientific interest in first-trimester prenatal diagnosis.

Chorionic villus sampling (CVS) involves the aspiration of the chorion frondosum between 10 and 11 weeks' gestation (Fig. 19–2). The fact that the procedure is performed early is advantageous, because most women at this point do not have external manifestations of pregnancy and have not yet perceived fetal movement. The chorionic villi are composed of syncytiotrophoblast and mesenchymal core cells that are actively growing and dividing. In contrast to the dying epithelial cells shed into the amniotic fluid, chorionic villus cells do not require prolonged culture to provide enough mitoses for a cytogenetic diagnosis. Karyotype results are generally available within 1 week of the procedure. Initially, direct preparations derived from syncytiotrophoblast were used for analysis, but the number of apparently

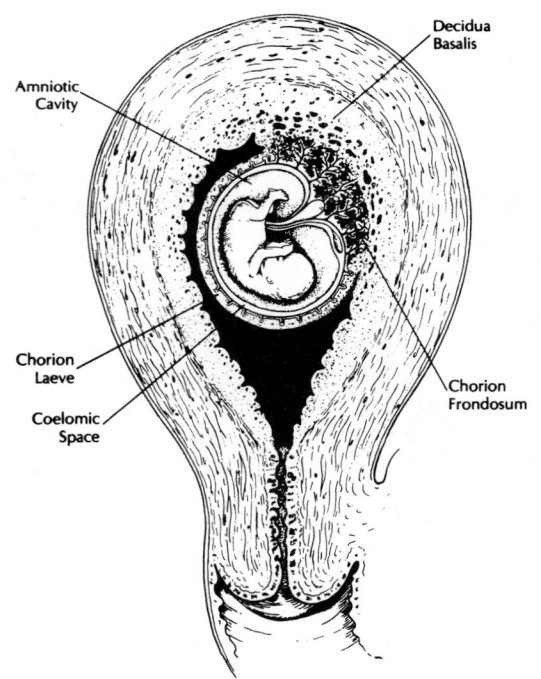

FIGURE 19–2. A pregnant uterus containing a fetus at about 9 weeks' gestation. The chorion frondosum, if biopsied, can provide fetal cells for chromosome, enzyme, or DNA analysis. (From Jackson LG: First trimester diagnosis of fetal genetic disorders. Hosp Prac March 15, 1985, p 40.)

mosaic abnormal results proved unacceptable. Cultured preparations derived from the cell of the mesenchymal core are more closely related in embryonic origin to the actual fetus (Bianchi et al, 1993). It is currently recommended that both direct and cultured preparations be used for cytogenetic analysis. *Mosaicism*, defined as the presence of two or more cell lines carrying different chromosomal constitutions, is a true biologic (not technical) problem in CVS. In several large studies, 0.8% to 1.7% of 1000 cases had a chromosome abnormality that was present in the villus but not in the fetus (Hogge et al, 1986; Ledbetter et al, 1992). This has led to the observation that postzygotic nondisjunction is more common than was previously suspected.

The indications for CVS are the same as those for amniocentesis with two exceptions: neural tube defects cannot be diagnosed by this procedure and AFP or other serum screening is not routinely offered at this early point in gestation. Furthermore, evidence shows that the feto-maternal hemorrhage associated with placental biopsy results in elevated maternal serum AFP immediately after the procedure (Brambati et al, 1988).

CVS is performed transcervically or transabdominally. With the transcervical technique, the inherent risks of fetal and maternal infection appear to be greater because it is impossible to sterilize the cervix. Under ultrasonic guidance, a flexible catheter is passed through the endocervix and placed into the chorion frondosum. A small segment of placenta is then aspirated into sterile tissue culture medium and the catheter is withdrawn (Jackson, 1985). In contrast, the transabdominal technique uses a needle to obtain villus material; sterilization of the skin surface is straightforward (Brambati et al, 1988). With either method, approximately 10 to 50 mg of tissue is obtained. Subsequently, the villi are dissected from maternal decidua and processed for tissue culture or DNA extraction.

The safety and accuracy of these techniques are being closely monitored. A randomized National Institutes of Health clinical trial compared amniocentesis with CVS (Rhoads et al, 1989). A consensus conference was held by the Centers for Disease Control and Prevention and NIH to summarize worldwide experience. After adjustment for confounding factors such as gestational age, the risk of miscarriage after CVS is on the order of 0.5% to 1.0% (Centers for Disease Control and Prevention, 1995).

The advantages and disadvantages of CVS are summarized in Table 19–3. For patients at high risk for single gene disorders amenable to DNA diagnosis (e.g., cystic fibrosis, sickle cell anemia, or Duchenne muscular dystrophy), CVS is probably the preferred prenatal diagnostic method. On the other hand, for patients with relatively low risk (e.g., a 35-year-old woman being tested for chromosome abnormalities), an amniocentesis may be more appropriate. There have been a few reports of serious maternal sepsis and transient bacteremia associated with transcervical CVS (Barela et al, 1986; Blakemore et al, 1985; Silverman et al, 1994). The 1% incidence of mosaicism in villus samples may necessitate further invasive techniques such as amniocentesis or cordocentesis to confirm or refute diagnoses. The biggest concern regarding CVS is the risk of limb deficiencies in infants whose mothers underwent the procedure.

TABLE 19-3

Chorionic Villus Sampling Versus Amniocentesis

Advantages
  Performed in first trimester; results available quickly
  Cells obtained are mitotically active
  Amount of tissue obtained is preferable for DNA analysis
  Placental mosaicism is detected
Disadvantages
  Miscarriage rate slightly higher
  Increased fetomaternal hemorrhage following procedure
  Risk of serious maternal infection
  Risk of fetal limb and jaw malformations

The risk of limb malformations was suggested by a number of publications that described an increased incidence of transverse limb anomalies and the hypoglossia-hypodactyly syndrome in infants whose mothers had undergone chorionic villus sampling (Burton et al, 1992; Firth et al, 1991, 1994; Hsieh et al, 1995). The overall rate of non–syndrome-related transverse limb deficiency from 65 centers performing CVS is 7.4 per 10,000 procedures (Centers for Disease Control and Prevention, 1995). This number is reasonably similar to population-based registries that monitor infants with all limb deficiencies and give a rate of 5 to 6 per 10,000 live births (Centers for Disease Control and Prevention, 1995). Of concern, however, are studies in which cases of limb malformation were classified to match the phenotype of CVS-exposed infants with limb deficiencies. In these studies, a background rate of 1.5 to 2.3 per 10,000 live births was found, suggesting that CVS does increase the risk for limb malformations (Centers for Disease Control and Prevention, 1995). Factors likely to influence the rate of limb malformations include gestational age (risk of limb deficiencies being greatest at less than or equal to 9 weeks of gestation and decreased at 10 weeks of gestation or after), type of catheter used, and operator experience. The overall risk of limb deficiency appears to be on the order of 1:3000 procedures (Centers for Disease Control and Prevention, 1995). Furthermore, an increased incidence of hemangioma has been suggested in infants born following CVS (Burton et al, 1995).

CORDOCENTESIS

Percutaneous umbilical blood sampling or cordocentesis was first described as a means of obtaining fetal immunoglobulin M (IgM) measurements in the prenatal diagnosis of congenital toxoplasmosis (Daffos et al, 1985). Under continuous ultrasonographic imaging, the insertion site of the umbilical cord into the placenta is identified. Using a 20-gauge needle, the umbilical vein in punctured, the sample is withdrawn, and the umbilical cord is observed for signs of hemorrhage. The technique has been used diagnostically in many clinical settings (Forestier et al, 1988) (Table 19–4). With regard to genetic diagnosis, the lymphocytes are a source of cells for a rapid karyotype. This is helpful in two situations: (1) when anomalies have been noted on ultrasonographic examination but it is too late in

gestation to perform an amniocentesis (antenatal diagnosis of trisomy 13 or 18 influences delivery room management), and (2) for confirmation of a fetal karyotype when amniocentesis or CVS has shown mosaicism (Gosden et al, 1988).

PREIMPLANTATION GENETIC DIAGNOSIS

The desire to avoid termination of pregnancy for fetuses affected with genetic disease has led to the development of techniques of preimplantation diagnosis. In a limited number of laboratories worldwide, it is possible to analyze the DNA or chromosomal constitution from the polar body of the oocyte, a blastomere, or a blastocyst. The underlying rationale is that if disease-causing genes are identified in the embryo, the embryo will not be replaced into the uterus for implantation. To perform preimplantation genetic diagnosis, various forms of assisted reproductive technology are necessary. As of the end of 1995, in a worldwide survey, only approximately 15% of couples with normal fertility who undergo these preimplantation genetic diagnostic procedures have had a "take home" baby (Harper, 1996). Furthermore, in 3 of the 34 babies born following this technique, a diagnostic error was made (Harper, 1996). Despite these concerns, impressive advances in the scope and capacity of single cell genetic analysis indicate the potential promise of this form of diagnosis (Handyside et al, 1992; Kristjansson et al, 1994).

FETAL CELLS IN MATERNAL BLOOD

All nucleated fetal cells from the same individual contain identical genetic information. As a result, research efforts are currently focused on noninvasive methods for fetal genetic diagnosis. An attractive potential population are the rare fetal cells that cross the placenta and circulate within the mother. The fetal cell types currently being studied include the trophoblast (Johansen et al, 1995) and nucleated erythrocyte (Bianchi et al, 1990). Genetic diagnoses that have already been made successfully in fetal cells isolated from maternal blood include trisomies 18 and 21, triploidy, Klinefelter syndrome (47, XXY), exclusion of beta globin mutations, inheritance of HLA-DR and DQ alpha types, and Rhesus D genotype (Bianchi, 1995; Simpson and Elias, 1993). Based on these encouraging preliminary results, the National Institutes of Child Health and Human Development is sponsoring a multicenter clinical evaluation designed to evaluate cytogenetic accuracy of fetal cells in maternal blood as compared with amniocentesis or CVS (de la Cruz et al, 1995).

TABLE 19-4

Indications for Fetal Blood Sampling

Hemoglobinopathies	Acid-base abnormalities
Bleeding disorders	Fetal blood type incompatibility
Immunodeficiency	Metabolic disorders
Congenital infection	Chromosome abnormalities

REFERENCES

Bakketeig LS, Eik-Neis SH, Jacobsen G, et al: Randomised controlled trial of ultrasonographic screening in pregnancy. Lancet 2:207, 1984.

Barela AL, Kleinman GE, Golditch IM, et al: Septic shock with renal failure after chorionic villus sampling. Am J Obstet Gynecol 154:1100, 1986.

Barss VA, Benacerraf BR, Frigoletto FD: Antenatal sonographic diagnosis of fetal gastrointestinal malformations. Pediatrics 76:445, 1985.

Benacerraf BR, Gelman R, Frigoletto FD: Sonographic identification of second trimester fetuses with Down's syndrome. N Engl J Med 317:1371, 1987.

Bergstrand CG: Alphafetoprotein in paediatrics: Acta Paediatr Scand 75:1, 1986.

Bianchi DW: Prenatal diagnosis by analysis of fetal cells in maternal blood. J Pediatr 127:847, 1995.

Bianchi DW, Flint AF, Pizzimenti MF, et al: Isolation of fetal DNA from nucleated erythrocytes in maternal blood. Proc Natl Acad Sci U S A 87:3279, 1990.

Bianchi DW, Wilkins-Haug LE, Enders AC, Hay ED: Origin of extraembryonic mesoderm: Relevance to chorionic villus sampling. Am J Med Genet 46:542–550, 1993.

Birnholz JC: Determination of fetal sex. N Engl J Med 309:942, 1983.

Blakemore KJ, Mahoney MJ, Hobbins JC: Infection and chorionic villus sampling. Lancet 2:338, 1985.

Bogart MH, Pandian MR, Hobbins JC: Abnormal maternal serum chorionic gonadotropin levels in pregnancies with fetal chromosome abnormalities. Prenat Diagn 7:623, 1987.

Brambati B, Lanzani A, Oldrini A: Transabdominal chorionic villus sampling. Clinical experience of 1,159 cases. Prenat Diagn 8:609, 1988.

Brambati B, Tului L, Shrimanker K, et al: Serum PAPP-A and free β-hCG are first-trimester screening markers for Down syndrome. Prenat Diagn 14:1043–1047, 1994.

Brock DJH, Sutcliffe RG: Alpha feto protein in the antenatal diagnosis of anencephaly and spina bifida. Lancet 2:197, 1972.

Burton BK, Dillard RG: Outcome in infants born to mothers with unexplained elevations of maternal serum alphafetoprotein. Pediatrics 77:582, 1986.

Burton BK, Schulz CJ, Angle B, et al: An increased incidence of haemangiomas in infants born following chorionic villus sampling (CVS). Prenat Diagn 15:209–214, 1995.

Burton BK, Schulz CJ, Burd LI: Limb anomalies associated with chorionic villus sampling. Obstet Gynecol 79:726–730, 1992.

Campbell S, Pearce JM: Ultrasound visualization of congenital malformations. Br Med Bull 39:322, 1983.

Centers for Disease Control and Prevention: Chorionic villus sampling and amniocentesis: Recommendations for prenatal counseling. MMWR Morb Mortal Wkly Rep 44:1–12, 1995.

Chervenak FA, Isaacson G, Blakemore KJ: Fetal cystic hygroma. Cause and natural history. N Engl J Med 309:822, 1983.

Crandall BF: Alpha-fetoprotein: The diagnosis of neural tube defects. Pediatr Ann 10:38, 1981.

Crandall BF, Robertson RD, Lebherz TB: Maternal serum alpha-fetoprotein screening for the detection of neural tube defects. West J Med 138:524, 1983.

Crane JP, LeFevre ML, Winborn RC: A randomized trial of prenatal ultrasonographic screening: Impact on the detection, management, and outcome of anomalous fetuses. Am J Obstet Gynecol 171:392–399, 1994.

Daffos F, Capella-Pavlovsky M, Forestier F: Fetal blood sampling during pregnancy with use of a needle guided by ultrasound: A study of 606 consecutive cases. Am J Obstet Gynecol 153:655, 1985.

de la Cruz F, Shifrin H, Elias S, et al: Prenatal diagnosis by use of fetal cells isolated from maternal blood. Am J Obstet Gynecol 173:1354–1355, 1995.

Dimaio MS, Baumgarten A, Greenstein RM, et al: Screening for fetal Down's syndrome in pregnancy by measuring maternal serum alphafetoprotein levels. N Engl J Med 317:342, 1987.

Eik-Neis SH, Okland O, Aure JC, et al: Ultrasound screening in pregnancy: A randomised controlled trial. Lancet 1:1347, 1984.

Elejalde BR, Elejalde MM: The prenatal growth of the human body determined by the measurement of bones and organs by ultrasonography. Am J Med Genet 24:575, 1986.

Ewigman BG, Crane JP, Frigoletto FD, et al: Effect of prenatal ultrasound screening on perinatal outcome. N Engl J Med 329:821–827, 1993.

Ferguson-Smith MA: The reduction of anencephalic and spina bifida births by maternal serum alpha-fetoprotein screening. Br Med Bull 39:365, 1983.

Firth HV, Boyd PA, Chamberlain PF, et al: Limb abnormalities and chorion villus sampling. Lancet 338:51, 1991.

Firth HV, Chamberlain PF, MacKenzie IZ, et al: Analyses of limb reduction defects in babies exposed to chorionic villus sampling. Lancet 343:1069–1071, 1994.

Fletcher JC, Evans MI: Maternal bonding in early fetal ultrasound examinations. N Engl J Med 308:392, 1983.

Forestier F, Cox WJ, Daffos F, et al: The assessment of fetal blood samples. Am J Obstet Gynecol 158:1184, 1988.

Golbus MS, Longman WD, Epstein CJ, et al: Prenatal genetic diagnosis in 3,000 amniocenteses. N Engl J Med 300:157, 1979.

Gosden CM: Amniotic fluid cell types and culture. Br Med Bull 39:348, 1983.

Gosden C, Nicolaides KH, Rodeck CH: Fetal blood sampling in investigation of chromosome mosaicism in amniotic fluid cell culture. Lancet 1:613, 1988.

Griffiths DM, Gough MH: Dilemmas after ultrasonographic diagnosis of fetal abnormality. Lancet 1:623, 1985.

Handyside AH, Lesko JG, Tarín JJ, et al: Birth of a normal girl after in vitro fertilization and preimplantation diagnostic testing for cystic fibrosis. N Engl J Med 327:905–909, 1992.

Hanson FW, Zorn EM, Tennant FR: Amniocentesis before 15 weeks' gestation: Outcome, risks, and technical problems. Am J Obstet Gynecol 156:1524, 1987.

Harper J: Preimplantation diagnosis of inherited disease by embryo biopsy: An update of the world figures. J Assist Reprod Genet 13:90, 1996.

Hayashi M, Kozu H: Maternal urinary β-core fragment of hCG/creatinine ratios and fetal chromosomal abnormalities in the second trimester of pregnancy. Prenat Diagn 15:11–16, 1995.

Hill LM, Breckle R, Gehrking WC: The prenatal detection of congenital malformations by ultrasonography. Mayo Clin Proc 58:805, 1983.

Hogge WA, Schonberg SA, Golbus MS: Chorionic villus sampling: Experience of the first 1,000 cases. Am J Obstet Gynecol 154:1249, 1986.

Hsieh F-J, Shyu M-K, Sheu B-C, et al: Limb defects after chorionic villus sampling. Obstet Gynecol 85:84–88, 1995.

Jackson LG: First trimester diagnosis of fetal genetic disorders. Hosp Prac March 15, 1985, p 39.

Johansen M, Knight M, Maher EJ, et al: An investigation of methods for enriching trophoblast from maternal blood. Prenat Diagn 15:921–932, 1995.

Kazy Z, Rozovsky IS, Bakharev VA: Chorion biopsy in early pregnancy: A method of early prenatal diagnosis for inherited disorders. Prenat Diagn 2:39, 1982.

Kristjansson K, Chong SS, Van den Veyver IB: Preimplantation single cell analyses of dystrophin gene deletions using whole genome amplification. Nat Genet 6:19–23, 1994.

Ledbetter DH, Zachary JM, Simpson JL, et al: Cytogenetic results from the U. S. collaborative study on CVS. Prenat Diagn 12:317–345, 1992.

Librach CL, Hogdall CK, Doran TA: Weights of fetuses with autosomal trisomies at termination of pregnancy: An investigation of the etiologic factors of low serum alphafetoprotein values. Am J Obstet Gynecol 158:290, 1988.

Merkatz IR, Nitowsky HM, Macri JN, et al: An association between low maternal serum alphafetoprotein and fetal chromosome abnormalities. Am J Obstet Gynecol 148:886, 1984.

National Institute of Child Health and Human Development (NICHHD) National Registry: Midtrimester amniocentesis for prenatal diagnosis: Safety and accuracy. JAMA 236:1471, 1976.

Nelson K, Holmes LB: Malformations due to presumed spontaneous mutations in newborn infants. N Engl J Med 320:19, 1989.

Nevin J, Nevin N, Dornan JC, et al: Early amniocentesis: Experience of 222 consecutive patients, 1987–1988. Prenat Diagn 10:79, 1990.

Norton ME: Biochemical and ultrasound screening for chromosomal abnormalities. Semin Perinat 18:256–265, 1994.

Palomaki GE, Haddow JE: Maternal serum alphafetoprotein, age, and Down syndrome risk. Am J Obstet Gynecol 156:460, 1987.

Rhoads G, Jackson L, Schlesselman S, et al: The safety and efficacy of chorionic villus sampling for early prenatal diagnosis of cytogenetic abnormalities. N Engl J Med 320:609, 1989.

Rose NC, Mennuti MT: Maternal serum screening for neural tube defects and fetal chromosome abnormalities. West J Med 159:312–317, 1993.

Rutledge JC, Weinberg AG, Friedman JM: Anatomic correlates of ultrasonographic prenatal diagnosis. Prenat Diagn 6:51, 1986.

Sabbagha RE, Sheikh Z, Tamura R, et al: Predictive value, sensitivity, and specificity of ultrasonic targeted imaging for fetal anomalies in gravid women at high risk for birth defects. Am J Obstet Gynecol 152:822, 1985.

Saul RA, Stevenson RE, Rogers RC, et al: Growth references from conception to adulthood. Proc Greenwood Genet Ctr Suppl 1, 1988.

Silverman NS, Sullivan MW, Jungkind DL, et al: Incidence of bacteremia associated with chorionic villus sampling. Obstet Gynecol 84:1021–1024, 1994.

Simpson JL, Elias S: Isolating fetal cells from maternal blood. Advances in prenatal diagnosis through molecular technology. JAMA 270:2357–2361, 1993.

Simpson NE, Dallaire L, Miller JR, et al: Prenatal diagnosis of genetic disease in Canada: Report of a collaborative study. Can Med Assoc J 115:739, 1976.

Verjaal M, Leschot NJ: Risk of amniocentesis and laboratory findings in a series of 1,500 prenatal diagnoses. Prenat Diagn 1:173, 1981.

CHAPTER 20

Genetic Examination of the Newborn Infant

Diana W. Bianchi

Congenital anomalies have surpassed prematurity as the leading cause of perinatal mortality (Centers for Disease Control, 1989). The widespread use of prenatal sonographic examination and subsequent referral of fetuses with anomalies to tertiary medical centers have markedly changed the types of patients who present to newborn intensive care units (Nichols and Bianchi, 1996). Practitioners of neonatal care need to know how to perform a genetic examination of the newborn infant because there is an increased percentage of patients with congenital anomalies in the newborn nursery. The incidence of congenital anomalies is 2% in all live births, but increases significantly to 16% in newborns who weigh less than 1500 g at birth (Mili et al, 1991). In a study of 196 infant deaths that occurred over a 5-year period in a regional neonatal intensive care unit, almost one fourth were due to genetic disorders (Hudome et al, 1994).

This chapter emphasizes the components of the genetic examination of a newborn infant. A genetic examination differs significantly from the traditional neonatal cardiopulmonary examination. Two caveats exist for the individual performing a genetic examination of the newborn infant. First, any infant who is nasotracheally intubated and on mechanical ventilation usually has adhesive tape obscuring the entire midface. Physical examination of the midface is a critical component of the dysmorphologic examination. It is difficult to make a definitive physical diagnosis in any infant who is intubated. Second, the muscular paralysis achieved by pancuronium bromide sedation generally results in third spacing of fluids and severe facial edema. This can result in a temporary distortion of facial features, and a perfectly normal infant can appear to have the facial flattening that is characteristic of Down syndrome. The dysmorphologic examination of a newborn infant who is receiving pancuronium bromide should be postponed until the drug has been discontinued and diuresis has occurred.

The definition of a birth defect is a congenital malformation that has medical, surgical, or cosmetic significance for the child (Marden et al, 1964). The origins of major malformations presenting in the newborn period, as obtained from a large database of more than 69,000 newborns, are listed in Table 20–1. Most birth defects have no known cause. Major anomalies are seldom overlooked in the newborn nursery. Often, however, the diagnosis of a genetic disease is suggested by the presence of multiple minor abnormalities (Leppig et al, 1987; Mehes et al, 1973). On physical examination of the affected infant, it is important to ascertain whether the abnormalities are due to malformation, deformation, or disruption (Spranger et al, 1982). A *malformation* implies that there was an underlying genetic or developmental abnormality in the initial formation of the organ or tissue. A *deformation* implies that the initial tissue or organ was normally formed, but it has been subjected to unusual forces, which have deformed

the tissue. In *disruption*, the tissue was normally formed, but subsequently was subjected to breakdown from a teratogenic or infectious agent.

APPROACH TO THE DYSMORPHIC INFANT

It is essential to obtain a maternal and family history in any newborn suspected to have genetic disease. Often, the infant arrives in the nursery with only a short delivery room note; little prenatal information is available. It is worthwhile to obtain maternal medical records or to speak directly with the mother regarding her history. Of specific importance is the description of any maternal medical problems, drug or infectious exposures, or the results of screening tests such as maternal serum alpha-fetoprotein levels (see Chapter 13). It is important to obtain a relevant family history firsthand by speaking to parents and grandparents, if possible. Even though the mother's initial obstetric history may have been unremarkable, the birth of an infant with malformations may later elicit additional (perhaps previously unknown) information from other family members.

On review of the delivery room events, it is important to note the position of fetal presentation and whether fetal distress was present during labor and delivery. Review of records indicates placental appearance and pathologic condition, and the length of the umbilical cord. The length of the umbilical cord is an indirect reflection of fetal neuromuscular activity in utero (Miller et al, 1981; Moessinger et al, 1982; Naeye, 1985). A short umbilical cord is associated with limitation of intrauterine space, either because of abnormalities in uterine anatomy or lack of amniotic fluid. It can also indicate severe fetal movement disorders.

TABLE 20–1

Major Malformations in a Large Newborn Survey

	Number	Percent of Total
Single gene disorder	48	4.1
Chromosome abnormality	157	10.1
Familial	225	14.4
Multifactorial	356	22.8
Teratogens	49	4.1
Uterine factors	39	2.5
Twinning	6	0.4
Unknown	669	43.1
Total (of 69,227 infants)	**1549**	**100%**

From Nelson K, Holmes LB: Malformations due to presumed spontaneous mutations in newborn infants. N Engl J Med 320:19–23, 1989. Copyright 1989 Massachusetts Medical Society. All rights reserved.

A short umbilical cord is also associated with trisomy 21 (Moessinger et al, 1986).

The fetal position in utero is important. Breech position is associated with an increased risk of underlying central nervous system abnormality. This fact may assume additional clinical importance if other findings suggest brain abnormalities.

PHYSICAL EXAMINATION

A number of references provide normal standards for anthropometric measurements of the newborn infant. Two references specifically address the differences between premature and full-term infants (Merlob et al, 1984; Saul et al, 1988). It is important to measure physical features of the newborn to provide objective evidence of dysmorphism.

The physical examination of the newborn infant who has suspected genetic disease begins with observation of the infant on a bed to obtain an immediate impression of newborn position, muscular tone, perfusion, and extent of physical activity. Typically, the physical examination begins at the top of the baby's head with an inspection of the hair whorl (Fig. 20–1). The hair whorls are an indication of forces and tension that were applied to the developing fetal scalp, resulting from an underlying expansion in brain growth that occurred at approximately 16 to 18 weeks of gestation (Smith and Gong, 1973). The hair whorl, therefore, provides an indirect assessment of brain growth occurring during the early second trimester. Infants who have profound central nervous system abnormalities have a hair

whorl that is more centrally placed than normal. The majority of newborn infants have a hair whorl that is relatively posterior on the occiput and may be slightly to the right or left of midline. Inspection of the infant's scalp also allows an opportunity to search for cutis aplasia. This finding is typically seen in trisomy 13, but may be mistaken for lesions resulting from fetal scalp electrode placement. The examination of the head should be followed by palpation of the fontanels and the sutures, with focus on detection of craniosynostosis (premature suture fusion) or abnormally large sutures. Subsequently, the face and occiput should be examined. The facial profile is important in the diagnosis of many syndromes. A flattened facial profile is typical of Down syndrome. A prominent occiput is typical of trisomy 18.

On inspection of the face, the eyes should be measured with respect to the inner and outer canthal distances, and the intrapupillary distance should be measured. These measurements can be compared with the normal standards in the references previously cited. Visual inspection of the eyes reveals microphthalmia or anophthalmia. Any abnormalities in the palpebral fissures (eyelid openings) should be apparent on direct inspection. Inspection of midface reveals hypoplasia or a flattened nasal bridge, or, conversely, a prominent midface. The philtrum (space between the base of the nose and top of the lip) can be measured in all infants and compared with normal standards. A smooth philtrum is characteristic of fetal alcohol effects. Long philtrums are characteristic of Williams and FG syndromes (Fig. 20–2). Inspection of the mouth reveals evidence of

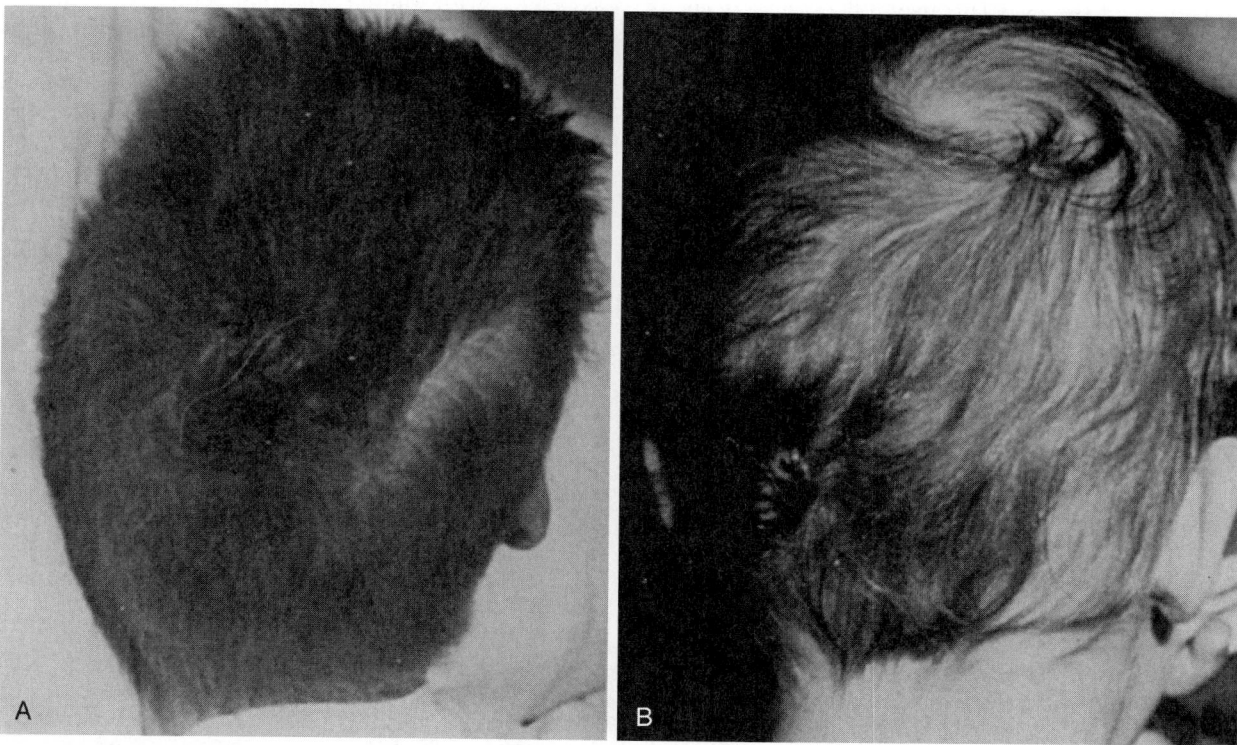

FIGURE 20–1. Photograph demonstrating abnormal scalp hair patterns in two children with retardation. The normal position of the hair whorl is usually more posteriorly placed than it is in the infant with Down syndrome shown in *B*. (Reprinted with permission from Smith DW, Gong BT: Scalp hair patterning as a clue to early fetal brain development. J Pediatr 83:379, 1973.)

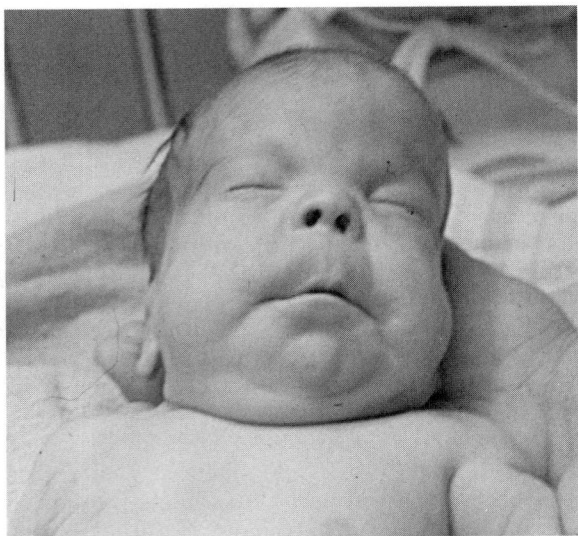

FIGURE 20–2. Unusually long philtrum in an infant with FG syndrome. Note also the thin lips. (From Bianchi DW: FG syndrome in a premature male. Am J Med Genet 19:383–386, 1984.)

cleft lip, cleft palate, or alveolar ridge abnormalities. The ears should be inspected and measured at their greatest vertical length. A term newborn's ear length should be more than 3 cm. Small ears are one of the hallmarks of trisomy 21. The term *low set ears*, although frequently used, is a relatively nonspecific finding. This term refers to the top of the ear running at a lower level than the outer canthal opening of the eye. This may reflect some delay in development, because the ears normally migrate up the neck during early embryonic life. Examination of the tongue reveals whether it is enlarged. A large tongue is seen in Beckwith-Wiedemann syndrome and glycogen storage disease (Fig. 20–3). In trisomy 21, the tongue is not enlarged. The apparent macroglossia is due to neuromuscular underdevelopment of the entire oral region. Inspection of the neck should reveal webbing or an increased size of the nuchal fat pad.

When examining the newborn infant's back, evidence should be sought for spinal abnormalities, clefts, tufts, or spinal dimples. A thorough examination of the chest includes listening to the breath and heart sounds. The position of the nipples may indicate underlying chest abnormalities. Normal standards also exist for chest circumference and internipple distance. Palpation of the abdomen may reveal kidney, liver, or spleen enlargement. The genitalia should be closely examined, because minor abnormalities may easily go unnoticed. For example, in trisomy 21, there is frequently hypoplasia of the labia minora in females. Micropenis is a frequent finding in males with trisomy 13. The normal appearance of the genitalia changes with gestational age.

Condition of the extremities is important in the diagnosis of genetic syndromes. Special attention should be paid to examination of the digits, flexion creases, and joints. Development of the nails is a reflection of the underlying terminal phalanx. If nail hypoplasia is present, consideration should be given to the radiographic examination of the affected extremity. Postaxial abnormalities refer to the ulnar side the hand; preaxial abnormalities refer to the radial side. Preaxial polydactyly is associated with disorders of the bone marrow. Postaxial polydactyly is a finding in trisomy 13, Meckel-Gruber syndrome, Ellis-van Creveld dwarfism, and other syndromes. Isolated postaxial polydactyly in a black infant is common. This is a single gene defect, inherited in an autosomal dominant fashion and found in 1% of black families. The following terms describe different digital abnormalities: clinodactyly (incurving of the digit caused by underlying hypoplasia of the middle phalanx), camptodactyly (bent digits caused by flexion contractures), arachnodactyly (long, spidery digits commonly associated with Marfan syndrome) (Fig. 20–4), brachydactyly (shortened digits), and syndactyly (apparent fusion of the digits at the bony or cutaneous level). The skin should be examined for birthmarks, abnormalities in pigmentation, or scarring. Finally, the neurologic examination is extremely important.

A thorough physical examination may reveal numerous "subtle" signs that may be helpful in establishing a genetic diagnosis. The presence of three or more minor malformations has been associated with a greatly increased risk for underlying major malformations (Leppig et al, 1987; Mehes et al, 1973).

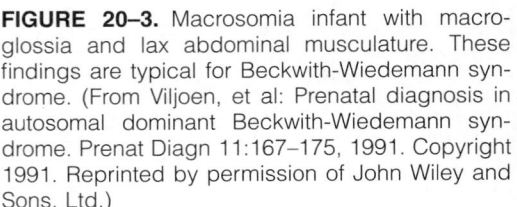

FIGURE 20–3. Macrosomia infant with macroglossia and lax abdominal musculature. These findings are typical for Beckwith-Wiedemann syndrome. (From Viljoen, et al: Prenatal diagnosis in autosomal dominant Beckwith-Wiedemann syndrome. Prenat Diagn 11:167–175, 1991. Copyright 1991. Reprinted by permission of John Wiley and Sons, Ltd.)

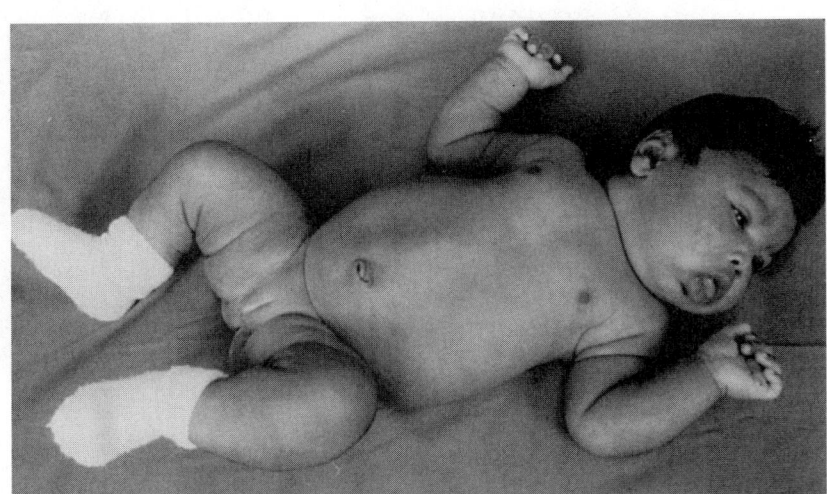

LABORATORY AND OTHER STUDIES

Although chromosome abnormalities only account for 10% of the cases of major malformations presenting in the newborn period (see Table 20–1), the chromosome analysis is the most commonly obtained clinical laboratory test in the newborn nursery. Most infants with birth defects have a normal karyotype. Because the karyotype could be a diagnostic test, however, it is worthwhile to perform it in an infant with a birth defect. This should be performed by obtaining a sample of peripheral blood in a green top tube that contains sodium heparin as the anticoagulant. The chromosome analysis can be performed on only 1 to 2 mL of blood kept at room temperature. In a dying infant with multiple malformations, it is also worthwhile to obtain a sterile skin biopsy sample to establish a fibroblast culture if the peripheral blood chromosomes cannot be analyzed. For disorders that have, or are suspected to have, an underlying DNA abnormality, it is also helpful to consider banking blood or fibroblasts for future DNA studies. Because an increasing number of disorders are being understood at the molecular level, many laboratories freeze and store tissue samples for future DNA analysis.

Other postnatal studies that may help in establishing a genetic diagnosis include postnatal sonographic examination of the head or abdomen, radiographs (especially for the diagnosis of skeletal dysplasias), computed tomography or magnetic resonance imaging scans that delineate central nervous system anatomy, TORCH (toxoplasmosis, rubella, cytomegalovirus, and herpes simplex) titers to establish the presence of perinatal infection, and metabolic studies if an inborn error of metabolism is suspected. Ophthalmologic examination is sometimes useful in the setting of suspected infection or central nervous system abnormalities.

DIAGNOSIS AND FOLLOW-UP

Resources available for clinicians trying to establish a genetic diagnosis are discussed in Chapter 29. Once a genetic diagnosis has been made in the infant, a meeting with the family is recommended for genetic counseling to provide further information regarding the specific condition. During the genetic counseling session, the expected prognosis, potential medical and surgical therapy, and recurrence risk are usually discussed. It is often helpful to follow up this session by writing a letter to the family. In the event of perinatal death, autopsy is recommended for histologic studies and to detect additional malformations. Follow-up after perinatal death is often neglected in a tertiary referral center. It is important to designate one individual to complete follow-up studies for recurrence risk counseling for the family. At my center, we make a special effort to ensure that all patients who have had a perinatal loss have a follow-up meeting with members of the clinical genetics team. In these sessions, the patient is also advised regarding the availability of future prenatal diagnosis for the specific condition.

The optimal diagnosis and management of the newborn infant with suspected genetic disease includes a multidisci-

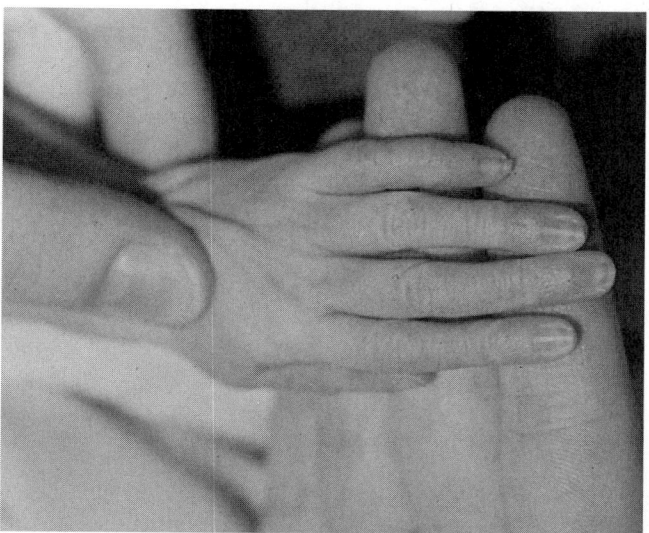

FIGURE 20–4. Arachnodactyly (exceptionally long, "spidery" fingers) in an infant with Marfan syndrome.

plinary team approach with participation of specialists in maternal fetal medicine, clinical genetics, neonatology, pediatric surgery, and the pediatric subspecialties.

REFERENCES

Centers for Disease Control: Contribution of birth defects to infant mortality—United States, 1986. MMWR Morb Mortal Wkly Rep 38:633–635, 1989.

Hudome SM, Kirby RS, Senner JW, Cunniff C: Contribution of genetic disorders to neonatal mortality in a regional intensive care setting. Am J Perinatol 11:100–103, 1994.

Leppig KA, Werler MM, Cann CI, et al: Predictive value of minor anomalies. I. Association with major malformations. J Pediatr 110:530–537, 1987.

Marden PM, Smith DW, McDonald MJ: Congenital anomalies in the newborn infant, including minor variations. J Pediatr 64:357–371, 1964.

Mehes K, Mestyean J, Knoch V, Vinceller M: Minor malformations in the neonate. Helv Paediatr Acta 28:477–483, 1973.

Merlob P, Sivan Y, Reisner SH: Anthropometric measurements of the newborn infant (27 to 41 gestational weeks). Birth Defects: Original Article Series 20:1–52, 1984.

Mili F, Edmonds LD, Khoury MJ, et al: Prevalence of birth defects among low-birth weight infants: A population study. Am J Dis Child 145:1313–1318, 1991.

Miller ME, Higginbottom M, Smith DW: Short umbilical cord: Its origin and relevance. Pediatrics 67:618–621, 1981.

Moessinger AC, Blanc WA, Marone PA, et al: Umbilical cord length as an index of fetal activity: Experimental study and clinical implications. Pediatr Res 16:109–112, 1982.

Moessinger AC, Mills JL, Harley EE, et al: Umbilical cord length in Down syndrome. Am J Dis Child 140:1276–1277, 1986.

Naeye RL: Umbilical cord length: Clinical significance. J Pediatr 107:278–281, 1985.

Nichols VG, Bianchi DW: Prenatal pediatrics: Traditional specialty definitions no longer apply. Pediatrics 97:729, 1996.

Saul RA, Stevenson RE, Rogers EC, et al: Growth references from conception to adulthood. Proc Greenwood Genet Center Suppl 1:1–214, 1988.

Smith DW, Gong BT: Scalp hair patterning as a clue to early fetal brain development. J Pediatr 83:374–380, 1973.

Spranger J, Benirschke K, Hall JG, et al: Errors of morphogenesis: Concepts and terms. J Pediatr 100:160–165, 1982.

Genetics of Common Problems Presenting in the Newborn

Barbara Shephard and Kenneth G. Kupke

In this chapter, common clinical problems of the newborn are discussed from a genetics perspective.

TWINNING
Epidemiology

Twinning is an unusual event of early development. There are two types: monozygotic (MZ) and dizygotic (DZ). In humans, the conventionally quoted overall estimate of twinning frequency is approximately 1 in 80 births. This is an underestimate because of the occurrence of "vanishing twins" that are either not identified or not registered as a multiple gestation in birth statistics. The incidence of multiple gestation varies greatly among different human races and environments. This variation is primarily due to differences in DZ twinning, as the incidence of MZ twinning is fairly constant in all populations.

MZ twins account for approximately 30% of all twins, and DZ twins account for about 70%. MZ twinning occurs sporadically, with no evidence of heritability. The incidence is approximately 1 in 260 births. The rate of DZ twinning, on the other hand, shows considerable racial and ethnic variation, being approximately 1 in 500 in Asians, 1 in 125 in whites, and as high as 1 in 20 in some African populations. There is a familial tendency to DZ twinning. The recurrence risk for a woman who has given birth to DZ twins is significantly greater than the general population risk. Other factors believed to influence the chance of DZ twinning are maternal age, parity, and availability of in vitro fertilization.

Pathogenesis

MZ twins, commonly referred to as "identical" twins, develop from a single fertilized ovum, carry identical genetic information, and are hence of the same sex. Approximately one half of MZ twin pairs are male, and one half are female. They result from splitting of the zygote sometime during the 14 days following fertilization. Placentation depends on when during this period the division takes place (Fig. 21–1).

If separation is early, at the two-cell stage, two separate zygotes develop, each with its own placenta and amniotic sac (dichorionic-diamniotic; approximately 35% of MZ twins). The separate placentas may be fused or separate (see also Chapter 6). More commonly, the inner cell mass splits within the same blastocyst cavity. These embryos share a placenta but have separate amniotic cavities (monochorionic, diamniotic; approximately 65% of MZ twins). Although the blood supply to each twin is usually well balanced, a variety of vascular anastomoses within the single placenta may occur.

Later separation of the embryo rarely occurs, resulting in the formation of twins with a single placenta and amnion sac (monochorionic, monoamniotic; <1% of MZ twins.) The splitting of the embryo during later stages of development may result in incomplete separation, giving rise to the formation of conjoined twins, an exceedingly rare phenomenon.

The etiology of MZ twinning is not known. Theories considered include that of "ovopathy," an error in the ovum itself, related to postovulatory aging of the oocyte. Delayed fertilization of an older oocyte may render the zygote more vulnerable to disruption. Alternatively, unequal X chromosome inactivation of distinct cellular clusters within a female embryo has been postulated to possibly influence separation of groups of cells and thus MZ twinning. Experimental work in animal models is ongoing.

Unexpectedly, the number of MZ twins is abnormally high in pregnancies conceived after in vitro fertilization (IVF) (Edwards et al, 1986). In addition, dichorionic-diamniotic pairs, indicating early separation, are overrepresented. Injury to the zona pellucida is postulated as an etiologic factor. These clinical observations have stimulated study and may provide insight into the MZ twinning phenomenon.

DZ twins, often called "fraternal," are more common. They result from the fertilization of two simultaneously ovulated oocytes by two different spermatozoa. The genetic constitution is therefore that of any two siblings; approximately 50% of genes are shared. Each twin develops its own placenta, which may or may not be fused, and amnion. Vascular anastomoses between placentas do not occur.

DZ twinning requires double ovulation. The growth and maturation of ovarian follicles leading to ovulation are dependent on gonadotropin secretion. Elevated levels of pituitary gonadotropins, particularly follicle-stimulating hormone, have been demonstrated in various populations of mothers of DZ twins (Martin et al, 1984; Milham, 1964) and in populations that have a high frequency of DZ twinning (Nylander, 1973). Increasing maternal age to a peak at around 35 years is associated with both increasing levels of pituitary gonadotropins and of DZ twinning. It is possible that there is a genetic predisposition to the production of gonadotrophins by mothers of twins, although this relationship has not been well studied. Environmental factors are also likely to be involved. Certainly the increased use of ovulatory agents for treatment of infertility has increased the number of DZ twin gestations.

Congenital Malformations

An increased prevalence of anomalies at birth in twins, when compared with singletons, has been demonstrated in

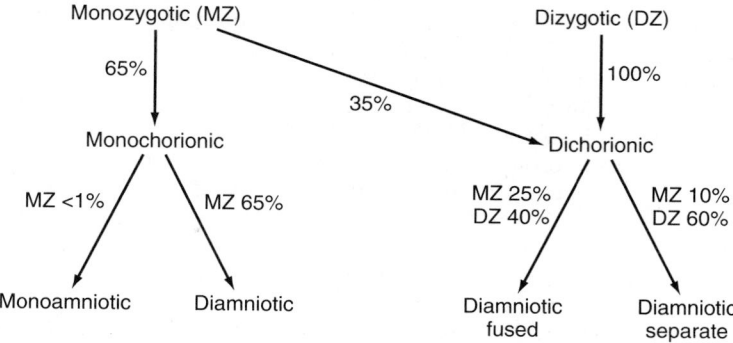

FIGURE 21–1. Twin placentation. Of monozygotic (MZ) twins, approximately 65% have monochorionic placentation, and almost all are diamniotic; 25% have dichorionic-diamniotic fused; and 10% have dichorionic-diamniotic separate placentas. Dizygotic (DZ) twins have dichorionic placentation; approximately 60% are dichorionic-diamniotic separate, and 40% have dichorionic-diamniotic fused placentas.

several large series (Myrianthopoulos, 1976). In studies of malformations in twins where zygosity has been established, the increase has been found to be primarily due to higher prevalence in MZ twins. Further, among twins known to be MZ, the occurrence of congenital malformations shows a significant association with zygosity but not with placentation.

The structural defects seen fall into three categories (McCulloch, 1988). First, there are deformations imposed by the constraint of limited intrauterine space, which, as expected, are as common in MZ as DZ twins. Second, disruption of normal blood flow due to placental vascular communications in monochorionic (and hence MZ) twins can occur and give rise most commonly to anomalies of the central nervous, cardiovascular, and gastrointestinal systems. The most extreme example of this is the formation of an acardiac fetus, believed to result from artery-to-artery anastomoses between twin fetuses (Schinzel et al, 1979). Early in gestation the pressure in the artery of one twin exceeds that in the artery of the other. The circulation in the recipient twin is reversed, with blood entering the recipient through an umbilical artery and leaving through the umbilical vein, draining into vein-to-vein anastomoses. Severe structural defects in the recipient result, including acardia. The normal or "pump" twin must provide circulation for itself as well as its acardiac sibling and can develop cardiac hypertrophy, congestive heart failure, or hydrops fetalis. Vascular disruption lesions represent only a small portion of total malformations found in twins.

Structural malformations due to early defects of morphogenesis, the third category, are found more commonly in MZ twins. The etiology is believed to be closely related to the MZ twinning process itself. The factor responsible for zygotic separation may inflict further developmental damage during embryogenesis (Schinzel et al, 1979). Alternatively, embryos disrupted by splitting may be more vulnerable to teratogenic influences.

MZ twins are often discordant for congenital malformations, although less often than DZ twins, despite genetic equivalence. Determination of zygosity should not be based on phenotypic similarity or differences. For heritable abnormalities with known genetic etiologies, however, such as Down syndrome, concordance in MZ twins approaches 100%.

Zygosity Determination

Zygosity determination may be desired for any number of reasons, including for estimating the genetic prognosis in a twin of a patient with a genetic disease, for transplantation needs, for research purposes, or to gratify normal curiosity. From simple observations of sex and placentation, the zygosity of approximately half of all twins can be determined at birth: different-sex twins are dizygous (approximately 35%) and twins with a monochorionic placenta are monozygous (approximately 20%). Molecular diagnosis is the method of choice in the remainder, looking for differences in the large number of DNA markers available for testing. Twins who are not MZ are virtually certain to show different polymorphisms inherited from each parent. As discussed, determination of zygosity should not be based on phenotypic appearance.

Prenatally, the determination of zygosity and chorionicity is important in the management of pregnancy when it is complicated by discordant growth, single intrauterine fetal demise, and discordant congenital anomalies, and because perinatal morbidity and mortality are greatly increased for monochorionic compared with dichorionic twins. Ultrasound examination can establish the diagnosis of chorionicity with absolute certainty when there are two placentas or when the fetuses are of the opposite sex. Although methods of sonographically examining the dividing membrane to assess chorionicity are helpful, they are not completely reliable (D'Alton and Simpson, 1995). Amniocentesis for molecular evaluation of DNA markers can be performed to determine zygosity when it cannot be established by ultrasound examination.

CLEFT LIP AND PALATE

Clefting of the lip and palate are relatively common congenital anomalies of heterogeneous etiology. Cleft lip with or without cleft palate (CL[P]) occurs in approximately 1 in 1000 whites, 1 in 600 Asians, 1 in 2500 blacks, and 1 in 280 Native Americans (Gorlin et al, 1990). Isolated cleft palate (CP) occurs in about 1 in 2000 whites and 1 in 1250 blacks. CL(P) is more common in males, whereas CP is more common in females.

Isolated CL(P) is generally considered etiologically distinct from isolated CP (Fraser, 1980). Lip closure in the developing embryo is dependent on the midline fusion of three mesodermal tissues—the maxillary, lateral nasal, and median nasal processes. The merger of these tissues is complete by 35 days of gestation. Failure of fusion results in a cleft lip, which can be partial or complete, unilateral or bilateral. The secondary palate is created by the midline fusion of the palatal shelves, which are derived from the maxillary processes, occurring by 9 weeks of gestation. Failure of this union results in CP, which can be partial or complete. When cleft lip occurs primarily, the migrating palatal shelves may become secondarily obstructed by the tongue, which is restricted by the prolabium.

Of all cases of orofacial clefting, about 50% involve both the lip and palate, 25% involve the lip only, and 25% involve the palate only. Cleft lip is unilateral in 80% of cases and bilateral in 20%. Associated CP occurs in 70% of unilateral and 85% of bilateral cases of cleft lip. Other birth defects are present in about 7% to 13% of patients with cleft lip alone, 11% to 14% of patients with cleft lip and palate, and 35% to 50% of patients with CP (Shprintzen et al, 1985). There are many multiple-malformation syndromes associated with cleft lip and CP (Table 21–1). For this reason, a newborn with orofacial clefting requires a thorough evaluation to exclude a syndromic diagnosis and to provide accurate recurrence risk counseling. In some conditions, the other defects are obvious, but in others, such as van der Woude syndrome, the findings may be rather inconspicuous.

In van der Woude syndrome, an autosomal dominant condition, lower lip pits may be the only manifestation present in family members who carry the trait. Most cases of isolated CP and CL(P) conform to a multifactorial basis of inheritance in which genetic and environmental factors interact to cause clefting once a threshold effect is reached. Rare families with autosomal dominant clefting have also been reported. In genetic counseling, the empiric recurrence risks vary with the number of affected people in the family and their relationship to the offspring at risk (Table 21–2).

CONGENITAL HEART DISEASE

Congenital heart disease (CHD) is the most common type of birth defect, occurring in about 1 in 140 newborns (see also Part IX). CHD accounts for about 50% of children dying of birth defects, and approximately 15% of infantile deaths are due to CHD.

Cardiovascular embryology involves the expression of many genes for normal cardiovascular formation. Cardiac development is sensitive to genetic and environmental effects during the embryonic period, from the 2nd to the 8th week of gestation. Maldevelopment may occur from insults during this period or due to persistence of fetal structures. Many different anatomic types of CHD exist, reflecting the complexity of this process.

TABLE 21–1

Select Syndromes Associated with Cleft Lip and Palate

Syndrome	Inheritance	Features
Cleft Lip With or Without Cleft Palate		
Amniotic rupture sequence	Sporadic	Constriction rings, limb defects, unusual clefts
Frontonasal dysplasia	XLD	Frontal bossing, hypertelorism, bifid or broad nose, skeletal abnormalities
EEC syndrome	AD	Absent fingers or toes, ectodermal dysplasia, oligodontia
Opitz G syndrome	AD	Hypertelorism; hypospadias; cryptorchidism; high, broad nasal bridge
Meckel-Gruber syndrome	AR	Polydactyly, polycystic kidneys, encephalocele, CHD
Oral-facial-digital syndrome type 1	XLD	Milia, hyperplastic frenula, lobed or bifid tongue, digital defects, cleft lip, cleft palate, polycystic kidneys
Short rib-polydactyly syndrome type 1	AR	Polydactyly, short ribs and limbs, GU anomalies, tibia hypoplasia
Trisomy 13		Chromosomal polydactyly, scalp defect, micro-ophthalmia, CHD, renal anomaly
Van der Woude syndrome	AD	Lower lip pits
Cleft Palate Only		
Apert syndrome	AD	Craniosynostosis, proptosis, hypertelorism, maxillary hypoplasia, syndactyly of hands and feet, MR
Diastrophic dysplasia	AR (DTDST)	Dwarfism, scoliosis, "hitchhiker" thumb, talipes equinovarus, ear anomalies, hip dysplasia
Fryns syndrome	AR	Micrognathia, pulmonary hypoplasia, diaphragmatic hernia, nail hypoplasia, CHD, renal and brain anomalies
Kniest dysplasia	AD (COL2A1)	Skeletal dysplasia, round facies, talipes equinovarus, prominent joints, myopia, retinal detachment
Larsen syndrome	AD	Flat facies, hypertelorism, multiple joint dislocations, cylindrical fingers, numerous carpal bones
Mandibulofacial dysostosis	AD (5q31–33)	Micrognathia, mandibular hypoplasia, ear anomalies, down-slanting palpebral fissures, conductive hearing loss
Otopalatodigital syndrome type 1	XLR (Xq28)	Frontal bossing, hearing loss, broad terminal phalanges, syndactyly, abnormal facies
Stickler syndrome	AD (COL2A1) (COL11A2)	Micrognathia, myopia, retinal detachment, degenerative arthritis, conductive hearing loss, marfanoid habitus
Velocardiofacial syndrome	AD (22q11.2)	Prominent straight nose, CHD, hypernasal speech, learning disabilities, DiGeorge sequence

AD, autosomal dominant; AR, autosomal recessive; XLD, X-linked dominant; XLR, X-linked recessive; CHD, congestive heart disease; GU, genitourinary; MR, mental retardation.

TABLE 21–2

Empiric Recurrence Risks (%) for Sibling or Offspring of Patients with Isolated Nonsyndromic Cleft Lip and Palate (CL[P]) and Cleft Palate (CP)

Affected Individual(s)	CL(P)	CP
1 sibling	4.3	3.6
2 siblings	14.0	13.3
1 parent	4.1	3.3
1 parent, 1 sibling	12.2	10.5
1 parent, 2 siblings	25.5	23.6
2 parents	37.1	27.6

Adapted from Tolarova M, Morton NE: Cleft lip and palate—recurrence risk and genetic counseling. Acta Chir Plast 17:97–111, 1975.

Approximately 20% to 45% of patients with CHD have one or more other congenital anomalies, and about 10% of patients with CHD have a syndromic diagnosis. Newborns with CHD should be carefully examined for evidence of dysmorphic features or other birth defects. If present, a chromosome analysis is indicated, and additional studies such as fluorescence in situ hybridization (FISH), DNA analysis, and metabolic testing may be required.

Specific types of CHD result from a myriad of chromosome, monogenic, environmental, and multifactorial effects on cardiac embryologic development (Table 21–3). The underlying basis of CHD is attributable to chromosome abnormalities in 5% to 6% of cases, single gene disorders in 3% to 5%, and environmental factors in 2%. The remaining 85% to 90% of cases of CHD have no definable cause and are usually considered multifactorial in origin.

Recently a deletion of chromosome 22q11 has been shown to be associated with three conditions associated with CHD: DiGeorge syndrome, velocardiofacial syndrome, and conotruncal anomaly face syndrome (Driscoll et al, 1993; Kelly et al, 1993). FISH studies reveal a 22q11 deletion in about 90% of patients with DiGeorge syndrome and 75% of patients with velocardiofacial syndrome. The acronym *CATCH 22* has been termed to denote the phenotype associated with this deletion: *C*ardiac defect, *A*bnormal facies, *T*-cell defect, *C*left palate, *H*ypocalcemia. Even among patients with nonsyndromic conotruncal anomalies, approximately 20% to 30% have demonstrable 22q11 deletions (Goldmuntz et al, 1993). For this reason 22q11 FISH

TABLE 21–3

Select Syndromes Associated with Congenital Heart Disease

Etiology	Cardiac Features	Etiology	Cardiac Features
Chromosome		**Single Gene** *(Continued)*	
Trisomy 21	AVC, VSD, ASD, ASCA	Smith-Lemli-Opitz type 1	ASD, AVC, TOF, CoA
Trisomy 18	VSD, AVC, DORV, BAV, HLHS	Thanatophoric dysplasia	ASD, PDA
Trisomy 13	ASD, VSD, PDA	Treacher Collins	VSD, PDA, ASD
Tetrasomy 22p (cat-eye syndrome)	TAPVR	Tuberous sclerosis	Rhabdomyomata, angiomata
Tetrasomy 12p (Pallister Killian syndrome)	VSD, CoA, ASD, PDA, AS	Zellweger	PDA, VSD
		Environmental	
45,X (Turner syndrome)	CoA, HLHS, AS, ASD, VSD, MVP, BAV	Hydantoin	PS, AS, CoA, PDA
		Maternal diabetes mellitus	VSD, CoA, TGA
Cri du chat (deletion 5p)	VSD, PDA, ASD	Maternal SLE	Complete heart block
Wolf-Hirschhorn (deletion 4p)	ASD, VSD	Maternal alcohol abuse	VSD, ASD, PDA, TOF
Williams (deletion 7q/elastin)	SVAS, PPS	Maternal PKU	TOF, VSD, PDA, HLHS
Alagille (deletion 20p)	PPS	Congenital CMV	MS, PS, ASD
DiGeorge (deletion 22q)	IAA, TOF, TArt	Congenital rubella	PDA, PPS, ASD, VSD
Velocardiofacial (deletion 22q)	TOF, VSD	Lithium	Ebstein anomaly, TA, ASD
Single Gene		Retinoic acid	IAA, TOF, TArt, VSD
Adams-Oliver	VSD, PS, TOF, CoA	Trimethadione	TGA, TOF, HLHS
Apert	PS, VSD	Vitamin A	TArt, TGA, ASD, VSD, TOF
Ellis–van Creveld	ASD, AVC, SA	**Unknown**	
FG	VSD, PS, HLHS	Laterality sequence (asplenia/polysplenia)	DC, TGA, TAPVR, TArt, AVC
Holt-Oram	ASD, VSD, AVC	CHARGE association	VSD, AVC, TOF
Kartagener	Dextrocardia	Goldenhar	VSD, TOF, ASD
Marfan	Aortic dilatation, valve incompetence	Klippel-Feil	ASD, VSD
Noonan	Valvular PS, CM	VACTERL association	VSD, various defects
Neurofibromatosis type 1	PS, neurofibromata		
Osteogenesis imperfecta	MVP, AR		

AR, aortic regurgitation; AS, aortic stenosis; ASCA, aberrant subclavian artery; ASD, atrial septal defect; AVC, atrioventricular canal; BAV, bicuspid aortic valve; CoA, coarctation of the aorta; CM, cardiomyopathy; DC, dextrocardia; DORV, double-outlet right ventricle; HLHS, hypoplastic left heart syndrome; IAA, interrupted aortic arch; MVP, mitral valve prolapse; MS, mitral stenosis; PDA, patent ductus arteriosus; PS, pulmonic stenosis; PPS, peripheral pulmonic stenosis; SA, common atrium; SVAS, supravalvular aortic stenosis; TA, tricuspid atresia; TArt, truncus arteriosus; TAPVR, total anomalous pulmonary venous return; TGA, transposition of great arteries; TOF, tetralogy of Fallot; VSD, ventricular septal defect.

TABLE 21–4

Empiric Recurrence Risks for Isolated Nonsyndromic Congenital Heart Disease

Affected Relative	Recurrence Risk (%)
Half-sibling or second-degree relative	1–2
One sibling	2–3
Two siblings	10
Father	2–3
Mother	5
>Two affected first-degree relatives	50

analysis is indicated for patients with tetralogy of Fallot, truncus arteriosus, aortic arch anomalies, or phenotypic features of DiGeorge or velocardiofacial syndromes.

Isolated nonsyndromic cardiac malformations are generally considered multifactorial, unless the family history indicates a specific mendelian pattern of inheritance. After one affected child with isolated nonsyndromic CHD, the recurrence risk for a sibling is 2% to 3% (Nora and Nora, 1983). The risk to the offspring is twofold to threefold greater if the mother has CHD than if the father has CHD (Nora and Nora, 1987). Recurrence risks are based on empiric data for isolated nonsyndromic CHD (Table 21–4).

HYPOTONIA

Neonatal hypotonia that persists after delivery is a serious physical finding that merits a careful search for its explanation. The list of causes is vast, and on that list are a large number of heritable conditions. Both central hypotonia (arising from disorders of the brain or spinal cord) and peripheral hypotonia (arising from disorders of the peripheral nervous system or motor unit) can be a presenting sign in genetic diseases of the newborn. Attempts to distinguish between the two can help narrow down diagnostic possibilities. Genetic diseases causing neonatal hypotonia can be found with all modes of inheritance (Table 21–5) (DiMario, 1989). A careful, thorough family history is essential. When possible, examination of family members may offer important clues to a diagnosis.

Chromosome aberrations that can be associated with a floppy baby include trisomy 21, in which hypotonia is present in 95%, Miller-Dieker syndrome due to microdeletion at chromosome 17p13.3, and Prader-Willi syndrome due to absence of paternal chromosome 15q11. These infants are dysmorphic. Infants with Down syndrome have a well-known facial appearance with midface hypoplasia; epicanthal folds; and small, posteriorly rotated ears, among other findings. Infants with Miller-Dieker syndrome are microcephalic but are less obviously dysmorphic. They have forehead furrowing, a small nose with anteverted nostrils, upslanting palpebral fissures, and a thin upper lip. Computed tomographic (CT) imaging reveals the lissencephaly that makes this diagnosis. Patients with Prader-Willi syndrome may appear only slightly dysmorphic and can be missed if the diagnosis is not considered during the evaluation of hypotonia. Karyotype analysis and pertinent FISH studies should be performed on all hypotonic infants with a dysmorphic appearance (see also Chapters 25 and 69).

The most well-known and most serious autosomal recessive disease giving rise to neonatal hypotonia is spinal muscular atrophy (SMA), or Werdnig-Hoffmann disease. In its most fulminant form, newborns are profoundly weak

TABLE 21–5

Heritable Disorders Associated with Neonatal Hypotonia

Autosomal Dominant Transmission

Achondroplasia
Central core myopathy
Congenital fiber-type disproportion
Congenital hypomyelinating neuropathy
Congenital myotonic dystrophy
Ehlers-Danlos syndrome (I, II, III, IV, VII, VIII)
Hereditary motor-sensory neuropathy
Marfan syndrome
Minicore myopathy
Myotubular myopathy
Nemaline myopathy

Autosomal Recessive Transmission

Acid maltase deficiency (Pompe disease)
Amino acid dysmetabolism
Carnitine deficiency
Congenital fiber-type disproportion
Central core myopathy
Congenital muscular dystrophy
Congenital myasthenia syndrome
Ehlers-Danlos syndrome (VI)
Lissencephaly

Myophosphorylase deficiency (McArdle disease)
Myotubular myopathy
Nemaline myopathy
Organic acid dysmetabolism
Peroxisomal disorders
Phosphofructokinase deficiency
Pyruvate dysmetabolism (Leigh disease)
Spinal muscular atrophy (Werdnig-Hoffmann disease)

X-Linked Transmission

Cerebro-oculo-renal syndrome (Lowe syndrome)
Ehlers-Danlos syndrome (V)
Kinky hair disease (Menkes disease)
Mucopolysaccharidosis (Hunter syndrome)
Myotubular myopathy

Nonmendelian Transmission

Chromosome aberrations
Down syndrome (trisomy 21)
Miller-Dieker syndrome (17 deletion)
Prader-Willi syndrome (15q deletion)
Cytoplasmic DNA abnormalities
Mitochondrial myopathies

Adapted from DiMario FJ: Genetic diseases in the etiology of the floppy infant. Rhode Island Med J 72:357–359, 1989.

and floppy, sometimes prenatally. The history of decreased fetal activity can sometimes be elicited. Tendon reflexes are weak or absent. The infants, however, are alert and sociable. Tongue fasciculations and tremors may be present. The carrier frequency for this disease is high, 1 in 80; therefore, although family history should be searched for consanguinity, it need not be present. SMA occurs in 1 in 20,000 to 25,000 newborns. The gene for SMA has been mapped to chromosome 5q11.2-13.3 (Brzustowicz et al, 1990), and DNA diagnosis is available.

Inborn errors of metabolism are frequently associated with neonatal hypotonia. The presence of acidosis or hepatomegaly, or both, should alert the clinician to this diagnostic possibility in a hypotonic infant. Many heritable metabolic disorders have autosomal recessive inheritance, and some, such as carnitine deficiency, are treatable. (See also Chapter 25.)

About 15% of babies born to mothers with myasthenia gravis are born with transient myasthenia gravis of the newborn, demonstrating severe hypotonia and weakness, facial diplegia, and pooling of oral secretions. These are manifestations of the mother's disease and treatment and are usually gone within 6 weeks (Plauche, 1991). Some infants benefit from treatment with anticholinesterase drugs while symptomatic.

In general, if complete family, pregnancy, and birth histories and physical examination fail to disclose a cause for hypotonia, close surveillance of these infants, often by a geneticist or neurologist in addition to the primary care provider, is imperative to allow prompt diagnosis of evolving disease. The disease may have neonatal hypotonia as the presenting feature, and it may have important genetic implications for the family.

CONGENITAL DISLOCATION OF THE HIP

Congenital dislocation of the hip (CDH) is a common birth defect inherited as an isolated multifactorial trait or as a feature of a multiple-malformation syndrome. As an isolated condition, its incidence varies widely among different ethnic populations, ranging from about 1 in 1000 whites to 1 in 5000 blacks to 1 in 26 Native Americans in the southwestern United States (Woolf, 1968). The highest frequency occurs among ethnic groups who "swaddle" their infants, such as Laplanders and Native Americans.

Other associated risk factors include breech presentation, firstborn status, and female sex. The fourfold to sixfold female-to-male predilection is believed to occur due to hormone-induced joint laxity. Other genetic factors include ligamentous laxity and shallowness of the acetabulum (Carter and Wilkinson, 1964; Czeizel et al, 1975).

Many syndromes have been described in which CDH is a common feature, including connective tissue disorders such as skeletal dysplasias, Marfan syndrome, Ehlers-Danlos syndrome, and Larsen syndrome, as well as neuromuscular disorders such as Pena-Shokeir syndrome type I, congenital muscular dystrophies, and neural tube defects.

Isolated CDH shows aggregation among first-degree relatives in families, demonstrating multifactorial inheritance. MZ twins display about a 50% concordance rate compared with 5% among DZ twins (Czeizel et al, 1975; Idelberger, 1951; Kambara and Sasakawa, 1954; Wynne-

TABLE 21–6

Recurrence Risks (%) for Congenital Dislocation of the Hip

Affected Relative	Recurrence Risk		
	Overall	Males	Females
One sibling	6	1	11
One parent	12	6	17
One parent, one sibling	36	—	—
Second-degree relative	1	—	—

Adapted from Wynne-Davies R: A family study of neonatal and late-diagnosis congenital dislocation of the hip. J Med Genet 7:315–333, 1970.

Davies, 1970). Empiric recurrence risks are reported in Table 21–6.

PIERRE ROBIN SEQUENCE AND MICROGNATHIA

Descriptions of infants born with the triad of micrognathia, CP, and respiratory obstruction were published as early as 1822 (Sadewitz, 1992). In 1923, however, French stomatologist Pierre Robin introduced the term *glossoptosis* to describe the tendency for the tongue to fall back into the airway, causing pharyngeal obstruction. He did not mention CP as a problem in children with micrognathia until his second report in 1934 (Robin, 1923; Robin, 1934). Pierre Robin sequence is now a well-recognized congenital condition involving a combination of micrognathia and/or retrognathia and glossoptosis causing upper airway obstruction, with or without a typically U-shaped CP. The designation *sequence* signifies the theory that the mandibular abnormality gives rise to the secondary problems of CP and airway obstruction. It is hypothesized that abnormal embryologic development of the mandible occurs between 7 and 11 weeks' postconception, resulting in a high tongue position in the nasopharynx that interferes with the medial growth of the lateral palatal shelves toward midline fusion. A U-shaped palatal cleft is created, and the upper airway becomes obstructed because of glossoptosis (Elliott et al, 1995).

Possible mechanisms that may lead to the arrest of mandibular development include positional deformation from intrauterine constriction, intrinsic mandibular hypoplasia, and neurologic abnormalities that inhibit normal fetal mandibular movements such as swallowing (Sherer et al, 1995). As such, the mechanisms that lead to the occurrence of Robin sequence are variable. In a study of 100 consecutive cases referred with the triad of findings associated with Robin sequence, only 17% were considered nonsyndromic. Eighty percent of children had other anomalies, and many had associated syndromes (Shprintzen, 1992). The most common were Stickler syndrome in 34%, velocardiofacial syndrome in 11%, and fetal alcohol syndrome in 10%. The importance of making the underlying syndrome diagnosis cannot be overemphasized. Patients with Stickler syndrome have normal intellect but may have severe ocular abnormalities. Stickler syndrome is an autosomal dominant disorder. Patients with velocardiofacial syndrome usually have cognitive impairment and heart malformations, and they may develop psychiatric illness. Affected patients have a deletion of chromosome 22 and transmit the disease in an autosomal dominant fashion. Isolated Robin sequence appears to be sporadic, but when part of another syndrome it follows the inheritance pattern of the associated disorder.

Elliott and associates (1995) retrospectively reviewed 55 patients with confirmed Pierre Robin sequence to determine the associated presence of pediatric conditions such as respiratory distress, feeding difficulties, and middle ear pathology. Respiratory problems, often from airway obstruction, were present in 55% of patients. Respiratory difficulties may not be apparent immediately after birth but may develop sometime during the first week. Various treatment strategies are employed, including positioning, glossopexy, and tracheostomy placement. Fifty-five percent of patients had feeding difficulties, related more often to the airway obstruction and respiratory difficulties than to the palatal clefts. Many infants in this study needed feeding assistance to support nutrition until they were able to maintain sufficient caloric intake with oral feeds. Most (90%) of the patients reviewed had recurrent otitis media, most eventually requiring myringotomy tube placement. Careful monitoring for middle ear disease is crucial to prevent hearing loss and speech delay. The presence of an associated syndrome did not alter the prevalence of these medical problems.

In addition to the Robin sequence, there are more than 70 syndromes or conditions in which micrognathia is a prominent feature. Facial defects are commonly found in association with many chromosome abnormalities and genetic syndromes. When diagnosed prenatally, the risk of associated abnormalities in the presence of micrognathia is high. Nicolaides and colleagues (1992) studied 2086 high-risk obstetric patients, referred because of ultrasonographically detected fetal malformations and/or growth retardation, for the incidence of facial defects and the pattern of associated malformations and chromosome abnormalities. Fifty-six patients had the finding of fetal micrognathia, defined subjectively as the presence of a prominent upper lip and small chin. Thirty-seven (66%) of the 56 were found to have chromosome aneuploidy, most commonly trisomy 18 and triploidy. In all cases of micrognathia, additional malformations or growth retardation were present. Among the chromosomally normal fetuses with micrognathia, the outcome was also poor, with only 1 of 19 surviving. Although theirs was a high-risk population, and prenatal ultrasound examination probably selects for more severe micrognathia that is significant enough to be detectable, the risk is clearly high for these fetuses. Other investigators who examined lower-risk populations have similarly reported micrognathia to be a common anomaly found in aneuploid fetuses, also in association with other major malformations (Bromley and Benacerraf, 1994; Turner and Twining, 1993).

The increasing recognition of micrognathia as an important marker for fetal genetic abnormality has prompted some investigators to establish fetal mandible measurement standards (Otto and Platt, 1991; Watson and Katz, 1993). One commonly accepted standard does not yet exist. Nonetheless, the currently available data indicate that the presence of micrognathia should prompt the search for other abnormalities, both in utero and after birth, and consideration of karyotype examination. Genetic counseling should be offered when fetal micrognathia and other sonographic findings are found.

ARTHROGRYPOSIS

Arthrogryposis refers to multiple congenital joint contractures that are nonprogressive and involve more than one area of the body. Arthrogryposis is found in a large heterogeneous group of disorders; more than 150 different syndromic conditions have been reported.

Multiple joint contractures occur at birth following any cause of limitation of movement in utero (Table 21–7). There are five etiologic causes: (1) neuropathy, either central or peripheral; (2) myopathy; (3) abnormal connective tissue involving joints; (4) in utero restraint; and (5) maternal illness (Hall, 1985). Neuropathies account for 90% to 95% of cases and myopathies for 5% to 10% (Banker, 1986).

The delivery of arthrogrypotic babies is often abnormal; breech and transverse lie are much more common leading to cesarean delivery. Fractures occur during the delivery in 5% to 10% of cases (Goldberg, 1987).

The newborn examination of a newborn with arthrogryposis should include a thorough description of the pattern of joint involvement (distal versus proximal), type of contracture (in flexion or extension), severity of limitation to motion, and characteristic position at rest. Photographs are helpful for accurate documentation. Other salient physical findings may include dimpling over the contractures, skin webbing across joints, abnormal tendon attachments, hernias, and diminished subcutaneous tissue. A careful neurologic examination and a description of the muscle mass and texture are important.

Laboratory studies may include radiographs of skeletal abnormalities and any ankylotic joints, cranial CT or ultrasonography, and visceral ultrasonography. Karyotyping should be done if there are dysmorphic features, brain or eye findings, or multiple organs involved. Muscle biopsy,

---

TABLE 21–7

Examples of Different Causes of Arthrogryposis

Neuropathy	Diastrophic dysplasia
Trisomy 18	Kniest dysplasia
Fetal alcohol syndrome	Multiple pterygium syndrome
Fryns syndrome	Freeman-Sheldon syndrome
Smith-Lemli-Opitz syndrome	Neonatal Marfan syndrome
Zellweger syndrome	**In Utero Constraint**
Congenital myasthenia gravis	
Miller-Dieker syndrome	Twins
Myopathy	Amniotic band sequence
	Oligohydramnios
Amyoplasia	
Nemaline myopathy	**Maternal Illness**
Schwartz-Jampel syndrome	
Abnormal Connective Tissue	Hyperthermia
	Myasthenia gravis
Larsen syndrome	Myotonic dystrophy
	Multiple sclerosis

electromyography, and nerve conduction studies may be performed in normal and abnormal areas. An ophthalmologic examination is usually indicated to exclude a variety of eye abnormalities.

The differential diagnosis of arthrogryposis is quite extensive, and the diagnostic evaluation should involve a geneticist and a neurologist.

Amyoplasia is considered the most common condition causing arthrogryposis, accounting for about one third of cases (Hall et al, 1983). In amyoplasia, all limbs are usually affected and muscle is replaced with fatty tissue and fibrous bands. The major joints are fusiform or cylindrical and firmly fixed. Sensation and cognitive development are normal. Abdominal wall defects occur in about 10% of patients, and 5% have evidence of amniotic bands with digital defects. Early physical therapy is essential to improve range of motion, and orthopedic surgery is often necessary. This condition is sporadic and most likely occurs from vascular compromise during midpregnancy.

POLYDACTYLY

Polydactyly, extra digits of the hands and feet, can be classified into two major types: postaxial (arising from the ulnar ray during limb development) and preaxial (arising from the radial ray). Postaxial extra digits may be well formed, articulating with the fifth or an extra metacarpal (type A) or not well formed, appearing more like a skin tag (type B). There are four types of preaxial polydactyly recognized: I, polydactyly of the thumb or great toe; II, polydactyly of a triphalangeal thumb; III, polydactyly of the index finger, with or without absent thumb; and IV, polysyndactyly (Temtamy and McKusick, 1978).

Postaxial polydactyly is far more common and occurs 10 times more frequently in blacks than in whites (Frazier, 1960). It may occur in 3 to 4 in 1000 births, and much higher frequencies have been published in some countries, such as 17 to 27 in 1000 in Nigeria (Scott-Emuakpor and Madueke, 1976). When isolated, postaxial polydactyly is an autosomal dominant trait. It may be associated with genetic syndromes, however, in which case it follows the inheritance pattern of the syndrome. Postaxial polydactyly is a frequent finding in trisomy 13, and in Meckel syndrome, an autosomal recessive disorder characterized by encephalocele and cystic dysplastic kidneys. Other syndromes that feature postaxial polydactyly include oral-facial-digital syndrome type II (Mohr), Pallister-Hall syndrome, and short rib polydactyly syndrome.

Preaxial polydactyly may occur as infrequently as 8 in 100,000 births and is much more likely to be present as part of a syndrome. It is more often unilateral. It is two to four times more frequent in the Native American population than in whites or blacks (Bingle and Niswander, 1975). Thumb polydactyly, type I, may be as subtle as broadening of the distal phalanx, as seen in Rubinstein-Taybi syndrome, or it may be a full duplication.

Embryologically, upper and lower limb buds appear between 26 and 30 days after fertilization. Upper limb development precedes lower limb by a few days. Mesenchymal cells at the margin of the paddle-shaped bud induce the overlying ectoderm to form the apical ectodermal ridge, which is essential for the proper elongation and differentia-

tion into separate digits and for the formation of cartilage, bone, and muscle. Separate digits are distinguishable, then separate, between 41 and 55 days. Programmed cell death must occur for appropriate separation into distinct digits.

Numerous homeobox genes are known to be expressed in various cell groups of the developing limb, guiding the developmental processes (Winter and Tickle, 1993). Cells in the limb bud receive positional information, which allows them to differentiate into specific cell types and structures with anteroposterior and dorsoventral axes. Positional information is believed to be gained from chemical gradients set up by morphogen diffusion from specific groups of cells. Retinoids are probably important morphogens in limb bud development. It is likely that mutations involving *HOX* genes, growth factors, and morphogen receptors give rise to abnormalities of limb development. Candidate genes have been identified, and study of the molecular genetics of limb anomalies is ongoing.

Some disorders that include limb defects have highly variable expression. The recurrence risk for polydactyly depends on the etiology. The recurrence risk when the affected patient has a new mutation is different than when inherited from a parent. Careful family history, and, whenever possible, examination of family members for subtle hand and foot abnormalities are important.

AURICULAR TAGS AND SINUSES

Auricular tags and sinuses are relatively common mild malformations, each occurring in about 1% of newborns (Melnick and Myrianthopoulos, 1979). More than 90% of cases are isolated and are usually unilateral. The birth prevalence of ear sinuses is somewhat greater for Asians and blacks than for whites. As isolated anomalies, ear tags and sinuses do segregate independently as autosomal dominant traits in some families.

Auricular tags are skin-covered nodules or appendages that often contain cartilage and represent remnants of the hillock of His. They are typically located anterior to the pinna but may be present anywhere along an arclike line from the temple to just below the tragus, conforming to the junction between the first and second branchial arches (Altmann, 1951). They may also be situated anterior to the tragus down to the angle of the mouth, corresponding embryologically to the fusion of the mandibular and maxillary portions of the first branchial arch.

Ear tags may exist as a part of a multiple malformation condition, such as the oculo-auriculo-vertebral spectrum (Goldenhar syndrome), Towne-Brocks syndrome, Treacher Collins syndrome, cat-eye syndrome, Wolf-Hirschhorn (4p-) syndrome, and cri du chat (5p-) syndrome.

Auricular sinuses are usually shallow dimples, pits, or depressions of 1 to 3 mm in diameter, most commonly located on the anterior margin of the ascending helix or, less commonly, in the preauricular region. The rarest location is posterior to the auricle at the site of its attachment. Auricular sinuses are twice as common in females as males. Although ear sinuses are usually isolated anomalies, they are associated with several multiple malformation syndromes, including oculo-auriculo-vertebral spectrum, Beckwith-Wiedemann syndrome, branchio-oto-renal (Melnick-Fraser) syndrome, Peters-plus syndrome, and various chromosome aberrations.

Preauricular pits and ear tags may coexist in a number of syndromes, including oculo-auriculo-vertebral spectrum (Goldenhar syndrome), cervico-oculo-acoustic (Wildervanck) syndrome, and mandibulofacial dysostosis (Treacher Collins syndrome).

Hearing loss is associated with both ear tags and sinuses. In approximately 13% of isolated cases of ear tags, mild to moderate sensorineural hearing loss is present (Kankkunen and Thiringer, 1987). Conductive and sensorineural hearing loss have also been described with ear sinuses. Hearing screening tests are warranted for patients presenting with either of these anomalies.

REFERENCES

Altmann F: Malformations of the auricle and external auditory meatus. Arch Otolaryngol 54:115, 1951.

Banker BQ: Arthrogryposis multiplex congenita: Spectrum of pathologic changes. Hum Pathol 17:656–671, 1986.

Bingle GJ, Niswander JD: Polydactyly in the American Indian. Am J Hum Genet 27:91–99, 1975.

Bromley B, Benacerraf BR: Fetal micrognathia: Associated anomalies and outcome. J Ultrasound Med 13:529–533, 1994.

Brzustowicz LM, Lehner T, Castilla LH: Genetic mapping of chronic childhood-onset spinal muscular atrophy to chromosome 5q11.2-13.3. Nature 344:540–541, 1990.

Carter CO, Wilkinson JA: Genetic and environmental factors in the etiology of congenital dislocation of the hip. Clin Orthop Rel Res 33:119–128, 1964.

Czeizel A, Szentpeley J, Tusnady G, Vizkelety T: Two-family study on congenital dislocation of the hip after early orthopaedic screening in Hungary. J Med Genet 12:125–150, 1975.

D'Alton ME, Simpson LL: Syndromes in twins. Semin Perinatol 19:375–386, 1995.

DiMario FJ: Genetic diseases in the etiology of the floppy infant. Rhode Island Med J 72:357–359, 1989.

Driscoll DA, Salvin J, Sellinger B, et al: Prevalence of 22q microdeletions in DiGeorge and velocardiofacial syndromes: Implications for genetic counseling and prenatal diagnosis. J Med Genet 30:813–817, 1993.

Edwards RG, Mettler L, Walters DE: Identical twins and in vitro fertilization. J In Vitro Fert Embryo Transfer 3:114, 1986.

Elliott MA, Studen-Pavlovich DA, Ranalli DN: Prevalence of selected pediatric conditions in children with Pierre Robin sequence. Pediatr Dentistry 17:106–111, 1995.

Fraser FC: The genetics of cleft lip and palate—yet another look. *In* Pratt R, Christiansen L (Eds): Current Research Trends in Prenatal Craniofacial Development. Amsterdam, Elsevier/North-Holland, 1980.

Frazier TM: A note on race-specific congenital malformation rates. Am J Obstet Gynecol 80:184–185, 1960.

Goldberg M: Arthrogryposis multiplex congenita and arthrogryposis syndromes. *In* The Dysmorphic Child: An Orthopedic Perspective. New York, Raven Press, 1987.

Goldmuntz E, Driscoll D, Budarf ML, et al: Microdeletion of chromosomal region 22q11 in patients with congenital cardiac defects. J Med Genet 20:807–812, 1993.

Gorlin RJ, Cohen MM, Levin LS: Syndromes of the Head and Neck, 3rd ed. New York, Oxford University Press, 1990.

Hall JG: Genetic aspects of arthrogryposis. Clin Orthop Rel Res 84:44–53, 1985.

Hall JG, Reed SD, Driscoll EP: Amyoplasia: A common sporadic condition with congenital contractures. Am J Med Genet 15:571–590, 1983.

Idelberger K: Die Erbpathologic der Sogenannten Angeborenen Huftverrenkung. Berlin, Urban & Schwarzenber, 1951.

Kambara H, Sasakawa Y: On twins with congenital dislocation of the hip. J Bone Joint Surg (Am) 36:186–187, 1954.

Kankkunen A, Thiringer K: Hearing impairment in connection with preauricular tags. Acta Paediatr Scand 76:143, 1987.

Kelly D, Goldberg R, Wilson D, et al: Confirmation that velocardiofacial syndrome is associated with haplo insufficiency of genes at chromosome 22q11. Am J Med Genet 45:308–312, 1993.

Martin NG, Beaini JL, Olsen ME, et al: Gonadotropin levels in mothers who have had two sets of twins. Acta Genet Med Gemellol (Roma) 33:1331, 1984.

McCulloch K: Neonatal problems in twins. Clin Perinatol 15:141–158, 1988.

Melnick M, Myrianthopoulos NC: External ear malformations: Epidemiology, genetics, and natural history. Birth Defects 15:1, 1979.

Milham S Jr: Pituitary gonadotropin and dizygotic twinning. Lancet 2:566, 1964.

Myrianthopoulos NC: Congenital malformations in twins. Acta Genet Med Gemellol (Roma) 25:331, 1976.

Nicolaides EK, Snijders RJM, Gosden CM, et al: Ultrasonographically detectable markers of fetal chromosomal abnormalities. Lancet 340:704–707, 1992.

Nicolaides KH, Salveson DR, Snijders RJM, et al: Fetal facial defects: Associated malformations and chromosomal abnormalities. Fetal Diagn Ther 8:1–9, 1993.

Nora JJ, Nora AH: Maternal transmission of congenital heart diseases: New recurrence risk figures and the question of cytoplasmic inheritance and vulnerability to teratogens. Am J Cardiol 59:459–463, 1987.

Nora JJ, Nora AH: Genetic epidemiology of congenital heart diseases. Prog Med Genet 5:91–137, 1983.

Nylander PPS: Serum levels of gonadotropins in relation to multiple pregnancy in Nigeria. J Obstet Gynaecol Br Commonw 80:651, 1973.

Otto C, Platt LD: The fetal mandible measurement: An objective determination of fetal jaw size. Ultrasound Obstet Gynecol 1:12–17, 1991.

Plauche WC: Myasthenia gravis in mothers and their newborns. Clin Obstet Gynecol 34:82–99, 1991.

Robin P: La chute de la base de la langue consideree comme une nouvelle cause de gene dans la respiration naso-pharyngienne. Bull Acad Natl Med 89:37–41, 1923.

Robin P: Glossoptosis due to atresia and hypotrophy of the mandible. Am J Dis Child 48:541–547, 1934.

Sadewitz VL: Robin sequence: Changes in thinking leading to changes in patient care. Cleft Palate-Craniofacial J 29:246–253, 1992.

Schinzel AA, Smith DW, Miller JR: Monozygotic twinning and structural defects. J Pediatr 95:921, 1979.

Scott-Emuakpor AB, Madueke EDN: The study of genetic variation in Nigeria: II. The genetics of polydactyly. Hum Hered 26:198–202, 1976.

Sherer DM, Metlay LA, Woods JR: Lack of mandibular movement manifested by absent fetal swallowing: A possible factor in the pathogenesis of micrognathia. Am J Perinatol 12:30–33, 1995.

Shprintzen RJ: The implications of the diagnosis of Robin sequence. Cleft Palate-Craniofacial J 29:205–209, 1992.

Shprintzen RJ, Schmatz RH, Daniller A, et al: Morphologic significance of bifid uvula. Pediatrics 75:553–561, 1985.

Temtamy SA, McKusick VA: The Genetics of Hand Malformations. New York, Alan R Liss, 1978.

Tolorova M, Morton NE: Cleft lip and palate–recurrence risk and genetic counseling. Acta Chir Plast 17:97–111, 1975.

Turner GM, Twining P: The facial profile in the diagnosis of fetal anomalies. Clin Radiol 1993; 47:380.

Watson WJ, Katz VL: Sonographic measurement of the fetal mandible: Standards for normal pregnancy. Am J Perinatol 10:226–228, 1993.

Winter RM, Tickle C: Syndactylies and polydactylies: Embryological overview and suggested classification. Eur J Hum Genet 1:96–104, 1993.

Woolf CM, Koehn JH, Coleman SS: Congenital hip disease in Utah: The influence of genetic and nongenetic factors. Am J Hum Genet 20:430–439, 1968.

Wynne-Davies R: A family study of neonatal and late-diagnosis congenital dislocation of the hip. J Med Genet 7:315–333, 1970.

CHAPTER 22

Specific Genetic Disorders Presenting in the Newborn

Barbara Shephard and Kenneth G. Kupke

THE HUMAN KARYOTYPE

Human chromosomes were first visualized in 1956, and subsequently many clinical disorders were discovered to be based on chromosome abnormalities. Down syndrome due to trisomy 21 was the first human chromosome disorder to be described (Lejeune et al, 1959). Since then, many different chromosome aberrations have been elucidated, most with stereotypic phenotypes that constitute syndrome complexes.

The human karyotype normally consists of 46 chromosomes with 22 pairs of autosomes and two sex chromosomes, either two X chromosomes, or an X and a Y chromosome (Fig. 22–1). During spermatogenesis and oogenesis, the diploid cell containing 46 chromosomes undergoes a chromosome reduction process to a haploid cell containing 23 chromosomes. During this process of meiosis, the homologous chromosomes pair off, exchange genetic material by crossing over, and separate to respective poles of the cell. The diploid state is then re-established at the time of fertilization.

Human chromosomes demonstrate a distinctive size, a centromeric position, and a banding pattern after staining with dyes. Each chromosome is routinely identified by number, using standard international nomenclature for cytogenetic findings (ISCN, 1995). The autosomes are generally numbered from largest to smallest, number 1 to 22.

Chromosomes are linear structures with two arms joined by the centromere. The short arm is designated p (for petit), and the long arm is called q. During the early cell cycle, each chromosome is present as a single structure called a *chromatid*. After chromosome replication, two sister chromatids are formed, each containing the same genetic material.

The major components of chromatin are DNA and protein. Each chromosome's DNA comprises tens of millions of base pairs. The proteins, both histone and nonhistone, provide the structural integrity of the chromosome for compacting the DNA. Chromatin has two differently condensed forms: highly condensed heterochromatin and less condensed euchromatin. Euchromatin contains the coding DNA (genes), whereas heterochromatin generally contains noncoding DNA. The terminals of the p and q arms are termed *telomeres*, which contain specialized DNA for preventing fusion with chromatin of other chromosomes. The centromeres also contain specialized DNA, which during mitosis provides for a site for anchoring the spindle apparatus to permit the separation of paired chromatids to opposite poles of the cell.

Chromosomes are analyzed under the light microscope at about ×1000 magnification. In nondividing cells the chromosomes are extended and cannot be distinguished. During mitosis, the chromosomes condense and become visible with staining. For this reason chromosome analysis is possible only for cells mitotically stimulated in culture (such as blood lymphocytes, skin fibroblasts, amniocytes, and chorionic villus) or for cells derived from tissues undergoing rapid cell division in vivo (such as bone marrow and chorionic villus). Several different staining methods have been developed to demonstrate different characteristics of the chromosomes. G-banding (Giemsa) remains the standard cytogenetic method, permitting the identification of every human chromosome and providing a minimum resolution of 400 bands distributed among the 23 pairs. High-resolution analyses of up to 800 bands may be necessary in some circumstances to rule out a subtle abnormality, which may not be resolvable at 400 bands. Other staining methods include Q banding (fluorescent quinacrine), R banding (reverse), C banding (centromeric), NOR staining (nucleolar organizing region), distamycin/DAPI staining, and replication banding.

Chromosome Abnormalities

Chromosome abnormalities occur in approximately 1 in 120 newborns, of which about one half of patients are phenotypically abnormal. The frequency of different chromosome aberrations is shown in Table 22–1 (Hook, 1992; Jacobs et al, 1992).

Most chromosomally abnormal conceptuses die prior to delivery (Boué et al, 1973). Approximately 25% of human blastocysts at the 10-cell stage have chromosome anomalies. Many of these conceptuses do not implant properly and are aborted before the pregnancy is clinically appreciated. Fifteen percent of recognized human pregnancies are spontaneously miscarried, and about 50% are attributed to chromosome abnormalities. Those rare chromosomally abnormal fetuses surviving the pregnancy have genetic imbalances small enough to permit adequate embryogenesis and fetal survival.

Aneuploidy

Aneuploidy refers to a genetic imbalance occurring because of a gain or a loss of chromosome material, either completely or partially. The classic aneuploidy syndromes involve trisomy or monosomy of complete chromosomes. The most commonly recognized human aneuploidy conditions are autosomal trisomies 8, 9, 13, 18, and 21 and sex chromosome aneuploidies XXX, XXY, XYY, and 45,X. Trisomy and monosomy both occur from an error in chromosome separation during meiosis or mitosis, termed *non-disjunction*.

In meiotic nondisjunction, the pair of homologs fail to separate, leading to 2:0 segregation in which one daughter cell possesses both of the chromosomes (disomic) and the other cell has none (nullisomic). This pathologic process

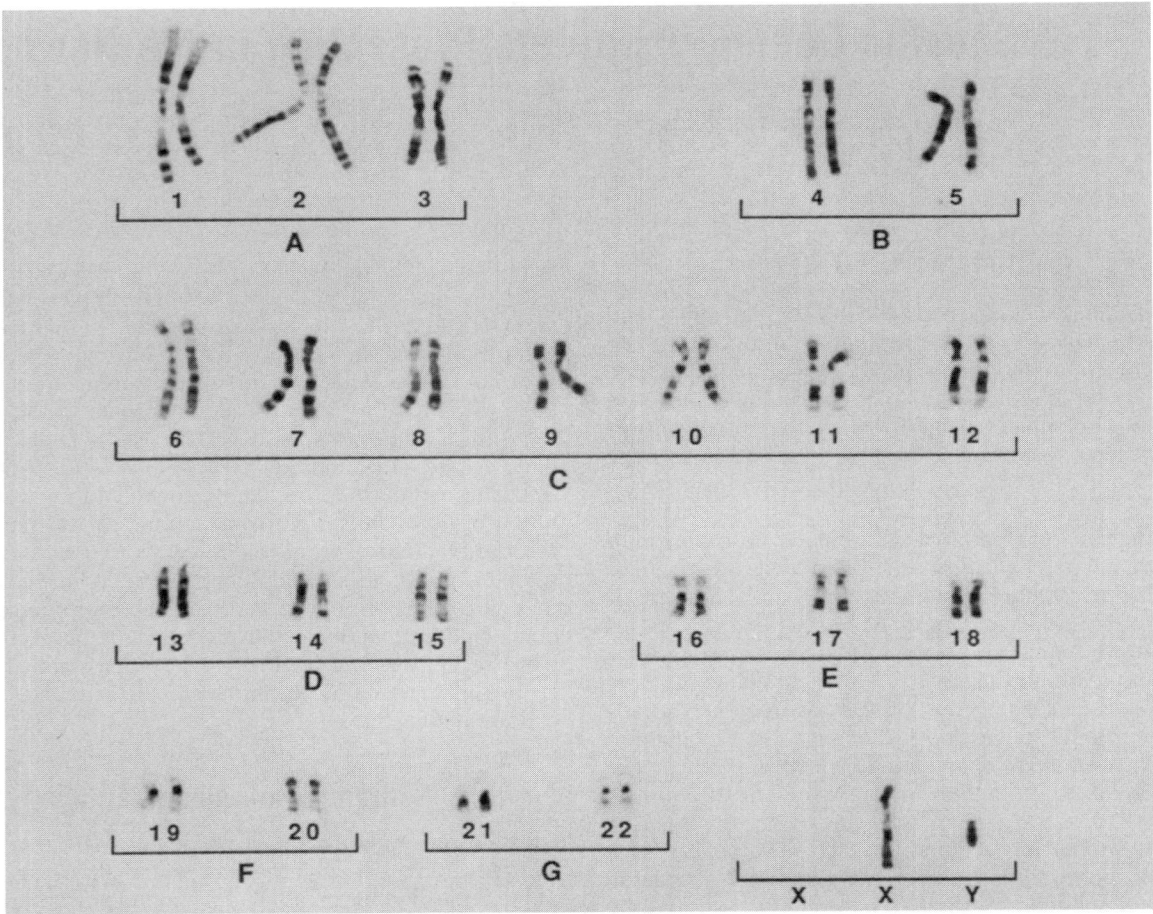

FIGURE 22–1. G-banded human male karyotype. The 46 chromosomes are arranged into 23 pairs, each with a specific banding pattern.

may occur during the first or second gametic cell division (meiosis I or II). Most meiotic nondisjunction in humans occurs in oogenesis in maternal meiosis I. For the trisomies of acrocentric chromosomes (numbers 13 to 15, 21 to 22) and XXX about 90% are of maternal origin, and roughly 75% arise in meiosis I (MacDonald et al, 1994; Zaragoza et al, 1994). In trisomy 18, maternal nondisjunction, mainly in meiosis II, is the predominant mechanism (Fisher et al, 1995; Kupke and Muller, 1989). Triploidy, 69,XXX or 69,XXY, may occur from retention of the polar body of the ovum as one basis, thereby representing total chromosome nondisjunction (Martin et al, 1991; Mueller et al, 1993). Other cases of triploidy are the result of double fertilization of a single ovum.

Studies of sperm indicate that approximately 3% to 4% are aneuploid owing to nondisjunction (Martin et al, 1991). The proportion of aneuploid ova has been more difficult to investigate but has ranged from 4% to 20% (Hassold et al, 1993; Kamiguchi et al, 1993; Martin et al, 1991). Meiotic nondisjunction increases significantly with maternal age for trisomy 13, 16, 18, 21, 47,XXX, and 47,XXY, which has led to the routine offering of prenatal karyotyping to all women 35 years of age and older (Ferguson-Smith and Yates, 1984; Hook and Cross, 1982). The underlying biologic mechanism for the maternal age effect still remains to be elucidated.

In mitotic nondisjunction, two cell lines are created, one trisomic and the other monosomic. The monosomic cell line is usually nonviable, leaving a potentially viable trisomic cell line. If the nondisjunctional event occurs after the first postzygotic cleavage, cells containing a normal chromosome number may also exist. The coexistence of two or more cell lines of differing chromosome constitution is termed *mosaicism.*

Other types of partial aneuploidy occur from gains or losses of chromosome segments. These conditions may occur sporadically without known mechanisms or may be a consequence of a balanced chromosome translocation in one of the parents. Translocations involve rearrangements of chromosome material between two nonhomologous chromosomes. If no loss or gain of genetic material occurs, the individual is genetically balanced and remains phenotypically normal. The offspring of balanced translocation carriers are at increased risk for unbalanced rearrangements during meiosis, often leading to spontaneous miscarriage or a liveborn with birth defects, dysmorphism, and developmental disabilities.

Trisomy 21 (Down Syndrome)

Down syndrome is the most common autosomal trisomy compatible with live birth, occurring in about 1 in 700 to

TABLE 22–1

Frequency of Chromosome Abnormalities in Newborns

Chromosome Abnormality	Frequency (per 1000)
Autosomol trisomies	
Trisomy 13	0.08
Trisomy 18	0.15
Trisomy 21	1.2
Triploidy	0.02
Sex chromosome aneuploidy, male	
XXY	1.2
XYY	1.2
Other	0.15
Sex chromosome aneuploidy, female	
45,X and X/XX	0.3
XXX	1.1
Structural rearrangement, unbalanced	0.3
Extra structurally abnormal chromosome	0.4
Structural rearrangement, balanced	
Reciprocal	2.5
Robertsonian	1.0
Pericentric inversion	0.8

Adapted from Hook EB: Chromosome abnormalities: Prevalence, risks, and recurrence. In Brock DJH, Rodeck CH, Ferguson-Smith MA (Eds): Prenatal Diagnosis and Screening. Edinburgh, Churchill Livingstone, 1992, pp 351–392; and Jacobs PA, Browne C, Gregson N, et al: Estimates of the frequency of chromosome abnormalities detectable in unselected newborns using moderate levels of banding. J Med Genet 29:103–108, 1992.

800 newborns (Hook, 1992; Smith and Berg, 1976). Trisomy 21 due to meiotic nondisjunction provides the underlying basis in 92% to 95% of liveborns with Down syndrome, and translocation Down syndrome with 46 chromosomes accounts for 3% to 5% of cases. In most cases of translocation Down syndrome, one parent has a balanced robertsonian translocation between chromosome 21 and another acrocentric chromosome, most commonly chromosome 14. In approximately 3% of Down syndrome, mitotic nondisjunction occurs leading to trisomy 21 mosaicism.

Many fetuses with Down syndrome are now diagnosed by prenatal karyotyping initiated because of advanced maternal age or abnormal maternal serum analyte screening (triple test) or fetal ultrasonographic findings. Many prenatal ultrasound findings are associated with Down syndrome, including atrioventricular canal defect, the "double-bubble" sign of duodenal atresia, short femur or humerus lengths, nuchal thickening or translucency, echogenic small bowel, choroid plexus cysts, cerebral ventriculomegaly, hydronephrosis, nonimmune hydrops, fifth-finger clinodactyly, and cholecystomegaly.

If not prenatally diagnosed, most patients with Down syndrome are usually recognized at birth owing to the constellation of physical findings (Fig. 22–2). Although no one physical feature is pathognomonic, a number of clinical signs are usually present in affected babies, allowing the nurse or midwife to frequently suspect the diagnosis first. Common neonatal features include a rounded head, third fontanelle, brachycephaly, upslanted palpebral fissures, epicanthal folds, Brushfield spots, midfacial hypoplasia, flat-tened nasal root, small dysplastic pinnae, a large tongue in a small mouth, short neck, transverse palmar creases, brachydactyly, fifth-finger clinodactyly, a wide gap between the first and second toe, and hypotonia.

Diagnostic scoring systems have been devised (Hall, 1966; Rex and Preus, 1982). In Table 22–2, six or more out of 10 signs are considered virtually diagnostic in the newborn. In some cases, the diagnosis may be difficult because the features may be subtle or confounded by other factors such as prematurity and ethnic background.

Whenever the diagnosis is suspected, an immediate karyotype is indicated to definitively confirm or rule out the condition. The parents should be informed of the level of clinical suspicion and the need for a confirmatory cytogenetic study.

Numerous birth defects have been described in association with Down syndrome (Kallen et al, 1996). Congenital heart disease comprises the common major malformation in Down syndrome, occurring in about 45% of babies (Rehder, 1981). The most frequently observed cardiac lesion is the atrioventricular canal defect; other lesions include ventricular septal defect (VSD), atrial septal defect (ASD), patent ductus arteriosus (PDA), and tetralogy of Fallot. An echocardiogram is indicated for all patients with Down syndrome, since the diagnosis of congenital heart disease may be missed by routine diagnostic means. The medical and surgical treatment of the heart lesions are the same as for chromosomally normal infants.

Gastrointestinal malformations also occur more commonly in Down syndrome. Approximately 2% to 5% of patients have duodenal atresia, and 2% have Hirschsprung disease. Other rarer associated anomalies include tracheoesophageal fistula, esophageal atresia, omphalocele, annular pancreas, duodenal web, distal small bowel atresia, microcolon, and anorectal anomalies.

Hearing loss of heterogenous origin may be present to some degree in 40% to 75% of patients with Down syndrome (Roizen et al, 1993). Middle ear disease is the most common cause of hearing problems.

Strabismus, myopia, cataracts, and glaucoma occur more frequently in Down syndrome, with 61% of patients requiring ongoing ophthalmologic care (Roizen et al, 1994). A pediatric eye evaluation at 6 months or less and annually thereafter is recommended.

Atlantoaxial subluxation is an infrequent but serious complication of Down syndrome; cord compression and neurologic symptoms may result (Anonymous, 1995). Generalized ligamentous laxity is considered the basis for the atlantoaxial instability. The radiographic signs of instability (gap >4 mm) have poor predictive value and generally do not merit treatment. Flexion-extension radiographs are recommended prior to anesthesia and the initiation of high-risk sports.

Growth problems occur in virtually all patients with Down syndrome. At birth, the mean weight, length, and head circumference range between 10% to 15% (Clementi et al, 1990). After infancy the growth velocity falls off so that linear growth retardation is the norm by 3 years of age. Growth curves for Down syndrome children have been published (Cronk et al, 1988). Growth hormone has been used to treat short stature in some patients who do not have growth hormone deficiency. This controversial

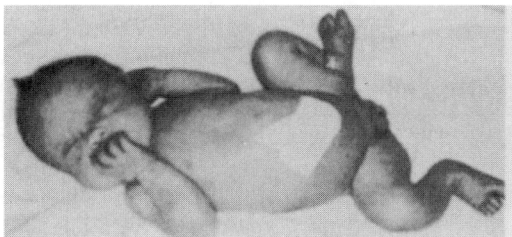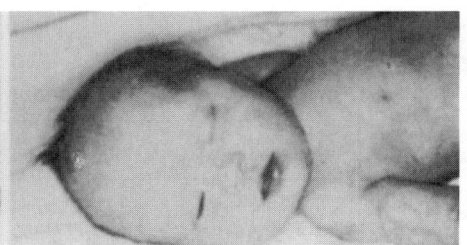

FIGURE 22–2. Newborn with Down syndrome (trisomy 21) illustrating some of the characteristic facial features, including upslanting palpebral fissures and flat facial profile.

treatment has shown some favorable short-term results. As adults, obesity is a common problem, occurring in 96% of females and 71% of males (Bell and Bhate, 1992).

Approximately 5% of patients with Down syndrome develop hypothyroidism; almost one third of patients have demonstrable thyroid autoantibodies (Dinani and Carpenter, 1990; Pueschel and Pezullo, 1985). The thyroid dysfunction may occur at any age, and newborn screening followed by regular thyroid screening is indicated.

Approximately 1 in 150 children with Down syndrome develop acute lymphoblastic leukemia (Fong and Brodeur, 1987). Transient myeloproliferative disorder associated with splenomegaly and hepatic fibrosis may occur at birth and usually resolves spontaneously in the first year of life. Neonatal thrombocytopenia is also associated with Down syndrome.

Children with Down syndrome show a great deal of developmental variability. Language and motor delay become more pronounced during the second year of life. The degree of central hypotonia is correlated to some degree with later cognitive and motor development (Gath and Gumley, 1984). I.Q. testing has revealed an extremely wide range, from 20 to 85 (Carr, 1995). Most children attain the learning ability of a 6- to 8-year-old child, but some patients may exceed this level. The popular Down syndrome stereotype of a happy, affectionate, pleasant, music-loving person with moderate intellectual handicaps does not accurately reflect the great variety of personalities, including behavioral and psychologic problems, in these patients (Pueschel et al, 1991). Epilepsy occurs in 5% to 10% of patients with Down syndrome, with peak onsets in infancy and late adulthood.

TABLE 22–2

Ten Cardinal Signs of Down Syndrome in a Newborn

Sign	Frequency (%) In Affected Newborn
Poor Moro reflex	85
Hypotonia	80
Flat facial profile	90
Upslanted palpebral fissures	80
Morphologically simple, small, round ears	60
Redundant loose neck skin	80
Transverse palmar crease	45
Hyperextensible large joints	80
Abnormal pelvic radiograph	70
Fifth-finger clinodactyly	60

Adapted from Hall B: Mongolism in newborns. Clin Pediatr (Phila) 5:4, 1966.

If a child with Down syndrome survives the infancy period, the prognosis for long-term survival is generally good; however, a shortened life span is still likely. About 44% of patients survive to 60 years of age and about 14% to 68 years (Baird and Sadovnick, 1989). Beyond 40 years of age, virtually all patients display neuropathologic features of Alzheimer disease, but most patients do not develop frank dementia (Dalton and Wisniewski, 1990).

For complete or mosaic trisomy 21, it is unnecessary to obtain parental chromosome analyses since in virtually all cases their karyotypes will be normal. After a child with trisomy 21 is born to a mother, her risk of recurrence for Down syndrome at the time of amniocentesis is about 1% greater than her age-specific risk (Hook, 1992). For younger mothers, this increase over the age-specific risk is significant, whereas for older mothers, the increased risk is only incremental.

For de novo Down syndrome translocation, the recurrence risk is less than 1%. In the case of a mother carrying a familial robertsonian translocation, the risk for translocation Down syndrome is about 15% at amniocentesis and 10% at birth. For male translocation carriers, the recurrence risk is small, at about 1%.

Trisomy 18 (Edwards Syndrome)

Trisomy 18 occurs in about 1 in 6000 live births, with a 3:1 female:male preponderance. It carries a high intrauterine mortality rate (Carothers, 1994; Goldstein and Nielsen, 1988). It is estimated that only 5% of trisomy 18 conceptuses survive to live birth, and 30% of fetuses diagnosed by mid-trimester amniocentesis succumb during the rest of the pregnancy (Hook, 1992).

Prenatal ultrasonography may provide important clues to the diagnosis of trisomy 18. Reported findings include growth retardation, oligohydramnios or polyhydramnios, heart defects, exomphalos, myelomeningocele, clenched fists, and radial limb anomalies. The combination of intrauterine growth retardation with any major birth defect should raise suspicion for trisomy 18. Maternal serum analyte screening has also been shown to be useful for the detection of trisomy 18; alpha-fetoprotein, uE3, and total human chorionic gonadotropin all demonstrate lower values than the normal population. The mid-trimester triple test can detect 66% of cases of trisomy 18 with a 0.4% false-positive rate (Palomaki et al, 1992).

At birth, physical findings are usually diagnostic of trisomy 18 (Fig. 22–3). Common features include intrauterine growth retardation (1500 to 2500 g near term); small, narrow cranium; prominent occiput; open metopic suture; low-set, posteriorly rotated, primitive pinnae; small mouth; micrognathia; short sternum; characteristic overlapping

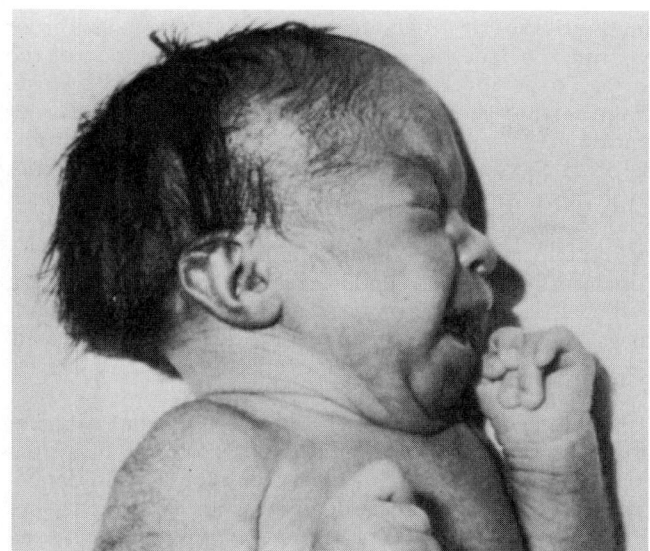

FIGURE 22–3. Newborn with trisomy 18, with prominent occiput, characteristic facial appearance, and clenched hands.

digits; hypoplastic fingernails; short, dorsiflexed great toes; and prominent heels with convex soles, termed *rocker-bottom feet.*

Many different major malformations are associated with trisomy 18. More common defects include congenital heart disease (ASD, VSD, PDA, pulmonic stenosis, coarctation), cleft palate, talipes equinovarus, omphalocele, colonic malrotation, renal anomalies, myelomeningocele, brain anomalies, choanal atresia, eye anomalies, vertebral anomalies, radial ray defects, hypospadias, and cryptorchidism.

Approximately 90% or more of babies with trisomy 18 die by 6 months of age, and about 5% are alive at 1 year (Root and Carey, 1994). Female survivors significantly outnumber males. The major causes of death include central apnea, infection, and congestive heart failure (Embleton et al, 1996). In the newborn period poor feeding is almost universal, so that gavage tube feeding is generally required.

Once the diagnosis is cytogenetically confirmed, the extremely poor prognosis should be fully explained to the parents. The caregivers should discuss the inappropriateness of aggressive life-sustaining therapies, which may inflict discomfort on the patient. Given the significantly shortened life span of such patients, most parents and providers jointly decide to forego heroic medical and surgical interventions. Arrangements to care for the baby at home may be considered if adequate medical, social, and emotional supports exist.

Rare long-term survivors with trisomy 18 have been described; profound somatic growth and mental retardation are the rule. In some patients, cardiac surgery has been performed, but this intervention has not been shown to improve outcome (Embleton et al, 1996). Overall development does not progress much beyond that of a 6-month-old infant (Baty et al, 1994b). Malignant tumors, such as Wilms tumor, hepatoblastoma, and neurogenetic tumors, have been described in some survivors (Dasouki and Barr, 1987; Karayalcin et al, 1981).

There are rare anecdotal reports of recurrences of trisomy 18, as well as the occurrence of other autosomal trisomies following trisomy 18 (Baty et al, 1994a; Pauli et al, 1978). In relatively small series of trisomy 18 index cases, this phenomenon appears extremely uncommon. Nonetheless, it is postulated that some women have a general predisposition to aneuploidy. In the case of young mothers, it is common practice to add a 1% risk to the maternal age–specific risk when estimating the recurrence risk of a viable autosomal trisomy (Hook, 1992).

Trisomy 13 (Patau Syndrome)

Trisomy 13 has a birth frequency of 1 in 12,500 to 21,000 newborns, and it is estimated that only 2.5% of trisomy 13 conceptuses survive to birth (Carothers, 1994; Hook, 1992).

Approximately 50% of cases of trisomy 13 can be diagnosed prenatally by using maternal age, maternal serum screening, and routine fetal ultrasonography (Abramsky and Chapple, 1993). Prenatal ultrasound has the potential to visualize many of the major associated malformations, including holoprosencephaly, anophthalmia, facial clefting, nasal deformities, congenital heart disease, renal anomalies, omphalocele, and polydactyly.

In the newborn, the diagnosis is suggested by the presence of postaxial polydactyly, microcephaly, eye anomalies, cleft lip and palate, scalp defects, congenital heart disease, and renal anomalies (Fig. 22–4).

Varying degrees of holoprosencephaly are present in 60% of patients, and seizures are quite common. Microcephaly is quite common, and the sutures are usually split with large fontanels. Microphthalmia, colobomas of the iris, abnormal ears, capillary hemangiomata, and cleft lip and/or palate are common facial findings. Localized scalp defects (cutis aplasia) in the parieto-occipital area are present in about 50% of cases. Approximately 80% of patients have some form of congenital heart disease, most commonly VSD, ASD, PDA, and dextrocardia. Typical limb findings are transverse palmar creases, postaxial polydactyly, camptylodactyly, and hyperconvex narrow fingernails.

Survival is extremely limited with 80% of babies dying in the neonatal period and 3% surviving to 6 months of age (Goldstein and Nielsen, 1988). Physical and mental development is severely delayed (Zoll et al, 1993). Patients are often blind and deaf, experience refractory epilepsy, and have feeding difficulties.

In the newborn period, management issues are similar to those of trisomy 18, in that decisions must be mutually reached regarding the goals of medical interventions. The dismal prognosis dictates that focus should be directed toward comfort measures and quality-of-life issues.

As in trisomy 18, the data on recurrences after having one child with trisomy 13 are incomplete, but available data suggest that recurrences are extremely rare (Baty et al, 1994a). Nonetheless, a maternal age–related risk plus 1% is usually offered for the recurrence risk of any viable autosomal trisomy (Hook, 1992).

Turner Syndrome (45,X)

Turner syndrome occurs in about 1 in 2500 female newborns, for which 45,X accounts for 40% to 60% of cases.

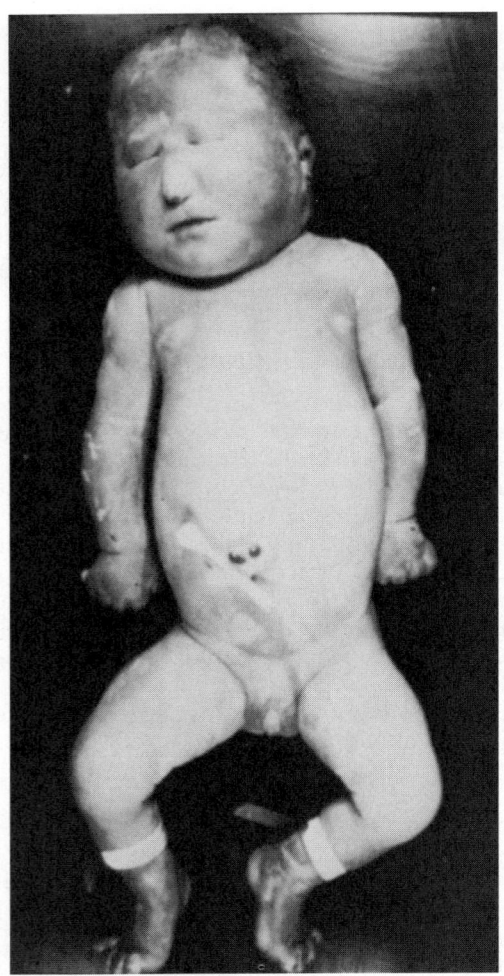

FIGURE 22–4. Stillborn with trisomy 13. The facial appearance is that of cebocephaly, which is associated with holoprosencephaly. There is an extra digit on the ulnar border of the right hand.

Other causes are predominantly due to X chromosome deletions, isochromosomes, or translocations. Only 0.1% of 45,X conceptuses are carried to live birth, whereas 99.9% are spontaneously aborted. Studies of parental origin indicate that in 80% of 45,X patients, the paternal X is lost.

Two active X chromosomes are normally required in early embryogenesis. One X chromosome subsequently becomes inactivated and produces the Barr body, whereas the other X chromosome remains completely active. The inactive X chromosome is not completely inoperative in that several discrete areas along the chromosome still express genes. One such active area on Xq produces the inactive specific transcript (X-IST), which is paradoxically not produced by the active X chromosome. This gene is most likely the inactivation center controlling the overall process of X inactivation (Brown et al, 1991).

The cardinal signs of Turner syndrome include short stature, mild craniofacial abnormalities (epicanthal folds, high-arched palate), strabismus, auditory defects, a webbed or short neck, shield chest, renal anomalies, pigmented nevi, lymphedema of hand and feet, nail hypoplasia, primary amenorrhea, and congenital heart disease (Ferguson-

Smith, 1965). The types of heart defects seen in Turner syndrome include bicuspid aortic valve, coarctation of the aorta, valvar aortic stenosis, and mitral valve prolapse. There is wide phenotypic variation in patients with Turner syndrome. The ultimate adult height in Turner syndrome is 135 to 150 cm. Delayed secondary sexual characteristics results from primary ovarian failure with lack of estrogen production.

Mental retardation is not a feature of Turner syndrome. Perceptual and spatial thinking may be impaired, however, leading to somewhat lower mean performance I.Q. Language as well as fine and gross motor skills may be delayed. Personality traits may be characterized by lack of aggressiveness, immaturity, shyness, and compliance.

Other medical problems later in life include a higher risk for autoimmune thyroiditis, hypothyroidism, hypertension, obesity, intestinal telangiectasia, non–insulin-dependent diabetes, osteoporosis, deafness, and aortic aneurysms.

Growth hormone therapy is commonly now used to treat short stature beginning at age 4 to 6 years. Cyclic hormonal therapy with estrogens and progesterone is usually initiated at puberty for the development of secondary sex characteristics, menses, and the prevention of osteoporosis. Infertility is highly likely secondary to primary ovarian failure (streak gonads), but assisted reproduction with in vitro fertilization of donated oocytes in hormonally treated patients has been successfully performed.

47,XXX

With a birth prevalence of 1 in 1200 female newborns, the XXX syndrome has no specific phenotype in the newborn period. There is a higher rate of minor anomalies, such as clinodactyly, ear anomalies, and epicanthal folds (Robinson et al, 1990a). Many display taller stature with disproportionate leg lengths relative to trunk height. The average I.Q. is normal in the 85 to 90 range, with wide variations. Speech delay, neuromotor incoordination, and learning disabilities are more common. Although about 60% of 47,XXX females require special education in high school, some attended college and are highly competent adults. Personality traits such as shyness, immaturity, passivity, mild depression, and conduct disorders are also more commonly reported. Most patients undergo normal puberty, have normal reproductive capacity, and cope well as adults.

47,XXY

Klinefelter syndrome occurs in about 1 in 600 male newborns and is the most common cause of hypogonadism in males. Maternal and paternal meiotic nondisjunction contribute equally as the underlying mechanism. In the newborn there is no significant dysmorphic pattern, although fifth-finger clinodactyly occurs in about 25% of patients. The major features noted later include tall stature, hypogonadism, infertility, light facial hair, and an increased risk for developmental problems. Gynecomastia occurs in 15% to 30% of patients. The mean I.Q. is 85 to 90, with most patients falling in the normal range. Learning disabilities, especially those involving reading, expressive language, and auditory processing, are common (Robinson et al, 1990a). Behavioral problems may also exist, including immaturity, shyness, unassertiveness, low frustration tolerance, and poor peer relations. The onset of puberty is normal and the sexual orientation is generally heterosexual. Testosterone therapy in adolescence is indicated to promote secondary sexual characteristics.

47,XYY

The 47,XYY karyotype occurs in about 1 in 1000 male newborns and there is no recognizable physical phenotype. The 47,XYY syndrome originates from paternal nondisjunction in meiosis II. Although preliminary reports invoked the supernumerary Y chromosome as the basis for criminal behavior in some mentally retarded persons, prospective studies have not shown an increased risk of frank mental retardation or severe behavioral problems (Robinson et al, 1990a, 1990b). There is an increased risk of hyperactivity, low impulse control, distractibility, and expressive and receptive language problems. Boys with 47,XYY have accelerated linear growth, becoming taller adults. Reproductive ability is not affected.

Triploidy

Triploidy occurs when the karyotype contains three copies of each chromosome: 69,XXX or 69,XXY. Approximately 15% of cytogenetically abnormal abortuses are triploid. Cytogenetic mechanisms include fertilization of one egg by two sperm (dispermy) and complete failure of nondisjunction in maternal meiosis. Most triploid conceptuses are spontaneous aborted, and of those live born, death in infancy is the rule. Patients with diploid-triploid mosaicism, known as *mixoploidy,* may survive with varying degrees of severity. A number of birth defects are associated with triploidy, including a large cystic placenta, low birth weight, hydrocephalus, neural tube defects, microphthalmia, colobomata, malformed ears, 2-3 syndactyly, cardiac septal defects, and ambiguous genitalia.

DELETION/CONTIGUOUS GENE SYNDROMES

Cri du Chat (5p−)

Partial deletion of 5p results in the cri du chat syndrome, named for the distinctive cry of a mewing cat in affected infants (Lejeune et al, 1963). The birth incidence is approximately 1 in 50,000 newborns (Niebuhr, 1978a). In the newborn period, patients present with the characteristic cry, low birth weight, microcephaly, craniofacial dysmorphism (round face, hypertelorism, downward-slanted palpebral fissures, epicanthal folds, and broad nasal bridge), and hypotonia. Approximately one third of patients have variable types of congenital heart disease, including ASD, VSD, and tetralogy of Fallot.

Over the first year of life, the catlike cry disappears and development progresses slowly. Mental retardation is generally severe, with reported I.Q. levels below 50 in infancy and below 20 in adulthood. Special education has been reported to be beneficial, with some adult patients reaching the developmental level of a normal 5- to 6-year-old child (Wilkins et al, 1980). Failure to thrive commonly occurs, and most patients survive to adulthood.

The cri du chat phenotype results from a deletion of the critical region of 5p15.2-p15.3 (Overhauser et al, 1986). De novo deletions account for 85% to 90% of cases; 10% to 15% occur due to malsegregation of parental balanced translocations (Niebuhr, 1978b). Fine molecular mapping of the critical region is now in progress to determine which of the estimated 100 genes in the critical region are responsible for specific phenotypic features (Simmons et al, 1995).

Lissencephaly/Miller-Dieker Syndrome (17p−)

The distal deletion of chromosome 17p leads to Miller-Dieker syndrome, characterized by facial dysmorphism and a severe neuronal migrational defect. Moreover, patients with isolated lissencephaly may also have deletions in the same region.

In Miller-Dieker syndrome, Type I lissencephaly is present, in which the surface of the brain is smooth without gyri. The craniofacial features include bitemporal hollowness, midfacial hypoplasia, a short nose with anteverted nostrils, micrognathia, and a protuberant upper lip with a thin vermilion border. Polyhydramnios is common during pregnancy owing to poor fetal swallowing. Postnatal growth retardation, seizures, profound mental retardation, and spasticity occur in most patients (Dieker et al, 1969; Miller, 1963). The disorder carries a significant mortality rate in childhood (Dobyns et al, 1991).

A microdeletion of the critical region, band 17p13.3, results in Miller-Dieker syndrome and will be visible by high-resolution methods in only about 50% of cases. Using cytogenetic and molecular techniques, 17p13 deletions are detectable in about 90% of patients with Miller-Dieker syndrome and 15% of patients with isolated lissencephaly (Kuwano et al, 1991). A brain morphogenesis gene *LIS1* has been isolated from this region and is deleted in patients with Miller-Dieker syndrome and isolated lissencephaly (Reiner et al, 1993). The diagnosis may be confirmed by either fluorescent in situ hybridization (FISH) analysis, polymorphic DNA markers, or direct *LIS1* mutational analysis. FISH probes for the 17p13 region are commercially available; most cytogenetic laboratories routinely offer specific testing for this condition.

Parental balanced translocations or pericentric inversions can account for recurrences in families, which previously were erroneously assumed to be due to an autosomal recessive trait.

DiGeorge/Velocardiofacial Syndromes (22q−)

The DiGeorge and the velocardiofacial (Sprintzen) syndrome (VCFS) were previously regarded as separate entities but have since shown phenotypic overlap when it was discovered that they contain deletions in the same 22q region (Driscoll et al, 1992a, 1992b).

In classic DiGeorge syndrome there is aplasia or hypoplasia of the thymus and parathyroid glands, congenital heart disease, and dysmorphic facies. Hypoparathyroidism leads to neonatal hypocalcemia and possibly seizures. Thymic hypoplasia results in a T-cell deficiency, with increased susceptibility to infections. The congenital heart defects are predominantly conotruncal, including tetralogy of Fallot, truncus arteriosus, interrupted aortic arch, right-sided aortic arch, and septal defects. The craniofacial findings include low-set ears, micrognathia, cleft palate, bifid uvula, and hypertelorism with short palpebral fissures.

VCFS is considered to be an autosomal dominant condition with cleft palate, cardiac defects, speech and language difficulties, and typical facies. Some patients with VCFS have additional features found in DiGeorge syndrome, namely neonatal hypocalcemia and lymphoid hypoplasia. Twenty percent of patients with VCFS demonstrate cytogenetic deletions of chromosome 22q by high-resolution techniques. Using FISH analysis, more than 80% of patients with VCFS have deletions. About 90% of cases of 22q deletions are de novo.

Approximately 15% to 20% of patients with DiGeorge syndrome have chromosome abnormalities, mainly involving chromosome 22. Additionally, FISH or DNA dosage studies now demonstrate 22q deletions in about 90% of patients with DiGeorge (Driscoll et al, 1992a).

DiGeorge syndrome and VCFS are now considered different manifestations of the same disorder, a loss of contiguous genes in the same region. The range of phenotype is quite wide and subtle dysmorphic features may be overlooked. In familial cases one parent may show features of predominantly VCFS but have a child with classic DiGeorge phenotype (Desmaze et al, 1993). The basis for the apparent autosomal dominant inheritance in VCFS has been shown to be due to the inheritance of a chromosome deletion from one of the parents.

Wolf-Hirschhorn Syndrome, 4p(−)

Infants with the Wolf-Hirschhorn syndrome, due to distal deletion of the short arm of chromosome 4, have dysmorphic features evident at birth. Prenatal ultrasound findings can also suggest the diagnosis. This clinical entity was first delineated in 1965 when Hirschhorn and Cooper (1961) cited a case with midline fusion defects and a deletion of a group B chromosome, and Wolf and colleagues (1965) described a similar case and were able to show that the deletion was of chromosome 4.

Hallmarks of this syndrome include growth restriction of prenatal onset, typical craniofacial malformations, microcephaly, and midline closure defects, including scalp defects, cleft lip and/or palate, cardiac septal defects, and hypospadias. The facial features, described as the "Greek helmet facies," consist of ocular hypertelorism with epicanthal folds; high forehead with prominent glabella; and a long, straight, beaked nose with broad nasal bridge. The ears are simple, large, and low set. Hypotonia is common, as is the history of poor fetal movement.

Approximately a third of infants with Wolf-Hirschhorn syndrome die in the first year, but some have lived to adulthood. Severe growth and mental retardation is invariable, and those that survive usually develop seizures.

The estimated case frequency is 1 in 50,000 births (Lurie et al, 1980). Some describe a female-to-male predilection. Most cases are due to a de novo deletion of 4pter, but 10% to 15% may be the result of translocation, making the study of parental karyotypes imperative for recurrence risk counseling (Lurie et al, 1980). The critical region has been mapped to 4p16 (McKeown et al, 1987). Most dele-

tions are apparent on routine karyotype, but small deletions, beyond the resolution of standard cytogenetic techniques, have been described. Diagnosis by FISH analysis is available. A homeobox gene, *HOX7,* has been mapped to 4p16.1 and has been proposed as a candidate gene for the Wolf-Hirschhorn syndrome (Ivens et al, 1990).

Wilms Tumor–Aniridia (WAGR)

In 1964, Miller and coworkers reported an association between aniridia, a congenital abnormality of the iris, and Wilms tumor (Miller et al, 1964). Later, the constellation of aniridia, genitourinary malformations, and mental retardation was found to be associated with a high probability of the development of Wilms tumor. Now known as the WAGR syndrome—Wilms tumor with Aniridia, Genitourinary malformations, and mental Retardation—it is another example of a contiguous gene syndrome. This constellation is associated with an interstitial deletion within the short arm of chromosome 11 at band 13 (Riccardi et al, 1978).

The WAGR deletion encompasses a number of contiguous genes, including the aniridia gene *PAX6* and Wilms tumor suppressor gene *WT1.* Loss of one allele of the *PAX6* gene is responsible for aniridia (Ton et al, 1991), whereas loss or mutation of one *WT1* allele results in the genitourinary defects (Pelletier et al, 1991) and is the first event required for the development of Wilms tumor.

Any combination of these developmental anomalies has been described, and deletions have been associated with every combination of these symptoms. When a deletion is found, aniridia is the most consistent finding and Wilms tumor the least frequent. The genitourinary abnormalities can range from simple hypospadias to ambiguous genitalia.

Isolated aniridia is usually inherited in an autosomal dominant fashion, with complete penetrance and little variability of expression. When sporadic aniridia is encountered, DNA analysis is warranted to look for the 11p deletion. If present, surveillance for the development of Wilms tumor is indicated, as is early developmental intervention, because of the high likelihood of mental retardation in these patients.

Although it accounts for approximately 8% of all childhood malignancies, the diagnosis of Wilms tumor in the newborn is rare (see Chapter 104). When found, it is usually as a unilateral, asymptomatic abdominal mass. Hypertension, microscopic hematuria, and, rarely, gross hematuria can be found.

Williams Syndrome

Another example of a contiguous gene deletion syndrome is Williams syndrome, caused by a microdeletion of the elastin *(ELN)* gene on chromosome 7. In patients with this disorder, a spectrum of abnormalities may be present, some of which may be apparent at birth. The most characteristic findings are distinctive facial features, growth and mental deficiency, cardiovascular anomalies, and infantile hypercalcemia in some cases (Beuren et al, 1962; Fanconi et al, 1952; Williams et al, 1961). Williams syndrome usually occurs sporadically, but it can be inherited as an autosomal dominant disorder. The estimated incidence is 1 in 20,000 to 50,000 live births.

Many infants with Williams syndrome are born small for

gestational age with mild microcephaly. The typical facial features of flat midface with depressed nasal bridge; anteverted nostrils; long philtrum; thick lips; a large, open mouth; and a stellate or lacy iris pattern may not be obvious at birth but become more striking with age. Most infants have a cardiovascular abnormality. Supravalvular aortic stenosis is the most common and is present in more than 50% of cases. Pulmonary artery stenoses are also characteristic, and other defects can be found. Hypercalcemia is present in only 5% to 10% of cases but can be severe, symptomatic, and persist into late infancy. Umbilical or inguinal hernias are more common than in the general population.

Feeding and growth are problematic during infancy, and these babies tend to be irritable and colicky. With age, Williams syndrome patients are more likely to develop strabismus, a hoarse voice, hypertension, and joint limitations (Morris et al, 1988). Most are mildly to moderately mentally retarded, but language skills are often disproportionately advanced and can mask the extent of the retardation. A characteristic, gregarious, "cocktail party personality" is described in these children. Although gross motor development is preserved, visual-motor integration is particularly impaired. Learning disabilities, most notably attention deficit disorders, are common.

Isolated supravalvular aortic stenosis (SVAS) also exists as a distinct, autosomal dominant trait. Linkage between this trait and *ELN*, which had been mapped to 7q11.23 in 1991 (Fazio et al, 1991), was identified in 1993 (Ewart et al, 1993). This led to the hypothesis that *ELN* was involved in the pathogenesis of Williams syndrome. When studied, it was found that most WS patients are missing one copy (hemizygous) of *ELN* (Ewart et al, 1993). Deletions in both the maternally and the paternally derived chromosome 7 have been found with no apparent predominance. In Williams syndrome, the microdeletion (submicroscopic, i.e., not visible by even high-resolution cytogenetic techniques) appears to be of the entire gene plus flanking DNA. SVAS mutations which have been defined involve only part of the gene.

Many of the features demonstrated by Williams syndrome patients can be well explained by the disruption of elastin, a major component of elastic tissue. Other features, such as the developmental and behavioral problems and hypercalcemia, cannot. It is likely that the deletion includes neighboring genes responsible for these other findings. The calcitonin receptor gene is also located on the long arm of chromosome 7 but not near enough to *ELN* to be included in the microdeletions seen (Perez-Juardo et al, 1994). The *ELN* deletion is found in more than 90% of patients with Williams syndrome. Because of this, diagnosis is now much easier to make in the newborn period. A low threshold for testing the infant with supravalvular aortic stenosis, unexplained hypercalcemia, or unusual facial features suggestive of Williams syndrome allows early diagnosis and thereby close and timely medical and developmental follow-up and intervention.

Extra Structurally Abnormal Chromosome

Marker chromosomes, or extra structurally abnormal chromosomes (ESACs), are small 47th chromosomes occurring with an estimated birth prevalence of 0.60% (Sachs et al, 1987). By definition, these chromosomes cannot be characterized by standard cytogenetic analysis owing to the paucity of bands represented. ESACs are heterogeneous in size and origin. An ESAC may or may not exert phenotypic effects, depending on whether critical coding regions are contained in the marker. Further definition of an ESAC is performed by FISH with chromosome-specific probes.

Inverted duplicated chromosome 15, denoted as *inv dup (15)*, accounts for about 40% of ESACs. These chromosomes are dicentric and bisatellited and contain two copies of the p arm, centromere, and proximal long arm. They have been described in normal and mentally retarded patients, who may have epilepsy, autistic features, and mild physical abnormalities (Robinson et al, 1993).

Once an ESAC is identified in a patient, it is important to determine if its origin is de novo or familial. De novo markers carry a higher risk for phenotypic abnormalities than familial markers. Likewise the chromosome origin of the ESAC also is correlated with the likelihood of a phenotypic effect.

Cat-Eye Syndrome

The cat-eye syndrome involves a distinctive clinical phenotype associated with an ESAC derived from chromosome 22 (Mears et al, 1994). In addition to the coloboma of the iris for which the syndrome is named, other clinical features include preauricular tags or sinuses, imperforate anus, congenital heart disease, renal anomalies, and mild to moderate developmental handicaps. More than one third of patients have heart defects, including total anomalous pulmonary venous return and persistence of the left superior vena cava.

The extra chromosome contains the region from 22pter to 22q11 and is often an inverted duplication. Trisomy or tetrasomy for this region results in the cat-eye phenotype. Although most cases occur de novo, there have been cases described with familial transmission, including mosaicism (Urioste et al, 1994). In such instances, the phenotype may be extremely variable.

Imprinting and Uniparental Disomy
Prader Willi Syndrome/Angelman Syndrome

Our understanding of the transmission of chromosomes and genetic information from one generation to the next has been revolutionized in the past decade. Extensive study of various mouse genetic processes and of several human disease phenotypes has revealed the phenomena of genomic imprinting and uniparental disomy.

Genomic imprinting is present when genetic material (whole chromosome, chromosome region, or gene) is expressed differentially depending on whether it is of paternal or maternal origin or passed through the male or the female germline. For example, in a number of genetic disorders, the expression of the disease phenotype depends on whether it has been inherited from the mother or the father. Differences may include severity of disease, age of onset, or even major clinical characteristics. These imprinted genes are functionally modified, not mutated. They are molecularly marked in such a way that a cell can differentiate between the maternal and the paternal gene copy. The precise molecular mechanism of imprinting is not completely understood, but differential DNA methylation, DNA replication, and transcriptional regulation are areas of vigorous study in both the mouse and the human.

A person normally inherits one copy of each chromosome from each parent. Uniparental disomy is the condition in which both copies of a chromosome are inherited from the same parent. Uniparental isodisomy exists if they are copies of the same homologue, and uniparental heterodisomy if two different homologues are inherited, for example, one of each paternal chromosome 11. Uniparental disomy can involve either autosomes or the sex chromosomes. This condition is clinically important when the chromosomes involved are imprinted or contain imprinted regions. Advanced maternal age has been associated with the occurrence of uniparental disomy.

Three genetic disorders that can present in the neonatal period are now known to involve imprinted genes and can arise by uniparental disomy of these imprinted genes.

Prader-Willi syndrome (PWS) (Prader et al, 1956) is a dysmorphic syndrome that principally affects the central nervous system (CNS). It results from loss of activity of a gene or several genes of the proximal long arm of paternal chromosome 15 (Ledbetter et al, 1981, 1989). This loss can arise either by deletion or disruption of the gene(s) or by complete absence of this genetic region because of maternal uniparental disomy (Nicholls et al, 1989a, 1989b).

Newborns with PWS are most notably hypotonic with a weak, sometimes absent cry. The hypotonia is truncal and the limbs can have better, even normal tone. Hyporeflexia is typical. Because of the hypotonia and poor sucking and swallowing reflexes, these infants feed poorly and almost invariably require gavage feeding for some or all of their intake. They tend to be quiet, sleepy babies. Failure to thrive is a concern in the first several months. Subtle dysmorphic craniofacial features include a narrow forehead, almond-shaped eyes, and thin down-turned lips with a small mouth. "Sticky" saliva has been described in these infants. The external genitalia are often underdeveloped. In boys, cryptorchidism and a small penis, and in girls, labial hypoplasia can be seen. Although hands and feet are described as small for age in older infants and children, this is not yet apparent in newborns. Hypopigmentation relative to other family members is noted in about 75% of patients. Strabismus is a frequent finding. Hypothermia and excessive perspiration have also been described.

Mothers of newborns with PWS often describe diminished and delayed onset of fetal activity during pregnancy, especially if they have had prior pregnancies. Breech positioning, perinatal depression, and asphyxia are overrepresented in these infants, likely because of their profound hypotonia. There may be mild prenatal growth restriction, with a mean birth weight of about 2.8 kg at term.

The hypotonia, and concurrently the feeding problems, begin to improve by around 6 months of age. Motor activity gradually increases. Growth remains poor, however, and signs of developmental delay, particularly gross motor and speech, become apparent later. Sometime between 1 and 3 years of age is when most children with PWS develop their insatiable appetite and uncontrollable hyperphagia, with consequent obesity if not restricted. It is a life-long

problem, and many behavioral problems, such as low frustration threshold and severe temper outbursts, surround food aquisition. Older children manifest self-abuse activities of itching, scratching, and skin picking. They seem to have a high pain threshold. Dysmorphic features, hypopigmentation, genital hypoplasia, and small size of hands and particularly feet are more obvious with time. Plethoric obesity becomes the most striking feature in children. Severe intellectual impairment is unusual, and patients with PWS and normal intelligence have been reported. Most, however, fall into the mild to moderate retardation range. It can be difficult to sort out intellectual from behavioral impairments.

Prader, Labhart, and Willi first described this syndrome in 1956 (Prader et al, 1956). After several reports of translocations involving chromosome 15 were described in patients with PWS, Ledbetter described a deletion of 15q11-13 in four of five patients with the syndrome (Ledbetter et al, 1981). Nicholls then described maternal heterodisomy in patients with PWS in whom a deletion was not detected, indicating that the gene involved is imprinted (Nicholls et al, 1989a, 1989b). Not long after, Knoll and associates (1989) reported that a deletion in the same region of the maternal chromosome 15 gives rise to Angelman syndrome.

It is estimated that 60% to 70% of patients with PWS have a 15q11-13 deletion. Approximately 20% have been found to have maternal uniparental disomy. A small proportion have translocations involving the critical region of chromosome 15, and in the others, no chromosome abnormality can be found. The syndrome is almost always sporadic. However, familial cases have been reported. Controversy exists regarding recurrence risks, but it is clear that when a de novo deletion is found, this risk is negligible. The recurrence risk in nondeleted families has been estimated at 1 in 1000 (Kennerknecht, 1992).

One clinically significant difference has been reported between cytogenetically deleted and nondeleted patients with PWS. Those patients with deletions are the patients who are hypopigmented. Hypopigmentation is a manifestation shared by both PWS and Angelman syndrome. In Angelman syndrome the patients with deletions are also those with hypopigmentation. This can be explained on a molecular basis by the presence of a gene (the "P" gene) in the PWS/AS deletion region, which may be responsible for the hypopigmentation seen in both syndromes (Rinchik et al, 1993).

Angelman syndrome is a neurogenetic disorder that is less likely to be recognized in the newborn period. It was first described in 1965 by an English pediatrician, Dr. Harry Angelman (Angelman, 1965). The term *happy puppet syndrome* was coined (Bower and Jeavons, 1967) and widely used but has fallen out of favor in more recent years (Williams and Frias, 1982). Characteristic features of Angelman syndrome are not usually apparent in the newborn. As they grow older, characteristic appearance and behavioral and developmental features become apparent. The most common age of diagnosis is between 3 and 7 years.

Newborns with Angelman syndrome are usually appropriately grown and well-formed at birth and not usually recognized as dysmorphic as newborns. They grow to resemble each other, however. Typical features are microcephaly with occipital flattening, prognathia, and macrostomia. There is frequent protrusion of the tongue and widely spaced teeth. Movements are tremulous and jerky. The irregular voluntary movements delay gross motor milestones and may be severe enough to prevent ambulation. When possible, gait is characteristically wide based, with uplifted arms and a "flapping" position of hands. Mental retardation is in the severe range, and conversational speech does not develop, although some children can use a few words. The excessive laughter so typically associated with this syndrome may be paroxysmal episodes of pronounced laughter or, in others, a predominantly happy grimace and disposition. Most children with Angelman syndrome develop seizures, most before 3 years of age. Electroencephalographic (EEG) findings are characteristic, with high-amplitude spike and slow waves at 2 to 3 Hz. Other EEG abnormalities can be seen as well. Structural brain abnormalities have not been described, other than atrophic changes.

This syndrome shares a unique genetic relationship with PWS. After years of normal karyotype examinations in patients with Angelman syndrome, an association with a deletion in the long arm of chromosome 15 was found when higher-resolution banding methods became available. Detected deletions have been shown to be in the same region as the deletion that gives rise to PWS, 15q11-13 (Pembrey et al, 1988, 1989). However, in patients with Angelman syndrome, the deletion is in the maternally derived chromosome 15, whereas it is in the paternally derived chromosome in deleted patients with PWS (Knoll et al, 1989). Although suspected initially to be the identical deletion, further study has demonstrated that the two genetic loci are distinct (Hamabe et al, 1991). Region 15q11-13 appears to contain different imprinted genes for each of these clinically distinct disorders. The Prader-Willi gene(s) is active only on the paternal chromosome 15, and the Angelman gene(s) is active only on the maternal chromosome 15.

Paternal uniparental disomy of chromosome 15 has been found in patients with Angelman syndrome but less frequently than maternal disomy is found in patients with PWS (Malcolm et al, 1991). An estimated 3% to 5% of cases of Angelman syndrome may be due to uniparental disomy. For approximately 20% of patients studied, neither a deletion nor uniparental disomy has been detected. The molecular mechanism of their disease is unknown.

The recurrence risk for Angelman syndrome is negligible when a de novo deletion or uniparental disomy is found. Rare familial cases have been reported when biparental inheritance of apparently normal chromosomes has been found. These cases present genetic counseling difficulties, and accurate prenatal diagnosis is not currently available.

Beckwith-Wiedemann Syndrome

Genomic imprinting affects the inheritance pattern of Beckwith-Wiedemann syndrome (Beckwith, 1963; Wiedemann, 1964), a common overgrowth syndrome that usually presents in the neonatal period. It is estimated to occur in one in approximately 14,000 births, but underdiagnosis is possible, because the severity of findings is variable and the diagnosis is more difficult to make at ages beyond childhood. The characteristic triad of findings in infants with Beckwith-Wiedemann syndrome include macrosomia, abdominal wall defect, and macroglossia (Elliott et al, 1994; Pettenati et al, 1986).

Most infants are large for gestational age with weight appropriate for length, unlike infants of diabetic mothers who are more likely to be overweight for their length. They then grow along their growth curve usually at or above the 95th percentile. Advanced bone age is usually present. In a few patients, overgrowth may be asymmetric, resulting in hemihypertrophy. Visceromegaly is a frequent manifestation of overgrowth in affected patients. Histologically, cytomegaly of the various tissues of the adrenal gland, pancreas, kidney, liver, and spleen can be found.

The most distinctive facial feature of Beckwith-Wiedemann syndrome is macroglossia, which nearly all described patients exhibit. Slitlike linear creases of the earlobe and indentations of the posterior helix are characteristic ear findings. Facial nevus flammeus and prominent eyes with infraorbital creases are often seen.

Hypoglycemia, often severe and recalcitrant, is a neonatal problem in at least one third of cases. Prompt recognition and testing is important in infants manifesting other findings suggestive of Beckwith-Wiedemann syndrome to minimize the short- and long-term sequelae of this complication. Hypoglycemia responds to therapy but may persist for months, spontaneously resolving during infancy.

Abdominal wall defects are common and may vary from an omphalocele to umbilical hernia or simple diastasis recti. Early visceromegaly of abdominal organs is postulated to disrupt return of the intestine to the abdominal cavity in early embryogenesis, giving rise to abdominal wall abnormalities. Prune belly, inguinal hernia, and diaphragmatic eventration have also been described in patients with Beckwith-Wiedemann syndrome.

Prenatal diagnosis of Beckwith-Wiedemann syndrome has been reported (Weinstein and Anderson, 1980). Prenatal findings to suggest the diagnosis include polyhydramnios, visceromegaly, macrosomia, and abdominal wall defect, often with elevated alpha-fetoprotein levels.

Patients with Beckwith-Wiedemann syndrome are at increased risk of childhood malignant tumor development, mostly intra-abdominal tumors, most commonly Wilms tumor. Estimated risk is 5% to 10%; those with hemihypertrophy are at increased risk. Close surveillance with a combination of abdominal examinations and abdominal ultrasound examinations is needed (Andrews and Amparo, 1993). Most centers perform sonographic examinations at 3-month intervals in infants and toddlers, 6-month intervals in early childhood, then yearly to age 12 and occasionally through adolescence. Baseline and yearly alpha-fetoprotein levels are also advocated.

Most cases of Beckwith-Wiedemann syndrome appear to be sporadic, but 5% to 15% may be familial. In familial cases, the mode of inheritance appears to be autosomal dominant with reduced penetrance and variable expressivity. Diagnostic features of Beckwith-Wiedemann syndrome are less prominent with advancing age, which implies that many "sporadic" cases may in fact be familial. Familial cases are more often transmitted from mother to offspring than from father. Penetrance is much lower when paternally inherited. Decreased reproductive fitness of affected fathers is also postulated.

Genomic imprinting appears to be important in the inheritance of Beckwith-Wiedemann syndrome. Linkage studies in familial cases have mapped the gene for Beckwith-Wiedemann syndrome to chromosome 11p15.5 (Ping et al, 1989). Also located in this region is the insulin-like growth factor Type 2 (IGF2), the product of which is an important fetal growth factor. This region is known to be subject to imprinting such that the maternal allele is not expressed. Maternal suppressor genes may be present in the same region balancing the growth effect of IGF2 expression. Overexpression of the paternal allele or underexpression of the maternal allele can result in the overgrowth and even the propensity for tumor formation seen in Beckwith-Wiedemann syndrome. Imprinting appears to be involved in sporadic cases as well: paternal uniparental disomy has been reported to occur in approximately 20% of sporadic cases (Slatter et al, 1994).

Mild to moderate mental retardation was reported more commonly in early reports of the syndrome. More recent series suggest that the intelligence is usually normal (Elliott et al, 1994). Unrecognized hypoglycemia and morbidity related to premature delivery, which is more common, may have contributed to these earlier reports. Once recovered from the problems of the neonatal period, and in the absence of malignant tumors, children and adults with Beckwith-Wiedemann syndrome can lead normal lives.

Prompt recognition of this diagnosis in the newborn is important to provide early detection and treatment of anticipated neonatal and childhood complications.

SINGLE GENE DISORDERS
Cystic Fibrosis

Cystic fibrosis is an autosomal recessive disease caused by mutations of a gene located on the long arm of chromosome 7. Although it is often not clinically symptomatic in newborns, a variety of circumstances arise for which cystic fibrosis testing is desired or indicated in the perinatal period. An understanding of the genetic mechanisms of disease, the testing available, and the implications of results is vital to accurate diagnosis and counseling.

The clinical manifestations of cystic fibrosis are related to the build-up of abnormal, viscous mucus in a variety of organ systems. Principally affected are the lungs, pancreas, intestine, and reproductive tract. Most of the morbidity and mortality of the disease are from pulmonary manifestations of chronic bronchiectasis and infection.

Meconium ileus is the most common manifestation in the newborn infant and is present in 10% to 15% of patients with cystic fibrosis (Rosenstein and Langbaum, 1980). They present with signs of small bowel obstruction within 24 to 48 hours, with failure to pass meconium, abdominal distention, and vomiting. Associated intestinal atresias may or may not be present. Occasionally meconium ileus is complicated by prenatal bowel perforation, in which case newborns may present with symptoms of an acute abdomen and peritonitis. Nonsurgical treatment of simple meconium ileus with a hypertonic contrast enema is often successful in liberating the abnormal meconium and meco-

nium plugs. Although there are other causes, a high percentage of patients with meconium plugs, when tested, will be identified as having cystic fibrosis (Rosenstein, 1978) and should be tested. Furthermore, prenatal sonographic findings suggestive of intestinal obstruction or peritonitis or of echogenic-appearing fetal bowel should prompt consideration of cystic fibrosis testing (Dicke and Crane, 1992; MacGregor et al, 1995).

Although not evident in the immediate neonatal period, symptoms of pancreatic exocrine insufficiency may begin as early as 4 to 6 weeks of life, presenting with diarrhea, edema, hypoproteinemia, and failure to thrive. Cholestasis from inspissated bile in bile ducts may be another presenting feature.

The incidence of cystic fibrosis is different in different ethnic populations. It is most common in people of northern European descent, with an incidence of approximately 1 in 2500. It is far less common in blacks (only 3% of all cystic fibrosis patients), and Asians (<1% of all patients with cystic fibrosis). Cystic fibrosis carriers are asymptomatic. Four percent (1 in 25) of whites in the United States are estimated to be carriers. This is a high carrier frequency, but it is still low enough that most children with cystic fibrosis are born to couples with no family history of the disease (Friderici, 1997).

The standard sweat test, or quantitative pilocarpine iontophoresis, remains the gold standard for the diagnosis of cystic fibrosis. It tests for concentrations of chloride or sodium in sweat. It is reliable only in the hands of a cystic fibrosis center that performs the technique on a regular basis. Both false-positive and false-negative results occur from suboptimal technique. Sweat testing in infants should be delayed until at least 48 hours of life. Collection of an adequate quantity of sweat can be a limitation to infant testing, particularly in low-birth-weight infants. Most centers require a minimum of 75 to 100 mg of sweat to conduct the test. Persistently elevated concentrations of electrolytes in sweat plus characteristic clinical findings or a family history are considered diagnostic for cystic fibrosis.

Genotyping is now an important, powerful diagnostic tool for cystic fibrosis. Mutation analysis of patients already known to have cystic fibrosis may provide information that will allow risk assessment for family members. Genotyping can detect asymptomatic carriers. It has provided the possibility of prenatal testing for at-risk families. It can be performed on infants for whom sweat testing is not possible, such as premature or critically ill infants. In some cases, genotype analysis may be helpful in predicting phenotype. Furthermore, DNA needed for testing can be easily prepared from blood, buccal samples, or amniocytes.

The cystic fibrosis gene was localized to chromosome 7 in 1985 (Tsui et al, 1985). In 1989, the gene was cloned by a large group of collaborators (Kerem et al, 1989; Riordan et al, 1989; Rommens et al, 1989). The gene codes for a very large protein named the *cystic fibrosis transmembrane conductance regulator* (CFTR), which is responsible for the transport of chloride ions across cell membranes. Abnormal electrolyte concentration of secretions is responsible for the primary manifestations of the disease. Since 1989, more than 600 mutations of the gene have been reported (Wallis, 1997). However, one mutation, delta-F508, is responsible for approximately 70% of all mutations. As is the incidence of the disease, the frequency of CFTR mutation alleles is highly dependent on ethnic origin. For example, delta-F508 accounts for only 30% of CFTR mutations in Ashkenazi Jews (Alton, 1995).

Currently commercially available DNA primers probes can test for approximately 70 of the most common cystic fibrosis mutations, which can identify approximately 90% of all cystic fibrosis genes in most populations. This means, however, that failure to find two abnormal genes does not rule out the disease because not all mutations are investigated. In approximately 1% of those with the disease, no abnormal gene can be found, and in about 18%, only one mutation will be identified. Carrier testing for relatives of a patient with cystic fibrosis is also dependent on the available mutation information of the affected patient and the degree of relatedness to the patient with cystic fibrosis. Cystic fibrosis genotyping, including carrier testing, should be conducted in concert with appropriate genetic counseling.

For families with cystic fibrosis whose mutations are not detectable by currently available testing, linkage analysis may be helpful. It requires sampling from an affected patient and several family members. By looking for markers known to be located close to, or within, the *CFTR* gene, family members having the chromosome with a mutation can be determined, often with a great deal of confidence. Although linkage analysis requires the participation of multiple family members, it does not require knowledge of the specific mutation.

Cystic fibrosis is a common, devastating disease. Although most common in whites, no ethnic group is known to be exempt. Nonwhite children may, in fact, be at greater risk for delayed diagnosis if it is not considered. A combination of sweat testing, genotyping, and linkage analysis satisfies most diagnostic needs of the perinatal period, including carrier testing. An understanding of the limitations of the various tests is imperative for accurate diagnosis and counseling.

Marfan Syndrome

Marfan syndrome (Marfan et al, 1896) is a hereditary disorder of connective tissue with the predominant clinical effects seen in the skeletal, ocular, and cardiovascular systems. There is wide variability in clinical features and severity, even within families. Prevalence is estimated to be 1 to 2 in 10,000 of the U.S. population, with no recognized ethnic or geographic predilection. The inheritance pattern is autosomal dominant, but in 15% to 35% of cases, there is no family history of Marfan syndrome, the disease presumably arising from a new mutation in the parental germline. These sporadic cases appear to be more severely affected and also seem to be overrepresented in infants; however, they may merely be more easily detected in the neonatal period. Although the disease is infrequently diagnosed in infancy, a neonatal form of the syndrome can be seen. This infantile form can be more severe and more rapidly progressive; thus, early recognition is important.

Clinical findings in the skeletal system are long, slender fingers and toes, out of proportion to the length of the hands and feet (arachnodactyly); long, slender limbs relative to the body (dolichostenomelia); and anterior chest deformities of either pectus excavatum or pectus carinatum. Dolichocephaly, a high-arched palate, joint laxity, and flexion contractures can be seen. There is also a tendency toward development of kyphoscoliosis.

The cardinal ocular feature is ectopia lentis, with the lens usually anteriorly dislocated. Myopia is also common, and abnormalities of the cornea or iris can be present. Ectopia lentis has not been reported in a newborn with Marfan syndrome.

Involvement of the cardiovascular system is responsible for 90% of deaths related to Marfan syndrome. Progressive widening of the aortic root and mitral annulus can lead to mitral valve prolapse, often with regurgitation, aortic valve incompetence, and/or aneurysms or dissections of the ascending aorta. In infants with Marfan syndrome, the cardiac abnormalities are frequently found in the neonatal period.

Other systems can be involved as well. Spontaneous pneumothoraces due to pulmonary blebs, striae distensiae (stretch marks) without obvious cause, hernias, and dural ectasia (which is very specific to this disorder and therefore diagnostically important) are seen in older children and adults with Marfan syndrome.

Infants with Marfan syndrome have been described to have a characteristic facies with large, deep-set eyes; malar hypoplasia; megalocornea; and frontal bossing. Some authors have described the appearance as a "worried" or "old man" look. They may also have large, floppy ears and micrognathia.

Diagnosis in infancy seems to predict greater morbidity and mortality. In one series (Morse et al, 1990), most infants diagnosed had serious cardiac pathology. Three of 22 died in the first year. Many of these patients did not have obvious physical findings of cardiovascular compromise. Prompt recognition and liberal use of echocardiography in suspected cases, whether or not a family history is present, was advocated.

The genetic defect responsible has been elucidated in the last few years (Francke et al, 1993). All cases of true Marfan syndrome appear to be due to a mutation in the fibrillin gene *(FBN1)*, which is located on the long arm of chromosome 15. The disease was first linked to this locus in Finland in 1990 (Kainulainen et al, 1990). At nearly the same time in other laboratories, the gene that codes for fibrillin was localized to the same region of chromosome 15 (Magenis et al, 1991). The causal link was finally made in 1991, when two unrelated children severely affected with Marfan syndrome were found to have an *FBN1* mutation while their unaffected parents did not (Dietz, 1991).

Fibrillin is a large glycoprotein constituent of microfibrils, which are structural components of elastic tissue. More than 20 mutations of the very large fibrillin gene have now been found (McGookey et al, 1990; Milewicz et al, 1992); so far, most mutations are specific to families. The number of different Marfan syndrome mutations existing in the population is expected to be large. Until most or all are known, diagnosis of the syndrome will be made based on diagnostic criteria. However, the ability to exclude the presence of a specific mutation known to be segregating in a particular family may be possible for at-risk people. Even if the molecular defect is known, however, no accurate prediction of clinical manifestations or disease course can be made owing to the wide phenotypic variation seen in Marfan syndrome, even within families.

In the absence of a family history, involvement of the skeletal system plus two other systems, with at least one major manifestation (aortic root dilatation, aortic dissection, ectopia lentis, dural ectasia) is needed to make the diagnosis of Marfan syndrome (Beighton et al, 1988). If a positive family history is obtained, the involvement of at least two systems, preferably with one major manifestation, is sufficient. Other disorders in the differential diagnosis should be ruled out, most notably homocystinuria. This is an autosomal recessive enzymatic defect that leads to an accumulation of homocysteine and methionine and a deficiency of cystathionene and cystine. Patients have a slim skeletal build, arachnodactyly, lens subluxation, and myopia, but vascular thromboses, mental retardation, and seizures can also be present. A normal urine amino acid profile rules it out. Congenital contractural arachnodactyly (sometimes known as *Beal syndrome*) has similar skeletal system abnormalities but without other system involvement. Some speculate that the original 5-year-old patient described by the French pediatrician Antoine Marfan in 1896 in fact had this and not what we now call Marfan syndrome, since a description of her at age 11 fails to mention other system involvement.

The natural history of Marfan syndrome has improved greatly with the widespread availability of noninvasive echocardiography (Morse et al, 1990). Following the aortic root dilatation closely allows early intervention, both medical and surgical, prior to catastrophic complications. Beta-blocking agents are used in adults and older children to retard further aortic enlargement with subsequent valvular compromise and possible dissection, although early initiation of these agents in infants has not been reported. Infants with Marfan syndrome with significant valve incompetence need treatment for congestive heart failure with diuretics, digoxin, or afterload-reducing agents. Antibiotic prophylaxis for dental work and other procedures with the risk of transient bacteremia is indicated. The surgical interventions of aortic or mitral valve replacement and aortic root replacement to prevent often fatal aortic dissection have improved the natural history of this disease, which at one time carried a life expectancy of approximately 32 years. Again, published experience of these procedures in infants does not yet exist.

Until molecular diagnosis is widely available, careful family history taking and a low threshold for echocardiographic examinations in suspected cases will allow earlier diagnosis, close follow-up, and early treatment of infants with Marfan syndrome.

Meckel Syndrome

The classic combination of congenital anomalies in patients with Meckel syndrome is occipital encephalocele, polydactyly, and polycystic kidneys. Gruber named this syndrome *dysencephalia splanchnocystica* (Gruber, 1934). The much earlier description of the syndrome by Meckel (Meckel, 1822) was publicized years later (Opitz and Howe, 1969), leading to the current designation of Meckel syndrome. Other prominent features include hepatic fibrosis with bile duct proliferation, cleft lip and/or palate, and genitourinary

abnormalities. The syndrome is lethal in the perinatal period and has an autosomal recessive pattern of inheritance. It can frequently be confused with trisomy 13 before karyotype results become available.

Other CNS abnormalities may be hydrocephalus, absence of olfactory lobes, or Dandy-Walker malformation. Microcephaly with marked sloping of the forehead is common. The polydactyly is usually postaxial (ulnar) and usually bilateral. Hands are more often affected than feet, but all four limbs may be abnormal. Nearly all males have hypoplastic penis and cryptorchidism.

Although attempts have been made to delineate diagnostic criteria (Fraser and Lytwyn, 1981; Salonen et al, 1984; Wright et al, 1994), no single malformation is invariably present. Wide variability of phenotypic manifestations can make diagnosis difficult. Two thirds demonstrate the triad of encephalocele, polydactyly, and polycystic kidneys, but others have only one or two of these findings. Even affected siblings may not have identical findings. Prenatal diagnosis is possible by sonographic findings and by elevated alpha-fetoprotein levels when an encephalocele is present. In a family at risk, diagnosis at 13 weeks has been reported (Pachi et al, 1989).

Disease frequency varies in different parts of the world, ranging from an estimated 1 in 3000 to 50,000 births. The locus for Meckel syndrome has been mapped to chromosome 17q21-q24 (Paavola et al, 1995).

Noonan Syndrome

The first published illustration of what is now known as Noonan syndrome was by Kobylinski in 1883. The clinical findings were then described by Noonan and Ehmke (1963), and the eponym Noonan syndrome began to be used thereafter (Noonan, 1968). This fairly common disorder is characterized by short stature, various congenital heart defects, broad or webbed neck, chest deformity, and a characteristic facial appearance that may be apparent in the newborn period. The incidence has been estimated to be 1 in 1000 to 2500 live births (Noonan, 1994). Noonan syndrome exhibits autosomal dominant inheritance, but as many as half of the cases may be sporadic. Diagnosis in family members may be difficult because of great phenotypic variability; thus, the proportion of sporadic cases is not precisely known. Careful examination of parents and their infant and childhood photos is important. A parent who may have a very mild form of Noonan syndrome has a 50% chance of having another child with the syndrome, whereas a sporadic case carries a very low recurrence risk for the parents.

The typical appearance changes with age. In the newborn period findings may be more subtle but may include a broad, sloping forehead; ocular hypertelorism; antimongoloid slant of the palpebral fissures; and a deeply grooved philtrum. The ears are thick, low-set, and posteriorly angulated. Mild retrognathia may be present. There is frequently a prenatal history of cystic hygroma, polyhydramnios, or hydrops fetalis, and the infant may be born edematous or hydropic. Excess nuchal skin or even webbing may be present, similar to Turner syndrome. Later in infancy, the eyes, still hyperteloric, appear prominent with thick, hooded eyelids, epicanthal folds, and ptosis. The nasal bridge is wide and depressed. Anterior chest deformities, pectus excavatum or carinatum, may be present. In childhood, the face is triangularly shaped, and the eyes are less prominent but neck webbing may become more prominent.

Other system involvement is common. Infants with Noonan syndrome may have early feeding problems, or even failure to thrive, which resolve. Although weight and length are usually normal at birth, short stature develops in the majority.

About half of patients have a cardiac problem. Pulmonary valve stenosis is the most characteristic, but hypertrophic cardiomyopathy is also seen, and many other structural defects can be found. Anterior chest deformities are common, and scoliosis develops in some. Many males with Noonan syndrome have unilateral or bilateral cryptorchidism, which is likely the reason for increased male infertility among patients. Females with Noonan syndrome have normal genitalia and usually normal fertility. A variety of neurologic problems have been reported, including seizures, hearing deficit, peripheral neuropathy, and schwannomas. Hair may be abnormally sparse or curly, and skin may have nevi, freckles, or café au lait spots, which may be difficult to distinguish from other neurocutaneous disorders. Bleeding problems have been found. When present, developmental delay, both motor and cognitive, are mild, and many children with Noonan syndrome have normal development.

The diagnosis of Noonan syndrome is currently based on clinical presentation. The karyotype is normal. Turner syndrome must be ruled out in females, and other syndromes in the differential, depending on the features of the individual case, may include fetal alcohol syndrome, Aarskog syndrome, neurofibromatosis type 1, LEOPARD* syndrome, Watson syndrome, or Williams syndrome.

Although molecular diagnosis and prenatal diagnosis are not yet available, a group in London (Jamieson et al, 1994) recently reported localizing the gene to a region of the long arm of chromosome 12, using linkage analysis of a large Dutch kindred with autosomal dominant Noonan syndrome.

Definitive diagnosis may not be possible in the early newborn period, but those suspected should be followed closely for the evolution of characteristic facial features as well as for surveillance for the multisystem problems that can occur. Making the diagnosis is important for anticipatory testing for and treatment of these problems, for providing early developmental assessment and enhancement interventions, and for family genetic counseling.

Surfactant Protein B Deficiency

Surfactant protein B (SP-B) deficiency is an inherited disease of full-term newborn infants that leads to lethal respiratory failure within the first year of life. It is refractory to mechanical ventilation, exogenous surfactant therapy, glucocorticoid induction of SP-B production, and extracorporeal membrane oxygenation (Hamvas et al, 1995). This

---

*LEOPARD = *l*entigines, *e*lectrocardiogram abnormalities, *o*cular hypertelorism, *p*ulmonary stenosis, *a*bnormal genitalia, *r*etardation of growth, and *d*eafness.

inborn error of surfactant metabolism causes what has been known as *congenital alveolar proteinosis,* an uncommon cause of respiratory failure in full-term newborns who have chest radiographs similar to that of the premature infant with surfactant deficiency but a severely progressive course ultimately leading to death. A family history of similar disease in siblings is frequently found. In 1993, the absence of SP-B protein was demonstrated in the lung of three infants (in a family) who died of congenital alveolar proteinosis (Nogee et al, 1993) (see also Chapter 48).

Rubinstein-Taybi Syndrome

First described in 1963 (Rubinstein and Taybi, 1963), Rubinstein-Taybi syndrome is characterized by dysmorphic facies, broad thumbs and great toes, growth retardation, and mental deficiency. Only recently has the genetic basis for Rubinstein-Taybi syndrome been elucidated. Prevalence in the general population is roughly estimated to range from 1 in 300,000 to 700,000.

When typical features are present, newborns with Rubinstein-Taybi syndrome can be readily recognized. The facial features change with age, in fact, and diagnosis can be more difficult later in infancy. Classic craniofacial appearance includes puffiness; down-slanting palpebral features; epicanthal folds; a prominent and/or beaked nose with nasal septum sometimes extending below the alae; and a narrow, high-arched palate. Patients can have a grimacing smile. They are frequently microcephalic. The ears are low set and often malformed. There is abundant dark hair with low anterior and posterior hairlines. Eyebrows are heavy and eyelashes are long.

Broad thumbs and/or halluces are present in almost all reported cases. Angulation deformities of thumbs may be found as well. The terminal phalanges of other fingers can also be broad, but less so. Significant dermatoglyphic findings are excess dermal ridge patterning in the thenar and first interdigital areas of the palm. There is a tendency toward keloid formation. Most of the males have cryptorchidism. Congenital heart defects, including PDA, VSD, and pulmonic stenosis, have been reported in about a third of the patients.

All patients have mental retardation, most severe, with expressive speech most prominently delayed. Seizures and absence of the corpus callosum have been reported.

Most reported cases are sporadic, and a recurrence risk of approximately 1% in families with one affected child is accepted. After several reports of patients with Rubinstein-Taybi syndrome having translocations and microdeletions involving chromosome 16, the localization of the gene for Rubinstein-Taybi was confirmed on the short arm, at 16p13.3 (Lacombe et al, 1992). Recently, it was shown that this region contains the gene for the human CREB binding protein, involved in cyclic-adenosine triphosphate–regulated gene expression (Petrij et al, 1995). De novo point mutations in this gene were demonstrated as a cause of Rubinstein-Taybi syndrome, implying that it is not a contiguous gene syndrome but rather the result of disruption of this single gene. Uniparental disomy has not been found (Hennekam et al, 1993). The molecular pathology of this disease is under intense study.

DISORDERS OF UNKNOWN ETIOLOGY
CHARGE Association

First defined by Pagon, the CHARGE association is a constellation of nonrandomly associated malformations that occur together in varying combinations. The malformations include *c*oloboma, *h*eart disease, *a*tresia choanae, *r*etarded *g*rowth and development and/or CNS anomalies, *g*enital anomalies, and *e*ar anomalies and/or deafness (Hall, 1979; Pagon et al, 1981). Criteria used "arbitrarily" by Pagon for diagnosis were the presence of either choanal atresia or ocular coloboma or both, and a total of at least four of the seven most common findings, with retardation and CNS anomalies considered separately. As the diagnosis of an association serves to alert clinicians to look for other, perhaps occult, associated anomalies, attempts to further delineate minimal diagnostic criteria have not been reported.

The coloboma may be unilateral or bilateral and of the iris, retina, or disc, and degree of visual impairment depends on the defect. The most common heart defect is tetralogy of Fallot, and other conotruncal defects are seen. ASD is also common (Wyse et al, 1993). Choanal atresia may be bony or membranous, unilateral or bilateral. Growth deficiency is postnatal, and mental retardation is extremely likely, although variable in severity. CNS anomalies have included arrhinencephaly, holoprosencephaly, Dandy-Walker malformation, and agenesis of the corpus callosum. Males usually have genital hypoplasia that may respond to androgen therapy (Pardo and Chua, 1985). Typical ears are low set and posteriorly rotated and have abnormal pinnae. Deafness, ranging from mild to profound, is common (Davenport et al, 1986).

Many other anomalies have been reported in patients with CHARGE association. Phenotypic overlap exists with several known malformation syndromes, most notably cat-eye syndrome, trisomy 13 and 18, and 4p- (Wolf-Hirschhorn) syndrome. In addition, the VACTERL association (see following section) needs to be considered in the differential. Choanal and coloboma abnormalities are less common in VACTERL, and skeletal anomalies are less common in CHARGE.

The causes of this association are unknown and possibly heterogeneous. The malformations seen suggest disruption of development between days 35 and 45 of gestation. Most cases are sporadic, but familial cases have been reported. Newborns with some features of CHARGE should have ophthalmologic evaluation, karyotype examination, hearing evaluation, and imaging of the CNS and genitourinary system.

VACTERL Association

The nonrandom tendency for five types of birth defects to associate together was described in 1972 (Quan et al, 1972). VATER is the acronym that was used to delineate these defects: *v*ertebral defects, *a*nal atresia, *t*racheoesophageal fistula with *e*sophageal atresia, *r*enal defects, and radial limb dysplasia. The association was subsequently expanded to include congenital cardiac disease and other limb defects (Khoury et al, 1983; Temtamy and Miller, 1974) and is now more commonly referred to as the *VACTERL association*. Although each of these defects may occur as isolated anomalies, they frequently occur in varying combination. The probability of the simultaneous occurrence of any three of these defects in the same person, based on their individual incidences, is so unlikely that it suggests a nonrandom association. Patients exhibiting any three or more of these defects, when other chromosome, single-gene, or recognized syndrome disorders are ruled out, are considered VACTERL cases.

This combination of anomalies is not believed to represent a discrete single etiologic syndrome. Rather, a common type of defect in differentiating mesoderm involved in the early development of these separate tissues is suggested as the basis for the association. The proposed defect would occur prior to the 35th day of gestation, because all of the involved mesodermal processes are near completion by that time. Although teratogenic influences have been speculated, no recognized teratogen has been proven. Nearly all cases have been sporadic, and no chromosome abnormalities have been found. The incidence of VACTERL has been estimated at 1.6 in 10,000 live births in one large series (Khoury et al, 1983).

The most common vertebral anomaly is hemivertebrae, but other anomalies can be seen. Most, but not all, patients with tracheoesophageal fistula also have esophageal atresia. Although the association was first described as having specifically radial limb anomalies, patients with VACTERL have been reported with a variety of upper limb anomalies, including preaxial polydactyly, a proximally placed thumb, and even humeral hypoplasia. The renal malformation is most commonly renal agenesis, either unilateral or bilateral, but combinations of other renal anomalies can be seen. A cardiac anomaly is the least specific of the findings, VSD being the most common. In fact, it has been recently suggested that the association of cardiac defects with other VACTERL components is not more frequent than with any other birth defects (Rittler et al, 1996). A variety of anomalies not considered components of the VACTERL association have been reported in patients with VACTERL, including single umbilical artery, inguinal hernia, hydrocephalus secondary to aqueductal stenosis, urogenital malformation, other gastrointestinal atresias, cleft lip and/or palate, and choanal atresia (Weaver et al, 1986).

When a diagnosis of VACTERL defects is made, an infant needs to be assessed more carefully for the presence of other components of the association. This is the importance of making the diagnosis. Other etiologies for the combination of defects need to be ruled out by clinical, chromosome, and DNA evaluation as indicated. An ophthalmologic examination should be considered because there is overlap between the VACTERL and CHARGE associations. As many as one third of infants with multiple defects including three or more of the VACTERL components may be shown to have other recognized disorders (Khoury et al, 1983). If other disorders are ruled out, the prognosis for this association is directly related to the prognosis of the involved defects. There have been no reports of hearing, developmental, or growth abnormalities unrelated to the specific defects known to be present, most of which are treatable.

Goldenhar Syndrome

Goldenhar syndrome is a complex, heterogeneous combination of abnormalities most classically involving the face, ears, and eyes that is also referred to as oculo-auriculo-vertebral spectrum and hemifacial microsomia (Goldenhar, 1952; Gorlin et al, 1963). The hallmark features are unilateral deformity of the external ear and hypoplasia of the ipsilateral half of the face. Epibulbar dermoids and vertebral anomalies were present in Goldenhar's original description. Coloboma of the upper eyelid is common. There is an extremely wide variety of anomalies included in this diagnosis, and more than one disorder may be found to account for this heterogeneity. Most cases are sporadic, but families demonstrating apparent autosomal dominant transmission have been reported. Most reported monozygotic twins are discordantly affected. The best estimates of incidence are between 1 in 3500 and 1 in 5000 live births with a slight (3:2) male predilection (Hamabe et al, 1991; Nicholls et al, 1989a, 1989b). Family recurrence risk is estimated to be 1% to 2%. Many chromosome aberrations have been described in association with this syndrome (Kobrynski et al, 1993), but the genetic etiology remains unknown.

The facial asymmetry is marked and obvious in some, but subtle in many. The asymmetry may not be apparent in the newborn period but can become evident with growth. Careful follow-up of infants with other presumably isolated features is warranted. Macrostomia is often present.

Ear abnormalities range from complete anotia to a mildly dysmorphic pinna. Preauricular tags are extremely common. Supernumerary ear tags may occur in a line from the tragus to the angle of the mouth. Preauricular sinuses can also be seen. Although bilateral ear abnormalities may be found, they are usually asymmetric in their severity.

Epibulbar dermoids or lipodermoids, when present, occur most often at the inferotemporal quadrant at the limbus. They may be unilateral or bilateral. Coloboma, when present, is of the upper lid, helping to distinguish from other syndromes demonstrating lower lid coloboma. Other eye abnormalities, including microphthalmia, are infrequently present.

Abnormalities are not limited to the facial region. Vertebral and other skeletal anomalies, cardiac defects, and renal malformations of varying severity can be present and should be sought.

This disorder, with low recurrence risk, must be distinguished from phenotypically similar syndromes with other modes of inheritance, such as Treacher-Collins syndrome, which tends to have more symmetric abnormalities and down-slanting palpebral fissures not typically seen in Goldenhar, and branchio-oto-renal syndrome, also with autosomal dominant inheritance. Many features of Goldenhar syndrome may occur as isolated findings, including hemifacial microsomia, preauricular skin tags and sinuses, and epibulbar dermoids. However, given the wide phenotypic spectrum of this disorder, longitudinal follow-up of patients believed to have isolated findings is prudent.

Klippel-Trenaunay-Weber Syndrome

Klippel and Trenaunay first described the combination of cutaneous angiomata, varicose veins, and enlargement of bone and soft tissue in 1900 (Klippel and Trenaunay, 1900). In 1907, Parks-Weber added arteriovenous communications to the constellation (Weber, 1907). The syndrome is accepted to be one entity, and is variably referred to as *Klippel-Trenaunay* and *Klippel-Trenaunay-Weber syndrome*. When the craniofacial area or the CNS is involved, Sturge-Weber angiomatosis is present, sometimes in addition to Klippel-Trenaunay-Weber. These two may be the same basic disorder, differing only in the location of involvement.

Unilateral leg hypertrophy is the most frequent finding. Occasionally more than one limb or other body area may be enlarged. Limb circumference or length or both are increased. The hypertrophy is usually evident at birth but may occur later. Imaging studies of affected limbs, including radiographic, sonographic, and magnetic resonance examinations, show enlargement of subcutaneous tissue, muscle, bone, or any combination thereof. Macrodactyly, clinodactyly, and syndactyly can be seen on severely affected extremities and when joints are involved.

A variety of vascular anomalies can be seen, most commonly macular capillary hemangiomata and venous varicosities. Other manifestations can be cavernous hemangiomata and lymphangiomatous and deep vein anomalies, including atresia, hypoplasia, valvular incompetence, and aneurysms. Arteriovenous fistulas can be found. The skin findings are typically on the affected hypertrophied limb but may extend to or be also present on the buttocks, lower back, flank, and lateral chest. Involvement of the upper limbs, abdomen, neck, and face have been reported. Viscera are sometimes involved. Hemangiomatous lesions of the gastrointestinal tract, urinary tract, pleura, and genitalia have been reported.

Almost all cases are sporadic. Reports of familial cases do exist and also of family members who have increased incidence of isolated hemihypertrophy or nevi flammei (Aelvoet et al, 1992). Prenatal diagnosis based on sonographic findings has been reported, as early as 19 weeks' gestation (Hatjus et al, 1981; Jorgenson et al, 1994).

Most patients with Klippel-Trenaunay-Weber have normal mentality, if intracranial angiomata are not involved. However, significant morbidity, including disfigurement, pain, decreased limb function, thrombocytopenia, disseminated intravascular coagulopathy, and bleeding, is suffered by some (Samuel and Spitz, 1995). Attempts at symptomatic treatment have included compression stockings, systemic steroid administration, vessel embolization, radiation therapy, and surgical resection in severe cases.

Acknowledgments

The section on chromosome abnormalities incorporates material from the previous edition of this textbook written by Bruce R. Korf, MD, PhD.

REFERENCES

Abramsky L, Chapple J: Room for improvement? Detecting autosomal trisomies without serum screening. Public Health 107:349–354, 1993.
Aelvoet GE, Jorens PG, Roelen LM: Genetic aspects of the Klippel-Trenaunay syndrome. Br J Dermatol 126:603–607, 1992.
Alton EW: Gene therapy for cystic fibrosis. J Inherit Dis 18:501–507, 1995.
Andrews MW, Amparo EG: Wilms' tumor in patients with Beckwith-Wiedemann syndrome: Onset detected with 3-month serial sonography. Am J Roentgenol 160:139–140, 1993.
Angelman H: "Puppet children": A report of three cases. Dev Med Child Neurol 7:681–683, 1965.

Anonymous: Atlantoaxial instability in Down syndrome: Subject review—American Academy of Pediatrics Committee on Sports Medicine and Fitness. Pediatrics 96:151–154, 1995.

Baird PA, Sadovnick AD: Life tables for Down syndrome. Hum Genet 82:291–292, 1989.

Barker D, Wright E, Nguyen K, et al: Gene for von Recklinghausen neurofibromatosis is in the pericentric region of chromosome 17. Science 236:1100–1102, 1987.

Baty BJ, Blackburn BL, Carey JC: Natural history of trisomy 18 and 13: I. Growth, physical assessment, medical histories, survival, and recurrence risk. Am J Med Genet 49:175–188, 1994a.

Baty BJ, Jorde LJ, Blackburn BL, et al: The natural history of trisomy 18 and 13: II. Psychomotor development. Am J Med Genet 49:189–194, 1994b.

Beckwith JB: Extreme cytomegaly of the adrenal fetal cortex, omphalocele, hyperplasia of the kidneys and pancreas, and Leydig cell hyperplasia—another syndrome? Presented at the Annual Meeting of Western Society for Pediatric Research, Los Angeles, CA, 1963.

Beighton P, de Paepe A, Danks D: International nosology of heritable disorders of connective tissue—Berlin, 1986. Am J Med Genet 29:581–594, 1988.

Bell AJ, Bhate MS: Prevalence of overweight and obesity in Down's syndrome and other mental handicapped adults living in the community. J Intellect Disabil Res 36:359–364, 1992.

Beuren AJ, et al: Supravalvular aortic stenosis in association with mental retardation and a certain facial appearance. Circulation 26:1235–1240, 1962.

Boles DJ, Bodurtha J, Nance WE: Goldenhar complex in discordant monozygotic twins: A case report and review of the literature. Am J Med Genet 28:103–109, 1987.

Boué J, Boué A, Lazar P: The epidemiology of human spontaneous abortions with chromosomal anomalies. *In* Blanda RJ (Ed): Aging Gametes. Basel, S Karger, 1973, pp 330–338.

Bower BD, Jeavons PM: The "happy puppet" syndrome. Arch Dis Child 42:298–301, 1967.

Brown CJ, Lafreniere RG, Powers VE, et al: Localization of the X-inactivation centre on the human X chromosome in Xq13. Nature 349:82–84, 1991.

Carothers AD: A cytogenetic register of trisomies in Scotland: Results of the first two years (1989–1990). Clin Genet 46:405–409, 1994.

Carr J: Down's Syndrome: Children Growing Up. Cambridge, Cambridge University Press, 1995.

Clementi M, Calzolari E, Turolla L, et al: Neonatal growth patterns in a population of consecutively born Down syndrome children. Am J Med Genet Suppl 7:71–74, 1990.

Cronk C, Crocker AC, Pueschel SM, et al: Growth charts for children with Down syndrome: One month to 18 years. Pediatrics 81:102–110, 1988.

Dalton A, Wisniewski H: Down syndrome and dementia of Alzheimer disease. Int Rev Psychiatry 2:41–50, 1990.

Dasouki M, Barr M: Trisomy 18 and hepatic neoplasia. Am J Med Genet 27:203–205, 1987.

Davenport SLH, Hefner MA, Mitchell JA: The spectrum of clinical features in CHARGE syndrome. Clin Genet 29:298–310, 1986.

Desmaze C, Prieur M, Amblard F, et al: Physical mapping by FISH of the DiGeorge critical region (DGCR): Involvement of the region in familial cases. Am J Hum Genet 53:1239–1249, 1993.

Dicke JM, Crane JP: Sonographically detected hyperechoic fetal bowel: Significance and implications for pregnancy management. Obstet Gynecol 80:778–782, 1992.

Dieker H, Edwards RH, ZuRhien GM, et al: The Lissencephaly syndrome. Birth Defects 5:53, 1969.

Dietz HC: Marfan syndrome caused by a recurrent de novo missense mutation in the fibrillin gene. Nature 352:337–339, 1991.

Dietz HC, Pyeritz RE, Hall BD, et al: The Marfan syndrome locus: Confirmation of assignment to chromosome 15 and identification of tightly linked markers at 15q15-q21.3. Genomics 9:355–361, 1991.

Dinani S, Carpenter S: Down's syndrome and thyroid disorder. J Ment Def Res 34:187–193, 1990.

Dobyns WB, Curry CJR, Hoyme HE: Clinical and molecular diagnosis of Miller-Dieker syndrome. Am J Hum Genet 48:584–594, 1991.

Driscoll DA, Budarf ML, Emanuel B: A genetic etiology for DiGeorge syndrome: Consistent deletions and microdeletions of 22q11. Am J Hum Genet 150:924–933, 1992a.

Driscoll DA, Spinner NB, Budarf ML, et al: Deletions and microdeletions of 22q11.2 in velocardiofacial syndrome. Am J Med Genet 14:261–268, 1992b.

Elliott M, Bayly R, Cole T, et al: Clinical features and natural history of Beckwith-Wiedemann syndrome: Presentation of 74 new cases. Clin Genet 46:168–74, 1994.

Embleton ND, Wyllie JP, Wright MJ, et al: Natural history of trisomy 18. Arch Dis Child Fetal Neonatal Ed 75:f38–41, 1996.

Ewart AK, Morris CA, Atkinson D, et al: Hemizygosity at the elastin locus in a developmental disorder, Williams syndrome. Nat Genet 5:11–16, 1993.

Fanconi G, et al: Chronische Hypercalcamie, kombiniert mit Osteosklerose, Hyperazotamie, Minderwuchs und knogenitalin Missbildungen. Helv Paediatr Acta 7:314–334, 1952.

Fazio MJ, Mattei M-G, Passage E, et al: Human elastin gene: New evidence for localization to the long arm of chromosome 7. Am J Hum Genet 48:696–703, 1991.

Ferguson-Smith MA: Karyotype-phenotype correlations in gonadal dysgenesis and their bearing on the pathogenesis of malformations. J Med Genet 2:142–155, 1965.

Ferguson-Smith MA, Yates JRW: Maternal-age–specific rates for chromosome aberrations and factors influencing them: Report of a collaborative European study of 52,965 amniocenteses. Prenat Diagn 4(Spec issue):5–44, 1984.

Fisher JM, Harvey JF, Morton NE, et al: Trisomy 18: Studies of the parent and cell division of origin and the effect of aberrant recombination on nondisjunction. Am J Hum Genet 56:669–675, 1995.

Fong C-T, Brodeur GM: Down's syndrome and leukemia: Epidemiology, genetics, cytogenetics, and mechanism of leukemogenesis. Cancer Genet Cytogenet 28:55–76, 1987.

Francke U, Furthmayr H: Genes and gene products involved in Marfan syndrome. Semin Thoracic Cardiovasc Surg 5:3–10, 1993.

Fraser FC, Lytwyn A: Spectrum of anomalies in the Meckel syndrome, or "Maybe there is a malformation syndrome with at least one constant anomaly." Am J Med Genet 9:67–73, 1981.

Friderici KH: Molecular diagnostics for cystic fibrosis. Clin Lab Med 17:59–72, 1997.

Gath A, Gumley D: Down's syndrome and the family: Follow-up of children first seen in infancy. Dev Med Child Neurol 26:500, 1984.

Goldenhar M: Associations malformatives de l'oeil et de l'oreille, En particulier, le syndrome: dermoide epibulbaire-appendices auriculaires—fistula auris congenita et ses relations avec la dysostose mandibulo-faciale. J Genet Hum 1:243–282, 1952.

Goldstein H, Nielsen KG: Rates and survival of individuals with trisomy 13 and 18. Clin Genet 34:366–372, 1988.

Gorlin RJ, Jue KL, Jacovsen B, et al: Oculoauriculovertebral dysplasia. J Pediat 63:991–999, 1963.

Grabb WC: The first and second branchial arch syndrome. Plas Reconstr Surg 36:485–508, 1965.

Gruber GB: Beitraege zur Frage "gekoppelter" Missbildungen. (Akrocephalo-Syndactylie and Dysencephalia splanchnocystica). Beitr Pathol Anat 93:459–476, 1934.

Hall B: Mongolism in newborns. Clin Pediatr (Phila) 5:4, 1966.

Hall BD: Choanal atresia and associated multiple anomalies. J Pediat 95:395–398, 1979.

Hamabe J, Kuroki Y, Imaizumi K, et al: DNA deletion and its parental origin in Angelman syndrome patients. Am J Med Genet 41:64–68, 1991.

Hassold T, Hunt PA, Sherman S: Trisomy in humans: Incidence, origin, and etiology. Curr Opin Genet Devel 3:398–403, 1993.

Hatjus CG, Philip AG, Anderson GG, et al: The in utero ultrasonographic appearance of Klippel-Trenaunay-Weber syndrome. Am J Obstet Gynecol 139:972–974, 1981.

Hennekam RCM, Tilanus M, Hamel BCJ, et al: Deletion at chromosome 16p13.3 as a cause of Rubinstein-Taybi syndrome: Clinical aspects. Am J Hum Genet 52:255–262, 1993.

Hirschhorn K, Cooper HL: Apparent deletion of short arms of one chromosome (4 or 5) in a child with defects of midline fusion. Hum Chromosome Newsl 4:14, 1961.

Hook EB: Chromosome abnormalities: Prevalence, risks, and recurrence. *In* Brock DJH, Rodeck CH, Ferguson-Smith MA (Eds): Prenatal Diagnosis and Screening. Edinburgh, Churchill Livingstone, 1992, pp 351–392.

Hook EB, Cross PK: Interpretation of recent data pertinent to genetic counseling for Down syndrome: Maternal-age–specific rates, temporal trends, adjustments for paternal age, recurrence risks, risks other than cytogenetic abnormalities, recurrence risk after remarriage. In Willey AM, Carter TP, Kelly S, et al (Eds): Clinical Genetics: Problems in

Diagnosis and Counseling. New York, Academic Press, 1982, pp 119–139.

ISCN, Mitelman F (Ed): An International System for Human Cytogenetic Nomenclature. Basel, S Karger, 1995.

Ivens A, Flavin N, Williamson R, et al: The human homeobox gene *HOX* 7 maps to chromosome 4p16.1 and may be implicated in Wolf-Hirschhorn syndrome. Hum Genet 84:473–476, 1990.

Jacobs PA, Browne C, Gregson N, et al: Estimates of the frequency of chromosome abnormalities detectable in unselected newborns using moderate levels of banding. J Med Genet 29:103–108, 1992.

Jamieson CR, van der Burgt I, Brady AF, et al: Mapping a gene for Noonan syndrome to the long arm of chromosome 12. Nature Genetics 8:357–60, 1994.

Jorgenson RJ, Darby B, Patterson R, et al: Prenatal diagnosis of the Klippel-Trenaunay-Weber syndrome. Prenatal Diag 14:989–992, 1994.

Kainulainen K, Pulkkinen L, Savolianen A, et al: Location on chromosome 15 of the gene defect causing Marfan syndrome. N Engl J Med 323:935–939, 1990.

Kallen B, Mastrioacovo P, Robert E: Major congenital malformations in Down syndrome. Am J Med Genet 65:160–166, 1996.

Kamiguchi Y, Rosenbusch B, Sterzik K, et al: Chromosomal analysis of unfertilized human oocytes prepared by a gradual fixation-air drying method. Hum Genet 90:533–541, 1993.

Karayalcin G, Shanske A, Honigman R: Wilms' tumor in a 13-year-old girl with trisomy 18. Am J Dis Child 135:665–667, 1981.

Kennerknecht I: Differentiated recurrence risk estimations in the Prader-Willi syndrome. Clin Genet 41:303–308, 1992.

Kerem B, Rommens JM, Cuchanan JA, et al: Identification of the cystic fibrosis gene: Genetic analysis. Science 245:1073–1080, 1989. [One of three papers reporting cloning of the gene]

Khoury MJ, Cordero JF, Greenberg F, et al: A population study of the VACTERL association: Evidence for its etiologic heterogeneity. Pediatrics 71:815–820, 1983.

Klippel M, Trenaunay P: Du naevus variqueux osteohypertrophique. Arch Gen Med 185:641–672, 1900.

Knoll JHM, Nicholls RD, Magenis RE, et al: Angelman and Prader-Willi syndromes share a common chromosome 15 deletion but differ in parental origin of the deletion. Am J Med Genet 32:285–290, 1989.

Kobrynski L, Chitayat D, Azhed L, et al: Trisomy 22 and facio-auriculo-vertebral (Goldenhar) sequence. Am J Med Genet 46:68–71, 1993.

Kobylinski O: Ueber Eine Flughoutahnbiche Ausbreitung. Am Halse Arch Anthropol 14:342–348, 1883.

Kupke KG, Muller U: Parental origin of the extra chromosome in trisomy 18. Am J Hum Genet 45:599–605, 1989.

Kuwano A, Ledbetter SA, Dobyns WB, et al: Detection of deletions and cryptic translocations in Miller-Dieker syndrome by in situ hybridization. Am J Hum Genet 49:707–714, 1991.

Lacombe D, Saura R, Taine L, et al: Confirmation of assignment of a locus for Rubinstein-Taybi syndrome gene to 16p13.3. Am J Med Genet 44:126–128, 1992.

Ledbetter DH, Riccardi VM, Airhart SD, et al: Deletions of chromosome 15 as a cause of the Prader-Willi syndrome. N Engl J Med 304:325–329, 1981.

Ledbetter DH, Riccardi VM, Youngbloom SA, et al: Deletion (15q) as a cause of the Prader-Willi syndrome (PWS). Am J Hum Genet 32:77A, 1989.

Lejeune J, Gautier M, Turpin R: Etudes des chromosomes somatiques de neuf enfants mongoliens. Comp Rend Acad Sci 248:1721–1722, 1959.

Lejeune J, Lafourcade, J, Berger R, et al: Trois cas de deletion partielle du bras cort d'n chromosome 5. Comp Rend Acad Sci 257:3098–3102, 1963.

Lurie IW, Lazjuk GI, Ussova YI, et al: The Wolf-Hirschhorn syndrome: I. Genetics. Clin Genet 17:375–384, 1980.

MacDonald M, Hassold T, Harvey J, et al: The origin of 47,XXY and 47,XXX aneuploidy: Heterogeneous mechanisms and role of aberrant recombination. Hum Mol Genet 3:1365–1371, 1994.

MacGregor SN, Tamura R, Sabbagha R, et al: Isolated hyperechoic fetal bowel: Significance and implications for management. Am J Obstet Gynecol 173:1254–1258, 1995.

Magenis RE, Maslen CL, Smith L, et al: Localization of the fibrillin (FBN) gene to chromosome 15, band q21.1. Genomics 11:346–351, 1991.

Malcolm S, Clayton-Smith J, Nichols M, et al: Uniparental paternal disomy in Angelman's syndrome. Lancet 337:694–697, 1991.

Marfan AB: Un cas de deformation congenitale des quatre membres plus

prononcee aux extremites caracterisee par allongement des os avec un certain degre d'amincissement. Bull Mem Soc Med Hop Paris 13:320–326, 1896.

Martin RH, Ko E, Rademaker A: Distribution of aneuploidy in human gametes: Comparison between human sperm and oocytes. Am J Med Genet 39:321–331, 1991.

McGookey DJ, Pyeritz RE, Byers PH: Marfan syndrome: Altered synthesis, secretion, or extracellular matrix incorporation of fibrillin. Am J Hum Genet 47:A67, 1990.

McKeown C, Read AP, Dodge A, et al: Wolf-Hirschhorn locus is distal to D4S10 on short arm of chromosome 4. J Med Genet 24:410–512, 1987.

Mears AJ, Duncan AMV, Budarf ML, et al: Molecular characterization of the marker chromosome associated with cat-eye syndrome. Am J Hum Genet 55:134–142, 1994.

Meckel JF: Beschribung zweier, durch sehr aehnliche Bildungsabweichungen enstellter Geschwister. Dtsch Arch Physiol 7:99–172, 1822.

Milewicz DM, Pyeritz RE, Crawford ES, et al: Marfan syndrome: Defective synthesis, secretion, and extracellular matrix formation of fibrillin by cultured dermal fibroblasts. J Clin Invest 89:79–86, 1992.

Miller JQ: Lissencephaly in two siblings. Neurology 13:841–850, 1963.

Miller RW, Fraumeni JF, Manning MD: Association of Wilms' tumor with aniridia, hemihypertrophy, and other congenital anomalies. N Engl J Med 270:922, 1964.

Morris CA, Demsey SA, Leonard CO, et al: Natural history of Williams syndrome: Physical characteristics. J Pediatr 113:318–326, 1988.

Morse RP, Rockenmacher S, Pyeritz RE, et al: Diagnosis and management of infantile Marfan syndrome. Pediatrics 86:888–895, 1990.

Mueller U, Weber JL, Berry P, et al: Second polar body incorporation into a blastomere results in 46,XX/69,XXX mixoploidy. J Med Genet 30:597–600, 1993.

National Institutes of Health: Consensus Development Conference Statement: Neurofibromatosis. Neurofibromatosis 1:172–178, 1988.

Nicholls RD, Knoll JHM, Butler MG, et al: Genetic imprinting suggested by maternal heterodisomy in non-deletion Prader-Willi syndrome. Nature 342:281–285, 1989a.

Nicholls RD, Knoll JHM, Butler MG, et al: Uniparental disomy for chromosome 15 in the Prader-Willi syndrome. Am J Hum Genet 45:A209, 1989b.

Niebuhr E: The cri du chat syndrome: Epidemiology, cytogenetics, and clinical features. Hum Genet 144:227–275, 1978a.

Niebuhr E: Cytologic observations in 35 individuals with a 5p- karyotype. Hum Genet 142:146–156, 1978b.

Nogee LM, deMello DE, Dehner LP, et al: Deficiency of pulmonary surfactant protein B in congenital alveolar proteinosis. N Engl J Med 328:406–410, 1993.

Nogee LM, Gernier G, Singer L, et al: A mutation in the surfactant protein B gene responsible for fatal neonatal respiratory disease in multiple kindreds. J Clin Invest 93:1860–1863, 1994.

Noonan JA: Noonan syndrome: An update and review for the primary pediatrician. Clin Pediatr (Phila) 33:548–555, 1994.

Noonan JA: Hypertelorism with Turner phenotype: A new syndrome with associated congenital heart disease. Am J Dis Child 116:373–380, 1968.

Noonan JA, Ehmke DA: Associated noncardiac malformations in children with congenital heart disease. J Pediatr 63:468–470, 1963.

Opitz JM, Howe JJ: The Meckel syndrome (dysencephalia splanchnocystica, the Gruber syndrome). Birth Defects 2:167–179, 1969.

Overhauser J, Beaudet AL, Wasmuth JJ: A fine structure physical map of the short arm of chromosome 5. Am J Hum Genet 39:562–572, 1986.

Paavola P, Salonen R, Weissenbach J, et al: The locus for Meckel syndrome with multiple congenital anomalies maps to chromosome 17q21-q24. Nature Genet 11:213–215, 1995.

Pachi A, Giancotti A, Torcia F, et al: Meckel-Gruber syndrome: Ultrasonographic diagnosis at 13 weeks' gestational age in an at-risk case. Prenat Diag 9:187–190, 1989.

Pagon RA, Graham JM Jr, Zonana J, et al: Coloboma, congenital heart disease, and choanal atresia with multiple anomalies: CHARGE association. J Pediatr 99:223–227, 1981.

Palomaki GE, Knight GJ, McCarthy MT, et al: Maternal serum screening for fetal Down syndrome in the United States—a 1992 survey. Am J Obstet Gynecol 169:1558–1562, 1992.

Pardo JM, Chua C: The CHARGE association in a male newborn infant. Clin Pediatr (Phila) 24:531, 1985.

Pauli RM, Pagon RA, Hall JG: Trisomy 18 in sibs and maternal chromosome 9 variant. Birth Defects 14:297–301, 1978.

Pelletier J, Bruening W, Li FP, et al: WT1 mutations contribute to abnormal genital system development and hereditary Wilms' tumour. Nature 353:431, 1991.

Pembrey M, Fennell SJ, van den Berghe J, et al: The association of Angelman's syndrome with deletions within 15q11-13. J Med Genet 26:73–77, 1989.

Perez-Juardo LA, Peoples R, Kaplan P, et al: Deletion and candidate genes in Williams syndrome. Am J Hum Genet 55:A42, 1994.

Petrij F, Giles RH, Dauwerse HG, et al: Rubinstein-Taybi syndrome caused by mutations in the transcriptional co-activator CBP. Nature 346:348–351, 1995.

Pettenati MJ, Haines JL, Higgins RR, et al: Wiedemann-Beckwith syndrome: Presentation of clinical and cytogenetic data on 22 new cases and review of the literature. Hum Genet 74:143–154, 1986.

Ping AJ, Reeve AE, Law DJ, et al: Genetic linkage of Beckwith-Wiedemann syndrome to 11p15. Am J Hum Genet 44:720–723, 1989.

Poswillo D: Otomandibular deformity: Pathogenesis as a guide to reconstruction. J Maxillofac Surg 2:54–72, 1974.

Prader A, Labhart A, Willi H: Ein Syndrom von Adipositas, Kleinwuchs, Kryptorchismus, und Oligophrenie nach Myatonieartigem Zustand in Neugeborenalter. Schweiz Med Wochenschr 86:1260–1261, 1956.

Pueschel SM, Bernier JC, Pezzullo JC: Behavioural observations in children with Down's syndrome. J Ment Defic Res 35:502–511, 1991.

Pueschel SM, Pezzullo JC: Thyroid dysfunction in Down syndrome. Am J Dis Child 139:636–639, 1985.

Quan L, Smith DW: The VATER association: Vertebral defects, anal atresia, tracheoesophageal atresia, radial dysplasia. Birth Defects 8:75–78, 1972.

Rehder H: Pathology of trisomy 21—with particular reference to persistent common atrioventriular canal of the heart. *In* Burgio GR, Fraccaro M, Tiepolo L, et al (Eds): Trisomy 21. Berlin, Springer-Verlag, 1981, p 57.

Reiner O, Carrozzo R, Shen Y, et al: Isolation of a Miller-Dieker lissencephaly gene containing G protein β subunit-like repeats. Nature 364:717–721, 1993.

Rex AP, Preus M: A diagnostic index for Down syndrome. J Pediatr 100:903–906, 1982.

Riccardi VM, Sujansky E, Smith MA, et al: Chromosomal imbalance in the Aniridia-Wilms' tumor association: 11p interstitial deletion. Pediatrics 61:604–610, 1978.

Rinchik EM, Bultman SJ, Horsthema B, et al: A gene for the mouse pink-eyed dilution locus and for human type II oculocutaneous albinism. Nature 361:72–76, 1993.

Riordan JR, Rommens JM, Kerem B, et al: Identification of cystic fibrosis gene: Cloning and characterization of complementary DNA. Science 245:1066–1073, 1989. [One of three papers reporting cloning of the gene]

Rittler M, Paz JE, Castilla EE: VACTERL association: Epidemiologic definition and delineation. Am J Med Genet 63:529–536, 1996.

Robinson A, Bender BG, Linden MG: Summary of clinical findings in children and young adults with sex chromosome anomalies. Birth Defects 126:225–228, 1990a.

Robinson A, Bender BG, Linden MG, et al: Sex chromosome aneuploidy: The Denver Prospective Study. Birth Defects 126:59–115, 1990b.

Robinson WP, Binkert F, Gine R, et al: Clinical and molecular analysis of five inv dup(15) patients. Eur J Hum Genet 1:37–50, 1993.

Roizen NJ, Mets BM, Blondis TA: Ophthalmic disorders in children with Down syndrome. Dev Med Child Neurol 36:594–600, 1994.

Roizen NJ, Wolters C, Nicol T, et al: Hearing loss in children with Down syndrome. J Pediatr 123(Suppl):S9–S12, 1993.

Rommens JM, Iannuzzi MC, Kerem B, et al: Identification of the cystic fibrosis gene: Chromosome walking and jumping. Science 245:1059–1065, 1989. [One of three papers reporting cloning of the gene]

Rosenstein BJ: Cystic fibrosis presenting with the meconium plug syndrome. Am J Dis Child 132:167, 1978.

Rosenstein BJ, Langbaum TS: Incidence of meconium abnormalities in newborn infants with cystic fibrosis. Am J Dis Child 134:72, 1980.

Root S, Carey JC: Survival in trisomy 18. Am J Med Genet 49:170–174, 1994.

Rubinstein JH, Taybi H: Broad thumbs and toes and facial abnormalities: A possible mental retardation syndrome. Am J Dis Child 105:588–603, 1963.

Sachs ES, Van Hemel JO, Den Hollander JC, et al: Marker chromosomes in a series of 10,000 prenatal diagnoses: Cytogenetic and follow-up studies. Prenat Diagn 7:81–89, 1987.

Salonen R: The Meckel syndrome: Clinicopathological findings in 67 patients. Am J Med Genet 18:671–689, 1984.

Samuel M, Spitz L: Klippel-Trenaunay syndrome: Clinical features, complications, and management in children. Br J Surg 82:757–761, 1995.

Simmons AD, Goodart SA, Gallardo TD, et al: Five novel genes from the cri du chat critical region isolated by direct selection. Hum Mol Genet 4:295–302, 1995.

Slatter RE, Elliott M, Welham K, et al: Mosaic uniparental disomy in Beckwith-Wiedemann syndrome. J Med Genet 31:749–753, 1994.

Smith GF, Berg JM: Down's Anomaly, 2nd ed. Edinburgh, Churchill Livingstone, 1976.

Temtamy SA, Miller JD: Extending the scope of the VATER association: Definition of the VATER syndrome. J Pediatr 85:345–349, 1974.

Ton CC, Hirvonen H, Miwa H, et al: Positional cloning and characterization of a paired box—and homeobox—containing gene from the aniridia region. Cell 67:1059–1074, 1991.

Tsui L-C, Buchwald M, Barker D, et al: Cystic fibrosis locus defined a genetically linked polymorphic DNA maker. Science 230:1054–1057, 1985. [The gene discovered to be located on chromosome 7]

Urioste M, Visedo G, Sanchis A, et al: Dynamic mosaicism involving an unstable supernumerary der(22) chromosome in cat-eye syndrome. Am J Med Genet 49:77–82, 1994.

Wallis C: Diagnosing cystic fibrosis: Blood, sweat, tears. Arch Dis Child 76:85–88, 1997.

Weaver KK, Mapstone CL, Yu P: The VATER association: Analysis of 46 patients. Am J Dis Child 140:225–229, 1986.

Weber FP: Angioma formation in connection with hypertrophy of limbs and hemihypertrophy. Br J Dermatol 19:231–235, 1907.

Weinstein L, Anderson C: In utero diagnosis of Beckwith-Wiedemann syndrome by ultrasound. Radiology 134:474, 1980.

Weng EY, Mortier GR, Graham JM: Beckwith-Wiedemann syndrome. Clin Pediatr (Phila) 34:317–326, 1995.

Wiedemann HR: Complexe malformatif famililial avec hernie ombilicale et macroglossie—un "syndrome nouveau"? J Genet Hum 13:232–233, 1964.

Wilkins LE, Brown JA, Wolf B: Psychomotor development in 65 home-reared children with cri du chat syndrome. J Pediatr 97:401–405, 1980.

Williams CA, Frias JL: The Angelman ("happy puppet") syndrome. Am J Med Genet 11:453–460, 1982.

Williams JCP, Barratt-Boyes BG, Lowe JB: Supravalvular aortic stenosis. Circulation 24:1311–1318, 1961.

Wolf U, Reinwein, H: Klinische and cytogenetische Differentialdiagnose der Defizienzen an den kurzen Armen der B-Chromosomen. A Kinderheilkd 98:235, 1967.

Wolf U, Reinwein H, Porsch R, et al: Defizienz an den kurzen Armen eines chromosoms Nr. 4. Hum Genet 1:397, 1965.

Wright C, Healicon R, English C, et al: Meckel syndrome: What are the minimum diagnostic criteria? J Med Genet 31:482–485, 1994. [diagnostic criteria]

Wyse RKH, Al-Mahdawi S, Burn J, et al: Congenital heart disease in CHARGE association. Pediatr Cardiol 14:75–81, 1993.

Zaragoza MV, Jacobs PA, James RS, et al: Nondisjunction of human acrocentric chromosomes: Studies of 432 trisomic fetuses and liveborns. Hum Genet 94:411–417, 1994.

Zoll B, Wolf J, Lensing-Hebben D, et al: Trisomy 13 with an 11-year survival. Clin Genet 43:46–50, 1993.

CHAPTER 23

Human Teratogens

Kenneth G. Kupke

Teratogens are environmental agents or maternal factors that cause a physical or functional alteration in the offspring. In the evaluation of every newborn, a thorough pregnancy history should be obtained to determine whether a potentially harmful exposure has occurred. It is important to obtain accurate information about the nature of the exposure, specifically the duration, dosage, and timing in gestation. Once these data are obtained, a careful review of the literature permits conclusions to be made about the risks posed to the particular pregnancy. In many exposures, the analysis is inconclusive because there is a lack of sufficient studies of human teratogenicity. The examination of the prenatally exposed newborn may permit the caregiver to identify physical stigmata associated with a particular teratogen and thereby establish a diagnosis. More often, the physical examination is normal, and the parents can be given reassuring information, which may alleviate the anxiety that often surrounds a prenatal exposure.

There are several recognized human teratogens (Table 23–1). Many others remain suspected, but are unproven. Definitive proof of teratogenicity in humans may be diffi-

cult to obtain because there are inherent hazards of interpreting retrospective human data and extrapolation from animal experiments. In general, a teratogenic agent fulfills the following criteria: (1) it is present during critical periods of development, (2) it produces congenital defects in experimental animals at a higher rate than in control subjects, and (3) it acts in an unaltered form on the embryo–fetus through the placenta (Shepard, 1995).

The timing of exposure plays an important role in the teratogenicity of an agent. The preimplantation period, from conception to the end of the second week, is generally considered a time of apparent immunity to teratogens. It is believed that a significant toxic exposure to the embryo during this time period prevents proper implantation, leading to an unnoticed spontaneous miscarriage. Alternatively, some researchers have argued that toxic levels cannot accumulate in the unimplanted embryo. Regardless of the basis, this concept of an "all or nothing" teratogenic effect at this stage of gestation has important counseling implications. The embryonic period, from the 2nd through the 8th weeks of gestation, remains the most important time with respect to the development of malformations, because this is the critical period of organogenesis. Cellular migration and differentiation into organ systems are occurring and are vulnerable to the effects of exogenous insults. The fetal period, from the 9th week of gestation until delivery, remains a period in which malformations may also occur, but it is also the time when agents may exert functional or behavioral effects on the developing human.

Many teratogens display critical "windows of action," that is, teratogenic effects only occur if the embryo–fetus has been exposed during a narrow period of time. For example, the sedative thalidomide was found to cause birth defects only if the exposure occurred between 21 and 40 days after conception (Lenz and Knapp, 1962).

Most drugs, chemicals, and environmental agents freely cross the placenta into the developing embryo–fetus. For each teratogen, however, there is a theoretical specific dose threshold above which deleterious effects occur. The level of the dose threshold is usually significantly lower than that which would cause symptoms in the adult (Hoyme, 1990). In most cases, a specific dose threshold has not been established in humans.

MATERNAL CONDITIONS
Diabetes Mellitus

Congenital anomalies remain a significant cause of perinatal morbidity and mortality among infants of diabetic mothers. Infants of insulin-dependent diabetic mothers carry an overall threefold to fourfold increased risk of major birth defects, corresponding to an absolute risk of 6% to 9%, depending on the study (Greene, 1993). The prevalence of

---

TABLE 23–1

Known Human Teratogens

Radiation	Drugs and environmental chemicals
Infections	*(Continued)*
Cytomegalovirus	Busulfan
Herpes simplex virus	Captopril
Parvovirus B-19	Chlorobiphenyls
Rubella	Cocaine
Syphilis	Coumarin
Toxoplasmosis	Cyclophosphamide
Varicella	Diethylstilbestrol
Venezuelan equine	Diphenlyhydantoin
encephalitis virus	Enalapril
Maternal conditions	Etretinate
Alcoholism	Iodides
Chorionic villus sampling	Lithium
Hypothyroidism	Mercury, organic
Diabetes mellitus	Methylene blue
Folic acid deficiency	Methimazole
Hyperthermia	Penicillamine
Phenylketonuria	1,3-*cis*-Retinoic acid
Rheumatic heart disease	Tetracycline
Virilizing tumors	Thalidomide
Drugs and environmental	Toluene
chemicals	Trimethadione
Aminopterin	Valproic acid
Androgenic hormones	

From Shepard TH: Catalog of Teratogenic Agents, 8th ed. Baltimore, Johns Hopkins University Press, 1995. © 1995, The Johns Hopkins University Press.

major anomalies is higher among women with more severe diabetes. Women with vascular disease (classes D and F) have shown the highest rate of offspring with malformations (Mills, 1982; Pedersen et al, 1964). Non-insulin-dependent and gestational diabetic mothers do not appear to have an increased risk for offspring with malformations (see also Chapter 7).

There has been controversy regarding the risk for anomalies based on degree of glycemic control, as judged by first-trimester hemoglobin A1C levels. In the Diabetes in Early Pregnancy (DIEP) study, there was no correlation between the risk for anomalies and the first trimester glycosylated hemoglobin level (Mills et al, 1988). A subsequent study, however, did show a striking relation between hemoglobin A1C levels and the risk for a malformed baby (Greene et al, 1989). For women with an HbA1C level greater than 12 standard deviations above the nondiabetic mean, the risk of malformations was 36%, compared with a 3.1% rate among the best controlled patients, in which the level was 6 standard deviations above the mean. It has been suggested that the DIEP patients were under much better metabolic control at the time of enrollment, which occurred before 21 days' postconception; therefore, they had a lower risk for malformations than a more representative sample of pregnant diabetic mothers. Future studies may address whether programs designed to optimize preconceptional glucose control can reduce the risk of malformations.

Most types of congenital anomalies among infants of diabetic mothers are usually nonspecific and involve a variety of different organ systems. Congenital malformations include varying types of congenital heart disease, hydrocephalus, neural tube defects, anencephaly, holoprosencephaly, renal agenesis, ureteral and urethral anomalies, anal atresia, small left colon syndrome, and vertebral abnormalities.

Caudal regression syndrome (or sacral agenesis) is a rare condition; 16% of cases have been associated with maternal diabetes mellitus (Passarge and Lenz, 1965). The condition occurs from a defect in the caudal axis, resulting in variable fusion of the lower limbs, absence of caudal structures (sacrum, vertebrae, kidney, genitalia, bladder), imperforate anus, and single umbilical artery.

The femoral hypoplasia–unusual facies syndrome is notable for cleft palate, distinctive facies, hypoplastic or aplastic femurs, micrognathia, and vertebral abnormalities. Approximately 35% of cases occur in infants of diabetic mothers (Johnson et al, 1982).

Phenylketonuria

Approximately 6000 women with phenylketonuria (PKU) are of child-bearing age in the United States. Many of these women were given phenylalanine-restricted diets in childhood, thereby preventing mental retardation. Many patients have relaxed their dietary restrictions after childhood, thereby allowing serum phenylalanine levels to elevate to high levels.

Untreated hyperphenylalanemic mothers with PKU demonstrate a high rate of spontaneous abortions and their offspring have a high rate of intrauterine growth retardation (IUGR), microcephaly, congenital heart disease, and

mental retardation (Lenke and Levy, 1980). Adverse effects can be prevented by dietary restriction of phenylalanine beginning before conception and continuing during the pregnancy (Drogari et al, 1987; Rohr et al, 1987). The risk of congenital malformations correlates with the level of maternal hyperphenylalanemia during the first trimester. Women with phenylalanine levels exceeding 1200 μM/dL have a 90% risk of having a fetus with microcephaly and IUGR compared with a negligible risk if the level is less than 360 μM/dL. Maternal treatment that begins later in pregnancy does not significantly improve fetal outcome (Platt et al, 1992).

Myasthenia Gravis

In maternal myasthenia gravis, an IgG-mediated autoimmune disorder, antibodies attack the acetylcholine receptor at the neuromuscular junction. Transitory neonatal myasthenia develops in approximately 12% of infants of mothers with myasthenic gravis because IgG is transmitted transplacentally (Namba et al, 1970). Symptoms of neonatal myasthenia include feeding difficulties, respiratory problems, hypotonia, weakness, ptosis, and ophthalmoplegia. The symptoms may be present soon after birth or may be delayed for several days. A diagnostic challenge test with edrophonium chloride (Tensilon) results in temporary improvement. Cholinesterase inhibitors, such as neostigmine methyl sulfate, can be helpful in treatment (see Chapter 69).

Thyroid Disease

Maternal hypothyroidism increases the risk for miscarriage, stillbirth, and preterm delivery. There is no increased rate of congenital anomalies in the offspring of hypothyroid mothers (Khoury et al, 1989).

Maternal autoimmune hyperthyroidism also increases the risk for spontaneous abortion and prematurity, as well as low birth weight. Hyperthyroid women may have a somewhat increased risk for infants with congenital malformations.

Fetal thyrotoxicosis may occur in mothers with Graves disease because thyroid-stimulating immunoglobulins are transferred transplacentally. This diagnosis should be suspected in any pregnant woman with Graves disease, regardless of her thyroid status. Fetal thyrotoxicosis is associated with IUGR, goiter, exophthalmos, tachycardia, irritability, and congestive heart failure (see Chapter 102).

Systemic Lupus Erythematosus

Maternal systemic lupus erythematosus carries an increased risk of spontaneous abortion, prematurity, and stillbirth (Hayslett, 1992). The observed increased fetal loss rate is postulated to be due to several mechanisms, including active decidual vasculitis, trophoblast-reactive lymphocytotoxic antibody, anti-Ro/SSA and anti-La/SSB antibodies causing destruction of the fetal cardiac conduction system, and lupus anticoagulant and anticardiolipin antibody (Gladman and Urowitz, 1995).

Transplacentally acquired IgG can cause the neonatal

lupus syndrome, which is characterized by a photosensitive rash, hematologic abnormalities, and congenital heart block. The condition generally resolves by 9 months of age.

Virilizing Tumors

Masculinization of the newborn female genitalia may result from transplacental androgen exposure from maternal virilizing tumors. Such tumors include Leydig cell tumors, adrenal rest tumors, granulosa cell tumors, leuteomas, and Krukenberg tumors.

RECREATIONAL DRUGS
Alcohol

Exposure of the fetus to alcohol can result in devastating effects of the fetal alcohol syndrome (FAS). FAS occurs with an incidence of 0.5 to 3.0 per 1000 live births and is considered the leading cause of mental retardation (Day and Richardson, 1991) (see Chapter 10).

Full-blown FAS occurs in 30% to 40% of the offspring of mothers who consume greater than 2 ounces of absolute alcohol per day during the first trimester. Binge drinking and lesser amounts of alcohol consumption have also been associated with FAS, but there is little evidence that FAS can occur with intake of less than 1 ounce of absolute alcohol per day. Nonetheless, because subtle effects of alcohol may occur at low levels of intake, complete abstinence during pregnancy clearly remains the safest approach.

FAS is characterized by prenatal and postnatal growth retardation, abnormal central nervous system function, and distinctive craniofacial dysmorphism. Common craniofacial features among affected children include microcephaly, short palpebral fissures, a poorly developed philtrum, thin upper lip, and flat maxilla. Less common features include epicanthal folds, microphthalmia, strabismus, ptosis, cleft lip and palate, and posteriorly rotated ears. Neurologic involvement includes developmental delay, hyperactivity, learning and language disabilities, behavioral problems, and sleep disturbances. Approximately 85% of children with FAS are mentally retarded (Streissguth et al, 1978). Congenital heart disease, ventricular septal defects, is also more common in FAS children.

The diagnosis of FAS should be confined to individuals displaying characteristic craniofacial findings, growth retardation, and neurologic symptoms. The phrase *fetal alcohol effects* (FAE) refers to any condition attributable to prenatal alcohol exposure, but without the classic triad described for FAS. Recently, there has been an argument put forth to abandon the term FAE because it is imprecise, stigmatizes the mothers, and presupposes that alcohol is the major or sole source of a child's problems (Aase et al, 1995).

Tobacco

Maternal smoking has been associated with a number of adverse effects on the developing fetus. Although the number of women who smoke has declined steadily over the past 2 decades, approximately 16% of women still smoke during pregnancy (Guyer et al, 1995). A variety of toxic agents are present in cigarette smoke, including carbon monoxide, hydrogen cyanide, ammonia, nicotine, and carcinogenic compounds (Werler et al, 1986) (see Chapter 10).

Infants of smoking women have lower birth weights by an average of 150 to 250 g than infants of nonsmokers. Moreover, smoking women have twice the rate of infants with birth weights of less than 2500 g, as nonsmoking women. The weight reduction observed in these babies depends on the number of cigarettes smoked and is independent of other factors. There is also evidence that passive exposure to cigarette smoke increases the risk for lower birth weight fetuses among nonsmoking women. The growth retardation effects of smoking are most operative after 16 weeks of gestation. If mothers quit smoking within the first trimester, most of the effects of smoking on preterm delivery and low birth weight are eliminated.

Cocaine

Cocaine abuse has become a significant public health problem in the United States during the past decade. Some large city hospitals report up to a 20% rate of cocaine use during pregnancy compared with a 1.4% rate in residential areas. Cocaine and alcohol are the two most commonly abused substances during pregnancy (see Chapter 10).

The length of gestation and neonatal head circumference are reduced among cocaine-exposed fetuses (Bateman et al, 1993). Congenital malformations occur more commonly in prenatally exposed newborns. Genitourinary tract anomalies, such as renal agenesis and hydronephrosis, and congenital heart disease are increased in frequency (Chavez et al, 1989; Lipshultz et al, 1991).

Narcotics

Narcotic analgesics, such as heroin, meperidine, and methadone, readily cross the placenta and cause fetal addiction with repeated use. Illicit use of narcotics during pregnancy results in fetal effects resulting from the maternal-fetal addiction to narcotics, simultaneous exposure to other abused chemical substances, associated maternal diseases (e.g., AIDS, hepatitis, syphilis), and life-style problems of the addict. Narcotic exposure alone does not generally increase the risk for congenital malformations (see Chapter 10).

ENVIRONMENTAL EXPOSURES
Hyperthermia

Several preliminary studies showed an association between high maternal temperature in the first trimester and neural tube defects, microphthalmia, and microcephaly (Chance and Smith, 1978; Miller et al, 1978; Shiota, 1982). A prospective follow-up study also demonstrated an increased relative risk for neural tube defects in women with hyperthermia during the first 2 to 3 months of gestation (Milunsky et al, 1992). The relative risk for a neural tube defect was 1.8 for fever and sauna use and 2.8 for hot tub exposure.

Lead

Acute lead poisoning during pregnancy increases the risk for spontaneous abortions and stillborns. Several cases of congenital lead intoxication have been described in which mothers ingested large amounts of lead. In all cases, the mothers and babies demonstrated toxic levels of lead (Karlog and Moller, 1958; Timpo et al, 1979). Anemia, bone changes and neurologic deficits were common findings in these infants. There is no increased risk of malformations among infants with higher umbilical blood lead levels (Needleman et al, 1984). Low-level lead exposure does not affect fertility or fetal survival (Earnhart, 1992). Deleterious neurodevelopmental effects have, however, been demonstrated for lower cord blood levels than the currently accepted Centers for Disease Control and Prevention upper limit of 25 μg/dL. In a prospective cohort study of 249 infants stratified by cord blood lead levels, Bayley Mental Developmental Indices at 6 through 24 months were 4 to 8 points lower for babies with "higher" cord levels (mean 14.8 μg/dL) than those with "low" (mean 1.8 μg/dL) or "medium" levels (mean 6.5 μg/dL).

Methyl Mercury

Methyl mercury is highly toxic to the developing fetal brain. Maternal poisoning results in cerebral palsy, mental retardation, microcephaly, and visual defects. This condition, known as congenital Minimata disease, was first described in Japan from 1953 to 1971 because there was mercury contamination of ingested fish from Minimata Bay (Harada, 1978). In this outbreak, pregnant women with affected infants were either asymptomatic or had only mild paresthesias. The risk of congenital methyl mercury intoxication has led to the recommendation that women of childbearing age avoid any occupational or environmental exposure to methyl mercury.

Radiation

Ionizing radiation has been clearly shown to be injurious to the developing fetus, but dosage and timing play critical roles in the effects. Natural background radiation in the United States exposes the embryo or fetus to approximately 80 mrems/year, a low-level amount that is considered to be insignificant for the incidence of miscarriage, growth retardation, or congenital malformations (Committee on the Biological Effects of Ionizing Radiation, 1980).

The prenatal effects of high-dose ionizing radiation have been studied extensively in the exposed offspring of the Japanese atomic bomb survivors (Otake and Schull, 1984). First trimester exposures exceeding 10 rads resulted in higher rates of microcephaly and mental retardation occurring in a dose-dependent fashion, with the greatest risk at 8 to 15 weeks of gestation. Even among otherwise healthy children exposed prenatally at 8 to 26 weeks, decrements in academic performance have been observed (Mole, 1987).

Other harmful effects of radiation include infertility, birth weight reduction, and pregnancy loss. High-dose (>100 rads) exposure during embryonic development has also been associated with a number of birth defects, including hydrocephalus, microphthalmia, coloboma, optic atrophy, spina bifida, cleft palate, club feet, hypophalangism, genital abnormalities, and growth retardation (Brent, 1980). A somewhat higher rate of malignancies, particularly leukemia, has been variably observed among prenatally exposed offspring, but this effect has not been found in the children of Japanese atomic bomb survivors.

Current diagnostic radiologic procedures generally result in an exposure of 20 to 5000 mrads. Although no absolute minimal threshold dose of irradiation has been definitively determined, the National Council of Radiation Protection recommends that 500 mrems be the maximal permissible fetal dose.

MATERNAL INFECTIONS
Herpes Simplex Virus Types I and II

Congenital herpes simplex virus infections may result in IUGR, microcephaly, hydranencephaly, intracranial calcifications, microphthalmia, chorioretinitis, a vesicular or bullous rash, scarring skin lesions, and prematurity (Baldwin and Whitely, 1989). Congenital infections may occur following either a primary or recurrent maternal infection. In many instances the maternal infection is completely asymptomatic or subclinical (Hutto et al, 1987) (see Chapter 42).

Cytomegalovirus

Congenital cytomegalovirus (CMV) infections occur mainly after primary infections, with a fetal attack rate of approximately 50% (Yow et al, 1988). Occasionally recurrent CMV infection leads to congenital infection.

Classic signs of congenital infection include IUGR, microcephaly, hepatosplenomegaly, thrombocytopenia, intracranial calcifications, chorioretinitis, seizures, blindness, and optic atrophy. In a large prospective study of CMV infections, approximately 8% of congenitally infected infants were symptomatic at birth (Stagno et al, 1986). An additional 13% of congenitally infected infants, who were asymptomatic at birth, demonstrated severe sensorineural hearing loss during the first few years of life. The sensorineural hearing loss is often progressive and requires longitudinal audiologic evaluation (Williamson et al, 1992).

Varicella

Fetal varicella syndrome occurs in the offspring of less than 1% of women infected during pregnancy, almost exclusively among those mothers infected before 20 weeks' gestation (Enders et al, 1994). Major findings in newborns include limb defects and cicatricial skin lesions conforming to a dermatomal pattern. A variety of neurologic abnormalities have also been reported, including bulbar dysphagia, mental retardation, seizures, optic atrophy, phrenic nerve palsy, microcephaly, hydrocephalus, Horner syndrome, and limb weakness (Alkalay et al, 1987). Eye abnormalities are also commonly seen, namely chorioretinitis, nystagmus, microphthalmos, anisocoria, and cataracts. Gastrointestinal and genitourinary anomalies have occasionally been reported.

Diagnostic criteria for fetal varicella syndrome include (1) evidence of maternal varicella-zoster infection, (2) congenital skin lesions corresponding to a dermatomal distribution, and (3) serologic proof of persisting infection in the neonate.

Maternal zoster infections do not pose a risk to the developing fetus (Brazin et al, 1979).

Rubella

Congenital rubella syndrome occurs after maternal rubella infection during the first 16 weeks of pregnancy (Cooper et al, 1969; Miller et al, 1982). The fetal attack rate is greater than 90% in the first 8 weeks and falls progressively thereafter.

Common neonatal manifestations include IUGR, sensorineural hearing loss, congenital heart disease, cataracts, retinopathy, glaucoma, microphthalmos, microcephaly, encephalitis, hepatosplenomegaly, thrombocytopenia, and characteristic long bone changes seen on radiograph. Long-term problems include postnatal growth retardation, mental retardation, recurrent infections, visual handicaps, and late-onset endocrinopathies (e.g., diabetes, hypothyroidism, hyperthyroidism, and growth hormone deficiency). Skin manifestations include petechiae, purpura, and signs of cutaneous extramedullary hematopoiesis. The types of congenital heart disease are patent ductus arteriosus, pulmonary artery stenosis, valvar pulmonic stenosis, valvar aortic stenosis, aberrant right subclavian artery, and ventricular septal defect. Neonatal myocarditis with ischemic electrocardiographic changes have also been described (Korones et al, 1965).

Infants with congenital rubella may shed virus for several months and typically demonstrate high rubella-specific IgM and IgG antibody titers.

Syphilis

The fetus may acquire a congenital treponemal infection from a mother with untreated primary, secondary, or latent syphilis. Untreated primary or secondary syphilis carries the highest risk for stillbirth, prematurity, and congenital infection.

Most newborns with congenital syphilis are completely asymptomatic at birth and symptoms develop later. Approximately 5% to 27% of luetic newborns show findings at birth, including a maculopapular rash, hepatosplenomegaly, jaundice, joint swelling, lymphadenopathy, anemia, and snuffles. The saddle nose deformity results from destruction of the cartilage of the nasal septum. Typical radiographic changes include periosteal reaction, osteitis, and metaphyseal lucencies (Hira, 1985). Ocular manifestations include chorioretinitis, uveitis, iridocyclitis, and keratitis. Hydrops fetalis has also been reported (Tan, 1973). When clinical manifestations occur at less than 4 weeks of age, there is a higher mortality rate of 54% compared with 9% at greater than 4 weeks.

Toxoplasmosis

Acute maternal toxoplasmosis occurs in 0.2% to 0.7% of pregnancies and carries a 13% risk of overt congenital disease and 26% risk of subclinical infection (Desmonts and Courveur, 1979; Kimball et al, 1971). The earlier in gestation in which the acute infection occurs, the lower is the risk of transmission to the fetus, but the higher is the risk of more severe consequences to the fetus. Prenatal treatment of acute toxoplasmosis in pregnant mothers with spiramycin and sulfonamides reduces the deleterious effects on the fetus.

Clinical manifestations at birth or in later infancy include hydrocephalus, chorioretinitis, intracranial calcifications, seizures, microcephaly, meningoencephalitis, hepatosplenomegaly, and nephrotic syndrome. Patients with subclinical congenital infection are at risk for the development of chorioretinitis, visual loss, sensorineural hearing loss, and lower intelligence quotient (IQ) (Sever et al, 1988; Stagno et al, 1977; Wilson et al, 1980).

Serologic diagnosis of congenital toxoplasmosis includes the presence of specific toxoplasmosis IgM in cord blood, or a fourfold or greater elevation of toxoplasmosis-specific IgG relative to that of the mother.

Human Immunodeficiency Virus

Congenital human immunodeficiency virus (HIV) infection may occur from transplacental or perinatal transmission of virus from an HIV-infected mother. The frequency of viral transmission to the baby is approximately 50% (Falloon et al, 1988).

HIV-infected infants are generally normal at birth. Occasionally lymphadenopathy, hepatosplenomegaly, failure to thrive, or severe infections may present in the newborn period, but generally symptoms do not develop before 4 to 6 months of age. An earlier report of a characteristic dysmorphic syndrome of HIV embryopathy has not been confirmed in subsequent larger studies, making its existence doubtful (European Collaborative Study, 1991; Marion et al, 1986; Qazi, 1988).

No congenital anomalies appear to be associated with congenital HIV infection (see Chapter 41).

MATERNAL MEDICATIONS

Drug use during pregnancy is a common occurrence, as was shown in a recent World Health Organization international survey of 14,778 pregnant women. In this study, 86% of women took medications during pregnancy for an average of 2.9 prescriptions. Over-the-counter preparations were not included, but presumably were an additional source of exposures.

The Food and Drug Administration assigns drugs to one of five risk factor categories—A, B, C, D, or X—based on the level of fetal risk posed by the drug (Table 23–2). The category assignments are based on review of the literature relative to the particular drug and are helpful to rapidly classify the risk of exposure to a specific drug during pregnancy.

Phenytoin (Class D)

Several studies have indicated that phenytoin use during pregnancy is associated with a twofold to threefold eleva-

TABLE 23-2

Fetal Risk Factor Categories

Category A	No risk demonstrated in controlled studies in women.
Category B	Either (1) animal reproduction studies have shown no risk, but there are no controlled human studies, or (2) animal studies have shown an adverse effect, but have not been confirmed in controlled studies in women.
Category C	Either (1) animal studies have revealed adverse effects on the fetus, but there are no controlled studies in women, or (2) there are no available studies in animals or humans.
Category D	There is positive evidence of human fetal risk, but the benefits from use in pregnant women may be acceptable despite the risk.
Category X	Studies in animals or humans have demonstrated fetal abnormalities, or there is evidence of fetal risk based on human experience, or both. The risk of the use of the drug clearly outweighs any possible benefit. The drug is contraindicated in women who are or may become pregnant.

Adapted from Federal Register, 1980.

tion in the rate of nonspecific congenital malformations relative to the general population. It remains unclear, however, whether this increased risk is related to the drug itself, the underlying epilepsy, or genetic factors.

The fetal hydantoin syndrome consists of a typical craniofacial appearance and hypoplasia of the distal phalanges and nails (Hanson, 1986; Meadow, 1968). Approximately 5% to 10% of prenatally exposed infants show signs of the fetal hydantoin syndrome. Typical craniofacial features include ocular hypertelorism, a broad nasal bridge, wide fontanels, a low-set hairline, a broad alveolar ridge, epicanthal folds, ptosis, and coarse scalp hair. Growth retardation, cleft lip and palate, congenital heart disease, and cognitive deficits have also been associated with the fetal hydantoin syndrome.

In prenatally exposed children who do not display the fetal hydantoin syndrome, mental retardation is not more common (Adams, 1990; Dessens et al, 1994).

Phenytoin, like many other drugs, is metabolized by the hepatic P450 cytochrome system. Epoxide metabolites occur as intermediate compounds and may mediate the teratogenic effects of phenytoin. The risk for adverse effects may depend on genetically determined fetal levels of epoxide hydrolase (Buehler, 1990). Fetuses with low activity levels of epoxide hydrolase may be at more risk for fetal hydantoin syndrome compared with those fetuses with intermediate or high levels of the enzyme due to the accumulation to toxic epoxide compounds.

Maternal phenytoin has been infrequently associated with early hemorrhagic disease of the newborn, occurring during the first day of life. A depletion of vitamin K–dependent clotting factors or thrombocytopenia has been described as a possible mechanism for this problem. Routine postnatal administration of vitamin K and close observation are currently recommended for prenatally exposed infants.

Valproic Acid (Class D)

Maternal use of valproic acid during pregnancy poses risks to the fetus, including congenital anomalies, IUGR, psychomotor retardation, and hepatotoxicity. Neural tube defects, mainly in the lumbosacral area, develop in approximately 1% to 2% of fetuses exposed between the 17th and 30th postconceptional day (Lammer et al, 1987). The craniofacial dysmorphism of valproic acid embryopathy is distinctive, with trigonocephaly (premature fusion of the metopic suture), brachycephaly, bifrontal narrowing, epicanthal folds, low-set rotated ears, depressed nasal bridge, anteverted nostrils, hypertelorism, thin upper vermillion border, downturned corners of the mouth, and microstomia. A number of other minor and major anomalies have been associated with prenatal valproate exposure, including congenital heart disease, cleft lip and palate, hydrocephalus, urogenital anomalies, radial ray abnormalities, vertebral anomalies, and talipes equinovarus (Ardinger et al, 1988).

Coumarin (Class D)

The use of coumarin (warfarin) for anticoagulation during pregnancy may cause a variety of problems for the developing fetus (Hall et al, 1980; Pauli et al, 1976). First-trimester exposure may result in the fetal warfarin syndrome, characterized mainly by chondrodysplasia punctata (stippled epiphyses in the axial skeleton, proximal femurs, and calcanei), nasal hypoplasia, and neonatal respiratory distress caused by upper airway obstruction. Eye anomalies (optic atrophy, microphthalmia) and central nervous system abnormalities such as agenesis of the corpus callosum, Dandy-Walker malformation, deafness, seizures, and developmental delay may occur after second or third trimester exposure to coumarin. Other problems include IUGR, scoliosis, congenital heart disease, and higher rates of miscarriage, stillborns, and neonatal death. Neonatal hemorrhage has occurred rarely following third trimester use.

Antithyroid Agents (Class D)

Propylthiouracil, methimazole, and carbamizole are thioamides used for the treatment of hyperthyroidism. Cutis aplasia has been occasionally associated with the use of methimazole and carbamizole during pregnancy (Van Dijke et al, 1987). Treatment of maternal hyperthyroidism with antithyroid agents may result in transient neonatal hypothyroidism, which usually resolves in the first week of life (Low et al, 1978). Occasionally small goiters have been seen in newborns prenatally exposed to these medications.

Diethylstilbestrol (Class X)

Diethylstilbestrol (DES), a synthetic estrogen, was used widely between 1940 and 1971 to treat a variety of obstetric problems. Prenatal exposure to DES carries significant risks to the reproductive tracts of both males and females. Among exposed women there is a high rate of vaginal adenosis, occurring in the majority of women exposed before the 9th week of gestation (Herbst et al, 1975). The rate of vaginal and cervical dysplasia and carcinoma in situ is elevated approximately twofold to fourfold and there have been many reports of clear cell carcinoma associated with DES exposure for a risk between 1.4 and 14 per 1000 (Robboy et al, 1984). Structural defects of the genital tract occur in approximately 25% of exposed women and include a variety of anomalies, such as fornix abnormalities, cervical collars, cervical hypoplasia, vaginal septae, uterine anomalies, and fallopian tube defects (Jefferies et al, 1984). There are also increased rates of spontaneous abortions, premature births, infertility, and ectopic pregnancies among DES-exposed women (Barnes et al, 1980).

Males exposed prenatally demonstrate a higher rate than normal of epididymal cysts, varicoceles, hypotrophic testes, microphallus, and altered semen (Gill et al, 1977).

Retinoic Acid (Class X)

Isotretinoin (Accutane) is a vitamin A analog used for the treatment of severe recalcitrant acne. It has been well demonstrated to be a potent human teratogen. The retinoic acid embryopathy encompasses a characteristic pattern of malformations, including the variable presence of craniofacial dysmorphism (microtia and anotia, low-set ears, micrognathia, narrow sloping forehead, hypertelorism, depressed nasal bridge, cleft palate), congenital heart disease (mainly conotruncal defects), central nervous system abnormalities (hydrocephalus, facial palsy, structural brain defects, microphthalmia, optic nerve hypoplasia, retinal defects), and thymic abnormalities (Lammer et al, 1985, 1987). There is also a high rate of associated spontaneous abortion in exposed pregnancies.

Prior to isotretinoin use, women of child-bearing age should have a negative pregnancy test to prevent this devastating condition from occurring (Public Affairs Committee, The Teratology Society, 1991). Many isotretinoin exposures, however, occur through nonprescriptive sharing of the drug among friends or family members with acne.

Etretinate (Tegison) is a synthetic vitamin A derivative used for the treatment of severe psoriasis. This drug has an extremely long half-life, remaining in adipose tissues for many months and potentially for years. Its use in pregnancy is also associated with a significantly increased risk for malformations, including neural tube defects, craniofacial dysmorphism, and skeletal anomalies. The length of time to avoid a pregnancy following discontinuation of treatment remains largely unknown because of its variable excretion pattern. For this reason the drug is contraindicated for both pregnant women and those likely to become pregnant (Lammer, 1988).

Tretinoin (Retin-A) is used only topically for severe acne and has not been associated with human malformations, presumably because of its low level of absorption (Kligman, 1988).

Corticosteroids

Corticosteroid use during pregnancy is not associated with an increase in birth defects. Betamethasone has been extensively studied due to its beneficial effects on reducing the incidence and severity of both respiratory distress syndrome and intraventricular hemorrhage and improving survival. There does not appear to be an increased risk of infection, glucose intolerance, or adrenal suppression following antenatal steroid treatment for fetal maturation. (NIH Conference Statement, 1994). Likewise, other corticosteroids, such as cortisone and prednisone pose minimal risks to the developing fetus.

Tetracycline

Maternal tetracycline use beginning after the fourth month of pregnancy often results in a yellow-brown discoloration of the deciduous teeth among exposed offspring. This permanent discoloration results from the chelation of tetracycline to calcium orthophosphate with incorporation of this complex into developing teeth and bone (Stewart, 1964). Permanent teeth are generally not affected, although if tetracycline is used close to term, some discoloration of permanent crowns may occur.

Lithium

First-trimester exposure to lithium has been associated with an increased risk for congenital heart disease, based on retrospective studies (Weinstein, 1977). Ebstein anomaly, in particular, has been reported more commonly among the offspring of women taking lithium. In a prospective study of 148 pregnant women taking lithium in the first trimester, one baby was born with Ebstein anomaly, which has an incidence of 1 per 20,000 in the general population (Jacobsen et al, 1992). Prenatal level II ultrasonography and fetal echocardiography are recommended for monitoring lithium-exposed pregnancies.

Lithium toxicity may occur in the fetus and newborn because of its direct systemic effects, which are self-limited once lithium has been renally cleared, generally in the first few weeks of life. Clinical manifestations include polyhydramnios, arrhythmias, congestive heart failure, shock, goiter with hypothyroidism, gastrointestinal bleeding, diabetes insipidus, hypotonia, and seizures (Ang et al, 1990; Krause et al, 1990).

Trimethadione (Class D)

Trimethadione is an anticonvulsant used to treat petit mal seizures and has been shown to be teratogenic in humans with a variety of associated congenital anomalies. The fetal trimethadione syndrome includes prenatal and postnatal growth retardation, craniofacial dysmorphism (abnormal ears, high arched palate, microcephaly, cleft palate, short nose with anteverted nares, mild synophrys), congenital heart disease, genitourinary anomalies, and mental retardation (Feldman et al, 1977; Zackai et al, 1975).

Antineoplastic Agents (Class D)

Antineoplastic agents, such as cyclophosphamide, vincristine, and doxorubicin, have been reported in association with congenital malformations, low birth weight, and higher rates of fetal loss (Gililland et al, 1983; Karp et al, 1983; Kirshon et al, 1988). There also appears to be a somewhat increased risk of adverse fetal outcome for occupational exposure to cytotoxic agents during the first trimester (Jeffrey, 1987).

Folic Acid Antagonists (Class D)

Methotrexate and aminopterin, folic acid antagonists, are associated with spontaneous miscarriage and multiple congenital anomalies when exposure occurs during the first trimester. Intrauterine growth retardation and a variety of congenital malformations have been reported (Milunsky et al, 1968). Defects include craniosynostosis, absence of frontal bones, hypertelorism, prominent eyes, abnormal ears, micrognathia, and digital anomalies.

Vitamin A (Class X if Used in Excess)

Vitamin A is a fat-soluble essential vitamin required for the maintenance of normal epithelial tissue, vision, bone growth, and reproduction. The current recommended daily allowance (RDA) is approximately 2700 IU of vitamin A per day. Vitamin A has clearly been shown to be teratogenic in animals (Cohlan, 1953). There have been several case reports in humans involving high dose (>25,000 IU/day) exposure and birth defects in patterns similar to retinoic acid embryopathy (Rosa et al, 1986) as well as case-controlled studies (Martinez-Frias et al, 1990; Werler et al, 1990).

A recent prospective study of 22,000 pregnant women showed an increased risk of malformations among prenatally exposed infants of women ingesting more than 10,000 IU/day (Rothman et al, 1995). The predominant birth malformations involved cranial-neural crest defects and neural tube closure. For women with this level of intake, it was estimated that 1 of 57 babies is born with a birth defect attributable to vitamin A exposure.

Penicillamine (Class D)

Penicillamine is a chelating agent used in the treatment of Wilson disease, cystinuria, and rheumatoid arthritis. There have been several reports of a connective tissue disorder in prenatally exposed neonates, characterized by cutis laxa, joint laxity, inguinal hernias, and, in one case, bowel perforation (Solomon et al, 1977). The absolute risk for fetal effects has not been established, however, and there remains controversy regarding whether penicillamine therapy should be discontinued during pregnancy (Miehle, 1988).

REFERENCES

Aase JM, Jones KL, Clarren SK: Do we need the term "FAE?" Pediatrics 95:428–430, 1995.

Adams J, Vorhees CV, Middaugh LD: Developmental neurotoxicity of anticonvulsants: Human and animal evidence on phenytoin. Neurotoxical Teratol 12:203–214, 1990.

Alkalay Al, Pomerance JJ, Rimoin DL: Fetal varicella syndrome. J Pediatr 111:320–321, 1987.

Ang MR, Thorp JA, Parisi VM: Maternal lithium therapy and polyhydramnios. Obstet Gynecol 76:517–519, 1990.

Ardinger HH, Atkin JF, Blackstone D, et al: Verification of the fetal valproate syndrome phenotype. Am J Med Genet 29:171–185, 1988.

Baldwin S, Whitely RS: Intrauterine herpes simplex virus infection. Teratology 39:1–10, 1989.

Barnes AB, Colton T, Gundersen J, et al: Fertility and outcome of pregnancy in women exposed in utero to diethylstilbestrol. N Engl J Med 205:609–613, 1980.

Bateman DA, Ng SKC, Hansen CA, et al: The effects of intrauterine cocaine exposure in newborns. Am J Public Health 83:190–193, 1993.

Brazin SA, Simkovich JW, Johnson WT: Herpes zoster during pregnancy. Obstet Gynecol 53:175–181, 1979.

Brent RL. Radiation teratogenesis. Teratology 21:281–298, 1980.

Buehler BA, Deliment D, Van Waes M, et al: Prenatal prediction of risk of the fetal hydantoin syndrome. N Engl J Med 322:1567–1572, 1990.

Chance PF, Smith DW. Hyperthermia and meningomyelocele and anencephaly. Lancet 1:769–770, 1978.

Chasnoff IF, Burns KA, Burns WJ: Cocaine use in pregnancy: Perinatal morbidity and mortality. Neurotoxicol Teratol 9:291–293, 1987.

Chavez GG, Mulinare J, Cordero JF: Maternal cocaine use during early pregnancy as a risk factor for congenital urogenital anomalies. JAMA 262:795–799, 1989.

Cohlan SQ. Excessive intake of vitamin A as a cause of congenital anomalies in the rat. Science 117:535–536, 1953.

Committee on the Biological Effects of Ionizing Radiation, Division of Medical Sciences, Assembly of Life Sciences, National Research Council: The Effects on Populations of Exposure to Low Levels of Ionizing Radiation (BEIRIII). Washington, DC; National Academy of Sciences, 1980.

Cooper LZ, Ziring PR, Ockerse AB, et al: Rubella. Clinical manifestations and management. Am J Dis Child 118:18–29, 1969.

Day NL, Richardson GA: Prenatal alcohol exposure: A continuum of effects. Semin Perinatol 15:271, 1991.

Desmonts G, Couvreur J: Congenital toxoplasmosis: A prospective study of the offspring of 542 women who acquired toxoplasmosis during pregnancy. Pathophysiology of congenital disease. In Thalhammer O, Baumgarten K, Pollak A (Eds): Perinatal Medicine, 6th European Congress. Stuttgart, Germany, Georg Thieme Verlag, 1975, pp 51–60.

Dessens AB, Boer K, Koppe JG, et al: Studies on long-lasting consequences of prenatal exposure to anticonvulsants drugs. Acta Paediatr Suppl 404:54–64, 1994.

Drogari E, Beasley M, Smith I, et al: Timing of strict diet in relation to fetal damage in maternal phenylketonuria. Lancet 2:927–934, 1987.

Earnhart CB: A critical review of low-level prenatal lead exposure in the human: 1. Effects on the fetus and newborn. Reproductive Toxicol 6:9–19, 1992.

Enders G, Miller E, Cradock-Warren J, et al: Consequences of varicella and herpes zoster in pregnancy: Prospective study of 1739 cases. Lancet 343:1548–1551, 1994.

European Collaborative Study: Children born to women with HIV-1 infection: Natural history and risk of transmission. Lancet 337:253–260, 1991.

Falloon J, Eddy J, Roper M, et al: AIDS in pediatric population. In AIDS: Etiology, Diagnosis, Treatment, Prevention, 2nd ed. Philadelphia: JB Lippincott, pp 339–351, 1988.

Feldman GL, Weaver DD, Lovrien EW: The fetal trimethadione syndrome. Am J Dis Child 131:1389–1392, 1977.

Gililland J, Weinstein L: The effects of cancer chemotherapeutic agents on the developing fetus. Obstet Gynecol Surv 38:6–13, 1983.

Gill WB, Schumacher GFB, Bibbo M. Pathological semen and anatomical abnormalities of the genital tract in human male subjects exposed to diethylstilbestrol in utero. J Urol 117:477–480, 1977.

Gladman DD, Urowitz MB: Rheumatic disease in pregnancy. In Burrow GN, Ferris TF (Eds): Medical Complications of Pregnancy, 4th ed. Philadelphia, WB Saunders, 1995, p 512.

Greene MF: Prevention and diagnosis of congenital anomalies in diabetic pregnancies. Clin Perinatol 20:533–547, 1993.

Greene MF, Hare JW, Cloherty JP, et al: First trimester hemoglobin A1 and risk for major malformation and spontaneous abortion in diabetic pregnancy. Teratology 39:225–231, 1989.

Guyer B, Shobino DM, Ventura JJ, Singh GP: Annual summary of vital statistics. Pediatrics 96:1029–1039, 1995.

Hall JG, Pauli RM, Wilson KM: Maternal and fetal sequelae of anticoagulation during pregnancy. Am J Med 68:122–140, 1980.

Hanson JW. Teratogen update: Fetal hydantoin effects. Teratology 33:349–353, 1986.

Harada M. Congenital Minimata disease: Intrauterine methyl mercury poisoning. Teratology 18:285–288, 1978.

Hayslett JP: The effect of systemic lupus erythematosus on pregnancy and pregnancy outcome. Am J Reprod Immunol 28:199, 1992.

Herbst Al, Poskanzer DC, Robboy SJ, et al: Prenatal exposure to stilbestrol: A prospective comparison of exposed female offspring with unexposed controls. N Engl J Med 292:334–339, 1975.

Hira SK, Bhat GH, Patel JB, et al: Early congenital syphilis: Clinicoradiographic features in 202 patients. Sex Transm Dis 12:177–183, 1985.

Hoyme HE. Teratogenically induced fetal anomalies. Clin Perinatol 17(3):547–567, 1990

Hutto C, Arvin A, Jacobs R, et al: Intrauterine herpes simplex virus infection. J Pediatr 110:97–101, 1987.

Jacobson SJ, Jones K, Johnson K, et al: Prospective multicentre study of pregnancy outcome after lithium exposure during first trimester. Lancet 339:530–533, 1992.

Jefferies JA, Robboy SJ, O'Brien PC, et al: Structural anomalies of the cervix and vagina in women enrolled in the Diethylstilbestrol Adenosis (DESAD) project. Am J Obstet Gynecol 148:59–66, 1984.

Jeffrey LP, Chairman, National Study Commission on Cytotoxic Exposure: Position statement. The handling of cytotoxic agents by women who are pregnant, attempting to conceive, or breast feeding. January 12, 1987.

Johnson JP, Carey JC, Gooch WM III, et al: Femoral hypoplasia–unusual facies syndrome in infants of diabetic mothers. J Pediatr 102:866–872, 1982.

Karlog O, Moller KO. Three cases of acute lead poisoning. Analyses of organs for lead, and observations on polarographic lead determinations. Acta Pharmacol Toxicol 15:8–16, 1958.

Karp GI, Von Oeyen P, Valone F, et al: Doxorubicin in pregnancy: Possible transplacental passage. Cancer Treat Rep 67:773–777, 1983.

Khoury M, Becerra J, d'Almada P: Maternal thyroid disease and the risk of birth defects in offspring: A population-based case control study. Paediatr Perinatol Epidemiol 3:402, 1989.

Kimball AC, Kean BH, Fuchs F: Congenital toxoplasmosis: A prospective study of 4048 obstetric patients. Am J Obstet Gynecol 111:211–218, 1971.

Kirshon B, Wasserstrum N, Willis R, et al: Teratogenic effects of first-trimester cyclophosphamide therapy. Obstet Gynecol 72:462–464, 1988.

Kligman AM. Question and answers: Is topical tretinoin teratogenic? JAMA 259:2918, 1988.

Korones SB, Ainger LE, Monif GRG, et al: Congenital rubella syndrome: Study of 22 patients with myocardial damage. Am J Dis Child 110:434–444, 1965.

Krause S, Ebbesen F, Lange AP: Polyhydramnios with maternal lithium treatment. Obstet Gynecol 75:504–506, 1990.

Lammer EJ Chen DT, Hoar RM et al. Retinoic acid embryopathy. N Engl J Med 313:837–841, 1985.

Lammer EJ, Hayes AM, Schunior A, et al: Risk for major malformation among human fetuses exposed to isotretinoin (13-*cis*-retinoic acid). Teratology 35:68A, 1987a.

Lammer EJ, Sever LE, Oakley GP Jr. Teratogen update: Valproic acid. Teratology 35:465–473, 1987b.

Lammer EJ. Embryopathy in infant conceived one year after termination of maternal etretinate. Lancet 2:1080–1081, 1988.

Lenke RR, Levy HL: Maternal phenylketonuria and hyperphenylalaninemia. N Engl J Med 303:1202–1208, 1980.

Lenz W, Knapp K. Thalidomide embryopathy. Arch Environ Health 5:100–105, 1962.

Lipshultz SE, Frassica JJ, Orav EJ: Cardiovascular abnormalities in infants prenatally exposed to cocaine. J Pediatr 118:44–51, 1991.

Low L, Ratcliffe W, Alexander W: Intrauterine hypothyroidism due to antithyroid-drug therapy for thyrotoxicosis during pregnancy. Lancet 2:370–371, 1978.

Malloy MH, Hoffman HJ, Peterson DR: Sudden infant death syndrome and maternal smoking. Am J Public Health 82:1380, 1992.

Marion R, Wiznia A, Hucheon RG, et al: AIDS embryopathy: A new dysmorphic syndrome in children with AIDS. Pediatr Res 20:339A, 1986.

Martinez-Frias ML, Salvador J: Epidemiological aspects of prenatal exposure to high doses of vitamin A in Spain. Eur J Epidemiol 6:118–123, 1990.

Meadow SR: Anticonvulsant drugs and congenital abnormalities. Lancet 2:1296, 1968.

Miehle W. Current aspects of D-penicillamine and pregnancy. Z Rheumatol 47(Suppl 1):20–23, 1988.

Miller E, Cradock-Watson JE, Pollack TM: Consequences of confirmed maternal rubella at successive stages of pregnancy. Lancet 2:781–784, 1982.

Miller P, Smith DW, Shepard TH: Hyperthermia as one possible etiology of anencephaly. Lancet 1:519, 1978.

Mills JI. Malformations in infants of diabetic mothers. Teratology 25:385–394, 1982.

Mills JL, Knopp RH, Simpson JL, et al: Lack of relation of increased malformation rates in infants of diabetic mothers to glycemic control during organogenesis. N Engl J Med 318:671–676, 1988.

Milunsky A, Graef JW, Gaynor MF: Methotrexate-induced congenital malformations with a review of the literature. J Pediatr 72:790–795, 1968.

Milunsky A, Ulcickas M, Rothman KJ, et al: Maternal heat exposure and neural tube defects. JAMA 268:882–885, 1992.

Mole RH. Irradiation of the embryo and fetus. Br J Radiol 60:17–31, 1987.

Namba T, Brown SB, Groh D: Neonatal myasthemia gravis: Report of two cases and a review of the literature. Pediatrics 45:488–504, 1970.

National Institutes of Health Consensus Development Conference Statement: Effect of corticosteroids for fetal maturation on perinatal outcomes. February 28 to March 2, 1994, Bethesda, MD.

Needleman HL, Rabinowitz M, Leviton A, et al: The relationship between prenatal exposure to lead and congenital anomalies. JAMA 251:2956–2959, 1984.

Otake M, Schull MJ. In utero exposure to A-bomb radiation and mental retardation: A reassessment. Br J Radiol 57:409–414, 1984.

Passarge E, Lenz W: Syndrome of caudal regression in infants of diabetic mothers: Observations of further cases. Pediatr 35:672, 1965.

Pauli RM, Madden JD, Kranzler KJ, et al: Warfarin therapy initiated during pregnancy and phenotypic chondrodysplasia punctata. J Pediatr 88:506–508, 1976.

Pedersen LM, Tygstup I, Pedersen JF: Congenital malformations in newborn infants of diabetic mothers. Correlation with maternal diabetic vascular complications. Lancet 1:1124–1126, 1964.

Platt LD, Koch R, Azen C, et al: Maternal phenylketonuria collaborative study, obstetric aspects and outcome: The first six years. Am J Obstet Gynecol 166:1150–1162, 1992.

Public Affairs Committee, Teratology Society position paper: Recommendations for isotretinoin use in women of childbearing potential. Teratology 44:1–6, 1991.

Qazi QH, Sheikh TM, Fikrig S, et al: Lack of evidence for craniofacial dysmorphism in perinatal human immunodeficiency virus infection. J Pediatr 112:7–11, 1988.

Robboy SJ, Noller KL, O'Brien P, et al: Increased incidence of cervical and vaginal dysplasia in 398 diethylstilbestrol-exposed young women. Experience of the National Collaborative Diethylstilbestrol Adenosis Project. JAMA 252:2979–2983, 1984.

Rohr FJ, Doherty LB, Waisbren SE, et al: New England maternal PKU project; prospective study of untreated and treated pregnancies and their outcomes. J Pediatr 110:391–398, 1987.

Rosa FW, Wilk AI, Kelsey FO: Teratogen update: Vitamin A congeners. Teratology 33:355–364, 1986.

Rothman KJ, Moore LL, Singer MR, et al: Teratogenicity of high vitamin A intake. N Engl J Med 333:1369–1373, 1995.

Sever JL, Ellenberg JH, Ley AC, et al: Toxoplasmosis: Maternal and pediatric findings in 23,000 pregnancies. Pediatrics 82:181–192, 1988.

Shepard TH: Catalog of Teratogenic Agents, 8th ed. Baltimore: Johns Hopkins University Press, 1995.

Shiota K: Neural tube defects and maternal hyperthermia in early pregnancy: Epidemiology in a human embryo population. Am J Med Genet 12:281–288, 1982.

Solomon L, Abrams G, Dinner M, et al: Neonatal abnormalities associated with D-penicillamine treatment during pregnancy. N Engl J Med 296:54–55, 1977.

Stagno S, Pass RF, Cloud BG: Primary cytomegalovirus infection in pregnancy. JAMA 256:1906, 1986.

Stagno S, Reynolds DW, Amos CS, et al: Auditory and visual defects resulting from symptomatic and subclinical congenital cytomegaloviral and *Toxoplasma* infections. Pediatrics 59:669–678, 1977.

Stewart DJ. The effects of tetracyclines upon the dentition. Br J Dermatol 76:374–378, 1964.

Streissguth AP, Herman CS, Smith DW. Intelligence, behavior, and dysmorphogenesis in the fetal alcohol syndrome: A report on 20 patients. J Pediatr 92:363–367, 1978.

Tan KL: The reemergence of early congenital syphilis. Acta Paediatr Scand 62:601–607, 1973.

Timpo AE, Amin JS, Casalino MD, et al: Congenital lead intoxication. J Pediatr 94:765–767, 1979.

Van Dijke CP, Heydendael RJ, De Kleine JM: Methimazole, carbimazole and congenital skin defects. Ann Intern Med 106:60–61, 1987.

Weinstein MR: Recent advances in clinical psychopharmacology. I. Lithium carbonate. Hosp Form 12:759–762, 1977.

Werler MM, Pober BR, Holmes LB: Smoking and pregnancy. *In* Sever JL, Brent RL (Eds): Teratogen Update. Environmentally Induced Birth Defects Risks. New York, Alan R Liss, pp 131–139, 1986.

Werler MW, Lammer EJ, Rosenberg L, et al: Maternal vitamin A supplementation in relation to selected birth defects. Teratology 42:497–503, 1990.

Williamson WD, Demmler GJ, Percy AK, et al: Progressive hearing loss in infants with asymptomatic congenital cytomegalovirus infection. Pediatrics 90:862–866, 1992.

Wilson CB, Remington JS, Stagno S, et al: Development of adverse sequelae in children born with subclinical *Toxoplasma* infection. Pediatrics 66:767–774, 1980.

Yow MD, Williamson DW, Leeds IJ, et al: Epidemiological characteristics of cytomegalovirus infection in mothers and their infants. Am J Obstet Gynecol 158:1189–1195, 1988.

Zackai EH, Melman WJ, Neiderer B, et al: The fetal trimethadione syndrome. J Pediatr 87:280–284, 1975.

CHAPTER 24

Introduction to the Metabolic or Biochemical Genetic Diseases

Gerard T. Berry

For the sake of simplicity, genetic diseases may be divided into the chromosome disorders, the contiguous gene deletion syndromes, the single gene defects, and the polygenic disorders. Biochemical genetic disease is almost always the consequence of a single gene defect, and most inborn errors of metabolism are inherited as autosomal recessive traits. However, not all biochemical genetic disorders are usually thought of as metabolic diseases. For the clinician caring for sick newborns, one tends to consider metabolic diseases in terms of certain well-recognized clinical presentations: the catastrophically ill, comatose newborn infant; the baby with failure to thrive, recurrent feeding problems and emesis, hypotonia, or seizures; and the infant with physical stigmata such as hepatosplenomegaly, characteristic of the storage diseases. Acidosis, ketosis, hypoglycemia, or hyperammonemia frequently alerts the pediatrician or neonatologist to initiate a workup for a metabolic disorder in the infant with life-threatening disease. In contrast, cystic fibrosis, a biochemical genetic disorder, has little in common with these kinds of inborn errors, except perhaps autosomal recessive transmission. The examples of the inborn errors offered in Chapters 25 through 27 help clarify this clinical nosologic concept. A list of general references or reviews that emphasize the genetic metabolic diseases is provided at the end of this chapter.

The purpose of this section is to review the biochemical genetic diseases and, specifically, the metabolic diseases that present in the extended newborn period, considering the appropriate laboratory testing to diagnose and therapeutic modalities to treat these disorders. With the exception of some rare contiguous gene deletion syndromes, the non–single gene defects such as the chromosome and polygenic genetic disorders are not causes of metabolic disease. Yet, as discussed in the context of biochemical genetic diseases producing dysmorphism, the distinction between what constitutes classic clinical genetics and metabolic diseases is becoming blurred. Although a few metabolic disorders are inherited as X-linked traits, autosomal dominant inheritance is not considered common, particularly in the group of inborn errors that can be readily detected by measuring the levels of chemicals such as amino and organic acids in body fluids. The biochemical genetic defects due to expansion of trinucleotide repeats such as the fragile X syndrome and disorders due to mitochondrial DNA mutations rarely present during the newborn period. Defects in the "imprinting" of a single parental gene of maternal or paternal origin, such as in Prader-Willi, Angelman, and Beckwith-Wiedmann syndromes, are covered in other chapters. In general, metabolic diseases in the newborn are the consequence of the malfunctioning of both the maternally and the paternally inherited alleles at one specific gene locus. Some biochemical genetic dis-

eases transmitted in such an autosomal recessive manner are not covered in this section because of the unique involvement of one organ or physiologic system that places that disease within a particular subspecialty. Examples include cystic fibrosis, disorders of hemostasis and coagulation, methemoglobinemias, and immunodeficiencies. Other metabolic disorders such as familial hyperinsulinism, congenital adrenal hyperplasia, and Crigler-Najjar syndrome are thoroughly discussed in other chapters.

Of the approximately 9000 genetic diseases or polymorphic traits that follow a mendelian inheritance pattern, more than 400 are considered biochemical genetic diseases and have been defined at the protein and/or gene level. As discussed earlier, not all present during the newborn period. Almost 40 inborn errors of amino and/or organic acid or ammonia metabolism can be recognized in the first weeks or months of life. The primary lactic acidoses are rare, as are the storage, peroxisomal, and connective tissue diseases that individually number few. Aside from hyperinsulinism, galactosemia is the most common of the defects in carbohydrate metabolism. Because of the number and rarity of these metabolic diseases (Table 24–1), a practical general approach to patients with a potential metabolic disease is essential. For the clinician, it is helpful to focus not on the individual diseases, except when characteristic syndromes are readily recognizable, but on the different general modes of presentation and the classes or types of inborn errors that fit a particular mode of presentation.

In general, the metabolic diseases affecting the newborn can be divided into those involving complex molecules such as the storage diseases and those concerning the intermediary metabolism of small molecules such as glucose, pyruvate, lactate, amino acids, organic acids, ammonia, and mitochondrial respiration and oxidative phosphorylation. Overwhelming, acute, life-threatening illness is the outstanding feature of the group of metabolic diseases

TABLE 24–1

Inborn Errors of Metabolism with Newborn Presentation

Amino acid disorders
Organic acid disorders
Disorders of ammonia metabolism
Disorders of carbohydrate metabolism
Disorders of gluconeogenesis/hypoglycemia
Primary lactic acidoses
Disorders of vitamin/metal metabolism
Storage diseases
Peroxisomal disorders
Connective tissue diseases

TABLE 24–2

Metabolic Diseases with Newborn Coma Secondary to Toxic Metabolite Accumulation or Mitochondrial Failure

Galactosemia
Inborn errors of ammonia metabolism
  Ornithine transcarbamylase deficiency
  Argininosuccinic aciduria
  Citrullinemia
  Carbamylphosphate synthetase deficiency
Maple syrup urine disease
Nonketotic hyperglycinemia
Methylmalonic acidemia ± homocystinuria
Propionic acidemia
Isovaleric acidemia
Multiple carboxylase deficiency
Glutaric aciduria type 2
Fatty acid oxidation defects
  Short-chain acyl-CoA dehydrogenase deficiency
  Medium-chain acyl-CoA dehydrogenase deficiency°
  Very-long-chain acyl-CoA dehydrogenase deficiency
  Long-chain 3-hydroxy acyl-CoA dehydrogenase deficiency
  Carnitine transporter deficiency
  Carnitine translocase deficiency
  Carnitine palmitoyltransferase I and II deficiencies
Primary lactic acidosis
  Pyruvate dehydrogenase deficiency
  Pyruvate carboxylase deficiency
  Mitochondrial respiratory chain or electron transport
    chain defects

°Rare cause of sudden infant death syndrome.

involving metabolism of small molecules. Acute encephalopathy may be due to the buildup of metabolic poisons such as ammonia and organic acids (Table 24–2), to hypoglycemia (Table 24–3), or to the failure to convert glucose to CO_2 and H_2O associated with diminished mitochondrial adenosine triphosphate formation and lactate buildup (see Table 24–2). As is well known to neonatologists and pediatricians, the newborn or young infant has a limited array of responses to acute, severe illness with encephalopathy. The signs are nonspecific and include poor feeding, spitting up, lethargy, skin color changes, hypothermia, and poor weight gain. In fact, few newborn infants suspected of a metabolic disease should have escaped a workup for sepsis. In many of these diseases, respiratory distress is also a presenting feature because of the presence of an acid-base disturbance. Metabolic acidosis and hyperammonemia both produce hyperventilation. During the progression of meta-

TABLE 24–3

Metabolic Diseases with Newborn Coma Secondary to Hypoglycemia

Hyperinsulinism
3-Hydroxy-3-methylglutaryl-CoA lyase deficiency
Fructose-1,6-diphosphatase deficiency
Hereditary fructose intolerance
Glycogen storage disease type I

TABLE 24–4

Modes of Presentation of Metabolic Diseases

Acute life-threatening illness with coma
Seizures
Respiratory distress
Feeding problems and poor growth
Developmental delay or failure with hypotonia
Unique or characteristic findings on physical examination
Dysmorphic features or multiple malformations
Hydrops fetalis or neonatal ascites
Persistent diarrhea

bolic coma, cerebral edema or other complications such as intracranial hemorrhages may develop in the patient, which makes it more difficult to establish the diagnosis.

Because a specific metabolic disorder may be associated with different amounts of residual enzyme activity, as the exact gene mutations often vary from patient to patient, or because different rates of protein ingestion lead to a variable accumulation of amino or organic acids, there may be different modes of presentation even for the same metabolic disorder. Examples of the different modes of presentation are shown in Table 24–4. A characteristic odor may provide the clue to the presence of phenylketonuria (musty), maple syrup urine disease (maple syrup), isovaleric aciduria (sweaty socks), and glutaric aciduria Type 2 (sweaty socks). Often the physical examination is not specifically helpful in those metabolic diseases involving small molecules. Conversely, the diseases involving cellular processing of complex molecules such as the storage diseases usually are associated with characteristic or unique findings on physical examination (Table 24–5). Although there are exceptions to both of these rules, this represents an easy and diagnostically helpful way to think about these rare disorders of metabolism. The characteristic unique or physical findings that underscore the complex molecule diseases, as well as those that may be detected in the diverse group of small molecule disorders, are outlined in Table 24–6. With regard to Table 24–4, note that feeding problems and poor growth, as well as developmental delay, may be seen in both categories of metabolic disease. Characteristic or unique laboratory or diagnostic testing findings seen in some of these illnesses are noted in Table 24–7. Measurements such as blood pH, total CO_2 content, glucose, ammonia, and amino acids are not particularly helpful in the evaluation of these infants with abnormalities in the metabolism of complex molecules whose workup must be dictated by the history and important findings on physical examination. The enigmatic picture of hydrops fetalis, al-

TABLE 24–5

Metabolic Diseases in Which Physical Examination Is Usually Helpful in Diagnosis

Storage diseases
Peroxisomal diseases
Connective tissue diseases

TABLE 24-6

Unique or Characteristic Physical Findings in Inborn Errors*

Hepatomegaly
Hereditary galactosemia
Glycogen storage disease type 1
Hereditary fructose intolerance
Fructose-1,6-bisphosphatase deficiency
Methylmalonic acidemia
Propionic acidemia
Glutaric acidemia type 2
Very-long-chain acyl-CoA dehydrogenase deficiency
Medium-chain acyl-CoA dehydrogenase deficiency
Short-chain acyl-CoA dehydrogenase deficiency
Long-chain 3-hydroxy acyl-CoA dehydrogenase deficiency
Carnitine transporter defect
Carnitine palmitoyltransferase type I deficiency
Carnitine palmitoyltransferase type II deficiency
Acyl carnitine translocase deficiency
3-Hydroxy-3-methylglutaryl CoA lyase deficiency
Phosphoenolpyruvate carboxykinase deficiency
Mitochondrial respiratory/electron transport chain defects
Hereditary tyrosinemia type 1
Argininosuccinicaciduria
Alpha$_1$ antitrypsin deficiency
Smith-Lemli-Opitz syndrome
Zellweger disease
Neonatal adrenoleukodystrophy
Niemann-Pick type C disease

Hepatosplenomegaly
G$_{M1}$ gangliosidosis
I-cell disease
Gaucher disease type 2
Niemann-Pick disease type A
Niemann-Pick disease type C
Galactosialidosis
Sialidosis
Mucopolysaccharidosis type VII
Wolman disease

Macrocephaly
Glutaric acidemia type 1
Canavan disease

Microcephaly
Short-chain acyl-CoA dehydrogenase deficiency
Mitochondrial respiratory/electron transport chain defects
Leigh disease

Coarse Facial Features
G$_{M1}$ gangliosidosis
I-cell disease
Mucopolysaccharidosis type VII
Sialidosis
Galactosialidosis

Macroglossia
Pompe disease
G$_{M1}$ gangliosidosis

Dystonia or Extrapyramidal Signs
Gaucher disease type 2
Glutaric acidemia type 1
Krabbe disease
Crigler-Najjar syndrome
Phenylketonuria due to a biopterin defect

Macular "Cherry Red Spot"
G$_{M1}$ gangliosidosis
Galactosialidosis
Niemann-Pick disease type A
Tay-Sachs disease (G$_{M2}$ gangliosidosis)

Retinitis Pigmentosa
Mitochondrial respiratory/electron transport chain defects
Methylmalonic acidemia/homocystinuria
Sjögren-Larsson syndrome
Zellweger disease
Neonatal adrenoleukodystrophy
Infantile Refsum disease
Abetalipoproteinemia
Long-chain 3-hydroxy acyl-CoA dehydrogenase deficiency

Otic Atrophy or Hypoplasia
Pyruvate dehydrogenase complex deficiency
Leigh disease
Zellweger disease

Corneal Clouding or Opacities
I-cell disease
Steroid sulfatase deficiency

Cataracts
Hereditary galactosemia
Lowe syndrome
Mitochondrial respiratory/electron transport chain defects
Zellweger disease
Rhizomelic chondrodysplasia punctata
Mevalonic aciduria

Dislocated Lens
Methionine synthetase deficiency
Sulfite oxidase deficiency

Bone or Limb Deformities/Contractures
Storage, peroxisomal, or connective tissue disorders

Thick Skin
I-cell disease
G$_{M2}$ gangliosidosis
Mucopolysaccharidosis type VII
Sialidosis
Galactosialidosis

Skin Nodules
Ceramidase deficiency

Desquamating, Eczematous, or Vesiculobullous Skin Lesions
Acrodermatitis enteropathica
Multiple carboxylase deficiency
Methylmalonic acidemia
Propionic acidemia
Hepatoerythropoietic porphyria
Congenital erythropoietic porphyria

Ichthyosis
Gaucher disease type 2
Sjögren-Larsson syndrome
Steroid sulfatase deficiency

Alopecia
Multiple carboxylase deficiency

Steely or Kinky Hair
Menkes disease

Persistent Diarrhea
Glucose galactose malabsorption
Congenital lactase deficiency
Congenital chloride diarrhea
Sucrase isomaltase deficiency
Acrodermatitis enteropathica
Congenital folate malabsorption
Wolman disease
Hereditary galactosemia

*For discussion of specific disorders, see Chapters 25 through 27.

TABLE 24–7

Characteristic or Unique Laboratory or Diagnostic Testing Outcomes in Inborn Errors

Metabolic Acidosis ± Increased Anion Gap
Methylmalonic acidemia
Propionic acidemia
Isovaleric acidemia
Multiple carboxylase deficiency
Maple syrup urine disease
Glutaric acidemia type 1
Glutaric acidemia type 2
Short-chain acyl-CoA dehydrogenase deficiency
Long-chain 3-hydroxy acyl-CoA dehydrogenase deficiency
Ketothiolase deficiency
Acetoacetate-CoA ligase deficiency
3-Hydroxy-3-methylglutaryl-CoA lyase deficiency
Pyruvate dehydrogenase complex deficiency
Pyruvate carboxylase deficiency
Phosphoenolpyruvate carboxykinase deficiency
Mitochondrial respiratory/electron transport chain defects
Leigh disease
Hereditary galactosemia
Glycogen storage disease type 1
Hereditary fructose intolerance
Fructose-1,6-diphosphatase deficiency
Hereditary tyrosinemia type 1
Respiratory Alkalosis
Ornithine transcarbamylase deficiency
Carbamylphosphate synthetase deficiency
Argininosuccinicaciduria
Citrullinemia
Hyperammonemia
Ornithine transcarbamylase deficiency
Carbamylphosphate synthetase deficiency
Argininosuccinicaciduria
Citrullinemia
Methylmalonic acidemia
Propionic acidemia
Isovaleric acidemia
Multiple carboxylase deficiency
Glutaric acidemia type 2
Very-long-chain acyl-CoA dehydrogenase deficiency
Medium-chain acyl-CoA dehydrogenase deficiency
Short-chain acyl-CoA dehydrogenase deficiency
Acylcarnitine translocase deficiency
Ketosis
Methylmalonic acidemia
Propionic acidemia
Isovaleric acidemia
Multiple carboxylase deficiency
Maple syrup urine disease
Glutaric acidemia type 2
Short-chain acyl-CoA dehydrogenase deficiency
Ketothiolase deficiency
Acetoacetate-CoA ligase deficiency
Pyruvate carboxylase deficiency
Glycogen storage disease type 1
Fructose-1,6-diphosphatase deficiency
Lactic Acidosis
Methylmalonic acidemia
Propionic acidemia
Isovaleric acidemia
Multiple carboxylase deficiency
Glutaric acidemia type 2
Short-chain acyl-CoA dehydrogenase deficiency
Long-chain 3-hydroxy acyl-CoA dehydrogenase deficiency
Ketothiolase deficiency

Lactic Acidosis (*Continued*)
Acetoacetate-CoA ligase deficiency
3-Hydroxy-3-methylglutaryl-CoA lyase deficiency
Pyruvate dehydrogenase complex deficiency
Pyruvate carboxylase deficiency
Phosphoenolpyruvate carboxykinase deficiency
Mitochondrial respiratory/electron transport chain defects
Leigh disease
Glycogen storage disease type 1
Hereditary fructose intolerance
Fructose-1,6-diphosphatase deficiency
Hypoglycemia
Hyperinsulinism
Glycogen storage disease type 1
Hereditary fructose intolerance
Fructose-1,6-diphosphatase deficiency
Glutaric acidemia type 1
Glutaric acidemia type 2
Very-long-chain acyl-CoA dehydrogenase deficiency
Medium-chain acyl-CoA dehydrogenase deficiency
Short-chain acyl-CoA dehydrogenase deficiency
Long-chain 3-hydroxy acyl-CoA dehydrogenase deficiency
Carnitine transporter defect
Carnitine palmitoyltransferase type I deficiency
Carnitine palmitoyltransferase type II deficiency
Acyl carnitine translocase deficiency
Ketothiolase deficiency
Acetoacetate-CoA ligase deficiency
3-Hydroxy-3-methylglutaryl-CoA lyase deficiency
Hereditary galactosemia
Neonatal hemochromatosis
Mitochondrial respiratory/electron transport chain defects
Lipemia
Glycogen storage disease type 1
Positive Urinary-Reducing Substances
Hereditary galactosemia
Hereditary fructose intolerance
Essential fructosuria
Lowe syndrome
Discolored Urine
Congenital erythropoietic porphyria
Alkaptonuria
Tryptophan malabsorption
Leukopenia
Methylmalonic acidemia
Propionic acidemia
Isovaleric acidemia
Multiple carboxylase deficiency
Glycogen storage disease type 1B
Mevalonic aciduria
Barth syndrome
Pearson syndrome
Thrombocytopenia
Methylmalonic acidemia
Propionic acidemia
Isovaleric acidemia
Multiple carboxylase deficiency
Pearson syndrome
Mevalonic aciduria
Anemia
Alpha$_1$-antitrypsin deficiency
Methylmalonic acidemia/homocystinuria/vitamin B$_{12}$ defects
Propionic acidemia
Isovaleric acidemia

TABLE 24–7

Characteristic or Unique Laboratory or Diagnostic Testing Outcomes in Inborn Errors *Continued*

Anemia (*Continued*)
   Multiple carboxylase deficiency
   Wolman disease
   Pearson syndrome
   Neonatal hemochromatosis
   Abetalipoproteinemia
   Mevalonic aciduria
   Hereditary galactosemia
Prolonged Prothrombin and Partial Thromboplastin Times
   Hereditary galactosemia
   Hereditary fructose intolerance
   Alpha$_1$-antitrypsin deficiency
   Neonatal hemochromatosis
   Hereditary tyrosinemia type 1
Vacuolated Lymphocytes or Neutrophils
   Storage diseases
Acanthocytosis
   Abetalipoproteinemia
   Wolman disease
Cardiomegaly
   Pompe disease
   Barth syndrome
   Carnitine palmitoyltransferase type II deficiency
   Carbohydrate-deficient glycoprotein syndrome
Electrocardiographic Abnormalities
   Pompe disease (short PR interval, large QRS)
   Acyl carnitine translocase deficiency
   Very-long-chain acyl-CoA dehydrogenase deficiency
   Long-chain 3-hydroxy acyl-CoA dehydrogenase deficiency
   Carnitine palmitoyltransferase type II deficiency
Ventricular Hypertrophy
   Pompe disease
   Propionic acidemia
   Isovaleric acidemia
   Multiple carboxylase deficiency
   Glutaric acidemia type 2
   Very-long-chain acyl-CoA dehydrogenase deficiency
   Long-chain 3-hydroxy acyl-CoA dehydrogenase deficiency
   Carnitine transporter defect

Ventricular Hypertrophy (*Continued*)
   Carnitine palmitoyltransferase type II deficiency
   Acyl carnitine translocase deficiency
   Ketothiolase deficiency
   Mitochondrial respiratory/electron transport chain defects
   Leigh disease
Dysostosis Multiplex
   G$_{MI}$ gangliosidosis
   Mucopolysaccharidosis type VII
   I-cell disease
   Sialidosis
   Galactosialidosis
Stippled Calcifications of Patellae
   Zellweger disease
Adrenal Calcifications
   Wolman disease
Rhizomelism
   Rhizomelic chondrodysplasia punctata
Pili Torti
   Menkes disease
Trichorrhexis Nodosa
   Argininosuccinicaciduria
Basal Ganglia Lesions on MRI
   Methylmalonic acidemia
   Propionic acidemia
   Pyruvate dehydrogenase complex deficiency
   Mitochondrial respiratory/electron transport chain defects
   Leigh disease
   Krabbe disease
Cerebellar Atrophy or Hypoplasia
   Pyruvate dehydrogenase complex deficiency
   Mitochondrial respiratory/electron transport chain defects
   Leigh disease
   Carbohydrate-deficient glycoprotein syndrome
Agenesis of Corpus Callosum
   Pyruvate dehydrogenase complex deficiency
   Pyruvate carboxylase deficiency
   Mitochondrial respiratory/electron transport chain defects

though uncommon as a mode of presentation, is exclusively associated with the storage diseases. Neurologic signs including seizures may also be seen in the storage diseases. Congenital chloride malabsorption, glucose-galactose malabsorption, and acrodermatitis enteropathica may present with congenital and/or persistent diarrhea.

Severe liver disease with jaundice or elevated serum transaminase determinations is characteristic of a few metabolic diseases. These are outlined in Table 24–8. Of these disorders, only alpha$_1$-antitrypsin deficiency, the peroxisomal disorders, such as Zellweger disease and neonatal adrenoleukodystrophy, and Niemann-Pick type C disease are secondary to impaired disposition of complex molecules. Mild or transient liver function test abnormalities may also be seen in the glycogen storage diseases, fructose-1,6-bisphosphatase deficiency, and hyperammonemic conditions, but bridging fibrosis is not usually detected. A renal tubulopathy may also be detected in galactosemia, hereditary fructose intolerance, tyrosinemia type 1, and the mitochondrial respiratory chain or electron transport chain

deficiencies. Hyperchloremic metabolic acidosis, therefore, may be an important clue to their presence.

Significantly, it is now recognized that some patients with multiple malformations may have a metabolic disease. The best example is Smith-Lemli-Opitz syndrome. Congenital craniofacial dysmorphic features, microcephaly, limb malformations, and progressive liver disease are secondary to a deficiency of the enzyme 7-dehydrocholesterol reductase. Another example of an autosomal recessive disorder resulting in malformations is Zellweger disease. In its classic form, the cellular organelle, the peroxisome, is not formed, resulting in multiple enzyme deficiencies such as those involved in very-long-chain fatty acid oxidation and plasmalogen biosynthesis. As a consequence, the brain, cranium, face, long bones, and kidney fail to develop normally. A list of the different metabolic diseases that can, but do not, always produce congenital dysmorphism or malformations is shown in Table 24–9. It is important, when confronted with an infant with these types of findings, that the physician not assume that a chromosome

TABLE 24–8

Newborn Metabolic Disorders with Severe Hepatocellular Disease Potentially Leading to Cirrhosis

Hereditary galactosemia
Hereditary fructose intolerance
Tyrosinemia type 1
Newborn iron storage disease
Alpha$_1$-antitrypsin deficiency
Long-chain acyl-CoA dehydrogenase deficiency
Long-chain 3-hydroxy acyl-CoA dehydrogenase deficiency
Mitochondrial respiratory/electron transport chain defects
Smith-Lemli-Opitz syndrome
Zellweger disease
Neonatal adrenoleukodystrophy
Niemann-Pick type C disease

disorder is the cause or that congenital disease excludes a single gene defect.

In the next four chapters, various inborn errors of metabolism, including key clinical and laboratory findings, sophisticated biochemical and molecular diagnostic testing, therapy, and newborn screening are discussed. It is impractical to exhaustively cover all known biochemical genetic diseases and still provide useful and readily accessible information for the clinician. For this reason, the succeeding chapters focus on the major categories of disease as discussed earlier.

TABLE 24–9

Metabolic Diseases with Congenital Malformation(s) or Dysmorphic Features

Smith-Lemli-Opitz syndrome
Zellweger disease
Neonatal adrenoleukodystrophy
Rhizomelic chondrodysplasia punctata
Glutaric aciduria type 2
Glutaric aciduria type 1
Primary lactic acidoses
    Pyruvate dehydrogenase deficiency
    Pyruvate carboxylase deficiency
    Mitochondrial respiratory/electron transport
      chain defects
Mevalonic aciduria
I-cell disease
Galactosialidosis
Neuraminidase deficiency
Sialic acid storage disease
Menke disease
Nonketotic hyperglycinemia
Lowe syndrome

In Chapter 25, the metabolic defects involving small and simple molecules such as glucose, galactose, amino and organic acids, ammonia, and lactate are reviewed. These include the inborn errors that can produce acute, life-threatening disease with coma in the newborn infant. In Chapter 26, the storage diseases that present in the extended neonatal period are reviewed. This includes the disorders that involve handling of complex molecules. The lysosomal enzyme deficiencies are the most notable members of the group. These include the storage diseases that may present as non–immune hydrops fetalis. Because physical examination is the key to the diagnosis of complex molecule diseases, the defects in peroxisomal metabolism such as Zellweger disease and Smith-Lemli-Opitz syndrome are also included in the chapter on storage diseases. In Chapter 27, the connective tissue diseases that involve metabolism of the complex molecules, collagen, fibrillin, and elastin and the osteochondrodystrophies that present in the newborn period are reviewed. Finally, in Chapter 28, the state of newborn screening, including metabolic diseases, is reviewed. Most metabolic diseases discussed in Chapters 25 through 27 are not detected in the newborn screening programs currently in place. Accordingly, another purpose of this section is to help the clinician develop a conceptual framework to fashion a useful and practical approach to diagnostic testing.

REFERENCES

Berry GT: Metabolism. *In* Polin RA, Ditmer MF (Eds): Pediatric Secrets, 2nd ed. Philadelphia, Henley & Belfus, 1996, pp 309–326.
Cohn RM, Roth KS: Metabolic Disease: A Guide to Early Recognition. Philadelphia, WB Saunders, 1983.
Fernandes J, Saudubray J-M, van den Berghe G (Eds): Inborn Metabolic Diseases: Diagnosis and Treatment, 2nd ed. Berlin, Springer-Verlag, 1995.
Jones KL: Smith's Recognizable Patterns of Human Malformation, 5th ed. Philadelphia, WB Saunders, 1997.
Lyon G, Adams RD, Kolodny EH (Eds): Neurology of Hereditary Metabolic Diseases of Children, 2nd ed. New York, McGraw-Hill, 1996.
McKusick VA: Mendelian Inheritance in Man: Catalogs of Human Genes and Genetic Disorders, 11th ed. Johns Hopkins University Press, Baltimore, 1994.
Nyhan WL, Sakati NO: Diagnostic Recognition of Genetic Disease. Philadelphia, Lea & Febiger, 1987.
Online Mendelian Inheritance in Man, OMIM (TM). Center for Medical Genetics, Johns Hopkins University (Baltimore, MD) and National Center for Biotechnology Information, National Library of Medicine (Bethesda, MD), 1996. World Wide Web URL: http://www.ncbi.nln.nih.gov/Omim/
Saudubray J-M, Charpentier C: Clinical phenotypes: Diagnosis/algorithms. *In* Scriver CR, Beaudet AL, Sly WS, et al (Eds): The Metabolic and Molecular Bases of Inherited Disease, 7th ed, vol 1. New York, McGraw-Hill 1995, pp 327–400.
Saudubray J-M, Ogier de Baulny H, Charpentier C: Clinical approach to inherited metabolic disorders. *In* Fernandes J, Saudubray JM, van den Berghe G (Eds): Inborn Metabolic Diseases: Diagnosis and Treatment, 2nd ed. Berlin, Springer-Verlag, pp 3–39, 1995.
Scriver CR, Beaudet AL, Sly WS, et al (Eds): The Metabolic and Molecular Bases of Inherited Disease, 7th ed. New York, McGraw-Hill, 1995.

CHAPTER 25

Inborn Errors of Carbohydrate, Ammonia, Amino Acid, and Organic Acid Metabolism

Gerard T. Berry

The inborn errors of carbohydrate, ammonia, amino acid, and organic acid metabolism have one factor in common: all may be associated with acute, life-threatening disease during the newborn period. The most notable exception in this broad group of small-molecule disorders is phenylketonuria (PKU). There are often few signs secondary to classic PKU in the first 6 months of life, underscoring the importance of newborn screening in establishing the diagnosis of this disease. As discussed in Chapter 24, a single biochemical genetic defect may be associated with more than one mode of presentation. This chapter presents the most common phenotype for each disorder. The disorders that comprise each group are outlined in Tables 25–1 to 25–4. The interrelationships among the major metabolites, biochemical cycles, and organelle pathways in the most critical facets of intermediary metabolism are simplified and depicted in Figure 25–1. The primary lactic acidosis and mitochondrial respiratory chain disorders, as well as the defects in fatty acid oxidation, are included in the section on inborn errors of organic acid metabolism.

INBORN ERRORS OF CARBOHYDRATE METABOLISM

Hereditary Galactosemia

Galactose-1-Phosphate-Uridyltransferase (GALT) Deficiency

Galactose-1-Phosphate + Uridine Diphosphate (UDP)
Glucose (UDPglucose) $\xrightarrow{\text{GALT}}$ UDPgalactose +
Glucose-1-Phosphate

Enzyme: Homodimer
Gene Location: Chromosome 9p13
Frequency: 1/35,000–60,000

CASE STUDY 1

A gravida 3, para 2 mother delivered a 10 lb, 3 oz male infant. On discharge from the nursery, the mother continued breast-feeding. The baby was noted to be jaundiced, with a total serum bilirubin of 28 mg/dL on day 4. He was readmitted to the local hospital, intravenous fluids were administered, and phototherapy was instituted. A sepsis workup was performed, and the infant was treated with ampicillin. A repeat serum total bilirubin was 24 mg/dL with a direct bilirubin of 1 mg/dL, and 3+ reducing substances were detected in a urine specimen. Because galactosemia was suspected, the baby was switched to Nutramigen formula. Serum

aspartate transaminase (AST) was 232 and gamma-glutamyl-transferase (GGT) was 132. On day 7, a trial of breast-feeding was resumed and urinary reducing substances again became positive. On day 8, a bleeding diathesis was noted and the prothrombin time (PT) and partial thromboplastin time (PTT) were greater than 30 and 150 minutes, respectively. Only a urine culture revealed the growth of *Escherichia coli*. The breast-feeding was again discontinued and ProSobee formula was started. A Beutler fluorescent spot test performed on a filter paper specimen revealed no fluorescence compatible with a diagnosis of hereditary galactosemia secondary to GALT deficiency. The infant's jaundice and laboratory abnormalities disappeared with the soy-based lactose-free formula regimen.

Following discharge, a repeat blood specimen was obtained for confirmation of the enzyme deficiency. However, instead of a quantitation of erythrocyte GALT activity, an erythrocyte galactokinase (GALK) analysis was performed by a commercial laboratory that not unexpectedly revealed normal activity. Although the parents were reassured by the testing result that the diagnosis of galactosemia was incorrect, they continued to administer the lactose-free formula. Over the next year of life, the infant demonstrated normal growth and development.

Subsequently, the mother became pregnant and delivered a female infant who was started on breast-feeding because the parents believed that galactosemia had been dismissed in the older infant. The newborn female infant began to develop jaundice with vomiting. Despite the use of broad-spectrum antibiotics, she died of *E. coli* sepsis on day 13. A Beutler fluorescent spot test revealed no GALT activity compatible with classic galactosemia. Quantitation of erythrocyte GALT activity in the male confirmed the severe reduction in enzyme activity, and a GALT molecular analysis on DNA extracted from blood showed that the two siblings were homoallelic for the most common GALT gene defect, the Q188R mutation.

The three enzymes of the galactose metabolic pathway that are responsible for the rapid hepatic conversion of galactose to glucose following ingestion of dietary lactose are GALK, GALT, and UDP galactose-4-epimerase (Fig. 25–2). All three enzymes have been associated with inborn errors of galactose metabolism (Segal and Berry, 1996). However, when one refers to the disease galactosemia or hereditary galactosemia in clinical medicine, the reference is usually to GALT deficiency. This is the most common of

TABLE 25–1

Inborn Errors of Carbohydrate Metabolism

Hereditary galactosemia
Glycogen storage diseases
Hereditary fructose intolerance
Fructose-1,6-bisphosphatase deficiency

TABLE 25–3

Inborn Errors of Amino Acid Metabolism

Maple syrup urine disease
Hereditary tyrosinemia type 1
Nonketotic hyperglycinemia
Methionine synthetase deficiency
Phenylketonuria

these disorders and probably the most common of the inborn errors of carbohydrate metabolism that come to clinical attention in the newborn period. The clinical syndrome of transferase-deficiency galactosemia has changed in the past 15 years since the advent of newborn screening for galactosemia. In the past, a severe multiorgan toxicity syndrome was a much more common occurrence, associated with weeks of unlimited intake of lactose in the proprietary formula or breast milk. However, as Case Study 1 illustrates, the disease can be devastating even in the first 1 or 2 weeks of life because of *E. coli* sepsis.

The most common initial clinical sign is poor growth; vomiting and poor feeding also occur in most of the patients. Jaundice may be present in the first few weeks of life and persist. Initially the jaundice may be due to indirect hyperbilirubinemia, only later to be associated with an elevation of direct bilirubin as well. While on lactose, many infants with galactosemia present in the first 2 to 3 weeks with only poor feeding and growth, jaundice, and mild irritability or lethargy. With continual ingestion, multiorgan toxicity syndrome ensues, associated with liver disease that may progress to cirrhosis with portal hypertension, splenomegaly, ascites, renal tubular dysfunction, sometimes the full-blown renal Fanconi syndrome, anemia primarily due to decreased red blood cell (RBC) survival, lethargy, and brain edema associated with a bulging fontanel. Two clinical phenomena deserve further mention: cataracts and *E. coli* sepsis. Cataracts may be evident in the first few weeks of life but often they are detected after 2 weeks of age. However, some infants are born with congenital cataracts that are associated with abnormalities of the embryonal lens: these are central in nature and require slit-lamp examination for documentation. *E. coli* sepsis is the most devastating complication in the newborn period; the mortality rate is higher than 50%. The reason that *E. coli* or gram-negative bacteria are unique for newborns with GALT deficiency remains unknown.

After initiation of a lactose-free diet in the newborn period, usually the problems related to liver and kidney

disease, anemia, and brain edema disappear unless there has been severe organ damage such as hepatic cirrhosis. Most infants begin to grow and develop at a normal rate. However, we know now that even prospectively treated patients may manifest long-term complications. They relate to speech defects, delays in language acquisition, learning problems in school, and hypergonadotropic hypogonadism in most of the females. The cause of these so-called dietary-independent complications is unknown. Patients with galactosemia must stay on a lactose-restricted diet for their entire lives. When the infant is initially diagnosed, either through the newborn screening program or because of the recognition of clinical signs, blood galactose levels may be as high as 5 to 20 mM, RBC galactose-1-phosphate level is significantly elevated, as are urine galactitol levels. During this phase of severe hypergalactosemia, positive reducing

TABLE 25–2

Inborn Errors of Ammonia Metabolism

Ornithine transcarbamylase deficiency
Argininosuccinicaciduria
Citrullinemia
Carbamylphosphate synthetase deficiency
Transient hyperammonemia of the newborn

TABLE 25–4

Inborn Errors of Organic Acid Metabolism

Methylmalonic acidemia
Propionic acidemia
Isovaleric acidemia
Multiple carboxylase deficiency
Glutaric acidemia type 1

Fatty acid oxidation disorders
  Glutaric acidemia type 2
  Very-long-chain acyl-CoA dehydrogenase deficiency
  Medium-chain acyl-CoA dehydrogenase deficiency
  Short-chain acyl-CoA dehydrogenase deficiency
  Long-chain 3-hydroxy acyl-CoA dehydrogenase deficiency
  Carnitine transporter defect
  Carnitine palmitoyltransferase type I deficiency
  Carnitine palmitoyltransferase type II deficiency
  Acylcarnitine translocase deficiency

Defects in ketone metabolism
  Ketothiolase deficiency
  Succinyl-CoA: 3-ketoacid-CoA transferase deficiency
  3-Hydroxy-3-methylglutaryl-CoA lyase deficiency

Primary lactic acidoses
  Pyruvate dehydrogenase complex deficiency
  Pyruvate carboxylase deficiency
  Phosphoenolpyruvate carboxykinase deficiency
  Mitochondrial respiratory/electron transport chain defects
    Barth syndrome
    Pearson syndrome
    Leigh disease

CoA, coenzyme A.

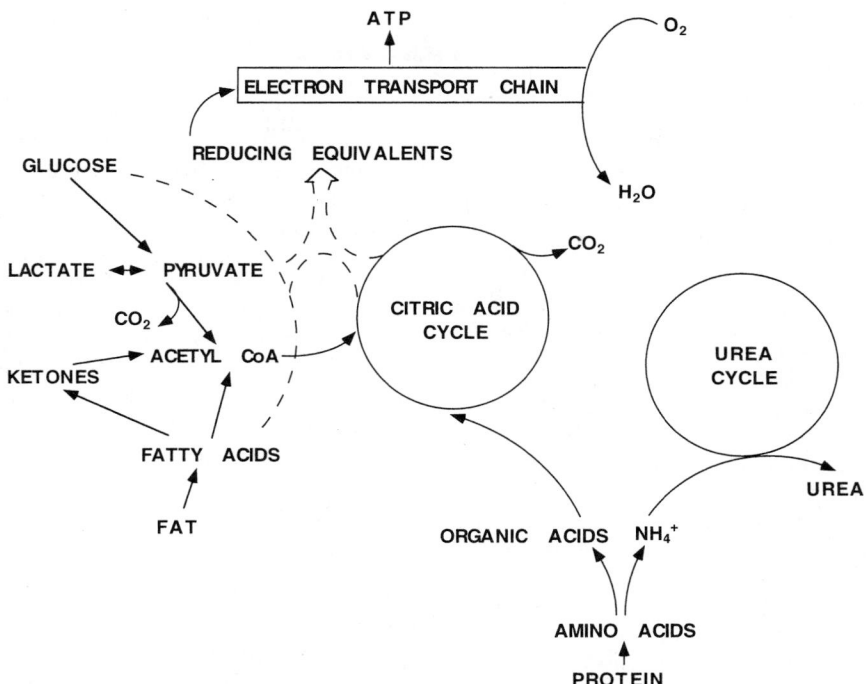

FIGURE 25–1. Intermediary metabolism interactions among the glycolytic, citric acid, mitochondrial respiratory/electron transport chain (ETC), amino acid, organic acid, and urea cycle pathways. Defects in these primarily catabolic pathways are the chief source of inborn errors of metabolism that involve the small, simple—not the large—complex molecules. ATP, adenosine triphosphate. (Adapted from Cowett RM [Ed]: Principles of Perinatal-Neonatal Metabolism, 2nd ed. New York, Springer-Verlag, 1998, p 800.)

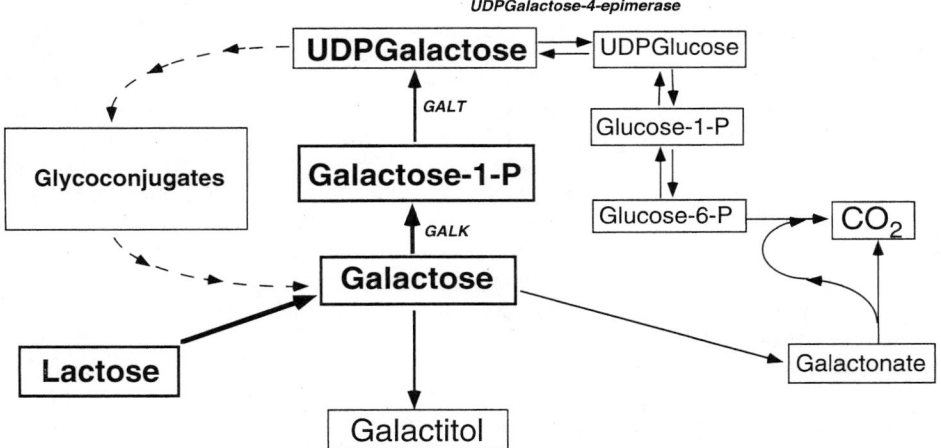

FIGURE 25–2. The important reactions in the galactose metabolic pathway are shown in relation to exogenous, via lactose primarily, and endogenous de novo synthesis of galactose. The reactions catalyzed by enzymes that have not been well delineated or are purported to exist are shown by broken or dotted lines. Carbon skeletons exit the galactose pool via galactokinase (GALK)-mediated conversion to galactose-1-phosphate (galactose-1-P), aldose reductase–mediated conversion to galactitol, and as galactonate. In patients with severe galactose-1-P-uridyltransferase (GALT) deficiency, there is little or no conversion of galactose-1-P to uridine diphosphate galactose (UDPgalactose). The epimerization of UDPglucose to UDPgalactose by UDPgalactose-4-epimerase, the utilization of UDPgalactose in the synthesis of glycoconjugates such as glycoproteins, and their subsequent degradation may constitute the pathways of de novo synthesis of galactose. (Adapted from Berry GT, Nissim I, Gibson JB, et al: Quantitative assessment of whole body galactose metabolism in galactosemic patients. Eur J Pediatr 156:S44, 1997.)

substances are present in the urine. One of the first abnormalities to be detected—albuminuria—reflects a poorly understood renal glomerular component. This develops within 24 to 48 hours of ingestion of lactose and disappears as quickly following galactose elimination. In addition to hyperbilirubinemia there may be mild to severe elevations of serum alanine transferase (ALT) and AST levels and various abnormalities related to renal tubular dysfunction, such as hyperchloremic metabolic acidosis, hypophosphatemia, glucosuria, and generalized aminoaciduria. Vitreous hemorrhages are newly recognized complications in the newborn period. After the patient is placed on a lactose-free diet, the RBC galactose-1-phosphate levels in patients with classic galactosemia fall but never return to the normal range and remain mildly elevated for the lifetime of the patient. This is also true for the urinary metabolite galactitol and may be related to endogenous galactose production (Berry et al, 1995).

The deficiency of the enzyme GALT may be detected in RBCs in patients with most common forms of galactosemia. The newborn screening programs in various states use either an enzymatic and/or a metabolite screening method. When metabolites are assayed, the level of galactose-1-phosphate or total galactose and galactose-1-phosphate in RBCs are usually measured. Most of the gene defects that produce galactosemia are now known; therefore, some patients or siblings may be screened for the disease or for being a carrier by genotype analyses. Liver disease of any cause and congenital hepatic vascular shunts may lead to impaired galactose tolerance and a positive newborn screening test for galactosemia (Gitzelmann et al, 1992; Matsumoto et al, 1993).

Glycogen Storage Diseases

The glycogen storage diseases (GSD) may be divided between those types that primarily affect the liver and those that affect striated muscle (Chen and Burchell, 1995; Cornblath and Schwartz, 1991; Fernandes, 1989; Hirschhorn, 1995). With some forms, such as GSD type 3, or debrancher disease, both striated muscle as well as the liver may be affected. According to European prevalence data, the overall frequency of GSD is 1 in 20,000 to 25,000 (Chen and Burchell, 1995). With the exception of GSD type 2, or Pompe disease (a lysosomal defect), most of the patients with glycogenosis do not come to clinical attention in the newborn period. As the following report of GSD type 1a illustrates, however, there are exceptions. Patients with the three most common forms of GSD—types I, III, and VI—have a phenotype that mimics a small-molecule disorder because glucose homeostasis is affected.

Glucose-6-Phosphatase Deficiency

Glucose-6-Phosphate + H_2O → Glucose + Phosphate

Enzyme: Heterodimer (Catalytic and Regulatory Subunit)
Catalytic Subunit Gene Location: Chromosome 17
Frequency: 1/100,000

CASE STUDY 2

A 6 lb, 11 oz male infant was born to consanguineous Lebanese parents. Despite hypoglycemia for which he received intravenous glucose in the first 48 hours of life, the baby was discharged from the newborn nursery on day 2. He was fed Carnation Good Start formula. At 10 weeks of age, he developed gastroenteritis and was treated with Pedialyte at home. He was subsequently admitted to a local hospital because of respiratory distress associated with fever and lethargy. Laboratory studies revealed a blood glucose of 5 mg/dL, serum total CO_2 of 5 mEq/L, an increased anion gap, and 3+ ketonuria. A chest radiograph was normal. The baby was intubated, placed on ventilatory support and given intravenous fluids with glucose, sodium bicarbonate, and antibiotics. He was subsequently transferred to the neonatal intensive care unit (NICU) at Children's Hospital of Philadelphia. On physical examination, the patient was lethargic with generalized hypotonia and the liver was enlarged. The liver edge was full, rounded, and palpated 7 cm below the right costal margin with a span >10 cm. A liver ultrasound revealed hepatomegaly with a coarsened echogenic texture. On the day of admission, a seizure was detected, associated with focal leg and jaw twitching and an increase in blood pressure. There was no recurrence following phenobarbital administration, which was later discontinued. Urine organic acid quantitation revealed increased excretion of 3-hydroxybutyrate, acetoacetate, and lactate. A plasma amino acid quantitation showed alanine to be elevated at 769 μM (normal 88 to 440). After correction of the acid-base imbalance and hypoglycemia, he appeared to stabilize on intravenous fluids with glucose. He was subsequently restarted on a proprietary formula, the Carnation Good Start formula. A sepsis workup proved negative. Antibiotics were discontinued. A head magnetic resonance imaging (MRI) scan was normal. Subsequently, a Destrostix was found to be 46 mg/dL 4 hours after a feeding. The blood lactate level was slightly increased at 2.2 mM (normal <2.0). The liver remained enlarged and a liver biopsy was performed. The histologic examination revealed microsteatosis. A periodic acid–Schiff (PAS) stain was positive but sensitive to diastase. Electron microscopy revealed increased glycogen. The glycogen content in the liver was increased at 6.8% (control, 2.3%). Glucose-6-phosphatase activity was measured in frozen liver homogenate and found to be markedly decreased (0.4 units; control, 3.8 units) compatible with glucose-6-phosphatase deficiency, specifically glycogen storage disease type 1A. A fasting study was performed that demonstrated that the infant developed a blood glucose level in the 40 mg/dL range or lower 4 hours after a bottle feeding. This was associated with an increase in blood lactate levels. The serum uric acid and triglyceride levels were also elevated. The baby was stabilized on ProSobee formula given every 2 hours during the day and a continuous glucose infusion administered at night via nasogastric tube. The baby was discharged on this regimen. The parents were instructed on home glucose monitoring. On discharge the liver remained palpable to the level of the umbilicus, but the spleen was not enlarged. There were no further episodes of symptomatic hypoglycemia. By 4 months of age, the weight was at the 95th percentile and the length at the 90th percentile.

GSD type 1 is due to a decreased activity of glucose-6-phosphatase, the enzyme that is perched at the terminus of both glycogenolysis and gluconeogenesis. Several different biochemical abnormalities can result in this phenotype, now classified as GSD types 1a, 1b, and 1c. The enzyme that resides on the anticytoplasmic side of internal membrane spaces of the hepatocyte catalyzes the hydrolysis of glucose-6-phosphate to glucose and phosphate. Impairments in the transport of either glucose-6-phosphate or phosphate may result in decreased function of this enzyme. The major clinical findings are poor growth and enlarged abdominal girth, hepatomegaly, and any of the signs that may be related to hypoglycemia. The major laboratory findings are fasting hypoglycemia, ketosis, lactic acidosis, hyperlipidemia (specifically, hypertriglyceridemia), and hyperuricemia. In patients with type 1b disease due to a defect in the microsomal transporter of glucose-6-phosphate, there may be a history of recurrent infections owing to neutropenia and defective neutrophil function. Diagnosis is based on hepatic enzyme analyses or, in some instances, molecular diagnostic testing (Burchell and Waddell, 1993; Chen and Burchell, 1995). The most important aspect of therapy is to prevent brain damage from hypoglycemia and growth failure. The mainstay of therapy is frequent feedings and restriction of lactose and sucrose (Chen and Burchell, 1995; Fernandes, 1989). The use of continuous nasogastric feedings or uncooked cornstarch, particularly during the night, has significantly improved the care of these children, and although it does not correct all the biochemical perturbations, it does improve growth and can prevent hypoglycemic spells.

Lysosomal α-Glucosidase Deficiency

$$Glycogen_{(n)} + H_2O \rightarrow Glycogen_{(n-1)} + Glucose$$

Enzyme: α-1,4-Glucosidase Monomer
Location: Chromosome 17 q23
Frequency: 1/100,000

GSD type 2, or Pompe disease, is a deficiency of the lysosomal enzyme alpha-glucosidase. In the newborn period the main clinical finding relates to heart disease. There is usually marked cardiomegaly and a typical abnormal electrocardiogram, with biventricular hypertrophy and a short PR interval. Decreased cardiac output may lead to heart failure and passive congestion. Infants may also have generalized hypotonia not just because of heart failure but also because of skeletal myopathy. There is increased deposition of glycogen within striated muscle. Except because of passive congestion, the liver is not usually enlarged. Diagnosis is based on muscle enzyme analysis

(Hirschhorn, 1995). Cardiac transplantation has been performed to prevent death in infancy.

Hereditary Fructose Intolerance
Fructose-1,6-Bisphosphate Aldolase B Deficiency

Fructose-1-Phosphate + H$_2$O →
  Dihydroxyacetone Phosphate + Glyceraldehyde

Enzyme: Homotetramer
Gene Location: Chromosome 9q13-q32
Frequency: Very Rare, Except Approximately 1/20,000 in Swiss

Hereditary fructose intolerance is secondary to a deficiency of the enzyme fructose-1,6-bisphosphate aldolase (Cornblath and Schwartz, 1991; Gitzelmann et al, 1995). There are different isoforms of aldolases in human tissues. The enzyme deficient in this disease results in an impairment in the conversion of fructose-1-phosphate to glyceraldehyde and dihydroxyacetone phosphate and, to a much lesser degree, fructose-1,6-bisphosphate to glyceraldehyde-3-phosphate and dihydroxyacetone phosphate. It is inherited as an autosomal recessive trait. Manifestations of clinical disease depend on sucrose or fructose ingestion. Thus, it usually does not come to clinical attention in the newborn period unless fruits are started early in the diet or the patients are placed on a formula that contains sucrose or fructose. The major clinical findings include poor feeding, vomiting, loose stools, poor growth, hepatomegaly, and any sign that could be related to hypoglycemia. Classically, the infants become ill soon after ingesting fructose. The acute signs may include pallor and lethargy, an altered state of central nervous system (CNS) function due to hypoglycemia. The major laboratory findings consist of hypoglycemia; hypophosphatemia; elevations of serum ALT and AST, including any of the findings that may be associated with hepatocellular disease per se; and reducing substances in the urine. The liver disease may be severe. Patients may be jaundiced with hyperbilirubinemia. There may be a bleeding diathesis. In addition to liver disease, renal tubular dysfunction may lead to full-blown renal Fanconi syndrome. Thus, one may detect metabolic acidosis due to a renal tubular acidosis, hypophosphatemia, impaired urate handling, spillage of glucose as well as fructose into the urine, and generalized aminoaciduria. It is believed that the severity of the clinical findings is related to the amount of fructose ingested. Infants, however, probably because of decreased intake, may manifest only the signs of poor growth and have few findings related to liver disease, except perhaps intermittent hypertransaminasemia. The suspicion of the physician is crucial in establishing the diagnosis. An intravenous fructose test may be performed under controlled circumstances, such as in the NICU or clinical research center, to determine whether after 15 to 30 minutes of fructose administration there is a decrease in serum phosphate and glucose levels and an elevation in the serum AST and ALT levels. In the past, diagnosis depended on enzyme analysis, but molecular diagnostic testing is more available now. The treatment consists of elimination of dietary fructose and sucrose.

Fructose-1,6-Bisphosphatase Deficiency

Fructose-1,6-Bisphosphatase Deficiency

Fructose-1,6-Bisphosphate + H_2O →
$$\text{Fructose-6-Phosphate + Phosphate}$$

Enzyme: Homotetramer
Gene Location: Unknown
Frequency: Very Rare

The deficiency of the enzyme fructose-1,6-bisphosphatase results in an inability to hydrolyze fructose-1,6-bisphosphate to fructose-6-phosphate (Baker and Winegrad, 1970; Gitzelmann et al, 1995). This is a key enzyme in gluconeogenesis. The main clinical features of this disease are hypoglycemia and the signs related to glucose deprivation in the CNS. The disease is primarily brought on by fasting, not by fructose ingestion, although fructose may exacerbate the abnormalities induced by fasting adaptation. Enlargement of the liver due to diffuse steatosis may be present only during periods of fasting and enhanced gluconeogenesis. The laboratory findings consists of hypoglycemia, ketosis, and lactic acidosis. The acidosis due to accumulation of lactic, 3-hydroxybutyric, and acetoacetic acids may be severe in this disease. Diagnosis depends on enzymatic analysis. The therapy primarily consists of avoidance of fasting.

INBORN ERRORS OF AMMONIA METABOLISM
Ornithine Transcarbamylase (OTC) Deficiency

$$\text{Ornithine + Carbamylphosphate} \xrightarrow{\text{OTC}} \text{Citrulline}$$

Enzyme: Homotrimer
Gene Location: Chromosome X p21.1
Frequency: 1/70,000–100,000

Argininosuccinate Lyase (ASAL) Deficiency

$$\text{Argininosuccinate} \xrightarrow{\text{ASAL}} \text{Arginine + Fumarate}$$

Enzyme: Homotetramer
Gene Location: Chromosome 7 cen-p21
Frequency: 1/70,000–100,000

Argininosuccinate Synthetase (ASAS) Deficiency

$$\text{Citrulline + Aspartate} \xrightarrow{\text{ASAS}} \text{Argininosuccinate}$$

Enzyme: Homotetramer
Gene Location: Chromosome 9q34
Frequency: 1/70,000–100,000

Carbamylphosphate Synthetase I (CPSI) Deficiency

NH_3 + Adenosine triphosphate (ATP) +
$$HCO_3 \xrightarrow{\text{CPSI}} \text{Carbamylphosphate}$$

Enzyme: Homodimer
Gene Location: Chromosome 2p
Frequency: 1/70,000–100,000

| CASE STUDY 3 |

A male infant born at term following an uncomplicated pregnancy, labor, and delivery was noted to be lethargic with poor feeding at 2 days of age. Laboratory studies showed his plasma ammonium level to be >1500 µM. A plasma amino acid quantitation revealed a massively elevated level of glutamine (2640 µM, normal 422 to 849) and alanine (2540 µM, normal 120 to 449) and an undetectable level of citrulline. The most likely diagnosis was the X-linked disease ornithine transcarbamylase (OTC) deficiency in a male infant. Because of hyperammonemic coma, arrangements were immediately made for hemodialysis. Prior to catheter placements, the infant was administered an intravenous bolus of sodium benzoate and sodium phenylacetate, both at 250 mg/kg per 24 hours. Intravenous arginine hydrochloride at 400 mg/kg per 24 hours was administered as a continuous infusion. In addition, the infant was given 10% glucose intravenously to suppress catabolism. The medications were continued during hemodialysis. After several hours of hemodialysis, the plasma ammonium level had reduced to the 200-µM range and peritoneal dialysis was instituted. There was a more gradual attainment of normalization of the plasma alanine and glutamine levels. After 3 days of peritoneal dialysis therapy, the plasma ammonium levels were within the normal range. There was resolution of the severe encephalopathy. The infant was discharged at 2½ weeks of age on a very-low-protein diet (0.7 g/kg per day) with supplementation of essential amino acids (0.7 g/kg per day), oral sodium benzoate (250 mg/kg per day), sodium phenylacetate (250 mg/kg per day) and arginine (174 mg/kg per day). The infant suffered no further episodes of hyperammonemia during the first year of life, and at 15 months of age underwent a liver transplantation. The OTC activity in the liver that was removed was undetectable. An analysis of genomic DNA revealed a CGA to CAA mutation in codon 141 of exon 5 of the OTC gene, thus producing an arginine to glutamine substitution (R141Q), which is a severe mutation involving the active site of the OTC enzyme. Following transplantation the therapy was discontinued, and while the patient has been on a regular protein diet, plasma ammonium levels have completely normalized. Plasma citrulline levels remained undetectable.

Genetic diseases involving each of the five enzymes of the hepatic mitochondrial urea cycle have been described (Brusilow and Horwich, 1995). In the urea cycle, carbamylphosphate, which carries the nitrogen atom from ammonia, condenses with ornithine to form citrulline in a reaction catalyzed by the enzyme ornithine transcarbamylase (OTC), which is the most common defect among the inborn errors of the urea cycle. Citrulline subsequently interacts with aspartate to form argininosuccinate (ASA) and, in the process, another waste nitrogen atom is shuttled into the urea cycle substrate. Arginine is formed from ASA and the terminal enzyme in this cycle, arginase, converts arginine to urea for urinary excretion while regenerating ornithine to complete the cycle (Fig. 25–3). The first step in this cycle involves the synthesis of carbamylphosphate, and this reaction, catalyzed by carbamylphosphate synthetase type I (CPS-I), requires an activator, N-acetylglutamate, which is synthesized from acetyl coenzyme A (CoA) and glutamate via the enzyme N-acetylglutamate synthetase (NAGS). Rare patients may have reduced activity of NAGS. With the exception of arginase deficiency, each of these enzymes has been associated with disease in the newborn period. Clinical presentation in the newborn period is similar for all these defects (Batshaw, 1984). Almost all the infants are well in the first 12 to 24 hours of life and then begin to manifest poor feeding, vomiting, hyperventilation, lethargy, and coma, usually with seizures. When these diseases are untreated, they are almost always fatal. The treatment requires specific therapy to lower the waste nitrogen burden, including the toxic substance ammonia. Additional clinical findings include increased intracranial pressure. As with maple syrup urine disease (MSUD) the severe encephalopathic and life-threatening features may be related to brain edema. Chronic hepatomegaly has been reported in patients with argininosuccinicaciduria, whereas in the other urea cycle disorders, hepatomegaly is evident only during hyperammonemic episodes. Histologic examination of the liver shows modest fatty infiltration and fibrosis. Children with argininosuccinicaciduria may also manifest a specific abnormality of the hair, termed *trichorrhexis nodosa*.

The main laboratory finding in the urea cycle enzyme defects (UCEDs) is an elevated plasma ammonium level. Plasma ammonium levels may vary in different laboratories. In general, however, with automated chemistry testing for ammonia, the normal plasma values in older infants, children, and adults range between 10 and 35 μmol/L. However, in the Clinical Chemistry Laboratory at Children's Hospital of Philadelphia, the normal plasma ammonium value in newborns may be as high as 110 μmol/L. In patients with newborn-onset UCEDs, the plasma ammonium levels are often higher than 1000 or 2000 μmol/L when they are acutely ill. Patients with UCED usually do not have metabolic acidosis unless they are in a terminal state with vascular collapse or respiratory failure. Instead, the characteristic acid-base abnormality associated with hyperammonemia is respiratory alkalosis due to the effect of ammonia on the respiratory control centers in the brain stem. The various UCEDs can usually be distinguished by the pattern and levels of plasma amino acids. Because citrulline is the product of the CPS-I and OTC reactions and the substrate for argininosuccinate synthetase (ASAS), its value is critical. In newborn-onset CPS-I and OTC deficiencies, plasma citrulline concentrations are zero to trace. With *OTC deficiency* there is increased urinary orotate excretion secondary to carbamylphosphate accumulation and pyrimidine synthesis. With *CPS-I deficiency*, carbamylphosphate production is decreased or absent and orotate excretion is decreased. Theoretically, a defect in

the production of the activator of CPS-I, namely NAG, resembles a partial CPS-I deficiency. In citrullinemia, the plasma citrulline concentrations are markedly elevated. With argininosuccinicaciduria, plasma citrulline concentration is moderately elevated in the 100 to 300 μmol/L range and can be readily detected during an analysis of plasma by amino acid column chromatography.

Because infants with these disorders have an impaired ability to excrete waste nitrogen as urea, therapy initially centered around the reduction of nitrogen intake by decreasing dietary protein and providing essential amino acids or the ketoacid analogues. This approach theoretically permits adequate growth without an excess nitrogen load. Excessive protein leads to hyperammonemia. However, too great a restriction of protein during long-term therapy leads to poor growth. Actually, this approach fails when the patient is in negative nitrogen balance, as occurs in the catastrophically ill infant presenting in the first week of life with massive hyperammonemia. For such an infant with hyperammonemia and coma, the mainstay of therapy is dialysis treatment. Hemodialysis is the most effective way of reducing plasma ammonium levels because the clearance of ammonia is greatest (Rutledge et al, 1990). Next in efficacy is continuous arteriovenous hemofiltration (CAVH) (Thompson et al, 1991). Although the clearance rate is not as great as with hemodialysis, it has the added benefit of not being administered intermittently and there is less likelihood of major swings in intravascular volume that may exacerbate an already catabolic state. Ammonia clearance with peritoneal dialysis is only approximately one tenth that of CAVH and is not recommended for specific UCED therapy in the newborn period.

While the intensive care personnel are waiting for dialysis therapy to be instituted, alternate waste nitrogen therapy (Brusilow and Batshaw, 1979; Brusilow et al, 1979; Brusilow 1991) using intravenous sodium benzoate, sodium phenylacetate, and for patients with ASAS and ASAL deficiencies, arginine hydrochloride should be initiated.[*] In addition, patients with OTC and CPS-I deficiency should also receive intravenous arginine hydrochloride, since body arginine pools can begin to deplete as arginine becomes an essential amino acid with a complete block in cycle function (Brusilow, 1984). The plasma arginine levels are usually low in all sick newborns with UCED. Unless corrected, arginine deficiency accentuates the hyperammonemia by promoting negative nitrogen balance and, theoretically, by failing to provide its usual stimulation of NAGS. A second role of arginine is to stimulate alternate pathways of waste nitrogen excretion. It does so by promoting synthesis and excretion of citrulline and ASA in citrullinemia and argininosuccinicaciduria, respectively. Argininosuccinate contains both waste nitrogen atoms destined for excretion as urea. It has a renal clearance rate equal to the glomerular filtration rate, provided it is continuously synthesized and excreted. Accordingly, ASA should serve as an effective substitute for urea as a waste nitrogen product.

Like ASA, citrulline can be a means to excrete waste nitrogen, but it contains only the one nitrogen atom derived from ammonium, lacking the second nitrogen derived from

---

[*]The medications as well as the proper doses for a bolus and 24-hour sustaining infusion are available from Ucyclyd Pharma (Hunt Valley, MD).

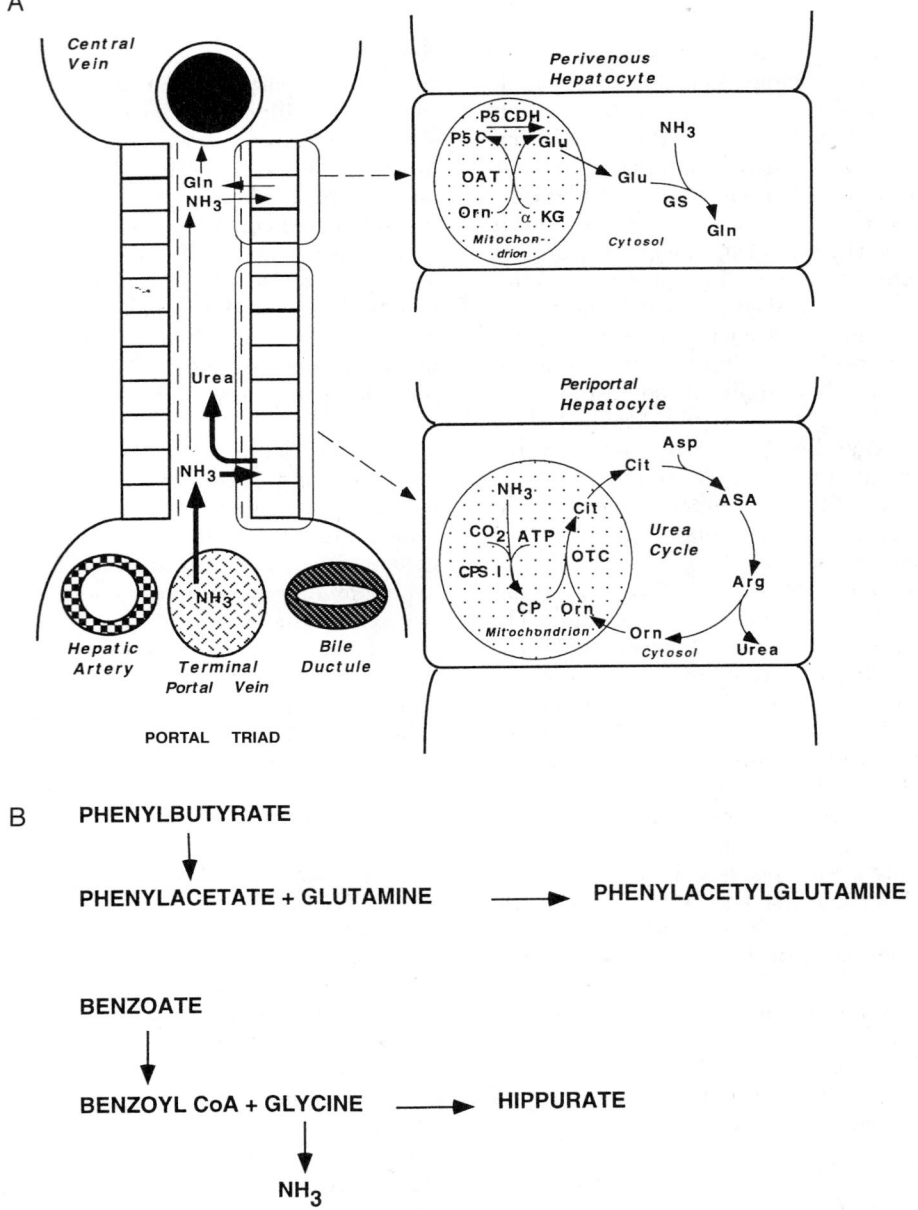

A

B

PHENYLBUTYRATE

PHENYLACETATE + GLUTAMINE ──────► **PHENYLACETYLGLUTAMINE**

BENZOATE

BENZOYL CoA + GLYCINE ──────► **HIPPURATE**

NH_3

FIGURE 25–3. *A,* Depicted is the nonhomogeneous distribution of enzymes involved in ammonia metabolism in the hepatocytes of an acinar sinusoid as they are linearly distributed from the portal triad to the region of the central vein or terminal hepatic venule. The specific enzymatic reactions are shown for an individual periportal and perivenous hepatocyte. The glutamine synthetase (GS) and ornithine aminotransferase (OAT) enzyme activities are expressed exclusively in the one to three cell layers surrounding the central vein, that is, the region of zone 3 of the liver lobule, whereas the urea cycle enzymes are concentrated within the periportal hepatocytes. However, the urea cycle enzyme activities are higher in zone 1 immediately surrounding the portal triad than in the middle zone 2. The hepatocytes are shown as squares, the hepatic mitochondria as shaded circles, and the lining of the space of Disse as the interrupted lines on either side of the linear array of hepatocytes. The abbreviations used to denote the metabolites or enzymes are as follows: NH_3, ammonia; CO_2, CO_2 or bicarbonate; ATP, adenosine triphosphate; CP, carbamyl phosphate; Orn, ornithine; Cit, citrulline; Asp, aspartate; ASA, argininosuccinate; Arg, arginine; α-KG, alpha-ketoglutarate; P5C, pyrroline 5-carboxylate; Glu, glutamate; Gln, glutamine; CPS-I, carbamyl phosphate synthetase type 1; OAT, ornithine aminotransferase; P5CDH, pyrroline-5-carboxylate dehydrogenase; and GS, glutamine synthetase. *B,* The medications, sodium phenylacetate or phenylbutyrate and sodium benzoate, promote alternate waste nitrogen disposal by participating in these two mitochondrial reactions. (Adapted from Tuchman M, Lichenstein GR, Rajagopal BS, et al: Hepatic glutamine synthetase deficiency in fatal hyperammonemia after lung transplantation. Ann Intern Med 127:447, 1997.)

aspartate. Citrulline also has a more limited urinary excretory capacity than ASA. Thus, therapy with arginine is less effective for citrullinemia. With citrullinemia and the other urea cycle disorders, arginine therapy is combined with sodium benzoate and sodium phenylacetate, both of which promote excretion of waste nitrogen. Sodium benzoate is conjugated with glycine to form hippurate, which is cleared by the kidney at five times the glomerular filtration rate (see Fig. 25–3). Theoretically, 1 mol of waste nitrogen is synthesized and excreted as hippurate for each mole of benzoate ingested. The hippurate synthetic mechanism resides primarily in the hepatic mitochondria and depends on an intact mitochondrial energy system for adenosine triphosphate (ATP) synthesis. The glycine consumed in this reaction can be replaced by either serine or the glycine cleavage pathway. Sodium phenylacetate, as well as sodium phenylbutyrate, which is used for chronic therapy in the absence of sodium benzoate, conjugates with glutamine to form phenylacetylglutamine, which is excreted by the kidney (see Fig. 25–3). Sodium phenylbutyrate is converted to phenylacetate in the liver. Glutamine contains two nitrogen atoms, whereas glycine contains one. Two moles of waste nitrogen are removed for each mole of phenylacetate administered. This acetylation reaction occurs in the kidney and the liver.

The outcome for patients with severe newborn-onset CPS-I and OTC deficiency is poor. Sometimes, even dialysis therapy cannot rescue severely affected male infants with X-linked OTC deficiency in the first few days of life. Prospectively administered alternate pathway therapy in conjunction with high-calorie administration usually prevents death and severe hyperammonemia in these patients. Even after institution of successful therapy, the morbidity and mortality are high in such patients. At the present time, liver transplantation is recommended for patients with CPS and OTC deficiencies who present in the newborn period and have almost no residual enzyme activity. Alternate pathway therapy has led to a 92% 1-year survival rate in newborns who recover from hyperammonemic coma, but most of the survivors are mentally retarded (Msall et al, 1984). There is a significant correlation between the duration of newborn hyperammonemic coma and the D.Q. score at 12 months of age (Msall et al, 1984). Four of five reported children whose duration of coma was 2 days or less had normal I.Q. scores, whereas all seven children whose duration of coma was 5 days or longer were severely mentally retarded. This fact points to the devastating effects of prolonged newborn hyperammonemic coma and the importance of early diagnosis and treatment. Mutational analysis of DNA is available for most of these disorders (Brusilow and Horwich, 1995). If the lesion in a particular family is known, prenatal diagnosis using direct DNA analysis is also feasible. With the exception of OTC deficiency, all the UCEDs are inherited as autosomal recessive traits.

Transient Hyperammonemia of the Newborn

Transient hyperammonia of the newborn (THAN) is a distinct clinical syndrome that was first identified by Ballard and colleagues in 1978. The disease usually develops in premature infants during the course of treatment for respiratory distress syndrome. The plasma ammonium level may be enormously elevated, as high as that found in any of the patients with the most severe type of UCED. Its onset is usually in the first 24 hours after birth when the infant is undergoing mechanical ventilatory support. The babies can manifest all the signs associated with hyperammonemic coma. The diagnosis may be difficult to determine, however, because many of these same infants are receiving sedatives and muscle relaxants to optimize therapy of their life-threatening pulmonary disease. Important clues are the absence of deep tendon reflexes, absence of the normal newborn reflexes, and decreased or absent response to painful stimuli. As with hyperammonemic coma in the UCED, this medical emergency requires dialysis therapy.

The cause of this disease is unknown. The plasma amino acid levels are similar to those found in CPS-I or OTC deficiency. Investigators have hypothesized that the disorder may be caused by impaired hepatic mitochondrial energy production or shunting of portal blood away from the liver, such as in patent ductus venosis. However, patients with congenital portal shunting defects have been described with disturbances in liver function such as impaired galactose metabolism but who are not premature and who do not have life-threatening hyperammonemia (Gitzelmann et al, 1992; Matsumoto et al, 1993). The mortality rate in THAN is high. If the patients can be treated early and aggressively, they may survive the episode. There is no evidence that any of the survivors have suffered any further episodes of hyperammonemia; nor has there been any further evidence of impaired ammonia metabolism.

INBORN ERRORS OF AMINO ACID METABOLISM
Maple Syrup Urine Disease
Branched-Chain 2-Keto Dehydrogenase (BCKAD) Complex Deficiency

Leucine $\longleftrightarrow$ 2-Ketoisocaproate $\xrightarrow{\text{BCKAD}}$ Isovalerlyl-CoA

Isoleucine $\longleftrightarrow$ 2-Keto-3-Methylvalerate $\xrightarrow{\text{BCKAD}}$

2-Methylbutyryl-CoA

Valine $\longleftrightarrow$ 2-Ketoisovalerate $\xrightarrow{\text{BCKAD}}$ Isobutyryl-CoA

Enzyme: 6 Subunits
    BCKA Decarboxylase Subunits (E_1)
      2 α Subunits
      2 β Subunits
    1 Dihydrolipoyl Transacylase (E_2) Subunit
    1 Dihydrolipoyl Dehydrogenase (E_3) Subunit
    1 BCKAD Kinase Subunit
    1 BCKAD Phosphatase Subunit

Gene Locations: $E_1\alpha$ on Chromosome 1q13.1-q13.2
               $E_1\beta$ on Chromosome 6p21-p22
               E_2 on Chromosome 2p31
               E_3 on Chromosome 7q31-q32

Frequency: For MSUD, 1/185,000, Except for $E_1\alpha$ Deficiency, Approximately 1/176 in Pennsylvania Mennonites

MSUD is a rare inborn error of amino acid metabolism (Chuang and Shih, 1995; Menkes et al, 1954). It is inherited as an autosomal recessive trait and secondary to a deficiency of the enzyme BCKAD complex. This enzyme catalyzes the conversion of each of the 3-ketoacid derivatives of the branched-chain amino acids into their decarboxylated coenzyme metabolites within the mitochondria (Fig. 25–4). The disease occurs in fewer than 1 in 200,000 newborn infants around the world, but in the Mennonite communities of the United States it has a frequency somewhat higher than 1 in 200 due to a founder effect for a point mutation in the $E_1\alpha$ gene. In most of the patients around the world, as well as in the Mennonite community, the classic form of the disease occurs. This is associated with severe and catastrophic illness in the newborn period and usually results in death without specific medical intervention. Typically, the infants are well at birth and only after 2 or 3 days of ingestion of breast milk or formula do the babies begin to manifest poor feeding and spitting up. Lethargy becomes evident; the cry may be shrill and high pitched. There may be hypotonia alternating with hypertonia and ophistotonic posturing. The odor of maple syrup may be detected in the saliva, on the breath, in the urine and feces, and in cerumen obtained from the ear. The babies become more and more obtunded and eventually lapse into a deep coma. The anterior fontanel may be bulging. Seizures may develop. The life-threatening encephalopathic features may simply be related to brain edema (Lungarotti et al, 1982; Riviello et al, 1991). Laboratory findings consist of metabolic acidosis. The anion gap may be raised but not necessarily so. There is almost always ketonuria. The plasma ammonium levels are not usually elevated. The complete blood count (CBC) is not usually abnormal. The levels of the plasma branched-chain amino acids, leucine, isoleucine, and valine, are elevated, with striking elevation in leucine. The normal range for plasma leucine, isoleucine, and valine in the newborn period is 29 to 152, 11 to 87, and 71 to 236 μmol/L (or 0.4 to 2.0, 0.1 to 1.1, and 0.8 to 2.8 mg/dL), respectively. In these patients who are critically ill, the leucine levels may range between 1.9 and 6.9 mM (or 25 and 90 mg/dL). In the past, almost every newborn infant who was recognized to have MSUD and was in a severely decompensated state received peritoneal dialysis in a tertiary care center. The treatment was successful in most instances, but it did not allow for as rapid a rate of reduction in plasma branched-chain amino acid levels as with hemodialysis or CAVH (Rutledge et al, 1990; Thompson et al, 1991).

It is now clear that a nutritional approach works just as well as peritoneal dialysis in newborns (Berry et al, 1991;

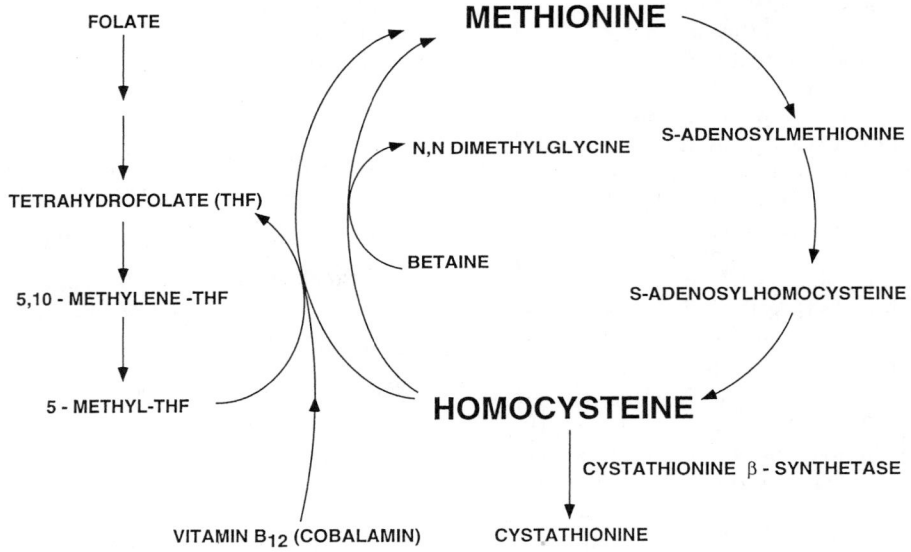

FIGURE 25–4. The pathways, metabolites, and vitamin cofactors important in the interconversion of methionine and homocysteine are shown in this abbreviated scheme of the transsulfuration pathway. In a methyl-transfer reaction, homocysteine is converted to methionine; the reaction is catalyzed by a cobalamin-containing enzyme, 5-methyl-tetrahydrofolate-homocysteine methyltransferase or methionine syntase. An alternate reaction involves betaine-homocysteine methyltransferase. Thus, vitamin B₁₂, as well as folate, are important vitamins in homocysteine and methionine metabolism. The 5,10-methylene tetrahydrofolate (THF) derived from dietary folate is converted to 5-methyl THF by the enzyme 5,10-methylene THF reductase. In classic homocystinuria the deficient enzyme is the cystathione β-synthetase, which catalyzes the conversion of homocysteine to cystathione, a precursor of cysteine. This pathway is readily operative in the adult so that cysteine is a nonessential amino acid. In newborn infants, however, synthesis of cysteine does not occur at the same rate as in adults. Adenosylmethionine-dependent methyl transfer may be extremely important in the central nervous system. Most of the patients who come to clinical attention in the newborn period have defects in the remethylation of homocysteine to methionine, and thus these patients may have a severe deficiency of adenosylmethionine in the brain and spinal cord.

Parini et al, 1993; Shih et al, 1975; Townsend and Kerr, 1982). This includes the use of a branched-chain amino acid–free modified parenteral nutrition therapy for infants as well as older children with acute metabolic decompensation (Berry et al, 1991). Usually, insulin therapy is also necessary to curtail the effects of catabolic stress (Berry et al, 1991; Wendel et al, 1982). Based on the rate of plasma leucine decline, we have found that this nutritional therapy is comparable to peritoneal dialysis when the plasma leucine levels are as high as 25 to 40 mg/dL. It is unclear, however, whether it is more beneficial to achieve a greater rate of reduction of the plasma branched-chain amino acids and their corresponding branched-chain ketoacids (BCKAs) by using CAVH or hemodialysis when the levels of leucine are in the 60 to 90 mg/dL range. Most patients who are successfully treated by 7 days of age do not have mental retardation. Patients whose diagnosis and therapy, however, are delayed, or perhaps even in those diagnosed in the first week of life but who have suffered such severe damage because of increased intracranial pressure, often have substantial decreases in their developmental quotient or I.Q., as well as signs compatible with spastic diplegia or quadriplegia.

The mainstay of long-term therapy for patients who survive the newborn period is a special formula devoid of the branched-chain amino acids. The amount of branched-chain amino acids necessary to sustain growth but maintain the plasma, leucine, isoleucine, and valine levels in the normal range is supplied with a regular proprietary formula in limited amounts. In the first week of life, this is about 100 mg of leucine per kilogram of body weight daily and 50 mg/kg daily of both isoleucine and valine. The branched-chain amino acid requirements and thus the rates of utilization of the branched-chain amino acids for protein accretion drop rapidly in the first year of life in conjunction with the decline in growth velocity in young infants. As with PKU, it is imperative that the administration of the special amino acid formula be carefully monitored with frequent plasma amino acid quantitations. One of the most common errors made in the treatment of MSUD is the failure to administer adequate amounts of supplemental isoleucine and valine solutions to maintain the normal plasma levels, because proprietary formulas alone do not always meet the needs of each growing baby (i.e., the adequate amounts of each branched-chain amino acid are not met by a formula alone). Deficiency of branched-chain amino acids may result in a severe exfoliative rash and anemia. The rash may mimic that of severe acrodermatitis enteropathica (Diliberti et al, 1973; Giacoia and Berry, 1993). As with many of the inborn errors of amino acid, organic acid, and ammonia metabolism, the infant under previous well control and in metabolic balance on diet therapy requires that protein administration be discontinued during periods of intercurrent infections because catabolism, possibly driven by counter-regulatory hormones or cytokines, triggers metabolic decompensation through release of BCKA from skeletal muscle. Metabolic decompensation is further exacerbated by poor nutritional intake. It is imperative that during these times adequate amounts of calories and fluids be maintained to prevent the crisis from escalating into a medical emergency. In selected instances, a molecular diagnosis may be undertaken and

is especially useful in targeted populations such as the Mennonites. Rarely, patients may have a defect in the E_2 component (Danner et al, 1985) or, as discussed in the following section, in the E_3 component.

Hereditary Tyrosinemia Type 1
Fumarylacetoacetate Hydrolase (FAH) Deficiency

$$\text{Fumarylacetoacetate} \xrightarrow{\text{FAH}} \text{Fumarate + Acetoacetate}$$

Enzyme: Homodimer
Gene Location: Chromosome 15q23-q25
Frequency: Very Rare, Except in French-Canadians in Quebec

Tyrosinemia type 1 is due to a deficiency of the enzyme FAH (Lindblad et al, 1977; Mitchell et al, 1995). This enzymatic reaction is distal in the phenylalanine and tyrosine pathway, and the disorder is actually an inborn error of organic acid metabolism, with hypertyrosinemia being a secondary and variable biochemical effect. This is a rare disease inherited in an autosomal recessive manner. The highest incidence is found in those of French-Canadian ancestry due to a founder effect (De Bracketeer and Larochelle, 1990). Two clinical phenotypes may be detected. The first occurs in early infancy and is a severe, usually fatal disease in which liver disease dominates the clinical picture. The second is a more chronic phenotype, with patients presenting with hypophosphatemic rickets related to renal Fanconi syndrome. These patients usually also have evidence of liver disease, albeit milder. Most of the patients with the severe liver disease phenotype do not come to clinical attention in the newborn period. Careful search, however, may reveal the laboratory findings compatible with this disease even in newborn infants (Hostetter et al, 1983). When the disease does present in the newborn period, the abnormalities are related to liver disease. Like hereditary fructose intolerance and hereditary galactosemia, this is one of the inborn errors of metabolism in which hepatocellular disease is also associated with renal Fanconi syndrome. In the phenotype seen in early infancy, the clinical findings include hepatomegaly, bleeding from coagulation defects, and jaundice. Ascites is not uncommon. The laboratory findings consist of abnormal liver function tests with increased serum AST, ALT, and direct and indirect bilirubin; prolonged PT and PTT; and the findings related to renal Fanconi syndrome, such as glycosuria, hypophosphatemia, hypouricemia, proteinuria due to beta$_2$-microglobulin hyperexcretion, and generalized aminoaciduria and organic aciduria.

More specific laboratory abnormalities consist of an increase in serum alpha-fetoprotein levels. In fact, these levels may even be elevated in cord blood (Hostetter et al, 1983). There may be an increase in tyrosine in plasma. However, the hypertyrosinemia is due to a secondary impairment in the function of the liver enzyme, *p*-hydroxyphenylpyruvic acid oxidase, and is not seen in all patients at all times. This also is true for the hypermethioninemia. Some patients may have only hypertyrosinemia or only hypermethioninemia. The most important metabolites are those related to the substrate, fumarylacetylacetic acid, whose handling is defective. This includes increased levels of the diagnostic metabolite succinylacetone, which can be detected on urine organic acid quantitation by gas chromatography–mass spectrometry (GC-MS) and in RBCs by the delta-aminolevulinic acid dehydratase inhibition assay. One must be careful about the interpretation of these tests. My colleagues and I have encountered patients who, because of the severity of their illness and poor dietary intake or who were on intravenous fluids, had elevations neither of methionine nor tyrosine in plasma and only minute amounts of succinylacetone detectable in urine or RBCs. I suggest that any infant with severe liver disease and renal Fanconi syndrome that is not obviously due to other causes have succinylacetone and/or FAH activity measured in RBCs, even if the urinary succinylacetone metabolites cannot be detected by GS-MS. In the past, most of the infants with the hepatic form of tyrosinemia type 1 died in early to late infancy. It is now recommended that patients with this disease receive a liver transplantation. However, a new medical therapy has been developed using the agent 2-(2-nitro-4-trifluoromethylbenzoyl)-1,3-cyclohexanedione (NTBC), which inhibits *p*-hydroxyphenylpyruvate dioxygenase (Lindstedt et al, 1992), thus blocking the conversion of *p*-hydroxyphenylpyruvate, the transamination product of tyrosine, to fumarylacetoacetate and thereby retarding the synthesis and accumulation of succinylacetate and succinylacetone. Therapy has been used successfully to improve liver and renal function, as well as normalize or improve the various laboratory abnormalities. It is unclear, however, whether this therapy will eliminate the need for liver transplantation.

One of the most devastating complications for older infants who have become stabilized is the development of hepatocellular carcinoma. This is quite prevalent in tyrosinemia, and most patients who survive infancy or those with a chronic phenotype succumb to this complication. Unfortunately, several older infants who have been successfully transplanted had pulmonary metastases from liver cancer at the time of the transplant and did not survive. It is recommended that NTBC therapy be started in infants who are acutely ill while they are waiting a liver for transplantation. There is no effect on the CNS in this disease other than as a secondary complication of the severe liver disease. So far, most of the liver transplantations have been successful, and the patients have done well on immunosuppressive therapy with only minimal persistent evidence of renal tubular dysfunction while on a normal diet.

This entity is not to be confused with transient *tyrosinemia* of the newborn, which is prevalent in prematures, probably the most common disturbance of amino acid metabolism in humans, secondary to a delayed maturation of *p*-hydroxyphenylpyruvate dioxygenase activity (Levine et al, 1939; Mitchell et al, 1995) or *hypertyrosinemia* secondary to liver disease, per se (David et al, 1970).

Nonketotic Hyperglycinemia
Glycine Cleavage Complex (GCC) Deficiency

$$\text{Glycine} + \text{Tetrahydrofolate} \xrightarrow{\text{GCC}} CO_2 +$$
$$NH_3 + \text{Methylenetetrahydrofolate}$$

Enzyme Complex: 4 Subunits
  1 Pyridoxal-Phosphate–Dependent Glycine Decarboxylase P Protein
  1 Lipoate-Containing Hydrogen Carrier H Protein
  1 Tetrahydrofolate-Dependent T Protein
  1 Lipoamide Dehydrogenase L Protein
P Protein Gene Location: Chromosome 9p13
Frequency: 1/250,000, Except 1/12,000 for P Protein Gene Mutation in Finns

Nonketotic hyperglycinemia is a rare defect of glycine metabolism (Gerritsen et al, 1965; Hamosh et al, 1995; Tada and Hayasaka, 1987). Inherited as an autosomal recessive trait, it is due to deficient activity of the glycine cleavage enzyme complex (GCC). Its frequency is fewer than 1 in 200,000 newborn infants. Although several variant forms exist, most infants who come to clinical attention in the newborn period, presumably most patients with this disease, have a severe catastrophic type of disease that mimics the most acute forms of ammonia, amino acids, or organic acid metabolism. The infants, usually well at birth, begin to manifest hypotonia and seizures after 12 to 36 hours. Quickly, they become comatose and there is a loss of all the newborn reflexes, as well as the deep tendon reflexes. The clinical findings predominantly relate to those associated with CNS intoxication. The electroencephalogram (EEG) usually shows a characteristic pattern of spike and slow waves. The babies may manifest hiccups owing to diaphragmatic spasms. The main laboratory finding is a massively elevated level of serum glycine. The urine glycine is usually also elevated. The cerebrospinal fluid (CSF) glycine is also elevated and out of proportion to the degree of elevation in blood. The amino acid serine, which is also a product of the defective enzyme reaction, is depressed in plasma and there is a corresponding increase in the glycine-to-serine ratio in body fluids. Prenatal CNS lesions have been reported (Dobyns, 1989). The pathophysiology of this brain disease is not well understood; it is believed that glycine may interfere with the activity of specific chloride channels, thus perturbing the membrane potential and depolarization of neurons. There also appears to be an impairment in alpha-motor neuron outflow tract activity producing a clinical state that mimics Werdnig-Hoffmann disease. Uncommonly, the plasma ammonium levels may be elevated. However, no acidosis or ketosis is seen in this disease, thus the old name of *nonketotic hyperglycinemia*. Many of the disorders of organic acid metabolism such as methylmalonic acidemia and propionic acidemia are also associated with elevations of plasma glycine, presumably due to a secondary impairment in the GCC, and have been referred to in the past as the *ketotic hyperglycinemia syndromes*. Although many therapies have been tried in this disease, such as protein restriction, benzoate to trap glycine as the byproduct hippurate, strychnine to affect the lower motor neuron function, and dextromethorphan to block *N*-methyl-D-aspartate (NMDA) receptors, there is no effective therapy. Most of the babies die in the newborn period despite medical support with assisted ventilation. A transient form of nonketotic hyperglycemia (NKH) has also been reported in newborns (Luder et al, 1989; Schiffman et al, 1989). Valproate may result in hyperglycinemia due to secondary inhibition of the GCC, as is postulated to explain secondary hyperglycinemia in the disorders of organic acid metabolism such as propionic acidemia.

Methionine Synthetase Deficiency

In humans, the essential amino acid methionine is converted to homocysteine and in the process a methyl group is transferred to an acceptor molecule from *S*-adenosyl-methionine that serves as a donor for methyl groups in many different reactions (see Fig. 25–4) (Mudd et al, 1995). Subsequently, the homocysteine may either be completely metabolized through the cysteine pathway to sulfate or it may be remethylated back to methionine. Defective methionine remethylation or a deficiency in methionine synthetase leads to an uncommon remethylation form of homocystinuria. Patients with classic homocystinuria, due to a deficiency of the cystathionine beta-synthase enzyme, rarely manifest signs in early infancy (Mudd et al, 1995). In contrast, patients with methionine synthetase deficiency or methionine remethylation defect may come to clinical attention in the newborn period (Fenton and Rosenberg, 1995b). The patients may have either an abnormality in vitamin B_{12} metabolism, which may also produce methylmalonic acidemia as well as homocystinuria, or an isolated defect in folate metabolism or the methionine synthetase enzyme (Rosenblatt, 1995). In this reaction, the methyl group from 5-methyltetrahydrofolate, which is derived from 5,10-methylene tetrahydrofolate, is transferred to methylcobalamin and subsequently to homocysteine. The clinical findings associated with methionine synthetase deficiency are poor growth and development. There may be severe cortical atrophy and possible brain lesions owing to thromboses of the arteries or veins, as in classic homocystinuria. The laboratory findings consist of an elevation in plasma homocysteine levels and a normal or decreased level of methionine. Often the levels of homocysteine are not as elevated as in classic cystathionine beta-synthetase deficiency. If there is a defect in folate or vitamin B_{12} metabolism that produces secondary impairment in methionine and synthetase activity, there may also be megaloblastic anemia. Some patients with a defect in cobalamin metabolism may respond to megadose therapy with hydroxycobalamin. The treatment of the methionine synthetase deficiency is methionine supplementation to restore methionine levels in plasma to normal and to restore CNS pools of methionine, which may be critical in one carbon transfer reaction within the CNS. One can also retard homocysteine accumulation as well as restore methionine levels by administering betaine, which can enhance remethylation of homocysteine to methionine through the alternate betaine methyltransferase pathway. Some investigators have also used pharmacologic doses of cobalamin, folate, and pyridoxine to stimulate flux either through the methionine synthetase or the classic homocysteine pathway. Unfortunately, if infants with this type of disorder are not treated early, there is usually a permanent and devastating effect on cognitive and motor function.

Phenylketonuria
Phenylalanine Hydroxylase (PAH) Deficiency

$$\text{Phenylalanine} + O_2 + \text{Tetrahydrobiopterin} \xrightarrow{\text{PAH}} \text{Tyrosine} + \text{Biopterin} + H_2O$$

Enzyme: Multimer, Identical Subunits
Gene Location: Chromosome 12q22-q24.1
Frequency: 1/10,000

CASE STUDY 4

The patient was the 8 lb, 1 oz product of a full-term uncomplicated gestation. Apgar scores were 8^1, 8^5. The newborn period passed without difficulty. He developed bronchiolitis at 5 months of age. During the hospitalization, no neurologic abnormalities were detected on physical examination. Parents reported that he walked at 1½ years of age.

At 4 years of age, he was referred for neurologic evaluation because of lack of speech development. A behavioral problem was evident: he was noted to be hyperactive. In addition, he was not toilet trained, was unable to feed or undress himself, related poorly to other people, and occasionally engaged in rocking and head banging. On physical examination, the right toe showed a plantar extension response. An EEG revealed discharges consistent with seizure activity and he was started on phenytoin.

At 6 years of age, since this blonde-haired, blue-eyed boy with eczema of the palms had a chronic, nonprogressive encephalopathy manifested by severe mental retardation and idiopathic seizure disorder, a plasma sample was submitted for amino acid column chromatography analysis. The plasma phenylalanine level was 23 mg/dL (normal: 0.4 to 1.6). A urinary ferric chloride test was positive for phenylketonuric derivatives despite the absence of a musty or mousy odor. The original newborn filter paper screen for PKU had been omitted.

PKU is the most common inborn error of amino acid metabolism that can result in mental retardation (Scriver et al, 1995). It is due to a defect in the activity of the enzyme phenylalanine hydroxylase (PAH), which converts phenylalanine to tyrosine, a reaction that resides primarily in the liver. Thus, in PKU it is the deficiency of this liver enzyme that results in brain disease. Because of the paucity of findings in the newborn period or even early infancy, PKU usually went undiagnosed in the prescreening era. As discussed in Chapter 28, newborn screening has enabled us to routinely prevent mental retardation from PKU. It is important for physicians caring for newborns to be aware of the pitfalls of screening that are outlined in Chapter 28. This disease, inherited as an autosomal recessive trait, has an overall frequency of about 1 in 12,000 newborns. It exemplifies the interaction of a gene and the manipulable environment (i.e., diet) in the expression of a disease (Scriver and Clow, 1980a, 1980b).

Case Study 4 illustrates that patients may easily escape detection, even during childhood. After birth, the baby with PKU who was ingesting adequate amounts of breast milk or a proprietary formula will experience a gradual and persistent increase in plasma phenylalanine levels. The cutoff for newborn screening in most states is 4 mg/dL, with the upper range of normal being approximately 2 mg/dL. In the first 24 hours most infants with PKU readily exceed the 4 mg/dL cutoff, and by the end of the first week of life the levels are usually between 20 and 40 mg/dL. At that time the derivatives of phenylalanine, the so-called phenylketonuric compounds, are excreted in urine in excess and the increased excretion of phenylpyruvic acid gives rise to the positive ferric chloride test in which the urine turns green. The odor in PKU is due to increased production of the derivative phenylacetic acid, which has a musty or mousy odor. This may be detected when the levels of phenylalanine exceed 10 to 15 mg/dL, but it is not always detected in every patient. In the first 6 months of life, the affected babies may have difficulties with feeding and vomiting. In some instances, the persistent vomiting has been associated with the diagnosis of pyloric stenosis for which corrective surgery has been performed, perhaps inappropriately. Developmental delay is usually evident in the second 6 months of life. Patients may have seizures, sometimes infantile spasms in early infancy associated with a hypsarrhythmic EEG pattern. Persistent elevation of plasma phenylalanine levels above 10 mg/dL is sufficient to result in mental retardation. The mechanism of brain disease in PKU is still unknown. It may be related to the effect of high phenylalanine levels on transport of amino acids across the blood-brain barrier and then into brain neurons or glial elements. The plasma levels of tyrosine may be decreased and especially in those patients with no tyrosine supplementation in the special amino acid powder used as a daily nutrient. For many years investigators have speculated that hypotyrosinemia may also play a role in the CNS deficits since tyrosine (only a liver enzyme) cannot be synthesized within the CNS by PAH. Older infants often exhibit long tract findings such as spastic quadriparesis or spastic quadriplegia. There is postnatal acquired microcephaly in the untreated infant and there may also be severe behavioral problems. Average findings consist of elevated serum plasma phenylalanine levels, normal or subnormal plasma tyrosine levels, and increased urinary excretion of phenylpyruvic acid, phenyllactic acid, and phenylacetic acid.

The mainstay of therapy is a low-protein diet and the use of a special formula in which phenylalanine is absent. The patients must receive an adequate amount of phenylalanine from proprietary formulas, and later from table foods using a phenylalanine exchange system, allowing for the normal daily utilization of phenylalanine for protein synthesis while maintaining plasma phenylalanine levels in a range as close as possible to normal. Deviations from normality in plasma are believed to be associated with chronic, perhaps even acute, effects on CNS function and testing performance. Thus, the diet should be one for life. The phenylalanine hydroxylase gene has been cloned and sequenced, and the mutations that are responsible for most abnormalities in humans are known. DNA sequencing and mutational analysis may be used to determine carriers in families and to provide a scientific rationale during family counseling.

There are some rare patients with hyperphenylaninemia who have a most severe disease, not because of the deficiency of the phenylalanine hydroxylase apoenzyme but rather because of deficiency of the active cofactor of this enzyme, which is tetrahydrobiopterin. There are several defects in the metabolism of biopterin that can produce this type of hyperphenylalaninemia. Patients with these uncommon types of PKU usually come to attention in the newborn period because of severe seizure activity. Patients with the biopterin deficiency can have evidence of severe brain damage despite treatment with a low-phenylalanine diet. This may be related to deficiencies of other neurotransmitters whose synthesis is also dependent on adequate levels of tetrahydrobiopterin. These various other defects such as the dihydropteridine reductase, 6-pyruvoyl tetrahydropterin synthetase, and the guanosine triphosphate cyclohydrolase deficiencies can be ascertained by urinary measurement of neopterin and biopterin in urine.

INBORN ERRORS OF ORGANIC ACID METABOLISM

Defects in the catabolism of the branched-chain amino acids are responsible for most of the disorders of organic acid metabolism (Fig. 25–5). Typical examples are methylmalonic, propionic, and isovaleric acidemia. An organic acid is any organic compound that contains a carboxy functional group but no alpha-amino group as in an amino acid. In this section we consider the disorders of fatty acid oxidation, ketone body metabolism, and lactic acid metabolism, as well as the more classic inherited defects in organic acid metabolism. What is true for all these disorders is that the ability to establish a diagnosis depends primarily on the suspicion of the clinician caring for the sick infant. Most of the disorders also require sophisticated testing such as GC-MS to identify the specific organic compound responsible for the toxic syndrome. As discussed earlier, acidosis and encephalopathy are usually the hallmarks of these syndromes when they present in the newborn period.

Methylmalonic Acidemia
L-Methylmalonyl-CoA Mutase (MCM) Deficiency

$$\text{L-Methylmalonyl CoA} \xrightarrow[\substack{\text{adenosylcobalamin} \\ \text{(or vitamin B}_{12})}]{\text{MCM}} \text{Succinyl-CoA}$$

Enzyme: Homodimer
Gene Location: 6p12-p21.2
Frequency: 1/20,000

CASE STUDY 5

The 2954-g male was the product of an uncomplicated pregnancy and delivery. He was discharged on breast-feeds and on day 4 begin to feed less and sleep more. On day 5, the parents noted him to be unarousable at times and to be breathing fast. He was brought to the local hospital when he was found to be obtunded and severely tachypneic. A sepsis workup was performed and antibiotics were administered. A serum total CO_2 was 6 mEq/L. The urine ketones were strongly positive. An arterial blood pH was 7.15, the P_{CO_2} 40 mm Hg, and the P_{O_2} 62 mm Hg. Because of impending respiratory failure, he was intubated and placed on mechanical ventilation. Despite the use of intravenous fluids with glucose and sodium bicarbonate, he remained comatose, and by day 8 his pupils were not reactive to light and he was unresponsive to painful stimuli. A plasma NH_4^+ level was 2059 µM. By this time, the results of the newborn screen performed on day 2 using the technology of tandem-mass spectrometry on filter paper cards revealed elevated levels of propionylcarnitine in blood. Subsequently, GC-MS analysis of urine revealed a massive increase in methylmalonic acid along with the other metabolites such as 3-hydroxypropionate, propionylglycine, and methylcitrate, confirming the diagnosis of methylmalonic acidemia. Because of the terminal neurologic condition, dialysis therapy was not instituted and life support was withdrawn; the baby died on day 9.

Methylmalonic acidemia, along with propionic acidemia, is the most common of the disorders of organic acid metabolism (Fenton and Rosenberg, 1995a, 1995b). Although

more than one enzyme defect may result in methylmalonic acidemia, all are inherited as autosomal recessive traits. The enzyme that is most often deficient is L-methylmalonyl-CoA mutase (see Fig. 25–5). This enzyme is present in mitochondria, and it depends on adenosyl-cobalamin for activity. Impaired function may result from either a mutation of the L-methylmalonyl-CoA mutase apoenzyme or deficient availability of the adenosyl form of vitamin B_{12}. The latter may result from impaired cellular metabolism of vitamin B_{12}, including defective activity of the enzyme adenosyl-cobalamin synthetase. Some patients, but not usually newborn infants with methylmalonic acidemia, are responsive to pharmacologic therapy with vitamin B_{12}. Methylmalonic acidemia, therefore, is one of the important disorders that can be considered to be a vitamin-responsive inborn error of metabolism. Because of the deficient activity of L-methylmalonyl-CoA mutase, the substrate L-methylmalonyl CoA accumulates in mitochondria and is subsequently hydrolyzed to methylmalonic acid. Because methylmalonic acid is capable of diffusing out of cells in which it is being produced, it may be detected in excess in the blood, CSF, and urine of patients with these various forms of the disease. The precursors of L-methylmalonyl

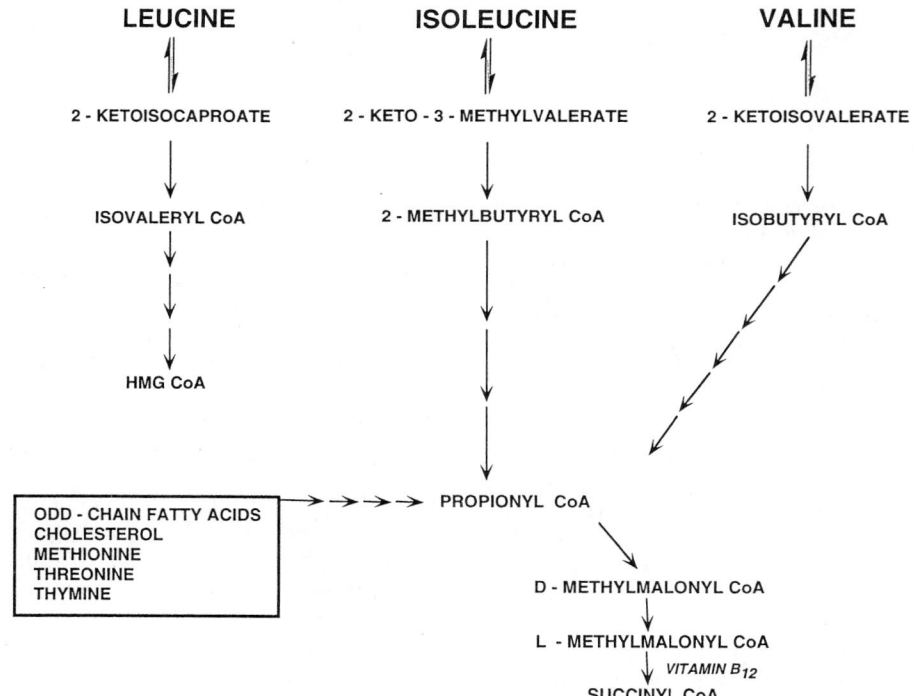

FIGURE 25–5. The branched-chain amino acids leucine, isoleucine, and valine are reversibly transaminated to their corresponding 2-keto analogues, which are the substrates for the single decarboxylase (branched-chain 2-keto dehydrogenase) ([BCKAD]) enzyme deficient in maple syrup urine disease. Reduced activity of isovaleryl coenzyme A (CoA) dehydrogenase, the next enzyme in the leucine degradative pathway, is the cause of isovaleric acidemia. The immediate precursor of ketones, 3-hydroxy-3-methylglutaryl CoA (HMG-CoA), is the final product of the leucine catabolic pathway. However, its production more strongly depends on oxidation of fatty acids as in ketogenesis and in cholesterol biosynthesis. Propionyl CoA, which accumulates in both propionic and methylmalonic acidemia, may be synthesized from isoleucine, valine, odd-chain fatty acids, cholesterol, methionine, threonine, and thymine. The adenosyl form of vitamin B_{12} is the important cofactor in the L-methylmalonyl CoA mutase-catalyzed conversion of L-methylmalonyl CoA to the citric acid cycle intermediate, succinyl CoA.

CoA are the branched-chain amino acids, isoleucine, and valine, as well as methionine, threonine, thymine, and odd-chain fatty acids (see Fig. 25–5).

There are many different phenotypes of methylmalonic acidemia. They range from severe catastrophic newborn-onset disease in the first week of life to an almost benign form that has been detected in adults with partial L-methylmalonyl-CoA mutase deficiency. The phenotypes are the newborn-onset type, the intermediate variety with onset in early and late infancy, the intermittent form with onset usually in late infancy and childhood, and an adult or benign phenotype. Most patients who present in the newborn period have a severe phenotype. In some of the patients who present in the first week of life with catastrophic illness, even dialysis therapy is not effective, possibly because of a delay in diagnosis and treatment. The most striking presentation is in the second or third day of life. The baby is usually well at birth, as in the UCEDs, but then gradually begins to manifest problems with feeding, vomiting, lethargy, and perhaps seizures. There may be respiratory distress as a manifestation of metabolic acidosis. The liver may be enlarged as a consequence of diffuse steatosis. The important laboratory findings include a metabolic acidosis usually associated with an increased anion gap, ketosis, and hyperammonemia. The elevation of plasma ammonium levels may be as high as in the severe newborn-onset hyperammonemic syndromes. Since ketonuria is relatively uncommon in newborn infants, even in stressed infants with hypoglycemia because of poor feeding, and because diabetes mellitus is so uncommon in the newborn period, the physician caring for newborn infants must always consider an inborn error of organic acid metabolism when confronted with the acutely ill baby with ketosis. Other laboratory findings include thrombocytopenia, leukopenia, and anemia due to effects of the metabolite on the hematopoietic elements in bone marrow. Older patients with methylmalonic acidemia during crisis have suffered acute pancreatitis as well as devastating lesions to the basal ganglia. Plasma amino acid analysis may reveal elevations of several amino acids such as glycine and alanine. Secondary carnitine deficiency with elevated levels of carnitine esters is expected (Chalmers et al, 1984). Methylmalonic acid may be detected in urine by performing GC in conjunction with MS. The diagnosis can be confirmed by assaying the activity of L-methylmalonyl-CoA mutase enzyme in cultured skin fibroblasts. In addition, the various other disturbances in vitamin B_{12} metabolism can also be studied by analyzing skin fibroblasts in culture. The treatment of acute disease consists of protein restriction; empirical therapy with vitamin B_{12} (1 mg IM per day); intravenous fluids with 10% glucose and sodium bicarbonate to correct dehydration; electrolyte imbalance and acidosis; high-calorie feeds via a nasogastric tube; and, often, dialysis. The use of carnitine, 25 to 200 mg/kg/day, intravenously or orally, is controversial. The treatment of the chronic state centers around the judicious use of a low-protein diet and alkali to eliminate any acid-base imbalance.

Propionic Acidemia
Propionyl CoA Carboxylase (PCC) Deficiency

$$\text{Propionyl CoA} + \text{ATP} + \text{HCO}_3 \xrightarrow[\text{biotin}]{\text{PCC}} \text{D-Methylmalonyl CoA}$$
$$+ \text{ AMP} + \text{Pyrophosphate}$$

Enzyme: 6 α Subunits
       6 β Subunits
α Subunit Gene Location: 13q32
β Subunit Gene Location: 3q13.3-q22
Frequency: Rare

Propionic acidemia was the first classic defect in organic acid metabolism to be described in humans (Fenton and Rosenberg, 1995). The first patient described by Childs and colleagues in 1961 was sick on the first day of life with severe metabolic acidosis and ketosis. He responded to massive alkali therapy and survived the newborn period. He subsequently suffered multiple episodes of recurrent attacks of metabolic decompensation with ketoacidosis usually precipitated by infections or protein ingestion; he also had developmental delay, a seizure disorder, and episodic neutropenia and thrombocytopenia. He died at age 7. His sister also developed ketosis and metabolic acidosis in the first week of life, but because of better control of her disease there were few severe episodes of decompensation in the first and second decades of life.

Propionic acidemia is due to a selective deficiency of propionyl-CoA carboxylase and is inherited as an autosomal recessive trait. This disorder was originally called *ketotic hyperglycinemia* because of the elevation of plasma glycine levels in conjunction with ketosis. The precursors of propionyl CoA include the amino acids, isoleucine, and valine, plus methionine, threonine, the pyrimidine compound, thymine, and odd-chain fatty acids (see Fig. 25–5). Of the several hundred patients described with this disease, most present in the newborn period with poor feeding, vomiting, lethargy, and hypotonia. Not uncommonly, the patients manifest seizures and hepatomegaly due to steatosis. The metabolic acidosis may be severe with or without an increase in the anion gap. Ketosis is almost always present. Patients who survive may often manifest choreoathetosis because of persistent damage to the basal ganglia. Usually episodes of metabolic decompensation characterized by acidosis and ketosis can be precipitated by excessive protein intake or infection. These type of episodes may result in permanent neurologic damage. Subsequent findings may, therefore, include developmental delay, seizures, cerebral atrophy, and EEG abnormalities. During the acute attacks, leukopenia, thrombocytopenia, and less rarely anemia, probably due to suppression of maturation of bone marrow hematopoietic precursors, may occur.

The diagnosis may be confirmed by GC-MS analysis of urine in an organic acid quantitation. The urine has excess concentrations of various propionate metabolites such as methylcitrate, propionylglycine, 2-methyl-3-hydroxybutyrate, 2-methylacetoacetate, and several other more rare compounds. The plasma glycine level may be elevated, and during acute attacks the plasma ammonium level is frequently increased. The enzyme activity propionyl-CoA carboxylase may be assayed in white blood cells (WBCs) or extracts of cultured skin fibroblasts for definitive diagnosis. Several mutations have been identified in the genes that encode the two nonidentical subunits (alpha and beta) of the propionyl-CoA carboxylase enzyme.

Therapy consists of a low-protein diet and adequate calories. As in L-methylmalonyl there is secondary carnitine deficiency with elevated levels of propionylcarnitine. The use of L-carnitine to relieve a deficiency of free carnitine and promote increased urinary excretion of propionylcarnitine to lower mitochondrial propionyl CoA levels is controversial. It has never been shown to unequivocally result in an improvement in the clinical state. Because gut bacteria can also contribute to propionate production, antimicrobial therapy with metronidazole has been used during an acute attack. In the acutely ill infant in the newborn period, the immediate treatment consists of elimination of protein administration or total parenteral nutrition; administration of an adequate amount of calories (10% glucose intravenously and/or administration of nonprotein formulas, such as Mead-Johnson 80056 or Ross Prophree products, via nasogastric tube infusion); alkali to eliminate metabolic acidosis; and platelet transfusion, if warranted, because of thrombocytopenia. Often because of the severe acidosis and coma, patients may require dialysis therapy. It is unclear whether administration of sodium benzoate and sodium phenylacetate as in the treatment of hyperammonemia associated with UCEDs is of benefit to the patient with secondary hyperammonemia. Several patients with propionic acidemia have undergone liver transplantation with mixed success. Most of the patients with severe newborn-onset disease do not survive the first decade of life.

Isovaleric Acidemia

Isovaleryl-CoA Dehydrogenase (IVCD) Deficiency

Isovaleryl CoA $\xrightarrow{\text{IVCD}}$ 3-Methylcrotonyl CoA

Enzyme: Homotetramer
Gene Location: Chromosome 15q14-q15
Frequency: Very Rare

Isovaleric acidemia is caused by a selective deficiency of the enzyme isovaleryl-CoA dehydrogenase (Sweetman and Williams, 1995; Tanaka et al, 1966). It is inherited as an autosomal recessive trait. There are two major phenotypes: an acute form that presents with catastrophic disease in the newborn period and a late-onset type characterized by chronic, intermittent episodes of metabolic decompensation. In the acute form the infants become extremely sick in the first week of life. There is usually a history of poor feeding, vomiting, lethargy, and often seizures. The characteristic odor of sweaty feet or rancid cheese due to isovaleric acid is noted. Metabolic acidosis usually with an elevated anion gap and ketosis is present. There may be secondary hyperammonemia, thrombocytopenia, neutropenia, and sometimes anemia, resulting in pancytopenia. The babies usually lapse into a coma. Dialysis therapy may be necessary. As with other organic acid disorders for which an amino acid determines organic acid production (see Fig. 25–5), treatment also consists of protein or total parenteral nutrition restriction, intravenous fluids with glucose and perhaps sodium bicarbonate, protein-free formula with calories via nasogastric tube administration, and glycine 250 mg/kg/day (Cohn et al, 1978). Intravenous L-carnitine may be beneficial. In the chronic, intermittent form, the patients have repeated episodes of metabolic decompensation

precipitated by infections or protein intake. Some of these episodes may mimic Reye syndrome. The same principles are applied to therapy for acute metabolic decompensation beyond the newborn period: no protein, calories, alkali to correct acidosis, glycine (Krieger and Tanaka, 1976; Naglak et al, 1988; Velazquez and Prieto, 1980), and L-carnitine (De Sousa et al, 1986; Roe et al, 1984). The mainstay of chronic therapy is a low-protein diet. Patients may benefit from the chronic administration of glycine (Berry et al, 1988), which enhances the production of the nontoxic compound isovalerylglycine and that serves to reduce the free levels of isovaleric acid in body fluids (Krieger and Tanaka, 1976; Yudkoff et al, 1978). In addition, carnitine administration may augment the excretion of isovalerylcarnitine (Berry et al, 1988; Mayatepek et al, 1991); the benefit of carnitine treatment in the chronic state, however, remains unknown. Most patients with late-onset type of disease are mentally retarded. In contrast, most of the patients with the acute phenotype are not severely retarded, but most have not survived the newborn period, attesting to the severe toxic nature of this organic acid disorder in the newborn period. The diagnosis may be made by measuring markedly increased levels of isovalerylglycine in urine. There is usually also increased excretion of 3-hydroxyisovaleric acid. The enzyme isoveryl-CoA dehydrogenase can be assayed in extracts of cultured skin fibroblasts. The gene has been identified and assigned to human chromosome 15. Various mutations have been described.

Multiple Carboxylase Deficiency

There are two specific forms of multiple carboxylase deficiency (Wolf, 1995). The first is holocarboxylase synthetase deficiency and the second is biotinidase deficiency. All the carboxylase enzymes such as propionyl-CoA carboxylase, pyruvate carboxylase, 3-methylcrotonyl-CoA carboxylase, and acetyl-CoA carboxylase require covalent linkage with biotin for normal activity. In the first type, holocarboxylase synthetase, the enzyme that accomplishes the addition of biotin to these various carboxylases is deficient. In the second form, the absence of the enzyme biotinidase does not allow for biotin recycling after a carboxylase enzyme is degraded and hydrolyzed. The biotinidase deficiency does not usually present in the newborn period. However, patients with the holocarboxylase synthetase deficiency have a severe disease and are characteristically catastrophically ill in the newborn period. Fewer than 20 cases have been reported (Michalski et al, 1989). They have severe metabolic acidosis with lactic acidosis and are in coma. As with the biotinidase deficiency, biotin administration is lifesaving. This is one of the few disorders of organic acid metabolism for which the administration of a vitamin in megadoses produces a dramatic turnabout in the clinical and laboratory findings. Diagnosis depends on GC-MS analysis of urine and the demonstration of markedly increased levels of lactate, 3-methylcrotonylglycine, and propionate metabolites. In most patients the affinity of the holocarboxylase synthetase enzyme for biotin is diminished and to normalize or improve the biochemical disturbances, patients require between 10 and 60 mg of biotin daily. The enzyme deficiency may be confirmed in cultured skin fibroblasts. The disorder is inherited as an autosomal recessive trait. There are also rare cases of isolated 3-methylcrotonyl-CoA carboxylase deficiency; these patients usually do not come to clinical attention until after early infancy. Of great interest, however, is our new understanding that previously asymptomatic women have developed "acute fatty liver of pregnancy" syndrome. Recurrent episodes of this potentially lethal syndrome has now also been reported in heterozygous mothers who were carrying infants with fatty acid oxidation defects (Schoeman et al, 1991).

Glutaric Acidemia Type 1

Glutaryl-CoA Dehydrogenase (GCDH) Deficiency

$$\text{Glutaryl-CoA} + \text{Flavin adenine dinucleotide (FAD)} \xrightarrow{\text{GDCH}}$$
$$\text{Crotonyl CoA} + CO_2 + FADH_2$$

Enzyme: Homotetramer
Gene Location: Chromosome 19p13.2
Frequency: Very Rare, Except in Saulteaux-Ojibway
    Canadian Indians and Pennsylvania Old-Order
    Amish

An isolated deficiency of GCDH causes glutaric acidemia type 1 (GA-1) (Goodman and Frerman, 1995; Goodman et al, 1975). Multiple phenotypes are known. In the most dramatic presentation, which accounts for less than half of the known patients with GA-1, the illness develops acutely in the first year of life, usually following an infection. Acute encephalopathy is followed by the development of what appears to be a severe form of extrapyramidal cerebral palsy (Hoffmann et al, 1991). In essence, these infants had developed bilateral damage to the caudate and putamen in the basal ganglia, resulting in an incapacitating dystonic syndrome. Some patients have a slowly progressive course with developmental delay, hypotonia, dystonia, and dyskinesia in the first couple years of life. Other patients are relatively asymptomatic. In general, this is not a disorder that is associated with acute disease in the newborn period. However, macrocephaly at birth is common (Iafolla and Kahler, 1989). The etiology of any of the CNS lesions is unknown. The MRI scan of the head typically shows bilateral widening of the sylvian fissures associated with hypo-opercularization, resulting in the "bat wing" appearance. Sometimes the fluid accumulation mimics subdural hygromas, and a few patients have actually been noted to have subdural hematomas. The congenital nature of these findings suggests that GA-1 has its onset in utero and affects CNS development. Usually infants do not develop bilateral damage to the basal ganglia in the newborn period. Diagnosis depends on the demonstration of glutaric acid and 3-hydroxyglutaric acid in urine and is confirmed by the demonstration of deficient GCDH activity or protein levels on Western analysis in cultured fibroblasts. It is a rare disorder but especially common in the Saulteaux-Ojibway Indians in Canada (Greenberg et al, 1993) and in the Old-Order Amish of Lancaster County, Pennsylvania (Morton et al, 1991). A low-protein diet may help in the treatment of these patients; acute illnesses, usually viral in nature, should be treated vigorously with fluids containing glucose and adequate amounts of calories to prevent catab-

olism. Bicarbonate may be necessary to correct acid-base imbalance. Carnitine has also been used to reduce mitochondrial glutaryl-CoA levels.

Fatty Acid Oxidation Disorders

Glutaric Acidemia Type 2

The first disorder to be considered is glutaric acidemia type 2 (GA-2), due to multiple acyl-CoA dehydrogenase deficiency (Frerman and Goodman, 1995; Przyrembel et al, 1976). The mitochondrial acyl-CoA dehydrogenases include the very-long-chain acyl-CoA dehydrogenase, the medium-chain acyl-CoA dehydrogenase, the short-chain acyl-CoA dehydrogenase (all of which are involved in fatty acid oxidation), the isovaleryl-CoA dehydrogenase and 2-methylbutaryl-CoA dehydrogenase (important in branched-chain amino acid catabolism), glutaryl-CoA dehydrogenase (important in lysine, hydroxylysine, and tryptophan metabolism), and the dimethylglycine and sarcosine dehydrogenases (important in choline degradation). All these dehydrogenase proteins have in common the binding of a protein called *electron transfer flavoprotein* (ETF). This protein is responsible for accepting the electrons in any of these oxidative dehydrogenation reactions, and it is a deficiency of either ETF or the ETF dehydrogenase enzyme, responsible for further transferring the electrons from ETF to coenzyme Q_{10} within the mitochondria, that causes GA-2. There are essentially three phenotypes of GA-2: (1) a newborn-onset type with congenital anomalies; (2) a newborn-onset type without anomalies; and (3) a milder or later-onset type, sometimes called *mild acyl-CoA dehydrogenase deficiency* or *ethylmalonic adipic aciduria*.

Patients with GA-2 who have multiple malformations are often premature; severe disease is usually evident in the first week of life (Lehnert et al, 1982). The patients develop hypotonia, encephalopathy, hepatomegaly, hypoglycemia, and metabolic acidosis; often the odor of isovaleric acid (IVA) is present since these patients also have a defect in metabolism of isovaleryl CoA as in isolated IVA. There may be facial dysmorphism consisting of a high forehead, low-set ears, hypertelorism, and a hypoplastic mid-face. The kidneys may be palpably enlarged associated with large renal cysts (Böhm et al, 1982), rocker-bottom feet, muscular defects of the inferior abdominal wall, and anomalies of the external genitalia, including hypospadias and cordee. Most of the patients with this disease do not survive the first weeks of life. In some, the malformations are not so noticeable and only renal cysts are identified at autopsy. Infants without the congenital abnormalities usually present in the first 24 to 48 hours of life with hypotonia, tachypnea due to a metabolic acidosis, liver enlargement, hypoglycemia, and the sweaty feet odor. Some of these patients develop cardiomyopathy. In contrast, some of these infants can survive the newborn period. The phenotype in the third form is quite variable. Some patients are relatively disease free and have intermittent episodes of vomiting, dehydration, hypoglycemia, and acidosis during childhood or adult life. In some, there may be hepatomegaly and muscle disease.

Laboratory studies in patients with the newborn-onset type usually show severe metabolic acidosis with lactic acidosis and increased anion gap, mild to moderate hyperammonemia, and hypoglycemia without a moderate or large ketonuria. The liver function test may be abnormal with increases in the serum transaminases and prolongation of the PT and PTT. A chest radiograph may show heart enlargement because of hypertrophic cardiomyopathy. Abdominal ultrasound or computed tomographic scan may reveal the renal cysts. The diagnosis is made by finding the characteristic pattern of organic acid metabolites on urine GC-MS analysis. This includes glutarate; ethylmalonate; 3-hydroxyisovalerate; 2-hydroxyglutarate; 5-hydroxyhexanoate; adipic, suberic, sebacic, and dodecanedioic acids; isovalerylglycine; isobutyrylglycine; and 2-methylbutyrylglycine. The ketones, acetoacetic acid, and 3-hydroxybutyric acid usually are not present or only minimally elevated if present and inappropriate for the degree of fatty acid metabolites that indicate free fatty acid mobilization and the potential for enhanced ketogenesis. The renal cystic disease may also be associated with evidence of impaired renal tubular function. Generalized aminoaciduria may be present. The amino-containing compound sarcosine may be elevated in serum as well as in urine. There may be secondary carnitine deficiency, and abnormal carnitine esters such as isovalerylcarnitine and butyrylcarnitine can be detected in blood. The ETF and ETF dehydrogenase deficiency may be detected by using specific antibodies on Western analysis of cultured skin fibroblasts or by performing the functional assays in skin cells. Prenatal diagnosis can be performed by demonstrating glutarate in amniotic fluid or by performing the dehydrogenase assays in cultured amniocytes. The ETF and the alpha and beta subunits of the ETF dehydrogenase genes have been cloned and sequenced. Several mutations of the alpha subunit of the ETF dehydrogenase have been described. In the future, in certain families, mutational analysis of DNA from the probands, as well as other family members, may be performed to establish the diagnosis or to perform prenatal testing using chorionic villus samples or cultured amniotic cells. A complete deficiency of the ETF dehydrogenase is often associated with the newborn type with congenital anomalies. Although treatment with intravenous glucose, riboflavin, carnitine, and diets low in protein and fat generally have not been successful, for the catastrophically ill newborn infant, there has been some success in patients with milder or later-onset disease. Although riboflavin is suggested to be administered to the newborn with severe disease, riboflavin at a dosage of 100 to 300 mg/day has been effective in only a few older patients (Gregersen et al, 1982; Harpey et al, 1983). The rationale behind this therapy is that riboflavin, being a precursor of FAD, may increase the concentrations of FAD and allow for better interaction with a mutated and defective ETF or ETF dehydrogenase proteins. Finally, some artificial electron acceptors such as methylene blue have been used in the newborn period without success.

Very-Long-Chain Acyl-CoA Dehydrogenase, Medium-Chain Acyl-CoA Dehydrogenase, and Short-Chain Acyl-CoA Dehydrogenase Deficiencies

The defects in fatty acid oxidation have been associated with coma, hypoglycemia, liver disease, cardiomyopathy, and skeletal myopathy (Roe and Coates, 1995; Saudubray et al, 1997; Stanley, 1987). All these defects involve abnormalities in the enzymes that participate in or facilitate the mitochondrial beta oxidation of fatty acids. In general, the pathophysiology associated with these disorders has the potential to place the patient in a life-threatening condition when there is a state of catabolism and enhanced liberation of free fatty acids by adipose stores.

Medium-Chain Acyl-CoA Dehydrogenase Deficiency

Medium-Chain Acyl-CoA Dehydrogenase (MCAD) Deficiency

$$R\text{-}CH=CH\text{-}\overset{\displaystyle O}{\overset{\|}{C}}\text{-}S\ CoA\ +\ FAD\ \xrightarrow{\ MCAD\ }$$

$$R\text{-}CH=CH\text{-}\overset{\displaystyle O}{\overset{\|}{C}}\text{-}S\ CoA\ +\ FADH_2$$

Enzyme: Homotetramer
Gene Location: Chromosome 1p31
Frequency: Approximately 1/20,000

The most common of these disorders is the MCAD deficiency (Roe and Coates, 1995). More than 200 patients with this disorder have been described. Most patients do not present until late infancy. The typical patient is an older infant who, following an infection, develops anorexia, vomiting, dehydration, lethargy, and hypoglycemia that may be associated with seizures. Similarly, older patients have features that mimic Reye syndrome and can die because of brain edema. Onset of symptoms in the newborn period is rare. However, some patients in the extended newborn period or in the first 6 months of life were originally believed to have sudden infant death syndrome (Ding et al, 1991; Mowat et al, 1984) but in retrospect turned out to have nonketotic hypoglycemia with coma following the development of fasting associated with an infection. In MCAD deficiency, there is a high mortality rate associated with the initial episode. The laboratory studies usually reveal hypoglycemia and an absence of moderate to large ketones in urine that would be expected to accompany hypoglycemia. The plasma ammonium level may be mildly elevated, the liver may be enlarged, and the serum ALT and AST levels may be slightly increased. During an acute episode, urine GC-MS analysis of organic acids characteristically shows increased levels of adipic, suberic, and sebacic acids, as well as the unsaturated analogues of these medium-chain dicarboxylic acids. Increased urinary excretion of dicarboxylic acids is common in many of the defects of carnitine or fatty acid metabolism. However, this is not pathognomic of a disorder of fat metabolism because infants fed medium-chain triglyceride–enriched formulas also manifest dicarboxylic aciduria (Whyte et al, 1986). Fatty acid analysis of plasma from patients with MCAD deficiency reveals increased levels of octanoic and 4-decenedioic acids. Urine also contains glycine conjugates such as suberylglycine and hexanoylglycine. A secondary carnitine deficiency can be present, and the acylcarnitines analyzed by tandem MS have increased concentrations of 4-, 5-, 6-,

8-, and 10-carbon monounsaturate acylcarnitine species. The MCAD enzyme may be assayed in cultured skin fibroblasts. The MCAD gene has been cloned and sequenced, and several mutations have been identified. The most conspicuous one is the *R329E*, a highly prevalent mutation in people of Northern European ancestry. The main treatment is the avoidance of fasting, and if an episode occurs with hypoglycemia or encephalopathy, the quick response with intravenous glucose and calorie support. Because of the possibility of the development of brain edema, patients may need to be aggressively treated if obtunded to relieve increased intracranial pressure. Avoidance of free fatty acid mobilization during relative insulin deficiency and catabolic stress and prevention of hypoglycemia are the cornerstones of therapy.

Very-Long-Chain Acyl-CoA Dehydrogenase Deficiency

Most of the patients who were previously diagnosed as having long-chain acyl-CoA dehydrogenase (LCAD) deficiency (Hale et al, 1985; Roe and Coates, 1995) actually had very-long-chain acyl-CoA dehydrogenase deficiency (Yamaguchi et al, 1993). Patients with this disease may be ill in the newborn period because of liver disease with hypoglycemia, cardiomyopathy, and skeletal myopathy (Treem et al, 1991). The membrane-bound very-long-chain acyl-Co dehydrogenase, as opposed to the soluble LCAD, whose specific metabolic role is unknown, is the main enzyme for initiating the oxidation of free fatty acids that are derived from adipose stores. This includes palmitic, stearic, and oleic acids. The fasting state may include coma. Even in its absence, however, the patients may exhibit hypotonia, hepatomegaly, and cardiomegaly. With an acute metabolic decompensation, urine organic acid analysis may reveal dicarboxylic aciduria. However, acylglycine excretion is not usually present. There may be a secondary carnitine deficiency with increased concentrations of the long-chain fatty acids bound to carnitine. This disorder may be fatal; sudden death in early infancy has been reported. Therapy is directed toward replenishment of glucose, calorie administration, and treatment of any potential brain edema. The myopathy and cardiomyopathy, however, may proceed even in the absence of fasting. Most investigators suggest a reduction in dietary fat intake or supplementation in medium-chain triglyceride. However, it is important not to provoke an essential fatty acid deficiency by too severe dietary fat restriction. Diagnosis can be made enzymatically in cultured skin fibroblasts.

Short-Chain Acyl-CoA Dehydrogenase Deficiency

The short-chain acyl-CoA dehydrogenase (SCAD) deficiency is a rare disorder (Amendt et al, 1987; Roe and Coates, 1995). Only a few patients have been reported. One patient manifested severe newborn-onset disease with feeding problems and vomiting, lethargy, and hypotonia in the first week of life. Laboratory findings revealed metabolic acidosis, hypoglycemia, and moderate hyperammonemia. The organic analysis showed increased levels of lactate, ketone bodies, butyrate, ethylmalonate, and adipic acid. The patient died at 6 days of age. Postmortem exami-

nation showed brain edema, hepatosplenomegaly with steatosis, cholestasis, and focal hepatocellular necrosis. Other cases, however, suggest a disease associated with neurologic abnormalities with later onset, as well as neuromuscular disease in adults. Diagnosis can be made by assaying the SCAD enzyme in cultured skin fibroblasts. The human gene has been cloned and sequenced and mutations have been described. This should enable a more rapid genetic diagnosis as well as make prenatal diagnosis feasible.

Long-Chain 3-Hydroxy Acyl-CoA Dehydrogenase Deficiency

The long-chain 3-hydroxy acyl-CoA dehydrogenase (LCHAD) deficiency is associated with acute illness, fasting-induced hypoketosis, hypoglycemia, cardiomegaly, and muscle weakness (Bertini et al, 1992; Duran et al, 1991; Roe and Coates, 1995). As with long-chain fatty acid oxidative abnormalities, some older patients may have episodes of illness associated with elevated serum creatine phosphokinase levels and myoglobinuria. A few patients have had sensory motor neuropathy and pigmentary retinopathy (Bertini et al, 1992). Half of the patients have not survived. Some patients may develop severe liver disease with fibrosis in addition to necrosis and steatosis. Women who are carriers for this disease may also develop acute fatty liver of pregnancy syndrome. The diagnosis may be suggested by the demonstration of 3-hydroxydicarboxylic acids on urine organic analysis. However, some patients with liver disease, per se, may also manifest 3-hydroxydicarboxylic aciduria. The demonstration of an enzyme deficiency in fibroblasts may be difficult in some patients. The specific LCHAD defect was demonstrated in cultured skin fibroblasts by using an antibody directed against its analogous activity associated with the short-chain 3-hydroxy acyl-CoA dehydrogenase. Treatment of this disorder has involved frequent high-carbohydrate feedings, dietary fat restriction, and supplementation with uncooked cornstarch. Medium-chain triglyceride may be helpful. Carnitine and riboflavin have also been tried without benefit. The treatment of the acute episode is, as in the other defects of fatty acid oxidation, associated with hypoglycemia and potential brain swelling. Liver and neurologic disease may progress despite any intervention.

Carnitine Transporter Defect, Carnitine Palmitoyltransferase I and II and Acylcarnitine Translocase Deficiencies

Carnitine is essential for fatty acid oxidation because transport of long-chain fatty acids into mitochondria is dependent on an adequate amount of carnitine and the presence of two enzymes that covalently link carnitine to the fatty acid or remove the linkage and one transporter that carries it across the inner mitochondrial membrane (Roe and Coates, 1995; Stanley, 1987). These include carnitine palmitoyltransferase I and II and a carnitine translocase. Cellular levels of carnitine in turn are dependent on a sodium-dependent carnitine transporter. Primary carnitine deficiency is probably associated only with the carnitine transporter defect (Treem et al, 1988). Since the first report of the carnitine transporter defect in 1988, more than 25 cases have been reported. However, many other cases previously reported as having cardiomyopathy or Reye syndrome may have had the transporter defect (Waber et al, 1982). Patients with the transporter defect may present in infancy or in childhood. Earliest reports concern the extended newborn period or early infancy. The disease is characterized by hypoketotic hypoglycemia, hyperammonemia, elevated transaminases, cardiomyopathy, and skeletal muscle weakness. In some of the older patients, cardiomyopathy may be the presenting sign. The characteristic laboratory finding in this disease is extremely low plasma carnitine levels. The total carnitine levels are usually less than 10 μM in plasma. A dicarboxylic aciduria is not usually evident on urine organic acid analysis. This is probably the only disorder in which pharmacologic administration of carnitine has dramatic effects on the clinical and laboratory abnormalities. The treatment is 100 to 200 mg of L-carnitine/kg/day.

Carnitine Palmitoyltransferase Type I Deficiency

Carnitine palmitoyltransferase I (CPT-I) is responsible for covalently linking long-chain fatty acids such as palmitate to carnitine. Although one patient presented in the newborn period, most come to attention in early to late infancy (Roe and Coates, 1995). The clinical findings include hypoketotic hypoglycemia, encephalopathy, and hepatomegaly; there is usually no evidence of cardiomyopathy or skeletal myopathy in CPT-I deficiency. Renal tubular acidosis, due to impaired distal hydrogen ion secretion, has been reported in two patients. Characteristic laboratory findings include the absence of dicarboxylic aciduria and high plasma total and free carnitine levels. However, the plasma acyl carnitine profile is not abnormal. The definitive diagnosis rests on measuring CPT-I enzyme activity in cultured skin fibroblasts. Frequent feeding, reduction of dietary fat, medium-chain triglyceride oil supplementation, and avoidance of fasting all have been beneficial in the long-term management of these patients.

Acylcarnitine Translocase Deficiency

Acylcarnitine translocase deficiency is an exceedingly rare defect. It was initially reported in a male infant who suffered a cardiac arrest at 36 hours of age associated with fasting stress and ventricular dysrhythmias (Stanley et al, 1992). Because of the failure to transport long-chain acylcarnitines across the intermitochondrial membrane following the synthesis by CPT-I, the patient had very low total plasma carnitine levels of which most was long-chain esterified carnitine, recurrent episodes of hypoglycemia, vomiting, gastroesophageal reflux, and mild chronic hyperammonemia. There was also severe skeletal myopathy and mild hypertrophic cardiomyopathy. The continuous nasogastric feeding of a low-fat, high-carbohydrate formula failed to normalize the clinical abnormalities and the patient died at 3 years of age. At that time, he had also developed liver failure. Pathophysiology in this patient suggests that accumulation of long-chain acylcarnitine species may be toxic for several organs, including the heart, liver, and skeletal muscle. In addition, the acute development of

ventricular dysrhythmias may be related to their accumulation in cardiac tissue.

Carnitine Palmitoyltransferase Type II Deficiency

There are two phenotypes of CPT-II deficiency (Roe and Coates, 1995). The enzyme is responsible for the hydrolysis of the long-chain fatty acid bound to carnitine following transport across the intermitochondrial membrane. Most of the patients reported with CPT-II deficiency have a mild deficiency of the enzyme and present in adulthood with episodes of muscle weakness and myoglobinuria brought on by prolonged exercise. The other phenotype is caused by a more serious enzyme defect and presents in early infancy. The first detailed report was of a 3-month-old boy with hypoketotic hypoglycemia, coma, seizures, hepatomegaly, cardiomegaly, cardiac arrhythmias associated with an increase in long-chain acylcarnitine levels in tissues, and the absence of urinary dicarboxylic aciduria (Demaugre et al, 1991). The enzyme is also expressed in renal tissue, as well as in skeletal muscle. Renal dysgenesis has been noted in three patients (Zinn et al, 1991). Reports of onset in the newborn period (Hug et al, 1991) and in later infancy have been recorded. The gene for the human CPT-II is on chromosome 1. Several mutations have been described. Decreased activity of the CPT-II enzyme may be demonstrated in cultured skin fibroblasts.

Defects in Ketone Metabolism

After long-chain fatty acids are broken down to medium-chain fatty acids and finally to short-chain fatty acids such as acetoacetyl CoA, in the liver they must be converted to 3-hydroxy-3-methylglutaryl CoA (HMG-CoA), before hydrolysis to acetoacetate. Depending on the mitochondrial redox potential, that is, the ratio of the reduced form of nicotinamide adenine dinucleotide to its oxidized form (NADH/NAD$^+$), some of the acetoacetate is converted to 3-hydroxybutyrate, and both ketone bodies are transported out of liver mitochondria and hepatocytes into blood where they may be used by other tissues, especially brain. Acetoacetyl CoA derived from the last turn of the beta oxidation spiral together with acetyl CoA forms HMG-CoA in a reaction catalyzed by HMG-CoA synthetase. Normally acetoacetyl CoA can also be hydrolyzed to acetyl CoA by the mitochondrial acetoacetyl-CoA thiolase. Patients with a deficiency of this thiolase do not have a defect in ketone body synthesis but rather have metabolic acidosis associated with excess ketosis (Cornblath et al, 1971; Daum et al, 1971; Sweetman and Williams, 1995). The clinical features are variable. Severe acute metabolic decompensation has been reported in infants, but there are also asymptomatic adults. The episodes are heralded by fasting or increased protein intake, because isoleucine is a precursor of 2-methylacetoacetyl CoA, which is also a substrate for the mitochondrial acetoacetyl-CoA thiolase enzyme. Thus, this block leads to a defect in the distal catabolism of isoleucine and in the processing of the precursor of ketone body formation, namely, acetoacetyl CoA. Cardiomyopathy has been identified in rare patients. The characteristic urinary metabolite pattern detected on urine organic acid quantitation centers around the presence of the isoleucine metabolites such as 2-methylacetoacetate, 2-methyl-3-hydroxybutyrate, and tiglylglycine. During acute decompensation, lactate, as well as the traditional ketone bodies, is detected in excess amounts in the urine. Some older children have been mistakenly identified as having ketotic hypoglycemia. The amino acid glycine may be elevated in plasma. Deficiency in the mitochondrial acetoacetyl-CoA thiolase can be demonstrated in cultured skin fibroblasts. The gene has been cloned and sequenced. Several mutations have been identified. Treatment of the acute episodes consists of intravenous glucose and administration of alkali to correct metabolic acidosis, which may be severe. Long-term therapy consists of protein restriction and avoidance of fasting.

The synthesis of acetoacetate from HMG-CoA is dependent on the HMG-CoA lyase enzyme. A deficiency of this enzyme represents the most profound defect in ketone body synthesis (Gibson et al, 1988; Sweetman and Williams, 1995). About one third of the patients with this disease present in the first week of life. The onset is dramatic and the disease is catastrophic as characterized by vomiting, lethargy, coma, seizures, hepatomegaly, hypoglycemia, little or no ketones in the urine, and hyperammonemia. Most of the complications are related to the severe effects of hypoglycemia on the CNS, in addition to the acidemia, which may be profound. The characteristic urine metabolites detected by GC-MS analysis are 3-hydroxy-3-methylglutaric acid, 3-methylglutaconic acid, and 3-hydroxyisovaleric acid. Only small, inappropriate amounts of acetoacetic acid and 3-hydroxybutyric acid may be detected. Lactate levels may be elevated during the acute metabolic decompensation. Inherited as an autosomal recessive trait, the HMG-CoA lyase deficiency can be demonstrated in cultured skin fibroblasts. Treatment of the acute episode consists of administration of intravenous glucose and alkali to correct the metabolic acidosis. Most chronic therapy consists of a high-carbohydrate diet. Some patients are placed on a protein-restricted diet, but the most important element in long-term care is the avoidance of fasting.

The last defect to be discussed in the area of disturbances in ketone body metabolism is the succinyl-CoA: 3-ketoacid-CoA transferase deficiency (Cornblath et al, 1971; Sweetman and Williams, 1995). In this disease, the ketone bodies, acetoacetic acid, and 3-hydroxybutyric acid are synthesized adequately in the liver, but in the extrahepatic tissues they cannot be metabolized because of the failure of activation of acetoacetate to acetoacetyl CoA by the transferase enzyme. Conversion to a CoA derivative is required for hydrolysis to acetyl CoA for final metabolism in the Krebs citric acid cycle. This is a rare disorder, and most of the patients who have presented in the newborn period have not survived. Such patients usually exhibit severe ketolactic acidosis. The hallmark of this disease is that ketosis never disappears, even after correction of the overt metabolic acidosis and the institution of frequent feedings with the avoidance of fasting. Plasma levels of acetoacetate and 3-hydroxybutyrate are always mild to moderately elevated, resulting in intermittent ketonuria. The most important aspect of therapy is the avoidance of fasting, during which time acidosis and ketosis can be overwhelming. The gene that encodes this enzyme has been cloned, and several mutations have been detected.

Primary Lactic Acidosis

The term *primary lactic acidosis* (PLA) refers to those diseases in which impaired lactate metabolism is due to a defect in the mitochondrial respiratory or ETC, the tricarboxylic acid (TCA) (Krebs) cycle, the accessory components that support mitochondrial function and shuttling of reducing equivalents, or when there is a primary defect in pyruvate metabolism that secondarily leads to impaired lactate handling (see Fig. 25–1) (Shoffner and Wallace, 1995; Robinson, 1995). However, there are only a handful of reports on inborn errors of the TCA cycle (Blass et al, 1972). Most of the information on PLA focuses on mitochondrial ETC, pyruvate dehydrogenase (PDH) complex, and pyruvate carboxylase (PC) defects, all of which have been masterfully reviewed by Shoffner and Wallace (1995) and Robinson (1995). The approach taken in this section has been influenced by their reviews, as well as by the pioneering work of DeVivo, DiMauro, Blass, Brown, Holt, and Kerr, to which the reader is directed for details that cannot be included because they are beyond the scope of this chapter.

Some patients present with overwhelming lactic acidosis. In others, lactate may only be elevated in CSF, a "cerebral" lactic acidosis syndrome (Brown et al, 1988). Depending on the nature of the enzyme deficiency, lactate and pyruvate, as well as alanine, can be elevated in blood. The ratio of blood lactate to pyruvate (L/P ratio) can be helpful in distinguishing the different types of inborn errors. For example, the L/P ratio is often normal (10 to 20) in the PDH and PC deficiencies but elevated in an ETC defect.

Pyruvate Dehydrogenase Deficiency

Pyruvate Dehydrogenase (PDH) Complex Deficiency

$$\text{Pyruvate} + \text{CoA} \xrightarrow{\text{PDH}} \text{Acetyl CoA} + CO_2$$

Enzyme: 12 Subunits per Functional Component
4 Pyruvate Decarboxylase (E_1) Subunits
2 $E_1\alpha$ Subunits
2 $E_1\beta$ Subunits
1 Dihydrolipoyl Transacylase (E_2) Subunit
1 X-lipoate component
2 Dihydrolipoyl Dehydrogenase (E_3) Subunits
2 PDH Kinase Subunits
2 PDH Phosphatase Subunits

Gene Location: $E_1\alpha$ on Chromosome X p22.1-22.2
$E_1\beta$ on Chromosome 3 p13-q23
E_3 on Chromosome 7 q31-32

Frequency: <1/250,000

CASE STUDY 6

The male infant, the product of a 36-week gestation, was delivered by caesarean section because of breech presentation. He required assistance with ventilation at birth. The Apgar scores were 5 and 9 at 1 and 5 minutes, respectively. At 1 hour of life, the infant developed generalized seizures. An arterial blood pH was 7.38 and P_{CO_2} was 13 mm Hg. The serum total CO_2 was 5 mmol/L and glucose was 76 mg/dL. Blood lactate and pyruvate were 9.93 mmol/L (normal ≤ 2.0) and 0.53 mmol/L (normal ≤ 0.20), respectively; the lactate/pyruvate ratio was 18.8 (normal ≤ 20).

On physical examination, the infant was lethargic and hypotonic. His weight (1770 g) and length (42 cm) were below the 3rd percentile, and head circumference (31 cm) was below the 10th percentile. Several minor craniofacial abnormalities including hypertelorism, micrognathia, and low-set posteriorly rotated ears were detected. He also had a pectus excavatum, first-degree hypospadius, and rocker-bottom feet. There were few spontaneous movements, but he responded to tactile stimulation with withdrawal. Neurologic findings included bilateral ptosis, bifacial palsy, and weak bulbar function.

The metabolic acidosis persisted, necessitating large amounts of intravenous sodium bicarbonate, and on day 2, the infant required mechanical ventilation. By the third day of life, the baby was completely unresponsive. An EEG showed a burst suppression pattern and a head CT revealed bilateral Grade II intraventricular hemorrhages, a subarachnoid hemorrhage, and agenesis of the corpus callosum. Phenobarbital was started. The infant had received only intravenous glucose since his initial resuscitation. Prior to initiation of total parenteral nutrition with triglycerides at 1 week of age, the neonatal reflexes, doll's eye, and pupillary light reflexes were absent.

Over the next few days, the infant's level of consciousness improved, he was weaned off the ventilator, and the metabolic acidosis resolved. The phenobarbital was eventually discontinued. Analysis of organic acids in urine by gas chromotography revealed increased lactate excretion. Prior to discharge at 1 month of age on a proprietary formula, the baby had had several episodes of bradycardia and was still hypotonic.

Over the next several months, the baby failed to grow despite adequate caloric intake. The metabolic acidosis had returned and was associated with elevated blood lactate levels. He required more than 4 mEq of sodium bicarbonate per kilogram per day for partial correction. The infant was administered a high-fat diet and megadoses of thiamine hydrochloride. Despite normalization of blood lactate, there was no clinical improvement. At 7 months his length, weight, and head circumference were less than 5th percentile.

He remained extremely hypotonic, did not appear to have vision, and had normal reflexes in the upper limbs but none in the lower extremities. He was resuscitated from a respiratory arrest at 7 months, but at 8 months he died of a nocturnal primary respiratory arrest.

In cultured skin fibroblasts, there was 20% residual activity of the PDH complex. Western blot analysis revealed trace amounts of both $E_1\alpha$ and $E_1\beta$ subunits, but only the $E_1\alpha$ peptide had abnormal electrophoretic mobility.

The most common cause of a primary defect in pyruvate metabolism is PDH complex deficiency (Robinson, 1995). This complex is located in the mitochondria and is made up of several components, including the $E_1\alpha$ and $E_1\beta$ subunits, the E_2 subunit, the E_3 subunit, the X-lipoate subunit, and the PDH phosphatase and kinase components. Most mutations have been reported in the E_1 subunit (Robinson et al, 1987). Unlike the other components, the $E_1\alpha$ subunit is encoded on the X chromosome. Because of the key importance of the PDH complex in energy metabolism, even partial defects may be associated with severe CNS disease. In addition, even though the $E_1\alpha$ subunit defect is an X-linked disease, many females are also affected, so this can be considered a dominant mutation. All the other defects are inherited as autosomal recessive disorders.

There are several different phenotypes of PDH complex deficiency, based on the severity of the enzyme deficiency. Most of the patients with less than 20% residual enzyme activity in cultured skin fibroblasts present in the newborn period with overwhelming lactic acidosis (Farrel et al, 1975; Federico et al, 1990; Robinson et al, 1987; Stromme et al, 1976). Some patients, but perhaps those without life-threatening acidosis, even have congenital lesions associated with cystic lesions in the cerebral hemisphere; cerebral atrophy; cystic lesions in the basal ganglia; and facial dysmorphism, including features that resemble fetal alcohol syndrome, such as a narrowed head, frontal bossing, wide nasal bridge and upturned nose, a long poorly developed philtrum, and flared nostrils. In addition, there may be partial or complete agenesis of the corpus callosum and impaired migration of neurons within the cerebral hemispheres, identified as heterotopic dysplasia on neuropathologic examination of brain tissue. Patients with less severe defects manifest progressive psychomotor retardation (Miyabayashi et al, 1985), including the entity termed *Leigh disease*, or *subacute necrotizing encephalomyelopathy* (SNE) (DeVivo et al, 1979), as discussed later, and older patients such as males with variant lesions may manifest only intermittent ataxia during childhood (Blass et al, 1970) with a mild or intermittent lactic acidosis. Secondary hyperammonemia has been detected (Brown et al, 1987).

The $E_1\alpha$ subunit gene on the X chromosome has been cloned and sequenced, and multiple mutations have been identified. The E_2 and protein X-lipoate defects are rare and usually result in chronic psychomotor retardation syndrome in late infancy and childhood (Robinson et al, 1990). The E_3 subunit defect is a unique syndrome (Taylor et al, 1978), because the subunit is important not only in the PDH complex but also in the branched-chain ketoacid dehydrogenase (BCKAD) complex and the alpha-ketoglutarate dehydrogenase (KGDH) complex. Thus, these patients have multiple deficiencies involving the branched-chain amino acid as in MSUD, as well as Krebs cycle metabolites indicative of a block in the TCA cycle. Most of the patients present later than the newborn period and have severe progressive neurodegenerative disease. The key laboratory findings are elevations of lactic acid in blood, branched-chain amino acids in plasma, and alpha-ketoglutarate in urine on urine organic acid testing. PDH phosphatase deficiency is a rare cause of congenital lactic acidosis (Robinson and Sherwood, 1975). There is no effective treatment for any of these defects in PDH complex metabolism that present in the newborn period. A response to thiamine megatherapy has been reported in a few patients. Metabolic imbalance in the patient with PDH deficiency, as well as in other PLA defects, may be further compromised by high- or selective-carbohydrate feedings. There has been some success in reducing lactate accumulation with the use of a ketogenic diet. Dichloracetate, an inhibitor of the PDH kinase, is being studied as a treatment for several PLAs (Kuroda et al, 1986; McCormick et al, 1985; Stacpoole et al, 1983).

Pyruvate Carboxylase Deficiency

Pyruvate Carboxylase (PC) Deficiency

$$\text{Pyruvate + ATP + HCO}_3 \xrightarrow{\text{PC}} \text{Oxaloacetate + AMP + PP}_1$$

Enzyme: Homotetramer
Gene Location: Chromosome 11q13
Frequency: 1/250,000

There are three types of PC deficiency (Robinson, 1995; Robinson et al, 1984). Type A is characterized by lactic acidosis in the newborn period and delayed development (DeVivo et al, 1977). However, the disease is of a chronic nature. In the catastrophic form of the disease, type B, the infant is acutely ill, usually in the first week of life with encephalopathy, severe metabolic acidosis with lactic acidosis, and hyperammonemia (Saudubray et al, 1976). The mortality rate in this form is high. In one case, referred to as type C, the patient presented with mild episodic metabolic acidosis and lactic acidosis, but with no evidence of CNS dysfunction (Van Coster et al, 1991).

As discussed earlier, PC is a biotin-containing enzyme. Most of the patients presenting with a type B form of PC deficiency were of French or English origin. Unlike patients with a type A defect, in whom the blood L/P ratio is normal because both lactate and pyruvate are comparably elevated, patients with the B defect form often have an elevated L/P ratio. Because of the importance of the PC product oxaloacetate in providing adequate cellular levels of aspartate, citrulline metabolism in the urea cycle is defective, leading to elevations of citrulline, as well as plasma ammonium concentrations. Although PC is also an important enzyme in gluconeogenesis, hypoglycemia has not been a frequently reported finding. The liver may be enlarged. There is no effective treatment for PC deficiency when it is associated with progressive neurodegeneration. The gene that encodes the PC subunits, of which four combine to make an active enzyme, has been cloned and sequenced. Several mutations have been identified. PC deficiency may be detected in cultured skin fibroblasts or in liver biopsy samples.

Phosphoenolpyruvate Carboxykinase Deficiency

Phosphoenolpyruvate carboxykinase (PEPCK) enzyme also functions in gluconeogenesis, and there are two forms in liver: one in the cytosol and the other in the mitochondrial compartment. Only three cases of PEPCK deficiency have been documented (Robinson, 1995). In each, the activity of PEPCK was found to be deficient in liver tissue. Patients do not usually come to attention until childhood with hypotonia, failure to thrive, hepatomegaly, lactic acidosis, and hypoglycemia. One patient had a more severe phenotype associated with severe liver disease and died at 6 months of age (Clayton et al, 1986). The accuracy of the diagnosis of PEPCK in some other patients is in question. Although there is no adequate experience on which to identify the optimal therapy for these patients, it is reasonable to assume that frequent feedings and avoiding of fasting are important in avoiding severe metabolic imbalance.

Mitochondrial Respiratory Chain or Electron Transport Chain Defects

Oxidative phosphorylation is the key process performed by the mitochondria of cells. Any inborn error of metabolism that involves the tightly coupled and regulated process of mitochondrial energy metabolism may have profound effects on health and disease because oxidative phosphorylation is the process by which we convert food into energy. The various derivatives of foodstuffs such as pyruvate and fatty acids are converted to CO_2 in mitochondria. The energy derived from such controlled chemical combustion is harnessed by allowing the reducing equivalences (in the form of NADH or $FADH_2$, which are derived from such metabolism) to combine with oxygen to form H_2O, and in the process the synthesis of ATP is coupled to the orderly flow of electrons down the respiratory chain components.

There are several important components in the mitochondrial respiratory chain, including complex 1 (NADH dehydrogenase); complex 2 (ETF dehydrogenase); complex 3 (cytochrome b, c_1) and the terminal complex in this chain; and complex 4, which is cytochrome c oxidase (Shoffner and Wallace, 1995). In addition, there is a complex 5 or ATP synthetase and an adenine nucleotide translocase, which permits transport of adenosine diphosphate (ADP) into and ATP out of the mitochondria. Complex 2 is involved primarily in fatty acid oxidation and oxidation of succinate derived from the Krebs cycle, as the reducing equivalents extracted from fatty acids, glutaric acid, and succinate flow from ETF into complex 2. The polypeptides that comprise these various complexes are derived from both the nuclear genes, as well as the genes on mitochondrial DNA (mtDNA). Except for complex 2, mtDNA is important in production of the subunits of all the respiratory chain complexes. PLA involving the ETC components has been associated with both nuclear and mtDNA mutations.

Based on molecular diagnostic testing, the oxidative phosphorylation diseases can be divided into four genetic groups: (1) nuclear DNA mutations; (2) mtDNA point mutations; (3) mtDNA deletions and duplications; and (4) unidentified genetic defects (Shoffner and Wallace, 1995). The relationship between phenotype and mtDNA mutations is not straightforward, probably because of the phenomenon of heteroplasmy. Mitochondria with their unique mtDNA are inherited solely from the mother (Hutchinson et al, 1974). Random segregation of mitochondria having mtDNA mutations leads to heteroplasmy and, ultimately, a variable concentration of defective mitochondria within cells and among tissues (Shoffner and Wallace, 1995). Most of our understanding of the detailed molecular mechanisms that contribute to or produce the ETC gene disturbances concern the mtDNA mutations. However, with the exception of the neurogenic muscle weakness, ataxia, retinitis pigmentosa (NARP) mutation, few of the primary mtDNA defects, as exemplified by the MELAS (*m*itochondrial *e*ncephalopathy, *l*actic acidosis, *a*nd *s*troke-like episodes) (Goto et al, 1990; Ciafaloni et al, 1992), MERRF (*m*yoclonic *e*pilepsy and *r*agged-*r*ed *f*iber) (Noer et al, 1991), Leber hereditary optic neuropathy (Wallace et al, 1988), and sporadic deletion syndromes (Holt et al, 1988), actually present in the newborn period. The diseases that affect young infants are benign infantile mitochondrial myopathy and/or cardiomyopathy, lethal infantile mitochondrial disease, Barth syndrome, SNE or Leigh disease, Pearson syndrome, Alpers disease, lethal infantile cardiomyopathies of unknown etiology, and the most dramatic form with presentation often in the first few days of life during which an acid-base disturbance dominates the clinical picture.

Benign Infantile Mitochondrial Myopathy and/or Cardiomyopathy

Benign infantile mitochondrial myopathy is associated with congenital hypotonia and weakness at birth, feeding difficulties, respiratory difficulties, and lactic acidosis. In this poorly understood, developmental-like disorder, only skeletal muscle appears to be affected, and histochemical analyses reveal a cytochrome *c* oxidase deficiency that returns to normal levels after 1 to 3 years of age (DiMauro et al, 1983; Jerusalem et al, 1973; Roodhooft et al, 1986; Tritschler et al, 1991; Zeviani et al, 1987). It is believed that a nuclear DNA mutation in a gene important in a fetal isoform of an ETC polypeptide specific for muscle oxidative phosphorylation is the cause of this problem and that a developmental switch from the defective fetal gene to the adult form may be responsible for the gradual improvement. This disorder may be an inherited autosomal recessive or autosomal dominant fashion and is the only example of a developmental defect in oxidative phosphorylation that is probably nuclear encoded and in which the treatment is only support during the early newborn period to prevent death from respiratory disease.

The form also associated with cardiomyopathy may just be a variant of the benign isolated myopathy and involves striated muscle in both skeletal and cardiac muscle. Presentation is in the newborn period with lactic acidosis and a cardiomyopathy that improves during the first year of life. The exact gene defect is unknown. More attention needs to be paid to these two disease entities because with early optimal medical care, these infants may have excellent prognoses.

Lethal Infantile Mitochondrial Disease

Infants with lethal infantile mitochondrial disease are severely ill in the first few weeks of life or in the extended newborn period (DiMauro et al, 1980; Zeviani et al, 1986). They present with hypotonia, muscle weakness, failure to thrive, and severe lactic acidosis. Death occurs by 6 months

of age and almost always is associated with overwhelming lactic acidosis. Skeletal muscle shows lipid and glycogen accumulation and abnormally shaped mitochondria on electron microscopic examination. Hepatic dysfunction may be a prominent finding in these patients. Generalized proximal renal tubular dysfunction may occur, leading to full-blown renal Fanconi syndrome (DiMauro et al, 1980; Heinman et al 1982; Zeviani et al, 1986). The ETC defects reported in these patients include defects in complexes 1, 3, and 4, (Birch-Machin et al, 1989; Moreadith et al, 1984; Robinson et al, 1985; Sengers et al, 1984; Shoffner and Wallace, 1995; Zheng et al, 1989). Original reports concerned infants with a phenotype resembling severe Wernig-Hoffman disease with cytochrome *c* oxidase deficiency and renal Fanconi syndrome (DiMauro et al 1980; Heiman et al, 1982). This is probably more than one disease. Some studies have suggested that the cause is tissue-specific depletions of mtDNA (Boustany et al, 1983). The cause of the depletion is believed to be a nuclear-encoded gene, perhaps inherited as an autosomal recessive trait. In addition, some patients may have selective cytochrome *c* oxidase deficiency owing to a defective nuclear-encoded complex 4 gene.

Barth Syndrome

Barth syndrome is an X-linked disorder associated with cardiomyopathy, skeletal muscle disease, and neutropenia (Barth et al, 1983; Neustein et al, 1979). Skeletal muscle shows abnormal mitochondrial morphology. Important laboratory findings include decreased plasma free carnitine, increased urinary excretion of 3-methylglutaconate on GC-MS analysis of urine organic acids, and decreased levels of serum cholesterol in early infancy (Kelley et al, 1991). Positional cloning identified a gene for this disorder, on Xq28. Several mutations have been identified. The function of the gene product is unknown. Investigators have speculated that this may represent a defect in the mevalonate/polyisoprenoid pathway since, theoretically, 3-methylglutaconate may be derived from a mevalonate shunt pathway in conversion of HMG-CoA to the end products of the pathway, which include cholesterol. If a deficient polyisoprenoid metabolite perturbs mitochondrial structures and function, this would be the example of a disease in which neither the mtDNA nor the nuclear ETC genes are mutated. Patients must be supported during the newborn and early infancy periods. Investigators speculate that if severe cholesterol deficiency can be avoided, the infants may survive and be relatively free of cardiomyopathy during the childhood years. However, infants with a bona fide defect in the polyisoprenoid pathway, namely, mevalonic aciduria, present with a phenotype that more resembles a storage disease (Hoffmann et al, 1986). Furthermore, not all patients with 3-methylglutaconic aciduria have Barth syndrome—a few have isolated leucine-dependent 3-methylglutaconyl-CoA hydratase deficiency, but most suffer from ill-defined mitochondropathies (Gibson et al, 1993).

Subacute Necrotizing Encephalomyelopathy or Leigh Disease

Probably because of a failure to recognize the clinical signs, infants with SNE or Leigh disease usually come to clinical attention after the newborn period. This disease is best characterized as a progressive neurodegenerative disorder with severe hypotonia, seizures, extrapyramidal movement disorders, optic atrophy, and defects in automatic ventilation or respiratory control (Pincus, 1972). It is clear that there are many causes of SNE. As discussed earlier, PDH complex deficiency may lead to Leigh disease. Patients with defects in the ETC have also been reported with findings compatible with SNE. Many neuropathologists believe that the diagnosis of SNE depends on an analysis of CNS tissue at autopsy. However, MRI scanning characteristically reveals bilateral symmetrical lesions of the basal ganglia. There is no effective treatment for this disease. It is possible that most of the patients with Leigh disease have disturbances in nuclear-encoded genes. Although, as discussed later, the NARP lesion due to a group II mtDNA mutation is one important cause in early infancy. Clearly, this is not one disease entity because the specific neuropathologic findings of SNE have also been reported in a patient with Menke disease in which there exists a secondary ETC complex 4 deficiency, because copper is an important metal cofactor of cytochrome *c* oxidase.

The following clinical findings have been noted in infants with SNE: optic atrophy, ophthalmoplegia, nystagmus, respiratory abnormalities, ataxia, hypotonia, spasticity, seizures, developmental delay, psychomotor retardation, myopathy, and renal tubular dysfunction. Some patients may manifest hypertrophic cardiomyopathy, liver dysfunction, and microcephaly. The neuropathologic lesions include demyelination, gliosis, necrosis, relative neuronal sparing, and capillary proliferation in specific brain lesions. There are lesions of the basal ganglia, bilaterally symmetrical in nature, brain stem, cerebellum, and, to a much lesser degree, the cerebral cortex. Commonly, the elevation in blood lactate is only slight to moderate, as well as intermittent, in this diverse group of patients. In some instances, lactate levels may be elevated only in the CSF. The most commonly reported biochemical abnormalities are cytochrome *c* oxidase or complex 4 (DiMauro et al, 1987; Hoganson et al, 1984; Miranda et al, 1989; Willems et al, 1977), NADH dehydrogenase or complex 1 (Hoppel et al, 1987), and PDH deficiency. In a few rare patients, the abnormality in oxidative phosphorylation has been reported to be secondary to the NARP mutation. This involves a T-C transition at bp 8993 of the adenosine triphosphatase (ATPase) 6 gene changing a leucine to a proline at position 156 in the ATPase 6 polypeptide. Investigators have speculated that defects such as the cytochrome *c* oxidase and the NADH dehydrogenase when associated with the neuropathology of Leigh disease are due to nuclear gene mutations (Miranda et al, 1989) and not to mtDNA gene defects such as the NARP point mutation in the ATPase 6 gene (Santorelli et al, 1993; Shoffner et al, 1992; Tatuch et al, 1992).

The diseases in group III, exemplified by the Kearns-Sayre and chronic progressive external ophthalmoplegia syndromes (Shoffner and Wallace, 1995), are not familial and are due to mtDNA deletions (Moraes et al, 1989) or duplications (Poulton et al, 1989) that are spontaneous mutations. These disorders do not usually come to clinical attention in infancy. The only example of such a mutation presenting in early infancy is the Pearson syndrome (Cor-

mier et al, 1991; Rotig et al, 1989). This is a systemic disorder that primarily affects the hematopoietic system and pancreas function. The characteristics are severe macrocytic anemia with varying degrees of neutropenia and thrombocytopenia. Bone marrow examination shows normal cellularity but extensive vacuolization of erythroid and myeloid precursors, hemosiderosis, and ringed sideroblasts. This disease of the bone marrow may lead to death in infancy. However, patients who are able to recover or who benefit from aggressive therapy may develop other signs of this systemic disorder in late infancy or childhood such as poor growth, pancreas dysfunction, mitochondrial myopathy, lactic acidosis, and progressive neurologic damage (Majander et al, 1991; Nelson et al, 1992).

A number of diseases have been believed to be caused by mitochondrial respiratory chain problems, but the specific mutations are unknown. These constitute the class IV mutations, or the disorders of unknown inheritance (Shoffner and Wallace, 1995). Alpers disease is one such example. It has also been called *progressive infantile poliodystrophy*. In this progressive disease the infants and children develop progressive cerebral cortical damage, sometimes also involving the cerebellum, basal ganglia, and brain stem; in some, liver disease may progress to cirrhosis. The neuropathologic lesions include spongiform or microcystic cerebral degeneration, gliosis, necrosis, and capillary proliferation (Sandbank and Lerman, 1972). Seizures are prominent, including myoclonus. Laboratory abnormalities have included abnormal NADH oxidation or complex 1 defects, impaired pyruvate handling, and PDH complex deficiency, TCA cycle malfunction, and decreased mitochondrial cytochrome $a + a_3$ content (Prick et al, 1983). The diversity of these findings suggests that this may be more than one disease. Finally, some patients in this "wastebasket" category have manifested lethal infantile cardiomyopathy associated with cardiac failure and cardiac dysrrhythmias, including Wolff-Parkinson-White syndrome. The pathologic abnormalities have included a reduced number of myofibrils, cardiac fibers with increased lipid and glycogen, and abnormal number of mitochondria. Both cytochrome *b* and cytochrome $c + c_1$ deficiencies have been reported. The exact gene defects remain unknown.

Early Lethal Lactic Acidosis

In an unknown fraction of patients with primary disturbances in mitochondrial oxidative phosphorylation or ETC defects, massive lactic acidosis develops within 24 to 72 hours after birth. Not uncommonly, it is untreatable, because it is relentless and unresponsive to alkali therapy. Dialysis is a remedy but not a cure. Often, these infants have no obvious organ damage early in the course or evidence of malformations. This is also true for the PDH complex deficiency, which is probably a more common cause of overwhelming acidosis in the first week of life. In addition, acidemia, per se, can easily explain the coma or impaired cardiac contractility that may be encountered. Some infants have survived with aggressive therapy. Anecdotal reports also suggest the existence of a transient disease process. The care of babies with these different forms of severe lactic acidosis almost always brings an ethical and moral dilemma to the forefront for the physicians and nurses of the NICU, as well as for the babies' families. To further complicate the issues, enzymatic and molecular analyses are usually not immediately available. The disease in most patients probably remains idiopathic and no DNA mutation, nuclear or mitochondrial, can be identified. A rigid approach to care is impractical and unwise. Decisions regarding management need to be individualized because the mitochondrial dysfunction and resultant pathophysiology may vary among infants.

REFERENCES

Amendt BA, Green C, Sweetman L, et al: Short-chain acyl-coenzyme A dehydrogenase deficiency: Clinical and biochemical studies in two patients. J Clin Invest 79:1303, 1987.

Baker L, Winegrad AI: Fasting hypoglycaemia and metabolic acidosis associated with deficiency of hepatic fructose-1,6-diphosphatase activity. Lancet 2:13, 1970.

Ballard RA, Vinocur B, Reynolds JW, et al: Transient hyperammonemia of the preterm infant. N Engl J Med 299:920, 1978.

Barth PG, Scholte HR, Berden JA, et al: An X-linked mitochondrial disease affecting cardiac muscle, skeletal muscle, and neutrophil leucocytes. J Neurol Sci 62:327, 1983.

Batshaw ML: Hyperammonemia. Curr Prob Pediatr 14:1, 1984.

Berry GT, Heidenreich R, Kaplan P, et al: Branched-chain amino acid–free parenteral nutrition in the treatment of acute metabolic decompensation in patients with maple syrup urine disease. N Engl J Med 324:175, 1991.

Berry GT, Nissim I, Zhiping L, et al: Endogenous synthesis of galactose in normal man and patients with hereditary galactosaemia. Lancet 346:1073, 1995.

Berry GT, Yudkoff M, Segal S: Isovaleric acidemia: Medical and neurodevelopmental effects of long-term therapy. J Pediatr 113:58, 1988.

Bertini E, Dionisi-Vici C, Garavaglia B, et al: Peripheral sensory-motor polyneuropathy, pigmentary retinopathy, and fatal cardiomyopathy in long-chain 3-hydroxyacyl-CoA dehydrogenase deficiency. Eur J Pediatr 151:121, 1992.

Birch-Machin MA, Shepherd IM, Watmough NJ, et al: Fatal lactic acidosis in infancy with a defect of complex III of the respiratory chain. Pediatr Res 25:553, 1989.

Blass JP, Avigan J, Uhlendorf BW: A defect of pyruvate decarboxylase in a child with an intermittent movement disorder. J Clin Invest 49:423, 1970.

Blass JP, Schulman JD, Young DS, et al: An inherited defect affecting the tricarboxylic acid cycle in a patient with congenital lacticacidosis. J Clin Invest 51:1845, 1972.

Böhm N, Uy J, Kiessling M, et al: Multiple acyl-CoA dehydrogenation deficiency (glutaric aciduria type II), congenital polycystic kidneys, and symmetric warty degeneration of the cerebral cortex in two newborn brothers: II. Morphology and pathogenesis. Eur J Pediatr 139:60, 1982.

Boustany RN, Aprille JR, Halperin J, et al: Mitochondrial cytochrome deficiency presenting as a myopathy with hypotonia, external ophthalmoplegia, and lactic acidosis in an infant and as fatal hepatopathy in a second cousin. Ann Neurol 14:462, 1983.

Brown GK, Haan EA, Kirby DM, et al: "Cerebral" lactic acidosis: Defects in pyruvate metabolism with profound brain damage and minimal systemic acidosis. Eur J Pediatr 147:10, 1988.

Brown GK, Scholem RD, Hunt SM, et al: Hyperammonemia and lactic acidosis in a patient with pyruvate dehydrogenase deficiency. J Inherit Metab Dis 10:359, 1987.

Brusilow SW: Arginine, an indispensable amino acid for patients with inborn errors of urea synthesis. J Clin Invest 74:2144, 1984.

Brusilow SW: Treatment of urea cycle disorders. In Desnick RJ (ed): Treatment of Genetic Disease. New York, Churchill Livingstone, 1991, p 79.

Brusilow SW, Batashaw ML: Arginine therapy of argininosuccinase deficiency. Lancet 1:124, 1979.

Brusilow SW, Horwich AL: Urea cycle enzymes. In Scriver CR, Beaudet AL, Sly WS, et al (Eds): The Metabolic and Molecular Bases of Inherited Disease, 7th ed. New York, McGraw-Hill, 1995, p 1187.

Brusilow SW, Valle DL, Batshaw ML: New pathways of nitrogen excretion in inborn errors of urea synthesis. Lancet 2:452, 1979.

Budd MA, Tanaka K, Holmes LB, et al: Isovaleric acidemia: Clinical features of a new genetic defect of leucine metabolism. N Engl J Med 277:321, 1967.

Burchell A, Waddell ID: The molecular basis of the genetic deficiencies of five of the components of the glucose-6-phosphatase system: Improved diagnosis. Eur J Pediatr (suppl 1) 152:518, 1993.

Chalmers RA, Roe CR, Stacey TE, et al: Urinary excretion of L-carnitine and acylcarnitines by patients with disorders of organic acid metabolism: Evidence for secondary insufficiency of L-carnitine. Pediatr Res 18:1325, 1984.

Chen Y-T, Burchell A: Glycogen storage diseases. In Scriver CR, Beaudet AL, Sly WS, et al (Eds): The Metabolic and Molecular Bases of Inherited Disease, 7th ed. New York, McGraw-Hill, 1995, p 935.

Childs B, Nyhan WL, Borden M, et al: Idiopathic hyperglycinemia and hyperglycinuria, a new disorder of amino acid metabolism. Pediatrics 27:522, 1961.

Chuang DT, Shih VE: Disorders of branched-chain amino acid and keto acid metabolism. In Scriver CR, Beaudet AL, Sly WS, et al (Eds): The Metabolic and Molecular Bases of Inherited Disease, 7th ed. New York, McGraw-Hill, 1995, p 1239.

Ciafaloni E, Ricci E, Shanske S, et al: MELAS: Clinical features, biochemistry, and molecular genetics. Ann Neurol 31:391, 1992.

Clayton PT, Hyland K, Brand M, et al: Mitochondrial phosphoenolypyruvate carboxykinase deficiency. Eur J Pediatr 145:46, 1986.

Cohn RM, Yudkoff M, Rothman R, et al: Isovaleric acidemia: Use of glycine therapy in neonates. N Engl J Med 299:996, 1978.

Cormier V, Rotig A, Bonnefont JP, et al: Pearson's syndrome— pancytopenia with exocrine pancreatic insufficiency: New mitochondrial disease in the first year of childhood. Arch Fr Pediatr 48:171, 1991.

Cornblath M, Gingell RL, Fleming GA, et al: A new syndrome of ketoacidosis in infancy. J Pediatr 79:413, 1971.

Cornblath M, Schwartz R: Disorders of glycogen metabolism. In Disorders of Carbohydrate Metabolism in Infancy, 3rd ed. Boston, Blackwell Scientific, 1991, p 247.

Danner DJ, Armstrong N, Heffelfinger SC, et al: Absence of branched-chain acyltransferase as a cause of maple syrup urine disease. J Clin Invest 75:858, 1985.

Daum RS, Lamm PH, Mamer OA, et al: A "new" disorder of isoleucine metabolism. Lancet 2:1289, 1971.

David M, Michel M, Collombel C, et al: Transient hypertyrosinemia secondary to hepatic involvement: two cases of different etiologies (galactosemia, hepatitis). Pediatrie 25:459, 1970.

De Bracketeer M, Larochelle J: Genetic epidemiology of hereditary tyrosinemia in Quebec and in Saguenay-Lac St-Jean. Am J Hum Genet 47:302, 1990.

Demaugre F, Bonnefont J-P, Colonna M, et al: Infantile form of carnitine palmitoyltransferase II deficiency with hepatomuscular symptoms and sudden death: Physiopathological approach to carnitine palmitoyltransferase II deficiencies. J Clin Invest 87:859, 1991.

De Sousa C, Chalmers RA, Stacey TE, et al: The response to L-carnitine and glycine therapy in isovaleric acidaemia. Eur J Pediatr 144:451, 1986.

DeVivo D, Haymond MW, Leckie MP, et al: Clinical and biochemical implications of pyruvate carboxylase deficiency. J Clin Endocrinol Metab 45:1281, 1977.

DeVivo DC, Haymond MW, Obert KA, et al: Defective activation of the pyruvate dehydrogenase complex in subacute necrotizing encephalomyelopathy (Leigh disease). Ann Neurol 6:483, 1979.

Diliberti JH, DiGeorge AM, Auerbach VH: Abnormal leucine/isoleucine ratio and the etiology of acrodermatitis enteropathica–like rash in maple syrup urine (MSUD). Pediatr Res 7:154, 1973.

DiMauro S, DiMauro PMM: Muscle carnitine palmityltransferase deficiency and myoglobinuria. Science 182:929, 1973.

DiMauro S, Lombes A, Nakase H, et al: Cytochrome C oxidase deficiency in Leigh syndrome. Ann Neurol 22:498, 1987.

DiMauro S, Mendell JR, Sahenk Z, et al: Fatal infantile mitochondrial myopathy and renal dysfunction due to cytochrome-C-oxidase deficiency. Neurology 30:795, 1980.

DiMauro S, Nicholson JF, Hays AP, et al: Benign infantile mitochondrial myopathy due to reversible cytochrome C oxidase deficiency. Ann Neurol 14:226, 1983.

Ding J-H, Roe CR, Iafolla AK, et al: Medium-chain acyl-coenzyme A dehydrogenase deficiency and sudden infant death. N Engl J Med 325:61, 1991.

Dobyns WB: Agenesis of the corpus callosum and gyral malformations are frequent manifestations of nonketotic hyperglycinemia. Neurology 39:817, 1989.

Duran M, Wanders RJA, de Jager JP, et al: 3-Hydroxydicarboxylic aciduria due to long-chain 3-hydroxyacyl-coenzyme A dehydrogenase deficiency associated with sudden neonatal death: Protective effect of medium-chain triglyceride treatment. Eur J Pediatr 150:190, 1991.

Farrel DF, Clark AF, Scott CR, et al: Absence of pyruvate decarboxylase activity in man: A cause of congenital lacticacidosis. Science 187:1082, 1975.

Federico A, Doti MT, Fabrizi GM, et al: Congenital lactic acidosis due to a defect of pyruvate dehydrogenase complex (E_1). Eur Neurol 30:123, 1990.

Fenton WA, Rosenberg LE: Disorders of propionate and methylmalonate metabolism. *In* Scriver CR, Beaudet AL, Sly WS, et al (Eds): The Metabolic and Molecular Bases of Inherited Disease, 7th ed. New York, McGraw-Hill, 1995a, p 1423.

Fenton WA, Rosenberg LE: Inherited disorders of cobalamin transport and metabolism. *In* Scriver CR, Beaudet AL, Sly WS, et al (Eds): The Metabolic and Molecular Bases of Inherited Disease, 7th ed. 1995b, p 3129.

Fernandes J, Chen Y-T: Glycogen storage diseases. *In* Fernandes J, Saudubray J-M, van den Berghe G (Eds): Inborn Metabolic Diseases: Diagnosis and Treatment, 2nd ed. Berlin, Springer-Verlag, 1995, p 71.

Fernandes J, Leonard JV, Moses SW, et al: Glycogen storage disease: Recommendations for treatment. Eur J Pediatr 147:226, 1988.

Fiser RHJR, Melsher HL, Fisher DA: Hepatic phosphoenolpyruvate carboxylase (PEPCK) deficiency: A new cause of hypoglycemia in childhood. Pediatr Res 10:60, 1974.

Frerman FE, Goodman SI: Nuclear-encoded defects of the mitochondrial respiratory chain, including glutaric acidemia type II. *In* Scriver CR, Beaudet AL, Sly WS, et al (Eds): The Metabolic and Molecular Bases of Inherited Disease, 7th ed. New York, McGraw-Hill, 1995, p 1611.

Gerritsen T, Kaveggia E, Waisman HA: A new type of idiopathic hyperglycinemia with hypooxaluria. Pediatrics 36:882, 1965.

Giacoia GP, Berry GT: Acrodermatitis enteropathica–like syndrome secondary to isoleucine deficiency during treatment of maple syrup urine disease. Am J Dis Child 147:954, 1993.

Gibson KM, Breuer J, Nyhan WL: 3-Hydroxy-3-methylglutaryl-coenzyme A lyase deficiency: Review of 18 reported patients. Eur J Pediatr 148:180, 1988.

Gibson KM, Elpeleg ON, Jakobs C, et al: Multiple syndromes of 3-methylglutaconic aciduria. Pediatr Neurol 9:120, 1993.

Gitzelmann R, Arbenz UV, Willi UV: Hypergalactosaemia and portosystemic encephalopathy due to persistence of ductus venosus Arantii. Eur J Pediatr 151:564, 1992.

Gitzelmann R, Steinmann B, Van den Berghe G: Disorders of fructose metabolism. *In* Scriver CR, Beaudet AL, Sly WS, et al (Eds): The Metabolic and Molecular Bases of Inherited Disease, 7th edition. New York, McGraw-Hill, 1995, p 905.

Goodman SI, Frerman FE: Organic acidemias due to defects in lysine oxidation: 2-ketoadipic acidemia and glutaric acidemia. *In* Scriver CR, Beaudet AL, Sly WS, et al (Eds): The Metabolic and Molecular Bases of Inherited Disease, 7th ed. New York, McGraw-Hill, 1995, p 1451.

Goodman SI, Markey SP, Moe PG, et al: Glutaric aciduria—A "new" disorder of amino acid metabolism. Biochem Med 12:12, 1975.

Goto Y, Nonaka I, Horai S: A mutation in the tRNA (Leu) (UUR) gene associated with the MELAS subgroup of mitochondrial encephalomyopathies. Nature 348:651, 1990.

Gregersen G, Wintzensen H, Kolvraa S, et al: C_6-C_{10}-Dicarboxylic aciduria: Investigations of a patient with riboflavin-responsive multiple acyl-CoA dehydrogenation defects. Pediatr Res 16:861, 1982.

Hale DE, Batshaw ML, Coates PM, et al: Long-chain acyl-coenzyme A dehydrogenase deficiency: An inherited cause of nonketotic hypoglycemia. Pediatr Res 19:666, 1985.

Hamosh A, Johnston MV, Valle D: Nonketotic hyperglycinemia. *In* Scriver CR, Beaudet AL, Sly WS, et al (Eds): The Metabolic and Molecular Bases of Inherited Disease, 7th ed. New York, McGraw-Hill, 1995, p 1337.

Harpey JP, Charpentier C, Goodman SI, et al: Multiple acyl-CoA dehydrogenase deficiency occurring in pregnancy and caused by a defect in riboflavin metabolism in the mother. J Pediatr 103:394, 1983.

Heiman PTD, Bonilla E, DiMauro S, et al: Cytochrome-C-oxidase deficiency in a floppy infant. Neurology 328:898, 1982.

Hirschhorn R: Glycogen storage disease type II: Acid a-glucosidase (acid maltase) deficiency. *In* Scriver CR, Beaudet AL, Sly WS, et al (Eds):

The Metabolic and Molecular Bases of Inherited Disease, 7th ed. New York, McGraw-Hill, 1995, p 2443.

Hoffmann G, Gibson KM, Brandt IK, et al: Mevalonic aciduria—an inborn error of cholesterol and nonsterol isoprene biosynthesis in man. N Engl J Med 314:1610, 1986.

Hoffmann GF, Trefz FK, Barth PG, et al: Glutaryl-CoA dehydrogenase deficiency: A distinct encephalopathy. Pediatrics 88:1194, 1991.

Hoganson GE, Paulson DJ, Chun R, et al: Deficiency of muscle cytochrome C oxidase in Leigh's disease. Pediatr Res 18:222, 1984.

Holt IJ, Harding AE, Morgan-Hughes JA: Deletions of muscle mitochondrial DNA in patients with mitochondrial myopathies. Nature 331:717, 1988.

Hommes FA, Bendien K, Elema JD, et al: Two cases of phosphoenolpyruvate carboxykinase deficiency. Acta Paediatr Scand 65:233, 1976.

Hoppel CL, Kerr DS, Dahms B, et al: Deficiency of the reduced nicotinamide adenine dinucleotide dehydrogenase component of complex I of mitochondrial electron transport: Fatal infantile lactic acidosis and hypermetabolism with skeletal-cardiac myopathy and encephalopathy. J Clin Invest 80:71, 1987.

Hostetter MK, Levy HL, Winter HS, et al: Evidence for liver disease preceding amino acid abnormalities in hereditary tyrosinemia. N Engl J Med 308:1265, 1983.

Hug G, Bove KE, Soukup S: Lethal neonatal multiorgan deficiency of carnitine palmitoyltransferase II. N Engl J Med 325:1862, 1991.

Hutchinson CAI, Newbold JA, Potter SS, et al: Maternal inheritance of mammalian mitochondrial DNA. Nature 251:536, 1974.

Iafolla AK, Kahler SG: Megaloencephaly in the neonatal period as the initial manifestation of glutaric aciduria type I. J Pediatr 114:1004, 1989.

Jerusalem F, Angelini C, Engel A, et al: Mitochondria-lipid-glycogen (MLG) disease of muscle: A morphologically regressive congenital myopathy. Arch Neurol 29:162, 1973.

Kelley RI, Cheatham JP, Clark BJ, et al: X-linked dilated cardiomyopathy with neutropenia, growth retardation, and 3-methylglutaconic aciduria. J Pediatr 119:738, 1991.

Krieger I, Tanaka K: Therapeutic effects of glycine in isovaleric acidemia. Pediatr Res 10:25, 1976.

Kuroda Y, Ito M, Toshima K, et al: Treatment of chronic congenital lacticacidosis by oral administration of dichloroacetate. J Inherit Metab Dis 9:244, 1986.

Lehnert W, Wendel U, Lindenmaier S, et al: Multiple acyl-CoA dehydrogenation deficiency (glutaric aciduria type II), congenital polycystic kidneys, and symmetric warty dysplasia of the cerebral cortex in two brothers: I. Clinical, metabolical, and biochemical findings. Eur J Pediatr 139:56, 1982.

Levine SZ, Marples E, Gordon HH: A defect in the metabolism of aromatic amino acids in premature infants: The role of vitamin C. Science 90:620, 1939.

Lindblad B, Lindstedt S, Steen G: On the enzyme defects in hereditary tyrosinemia. Proc Natl Acad Sci USA 74:4641, 1977.

Lindstedt S, Holme E, Lock EA, et al: Treatment of hereditary tyrosinaemia type I by inhibition of 4-hydroxyphenylpyruvate dioxygenase. Lancet 340:813, 1992.

Luder AS, Davidson A, Goodman SI, et al: Transient nonketotic hyperglycinemia in neonates. J Pediatr 114:1013, 1989.

Lungarotti MS, Calabro A, Signorini E, et al: Cerebral edema in maple syrup urine disease. Am J Dis Child 136:648, 1982.

Majander A, Suomalainen A, Vettenranta K, et al: Congenital hypoplastic anemia, diabetes, and severe renal tubular dysfunction associated with a mitochondrial DNA deletion. Pediatr Res 30:327, 1991.

Matsumoto T, Ikano R, Sakura N, et al: Hypergalactaosaemia in a patient with portal-hepatic venous and hepatic arteriovenous shunts detected by neonatal screening. Eur J Pediatr 152:990, 1993.

Mayatepek E, Kurczynski TW, Hoppel CL: Long-term L-carnitine treatment in isovaleric acidemia. Pediatr Neurol 7:137, 1991.

McCormick K, Viscardi RM, Robinson BH, et al: Partial pyruvate decarboxylase deficiency with profound lacticacidosis and hyperammonemia: Responses to dichloroacetate and benzoate. Am J Med Genet 22:291, 1985.

Menkes JH, Hurst PL, Craig JM: A new syndrome: Progressive familial infantile cerebral dysfunction associated with an unusual urinary substance. Pediatrics 14:462, 1954.

Michalski AJ, Berry GT, Segal S: Holocarboxylase synthetase deficiency: Nine-year follow-up of a case and a review of the literature. J Inherit Metab Dis 12:312, 1989.

Middleton B, Day R, Lombes A, et al: Infantile ketoacidosis associated with decreased activity of succinyl-CoA: 3-ketoacid CoA-transferase. J Inherit Metab Dis 10(Suppl 2):273, 1987.

Miranda DF, Ishii S, DiMauro S, et al: Cytochrome C oxidase (COX) deficiency in Leigh's syndrome: Genetic evidence for a nuclear DNA-encoded mutation. Neurology 39:697, 1989.

Mitchell GA, Lambert M, Tanguay RM: Hypertyrosinemia. *In* Scriver CR, Beaudet AL, Sly WS, et al (Eds): The Metabolic and Molecular Bases of Inherited Disease, 7th ed. New York, McGraw-Hill, 1995, p 1077.

Miyabayashi S, Ito T, Narisawa K, et al: Biochemical study in 28 children with lactic acidosis in relation to Leigh's encephalomyelopathy. Eur J Pediatr 143:278, 1985.

Morales CT, DiMauro S, Zeviani M, et al: Mitochondrial DNA deletions in progressive external ophthalmoplegia and Kearns-Sayre syndrome. N Engl J Med 320:1293, 1989.

Moreadith RW, Batshaw ML, Ohnishi T, et al: Deficiency of the iron-sulfur clusters of mitochondrial-reduced nicotinamide-adenine dinu-cleotide-ubiquinone oxidoreductase (complex I) in an infant with congenital lactic acidosis. J Clin Invest 74:685, 1984.

Morton DH, Bennett MJ, Seargeant LE, et al: Glutaric aciduria type I: A cause of episodic encephalopathy and spastic paralysis in the Amish of Lancaster County, Pennsylvania. Am J Med Genet 41:89, 1991.

Mowat AJ, Bennett MJ, Variend S, et al: Deficiency of medium chain fatty acyl coenzyme A dehydrogenase presenting as the sudden infant death syndrome. Br Med J 288:976, 1984.

Msall M, Batshaw ML, Suss R, et al: Neurologic outcome in children with inborn errors of urea synthesis. N Engl J Med 310:1500, 1984.

Mudd SH, Levy HL, Skovby F: Disorders of trans-sulfuration. *In* Scriver CR, Beaudet AL, Sly WS, et al (Eds): The Metabolic and Molecular Bases of Inherited Disease, 7th ed. New York, McGraw-Hill, 1995, p 1279.

Munnich A, Saudubray JM, Taylor J, et al: Congenital lactic acidosis, alpha-ketoglutaric aciduria and variant form of maple syrup urine disease due to a single enzyme defect: Dihydrolipoyl dehydrogenase deficiency. Acta Paediatr Scand 71:161, 1982.

Naglak M, Salvo R, Madsen K, et al: The treatment of isovaleric acidemia with glycine supplement. Pediatr Res 24:9, 1988.

Nelson I, Bonne G, Degoul F, et al: Kearns-Sayre syndrome with sid-eroblastic anemia: Molecular investigations. Neuropediatrics 23:199, 1992.

Neustein HB, Lurie PR, Dahms B, et al: An X-linked cardiomyopathy with abnormal mitochondrial. Pediatrics 64:24, 1979.

Noer AS, Sudoyo H, Lertrit P, et al: A tRNA (Lys) mutation in the mtDNA is the causal genetic lesion underlying myoclonic epilepsy and ragged-red fiber (MERRF) syndrome. Am J Hum Genet 49:715, 1991.

Parini R, Sereni LP, Bagozzi DC, et al: Nasogastric drip feeding as the only treatment of neonatal maple syrup urine disease. Pediatrics 92:280, 1993.

Pincus JH: Subacute necrotizing encephalomyelopathy (Leigh's disease): A consideration of clinical features and etiology. Dev Med Child Neurol 14:87, 1972.

Poulton J, Deadman ME, Gardiner RM: Duplications of mitochondrial DNA in mitochondrial myopathy. Lancet 1:236, 1989.

Prick MJJ, Gabreels FJM, Trijbels JMF, et al: Progressive poliodystrophy (Alpers disease) with a defect in cytochrome aa3 in muscle: A report of two unrelated patients. Clin Neurol Neurosurg 85:57, 1983.

Przyrembel H, Wendel U, Becker K, et al: Glutaric aciduria type II: Report on a previously undescribed metabolic disorder. Clin Chim Acta 66:227, 1976.

Riviello JJ Jr, Rezvani I, diGeorge AM, et al: Cerebral edema causing death in children with maple syrup urine disease. J Pediatr 119:42, 1991.

Robinson BH: Lactic acidemia (disorders of pyruvate carboxylase, pyruvate dehydrogenase). *In* Scriver CR, Beaudet AL, Sly WS, et al (Eds): The Metabolic and Molecular Bases of Inherited Disease, 7th ed. New York, McGraw-Hill, 1995, p 1479.

Robinson BH: Lactic acidemia: Biochemical, clinical and genetic considerations. *In* Harris H, Hirscborn K (Eds): Advances in Human Genetics. New York, Plenum, 1989.

Robinson BH, MacKay N, Petrova-Benedict R, et al: Defects in the E2 lipoyl transacetylase and the X-lipoyl containing component of the pyruvate dehydrogenase complex in patients with lactic acidemia. J Clin Invest 85:1821, 1990.

Robinson BH, MacMillan H, Petrova-Benedict R, et al: Variable clinical presentation in patients with deficiency of the pyruvate dehydrogenase complex: A review of 30 cases with a defect in the E1 component of the complex. J Pediatr 111:525, 1987.

Robinson BH, McKay N, Goodyer P, et al: Defective intramitochondrial NADH oxidation in skin fibroblasts from an infant with fatal neonatal lacticacidemia. Am J Hum Genet 37:938, 1985.

Robinson BH, Oei J, Sherwood WG, et al: The molecular basis for the two different clinical presentations of classical pyruvate carboxylase deficiency. Am J Hum Genet 36:283, 1984.

Robinson BH, Sherwood WG: Pyruvate dehydrogenase phosphatase deficiency: A cause of chronic congenital lacticacidosis in infancy. Pediatr Res 9:935, 1975.

Roe CR, Coates PM: Mitochondrial fatty acid oxidation disorders. *In* Scriver CR, Beaudet AL, Sly WS, et al (Eds): The Metabolic and Molecular Bases of Inherited Disease, 7th ed. New York, McGraw-Hill, 1995, p 1501.

Roe CR, Millington DS, Maltby DA, et al: L-carnitine therapy in isovaleric acidemia. J Clin Invest 74:2290, 1984.

Roodhooft AM, Van AKJ, Martin JJ, et al: Benign mitochondrial myopathy with deficiency of NADH-CoQ reductase and cytochrome *c* oxidase. Neuropediatrics 17:221, 1986.

Rosenblatt DS: Inherited disorders of folate transport and metabolism. *In* Scriver CR, Beaudet AL, Sly WS, et al (Eds): The Metabolic and Molecular Bases of Inherited Disease, 7th ed. New York, McGraw-Hill, 1995, p 3111.

Rotig A, Colonna M, Blanche S, et al: Mitochondrial DNA deletions in Pearson's marrow/pancreas syndrome. Lancet 1:902, 1989.

Rutledge SL, Havens PL, Haymond MW, et al: Neonatal hemodialysis: Effective therapy for the encephalopathy of inborn errors of metabolism. J Pediatr 116:125, 1990.

Sandbank U, Lerman P: Progressive cerebral poliodystrophy: Alpers disease—disorganized giant neuronal mitochondria on electron microscopy. J Neurol Neurosurg Psychiatry 35:749, 1972.

Santorelli FM, Shanske S, Jain KD, et al: A new mtDNA mutation in the ATPase 6 gene in a child with Leigh syndrome. Neurology 43:A171, 1993.

Saudubray JM, Marsac C, Charpentier C, et al: Neonatal congenital lactic acidosis with pyruvate carboxylase deficiency in two siblings. Acta Paediatr Scand 65:717, 1976.

Saudubray J-M, Martin D, Poggi-Travert F, et al: Clinical presentations of inherited mitochondrial fatty acid oxidation disorders: An update. Int Pediatr 12:34, 1997.

Schiffman R, Kaye EM, Willis JK III, et al: Transient neonatal hyperglycinemia. Ann Neurol 25:201, 1989.

Schoeman MN, Batey RG, Wilcken B: Recurrent acute fatty liver of pregnancy associated with a fatty acid oxidation defect in the offspring. Gastroenterology 100:544, 1991.

Scriver CR, Clow CL: Phenylketonuria: Epitome of human biochemical genetics: I. N Engl J Med 303:1336, 1980a.

Scriver CR, Clow CL: Phenylketonuria: Epitome of human biochemical genetics: II. N Engl J Med 303:1394, 1980b.

Scriver CR, Kaufman S, Eisensmith RC, et al: The hyperphenylalanin-emias. *In* Scriver CR, Beaudet AL, Sly WS, et al (Eds): The Metabolic and Molecular Bases of Inherited Disease, 7th ed. New York, McGraw-Hill, 1995, p 1015.

Segal S, Berry, GT: Disorders of galactose metabolism. *In* Scriver CR, Beaudet AL, Sly WS, et al (Eds): The Metabolic and Molecular Bases of Inherited Disease, 7th ed. New York, McGraw-Hill, 1996, p 967.

Sengers RCX, Trijbels JMF, Bakkeren JAJM, et al: Deficiency of cytochromes b and aa3 in muscle from a floppy infant with cytochrome C oxidase deficiency. Eur J Pediatr 141:178, 1984.

Shih VE, Herrin JT, Erickson AM: Hyperalimentation and peritoneal dialysis during acute metabolic decompensation in maple syrup urine disease. Pediatr Res 9:355, 1975.

Shoffner JM, Fernhoff PM, Krawiecki NS, et al: Subacute necrotizing encephalopathy: Oxidative phosphorylation defects and the ATPase 6 point mutation. Neurology 42:2168, 1992.

Shoffner JM, Wallace DC: Oxidative phosphorylation diseases. *In* Scriver CR, Beaudet Al, Sly WS, et al (Eds): The Metabolic and Molecular Bases of Inherited Disease, 7th ed. New York, McGraw-Hill, 1995, p 1535.

Stacpoole PW, Harman EM, Curry SH, et al: Treatment of lactic acidosis with dichloroacetate. N Engl J Med 309:390, 1983.

Stanley CA: New genetic defects in mitochondrial fatty acid oxidation and carnitine deficiency. Adv Pediatr 34:59, 1987.

Stanley CA, Hale DE, Berry GT, et al: A deficiency of carnitine-acylcarnitine translocase in the inner mitochondrial membrane. N Engl J Med 327:19, 1992.

Stromme JH, Borud O, Moe PJ: Fatal lactic acidosis in a newborn attributable to a congenital defect of pyruvate dehydrogenase. Pediatr Res 10:60, 1976.

Sweetman L, Williams JC: Branched-chain organic acidurias. *In* Scriver CR, Beaudet Al, Sly WS, et al (Eds): The Metabolic and Molecular Bases of Inherited Disease, 7th ed. New York, McGraw-Hill, 1995, p 1387.

Tada K, Hayasaka K: Nonketotic hyperglycinaemia: Clinical and biochemical aspects. Eur J Pediatr 146:221, 1987.

Tanaka K, Budd MA, Efron ML, et al: Isovaleric acidemia: A new genetic defect of leucine metabolism. Proc Natl Acad Sci USA 56:236, 1966.

Tatuch Y, Chrisrodoulou J, Feigenbaum A, et al: Heteroplasmic mitochondrial DNA mutation (T to G) at 8993 can cause Leigh disease when the percentage of abnormal mtDNA is high. Am J Hum Genet 50:852, 1992.

Taylor J, Robinson BH, Sherwood WG: A defect in branched-chain amino acid metabolism in a patient with congenital lacticacidosis due to dihydrolipoyl dehydrogenase deficiency. Pediatr Res 12:60, 1978.

Thompson GN, Butt WW, Shann FA, et al: Continuous venovenous hemofiltration in the management of acute decompensation in inborn errors of metabolism. J Pediatr 118:879, 1991.

Townsend I, Kerr DS: Total parenteral nutrition therapy of toxic maple syrup urine disease. Am J Clin Nutr 36:359, 1982.

Treem WR, Stanley CA, Finegold DN, et al: Primary carnitine deficiency due to a failure of carnitine transport in kidney, muscle, and fibroblasts. N Engl J Med 319:1331, 1988.

Treem WR, Stanley CA, Hale DE, et al: Hypoglycemia, hypotonia, and cardiomyopathy: The evolving clinical picture of long-chain acyl-CoA dehydrogenase deficiency. Pediatrics 87:328, 1991.

Tritschler HJ, Bonilla E, Lombes A, et al: Differential diagnosis of fatal and benign cytochrome C oxidase–deficient myopathies of infancy: An immunohistochemical approach. Neurology 41:300, 1991.

Van Biervliet JPGM, Bruinvis L, Ketting D, et al: Hereditary mitochondrial myopathy with lactic acidemia, a DeToni-Fanconi-Debre syndrome and a defective respiratory chain in voluntary striated muscles. Pediatr Res 11:1088, 1977.

Van Coster RN, Fernhoff PM, DeVivo DC: Pyruvate carboxylase deficiency: A benign variant with normal development. Pediatr Res 30:1, 1991.

Velazquez A, Prieto EC: Glycine in acute management of isovaleric acidemia. Lancet 1:313, 1980.

Waber LJ, Valle D, Neill C, et al: Carnitine deficiency presenting as familial cardiomyopathy: A treatable defect in carnitine transport. J Pediatr 101:700, 1982.

Wallace DC, Singh G, Lott MT, et al: Mitochondrial DNA mutation associated with Leber's hereditary optic neuropathy. Science 242:1427, 1988.

Wendel U, Langenbeck U, Lombeck I, et al: Maple syrup urine disease: Therapeutic use of insulin in catabolic states. Eur J Pediatr 139:172, 1982.

Whyte RK, Whelan D, Hill R, et al: Excretion of dicarboxylic and w-1 hydroxy fatty acids by low-birth-weight infants fed with medium-chain triglycerides. Pediatr Res 20:122, 1986.

Willems JL, Monnens LAH, Trijbels LMF, et al: Leigh's encephalomyelopathy in a patient with cytochrome *c* oxidase deficiency in muscle tissue. Pediatrics 60:850, 1977.

Wolf B: Disorders of biotin metabolism. *In* Scriver CR, Beaudet A, Sly WS, et al (Eds): The Metabolic and Molecular Bases of Inherited Disease, 7th ed. New York, McGraw-Hill, 1995, p 3151.

Yamaguchi S, Indo Y, Coates PM, et al: Identification of very-long-chain acyl-CoA dehydrogenase deficiency in three patients previously diagnosed with long-chain acyl-CoA dehydrogenase deficiency. Pediatr Res 34:111, 1993.

Yudkoff M, Cohn RM, Pushak R, et al: Glycine therapy in isovaleric acidemia. J Pediatr 92:813, 1978.

Zeviani M, Peterson P, Servidei S, et al: Benign reversible muscle cytochrome C oxidase deficiency: A second case. Neurology 37:64, 1987.

Zeviani M, Van Dyke DH, Servidei S, et al: Myopathy and fatal cardiopathy due to cytochrome C oxidase deficiency. Arch Neurol 43:1198, 1986.

Zheng X, Shoffner JM, Lott MT, et al: Evidence in a lethal infantile mitochondrial disease for a nuclear mutation affecting respiratory complexes I and IV. Neurology 39:1203, 1989.

Zinn AB, Zurcher VL, Kraus F, et al: Carnitine palmitoyltransferase B (CPT B) deficiency: A heritable cause of neonatal cardiomyopathy and dysgenesis of the kidney. Pediatr Res 29:73A, 1991.

CHAPTER 26

Lysosomal Storage and Peroxisomal Disorders Presenting in the Newborn

Janet A. Thomas, Carol L. Greene and Robert M. Cohn

Lysosomal storage diseases, peroxisomal disorders, and Smith-Lemli-Opitz syndrome (SLO) are single gene disorders, most of which demonstrate autosomal recessive inheritance. The incidence of peroxisomal disorders is estimated to be approximately 1/25,000 to 1/50,000. No collective estimate of frequency for the many disorders of lysosomal dysfunction exists, but individual diseases affect less than 1/100,000 births in the general population. The most current estimate of SLO is 1/20,000. These three categories of metabolic diseases involve molecules important in cell membranes and share overlapping clinical presentations. Clinical presentations are heterogeneous, with a broad range of age of presentation and severity of symptoms. All are chronic and progressive. Age of onset varies from prenatal to adulthood, and severity may range from severe disability and early death to nearly normal life-style and life span. For each condition, interfamilial variability is greater than intrafamilial variability. The genetic and clinical characteristics are presented in Table 26–1.

Important presentations that should lead the neonatologist to consider these disorders in the differential diagnosis are the following:

1. "In utero infection"—hepatosplenomegaly and hepatitis, possibly with extramedullary hematopoiesis
2. Nonimmune hydrops fetalis
3. Neurologic only—early and often difficult to control seizures, hypertonia or hypotonia, with or without altered head size, and with or without eye findings
4. Coarse features with bone changes, dysostosis multiplex, or osteoporosis
5. Dysmorphic facial features with or without major malformations
6. Rarely, known family history or positive prenatal diagnosis

Only for the last three presentations are these conditions likely to be considered early in the differential diagnosis. Most babies with these conditions are born to healthy, nonconsanguineous couples with normal family histories, and these disorders are usually considered late, if at all, as in the following example.

CASE STUDY

CJ was the 2200-g product of a 32-week gestation born to a 24-year-old G3P2 mother by cesarean section for fetal distress. Pregnancy was complicated by the finding on ultrasound of fetal hydrops and ascites and possible hepatosplenomegaly at 24 weeks' gestation. Fetal blood sampling showed a hematocrit of 31 and elevated gamma-glutamyl-transferase (GGT) and aspartate transaminase (AST). Viral studies were negative and chromosomes were normal. At delivery, the infant was limp and blue with a heart rate of 60 beats/min. Examination and chest radiograph revealed marked abdominal distention, hepatosplenomegaly, multiple petechiae and bruises, a bell-shaped thorax, generalized hypotonia, talipes equinovarus, contractures at the knees, a large heart, and hazy lung fields with low volumes. She rapidly developed disseminated intravascular coagulopathy and evidence of liver disease with elevated AST, GGT, and increasing hyperbilirubinemia. She was maintained on a ventilator and treated with antibiotics for suspected sepsis.

Evaluation for bacterial and viral agents was negative. Metabolic studies, including ammonia, lactate, very-long-chain fatty acids (VLCFAs), and urine amino and organic acids, were unremarkable. The white blood cells were noted to have marked toxic granularity consistent with overwhelming bacterial sepsis or metabolic storage disease.

The patient experienced continued cardiorespiratory deterioration, developed bilateral pneumothoraces and pneumopericardium, and died on her third day of life. Consent for autopsy was obtained from the family. A standard autopsy was performed and revealed the presence of large, membrane-bound vacuoles within hepatocytes, endothelial cells, pericytes, and bone marrow stromal cells, typical of a metabolic storage disorder. Similar cells were also found within the placenta. There was no evidence of an infectious etiology. Unfortunately, since a lysosomal storage disorder was not considered as a possible etiology at the time of death, no frozen tissue or cultured fibroblasts were available to pursue the diagnosis. As a result of efforts by a research laboratory and the recurrence of disease in the couple's subsequent pregnancy, a diagnosis of beta-glucuronidase deficiency, or mucopolysaccharidosis type VII, was confirmed.

Lysosomal storage diseases as a group and individually are addressed in the first part of this chapter. Following are sections on peroxisomal disorders and SLO.

LYSOSOMAL STORAGE DISORDERS

In this section, we first consider lysosomes in general, then the neonatal clinical presentation of individual diseases.

TABLE 26–1

Lysosomal Storage Disorders Presenting in the Newborn Period: Genetic and Clinical Characteristics of Neonatal Presentation

	Onset	Facies	Neurologic Findings	Distinctive Features	Eye Findings	Cardiovascular Findings	Dysostosis Multiplex	Hepatomegaly/Splenomegaly	Defect	Gene Location and Molecular Findings	Ethnic Predilection
Niemann-Pick Type IA	Early infancy	Frontal bossing	Difficulty feeding, apathy, deafness, blindness, hypotonia	Brownish-yellow skin, xanthomas	Cherry-red spot (50%)	–	–	+/+/+	Sphingomyelinase deficiency	ASM gene at 11p15.1-p15.4; 3 of 12 mutations account for ~92% of mutant alleles in the Ashkenazi population	1/40,000 in Ashkenazi Jews with carrier frequency of 1/60
Niemann-Pick Type II	Birth–3 mo	Normal	Developmental delay, vertical gaze paralysis, hypotonia, later spasticity	–	–	–	–	+/+ +	Abnormal cholesterol esterification	Chromosome 18; possible second gene elsewhere	Increased in French Canadians of Nova Scotia and Spanish Americans in southwest United States
Gaucher Disease Type 2	In utero–6 mo	Normal	Poor suck and swallow, weak cry, squint, trismus, strabismus, opsiclonus, hypertonic, later flaccid	Congenital ichthyosis, collodion skin	–		–	+/+ +	Glucocerebrosidase deficiency	1q21; large number of mutations known; five mutations account for ~97% of mutant alleles in the Ashkenazi population, but only ~75% in the non-Jewish population	Panethnic
Krabbe Disease	3–6 mo	Normal	Irritability, tonic spasms with light or noise stimulation, seizures, hypertonia, later flaccidity	Increased CSF protein	Optic atrophy	–	–	–/–	Galactocerebrosidase deficiency	14q24.3-q32.1	Increased in Scandinavian countries and in a large Druze kindred in Israel
G$_{M1}$ Gangliosidosis	Birth	Coarse	Poor suck, weak cry, lethargy, exaggerated startle, blindness, hypotonia, later spasticity	Gingival hypertrophy, edema, rashes	Cherry-red spot (50%)	–	+	+/+	Beta-galactosidase deficiency	3pter-p21; heterogeneous mutations	Panethnic
Farber Type I	2 wk–4 mo	Normal	Progressive psychomotor impairment, seizures, decreased reflexes, hypotonia	Joint swelling with nodules, hoarseness, lung disease, contractures, fever, granulomas, dysphagia, vomiting, increased CSF protein	Grayish opacification surrounding retina in some patients, subtle cherry-red spot	Occasional	–	Hepatomegaly (50%), splenomegaly less frequent	Lysosomal acid ceramidase	Unknown	Panethnic

Disease	Age at onset	Facial appearance	Neurologic	Visceral/somatic	Ocular	Skeletal	Cardiac	HSM	Defect	Gene	Ethnic distribution
Farber Types II and III	Birth–9 mo (≤20 mo)	Normal		Joint swelling with nodules, hoarseness	Normal macula, +/- corneal opacities	–	–	HSM less frequent than type I	Lysosomal acid ceramidase	Unknown	Panethnic
Farber Type IV (neonatal)	Birth	Normal		Nodules not consistent findings	Corneal opacities (1/3)	–	–	+++/++	Lysosomal acid ceramidase	Unknown	Panethnic
Congenital Sialidosis	In utero–birth	Coarse, edema	Mental retardation, hypotonia	Neonatal ascites, inguinal hernias, renal disease	Corneal clouding	+	–	+/+	Neuraminidase deficiency	10pter-q23	Panethnic
Galactosialidosis	In utero–birth	Coarse	Mental retardation, occasional deafness, hypotonia	Ascites, edema, inguinal hernias, renal disease, telangiectasias	Cherry-red spot, corneal clouding	+	Cardiomegaly progressing to failure	+/+	Absence of a protective protein that safeguards neuraminidase and beta-galactosidase from premature degradation	20q13.1	Panethnic
Wolman Disease	First weeks of life	Normal	Mental deterioration	Vomiting, diarrhea, steatorrhea, abdominal distention, failure to thrive, anemia, adrenal calcifications			–	+/+	Lysosomal acid lipase deficiency	10q23.2-q23.3	Increased in Iranian Jews and in non-Jewish and Arab populations of Galilee
Infantile Sialic Acid Storage Disease	In utero–birth	Coarse, dysmorphic	Mental retardation, hypotonia	Ascites, anemia, diarrhea, failure to thrive		+	Congestive heart failure	+/+	Defective transport of sialic acid out of the lysosome	6q	Panethnic
I-Cell Disease	In utero–birth	Coarse	Mental retardation, +/- deafness	Gingival hyperplasia, restricted joint mobility, hernias	Corneal clouding	++	Valvular disease, congestive heart failure, cor pulmonale	+++/+++	Lysosomal enzymes lack mannose-6-PO$_4$ recognition marker and fail to enter the lysosome	Unknown	Panethnic
Mucolipidosis Type IV	Birth–3 mo	Normal	Mental retardation		Severe corneal clouding, retinal degeneration, blindness	–	–	–/–	Unknown, some patients with partial deficiency of ganglioside sialidase	Unknown	Increased in Ashkenazi Jews
Mucopolysaccharidosis Type VII	In utero–childhood	Variable coarseness	Mild–severe mental retardation	Hernias	Variable corneal clouding	++	Variable	Variable	Beta-glucuronidase deficiency	GUSB gene at 7q21.1-q22	Panethnic
Carbohydrate Deficient Glycoprotein Syndrome	Birth	Dysmorphic	Mental retardation, ataxia, peripheral neuropathy, strokelike episodes, hypotonia	Inverted nipples, abnormal fat distribution, thrombotic disease, liver dysfunction, multicystic kidneys, hypogonadism	Strabismus, esotropia, retinitis pigmentosa	–	Pericardial effusions, cardiomyopathy	+/+ or ++/++	Defect in the addition of N-linked carbohydrates to glycoproteins	Type II disease gene at 14q21	Increased in Scandinavian populations

CSF, cerebrospinal fluid; HSM, hepatosplenomegaly.

–, not seen; +, typically present, usually not severe; ++, usually present, and moderately severe; +++, always present, usually severe.

Diagnosis and treatment are discussed at the end of the section, followed by a discussion of carbohydrate-deficient glycoprotein syndrome.

Lysosomes are single membrane-bound intracellular organelles, which contain enzymes called *hydrolases.* These lysosomal enzymes are responsible for splitting large molecules into simple, low-molecular-weight compounds, which can be recycled. The material digested by lysosomes is either exogenous material taken up by endocytosis, or endogenous material separated from other intracellular materials by autophagy. The common element of all compounds digested by lysosomal enzymes is that they contain a carbohydrate portion attached to a protein or lipid. These glycoconjugates include glycoproteins, glycosaminoglycans, and glycolipids.

Glycolipids are large molecules with carbohydrates attached to a lipid moiety. Sphingolipids, globosides, gangliosides, cerebrosides, and lipid sulfates all are glycolipids. The different classes of glycolipids are primarily distinguished from each other by different polar groups at C1. Sphingolipids are complex membrane lipids composed of one molecule each of the amino alcohol sphingosine, a long-chain fatty acid, and various polar head groups attached by a beta-glycosidic linkage. Sphingolipids occur in the blood and nearly all tissues of the body, with the highest concentration found in the white matter of the central nervous system. Additionally, various sphingolipids are components of the plasma membrane of practically all cells. The core structure of the natural sphingolipids is ceramide, a long-chain fatty acid amide derivative of sphingosine. Free ceramide is an intermediate in the biosynthesis and catabolism of glycosphingolipids and sphingomyelin and makes up 16% to 20% of the normal lipid content of the stratum corneum of the skin. Sphingomyelin, a ceramide phosphocholine, is one of the principal structural lipids of the membranes of nervous tissue.

Cerebrosides, a group of ceramide monohexosides, have a single sugar, either glucose or galactose, and an additional sulfate group on galactose. The two most common cerebrosides are galactocerebroside and glucocerebroside. The largest concentration of galactocerebroside is found in the brain. Glucocerebroside is an intermediate in the synthesis and degradation of more complex glycosphingolipids.

Gangliosides, the most complex class of glycolipids, contain several sugar units and one or more sialic acid residues. Gangliosides are normal components of cell membranes and are found in high concentrations in the ganglion cells of the central nervous system, particularly in the nerve endings and dendrites. G_{MI} is the major ganglioside in the brain of vertebrates. Gangliosides function as receptors for toxic agents, hormones, and certain viruses; are involved in cell differentiation; and may also play a role in cell-cell interaction by providing specific recognition determinants on the surface of the cells.

Globosides, ceramide oligosaccharides, are a family of cerebrosides that contain two or more sugar residues, usually galactose, glucose, or *N*-acetylgalactosamine. Glycosaminoglycans and oligosaccharides are essential constituents of connective tissue, parenchymal organs, cartilage, and the nervous system. Glycosaminoglycans, also called *mucopolysaccharides,* are complex heterosaccharides consisting of long sugar chains rich in sulfate groups. The polymeric chains are bound to specific proteins (core proteins). Glycoproteins contain oligosaccharide chains (long sugar molecules) attached covalently to a peptide core. Glycosylation occurs in the endoplasmic reticulum and the Golgi apparatus. Most glycoproteins are secreted from cells and include transport proteins, glycoprotein hormones, complement factors, enzymes, and enzyme inhibitors. There is extensive diversity in the composition and structure of the oligosaccharides.

The degradation of glycolipids, glycosaminoglycans, and glycoproteins takes place especially within the lysosomes of phagocytic cells, related to histiocytes and macrophages, in any tissue or organ. A series of hydrolytic enzymes cleaves specific bonds resulting in the sequential, stepwise removal of constituents such as sugars and sulfate, degrading the complex glycoconjugates to the level of their basic building blocks. Lysosomal storage diseases most commonly result when an inherited defect causes significantly decreased activity in one of these hydrolases. Other causes include failure of transport of enzyme, substrate, or product. Whatever the specific etiology, incompletely metabolized molecules accumulate, especially within the tissue responsible for the catabolism of the glycoconjugate. Additional excess storage material maybe excreted in the urine.

Lysosomal storage diseases are classified according to the stored compound. Clinical phenotype partially depends on the type and amount of storage substance. Disorders were selected for discussion in this chapter if there is known presentation in the neonatal period.

Clinical Presentations (see Table 26–1)

Niemann-Pick Type IA (Acute, Sphingomyelinase Deficient)

In a recent classification, the former types A and B were regrouped as type I, while former types C and D were regrouped as type II.

Etiology. Niemann-Pick Type IA is caused by a deficiency of sphingomyelinase. Sphingomyelinase catalyzes the breakdown of sphingomyelin to ceramide and phosphocholine, and deficiency results in sphingomyelin storage within lysosomes. Cholesterol is also stored, suggesting that its metabolism is tied to that of sphingomyelin. Sphingomyelin normally makes up 5% to 20% of phospholipid in the liver, spleen, and brain. In these disorders, it may make up to 70% of the phospholipids. Patients with Niemann-Pick Type IA usually have less than 5% of normal enzyme activity.

Clinical Features. The onset of clinical features of this disorder may begin in utero or up to 1 year of age. These infants usually present with massive hepatosplenomegaly (hepatomegaly greater than splenomegaly), constipation, feeding difficulties, and vomiting with consequent failure to thrive. Patients eventually appear strikingly emaciated with a protuberant abdomen and thin extremities. Neurologic disease is evident by 6 months of age with hypotonia, decreased or absent deep tendon reflexes, and weakness. Later, loss of motor skills, spasticity and rigidity, and loss of vision and hearing occur. Seizures are rare. A retinal cherry-red spot is present in about half of the cases and the electroretinogram is abnormal. Respiratory infections are common. The skin may have an ochre or brownish-yellow color and xanthomas have been observed. Radiographically, widening of the medullary cavities, cortical thinning of the long bones, and osteoporosis are seen. In the brain and spinal cord neuronal storage is widespread, leading to cytoplasmic swelling together with atrophy of the cerebellum. Bone marrow and tissue biopsy may reveal foam cells or sea blue histiocytes, which represent lipid laden cells of the monocyte-macrophage system. Similarly, vacuolated lymphocytes or monocytes may be present in the peripheral blood. Tissue cholesterol levels may be 3 to 10 times normal, and patients may have a microcytic anemia and thrombocytopenia. Death occurs by 2 to 3 years of age.

Niemann-Pick C (Type II)

Etiology. Niemann-Pick Type II is due to an error in the intracellular transport of exogenous low-density lipoprotein (LDL)-derived cholesterol, which leads to impaired esterification of cholesterol and trapping of unesterified cholesterol in lysosomes. The primary defect is abnormal cholesterol esterification, but the enzyme responsible for cholesterol esterification, acyl–CoA:cholesterol acyltransferase (ACAT), is not deficient. The storage of sphingomyelin is secondary. It has been suggested that the defect is in the transport of cholesterol out of the lysosome resulting in cholesterol being unavailable to ACAT (Natowicz et al, 1995). Sphingomyelinase activity appears normal or elevated in most tissues but partially deficient (60% to 70%) in fibroblasts from most patients. Storage of sphingomyelin in tissues is much less than in Niemann-Pick Type I and is accompanied by additional storage of unesterified cholesterol, phospholipids, and glycolipids in the liver and spleen. Only glycolipids are increased in the brain.

Clinical Features. The age of onset, clinical features, and natural history of Niemann-Pick Type II are highly variable. The disease may have its onset from birth to 18 years of age. In the neonatal period 50% of children have conjugated hyperbilirubinemia, which usually resolves spontaneously to be followed by neurologic symptoms later in childhood. In the severe infantile form, hepatosplenomegaly is common, accompanied by hypotonia and delayed motor development. Further mental regression is usually evident by the age of 1 to 1.5 years, associated with behavior problems, vertical supranuclear ophthalmoplegia, progressive ataxia, dystonia, spasticity, dementia, drooling, dysphagia, and dysarthria. Seizures are rare. Foam cells and sea blue histiocytes may be found in many tissues. Neuronal storage with cytoplasmic ballooning, inclusions, meganeurites, and axonal spheroids are also seen. Death may occur in infancy or as late as the third decade. Niemann-Pick Type II may also present as fatal neonatal liver disease, often misdiagnosed as fetal hepatitis.

Gaucher Disease Type 2 (Acute Neuropathic)

Etiology. Three types of Gaucher disease have been defined. Type 1, nonneuropathic, is the most common type and is distinguished from types 2 and 3 by the lack of central nervous system involvement. Type 1 disease most commonly presents in early childhood, but it may present in adulthood. Type 2 disease, acute neuropathic, is characterized by infantile onset of severe central nervous system involvement. Type 3 disease, subacute neuropathic, is also late onset with slow neurologic progression. Almost all types of Gaucher disease are caused by a deficiency of lysosomal glucocerebrosidase and result in the storage of glucocerebroside in visceral organs; the brain is affected in types 2 and 3. The enzyme splits glucose from cerebroside, yielding ceramide and glucose. A few patients have a deficiency of saposin C, a cohydrolase required by glucocerebrosidase.

Clinical Features. Typically, Gaucher disease type 2 has its onset at approximately 3 months of age with hepatosplenomegaly (splenomegaly predominates) with subsequent neurologic deterioration. Hydrops fetalis, congenital ichthyosis, and collodion skin babies, however, are well-described presentations (Fujimoto et al, 1995; Ince et al, 1995; Lipson et al, 1991; Liu et al, 1988; Sherer et al, 1993; Sidransky et al, 1992). In a review of 18 cases of Gaucher patients presenting in the newborn period, Sidransky and associates (1992) found 8 of 18 patients to have associated dermatologic findings and 6 to 18 patients to have presented with hydrops. The etiology of the association of such findings and Gaucher disease is unclear, although the enzyme deficiency appears to be directly responsible (Sidransky et al, 1992). Ceramides have been shown to be major components of the intracellular bilayers in epidermal stratum corneum and play an important role in skin homeostasis (Fujimoto et al, 1995). Thus, Gaucher disease should be considered in the differential diagnosis of infants presenting with hydrops fetalis and congenital ichthyosis. For the subset of patients presenting prenatally or at birth, death frequently occurs within hours to days, or at least within 2 to 3 months.

Krabbe Disease (Globoid Cell Leukodystrophy)

Etiology. The name of this disorder, *globoid cell leukodystrophy,* is derived from the presence of large numbers of multinuclear macrophages in the cerebral white matter that contain undigested galactocerebroside. Disease is caused by a deficiency of lysosomal galactocerebroside beta-galactosidase, which normally degrades galactocerebroside to ceramide and galactose. Deficiency of the enzyme results in storage of galactocerebroside. Galactocerebroside is present almost exclusively in myelin sheaths. It has been postulated that accumulation of a toxic metabolite, psychosine, also a substrate for the enzyme, leads to early destruction of the oligodendroglia. Impaired catabolism of galactosylceramide is also important in the pathogenesis of the disease.

Clinical Features. Age of onset ranges from the first weeks of life to adulthood. Infantile Krabbe disease typically has its onset between 3 and 6 months of age, but there are cases of very early onset with neurologic symptoms evident within weeks after birth. Symptoms and signs are confined to the nervous system; no visceral involvement is present. The clinical course has been divided into three stages. In stage I, patients present with hyperirritability, vomiting, episodic fevers, hyperesthesia, tonic spasms on light or noise stimulation, stiffness, and seizures after appearing relatively normal after birth. Peripheral neuropathy is present, but reflexes are increased. Stage II is marked by central nervous system deterioration and hypertonia that progresses to hypotonia and flaccidity. Deep tendon reflexes are eventually lost. Patients in stage III are decerebrate, deaf, and blind with hyperpyrexia, hypersalivation, and frequent seizures. Routine laboratory findings are unremarkable with the exception of elevated cerebrospinal fluid protein. Cerebral atrophy and demyelination become evident in the central nervous system, and segmental demyelination, axonal degeneration, fibrosis, and macrophage infiltration are common in the peripheral nervous system. The segmental demyelination of peripheral nerves is demonstrated by the finding of decreased motor nerve conduction. The white matter is severely depleted of all lipids, especially glycolipids, and nerve and brain biopsies show globoid cells. Death from hyperpyrexia, respiratory complications, or aspiration occurs at a median age of 13 months.

G_{M1} Gangliosidosis

Etiology. Infantile G_{M1} gangliosidosis is caused by deficiency of lysosomal beta-galactosidase. The enzyme cleaves the terminal galactose in a beta linkage from oligosaccharides, keratan sulfate, and G_{M1} ganglioside. Deficiency of the enzyme results in storage of G_{M1} ganglioside and oligosaccharides. Clinical severity correlates with the degree of substrate storage and residual enzyme activity. The same enzyme is deficient in Morquio disease type B.

Clinical Features. Onset of symptoms ranges from prenatal to adult life. Infantile, or type 1 G_{M1} gangliosidosis may be evident at birth with coarse and thick skin, hirsutism on the forehead and neck, and coarse facial features consisting of a puffy face, frontal bossing, depressed nasal bridge, maxillary hyperplasia, large and low-set ears, wide upper lip, moderate macroglossia, and gingival hypertrophy. These dysmorphic features, however, are not always obvious in the neonate. A retinal cherry-red spot is seen in 50% of patients, and corneal clouding is often observed. Shortly after birth, or by 3 to 6 months of age, failure to thrive and hepatosplenomegaly become evident, as does neurologic involvement with poor development, hyper-reflexia, hypotonia, and seizures. Cranial imaging reveals diffuse atrophy of the brain, enlargement of the ventricular system, and evidence of myelin loss in the white matter. The neurologic deterioration is progressive, resulting in generalized rigidity and spasticity and sensorimotor and psychointellectual dysfunction. By 6 months of age, skeletal features are present, including kyphoscoliosis and stiff joints with generalized contractures, and striking bone changes are seen with vertebral beaking in the thoracolumbar region, broadening of the shafts of the long bones with distal and proximal tapering, and widening of the metacarpal shafts with proximal pinching of the four lateral metacarpals. Tissue biopsies demonstrate neurons filled with membranous cytoplasmic bodies and various types of inclusions, as well as foam cells in the bone marrow. Death generally occurs before 2 years of age. A severe neonatal-

onset type has also been described with cardiomyopathy (Kohlschütter et al, 1982).

Farber Lipogranulomatosis

Etiology. Farber lipogranulomatosis results from a deficiency of lysosomal acid ceramidase. Ceramidase catalyzes the degradation of ceramide to its long-chain base, sphingosine, and a fatty acid. Clinical disease is a consequence of storage of ceramide in various organs and body fluids.

Clinical Features. Four types of Farber lipogranulomatosis may present in the neonatal period. Type I, classic disease, is a unique disorder with onset from approximately 2 weeks to 4 months of age. Patients present with hoarseness progressing to aphonia, feeding and respiratory difficulties, poor weight gain, and intermittent fever due to granuloma formation and swelling of the epiglottis and larynx. Palpable nodules appear over joints and pressure points and joints become painful and swollen. Later, joint contractures and pulmonary disease appear. Liver and cardiac involvement may occur and patients may have a subtle retinal cherry-red spot. Severe and progressive psychomotor impairment may occur, as well as seizures, decreased deep tendon reflexes, hypotonia, and muscle atrophy. Death occurs in early infancy usually due to pulmonary disease.

Type 2, intermediate, presents from birth to 9 months of age with joint and laryngeal involvement and nodules. Death is in early childhood. Type 3 disease, mild, presents slightly later, from approximately 2 months to 20 months of age, with survival into the third decade. Clinically, both types 2 and 3 are dominated by subcutaneous nodules, joint deformity, and laryngeal involvement. Liver and pulmonary involvement may be absent. Two thirds of patients have a normal intelligence quotient. Type 4, neonatal visceral, presents at birth with hepatosplenomegaly due to massive histiocyte infiltration of the liver and spleen, with infiltration also in the lungs, thymus, and lymphocytes. Subcutaneous nodules and laryngeal involvement may be subtle. Death occurs by 6 months of age. In all types, tissue biopsies show granulomatous infiltration, foam cells, and lysosomes with comma-shaped, curvilinear tubular structures, called *Farber bodies*. Cerebrospinal fluid protein may be elevated in patients with type I disease.

Sialidosis

Etiology. Sialidosis is caused by a deficiency of neuraminidase, which is responsible for the cleavage of terminal sialyl linkages of several oligosaccharides and glycopeptides. The defect results in the multisystem lysosomal accumulation of sugars rich in sialic acid.

Clinical Features. Type I sialidosis is characterized by retinal cherry-red spots and generalized myoclonus with onset generally in the second decade of life. Type II is distinguished from type I by the early onset of a progressive, severe phenotype with somatic features. Type II is often subdivided into juvenile, infantile, and congenital forms. Congenital sialidosis has onset in utero and presents at birth with coarse features, facial edema, hepatosplenomegaly, ascites, hernias, and hypotonia, and occasionally frank hydrops fetalis. Radiographs reveal dysostosis multiplex and epiphyseal stippling. Delayed mental development is quickly apparent. Recurrent infections may occur. Most patients are stillborn or die prior to 1 year of age. The infantile form has onset from 0 to 12 months of age with coarse features, organomegaly, dysostosis multiplex, retinal cherry-red spot, and mental retardation. Death occurs by the second or third decade. In both types, vacuolated cells can be seen in almost all tissues and bone marrow foam cells are present.

Galactosialidosis

Etiology. Galactosialidosis results from a deficiency of two lysosomal enzymes, neuraminidase and beta-galactosidase. The primary defect in galactosialidosis is believed to be in a protective protein that forms a complex with the two enzymes and safeguards them from premature degradation. The protective protein has catalytic as well as protective functions, and the two functions appear to be distinct. Deficiency of the enzymes results in the accumulation of sialyloligosaccharides in tissue lysosomes and in excretion in body fluids.

Clinical Features. Galactosialidosis has been divided into three phenotypic subtypes based on age of onset and severity of clinical manifestations. Most patients present in adolescence and adulthood, but early infantile and late infantile presentations occur. Patients with early infantile galactosialidosis present between birth and 3 months of age with ascites, edema, coarse facial features, inguinal hernias, proteinuria, hypotonia, and telangiectasias, and occasionally frank hydrops fetalis. Patients subsequently develop organomegaly, including cardiomegaly progressing to cardiac failure, psychomotor delay, and skeletal changes, particularly in the spine. Ocular abnormalities, including corneal clouding and retinal cherry-red spots, may occur. Death occurs at an average age of 8 months usually due to cardiac and renal failure. Galactosialidosis may be an etiology of recurrent fetal loss or recurrent hydrops fetalis.

Late infantile galactosialidosis presents in the first months of life with coarse facial features, hepatosplenomegaly, and skeletal changes consistent with dysostosis multiple. Cherry-red spots and corneal clouding may also be present. Neurologic involvement may be absent or mild. Valvular heart disease is a common feature, as is growth retardation, partially due to spinal involvement, and often associated with muscular atrophy. Early death is not a feature of the late infantile form. In all forms of galactosialidosis vacuolated cells in blood smears and foam cells in bone marrow are present.

Wolman Disease

Etiology. Wolman disease is caused by lysosomal acid lipase deficiency, an enzyme involved in cellular cholesterol homeostasis and responsible for the hydrolysis of cholesterol esters and triglycerides. The result of the enzyme deficiency is the defective release of free cholesterol from lysosomes, which leads to up regulation of the LDL receptors and 3-hydroxy-3-methylglutaryl-CoA reductase activity.

This causes increased de novo synthesis of cholesterol and activation of receptor-mediated endocytosis of LDL leading to further deposition of lipid in the lysosomes. The result is the accumulation of cholesterol esters and triglycerides in most tissues of the body, including the liver, spleen, lymph nodes, heart, blood vessels, and brain. An extreme degree of lipid storage occurs in the cells of the small intestine, particularly in the mucosa. Additionally, the neurons of the myenteric plexus demonstrate a large degree of storage, with evidence of neuronal cell death, which may account for the prominence of gastrointestinal symptoms (Wolman, 1995).

Clinical Features. Patients present within weeks of birth with evidence of malnutrition and malabsorption, including symptoms of vomiting, diarrhea, steatorrhea, failure to thrive, abdominal distention, and hepatosplenomegaly. Adrenal calcifications may be seen on radiographs and adrenal insufficiency occurs. The presence of adrenal calcifications associated with hepatosplenomegaly and gastrointestinal symptoms is strongly suggestive of Wolman disease. Later, mental deterioration becomes apparent. Laboratory findings include anemia secondary to foam cell infiltration of the bone marrow and evidence of adrenal insufficiency. Serum cholesterol level is normal. Death usually occurs before 1 year of age.

Infantile Sialic Acid Storage Disease

Etiology. A defective lysosomal sialic acid transporter that is responsible for the efflux of sialic acid and other acidic monosaccharides from the lysosomal compartment is the cause of infantile sialic acid storage disease. The defective transporter results in increased storage of free sialic acid and glucuronic acid within the lysosomes and increased sialic acid excretion.

Clinical Features. Infantile sialic acid storage disease often presents at birth with mildly coarse features, hepatosplenomegaly, ascites, hypopigmentation, and generalized hypotonia. Mild dysostosis multiplex may be seen on radiographs. Failure to thrive and severe mental and motor retardation soon appear. Vacuolated cells are seen on tissue biopsy, and electron microscopy reveals swollen lysosomes, filled with finely granular material. Central nervous system changes include myelin loss, axonal spheroids, gliosis, and neuronal storage. Death occurs in early childhood. Infantile sialic acid storage disease may also present with fetal ascites or nonimmune fetal hydrops.

I-Cell Disease (Mucolipidosis Type II)

Etiology. In normal cells, targeting of the enzymes to the lysosomes is mediated by receptors that bind a mannose-6-phosphate recognition marker on the enzyme. The recognition marker is synthesized in a two-step reaction in the Golgi complex, and it is the enzyme that catalyzes the first step of this process, UDP-*N*-acetylglucosamine:lysosomal enzyme *N*-acetylglucosaminyl-1-phosphotransferase, that is defective in I-cell disease. As a result, the enzymes lack the mannose-6-phosphate recognition signal, and the newly synthesized lysosomal enzymes are secreted into the extracellular matrix instead of being targeted to the lysosome. Consequently, multiple lysosomal enzymes are found in the plasma in 10 to 20 times their normal concentrations. Affected cells, especially fibroblasts, show dense inclusions of storage material that probably includes oligosaccharides, glycosaminoglycans, and lipids. These are the "inclusion bodies" from which the disease derives its name.

Clinical Features. I-cell disease may present at birth with coarse features, corneal clouding, organomegaly, hypotonia, and gingival hyperplasia. Birth weight and length are often below normal. Kyphoscoliosis, lumbar gibbus, and restricted joint movement are often present, and there may be hip dislocation, fractures, hernias, or bilateral talipes equinovarus. Dysostosis multiplex may be seen on radiographs. Severe psychomotor retardation, evident by 6 months of age, and progressive failure to thrive occur. The facial features become progressively more coarse with a high forehead, puffy eyelids, epicanthal folds, flat nasal bridge, anteverted nares, and macroglossia. Linear growth slows during the first year of life and halts completely thereafter. The skeletal involvement is also progressive with the development of increasing joint immobility and claw-hand deformities. Respiratory infections, otitis media, and cardiac involvement are frequent complications. Death usually occurs in the first decade of life owing to cardiorespiratory complications.

Mucolipidosis Type IV

Etiology. Mucolipidosis type IV is associated with a partial deficiency of the lysosomal enzyme, ganglioside sialidase, but it is not certain that this is the root cause of this disorder, Nevertheless, deficiency of this enzyme causes lysosomal storage of gangliosides and glycosaminoglycans.

Clinical Features. This disorder has its onset from infancy to 5 years of age, with corneal clouding, retinal degeneration, blindness, and mental retardation. Cytoplasmic inclusions are noted in conjunctiva, fibroblasts, liver, and spleen.

Mucopolysaccharidosis Type VII (Sly Disease)

Etiology. Sly disease is a member of a group of lysosomal storage disorders that are caused by deficiency of enzymes catalyzing the stepwise degradation of glycosaminoglycans. Skeletal and neurologic involvement are variable. There is a wide spectrum of clinical severity among the mucopolysaccharidoses and even within a single enzyme deficiency. Most of these disorders present in childhood, but type VII is included in this chapter because of its well-recognized neonatal and infantile presentation. Sly disease is caused by beta-glucuronidase deficiency and results in lysosomal accumulation of glycosaminoglycans, including dermatan sulfate, heparan sulfate, and chondroitin sulfates, causing cell, tissue, and organ dysfunction.

Clinical Features. Sly disease may present with a wide spectrum of severity. Patients with early-onset or the neonatal form may present with coarse features, hepatosplenomegaly, moderate dysostosis multiplex, hernias, and nonprogressive mental retardation. Corneal clouding is a

variable finding. Frequent episodes of pneumonia during the first year of life are common. Short stature becomes evident. Granulocytes show coarse metachromic granules. A severe neonatal form has been recognized associated with hydrops fetalis, and frequently early death. Milder forms with later-onset disease are also known.

Diagnosis, Management, and Prognosis

Recognition of lysosomal storage disorders in the newborn period can be difficult since they often mimic more common causes of illness in newborns, such as respiratory distress, nonimmune hydrops fetalis, liver disease, or sepsis. The initial step in the diagnosis of these disorders is, therefore, to consider them in the differential diagnosis of a sick or unusual-appearing newborn. At times, the phenotype may suggest a specific diagnosis, such as respiratory distress and painful, swollen joints in Farber lipogranulomatosis; or gastrointestinal symptoms, hepatosplenomegaly, and adrenal calcifications in Wolman disease. Subtle dysmorphic features, coarsening of features, or radiographic evidence of dysostosis multiplex are also strong indications that lysosomal storage disorders should be considered. Routine laboratory analysis is often normal or nonspecific. These infants do not have episodes of acute metabolic decompensation. Anemia and thrombocytopenia may be seen owing to bone marrow involvement, and vacuolated cells may be seen in peripheral blood. Elevated cerebrospinal fluid protein is seen in Krabbe disease and Farber lipogranulomatosis type I.

Directed analysis of urine is usually the first diagnostic step. One- or two-dimensional electrophoresis or thin-layer chromatography can detect excess excretion of urine glycosaminoglycans, oligosaccharides, or free sialic acid, but all urinary tests for the diagnosis of lysosomal storage disorders can give false-negative results. Examination of the bone marrow or other tissues may reveal storage macrophages in Gaucher disease and in Niemann-Pick types I and II. Small skin biopsies or conjunctival biopsies may demonstrate storage within lysosomes in most of these disorders. Definitive diagnosis for all lysosomal storage disorders, with the exception of Niemann-Pick type II, is confirmed by enzymatic assay in serum, leukocytes, and fibroblasts. The diagnosis of Niemann-Pick type II requires measurement of cellular cholesterol esterification and documentation of a characteristic pattern of filipin-cholesterol staining in cultured fibroblasts during LDL uptake. Analysis of DNA mutations may be helpful for the diagnosis of Gaucher disease. Additionally, prenatal diagnosis is available for lysosomal storage disorders by use of enzyme assays performed on amniocytes or chorionic villus cells or by measuring elevated levels of stored substrate in cultured cells or amniotic fluid.

These conditions need to also be considered in the dying infant, and the neonatologist must be prepared to request the appropriate samples for diagnosis at the time of death. In the surviving patients, treatment and management must be considered. All of these disorders are chronic and progressive conditions for which there is no curative treatment. Gene transfer therapy holds promise but is not currently available for lysosomal storage disorders. Most current medical management is supportive and palliative.

Patients must be continually reassessed for evidence of disease progression and associated complications. These complications, which may include hydrocephalus, valvular heart disease, joint limitation, and obstructive airway disease, present at variable ages. For several disorders, particularly neonatal Gaucher disease and Niemann-Pick Type II, splenectomy may be indicated to improve severe anemia and thrombocytopenia. This procedure, however, enhances the risk of serious infections and may accelerate the progression of the disease at other sites. Patients with Krabbe disease may suffer from significant pain from radiculopathy and spasms, and alleviation of that pain is important for the comfort of the patient. The administration of the glutamic acid transaminase inhibitor, vigabatrin, has been used in a small number of patients with Krabbe disease, since part of the pathology may be caused by a secondary deficiency of gamma-aminobutyric acid (Barth, 1995).

Enzyme replacement therapy is available for Gaucher disease. Alglucerase (Ceredase), replacement enzyme purified from placentas, and imiglucerase (Cerezyme), recombinant enzyme, are available for use in affected patients. Although enzyme replacement therapy has successfully reversed many of the systemic manifestations of the disease, it has been suggested that enzyme replacement therapy should not be given to patients with Gaucher disease type 2 who have already developed severe neurologic signs, since no substantial improvement has been demonstrated to occur in the neurologic symptoms of patients treated (Erikson et al, 1993; NIH Technology Assessment Panel, 1996).

Bone marrow transplantation has been tried for a variety of lysosomal storage disorders. The rationale for the procedure is that circulating blood cells derived from the transplanted marrow become a source of the missing enzyme. In disorders of glycosaminoglycans, results show that, after successful engraftment, leukocyte and liver tissue enzyme activity normalizes, organomegaly decreases, and joint mobility increases. Skeletal abnormalities stabilize but do not improve. Whether brain function can be improved in patients with central nervous system disease remains questionable. Some patients maintained their learning capability or intelligence quotient, while others continued to deteriorate. Clinical experience and studies in animal models indicate that bone marrow transplantation before the onset of neurologic symptoms can prevent or delay the occurrence of symptoms, whereas there is no clear benefit if transplantation is done when symptoms are already present (Hoogerbrugge et al, 1995). Bone marrow transplantation in patients with nonneuropathic Gaucher disease may result in complete disappearance of all symptoms. The procedure, however, is associated with a 9% to 25% mortality rate (Hoogerbrugge et al, 1995). This risk has to be balanced against life-long enzyme replacement therapy. Currently, it is unclear to what extent patients with Gaucher disease with associated neurologic disease, Types 2 and 3 disease, would benefit from transplantation. Bone marrow transplantation has also been attempted in a small number of patients with infantile Krabbe disease, Farber lipogranulomatosis, and Niemann-Pick Type IA. The outcome after transplantation for these few patients has been poor, with continued disease progression and death. Lysosomal storage diseases are not all equally amenable to bone marrow transplantation, and the use of bone marrow transplantation as a treatment modality for most lysosomal storage disorders remains uncertain. In a small number of cases, bone marrow transplantation has been performed in utero following prenatal diagnosis showing an affected infant, and experimental protocols are available for families who wish to pursue this option.

A dietary protocol proposed for the treatment of Wolman disease has as its goal of therapy lessened accumulation of storage material in the intestine and phagocytes. Diet should be started as soon as the diagnosis of Wolman disease is suspected and consists of discontinuing breast-feeding or feeding with a formula containing triglycerides and cholesterol esters, and keeping the infant on a fatty ester-free diet (Wolman, 1995). The diet should include all the necessary vitamins, including the fat-soluble vitamins. In addition, daily smearing of the skin of a different extremity with a small amount (10 to 50 μL) of sunflower or safflower oil or preferably soy, canola, flax, cod liver, or algal oil is required for the prevention of essential fatty acid deficiency, which complicates the restricted diet (Wolman, 1995). The absorption of fatty acids through the skin spares the gastrointestinal tract from accumulation and is associated with the formation of phospholipids and triglycerides (Wolman, 1995). Preliminarily, results suggest that treatment appears to halt disease progression.

Carbohydrate-Deficient Glycoprotein Syndrome

Etiology. The carbohydrate-deficient glycoprotein syndromes (CDGSs) are a group of disorders that can also be loosely classified as lysosomal storage diseases. In these conditions liver pathology is characterized by fibrosis, and electron microscopy shows myelin-like and granular lysosomal inclusions as well as abnormalities of the endoplasmic reticulum in hepatocytes. These disorders are due to the partial deficiency of carbohydrates on many glycoproteins with evidence of a defect in the addition of *N*-linked carbohydrates. Abnormalities of all classes of glycoproteins have been identified in CDGS. The basic defect in CDGS Type I has been suggested to be a deficiency of the enzyme, phosphomannomutase, an enzyme required for the early steps of protein glycosylation (van Schaftingen and Jaeken, 1995). Autosomal recessive inheritance is most likely. Type II disease is also an autosomal recessive disorder due to a deficiency of the enzyme, *N*-acetylglucosaminyltransferase II, a Golgi enzyme important in the later stages of glycosylation. The basic defect in CDGS type III remains unclear.

Clinical Features. Patients with CDGS type I present at birth with dysmorphic features, including high nasal bridge, prominent jaw, large ears, and inverted nipples, feeding difficulties and subsequent growth failure, hypotonia, lipocutaneous abnormalities, and mild to moderate hepatomegaly. The clinical progression of this disorder is divided into four stages. In stage I, the infantile, multisystem stage, patients demonstrate evidence of multisystem involvement, including strokelike episodes, thrombotic disease, liver dysfunction, pericardial effusions and cardiomyopathy, proteinuria, and retinal degeneration. Mental retardation, peripheral neuropathy, and decreased nerve conduction velocities are present. Strabismus and alternating esotropia are present in nearly all patients, and retinitis pigmentosa and abnormalities of the electroretinogram are present in most. Cranial imaging reveals varying degrees of cerebral, cerebellar, and brain stem hypoplasia. Electroencephalogram results are usually normal. Liver biopsies typically reveal steatosis and fibrosis, and multicystic changes in the kidneys have been noted. Stage II, the childhood stage, is characterized by ataxia and mental retardation. Skeletal abnormalities may become more prominent and consist of contractures, kyphoscoliosis, pectus carinatum, and short stature. Stage III, generally occurring in the teenage years, is characterized primarily by lower extremity atrophy. Adulthood, or stage IV, is characterized by hypogonadism. In general, patients have an extroverted disposition and happy appearance. About 20% of patients die during the first year of life owing to severe infection, liver failure, or cardiac insufficiency.

Two patients have been described with CDGS type II and differ from type I in the absence of cerebellar hypoplasia, peripheral neuropathy, and lysosomal inclusions in the liver. Special features of type III, also only described in two patients, include infantile spasms, severe cerebral atrophy, and pigmentary skin changes. A new variant recently described involved a patient with neonatal cataracts and involvement of the spinal cord (Jaeken, 1995).

The presence of carbohydrate-deficient transferrin in serum and cerebrospinal fluid is a distinctive biochemical feature of these disorders. Normal serum transferrin is mainly composed of tetrasialotransferrin. Patients have prominent increases in asialotransferrin and disialotransferrin, and a pronounced decrease of tetrasialotransferrins, pentasialotransferrins, and hexasialotransferrins. Additionally, low serum levels of thyroxine-binding globulin, haptoglobin, transcortin, apolipoprotein B, cholesterol, coagulation factors, and various peptide and glycopeptide hormones have repeatedly been reported.

Diagnosis. Diagnosis of CDGS requires isoelectric focusing to analyze transferrin and quantitation of carbohydrate-deficient transferrin. Similar transferrin changes are also found in people with chronic alcoholism and galactosemia. Patients with CDGS can often be detected through neonatal screening for congenital hypothyroidism because of an associated thyroid-binding globulin deficiency and an increased thyroid-stimulating hormone level. Prenatal diagnosis is not available.

Treatment and Management. The treatment and management of CDGS is primarily supportive and palliative. There is no curative or corrective treatment. In infancy, evidence of multisystem involvement and the resulting complications must be treated promptly.

DISORDERS OF PEROXISOME BIOGENESIS

In this section we first consider peroxisomes in general, then the clinical presentation of individual disorders of peroxisome biogenesis. Diagnosis and treatment are discussed at the end of the section.

Peroxisomes are single membrane-bound cellular organelles that contain no internal structure or DNA and are characterized by an electron-dense core and a homogeneous matrix. Peroxisomes are found in all cells and tissues except mature erythrocytes and are in highest concentration in the liver and kidney. They are formed by growth and division of preexisting peroxisomes and are randomly destroyed by autophagy. Their half-life is 1.5 to 2 days. Peroxisomal proteins are encoded by nuclear genes, synthesized in the cytosol, and imported post-translationally into the peroxisome. Import is mediated by receptors and requires adenosine triphosphate hydrolysis. Peroxisomes contain enzymes that use oxygen to oxidize a variety of substrates, thereby forming peroxide. The peroxide is decomposed within the organelle by the enzyme catalase to water and oxygen. This process protects the cell against peroxide damage by compartmentalization of peroxide metabolism within the organelle. Peroxisomes may also function to dispose of excess reducing equivalents and may contribute to thermogenesis producing heat from cellular respiration.

More than 50 enzymes have been found within peroxisomes. The proteins have multiple functions, both synthetic and degradative. The primary synthetic functions include plasmalogen synthesis and bile acid formation. Plasmalogens constitute 5% to 20% of the phospholipids in cell membranes and 80% to 90% of the phospholipids in myelin. They are also involved in platelet activation and may also protect cells against oxidative stress. Degradative functions include the following: beta-oxidation of VLCFA ($\geq C26$), fatty acids (down to C8–C6), long-chain dicarboxylic acids, prostaglandins, and polyunsaturated fatty acids; oxidation of bile acid intermediates, pipecolic acid and glutaric acid (intermediates in lysine catabolism), and phytanic acid; deamination of D and L amino acids; metabolism of glycolate to glyoxylate; polyamine degradation (spermine and spermidine); and ethanol clearance.

Peroxisomal disorders constitute a clinically and biochemically heterogeneous group of inherited diseases that result from the absence or dysfunction of one or more peroxisomal enzymes. Pathophysiology apparently involves deficiency of necessary products of peroxisomal metabolism, or excess unmetabolized substrates. Disorders with similar biochemical defects may have markedly different clinical features, and disorders with similar clinical features may be associated with different biochemical findings. Peroxisomal disorders have been divided into three groups (Brown et al, 1993). Group 1 disorders result from the dysfunction of multiple enzymes owing to errors in peroxisome assembly. Group 2 disorders result from the dysfunction of a single peroxisomal enzyme. The peroxisomes are structurally intact. Group 3 disorders are characterized by peroxisomes of normal density but the presence of multiple enzyme deficiencies. General features of peroxisomal disorders may include dysmorphic craniofacial features; neurologic dysfunction, primarily consisting of severe hypotonia, possibly associated with hypertonia of the extremities and seizures; and hepatodigestive dysfunction, including hepatomegaly, cholestasis, and prolonged hyperbilirubinemia, each of which may present or be evident in the newborn period. Rhizomelic shortening of the limbs, stippled calcifications of epiphyses, renal cysts, and abnormalities in neuronal migration may also be seen.

Discussed here are peroxisomal disorders that may present in the newborn period. Zellweger syndrome is the prototype of neonatal peroxisomal disease. It is a disorder of peroxisome biogenesis (group 1) due to failure to import newly synthesized peroxisomal proteins into the peroxisome. The proteins remain in the cytosol, where they are rapidly degraded. In this condition, peroxisomes are absent from liver hepatocytes or exist as "ghosts." Neonatal adrenoleukodystrophy and infantile Refsum disease are also disorders of peroxisome biogenesis and, like Zellweger syndrome, disruption of function of more than one peroxisomal enzyme is demonstrable. A few residual peroxisomes, however, may be seen in the liver. These disorders represent a continuum of clinical severity. Rhizomelic chondrodysplasia punctata is caused by a defect in a subset of peroxisomal enzymes (group 3). Liver peroxisomes are demonstrable and normal in number, but their distribution and structure are abnormal.

Clinical Presentations (Table 26–2)

Zellweger Syndrome

Clinical Features. Zellweger syndrome is most often evident at birth with dysmorphic facial features, including large fontanels, high forehead, flat occiput, epicanthus, hypertelorism, up-slanting palpebral fissures, hypoplastic supraorbital ridges, abnormal ears, severe weakness and hypotonia, hepatomegaly, multicystic kidneys, and congenital heart disease. Seizures, feeding difficulties, and postnatal growth failure soon manifest. Ophthalmologic examination may reveal cataracts, corneal clouding, glaucoma, optic atrophy, retinitis pigmentosa, and Brushfield spots. Somatic sensory evoked responses and electroretinograms are abnormal. Hearing assessment often reveals an abnormal brain stem auditory evoked response consistent with sensorineural hearing loss. Skeletal radiographs demonstrate epiphyseal stippling, and cranial imaging reveals leukodystrophy and neuronal migration abnormalities. Later, hepatic cirrhosis and severe psychomotor retardation occur. Laboratory analysis may reveal abnormal liver function tests, hyperbilirubinemia, or hypoprothrombinemia. Death usually occurs within the first year of life, with an average life span of 12.5 weeks.

Neonatal Adrenoleukodystrophy

Clinical Features. Clinically, neonatal adrenoleukodystrophy is similar to, but less severe, than Zellweger syndrome. Differences include less dysmorphology, absence of chondrodysplasia punctata and renal cysts, and less neuronal and gray matter changes. The patients, however, may have striking white matter disease and often demonstrate degenerative changes in the adrenal glands. Patients with neonatal adrenoleukodystrophy show slow psychomotor development, followed by neurodegeneration that usually begins before the end of the first year of life. Disease progression is slower than that observed in Zellweger syndrome, and longer survival is usual, to an average of approximately 15 months of age.

Infantile Refsum Disease

Clinical Features. Patients with infantile Refsum disease also present at birth with relatively mild dysmorphic features, such as epicanthic folds, midface hypoplasia and low-set ears, and mild hypotonia. Early neurodevelopment is normal, possibly up to 6 months of age, but then slow deterioration follows. Later, sensorineural hearing loss (100%), anosmia, retinitis pigmentosa, hepatomegaly with impaired function, and severe mental retardation are evident. Patients learn to walk, although their gait may be

---

TABLE 26–2

Peroxisomal Disorders Presenting in the Newborn Period

	Zellweger Syndrome	Neonatal Adrenoleukodystrophy	Infantile Refsum Disease	Rhizomelic Chondrodysplasia Punctata
Onset	Birth	Birth–3 months	Birth–6 months	Birth
Facies	High forehead, large fontanels, upslanting palpebral fissures, hypoplasic supraorbital ridges, epicanthic folds, micrognathia, abnormal ears	Milder features of Zellweger syndrome	Epicanthic folds, midface hypoplasia, low-set ears	Depressed nasal bridge, hypertelorism, microcephaly
Neurologic Findings	Weakness, hypotonia, seizures, psychomotor retardation, sensorineural hearing loss	Hypotonia, seizures, slow psychomotor development and neurodegeneration	Mild hypotonia, normal early development followed by degeneration, ataxia, sensorineural hearing loss	Severe psychomotor retardation
Ophthalmologic Findings	Cataracts, glaucoma, corneal clouding, retinitis pigmentosa, optic nerve dysplasia, Brushfield spots	Retinopathy	Retinitis pigmentosa	Cataracts
Other	Hepatomegaly, multicystic kidneys, congenital heart disease, growth failure, chondrodysplasia punctata	Impaired adrenal function	Hepatomegaly, anosmia, diarrhea	Severe shortening of proximal limbs, joint contractures, ichthyosis
Diagnosis	↑ plasma VLCFA, phytanic acid, pipecolic acid, and bile acid intermediates; ↓ plasmalogens	Same as Zellweger syndrome	Same as Zellweger syndrome	↑ phytanic and pipecolic acids, ↓ plasmalogens, normal VLCFA and bile acid intermediates

VLCFA, very-long-chain fatty acid.

ataxic and broad-based. Diarrhea and failure to thrive may also occur. Chondrodysplasia punctata and renal cysts are absent. Neuronal migration defects are minor and adrenal hypoplasia occurs. The life span of patients with infantile Refsum disease is longer, lasting from 3 to 11 years.

Rhizomelic Chondrodysplasia Punctata

Clinical Features. Patients with rhizomelic chondrodysplasia punctata present at birth with facial dysmorphia, microcephaly, cataracts, rhizomelic shortening of the extremities with prominent stippling, and coronal clefting of vertebral bodies. The chondrodysplasia punctata is more widespread than in Zellweger syndrome and may involve extraskeletal tissues. Infants with this disorder have severe psychomotor retardation from birth onward and severe failure to thrive. Additionally, patients may have joint contractures, and 25% develop ichthyosis. Neuronal migration is normal. Life span is usually less than 1 year.

Diagnosis, Management, and Prognosis

The key to the diagnosis of peroxisomal disease is a high index of suspicion. Peroxisomal disorders should be considered in newborns with dysmorphic facial features, skeletal abnormalities, shortened proximal limbs, neurologic abnormalities, ocular abnormalities, and hepatic abnormalities. Babies with abnormal visual, hearing, or somatosensory evoked potentials should also be considered for these diagnoses.

Peroxisomal disorders are not associated with acute metabolic derangements or abnormal routine laboratory tests. Measurement of VLCFA, phytanic acid, pipecolic acid, bile acid intermediates, and plasmalogens is required for diagnosis. Zellweger syndrome is associated with elevated levels of VLCFA, phytanic acid, pipecolic acid, and bile acid intermediates, and a decreased level of plasmalogen synthesis. Neonatal adrenoleukodystrophy and infantile Refsum disease have similar biochemical findings; however, the defect in plasmalogen synthesis and the degree of VLCFA accumulation are less severe. Rhizomelic chondrodysplasia punctata has elevated phytanic and pipecolic acids levels, decreased plasmalogen levels, and normal VLCFA and bile acid intermediate levels. Thus, screening using only levels of VLCFA will fail to detect rhizomelic chondrodysplasia punctata. Abnormalities in phytanic acid and plasmalogens are age dependent. The elevation of phytanic acid may not be demonstrable in young infants, and the reduction in red blood cell plasmalogen levels may not be evident in children who are more than 20 weeks old (Lazarow and Moser, 1995). A liver biopsy, to assess the presence or absence and structure of peroxisomes, may be a useful adjunct diagnostic tool. Definitive diagnosis for all types of peroxisomal disease requires cultured skin fibroblasts for measurement of VLCFA levels and their beta-oxidation, and, as needed, assay of the peroxisomal steps of plasmalogen synthesis, phytanic acid oxidation, the subcellular localization of catalase, enzyme assays, and immunocytochemistry studies. Prenatal diagnosis is available using a variety of methods.

Treatment for all peroxisomal disorders presenting in the newborn period remains supportive. These disorders are chronic, progressive disorders with no presently available curative therapy. Two therapeutic trials have been attempted in patients with Zellweger syndrome and neonatal adrenoleukodystrophy. Setchell and associates (1992) described the effects of administration of primary bile acids on the liver function in a 6-month-old infant with Zellweger syndrome. The effects of treatment included the normalization of serum bilirubin and liver enzyme levels and a decrease in hepatic inflammation, bile duct proliferation, and canalicular plugs (Setchell et al, 1992). In addition, the patient demonstrated an improvement in growth and neurologic function (Setchell et al, 1992). Martinez (1992) reported the use of docosahexaenoic acid ethyl ester in two patients with neonatal adrenoleukodystrophy. Both patients had an increase in erythrocyte omega fatty acid levels and plasmalogens accompanied by significant clinical improvement, including improved alertness, motor performance, vocabulary, and visual evoked responses (Martinez, 1992). In addition, a "triple" dietary approach has been proposed that includes the oral administration of ether lipids, decreased phytanic acid intake, and the oral administration of glyceryl trioleate and glyceryl trierucate (Lorenzo's oil) (Lazarow and Moser, 1995). This approach is now being tested in patients with mild forms of disordered peroxisomal biogenesis. Hence, future treatment protocols may be available for infants affected with peroxisomal disease, but long-term outcome remains unknown.

SMITH-LEMLI-OPITZ SYNDROME

Etiology. SLO is a well-recognized autosomal recessive malformation syndrome, with an estimated incidence of approximately 1/20,000. In recent years, due to the identification of an underlying biochemical defect, SLO has been "reclassified" as an inborn error of metabolism. In 1993 it was discovered that SLO is caused by a defect in cholesterol biosynthesis that results in low levels of cholesterol and elevated levels of 7-dehydrocholesterol and its isomer, 8-dehydrocholesterol. Patients have markedly reduced activity of the enzyme 7-dehydrocholesterol reductase, the enzyme responsible for the conversion of 7-dehydrocholesterol to cholesterol (Salen et al, 1995). Patients are also noted to be deficient in bile acids, which can interfere with absorption of dietary lipids (Natowicz and Evans, 1994). Cholesterol is an important component of myelin and other cell membranes, and a defect in cholesterol synthesis may explain some of the clinical features of SLO.

Clinical Features. SLO is often evident at birth with microcephaly and facial dysmorphism, including bitemporal narrowing, ptosis, epicanthic folds, anteverted nares, broad nasal tip, prominent lateral palatine ridges, micrognathia, and low-set ears. Other features include 2 to 3 syndactyly of the toes, small proximally placed thumbs, and occasionally postaxial polydactyly and cataracts. Males usually have hypospadias, cryptorchidism, and a hypoplastic scrotum. Pyloric stenosis, cleft palate, pancreatic anomalies, and lung segmentation defects have also been reported (Baraitser and Winter, 1996). Hypotonia, progressing to hypertonia, and moderate to severe mental deficiency are also present. Feeding difficulties and vomiting are frequent problems in infancy. Irritable behavior and shrill screaming may also pose problems during infancy. Cranial imaging studies reveal (and autopsy confirms) defects in brain morphogenesis, including hypoplasia of the frontal lobes, cerebellum, and brain stem; dilated ventricles; irregular gyral patterns; and irregular neuronal organization. Approximately 20% of patients die within the first year of life. In other patients, life span may exceed 30 years. Life expectancy appears to correlate inversely with the number and severity of organ defects and with the kinds and numbers of limb, facial, and genital abnormalities (Tint et al, 1995).

Some patients have a severe lethal form of SLO, type II. In this form, the external genitalia of male infants may be ambiguous or female. Postaxial polydactyly of the hands, valgus deformity of the feet with syndactyly of several toes, cleft palate, and hypoplasia of the anterior portion of the tongue are common. Other findings may include unilobar lungs, hypoplastic kidneys, agenesis of the gallbladder, cerebellar hypoplasia, cardiac defects, and enlarged pancreatic islets with giant cells.

Diagnosis. The diagnosis of SLO types I and II is based on the findings of low levels of plasma cholesterol and elevated levels of 7-dehydrocholesterol and 8-dehydrocholesterol. The biochemical defect and findings are the same for both types. The difference between type I and type II appears to be one of degree: the enzyme defect is more severe and the block is more complete in patients with type II disease (Tint et al, 1995).

Treatment. The goal of therapy for SLO is twofold: (1) to increase the level of cholesterol in plasma and other body fluids, and (2) to decrease the level of 7-dehydrocholesterol. Treatment consists of providing exogenous cholesterol, either in the form of dietary cholesterol or cholesterol suspension, to replenish body stores of cholesterol and to down-regulate the patient's endogenous cholesterol synthesis, thus decreasing the amount of 7-dehydrocholesterol produced. A goal of cholesterol supplementation of 20 to 60 mg/kg per day was initially advocated, but doses higher than 300 mg/kg per day have been used without adverse outcome (Irons et al, 1995; Irons, personal communication). Provision of bile acids to facilitate adequate absorption of the dietary cholesterol is controversial. In infants with SLO, the use of breast milk should be encouraged since breast milk supplies approximately 133 mg/L of cholesterol (Irons et al, 1995).

Although the outcome remains largely unknown, therapy does appear to increase plasma cholesterol levels, decrease 7-dehydrocholesterol levels, and improve irritability, behavior, and growth (Irons et al, 1995). Parents report children to be more alert, active, and happier during therapy. Gain of developmental skills may be noted, and improvement in hypotonia may occur. Similar improvement has been noted in patients treated with cholesterol supplementation alone or cholesterol and bile acids. Therapy appears well tolerated. For maximal benefit, it is likely that treatment will need to begin prenatally, since SLO demonstrates many features consistent with in utero involvement of the disease process. Treatment should otherwise begin as soon as possible in the neonatal period or as soon as the diagnosis is confirmed.

REFERENCES

Baraitser M, Winter RM: Color Atlas of Congenital Malformation Syndromes. London, Mosby-Wolfe, 1996, p 61.

Barth PG: Sphingolipids. *In* Fernandes J, Saudubray J-M, van den Berghe G (Eds): Inborn Metabolic Diseases: Diagnosis and Treatment, 2nd ed. Berlin, Springer-Verlag, 1995, pp 375–382.

Brown FR, Voigt R, Singh AK, et al: Peroxisomal disorders: Neurodevelopmental and biochemical aspects. Am J Dis Child 147:617–626, 1993.

Erikson A, Johansson K, Mansson J-E, et al: Enzyme replacement therapy of infantile Gaucher disease. Neuropediatrics 24:237–238, 1993.

Fujimoto A, Tayebi N, Sidransky E: Congenital ichthyosis preceding neurologic symptoms in two sibs with type 2 Gaucher disease. Am J Med Genet 59:356–358, 1995.

Hoogerbrugge PM, Brouwer OF, Bordigoni P, et al: Allogenic bone marrow transplantation for lysosomal storage diseases. Lancet 345:1398–1402, 1995.

Ince Z, Coban A, Peker O, et al: Gaucher disease associated with congenital ichthyosis in the neonate. Eur J Pediatr 154(5):418, 1995.

Irons M, Elias ER, Abuelo D, et al: Clinical features of the Smith-Lemli-Opitz syndrome and treatment of the cholesterol metabolic defect. Int Pediatr 10(1):28–32, 1995.

Jaeken J: Carbohydrate-deficient glycoprotein syndromes. *In* Fernandes J, Saudubray J-M, van den Berghe G (Eds): Inborn Metabolic Diseases: Diagnosis and Treatment, 2nd ed. Berlin, Springer-Verlag, 1995, pp 395–397.

Kohlschütter A, Sieg K, Schulte FJ, et al: Infantile cardiomyopathy and neuromyopathy with beta-galactosidase deficiency. Eur J Pediatr 139:75–81, 1982.

Lazarow PB, Moser HW: Disorders of peroxisome biogenesis. *In* Scriver CR, Beaudet AL, Sly WS, Valle D (Eds): The Metabolic and Molecular Bases of Inherited Disease, 7th ed. New York, McGraw-Hill, 1995, pp 2287–2324.

Lipson AH, Rogers M, Berry A: Collodion babies with Gaucher's disease: A further case. Arch Dis Child 66:667, 1991.

Liu K, Commens C, Choong R, et al: Collodion babies with Gaucher's disease. Arch Dis Child 63:854–856, 1988.

Martinez M: Treatment with docosahexaenoic acid favorably modifies the fatty acid composition or erythrocytes in peroxisomal patients. *In* Coates PM, Tanaka K (Eds): New Developments in Fatty Acid Oxidation. New York, Wiley-Liss, 1992, pp 389–397.

Natowicz MR, Evans JE: Abnormal bile acids in the Smith-Lemli-Opitz syndrome. Am J Med Genet 50:364–367, 1994.

Natowicz MR, Stoler JM, Prence EM, et al: Marked heterogeneity in Niemann-Pick disease, type C: Clinical and ultrastructural findings. Clin Pediatr 34(4):190–197, 1995.

NIH Technology Assessment Panel on Gaucher Disease: Gaucher disease: Current issues in diagnosis and treatment. JAMA 275(7):548–553, 1996.

Salen G, Shefer S, Batta AK, et al: Biochemical abnormalities in the Smith-Lemli-Opitz syndrome. Int Pediatr 10(1):33–36, 1995.

Setchell KDR, Bragetti P, Zimmer-Nechemias L, et al: Oral bile acid treatment and the patient with Zellweger syndrome. Hepatology 15:198–207, 1992.

Sherer DM, Metlay LA, Sinkin RA, et al: Congenital ichthyosis with restrictive dermopathy and Gaucher disease: A new syndrome with associated prenatal diagnostic and pathology findings. Obstet Gynecol 81:842–844, 1993.

Sidransky E, Sherer DM, Ginns El: Gaucher disease in the neonate: A distinct Gaucher phenotype is analogous to a mouse model created by targeted disruption of the glucocerebrosidase gene. Pediatr Res 32(4):494–498, 1992.

Tint GS, Salen G, Batta AK, et al: Correlation of severity and outcome with plasma sterol levels in variants of the Smith-Lemli-Opitz syndrome. J Pediatr 127:82–87, 1995.

van Schaftingen E, Jaeken J: Phosphomannomutase deficiency as a cause of carbohydrate-deficient glycoprotein syndrome type I. FEBS Letters 377:318–320, 1995.

Wolman M: Wolman disease and its treatment. Clin Pediatr 34(4):207–212, 1995.

Connective Tissue Disorders and Skeletal Dysplasias

Paige Kaplan

The *skeletal dysplasias*, or osteochondrodysplasias, are disorders of the development and growth of cartilage and bone. They have been classified into 24 groups based on radiologic criteria (Beighton et al, 1992). Other classifications vary according to etiologic, clinical, and pathologic as well as radiologic criteria and may be confusing; for example, osteogenesis imperfecta (OI) can be classified as either a skeletal dysplasia or a connective tissue disorder. With recent advances in molecular knowledge, several groups of dysplasias that have mutations in the same genes have been identified. In some of these disorders, clinical similarities had been noted previously, for example, achondroplasia, hypochondroplasia, and thanatophoric dysplasia, all of which are due to mutations in the fibroblast growth factor receptor 3 (*FGFR3*) gene (Francomano et al, 1994; Le Merrer et al, 1994; Rousseau et al, 1995; Tavormina et al, 1995). Another group of disorders with mutations in the same gene comprises, from mildest to most severe, Kniest, spondyloepiphyseal dysplasias, spondyloepimetaphyseal dysplasia, Stickler syndrome, hypochondrogenesis, and achondrogenesis Type II. These are caused by mutations in the gene for collagen Type II, *COL2A1* (Rousseau et al, 1995; Spranger et al, 1994; Wilkin et al, 1994; Winterpacht et al, 1993), encoded on chromosome 12q13.11-q13.2. In other disorders, the common cause was not as obvious: diastrophic dysplasia (the mildest), atelosteogenesis Type II, and achondrogenesis Type 1B (the most severe) were found to be caused by mutations in the diastrophic dysplasia sulfate transporter (*DTDST*) gene, on chromosome 5q31-q34 (Hastbacka et al, 1994, 1996; Kaitila et al, 1989; Rousseau et al, 1995; Superti-Furga et al, 1996). This affects the transport of sulfate to proteoglycans (mucopolysaccharides), especially chondroitin sulfate–containing proteoglycans prevalent in cartilage.

With the increasing use and accuracy of ultrasonography for prenatal care, a greater number of osteochondrodysplasias are diagnosed in the second trimester (Gordienko et al, 1996; Rasmussen et al, 1996). In one series (Rasmussen et al, 1996) of 126,316 deliveries monitored over 15 years, the incidence was 2.14/10,000. This chapter focuses on several of the more common dysplasias and connective tissue disorders that manifest prenatally or perinatally (Gordienko et al, 1996; Rasmussen et al, 1996) but is not exhaustive (Table 27–1). The osteochondrodysplasias are reviewed extensively by Rimoin and Lachman (1996) according to the International Classification and by Spranger and Maroteaux (1990).

Precise diagnoses are important for prognosis, acute and chronic management, and genetic counseling regarding other possible affected family members. Most skeletal dysplasias cause short stature, which may be proportionate or disproportionate. In considering a diagnosis, it is important to know whether the skull, vertebrae (trunk), ribs, or limbs are affected. If the limbs are disproportionately shortened compared with the trunk, there may be segmental (disproportionate) or proportionate involvement of the three parts of the limbs: upper arms and thighs (rhizomelic), forearms and legs (mesomelic), or hands and feet (acromelic). Accurate measurements of length on a rigid board, arm span, and head and chest circumferences are essential and must be plotted on standard growth curves. Very large heads occur in achondroplasia and thanatophoric dysplasia. Cloverleaf skull deformity is present in thanatophoric and, occasionally, diastrophic dysplasias. A relatively long chest is seen in asphyxiating thoracic dystrophy. The hand in achondroplasia is short with trident fingers; distinctive "hitchhiker" thumbs occur in diastrophic dysplasia. Deformations of feet ("clubfeet") occur in diastrophic, Kniest syndrome, spondyloepiphyseal dysplasias, and OI II. Multiple joint dislocations occur in Larsen and Ehlers-Danlos Type VII syndromes and atelosteogenesis.

The presence of other abnormalities can be valuable clues to diagnosis. Cleft palate or uvula can occur in campomelic, Kniest, spondyloepiphyseal, short-rib polydactyly (Majewski), atelosteogenesis Types I and II, hypochondrogenesis, and diastrophic dysplasias. Congenital cataracts occur in chondrodysplasia punctata. Congenital cardiac defects occur in short-rib polydactyly dysplasias (conotruncal malformations in Type I and transposition of the great arteries in Type II). Postaxial polydactyly occurs in short-rib polydactyly and thoracic asphyxiating and chondroectodermal dysplasias; occasionally, preaxial polydactyly also occurs in the short rib dysplasias.

Radiographs of the entire skeleton, including hands and feet, are essential for accurate diagnosis. If the infant or fetus dies, cartilage and skin fibroblasts should be obtained for histochemical tests and molecular-gene mutation analysis as well as photographs. Detailed family history and measurements of family members may be helpful; milder affected members might have gone undiagnosed.

The *connective tissues* in the matrix are the supporting and connecting structures for the cell. There are a large number of different molecules, including collagen (at least 16 types), elastin, fibrillin (2 types), and microfibril-associated glycoproteins. These are components of tissues such as bone, cartilage, vascular media, tendon, skin, basement membranes in the renal glomeruli and other organs, and the suspensory ligament of the lens. The heritable disorders of connective tissue are varied, may be very dissimilar, and may manifest in utero or at any age postnatally. Most are rare, but some of the more common conditions that manifest at birth are discussed. Early diagnosis optimizes the management and prognosis for the infant and family.

OSTEOGENESIS IMPERFECTA TYPES II AND III

OI is characterized by increased bone fragility. It can be classified as a connective tissue disorder or skeletal dyspla-

TABLE 27–1

Most Frequent Types of Osteochondrodysplasias Detected Prenatally and Perinatally

Dysplasia	No. Cases (%)	
	Gordienko et al, 1996	**Rasmussen et al, 1996**
Thanatophoric	3 (8)	5 (20)
Osteogenesis imperfecta Type II	10 (26)	3 (12)
Osteogenesis imperfecta Type III		2 (7)
Achondroplasia	5 (13)	3 (11)
Spondyloepiphyseal dysplasia congenita		3 (11)
Campomelic	2 (5)	2 (7)
Short-rib polydactyly I	2 (5)	1 (4)
Short-rib polydactyly II	2 (5)	1 (4)
Other diagnoses	15 (38)	3 (11)
No diagnoses	—	4 (13)
Total no. cases	39	27

Adapted from Gordienko IY, Grechanina EY, Sopko NI, et al: Prenatal diagnosis of osteochondrodysplasias in high risk pregnancy. Am J Med Genet 63:90, 1996; and Rasmussen SA, Bieber FR, Benacerraf BR, et al: Epidemiology of osteochondrodysplasias. Changing trends due to advances in prenatal diagnosis. Am J Med Genet 61:49, 1996. Copyright ©1996. Reprinted by permission of Wiley-Liss, Inc., a division of John Wiley & Sons, Inc.

sia. There are four clinical types: Types II and III are the most severe, manifesting pre- and perinatally. OI Type I rarely causes prenatal or perinatal fractures.

Etiology. OI is caused by abnormalities in Type I collagen, which is composed of three polypeptide chains—two alpha-1 (I) and one alpha-2 (I) fibrils, coiled in a triple helix (Byers, 1993; Byers et al, 1988, 1991). There are two genes, *COL1A1* and *COLIA2*, on chromosomes 17q21 and 7q22.1, respectively, that encode the chains. Mutations in either of the genes result in abnormal collagen. In Type I OI, there is secretion of normal collagen but only half as much as usual, with a milder phenotype. In the other types, the altered procollagen chains are incorporated into the helix, causing 50% to 75% collagen fibers to be abnormal, resulting in more severe phenotypes (Byers, 1993). Most, if not all, OI is inherited as an autosomal dominant trait.

OI Type II (perinatal lethal type) is estimated to affect 1/20,000 to 60,000 infants. Affected infants may be born prematurely, with low weight and disproportionately short stature. The limbs are short and bowed with extra, circular skin creases; the hips are abducted and flexed. The head is soft and boggy, and minimal calvarial bone can be felt. The sclerae are dark blue, the nose may be prominent, and the chest is narrow. The infant cries with handling because there are many fractures at different stages of healing. Sixty percent are stillborn or die during the first day of life and 80% die by 1 month (Byers et al, 1988). With the increasing use of ultrasonography, fetuses may be detected in the early second trimester because of short and bowed or angulated limbs and narrow thoraces (Fig. 27–1A).

Prenatal histochemical or molecular diagnosis is possible by analysis of chorionic villi or amniocytes, if the previously affected sibling's mutation is known, but may not be 100%. *Radiologically,* the femurs are short, broad, and "telescoped" or "crumpled"; the tibias are short and bowed, and fibulas may be thin (Fig. 27–1B). There is minimal or no calvarial mineralization, with occasional wormian bones (small islands of bone in the suture spaces). The vertebrae

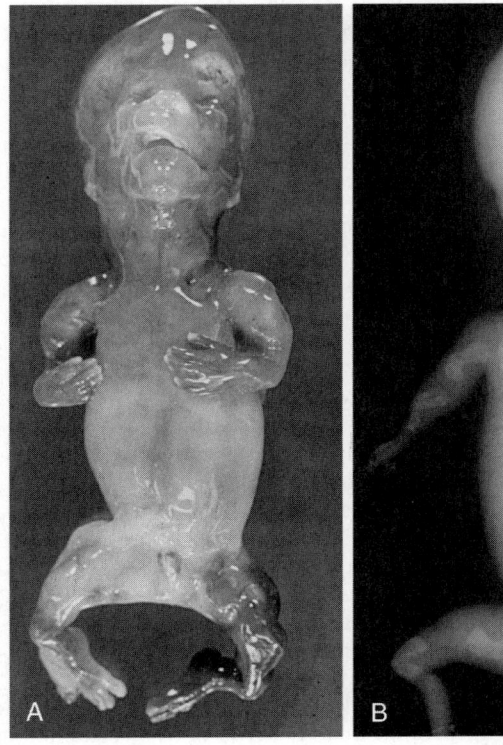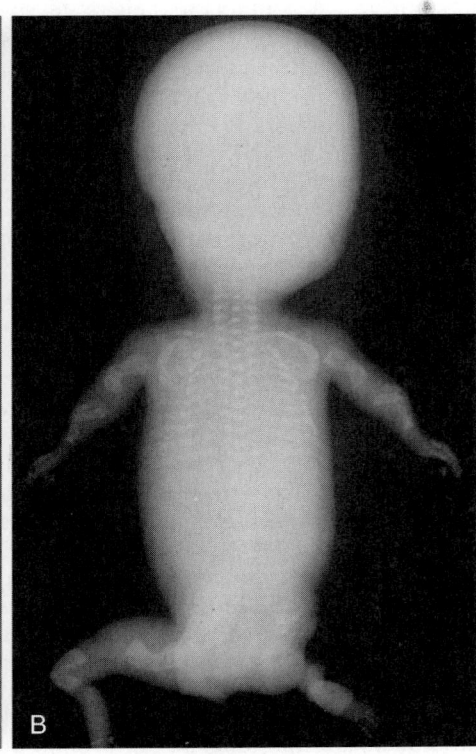

FIGURE 27–1. Osteogenesis imperfecta Type II. *A,* 14-Week fetus. The calvarium is deformed; limbs are angulated and deformed from multiple fractures. *B,* Radiograph of fetus (14 weeks) showing absence of ossification in calvarium, short telescoped/crumpled humeri and femurs, short and wavy ribs.

are very flat (platyspondyly). The ribs are short, wavy, and thin or broad, with "beading" from callus formation.

OI Type III (progressive deforming type) may manifest prenatally and perinatally as well as in the first 2 years of life (Byers, 1993). Prenatal and perinatal clinical features are similar to but less severe than those in OI Type II (Fig. 27–2A). Perinatal death is common. If not present at birth, fractures and deformations of the limbs develop in the first and second years. The highest frequency of fractures in OI, up to 200, occur in Type III. Extremely short stature, with adult heights of 92 to 108 cm, may result from micro-

fractures in the growth plates. The head may be large because the calvarium is soft with a large anterior fontanel. The sclerae may be blue at first but are white by puberty. The head assumes a triangular shape, with bossed, broad forehead and tapered, pointed chin. Later in childhood, dentinogenesis imperfecta and hearing loss may develop. Severe kyphoscoliosis may develop, leading to cardiopulmonary compromise, the major cause of early death. *Radiologically* (Fig. 27–2B), the long bones are thin and gracile with healing fractures incurred in utero, bowing, and deformations. The femurs are short and deformed but not crum-

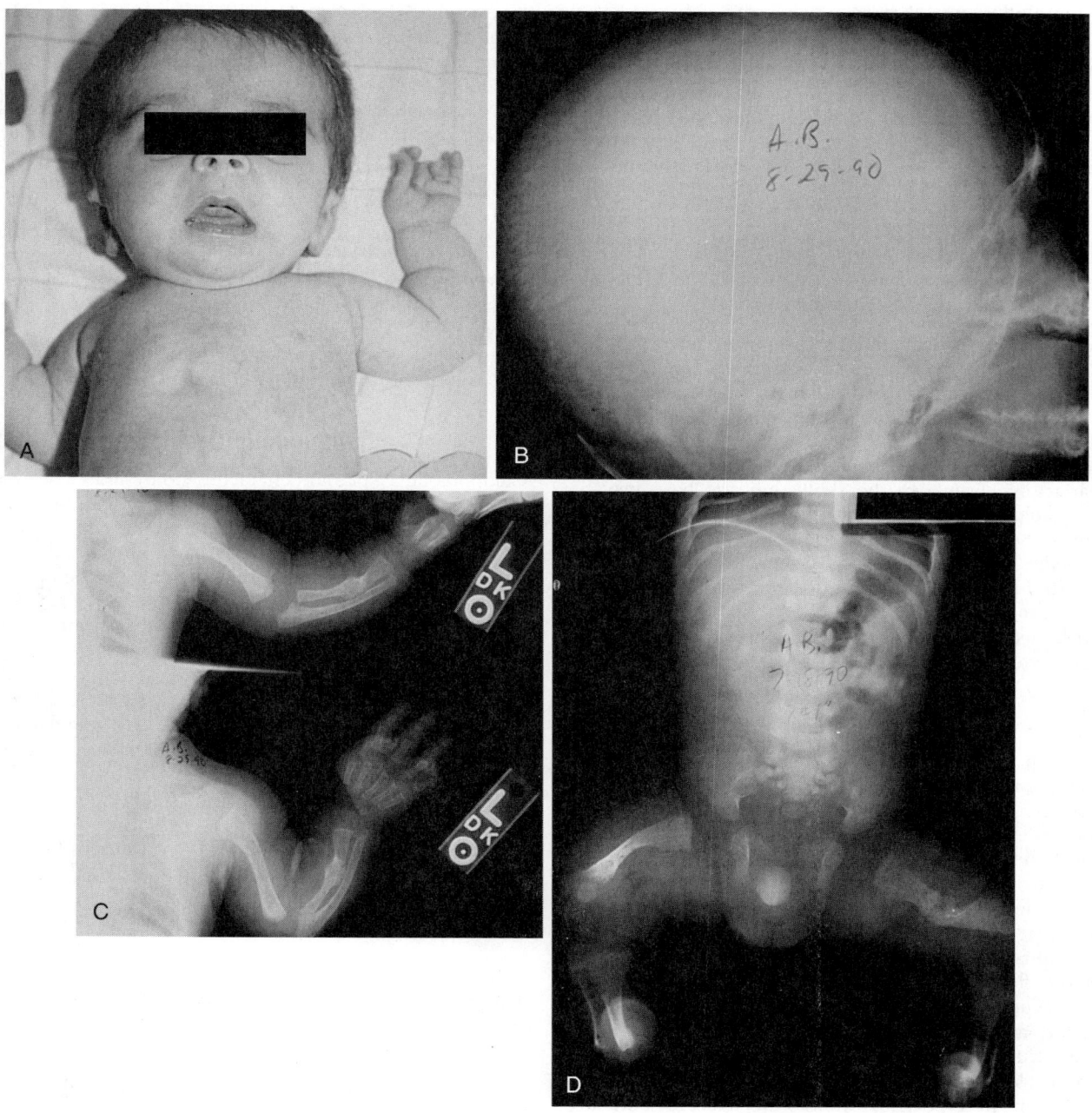

FIGURE 27–2. Osteogenesis imperfecta Type III. *A,* Neonate with normal face, short neck, slightly short limbs. *B,* Radiograph shows calvarium is undermineralized with wormian bones. *C,* Radiograph shows upper limbs: bowed humeri, callus in ulnae. *D,* Radiograph shows lower limbs: moderately short, thick femora, angulated tibias and fibulas.

pled as in OI Type II (Fig. 27–2C). The calvarium is undermineralized with wormian bones and large anterior fontanel (Fig. 27–2D). The ribs are thin and gracile.

Inheritance. The affected fetus or infant with OI Type II or III is usually a sporadic occurrence in a family, but there is a risk of recurrence of approximately 6% in subsequent siblings because the gene mutation might be present in some of a parent's somatic cells or germline (parental mosaicism) (Byers et al, 1988). The parent is usually asymptomatic but may have minimal manifestation such as short stature. *Prenatal diagnosis* is possible with ultrasonography and gene mutation analysis.

Differential Diagnosis. The lethal skeletal dysplasias can be diagnosed in the first half of pregnancy with ultrasonography. It may be difficult to differentiate the dysplasias; therefore, experienced ultrasonographers are required for accurate diagnoses. The types of dysplasias include the following:

1. Thanatophoric dysplasia (see Fig. 27–3)
2. Campomelic dysplasia (see Fig. 27–4)
3. Achondrogenesis Type IA (see Fig. 27–5)
4. Perinatal hypophosphatasia (Whyte, 1995)

Perinatal hypophosphatasia, caused by deficient alkaline phosphatase (ALP), occurs in approximately 1/100,000 live births; neonatal death is usual and in utero death can occur. It is characterized by polyhydramnios, short deformed limbs, and a soft skull. The entire skeleton is undermineralized, so that many bones cannot be visualized and may appear to be absent. In the skull, only the base may be seen radiologically. There may be rachitic changes and fractures. Serum ALP is very low. The gene for tissue nonspecific ALP is mutant and is on chromosome 1p34-p36.1. Its *inheritance* is autosomal recessive; each subsequent sibling has a 25% risk. *Prenatal diagnosis* is optimized by using ultrasonography and assay of ALP activity in amniocytes.

Thanatophoric Dysplasia

Thanatophoric dysplasia is one of the most common lethal dysplasias (Rimoin and Lachman, 1996; Spranger and Maroteaux, 1990), occurring in 1/35,000 births. It is characterized by extremely short limbs, long narrow trunk, large head with bulging forehead, prominent eyes, flat nose bridge, wide fontanel, and occasionally cloverleaf skull deformity (Fig. 27–3A). Death occurs in the neonatal period from respiratory insufficiency. *Radiologically,* the femurs are short, flared at the metaphyses, with a medial spike, bowed (Type I) or straight (Type II); other long bones are also short and bowed (Fig. 27–3B and C) (Table 27–2). The calvarium is large with a short base and small foramen magnum; cloverleaf skull is sometimes present in Type I and is severe in Type II. Vertebrae are flat with notching of superior and inferior aspects on lateral views; lumbar vertebrae have an inverted-U appearance on anteroposterior views. Ribs are short, cupped, and splayed anteriorly (Tavormina et al, 1995).

Differential Diagnosis

1. OI Types II and III
2. Achondroplasia (see later discussion)
3. Achondrogenesis and hypochondrogenesis

Etiology. Thanatophoric dysplasia Types I and II are caused by distinct mutations in the gene for *FGFR3*. *FGFR3* is located at chromosome 4p16.3 and is the same gene that causes achondroplasia and hypochondroplasia (Francomano et al, 1994; Le Merrer et al, 1994). In thanatophoric dysplasia Type I, most mutations have been in the extracellular domain, with single amino acid substitutions by cysteine (Rousseau et al, 1995; Tavormina et al, 1995). In all studied cases of thanatophoric dysplasia Type II, the lysine at nucleotide 650 has been substituted by glutamate (lys650glu) (Tavormina et al, 1995). In achondroplasia, more than 98% have substitution of the same amino acid, glycine, by arginine (Gly380Arg) (Shiang et al, 1994). In several patients with hypochondroplasia, mutations have been found at one specific nucleotide coding for asparagine, which has been substituted by lysine (Asp540Lys) (Bellus, McIntosh, et al, 1995; Bellus, Szabo, et al, 1995).

Inheritance. Most cases of thanatophoric dysplasia as well as achondroplasia and hypochondroplasia occur sporadically, resulting from new autosomal dominant mutations. There is a low risk of recurrence in siblings of a sporadic case, because of possible parental mosaicism.

Campomelic Dysplasia

Campomelic dysplasia is characterized by short stature with relatively long, slender thighs and upper arms, short bowed legs with dimples in midshaft, large dolichocephalic skull, cleft soft palate, micrognathia, narrow chest, and external genital abnormalities (from mild anomalies to complete sex reversal in XY males) (Houston et al, 1983) (Fig. 27–4A and B). The ribs may be thin and wavy, with only 11 pairs. Death results from respiratory compromise.

Radiology. In the second trimester, with ultrasonography, the limbs may appear short, bowed, and angulated and may be mistaken for OI (Fig. 27–4C). However, it is distinguishable because the calvarium is better ossified, the palate may be cleft, and the chin is small.

Etiology. The mutant gene, *SOX9* (a transcription factor gene) is located at chromosome 17q24.1-25.1 (Tommerup, 1993).

Inheritance

This is an autosomal dominant trait. Most cases are new sporadic occurrences in a family.

Achondrogenesis Types IA and IB

Achondrogenesis Types IA and IB (Borochowitz et al, 1988) are similar, characterized by short stature, extremely short limbs (with "flipper" hands in Type IA), relatively large head with round face, short nose, small mouth, soft

TABLE 27–2

Skeletal Dysplasias Manifesting Prenatally or Perinatally

Dysplasia Name	Skeletal Features	Nonskeletal Features	Radiographic Features	Inheritance, Gene, Chromosome	Comments
Lethal					
Thanatophoric	Large cranium, "proptosis," flat nose bridge, narrow chest, limbs very short (all segments)	Polyhydramnios, hydrocephalus, brain anomalies, congenital cardiac abnormalities	Large calvarium, short base, small magnum foramen, cloverleaf skull; ribs short, splayed, cupped; vertebrae small and flat, U-shaped; pelvis short, small, flat; limbs short, bowed, metaphyseal flare with spike	AD; most new mutations; *FGFR3*; 4p16.3	Same gene as achondroplasia, hypochondroplasia
Campomelic	Large cranium, small face, nose bridge flat, chin small, (cleft soft palate); small, narrow chest; limbs: bowed thighs and legs, dimple on leg	Polyhydramnios, congenital cardiac abnormalities, female external genitalia in XY males	Large dolichocephalic calvarium, shallow orbits; ribs short and wavy, often 11 pairs; vertebrae small, flat; pelvis tall and narrow; limbs relatively long; thin, bowed femurs; short tibias	AD; most new mutations; *SOX9*; 17q24.1-q25.1	
Achondrogenesis Type I	Soft cranium; round face; short, round chest; limbs very short	Polyhydramnios	Poorly ossified calvarium; ribs short, fractures (beading); vertebrae nonossified; pelvis small; limbs: short, broad femurs with metaphyseal spikes; short broad tibias and fibulas		
Short-rib polydactyly Types I/III	Hydropic appearance; round, flat face; micrognathia; extremely narrow chest; limbs very short; postaxial polydactyly	Cardiac, renal, anal malformations	Normal calvarium; ribs very short, horizontal; vertebrae flat, wide intervertebral disc spaces; pelvis small; limbs short; lateral and medial metaphyseal spurs	AR	
Short-rib polydactyly Type II	Hydropic; face short, flat nose, cleft lip-palate, low-set ears; narrow chest, protuberant abdomen; limbs moderately short	Cardiac, renal (dysplastic kidneys), respiratory malformations	Ribs very short, horizontal; vertebrae and pelvis normal; limbs short; round metaphyses; premature epiphyseal ossification; polydactyly	AR	
Asphyxiating thoracic dystrophy	Face normal; narrow, long chest; limbs: variable shortening	Lethal pulmonary insufficiency	Calvarium and vertebrae normal; ribs very short, anterior cupping; limbs short; wide proximal femoral metaphysis; premature ossification proximal femoral epiphysis	AR	If newborn period is survived, renal disease (proteinuria, hypertension)
Atelosteogenesis Type I (Fig. 27–9)	Face flat; cleft palate, micrognathia; very narrow chest; limbs very short (rhizomelic); equinovalgus deformities; joint dislocations	Premature; stillbirth	Vertebrae flat; coronal and sagittal clefts; scoliosis; ribs short (11 pairs); pelvis small; enlarged sacrosciatic notch; limbs: short "drumstick" humerus; absent fibulas; short metacarpals, triangular first metacarpals, dysharmonic ossification of hand bones; dislocated knees	? (sporadic)	Similar to boomerang dysplasia
Atelosteogenesis Type II	Face-cleft palate; narrow chest; limbs: short, dislocations; equinovarus deformities; gap between first and second digits	Laryngeal stenosis; patent foramen ovale	Vertebrae occasional coronal and sagittal clefts; ribs short; Pelvis: normal sacrosciatic notch; limbs: short "dumbell" humeri and femurs, small fibulas; large second and third metacarpals; small round midphalanges	AR; *DTDST*; 5q31-q34	Same gene as diastrophic dysplasia (milder disease) and achondrogenesis Type IB (more severe disease)

Table continued on following page

TABLE 27–2

Skeletal Dysplasias Manifesting Prenatally or Perinatally *Continued*

Dysplasia Name	Skeletal Features	Nonskeletal Features	Radiographic Features	Inheritance, Gene, Chromosome	Comments
Dyssegmental (Silverman-Handmaker)	Face: flat midface, flat orbits, cleft palate, micrognathia; short neck; narrow chest; limbs: extremely small	Encephalocele; cardiac: patent ductus arteriosus	Cranium: midface hypoplasia; vertebrae variable sizes; coronal and sagittal clefts; ribs very short and flared; scapulae round, abnormal shape; limbs: very short, broad, bowed long bones; small first metacarpals; pelvis: small and round	AR	Resembles dyssegmental (Rolland-Desbuquois) (less severe) and Kniest syndrome
Chondrodysplasia punctata, rhizomelic type (Fig. 27–10)	Face flat; very flat nose bridge and tip; limbs: proximal shortening	Cataracts; joint contractures; skin: icthyosiform erythroderma	Vertebrae: wide coronal clefts; limbs: short humeri and femurs; stippled epiphyses of long bones and pelvis and peroxisomal periarticular areas; pelvis: trapezoid ilia	AR	Infant who survives newborn period can live a few years; severe growth and mental retardation
Nonlethal					
Achondroplasia	Large cranium; face: bossed forehead, flat nose bridge, prominent chin, short neck; chest slightly narrow; limbs: proximal shortening, short trident hands; short proximal and middle phalanges; later genu varum; thoracolumbar kyphosis; lumbar lordosis	Hypotonia: delayed motor milestones; spinal stenosis causes spinal compression; small foramen magnum can cause hydrocephalus; short: mean adult heights; for males, 131 cm; for females, 124 cm	Calvarium large, small foramen magnum, short base; vertebrae: diminished lumbosacral interpedicular space, short pedicles; ribs: short, anterior cupping; limbs: short humeri and femurs; relatively long fibulas; metaphyseal flare; pelvis: small iliac wings	AD; most are new mutations, associated with advanced paternal age *FGFR3* 4p16.3	Same gene as hypochondroplasia (milder) and thanatophoric dysplasia (very severe) Hypochondroplasia is usually not apparent until 1–2 yrs
Diastrophic dysplasia (Fig. 27–11)	Normal cranium; face: cleft palate, micrognathia; chest: normal at birth; limbs: very short; thumbs proximally placed and adducted ("hitchhiker thumb"); severe equinovarus of feet; limited movement at many joints	External ears: cystic masses in infancy ("cauliflower" ears); deafness caused by lack or fusion of ossicles; narrow external canal; scoliosis in childhood	Ribs: premature ossification of cartilage; vertebrae: narrow L1–L5 interpedicular spaces; scoliosis; limbs: short; disproportionately short ulna and fibula (mesomelic); broad flared metaphyses; ovoid first metacarpals; variable symphalangism of proximal interphalangeal joints; irregular delayed epiphyseal ossification except carpals accelerated	AR *DTDST* 5q31.3-q34	Intrafamilial variability Normal life span if scoliosis does not impair respiratory function; normal intelligence
Kniest syndrome	Large cranium; face: flat, "large" eyes, flat nasal bridge, cleft palate; trunk: short; limbs: proximal shortening (more severe in lower limbs), enlarged joints, flexion contractures	Infancy: tracheomalacia; childhood: myopia and retinal detachment; hearing loss; delayed motor development; normal intelligence	Calvarium: frontal and maxillary hypoplasia, shallow orbits; ribs: slightly short; vertebrae: flat, coronal clefts; anisospondyly (different sizes); pelvis: small, irregular acetabular roof; limbs: short; metaphyses broad and flared ("dumbbell"), lateral bowing of femurs and upper tibias; tubular bones of hands and feet; slightly short and broad/normal; epiphyses at knees not ossified	AD *COL2A1* 12q13.11q13.2	Same gene as some spondyloepiphyseal dysplasias, spondyloepimetaphyseal dysplasia, Stickler, hypochondrogenesis, achondrogenesis Type II (most severe)

AD, autosomal dominant; FGFR3, fibroblast growth factor receptor 3; AR, autosomal recessive; DTDST, diastrophic dysplasia sulfate transporter.

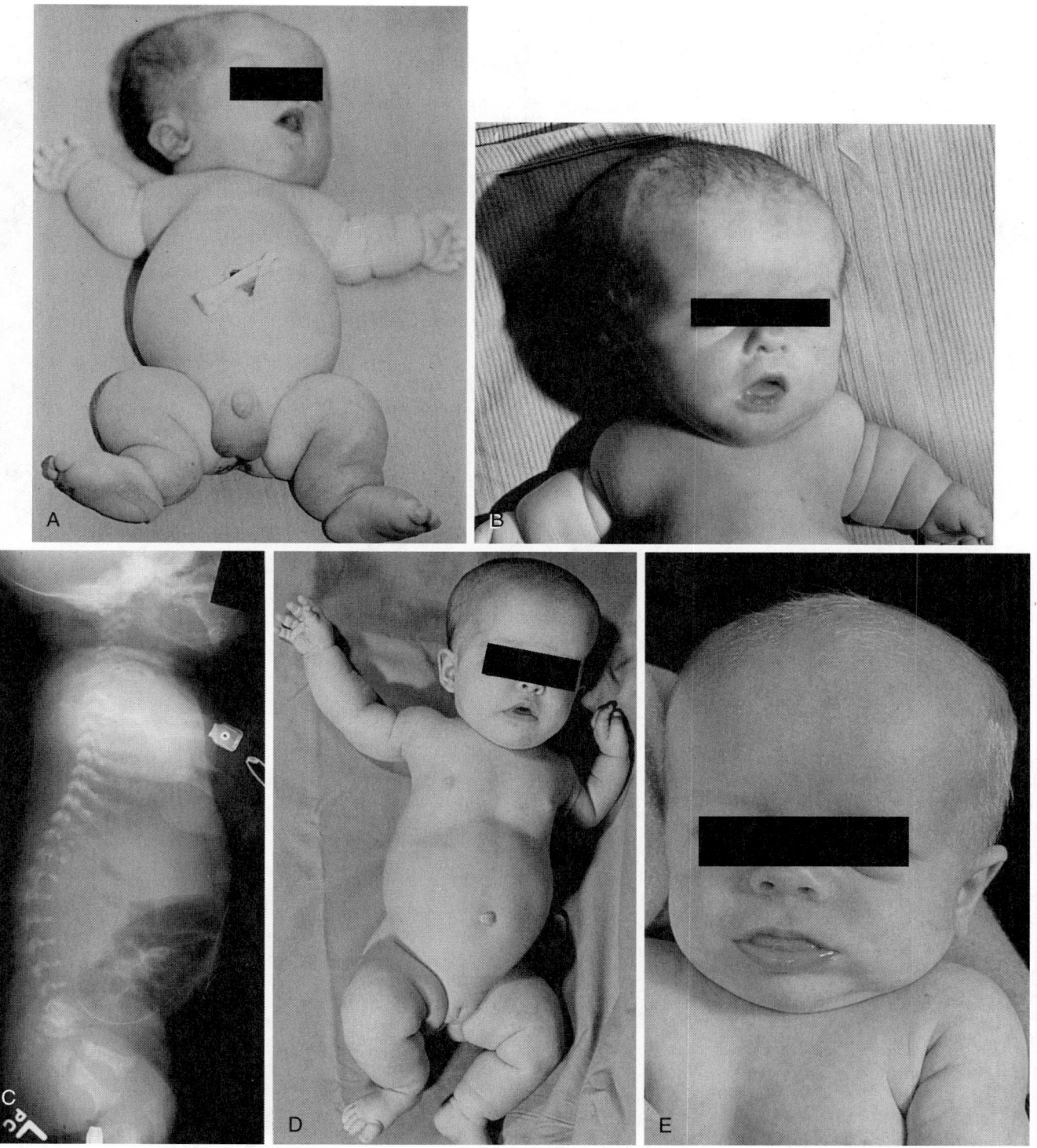

FIGURE 27–3. Thanatophoric dysplasia *(A–C)* and achondroplasia *(D, E). A,* Neonate with thanatophoric dysplasia has large head, narrow chest, very short limbs and extra creases on limbs, short hands with trident fingers, angulated abducted thighs. (Courtesy Montreal Children's Hospital, Montreal, Quebec, Canada.) *B,* Neonate with thanatophoric dysplasia has face with bossed forehead, flat nose bridge, short neck, very short limbs with extra creases and trident fingers. (Courtesy Montreal Children's Hospital, Montreal, Quebec, Canada). *C,* Radiograph shows thanatophoric dysplasia with large calvarium, short ribs with anterior splaying, short bowed femurs with medial metaphyseal spike. *D,* Infant with achondroplasia showing bossed forehead and proximal limb shortening. (Courtesy Charles I. Scott, M.D., Al Dupont Institute, Wilmington, DE.) *E,* Infant with achondroplasia showing bossed forehead and flat nasal bridge. (Courtesy Charles I. Scott, M.D., Al DuPont Institute, Wilmington, DE.)

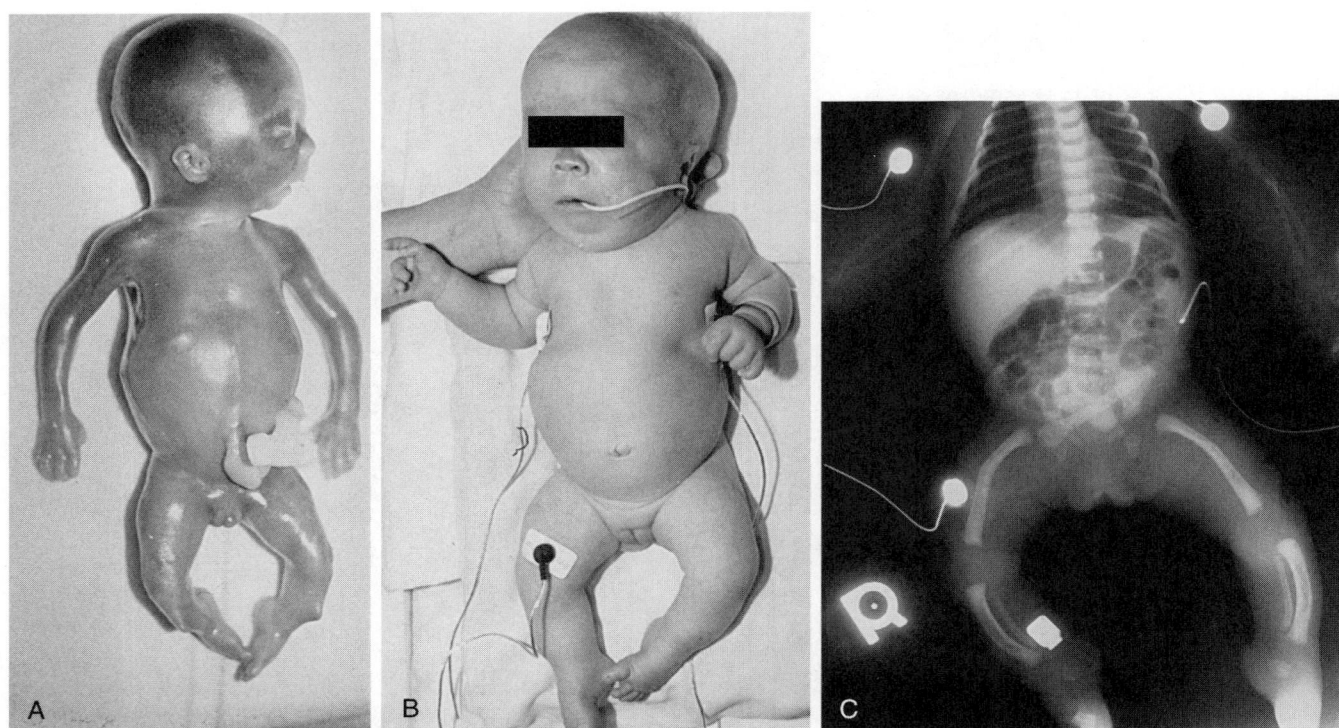

FIGURE 27–4. Campomelic dysplasia. *A,* 46XY "female" 22-week-old fetus with normal head, long philtrum, micrognathia, low-set ears, mild narrowing of chest, proximally placed thumbs, and bowed or angulated lower limbs resembling osteogenesis imperfecta Type II but less shortened; the external genitalia are female. *B,* Neonate with long-limb form, with relatively large head, micrognathia, narrow chest, bowing of lower limbs with characteristic dimpling of lower leg. *C,* Radiograph shows narrow chest; relatively long, thin limb bones with bowing of femurs and tibias; long, narrow pelvis.

skull, and very short neck. Polyhydramnios during pregnancy, premature delivery, and hydrops are common. The infant is stillborn or dies within hours of birth.

Radiology

The long bones are extremely short, with square, globular, or triangular shapes and medial spikes of metaphyses of femurs (Fig. 27–5A and B). The calvarium is poorly ossified, the vertebrae are unossified (Type IA) or poorly ossified (Type IB), and the ribs are short (with multiple fractures and callus [beading] in Type IA). Its pattern of *inheritance* and *cause* are unknown.

Differential Diagnosis. Achondrogenesis Type II and hypochondrogenesis are the same condition, caused by different mutations in the same gene for Type II collagen but with variable phenotypic expression. The short staure, limb, calvarial, and vertebral abnormalities are somewhat less severe than in achondrogenesis Type I, but there is also hydrops, with stillbirth, or death within hours after birth. Cleft palate may occur in hypochondrogenesis (Fig. 27–5C). Its *inheritance* pattern is autosomal dominant, usually a new sporadic mutation.

ACHONDROPLASIA

Achondroplasia is the most common of the nonlethal chondrodysplasias: it affects 1 in 15,000 live births. It is charac-

terized at birth by short limbs, particularly rhizomelic (proximal) and acromelic (hands) with trident fingers, large head with frontal prominence, flat nose bridge, flat midface, long narrow trunk, and thoracolumbar gibbous deformity (see Fig. 27–3D and E). The lateral cerebral ventricles may be large, but hydrocephalus is not common, although it is more prevalent than in the general population. The child is hypotonic; together with the large head, this results in delayed motor milestones. Most achondroplastic children have normal intelligence. However, development can be impaired if there is hydrocephalus, which can result from perinatal bleeds associated with vaginal deliveries, or impaired respiratory function (Hecht et al, 1991). The foramen magnum and the lumbar spinal canal may be narrow, causing compression of the spinal cord. Compression of the lower brain stem and cervical spinal cord can lead to hypotonia, retardation, quadriparesis, obstructive or central apnea, and sudden death (Pauli et al, 1984). Perinatal death is unusual; most deaths occur between 2 and 5 months, often during the day, and may be precipitated by sleeping upright without support for the head. In the infants with sudden death, the head circumference is usually not larger than average for achondroplasia, neurologic state is not abnormal, and development is average. Radiologic imaging of the skull and brain is recommended for monitoring; surgical decompression of foramen magnum or lumbar stenosis may prevent neurologic damage. In older people, untreated spinal stenosis can cause

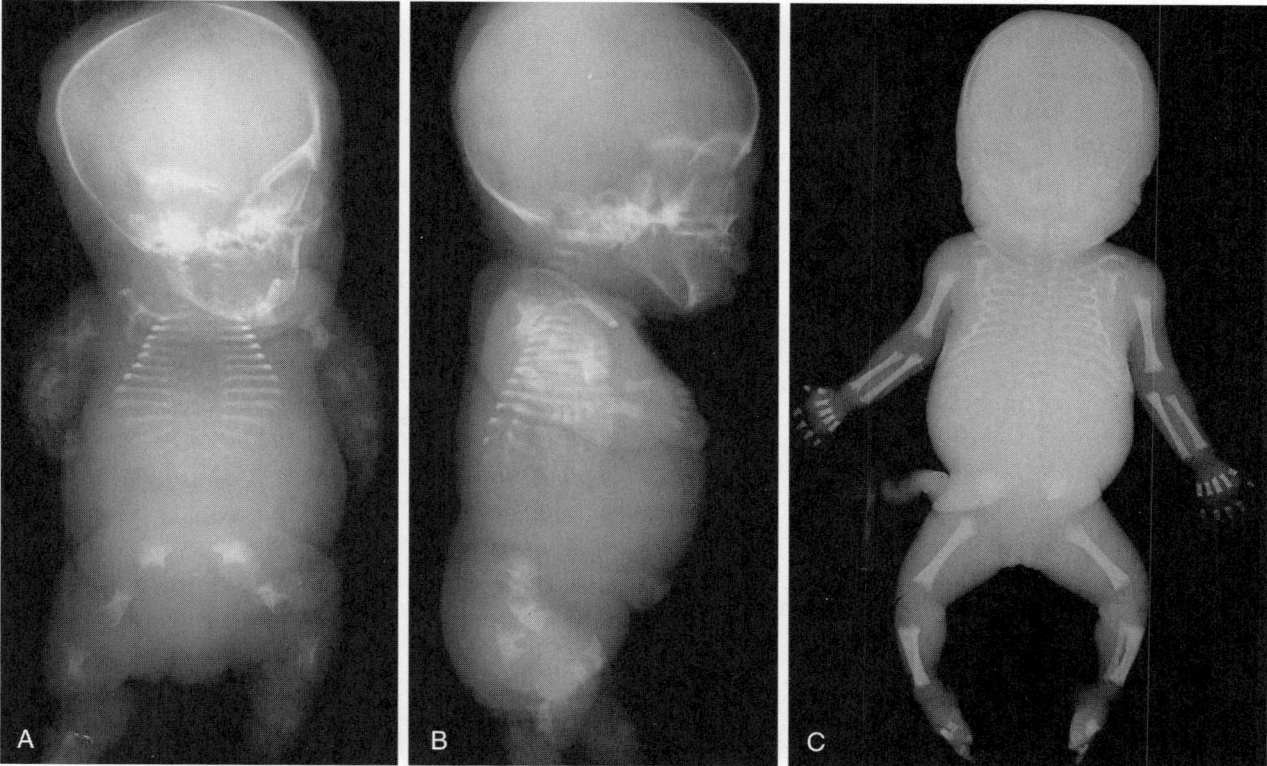

FIGURE 27–5. *A* and *B,* Radiographs showing characteristics of achondrogenesis Type I: cervical, thoracic, and lumbar vertebral bodies are not ossified, sacrum is unossified, ribs are short, limbs are extremely short with medial femoral metaphyseal spikes. *C,* Radiograph showing hypochondrogenesis in a midgestation fetus with underossified calvarium and vertebral bodies (although better ossified than in achondrogenesis), unossified pubis, longer limb bones but irregular metaphyses, short ribs, and narrow thorax. (Courtesy Elaine Zackai, MD, Children's Hospital of Philadelphia, PA.)

paresthesias, numbness, bladder and bowel incontinence, and impotence. Standard growth curves for achondroplasia (Horton et al, 1978) should be used routinely; deviation from the expected should alert the physician to a possible new complication such as hydrocephalus. Average adult height is 118 to 145 cm (males) and 112 to 136 cm (females). A controversial surgical technique to lengthen limbs, the Ilizarov method (Ilizarov, 1988) can add as much as 25 cm. It is used in adolescents. Pins are inserted into the limbs on either side of epiphyses or fractured bone with callus formation, and the areas are stretched by millimeters daily.

Radiology. The proximal long bones, humeri and femurs, are short. Fibulas are longer than tibias. Calvarium is large with small foramen magnum and short base. Vertebrae have short pedicles, with narrowed interpedicular spaces between lumbar vertebrae. Pelvis has small, round iliac wings and flat acetabular roofs.

Inheritance

The inheritance pattern is autosomal dominant. Approximately 90% are new mutations with advanced paternal age.

Etiology

The cause is a mutation of the *FGFR3* gene, encoded on chromosome 4p16.3. The same gene is mutated, at different sites, in hypochondroplasia and thanatophoric dysplasia.

Differential Diagnosis

1. Thanatophoric dysplasia
2. Hypochondroplasia (this is usually not apparent at birth; the face is normal; final height is greater)

CONGENITAL (NEONATAL, INFANTILE) MARFAN SYNDROME

Congenital Marfan syndrome (cMFS) is the most severe form of Marfan syndrome and is caused by mutations in the same gene associated with classic Marfan syndrome (Dietz et al, 1991). The affected neonate has a long, thin body with an aged appearance because of lack of subcutaneous tissue and wrinkled, sagging skin (cutis laxa) (Morse et al, 1990) (Fig. 27–6A). The characteristic facies has dolichocephaly, deep-set eyes with large or small corneas (and occasionally cataracts), high nose bridge, high palate, small pointed chin with a horizontal skin crease, and large simple or crumpled ears (Fig. 27–6B and C). The fingers

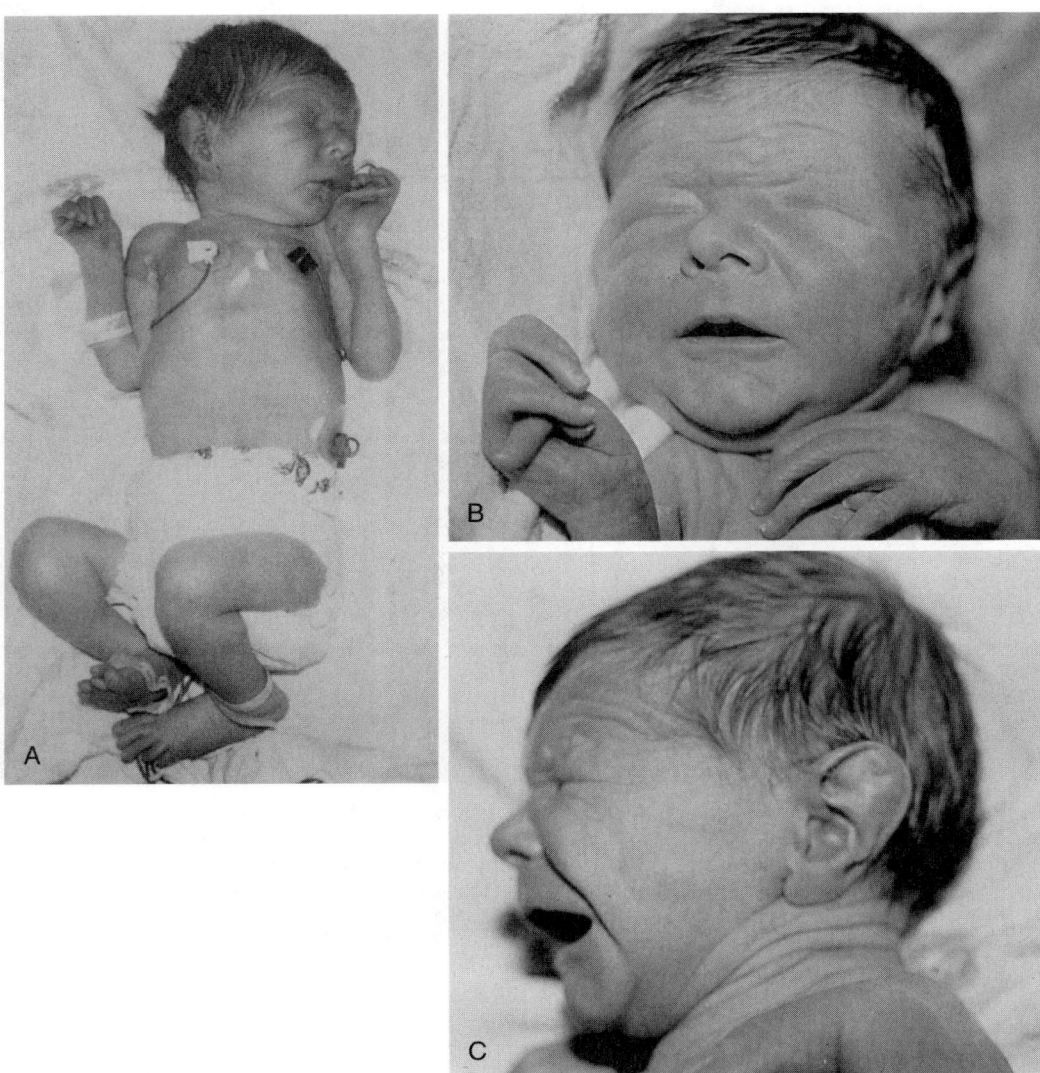

FIGURE 27–6. Congenital Marfan syndrome. *A,* Neonate with long thin trunk and limbs (particularly the feet), lack of adipose tissue, and multiple skin creases giving an aged appearance. Ears are large and simple, chin is small with horizontal crease. Flexion contractures at joints. *B,* Neonate's face showing laxity of skin, typical horizontal chin crease, pointed chin; the fingers are long with adduction contractures of thumbs, which extend past edge of palm, and floppy wrists. *C,* Lateral view of neonate's head showing simple "large" ears and redundant skin on neck.

and toes are long and thin (arachnodactyly). Some joints are hyperextensible and others have flexion contractures, causing equinovarus or equinovalgus, dislocated hips, or adducted thumbs. The infant tends to be hypotonic, with low muscle mass. Occasional features include diaphragmatic or inguinal hernias and retinal detachment. Lenses are usually not subluxated at birth. The most important cause of morbidity and mortality is severe cardiovascular disease, which affects almost every neonate with cMFS: mitral and tricuspid valve prolapse and insufficiency and aortic root dilation. The ascending aorta may be dilated and tortuous. Congestive cardiac failure develops; most infants die in the 1st year. Survivors have continuing hypotonia, contractures, and an inability to walk and require repeated surgery.

Inheritance. Marfan syndrome is an autosomal dominant disorder. Most neonates with cMFS are sporadic occurrences in a family (Dietz et al, 1991; Godfrey et al, 1995; Morse et al, 1990). However, there is one well-documented neonate with cMFS whose father had classic Marfan syndrome except for average height (Lopes et al, 1995). Routine ultrasonography at 34 weeks' gestation showed oligohydramnios and cardiomegaly. Fetal echocardiography showed the typical severe features and pleural effusion.

Etiology. cMFS is caused by abnormalities of a connective tissue, fibrillin, which is encoded by the gene fibrillin 1 (*FBN1*) on the long arm of chromosome 15 (15q21.1) (Dietz et al, 1991; Godfrey et al, 1995). Fibrillin, together with other proteins (microfibril-associated glycoproteins), is a component of microfibrils, which form linear bundles in the matrices of many tissues, such as aorta, periosteum, perichondrium, cartilage, tendons, muscle, pleura, and meninges. Microfibrils have several functions: (1) scaffolding, onto which elastin is deposited, for example, in the tunica media of the aorta; (2) scaffolding for nonelastic tissues, for example, the ciliary zonule of the eye, periodontal ligament, and mesangium of renal glomeruli; and (3) connections between elastin and other matrix components, for example, in the skin between elastin bundles and the dermoid-epidermoid junction.

Tests. Blood and skin should be obtained for gene mutation studies in lymphocytes and skin fibroblasts, although it has not been possible to detect the mutation in each case.

Prenatal Diagnosis

If the gene mutation is known, prenatal diagnosis by chorionic villous biopsy and amniocentesis is feasible. Prenatal detection by ultrasonography is possible in the second half of pregnancy. It is not known whether the cardiovascular and joint abnormalities are detectable before 20 weeks' gestation.

Differential Diagnosis

1. Beals congenital contractural arachnodactyly (CCA) syndrome is exhibited by a similar thin, wasted appearance with minimal muscle and fat mass and contractures of large and small joints (Fig. 27–7A). Cardiovascular involvement is usually limited to mitral valve prolapse, contractures improve to some degree with time, and life span is normal. CCA is an autosomal dominant condition caused by mutations in fibrillin 2 (*FBN2*) gene on chromosome 5 (5q23-31).

2. In cutis laxa syndrome, the autosomal recessive form is severe and can manifest at birth with loose, sagging skin, pulmonary emphysema, and gastrointestinal and urinary tract diverticula (Fig. 27–7B). There is no cardiovascular abnormality as occurs in Marfan syndrome.

WILLIAMS SYNDROME

Williams syndrome is difficult to diagnose in the newborn period, but the astute clinicians note an irritable infant with a coarse "swollen" face with periorbital fullness and thick lips who may have a cardiac murmur (Morris et al, 1988) (Fig. 27–8A and B). Supravalvar aortic stenosis and peripheral pulmonic stenosis may manifest in the newborn period, with occasional atrial or ventricular septal defects and, rarely, coarctation of the aorta. The presence of such an unusual vascular lesion, supravalvar aortic stenosis, should bring to mind the possibility of either isolated autosomal dominant supravalvar aortic stenosis or Williams syndrome. Supravalvar aortic stenosis affects more than 50% of children with Williams syndrome. Gestation is usually approximately 42 weeks, with birth weight and length in the lower half of or below the normal growth curves. The facies in infancy may be coarse or fine, with periorbital fullness, medial flare to the eyebrows, frequent blue irises with a stellate pattern, epicanthic folds, flat nose bridge with full nasal tip and anteverted nares, long or undefined philtrum, chubby "low-set" cheeks, small chin, and large ears (Fig. 27–8C and D). The lips may be thick at birth or thicken later; the "Cupid's bow" is diminished or absent. The head may be dolichocephalic (increased anteroposterior diameter) and the hair curly. Clinodactyly (incurving) of the fifth fingers is common. The skin is very soft, with fine creases on the palms, and ages prematurely. There is

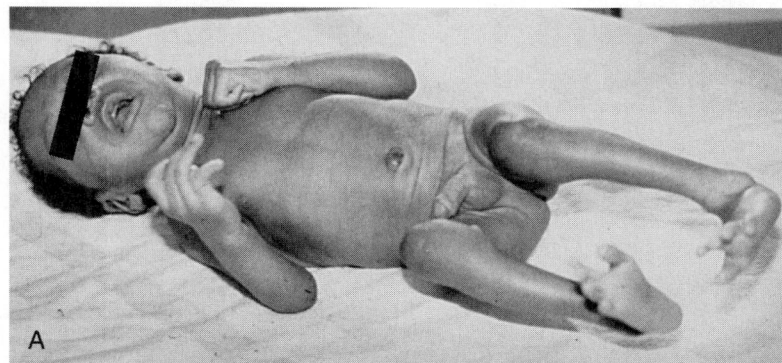

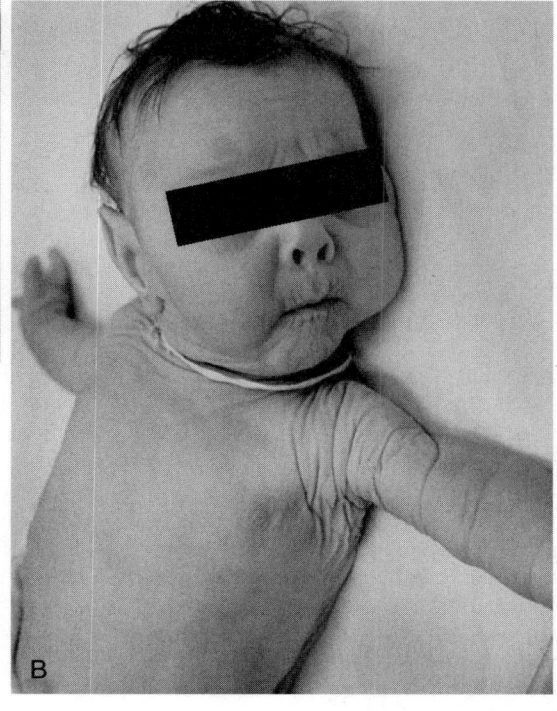

FIGURE 27–7. *A,* Congenital contractural arachnodactyly (Beals syndrome). Infant with long, thin trunk and limbs; contractures of joints, crumpled ears. *B,* Cutis laxa. (Courtesy Montreal Children's Hospital, Montreal, Quebec, Canada.)

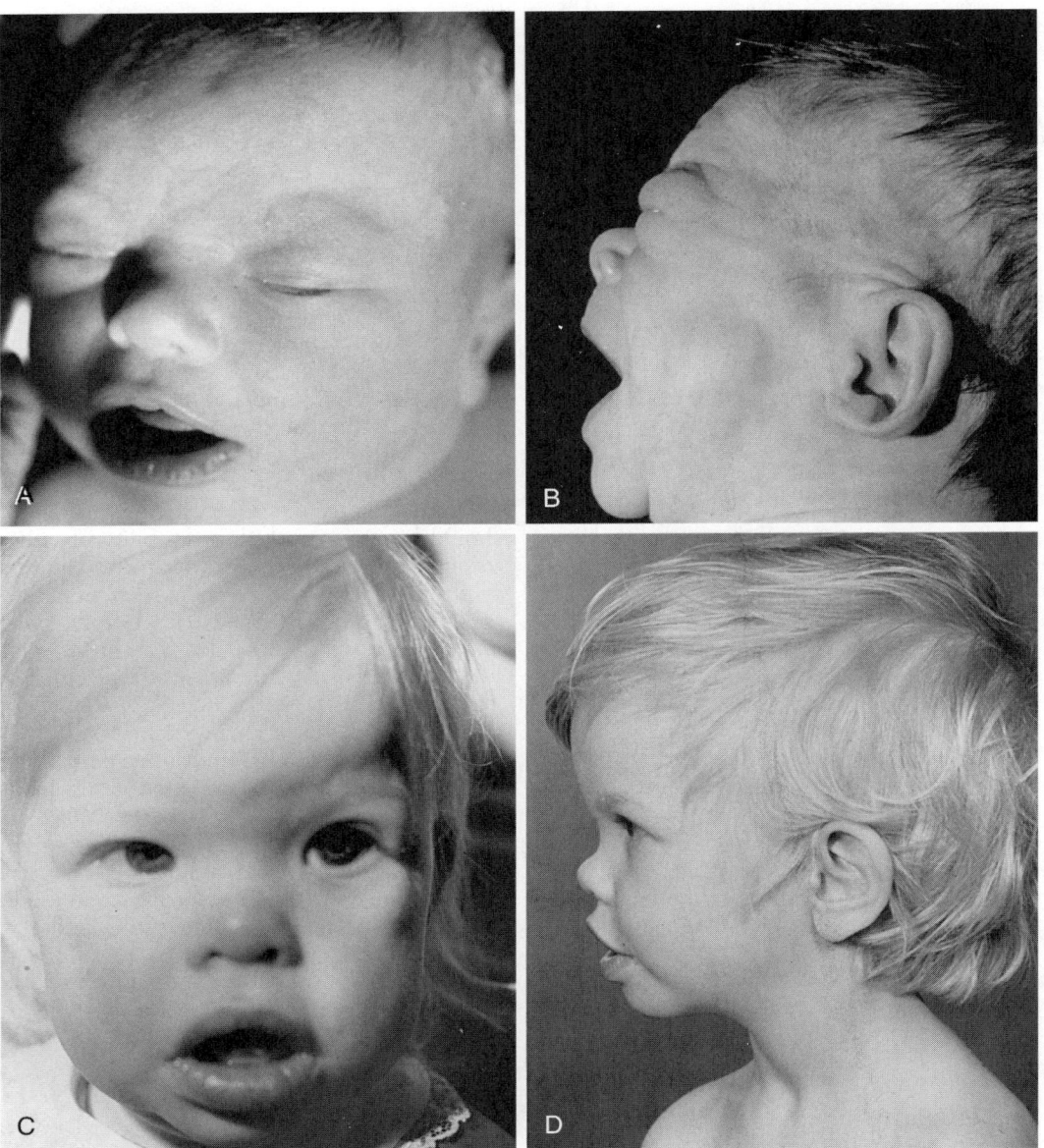

FIGURE 27–8. Williams syndrome. *A,* Neonate showing coarse face, periorbital fullness, wide mouth, and thick lips with decreased Cupid's bow. *B,* Neonate profile showing periorbital fullness, flat nasal bridge with full tip, and prominent cheeks. *C,* Infant showing periorbital fullness, flat nasal bridge, thick lips with decreased Cupid's bow, pouty lower lip, and "low-set" full cheeks. *D,* Infant profile showing dolichocephaly (increased anteroposterior diameter of head), higher nasal bridge than in neonate, full nasal tip, pouty lower lip, long neck, sloping shoulders, and part of pectus excavatum.

occasional inability to pronate and supinate the forearm. The limbs are short compared with the trunk but this characteristic may not be obvious in the newborn period. Mild hypotonia is common. Frequent vomiting starts soon after birth, and it is not unusual for the infant to scream most of the day and refuse feedings. This may be due to gastroesophageal reflux, causing esophagitis, or hypercalcemia. The irritability can persist for most of the first year. Moderate global developmental delay with a specific pattern of strengths and weaknesses is usual; rare individuals have normal intelligence quotient or severe retardation. Strengths include good expressive language, recognition

of faces, friendliness (which may be inappropriate), and sometimes short-term memory. These qualities can mask for the casual acquaintance the difficulties with visuomotor abilities such as writing and drawing figures, mathematical reasoning, understanding money, and subtle social interactions. The voice is deep and hoarse. Hyperactivity is common and can be controlled with methylphenidate and similar drugs, improving learning and performance (Power et al, 1997). Narrowing (stenosis or coarctation) of other vessels, including the aortic, renal, and cerebral arteries, may occur (Kaplan et al, 1995). Hypertension may develop because of arterial stenosis or renal disease. Life span may be shortened by cardiac or renal failure. Cardiac failure is less common than a decade ago because of earlier diagnosis and cardiac intervention with medications or surgery. Diverticulosis of bowel (associated with chronic constipation) and bladder (associated with chronic dyssynergia of bladder emptying) may develop in adolescence or adulthood (Schulman et al, 1996). Contractures can impair daily function (Kaplan et al, 1989). Rarely, renal failure develops (Pober et al, 1993).

Etiology. Williams syndrome is a contiguous gene deletion syndrome resulting from a deletion at 7q11.23 on one chromosome 7 only (Ewart et al, 1993). At least nine genes have been deleted, including elastin (Ewart et al, 1993) and replication factor C subunit 2 (Peoples et al, 1996), and LIM kinase 1 (Frangiskakis et al, 1996). The lack of elastin accounts for many features such as arterial narrowing, diverticula, skin and joint problems, some facial characteristics, and deep voice. The replication factor may

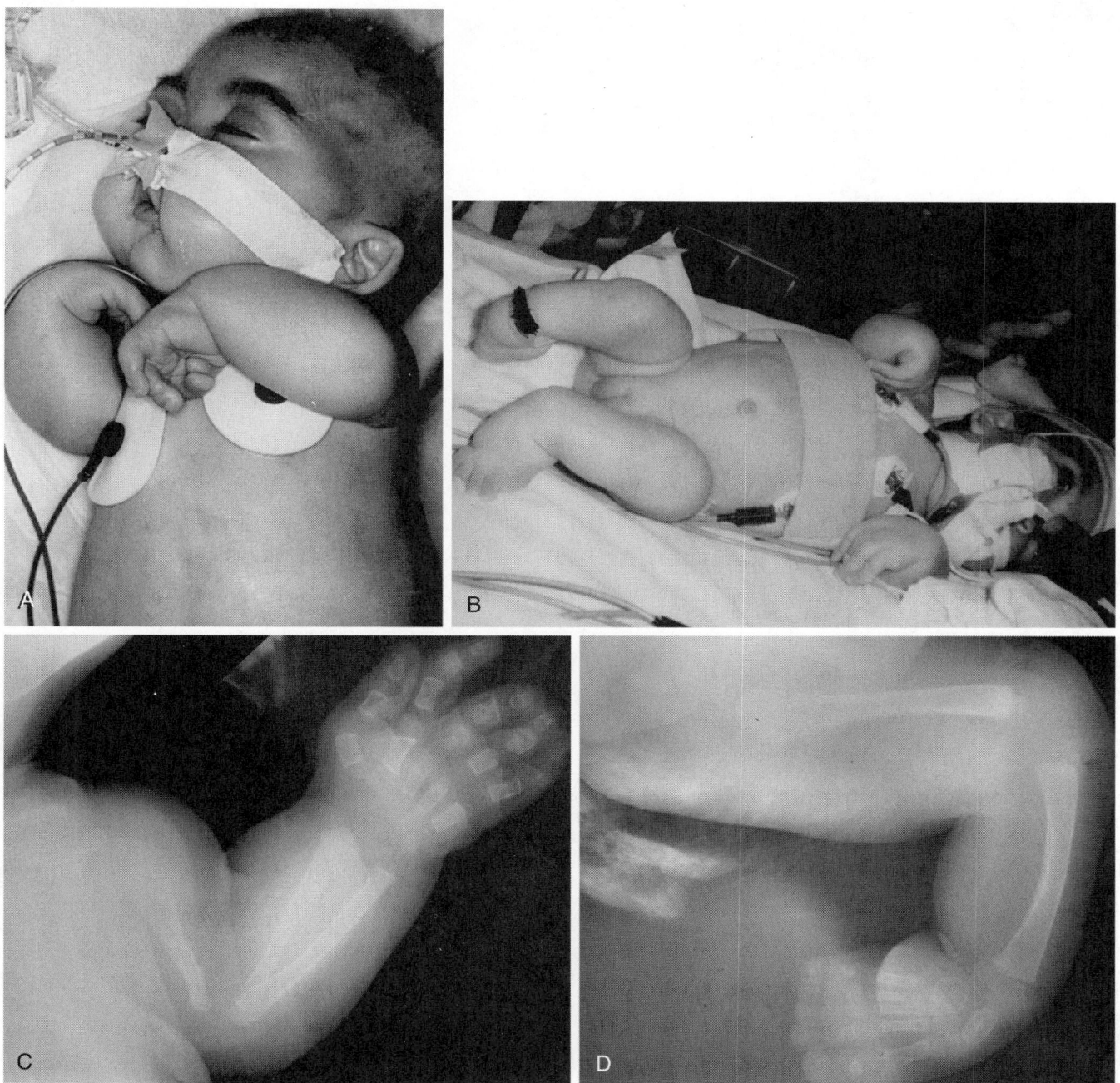

FIGURE 27–9. Atelosteogenesis (see Table 27–2). *A* and *B*, Infant with proximal limb shortening and equinovalgus deformities of hands and feet. *C*, Radiograph of upper limb showing distal tapering of humerus; metacarpals and phalanges are short and broad or irregular. *D*, Radiograph of lower limb showing "clubbing" of foot; fibula is not visualized and may be hypoplastic or absent. (Courtesy Charles I. Scott, MD, AI DuPont Institute, Wilmington, DE.)

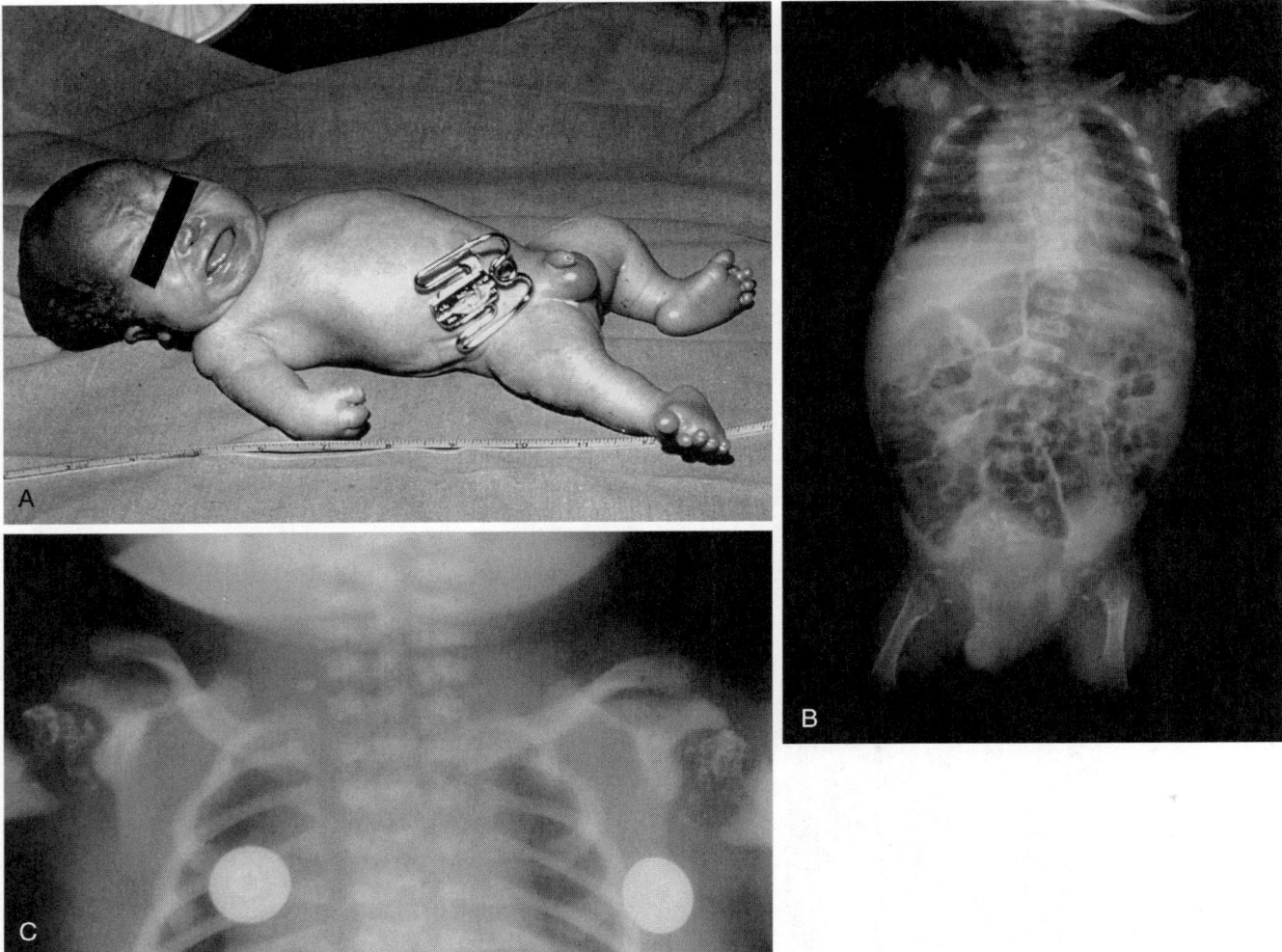

FIGURE 27–10. Chondrodysplasia punctata, rhizomelic type (see Table 27–2). *A,* Neonate with flat face, very flat nasal bridge, marked shortening of limbs (especially proximally), and joint contractures. *B,* Radiograph shows shortening of humeri and femora; stippled epiphyses. *C,* Radiograph shows stippling of shoulder joints. (Courtesy Charles I. Scott, MD, Al DuPont Institute, Wilmington, DE.)

be important for cell growth. The LIM kinase appears to be linked to the visuomotor dysfunction. The frequency of deletion in chromosomes of maternal and paternal origin is the same, but there may be more severe growth retardation when the parent-of-origin deletion is maternal (Perez Jurado et al, 1996). The deletion can be demonstrated with fluorescent-in-situ hybridization (FISH) using a probe that includes the elastin gene and extends beyond the 3′ and 5′ borders.

Inheritance. Most cases are sporadic occurrences in a family, but we have become aware of one sibling pair with Williams syndrome with neither parent affected (CI Scott Jr, personal communication, 1997). This could be due to germline mosaicism in one parent; the risk for recurrence in a sibling of a sporadic case is approximately 5%, based on experience elsewhere (Byers et al, 1988). Each child of a person with Williams syndrome has a 50% chance of inheriting the chromosome 7 with the deletion and manifesting the disorder (Morris et al, 1993).

Prenatal Diagnosis. Prenatal diagnosis is established with FISH of chorionic villus cells and amniocytes

Differential Diagnosis (newborn)

1. Lysosomal storage disease, particularly G_{M1} gangliosidosis or mucolipidosis Type II (I cell disease), may have coarse facial features and joint contractures in the newborn period. There may be cardiomyopathy but not arterial narrowing and other features.
2. Noonan syndrome may have coarse features and valvar pulmonic stenosis but not usually peripheral pulmonic stenosis.
3. Autosomal dominant supravalvar aortic stenosis is not associated with all the other features of Williams syndrome. Often there are other affected family members.

EHLERS-DANLOS SYNDROMES

There are at least eight types of Ehlers-Danlos syndrome characterized by varying degrees and extent of joint and

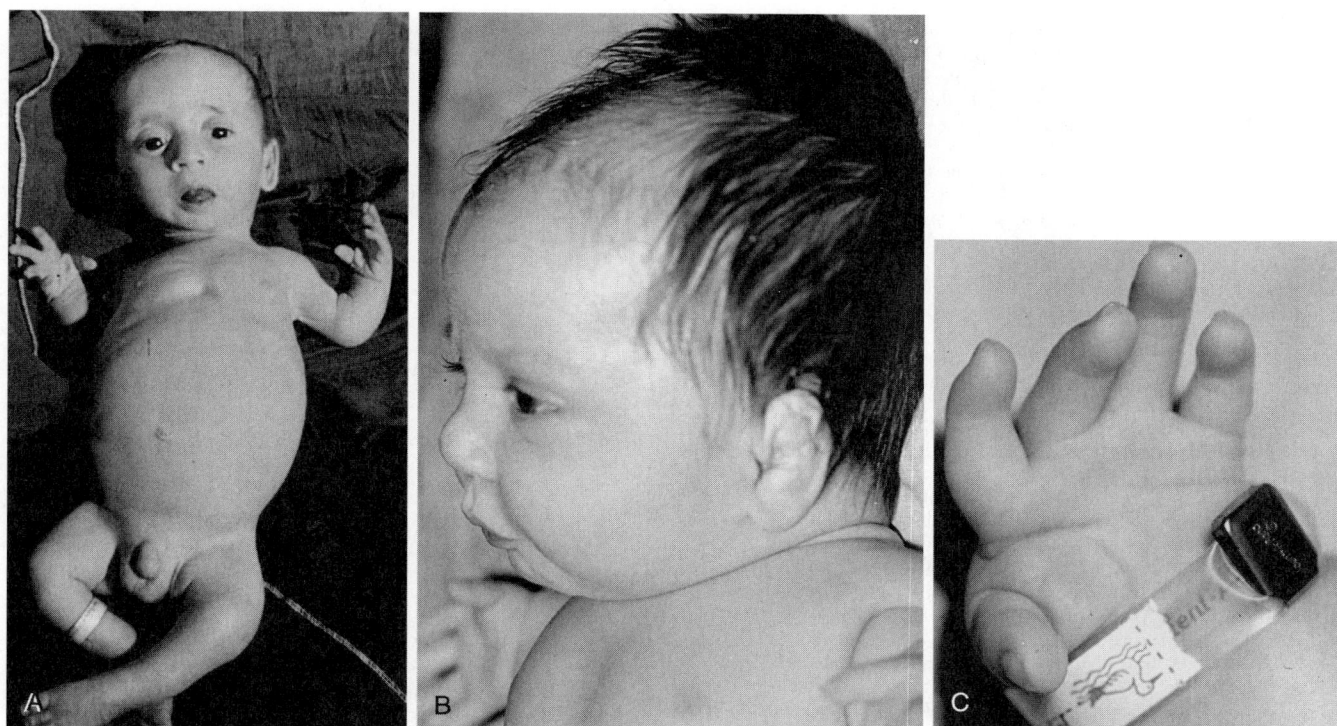

FIGURE 27–11. Diastrophic dysplasia (see Table 27–2). *A,* Infant with prominent eyes, small chin, slightly narrow chest, proximally placed angulated thumbs, and short limbs. *B,* Neonate profile showing small chin, swollen ears, and short neck. Note proximally placed angulated thumb. *C,* View of neonate's hand showing proximally placed angulated thumb, mild syndactyly.

skin hypermobility, excessive bruising, thin wide scars, and fragility of tissues (Steinmann et al, 1993). Types I and VII are the most likely to manifest in the newborn period. Type I is characterized by premature delivery of a fetus with Ehlers-Danlos syndrome as a result of rupture of the amniotic membranes. The infant may be floppy and in breech position. There may be joint laxity and instability. In Type VII, the major involvement is in the ligaments and joint capsules. Large and small joints are hypermobile and dislocatable; severe congenital dislocation of hips occurs. Dislocations are recurrent.

In Type IV Ehlers-Danlos syndrome, the greatest danger is to the pregnant affected woman, for whom there is a high risk of uterine rupture. Although there is a 50% risk of the fetus being affected, the problems of blood loss and prematurity are more important in the newborn period than the disorder itself.

Etiology. Recently, collagen Type V has been implicated in causing (some) cases of Types I and II Ehlers-Danlos syndrome (Burrows et al, 1996; De Paepe et al, 1997). Type IV is caused by mutations in collagen Type III. Type VII is caused by a deleted exon 6 in the alpha-1 (COL1A1) or alpha-2 chain (COL1A2) of Type I collagen.

Inheritance. The types discussed here are inherited as autosomal dominant traits. Each child of an affected person has a 50% chance of inheriting and manifesting the disorder.

Prenatal Diagnosis. If the molecular defect has been characterized, chorionic villus sampling or amniocentesis is feasible. This has been difficult for Type I until recently because the connective tissue had not been known. However, amniocentesis in an fetus affected with Type I may cause amniotic tears and fluid leaking.

OTHER SKELETAL DYSPLASIA

For additional skeletal dysplasias, see Table 27–2. The dysplasias discussed in the table as well as illustrated include atelosteogenesis (Fig. 27–9), chondrodysplasia (Fig. 27–10), and diastrophic dysplasia (Fig. 27–11).

REFERENCES

Beighton P, Giedion A, Gorlin R, et al: International classification of osteochondrodysplasias. Am J Med Genet 44:223, 1992.

Bellus GA, McIntosh I, Smith EA, et al: A recurrent mutation in the tyrosine kinase domain of fibroblast growth factor receptor 3 causes hypochondroplasia. Nat Genet 10:357, 1995.

Bellus GA, Szabo JK, McIntosh I, et al: Hypochondroplasia: A second recurrent mutation of fibroblast growth factor receptor 3 (FGFR3) at nucleotide 1620. Am J Hum Genet 57:47, 1995.

Borochowitz Z, Lachman R, Adomian GE, et al: Achondrogenesis type I: Delineation of further heterogeneity and identification of two distinct subgroups. J Pediatr 112:23, 1988.

Burrows NP, Nicholls AC, Yates JRC, et al: The gene encoding collagen alpha 1(V) (COL5A1) is linked to mixed Ehlers-Danlos syndrome type I/II. J Invest Dermatol 106:1273, 1996.

Byers PH: Osteogenesis imperfecta. *In* Royce PM, Steinmann B (Eds):

Connective Tissue and Its Heritable Disorders: Medical and Genetic Aspects. New York, Wiley-Liss, 1993, pp 317–350.

Byers PH, Tsipouras P, Bonadio JF, et al: Perinatal lethal osteogenesis imperfecta (OI Type II): A biochemically heterogeneous disorder usually due to new mutations in the genes for type I collagen. Am J Hum Genet 42:37, 1988.

Byers PH, Wallis GA, Willing MC: Osteogenesis imperfecta: Translation of mutation to phenotype. J Med Genet 28:433, 1991.

De Paepe A, Nuytinck L, Hausser I, et al: Mutations in the COL5A1 gene are causal in the Ehlers-Danlos syndromes I and II. Am J Hum Genet 60:547, 1997.

Dietz HC, Cutting GR, Pyeritz RE, et al: Marfan syndrome caused by a recurrent de novo missense mutation in the fibrillin gene. Nature 352:337, 1991.

Ewart AE, Morris CA, Atkinson D, et al: Hemizygosity at the elastin locus in a developmental disorder: Williams syndrome. Nat Genet 5:11, 1993.

Francomano CA, Ortiz de Luna RI, Hefferon TW, et al: Localization of the achondroplasia gene to the distal 2.5 Mb of human chromosome 4p. Hum Mol Genet 3:787, 1994.

Frangiskakis JM, Ewart AK, Morris CA, et al: LIM-kinase 1 hemizygosity implicated in impaired visuospatial constructive cognition. Cell 86:1, 1996.

Godfrey M, Raghunath M, Cisler J, et al: Abnormal morphology of fibrillin microfibrils in fibroblast cultures from patients with neonatal Marfan syndrome. Am J Pathol 146:1414, 1995.

Gordienko IY, Grechanina EY, Sopko NI, et al: Prenatal diagnosis of osteochondrodysplasias in high risk pregnancy. Am J Med Genet 63:90, 1996.

Hastbacka J, de la Chapelle A, Mahtani MM, et al: The diastrophic dysplasia gene encodes a novel sulfate transporter: Positional cloning by fine-structure linkage dysequilibrium mapping. Cell 78:1078, 1994.

Hastbacka J, Superti-Furga A, Wilcox W, et al: Atelosteogenesis type II is caused by mutations of the diastrophic dysplasia sulfate transporter gene (DTDST): Evidence for a phenotypic series involving three chondrodysplasias. Am J Hum Genet 58:255, 1996.

Hecht JT, Thompson NM, Weir T, et al: Cognitive and motor skills in achondroplastic infants: Neurologic and respiratory correlates. Am J Hum Genet 41:208, 1991.

Horton WA, Rotter JI, Rimoin DL, et al: Standard curves for achondroplasia. J Pediatr 93:435, 1978.

Houston CS, Opitz JM, Spranger JW, et al: The campomelic syndrome: Review, report of 17 cases and follow-up of the currently 17-year old boy first reported by Maroteaux et al in 1971. Am J Med Genet 15:3, 1983.

Ilizarov GA: The possibilities offered by our method for lengthening various segments in upper and lower limbs. In Nicoletti B, Kopits SE, Ascani E, McKusick VA (Eds): Human achondroplasia, a multidisciplinary approach. New York, Plenum Press, 1988, pp 323–324.

Kaitila I, Marttinnen E, Merikanto J, et al: Clinical expression and course of diastrophic dysplasia. Am J Med Genet 34:141, 1989.

Kaplan P, Kirschner M, Watters G, et al: Contractures in patients with Williams syndrome. Pediatrics 84:895, 1989.

Kaplan P, Levinson M, Kaplan BS: Cerebral artery stenoses in Williams syndrome cause strokes in childhood. J Pediatr 126:943, 1995.

Le Merrer M, Rousseau F, Legeai-Mallet L, et al: A gene for achondroplasia-hypochondroplasia maps to chromosome 4p. Nat Genet 6:314, 1994.

Lopes LM, Cha SC, De Moraes EA, Zugaib M: Echocardiographic diagnosis of fetal Marfan syndrome at 34 weeks gestation. Prenat Diagn 15:183, 1995.

Morris C, Thomas IT, Greenberg F: Williams syndrome: Autosomal dominant inheritance. Am J Med Genet 47:478, 1993.

Morris CA, Demsey SA, Leonard CO, et al: Natural history of Williams syndrome: Physical characteristics. J Pediatr 113:318, 1988.

Morse RP, Rockenmacher S, Pyeritz RE, et al: Diagnosis and management of infantile Marfan syndrome. Pediatrics 86:888, 1990.

Pauli RM, Scott CI, Wassman ER Jr, et al: Apnea and sudden unexpected death in infants with achondroplasia. J Pediatr 104:342, 1984.

Peoples R, Perez Jurado LA, Wang Y-K, et al: The gene for replication factor C subunit 2 (RFC2) is within the 7q11.23 Williams syndrome deletion. Am J Hum Genet 58:1370, 1996.

Perez Juardo LA, Peoples R, Kaplan P, et al: Molecular definition of the chromosome 7 deletion in Williams syndrome and parent-of-origin effects on growth. Am J Hum Genet 59:781, 1996.

Pober BR, Lacro RU, Rice C, et al: Renal findings in 40 individuals with Williams syndrome. Am J Med Genet 46:271, 1993.

Power TJ, Blum NJ, Jones S, et al: Brief report: Response to methylphenidate in two children with Williams syndrome. J Autism Dev Disord 27:79, 1997.

Rasmussen SA, Bieber FR, Benacerraf BR, et al: Epidemiology of osteochondrodysplasias: Changing trends due to advances in prenatal diagnosis. Am J Med Genet 61:49, 1996.

Rimoin DL, Lachman RS: Chondrodysplasias. In Rimoin DL, Pyeritz R (Eds): Emery & Rimoin's Principles and Practice of Medical Genetics, 3rd ed. 1997, New York, Churchill Livingstone, p 2779.

Rousseau F, Saugier P, Le Merrer M, et al: Stop codon FGFR3 mutations in thanatophoric dysplasia type I. Nat Genet 10:11, 1995.

Schulman SL, Zderic S, Kaplan P: Increased prevalence of urinary symptoms and voiding dysfunction in Williams syndrome. J Pediatr 129:466, 1996.

Shiang R, Thompson LM, Zhu Y-Z, et al: Mutations in the transmembrane domain of FGFR3 cause the most common genetic form of dwarfism, achondroplasia. Cell 78:335, 1994.

Spranger J, Maroteaux P: The lethal osteochondrodysplasias. Adv Hum Genet 19:1, 1990.

Spranger J, Winterpacht A, Zabel R: The type II collagenopathies: A spectrum of chondrodysplasias. Eur J Pediatr 153:56, 1994.

Steinmann B, Royce PM, Superti-Furga A: The Ehlers Danlos syndrome. In Royce PM, Steinmann B (Eds): Connective Tissue and Its Heritable Disorders: Medical and Genetic Aspects. New York, Wiley-Liss, 1993, pp 351–407.

Superti-Furga A, Hastbacka A, Wilcox W, et al: Achondrogenesis type IB is caused by mutations in the diastrophic dysplasia sulfate transporter gene. Nat Genet 12:100, 1996.

Tavormina P, Shiang R, Thompson L, et al: Thanatophoric dysplasia (types I and II) caused by distinct mutations in the fibroblast growth factor receptor 3. Nat Genet 9:321, 1995.

Tommerup N: Assignment of an autosomal sex reversal locus (SRA1) and campomelic dysplasia (CMPD1) to 17q24.3-q25.1. Nat Genet 4:170, 1993.

Whyte MP: Hypophosphatasia. In Scriver CR, Beaudet AL, Sly WS, Valle D (Eds): The Metabolic and Molecular Bases of Inherited Disease, 7th ed, vol III. New York, McGraw-Hill, 1995, pp 4095–4111.

Wilkin DJ, Rogaert R, Lachman RS, et al: A single amino acid substitution (G103D) in the type II collagen triple helix produces Kniest dysplasia. Hum Mol Genet 3:1999, 1994.

Winterpacht A, Hilbert M, Schwarze U, et al: Kniest and Stickler dysplasia phenotypes caused by collagen type II gene (COL2A1) defect. Nat Genet 3:323, 1993.

CHAPTER 28

Newborn Screening

Sook Z. Kim and Harvey L. Levy

Newborn screening is primarily directed at disorders in which the clinical complications develop postnatally rather than prenatally. In metabolic disorders, these complications (phenotype) result from biochemical abnormalities that appear after birth when the infant is no longer protected by fetal-maternal exchange. The infant with phenylketonuria (PKU), for instance, has a normal blood phenylalanine level at birth but within a few hours develops hyperphenylalaninemia. If this and other biochemical abnormalities of PKU are not corrected or at least controlled by dietary treatment, the infant begins to show signs of developmental delay and, subsequently, becomes mentally retarded. If dietary therapy begins during the first weeks of life and the blood phenylalanine level is controlled, mental retardation is prevented (Levy and Cornien, 1994).

PKU was the first metabolic disorder known to benefit from early dietary therapy. This fact was established by the mid-1950s. By the late 1950s, it was evident that the diet could prevent mental retardation. Detecting PKU in all affected infants before irreversible brain damage occurred then became the challenge. This meant neonatal screening for a biochemical marker of the disease.

In 1962, Guthrie developed a simple bacterial assay for phenylalanine that required only a small amount of whole blood soaked into filter paper (Guthrie and Susi, 1963). Thus, infants in newborn nurseries could be routinely tested for PKU from blood specimens obtained by lancing the heel and blotting the drops of blood onto a filter paper card. This filter paper blood specimen could be mailed to a central laboratory for PKU testing. An increased phenylalanine concentration in the specimen suggested PKU in the infant.

By the mid-1960s, many states had established routine newborn screening programs for PKU using the Guthrie test. Infants with PKU were identified in larger numbers than anticipated and were showing normal development while on treatment (O'Flynn, 1992). The success of PKU screening led to the addition of tests for other metabolic disorders, including galactosemia, maple syrup urine disease (MSUD), and homocystinuria—all of which are inborn errors of metabolism similar in principle to PKU (Irons, 1993). These additional tests could be applied to the same blood specimen obtained for PKU screening. Later a test for an endocrine disorder, congenital hypothyroidism, was added. More recently, tests for other disorders, such as the hemoglobinopathies, congenital adrenal hyperplasia (CAH), biotinidase deficiency, cystic fibrosis, glucose-6-phosphate dehydrogenase deficiency, the organic acid and fatty acid oxidation disorders, and congenital toxoplasmosis, have been added. Furthermore, urine soaked into filter paper has been used to screen for neuroblastoma. Thus, newborn screening is not only expanding within the field of metabolic disorders but also is beginning to include screening for nonmetabolic genetic disorders, infectious diseases, and cancer. Table 28–1 lists the frequencies of the disorders for which newborn screening is currently performed or considered.

SCREENING PROGRAMS
Specimen

The blood specimen is obtained from the heel of the infant (Fig. 28–1). This simple specimen, conceived and introduced by Guthrie, has had an enormous impact on newborn screening. The specimen is not only easily obtained but also is easily and inexpensively sent by mail to a central testing facility. There are no complications in obtaining this specimen from the newborn, contrary to early fears that this would lead to infection or result in excessive bleeding.

Specimen Collection Procedure

The blood specimen should be obtained from the lateral or the medial side of the heel (Fig. 28–2), avoiding the central part of the heel. Blood should be applied to only one side of the filter paper card but should fully saturate each circle on the card. Contamination of the filter paper specimen with iodine, alcohol, petroleum jelly, stool, urine, milk, or a substance such as oil from the fingers can adversely affect the results of the screening tests. Also, exposure to heat and humidity can inactivate enzymes and produce false results. The specimen should be dried in air at room temperature for at least 3 hours before being placed in an envelope.

Timing of the Collection

The specimen should be obtained from every newborn infant before nursery discharge or by the 4th day of life (whichever is first). With the practice of early nursery discharge, often during the 1st or 2nd day of life, there is concern that some infants with metabolic disorders will not have ingested sufficient protein for an amino acid elevation to occur and, therefore, may not be identified. Lack of amino acid elevation is unlikely for severe forms of PKU but could occur in mild PKU and in disorders such as homocystinuria. In addition, an early specimen could result in missing an infant with congenital hypothyroidism in programs that use a low thyroxine (T_4) level as the indicator of this disorder. Consequently, to be certain that an infant with a disorder is not missed, a repeat blood specimen should be obtained no later than 2 weeks of age from infants whose initial specimen was obtained within the first 24 hours of life.

Special circumstances require specific attention to newborn blood specimen collection. In a newborn who is to receive a blood transfusion, a screening specimen should

TABLE 28–1

Approximate Frequencies in the United States of Disorders Included in or Considered for Newborn Screening

Disorder	Frequency
Congenital hypothyroidism	1 : 4000
Phenylketonuria	1 : 12,000
Galactosemia	1 : 60,000
Maple syrup urine disease	1 : 200,000
Homocystinuria	1 : 200,000
Biotinidase deficiency	1 : 70,000
Congenital adrenal hyperplasia	1 : 19,000
Sickle cell disease	1 : 4000
Cystic fibrosis	1 : 4000
Duchenne muscular dystrophy	1 : 8000°
Congenital toxoplasmosis	1 : 10,000
Hyperlipidemia	1 : 500
Alpha₁-antitrypsin deficiency	1 : 8000
Neuroblastoma	1 : 4000

°For males, 1 : 4000.

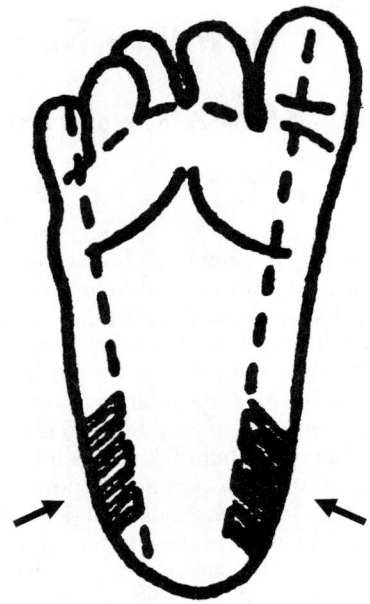

FIGURE 28–2. Hatched areas at medial and lateral sides of the heel indicate the proper sites for heel stick in the newborn.

be collected before transfusion and a repeat specimen 2 days after the transfusion. This latter specimen is for metabolite testing because the pretransfusion specimen might have been obtained within the first 24 hours of life. In addition, a third screening specimen should be obtained 2 months after the transfusion, when most of the donor red cells have been replaced. This practice ensures reliable testing for analytes present in red cells, should a pretransfusion specimen not have been obtained. Infants transferred to a neonatal intensive care unit should have a blood specimen collected before transfer, regardless of age, and a second specimen collected in the neonatal intensive care unit by 4 days of age. This dual collection avoids the possibility that a newborn specimen will not have been obtained in the turmoil that frequently accompanies hospital transfer.

Screening Laboratory

Newborn screening tests are usually performed in a centralized state, provincial, or regional laboratory. In the United States, for example, the blood specimen is usually

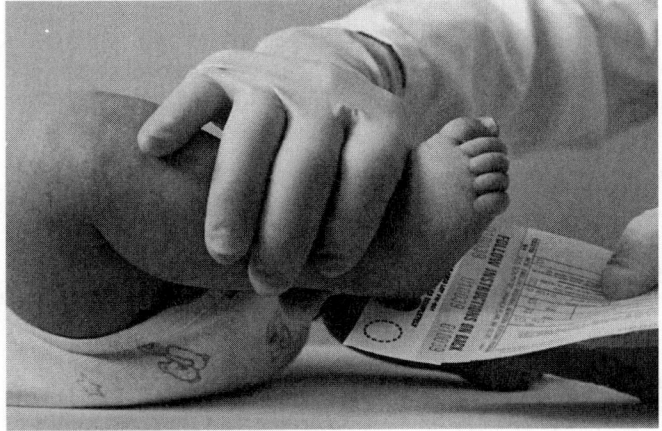

FIGURE 28–1. Collection of the filter paper blood specimen from the heel of a newborn for routine newborn screening.

sent to the state newborn screening program. It may be tested in the state laboratory in which the program is housed or sent to a neighboring state laboratory that serves as the regional testing facility. A few states contract with private laboratories or large medical center laboratories to conduct the testing. The screening laboratory performs the basic screening tests and notifies the attending physician or birth hospital (or collaborating state program) of abnormal results. Some screening laboratories also perform confirmatory testing.

Screening Tests

The testing procedure begins with the punching of small discs (each usually 3 mm in diameter) from the filter paper specimen. This process may be performed manually with a paper punch or semiautomatically with a quadratic punch indexer machine. In the bacterial assays for PKU and other inborn errors of metabolism (galactosemia, homocystinuria, and MSUD), the discs are placed on agar or silica gels that contain bacteria, growth media, and other necessary factors. The constituents of each bacterial plate are directed for response to a particular metabolite, and the amount of bacterial growth around the disc is proportional to the concentration of the metabolite in the blood. For instance, in the Guthrie test for PKU, the disc from the blood specimen of an affected newborn is surrounded by a large zone of bacterial growth indicating increased phenylalanine (Fig. 28–3). PKU and galactosemia can also be screened by chemical assays that measure phenylalanine and galactose. Radioimmunoassays or enzyme-linked immunosorbent assays (ELISA) are used to test for congenital hypothyroidism and CAH. The discs are placed in test tubes for these procedures. Hemoglobin electrophoresis of blood eluted from the filter paper disc is employed for sickle cell disease screening. An enzyme assay is often used to screen for

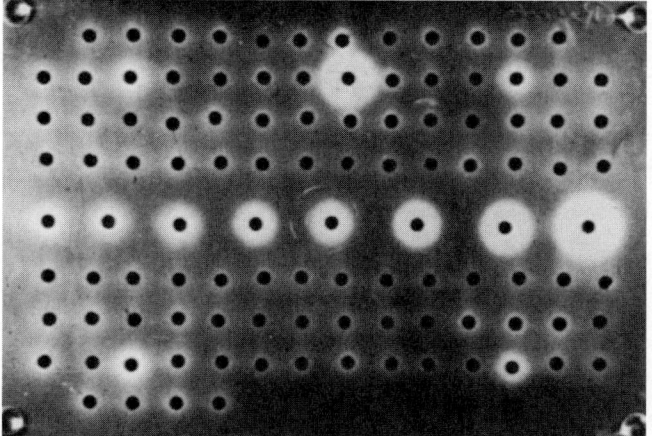

FIGURE 28–3. Guthrie bacterial assay for phenylalanine that identifies phenylketonuria in the newborn. Small discs from the filter paper blood specimen are placed on the agar gel of the assay plate. Note the large growth around the disc in the center of the second row from the top, which indicated phenylketonuria in this infant. The center row of discs are control specimens containing increasing amounts of phenylalanine from 2 mg/dL (a normal value) on the left to 20 mg/dL on the right. The remaining discs are from normal newborns and are surrounded by growth zones smaller than or no larger than that surrounding the 2-mg/dL control disc.

galactosemia and always used to screen for biotinidase deficiency. Enzyme immunoassays, including ELISA methods, are now readily available and are in more frequent use for the screening of congenital toxoplasmosis, neuroblastoma, and human immunodeficiency virus (HIV) seropositivity and even as a specific assay for sickle cell disease. An especially valuable test recently introduced into newborn screening is tandem mass spectrometry. This technology allows for the identification of most amino acid disorders and many disorders of organic acids and fatty acids using only one or two discs from the filter paper blood specimen.

Secondary Tests

An abnormal finding in a newborn screening test is not diagnostic of a disorder. Abnormalities in the newborn specimen can be transient or produced by artifacts. Accordingly, when an abnormality is identified, additional tests are often performed by the screening laboratory to substantiate the original finding. This includes retesting the original specimen for the analyte that was abnormal. In some laboratories, procedures such as high-performance liquid chromatography are used to confirm the original bacterial assay finding of an increased amino acid level.

In screening for congenital hypothyroidism, the original newborn blood specimen in which a low T_4 level was found is further tested by immunoassay for thyroid-stimulating hormone (TSH) to determine whether TSH is increased, indicating congenital hypothyroidism, or is normal, which suggests transient low T_4 or thyroxine-binding globulin deficiency. Confirmation of PKU, galactosemia, or other inborn errors of metabolism requires additional specimens. Consequently a repeat blood specimen (filter paper or

plasma) and, on occasion, a urine specimen are necessary for specific testing when the newborn blood specimen suggests an abnormality of this type.

DNA analysis may be used for the confirmation of several disorders identified by newborn screening. The combination of gene amplification by the polymerase chain reaction and either hybridization with specific oligonucleotide probes or analysis using restriction enzymes and band staining allows for the application of DNA analysis to the blood filter paper specimen. Currently, this type of procedure is used for identifying one or more of the mutations associated with cystic fibrosis as the second tier in cystic fibrosis screening to sort those infants with probable cystic fibrosis from the many other infants with increased immunoreactive trypsinogen but who do not have cystic fibrosis (Wilcken, 1993). Studies are currently being conducted in the use of similar DNA techniques for secondary screening of galactosemia and PKU (Fig. 28–4).

Physician Contact

The pediatrician or other physician of record should be contacted immediately when the newborn blood specimen illustrates such a striking abnormality that a metabolic disorder is strongly suspected. Table 28–2 indicates the possible disorder or other reason for abnormal screening result and initial action to be taken when the physician is contacted. For instance, a low T_4 level combined with an elevated TSH concentration indicates congenital hypothyroidism; a markedly elevated level of phenylalanine, galactose, methionine, or leucine indicates, respectively, the probability of PKU, galactosemia, homocystinuria, or MSUD. If the infant is well, confirmatory testing should be performed, and if a disorder is confirmed, the infant

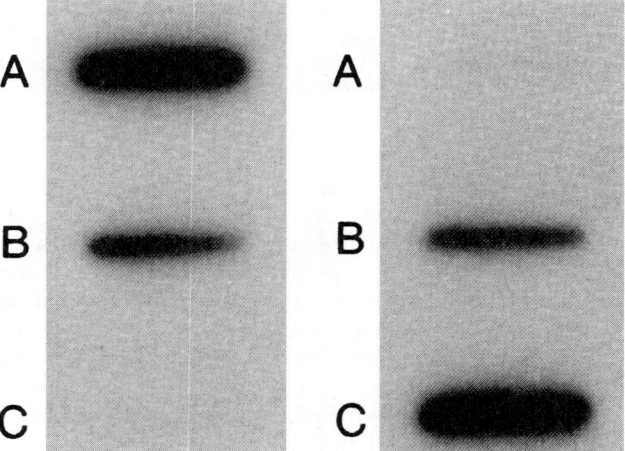

FIGURE 28–4. DNA analysis from dried blood specimen used in newborn screening. The technique illustrated here is slot-blot hybridization analysis of phenylalanine hydroxylase gene using allele-specific oligonucleotide probes. Infant *A* is normal. Infant *B* carries a normal allele and an allele for the R408W mutation and thus is a phenylketonuria carrier. Infant *C* has phenylketonuria and is homozygous for the R408W mutation.

TABLE 28–2

Abnormal Newborn Screening Results: Possible Implications and Initial Action to Be Taken

Newborn Screening Finding	Differential Diagnosis	Initial Action
↑ Phenylalanine	PKU, non-PKU hyperphenylalaninemia, pterin defect, galactosemia, transient hyperphenylalaninemia	Repeat blood specimen
↓ T₄, ↑ TSH	Congenital hypothyroidism, iodine exposure	Repeat blood specimen or thyroid function testing, begin thyroxine treatment
↓ T₄, normal TSH	Maternal hyperthyroidism, thyroxine-binding globulin deficiency, secondary hypothyroidism, congenital hypothyroidism with delayed TSH elevation	Repeat blood specimen
↑ Galactose (-1-P)	Galactosemia, liver disease, portosystemic shunt, transferase deficiency variant (Duarte), transient	Clinical evaluation, urine for reducing substance, repeat blood specimen. If reducing substance positive, begin lactose-free formula
↓ Galactose-1-phosphate uridyltransferase°	Galactosemia, transferase deficiency variant (Duarte), transient	Clinical evaluation, urine for reducing substance, repeat blood specimen. If reducing substance positive, begin lactose-free formula
↑ Methionine	Homocystinuria, isolated hypermethioninemia, liver dysfunction, tyrosinemia Type I, transient hypermethioninemia	Repeat blood and urine specimen
↑ Leucine	Maple syrup urine disease, transient elevation	Clinical evaluation including urine for ketones, acid-base status, amino acid studies, immediate neonatal intensive care unit care if urine ketones positive
↑ Tyrosine	Tyrosinemia Type I or Type II, transient tyrosinemia, liver disease	Repeat blood specimen
↑ 17 alpha-hydroxyprogesterone	Congenital adrenal hyperplasia, prematurity, transient (residual fetal adrenal cortex), stress in neonatal period, early specimen collection	Clinical evaluation including genital examination, serum electrolytes, repeat blood specimen
S-hemoglobin	Sickle cell disease, sickle cell trait	Hemoglobin electrophoresis
↑ Trypsinogen	Cystic fibrosis, transient, intestinal anomalies, perinatal stress, trisomies 13 and 18, renal failure	Repeat blood specimen, possible sweat test
↑ Creatinine phosphokinase	Duchenne muscular dystrophy, other type of muscular dystrophy, birth trauma, invasive procedure	Repeat blood test
↓ Biotinidase	Biotinidase deficiency	Serum biotinidase assay, biotin therapy
↓ G-6-PD	G-6-PD deficiency	Complete blood count, bilirubin determination
↓ Alpha₁-antitrypsin	Alpha₁-antitrypsin deficiency	Confirmatory test
Toxoplasma antibody (IgM)	Congenital toxoplasmosis	Infectious disease consultation
HIV antibody (IgG)	Maternally transmitted HIV, possible AIDS	Infectious disease consultation
↑ Urine vanillylmandellic acid, homovanillic acid	Neuroblastoma, other catecholamine-secreting tumors, transient elevation	Repeat urine test

°Often reported by screening laboratories as the result of the Beutler test.

PKU, phenylketonuria; T₄, thyroxine; TSH, thyroid-stimulating hormone; G-6-PD, glucose-6-phosphate dehydrogenase; HIV, human immunodeficiency virus; AIDS, acquired immunodeficiency syndrome.

should be evaluated at a center that specializes in metabolic disorders. If the infant is ill, he or she should be admitted to a special care nursery, preferably in a center that has a pediatric metabolic unit experienced in the diagnosis and treatment of inborn errors of metabolism and related disorders. Specimens for confirmatory testing should be collected, and therapy for the illness should be initiated without delay.

Less striking abnormalities found by newborn screening are followed up by a letter to the physician from the screening program requesting a repeat specimen. The physician should be notified of these results as soon as possible.

Most infants with a positive screening result, particularly when this result is only mildly or moderately abnormal, do not have a disorder. Transient or nonspecific abnormalities are quite frequent. Although all infants with an abnormal screening result must have repeat testing, the families should be informed that an initial positive result may have no medical implications. This can alleviate excessive anxiety and prevent unnecessary diagnostic procedures and treatment.

The physician should contact the screening laboratory whenever the results of repeat testing have not been received or when an infant has symptoms that suggest a metabolic disorder or any other disorder for which screening may be conducted. The screening laboratory can check the results in the newborn specimen. If the newborn specimens are saved, the laboratory may wish to repeat the tests in that specimen.

DISORDERS MOST FREQUENTLY SCREENED
Phenylketonuria

This metabolic disorder should always be identified by newborn screening. Most newborns with an elevated blood phenylalanine level have PKU, a variant such as non-PKU hyperphenylalaninemia, a pterin defect with secondary hyperphenylalaninemia, or a transient elevation of phenylalanine. Infants with severe liver disease or who are acutely ill from galactosemia may also have an increased concentration of phenylalanine.

Urine screening, either by ferric chloride testing for phenylketone identification or by Guthrie bacterial assay, should never be used to identify PKU in the newborn. Phenylketones usually do not appear in sufficient quantity in the urine to be identifiable by the ferric chloride test until the infant is 2 months old or older. Increased phenylalanine may also not be detectable in urine because phenylalanine is readily reabsorbed by the kidney. Moreover, the urine of the newborn infant is usually dilute, further reducing the phenylalanine concentration.

Treatment for PKU should never be given on the basis of a positive screening test alone. The dietary therapy is complicated and can be hazardous to an infant who does not have PKU. Only after repeat testing and confirmation of PKU should treatment be given and then only in collaboration with or directly by a metabolic center.

Congenital Hypothyroidism

Congenital hypothyroidism is the most frequent disorder identified by routine newborn screening. It occurs in 1:3000 to 1:5000 screened infants (Dussault, 1993). This may be compared with the PKU frequency of 1:12,000.

Two different approaches are used to screen for congenital hypothyroidism. One is primary screening for low T_4 with secondary screening for high TSH. The other is primary screening for high TSH, often with secondary screening for low T_4. Either procedure reliably identifies congenital hypothyroidism. Nevertheless, affected infants can be missed. This may be due to lack of the marker (either low T_4 or high TSH). Specifically the T_4 level during the first 24 hours of life in an infant with congenital hypothyroidism might not yet be sufficiently decreased for identification, owing to an ectopic thyroid gland or to persistence of maternally transmitted T_4. In addition, the premature infant with congenital hypothyroidism can have a lag of 2 weeks or more in developing an elevated TSH level.

False-positive results occur with a frequency of approximately 0.1% to 0.2%. These infants transiently have low T_4 or elevated TSH. Many of those with low T_4 are premature infants with a normal TSH concentration or infants with perinatal stress and elevated TSH. To avoid missing congenital hypothyroidism, screening programs require a repeat blood specimen from each of these infants.

Infants with a positive screening test should not be labeled *congenital hypothyroidism* or treated for this disorder until confirmatory testing is in progress. This is especially true if the TSH concentration reported by the screening program is normal. In addition to prematurity, a low T_4 with normal TSH can result from thyroxine-binding globulin deficiency (Mandel et al, 1993) or hypothyroidism secondary to pituitary deficiency.

Galactosemia

Newborn screening for this disorder is advisable. Without routine newborn screening, 20% of affected infants may die without being diagnosed or remain undiagnosed until they become terminally ill with sepsis (Levy and Hammersen, 1978). In addition, another disorder of galactose metabolism, galactokinase deficiency, may not be identified until the development of irreversible cataracts.

Some screening programs use a metabolite assay for *total* galactose (galactose and galactose-1-phosphate) to detect galactosemia. Other programs screen the newborn specimen by a specific enzyme assay for activity of galactose-1-phosphate uridyltransferase, which is deficient in galactosemia. The enzyme assay identifies only galactosemia, whereas the metabolite assay identifies galactokinase and epimerase deficiencies as well as galactosemia. Several conditions other than the galactose metabolic disorders can produce increased galactose. These include severe neonatal liver disease, portosystemic shunting as a result of anomalies, and partial galactose-1-phosphate uridyltransferase deficiency.

The most rapid confirmatory test for a positive result in galactosemia screening is urine testing for reducing substance. In almost all cases of galactosemia, this test produces a strongly positive reaction. This is also true in galactokinase deficiency. If the urine contains reducing substance and the infant has clinical signs of galactosemia, a blood specimen for confirmatory testing should be immediately collected and milk feeding (breast or formula) discontinued. The confirmatory tests should include the measurement of blood galactose and galactose-1-phosphate and of galactose-1-phosphate uridyltransferase activity (Beutler, 1991). If the urine is negative for reducing substance, the newborn screening result is likely to be false-positive or to indicate a galactose-1-phosphate uridyltransferase enzyme variant, probably one that is benign. Nevertheless, repeat blood testing should be performed.

Homocystinuria

The newborn blood screening marker for detection of homocystinuria is an increased level of methionine. This screening test is included in some programs, and affected newborns have been detected. Infants with homocystinuria have also been missed, however, usually because their blood methionine concentration was not increased at the time the newborn specimen was collected (Whiteman et al, 1979). In addition, methionine is not increased in some forms of homocystinuria.

A high methionine level by itself is not diagnostic of homocystinuria. Liver disease can produce a strikingly increased methionine as can a metabolic disorder known as isolated hypermethioninemia, which may be benign. Tyrosinemia Type I (hereditary tyrosinemia) is also associated with high methionine. Furthermore, transient hypermethioninemia may occur in newborn infants. The initial action required for a newborn screening report of increased methionine is collection and submission of a repeat blood specimen. If the methionine level is again increased, quantitative amino acid analysis of plasma and urine should be performed. In the homocystinuric infant, homocystine is usually detectable in plasma and urine, methionine is usually increased in plasma, and cystine is reduced. In isolated hypermethioninemia, methionine is markedly increased in plasma, but there is no detectable homocystine in plasma or urine, and the plasma cystine concentration is normal.

Treatment of homocystinuria is complicated and should be administered and monitored by a metabolic center. The treatment is dietary and consists of a special formula and low-protein foods as well as other nutrient considerations.

Maple Syrup Urine Disease

The marker for MSUD is increased leucine in the newborn blood specimen. Newborns with classic MSUD almost always have at least a fourfold elevation of leucine. Transient increases in the blood leucine concentration are infrequent and usually no more than twice the normal concentration.

MSUD can be a fulminant disease associated with severe ketoacidosis and profound neurologic effects. Consequently the finding of a substantially increased leucine level in the newborn blood specimen should prompt an immediate call from the screening program to the attending physician. If the infant is ill, confirmatory plasma and urine specimens should be obtained and emergency therapy initiated. If the infant has MSUD, the plasma contains markedly increased concentrations of leucine, isoleucine, and valine (the branched-chain amino acids). In addition, the urine is strongly positive for ketones and contains large quantities of the branched-chain ketoacids and amino acids. The characteristic odor reminiscent of maple syrup may not yet be present.

Milder variants of MSUD can be missed in newborn screening. The newborn with the intermediate variant may not have an elevated blood leucine level, or the increase may be mild and overlooked. In the intermittent variant, the blood leucine concentration is normal in the newborn period and elevated only in later infancy or childhood during acute metabolic episodes precipitated by febrile illness or surgery.

Congenital Adrenal Hyperplasia

A decidedly increased level of 17-alpha-hydroxyprogesterone (17-OHP) suggests CAH owing to 21-hydroxylase deficiency. Infants with the salt-losing form of this disorder can die precipitously, often without a specific diagnosis. The clinical diagnosis may be suspected in the female newborn because of ambiguous genitalia but is rarely suspected on clinical grounds in male newborns or in females with atypical forms of CAH in which ambiguous genitalia may not occur. Even females with ambiguous genitalia may be clinically unrecognized in infancy, if the ambiguity is not obvious, or may be gender misassigned as males, if the ambiguity is advanced. Because accurate gender assignment and initiation of hormone therapy as soon as possible are critical to a favorable prognosis in CAH, newborn screening in leading to early diagnosis and prompt therapy is important. Consequently, screening for CAH has been added to routine newborn screening in a number of programs in North America, Europe, and Asia (Pang and Clark, 1993).

False-positive results in newborn screening for CAH are relatively frequent, often at a rate as high as 0.6%. Prematurity and low birth weight are the most common causes (Saedi et al, 1996). The elevated level may be truly 17-OHP or may be due to cross-reacting steroids. These steroids are produced by residual fetal adrenal cortex or result from decreased metabolic clearance by an immature liver. Perinatal stress and early specimen collection (within the first 24 hours of life) are frequent causes of high 17-OHP.

Repeat blood specimens are required from all infants with increased 17-OHP. If CAH seems likely on clinical grounds, serum electrolytes should be measured, and if this reveals hyponatremia and hyperkalemia, the electrolyte imbalance should be immediately corrected with intravenous fluids. In addition, pediatric endocrinology consultation should be sought.

Biotinidase Deficiency

Biotin recycling is necessary for maintaining sufficient intracellular biotin to activate carboxylase enzymes. Biotinidase is a key enzyme in biotin recycling. Lack of biotinidase activity results in carboxylase inactivities and an organic acid disorder known as *multiple carboxylase deficiency* (Wolf and Heard, 1992). The clinical features of the disorder include developmental delay, seizures, hearing loss, alopecia, and dermatitis. The developmental delay and seizures usually present at 3 to 4 months of age. Death during infancy has also been reported.

The initiation of biotin therapy in early infancy, when the disorder is presymptomatic, prevents all of the features of biotinidase deficiency. For this reason, a screening test has been developed and added to the newborn blood specimen in a number of newborn screening programs throughout the world (Hart et al, 1992). The frequency of identified newborns in these programs has a wide range, from 1:30,000 to 1:235,000. The average frequency is about 1:70,000. Almost all infants have been asymptomatic when identified and have remained normal on biotin treatment.

Sickle Cell Disease

In a number of state newborn screening programs, the blood specimen is tested for hemoglobin abnormalities. The major goal of this testing is to identify infants with sickle cell disease so that they can be given penicillin prophylaxis to prevent pneumococcal septicemia. Additional benefits of early detection include early referral to a comprehensive sickle cell program and early education and genetic counseling for parents (Smith and Kinney, 1993).

Sickle cell screening is usually performed by hemoglobin electrophoresis of blood eluted from a disc of the newborn specimen. This procedure identifies not only sickle cell disease, but also sickle cell trait and the presence of several other abnormal hemoglobins. Other than sickle cell disease, most of these abnormalities are benign. Consequently, whenever a hemoglobin abnormality is found by screening, it is important to perform confirmatory testing. This testing is especially critical in differentiating the frequent and benign sickle cell trait from the much rarer sickle cell disease. For instance, sickle cell disease (homozygosity for S hemoglobin) affects approximately 1:600 of the black population, whereas sickle cell trait (carrier status for S hemoglobin) is present in 1:12 blacks. Infants with sickle cell trait do not develop complications and should not be stigmatized as having sickle cell disease.

When sickle cell disease is confirmed, the infant should be started on penicillin prophylaxis as soon as possible and referred to a sickle cell disease center or hematologist. This combination of screening and careful follow-up has been effective. In Massachusetts, for instance, no infant with sickle cell disease is known to have developed pneumococcal sepsis since newborn screening for hemoglobinopathies began.

OTHER DISORDERS SCREENED
Cystic Fibrosis

The frequency and severity of cystic fibrosis explain its consideration for routine newborn detection. Similar to sickle cell disease, therapy that can prevent the ultimate complications is not yet available. Again similar to sickle cell disease, however, there is benefit from early and usually presymptomatic diagnosis. This benefit includes early nutritional therapy, pancreatic enzyme replacement, and antibiotic prophylaxis for pulmonary infection. Other benefits of newborn screening include identifying the genetic *set-up* for producing additional children with cystic fibrosis before subsequent pregnancies occur and, through presymptomatic identification, allowing the family to avoid months or years of delay in the correct diagnosis of a child with chronic respiratory problems or poor growth (Farrell and Mischler, 1992; Wilcken, 1993).

The analyte marker in newborn screening for cystic fibrosis is increased immunoreactive trypsinogen (IRT) in the newborn blood specimen. Increased IRT can also occur in normal newborns as a transient finding as a result of perinatal stress or for unknown reasons. Consequently the false-positive rate in cystic fibrosis screening is relatively high. To reduce this rate, screening programs have adopted a *second-tier* DNA analysis for one or more of the mutations associated with cystic fibrosis in specimens with increased IRT (Ferec et al, 1995). Despite this expanded approach to screening detection, a substantial number of infants who do not have cystic fibrosis must have a sweat test before the diagnosis of cystic fibrosis can be eliminated. Because of this relatively high false-positive rate and the need for a somewhat interventive test for follow-up, screening for cystic fibrosis has not yet been adopted by most programs.

Congenital Toxoplasmosis

Screening for congenital toxoplasmosis has been added to the newborn blood specimen in two states, Massachusetts and New Hampshire. The test is an ELISA that captures *Toxoplasma*-specific gamma M immunoglobulin (IgM) antibodies. The objective is to identify the majority of newborns with prenatally acquired toxoplasmosis who are asymptomatic at birth. It is believed that many, or perhaps most, of these infants develop neurologic sequelae or hearing loss or suffer recurrent chorioretinitis with progressive visual impairment and blindness unless treated in early infancy. Treatment with sulfadiazine, pyrimethamine, and leucovorin (folinic acid) is effective against actively multiplying parasites and may prevent the development of these clinical sequelae. Among 1 million newborns screened for congenital toxoplasmosis, the frequency has been about 1:10,000. Most of these infants were asymptomatic and, on treatment, have remained asymptomatic (Guerina et al, 1994).

Medium-Chain Acyl-Coenzyme A Dehydrogenase Deficiency

Medium-chain acyl-coenzyme A (CoA) dehydrogenase deficiency is the most frequent disorder of fatty acid oxidation, occurring in 1:10,000 to 1:20,000 individuals. Under conditions of fasting or stress, these infants can develop hypoketotic hypoglycemia and metabolic acidosis, hepatomegaly, and hyperammonemia. The presentation can be identical to Reye syndrome. Sudden infant death can occur. The mainstay of treatment is prevention of metabolic episodes by avoidance of fasting and restricting fat intake. This treatment is effective in allowing these children to maintain a normal life. Consequently, screening for medium-chain acyl-CoA dehydrogenase deficiency would be a valuable addition to newborn screening. Two methods are available. One is a direct analysis for the specific genetic mutation that is present in greater than 90% of affected individuals. The other is an analysis for the major metabolites that accumulate. Either method can be performed on the newborn blood specimen. Presently a newborn screening program in Pennsylvania includes this disorder using tandem mass spectrometry to identify increased metabolites. Among the first 80,000 infants screened, 9 (1:9000) were found to have medium-chain acyl-CoA dehydrogenase deficiency (Ziadeh et al, 1995).

Duchenne Muscular Dystrophy

Duchenne muscular dystrophy is an X-linked recessive muscle disorder that affects approximately 1:4000 male infants. It is progressive and produces profound muscle weakness leading to early death. It can be detected by newborn screening. The screening test is an assay that identifies increased creatinine phosphokinase activity. Several areas in France and Germany and a large screening program in Manitoba include this test (van Ommen and Scheurbrant, 1993). Increased creatinine phosphokinase, however, is not specific for Duchenne muscular dystrophy but also occurs in other muscular dystrophies and transiently in infants with perinatal stress or muscle trauma. Both the gene and the protein (dystrophin) defects in this disorder have been identified, but there is as yet no therapy that prevents the clinical manifestations. Nevertheless, presymptomatic diagnosis can lead to early information for these families and allow them to obtain support in preparing for the disabilities in the affected child. In addition, these families can receive genetic counseling before subsequent pregnancies.

Neuroblastoma

Neuroblastoma is the most frequent solid tumor of childhood, accounting for a significant number of deaths in preschool children. It is characterized by the excretion of increased vanillylmandelic acid (VMA) and homovanillic acid (HVA). In Japan and in several European programs, screening for neuroblastoma is conducted with filter paper urine specimens collected when the infant is 6 months old. VMA and HVA are measured by high-performance liquid chromatography in the urine eluted from the paper (Sawada, 1992). In Quebec, Canada, filter paper urine specimens collected at 3 weeks and again at 6 months of age are initially screened for VMA and HVA by thin-layer chromatography with confirmatory follow-up by gas chromatography–mass spectrometry. Both types of screening have resulted in the early detection of neuroblastoma in many clinically normal infants. In most, the tumor was localized and could be completely removed at surgery. These infants have remained well. Only a few infants already had advanced and inoperable cancer.

A study of the program in Quebec, however, has shown that the screening has not reduced the mortality rate from neuroblastoma. Notably, most children clinically diagnosed with poor prognosis disease have had false-negative screening results, whereas most of the infants identified by screening have had good prognosis neuroblastoma, which either spontaneously regresses or can be effectively treated after clinical detection (Woods et al, 1996) and probably does not require detection by screening. Consequently, screening for neuroblastoma may not only be unnecessary, but may also cause inappropriate intervention. In Japan, however, screening continues in the belief that it has significantly reduced the mortality from neuroblastoma. Debate on this subject continues.

Alpha$_1$-Antitrypsin Deficiency

In the 1970s, there was much interest in newborn screening for alpha$_1$-antitrypsin deficiency. The association of this deficiency with infantile cirrhosis in infants and obstructive lung disease in young adults had been discovered in the 1960s, and it seemed that presymptomatic identification such as in newborns could lead to measures that might at least reduce the risk of lung disease. The prophylactic measures that were suggested included the avoidance of areas in which the air is polluted or smoke filled. In Sweden, 200,000 infants were screened by electroimmunoassay applied to the newborn blood specimen, and approximately 1:2000 were found to have PiZZ, the type of alpha$_1$-antitrypsin deficiency associated with disease. Only three of these infants, however, developed cirrhosis; it is still too early to determine the frequency of lung disease in this identified population (Sveger, 1994). Uncertainty over the risk of disease, even in PiZZ alpha$_1$-antitrypsin–deficient individuals, and the absence of clearly preventive therapy for either the hepatic or pulmonary sequelae caused the interest in newborn screening for alpha$_1$-antitrypsin deficiency to wane. Presently, no newborn screening programs include this disorder.

Human Immunodeficiency Virus

A high percentage of newborns infected by HIV from the mother develop acquired immunodeficiency syndrome (AIDS). To determine the frequency and distribution of HIV seropositivity in pregnant women as reflective of the general population, newborn blood specimens were tested for HIV-specific IgG in most newborn screening programs in the United States. This screening was anonymous, and consequently the affected infants and their mothers were not identified (Grady, 1994). There is a movement in the United States to require routine newborn screening of HIV for the identification and treatment of affected infants. This movement is controversial. Only in New York state is there such linked newborn screening, but a parent must provide informed consent for the result to be diagnosed.

Hyperlipidemia

Recognition that hyperlipidemia, particularly increased low-density lipoprotein, is a major cause of premature cardiovascular disease has led to an interest in general population screening so as to identify those at risk. Although most of this interest has focused on children and adolescents, screening of the newborn has been considered. Evidence that hyperlipidemia can be controlled with medication as well as diet has increased this interest (Hunninghake et al, 1993). Until recently, however, there was no reliable marker for newborn screening. For instance, the cholesterol level varies widely in early infancy and was found not to correlate with later serum cholesterol levels. Investigators are now studying increased apolipoprotein B in the newborn as a marker for genetically determined hyperlipoproteinemia (Bangert et al, 1992). Apolipoprotein B, the major carrier of low-density lipoproteins, can be measured in the newborn blood specimen by an ELISA method. This could become an important addition to routine newborn screening.

OTHER SCREENING
Cord Blood

Umbilical cord blood can be screened for maternal metabolic disorders that secondarily affect the fetus and produce neonatal abnormalities. Paramount among these abnormalities is maternal PKU. Cord blood contains the increased phenylalanine transferred from the mother. Disorders intrinsic to the infant can also be screened in cord blood when the abnormality is present in erythrocytes. Among these disorders is galactosemia, in which cord blood has increased galactose-1-phosphate and no activity of galactose-1-phosphate uridyltransferase.

Routine cord blood screening was conducted in Massachusetts for more than 10 years. A filter paper card was soaked with umbilical cord blood at delivery of the infant and sent to the state screening laboratory. Initially, this specimen was screened for galactosemia and maternal PKU. Subsequently, galactosemia screening was discontinued because this disease could be effectively screened in the newborn blood specimen. Screening for maternal PKU continued, and screening for other maternal metabolic disorders, such as maternal histidinemia, was added. This screening led to valuable genetic and biochemical information about these disorders and their relation to the fetus. The information was of limited value to the families, however, and cord blood screening has been discontinued.

Cord blood is currently used for congenital hypothyroidism screening in several newborn screening programs (Fernandez-Iglesias et al, 1995). This specimen may be collected in filter paper or submitted as a tube of cord serum. If TSH elevation is the indicator, this may constitute effective screening for congenital hypothyroidism. A newborn blood specimen must then be collected for PKU screening, however, because in PKU (as distinguished from maternal PKU) the phenylalanine level in cord blood is normal and does not become elevated until at least several hours after birth.

SPECIFIC ISSUES OF NEWBORN SCREENING
Specimen Collection
Routine Follow-Up (Repeat) Screening

Obtaining a second or follow-up blood specimen from all infants was recommended when newborn screening began and was common practice in most screening programs during the 1960s. After several years, however, it became apparent that few infants with PKU were identified through the use of this specimen, and some screening programs abandoned the practice. A number of programs still require or at least strongly recommend a second specimen from all newborns. These programs report that an occasional infant who was normal on initial testing is identified with hyperphenylalaninemia, congenital hypothyroidism, or CAH by the second specimen. Whether these infants have significant forms of these disorders is unclear. Consequently the need for routine repeat screening is an issue in newborn screening.

Informed Consent

During the 1970s, there was lively discussion about the need for informed consent for newborn screening. Advocates argued that parents should decide whether newborn screening is to be performed and that public health laws mandating newborn screening are intrusive. This advocacy has waned, primarily because of the virtually insurmountable difficulty in obtaining truly informed consent from the parents of all newborn infants.

The issue of informed consent has implications that go beyond practicality. A major question is whether specific informed consent should be required for routine newborn screening when it is not required for other newborn tests (e.g., serum bilirubin) that are often necessary. There seems to be a consensus that mandatory screening without specific informed consent is justifiable for disorders such as congenital hypothyroidism and PKU that cause mental retardation and for which there is proven preventive treatment. As it becomes possible to use the newborn specimen to screen for many other abnormalities, however, particularly genetic disorders in which the phenotype may be variable and for which there may be little or no treatment and, most recently, for HIV seropositivity, the issue of informed consent has once again become prominent.

Screening Programs
Central Laboratories

Newborn screening should be conducted by relatively few, large centralized laboratories rather than by many small laboratories. This usually means that a single state laboratory or a regional laboratory serving several states should perform the screening. The mass analysis that results from centralized screening decreases costs and enhances accuracy because there is much greater exposure to and, thus, familiarity with abnormal results. Perhaps most important, a large central laboratory can include, in addition to an experienced technical staff, professional and administrative units that can continually monitor the process of specimen collection and repeat testing.

Missed Cases

Infants with PKU, congenital hypothyroidism, and other screened disorders have been missed in newborn screening. Laboratory or program error is the usual cause of these missed cases (Holtzman et al, 1986). In some instances, a specimen was never collected, particularly when the infant was transferred to another hospital. In other instances, mistakes occurred because the laboratory was not properly supervised. Thus, physicians must exercise clinical judgment and not fall into the trap of excluding a diagnosis because an infant has presumably been screened. Specific testing for metabolic and endocrine disorders should be performed in any infant or child with symptoms that suggest the presence of such a disorder, regardless of the assumed or actual newborn screening result.

Metabolic Disorders Not Screened

A frequent error is the assumption that routine newborn screening covers metabolic and congenital endocrine disorders and that a normal screening result excludes these disorders. Actually, most screening programs in North America test only for PKU and congenital hypothyroidism. This is also true for some programs in other parts of the world. Other programs in the United States and many in Europe and Japan include screening for several metabolic disorders as well as for CAH, in addition to PKU and congenital hypothyroidism. Nevertheless, most metabolic disorders are not covered by newborn screening. All infants and children with symptoms that suggest a metabolic diagnosis should undergo specific testing.

REFERENCES

AAP Section on Endocrinology and Committee on Genetics, and American Thyroid Association Committee on Public Health: Newborn screening for congenital hypothyroidism: Recommended guidelines. Pediatrics 91:1203, 1993.

Al-Jurayyan NAM, Al-Nuaim AA, El-Desouki MI, et al: Neonatal screening for congenital hypothyroidism in Saudi Arabia: Results of screening the first 1 million newborns. Screening 4:213, 1996.

Bangert SK, Eldridge PH, Peters TJ: Neonatal screening for familial hypercholesterolemia by immunoturbidimetric assay of apolipoprotein B in dried blood spots. Clin Chim Acta 213:95, 1992.

Beutler E: Galactosemia: Screening and diagnosis. Clin Biochem 24:293, 1991.

Buist NRM, Tuerck JM: The practitioner's role in newborn screening. Pediatr Clin North Am 39:199, 1992.

Committee on Genetics, American Academy of Pediatrics: Newborn screening fact sheets. Pediatrics 83:449, 1989.

Committee on Genetics, American Academy of Pediatrics: Issues in newborn screening. Pediatrics 89:345, 1992.

Dussault JH: Neonatal screening for congenital hypothyroidism. Clin Lab Med 13:645, 1993.

Farrell PM, Mischler EH: Newborn screening for cystic fibrosis. Adv Pediatr 39:35, 1992.

Ferec C, Verlingue C, Parent P, et al: Neonatal screening for cystic fibrosis: Result of a pilot study using both immunoreactive trypsinogen and cystic fibrosis gene mutation analyses. Hum Genet 96:542, 1995.

Fernandez-Iglesias C, Florez IG, Rodriguez-Gonzalez MC, et al: Neonatal screening for phenylketonuria and congenital hypothyroidism in Principado de Asturias (Spain) using two types of blood samples. Screening 4:131, 1995.

Forman DT, Bankson DD, Highsmith WE: Neonatal screening for biotinidase deficiency. Ann Clin Lab Sci 22:144, 1992.

Grady GF: HIV mass screening of infants and mothers: Historical, technical, and practical issues. Acta Paediatr 400(suppl):39, 1994.

Grant DB: Congenital hypothyroidism: Optimal management in the light of 15 years' experience of screening. Arch Dis Child 72:85, 1995.

Guerina NG, Hsu, H-W, Meissner HC, et al: Neonatal serologic screening and early treatment for congenital *Toxoplasma gondii* infection. N Engl J Med 330:1858, 1994.

Guldberg P, Levy HL, Hanley WB, et al: Phenylalanine hydroxylase gene mutations in the United States: Report from the Maternal PKU Collaborative Study. Am J Hum Genet 59:84, 1996.

Guthrie R, Susi A: A simple phenylalanine method for detecting phenylketonuria in large populations of newborn infants. Pediatrics 32:338, 1963.

Hart PS, Barnstein BO, McVoy JRS, et al: Comparison of profound biotinidase deficiency in children ascertained clinically and by newborn screening using simple methods of accurately determining residual biotinidase activity. Biochem Med Metab Biol 48:41, 1992.

Health Department: Pitfalls in metabolic screening. J Okla State Med Assoc 87:74, 1994.

Heeley AF, Bangert SK: The neonatal detection of cystic fibrosis by measurement of immunoreactive trypsin in blood. Ann Clin Biochem 29:361, 1992.

Heeley AF, Fagan DG: Trisomy 18, cystic fibrosis, and blood immunoreactive trypsin. Lancet 1:169, 1984.

Holtzman C, Slazyk WE, Cordero JF, et al: Descriptive epidemiology of missed cases of phenylketonuria and congenital hypothyroidism. Pediatrics 78:553, 1986.

Hunninghake DB, Stein EA, Dujovne CA, et al: The efficacy of intensive dietary therapy alone or combined with Lovastatin in outpatients with hypercholesterolemia. N Engl J Med 328:1213, 1993.

Irons M: Screening for metabolic disorders: How are we doing? Pediatr Clin North Am 40:1073, 1993.

Kelnar CJH: Congenital adrenal hyperplasia (CAH)—the place for prenatal treatment and neonatal screening. Early Hum Dev 35:81, 1993.

Levy HL, Cornier AS: Current approaches to genetic metabolic screening in newborns. Curr Opin Pediatr 6:707, 1994.

Levy HL, Hammersen G: Newborn screening for galactosemia and other galactose metabolic defects. J Pediatr 92:871, 1978.

MacMillan DR, Mabry CC: Differences in screening and confirmatory thyroid profiles in congenital hypothyroid subtypes: Implications for missed cases. J Perinatol 15:126, 1995.

Mandel S, Hanna C, Boston B, et al: Thyroxine-binding globulin deficiency detected by newborn screening. J Pediatr 122:227, 1993.

Masson J, Lemonnier F, Travert J, et al: Neonatal concentration of apolipoproteins B and A-1 measured by radioimmunoassay in dried blood spots. Screening 3:11, 1994.

O'Flynn ME: Newborn screening for phenylketonuria: Thirty years of progress. Curr Prob Pediatr 22:159, 1992.

Ohkubo S, Shimozawa K, Matsumoto M, et al: Analysis of blood spot 17 α-hydroxyprogesterone concentration in premature infants—proposal for cut-off limits in screening for congenital adrenal hyperplasia. Acta Paediatr Jpn 34:126, 1992.

Pang S, Clark A: Congenital adrenal hyperplasia due to 21-hydroxylase deficiency: Newborn screening and its relationship to the diagnosis and treatment of the disorder. Screening 2:105, 1993.

Pollitt RJ: Neonatal screening. J Clin Pathol 46:497, 1993.

Rock MJ, Mischler EH, Farrell PM, et al: Immunoreactive trypsinogen screening for cystic fibrosis: Characterization of infants with a false-positive screening test. Pediatr Pulmonol 6:42, 1989.

Saedi SA, Dean H, Dent W, et al: Screening for congenital adrenal hyperplasia: The Delfia screening test overestimates serum 17-hydroxyprogesterone in preterm infants. Pediatrics 97:100, 1996.

Sawada T: Screening infants for neuroblastoma in Japan. Screening 1:253, 1992.

Schweitzer S: Newborn mass screening for galactosemia. Eur J Pediatr 154(suppl 2):S37, 1995.

Slyper AH, Shaker JL: Neonatal hypothyroxinemia with normal thyrotropin: Clue to maternal Graves' disease. Clin Pediatr 32:121, 1993.

Smith JA, Kinney T: Clinical practice guidelines, quick reference guide for clinician: Sickle cell disease: Screening and management in newborns and infants. Am Fam Physician 48:95, 1993.

Sveger T: Screening for α₁-antitrypsin deficiency. Acta Paediatr 393(suppl):18, 1994.

Therrell BL, Panny SR, Davidson A, et al: U.S. newborn screening system guidelines: Statement of the council of regional networks for genetic services. Screening 1:135, 1992.

van Ommen JB, Scheurbrant G: Neonatal screening for muscular dystrophy. Neuromusc Disord 3:231, 1993.

West R, Ashcraft P, Becton D: Newborn screening for hemoglobinopathies in Arkansas: First two years' experience. J Ark Med Soc 88:382, 1992.

Whiteman PD, Clayton BE, Ersser RS, et al: Changing incidence of neonatal hypermethioninaemia: Implications for the detection of homocystinuria. Arch Dis Child 54:593, 1979.

Wilcken B: Newborn screening for cystic fibrosis: Its evolution and a review of the current situation. Screening 2:43, 1993.

Wolf B, Heard GS: Biotinidase deficiency. Adv Pediatr 38:1, 1992.

Woods WG, Tuchman M, Robison LL, et al: A population-based study of the usefulness of screening for neuroblastoma. Lancet 348:1682, 1996.

Ziadeh R, Hoffman EP, Finegold DN, et al: Medium chain acyl-CoA dehydrogenase deficiency in Pennsylvania: Neonatal screening shows high incidence and unexpected mutation frequencies. Pediatr Res 37:675, 1995.

CHAPTER 29

Other Resources for Genetic Diagnosis

Robert J. Vosatka

The tremendous amount of information on the genetic basis of disease has made it virtually impossible for the clinician to remain current on the ever-increasing relevance of genetics to diagnosis, counseling, and therapy. To aid in understanding the reasons for this tremendous expansion and its impact on clinical medicine, particularly in the newborn, an overview of the history of gene mapping is presented.

The importance of genetics to clinical newborn medicine will only increase over the next few years. This chapter introduces the clinician to new modes of information retrieval as well as existing references that can be clinically useful and may be essential for appropriate and timely clinical care of patients.

HISTORY

The concept that human traits could serve as milestones on a map of the human genome can be attributed to Victor McKusick, the father of modern genetics. Although many traits with a recognizable pattern of mendelian inheritance are diseases, many nondisease phenotypes comprise the traits listed in the *Mendelian Inheritance in Man* catalog (McKusick, 1994).

Advances in different chromosomal and genetic mapping techniques have led to a near exponential growth in the number of genes mapped (Fig. 29–1). A historical overview allows not only an understanding of modern approaches to disease gene mapping but also an understanding of the broad armamentarium available to pursue genetic diagnosis in utero or shortly after birth.

The first disease genes were mapped based on readily discernible features such as gender.

Sex Linked

Traits that map to the human X chromosome are transmitted from carrier females to their male offspring. Even though females can express some X-linked traits, most phenotypically identifiable individuals with an allele for an X-linked trait are male. Identification of phenotypes and their relationship to the gender of the affected or carrier individuals does not require any sophisticated techniques to follow the inheritance pattern. Nonetheless, the unambiguous formal mapping of a trait to the X chromosome can be a difficult task, requiring a large number of informative pedigrees.

Cell Surface Antigens

The identification and mapping of cell surface antigens allowed a broader approach to the mapping of mendelian traits. No longer were only sex-linked traits open to a linkage-based genetic approach. Inheritance patterns of traits (or cell surface markers themselves) could be mapped based on extensive analysis of human pedigrees. All that was required to consider a mapping project based on a cell surface marker, or polymorphism, was the presence of a cell surface marker that was present on some subset of the population.

The dramatic increase in the number of loci mapped by cell surface markers caused a rapid increase in the density of markers throughout the genome. As markers became more widely distributed across the human genome, mapping projects became more productive, with improved tools being used to exclude or include a chromosomal region as being linked to a genetic trait.

Heterokaryon Analysis

In the 1960s, the ability to grow cells in culture and to fuse cells from different species allowed the possibility of constructing genetic tools that did not previously exist in nature. Heterokaryons, cells that are the product of a fusion of two different cell types, can be produced from the fusion of cells from individuals with or without a genetic trait, or between cells of human origin and those of other species. These heterokaryons often only contained one or a few human chromosomes together with a full

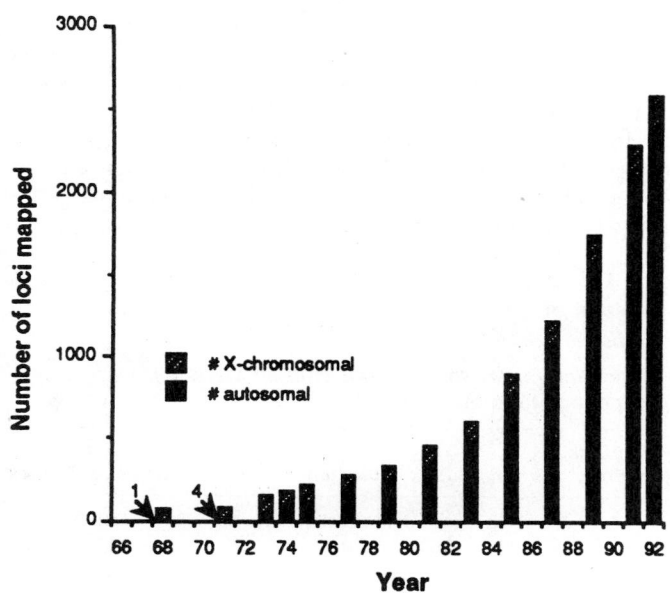

FIGURE 29–1. The expansion of knowledge of human genetic traits is evident from the rapid increase in the number of loci mapped to human chromosomes. (From McKusick VA: Mendelian Inheritance in Man, 11th ed. Baltimore, Johns Hopkins University Press, 1994. ©1994, The Johns Hopkins University Press.)

complement of chromosomes from another species. As long as an identifiable marker (e.g., an enzymatic activity) could be followed in the cells, the inheritance of the marker could be correlated with the human chromosome or chromosome fragments that were present in a particular heterokaryon.

Restriction Fragment Length Polymorphism

David Botstein and colleagues (1980) first conceived of the possibility of using anonymous pieces of DNA to construct a complete map of the human genome. The concept of restriction fragment length polymorphism (RFLP) based diagnosis quickly introduced a method to study the inheritance patterns of sequences of DNA. No longer did a sequence of DNA need to be "expressed." That is, no longer did the DNA need to encode a molecule of RNA or a protein to be detected. The sequence of the DNA itself could be a new milestone in the genome. The number of markers skyrocketed, such that, there are currently markers for nearly every part of every chromosome, including the mitochondrial chromosome.

CONVENTIONAL RESOURCES
Texts
Mendelian Inheritance in Man

Mendelian Inheritance in Man (McKusick, 1994) is the standard reference for cataloging genetic traits based on their reported inheritance patterns. The text defines what has been referred to as "the morbid anatomy of the human genome," or the assignment of disease genes according to their location on different human chromosomes. The text is divided into five parts. Each entry has a unique identifying number that may be preceded by an asterisk (*) or number symbol (#). The first digit of the identifying number denotes the pattern of inheritance (Table 29–1). Those traits whose identifying number is preceded by an asterisk are those that, in the opinion of McKusick or the editorial staff, have sufficient clinical or other data to support the proposed mode of inheritance. Entries preceded by a number symbol denote entries for which two or more genes may be responsible for the phenotype. Decimal entries

TABLE 29–1

Mendelian Inheritance in Man, Human Traits by Proposed Mode of Inheritance

First Digit of Entry	Mode of Inheritance	Number of Entries
1	Autosomal dominant	4458
2	Autosomal recessive	1730
3	X-linked	412
4	Y-linked	19
5	Mitochondrial	59

From McKusick VA: Mendelian Inheritance in Man, 11th ed. Baltimore, Johns Hopkins University Press, 1994. © 1994, The Johns Hopkins University Press.

describe traits for which the molecular basis is established and for which alternative alleles have been reported for a particular gene locus. The first digit of each entry indicates the proposed mode of inheritance of each reported trait. Table 29–1 lists the modes of inheritance and number of entries given in the 11th edition of the text.

Pictorial Texts of Genetic Syndromes

Several texts are available with large numbers of photographs demonstrating subtle aspects of various genetic diseases and congenital malformations. *Smith's Recognizable Patterns of Human Malformation* (Jones, 1988) provides a comprehensive overview of a large number of phenotypes likely to be encountered in the newborn period and beyond. Its accompanying text has only limited information. More frequently updated resources, such as those found in the McKusick database and recent journal articles, should be consulted to provide accurate information in this rapidly advancing field. *Syndromes of the Head and Neck* (Gorlin, 1990) focuses on facial features that may provide clues to a morphologic diagnosis. Together, these texts provide pictorial references that can be useful as an aid to diagnosis of congenital disorders. A third reference that also provides a large number of photographs is the *Birth Defects Encyclopedia* (Buyse, 1990). The text (but not photographs) can be updated electronically. (See Computer-Based Resources.) Frequent and extensive reviews of the photographs in these references are necessary to make these texts truly useful. P.O.S.S.U.M., a computer-based reference, may be more helpful in directing a clinician to relevant photographs of patients with congenital and genetic disorders.

Catalogue of Unbalanced Chromosome Aberrations in Man

The text by Schinzel (1984) is useful for interpreting abnormal karyotypes. Here, structural abnormalities are cataloged by the chromosome involved. The discussion and references may be helpful in interpreting the significance and relevance of an abnormal karyotype in a clinical situation. The text is supplemented by large numbers of references and accompanying photographs. These photographs are perhaps more helpful once an abnormal karyotype has been identified than in initially establishing a diagnosis. If a suspicion exists that a congenital anomaly could be caused by an abnormal karyotype, a karyotype should be obtained.

The Metabolic Basis of Inherited Disease

The Metabolic Basis of Inherited Disease (Scriver et al, 1994) provides a comprehensive discussion of current information regarding metabolic diseases, many of which are relevant to the neonatal intensive care unit. Complete descriptions of the biochemistry, pathophysiology, molecular biology, molecular diagnosis, and treatment are considered. The text is frequently updated and the current edition is in three volumes containing more than 3000 pages and includes extensive citations to the relevant literature. This text can often be more helpful in educating a clinician in the details of a specific diagnosis than more general texts.

Drugs in Pregnancy and Lactation

It is important to recognize that not all abnormalities present at birth have a genetic origin. *Drugs in Pregnancy and Lactation* (Briggs, 1994) provides a comprehensive review of the potential teratogenic effects of a large number of substances to which a woman may be exposed during pregnancy.

COMPUTER-BASED RESOURCES
Online Mendelian Inheritance in Man

The increasing complexity of the genetic map requires a genetic database. In 1966 Victor McKusick published the first edition of McKusick's *Mendelian Inheritance in Man* in which he cataloged approximately 1000 traits in humans that were inherited in a mendelian fashion. This effort at cataloging human traits began to put markers on the human gene map, in that each genetic trait corresponded to a single physical location in the human genome. The physical mapping of these loci to particular locations in the human genome lagged behind the identification of the individual traits (see Fig. 29–1).

Beginning in 1993, *Mendelian Inheritance in Man* has been compiled as a computerized compendium and is updated daily. Beginning in 1985, the number of entries in *Mendelian Inheritance in Man* approached 4000. The database subsequently became available via the then primitive Internet. Files were initially available only through more difficult ways of access called file transfer protocols. Recently, however, with the increased use and interest in the Internet, access to these ever-expanding files is readily available, often within the neonatal intensive care unit through hospital computers with Internet access. Frequent updating of the database and the great amount of information available has necessitated that 12 expert subject editors be responsible for different sections of the book. Access is available through the Internet via the worldwide web through the genome database at the citation http://gdbwww.gdb.org. This setup makes access to this tremendous amount of data even more readily available to the clinician on a regular basis. These archives can be searched for specific terms and combinations of terms, allowing rapid location of the information of interest. Many entries not only include descriptions of very detailed aspects of the genetics but also include certain key features related to the diagnosis that can help the clinician sort out the differential diagnosis. The current on-line version also includes color photographs of patients or relevant clinical features and audio excerpts from clinical disorders that have sounds related to them, for example, the high-pitched, catlike cry associated with cri du chat syndrome.

The multimedia enhancements of *Mendelian Inheritance in Man* are expected to increase in the future. There are also video clips available on-line of disorders with primarily movement disorders, such as the choreiform movements that are characteristic of Huntington disease.

Birth Defects Encyclopedia

The *Birth Defects Encyclopedia* (Buyse, 1990) is available as an electronic supplement to the text. Current information on genetic disorders discussed in the text can be retrieved by FAX directly from the regularly updated database. Like the McKusick database, this resource can potentially provide timely information helpful in the diagnosis and treatment of genetic disorders. Instructions are provided in the text and require the text entry number to access updated information by FAX.

Picture of Standard Syndromes and Undiagnosed Malformations

Unlike the McKusick and Buyse databases, the *Picture of Standard Syndromes and Undiagnosed Malformations* (P.O.S.S.U.M.) database has no textual equivalent. It contains an extensive searching system on a floppy disk that allows the informed user to search for disorders based on greater than 1000 different clinical traits. It is useful to assist the physician in considering relevant diagnoses in a particular patient. Brief descriptions of disorders and references to the primary literature are included. Although the computerized differential diagnosis searching technique can be used alone, the P.O.S.S.U.M. system also allows access to digitalized photographs of patients with the cited disorders to allow comparison of subtle phenotypic traits to those exhibited by a patient of interest. The P.O.S.S.U.M. system also includes photographs of more than 250 patients with a variety of undiagnosed malformations. These may allow the diagnosis and inclusion of hitherto unknown morphologic syndromes.

REFERENCES

Botstein D, White RL, Skolnick M, Davis RW: Construction of a genetic linkage map in man using restriction fragment length polymorphisms. Am J Human Genet 32:314–331, 1980.

Briggs GG, Freeman RK, Yaffe SJ: Drugs in pregnancy and lactation, 4th ed. Baltimore, Williams & Wilkins, 1994.

Buyse ML: Birth Defects Encyclopedia. Dover, MA, Center for Birth Defects Information Services, 1990.

Jones KL: Smith's Recognizable Patterns of Human Malformation, 4th ed. Philadelphia, WB Saunders, 1988.

Gorlin RJ: Syndromes of the Head and Neck, 3rd ed. New York, Oxford University Press, 1990.

McKusick VA: Mendelian Inheritance in Man, 11th ed. Baltimore, Johns Hopkins University, 1994.

Scriver CR, Beaudet AL, Sly WS, Valle D: The Metabolic Basis of Inherited Disease, 7th ed. New York, McGraw-Hill, 1994.

Schinzel A: Catalogue of Unbalanced Chromosome Aberrations in Man. Berlin, Walter de Gruyter, 1984.

CHAPTER 30

Resuscitation in the Delivery Room

Roberta A. Ballard

PHYSIOLOGY OF BIRTH

During normal gestation, labor, and delivery, powerful biochemical and mechanical forces act upon the fetus to prepare it to adapt to extrauterine life. However, a myriad of adverse circumstances—genetic, maternal, and fetal—that vary in duration, degree, and implication for outcome can occur during the antepartum and intrapartum periods and impair the infant's ability to make this adaptation successfully. Hence, there is a need for resuscitative efforts to assist in this process. The approach to the resuscitation of any infant depends on a keen appreciation of the historical factors behind the need, an understanding of the physiologic mechanisms of adaptation, and sensitivity to the individual infant's responses, as well as skill in resuscitative techniques. Thus, successful resuscitation depends on much more than the "mechanical" application of practiced routines; it requires a clear understanding of basic physiologic principles and excellent assessment skills as well as the essential equipment and practiced teamwork.

"Stress" of Birth

As pointed out by Lagercrantz and Slotkin (1986), "At first thought, being born would seem to be a terrible and dangerous ordeal. The human fetus is squeezed through the birth canal for several hours, during which the head sustains considerable pressure, and the infant is intermittently deprived of oxygen. . . . then delivered from a warm, dark, sheltered environment into a cold, bright hospital room . . . (in response) the fetus produces unusually high levels of the "stress" hormones, adrenalin and noradrenalin, . . . typically used to prepare the body to fight or flee from a perceived threat to survival." Surely, the process of labor and delivery is the time of greatest jeopardy that occurs during life, but would avoidance of this stress and the consequent elevation of catecholamine levels lead to better outcomes? Catecholamines clearly contribute to the regulation of many processes important to the infant's adaptation at birth, including resorption of lung liquid, release of surfactant into the alveoli, mobilization of readily usable fuel for nutrition, defense against cold stress, and modulation of cardiac output to ensure the preferential flow of blood to vital organs, such as the heart and brain. Perhaps, as some researchers have suggested, elevated levels of catecholamines even promote attachment between mother and child by increasing the appearance of alertness of the infant (Fig. 30–1).

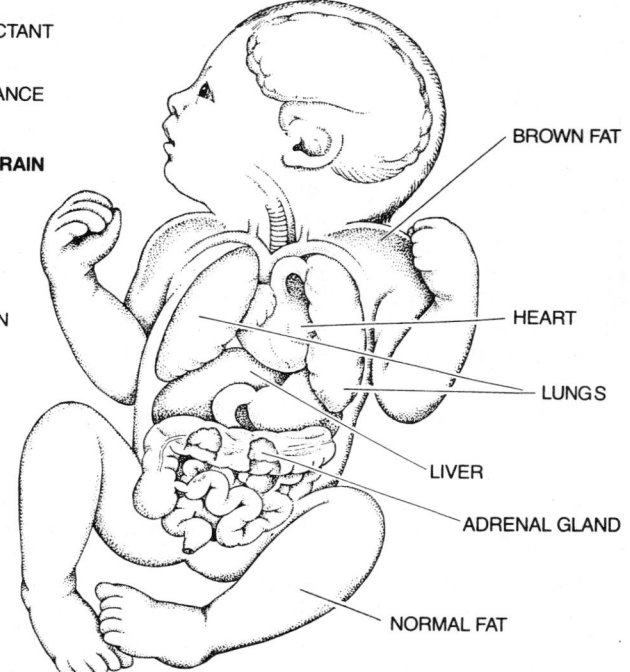

IMPROVES BREATHING
INCREASES LUNG SURFACTANT
INCREASES LUNG-LIQUID
   ABSORPTION
IMPROVES LUNG COMPLIANCE
DILATES BRONCHIOLES

PROTECTS HEART AND BRAIN
INCREASES BLOOD FLOW
   TO VITAL ORGANS

MOBILIZES FUEL
BREAKS DOWN NORMAL
   FAT INTO FATTY ACIDS
BREAKS DOWN GLYCOGEN
   (IN LIVER) TO GLUCOSE
STIMULATES NEW
   PRODUCTION OF
   GLUCOSE BY LIVER

FACILITATES BONDING?
DILATES PUPILS
APPEARS TO INCREASE
   ALERTNESS

BROWN FAT

HEART

LUNGS

LIVER

ADRENAL GLAND

NORMAL FAT

FIGURE 30–1. Adaptational effects of a catecholamine surge during delivery include promotion of normal breathing, alteration of blood flow to protect the heart and brain against potential asphyxia, immediate mobilization of fuel for energy and, possibly, enhancement of maternal-infant attachment. (From Lagercrantz H, Slotkin TA: The "stress" of being born. Sci Am 254:100, 1986. Copyright © 1986 by Scientific American, Inc. All rights reserved.)

The normal preterm infant has lower catecholamine levels at birth than the normal term infant, which contributes to the disadvantages of preterm infants in establishing ventilation and maintaining temperature. In both term and preterm infants, catecholamine levels are higher with delivery after labor and also higher in girls than in boys. Levels are proportionally very much higher in each of these groups when there is asphyxia (Greenough et al, 1987; Newnham et al, 1984). The endogenous opiate peptides (enkephalins and endorphins) also probably modulate the cardiovascular response to stress and play a role in the infant's adaptation at birth (Martinez et al, 1988). It is hoped that increased understanding of the interaction of these and other agents will eventually allow optimal preparation of the fetus for labor. This understanding may also provide insight on which interventions to use during labor and at birth to ensure an optimal outcome.

Transition from Fetal to Neonatal Circulation

Prior to birth, the placenta serves as the gas-exchange organ for the fetus and provides a low-resistance "shunt" compared with the high resistance of the fetus's peripheral circulation. As a result, the fetus normally has two large right-to-left shunts: one from the right atrium to the left atrium through the foramen ovale, and the second from the pulmonary artery to the aorta across the ductus arteriosus (Fig. 30–2). In utero, as a result of constricted pulmonary arterioles that produce high pulmonary vascular resistance, only a small percentage of the fetal cardiac output flows through the lungs. The fetus accommodates well to a normal PO_2 of 20 to 25 mm Hg in its best-oxygenated blood, which comes through the umbilical vein from the placenta. As a result of the right-to-left shunts through the foramen ovale and the ductus arteriosus, the best-oxygenated blood streams from the umbilical vein to the inferior vena cava, through the foramen ovale into the left atrium and ventricle, and then out the aorta, thus supplying best-oxygenated blood to the brain and myocardium of the fetus (see Fig. 30–2).

At delivery, two major changes occur in this system. First, the umbilical cord is clamped, eliminating the placenta as a gas exchange organ as well as a low-resistance "shunt." Second, respiration is initiated by the fetus. Expansion of the lungs results in a marked decrease in pulmonary vascular resistance that is furthered by the increased level of oxygenation that occurs as the infant begins to breathe (Fig. 30–3). With these changes, the flow of blood to the left atrium via the pulmonary veins increases, so that left atrial pressure exceeds right atrial pressure and functionally closes the foramen ovale. When pulmonary vascular resistance decreases to a level lower than the systemic vascular pressure, the ductus arteriosus is functionally closed.

At birth, the lungs normally are partially filled with fluid. Therefore, the initial breaths taken by the infant must inflate the lungs and effect a change in vascular pressures so that lung water is absorbed into the pulmonary arterial system and cleared from the lung. At the same time, inflation is a powerful mechanism for the release of pulmonary surface active material, which increases compliance of

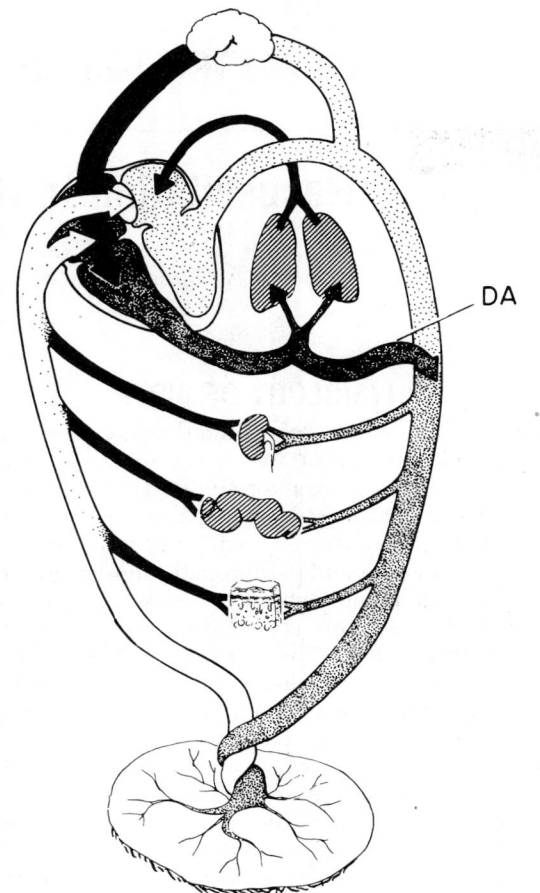

FIGURE 30–2. The fetal circulation. Oxygenated blood leaves the placenta by way of the umbilical vein (vessel without stippling). It flows into the portal sinus in the liver (not shown), and a variable portion of it perfuses the liver. The remainder passes from the portal sinus through the ductus venosus into the inferior vena cava, where it joins blood from the viscera (represented by kidney, gut, and skin). About half of the inferior vena cava flow passes through the foramen ovale to the left atrium, where it mixes with a small amount of pulmonary venous blood. This relatively well-oxygenated blood (light stippling) supplies the heart and brain by way of the ascending aorta. The other half of the inferior vena cava stream mixes with superior vena cava blood and enters the right ventricle (blood in the right atrium and ventricle has little oxygen, which is denoted by heavy stippling). Because the pulmonary arterioles are constricted, most of the blood in the main pulmonary artery flows through the ductus arteriosus (DA) so that the descending aorta's blood has less oxygen (heavy stippling) than blood in the ascending aorta (light stippling). (From Avery GN: Neonatology. Philadelphia, JB Lippincott, 1987.)

the lung and enables stabilization of functional residual capacity (Massaro and Massaro, 1983; Taeusch et al, 1974).

Fetal Reserve

Because the fetus is normally relatively hypoxemic (PO_2 of 20 to 24 mm Hg) and during labor is subjected to stresses associated with both increased oxygen consumption and interrupted gas exchange, the fetus is at particular risk for occur in the minutes following birth and the infant is unable to establish ventilation and pulmonary perfusion, a progressive cycle of worsening hypoxemia, hypercapnia, and metabolic acidemia evolves. Pulmonary vascular resistance remains high, the ductus arteriosus remains widely patent (Fig. 30–4), and right-to-left shunting through the foramen ovale also persists. Once this process begins, it tends to be self-perpetuating and may result in serious tissue hypoxia, ischemia, and acidosis, which ultimately may lead to irreversible organ damage. Asphyxia may be caused by maternal, placental, or fetal factors that reduce the fetal reserve (Table 30–1). The duration of asphyxia is critical to the outcome of the infant, so it is important to evaluate rapidly all of the factors contributing to the asphyxia and to interrupt the process as early as possible.

Figure 30–5 demonstrates the classic cardiopulmonary

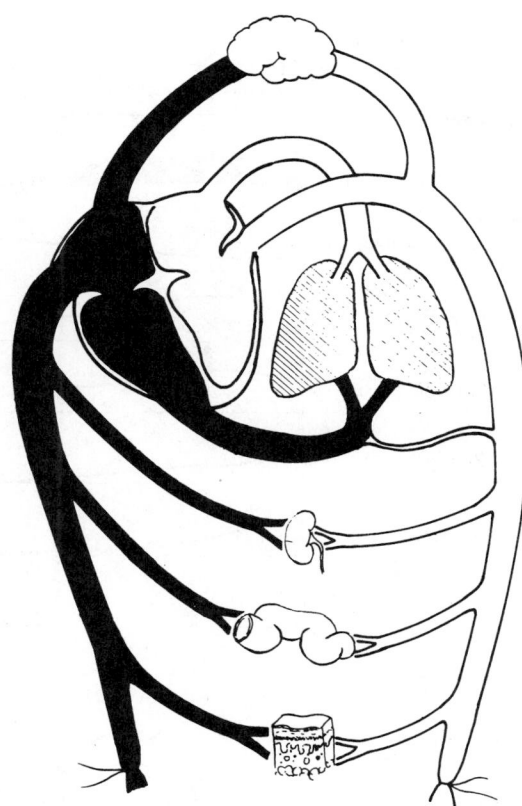

FIGURE 30–3. The circulation in the normal newborn. After expansion of the lungs and ligation of the umbilical cord, pulmonary blood flow increases and left atrial and systemic arterial pressures increase while pulmonary arterial and right heart pressures decrease. When the left atrial pressure exceeds right atrial pressure, the foramen ovale closes so that all of the inferior and superior vena cava blood leaves the right atrium, enters the right ventricle, and is pumped through the pulmonary artery toward the lung. With the increase in systemic arterial pressure and decrease in pulmonary arterial pressure, flow through the ductus arteriosus becomes left to right, and the ductus constricts and closes. The course of the circulation is the same as in the adult. (From Avery GN: Neonatology. Philadelphia, JB Lippincott, 1987.)

asphyxia at the time of birth. However, the fetus has several compensatory mechanisms that help protect it: fetal hemoglobin has greater oxygen affinity than adult hemoglobin, fetal tissues have an increased ability to extract oxygen, and the fetus has greater tissue resistance to acidosis than does the adult. In addition, the fetus has mechanisms that compensate for asphyxia. These include bradycardia and the "diving reflex" (similar to that found in diving mammals), which allows a preferential distribution of blood flow to the brain, adrenal glands, and heart and away from the lungs, gut, liver, spleen, kidney, and carcass. The fetus is also capable of decreasing oxygen consumption and switching to anaerobic glycolysis, as long as liver glycogen stores are adequate.

ASPHYXIA
Physiology

Asphyxia is defined as a combination of *hypoxemia, hypercapnia,* and *metabolic acidemia.* If lung expansion does not

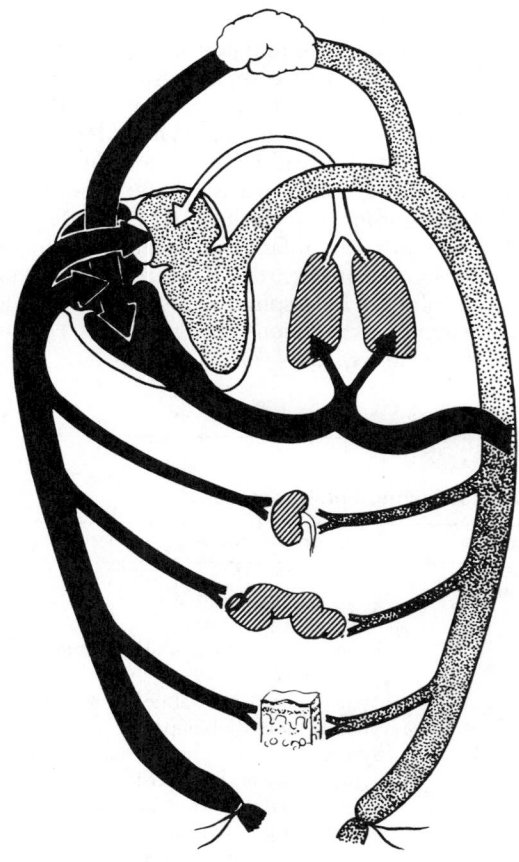

FIGURE 30–4. The circulation in an asphyxiated newborn with incomplete expansion of the lungs. Pulmonary vascular resistance is high, pulmonary blood flow is low (normal number of pulmonary veins), and flow through the ductus arteriosus is high. With little pulmonary arterial flow, left atrial pressure decreases below right atrial pressure, the foramen ovale opens, and vena caval blood flows through the foramen into the left atrium. Partially venous blood goes to the brain via the ascending aorta. The blood of the descending aorta that goes to the viscera has less oxygen than that of the ascending aorta (heavy stippling) because of the reverse flow through the ductus arteriosus. Thus, the circulation is the same as in the fetus except that there is less well-oxygenated blood in the inferior vena cava and umbilical vein. (From Avery GN: Neonatology. Philadelphia, JB Lippincott, 1987.)

changes seen in the animal model of asphyxia, as described by Dawes (1968). The initial phase of asphyxia is marked by increased respiratory effort (*primary hyperpnea*). This is followed by *primary apnea*, which lasts approximately 1 minute. Rhythmic gasping then begins and is maintained at a rate of 8 to 10 gasps per minute for several minutes, after which the gasps become weaker and slower until they cease, which is called *secondary apnea*. Some variation occurs in the period of gasping as a result of prior maternal and fetal medications or conditions that may have affected the infant's level of asphyxia at the moment of birth.

Delivery Room Assessment

When called to the delivery room to care for an infant who has failed to establish normal ventilation, the physician must rapidly determine whether the infant's problem (1) is due to asphyxia that began because of maternal and fetal conditions before or during labor and delivery or (2) represents a condition that was initiated in the newborn infant following birth. In the first case, the asphyxia represents a process that must be interrupted rapidly and that should respond to standard resuscitation. When the infant does not respond, it usually indicates severe fetal acidemia (Perlman and Risser, 1995). In the latter case, the infant was probably vigorous at birth and then, in attempting to establish respiration, the infant underwent development of apnea, cyanosis, or bradycardia. Differential diagnosis in the second infant with asphyxia after delivery requires rapid assessment of conditions that might be causing obstruction of the airway.

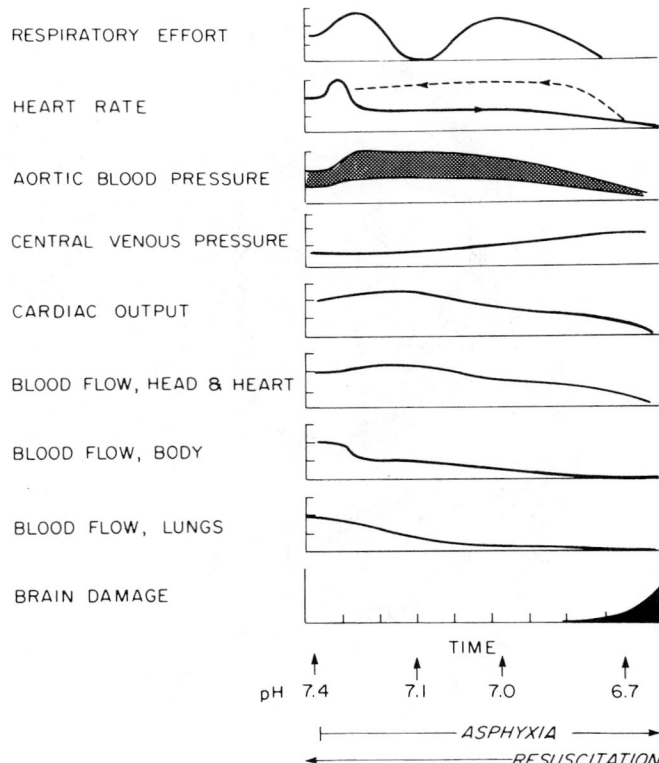

FIGURE 30–5. The sequence of cardiopulmonary changes with asphyxia and resuscitation. Time is on the horizontal axis. Asphyxia progresses from left to right; resuscitation proceeds from right to left. Units of time are not given. If there is complete interruption of respiratory gas exchange, the entire process of asphyxia from extreme left to right could occur in about 10 minutes. It could take much longer with an asphyxiating process that only partly interrupts gas exchange or does so completely, but only for repeated brief periods. With resuscitation, the process reverses, beginning at the point to which asphyxia has proceeded. (Adapted from Dawes G: Foetal and Neonatal Physiology. Chicago, Year Book Publishers, 1968, and Avery GN: Neonatology. Philadelphia, JB Lippincott, 1987.)

Obstruction of the airway may be due to (1) meconium aspiration or severe pneumonia that will respond to suctioning, (2) intrathoracic malformations that interfere with ventilation, for example, cystic adenomatoid malformation and diaphragmatic hernia, (3) congenital malformations of the airway, such as laryngeal web or (4) severe congenital heart disease with an intact foramen ovale. In addition, pneumothorax should always be considered in an infant who is initially vigorous at birth. If asphyxia is due to malformations, standard resuscitation and establishment of ventilation must be accompanied by interventions to correct the underlying cause.

Universal Prerequisites for Resuscitation
Skilled Personnel

In the United States, 3.7 million babies per year are born in 5000 hospitals with delivery services. Ninety percent of these hospitals are small, Level 1 services; 5% are Level 2; and another 5% are Level 3 (Bloom and Cropley, 1987).

TABLE 30–1

Conditions Affecting Fetal Reserve

Determinants	Common Disorders
Maternal	
Infection	Amnionitis
Lungs	Pneumonia, asthma, adult respiratory distress syndrome
Heart	Arrhythmia, structural defect, failure
Blood	Anemia, hemoglobinopathy
Blood vessels	Systemic lupus erythematosus, diabetes, hypertension, hypotension
Uterus	Hypertonus, malformation, rupture
Other	Genetic, drugs, deformities, preterm labor, multiple gestation, abnormal fetal presentation
Placental	
Age	Postmaturity
Size, morphology	Abruptio placentae, placenta previa
Fetal	
Umbilical cord	Knot, entanglement, prolapse, compression, thrombosis
Blood	Anemia
Metabolic	Inborn error, aneuploidy
Other	Infection, hydrops, malformations, multiple gestation

Adapted from Jacobs M, Phibbs R: Prevention, recognition, and treatment of perinatal asphyxia. Clin Perinatol 16(4):785, 1989.

Thus, most infants are born in hospitals that do not have sophisticated perinatal programs. In their combined program for neonatal resuscitation, the American Heart Association (AHA) and the American Academy of Pediatrics (AAP) emphasize the basic principle that effective resuscitation must begin with the awareness that *well-trained personnel must be immediately available in any setting where an infant is likely to be delivered.*° Identification and training of staff is, therefore, the first step in preparation for neonatal resuscitation. The second step is close communication between obstetricians and pediatricians to identify high-risk women before labor if possible, to prevent abnormal labors, and to focus planning for the resuscitation of infants thus identified. Understanding the special needs of different kinds of infants enables caregivers to anticipate and prepare for various types of resuscitation appropriately.

Resuscitation of the newborn is best done in the delivery room or immediately adjacent to it, so that the time lapse between delivery and initiation of resuscitation is minimized.

Equipment

The equipment that should be available for neonatal resuscitation is listed in Table 30–2 and is divided into (1) items needed in every institution for resuscitation of low-risk term infants with unexpected problems and (2) additional equipment required for resuscitation of high-risk or known preterm infants.

MANAGEMENT AT DELIVERY
Assessment of Degree of Asphyxia

The Apgar score (Table 30–3) was originally introduced to help quantitate the initial evaluation of newborn infants. Apgar scores should be assigned at 1, 5, and 10 minutes, and, if the infant still requires resuscitation, at 15 and 20 minutes as well. The scoring process requires the discipline to evaluate several aspects of the infant at once within the 1st minute of life. It serves as a framework around which to gear resuscitative efforts, because the score is an indicator of responsiveness to therapy as well as a way of defining infants who are at high risk for further difficulty. The score at 5 minutes and later is more predictive of survival and neurologic status than the 1-minute score, because the ability to interrupt and reverse the process indicates not only successful intervention but also that the process was not established for a long period in utero.

Overview of Resuscitation

Initial resuscitation of the depressed newborn always includes maintenance of body temperature and rapidly drying and placing the infant under a radiant heater. Clearing the airway is essential; this may be done using a bulb syringe, or, in the case of the infant born through thick

---

°The American College of Obstetrics and Gynecology, the American Society of Anesthesiology, the American Academy of Family Physicians, and the Canadian Pediatric Society have also stated their support for this principle.

TABLE 30–2

Equipment for Neonatal Resuscitation

Low-Risk and Term Infants

Radiant warmer to maintain temperature control
Stethoscope
Source of warm, humidified oxygen with flow meter
Bulb syringe
Suction source
Suction catheter and meconium aspirator
Nasogastric tube and syringe
Oral airway
Apparatus for bag and mask ventilation of infant, either anesthesia bag or Ambu bag with masks for different-sized infants
Laryngoscope with pencil handle
Endotracheal tubes (Portex)—sizes 2.5, 3.0, 3.5, 4.0, and stylet
Sterile gloves
Tape
Scissors
Fluids (D_5W, $D_{10}W$, normal saline)
Medications (naloxone hydrochloride [Narcan], sodium bicarbonate, atropine, calcium gluconate, epinephrine)
Clock or stopwatch
Tubes for obtaining blood gases or other samples
Equipment for placing umbilical catheter
Equipment for microtechnique for measuring blood gases
Portable radiographic equipment

High-Risk and Preterm Infants

All of the equipment listed, plus
Spotlight
Manometer for gauging pressure being used in ventilation
Blender for delivering oxygen in concentrations ranging from room air to 100%, with heated nebulizer
Oxygen analyzer
Electrocardiographic electrodes
Heart rate monitoring equipment
Blood pressure monitoring equipment
Hemoglobin saturation monitor
Blood gas syringes, heparinized and ready to use
Blood gas laboratory immediately available (10-minute processing time)
Volume expander (normal saline preferred) and/or blood available on emergency basis
Umbilical artery and vein catheters set up and ready to insert, with vascular pressure monitor
Gowns, masks, hats, for sterile procedure
Emergency medications with estimated dosages calculated

---

particulate material, by endotracheal suction. The infant is placed on an open bed near a table with all of the resuscitative equipment (see Table 30–2) available and then assessed for further intervention. A double-clamped segment of umbilical cord should be obtained for cord blood gas analysis.

American Heart Association–American Academy of Pediatrics Approach to Resuscitation

The AHA-AAP approach to resuscitation of the newborn takes the same type of clinical information that is gathered

TABLE 30–3

Apgar Scoring System

Features Evaluated	0 Points	1 Point	2 Points
Heart rate	0	<100	>100
Respiratory effort	Apnea	Irregular, shallow, or gasping respirations	Vigorous and crying
Color	Pale, blue	Pale or blue extremities	Pink
Muscle tone	Absent	Weak, passive tone	Active movement
Reflex irritability	Absent	Grimace	Active avoidance

from the Apgar score and uses it to develop a schema for approaching resuscitation of the term infant (Fig. 30–6). Even though these are guidelines developed by experienced physicians, they have not undergone any clinical trials. Recently, concerns have been raised about the value of resuscitation with 100% oxygen versus room air (Ramji et al, 1993; Rootwelt et al, 1992) as well as the need for chest compressions and medications (Davis, 1993; Perlman and Risser, 1995).

Infants with an Apgar Score of 7 or More

Vigorous infants generally do not require resuscitation other than perhaps a brief period of oxygen blown over the face. In approaching these infants who are not at risk for retrolental fibroplasia, it is important to remember (1) that administration of oxygen is accompanied by decreased pulmonary vascular resistance and increased pulmonary blood flow, and (2) that at birth, the newborn infant's lungs are normally full of fluid, which is cleared by resorption into the pulmonary arterial system. Excessive suctioning of clear fluid from the nasopharynx is not helpful and may contribute to atelectasis.

Infants with an Apgar Score of 4 to 6

Infants with an Apgar score of 4 to 6 require stimulation and often administration of oxygen by face mask; in addition, they may require some use of bag and mask ventilation to expand the lungs. Most infants respond to these measures and begin spontaneous respiration. It is important to empty the stomach of any infant who is receiving bag and mask ventilation.

Infants with an Apgar Score of 1 to 3

Infants with an Apgar score of 1 to 3 usually require intubation and expansion of the lung. However, if staff skilled in intubation and the appropriate equipment are not immediately available, initial bag and mask ventilation usually is adequate to sustain the infant. Further resuscitative steps depend on the heart rate response to ventilation.

Infants with an Apgar Score of 0

Virtually no live born infant should be assigned a score of 0, and resuscitation of an infant who truly has an Apgar score of 0, indicative of cardiac arrest before delivery, is probably a subject for ethical discussion. However, it is

frequently impossible in the excitement that surrounds the delivery of an asphyxiated infant to make absolutely certain that there is no heartbeat, and, in such circumstances, resuscitation should proceed immediately as for an infant with an Apgar score of 1 to 3, with the addition of cardiac compression.

The primer for resuscitation techniques is the manual prepared by the American Heart Association in conjunction with the American Academy of Pediatrics (Bloom and Cropley, 1994). It provides complete, well-illustrated instructions on how to proceed with mask ventilation, intubation, and cardiac compressions if necessary. Figure 30–7 shows the landmarks of the larynx that should be visualized for successful intubation of the newborn. If an infant does not respond to adequate ventilation and cardiac compression with an increase in heart rate to greater than 80 after 30 seconds of positive-pressure insufflation, then the administration of medications should be considered. However, the most likely explanation for failure to respond is inadequate ventilatory support. Figure 30–8 contains the chart developed by the AHA-AAP for administration of drugs, including epinephrine, volume expanders, sodium bicarbonate, dopamine, and naloxone. Table 30–4 provides the recommended drug dosages for neonatal resuscitation.

Expansion of the Lungs

Usually, the only requirement for initiation of resuscitation of the newborn is adequate expansion of the lung. The airway must be cleared before attempts to expand the lung are made. Initial inflation of the gasless, fluid-filled lung is best accomplished by application of a relatively high inflation pressure (sufficient to move the chest, usually 25 to 40 cm H_2O) over a relatively long time (0.5 to 1 second). The object is to inflate the lung as well as to trap some gas during exhalation, thereby creating a functional residual capacity. This process occurs over a series of breaths. The term infant with a strong chest wall and larger terminal airways is better able to generate the necessary forces to achieve lung inflation than is the premature infant who may need to be assisted. Lung inflation also stimulates surfactant secretion in mature lungs, and this response is enhanced by large-volume inflation. No attempt at intubation should last longer than 30 to 45 seconds before returning to bag and mask ventilation to support the child.

Administration of Epinephrine

If the infant does not respond to intubation and ventilation with an increase in heart rate, and it is certain that the

Overview of
Resuscitation in the Delivery Room

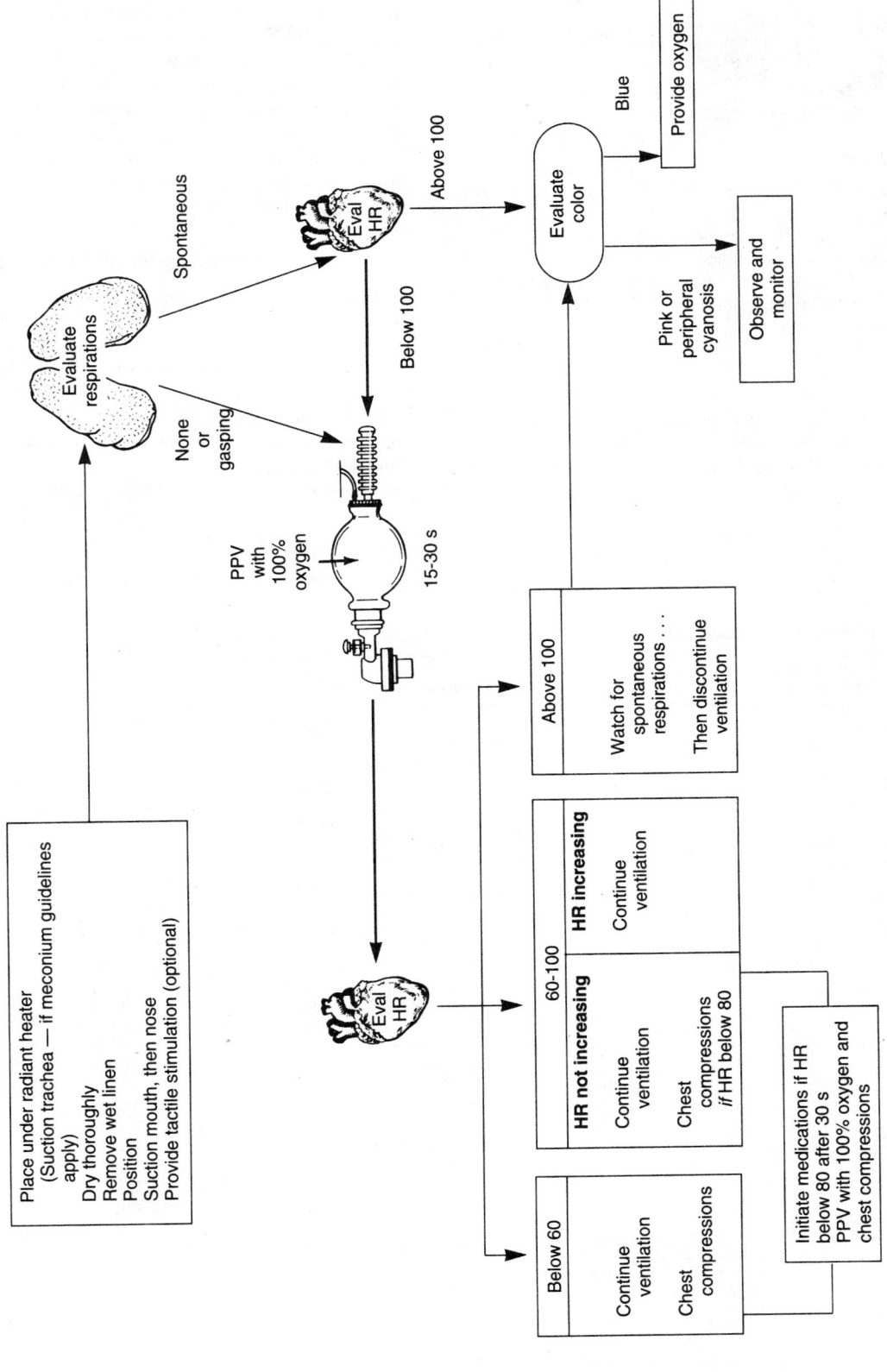

FIGURE 30-6. Overview of resuscitation in the delivery room. (From Bloom RS, Cropley C: American Heart Association–American Academy of Pediatrics Textbook of Neonatal Resuscitation. Dallas, American Heart Association National Center, 1994. Reproduced with permission. © Textbook of Neonatal Resuscitation, 1994 Copyright American Heart Association.)

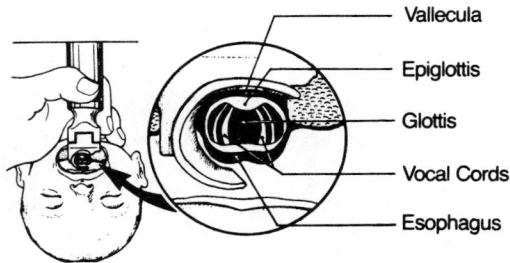

Vallecula

Epiglottis

Glottis

Vocal Cords

Esophagus

FIGURE 30–7. Landmarks of the larynx that should be visualized for intubation of the newborn. (From Bloom RS, Cropley C: American Heart Association–American Academy of Pediatrics Textbook of Neonatal Resuscitation. Dallas, American Heart Association National Center, 1994. Reproduced with permission. © Textbook of Neonatal Resuscitation, 1994. Copyright American Heart Association.)

endotracheal tube is in good position, epinephrine should be administered either endotracheally or preferably intravenously (McCrirrick and Kestin, 1992; Perlman and Risse, 1995).

Umbilical Vessel Catheterization

In the high-risk or significantly asphyxiated infant, it is important to place an umbilical catheter, preferably in the umbilical artery (although frequently a venous catheter can be placed more rapidly), to obtain arterial blood gases and other samples as well as to monitor arterial pressure. Changes in arterial pulse pressure and mean pressure can thus be followed up during the resuscitation, providing important indicators of cardiovascular responsiveness. In addition, appropriate medications can be administered easily through the catheter.

Correcting Metabolic Acidosis

Whenever possible, samples for cord blood gas determination should be obtained. In addition, the infant's blood gases should be measured immediately and the results known before the infusion of sodium bicarbonate. No bicarbonate should be given unless ventilation has been established and $PaCO_2$ is normal or low. The most severely asphyxiated infants are those with an arterial pH of 7.0 or less and a calculated base deficit of 25 mEq/L or greater in the presence of a marked elevation of $PaCO_2$. By means

TABLE 30–4

Medications for Neonatal Resuscitation

Medication	Concentration to Administer	Preparation	Dosage/Route	Total Dose/Infant			Rate/Precautions
Epinephrine	1:10,000	1 mL	0.1–0.3 mL/kg IV or ET	**Weight** 1 kg 2 kg 3 kg 4 kg	**Total mL** 0.1–0.3 mL 0.2–0.6 mL 0.3–0.9 mL 0.4–1.2 mL		Give rapidly May dilute with normal saline to 1–2 mL if giving ET
Volume expanders	5% Albumin–saline Normal saline Ringer's lactate		10 mL/kg IV	**Weight** 1 kg 2 kg 3 kg 4 kg	**Total mL** 10 mL 20 mL 30 mL 40 mL		Give over 5–10 minutes
Sodium bicarbonate	0.5 mEq/mL (4.2% solution)	20 mL or two 10-mL prefilled syringes	2 mEq/kg IV	**Weight** 1 kg 2 kg 3 kg 4 kg	**Total Dose** 2 mEq 4 mEq 6 mEq 8 mEq	**Total mL** 4 mL 8 mL 12 mL 16 mL	Give *slowly*, over at least 2 minutes Give only if infant is being effectively ventilated
Naloxone hydrochloride	0.4 mg/mL	1 mL	0.1 mg/kg (0.25 mL/kg) IV, ET IM, SQ	**Weight** 1 kg 2 kg 3 kg 4 kg	**Total Dose** 0.1 mg 0.2 mg 0.3 mg 0.4 mg	**Total mL** 0.25 mL 0.50 mL 0.75 mL 1.00 mL	Give rapidly IV, ET preferred IM, SQ acceptable
	1.0 mg/mL	1 mL	0.1 mL/kg (0.1 mL/kg) IV, ET IM, SQ	1 kg 2 kg 3 kg 4 kg	0.1 mg 0.2 mg 0.3 mg 0.4 mg	0.1 mL 0.2 mL 0.3 mL 0.4 mL	
Dopamine	$$6 \times \frac{Weight\ (kg) \times Desired\ dose\ (\mu g/kg/min)}{Desired\ fluid\ (mL/h)} = \frac{mg\ of\ dopamine}{per\ 100\ mL\ of\ solution}$$		Begin at 5 µg/ kg/min (may increase to 20 µg/kg/ min if necessary)° IV	**Weight** 1 kg 2 kg 3 kg 4 kg	**Total µg/min** 5–20 µg/min 10–40 µg/min 15–60 µg/min 20–80 µg/min		Give as a continuous infusion using an infusion pump Monitor heart rate and blood pressure closely Seek consultation

°There is evidence that 2–3 µg/kg/min may be adequate in many infants (Seri, 1995).

IM, intramuscular; ET, endotracheal; IV, intravenous; SQ, subcutaneous.

From Bloom RS, Cropley CS: American Heart Association–American Academy of Pediatrics Textbook of Neonatal Resuscitation. Dallas, American Heart Association National Center, 1994. Reproduced with permission. Copyright American Heart Association.

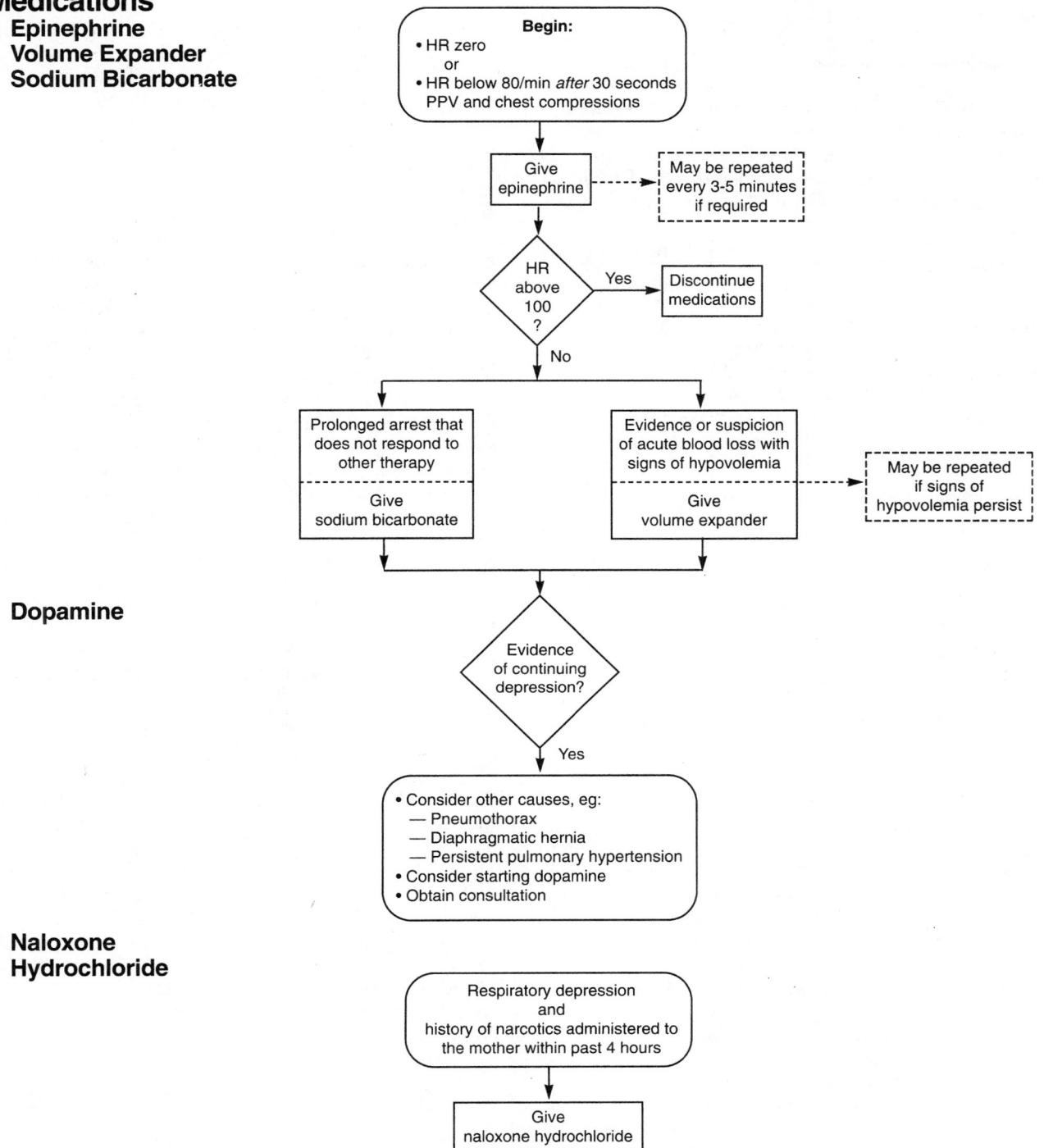

FIGURE 30–8. Schedule for administration of drugs for resuscitation of the newborn. (From Bloom RS, Cropley C: American Heart Association–American Academy of Pediatrics Textbook of Neonatal Resuscitation. Dallas, American Heart Association National Center, 1994. Reproduced with permission. © Textbook of Neonatal Resuscitation, 1994. Copyright American Heart Association.)

of artificial ventilation alone, this calculated deficit can be reduced by approximately 10 mEq/L if the infant's circulation is normal and oxygenation is achieved. This effect results from a significant bicarbonate shift that occurs when $PaCO_2$ exceeds 70 mm Hg and therefore must be taken into consideration in calculations for correcting base deficit. Some additional correction occurs with ventilation at pH levels above 7.0, and therefore, the dose of bicarbonate administered should always be no more than one fourth of the initially calculated value. Blood gas studies should be repeated before giving additional increments of bicarbonate. The equation for calculation of base replacement is:

$$mEq\ Base = \frac{0.3 \times weight\ in\ kg \times base\ deficit\ in\ mEq/L}{4}$$

Bicarbonate should always be diluted 1:1 with sterile water and administered very slowly. Arterial blood pressure should be measured both before and after bicarbonate is given, because the administration of sodium bicarbonate may unmask hypovolemia that has not been apparent because of peripheral vasoconstriction.

Support of the Cardiovascular System

Many conditions that produce asphyxia or preterm birth may be associated with loss of a large volume of blood, and the asphyxiated infant is even less able to compensate for large losses of blood volume than the normal infant. However, most asphyxiated infants are *not* hypovolemic, and it is often a challenge to assess the infant's circulatory status to determine whether hypovolemia is the cause of hypotension or whether the infant is suffering cardiovascular depression because of some other problem. Physiologic variables to be remembered are as follows:

1. There is an association of falsely high arterial blood pressure readings with acidosis (which may respond to sodium bicarbonate administration).
2. There is an association of hypocapnia with hypotension, so that infants who are being overventilated may have falsely low arterial blood pressure readings.
3. An infant with normal blood pressure who has poor perfusion may be maximally vasoconstricted; therefore, significant hypotension may be masked.
4. An infant who is distressed and in pain may have a falsely elevated blood pressure level.
5. The normal range of blood pressure for very small premature infants may be low (see Appendix 3). The physician should assume that the blood pressure is normal in infants with good oxygenation and good peripheral perfusion and no signs of circulatory collapse, particularly if the infant passes urine. In the infant who is not voiding, use of low-dose dopamine (2–5 μg/kg per minute) may help establish normotension.
6. Monitoring an infant's hematocrit levels over time can be enormously helpful. A decrease in hematocrit during the first 2 hours after birth may be an indication of hypovolemia, because infants have the ability to mobilize fluid rapidly.
7. Preterm newborn infants ordinarily do not exhibit

tachycardia as a sign of shock; therefore, a rapid heart rate generally is not useful as an indicator of volume status.

Support of the circulatory system and treatment of hypovolemic shock may be accomplished by the administration of small (10 mL/kg) transfusions of packed red blood cells. However, it is usually appropriate to give an initial infusion of 10 mL/kg of normal saline and to note the infant's response in blood pressure, peripheral perfusion, and oxygenation. Five percent albumin in saline may also be used while awaiting the availability of packed red cells. In administering volume replacement, it is of the utmost importance that it be given slowly, because some vascular beds (particularly those of the brain) may already be maximally dilated in response to systemic hypotension, and excessive pressure may be transmitted to the fragile capillaries, leading to intracranial hemorrhage.

In infants who have had prolonged or severe asphyxia, myocardial failure resulting from poor contractility may occur, evidenced by hypotension that persists after initial resuscitation. Such infants may respond to dopamine at a starting dose of 2.5 to 5 μg/kg per minute and increased as needed up to 15 to 20 μg/kg per minute to produce an adequate response. Rarely, dobutamine may be added at 5 μg/kg per minute (up to 15 μg/kg per minute). It may be useful in these infants to pass a second umbilical catheter through the umbilical vein, via the ductus venosus, into the right atrium to monitor central venous pressure in addition to arterial pressure.

Continuation of Support after Resuscitation

One of the factors essential to successful resuscitation is the ability to identify the infant who has continuing difficulties after resuscitation and, thus, to facilitate prevention of a relapse. This applies particularly to the premature infant with respiratory distress syndrome who initially responds favorably to treatment with ventilation and sodium bicarbonate but then requires continued cardiorespiratory support to prevent respiratory distress from becoming severe and causing another cycle of hypoxia and acidosis. Another example is in the infant born after undergoing an episode of fetal distress, who may have reactive pulmonary vasculature. If such an infant is allowed to become hypoxic, pulmonary vasoconstriction may occur (or worsen) and progress to persistent pulmonary hypertension of the newborn.

THINGS TO AVOID IN RESUSCITATION

Successful resuscitation of a newborn infant involves not only interrupting the cycle of hypoxia and acidemia and bringing the infant back toward the physiologic norm but also avoiding iatrogenic damage. There are, therefore, some important "rules" of resuscitation:

1. *Don't panic if an endotracheal tube cannot be placed immediately.* Concentrate on bag and mask ventilation and call for help. Do not assume that medication is a substitute for ventilation.
2. *Don't do excessive suctioning of clear fluid from the*

infant's nasopharynx. Fluid is normally absorbed into the lungs.

3. *Don't use excessive oxygen concentrations to resuscitate the premature infant unless the infant clearly requires it.*

4. *Don't use too much ventilatory pressure to expand the infant's lungs.* Initially this may briefly be significantly higher than it is within just 15 to 30 minutes after birth. Use good clinical judgment. Watch the infant's chest and listen to breath sounds. Try reducing ventilation with hand ventilation to ensure that the lowest pressure necessary is being used. Excessive pressure on lungs that are normalizing may decrease venous return to the heart and decrease cardiac output and cause injury to lung tissue.

5. *Avoid hypocapnia.* There is evidence that even brief overdistention of the lung may increase risk of bronchopulmonary dysplasia (Garland et al, 1995).

6. *Don't give volume or sodium bicarbonate automatically.* Each of these agents has been associated with production of intracranial hemorrhage in animal models.

7. *Don't focus or rely too heavily on cardiac resuscitation,* because, by far, the most likely problem in neonatal resuscitation is the need for ventilatory support.

8. *Don't withhold oxygen from the term or post-term infant with meconium aspiration or asphyxia,* who needs it because these infants may have reactive pulmonary blood vessels and pulmonary vasoconstriction may develop if oxygen administration is not generous.

SPECIAL CONDITIONS REQUIRING ATTENTION DURING RESUSCITATION
Extremely Premature Infant (<1000 g)

Resuscitation of the very premature infant begins in utero; therefore, whenever possible, such infants should be born in a perinatal center with skilled staff from the obstetric, anesthetic, and neonatal teams in attendance. The fragility of these infants requires gentleness in handling and a high level of skill in the staff performing the resuscitation. Because of their relatively large surface area, attention to immediate drying and temperature control is of even greater importance for these infants than for the normal newborn. When possible, they should be moved to a small warm room adjacent to the delivery room and carefully dried and placed under a radiant warmer for resuscitation. It is essential that the gas used for very small infants, even for resuscitation, be warmed and humidified. Many of these infants require immediate intubation as part of their resuscitation, and, in many centers, such infants are intubated routinely to enhance the clearance of lung water and the release of surfactant. If infants are intubated routinely, it is of great importance to avoid overventilation, which may cause interstitial emphysema or pneumothoraces as well as interfere with cardiac output. Other centers observe tiny infants briefly and provide respiratory support, particularly in the form of oxygen and continuous distending pressure via nasal prongs, if there is any evidence of respiratory deterioration. Particularly if the infants are known to be surfactant deficient, it would appear appropriate to initially intubate these tiny infants, give them surfactant, and then carefully evaluate their status to determine whether further respiratory support is needed. In resuscitating very small infants, it is also important to avoid hyperoxia; therefore, it is recommended that the oxygen blender be set at 40% when resuscitation is begun, then turned down as rapidly as possible, and thereafter increased only if the infant has clinical signs of cyanosis.

Most of these tiny infants also benefit from having an umbilical artery catheter placed so that the initial monitoring of their blood gases does not require painful procedures for obtaining blood or for the administration of fluid, drugs, or volume. At many centers, umbilical venous lines are also placed. Arterial blood pressure monitoring is important in this group of infants as an adjunct to assessing adequacy of circulating blood volume. The range of mean blood pressure for the tiny infant is wide and initially may be as low as 28 to 30 mm Hg. In an infant who is well oxygenated at low inspired oxygen concentrations and who has good peripheral perfusion, low blood pressure alone should never be used as the basis for volume administration. These infants should, however, have initial blood pressure support with low-dose dopamine (2 to 5 µg/kg per minute). Careful administration and monitoring of blood glucose concentrations are also critical.

Finally, it is important to move these infants from the resuscitation area to the nursery with as little disruption of their support systems as possible. Therefore, a resuscitation bed that is fully equipped to be moved from the delivery area to the nursery is essential to maintain stabilization. It also enables continuous observation of these fragile infants whose course may change rapidly during the first few hours after birth.

Meconium Aspiration

It is estimated that approximately 11% of all pregnancies are complicated by passage of meconium and that 2% of infants have some degree of aspiration syndrome, ranging from some minor initial tachypnea to very severe meconium aspiration pneumonia with pulmonary hypertension. There are two reasons why it is essential that skilled personnel are present at the delivery of an infant born through meconium:

1. It is critical that any *particulate* matter be removed from the infant's airway as rapidly as possible. A combined approach of suctioning of the nasopharynx on the perineum, followed by intubation and gentle tracheal suction, appears to be the most effective procedure for preventing obstruction of the airway and pneumonitis. It is *not* necessary to intubate an infant who is simply born through fluid that is stained with meconium but does not contain particulate material. Unnecessary intubation can cause iatrogenic damage. The most severe meconium aspiration pneumonias occur when an infant has passed a large amount of meconium in utero and is asphyxiated and gasping, thus moving large amounts of meconium into the thoracic airways before birth.

2. The passage of meconium indicates that an infant has been in trouble at some period in time. This group of infants is more susceptible to having reactive pulmonary vessels, which may reconstrict with hypoxia. They require careful initial evaluation and close observation to ensure that oxygenation is adequate and to prevent the gradual development of hypoxia and consequent pulmonary vasoconstriction, setting off the cycle that ultimately may result in persistent pulmonary hypertension of the newborn.

Hydrops

The evaluation and resuscitation of the infant with hydrops, as for very small premature infants, begins with interdisciplinary management by the perinatal team to assess the fetus and to arrive at decisions as to optimal time of delivery (see also Chapter 11). It is always appropriate to administer antenatal corticosteroids before delivery of these infants. Ultrasound evaluation is recommended to determine whether the infant would benefit from removal of excessive fluid from either the abdominal or thoracic cavity before delivery. In preparing for resuscitation of a hydropic infant, it is critical that equipment be set up and a member of the team assigned to perform either paracentesis or thoracentesis, or both, immediately after the birth, if the amount of fluid should interfere with the ability to ventilate the infant. In addition, it is essential to have packed red cells available at the resuscitation site if the cause of the hydrops is related to anemia. Hydropic infants have extremely stiff lungs and may require high ventilatory pressures, including high end-expiratory pressure, for initial stabilization. It is usually necessary to continue administering oxygen at high pressures until the infant begins to mobilize and clear fluid. It is always appropriate to administer surfactant as soon as possible after delivery. In severe cases, it may also be appropriate to have a dose of diuretic already drawn up and ready to administer in the delivery room. It is always appropriate to catheterize both the umbilical vein and umbilical artery so that central venous pressure, as well as systemic pressures, can be measured for evaluation of volume status. In addition, for severely anemic infants, the hematocrit can be augmented by immediate, isovolemic exchange transfusion through the two catheters. Staff should be aware that skin electrodes and saturation monitors frequently do not function accurately when used for infants with hydrops.

Infants with Severe Malformations

Sometimes the resuscitation team is faced with an infant who has severe malformations. Resuscitation should proceed in a normal fashion unless (1) the staff present at the delivery have enough experience and skill to recognize that the malformations are associated with conditions incompatible with life, and (2) there has been some foreknowledge of the possibility of malformations and the family has requested that there be no resuscitation of a severely malformed infant. Otherwise, it is appropriate to proceed with the resuscitation and stabilize the infant so that an accurate diagnosis can be made and the family can see the baby and participate in further decision-making about their child.

CONTROVERSIES IN RESUSCITATION
Administration of Sodium Bicarbonate

The routine use of sodium bicarbonate to treat asphyxiation in infants is clearly fraught with danger ranging from problems associated with hypernatremia and high osmotic load to those related to rapid shifts in volume and circulatory status of the infant. Complete avoidance of sodium bicarbonate, however, may delay an infant's recovery from severe asphyxia. Therefore, it is probably most reasonable to give bicarbonate with extreme caution.

Intubation of the Extremely Low-Birth-Weight Infant

Although many centers have adopted a policy to intubate and ventilate at birth all infants weighing less than 1000 g, there remains some controversy. Other centers prefer to stabilize and watch vigorous, extremely low-birth-weight infants (James, 1987) and only give respiratory support if signs of respiratory distress syndrome develop. Such centers recommend that an infant who is having retractions and other signs of distress have nasal prongs inserted for continuous positive airway pressure and oxygen administration to facilitate stabilization of the chest wall. As discussed previously, however, it has become standard procedure to give extremely low-birth-weight infants surfactant if they have any early evidence of distress, in which case intubation is necessary.

Resuscitation with Room Air Versus 100% Oxygen

Saugstad (1990) and others (Ramji et al, 1993; Saugstad, 1996) have recently raised concerns about the possibility that oxygen radicals produced in excess in the posthypoxic reoxygenation period may cause tissue damage, particularly to the brain. Animal data and some preliminary human clinical studies suggest that resuscitation with room air may be both effective and possibly even safer than with 100% oxygen.

Duration of Resuscitation

Resuscitation should rarely be continued beyond 15 to 20 minutes in an infant whose initial Apgar score is truly 0 and who does not respond rapidly to adequate ventilation, appropriate cardiac compression, and drugs. In infants who respond after this period of time, the incidence of death or very severe, irreversible, neurologic damage is unacceptably high.

LONG-TERM OUTCOME

The two central questions to be considered in thinking about the outcome of an infant after perinatal asphyxia are as follows:

1. What is the contribution of perinatal asphyxia to mental retardation and cerebral palsy in the population?

Prevalence Rate of Cerebral Palsy by Apgar Score and Birth Weight

Apgar Score	Infants < 2500 g			Infants > 2500 g		
	Mortality in 1st Year (Percent)	Percent of Survivors with Cerebral Palsy	Number of Cerebral Palsy Cases	Mortality in 1st Year (Percent)	Percent of Survivors with Cerebral Palsy	Number of Cerebral Palsy Cases
7–10 @ 1 minute	3.8	0.6	13	<1	0.2	53
0–3 @ 1 minute	50	2.9	9	6	1.5	22
0–3 @ 5 minutes	75	6.7	5	15	4.7	13
0–3 @ 10 minutes	85	3.7	1	34	16.7	11
0–3 @ 15 minutes	92	0	0	52	36.0	9
0–3 @ 20 minutes	96	0	0	59	57.1	8

Modified from Nelson KB, Ellenberg JH: Apgar scores as predictors of chronic neurologic disability. Pediatrics 68:36, 1981. Reproduced by permission of Pediatrics.

2. How often does documented perinatal asphyxia result in cerebral palsy and mental retardation?

Severe mental retardation without cerebral palsy does not appear to be related to perinatal asphyxia (Paneth and Stark, 1983), and only 10% to 15% of children with mental retardation were subject to perinatal asphyxia. In addition, at least 50% of infants with cerebral palsy had no documented respiratory depression at the time of birth.

The attempt to delineate which cases of perinatal asphyxia lead to cerebral palsy began in 1862 when Little noted the association of suboptimal perinatal events with subsequent poor neurologic outcome. A number of studies since that time have attempted to relate outcome to Apgar score, to the interval between birth and spontaneous respiration, and to various biochemical and biophysical markers of oxygen deprivation. The Collaborative Perinatal Project, conducted from 1959 to 1966 (Niswander et al, 1975), reported on the outcome of 49,000 infants as correlated with Apgar scores (Table 30–5). The conclusions of this study were that low Apgar scores are risk factors for cerebral palsy; however,

1. Fifty-five percent of children with cerebral palsy had Apgar scores of 7 to 10 at 1 minute.
2. Seventy-three percent of children with cerebral palsy had Apgar scores of 7 to 10 at 5 minutes.
3. Of 99 children who had Apgar scores of 0 to 3 at 10, 15, or 20 minutes, only 12 (12%) had cerebral palsy. However, the mortality rate in the last group was more than 50% in infants weighing more than 2500 g and more than 90% in infants of less than 2500 g.
4. Eleven of the 12 infants with cerebral palsy were mentally retarded.

Hypoxic Ischemic Encephalopathy

Sarnat and Sarnat (1975) developed a clinical staging system for evaluating hypoxic-ischemic encephalopathy (HIE) (Table 30–6), and Robertson and Finer (1985) reported on

Clinical Staging of Posthypoxic Encephalopathy

Factor	Stage I	Stage II	Stage III
Level of consciousness	Alert	Lethargic	Comatose
Muscle tone	Normal	Hypotonic	Flaccid
Tendon reflexes	Increased	Present	Depressed or absent
Myoclonus	Present	Present	Absent
Complex reflexes			
Sucking	Active	Weak	Absent
Moro response	Exaggerated	Incomplete	Absent
Grasping	Normal to exaggerated	Exaggerated	Absent
Oculocephalic response (doll's eyes)	Normal	Overreactive	Reduced or absent
Autonomic function			
Pupils	Dilated	Constricted	Variable or fixed
Respiration	Regular	Variations in rate and depth, periodic	Ataxic, apneic
Heart rate	Normal or tachycardia	Bradycardia	Bradycardia
Seizures	None	Common	Uncommon
Electroencephalogram	Normal	Low voltage, periodic and/or paroxysmal	Periodic or isoelectric

Modified from Sarnat HB, Sarnat MS: Neonatal encephalopathy following fetal distress. Arch Neurol 33:696, 1975. Copyright 1975, American Medical Association.

TABLE 30–7

Outcome 3 to 5 Years after Hypoxic-Ischemic Encephalopathy (HIE)

Severity of HIE	Number of Infants	Information Available at 3 to 5 Years	Number of Deaths	Outcome at 3 to 5 Years (Survivors)	
				Normal	**Handicapped**
Mild	79	69	0	69	0
Moderate	119	103	6°	75	22
Severe†	28	28	21	0	7
Total	226	200	27	144	29
				% Survivors	
Percent	100	88.5	13.5	83.2	16/8

°One death was due to an unrelated accident.
†All infants died or became handicapped.
 Classification from Sarnat HB, Sarnat MS: Neonatal encepalopathy following fetal distress. Arch Neurol 33:696, 1975. Adapted from Robertson C, Finer N: Term infants with hypoxic-ischemic encephalopathy: Outcome at 3–5 years. Dev Med Child Neurol 27:473, 1985.

the follow-up of infants after HIE (Table 30–7). Robertson and Finer found that 100% of infants with severe HIE either died or had significant handicap. Among those with moderate HIE, 26% died or were handicapped; among those with mild HIE, none died subsequently or were handicapped. Robertson and associates (1989) also noted no difference in school performance (at 8 years of age) between neurologically unimpaired children who suffered mild or moderate HIE and a matched peer group.

Holden and colleagues (1982) noted that the incidence of seizures was associated with a 17-fold increase in the likelihood of cerebral palsy compared with that found in infants without seizures. Evaluation using a modified Amiel-Tison examination (1973) at the time of discharge (around 2 weeks of age) can be predictive of abnormal outcome (Piecuch et al., 1987). Others (Perlman and Tack, 1988) have attempted to use injury to other organs as an indicator to help predict eventual outcome. They found that oliguria in the perinatal period was significantly associated with signs of HIE, including seizures, death, and long-term neurologic deficit. In general, it can be assumed that an infant who has experienced an asphyxial event severe enough to produce permanent brain damage will have evidence of significant damage to other organs within hours to days after birth.

Sunshine (1989) concluded that infants with perinatal asphyxia should be evaluated for structural abnormalities with current imaging techniques and that, if identified, an attempt should be made to determine whether the abnormalities can be explained on the basis of intrapartum asphyxia or are developmental aberrations or abnormalities that occurred before labor. In addition, he pointed out that infants who are small for gestational age comprise a significant percentage of the total patients who experience neonatal asphyxia, HIE, and seizures as well as cerebral palsy. Therefore, attempts to improve outcome should focus on recognition of infants who are small for gestational age and on possible types of intervention in pregnancies complicated by intrauterine growth retardation. Others have attempted to predict the degree of perinatal brain damage by measurement of substances presumed to be released in response to hypoxia and acidemia, including vasopressin, erythropoietin, and hypoxanthine. Whether cerebral palsy and mental retardation can result from perinatal asphyxia in the absence of neonatal encephalopathy is unknown, but it is unlikely. Many infants with moderate degrees of perinatal asphyxia do not exhibit encephalopathy, whereas others with similar degrees of fetal distress have severe encephalopathy.

The most accurate prediction comes from a full knowledge of perinatal and neonatal events, combined with biochemical and imaging studies and careful repeated clinical evaluations in the first years of life.

REFERENCES

American Academy of Pediatrics Committee on Drugs: Emergency drug doses for infants and children. Pediatrics 81:462, 1988.
Amiel-Tison C: Neurologic disorders in neonates associated with abnormalities of pregnancy and birth. Curr Probl Pediatr 3:1, 1973.
Apgar V: A proposal for new method for evaluation of the newborn infant. Anesth Analg 32:260, 1953.
Blair E, Stanley J: Intrapartum asphyxia: A rare cause of cerebral palsy. J Pediatr 112:515, 1988.
Bloom RS, Cropley CS: American Heart Association–American Academy of Pediatrics Textbook of Neonatal Resuscitation. Dallas, American Heart Association National Center, 1994.
Cabal LA, Devaskar U, Siassi B, et al: Cardiogenic shock associated with perinatal asphyxia in preterm infants. J Pediatr 96:705, 1980.
Carson BS, Lasey BW, Bowes WA, et al: Combined obstetric and pediatric approach to prevent meconium aspiration syndrome. Am J Obstet Gyencol 126:712, 1976.
Corbet A, Cregan J, Frink J: Distention-produced phospholipid secretion in postmortem in situ lungs of newborn rabbits. Am Rev Respir Dis 128:695, 1983.
Cunningham AS, Lawson EE, Martin RJ, Pildes RS: Tracheal suction and meconium: A proposed standard of care. (Discussion) J Pediatr 116:153, 1990.
Dale HH, Evans CL: Effects on the circulation of changes in carbon dioxide content of the blood. J Physiol 56:125, 1972.
Davis DJ: How aggressive should delivery room cardiopulmonary resuscitation be for extremely low-birth-weight neonates? Pediatrics 92:447–450, 1993.
Dawes G: Foetal and Neonatal Physiology. Chicago, Year Book Publishers, 1968.
Drew JH: Immediate intubation at birth of the very low birth weight infant: Effect on survival. Am J Dis Child 136:207, 1982.

Ellis WG, Goetzman BW, Lindenberg JA: Neuropathologic documentation of prenatal brain damage. Am J Dis Child 12:858, 1988.

Falcilia HS: Failure to prevent meconium aspiration syndrome. Obstet Gynecol 71:349, 1988.

Garland JS, Buck RK, Allred EN, Leviton A: Hypocarbia before surfactant therapy appears to increase bronchopulmonary dysplasia risk in infants with respiratory distress syndrome. Arch Pediatr Adolesc Med 149:617–623, 1995.

Greenough H, Lagercrantz H, Pool J, et al: Plasma catecholamine levels in preterm infants: Effect of birth asphyxia and Apgar score. Acta Paediatr Scand 76:54, 1987.

Gregory GA, Gooding CA, Phibbs RH, et al: Meconium aspiration in infants: A prospective study. J Pediatr 85:807, 1974.

Hack MN, Fanaroff AA: Changes in the delivery room care of the extremely small infant (less than 750 g). Effects on morbidity and outcome. N Engl J Med 314:660, 1986.

James LS: Emergencies in the delivery room. In Fanaroff AA, Martin RJ (Eds): Neonatal-Perinatal Medicine, 4th ed. St Louis, CV Mosby, 1987, pp 360–378.

Karlberg P: The adaptive changes in the immediate postnatal period, with particular reference to respiration. J Pediatr 56:585, 1960.

Kitterman JA, Phibbs RH, Tooley WH: Catheterization of umbilical vessels in newborn infants. Pediatr Clin North Am 17:895, 1970.

Lagercrantz H, Slotkin TA: The "stress" of being born. Sci Am 254:100, 1986.

Lindemann R: Resuscitation of the newborn with endotracheal administration of epinephrine. Acta Paediatr Scand 73:210, 1984.

Linder N, Aranda JV, Tsur M, et al: Need for endotracheal intubation and suction in meconium-stained neonates. J Pediatr 112:613–615, 1988.

Little WJ: On the influence of abnormal parturition, difficult labours, premature birth, and asphyxia neonatorum on the mental and physical condition of the child, especially in relation to deformities. Trans Obstet Soc (London) 3:293, 1861–1862.

Martinez A, Padbury J, Shames L, et al: Naloxone potentiates epinephrine release during hypoxia in fetal sheep: Dose response and cardiovascular effects. Pediatr Res 23:343, 1988.

Massaro GD, Massaro D: Morphologic evidence that large inflations of the lung stimulate secretion of surfactant. Ann Rev Respir Dis 127:235, 1983.

McCrirrick A, Kestin I: Haemodynamic effects of tracheal compared with intravenous adrenaline. Lancet 340:868–870, 1992.

Nelson KB: What proportion of cerebral palsy is related to birth asphyxia? J Pediatr 112:572, 1988.

Newnham JP, Marshall CL, Padbury JF, et al: Fetal catecholamine release with preterm delivery. Am J Obstet Gynecol 149:888, 1984.

Niswander KR, Gordon M, Drage JS: The effect of intrauterine hypoxia on the child surviving to 4 years. Am J Obstet Gynecol 121:892, 1975.

Paneth N, Fox HE: The relationship of Apgar score to neurologic handicap: A survey of clinicians. Obstet Gynecol 61:547, 1983.

Paneth N, Stark RI: Cerebral palsy and mental retardation in relation to indicators in perinatal asphyxia. Am J Obstet Gynecol 147:960, 1983.

Perlman JM, Risser R: Cardiopulmonary resuscitation in the delivery room. Arch Pediatr Adolesc Med 149:2025, 1995.

Perlman JM, Tack ED: Renal injury in the asphyxiated newborn infant: Relationship to neurologic outcome. J Pediatr 113:875, 1988.

Phibbs RH: Delivery room management of the newborn. In Avery, GB (Ed): Neonatology, 3rd ed. Philadelphia, JB Lippincott, 1985, pp 215–234.

Piecuch R, Leonard C, et al: Predicting neurodevelopmental outcome in infants with severe perinatal asphyxia. Pediatr Res 21:401A, 1987.

Ramji S, Ahuja S, Thirupuram S, et al: Resuscitation of asphyxic newborn infants with room air or 100% oxygen. Pediatr Res 34:809–812, 1993.

Robertson C, Finer N: Term infants with hypoxic-ischemic encephalopathy: Outcome at 3–5 years. Dev Med Child Neurol 27:473, 1985.

Robertson CMT, Finer NN, Grace MGA: School performance of survivors of neonatal encephalopathy associated with birth asphyxia at term. J Pediatr 114:753, 1989.

Rootwelt T, Loberg EM, Moen A, Saugstad OS: Hypoxemia and reoxygenation with 21% or 100% oxygen in newborn pigs: Changes in blood pressure, base deficit and hypoxanthine and brain morphology. Pediatr Res 32:107–113, 1992.

Rosen MG: Factors during labor and delivery that influence brain disorders. In Freeman JM (Ed): Prenatal and Perinatal Factors Associated with Brain Disorders. Bethesda, MD, NIH Publication No. 85–1149, April, 1985, pp 237–262.

Rossi EM, Philipson EH, Williams TG, et al: Meconium aspiration syndrome: Intrapartum and neonatal attributes. Am J Obstet Gynecol 161:1106–1110, 1989.

Ruth V, Sutti-Ramo I, Granstrom M-L, et al: Prediction of perinatal brain damage by cord plasma vasopressin, erythropoietin and hypoxanthine levels. J Pediatr 113:880, 1988.

Sarnat HB, Sarnat MS: Neonatal encephalopathy following fetal distress. Arch Neurol 33:696, 1975.

Saugstad OD: Oxygen toxicity in the neonatal period. Acta Paediatr Scand 79:881–892, 1990.

Saugstad OD: Resuscitation of newborn infants; do we need new guidelines? Prenatal Neonatal Med 1:26–28, 1996.

Seri I: Cardiovascular, renal, and endocrine actions of dopamine in neonates and children: Medical progress. J Pediatr 126:333–344, 1995.

Sola A, Spitzer AR, Morin FC, et al: Effects of arterial carbon dioxide tension on the newborn lamb's cardiovascular responses to rapid hemorrhage. Pediatr Res 17:70, 1983.

Strang LB: Neonatal Respiration: Physiological and Clinical Studies. Oxford, Blackwell Scientific, 1977.

Sunshine P: Epidemiology of perinatal asphyxia. In Stevenson DK, Sunshine P (Eds): Fetal and Neonatal Brain Injury. Philadelphia, BC Decker, 1989.

Taeusch HW, Wyszogrodski I, Wang NS, et al: Pulmonary pressure-volume relationships in premature fetal and newborn rabbits. J Appl Physiol 37:809, 1974.

Thiebault DW, Hall TK, Sheehan MB, et al: Postasphyxial lung disease in newborn infants with severe perinatal acidosis. Am J Obstet Gynecol 150:393, 1984.

Vyas H, Millner AD, Hopkin IE, et al: Physiologic responses to prolonged and slow-rise inflation in the resuscitation of the asphyxiated newborn infant. J Pediatr 99:635, 1981.

Walters DV, Olver RE: The role of catecholamines in lung liquid absorption at birth. Pediatr Res 12:239, 1978.

Weil MH, Rackrow EC, Trevino R, et al: Difference in acid base state between venous and arterial blood during cardiopulmonary resuscitaton. N Engl J Med 315:153, 1986.

Wiswell TE, Tuggle JM, Turner BS: Meconium aspiration syndrome: Have we made a difference? Pediatrics 85:715–721, 1990.

CHAPTER 31

Initial Evaluation

HISTORY AND PHYSICAL EXAMINATION OF THE NEWBORN

H. William Taeusch and Susan Sniderman

Most newborns infants are normal, that is free from disease or birth defects. Most are able to adapt easily to extrauterine life. Most parents, while having some degree of ambivalence, are excited by their newborn child and are able to care for the infant. When this scenario pertains, physicians must offer parents support and information about the major issues, risks, and achievements that they can expect for their infant over the next few months.

When an infant is born prematurely or is found to have anomalies or illnesses, the history and physical examination may have to be done concurrently with informing the parents of the infant's problems and likely course.

Specifics of the examination of various systems are given throughout this book. Therefore, the points relevant to newborns, particularly sick and anomalous infants, are emphasized in this chapter.

EMERGENCY ASSESSMENT

Assessment of the newborn includes routine evaluation of a healthy full-term infant nearing the time of discharge or emergency assessment of a gray, evidently lifeless, 500-g newborn in the delivery room. The impressions gained in the first seconds and minutes often dictate the speed with which further assessment and treatment must occur. A rapid assessment including both a brief history and physical examination is warranted whenever an infant has an acute change in status. The evaluation should not impede attention to the infant's immediate needs. It is a novice's mistake to suspect overwhelming sepsis, then to take several hours to do the history and physical examination and a leisurely lumbar puncture before ensuring that antibiotics have been given to the infant. Another mistake is to wait for a chest radiograph to be obtained when an infant has hypotension with a clinically evident tension pneumothorax. A third mistake is to allow an infant to suffer thermal and oxygen insufficiency while hidden under sterile drapes during a protracted insertion of an umbilical artery catheter. A list of perinatal and postnatal conditions necessitating emergency assessment is given in Table 31–1. Delivery room assessment and resuscitation are discussed in Chapter 30.

HISTORY

The first interview with the parents should occur, whenever possible, before birth. With rapidly expanding genetic diagnostic capabilities and identification of high-risk fetuses with prenatal ultrasonography, the need for pediatricians to meet with the parents before birth is increasing in frequency.

The first evaluation of the newborn infant is often said to be the most important routine examination that a person receives in his or her lifetime. If the infant is sick or has anomalies, this statement is particularly pertinent. However, for well infants, remarkably few studies have examined which elements of the initial history and physical examination are most important and which professional personnel should conduct them. If the infant is born at term with no complications, the parents are delighted with the good news. If the infant requires intensive care (approximately 3% of live births), the tendency to focus on ventilators, monitors, laboratory tests, radiographs, and ultrasounds makes it difficult for the parents to focus on more mundane but possibly very important and pertinent medical history. Frequently, infants enter the neonatal intensive care unit (NICU) without the parents having been able to anticipate this occurrence. When the parents first visit the NICU, they confront a strange environment in which the life of their infant is entrusted to nurses and doctors not known to them. Both parents may be exhausted and anxious in the hours after the delivery, at the time they become aware that the infant is seriously ill. Some parents are fatalistic and accept opinions about diagnosis and prognosis less out of trust than a belief that they can little affect events. Others attempt to exert control over the caregivers in the belief that their infant's plight can be fixed if they (the parents) can only force the correct decisions and treatments to be made.

Therefore, the style with which the initial interview is conducted must be adapted to the parents' needs as well as to those of the infant, and the interview serves several purposes. First, it allows the collection of information that affects the management of the infant. Second, a therapeutic bond may be formed with the parents, the first stage in enlisting them as allies rather than adversaries in the days, weeks, and possibly months ahead while the infant is in the NICU. Third, an initial assessment of the adequacy of the home and the parents with regard to the care of the infant can be made. Fourth, the interview provides the opportunity for the parents to receive an initial report on the status of the infant.

If the infant is being transferred to another hospital, giving the mother a belonging of the infant (e.g., a bracelet or Polaroid picture) can help her to contend with the birth and immediate loss (to the NICU) of her infant. Realistically allaying parental anxiety about their infant's condition on the first interview is often not possible, but the manner and conduct of the history-taking can help the parents feel that their infant will receive competent care. Frightening though the illness or anomaly may be, the parents' conception of their infant's problem may be even more frightening, thus some reassurance can be offered in

TABLE 31–1

Neonatal Conditions Requiring Emergency Assessment

Probably lethal conditions	Anencephaly or hydranencephaly, severe hydrops with hypoplastic lungs, extremely low birth weight (previability), known 13 and 18 trisomies, and nonresponsiveness to resuscitation
Respiratory conditions	
Airway obstruction	Mucus, meconium, kinked endotracheal tube, webs, cysts, large tongue, stenosis, tumors, and vascular rings
Space-occupying lesions	Pneumothorax, pleural effusions, tracheoesophageal fistula, diaphragmatic hernia, adenomatoid malformation, and tumors
Insufficient respiratory drive	Immaturity, asphyxia, maternal drugs, central nervous system depression, and neuromuscular disease
Parenchymal disease	Respiratory distress syndrome, meconium aspiration pneumonia, infectious pneumonitis, and hypoplastic lungs
Cardiovascular conditions	Hypovolemia or hypotension, bradycardia or other arrhythmia, hydrops and congestive heart failure, decreased pulmonary blood flow due to structural cyanotic congenital heart disease or persistent pulmonary hypertension, and anemia or hyperviscosity

most cases, especially after the parents have seen their infant. Novice caregivers, as a symptom of their own insecurity, may emphasize data in these discussions. This tactic, particularly at the first meeting, usually does more harm than good. The error of the opposite approach is to patronize the parents in an abbreviated interview. The worst mistake is to minimize contact with the parents altogether.

Usually, parents are justly intolerant of the professional who waits until after all history-taking, examinations, and laboratory data are in hand before giving them any notion of the problems. It may be wise to start an interview with an overview and follow with the history-taking. At the conclusion of the interview, the clinician should outline the next steps (diagnostic and therapeutic), describe real and potential problems, seek questions from the parents, and close with plans for the next contact.

The initial history and physical examination are screening tools. All systems and areas of the body are evaluated in a feed-forward mode; that is, if the initial screen is positive (e.g., with the heart or lungs), then that system immediately receives a more thorough evaluation, not only through the physical examination, but also through expansion of the history and laboratory examinations. The equally weighted and relentlessly thorough history and physical examination of the compulsive novice are rightfully replaced by a balanced examination suitable for the individual circumstances of the infant.

The examiner, throughout the history and physical examination, seeks answers to a series of questions, the first and most important of which is whether the infant is acutely ill. Next, the examiner seeks whether there is a problem with regard to the following:

- Any specific organ system
- Infection
- Inadequate oxygen or nutrients (acute or chronic)
- Abnormal in utero environment
- Growth
- Anomalies or genetic disease
- Trauma
- Maturity
- Transition from in utero existence
- Home environment

The history, physical examination, and laboratory evaluations are never complete with sick infants in an intensive care setting. Information is constantly being compiled from diagnostic studies, physicians, nurses, respiratory therapists, family members, and so forth. Integration of these data with clear and appropriate communication is one of the hardest tasks to learn. One of the best techniques is the use of careful, succinct, system- or problem-oriented, dated, and timed notes in the infant's hospital chart, including information about what has been told to the parents and their particular concerns.

MATERNAL HISTORY

The history of the newborn is principally the history of the mother's pregnancy, general health, and prior pregnancies. Table 31–2 outlines the array of maternal conditions that can affect the newborn. Maternal influences on the fetus are thoroughly reviewed by Creasy and Resnick (1989).

The major problem of newborns throughout the world is that of low birth weight and prematurity. The complex and interrelated risk factors for low birth weight are summarized in Table 31–3, and each of these factors is important. If present in the maternal history, their relative weight has to be individualized because none of the items listed is necessarily associated with preterm delivery.

Prenatal Care

The reasons why only some women receive prenatal care are of vital interest. Even though birth weight–specific mortality in the United States is among the world's lowest, the high neonatal mortality rate is directly related to a high rate of low-birth-weight deliveries. Deficient or absent prenatal care is associated with an increased risk of prematurity. All people who care for mothers and infants share a responsibility for disseminating these facts and uncovering and correcting the causes of late or absent prenatal care.

Duration of Pregnancy

Estimates of gestational length should be obtained from the date of the mother's last menstrual period, date of quickening, that is, when the mother first feels the fetus move (16 to 18 weeks), and the first occurrence of fetal heart sounds (14 to 16 weeks with a fetoscope) and ultrasound measurements. Nägele's rule is used to estimate the time of term delivery by subtracting 3 calendar months from the 1st day of the last menstrual period and adding 7 days. The fundus is usually at the umbilicus by the 5th month after the last menstrual period.

TABLE 31–2

Maternal History

Social, educational, and economic factors
  Age, race, primary language, work, stress, education, religion, reasons for becoming pregnant, preparation for infant care, home support, health care access, and history of child abuse
Behavioral factors and habits
  Smoking, drugs, alcohol, and exercise (duration and amount)
Exposure to toxins or teratogens
  Radiation, radiochemicals, hormones (including diethylstilbestrol), thyroid suppressants, aminopterin, anticancer agents, mercury, chlorobiphenyls and other organic substances, hydantoins, coumarin, and Accutane
Nutrition
  Diet, vitamin and mineral supplements, and weight gain
Genetic/familial disorders (See Table 31–4)
Chronic medical problems predating pregnancy outcome of prior pregnancies
  Fetal death, twins, prematurity, blood group incompatibilities, and birth weight or gestational age of prior children
Prenatal care
  Number of visits, trimester of first visit, ultrasound examinations.
Problems of current pregnancy°
  Central nervous system or psychiatric, endocrine (diabetes, thyroid status, or thyroid medication), metabolic (cholestasis), cardiopulmonary (mitral insufficiency or asthma), hypertensive disorders, preeclampsia, hematologic (anemia, Rh incompatibility, and idiopathic or alloimmune thrombocytopenia), third-trimester bleeding (placenta previa, abruptio placentae, or ruptured uterus), immunologic (lupus), surgery or trauma, infections, medications (tocolytics, glucocorticoids, antibiotics, or antihypertensives), renal, neoplastic, and reproductive (incompetent cervix and hydramnios or oligohydramnios)
Special tests during pregnancy
  Ultrasound examinations, karyotyping, alpha-fetoprotein, chorionic villus biopsy, percutaneous umbilical blood sampling of the fetus, stress and nonstress testing, amniotic fluid testing for bilirubin, fetal lung maturity, and biophysical profile
Infection screening
  Rubella, syphilis, acquired immunodeficiency syndrome, toxoplasmosis, herpes, hepatitis B, cytomegalovirus, tuberculosis, and gonorrhea (for close contacts as well as mother)
Onset and events of labor
  Fetal heart rate monitoring, fetal scalp pH, meconium, rupture of membranes, amnioinfusion, fever, maternal oxygen, vena cava decompression, blood pressure, ventilation, analgesia or anesthesia, other medications, and duration of stages of labor (1 = onset to full cervical dilation, 2 = dilation to delivery, and 3 = delivery to delivery of placenta), and mode of delivery

°Pregnancy-associated diseases and fetal exposure to tobacco, marijuana, alcohol, or illicit drugs are included on the U.S. Standard Certificates of Live Birth and Fetal Death (Freedman et al, 1988).

Genetic and Familial Factors

A history of genetic and familial disorders is becoming increasingly important as diagnosis of genetic disease of the fetus during pregnancy becomes more widely available (see Part IV). Table 31–4 illustrates a screening history adapted from the one recommended by the American College of Obstetricians and Gynecologists.

Complications of Pregnancy

Complications of pregnancy (e.g., gestational diabetes mellitus, preeclampsia) may place the fetus at risk for specific abnormalities after birth such as hypoglycemia or intrauterine growth retardation. Medications used to treat other complications may be important because they may have certain effects on the fetus (e.g., hydantoin causes dysmorphic features; diuretics may cause fetal thrombocytopenia). Even though they may be subclinical in the mother, infectious illnesses may lead to the birth of an infant with evidence of chronic in utero infection.

TABLE 31–3

Principal Risk Factors for Low Birth Weight

  I. Demographic risks
    A. Age (<18 or >35)
    B. Ethnicity
    C. Low socioeconomic status
    D. Unmarried
    E. Low level of education
 II. Medical risks predating pregnancy
    A. Parity (0 or >4)
    B. Low weight for height
    C. Genitourinary problems, renal insufficiency, or surgery
    D. Selected diseases, e.g., diabetes and hypertension
    E. Nonimmune status, e.g., rubella
    F. Poor obstetric history, including previous low-birth-weight baby or multiple abortions
    G. Maternal genetic factors, e.g., the mother herself was a low-birth-weight infant
III. Medical risks in current pregnancy
    A. Multiple pregnancy
    B. Poor weight gain
    C. Short interpregnancy interval
    D. Hypotension
    E. Hypertension, preeclampsia, or toxemia
    F. Infections, e.g., rubella, symptomatic bacteriuria, or cytomegalovirus infection
    G. First- or second-trimester bleeding
    H. Placental problems, such as placenta previa or abruptio placentae
    I. Hyperemesis
    J. Oligohydramnios or polyhydramnios
    K. Anemia or abnormal hemoglobin
    L. Isoimmunization
    M. Fetal anomalies
    N. Incompetent cervix
    O. Spontaneous premature rupture of membranes
IV. Behavioral and environmental risks
    A. Smoking
    B. Poor nutritional status
    C. Alcohol and other substance abuse, particularly cocaine
    D. Diethylstilbestrol exposure and exposure to other toxins
    E. High altitude
 V. Health care risks
    A. Insufficient prenatal care
    B. Iatrogenic prematurity
VI. Other possible correlates of premature labor
    A. Physical and psychosocial stress or abuse
    B. Uterine irritability
    C. Cervical changes before labor
    D. Infections, e.g., with *Mycoplasma* and *Chlamydia*
    E. Plasma volume
    F. Progesterone
    G. Immune interactions between the mother and fetus

Adapted from Institute of Medicine Committee to Study the Prevention of Low Birthweight: Preventing Low Birthweight. Washington, DC, National Academy Press, 1985.

TABLE 31–4

Maternal Prenatal Genetic Screen

1. Are you over 34 years of age?
2. Has anyone in your family or the father's family had: Down syndrome ("mongolism"), chromosome problems or abnormalities, back (midline) defects at birth or later in life (spina bifida), prolonged or excessive bleeding (hemophilia), muscle weakness problems (muscular dystrophy), or childhood lung problems (cystic fibrosis)?
3. Do you or does the baby's father have a birth defect? Do family members of you or the father have birth defects of any kind?
4. Have any members of your family, the father's family, or any of your prior infants had other problems that were inherited or "passed down" through family members to their children?
5. Do you or the baby's father have any close relatives with mental retardation or trouble learning in school?
6. Have you or the father ever been tested for these genetic problems [relevant to specific ethnic group]: Tay-Sachs disease, sickle cell trait or disease, or beta-thalassemia?
7. Have you lost any early pregnancies (miscarriages)?

Adapted from American College of Obstetricians and Gynecologists: Antenatal Diagnosis of Genetic Disorders. ACOG Technical Bulletin No. 108. Washington, DC, ACOG, 1987, p 3.

General Health of Mother

In the same way, long-term chronic diseases in the mother may have important consequences for her infant. A mother with systemic lupus erythematosus may have certain antibodies that may cause heart block in the fetus, or a mother with long-standing renal disease may have a growth-retarded infant. Even diseases that have resolved in the mother (e.g., Graves' disease and idiopathic thrombocytopenic purpura) may continue to affect the fetus because of the presence of serum factors that persist and cross the placenta, causing problems in the fetus and newborn infant.

Onset and Events of Labor

The timing and events that occur around the onset of labor are important. Examples include a car accident, premature rupture of membranes, or sharp, near-continuous low back pain with vaginal bleeding. Indications for risk of acute infections to the fetus should be sought. Has the mother had a recent infection? Did she have a fever around the time of delivery? Has she received antibiotics? How long did labor last and how long were the membranes ruptured?

The fetal heart rate in conjunction with uterine contractions is the best signal during labor of the condition of the fetus (see Chapter 13). Adjuncts include use of fetal scalp pH.

The presentation of the fetus in the birth canal and the route of delivery are of obvious importance. Breech position occurs in 8% of women in labor. In approximately 25% of breech deliveries, conditions such as placenta previa, malformations of the fetus or uterus, twinning, or premature labor may coexist. Risks of vaginal delivery for the fetus in the breech position include prolapse of the cord, trapping of the head at the level of the cervix, asphyxia, trauma, and congenital hip dysplasia.

Amniotic Fluid

The infant at term is immersed in about 1 L of amniotic fluid. Its sources are fetal urine, lung secretions, and transudate from surrounding membranes. Before birth, ultrasound assessment of amniotic fluid volume is part of the biophysical profile. Although standards vary, normal volumes are associated with one or more pockets of fluid with a total vertical diameter of greater than 4 cm. Oligohydramnios is indicated by less than 500 mL of fluid. Polyhydramnios indicates more than 2 L of fluid at birth. Near term, the fetus drinks approximately 125 mL/kg body weight of amniotic fluid per day (equivalent to volume of postnatal milk intake). The fluid has a pH of 7.2 and is alkaline with respect to vaginal fluid. Therefore leakage of amniotic fluid from the vagina can be tested by checking the pH of the fluid.

Oligohydramnios or polyhydramnios is most common when fetal swallowing or micturition is increased or decreased. Either condition can be a matter of degree and is best assessed with fetal ultrasound. Phelan and colleagues (1987) describe the simplest method in which the largest pocket of fluid visualized by ultrasound in each of four uterine quadrants is summed. If the sum is less than 6 cm, oligohydramnios is diagnosed. Causes of oligohydramnios include conditions in which there is decreased urination (e.g., bilateral cystic dysplastic kidneys, posterior urethral valves, maternal indomethacin use), severe placental insufficiency, and chronic leaking of amniotic fluid resulting from premature membrane rupture. The consequences of oligohydramnios include joint contractures and limb deformities, lung hypoplasia, and Potter facies. Conditions listed in Table 31–5 are associated with polyhydramnios. High intestinal obstruction and anencephaly (presumably caused by decreased clearance of amniotic fluid by swallowing) are the most common.

TABLE 31–5

Conditions Associated with Polyhydramnios

Agnathia
Anencephaly and other central nervous system defects
Beckwith-Wiedemann syndrome
Chylothorax
Conjoined twins
Cystic adenomatoid malformation of the lung
Diaphragmatic hernia
Fetal akinesia
Fetal death
Hydrops
Gastroschisis
Hemangioma
Maternal diabetes
Obstructive teratoma
Trisomies
Tumors of the lungs, placenta, or ovaries
Umbilical cord compression
Upper gastrointestinal obstruction (e.g., duodenal atresia)
Werdnig-Hoffmann disease

Timing of Umbilical Cord Clamping

Many events affect the relative volume of blood left in the newborn versus the placenta after birth. Prenatal asphyxia shifts blood from the placenta to the fetus, and, in these cases, because of the need to suction meconium and resuscitate the infant, no delay in cord clamping appears to be useful. In normal infants, if the cord is clamped within 5 seconds of delivery before a contraction compresses the placenta and if the infant is held well above the mother's introitus before cord clamping, then the infant may be hypovolemic. In contrast, if the obstetrician zealously "strips" the cord toward the infant and delays clamping it, the resulting shift of blood volume from the placenta to the newborn may result in polycythemia, delayed absorption of lung fluid, and hyperbilirubinemia. Despite years of research, there is little consensus on the optimal timing of cord clamping. In the absence of asphyxia or isoimmunization, 30 to 45 seconds is a reasonable period to lapse while the infant is held at the level of the introitus. This interval usually allows for an inspiratory gasp on the part of the newborn and a uterine contraction on the part of the mother—both occurrences favor transfer of blood from the placenta to the newborn (Table 31–6). The obstetrician can suction the nares and oropharynx during this period. Few pediatricians and obstetricians note the timing and nature of the separation of the newborn infant from the placenta, although it would be helpful in infants with anemia or polycythemia.

Blood volumes are between 85 and 100 mL/kg of body weight in term infants and up to 110 mL/kg in preterm infants. Values can be 35% higher with large shifts of blood volume from the placenta. At term, 75 to 100 mL (20 to 35 mL/kg) of blood is available to the newborn from the placenta.

PLACENTA AND UMBILICAL CORD

The problems of the placenta are discussed in Chapter 6. The placenta at term (cord and membranes excised 2 cm from the insertion) weighs between 400 and 500 g, with approximately 50% the weight representing maternal blood

and approximately 15% composed of fetal blood. When the fetal-placental weight ratio at birth is greater than 10, it implies that nutrient delivery and gas exchange may have been suboptimal. The cord may demonstrate one umbilical artery (0.7% of live births), true knots, evidence of vascular rupture, cord compression, hematoma, or edema. In some infants with intrauterine growth retardation, the cord and chorionic plate may be stained greenish-brown, the cord may be long and thin, and diminished Wharton jelly may be present. The insertion of the cord may be central or marginal, or incorporated into the membranes (velamentous), sometimes with vasa praevia (splitting of the vessels in the membranes before insertion into the placenta). The umbilical cord is usually greater than 40 cm in length at term, and shorter cords may indicate relative fetal akinesia from a variety of causes, the inference being that fetal activity contributes to lengthening of the cord. Amniotic membranes may show evidence of banding or thickening, often in association with amniotic fluid infection. In twins, there may be no membrane between cord insertions (monochorionic, monoamniotic), a thin transparent membrane (diamniotic), or a thick but separable opaque membrane (dichorionic, diamniotic).

PHYSICAL EXAMINATION

The examiner always faces the dilemma of needing to be thorough versus needing to be gentle and quick so as not to destabilize the smallest and sickest infants. The physical examination of newborn infants is tailored to fit both the gestation and the postnatal age of an infant. The evaluation in the delivery room of a gasping 25-week premature infant is different from the routine examination at 12 hours of age of a full-term infant in the well baby nursery. (Compare Figures 31–1, 31–2, and 31–3 with the full-term infants in subsequent figures, then look at Figure 31–4.) The clinician needs patience to return frequently to do parts of the examination in order to stay within the limits of an infant's tolerance. It is fruitless to examine the abdomen of a crying infant and risky to do the same examination after a full feeding. At the same time, it is embarrassing to miss an imperforate anus or extra digits in an infant whose respiratory problems have captivated initial interest. An outline of a complete history and physical examination is given in Table 31–7.

Nosocomial Infection

Before touching an infant for any purpose, hand-washing should be carried out after removal of rings and watches. The hand-washing should occur immediately before and immediately after the examination. A "low level of mysophobia" is prevalent among nursery personnel, and this no doubt contributes to the nosocomial infection rate that approaches 50% for small sick infants who have spent more than several months in an NICU. If the prevalence of hand-washing is suboptimal in most nurseries, the use of insufficiently cleaned stethoscopes and other equipment is ever present. With concern provoked by the prevalence of acquired immunodeficiency syndrome (AIDS), many nurseries use universal precautions, meaning that a fresh gown and gloves are used for each direct contact of each

---

TABLE 31–6

Factors Determining Neonatal and Placental Blood Volume

Prenatal drugs (e.g., ergot derivatives)
Maternal vascular disease (preeclampsia or diabetes)
Placental and fetal size
Maternal hypotension
Fetal asphyxia or placental insufficiency
Rate of umbilical artery constriction
Position of fetus relative to placenta
Uterine contractions (frequency, amplitude, duration, and baseline)
Time of cord clamping
Neonatal cardiac output
Fetal blood volume (hydrops)
Time of placental separation
Route of delivery
Cord compression
Timing of first breaths relative to cord clamping

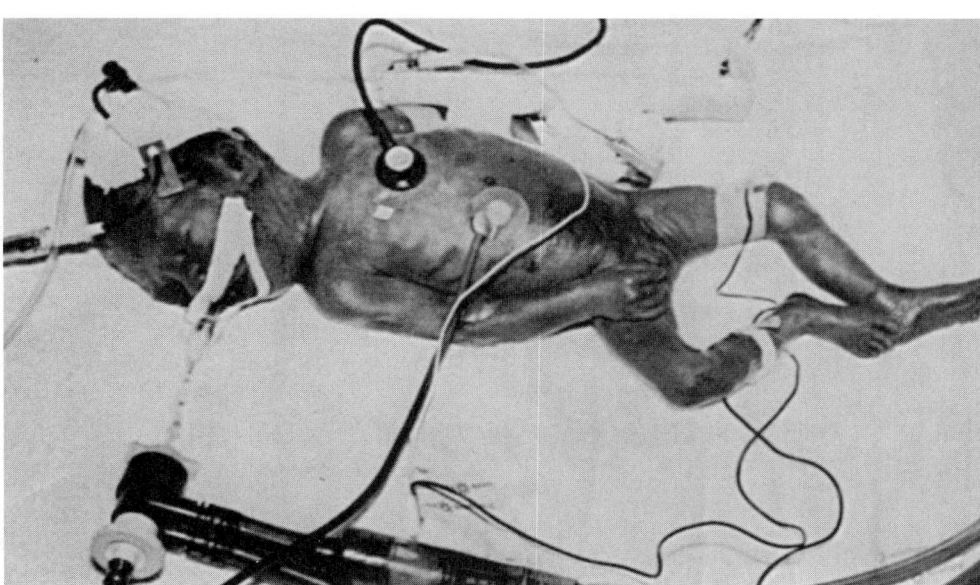

FIGURE 31–1. The problems of physical examination are illustrated by comparing this 25-week, 710-g infant (A.W.) with respiratory distress syndrome with the full-term newborn in Figure 31–5. The story of this premature infant is the subject of a book entitled *Born Early.* (From *Born Early: The Story of a Premature Baby,* by Mary Ellen Avery, MD, and Georgia Litwack. Copyright © 1983 by Mary Ellen Avery, MD, and Georgia Litwack. By permission of Little, Brown and Company.)

patient, whether or not direct handling of bodily fluids occurs. Reason dictates that patients should receive at least the same protection against common nosocomial bacteria as caregivers afford themselves against the much smaller risk of AIDS.

Vital Signs

Vital signs are usually assigned the first place in write-ups of the physical examination. For small sick newborns, single measurements are less important than trends, and these

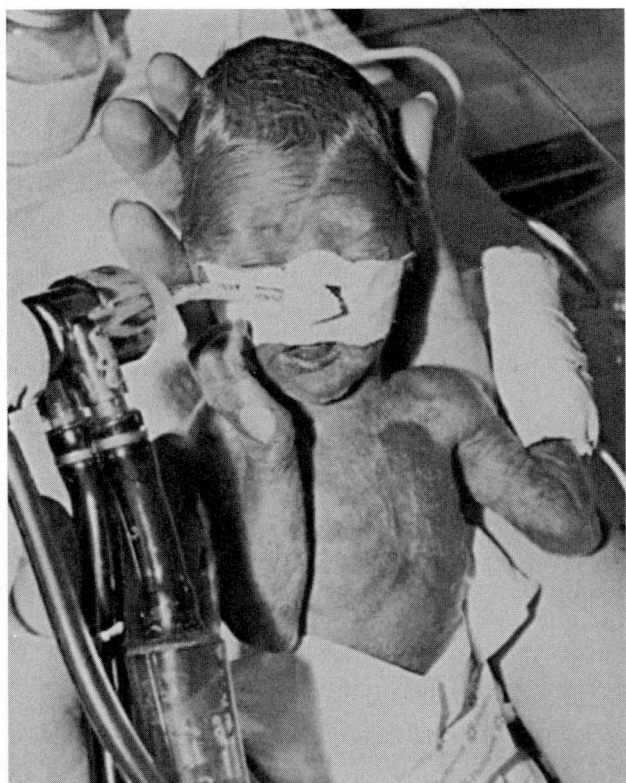

FIGURE 31–2. The infant (A.W.) is shown after the first week of life. Note the size of the skull relative to the adult hand supporting the head. Abundant lanugo hair is evident. (Courtesy of G. Litwack.)

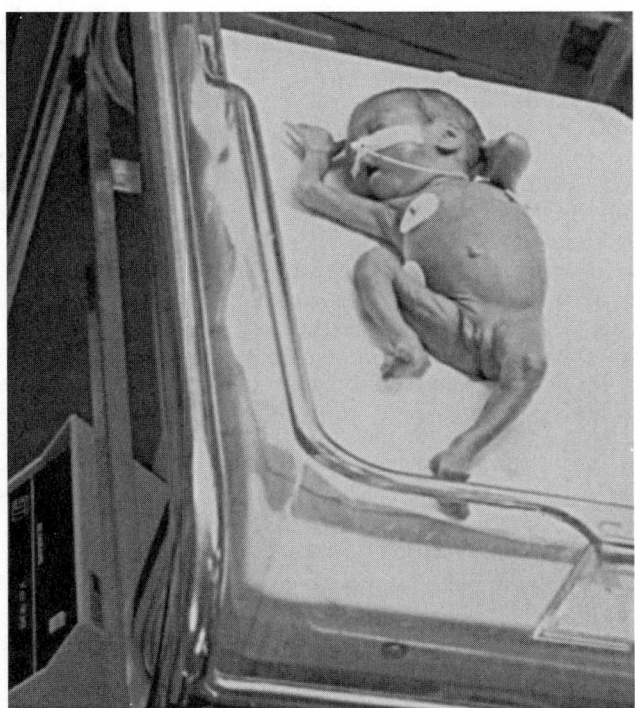

FIGURE 31–3. The infant (A.W.) at 6 weeks of age and 850 g. She required 33 days of ventilator support and had surgical ligation of a patent ductus arteriosus. With the head to the right, the infant manifests a strong spontaneous tonic neck reflex posture. The infant required an incubator for temperature control but is shown here during a weight measurement. (Courtesy of G. Litwack.)

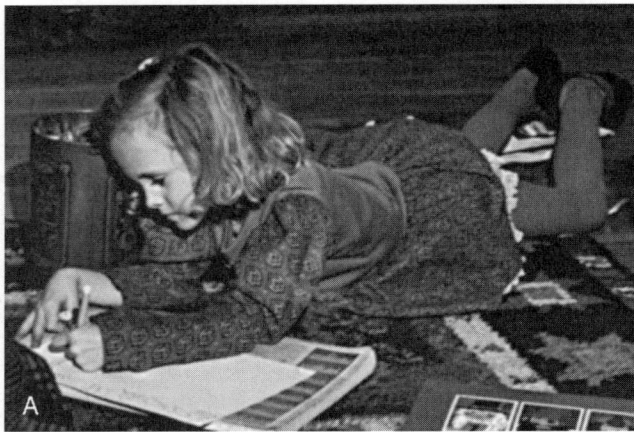
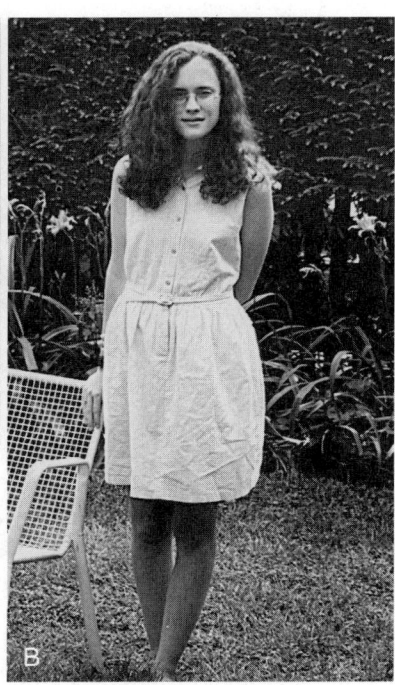

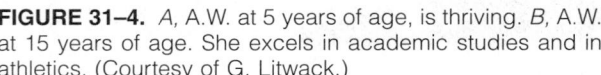

FIGURE 31–4. *A,* A.W. at 5 years of age, is thriving. *B,* A.W. at 15 years of age. She excels in academic studies and in athletics. (Courtesy of G. Litwack.)

can be recorded as such. For example, "Axillary temperature was 34° C at 20:05 on arrival in the NICU and was 36.8° C after 2 hours in the servo-controlled overhead warmer supplemented with heat lamps." Without a good indication of the times of the measurements, vital signs for newborns have little meaning. Temperature for the most part is measured in the axilla using electronic thermometers with disposable tips (see Chapter 33). Rectal temperatures, because of the greater risk of trauma or perforation, are useful only when core temperature may be in question. When the infant's temperature is more than 37.5° C, it is important to assess whether this elevation is a fever associated with infection of whether it is related to an overly warm environment or excessive bundling. If the core temperature is elevated but the extremities are cool, sepsis is likely. When the extremities are warm, the cause is likely to be environmental or rarely "warm shock."

For all spontaneously breathing infants, term and premature, respiratory rates normally fall within a range of 40 to 60 breaths/min by 1 hour of age. Rarely, a term infant has a persisting respiratory rate of 100 on the 2nd day of life with no evident clinical, radiographic, or laboratory abnormality. In these cases, the respiratory rate becomes normal by the end of the 1st week. Persistent bradypnea is rare, seen only in extremely premature infants who are ill, infants whose respiratory drive is depressed from maternal narcotic administration, or in those with persisting central hypoventilation (Ondine's curse). Apneic episodes and periodic breathing should be described. In recording observations, description rather than opinion is preferable, for example, "The infant had about six respiratory pauses of 4 to 7 seconds each without bradycardia or evident desaturation during a 5-minute period while lying undisturbed in apparent REM sleep."

Blood pressure is not usually routinely measured in well infants, and the cost–benefit analysis of this procedure for normal infants is unknown. For sick infants, blood pressure is assessed, for example, by direct intra-arterial measurement, oscillometry, auscultation, and Doppler flow. Intra-arterial catheters permit continuous blood pressure monitoring as a matter of routine. Infants being evaluated for a heart problem should have blood pressure measured in all four extremities to check primarily for problems of juxtaductal coarctation and left ventricular and outflow tract hypoplasia. Blood pressure correlates directly with gestational age and birth weight. In general, hypotension must be considered for blood pressures below 35/25 with means of less than 30 in infants weighing less than 1000 g. In the first 12 hours, mean blood pressures as low as 23 may not be abnormal in the smallest liveborn infants (although the definition of "normal" in this group is a conundrum). In the smallest, sickest newborns, blood pressures are usually measured intra-arterially with transducers that often receive suboptimal calibration. The transducer must be at the level of the ventricles, and, with lower blood pressures, errors with leveling may cause large errors in blood pressure readings. Trends in blood pressure, skin perfusion, recent clinical events, urine output, and arterial pH are essential inputs for the diagnosis of clinically significant hypotension. Hypertension is a consideration with mean pressures of more than 50 to 70 mm Hg in preterm or term infants (see Appendix 3).

Weight, Length, and Head Circumference

Weight should be measured in grams for greatest accuracy. For infants from 500 to 800 g birth weight, differences of only 100 g are associated with differences in mortality of 50%. Length is more easily measured with an inflexible meter rule beside the baby rather than with a flexible measuring tape. Measurements of length carried out by one person using a measuring tape on a squirming infant are commonly inaccurate by several centimeters. The tonic neck reflex can occasionally help in straightening the leg during the measurement. The "ponderal index" (weight in grams × 100 divided by the length in cubic centimeters) may be useful in identifying the occasional baby who is underweight for length and therefore small for gestational age, who nonetheless is not so identified by standard weight, gestation, and length norms. Head circumference is determined by placing a soft tape measure just above the eyebrows and finding the largest circumference over the occiput (Fig. 31–5).

Gestational Age Assessment

Gestational age assessment is best done by recording all the available data, that is, by recording gestation duration

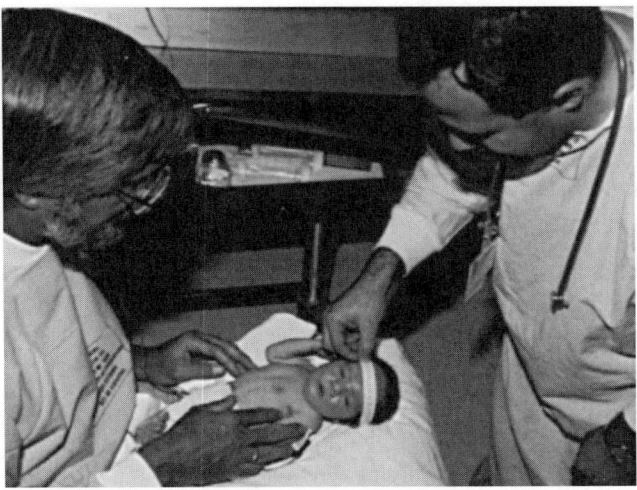

FIGURE 31–5. Positioning of tape for head circumference measurement.

based on last menstrual period, prenatal ultrasound estimates, and, after birth, the gestation that matches the 50th percentile for head circumference, length, and weight and the estimate of gestation based on physical characteristics. These indicators can be combined to give an "obstetric" estimate of gestation and a "pediatric" estimate of gestation that can be combined into a "clinical" estimate. We believe that the physical assessments of gestation have been overemphasized because the skin and the central nervous system, which contribute the most to the score, can be affected by factors other than the duration of gestation, such as respiratory distress, asphyxia, and antenatal steroid therapy. The scoring examination by Ballard (1991) is one of the simplest and should be consulted for detailed assessments (see Appendix 3). In terms of weight, as a rule of thumb, 24-week infants are about 600 g (usual limit of viability), 28-week infants are 1200 g (600 × 2), and 33-week infants are 1800 g (600 × 3).

Overall Appearance

Observing the infant is the most important aspect of the physical examination. It is best performed with the infant quiet and nude. Occasionally, the two states are incompatible, in which case the infant can usually be quieted by rocking to-and-fro while the examiner makes faces and babbles. This time-honored method usually catches the surprised attention of the infant (and other personnel who happen by). The state of alertness, the muscle tone, the activity, obvious anomalies or injuries, respiration, and the skin are assessed during inspection. The infant may appear sick or well, responsive or lethargic. The muscle tone in a term infant should be sufficient for the hips, knees, and elbows to be flexed while the infant is lying supine or prone. Some spontaneous movements should be evident, and the well infant should appear alert at some point during the examination, unless the examiner is an extraordinarily boring person. The color should be pink, rather than sallow and pale or blue. Cyanosis may be generalized or limited to the distal extremities or to the lower part of

---

TABLE 31–7

History and Physical Examination Outline

Time and date of history
Address and telephone numbers for day and night contact
Maternal history (See Table 31–2)
Neonatal course
    Delivery room events, resuscitation, Apgar scores, cord blood gases, evident anomalies, maternal condition after birth, gross appearance of placenta, results of initial laboratory tests, and other events before the physical examination
Newborn physical examination
    Date and time of examination
    Weight and gross appearance of placenta
    Vital signs
    Overall appearance, symmetry, and general proportions
    Assessment of gestational length
    Height, weight, head circumference, and growth percentile
    Skin: bands, rash, birthmarks, tumors, and angiomas
    Head: size, shape, sutures, fontanels, and pressure
    Ears: tags, anatomy of folds, and placement on skull
    Eyes: size, spacing, colobomas, and cataracts
    Mouth: filtrum, size, and clefts
    Neck: fistulas and swellings
    Lungs and chest: malformations or air entry
    Heart and vascular: pulses, rhythm, murmurs, and point of maximal intensity
    Abdomen: cord, vessels, masses, distention, scaphoid, bowel sounds, and musculature
    Extremities: extra digits, bands, duplications, or fusions
    Spine: scoliosis, sinus, or masses
    Genitourinary and anus
    Musculoskeletal: range of motion, movement, or pain
    Neurologic: movement, responses, tone, sensorium, cranial nerves, and reflexes
Impressions/problems
Common laboratory results
    Initial neonatal blood gases and oxygen saturation, and FiO_2
    Complete blood count and hematocrit
    Blood sugar (Dextrostix)
    Cultures taken: blood or cerebrospinal fluid
    Screenings: syphilis, rubella, human immunodeficiency virus, hepatitis, tuberculosis, genetic and metabolic diseases, and illicit drugs
Initial radiography and imaging results
Plan
Signature and title

the body, as is seen occasionally with massive right-to-left shunting through a ductus arteriosus. When only the hands and feet are blue, the infant may be cold with resulting peripheral vasoconstriction. This appearance is called acrocyanosis.

The appearance of the small premature infant after stabilization is different from this description. The 900-g infant with respiratory distress syndrome may be intubated or ventilated and have an arterial line or peripheral intravenous lines in place. He or she usually has a thermistor attached for temperature regulation and leads attached for cardiac and respiratory monitoring. This infant may also be sedated or paralyzed by muscle relaxants. Regardless, the infant is usually flaccid and minimally responsive. The infant may be covered in various ways to minimize heat loss and restrained to maintain the vascular lines. Stimulation during the examination may cause arterial desaturation, silent crying attempts around the endotracheal tube, decreased blood pressure, tachycardia or bradycardia, and decreased skin perfusion. In these cases, continual information on gas exchange, blood pressure, temperature, ventilation, and heart rate is gained at the price of access to the infant, which in any case can be harmful, especially if the examination is lengthy and/or inept. Nonetheless, a careful head-to-foot examination can be gently and quickly carried out by one or two (not four or five) examiners. The cardiac and pulmonary examinations are often difficult because of ventilator noise (water accumulation in the inspiratory tube) and because of difficulties obtaining a good seal on the chest of premature babies with stethoscope bells designed for larger babies. The examination of the abdomen using a single index finger is often easier than the examination of full-term infants because of the thinness and diminished tone of the anterior abdominal wall.

Anomalies and birth injuries are often apparent on inspection. When observing the infant, it is important to look carefully at the facial features and the shape of the ears and head to see whether there are any obviously dysmorphic or malformed features. Are there any obvious anomalies? Is the infant well proportioned or are the limbs short or long compared to the trunk? If any anomaly or dysmorphic feature is noted, a search should begin for other major or minor abnormalities that may help lead to diagnosis of isolated malformations, a malformation sequence or syndrome, or a deformation or disruption caused by external environmental factors. Malformations, deformations, and chromosome problems are discussed in Part IV. The most common anomalies are listed in Table 31–8. Birth injuries are often apparent by observing lack of motion or asymmetries of movement of the limbs or face. There may be obvious pain when an extremity or clavicle is palpated and bruising may be apparent after a few hours of life. Birth injuries occur with greater frequency in breech deliveries and with other abnormal presentations. The most common birth injuries are listed in Table 31–9.

The chest should be inspected for symmetry. A prominent left chest may indicate cardiac hypertrophy from an obstructive lesion. A visible cardiac impulse may indicate a patent ductus arteriosus with left-to-right shunt. A small chest with the infant manifesting respiratory distress or

TABLE 31-8

Most Common Anomalies Noted on the Initial Examination

Anomaly	Frequency (live births)
Skin tags	10–15/1000
Polydactyly	10–15/1000
Cleft lip or palate	1–4/1000
Congenital heart defects	1–4/1000
Congenital hip dislocation	1–4/1000
Down syndrome	1–4/1000*
Talipes equinovarus	1–4/1000
Spina bifidas, anencephaly, or encephalocele	1–4/10,000

*Increases with maternal age older than 33 years.

failure may indicate pulmonary hypoplasia or, in a more severe form, asphyxiating thoracic dystrophy.

Much information is obtained by watching the infant breathe. Regular respiratory movements of less than 60 breaths/min without suprasternal, intercostal, or subcostal retractions make pulmonary disease unlikely. Apneic spells and periodic breathing can be observed.

Inspection by System

After the clinician gains a general impression of the infant's status and is convinced that emergency intervention (intubation, relief of pneumothorax, or transfusion) is unnecessary, the clinician may continue observation of the infant by system, usually starting at the head and working caudad. Then the examination is repeated with palpation, auscultation, reflex testing, the shining of lights into various orifices, and finally, range of motion. Auscultation and abdominal examination require a quiet if not cooperative infant. The hip examination and the Moro reflex testing should be the finale because these assessments frequently leave the infant displeased with the whole concept of being examined.

TABLE 31-9

Most Frequent Birth Injuries and Insults

Decreased gas exchange: placental insufficiency, prolapsed cord, or premature placental separation*
Broken clavicle
Facial palsy
Brachial plexus injuries (especially Erb's palsy)
Fractures of the humerus or skull
Ruptured internal organs
Testicular trauma
Fat necrosis
Lacerations or scalpel injury and cephalohematoma
Scalp lesions from fetal scalp electrode or forceps
Umbilical cord accidents

*Acute prepartum asphyxia of sufficient duration and severity to be associated with hypoxic-ischemic encephalopathy. The incidence for each of these conditions is roughly 1–3/1000 live births.

The Cry

As the clinician performs various parts of the newborn examination, he or she should listen for the infant's cry. Is it husky, loud, and sustained or is it shrill and high-pitched indicating a possible central nervous system abnormality? The cry may be low pitched and husky in hypothyroidism, or it may be hoarse with vocal cord injury or recurrent laryngeal nerve palsy. A weak whimper may indicate overwhelming sepsis or neuromuscular disease. Inspiratory stridor from airway obstruction may be heard only when the infant is crying. Complete aphonia usually indicates bilateral vocal cord injury or paralysis.

Skin

Vernix usually covers the skin especially in the skinfolds of the axillae, neck, and groin at birth. Post-term infants characteristically have little vernix, and the skin is dry, cracked, and wrinkled. The texture of the skin is evaluated with regard to scaliness, elasticity, thickness, and local or generalized edema. Hemangiomas, nevi, and urticarial, pustular, vesicular, or nodular rashes are sought. Particularly in infants with vascular catheters, evidence of partial or complete arterial or venous obstruction should be sought at regular intervals. Dermal sinuses occur in the midline of the back from occiput to coccyx and near the ears and in the neck. Dimples, sinuses, hirsute areas, or cystic swellings suggest the presence of cranial or vertebral sinuses or underlying defects. Preterm infants may have fine downy hair (lanugo) over the shoulders, back, thighs, forehead, and ears. This regresses as they mature over weeks.

Ecchymoses or petechiae may relate to birth trauma and may herald a more-than-normal degree of hyperbilirubinemia as the blood products break down and are absorbed over 24 to 36 hours. Generalized and recurring petechiae, especially those not on the head and necklace region, may signify serious infectious or hematologic problems.

Common findings include milia, white papules less than 1 mm, that are scattered across the forehead. These and white vesicles with a red base (erythema toxicum) are transient and benign. In black infants, a similar but more dramatic benign condition is transient neonatal pustular melanosis. These conditions at times are impossible to differentiate from infectious pustules by inspection. Jaundice in the 3rd day of life or later is common, but jaundice that is evident on the 1st day of life is unusual and needs laboratory investigation.

Head

The most common findings after birth are caput succedaneum and cephalohematoma. The first is edema of the scalp skin and crosses suture lines. Cephalohematomas are subperiosteal and therefore do not cross suture lines. Frequently, the clinician gains the impression of a depressed skull fracture as the rim of a cephalohematoma is palpated. This (false) perception is so common that we do not routinely obtain skull radiographs of an infant with a cephalohematoma unless other worrisome signs are present

as well. Rarely, subgaleal hemorrhage may occur especially after a birth assisted with vacuum extraction. The hemorrhage is under the aponeurosis but above the periosteum. The swelling crosses suture lines and can be differentiated from a caput by its firmness and other signs of loss of blood from the intravascular space. In the first day of life, molding of the head from descent through the birth canal may be present, and the skull plates are overriding. After a few days, the clinician can better estimate the size of the fontanels and their flatness, fullness, or tenseness and the width of suture lines (Faix, 1982; Popich and Smith, 1972). Fontanels may tense normally with vigorous crying. A bulging or tense fontanel has a feel by palpation nearly equivalent to bone. In contrast, a full fontanel may be normal and is easily distinguished by palpation from bone. The clinician can note the fusion of the sagittal, metopic, or coronal sutures—totally, partially, or unilaterally. Large fontanels and split sutures are most often a normal variant, but they can be associated with increased intracranial pressure or conditions that impair bone growth. Likewise, small fontanels and overriding sutures are generally of little significance but may be associated with conditions in which brain growth has been retarded (Table 31–10). A small (third) fontanel anterior to the posterior fontanel is occasionally found and is associated with Down syndrome or hypothyroidism. Unusual whorls or other hair patterns or asymmetries of the skull may indicate problems in global or regional brain development.

Craniotabes is a demineralized area or softening of the skull. When this is appreciated to a mild degree near the suture lines in newborn infants, it is commonly a normal variant. When it is present over most of the skull, it may be associated with conditions in which calcification has been deficient (e.g., syphilis or osteogenesis imperfecta). By contrast, craniosynostosis is a condition wherein sutures are fused, thereby brain growth is constrained.

Transillumination is useful for detecting severe hydrocephaly and hydranencephaly before obtaining an ultrasound examination. The heads of premature infants normally have a greater degree of transillumination than the heads of term infants.

TABLE 31–10

Disorders Sometimes Associated with Abnormal Fontanel Size

Too large
    Skeletal disorders (e.g., hypophosphatasia or
      osteogenesis imperfecta)
    Chromosome abnormalities
    Hypothyroidism
    Increased intracranial pressure or hydrocephalus
Too small
    Hyperthyroidism
    Craniosynostosis
    Microcephaly
Third fontanel
    Down syndrome
    Hypothyroidism

Eyes

Eyes are difficult to examine in the newborn especially when instillation of silver nitrate has occurred. Its use, which is currently not preferred over other antibacterials, is associated with swelling and conjunctivitis during the first 36 hours of life. Often a soothed infant with to-and-fro rocking during which the head is elevated, spontaneously opens his or her eyes, allowing inspection and the ability to assess visual tracking of the examiner's face or a bright object as it moves from side to side (Fig. 31–6). Gross vision can also be assessed by observing whether the infant turns to a diffuse light. Pupils should be equal, reactive to light, and symmetric. The corneae should be clear. The pupil can be inspected with a light and the pink retina (red reflex) discerned to rule out lenticular, anterior, or posterior chamber opacities. (With the ophthalmoscope about 6 inches from the infant, the clinician uses the +10 diopter lens.) Fixed strabismus should be absent, and the eye movements for the most part should be coordinated. Eye movements can be assessed by checking for oculovestibular nystagmus by holding the infant under the axillae facing the examiner while the examiner turns in a circle. The infant's eyes have a slow deviation in the direction of spin with quick movements in the opposite direction. If other disease is present or a more complete examination is indicated, then the eyes should be dilated for a complete retinal examination.

Ears

The ears are examined for placement and deformation. Low-set and/or posteriorly rotated ears may be associated with other more major anomalies. Usually, the tips of the ears are cephalad to a circumferential line around the skull through the inner and outer canthus of both eyes. Gross hearing is assessed by observing whether the infant blinks to a loud noise (hand clap) and whether the infant attends

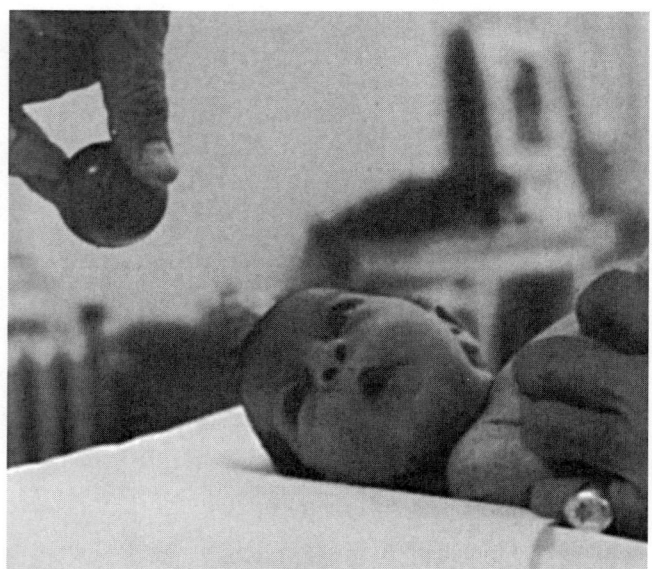

FIGURE 31–6. Head turning to follow ball. (Courtesy of Dr. B. Brazelton.)

to an unusual sound (ringing a bell or tuning fork). More formal hearing screening for all newborns has recently been recommended (see Laboratory Screening). In the immediate newborn period, the ear canals are usually occluded by vernix and are not routinely examined.

Mouth and Lower Face

The lips may be good indicators of whether the infant is cyanotic. Retention cysts on the alveolar ridge may appear like teeth; natal teeth occur rarely and are usually shed in a few days. Retention cysts are called Epstein pearls, and these disappear in a few weeks. The frenulum, which in years past was occasionally cut to prevent "tongue-tie," can usually be ignored. The palate is examined for cleft, the tongue for size, and the sublingual area for masses. Both corners of the mouth should move symmetrically when the infant cries or grimaces, and asymmetry is most usually caused by a seventh cranial nerve palsy. A long philtrum, thin upper lip, cleft lip, cleft palate, and small jaw are other significant findings associated with abnormal fetal development sometimes caused by chromosome abnormalities, alcohol, or other fetal toxins.

Nose

Patency of each naris can be checked by listening at the orifice while the other naris is occluded with the mouth closed. Newborn infants breathe preferentially through the nose so that bilateral choanal atresia may cause severe respiratory distress. Flaring of the nostrils occurs whenever respiratory effort is increased regardless of cause.

Almost half of all infants have nonfunctional nasolacrimal ducts for 1 to 5 days. Swelling is common at the inner canthal region, but infection (dacryocystitis) is rare. More than 80% open spontaneously by age 3 months.

Neck

The neck of the newborn always seems short. Very short and webbed necks may be associated with Klippel-Feil or Turner syndrome. The neck is palpated for cysts or masses. A thyroglossal duct cyst is usually palpable in the midline and retracts with tongue protrusion. The infant may have congenital muscular torticollis with or without a fibrous mass in the sternocleidomastoid muscle, associated with head tilt. A cystic hygroma is a spongy mass that may increase with increased intrathoracic pressure and may transilluminate. Hemangiomas are similar to hygromas upon palpation but frequently are associated with skin discoloration. Branchial cleft cysts may have associated fistulae. They are palpable anterior to the sternocleidomastoid and may retract with swallowing. Thyroid masses are usually visible and easily palpable with the head extended.

Chest and Lungs

The circumference of the chest of the newborn is roughly equivalent to that of the head. Continued inspection of the chest may reveal a protruding xiphisternum (pectus carinatum), which is usually a normal variant. In contrast, a pectus excavatum deformity may be present at birth or associated with prolonged low-compliance respiration.

While the infant is breathing, nasal flaring may be present along with retractions and "grunting," which is partial glottic closure at the first part of expiration. Suprasternal retractions and gasping, as opposed to substernal retractions, may indicate upper airway obstruction, and laryngoscopy should be performed rapidly. Almost any cardiopulmonary disease in the newborn period reduces lung compliance and is associated with subcostal retractions. The appearance of flaring, grunting, tachypnea, and retractions is called respiratory distress. Respiratory distress may be associated with pneumonia, delayed resorption of lung fluid, respiratory distress syndrome, or any number of cardiorespiratory problems.

Asymmetry of the chest may indicate fetal obstructive cardiac anomalies, a tension pneumothorax, or other forms of air trapping or mass lesions.

The nipples and underlying breast tissue are usually 1 cm in diameter in term infants, both boys and girls, and these may be asymmetric. Under maternal hormonal influence, the breast bud may become as large as 3 to 4 cm and may excrete a watery whitish fluid for a few days or weeks ("witch's" milk). The enlargement occurs in both sexes, and is usually symmetric. Redness or asymmetry indicates probable infection, which requires the administration of antibiotics. Widely spaced nipples and accessory nipples should be noted.

Single-finger percussion can be useful for detection of consolidated pneumonias or pleural effusions. Suspicion of clinically significant pneumothorax should lead to instant confirmatory checks of blood pressure, auscultation, transillumination, emergency pleural taps, and chest radiographs. Transillumination is carried out with high-energy fiberoptic transillumination devices in a darkened room. Some practice is necessary before the examiner can clearly distinguish the normal from excessive coronas of pink transillumination around the closely applied light source.

Auscultation of the lungs is best carried out with a cleaned and warmed stethoscope bell. Rhonchi can be inspiratory or expiratory. Inspiratory stridor implies large airway obstruction, and expiratory prolongation indicates small airway obstruction. Rales are moist crackling sounds emulated by licking a thumb and forefinger and separating them close to one's ear. The burst of fine crackles on separation of the thumb and forefinger is of the same quality and intensity as rales in the newborn. Gurgling and bubbling sounds come from secretions in large airways and often indicate the need for tracheal suctioning. Harsher bubbling sounds may be from water accumulating in the tubing of a ventilator. Listening alternately in the right and left axillae may indicate diminished breath sounds on either the right or the left. These asymmetries may indicate unilateral pneumothorax or that an endotracheal tube has inadvertently advanced into the right mainstem bronchus. Rarely, bowel sounds may be heard high in the chest in the absence of breath sounds. If so, diaphragmatic hernia is suspected, and emergency radiologic examination and surgical consultation are necessary. Meanwhile, a nasogastric tube should be inserted to prevent distention of stomach and bowel within the chest cavity.

Heart and Vascular System

The most common cardiac conditions in the newborn period include perinatal adaptations involving the ductus arteriosus (see Chapter 61), with right-to-left shunting through the ductus of term infants and persistent pulmonary hypertension and left-to-right shunting through the ductus of premature infants. Significant structural heart anomalies are diagnosed in the 1st week of life in about 1% of live births. The most common serious anomalies recognized in the first week of life are ventricular septal defects, patent ductus arteriosus, transpositions, hypoplastic left heart syndromes, tetralogy of Fallot, and coarctations. The most common findings for an infant with heart disease in the newborn period are tachypnea and/or cyanosis—"an increased O_2 requirement." These findings are associated with the most common pathophysiologic conditions associated with congenital heart disease: low output, congestive heart failure from shunts, obstruction to outflow, and insufficient pulmonary blood flow. The general appearance can often signal a cardiac problem, for example, the shocky underperfused infant on the 3rd day of life with a hypoplastic left ventricle versus the contented cyanotic infant in no distress with transposition of the great vessels. Other aspects of heart disease detectable from general inspection are the severity of signs, hypertrophy of the left chest, and, rarely, venous engorgement (e.g., in an infant with thrombosis of a central venous line leading to a vena cava syndrome).

Auscultation

The clinician should listen for cardiovascular problems first in "noncardiac" areas such as the axilla (peripheral pulmonic stenosis), the neck (aortic obstruction), and the head and liver (arteriovenous malformations). Timing of the onset of murmurs is important. Frequently, murmurs that depend on pulmonary vascular tone (e.g., left-to-right shunt through a patent ductus arteriosus) may not be heard until pulmonary vascular resistance has decreased in the 2nd to 3rd day of life in an infant with respiratory distress syndrome or within 12 hours of birth in a normal full-term infant. The murmur of tricuspid insufficiency associated with a dilated heart after severe perinatal asphyxia may be present only in the first hours of life. Obstructive murmurs characteristically are heard from birth unless low cardiac output is present. Other characteristics that are important to note are the site where they are heard best, the timing of the murmur with regard to systole and diastole, the quality, and the loudness. The murmurs that are of low intensity, that occur near the sternum or only in noncardiac areas, and that occur early in systole, are often innocent.

A detailed history and physical examination, including four-extremity blood pressures, a chest radiograph, blood gases, electrocardiogram, and ultrasound examination, are usually sufficient to clarify whether congenital heart disease is present. Neonatologists and pediatricians who frequently care for newborns should be able to screen the heart with ultrasound as well as with chest radiographs, electrocardiograms, and auscultation.

CASE STUDY 1

Baby B was transferred to the NICU at 6 hours of age because of tachypnea. The history of pregnancy and delivery was unremarkable. On examination the infant was a well-formed full-term infant breathing at a rate of 78/minute. Lungs had occasional rales. The heart rate was 180/minute. A gallop rhythm was heard but no murmurs. The liver was palpable 4 cm below the costal margin and was thought to be enlarged. The physical findings suggested heart failure, which was confirmed by a chest radiograph that showed an enlarged heart and pulmonary congestion. Arterial blood gases in 30% oxygen revealed a PaO_2 of 68, a PCO_2 of 48, and a pH of 7.2 with a base deficit. An electrocardiogram indicated a modest reduction of voltage in all leads. Ultrasound examination of the heart revealed a large heart with poor contractility. A number of diagnoses were entertained including various cardiomyopathies, pericardial effusion, and anomalous pulmonary venous drainage with obstruction. The infant was taken for cardiac catheterization where a large and inoperable arteriovenous malformation of the brain was diagnosed after injection of dye for cardiac angiography. After the infant returned to the unit, a large bruit was easily heard with the stethoscope applied to the anterior fontanel or to the skull lateral to the eyes.

This case serves as a reminder that heart failure may occur from arteriovenous fistulas anywhere in the body.

Abdomen

The abdomen is assessed by inspection and palpation for organomegaly, masses, inflammation, and distention. Unusual flatness or a scaphoid shape to the abdomen may be associated with congenital diaphragmatic hernia. Examination by inspection, palpation, auscultation, transillumination, and ultrasound examination can usually discriminate between air within or outside the gastrointestinal tract and enlarged viscus or viscera, or a cystic or solid tumor. Normally, the examiner palpates a 1- to 2-cm liver edge below the right costal margin, a spleen tip overlying the stomach, and the lower pole of the left kidney in the pelvic gutter (Fig. 31–7). The examiner also looks for dilated veins on the abdominal wall indicating venous distention. Visible gastric or bowel patterns may be considered a certain sign of ileus or other obstruction. The umbilical stump should be examined for bleeding, abnormal vessels, increased or decreased Wharton jelly, meconium staining, polyps, granuloma, exudative discharge, or other evidence of inflammation (redness, tenderness, edema of abdominal wall, induration) or abnormal communication with intra-abdominal viscera. Omphaloceles and gastroschisis are readily apparent, but small umbilical hernias and diastasis recti abdominis may be less so.

Abdominal masses occur in approximately 1 of 1000 live births (Table 31–11). Evaluation is carried out by history, physical examination, ultrasound, and radiography. Some masses are transitory and of little significance (e.g., intra-luminal stool, gaseous dilation of the stomach or colon, distended bladder, or large but normal kidneys) (Table 31–12).

Genital System

Maturation of the genitalia is apparent over the last 3 months of gestation, and these changes serve as one index

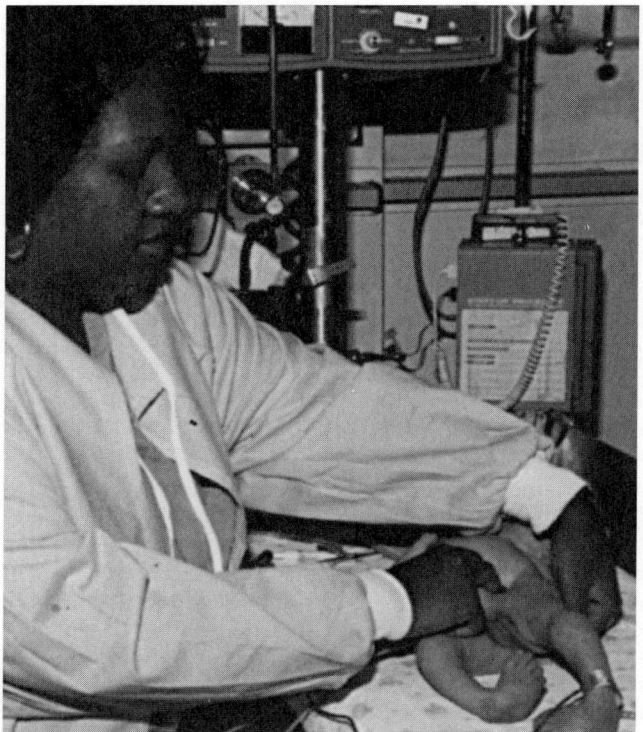

FIGURE 31–7. Abdominal palpation is carried out using counterpressure in the flank with one hand. The lower pole of each kidney is usually palpable with this technique in the first days of life before abdominal muscle tone increases. Note the bilateral clubfeet.

on scoring of physical attributes for gestational age assignment. There is a surprising range of differences that nonetheless fall within the normal range. For a discussion of ambiguous genitalia, see Chapter 101. Penile length and clitoral size are assessed. A clear white mucus is often present in the vagina of term infants for the first few days

TABLE 31–11

Most Common Congenital Abdominal Masses

Renal (55% of total abdominal masses)	**Liver and biliary** (5%)
Hydronephrosis	Cysts
Multicystic or polycystic kidneys	Tumors
Renal malformations	**Retroperitoneal** (5%)
Renal vein thrombosis	Solid tumors
Renal neoplasms	Anterior meningomyelocele
Genital (15%)	**Adrenal** (5%)
Hydrometrocolpos	Hemorrhage
Ovarian cyst	Neuroblastoma
Gastrointestinal (15%)	
Obstructions	
Cysts or tumors	
Duplications	

Data from Griscom NT: The roentgenology of neonatal abdominal masses. AJR Am J Roentgenol 93:447, 1965, and Kirks D: Radiol Clin North Am 19:527, 1981.

TABLE 31–12

Common Findings of Little Clinical Significance*

Head: caput succedaneum, cephalohematoma, asymmetries, bony protrusions, or molding
Ears: skin tags
Eyes: position (close-set) or conjunctival hemorrhage
Nose: asymmetric nares
Mouth: ranula, sucking calluses, epulis, frenulum, natal teeth, or Epstein pearls
Face: unusual features not consistent with known syndromes
Skin: sparse petechiae on the head, erythema toxicum, mongolian spot, nevus flammeus, telangiectasia, nevi, inclusion cysts, bruises, prominent lanugo or vernix, milia, miliaria, dark pigmentation over genital skin, mild jaundice after 2nd day, peeling of skin, skin tags, or sacrococcygeal dimple
Neck: relative absence
Chest: nipple spacing, extra nipples, breast hypertrophy, witch's milk
Umbilicus: erythema or umbilicus cutis
Abdomen: evanescent masses
Heart: evanescent murmurs and adventitious sounds
Genitalia: mild hypospadias, prominent labia, mucous secretion, transient vaginal blood, or phimosis
Extremities: extra digits, syndactyly, hips tight to abduction, or neck in extension after breech delivery
Neurologic system: transient tone asymmetries or abnormality, jitters, or sudden jerky movements

*Some of the items on this list may be associated with significant disease, e.g., jitteriness may be associated with metabolic problems or drug withdrawal. However, when findings on this list are mild and transient, they are most frequently not associated with significant disease. When in doubt, it is prudent to ask for another opinion and follow up.

as a result of estrogens from the mother. The location of the urethral meatus and presence or absence of palpable gonads are noted, and inguinal hernias are sought. Most "congenital" hernias have an onset in appearance only after a month or two, and these are most common in premature infants. The anus should be checked for patency and distance from the genitalia. The perineum should be checked for palpable masses. Rarely, with variants of imperforate anus with fistula, stool exudes from the vagina.

Musculoskeletal System

The musculoskeletal system is assessed by observation and palpation for obvious trauma, inflammation, or malformation. The most common alterations in the musculoskeletal system are deformations caused by adverse mechanical forces in utero. Oligohydramnios that limits fetal movement and neuromuscular problems of the fetus can both be associated with multiple contractures known as arthrogryposis. Most positional deformities are mild and resolve with time. The hips deserve special attention because the physical examination is the only method of detecting problems before permanent damage has occurred by 1 year of age or so. Examination of the hips should be undertaken repeatedly in the 1st year of life because a dislocation may not be demonstrable for several months after birth (Place et al, 1978).

Developmental dysplasia of the hip (DDH) occurs in about 1 of 800 live births, more commonly in whites and females. Maternal hormones during pregnancy may contribute to joint capsule laxity particularly in the female fetus. The condition represents a spectrum of conditions from the dislocatable hip found in approximately 5 of 100 live births to the fixed dislocation that may occur in the second trimester associated with some forms of arthrogryposis. It is found more frequently in infants delivered by breech and in those with a positive family history for DDH. In utero conditions that limit hip movement as well as specific syndromes and chromosome disorders may be associated with hip dislocation. It is often unilateral, occurring more commonly in the left hip, for reasons that are unclear.

There are two major tests (with a number of variations) for determining whether the femoral head is fixed in the acetabulum (Fig. 31–8). The Barlow test determines whether the femoral head can be dislocated posteriorly. As the knees are brought together (adducted) or held in midabduction, the examiner pushes laterally on the upper inner thigh (lesser trochanter). A click or clunk indicates that the femoral head slips over the lateral ridge of the acetabulum during this maneuver. With the examiner's fingers on the greater trochanter, the hip can be alternately pushed into and out of the acetabulum by alternating pressure with the thumb or the fingers. The Ortolani test is carried out by abducting the flexed hips while the examiner pushes upward on the posterior proximal femur. The hips are adducted and flexed to 90 degrees; downward pressure is exerted on the knee while the hips are simultaneously abducted. A positive test occurs with a click or clunk as the laterally dislocated femoral head is pushed over the acetabular ridge into the acetabulum. A modification of the Barlow maneuver is to move the thigh anteriorly and posteriorly while holding the midthigh firmly with one hand and stabilizing the pelvis with the other. With this maneuver, the femoral head can alternately be dislocated and relocated, and in our experience, this test has been successful where the Ortolani maneuver has not (see Fig. 31–8).

Fixed dislocations that occurred early in fetal life can often not be detected by the tests described because the femoral head is locked outside of the acetabulum because of joint capsule contractures. The diagnosis is made by palpation of the femoral head posteriorly and by detecting limitation of hip mobility, in association with other problems such as spina bifida or arthrogryposis. The sine qua non for diagnosis of DDH is real-time ultrasound examination (Aronsson, 1994). (For a fuller discussion of DDH, including a discussion of Galeazzi's and Klisic's signs, see Morrissy, 1990.)

The four extremities should be checked for fractures and the joints for hypermobility or hypomobility. A hypotonic arm or wrist drop implies brachial palsy on the affected side. The digits should be examined for polydactylism, syndactylism, edema, unusual skin ridge whorls and creases, nail growth, and unusual digit placement or contractures. Amputations or other evidence of amniotic bands may be present. A variety of malformations of the lower extremities are common. Genu recurvatum is characterized by abnormal hyperextensibility of the knee joint. The number of females who are affected is significantly greater than the number of males. Many more babies with genu

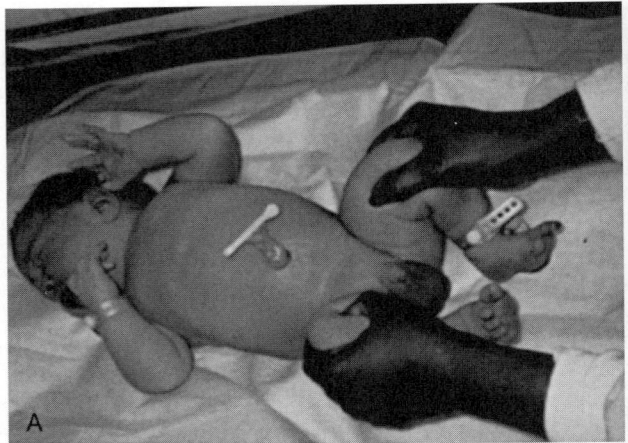
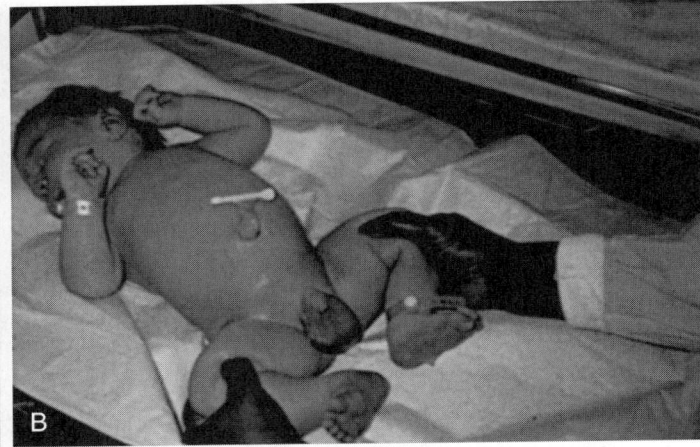
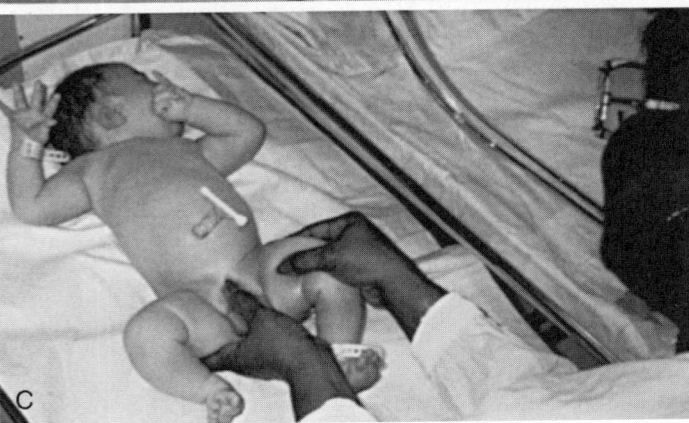

FIGURE 31–8. *A,* The hips are checked with the Ortolani maneuver. The examiner's second and third fingers press up against the heads of the femurs, and the hands press the shafts of the femurs toward the mattress while simultaneously abducting the hips. A palpable "clunk" during this maneuver indicates that the femoral head has slipped over the lip of the acetabulum and is dislocatable. *B,* Shows full abduction. *C,* For the Barlow maneuver, the examiner stabilizes the pelvis with her left hand and attempts to move the shaft of the femur upward and downward without flexing the hip. This maneuver checks whether the femoral head can be displaced posteriorly out of the acetabulum; instability of the femoral head is palpable during this maneuver with congenitally dislocated hips.

recurvatum present by the breech position than is to be expected. The disorder may also occur as a feature in a number of disorders, such as the Ehlers-Danlos, Marfan, Klinefelter, and Turner syndromes, but usually it occurs as an in utero deformation not associated with other conditions. The extended leg or both legs describe a concave arc when hyperextended at the knee. Hyperextensibility is mild or severe; that is, the arc is shallow or deep. In severe cases, there may be actual posterior dislocation of the knee. Nothing need be done for cases of mild or moderate severity. Posterior splinting or, rarely, casting for 2 to 4 weeks is indicated for the most severe forms.

Pes calcaneovalgus is the absolutely flat and sometimes slightly convex foot that often lies at rest dorsiflexed at an acute angle to the foreleg. When gentle pressure is applied to the sole of the foot, dorsiflexion increases easily until its dorsal surface lies in contact with the shin.

These feet should be casted in the equinovarus position for 4 to 6 weeks, and this therapy should be repeated several times if necessary. Continued treatment may be needed for several years.

In pes metatarsovarus, the heel and posterior half of the foot appear normal, but the forefoot angulates sharply inward. Thus, the outer border of the foot is convex, whereas its inner border is concave. If the foot can be straightened by gentle traction, with the thumb held firmly over the apex of the convexity, no immediate treatment is needed. If, however, the angulation is difficult or impossi-

ble to overcome, casting is probably indicated. Later use of corrective shoes may or may not be necessary.

Pes equinovarus is the classic clubfoot with sharp and tight hyperextension and incurving of the entire foot. It is often a solitary defect but not infrequently it is associated with congenital dislocation of the hip, myelomeningocele, arthrogryposis, or other defects. It requires immediate and long-term orthopedic care. Most cases can be corrected by

---

TABLE 31–13

Outline of Neurologic Screening Examination

Appearance
Behavior, state, cry, abnormal movements
Visual responses
Hearing responses
Head size and shape
Active and passive tone of major muscle groups:
    Neck, shoulders, and upper extremities (pull
        to sit–traction response, vertical sling)
    Trunk (horizontal suspension)
    Lower extremities
Cranial nerves
Primitive neonatal reflexes (grasp, root, suck,
    Moro, withdrawal, tonic neck reflex)
Deep tendon reflexes

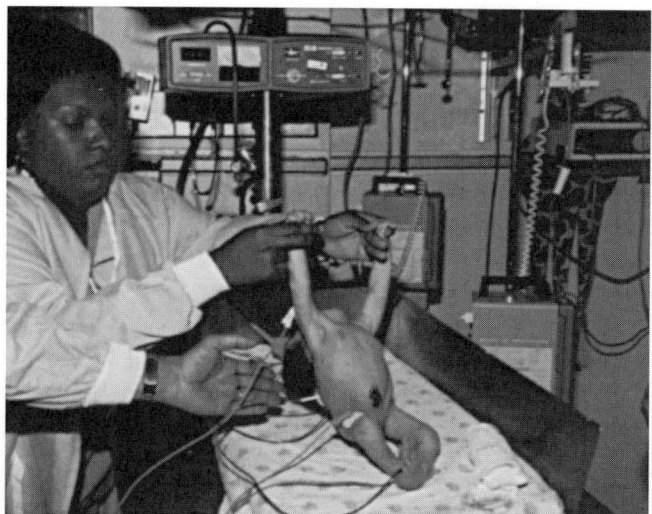

FIGURE 31–9. Tone of the neck flexors is assessed by pulling the infant off the mattress by both hands. In this infant marked head lag is present.

casting and subsequent shoe corrections. A few cases require open operation.

Neurologic System

The neurologic examination is discussed in detail in Chapter 69. For most infants, the aim is to find whether a neurologic problem exists (Table 31–13). If so, the examination can be expanded to fully describe the findings. For a paralyzed 800-g infant on a ventilator, a complete neurologic examination is impossible. Nonetheless, it should not be deferred completely. For example, attention to head size, shape, or abnormality, fontanel size and pressure, pupil size and equality, lability of blood gases and blood pressure, variability of heart rate, and limb muscle mass are all available information about an infant's central nervous system status.

The quality and quantity of spontaneous movements are the best indicators of neuromuscular function and are assessed by inspection. Decreased tone may be one of the first detectable abnormalities in a full-term infant with sepsis. Tone is gestation- and illness-dependent, with smaller and sick infants having decreased tone. Tone may also differ in different muscle groups. The range of passive rotation of the neck is checked by turning the head to the left and right. Flexor tone in the neck and arms is assessed by pulling the infant toward a sitting position (Fig. 31–9). Extensor tone in the neck is evaluated by holding the infant prone. Shoulder tone is assessed by holding the infant in a vertical sling, that is, under the axillae, and by the scarf maneuver (Fig. 31–10). Tone in the lower extremities is checked by the hip examination and by the heel-to-ear maneuver.

An array of primitive reflexes are present in the term newborn infant, but their expression is highly dependent on state—the most optimal being a sleepy awake state. Premature infants have diminished responses with decreasing gestational age, although this belief may be confounded by the increasing frequency of illness with decreasing gestation and the fact that sick infants respond poorly to elicitation of these reflexes. The Moro and the tonic neck reflex disappear by 6 months of age, but others (e.g., the parachute and Landau reflexes) make their appearance as these wane.

The most obvious primitive reflex of the newborn is the Moro. The infant can be supported behind the upper back by the examiner's hand, then dropped back 1 cm or so to the mattress. The arms are flung open followed by a flexion and an adduction (i.e., an "embrace"). The eyes open, as if in surprise, and the baby commonly emits a lusty cry making this reflex a good stopping point for the examination. The grasp reflex can be elicited in both hands and feet by placing a thumb on the infant's palm. With palmar pressure, the infant may open his or her mouth and yawn

FIGURE 31–10. The infant is held in a vertical sling. Muscle tone of the shoulder girdle is assessed with this maneuver. Extensor tone of the neck is checked. The infant may follow the face of the examiner. In older infants, "scissoring" of the lower extremities is suggestive of increased tone. With the infant held in this position while the examiner turns in a circle, oculovestibular nystagmus can be assessed.

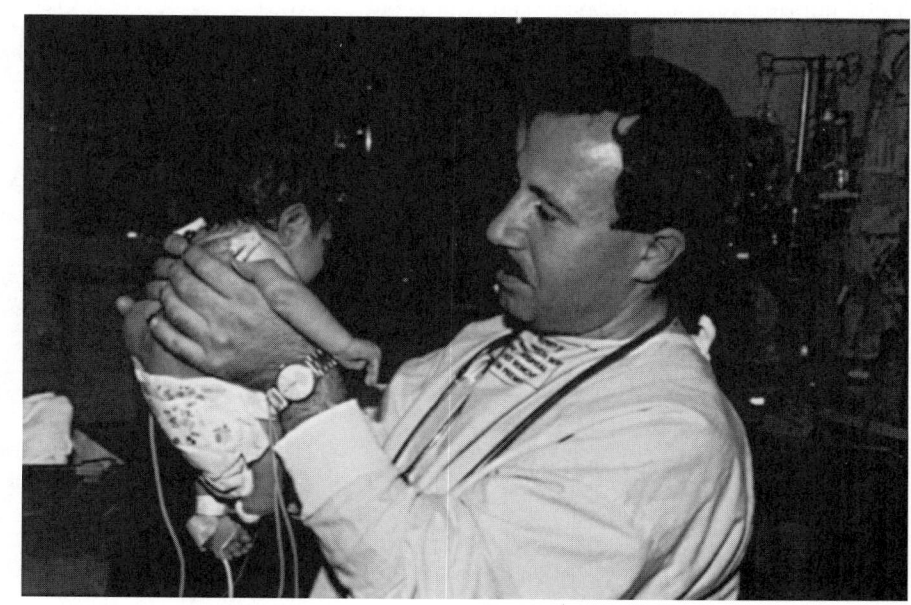

(palmar-mental reflex). When the dorsum of the foot is stimulated, the infant lifts the stimulated foot and places it on a surface (placing). By allowing the plantar surface of the other foot to contact a table top, the infant makes crude sequential walking movements (stepping). The tonic neck reflex is obtained by rotating the infant's head to the right or left while maintaining the supine infant's shoulders flat. The arm and leg to the side of the occiput flex, and the contralateral arm and leg extend (fencer's stance). When the infant is supported prone by the examiner's hand, tickling the area of the lateral spine causes the buttocks to swing to the side of stimulation (trunk incurvation reflex). Holding the infant in the same position and running a finger from the base of the spine toward the neck elicits spinal extension and, with a full bladder, micturition. Light pressure applied with the examiner's fingers to the soles of the feet causes the legs to extend (magnet reflex). Extending one of the infant's legs while the infant is supine and stimulating the plantar surface of the same foot causes the contralateral leg to flex, adduct, and extend (crossed extension reflex).

The deep tendon reflexes are best assessed using the tap of the examiner's index finger.

Other physical findings of clinical significance are listed in Table 31–14. Table 31–15 lists the various evaluations for a "typical" high-risk premature infant during hospitalization.

ULTRASOUND EXAMINATION

Whenever a problem is defined with anomalies or with the head, heart, abdomen, or kidneys, the physician should conduct a screening ultrasound examination. While the physician of newborns may not be an expert in imaging technique, he or she should be capable of doing a screening examination in the same way one carries out auscultation of the heart even when one is not a cardiologist. In this, obstetricians subspecializing in perinatology have surpassed neonatologists in their proficiency with ultrasound screening. Using a 5-MHz sector scanner, the examiner can gain useful information using only gain and depth controls (Walther and Leighton, 1996).

Head

The head is examined in the coronal and parasagittal planes through the anterior fontanel. Ventricular size and the presence or absence of paraventricular and intraventricular

---

TABLE 31–14

Common Physical Findings of Clinical Significance

Apnea	Heart murmurs
Tachypnea	Organomegaly
Grunting	Evident anomalies other than ears
Bradycardia	and digits
Cyanosis	Jaundice
Hypotonia	Plethora or pallor
Decreased breath sounds	Diffuse petechiae

TABLE 31–15

Changing Issues During Hospitalization of a "Typical" High-Risk Premature Infant

Initial evaluation
  Major malformations
  Severe cardiopulmonary conditions
  Viability
  Postasphyxial complications
  Hypotension
  Intrauterine growth and length of gestation
  Meeting with parents
Midweek evaluation
  Patent ductus arteriosus
  Intraventricular hemorrhage
  Pneumothoraces and air leaks
  Jaundice
  Culture reports
  Meeting with parents
First-week evaluation
  Metabolic
  Renal
  Gastrointestinal issues, necrotizing enterocolitis
  Intraventricular hemorrhage
  Meeting with parents
First-month evaluation
  Chronic lung disease
  Cystic periventricular lesions or ventricular enlargement
  Retinopathy
  Nutritional status
  Nosocomial infection
  Meeting with parents
Intermediate care evaluations
  Parental issues
  Anemia
  Feeding
  Hydrocephalus
  Growth
  Chronic central nervous system disability
  Apnea
Before-discharge evaluations
  Meeting with parents
  Special needs, e.g., home oxygen
  Primary care versus specialty medical follow-up planning
  Other support services
  Review of hospital course and global follow-up plans

---

blood are noted. A large degree of ventricular enlargement can be appreciated even by the relatively untrained examiner.

Heart

The examiner should be able to identify all four chambers of the heart by aiming the probe, held in a transverse plane, cephalad from the substernal area. Atria are smaller than the ventricles and are symmetric. At birth, the ventricles appear equally sized. Good contractility can be appreciated. Pericardial fluid may be noted by the presence of an echo-free area around the heart that is surrounded by the echo-dense pericardium.

Renal System

The paravertebral areas and the locale of the bladder are examined. Size, shape, and presence of large cysts or dilated collection systems are noted. The bladder can be visualized if filled with urine.

LABORATORY SCREENING

At the time of the initial history and physical examination, the infant should be screened for a number of conditions that depend on the characteristics of the population being served. For example, in an inner-city population, we tend to screen particularly for the following conditions:

Hematocrit, Rh, Blood Type, and Direct Antiglobulin Test (DAT, Direct Coombs' Test). We take heelstick blood on all live born infants. In our inner-city population with greater risk of poor placentation and less than optimal use of prenatal care, we find about a 4% risk of clinical polycythemia (one central hematocrit > 65% with symptoms, or > 70% even in absence of symptoms).

Hearing Screening. Only 50% of infants with significant hearing loss have identifiable risk factors. Fifty percent of hearing loss in newborns is genetic, with over half of these being autosomal recessive. Nongenetic causes of hearing loss include fetal infection, teratogens, maternal disease, and perinatal events such as asphyxia, hyperbilirubinemia, and meningitis. Behavioral testing of hearing is crude in the newborn. Therefore, we follow the American Academy of Pediatrics (AAP) recommendation by screening all newborns with automated auditory brainstem response (ABR), a technique using three scalp electrodes that record brain waves and wave form responses to auditory stimulation, thereby providing information on pathways from the outer ear to the cortex. Sensitivity is 100% and specificity is 96%. Depending on the cause and extent of hearing loss, language acquisition may be improved by fitting newborns with a hearing aid as early as 1 to 3 months. (American Academy of Pediatrics, 1995; Eilers and Oller, 1994; Kuhl, 1993; Stewart, 1997).

Syphilis. Standard immunologic tests for syphilis are a routine part of prenatal care in the United States. Because it is possible for exposure to occur between the first trimester and delivery, mothers or infants of high-risk populations should be screened at delivery as well.

Human Immunodeficiency Virus. We offer testing for the human immunodeficiency virus (HIV) antibody to the newborn of any mother who has not had recent HIV testing during pregnancy. Risk varies widely in different geographic areas.

Hepatitis B. We screen all mothers for hepatitis B with increased attention to those at special risk, for example, those involved in prostitution or those from high-risk areas (Asia, Africa, Pacific islands, or inner cities of the United States) and those with occupational exposure to blood products, those who have been rejected for blood donation, those who have received multiple frequent blood transfusion, intravenous IV drug users, those who have had no prenatal care, or those with a positive history of liver disease or who live with family members with liver disease or on dialysis. Current risk estimates for infants born in Los Angeles are approximately 3 per 1000 live births (hepatitis data courtesy of L. Mascola, Los Angeles Department of Health Services). We administer hepatitis vaccine to all newborns according to current AAP recommendations. If the mother is hepatitis B–positive, then hepatitis immune globulin is administered in addition to the vaccine.

Drug Abuse. Toxicology screens are carried out on urine for newborns whose mothers have an illicit drug history, who received little prenatal care, and (for our inner-city population) on all NICU admissions. The screen used in our hospital identifies metabolites of amphetamines, phencyclidine (angel dust), opiates, and cocaine. It does not identify alcohol or cannabis. Approximately 12% of inner-city infants admitted to NICUs test positive for illicit drugs (see Chapter 10).

Tuberculosis. Mothers in high-risk groups should be skin-tested near delivery, and positive results should be followed up with a chest radiograph and a careful history for tuberculosis exposure and treatment.

Metabolic Diseases. All states screen newborns for phenylketonuria and hypothyroidism (although different screening tools are used for hypothyroidism). Most screen for galactosemia and hemoglobinopathies (such as sickle cell disease). Less than half the states screen for branched-chain aminoacidemia, biotinidase deficiency, congenital adrenal hyperplasia, and homocystinuria. Only a few states currently screen for cystic fibrosis and toxoplasmosis (Stoddard and Farrell, 1997).

WELL BABY CARE

The principles of routine care for normal infants are those of screening for disease, prophylaxis for common problems (eye care and vitamin K_1 oxide), education when needed about infant care, and anticipatory guidance. The initial and discharge history and examinations are truncated versions. A welcome current trend "demedicalizes" routine delivery and postpartum care. This concept means delivery in a "homey," rather than an operating room setting. More choices are offered to the parents concerning issues of childbirth, such as anesthesia and route and timing of delivery. The infant and mother are kept together as much as possible after birth. Fathers are often present during delivery, and liberal visiting policies that allow children to see their mother and new sibling are encouraged. Both before and after birth, nonmedically oriented classes are offered for discussing problems of both the mother and the infant. Forces in favor of these trends come from parents and (with regard to shorter hospital stays) financial considerations. Forces against these trends stem from administrative difficulties in handling the desires of parents and concerns about cross-infection.

How long should a mother and newborn stay in the hospital after delivery? Nobody knows. Since the last edition of this book, "managed care" has, to an increasing degree, replaced "fee for service" as a medical reimbursement scheme in the United States. This change has provided a new impetus to find ways of reducing medical costs. Discharging mothers and newborn infants sooner after delivery is believed to be one way of achieving this goal. In California, the current norm is a hospital stay of 24 hours for a mother and infant after a vaginal delivery, and 3 days after a cesarean section. Although the benefit for cost savings in the short term appears obvious, it is not known whether this practice carries significant increased risk, especially for inner-city women and their infants (Braveman, 1995). Lee (1995) found that readmission rates for infants nearly doubled since the length of stay after delivery has halved (Lee, 1995). Readmissions were largely for jaundice and poor milk intake. Table 31–16 lists questions for which answers are needed before discharge of the mother and infant. The length of the list illustrates the difficulties presented by discharge of the mother within 24 hours of delivery.

In most United States hospitals, in the delivery room, the newborn's eyes are instilled with erythromycin or 1% silver nitrate drops from single-use containers for prophylaxis of gonococcal eye infection. Vitamin K_1 oxide, 0.5 to 1.0 mg is given intramuscularly to prevent hemorrhagic disease of the newborn. The infant is then bathed with a nonmedicated mild soap. No antiseptic is routinely applied to the umbilical cord stump.

DISCHARGE PLANNING

Discharge from the intermediate care unit for premature infants can take place when the parents have made adequate preparations (actual and psychological) for the care of the infant. Meeting this need may take weeks of preparation on the part of the staff and may include arranging in-home support and equipment, teaching feeding and medication techniques, and providing anticipatory guidance. Other criteria for discharge include adequate feeding and weight gain, and physiologic stability (e.g., absence of apnea and steady body temperature).

Detailed recording of the major events of the infant's stay—diagnoses, results of meetings with parents and case conferences, most recent evaluations, medications, and future needs—all should be summarized, and the information disseminated appropriately.

Most importantly, the primary physician should know the parents and the infant well by the time of discharge, so that trust and confidence exist on both sides.

Discharge Summary

An array of computerized data collection systems are available and should soon permit vastly improved information transfer, freeing physicians from the tyranny of the handwritten medical record. We currently use a custom-programmed FoxPro database for data entry and retrieval including daily hospital notes for a hospital delivery service of 1700 inner-city births per year including well babies, intermediate care babies, and babies requiring intensive care.

FOLLOW-UP CARE

A variety of support groups are available for parents of infants with special problems. Pediatric follow-up care for normal infants is detailed in the *Guidelines for Health Supervision* published by the American Academy of Pediatrics and in standard pediatric texts (Avery and First, 1989). California has recently published detailed infant and child health assessment guidelines (Children's Medical Services, 1997). Follow-up care of high-risk infants is described in detail by Ballard (1988) and by Taeusch and Yogman (1987). Current changes in immunization recommendations (see Appendix 4) can be ascertained via the Centers for Disease Control and Prevention home page and the most recent Academy of Pediatrics Red Book (1997).

TABLE 31–16

Screening for Newborns

Maternal questions
  Have maternal factors affected the fetus or newborn?
    Behaviors
    Illness
    Trauma
    Surgery
  What is the mother's general physical and mental health?

Newborn infant questions
  Has the infant received good obstetric care?
  Does the infant need cardiopulmonary resuscitation?
  Does the infant have an acute or chronic infection?
  Does the infant need acute therapy?
  Does the infant have anomalies?
  Is the infant hypovolemic?
  Is the infant in pain?
  Is the infant well?
  What is the gestation?
  Is the infant of the appropriate size for gestation and, if not, to what degree and for what reason?
  Is it likely that the infant has genetic disease?
  Does the infant have difficulty with acute perinatal adaptations?
  Is there evidence of intoxication or illicit drug exposure?
  Have the parents reached an informed decision regarding circumcision?
  What is the infant's temperament?
  What is the infant's name?
  Is the infant feeding and eliminating normally?

Questions concerning future well-being
  Does the infant have a medical "home"?
  What is the health insurance, if any? Do the parents need help with this issue?
  Is the mother or family able to contend with a minor or major problem with the baby soon after discharge?
  Is the mother or family able to provide usual care for the baby? Are the parents prepared for the baby at home? Have the siblings been prepared for the arrival of a new baby?
  Is the initial maternal–infant interaction appropriate?
  Will the mother breast-feed the infant? Does she know where to get support?
  Does the mother have other emotional support and help after discharge?
  Is the mother aware of where to get postpartum care for herself?
  Is she aware of family planning choices?
  Are the parents aware of customary newborn prophylaxis and screening, e.g., eye care, vitamin K, screening for metabolic errors, hepatitis immunization, and hearing screening?
  Have the mother and father had opportunity to discuss questions, problems, and issues?
  Is a clear discharge plan in place?
  Do the parents have a copy of the pertinent birth records?
  Is the infant at risk of abuse?
  Have the parents received anticipatory guidance with regard to feeding problems, jaundice, infection signs, car seats, falls, plan for health supervision, and sleeping position (on the back to reduce risk of sudden infant death syndrome)?

REFERENCES

American Academy of Pediatrics, Committee on Infectious Diseases: Red Book, 24th ed. Elk Grove, IL, American Academy of Pediatrics, 1997.

American Academy of Pediatrics, Joint Committee on Infant Hearing. Pediatrics 99:330–334, 1995.

Aronsson DD, Goldberg MJ, Kling TF, Roy DR: Developmental dysplasia of the hip. Pediatrics 94:201–208, 1994.

Avery G: Neonatology: Pathophysiology and Management of the Newborn, 3rd ed. Philadelphia, JB Lippincott, 1987.

Avery M, First L: Pediatric Medicine. Baltimore, Williams & Wilkins, 1989.

Avery M, Litwack G: Born Early. Boston, Little, Brown, 1983.

Ballard JL, Khoury JC, Wedig K, et al: New Ballard score expanded to include extremely premature infants. J Pediat 119:417–423, 1991.

Ballard R: Pediatric Care of the ICN Graduate. Philadelphia, WB Saunders, 1988.

Balsan MJ, Holyman IR: Slide Atlas of Pediatric Physical Diagnosis: 2 Neonatology. Gower Med Pub NY, 1992.

Barness L: Manual of Pediatric Physical Diagnosis. 4th ed. Chicago, Year Book, 1976.

Bates B: A Guide to Physical Diagnosis and History Taking. 4th ed. Philadelphia, JB Lippincott, 1987.

Boylan P, Parisi V: An overview of hydramnios. Sem Perinatol 10:136, 1986.

Braveman P, Egerter S, Pearl M, Marchi K, et al: Problems associated with early discharge of newborn infants. Pediatrics 96:716–726, 1995.

CDC home page: http://www.cdc.gov/nip/child.htm

Children's Medical Services: Health Assessment Guidelines of the Child Health and Disability Prevention Program. Department of Health Services, 714/744 P Street, PO Box 942732, Sacramento, CA 94234-7320, 1997.

Cloherty J, Stark A: Manual of Neonatal Care. 2nd ed. Boston, Little, Brown, 1985.

Coen R, Koffler H: Primary Care of the Newborn. Boston, Little, Brown, 1987.

Creasy R, Resnick R: Maternal-Fetal Medicine: Principles and Practice, 2nd ed. Philadelphia, WB Saunders, 1989.

Crelin E: Anatomy of the Newborn—an Atlas. Philadelphia, Lea & Febiger, 1969.

Duncan R: Cedars Sinai Teaching Files: Detailed Newborn Exam. http://www.csmc.edu.neonatology/syllabus.exam.nursery.html.

Dunn P, Evans T, Thearle M, et al: Congenital dislocation of the hip: Early and late diagnosis and management compared. Arch Dis Child 60:407, 1985.

Eden R, Boehm F: Assessment and Care of the Fetus. Norwalk, Conn, Appleton & Lange, 1990.

Eilers RE, Oller DK: Infant vocalizations and the early diagnosis of severe hearing impairment. J Pediatr 582:248–263, 1994.

Ekelem I, Taeusch HW: Defining quality of care indicators for the neonatal intensive care unit. J Natl Med Assoc 82:345, 1990.

Faix R: Fontanel size in black and white infants. J Pediatr 100:304, 1982.

Fanaroff A, Martin R: Neonatal-Perinatal Medicine. St. Louis, CV Mosby, 1987.

Fenichel G: Neurological exam of the newborn. Int. Pediatrics 9:77, 1994.

Freedman MA, Gay GA, Brookert JE, et al: The 1989 revisions of the U.S. Standard Certificates of Live Birth and Death and the U.S. Standard Report of Fetal Death. Am J Public Health 78:168–171, 1988.

Gottfried A, Garter J: Infant Stress under Intensive Care: Environmental Neonatology. Baltimore, University Park Press, 1985.

Graham J: Smith's Recognizable Patterns of Human Deformation. Philadelphia, WB Saunders Company, 1988.

Gruebel-Lee D.: Disorders of the Hip. Philadelphia, JB Lippincott, 1983.

Hoeckelman R.: The physical examination of infants and children. *In* Bates B (Ed): A Guide to Physical Exam and History Taking. 4th ed. Philadelphia, JB Lippincott, 1987, pp 525–598.

Illingworth R: The Development of the Infant and Young Child. 2nd ed. Baltimore, Williams & Wilkins, 1963.

Kuhl PK: Development of speech perception. Ann NY Acad Sci 582:248–263, 1993.

Larson E: A causal link between hand washing and risk of infection? Examination of the evidence. Infect Control 9:28, 1988.

Lee KS, Perlman M, Ballantyne M, Elliott I, et al: Association between duration of neonatal hospital stay and readmission rate. J Pediatr 127:758–766, 1995.

Levene M, Bennett M, Punt J: Fetal and Neonatal Neurology and Neurosurgery. Edinburgh, Churchill Livingstone, 1989.

Lovery JP: Human Placenta, Clinical Perspectives. Rockville, Md, Aspen, 1987.

Mehes K: Head measurements in newborn infants. J Craniofac Genet Dev Biol 7:295, 1987.

Morrissy RT: Lovell and Winter's Pediatric Orthopedics, 3rd ed. Philadelphia, JB Lippincott, 1990.

Oski F, DeAngelis C, Feigin R, et al: Principles and Practice of Pediatrics. Philadelphia, JB Lippincott, 1990.

Phelan J, Smith C, Broussard P, et al: Amniotic fluid volume assessment using the four quadrant technique in the pregnancy between 36 and 42 weeks gestation. J Reprod Med 32:540, 1987.

Place M, Parkin PM, Fitton M: Effectiveness of neonatal screening for congenital dislocation of the hip. Lancet 2:249, 1978.

Popich G, Smith D: Fontanels, range of normal size. J Pediatr 80:749, 1972.

Raymond GV, Holmes LB: Head circumference standards in neonates. J Child Neurol 9:63–66, 1994.

Roberton N: Textbook of Neonatology, Edinburgh, Churchill Livingstone, 1987.

Scanlon J: A System of Newborn Physical Exam. Baltimore, University Park Press, 1979.

Schwartz M, Shaul D: Abdominal masses in the newborn. Pediatr Rev 11:172, 1989.

Staheli L: Management of congenital hip dysplasia. Pediatr Ann 18:24, 1989.

Stewart J, Codirector, Newborn Hearing Sceening Program, Beth Israel Deaconess Medical Center, Boston. Personal communication, 1997.

Stoddard JJ, Farrell PM: State-to-state variations in newborn screening policies. Arch Pediatr Adolesc Med 151:561–564, 1997.

Taeusch HW, Yogman Y: Follow-up Management of the High-Risk Infant. Boston, Little, Brown, 1987.

Versmold HT, Kitterman JA, Phibbs RH, et al: Aortic blood pressure during the first 12 hours of life in infants with birth weight 610 to 4220 grams. Pediatrics 67:607–613, 1981.

Volpe J (Ed): Neonatal neurology (Preface). Clin Perinatol 16:xi, 1989.

Vulliamy D, Johnston P: The Newborn Child. 6th ed. Edinburgh, Churchill Livingstone, 1987.

Walther FJ, Leighton JO: Diagnostic ultrasound screening of infants. *In* Pediatric and Neonatal Tests and Procedures. Philadelphia, WB Saunders, 1996, pp 387–405.

Yu V, Wood C: Prematurity. Edinburgh, Churchill Livingstone, 1987.

Ziai M, Clarke T, Merritt A: Assessment of the Newborn—A Guide for the Practitioner. Boston, Little, Brown, 1984.

Zitelli BJ, Davis HW: Slide Atlas of Pediatric Physical Diagnosis. St. Louis, CV Mosby, 1992.

CHAPTER 32

Behavioral Assessment of the Newborn

Peter A. Gorski

Thanks to the advanced state of contemporary neonatal medicine, scientific and clinical attention is increasingly directed toward functional understanding and support of the developing brain and central nervous system (CNS) of newborn infants. In modern neonatal intensive care units, infants who survive deliveries after only 24 to 26 weeks' gestation can be cared for. Such infants face months of hospitalization, even in the absence of life-threatening physiologic instability. While providing necessary pulmonary, cardiac, nutritional, and metabolic support, the nursery should also offer a balance of sensory stimulation and protection for the immature brain and nervous system of these smallest newborns.

The science of brain–behavior relationships has exploded with insights into the nature of neonatal neurologic functioning—infant behavior. Normal or disturbed behavior may point to healthy or affected areas and mechanisms in the CNS (Pearson and Dietrich, 1985). As a result, research is beginning to inform clinical practice about the effects on infant neurobehavioral outcome from sensory patterns and caregiving protocols in the hospital environment.

BIOLOGICAL FOUNDATIONS OF NEONATAL BEHAVIOR
Intrinsic Activity Cycles

Much research has concentrated on the search for a basic cycle of human movement, rest, and alerting that might describe a fundamental characteristic of behavioral organization and underlying brain activity that exists from early fetal life. Robertson (1987) has documented the existence of spontaneous motility cycles in human newborns across all behavioral states of sleep and wakefulness. This cyclic variation in spontaneous movement every 1 to 10 minutes is observed in utero in human fetuses during the second half of gestation and perhaps earlier (deVries et al, 1982, 1985). These patterns of human cyclic motility are weaker and less regular during less organized behavioral states of active sleep and may be influenced by alterations in the metabolic environment of the fetus and newborn (Robertson and Dierker, 1986). Most importantly, the finding of remarkable stability of these cycles of spontaneous movement from midgestation through the first 10 weeks of postterm life adds evidence for a dramatic shift in brain organization and behavioral self-regulation, not at the time of birth at 40 weeks, but after 50 postconceptual weeks. Previous studies of electrophysiologic organization of the CNS, structural maturation of the cerebral cortex, and behavioral development of infant crying and sleep patterns indicate relative CNS immaturity during the first 2 to 4 months postterm with respect to fundamental organization of cortical activity as well as of higher perceptual and cognitive processes (Brazelton, 1962; Conel, 1947; Parmelee et al, 1964). Therefore, despite the substantial environmental and physiologic changes that accompany birth, the human fetus and newborn share basic continuities of behavior and responsiveness.

In general, healthy full-term infants display a regular series of distinct states over a period of time. These were first described and systematized by Wolff (1959 and 1966). A number of other classification schemes have been published (Brazelton, 1984; Prechtl, 1974; Thoman, 1985). As an example, Brazelton has proposed a system with the following six states: (1) quiet sleep, (2) active sleep, (3) drowsiness, (4) alert inactivity, (5) active awake, and (6) crying. Each state can be distinguished on the basis of a number of distinct clusters of behavior (Table 32–1).

TABLE 32–1

Neonatal State Classification Scale

State	Characteristics
Quiet sleep	Regular breathing, eyes closed; spontaneous activity confined to startles and jerky movements at regular intervals. Responses to external stimuli are partially inhibited, and any response is likely to be delayed. No eye movements, and state changes are less likely after stimuli or startles than in other states.
Active sleep	Irregular breathing patterns, sucking movements, eyes closed but rapid eye movements can be detected underneath the closed lids. Infants also have some low-level and irregular motor activity. Startles occur in response to external stimuli and can produce a change of state.
Drowsiness	While the newborn is semidozing, eyes may be open or closed; eyelids often flutter; activity level variable and interspersed with mild startles. Drowsy newborns are responsive to sensory stimuli but with some delay, and state change frequently follows stimulation.
Alert inactivity	A bright alert look, with attention focused on sources of auditory or visual stimuli; motor activity is inhibited while attending to stimuli.
Active awake	Eyes open, considerable motor activity, thrusting movements of extremities, and occasional startles set off by activity; reactive to external stimulation with an increase in startles or motor activity. Discrete responses are difficult to distinguish due to general high activity level.
Crying	Intense irritability in the form of sustained crying, and jerky limb movement. This state is difficult to break through with stimulation.

Data from Brazelton TB: Neonatal Behavioral Assessment Scale, 2nd ed. London, Heinemann, 1984.

The study of behavioral states in infants has attracted wide interest as an indicator of the functional integrity of the CNS during the fetal, neonatal, and infant periods of development. Maturational changes in sleep-wake cycles have been studied, and neonatal state periodicities have been correlated with later neurodevelopmental, especially mental, outcome. These investigations have found that earlier maturation of electrophysiologic and behavioral patterns of quiet sleep in the neonatal period predict higher performance on cognitive tests at preschool and school age (Anders and Keener, 1985; Beckwith and Parmelee, 1986; Nijhuis et al, 1982; Thoman et al, 1981; Whitney and Thoman, 1993).

While sleeping and waking states in infancy reflect the competency of the CNS, they also modulate the infant's interactions with the external environment. A number of studies have documented the influence that an infant's state has on his or her response to stimulation; the response may be different, depending on whether the infant is in a sleep, drowsy, or alert state. For example, a visual stimulus that captures the attention of a quietly awake infant does not elicit a response from a more aroused, crying infant. Indeed, this arousal distinction applies not only between states but also within a particular state. A newborn infant displays a different pattern of responsiveness at the beginning of an alert period compared with the end of the period. This difference is analogous to the daytime pattern of adults who commonly go through periods of higher and lower arousal while awake. This pattern, called the basic rest-activity cycle (BRAC) by Aserinsky and Kleitman (1955), is distinct from the sleep-wake cycle and is theoretically related to the cyclic activity of the autonomic nervous system (ANS). The ANS mediates the infant's responsivity to the external environment and regulates a number of homeostatic functions.

Among the ANS effects on homeostatic processes are its effects on cardiac and respiratory functions. The effect of the ANS on cardiac activity develops prenatally and through the 1st year of life. When cardiac activity first appears in the embryo, it shows no beat-to-beat variability, even during periods of increased movement (Berg and Berg, 1979). As the fetus develops, heart rate (HR) becomes more responsive to increased movement. The average HR of a full-term infant is between 120 and 160 beats per minute (Ashton and Connolly, 1971). Both the average and the variability of HR are affected by the behavioral state of the infant, with higher, more variable rates seen in the more active states and lower, more regular rates found in the quiet states. During the first 2 to 3 months after birth, both the mean HR and the HR variability increase, followed by a decrease in both rate and variability between 3 and 6 months (Harper et al, 1976). In addition, the increase in HR variability is increasingly regulated by input from the ANS.

Respiratory activity, although not under direct ANS control, shows a pattern of development that is similar to that seen in cardiac activity. Before 30 weeks' gestational age, preterm infants show a constant semiregular pattern of respiration that is not affected by increased motor activity (Dreyfus-Brisac, 1968). By 40 weeks, respiration becomes more related to body activity, with quiet periods becoming more strongly associated with periods of regular respiration

(Parmelee et al, 1967). In addition, the proportion of irregular to regular respirations decreases across the first 8 months of life (Parmelee et al, 1972).

Apnea and bradycardia are phenomena that may also demonstrate relative lack of organization of nervous system control over respiratory and cardiac functions, respectively. The decrease in frequency of apnea and bradycardia with increasing age parallels maturational changes in the structure and function of the infant's nervous system (Bronson, 1982). Parmelee and colleagues (1972) demonstrated that such changes in respiratory patterns were concurrent with changes in eye movement and body movement patterns, which appear to reflect the maturation of inhibitory cortical mechanisms in infants. Recent data from extensive population studies in Great Britain demonstrate the common occurrence of apnea without oxygen desaturation in healthy infants (Poets et al, 1993). Only a small minority of apneic pauses seemingly affect blood gas homeostasis, suggesting that recording breathing signals without monitoring oxygenation may provide little information about the maturation of respiratory control.

Neonatal behavioral and psychophysiologic measures of state organization and cardiac variability are among the most frequently applied methods in neonatal behavioral research. These techniques highlight maturational differences between preterm and term infants that could affect their responses to treatment practices. Consistent differences in the sleep characteristics of preterm infants distinguish them from full-term infants when tested at the same conceptual ages. Preterms have been found to have relatively longer bouts of quiet sleep, more movement in sleep states, more frequent rapid eye movement episodes, and less consistent combinations of behavioral and physiologic criteria used to define infant sleep states (Anders and Keener, 1985; Davis and Thoman, 1987; Parmelee et al, 1967).

Less consensus exists across studies of waking behavior in preterm and full-term infants. Some researchers report less alert time in preterm infants when compared with full-term infants at the same postconception ages (DiVitto and Goldberg, 1979; Lester et al, 1976). Other researchers find them to be equally alert (Paludetto et al, 1982; Telzrow et al, 1982). Still other investigators find preterm infants to be more alert (Palmer et al, 1982). Similar discrepancies are reported with respect to irritability and arousal levels (Aylward, 1982; Howard et al, 1976; McGehee and Eckerman, 1983; Michaelis et al, 1973).

Taken together, the findings suggest that the underlying difference in CNS organization between premature and full-term infants lies in an unevenness in the development of premature infants. Aspects of greater CNS maturity (more alertness and less sleep) coexist with characteristics of less CNS maturity (more nonalert waking activity and more frequent sleep-wake transitions). As Davis and Thoman (1987) conclude, premature infants exhibit irregular state development as compared with full-term infants, rather than either increased maturity or immaturity. These early neurobehavioral differences between infants of different gestational ages could reflect significant changes in brain organization that may continue throughout childhood development. Such functional differences may affect specific perceptual, cognitive, or emotional processes rather than intelligence. Current long-term follow-up studies of preterm infants tend to find that the mental development and neurologic status of medically uncompromised preterm infants at school age does not differ from that of full-terms (Bakeman and Brown, 1980; Saint-Anne Dargassies, 1979), yet these same children are more likely to show visual-motor and spatial difficulties, with associated school under-achievement (Hunt et al, 1982; Klein et al, 1985). Infants who experience severe perinatal medical complications, such as bronchopulmonary dysplasia or severe intracranial hemorrhage, are more vulnerable to continued long-term neurodevelopmental disabilities (Brazy et al, 1991; Vohr et al, 1991).

The infant cry state is itself attracting interest in the effort to develop predictive measures of CNS functioning (Lester, 1987). The association of unusual cry features with conditions related to nervous system damage has been recognized for years. Early research demonstrated the association of cry features, such as unusually high pitch and short duration, with brain damage as well as with illnesses that affect the nervous system and prenatal drug exposure. The cry characteristics were generally not key diagnostic criteria in these cases but served to substantiate a previous diagnosis.

Analysis of cries may serve a useful diagnostic function. The cry characteristics of full-term infants with prenatal and perinatal complications and infants who show signs of inadequate prenatal nutrition, for example, have been found to be much like those found among infants with more obvious signs of nervous system problems (Zeskind and Lester, 1978, 1981). Successful prediction of developmental outcome from neonatal cry analyses corroborates a relation between the characteristics of the infant's cry and the functional integrity of the infant's nervous system (Lester, 1987).

Physiologic measures of autonomic regulation are linked to maturational and developmental characteristics of CNS organization in full-term and high-risk infants. Furthermore, research identifies correlations between behavioral and physiologic indices of neurodevelopment. Neural control of heart rate patterns through parasympathetic pathways may be a marker of CNS integrity and reactivity (Porges et al, 1982). In particular, vagal activity, or respiratory arrhythmia, has been linked to CNS maturation, cognitive outcome following high-risk birth, intrinsic temperamental characteristics of individual children, and emotional adaptation to stress in the parent-infant relationship (Coll et al, 1984; Field et al, 1988; Fox and Porges, 1985; Lester et al, 1990; Porges, 1983). Recent research examining the pituitary-adrenal stress response of infants demonstrates prolonged elevations of salivary cortisol in 1 year olds scored as insecurely attached to their mothers (Spangler and Grossmann, 1993).

Sensory-Perceptual Functions

Sensory systems undergo rather rapid changes during the last trimester of pregnancy and the first several months after birth. Prenatally, the various senses begin to differentiate at separate times and then continue to develop at different rates through postnatal life. Estimation of the functional onset of a given sensory system is complicated by a number of factors. First, because peripheral structures mature before central ones, responsiveness in peripheral structures does not necessarily indicate that the full system is functional. Second, because a variety of methods (i.e., histologic, electrophysiologic, and behavioral) have been used to determine the onset of function, discrepancies in the estimation of actual time of functional onset may result. Despite these problems, there appears to be an orderly sequence in the functional development of the sensory systems of human infants. This sequence is cutaneous (tactile), vestibular, auditory, and visual across a variety of species, including the human (Gottlieb, 1971).

The path from first onset to functional maturity is marked by changes in the ability of the system to respond to stimulation and by shifts in the system's organization (Turkewitz et al, 1983). Because the tactile, visual, and auditory senses are the avenues of communication between the infant and the world, a brief outline of some key aspects of development in these systems follows.

Cutaneous (Tactile) System

The earliest signs of human behavior appear as the reaction of a fetus to touch. Hooker's (1952) classic studies demonstrate that before 7½ weeks' gestational age, the human embryo shows no evidence of reflex activity, and no area of the skin is sensitive to tactile stimulation. During the next 7 weeks, however, almost the entire body surface becomes sensitive to touch, beginning with the lips and ending with the feet and legs. (The top and back of the head remain insensitive until birth.) Thus, responses to somesthetic stimulation are the first human behaviors to develop, followed approximately 2 weeks later by responses to vestibular and proprioceptive stimulation. Being the first, it may prepare the organism for subsequent organization around environmental input and thus have fundamental importance for later development (Carmichael, 1954; Montagu, 1971).

Early tactile contact during infancy may influence growth rates, adaptability, learning, activity level, exploratory behavior, attachment, sociability, ability to withstand stress, and immunologic development (Brown, 1984; Field et al, 1986). Whether the human newborn is sensitive to pain stimuli induced by medical procedures, such as common heel sticks for blood or invasive surgical operations, has been debated (Anand and Hickey, 1987; Owens and Todt, 1984) (see Chapter 16). Neuroanatomic and physiologic studies declare the early fetal development of sensory nerve tract fibers responsive to pain (Anand and Hickey, 1987; Swafford and Allan, 1968). Neonatal circumcision has been the prototypic subject for demonstrating infant behavioral, physiologic, and humoral responses to pain stimulation (Dixon et al, 1984; Gunnar et al, 1981; Williamson and Williamson, 1983). Non-nutritive sucking on pacifiers and parenteral use of sedatives and analgesics diminish irritable behavior and blunt heart rate and mean arterial pressure changes during and immediately following painful medical procedures (Anand et al, 1987; Anderson et al, 1983; Field and Goldson, 1984; Gunnar et al, 1984). Such interventions may help maintain physiologic homeostasis during stressful procedures. Preterm infants, in particular, may benefit from the resultant stability of cerebral and possibly pulmonary blood flow (Brazy, 1988; Perlman and Volpe, 1985). The potential for preventing some of the occurrences and consequences of intracranial hemorrhage or acute pulmonary vasoconstriction could have enormous impact on the developmental outcome of high-risk infants, and prevention may, in part, depend on increased recognition and control of pain in newborn infants.

Auditory System

The auditory system becomes functional between the 25th and 27th week of gestation (Grimwade et al, 1971; Rubel, 1985; Starr et al, 1977). Moreover, sound is capable of penetrating the abdominal wall as well as the amniotic sac (Armitage et al, 1980; Bench, 1968; Bench et al, 1979). Low-frequency sounds (below 1000 Hz) pass most easily through the abdominal wall; as the frequency of the sounds increases, the intensity of the sound becomes progressively attenuated. Once the sound passes through the abdominal wall, its spectral composition is further altered because the sound-conducting medium is aquatic. From a functional standpoint, the auditory system is initially responsive to low and middle frequencies, and, as development progresses, sensitivity to higher frequencies increases. These changes have been shown to be related to the growth of the basilar membrane, although more central changes may be responsible for them as well (Hecox and Deegan, 1985; Rubel, 1985). During development of the fetus, the overall intensity of sound necessary for a response decreases. Roughly speaking, the infant's sensitivity to sounds is approximately 15 to 20 decibels lower than that of an adult, although these thresholds change during the first months of life.

Primary sounds probably available to the mammalian fetus are cardiovascular sounds. However, both internal sounds generated by the mother and externally generated sounds are clearly audible (Armitage et al, 1980). Thus, the fetus is exposed to internal and external sounds whose characteristics change during gestation because there are changes in both the properties of the auditory environment of the mother and in the auditory structures. Such exposure to sound during gestation may permit the infant to recognize the mother's voice right after birth. Infants younger than 30 hours of age preferentially suck on a non-nutritive pacifier that triggers a recording of their mother's voice rather than a stranger's voice (De Casper and Fifer, 1980).

From a behavioral standpoint, the full-term newborn is able to orient toward nonaversive sources of auditory stimulation by turning the head and eyes toward the sound and to turn away from an intense, aversive stimulus (Muir and Field, 1979; Turkewitz et al, 1966). This orienting behavior, characterized by a fairly long latency (7 to 8 seconds), gradually declines over the first 4 months of life and then reemerges by the 5th month as a short latency response (Muir and Clifton, 1985).

In addition to these basic auditory capacities, the young infant can discriminate basic sounds of spoken language. Such an ability is crucial for the acquisition of language because a linguistic system consists of a set of distinct classes of sounds, known as phonemes (e.g., "ba" and "pa"), that signal to the listener differences in meaning. The general findings from numerous studies are that similar to adults, infants are able to distinguish between phonemes that belong to different categories (Aslin et al, 1983). Moreover, the set of phonemes that infants are able to discriminate either diminishes or changes once they are exposed to their native linguistic environment.

Visual System

The visual system offers an interesting paradox. On the one hand, it is the last system to start functioning during gestation and the least well-developed at birth. On the other hand, it is the system that is usually dominant in a person's everyday interactions with the environment and, as a result, has been the most investigated.

The retina differentiates during the first trimester of gestation. The retina consists of the fovea, located in the central region, as well as rods and other peripheral structures. The fovea is composed of cones whose primary function is to mediate detail and color vision. The rods detect changes in brightness and movement. Although differentiation of the foveal region occurs first, at birth, the foveal region is quite immature and different from the adult fovea, whereas the periphery is fairly similar to the adult periphery (Abramov et al, 1982).

The other major structures in the visual pathway also change considerably during postnatal development. The lateral geniculate nucleus (LGN) of the thalamus, a relay station between the eye and the visual cortex, undergoes important physiologic and anatomic changes. In primates, the LGN becomes more responsive with development. The most significant changes, however, occur in the visual cortex where the neurons undergo marked morphologic changes. These changes, which peak at 6 months postterm, consist of the growth and arborization of a large number of dendrites, presumably accompanied by synaptogenesis. In addition, the visual pathway is gradually myelinated. Myelination of the optic nerve is completed by 3 months of age and that of the visual cortex is completed somewhat later (Yakovlev and LeCours, 1967).

Nearly all basic functions of the visual system exhibit marked changes in the first 3 to 6 months of life. Accommodation (i.e., ability to focus objects) is poor between birth and 1 month of age and then improves through the 3rd month (Banks, 1980). In the 1st month, infants tend to overaccommodate distant objects and underaccommodate near objects. Smooth-pursuit eye movements display similar changes. Before 6 weeks of age, infants do not display smooth pursuit of a moving target, but track it with jerky (saccadic) eye movements. By the 8th week, smooth pursuit appears and improves thereafter until the 3rd month when no saccades are present (Aslin, 1981).

One of the most important functions of the visual system is to detect patterned information. A traditional measure of the system's ability to do so has been visual acuity. Acuity is poor at birth and improves rapidly over the first 6 months of life. Acuity in a newborn infant is roughly equivalent to a Snellen value of 20/600, which is 30 times lower than normal adult acuity. There is also a steady increase in the range of detectable spatial frequencies and contrasts over the first 6 months of life. Thus, young infants are sensitive to only a fraction of the patterned information that adults are sensitive to and are able to perceive best only those objects that are close to them and that have high contrast (Banks and Salapatek, 1983).

Despite these limitations, young infants can fixate visually with a variety of stimuli with attributes such as intensity, number and size of elements, pattern, and flicker. Response to color is a somewhat controversial topic, but the most conservative estimate is that, by 2 months of age, infants probably possess red and green cones but lack blue cones and are therefore, at least dichromats; by 3 months, it is less likely that they have a blue insensitivity (Banks, 1983; Fantz and Nevis, 1967; Lewkowicz, 1985).

Temperament

The preceding discussion highlighted aspects of behavioral and neurobiological development that are common to all human infants. Differences in development were noted to be caused by idiosyncrasies of gestational age at birth or other medical risk factors. How then, can the range and stability of differences in the behavior of infants born at the same gestation and with similar medical courses be accounted for? The pattern of behavioral and psychophysiologic responses to animate and inanimate stimuli that characterize each newborn is often referred to as temperament. Temperament describes the style without supplying the explanation of individual patterns of behavior.

Researchers tend to agree that temperamental dimensions reflect behavioral styles rather than discrete behavioral acts, have biological underpinnings, and enjoy continuity of expression relative to other aspects of behavior (Goldsmith et al, 1987; Tirosh et al, 1992). Infancy is commonly regarded as the time of clearest expression of temperamental characteristics, before the link between temperament and behavior becomes more complex as the child matures.

Disagreements exist about the extent to which an infant's behavior can be attributed to temperament, whether temperament is stable within individuals regardless of social contexts, and the nature of its inheritance (Goldsmith et al, 1987). Formal neonatal behavioral examination, standardized psychological assessment, and parents' reports all identify behavioral traits that together compose an image of the nature each infant brings into interaction with the caregiving world (Brazelton, 1984; Carey and McDevitt, 1978; Rothbart, 1981; Thomas et al, 1963). According to Chess and Thomas (1986), caregivers learn to relate to infants through nine behavioral categories of individual differences that comprise temperament (Table 32–2).

Chess and Thomas (1986) describe three functionally significant temperamental constellations that emerged from their sample during the New York Longitudinal Study. Perinatal medical risks were distributed equally across the three groups of children, and, thus, did not appear to determine temperament. About 40% of all children were characterized by early and sustained rhythmicity, predominantly positive mood, mild intensity of reactions, positive approach to new stimuli, and positive adaptability over repeated exposures to change. About 10% of the sample were infants and children with irregular behavior, intense and predominantly negative expressions, negative withdrawal from new stimuli, and difficulty adapting to change even over time. Another 15% were somewhere in between

TABLE 32–2

Temperament Categories

Category	Description
Activity level	The motor level of a child's functioning. The ratio of active to inactive periods each day (e.g., infant may move often even during sleep).
Intensity of reaction	The general magnitude of response, regardless of affective direction (e.g., cries loudly for all needs, also vocalizes with audible vigor).
Quality of mood	The predominance of contented, positive behavior versus irritable, negative disposition, regardless of intensity (e.g., generally calm, smiling, easily engaged versus fussy).
Rhythmicity or regularity	The predictability or unpredictability of biological or behavioral patterns (e.g., sleep-wake cycle, hunger, feeding pattern, elimination schedule, crying, and alerting).
Threshold of responsiveness	The amount of stimulation required to elicit a response (e.g., rapidity of buildup to full cry when handled).
Approach or withdrawal	The initial response to a new stimulus (e.g., new food, toy, person, or room). Responses are observed through mood (e.g., smiling, grimacing, or crying) or activity (e.g., in infants, by calming, squirming, or spitting).
Adaptability	The eventual response to a new or changed environment or condition (e.g., acceptance of bottle or babysitter).
Attention span and persistence	Two related categories describing the duration of effort at a task or activity and the continuation at task, despite attention to distractions (e.g., prolonged visual fixation and orienting).
Distractibility	The infant's susceptibility to changing attention or activity when presented with interfering stimuli (e.g., diverted from visual attention by extraneous sound stimulus).

Adapted from Chess S, Thomas A: Temperament in Clinical Practice. New York, Guilford Press, 1986, pp 273–278.

the two. These infants were distinguished by mildly negative initial withdrawal from new stimuli with slow, yet eventual adaptability after repeated contact. Thirty-five percent of their sample could not readily be classified into those "easy," "difficult," or "slow-to-warm up" personalities.

Caregivers and children bring their individual temperaments into the relationship they create with each other. Similarities or differences can produce understanding and comfort or confusion and conflict. Whether stable or changed over time, temperament influences the ease, harmony, and pleasure between the child and his environment at each stage of development. In return, the child continuously learns to find those environments and relationships that best support his or her needs and style. These lessons begin immediately through the new relationship between newborn infant and parent. The neonatal period serves to launch parents' perceptions and infants' expectations in the direction of contented anticipation of the future or toward frustration and learned helplessness (Goldberg, 1979; Seligman, 1975; Sroufe, 1986).

ENVIRONMENTAL INFLUENCES

The preceding sections discussed the genetically influenced biologic foundations of behavior in human infants. This structural and functional development unfolds throughout the prenatal and neonatal period. Concurrently, the developing brain and nervous system are constantly exposed and responsive to various conditions, substances, and stimuli from the external environment. The course of behavioral development may be altered accordingly. This section illustrates some of the better-known sources of environmental influence on the emerging behavioral organization of infants.

In Utero Drug Exposure

There has been long-standing concern as to the behavioral effects of narcotic drugs on the developing fetus. Heroin-addicted newborns are at high risk for sleep disturbances (as measured by electroencephalograms), growth retardation, CNS irritability associated with narcotic withdrawal, sudden infant death syndrome, and behavioral disorganization of state and alerting and motor processes (Chavez et al, 1979; Desmond and Wilson, 1975; Strauss et al, 1975). Similar findings have been reported for infants prenatally exposed to numerous other narcotic as well as nonnarcotic drugs (Chasnoff et al, 1982, 1983; Doberczak et al, 1987; Ward et al, 1986). Quality of prenatal care, maternal nutrition, and home environment compound, or even exceed, the developmental risks associated with maternal drug addiction (Lifschitz et al, 1985).

The potential neurodevelopmental and behavioral effects of cocaine on the human infant are of serious concern, ranging from perinatal cerebral infarction to intrauterine growth retardation, abnormal sleep and feeding patterns, irritability, and tremulousness (Chasnoff et al, 1986; Chasnoff 1988; Chiriboga et al, 1993; Dixon et al, 1990; Mayes et al, 1993; Oro and Dixon, 1987). More recently, studies find that cocaine may have less direct neurobehavioral teratogenicity than associated or synergistic influence along with an impoverished, depressed, polydrug caregiving environment (Brooks-Gunn et al, 1994; Coles and Platzman, 1993; Singer et al, 1994; Volpe, 1992; Zuckerman and Frank, 1992).

Other substances that cross the placental circulation may contribute to neonatal behavioral disturbances and later developmental dysfunction. These include, among others, alcohol, caffeine, and compounds in cigarette smoke (Clarren and Smith, 1978; Emory et al, 1988; MacArthur and Knox, 1988; Shaywitz et al, 1981). Often, the extent to which the drugs directly cause long-term CNS damage, whether they act primarily to contribute to hypoxic ischemic conditions, or whether they serve as a proxy for a suboptimal home environment cannot be ascertained (see Chapter 10).

Maternal Stress

Studies of the psychobiology of stress during pregnancy warn of possible noradrenergic and cholinergic perturba-

tions resultant from severe psychological stress (Moyer et al, 1977). Such biochemical alterations during fetal development may in turn modify neuroanatomic and physiologic organization, resulting in neonatal behavioral disorders and developmental risk (Herrenkohl, 1986).

Perinatal Environmental Influences

Compounds that create regional depression of sensory pathways during labor may cross the placental circulation and could cause CNS depression in the delivered newborn. However, studies that carefully control for the effects of parity and length of labor indicate that, when applied in tightly controlled dosage, using the minimum quantities needed to achieve anesthesia, behavioral signs of neurologic depression are minimal and short-lived (Kraemer et al, 1972; Tronick et al, 1976). This finding has been replicated across studies that tested the effects of a variety of drugs and routes of administration (Lester et al, 1982; Murray et al, 1981; Sepkoski et al, 1992). Current clinical concern, however, centers on the possibly disorganizing effect of obstetric medication on newborn sucking and feeding (Kuhnert et al, 1985; Sanders-Phillips et al, 1988).

Neonatal medical procedures may themselves affect newborn behavior during the first days or weeks of life. For example, research on the disorganizing effects of phototherapy cautions about the prudent use of this therapeutic intervention in cases of mild-to-moderate nonhemolytic hyperbilirubinemia (Ju and Lin, 1991).

After birth, infants are placed in any number of physical environments. Each caregiving locale presents a unique combination and pattern of sensory stimuli. The newborn's response and adaptation depend on the nature of the interaction between the infant's biobehavioral capacities and the sensory characteristics of the caregiving environment. Public attention has long been directed at alternative birthing environments in and out of hospital for full-term low-risk infants (Ballard et al, 1985). Well-timed social support can further improve pregnancy outcomes for mother and newborn (Kennell et al, 1991). Meanwhile, professionals who treat high-risk and prematurely born infants have begun to investigate the sources and neurobehavioral impact of sensory stimulation intrinsic to the physical and human environment of neonatal intensive care units (NICUs).

Environment of the Neonatal Intensive Care Unit

Consequent to recent technological breakthroughs in neonatal medicine, neonatal mortality has dramatically decreased in the past half decade. The exogenous administration of natural or synthetic surfactant offers hope for even more accelerated progress toward reducing neonatal mortality and morbidity. NICUs are increasingly populated by tiny newborns (<1000 g) who breathe spontaneously, oxygenate effectively, and are likely to survive well beyond the neonatal period. However, the physiologic immaturity of all their organ systems aside from their pulmonary alveoli demands prolonged hospitalization in high-risk neonatal medical centers. These infants are often medically stable, yet fragile, and their CNSs are appropriately immature given their gestational age at birth. Hospitalized for weeks or months during the critical period of preterm neurologic organization previously discussed in this chapter, these infants are chronically exposed to potentially positive or negative conditions in their environment. Evidence links acute fluctuations of systemic hemodynamics with environmental events and caregiver interventions (Gorski et al, 1984; Gorski and Huntington, 1988; Linn et al, 1985b; Long et al, 1980). Moreover, modern methods of monitoring cerebral blood flow, intracranial pressure changes, and brain oxygenation identify a direct relationship between central hypoxemia, apnea, bradycardia, and cerebral circulation and autoregulation (Brazy, 1988; Perlman and Volpe, 1985; Perlman et al, 1984).

Over the past decade, investigators have systematically examined characteristics of NICUs, caregiving protocols including patterns of medical and social intervention, and infant behavioral and physiologic responses in interaction with this level of care (Gaiter, 1985; Gorski et al, 1979, 1983; Gottfried, 1985; Gottfried et al, 1981; High and Gorski, 1985; Lawson et al, 1977; Linn et al, 1985a). Because these studies did not impose changes in caregiver behavior, they provide representative views of the sensory conditions normally experienced by premature infants in a NICU. For example, results have depicted the NICU environment as one which provides both sensory overload and deprivation (High and Gorski, 1985). These studies found that infants experience a bombardment of stimuli from sheer numbers of different caregivers and procedures each day. At the same time, however, little social contact and long intervals of social isolation also characterize the nature of caregiver–infant interaction in NICUs. They also discovered an absence of temporal contingency between the sleep or awake state of infants in a NICU and the onset of either medical or, surprisingly, social interventions by NICU caregivers. These dissociated sensory experiences in the neonatal period might theoretically relate to subsequent developmental deficits of cross-sensory and sensory-motor integration in premature infants (Rose et al, 1978).

How and to what extent can caregivers influence developmental outcome by manipulating the NICU environment? Some investigators started from the theoretical premise that the NICU environment deprives infants of necessary stimulation and therefore tested the effects of supplemental sensory input (Bernbaum et al, 1983; Field et al, 1982, 1986; Katz, 1971; Korner et al, 1975, 1978; Korner and Schneider, 1983; Leib et al, 1980; Resnick et al, 1987; White and Labarba, 1976). Positive results from these studies include increased formula intake and weight gain; better motor, visual, and auditory functioning; altered sleep patterns; decreased apnea; and improved scores on developmental testing after hospital discharge. Other researchers who professed a belief that the NICU bombards infants with constant overstimulation designed methods of protecting infants from potentially damaging responses to sensory inputs from the environment while at the same time offering stimuli contingent with the infant's activity or physiologic status (Als et al, 1986; Barnard and Bee, 1983; Thoman and Graham, 1986). Their positive results include earlier weaning from ventilatory support, improved devel-

opmental scores on follow-up, enhanced motor organization, and increased time in quiet sleep (Als et al, 1994).

Neonatal behavioral intervention programs represent a proactive effort to consider and support infant and family development at the beginning of extrauterine life. Methodologic weaknesses pervade the literature and weaken the generalizability and efficacy of current research in this field (Gilkerson et al, 1990). Common limitations include small sample sizes, insufficient demographic data to ensure subject comparability before intervention, limited descriptions of routine and experimental protocols, simultaneous use of multiple interventions, limited involvement of parents, and short-term follow-up periods.

Much useful and positive experience also has resulted from these investigations. The work has advanced concern for the effects of the NICU environment on brain growth and behavior, while providing further explanation for the nearly universal discrepancy in function between premature and full-term infants when tested at the same postconceptual age during infancy (Als et al, 1988; Aylward, 1982; Duffy et al, 1990; Majnemer et al, 1992).

Non-Nutritive Sucking

Stimulating non-nutritive sucking during gavage feedings has been used as a method of influencing neuromaturation through learned experience. Contemporary research on preterm human infants documents the benefits of this practice on a wide range of physiologic processes and health outcomes. For example, compared with control group infants, infants who were gavage-fed while simultaneously using a pacifier had fewer tube feedings, earlier onset of successful bottle and breast-feeding, a higher average daily weight gain, earlier discharge from hospital, and lower hospital care costs (Burroughs et al, 1981; Field et al, 1982).

Bernbaum and coworkers (1983) found that non-nutritive sucking during gavage feeding accelerated the maturation of the sucking reflex, decreased intestinal transit time, and led to more efficient use of calories absorbed. Woodson and Hamilton (1988) linked improved growth in preterm infants to the finding that non-nutritive sucking sustains reduced heart rates. The behavioral calming effect produced during non-nutritive sucking may rechannel calorie consumption from aroused states, crying, and motor activity to sleep and growth.

THE SOCIAL SIGNIFICANCE OF NEONATAL BEHAVIOR

This chapter has reviewed evidence for the newborn's competence to perceive, respond to, and communicate with its environment. Newborns help adults succeed as caregivers by being readable, predictable, and responsive. No longer can professionals allow parents to feel totally responsible for all their infant's actions. The newborn, once thought to be a "blank slate to be written upon by his environment, his world a blooming, buzzing confusion" (James, 1890), has become respected as a social partner who can effectively engage and, to some extent, guide caregivers to support his or her growth and development.

Not all infants are born after a complete intrauterine gestation, without a CNS condition or behavioral dysfunction. Premature infants are generally less alert, less active, and less responsive than full-term infants during the neonatal period and the first few months of infancy (Brown and Bakeman, 1979; DiVitto and Goldberg, 1979). These infants challenge their caregivers to be more active in initiating social interaction or, paradoxically, less intrusive and more sensitive of their lower sensory thresholds (Beckwith and Cohen, 1978; Field, 1977). Whereas healthy full-terms quickly and consistently reward their parents for providing a satisfying or organizing response, premature infants and their parents risk repeated frustration and interactive failures. For example, when a caregiver holds and talks to an alert full-term newborn, the infant may calmly inhibit body movements and smoothly follow the adult's face while maintaining healthy skin color and breathing patterns. In contrast, the same social stimulation might exceed premature infants' sensory threshold, causing them to startle, avert their gaze, and become cyanotic or tachypneic (Gorski, 1983).

Premature delivery and the NICU experience can themselves foster unique psychological stress on preterm parents. If the family of a high-risk infant is burdened further by social isolation, serious marital problems, a history of child abuse or neglect, or emotional depression, the parents may not be able to cope with the added stress of a behaviorally disorganized infant. Without professional intervention, such infants may be at increased risk for maltreatment (Hunter et al, 1978; Klein and Stern, 1971). Although few families are incapacitated to the point of actively harming their infants, many parents of medically vulnerable newborns continue to anxiously overprotect their infants long after such restriction is warranted and healthy (Gorski, 1988; Green and Solnit, 1964). Early intervention that provides emotional support and developmental counseling for parents of high-risk newborns at home and in hospital can help prevent negative outcomes and foster positive infant growth and family relationships (Gilkerson et al, 1990; Olds et al, 1994; Rauh et al, 1990). Neonatal healthcare professionals have an opportunity to note the psychological condition of the parents in addition to the medical status and behavior of the newborn. By offering attention and support to the family as well as to the newborn, caregivers can contribute most effectively to the quality of infant health and development following high-risk birth.

REFERENCES

Abramov I, Gordon J, Hendrickson A, et al: The retina of the newborn human infant. Science 217:265–267, 1982.

Als H, Duffy FH, McAnulty GB: Behavioral differences between preterm and full-term newborns as measured with the APIB system scores: I. Inf Behav Dev 11:305–318, 1988.

Als H, Lawhon G, Brown E: Individualized behavioral and environmental care for the very low birthweight preterm infant at high risk for bronchopulmonary dysplasia: Neonatal intensive care unit and developmental outcome. Pediatrics 78:1123–1132, 1986.

Als H, Lawhon G, Brown E, et al: Individualized developmental care for the very low birthweight preterm infant: Medical and neurofunctional effects. JAMA 272:853–858, 1994.

Anand KJS, Hickey PR: Pain and its effects in the human neonate and fetus. N Engl J Med 317:1321–1329, 1987.

Anand KJS, Sippell WG, Aynsley-Green A: Randomized trial of fentanyl anaesthesia in preterm babies undergoing surgery: Effects on the stress response. Lancet 1:243–248, 1987.

Anders TF, Keener MA: Developmental course of nighttime sleep-wake patterns in full-term and premature infants during the first year of life. I. Sleep 8:173–192, 1985.

Anderson GC, Burroughs AK, Measel CP: Nonnutritive sucking opportunities: A safe and effective treatment for preterm neonates. *In* Field T, Sostek A (Eds): Infants Born at Risk. New York, Grune & Stratton, 1983, pp 129–146.

Armitage SE, Baldwin BA, Vince MA: The fetal environment of sheep. Science 208:1173–1174, 1980.

Aserinsky E, Kleitman N: A motility cycle in infants as manifested by ocular and gross bodily activity. J Appl Physiol 8:11–18, 1955.

Ashton R, Connolly K: The relation of respiration and heart rate to sleep states in the human newborn. Dev Med Child Neurol 13:180–187, 1971.

Aslin RN: Development of smooth pursuit in human infants. *In* Fisher DF, Monty RA, Sanders JW (Eds): Eye Movements: Cognition and Visual Perception. Hillsdale, NJ, Erlbaum, 1981.

Aslin RN, Pisoni DB, Jusczyk PW: Auditory development and speech perception in infancy. *In* Haith MM, Campos JJ (Eds): Handbook of Child Psychology: Infancy and Developmental Psychobiology, vol 2. New York, John Wiley, 1983, pp 573–687.

Aylward GP: Forty-week full-term and preterm neurologic differences. *In* Lipsitt LP, Field TM (Eds): Infant Behavior and Development: Perinatal Risk and Newborn Behavior. Norwood, NJ, Ablex, 1982, pp 67–83.

Bakeman R, Brown JV: Early Interaction: Consequences for social and mental development at three years. Child Dev 51:437–447, 1980.

Ballard RA, Ferris CB, Clyman RI, et al: The hospital alternative birth center: Is it safe? Experience in 1000 cases from 1976–1980. J Perinatol 5(3):61–64, 1985.

Banks MS: The development of visual accommodation during early infancy. Child Dev 51:646–666, 1980.

Banks MS, Salapatek P: Infant visual perception. *In* Haith MM, Campos JJ (Eds): Handbook of Child Psychology: Infancy and Developmental Psychobiology, vol 2. New York, John Wiley, 1983, pp 435–571.

Barnard K, Bee H: The impact of temporally patterned stimulation on the development of preterm infants. Child Dev 54:1156–1167, 1983.

Beckwith L, Cohen SE: Preterm birth: Hazardous obstetrical and postnatal events as related to caregiver-infant behavior. Inf Behav Dev 1:403–411, 1978.

Beckwith L, Parmelee AH: EEG patterns of preterm infants, home environment, and later IQ. Child Dev 57:777–789, 1986.

Bench J: Sound transmission to the human fetus through the maternal abdominal wall. J Genet Psychol 113:85–87, 1968.

Bench J, Anderson J, Hoare M: Measurement system for fetal audiometry. J Acoust Soc Am 47:1602–1606, 1979.

Berg WK, Berg KM: Psychophysiologic development in infancy: State, sensory function, and attention. *In* Osofsky JD (Ed): Handbook of Infant Development. New York, John Wiley, 1979, pp 283–343.

Bernbaum J, Pereira G, Watkins J: Nonnutritive sucking during gavage feeding enhances growth and maturation in premature infants. Pediatrics 71:41–45, 1983.

Brazelton TB: Crying in infancy. Pediatrics 4:579–588, 1962.

Brazelton TB: Neonatal Behavioral Assessment Scale, 2nd ed. London, Heinemann, 1984.

Brazy JE: Effects of crying on cerebral blood volume and cytochrome aa$_3$. J Pediatr 112:457–461, 1988.

Brazy JE, Eckerman CO, Oehler JM, et al: Nursery neurobiologic risk score: Important factors in predicting outcome in very low birth weight infants. J Pediatr 118:783–792, 1991.

Bronson GW: Structure, status and characteristics of the nervous system at birth. *In* Stratton P (Ed): Psychobiology of the Human Newborn. Chichester, John Wiley, 1982, pp 99–118.

Brooks-Gunn J, McCarton C, Hawley T: Effects of in utero drug exposure on children's development. Arch Pediatr Adolesc Med 148:33–39, 1994.

Brown CC (Ed): The Many Facets of Touch. Skillman, NJ, Johnson & Johnson, 1984.

Brown JV, Bakeman R: Relationships of human mothers with their infants during the first year of life: Effects of prematurity. *In* Bell RW, Smotherman WP (Eds): Maternal Influences and Early Behavior. Holliswood, NY, Spectrum, 1979.

Burroughs AK, Anderson GC, Patel MK, et al: Relation of nonnutritive sucking pressures to t$_c$PO$_2$ and gestational age in preterm infants. Perinat Neonatol 5:54–62, 1981.

Carey WB, McDevitt SC: Revision of the infant temperament questionnaire. Pediatrics 61:735–739, 1978.

Carmichael L: The onset and early development of behavior. *In* Carmichael L (Ed): Manual of Child Psychology. New York, John Wiley, 1954.

Chasnoff IJ: Newborn infants with drug withdrawal symptoms. Pediatr Rev 9:273–277, 1988.

Chasnoff IJ, Bussey ME, Savich R, et al: Perinatal cerebral infarction and maternal cocaine use. J Pediatr 108:456–459, 1986.

Chasnoff IJ, Hatcher R, Burns WJ: Polydrug- and methadone-addicted newborns: A continuum of impairment? Pediatrics 70:210–213, 1982.

Chasnoff IJ, Hatcher R, Burns WJ, et al: Pentazocine and tripelennamine ("t's and blue's"): Effects on the fetus and newborn. Dev Pharm Ther 6:162–169, 1983.

Chavez CJ, Ostrea EM, Stryker JC, et al: Sudden infant death syndrome among infants of drug-dependent mothers. J Pediatr 95:407–409, 1979.

Chess S, Thomas A: Temperament in Clinical Practice. New York, Guilford Press, 1986, pp 273–281.

Chiriboga CA, Bateman DA, Brust JC, Hauser WA: Neurologic findings in neonates with intrauterine cocaine exposure. Pediatr Neurol 9:115–119, 1993.

Clarren SK, Smith DW: The fetal alcohol syndrome. N Engl J Med 298:1063–1067, 1978.

Coles CD, Platzman KA. Behavioral development in children prenatally exposed to drugs and alcohol. Int J Addict 28:1393–1433, 1993.

Coll CG, Kagan J, Resnick SJ: Behavioral inhibition in young children. Child Dev 55:1005–1019, 1984.

Conel JL: The Postnatal Development of the Human Cerebral Cortex. Cambridge, MA, Harvard University Press, 1947.

Davis DH, Thoman EB: Behavioral states of premature infants: Implications for neural and behavioral development. Dev Psychobiol 20(1):25–38, 1987.

De Casper AJ, Fifer WP: Of human bonding: Newborns prefer their mother's voices. Science 208:1174–1176, 1980.

Desmond MM, Wilson GS: Neonatal abstinence syndrome: Recognition and diagnosis. Addict Dis 2:113–121, 1975.

deVries JIP, Vissar GHA, Prechtl HFR: The emergence of fetal behaviour. I. Qualitative aspects. Early Hum Dev 7:301–322, 1982.

deVries JIP, Visser GHA, Prechtl HFR: The emergence of fetal behaviour. II. Quantitative aspects. Early Hum Dev 12:99–120, 1985.

DiVitto B, Goldberg S: The effects of newborn medical status on early parent-infant interaction. *In* Field TM, Sostek AS, Goldberg S, Shuman HH (Eds): Infants Born At Risk. New York, Spectrum, 1979.

Dixon SD, Bresnahan K, Zuckerman B: Cocaine babies: Meeting the challenge of management. Contemp Pediatr 7(6):70–92, 1990.

Dixon S, Snyder J, Holve R, et al: Behavioral effects of circumcision with and without anesthesia. J Dev Behav Pediatr 5:246–250, 1984.

Doberczak TM, Thornton JC, Berstein J, et al: Impact of maternal drug dependency on birth weight and head circumference of offspring. Am J Dis Child 141:1163–1167, 1987.

Dreyfus-Brisac C: Sleep ontogenesis in early human prematures from 24 to 27 weeks conceptional age. Dev Psychobiol 1:162–169, 1968.

Duffy FH, Als H, McAnulty GB: Behavioral and electrophysiological evidence for gestational age effects in healthy preterm and fulterm infants studied two weeks after expected due date. Child Dev 61:271–286, 1990.

Emory EK, Konopka S, Hronsky S, et al: Salivary caffeine and neonatal behavior: Assay modification and functional significance. Psychopharm Bull 94:64–68, 1988.

Fantz RL, Nevis S: Pattern preferences and perceptual-cognitive development in early infancy. Merrill-Palmer Q 13:77–108, 1967.

Field TM: Effects of early separation, interactive deficits, and experimental manipulations on mother-infant interaction. Child Dev 48:763–771, 1977.

Field TM, Goldson E: Pacifying effects of nonnutritive sucking on term and preterm neonates during heelstick procedures. Pediatrics 74:1012–1015, 1984.

Field TM, Healy B, Goldstein R, et al: Infants of depressed mothers show "depressed" behavior even with nondepressed adults. Child Dev 59:1569–1579, 1988.

Field TM, Ignatoff E, Stringer S, et al: Nonnutritive sucking during tube feedings: Effects on preterm neonates in an intensive care unit. Pediatrics 70:381–384, 1982.

Field TM, Schanberg SM, Scafidi F, et al: Tactile/kinesthetic stimulation effects in preterm neonates. Pediatrics 47:654–658, 1986.

Fox NA, Porges SW: The relation between neonatal heart period patterns and developmental outcome. Child Dev 56:28–37, 1985.

Gaiter JL: Nursery environments: The behavior and caregiving experiences of full-term and preterm newborns. *In* Gottfried AW, Gaiter JL (Eds): Infant Stress Under Intensive Care. Baltimore, University Park Press, 1985, pp 55–81.

Gilkerson L, Gorski PA, Panitz P: Hospital-based intervention for preterm infants and their families. *In* Meisels SJ, Shonkoff JP (Eds): Handbook of Early Intervention: Theory, Practice, and Analysis. Cambridge, Cambridge University Press, 1990.

Goldberg S: Premature birth: Consequences for the parent-infant relationship. Am Sci 67:214–220, 1979.

Goldsmith HH, Buss AH, Plomin R, et al: Roundtable: What is temperament? Four approaches. Child Dev 58:505–529, 1987.

Gorski PA: Premature infant behavioral and physiological responses to caregiving interventions in the intensive care nursery. *In* Call JD, Galenson E, Tyson RL (Eds): Frontiers of Infant Psychiatry. New York, Basic Books, 1983, pp 256–263.

Gorski PA: Fostering family development following preterm hospitalization. *In* Ballard RA (Ed): Pediatric Care of the ICN Graduate. Philadelphia, WB Saunders, 1988, pp 27–32.

Gorski PA, Davison MF, Brazelton TB: Stages of behavioral organization in the high-risk neonate: Theoretical and clinical considerations. Semin Perinat 3:61–72, 1979.

Gorski PA, Hole WT, Leonard CH, et al: Direct computer recording of premature infants and nursery care. Pediatrics 72:198–202, 1983.

Gorski PA, Huntington L: Physiological measures relative to tactile stimulation in hospitalized preterm infants. Pediatr Res 23:210A, 1988.

Gorski PA, Leonard C, Sweet D, et al: Caring for immature infants—A touchy subject. *In* Brown CC (Ed): The Many Facets of Touch. Skillman, NJ, Johnson & Johnson, 1984, pp 84–91.

Gottfried AW: Environment of newborn infants in special care units. *In* Gottfried AW, Gaiter JL (Eds): Infant Stress Under Intensive Care. Baltimore, University Park Press, 1985, pp 23–54.

Gottfried AW, Wallace-Lande P, Sherman-Brown S, et al: Physical and social environment of newborn infants in special care units. Science 214:673–675, 1981.

Gottlieb G: Ontogenesis of sensory function in birds and mammals. *In* Tobach E, Aronson LR, Shaw E (Eds): The Biopsychology of Development. New York, Academic Press, 1971, pp 67–126.

Green M, Solnit A: Reactions to the threatened loss of a child: A vulnerable child syndrome. Pediatrics 34:58–66, 1964.

Grimwade JC, Walker DW, Bartlett M, et al: Human fetal heart rate changes and movement in response to sound and vibration. Am J Obstet Gynecol 109:86–90, 1971.

Gunnar MR, Fisch RO, Kovsvilc S, et al: The effects of circumcision on serum cortisol and behavior. Psychoneuroendocrinology 6:269–275, 1981.

Gunnar MR, Fisch RO, Malone S: The effects of a pacifying stimulus on behavioral and adrenocortical responses to circumcision in the newborn. J Am Acad Child Psych 23:34–38, 1984.

Harper RM, Hoppenbrowers T, Sterman MB, et al: Polygraphic studies of normal infants during the first six months of life. 1. Heart rate as a function of state. Pediatr Res 10:945–951, 1976.

Hecox KE, Deegan DM: Methodological issues in the study of auditory development. *In* Gottlieb G, Krasnegor NA (Eds): Measurement of Audition and Vision in the First Year of Postnatal Life: A Methodological Overview. Norwood, NJ, Ablex, 1985, pp 391–418.

Herrenkohl LR: Prenatal stress disrupts reproductive behavior and physiology in offspring. Ann NY Acad Sci 474:120–128, 1986.

High PC, Gorski PA: Recording environmental influences on infant development in the intensive care nursery. *In* Gottfried AW, Gaiter JL (Eds): Infant Stress Under Intensive Care. Baltimore, University Park Press, 1985, pp 131–155.

Hooker D: The Prenatal Origins of Behavior. Lawrence, KS, University of Kansas Press, 1952.

Howard J, Parmelee AH, Kopp CB, et al: A neurologic comparison of pre-term and full-term infants at term conceptional age. J Pediatr 88:995–1002, 1976.

Hunt JV, Tooley WH, Harvin D: Learning disabilities in children with birth weights ≤1500 grams. Semin Perinatol 6:280–287, 1982.

Hunter RS, Kilstrom W, Kraybill EN, et al: Antecedents of child abuse and neglect in premature infants: A prospective study in a newborn intensive care unit. Pediatrics 61:629–635, 1978.

James W: Principles of Psychology, vol I. Burkhardt F (Ed). Cambridge, Harvard University Press, 1981 [1890].

Ju SH, Lin CH: The effect of moderate non-hemolytic jaundice and phototherapy on newborn behavior. Acta Paediatr Sin 32:31–41, 1991.

Katz V: Auditory stimulation and developmental behavior of one premature infant. Nurs Res 20:196–201, 1971.

Kennell J, Klaus M, McGrath S, et al: Continuous emotional support during labor in a U. S. hospital. JAMA 265:2197–2201, 1991.

Klein M, Stern L: Low birth weight and the battered child syndrome. Am J Dis Child 122:15–18, 1971.

Klein M, Hack M, Gallagher J, et al: Preschool performance of children with normal intelligence who were very low birth weight infants. Pediatrics 75:531–537, 1985.

Korner AF: State as variable, as obstacle, and as mediator of stimulation in infant research. Merrill-Palmer Q 18:77–94, 1972.

Korner AF, Van den Hoed J: Reduction of sleep apnea and bradycardia in preterm infants on oscillating water beds: A controlled polygraphic study. Pediatrics 61:528–533, 1978.

Korner AF, Kraemer H, Haffner E: Effects of waterbed flotation in premature infants: A pilot study. Pediatrics 5:361–365, 1975.

Korner AF, Schneider P: Effects of vestibular-proprioceptive stimulation on the neurobehavioral development of preterm infants: A pilot study. Neuropediatrics 14:170–175, 1983.

Kraemer H, Korner AF, Thoman EB: Methodological considerations in evaluating the influence of drugs used during labor and delivery on the behavior of the newborn. Dev Psychol 6:128–134, 1972.

Kuhnert BR, Linn PL, Kuhnert PM: Obstetric medication and neonatal behavior: Current controversies. Clin Perinatol 12:423–440, 1985.

Lawson K, Daum C, Turkewitz G: Environmental characteristics of a neonatal intensive care unit. Child Dev 48:1633–1639, 1977.

Leib S, Benfield G, Guidubaldi J: Effects of early intervention and stimulation on the preterm infant. Pediatrics 66:83–89, 1980.

Lester BM: Developmental outcome prediction from acoustic cry analysis in term and preterm infants. Pediatrics 80:529–534, 1987.

Lester BM, Als H, Brazelton TB: Regional obstetric anesthesia and newborn behavior: A reanalysis toward synergistic effects. Child Dev 53:687–692, 1982.

Lester BM, Boukydis CF, McGrath M, et al: Behavioral and psychophysiologic assessment of the preterm infant. Clin Perinatol 17:155–171, 1990.

Lester BM, Emory EK, Hoffman SL, et al: A multivariate study of the effects of high-risk factors on performance on the Brazelton Neonatal Assessment Scale. Child Dev 47:515–517, 1976.

Lewkowicz DJ: Developmental changes in infants' response to temporal frequency. Dev Psychol 21:858–865, 1985.

Lifschitz MH, Wilson GS, Smith EO, et al: Factors affecting head growth and intellectual function in children of drug addicts. Pediatrics 75:269–274, 1985.

Linn PL, Horowitz FD, Buddin BJ, et al: An ecological description of a neonatal intensive care unit. *In* Gottfried AW, Gaiter JL (Eds): Infant Stress Under Intensive Care. Baltimore, University Park Press, 1985a, pp 83–111.

Linn PL, Horowitz FD, Fox HA: Stimulation in the NICU: Is more necessarily better? Clin Perinat 12:407–422, 1985b.

Long J, Lucey J, Philip A: Noise and hypoxemia in the intensive care nursery. Pediatrics 65:143–145, 1980.

MacArthur C, Knox EG: Smoking in pregnancy: Effects of stopping at different stages. Br J Obstet Gynaecol 95:551–555, 1988.

Majnemer A, Brownstein A, Kadanoff R, et al: A comparison of neurobehavioral performance of healthy term and low-risk preterm infants at term. Dev Med Child Neurol 34:417–424, 1992.

Mayes LC, Granger RH, Frank MA, et al: Neurobehavioral profiles of neonates exposed to cocaine prenatally. Pediatrics 91:778–783, 1993.

McGehee LJ, Eckerman CO: The preterm infant as a social partner: Responsive but unreadable. Infant Behav Dev 6:467–470, 1983.

Michaelis R, Parmelee AH, Stern E, et al: Activity states in premature and term infants. Dev Psychobiol 6:209–215, 1973.

Montagu A: Touching: The Human Significance of the Skin. New York, Columbia University Press, 1971.

Moyer JA, Herrenkohl LR, Jacobowitz DM: Effects of stress during pregnancy on catecholamines in discrete brain regions. Brain Res 121:385–393, 1977.

Muir D, Clifton RK: Infants' orientation to the location of sound sources. *In* Gottlieb G, Krasnegor NA (Eds): Measurement of Audition and Vision in the First Year of Postnatal Life: A Methodological Overview. Norwood, NJ, Ablex, 1985, pp 167–194.

Muir D, Field J: Newborn infants orient to sounds. Child Dev 50:431–436, 1979.

Murray AD, Dolby RM, Nation RL, et al: Effects of epidural anesthesia on newborns and their mothers. Child Dev 52:71–82, 1981.

Nijhuis J, Prechtl H, Martin C, et al: Are there behavioral states in the human fetus? Early Hum Dev 6:177–195, 1982.

Olds DI, Henderson CR, Kitzman H: Does prenatal and infancy nurse home visitation have enduring effects on qualities of parental caregiving and child health at 25 to 50 months of life? Pediatrics 93:89–98, 1994.

Oro AS, Dixon SD: Perinatal cocaine and methamphetamine exposure: Maternal and neonatal correlates. J Pediatr 111:571–578, 1987.

Owens ME, Todt EH: Pain in infancy: Neonatal reaction to a heel lance. Pain 20:77–86, 1984.

Palmer PG, Dubowitz LMS, Verghote M, et al: Neurological and neurobehavioural differences between preterm infants at term and full-term newborn infants. Neuropediatrics 13:183–189, 1982.

Paludetto R, Mansi G, Rinaldi P, et al: Behavior of preterm newborns reaching term without any serious disorder. Early Human Dev 6:357–363, 1982.

Parmelee AH, Stern E, Harris MA: Maturation of states in premature and young infants. Neuropediatrie 3:294–304, 1972.

Parmelee AH, Wenner WH, Akiyama Y, et al: Sleep states in premature infants. Dev Med Child Neurol 9:70–77, 1967.

Parmelee AH, Wenner WH, Schulz HR: Infant sleep patterns from birth to 16 weeks of age. J Pediatr 65:576–582, 1964.

Pearson DT, Dietrich KN: The behavioral toxicology and teratology of childhood: Models, methods, and implications for intervention. Neurotoxicology 6:165–182, 1985.

Perlman JM, McMenamin JB, Volpe JJ: Fluctuating cerebral blood-flow velocity in respiratory-distress syndrome. N Engl J Med 310:204–209, 1984.

Perlman JM, Volpe JJ: Episodes of apnea and bradycardia in the preterm newborn: Impact on cerebral circulation. Pediatrics 76:333–338, 1985.

Poets CF, Stebbens VA, Samuels MP, Southall DP: Oxygen saturation and breathing patterns in children. Pediatrics 92:686–690, 1993.

Pomerleau-Malcuit A, Clifton RK: Neonatal heart rate response to tactile, auditory, and vestibular stimulation in different states. Child Dev 44:485–496, 1973.

Porges SW: Heart rate patterns in neonates: A potential diagnostic window to the brain. *In* Field TM, Sostek AS (Eds): Infants Born at Risk. New York, Grune & Stratton, 1983, pp 3–22.

Porges SW, McCabe PM, Yongue BG: Respiratory-heart rate interactions: Psychophysiological implications for pathophysiology and behavior. *In* Cacippo JT, Petty RE (Eds): Perspectives in Cardiovascular Psychophysiology. New York, Guilford Press, 1982, pp 233–260.

Prechtl HFR: The behavioral states of the newborn infant: A review. Brain Research 76:1304–1311, 1974.

Rauh VA, Nurcombe B, Achenbach T, Howell C: The mother-infant transaction program. The content and implications of an intervention for the mothers of low-birthweight infants. Clin Perinatol 17:31–45, 1990.

Resnick M, Eyler F, Nelson R: Developmental intervention for low birth weight infants: Improved early developmental outcome. Pediatrics 80:68–74, 1987.

Robertson SS: Cyclic motor activity in the human fetus after midgestation. Dev Psychobiol 18:411–419, 1985.

Robertson SS: Human cyclic motility: Fetal-newborn continuities and newborn state differences. Dev Psychobiol 20:425–442, 1987.

Robertson SS, Dierker LJ: The development of cyclic motility in fetuses of diabetic mothers. Dev Psychobiol 19:223–234, 1986.

Rose SA, Gottfried AW, Bridger WH: Cross-modal transfer in infants: Relationship to prematurity and socioeconomic background. Dev Psychol 14:643–652, 1978.

Rothbart MK: Measurement of temperament in infancy. Child Dev 52:569–578, 1981.

Rubel EW: Auditory system development. *In* Gottlieb G, Krasnegor NA (Eds): Measurement of Audition and Vision in the First Year of Postnatal Life: A Methodological Overview. Norwood, NJ, Ablex, 1985, pp 53–89.

Saint-Anne Dargassies S: Normality and normalization as seen in a long-term neurological follow-up of 286 truly premature infants. Neuropediatr 10:226–244, 1979.

Sanders-Phillips K, Strauss ME, Gutberlet RL: The effect of obstetric medication on newborn infant feeding behavior. Infant Behav Dev 11:251–263, 1988.

Seligman MR: Helplessness: On Development, Depression, and Death. San Francisco, WH Freeman, 1975.

Sepkoski CM, Lester BM, Ostheimer GW, Brazelton TB: The effects of maternal epidural anesthesia on neonatal behavior during the first month. Dev Med Child Neurol 34:1072–1080, 1992.

Shaywitz SE, Capanilo BK, Hodgson ES: Developmental language disability as a consequence of prenatal exposure to ethanol. Pediatrics 68:850–855, 1981.

Singer LT, Yamashita TS, Hawkins S, et al: Increased incidence of intraventricular hemorrhage and developmental delay in cocaine-exposed, very low birth weight infants. J Pediatr 124:765–771, 1994.

Spangler G, Grossmann KE: Biobehavioral organization in securely and insecurely attached infants. Child Dev 64:1439–1450, 1993.

Sroufe A: Attachment and the construction of relationships. *In* Hartup WW, Rubin Z (Eds): Relationships and Development. Hillsdale, NJ, Erlbaum, 1986, pp 51–71.

Starr A, Amlie RN, Martin WH, et al: Development of auditory function in newborn infants revealed by auditory brainstem potentials. Pediatrics 60:831–839, 1977.

Strauss ME, Lessen-Firestine JK, Starr RH, et al: Behavior of narcotic-addicted newborns. Child Dev 46:887–893, 1975.

Swafford LI, Allan D: Pain relief in the pediatric patient. Med Clin North Am 52:131–136, 1968.

Telzrow RW, Kang RR, Mitchell SK, et al: An assessment of the behavior of the preterm infant at 40 weeks conceptional age. *In* Lipsitt LP, Field TM (Eds): Infant Behavior and Development: Perinatal Risk and Newborn Behavior. Norwood, NJ, Ablex, 1982, pp 85–96.

Thoman EB: Sleep and Waking States of the Neonate (revised edition), 1985. (Available from E. B. Thoman, Dept. of Psychology/Behavioral Neuroscience, 3107 Horsebarn Hill Rd, University of Connecticut, Storrs, CT 06269-4154).

Thoman EB, Denenberg VH, Sieval J, et al: State organization in neonates: Developmental inconsistency indicates risk for developmental dysfunction. Neuropediatr 12:45–54, 1981.

Thoman EB, Graham S: Self-regulation of stimulation by premature infants. Pediatrics 78:855–860, 1986.

Thomas A, Chess S, Birch HG, et al: Behavioral Individuality in Early Childhood. New York, New York University Press, 1963.

Tirosh E, Harel J, Abadi J, et al: Relationship between neonatal behavior and subsequent temperament. Acta Paediatr 81:829–831, 1992.

Tronick E, Wise S, Als H, et al: Regional obstetric anesthesia and newborn behavior: Effect over the first ten days of life. Pediatrics 58:94–100, 1976.

Turkewitz G, Birch HG, Moreau T, et al: Effect of intensity of auditory stimulation on directional eye movements in the human neonate. Anim Behav 14:93–101, 1966.

Turkewitz G, Lewkowicz DJ, Gardner JM: Determinants of infant perception. *In* Rosenblatt J, Beer C, Hinde R, et al (Eds): Advances in the Study of Behavior. New York, Academic Press, 1983, pp 39–62.

Vohr BR, Coll CG, Lobato D, et al: Neurodevelopmental and medical status of low-birthweight survivors of bronchopulmonary dysplasia at 10 to 12 years of age. Dev Med Child Neurol 33:690–697, 1991.

Volpe JJ: Effect of cocaine use on the fetus. N Engl J Med 327:399–407, 1992.

Ward SLD, Schuetz S, Krishna V, et al: Abnormal sleeping ventilatory pattern in infants of substance-abusing mothers. Am J Dis Child 140:1915–1920, 1986.

White J, Labarba R: The effects of tactile and kinesthetic stimulation on neonatal development in the premature infant. Dev Psychobiol 9:569–577, 1976.

Whitney MP, Thoman EB: Early sleep patterns of premature infants are differentially related to later developmental disabilities. J Dev Behav Pediatr 14(2):71–80, 1993.

Williamson PS, Williamson ML: Physiologic stress reduction by a local anesthetic during newborn circumcision. Pediatrics 71:36–40, 1983.

Wolff PH: Observations on newborn infants. Psychosom Med 221:110–118, 1959.

Wolff PH: The causes, controls, and organization of behavior in the neonate. Psychol Issues 5:1–105, 1966.

Woodson R, Hamilton C: The effect of nonnutritive sucking on heart rate in preterm infants. Dev Psychobiol 21:207–213, 1988.

Yakovlev PI, LeCours A: The myelogenetic cycles of regional maturation of the brain. *In* Minkowski A (Ed): Regional Development of the Brain in Early Life. Philadelphia, FA Davis, 1967, pp 3–65.

Zeskind PS, Lester BM: Acoustic features and auditory perceptions of the cries of newborns with prenatal and perinatal complications. Child Dev 49:580–589, 1978.

Zeskind PS, Lester BM: Cry features of newborns with differential patterns of fetal growth. Child Dev 51:207–212, 1981.

Zuckerman B, Frank DA: Prenatal cocaine exposure: Nine years later. J Pediatr 124:731–733, 1994.

Temperature Regulation of the Premature Infant

Stephen Baumgart

The human newborn is considered homeothermic. Morbidity (i.e., poor brain and somatic growth) and mortality rates increase when core body temperature is permitted to decline much below 36° C (96.8° F). Moreover, even premature newborns respond adaptively to changes in their environment. Response to cold stress, however, may be insufficient to maintain core body temperature in premature infants and render them functionally poikilothermic, even in moderately temperate environments.

COLD STRESS: THE PROBLEM

The newborn frequently encounters the problem of severe heat loss for several reasons. First, the baby's exposed surface is much larger than the adult's relative to metabolically active body mass (Table 33–1). Especially for the very-low-birth-weight infant, the heat-dissipating area is five to six times greater proportionate to that of the adult. Second, the tiny baby's small size presents a much smaller heat sink to store thermal reserve. Finally, the radius of curvature of the body is less than in the adult, resulting in a thinner protective boundary layer of warm, humidified air.

Aside from these geometric considerations, characteristics of the premature infant's skin contribute to the problem of excessive heat loss. Especially in premature babies, the skin and subcutaneous fascia provide little insulation against the flow of heat from the core to the surface. Moreover, the lack of a keratinized epidermal barrier exposes infants to vastly increased evaporative heat loss. In very-low-birth-weight infants (<1.0 kg), water lost to evaporation may be 8 to 10 times more than adult quantities. For these reasons, a major problem confronting small premature infants from birth is cold stress.

PHYSICAL ROUTES OF HEAT LOSS
Convection

Convective heat loss in newborns occurs when ambient air temperature is less than the infant's skin temperature. Convective heat loss includes (1) natural convection (passage of heat from the skin to the ambient still air), and (2) forced convection, in which mass movement of air over the infant conveys heat away from the skin. The quantity of heat lost is proportional to the difference between air and skin temperatures, and to air speed. The effect of forced convection in disrupting the microenvironment of warm, humid air layered near an infant's skin usually is not appreciated in the nursery, where drafts, air turbulence, and consequently heat loss may occur even within the relatively protective environment of an incubator.

Evaporation

Passive transcutaneous evaporation of water from a newborn's skin (termed insensible water loss) results in the dissipation of 0.58 kcal/mL latent heat. As shown in Figure 33–1, transcutaneous water loss increases exponentially with decreasing size and gestation. The tiniest premature baby, least able to tolerate cold stress, may incur evaporative loss in excess of 4 kcal/hour. Evaporation is enhanced by low vapor pressure (high temperature and low relative humidity) and air turbulence. The highest evaporative losses occur on the 1st days of life, and, during the 1st week of life in infants of 25 to 27 weeks' gestation, evaporative heat losses may be higher than radiant losses (Hammarlund et al, 1986).

Radiation

Radiant heat loss constitutes the transfer of heat from an infant's warm skin via infrared electromagnetic waves to the cooler surrounding walls. Radiant heat loss is proportional to the difference between skin and surrounding wall temperatures. An infant's posture may also affect radiant heat loss by increasing or reducing the effective radiating surface area of the baby exposed outward. In a humid environment (relative humidity 50%), babies experience an ambient temperature (termed *operant temperature*) determined 60% by wall temperature and 40% by air temperature.

TABLE **33–1**

Body Surface Area to Body Mass Ratio

	Body Weight (kg)	Surface Area (m²)	Ratio (cm²/kg)
Adult	70	1.73	250
Premature infant	1.5	0.13	870
Very premature infant	0.5	0.07	1400

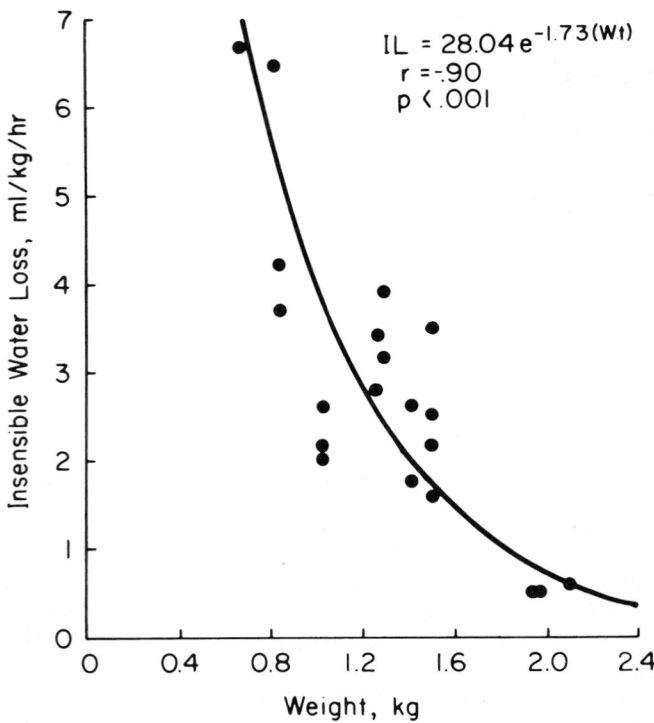

$$IL = 28.04\,e^{-1.73(Wt)}$$
$$r = -.90$$
$$p < .001$$

FIGURE 33–1. Exponential increase in evaporative water loss from skin of very-low-birth-weight infants nurtured under radiant warmers. (Adapted with permission from Baumgart S, Langman CB, Sosulski R, et al: Fluid, electrolyte and glucose maintenance in the very-low-birth-weight infant. Clin Pediatr 21(4):199–205, 1982.)

Conduction

Conductive heat loss to cooler surfaces in contact with an infant's skin depends on the material of the surface and its temperature. Usually, babies are nursed on insulating mattresses and blankets that minimize conductive heat loss.

PHYSIOLOGY OF COLD RESPONSE
Afferents

Homeothermic response to a cold environment begins with sensation of temperature. Traditional physiology identifies two temperature-sensitive sites: the hypothalamus and the skin. Sensation of cold by neonatal skin triggers a cold-adaptive response long before core sensors in the hypothalamus become chilled. Some investigators conjecture that neonatal cold reception resides primarily in the skin, whereas warm reception resides in the hypothalamus. Both sensors are probably integrated, however, because cold sensory response is inhibited by core sensor hyperthermia and vice versa. Peripheral skin cold sensation is teleologically important, because early detection of heat loss from the skin aids in the infant's timely response for maintaining core temperature.

Central Regulation

Integration of multiple skin and hypothalamic temperature inputs probably occurs in the hypothalamus. No single control temperature seems to exist, however. Under different environmental conditions, temperature of the skin may fluctuate 8° to 10° C and temperature of the hypothalamus may vary ±0.5° C. There exist also diurnal temperature fluctuations, variations with general sympathetic tone, and blunted regulation with asphyxia, hypoxemia, and other central nervous system defects. Premature infants may regulate core temperature near 37.5° C (99.4° F), whereas term infants may respond to maintain 36.5° C (97.7° F). Because important thermoregulatory processes are triggered by as little as 0.5° C, deviation at any temperature-sensitive site is important.

Efferents

The effector limb of the neonatal thermal response is mediated primarily by the sympathetic nervous system, although infant motor behavior may also be involved. The earliest maturing response is vasoconstriction in deep dermal arterioles, resulting in reduced flow of warm blood from the infant's core to the exposed periphery. Additionally, reduction of blood flow effectively places a layer of insulating fat between the core and the exposed skin in the term infant. Reduced fat content in low-birth-weight babies, however, decreases the effective insulating properties of this mechanism. Vasoconstriction nevertheless remains the newborn's first line of defense, and the response is present even in the most premature infant.

Brown fat constitutes a second sympathetic effector organ that provides a metabolic source of nonshivering thermogenesis (babies do not shiver like adults do to generate heat). Brown fat located in axillary, mediastinal, perinephric, and other regions of the newborn is especially enervated and equipped with an abundance of mitochondria to hydrolyze and re-esterify triglycerides and to oxidize free fatty acids. In the term infant, these reactions are exothermic and increase metabolic rate by twofold or more. Preterm babies, however, have little brown fat and may not be capable of more than a 25% increase in metabolic rate despite the most severe cold stress (Hull, 1966).

Finally, recent evidence suggests that control of voluntary muscle tone, posture, and increased motor activity with agitation may serve to augment heat production in skeletal muscle via glycogenolysis and glucose oxidation. Clinical observations of infant posture, behavior, and skin perfusion, and measurements of skin and core temperatures may ultimately provide the most useful guidelines for assessing infant comfort during incubation.

MODERN INCUBATION

The lifesaving requirement of an appropriate thermal environment was demonstrated conclusively by Day and colleagues in 1964 and further defined by Silverman and associates (1966). Minor changes in heat balance exact an oxygen cost and an increased metabolic rate that can only be met by increased ventilation or increased inspired oxygen and appropriate cardiovascular response.

Thermal Neutral Zone

The thermal neutral zone is a narrow range of environmental temperatures within which newborn babies do not alter

FIGURE 33–2. The range of temperature needed to provide neutral environmental conditions for a baby lying naked on a warm mattress in draft-free surroundings of moderate humidity (50% saturation) when mean radiant temperature is the same as air temperature. The hatched areas show the average neutral temperature range for a healthy baby weighing 1 kg or 2 kg at birth. Optimum temperature probably approximates the lower limit of neutral range as defined here. Approximately 1° C should be added to these operative temperatures to derive the appropriate neutral air temperature for a single-walled incubator when room temperature is less than 27° C (80° F), and more should be added if room temperature is very much less. (From Hey EN, Katz G: The optimum thermal environment for naked babies. Arch Dis Child 45:328,1970.)

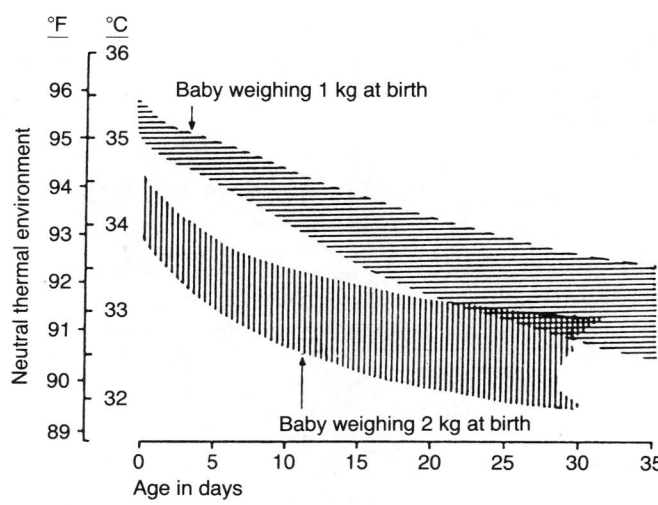

their metabolic rate in response to either peripheral cold stimulation or core hyperthermia. Rather, infants regulate temperature through vasomotor tone alone. A range of "critical" environmental temperatures relevant to modern incubators was identified by Hey and Katz (1970) (Fig. 33–2 and Table 33–2). Below this range, an increase in the infant's minimal metabolic rate was observed. This range, therefore, was defined as the optimal incubator temperature. Several important considerations in regulating incubator temperature were included in these studies: (1) incubator wall temperature was maintained identical to air temperature, (2) relative humidity was controlled near 50%, and (3) the environment was maintained in a steady state, uninterrupted by turbulence.

Many modern incubators, however, incorporate a single-walled design that results in higher radiant heat loss because the incubator's outside wall is exposed to cooler room air. Moreover, many nurseries do not humidify incubators artificially, fearing the occurrence of bacterial colonization. Finally, the incubator's steady state is frequently interrupted for nursing and medical procedures that require that doors be open to care for the infant. Although a useful concept, the thermal neutral zone must be rigorously

defined in practical terms. Silverman and colleagues (1966) used a modified concept of the thermal neutral zone to simplify clinical application. Reasoning that infants sense environmental temperature first on the skin, electronic negative-feedback (servocontrolled) regulation of the incubator heater in response to skin temperature was used. These authors demonstrated minimal metabolic expenditure near 36.5° C (97.7° F) abdominal skin temperature measured by a shielded thermistor in a less rigidly defined incubator environment. The importance of frequently checking core temperatures (axillary or rectal) must be emphasized, however, before delegating the infant's environment to such thermostatic control. In addition, Chessex and associates (1988) have demonstrated that incubator temperature may vary by more than 2° C when skin temperature servocontrol rather than air temperature control is used.

Finally, with the modern use of open radiant warmer beds (improving the means of access to the critically ill premature infant without interrupting heat delivery), skin temperature servocontrol has become the only practical method for approximating the thermal neutral zone (Malin and Baumgart, 1987). These variations in incubator design

---

TABLE 33–2

Mean Temperature Needed to Provide Thermal Neutrality for a Healthy Baby Nursed Naked in Draft-Free Surroundings of Uniform Temperature and Moderate Humidity after Birth

| Birth Weight (kg) | Operative Environmental Temperature* | | | | | | |
	35°C		34°C		33°C		32°C
1.0	For 10 days	→	After 10 days	→	After 3 weeks	→	After 5 weeks
1.5	—		For 10 days	→	After 10 days	→	After 4 weeks
2.0	—		For 2 days	→	After 2 days	→	After 3 weeks
>2.5	—				For 2 days	→	After 2 days

*To estimate operative temperature in a single-walled incubator, subtract 1° C from incubator air temperature for every 7° C by which this temperature exceeds room temperature.

Data from Hey E: Thermal neutrality. Br Med Bull 31:72, 1975.

and technique, and the extension of infant warming to include very-low-birth-weight, critically ill premature babies have generated new problems for determining a universally accepted optimal environment.

Partitioning Infant Heat Losses and Heat Gains

Wheldon and Rutter (1983) demonstrated the special problems encountered in incubating very-low-birth-weight infants in a convection-warmed, closed-hood incubator environment (Fig. 33–3). The top graph demonstrates the thermal balance achieved by a series of 12 infants (mean weight 1.58 kg). Heat losses to radiation (R), convection (C) and evaporation (E) are modest, and their sum (Σ) is balanced by the infant's metabolic heat production (M). Used in this fashion, the incubator reduces physical heat losses such that the infant's minimal metabolism (larger than any single avenue of heat loss) delicately balances

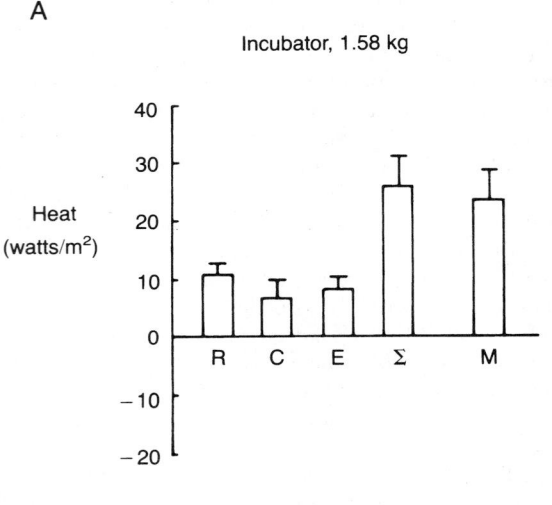

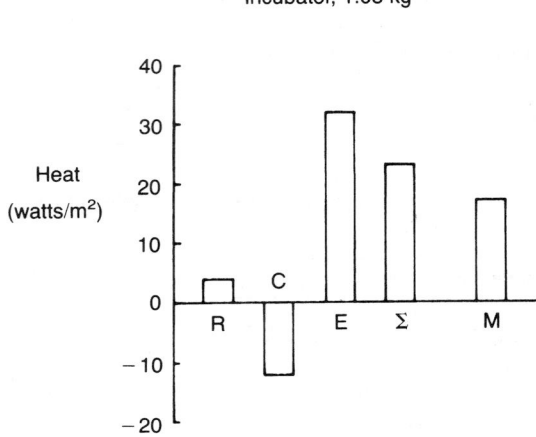

FIGURE 33–3. *A,* Partition of heat losses and gains in 12 premature infants nursed within incubators. *B,* Partition in a 1.08-kg low-birth-weight newborn. (From Wheldon AE, Rutter N: The heat balance of small babies nursed in incubators and under radiant warmers. Early Hum Dev 6:131–143, 1982.)

minimal physical heat losses caused by radiation with the thermal environment.

In contrast, a very-low-birth-weight subject (1.08 kg) is evaluated in the bottom portion of Figure 33–3. As the incubator servocontrol increases warming power (to accommodate massive evaporative heat loss), convective "loss" becomes a net "gain" (negative histogram bar). Radiant loss is diminished by warm walls inside the incubator. These conditions differ strikingly from those discussed previously: (1) the incubator truly warms the infant rather than modestly attenuating convective heat loss and (2) evaporative heat loss vastly exceeds the infant's metabolism. The very small infant's body temperature is balanced, therefore, between opposing physical parameters of evaporative and convective heat transfer: metabolism plays a secondary role.

The modern use of radiant warmers that are servocontrolled to maintain infant abdominal skin temperature between 36.5° and 37° C (97.7° to 98.6° F) also demonstrates the opposition of physical forces described earlier. Figure 33–4 (Baumgart, 1990) demonstrates the heat balance partition for 10 critically ill premature infants (mean weight 1.39 kg) nursed on open radiant warmer beds. Because ambient room air temperature is almost 10° C cooler than air inside an incubator, convective heat loss is nearly double the infant's metabolic heat production. Evaporation adds to the net physical heat loss. Additionally, small amounts of heat are lost to conduction and radiation (to cooler room walls). The infant's metabolism provides only one third of the energy required to maintain body temperature, whereas the remainder is supplied by the servocontrolled radiant heat source. In this instance, radiant warming (not convection as in the incubator discussed earlier) delicately balances the infant's physical temperature environment. Wheldon and Rutter (1982) have demonstrated similar results in their studies.

Altering the Partition of Heat Balance

During the 1980s, several investigators proposed the use of a variety of heat shields to reduce the opposition of large physical heat losses and gains in incubators and under radiant warmers. Double-walled incubators reduce infant radiant heat loss by warming the interior wall via convection. Thin transparent plastic films have been proposed as blankets or tents over infants within incubators or under radiant warmers to reduce evaporation and convective turbulence by preserving the warm, humid microenvironment layered near the infant's skin. The possibility of a semipermeable membrane adherent to an infant's torso as an artificial barrier has also been investigated in this regard. These techniques, although occasionally useful, bear the risk of disrupting the heat partition unpredictably. Cases of hyperthermia have been reported. Their use should be restricted to carefully monitored settings where rigorous attention is given to all aspects of achieving safe thermal balance.

CONCLUSION

The very-low-birth-weight premature newborn is extremely vulnerable to harsh fluctuations in physical environment. These infants require frequent assessments of skin, core,

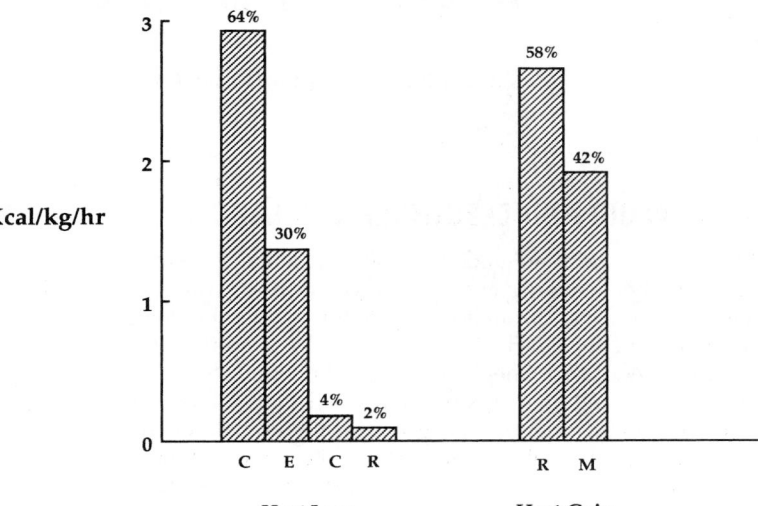

FIGURE 33–4. Partitional calorimetry in 10 critically ill low-birth-weight premature newborns nursed under open radiant warmers. (From Baumgart S: Radiant heat loss vs. radiant heat gain in premature neonates under radiant warmers. Biol Neonate 57:10–20, 1990. Reproduced with permission of S. Karger AG, Basel.)

and air temperatures and relative humidity to design an optimal strategy for thermal regulation. In caring for smaller babies, heat replacement is often required, and refinement of techniques to accomplish replacement without inducing hyperthermia is needed.

REFERENCES

Baumgart S: Reduction of oxygen consumption, insensible water loss and radiant heat demand with use of a plastic blanket for low-birth-weight infants under radiant warmers. Pediatrics 74:1022–1028, 1984.

Baumgart S: Partitioning of heat losses and gains in premature newborn infants under radiant warmers. Pediatrics 75:89–99, 1985.

Baumgart S: Radiant heat loss vs. radiant heat gain in premature neonates under radiant warmers. Biol Neonate 57:10–20, 1990.

Baumgart S, Fox WW, Polin RA: Physiologic implications of two different heat shields for infants under radiant warmers. J Pediatr 100:787–790, 1982.

Bell EF, Rios GR: A double-walled incubator alters the partition of body heat loss of premature infants. Pediatr Res 17:135–140, 1983.

Bell EF, Rios GR: Air versus skin temperature servocontrol of infant incubators. J Pediatr 103:954–959, 1983.

Bell EF, Weinstein MR, Oh W: Heat balance in premature infants: Comparative effects of convectively heated incubator and radiant warmer, with and without plastic heat shield. J Pediatr 96:460–465, 1980.

Bruck K: Heat production and temperature regulation. *In* Stave U (Ed): Perinatal Physiology. New York, Plenum Publishing, 1978, pp 455–498.

Chessex P, Blouet S, Vaucher J: Environmental temperature control in very low birth weight infants (<1000 gms) cared for in double-walled incubators. J Pediatr 113:373, 1988.

Hammarlund K, Strömberg B, Sedin G: Heat loss from the skin of preterm and full-term newborn infants during the first weeks after birth. Biol Neonate 50:1–10, 1986.

Hey EN, Katz G: The optimum thermal environment for naked babies. Arch Dis Child 45:328–334, 1970.

Hull D: Brown adipose tissue. Br Med Bull 22:92, 1966.

Knauth A, Gordin P, McNelis W, Baumgart S: A semipermeable polyurethane membrane as an artificial skin for the premature neonate. Pediatrics 83:945, 1988.

Malin S, Baumgart S: Optimal thermal management for low birth weight infants nursed under high-power radiant warmers. Pediatrics 79:47–54, 1987.

Marks KH, Lee CA, Bolan CD, Maisels MJ: Oxygen consumption and temperature control of premature infants in a double-wall incubator. Pediatrics 68:93–98, 1981.

Mayfield SR, Bhatia J, Nakamura KT, et al: Temperature measurement in term and preterm neonates. J Pediatr 104:271–275, 1984.

Okken A, Blijham C, Franz W, Bohn E: Effects of forced convection of heated air on insensible water loss and heat loss in preterm infants in incubators. J Pediatr 101:108–112, 1982.

Scopes JW: Thermoregulation in the Newborn. *In* Avery CB (Ed): Neonatology, Pathophysiology and Management of the Newborn, 2nd ed. Philadelphia, JB Lippincott, 1981, pp 171–181.

Silverman WA, Sinclair JC, Agate FJ: The oxygen cost of minor changes in heat balance of small newborn infants. Acta Paediatr Scand 55:294, 1966.

Wheldon AE, Rutter N: The heat balance of small babies nursed in incubators and under radiant warmers. Early Hum Dev 6:131–143, 1982.

SUGGESTED READINGS

Dawkins MJR, Hull D: The production of heat by fat. Sci Am 213:62, 1965.

Day RL, Caliguiri L, Kaminski C, et al: Body temperature and survival of premature infants. Pediatrics 34:171, 1964.

CHAPTER 34

Acid-Base, Fluid, and Electrolyte Management

Istvan Seri and Jacquelyn Evans

FLUID AND ELECTROLYTE BALANCE

Maintenance of fluid and electrolyte balance is essential for normal cell and organ function both during intrauterine development and throughout extrauterine life. Pathologic conditions in the newborn often lead to disruption of the complex regulatory mechanisms of fluid and electrolyte homeostasis and may result in irreversible cell damage. Thus, thorough understanding of the physiologic changes in fluid and electrolyte homeostasis during development and provision of appropriate fluid and electrolyte therapy based on the principles of developmental fluid and electrolyte physiology are among the cornerstones of modern neonatal intensive care.

Developmental Changes in Body Composition, Fluid Compartments, and Organ Function Affecting Prenatal, Perinatal, and Postnatal Fluid and Electrolyte Balance

Protection of the intracellular milieu implies that the organism must be able to monitor and correct changes in the composition and volume of the extracellular fluid compartment resulting from its interaction with the ever-changing environment. Recognition of this basic physiologic requirement and advances in understanding of the developmental changes in body composition, fluid compartments, and organ functions regulating fluid and electrolyte balance have resulted in the emergence of the modern principles of neonatal fluid and electrolyte therapy.

Developmental Changes in Body Composition and Fluid Compartments

Dynamic changes occur in body composition and fluid distribution during intrauterine life, labor and delivery, and the early postnatal period. Thereafter the pace of change in body composition and fluid distribution gradually decreases, with more subtle changes taking place especially after the 1st year of life (Friis-Hansen, 1961).

Changes During Intrauterine Development

In early gestation, body composition is characterized by a high proportion of total body water and a large extracellular compartment (Friis-Hansen, 1983). There also appears to be a prolactin-mediated increase in the water-binding capacity of fetal cells and perhaps the interstitium, which contributes to the maintenance of increased total fetal body water content (Coulter, 1983). As gestation advances, the rapid cellular growth, accretion of body solids, and fat deposition result in gradual decreases in total body water content and extracellular water volume while the intracellu-

lar fluid compartment increases (Friis-Hansen, 1983). In the 16-week fetus, total body water represents approximately 94% of total body weight with roughly two thirds of the total body water being distributed in the extracellular compartment and one third in the intracellular compartment. In the full-term newborn, total body water is only about 75% of total body weight with almost half of it located in the intracellular space (Fig. 34–1). Thus, infants born prematurely are in a state of total body water excess and extracellular volume expansion compared to their full-term counterparts with the majority of the expanded extracellular volume being distributed in the interstitium (Brace, 1992).

During intrauterine development, the placenta provides ample supply of nutrients and electrolytes for the fetus. To maintain normal fetal weight gain, especially during the third trimester when an acceleration of fetal mass accumulation occurs, the fetus must be in a positive electrolyte balance.

Changes During Labor and Delivery

Additional, more acute changes in total body water and its distribution take place during labor and delivery. Arterial blood pressure increases a few days before delivery in response to increases in catecholamine, vasopressin, and cortisol plasma concentrations and translocation of blood from the placenta into the fetus. The rise in arterial blood pressure and the changes in the fetal hormonal milieu along with the borderline intrapartum hypoxia-induced increase in capillary permeability result in a shift of fluid

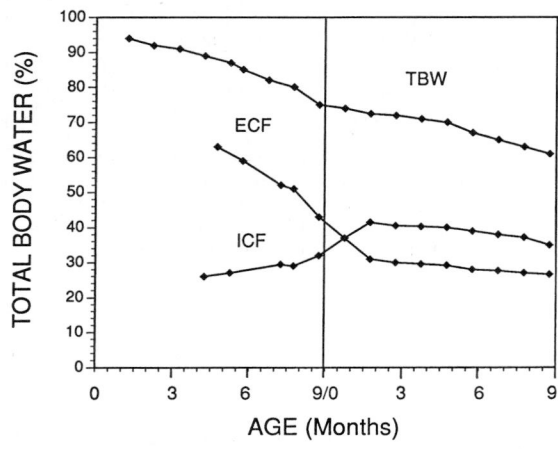

FIGURE 34–1. Total body water (TBW) content and its distribution between the extracellular fluid (ECF) and intracellular fluid (ICF) compartments in the human fetus, newborn, and infant from conception until 9 months of age. The data represent average values from Friis-Hansen (1961).

from the intravascular to the interstitial compartment. This fluid shift results in an approximately 25% reduction in circulating plasma volume in the human fetus during labor and delivery (Brace, 1992). Because the expanded interstitial fluid is not immediately accessible for filtration and excretion by the kidneys after birth, it may serve as a source of volume supply until maternal milk production becomes adequate. Thus, the translocation of fluid from the intravascular to the interstitial compartment during labor and delivery is part of the physiologic adaptation for the transition to extrauterine life. The postnatal increase in oxygenation and the concurrent changes in vasoactive hormone production then restore capillary membrane integrity and favor absorption of interstitial fluid into the intravascular compartment. The ensuing gradual movement of fluid from the expanded interstitial space into the vessels aids in maintaining intravascular volume during the first 24 to 48 hours when oral fluid intake may be limited. Prematurity or pathologic conditions may disrupt this delicate process, however, and interfere with the physiologic contraction of the extracellular fluid compartment in the immediate postnatal period.

In the fetus, body composition and fluid balance depend on the electrolyte and water exchange between the mother, fetus, and amniotic space (Brace, 1992). Therefore, several antenatal events influencing this exchange may exert significant effects on the postnatal fluid balance. Maternal indomethacin treatment or excessive intravenous fluid administration during labor may result in neonatal hyponatremia with an expanded extracellular water content (Heijden et al, 1988). Hydrops fetalis is the ultimate example of extreme fetal extracellular volume expansion. Placental insufficiency or maternal diuretic therapy may impair fetal hydration leading to decreases in extracellular volume, urine output, and amniotic fluid volume (Brace, 1992). Such newborns have attenuated postnatal diuresis and weight loss and initially require increased fluid intake to correct the state of prenatal dehydration. Finally, there is no evidence that the mode of delivery influences neonatal extracellular water content (Cheek et al, 1982).

The timing of cord clamping after delivery is another important factor significantly affecting total circulating blood volume and extracellular volume in the newborn. Immediate clamping of the cord results in an average hematocrit of 48% to 51%, and there is little change in the newborn's hematocrit over the next days (Linderkamp, 1982). If the cord is clamped only 3 to 4 minutes after delivery with the newborn being positioned at or below the level of the placenta, however, 25 to 50 mL/kg of blood is transfused into the newborn representing an approximately 25% to 50% increase in the total blood volume (Linderkamp, 1982). Because in these cases the increased transcapillary hydrostatic pressure forces an additional 25 to 30 mL/kg of intravascular fluid out into the interstitium, hematocrit gradually increases to 60% to 65% or higher over the first 3 to 4 hours of life (Brace, 1992; Linderkamp, 1982). Thus, if the newborn is suspected to have received a prolonged placental transfusion and the initial hematocrit is between 60% to 65%, the hematocrit should be checked again 4 to 6 hours later. The effects of the timing of cord clamping on intravascular and extracellular volumes are modified by the presence of asphyxia and neonatal breathing.

Changes in the Postnatal Period

During the first few days and weeks of life, gestational and postnatal age, the presence or absence of pathologic conditions, the immediate environment, and the type of nutrition have the most important effects on the pace of further change in body composition, total body water content, and its distribution. During the early transitional period, the healthy newborn loses weight. It is generally accepted that the postnatal weight loss is primarily due to the contraction of the expanded extracellular fluid compartment and that it approximates the total body fluid loss (Shaffer et al, 1986). Water loss from the intracellular space may also contribute to the physiologic weight loss (Coulter, 1983), especially if rapid changes in serum osmolality occur. Such changes in serum osmolality may be seen in extremely low-birth-weight infants with increased transepidermal water losses (Costarino and Baumgart, 1991; Sedin, 1995).

Although the exact mechanisms of the extracellular fluid contraction are unknown, several studies have suggested that atrial natriuretic peptide may play a role in this process (Ronconi et al, 1995; Rozycki and Baumgart, 1991; Tulassay et al, 1987). The postnatal increase in capillary membrane integrity favors absorption of the interstitial fluid into the intravascular compartment. The ensuing increase in circulating blood volume stimulates atrial natriuretic peptide release from the heart, which, in turn, may contribute to the postnatal enhancement of renal sodium and water excretion (Sagnella and MacGregor, 1984). In addition, the concomitant decrease in the release of vasoconstrictive and antidiuretic hormones also may play a role in the postnatal extracellular volume contraction.

The total body water excess and extracellular volume expansion of preterm infants imply that their negative water and sodium balance during the first 5 to 10 days of life (Shaffer and Meade, 1989) (Fig. 34–2) represents an appropriate adaptation to extrauterine life and should not be compensated for by increased fluid administration and sodium supplementation. If this principle is not followed and a positive fluid balance (i.e., weight gain) is achieved during the transitional period, preterm infants are at higher risk to present with a more severe course of hyaline membrane disease (Shaffer and Weismann, 1992) as well as with an increased incidence of patent ductus arteriosus (Bell et al, 1980), congestive heart failure (Bell et al, 1980), pulmonary edema (Shaffer and Weismann, 1992), necrotizing enterocolitis (Bell, 1979), and bronchopulmonary dysplasia (Van Marter et al, 1990). Only thorough understanding of the principles of developmental fluid and electrolyte physiology enables the clinician to adjust fluid and caloric requirements appropriately during the transitional period in the sick term and preterm newborn and thus minimize the impact of abnormalities in postnatal fluid and electrolyte homeostasis on different short-term and long-term outcome measures (see section on fluid and electrolyte management).

Healthy full-term newborns lose an average of 5% to 10% of their body weight during the first 4 to 7 days of life (Brace, 1992). Thereafter they establish a steady weight

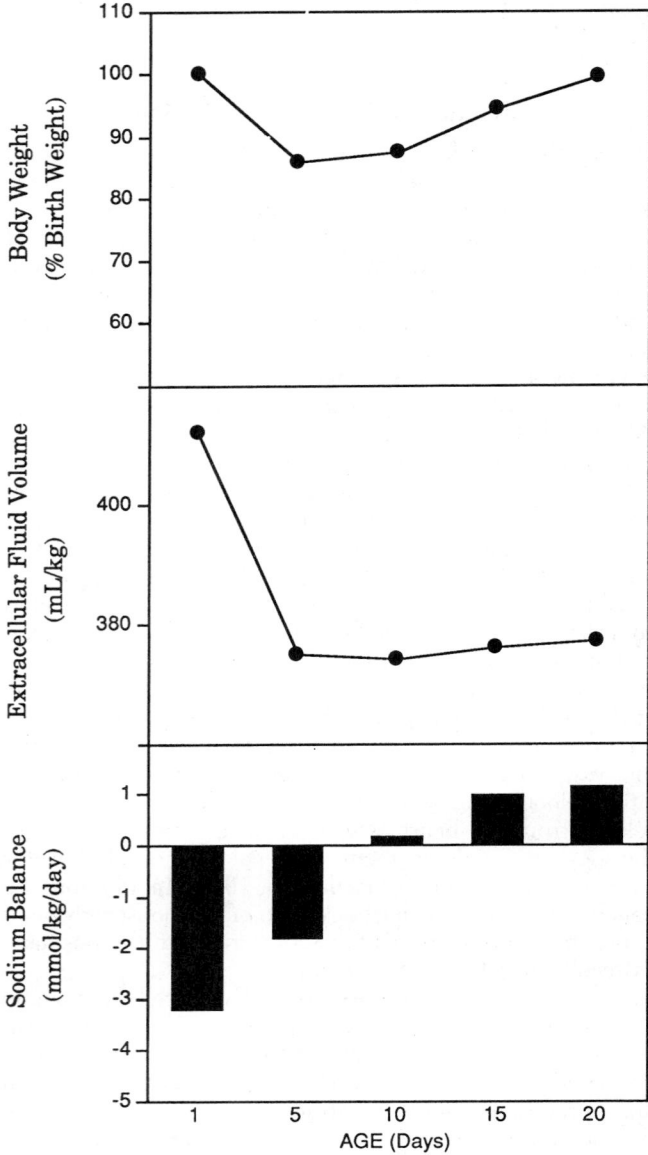

FIGURE 34–2. Postnatal changes in body weight (expressed in percent of birth weight), extracellular fluid volume (estimated by the bromide dilution method), and sodium balance (defined as the difference between sodium intake and urinary sodium excretion). (From Shaffer SG, Weismann DN: Fluid requirements in the preterm infant. Clin Perinatol 19:233, 1992.)

gain pattern. Because preterm infants have an increased total body water content and extracellular volume, they lose on average 15% of their body weight during transition (Shaffer and Weismann, 1992), and depending on the degree of prematurity and associated pathologic conditions, these newborns regain their birth weight only by 10 to 20 days after birth. Because total body water content at birth is also influenced by factors other than maturity (see earlier), however, physiologic weight loss may significantly differ among patients of the same gestational age, and there is no established optimal rate or extent of weight loss in infants born prematurely.

The healthy term infant is born after having developed

adequate macromineral stores. Following the extracellular volume contraction, these infants maintain an appropriate positive macromineral balance and steadily gain weight. Preterm infants, especially those born before the third trimester, have missed the period of intrauterine life when the highest rate of macromineral retention takes place. To achieve and maintain normal growth, these newborns must be in a positive macromineral balance after their transitional period. Certain pathologic conditions and the long-term administration of diuretics, however, may hinder their ability to achieve a positive macromineral balance and thus appropriate growth rate.

Physiology of Regulation of Body Composition and Fluid Compartments

Although human cells have the ability to adjust their intracellular composition, ultimate regulation of the intracellular volume and osmolality relies on the control of the extracellular compartment. Therefore, the human body must be able to monitor the volume and osmolality of the extracellular compartment and to correct the changes resulting from its interaction with the environment.

Regulation of Intracellular Solute and Water Compartment

The major intracellular solutes are the cellular proteins necessary for cell function, the organic phosphates associated with cellular energy production and storage, and the equivalent cations balancing the phosphate and protein anions. As a result of the activity of the cell membrane-bound sodium-potassium (Na^+-K^+) pump, potassium is the major intracellular cation, and sodium is the major extracellular cation. The energy derived from the concentration differences for sodium and potassium between the intracellular and extracellular compartments is used for cellular work.

Because changes in osmolality of the extracellular compartment are reflected as net movements of water in or out of the cell, regulation of extracellular fluid concentration ultimately controls the osmolality and size of the intracellular compartment. This physiologic principle must be kept in mind by the neonatologist when managing sick term and preterm newborns with disturbances of sodium homeostasis. Rapid changes in serum sodium concentration and thus in extracellular osmolality directly affect the osmolality and size of the intracellular compartment and may lead to irreversible cell damage, especially in the central nervous system (see later).

Regulation of the Intracellular/Extracellular Interface: The Interstitial Compartment

There are small but important differences in the composition of the interstitial and intravascular fluid compartments that allow the movement of water, solute, and nutrients from the blood into the interstitium and the transport of cellular waste products into the circulation for final elimination. The tightly regulated differences in the composition of the interstitium and the intravascular fluid space result from the interaction of the intravascular and interstitial hydrostatic and oncotic pressures (Starling, 1896). According to this principle, water movement across the capillary wall can be described by the following equation:

$$J_V = K_F [(P_C - P_T) - \delta (\pi_P - \pi_T)]$$

where J_V = the net flow across the capillary, K_F = filtration coefficient, P_C = capillary hydrostatic pressure, P_T = interstitial hydrostatic pressure, δ = protein reflection coefficient, π_P = plasma oncotic pressure, and π_T = interstitial oncotic pressure. Thus, the movement of fluid out of the capillary is determined by the product of the water permeability characteristics of the capillary wall (K_F) and the net driving pressure $[(P_C - P_T) - \delta(\pi_P - \pi_T)]$ that forces fluid out from the capillary. The net driving pressure is the difference between the hydrostatic ($P_C - P_T$) and oncotic ($\pi_P - \pi_T$) pressures on either side of the capillary wall (Fig. 34–3).

Under physiologic conditions, the balance of these forces results in a small amount of fluid leaving the plasma at the arterial end of the capillary circulation. As capillary hydrostatic pressure falls and plasma oncotic pressure increases along the capillary bed, filtration ceases, and much of the filtered fluid re-enters at the venous end of the capillary circulation. The difference between the filtered and reabsorbed fluid is cleared from the interstitium by the lymphatic system (Taylor, 1981). The reflection coefficient (δ) describes the protein permeability characteristics of the capillary wall, which is tissue specific. In tissues with capillaries that are virtually impermeable to proteins (e.g., brain, skin: $\delta = 0.8$), the oncotic pressure difference plays an important role in counterbalancing the tendency of the

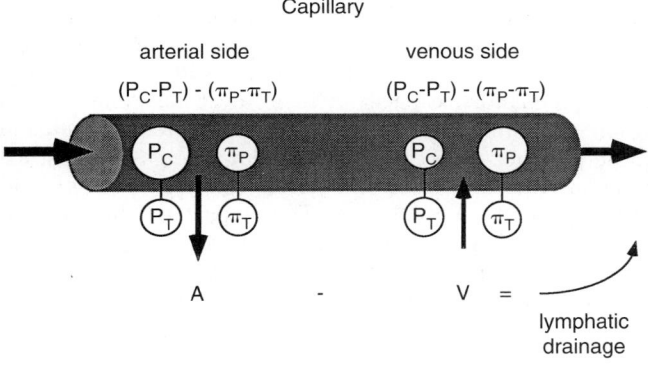

Capillary

arterial side
$(P_C{-}P_T) - (\pi_P{-}\pi_T)$

venous side
$(P_C{-}P_T) - (\pi_P{-}\pi_T)$

A - V = lymphatic drainage

FIGURE 34–3. Filtration and reabsorption of fluid along the capillary under physiologic conditions. Movement of fluid across the capillary is determined by the direction of the net driving pressure $[(P_C - P_T) - (\pi_P - \pi_T)]$ and the water and protein permeability characteristics of the capillary wall. At the arterial end of the capillary, intracapillary hydrostatic pressure (P_C) is high, and plasma oncotic pressure (π_P) is relatively low resulting in a net movement of fluid out of the capillary. As filtration of the protein-poor fluid continues along the capillary, plasma oncotic pressure rises, and intracapillary hydrostatic pressure drops. Therefore, on the venous side, fluid moves from the interstitium into the capillary so that most of the filtered fluid is reabsorbed at the end of the capillary bed. The small amount of fluid remaining in the interstitium (A − V) is drained by the lymphatic system. Interstitial hydrostatic (P_T) and oncotic (π_T) pressures remain virtually unchanged along the capillary bed. See text for details.

TABLE 34–1

Mechanisms Promoting Fluid Accumulation in the Interstitial Compartment

Conditions Favoring Fluid Accumulation in the Interstitial Space by Causing a Disequilibrium Between Filtration and Reabsorption of Fluid by the Capillaries

Increased hydrostatic pressure gradient
  Elevated capillary hydrostatic pressure
    Increased cardiac output
    Venous obstruction
  Decreased tissue hydrostatic pressure
    Conditions associated with changes in the properties of the interstitial gel (edematous states, hormonal effects including that of prolactin)
Decreased oncotic pressure gradient
  Decreased capillary oncotic pressure
    Prematurity, hyaline membrane disease
    Malnutrition, liver dysfunction
    Nephrotic syndrome
  Increased interstitial oncotic pressure is usually the result of increased capillary permeability (see below)
Elevation of the filtration coefficient
  Increased capillary permeability
    Organs with large-pore capillary endothelium (liver, spleen)
    State of maturity (preterm infants > term newborns > adults)
    Production of proinflammatory cytokines (sepsis, anaphylaxis, hypoxic tissue injury, tissue ischemia, ischemia-reperfusion, soft tissue trauma, extracorporeal membrane oxygenation)
  Increased capillary surface area
    Vasodilation

Conditions Associated with Decreased Lymphatic Drainage

Decreased muscle movement
  Neuromuscular blockade and/or heavy sedation
  Central and/or peripheral nervous system pathology
Obstruction of lymphatic flow
  Increased central venous pressure
  Scar tissue formation (bronchopulmonary dysplasia)
  Mechanical obstruction (high mean airway pressure in mechanically ventilated newborns, dressings)

Modified from Costarino AT, Baumgart S: Neonatal water metabolism. *In* Cowett RM (Ed): Principles of Perinatal/Neonatal Metabolism. New York, Springer Verlag, 1991, pp 623–649.

hydrostatic forces to move fluid out from the capillaries. In tissues with high capillary permeability to protein (e.g., liver, spleen: $\delta = 0.2$), the lymphatic circulation plays a more important role in regulating the volume of the interstitial fluid compartment.

In the healthy full-term newborn, hydrostatic and oncotic pressures are well balanced, being roughly half of those in the adult (Sola and Gregory, 1981). Pathologic conditions readily disturb the delicate balance between the hydrostatic and oncotic forces and result in an expansion of the interstitial compartment at the expense of the intravascular volume. The increased interstitial fluid volume (edema) then further affects tissue perfusion by altering the normal function of the extracellular/intracellular interface. Table 34–1 summarizes the conditions resulting in increased edema formation in the newborn.

There also are some important developmentally regulated differences between the newborn and the adult concerning the pathomechanisms of edema formation. Capillary permeability to proteins is increased during the early stages of development, which is reflected by a decreased tissue-specific protein reflection coefficient (δ) in the fetus and newborn compared to that in the adult (Brace, 1992; Gold and Brace, 1988). Because neonatal capillary permeability is further increased under pathologic conditions (see Table 34–1), interstitial protein concentration may approach that of the intravascular space favoring further intravascular volume depletion and interstitial volume expansion. When such newborns are treated with frequent albumin boluses, much of the infused albumin leaks out into the interstitium creating a cycle of intravascular volume depletion and edema formation. If the cycle is not interrupted, such cases may result in the formation of anasarca with extremely poor prognosis. As mentioned earlier, when the permeability of the capillary endothelium to protein is increased, the final balance between fluid filtration and reabsorption is more dependent on an effective lymphatic drainage (Taylor, 1981). Lymph flow in the newborn is readily disrupted by even a small elevation in venous pressure (Brace, 1992); pathologic conditions and therapeutic maneuvers increasing venous pressure are frequently associated with decreased lymphatic clearance and thus edema formation in the sick infant.

The sick newborn has a limited capacity to maintain appropriate intravascular volume and to regulate the volume and composition of the interstitium. The ensuing intravascular hypovolemia and edema formation result in vasoconstriction and disturbances in tissue perfusion and cellular function with further impairments in the regulation of extracellular volume distribution.

Regulation of Extracellular Solute and Water Compartment

The regulation of the volume and osmolality of the extracellular compartment ensures the integrity of the circulation and maintains the osmolality of the extracellular compartment within 2% of the osmolar set-point between 275 and 290 mOsm (Robertson and Berl, 1986). Blood pressure and serum sodium concentration (i.e., osmolality) are monitored by baroreceptors and osmoreceptors. The effector limb of the regulatory system consists of the heart, the vascular bed, the kidneys, and the gastrointestinal intake of fluid in response to thirst. The last part of the effector system is inactive in the critically ill term and preterm newborn, whose fluid intake is completely controlled by the caregivers. By regulating the function of the effector organs, several hormones play a role in the control of the extracellular compartment, including the renin-angiotensin-aldosterone system, vasopressin, atrial natriuretic peptide, and catecholamines.

Because volume changes in the extracellular compartment must be reflected by similar changes in the intravascular volume for effective operation of the regulatory mechanisms, regulation of the extracellular compartment relies on intact cardiovascular function as well as on the integrity of the capillary endothelium (Robertson and Berl, 1986). For instance, under physiologic conditions, an increase in the extracellular volume is reflected by an increase in the circulating plasma volume leading to increases in blood pressure and organ blood flow. The ensuing increase in urine output returns the extracellular volume to normal.

In critically ill newborns, the capillary leak and decreased myocardial responsiveness resulting from immaturity and the underlying pathologic condition limit the increase in the circulating blood volume in cases of extracellular volume expansion. Thus, especially in sick preterm infants, blood pressure may increase only transiently, and renal blood flow and glomerular filtration rate remain low after volume boluses as fluid rapidly leaks out into the interstitium. By causing peripheral vasodilation, inappropriate central regulation of vascular tone further decreases effective circulating blood volume. With the concomitant release of catecholamines, vasopressin, and renin-angiotensin-aldosterone, renal tubular sodium and water reabsorption continue to be favored to increase diminished intravascular volume. This compensatory mechanism, however, fails as the retained fluid continues to leak out from the intravascular space into the interstitium further compromising tissue perfusion. This interstitial fluid accumulation leads to impaired gas exchange in the lungs resulting in hypoxia with further increases in capillary leak. Thus, unless interrupted by appropriate therapeutic measures (see later), a vicious cycle with further deterioration rather than an effective extracellular volume regulation occurs in the sick preterm and term newborn.

Maturation of Organs Regulating Body Composition and Fluid Compartments

The heart, the kidneys, the skin, and the endocrine system play the most important role in the regulation of extracellular (and thus intracellular) fluid and electrolyte balance in the newborn. Immaturity of these organ systems, especially in the very-low-birth-weight infant, results in a compromised regulatory capacity, which must be remembered when estimating daily fluid and electrolyte requirements in these patients. Other organs, including the gastrointestinal tract, are also involved in the physiologic regulation of fluid and electrolyte homeostasis. The impact of the maturational state of these organs, however, is less significant on fluid and electrolyte management in the critically ill preterm and term newborn.

Maturation of the Cardiovascular System

There is a direct relationship between the degree of maturity and the ability of the neonatal heart to respond to acute volume loading (Baylen et al, 1986). The blunted Starling response of the immature myocardium results from its decreased content of contractile elements and incomplete sympathetic innervation (Mahony, 1995). Because central vasoregulation and endothelial integrity are also developmentally regulated (Brace, 1992; Gold and Brace, 1988), an appropriate effective intravascular volume is seldom maintained in a critically ill preterm infant. Because regulation of the extracellular volume requires the maintenance of an adequate effective circulating blood volume, the immaturity of the cardiovascular system contributes to the limited capacity of sick preterm infants to regulate the total volume of their extracellular compartment effectively.

Maturation of Renal Function

The kidney plays a crucial role in the physiologic control of fluid and electrolyte balance. It regulates extracellular volume by the selective reabsorption of sodium and osmolality by the selective reabsorption of water. In the fetus, nephrogenesis is incomplete until 34 to 36 weeks of gestation (see Chapter 91). Thus, in addition to immaturity of their tubular functions, preterm infants have a decreased number of glomeruli, and the postnatal increase in renal blood flow and glomerular filtration rate is attenuated compared to the that of the full-term newborn. Tubular immaturity in preterm infants is reflected by their increased sodium, bicarbonate, and free water excretion and decreased renal concentrating capacity (Jones and Chesney, 1992) (see also Chapter 91).

Some aspects of developmental renal physiology significantly influence the clinical management of the sick newborn. Because prenatal steroid administration accelerates maturation of renal function (van den Anker et al, 1994), preterm infants treated with steroids in utero have an improved capacity to regulate postnatal extracellular fluid contraction, which may facilitate pulmonary recovery. Furthermore, immaturity of renal function renders preterm infants susceptible to both sodium losses and sodium and volume overloading (El-Dahr and Chevalier, 1990). Sodium losses occur despite the low glomerular filtration rate and are mainly due to the immaturity of the tubular membrane transport processes and their hormonal regulation. The high urinary sodium excretion may be of clinical benefit during the period of transition because it promotes contraction of the expanded extracellular volume. Because sodium retention is necessary for normal growth, however, a negative sodium balance beyond the first 1 to 2 weeks of life may hinder appropriate weight gain (Sulyok et al, 1985). The inability of the preterm infant to respond promptly to a sodium or volume load results in a tendency of extracellular volume expansion with edema formation. This volume expansion is the consequence of the limited glomerular filtration rate, and it occurs despite the preterm infant's ability to produce a dilute urine (El-Dahr and Chevalier, 1990).

Maturation of the Skin

Although term infants have a well-developed cornified layer of the epidermis, extremely immature newborns have only two to three cell layers in the epidermis (Cartridge-Patrick and Rutter, 1992). Because of the lack of an effective barrier to diffusion of water through the immature skin, transepidermal free water losses in the immature infant may be extremely high during the first few days of life. Gestational age, postnatal age, pattern of intrauterine growth, and environmental factors play a crucial role in the magnitude of transepidermal free water losses (Fig. 34–4). Although skin cornification rapidly increases even in the extremely immature 23- to 26-week preterm infant during the first few days of life, full maturation of the epidermis occurs only after 28 days of postnatal age (Sedin, 1995). In

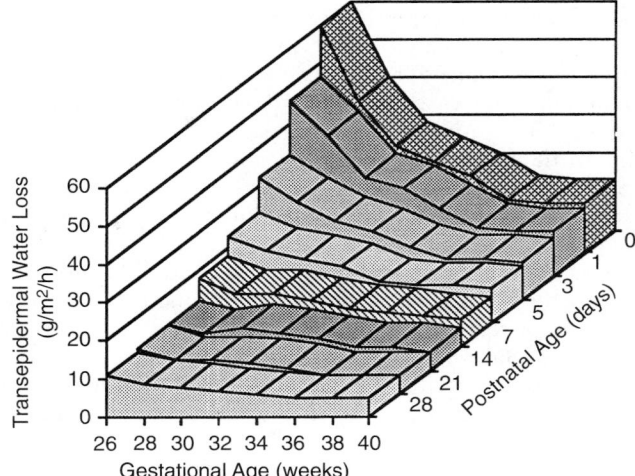

FIGURE 34–4. Transepidermal water loss in relation to gestational age during the first 28 days of life in appropriate-for-gestational-age infants. There is an exponential relationship between transepidermal water loss and gestational age, with the water loss being higher in the preterm infants than in full-term newborns. Transepidermal water loss is also significantly affected by postnatal age especially in the immature preterm newborn. The measurements were performed at an ambient air humidity of 50% and with the infants calm and quiet. (From Hammarlund K, Sedin G, Strömberg B: Transepidermal water loss in newborn infants: VIII. Relation to gestational age and post-natal age in appropriate and small for gestational age infants. Acta Paediatr Scand 72:721, 1983.)

addition to advancing gestational and postnatal age, chronic intrauterine stress (Hammarlund et al, 1983) and prenatal steroid treatment (Aszterbaum et al, 1993) enhance maturation of the skin.

Because regulation of extracellular fluid volume and osmolality ultimately controls the intracellular compartment, increases in free water losses through the immature skin in the very-low-birth-weight infant may result in early postnatal hypertonic dehydration with rapid changes in intracellular volume and osmolality. In many organs, especially in the brain, the abrupt changes in intracellular volume and osmolality may lead to cell dysfunction and ultimately to cell death (see later).

Maturation of End-Organ Responsiveness to Hormones Involved in the Regulation of Fluid and Electrolyte Balance

Several hormones, including but not limited to the renin-angiotensin-aldosterone system, vasopressin, atrial natriuretic peptide, and dopamine and noradrenaline, directly regulate the volume or the composition (or both) of the extracellular compartment. These hormones exert their effects mainly by altering renal sodium and water excretion and by inducing changes in systemic vascular resistance and myocardial contractility. Other hormones, including the prostaglandins, bradykinin, and prolactin, modulate the actions of many of the regulatory hormones.

Renin-Angiotensin-Aldosterone System. Decreases in renal capillary blood flow and tubular sodium delivery to the juxtaglomerular apparatus stimulate renin secretion, which, in turn, initiates the production of angiotensin. Angiotensin induces vasoconstriction, increased tubular sodium and water reabsorption, and aldosterone release (Riordan, 1995). Aldosterone increases potassium secretion and further enhances sodium reabsorption in the distal tubule. Thus, the primary function of this system is to protect the volume of the extracellular compartment and maintain adequate tissue perfusion (Bailie, 1992). Its effectiveness in the newborn is somewhat limited, however, by the decreased responsiveness of the immature kidney to the sodium-retaining and water-retaining effects of these hormones (Sulyok et al, 1985). This insensitivity is also one of the reasons why this system remains activated for several weeks to months, especially in the more immature or the critically ill newborn (Sulyok et al, 1979).

Vasodilatory and natriuretic prostaglandins generated in the kidney (Gleason, 1987) are the main counter-regulatory hormones balancing the renal actions of renin-angiotensin-aldosterone. Therefore, when prostaglandin production is inhibited by indomethacin, unopposed vasoconstrictive and sodium-retentive actions of the activated renin-angiotensin-aldosterone system contribute to the development of the drug-induced renal failure in the preterm infant (Gleason, 1987; Seri, 1995).

Vasopressin (Antidiuretic Hormone). The increase in serum osmolality is a much more potent stimulus for vasopressin secretion than the decrease in systemic blood pressure. This fact indicates that vasopressin is more important for maintaining the osmolality of the extracellular compartment than it is for regulating total extracellular volume and effective circulating blood volume. By midgestation, the fetus is able to respond to both osmotic and baroreceptor stimulation as well as to hypoxia with increased vasopressin release (Leake, 1992). The primary renal action of vasopressin is to increase free water reabsorption selectively via the insertion of water channels into the luminal membrane of the distal tubular and collecting duct epithelium (Elliott et al, 1996). The hormone-induced free water retention is counterbalanced by locally generated prostaglandins (Gleason, 1987). Indomethacin administration abolishes this regulatory effect, and the unopposed vasopressin-induced free water reabsorption contributes to the development of the drug-induced renal side effects (Gleason, 1987; Seri, 1995).

The primary cardiovascular action of the hormone is peripheral vasoconstriction resulting in blood pressure elevation and redistribution of blood flow (Leake, 1992). Plasma levels of vasopressin are markedly elevated in the newborn, especially following vaginal delivery, and its cardiovascular actions facilitate neonatal adaptation. The high vasopressin levels are also in part responsible for the diminished urine output of the healthy term newborn during the 1st day of life.

Under certain pathologic conditions, the dysregulated release of, and/or the end-organ unresponsiveness to, vasopressin significantly affect renal and cardiovascular functions in the sick preterm and term infant. In the syndrome of inappropriate secretion of antidiuretic hormone (SIADH), an uncontrolled release of vasopressin occurs in sick preterm and term infants. SIADH may be associated with birth asphyxia, intracerebral hemorrhage, respiratory distress syndrome, pneumothorax, and use of continuous positive-pressure ventilation (El-Dahr and Chevalier, 1990; Leake, 1992). The syndrome is characterized by renal free water retention with decreased serum sodium values and serum osmolality as well as by oliguria, increased urine concentration, and weight gain with edema formation. Because urinary concentrating capacity of the newborn is limited, a less than maximally diluted urine satisfies the diagnosis of SIADH in the presence of the other symptoms. The treatment is based on fluid and sodium restriction, despite the oliguria and hyponatremia, as well as appropriate circulatory and ventilatory support. The clinician must remember that total body sodium is normal and total body water is elevated in these cases and that it is particularly dangerous to treat the hyponatremia caused by free water retention with large amounts of sodium. Because of more immature renal function, extremely low-birth-weight infants during the first few weeks of life usually do not present with the full-blown syndrome despite sometimes excessively high plasma vasopressin levels.

Diminished vasopressin secretion or complete unresponsiveness of the renal tubules results in polyuria, diluted urine production, and increased serum osmolality (Leake, 1992). The treatment of these newborns consists of provision of adequate free water intake. During the first few weeks of life, hemodynamically stable, extremely immature infants produce a dilute urine and may become polyuric despite appropriate vasopressin production because of renal tubular immaturity. As tubular functions mature, concentrating capacity gradually improves from the 2nd to 4th week of life. It takes years, however, for the developing kidney to reach the concentrating capacity of that of the adult.

Atrial Natriuretic Peptide. Via its direct vasodilatory and renal natriuretic actions, atrial natriuretic peptide regulates the volume of the extracellular compartment in the fetus and newborn in a fashion opposite to that of the renin-angiotensin-aldosterone system (Iwamoto, 1992; Needleman and Greenwald, 1986). This opposing action is further reflected by the direct inhibitory effect of atrial natriuretic peptide on renin production and aldosterone release (Christensen, 1993). The stretch of the atrial wall caused by an increase in the circulating blood volume is the most potent stimulus for the release of this hormone. During early development, atrial natriuretic peptide is produced by all the chambers of the heart, and plasma levels are high in the fetus (Christensen, 1993).

There are a few specific conditions in which the actions of atrial natriuretic peptide are directly relevant for the neonatologist. For instance, the hormone is involved in the regulation of both the fluid shifts during labor (Brace, 1992) and the extracellular volume contraction during postnatal transition (Ronconi et al, 1995; Rozycki and Baumgart, 1991; Tulassay et al, 1987). Furthermore, the oliguric effects of positive end-expiratory pressure ventilation are in part due to a decrease in atrial natriuretic peptide secretion (Christensen, 1993) along with the enhanced release of vasopressin (El-Dahr and Chevalier, 1990).

Dopamine, Noradrenaline, and Adrenaline. Dopamine, produced in the renal proximal tubule cells and the dopaminergic nerve endings of the kidneys, regulates total extra-cellular fluid volume by enhancing sodium excretion and selectively increasing blood flow to the kidney (Seri, 1995). In general, adrenaline and locally produced noradrenaline exert opposite renal vascular and tubular effects in the fetus and newborn (Robillard et al, 1990). Both the dopa-minergic and the alpha-adrenergic systems appear to be functionally mature even in the preterm newborn as evidenced by their cardiovascular and renal response to dopamine treatment (Seri, 1995).

Prostaglandins. Prostaglandins play a well-documented counter-regulatory role for the renal vascular and tubular effects of renin-angiotensin-aldosterone and vasopressin (Gleason, 1987). The inhibition of these actions of prostaglandins by indomethacin results in clinically important and sometimes detrimental renal vascular and tubular effects in the preterm infant (see later). The actions of prostaglandins modulating the effects of the other regulatory hormones of the neonatal fluid and electrolyte homeostasis are less well studied.

Kallikrein-Kinin System. The renal cortical enzyme, kallikrein, catalyzes the formation of the vasodilator and natriuretic hormone bradykinin. The kallikrein-kinin system is activated at birth and stimulates renal prostaglandin production. Bradykinin also antagonizes the renal actions of vasopressin, renin, and angiotensin.

Prolactin. Prolactin plays a permissive role in the regulation of fetal and neonatal water homeostasis (Coulter, 1983; Pullano et al, 1989). The high fetal plasma prolactin levels contribute to the increased tissue water content of the fetus. Interestingly, postnatal prolactin levels remain high in the preterm newborn until the 40th postconceptional week (Perlman et al, 1978). Dopamine inhibits prolactin secretion in the preterm and term newborn (de Zegher et al, 1993; Seri et al, 1985) resulting in a decreased water-binding capacity of the tissues (Coulter, 1983). A clinical significance for this hypolactotropic effect in the dopamine-treated edematous preterm infant remains to be demonstrated.

Fluid and Electrolyte Management in Preterm and Term Newborns

Patient Evaluation

Maternal conditions during pregnancy, drug and fluid administration to the mother during labor and delivery, and specific fetal and neonatal conditions all affect the fluid and electrolyte balance of the newborn and should be taken into consideration when prescribing the initial daily fluid intake. Clinical evaluation of the newborn's fluid and electrolyte status should be based on clinical signs of dehydration or edema formation and on accurate serial measurements of body weight. Laboratory studies aiding in daily fluid and electrolyte management include serial measurements of serum electrolytes, blood urea nitrogen (BUN), serum creatinine, serum albumin, and serum osmolality. The frequency of monitoring depends on the

degree of immaturity, the severity of the fluid and electrolyte disturbance, and the severity of the underlying pathologic conditions.

General Principles of Fluid and Electrolyte Management

The most important principle of fluid and electrolyte management of the sick preterm and term infant is to find means to prevent or at least to decrease the likelihood of significant pulmonary and extrapulmonary edema formation. The measures to achieve this goal include provision of a negative fluid and electrolyte balance during the 1st week of life by restriction of fluid and salt administration, avoidance of excessive fluid intake during the rest of the first months of life, early closure of the ductus arteriosus, use of blood transfusions rather than that of colloid or crystalloid boluses for volume support if appropriate, and provision of sufficient nutrition. Because peripheral vasodilation as a result of disturbed regulation of vascular tone almost always contributes to the development of hypotension in the sick newborn, early administration of low to moderate doses of dopamine may further decrease the need for volume boluses, and, via its renal and hormonal effects, dopamine may facilitate the process of extracellular volume contraction (Seri, 1995).

Water and electrolyte requirements depend on the daily losses and the state of metabolic activity. Water requirement should be estimated based on the volume status and the sensible and insensible losses in the given infant. Because abrupt alterations in serum sodium concentration are associated with similar changes in serum osmolality, they may result in severe central nervous system sequalae.

Hyponatremia (<130 mEq/L) is most frequently caused by excessive free water administration or retention in the sick preterm and term newborn. In these cases, the diagnosis is based on the clinical signs of edema and weight gain and on the history of increased free water administration and medical conditions associated with enhanced vasopressin production. The appropriate restriction of free water intake is the treatment of choice in these cases. Less frequently, hyponatremia develops secondary to increased renal sodium losses. This may occur in the immature preterm infant with improving cardiovascular status and renal perfusion after the immediate postnatal period and in the recovering term infant following a cardiovascular and renal compromise. These infants usually lose weight, and supplementation of the calculated sodium deficit and that of the ongoing sodium losses leads to normalization of serum sodium concentration.

Hypernatremia (>150 mEq/L) most frequently occurs in the extremely immature newborn as a result of excessive transepidermal free water losses. The diagnosis is based on the attendant decrease in body weight and clinical signs of severe extracellular volume contraction. The treatment of choice is the replacement of free water losses. Hypernatremia may also develop in response to excessive sodium supplementation, mainly in the sick newborn receiving repeated volume boluses for cardiovascular support. In these cases, clinical signs of edema, increased body weight, and history of volume boluses help to establish the diagnosis. Management is more complex in these cases because the underlying severe illness and cardiovascular compromise limit the physician's ability to restrict fluid (and sodium) boluses. Appropriate fluid and sodium restriction and early support of cardiovascular and renal functions with dopamine may be of value in these patients by buying time to allow recovery from the underlying pathologic process.

In the critically ill infant, the cause of the serum sodium abnormality may be multifactorial and the treatment less straightforward. Thorough analysis of the medical history and the changes in clinical signs, laboratory findings, and body weight usually aid in determining the major causative factor and thus the treatment of the more complex cases of serum sodium abnormality. Because serum sodium concentration is the major determinant of serum osmolality, correction of its abnormalities should be carried out in a stepwise manner by limiting the changes in serum sodium concentration to 10 mEq/L per 24 hours or less.

The following calculations may be used to govern fluid and electrolyte replacement therapy in newborns with abnormal fluid and electrolyte status. Sodium deficit (or excess) may be calculated using the formula:

$$\text{Na}^+ \text{ deficit (or excess)} = (0.6 \times \text{BW}) \times ([\text{Na}^+]_{\text{desired}} - [\text{Na}^+]_{\text{actual}})$$

In this formula, sodium deficit (or excess) and body weight (BW) are expressed in mEq/L and kg, and $(0.6 \times \text{BW})$ is the estimation of the extracellular volume. Similarly, free water deficit (or excess) may be calculated as:

$$\text{H}_2\text{O deficit (or excess)} = (0.6 \times \text{BW}) \times ([\text{Na}^+]_{\text{desired}}/[\text{Na}^+]_{\text{actual}} - 1)$$

In this formula, H_2O deficit (or excess) and body weight (BW) are given in L and kg, and $(0.6 \times \text{BW})$ is the estimation of the extracellular volume. Finally, serum osmolality may be calculated by the formula:

$$\text{Serum osmolality} = 2[\text{Na}^+_{\text{plasma}}] + \text{BUN}/2.8 + \text{blood glucose}/18$$

Serum osmolality, $[\text{Na}^+_{\text{plasma}}]$, BUN, and blood glucose should be expressed in mOsm/L, mEq/L, mg/dL, and mg/dL. Although use of the above-listed calculations has limitations, these formulas may be helpful in the initiation of the appropriate therapeutic measure, while strict monitoring of the changes in the clinical condition, body weight, and laboratory findings provide the ultimate guidance in clinical management.

Water Requirements

To estimate the daily free water requirements of the sick newborn appropriately, all sources of water losses must be taken into account, which include the insensible, sensible, and surgical water losses. Free water losses occurring through the skin and the respiratory tract are considered insensible losses, whereas sensible water losses are comprised of urinary and fecal free water losses.

Insensible Losses

As described in the section on the maturation of the skin, gestational age, postnatal age, and environmental factors determine the amount of daily insensible water losses through the skin (see Fig. 34–4). During the first few days of life, transepidermal water losses may be 15 times higher in extremely premature infants born at 24 to 26 weeks of gestation than in full-term newborns (Sedin, 1995). Although the skin rapidly matures in the early postnatal period even in extremely immature infants, insensible water losses in these infants is still somewhat higher at the end of the first months of life than those of their full-term counterparts. Among the environmental factors, ambient humidity has the greatest impact on transepidermal water loss. In extremely immature newborns, an increase in the ambient humidity of the isolette from 20% to 80% decreases the transepidermal water loss by approximately 75% (Sedin, 1995). The difference in daily free water losses between the 20% and 80% ambient humidity is around 150 mL/kg. The use of an open radiant warmer more than doubles transepidermal water losses. If a plastic heat shield is applied while the infant is under the warmer, however, transepidermal water loss may be decreased by 30% to 50% (Costarino and Baumgart, 1991). At low ambient humidity, phototherapy increases transepidermal water losses by approximately 30%. In infants older than 28 weeks, phototherapy does not increase the transepidermal water loss if the ambient humidity is 50% in the isolette (Sedin, 1995). Other factors, including activity, air flow, and prenatal steroid treatment, also influence the magnitude of transepidermal free water losses (Aszterbaum et al, 1993; Sedin, 1995).

Insensible water losses from the respiratory tract depend mainly on the temperature and humidity of the inspired gas mixture and on the respiratory rate, tidal volume, and dead space ventilation. In a healthy full-term newborn, the water loss through the respiratory tract is approximately half of the total insensible water loss if the ambient air temperature is 32.5°C and humidity is 50% (Sedin, 1995). The respiratory water loss in critically ill preterm and full-term infants on mechanical ventilation is zero if the gas mixture is saturated with water at body temperature.

Sensible Losses

Free water loss in the urine is the most important form of sensible water loss. Smaller preterm infants without systemic hypotension and prerenal renal failure usually lose 30 to 40 mL/kg per day water in the urine during the 1st day of life and around 120 mL/kg per day on the 3rd day after birth. In stable, more mature preterm infants born after the 28th week of gestation, the values are around 90 and 150 mL/kg per day. Because of their renal immaturity, preterm newborns have a tendency to produce dilute urine, which increases their obligatory free water losses.

Water losses in the stool are less significant and amount to approximately 10 and 7 mL/kg per day in term and preterm infants during the 1st week of life (Sedin, 1995). Water losses in the stool increase thereafter and are influenced by the type of feeding and the frequency of stooling.

Surgical Losses

The most frequently encountered surgical water losses occur when a nasogastric tube is placed under continuous suction to provide relief for the gastrointestinal tract with conditions such as necrotizing enterocolitis and postoperative management after abdominal surgery. Because these losses may be significant, their replacement every 8 to 12 hours is necessary to maintain appropriate water and electrolyte balance. Because free water retention often develops after surgery, full replacement of the nasogastric free water loss is not recommended. The composition of the replacement solution depends on the electrolyte concentration of the fluid loss. Gastric fluid usually contains 50 to 60 mEq/L of sodium chloride, and it should also be replaced.

Electrolyte Requirements

Because among the electrolytes sodium, potassium, chloride, and bicarbonate have the most profound effect on total body water volume and fluid balance, the requirements for these electrolytes only are considered here.

Sodium and Its Anions

In the preterm infant, sodium chloride supplementation should be started only after the completion of the postnatal extracellular volume contraction. In general, as long as the infant's fluid balance is stable, daily sodium requirement does not exceed 3 to 4 mEq/kg per day, and provision of this amount usually ensures a positive sodium balance necessary for adequate growth. Extreme prematurity and pathologic conditions associated with delayed transition or disturbed fluid and electrolyte balance may significantly reduce or increase the infant's daily sodium requirement. Newborns recovering from an acute renal insult or preterm infants with immature proximal tubule functions who are in a state of extracellular volume expansion (Ramiro-Taolentino et al, 1996) may require daily sodium bicarbonate supplementation to compensate for their increased renal bicarbonate losses.

Potassium

In the early postnatal period, newborns, especially immature preterm infants, have higher serum potassium concentrations than older age groups. The cause of the relative hyperkalemia of the newborn is multifactorial and includes developmentally regulated differences in renal functions, Na^+/K^+-ATPase activity, and hormonal milieu. In general, potassium chloride supplementation should be started after urine output has been established, usually during the 2nd day of life. In the majority of cases, potassium requirement is 2 to 3 mEq/kg per day. After the completion of the postnatal volume contraction, however, preterm infants may require more potassium because of increased plasma aldosterone concentrations, prostaglandin excretion, disproportionately high urine flow rates, and use of diuretics.

Clinical Conditions Associated with Fluid and Electrolyte Disturbances

Extreme Prematurity

Infants born between 23 and 27 weeks of gestation are at a particular risk to develop acute abnormalities of fluid and electrolyte status in the immediate postnatal period. Their transepidermal water loss is much higher than that in the more mature preterm newborn (see Fig. 34–4), and it is difficult to maintain water balance unless the excessive losses are prevented. These infants, when cared for in an open warmer without the use of a plastic heat shield, may lose 150 to 300 mL/kg per day free water through their skin during the first 3 to 5 days of life. Although the insensible water loss primarily affects extracellular volume, the intracellular compartment ultimately shares the loss of free water as osmotic pressure in the extracellular compartment rises. As water leaves the cells, intracellular osmolality increases, and cell volume decreases. In many organs, including the central nervous system, these changes stimulate the generation of osmoprotective amino acids (*idiogenic osmoles*). These molecules selectively increase intracellular osmolality and thus prevent further intracellular water and volume losses. This protective mechanism has significant clinical implications for the rate at which hypernatremia should be corrected. If large amounts of idiogenic osmoles have been generated, a rapid lowering of the extracellular sodium concentration places the infant at high risk for development of acute cerebral edema. This iatrogenic central nervous system compromise then further increases the high underlying risk for neurologic sequelae in the immature preterm newborn, including the development of periventricular leukomalacia. Because effective generation of idiogenic osmoles takes several days, however, a more rapid decrease in serum sodium concentration during the first 2 days of life may, at least in theory, be less harmful than that after a more prolonged period of hypernatremia. Nevertheless, the decrease in serum sodium concentration should not exceed 10 mEq/L per 24 hours during the correction of hypernatremia in the immature newborn.

Because serum sodium concentration is a reliable clinical indicator of extracellular osmolality, monitoring of serum sodium concentration every 6 to 8 hours during the first 2 to 3 days of life coupled with daily measurements of body weight provides valuable information and appropriate guidance for the fluid and electrolyte management of the extremely immature preterm newborn. The critically ill, extremely immature infant may tolerate daily measurements of body weight only if a built-in scale is available in the incubator or on the radiant warmer. Serum osmolality should be directly measured in cases in which calculated serum osmolality is greater than 300 to 320 mOsm/L.

Because immature newborns cared for in an incubator with an ambient air humidity of 50% to 80% require significantly less free water and less frequent serum electrolyte and osmolality measurements (Sedin, 1995), open radiant warmers should be used only for critically ill, extremely labile preterm infants requiring frequent hands-on medical management. In these cases, the use of a protective plastic heat shield decreases excessive evaporative losses, and total daily fluid intake may be started at 80 to 100 mL/kg per day with 5% dextrose in water. Daily fluid intake is then increased by 10 to 30 mL/kg per day every 6 to 8 hours if serum sodium concentration rises from the baseline, with the goal being to maintain serum sodium concentration below 150 mEq/L. As skin integrity increases during the course of the 2nd to 3rd days, serum sodium concentration starts to decrease. At this time, a significant stepwise limitation of total fluid intake is obligatory to allow for a complete contraction of the extracellular volume to occur and to minimize the possibility of free water overload with its attendant risks for the development of ductal patency, pulmonary edema, and worsening underlying lung disease. Prenatal steroid administration may also decrease the rate of transepidermal water evaporation during the immediate postnatal period.

Potassium chloride supplementation may be started as soon as urine output has been established and serum potassium is below 5 mEq/L. Because extremely premature infants are at risk for the development of both oliguric and nonoliguric hyperkalemia, serum potassium should be monitored closely and potassium chloride supplementation discontinued if changes in serum potassium values or in renal function indicate. Critically ill, extremely immature newborns usually receive excess sodium with volume boluses, medications, and maintenance infusion of arterial lines. Therefore, extra sodium supplementation should not be started during the first few days of life to prevent an increase in total body sodium and thus extracellular volume. Many critically ill infants, however, retain their originally high extracellular volume during the course of the disease even when sodium and water intake are restricted. Such preterm newborns also tend to lose more bicarbonate in the urine. Interestingly, despite the immaturity of their renal functions, proximal tubular bicarbonate reabsorption may be appropriate even in the very-low-birth-weight infant as long as extracellular volume contraction takes place (Ramiro-Tolentino et al, 1996). Therefore, it appears that the presence of extracellular volume expansion is necessary for the manifestation of the renal bicarbonate wasting in these infants. Moreover, the diagnosis of functional proximal tubular acidosis in such cases should not rely solely on the finding of an alkaline urine pH because the distal tubular function is usually mature enough to acidify the urine once serum bicarbonate has decreased to its new threshold. Daily supplementation of bicarbonate in the form of sodium acetate or potassium acetate normalizes blood pH and serum bicarbonate in these infants and increases urine pH, aiding in the diagnosis. Once extracellular volume contraction occurs, these newborns generally achieve a positive bicarbonate balance (Ramiro-Tolentino et al, 1996), and supplementation therapy becomes unnecessary.

Other general guidelines in the fluid and electrolyte management of the immature preterm infant during the 1st week of life include calculation of fluid balance and estimation of sodium balance every day; testing of all urine samples for glucose, albumin, hemoglobin, and osmolality or specific gravity; and daily analyses of serum electrolytes, BUN, creatinine, and blood glucose. The frequency of testing and addition of other tests, including the measurement of serum albumin concentration and osmolality, depend on the clinical status, severity of underlying disease, and fluid and electrolyte disturbance of the given patient.

Respiratory Distress Syndrome

There is a well-established relationship between fluid and electrolyte balance and respiratory distress syndrome. Surfactant deficiency results in pulmonary atelectasis, elevated

pulmonary vascular resistance, poor lung compliance, and decreased lymphatic drainage. In addition, preterm infants have low plasma oncotic pressures and suffer pulmonary capillary endothelial injury from mechanical ventilation, oxygen administration, and perinatal hypoxia (Jefferies et al, 1984; Sola and Gregory, 1981). These abnormalities alter the balance of the Starling forces in the pulmonary microcirculation leading to interstitial edema formation with further impairment in pulmonary functions (see also Chapter 50).

If replacement surfactant is not administered, an improvement in pulmonary function occurs during the 3rd to 4th day of life. A period of brisk diuresis usually precedes pulmonary recovery and is characterized by small increases in glomerular filtration rate and sodium clearance and a larger rise in free water clearance (Costarino and Baumgart, 1991). Although the exact mechanism of the diuresis is not known, it is likely that improving endogenous surfactant production and capillary integrity promotes the recovery of the pulmonary capillary endothelium and lymphatic drainage. The ensuing changes in Starling forces now promote reabsorption of the hypotonic interstitial lung fluid into the circulation, and a delayed *physiologic diuresis* takes place. Because significant improvements in lung function occur only after the majority of the excess free water is excreted (Costarino and Baumgart, 1991), daily fluid intake should be restricted to allow for the extracellular volume contraction to take place. If this principle is not followed and a positive fluid balance is achieved, preterm infants with hyaline membrane disease are at higher risk to run a more severe course of acute lung disease as well as to present with an increase in the incidence of patent ductus arteriosus, congestive heart failure, and necrotizing enterocolitis and with a higher incidence and increased severity of ensuing chronic lung disease.

Prenatal steroid administration and postnatal surfactant administration have altered the course and clinical presentation of hyaline membrane disease (Ballard and Ballard, 1995; Ishisaka, 1996; Kari et al, 1994). Antenatal steroid administration accelerates maturation of organs, including those involved in the regulation of fluid and electrolyte balance (Ballard and Ballard, 1995), and the use of exogenous surfactant decreases pulmonary capillary leak and edema formation (Carlton et al, 1995). Furthermore, surfactant administration does not alter the rate and timing of ductal closure (Reller et al, 1993), although it may acutely affect the pattern of shunting through the ductus arteriosus (Kaapa et al, 1993). Thus, these interventions generally enhance extracellular volume contraction and aid in the stabilization of fluid and electrolyte homeostasis in preterm newborns with hyaline membrane disease. Maintenance of a negative water and sodium balance during the first few days of life, however, remains the cornerstone of fluid and electrolyte management in these infants (Tammela, 1995; Van Marter et al, 1990).

Based on the above-discussed events in the pathophysiology of pulmonary edema formation in infants with hyaline membrane disease, the use of furosemide has long been suggested to promote a negative fluid balance and inhibit directly pulmonary epithelial transport processes involved in edema formation in the lungs (Green et al, 1988; Yeh et al, 1984). Furosemide, however, induces only short-term improvements in pulmonary function in these patients, and no beneficial effects on long-term morbidity or mortality could be documented. Moreover, prophylactic use of the drug during the first days of life may lead to intravascular volume depletion with hypotension, tachycardia, and decreased peripheral perfusion as well as to acute and chronic disturbances in serum electrolytes and thus osmolality (Green et al, 1988; Schaffer and Weismann, 1992; Yeh et al, 1984). Furthermore, long-term administration of furosemide is associated with an increased incidence of patent ductus arteriosus (Green et al, 1983). Therefore, use of furosemide during this period should be restricted to cases with oliguria of renal origin when intravascular volume appears to be adequate.

Bronchopulmonary Dysplasia

Low gestational age and birth weight; lack of prenatal steroid administration; severe hyaline membrane disease with oxygen toxicity, barotrauma, air leak, inflammation, and patent ductus arteriosus; and insufficient nutrition are among the known causative factors for the development of bronchopulmonary dysplasia (see also Chapter 55). In addition, a high fluid and salt intake during the first weeks of life has also been shown to increase the incidence and severity of chronic lung disease. Excess fluid and electrolyte intake is of practical importance since it is controlled by the caregiver.

Newborns who develop bronchopulmonary dysplasia following hyaline membrane disease continue to retain excess interstitial lung fluid owing to the nonspecific inflammatory process–induced increase in pulmonary capillary permeability, high capillary hydrostatic and low oncotic pressures, and insufficient lymphatic drainage (Abman and Groothius, 1994; Jefferies et al, 1984). Administration of excessive fluid boluses and a positive fluid and sodium balance during the first few days of life promote lung fluid accumulation and ductal patency and are associated with an increased incidence and severity of bronchopulmonary dysplasia (Costarino and Baumgart, 1991; Van Marter et al, 1990). Interestingly a strict fluid restriction may offer further benefit over a less limited fluid intake if it is maintained during the entire 1st month of life (Tammela and Koivisto, 1992). According to this study, a fluid intake that advances gradually from 50 mL/kg per day to 120 mL/kg per day during the 1st week and is limited to 150 mL/kg per day during the following 3 weeks decreases the risk for pulmonary air leak and necrotizing enterocolitis and is associated with an increased survival without bronchopulmonary dysplasia when compared to a more liberal fluid administration (80 mL/kg per day advancing to 150 mL/kg per day during the 1st week and 200 mL/kg per day thereafter).

The beneficial effects of the lower fluid intake occur despite the achievement of an early negative fluid balance of similar magnitude and the provision of identical nutritional support in both groups. Therefore, the length of time over which the fluid restriction is applied may also contribute to the benefits of the strict fluid intake. In addition, by reducing the occurrence of hypernatremia and the subsequent excessive administration of parenteral fluids, restriction of salt intake during the first 5 days

of life may also decrease the risk for development of bronchopulmonary dysplasia (Costarino et al, 1992).

In infants with evolving or full-blown bronchopulmonary dysplasia, pulmonary edema impairs lung function and gas exchange. The ensuing increase in ventilatory support results in further damage and a vicious cycle develops. Therapeutic measures aimed at decreasing the interstitial and peribronchiolar pulmonary edema include fluid restriction; diuretic and steroid treatment; and provision of sufficient nutrition to meet the patient's increased metabolic energy demand, especially when steroids are administered (Kurzner et al, 1988). In infants with evolving or established bronchopulmonary dysplasia, restriction of daily fluid intake to 120 to 140 mL/kg usually allows the provision of appropriate nutrition, and long-term diuretic treatment improves their outcome (Albersheim et al, 1989).

Furosemide, the most frequently used diuretic in the treatment of bronchopulmonary dysplasia, directly reduces pulmonary interstitial water in addition to decreasing total body and extracellular water content (O'Donovan and Bell, 1989). Furosemide exerts these effects via its complex renal, cardiovascular, and pulmonary actions (Wahlig et al, 1992). In the kidney, the drug induces diuresis by inhibiting tubular chloride transport, thereby decreasing attendant sodium and potassium reabsorption. Furosemide also enhances free water excretion by inhibiting carbonic anhydrase activity in the proximal tubule and by attenuating the antidiuretic effects of vasopressin. Finally, the drug-induced increases in renal blood flow and glomerular filtration rate also contribute to its diuretic effects. Among its cardiovascular actions, the reduction of the right ventricular end-diastolic and pulmonary arterial pressure and the increase in venous capacitance directly contribute to drug-induced decreases in lung fluid filtration. In the lungs, furosemide inhibits chloride transport across the airway epithelium, which reduces airway reactivity and edema formation. Some of its renal and cardiovascular effects are mediated by the drug-induced stimulation of prostaglandin synthesis. In the long-term treatment of bronchopulmonary dysplasia, furosemide may be administered daily or every other day providing the same dose in milligrams per kilograms per day. The alternate-day dosage schedule may decrease the incidence of untoward effects on electrolyte homeostasis (Rush et al, 1990). Side effects of long-term furosemide administration include hypochloremic alkalosis, hyponatremia, hypokalemia, hypomagnesemia, hypocalcemia with nephrocalcinosis, formation of gallbladder stones, bone demineralization, and ototoxicity (Shaffer and Weismann, 1992; Wahlig et al, 1992).

Although less effective than furosemide in directly improving pulmonary functions, thiazide diuretics are useful in the medical management of infants with bronchopulmonary dysplasia (Albersheim et al, 1989; Kao et al, 1994). In milder forms of the disease, long-term administration of hydrochlorothiazide or chlorothiazide is associated with fewer untoward effects on electrolyte homeostasis and perhaps bone metabolism than furosemide. Thiazide diuretics have also been widely used in combination with spironolactone, although no study has convincingly demonstrated an advantage of the addition of this potassium-sparing aldosterone antagonist diuretic to hydrochlorothiazide or chlorothiazide in preterm infants with bronchopulmonary dysplasia. In more severe cases, the addition of the calcium-sparing chlorothiazide to furosemide may further diminish pulmonary interstitial edema formation and offers the additional benefit of attenuating the calciuric and thus osteopenic side effects of long-term furosemide therapy. In contrast, the addition of hydrochlorothiazide to furosemide is less effective in preventing the furosemide-induced disturbance in calcium homeostasis (Atkinson et al, 1988).

Although chlorothiazide primarily inhibits coupled sodium/chloride transport in the distal tubule, it also affects proximal tubule fluid reabsorption (Puschett, 1994; Wahlig et al, 1992). Thus, in very-low-birth-weight infants with disproportionately immature proximal tubular functions, the drug may cause excessive urinary sodium losses and severe hyponatremia. Therefore, it is prudent to start chlorothiazide below the recommended dose, at around 5 to 10 mg/kg per day, and monitor serum electrolytes closely as the dose of the drug is being increased daily in a stepwise manner. Interestingly, thiazide diuretics can cause the depletion of magnesium in the central nervous system and result in the development of intracellular alkalosis. These effects may serve as the cellular mechanisms for the suggested contribution of long-term chlorothiazide use to poor neurologic outcome in some infants with bronchopulmonary dysplasia.

Replacement of electrolyte losses induced by diuretics requires understanding of the developmental physiology of fluid and electrolyte homeostasis and that of the pharmacology of the diuretics applied. Significant amounts of sodium, potassium, chloride, calcium, and phosphorus are lost in the urine in these infants. Sodium and chloride losses are readily reflected by hyponatremia and hypochloremia, but serum potassium concentration may be maintained in the normal range for quite a while at the expense of intracellular potassium. The excess chloride loss triggers bicarbonate retention leading to progressive metabolic alkalosis. Furthermore, owing to the decreased intracellular potassium stores, the kidneys' ability to retain hydrogen ions is impaired, and the metabolic alkalosis becomes even more severe. Because newborns with bronchopulmonary dysplasia originally have a compensated respiratory acidosis, the development of the diuretic-induced metabolic alkalosis may go unrecognized as the infant retains more carbon dioxide in compensation. If the metabolic alkalosis–induced primary increase in the blood pH is ignored, the rise in carbon dioxide inappropriately triggers an increase in the ventilatory support by the unsuspecting physician, causing further lung injury, and the cycle continues. Therefore, it must be remembered that in hypercapnic newborns who are receiving diuretic treatment, a normal or elevated pH always indicates potassium chloride depletion and metabolic alkalosis.

Diuretic-induced hypochloremic metabolic alkalosis is also associated with growth failure and may be a contributing factor of poor outcome in infants with bronchopulmonary dysplasia (Perlman et al, 1986). Growth failure is caused most likely by the decrease in cell proliferation and diminished DNA and protein synthesis in response to intracellular alkalosis (Heinly and Wassner, 1994). Chronic hyponatremia with a negative sodium balance may further hinder appropriate growth in these infants (Sulyok et al, 1985).

Thus, appropriate electrolyte replacement is one of the cornerstones of management of infants with bronchopulmonary dysplasia. Supplementation therapy should be started with potassium chloride administration at the time of the initiation of long-term diuretic treatment. In the majority of cases, 3 to 7 mEq/kg per day potassium chloride is required to maintain serum chloride concentrations greater than 95 mEq/L with normal serum potassium values. The patient's renal function and, at least theoretically, the use of spironolactone may limit the amount of daily potassium chloride supplementation. By stimulating $Na^+,K^+/ATPase$ activity, potassium supplementation also leads to decreases in the intracellular sodium content, whereas extracellular sodium remains regulated by diuretic management. Therefore, preterm infants treated with diuretics and potassium chloride supplementation have a lower total body sodium than those without appropriate potassium supplementation when their serum sodium concentrations are identical. Because total body sodium regulates extracellular volume, these infants may be less prone to retain excessive amounts of interstitial fluids. Sodium supplementation should be adjusted so that serum sodium concentrations remain in the 130 to 135 mEq/L range. If serum sodium concentration can be maintained only by excessive daily sodium supplementation (>5 to 6 mEq/kg/day), a readjustment of the dose or the medications used in diuretic therapy should be considered.

Some previously critically ill, immature preterm newborns may continue to lose excess amounts of bicarbonate secondary to a renal insult during the acute phase of disease associated with a delay in the maturation of proximal tubular functions. In infants with bronchopulmonary dysplasia on diuretic therapy, however, this is seldom a problem.

Calcium and phosphate losses induced by long-term diuretic treatment must also be replaced because these minerals are essential for bone mineralization and normal growth. In the majority of cases, appropriately fortified preterm formulas provide adequate supplementation of these macrominerals as well as that of vitamin D, especially if furosemide is used on an alternate-day dosage schedule or in combination with chlorothiazide.

Shock and Edema

In the uncompensated phase of shock, blood pressure is low, effective circulating blood volume is usually decreased, transcapillary hydrostatic pressure is elevated, and capillary integrity and lymphatic drainage are impaired resulting in edema formation and increased interstitial compliance. The latter further enhances fluid accumulation in the interstitium. The changes in the effective circulating blood volume also trigger the release of antidiuretic hormones, including the catecholamines, renin-angiotensin-aldosterone, and vasopressin, resulting in sodium and free water retention. The specific cause of shock (infection, asphyxia, intraventricular hemorrhage) may independently contribute to the above-described chain of events further compromising fluid and electrolyte balance. In these infants, treatment is directed at normalizing tissue perfusion and oxygen delivery by restoring effective intravascular volume, cardiac output, and renal function with the use of pressor and inotropic support as well as with the judicious use of volume expanders. In shock refractory to the aforementioned management, early initiation of stress-dose steroid treatment may help break the cycle by improving capillary integrity and thus effective circulating blood volume and by potentiating the cardiovascular response to pressors and inotropic agents.

Patent Ductus Arteriosus

Patent ductus arteriosus significantly increases morbidity and mortality, especially in the very-low-birth-weight preterm infant. Several conditions, including hypoxemia, unstable cardiovascular status, acute deterioration, and increases in extracellular volume and ductal prostaglandin synthesis, have been recognized to promote the patency of the ductus arteriosus (Hammerman, 1995) (see Chapter 61). Accordingly, clinical management aimed at preventing the occurrence of ductal patency includes interventions keeping the cardiovascular status and oxygenation stable, restricting fluid intake, and maintaining low levels of local prostaglandin synthesis by indomethacin (Clyman, 1996). Indomethacin administration is indicated mostly during the first 2 weeks of life because ductal sensitivity to prostaglandins rapidly diminishes thereafter (Clyman, 1996).

In the sick preterm infant, indomethacin administration is almost always associated with clinically significant, although mostly transient, renal side effects. If not recognized and treated promptly, however, these untoward renal actions may alter the infant's fluid and electrolyte balance and could potentially decrease the effectiveness of indomethacin treatment. Because of the high levels of vasoconstricting and sodium-retaining and water-retaining hormones in the immediate neonatal period, renal prostaglandin production is increased to counterbalance the renal actions of these hormones (Gleason, 1987). Thus, compared to the renal function of the adult, the neonatal kidney is more dependent on the increased production of vasodilatory and natriuretic prostaglandins, which renders it more sensitive to the actions of indomethacin (Gleason, 1987).

In the indomethacin-treated newborn, the unopposed renal vasoconstriction and sodium and water reabsorption lead to decreases in renal blood flow and glomerular filtration rate and to increases in sodium and free water reabsorption. These side effects occur despite the decreasing left-to-right shunt through the closing ductus. Characteristic clinical findings include increases in serum creatinine levels, oliguria, and hyponatremia. Hyponatremia occurs because the free water retention caused by the unopposed renal actions of high plasma vasopressin levels is out of proportion to the angiotensin-induced and noradrenaline-induced sodium retention. This pattern of renal response is most likely due to the preterm infant's more mature distal tubular function compared to that of the proximal tubule (Lumbers et al, 1988) and results in an expanded but somewhat hypotonic extracellular space. Therefore, treatment must focus on maintaining an appropriately restricted fluid intake and avoiding extra sodium supplementation. As the prostaglandin-inhibitory effects of indomethacin diminish after the last dose, renal prostaglandin production returns to normal, and the retained sodium

and excess free water are rapidly excreted, especially with improvement in cardiovascular status as the ductus closes.

Because furosemide treatment increases prostaglandin production, the drug may be used to attenuate the renal side effects of indomethacin if the intravascular volume is judged to be adequate (Yeh et al, 1982). Because long-term furosemide administration increases the incidence of ductal patency (Green et al, 1983), however, routine and extensive use of the drug may not be prudent in preterm infants treated with indomethacin owing to the theoretical risk of reopening the ductus arteriosus (Seri, 1995). In cases of hemodynamic instability or to avoid the potential impact of furosemide on ductal closure, dopamine infusion may be used to support the cardiovascular status and attenuate the indomethacin-induced oliguria (Cochran et al, 1989; Seri et al, 1984, 1993). The efficacy and clinical significance of these interventions have not yet been systematically evaluated (Fajardo et al, 1992; Seri, 1995).

Growing Premature Infant with Negative Sodium Balance

The 2- to 6-week-old growing preterm newborn without significant chronic lung disease and diuretic treatment may present with hyponatremia (serum sodium concentration 125 to 129 mEq/L) as a result of a relative sodium deficiency (Sulyok et al, 1979, 1985). Despite low total body sodium and high activity of sodium-retaining hormones, these infants continue to lose sodium in the urine mainly because of immaturity of renal function. Although these infants usually are in a positive sodium balance, it is insufficient to keep up with the increased sodium demand of their growth. The treatment of this condition is to provide extra sodium supplementation in the form of sodium chloride (usually 2 to 4 mEq/kg/day) to keep serum sodium values higher than 130 mEq/L.

Surgical Conditions

Surgery has a major impact on metabolism and fluid and electrolyte balance in the newborn. Preterm infants with acute or chronic lung disease are especially sensitive and respond to surgical procedures with significant catabolic responses, increases in capillary permeability with the attendant shift of fluid into the interstitial space, and sodium and free water retention (John et al, 1989). Sodium and free water retention is secondary to the decrease in effective circulating blood volume and the increased plasma levels of sodium-retaining and water-retaining hormones, including catecholamines, renin-angiotensin-aldosterone, and vasopressin. Preoperative management has a significant impact on outcome and should be aimed at maintaining adequate effective circulating blood volume and cardiovascular and renal function. In preterm infants who are receiving or have completed long-term dexamethasone treatment for bronchopulmonary dysplasia, provision of stress doses of steroids should be considered. In the postoperative period, maintenance of the integrity of the cardiovascular system with the judicious use of volume expanders and pressor support, prompt correction of any acute acid-base disorder, meticulous replacement of ongoing surgical and nonsurgical fluid and electrolyte losses, close monitoring, and intense communication between the neonatal and surgical teams are essential to ensure successful outcome. As capillary integrity improves, reabsorption and excretion of the expanded interstitial fluid volume takes place with normalization in the secretion of hormones regulating fluid and electrolyte balance. At this time, the provision of maximized nutritional support becomes essential to restore the anabolic state and growth of the infant.

ACID-BASE BALANCE
Physiology of Acid-Base Balance Regulation

As in adults, newborns must maintain their extracellular pH, or hydrogen ion concentration, within a narrow range. A normal pH is essential for intact functioning of all enzymatic processes and therefore the intact functioning of all organ systems of the body. Newborns are subjected to many stresses that may affect their acid-base balance. In addition, infants, especially when they are premature, are limited in their ability to compensate for acid-base alterations. Therefore, acid-base disturbances are common in the neonatal period. An understanding of the principles of acid-base regulation is essential for proper diagnosis and treatment of these disturbances.

In the healthy human, the normal range of extracellular fluid hydrogen ion concentration is 35 to 45 mEq/L. As pH is defined as the negative logarithm of hydrogen ion concentration ($pH = -\log[H^+]$), these values of hydrogen ion concentration correspond to a pH range of 7.35 to 7.45. Acidosis is a shift downward in pH below 7.35, and alkalosis is a shift upward in pH above 7.45. Alterations in normal pH are resisted by complex physiologic regulatory mechanisms. The main systems that maintain pH include the body's buffer systems, the respiratory system, and the kidneys. Some of these systems respond acutely to sudden alterations in hydrogen ion concentration, whereas others respond more slowly to changes but maintain long-term the overall balance between acid and base production, intake, metabolism, and excretion.

The systems that respond acutely in the physiologic regulation of acid-base balance include the various intracellular and extracellular buffers as well as the lungs. A buffer is a substance that can minimize changes in pH when acid or base is added to the system. The extracellular buffers, which include the bicarbonate-carbonic acid system, phosphates, and plasma proteins, act rapidly to return the extracellular pH toward normal. The intracellular buffers, which include hemoglobin, organic phosphates, and bone apatite, act more slowly, taking several hours to reach maximum capacity.

The most important extracellular buffer is the plasma bicarbonate–carbonic acid buffer system, in which the acid component (carbonic acid [H_2CO_3]) is regulated by the lungs, and the base component (bicarbonate [HCO_3^-]) is regulated by the kidneys. The buffer equation is:

$$H^+ + HCO_3^- \leftrightarrow H_2CO_3 \leftrightarrow H_2O + (CO_2)_d \uparrow$$

At equilibrium, the amount of dissolved carbon dioxide [$(CO_2)_d$] exceeds that of H_2CO_3 by a factor of 800:1; thus, for practical purposes, $(CO_2)_d$ and H_2CO_3 can be treated interchangeably. The fact that CO_2 excretion can be con-

trolled by the respiratory system markedly improves the efficiency of this buffer system at physiologic pH. The enzyme carbonic anhydrase allows rapid interconversion of H_2CO_3 to H_2O and CO_2. If the hydrogen ion (H^+) concentration increases for any reason, hydrogen combines with HCO_3^-, driving the buffer reaction toward increased production of H_2CO_3 and CO_2. CO_2 crosses the blood-brain barrier and stimulates central nervous system chemoreceptors, leading to increased alveolar ventilation and decreased concentration of extracellular CO_2. This respiratory compensation begins within minutes after a pH change and is complete within 12 to 24 hours. A similar compensation occurs in response to decrease in H^+ concentration, with a decreased HCO_3^- concentration leading to decreased alveolar ventilation and increased extracellular CO_2.

The relationship of the two components of the bicarbonate–carbonic acid buffer system to pH is expressed by the Henderson-Hasselbalch equation:

$$pH = pK^+ \log ([HCO_3^-]/[H_2CO_3])$$

Because H_2CO_3 is in equilibrium with the dissolved CO_2 in the plasma, and because the amount of *dissolved* CO_2 depends on the *partial pressure* of CO_2, the equation can be modified as:

$$pH = pK' + \log ([HCO_3^-]/0.03 \times P_{CO_2})$$

Both the original and the modified equations are clinically difficult to use. Therefore, the modified Henderson-Hasselbalch equation can be rewritten as the Henderson equation without logarithms for an easier clinical use:

$$[H^+] = 24 \times (P_{CO_2}/[HCO_3^-])$$

This latter equation clearly points out the clinically most important aspect of acid-base regulation by the bicarbonate–carbonic acid buffer system, that the change in the ratio of P_{CO_2} to HCO_3^- concentration, and not their absolute values, determines the direction of change in H^+ concentration and thus in pH. The status of the carbonic acid–bicarbonate buffer system can be easily monitored by repeated blood gas measurements, making understanding of this buffer system important in clinical care.

The system that responds more slowly in the physiologic regulation of acid-base balance is the renal system. There must be a long-term balance between net acid increase owing to intake and production and net acid decrease owing to excretion and metabolism. Although formula and protein-containing intravenous fluids contain small amounts of preformed acid, most of the daily acid load results from metabolism. Although a large amount of the acid produced is in the form of the *volatile* H_2CO_3 that can be excreted in the lungs, *nonvolatile* or *fixed* acids are also produced, which must be excreted through the kidneys. Nonvolatile acids normally include sulfuric acid produced in the metabolism of the amino acids methionine and cysteine as well as smaller contributions from phosphoric acid, lactic acid, hydrochloric acid, and incompletely oxidized organic acids. In addition to excretion of nonvolatile acids, however, the kidneys play a role in long-term acid-base regulation by controlling renal HCO_3^- excretion.

Two regions of the kidney act to achieve urinary acidification, the proximal tubule and the collecting tubule. The proximal tubule acidifies the urine by two mechanisms.

The first mechanism is the reabsorption of any HCO_3^- already present in the blood that is being constantly filtered through the glomeruli. The proximal tubule reabsorbs 60% to 80% of all filtered HCO_3^- and performs this role by an exchange of Na^+ for H^+ across the luminal membrane of the proximal tubular cells via the Na^+/H^+ exchanger. The excreted H^+ combines with filtered HCO_3^-, producing H_2CO_3 by the activity of carbonic anhydrase in the cellular brush border. The H_2CO_3 is then quickly converted to CO_2, which crosses into the tubular cell, where HCO_3^- is regenerated and reabsorbed back into the bloodstream, probably in exchange for chloride (Cl^-). The regenerated H^+ ion re-enters the cycle at the Na^+/H^+ exchanger.

The second mechanism by which the proximal tubule acidifies urine is by the production of ammonia (NH_3). Inside the tubular cell, NH_3 is produced by the deamination of glutamine. The NH_3 is secreted into the tubular lumen, where it combines with and "traps" free H^+ to form ammonium (NH_4^+).

The remaining urinary acidification occurs mostly in the collecting tubule. H^+ secretion in this region of the kidney is sufficient to combine with or *titrate* any remaining filtered HCO_3^- or any filtered anions, such as phosphate and sulfate. Hydrogenated phosphate and sulfate anions produce the *titratable acid* of the urine. The collecting tubule also takes up NH_3 from the medullary interstitium and secretes it into the urine, where again it can combine with and trap H^+ as NH_4^+. This urinary NH_4^+ can act as a cation and be excreted with urinary anions such as Cl^-, PO_4^-, and SO_4^-, thereby preventing loss of cations such as Na^+, Ca^{++}, and K^+. Total acid secretion in the kidney can be represented by:

$$\text{titratable acid} + NH_4^+ - HCO_3^-$$

and under normal conditions should equal the net production of acid from diet and metabolism that is not excreted in the form of CO_2 through the lungs.

In adults, the steady state for renal compensation for respiratory alkalosis is reached within 1 to 2 days and for respiratory acidosis within 3 to 5 days. Newborns are able to compensate for acidemia through the above-described renal mechanisms, although renal response to acid loads is limited, especially in premature infants under 34 weeks' gestation. Reabsorption of HCO_3^- in the proximal tubule and distal tubular acidification are also decreased, with a fairly rapid gestational age–dependent maturation of these functions postnatally (Jones and Chesney, 1992) (see Chapter 91).

To accomplish the tight regulation of pH necessary for survival, H^+ generated in the form of the volatile acid, H_2CO_3 are excreted by the lungs as CO_2. H^+ generated in the form of nonvolatile acids are buffered rapidly by extracellular HCO_3^- and more slowly by intracellular buffers. HCO_3^- is then replenished by the kidneys via the reabsorption of much of the filtered HCO_3^- and by the excretion of H^+ in the urine as NH_4^+ and titratable acids.

Disturbances of Acid-Base Balance in the Newborn
General Principles

The carbonic acid–bicarbonate buffer system is the reference base for acid-base equilibrium, and the status of this system can be monitored by blood gas measurements. Therefore, the blood gas should be the starting point for the evaluation of any acid-base disorder. In the blood gas measurement, the pH and $PaCO_2$ are directly measured, and from these the HCO_3^- is calculated.

The whole blood buffer base, defined as the conjugate sum of the HCO_3^- and non-HCO_3^- buffer systems, is the other important blood gas value used in evaluating acid-base disturbances. The difference between the observed whole-blood buffer base of any blood gas sample and the expected normal buffer base of that sample is called the *base excess* or *deficit*. The base excess and deficit give an accurate measure of the amount of strong base and acid, respectively, that have been added to the extracellular fluid. For example, a base excess of 10 mEq/L indicates the addition of 10 mEq of base per liter (or loss of 10 mEq of H^+ per liter). A base deficit of 10 mEq/L indicates addition of a similar amount of strong acid (or loss of base).

Acid-base disorders are classified according to their cause as being either *metabolic* or *respiratory*. *Metabolic acidosis* occurs as a result of accumulation of increased amounts of nonvolatile acid or decreased amounts of HCO_3^- in the extracellular fluid. *Metabolic alkalosis* occurs as a result of increased HCO_3^- amounts in the extracellular fluid. *Respiratory acidosis* is due to hypoventilation and decreased excretion of volatile acid (CO_2), whereas *respiratory alkalosis* is due to hyperventilation and increased excretion of volatile acid (CO_2).

Acid-base disorders are also classified according to the number of causes giving rise to the disorder. When only one primary acid-base abnormality and its compensatory mechanisms occur, the disorder is classified as a *simple acid-base disorder*. When a combination of simple acid-base disturbances occurs, the patient has a *mixed acid-base disorder*. Because secondary physiologic regulatory mechanisms ameliorate the alteration in pH caused by primary disturbances, it sometimes is difficult to differentiate simple from mixed disorders or even a simple disorder from its resulting compensation. One important principle that allows determination of primary acid-base disturbance is that the compensatory regulatory mechanisms do not completely normalize the pH. Nomograms, such as the one in Figure 34–5, can help in the diagnosis of the primary disturbance. The nomogram describes the 95% confidence limits of the expected compensatory response to a primary abnormality in either $PaCO_2$ or HCO_3^-. Table 34–2 summarizes the expected respiratory and metabolic compensation for primary acid-base disorders (Brewer, 1990). If the compensation in a given patient differs from that predicted in Figure 34–5 or Table 34–2, the patient either has not had enough time to compensate for a simple acid-base disturbance or has a mixed acid-base disorder. Furthermore, the complete correction of an acid-base disturbance occurs only when the underlying process responsible for the abnormality has been effectively treated.

The analysis of the blood gas values must be considered in light of the patient's history and physical findings and with an understanding of expected compensatory responses to identify the primary disturbance. Further laboratory evaluation is indicated if the problem is not immediately obvious or if the response to therapy is not as expected. The evaluation of the acid-base disturbance should always

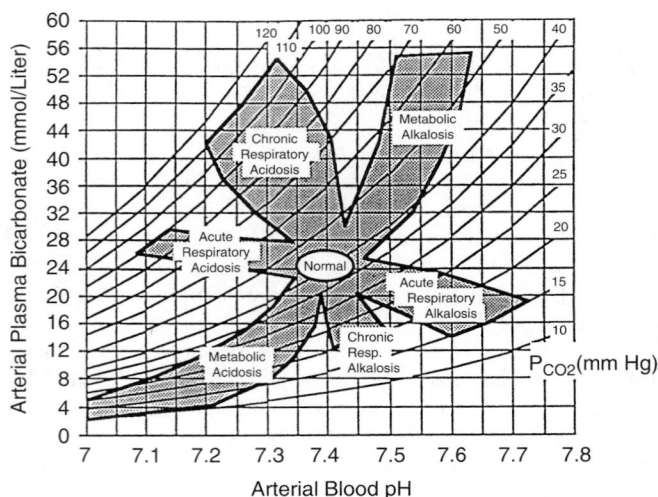

FIGURE 34–5. Acid-base diagram illustrating the 95% confidence limits for compensatory responses to primary acid-base disorders. (From Cogan MG, Rector FC Jr: Acid-base disorders. *In* Brenner BM, Rector FC Jr [Eds]: The Kidney. Philadelphia, WB Saunders, 1986.)

involve efforts to determine the underlying cause of the disturbance because adequate treatment requires correction of the underlying disorder, if possible.

Metabolic Acidosis

Metabolic acidosis is a common problem, particularly in the critically ill newborn. Metabolic acidosis occurs when the fall in pH is caused by the accumulation of acid other than H_2CO_3 by the extracellular fluid resulting in loss of available HCO_3^- or by the direct loss of HCO_3^- from body fluids. Cases of metabolic acidosis are divided into those with an *elevated anion gap* and those with a *normal anion gap*.

The anion gap reflects the unaccounted for acidic anions and certain cations in the extracellular fluid. The unmeasured anions normally include the serum proteins, phosphates, sulfates, and organic acids, whereas the unac-

counted for cations are the serum potassium, calcium, and magnesium. Thus, in clinical practice, the anion gap is estimated using the following formula:

$$\text{Anion gap} = [\text{Na}^+]_{serum} - ([\text{Cl}^-]_{serum} + [\text{HCO}_3^-]_{serum})$$

The normal range of the serum anion gap in newborns is 8 to 16 mEq/L, with slightly higher values in very premature newborns. Accumulation of strong acids owing to increased intake or production or to decreased excretion results in an increased anion gap acidosis, whereas loss of HCO_3^- or accumulation of H^+ results in a normal anion gap acidosis. A decrease in serum potassium, calcium, and magnesium concentrations; an increase in serum protein concentration; or a falsely elevated serum sodium concentration may also result in an increased anion gap in the absence of metabolic acidosis.

An increased anion gap metabolic acidosis in the newborn is most frequently due to lactic acidosis secondary to tissue hypoxia as seen in asphyxia, hypothermia, severe respiratory distress, sepsis, and many other severe neonatal illnesses. Other important, but much less frequent causes of an increased anion gap metabolic acidosis in the neonatal period are outlined in Table 34–3 and include inborn errors of metabolism, renal failure, and intake of toxins. Table 34–4 lists inborn errors of metabolism that can present with increased anion gap metabolic acidosis in the newborn period.

The syndrome of late metabolic acidosis of prematurity was first described in the 1960s, in which otherwise healthy premature infants at several weeks of age developed mild to moderate increased anion gap acidosis and decreased growth. All the infants were receiving high-protein cow's milk formula, and they demonstrated increased net acid excretion compared to controls. This type of late metabolic acidosis is now rarely seen, probably because of the use of special premature formulas and changes in regular formulas with decreased casein:whey ratios and lower fixed acid loads.

A normal anion gap metabolic acidosis most frequently occurs in the newborn as a result of HCO_3^- loss from the extracellular space through the kidneys or the gastrointestinal tract. Hyperchloremia develops with the HCO_3^- loss because a proportionate increase in serum chloride concen-

TABLE 34–2

Expected Compensatory Mechanisms Operating in Primary Acid-Base Disorders

Acid-Base Disorder	Primary Event	Compensation	Rate of Compensation
Metabolic acidosis			
Normal anion gap	↓ [HCO₃⁻]	↓ PCO₂	For 1 mEq/L ↓ [HCO₃⁻], PCO₂ ↓ by 1–1.5 mm Hg
Increased anion gap	↑ Acid production ↑ Acid intake	↓ PCO₂	For 1 mEq/L ↓ [HCO₃⁻], PCO₂ ↓ by 1–1.5 mm Hg
Metabolic alkalosis	↑ [HCO₃⁻]	↑ PCO₂	For 1 mEq/L ↑ [HCO₃⁻], PCO₂ ↑ by 0.5–1 mm Hg
Respiratory acidosis			
Acute (<12–24 h)	↑ PCO₂	↑ [HCO₃⁻]	For 10 mm Hg ↑ PCO₂, [HCO₃⁻] ↑ by 1 mEq/L
Chronic (3–5 d)	↑ PCO₂	↑↑ [HCO₃⁻]	For 10 mm Hg ↑ PCO₂, [HCO₃⁻] ↑ by 4 mEq/L
Respiratory alkalosis			
Acute (<12 h)	↓ PCO₂	↓ [HCO₃⁻]	For 10 mm Hg ↓ PCO₂, [HCO₃⁻] ↓ by 1–3 mEq/L
Chronic (1–2 d)	↓ PCO₂	↓↓ [HCO₃⁻]	For 10 mm Hg ↓ PCO₂, [HCO₃⁻] ↓ by 2–5 mEq/L

Modified from Brewer ED: Disorders of acid-base balance. Pediatr Clin North Am 37:430, 1990.

TABLE 34–3

Common Causes of Metabolic Acidosis

Increased Anion Gap	Normal Anion Gap
Lactic acidosis due to tissue hypoxia + Asphyxia, hypothermia, shock + Sepsis, respiratory distress syndrome Inborn errors of metabolism + Congenital lactic acidosis + Organic acidosis Renal failure Late metabolic acidosis Toxins (e.g., benzyl alcohol)	Renal bicarbonate loss + Bicarbonate wasting owing to immaturity + Renal tubular acidosis + Carbonic anhydrase inhibitors Gastrointestinal bicarbonate loss + Small bowel drainage: ileostomy, fistula + Diarrhea Extracellular volume expansion with bicarbonate dilution Aldosterone deficiency Excessive chloride in intravenous fluids

tration must occur to maintain the ionic balance and/or to correct the volume depletion in the extracellular compartment. The most common cause of normal anion gap metabolic acidosis in the preterm newborn is a mild, developmentally regulated, proximal renal tubular acidosis with renal HCO_3^- wasting. In these infants, the serum HCO_3^- usually stabilizes at 14 to 18 mEq/L in the early postnatal period. The urinary pH is normal once the serum HCO_3^- falls to this level because the impairment in proximal tubular HCO_3^- reabsorption is not associated with an impaired distal tubular acidification of similar magnitude (Jones and Chesney, 1992). The diagnosis of this temporary cause of acidosis can be established by the recurrence of a urinary alkaline pH when serum HCO_3^- is raised above the threshold after HCO_3^- or acetate supplementation. Even term newborns have a lower renal threshold for HCO_3^-, with normal plasma HCO_3^- levels in the range of 17 to 21 mEq/L. In most infants, plasma HCO_3^- increases to adult levels over the first year as the proximal tubule matures. Other common causes of normal anion gap metabolic acidosis seen in neonatal intensive care units include gastrointestinal HCO_3^- losses often owing to increased ileostomy drainage, diuretic treatment with carbonic anhydrase inhibitors, and dilutional acidosis with rapid expansion of the extracellular space using non-HCO_3^- solutions in the hypovolemic newborn (see Table 34–3).

TABLE 34–4

Inborn Errors of Metabolism Associated with Metabolic Acidosis

Primary lactic acidosis
Organic acidemias
Pyruvate carboxylase deficiency
Pyruvate dehydrogenase deficiency
Galactosemia
Hereditary fructose intolerance
Type I glycogen storage disease

The presence of metabolic acidosis in the newborn should be suspected from the clinical presentation and the history of predisposing conditions, including perinatal depression, respiratory distress, blood or volume loss, sepsis, and congenital heart disease associated with poor systemic perfusion or cyanosis. Metabolic acidosis is confirmed by blood gas measurements. The cause of metabolic acidosis is often readily discernible from the history and physical examination; specific laboratory evaluation of electrolytes, renal function, lactate, and serum and urine amino acids may be undertaken, depending on the diagnosis clinically suspected. Figure 34–6 is a simple flow diagram outlining an approach to diagnosis.

The morbidity and mortality of metabolic acidosis depend on the severity of the acidosis and the responsiveness of the underlying pathologic process to clinical management. Because experimental data suggest that even a very low pH is compatible with neurologically intact survival (von Planta et al, 1993), and because a clear benefit of buffer therapy in the management of metabolic acidosis has not been demonstrated (Basir et al, 1996; Brewer, 1990; Nudel et al, 1993), indications for the use of buffers in newborns remain uncertain. At present, the judicious use of temporizing buffer therapy aimed at increasing the arterial pH to 7.25 to 7.30 in cases of severe acidosis is recommended and practiced by most neonatologists to avoid the complications of acidosis per se (Brewer, 1990; von Planta et al, 1993), which include arteriolar vasoconstriction followed by dilation, depression of cardiac contractility, systemic hypotension, pulmonary edema, and arrhythmias. This practice is supported by findings on the cardiovascular effects of sodium bicarbonate in preterm newborns with an arterial pH of less than 7.25 and term newborns with an arterial pH of less than 7.30 (Fanconi et al, 1993). The use of sodium bicarbonate in this study induced an increase in myocardial contractility and a reduction in afterload.

Sodium bicarbonate is the most widely used buffer in the treatment of metabolic acidosis in the neonatal period (see also Chapter 30). Bicarbonate should not be given if ventilation is inadequate because its administration results in an increase in $PaCO_2$ with no improvement in pH. There-

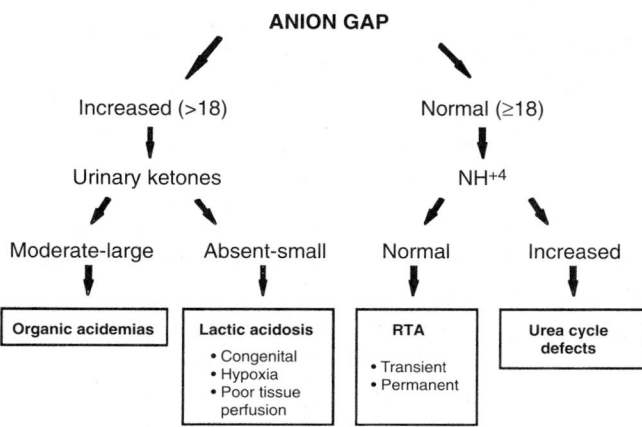

FIGURE 34–6. Flow diagram outlining a diagnostic approach in cases of increased anion gap and normal anion gap metabolic acidosis in the newborn. RTA, renal tubular acidosis.

fore, sodium bicarbonate should be administered slowly and in its diluted form only to newborns with documented metabolic acidosis and adequate alveolar ventilation. Once a blood gas measurement has been obtained, the dose of sodium bicarbonate required to correct the pH can be estimated using the following formula:

$$\text{Dose of NaHCO}_3 \text{ (mEq)} = \text{base deficit (mEq/L)} \times \text{body weight (kg)} \times 0.3$$

Sodium bicarbonate is confined mostly to the extracellular fluid compartment, and the 0.3 value in the formula represents its volume of distribution. Most clinicians would use half of the calculated total correction dose for initial therapy to avoid overcorrection of metabolic acidosis. Subsequent doses of sodium bicarbonate are then based on the results of repeated blood gas measurements.

In certain clinical situations, tromethamine (Tham) may be used as an alternative buffer to sodium bicarbonate. The theoretical advantages of tromethamine over sodium bicarbonate in the treatment of metabolic acidosis of the newborn include its more rapid intracellular buffering capability, its ability to lower $PaCO_2$ levels directly, and the lack of an increase in the sodium load (Schneiderman et al, 1993). Tromethamine lowers $PaCO_2$ by directly reacting with plasma CO_2, resulting in formation of cations and one HCO_3^- ion per one molecule of tromethamine. Because the cations are excreted by the kidneys, oliguria is a contraindication to the repeated use of this buffer. Tromethamine administration also has been associated with the development of acute respiratory depression, most likely secondary to an abrupt decrease in $PaCO_2$ levels as well as from rapid intracellular correction of acidosis in the cells of the respiratory center (Robertson, 1970). Furthermore, especially when large doses of tromethamine are administered, dilutional hyponatremia, hypoglycemia, hyperkalemia, an increase in hemoglobin oxygen affinity, and diuresis followed by oliguria may occur. Because the solution is hyperosmolal, and because rapid infusion of tromethamine may also lower blood pressure and intracranial pressure (Duthie et al, 1994), slow infusion rates are recommended.

Despite these disadvantages, tromethamine has a major advantage over sodium bicarbonate in that it acts to increase pH by lowering $PaCO_2$. Therefore, *tromethamine is the recommended buffer therapy in life-threatening situations of combined metabolic and respiratory acidosis.* Some centers also use tromethamine as initial therapy for neonatal resuscitation until adequate ventilation is documented by blood gas measurements. The suggested initial dose is 1 to 2 mEq/kg or 3.5 to 6 mL/kg intravenously using the 0.3 M solution, with the rate of administration not exceeding 1 mL/kg per minute. Once a blood gas measurement has been obtained, the dose of tromethamine required to increase the pH can be estimated using the following formula:

$$\text{Dose of tromethamine in mL} = \text{base deficit (mEq/L)} \times \text{body weight (kg)}$$

A third buffer, dichloroacetate, has been successfully used in critically ill adults as an alternative to sodium bicarbonate or tromethamine. Dichloroacetate enhances cardiac output and increases oxidation of pyruvate and lactate by the stimulation of pyruvate dehydrogenase activity (Brewer, 1990). Because there is only limited experimental information available regarding its effectiveness in the newborn period, however, its use cannot be recommended at this time (Nudel et al, 1993).

Regardless of the buffer used, care should be taken not to overtreat, to minimize adverse effects of the buffer itself and of rapid swings in pH. In most conditions, correcting the pH to 7.25 to 7.30 is adequate. In addition, the recommendations for buffer treatment in metabolic acidosis, although widely practiced, are largely empiric without the backing of substantial experimental evidence.

Finally, during the correction of metabolic acidosis, particular attention should be paid to ensure an appropriate potassium balance. Because potassium moves from the intracellular space to the extracellular space in exchange for H^+ when acidosis occurs, the presence of a total body potassium deficit may not be appreciated during metabolic acidosis. Hypokalemia may become evident only as the pH increases and potassium returns to the intracellular space. Furthermore, the acidosis cannot be completely corrected until the potassium stores are restored. Therefore, close monitoring of serum electrolytes and, if necessary, potassium supplementation are important during the correction of metabolic acidosis in the sick newborn.

Respiratory Acidosis

Respiratory acidosis occurs when a primary increase in $PaCO_2$ develops secondary to impairments in alveolar ventilation resulting in an arterial pH of less than 7.35. Primary respiratory acidosis is a common problem in the newborn, and causes include hyaline membrane disease, pneumonia owing to infection or aspiration, patent ductus arteriosus with pulmonary edema, bronchopulmonary dysplasia, pleural effusion, pneumothorax, and pulmonary hypoplasia. The initial increase in $PaCO_2$ is buffered by the non-HCO_3^- intracellular buffers without noticeable renal compensation for at least 12 to 24 hours (see Table 34–2). Renal metabolic compensation reaches its maximum levels within 3 to 5 days, and its effectiveness in the newborn is influenced mainly by the functional maturity of proximal tubular HCO_3^- transport.

Management of respiratory acidosis is directed toward improving alveolar ventilation and treating the underlying disorder. In the sick newborn, adequate ventilation often must be provided by mechanical ventilation. In severe respiratory acidosis, tromethamine, because it lowers CO_2, may be used to raise pH. Tromethamine, however, produces only a transient decrease in $PaCO_2$, and toxic doses would quickly be reached if it were used to buffer all the CO_2 produced by metabolism over any sustained period of time. Therefore, tromethamine should be used only as a temporizing measure in severe respiratory acidosis until alveolar ventilation can be improved. More detailed management of respiratory disorders is reviewed in Chapters 50 and 51.

Metabolic Alkalosis

Metabolic alkalosis is characterized by a primary increase in the extracellular HCO_3^- concentration sufficient to raise the arterial pH above 7.45. In the newborn, metabolic alkalosis occurs when there is a loss of H^+, a gain of HCO_3^-, or a depletion of the extracellular volume with the loss of more chloride than HCO_3^-. It is important to understand that metabolic alkalosis generated by any of these mechanisms can be maintained only when factors limiting the renal excretion of HCO_3^- are also present.

Metabolic alkalosis can result from a *loss of H^+* from the body, either from the gastrointestinal tract or the kidneys, which induces an equivalent rise in the extracellular HCO_3^- concentration. The most common causes of this type of metabolic alkalosis in the newborn period are continuous nasogastric aspiration, persistent vomiting, and diuretic treatment. Less frequent causes of H^+ losses include congenital chloride-wasting diarrhea, certain forms of congenital adrenal hyperplasia, hyperaldosteronism, posthypercapnia, and Bartter syndrome.

Metabolic alkalosis can also result from a *gain of HCO_3^-*, such as occurs during the administration of buffer solutions to the newborn. In certain situations, the creation of a metabolic alkalosis is intentional, for example, in the use of sodium bicarbonate or tromethamine to raise pH and thus to decrease pulmonary vasoreactivity in infants with persistent pulmonary hypertension. At other times, however, iatrogenically produced metabolic alkalosis is unintentional and due to chronic excessive administration of HCO_3^-, lactate, citrate, or acetate in intravenous fluids. Because excretion of HCO_3^- is normally not limited in the newborn, metabolic alkalosis resulting from HCO_3^- gain alone should rapidly resolve following the discontinuation of HCO_3^- administration.

Metabolic alkalosis can also result from a *loss of extracellular fluid* containing disproportionally more chloride than HCO_3^-, so-called contraction alkalosis. During the diuretic phase of normal postnatal adaptation, preterm and term newborns retain relatively more HCO_3^- than chloride (Ramiro-Tolentino et al, 1996). The obvious clinical benefits of allowing this physiologic extracellular volume contraction to occur, especially in the critically ill newborn, clearly outweigh the clinical importance of a mild contraction alkalosis developing after recovery. No specific treatment is needed in such cases because with the stabilization of the extracellular volume and renal function after recovery, acid-base balance rapidly returns to normal. Contraction alkalosis due to other causes, however, may require treatment as discussed subsequently.

For metabolic alkalosis to persist, *factors limiting the renal excretion of HCO_3^-* must be present. The kidneys are usually effective in excreting excess HCO_3^-, but this ability can be limited under certain conditions, including a decreased glomerular filtration rate, an increased aldosterone production, and the more common clinical situation of volume contraction–triggered metabolic alkalosis with potassium deficiency. In the last-mentioned condition, there is a direct stimulation of Na^+ reabsorption coupled to H^+ loss in the proximal tubule, and an indirect stimulation of H^+ loss in the distal nephron by the increased activity of the renin-angiotensin-aldosterone system. Contraction alkalosis responds to saline administration to replete the intravascular volume and potassium supplementation. In the other disorders, however, the primary problem of reduced glomerular filtration rate or elevated aldosterone must be treated for the alkalosis to resolve.

One of the most frequently encountered clinical scenarios of chronic metabolic alkalosis actually occurs most often in the form of a mixed acid-base disorder in preterm newborns with bronchopulmonary dysplasia on long-term diuretic treatment. These newborns initially have a chronic respiratory acidosis that is partially compensated by renal HCO_3^- retention. Prolonged or aggressive diuretic use can lead to total-body potassium depletion and contraction of the extracellular volume, thus exacerbating the metabolic alkalosis. By stimulating proximal tubular Na^+ reabsorption and thus H^+ loss, distal tubular H^+ secretion, and renal ammonium production, the diuretic-induced hypokalemia contributes to the severity and maintenance of the metabolic alkalosis in these newborns. Furthermore, metabolic alkalosis per se worsens hypokalemia because potassium replaces intracellular hydrogen as the latter shifts into the extracellular space. Although serum potassium may be decreased, the serum levels in these newborns do not accurately reflect the degree of total-body potassium deficit because potassium is primarily an intracellular ion. In addition, the condition is often accompanied by marked hypochloremia and hyponatremia. Hyponatremia occurs in part because sodium shifts into the intracellular space to compensate for the depleted intracellular potassium. If the alkalosis is severe, alkalemia (pH >7.45) can supervene and result in hypoventilation. In this situation, potassium chloride and not sodium chloride supplementation reverses hyponatremia and hypochloremia, corrects hypokalemia and metabolic alkalosis, and increases the effectiveness of diuretic therapy. Because chloride deficiency is the predominant cause for the increased pH, ammonium chloride or arginine chloride also corrects the alkalosis. Because these agents do not affect the other electrolyte imbalances, they should not be used as the only therapy.

It is important to keep ahead of the potassium losses in infants on long-term diuretics, rather than attempt to replace potassium after intracellular depletion has occurred. Because the rate of potassium repletion is limited by the rate at which potassium moves intracellularly, correction of total body potassium deficits can take days to weeks. In addition, there is also a risk of acute hyperkalemia if serum potassium levels are driven too high during repletion, particularly in newborns in whom an acute respiratory deterioration may occur, with worsened respiratory acidosis and the subsequent movement of potassium from the intracellular to the extracellular space. The routine use of potassium chloride supplementation and close monitoring of serum sodium, chloride, and potassium are therefore recommended during long-term diuretic therapy to prevent these common iatrogenic problems (see the section on bronchopulmonary dysplasia in this chapter and also Chapter 55).

Respiratory Alkalosis

When a primary decrease in $Paco_2$ results in an increase in the arterial pH beyond 7.45, respiratory alkalosis develops. The initial hypocapnia is acutely titrated by the intracellular buffers, and metabolic compensation by the kidneys returns pH toward normal within 1 to 2 days (see Table 34–2). Interestingly, this is the only simple acid-base disorder in which, at least in the adult, the pH may completely be normalized by the compensatory mechanisms (Brewer, 1990). The cause of respiratory alkalosis is hyperventilation, which in the spontaneously breathing newborn is most often caused by fever, sepsis, retained fetal lung fluid, mild aspiration pneumonia, or central nervous system disorders. In the neonatal intensive care unit, the most frequent cause of respiratory alkalosis is increased alveolar ventilation secondary to hyperventilation of the intubated newborn. Because findings suggest an association between hypocapnia and the development of periventricular leukomalacia (Wiswell et al, 1996) and bronchopulmonary dysplasia (Garland et al, 1995) in ventilated preterm infants, avoidance of hyperventilation during resuscitation and mechanical ventilation appears to be of utmost importance in the management of the sick preterm newborn. The treatment of neonatal respiratory alkalosis consists of the specific management of the underlying process causing hyperventilation.

REFERENCES

Abman SH, Groothius JR: Pathophysiology and treatment of bronchopulmonary dysplasia: Current issues. Pediatr Clin North Am 41:277, 1994.

Albersheim SG, Solimano AJ, Sharma AK, et al: Randomized, double-blind, controlled trial of long-term diuretic therapy for bronchopulmonary dysplasia. J Pediatr 115:615, 1989.

Aszterbaum M, Feingold KR, Menon GK, Williams ML: Glucocorticoids accelerate fetal maturation of the epidermal permeability barrier in the rat. J Clin Invest 91:2703, 1993.

Atkinson SA, Shah JK, McGee C, et al: Mineral excretion in premature infants receiving various diuretic therapies. J Pediatr 113:540, 1988.

Bailie MD: Development of the endocrine function of the kidney. Clin Perinatol 19:59, 1992.

Ballard PL, Ballard RA: Scientific basis and therapeutic regimens for use of antenatal glucocorticoids. Am J Obstet Gynecol 173:254, 1995.

Basir MA, Bhatia J, Brudno DS, et al: Effects of Carbicarb and sodium bicarbonate on hypoxic lactic acidosis in newborn pigs. J Invest Med 44:70, 1996.

Baylen BG, Ogata H, Ikegami M, et al: Left ventricular performance and contractility before and after volume infusion: A comparative study in preterm and full-term newborns. Circulation 73:1042, 1986.

Bell EF: High-volume fluid intake predisposes premature infants to necrotizing enterocolitis. Lancet 2:90, 1979.

Bell EF, Warburton D, Stonestreet BS, Oh W: Effect of fluid administration on the development of symptomatic patent ductus arteriosus and congestive heart failure in premature infants. N Engl J Med 302:598, 1980.

Brace RA: Fluid distribution in the fetus and newborn. In Polin RA, Fox WW (Eds): Fetal and Neonatal Physiology. Philadelphia, WB Saunders, 1992, pp 1288–1298.

Brewer ED: Disorders of acid-base balance. Pediatr Clin North Am 37:430, 1990.

Carlton DP, Cho SC, Davis P, et al: Surfactant treatment at birth reduces lung vascular injury and edema in preterm lambs. Pediatr Res 37:265, 1995.

Cartridge-Patrick HT, Rutter N: Skin barrier function. In Polin RA, Fox WW (Eds): Fetal and Neonatal Physiology. Philadelphia, WB Saunders, 1992, pp 569–585.

Cheek DB, Wishart J, MacLennan AH, et al: Hydration in the first 24 hours of postnatal life in normal infants born vaginally or by caesarean section. Early Hum Dev 7:323, 1982.

Christensen G: Cardiovascular and renal effects of atrial natriuretic factor. Scand J Clin Lab Invest 53:203, 1993.

Clyman RI: Recommendations for the postnatal use of indomethacin: An analysis of four separate treatment strategies. J Pediatr 128:601, 1996.

Cochran J, Reddy R, Devaskar U: Effect of indomethacin vs indomethacin + dopamine on serum BUN and creatinine, urinary output and the closure of patent ductus arteriosus in preterm newborns with hyaline membrane disease. Pediatr Res 25:211A, 1989.

Cogan MG, Rector FC Jr: Acid-base disorders. In Brenner BM, Rector FC Jr (Eds): The Kidney. Philadelphia, WB Saunders, 1986, p 473.

Costarino AT, Baumgart S: Neonatal water metabolism. In Cowett RM (Ed): Principles of Perinatal/Neonatal Metabolism. New York, Springer Verlag, 1991, pp 623–649.

Costarino AT, Gruskay JA, Corcoran L, et al: Sodium restriction versus daily maintenance replacement in very low birth weight premature newborns: A randomized, blind therapeutic trial. J Pediatr 120:99, 1992.

Coulter DM: Prolactin: A hormonal regulator of the neonatal tissue water reservoir. Pediatr Res 17:665, 1983.

de Zegher F, Van den Berghe G, Devlieger H, et al: Dopamine inhibits growth hormone and prolactin secretion in the human newborn. Pediatr Res 34:642, 1993.

Duthie SE, Goulin GD, Zornow MH, et al: Effects of THAM and sodium bicarbonate on intracranial pressure and mean arterial pressure in an animal model of focal cerebral injury. J Neurosurg Anesthesiol 6:201, 1994.

El-Dahr SS, Chevalier RL: Special needs of the newborn infant in fluid therapy. Pediatr Clin North Am 37:323, 1990.

Elliot S, Goldsmith P, Knepper M, et al: Urinary excretion of aquaporin-2 in humans: A potential marker of collecting duct responsiveness to vasopressin. J Am Soc Nephrol 7:403, 1996.

Fajardo CA, Whyte RK, Steele BT: Effect of dopamine on failure of indomethacin to close the patent ductus arteriosus. J Pediatr 121:771, 1992.

Fanconi S, Burger R, Ghelfi D, et al: Hemodynamic effects of sodium bicarbonate in critically ill newborns. Intens Care Med 19:65, 1993.

Friis-Hansen B: Body water compartments in children: Changes during growth and related changes in body composition. Pediatrics 28:169, 1961.

Friis-Hansen B: Water distribution in the foetus and newborn infant. Acta Paediatr Scand 305(suppl):7, 1983.

Garland JS, Buck RK, Allred EN, et al: Hypocarbia before surfactant therapy appears to increase bronchopulmonary dysplasia risk in infants with respiratory distress syndrome. Arch Pediatr Adolesc Med 149:617, 1995.

Gleason CA: Prostaglandins and the developing kidney. Semin Perinatol 11:12, 1987.

Gold PS, Brace RA: Fetal whole-body permeability-surface area product and reflection coefficient for plasma proteins. Microvasc Res 36:262, 1988.

Green TP, Thompson TR, Johnson D, et al: Furosemide promotes patent ductus arteriosus in premature infants with the respiratory distress syndrome. N Engl J Med 308:743, 1983.

Green TP, Johnson DE, Bass JL, et al: Prophylactic furosemide in severe respiratory distress syndrome: Blinded prospective study. J Pediatr 112:605, 1988.

Hammarlund K, Sedin G, Strömberg B: Transepidermal water loss in newborn infants: VIII. Relation to gestational age and post-natal age in appropriate and small for gestational age infants. Acta Paediatr Scand 72:721, 1983.

Hammerman C: Patent ductus arteriosus: Clinical relevance of prostaglandins and prostaglandin inhibitors in PDA pathophysiology and treatment. Clin Perinatol 22:457, 1995.

Heijden AJ, Provoost AP, Nauta J, et al: Renal functional impairment in preterm newborns related to intrauterine indomethacin exposure. Pediatr Res 24:644, 1988.

Heinly MM, Wassner SJ: The effect of isolated chloride depletion on growth and protein turnover in young rats. Pediatr Nephrol 8:555, 1994.

Ishisaka DY: Exogenous surfactant use in newborns. Ann Pharmacother 30:389, 1996.

Iwamoto HS: Endocrine regulation of the fetal circulation. In Polin RA, Fox WW (Eds): Fetal and Neonatal Physiology. Philadelphia, WB Saunders, 1992, pp 646–655.

Jefferies AL, Coates G, O'Brodovich H: Pulmonary epithelial permeability in hyaline membrane disease. N Engl J Med 31:1075, 1984.

John E, Klavdianou M, Vidyasagar D: Electrolyte problems in neonatal surgical patients. Clin Perinatol 16:219, 1989.

Jones DP, Chesney RW: Development of tubular function. Clin Perinatol 19:33, 1992.

Kaapa P, Seppanen M, Kero P, et al: Pulmonary hemodynamics after synthetic surfactant replacement in neonatal respiratory distress syndrome. J Pediatr 123:115, 1993.

Kao LC, Durand DJ, McCrea RC, et al: Randomized trial of long-term diuretic therapy for infants with oxygen-dependent bronchopulmonary dysplasia. J Pediatr 124:772, 1994.

Kari MA, Hallman M, Eronen M, et al: Prenatal dexamethasone treatment in conjunction with rescue therapy of human surfactant: A randomized placebo-controlled multicenter study. Pediatrics 93:730, 1994.

Kurzner SI, Garg M, Bautista DB, et al: Growth failure in bronchopulmonary dysplasia: Elevated metabolic rates and pulmonary mechanics. J Pediatr 112:73, 1988.

Leake RD: Fetal and neonatal neurohypophyseal hormones. In Polin RA, Fox WW (Eds): Fetal and Neonatal Physiology. Philadelphia, WB Saunders, 1992, pp 1815–1819.

Linderkamp O: Placental transfusion: Determinants and effects. Clin Perinatol 9:559, 1982.

Lou HC, Skov H, Pedersen H: Low cerebral blood flow: A risk factor in the newborn. J Pediatr 95:606, 1979.

Lumbers ER, Hill KJ, Bennett VJ: Proximal and distal tubular activity in chronically catheterized fetal sheep compared with the adult. Can J Physiol Pharmacol 66:697, 1988.

Mahony L: Development of myocardial structure and function. In Emmanouilides GC, Riemenschneider TA, Allen HD, Gutgesell HP (Eds): Heart Disease in Infants, Children, and Adolescents Including the Fetus and the Young Adult. Baltimore, Williams & Wilkins, 1995, pp 17–28.

Needleman P, Greenwald JE: Atriopeptin: A cardiac hormone intimately involved in fluid, electrolyte, and blood pressure regulation. N Engl J Med 314:828, 1986.

Nudel DB, Camara A, Levine M: Comparative effects of bicarbonate, tris-(hydroxymethyl)aminomethane and dichloroacetate in newborn swine with normoxic lactic acidosis. Dev Pharmacol Ther 20:20, 1993.

O'Donovan HB, Bell EF: Effects of furosemide on body water compartments in infants with bronchopulmonary dysplasia. Pediatr Res 26:121, 1989.

Papile LA, Burstein J, Burstein R, et al: Relationship of intravenous sodium bicarbonate infusions and cerebral intraventricular hemorrhage. J Pediatr 93:834, 1978.

Perlman M, Schenker J, Glassman M, Ben-David M: Prolonged hyperprolactinemia in preterm infants. J Clin Endocrinol Metab 47:894, 1978.

Perlman JF, Moore V, Siegel MJ, Dawson J: Is chloride depletion an important contributing cause of death in infants with bronchopulmonary dysplasia? Pediatrics 77:212, 1986.

Pullano JG, Cohen-Addad N, Apuzzio JJ, et al: Water and salt conservation in the human fetus and newborn: I. Evidence for a role of fetal prolactin. J Clin Endocrinol Metab 69:1180, 1989.

Puschett JB: Pharmacological classification and renal actions of diuretics. Cardiology 84(suppl 2):4, 1994.

Ramiro-Tolentino SB, Markarian K, Kleinman LI: Renal bicarbonate excretion in extremely low birth weight infants. Pediatrics 98:256, 1996.

Reller MD, Rice MJ, McDonald RW: Review of studies evaluating ductal patency in the premature infant. J Pediatr 122:S59, 1993.

Riordan JF: Angiotensin II: Biosynthesis, molecular recognition, and signal transduction. Cell Mol Neurobiol 15:637, 1995.

Robertson GL, Berl T: Water metabolism. In Brenner BM, Rector FC (Eds): The Kidney. Philadelphia, WB Saunders, 1986, pp 385–431.

Robertson NR: Apnea after THAM administration in the newborn. Arch Dis Child 45:306, 1970.

Robillard JE, Smith FG, Nakamura KT, et al: Neural control of renal hemodynamics and function during development. Pediatr Nephrol 4:436, 1990.

Ronconi M, Fortunato A, Soffiati G, et al: Vasopressin, atrial natriuretic factor and renal water homeostasis in premature newborn infants with respiratory distress syndrome. J Perinat Med 23:307, 1995.

Rozycki HJ, Baumgart S: Atrial natriuretic factor and postnatal diuresis in respiratory distress syndrome. Arch Dis Child 662:43, 1991.

Rush MG, Engelhardt B, Parker RA, Hazinski TA: Double-blind, placebo-controlled trial of alternate-day furosemide therapy in infants with chronic bronchopulmonary dysplasia. J Pediatr 117:112, 1990.

Sagnella GA, MacGregor GA: Cardiac peptides and the control of sodium excretion. Nature 309:666, 1984.

Schneiderman R, Rosenkrantz TS, Knox I, et al: Effects of a continuous infusion of tris(hydroxymethyl)aminomethane on acidosis, oxygen affinity, and serum osmolality. Biol Newborn 64:287, 1993.

Sedin G: Fluid management in the extremely preterm infant. In Hansen TN, McIntosh N (Eds): Current Topics in Neonatology. London, WB Saunders, 1995, pp 50–66.

Seri I: Cardiovascular, renal, and endocrine actions of dopamine in newborns and children. J Pediatr 126:333, 1995.

Seri I, Rudas G, Bors ZS, et al: Effects of low-dose dopamine on cardiovascular and renal functions, cerebral blood flow, and plasma catecholamine levels in sick preterm newborns. Pediatr Res 34:742, 1993.

Seri I, Tulassay T, Kiszel J, Csömör S: The use of dopamine for the prevention of the renal side effects of indomethacin in premature infants with patent ductus arteriosus. Int J Pediatr Nephrol 5:209, 1984.

Seri I, Tulassay T, Kiszel J, et al: Effect of low-dose dopamine infusion on prolactin and thyrotropin secretion in preterm infants with hyaline membrane disease. Biol Newborn 47:317, 1985.

Shaffer SG, Bradt SK, Hall RT: Postnatal changes in total body water and extracellular volume in the preterm infant with respiratory distress syndrome. J Pediatr 109:509, 1986.

Shaffer SG, Meade VM: Sodium balance and extracellular volume regulation in very low birth weight infants. J Pediatr 115:285, 1989.

Shaffer SG, Weismann DN: Fluid requirements in the preterm infant. Clin Perinatol 19:233, 1992.

Sola A, Gregory GA: Colloid osmotic pressure of normal newborns and premature infants. Crit Care Med 9:568, 1981.

Starling EH: On the absorption of fluid from the connective tissue spaces. J Physiol (London) 19:312, 1896.

Sulyok E, Kovacs L, Lichardus B, et al: Late hyponatremia in premature infants: Role of aldosterone and arginine vasopressin. J Pediatr 106:990, 1985.

Sulyok E, Nemeth M, Tenyi I, et al: Relationship between maturity, electrolyte balance and the function of the renin-angiotensin-aldosterone system in newborn infants. Biol Newborn 35:60, 1979.

Tammela OK, Koivisto ME: Fluid restriction for preventing bronchopulmonary dysplasia? Reduced fluid intake during the first weeks of life improves the outcome of low-birth-weight infants. Acta Paediatr 81:207, 1992.

Tammela OKT: Appropriate fluid regimens to prevent bronchopulmonary dysplasia. Eur J Pediatr 154:S15, 1995.

Taylor AE: Capillary fluid filtration. Circ Res 49:557, 1981.

Tulassay T, Seri I, Rascher W: The role of atrial natriuretic peptide in extra-cellular volume contraction after birth. Acta Paediatr Scand 76:144, 1987.

van den Anker JN, Hop WCJ, de Groot R, et al: Effects of prenatal exposure to betamethasone and indomethacin on the glomerular filtration rate in the preterm infant. Pediatr Res 36:578, 1994.

Van Marter LJ, Leviton A, Allred EN, et al: Hydration during the first days of life and the risk of bronchopulmonary dysplasia in low birth weight infants. J Pediatr 116:942, 1990.

von Planta M, Bar-Joseph G, Wiklund L, et al: Pathophysiologic and therapeutic implications of acid-base changes during CPR. Ann Emerg Med 22:404, 1993.

Wahlig TM, Thompson TR, Sinaiko AR: Drug use in the newborn. Clin Perinatol 19:251, 1992.

Wiswell TE, Graziani LJ, Kornhauser MS, et al: Effects of hypocarbia on the development of cystic periventricular leukomalacia in premature infants treated with high-frequency jet ventilation. Pediatrics 98:918, 1996.

Yeh TF, Shibli A, Leu ST, et al: Early furosemide therapy in premature infants (less than or equal to 2000 gm) with respiratory distress syndrome: A randomized controlled trial. J Pediatr 105:603, 1984.

Yeh TF, Wilks A, Singh J, et al: Furosemide prevents the renal side effects of indomethacin therapy in premature infants with patent ductus arteriosus. J Pediatr 101:433, 1982.

CHAPTER 35

Issues in Nursing Care of the Newborn

Peggy Gordin

The care of newborn infants was historically managed by nurses and midwives in the home. Gradually, during the 1930s and 1940s, childbirth moved into the hospital setting, and the hospital newborn nursery became the setting for neonatal care. Until the 1960s, there was little that could be done to save infants who were born prematurely, with major congenital anomalies, or with other illnesses. With the development of neonatal intensive care units (NICUs) in the late 1960s and early 1970s, it was natural that nurses would develop a significant role in the care of these very sick infants. In fact, the tremendous growth of critical care units for all age groups and specialty populations has led to changes in the relationship between nurses and physicians. The vast amount of work generated by the application of technology in the care of critically ill patients could be managed only by a more collegial, interdependent nurse-physician relationship. This is most apparent in neonatal intensive care.

Research on patient outcomes reveals that the interaction and coordination of intensive care unit staff are the most important factors influencing mortality rates (Fagin, 1992; Knaus et al, 1986). The intensive care nurse is often a proxy for the physician in the ongoing monitoring needed by critically ill patients, requiring a high degree of training and clinical expertise. The degree to which physicians respect and listen to nurses' concerns about a patient often influences the timeliness of diagnosis and definitive intervention. This is particularly true for sick newborns who are totally dependent on their caregivers to recognize signs of distress and illness.

An additional role of the nursing staff in a NICU is to collaborate with the medical staff to create systems that allow for efficient and proper care delivery. This is generally done through the establishment of unit policies, procedures, and protocols that define specific caregiving practices. These systems allow all the professionals working in the unit to function in coordination with clear understanding of everyone's role. With well-defined care protocols, physicians do not need to write orders for every detail of care. In addition, the unit practice guidelines help to ensure that care is consistent with published standards of practice and may reduce the risk of adverse occurrences.

SPECIFIC NURSING CARE ISSUES
Family-Centered Care

Early premature and newborn nurseries had strict infection control policies that isolated infants from their families. This paralleled the movement of health care out of the home environment and into the technologically focused hospital. In the 1970s, work by Klaus and Kennell (1976) on maternal-infant bonding pointed out the problems created by these policies that separated parents from their newborn infant, and NICUs began to open up their doors.

Over the last decade, neonatologists, neonatal nurses, and social workers have heard from parents who have experienced a NICU stay that attempts at family-centered care have fallen short of their needs (Harrison, 1993). In addition, many parents have expressed concerns regarding their experiences with pain management, informed consent procedures, and the overall ethics of some NICU procedures (Harrison, 1993).

In response to these concerns, many NICUs are revising their policies not only to allow parents free access to their infant but also to define clearly the importance of the parent as a member of the caregiving team. Implementation of this cultural change in a NICU requires extensive collaboration between the medical and nursing staff of the unit. Nurses and physicians alike must challenge long-held assumptions regarding appropriate visiting policies and roles of parents in the unit. Communication with parents can be enhanced by collaboration between physicians and nurses so that consistent messages are conveyed and the plan of care is supported by each caregiver.

Early and consistent involvement of parents in caretaking activities may promote earlier discharge, in addition to better family adaptation to the birth of a sick or premature infant (Kenner, 1990). Nurses are key in helping parents learn to understand their infant's behavior and ways to handle their infant so that physiologic stability is maintained (Griffen, 1990).

Developmental Care

Another trend in neonatal intensive care is the movement toward a nursery environment and caregiving approach designed to minimize stress and support the infant's own efforts toward self-regulation. Specific interventions include regulation of the amount of light and noise in the nursery, use of swaddling and special positioning techniques that promote enhanced behavioral organization, and structuring of all caregiving procedures to promote infant coping. The use of such an individualized developmental approach to care has shown promise as a means to improve neurodevelopmental outcomes in very-low-birth-weight preterm infants (Als et al, 1986, 1994). The implementation of such an approach to care is primarily the responsibility of the NICU nursing staff. Other professionals must support these practices, but the nurse interacts with the infant the most and has most of the control over the infant's environment. Nurses also teach the parents to provide care that is appropriate for the infant's developmental age and individual temperament.

Pain Assessment and Management

No discussion of the role of nursing in developmental care would be complete without mention of pain management.

In the past, the newborn was considered incapable of pain perception because of neurologic immaturity. More recent studies (Anand and Carr, 1989; Anand and Hickey, 1987; Marshall, 1989) have led to general recognition that preterm and term newborns have full nociceptive capabilities and dramatic changes in how pain is managed in NICUs. Neonatal nurses have expertise in assessing for signs of pain, applying nonpharmacologic interventions (similar to those used to promote behavioral organization), and administering and monitoring pain medication. The plan for pain management in a particular infant should be developed and monitored collaboratively to ensure that effective pain relief is achieved in the safest manner possible.

Infants receiving intravenous opiates should be closely monitored for respiratory depression, and equipment for airway management and ventilation must be immediately available. In ventilated infants who have obvious cause for frequent or prolonged pain, around-the-clock administration or continuous infusion of low-dose opioid analgesics is safe and effective for pain relief (Franck and Gregory, 1993). When discontinuing opiates, the dose should be gradually tapered while maintaining the same interval between doses, to avoid withdrawal syndrome (Franck and Gregory, 1993). Although patients who receive more than a few doses of opioid analgesics develop physical dependence and tolerance to the drug (Franck and Gregory, 1993), the use of the term *addicted* is discouraged when referring to these known physiologic side effects of narcotics. Addiction implies a chronic social problem associated with drug-seeking and antisocial behavior, making this an upsetting term for a parent to hear and inappropriate to apply to a newborn. The use of appropriate terminology as well as pharmacologically correct dosing and weaning protocols helps dispel the common misconceptions held by parents and caregivers regarding the use of narcotics for pain management.

Airway Management

Procedures for stabilization and maintenance of artificial airways are an important responsibility of the nursing staff working in a NICU. Endotracheal suctioning is a necessary but potentially risky procedure that has been associated with hypoxemia, airway tissue trauma (Grylack and Anderson, 1984; Kleiber et al, 1988), pneumothorax (Anderson and Chandra, 1976), and cerebral blood flow changes (Perlman and Volpe, 1983). A review of current literature regarding various techniques for suctioning supports the following recommendations:

1. Suctioning should be done only when necessary, based on signs of airway secretions. Depending on the infant's disease process and mode of support, suctioning may be done as infrequently as every 12 hours or as frequently as several times an hour (Hodge, 1991).
2. Atelectasis and subsequent hypoxemia may be somewhat ameliorated by the use of a closed suctioning system (Ballard Medical Products, Draper, UT) or a side-port endotracheal tube adaptor (Zmora and Merritt, 1980). If these devices are not available or desired, the lung should be re-expanded after suctioning by manual ventilation or additional breaths via the ventilator. Enough inflating pressure and positive end-expiratory pressure should be used to re-recruit alveoli that may have collapsed during suctioning, but overdistention of the lungs is to be avoided. A 10% to 20% increase in the fraction of inspired oxygen and inflating pressure is recommended as a guideline; however, an individualized approach based on the infant's response to suctioning and manual ventilation should determine the actual settings used (Hodge, 1991).
3. Adequate airway humidification is the most effective means of treating secretions that are thick and difficult to remove. The suction catheter should not be inserted more than 1 cm beyond the tip of the endotracheal tube. Suction catheters that are precalibrated in centimeter increments are commercially available. The exact length of the cut endotracheal tube, plus the additional distance added by the adapter, is used to determine the distance for suction catheter insertion (Hodge, 1991; Kleiber et al, 1988).

In addition to proper suctioning procedures, proper stabilization and positioning of artificial airways are important safety precautions. Endotracheal tubes must be securely held in position to prevent movement and friction against the fragile tracheal endothelium. Tubing connecting the patient to the ventilator must be kept free from condensation and positioned below the connection to the endotracheal tube so that water cannot flow into the airway.

Skin Care

The skin of preterm infants is permeable and fragile particularly in the first week after birth. Meticulous care is required to prevent injury from tape and chemicals that are associated with the use of NICU equipment. Special cardiorespiratory monitoring leads are available that use either a pectin-based wafer (such as Stomahesive) or gel for adhesion. These types of leads can be applied, removed, and reapplied without injury to the delicate skin of very-low-birth-weight infants. Protective barriers such as pectin-based wafers (Stomahesive) may also be applied to the skin before placing tape to secure umbilical catheters, temperature probes, or endotracheal tubes to prevent epidermal stripping with tape removal (Lund et al, 1984).

Skin preparations containing alcohol, iodine, or other chemicals must be used with extreme care in newborns because of the risk of burns and systemic absorption. Benzoin should not be used under any type of adhesive product because it increases the adhesion between the epidermis and the adhesive, making epidermal stripping more likely. Adhesive removers are not recommended for use in newborns, but if they are to be used in the NICU, the ingredients should be checked carefully for substances that can be absorbed rapidly and prove toxic to a preterm infant. A nontoxic medical adhesive remover, used sparingly and removed immediately with clear water, may be of benefit to reduce the duration of a procedure such as changing endotracheal tube tapes.

Medication Administration Procedures

Medication administration is an important area for collaborative practice in the NICU. Pharmacokinetics in preterm and term newborns are constantly undergoing maturational changes, leading to the need to rely on drug levels to determine effective therapy for many medications. In addition, medication administration in the neonatal population is complicated by the tiny fluid volumes allowed for drug delivery and the low intravenous flow rates used in this population (Weatherstone and Leff, 1992). It has been shown that the procedures used by nursing staff to administer intravenous medications (particularly antibiotics) can significantly affect drug pharmacokinetics (Gould and Roberts, 1979; Nahata, 1987) and thus the incidence of side effects or complications associated with a particular drug.

The length and diameter of drug administration tubing, intravenous flow rate, and point of drug solution entry into the patient intravenous line can dramatically affect the delivery medications given intravenous piggyback (Gauger and Carey, 1986; Kubajak et al, 1988; Leff and Roberts, 1992). Because of the effects of laminar flow, studies have shown that it takes two to three times the volume of the tubing that the medication must travel to flush the dose into the patient (Leff and Roberts, 1992). In some cases, an entire dose may be discarded when the intravenous tubing is changed, if the medication is delivered fairly distal to the patient at a low flow rate.

These problems can be minimized if NICUs develop medication administration procedures that include the following characteristics:

1. The medication is delivered into the intravenous tubing as close as possible to the patient.
2. Microbore tubing is used to minimize the volume of fluid required to flush the medication into the patient.
3. Medication delivery rate is controlled independently of the primary intravenous flow rate through the use of an infusion pump.
4. The medication administration system should accommodate to all the various forms of intravenous access used in the NICU without increasing the risk for infection (e.g., maintain a closed system for central lines or lines containing parenteral nutrition solutions).

ADVANCED-PRACTICE NURSING ROLES IN NEONATAL INTENSIVE CARE UNITS
Neonatal Nurse Practitioners

During the 1970s and 1980s, the limited number of neonatologists and the development of regionalized perinatal care led to the evolution of expanded nursing roles in which specially trained nurses assumed responsibility for care that was previously the exclusive province of physicians. Nurses were increasingly relied on to perform newborn resuscitation in the delivery room, transport, and primary patient management in the NICU. Their practice included writing medical care orders; writing progress notes; and performing various invasive procedures such as intubation, chest tube placement, umbilical catheter placement, and lumbar puncture. This expanded role was initially identified by a number of titles, but the term *neonatal nurse practitioner* is now the accepted title endorsed by professional nursing organizations. By the early 1980s, neonatal nurse practitioners were present in 57% of all tertiary neonatal units (Harper et al, 1982).

More recently, the intensive care needs of sick newborns and the vast array of technology used in the NICU have been targeted as a tremendous cost burden on the health-care system. Health-care professionals are challenged to provide more cost-effective care while continuing to improve the outcomes for patients. In addition, pediatric residency training programs have shifted their focus to primary care, limiting the number of staff available to provide direct care in teaching hospital NICUs. These changes have served only to increase further the demand for neonatal nurse practitioners.

The education and credentialing of neonatal nurse practitioners have been the subjects of much debate and change over the past 15 years. The early practitioners were often trained by neonatologists in their unit for a specific role. These nurses had no recognized documentation of their training or any specific credential. In the late 1970s and early 1980s, a number of more formal neonatal nurse practitioner training programs were established ranging from a 9- to 12-month certificate program offered by a hospital to a 2-year university-based graduate program. In the mid-1980s, the Nurses Association of the American College of Obstetricians and Gynecologists (NAACOG) Certification Corporation (now known as National Certification Corporation [NCC]) developed a certification examination for neonatal nurse practitioners, providing a nationally recognized credential for these advanced-practice nurses. This is a voluntary specialty certification, but candidates must meet certain didactic and clinical criteria to be eligible to sit for the examination, and certification status must be renewed every 3 years through continuing education or reexamination (NCC, 1995).

In 1992, the National Association of Neonatal Nurses (NANN) published a position paper recommending that credentialing for the neonatal nurse practitioner role require graduate-level education, with a grandfathering mechanism for nurses currently prepared by certificate programs (NANN, 1992). At present, however, the NCC examination still allows neonatal nurse practitioners who have completed an accredited certificate program to sit for the certification examination because there are still a limited number of graduate neonatal nurse practitioner programs. Neonatal nurse practitioners are generally licensed in each state through the same mechanism as other nurse practitioners.

Other Neonatal Nursing Roles

Several other significant leadership roles may be encountered in a NICU. These roles may include management, education, or clinical practice as their focus. Depending on the size of the unit and number of staff working there, any combination of the following positions may be important in ensuring a smooth-functioning unit that delivers high-quality patient care.

The nurse manager, head nurse, or unit director usually

has the responsibility for overseeing all aspects of the NICU's operations and staff. Depending on the educational background and hospital organizational structure, this individual may be responsible for supervising advanced-practice nursing staff or may be considered a peer to those personnel. In either instance, a strong working relationship with the other leadership personnel in the unit is essential for a manager to be effective.

The unit may also have a clinical nurse specialist, educator, or similarly titled person who is a masters-prepared nurse with a strong clinical background in neonatal intensive care. Generally this is the person who is responsible for working with the nursing staff to develop procedures, protocols, and patient care standards. Orientation of new staff may also be part of this person's job, in collaboration with the nurse manager and senior staff nurses. Some clinical nurse specialists have particular areas of focus in their unit, such as discharge planning or developmental care, but they are generally expected to oversee all aspects of clinical practice.

Finally, NICUs may use nurses who are trained to be nurse practitioners or clinical specialists in roles such as transport and neonatal follow-up. Sometimes it is not only education and credentials but also a specific job description that determines the roles played by various personnel in a NICU. Neonatal units have needs as varied as their patient populations. Through ongoing planning and a collaborative relationship between nursing and medicine, the optimal team and approach to patient care for a particular NICU can be developed.

REFERENCES

Als H, Lawhon G, Brown E, et al: Individualized behavioral and environmental care for the very-low-birth-weight infant at high risk for bronchopulmonary dysplasia: Neonatal intensive care unit and developmental outcome. Pediatrics 78:1123, 1986.

Als H, Lawhon G, Duffy FH, et al: Individualized developmental care for the very-low-birth-weight preterm infant. JAMA 272:853, 1994.

Anand KJS, Carr DB: The neuroanatomy, neurophysiology, and neurochemistry of pain, stress, and analgesia in newborns and children. Pediatr Clin North Am 36:795, 1989.

Anand KJS, Hickey PR: Pain and its effects in the human neonate and fetus. N Engl J Med 31:1321, 1987.

Anderson KD, Chandra R: Pneumothorax secondary to perforation of sequential bronchi by suction catheters. J Pediatr Surg 11:687, 1976.

Fagin CM: Collaboration between nurses and physicians: No longer a choice. Acad Med 67:295, 1992.

Franck LS, Gregory GA: Clinical evaluation and treatment of infant pain in the neonatal intensive care unit. *In* Schechter NL, Berde CB, Yaster M (Eds): Pain in Infants, Children, and Adolescents. Baltimore, Williams & Wilkins, 1993, pp 519–535.

Gauger LJ, Cary JD: The theory and practice of retrograde infusion: Influence of tube diameter on drug delivery. Drug Intell Clin Pharm 20:616, 1986.

Gould T, Roberts R: Therapeutic problems arising from the use of intravenous route for drug administration. J Pediatr 95:465, 1979.

Griffen T: Nurse barriers to parenting in the special care nursery. J Perinat Neonat Nurs 4:56, 1990.

Grylack LJ, Anderson KD: Diagnosis and treatment of traumatic granuloma in tracheobronchial tree of newborn with history of chronic intubation. J Pediatr Surg 19:200, 1984.

Harper RG, Little GA, Sia CG: Scope of nursing practice in level III NICUs. Pediatrics 70:875, 1982.

Harrison H: The principles for family-centered neonatal care. Pediatrics 92:643, 1993.

Hodge D: Endotracheal suctioning and the infant: A nursing care protocol to decrease complications. Neonatal Network 9:7, 1991.

Kenner C: Caring for the NICU parent. J Perinat Neonat Nurs 4:78, 1990.

Klaus MH, Kennell JH: Maternal-Infant Bonding. St. Louis, CV Mosby, 1976.

Kleiber C, Krutzfield N, Rose EF: Acute histologic changes in the tracheobronchial tree associated with different suction catheter insertion techniques. Heart Lung 17:10, 1988.

Knaus WA, Draper EA, Wagner DP, Zimmerman JE: An evaluation of outcome from intensive care in major medical centers. Ann Intern Med 104:410, 1986.

Kubajak CAM, Leff RD, Roberts RJ: Influence of physical characteristics of intravenous systems on drug delivery. Dev Pharmacol Ther 11:189, 1988.

Leff RD, Roberts RJ: Practical Aspects of Intravenous Drug Administration. Bethesda, MD, American Society of Hospital Pharmacists, 1992.

Lund C, Kuller JM, Tobin C, et al: Evaluation of a pectin-based barrier under tape to protect neonatal skin. J Obstet Gynecol Neonatal Nurs 13:39, 1984.

Marshall RE: Neonatal pain associated with caregiving procedures. Pediatr Clin North Am 36:885, 1989.

Nahata MC: Effect of intravenous drug delivery systems on pharmacokinetic monitoring. Am J Hosp Pharm 44:2538, 1987.

National Association of Neonatal Nurses (NANN): Neonatal Nurse Practitioners: Standards of Education and Practice. Petaluma, CA, NANN, 1992.

National Certification Corporation for the Obstetric, Gynecologic, and Neonatal Nursing Specialties (NCC): 1995 Certification Program. Chicago, NCC, 1995.

Perlman JM, Volpe JJ: Suctioning in the preterm infant: Effects on cerebral blood flow velocity, intracranial pressure, and arterial blood pressure. Pediatrics 72:329, 1983.

Weatherstone KB, Leff RD: Intravenous drug delivery considerations for newborn infants. Semin Perinatol 16:41, 1992.

Zmora E, Merritt TA: Use of side-hole endotracheal tube adapter for tracheal aspiration. Am J Dis Child 134:250, 1980.

CHAPTER 36

Caring for Parents of Infants in Intensive Care

Stephanie A. Berman

The extraordinary advances in neonatal care have made it possible for increasing numbers of sick and preterm infants to be treated successfully. Most of these children eventually go on to normal and productive lives. Many, however, require additional help and services after discharge home, and some die in the days and months after birth. For each infant who dies or is disabled, as well as for those whose lives become a testimony to the success of neonatology, there is a family whose life is forever altered. For each neonate who is rescued by a sophisticated neonatal transport team and whisked away to a high-risk tertiary unit, there is a bereft mother left behind at the referring hospital. She and other concerned family members watch as the care of their fragile newborn is assumed by health-care providers introduced to them just moments before. The intimacy of their childbirth has become a medical emergency shared with strangers.

In the days that follow, parents need to adjust to an environment that is totally foreign to them and to a specialized language that few have heard before. Many are in unfamiliar cities and hospitals. Most worry about their other children, work, home, and insurance. The demands on a family whose baby is in intensive care are incalculable. Parents find themselves dependent on people they do not know for problems they do not understand. The response is, predictably, a loss of parenting control and a suspension of normalcy.

How families adapt to these abrupt changes depends to an important extent on the particular combination of coping skills and mechanisms they bring to this situation and its confounding problems. How the neonatal team can work together to help families identify and enhance these coping strengths is the subject of this chapter.

One of the difficulties confronting a family is the sheer number of people with whom they must interact in the course of their baby's hospitalization. This is especially problematic at regional tertiary centers, which are often teaching hospitals. For parents of an infant transferred to a tertiary care center, just the first 48 hours entails interaction with the physicians and nurses at the delivery; the nurse, doctor, and paramedics on the transport team; the neonatologist, resident and fellow at the center; and some six shifts of nurses and respiratory therapists along with social workers, billing staff, and others.

In contrast to a private pediatric practice, in which the family has a close and trusting relationship with one physician, who orchestrates care and relates personally to them, neonatal intensive care requires a team approach to meet all of the family's needs. Ideally, the team members from different disciplines and perspectives work together to address the special needs intrinsic to the family's current crisis (Miles, 1979). Guidelines for supporting the families of high-risk infants are summarized in Table 36–1.

TEAM GOALS

Team goals for families remain relatively constant regardless of a baby's medical course and the length of stay. They are, in essence, to help families cope with their transient dependence on the medical care providers and to work toward the parents' independence and assumption of responsibility for their infant's care. Restoring parental control depends in part on the team's willingness to empower families. Communicating information, sharing decision

---

TABLE 36–1

Guidelines for Supporting Families of High-Risk Infants

Goals

1. To enable the family to cope with transient dependence on the medical care team
2. To enable parents to assume responsibility for the care of their newborn at discharge

Strategies

Antepartum Approaches

1. Coordinate information among team members
2. Provide concrete information to family
3. Introduce neonatal team
4. Orient family to the intensive care nursery

Intensive Care Nursery

1. Coordinate information and assign responsibility for communication
2. Meet with the family outside the unit (e.g., neonatologist, social worker, primary nurse, and resident)
3. Encourage family to participate in the infant's care
4. Recognize stresses and coping strengths, and offer opportunities for counseling and support

Preparing for Outcome

Discharge Home

1. Coordinate follow-up plan and family meeting with team members
2. Identify resources (e.g., medical needs, follow-up care, family support, and public health)
3. Arrange rooming-in before discharge
4. Follow up with a telephone call after discharge to assess adjustment

Death

1. Prepare family for the possibility of a fatal outcome
2. Provide parenting opportunities (holding, extended visits, and privacy)
3. Mobilize family support (e.g., extended family and clergy)
4. Support the family's pace in decision making (e.g., postmortem examination and funeral plans)
5. Offer resources (e.g., reading lists, support groups, and a staff resource person)
6. Follow up with a telephone call to assess adjustment
7. Arrange a death conference

making, and providing ongoing supportive care are the seminal elements for achieving this end. When the parents can master the crisis of having a sick or preterm baby, parents' feelings of self-worth are enhanced, and they can later resume their independence and their role as parents with increased confidence (Minde, 1984).

Teaching hospitals bring together medical providers with different levels of training, who are disparate in their abilities to work with families. The team approach of providing for the emotional and educational needs of families affords abundant opportunities for teaching through role modeling. Because parents are often isolated from friends and families, they rely on members of the health-care team for support. Whether it is the primary nurse, the neonatologist, or social worker on whom the parents come to depend most depends largely on "chemistry" and timing.

In a teaching center, where residents and neonatologists rotate on and off services, primary nurses are often the care providers with whom parents spend the most time and develop the strongest bond (Etzler, 1984). In units where a social worker is consistently available, the nurse and social worker can identify daily signs of family dysfunction and strength. Problems can be shared with team members, and approaches to solving them planned.

INTERVENTION STRATEGIES
Antepartum Period

Normal pregnancy is accompanied by physical and psychological changes that require adaptation by the parents, particularly with regard to their expectations about the infant. When there is a prospect of fetal abnormality, illness, or death, parents must readjust to these new circumstances. Their successful readjustment depends on having a clear understanding of the risks to the mother, fetus, and newborn as well as the support systems and problem-solving skills available.

Providing Information

The most available strategy for adaptation to a threatening event is understanding. Concrete information about the status of a high-risk fetus should be shared with a family. Parents usually want to hear the news together; sometimes, they want a friend or relative with them as well. When presented with information about potential problems that are technical and complicated, parents are often scared and distracted. They experience a flagging sense of control; everyone seems to know more about the mother's pregnancy and their baby than they do. Coordination of communications is important; team members need to share what has been discussed with the family, identify needs for follow-up, and assign responsibility for carrying out these tasks.

Introducing the Neonatal Team

Obstetric staff should introduce the family to appropriate members of the neonatal team who can prepare families for their baby's admission to the neonatal intensive care unit (NICU).

Orientation

When there is time before delivery, orienting the family to the NICU can ready them for the events to come. Parents often appreciate talking with different team members, each reinforcing information from a different vantage point and adding perspective to the anticipated birth. When a prospective mother can be moved, a wheelchair visit to the nursery provides a critical desensitizing step. The sight of a preterm infant on a respirator or with multiple intravenous lines, although unsettling at first, helps prepare a family for what they may likely see later. Similarly, the sounds of monitors are far less distracting if they have been experienced and explained. Once the baby has been delivered, parents who have been introduced to the nursery have some conceptual and factual framework to help them assess and cope with their baby's presence there.

Neonatal Period

Physicians in a NICU are often pressed for time. Interruptions are the norm. A sick preterm infant frequently has a variable course. When parents hear a working diagnosis from a physician who stops by the bedside and the next day they hear from a nurse about information conveyed "at report," they sometimes feel they are receiving piecemeal and even conflicting information. When they receive information from residents unfamiliar to them and sometimes even to the problems they are attempting to explain, confusion and even alarm ensue.

Primary Caregivers

When an infant is likely to remain hospitalized for an extended period, it is helpful if parents can identify staff members who will be involved with them throughout the baby's NICU stay. A nurse, senior physician, or social worker can fulfill the "primary caregiver" role. Primary caregivers maintain contact with the family and join in some, if not all, of the family meetings, even at times when they are not directly involved in the infant's daily care. They provide continuity for the parents and for the infant's day-to-day providers, helping both the family and providers remain focused on long-term goals for the infant's care.

Family Meeting

Meeting with families outside the nursery environment and together with other members of the care team can be a most efficient mode of transmitting information. Family meetings are an opportunity to meet at a fixed point in time, to clarify what has happened, and to discuss anticipated events. They provide a chance to assess a family's level of understanding and to identify issues that require review or elucidation. Once the parents grasp and integrate the medical information they receive, they can actively participate in decision making and regain a sense of control over their circumstances.

Family meetings are cumbersome in that they require scheduling and organizing. At their best, however, they provide a common perspective for families and caregivers. They provide an overview of an infant's condition and also an opportunity for trainees to learn (by observing) styles of conveying technical information to parents.

It is useful when team members from different disciplines meet together with a family, so that all have a uniform understanding of the information conveyed. They then can better reinforce, explain, and exemplify consistent information to families. When a family hears consistent information from their baby's nurse and more than one of the physicians, they are less anxious as well as less inclined to feel dependent on one individual, who may rotate off service and leave the family without needed support.

Family meetings are also times to prepare for potential long-term disability or to brace parents for their infant's death. Miles and Carter (1982) defined voids in communication as "not stating what was wrong with the child, not communicating how sick the child was, not telling parents about tests and treatments, not talking with them, not giving emotional support, not encouraging repeated questioning, staff not telling their names or who they were, and suddenly sending parents out of the room without explanation." Family meetings can eliminate these problems. Issues that families are reluctant to raise can be broached by one of the team members, and parents' concerns can be revealed in a nonjudgmental and supportive atmosphere.

A family meeting should be organized soon after an infant's admission to the nursery. When an infant's course is unstable and the outcome is uncertain, the primary team may need to meet with parents every few days. Soon after each meeting, a summarizing note should be placed in the chart.

Parents vary widely in their ability to cope with the crisis of having a sick or preterm infant. Many experience persistent feelings of guilt and anxiety. Sometimes they become withdrawn and unavailable and thwart staff efforts to maintain open communication (Leander and Pettett, 1986). Supportive intervention by the NICU social worker can meet the needs of families burdened with such feelings. Parents appreciate interaction with a team member whose primary focus and skills are to meet their needs apart from the needs of the infant.

Sometimes normal feelings of guilt are exacerbated by the reality of a pregnancy and birth complicated by maternal drug and alcohol abuse, heavy smoking, or other potentially adverse activities. Mothers of infants born under such circumstances face disapproval from friends and family and often from hospital staff as well. Social service intervention is imperative here, and referral to child protective services is mandatory in most cases of documented drug abuse.

How families express their stress also varies widely. Medical care providers, by refraining from judgment, give family members opportunities to express their distress within the context of their personal coping styles. If, when interacting with families, staff appear to be overly judgmental, communication and trust can be jeopardized. Compassion, empathy, and understanding can enhance a family's ability to adjust. Facilitating adjustment, that is, helping the family resume its customary level of mental health, is the focus of support for families (Baird, 1979).

Sometimes perinatal crises trigger underlying problems that result in depression and inability to function, and a parent with fragile mental health may decompensate. For such families, perinatal social workers may make referrals to outside mental health professionals. In general, depression and disequilibrium are a part of the grieving process that accompanies the loss of a normal pregnancy and the idealized baby. With support and open communication, most parents adjust. Information about peer support groups, social services available from hospital staff, and outside mental health resources should be communicated to families. Parents can best decide when and if they need outside help. Reinforcing the family's own coping systems helps them marshal confidence in their ability to assume control of their lives after the immediate medical crisis (Baird, 1979).

DISCHARGE HOME

Discharge home, especially from a tertiary care nursery, creates anxiety and fear for parents. Discharge signals resumption of parental control, but it also marks a disengagement from the experts and monitors and the hospital structure. When a NICU has unlimited visiting policies, many parents involve themselves quite early in routine infant care. Coupled with frequent visits and ongoing staff interaction, these parents are preparing themselves to care for their baby at home. Parents who have been unable to visit frequently are less prepared for the infant's discharge.

Ideally, a family discharge meeting can be held 7 to 10 days before the baby's proposed departure. Concerns can be reviewed, a discharge plan can be formulated, and parents can have time to organize their lives to accommodate the arrival of their infant. Parents should be offered a chance to room-in overnight with their baby before discharge (Minde, 1984).

Resources for follow-up at home should be discussed. A public health nurse, together with the baby's pediatrician, can assess needs over time and introduce additional programs and resources gradually, if they become needed. At this time, parents find local community resources helpful. The name of a contact family of a recent premature or sick baby already at home may be helpful.

Choices for follow-up resources should be presented. Familes vary in their desire for independence and privacy as they leave the nursery experience. The most successful discharge plan is one formulated in conjunction with the parents. Sometimes, in their eagerness to coordinate a thorough and comprehensive discharge plan, caregivers overwhelm families. Parents may surmise that staff members think them unready to assume full charge of their recovering infant. Some families are reassured by numerous, closely spaced follow-up appointments. Others need time to adjust at home and to know their infant before they begin to relate to a new cast of medical providers. Interviewing and choosing a private pediatrician while their infant is still in the NICU are important steps for parents in resuming control. A predischarge and an early postdischarge visit with the baby's pediatrician are essential and usually arranged as part of the discharge plan. Choices should be presented about follow-up resources and the timing of referrals.

The transition of an infant's care from hospital to family and community can be smoothed by the care team's ability to give control back to the parents. When a family has been kept well informed and involved in decision making during the hospital course, they feel trusted by staff and confident in their ability to carry out their parenting responsibilities. Comprehensive follow-up of high-risk infants and their families is essential (Ballard, 1988; Taeusch and Yogman, 1987).

NEONATAL DEATH

Parents need to know as soon as the staff expect that their baby may die. Most infants who come to a high-risk center are gravely ill for a time. Whereas experienced staff are accustomed to working with fragile newborns, parents often have no way to gauge the severity of their child's condition. The medical care team needs to share the benefit of their experience and perspective in the interest of parental orientation. The challenge is to prepare a family for the possibility of death without extinguishing hope. It requires sharing with parents confidence in neonatal medicine while recognizing its limitations; in other words, honestly telling a family that the best efforts possible might not be enough. Parents need as much time as possible to prepare for the loss of their infant. It is the first essential step in the long and arduous process of grieving. It is not unusual for some of the parents' initial anger at the thought of losing their infant to be displaced to the health-care team. It is essential that staff recognize this displacement and resist a defensive reaction. In addition, staff must often deal with their own sense of failure and loss of control when an infant dies, making it doubly hard to work supportively with the parents.

When a baby is dying, opportunities for the parents to participate in the infant's care can be offered. Separated from their baby by machines and tubes and monitors, most parents have been unable to hold or be alone with their newborn. They are apprehensive but grateful to be with their dying baby.

The circumstances of an infant's death need to be coordinated by health team members and choices for parent interaction with their infant need to be offered. The presence of extended family or clergy needs to be considered, as does the gathering of keepsakes and mementos. When death is precipitous, parents need to know they still can see and hold their infant.

> Freed in death from the intravenous lines, endotracheal tube, and monitoring systems, the final image of the baby is often one of relative or restored peace, comfort, and tranquility. The calmer memory lasts forever and possibly helps start the parents' huge, long-term effort to cope and eventually to adapt their lives to their loss.
>
> *Gorski, 1988*

Follow-Up After Death

Bringing the family back to meet with staff after the death of an infant is a major therapeutic step in moving the parents toward resolution of their grief. While the timing of the conference varies with availability of family, staff, and autopsy results, 6 to 8 weeks seems optimal. It is a

time when parents are beginning to reorganize their lives, when the mother's postpartum recovery is well along, and when the numbness and anguish of the nursery experience have begun to ease. Parents want to know more about their baby's death and its implications for future pregnancies. Sometimes they have questions and misunderstandings. Often, they simply want to make contact with those who knew their child.

These follow-up conferences are also important for staff. Those who can attend are able to share with the parents their observations and have opportunities for clarification and closure. It is a chance to hear from families when they have re-established equilibrium and order in their lives and thoughts. It is a chance to express gratitude or vent frustration. Lastly, it is a chance to reintroduce information about support resources, which range from reading lists on dying and grieving to referrals to peer support groups and mental health professionals. Families need reassurance that grieving is a long-term adaptive process that takes different forms and disrupts their lives for even a year or more. How they cope with this task depends in part on support from partners, family, and community. They need to know that it is normal that their loss may destabilize them for a time and that their lives will be disrupted after the loss of a child. Armed with opportunities for outside help and support from those around them, parents can evaluate how their lives are going and decide for themselves whether additional outside intervention will lessen their stress. Parents can control their time of grieving and the form it takes in their lives.

REFERENCES

Affleck G, Tennen H: The effect of newborn intensive care on parents' psychological well-being. Children's Health Care 20:6–14, 1991.

Affleck G, Tennen H, Rowe J: Mothers, fathers, and the crisis of newborn intensive care. Infant Mental Health J 11:12–20, 1990.

Avery ME, Litwack G: Born Early: The Story of a Premature Baby. Boston, Little, Brown, 1983.

Baird SF: Crisis intervention strategies. *In* Johnson SH (Ed): High-Risk Parenting: Nursing Assessment and Strategies for Assessment. Philadelphia, JB Lippincott, 1979, pp 299–311.

Ballard RA (Ed): Pediatric Care of the ICN Graduate. Philadelphia, WB Saunders, 1988.

Berman SA: Support of the family whose infant dies. *In* Ballard RA (Ed): Pediatric Care of the ICN Graduate. Philadelphia, WB Saunders, 1988, pp 218–285.

Cagan J: Weaning parents from intensive care unit care. Matern Child Nurs 13:275, 1988.

Consolvo CA: Relieving parental anxiety in the Care-By-Parent Unit. J Obstet Gynecol Neonatal Nurs 15:154, 1986.

Crnic KA, Greenberg MT, Ragozin AS, et al: Effects of stress and social support on mothers and premature and full-term infants. Child Dev 54:209–217, 1983.

Cronenwett LR: Network structure, social support, and psychological outcomes of pregnancy. Nurs Res 34:93–99, 1985.

Etzler CA: Parents' reactions to pediatric critical care settings: A review of the literature. Issues in Comprehensive Pediatr Nurs 7:319, 1984.

Gelkerson L, Gorski P, Panitz P: Hospital-based intervention for preterm infants and their families. *In* Meisels ST, Shankoff TP (Eds): Handbook of Early Childhood Intervention. Cambridge, Cambridge University Press, 1990, pp 445–568.

Goodman JR, Sauve RS: High risk infant: Concerns of the mother after discharge. Birth 12:235, 1985.

Gorski PA: Comment. *In* Ballard RA (Ed): Pediatric Care of the ICN Graduate. Philadelphia WB Saunders, 1988, p 282.

Leander K, Pettett G: Parental response to the birth of a high-risk neonate: Dynamics and management. Phys Occupat Ther Pediatr 6:205, 1986.

Miles MS: Counseling strategies. *In* Johnson SH (Ed): High-Risk Parenting: Nursing Assessment and Strategies for Assessment. Philadelphia, JB Lippincott, 1979, pp 283–298.

Miles MS: Parents of critically ill premature infants: Sources of stress. Crit Care Nurs Q 12:69–74, 1989.

Miles MS, Carter MC: Sources of parental stress in pediatric intensive care units. Children's Health Care 11:65, 1982.

Miles MS, Spicher C, Hassanein RS: Maternal and paternal stress reactions when a child is hospitalized in a pediatric intensive care unit. Issues Comprehensive Pediatr Nurs 7:333, 1984.

Minde KK: The impact of prematurity on the later behavior of children and their families. Clin Perinatol 11:227, 1984.

Petrick JM: Postpartum depression: Identification of high-risk mothers. JOGN Nurs 13:37, 1984.

Sims-Jones N: Back to the theories: Another way to view mothers of prematures. Matern Child Nurs J 11:394, 1986.

Taeusch HW, Yogman MW: Follow-up Management of the High-Risk Infant. Boston, Little, Brown, 1987.

Wohlreich MM: Psychiatric aspects of high-risk pregnancy. Psychiatr Clin North Am 10:53, 1986.

Wolterman MC, Miller M: Caring for parents in crisis. Nurs Forum 22:34, 1985.

Zeskind PS, Iacino R: Effects of maternal visitation to preterm infants in the neonatal intensive care unit. Child Dev 55:1887, 1984.

Pharmacologic Principles and Practicalities

Robert M. Ward

The rapid application of new drug therapy in the neonatal intensive care unit (NICU) has made pharmacology in the newborn increasingly complex. Accompanying that complexity is the realization that, even though drug treatment of newborns may be curative, it may also induce significant problems. Potential morbidity and mortality associated with drug treatment of newborns must be recognized and weighed against the expected benefits.

Drug therapy of newborns follows basic principles of pharmacology superimposed on dynamic, developmental changes during the newborn period. Patients cared for in the NICU are exposed to a wide variety of drugs, many of which are incompletely studied in newborns. Therapeutic drug monitoring is often an integral part of this drug exposure in the NICU. The effective use of drug concentration measurements requires a working knowledge of pharmacokinetics and thoughtful consideration of when such measurements are appropriate and helpful.

Perinatal Drug Exposure

Repeated warnings about fetal drug exposure were issued to physicians and the public after recognition of the teratogenic effects of thalidomide in the 1960s. Despite these warnings, drug exposure of the human fetus and newborn increased during subsequent decades and remains extensive today. The average number of drugs ingested during pregnancy increased from three in the 1950s to 11 in the 1970s (Ward and Green, 1988). Virtually all drugs administered to the pregnant woman reach the fetus, but careful interpretation is needed because fetal drug concentrations and effects vary widely from insignificant to life-threatening (Ward et al, 1980, 1988).

For hospitalized newborns, a similar pattern of increasing drug exposure is evident. Serial observations from the same NICU reveal almost a doubling of the average number of drugs administered to newborns in less than a decade, from 3.4 per patient during 1974 to 1975 (Aranda et al, 1976) to 6.2 per patient during 1977 to 1981 (Aranda et al, 1982a). Unfortunately, drug exposure among NICU patients is disproportionately greater in the most susceptible (and least studied) patients—the most immature newborns and those with multiple organ dysfunction (Aranda, 1983).

Drug-Induced Illness

The extensive exposure of newborns to drugs in the NICU is not benign. During their NICU hospitalization, 30% of newborns sustain one or more adverse drug reactions, of which 14.7% are fatal or life threatening (Aranda et al, 1982b). The causes of this NICU "epidemic" of drug-related morbidity and mortality are complex. Pharmaco-

logic studies in pediatric patients are difficult because of a variety of problems from ethics to study design (Ward and Green, 1988). The difficulty of studying therapeutics in the newborn has created a situation in which a plethora of drugs is administered with a paucity of pharmacologic data. The smaller and more immature newborns, who are now surviving, lack gestational age-appropriate pharmacologic data about efficacy, dose-response, and kinetics for most drugs they receive. Furthermore, drug-induced illness is seldom considered in newborns. Failure to recognize drug-induced illness in the newborn often leads to further pharmacologic treatment as the first approach to correct unrecognized drug-induced problems. This may reflect an expectation that drug therapy is usually effective and safe. The observations of Aranda suggest the opposite. Prudent management of newborns must recognize and weigh the potential benefits of unstudied drug therapy against potential drug-induced morbidity and mortality. Some examples from the history of drug-induced mortality and morbidity in newborns should serve as a reminder of how more harm than good may accrue from uncontrolled or unstudied drug therapy in the NICU.

Lessons from Chloramphenicol

Chloramphenicol was released for use in the 1940s and reports of its efficacy for treatment of *Salmonella* infections included pediatric patients. The manufacturer recommended dosages of 50 to 100 mg/kg/day for patients ≤15 kg. In 1959, when Sutherland reported three cases of sudden death in newborns treated with high dosages of chloramphenicol (up to 230 mg/kg per day), the drug was considered "well tolerated and nontoxic." Later in 1959, Burns and colleagues reported the disturbing results of a controlled trial of four prophylactic treatment regimens for newborn sepsis: (1) no treatment, (2) chloramphenicol alone, (3) penicillin and streptomycin, and (4) penicillin, streptomycin, and chloramphenicol. Groups 2 and 4, which received chloramphenicol (100 to 165 mg/kg per day), had overall mortality rates of 60% and 68%, respectively, whereas groups 1 and 3 had mortality rates of 19% and 18%, respectively. The deaths of these newborns demonstrated the stereotyped sequence of symptoms and signs caused by chloramphenicol, designated the "gray syndrome," which included abdominal distention with or without emesis, poor peripheral perfusion and cyanosis, vasomotor collapse, irregular respirations, and death within hours of the onset of these symptoms. One year later, Weiss and coworkers (1960) attributed the gray syndrome in newborns to high concentrations of chloramphenicol secondary to its prolonged half-life in newborns who received dosages of more than 100 mg/kg per day, which are usually used in older children. They recommended maximum dosages of 50 mg/kg per day in term infants younger than 1 month of age, half that dose for premature infants, and careful monitoring of chloramphenicol blood concentrations.

The discovery and explanation of chloramphenicol toxicity in newborns illustrate several important aspects of neonatal pharmacology. Because chloramphenicol was considered well tolerated in older children and adults, it was regarded as nontoxic for newborns. Chloramphenicol was so effective in newborns that higher dosages were used without pharmacokinetic study. Higher doses were administered to newborns despite recognition that its clearance required glucuronide conjugation, which was known to be immature in newborns. The unexpected finding that chloramphenicol in doses of 100 to 165 mg/kg per day could be lethal to newborns was demonstrated because this study included appropriate control groups. In fact, because the mortality rate from the most effective antibiotic treatment regimen was equivalent to no antibiotic treatment, Burns and associates (1959) discontinued prophylactic use of antibiotics in the nursery. Similar pharmacologic comparisons are needed. Even more, thoughtful consideration should be given to the response to therapeutic failure. Fewer drugs and lower dosages may be safer and more effective than additional drugs in higher dosages.

Reduction and Prevention of Medication Errors in Newborn Care

Drug treatment is one of the most frequent procedures used in the care of sick newborns. At Primary Children's Medical Center 35-bed NICU (Salt Lake City, UT) with an average of 785 patient-days per month, patients receive an average of 8700 (range 6990 to 11,290) doses of medications, pharmacy-formulated intravenous solutions, and aerosols each month (unpublished observations). These are usually prepared by pharmacists and administered by nurses, respiratory therapists, and (rarely) physicians. In such a large and complex system that produces so many drug treatments per month, errors are virtually inevitable despite several levels of prospective and redundant reviews by nurses, pharmacists, and NICU unit secretaries involved in the drug treatment process. At Primary Children's NICU, the medication error rate averages 0.04% for nurses and pharmacists and 0.07% for physicians (unpublished observations). Many errors are inconsequential, whereas others produce serious adverse effects. Medication errors incur significant costs, ranging from the obvious ones of direct patient injury, prolonged hospital stays, and additional corrective treatments to the more subtle costs associated with monitoring and regulation of medication use within hospitals (Proceedings, 1995).

In a study of 393 malpractice claims reported to the Physician Insurers Association of America (PIAA), the second most frequent cause of malpractice claims was drug errors (Physician Insurers Association of America, 1993). Among 16 medical specialties with two or more claims, pediatric practice ranked 6th in the number of claims, yet it had the 3rd highest average cost/indemnity. The most frequent medications involved in all claims were antibiotics, glucocorticoids, narcotic/non-narcotic analgesics, and narcotic antagonists. In pediatric practice, the medications involved most frequently were vaccines (DPT) and bronchodilators (theophylline). In the PIAA review, the five most frequent causes of drug errors were as follows (Physician Insurers Association of America, 1993):

- Incorrect doses
- Medications that were inappropriate for the medical condition
- Failure to monitor for drug side effects
- Failure of communication between physician and patient
- Failure to monitor drug levels

The primary opportunity for prevention of these five most frequent errors rests with the prescribing physician. Additional information as well as additional time for communication and documentation may be needed.

Physician prescriptions and drug orders are a means of communicating, yet too little attention is often devoted to making these legible, clear, and unambiguous (American Society of Hospital Pharmacists, 1993). The following steps may help ensure that medication orders communicate more effectively:

- Write out instructions rather than use abbreviations.
- Avoid vague instructions (e.g., "take as directed").
- Specify exact dosage strengths.
- Avoid abbreviations of drug names (e.g., MS for morphine sulfate or magnesium sulfate)
- Ensure that prescriptions and signatures are legible, even if it means printing the prescriber's name that corresponds to the signature.

The process for ordering, preparing, dispensing, and administering medications in an intensive care unit with acutely ill patients is often complicated and may directly contribute to errors. The frequency of those errors, however, may be reduced in almost every NICU. Although complex and expensive computerized systems may help to reduce medication errors, caregivers can take steps that are completely within their control to reduce medication errors without waiting for changes in the entire pharmacy process within the hospital (American Society of Hospital Pharmacists, 1993).

PRINCIPLES OF NEONATAL THERAPEUTICS

A thorough understanding of factors that affect drug concentrations helps in planning accurate therapy and in identifying the causes of therapeutic failure. Many of these factors are not chosen consciously in a therapeutic plan but have tremendous impact on its effectiveness. Pharmacokinetics and pharmacodynamics in newborns follow the same general principles that govern drug actions in patients of any age: diagnosis, drug selection and administration, absorption, distribution, metabolism, and excretion. When applied to the newborn, these principles must accommodate several unique physiologic and pharmacologic features of the newborn, as outlined in Table 37–1.

Diagnosis

Effective treatment begins with an accurate diagnosis and accurate assessment of symptoms. Although this applies to

TABLE 37–1

Pharmacologic Principles and Pitfalls in Management of the Very-Low-Birth-Weight Infant

I. *Diagnosis*
   A. Limited diagnostic procedures
II. *Absorption*
   A. Intravenous
      1. Drug injection away from patient
      2. Uneven mixing of drugs and intravenous fluids
      3. Delayed administration due to very low flow
      4. Part of the dose discarded with tubing changes
   B. Intramuscular
      1. Poor perfusion limits absorption
      2. Danger of sclerosis or abscess formation
      3. Depot effect
   C. Oral
      1. Poorly studied
      2. Affected by delayed gastric emptying
      3. Potentially affected by reflux
      4. Passive venous congestion may occur with chronic lung disease, decreasing absorption
III. *Distribution* (affected by):
   A. Higher (85%) total body water (versus 65% in adults)
   B. Lower body fat, i.e., about 1% body weight (versus 15% in term infants)
   C. Low protein concentration
   D. Decreased protein affinity for drugs
IV. *Metabolism*
   A. Half-life prolonged and unpredictable
   B. Total body clearance decreased
   C. Affected by nutrition, illness, and drug interaction
   D. Affected by maturational changes
V. *Excretion*
   A. Decreased renal function, both glomerular filtration rate and tubular secretion

all areas of therapeutics, treatment in newborns presents special diagnostic challenges because their small size and fragility may preclude useful, but inordinately invasive, diagnostic procedures. For example, many small immature newborns with chronic lung disease are given treatment for "bronchospasm" after decreased air entry associated with desaturation and abnormal breath sounds is observed. Relief of these symptoms with aerosolized bronchodilators may be interpreted as confirmation of the diagnosis. Although this may be correct, increased humidity, chest physiotherapy, or movement of the endotracheal tube bevel away from a pliable tracheal wall during an aerosol treatment may account for the improvement. Evaluation of ineffective therapy should include reconsideration of the diagnosis.

Absorption

Although most types of drug therapy for acute problems include *intravenous administration* to ensure drug delivery to the site of action, this may *not* be reliable in newborns (Roberts, 1984). Drugs are often injected away from newborns "up the IV line" through a Y-site injection port with the expectation that the preset flow rate will deliver the drug over an appropriate infusion time. Intravenous infu-

sion rates for very-low-birth-weight infants may be less than 2 mL/hour, sometimes divided between two infusion sites. Consequently, a drug injected away from the infant may infuse so slowly that it does not reach the circulation for several hours and then enters over a prolonged period. Gould and Roberts (1979) estimated that as much as 36% of the total daily dose may be discarded when the intravenous solution tubing is changed. Infusion solution filters may also prevent drug delivery by direct adsorption of the drug or by allowing a heavier drug to settle in the filtration chamber and mix slowly with the infusion solution. For drug therapy in which the driving force for tissue entry is a concentration gradient between the circulation and the tissue (e.g., in meningitis), sustained low drug concentrations may provide suboptimal therapy.

Intramuscular administration of drugs to newborns is suboptimal and generally used when there is difficulty maintaining intravenous access. Absorption of drugs from an intramuscular injection site is directly related to muscle perfusion. Patients with hypothermia or shock are unlikely to absorb intramuscular doses effectively. Intramuscular administration of drugs may sclerose tissue or create large intramuscular collections of drugs, which are absorbed slowly, producing a "depot effect" in which serum concentrations increase slowly over a prolonged period. Intramuscular drug administration to newborns, especially for multiple doses, should be avoided because it may not deliver effective drug concentrations to the site of action and may cause disfiguring sterile abscesses in the limited muscle mass of small newborns.

Even though *oral administration* of drugs is preferred for treatment of chronic illnesses in newborns, this route is not well studied. In adults, less drug is usually absorbed from the stomach than from the intestinal tract because of its smaller surface area. Delayed gastric emptying postpones reaching peak serum drug concentrations and prolongs the absorption phase while elimination continues. Many newborns experience gastroesophageal reflux associated with delayed gastric emptying, which may alter drug bioavailability. Passive venous congestion of the intestinal tract from elevated right atrial pressures decreases drug absorption in adults and may do so in premature infants with severe bronchopulmonary dysplasia complicated by cor pulmonale (Peterson et al, 1980). The administration of medications to newborns in small volumes of formula or during continuous gastric feedings may also alter drug absorption. The possible effects of feeding patterns on drug absorption and action must be considered when enteral drug therapy fails.

Distribution

In pharmacokinetics, distribution is the partitioning of drugs among various body fluids, organs, and tissues. The distribution of a drug within the body is determined by several factors including organ blood flow, pH and composition of body fluids and tissues, physical and chemical properties of the drug (e.g., lipid solubility, molecular weight, and ionization constant), and the extent of drug binding to plasma proteins and other macromolecules (Ward et al, 1980).

Important differences among premature infants, children, and adults affect the distribution of drugs. Total body water varies from 85% in premature newborns to 75% in term newborns to 65% in adults (Boreus, 1982). Conversely, body fat content varies from ≤1% in premature infants to 15% in term newborns (Mirkin, 1978). This changes the distribution of many drugs, especially polar, water-soluble drugs, such as the aminoglycosides. Protein binding of drugs in the circulation is decreased in the premature newborn through a decrease in the total amount of circulating protein and through decreased binding affinity by the protein itself. With rare exception, only the free (not bound to protein) drug molecules are "active," that is, cross membranes, exert pharmacologic actions, and undergo metabolism and excretion. Clinical measurements of serum or plasma drug concentrations usually reflect total circulating drug concentrations, which include both free and protein-bound drug. Thus, total circulating drug concentrations in the newborn, which are low by adult standards, may represent free drug concentrations that are equivalent to those of the adult because of the decreased protein binding in the newborn.

Metabolism

Many drugs require metabolic conversion before elimination from the body. Biotransformation of a drug usually produces a more polar, less lipid-soluble molecule that can then be eliminated rapidly by renal, biliary, or other routes of excretion. Drug biotransformation is classified into two broad categories: (1) nonsynthetic (Phase I) reactions, which include oxidation, reduction, and hydrolysis, and (2) synthetic or conjugation (Phase II) reactions, which include glucuronidation, sulfation, and acetylation. Although the liver is considered the major organ responsible for drug biotransformation, many other organs carry out drug metabolism.

For most drugs in the newborn, the half-life is prolonged and total body clearance is decreased. Important variations occur, however, among drug classes and among individuals. Glucuronide conjugation of bilirubin is usually low at birth unless this enzyme has been induced in utero through maternal exposure to drugs, cigarette smoke, or other inducing agents (Ward et al, 1980). In contrast, conjugation through sulfation is usually active at birth. Various factors after birth, such as nutrition, illness, or drug interactions, may hasten or retard the maturation of enzymes and organs responsible for drug metabolism in the newborn. Maturational changes in hepatic blood flow, drug transport into hepatocytes, synthesis of serum proteins, protein binding of drugs, and biliary secretion—alone and in combination—confound accurate predictions about drug metabolism after birth, which leads to empiric dose adjustments (Morselli et al, 1980). These factors must be restudied in the very immature, very-low-birth-weight infant.

Excretion

Another major pathway for drug elimination from the body is renal excretion of metabolized and unchanged drug. Neonatal renal function is diminished both in absolute terms and when normalized to body weight or surface area.

The neonatal glomerular filtration rate averages about 30% of the adult rate per unit surface area. Glomerular function increases steadily after birth whereas tubular function matures more slowly, causing a glomerular and tubular imbalance (Aperia et al, 1981). The postnatal increase in glomerular function reflects increased cardiac output, decreased renal vascular resistance, redistribution of intrarenal blood flow, and changes in intrinsic glomerular basement membrane permeability (Morselli et al, 1980). The dynamics of neonatal renal function markedly influence drug excretion. The rate of change of renal function and its susceptibility to hypoxemia, nephrotoxic drugs, and underperfusion confound predictions of drug elimination rates, which must be measured empirically.

PHARMACOKINETIC PRINCIPLES

Pharmacokinetics describes the time course of changes in drug concentrations within the body. Although rates of change are often described with differential equations, concepts useful at the bedside are emphasized here. More detailed mathematical discussions of pharmacokinetics are presented elsewhere (Gibaldi and Perrier, 1982; Greenblatt and Koch-Weser, 1975a and 1975b; Notari, 1980).

Compartment

In pharmacokinetics, compartment refers to fluid and tissue spaces into which drugs penetrate. These compartments may or may not be equivalent to anatomic or physiologic fluid volumes. In the simplest case, the compartment may correspond to the vascular space and equal the volume of a real body fluid, blood. Large or quite polar molecules may be confined to this central compartment until they are eliminated by excretion or metabolism. Many drugs, however, diffuse reversibly out of the central compartment into tissues or other fluid spaces, referred to generically as peripheral or tissue compartments. Such compartments are seldom sampled directly, but their involvement in kinetic processes may be recognized from the graphic or mathematical description of the kinetics of a drug.

Apparent Volume of Distribution

The apparent volume of distribution might be better termed "volume of dilution" because it is a mathematical description of the volume (L or L/kg) required for dilution of a dose (mg or mg/kg) to produce the observed circulating drug concentration (mg/L or μg/mL). (To simplify cancellation of units, concentrations are expressed here as mg/L, which is the same as μg/mL, the more conventional units for drug concentrations.)

$$\text{Concentration (mg/L)} = \frac{\text{Dose (mg/kg)}}{\text{Apparent volume of distribution (L/kg)}}$$

For many drugs, the volume of distribution does not correspond to a specific physiologic body fluid or tissue, hence the term "apparent." In fact, the volume of distribution for drugs that are bound extensively in tissues may exceed 1.00 L/kg, a physiologic impossibility that emphasizes the arithmetic, nonphysiologic nature of the apparent volume of distribution. The calculation of distribution volume is outlined later.

First-Order Kinetics

Removal of most drugs from the body can be described by first-order (exponential or proportional) kinetics, in which a constant proportion or percentage of a drug is removed over time, rather than a constant amount over time. For drugs exhibiting first-order kinetics, the higher the concentration, the greater the amount removed. The following equations describe the concentration (C) of a drug whose first-order kinetics have a rate constant, k (min^{-1}), at time (t) and an initial concentration of C_0.

In differential form, the change in C with time is:

$$\frac{dC}{dt} = -kC$$

In exponential form, C at time t is:

$$C_t = C_0 e^{-kt}$$

If integrated, C at time t is expressed as the natural logarithm (ln):

$$\ln C_t = \ln C_0 - kt$$

The latter equation fits the equation of a straight line so that a graph that plots $\ln C_t$ versus t has an intercept of $\ln C_0$ at t = 0 and a slope of $-k$, the rate constant for the change in concentration, which can be used to calculate the half-life and dosages. Multiple rate constants in more complex equations are distinguished with the letter k and numbered subscripts or with Greek letters.

Half-Life

The drug half-life ($t_{1/2}$) is the time required for a drug concentration to decrease by 50%. Half-life is a first-order kinetic process because the same proportion, 50%, of the drug is removed during equal time periods. Half-life can be determined mathematically from the elimination rate constant, k:

$$t_{1/2} = \frac{\text{natural logarithm 2}}{k} = \frac{0.693}{k}$$

Figure 37–1 illustrates a graphic method for determination of half-life. Drug concentrations measured serially are graphed on semilogarithmic axes, and the best-fit line is determined either visually or by linear regression analysis. In this illustration of first-order kinetics, the concentration decreases 50% (from 800 to 400) during the 1st hour and decreases another 50% (from 400 to 200) during the 2nd hour. Thus, the half-life is 1 hour. More drug is removed during one half-life at higher concentrations, although the proportion removed remains constant. The exponential equation for this graph is C = $800e^{-0.0116t}$, where k = 0.0116/minute and C_0 = 800, allowing a mathematical

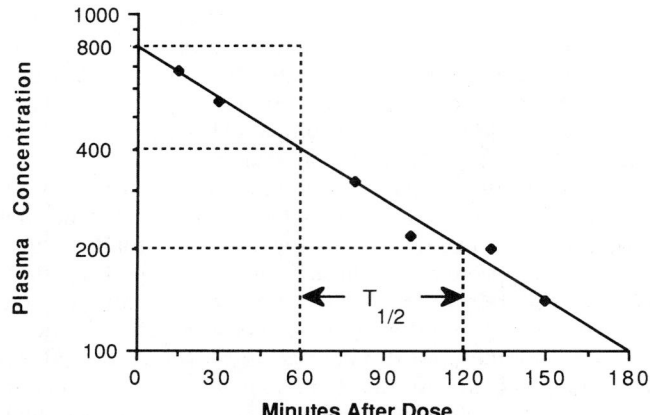

FIGURE 37–1. Apparent single-compartment, first-order plasma drug disappearance curve illustrating graphic determination of half-life from best-fit line of serial plasma concentrations.

calculation of half-life using the equation previously described.

$$t_{1/2} = \frac{0.693}{k(\text{minute}^{-1})} = \frac{0.693}{0.0116/\text{minute}} = 60 \text{ minutes}$$

Multicompartment, First-Order Kinetics

The rate of removal of many drugs from the circulation is biphasic. The initial rapid decrease in concentration is the distribution (α) phase, often lasting 15 to 45 minutes, which is followed by a sustained slower rate of removal, the elimination (β) phase. Such biphasic processes are best visualized from semilogarithmic graphs of concentration versus time. When such semilogarithmic graphs reveal kinetics that best fit two straight lines, the kinetics are described as biexponential or two-compartment, first-order (Fig. 37–2). Two exponential terms are needed to describe such changes in concentration:

$$C = Ae^{-\alpha t} + Be^{-\beta t}$$

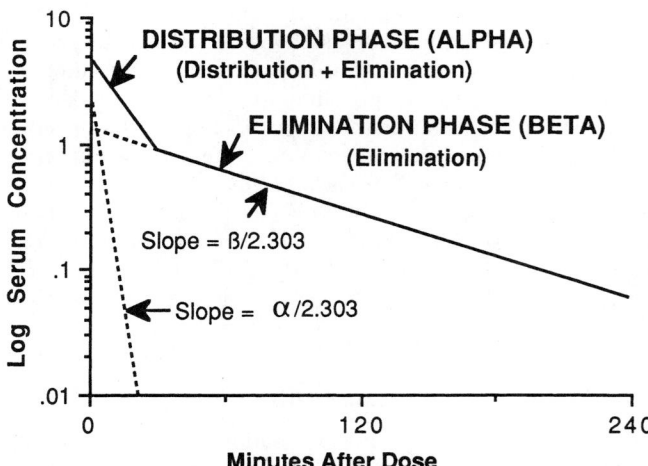

FIGURE 37–2. Multicompartment serum drug disappearance curve.

In this equation, the rate constant for distribution is designated α to discriminate it from the rate constant for elimination (β), where A and B are the time = 0 intercepts for the lines describing distribution and elimination, respectively. Division by 2.303 converts logarithms to natural logarithms.

After an intravenous dose, drug loss from the vascular space during the distribution phase occurs through both distribution and elimination (see Fig. 37–2). The rate constant of distribution (α) can be determined by plotting the difference between the total amount of drug lost initially and the amount of drug lost through elimination (Greenblatt et al, 1975a). This produces the line with the steeper slope (equal to α) below the serum concentration graph in Figure 37–2. The single slope of the distribution phase and of the elimination phase does not imply that distribution or elimination occurs through a single process. The observed rates usually represent the summation of several simultaneous processes, each with differing rates, occurring in various tissues.

When the time course of drug elimination is observed for prolonged periods, a third rate of elimination, or γ phase, may be observed which is usually attributed to elimination of drug that has reequilibrated from deep tissue compartments back into the plasma. Such kinetics are designated *three-compartment* and *first-order.* The kinetics of a drug are expressed with the smallest number of compartments that accurately describes its concentration changes over time.

Apparent Single-Compartment, First-Order Kinetics

When a semilogarithmic graph of concentration versus time reveals a single slope with no distribution phase, the kinetics are characterized as "apparent" first-order (see Fig. 37–1). This may occur when a drug remains entirely within the vascular space or central compartment or when a drug passes very rapidly back and forth between the circulation and peripheral sites until it is metabolized or excreted by first-order kinetics. The adjective "apparent" is used because careful study often reveals distribution does occur although the kinetic curve has only a single slope. Single-compartment kinetics implies that the drug rapidly and completely distributes homogeneously throughout the body, which rarely occurs clinically.

In many pharmacokinetic studies in newborns, blood samples are not obtained early enough to calculate the distribution phase, and the kinetics are described as single compartment. If sampling begins after the distribution phase, the concentration time points may fit a first-order, single-compartment model, which determines the elimination rate constant (β). The kinetics cannot be assumed, however, to fit a single-compartment model from such a limited study. The most accurate approach to kinetic analysis, "noncompartmental analysis," makes no assumptions about the number of compartments (Gibaldi and Perrier, 1982; Notari, 1980).

Zero-Order Kinetics

Some drugs demonstrate zero-order kinetics in which a constant amount of drug is removed over time, rather than

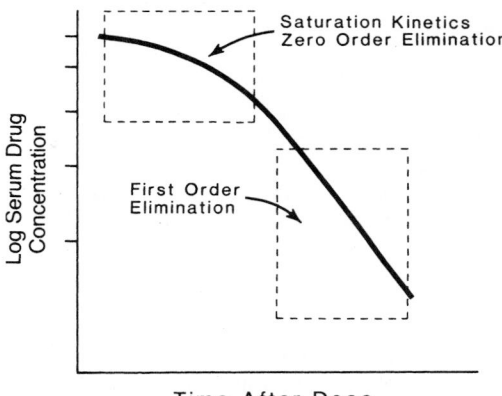

FIGURE 37–3. Representation of saturation, or zero-order (serum concentration–dependent), and first-order (serum concentration–independent) pharmacokinetics.

a constant proportion or percentage. This relationship can be expressed as $dC/dt = -k$. It is important to understand when zero-order kinetics occurs, how to recognize it, and how it affects drug concentrations. Zero-order kinetics is sometimes referred to as "saturation kinetics" because it may occur when excess amounts of drug completely saturate enzymes or transport systems so that they metabolize or transport only a constant amount of drug over time. Zero-order processes produce a curvilinear shape in a semilogarithmic graph of concentrations versus time (Fig. 37–3). When drug concentrations are high from inappropriate dosing or a drug overdose, kinetics may be zero-order, followed by first-order kinetics at lower concentrations. For drugs exhibiting zero-order kinetics, small increments in dose may cause disproportionately large increments in serum concentration. Certain drugs administered to newborns exhibit zero-order kinetics at therapeutic doses and concentrations and need to be recognized for their potential accumulation (Table 37–2).

Target Drug Concentration Strategy

Drug treatment of newborns frequently uses the target drug concentration strategy (Table 37–3) in which drug therapy corrects a specific problem by producing an effective concentration of free drug at a specific site of action (Sheiner et al, 1978). The target site of drug action is usually inaccessible for monitoring concentrations.

The requirements for effective and accurate application of the target drug concentration treatment in adults have been discussed by Spector and colleagues (1988). When applied to newborns, these requirements highlight the spe-

TABLE 37–2

Drugs that Demonstrate Saturation Kinetics with Therapeutic Doses in Newborns

Caffeine	Furosemide
Chloramphenicol	Indomethacin
Diazepam	Phenytoin

TABLE 37–3

Target Drug Concentration Strategy

Drug dose	→	Plasma total drug concentration	↔	Plasma unbound drug concentration	↔	Target site unbound drug concentration	→	Desired pharmacologic effect

Data from Sheiner LB, Tozer TN: Clinical pharmacokinetics: The use of plasma concentrations of drugs. *In* Melmon KL, Morrelli, HF (Eds): Clinical Pharmacology: Basic Principles in Therapeutics, 2nd ed. New York, Macmillan, 1978, p 71.

cial problems of drug therapy in these patients and the special circumstances in which clinical drug concentration monitoring is appropriate. Some of these requirements include the following:

1. An available analytic procedure for accurate measurement of drug concentrations in small volumes of blood
2. A wide variation in pharmacokinetics among individuals with the knowledge that population-based kinetics do not accurately predict individual kinetics
3. Drug effects that are proportional to plasma drug concentrations
4. A narrow concentration range between efficacy and toxicity (narrow therapeutic index)
5. Constant pharmacologic effect over time in which tolerance does not develop
6. Clinical studies that have determined the therapeutic and toxic drug concentration ranges

Therapeutic Drug Monitoring

Table 37–3 illustrates the basic assumptions of therapeutic drug monitoring: that total plasma drug concentrations correlate with dose as well as with circulating unbound drug concentrations and unbound drug concentration at the site of action. Clinical measurements of drug concentrations usually include both bound and unbound drug, while the active portion is that which is unbound (see Distribution). There are two broad indications for monitoring drug concentrations: (1) attainment of effective concentrations and (2) avoidance of toxic concentrations. As pointed out by Kauffman (1981), drug concentration ranges are not absolute reflections of effective therapy. Patient response, not a specific drug concentration range, is the end point of therapy.

Although concentrations of aminoglycoside antibiotics, such as gentamicin, are monitored frequently in newborns, toxicity is rare in newborns compared with adults (McCracken, 1986). Because of the limited evidence of toxicity in newborns, it is more important to measure aminoglycoside concentrations to achieve effective concentrations for treatment of culture-proven infections than to avoid toxicity. In newborns with serious therapeutic problems, measurement of serum drug concentrations should be used to achieve effective concentrations as well as to avoid toxicity. When the desired concentration range and kinetic parameters are known, doses may be estimated to reach that concentration with single bolus doses or bolus doses followed by continuous infusions.

Kinetic Dosing

The following equations can be used both to guide dosing and to derive kinetic parameters for individual patients.

Where C = concentration and Vd = volume of distribution:

$$\text{Dose} = \Delta C \cdot Vd = [C \text{ desired} - C \text{ initial}] \cdot VD$$
$$(\text{mg/kg}) = (\text{mg/L})(\text{L/kg}) = \qquad (\text{mg/L}) \qquad (\text{L/kg})$$

This equation may be used to estimate dosage changes needed to increase or decrease concentration. For the first dose, the starting concentration is zero; for doses after the first, the calculation of distribution volume should use the change (Δ) in concentration from the preceding trough to the peak associated with that dose. To reach a desired concentration rapidly, a loading dose can be administered followed by a sustaining infusion. The equation for calculation of infusion doses to maintain a constant concentration is shown below.

Where C = concentration, Vd = volume of distribution, and k = rate constant of elimination:

$$\text{Infusion rate} = k \cdot Vd \cdot C$$
$$(\text{mg/kg} \cdot \text{minute}^{-1}) \quad (\text{minute}^{-1}) \quad (\text{L/kg}) \quad (\text{mg/L})$$

Steady state is reached when tissues are in equilibrium and the amount of drug removed equals the amount of drug infused. The time to reach a steady state depends on the elimination half-life and is *not* shortened by the administration of a loading dose.

Repetitive Dosing and the "Plateau Principle"

During the typical course of drug therapy, drug doses are administered before complete elimination of the previous dose, and the kinetics are more complex (Greenblatt et al, 1975b). During repeated administration, the peak and trough levels after each dose increase for a time. Steady state, or plateau, concentrations are reached when the amount of drug eliminated equals the amount of drug administered during each dosing interval. During repetitive dosing, the steady-state concentrations achieved are related to the half-life, dose, and dosing interval relative to the half-life (Greenblatt et al, 1975b).

Figure 37–4 illustrates a hypothetical concentration-time curve for a drug with a half-life of 4 hours administered orally every 4 hours, so the dosing interval corresponds to one half-life. Several important principles of pharmacoki-

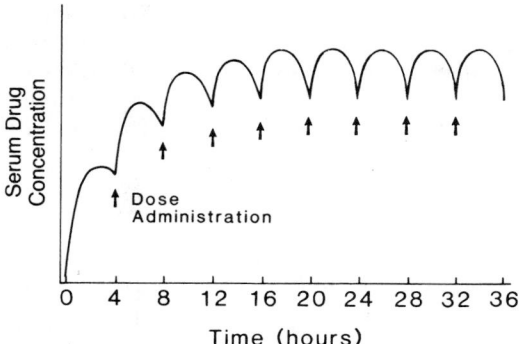

FIGURE 37–4. Representation of multiple dosing with accumulation of serum drug levels to steady-state concentration.

netics are illustrated in this figure, with the mathematics described in detail elsewhere (Greenblatt et al, 1975b). Drug concentrations increase and decrease with drug administration (absorption) and elimination. For dosing intervals of one half-life, accumulation is 88% complete after the third dose, 94% complete after the fourth dose, and 97% complete after the fifth dose. At steady state, the peak and trough concentrations between doses are the same after each dose. If a drug is administered with a dosing interval equal to one half-life, the steady-state peak and trough concentrations are two times those reached after the first dose. If the dosing interval is shortened to half of a half-life, the concentration decreases less before the next dose, more total drug is administered per day, and the steady-state peak and trough concentrations are considerably higher (3.4 times the peak and trough concentrations after the first dose). Thus, the shorter the dosing interval-to–half-life ratio, the greater the degree of drug accumulation. As noted during infusions, the *length of time* required to reach steady-state concentrations depends primarily on the elimination half-life, not the dosing interval.

If the time to reach a therapeutic concentration is excessive, a loading dose can be administered, based on the desired concentration and estimated distribution volume. Care must be exercised with such doses because toxic concentrations may be reached if the patient has a decreased distribution volume or if certain tissues preferentially absorb the particular drug. Digoxin exhibits the latter problem, so the loading dose is usually divided into two or three smaller doses to decrease toxicity while shortening the time to reach a therapeutic concentration.

PHARMACOKINETIC PRACTICALITIES
Dose Adjustments

Gentamicin and phenobarbital can be used to illustrate the practical application of the principles of pharmacokinetics and therapeutic drug monitoring already outlined. The calculations may be carried out at the bedside with standard arithmetic calculators.

Gentamicin

Assume that optimal gentamicin concentrations are 10 µg/mL ≥ peak ≥ 6 µg/mL; 2 µg/mL ≥ trough ≥ 0.5 µg/mL.

Gentamicin peak concentration was 5.0 µg/mL, and 18 hours later the trough was 2.5 µg/mL after the fourth 2.5 mg/kg dose was administered intravenously to an edematous premature newborn. It is apparent that the distribution volume is greater than predicted because the peak concentration is lower than anticipated, and the half-life is longer than anticipated because the trough is higher than expected. The times of drug infusion and blood sampling were confirmed (an important step), so the half-life is 18 hours because the concentration decreases 50% from 5.0 to 2.5 µg/mL in 18 hours. (This assumes that the kinetics are linear and first-order.)

$$\begin{array}{l}\text{Volume of} \\ \text{distribution} \\ \text{(mL/kg)}\end{array} = \frac{\text{Dose (mg/kg)}}{\Delta \text{ Concentration (µg/mL)} \cdot 1 \text{ mg/1000 µg}}$$

$$= \frac{2.5 \text{ mg/kg} \cdot 1000 \text{ µg/mg}}{(5.0 - 2.5)\ (\text{µg/mL})}$$

$$= 1000 \text{ mL/kg}$$

To ensure a trough concentration of 2.0 µg/mL or less, doses are administered every two half-lives or every 36 hours. When two half-lives have passed after the fourth dose, the gentamicin concentration should be about 1.25 µg/mL (50% of 2.5 µg/mL). To increase the concentration from the 1.25 µg/mL trough to >6 µg/mL requires a concentration difference of ≥4.75-µg/mL. A dose of 4.75 mg/kg is selected and estimated to produce a peak concentration of 6 µg/mL. In one half-life, this concentration will decrease to 3.0 µg/mL, and in two half-lives or 36 hours, to 1.5 µg/mL. Another 4.75-mg/kg dose will increase the peak to 6.25 µg/mL, which will decrease to 3.12 µg/mL in one half-life and to 1.6 µg/mL in two half-lives. The variation between the peak and trough concentrations after the last dose is within the measurement error for gentamicin and should achieve the optimum concentrations defined above.

Phenobarbital

Seizures that were hard to control developed in a 3.6-kg asphyxiated newborn. Seizures continued after two 20-mg/kg phenobarbital doses until an additional 10-mg/kg dose was administered. A maintenance dose of 7 mg/kg per day was started 24 hours after the loading doses were administered. At 10 days, this child was increasingly somnolent. A phenobarbital level drawn 2 hours after the oral maintenance dose was 50 µg/mL. Additional doses were held, and the phenobarbital concentration was checked daily, as follows: 24 hours = 40 µg/mL; 48 hours = 31 µg/mL; 72 hours = 25 µg/mL; 96 hours = 21 µg/mL. The maintenance dose (7 mg/kg) was resumed immediately after the 21 µg/mL concentration was measured and produced a concentration of 30 µg/mL. These concentrations and dosages can be used to calculate the volume of distribution and a dose to maintain the phenobarbital concentration between 20 and 30 µg/mL.

$$\text{Volume of distribution (L/kg)} = \frac{\text{Dose (mg/kg)}}{\Delta \text{Concentration (}\mu\text{g/mL)} = \text{mg/L)}}$$

$$= \frac{7.0 \text{ (mg/kg)}}{(30-21) \text{ (mg/L)}}$$

$$= \frac{7 \text{ (mg/kg)}}{9 \text{ (mg/L)}}$$

$$= 0.78 \text{ L/kg}$$

Half-life can be determined from inspection because the concentration decreased from 50 to 25 μg/mL in 72 hours. Thus, it should take 72 hours for the concentration to decrease by 15 μg/mL from 30 to 15 μg/mL. The concentration will decrease approximately 5 μg/mL every 24 hours, or one third of a half-life. Dividing the half-life into fractions is an approximation because it estimates the change in concentration as linear rather than exponential. To be more accurate, the concentration decreases 59% in half of one half-life. Although this approximation violates certain principles of pharmacokinetics, it allows estimation of the change in concentration for each one third of a half-life as one third of the change during one half-life. Thus, the concentration decreases about 5 μg/mL in 24 hours. The following approach can be used to estimate the daily phenobarbital dose needed to return the concentration to 30 μg/mL, a change in concentration of 5 μg/mL.

$$\Delta \text{Concentration (mg/L)} = \frac{\text{Dose (mg/kg)}}{\text{Volume of distribution (L/kg)}}$$

$$5 \text{ (mg/L)} = \frac{\text{Dose (mg/kg)}}{(0.78) \text{ (L/kg)}}$$

$$3.9 \text{ mg/kg} = \text{Dose (mg/kg)}$$

BREAST-MILK DRUG EXCRETION

The excretion of drugs in breast milk remains a source of confusion and concern for many physicians and families. Newer analytic techniques and more thorough pharmacokinetic studies have improved the available data in this area of neonatal pharmacology. The available data regarding drug exposure of the newborn through human milk have been organized recently by decreasing levels of concern, from drugs that are clearly contraindicated during nursing to those that are of concern pharmacologically to those that have not been associated with problems during nursing. The list of drugs clearly contraindicated during nursing is surprisingly short (see Appendix 1).

SUMMARY

The extensive drug exposure of the sick newborn in the NICU is dangerous because of the frequency of adverse, sometimes fatal, drug reactions. Unfortunately, in the rapidly changing fetus and newborn, drug therapy is often empiric owing to a lack of gestational age–appropriate kinetic data. Methods appropriate for the study of therapeutics in newborns present unique difficulties, but a re-

view by Ward and Green (1988) may provide assistance for investigators. Drug therapy of newborns requires practical application of the principles of pharmacokinetics and pharmacodynamics that describe the processes of drug absorption, distribution, metabolism, and excretion to estimate and individualize dosages.

REFERENCES

American Society of Hospital Pharmacists: ASHP guidelines on preventing medication errors in hospitals. Am J Hosp Pharm 50:305, 1993.

Aperia A, Broberger O, Elinder G, et al: Postnatal development of renal function in pre-term and full-term infants. Acta Paediatr Scand 70:183, 1981.

Aranda JV, Cohen S, Neims AH: Drug utilization in a newborn intensive care unit. J Pediatr 89:315, 1976.

Aranda JV, Collinge JM, Clarkson S: Epidemiologic aspects of drug utilization in a newborn intensive care unit. Semin Perinatol 6:148, 1982a.

Aranda JV, Portuguez-Malavasi A, Collinge JM, et al: Epidemiology of adverse drug reactions in the newborn. Dev Pharmacol Ther 5:173, 1982b.

Aranda JV: Factors associated with adverse drug reactions in the newborn. Pediatr Pharmacol 3:245, 1983.

Boreus LO: Principles of Pediatric Pharmacology. New York, Churchill Livingstone, 1982.

Burns LE, Hodgman JE, Cass AB: Fatal circulatory collapse in premature infants receiving chloramphenicol. N Engl J Med 261:1318, 1959.

Gibaldi M, Perrier D: Pharmacokinetics, 2nd ed. New York, Marcel Dekker, 1982.

Gould T, Roberts RJ: Therapeutic problems arising from the use of the intravenous route for drug administration. J Pediatr 95:465, 1979.

Greenblatt DJ, Koch-Weser J: Clinical pharmacokinetics (First of two parts). N Engl J Med 293:702, 1975a.

Greenblatt DJ, Koch-Weser J: Clinical pharmacokinetics (Second of two parts). N Engl J Med 293:964, 1975b.

Kauffman RE: The clinical interpretation and application of drug concentration data. Pediatr Clin North Am 28:35, 1981.

McCracken GH: Aminoglycoside toxicity in infants and children. Am J Med 80(Suppl. 6B):172, 1986.

Mirkin BL: Pharmacodynamics and drug disposition in pregnant women, in neonates, and in children. In Melmon KL, Morrelli HF (Eds): Clinical Pharmacology: Basic Principles in Therapeutics, 2nd ed. New York, Macmillan, 1978, p 127.

Morselli PL, Franco-Morselli R, Bossi L: Clinical pharmacokinetics in newborns and infants: Age-related differences and therapeutic implications. Clin Pharmacokinet 5:485, 1980.

Notari RE: Biopharmaceutics and Clinical Pharmacokinetics, 3rd ed. New York, Marcel Dekker, 1980.

Peterson RG, Simmons MA, Rumack BH, et al: Pharmacology of furosemide in the premature newborn infant. J Pediatr 97:139, 1980.

Physician Insurers Association of America: Medication Error Study. Washington, DC, June, 1993.

Proceedings: Understanding and preventing drug misadventures. Am J Health Syst Pharm 52:369, 1995.

Roberts RJ: Drug Therapy in Infants: Pharmacologic Principles and Clinical Experience. Philadelphia, WB Saunders, 1984, p 3.

Sheiner LB, Tozer TN: Clinical pharmacokinetics: The use of plasma concentrations of drugs. In Melmon KL, Morrelli HF (Eds): Clinical Pharmacology: Basic Principles in Therapeutics, 2nd ed. New York, Macmillan, 1978, p 71.

Spector R, Park GD, Johnson GF, et al: Therapeutic drug monitoring. Clin Pharmacol Ther 43:345, 1988.

Sutherland JM: Fatal cardiovascular collapse, of infants receiving large amounts of chloramphenicol. J Dis Child 13:761, 1959.

Ward RM, Singh S, Mirkin BL: Fetal clinical pharmacology. In Avery GS (Ed): Drug Treatment: Principles and Practice of Clinical Pharmacology and Therapeutics. 2nd ed. New York, Adis Press, 1980, p 76.

Ward RM, Green TP: Developmental pharmacology and toxicology: Principles of study design and problems of methodology. Pharmacol Ther 36:309, 1988.

Weiss CF, Glazko AJ, Weston JK: Chloramphenicol in the newborn infant: A physiologic explanation of its toxicity when given in excessive doses. N Engl J Med 262:787, 1960.

CHAPTER 38

Outcome and Follow-Up of High-Risk Infants

Marilee C. Allen

RISK OF NEURODEVELOPMENTAL DISABILITY

"Will my child survive?" "What kind of life will my child have?" These are the two questions most frequently asked by parents of infants in a neonatal intensive care unit (NICU). As difficult as it is to predict survival of a sick or very-preterm infant, it is far more difficult to answer questions regarding quality of life for the infant who survives. How much recovery will there be? Will the child develop further complications? Most important, how will this early illness affect or predict the child's neurologic, sensory, and cognitive development?

Only a few conditions (e.g., some chromosome disorders or dysmorphic syndromes) carry certain knowledge of disability, and many of these are associated with shortened life span (see Part IV). For most conditions requiring neonatal intensive care, it is difficult to define the full extent (if any) of damage to or malformation of the infant's organ systems. In addition, the newborn has a remarkable potential for recovery. Few factors hindering or contributing to this recovery have been identified. Predicting the outcome of individuals is therefore difficult.

How is quality of life defined? What is abnormal outcome? The World Health Organization has differentiated the words *impairment*, *disability*, and *handicap* (International Classification of Impairments, Disabilities, and Handicaps, 1980). An *impairment* is a structural, psychological, or physical abnormality; a *disability* is a restriction or inability to perform normally because of impairment; and a *handicap* is a disadvantage in society because of a disability. Most commonly, *high risk* refers to the likelihood of neurodevelopmental disability, which is a group of interrelated, chronic, nonprogressive disorders of the central nervous system caused by injury to or malformation of the developing brain. They form a spectrum, from cerebral palsy (motor impairment) to mental retardation (cognitive impairment), to sensory impairment, and to the more subtle disorders of central nervous system function (Table 38–1). These more subtle disorders of higher cortical function include language disorder, learning disability, minor neuromotor dysfunction, attention deficits, hyperactivity, and behavior problems. Most children with neurodevelopmental disabilities were full-term, were not in a NICU, and had no or few perinatal risk factors (Blair and Stanley, 1988; Ellenberg and Nelson, 1988; Freeman, 1985; Kuban and Leviton, 1994; Louhiala, 1995; Sabel et al, 1976) (see Table 38–1).

Although preterm infants and sick full-term infants have an increased risk of neurodevelopmental disabilities compared with the general population, most do not develop major disability and are quite functional. Most children with disability manifest initial developmental delay, but some have functional limitations without delay in milestone attainment (e.g., the child with a right spastic hemiplegia who walks on time but limps and has a left mature pincer grasp but only a raking grasp on the right). In addition, some children may have developmental delay because of complex medical conditions but do not develop disability (e.g., a child with chronic lung disease who has mild hypotonia and initial motor delay but catches up once the lung disease improves).

A large number of perinatal and demographic risk factors for neurodevelopmental disabilities have been identified. They are so numerous that it is helpful to group them by category (Table 38–2). Not all perinatal and demographic risk factors are equally predictive of developmental disability (Leonard et al, 1990; Skouteli et al, 1985; Stewart et al, 1987; Vohr et al, 1992). A number of obstetric conditions (e.g., abruptio placentae, maternal antepartum hemorrhage, fetal distress during labor) may be catastrophic, leading to death or disability. Prompt intervention may circumvent this. Consequently, obstetric risk factors are weak predictors of neurodevelopmental disability. Associated neonatal conditions (e.g., severe hypoxic-ischemic encephalopathy) are better predictors of outcome than either preceding obstetric conditions or measures of the infant's condition at the time of birth (e.g., Apgar scores, need for resuscitation) (Ellenberg and Nelson, 1988; Nelson and Leviton, 1991; Robertson and Finer, 1985; Skouteli et al, 1985; Yeo and Tudehope, 1994).

Different risk factors predict different neurodevelopmental disabilities. Socioeconomic status is strongly related to cognition but has little effect on cerebral palsy (except as it may be related to preterm birth, intrauterine growth retardation, and other biologic risk factors) (Dammann et al, 1996; Drillien et al, 1980; Forfar et al, 1994; Hack et al, 1994; Louhiala, 1995; Low et al, 1982; Ross et al, 1991; Vohr et al, 1992; Weisglas-Kuperus et al, 1993). Severity is also important to consider: The more severe the hypoxic-ischemic encephalopathy, the more extensive the neuroimaging abnormalities, or the greater number of abnormalities on neurodevelopmental examination, the higher the risk of disability (Allen and Capute, 1989; Aziz et al, 1995; Robertson and Finer, 1985; Rogers et al, 1994; Roth et al, 1993; Rutherford et al, 1994; Stewart et al, 1987). Size and location of intraparenchymal cysts predict both likelihood and type of cerebral palsy (Fawer et al, 1987; Rogers et al, 1994) (see Part X).

Multiple risk factors increase the risk of developmental disability, either by additive or multiplicative effects. The effects of prematurity and intrauterine growth retardation on cognition are greatest in infants with low socioeconomic status (Dammann et al, 1996; Drillien et al, 1980; Forfar et al, 1994; Hack et al, 1994; Low et al, 1992; Ross et al, 1991; Vohr et al, 1992). Abnormalities on cranial ultrasonography and neonatal neurodevelopmental examination are powerful predictors of neurodevelopmental disability in very-preterm infants (Dubowitz et al, 1984; Stewart et

TABLE 38-1

Prevalence of Neurodevelopmental Disabilities in the General Population

Disability	Descriptor	Prevalence (%)*
Major disability	CP + MR†	2–3
Cerebral palsy	Motor impairment	0.1–0.3
Mental retardation	I.Q.‡ <70	1–2
Mild mental retardation	I.Q. 50–70	1.5
Severe mental retardation	I.Q. <50	0.5
Sensory impairments		
Visual impairment	Severe	0.4–0.6
Hearing impairment	Severe	1.5–2.0
Disorders of higher cortical function		
Language delay/speech defects		4–11
Learning disability		5–10
Attention-deficit disorder		6–20
Minor neuromotor dysfunction		5–15

*Prevalence figures adapted from Boyle CA, Decoufle P, Yeargin-Allsopp M. Prevalence and health impact of developmental disabilities in U.S children. Reproduced by permission of PEDIATRICS, Vol 93, Pages 399–403, 1994.

†CP + MR, Cerebral palsy and mental retardation.

‡I.Q., Intelligence quotient (2 SD below the mean varies by test, may be 68 or 70).

al, 1988; Weisglas-Kuperus et al, 1992). The most immature infants have the highest incidence of severe abnormalities on cranial ultrasonography, chronic lung disease, and neurodevelopmental disability (Allen et al, 1993; Aziz et al, 1995; Hack et al, 1994; Regev et al, 1995). The fact that many sick infants have multiple risk factors contributes to the difficulty of attributing risk to individual factors.

Neither risk nor statistical association implies causation (Forfar et al, 1994; Freeman, 1985; Kuban and Leviton, 1994; Nelson and Leviton, 1991). In a comprehensive long-term follow-up study of preterm infants, Drillien and colleagues (1980) found that preterm infants "who showed no evidence of early intrauterine insult and who were neurologically normal in the first year of life were largely indistinguishable from control children reared in similar homes." Prematurity, intrauterine growth retardation, or poor respiratory effort at birth all may be caused by some insult or malformation that occurred prenatally. An abnormal fetus may grow poorly, may precipitate preterm delivery, may not descend properly, or may not breathe immediately at birth. After delivery, the infant may be small or immature (or both), with low Apgar scores, poor feeding, or an abnormal neurodevelopmental examination. All these factors are predictive of outcome, but it is the fetal abnormality that causes the infant's disability. Unfortunately, prenatal injury or subtle central nervous system malformations cannot be adequately assessed. The cause of a child's neurodevelopmental disability is often difficult to determine (see Part X).

Although risk factors cannot be used to diagnose developmental disability, the absence of significant risk factors is reassuring. Because there is always a baseline incidence of neurodevelopmental disability (see Table 38–1), pediatricians should monitor the development of all children during infancy and childhood. Nevertheless, absence of significant risk factors, normal neuroimaging studies, and normal neurodevelopmental examinations can be used to help alleviate parental anxiety related to having an infant in a NICU (Allen and Capute, 1989; Dubowitz et al, 1984; Robertson and Finer, 1985; Rutherford et al, 1994; Stewart et al, 1988; Weisglas-Kuperus et al, 1992). Mildly increased risk, which should be acknowledged, must be put into perspective for parents. Parents of infants with significant or multiple risk factors should be offered focused developmental follow-up and support, especially during those critical early years. Comprehensive, developmentally based follow-up ensures early diagnosis of neurodevelopmental disability, helps to shape early intervention strategies to

TABLE 38-2

Categories of Perinatal Risk Factors

Background characteristics
   Socioeconomic status/social class, parental education, race

Obstetric/prenatal complications
   Maternal acute or chronic illness, maternal ingestion of drugs, congenital infection, multiple gestation, labor or delivery complications (e.g., abruptio placentae, prolapsed cord), placental abnormalities

Physical characteristics
   Prematurity, postmaturity, small for gestational age/intrauterine growth retardation, gender, microcephaly, congenital anomalies, dysmorphic features

Condition at birth
   Apgar scores, cord pH, meconium staining, need for and response to resuscitation

Neonatal complications
   Hypoxia, acidosis, hypotension/shock, apnea and bradycardia, chronic lung disease, sepsis, meningitis, seizures, hypoxic-ischemic encephalopathy

Measures of central nervous system structure and function
   Intraventricular hemorrhage, intraparenchymal hemorrhage, ventricular dilation, cortical atrophy, intraparenchymal cysts or echodensities (periventricular leukomalacia), burst-suppression pattern on electroencephalogram, abnormal neonatal neurodevelopmental examination

meet the infant's and family's evolving needs, and provides parents with continuity and ongoing support during their difficult period of uncertainty and adjustment.

Uncertainty regarding a child's outcome is difficult for both parents and professionals. Experience with other infants and a knowledge of the literature help the clinician to describe the range of outcomes and to some degree their likelihood, based on the circumstances surrounding an individual infant. Helping parents to recognize and cope with their fears allows them to develop a realistic plan for the future, including identifying family and community resources.

NEURODEVELOPMENTAL OUTCOME

This section describes the outcome for several groups of high-risk infants cared for in NICUs. The reported incidences of disability vary from study to study because of a number of factors: variations in study criteria, ethnic and demographic composition of the populations, obstetric and neonatal care practices, follow-up rate, length of follow-up, and how outcome was assessed. High follow-up rates are preferable, but they are difficult to attain. Low follow-up rates raise the concern that bias was introduced when infants did not return for follow-up, either because of impairment or because they had no problems.

How the children are followed, and for how long, affects what neurodevelopmental disabilities are reported. Studies that follow infants to 1 year focus on the major disabilities (cerebral palsy and mental retardation) but are inadequate for assessing mild cerebral palsy, mild mental retardation, or borderline intelligence. Although diagnostic accuracy improves at 18 to 24 months, the follow-up rate is generally lower. Mild to moderate sensory impairments may be missed if specific evaluations of hearing and vision are not performed. Follow-up from 2 to 6 years can begin to describe minor neuromotor dysfunction, behavior problems, attention deficits, and language delay. Questions about learning disability and other school-related problems, however, require follow-up to school age.

Longitudinal studies have found an increased incidence of school problems the longer the children are followed (Hunt et al, 1982; Saigal et al, 1984, 1990, 1991, 1994; Victorian Infant Collaborative Study Group, 1991). This finding suggests that the younger child with more subtle impairments often has some ability to compensate for learning difficulties or inefficiencies. In the higher grades, the work becomes more complex, and efficiency becomes important in completing work and test-taking. The child with subtle impairments may at this point begin to demonstrate learning disability.

Preterm Infants

Most prematurity follow-up studies report outcome related to birth weight because it is more reliably measured than gestational age (Tables 38–3 and 38–4). Very-low-birth-weight (VLBW) infants have birth weights below 1500 g (3 pounds, 5 ounces), extremely low-birth-weight (ELBW) infants have birth weights below 1000 g (2 pounds, 3 ounces), and incredibly-low-birth-weight (ILBW) infants have birth weights below 750 to 800 g (1 pound, 1 ounce).

Major Disability

Although preterm infants have a higher incidence of all neurodevelopmental disabilities than full-term infants, most preterm infants are free of major disability (cerebral palsy or mental retardation) (see Table 38–3). In a meta-analysis of 110 studies published between 1960 and 1990, the median incidence of cerebral palsy in VLBW infants was 7.7%, with a range of 0% to 50% (Escobar et al, 1991). The improved survival of large numbers of extremely preterm infants appears to have led to a modest rise in the prevalence of cerebral palsy (Bhushan et al, 1993; Kuban and Leviton, 1994). Multiple disability occurs in 1.2% to 4.5% of infants with birth weights below 1500 g, 14% to 16% with birth weights below 800 g, and 8% to 13% of infants born before 28 weeks' gestation.

One difficulty with reporting the incidence of cerebral palsy in these studies is variability in definition of cerebral palsy. The most common type of cerebral palsy in VLBW children is spastic diplegia, and it is frequently mild. There is no uniform agreement on whether the child with tight heel cords and hyper-reflexia who toe walks initially but walks by age 2 should be classified as having cerebral palsy (versus mild motor impairment, called here *minor neuromotor dysfunction*). Although some children require physical therapy and even bracing (frequently ankle-foot orthoses), most have little, if any, functional motor impairment at school age (Kitchen et al, 1987; Scottish Low Birthweight Study Group, 1992). They are at higher risk for school and behavior problems, which may be far more devastating than their mild cerebral palsy (Dammann et al, 1996; Drillien et al, 1980; Khadilkar et al, 1993; Marlow et al, 1989; Vohr and Garcia-Coll, 1985; Weisglas-Kuperus et al, 1994).

Populations of preterm children demonstrate a normal range of intelligence. Although only some studies have shown that VLBW and ELBW children have lower intelligence quotients (I.Q.s) than full-term control subjects, a meta-analysis of 80 studies published between 1979 and 1989 found that the mean I.Q./developmental quotient (D.Q.) for low-birth-weight (LBW) children with birth weight below 2500 g was 97.8 ± 6.2, significantly lower than that of full-term control subjects (103.8 ± 8.2) (Aylward et al, 1989). The six-point I.Q. difference, which was statistically significant only when all LBW children were grouped together, may not be clinically meaningful. It represents *more* children, however, with mental retardation, borderline intelligence, or low average intelligence who have difficulties functioning at school and in society.

In VLBW infants, lower birth weight carries a higher mortality rate but not necessarily a higher incidence of neurodevelopmental disability (Aziz et al, 1995; Forfar et al, 1994; Regev et al, 1995; Saigal et al, 1982, 1984; Thompson et al, 1993; van Zeben-van der Aa et al, 1989). Nevertheless, infants born at the limit of viability appear to have an increased incidence both of perinatal complications and of major disability (Allen et al, 1993; Synnes et al, 1994; Whyte et al, 1993). Only 43% to 81% of infants with birth weights below 750 to 800 g have no abnormalities on follow-up during infancy and preschool years (see Table 38–4). Hack and colleagues (1994) found that preterm children with birth weights below 750 g who were followed

TABLE 38–3

Neurodevelopmental Disability in Preterm Children

Study	Follow-Up Age°	No.	Cerebral Palsy (%)	Mental Retardation (%)	Hearing Loss (%)	Visual Impairment (%)	Learning Disability (%)†
Gestational Age <33 weeks							
Roth, 1993	7–10	206	6	6	4	1	5
Gross, 1992	4	125	9	9	1	1	—
Birth Weight <1750 g							
SLBSG, 1992	4.5	611	5	—	2	1	—
Birth Weight ≤1500 g							
Klein, 1985	5	80	5	5	—	—	10
Kitchen, 1986	2	146	11	4	1	1	—
Van Zeben-van der Aa, 1989	2	944	6	6	0.1	0.1	—
Grogaard, 1990	1.5	462	7.6	6.5	5.4	5.5	—
Ross, 1991	7–8	88	14	8	1	—	48
Hall, 1995	8	324	—	—	—	—	21
Birth Weight ≤1250 g							
Thompson, 1993	2	96	6	4	?1	0	—
Aziz, 1995	1	646	9	5	1	3	—
Robertson, 1994	1	163	7	2	1	1	—
Birth Weight ≤1000 g							
Lefebvre, 1988	5–7	44	9	6.5	6	11	35
VISCG, 1991	8	88	9	—	6	11	23
Teplin, 1991	6	28	11	14	7	12	—
Saigal, 1991	8	129	8‡	8	6	7	52
SMSG, 1994	2	429	9	—	—	4	—

°Age in years at time of follow-up.
†Learning disability, required special education, or failed grade(s).
‡Cerebral palsy rate from Saigal, 1990, study of 78 followed to age 5.
SLBSG, Scottish Low Birthweight Study Group; VISCG, Victorian Infant Collaborative Study Group; SMSG, Survanta Multidose Study Group.

to school age had higher rates of cerebral palsy (9% versus 6%) and mental retardation (21% versus 8%) and lower I.Q.s (Kaufman Assessment Battery Mental Processing Composite Score, 87 ± 15 versus 93 ± 14) than children with birth weights 750 to 1499 g.

The evidence is even stronger when outcome is viewed in terms of gestational age: Only 24% to 68% of infants born before 28 weeks' gestation have no abnormalities on follow-up. As many as 50% to 67% of children born at 23 weeks' gestation develop major disability or sensory impairment (or both), as do 30% to 40% born at 24 to 26 weeks' gestation. Although there are only anecdotal reports of survival at 22 weeks' gestation in the United States, a report from Japan noted that *none* of five survivors born at 22 weeks' gestation were normal at 1 year (Ishizuka, 1990; Nishida, 1993).

Sensory Impairments

Both hearing and visual impairments are more common in the most immature infants. Retinopathy of prematurity causes severe visual impairment in 0.1% to 5.5% of VLBW children, 4% to 12% of ELBW children, and 4% to 25% of ILBW children (Keith and Doyle, 1995) (see Tables 38–3 and 38–4). Myopia is common, occurring in 8% to 21% of VLBW children, and it may be severe (Britton et al, 1981; Hack et al, 1994; Hirata et al, 1983; Kitchen et

al, 1980; LaPine et al, 1995; Lefebvre et al, 1988; Saigal et al, 1982, 1984; Scottish Low Birthweight Study Group, 1992; Teplin et al, 1991). Strabismus is also a common finding in preterm infants and may require surgical correction (Kitchen et al, 1980; Saigal et al, 1984; Scottish Low Birthweight Study Group, 1992; Teplin et al, 1991). Some degree of hearing impairment occurs in 1% to 5% of VLBW infants and in 5% to 20% ILBW infants (Kitchen et al, 1980; Robertson et al, 1994) (see Tables 38–3 and 38–4). Hearing impairment is important to diagnose as early as possible, before language acquisition.

Function at School Age

Most (95%) of VLBW children attend regular schools, but 10% to 48% of VLBW children and 20% to 50% of ELBW children have diagnosed learning disability, require special education, or have failed grades (see Table 38–3). Despite normal intelligence, children with learning disability may have difficulties in processing complex language, in perceiving symbols, or with the fine motor control involved in drawing and writing. When compared with full-term control subjects, VLBW, ELBW, and ILBW children have higher incidences of minor neuromotor dysfunction, language delay, visual-perceptual problems, reading disability, difficulties with arithmetic, and behavior problems (Hall et al, 1995; Marlow et al, 1989; McCormick et al, 1996; Ross

TABLE 38-4

Neurodevelopmental Disability in Incredibly-Low-Birth-Weight Children

Study	Follow-up Age°	No.	Birth Years†	CP (%)‡	MR (%)§	BIQ (%)**	Deaf (%)	Blind (%)	Normal (%)
Birth Weight ≤ 800 g									
Britton, 1981	1–2	37	74–77	14	22	24	5	8	51
Bennett, 1983	0.5–3	16	77–80	6	6	12	0	0	51
Buckwald, 1984	1	54	77–81	6	28	22	—	6	43
Hoffman, 1990	0.5–4	38	83–85	—	16	29	—	—	50
LaPine, 1995	0.3–4	78	86–90	—	—	—	1	5	78
Perlman, 1995	1.5	120	80–89	7	10	—	4	13	70
Birth Weight ≤750 g									
Hirata, 1983	1.8–7	18	75–80	11	17	22	5	—	67
Hack, 1989	1.6	32	82–88	9	3	6	—	13	78
Ferrara, 1991	1	32	88–89	3	—	—	—	9	59
Hack, 1994	6.7	68	82–86	9	21	29	1.5	6	50
Gestational Age <28 weeks									
Nwaesei, 1987	2–4	25	80–82	8	8	24	4	4	68
Walker, 1987	2	24	80–84	17	4	—	—	8	67
Msall, 1992	4.4	153	83–86	5	10	—	—	1	24
Gestational Age <26–27 weeks									
Whyte, 1993	2	322	82–87	16	13	15	3	7	61
Synnes, 1994	1.5	129	83–89	26	15	—	3	15	64
Gestational Age <25 weeks									
Whyte, 1993	2	61	82–87	15††	20	—	10	21	43
Synnes, 1994	1.5	52	83–89	33	19	—	4	12	58
Gestational Age 23 weeks									
Ishizuka, 1990	1	49	86–88	—	—	—	—	—	48
Whyte, 1993	2	12	82–87	16¶	8	—	0	11	50
Synnes, 1994	1.5	9	83–89	33	11	—	0	22	33

°Follow-up age: age at follow-up examination, either range or mean age at follow-up, when range not given.
†Birth years: years during which study samples were born (e.g., 1974–1977).
‡CP, cerebral palsy; sometimes reported as severe neurologic impairment.
§MR, mental retardation; with developmental or intelligence quotient <68 or 70.
**BIQ, borderline intelligence; with developmental or intelligence quotient 68 or 70 to 80 or 85.
††Only severe cerebral palsy was reported.

et al, 1990, 1991; Teplin et al, 1991). These differences persisted even when only preterm children with normal intelligence and no neurologic impairments were included in the data analysis (Klein et al, 1985; Largo et al, 1986; Saigal et al, 1991). Hack and colleagues (1994) found that ILBW children had worse language processing, gross motor function, visual motor abilities, attention, academic achievement, behavior, and social skills than children with birth weights 750 to 1499 g.

Visual-perceptual abnormalities, sensorimotor integration problems, and minor neuromotor dysfunction are often striking findings in preschool and school-age preterm children (Dammann et al, 1996; Drillien et al, 1980; Klein et al, 1985; Saigal et al, 1991; Weisglas-Kuperus et al, 1994). Many preterm children have initial motor delays and persistent mild abnormalities on examination, including asymmetries, tight heel cords, and trunk and upper extremity hypotonia. These findings are consistent with minor neuromotor dysfunction. Children who have neuromotor abnormalities during the first 1 to 2 years who do not develop cerebral palsy (called *transient dystonia* by Drillien and colleagues) have a high incidence of associated school and behavior problems (Drillien et al, 1980; Khadilkar et

al, 1993; Vohr and Garcia-Coll, 1985). In addition, subtle residual motor impairments can lead to many day-to-day problems, including problems with dressing, using playground equipment, and cutting with scissors and poor handwriting. Saigal and coworkers (1994) found that most (86%) 8-year-old ELBW children had some functional limitation that involved cognition, sensation, mobility, or self-care in comparison with 50% of full-term control subjects ($P < 0.0005$).

All these subtle central nervous system abnormalities can have a devastating impact on self-esteem, peer relationships, and school performance. Early recognition and intervention aim to help the child to become more functional in his or her daily life. By improving the child's ability to cope with the demands of school and playground, many secondary social and emotional problems can be prevented or ameliorated.

Small-for-Gestational-Age Infants

The term *small for gestational age* (SGA) is an arbitrary classification that refers to an infant whose intrauterine growth is less than expected for gestational age at birth. It is, in fact, a heterogeneous category, with a wide range of causes, risk of perinatal complications, and outcomes (Allen, 1992). Small size at birth may be due to parental (especially maternal) small size; insult or injury to the fetus; fetal maldevelopment; or deprivation of supply of oxygen or nutrients because of placental insufficiency, maternal ingestion (e.g., cigarettes, alcohol, narcotics), or maternal illness. Degree of risk for death, perinatal complications, and neurodevelopmental disability varies with the cause of the intrauterine growth retardation, timing of the insult (if any), and the perinatal complications that the child encounters (Allen, 1992).

The SGA infant whose mother is small is likely to be only mildly growth retarded and have no increased risk. The child with trisomy 18 is likely to have poor fetal growth early in pregnancy and die within the first several months or develop multiple severe neurodevelopmental disabilities. The SGA infant with fetal alcohol syndrome has prenatal and postnatal growth deficiency and an increased risk of congenital anomalies (e.g., characteristic facies, joint anomalies, ventricular septal defect) and central nervous system dysfunction (e.g., mild to moderate mental retardation, tremors, fine motor incoordination, hyperactivity).

Fetal deprivation of supply of oxygen or nutrients, owing to maternal or placental factors (or both), generally presents later in pregnancy (after 27 or 28 weeks' gestation) and causes asymmetric growth retardation. As Warshaw (1985) has suggested,

> Rather than representing serious pathology, therefore, intrauterine growth retardation can be viewed as an adaptation in which the size of the fetus may be appropriate to the availability of nutrients. Low birth weight may improve the chances for survival with good outcome. The fetus exhibiting intrauterine growth retardation may represent a successful adaptation to a substrate-deficient intrauterine environment.

Although it may be an effective human adaptation to adverse circumstances, there are consequences to this strategy: an increased risk of perinatal complications that can affect survival and outcome (e.g., perinatal asphyxia, hypoglycemia), of hypertension later in life, of short stature, and of neurodevelopmental disabilities (Low et al, 1978, 1982, 1992; Neligan, 1976; Parkinson et al, 1981, 1986; Pena et al, 1988; Wocadlo and Rieger, 1994).

Studies that report developmental outcome of SGA infants generally exclude infants with congenital anomalies, genetic syndromes, or congenital infections. They follow primarily infants with placental insufficiency or unknown cause of intrauterine growth retardation, and they distinguish between the full-term and preterm SGA infant.

Full-Term Small-for-Gestational-Age Infants

Although early neuromotor abnormalities (e.g., abnormal muscle tone, jitteriness) may make it more difficult to care for full-term SGA infants, this population group does not appear to have an increased incidence of major disability or sensory impairment (Fitzhardinge and Steven, 1972; Leijon et al, 1980; Low et al, 1978, 1982; Neligan, 1976; Parkinson et al, 1981; Paz et al, 1995; Westwood et al, 1983). Some have found a lower mean I.Q. in school-age

SGA children, and this lower IQ is generally associated with socioeconomic status or gender (i.e., boys) (Fitzhardinge and Steven, 1972; Low et al, 1992; Neligan, 1976; Paz et al, 1995; Westwood et al, 1983). Studies of populations of children with mental retardation demonstrate a disproportionately greater number of SGA children than expected, although the studies do not differentiate among causes of intrauterine growth retardation (Louhiala, 1995; Sabel et al, 1976).

Speech and language problems, hyperactivity, attention deficit, learning disability, and minor neuromotor dysfunction are more frequent in full-term SGA children than in appropriate-for-gestational-age (AGA) children (Fitzhardinge and Steven, 1972; Low et al, 1992; Neligan, 1976; Paz et al, 1995). Learning deficits or academic failure occurs in as many as 45% to 50% of full-term male SGA school-age children with normal intelligence (Fitzhardinge and Steven, 1972; Low et al, 1992; Paz et al, 1995). Even if there is no evidence of congenital infection or anomalies, the earlier the growth retardation (e.g., noted before 26 weeks' gestation), the higher the incidence of lower I.Q.s, academic difficulties, behavior problems, and attention deficits (Parkinson et al, 1981, 1986).

Preterm Small-for-Gestational-Age Infants

The preterm SGA infant has the disadvantages of both prematurity and intrauterine growth retardation (Matilainen et al, 1987; Pena et al, 1988; Robertson et al, 1990; Thompson et al, 1993; Wocadlo and Rieger, 1994). In addition to being vulnerable to the complications of both conditions, preterm SGA infants may be viewed as having more severe intrauterine growth retardation than most full-term SGA infants because they already manifest growth retardation at the time of their preterm birth.

Major disability occurs in 7% to 23% of preterm SGA children (Table 38–5). Most preterm SGA children have normal intelligence, but the mean I.Q. is often lower than in full-term AGA children and sometimes even preterm AGA children. In preterm children without major disability, minor neuromotor dysfunction, visual-perceptual abnormalities, academic difficulties, and behavior problems are far more common than in the general population (Matilainen et al, 1987; Vohr and Oh, 1983). Learning deficits occur in 36% to 50% of preterm SGA children at 8 to 11 years (Low et al, 1992; Robertson et al, 1990).

It is difficult to determine whether the prematurity or the intrauterine growth retardation makes the greatest contribution to adverse neurodevelopmental outcome. Preterm SGA children do *not* have a higher incidence of major disability when compared with preterm AGA infants matched for *birth weight* and socioeconomic status (Pena et al, 1988; Robertson et al, 1990; Sung et al, 1993; Vohr and Oh, 1983). Although preterm SGA children may initially have lower D.Q./I.Q.s to age 3, there is no difference in I.Q. between birth weight–matched groups at ages 4 and 5 years (Pena et al, 1988; Vohr and Oh, 1983).

There is less agreement when preterm SGA children are matched to preterm AGA children for *gestational age* and socioeconomic status (see Table 38–5). Pena and coworkers (1988) noted a higher incidence of major neurologic problems and a lower D.Q. in preterm SGA children

TABLE 38–5

Neurodevelopmental Outcome in Preterm Infants Small for Gestational Age (SGA) Versus Appropriate for Gestational Age (AGA)

Study	Follow-up Age (years)	No.	SGA Infants MD (%)[*]	SGA Infants D.Q./I.Q.[†]	Birth Weight MD (%)	Birth Weight D.Q./I.Q.	Gestational Age MD (%)	Gestational Age D.Q./I.Q.
Vohr, 1983	5	21	15	n.s.[‡]	12	n.s.[‡]	—	—
Pena, 1988	0.8/1[§]	35	23	88	26	88	5	99[°°]
Robertson, 1990	8	36	17	102	22	102	14	101
Sung, 1993	3	27	7	87	4	82	26	102[°°]
Wocadlo, 1994	1	18	22	—	22	—	—	—

°MD, major disability or neurologic impairment, as defined by authors; generally cerebral palsy and mental retardation and occasionally includes severe sensory impairment.
†D.Q./I.Q., mean developmental quotient (D.Q.) or intelligence quotient (I.Q.).
‡n.s., not significantly different, means not specifically stated.
§0.8/1: D.Q. at 40 weeks from term; neurologic outcome determined at 1 year from term.
°°Significantly different from SGA infants, at least at *P*<0.05 level.

at 1 year, whereas Sung and colleagues (1993) found only a lower mean I.Q. at age 3. Robertson and associates (1990) found only an increased incidence of hyperactivity in 8-year-old preterm SGA children when compared with preterm AGA and full-term control groups. All preterm groups scored worse than full-term control groups, however, on measures of growth, intellectual function, visual-motor integration abilities, reading, arithmetic, and behavior.

The risk of neurodevelopmental disability seems to be related more to size at birth than to maturity. Although both factors confer significant risk, prematurity appears to have a greater influence than intrauterine growth retardation on outcome. Long-term follow-up to school age is important for children with prematurity, intrauterine growth retardation, or both.

Sick Full-Term Infant

The full-term infant may require neonatal intensive care for a variety of reasons, including complications of intrauterine growth retardation, perinatal asphyxia, maternal substance abuse, congenital anomalies, or infection. It is most difficult to predict outcome in infants with poorly understood illness: the newborn with sluggish but eventually good response in the delivery room, the newborn who appears septic but has negative cultures, the newborn who does not feed well initially, and others with undefined illness. Under most circumstances, these children will do well, but for some, initial illness may be a sign of central nervous system disorder or systemic illness that contributes to abnormal outcome. Maternal substance abuse or congenital anomalies may underlie conditions that require neonatal intensive care, thereby adding to risk for disability (see Parts III and V).

One recurring scenario in the NICU is the full-term infant with either subtle or florid signs of perinatal asphyxia (see Parts V and X). Increasing attention to the difficulties of recognizing and defining asphyxia has led to an appreciation of the complexities of determining causes, effects, and outcomes (Ellenberg and Nelson, 1988; Freeman, 1985;

Kuban and Leviton, 1994; Nelson and Leviton, 1991). Because the extent and often the nature of an asphyxiating insult cannot be determined, perinatal asphyxia is described by the effect on the infant (e.g., low Apgar scores, low cord pH, resuscitation required, neonatal signs and symptoms of hypoxic ischemic encephalopathy [HIE]).

Major disability occurs in 11% to 25% of survivors of severe perinatal asphyxia and tends to be severe, including severe mental retardation, spastic quadriplegia or mixed cerebral palsy, microcephaly, seizure disorder, cortical blindness, and hearing impairment (Ishikawa et al, 1987; Robertson and Finer, 1985; Yeo and Tudehope, 1994). Severity of HIE is the best predictor of neurodevelopmental outcome (Robertson and Finer, 1985; Robertson et al, 1989; Yeo and Tudehope, 1994). All infants with severe HIE die or develop major disability. Children with moderate HIE have an increased incidence (21%) of major disability. Even those without major disability have lower scores on tests of intelligence, visual-motor integration, vocabulary, reading, spelling, and arithmetic than either healthy peers or children with mild HIE.

Infants with persistent pulmonary hypertension also have a higher risk of major disability (13% to 24%) and mild impairments (minor neuromotor dysfunction, borderline intelligence, and attention problems) in up to 30% (Bifano and Pfannenstiel, 1988; John et al, 1988; Marron et al, 1992; Walsh-Sukys et al, 1994) (see Part VIII). When specifically tested, children with persistent pulmonary hypertension can have a high incidence of hearing loss (20% to 53%), which is associated with alkalosis and duration of ventilation (Sell et al, 1985; Hendricks-Munoz and Walton, 1988). This hearing loss can be progressive, which highlights the need for serial audiologic evaluations in addition to neurodevelopmental follow-up of this population.

Neonates treated with extracorporeal membrane oxygenation (ECMO) have a variety of life-threatening conditions that carry an increased risk of neurodevelopmental disability. Two percent to 26% of survivors of ECMO develop major disability, and 3% to 21% develop hearing impairment (Table 38–6). Mild disability, including border-

TABLE 38–6

Neurodevelopmental Disability in Children Treated with Extracorporeal Membrane Oxygenation

Study	No.	Follow-up Age (years)	Major* Disability (%)	Mild† Disability (%)	No Disability (%)
Adolph, 1990	57	0.5–4	2	19	79
Hofkosh, 1991	67	0.5–10	11	25	64
Schumacher, 1991	80	1–7	8	12	80
Glass, 1995	103	5	16	49†	35
Wildin, 1994	25	2	20°	8	72
Walsh-Sukys, 1995	38	1.6	26°	—	74

°Major disability generally means cerebral palsy (severe neurologic impairment) or mental retardation (I.Q. <70), but some studies include I.Q. <80. Authors may also have included severe sensory impairment (blind or deaf).

†Mild disability includes sensory impairment and borderline intelligence (except as noted above), language delay, and, in Glass, 1995, evidence suggestive of learning disability.

line intelligence, language delay, visual impairment, and minor neuromotor dysfunction, occurs in 8% to 49%. Glass and colleagues (1995) found that 5-year-old ECMO survivors had an 11% incidence of mental retardation (1% profound mental retardation), 5% cerebral palsy (most had mild cerebral palsy), 2% severe learning disabilities, and a lower mean I.Q. than 37 healthy control children (96 versus 115, $P < 0.001$). Adverse neurodevelopmental outcome is associated with lower birth weight, sepsis, congenital diaphragmatic hernia, and abnormal neuroimaging studies (Bernbaum et al, 1995; Bulas et al, 1995; Lago et al, 1995; Revenis et al, 1992; Robertson et al, 1995; Stolar et al, 1995; Taylor et al, 1989).

HEALTH AND GROWTH

Although NICU infants are much improved at the time of discharge, many have lingering medical problems that require close follow-up by their primary care providers. They remain vulnerable to infections, further complications, difficulty feeding, and poor growth. Rehospitalization for illness (especially respiratory illness) or surgery (e.g., umbilical hernia repair, gastrostomy, Nissen fundoplication) is common (Combs-Orme et al, 1988; Lefebvre et al, 1988; Survanta Multidose Study Group, 1994; Teplin et al, 1991).

Adequate nutrition is essential for growth of the developing infant, especially for brain growth. Good weight gain, linear growth, and head growth are good measures of nutrition. Preterm infants are frequently below the 5th percentile for chronologic age, but they should grow along their own parallel curve, and some growth curves specific to LBW infants have been developed (Casey et al, 1991). Although most infants catch up in their growth within several years, some infants with extreme prematurity, intrauterine growth retardation, severe neonatal illness, or syndromes such as fetal alcohol syndrome always remain small for their age.

Infants who fall off their growth curves should be evaluated for undetected or inadequately treated gastrointestinal, pulmonary, urologic, or cardiac conditions. Gastroesophageal reflux can lead to discomfort from esophagitis, irritability, extensor posturing, and poor growth. Some children with genetic syndromes or who were critically ill as newborns demonstrate decreased appetite, food refusal, and poor growth. Oromotor dysfunction, with poorly coordinated suck and swallow, must be considered in NICU newborns with poor growth, food refusal behaviors, or neurologic abnormalities. Infants with chronic lung disease or congestive heart failure may tire with feedings and require frequent interruptions owing to exercise intolerance.

An oromotor evaluation by an occupational therapist or speech pathologist may include a radiographic swallow study to pinpoint the problem, decide if oral feeding is safe, and determine how the infant handles liquids versus solid foods. The cause of the feeding problem determines treatment: positioning, thickening liquids, medications, and possibly surgery for infants with gastroesophageal reflux; calorically dense food for poor appetite and growth; behavior management program for food refusal behavior not due to organic causes; supplemental oxygen for children with intermittent hypoxia; and gastrostomy for children who chronically aspirate, have severe oromotor dysfunction, or have food refusal unresponsive to behavioral interventions. Children fed totally or primarily by gastrostomy require an oromotor stimulation program to maintain feeding skills and prevent oromotor hypersensitivity. When NICU infants are discharged with gastrostomy, continuous feedings, special formulas, or dietary supplements, they require specific nutritional or gastrointestinal follow-up to address changing needs and parental concerns.

Chronic lung disease (i.e., bronchopulmonary dysplasia) occurs in 11% to 40% of VLBW preterm infants, 7% to 9% of more mature preterm infants, 7% to 35% of full-term infants with persistent pulmonary hypertension, 15% to 40% of infants treated with ECMO, and 63% of infants with congenital diaphragmatic hernia (Bernbaum et al, 1995; Bifano and Pfannenstiel, 1988; Ferrara et al, 1991; Glass et al, 1995; Hack et al, 1994; Revenis et al, 1992; Survanta Multidose Study Group, 1994, Walsh-Sukys et al, 1994). These children are vulnerable to respiratory infections, and they frequently require bronchodilators, oxygen supplement, or diuretics. The experienced clinician uses clinical history, physical examination, evidence of growth, signs of exercise intolerance, and pulse oximetry (especially during feeding and sleep) in making decisions regarding tapering oxygen supplements and diuretics. Infants who are well oxygenated at rest may be relying on their reserves and have difficulties when nipple feeding or sleeping. Some infants with chronic lung disease have transient increases in oxygen requirements during periods of accelerated growth.

Developmental interventions for medically fragile infants should be home based whenever possible to reduce the risks of infection. Infants should be shielded from friends and family with infectious illnesses. Therapists who provide early intervention should be skilled in working with these infants, should recognize the signs of exercise intolerance or increasing distress, and should have been trained in how to respond promptly in an emergency (e.g., cardiopulmonary resuscitation training). Infants on supplemental oxygen may need an increase in oxygen when handled.

Preterm infants and other high-risk infants need the protection from childhood illnesses that is conferred by immunization. Immunizations should be given according to the recommended schedule (American Academy of Pediatrics, 1994). Even in extremely preterm infants, full doses and chronologic age should be used. Infants who are still in the NICU or who are immunocompromised (or have immunocompromised family members) should not be given live viral vaccines. Pertussis protection should be deferred only for infants with signs of neurologic deterioration or uncontrolled seizure disorder, although it may be postponed pending diagnostic evaluation in a child with recent onset of seizures.

FOLLOW-UP OF THE HIGH-RISK INFANT

The high-risk NICU infant's medical problems, increased risk of neurodevelopmental disability, and uncertainty regarding outcome necessitate long-term follow-up.

Importance of Discharge Planning

Good discharge planning aims to smooth the infant's transition from hospital to home and to provide the health, developmental, and parental supports needed by infant and family. A parent conference that reviews the infant's hospital course and plans for discharge provides an opportunity to discuss the infant's risk status, to assess the parent's understanding, to appreciate the infant's progress, and to begin to make plans for discharge home. When reviewing the infant's various risk factors, an honest but sensitive discussion puts the infant's risk for neurodevelopmental disabilities into perspective, giving the range of possible outcomes. Parents should be reassured whenever possible, given the opportunity to hope, and given perspective about their infant's risks.

Discharge teaching includes well-baby care (for first-time parents); techniques of cardiopulmonary resuscitation (useful for all parents); use of any special equipment or medication; and recommendations regarding infant car seats, bedding, feeding, positioning, and handling. Plans for follow-up after hospital discharge should address both the infant's and the family's special needs. All infants discharged from a NICU should have a designated primary care provider who can follow the infant closely and address the infant's special needs as they emerge. Preterm infants

with retinopathy of prematurity, incompletely vascularized retinas, congenital infection, or cortical abnormalities require ophthalmologic follow-up. Infants who failed or did not receive audiologic screening require audiologic follow-up. Infants with specific medical conditions may require pediatric surgical, pulmonary, gastrointestinal, nutritional, cardiologic, neurologic, orthopedic, or other subspecialty follow-up.

Comprehensive Developmental Follow-Up

Criteria for referral of high-risk NICU infants for comprehensive developmental follow-up vary widely, based on available resources, funding, geography, and family needs. Ideally all NICU infants should be viewed as high risk and offered comprehensive developmental follow-up through school age. Incentives for families to return for follow-up encourage high follow-up rates, thereby providing NICUs with accurate outcome data for specific conditions. Close relationships between a NICU follow-up clinic and community health, educational, and social services promote coordination of intervention services based on the child's and family's needs. Limited resources and funding, organizational difficulties, and time constraints all interfere with ideal comprehensive, coordinated, family-focused follow-up and intervention efforts. Although often considered to be dispensable, developmental follow-up and early intervention should be viewed as an essential part of the continuum of care provided to high-risk infants and their families.

The goals of comprehensive, coordinated developmental follow-up are to help the family optimize the child's growth and development; to help integrate the child into the family, school, and community; and to intervene when possible to reduce future medical, social, and emotional costs. These goals are promoted by the recognition that each child is an individual with unique qualities, strengths, impairments, and abilities and that each family differs in background, social supports, finances, and personal coping mechanisms.

Follow-up is a dynamic process that evolves as the child grows, develops, and increasingly interacts with his or her environment. Recognition of impairments, disabilities, and handicaps relies on parental reports, an appreciation of individual variability in the normal pattern of development over time, and the examiner's assessment skills and ability to determine the significance of abnormalities or deviations from the normal pattern. Once recognized, problems should be discussed with parents, including a nonmedical definition of specific diagnoses (e.g., cerebral palsy, learning disability) and identification of specific intervention strategies.

Assessing the development of the high-risk infant relies on the basic tools of medicine: the history and the physical examination. The focus of the developmental history is to obtain information about the infant's behavior (e.g., sleep, feeding, temperament, behavior problems) and developmental milestone acquisition. The physical examination is expanded to a neurodevelopmental examination that includes an assessment of posture, muscle tone, reflexes, and functional abilities.

The developmental milestones should be viewed in terms of the major streams of development: gross motor, fine motor, adaptive, and language abilities (Tables 38–7 and 38–8). Gross and fine motor abilities are used to assess motor development and to screen for cerebral palsy and minor neuromotor dysfunction. Children with cerebral palsy generally have significant motor delay and persistent neuromotor abnormalities. Children with minor neuromotor dysfunction have milder or no delay and mild neuromotor abnormalities on examination. Delay in adaptive, or self-help, skills may be seen with mental retardation, cerebral palsy, minor neuromotor dysfunction, or environmental or behavioral causes (e.g., mother did not introduce a fork or took it away). Delay in language abilities can signal mental retardation, hearing impairment, or language disorder and requires an audiologic evaluation.

Assessing milestone acquisition in preterm infants raises the controversial question of whether to correct for the degree of prematurity. This issue is most important early in life and in extremely preterm infants. Consider this example: An infant born at 27 weeks' gestation is now 6 months old and not yet rolling over but is unfisted, plays with her hands in midline, and can support herself on her forearms in prone (see Table 38–7). Her motor quotient (i.e., developmental age divided by her chronologic age) is 50 (i.e., 50% of normal, therefore delayed). If one corrects for degree of prematurity (using her term age equivalent/ adjusted age/corrected age), her motor quotient is 100 (i.e., normal). Her developmental status at this age is determined by whether one corrects for degree of prematurity. At 5 years, correction is no longer important because children 57 and 60 months old do not significantly differ.

When considering correction for degree of prematurity, one should evaluate each stream of development separately because they may differ in responsiveness to environmental stimulation. Earlier exposure to the extrauterine environment may have greater effect on the development of language than on motor development. Language, a component of cognition, may be accelerated by early extrauterine experience (Eilers et al, 1993).

Traditionally, psychologists do correct for degree of prematurity in preterm infants when assessing cognition. They do not agree on full versus partial correction or on how long to correct: for 1 year, 2 years, or indefinitely (Barrera et al, 1987; Den Ouden et al, 1991; Mauk and Ting, 1987; Siegel, 1983). There is some concern that correcting for degree of prematurity overestimates a child's cognitive abilities and may fail to identify those infants who would benefit from community services (Den Ouden et al, 1991; Miller et al, 1984; Thompson et al, 1993). Because this issue remains controversial, infant cognitive assessments are imprecise, and it is unlikely that infant development

TABLE 38–7

Gross and Fine Motor Milestone Attainment

Milestone	Motor Milestone Attainment (in months)	
	Mean Age°	Delay Criterion†
Gross Motor Abilities		
Roll over prone to supine	3.6	5.5
Roll over supine to prone	4.8	7.25
Sit with arm support‡	5.3	8.0
Sit without arm support§	6.3	9.5
Creep°°	6.7	10.25
Come to sit††	7.5	11.25
Crawl‡‡	7.8	11.75
Pull to stand on furniture	8.1	12.25
Cruise§§	8.8	13.25
Walk independently	11.7	17.25
Walk backwards	14.3	
Run	14.8	
Fine Motor Abilities		
Unfisted	3	
Brings hands to midline	3	
Unilateral reach and grasp	4	
Transfers object from hand to hand	5	
Raking grasp	6	
Three-finger grasp (picks up pellets)	8	
Mature pincer grasp	11	
Good voluntary release	12	

°Gross motor milestone mean ages of attainment from a longitudinal study of 381 normal full-term children, followed from birth to 2 years (Capute et al, 1985).
†Delay criteria from Allen and Alexander, 1994.
‡*Sit with arm support* uses arms to maintain balance in sitting but not propped up with pillows.
§*Sit without arm support* means good independent sitting, without using arms for balance.
°°*Creep* means pulling self forward on abdomen, using arms and legs for propulsion.
††*Come to sit* means independently getting into a sitting position from supine or prone, without pulling up on furniture.
‡‡*Crawl* means good reciprocal crawl, up on hands and knees.
§§*Cruise* means walking holding onto furniture.

TABLE 38–8

Language Milestone Attainment

Milestone	Milestone Attainment: Mean Age (months)	Standard Deviation
Alert to sound°	0.25	0.3
Social smile°	1.2	0.5
Coo (musical vowel sounds)	1.5	0.6
Orient (turn) to voice°	2.8	1.2
Say "ah-goo"	4.0	1.6
Make raspberry (razz, "Bronx cheer")	4.4	1.6
Babble (repetitive consonant sound)	6.3	1.4
"Mama"/"Dada" indiscriminately	7.7	1.7
Gesture language (e.g., peekaboo)°	8.6	1.5
"Dada" discriminately	10.5	2.5
"Mama" discriminately	11.1	2.7
Follow one-step command with gesture°	11.1	1.7
First meaningful word (not a name)	11.3	2.3
Immature jargon (no words)	12.2	2.1
Second meaningful word (no names)	12.4	2.2
Third meaningful word (no names)	13.2	2.2
Follow one-step command without gesture°	13.6	2.1
Use four to six words (not including names)	14.7	2.5
Mature jargon (includes words)	16.5	2.9
Point to five body parts when asked°	16.7	2.8
Use 7- to 10-word vocabulary	16.9	2.9
Use novel two-word combinations	19.2	3.0
Use two- to three-word sentences	20.9	3.0
Use 50-word vocabulary	20.9	3.2

°Receptive language milestones; the remainder are expressive language milestones.
Data from Clinical Linguistic and Auditory Milestone Scale (CLAMS), Capute and Accardo (1978) and Capute et al (1986a).

suddenly accelerates at 1 to 2 years; calculating both ages and discussing the child's cognitive performance in terms of both calculations are recommended (Barrera et al, 1987). Preterm children with language or cognitive abilities consistently below their age corrected for degree of prematurity should be referred for multidisciplinary evaluation and possibly early intervention.

Using age of attainment of the motor milestones is a quick, practical, and inexpensive method of identifying infants at highest risk of cerebral palsy (Allen and Alexander, 1992, 1994, 1997). It is most effective when a history of motor milestone attainment is obtained at each child care visit, when correcting for degree of prematurity, and when using 50% delay criteria (see Table 38–7). There is strong evidence that one should correct for degree of prematurity when evaluating motor development throughout infancy (Allen and Alexander, 1990, 1992, 1994, 1997; Palisano, 1986). Correction for degree of prematurity led to much better specificity and positive predictive values for cerebral palsy than chronologic age (Allen and Alexander, 1992). Infants identified as demonstrating motor delay warrant a comprehensive neurodevelopmental examination, multidisciplinary evaluation, and often referral for physical and occupational therapy.

Language assessments such as the Clinical Linguistic and Auditory Milestone Scale (CLAMS) (see Table 38–8) can be used to follow language development and to screen for cognitive delays (Capute and Accardo, 1978; Capute et al, 1986a, 1986b; Rossman et al, 1994; Wachtel et al, 1994).

Infants identified as having language delays should then be referred for both hearing assessment and neuropsychologic testing. Many follow-up clinics rely on neuropsychologists to assess the cognition of high-risk infants, either with sequential assessments or with one or two carefully timed assessments (e.g., at 12, 18, or 24 months). A number of frequently used cognitive tests developed for use in infants and children are listed in Table 38–9.

Referral for Multidisciplinary Evaluation and Early Intervention Services

Infants with identified developmental delays should be referred for a multidisciplinary evaluation that assesses all aspects of development. Brain injury is more likely to be diffuse than focal, and more than one stream of development may be affected. Although the most obvious abnormality is first identified, this may not be the most disabling of the child's problems. A preterm infant who presents with delayed walking and tight heel cords may be diagnosed with mild spastic diplegia. This child has an excellent prognosis for walking, running, and good motor function. Problems associated with cerebral palsy (e.g., learning disability, myopia, attention deficit) may have far more impact on the child's quality of life and adult functioning than the presenting motor impairment.

Part H of Public Law 99-157 passed by the U.S. Congress in 1986 followed by the Individuals with Disabilities Education Act (IDEA, PL 101-476 and 102-119) in 1990

TABLE 38–9

Cognitive Tests for Infants and Children

Test	Age Range	Score	Reference
Bayley Scales of Infant Development—Second Edition (BSID-II)	1–42 mo	MDI°	Bayley, 1993
Clinical Adaptive Text/Clinical Linguistic and Auditory Milestone Scale (CAT/CLAMS)	Newborn–35 mo	CAT DQ† CLAMS DQ†	Capute, 1978 Capute, 1986a Wachtel, 1994
Gesell Developmental Schedules (Gesell)	1–36 mo	DQ†	Knoblach, 1980
Stanford-Binet Intelligence Scale—Fourth Edition	2 yr–adult	Composite score	Thorndike, 1986
McCarthy Scales of Children's Abilities	2.5–3.5 yr	GCI‡	McCarthy, 1972
Kaufman Assessment Battery for Children (K-ABC)	2.5–12 yr	Composite score	Kaufman
Wechsler Preschool and Primary Scale of Intelligence—Revised (WPPSI-R)	3–7.25 yr	FS IQ VIQ, PIQ§	Wechsler, 1989
Wechsler Intelligence Scale for Children—Third Edition (WISC-III)	6–16 yr	FS IQ VIQ, PIQ§	Wechsler, 1993

°MDI, mental developmental index. The Bayley also has a motor and behavior scale.
†DQ, developmental quotient, including both a CLAMS DQ and CAT DQ.
‡GCI, general cognitive index, a composite of the verbal, perceptual/performance and quantitativie scales.
§FS IQ, full-scale intelligence quotient; VIQ, verbal intelligence quotient; PIQ, performance intelligence quotient. The Wechsler tests have 13 subtests that compose its verbal and performance scales, and these two scales are combined to give the full-scale IQ.

encouraged, then required, states to provide a comprehensive, coordinated interagency system of early intervention services for infants and toddlers with developmental delay and with conditions that lead to developmental delay (e.g., Down syndrome, fetal alcohol syndrome). Some states also provide services for high-risk infants and their families. Infants may be referred by NICUs, NICU follow-up clinics, pediatricians, or families. Each child who is referred is entitled to a multidisciplinary assessment and a service coordinator to help coordinate the assessment and services. If the child is eligible for the program, the parents, service coordinator, and multidisciplinary team devise an individualized family service plan, which identifies the child's and family's needs and what services will be put into place to address these needs. This program recognizes the importance of (1) viewing each child as a unique individual, (2) evaluating not only needs but also strengths, (3) including the family in the planning process, and (4) coordinating all intervention services.

Early intervention strategies minimize secondary complications and provide much needed parental support in coping with disability or uncertainty. The choice of interventions is determined by the individual child's developmental profile and health, the needs of the family, and available resources. Programs or services that enable the family to meet the child's needs better (e.g., drug counseling, transportation, parent support groups) are also identified.

Although a number of studies have demonstrated beneficial effects of early intervention programs, there is no proof that early intervention prevents neurodevelopmental disability (Achenbach et al, 1993; Bennett and Guralnick, 1991; Brooks-Gunn et al, 1994; Infant Health and Developmental Program, 1990; Palmer et al, 1988; Piper et al, 1986; Ramey et al, 1992; Rothberg et al, 1991). One difficulty is the use of the global term *early intervention*, which covers many different intervention strategies. Early intervention can be as nonspecific as providing social work

support and parent classes on infant development or as specific as a physical therapy intervention aimed at facilitating coming to a sitting position from supine in a child with the prerequisite skills and postural reactions. Early intervention for a child with severe spastic quadriplegia would include recommendations for positioning and handling the child and providing adaptive equipment for sitting, traveling, eating, and communication. Designing good intervention trials that evaluate the efficacy of specific intervention strategies is complicated by the fact that each individual is so unique. This makes it difficult to define study sample criteria and outcomes and to match disabled children for randomization.

Nevertheless, each intervention strategy must be evaluated as to efficacy in a well-defined population. Both hearing and visual impairments are responsive to early intervention services that can dramatically improve the child's functioning and quality of life, especially if begun early. Infants with severe hearing impairments may benefit from hearing aids, sign language, specific educational interventions using multiple sensory modalities, and parental support. Studies have shown that a focused educational intervention for preterm infants has beneficial initial effects on cognition and behavior, although long-term benefits have not been proven (Achenbach et al, 1993; Brooks-Gunn et al, 1994; Infant Health and Developmental Program, 1990; Ramey et al, 1992). Few early intervention studies have evaluated whether there is an effect on function at school or at home. These functional abilities may be not only the most responsive to early intervention but also the most important outcome variables.

SUMMARY

Although children who required neonatal intensive care have a higher incidence of neurodevelopmental disabilities and health sequelae, most survivors are healthy and function well. The likelihood, type, and severity of disability vary with the condition requiring neonatal intensive care, with various perinatal and demographic risk factors, and perhaps with developmental supports for the child and social supports for the family. It is impossible to diagnose neurodevelopmental disabilities with certainty in the neonatal period. Absence of risk factors and neurologic abnormalities is reassuring. Multiple or severe risk factors can identify infants at high risk for disability.

The uncertainty regarding an infant's outcome and the dynamic nature of early infant and child development necessitate careful medical and developmental follow-up of high-risk NICU infants during infancy and childhood. Survival is not the only goal of neonatal intensive care. Because the NICU is but the first step in an infant's life, follow-up (or perhaps follow-through) is an important component of the continuum of care that should be offered to high-risk infants. The goals of follow-up are to assist the family to optimize the child's growth and development so that the child is as functional as possible and to help integrate the child into the family, school, and community.

REFERENCES

Achenbach TM, Howell CT, Aoki MF, et al: Nine-year outcome of the Vermont Intervention Program for Low Birthweight Infants. Pediatrics 91:45, 1993.

Adolph V, Ekelund C, Smith C, et al: Developmental outcome of neonates treated with extracorporeal membrane oxygenation. J Pediatr Surg 25:43, 1990.

Allen MC: Developmental implications of intrauterine growth retardation. Inf Young Children 5:13, 1992.

Allen MC: The high-risk infant. Pediatr Clin North Am 40:479, 1993.

Allen MC, Alexander GR: Gross motor milestones in preterm infants: Correction for degree of prematurity. J Pediatr 116:955, 1990.

Allen MC, Alexander GR: Using gross motor milestones to identify very-preterm infants at risk for cerebral palsy. Dev Med Child Neurol 34:226, 1992.

Allen MC, Alexander GR: Screening for cerebral palsy in preterm infants: Delay criteria for motor milestone attainment. J Perinatol 14:190, 1994.

Allen MC, Alexander GR: Using motor milestones as a multistep process to screen preterm infants for cerebral palsy. Dev Med Child Neurol 39:12, 1997.

Allen MC, Capute AJ: Neonatal neurodevelopmental examination as a predictor of neuromotor outcome in premature infants. Pediatrics 83:498, 1989.

Allen MC, Donohue PK, Dusman AE: The limit of viability: Neonatal outcome of infants born at 22–25 weeks' gestation. N Engl J Med 329:1597, 1993.

American Academy of Pediatrics: 1994 Red Book: Report of the Committee on Infectious Diseases. Elk Grove Village, IL, American Academy of Pediatrics, 1994.

Aylward GP, Pfeiffer SI, Wright A, et al: Outcome studies of low-birth-weight infants published in the last decade: A meta-analysis. J Pediatr 115:515, 1989.

Aziz K, Vickar DB, Sauve RS, et al: Province-based study of neurologic disability of children weighing 500 through 1249 g at birth in relation to neonatal cerebral ultrasound findings. Pediatrics 95:837, 1995.

Barrera ME, Rosenbaum PL, Cunningham CE: Corrected and uncorrected Bayley scores: Longitudinal developmental patterns in low- and high-birth-weight preterm infants. Inf Behav Dev 10:337, 1987.

Bayley N: The Bayley Scales of Infant Development—Second Edition Manual. San Antonio, TX, Psychological Corporation, 1993.

Bennett FC, Robinson NM, Sells CJ: Growth and development of infants weighing less than 800 g at birth. Pediatrics 71:319, 1983.

Bennett RC, Guralnick MJ: Effectiveness of developmental intervention in the first five years of life. Pediatr Clin North Am 38:1513, 1991.

Bernbaum J, Schwartz IP, Gerdes M, et al: Survivors of extracorporeal membrane oxygenation at 1 year of age: The relationship of primary diagnosis with health and neurodevelopmental sequelae. Pediatrics 96:907, 1995.

Bhushan V, Paneth N, Kiely JL: Impact on improved survival of very-low-birth-weight infants on recent secular trends in the prevalence of cerebral palsy. Pediatrics 91:1094, 1993.

Bifano EM, Pfannenstiel A: Duration of hyperventilation and outcome in infants with persistent pulmonary hypertension. Pediatrics 81:657, 1988.

Blair E, Stanley F: Intrapartum asphyxia: A rare cause of cerebral palsy. J Pediatr 112:515, 1988.

Britton SG, Fitzhardinge PM, Ashby S: Is intensive care justified for infants weighing less than 801 gm at birth? J Pediatr 99:937, 1981.

Brooks-Gunn J, McCarton CM, Casey PH, et al: Early intervention in low-birth-weight premature infants: Results through age 5 years from the Infant Health and Development Program. JAMA 272:1257, 1994.

Buckwald S, Zorn WA, Egan EA: Mortality and follow-up data for neonates weighing 500 to 800 g at birth. Am J Dis Child 138:779, 1984.

Bulas DI, Glass P, O'Donnell RM, et al: Neonates treated with ECMO: Predictive value of early CT and US neuroimaging findings on short-term neurodevelopmental outcome. Radiology 195:407, 1995.

Capute AJ, Accardo PJ: Linguistic and auditory milestones during the first two years of life: A language inventory for the practitioner. Clin Pediatr 17:847, 1978.

Capute AJ, Accardo PJ (Eds): Developmental Disabilities in Infancy and Childhood, vols I and II, 2nd ed. Baltimore, Paul H. Brookes Publishing, 1996.

Capute AJ, Palmer FB, Shapiro BK, et al: Clinical Linguistic and Auditory Milestone Scale: Prediction of cognition in infancy. Dev Med Child Neurol 28:762, 1986a.

Capute AJ, Shapiro BK, Palmer FB, et al: Normal gross motor development: The influences of race, sex, and socioeconomic status. Dev Med Child Neurol 27:635, 1985.

Capute AJ, Shapiro BK, Wachtel RC, et al: The Clinical Linguistic and Auditory Milestone Scale (CLAMS): Identification of cognitive defects in motor delayed children. Am J Dis Child 140:694, 1986b.

Casey PH, Kraemer HC, Bernbaum J, et al: Growth status and growth rates of a varied sample of low-birth-weight, preterm infants: A longitudinal cohort from birth to three years of age. J Pediatr 119:599, 1991.

Combs-Orme T, Fishbein J, Summerville C, Evans MG: Rehospitalization of very-low-birth-weight infants. Am J Dis Child 142:1109, 1988.

Dammann O, Walther H, Allers B, et al: Development of a regional cohort of very-low-birth-weight children at six years: Cognitive abilities are associated with neurological disability and social background. Dev Med Child Neurol 38:97, 1996.

Den Ouden L, Rijken M, Brand R, et al: Is it correct to correct? Developmental milestones in 555 "normal" preterm infants compared with term infants. J Pediatr 118:399, 1991.

Drillien CM, Thomson AJM, Burgoyne K: Low-birthweight children at early school-age: A longitudinal study. Dev Med Child Neurol 22:26, 1980.

Dubowitz LMS, Dubowitz V, Palmer PG, et al: Correlation of neurologic assessment in the preterm newborn infant with outcome at 1 year. J Pediatr 105:452, 1984.

Eilers RE, Oller DK, Levine S, et al: The role of prematurity and socioeconomic status in the onset of canonical babbling in infants. Inf Behav Dev 16:297, 1993.

Ellenberg JH, Nelson KB: Cluster of perinatal events identifying infants at high risk for death or disability. J Pediatr 113:546, 1988.

Escobar GJ, Littenberg B, Petitti DB: Outcome among surviving very-low-birth-weight infants: A meta-analysis. Arch Dis Child 66:204, 1991.

Fawer C, Diebold P, Calame A: Periventricular leucomalacia and neurodevelopmental outcome in preterm infants. Arch Dis Child 62:30, 1987.

Ferrara TB, Hoekstra RE, Couser RJ, et al: Effects of surfactant therapy on outcome of infants with birth weights 600 to 750 g. J Pediatr 119:455, 1991.

Fitzhardinge PM, Steven EM: The small-for-date infant: II. Neurological and intellectual sequelae. Pediatrics 49:50, 1972.

Forfar JO, Hume R, McPhail FM, et al: Low birth weight: A 10-year outcome study of the continuum of reproductive casualty. Dev Med Child Neurol 36:1037, 1994.

Freeman JM: Prenatal and Perinatal Factors Associated with Brain Disorders. National Institutes of Health Publication No. 85-1149. Bethesda, MD, U.S. Department of Health and Human Services, 1985.

Glass P, Wagner AE, Papero PH, et al: Neurodevelopmental status at age five years of neonates treated with extracorporeal membrane oxygenation. J Pediatr 127:447, 1995.

Grogaard JB, Lindstrom DP, Parker RA, et al: Increased survival rate in very-low-birth-weight infants (1500 g or less): No association with increased incidence of handicaps. J Pediatr 117:139, 1990.

Gross SJ, Slagle TA, D'Eugenio DB, et al: Impact of a matched term control group on interpretation of developmental performance in preterm infants. Pediatrics 90:681, 1992.

Hack M, Fanaroff AA: Outcome of extremely low-birth-weight infants between 1982 and 1988. N Engl J Med 321:1642, 1989.

Hack M, Taylor HG, Klein N, et al: School-age outcomes in children with birth weights under 750 g. N Engl J Med 331:753, 1994.

Hall A, McLeod A, Counsell C, et al: School attainment, cognitive ability, and motor function in a total Scottish very-low-birth-weight population at eight years: A controlled study. Dev Med Child Neurol 37:1037, 1995.

Hendricks-Munoz KD, Walton JP: Hearing loss in infants with persistent fetal circulation. Pediatrics 81:650, 1988.

Hirata T, Epcar JT, Walsh A, et al: Survival and outcome of infants 501 to 750 gm: A six-year experience. J Pediatr 102:741, 1983.

Hoffman EL, Bennett FC: Birth weight less than 800 g: Changing outcomes and influences of gender and gestation number. Pediatrics 86:27, 1990.

Hofkosh D, Thompson AE, Nozza RJ, et al: Ten years of extracorporeal membrane oxygenation: Neurodevelopmental outcome. Pediatrics 87:549, 1991.

Hunt JV, Tooley WH, Harvin D: Learning disabilities in children with birth weight ≤1500 g. Semin Perinatol 6:280, 1982.

Infant Health and Developmental Program: Enhancing the outcomes of low-birth weight, premature infants: A multisite, randomized trial. JAMA 263:3035, 1990.

International Classification of Impairments, Disabilities, and Handicaps. Geneva, World Health Organization, 1980.

Ishikawa T, Ogawa Y, Kanayama M, et al: Long-term prognosis of asphyxiated full-term neonates with CNS complications. Brain Dev 9:48, 1987.

Ishizuka Y: Long-term survival of infants born less than 500 g or less than 24 weeks' gestation [in Japanese]. J Jpn Pediatr Soc 94:841, 1990.

John E, Roberts V, Burnard ED: Persistent pulmonary hypertension of the newborn treated with hyperventilation: Clinical features and outcome. Aust Paediatr J 24:357, 1988.

Kaufman AS, Kaufman NL: Kaufman Assessment Battery for Children (K-ABC). Circle Pines, MN, American Guidance Service.

Keith CG, Doyle LW: Retinopathy of prematurity in extremely low-birth-weight infants. Pediatrics 95:42, 1995.

Khadilkar V, Tudehope D, Burns Y, et al: The long-term neurodevelopmental outcome for very-low-birth-weight (VLBW) infants with "dystonic" signs at 4 months of age. J Pediatr Child Health 29:415, 1993.

Kitchen WH, Ford GW, Doyle LW, et al: Health and hospital readmissions of very-low-birth-weight and normal-birth-weight children. Am J Dis Child 144:213, 1990.

Kitchen WH, Ford GW, Rickards AL, et al: Children at birth weight <1000 g: Changing outcome between ages 2 and 5 years. J Pediatr 110:283, 1987.

Kitchen WH, Rickards A, Ryan MM, et al: Improved outcome to two years of very-low-birth-weight infants: Fact or artifact? Dev Med Child Neurol 28:479, 1986.

Kitchen WH, Ryan MM, Rickards A, et al: A longitudinal study of very-low-birth-weight infants: IV. An overview of performance at eight years. Dev Med Child Neurol 22:172, 1980.

Klein N, Hack M, Gallagher J, et al: Preschool performance of children with normal intelligence who were very-low-birth-weight infants. Pediatrics 75:531, 1985.

Knoblach H, Stevens F, Malone A: Manual of Developmental Diagnosis: The Administration and Interpretation of the Revised Gesell and Amatruda Developmental and Neurologic Examination. New York, Harper & Row, 1980.

Kuban KCK, Leviton A: Cerebral palsy. N Engl J Med 330:188, 1994.

Lago P, Rebsamen S, Clancy RR, et al: MRI, MRA, and neurodevelopmental outcome following neonatal ECMO. Pediatr Neurol 12:294, 1995.

LaPine TRL, Jackson JC, Bennett FC: Outcome of infants weighing less than 800 g at birth: 15 years' experience. Pediatrics 96:479, 1995.

Largo RH, Molinari L, Rinto LC, et al: Language development of term

and preterm children during the first five years of life. Dev Med Child Neurol 28:333, 1986.

Lefebvre F, Bard H, Veilleux A, et al: Outcome at school age of children with birth weights of 1000 g or less. Dev Med Child Neurol 30:170, 1988.

Leijon I, Billstrom G, Lind I: An 18-month follow-up study of growth-retarded neonates: Relation to biochemical tests of placental function in late pregnancy and neurobehavioural condition in the newborn period. Early Hum Dev 4:271, 1980.

Leonard CH, Clyman RI, Piecuch RE, et al: Effect of medical and social risk factors on outcome of prematurity and very low birth weight. J Pediatr 116:620, 1990.

Lloyd BW, Wheldall K, Perks D: Controlled study of intelligence and school performance of very-low-birth-weight children from a defined geographical area. Dev Med Child Neurol 30:36, 1988.

Louhiala P: Risk indicators of mental retardation: Changes between 1967 and 1981. Dev Med Child Neurol 37:631, 1995.

Low JA, Galbraith RS, Muir D, et al: Intrauterine growth retardation: A preliminary report of long-term morbidity. Am J Obstet Gynecol 130:534, 1978.

Low JA, Galbraith RS, Muir D, et al: Intrauterine growth retardation: A study of long-term morbidity. Am J Obstet Gynecol 142:670, 1982.

Low JA, Handley-Derry MH, Burke SO, et al: Association of intrauterine fetal growth retardation and learning deficits at age 9 to 11 years. Am J Obstet Gynecol 167:1499, 1992.

Marlow N, Roberts BL, Cooke RWI: Motor skills in extremely low-birth-weight children at the age of 6 years. Arch Dis Child 64:839, 1989.

Marron MJ, Crisafi MA, Driscoll JM Jr, et al: Hearing and neurodevelopmental outcome in survivors of persistent pulmonary hypertension of the newborn. Pediatrics 90:392, 1992.

Matilainen R, Heinonen K, Siren-Tiusanen H, et al: Neurodevelopmental screening of in utero growth-retarded prematurely born children before school age. Eur J Pediatr 146:453, 1987.

Mauk JE, Ting RY: Correction for prematurity: How much, how long? Am J Dis Child 141:373, 1987.

McCarthy DA: Manual for the McCarthy Scales of Children's Abilities. New York, Psychological Corporation, 1972.

McCormick MC, Workman-Daniels K, Brooks-Gunn J: The behavioral and emotional well-being of school-age children with different birth weights. Pediatrics 97:18, 1996.

Miller G, Dubowitz LMS, Palmer P: Follow-up of pre-term infants: Is correction of the developmental quotient for prematurity helpful? Early Hum Dev 9:137, 1984.

Msall ME, Buck GM, Rogers BT, et al: Kindergarten readiness after extreme prematurity. Am J Dis Child 146:1371, 1992.

Neligan GA: Born too soon or born too small: A follow-up study to seven years of age. Clinics in Developmental Medicine. London, Spastics International Medical Publications, 1976.

Nelson KB, Leviton A: How much of neonatal encephalopathy is due to birth asphyxia? Am J Dis Child 145:1325, 1991.

Nishida H: Outcome of infants born preterm, with special emphasis on extremely low-birth-weight infants. Bailliere's Clin Obstet Gynaecol 7:611, 1993.

Nwaesei CG, Young DC, Byrne JM, et al: Preterm birth at 23 to 26 weeks' gestation: Is active obstetric management justified? Am J Obstet Gynecol 157:890, 1987.

Palisano RJ: Use of chronological and adjusted ages to compare motor development of healthy preterm and fulltern infants. Dev Med Child Neurol 28:180, 1986.

Palmer FB, Shapiro BK, Wachtel RC, et al: The effects of physical therapy on cerebral palsy: A controlled trial in infants with spastic diplegia. N Engl J Med 318:803, 1988.

Parkinson CE, Scrivener R, Graves L, et al: Behavioural differences of school-age children who were small-for-dates babies. Dev Med Child Neurol 28:498, 1986.

Parkinson CE, Wallis S, Harvey D: School achievement and behaviour of children who were small-for-dates at birth. Dev Med Child Neurol 23:41, 1981.

Paz I, Gale R, Laor A, et al: The cognitive outcome of full-term small for gestational age infants at late adolescence. Obstet Gynecol 65:452, 1995.

Pena IC, Teberg AJ, Finello KM: The premature small-for-gestational-age infant during the first year of life: Comparison by birth weight and gestational age. J Pediatr 113:1066, 1988.

Perlman M, Claris O, Hao Y, et al: Secular changes in the outcomes to eighteen to twenty-four months of age of extremely low-birth-weight infants, with adjustment for changes in risk factors and severity of illness. J Pediatr 126:75, 1995.

Piper MC, Kunos I, Willis DM, et al: Early physical therapy effects on the high-risk infant: A randomized, controlled trial. Pediatrics 78:216, 1986.

Ramey CT, Bryant DM, Wasik BH, et al: Infant health and development program for low-birth-weight, premature infants: Program elements, family participation, and child intelligence. Pediatrics 89:454, 1992.

Regev R, Dolfin T, Ben-nun Y, et al: Survival rate and two-year outcome in very-low-birth-weight infants. Isr J Med Sci 31:309, 1995.

Revenis ME, Glass P, Short BL: Mortality and morbidity rates among lower-birth-weight infants (2000 to 2500 g) treated with extracorporeal membrane oxygenation. J Pediatr 121:452, 1992.

Robertson C, Sauve RS, Christianson HE: Province-based study of neurologic disability among survivors weighing 500 through 1249 g at birth. Pediatrics 93:636, 1994.

Robertson CM, Finer NN, Sauve RS, et al: Neurodevelopmental outcome after neonatal extracorporeal membrane oxygenation. Can Med Assoc J 152:1981, 1995.

Robertson CMT, Etches PC, Kyle JM: Eight-year school performance and growth of preterm, small-for-gestational-age infants: A comparative study with subjects matched for birth weight or for gestational age. J Pediatr 116:19, 1990.

Robertson CMT, Finer NN: Term infants with hypoxic-ischemic encephalopathy: Outcome at 3–5 years. Dev Med Child Neurol 27:473, 1985.

Robertson CMT, Finer NN, Grace MGA: School performance of survivors of neonatal encephalopathy associated with birth asphyxia at term. J Pediatr 114:753, 1989.

Rogers B, Msall M, Owens T, et al: Cystic periventricular leukomalacia and type of cerebral palsy in preterm infants. J Pediatr 125:S1, 1994.

Ross G, Lipper EG, Auld PAM: Social competence and behavior problems in premature children at school age. Pediatrics 86:391, 1990.

Ross G, Lipper E, Auld PAM: Educational status and school-related abilities of very-low-birth-weight premature children. Pediatrics 88:1125, 1991.

Rossman MJ, Hyman SL, Rorabaugh ML, et al: The CAT/CLAMS assessment for early intervention services. Clin Pediatr 33:404, 1994.

Roth SC, Baudin F, McCormick DC, et al: Relation between ultrasound appearance of the brain of very-preterm infants and neurodevelopmental impairment at eight years. Dev Med Child Neurol 35:755, 1993.

Rothberg AD, Goodman M, Jacklin LA, et al: Six-year follow-up of early physiotherapy intervention in very-low-birth-weight infants. Pediatrics 88:547, 1991.

Rutherford MA, Pennock JM, Dubowitz LMS: Cranial ultrasound and magnetic resonance imaging in hypoxic-ischemic encephalopathy: A comparison with outcome. Dev Med Child Neurol 36:813, 1994.

Sabel KG, Olegard E, Victorin L: Remaining sequelae with modern prenatal care. Pediatrics 57:652, 1976.

Saigal S, Rosenbaum P, Stoskopf B, et al: Follow-up of infants 501- to 1500-gm birth weight delivered to residents of a geographically defined region with perinatal intensive care facilities. J Pediatr 100:606, 1982.

Saigal S, Rosenbaum P, Stoskopf B, et al: Outcome in infants 501- to 1000-gm birth weight delivered to residents of the McMaster Health Region. J Pediatr 105:969, 1984.

Saigal S, Rosenbaum P, Stoskopf B, et al: Comprehensive assessment of the health status of extremely low-birth-weight children at eight years of age: Comparison with a reference group. J Pediatr 125:411, 1994.

Saigal S, Szatmari P, Rosenbaum P, et al: Intellectual and functional status at school entry of children who weighed 1000 g or less at birth: A regional perspective of births in the 1980s. J Pediatr 116:409, 1990.

Saigal S, Szatmari P, Rosenbaum P, et al: Cognitive abilities and school performance of extremely low-birth-weight children and matched term control children at age 8 years: A regional study. J Pediatr 118:751, 1991.

Schumacher RE, Palmer TW, Roloff DW, et al: Follow-up of infants treated with extracorporeal membrane oxygenation for newborn respiratory failure. Pediatrics 87:451, 1991.

Scottish Low Birthweight Study Group: The Scottish low birthweight study: I. Survival, growth, neuromotor and sensory impairment. Lancet 1:675, 1992.

Sell EF, Gaines JA, Gluckman C, et al: Persistent fetal circulation. Am J Dis Child 139:25, 1985.

Siegel LS: Correction for prematurity and its consequences for the assessment of the very-low-birth-weight infant. Child Dev 54:1176, 1983.

Skouteli HN, Eubowitz LMS, Levene MI, et al: Predictors for survival and normal neurodevelopmental outcome of infants weighing less than 1001 g at birth. Dev Med Child Neurol 27:588, 1985.

Stewart A, Hope PL, Hamilton P, et al: Prediction in very-preterm infants of satisfactory neurodevelopmental progress at 12 months. Dev Med Child Neurol 30:53, 1988.

Stewart AL, Reynolds EOR, Hope PL, et al: Probability of neurodevelopmental disorders estimated from ultrasound appearance of brains of very-preterm infants. Dev Med Child Neurol 29:3, 1987.

Stolar CJH, Crisafi MA, Driscoll YT: Neurocognitive outcome for neonates treated with extracorporeal membrane oxygenation: Are infants with congenital diaphragmatic hernia different? J Pediatr Surg 30:366, 1995.

Sung IK, Vohr B, Oh W: Growth and neurodevelopmental outcome of very-low-birth-weight infants with intrauterine growth retardation: Comparison with control subjects matched by birth weight and gestational age. J Pediatr 123:618, 1993.

Survanta Multidose Study Group: Two-year follow-up of infants treated for neonatal respiratory distress syndrome with bovine surfactant. J Pediatr 124:962, 1994.

Synnes AR, Ling EWY, Whitfield MF, et al: Perinatal outcomes of a large cohort of extremely low-gestational-age infants (23 to 28 completed weeks of gestation). J Pediatr 125:952, 1994.

Taylor GA, Fitz CR, Glass P, et al: CT of cerebrovascular injury after neonatal extracorporeal membrane oxygenation: Implications for neurodevelopmental outcome. AJR Am J Roentgenol 153:121, 1989.

Teplin SW, Burchinal M, Johnson-Martin N, et al: Neurodevelopmental, health, and growth status at age 6 years of children with birth weights less than 1001 g. J Pediatr 118:768, 1991.

Thompson CM, Buccimazza SS, Webster J, et al: Infants of less than 1250-g birth weight at Groote Schuur Hospital: Outcome at 1 and 2 years. Pediatrics 91:961, 1993.

Thorndike RL, Hagen EP, Sattler JM: Guide for Administering and Scoring the Stanford-Binet Intelligence Scale, 4th ed. Chicago, Riverside, 1986.

van Zeben-van der Aa TM, Verloove-Verhorick SP, Brand R, et al: Morbidity of very-low-birth-weight infants at corrected age of two years in a geographically defined population. Lancet 1:253, 1989.

Victorian Infant Collaborative Study Group: Eight-year outcome in infants with birth weight of 500 to 999 g: Continuing regional study of 1979 and 1980 births. J Pediatr 118:761, 1991.

Vohr B, Coll CG, Flanagan P, et al: Effects of intraventricular hemorrhage and socioeconomic status on perceptual, cognitive, and neurologic status of low-birth-weight infants at 5 years of age. J Pediatr 121:280, 1992.

Vohr BR, Garcia-Coll CT: Neurodevelopmental and school performance of very-low-birth-weight infants: A seven-year longitudinal study. Pediatrics 76:345, 1985.

Vohr BR, Oh W: Growth and development in preterm infants small for gestational age. J Pediatr 103:941, 1983.

Wachtel RC, Shapiro BK, Palmer FB, et al: A tool for the pediatric evaluation of infants and young children with developmental delay. Clin Pediatr 33:410, 1994.

Walker EM, Patel NB: Mortality and morbidity in infants born between 20 and 28 weeks' gestation. Br J Obstet Gynaecol 94:670, 1987.

Walsh-Sukys MC, Bauer RE, Cornell DJ, et al: Severe respiratory failure in neonates: Mortality and morbidity rates and neurodevelopmental outcomes. J Pediatr 125:104, 1994.

Warshaw JB: Intrauterine growth retardation: Adaptation or pathology? Pediatrics 76:998, 1985.

Wechsler D: Manual for the Wechsler Preschool and Primary Scale of Intelligence. New York, Psychological Corporation, 1989.

Wechsler D: Manual for the Wechsler Intelligence Scale for Children—III. New York, Psychological Corporation, 1993.

Weisglas-Kuperus N, Baerts W, Fetter WPF, et al: Neonatal cerebral ultrasound, neonatal neurology, and perinatal conditions as predictors of neurodevelopmental outcome in very-low birth-weight infants. Early Hum Dev 31:131, 1992.

Weisglas-Kuperus N, Baerts W, Fetter WPF, et al: Minor neurological dysfunction and quality of movement in relation to neonatal cerebral damage and subsequent development. Dev Med Child Neurol 36:727, 1994.

Weisglas-Kuperus N, Baerts W, Smrkovsky M, et al: Effects of biological and social factors on the cognitive development of very-low-birth-weight children. Pediatrics 92:658, 1993.

Westwood M, Kramer MS, Munz D, et al: Growth and development of full-term nonasphyxiated small-for-gestational-age newborns: Follow-up through adolescence. Pediatrics 71:376, 1983.

Whyte HE, Fitzhardinge PM, Shennan AT, et al: Extreme immaturity: Outcome of 568 pregnancies of 23 to 26 weeks' gestation. Obstet Gynecol 82:1, 1993.

Wildin SR, Landry SH, Zwischenberger JB: Prospective, controlled study of developmental outcome in survivors of extracorporeal membrane oxygenation: The first 24 months. Pediatrics 93:404, 1994.

Wocadlo C, Rieger I: Developmental outcome at 12 months corrected age for infants born less than 30 weeks' gestation: Influence of reduced intrauterine and postnatal growth. Early Hum Dev 39:127, 1994.

Yeo CL, Tudehope DI: Outcome of resuscitated apparently stillborn infants: A ten-year review. J Paediatr Child Health 30:129, 1994.

CHAPTER 39

Long-Term Costs of Perinatal Disabilities

Marie C. McCormick and Douglas Richardson

Increasingly, economic jargon predominates in many medical discussions with terms such as "cost-containment," "cost-benefit analysis," "providers," and "products." In such an era, outcomes of medical care must be considered in a broader context than simple survival to provide recognition of the broader implications of the consequences of clinical decisions. Thus, the concept of the long-term costs of perinatal disabilities makes explicit that, with the survival of neonates with disabling conditions, society incurs a long-term responsibility for support, with the scope of this support characterized in monetary terms or costs.

Precise estimates of the long-term costs of perinatal disabilities, however, involve a conceptualization of outcomes that is not familiar to clinicians and requires information that may not be readily available. For example, the economic concept of "cost" extends beyond the hospital and visit fees familiar to health care providers. In the complex medical environment, it is important to recognize a variety of costs, including travel time and lost wages. Furthermore, methods of assigning dollar amounts to these costs are not all equivalent. Much more difficult is the conceptualization and valuation of human "costs," or costs not directly related to the provision of medical and related services.

Beyond these issues, however, are issues related to the availability and timeliness of data on outcomes. To estimate long-term costs requires information on the nature and relevance of disabilities, as well as the types of services needed and the sources of payment for the services. Because interest in the economic implications of neonatal intensive care unit (NICU) graduates is fairly recent, the available data reflect traditional concerns about survival and more severe morbidity, not necessarily the more comprehensive information needed for estimating economic burden. In addition, neonatal intensive care is not a static intervention, but a changing package of services. Thus, the more complete data on longer term outcome may not reflect the current technologic methods.

Any discussion of short or longer term costs implicitly or explicitly addresses an assessment of the value or worth of NICU care. Evaluation of the merits of an intervention, however, must always involve a comparison, either of the relative costs of two interventions that achieve similar effects (cost-effectiveness analysis) or of the costs and benefits, both in dollars (cost-benefit analysis). The available methods of assigning dollar values to outcomes are even less clear than those for costs. The point is that, although identification of the costs of perinatal disabilities may have great importance in estimating the implications of changes in survival and morbidity rates for both the individual family and larger social units, knowledge of costs alone is not sufficient to assess the value of NICU care.

OVERVIEW OF DEFINITIONS

A number of methods may be used to estimate costs, but some general concerns pertain to all methods. First, when costs occur at different points in time, some adjustment must be made. A dollar spent immediately "costs" more than the same dollar spent a year later because of the interest accrued over that year. Thus, costs occurring over time are conventionally discounted to their net present value. Future benefits must be similarly discounted. This discounting is independent of inflation. Second, for many items, the best estimate of cost is simply the market price. Such estimation techniques are inadequate when the item has no price or is subsidized—for example, routine newborn metabolic screening. In such instances, the costs of the whole screening program are summed and divided by the number of samples processed to provide an average cost. Third, average cost may be quite an inaccurate estimate for nonaverage cases. For example, the resources consumed in caring for a critically ill neonate or a growing premature baby cannot both be described by the average per diem hospital costs. Yet such averages are often used because actual measurement of resource use is usually prohibitively expensive. Hospital charges (as distinct from hospital costs) are an important example of this distinction (Finkler, 1982). Distortions may be significant enough to change the conclusions of an economic analysis. Finally, implicit in what is tabulated as a cost is the viewpoint of the analysis. A very narrow viewpoint might be taken by a single insurance company setting a premium, a hospital considering opening a disabilities clinic, or a governmental agency. The most appropriate viewpoint for this discussion is a societal perspective, which includes costs incurred by all parties.

Direct Costs

To an economist, direct costs are those resources consumed in making a product. In the medical context, this product is an outcome such as a NICU graduate or the provision of a particular service, such as a day of hospitalization or an outpatient visit. Direct costs therefore include not only hospital bills, physician fees, office visit fees, laboratory test costs, rehabilitation services, and medication expenses (whether or not covered by insurance), but also parental out-of-pocket costs, such as for transportation, parking, and child-care for siblings during medical care for the NICU graduate. Also included are the incremental costs of providing specialized education services over those routinely incurred by the average child. Notably this analytic perspective does not take into consideration questions of equity in the distribution of costs or the ability to pay, issues which in themselves have important implications for social policy.

Indirect Costs

Indirect costs reflect foregone opportunities ("opportunity costs") such as wages lost when seeking medical treatment or convalescing. In the context of NICU graduates, indirect costs may be a significant cost or even the dominant cost if one parent fails to rejoin the work force for several years after the birth of a very premature infant. Such costs include the impact on other family members in terms of stress and divorce, limitations in geographic and job mobility, and activities of family members foregone because of the needs of the NICU graduate—issues for which monetary values may be difficult to assess. Indirect costs also include lost societal opportunities such as investment in other health or social programs.

Benefits

Two basic techniques have been used to assign dollar values to health benefits. The most common one is the human capital approach, which views health in terms of economic productivity. The dollar value assigned to a given health state is derived from the earnings that a person with that health state would generate. For a child, this approach would involve an estimate of lifetime earnings, either as a completely healthy individual, or at some reduced rate for those with handicap.

The second approach requires an estimate of how much an individual would be willing to pay to avoid death or some specified level of ill health. A variety of methodologic questions pertain to ascertaining and validating such assessments.

Besides the specific methodologic issues pertaining to each method, both have limited applicability in either children or the elderly. With the former approach, for example, a value to life and health beyond the market value of a livelihood cannot be estimated. In addition, the long delay between medical investment (i.e., neonatal intensive care) and the eventual revenues (wages upon entry into the work force) make such estimates extremely sensitive to the discount rates. In applying the latter, the opinions of the child cannot be directly ascertained until adolescence or adulthood many years after the event (Saigal et al, 1996).

For these and other reasons, much of clinical research tends to involve "cost-effectiveness" rather than "cost-benefit" comparisons. In the former, the object is to compare the costs (or charges) of achieving comparable clinical effects with the value of the "effect" assumed or established in some other context. Warner and Luce (1982) and Doubilet and coworkers (1986) provide more detailed discussions of these issues.

COSTS RELATED TO PERINATAL DISABILITIES

What is known about the costs related to perinatal disabilities? To address this topic completely would require detailed information on children with congenital malformations, on neonates suffering intrapartum catastrophes such as asphyxia, and on premature infants, but such detailed data do not exist. To illustrate the type of analysis required, this chapter focuses on the very-low-birth-weight (VLBW) infant (<1500 g), for whom more information is available.

However, non-VLBW children account for half of children receiving neonatal intensive care, and reports of their postdischarge experience are just beginning to emerge (Gray et al, 1996).

Direct Costs

Hospitalization

In the first years of life, VLBW infants experience higher rates of hospital use after discharge from the NICU. The percentage of such infants rehospitalized in the first year is between 30% and 40% with an average of two or more hospital episodes for each child hospitalized. In contrast, the rate is 8% to 10% for normal birth-weight infants who rarely have more than one admission. Close to half the admissions are for conditions that can be related specifically to perinatal and neonatal events, although others may be indirectly related to such events. The reported average length of stay for each hospitalization has varied from 5 to 9 days, although the range of variation is wide (Hack et al, 1981; McCormick et al, 1980; Morgan, 1985).

After the first year, the risk of subsequent hospitalization decreases to about 10% per year through early school age with evidence of relatively short lengths of stay for problems not necessarily related to perinatal events (Hack et al, 1983; Kitchen et al, 1990; McCormick et al, 1993; Yuksel and Greenough, 1994). Thus, by age 8 to 10 years, approximately 60% of VLBW infants will have experienced at least one hospitalization, and some children will have accumulated a substantial number of hospital days (Hack et al, 1983; Shankaran et al, 1988). These rates contrast with national data of rates of hospitalization of 34.2/1000 for children age 5 to 14 years (Butler et al, 1985). Estimates of the costs of hospital care for VLBW children vary, in part due to differences in estimates of daily charge rates, from $372 per day (Preventing, National Academy of Science, 1985) to $1500 (McCormick et al, 1991). The relative increase in costs of hospital care of VLBW compared to term infants also varies in these studies from twofold to 10-fold. Only Shankaran and coworkers (1988) have reported total hospital costs to 3 years of age, and VLBW children averaged $9902, exclusive of professional fees.

Outpatient Care

VLBW children also have increased use of ambulatory care in the first year, with 18.5 doctors' visits versus 9.3 for term infants, and with more of these visits to subspecialists or hospital clinics (McCormick et al, 1991; van Zeben-vander Aa et al, 1991). Data on doctors' visits in later years are not readily available, although trends in the first year show the visit rate becoming more comparable between VLBW and term infants (McCormick et al, 1991). Shankaran and colleagues (1988) have estimated the monthly costs for VLBW children in the first 3 years as ranging from $31 for children with no residual disabilities to $109 for severely disabled children, or totals of $1116 to $3924. National estimates for the same time period indicate that children past the first year average 3 to 4 visits per year at an annual cost of $177 (Butler et al, 1985). Information on use of ambulatory care by older children is not available, but

VLBW children are likely to use more care because they remain at risk for higher levels of morbidity (Hack et al, 1993; McCormick et al, 1992).

Other direct medical costs include equipment rental, home health care, renovations, diagnostic tests, and medications. Only one study on a small sample (McCormick et al, 1991) has attempted to estimate these costs. The generalizability of these results is very limited in an era with massive shifts of care to the home and a high degree of variability in the use of some postdischarge techniques such as apnea monitoring. Nonetheless, in this study, such expenditures added $1300 to the first-year costs of medical care. Finally, parents may experience direct, related nonmedical costs for obtaining care such as transportation and child-care. While the total dollars added are relatively small, the results suggest that parents of VLBW children do travel farther to obtain care and may require different types (i.e., more expensive) of child-care support.

Developmental and Educational Costs

VLBW children are eligible for early intervention services up to 3 years of age under Public Law 99-457 in most states. The actual duration and content of these services is highly variable, and no national cost estimates are available. In Massachusetts, the annual costs budgeted for early intervention services by the State Department of Public Health are up to $3200 per child (Ware J, personal communication, 1997).

Once the child enters school, some of the responsibility for providing special remedial services shifts to the educational system. In a study of three metropolitan school districts, the average annual expenditures for students with special needs averaged about twice that of regular education students in those schools ($7026 versus $3966) (Raphael et al, 1985). Expenditures varied by classification from the low of $5000 for children with speech impairment to close to twice that amount for children with physical, sensory, and other health impairments. Substantial variation occurred within special education classifications, with standard deviations of $2000 to $5000.

Recent studies reveal that approximately 40% of all VLBW children and 50% to 60% of those weighing less than 1000 g at birth have failed a grade or require special education early in elementary school (Klebanov et al, 1994; Klein, 1988; Saigal S et al, 1991). These studies reveal that the portion of children with severe impairments is similar to the portion estimated from infancy (i.e., 10% of all VLBW children, and few such children are among the most expensive group, those with technology dependence (Palfrey et al, 1991). Thus, most VLBW children fall within the less expensive categories. Moreover, not all educational difficulty can be attributed to perinatal events. VLBW children tend to come disproportionately from disadvantaged backgrounds, a factor that also contributes to their educational risk (Klebanov et al, 1994). The extent to which more intensive early educational intervention might ameliorate this risk is unclear, but one large trial suggests that there is potential for substantial benefit (McCormick et al, 1993).

In the most comprehensive assessment of direct costs to date, Lewitt and associates (1995) have estimated the incremental costs of a LBW child through 15 years of age in 1988 as at least $16,000 per child, with a total cost for all LBW children at different ages in 1988 as more than $5 billion. Of course, the incremental costs are higher the lower the birth weight. The annual incremental direct costs of LBW were about one third of those attributable to smoking and several times those of human immunodeficiency virus (HIV)/acquired immunodeficiency syndrome (AIDS). Even with the increased costs of treating HIV/AIDS with new protocols, the authors still concluded that the cost of LBW exceeded the current costs for HIV/AIDS.

Studies support the notion that VLBW children, on average, continue to require more medical care and educational support at somewhere between 2 to 4 times the costs for term infants. Several caveats pertain to these estimates, however. First, most of the studies reflect costs from the 1980s, so the estimates are likely to be low for current costs. For example, per capita personal health care expenditures increased from about $1500 in 1985 to $2500 in 1991, although the increase in costs for children is likely to be somewhat less because this overall increase would reflect aging of the population and increased intensity of services (Department of Health and Human Services, 1993). In the absence of national data, the estimates in this chapter are sometimes derived from very limited samples and do not encompass the full range of variation resulting from demographics, medical insurance coverage, and availability of public services. Even if modern intensive care is found to result in lower disability rates (a repeatedly projected but unfulfilled promise), the higher costs per disabled survivor will remain significant. The estimates do not reflect the fate of VLBW children in the current rapid shift to managed care and home services. Finally, because so little attention has been paid to postdischarge morbidity and needed services, the potential for reduction in costs by more organized approaches (e.g., case management) remains unexplored.

Indirect Costs

Where studies are limited with regard to direct costs, they are virtually nonexistent concerning indirect costs of having a VLBW infant. In the small study of McCormick and colleagues (1991), mothers of term infants were twice as likely as those of VLBW infants to be working shortly after delivery (a difference that did not achieve statistical significance), but they had also been twice as likely to have been working in the year before pregnancy. In a study of heavier low-birth-weight infants (Brooks-Gunn et al, 1994), nearly 75% of all mothers were working by the child's first birthday.

If frequent doctor's visits for health care and participation in physical therapy and other intervention programs requires one parent (usually the mother) to stay home, the failure of one parent to return to the work force would have implications for family income. Indirect evidence for this problem among the families of VLBW infants is provided by a study showing that an indicator of nursing burden (number of the child's activities of daily living limited by health problems) is the major predictor of family impact for VLBW children younger than 3 years of age (McCormick et al, 1986). This measure of family impact taps many of the dimensions of indirect costs noted above, including parental perceptions of need for more income, disruption of family activities, and social isolation due to the child's health problems, but does not provide a direct estimate of the specific costs. These results are supported by more recent work indicating that the increased stress of having a VLBW infant persists into the preschool period, especially among more disabled children (Cronin et al, 1995; McCormick et al, 1986). Despite the increased levels of direct and indirect costs, parents and the children themselves tend to place a high value on their quality of life and support intensive intervention for very preterm children (Cronin et al, 1995; Saigal et al, 1994, 1996).

In the longer term, indirect costs would include lost wages because the grown child failed to join the work force because of postdischarge death or severe disability, or they would include the reduction in future wages and job opportunities owing to the limited skills of children with moderate disabilities. Lost wages resulting from each infant death or severe handicap precluding work force participation range from $472,146 (4% discount rate) to $254,809 (6% discount rate). Based on the salaries of persons currently employed with disabilities, this same study estimates that disabled persons earn only 28% of wages of nondisabled persons over a lifetime, or a loss in earning for each disabled child of $338,815 (4% discount) to $162,396 (6%). The loss in maternal salaries for these same children is estimated at $36,088 to $54,132 per child (Chu, 1988). Clearly, these monetary losses represent only a part of the impact of the problems of VLBW infants. Moreover, these estimates are crude averages with wide variation and certainly may underestimate the costs for individual children.

The results are summarized in Table 39–1, which illustrates the relative increase in costs for a cohort of VLBW children; however, because there are far more healthy children born than VLBW children, VLBW children account for only a small fraction of total costs.

IMPLICATIONS

While increasing in volume, the information generated on the long-term costs of NICU graduates may still be flawed by methodologic problems (source of information, costs versus charges, analytic perspective) or rely on broad extrapolations requiring untested and sometimes disconcerting assumptions. Thus, perhaps the first implication of this overview is that more careful attention to these issues is needed. For the foreseeable future, NICU care will be required to sustain the lives of some fraction of the births in the United States, and accurate assessment of the longer term costs incurred by the survivors represents an important element in the ongoing examination of NICU care.

Part of that importance derives from pragmatic concerns about the short-term management of the NICU graduate.

TABLE 39–1

Summary of Estimates of Postdischarge Costs of Care: Very-Low-Birth-Weight versus General Population

	VLBW Children		General Population	
	Occurrence	**Cost/Occurrence**	**Occurrence**	**Cost/Occurrence**
Direct Costs				
Hospitalization°				
First year	30%–50% Average length of stay: 5–9 days per hospitalization	$600–$1500/d	8%–10% Average stay less than 5–9 days per hospitalization	$300–$400/d
Annually	10%	$300–$400/d	2%–4%	$300–$400/d
Doctor's visits				
First year	15–20	$30–60	9–10	$25
Annually	5–7	$30–60	4–5	$25
Other				
First year	—	$1300	—	$63
Annually	—		—	
Developmental and educational costs†				
Early intervention	—	$1000/yr up to 3 years	2% to 4%	$1000/yr up to 3 years
Special education				
Severely impaired	10%	$10,000/yr	2% to 4%	$10,000/yr
Mild–moderate	30%	$5000/yr	10%	$5000/yr
Indirect Costs‡				
Parental delay or failure to return to work	—	$36,000–$54,000/ child	—	$36,000–$54,000/ child
Foregone wages for grown child's reduced earning	10%	$160,000–$500,000	?2%	$160,000–$500,000

°Costs largely based on Shankaran et al (1988) and McCormick et al (1991).
†Costs largely based on Raphael et al (1985).
‡From Chu (1988).

Although it can be criticized, the available information on the first few years of life of VLBW children indicates a continuing need for relatively high levels of care, in large part due to the sequelae of prematurity and their management. Although most of these conditions resolve satisfactorily, the ability to provide needed care may be severely constrained if parents are unable to sustain the financial burden of frequent medical visits, equipment, and other medical needs.

Whatever the short-term costs, they pale in significance to the life-long costs of total or partial disability. The extent to which such disability can be prevented or ameliorated by postdischarge interventions becomes exceedingly important to the full realization of the gains achieved in the NICU.

Finally, the focus on cost should not obscure the fact that it is but one measure of outcome and may not even be the best measure. Current methods of cost-benefit analysis do better at estimating costs than benefits. Other values held by society may not be well characterized by techniques that rely on developing monetary estimates. The value of the survival of a child, even a child with special needs, is not solely an economic argument.

REFERENCES

Bloom BS, Knorr RS, Evans AE: The epidemiology of disease expenses. The costs of caring for children with cancer. JAMA 253:2393–2397, 1985.

Brooks-Gunn J, McCormick MC, Shapiro S, et al: Effects of early intervention on maternal employment, public assistance, and health insurance. Am J Public Health 84:924–931, 1994.

Butler JA, Winter WD, Singer JP, Wenger M: Medical care use and expenditure among children and youth in the United States: Analysis of a national probability sample. Pediatrics 76:495–507, 1985.

Chu RC: 1985 Indirect costs of infant mortality and low birth weight. Washington, DC: National Commission to Prevent Infant Mortality, 1988.

Cronin CMG, Shapiro CR, Casero OG, Cheang MS: The impact of very low-birth-weight infants on the family is long lasting. A matched control study. Arch Pediatr Adolesc Med 149:151–158, 1995.

Doubilet P, Weinstein MC, McNeil BJ: Use and misuse of the term "cost effective" in medicine. N Engl J Med 314:253–256, 1986.

Finkler SA: The distinction between costs and charges. Ann Intern Med 96:102–109, 1982.

Gray JE, McCormick MC, Richardson DK, et al: Normal birth weight intensive care unit survivors: Outcome assessment. Pediatrics 97:832–838, 1996.

Hack M, DeMonterice D, Merkatz IR, Fanaroff AA: Rehospitalization of the very-low-birth-weight infant. Continuum of perinatal and environmental morbidity. Am J Dis Child 135:263–266, 1981.

Hack M, Rivers A, Fanaroff AA: The very low birth weight infant: The broader spectrum of morbidity during infancy and early childhood. J Behav Dev Pediatr 4:243–249, 1983.

Hack M, Weissman B, Breslau N, et al: Health of very low birth weight children during their first eight years. J Pediatr 122:887–892, 1993.

Health United States 1992. DHHS Publication No (PHS) 93–1232. Hyattsville, MD: Department of Health and Human Services, 1993.

Kitchen WH, Ford GW, Doyle LW, et al: Health and hospital readmissions of very-low-birth-weight and normal-birth-weight children. Am J Dis Child 144:2213–2218, 1990.

Klebanov PK, Brooks-Gunn J, McCormick MC: School achievement and failure in very low birth weight children. J Devel Behav Pediatr 15:248–256, 1994.

Klein NK: Children who were very low birthweight: Cognitive abilities and classroom behavior at five years of age. J Spec Educ 22:41–54, 1988.

Lewitt EM, Baker LS, Corman H, et al: The direct costs of low birth weight. Future Child 5:35–56, 1995.

McCormick MC, Bernbaum JC, Eisenberg JM, et al: Costs incurred by parents of very low birth weight infants after the initial neonatal hospitalization. Pediatrics 88:533–541, 1991.

McCormick MC, Brooks-Gunn J, Workman-Daniels K, et al: The health and developmental status of very low birth weight children at school age. JAMA 267:2204–2208, 1992.

McCormick MC, McCarton C, Tonascia J, Brooks-Gunn J: Early educational intervention for very low birth weight infants. Results from the Infant Health and Development Program. Pediatrics 123:527–533, 1993.

McCormick MC, Shapiro S, Starfield BH: Rehospitalization in the first year of life for high-risk survivors. Pediatrics 66:991–999, 1980.

McCormick MC, Stemmler MM, Bernbaum JC, Farran AC: The very low birth weight transport goes home: Impact on the family. J Dev Behav Pediatr 7:217–223, 1986.

McCormick MC, Workman-Daniels K, Brooks-Gunn J, Peckham GJ: Hospitalization of very low birth weight children at school age. J Pediatr 122:360–365, 1993.

Morgan MEI: Late morbidity of very low birth weight infants. BMJ 291:171–173, 1985.

Palfrey JS, Walker DK, Haynie M, et al: Technology's children: Report of a statewide census of children dependent on medical supports. Pediatrics 87:611–618, 1991.

Preventing Low Birthweight. Washington, DC: National Academy of Sciences, 1985.

Raphael ES, Singer JD, Walker DK: Per pupil expenditures on special education in three metropolitan school districts. J Educ Finance 11(1):69–88, 1985.

Saigal S, Szatmari P, Rosenbaum P, et al: Cognitive abilities and school performance of extremely low birth weight children and matched term control children at 8 years. A regional study. J Pediatr 118:751–760, 1991.

Saigal S, Feeny D, Furlong W, et al: Comparison of health-related quality of life of extremely-low-birth-weight children and a reference group at age eight years. J Pediatr 125:418–25, 1994.

Saigal S, Feeny D, Rosenbaum P, et al: Self-perceived health status and health-related quality of life of extremely-low-birth-weight infants at adolescence. JAMA 276:453–459, 1996.

Shankaran S, Cohen SN, Lenver M, Zonia S: Medical care costs of high-risk infants after neonatal intensive care: A controlled study. Pediatrics 81:372–378, 1988.

Warner KE, Luce BR: Cost-Benefit and Cost-Effectiveness Analysis in Health Care. Principles, Practice and Potential. Ann Arbor: Health Administration Press, 1982.

van Zeben-vander Aa DM, Verloove-Vanhorick SP, Beaud R, Rueps JH: The use of health services in the first 2 years of life in a nationwide cohort of very preterm and/or low birthweight infants in the Netherlands: Rehospitalization and outpatient care. Paediatr Perinatal Epidemiol 5:11–16, 1991.

Yuksel B, Greenough A: Birth weight and hospital readmission of infants born prematurely. Arch Pediatr Adolesc Med 148:384–388, 1994.

PART VII

INFECTIONS AND IMMUNOLOGIC DEFENSE MECHANISMS

CHAPTER 40

Immunology

F. Sessions Cole

The contrasting functions of the fetal and neonatal immunologic responses, that is, preservation of fetal well-being as a semiallogenic graft versus adequate immunologic protection in a nonsterile extrauterine environment, are regulated by a host of incompletely understood developmental and genetic mechanisms. The diversity and importance of these mechanisms are suggested by the heterogeneity and frequency of the infectious problems encountered in newborns. Differences in immunologic responsiveness between adults and newborns should not be considered defects or abnormalities. Just as the ductus arteriosus, a cardiopulmonary necessity in the intrauterine environment, closes at different rates in different infants, human fetal and newborn infant immunologic response mechanisms are developmentally and genetically programmed to change from graft preservation to identification and destruction of invading pathogens at different rates.

Fortunately, systemic antimicrobial chemotherapy can control microbial invasion and permit adaptation of the infected infant's immunologic system to an extrauterine existence exposed to multiple potential pathogens. However, antibiotics coupled with advances in support technology do not ensure survival of infected infants: 10% to 50% of infants systemically infected with polysaccharide-encapsulated organisms die.

MATERNAL IMMUNOLOGY

The survival of a semiallogeneic graft (the fetoplacental unit) in the uterus requires multiple adaptive immunologic mechanisms. Medawar (1953), Billingham (1964), and Simmons (1967, 1969) have developed several hypotheses useful in understanding the mechanisms for survival of the human fetus, including:

1. The uterus is an immunologically privileged site.
2. The fetus is not antigenically mature.
3. The placenta provides a barrier to humoral and cellular maternal-fetal interaction.
4. The mother is immunosuppressed.
5. The immunologic response of the mother is altered during pregnancy to enhance fetal survival.

Since these hypotheses were developed, the first has been disproved (Bernard et al, 1978; Croy et al, 1993; De and Wood, 1991; Lala et al, 1983; Peel, 1989; Redline and Lu, 1989). Fetal antigenic maturity in eliciting a maternal immunologic response has been well documented (Beer and Billingham, 1976; Billington, 1987). The placenta pro-

vides multiple important functions for mother and fetus, but maternal immunologic recognition of the fetus is not required for normal placental function (Croy, 1993). The fact that pregnant women are healthy and display all appropriate immunologic defense mechanisms suggests strongly that pregnancy-induced, maternal immunosuppression is not necessary for successful pregnancy (Gill, 1992). The availability of genetically homogeneous murine lineages with altered immunologic responsiveness, the availability of reagents with which to evaluate regulation of expression of genes of the major histocompatibility complex (MHC), and greater understanding of the importance of cytokines have suggested that genetic and developmental mechanisms are responsible for successful human pregnancy (Beer and Billingham, 1976; Croy, 1993; Guilbert et al., 1993; Hunziker and Wegmann, 1989; Tangri et al, 1994; Wegmann et al, 1991).

Lack of genetic maternal-fetal histocompatibility appears to be important in maintaining pregnancy (Stern and Coulam, 1993). When couples share common alleles at the human lymphocyte antigen (HLA)-DR locus, recurrent spontaneous abortion has been observed, and the success of in vitro fertilization and tubal embryo transfer is reduced (Coulam et al, 1987; Faulk et al, 1978; Ho et al, 1994; Scott et al, 1987; Thomas et al, 1985). However, the contribution of immunologic recognition to this phenomenon has not been analogous to the role of immunologic recognition in transplantation rejection. In mice, embryo transfer between two noninterbreeding species of mice results in fetal lymphocyte infiltration and fetal resorption (Crepeau and Croy, 1988; Crepeau et al, 1989; Croy et al, 1982). However, when immunodeficient mice (*scid/scid*) were used in the same experiments, embryos were similarly nonviable (Crepeau and Croy, 1988). These data suggest that fetal death is not the result of rejection of the fetal allograft (Croy, 1993).

The possibility that maternal immunologic recognition is necessary for development of placental function (the immunotrophism hypothesis) has also been examined. The observation that *scid/scid* mice are fertile suggests that an antigen-specific immune response is not necessary for placental function (Croy, 1993). A double-mutant strain of mice has recently been developed to examine this question in greater detail. Breeding of *scid/scid* mice with mice that carry the *beige* (*bg*) mutation permits examination of the role of natural killer (NK) cell activity (Croy and Chapeau, 1990). The *bg* mutation selectively impairs NK cell function (Roder and Duwe, 1979). No infertility could be demonstrated. Recently, *scid/scid* mice bred with a different genetic background (CB-17) did not have a high rate of successful syngeneic pregnancies (Clark et al, 1994). The possibility of a tumor necrosis factor-alpha induced vasculopathy triggered by an unidentified infectious agent was raised in these studies. These observations suggest either that multiple redundant systems contribute to successful pregnancy outcome or that placental function does not require induction by immune recognition of lymphoid or cytokine functions (Croy, 1993; Ossa et al, 1994).

The importance of MHC molecules for successful pregnancy outcome has been documented in rodents and humans (Gill, 1983, 1993; Gill et al, 1983, 1993). The immunogenic stimulus of the fetal-placental unit has two sources: the unique antigenic structure of the placenta and transplacental passage of fetal cells, primarily lymphocytes (Beer et al, 1994; Gill, 1993; Schmidt and Orr, 1993). In humans and rodents, MHC Class II antigens and immunogenic determinants of MHC Class I molecules are not detectable on placental cell surfaces (Gill, 1993). A major role for the class I MHC molecule, HLA-G, a nonpolymorphic protein, has been postulated to prevent rejection of the trophoblast (Sargent, 1993; Schmidt and Orr, 1993). The antibody response elicited by the placenta and fetal lymphocytes is not destructive, possibly because of the expression of complement regulatory proteins on trophoblasts (Gill, 1993; Holmes and Simpson, 1992; Johnson, 1993; Vanderpuye et al, 1992). Two possible explanations for the importance of maternal-fetal disparity in MHC antigens for successful pregnancy outcome have been proposed. First, structural differences in MHC Class II antigens such as HLA-B, DR, and DQ result in complexes of maternal and fetal peptides, which reduce activation of maternal T lymphocytes (Gill, 1993). Second, associations of MHC disparity with successful pregnancy outcome may result from genes or genetic defects linked to the MHC genes. In this explanation, the sharing of MHC antigens may represent a marker for these linked genes (Gill, 1993). Currently, neither blocking antibodies nor compromise of maternal immunologic responsiveness appears to prevent rejection of the placenta (Gill, 1993; Sargent, 1993).

Abnormalities of maternal-fetal immunologic interaction can lead to spontaneous abortion or to morbidity or mortality for the fetus or newborn as seen in pregnancies complicated by rhesus (Rh) isoimmunization. Approximately 75% of Rh-negative women with Rh-incompatible fetuses give birth to unaffected or mildly affected infants (Baskett et al, 1986; Berlin et al, 1985; Eklund and Nevanlinna, 1986; Mills and Napier, 1988). The regulation of the maternal immunologic response suggested by this heterogeneity is complex. The genetic immunoregulation of this response has been studied by Raum and colleagues (1984). They demonstrated that a specific complotype of genetically determined allotypic variants of the second and fourth complement proteins of the classical pathway and factor B of the alternative complement pathway, all of which are encoded by genes within the MHC on the short arm of human chromosome 6, is tightly linked to a single extended haplotype, which is associated with fetal or neonatal morbidity and mortality. This observation suggests that maternal immunologic responsiveness to the Rh antigen is regulated by genes that are closely linked to the MHC.

Preconceptual or antenatal determination of the complotype of Rh-negative women might supplement utilization of measurement of maternal anti-Rh titer to assess fetal risk. Genetic and developmental regulation of maternal immunologic response to polysaccharide antigens also plays a role in determining risk of individual infants for systemic bacterial infection with polysaccharide-encapsulated organisms. Similar genetic markers may soon be available from studies of women in whose sequential infants group B streptococcal infection has developed within the first 3 months of life (Christensen and Christensen, 1988).

PLACENTAL IMMUNOLOGY

The placenta provides a regulatory barrier between maternal immunocompetent cells and semiallogenic fetal tissue. It also regulates maternal-fetal and fetal-maternal transfer of immunologically important factors (Gitlin et al, 1964; Gurka and Rocklin, 1987; Hunziker and Wegmann, 1986; Jacoby et al, 1984). To accomplish these complex functions, the placenta has a wealth of cell populations that provide considerable regulatory diversity. The hemochorial placenta of the human is a chimeric organ. Fetal villi covered with invasive trophoblasts erode into layers of maternal epithelium, stroma, and vessel endothelium. In addition to the various cell types of the decidua, there are multiple immunologically competent cells in the placenta including lymphocytes and macrophages. The importance of these cell types has been emphasized by the immunotrophism model that suggests that maternal immunologic recognition of fetal antigens induces production of cytokines that are necessary for placental growth and by the important roles of interleukin-1, interleukin-6, tumor necrosis factor-alpha, and other immunoregulatory cytokines in the initiation of parturition (Guilbert et al, 1993; Romero et al, 1992, 1994; Tangri et al, 1994).

Besides local production of factors that regulate fetal and maternal well-being, the placenta can regulate passage of maternal immunologic effectors to the fetus (Tongio et al, 1975). For example, while maternal IgG is transported efficiently beginning at 20 weeks' gestation, maternal antibody can also be bound and degraded by the placenta (Swinburne, 1970; Wegmann et al, 1980). On the basis of observations in rabbits and mice, there is considerable antibody-binding capacity in the placenta: radiolabeled maternal antibody is internalized and degraded by the placenta in 4 to 6 hours. Failure of this placental function may be due to elevated concentrations of maternal antibody that cannot be cleared by the placenta. Alternatively, specific antibodies may escape placental clearance and accumulate in the fetus because of a poorly understood lack of recognition of these antibodies.

In contrast with effector proteins, the placental barrier restricts access of cytotoxic cells to the fetus in normal pregnancy (Beer et al, 1994; Sargent, 1993). Evidence from infants with severe combined immunodeficiency (SCID) suggests that maternal T lymphocytes can cross the placenta and engraft in fetal bone marrow (Thompson et al, 1984). Whether aberrant regulation of maternal-fetal effector cell traffic plays a role in specific fetal or neonatal diseases, for example, intrauterine growth retardation, is poorly understood (Beer and Billingham, 1973; Beer et al, 1972). As understanding of the diverse immunologic functions of the placenta increases, more specific immunoregulatory clinical information will be derived from this important organ.

FETAL AND NEONATAL IMMUNOLOGY
Humoral Immunity
Complement

The complement system consists of approximately 2 dozen plasma and cell surface proteins (Table 40–1) that interact dynamically to regulate multiple functions of this immunologic effector system (Colten and Gitlin, 1995). These functions include cytolysis of bacteria, nonspecific opsonization, release of anaphylatoxins, solubilization of immune complexes, and induction of B-cell proliferation and differentiation. Activation of the complement cascade can occur via the classical or alternative pathway (Colten and Rosen, 1992; Davies, 1991; Johnston, 1993; Moore, 1994). The activation steps in these pathways have recently been reviewed (Colten and Gitlin, 1995). Several characteristics of this cascade are important for the fetal/neonatal immuno-

logic response. First, although the specificity of classical pathway activation results from interaction of antigens with antibodies of several isotypes, activation of the alternative pathway is antibody independent and may be initiated by structures such as endotoxin and polysaccharides frequently encountered among pathogenic organisms. For the fetus or infant who lacks type-specific IgG for immunologic recognition, the alternative pathway may be critical for triggering the effector functions of the complement cascade (Cole, 1987; Cole and Colten, 1984; Edwards, 1986; Stossel et al, 1973). Second, the enzymatic activation of the complement cascade permits prompt amplification of its functions: deposition of a single immunoglobulin molecule or C3b fragment can generate enzymatic cleavage of thousands of later-acting components and thus multiple complement activities (Pangburn and Muller-Eberhard, 1984). In addition, the alternative pathway may be amplified via a positive feedback activation mechanism, because C3b, an activation product of the alternative pathway C3 convertase, is a component of this convertase (Volanakis, 1988). Because of the importance of antibody-independent recognition for the immunologic responsiveness of the fetus and infant, the positive amplification loop of the alter-

TABLE 40–1

Proteins, Regulators, and Receptors of the Complement System

Complement Protein	Molecular Mass (Daltons)	Serum Concentration (μg/Ml)	
		Adult	**Newborn Infant (term)**
C1			
C1q	410	70	63
C1r	95	35	—
C1s	87	35	—
C2	110	25	18
B	93	200	110
D	24	1	0.5
C3	185	1500	700
C4	200	500	130
C5	190	75	48
C6	115	209	98
C7	115	65	—
C8	163	55	—
C9	71	60	—
C1 INH	104	150	—
P	224	25	—
C4-bp	500	150	50
I	88	35	17
H	155	500	300
S-protein	80	500	—
Membrane regulatory proteins			
Decay-accelerating factor (DAF)	70	—	—
Membrane cofactor protein (MCP)	58–63	—	—
Homologous restriction factor (HRF)	65	—	—
Membrane receptors and regulators			
Complement Receptor 1 (CR1)	190–250	—	—
Complement Receptor 2 (CR2)	140	—	—
Complement Receptor 3 (CR3)	260	—	—
C5D-R	45	—	—
C1q-R	70	—	—

From Colten HR, Gitlin JD: Immunoproteins. *In* Handin RI, Lux SE, Stossel TP (Eds): Blood: Principles and Practice of Hematology. Philadelphia, JB Lippincott, 1995.

native pathway is critical for rapid generation of complement effector functions without specific immunologic recognition.

Complement activation via either pathway occurs in two distinct phases, proteolysis and assembly. First, early-acting components of the classical (C1, C4, and C2) or alternative (factor B, factor D, and C3) pathway are activated by highly specific, limited proteolysis. Proteolytically activated components form specific enzymatic complexes composed of classical (C2a and C4b) or alternative (C3bBb) pathway components, which activate the third component of complement (C3). These two endopeptidases have identical substrate specificities: each cleaves the single peptide bond Arginine$_{77}$-Serine$_{78}$ of the alpha chain of C3 (Volanakis, 1988). The rates of formation and dissociation of both C3 convertases are regulated by multiple soluble (e.g., factor H, factor I, C4b-binding protein) and membrane-associated proteins (e.g., membrane cofactor protein, delay accelerating factor) (Schieren and Hansch, 1993). During activation of the early-acting classical components, small (8 to 10 kilodaltons) peptides are released by proteolytic cleavage from the second, third, and fourth components of complement. These fragments and an activation fragment of the fifth component of complement, C5a, have anaphylatoxin activities and modulate vascular permeability, smooth muscle reactivity, and chemotaxis of polymorphonuclear leukocytes and monocytes.

Upon activation of C3 by either convertase, the second phase of complement activation is initiated: the membrane attack complex is assembled by protein–protein interaction of terminal (C5 to C9) complement proteins (Muller-Eberhard, 1986). This complex alters membrane integrity via a transmembrane channel and thereby causes cytolysis of bacteria or cells.

Studies of fetal/neonatal complement have focused on quantification of serum concentrations of individual components, determining hepatic and extrahepatic synthesis rates, examining maternal-fetal transport of these proteins, and assessing specific effector functions of the classical and alternative pathways. In the human, Gitlin and Biasucci (1969) reported detectable concentrations of C3 (1% of adult levels) and C1 inhibitor (20% of adult levels) by immunochemical methods as early as 5 to 6 weeks of gestation. By 26 to 28 weeks' gestation, both C3 and C1 inhibitor concentration increased to 66% of adult levels. Since these studies, multiple investigators have demonstrated that functionally and immunochemically measured complement protein concentrations in cord blood increase with advancing gestational age and that they are only 50% to 75% of adult concentrations at full-term gestation (Davis et al, 1979; Fietta et al, 1987; Miyano et al, 1987; Shapiro et al, 1983; Strunk et al, 1979). The important roles of complement regulatory proteins, decay-accelerating factor (DAF), membrane cofactor protein (MCP), and CD59 have prompted more recent examination of the ontogeny of these proteins in the human fetus (Simpson et al, 1993).

To examine the possible mechanisms of this developmental increase in serum concentrations of complement proteins, Adinolphi (1967), Gitlin and Biasucci (1969), and Colten (1972) have studied the hepatic synthesis rates of individual complement proteins in the human liver obtained at different gestational ages. They have shown that C2, C3, C4, C5, factor H, and C1 inhibitor are synthesized by the human fetal liver: C3 and C1 inhibitor synthesis can be demonstrated as early as 4 to 5 weeks of gestation. A marked increase in C4 synthesis by the fetal liver occurs at approximately 15 weeks' gestation, coincident with an increase in serum concentration. The hepatic synthesis mechanisms that regulate this increase, either a change in the amount of C4 produced by individual hepatocytes or a change in the number of hepatocytes that produce C4, are not yet determined. Extrahepatic fetal synthesis of complement has been shown in the large and small intestines at 19 weeks of gestation (Colten et al, 1968) and in fetal monocytes obtained from cord blood (Sutton et al, 1986). An additional source of developmentally regulated complement proteins is the tissue fibroblast. Strunk and colleagues (1994) have demonstrated that regulation of endotoxin-induced synthesis of the third component of complement (C3) and factor B is pretranslationally regulated in the fetus, translationally regulated in the newborn, and transcriptionally regulated in the adult.

On the basis of studies of genetically determined, structurally distinct complement variants in maternal and cord serum, no transplacental passage from mother to fetus of C3, C4, factor B, or C6 has been observed (Colten et al, 1981; Propp and Alper, 1968). The presence of detectable amounts of C2 and C1 inhibitor in cord blood but not in the sera of mothers with genetic deficiencies of these proteins suggests that fetal-maternal transport of these components does not occur.

Regulation of complement effector functions in the fetus and newborn infant has not been as extensively examined. Opsonization of invading microorganisms without specific immunoglobulin recognition requires alternative pathway activation. For infants born prematurely or without organism-specific maternal IgG, alternative pathway activation provides a critical mechanism for triggering complement effector functions (Baker et al, 1986; Cole, 1987; Correa et al, 1994; Edwards, 1986). For example, Stossel and colleagues (1973) demonstrated opsonic deficiency in 6 of 40 cord sera examined because of decreased factor B concentrations, despite normal C3 and IgG levels. The functional contribution of the classical pathway to neonatal effector functions has been assessed using cord blood–mediated opsonophagocytosis by adult polymorphonuclear leukocytes of group B streptococci type Ia (Edwards et al, 1983). This serotype may be opsonized by classical pathway components in the absence of specific antibodies and thus permits evaluation of the function of classical pathway activation. In 8 of 20 neonatal sera examined, decreased bactericidal activity was detected and correlated with significantly lower functional activity of C1q and C4. These studies did not determine whether this decrease was mediated by an inhibitor of function or by an intrinsic change in functional activity of these components in neonatal sera. The importance of the terminal complement component C9 for cytolysis of multiple isolates of *Escherichia coli* was suggested by in vitro experiments in which killing of *E. coli* by neonatal serum samples was limited by C9 but not by other classical pathway components (Lassiter et al, 1992, 1994).

Even though lower serum concentrations of classical and alternative pathway complement proteins may contribute to enhanced susceptibility of infants to systemic infection, other complement functions important for fetal/neonatal well-being but not related to antimicrobial response may require decreased classical and alternative pathway activation. For example, reduced serum concentration of C4b-binding protein (8% to 35% of pooled adult plasma levels), a critical regulator of classical pathway C3 convertase activity, has been noted in fetal and neonatal sera (Fernandez et al, 1989; Malm et al, 1988; Melissari et al, 1988; Moalic et al, 1988). Lower C4b-binding protein concentration increases the functional anticoagulant activity of protein S with which it complexes and thereby contributes to decreased coagulation function of the fetus and newborn. Consideration of functions besides immunologic effector functions may be important in understanding the developmental regulation of complement component production.

Because of the low plasma concentrations of individual complement proteins, administration of purified, recombinant complement proteins has been considered as an adjunct to immunoglobulin replacement therapy and polymorphonuclear leukocyte transfusion in the treatment of neonatal systemic bacterial infection (Cairo et al, 1987; Hill et al, 1986; Kalli et al, 1994; Krause et al, 1989). While a provocative idea, this approach must be studied thoroughly to ensure that effector functions of complement activation in resting and uninfected tissues are not triggered in an unregulated fashion. Peripheral administration of one or more complement proteins might result in the unregulated activation of complement at tissue sites that would compromise rather than enhance neonatal survival. Consequences of such unregulated activation have been suggested by detection of the complement anaphylatoxin C5a in pulmonary effluent of infants with chronic pulmonary inflammation in whom bronchopulmonary dysplasia develops (Groneck et al, 1993a, 1994). Concern has also been raised that unregulated complement activation may occur in selected infants who undergo extracorporeal membrane oxygenation (Johnson, 1994).

Complement activation is the regulator of multiple effector functions of the host immunologic response. Further studies of the fetus and newborn infant will be aimed at understanding the developmental and genetic regulation of immunologic and nonimmunologic functions of this important group of plasma and cell surface proteins.

Immunoglobulin

Immunoglobulins are a heterogeneous group of proteins detectable in plasma and body fluids and on the surface of B lymphocytes. Whereas these proteins have multiple, diverse functions, they are classified as a family of proteins because of their capacity to act as antibodies, that is, recognize and bind specifically to antigens. The rapid advances in understanding molecular structure and regulation, genetic diversity, and differences in function of immunoglobulins have recently been reviewed (Colten and Gitlin, 1995; Davey et al, 1986; Davis et al, 1981; Waldmann et al, 1983). The functions of immunoglobulins relevant to fetal/neonatal immunity are summarized in Table 40–2.

There are five known classes of immunoglobulins: IgG, IgM, IgA, IgE, and IgD. The prototype immunoglobulin molecule consists of a pair of identical heavy chains that determine the immunoglobulin class in combination with a pair of identical light chains. The chains are linked by disulfide bonds and electrostatic forces. Each immunoglobulin molecule contains two identical domains with antigen-binding activity (Fab) and a third fragment (Fc) devoid of antibody activity. The antigen-binding activity involves sites on both the heavy and light chains, whereas sequences in the Fc region of the heavy chain are involved in mediating immunoglobulin effector functions. Functions of individual immunoglobulin classes are different but overlapping.

IgG

IgG is the most abundant immunoglobulin class in human serum and accounts for more than 75% of all antibody activity in this compartment. Its monomeric form circulates in plasma, has a molecular mass of approximately 155,000 daltons, and, in adults, approximately 45% of total body IgG is in the extravascular compartment. The human conceptus is able to produce IgG by 11 weeks of gestation (Gitlin and Biasucci, 1969; Martensson and Fudenberg, 1965). The importance of its contributions to immunologic function is illustrated by the clinical problems encountered in individuals who are genetically deficient in IgG production: these patients suffer with recurrent infections if not treated with immunoglobulin replacement therapy (Sorensen and Polmar, 1987). The observations by several investigators that infants in whom group B streptococcal sepsis develops have low concentrations of type-specific IgG prompted attempts at acute or prophylactic treatment with immunoglobulin replacement therapy (Stiehm et al, 1987). Although successful in some trials, replacement therapy in newborns has not proved as efficacious as in individuals with genetically determined hypogammaglobulinemia (Noya and Baker, 1989). This difference in part may be due to the fact that fetal/neonatal IgG synthesis is regulated by both developmental and genetic mechanisms (Cates et al, 1987).

The kinetics of IgG placental transport suggest both passive and active transport mechanisms. Because IgG transport begins at approximately 20 weeks' gestation, preterm infants are born with lower IgG concentrations than term infants or their mothers. The full-term infant has a complete repertoire of adult IgG antibodies. Thus, provided relevant maternal IgG has been transported to the fetus, newborns are not susceptible to most viral and bacterial infections (e.g., measles, rubella, varicella, group B *Streptococcus*, and *E. coli*) until transplacentally acquired antibody titers decrease to biologically nonprotective concentrations. The regulation of IgG production in preterm infants has been a topic of study for 4 decades (Ballow et al, 1986; Dancis et al, 1953). Although adults with antibody deficiency syndromes have increased frequency of infections when IgG concentrations decrease below 300 mg/dL, the serum IgG concentrations of many preterm infants decrease below 100 mg/dL apparently without consequences. These observations suggest that preterm infants have additional immunologic protective mechanisms or that regulation of IgG function is not accurately assessed by serum IgG concentrations alone in preterm infants. Recent

TABLE 40-2

Immunoglobulin Classes and Functions

| Immunoglobulin | Molecular Mass (Daltons) | Serum Concentration (µg/ML) | | Functions |
		Adult	Newborn Infant (term)	
IgG	155,000	1200	1200	• Neutralizes toxins. • Binds antigens. • Activates complement. • Promotes immune complex clearance or phagocytosis. • Mediates antibody-dependent cellular cytotoxicity.
IgM	>900,000	97	<20	• Activates complement. • Multivalent ligand binding. • Clearance of microorganisms.
IgA	160,000	250	ND	• Mucosal antigen recognition.
IgE	190,000	0.04	0.003	• Mediates hypersensitivity reactions.
IgD	180,000	2.2	0.1	• Identifies pre–B lymphocytes.

Adapted from Colten HR, Gitlin JD: Immunoproteins. *In* Handin RI, Lux SE, Stossel TP (Eds): Blood: Principles and Practice of Hematology. Philadelphia, JB Lippincott, 1995.

studies suggest that low serum concentrations of IgG in the newborn may result from reduced ability of neonatal B cells to undergo immunoglobulin isotype switching because of decreased or ineffective expression of the ligand for the B cell surface protein CD40 on activated cord blood T cells (Brugnoni et al, 1994; Fuleihan et al, 1994).

IgG functions in host defenses in several ways. It can neutralize a variety of toxins in plasma by direct binding. After antigen binding, IgG can activate the complement cascade via interaction with the early-acting complement components. The Fc portion of IgG can interact with cell surface receptors on mononuclear phagocytes and polymorphonuclear leukocytes and thereby promote clearance of immune complexes and phagocytosis of particles or microorganisms. Finally, the presence of IgG on specific target cell antigens (e.g., tumors or allogeneic transplant tissues) can mediate antibody-dependent cellular cytotoxicity, a mechanism through which lymphocyte subpopulations recognize nonself antigens.

IgM

IgM represents approximately 15% of normal adult immunoglobulin. IgM circulates in serum as a pentamer of disulfide-linked immunoglobulin molecules joined by a single cross-linking peptide. The size of IgM (molecular mass >900,000 daltons) restricts its distribution to the vascular compartment. Although the antibody-binding affinity of monomeric IgM is low, the multivalent structure of the molecule provides high pentameric antibody avidity. IgM synthesis has been detected in the human conceptus at 10½ weeks' gestation (Rosen and Janeway, 1964). Because maternal-fetal transport of IgM does not occur, elevated (>20 mg/dL) concentrations of IgM in the fetus or newborn are suggestive of intrauterine infection or immunologic stimulation (Alford et al, 1969; Stiehm et al, 1966). However, because it is technically difficult to distinguish IgM molecules with specificity for individual organisms,

diagnosis of infections by analysis for specific IgM antibody remains of limited usefulness.

IgM is important for fetal/neonatal host defenses for several reasons. First, the IgM molecule is the most efficient of any immunoglobulin isotype in activation of the classical pathway of complement. It thus can trigger multiple effector functions of this cascade. Second, its pentameric structure provides conformational flexibility to accommodate multivalent ligand binding. Third, because of its localization in the vascular compartment and its high efficiency in complement activation, IgM plays a prominent role in clearance from serum of invading microorganisms.

IgA

Although IgA accounts for approximately 10% of serum immunoglobulins, it is detectable in abundance in all external secretions. In serum, IgA is present as a monomer (molecular weight, 160,000 daltons), whereas in secretions it exists as a dimer (molecular weight, 500,000 daltons) attached to a J chain identical to that found in IgM. In addition to the structural difference between serum and mucosal IgA, IgA found in secretions is attached to an additional protein called the secretory component (SC). This protein is a proteolytic cleavage fragment of the receptor involved in the secretion of polymeric IgA onto mucosal surfaces and into bile. Secretory IgA produced locally on mucosal surfaces by plasma cells is thus readily distinguishable from serum IgA. Although not rigorously quantified, it is estimated that the amount of IgA produced daily exceeds immunoglobulin production of all isotypes combined. Despite its relative abundance, unlike IgM and IgG, IgA cannot activate the classical pathway of complement nor effectively opsonize for phagocytosis particles or microorganisms.

Although IgA is detectable on the surface of human fetal B cells at 12 weeks' gestation, adult concentrations of serum and secretory IgA are not achieved until approximately 10 years of age. Because serum IgA is not transplacentally transferred in significant amounts, IgA is almost undetectable in cord blood. Colostrum-derived secretory IgA may provide a source of IgA in both gastrointestinal tract and other secretions for the newborn infant. Unlike other immunoglobulin isotypes, amino acid sequences of the hinge region of the IgA-2 subclass confer partial resistance to bacterial proteases. IgA is thus more resistant than other immunoglobulin isotypes to proteolytic effects of gastric acidity. Although considerable investigation suggests that passive immunization with IgA does occur with breastfeeding in humans, the overall importance of IgA in host defenses is presently not well characterized.

IgE

The concentration of IgE is undetectable by standard immunochemical techniques and accounts for approximately 1/10,000 of the immunoglobulin in adult serum. It circulates in the monomeric form (molecular weight, 190,000 daltons). Structurally, IgE lacks a hinge region. It is produced by most lymphoid tissues in the body but in greatest amounts in the lung and gastrointestinal tract. It is not secreted, and its appearance in body fluids generally occurs only with induction of inflammation. IgE cannot activate complement nor act as an effective opsonin. Its primary function identified to date is to mediate immediate hypersensitivity reactions. Specifically, antigen-specific IgE triggers mast cell degranulation with resultant bronchoconstriction, tissue edema, and urticaria via interactions with IgE receptors on the mast cell surface. Because of the presence of IgE in lung secretions and its potential importance in mediating allergic pulmonary and gastrointestinal reactions, considerable interest has been recently focused on use of serum IgE concentrations to identify premature infants at risk for development of reactive airways disease or in the diagnosis of gastrointestinal hypersensitivity reactions (Bazaral et al, 1971; Jarrett, 1984).

IgD

Although IgD is found in trace quantities in adult human serum and has neither complement-activating activity nor the capacity to opsonize particles or microorganisms, approximately 50% of cord blood lymphocytes exhibit IgD on their cell surface (Colten and Gitlin, 1995). These pre–B lymphocytes express surface IgM and IgD simultaneously. Because of its wide distribution on B cells, IgD may play an important role in primary antigen recognition for the fetus and newborn infant.

Immunoglobulin Replacement Therapy

Klesius and coworkers (1973) suggested that lack of antibody to group B *Streptococcus* occurs in infants at risk for systemic infection with this organism. The maternal contribution to type-specific IgG was subsequently supported by the work of Hemming and associates (1976) and Baker and Kasper (1976). Animal and human studies have suggested that type-specific IgG can decrease mortality from systemic group B streptococcal infections. However, opsonization is not the sole mechanism of this protective

effect (Fischer, 1988). Strain- and species-specific differences in protective effects of IgG have been noted. In addition, timing of administration and dosage of IgG can affect outcome. Prenatal administration has only been attempted in a small number of cases (Morrell et al, 1986), but postnatal administration has been studied extensively. Although no major short-term adverse effects were noted, studies in the 1980s to test the efficacy of immunoglobulin replacement therapy to prevent or treat bacterial infection were generally inconclusive (Noya and Baker, 1989). Over the past 5 years, investigators have focused on assessment of intravenous immunoglobulin replacement to prevent nosocomial infections in preterm infants and to treat infection in infants.

Because of low serum immunoglobulin concentrations in preterm infants and concurrent increased susceptibility to infection, several investigators have proposed prophylactic administration of immunoglobulin to prevent antibody deficiency and nosocomial infection among preterm infants (Baker et al, 1992; Clapp et al, 1989; Fanaroff et al, 1994; Kinney et al, 1991; Magny et al, 1991; Weisman et al, 1994). With one exception (Baker et al, 1992), these well-designed, placebo-controlled studies have failed to show consistent benefit of this strategy using different preparations of immunoglobulin, different treatment groups, and different dosage regimens.

In septic infants, the results of immunoglobulin replacement have been difficult to interpret because of the complexities in study design associated with enrolling acutely ill infants and small numbers of enrolled infants. Sidiropoulos and colleagues (1986) and Haque and coworkers (1988) compared antibiotics alone to antibiotics plus intravenous immunoglobulin. Each study suggested therapeutic benefit, although neither was blinded nor placebo controlled. A small pilot study of 22 patients was reported by Christensen and associates (1991), which was placebo controlled, demonstrated no difference between placebo treated and immunoglobulin treated groups with respect to survival, but did demonstrate a marked increase in immature polymorphonuclear leukocytes in the immunoglobulin-treated group. In a study of prophylactic immunoglobulin therapy in infants who weighed 500 to 2000 g, Weisman and coworkers (1993a) randomized 31 infants to either placebo or immunoglobulin treatment. Five of 17 placebo-treated infants died during the first 7 days after birth, but none of 14 died who received immunoglobulin. Long-term survival was not significantly different in the two groups. Because group B *Streptococcus* is the most common causal organism of neonatal bacterial sepsis, and because there are varying amounts of antibody against this organism in standard immunoglobulin preparations, Weisman and coworkers (1993a) have developed hyperimmune immunoglobulin for use in treatment of infected infants by immunizing plasma donors. Administration of this immunoglobulin preparation to 20 newborns increased significantly serum group B *Streptococcus* type–specific opsonic activity. Human monoclonal antibodies against group B *Streptococcus*, *E. coli* K1, and *Neisseria meningitides* have also been reported, but no large clinical trials have been reported concerning efficacy of these preparations (Hill, 1993a; Weisman et al, 1993b). Cairo and colleagues (1992) compared neutrophil transfusions with immunoglobulin replacement therapy in 35 newborns with sepsis and observed better survival in the neutrophil-treated group. Recently, Whitley (1994) suggested the potential benefit of immunoglobulin therapy and concomitant administration of antiviral therapy for infants with herpes simplex encephalitis or disseminated infection. These studies suggest that intravenous immunoglobulin is more appropriate as a therapeutic agent for infants with established infection than as a preventive strategy, but further studies are required to document efficacy (Hill, 1993; Weisman et al, 1993b).

Besides prophylactic or acute treatment of systemic infection, immunoglobulin replacement therapy has been used in other clinical situations. Oral immunoglobulin administration with a preparation that contains IgG and IgA has been proposed for prevention of necrotizing enterocolitis (Eibl et al, 1988). Necrotizing enterocolitis did not develop in any of 88 preterm infants who received 600 mg of an oral IgG-IgA preparation daily for 28 days, whereas necrotizing enterocolitis developed in 6 of 91 concurrent control infants. Confirmation was by x-ray examination (pneumatosis, pneumoperitoneum, or hepatic portal vein gas) or histopathologic examination of specimens obtained during surgery or autopsy. Similar results have been reported in an Italian study of 132 Italian infants with birth weight less than 1500 g (Rubaltelli et al, 1991). Intravenous immunoglobulin has also been used with some success in small numbers of infants with neonatal isoimmune thrombocytopenia (Massey et al, 1987). Although immunoglobulin replacement therapy may be a promising intervention in selected clinical circumstances, its role in the newborn in acute treatment of or prophylaxis for systemic infections, prevention of necrotizing enterocolitis, or treatment of isoimmune thrombocytopenia warrants further study (Noya and Baker, 1989).

Cellular Immunity

The newborn infant, especially the preterm infant, is at increased risk for development of a considerable spectrum of opportunistic infections, including *Candida albicans,* herpes simplex, and cytomegalovirus. Developmental and genetic differences between adults and infants in cell-mediated immunologic responsiveness account for this enhanced susceptibility. Considerable investigative interest has focused on the molecular, cellular, and functional definitions of these differences (Bellanti et al, 1994; Hogg et al, 1993; Krensky and Clayberger, 1994; Leung, 1994). This discussion focuses on those developmental aspects of cell-mediated immunity known to be important for fetal or neonatal responsiveness to opportunistic infections.

Lymphocytes

Lymphocytes play multiple critical roles in the cell-mediated immunologic response. Three lymphocytic lineages have been identified by cell surface and functional criteria: T, or thymus-dependent, lymphocytes, B, or bursa-derived, lymphocytes, and NK, or natural killer, lymphocytes (Abo et al, 1983; Baley and Schacter, 1985). T and B cells are known to differentiate from a stem cell common to other hematopoietic cells. Although not conclusively demonstrated, studies of children with SCID suggest that, in some of these patients, defective development of all three cells is observed, and thus a common lymphoid stem cell may exist (Thompson et al, 1984).

Immunocompetent cells capable of responding to foreign lymphocytes in the mixed lymphocyte reaction are found in the fetal liver at 5 weeks' gestation. Before 8 weeks' gestation, lymphocytes are not detectable in the fetal thymus. After 8 weeks, lymphoid follicles, T lymphocytes, and Hassall's corpuscles can be identified. By 12 to 14 weeks, T lymphocytes can be found in the fetal spleen (Timens et al, 1987). By 15 to 20 weeks, the fetus has readily detectable numbers of peripheral T lymphocytes.

B lymphocytes with surface IgM are first found in the fetal liver at 9 weeks' gestation and in the fetal spleen at 11 weeks (Owen et al, 1977; Timens et al, 1987). Antigen-specific antibody production can be detected in the human fetus by 20 weeks' gestation. Fetal spleen cells can synthesize in vitro IgM and IgG by 11 and 13 weeks' gestation, respectively.

Multiple studies have documented differences in the proportions of fetal/neonatal T lymphocyte subpopulations and B cells at different gestational ages and in a variety of perinatal disease states (Baker et al, 1987; Lilja et al, 1984; Pittard et al, 1985). In addition, functional differences between cord blood and adult T cells and B cells have been identified (Andersson et al, 1983; Bussel et al, 1988; Hauser et al, 1985; Hayward and Mori, 1984; Hicks et al, 1983; Jacoby and Oldstone, 1983; Nelson et al, 1986; Olding and Oldstone, 1974; Oldstone et al, 1977; Papadogiannakis and Johnsen, 1988; Pittard et al, 1984, 1989). Because of the potential importance of both of these areas to future immunologic treatment of newborns, each is reviewed here.

Although multiple functional and cell surface characteristics have been used to identify and study T lymphocytes, decreased mitogen-induced proliferation, decreased ability to induce immunoglobulin synthesis by B cells, presence of different proportions of helper and suppressor cell surface markers, and decreased capacity to produce lymphokines have all been shown to differentiate fetal/neonatal from adult T cells. Even though the in vivo significance of these differences has not been defined, the fetus and newborn infant can mount a cell-mediated immunologic response against certain antigens comparable to that of adults. Differences in the regulation of this responsiveness in the fetus and newborn are most likely the result of the necessity of preserving the fetus' immunologic role as a graft.

Availability of monoclonal antibodies directed at epitopes found on functionally distinct T-cell subsets has permitted identification of differences in T-cell regulation in certain common perinatal medical and infectious conditions (Ryhanen et al, 1984; Wilson et al, 1985). From a therapeutic perspective, the decreased production of lymphokines has considerable potential for clinical utilization. Specifically, Wilson and colleagues (1986), Winter and associates (1983), Frenkel and Bryson (1987), and Wakasugi and Virelizier (1985) have shown that neonatal T cells produce less interferon-gamma than adult T cells. Young and coworkers (1994) and Penix and colleagues (1993) have elucidated the molecular details of interferon-gamma regulation in newborn T cells: methylation status of a specific nucleotide motif in the 5′ regulatory region of the interferon-gamma gene correlates with transcription of the gene. These studies suggest that induction by interferon-gamma may play a major role in developmental regulation of immunologic responsiveness and may thereby provide an important reagent with which to enhance the capacity of infected infants to respond to invading microbes. Interferon-gamma might be used by systemic administration as has been done in adults with chronic granulomatous disease, leprosy, and acquired immunodeficiency syndrome (AIDS). However, an alternative in the neonatal period may be provided by in vitro activation of autologous lymphocytes, as has been used in adults with malignancies. Such an approach might avoid the unanticipatable developmental regulatory problems of systemic administration of a substance such as interferon-gamma with multiple, potentially deleterious effects. Similar approaches may be considered in specific infections with individual cytokines, for example, tumor necrosis factor-alpha and granulocyte/macrophage–colony-stimulating factor (Cairo, 1991; Wilson et al, 1993).

Considerable investigation has focused on the ontogeny of B lymphocytes (Bofill et al, 1985; Gathings et al, 1977; Pedersen et al, 1983; Pereira et al, 1982; Tedder et al, 1985a, 1985b). In the fetus, these cells are detectable during the first trimester, but their expression of immunoglobulins differs from that observed in adults. B-cell precursors (pre–B cells) are detectable in human fetal liver at 8 weeks' gestation and in the bone marrow at 12 weeks' gestation. By the 15th week of gestation, the proportions of fetal B cells that express different immunoglobulin heavy-chain isotypes are equivalent to those in adults. These cells exhibit intracytoplasmic heavy chains. They lack stable surface immunoglobulin molecules characteristic of mature B cells but are the precursors of IgM⁺ B lymphocytes. The generation of immunoglobulin isotype diversity within the B-cell lineage occurs in the fetus without apparent stimulation by multiple foreign antigens. However, a fetal/neonatal characteristic of B lymphocytes is their concurrent expression of two or three immunoglobulin isotypes. The molecular events that regulate isotype switching and diversity are being investigated. (For review, see Colten and Gitlin, [1995].)

Although the B cells of full-term and preterm infants can synthesize IgM, IgG, and IgA, the response of human infants to certain foreign antigens is qualitatively distinct from that of adults. For example, as noted in early studies of antibody responses to *Salmonella* organisms, infants can respond vigorously to protein H antigen but are incapable of responding to polysaccharide antigenic determinants (the O antigens of the cell wall). These differences appear to be due to both intrinsic differences in B cell responsiveness and increased suppressor T-cell activity in the fetus and newborn. Further understanding of the mechanisms that regulate B-cell function may permit individualized immunologic manipulation of antibody responsiveness specific for the developmental stages of preterm and full-term infants. For example, systemic administration of pharmacologic agents, for example, recombinant human cytokines, may permit enhanced B-cell or T-cell responsiveness to specific infectious agents. Alternatively, in vitro exposure

of autologous T or B cells to these cytokines may also permit focused immunoenhancing therapy.

Polymorphonuclear Neutrophils

As observed for T and B lymphocytes, neonatal polymorphonuclear neutrophils (PMN) are present at early stages of gestation but have different functional capacities than adult PMNs. Progenitor cells that are committed to maturation along granulocyte or macrophage cell lineages (granulocyte/macrophage colony-forming units, or CFU-GM) are detectable in the human fetal liver between 6 and 12 weeks' gestation in proportions comparable to those observed in adult bone marrow (Christensen, 1989). Human fetal blood has detectable CFU-GM from the 12th week of gestation to term (Christensen, 1989; Liang et al, 1988). Although these progenitor cells are detectable in the fetus and newborn infant, developmental differences in mature PMNs between adult and neonatal cells in signal transduction, cell surface protein expression, cytoskeletal rigidity, microfilament contraction, oxygen metabolism, and intracellular antioxidant mechanisms have all been demonstrated (Hill, 1987; Ricevuti and Mazzone, 1987). Besides intrinsic differences in PMN function, induction of specific functions as well as maturation of these cells are developmentally regulated by the availability in the microenvironment of specific inflammatory mediators and growth factors (Christensen, 1989; Vercellotti et al, 1987). For example, an activation product of the fifth component of complement, C5a, is a chemoattractant at sites of inflammation. Low concentrations of C5 in neonatal sera may not permit establishment of chemoattractant gradients at sites of inflammation in newborns comparable to those in adults. Differences between adult and fetal/neonatal PMN functions may thus reflect intrinsic cellular differences required for fetal well-being and differences in the availability or activity of substances that regulate PMN function.

The recognition that systemic bacterial infection in newborns is frequently accompanied by profound neutropenia prompted investigation of neutrophil kinetics in infected infants (Christensen et al, 1980, 1982; Santos et al, 1980). These studies have suggested diverse, developmentally specific regulatory mechanisms required for mobilization of the neutrophil response to infection. Lack of neutrophil precursors in bone marrow aspirates of infected infants and systemic neutropenia motivated several investigators to give neutropenic, infected infants neutrophil replacement therapy (Christensen and Rothstein, 1980). While successful in some cases, the results have not been uniformly beneficial (Cairo, 1987, 1989; Cairo et al, 1984, 1987; Menitove and Abrams, 1987; Stegagno et al, 1985). More recently, immunoglobulin replacement therapy treatment with recombinant cytokines has been observed to have beneficial effects on mobilization of neutrophils during bacterial sepsis (Christensen et al, 1991). This heterogeneity emphasizes the importance of individualizing immunologic interventions for the developmental stage of the infant and the invading microorganism being treated. In vitro treatment of neutrophil precursors in peripheral neonatal blood with recombinant cytokines as well as adjunctive therapy with immunoregulatory proteins may provide future options for this therapy (Cairo et al, 1991; Hill, 1993; Hill et al, 1991; Gillan et al, 1994).

Monocytes and Macrophages

Cells committed to phagocyte maturation (granulocyte or monocyte/macrophage) are detectable in the human fetal liver by the 6th week of gestation and in peripheral fetal blood by the 15th week. Unlike granulocytes, whose tissue half-life is hours to days, macrophages migrate into tissues and reside for weeks to months. In a tissue-specific fashion, these cells regulate availability of multiple factors, including proteases, antiproteases, prostaglandins, growth factors, reactive oxygen intermediates, and a considerable repertoire of monokines.

The importance of macrophages in the neonatal response to infectious agents has been documented in multiple studies. For example, increased antibody response and protection from lethal doses of *Listeria monocytogenes* were induced in newborn mice by administration of adult macrophages (Lu et al, 1979). Functional differences in chemotaxis and phagocytosis between adult and neonatal cells have been observed and most likely result from both intrinsic fetal/neonatal monocyte/macrophage characteristics and from nonmacrophage factors (e.g., decreased production of the lymphokine interferon gamma) (English et al, 1988; Stiehm et al, 1984; Van Furth et al, 1965; Van Tol et al, 1984). Inducible expression of individual complement proteins by lipopolysaccharide (LPS), a constituent of gram-negative cell walls, has also been shown to differ between adult and neonatal monocyte/macrophages (Strunk et al, 1994; Sutton et al, 1986). This difference suggests that, even though signal transduction mediated by LPS, LPS-induced transcription, and accumulation of mRNAs, which direct the synthesis of the third component of complement and factor B, are comparable in adult and neonatal cells, a translational regulatory mechanism does not permit these important inflammatory proteins to be synthesized by LPS-induced neonatal cells. This observation emphasizes the fact that fetal/neonatal monocytes/macrophages may have functions developmentally distinct from those of adult cells. For example, in utero, production of growth factors and removal of senescent cells during tissue remodeling may be critical to fetal development (Kannourakis et al, 1988). Concurrent induction of these functions and immunologic effector functions in fetal monocyte/macrophages would potentially elicit nonspecific inflammation in actively remodeling tissues.

Besides antibacterial functions, neonatal monocytes/macrophages contribute to tissue-specific regulation of the microenvironment in individual organs. For example, considerable attention has focused on the contributions of these cells to antioxidant defenses and to regulation of protease–antiprotease balance. Because of the importance in tissue injury and repair of these functions, tissue and injury-specific treatment by appropriately targeted and primed monocytes/macrophages may provide therapeutic options for treatment of a spectrum of problems, from oxygen toxicity in the lung to hemorrhage in the brain.

Specific Immunologic Deficiencies

The physician should attempt to differentiate infants with specific genetically regulated immunologic deficiencies from those with developmentally regulated, environmentally induced, or infection-related susceptibility to microbial invasion (Rosen, 1986; Rosen et al, 1984). The most common reason for increased immunologic susceptibility to infection besides prematurity is administration of corticosteroids for treatment or prevention of bronchopulmonary dysplasia. Both pulmonary and neurodevelopmental benefits have been described for this therapy (Abman and Groothius, 1994; Cummings et al, 1989). Even though the mechanisms that lead to steroid-induced amelioration of pulmonary disease have not been completely elucidated (see Chapter 55), pulmonary inflammatory response measured by concentrations of the anaphylatoxin C5a, leukotriene B4, interleukin 1, elastase-alpha-1-proteinase inhibitor, and a number of neutrophils is attenuated in steroid-treated infants (Groneck et al, 1993). Whereas shorter courses of steroids may reduce side effects, including immunosusceptibility, the availability of nebulized steroids may provide effective anti-inflammatory therapy with minimum toxicity (LaForce and Brudno, 1993).

A careful family history during an antenatal visit may be helpful in identifying relatives removed by as many as two to four generations with histories suggestive of genetic immunodeficiency. Availability of antenatal diagnostic techniques for several of these diseases permits consideration of treatment initiation immediately following or possibly before birth (Harland et al, 1988; Holzgreve et al, 1984; Perignon et al, 1987).

When a fetus at risk for a genetic form of SCID is identified, treatment should begin in the delivery room and be coordinated with antenatal diagnostic interventions. Specifically, cord blood should be obtained for white blood cell count and differential, lymphocyte subsets, karyotype (if not performed antenatally), mitogen stimulation studies, and immunoglobulin concentrations. Because the majority of these children do not become ill within the 1st week of life, care in an incubator should be provided, and staff should observe strict hand-washing technique.

Severe Combined Immunodeficiency

In the neonatal period, a morbilliform rash, probably the result of attenuated graft-versus-host disease from transplacental passage of maternal lymphocytes, may be the only symptom of SCID (Rosen, 1986). Over the first several months of life, failure to thrive characterized by intractable diarrhea, pneumonia, and persistent thrush, especially oral thrush, are the triad of findings most frequently seen in infants with this disease (Stephan et al, 1993). The diagnosis is established by profound lymphopenia (<1000 lymphocytes/mm^3) and an absence of T lymphocytes. T cells detectable in peripheral blood of affected infants shortly after birth may be either maternal T cells or circulating thymocytes. The thymus gland is not seen on chest radiographs. Histologically, the gland is composed of islands of endodermal cells that have not become lymphoid and contain no identifiable Hassall corpuscles. The pattern of inheritance of SCID can be either autosomal recessive or X-linked. Thus, 75% of patients with this disorder are male. Approximately 50% of the autosomal recessive cases result from a genetic deficiency of the enzyme adenosine deaminase (ADA). Although this enzyme is present in all mammalian cells, only lymphoid cells appear to be adversely affected.

If untreated, SCID is invariably fatal in the first few years of life. In 1968, Good and colleagues performed the first successful bone marrow transplantation in a patient with this disease (Gatti et al, 1968). Progress in transplantation biology permits successful use of parental haploidentical marrow with success for infants with all types of SCID. Besides increased susceptibility to opportunistic infections, these infants are also susceptible to development of graft-versus-host disease as a result of engraftment of maternal T lymphocytes acquired prenatally or postnatally as a result of T lymphocytes in transfused blood products (Pollack et al, 1982; Thompson et al, 1984). Thus, infants suspected of having this disorder should receive only irradiated blood products.

Wiskott-Aldrich Syndrome

Wiskott-Aldrich syndrome, another form of immunodeficiency, is characterized by severe eczema, thrombocytopenia, and susceptibility to opportunistic infection. It is inherited as a sex-linked recessive trait (Rosen, 1986). In untreated cases, children survive longer than infants with SCID (median survival, 5.7 years). T lymphocytes in these patients are decreased in number and in function. Decreased platelet size and decreased thrombopoiesis are also noted. These children are potentially treatable with bone marrow transplantation. Even though transplantation corrects the T-cell defects, thrombocytopenia persists. As in children with SCID, all blood products should be irradiated before administration to avoid T-cell engraftment and graft-versus-host disease.

DiGeorge Syndrome

The embryologic anlage of the thymus gland and the parathyroid gland is the endodermal epithelium of the third and fourth pharyngeal pouches. When normal development of these structures is disturbed, thymic and parathyroid hypoplasia can occur (Rosen, 1986). Infants with this disorder, DiGeorge syndrome, may exhibit abnormalities of calcium homeostasis during the neonatal period (hypocalcemia and tetany) and variable T-cell deficits, which appear to depend on the presence and number of small, normal-appearing ectopic thymic lobes. In addition, these infants have congenital conotruncal cardiac defects, low-set ears, midline facial clefts, hypomandibular abnormalities, and hypertelorism. Recently, the availability of methodology for performing gene dosage studies and more refined cytogenetic techniques (fluorescence in situ hybridization, or FISH) has permitted description of the CATCH 22 syndrome, a contiguous gene syndrome that includes DiGeorge syndrome (Hall, 1993). The CATCH acronym stands for *c*ardiac, *a*bnormal facies, *t*hymic hypoplasia, *c*left palate, and *h*ypocalcemia. This phenotype results from varying sized deletions on chromosome 22q11. In the nursery, identification of infants with congenital conotruncal abnormalities should prompt consideration of this syndrome. Fetal thymic implants can correct the immunologic deficits (Reinherz et al, 1981).

IMMUNIZATION
Maternal Immunization

Immunization before pregnancy has been effective in preventing several specific neonatal infections including diphtheria, pertussis, tetanus, hepatitis B, and rabies (ACOG Technical Bulletin, 1991; Centers for Disease Control and Prevention, 1994). For example, in developing countries, immunization during pregnancy with tetanus toxoid is a cost-effective method for preventing neonatal tetanus and for providing up to 10 years of protection for infants (Gill et al, 1991; Schofield, 1986). The benefits for both mother and infant from induction during pregnancy of maternal IgG antibody that can be transferred to the fetus and protect both the fetus and mother against postpartum morbidity and mortality are substantial (Insel et al, 1994; Linder and Ohel, 1994). However, maternal immunization, especially during pregnancy, is biologically distinct from immunization of nonpregnant individuals. Vaccine epitopes may be shared with vital fetal or placental tissues; therefore, vaccination may lead to unanticipated maternal or fetal morbidity. Maternal immunization may induce an antibody response in the fetus, as has been demonstrated with tetanus toxoid (Gill et al, 1983), and thereby induce potentially undesirable immunologic side effects (e.g., immunologic unresponsiveness or tolerance) in the infant. However, the increase in availability of potentially protective transplacentally transferred IgG through active maternal vaccination prompted the Institute of Medicine recently to recommend establishment of a program of active immunization to control early onset and late onset group B streptococcal disease in both infants and mothers (Institute of Medicine, 1985). Efforts to develop safe, effective vaccines for protection from group B streptococcal infections have encountered the same difficulties with immunogenicity and safety observed in the development of other vaccines that induce protection from polysaccharide-encapsulated organisms (Baker et al, 1988; Noya and Baker, 1992). Recently, the availability of conjugate vaccines, which include group B streptococcal polysaccharide antigens covalently linked either to tetanus toxoid or to a protein in the membrane of group B streptococci (beta C protein), (Madoff et al, 1994; Wessels et al, 1993) have shown considerable promise.

The indications for active vaccination during pregnancy rest on assessment of maternal risk of exposure, the maternal/fetal/neonatal risk of disease, and the risk from the immunizing agents (ACOG Technical Bulletin, 1991, Amstey, 1989; Centers for Disease Control and Prevention, 1994). In general, immunization with live viral vaccines during pregnancy is not recommended. Preferably, immunization with live viral vaccines are performed before pregnancy occurs. However, rare instances may occur in which live viral vaccine administration is indicated. For example, if a pregnant woman travels to an area of high risk for yellow fever, administration of that vaccine might be indicated because of the susceptibility of the mother and the fetus, the probability of exposure, and the risk of the mother and fetus from the disease. More common examples in the United States include influenza and polio virus vaccination. If a chronic maternal medical condition would be adversely affected by influenza, active immunization

TABLE 40–3

Summary of Recommendations for Immunization During Pregnancy

Live Virus Vaccines

- Measles—contraindicated.
- Mumps—contraindicated.
- Poliomyelitis—not routine; increased risk exposure.
- Rubella—contraindicated.
- Yellow fever—travel to high-risk areas only.

Inactivated Virus Vaccines

- Influenza—serious underlying diseases.
- Rabies—same as nonpregnant.
- Hepatitis B—pre- and postexposure for at-risk women.

Inactivated Bacterial Vaccines

- Cholera—to meet international travel requirements.
- Meningococcus—same as nonpregnant.
- Plague—selective vaccination of exposed persons.
- Typhoid—travel to endemic areas.
- Pneumococcus—same as nonpregnant.

Toxoids

- Tetanus-diphtheria—same as nonpregnant.

Hyperimmune Globulin

- Hepatitis B—postexposure prophylaxis given along with hepatitis B vaccine initially, then vaccine alone at 1 and 6 months.
- Rabies—postexposure prophylaxis.
- Tetanus—postexposure prophylaxis.
- Varicella—same as nonpregnant.

Pooled Immune Serum Globulins

- Hepatitis A—postexposure prophylaxis.
- Measles—postexposure prophylaxis.

Adapted from American College of Obstetricians and Gynecologists: Immunization During Pregnancy (Technical Bulletin No. 160). Washington, DC, ©ACOG, October 1991.

may be indicated during pregnancy. Similarly, if imminent exposure to live polio virus in an unprotected woman is anticipated, live oral polio virus vaccine may be used during pregnancy. If immunization can be completed before anticipated exposure, inactivated polio virus vaccine can be given. A summary of recommendations for immunizations during pregnancy is provided in Table 40–3.

For the pediatrician, maternal immunization represents an important preventive intervention. Breast-feeding does not adversely affect immunization and inactivated or killed vaccines pose no special risk for mothers who are breast-feeding or for their infants (Centers for Disease Control and Prevention, 1994). The availability of vaccines against polysaccharide-encapsulated organisms (e.g., *Haemophilus influenzae* type b and group B *Streptococcus*) may decrease morbidity and mortality from these diseases during the first 3 to 6 months of the infant's life (Amstey et al, 1985; Baker et al, 1988; Walsh and Hutchins, 1989). The possibility of decreasing the risks of development of hepatocellular carcinoma, cirrhosis, and chronic active hepatitis from perinatal transmission of hepatitis B through prenatal screening and active and passive immunization of the infant is substantial (Arevalho and Washington, 1988). The implications of maternal vaccination during pregnancy for preterm infants have not been studied.

Infant Immunization

Recent advances in understanding the developmental regulation of immunity have suggested that immunization during the neonatal period offers important advantages (Lawton, 1994). The recommendations of the American Academy of Pediatrics for immunization of infants are given in Table 40–4 and in Appendix 4. Immunization against *H. influenzae* type b should be considered for infants who are discharged from intensive care nurseries at or after 2 months of age. For the preterm infant, although different clinical approaches are used by practitioners, including decreasing the dosage of immunogen, postponing the first immunization until a corrected age of 2 months, or waiting for an arbitrary weight to be achieved by the infant (e.g., 10 pounds), the American Academy of Pediatrics recommends administering full-dose diphtheria, tetanus, and pertussis (DTP) immunization beginning at 2 months of age. These recommendations that no correction needs to be made for prematurity when initiating routine immunization in preterm infants have recently been supported by longitudinal evaluation of serum antibody response in preterm infants (Bernbaum et al, 1989; Conway et al, 1993).

The Committee on Infectious Diseases of the American Academy of Pediatrics and the Advisory Committee on Immunization Practices of the United States Public Health Service have recommended universal immunization of infants to reduce hepatitis B–associated morbidities (e.g., chronic hepatitis, hepatocellular carcinoma, cirrhosis) (Centers for Disease Control and Prevention, 1991, 1994; Committee on Infectious Diseases, 1992, 1994). All infants born to hepatitis B surface antigen (HBsAg)–negative women should begin hepatitis immunization schedule in the newborn period or within the first 2 months of life (AAP Committee on Infectious Diseases, 1994).

TABLE 40–4

Recommended Schedule of Hepatitis B Immunoprophylaxis to Prevent Perinatal Transmission

Vaccine Dose* and HBIG	Age
Infant Born to Mother Known to be HBsAg-Positive	
First	Birth (within 12 h)
HBIG†	Birth (within 12 h)
Second	1–2 mo
Third	6 mo
Infant Born to Mother Not Screened for HBsAg	
First‡	Birth (within 12 h)
HBIG†	If mother is found to be HBsAg-positive, give 0.5 mL as soon as possible, not later than 1 wk after birth
Second	1–2 mo
Third	6–18 mo§

*See Table 42–11 for appropriate vaccine dose.

†HBIG (0.5 mL) given intramuscularly at a site different from that used for vaccine.

‡First dose is same as that for infant of HBsAg-positive mother. Subsequent doses and schedules are determined by maternal HBsAg status.

§Infants of HBsAg-positive mothers should be vaccinated at 6 mo.

Used with permission of the American Academy of Pediatrics: Hepatitis B. *In* Peter G (Ed): 1997 Red Book: Report of the Committee on Infectious Diseases, 24th ed. Elk Grove Village, IL: American Academy of Pediatrics, 1997, p 258.

All infants regardless of gestational age at the time of birth whose mothers are HBsAg-positive should receive passive immunization within 12 hours of birth, and active immunization within 7 days of birth and at 1 and 6 months of age. Special efforts should be made to complete the hepatitis B vaccination schedule within 6 to 9 months in populations of infants with high rates of childhood hepatitis B infection (Peter, 1994). For premature infants with birth weights of less than 2000 g born to HBsAg-negative women, vaccination may be delayed until just before discharge or until 2 months of age when other immunizations are given. These infants do not need routine serologic testing after the third dose for anti-HBsAg. For infants whose mothers are HBsAg-negative but whose mothers have received active or passive immunization during pregnancy because of exposure to hepatitis B, recommendations include no treatment for the infant as long as the mother is HBsAg-negative at the time of birth. Yeast-derived recombinant hepatitis B vaccines have excellent safety records, induce minimum adverse reactions, and are highly immunogenic (Greenberg, 1993). The recommended dose of hepatitis B vaccine for infants varies by manufacturer and HBsAg status of the mother: for infants of HBsAg-negative mothers, 2.5 μg of recombivax HB and 10.0 μg of Engerix-B are recommended; for infants of HBsAg-positive mothers, 5.0 μg of Recombivax HB and 10.0 μg of Engerix-B are recommended. The need for booster doses and the feasibility of combining antigens in multivalent vaccines are currently under study. These guidelines for hepatitis immunization of infants have been developed for implementation for term and preterm infants. However, the extremely preterm infant whose mother is HBsAg-positive, a population seen with increasing frequency owing to the coincidence of intravenous drug abuse and carriage of HBsAg, has not been studied.

REFERENCES

Abman SH, Groothis JR: Pathophysiology and treatment of bronchopulmonary dysplasia. Pediatr Clin North Am 41:277, 1994.

Abo T, Miller CA, Gartland GL, et al: Differentiation stages of human natural killer cells in lymphoid tissues from fetal to adult life. J Exp Med 157:273, 1983.

ACOG Technical Bulletin: Immunization during pregnancy. 160, 1991.

Adinolfi M, Gardner B: Synthesis of beta-1-E and beta-1-C components of complement in human fetuses. Acta Paediatr Scand 56:450, 1967.

Alford CA, Blankenship WJ, Straumfjord JB, et al: The diagnostic significance of IgM globulin elevations in neonate infants with chronic intrauterine infections. Birth Defects 4:3, 1969.

Allen WR, Kydd JH, Antczak DR: Successful application of immunotherapy to a model of pregnancy failure in equids. In Clark DA, Croy BA (Eds): Reproductive Immunology. Amsterdam, Holland, Elsevier Science Publishers, 1986, p 253.

American Academy of Pediatrics: Hepatitis B. In Peter G (Ed): 1997 Red Book: Report of the Committee on Infectious Diseases, 24th ed. Elk Grove Village, IL: American Academy of Pediatrics, 1997.

American Academy of Pediatrics Committee on Infectious Diseases: Update on timing of hepatitis B vaccination for premature infants and for children with lapsed immunization. Pediatrics 94:403, 1994.

Amstey MS: Immunization in pregnancy. Contemp Ob/Gyn 34:15, 1989.

Amstey MS, Insel RA, Munoz J, et al: Fetal-neonatal passive immunization against Hemophilus influenzae type b. Am J Obstet Gynecol 153:607, 1985.

Andersson U, Britton S, De Ley M, et al: Evidence for the ontogenic precedence of suppressor T cell functions in the human neonate. Eur J Immunol 13:6, 1983.

Arevalho JA, Washington AE: Cost effectiveness of prenatal screening and immunization for hepatitis B virus. JAMA 259:365, 1988.

Baker CJ, Kasper DL: Correlation of maternal antibody deficiency with susceptibility to neonatal group B streptococcal infection N Engl J Med 294:753, 1976.

Baker CJ, Melish ME, Hall RT, et al: Intravenous immune globulin for the prevention of nosocomial infection in low-birth-weight neonates. The Multicenter Group for the Study of Immune Globulin in Neonates. N Engl J Med 327:213, 1992.

Baker CJ, Rench MA, Edwards MS, et al: Immunization of pregnant women with a polysaccharide vaccine of group B Streptococcus. N Engl J Med 319:1180, 1988.

Baker CJ, Webb BJ, Kasper DL, et al: The role of complement and antibody in opsonophagocytosis of type II group B streptococci. J Infect Dis 154:47, 1986.

Baker DA, Hameed C, Tejani N, et al: Lymphocyte subsets in the neonates of preeclamptic mothers. Am J Reprod Immunol 14:107, 1987.

Baley JE, Schacter BZ: Mechanisms of diminished natural killer cell activity in pregnant women and neonates. J Immunol 134:3042, 1985.

Ballow M, Cates KL, Rowe JC, et al: Development of the immune system in very low birth weight (less than 1500 g) premature infants: Concentrations of plasma immunoglobulins and patterns of infections. Pediatr Res 20:899, 1986.

Baskett TF, Parsons ML, Peddle LJ: The experience and effectiveness of the Nova Scotia Rh program, 1964–84. Can Med Assoc J 134:1259, 1986.

Bazaral M, Orgel HA, Hamburger RN: IgE levels in normal infants and mothers and an inheritance hypothesis. J Immunol 107:794, 1971.

Beer AE, Billingham RE: Maternally acquired runt disease. Science 179:240, 1973.

Beer AE, Billingham RE: The Immunobiology of Mammalian Reproduction. Englewood Cliffs, NJ, Prentice Hall, 1976.

Beer AE, Billingham RE, Yang SL: Maternally induced transplantation immunity, tolerance, and runt disease in rats. J Exp Med 135:808, 1972.

Beer AE, Kwak JY, Ruiz JE: The biological basis of passage of fetal cellular material into the maternal circulation. Ann NY Acad Sci 731:21, 1994.

Bellanti JA, Kadlec JV, Escobar-Gutierrez A: Cytokines and the immune response. Pediatr Clin North Am 41:597, 1994.

Berlin G, Selbing A, Ryden G: Rhesus haemolytic disease treated with high-dose intravenous immunoglobulin. Lancet 1:1153, 1985.

Bernard O, Schied M, Ripoche M, et al: Immunological studies of mouse decidual cells. I. Membrane markers of decidual cells in the days after implantation. J Exp Med 148:580, 1978.

Bernbaum J, Daft A, Samuelson S, Polin RA: Half-dose immunization for diphtheria, tetanus, pertussis: Response of preterm infants. Pediatrics 83:471, 1989.

Billingham RE: Transplantation immunity and the maternal-fetal relation. N Engl J Med 270:667, 1964.

Billington D: Evidence for trophoblast immunogenicity in the induction of maternal alloantibody formation in murine pregnancy. Reproductive immunology: Materno-fetal relationship. Colloque INSERM 154:17, 1987.

Bofill M, Janossy G, Janossa M, et al: Human B cell development. II. Subpopulations in the human fetus. J Immunol 134:1343, 1985.

Brugnoni D, Airo P, Graf D, et al: Ineffective expression of CD40 ligand on cord blood T cells may contribute to poor immunoglobulin production in the newborn. Eur J Immunol 24:1919, 1994.

Bussel JB, Cunningham-Rundles S, LaGamma EF, et al: Analysis of lymphocyte proliferative response subpopulations in very low birth weight infants and during the first eight weeks of life. Pediatr Res 23:457, 1988.

Cairo MS: Granulocyte transfusions in neonates with presumed sepsis. Pediatrics 80:738, 1987.

Cairo MS: Neutrophil host defense. Am J Dis Child 143:40, 1989.

Cairo MS: Cytokines: A new immunotherapy. Clin Perinatol 18:343, 1991.

Cairo MS, Rucker R, Bennetts GA, et al: Improved survival of neonates receiving leukocyte transfusions for sepsis. Pediatrics 74:887, 1984.

Cairo MS, Worcester C, Rucker R, et al: Role of circulating complement and polymorphonuclear leukocyte transfusion in treatment and outcome in critically ill neonates with sepsis. J Pediatr 110:935, 1987.

Cairo MS, VandeVen C, Toy C, et al: GM-CSF primes and modulates neonatal PMN motility: Up-regulation of C3bi (Mo1) expression with alteration in PMN adherence and aggregation. Am J Pediatr Hematol Oncol 13:249, 1991.

Cairo MS, Worchester CC, Rucker RW, et al: Randomized trial of granulocyte transfusions versus intravenous immune globulin therapy for neonatal neutropenia and sepsis. J Pediatr 120:281, 1992.

Cates KL, Goetz C, Rosenberg N, et al: Longitudinal development of specific and functional antibody in very low birth weight premature infants. Pediatr Res 23:14, 1988.

Centers for Disease Control: Diphtheria, tetanus, and pertussis: Guidelines for vaccine prophylaxis and other measures. Recommendations of the Advisory Committee on Immunization Practices (ACIP). MMWR Morb Mortal Wkly Rep 34:405, 1985.

Centers for Disease Control and Prevention: Hepatitis B virus: A comprehensive strategy for eliminating transmission in the United States through universal childhood vaccination: Recommendations of the Advisory Committee on Immunization Practices (ACIP). MMWR Morb Mortal Wkly Rep 40:1, 1991.

Christensen KK, Christensen P: IgG subclasses and neonatal infections with Group B streptococci. Monogr Allergy 23:138, 1988.

Christensen RD: Hematopoiesis in the fetus and neonate. Pediatr Res 26:531, 1989.

Christensen RD, Anstall HB, Rothstein G: Use of whole blood exchange transfusion to supply neutrophils to septic, neutropenic neonates. Transfusion 22:504, 1982.

Christensen RD, Brown MS, Hall DC, et al: Effect on neutrophil kinetics and serum opsonic capacity of intravenous administration of immune globulin to neonates with clinical signs of early-onset sepsis. J Pediatr 118:606, 1991.

Christensen RD, Rothstein GR: Exhaustion of mature marrow neutrophils in neonates with sepsis. J Pediatr 96:316, 1980.

Christensen RD, Shigeoka AO, Hill HH, et al: Circulating and storage neutrophil changes in experimental type II group B streptococcal sepsis. Pediatr Res 14:806, 1980.

Clapp DW, Kliegman RM, Baley JE, et al: Use of intravenously administered immune globulin to prevent nosocomial sepsis in low birth weight infants: Report of a pilot study. J Pediatr 115:973, 1989.

Clark DA, Quarrington C, Banwatt D, et al: Spontaneous abortion in immunodeficient SCID mice. Am J Reprod Immunol 32:15, 1994.

Cole FS: Complement function in the neonate. In Burgio GR, Hanson

LA, Ugazio AG (Eds): Immunology of the Neonate. Berlin, Springer Verlag, 1987, pp 76–82.

Cole FS, Colten HR: Complement. *In* Ogra PL (Ed): Neonatal Infections, Nutritional and Immunologic Interactions. New York, Grune & Stratton, 1984, pp 37–49.

Colten HR: Ontogeny of the human complement system: *In vitro* biosynsthesis of individual complement components by fetal tissues. J Cin Invest 51:725, 1972.

Colten HR, Alper CA, Rosen B: Genetics and biosynthesis of complement proteins. N Engl J Med 304:653, 1981.

Colten HR, Gitlin JD: Immunoproteins. *In* Handin RI, Lux SE, Stossel TP (Eds): Blood: Principles and Practice of Hematology. Philadelphia, JB Lippincott, 1995, pp 477–511.

Colten HR, Gordon JM, Borsos T, et al: Synthesis of the first component of human complement in vitro. J Exp Med 128:595, 1968.

Colten HR, Rosen FS: Complement deficiencies. Ann Rev Immunol 10:809, 1992.

Committee on Infectious Diseases: Update on timing of hepatitis B vaccination for premature infants and for children with lapsed immunization. Pediatrics 94:403, 1994.

Committee on Infectious Diseases: Universal hepatitis B immunization. Pediatrics 89:795, 1992.

Conway S, James J, Balfour A, Smithells R: Immunization of the preterm baby. J Infect 27:143, 1993.

Correa AG, Baker CJ, Schutze GE, Edwards MS: Immunoglobulin G enhances C3 degradation on coagulase-negative staphylococci. Infect Immunol 62:2362, 1994.

Crepeau MA, Croy BA: Evidence that specific cellular immunity cannot account for death of Mus caroli embryos transferred to Mus musculus with severe combined immune deficiency disease. Transplantation 45:1104, 1988.

Crepeau MA, Yamashiro S, Croy BA: Morphological demonstration of the failure of Mus caroli trophoblast in the Mus musculus uterus. J Reprod Fertil 86:277, 1989.

Croy BA: The application of SCID mouse technology to questions in reproductive biology. Lab Anim Sci 43:123, 1993.

Croy BA, Stewart CM, McBey A, Kiso Y: An immunohistologic analysis of uterine T cells between birth and puberty. J Reprod Immunol 23:223, 1993.

Croy BA, Rossant J, Clark DA: Histological and immunological studies of postimplantation death of Mus caroli embryos in the Mus musculus uterus. J Reprod Immunol 4:277, 1982.

Croy BA, Chapeau C: Evaluation of the pregnancy immunotrophism hypothesis by assessment of the reproductive performance of young adult mice of genotype scid/scid.bg/bg. J Reprod Fertil 88:231, 1990.

Cummings JJ, D'Eugenio DB, Gross SJ: Controlled trial of dexamethasone in preterm infants at risk for BPD. N Engl J Med 320:1505, 1989.

Coulam CB, Moore SB, O'Fallon WM: Association between major histocompatibility antigen and reproductive performance. Am J Reprod Immunol Microbiol 14:54, 1987.

Dancis J, Osborn JJ, Kunz HW: Studies of the immunology of the neonate infants, IV. Antibody formation in the premature infant. Pediatrics 12:151, 1953.

Davey MP, Bongiovanni KF, Kaulfersch W, et al: Immunoglobulin and T-cell receptor gene rearrangement and expression in human lymphoid leukemia cells at different stages of maturation. Proc Natl Acad Sci U S A 83:8759, 1986.

Davies KA: Complement. Baillieres Clin Haematol 4:927, 1991.

Davis CA, Vallota EH, Forristal J: Serum complement levels in infancy: Age related changes. Pediatr Res 13:1043, 1979.

Davis MM, Kim SR, Hood L: Immunoglobulin class switching: Developmentally regulated DNA rearrangements during differentiation. Cell 22:1, 1981.

De M, Wood GW: Analysis of the number and distribution of macrophages, lymphocytes, and granulocytes in the mouse uterus from implantation through parturition. J Leukoc Biol 50:381, 1991.

Edwards MS: Complement in neonatal infections: An overview. Pediatr Infect Dis 5:S168, 1986.

Edwards MS, Buffone GJ, Fuselier PA, et al: Deficient classical complement pathway activity in neonate sera. Pediatr Res 17:685, 1983.

Eibl MM, Wolf HM, Furnkranz H, et al: Prevention of necrotizing enterocolitis in low birth weight infants by IgA-IgG feeding. N Engl J Med 319:1, 1988.

Eklund J, Nevanlinna HR: Perinatal mortality from Rh(D) hemolytic disease in Finland, 1975–1984. Acta Obstet Gynecol Scand 65:187, 1986.

English BK, Burchett SK, English JD, et al: Production of lymphotoxin and tumor necrosis factor by human neonatal mononuclear cells. Pediatr Res 24:717, 1988.

Fanaroff AA, Korones SB, Wright LL, et al: A controlled trial of intravenous immune globulin to reduce nosocomial infections in very low birth weight infants. National Institute of Child Health and Human Development Neonatal Research Network. N Engl J Med 330:1107, 1994.

Faulk WP, Temple A, Lovins RE, et al: Antigens of human trophoblasts: A working hypothesis for their role in normal and abnormal pregnancies. Proc Natl Acad Sci U S A 75:1947, 1978.

Fernandez JA, Estelles A, Gilabert J, et al: Functional and immunologic protein S in normal pregnant women and in full-term neonates. Thromb Haemost 61:474–478, 1989.

Fietta A, Sacchi F, Bersani C, et al: Complement-dependent bactericidal activity for *E. coli* K12 in serum of preterm neonate infants. Acta Pediatr Scand 76:47, 1987.

Fischer GW: Immunoglobulin therapy in neonatal group B streptococcal infections: An overview. Pediatr Infect Dis 7:513, 1988.

Frenkel L, Bryson YJ: Ontogeny of phytohemagglutinin-induced gamma interferon by leukocytes of healthy infants and children: Evidence for decreased production in infants younger than two months of age. J Pediatr 111:97, 1987.

Fuleihan R, Ahern D, Geha RS: Decreased expression of the ligand for CD40 in newborn lymphocytes. Eur J Immunol 24:1925, 1994.

Gathings WE, Lawton AR, Cooper MD: Immunofluorescent studies of the development of pre–B cells, B lymphocytes and immunoglobulin isotype diversity in humans. Eur J Immunol 7:804, 1977.

Gatti RA, Meuwissen HJ, Allen HD, et al: Immunological reconstitution of sex-linked lymphopenic immunological deficiency. Lancet 2:1366, 1968.

Gill TJ III: Immunogenetics of spontaneous abortions in humans. Transplantation 35:1, 1983.

Gill TJ III: Reproductive immunology: A personal view. Am J Reprod Immunol 27:87, 1992.

Gill TJ III: Maternal-fetal interactions and disease. N Engl J Med 329:501, 1993.

Gill TJ III, Karasic RB, Antonicic J, Rabin BS: Long-term follow-up of children born to women immunized with tetanus toxoid during pregnancy. Am J Reprod Immunol 25:69, 1991.

Gill TJ, Repetti CF, Metlay LA, et al: Transplacental immunization of the human fetus to tetanus by immunization of the mother. J Clin Invest 72:987, 1983.

Gillan ER, Christensen RD, Suen Y, et al: A randomized, placebo-controlled trial of recombinant human granulocyte colony-stimulating factor administration in newborn infants with presumed sepsis: Significant induction of peripheral and bone marrow neutrophilia. Blood 84:1427, 1994.

Gitlin D, Biasucci A: Development of gamma G, gamma A, gamma M, beta1c/beta1a, C′1 esterase inhibitor, ceruloplasmin, transferrin, hemopexin, haptoglobin, fribrinogen, plasminogen, alpha-1-antitrypsin, orosomucoid beta-lipoprotein, alpha-1 macroglobulin and human prealbumin in the human conceptus. J Clin Invest 48:1433, 1969.

Gitlin D, Kumate J, Urrusti J, et al: The selectivity of the human placenta in the transfer of plasma proteins from mother to fetus. J Clin Invest 43:1938, 1964.

Greenberg DP: Pediatric experience with recombinant hepatitis B vaccines and relevant safety and imunogenicity studies. Pediatr Infect Dis J 12:438, 1993.

Groneck P, Gotze-Speer B, Oppermann M, et al: Association of pulmonary inflammation and increased microvascular permeability during the development of bronchopulmonary dysplasia: A sequential analysis of inflammatory mediators in respiratory fluids of high-risk preterm neonates. Pediatrics 93:712, 1994.

Groneck P, Oppermann M, Speer CP: Levels of complement anaphylatoxin C5a in pulmonary effluent fluid of infants at risk for chronic lung disease and effects of dexamethasone treatment. Pediatr Res 34:586, 1993a.

Groneck P, Reuss D, Goeze-Speer B, Speer CP: Effects of dexamethasone on chemotactic activity and inflammatory mediators in tracheobronchial aspirates of preterm infants at risk for chronic lung disease. J Pediatr 122:038, 1993b.

Guilbert L, Roberson SA, Wegmann TG: The trophoblast as an integral component of a macrophage-cytokine network. Immunol Cell Biol 71:49, 1993.

Gurka G, Rocklin RE: Reproductive immunology. JAMA 258:2983, 1987.

Hall J: CATCH 22. J Med Genet 30:801, 1993.

Haque KN, Zaidi MH, Bahakim H: IgM-enriched intravenous immuno-globulin therapy in neonatal sepsis. Am J Dis Child 142:1293, 1988.

Harland C, Shah T, Webster ADB, et al: Dipeptidyl peptidase IV—Subcellular localization, activity and kinetics in lymphocytes from control subjects, immunodeficient patients and cord blood. Clin Exp Immunol 74:201, 1988.

Hauser GJ, Zakuth V, Rosenberg H, et al: Interleukin-2 production by cord blood lymphocytes stimulated with mitogen and in the mixed leukocyte culture. J Clin Lab Immunol 16:37, 1985.

Hayward AR, Mori M: Human neonate autologous mixed lymphocyte response: Frequency and phenotype of responders and xenoantigen specificity. J Immunol 133:719, 1984.

Hemming VG, Hall RT, Rhodes PG, et al: Assessment of group B streptococcal opsonins in human and rabbit serum by neutrophil chemiluminescence. J Clin Invest 58:1379, 1976.

Hicks MJ, Jones JF, Thies AC, et al: Age-related changes in mitogen-induced lymphocyte function from birth to old age. Am J Clin Pathol 80:159, 1983.

Hill HR: Biochemical, structural, and functional abnormalities of poly-morphonuclear leukocytes in the neonate. Pediatr Res 22:375, 1987.

Hill HR: Intravenous immunoglobulin use in the neonate: Role in prophy-laxis and therapy of infection. Pediatr Infect Dis J 12:549, 1993a.

Hill HR: Modulation of host defenses with interferon-gamma in pediat-rics. J Infect Dis 167:23, 1993b.

Hill HR, Augustine NH, Jaffe HS: Human recombinant interferon gamma enhances neonatal polymorphonuclear leukocyte activation and move-ment, and increases free intracellular calcium. J Exp Med 173:767, 1991.

Hill HR, Shigeoka AO, Pincus S, et al: Intravenous IgG in combination with other modalities in the treatment of neonatal infection. Pediatr Infect Dis 5:S180, 1986.

Ho HN, Yang YS, Hsieh RP, et al: Sharing of human leukocyte antigens in couples with unexplained infertility affects the success of in vitro fertilization and tubal embryo transfer. Am J Obstet Gynecol 170:63, 1994.

Hogg N, Harvey J, Cabanas C, Landis RC: Control of leukocyte integrin activation. Am Rev Respir Dis 148:55, 1993.

Holmes CH, Simpson KL: Complement and pregnancy: New insights into the immunobiology of the fetomaternal relationship. Bailliers Clin Obstet Gynaecol 6:439, 1992.

Holzgreve B, Goldsmith PC, Holzgreve W, Golbus MS: A monoclonal antibody micromethod for studying fetal lymphocytes: Potential for prenatal diagnosis of inherited immunodeficiencies. J Reprod Immu-nol 6:341, 1984.

Hunziker RD, Wegmann TG: Placental immunoregulation. Crit Rev Im-munol 6:245, 1986.

Hunziker RD, Wegmann TG: Placental immunoregulation. Crit Rev Im-munol 6:245, 1989.

Insel RA, Amstey M, Woodin K, Pichichero M: Maternal immunization to prevent infectious disease in the neonate or infant. Int J Tech Assess Health Care 10:143, 1994.

Institute of Medicine, National Academy of Sciences: New vaccine devel-opment: Establishing priorities. Diseases of Importance in the United States, Vol. 1. Washington, DC, National Academy Press, 1985, p 424.

Jacoby DR, Olding LB, Oldstone MBA: Immunologic regulation of fetal-maternal balance. Adv Immunol 35:157, 1984.

Jacoby DR, Oldstone MBA: Delineation of suppressor and helper activity within the OKT4-defined T lymphocyte subset in human neonates. J Immunol 13:1765, 1983.

Jarrett EEE: Perinatal influences on IgE responses. Lancet 1:797, 1984.

Johnson PM: Immunobiology of the human placental trophoblast. Exp Clin Immunogenet 10:118, 1993.

Johnson RJ: Complement activation during extracorporeal therapy: Bio-chemistry, cell biology and clinical relevance. Nephrol Dial Transplant 2:36, 1994.

Johnston RB Jr: The complement system in host defense and inflamma-tion: The cutting edges of a double edged sword. Pediatr Infect Dis J 12:933, 1993.

Kalli KR, Hsu P, Fearon DT: Therapeutic uses of recombinant comple-ment protein inhibitors. Springer Semin Immunopathol 15:417, 1994.

Kannourakis G, Begley CG, Johnson GR, et al: Evidence for interactions between monocytes and natural killer cells in the regulation of in vitro hemopoiesis. J Immunol 140:2489, 1988.

Kinney J, Mundorf L, Gleason C, et al: Efficacy and pharmacokinetics of intravenous immune globulin administration to high risk neonates. Am J Dis Child 145:1233, 1991.

Klesius PH, Zimmerman RA, Matthews JH: Cellular and humoral im-mune response to group B streptococci. J Pediatr 83:926, 1973.

Krause PJ, Herson VC, Eisenfeld L, et al: Enhancement of neutrophil functions for treatment of neonatal infections. Pediatr Infect Dis 8:382, 1989.

Krensky AM, Clayberger C: Transplantation immunology. Pediatr Clin North Am 41:819, 1994.

LaForce WR, Brudno DS: Controlled trial of beclomethasone dipropio-nate by nebulization in oxygen and ventilator dependent infants. J Pediatr 122:285, 1993.

Lala PK, Chatterjee-Hasrouni S, Kearns M, et al: Immunobiology of the fetomaternal interface. Immunol Rev 75:87, 1983.

Lassiter HA, Watson SW, Seifring ML, Tanner JE: Complement factor 9 deficiency in serum of human neonates. J Infect Dis 166:53, 1992.

Lassiter HA, Wilson JL, Feldhoff RC, et al: Supplemental complement component C9 enhances the capacity of neonatal serum to kill multi-ple isolates of pathogenic *Escherichia coli*. Pediatr Res 35:389, 1994.

Lawton AR: Immunization of the neonate. Int J Tech Assess Health Care 10:154, 1994.

Leung DY: Mechanisms of the human allergic response. Clinical implica-tions. Pediatr Clin North Am 41:727, 1994.

Liang DC, Ma SW, Lin-Chu M, Lan CC: Granulocyte/macrophage col-ony-forming units from cord blood of premature and full-term neo-nates: Its role in ontogeny of human hemopoiesis. Pediatr Res 24:701, 1988.

Lilja G, Winbladh B, Vedin I, et al: Cord blood T lymphocyte subpopula-tions in premature and full-term infants. Int Arch Allergy Appl Immu-nol 75:273, 1984.

Linder N, Ohel G: In utero vaccination. Clin Perinatol 21:663, 1994.

Lu CY, Calamai EG, Unanue ER: A defect in the antigen presenting function of macrophages from neonatal milk. Nature 282:327, 1979.

Madoff LC, Paoletti LC, Tai JY, Kasper DL: Maternal immunization of mice with group B streptococcal type III polysaccharide-beta C pro-tein conjugate elicits protective antibody to multiple serotypes. J Clin Invest 94:286, 1994.

Magny JF, Bremard-Oury C, Brault D, et al: Intravenous immunoglobu-lin-therapy for prevention of infection in high-risk premature infants: Report of a multicenter, double-blind study. Pediatrics 88:437, 1991.

Malm J, Bennhagen R, Homberg L, et al: Plasma concentrations of C4b-binding protein and vitamin K–dependent protein S in term and preterm infants: Low levels of protein S-C4b–binding protein com-plexes. Br J Haematol 68:445, 1988.

Martensson L, Fudenberg HH: G_m genes and gamma globulin synthesis in the human fetus. J Immunol 94:514, 1965.

Massey GV, McWilliams NB, Mueller DG, et al: Intravenous immuno-globulin in treatment of neonatal isoimmune thrombocytopenia. J Pediatr 111(1):133, 1987.

Medawar PB: Some immunological and endocrinological problems raised by the evolution of viviparity in vertebrates. Symp Soc Exp Biol 7:320, 1953.

Melissari P, Nicolaides KH, Scully MF, et al: Protein S and C4b-binding protein in fetal and neonatal blood. Br J Haematol 70:199, 1988.

Menitove JE, Abrams RA: Granulocyte transfusions in neutropenic pa-tients. Crit Rev Oncol Hematol 7:89, 1987.

Mills L, Napier JAF: Massive feto-maternal haemorrhage: Effect of pas-sively administered anti-D in the prevention of Rh sensitization and haemolytic disease of the neonate. Br J Obstet Gynecol 45:1007, 1988.

Miyano A, Nakayama M, Fujita T, et al: Complement activation in fetuses: Assessment by the levels of complement components and split prod-ucts in cord blood. Diag Clin Immunol 5:86, 1987.

Miyawaki T, Seki H, Taga K, et al: Dissociated production of interleukin-2 and immune (gamma) interferon by phytohaemagglutinin stimulated lymphocytes in healthy infants. Clin Exp Immunol 59:505, 1985.

Moalic P, Gruel Y, Body G, et al: Levels and plasma distribution of free and C4b-BP-bound protein S in human fetuses and full-term neo-nates. Thromb Res 49:471, 1988.

Moore FD Jr: Therapeutic regulation of the complement system in acute injury states. Adv Immunol 56:267, 1994.

Morell A, Sidiropoulos D, Herrmann U, et al: IgG subclasses and antibod-ies to Group B streptococci in preterm neonates after intravenous infusion of immunoglobulin to the mothers. Pediatr Infect Dis 5:S195, 1986.

Muller-Eberhard HJ: The membrane attack complex of complement. Ann Rev Immunol 4:503, 1986.

Nelson DL, Kurman CC, Fritz ME, et al: The production of soluble and cellular interleukin-2 receptors by cord blood mononuclear cells following *in vitro* activation. Pediatr Res 20:136, 1986.

Noya FJD, Baker CJ: Intravenously administered immune globulin for premature infants: A time to wait. J Pediatr 115:969, 1989.

Noya FJD, Baker CJ: Prevention of group B streptococcal infection. Pediatr Infect 6:41, 1992.

Noya FJD, Rench MA, Garcia-Prats JA, et al: Disposition of an immunoglobulin intravenous preparation in very low birth weight neonates. J Pediatr 112:278, 1988.

Olding LB, Oldstone MBA: Lymphocytes from neonates abrogate mitosis of their mothers' lymphocytes. Nature 249:161, 1974.

Oldstone MBA, Tishon A, Moretta L: Active thymus-derived suppressor lymphocytes in human cord blood. Nature 269:333, 1977.

Ossa JE, Cadavid AP, Maldonado JG: Is the immune system necessary for placental reproduction? A hypothesis on the mechanisms of alloimmunotherapy in recurrent spontaneous abortion. Med Hypoth 42:193, 1994.

Owen JJT, Wright DE, Habu S, et al: Studies on the generation of B lymphocytes in fetal liver and bone marrow. J Immunol 118:2067, 1977.

Pangburn MD, Muller-Eberhard HJ: The alternative pathway of complement. Springer Semin Immunopathol 7:163, 1984.

Papadogiannakis N, Johnsen SA: Distinct mitogens reveal different mechanisms of suppressor activity in human cord blood. J Clin Lab Immunol 26:37, 1988.

Pedersen SA, Petersen J, Andersen V: Suppression of B lymphocytes in mature neonate infants. Acta Paediatr Scand 72:441, 1983.

Peel S: Granulated metrial gland cells. Adv Anat Embryol Cell Biol 115:1, 1989.

Penix L, Weaver WM, Pang Y, et al: Two essential regulatory elements in the human interferon gamma promoter confer activation specific expression in T cells. J Exp Med 178:1483, 1993.

Pereira S, Webster D, Platts-Mills T: Immature B cells in fetal development and immunodeficiency: Studies of IgM, IgG, IgA and IgD production *in vitro* using Epstein-Barr virus activation. Eur J Immunol 12:540, 1982.

Perignon JL, Durandy A, Peter MO, et al: Early prenatal diagnosis of inherited severe immunodeficiencies linked to enzyme deficiencies. J Pediatr 111:595, 1987.

Peter G: Summary of major changes in the 1994 Red Book: American Academy of Pediatrics Report of the Committee on Infectious Disease. Pediatrics 93:1000, 1994.

Pittard WB III, Miller K, Sorensen RU: Normal lymphocyte responses to mitogens in term and premature neonates following normal and abnormal intrauterine growth. Clin Immunol Immunopathol 30:178, 1984.

Pittard WB III, Miller KM, Sorensen RU: Perinatal influences on *in vitro* B lymphocyte differentiation in human neonates. Pediatr Res 19:655, 1985.

Pittard WB III, Schleich DM, Geddes KM, et al: Newborn lymphocyte subpopulations: The influence of labor. Am J Obstet Gynecol 160:151, 1989.

Pollack MS, Kirkpatrick D, Kapoor N, et al: Identification by HLA typing of intrauterine-derived maternal T cells in four patients with severe combined immunodeficiency. N Engl J Med 307:662, 1982.

Propp RP, Alper CA: C′3 synthesis in the human fetus and lack of transplacental passage. Science 162:672, 1968.

Raum DD, Awdeh ZL, Page PL, et al: MHC determinants of response to Rh immunization. J Immunol 132:157, 1984.

Redline RW, Lu CY: Localization of fetal major histocompatibility antigens and maternal leukocytes in the murine placenta. Implications for the maternal-fetal relationship. Lab Invest 61:27, 1989.

Reinherz EL, Cooper MD, Schlossman SF, et al: Abnormalities of T cell maturation and regulation in human beings with immunodeficiency disorders. J Clin Invest 68(3):699, 1981.

Reproductive immunology and immunogenetics. *In* Knobil E, Neill JD (Eds): The Physiology of Reproduction, 2nd ed. New York, Raven Press, 1994.

Ricevuti G, Mazzone A: Clinical aspects of neutrophil locomotion disorders. Biomed Pharmacother 41:355, 1987.

Roder JC, Duwe AW: The beige mutation in the mouse selectively impairs natural killer cell function. Nature 278:451, 1979.

Romero R, Mazor M, Munoz H, et al: The preterm labor syndrome. Ann N Y Acad Sci 734:414, 1994.

Romero R, Sepulveda W, Kenney JS, et al: Interleukin 6 determination in the detection of microbial invasion of the amniotic cavity. Ciba Foundation Symposium 167:205, 1992.

Rosen FS: Defects in cell-mediated immunity. J Immunol Immunopathol 41:1, 1986.

Rosen FS, Cooper MD, Wedgwood RJP: The primary immunodeficiencies. N Engl J Med 311:300, 1984.

Rosen FS, Janeway CA: Immunologic competence of the neonate infant. Pediatrics 33:159, 1964.

Rubaltelli FF, Benini F, Sala M: Prevention of necrotizing enterocolitis in neonates at risk by oral administration of monomeric IgG. Dev Pharmacol Ther 17:138, 1991.

Ryhanen P, Jouppila R, Lanning M, et al: Effect of segmental epidural analgesia on changes in peripheral blood leucocyte counts, lymphocyte subpopulations, and *in vitro* transformation in healthy parturients and their neonates. Gynecol Obstet Invest 17:202, 1984.

Santos JI, Shigeoka AO, Hill HH: Functional leukocyte administration in protection against experimental neonatal infection. Pediatr Res 14:1408, 1980.

Sargent IL: Maternal and fetal immune responses during pregnancy. Exp Clin Immunogenet 10:85, 1993.

Schieren G, Hansch GM: Membrane-associated proteins regulating the complement system: Functions and deficiencies. Int Rev Immunol 10:87, 1993.

Schmidt CM, Orr HT: Maternal/fetal interactions: The role of the MHC class I molecule HLA-G. Crit Rev Immunol 13:207, 1993.

Schofield F: Selective primary health care: Strategies for control of disease in the developing world. XXII. Tetanus: A preventative problem. Rev Infect Dis 8:144, 1986.

Scott JR, Rote NS, Branch DW: Immunologic aspects of recurrent abortion and fetal death. Obstet Gynecol 70:645, 1987.

Shapiro R, Beatty DW, Woods DL, et al: Complement activity in the cord blood of term neonates with the amniotic fluid infection syndrome. S Afr Med J 63:86, 1983.

Sidiropoulos D, Boehme U, Von Murlat G, et al: Immunoglobulin supplementation in prevention or treatment of neonatal sepsis. Pediatr Infect Dis 5:193, 1986.

Simmons RL: Histoincompatibility and the survival of the fetus: Current controversies. Transplant Proc 1:47, 1969.

Simmons RL, Russell PS: Immunologic interactions between mother and fetus. Adv Obstet Gynecol 1:38, 1967.

Simpson KL, Houlihan JM, Holmes CH: Complement regulatory proteins in early human fetal life: CD59, membrane co-factor protein (MCP) and decay-accelerating factor (DAF) are differentially expressed in the developing liver. Immunology 80:183, 1993.

Sorensen RU, Polmar SH: Immunoglobulin replacement therapy. Ann Clin Res 19:392, 1987.

Stegagno M, Pascone R, Colarizi P, et al: Immunologic follow-up of infants treated with granulocyte transfusion for neonatal sepsis. Pediatrics 76:508, 1985.

Steinbeck MJ, Roth JA: Neutrophil activation by recombinant cytokines. Rev Infect Dis 11:549, 1989.

Stephan JL, Vlekova V, LeDeist F, et al: Severe combined immunodeficiency: A retrospective single-center study of clinical presentation and outcome in 117 patients. J Pediatr 123:564, 1993.

Stern JJ, Coulam CB: Current status of immunologic recurrent pregnancy loss. Curr Opin Obstet Gynecol 5:252, 1993.

Stiehm ER, Ammann AJ, Cherry JD: Elevated cord macroglobulins in the diagnosis of intrauterine infections. N Engl J Med 275:971, 1966.

Stiehm ER, Ashida E, Kim KS, et al: Intravenous immunoglobulins as therapeutic agents. Ann Intern Med 107:367, 1987.

Stiehm ER, Sztein MB, Steeg PS, et al: Deficient DR antigen expression on human cord blood monocytes: Reversal with lymphokines. Clin Immunol Immunopathol 30:430, 1984.

Stossel TP, Alper CA, Rosen FS: Opsonic activity in neonate. Pediatrics 52:134, 1973.

Strunk RC, Fenton LJ, Gaines JA: Alternative pathway of complement activation in full term and premature infants. Pediatr Res 13:641, 1979.

Strunk RC, Fleischer JA, Katz Y, Cole FS: Developmentally regulated effects of lipopolysaccharide on biosynthesis of the third component of complement and factor B in human fibroblasts and monocytes. Immunology 82:314, 1994.

Sutton MB, Strunk RC, Cole FS: Regulation of synthesis of the third component of complement and factor B in cord blood monocytes by lipopolysaccharide. J Immunol 136:1366, 1986.

Swinburne LM: Leucocyte antigens and placental sponge. Lancet 2:592, 1970.

Tangri S, Wegmann TG, Lin H, Raghupathy R: Maternal antiplacental reactivity in natural, immunologically mediated fetal resorptions. J Immunol 152:4903, 1994.

Tedder TF, Clement LT, Cooper MD: Development and distribution of a human B cell subpopulation identified by the HB-4 monoclonal antibody. J Immunol 134:1539, 1985a.

Tedder TF, Clement LT, Cooper MD: Human lymphocyte differentiation antigens HB-10 and HB-11. I. Ontogeny of antigen expression. J Immunol 134:2983, 1985b.

Thomas ML, Harger JH, Wagener DK, et al: HLA sharing and spontaneous abortion in humans. Am J Obstet Gynecol 151:1053, 1985.

Thompson LF, O'Connor RD, Bastian JF: Phenotype and function of engrafted maternal T cells in patients with severe combined immunodeficiency. J Immunol 133:2513, 1984.

Timens W, Rozeboom T, Poppema S: Fetal and neonatal development of human spleen: An immunohistological study. Immunology 60:603, 1987.

Tongio MM, Mayer S, Lebel A: Transfer of HL-A antibodies from the mother to the child. Transplantation 20:163, 1975.

Vanderpuye OA, Labarrere CA, McIntyre JA: The complement system in human reproduction. Am J Reprod Immunol 27:145, 1992.

Van Furth R, Schuitt HRE, Hijmans W: The immunological development of the human fetus. J Exp Med 122:1173, 1965.

Van Tol MJD, Zijlstra J, Thomas CMG, et al: Distinct role of neonatal and adult monocytes in the regulation of the *in vitro* antigen-induced plaque-forming cell response in man. J Immunol 134:1902, 1984.

Vercellotti G, Stroncek D, Jacob HS: Granulocyte oxygen radicals as potential suppressors of hemopoiesis: Potentiating roles of lactoferrin and elastase; inhibitory role of oxygen radical scavengers. Blood Cells 13:199, 1987.

Volanakis JE: C3 convertases of complement. Year in Immunology 4:218, 1988.

Wakasugi N, Virelizier J-L: Defective interferon gamma production in the human neonate. I. Dysregulation rather than intrinsic abnormality. J Immunol 134(1):167, 1985.

Waldmann TA, Korsmeyer SJ, Hieter PA, et al: Regulation of the humoral immune response from immunoglobulin genes to regulatory T cell networks. Fed Proc 42:2498, 1983.

Walsh JA, Hutchins S: Group B streptococcal disease: Its importance in the developing world and prospect for prevention with vaccines. Pediatr Infect Dis 8:271, 1989.

Wegmann TG, Barrington LJ, Carlson GA, et al: Quantitation of the capacity of the mouse placenta to absorb monoclonal anti-fetal H-2K antibody. J Reprod Immunol 2:53, 1980.

Wegmann TG, Gill TJ, Nesbet-Brown E: Molecular and Cellular Immunobiology of the Maternal Fetal Interface. New York, Oxford University Press, 1991.

Weisman LE, Anthony BF, Hemming VG, Fischer GW: Comparison of group B streptococcal hyperimmune globulin and standard intravenously administered immune globulin in neonates. J Pediatr 122:929, 1993a.

Weisman LE, Cruess DF, Fischer GW: Standard versus hyperimmune intravenous immunoglobulin in preventing or treating neonatal bacterial infections. Clin Perinatol 20:211, 1993b.

Weisman LE, Stoll BJ, Kueser TJ, et al: Intravenous immune globulin prophylaxis of late-onset sepsis in premature neonates. J Pediatr 125:922, 1994.

Wessels MR, Paoletti LC, Rodewald AK, et al: Stimulation of protective antibodies against type Ia and Ib group B streptococci by a type Ia polysaccharide-tetanus toxoid conjugate vaccine. Infect Immunol 61:4760, 1993.

Whitley RJ: Neonatal herpes simplex virus infections: Is there a role for immunoglobulin in disease prevention and therapy? Pediatr Infect Dis J 13:432, 1994.

Wilson CB: Immunologic basis for increased susceptibility of the neonate to infection. J Pediatr 108(1):1, 1986.

Wilson CB, Penix L, Melvin A, Lewis DB: Lymphokine regulation and the role of abnormal regulation in immunodeficiency. Clin Immunol Immunopathol 67:25, 1993.

Wilson M, Rosen FS, Schlossman SF, et al: Ontogeny of human T and B lymphocytes during stressed and normal gestation: Phenotypic analysis of umbilical cord lymphocytes from term and preterm infants. J Immunol Immunopathol 37:1, 1985.

Wilson CB, Westall J, Johnston L, et al: Decreased production of interferon-gamma by human neonatal cells. J Clin Invest 77:860, 1986.

Winter HS, Gard SE, Fischer TJ, et al: Deficient lymphokine production of neonate lymphocytes. Pediatr Res 11:573, 1983.

Young HA, Ghosh P, Ye J, et al: Differentiation of the T helper phenotypes by analysis of the methylation state of the IFN-gamma gene. J Immunol 153:3603, 1994.

CHAPTER 41

Fetal/Newborn Human Immunodeficiency Virus Infection

F. Sessions Cole

Human immunodeficiency virus (HIV) infection, first described in 1981 (Gottlieb et al, 1981; Masur et al, 1981; Siegal et al, 1981) has reached epidemic proportions in the 46 countries of the western hemisphere, including the United States (Quinn et al, 1989; Chin, 1994). The prevalence of acquired immunodeficiency syndrome (AIDS) among U.S. residents older than 13 years of age was 223,000 in June 1996 (CDC, 1997). Approximately 80,000 new cases of AIDS are reported annually in the United States (Centers for Disease Control and Prevention, 1995a). Between 330,000 and 385,000 individuals are estimated to have died after diagnosis of AIDS between 1989 and 1994 (Centers for Disease Control and Prevention, 1992a). Although recent estimates of the lifetime cost of HIV/AIDS have been revised downward resulting from a reduction in the use of inpatient hospital resources to $119,274 per case (95% confidence intervals $105,760 to $132,789), the total cost of care for HIV and AIDS patients is conservatively estimated at $5 billion to $13 billion annually (Hellinger, 1993; Rogers, 1989; Winkenwerder et al, 1989). Recently, new case definitions for adults, adolescents, and children (13 years of age and younger) have been developed (Centers for Disease Control and Prevention, 1993a, 1994b, 1994c) and will prompt continued revisions in both incidence and cost estimates. The impact of new therapies, including zidovudine, on survival and health-care costs cannot be estimated.

Because of HIV screening of donated blood products and aggressive educational programs, the risk of new infection in hemophiliacs, in persons who receive blood transfusions, and in homosexual men has stabilized or declined. However, the risk of new infections remains high in intravenous drug users and in their heterosexual or homosexual partners (Centers for Disease Control and Prevention, 1993b). These facts have resulted in an increasing net seroprevalence rate during the first half of the 1990s among child-bearing women. This observation is consistent with the increasing risk of congenitally infected newborn infants.

EPIDEMIOLOGY AND NATURAL HISTORY OF PERINATAL HIV INFECTION
Epidemiology

Since the first reported cases of HIV infection in children in 1982, more than 5700 cases of pediatric AIDS (children 13 years of age or younger) have been reported to the Centers for Disease Control and Prevention (1982, 1994a). These cases represent only a fraction of the total seropositive pediatric population with the most severe clinical manifestations. Within the pediatric group diagnosed in the

1980s and early 1990s, the majority (approximately 80%) acquires HIV infection vertically from chronically infected mothers (Pizzo, 1990). With improved screening of blood products, this proportion increased to more than 95% of pediatric AIDS cases from perinatal infection in the 1990s. Among women screened without knowledge of risk status, observed seroprevalence rates range from less than 1% to 4.3% in inner-city hospitals of the northeast United States. Surveys of child-bearing women performed in nine states by anonymous testing blood routinely collected from newborns for diagnosis of hereditary metabolic disorders indicates statewide seroprevalence rates that range from 0.1% in California, Colorado, Michigan, New Mexico, and Texas and 0.2% in Massachusetts to 0.5% in Florida and New Jersey and 0.7% in New York (Centers for Disease Control, 1989; Hoff et al, 1988). Because the net seroprevalence rate among child-bearing women has been increasing, ongoing new infection of women in their child-bearing years has been occurring and will provide the most important contribution to increasing numbers of HIV seropositive children in the United States (Centers for Disease Control and Prevention, 1995a; Katz and Wilfert, 1989). Current estimates suggest that approximately 7000 HIV-infected women give birth annually in the United States and that 1000 to 2000 of their infants are congenitally infected (Rogers and Jaffe, 1994).

Women at high risk for acquiring HIV infection include those who received a blood transfusion before 1985, those who share needles for intravenous drug use, and those who have unprotected sexual intercourse with an infected partner. In 1992, the number of newly diagnosed AIDS cases among women infected through heterosexual contact exceeded those infected through intravenous drug use for the first time (Centers for Disease Control and Prevention, 1993b). Antenatal history-taking should include a careful transfusion history, history of intravenous drug use, and history of sexual contacts including bisexual or homosexual men, hemophiliacs, intravenous drug abusers, or males born in countries where heterosexual transmission of HIV is thought to play a major role (e.g., Haiti or central Africa). The risk of disease acquisition from a single heterosexual encounter with an infected partner is currently undefinable. The probability of HIV transmission during a single episode of unprotected vaginal or anal intercourse ranges from approximately 1 in 100 to 1 in 1000 (Chin, 1994). Although transmission occurs in both directions, the receptive partner has a greater likelihood of acquiring an HIV infection, a fact that increases risk among susceptible female partners. On the basis of studies of steady sexual partners of hemophiliacs or partners of patients with AIDS, repeated sexual contact may increase the risk of HIV transmission to 7% to 40% (Landesman, 1989). The latency period for the virus in the adult population is 7 to 9 years (Imagawa et al, 1989).

Universal prenatal testing has been a topic of considerable discussion. Currently, the American Academy of Pediatrics and the American College of Obstetricians and Gynecologists recommend HIV screening of pregnant women who are "at increased risk of HIV infection" (American Academy of Pediatrics Task Force on Pediatric AIDS, 1988; Frigoletto and Little, 1988). Rhame and Maki (1989) advocate universal prenatal testing for HIV, whereas Weiss and Thier (1988) have suggested screening before blood and tissue donation only. Availability of a therapeutic intervention (prenatal zidovudine) reduces significantly the risk of fetal/neonatal infection in HIV-infected pregnant women and has strengthened the case for universal prenatal screening (Connore et al, 1994; Rogers and Jaffe, 1994; Wilfert, 1994). In 1995 and 1996 more than 50 HIV-positive women delivered newborn infants after receiving zidovudine prenatally. None of the infants were found to be HIV positive after 8 months of follow-up (K. Beckerman, MD, personal communication). Because of the potential inaccuracy of risk histories as demonstrated in studies of perinatal transmission of hepatitis B virus (Centers for Disease Control, 1988), aggressive prenatal screening should continue to be considered among all pregnant women.

Because a substantial proportion of drug abuse is in inner-city areas, racial minority groups or the socioeconomically disadvantaged are most affected: of the HIV-infected children in the United States, approximately 48% are black and 22% are Hispanic (Pizzo, 1990; Centers for Disease Control and Prevention, 1995a). The congruence of the demographics of drug abuse and HIV infection suggests the importance of this route of infection: during the 1980s and early 1990s, drug abuse has been the numerically most significant high-risk group for fetal/neonatal infection. In one study, 76% of 59 infants with vertically transmitted HIV-infection had one or both parents who were intravenous drug abusers (Guinan and Hardy, 1987). However, the increasing contribution of infection among women through heterosexual contact will serve to amplify the epidemic among children (Bonkovsky, 1994; Centers for Disease Control and Prevention, 1994b).

Natural History

Currently, no prospective data are available concerning the route or timing of HIV infection during pregnancy or during the immediate postpartum period (Table 41–1).

Recovery of HIV from early gestation conceptuses, placenta, blood and amniotic fluid around the time of delivery, and breast milk suggests multiple possible perinatal routes of fetal/neonatal infection (Pizzo, 1990). Recent studies using viral culture have suggested that up to 50% of perinatal infections in infants occur late in pregnancy (Burgard et al, 1992; Mofenson, 1995; Soeiro et al, 1992) The contribution of breast-feeding to mother-infant transmission has not been evaluated rigorously in a prospective fashion. While HIV-infected women express anti-HIV secretory IgA in breast milk, the effect of these antibodies on HIV transmission remains unclear (Duprat et al, 1994). Current recommendations in the United States suggest that HIV-infected women avoid breast-feeding. In prospective studies of infants with seropositive and seronegative mothers in Zaire, Europe, Brazil, and the United States, a minimum vertical transmission rate of 15% to 30% has been observed (Connor et al, 1994; Cortes et al, 1989; Rogers et al, 1989; Ryder et al, 1989).

Because of antenatal transfer of HIV antibody of IgG isotype from mother to fetus, serologic status of an infant at birth is not a reliable indicator of infection. In addition, cord blood T-cell subset ratios and immunoglobulin concentrations have not been helpful in predicting subsequent development of HIV infection (Centers for Disease Control and Prevention, 1994d; Pizzo, 1990). Availability of molecular diagnostic methods as well as viral isolation methods from small amounts of plasma or small numbers of peripheral blood mononuclear cells permit more accurate categorization of infected infants at birth. This categorization is especially important for prognosis and for development of prophylactic pharmacologic interventions.

Immunologic classification of progression of HIV infection in adults has utilized $CD4^+$ T-lymphocyte counts as a principal indicator of disease severity. Depletion of $CD4^+$ T lymphocytes is a major consequence of HIV infection in adults and results in many of the severe manifestations of HIV infection (Centers for Disease Control and Prevention, 1994c). Because $CD4^+$ counts are developmentally regulated in infants and children (Denny et al, 1992; Erkeller-Yuksel et al, 1992; The European Collaborative Study, 1992; McKinney and Wilfert, 1992; Waecker et al, 1993) and because children are more susceptible to opportunistic infections at higher $CD4^+$ counts than adults (Connor et al, 1991; Kovacs et al, 1991; Leibovitz et al, 1990), age-specific values for $CD4^+$ counts have been developed by the Centers for Disease Control and Prevention for immunologic classification of disease severity, which use both absolute $CD4^+$ count and $CD4^+$ percent of total

---

TABLE 41–1

Perinatal Transmission of the Human Immunodeficiency Virus

Intrauterine Transmission (Rubella Model)	Intrapartum Transmission (Hepatitis Model)	Postpartum Transmission
• Virus found in 13- to 20-week fetus. • Infectivity of trophoblast cell lines. • Funisitis and chorioamnionitis of placenta. • Isolation of HIV from cord blood. • Craniofacial dysmorphic features.	• Exposure to blood during delivery (both vaginal and by cesarean). • Maternal-fetal transfusion during delivery.	• Number of definitive cases by breast-feeding is small, but transmission can occur. • No household cases reported to date.

Adapted from Pizzo PA: Pediatric AIDS: Problems within problems. J Infect Dis 161:316, 1990.

TABLE 41–2

Immunologic Categories Based on Age-Specific CD4+ T-Lymphocyte Counts and Percent of Total Lymphocytes

	Age of Child					
	<12 mos		1–5 y		6–12 y	
Immunologic Category	μL	(%)	μL	(%)	μL	(%)
1. No evidence of suppression	≥1500	(≥25)	≥1000	(≥25)	≥500	(≥25)
2. Evidence of moderate suppression	750–1499	(15–24)	500–999	(15–24)	200–499	(15–24)
3. Severe suppression	<750	(<15)	<500	(<15)	<200	(<15)

From Centers for Disease Control. Revised classification system for human immunodeficiency virus infection in children less than 13 years of age. MMWR Morb Mortal Wkly Rep 43:RR-12, 1994.

lymphocytes (Centers for Disease Control and Prevention, 1994c) (Table 41–2). Under this classification system, a child should not be reclassified to a less severe category even if subsequent CD4+ determinations improve.

Clinical categorization of HIV infection in children has been revised into four mutually exclusive clinical categories (Centers for Disease Control and Prevention, 1994c) (Table 41–3). The goal of this classification is to link prognosis and staging. All AIDS-defining conditions except lymphoid interstitial pneumonitis (LIP) are included in Category C. Exclusion of LIP from Category C is based on reports that suggest that the prognosis for HIV-infected children with

TABLE 41–3

Clinical Categories for Children with Human Immunodeficiency Virus Infection

Category N: Not symptomatic

Children who have no signs or symptoms considered to be the result of HIV infection or who have only one of the conditions listed in Category A.

Category A: Mildly symptomatic

Children with two or more of the conditions listed below but none of the conditions listed in Categories B and C.
  Lymphadenopathy (≥0.5 cm at more than two sites; bilateral = one site)
  Hepatomegaly
  Splenomegaly
  Dermatitis
  Parotitis
  Recurrent or persistent upper respiratory infection, sinusitis, or otitis media

Category B: Moderately symptomatic

Children who have symptomatic conditions other than those listed for Category A or C that are attributed to HIV infection. Examples of conditions in clinical Category B include but are not limited to:
  Anemia (<8 gm/dL), neutropenia (<1000/mL), or thrombocytopenia (<100,000/mL) persisting ≥30 days
  Bacterial meningitis, pneumonia, or sepsis (single episode)
  Candidiasis, oropharyngeal (thrush), persisting (>2 months) in children >6 months of age
  Cardiomyopathy
  Cytomegalovirus infection, with onset before 1 month of age
  Diarrhea, recurrent or chronic
  Hepatitis
  Herpes simplex virus (HSV) stomatitis, recurrent (more than two episodes within 1 year)
  HSV bronchitis, pneumonitis, or esophagitis with onset before 1 month of age
  Herpes zoster (shingles) involving at least two distinct episodes or more than one dermatome
  Leiomyosarcoma
  Lymphoid interstitial pneumonia (LIP) or pulmonary lymphoid hyperplasia complex
  Nephropathy
  Nocardiosis
  Persistent fever (lasting >1 month)
  Toxoplasmosis, onset before 1 month of age
  Varicella, disseminated (complicated chickenpox)

Category C: Severely symptomatic

Children who have any condition listed in the 1987 surveillance case definition for acquired immunodeficiency syndrome, with the exception of LIP.

Table continued on following page

TABLE 41–3

Clinical Categories for Children with Human Immunodeficiency Virus Infection *Continued*

Serious bacterial infections, multiple or recurrent (i.e., any combination of at least two culture-confirmed infections within a 2-year period), of the following types: septicemia, pneumonia, meningitis, bone or joint infection, or abscess of an internal organ or body cavity (excluding otitis media, superficial skin or mucosal abscesses, and indwelling catheter-related infections)

Candidiasis, esophageal or pulmonary (bronchi, trachea, lungs)

Coccidioidomycosis, disseminated (at site other than or in addition to lungs or cervical or hilar lymph nodes)

Cryptococcosis, extrapulmonary

Cryptosporidiosis or isosporiasis with diarrhea persisting >1 month

Cytomegalovirus disease with onset of symptoms at age >1 month (at a site other than liver, spleen, or lymph nodes)

Encephalopathy (at least one of the following progressive findings present for at least 2 months in the absence of a concurrent illness other than HIV infection that could explain the findings): (1) failure to attain or loss of developmental milestones or loss of intellectual ability, verified by standard developmental scale or neuropsychological tests; (2) impaired brain growth or acquired microcephaly demonstrated by head circumference measurements or brain atrophy demonstrated by computerized tomography or magnetic resonance imaging (serial imaging is required for children <2 years of age); (3) acquired symmetric motor deficit manifested by two or more of the following: paresis, pathologic reflexes, ataxia, or gait disturbance

Herpes simplex virus infection causing a mucocutaneous ulcer that persists for >1 month; or bronchitis, pneumonitis, or esophagitis for any duration affecting a child >1 month of age

Histoplasmosis, disseminated (at a site other than or in addition to lungs or cervical or hilar lymph nodes)

Kaposi's sarcoma

Lymphoma, primary, in brain

Lymphoma, small, noncleaved cell (Burkitt's), or immunoblastic or large cell lymphoma of B-cell or unknown immunologic phenotype

Mycobacterium tuberculosis, disseminated or extrapulmonary

Mycobacterium, other species or unidentified species, disseminated (at a site other than or in addition to lungs, skin, or cervical or hilar lymph nodes)

Mycobacterium avium complex or *Mycobacterium kansasii,* disseminated (at site other than or in addition to lungs, skin, or cervical or hilar lymph nodes)

Pneumocystis carinii pneumonia

Progressive multifocal leukoencephalopathy

Salmonella (nontyphoid) septicemia, recurrent

Toxoplasmosis of the brain with onset at >1 month of age

Wasting syndrome in the absence of a concurrent illness other than HIV infection that could explain the following findings: (1) persistent weight loss >10% of baseline, or (2) downward crossing of at least two of the following percentile lines on the weight-for-age chart (e.g., 95th, 75th, 50th, 25th, 5th) in a child ≥1 year of age, or (3) <5th percentile on weight-for-height chart on two consecutive measurements, ≥30 days apart, plus (4) chronic diarrhea (i.e., at least two loose stools per day for ≥30 days) or (5) documented fever (for ≥30 days, intermittent or constant)

From Centers for Disease Control. Revised classification system for human immunodeficiency virus infection in children less than 13 years of age. MMWR Morb Mortal Wkly Rep 43:RR-12, 1994.

LIP is better than for children with other AIDS-defining conditions (Blanche et al, 1990; de Martino et al, 1991; Tovo et al, 1992). Clinical classification should be based on signs and symptoms related to HIV infection, not to drug-related conditions (e.g., drug-related hepatitis or anemia). Finally, new definitions of HIV encephalopathy based on recommendations of the Working Group of the American Academy of Neurology AIDS Task Force (1991) and of HIV wasting syndrome replace the definitions published in the 1987 AIDS surveillance case definition for children (Table 41–3). The impact of the new classification system on numbers of children with AIDS has not been evaluated.

The frequency of spontaneous remission of perinatal HIV infection as described in a recent report of a 5-year-old child who had HIV-1 cultured from peripheral blood mononuclear cells twice during the first 60 days of life and who is currently seronegative with normal growth and development has not been determined (Bryson et al, 1995). The possibility that some infants are capable of clearing HIV infection has been proposed (Bryson et al, 1995; McIntosh and Burchett, 1995). If this phenomenon occurs

with detectable frequency, classification of infants of HIV seropositive mothers might need to be revised.

There is considerable heterogeneity of disease progression among infants who are HIV-infected (The European Collaborative Study, 1991). For example, among children who contracted HIV infection after receiving HIV-contaminated blood products at birth, disease progression has been slower than observed among HIV-seropositive infants infected via maternal-infant transmission (Albersheim et al, 1988; Ammann et al, 1983; Church and Isaacs, 1984; Saulsbury et al, 1987; Shannon et al, 1983). Approximately 5% of infants HIV infected at birth have a rapidly deteriorating course over the first 10 to 18 months of life. These children succumb to *Pneumocystis carinii* pneumonia, encephalopathy, or recurrent bacterial infection (Pahwa, 1988). Prevention of *P. carinii* pneumonia requires early identification of HIV-infected infants and initiation of antibiotic prophylaxis as soon as possible (Simonds et al, 1995). An additional 30% present with nonspecific findings including failure to thrive, persistent generalized lymphadenopathy, persistent oral candidiasis, and developmental delay. These children may be seropositive or seronegative. The indolent form of the disease is also characterized by cough, arterial desaturation, digital clubbing, and immunologic abnormalities (elevated immunoglobulins, abnormal T-cell numbers, and abnormal peripheral blood mononuclear cell mitogen responses) (Pahwa, 1988). Approximately 70% of newborns seropositive at birth are seronegative and free of symptoms by 18 to 24 months of age (Blanche et al, 1989). The availability of more sensitive molecular and viral isolation techniques to identify HIV-infected children permits more accurate categorization of and assessment of prognosis for these patients (Coombs et al, 1989; Rogers et al, 1989).

The impact of maternal HIV infection on pregnancy outcome in the United States has been difficult to assess because of multiple confounding factors, including drug abuse and malnutrition. However, in a study from Zaire where none of the women reported a history of intravenous drug abuse, low birth weight, prematurity, low ratio of head circumference to length, and chorioamnionitis were all more common among infants of HIV-positive mothers with AIDS than among infants of HIV-positive asymptomatic women or infants with seronegative mothers (Ryder et al, 1989). These problems substantially enhance the risk of death in the first year of life for infants born to seropositive mothers: 100 deaths (21%) occurred among 468 children of HIV-seropositive mothers and 23 deaths (3.8%) among 604 children of seronegative mothers. Based on these figures, Ryder and colleagues (1989) suggested that HIV infections will account for at least a 15% increase in infant mortality in Zaire. Educational interventions aimed at reproductive age women are targeted to reduce risk of

contracting HIV infection, to increase screening of pregnant women for HIV infection, and to increase availability of societal resources for children of HIV infected women; these are critical to attenuate the impact of the HIV epidemic on prognosis for children of the 1990s (Des Jarlais et al, 1994; Centers for Disease Control and Prevention, 1995b).

PATHOGENESIS OF HIV INFECTION

Human immunodeficiency virus type 1, previously known as lymphadenopathy-associated virus (LAV-1), human T-cell lymphotrophic virus type III (HTLV-III), or AIDS-related virus (ARV), is an RNA virus that has a lipid envelope and is approximately 100 nm in diameter (Zeichner, 1994). HIV is related to a family of nontransforming, cytopathic retroviruses (lentiviruses) based on direct comparisons of nucleotide sequence, morphologic characteristics, and in vitro comparisons (Ho et al, 1987) (Fig. 41–1). HIV-1 differs from other retroviruses in that it contains a distinctive set of proteins, *Tat* and *Rev*, that regulate the temporal pattern of gene expression and syncytium production (Zeichner, 1994). A brief overview of the viral life cycle (see Fig. 41–1A and 41–1B) and the roles of the major HIV genes (Table 41–4) follows (Zeichner, 1994).

The entry of HIV into host cells occurs through binding of gp120 to the cell surface antigen CD4. Study of gp120 has identified several distinct domains, including constant (C) regions and variable (V) regions. One part of the variable region forms a loop structure, termed the V3 loop, and plays a major role in mediating HIV binding. When

FIGURE 41–1. *A,* A schematic diagram of the HIV virion. The virion core, enclosed by p24 (CA) gag protein, contains the viral genome together with the associated NC gag-derived proteins, the pol-derived proteins, and lysine tRNA. The core is in turn surrounded by the membrane associated (MA) gag-derived protein and a lipid bilayer derived from the host cell plasma membrane. The gp41 transmembrane env-derived protein is anchored in the membrane, and the gp120 env-derived protein is noncovalently associated with gp41 outside the bilayer.

Illustration continued on following page

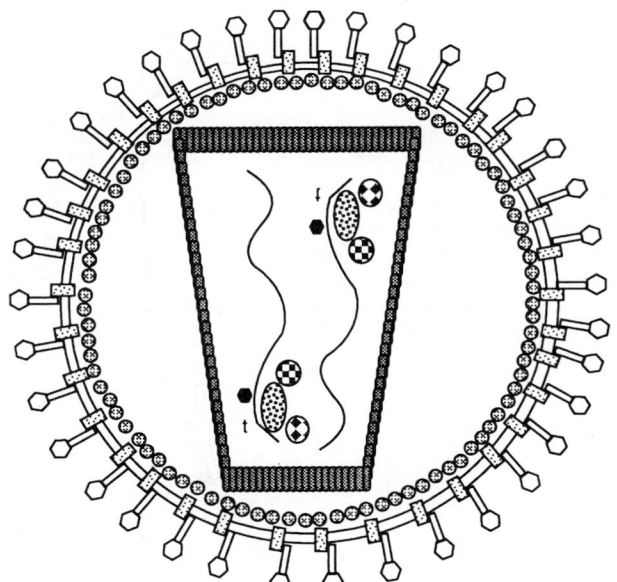

Gag Proteins	Pol Proteins	Env Proteins
p24 (CA)	p66,p51	gp120 (external;SU)
p16 (MA)	(Reverse	gp41 (transmembrane;TM)
p9 (NC)	Transcriptase/	
	RNase H; RT)	
Lys tRNA primer	p31 (integrase;IN)	
t	p10 (protease;PR)	

A

antibody directed against the V3 loop is present, binding is blocked and HIV infection inhibited. Efforts aimed at blocking this interaction with soluble CD4 antigen have been unsuccessful, largely because inhibitory concentrations have not been achieved in vivo. Besides mediating the interaction with CD4+ cells, gp120, along with a protein (gp 41), which is a second proteolytic product from the gp 120 precursor (gp 160), may play a critical role in vertical transmission of HIV-1 (Rubinstein et al, 1993; Ugen et al, 1992).

After membrane fusion occurs, reverse transcription, the defining feature of the retroviral life cycle, occurs. Because it is virus specific, the reverse transcriptase of HIV has been a primary focus for therapeutic agents like zidovudine, dideoxycytidine (ddC), and dideoxyinosine (ddI). Reverse transcription is a highly error prone process with misincorporation rates estimated at 1 per 1700 to 1 per 4000 bases. This error rate may contribute significantly to the rapidly mutating HIV genome.

After a cDNA copy of the viral genome is synthesized by reverse transcriptase, integration into host DNA occurs via the integrase protein, without the need for a high-energy cofactor or covalent intermediates. After integration, the viral genome is regulated and behaves much like a host cell gene. The regulatory sequences for the integrated HIV provirus are found in the long terminal repeat (LTR) region. This region interacts with host cell transcription factors (e.g., nuclear factor kappa B [NF-κB]) to permit low-level expression of HIV genes. This stage of viral gene expression is characterized by multiply spliced RNA transcripts encoding regulatory proteins, especially the potent viral stimulatory protein, *Tat*. Accumulation of *Tat* protein leads to a distinct increase in viral gene expression during the second stage of HIV gene regulation. In the final stage of HIV gene expression, the viral regulatory protein Rev induces production of unspliced or singly spliced RNA transcripts, which direct the synthesis of viral structural proteins, enzymes, and the viral genome.

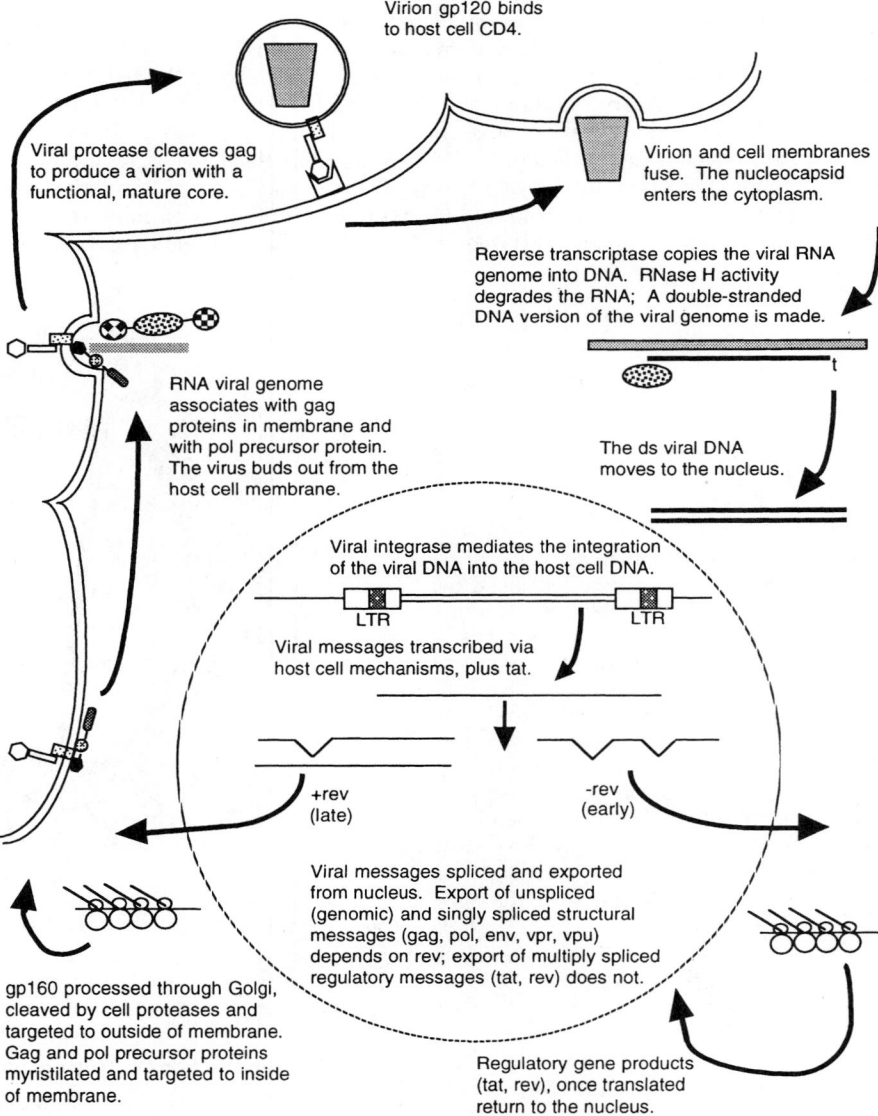

FIGURE 41–1 *Continued. B*, A schematic diagram of the viral life cycle. (*A* and *B* from Zeichner SL: The molecular biology of HIV: Insights into pathogenesis and targets for therapy. Clin Perinatol 21:39, 1994.)

Virion gp120 binds to host cell CD4.

Viral protease cleaves gag to produce a virion with a functional, mature core.

Virion and cell membranes fuse. The nucleocapsid enters the cytoplasm.

Reverse transcriptase copies the viral RNA genome into DNA. RNase H activity degrades the RNA; A double-stranded DNA version of the viral genome is made.

RNA viral genome associates with gag proteins in membrane and with pol precursor protein. The virus buds out from the host cell membrane.

The ds viral DNA moves to the nucleus.

Viral integrase mediates the integration of the viral DNA into the host cell DNA.

LTR   LTR

Viral messages transcribed via host cell mechanisms, plus tat.

+rev (late)

−rev (early)

Viral messages spliced and exported from nucleus. Export of unspliced (genomic) and singly spliced structural messages (gag, pol, env, vpr, vpu) depends on rev; export of multiply spliced regulatory messages (tat, rev) does not.

gp160 processed through Golgi, cleaved by cell proteases and targeted to outside of membrane. Gag and pol precursor proteins myristilated and targeted to inside of membrane.

Regulatory gene products (tat, rev), once translated return to the nucleus.

B

TABLE 41–4

Proteins of HIV: Functions and Inhibitors

Name[131]	Derived From	Size (kd)	Function	Location	Inhibitors
Structural Proteins					
p16 (MA)	gag (p55)	17	Membrane associated matrix protein	Inside viral membrane	Myristoylation inhibitors; zinc chelators; dominant negative gag mutants
p24 (CA)	gag (p55)	24	Viral core	Capsid	Protease inhibitors: block cleavage of gag and pol polyproteins
p9 (NC)	gag (p55)	9	Nucleocapsid	Inner virion core	
p6 (NC)	gag (p55)	6			
Protease (PR)	gag-pol polyprotein (Pr160)	10	Cleaves viral gag-pol polyprotein into final products; required for virion maturation	Functions in maturing virion	Protease inhibitors
Reverse transcriptase (RT)	gag-pol polyprotein (Pr160)	66; 51 (p14-function obscure, cleaved off p66)	DNA-directed RNA polymerase (reverse transcriptase); includes RNase H	Resides within virion; reverse transcriptase functions in cytoplasm	Nucleosides: AZT, ddI, ddC, 3TC Non-nucleosides; HEPT, TIBO, nevirapine, "L-drugs"
Integrase (IN)	gag-pol polyprotein (Pr160)	32	Catalyzes integration of viral cDNA into host DNA	Resides within virion; functions in nucleus	Integrase inhibitors
env (gp120) (SU)	env (gp160)	120	Binds CD4, mediates initial interaction of virus with target host cell	Virion envelope, associated with gp41	Soluble CD4, antibodies, intracellular protein processing inhibitors (modified CD4)
env (gp41) (TM)	env (gp160)	41	Anchored in virion membrane, noncovalently associated with gp120, mediates fusion of envelope with cell membrane	Virion envelope	Fusion inhibitors
Regulatory Proteins					
tat		16, 14	Potent transactivator of viral gene expression	Functions in nucleus	Tat inhibitors, TAR decoys, ribozymes
rev		19	Allows for export from nucleus of unspliced and singly splice mRNAs; regulates transition from early to late gene expression	Functions in nucleus	Transdominant rev mutants; ribozymes
Accessory Proteins					
vif		23	Increases virion infectivity; little effect on cell-to-cell infection		
vpu	Bicistronic vpu-env messages	16	Facilitates processing/export of env; inhibits formation of gp160-CD4 complexes	Perinuclear region: ?Golgi	
vpr		10, 15	Present in virion; modestly activates transcription	Virion	
nef		27, 25	Precise function unclear, but required for fully pathogenic virus in SIV model	Unknown	

The proteins that make up the HIV virion and the HIV proteins that function within the cell during infection are listed together with the larger precursor protein from which they are derived, their size (in kilodaltons, kd), their function in the viral life cycle, their location in the virion and in the cell, together with available and potential inhibitors.

From Zeichner SL: The molecular biology of HIV: Insights into pathogenesis and targets for therapy. Clin Perinatol 21:39, 1994.

HIV-2 is endemic to West Africa and results in an immunodeficiency syndrome similar to AIDS (Quinn, 1994). Recent migratory patterns of poor, rural, and young sexually active individuals to urban centers has contributed significantly to the spread of HIV-2 to Europe, India, and the Americas (Quinn, 1994). Because of reports of lower perinatal transmission of HIV-2 than HIV-1, differences in genetic regulation between the two viruses, and a paucity of therapeutic studies concerning HIV-2, the perinatal impact of HIV-2 is difficult to predict (Markovitz, 1993).

In adults, the diagnosis of HIV infection is usually predicated on a depletion of a subpopulation of helper/inducer T lymphocytes characterized by the presence on the cell surface of CD4 antigen. This abnormality results from the selective tropism of HIV for a $CD4^+$ subpopulation of lymphocytes. As might be anticipated from the developmentally distinct role that these cells play in immunologic responsiveness in infants, different immunologic abnormalities are seen in children.

While long-term prospective indicators are currently being studied, marked polyclonal hypergammaglobulinemia with elevations in IgG and variable elevations in IgA and IgM is a common finding in infants and children even in the early phases (ages 3 to 8 months) of the infection (Wilfert et al, 1994). Measurement of cord blood immunoglobulins alone has not been helpful in neonatal diagnosis. Depletion of $CD4^+$ lymphocytes with reversal of the T4/T8 ratio to less than 1 and decreased T-cell responsiveness to specific and nonspecific mitogens become evident later in the course of the infection. Prematurely born HIV-infected infants appear to manifest hypogammaglobulinemia as a feature of their immunodeficiency (Pahwa et al, 1987). These children may also have intracranial calcification. Serologic diagnostic tests may be negative in children with hypogammaglobulinemia after birth, so that viral isolation is required to establish the diagnosis.

Viral coinfection may enhance HIV replication in $CD4^+$ lymphocytes through several different mechanisms (Zeichner, 1994). For example, cytomegalovirus (CMV), herpes simplex virus, and hepatitis B virus can directly interact with the LTR region in the HIV genome to induce viral replication. Viral replication leads to death of $CD4^+$ lymphocytes. Loss of suppressor/cytotoxic T-cell regulation may facilitate HIV replication as well as allow latent Ebstein-Barr virus to replicate with consequent emergence of B-cell malignant lymphomas.

Syncytia formation, probably resulting from a lower surface density of CD4 molecules, and the relative refractoriness of HIV-induced cell death suggest that monocytes and macrophages may serve as significant reservoirs for the virus in the host and a vehicle for transport of HIV to multiple tissues including the central nervous system (Sattentau and Weiss, 1988). Among the defects observed in monocytes and macrophages from HIV-infected patients are the inability to migrate along chemotactic gradients and increased production of tumor necrosis factor. This latter abnormality may be critical in the pathogenesis of infant wasting syndrome.

DIAGNOSIS AND CLASSIFICATION OF HIV INFECTION

In adults, the diagnosis of HIV infection is made only after the presence of HIV antibody is repeatedly documented with a licensed enzyme immunoassay by identification of multiple virus-specific proteins (e.g., P24, P31, and either GP41 or GP160) by Western blot analysis (see Table 41–4) (Centers for Disease Control, 1993a). However, the serologic diagnosis of HIV infection in newborns is difficult because of the transplacental transport of maternal antibody to HIV (Church, 1994). An additional problem in utilization of Western blot techniques for diagnosis of HIV infection during infancy results from the inability to detect the HIV-specific proteins when excess maternally derived antibody is present. Because maternally derived antibody may persist for up to 18 months, the Centers for Disease Control and Prevention recommend serologic diagnosis of HIV infection only after the infant reaches 18 months of age (Simpson and Andiman, 1994). However, this test may also be unreliable after 18 months of age because some infants with HIV infection become hypogammaglobulinemic and may thus not be detectable by serologic testing. These concerns have prompted efforts to develop nonserologic methods with which to identify HIV infections on small amounts of blood.

Availability of sequence data for the genes that encode P24 antigen and GP41 transmembrane glycoprotein of HIV permitted Rogers and coworkers (1989) to use the polymerase chain reaction (PCR) to identify amplified HIV proviral sequences (Fig. 41–2). Five of seven infants in whom AIDS later developed (mean age 9.8 months) were detected by PCR in the neonatal period. However, the sensitivity of this method may be compromised by the inability to detect HIV that is transmitted during the intrapartum period, by its detection of proviral sequences in maternally derived lymphocytes, or by a frequency of viral sequences too low per cell to detect in the volume of blood or white blood cells obtained.

Besides PCR of proviral sequences, the other most sensitive and specific method for identifying HIV infection in infants born to infected mothers is virus culture (Burgard et al, 1992; Krivine et al, 1992; Rogers et al, 1989). Although potentially limited by detection of HIV in maternal blood and by technical requirements of HIV culture, this method has been useful in prospective studies of the natural history of vertically acquired HIV infection.

Whereas PCR and virus culture can identify approximately 30% to 50% of infected infants at birth and nearly 100% of infected infants by 3 to 6 months of age, other tests have been developed to provide lower cost, technically more feasible assays. The most useful of these is the p24-antigen assay, which, when modified to dissociate immune complexes of p24 antigen, has been used for early detection of HIV infection in infants (Miles et al, 1993; Rogers et al, 1991). Other laboratory assays including anti-HIV IgA and ELISPOT/in vitro antibody production (IVAP) are not commonly used and are less sensitive than viral culture or PCR (Centers for Disease Control, 1994c).

A new classification of clinical features of HIV infections in children younger than 13 years of age has recently been developed by the Centers for Disease Control and Prevention (1994c) (Table 41–5). The goals of the revised classification include staging to reflect prognosis, mutually exclusive classification categories, and balance of simplicity and medical accuracy. In the new classification system, HIV-infected children are classified on the basis of infec-

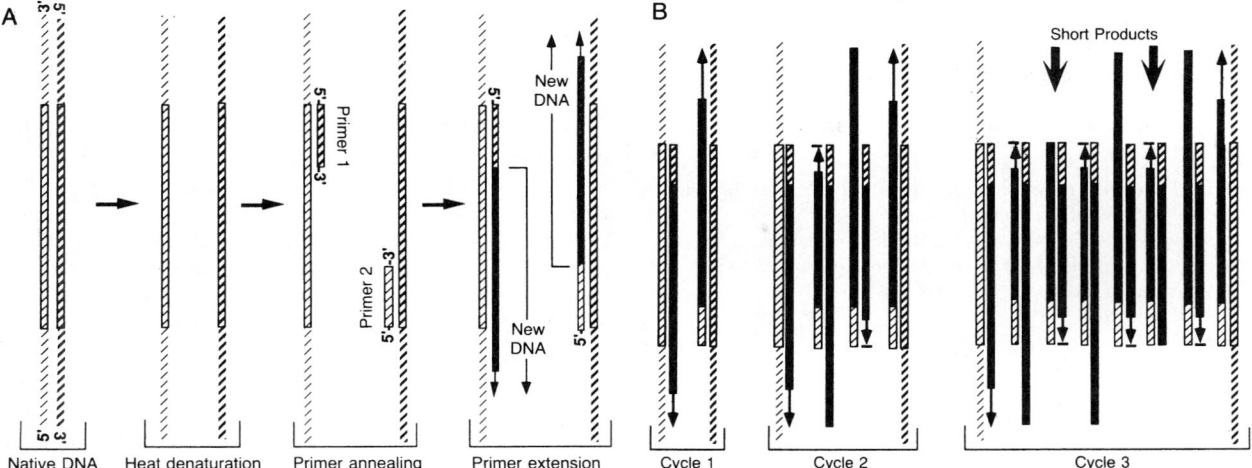

FIGURE 41–2. *A,* First round of the polymerase chain reaction. The basic polymerase chain reaction cycle consists of three steps performed in the same closed container but at different temperatures. The elevated temperature in the first step melts the double-stranded DNA into single strands. As the temperature is lowered for the second step, the two oppositely directed oligonucleotide primers anneal to complementary sequences on the target DNA, which acts as a template. During the third step, also performed at a lower temperature, the Taq polymerase enzymatically extends the primers covalently in the presence of excess deoxyribonucleoside triphosphates, the building blocks of new DNA synthesis. The native DNA target sequences, which will massively amplified as "short products" in the ensuing cycles, are boxed. The vector of action of the DNA polymerase is denoted by the arrows projecting from the newly synthesized DNA, indicated by the dark bars. *B,* Products at the end of the initial polymerase chain reaction cycles. A key element of the polymerase chain reaction is the repetitive thermocycling of the steps shown in *A.* At each cycle, the dark bars denote the accumulated DNA that has already been synthesized, and the currently synthesized DNA is indicated by the arrows that project in the direction of active DNA polymerization. Because the synthesized products of all previous cycles act as templates for all ensuing cycles, the number of short products increases geometrically at the completion of each cycle (the first three are shown). After the completion of the 30 or so cycles typical of the method, the ratio of short products to other DNA entities becomes so large that they appear to be the only detectable DNA in the reaction mixture. (From Eisenstein BI: Current concepts—The polymerase chain reaction: A new method of using molecular genetics for medical diagnosis. N Engl J Med 322:178, 1990.)

tion status, clinical status, and immunologic status, and cannot be reclassified into a less severe category even if the child's clinical or immunologic status improves (Tables 41–2, 41–6, and 41–7). The diagnosis of HIV infection in infants younger than 18 months of age requires positive results on two separate determinations (excluding cord blood) by HIV culture, PCR, or p24 antigen assay (Table 41–2).

TABLE 41–5

Pediatric Human Immunodeficiency Virus Classification*

	Clinical Categories			
Immunologic Categories	**N: No Signs/ Symptoms**	**A: Mild Signs/ Symptoms**	**B: Moderate Signs/ Symptoms†**	**C: Severe Signs/ Symptoms†**
1. No evidence of suppression	N1	A1	B1	C1
2. Evidence of moderate suppression	N2	A2	B2	C2
3. Severe suppression	N3	A3	B3	C3

*Children whose HIV infection status is not confirmed are classified by using the letter E (for perinatally exposed) placed before the appropriate classification code (e.g., EN2).

†Both Category C and lymphoid interstitial pneumonitis in Category B are reportable to state and local health departments as acquired immunodeficiency syndrome.

From Centers for Disease Control and Prevention. Revised classification system for human immunodeficiency virus infection in children less than 13 years of age. MMWR Morb Mortal Wkly Rep 43:RR-12, 1994.

Diagnosis of Human Immunodeficiency Virus Infection in Children

Diagnosis: HIV infected

I. A child <18 months of age who is known to be HIV seropositive or born to an HIV-infected mother and
  A. Has positive results on two separate determinations (excluding cord blood) from one or more of the following HIV detection tests:
    1. HIV culture
    2. HIV polymerase chain reaction
    3. HIV antigen (p24)
            OR
  B. Meets criteria for acquired immunodeficiency syndrome (AIDS) diagnosis based on the 1987 AIDS surveillance case definition

II. A child ≥18 months of age born to an HIV-infected mother or any child infected by blood, blood products, or other known modes of transmission (e.g., sexual contact) who
  A. Is HIV-antibody positive by repeatedly reactive enzyme immunoassay (EIA) and confirmatory test (e.g., Western blot or immunofluorescence assay [IFA])
            OR
  B. Meets any of the criteria in I.

Diagnosis: Perinatally Exposed (Prefix E)

A child who does not meet the criteria above who
  A. Is HIV seropositive by EIA and confirmatory test (e.g., Western blot or IFA) and is <18 months of age at the time of test
            OR
  B. Has unknown antibody status, but was born to a mother known to be infected with HIV

Diagnosis: Seroreverter (SR)

A child who is born to an HIV-infected mother and who:
  A. Has been documented as HIV-antibody negative (i.e., two or more negative EIA tests performed at 6–18 months of age or one negative EIA test after 18 months of age)
  B. Has had no other laboratory evidence of infection (has not had two positive viral detection tests, if performed)
            AND
  C. Has not had an AIDS-defining condition

From Centers for Disease Control and Prevention. Revised classification system for human immunodeficiency virus infection in children less than 13 years of age. MMWR Morb Mortal Wkly Rep 43:RR-12, 1994.

RISK OF HIV EXPOSURE TO PERINATAL HEALTH-CARE WORKERS

HIV infection among health-care workers results primarily from exposures that occur outside the health-care setting (Fahrner and Gerberding, 1993; Udasin and Gochfeld, 1994). Several prospective studies of health-care workers who have had needle-stick exposure to known HIV-positive patients suggest that the risk of seroconversion is approximately 0.4% (Centers for Disease Control, 1990). The risk of mucous membrane or skin exposure to HIV-infected blood is less than 0.4% (Centers for Disease Control and Prevention, 1992b; Marcus, 1988). Through June, 1994, surveillance by the Centers for Disease Control and Prevention (1994a) has identified 42 health-care workers who have documented occupational acquisition of AIDS/HIV

infection. Of these individuals, 36 had percutaneous exposure to fluid thought to contain HIV, 4 had mucocutaneous exposure, 1 had both percutaneous and mucutaneous exposures, and 1 had an unknown route of exposure. AIDS developed in 15 of these individuals. The specific health-care occupations of these individuals included 15 clinical laboratory technicians, 13 nurses, and 6 nonsurgical physicians. In addition, 88 health-care workers have possible occupational acquisition of AIDS/HIV infection. These individuals are reportedly without identifiable behavioral or transfusion risks for HIV infection, but HIV seroconversion specifically resulting from an occupational exposure was not documented.

The United States Department of Labor, Occupational Safety and Health Administration (OSHA) published final rules in December, 1991, which are intended to reduce or minimize occupational exposure to blood-borne pathogens, including HIV and hepatitis B (OSHA, 1991). These rules encourage the use of a combination of engineering and work practice controls, personal protective equipment, training, medical surveillance, hepatitis B vaccination, signs and labels that identify hazards, and other provisions including universal precautions for infection controls, a written exposure-control plan, and postexposure evaluation and testing for all employees who have exposure incidents (Fahrner and Gerberding, 1993). For perinatal services and nurseries, the following specific recommendations may be useful.

First, individuals likely to be exposed to blood or body fluids should be immunized with hepatitis B vaccine. Second, blood and body fluid precautions should be consistently used for all patients regardless of blood-borne infection status. These universal precautions do not apply to feces, nasal secretions, sputum, sweat, tears, urine, or vomitus unless contaminated with blood. Occupational exposure to human breast milk, semen, and vaginal secretions has not been implicated in transmission of HIV infection to health-care workers. Gloves should be worn by all individuals who handle newborns or placentas immediately

Recommendations for Routine Immunization of HIV-Infected Children in the United States

Vaccine	Known Asymptomatic HIV Infection	Symptomatic HIV Infection
Hepatitis B	Yes	Yes
DTP	Yes	Yes
IPV	Yes	Yes
MMR	Yes	Yes
Hib	Yes	Yes
Pneumococcal	Yes	Yes
Influenza	Yes	Yes
Varicella	No	No

DTP, diphtheria and tetanus toxoids and pertussis vaccine; IPV, inactivated poliovirus vaccine; MMR, live-virus measles, mumps, and rubella; Hib, *Haemophilus influenzae* type b conjugate.

Used with permission of the American Academy of Pediatrics. HIV infection and AIDS. *In* Peter G (Ed): 1997 Red Book: Report of the Committee on Infectious Diseases, 24th ed. Elk Grove Village, IL, American Academy of Pediatrics, 1997, p 294.

following birth. Hands should be washed immediately after gloves are removed and/or when skin surfaces are contaminated with blood. During resuscitation, regulated wall suction should be used. If mouth suction is necessary, traps should be installed to prevent direct aspiration. Infants of known seropositive mothers may be cared for in a normal nursery and do not require isolation. Gloves are not required for prevention of HIV transmission while changing diapers. Currently, data are insufficient to establish whether health-care workers who sustain an occupational exposure to HIV-infected blood are benefited by postexposure prophylaxis with zidovudine (Centers for Disease Control, 1990; Fahrner et al, 1992). However, most centers offer postexposure zidovudine prophylaxis (Henderson, 1991; Weiss, 1992). Even though various zidovudine prophylaxis regimens have been used, 200 mg five or six times daily for 4 to 6 weeks is a generally accepted protocol (Centers for Disease Control and Prevention, 1990). During all phases of follow-up, confidentiality of the worker and the source should be maintained.

Counseling for the exposed individual should provide the following:

1. The theoretical basis for postexposure prophylaxis (primarily data from animal studies).
2. The risk of the exposure.
3. The lack of definitive information concerning efficacy of zidovudine when used as postexposure prophylaxis in humans.
4. Data concerning toxicity.
5. Emphasizing the need for postexposure serologic testing regardless of zidovudine use (Centers for Disease Control, 1990).

TREATMENT AND MANAGEMENT OF HIV-INFECTED INFANTS

From a management perspective, infants seropositive for or infected with HIV are members of a family whose other members are immunocompromised and may soon die (Pizzo, 1990). Therefore, HIV has been called a killer of families, not just of the infected children or adults. Thus, good therapy for this disease must begin with multidisciplinary, supportive care (Fig. 41–3). Even though the physician plays an important role in this care, the needs of these children and families exceed the treatment capacity of a single discipline or individual. Nurses, social workers, physical therapists, educators, internists, infectious disease and neurology specialists, obstetricians, and many other professionals must be involved with the care of these children and families.

As in other areas of pediatrics, aggressive anticipatory care must be provided. Evaluation of the mother's health, family support systems, housing, and care providers for the infant should be carried out before birth. In certain circumstances, legal guardianship or foster care plans should be formalized before birth. Medical care of the infant should also be prevention oriented. Voluntary antenatal screening for HIV infection in pregnant women permits identification of pregnancies in which vertical HIV transmission is a potential complication. Zidovudine, a thymidine analogue that inhibits replication of HIV in vitro

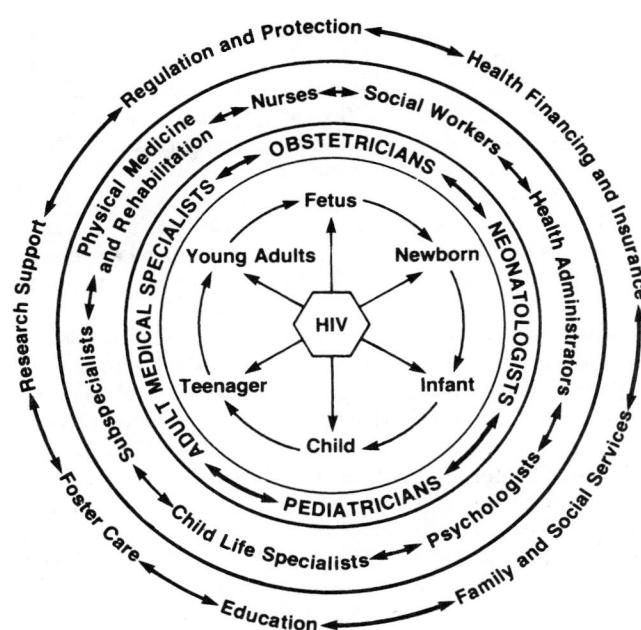

FIGURE 41–3. Pediatric AIDS represents a challenge to many facets of medicine and society. (From Pizzo PA: Pediatric AIDS: Problems within problems. J Infect Dis 161:315, 1990.)

by inhibiting the action of reverse transcriptase and possibly by other mechanisms, has been the best studied drug for interrupting vertical transmission (Yarchoan et al, 1989). In a placebo-controlled trial performed on 477 pregnant women, zidovudine treatment was shown to lower the risk of vertical transmission from 25.5% to 8.3% ($P = .00006$) (Connor et al, 1994). The treatment regimen used in this study consisted of zidovudine 100 mg orally five times a day beginning as early as 14 weeks of gestation plus intrapartum zidovudine (2 mg/kg of body weight given intravenously for 1 hour, followed by 1 mg/kg/hour until delivery) plus zidovudine for the infant (2 mg/kg orally every 6 hours for 6 weeks, beginning 8 to 12 hours after birth). The primary toxic effect on infants observed in this study was a statistically significant but clinically insignificant lower hemoglobin at birth in the zidovudine treated group. The United States Public Health Service has suggested that the results of this study, the potential long-term adverse effects of zidovudine for infants and women, and the needs of women and infants who receive this therapy be discussed with each HIV-infected pregnant woman to permit individualization for differing clinical situations (Centers for Disease Control and Prevention, 1994e). Only 9 of 239 infants in the zidovudine group had birth weights less than 2000 g. The applicability of these results to premature infants has not been rigorously evaluated. Because of the beneficial effects of this regimen on vertical HIV transmission, it was interrupted by the Data and Safety Monitoring Board of the National Institute of Allergy and Infectious Diseases (Bayer, 1994). The study lacked sufficient statistical power to evaluate possible teratogenic effects of antenatally administered zidovudine (Centers for Disease Control and Prevention, 1994e).

Recent data by the AIDS Clinical Trial Group Protocol

152 (ACTG 152) (1995) have suggested that another nucleoside, 2',3'-dideoxyinosine, either alone or in combination with zidovudine may be more effective in preventing clinical deterioration with less toxicity (McIntosh K, personal communication) in older children (3 months to 18 years). When administered as monotherapy in ACTG 152, the dose of ddI was 120 mg/m² administered every 12 hours and 90 mg/m² every 12 hours when combined with zidovudine (120 mg/m² every 6 hours). The potential applicability of these results to seropositive infants is under investigation.

Other prevention-oriented interventions should also be considered for HIV-infected infants (Connor and McSherry, 1994). Two double-blind, placebo-controlled trials have demonstrated that intravenous immunoglobulin (400 mg/kg body weight every 28 days) reduces serious and minor bacterial infections and hospitalizations in HIV-infected children with early or advanced disease independent of treatment with zidovudine (Mofenson et al, 1992; The National Institute of Child Health and Human Development Intravenous Immunoglobulin Study Group, 1991; Spector et al, 1994). Prophylactic intravenous immunoglobulin has been shown in earlier studies to increase numbers of inducer T cells, improve in vitro mitogen stimulation responses in peripheral blood mononuclear cells, and restore suppressor T-cell function (Calvelli and Rubinstein, 1986). Second, prophylaxis for *P. carinii* pneumonia (e.g., 75 mg/m² of trimethoprim and 375 mg/m² of sulfamethoxazole given twice daily three times per week on a Monday, Tuesday, and Wednesday) should be considered, because *P. carinii* pneumonia is rapidly fatal and frequently diagnosed in infants (Centers for Disease Control and Prevention, 1991; Simonds et al, 1995). Finally, immunizations should be administered as suggested in Table 41–7 (American Academy of Pediatrics, 1994). Killed poliomyelitis vaccine should be used. Exposure to varicella or measles should be treated with varicella zoster immune globulin or immune serum globulin, respectively. Family members should be screened for hepatitis B surface antigen, and HIV-positive children at risk should be vaccinated. Suspected infections should be aggressively diagnosed and treated. For example, treatment of severe thrush unresponsive to nystatin should be treated with ketoconazole (5 mg/kg/day) or severe, mucocutaneous herpes infections with oral (400 mg five times per day) or intravenous (5 to 10 mg/kg every 8 hours) acyclovir (Pahwa et al, 1990). Treatment of thrombocytopenia with intravenous immunoglobulin has not produced success comparable to that seen in immune thrombocytopenia (Pizzo, 1990). Steroids have been used with limited success. Lymphocytic interstitial pneumonia has been treated with steroids (5 mg of prednisone every other day with increased dosages during times of physiologic stress) and/or acyclovir. The latter is used because Epstein-Barr viral genome has been detected in approximately 75% of the lung biopsies from children with this manifestation of HIV infection. However, evaluation of these and other treatments for lymphocytic interstitial pneumonia is difficult without a better understanding of the natural history and biology of the disease.

CONCLUSION

Fetal and neonatal HIV infection remains a major health problem. Careful investigation of these infants will permit identification of improved treatment modalities and enhanced understanding of developmental and genetic immunoregulatory mechanisms. (Nahmias et al, 1994). Ultimately, prevention through education of high-risk groups along with palliative or curative therapies will permit control of this epidemic.

REFERENCES

ACTG Protocol 152: A randomized comparative trial of zidovudine (ZDV) versus 2',3' dideoxyinoaine (ddI) versus ZDV plus ddI in symptomatic HIV-infected children. ACTG 152 Executive Summary 1995, p 1.

American Academy of Pediatrics: HIV infection and AIDS. *In* Peter G (Ed): 1994 Red Book: Report of the Committee on Infectious Diseases, 23rd ed. Elk Grove Village, IL: American Academy of Pediatrics, 1994, p 264.

Albersheim SG, Smyth JA, Solimano A, et al: Passively acquired human immunodeficiency virus seropositivity in a neonate after hepatitis B immunoglobulin. J Pediatr 112(6):915, 1988.

American Academy of Pediatrics Task Force on Pediatric AIDS: Perinatal human immunodeficiency virus infection. Pediatrics 82:941, 1988.

Ammann AJ, Wara DW, Dritz S, et al: Acquired immunodeficiency in an infant: Possible transmission by means of blood products. Lancet 1:956, 1983.

Bayer R: Ethical challenges posed by zidovudine treatment to reduce vertical transmission of HIV. N Engl J Med 331:1223, 1994.

Blanche S, Rouzioux C, Moscato M-LG, et al: A prospective study of infants born to women seropositive for human immunodeficiency virus type 1. N Engl J Med 320:1643, 1989.

Blanche S, Tardieu M, Duliege AM, et al: Longitudinal study of 94 symptomatic infants with perinatally acquired human immunodeficiency virus infection. Am J Dis Child 144:1210, 1990.

Bonkovsky FO: Ethical issues in perinatal HIV. Clin Perinatol 21:15, 1994.

Bryson YJ, Pang S, Wei LS, et al: Clearance of HIV infection in a perinatally infected infant. N Engl J Med 332:833, 1995.

Burgard M, Mayaux MJ, Blanche S, et al: The use of viral culture and p24 antigen testing to diagnose human immunodeficiency virus infection in neonates. The HIV Infection in Newborns French Collaborative Study Group. N Engl J Med 327:1192, 1992.

Calvelli TA, Rubinstein A: Intravenous gamma-globulin in infant acquired immunodeficiency syndrome. Pediatr Infect Dis 5:S207, 1986.

Centers for Disease Control and Prevention: Unexplained immunodeficiency and opportunistic infection in infants—New York, New Jersey, California. MMWR Morb Mortal Wkly Rep 31:665, 1982.

Centers for Disease Control: Prevention of perinatal transmission of hepatitis B virus: Prenatal screening of all pregnant women for hepatitis B surface antigen. MMWR Morb Mortal Wkly Rep 37:341, 1988.

Centers for Disease Control: AIDS and human immunodeficiency virus infection in the United States: 1988 update. MMWR Morb Mortal Wkly Rep 38(S-4):1, 1989.

Centers for Disease Control: Public health service statement on management of occupational exposure to human immunodeficiency virus, including considerations regarding zidovudine postexposure use. MMWR Morb Mortal Wkly Rep 39:1, 1990.

Centers for Disease Control and Prevention: Guidelines for prophylaxis against *Pneumocystis carinii* pneumonia for children infected with human immunodeficiency virus. MMWR Morb Mortal Wkly Rep 40:1, 1991.

Centers for Disease Control and Prevention: Projections of the number of persons diagnosed with AIDS and the number of immunosuppressed HIV-infected persons—United States, 1992–1994. MMWR Morb Mortal Wkly Rep 41:RR-18, 1992a.

Centers for Disease Control and Prevention: Surveillance for occupationally acquired HIV infection—United States, 1981–1992. MMWR Morb Mortal Wkly Rep 41:823, 1992b.

Centers for Disease Control and Prevention: 1993 Revised classification system for HIV infection and expanded surveillance case definition for AIDS among adolescents and adults. MMWR Morb Mortal Wkly Rep 41:RR-17, 1993a.

Centers for Disease Control and Prevention: Update: Acquired immunodeficieny syndrome—United States, 1992. MMWR Morb Mortal Wkly Rep 42:547, 1993b.

Centers for Disease Control and Prevention: U.S. HIV and AIDS cases reported through June 1994. HIV/AIDS Surveillance Report 6:1, 1994a.

Centers for Disease Control and Prevention: Update: Trends in AIDS diagnosis and reporting under the expanded surveillance definition for adolescents and adults—United States, 1993. MMWR Morb Mortal Wkly Rep 43:826, 1994b.

Centers for Disease Control and Prevention: 1994 Revised classification system for human immunodeficiency virus infection in children less than 13 years of age. MMWR Morb Mortal Wkly Rep 43:RR-12, 1994c.

Centers for Disease Control and Prevention: Birth outcomes following zidovudine therapy in pregnant women. MMWR Morb Mortal Wkly Rep 43:409, 1994d.

Centers for Disease Control and Prevention: Recommendations of the U.S. Public Health Service Task Force on the use of zidovudine to reduce perinatal transmission of human immunodeficiency virus. MMWR Morb Mortal Wkly Rep 43:1, 1994e.

Centers for Disease Control and Prevention: Update—AIDS among young women—United States, 1994. MMWR Morb Mortal Wkly Rep 44:81, 1995a.

Centers for Disease Control and Prevention: HIV counseling and testing—United States, 1993. MMWR Morb Mortal Wkly Rep 44:169, 1995b.

Centers for Disease Control and Prevention: Update: Trends in AIDS incidence, deaths, and prevalence—United States, 1996. MMWR Morb Mortal Wkly Rep 46:165, 1997.

Chin J: The growing impact of the HIV/AIDS pandemic on children born to HIV-infected women. Perinatol AIDS 21:1, 1994.

Church JA: The diagnostic challenge of the child born "at risk" for HIV infection. Pediatr Clin North Am 41:715, 1994.

Church JA, Isaacs H: Transfusion-associated acquired immune deficiency syndrome in infants. J Pediatr 105:731, 1984.

Connor E, McSherry G: Treatment of HIV infection in infancy. Clin Perinatol 21:163, 1994.

Connor EM, Sperling RS, Gelber R, et al: Reduction of maternal-infant transmission of human immunodeficiency virus type 1 with zidovudine treatment. N Engl J Med 331:1173, 1994.

Connor E, Bagarazzi M, McSherry G, et al: Clinical and laboratory correlates of *Pneumocystis carinii* pneumonia in children infected with HIV. JAMA 265:1693, 1991.

Cooke M: Patient rights and physician responsibility: Four problems in AIDS care. AIDS Clin Rev 14:253, 1993.

Coombs RW, Collier AC, Allain JP, et al: Plasma viremia in human immunodeficiency virus infection. N Engl J Med 320:1626, 1989.

Cortes E, Detels R, Aboulafia D, et al: HIV-1, HIV-2, and HTLV-I infection in high-risk groups in Brazil. N Engl J Med 320:953, 1989.

de Martino M, Tovo PA, Galli L, et al: Prognostic significance of immunologic changes in 675 infants perinatally exposed to human immunodeficiency virus. J Pediatr 119:702, 1991.

Denny T, Yogev R, Gelman, et al: Lymphocyte subsets in healthy children during the first 5 years of life. JAMA 267:1484, 1992.

Des Jarlais DC, Padian NS, Winkelstein W: Targeted HIV-prevention programs. N Engl J Med 331:1451, 1994.

Duprat C, Mohammed Z, Datta P, et al: Human immunodeficiency virus type 1 IgA antibody in breast milk and serum. Pediatr Infect Dis J 13:603, 1994.

Eisenstein BI: Current concepts—The polymerase chain reaction: A new method of using molecular genetics for medical diagnosis. N Engl J Med 322:178, 1990.

Erkeller-Yuksel FM, Deneys V, Yuksel B, et al: Age-related changes in human blood lymphocyte sub-populations. J Pediatr 120:216, 1992.

The European Collaborative Study: Age-related standards for T-lymphocyte subsets based on uninfected children born to human immunodeficiency virus-1-infected women. Pediatr Infect Dis J 11:1018, 1992.

The European Collaborative Study: Children born to women with HIV-1 infection: Natural history and risk of transmission. Lancet 337:253, 1991.

Fahrner R, Beekmann SE, Koziol DE, et al: Safety of zidovudine as postexposure chemoprophylaxis to healthcare workers after occupational exposure to HIV (Abstract PoC 4132). *In* Poster Abstracts. VIII International Conference on AIDS, Amsterdam, The Netherlands, July 1992.

Fahrner R, Gerberding JL: Risk of HIV infection in health care workers. AIDS Clin Rev 13:239, 1993.

Frigoletto FD, Little GA (Eds): Guideline for Perinatal Care, 2nd ed. Elk Grove, IL, American Academy of Pediatrics, 1988.

Gottlieb MS, Schroff R, Schanker HM, et al: *Pneumocystis carinii* pneumonia and mucosal candidiasis in previously healthy homosexual men: Evidence of a new acquired cellular immunodeficiency. N Engl J Med 305:1425, 1981.

Guinan ME, Hardy A: Epidemiology of AIDS in women in the United States: 1981 through 1986. JAMA 257:2039, 1987.

Hellinger FJ: The lifetime cost of treating a person with HIV. JAMA 270:474, 1993.

Henderson DK: Postexposure chemoprophylaxis for occupational exposure to human immunodeficiency virus type 1: Current status and prospects for the future. Am J Med 91:312, 1991.

Ho DD, Pomerantz RJ, Kaplan JC: Pathogenesis of infection with human immunodeficiency virus. N Engl J Med 317:278, 1987.

Hoff R, Berardi VP, Weiblen BJ, et al: Seroprevalence of human immunodeficiency virus among child-bearing women: Estimation by testing samples of blood from newborns. N Engl J Med 318:525, 1988.

Hsu HW, Moye J Jr, Kunches L, et al: Perinatally acquired human immunodeficiency virus infection: Extent of clinical recognition in a population-based cohort. Massachusetts Pediatric HIV Surveillance Working Group. Pediatr Infect Dis J 11:941, 1992.

Imagawa DT, Lee MH, Wolinsky SM, et al: Human immunodeficiency virus type 1 infection in homosexual men who remain seronegative for prolonged periods. N Engl J Med 320:1458, 1989.

Katz SL, Wilfert CM: Human immunodeficiency virus infection of newborns. N Engl J Med 320:1687, 1989.

Kovacs A, Frederick T, Church J, et al: CD4 T-lymphocyte counts and *Pneumocystis carinii* pneumonia in pediatric HIV infection. JAMA 265;1698, 1991.

Krivine A, Firtion G, Cao L, et al: HIV replication during the first weeks of life. Lancet 339:1187, 1992.

Landesman SH: Human immunodeficiency virus infection in women: An overview. Semin Perinatol 13:2, 1989.

Leibovitz E, Riguad M, Pollack H, et al: *Pneumocystis carinii* pneumonia infants infected with the human immunodeficiency virus with more than 450 CD4 T lymphocytes per cubic millimeter. N Engl J Med 323:531, 1990.

Marcus R: CDC cooperative needlestick study group. Surveillance of health care workers exposed to blood from patients infected with human immunodeficiency virus. N Engl J Med 319:1118, 1988.

Markovitz DM: Infection with the human immunodeficiency virus type 2. Ann Intern Med 118:211, 1993.

Masur H, Michelis MA, Green JB, et al: An outbreak of community acquired *Pneumocystis carinii* pneumonia: An initial manifestation of cellular immune dysfunction. N Engl J Med 305:1431, 1981.

McIntosh K, Pitt J, Brambilla D, et al: Blood culture in the first 6 months of life for the diagnosis of vertically transmitted human immunodeficiency virus infection. The Women and Infants Transmission Study Group. J Infect Dis 170:996, 1994.

McIntosh K, Burchett SA: Clearance of HIV—Lessons from newborns. N Engl J Med 332:883, 1995.

McKinney RE, Wilfert CM: Lymphocyte subsets in children younger than 2 years old: Normal values in a population at risk for human immunodeficiency virus infection and diagnostic and prognostic application to infected children. Pediatr Infect Dis J 11:639, 1992.

Miles SA, Baldern E, Magpantay L, et al: Rapid serologic testing with immune-complex-dissociated HIV p24 antigen for early detection of HIV infection in neonates. N Engl J Med 328:297, 1993.

Mofenson LM: A critical review of studies evaluating the relationship of mode of delivery to perinatal transmission of human immunodeficiency virus. Pediatr Infect Dis J 14:169, 1995.

Mofenson LM, Moye J Jr, Bethel J, et al: Prophylactic intravenous immunoglobulin in HIV-infected children with CD4$^+$ counts of 0.2×10^9/L or more: Effect on viral, opportunistic, and bacterial infections. JAMA 268:483, 1992.

Nahmias A, Ibegbu C, Lee F, Spira T: The development of the immune system—Importance in the ascertainment of immunophenotypic changes in perinatal HIV infection. Clin Immunol Immunopathol 71:2, 1994.

The National Institute of Child Health and Human Development Intravenous Immunoglobulin Study Group. Intravenous immune globulin for the prevention of bacterial infections in children with symptomatic human immunodeficiency virus infection. N Engl J Med 325:73, 1991.

OSHA: Occupational exposure to bloodborne pathogens standard. Fed Reg 235:64175, 1991.

Pahwa S: Human immunodeficiency virus infection in children: Nature of immunodeficiency, clinical spectrum and management. Pediatr Infect Dis 7:S61, 1988.

Pahwa S, Chirmule N, Oyaizu N: Clinical and immunologic spectrum of HIV infection in infants and children and disease pathogenesis. Prog Clin Biol Res 325:393, 1990.

Pahwa R, Good R, Pahwa S: Prematurity, hypogammaglobulinemia, and neuropathy with human immunodeficiency virus (HIV) infection. Proc Natl Acad Sci U S A 84:3826, 1987.

Pizzo PA: Pediatric AIDS: Problems within problems. J Infect Dis 161:316, 1990.

Pizzo PA, Eddy J, Falloon J, et al: Effect of continuous intravenous infusion of zidovudine (AZT) in children with symptomatic HIV infection. N Engl J Med 319:889, 1988.

Popovic M, Sarngadharan MG, Read E, Gallo RC: Detection, isolation, and continuous production of cytopathic retroviruses (HTLV-III) from patients with AIDS and pre-AIDS. Science 224:497, 1984.

Quinn TC: Population migration and the spread of types 1 and 2 human immunodeficiency viruses. Proc Natl Acad Sci U S A 91:2407, 1994.

Quinn TC, Zacarias FRK, St John RK: AIDS in the Americas: An emerging public health crisis. N Engl J Med 320:1005, 1989.

Rhame FS, Maki DG: The case for wider use of testing for HIV infection. N Engl J Med 320:1248, 1989.

Rogers DE: Federal spending on AIDS—How much is enough? N Engl J Med 320:1623, 1989.

Rogers MF, Caldwell MB, Gwinn ML, Simonds RJ: Epidemiology of pediatric human immunodeficiency virus infection in the United States. Ann N Y Acad Sci 693:4, 1993.

Rogers MF, Jaffe HW: Reducing the risk of maternal-infant transmission of HIV: A door is opened. N Engl J Med 331:1222, 1994.

Rogers M, Ou CY, Kilbourne B, Schochetman G: Advances and problems in the diagnosis of human immunodeficiency virus infection in infants. Pediatr Infect Dis J 10:523, 1991.

Rogers MF, Ou CY, Rayfield M, et al: Use of the polymerase chain reaction for early detection of the proviral sequences of human immunodeficiency virus in infants born to seropositive mothers. N Engl J Med 320:1649, 1989.

Rubinstein A: Pediatric AIDS. Curr Probl Pediatr 16:361, 1986.

Rubinstein A, Goldstein H, Calvelli T, et al: Maternofetal transmission of human immunodeficiency virus-1: The role of antibodies to the V3 primary neutralizing domain. Pediatr Res 33:76, 1993.

Ruprecht RM, O'Brien LG, Rossoni LD, et al: Suppression of mouse viraemia and retroviral disease by 3'-azido-3'-deoxythymidine. Nature 323:467, 1986.

Ryder RW, Nsa W, Hassig SE, et al: Perinatal transmission of the human immunodeficiency virus type 1 to infants of seropositive women in Zaire. N Engl J Med 320:525, 1989.

Sattentau QJ, Weiss RA: The CD4 antigen: Physiological ligand and HIV receptor. Cell 52:631, 1988.

Saulsbury FT, Wykoff RF, Boyle RJ: Transfusion-acquired human immunodeficiency virus infection in twelve neonates: Epidemiologic, clinical and immunologic features. Pediatr Infect Dis 6:544, 1987.

Shannon K, Ball E, Wasserman RL, et al: Transfusion-associated cytomegalovirus infection and acquired immune deficiency syndrome in an infant. J Pediatr 103:859, 1983.

Siegal FP, Lopez C, Hammer GS, et al: Severe acquired immunodeficiency in male homosexuals, manifested by chronic perianal ulcerative herpes simplex lesions. N Engl J Med 305:1439, 1981.

Simonds RJ, Lindegren ML, Thomas P, et al: Prophylaxis against *Pneumocystis carinii* pneumonia among children with perinatally acquired human immunodeficiency virus infection in the United States. N Engl J Med 332:786, 1995.

Simpson BJ, Andimam WA: Difficulties in assigning human immunodeficiency virus-1 infection and seroreversion status in a cohort of HIV-exposed children using serologic criteria established by the CDC and Prevention. Pediatrics 93:840, 1994.

Soeiro R, Rubinstein A, Rashbaum WK, Lyman WD: Maternofetal transmission of AIDS: Frequency of human immunodeficiency virus type 1 nucleic acid sequences in human fetal DNA. J Infect Dis 166:699, 1992.

Spector SA, Gelber RD, McGrath N, et al: A controlled trial of intravenous immune globulin for the prevention of serious bacterial infections in children receiving zidovudine for advanced human immunodeficiency virus infection. N Engl J Med 331:1181, 1994.

Thomas PA, Lubin K, Milberg J, et al: Cohort comparison study of children whose mothers have acquired immunodeficiency syndrome and children of well inner city mothers. Pediatr Infect Dis 6:247, 1987.

Tovo PA, de Martino M, Gabiano C, et al: Prognostic factors and survival in children with perinatal HIV-1 infection. Lancet 339:1249, 1992.

Udasin IG, Gochfeld M: Implications of the Occupational Safety and Health Administration's bloodborne pathogen standard for the occupational health professional. J Occup Med 36:548, 1994.

Ugen KE, Goedert JJ, Boyer J, et al: Vertical transmission of human immunodeficiency virus (HIV) infection. Reactivity of maternal sera with glycoprotein 120 and 41 peptides from HIV type 1. J Clin Invest 89:1923, 1992.

Waecker NJ, Ascher DP, Robb ML, et al: Age adjusted CD4$^+$ lymphocyte parameters in HIV at risk uninfected children. Clin Infect Dis 17:123, 1993.

Weiss R, Thier SO: HIV testing is the answer—What's the question? N Engl J Med 319:1010, 1988.

Weiss SH: HIV infection and the healthcare worker. Med Clin North Am 76:269, 1992.

Wilfert CM: Mandatory screening of pregnant women for the human immunodeficiency virus. Clin Infect Dis 19:664, 1994.

Wilfert CM, Wilson C, Luzuriaga K, Epstein L: Pathogenesis of pediatric human immunodeficiency virus type 1 infection. J Infect Dis 170:286, 1994.

Winkenwerder W, Kessler AR, Stolec RM: Federal spending for illness caused by the human immunodeficiency virus. N Engl J Med 320:1598, 1989.

Working Group of the American Academy of Neurology AIDS Task Force: Nomenclature and research case definitions for neurologic manifestations of human immunodeficiency virus type 1 (HIV-1) infection. Neurology 41:778, 1991.

Yarchoan R, Mitsuya H, Myers C, et al: Clinical pharmacology A²3¹-azido-2¹,3¹-dideoxythymidine (zidovudine) and related dideoxynucleosides. N Engl J Med 321:726, 1989.

Zeichner SL: The molecular biology of HIV: Insights into pathogenesis and targets for therapy. Perinatol AIDS 21:39, 1994.

CHAPTER 42

Viral Infections of the Fetus and Newborn

F. Sessions Cole

The infant who is born with an infection acquired transplacentally during the first, second, or early third trimester may have what is termed "congenital infection." Although in rare instances these infections are due to herpes simplex virus, varicella-zoster virus, *Mycobacterium tuberculosis*, and *Listeria monocytogenes*, the most common causes are rubella virus, cytomegalovirus (CMV), *Toxoplasma gondii*, *Treponema pallidum*, human immunodeficiency virus (HIV), human parvovirus B19, and Epstein-Barr virus (EBV) (Kinney and Kumar, 1988; Stamos and Rowley, 1994). The first four organisms are the so-called and somewhat misnamed "TORCH" group. The confusion generated by this acronym arises because "H," or herpes simplex, so rarely belongs to the group and because syphilis and other infections are omitted (Stamos and Rowley, 1994). Because of the increasing frequency and interest in HIV, parvovirus, and EBV, Kinney and Kumar (1988) have recommended their inclusion in the "other" category of TORCH infections. Certain other organisms may cause intrauterine infection but are usually transmitted just before delivery. This pattern is characteristic of herpes simplex virus, enteroviruses, group B streptococci, *Listeria*, and others, but these intrauterine infections differ little from those caused by the same organisms when acquired either just after delivery or during the 1st week or so of extrauterine life. For this reason, they are usually classified as "perinatal" rather than "congenital" infections.

Despite the extraordinary biologic heterogeneity of the four TORCH organisms responsible for congenital infections, the syndromes they produce are remarkably similar. The literature was carefully reviewed by Kinney and Kumar in 1988 and Alpert and Plotkin in 1986 (Tables 42–1 and 42–2). The most common manifestations include hepatomegaly, splenomegaly, pneumonia, bone lesions, and anemia. Differentiating features of individual infections are discussed in this section (Stamos and Rowley, 1994). Neurologic morbidities of each infection have been reviewed (Bale and Murph, 1992).

The rational approach to the diagnosis of congenital infection includes information on the biology, epidemiology, and disease manifestations of each infection. Once the suspicion is raised, therefore, the differences rather than similarities among these diseases should be the object of analysis.

DIAGNOSTIC APPROACH

Because the incidence of congenital infection in the fetus and newborn infant is high (0.5% to 2.5%) (Alpert and Plotkin, 1986), and a significant number of congenitally infected infants are asymptomatic, a high index of suspicion plus a sensitive, specific, and cost-effective approach to diagnosis is used. Evaluation begins with complete family and maternal history, including information on birth weights and medical problems of siblings, drug use, sexual orientation of sexual partners, maternal travel history, and blood transfusion history. Common neonatal clinical features associated with congenital infection are listed in Table 42–3. No data are available to determine whether isolated findings or combinations of signs should prompt further evaluation. For example, whether the children born with a birth weight less than the third percentile for gestational age (small for gestational age [SGA]) without other signs should be evaluated is unclear. Studies from Sweden and Canada suggest that isolated growth retardation is not associated with congenital infection, but these studies had some methodologic flaws (Andersson et al, 1981; Primhak and Simpson, 1982). However, growth retardation has been described as the only manifestation of congenital infection with CMV, rubella, and toxoplasmosis (Alpert and Plotkin, 1986). The clinician must rely on the history and the physical examination to identify infants for further evaluation.

If an infant is suspected of having a congenital infection, the infection may be confirmed through total cord IgM determination, although its efficacy is the subject of debate (Alpert and Plotkin, 1986; Kinney and Kumar, 1988). Approximately 4% of newborn infants have elevated (>18 to 20 mg/dL) IgM in cord blood (Kinney and Kumar, 1988). Alford and associates (1969) showed that 42 of 123 infants with elevated IgM (>19.5 mg/dL) had identifiable infections. Although a normal IgM does not exclude perinatal or congenital infection, an elevated cord blood level of total IgM provides an indication for pursuing further diagnostic studies in the context of an unclear clinical picture. The nonspecific and specific diagnostic tests are outlined in Table 42–4. Establishment of the specific agent is important for prognostic evaluation and for possible treatment. An approach to the laboratory diagnosis is outlined in Figure 42–1. Serologic tests that are not specific for IgM antibody require maternal serum for interpretation.

CONGENITAL RUBELLA

Since 1941, when Gregg first made the association of maternal rubella and cataracts in infants, physicians have been aware of the teratogenicity of the rubella virus. Not until the epidemic of 1964 and 1965 in North America, however, were the multiple manifestations of the rubella syndrome fully appreciated and the later consequences well delineated. Since that time, the capacity to grow the virus in tissue culture has led rapidly to the development of vaccines and a reduction in incidence of congenital disease, at least in the United States. Although availability of vaccine has lowered the incidence of congenital rubella syndrome in the United States relative to other countries, failure to

TABLE 42–1

Incidence of Maternal and Fetal Infections Caused by Selected Organisms

Microorganism	Mother (Per 1000 Pregnancies)	Fetus (Per 1000 Live Births)
Cytomegalovirus	40–150	5–25
Rubella		
Epidemic	20–40	4–30
Interepidemic	0.1	0.5
Toxoplasma gondii	1.5–6.4	0.5 to 1
Herpes simplex	10–15	Rare
Treponema pallidum	0.2	0.1

From Alpert G, Plotkin SA: A practical guide to the diagnosis of congenital infections in the newborn infant. Pediatr Clin North Am 33:465, 1986.

vaccinate rather than vaccine failure continues to slow efforts to eradicate this problem (Centers for Disease Control and Prevention, 1991a. Between 1993 and 1994, the number of cases reported to the Centers for Disease Control and Prevention almost doubled (from 5 to 9), and the number of documented cases of rubella in older children or adults also increased from 192 to 225 (Centers for Disease Control and Prevention, 1995). In other parts of the world, congenital rubella syndrome continues to contribute significantly to pediatric morbidity and mortality.

Etiology

Maternal rubella infection that occurs within 1 month before conception and through the second trimester may be associated with disease in the infant. The classic findings of congenital rubella predominate when the onset of maternal

TABLE 42–2

Clinical Findings in Congenitally Infected Infants That Suggest a Specific Diagnosis

Congenital	Findings
Rubella	Eye—cataracts, cloudy cornea, pigmented retina Skin—"blueberry muffin" syndrome Bone—vertical striation Heart—malformation (ductus, pulmonary artery stenosis)
Cytomegalovirus	Microcephaly with periventricular calcifications; inguinal hernias in males; petechiae with thrombocytopenia
Toxoplasmosis	Hydrocephalus with generalized calcifications; chorioretinitis
Syphilis	Osteochondritis and periostitis, eczematoid skin rash, mucocutaneous lesions (snuffles)
Herpes	Skin vesicles, keratoconjunctivitis; acute central nervous system findings

Modified from Stagno S, Pass RF, Alford CA: Perinatal infections and maldevelopment. *In* Bloom AD, James LS (Eds): The Fetus and the Newborn, vol 17, series 1. New York, Alan R Liss, 1981. Copyright © 1981, Alan R. Liss, Inc. Reprinted by permission of Wiley-Liss, a division of John Wiley and Sons, Inc.

TABLE 42–3

Common Neonatal Clinical Features Associated with TORCH Agents

Growth retardation (hydrocephalus)
Hepatosplenomegaly
Jaundice (greater than 20% direct reacting)
Hemolytic anemia
Petechiae and ecchymoses
Microcephaly and hydrocephaly
Intracranial calcification
Pneumonitis
Myocarditis
Cardiac abnormalities (especially peripheral pulmonic stenosis [rubella])
Chorioretinitis
Keratoconjunctivitis
Cataracts
Glaucoma
Nonimmune hydrops

From Kinney JS, Kumar ML: Should we expand the TORCH complex? Clin Perinatol 15:727, 1988.

infection occurs during the first 8 weeks of gestation (Miller et al, 1982). Cataracts occur with maternal rubella before the 60th day after the 1st day of the last menstrual period; heart disease is found almost exclusively when maternal infection is before the 80th day (i.e., first trimester). Deafness, the most common manifestation, occurs, along with retinopathy as a consequence of both first and

TABLE 42–4

Diagnostic Approach to the Newborn Suspected of Being Congenitally Infected

Nonspecific Tests	Specific Tests
Complete blood and platelet counts	Viral culture* Oropharynx, urine, rectum
Lumbar puncture	Blood for HIV
Roentgenogram of long bones	Optional: cerebrospinal fluid, conjunctiva
Computed tomography scan of head	Smears of skin lesions FA stain
Ophthalmologic evaluation	Dark-field examination
Audiologic evaluation	Tzanck smear
	Serology
	Rubella: HAI, PHA, LA or Elisa screen for IgG antibody
	Toxoplasma: SF or IFA for IgG antibody
	Syphilis: VDRL or RPR
	Hepatitis B: HBsAg test
	Polymerase chain reaction: HIV test
	ELISA or Western blot: HIV test

*African green monkey kidney cell line must be inoculated.

HAI, hemagglutination inhibition; PHA, passive hemagglutination; LA, latex agglutination; SF, Sabin-Feldman dye test; IFA, immunofluorescence test; FA, fluorescent antibody.

From Alpert G, Plotkin SA: A practical guide to the diagnosis of congenital infections in the newborn infant. Pediatr Clin North Am 33:465, 1986.

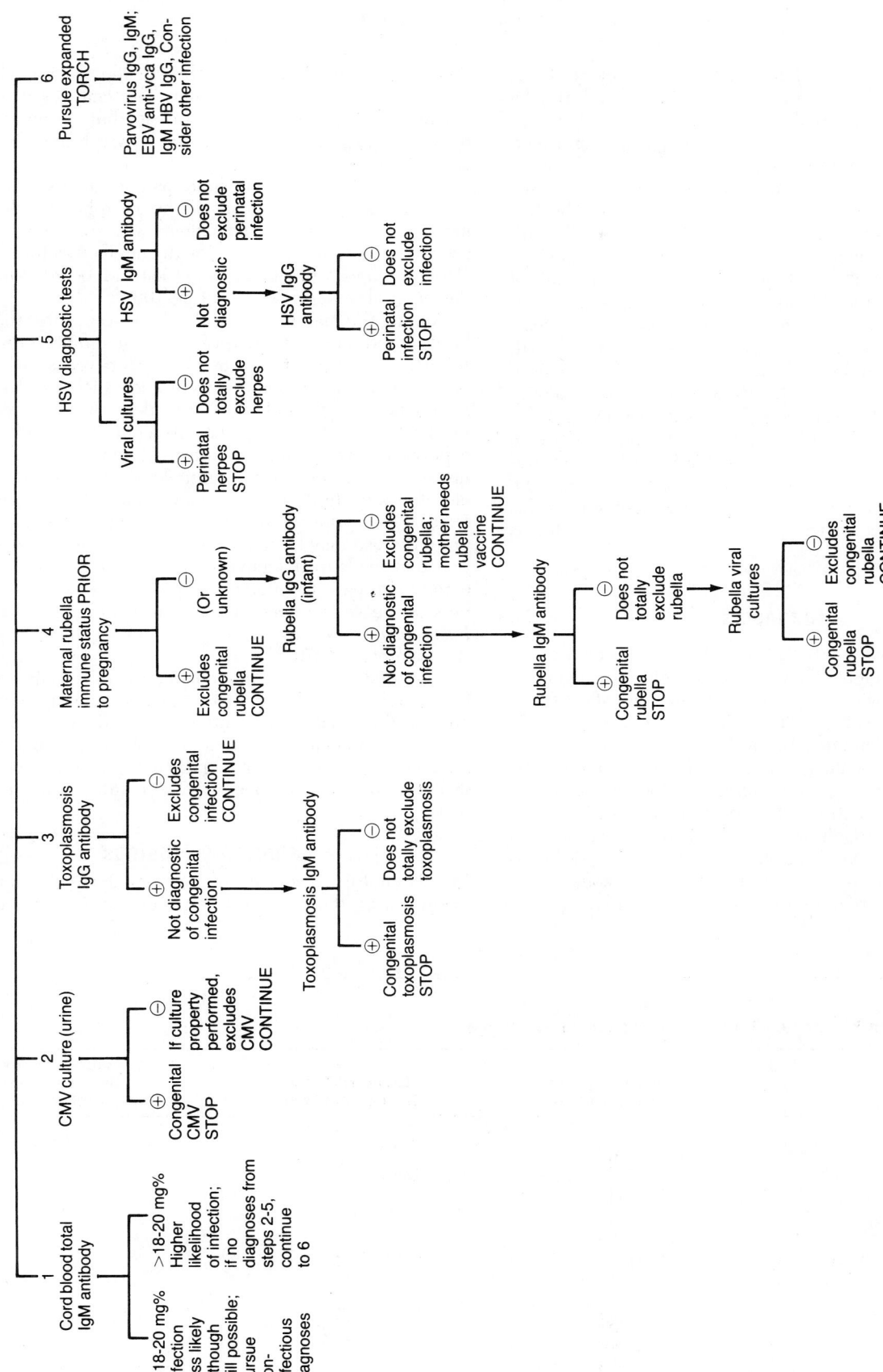

FIGURE 42–1. An approach to the laboratory diagnosis of suspected TORCH infection in the newborn. (From Kinney JS, Kumar ML: Should we expand the TORCH complex? Clin Perinatol 15:727, 1988.)

second trimester maternal infections (Miller et al, 1982; Ueda et al, 1979). The incidence of congenital rubella defects following maternal rubella varies widely between series. A study of 1016 women with serologically confirmed rubella infection at different stages of pregnancy who were followed prospectively provides the most convincing estimate of the risks of congenital rubella infection. The frequency of congenital infection after maternal rubella with a rash was more than 80% during the first 12 weeks of pregnancy, 54% at 13 to 14 weeks, and 25% at the end of the second trimester (Miller et al, 1982). Rubella-associated defects (primarily congenital heart disease and deafness) were observed in all infants infected before the 11th week (n = 9) and in 35% of infants (9 of 26 infants) whose infections occurred at 13 to 16 weeks (deafness alone) (Miller et al, 1982). The infected infant may excrete the virus for many months after birth despite the pressure of neutralizing antibody and, thus, pose a hazard to susceptible individuals in the environment. Only rarely can the virus be recovered by 1 year of age. An exception to this rule is the cataract, in which the virus may remain for as long as 3 years.

Diagnosis

Infants infected with rubella are usually born at term but are of low birth weight. They may show only a few manifestations of the disease, such as glaucoma or cataracts, or they may have a systemic illness characterized by purpuric lesions, hepatosplenomegaly, cardiac defects, pneumonia, and meningoencephalitis (Table 42–5). The skin lesions have been described as resembling a "blueberry muffin." These represent extramedullary hematopoietic tissue within the skin (Brough et al, 1967). Thrombocytopenia is commonly seen (Cooper et al, 1965). Osseous lesions include a large anterior fontanel and striking lesions in the long bones. Linear areas of radiolucency and increased

density are found in the metaphyses. The provisional zones of calcification are also irregular. The changes in rubella are not pathognomonic of the disease but resemble those of other congenital infections, such as cytomegalic inclusion disease.

The cardiac lesions include patent ductus arteriosus, septal defects, and stenosis of the peripheral pulmonary arteries. In one study of 18 patients with simple pulmonary artery stenosis, an association with rubella was found in 11 (Hodgson and Morgan-Capner, 1984). Myocardial necrosis has been observed (Cooper et al, 1969).

Among the manifestations that may occur after the newborn period (late-onset disease) are a generalized rash with seborrheic features that may persist for weeks, interstitial pneumonia (either acute or chronic) such as described by Phelan and Campbell (1969), defective hearing from involvement of the organ of Corti, central auditory imperception, or even complete autism. Infants with late-onset disease sometimes have immunologic abnormalities, with elevated total IgM and depressed total IgG (Soothill et al, 1966). The principal immunologic perturbation in late-onset disease may be defective cytotoxic effector cell function that leads to defective virus elimination and immune complex disease (Verder et al, 1986). These patients may be susceptible to infection with unusual organisms such as *Pneumocystis carinii* or to development of histiocytosis (Claman et al, 1970).

Longitudinal studies of somatic growth reveal that most infants remain smaller than average throughout infancy but grow at a normal rate. Stunting of growth was more common after rubella in the first 8 weeks of pregnancy than after later infection. A higher than expected incidence of diabetes mellitus has been reported after congenital rubella.

Laboratory Findings

The laboratory diagnosis of congenital rubella must be made during the 1st year of life, unless the virus can be

TABLE 42–5

Clinical Findings in 81 Infants with Congenital Rubella Syndrome

	Group 1: Expanded Rubella Syndrome	Group 2: Classic Rubella Syndrome	Group 3: History of Maternal Rubella, Presumably Normal Baby
Number of infants	34	37	10
Sex { Male	26	23	7
Female	8	14	3
Mean gestational age (weeks)	40.1	39.8	39.8
Mean birth weight (g)	2178	2533	3327
Purpura	78%	0	0
Thrombocytopenia (<140,000)	100%	0	0
Hepatomegaly	85%	81%	20%
Splenomegaly	76%	62%	10%
Cardiac defects	78%	86%	0
Eye defects	41%	54%	0
Full fontanel	69%	43%	0
Positive virus isolation	66%	25%	50%
Mortality	32%	8%	0

From Rudolph AJ, Singleton EB, Rosenberg HS, et al: Osseous manifestations of congenital rubella syndrome. Am J Dis Child *110*:416, 1965. Copyright 1965, American Medical Association.

recovered from an affected site such as the lens after that time. Both serologic and virus isolation may be helpful. If IgM antirubella titers are elevated at birth or shortly thereafter or if IgG antirubella titers remain high during the first year, the diagnosis of intrauterine infection is ensured (Alpert and Plotkin, 1986). Antirubella IgM can be determined with one of several immunofluorescence or enzyme immunoassays (Alpert and Plotkin, 1986). Not all congenitally infected infants have detectable IgM antirubella antibody in the 1st month of life (Alpert and Plotkin, 1986). If suspicion is high, repeat serologic examination and culture should be performed.

The virus is most often isolated from throat swabs but may also be found in the spinal fluid or urine. In late-onset disease, the virus is found in affected skin and lung.

Treatment

There is no specific therapy for congenital rubella. The infant may need a blood transfusion for anemia or active bleeding and general supportive measures. The best therapy is to ensure that women who are considering pregnancy are immune to rubella (ACOG Technical Bulletin, 1992a). Vaccination of nonimmune women during the postpartum period has become an established medical practice, although prolonged polyarticular arthritis, acute neurologic sequelae including carpal tunnel syndrome and multiple paresthesias, and chronic rubella viremia have been reported in these women (Tingle et al, 1985).

The problem of management of the pregnant woman who is exposed to or who contracts the disease should be resolved after weighing the known risks. If, at the time of exposure, serum antibody is detectable, then the fetus probably is protected completely. Routine postexposure rubella prophylaxis with immunoglobulin is not recommended, because efficacy has not been shown (ACOG Technical Bulletin, 1992a). Decisions about the interruption of pregnancy should be made only after maternal infection has been proved. An increase in antibody must be measured in two or more sera samples in the same laboratory on the same day; test variation may account for apparent antibody "rises" measured on different days.

Decisions concerning elective termination of pregnancy should also take into account the risk of rubella-associated damage to the fetus, which is highest when maternal infection occurs during the first 8 weeks of pregnancy.

Prognosis

The consequences of fetal rubella infection may not be evident at birth. Infection in the first or second trimester may lead to deafness or persistent growth retardation (Miller et al, 1982). Although infection in the third trimester may also lead to fetal growth retardation, this growth problem does not persist, suggesting that the mechanism of growth retardation among infants infected in the first or second trimester is different from that of infants infected in the third trimester (Miller et al, 1982). Hardy and coworkers (1966) followed up 123 infants with documented congenital rubella and found that 85% of them were not clinically suspect until after discharge from the nursery. Communication disorders, hearing defects, some mental or

motor retardation, and microcephaly by 1 to 3 years of age were among the major problems that were discovered after the newborn period. A predisposition to inguinal hernias was also noted.

Even in the absence of mental retardation, neuromuscular development is frequently abnormal. Desmond and coworkers (1978) followed up 29 children in this category and found that 25 of them were abnormal. Hearing loss, difficulties with balance and gait, learning deficits, and behavioral disturbances were found in more than one half of the affected children.

Weil and coworkers (1975) described an alarming report of chronic progressive panencephalitis with onset at age 11 years in a child who had congenital rubella. The patient was small for his age, with sensorineural hearing loss of 60 decibels at age 4 years. At age 11 years, he had the insidious onset of motor incoordination, ataxia, and myoclonic jerks, with progressive deterioration. Although this complication of congenital rubella must be rare, it emphasizes that the cause of subacute sclerosing panencephalitis need not be restricted to the measles virus.

Prevention

Live attenuated rubella virus vaccine is safe and effective (Lepow et al, 1968), although the duration of immunity is uncertain. Given as a single subcutaneous injection, it is recommended for children between 15 months of age and puberty and for women of childbearing age with negative findings on both a hemagglutination inhibition antibody test and a pregnancy test. It should be given only if the physician is assured that there is no likelihood of pregnancy for the next 2 months, because of the potential hazard to the fetus. (ACOG Technical Bulletin, 1992a). Although cases of congenital rubella syndrome have continued to occur in the United States, these cases appear to result from failure to vaccinate rather than vaccine failure (ACOG Technical Bulletin, 1992a).

Follow-up studies of a large number of women inadvertently immunized during or just before pregnancy have indicated that although the fetus is sometimes infected, there appear to be no or, at most, rare adverse consequences (Hayden et al, 1980). Even so, it appears advisable to administer vaccine only in the immediate postpartum period or when pregnancy can be avoided. A mild rubella-like illness is sometimes seen after immunization, with arthralgia occurring 10 days to 3 weeks after injection. Immunization in the postpartum period has infrequently led to polyarticular arthritis, neurologic symptoms, and chronic rubella viremia (Tingle et al, 1985).

CYTOMEGALOVIRUS

Although all aspects of CMV infections in utero and in the newborn period are not known, much has been learned about this ubiquitous and often confusing virus since its first cultivation in vitro in 1955 and since the recognition that it caused the devastating syndrome called *cytomegalic inclusion disease* (Weller, 1971; Weller et al, 1957). CMV infection at any age is usually asymptomatic. After a period of active replication, the virus usually becomes latent but retains the capability of reactivation under special circumstances. Such reactivation appears to occur frequently during pregnancy.

The fetus can be infected by either a newly acquired maternal infection (Davis et al, 1971) or a reactivated maternal infection (Stagno et al, 1982). The newly acquired maternal infection, although less common than the reactivated maternal infection, appears to carry a much higher risk of severe disease in the fetus. In reactivated infections, newborns are normal on examination and, if defects appear, they do not apparently do so until some time later in childhood. Follow-up studies of congenitally infected infants whose mothers were proved to be antibody positive before pregnancy are incomplete, and the prognosis of such infections, although clearly better than that of primary infections, is uncertain.

A newborn infant without congenital infection can be infected by his or her mother at the time of delivery, through breast milk, by acquisition from the nursery or home environment, or by transfusion of blood from a donor who is antibody positive (i.e., latently infected). Perinatal or postnatal acquisition from the mother appears to be benign and common. Postnatal acquisition from the environment is probably less common and may be benign, although lower respiratory illness may occur under these circumstances (Stagno et al, 1981). Acquisition from blood transfusion often results in severe, sometimes fatal, generalized disease in a setting in which maternal antibody is lacking (Yeager et al, 1981). Although neonatal intensive care units in the United States are providing CMV-negative blood for transfusion, antibody-negative women who require transfusion during pregnancy should also be considered for transfusion with CMV-negative blood (Onorato et al, 1985).

Incidence

Approximately 40,000 infants are born with congenital CMV infection annually in the United States (Griffiths, 1993; Stagno and Whitley, 1985). This infection rate (approximately 1%) is greater than that observed in England,

Denmark, and Sweden (approximately 0.3%) and comparable to that in Africa (1.4%) (Peckham, 1991; Starr et al, 1970). Twelve percent of congenitally infected infants die, and more than 90% have late complications (Stagno and Whitley, 1985; Griffiths, 1993), the most common of which is sensorineural hearing loss. Approximately 90% of congenitally infected infants are asymptomatic at birth (Griffiths, 1993; Kinney et al, 1985). Characteristics of CMV infection in pregnancy are given in Figure 42–2. The proportion of children and adults with detectable CMV antibody varies with age, geographic location, and socioeconomic status. In the United States, approximately 60% of adult women have complement-fixing antibody. The incidence of excretion in the cervix or urine appears to increase during pregnancy from 3% in the first trimester to as much as 12% at term, although such findings are variable. Congenital infection occurs more frequently (3.4% versus 1%) among women who were antibody positive before pregnancy (Stagno et al, 1977), a finding that implies either that most intrauterine infections result from reactivated maternal infections or that primary infections with different serotypes can occur in sequential pregnancies. Two babies infected in sequential pregnancies from a single mother were found to be excreting viruses that were identical by restriction endonuclease mapping (Stagno et al, 1977). The first of these infants had severe cytomegalic inclusion disease; the second, although excreting virus at birth, was clinically normal. Evidence suggests that a primary maternal CMV infection is more likely to cause congenital infection than a recurrent infection (Stagno et al, 1982).

The incidence of neonatal and postnatal infection is still higher than that of intrauterine infection. Approximately 50% of babies born to mothers excreting virus at term acquire infection in the first weeks of life (Reynolds et al, 1973). Many of these babies are infected through breast milk (Hayes et al, 1972). None, apparently, is affected adversely by the infection. All infants, regardless of the route of infection, excrete virus for a prolonged period, usually 1 year or more (Emanuel and Kenny, 1966). A longitudinal study of 10,218 Japanese women between

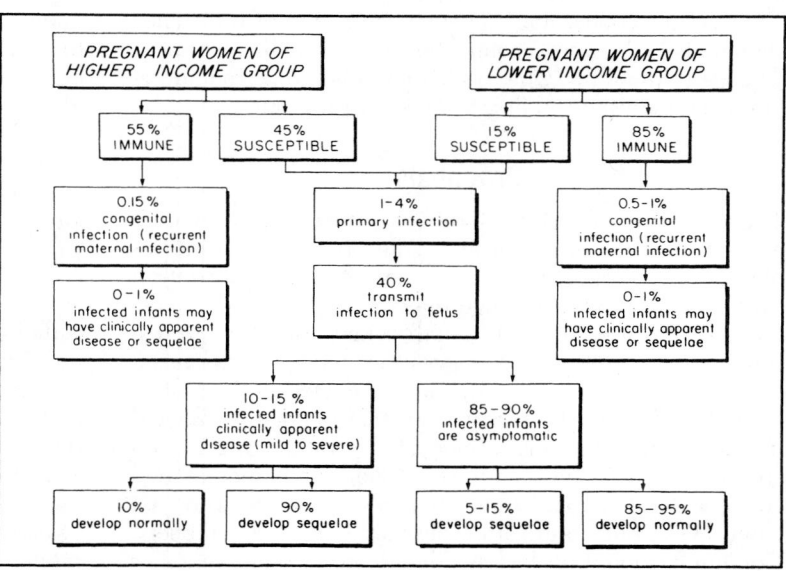

FIGURE 42–2. Characteristics of cytomegalovirus infection in pregnancy. (From Stagno S, Whitley RT: Herpesvirus infections of pregnancy. Part I: Cytomegalovirus and Epstein-Barr virus infections. N Engl J Med 313:1270, 1985. Reprinted by permission of the New England Journal of Medicine.)

1976 and 1990 used serologic methods to measure the reinfection rate during pregnancy of seropositive women (0.76%) and the primary infection rate during pregnancy of seronegative women (1.14%) (Hirota et al, 1992). None of 13 infants who had serologic evidence in cord blood of CMV infection or were shedding CMV had physical or mental retardation.

Although nosocomial infant-to-infant transmission of CMV has been reported, it most likely occurs infrequently (Adler et al, 1986; Spector, 1983; Yeager et al, 1983). However, nosocomial acquisition does occur. McCracken and associates (1969b) first reported the association between exchange blood transfusion and symptomatic CMV infection in the neonatal intensive care unit and, in the same year, King-Lewis and Gardner reported primary CMV disease following intrauterine transfusion. Luthardt and coworkers (1971) first suggested the connection between seropositive blood used for exchange transfusion and CMV acquisition by CMV seronegative recipients. These authors also suggested that such infections could be prevented by selection of CMV seronegative donors. Yeager and coworkers (1972) first pointed out the connection between blood transfusions and acquired CMV infection in newborn infants. Subsequently, Yeager and colleagues (1981) found that exclusive use of CMV seronegative blood eliminated CMV infection in seronegative infants. These observations were confirmed by other investigators (Adler, 1986). Frozen deglycerolized red blood cells may provide an alternative to blood taken from CMV seronegative donors but appears to be less effective in preventing CMV acquisition than blood from seronegative donors (Adler, 1986). Another useful approach is to filter out leukocytes, the site of latent CMV infection. Although the frequency of postnatal transfusion-acquired CMV has decreased with use of CMV-negative donors, a high index of suspicion must be maintained when pneumonia, hepatosplenomegaly, leukopenia, and thrombocytopenia develop and there are abnormal findings on liver function tests after 6 to 8 weeks of age in multiply transfused infants.

In addition to prenatal and postnatal transmission and infection through blood transfusion, the prevalence of CMV infection may be significantly increased in different populations by differences in prevalence of breast-feeding and child-rearing practices (Stagno and Cloud, 1994). In the United States, this impact may be greatest among women of upper socioeconomic status who send their children to day care centers and for day care center workers (Stagno and Cloud, 1994). If these seronegative women in the reproductive age range are exposed to increasing numbers of seropositive children, the risk of primary infection increases. In contrast, among women of low socioeconomic status, breast-feeding is less common as is use of day care. Thus, the proportion of seronegative, socioeconomically disadvantaged women increases (Stagno and Cloud, 1994).

Etiology

CMV is a member of the herpes virus family and has the largest DNA genome of any known virus (Adler, 1986). Although all strains are serologically related, there appear to be some variations in antigenicity, and it is not clear whether this heterogeneity affects the incidence of exoge-

nous reinfections. The virus differs from herpes simplex and varicella viruses in that it lacks the enzyme thymidine kinase, which renders it resistant to those antiviral agents that depend on this enzyme for their action, such as acyclovir.

As with rubella, it seems likely that the virus first infects the placenta and then the fetus and that the placenta functions as a relative barrier in this sequence.

Pathology

Characteristic multinuclear giant cells with both cytoplasmic and intranuclear inclusion bodies are found in many organs. Liver, lungs, brain, pancreas, and kidneys contain them in large numbers. Mononuclear cell infiltration and diffuse fibrosis may be intense. The brain contains areas of necrosis, often subependymal and periventricular, and glial overgrowth, containing heavy deposits of calcium. Petechiae and larger hemorrhages involve skin and serous surfaces.

Diagnosis

Infants infected with the virus are often prematurely delivered. In the classic form of the infection, cytomegalic inclusion disease, newborn infants have acute progressive disseminated disease. They show petechiae and ecchymoses and are jaundiced at birth, or jaundice appears within a few hours and becomes intense. The liver and spleen are enlarged and firm from the start and may increase in size for a number of days. Skull radiographs usually demonstrate periventricular calcifications. Temperature as high as 39° C (102° F to 103° F) may be found. Tachypnea and moderate dyspnea suggesting pulmonary involvement may appear. Pallor may or may not be striking. Puncture wounds bleed for many minutes, and hemorrhage from internal organs may cause death.

It is clear from prospective studies that most infants with congenital CMV infections are asymptomatic at birth and that milder manifestations of infections are more common than the aforementioned classic syndrome. Table 42–6 is a chart of the frequency of various clinical findings in 34 infants who were symptomatic by 2 weeks of age (Pass et al, 1980). Petechiae, hepatosplenomegaly, and jaundice were the most common signs at this age. Ten of the 34 infants died of their disease, most of them before 3 months of age, and all primarily because of severe neurologic impairment. Although microcephaly was seen in only half the infants at birth, a number of additional children became microcephalic as they grew older. In others, hearing or visual impairment developed, so that the proportion of surviving infants with sensorineural handicaps was increased to 91% at the time that the study was performed.

Uncommon findings at birth are cardiac defects and a number of gastrointestinal malformations. None of these has been systematically associated with CMV infection, however. Musculoskeletal abnormalities also occur, with indirect inguinal hernia being the most common.

Laboratory Investigations

The laboratory diagnosis of congenital CMV infection can be made with absolute certainty only through detection of

TABLE 42–6

Newborn Clinical Findings in 34 Patients with Congenital CMV Infection, All of Whom Were Symptomatic by 2 Weeks of Age

Abnormality	Positive/Total Examined (%)
Petechiae	27/34 (79)
Hepatosplenomegaly	25/34 (74)
Jaundice	20/32 (63)
Microcephaly°	17/34 (50)
Small for gestational age†	14/34 (41)
Prematurity‡	11/32 (34)
Inguinal hernia	5/19§ (26)
Chorioretinitis	4/34 (12)

°Less than tenth percentile based upon Colorado Intrauterine Growth Charts, for premature newborns or more than 2 SD below mean for term babies.

†Weight less than tenth percentile for gestational age.

‡Gestational age less than 38 weeks.

§Boys.

From Pass RF, et al: Outcome of symptomatic congenital cytomegalovirus infection: Results of long-term longitudinal follow-up. Pediatrics 66:758, 1980. Reproduced by permission of Pediatrics.

the virus in organs or culture specimens at birth or within the first 3 weeks of life. The most sensitive detection system is growth of the virus from urine in tissue culture (Kinney and Kumar, 1988). Serologic tests are often difficult to interpret, because, at the time of delivery, 50% to 75% of women have anti-CMV IgG, which is transplacentally transmitted to the infant, and even serial antibody titers cannot differentiate between congenital infection and perinatally acquired infection. No reliable CMV IgM assay is available (Kinney and Kumar, 1988). Molecular probes may permit rapid and specific diagnosis in the future (Chou and Merigan, 1983; Schrier et al, 1985). Careful consideration should be given to obtaining urine CMV cultures immediately after birth from those infants likely to receive blood transfusions or those who are at risk for enhanced immunosusceptibility. Such cultures would permit identification of infants who are congenitally infected and those who are postnatally infected. Prenatal diagnosis of congenital cytomegalovirus can be established by virus isolation from amniotic fluid obtained by amniocentesis (Grose et al, 1992). In recurrent infection during pregnancy, only 8% of infants have sequelae, and none should suffer mental retardation (Fowler et al, 1992; Grose et al, 1992). The results of such a culture in an asymptomatic infant should alert the physician to consider the need for hearing evaluation during childhood. If seroconversion occurs in a seronegative mother, a culture might be helpful to determine whether the fetus has been infected, although current data are insufficient to predict outcome of such a pregnancy with certainty (Boppana et al, 1992; Grose et al, 1992).

A presumptive diagnosis may sometimes be made after the infant is several months of age if virus is found and the clinical syndrome is classic. Other causes of congenital infection must be ruled out, because there is extensive overlap in the symptoms of several types of infections.

The principal types of abnormalities found on laboratory tests in infants with symptomatic CMV infection at birth

are listed in Table 42–7. Anemia (usually hemolytic) is also common.

The urine usually contains bile but no urobilin. Albumin is commonly present, as are some red and white blood cells. Sediment that has been dried, fixed, and stained with hematoxylin and eosin often demonstrates the characteristic inclusion bodies within desquamated renal epithelial cells (Fig. 42–3), so-called "owl's eye cells." Virus may be cultivated from the urine for an extended length of time.

Treatment

Attempts to treat CMV infection with idoxuridine, cytosine arabinoside, adenine arabinoside, and interferon inducers have failed. Transient reduction in the titer of virus excretion in the urine may be seen, but no clinical benefit has been detected. Corticosteroids and cytotoxic agents have been used without success. Transfusion is indicated for anemia. Multicenter trials are underway to examine the potential efficacy of gancyclovir (9-[2-hydroxy-1-(hydroxymethyl)ethoxymethyl]guanine), an acyclic nucleoside structurally related to acyclovir but with increased potency against CMV in vitro (Demmler, 1991; Shepp et al, 1985). In addition, alpha interferon (Hirsch et al, 1983) and CMV immune globulin (Bowden et al, 1988) are being studied.

Prognosis

Of infants who are symptomatic at birth, older studies suggested that approximately 25% die within the first 3 months (Pass et al, 1980; Weller and Hanshaw, 1962). Of the remainder, 60% to 75% have intellectual or developmental impairment (Berenberg and Nankervis, 1970), about one third have hearing loss, one third have neuromuscular disorders (spasticity or seizures), and a smaller

TABLE 42–7

Laboratory Abnormalities in Newborns with Symptomatic Congenital CMV Infection

Test	Abnormal/Total Examined (%)
Increased cord serum IgM (>20 mg/100 mL); range, 22–170	21/25 (84)
Atypical lymphocytosis (≥5%)°; range, 5%–42%	8/10 (80)
Elevated SGOT (>80 μU/mL)°; range 85–495	14/18 (79)
Thrombocytopenia (<100,000 platelets/mm³)†; range, 3000–66,000	17/28 (61)
Conjugated hyperbilirubinemia (direct serum bilirubin >2 mg/100 mL)†; range, 3–21	19‡/31 (61)
Increased CSF protein (>120 mg/100 mL)†; range, 130–198	9/19 (47)

°Determinations during first month of life.

†Determinations during first week of life.

‡One patient with jaundice had a maximum direct bilirubin of 1.2 mg/100 mL but was icteric within 24 hours of birth.

From Pass RF, Stagno S, Myers GJ, Alford CA: Outcome of symptomatic congenital cytomegalovirus infection: Results of long-term longitudinal follow-up. Pediatrics 66:758, 1980. Reproduced by permission of Pediatrics.

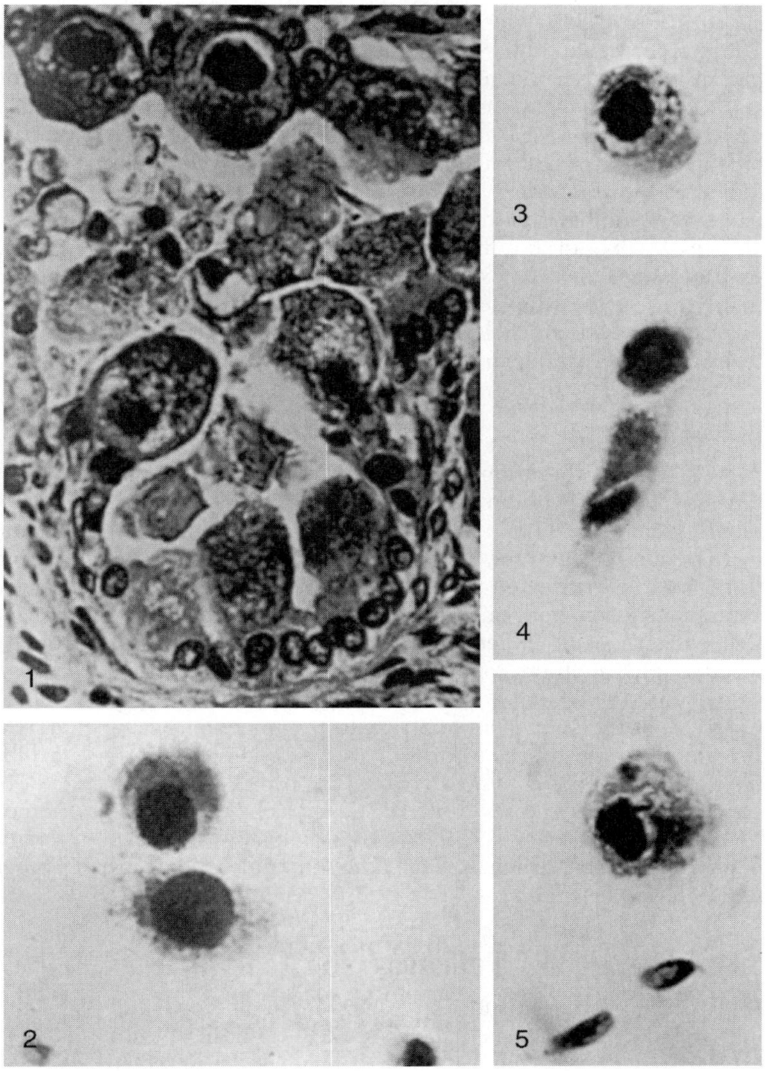

FIGURE 42–3. Renal tubule from a patient who died with cytomegalic inclusion disease. Note the intranuclear and intracytoplasmic inclusion bodies, with associated degeneration and desquamation of cells. Some of the necrotic cells appear as large masses of cytoplasm. *2, 3, 4,* Various types of cytomegalic cells observed in the urinary sediment from this infant. The shape of the cell in *3* suggests that it originated in the lower part of the collecting tubules or in the pelvis. In *4,* note the two small desquamated cells whose size corresponds to that of normal tubular cells. *5,* Cytomegalic cell and two normal cells from the gastric mucosa observed in the sediment from a gastric washing. Hematoxylin and eosin, × 782. (From Blanc WA: Am J Clin Pathol 28:46, 1957.)

proportion have visual impairment due to chorioretinitis. Only 10% to 25% are normal late in childhood, and those who demonstrated minimal abnormalities at birth have the greatest chance of being normal at long-term follow-up.

The fate of the congenitally infected infant who is normal at birth is still not clear. Two series (Hanshaw et al, 1976; Reynolds et al, 1974) indicate variable risks of deafness and reduction of intelligence quotient (IQ) scores. In both instances, however, the case finding method was measurement of cord IgM level; an increase in this value might be found only in more severely affected infants (possibly reflecting primary infection in the mother). In one other follow-up study (Kumar et al, 1973), the children were found to be normal at 4 years, but audiometric screening was not performed.

ENTEROVIRUS DISEASES

The enteroviruses of humans include polioviruses, coxsackieviruses A and B, and the echoviruses. Poliovirus infection of newborn infants has become rare. According to early accounts, however, severe, often fatal diseases developed in infants infected in the perinatal period, with a high incidence of paralysis occurring in the survivors. Refer to Bates (1955) and Cherry (1990) for further information.

Coxsackie A virus infections have been described only rarely; this review is limited to consideration of only those diseases associated with coxsackie B virus and echoviruses.

Incidence

All enterovirus infections are seasonal, occurring most frequently during the late summer and early autumn in temperate climates. The incidence varies from year to year, with outbreaks sometimes caused by a single coxsackie or echo serotype and sometimes by several (Sawyer et al, 1994). Disease in newborn infants is uncommon but reflects the frequency of infections in the population at large (Krajden and Middleton, 1983). It seems likely that severe disease in infants is seen with a frequency equal to or greater than that of perinatal herpes virus infection.

Etiology

It appears that any of the nonpolio enteroviruses can cause disease in the newborn infant. In a recent retrospective chart review of 24 newborn infant enteroviral infections in Toronto, 10 infants died, 12 had aseptic meningitis, and 5 had myocarditis (Krajden and Middleton, 1983). Of the 24 isolates, 7 were echovirus, 15 were coxsackie B virus, one was coxsackie A virus, and one was nontypable. A more recent review of 29 infants younger than 2 weeks old indicated more favorable outcomes: only 5 of these infants had severe multisystem disease, and all survived (Abzug et al, 1993). Two of the five infants had residual hepatic dysfunction. Types of coxsackie B virus are associated primarily with myocarditis and aseptic meningitis or combinations of the two (Kibrick and Benirschke, 1958). Echoviruses, however, are seen more often with severe nonspecific febrile illnesses with disseminated intravascular coagulation (Nagington et al, 1978), aseptic meningitis (Cramblett et al, 1973; Linnemann et al, 1974), or hepatitis (Modlin, 1980). With both groups of viruses, nonspecific febrile illnesses, with or without the presence of a rash, are commonly seen.

Infection takes place either just before or just after birth. Because infected infants have been delivered by cesarean section with intact membranes, it seems likely that transplacental infection has occurred. Regardless of whether the mother, a family member, or some other caretaker is the source of the infection, severe disease may result when the baby lacks antibody to the infecting strain. It is not clear why the newborn infant is so highly susceptible to overwhelming illness. Nursery outbreaks of both coxsackie B virus (Javett et al, 1956) and echovirus infections (Cramblett et al, 1973; Nagington et al, 1978) have been reported in which severe, and sometimes fatal, illnesses have occurred.

Pathology

In coxsackie B virus infections, myocardial necrosis and inflammation may be seen that is patchy or diffuse, with extensive infiltration by lymphocytes, mononuclear cells, histiocytes, and some polymorphonuclear leukocytes. Similar infiltrates are seen in the meninges in both coxsackie virus and echovirus infections. When liver or adrenal glands are involved, there is usually extensive hemorrhage as well as inflammation and necrosis.

Diagnosis

Viral culture from stool, nasopharynx, blood, urine, or cerebrospinal fluid remains the preferred diagnostic test. Serologic tests for enteroviruses have been reported (Swanink et al, 1993). When disease is acquired from the mother, an infant is characteristically well at birth, although premature delivery is more frequent in this group. The mother, however, may be febrile at this time. Fever, anorexia, and vomiting develop in the baby after an incubation period of 1 to 5 days. The onset of illness occurs in the 1st week of life in more than 50% of affected infants (Krajden and Middleton, 1983). At that point, the clinical evolution depends on the infecting virus and the extent of involvement.

In most instances, the disease is mild and self-limited. A rash may appear in some infants and aseptic meningitis in others. If myocarditis is present, the liver rapidly enlarges, the heart dilates, and the heart sounds become muffled. The echocardiogram and electrocardiogram show diffuse myocardial inflammation. Not infrequently, disseminated intravascular coagulation, refractory hypotension, and death follow rapidly. However, in many infants, myocardial involvement is temporary and recovery occurs over the course of several weeks.

The severity of central nervous system infection is also variable. Enteroviruses can produce overwhelming meningoencephalitis, sometimes with cranial nerve signs. It is more common, however, to see a moderate or mild meningitis characterized by only temporary irritability, lethargy, fever, and feeding difficulty. In a series of nine children with enteroviral meningitis and nine matched controls evaluated for sequelae at approximately 4 years of age, no differences in mean IQ level, head circumference, detectable sensorineuronal hearing loss, or intellectual functioning were detected (Wilfert et al, 1981). Receptive language functioning of the meningitis group was significantly less than that in control subjects. In a recent review of neonatal meningitis seen over a 15-year period in Galveston, Texas, enterovirus was the most common cause of meningitis in newborn infants older than 7 days and accounted for 33% of all cases of neonatal (<28 days of age) meningitis (Shattuck and Chonmaitree, 1992). Some infections, particularly those with echoviruses, are characterized by a rampant and overwhelming hepatitis (Modlin, 1980). Others are exhibited primarily in the form of pulmonary disease, and still others indicated by diarrhea and even necrotizing enterocolitis (Lake et al., 1976). Disseminated intravascular coagulation develops in virtually all instances of widespread, fulminant involvement.

Treatment

The symptoms of myocarditis and heart failure must be treated by slow digitalization, diuretics, and other supportive measures. Both plasma infusions and exchange transfusions have been attempted in overwhelming enterovirus infections with little evidence of beneficial effect. The use of steroids should be discouraged unless there is a clear rationale.

Prognosis

By the time disseminated intravascular coagulation has developed, the prognosis is grave. On the other hand, many infants with Coxsackie B virus myocarditis survive and the prognosis in such instances is probably closely related to early detection of the infection through electrocardiogram and viral diagnostic measures. Few long-term follow-up studies have been published, but the available information suggests that recovery is complete in most instances.

The prognosis following central nervous system involvement is also not clear. Most patients do well. However, a number of studies of infants under 3 months of age with aseptic meningitis have suggested that there may be some impairment of intellectual development when compared with carefully selected control groups (Farmer et al., 1975; Sells et al., 1975; Wilfert et al., 1981).

The following case illustrates the fulminant disease caused by Coxsackie B-2 virus.

CASE STUDY 1

A white male infant was born at term to a 35-year-old multiparous woman and weighed 3500 g. He did well at birth. On the 7th postnatal day, his mother became febrile. Four days later, the infant's temperature increased to 101.8° F, and tachypnea with cyanosis and grunting respiration developed. His heart rate increased to 198 beats per minute. Although the child appeared ill, physical examination did not identify an etiology for his illness. He was given ampicillin (200 mg/kg/day) and gentamicin (7.5 mg/kg/day) parenterally. Fever, tachypnea, and tachycardia persisted and hepatomegaly developed. Chest x-ray study and two-dimensional echocardiogram suggested biventricular cardiac failure, and digoxin was given at 5 mg/kg/day. Lumbar puncture revealed cerebrospinal fluid, which contained 2500 red blood cells and 1200 white blood cells/mm³ as well as an increased protein concentration (>120 mg/100 mL). Within 3 days, diarrhea, which was blood tinged, developed. Bacterial cultures of blood, cerebrospinal fluid, stool, urine, and nasopharynx revealed no pathogen. On the 13th day after presentation, the intractable hypotension and hypothermia (95.6° F) developed. Increasing hepatomegaly was noted. The child died within 24 hours thereafter. Antemortem and postmortem viral studies confirmed infection with coxsackie B-2 virus, which was grown from cerebrospinal fluid, blood, throat washings, and brain.

Comment

The onset of a febrile illness in this 11-day-old infant followed a similar illness in his mother. Tachycardia and heart failure developing in a previously normal heart suggested primary myocarditis, and cerebrospinal fluid alterations suggested encephalomyelitis. The combination of these two indicated generalized infection, with either a virus or *Toxoplasma* being the most likely pathogen. A virus appeared more probable in view of the simultaneous maternal illness and the absence of jaundice, hepatosplenomegaly, and thrombocytopenia.

HERPES SIMPLEX INFECTIONS

Herpes simplex viruses are classified into two types: Type 1 causes approximately 98% of oral infections (gingivostomatitis and pharyngitis), 7% to 50% of primary genital herpes, and almost 100% of encephalitis outside of the newborn period; Type 2 causes 90% of primary genital herpes, 99% of recurrent genital infections, and most cases of aseptic meningitis (Freij and Sever, 1988; Nahmias and Roizman, 1973). Seventy percent to 85% of neonatal herpes simplex infections are due to herpes Type 2 (Whitley, 1990; Whitley et al, 1980b). It is likely that most infections are acquired from the mother shortly before or at the time of delivery. Some, perhaps accounting for the slight excess

of cases resulting from Type 1 that are above the percentage found in the adult genital tract, must be acquired from other sources. Considering the frequency of labial herpes in the adult population, however, acquisition of herpes simplex from such lesions must be extremely rare.

Incidence

Genital herpes infections have been increasing steadily in incidence since the 1970s (Whitley, 1994). The frequency of neonatal disease has also increased (Prober et al, 1988). Neonatal disease frequency differs between populations according to socioeconomic status as well as incompletely understood immunologic factors (Nahmias et al, 1971, 1973; Whitley, 1990). Current estimates suggest an incidence of one case of neonatal herpes simplex infection in approximately 3500 deliveries (Whitley, 1993). Primary maternal genital herpes infections result in an attack rate of 50%, whereas recurrent maternal infection results in less than a 5% attack rate (Arvin, 1991; Prober et al, 1987).

Etiology and Pathogenesis

Most infants acquire the herpes simplex virus from the maternal genital tract at the time of delivery. Lesions have been reported to develop at the site of intrapartum monitoring electrodes on the infant's scalp. A smaller number of infants are infected several days before delivery and are born with clinically evident disease. There are some cases described of infants with a syndrome more closely resembling congenital viral infection who were probably infected in utero during the first or second trimester (Florman et al, 1973; Freij and Sever, 1988; South et al, 1969). Primary herpes simplex virus infections that occur during the first half of pregnancy are associated with an increased frequency of spontaneous abortions and stillbirths (Freij and Sever, 1988; Stagno and Whitley, 1985). Cases proved to have been acquired from individuals other than the mother, or even from the mother at any time other than during delivery, are rare (Linnemann et al, 1978; Yeager et al, 1983a).

The pathogenic mechanisms responsible for the newborn infant's susceptibility to herpes infection are not dependent on a single key difference between adult and infant but are the result of a spectrum of immunologic deficiencies (Arvin, 1991; Jenkins and Kohl, 1992). Among the currently identified cellular deficits are the inability of the neonatal macrophage to mediate early viral containment, the fact that unstimulated neonatal lymphocytes are permissive for herpes simplex virus infection, and a profound defect in natural killer cell cytotoxicity (Kohl, 1985). The contribution of transplacentally acquired antibody is unresolved and controversial (Arvin, 1991; Arvin and Prober, 1993; Kohl, 1991). Antibody dependent effector mechanisms, including antibody-dependent cellular cytotoxicity, which may rely on lymphocytes, macrophages, and polymorphonuclear leukocytes, may be responsible in different infants for the conflicting data concerning anti–herpes simplex virus antibody titers and protection from infection. The genetic and developmental regulatory mechanisms of these varied immunologic defects suggest different immunoregulatory interventions that are individualized for specific infants.

Pathology

Macroscopically, many viscera, but chiefly the liver, lungs, and adrenal glands, are riddled with pale yellow, firm, necrotic nodules, measuring 1 to 6 mm in diameter. Under the microscope, massive coagulation necrosis is seen to involve the parenchyma, stroma, and vessels in these areas. Necrotizing, calcifying lesions of the brain may also be found. Intranuclear eosinophilic inclusions as well as multinucleated giant cells, which represent the individual cell's response to viral infection, may be seen.

Diagnosis

Most infants are normal at birth and illness develops at 5 to 10 days of age. Approximately 40% of affected infants are less than 36 weeks' gestational age (Whitley and Hutto, 1985). Overt herpetic disease in the maternal genital tract is evident in only about one third of patients (Overall, 1994). In most of the remainder, the virus probably originates from an asymptomatic maternal genital infection.

The clinical manifestations of disease have been classified into two broad groups: disseminated and localized (Whitley, 1990). Within the disseminated group, two categories are recognized—those with and those without central nervous system involvement. Localized infections include those involving the central nervous system, with or without skin, eye, or mouth lesions, and those with isolated skin, eye, or oral cavity disease. Localized infections without central nervous system involvement represent approximately 20% of all cases of neonatal herpes (Whitley and Hutto, 1985). Despite undetectable central nervous system disease, in 25% of this group, neurologic abnormalities develop. Localized central nervous system disease with or without skin, eye, or oral cavity involvement is seen in approximately 33% of infants with neonatal herpes. The mortality rate in this group is from 17% to 50%, and 40% have long-term neurologic sequelae. Infants with disseminated disease represent approximately 50% of all neonatal herpes patients. Without antiviral therapy, 80% die and survivors have serious neurologic sequelae (Whitley and Hutto, 1985). With therapy, 15% to 20% die, but 40% to 55% suffer neurologic sequelae (Freij and Sever, 1988).

Disseminated disease usually begins toward the end of the 1st week of life. Skin vesicles may be the first or a later sign, but they do not appear at all in more than half of patients. Systemic symptoms, although insidious in onset, progress rapidly. Poor feeding, lethargy, and fever may be accompanied by irritability or convulsions if the central nervous system is involved. These symptoms are followed rapidly by jaundice, hypotension, disseminated intravascular coagulation, apnea, and shock. This form of disease is indistinguishable at its onset from both neonatal enterovirus infection and bacterial sepsis.

Localized disease may begin somewhat later, with most cases appearing in the 2nd week of life. When the central nervous system is the primary site of infection, the skin or eyes may or may not be involved; if not, then brain biopsy may be the only mode of diagnosis, as with encephalitis

in older subjects. The infants are lethargic, irritable, and tremulous, and seizures are frequent and difficult to control.

Eye infections usually take the form of keratoconjunctivitis or chorioretinitis. On the neonatal skin, herpes simplex virus produces the characteristic grouped vesicles seen in later life, although individual lesions may be large and even bullous and late lesions are typically eroded, flat, irregular ulcers with an erythematous base.

In disseminated disease, there is usually chemical evidence of hepatocellular injury. If the central nervous system is involved, the spinal fluid usually contains white cells (mostly lymphocytes) and sometimes demonstrates erythrocytes, and the protein level is usually elevated. Except when encephalitis is the only manifestation of disease, as discussed, herpes simplex virus is readily recovered from clinical samples. In the disseminated form, virus is present in blood, cerebrospinal fluid, conjunctivae, respiratory secretions, and urine. In the localized form, the virus can be found at the site of disease. Scrapings of skin vesicles show giant, multinucleated cells when stained with Wright or Giesma stain (the Tzanck smear), typical of either herpes or varicella virus infection. Demonstration of viral antigens in cytologic smears using monoclonal or polyclonal antibodies is a more sensitive tool than Tzanck smear (Alpert and Plotkin, 1986). Definitive microbiologic diagnosis, however, requires growth of the virus in tissue culture. Fortunately, herpes simplex virus can be detected by its cytopathic effect in 24 to 48 hours in most instances. When herpes neonatorum is suspected, viral cultures of the throat, conjunctival and cerebrospinal fluids, blood, and urine should all be obtained as should scrapings of any suspicious skin lesions. The mother's genital and respiratory tracts should also be sampled. Serologic assays are rarely helpful and are difficult to interpret in view of the cross-reactions between the two herpes serotypes.

Treatment and Prevention

If a mother has active genital herpes simplex infection at the time of delivery and if the membranes are either intact or have been ruptured for less than 4 hours, strong consideration should be given to delivery by cesarean section (Dwyer and Cunningham, 1993; Prober et al, 1992). The risk to the child is greatest if maternal infection is primary (i.e., if the mother has previously had no infection with either Type 1 or Type 2 virus). Recurrences, however, with infectious virus recoverable from the genital area at the time of delivery also pose a hazard.

When neonatal disease is suspected, every effort to establish a definitive diagnosis must be made as rapidly as possible. As soon as this diagnosis is suspected, the infant should receive adenine arabinoside (Vidarabine), 20 to 30 mg/kg/day administered intravenously over a 12-hour period for 10 days, or acyclovir, 10 to 30 mg/kg/day intravenously in every 8 to 12 hours, depending on the degree of renal impairment, for 10 to 14 days (Toltzis, 1991). This treatment has been shown to be effective in all forms of the disease, reducing (but by no means eliminating) both mortality and sequelae. The survival results of the Collaborative Antiviral Study Group trials for infants with central nervous system or disseminated disease are shown in Fig-

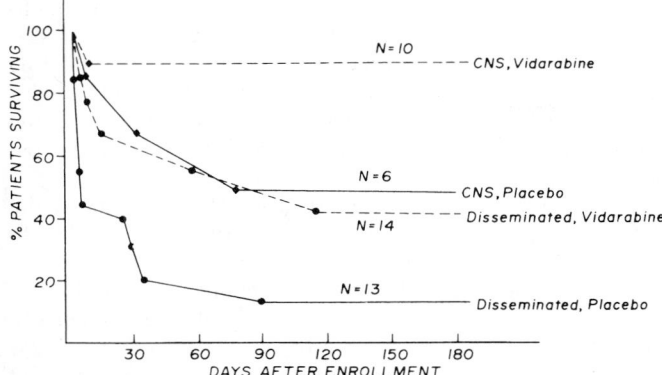

FIGURE 42–4. Outcome of herpes simplex virus infection in newborns according to type of disease and therapy. Points represent last death(s). (From Whitley RJ, Nahmias AJ, Visintine AM, et al: The natural history of herpes simplex virus infection of mother and newborn. Pediatrics 66:489, 1980. Reproduced by permission of Pediatrics.)

ure 42–4 (Whitley et al, 1980a). The mortality rate in infants with localized disease outside the central nervous system has always been close to zero. Recently, Whitley (1994b) suggested that concomitant administration of antiviral therapy with antibody to herpes simplex (humanized monoclonal antibodies, human monoclonal antibodies, or hyperimmune globulin) might improve outcome for infants with encephalitis or disseminated infection. This strategy has theoretical promise but is clinically untested. If cultures are negative, breast-feeding is safe (Grossman et al, 1981).

Prognosis

Even with antiviral treatment, the prognosis for survivors is not good. Microcephaly, spasticity, paralysis, seizures, deafness, or blindness develop in more than half of infants with disseminated disease. Those with skin involvement often have recurrent crops of skin vesicles for several years.

The following case illustrates a typical severe generalized herpes virus infection in an infant with disseminated disease.

CASE STUDY 2

After an uncomplicated pregnancy and delivery, a 5-day-old full-term female infant was admitted because of fever, anorexia, and lethargy. Immediately after the delivery, the mother had noted the onset of intense vaginal pain and itching. Physical examination revealed herpetic lesions about the genitalia. The child had done well during the first 4 days of life but then had a temperature of 102° F and anorexia. On physical examination, her temperature was 100.8° F, a large pustular lesion was noted on the left cheek, the liver was palpated 1.5 cm below the right costal margin, and the spleen was not palpable. The remainder of the physical examination was unremarkable. Her white blood cell count was 5600/mm³ with 73% polymorphonuclear

leukocytes. Her hemoglobin was 16.9 g/100 mL. Cultures of blood, urine, cerebrospinal fluid, and stool showed no bacterial pathogens. She was started on ampicillin and gentamicin.

Her fever persisted, and additional skin lesions were observed over the subsequent 3 days. A repeat lumbar puncture revealed 500 white blood cells/mm³ in her cerebrospinal fluid, consisting of 50% polymorphonuclear leukocytes and 50% mononuclear cells. Thrombocytopenia (<100,000 platelets/mm³) developed, and evidence of hepatocellular inflammation was noted. Hepatosplenomegaly increased. Generalized convulsions were noted on the 6th hospital day as were hematologic manifestations of disseminated intervascular coagulation. The infant died on the 17th day of life.

Autopsy showed extensive necrobiotic lesions characteristic of generalized herpes simplex infection in the liver, lungs, and adrenals. Herpes simplex virus was grown from the liver, lungs, and brain. Virus was also isolated from persistent vesicular lesions of the skin.

Comment

The infant was undoubtedly infected during parturition by contact with the mother's genital herpes. Skin lesions appeared on the 4th day, and new vesicles developed during the course. Unlike most instances of the disease, jaundice was never prominent. The liver and spleen were enlarged, and thrombocytopenia with bleeding and evidence of brain damage appeared. The virus was identified. Neutralizing antibodies were not found in appreciable quantities in the mother or child.

This case illustrates the course of herpes simplex infection before the advent of antiviral agents.

VARICELLA

There is some confusion about the term "congenital varicella" that would probably be best resolved by reserving this term for the rare cases transmitted to the fetus in the first or second trimester of pregnancy (Laforet and Lynch, 1947; Srabstein et al, 1974). Also called "congenital varicella" but probably better termed "neonatal varicella" are those cases of perinatal varicella beginning before or on the 10th day of life and, therefore, because of the incubation period of the disease, acquired in utero. The two syndromes are discussed by Brunell (1992) and Feldman (1986). Some cases (e.g., that described by Bai and John, 1979) fall somewhere in between.

Incidence

Varicella-zoster virus infections occur during pregnancy with a frequency of 7 per 10,000 pregnancies (Balducci et al, 1992; Brunell, 1992). Approximately 24 cases of congenital varicella are reported (Paryani and Arvin, 1986). On the basis of four carefully perfomed studies of varicella during pregnancy, the risk of symptomatic intrauterine varicella-zoster virus infection after maternal varicella during the first and second trimester is 2.0% to 4.9% (Enders,

1984; Enders et al, 1994; Paryani and Arvin, 1986; Siegel, 1973). Unlike mumps and rubella infection during the first trimester, first trimester varicella does not result in a detectable increase in fetal wastage (Brunell, 1992; Siegel and Fuerst, 1966). Paryani and Arvin (1986) reported that in 1 of 11 infants with maternal varicella during the second trimester herpes zoster developed during infancy, and 2 of 16 infants with maternal varicella during the third trimester had varicella at birth. For infants whose mothers contract varicella 5 days or less before delivery or up to 2 days after delivery, the infant attack rate is 17% to 31% (Brunell, 1992; Feldman, 1986; Meyers, 1974). In two of three infants whose mothers contracted the infection less than 10 days before delivery, varicella developed despite the administration of varicella zoster immune globulin at birth (Paryani and Arvin, 1986).

Etiology and Pathogenesis

The congenital varicella syndrome is acquired from a maternal varicella infection that occurs during the first or second trimester. The virus must be transmitted transplacentally during the viremia that precedes or accompanies the rash. In most situations, however, the fetus either is not infected at all or recovers fully in utero, because the syndrome itself is so rare and because varicella during pregnancy is not uncommon.

Neonatal varicella is also probably transplacentally acquired in most cases. Because the incubation period for varicella is between 10 and 21 days, those cases beginning in the first 10 days of life are considered to have been acquired in utero. The prognosis, however, differs markedly between those cases in which maternal illness began 5 or more days from delivery and those in which maternal illness occurred from 5 days before to 2 days after delivery. In the first group, neonatal disease usually begins with the first 4 days of life, and the prognosis is good. Of 27 cases cited by Gershon (1975), all survived. Presumably, maternal immunity has appeared before delivery and has been transferred to the baby before birth. In the second group, neonatal disease begins between 5 and 10 days after delivery (Brunell, 1966). Of the 23 cases described, 7 (30%) died if overwhelming varicella and two barely survived after severe disease. In those instances in which the infant's preillness antibody has been measured in severe disease, none has been found.

Presumably, the placenta acts as a partial barrier to infection at term as well as earlier during pregnancy. Only about one in six such maternal infections results in neonatal disease (Meyers, 1974).

Diagnosis

The rare cases of congenital varicella syndrome are characterized by the presence of unusual cicatrices, asymmetric muscular atrophy and limb hypoplasia, low birth weight, chronic encephalitis with cortical atrophy, and ophthalmitis (chorioretinitis, microphthalmia, atrophy, and cataracts) (Brunell, 1992; Feldman, 1986).

Neonatal varicella follows typical maternal varicella and thus can usually be anticipated. When the disease appears in the infant during the danger period (from 5 to 10 days of age), it resembles closely varicella in the immunodeficient or immunosuppressed host. Recurrent crops of skin vesicles develop over a prolonged period of time, reflecting the newborn infant's inability to control the infection. Visceral dissemination is common, with involvement of the liver, lung, and brain. Secondary bacterial infection may occur.

Disease that is evident at birth or that appears in the first 4 days of life is usually mild, presumably owing to modification of the illness by maternal immunity.

The laboratory may be helpful in confirming the diagnosis. Prenatal diagnosis has been performed on blood obtained by funicentesis by quantifying varicella-specific IgM with an immunofluorescent antibody assay (Cuthbertson et al, 1987). Similar serologic studies can be performed on infants (Paryani and Arvin, 1986). Scrapings of skin lesions, as with herpes simplex infections, show large multinucleated cells when stained with Wright or Giemsa stain (Tzanck smears). The virus can be grown in tissue culture from skin and visceral lesions.

Prevention and Treatment

Infants of mothers in whom varicella develops from 5 days before to 2 days after delivery should receive high-titered immune globulin as soon as possible (125 U) (American Academy of Pediatrics, 1994a; Centers for Disease Control and Prevention, 1984). Such preparations (zoster immune globulin, or varicella-zoster immune globulin) have been shown to prevent chicken pox in exposed older children (Brunell et al, 1969) and are available from regional blood centers of the American Red Cross Services. In approximately 50% of exposed and treated infants, varicella develops, but the disease often is less severe (American Academy of Pediatrics, 1994a). Follow-up of exposed and treated infants should include consideration of serologic testing (enzyme immunoassay, latex agglutination, or indirect fluorescent antibody) to determine whether asymptomatic infection has elicited immune protection (American Academy of Pediatrics, 1994a). Repeat exposure of exposed and treated infants in whom varicella did not develop more than 3 weeks after administration of varicella zoster immune globulin (VZIG) should prompt giving another dose of VZIG (American Academy of Pediatrics, 1994a). If special globulin preparations are not available, then standard immune serum globulin (0.5 to 1.0 mL/kg) should be given.

In the event of a significant exposure in a nursery situation, as defined by prolonged contact (greater than 20 minutes) with an infectious staff member, patient, or visitor, infants who have no maternal history of varicella and who have undetectable antivaricella titers should be considered candidates for VZIG. All infants less than 28 weeks' gestational age regardless of maternal history should be considered (American Academy of Pediatrics, 1994). The recommended dosage is 125 units/10 kg. Fractional doses are not recommended. However, little experience is available to guide treatment of extremely preterm infants. Currently, all infants should receive 125 units.

If severe disease develops, antiviral chemotherapy might be considered. Drugs that might be effective are adenine arabinoside (15 mg/kg/day) and acycloguanosine (acyclovir) (10 to 30 mg/kg/day) (Brunell, 1992).

VIRAL HEPATITIS

Owing to the alliance between molecular biology and virology and clinical medicine, dramatic advances were made during the 1980s in understanding the pathogenesis of viral hepatitis (Balistreri, 1988). The known forms of acute and chronic viral hepatitis and the antigens and antibodies associated with them are listed in Tables 42–8 and 42–9. Although hepatitis A virus has been nosocomially transmitted in the setting of a neonatal intensive care unit, and multiply transfused infants are at increased risk for non-A, non-B hepatitis, hepatitis B and hepatitis C are currently of greatest importance for the pediatrician (Krugman, 1992). This discussion focuses on perinatal hepatitis B and C infections.

The findings that perhaps are the most important to neonatologists pertain to the frequency with which hepatitis B is transmitted to infants at the time of birth, the short- and long-term consequences of these infections, the importance of increased surveillance for maternal hepatitis B carriage, and the availability of effective hepatitis B virus immunoprophylaxis (Krugman, 1988). The frequency of transmission depends primarily on the prevalence of the hepatitis B carrier state among women of child-bearing age.

In certain parts of the world and among certain ethnic groups, as many as 7% to 10% of all infants acquire hepatitis B infections at the time of birth, and a high proportion of these infections is chronic. The relationship of these infections to chronic liver failure and hepatic carcinoma in adult life has been noted (Balistreri, 1988; Beasley et al, 1981).

Incidence

The incidence of neonatal hepatitis B infection depends on a number of factors. Women with acute hepatitis B infection during the first or second trimester rarely transmit the virus to their infants (Krugman, 1988; Stevens, 1994). Besides the timing of the infection, the hepatitis B surface antigen (HBAg) carriage rate varies from 0.1% in the United States and Europe to 15% in Taiwan and parts of Africa, with intermediate rates in Japan, South America, and Southeast Asia. Transmission rates among immigrant women in western countries appear to parallel the rates in their country of origin (Krugman, 1988). Another factor is the potential of the infection to be transmitted from the mother at the time of delivery. This potential is great if symptomatic acute disease is present (60% to 70% transmission) (Gerety and Schweitzer, 1977). Infants of hepatitis B e antigen (HBeAg)-positive mothers have an 80% to 90% chance of becoming HBsAg carriers (Okada et al, 1976). Chronic neonatal infection occurs in less than 10% of infants of e antigen-negative mothers (Krugman, 1988). Transplacental leakage of HBeAg-positive maternal blood is the most likely source of intrauterine infection (Lin et al, 1987). The serologic and biochemical course of subclinical infection is outlined in Figure 42–5. Although HbsAg has been found in breast milk, breast-feeding does not appear

---

TABLE 42–8

Viral Hepatitis Types A, B, C, D, and E: Comparison of Clinical, Epidemiologic, and Immunologic Features

Features	Hepatitis A	Hepatitis B	Hepatitis C	Hepatitis D	Hepatitis E
Virus	HAV	HBV	HCV	HDV	HEV
Family	Picornavirus	Hepadnavirus	Flavivirus	Satellite	Calcivirus
Genome	RNA	DNA	RNA	RNA	RNA
Incubation period	15–40 d	50–180 d	1–5 mo	21–90 d	2–9 wk
Type of onset	Usually acute	Usually insidious	Usually insidious	Usually acute	Usually acute
Prodrome					
Arthritis and rash	Not present	May be present	May be present	Unknown	Not present
Mode of transmission					
Oral (fecal)	Usual	No	No	No	Usual
Parenteral	Rare	Usual	Usual	Usual	No
Other	Food or water borne	Intimate (sexual) contact Perinatal	Intimate (sexual) contact less common	Intimate (sexual) contact less common	Water-borne transmission in developing countries
Sequelae					
Carrier	No	Yes	Yes	Yes	No
Chronic hepatitis	No cases reported	Yes	Yes	Yes	No cases reported
Mortality rate	0.1%–0.2%	0.5%–2.0% in uncomplicated cases; may be higher in complicated cases	1%–2% in uncomplicated cases; may be higher in complicated cases	2%–20%	20% in pregnant woman; 1%–2% in general population
Immunity					
Homologous	Yes	Yes	Yes	Yes	Yes
Heterologous	No	No	No	No	No

From Krugman S. Viral hepatitis A–E—Prevention. Pediatr Rev 13:205, 1992.
Reproduced by permission of *Pediatrics in Review,* Vol 13, page 205, copyright 1992.

to have any influence, either positive or negative, on the rate of transmission (Beasley et al, 1975).

Etiology and Pathogenesis

Hepatitis B virus is the only representative of a unique group of DNA-containing viruses that infects the human host. The virus localizes primarily in hepatic parenchymal cells but circulates in the bloodstream, along with several subviral antigens, for periods of time ranging from a few days to many years. Despite either acute or persistent viremia in the mother, the virus rarely crosses the placenta and infection in the neonatal period occurs at or shortly after birth, probably by means of virus carried in maternal blood. Most infants born to mothers infected with hepatitis B virus have negative test results at birth and become HB $_s$Ag-positive during the first 3 months of life (Krugman, 1988, 1992; Mulligan and Stiehm, 1994; Shapiro, 1993).

Diagnosis

Infants with hepatitis B infection do not show clinical or chemical signs of disease at birth. The usual pattern is the development of chronic antigenemia with mild and often persistent enzyme elevations, beginning at 2 to 6 months of age (Mulligan and Stiehm, 1994). Occasionally, the anti-

genemia is entirely missed, and the child is merely found to have antibody to the surface antigen at 6 to 12 months of age. Sometimes, the infection becomes clinically manifest, with jaundice, fever, hepatomegaly, and anorexia, followed by either recovery or chronic active hepatitis. Rarely, fulminant hepatitis is seen (Delaplane et al, 1983).

Laboratory tests are essential in the diagnosis of hepatitis B infection. Evaluations of serum enzymes and of bilirubin reflect the extent of liver damage. There are several helpful serologic tests that identify the virus involved (Krugman, 1988) (Fig. 42–6). HB $_s$Ag appears early, usually before liver disease is found, and may disappear or persist. Antibody to the hepatitis B core antigen (anti-HBc) usually appears during or shortly after the acute disease and lasts for years. Hepatitis B e antigen appears concurrently with HBsAg and is indicative of an increased potential to transmit the infection. Antibody to hepatitis B e antigen appears approximately 2 to 4 weeks after the disappearance of e antigen. The last factor to appear, usually several weeks or even months after the illness (and never if HBsAg persists), is antibody to the surface antigen, or anti-HBs. It is very unusual for all three of these tests to yield negative results in the presence of hepatitis B infection.

Prevention and Treatment

In 1991, the Advisory Committee on Immunization Practices of the United States Public Health Service recom-

TABLE 42–9

The Hepatitis Viruses: Characteristics of Associated Antigens and Antibodies

	Definitions	Significance
Serologic Markers of Hepatitis A Virus (HAV)°		
Anti-HAV	Total antibody (IgM and IgG subclasses) directed against HAV	Indicates recent acute (IgM) or past HAV infection (Ig) Confirms past exposure and immunity towards HAV
Anti-HAV-IgM	IgM antibody to HAV	Indicates recent acute infection
Serologic Markers of Hepatitis B Virus (HBV)°		
HBsAg	Hepatitis B surface antigen—found on the surface of the intact virus and in serum as unattached particles (spherical or tubular)	Indicates infection with HBV (either acute or chronic)
HBcAg	Hepatitis B core antigen—found within the core of the intact virus	Not detectable in serum (found only in liver tissue)
HBeAg	Hepatitis B core antigen—(soluble antigen produced during self-cleavage of HBcAg)	Indicates active HBV infection Signifies high infectivity Persistence for 6–8 months suggests chronic carrier and/or chronic liver disease
Anti-HBs	Antibody to HBV surface antigen (HBsAg); subclasses	Indicates clinical recovery from HBV infection and immunity
	IgM (early and IgG)	Protective
Anti-HBc	Total antibody to HBV core antigen (HBcAg)	Indicates active HBV infection (acute and chronic)
Anti-HBc-IgM	IgM antibody to HBcAg	Early index of acute HBV infection Rises during acute phase then declines Not present in chronic HBV
Anti-HBe	Antibody to HBV e antigen (HBeAg)	Seroconversion (HBeAg to anti-HBe) indicates resolution
Serologic Markers of Hepatitis Delta Virus (HDV)°		
Anti-HDV	Total antibody to the hepatitis D (delta) virus	Indicates exposure to the delta agent (HDV) Patient may transmit HDV infection
HDV RNA	RNA of the hepatitis D (delta) virus	Present in serum

°These are detectable using sensitive and specific commercial serologic assays.
From Balistreri WF: Viral hepatitis. Pediatr Clin North Am 35:637, 1988.

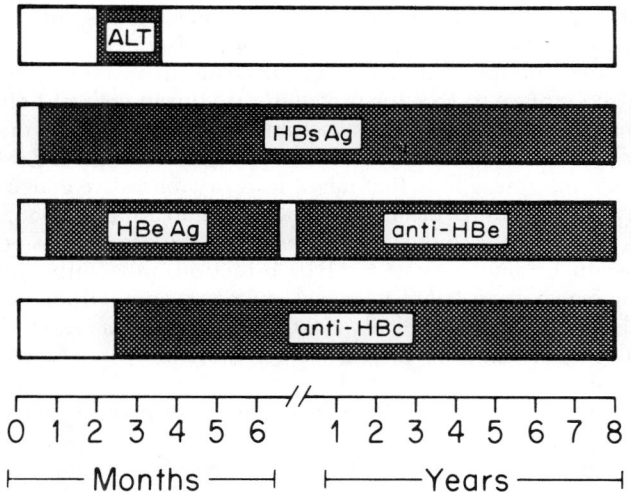

FIGURE 42–5. Serologic and biochemical course of subclinical hepatitis B infection progressing to asymptomatic chronic carrier state. (From Krugman S: Hepatitis B virus and the neonate. Ann N Y Acad Sci 549:129, 1988.)

mended universal childhood vaccination against hepatitis B virus to begin in the neonatal period intended to eliminate transmission of hepatitis B virus in the United States (Centers for Disease Control and Prevention, 1991b). Hepatitis B vaccination is recommended for all infants born to HBsAg-negative and -positive mothers. The three-dose vaccination schedule should be initiated in the neonatal period or by 2 months of age (Tables 42–10 and 42–11). The second dose is given 1 to 2 months after the first dose, and the third dose is given at 6 to 18 months of age (American Academy of Pediatrics, 1997). Vaccination may be delayed until just before hospital discharge in preterm (less than 2000 g birth weight) infants born to HbsAg-negative mothers. However, all infants born to HBsAg-positive women should receive both active and passive

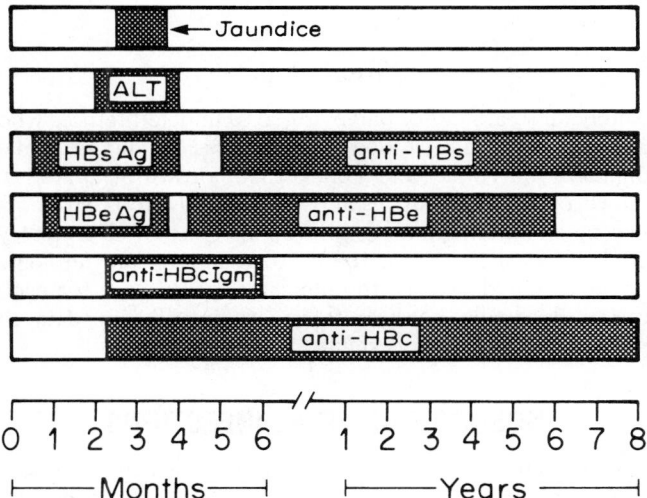

FIGURE 42–6. Chemical, serologic, and biochemical course of acute hepatitis B infection followed by recovery. (From Krugman S: Hepatitis B virus and the neonate. Ann N Y Acad Sci 549:129, 1988.)

TABLE 42–10

Recommended Schedule of Hepatitis B Immunoprophylaxis to Prevent Perinatal Transmission

Vaccine Dose* and HBIG	Age
Infant Born to Mother Known to be HBsAg-Positive	
First	Birth (within 12 h)
HBIG†	Birth (within 12 h)
Second	1–2 mo
Third	6 mo
Infant Born to Mother Not Screened for HBsAg	
First‡	Birth (within 12 h)
HBIG†	If mother is found to be HBsAg-positive, give 0.5 mL as soon as possible, not later than 1 wk after birth
Second	1–2 mo
Third	6–18 mo§

°See Table 42–11 for appropriate vaccine dose.

†HBIG (0.5 mL) given intramuscularly at a site different from that used for vaccine.

‡First dose is same as that for infant of HBsAg-positive mother. Subsequent doses and schedules are determined by maternal HBsAg status.

§Infants of HBsAg-positive mothers should be vaccinated at 6 mo.

Used with permission of the American Academy of Pediatrics: Hepatitis B. *In* Peter G (Ed): 1997 Red Book: Report of the Committee on Infectious Diseases, 24th ed. Elk Grove Village, IL: American Academy of Pediatrics, 1997, p 258.

vaccination. The dosage size of the two hepatitis B vaccines currently licensed in the United States are given in Table 42–10. The highest immunization failure rate (3 of 21 infants, or 14%) has been observed in infants of HBeAg-positive women (Farmer et al, 1987).

TABLE 42–11

Recommended Dosages of Hepatitis B Vaccines

	Vaccine*			
	Recombivax HB† Dose		Engerix-B‡ Dose	
	µg	(mL)	µg	(mL)
Infants of HBsAg-negative mothers and children <11 y	2.5	(0.5)§	10	(0.5)
Infants of HBsAg-positive mothers (HBIG [0.5 mL] also is recommended)	5	(1.0)§ (0.5)°°	10	(0.5)

°Vaccines should be stored at 2°C to 8°C. Freezing destroys effectiveness. Both vaccines are administered in a 3-dose schedule.

†Available from Merck & Co.

‡The Food and Drug Administration has approved this vaccine for use in an optional 4-dose schedule at 0, 1, 2, and 12 mo; available from SmithKline Beecham.

§Pediatric formulation.

°°Adult formulation.

Used with permission of the American Academy of Pediatrics: Hepatitis B. *In* Peter G (Ed): 1997 Red Book: Report of the Committee on Infectious Diseases, 24th ed. Elk Grove Village, IL: American Academy of Pediatrics, 1997, p 252.

For immunoprophylaxis to be successful, maternal screening is important (Cruz et al, 1987; Summers et al, 1987). The United States Public Health Service Immunization Practices Advisory Committee and the American College of Obstetricians and Gynecologists have recommended routine screening of all pregnant women (Centers for Disease Control and Prevention, 1988; ACOG, 1992b). In developing countries, such a strategy is neither feasible nor affordable. In areas where hepatitis B virus infection is hyperendemic, all newborn infants should be routinely immunized (Hsu et al, 1988; Krugman, 1988).

Hepatitis C

In 1989, hepatitis C virus (HCV) was found to be the main cause of non-A, non-B parenterally transmitted hepatitis and has been subsequently found to account for a significant portion of the cases of sporadic acute and chronic hepatitis (Gross and Persing, 1995). In contrast to hepatitis B virus, HCV is not easily transmitted by sexual contact. Risk factors for HCV infection include transfusion, especially with contaminated lots of intravenous immune globulin beginning in April 1993, intravenous drug use, frequent occupational exposure to blood products, and household or sexual contact with an infected person (Gross and Persing, 1995). The vertical transmission rate of HCV is low (10%) and correlates with the titer of HCV RNA in mothers (Lynch-Salamon and Combs, 1992; Ohto et al, 1994). Transmission of HCV in breast milk appears to be rare (Ogasawara et al, 1993), although large, prospective studies are not available. Treatment of potentially infected individuals with immune globulin has been equivocal at best. Because of exclusion of anti-HCV–positive persons by screening programs, immune globulin manufactured in the United States is unlikely to provide passive immunity against HCV. The risks and consequences of perinatal transmission have not been defined (A-Kader and Balistreri, 1993; American Academy of Pediatrics, 1994c). Other viral hepatitides may rarely complicate pregnancy (Simms and Duff, 1993).

HUMAN PARVOVIRUS B19

Considerable interest in the role of human parvovirus B19 infection in neonatal hydrops fetalis (nonimmune) and fetal aplastic crisis has developed since two cases of fetal deaths in humans associated with maternal B19 infection were reported (Kinney and Kumar, 1988).

Incidence, Etiology, and Pathogenesis

Approximately 30% to 60% of adults in the United States are seropositive for human parvovirus B19. A significant proportion of child-bearing women is thus presumably susceptible to human parvovirus B19 infection. Approximately 36 fetal deaths associated with maternal human parvovirus B19 infection have been reported as have approximately 130 cases in which the fetus survived and was normal at birth (Kinney and Kumar, 1988). Although large studies are not available, the overall risk of maternal exposure or infection to the fetus appears low (Berry et al, 1992; Sheikh

et al, 1992). Postexposure passive immunization is not currently recommended (Boley and Popek, 1993).

Two potential pathogenic mechanisms involve the recognized affinity of B19 for progenitor erythroid cells of bone marrow and the finding of nonimmune hydrops in several of the affected fetuses. The pathologic findings suggest bone marrow aplasia that might lead to progressive congestive heart failure and hydrops (Kinney and Kumar, 1988).

Two studies undertaken to examine the association between human parvovirus B19 infection and congenital anomalies have failed to reveal any connection (Kinney et al, 1988; Mortimer et al, 1983). A recent Japanese study suggested that 10% of cases of nonimmune hydrops fetalis (4 of 42 cases) are due to human parvovirus B19 infection (Yaegashi et al, 1994). Pathologic studies of parvovirus B19 infected human fetuses have suggested that myocardial inflammation and subendocardial fibroelastosis may contribute to fetal hydrops (Morey et al, 1992).

Diagnosis

The diagnosis can be made serologically or by viral culture. Both radioimmunoassays and enzyme-linked immunosorbent assays are available for detection of human parvovirus B19–specific IgG and IgM (Kinney and Kumar, 1988). Preliminary observations suggest that human parvovirus B19 IgM antibodies may have a shortened half-life (Anderson and Pattison, 1984). Virus can be cultured from tissue in suspension cultures of bone marrow cells from persons with hemolytic anemias. Electron microscopy has permitted visualization of parvovirus-like particles in peripheral blood. Finally, molecular probes can detect human parvovirus B19 DNA in tissues, serum, and urine (Kinney and Kumar, 1988).

Elevated maternal alpha-fetoprotein concentration may be a marker for an adverse outcome (Carrington et al, 1987). In the context of a human parvovirus B19 infection in a symptomatic, pregnant woman, rising weekly measurements of maternal serum alpha-fetoprotein may indicate that the fetus is infected.

Treatment

Antenatal treatment of parvovirus B19 infected fetuses who are hydropic has included fetal transfusion and maternal digitalization (Boley and Popek 1993; Brown et al, 1994). However, spontaneous resolution of fetal hydrops with normal neonatal outcome has also been reported (Humphrey et al, 1991; Sheikh et al, 1992). After appropriate serologic or molecular diagnosis, the clinician should care for each case individually because there are insufficient data to predict outcome with certainty.

NOSOCOMIAL VIRAL INFECTIONS

Nursery outbreaks of enterovirus infections can cause diseases ranging from mild, benign febrile illness to aseptic meningitis, myocarditis, and overwhelming generalized infections with disseminated intravascular coagulation (Cramblett et al, 1973; Javett et al, 1956; Nagington et al, 1978). Nursery-acquired herpes simplex infections are rare, and symptomatic nosocomial CMV infections appear to be largely confined to recipients of latently infected blood who themselves lack antibody. Two other groups of viruses, however, previously unrecognized as important pathogens in the newborn period, appear to be responsible for a significant proportion of nursery-acquired viral infections. These are the respiratory viruses and the viruses that cause diarrhea.

Respiratory Viruses

It seems likely that any one of the large number of respiratory viruses can cause symptomatic respiratory disease in newborn infants. The association has been described for rhinoviruses, adenoviruses, parainfluenza viruses, influenza virus, and respiratory syncytial virus. Adenovirus, rhinovirus, and parainfluenza virus infections are characterized by mild rhinorrhea under these conditions. Influenza virus infections are usually mild, but in the absence of maternally transmitted antibody they can be life threatening, with extensive pneumonia and hypoxia and a prolonged course. The most extensive nursery outbreaks, however, have been caused by respiratory syncytial virus (Berkovich and Taranko, 1964; Hall et al, 1979). Simultaneous outbreaks of respiratory syncytial virus and parainfluenza virus type B have also been reported (Meissner et al, 1984).

Respiratory syncytial virus is the major cause of viral pneumonia and bronchiolitis in infants and children. In temperate climates, it causes large annual epidemics during the cold months. Nosocomial infections are frequent during these times, with illness in the hospital staff probably being a major factor in its spread from infant to infant. Several nursery outbreaks have been described. In one of these outbreaks, cultures were obtained prospectively so that a full picture of the viral pathogenicity and epidemiology could be drawn (Hall et al, 1979). Twenty-three of 66 infants who were hospitalized for 6 or more days, and therefore at risk of nosocomial infection were infected. Only one was asymptomatic. Six had pneumonia, eight presented with upper respiratory infection, four had predominantly apneic spells, and four demonstrated nonspecific signs. Pneumonia and apnea were seen almost exclusively in infants older than 3 weeks of age, and nonspecific signs were most commonly observed in those younger than that. Four (17%) infants died, two unexpectedly, during the course of their infections. Infants in isolettes did not seem to be protected against acquiring infection. Eighteen of the 53 nursery personnel were infected during the outbreak. Eighty-three percent of these patients were symptomatic. Respiratory syncytial virus infection in preterm infants frequently appears to be associated with a new onset of apnea (Bruhn et al, 1977).

Treatment and prevention of respiratory syncytial virus infection in infants have attracted considerable attention during the 1990s because of the clinical and economic impact of these infections (Groothuis, 1994; Hall, 1994; Kinney et al, 1995; Levin, 1994; Meissner, 1994). After approval by the Food and Drug Administration in 1986, ribavirin was recommended by the American Academy of Pediatrics in 1993 as a safe and effective treatment of RSV. More recently the same group has limited its recommendation for ribavirin use to infants at high risk for severe or complicated RSV infection, infants who are severely ill, infants who are immunosuppressed, and those with chronic lung or cardiac disease (American Academy of Pediatrics, 1993, 1996). Treatment consists of nebulization of ribavirin by a small-particle aerosol generator supplied by the manufacturer into an oxygen hood, tent, or mask from a solution containing 20 mg of ribavirin per milliliter of water. The aerosol has been administered on various schedules for 3 to 5 days (e.g., 12 to 20 hours per day). After the promulgation of these recommendations, considerable debate has ensued concerning efficacy, safety, and potential impact on health care workers of ribarivirn therapy (Wald and Dashefsky, 1994).

Prevention efforts have focused on passive and active immunization. The efficacy of monthly prophylactic administration of respiratory syncytial virus immune globulin (750 mg/kg or 150 mg/kg) in 249 infants with cardiac disease or bronchopulmonary dysplasia was examined in a multicenter trial by Groothuis and colleagues (1993). In the high-dose group, there were fewer lower respiratory tract infections, fewer hospitalizations, fewer hospital days, fewer days in the intensive care unit, and less use of ribavirin. In the low-dose group, there was a significant reduction only in the number of days in the intensive care unit. The American Academy of Pediatrics Committee on Infectious Diseases has recently outlined indications for use of anti-RSV immune globulin (American Academy of Pediatrics Committee on Infectious Diseases, 1997a). The safety and efficacy of monthly prophylaxis with intravenous RSV immune globulin have recently been reported (American Academy of Pediatrics Committee on Infectious Diseases, 1997b). Standard immune globulin has not been shown to be efficacious for prevention of RSV infection in high-risk infants (Meissner et al, 1993). The prospects for infant or maternal immunization are under active investigation (Hall, 1994; Englund, 1994).

Nosocomial spread of RSV and other respiratory viruses can be minimized by emphasis on handwashing between contacts with patients. Without additional special precautions, an attack rate of approximately 26% has been observed (Madge et al, 1992). Use of cohort nursing and gowns and gloves for all contacts with RSV-infected children can reduce the risk of nosocomial RSV infection to 9.5% (Madge et al, 1992).

Viruses Causing Diarrhea

The best studied of the viruses that cause diarrhea are the rotaviruses. This important group of viruses, with at least four serotypes, is responsible for a large proportion of significant and sometimes severe diarrhea in infants 6 to 24 months of age. (Cohen, 1991; Greenberg et al, 1994; Haffejee, 1991; Taylor and Echeverria, 1993). Nursery-acquired infections are frequent in parts of the world where they have been sought; surprisingly, they appear to be benign in most infected infants. In certain nurseries in Sydney, Australia, and in London, 30% to 50% of 5-day-old babies excreted the virus (Chrystie et al, 1978; Murphy et al, 1977). However, more than 90% of these infected infants were asymptomatic. The remainder had loose stools and vomiting, but this proportion was only slightly greater than that found among uninfected infants.

A study from France suggested that over the first 2 years of life, 20% of children have rotaviral disease, 10% have asymptomatic infection, 20% are virus carriers, and 50% are not infected (Champsaur et al, 1984). Rotavirus vaccines have considerable promise for stimulating protective local and systemic immunity (Bernstein, 1995). Molecular characterization of rotavirus has been useful for taxonomic categorization and for identification of children who are excreting rotavirus (Taylor and Echeverria, 1993; Wilde et al, 1991).

REFERENCES

A-Kader HH, Balistreri WF: Hepatitis C virus: Implications to pediatric practice. Pediatr Infect Dis J 12:853, 1993.

Abzug MJ, Levin MJ, Rotbart HA: Profile of enterovirus disease in the first two weeks of life. Pediatr Infect Dis J 12:820, 1993.

ACOG: Rubella and Pregnancy. ACOG Technical Bulletin No. 171, 1992a.

ACOG: Maternal and fetal medicine: Guidelines for hepatitis B virus screening and vaccination during pregnancy. ACOG Comm Opin 111:1992b.

Adler SP: Nosocomial transmission of cytomegalovirus. Pediatr Infect Dis 5:239, 1986.

Adler SP, Bagett J, Wilson M, et al: Molecular epidemiology of cytomegalovirus in a nursery: Lack of evidence for nosocomial transmission. J Pediatr 108:117, 1986.

Alford CA, Schaefer J, Blankenship WJ, et al: Subclinical central nervous system disease of neonates: A prospective study of infants born with increased levels of IgM. J Pediatr 75:1169, 1969.

Alpert G, Plotkin SA: A practical guide to the diagnosis of congenital infections in the newborn infant. Pediatr Clin North Am 33:465, 1986.

American Academy of Pediatrics Committee on Infectious Diseases: Use of ribavirin in the treatment of respiratory syncytial virus infection. Pediatrics 92:501, 1993.

American Academy of Pediatrics Committee on Infectious Diseases: Reassessment of the indications for ribavirin therapy in respiratory syncytial virus infections. Pediatrics 97:137, 1997a.

American Academy of Pediatrics Committee on Infectious Diseases: Respiratory syncytial virus immune globulin intravenous: Indications for use. Pediatrics 99:645, 1997b.

American Academy of Pediatrics: Varicella zoster infections. *In* Peter G (Ed): 1997 Red Book: Report of the Committee on Infectious Diseases, 24th ed. Elk Grove Village, IL: American Academy of Pediatrics, 1997a.

American Academy of Pediatrics: Hepatitis B. *In* Peter G (Ed): 1997 Red Book: Report of the Committee on Infectious Diseases, 24th ed. Elk Grove Village, IL: American Academy of Pediatrics, 1997b.

American Academy of Pediatrics: Hepatitis C. *In* Peter G (Ed): 1997 Red Book: Report of the Committee on Infectious Diseases, 24th ed. Elk Grove Village, IL: American Academy of Pediatrics, 1997c.

Anderson MJ, Pattison JR: The human parvovirus: A brief review. Arch Virol 82:137, 1984.

Andersson B, Svenningsen NW, Nordenfelt E: Screening for viral infections in infants with poor intrauterine growth. Acta Paediatr Scand 70:673, 1981.

Arvin AM: Relationships between maternal immunity to herpes simplex virus and the risk of neonatal herpesvirus infection. Rev Infect Dis 13:953, 1991.

Arvin AM, Prober CG: Analysis of the epidemiology and pathogenesis of herpes simplex virus (HSV) infections in the pregnant women and infants using the HSV-2 glycoprotein G antibody assay. Infect Agents Dis 2:375, 1993.

Bai PVA, John TJ: Congenital skin ulcers following varicella in late pregnancy. J Pediatr 94:65, 1979.

Balducci J, Rodis JF, Rosengren S, et al: Pregnancy outcome following first-trimester varicella infection. Obstet Gynecol 79:5, 1992.

Bale JF, Murph JR: Congenital infections and the nervous system. Pediatr Neurol 39:669, 1992.

Balistreri WF: Viral hepatitis. Pediatr Clin North Am 35:637, 1988.

Bates T: Poliomyelitis in pregnancy, fetus and newborn. Am J Dis Child 90:189, 1955.

Beasley RP, Stevens CE, Shiao I-S, Meng H-C: Evidence against breast-feeding as a mechanism for vertical transmission of hepatitis B. Lancet 2:740, 1975.

Beasley RP, Lin C-C, Hwang L-Y, Chien C-S: Hepatocellular carcinoma and hepatitis B virus. Lancet 2:1129, 1981.

Berenberg W, Nankervis G: Long-term follow-up of cytomegalic inclusion disease of infancy. Pediatrics 46:403, 1970.

Berkovich S, Taranko L: Acute respiratory illness in the premature nursery associated with respiratory syncytial virus infections. Pediatrics 34:753, 1964.

Bernstein D, Glass R, Rodgers G, et al: Evaluation of Rhesus rotavirus vaccines in U.S. children. JAMA 273:1191, 1995.

Berry PJ, Gray ES, Porter HJ, Burton PA: Parvovirus infection of the human fetus and newborn. Semin Diagn Pathol 9:4, 1992.

Boley TJ, Popek EJ: Parvovirus infection in pregnancy. Semin Perinatol 17:410, 1993.

Boppana SB, Pass RF, Britt WJ, et al: Symptomatic congenital cytomegalovirus infection: Neonatal morbidity and mortality. Pediatr Infect Dis 11:93, 1992.

Bowden RA, Sayers M, Flournoy N, et al: Cytomegalovirus immune globulin and seronegative blood products to prevent primary cytomegalovirus infection after marrow transplantation. N Engl J Med 314:1006, 1986.

Brough AJ, Jones D, Page RH, Mizukami I: Dermal erythropoiesis in neonatal infants. Pediatrics 40:627, 1967.

Brown KE, Green SW, Antunez de Mayolo J, et al: Congenital anaemia after transplacental B19 parvovirus infection. Lancet 343:895, 1994.

Bruhn FW, Mokrohisky ST, McIntosh K: Apnea associated with respiratory syncytial virus infection in young infants. J Pediatr 90:382, 1977.

Brunell PA: Placental transfer of varicella zoster antibody. Pediatrics 38:1034, 1966.

Brunell PA: Varicella in pregnancy, the fetus, and the newborn: Problems in management. J Infect Dis 166:42, 1992.

Brunell PA, Ross A, Miller LH, et al: Prevention of varicella by zoster immune globulin. N Engl J Med 280:1191, 1969.

Carrington D, Gilmore DH, Whittle MJ, et al: Maternal serum alpha-fetoprotein: A marker of fetal aplastic crisis during intrauterine human parvovirus infection. Lancet 1:433, 1987.

Centers for Disease Control and Prevention: Varicella-zoster immune globulin distribution—United States and other countries, 1981–1983. MMWR Morb Mortal Wkly Rep 33:81, 1984.

Centers for Disease Control and Prevention: Rubella and congenital rubella—United States, 1984–1986. MMWR Morb Mortal Wkly Rep 36:664, 1987.

Centers for Disease Control and Prevention: Prevention of perinatal transmission of hepatitis B virus. MMWR Morb Mortal Wkly Rep 37:341, 1988.

Centers for Disease Control and Prevention: Rubella vaccination during pregnancy—United States, 1971–1988. MMWR Morb Mortal Wkly Rep 38:289, 1989a.

Centers for Disease Control and Prevention: Summary of notifiable diseases, United States. MMWR Morb Mortal Wkly Rep 38:8, 1989b.

Centers for Disease Control and Prevention: Increase in rubella and congenital rubella syndrome: United States 1988–1990. MMWR Morb Mortal Wkly Rep 40:93, 1991a.

Centers for Disease Control and Prevention: Hepatitis B virus: A comprehensive strategy for eliminating transmission in the United States through universal childhood vaccination. Recommendations of the Immunization Practices Advisory Committee (ACIP). MMWR Morb Mortal Wkly Rep 40:1, 1991b.

Centers for Disease Control and Prevention: Monthly Immunization Table. MMWR Morb Mortal Wkly Rep 44:99, 1995.

Champsaur H, Henry-Amar M, Goldszmidt D, et al: Rotavirus carriage, asymptomatic infection, and disease in the first two years of life. II. Serologic response. J Infect Dis 149:675, 1984.

Cherry JD: Enterovirus. *In* Remington JS, Klein JO (Eds): Infectious Diseases of the Fetus and Newborn Infant. Philadelphia, WB Saunders, 1990, pp 325–366.

Chou S, Merigan TC: Rapid detection and quantitation of human cytomegalovirus in urine through DNA hybridization. N Engl J Med 308:921, 1983.

Chrystie IL, Totterdell BM, Banatvala JE: Asymptomatic endemic rotavirus infections in the newborn. Lancet 1:1176, 1978.

Claman HN, Savatte V, Githens JH, Hathaway WE: Histiocytic reaction in dysgammaglobulinemia and congenital rubella. Pediatrics 46:89, 1970.

Cohen MB: Etiology and mechanisms of acute infectious diarrhea in infants in the United States. J Pediatr 118:34, 1991.

Cooper LZ, Green RH, et al: Neonatal thrombocytopenic purpura and other manifestations of rubella contracted in utero. Am J Dis Child 110:416, 1965.

Cooper LZ, Ziring PR, Ockerse AR, et al: Rubella: Clinical manifestation and management. Am J Dis Child 118:18, 1969.

Cramblett HG, Haynes RE, Azimi PH, et al: Nosocomial infection with echovirus type II in handicapped and premature infants. Pediatrics 51:603, 1973.

Cruz AC, Frentzen BH, Behnke M: Hepatitis B: A case for prenatal screening of all patients. Am J Obstet Gynecol 156:1180, 1987.

Cuthbertson G, Weiner CP, Giller RH, Grose C: Prenatal diagnosis of second-trimester congenital varicella syndrome by virus-specific immunoglobulin M J Pediatr 111:592, 1987.

Davis LE, Tweed GV, Stewart JA, et al: Cytomegalovirus mononucleosis in a first trimester pregnant female with transmission to the fetus. Pediatrics 48:200, 1971.

Delaplane D, Yogev R, Crussi F, et al: Fetal hepatitis B in early infancy: The importance of identifying HB₅Ag-positive pregnant women and providing immunoprophylaxis to their newborns. Pediatrics 72:176, 1983.

Demmler GJ: Summary of a workshop on surveillance for congenital cytomegalovirus disease. Rev Infect Dis 13:315, 1991.

Desmond MM, Fisher ES, Vorderman AL, et al: The longitudinal course of congenital rubella encephalitis in nonretarded children. J Pediatr 93:584, 1978.

Dudgeon JA: Congenital rubella. J Pediatr 87:1078, 1975.

Dwyer DE, Cunningham AL: Herpes simplex virus infection in pregnancy. Baillieres Clin Obstet Gynaecol 7:75, 1993.

Emanuel I, Kenny GE: Cytomegalic inclusion disease of infancy. Pediatrics 38:957, 1966.

Enders G: Varicella-Zoster virus infection in pregnancy. Prog Med Virol 29:166, 1984.

Enders G, Miller E, Cradock-Watson J, et al: Consequences of varicella and herpes zoster in pregnancy: Prospective study of 1739 cases. Lancet 343:1548, 1994.

Englund JA: Passive protection against respiratory syncytial virus disease in infants: The role of maternal antibody. Pediatr Infect Dis J 13:449, 1994.

Farmer K, Gunn T, Woodfield DG: A combination of hepatitis B vaccine and immunoglobulin does not protect all infants born to hepatitis B e antigen positive mothers. N Z Med J 100:412, 1987.

Farmer K, MacArthur BA, Clay MM: A follow-up study of 15 cases of neonatal meningoencephalitis due to coxsackie virus B5. J Pediatr 87:568, 1975.

Feldman S: Varicella zoster infections of the fetus, neonate, and immuno-compromised child. Curr Prob Pediatr 16:99, 1986.

Florman AL, Gershon AA, Blackett PR, Nahmias AJ: Intrauterine infection with herpes simplex virus: Resultant congenital malformations. JAMA 225:129, 1973.

Fowler KB, Stagno S, Pass RF, et al: The outcome of congenital cytomegalovirus infection in relation to maternal antibody status. N Engl J Med 326:663, 1992.

Freij BJ, Sever JL: Herpesvirus infections in pregnancy: Risks to embryo, fetus, and neonate. Clin Perinatol 15:203, 1988.

Gerety RJ, Schweitzer IL: Viral hepatitis type B during pregnancy, the neonatal period, and infancy. J Pediatr 90:368, 1977.

Gershon AA: Varicella in mother and infant: Problems old and new. *In* Krugman S, Gershon AA (Eds): Infections of the Fetus and the Newborn Infant. New York, Alan R Liss, 1975, pp 79–95.

Gilbert GL, Hayes K, Hudson IL, et al: Prevention of transfusion-acquired cytomegalovirus infection in infants by blood filtration to remove leucocytes. Lancet i:1228, 1989.

Greenberg HB, Clark HF, Offit PA: Rotavirus pathology and pathophysiology. Curr Topics Microbiol Immunol 185:255, 1994.

Gregg NM: Congenital cataract following German measles in the mother. Trans Ophthal Soc Austr 3:35, 1941.

Griffiths PD: Current management of cytomegalovirus disease. J Med Virol 1:106, 1993.

Groothuis JR: Role of antibody and use of respiratory syncytial virus (RSV) immune globulin to prevent severe RSV disease in high-risk children. J Pediatr 124:28, 1994.

Groothuis JR, Simoes EA, Levin MJ: Prophylactic administration of respiratory syncytial virus immune globulin to high-risk infants and young children. The Respiratory Syncytial Virus Immune Globulin Study Group. N Engl J Med 329:1524, 1993.

Grose C, Meehan T, Weiner CP: Perinatal diagnosis of congenital cytomegalovirus infection by virus isolation after amniocentesis. Pediatr Infect Dis J 11:605, 1992.

Gross JB, Persing DH: Hepatitis C: Advances in diagnosis. Mayo Clin Proc 70:296, 1995.

Grossman JH, Wallen UC, Sever JL: Management of genital herpes simplex virus infection during pregnancy. Obstet Gynecol 58:1, 1981.

Haffejee LE: Neonatal rotavirus infections. Rev Infect Dis 13:957, 1991.

Hall CB: Prospects for a respiratory syncytial virus vaccine. Science 265:1393, 1994.

Hall CB, Kopelman AE, Douglas RG Jr, et al: Neonatal respiratory syncytial virus infection. N Engl J Med 300:393, 1979.

Hanshaw JB, Scheiner AP, Moxley AW, et al: School failure and deafness after "silent" congenital cytomegalovirus infection. N Engl J Med 295:468, 1976.

Hardy JB, Monif GRG, Sever JL: Studies in congenital rubella. Baltimore 1964–65, II. Clin Virol Bull Hopkins Hosp 118:97, 1966.

Hayden GF, Herrmann KL, Buimovici-Klein E, et al: Subclinical congenital rubella infection associated with maternal rubella vaccination in early pregnancy. J Pediatr 96:869, 1980.

Hayes K, Danks DM, Gibas H, Jack I: Cytomegalovirus in human milk. N Engl J Med 287:177, 1972.

Hirota K, Muraguchi K, Watabe N, et al: Prospective study on maternal, intrauterine, and perinatal infections with cytomegalovirus in Japan during 1976–1990. J Med Virol 37:303, 1992.

Hirsch MS, Schooley RT, Cosimi AB, et al: Effects of interferon-α on cytomegalovirus reactivation syndromes in renal-transplant recipients. N Engl J Med 308:1489, 1983.

Hodgson J, Morgan-Capner P: Evaluation of a commercial antibody capture enzyme immunoassay for the detection of rubella specific IgM. J Clin Pathol 37:573, 1984.

Hsu H-M, Chen D-S, Chuang C-H, et al: Efficacy of a mass hepatitis B vaccination program in Taiwan. JAMA 260:2231, 1988.

Humphrey W, Magoon M, O'Shaughnessy R: Severe nonimmune hydrops secondary to parvovirus B-19 infection: Spontaneous reversal in utero and survival of a term infant. Obstet Gynecol 78:900, 1991.

Javett SN, Heymann S, Mundel B, et al: Myocarditis in the newborn infant. J Pediatr 48:1, 1956.

Jenkins M, Kohl S: New aspects of neonatal herpes. Infect Dis Clin North Am 6:57, 1992.

Kaplan KM, Cochi SL, Edmonds LD, et al: A profile of mothers giving birth to infants with congenital rubella syndrome. Am J Dis Child 144:118, 1990.

Kibrick S, Benirschke K: Severe generalized disease (encephalohepatomy-ocarditis) occurring in the newborn period due to infection with coxsackie virus, Group B. Pediatrics 22:857, 1958.

King-Lewis PA, Gardner SD: Congenital cytomegalic inclusion disease following intrauterine transfusion. BMJ 2:603, 1969.

Kinney JS, Anderson LJ, Farrar J, et al: Risk of adverse outcomes of pregnancy following human parvovirus B19 infection. J Infect Dis 157:663, 1988.

Kinney JS, Kumar ML: Should we expand the TORCH complex? Clin Perinatol 15:727, 1988.

Kinney JS, Onorato IM, Stewart JA, et al: Cytomegaloviral infection and disease. J Infect Dis 151:772, 1985.

Kinney JS, Robertsen CM, Johnson KM, et al: Seasonal respiratory viral infections. Impact on infants with chronic lung disease following discharge from the neonatal intensive care unit. Arch Pediatr Adolesc Med 149:81, 1995.

Kohl S: Herpes simplex virus immunology: Problems, progress, and promises. J Infect Dis 152:435, 1985.

Kohl S: Role of antibody-dependent cellular cytotoxicity in neonatal infection with herpes simplex virus. Rev Infect Dis 13:950, 1991.

Krajden S, Middleton PJ: Enterovirus infections in the neonate. Clin Pediatr 22:88, 1983.

Krugman S: Hepatitis B virus and the neonate. Ann N Y Acad Sci 549:129, 1988.

Krugman S: Viral hepatitis: A, B, C, D, and E—Prevention. Pediatr Rev 13:245, 1992.

Kumar ML, Nankervis GA, Gold E: Inapparent congenital cytomegalovirus infection: A follow-up study. N Engl J Med 288:1370, 1973.

Laforet EG, Lynch CC: Multiple congenital defects following maternal varicella. N Engl J Med 236:534, 1947.

Lake AM, Lauer BA, Clark JC, et al: Enterovirus infection in neonates. J Pediatr 89:787, 1976.

Lepow ML, Veronelli JA, Hostetler DD, et al: A trial with live attenuated rubella vaccine. Am J Dis Child 115:639, 1968.

Levin MJ: Treatment and prevention options for respiratory syncytial virus infections. J Pediatr 124:22, 1994.

Lin H-H, Lee T-Y, Chen D-S, et al: Transplacental leakage of HBeAg-positive maternal blood as the most likely route in causing intrauterine infection with hepatitis B virus. J Pediatr 111:877, 1987.

Linnemann CC Jr, Buchman TG, Light IJ, et al: Transmission of herpes simplex type 1 in a newborn nursery: Identification of viral isolates by DNA "fingerprinting." Lancet 1:964, 1978.

Linnemann CC, Steichen J, Sherman WG, Schiff GM: Febrile illness in early infancy associated with ECHO virus infection. J Pediatr 84:49, 1974.

Luthardt TH, Siebert H, Losel I, et al: Cytomegalievirus-infektionen bei Kindern mit Blutaustauschtransfusion in Neugeborenenalter. Klin Wochenschr 49:81, 1971.

Lynch-Salamon DI, Combs CA: Hepatitis C in obstetrics and gynecology. Obstet Gynecol 79:621, 1992.

Madge P, Paton JY, McColl JH, Mackie PL: Prospective controlled study of four infection-control procedures to prevent nosocomial infection with respiratory syncytial virus. Lancet 340:1079, 1992.

Maupas P, Chiron JP, Barin F, et al: Efficacy of hepatitis B vaccine in prevention of early HB$_s$Ag carrier state in children: Controlled trial in an endemic area (Senegal). Lancet 1:289, 1981.

McCracken GH, Hardy JB, Chen TC, et al: Serum immunoglobulin levels in newborn infants. II. Survey of cord and follow up sera from 123 infants with congenital rubella. J Pediatr 74:383, 1969a.

McCracken GH, Shinefield HR, Cobb K, et al: Congenital cytomegalic inclusion disease. Am J Dis Child 117:522, 1969b.

Meissner HC: Economic impact of viral respiratory disease in children. J Pediatr 124:17, 1994.

Meissner HC, Murray SA, Kiernan MA, et al: A simultaneous outbreak of respiratory syncytial virus and parainfluenza virus type 3 in a newborn nursery. J Pediatr 104:680, 1984.

Meissner HC, Fulton DR, Groothuis JR, et al: Controlled trial to evaluate protection of high-risk infants against respiratory syncytial virus disease by using standard intravenous immune globulin. Antimicrob Agents Chemo 37:1655, 1993.

Meyers JD: Congenital varicella in term infants: Risk reconsidered. J Infect Dis 129:215, 1974.

Miller E, Cradock-Watson JE, Pollock TM: Consequences of confirmed maternal rubella at successive stages of pregnancy. Lancet ii:781, 1982.

Modlin JF: Fatal echovirus II disease in premature neonates. Pediatrics 66:775, 1980.

Morey AL, Keeling JW, Porter HJ, Fleming KA: Clinical and histopathological features of parvovirus B19 infection in the human fetus. Br J Obstet Gynecol 99:566, 1992.

Mortimer PP, Cohen BJ, Buckley MM, et al: Human parvovirus and the fetus. Lancet 2:1012, 1985.

Mulligan MJ, Stiehm ER: Neonatal hepatitis B infection: Clinical and immunologic considerations. J Perinatol 14:2, 1994.

Murphy AM, Albrey MB, Crewe EB: Rotavirus infections in neonates. Lancet 2:1149, 1977.

Nagington J, Wreghitt TC, Gandy G, et al: Fatal echovirus II infections in outbreak in special-care baby unit. Lancet 2:725, 1978.

Nahmias AJ, Josey WE, Naib ZM, et al: Perinatal risk associated with maternal genital herpes simplex virus infection. Am J Obstet Gynecol 110:825, 1971.

Nahmias AJ, Roizman B: Infection with herpes-simplex viruses 1 and 2. N Engl J Med 289:667, 719, 781, 1973.

Ogasawara S, Kage M, Kosai KI, et al: Hepatitis C virus RNA in saliva and breastmilk of hepatitis C carrier mothers. Lancet 341:561, 1993.

Ohto H, Terazawa S, Sasaki N, et al: Transmission of hepatitis C virus from mothers to infants. N Engl J Med 330:744, 1994.

Okada K, Kamiyama I, Inomata M, et al. e Antigen and anti-e in the serum of asymptomatic carrier mothers as indicators of positive and negative transmission of hepatitis B virus to their infants. N Engl J Med 294:749, 1979.

Onorato IM, Morens DM, Martone WJ, Stansfield SK: Epidemiology of cytomegaloviral infections: Recommendations for prevention and control. Rev Infect Dis 7:479, 1985.

Overall JC Jr: Herpes simplex virus infection of the fetus and newborn. Pediatr Ann 23:131, 1994.

Overall JC, Glasgow LA: Virus infections of the fetus and newborn infant. J Pediatr 77:315, 1970.

Paryani SG, Arvin AM: Intrauterine infection with varicella zoster virus after maternal varicella. N Engl J Med 314:1542, 1986.

Pass RF, Stagno S, Myers GJ, Alford CA: Outcome of symptomatic congenital cytomegalovirus infection: Results of long-term longitudinal follow-up. Pediatrics 66:758, 1980.

Peckham C: Cytomegalovirus infection: Congenital and neonatal disease. Scand J Infect 78:82, 1991.

Phelan P, Campbell P: Pulmonary complications of rubella embryopathy. J Pediatr 75:202, 1969.

Prevent Study Group: Reduction of respiratory syncytial virus hospitalization among premature infants and infants with bronchopulmonary dysplasia using respiratory syncytial virus immune globulin prophylaxis. Pediatrics 99:93, 1997.

Primhak RA, Simpson RMD: Screening small for gestational age babies for congenital infection. Clin Pediatr 21:417, 1982.

Prober CG, Corey L, Brown ZA, et al: The management of pregnancies complicated by genital infections with herpes simplex virus. Clin Infect Dis 15:1031, 1992.

Prober CG, Hensleigh PA, Boucher FD, et al: Use of routine viral cultures at delivery to identify neonates exposed to herpes simplex virus. N Engl J Med 318:887, 1988.

Prober CG, Sullender WM, Yasukawa IL, et al: Low risk of herpes simplex virus infections in neonates exposed to the virus at the time of vaginal delivery to mothers with recurrent genital herpes simplex virus infections. N Engl J Med 316:240, 1987.

Reynolds DW, Stagno S, Hosty TS, et al: Maternal cytomegalovirus excretion and perinatal infection. N Engl J Med 289:1, 1973.

Reynolds DW, Stagno S, Stubbs KG, et al: Inapparent congenital cytomegalovirus infection with elevated cord IgM levels: Causal relation with auditory and mental deficiency. N Engl J Med 290:291, 1974.

Robino G, Perlman A, Togo Y, et al: Fatal neonatal infection due to coxsackie B2 virus. J Pediatr 61:911, 1962.

Rudolph AJ, Singleton EB, et al: Osseous manifestations of congenital rubella syndrome. Am J Dis Child 110:428, 1965.

Sawyer MH, Holland D, Aintablian N, et al: Diagnosis of enteroviral central nervous system infection by polymerase chain reaction during a large community outbreak. Pediatr Infect Dis J 13:177, 1994.

Schrier RD, Nelson JA, Oldstone MBA: Detection of human cytomegalovirus in peripheral blood lymphocytes in a natural infection. Science 230:1048, 1985.

Sells CJ, Carpenter RL, Ray GC: Sequelae of central nervous system enterovirus infections. N Engl J Med 293:1, 1975.

Shapiro CN: Epidemiology of hepatitis B. Pediatr Infect Dis J 12:433, 1993.

Shattuck KE, Chonmaitree T: The changing spectrum of neonatal meningitis over a fifteen-year period. Clin Pediatr 31:130, 1992.

Sheikh AU, Ernest JM, O'Shea M: Long-term outcome in fetal hydrops from parvovirus B19 infection. Am J Obstet Gynecol 167:337, 1992.

Shepp DH, Dandliker PS, de Miranda P, et al: Activity of 9-[2-hydroxy-1-(hydroxymethyl)ethoxymethyl]guanine in the treatment of cytomegalovirus pneumonia. Ann Intern Med 103:368, 1985.

Siegel M, Fuerst HT: Low birth weight and maternal virus diseases. JAMA 197:680, 1966.

Siegel M: Congenital malformations following chicken pox, measles, mumps, and hepatitis: Results of a cohort study. JAMA 276:1521, 1973.

Simms J, Duff P: Viral hepatitis in pregnancy. Semin Perinatol 17:384, 1993.

Skoldenberg B, Alestig K, Burman L, et al: Acyclovir versus vidarabine in herpes simplex encephalitis. Lancet 2:707, 1984.

Soothill JE, Hayes K, Dudgeon JA: The immunoglobulins in congenital rubella. Lancet 1:1385, 1966.

South MA, Thompkins WAF, Morris CR, et al: Congenital malformation of the central nervous system associated with genital type (type 2) herpes virus. J Pediatr 75:13, 1969.

Spector SA: Transmission of cytomegalovirus among infants in hospital documented by restriction-endonuclease analyses. Lancet 2:378, 1983.

Srabstein JC, Morris N, Larke RPB, et al: Is there a congenital varicella syndrome? J Pediatr 84:239, 1974.

Stagno S, Brasfield DM, Brown MB, et al: Infant pneumonitis associated with cytomegalovirus, Clamydia, Pneumocystis and Ureaplasma: A prospective study. Pediatrics 68:322, 1981.

Stagno S, Cloud GA: Working parents: The impact of day care and breast feeding on cytomegalovirus infections in offspring. Proc Natl Acad Sci U S A 91:2384, 1994.

Stagno S, Pass RF, Dworsky ME, et al: Congenital cytomegalovirus infection: The relative importance of primary and recurrent maternal infection. N Engl J Med 306:945, 1982.

Stagno S, Reynolds DW, Huang ES, et al: Congenital cytomegalovirus infection: Occurrence in an immune population. N Engl J Med 296:1254, 1977.

Stagno S, Whitley RJ: Herpesvirus infections of pregnancy. Part I: Cytomegalovirus and Epstein-Barr virus infections. N Engl J Med 313:1270, 1985.

Stagno S, Whitley RJ: Herpes-virus infections of pregnancy: II. Herpes simplex virus and varicella-zoster virus infections. N Engl J Med 313:1327, 1985.

Stamos JK, Rowley AH: Timely diagnosis of congenital infections. Pediatr Clin North Am 41:1017, 1994.

Starr JG, Bart RD Jr, Gold E: Inapparent congenital cytomegalovirus infection: Clinical and epidemiological characteristics in early infancy. N Engl J Med 282:1075, 1970.

Stevens CE: Inutero and perinatal transmission of hepatitis viruses. Pediatr Ann 23:152, 1994.

Summers PR, Biswas MK, Pastorek JG, et al: The pregnant hepatitis B carrier: Evidence favoring comprehensive antepartum screening. Obstet Gynecol 69:701, 1987.

Swanink CM, Veenstra L, Poort YA, et al: Coxsackievirus B1-based antibody-capture enzyme-linked immunosorbent assay for detection of immunoglobulin G (IgG), IgM, and IgA with broad specificity for enteroviruses. J Clin Microbiol 31:3240, 1993.

Taylor DN, Echeverria P: Diarrhoeal disease: Current concepts and future challenges. Molecular biological approaches to the epidemiology of diarrhoeal diseases in developing countries. Trans R Soc Trop Med Hyg 87:3, 1993.

Tingle AJ, Chantler JK, Pot KH, et al: Postpartum rubella immunization: Association with development of prolonged arthritis, neurologic sequelae, and chronic rubella viremia. J Infect Dis 152:606, 1985.

Toltzis P: Current issues in neonatal herpes simplex virus infection. Clin Perinatol 18:193, 1991.

Ueda K, Nishida Y, Oshina K, Shepard TH: Congenital rubella syndrome: Correlation of gestational age at time of maternal rubella with type of defect. J Pediatr 94:763, 1979.

Verder H, Dickmeiss E, Haahr S, et al: Late-onset rubella syndrome: Coexistence of immune complex disease and defective cytotoxic effector cell function. Clin Exp Immunol 63:367, 1986.

Visintine AM, Nahmias AJ, Josey WE: Genital herpes. Perinatal Care 2:32, 1978.

Wald ER, Dashefsky B: Ribavirin. Red Book Committee recommendations questioned. Pediatrics 93:672, 1994.

Weil ML, Itabashi H, Cremer NE, et al: Chronic progressive panencephalitis due to rubella virus simulating subacute sclerosing panencephalitis. N Engl J Med 292:994, 1975.

Weller TH: The cytomegaloviruses: Ubiquitous agents with protean clinical manifestations. Part I. N Engl J Med 285:203, 267, 1971.

Weller TH: The cytomegalovirus: Ubiquitous agents with protean clinical manifestations. Part II. N Engl J Med 266:1233, 1962.

Weller TH, Hanshaw JB: Virologic and clinical observations on cytomegalic inclusion disease. N Engl J Med 266:1233, 1962.

Weller TH, Macauley JC, Craig JM, et al: Isolation of intranuclear inclusion-producing agents from infants with illnesses resembling cytomegalic inclusion disease. Proc Soc Exp Biol Med 94:4, 1957.

Whitley RJ: Herpes simplex virus infections. *In* Remington JA, Klein JO (Eds): Infectious Diseases of the Fetus and Newborn Infant. Philadelphia, WB Saunders, 1990, pp 282–305.

Whitley RJ: Herpes simplex virus infections of women and their offspring: Implications for a developed society. Proc Natl Acad Sci U S A 91:2441, 1994a.

Whitley RJ: Neonatal herpes simplex virus infections: Is there a role for immunoglobulin in disease prevention and therapy? Pediatr Infect Dis J 13:432, 1994b.

Whitley RJ: Neonatal herpes simplex virus infections. J Med Virol 1:13, 1993.

Whitley RJ, Hutto C: Neonatal herpes simplex virus infections. Pediatr Rev 7:119, 1985.

Whitley RJ, Nahmias AJ, Soong S-J, et al: Vidarabine therapy of neonatal herpes simplex virus infections. Pediatrics 66:495, 1980a.

Whitley RJ, Nahmias AJ, Visintine AM, et al: The natural history of herpes simplex virus infection of mother and newborn. Pediatrics 66:489, 1980b.

Wilde J, Yolken R, Willoughby R, Eiden J: Improved detection of rotavirus shedding by polymerase chain reaction. Lancet 337:323, 1991.

Wilfert CM, Thompson RJ, Sunder TR, et al: Longitudinal assessment of children with enteroviral meningitis during the first three months of life. Pediatrics 67:811, 1981.

Yaegashi N, Okamura K, Yajima A, et al: The frequency of human parvovirus B19 infection in nonimmune hydrops fetalis. J Perinatol Med 22:159, 1994.

Yeager AS, Arvin AM, Urbani LJ, Kemp JA: The relationship of antibody to outcome in neonatal herpes simplex infections. Infect Immunol 29:532, 1980.

Yeager AS, Ashley RL, Corey L: Transmission of herpes simplex virus from father to neonate. J Pediatr 103:905, 1983a.

Yeager AS, Grumet FC, Hafleigh EB, et al: Prevention of transfusion-acquired cytomegalovirus infections in newborn infants. J Pediatr 98:281, 1981.

Yeager AS, Jacobs H, Clark J: Nursery-acquired cytomegalovirus infection in two premature infants. J Pediatr 81:332, 1972.

Yeager AS, Palumbo P, Malachowski B, et al: Sequelae of maternally derived cytomegalovirus infections in premature infants. J Pediatr 102:918, 1983b.

CHAPTER 43

Bacterial Infections of the Newborn

F. Sessions Cole[*]

Changes during the fetal and neonatal period affect the cause of bacterial infections, an infant's response to infection, the agents used for treatment, and the pharmacologic properties of antimicrobial agents. For example, absorption, distribution, metabolism, and excretion of drugs depend in part on the maturity and age of the infant. The administration of a particular drug is determined by the gestational and chronologic age of the infant and cannot be extrapolated from studies of normal adults. Failure to take these physiologic and metabolic factors into account when treating bacterial infection in infants may result in ineffective or toxic drug therapy.

USE OF ANTIBIOTICS IN NEWBORNS

The selection of antibiotic therapy in newborn infants depends on (1) general experience with infections in the nursery, (2) the susceptibility of commonly encountered bacterial pathogens, (3) the physician's familiarity with antibiotic pharmacokinetics in newborn infants, and (4) the physician's knowledge of maternal infections, course of labor, and antibiotic treatment administered to the mother. Pediatricians must know which are the most common organisms that cause disease in the nurseries and the current antimicrobial susceptibilities of these organisms. Moreover, it has been shown in many instances that the judicious use of antibiotics in nurseries limits the emergence and spread of resistant bacteria. Vertical transmission of organisms from the mother to the fetus must also be considered in the selection of antibiotics.

Generally, as few antibiotics as possible should be used to treat individual infections and, whenever possible, single-drug therapy should be used. Frequently, however, combining two drugs is good medical practice. This is true at the initiation of treatment before culture and sensitivity data are available to cover a wide range of likely bacterial species that cause newborn sepsis, or, sometimes, after the organism has been identified to incorporate antibiotic synergy in widespread and severe infections by bacteria that are difficult to eliminate with a single drug.

Bacterial sepsis is frequently suspected in newborn infants because of nonspecific symptoms and signs. Usually, cultures are obtained and antibiotics are administered only to reveal that, after 48 to 72 hours, the cultures are sterile. Not infrequently, the child improves during this interval. At this time, the pediatrician must use clinical judgment. If the cultures were obtained from the proper sites in the proper way and if the particular microbiology laboratory used is reliable, then it is usually wise to discontinue antibiotics and re-evaluate the child at frequent intervals

thereafter. However, if an infant's mother was given antibiotics and the infant has persuasive evidence of infection, then it is prudent to continue the antibiotics for at least 7 days. Sometimes, culture results are difficult to interpret (e.g., *Staphylococcus epidermidis* from a blood culture; gram-negative organisms from a tracheal aspirate in a long-term occupant of the nursery). In these instances, a knowledge of the pathogenicity of these organisms in newborn infants should be combined with information on the clinical appearance of the infant and other laboratory data so that a plan that minimizes the use of antibiotics can be developed.

Although antibiotics are commonly used to prevent infection of newborn infants, the efficacy of this approach is limited to a few well-defined circumstances (Rhodes and Henry, 1992). A good example of one such circumstance is the use of topical 2.5% solution of povidone-iodine to prevent ophthalmia neonatorum (Isenberg et al, 1995). However, when antibiotics are used as "broad coverage" against many potential pathogens for extended intervals, they are rarely effective. This type of chemoprophylaxis encourages the emergence of resistant strains among previously susceptible bacteria and causes the alteration of the normal bacterial flora of the gastrointestinal and respiratory tracts.

Table 43–1 is a guide for treating neonatal bacterial diseases. Modification of these schedules is necessary to take into account the gestational and chronologic age of the infant, the specific infectious agent that is suspected or documented, the tissue site being treated, the status of excretory (hepatic or renal) function of the infant, and the cardiopulmonary stability of the infant. Because of economic pressure from managed care organizations to reduce health-care costs, several strategies for identifying infants at risk for infection who require antibiotic therapy and for reducing duration of antibiotic therapy for high-risk infants have been proposed (Philip, 1981; Pourcyrous et al, 1993; Rodwell et al, 1988; Squire et al, 1982). Recently, Escobar and colleagues (1994) reviewed the charts of 214 infants who weighed more than 2500 g, who did not receive systemic antibiotics, and who did not become critically ill within 24 hours of admission to a special care nursery. Among these infants, eight had positive blood cultures for group B streptococcus, one had both positive blood and cerebrospinal fluid cultures for group B streptococcus, and two had positive viral cultures. Despite the lack of gram-negative isolates (atypical for most intensive care nurseries), the retrospective nature of the study, the lack of deaths resulting from systemic bacterial infection, and the small number of infants reviewed, these authors suggested that discontinuation of antibiotics within 24 hours was safe and could reduce hospital use. Larger-scale studies investigating the safety and efficacy of this sort of approach are in progress.

---

[*]This chapter includes some contributions from the previous authors, Drs. Alexander Schaffer, George H. McCracken, Jr., Jorge B. Howard, and Kenneth McIntosh.

TABLE 43–1

Dosage Recommendations for Antibiotics Commonly Used in Newborn Infants*

Drug	Route	Infants < 7 Days of Age			Infants > 7 Days of Age†
		< 30 Weeks' Gestation†	30–37 Weeks' Gestation†	> 37 Weeks' Gestation†	
Amikacin‡	IV, IM	7.5 q 24 hr	10.0 q 24 hr	7.5 q 12 hr	7.5–10.0 q 8–q 12 hr
Ampicillin§	IV, IM	50 q 12 hr	75 q 12 hr	100 q 12 hr	100 q 8 hr
Cefotaxime	IV, IM	50 q 12 hr	50 q 12 hr	50 q 8 hr	50 q 6 hr
Ceftazidime	IV, IM	30 q 12 hr	50 q 12 hr	50 q 8 hr	50 q 6 hr
Ceftriaxone	IV, IM	50 q 24 hr	75 q 24 hr	75 q 12 hr	75 q 12 hr
Chloramphenicol‡	IV	2.5 q 6 hr	5.0 q 6 hr	5.0 q 6 hr	12.5 q 6 hr
Clindamycin‡	IV	5.0 q 8 hr	7.5 q 8 hr	10 mg q 6 hr	10 mg q 6 hr
Erythromycin	IV	10 q 12 hr	15 q 12 hr	20 q 12 hr	20 q 12 hr
Gentamicin‡	IV, IM	2.5 q 24 hr	3.0 q 24 hr	2.5 q 12 hr	2.5 q 8–q 12 hr
Methicillin	IV	25 q 12 hr	35 q 12 hr	50 q 8 hr	50 q 6–q 8 hr
Nafcillin	IV	25 q 12 hr	35 q 12 hr	50 q 8 hr	50 q 6–q 8 hr
Oxacillin	IV	25 q 12 hr	35 q 12 hr	50 q 8 hr	50 q 6–18 hr
Penicillin G§	IV, IM	25,000 IU IV q 12 hr	50,000 IU IV q 12 hr	50,000 IU IV q 8 hr	50,000 IU IV q am
Piperacillin	IV, IM	50 q 12 hr	75 q 12 hr	100 q 8 hr	100 q 6 hr
Tobramycin‡	IV	2.5 q 24 hr	3.0 q 24 hr	2.5 q 12 hr	2.5 q 8–q 12 hr
Vancomycin‡	IV	18 q 24 hr	15 q 12 hr	10 q 8 hr	10 q 6 hr

°All dosages given represent approximate schedule for initiation of therapy. These dosages should be individualized for specific clinical situations.
†mg/kg per dose.
‡Dosage should be individually adjusted for each infant by monitoring serum drug concentrations.
§For meningitis, double recommended dosage.

PATHOGENESIS OF NEONATAL INFECTIONS

Throughout gestation, the infant is usually protected from bacterial infections by the chorioamniotic membranes, the placenta, and poorly understood antibacterial factors in amniotic fluid. Subclinical infections of the fetus, amniotic fluid, membranes, or placenta contribute significantly to the onset of preterm labor and the frequency of preterm birth (Gibbs et al, 1992). Most viruses, especially herpes simplex, cytomegalovirus, human immunodeficiency virus-1, and rubella can infect the fetus before membrane rupture (Kaplan, 1993). Under normal circumstances, at delivery and during the immediate neonatal period, the infant is exposed to many organisms, including aerobic and anaerobic bacteria, viruses, fungi, and protozoa. This encounter initiates colonization of the respiratory and gastrointestinal tracts (Sprunt, 1985). Most newborns establish their microbial flora without incident; however, occasionally disease caused by one of these organisms develops. The factors contributing to conversion from colonization to disease are not completely understood (Goldmann et al, 1983; Polin and St. Geme, 1992; Sprunt, 1985).

There appear to be four separate mechanisms by which bacteria reach the fetus or newborn to cause infection. First, certain bacteria (particularly *Treponema pallidum*, *Listeria monocytogenes*, and *Mycobacterium tuberculosis*) can reach the fetus through the maternal bloodstream, despite placental protective mechanisms, causing transplacental infection. This process is uncommon, but it leads either to congenital infection not unlike infections caused by certain viruses or *Toxoplasma* or to stillbirth resulting from overwhelming infection. Second, it seems likely that many early-onset group B streptococcal diseases are the result of infection that occurs immediately before delivery

(Noya and Baker, 1992). The bacteria appear to be acquired from the vagina or cervix through either ruptured or intact membranes, leading to amnionitis, pneumonitis, and premature delivery. The role of cytokines (e.g., interleukin 1, interleukin 6, and tumor necrosis factor alpha) in the induction of preterm labor has been investigated by Romero and colleagues (Hertelendy et al, 1993; Romero et al, 1993a, 1994a, 1994b). Despite the important contribution of subclinical intrauterine infection to preterm birth, recent trials come to different conclusions about antibiotic efficacy in reducing the risk of preterm labor (e.g., Romero et al, 1993b). Third, infection may occur during passage through the birth canal at the time of delivery. Gonococcal ophthalmia and most infections of *Escherichia coli* appear to develop in this manner. In some instances (e.g., late-onset group B streptococcal infection), colonization may occur at the time of birth. The mechanisms by which colonization contributes to late-onset (occurring weeks to months later) infection are poorly understood (Noya and Baker, 1992). Genetic and developmental immunoregulatory mechanisms are most likely involved. Finally, bacteria can be introduced after birth from the environment surrounding the baby, either in the nursery or at home.

The two most common bacterial pathogens in term infants in the first 28 days of life are the group B streptococcus and *E. coli*. These two organisms account for approximately 70% of systemic neonatal bacterial diseases. Either organism may be acquired from the mother during the intrapartum period, from the father, or nosocomially. The acute (early-onset [occurring within the first 7 days of life]) septicemic form of group B streptococcal disease may be caused by any of the group B serotypes (Ia, Ib, II, III, or V). The frequency of recovery of individual group B streptococcal serotypes that cause disease is approximately equal among serotypes I, II, and III and closely correlates with recovery of these organisms from the maternal genitourinary tract (Noya and Baker, 1992). Recently, two infants with invasive disease caused by the new serotype V organism have been described (Rench and Baker, 1993). Epidemiologic studies have shown that from 5% to 30% of pregnant women are vaginally or rectally colonized with group B streptococci. Approximately 50% of infants of colonized mothers are themselves asymptomatically colonized at birth, and a similar number acquire the organism without disease from the environment (Siegel et al, 1980; Yow et al, 1979). The major colonization sites in the infant are the skin, the nasopharynx, and the rectum. The group B streptococcus persists in the nasopharynx and rectum for weeks to months. It has been estimated that for every 100 infants colonized with group B streptococci, disease develops in one infant caused by this organism (Baker and Barrett, 1973). Therefore, colonization is not a sole indication for systemic antibiotic treatment (Evans et al, 1988).

Group B streptococcal meningitis is caused almost exclusively by organisms of serotype III. These organisms may be acquired from sources other than the mother. Clusters of three or four cases of meningitis caused by group B streptococci have occurred in nurseries during short time periods, suggesting nosocomial acquisition.

Certain studies have shown that approximately 80% of *E. coli* strains that cause neonatal meningitis possess a single, specific capsular polysaccharide antigen, which has been designated as K1 (Robbins et al, 1974). There are more than 100 recognized K antigens associated with *E. coli* strains. In contrast, approximately 40% of *E. coli* strains that cause neonatal septicemia possess K1 and only 10% to 15% of strains that cause septicemia and urinary tract infections in adults contain this antigen (Siitonen et al, 1993).

The reason for this association between K1 antigen and *E. coli* strains that cause neonatal meningitis and, to a lesser degree, septicemia is unknown. The K1 polysaccharide is chemically identical to that found in the capsule of group B meningococci. Animal studies have demonstrated that *E. coli* possessing K1 are highly virulent for mice and that this lethal effect can be completely prevented by the pretreatment of mice with minute amounts of specific K1 antibody (Robbins et al, 1974). Furthermore, the outcome of neonatal meningitis is directly correlated with the presence, concentration, and persistence of K1 antigen in the cerebrospinal fluid and blood of these infants (McCracken et al, 1974). Work by Edwards and associates (1982) with group B streptococci has suggested that a specific polysaccharide (sialic acid) found in the outer capsules of both K1 *E. coli* and group B streptococcus prevents the activation of the alternative complement pathway and thereby may account for the virulence of these organisms. Alternatively, lower concentrations of the ninth component of complement in infants or reduced recognition by neutrophils may account for enhanced virulence of these organisms (Lassiter et al, 1994; Ohman et al, 1995).

Extensive epidemiologic studies have shown that approximately 20% to 30% of newborn babies are colonized rectally with *E. coli* (Sarff et al, 1975). This percentage may increase to 50% during the 2nd and 3rd weeks of life (Peter and Nelson, 1978). 30% to 40% of normal infants and children demonstrate K1 organisms on rectal swab culture, as do nearly 50% of women at the time of delivery. Approximately two thirds of babies born to K1-positive mothers are colonized with the identical serotypes of *E. coli* K1. Vertical transmission of these organisms has been documented in 70% of newborns with *E. coli* K1 meningitis and is the major route of neonatal gastrointestinal colonization. The colonization to disease ratio for *E. coli* K1 is similar to that observed for group B streptococci; that is, approximately 100 to 200:1. Nosocomial infection with *E. coli* K1 has also been noted.

Although the pathogenesis of neonatal group B streptococcal and *E. coli* K1 disease has not been completely elucidated, a reasonable hypothesis can be proposed. While a lack of type-specific antibody has been associated with enhanced susceptibility to systemic bacterial infection in infants (Baker and Kasper, 1976), recent investigators have focused on differences in cytokine responses between infants and adults to explain enhanced susceptibility of infants. For example, Lee and coworkers (1993) and Schibler and colleagues (1993) have shown reduced production of granulocyte colony-stimulating factor in mononuclear cells isolated from infants. Tumor necrosis factor alpha has been detected in blood, urine, and cerebrospinal fluid from infants and is produced actively by mononuclear cells in response to group B streptococci (Williams et al, 1993). These observations suggest that induction of colony-stimulating factors or inhibition of tumor necrosis factor alpha may be important targets for recombinant cytokine replacement or immunotherapy (Cairo, 1991).

Although this discussion has centered on only two organisms that cause neonatal disease, considerable data support the importance of vertical transmission of other microorganisms during the intrapartum period. These include *Listeria monocytogenes*, anaerobic bacteria (Chow et al, 1974), *Chlamydia* (Frommell et al, 1979), *Candida albicans* (Kozinn et al, 1958), and viruses such as cytomegalovirus and *Herpesvirus hominis*.

SEPTICEMIA

Neonatal sepsis (Polin and St. Geme, 1992; Saez-Llorens and McCracken, 1993) is a disease of infants who are younger than 1 month of age, are clinically ill, and have positive blood cultures. The presence of clinical manifestations distinguishes this condition from the transient bacteremia observed in some healthy newborns.

The incidence of neonatal sepsis is between 1 and 4 cases per 1000 live births for full-term and premature infants, respectively. Among very-low-birth-weight infants who are undergoing prolonged hospitalization, the incidence increases dramatically to 300 per 1000 very-low-birth-weight infants. These incidence rates vary from nursery to nursery and depend on the presence of conditions that predispose infants to infection.

Diagnosis of Sepsis: Predisposing Factors

Although multiple factors have been associated with increased risk of bacterial infection within the first 7 days of life, the most important factors are the degree of prematurity of the infant and maternal medical conditions that may predispose the infant to fetal or neonatal infection (e.g., preterm labor, maternal genitourinary tract infection, or chorioamnionitis) (Polin and St. Geme, 1992). The more premature the infant, the higher the risk of infection. Maternal or fetal infection probably contributes to initiation of preterm labor and a significant proportion of preterm births. The considerable rates of morbidity and mortality associated with bacterial infection in the newborn infant have prompted multiple investigations to develop risk evaluation methods that use information on maternal infection, fetal problems, and the initial evaluation of the infant (Philip and Hewitt, 1980; Polin and St. Geme, 1992). Unfortunately, the spectrum of variables requires individualized decision-making for each patient. For example, duration of rupture of membranes before onset of labor, the latent period, or time before delivery has been investigated by several authors (Blackmon et al, 1986). None was able to demonstrate a significant difference in culture-proven sepsis with prolongation of the interval from rupture to delivery (Garite and Freeman, 1982). However, maternal medical risk factors should prompt suspicion of infection, more intense monitoring of vital signs, and active consideration of the need for cultures and antimicrobial therapy. Risk factors that should be considered in judging the probability that a child is infected are listed in Table 43–2.

Antenatal treatment of fetuses at risk for infection has improved infant outcome by decreasing the frequency of bacteremia (Noya and Baker, 1992). Boyer and Gotoff (1986) reported that bacteremia developed in none of 85 infants whose high-risk mothers received ampicillin developed bacteremia, whereas the disease did develop in 5 of 79 control subjects ($P = .024$). They suggested that selective

TABLE 43–2

Conditions that Increase the Risk of Systemic Bacterial Infection in Newborn Infants During the First 7 Days of Life

Family history of sibling with systemic bacterial disease under 3 months of age
Maternal conditions
  Premature or prolonged time between rupture of membranes and delivery
  Chorioamnionitis
  Urinary tract infection
Labor characteristics
  Preterm labor
  Fetal tachycardia without maternal fever, blood loss, hypotension, or tachycardia-inducing medication
Infant characteristics
  Apgar < 6 at 5 minutes
  Meconium-stained amniotic fluid
  Oxygen requirement
  Fever
  Neutropenia
  Male sex
  Congenital anomalies that cause breakdown of anatomic barriers to infection
  Polymorphonuclear leukocytes and intracellular organisms in gastric aspirate

TABLE 43–3

Clinical Signs of Bacterial Sepsis and Meningitis*

Clinical Sign	Percent of Infants with Sign	
	Sepsis	Meningitis
Hyperthermia	51	61
Hypothermia	15	—
Respiratory distress	33	47
Apnea	22	7
Cyanosis	24	—
Jaundice	35	28
Hepatomegaly	33	32
Anorexia	28	49
Vomiting	25	—
Abdominal distention	17	—
Diarrhea	11	17
Convulsions	—	40
Building or full fontanel	—	28
Nuchal rigidity	—	15

*Data from 455 infants studied at four medical centers.
From Klein JO: Current concepts of infectious diseases in the newborn infant. Curr Prob Pediatr 31:405–446, 1984.

intrapartum chemoprophylaxis can prevent early-onset neonatal group B streptococcal disease.

Among infants older than 7 days of age who require neonatal intensive care, maternal risk factors become less important in predicting the risk of sepsis than the degree of prematurity, the presence of central venous or arterial catheters, poor skin integrity, and malnutrition. Attempts at preventing infection in these high-risk infants through the use of systemic prophylactic antibiotics only increase the risk of selecting multiply resistant organisms and systemic opportunistic infection, especially with *Candida* species. As discussed later, the most common systemic isolate in this group is *Staphylococcus epidermidis*.

Diagnosis of Sepsis: Clinical Manifestations

The early signs and symptoms of septicemia in term or preterm infants younger than and older than 7 days of age are usually nonspecific. Early temperature imbalance with transient hyperthermia or hypothermia occurs in approximately 66% of septic infants (Table 43–3) (Bonadio, 1988). Respiratory distress or apnea occurs in 55% of septic infants. Other symptoms include tachycardia, lethargy, vomiting, or diarrhea, and unwillingness to breast-feed may be noted. Conjugated hyperbilirubinemia, petechiae, seizures, and hepatosplenomegaly are late signs that usually denote a poor prognosis. Severe unconjugated hyperbilirubinemia has recently been shown in a retrospective series of 306 infants to be rarely a single symptom of bacteremia or incipient sepsis (Maisels and Kring, 1992).

Although it is tempting to recommend a work-up for septicemia in all infants with nonspecific clinical manifestations, this approach is both impractical and unnecessary in many instances. A complete history and physical examination, longitudinal and regular (every 1 hour to every 4 hours) assessment of symptoms and vital signs, and clinical experience are the best guides in determining the timing and extent of evaluation. Infants who are deteriorating on the basis of clinical manifestations should be strongly considered for evaluation and treatment. For example, full-term infants who require increased ambient oxygen shortly after birth should be considered for evaluation and treatment if their respiratory distress does not improve or worsens by 6 hours of age.

Making the Diagnosis of Sepsis

The diagnosis of systemic bacterial infection must start with a careful evaluation of the infant's signs and symptoms, physical examination, information on longitudinal changes in vital signs and laboratory indicators, and history including maternal history and relevant recent nursery history. The diagnosis is predicated on recovery of the organism from the blood or other sites. Blood (usually a minimum of 0.5 mL) may be obtained from a peripheral vein or from the umbilical vessels immediately following sterile umbilical vessel catheterization (Paisley and Lauer, 1994). Femoral vein aspiration should be avoided because of both potential contamination with coliform organisms from the perineum and the danger of inadvertent penetration of the hip joint capsule. It is frequently helpful to obtain cultures from other sites (e.g., cerebrospinal fluid or urine) before initiating antimicrobial therapy. For example, using percutaneous bladder aspiration of urine for culture is frequently helpful in identifying the urinary tract as the focus of infection or in recovering antigens as evidence of bacteremia (e.g., latex agglutination test for group B streptococcus) (Hamoudi et al, 1983). In contrast, surface cultures or urine collected in urine bags does not provide useful information for determination of which antibiotic agent should be used, the duration of therapy, or the prognosis (Evans et al, 1988). Microscopic examination and culture of material obtained from gastric aspiration for leukocytes and bacteria has been advocated as a means of identifying infants who are at risk for development of systemic bacterial disease (Hamoudi et al, 1983). The presence of amniotic fluid infection increases the risk of systemic infection in a full-term infant from 1 to 5 per 1000 live births to 5 per 100 live births (Siegel and McCracken, 1981). However, the bacteriologic results of a gastric aspirate cannot be used as a sole indication for initiation or prolongation of antibiotic treatment (Borderon et al, 1994).

Measuring the peripheral white blood cell count and differential is a useful and rapid test, but it is nonspecific (Philip and Hewitt, 1980). If the total count is less than 5000 or if the band-to-neutrophil ratio exceeds 0.2 or 0.3, bacterial sepsis should be strongly considered, especially if the blood is drawn when the newborn is older than 12 hours of age. The normal range of white blood cell counts in newborn infants is wide, and this wide range should be taken into account in interpreting the values (Manroe et al, 1979). Other tests, such as sedimentation rate, C-reactive protein, haptoglobin concentration, and nitroblue tetrazolium have been extensively evaluated but are rarely more useful than the history, the physical examination, and careful longitudinal evaluation of the infant's status.

Etiology

Through the years, there has been a shift in the microorganisms responsible for neonatal septicemia and meningi-

tis. This is clearly illustrated by the experience at Yale-New Haven Hospital (Freedman et al, 1981; Thompson et al, 1992; Unhanand et al, 1993; Yagupsky et al, 1991). During the 1930s, group A streptococci were the predominant organisms. In the 1950s, staphylococci (largely of phage group I) became a major cause of nursery outbreaks throughout the world. *Pseudomonas* was prominent during the same decade, perhaps because of the introduction of respiratory support systems. Since the late 1950s, *E. coli* has been an important cause of neonatal sepsis. The dramatic increase in incidence of group B streptococcal infections is notable and has been reflected in other centers as well. Both group D streptococci and *Klebsiella* are pathogens that have been found relatively recently, the latter accounting for a high proportion of antibiotic-resistant organisms that colonize and infect babies in neonatal intensive care units (Goldmann et al, 1978). During the 1980s and 1990s, *S. epidermidis* has been recovered from systemic cultures with increasing frequency (Battisti et al, 1981; Huebner et al, 1994; Kumar and Delivoria-Papadopoulos, 1985; Tan et al, 1994). This organism is most commonly seen in infants who are premature and who have required prolonged maintenance with central vascular catheters, peritoneal dialysis, or thoracostomy tubes. In most intensive care nurseries, this organism is the most common nosocomial systemic isolate. The prevalence rates for a specific bacterial pathogen vary from nursery to nursery and may change rather abruptly. Knowledge of the most commonly isolated bacteria in a nursery or intensive care unit, coupled with the antimicrobial susceptibilities of these organisms, is invaluable in treating suspected neonatal sepsis.

Streptococcal Disease

The group B streptococcus is the most common gram-positive organism that causes septicemia and meningitis during the 1st month of life in infants older than 37 weeks' gestational age. Vertical transmission of this organism from mother to infant is one route of infection. Nosocomial acquisition of infection has been implicated in some nurseries and may be more common than was thought previously. The incidence of group B streptococcal disease has varied widely. However, despite this variability, group B streptococcus has been noted as an important neonatal pathogen since 1938 (Noya and Baker, 1992).

The most common clinical manifestations of group B streptococcal infections are septicemia, pneumonia, and meningitis, but other more localized syndromes also occur, including osteomyelitis and septic arthritis, otitis media, cellulitis, and conjunctivitis as well as asymptomatic bacteremia. Generalized disease takes two clinically and epidemiologically distinct forms, early- and late-onset infection (Yagupsky et al, 1991; Zangwill et al, 1992). By definition the early form occurs in the first 7 days of life, usually within hours of delivery (mean age 20 hours) and up to 50% of affected infants are symptomatic at birth. Infants with the early form of the disease usually deteriorate within hours of delivery and may exhibit unexplained apnea or tachypnea, respiratory distress with hypoxia, and shock (Noya and Baker, 1992). Chest roentgenograms reveal a diffuse pulmonary infiltrate that may be indistinguishable from the pathologic findings characteristic of hyaline membrane disease. In some instances, disease that occurs in utero may precipitate premature delivery. In a recent population-based analysis of group B streptococcal mortality, a mortality rate of 5.7% was noted in early-onset disease and 6.0% in late-onset disease (Zangwill et al, 1992). Significant racial disparity was noted in the frequency and impact of group B streptococcal disease in infancy. In black infants, the likelihood of developing early-onset disease and dying of this disease is two times that in white infants; development of late-onset disease is three times more likely in black infants (Zangwill et al, 1992). The increased rate of prematurity among black infants may account for this disparity. Pneumonitis is the primary finding on pathologic examination, and postmortem cultures of the lung, blood, cerebrospinal fluid yield group B organisms. Approximately 30% of infants have concomitant meningitis (Baker, 1986).

The late-onset meningitic form of disease is exhibited at 1 to 12 weeks of age and is indistinguishable from the other forms of purulent meningitis. Group B streptococci are grown from cultures of blood and cerebrospinal fluid, and the mortality rate is 20% to 40%. The principal organism appears to be serotype III. The pathogenesis is uncertain. Recurrent group B streptococcal infections have been consistently noted in approximately 1% of infected infants (Green et al, 1994; Zangwill et al, 1992). Data suggest that immunologic susceptibility may play as great a role in these recurrences as inadequate eradication of the organism, because recurrence has been associated with both the original infecting strain or a second acquired strain (Green et al, 1994).

Prevention

Considerable interest over the past 5 years has focused on strategies to prevent perinatal group B streptococcal infections (Baker, 1993; Mohle-Boetani et al, 1993; Noya and Baker, 1992). The American College of Obstetricians and Gynecologists (1992) and the American Academy of Pediatrics (1992) have each suggested different prevention strategies. Currently, individualized coordination of obstetric and pediatric approaches for each family and infant is required. Maternal immunization using a group B streptococcal type III polysaccharide-beta C-protein conjugate may prove to be a broadly useful prevention tool (Madoff et al, 1994).

Group A Streptococcal Disease

As described by Semmelweiss and Holmes, the group A streptococcus was the infectious cause of the most common, lethal perinatal infection of both mothers and infants in the late 19th century, puerperal fever (Busby and Rodin, 1976). During the 1970s and 1980s, this organism was a relatively infrequent cause of perinatal infection. However, group A streptococcal disease has been noted to be increasing in both adults and children over the past decade (Givner et al, 1991; Wheeler et al, 1991). The severity of disease caused by this organism in the newborn period varies from a low-grade, chronic omphalitis to fulminant septicemia and meningitis. Vertical transmission has been documented by molecular techniques (Bingen et al, 1992;

Panaro et al, 1993). Because of the explosive nature of outbreaks in nursery settings, surveillance for colonized infants is probably indicated at the time the organism is found or when infant infections are recognized (see the discussion of nosocomial infections).

Group D Streptococcal Disease

Group D streptococci include the enterococci and several other species, particularly *S. bovis*, which have been found in neonatal infection. Enterococci tend to be resistant to penicillin, and therefore ampicillin, with or without an aminoglycoside such as kanamycin or gentamicin, should be used. For nonenterococcal strains, penicillin may be adequate. The incidence of these infections appears to have increased in many centers, and they are recognized as often as, or more often than, those caused by *E. coli* (Siegel and McCracken, 1978). The clinical pattern of the disease is remarkably similar to that seen with group B streptococci (Alexander and Giacoia, 1978) and is frequently associated with complicated deliveries. With prompt and appropriate antibiotic therapy, however, prognosis appears to be somewhat better.

Infection with Streptococcus Viridans

Two reports (Broughton et al., 1981; Spigelblatt et al., 1985) have discussed the emergence of *Streptococcus viridans* as an important neonatal pathogen. In contrast to infants with systemic group B streptococcal infection, infants with *Streptococcus viridans* disease present later (mean age 3.5 days), exhibit leukopenia less frequently, and are less likely to have respiratory distress (Spigelblatt et al., 1985).

Staphylococcal Disease

In the 1950s, phage group I *Staphylococcus aureus* was the most common bacterial agent that caused septicemia in neonatal units. Its unique invasive properties caused disseminated disease with widespread manifestations, including neonatal mastitis, furunculosis, septic arthritis, osteomyelitis, and septicemia. Because infection of the bloodstream is usually secondary to local invasion, a careful search for the primary focus must be made in all septic babies. Microbial surveillance, intensified infection control measures, and increased local skin care have reduced colonization and disease rates caused by the group I organism.

In the 1970s, coagulase-positive staphylococcal disease in nurseries was caused by organisms of the phage II group (Melish and Glasgow, 1971). These organisms produce an exotoxin (exfoliatin) that causes intraepidermal cleavage through the granular cell layer resulting from disruption of desmosomes (Melish et al, 1972). Clinical disease may take one of several forms, which include bullous impetigo, toxic epidermal necrolysis, Ritter disease, and nonstreptococcal scarlatina. The initial findings in Ritter disease are intense, painful erythema that is similar to a severe sunburn. Over the next few hours, bullae may form that, when ruptured, leave a tender, weeping erythematous area. The characteristic desquamation of large epidermal sheets occurs approximately 3 to 5 days after the onset of the illness. A fine desquamation is commonly seen in the perioral region. Bullous impetigo has been the most common disease associated with nursery outbreaks of phage group II staphylococcal infections.

In the 1980s, two additional kinds of staphylococcal infections have been recognized as major contributors to nursery infections, namely methicillin-resistant *Staphylococcus aureus* (MRSA) and *S. epidermidis*. Since the early 1980s, adult surgical and medical intensive care units in the United States and other countries have noted an increase in nosocomially acquired and community-acquired MRSA (Bartokas et al, 1984; Fang et al, 1993; Saravolatz et al, 1982; Thompson and Wenzel, 1982; Wenzel, 1982). Similarly, MRSA outbreaks have been reported with increasing frequency in neonatal intensive care units (Back et al, 1993; Ish-Horowicz et al, 1992; Noel et al. 1992; Reboli et al, 1989). Although standard infection control measures including contact isolation, hand-washing with chlorhexidine, and cohorting are frequently used to control outbreaks, eradication of MRSA may require hand-washing with hexachlorophene (Reboli et al, 1989). The population at highest risk for colonization or infection include infants under 1500 g with long-standing central vascular catheters, thoracostomy tubes, or central nervous system shunts, or those infants undergoing prolonged hospitalization after surgical procedures (Storch and Rajagopazan, 1986). When colonization with MRSA is noted and clinical deterioration suggestive of systemic infection occurs, some authors have strongly suggested the inclusion of vancomycin in the initial antibiotic administration. Vancomycin has been shown to be effective therapy for systemic MRSA infection in both adults and children (Myers and Linnemann, 1982; Schaad et al, 1980). However, regular use of vancomycin may cause the development of vancomycin-resistant organisms. Decisions concerning the use of antibiotics must be individualized and predicated on the clinical condition and history of the infant, the microbiologic history of the nursery, and the contribution of indwelling catheters. Routine surveillance for MRSA in individual nurseries may be necessary if outbreaks or endemic colonization and infection are observed.

In conjunction with the emergence of MRSA as a major neonatal pathogen during the decade of the 1980s, coagulase-negative staphylococci, collectively known as *S. epidermidis*, have assumed considerable importance as troublesome nosocomial pathogens in the neonatal intensive care unit (St. Geme and Harris, 1991). Similar to MRSA, these organisms are most frequently isolated from the smallest and sickest infants, many of whom have indwelling central vascular catheters, thoracostomy tubes, or central nervous system shunts (Carlos et al, 1991; Gellert et al, 1993; Thompson et al, 1992). In contrast to MRSA infection, infants infected with coagulase-negative staphylococci have indolent presentations and infrequently metastatic focal infection develops. Although central venous catheters and contaminated hyperalimentation solutions have both been associated with *S. epidermidis* bacteremia, the surface hydrophobicity of the organism as well as opsonic differences in neonatal sera are more likely pathogenic mechanisms (St. Geme and Harris, 1991). In addition, after adherence to a hydrophobic polymer used in biomaterials (e.g.,

teflon), these organisms produce a thick layer of amorphous material called extracellular slime (Marrie and Costerton, 1984). This substance may permit the organism to escape phagocytosis by polymorphonuclear leukocytes (Johnson et al, 1986). Treatment of these infections is also complicated by the high frequency of penicillin- and gentamicin-resistant strains. Most strains remain sensitive to vancomycin. In some cases, removal of all vascular catheters in conjunction with the administration of a penicillin and aminoglycoside is sufficient for sterilizing the bloodstream. Use of vancomycin should be reserved for those infections that involve a catheter or anatomic site that cannot be readily removed or surgically approached (e.g., a heart valve) (Bryant, 1982), or that does not respond to initial antibiotic therapy. Persistent staphylococcal bacteremia unresponsive to vancomycin may be treated with intravenous rifampin (2.5 to 10 mg/kg every 12 hours for 10 days) (Tan et al, 1993). Epidemiologic studies of persistence and source of nosocomial *S. epidermidis* infections using restriction endonuclease analysis of plasmid DNA, genotyping, ribotyping, and arbitrarily primed polymerase chain reaction have been particularly useful in tracking spread of microbial strains and their mobile genetic elements (Back et al, 1993; Carlos et al, 1991; Fang et al, 1993; Noel et al, 1992; Patrick et al, 1992; Wanger et al, 1992).

Infection with *Listeria monocytogenes*

Listeria is a small, motile gram-positive rod that grows slowly in the laboratory and that can be mistaken for either corynebacteria or streptococci in Gram stains. It is a facultative intracellular parasite that is found widely in the animal kingdom, and infections in humans are sometimes seen as a result of contact with domestic animals or contaminated food. (Centers for Disease Control and Prevention, 1992; Cherubin et al, 1991; Jones et al, 1994; Schlech et al, 1983). As with group B streptococcal infections, there are two forms, early- and late-onset infection. Early-onset infections are acquired transplacentally or during passage through the vaginal canal. In such instances, fetal death and abortion may result or the child may be born with hepatosplenomegaly, disseminated disease, and granulomatous papules on the trunk and oral mucous membranes. This form of the disease has been called "granulomatosis infantisepticum." Perinatal complications are common in this group, and the prognosis is often grave (Teberg et al, 1987). A recent study in the United Kingdom suggested a mortality rate of 14% among infected infants (Jones et al, 1994). In the United States, the annual incidence of listeriosis is estimated to be 7.4 cases per 1 million population (Centers for Disease Control and Prevention, 1992). Between 30% and 50% of these cases occur among pregnant women or their newborn infants. For infants younger than 1 year of age, the annual incidence has been estimated to be approximately 5.2 per 100,000 population, considerably less frequent than group B streptococcal infection (180 per 100,000 population). Late-onset disease takes the form of meningitis (Visintine et al, 1977), which occurs usually in the 2nd week of life but also may occur as late as the 4th or 5th week. The cerebrospinal fluid is highly cellular, the glucose is almost always markedly depressed, and monocytes are often seen on the smear, although they are usually not the predominant cell type. Diagnosis is predicated on isolation of the organism, because serologic tests do not provide adequate sensitivity (Hudak et al, 1984). The early-onset type of listeriosis, as with group B streptococcal disease, reflects the genital colonization of the mother and can be one of several serotypes. Meningitis, on the other hand, is almost always caused by type IV B and is usually acquired from the environment (Albritton et al, 1976). The prognosis of the meningitic form is relatively good with regard to both survival and sequelae. Ampicillin plus gentamicin or kanamycin should be given for the first 5 to 7 days, followed by ampicillin alone to complete a 2-week course. The combination of ampicillin and an aminoglycoside has been shown to kill listeria more rapidly than either drug alone (Gordon et al, 1972). Follow-up studies suggest that newborn infants infected with *Listeria* at birth evidence little or no immunologic response to *Listeria* (opsonizing activity, anti-*Listeria* antibody titer, or lymphocyte proliferation in response to *Listeria*) at 1 year of age (Issekutz et al, 1984).

Infection with *Escherichia coli*

E. coli is the most common gram-negative bacteria that causes septicemia during the neonatal period. Approximately 40% of *E. coli* strains that cause septicemia possess K1 capsular antigen, and strains identical with that in blood can usually be identified in the patient's nasopharynx or rectal cultures (see previous discussion of pathogenesis of neonatal infections). The clinical features of *E. coli* septicemia are generally similar to those observed in infants with disease caused by other pathogens. Recent advances in understanding the role of regular antibiotic usage in the selection of specific resistance plasmids, the efficacy of immune globulin replacement therapy in the treatment of *E. coli* and other gram-negative infections, the development of specific molecular probes for identification and characterization of plasmids that encode resistance factors, and enhanced recognition of the importance of prevention through the use of vaccines and, in developing countries, through the provision of clear water, safe waste disposal, and hygiene education may act in concert over the decade of the 1990s to reduce the incidence of neonatal disease caused by *E. coli* (Bortolussi, 1986; Cates et al, 1988; Rennels and Levine, 1986; Shaio et al, 1989; Tullus and Berman, 1989).

Pseudomonas Septicemia

Pseudomonas septicemia may present with one or several characteristic violaceous papular lesions that, after several days, develop central necrosis. Although this condition is most commonly observed in *Pseudomonas* infection, it may also be associated with other pathogens. In the newborn who receives broad-spectrum antibiotics while in an environment that is potentially contaminated by bacteria from respirators or moist oxygen, is disease is likely to be caused by *Pseudomonas* species or other fastidious organisms.

Infection with Nontypable *Haemophilus influenzae*

Although fewer than 50 cases of neonatal sepsis resulting from nontypeable *Haemophilus influenzae* were reported between 1909 and 1981, during the decade of the 1980s this organism became a well-recognized neonatal pathogen that accounts in some centers for up to 7.9% of all cases of neonatal sepsis (Campognone and Singer, 1986; Eisenfeld et al, 1983; Grundmann et al, 1993; Verweij et al, 1993; Wallace et al, 1983). Pseudomonas may also cause nosocomial urinary tract infections in sick newborn infants (Davies et al, 1992). Infants infected with this organism generally present with fulminant infection, exhibit neutropenia, and are born prematurely. The most common biotypes recovered are biotype II and III (Campognone and Singer, 1986). Approximately 20% of *H. influenzae* isolates recovered from the newborns are encapsulated (biotype I) (Wallace et al, 1983; St. Geme, 1993). The increasing frequency of this organism should prompt consideration of ampicillin as one of the antibiotics included in the initial treatment of potentially septic newborn infants.

Therapy

Before the definitive diagnosis of septicemia is made and before the availability of microbial susceptibility studies, antibiotic therapy should be initiated using a combination that includes a penicillin and an aminoglycoside. The choice of antibiotics must be based on the historical experience of the nursery, the antimicrobial susceptibilities of bacteria recently isolated from both sick and healthy newborns, and the maternal history. For initial therapy, ampicillin in combination with gentamicin is a reasonable choice. Ampicillin is active in vitro against *L. monocytogenes* and enterococci as well as against many strains of *E. coli*. When the historical experience of the nursery or the physical findings suggest *Pseudomonas* infection, carbenicillin in combination with gentamicin should be used. Once the pathogen is identified and its antimicrobial susceptibilities are known, the most effective and least toxic drug or combination of drugs should be used. The aminoglycosides tobramycin and amikacin should not be used except in therapy of disease caused by kanamycin- and gentamicin-resistant gram-negative organisms to minimize the risk of aminoglycoside-resistant bacteria.

Additional immunoregulatory interventions including immune globulin replacement therapy, polymorphonuclear leukocyte transfusion, exchange transfusion, and treatment with recombinant cytokines have been used in specific clinical studies. They are reviewed in Chapter 40.

BACTERIAL MENINGITIS

The incidence of purulent meningitis of the newborn infant varies among institutions and is higher in those city hospitals in which prenatal care is suboptimal and in which complicated pregnancies and deliveries often result in high-risk premature births. Incidence rates are approximately two to four cases per 10,000 live births and may be as high as one case per 1000 live births in some nurseries. Within the 1st week of life, group B streptococci and *E. coli* strains account for approximately 70% of all cases and *Listeria monocytogenes* is seen in an additional 5% of infants (Shattuck and Chonmaitree, 1992; Synnott et al, 1994; Unhanand et al, 1994). Among infants who are hospitalized for longer than a week in neonatal intensive care units, *S.*

epidermidis represents the most frequent isolate. Occasionally, in *S. epidermidis* meningitis, biochemical and cellular indicators of infection in cerebrospinal fluid are absent, but cultures are positive (Gruskay et al, 1989).

Group B streptococcal meningitis usually manifests after the first several days of life, and the principal organism encountered in these infants is serotype III. The mortality rate is 20% to 40%. Streptococcal disease that occurs in the first 48 hours after delivery usually becomes manifest as acute respiratory distress with or without shock. Although the organism is frequently isolated from postmortem cerebrospinal fluid cultures taken from these infants, histologic evidence of meningeal inflammation may be lacking (Franciosi et al, 1973).

Approximately 80% of all types of *E. coli* that cause meningitis possess K1 antigen. The 018 and 07 somatic types and H6 and H7 flagellar types are most commonly associated with K1 strains cultured from cerebrospinal fluid (Sarff et al, 1975). The presence, concentration, and persistence of this capsular polysaccharide antigen in cerebrospinal fluid and blood of infants with meningitis correlate directly with the outcome of the disease (Franco et al, 1992). The concentration and persistence of interleukin 1 beta and tumor necrosis factor alpha, the principal mediators of meningeal inflammation, correlate with an adverse outcome (Dodge, 1994; McCracken et al, 1989; Mustafa et al, 1989; Velasco et al, 1991). The mortality rates for neonatal *E. coli* meningitis vary from 20% to 30% in some centers to 50% to 60% in others. These figures have been relatively constant despite improvements in overall perinatal mortality (Bell et al, 1989). This lack of improvement in outcome among infants with meningitis probably reflects the decrease in size and gestational age of infants who are receiving medical interventions in neonatal intensive care units and the emergence of different organisms with increased antibiotic resistance. In Sweden, where premature birth is less frequent than in other European countries and in the United States, neonatal bacterial meningitis occurred at a rate of 1.9 per 10,000 live births in 1983 (Bennhagen et al, 1987). In this report, a significant improvement in combined mortality and handicap rates from meningitis was observed between 1976 (34%) and 1983 (15%).

The epidemiology and clinical manifestations of *Listeria meningitis* are described previously in the discussion of septicemia. Rare cases of meningitis caused by *Campylobacter* have also been described, with onset at 1 to 22 days of age (Goossens et al, 1986; Torphy and Bond, 1979). In these reported cases, the disease closely resembled neonatal bacterial meningitis caused by other organisms.

Pathology

The pathologic findings are similar regardless of the bacterial etiology. The most consistent findings at necropsy of babies who die of meningitis are purulent exudate of the meninges and of the ependymal surfaces of the ventricles associated with vascular inflammation. The inflammatory response of newborns is similar to that observed in adults with meningitis, except that babies have a sparsity of plasma cells and lymphocytes during the subacute stage of meningeal reaction. Hydrocephalus and a noninfectious encephalopathy can be demonstrated in approximately 50%

of infants who die of meningitis. Subdural effusions occur rarely in newborns. In contrast, this complication of meningitis is common in infants 3 to 12 months of age. Varying degrees of phlebitis and arteritis of intracranial vessels can be found in all infants who die of meningitis. Thrombophlebitis with occlusion of veins may occur in the subependymal zones. K1 antigen has been demonstrated in brain tissue of infants who die of *E. coli* K1 infection.

Clinical Manifestations

The early signs and symptoms of neonatal meningitis are frequently indistinguishable from those of septicemia (see Table 43–3). Specific findings such as stiff neck and Kernig and Brudzinski signs are rarely found. Lethargy, feeding problems, and altered temperature are the most frequent presenting complaints, and respiratory distress, vomiting, diarrhea, and abdominal distention are common findings. A bulging fontanel may be a late sign of meningitis. Seizures are observed frequently and may be caused by direct central nervous system inflammation or may occur in association with hypoglycemia, hyponatremia, or hypocalcemia.

Diagnosis

The interpretation of cerebrospinal fluid cell counts in newborn infants may be difficult (Bonadio, 1988; Gruskay et al, 1989; Polk and Steele, 1988; Unhanand et al, 1993). During the first several days of life, as many as 32 white blood cells/mm^3 (mean, 8 cells/mm^3) may be found in cerebrospinal fluid of healthy or high-risk, uninfected babies. Approximately 60% of these cells are polymorphonuclear leukocytes. During the 1st week, the cell count slowly diminishes in full-term infants but may remain high or even increase in premature babies. Cell counts in the range of 0 to 10 cells/mm^3 are observed at 1 month of age. The cerebrospinal fluid protein concentration may be as high as 170 mg/100 mL, and the cerebrospinal fluid glucose to blood glucose percentage ratio is 44% to greater than 100% in both preterm and term infants. Thus, it is apparent that total evaluation of the cerebrospinal fluid examination is necessary to make an early diagnosis of neonatal meningitis. Although the cerebrospinal fluid cell counts and protein and sugar concentrations from normal infants overlap with those from infants with meningitis, less than 1% of babies with proven meningitis have totally normal results from a cerebrospinal fluid study on the initial lumbar tap (Sarff et al, 1976; Hristeva et al, 1993). Approximately 50% of all infants with positive cerebrospinal fluid cultures for bacteria have negative blood cultures (Shattuck and Chonmaitree, 1992).

Stained smears of cerebrospinal fluid must be examined carefully from every infant with suspected meningitis. Grossly clear fluid may contain few white blood cells and many bacteria. The stained smears from approximately 20% of newborns with proven meningitis are interpreted as showing no bacteria. As its name implies, *L. monocytogenes* commonly evokes a mononuclear cellular response in the cerebrospinal fluid.

Latex agglutination assays can also be helpful in the early identification of infants with meningitis and in infants with abnormal cerebrospinal fluid findings who have received systemic antibiotics before culture of cerebrospinal fluid. The disadvantage of these tests is the lack of the availability of antibiotic susceptibility testing to direct antimicrobial therapy. Blood and urine cultures should be obtained from every infant with suspected meningitis.

Therapy

Infants with meningitis require multisystem, aggressive management in the setting of an intensive care unit (Ashwal et al, 1994; Feigin et al, 1992; McCracken, 1992; Roos and Scheld, 1989). Besides requiring antibiotic administration, these infants frequently require mechanical ventilation, compulsive fluid management to minimize the effects of cerebral edema, seizure control, pressor support, and cardiopulmonary monitoring. The beneficial effects of early administration of dexamethasone in infants with bacterial meningitis have recently been described in a placebo-controlled, double-blind trial in 101 infants and children (Odio et al, 1991). Dexamethasone (0.15 mg/kg of body weight) was administered approximately 20 minutes before the first dose of antibiotics and continued every 6 hours for 4 days. The placebo group evidenced higher mean opening cerebrospinal pressure within 12 hours of therapy, greater concentrations of two cytokines (tumor necrosis factor alpha and platelet activating factor), which contribute to meningeal inflammation, and 3.8-fold greater risk of neurologic or audiologic sequelae ($P = .007$) than the dexamethasone treated group. The efficacy of this intervention may result from attenuation of induction of cytokines, which mediate meningeal inflammation (Velasco et al, 1991). The success of dexamethasone also suggests that other more specific therapies to reduce meningeal inflammation (e.g., anti-CD18 monoclonal antibodies) may be useful in improving outcome (Jafari and McCracken, 1994; Saez-Llorens et al, 1991). Selection of appropriate antibiotic therapy is based in part on the achievable cerebrospinal fluid levels of these drugs in relation to the susceptibility of the organisms that cause the disease. The highest kanamycin and gentamicin concentrations in cerebrospinal fluid are approximately 40% of the peak serum levels and are only equal to or slightly greater than the minimal inhibitory concentrations for disease-causing coliform bacteria. In contrast, cerebrospinal fluid penicillin and ampicillin concentrations may be only 10% of the corresponding peak serum levels, but these values are usually 10- to 100-fold higher than the greatest minimal inhibitory concentrations for group B streptococci and *L. monocytogenes*. The ability to attain spinal fluid antimicrobial activity that is many times greater than is necessary to inhibit the pathogen may explain the rapid sterilization of spinal fluid cultures from infants with gram-positive meningitis. Delayed sterilization of cerebrospinal fluid cultures from newborns with gram-negative meningitis may likewise be due to the low inhibitory and bactericidal spinal fluid concentrations. As a result of these considerations, the physician may find it necessary, in some infants with coliform meningitis, to alter the therapeutic regimens by adding a second antibiotic, selecting a different aminoglycoside, using one of the newer cephalosporin derivatives, or changing the route of administration. In addition, dosage and timing should be guided by renal, hepatic, and cardiopulmonary function. When possible, in-

dividualizing drug regimens based on regular measurement of serum drug concentrations permits the attainment of therapeutic antibiotic effects and the avoidance of toxicity. The Committee on Infectious Diseases of the American Academy of Pediatrics has recommended that if facilities for monitoring aminoglycoside or chloramphenicol pharmacokinetics are not available, these drugs should be avoided and cephalosporins (cefotaxime or ceftazidime) should be considered (Committee on Infectious Diseases, 1988).

In the United States, ampicillin and either gentamicin or kanamycin are recommended as the initial therapy for neonatal meningitis (American Academy of Pediatrics, 1994). The dosages of ampicillin are 100 mg/kg per day in two divided doses during the 1st week of life and 200 mg/kg per day in three divided doses thereafter. The dosages for gentamicin and kanamycin are the same as those used for septicemia (see Table 43–1). An alternative regimen of ampicillin and a cephalosporin (e.g., cefotaxime or ceftazidime) can be used, but frequent use of such a regimen may lead to emergence of cephalosporin-resistant gram-negative bacterial isolates (American Academy of Pediatrics, 1994). All infants should have a repeated spinal fluid examination and culture at 24 to 36 hours after initiation of therapy. If organisms are seen on methylene blue or gram-stained smears of the fluid, modification of the therapeutic regimen should be considered. In general, approximately 3 days are required to sterilize the cerebrospinal fluid in infants with gram-negative meningitis. In infants with gram-positive meningitis, sterilization is usually seen within 36 to 48 hours. Neuroimaging to exclude parameningeal foci should be considered in infants with persistently positive cerebrospinal fluid cultures who are receiving appropriate antibiotic coverage.

In infants with gram-negative meningitis whose cerebrospinal fluid is not sterilized within 3 days, some investigators have suggested use of intraventricular instillation of antibiotics (usually an aminoglycoside) via a surgically placed ventricular reservoir. With monitoring of ventricular fluid concentrations of the instilled antibiotic, this strategy is used until sterilization is achieved. This approach is predicated on the observation that ventriculitis develops, thus reducing accessibility of systemically administered antibiotics to the infected ventricles. However, in two large studies, neither intrathecal nor intraventricular antibiotics significantly improved either morbidity or mortality in infants with gram-negative meningitis (McCracken and Mize, 1976; McCracken et al, 1980). Chloramphenicol, because of its capacity to diffuse readily into the cerebrospinal fluid, has been used in neonatal meningitis, and, with frequent measurement of blood levels, is relatively safe (Krasinski et al, 1982).

Once the pathogen has been identified and the susceptibility studies are available, the single drug or combination of drugs that is most effective should be used (Klein, 1994). In general, penicillin or ampicillin is preferred for group B streptococcal infection, ampicillin with or without kanamycin or gentamicin for infection with *L. monocytogenes* and *Enterococcus*, ampicillin plus gentamicin or kanamycin for infection with coliform bacteria, and carbenicillin plus gentamicin for *Pseudomonas* infections. There is no precise method for determining the duration of antimicrobial therapy. A useful guide is to continue therapy for approximately

2 weeks after sterilization of cerebrospinal fluid cultures or for a minimum of 2 weeks for gram-positive meningitis and 3 weeks for gram-negative meningitis, whichever is longer (American Academy of Pediatrics, 1994).

Prognosis

The mortality in neonatal meningitis is high. The overall mortality rate is approximately 20% to 50%, depending on the etiologic agent, the high-risk factors predisposing the infant to illness, and the ability of nursery personnel and physicians to provide general supportive care. Short- and long-term sequelae of neonatal meningitis occur frequently (Dodge, 1994; Edwards et al, 1985; Franco et al, 1992; Unhanand et al, 1993). The complications include communicating or noncommunicating hydrocephalus, subdural effusions, ventriculitis, deafness, and blindness. Gross retardation may be obvious at discharge. However, many infants appear relatively normal at time of discharge, and only after prolonged and careful follow-up do perceptual difficulties, reading problems, or signs of minimal brain damage become apparent. Approximately 40% to 50% of survivors have some evidence of neurologic damage. Infants who survive neonatal meningitis should have regular audiology, language, and neurologic evaluations until matriculation into the school system (Edwards et al, 1985).

OTITIS MEDIA

Otitis media is infrequently diagnosed in newborn infants because of the paucity of clinical findings and the difficulty in examining the infant's tympanic membrane (Burton et al, 1993; Warren and Stool, 1971). The external canal is narrow and often filled with cheesy debris (Eavey, 1993). Because the healthy baby's membrane may appear thickened and dull, mobility of the drum by pneumoscopy should be used as the single most reliable indicator of middle ear infection.

Neonatal otitis media occurs most often in premature infants and in bottle-fed babies. The exact incidence of this disease is unknown, but it has been estimated to occur in approximately 1% to 5% of infants from birth to 6 weeks of age. The onset of illness is insidious, and the most common complaints are rhinorrhea, irritability, and failure to thrive. The presence of a fever greater than 38° C (100.4° F) and tugging of the affected ear are unusual.

It has been suggested that all newborn infants with suspected otitis media have needle aspiration of middle ear contents, because the pathogens associated with disease may be different from those encountered in infants after the first several months of life (Bland, 1972). However, a recent review of records of 37 newborn infants with otitis media revealed no bacterial isolates with resistant antibiotic sensitivities (Burton et al, 1993). These findings prompted the recommendation that newborn infants with otitis may receive empiric therapy and that tympanocentesis should be reserved for patients in whom medical treatment fails. Of special importance is the examination of the infant who has required prolonged oral or nasotracheal intubation (Derkay et al, 1989; Kinney et al, 1995). These children are at high risk for the development of eustachian tube dysfunction. The bacteriology of their infections is more

likely to reflect the hospital environment (Derkay et al, 1989). Recent preliminary data from children not born prematurely suggest that *S. epidermidis* is as important as *H. influenzae*, *S. pneumoniae*, and *Branhamella catarrhalis* in otitis media of early infancy (Casselbrant, 1989). Perinatal problems, especially prematurity, appear to increase the risk of otitis media in the first 6 months of life (Harma et al, 1989). The material obtained from aspiration is cultured in suitable media, and a stained smear is prepared for direct visualization of bacteria. *E. coli*, *S. aureus*, *Klebsiella pneumoniae*, and *S. epidermidis* cause approximately one half of the cases of otitis media outside of neonatal intensive care units. *Diplococcus pneumoniae* and *H. influenzae* are the most frequently encountered pathogens during the first 6 weeks of life, as they are during the entire period of infancy (Giebink, 1989). Selection of initial therapy is based on results of the gram-stained smear, nursery history, and previous organisms taken from the affected infant (Giebink et al, 1991; Berman, 1995). If organisms are not observed, oxacillin and gentamicin should be started and continued until results of cultures and susceptibility studies are available.

The importance of establishing the diagnosis and cause of otitis media in newborn infants and of using appropriate therapy cannot be overemphasized. A missed diagnosis and improper therapy may result in a chronic course of middle ear disease throughout infancy and, occasionally, extension of the infection to adjacent structures such as the mastoid or central nervous system.

DIARRHEAL DISEASE

Diarrheal disease during the neonatal period is usually brief and self-limited. Brief episodes of loose stools secondary to alterations of diet and feeding patterns, are common in young infants. Many infants have loose stools during an upper respiratory tract infection or as a systemic response to infection elsewhere. Modern sterilization practices and increased emphasis on infection control measures have significantly reduced the incidence of bacterial diarrhea in nurseries in developed countries.

Etiology and Pathogenesis

The primary route of infection for diarrheal disease is fecal-oral contamination. This disease is linked to both poverty and economic development (Glass et al, 1991).

Infectious diarrhea in newborns may be caused by bacteria, yeast (*Candida*), and viruses, but the most frequent of these agents is rotavirus (Cohen, 1991; Haffejee, 1991). Rotavirus infections in newborns differ from those observed in older infants in that most cases are asymptomatic (Greenberg et al, 1994). Although severe symptoms have been reported in rotavirus infected newborn infants (e.g., bowel perforation, necrotizing enterocolitis, and diarrhea), these manifestations are rare (Haffejee, 1991). Neonatal rotavirus infection provides significant immunologic protection against severe rotavirus disease later in childhood. Strains that infect newborn infants are characterized by a highly conserved outer capsid protein (VP4) that may play an important role in attenuated virulence of these strains.

The pathogenesis of bacterial diarrhea is complex and

depends on host factors as well as the particular bacterial species involved (Cohen, 1991; Glass et al, 1991). In nursery outbreaks of bacterial diarrhea, enteropathogenic *E. coli, Campylobacter jejuni,* and, much less commonly, *Shigella* and *Salmonella* have all been recognized (Guerrant et al, 1986). Although five types of *E. coli* can cause gastrointestinal infections, including enteropathogenic (EPEC), enterotoxigenic (ETEC), enteroinvasive (EIEC), enterohemorrhagic (EHEC), and enteroadherent (EAEC), ETEC and EPEC are important causes in nursery outbreaks (Cohen, 1991; Robins-Browne, 1987). ETEC strains produce well-characterized heat labile or heat stable enterotoxins (Robins-Browne, 1987). Enteropathogenic strains have been identified by serotype and display characteristic adhesive histology in cultured epithelial cells (Robins-Browne, 1987). The adherence factors are probably encoded on a 55- to 70-megadalton plasmid. The enteropathogenic strain may also express its pathogenicity through the production of at least one shiga-like enterotoxin. Molecular probes have been useful in detecting bacterial pathogens, including ETEC, EIEC, and EPEC, and in epidemiologic studies (Taylor and Echeverria, 1993).

Salmonellae produce diarrhea by mechanisms that are even less clearly understood (Rubin and Weinstein, 1977). Many species invade the mucosa without destroying it and set up an inflammatory reaction in the lamina propria. From there, particularly in newborn infants, the bloodstream may be invaded. Finally, *Campylobacter fetus* species *jejuni* (the form that most often causes diarrhea in older individuals) may sometimes be present in newborn infants and produce bloody diarrhea. The outcome is usually favorable (Anders et al, 1981; Karmali et al, 1984; Sartor and Anday, 1987). Both *Clostridium difficile* and *S. epidermidis* have been associated with a syndrome that resembles necrotizing enterocolitis (Grusky et al, 1986; Han et al, 1983; Mollitt et al, 1988). The specific pathogenic mechanisms of these agents have not been identified.

Clinical Manifestations

It is difficult to differentiate the causes of diarrhea in newborn infants on the basis of clinical findings only. As a general rule, diarrhea caused by enteropathogenic strains of *E. coli* is insidious in onset and is associated with 7 to 10 green, watery stools a day, but does not contain blood or mucus. The infants do not appear acutely ill. Complications are rare and are related primarily to dehydration and electrolyte disturbances. *Salmonella* gastroenteritis is usually associated with 5 to 10 foul-smelling loose green stools a day that rarely contain mucus or blood. Complications, which are unusual, include extraintestinal foci of infection such as septicemia, osteomyelitis, and septic arthritis. Shigellosis is rare in neonates, but when encountered, it is an acute illness associated with a profuse, watery, nonodorous diarrhea frequently containing blood and mucus. The infants may be very toxic, and illness in a small number of patients initially mimics meningitis or gram-negative shock. Suppurative complications are rare, but dehydration and electrolyte disturbances are common and need immediate and constant attention.

A useful procedure for differentiating enteropathogenic from enterotoxigenic diarrhea is examination of fecal material for polymorphonuclear cells. Feces from patients with dysentery have significant numbers of polymorphonuclear cells, whereas those from patients with enterotoxigenic disease have very few neutrophils. This test may be helpful in the selection of appropriate antimicrobial therapy.

Therapy

The most important aspect of therapy for infantile diarrhea is maintenance of hydration and electrolyte balance. As a rule, oral electrolyte solutions with a carbohydrate-to-sodium ratio less than 2:1 should be administered during the time of active diarrhea, and the infant should be examined and weighed frequently to ensure proper rehydration and to prevent complications (Williams et al, 1986). If sepsis or shock is suspected, intravenous fluids are needed. Estimation of fluid loss from diarrhea and vomiting should be carefully recorded and used as a basis for replacement therapy.

The selection of an antimicrobial agent depends in part on the mechanism of diarrhea (Edelman, 1985; Gorbach, 1987; Williams et al, 1986). An absorbable antibiotic such as ampicillin or chloramphenicol is indicated for disease caused by invasive bacteria, whereas orally administered nonabsorbable drugs such as neomycin or colistin sulfate should be used for noninvasive organisms that produce enterotoxin.

In the context of a nursery outbreak of bacterial diarrhea, all nursery infants with enteropathogenic *E. coli* should be considered for treatment with neomycin or colistin sulfate administered orally, whether or not they are symptomatic. Neomycin is administered orally in a dosage of 100 mg/kg per day in three or four divided doses. Colistin sulfate is administered in a dosage of 15 to 17 mg/kg per day orally in four divided doses. The duration of therapy is 3 to 5 days. Longer periods of therapy are unnecessary and may result in neomycin-induced steatorrhea (Nelson, 1971b). If enteropathogenic *E. coli* are isolated from stools of nonhospitalized, asymptomatic infants, it is usually not necessary to give antimicrobial agents to these infants; however, they should be followed up carefully.

All infants with *Salmonella* gastroenteritis should have blood cultures performed and be examined to determine whether the disease has developed at other sites, such as bones and joints. Newborn infants with symptomatic *Salmonella* infections should receive antimicrobial therapy if they are febrile or toxic or if their diarrhea is severe because there is greater potential for systemic infection in these patients. Older infants and children with *Salmonella* gastroenteritis and asymptomatic or minimally symptomatic newborn infants with positive stool cultures for *Salmonella* species should not receive antibiotics. In these patients, antimicrobial therapy may prolong gastrointestinal *Salmonella* carriage and does not significantly affect the clinical course of disease. When therapy is indicated in the newborn, ampicillin is the drug of choice and should be administered parenterally in a dosage of 50 to 100 mg/kg per day, divided into two or three doses. Therapy is continued for approximately 5 to 7 days.

Although shigellosis in the newborn infant is rare, it may be associated with high rates of morbidity and mortality. All newborns with symptomatic shigellosis should be treated with ampicillin in a dosage of 50 to 100 mg/kg per day, administered parenterally in two or three divided doses. The duration of therapy is approximately 5 days. In some hospitals, a significant percentage of ampicillin-resistant *Shigella* strains have been encountered. In these centers, trimethoprim-sulfamethoxazole is the initial drug of choice. The dosage is 10 mg trimethoprim and 50 mg sulfamethoxazole/kg per day in two divided doses for 5 days.

Any infant with diarrhea must be isolated from the other babies in the nursery. Surveillance of other infants in the unit and institution of infection control measures are also indicated (see discussion of nosocomial bacterial disease).

URINARY TRACT INFECTION

Improved methods of obtaining sterile specimens have made it possible to define more accurately the incidence of neonatal urinary tract infection. With bladder aspiration technique, bacteriuria may be demonstrated in approximately 1% of full-term infants and 3% of premature infants. Urinary tract infections are more common in babies born to bacteriuric mothers and in males during the neonatal period. After this period, these infections are more common in females and also in uncircumcised males (Wiswell and Roscelli, 1986).

Etiology

E. coli is the most common etiologic agent of urinary tract infections. Approximately 70% of *E. coli* strains belong to one of eight common somatic antigenic groups similar to those found in older patients. Renal parenchymal disease may be associated with one of several *E. coli* capsular types: K1, K2ac, K12, or K13 (Kaijser, 1972). *Klebsiella* and *Pseudomonas* species are encountered less frequently. *Proteus* species commonly cause urinary tract disease in infants with meningomyeloceles, and gram-positive bacteria, primarily *S. epidermidis*, are increasingly frequent causes of urinary tract infection.

The higher frequency of urinary tract infections in male infants suggests that the predominant pathogenesis at this age may differ from that in the older child or adult. Bacteremia, with seeding in a kidney that is in some way abnormal, may be responsible for at least some cases.

Clinical Manifestations

Most infants with significant bacteriuria are asymptomatic. In a prospective study of 1460 consecutive newborn infants in New Zealand in 1972, 9 of 14 bacteriuric infants were asymptomatic (Abbott, 1972). Similar findings have been reported in Sweden (Bergstrom et al, 1972). When symptoms are present, they are usually nonspecific and include poor weight gain, altered temperature, cyanosis or gray skin color, abdominal distention with or without vomiting, and loose stools. Conjugated hyperbilirubinemia, hepatomegaly, and thrombocytopenia may be observed in a few infants with urinary tract infection, and these findings are associated with septicemia, cholestatic hepatitis, or both in some babies. Localizing signs suggesting urinary tract involvement are unusual; when present, they usually consist of a weak urinary stream on voiding or an abdominal mass from bladder distention or hydronephrosis.

The diagnosis of urinary tract infection is made by examination and culture of a properly obtained specimen of urine (el-Dahr and Lewy, 1992; Landau et al, 1994). At any age but particularly in the neonatal period, during which diagnosis of urinary tract infection brings with it suggestions of renal or collecting system anomalies and bacteremia, the diagnosis is never made on the basis of urinalysis alone. A culture collected from a urine bag is not useful. The presence of bacteria, even in high numbers and in pure culture, may always be accounted for by contamination from the perineum.

At all ages, urinary tract infection may be present in the absence of leukocytes in the urine. The converse is also true, particularly when the urine is collected in a sterile plastic bag. Leukocytes or round epithelial cells (easily confused with leukocytes) are often found in urine samples collected in a urine bag, particularly after circumcision, in the absence of urinary tract infection. For these reasons, culture (or, for rapid screening, Gram stain) of urine obtained by suprapubic bladder aspiration or sterile bladder catheterization is the only certain means to diagnose urinary tract infection. In newborns, in whom restriction of fluid intake is not appropriate, greater than 10,000 organisms/mm^3 of a single species (rather than greater than 100,000 as is often thought) is diagnostic if the specimen is obtained by bladder puncture or catheterization. Moreover, concern about whether an infection is in the upper or lower urinary tract is rarely justified in the newborn infant, because either one carries with it concerns about urinary tract anomalies and bacteremia (el-Dahr and Lewy, 1992). Debate concerning the usefulness of dimercaptosuccinic acid (DMSA) renal scans in differentiating upper from lower tract infection has not provided a clear answer (Landau et al, 1994). Latex agglutination assays (e.g., for group B *streptococcal* infection) are sensitive and specific indicators of the presence of bacterial antigens but may not necessarily indicate a urinary tract infection. Consideration of a urinary tract infection in light of a positive latex agglutination test in the urine should include urinalysis, urine culture, and physical examination of the genitourinary system.

Therapy

All infants with suspected or proved urinary tract infections should have blood and urine cultures obtained before initiation of therapy. In general, antimicrobial agents should initially be given parenterally because septicemia may occur in association with urinary tract infection, and antibiotic absorption after oral administration may be erratic in newborn infants. Ampicillin plus kanamycin or gentamicin should be administered to symptomatic infants with bacteriuria before the receipt of results of cultures and susceptibility studies. Final antibiotic selection is based on these studies.

A repeat urine culture taken 48 to 72 hours after initiation of appropriate therapy should be sterile or show a substantial reduction in the bacterial count. Infants with persistent bacteriuria should be evaluated for resistant organisms, obstruction, or possible abscess formation. In the patient without complications, therapy is usually continued for 10 to 14 days. Blood urea nitrogen and serum creatinine levels as well as blood pressure should be determined at the initiation and completion of therapy. If there is evidence of renal failure, dosage and frequency of administration of these drugs, particularly the aminoglycosides, may need to be altered. Approximately 1 week after discontinuing therapy, a repeat urine culture is obtained. If the culture is positive, therapy is reinstated and a thorough investigation of the urinary tract is made to exclude obstruction or abscess formation.

All infants with culture-documented urinary tract infections should have radiologic or ultrasonic evaluation of the urinary tract. The usefulness of DMSA renal scans in evaluation of culture-documented urinary tract infection has not been conclusively determined. An excretory urogram or renal ultrasound is obtained at the onset of therapy to rule out the possibility of gross congenital abnormalities of the urinary system. If obstruction is demonstrated, urologic procedures to ensure proper drainage are necessary if therapy is to be successful. Voiding cystourethrography can be obtained within 2 weeks of the end of antibiotic therapy if reflux is suspected. Results are affected by previous bladder inflammation.

Prognosis

It is the physician's responsibility to be certain that newborn infants with culture-documented urinary tract infections do not have congenital abnormalities of the urinary system. In such patients, recurrent urinary tract infections are common, and physical growth may be retarded until definitive surgery has been performed. One must conduct careful, long-term follow-up studies in every patient to detect recurrent infections, many of which are asymptomatic (Smellie et al, 1983).

Prevention

The contribution of antenatal diagnosis of fetal hydronephrosis to the prevention of urinary tract infection has recently been evaluated (Daucher et al, 1992). Urinary tract infection developed in 13 of 413 infants who had fetal hydronephrosis in the first 6 months of life; 11 of the were formula-fed infants younger than 2 months of age, 10 of whom were males. In 10 infants for whom bacteriologic data were available, amoxicillin-resistant bacteria were the causative organisms. Individualized evaluation of infants with antentally diagnosed hydronephrosis provides an opportunity to reduce morbidity associated with urinary tract infection in the first 6 months of life.

SEPTIC ARTHRITIS AND OSTEOMYELITIS

During the neonatal period and throughout infancy, the epiphyseal plate is traversed by multiple small transepiphyseal vessels that provide a direct communication between the articular space and the metaphysis of the long bones (Ogden and Lister, 1975). Thus, infection of a metaphyseal site can spread across the growth plate to penetrate the epiphysis. Because these perforating vessels disappear at approximately 1 year of age, osteomyelitis is usually not associated with septic arthritis in older infants and children. There are two possible exceptions: osteomyelitis of the proximal femur and of the humerus. Infection of the epiphyseal cartilage may rupture through the periosteum and enter the joint space, producing purulent arthritis. Because the capsular articulations of the hip and shoulder are permanent, osteomyelitis and septic arthritis may coexist, making the origin of infection difficult to establish. Because the inflammatory process of osteomyelitis or of septic arthritis can occupy the epiphyseal and metaphyseal sides of the growth plate, ischemia and necrosis of the plate may occur, resulting in permanent damage (Peters et al, 1992).

Etiology

Group B streptococcus, *S. aureus*, and coliform bacteria are the most common etiologic agents (Asmar, 1992; Frederiksen et al, 1993). Prematurity, antecedent trauma (most commonly originating from a heel stick for blood sampling but also from infected cephalohematomas) (Blom and Vreede, 1993), umbilical vessel catheterization, respiratory tract disease, and femoral venipunctures have been implicated in the pathogenesis of these infections in some infants.

Clinical Manifestations

Initial signs and symptoms are usually nonspecific. Most infants are not brought to medical attention until local signs such as swelling, irritability, and decreased motion of an extremity become apparent. Fever may be observed, but normal temperature is found in most cases (Morrissy, 1989). Physical examination reveals swelling, localized pain on palpation, and resistance to movement of the affected extremity. These signs may be obscured in the term infant by subcutaneous fat and normal joint contractions soon after birth (Morrissy, 1989). Localized heat and fluctuation are late findings.

Although blood cultures are frequently positive, clinically the infants usually do not appear septic. An exception is group A beta-hemolytic streptococcal infection, in which the infant appears gravely ill.

Diagnosis

Blood cultures should be obtained from all infants with suspected osteomyelitis or septic arthritis. Latex agglutination assays on urine or joint fluid for group B *streptococcus* or other pathogens should be obtained. In infants with septic arthritis, a percutaneous needle aspiration of intra-articular pus should be performed; in osteomyelitis, direct needle aspiration of the affected periosteum and bone is attempted. If pus is obtained, the material should be examined with Gram stain and cultured. Preliminary identification of the pathogen from stained smears is helpful in the selection of initial antimicrobial therapy.

In patients with suspected septic arthritis, radiographs may be normal or may show widening of the arterial space and capsular swelling. Later in the course of the disease, subluxation and destruction of the joint are common. Early in the course of osteomyelitis, the normal radiographic water markings of the deep tissues adjacent to the affected bone are obliterated, indicating inflammation (Mok et al, 1982). Lifting of the periosteum from the bone may also be observed, but cortical destruction is unusual before the 2nd week of illness, and new bone formation is a late finding. Resolution of bone changes is considerably slower than clinical improvement (Weissberg et al, 1974). Because of the multifocal nature of musculoskeletal sepsis in the newborn infants, compulsive, sequential examinations of other joints and bones must be undertaken in the affected child (Morrissy, 1989). Two types of bone scan may be useful, technetium phosphate and gallium scans (Morrissy, 1989). Technetium scans reveal areas of increased blood flow and new bone formation, whereas gallium scans identify areas of white blood cell accumulation. Because of the higher radiation dose to the patient from gallium scans, technetium scans are recommended for aiding in the identification of silent sites of infection despite their lack of specificity in the newborn infant because of the normally high epiphyseal blood flow, small imaging window, and motion artifact (Morrissy, 1989).

Therapy

Selection of initial antimicrobial therapy is based on results of the examination of stained smears of aspirated purulent material and on the presence of associated clinical findings such as furuncles or cellulitis. If gram-positive cocci are observed, the administration of oxacillin should be started. Either kanamycin or gentamicin is indicated if gram-negative organisms are noted. If no organisms are seen or if doubt exists regarding their identification, oxacillin plus gentamicin or kanamycin should be administered until results of the cultures are available. Direct instillation of an antibiotic into the joint space is unnecessary because most drugs penetrate the inflamed synovium, and adequate concentrations are achieved in purulent material (Nelson, 1971). This also applies to treatment of osteomyelitis; direct instillation of antibiotics into acutely inflamed bone is unwarranted.

As a general rule, infection of the joint space and bone should be drained either by repeated aspiration or by surgery. Septic arthritis of the hip and shoulder is treated best with incision and drainage in order to prevent vascular compromise or extension of infection into the metaphysis. Orthopedic consultation should be obtained for all patients.

Parenteral antimicrobial therapy of neonatal musculoskeletal bacterial infections is continued for a minimum of 3 weeks. The use of oral antibiotics as a substitute for parenteral therapy during the 2nd and 3rd weeks of therapy is unwise because of the lack of experience with this route of administration in newborns. In general, systemic symptoms appear within several days of initiating therapy, although local signs such as heat, erythema, and swelling may persist for 4 to 7 days. The decision to discontinue therapy should be predicated on lack of systemic symptoms, sterile blood and joint fluid cultures, and improvement in the affected bone or joint. Full range of motion may not return to the involved limb for several months. Because of this problem, physical therapy should be insti-

tuted early in illness to prevent contractures. Complete resolution of the radiographic changes may take several months.

Prognosis

Death resulting from these diseases is rare. However, morbidity caused by growth plate damage may be considerable, particularly when a weight-bearing joint such as the hip or knee is involved. Contractures, muscle damage, limb-shortening, and angular deformity may be permanent.

OPHTHALMIA NEONATORUM

High prevalence rates of sexually transmitted diseases among women in labor have been observed to correlate with a high incidence of gonococcal and chlamydial ophthalmia neonatorum. In a prospective study of 3117 infants born in Kikuyu, Kenya, from 1991 to 1993, *Chlamydia trachomatis* was present in 7.7% of all infants, *S. aureus* in 6.0%, and *Neisseria gonorrhoeae* in 0.8% (Isenberg et al, 1995). *N. gonorrhoeae* is acquired during passage through the infected birth canal when the mucous membranes come in contact with infected secretions. Infection usually becomes apparent within the first 5 days of life and is initially characterized by a clear, watery discharge, which rapidly becomes purulent. This is associated with marked conjunctival hyperemia and chemosis. Both eyes are usually involved but not necessarily to the same degree. Untreated gonococcal ophthalmia may extend to involve the cornea (keratitis) and the anterior chamber of the eye. This extension may result in corneal perforation and blindness. Until the introduction of adequate prophylactic measures, ophthalmia neonatorum was the most frequent cause of acquired blindness in the United States. Any infant presenting with a conjunctival discharge should have the material stained and cultured for gonococcus and other bacterial agents. Demonstration of gram-negative intracellular diplococci on a stained smear is an indication for immediate antibiotic therapy before definitive laboratory diagnosis is made.

Differential Diagnosis

Conjunctivitis occurring in the 1st days of life can be either chemical or bacterial in nature. Chemical irritants such as 1% silver nitrate cause transient conjunctival hyperemia and a watery discharge, but this is not associated with a purulent discharge. Common bacterial agents associated with conjunctivitis in newborns are *Haemophilus* species, *C. trachomatis*, *S. aureus*, *N. gonorrhoeae*, and *S. pneumoniae* (de Toledo and Chandler, 1992; O'Hara, 1993). It is important to determine the specific cause in order to select appropriate therapy and to prevent permanent sequelae. Viral conjunctivitis in a single nursery infant is unusual.

Conjunctivitis that occurs during the 2nd or 3rd week of life may be caused by viral or bacterial agents. Viral conjunctivitis is frequently associated with other symptoms of respiratory tract disease, such as rhinorrhea, cough, and sore throat, and several individuals in the family may have simultaneous disease. In general, the discharge in viral conjunctivitis is watery or mucopurulent but rarely purulent. Preauricular adenopathy is common. Staphylococci, streptococci, and occasionally, gonococci cause conjunctivitis in this age group. Study of a smear of the purulent material is helpful in differentiating these etiologic agents. However, the presence of bacteria on a gram-stained smear of material is not necessarily related etiologically to the conjunctivitis. Normal inhabitants of the skin and mucous membranes, such as staphylococci, diphtheroids, and *Neisseria catarrhalis* may be observed.

Conjunctivitis caused by *Chlamydia* (inclusion blennorrhea) is a venereally transmitted disease that is observed in infants 5 to 14 days of age (de Toledo and Chandler, 1992; O'Hara, 1993). Clinical manifestations vary from mild conjunctivitis to intense inflammation and swelling of the lids associated with copious purulent discharge. Pseudomembrane formation and a diffuse "matte" injection of the tarsal conjunctiva are common. The cornea is rarely affected, and preauricular adenopathy is unusual. In the early stages of the disease, one eye may appear more swollen and infected than the other, but both eyes are almost invariably involved. Diagnosis is made by scraping the tarsal conjunctiva and culturing the material (Sandstrom et al, 1984). In addition, the conjunctival scraping should also be examined for typical cytoplasmic inclusions within epithelial cells, using Giemsa stain (Sandstrom et al, 1984). These inclusions are seen on smears of purulent discharge, and cultures of the discharge yield various bacteria that are not related etiologically to the clinical disease. Use of polymerase chain reaction with primers directed against the gene that encodes its major outer membrane protein and *C. trachomatis*–specific cryptic plasmid DNA has been shown to be equally specific and more sensitive than McCoy cell culture for detection of *C. trachomatis* from ocular specimens (Talley et al, 1994). Without treatment, the acute inflammation continues for several weeks, merging into a subacute phase of slight conjunctival infection with scant purulent material. Occasionally, chronicity develops, and some cases persist for more than a year.

Therapy

Ophthalmia neonatorum caused by *N. gonorrhoeae* should be treated with parenteral antimicrobial therapy. Because of the increased prevalence of penicillin-resistant *N. gonorrhoeae*, empiric therapy should include a penicillinase-resistant antimicrobial, for example, ceftriaxone (25 to 50 mg/kg per day intravenously or intramuscularly) given once. If hyperbilirubinemia is present, cefotaxime (50 to 100 mg/kg per day intravenously or intramuscularly in two divided doses) for 7 days is an alternative. If the infecting organism is penicillin sensitive, Crystalline penicillin G should be administered intravenously or intramuscularly in a dose of 50,000 to 75,000 units/kg per day in two divided doses for infants younger than 1 week and in three divided doses for infants older than 1 week of age. The duration of parenteral therapy is 7 to 10 days. In addition to systemic antibiotic therapy, the eyes should be washed immediately and at frequent intervals with saline solution followed by topical administration of chloramphenicol or tetracycline. Initially, local saline irrigations are given every 1 to 2 hours, and

gradually the interval is increased to every 6 to 12 hours as clinical improvement is noted. Patients with ophthalmia neonatorum should be isolated, and strict hand-washing techniques should be used because of the highly contagious nature of the exudate. Conjunctivitis caused by other bacterial agents should be treated parenterally with the single most appropriate agent as judged by susceptibility testing of the organism. Because the most likely source of ophthalmia neonatorum is the maternal genitourinary tract, detection of *N. gonorrhoeae* or *C. trachomatis* should prompt evaluation and treatment of the infant's mother and her sexual partners.

Inclusion blennorrhea is treated with the topical administration of 10% sulfacetamide or 1% tetracycline ointment applied every 3 to 4 hours for approximately 14 days. Marked reduction in swelling and discharge is observed within 24 hours of therapy.

Ophthalmia neonatorum is preventable. Recently, several studies have evaluated the relative effectiveness of 1% silver nitrate solution, 1% tetracycline ointment, 0.5% erythromycin ointment, and 2.5% solution of povidone-iodine for prevention of ophthalmia neonatorum (Bell et al, 1993; Foster and Klauss, 1995; Isenberg et al, 1995; Laga et al, 1988). Although each of these interventions is effective, povidone-iodine has antiviral activity and elicits few toxic effects (Isenberg et al, 1995; Foster and Klauss, 1995). None of these treatments should be irrigated with saline because this may reduce efficacy. Ophthalmic ointments containing chloramphenicol are also effective prophylactic agents. Bacitracin ophthalmic ointment is not effective. Penicillin drops are effective and produce less conjunctivitis than does silver nitrate, but their routine use is not recommended because of the remote risk of sensitization to the drug (Hammerschlag, 1988).

CUTANEOUS INFECTIONS

The most common bacteria that cause skin infections during the neonatal period are *S. aureus* and groups A and B streptococci (Wooldridge, 1991). Disease caused by *S. aureus* can assume several clinical forms, the most common of which are pustular lesions. These tend to concentrate in the periumbilical and diaper areas and rarely become invasive except when extensive areas are involved or when the use of monitoring devices, catheters, or other invasive procedures are necessary in gravely ill infants. The study of a stained smear and a culture of an intact lesion are usually helpful in identifying the pathogen. The organisms should be phage-typed (they usually belong to Group I) so that if additional cases are encountered in the same nursery, these infants and others in the unit can be evaluated for the possibility of a nosocomial staphylococcal outbreak. If these infections are caused by the same phage type of staphylococci prompt measures should be instituted to determine the source of infection and to prevent further colonization and disease.

Therapy of cutaneous staphylococcal disease depends on the extent of the lesions and the general clinical condition of the infant. The physician can manage small isolated pustules through local care using a mild cleansing agent or an antiseptic such as hexachlorophene or povidone-iodine. Infants with more extensive cutaneous involvement, systemic signs of infection, or both should be given parenteral antimicrobial agents. A penicillinase-resistant penicillin should be used initially; continuation of this drug depends on the results of sensitivity testing.

The second form of neonatal staphylococcal disease has been previously described (see discussion of septicemia in this chapter) and is referred to as the expanded scalded-skin syndrome.

Group A and group B beta-hemolytic streptococci occasionally cause disease in the nursery (Dillon, 1966). The most common manifestation is a low-grade omphalitis characterized by a wet, malodorous umbilical stump with minimal inflammation. Disseminated disease occurs secondary to invasion of the bloodstream or by direct extension to the peritoneal cavity by way of the umbilical vessels. Identification of one infant with group A streptococcal disease in a nursery necessitates surveillance by culture of the other infants and of the personnel in the unit. The organism is usually introduced into the nursery by personnel or parents who have an asymptomatic nasopharyngeal infection. When a nursery outbreak is suspected, specific M- and T-typing of the organism is useful in defining the source and spread of infection. Group B streptococci have been associated with cellulitis, impetiginous lesions, and small abscesses in a few newborn infants. Penicillin is the drug of choice for streptococcal infections.

Necrotizing fasciitis is an unusual disease of newborn infants. This disease is frequently associated with surgical procedures, birth trauma, or cutaneous infection (Wilson and Haltalin, 1973). Staphylococci, either alone or associated with streptococci, are usually causative, but other bacteria, including gram-negative enteric bacilli, can be cultured. In this condition, subcutaneous tissues, including muscle layers, are invaded and the organism spreads along the fascial planes. Overlying skin may appear violaceous and is edematous, which imparts a thick "woody" sensation on palpation. The borders of the lesion are usually indistinct when compared with those seen with erysipelas, which are raised and easily palpated. Extensive surgery involving resection of destroyed tissue is imperative in treating necrotizing fasciitis. Blood and tissue cultures should be obtained, and oxacillin and gentamicin are the drugs of choice for initial therapy. Necrotic, fatty tissue may combine with calcium, resulting in tetany and convulsions.

Breast Abscess

Breast abscesses are most frequently encountered during the 2nd or 3rd weeks of life and occur more commonly in females. The disease does not occur in premature infants, presumably because of underdevelopment of the mammary gland in these infants. Bilateral disease is rare.

The major presentation of neonatal breast abscess is localized swelling with or without accompanying erythema and warmth. Systemic manifestations are uncommon, and only 25% of these infants have low-grade fever. *S. aureus* is the major pathogen; coliform bacteria and group B streptococci are also encountered (Brook, 1991). The diagnosis of breast abscess is best made by needle aspiration of the affected site. The single most important aspect of management is prompt incision and drainage by a skilled surgeon. Oxacillin should be administered for approxi-

mately 5 days during the period of drainage. Experience with this condition in Dallas indicates that antimicrobial therapy plays a secondary role to adequate drainage (Rudoy and Nelson, 1975). Long-term follow-up studies suggest that some girls have diminished breast tissue on the affected side.

NOSOCOMIAL BACTERIAL INFECTIONS

Hospital-acquired (nosocomial) infections have become a significant problem in most hospitals and may affect 2% to 5% of all hospitalized patients (Goldmann et al, 1983; Milliken et al, 1988). In nurseries, nosocomial bacterial infections are of particular importance because of the unusual susceptibility of small infants to severe illness. This applies both to routine, short-stay nurseries and to intensive care nurseries, in which babies are frequently intubated and placed on respirators and require monitoring or hyperalimentation by means of central catheters. In short-stay nurseries, problems are most frequently due to gram-positive organisms, such as *S. aureus* and streptococci (groups A and B). In intensive care nurseries, many organisms may pose a threat: *S. aureus*, especially strains that are resistant to several antibiotics, are important; *S. epidermis* is the most frequently encountered organism; gram-negative enteric bacilli are frequently a hazard and are similarly often resistant to antibiotics. Fungi, particularly *Candida albicans*, and respiratory viruses, such as respiratory syncytial virus, are also seen.

In neonatal intensive care units, surveys have shown that as many as 15% of infants hospitalized over 48 hours acquire nosocomial infections from their environment, many of them more than once (Hemming et al, 1976; Thompson et al, 1992). In one such survey, surface conditions accounted for 40% of the total of nosocomial infections; pneumonia for 29%; bacteremia for 14%; and surgical, urinary tract, and central nervous system infections for many of the remainder. Staphylococci and gram-negative enteric bacilli were responsible for more than 90% of these infections (Hemming et al, 1976). It has been shown that scrupulous attention to such matters as staff-to-patient ratios, nursery design, and containment principles can assist in minimizing the infection rate (Goldmann et al, 1981, 1983). The American Hospital Association urges every hospital to establish an infection control committee, the functions of which are as follow: (1) routine surveillance and education of personnel in principles of infection control, and (2) prompt recognition and control of a nosocomial infection when it occurs. All hospitals should appoint an infection control practitioner to supervise and coordinate the infection control and surveillance programs (Garner et al, 1988; Sprunt, 1988).

When an infectious disease caused by the same organism appears in several infants from the same nursery over a short period of time, a nosocomial outbreak should be suspected. The sick infants must be isolated and cultured to identify the pathogen. If a specific, single pathogen is responsible for the outbreak, epidemiologic investigations facilitate the process of determining the source and mode of transmission of the infection. Molecular epidemiologic methods, including restriction endonuclease digestion analysis of plasmid DNA, arbitrarily primed polymerase chain reaction, and ribotyping, have been useful in tracing origins of outbreaks of bacterial infections and evaluating effectiveness of eradication strategies (Alos et al, 1992; Back et al, 1993; Bialkowska-Hobrzanska et al, 1993; Fang et al, 1993; Patrick et al, 1992). It is probably best for the infection control practitioner and the nursery director to obtain expert microbiologic assistance in these instances. The investigation of each outbreak and the control procedures that are consequently recommended are often matters that require multidisciplinary planning and coordination.

Recent challenges for nursery infection control have included standardizing reporting of nosocomial infections in neonatal intensive care units and tracking nosocomial infections among normal newborn infants who have short lengths of stay. Gaynes and coworkers (1991) have used data from 35 hospitals from the National Nosocomial Infections Surveillance System to suggest that comparisons between neonatal intensive care units are complicated by the variable degree of illness acuity in different units. These authors suggest using device-associated nosocomial infection rates, that is, using device-days (those hospital days during which a device was required for the infant) as the denominator to control for the duration of exposure to this primary risk factor between neonatal intensive care units to provide more meaningful basis for interhospital comparison. Shortened length of stay in normal nurseries has prompted the development of self-administered questionnaires to monitor nosocomial infection rates in mothers and infants (Holbrook et al, 1991). This problem may also be addressed by information systems that link private pediatricians' offices to a central repository of patient information.

The following discussions of specific bacterial infections are intended to familiarize the reader with some of the more common nosocomial infections encountered in nurseries. This section is not designed to be an exhaustive review of each or all nosocomial bacterial infections.

Staphylococcal Infection

Phage group I *S. aureus* (phage types 29, 52, 52A, 79, and 80) caused significant hospital disease in the late 1950s and early 1960s. Disease ranging from pustules and omphalitis to pneumonia, septicemia, and meningitis occurred in newborns during this period. Although the majority of infants are colonized with the epidemic strain during a staphylococcal outbreak, disease occurs in only a small percentage of these infants. Epidemic disease caused by phage group I organisms is still an important problem in many nurseries. In some nurseries, the disease re-emerged after 3% hexachlorophene bathing was discontinued. Disease is apparently milder than it was in the 1960s, but it is still widespread.

Disease caused by phage group II *S. aureus* (phage types 3A, 3B, 3C, 55, and 71) in newborn and young infants has been encountered. Clinical manifestations caused by this organism have been broadly classified into the expanded scalded-skin syndrome (Melish and Glasgow, 1971). Nursery epidemics of bullous impetigo caused by group II staphylococci have been reported (Anthony et al, 1972). The source of one outbreak was a member of the nursery staff, who was a carrier of the organism, whereas

an infant reservoir of infection and a change in bathing technique may have contributed to the other outbreaks. Contamination of the circumcision site may be an additional source of such infections.

When staphylococcal disease occurs in a nursery, the extent of infection must first be determined. Using molecular epidemiologic analysis and traditional methods to isolate infected patients and eradicate colonization from patients and staff, such outbreaks can be terminated (Back et al, 1993; Fang et al, 1993). However, the importance of handwashing between patients and attention to institution-specific practices are critical to containment and analytic strategies.

Personnel who are carriers in an epidemic situation and are implicated in spread should be treated. Bacitracin ointment is smeared on the mucosa of the anterior nares three times a day and hexachlorophene showers and shampoos should be taken daily for 3 days. If possible, carriers should be kept away from work until they are free of the organism.

In short-stay nurseries, staphylococcal infections are often clinically apparent only several days after the infants are discharged. For this reason, some reporting system that includes infants requiring care after discharge is essential (Holbrook et al, 1991).

It is often necessary for the physician to take certain precautionary measures before microbiologic and molecular characterization of the outbreak is available. Selection of one or several measures necessary to control a nursery epidemic must be individualized (Sutherland, 1973). The measures commonly used are as follows:

1. Isolation of all infants colonized with virulent *Staphylococcus*. It is advisable to form a cohort system in the nursery for exposed but as yet noncolonized infants and for all new admissions to the nursery. These separate cohorts are cared for by separate nursery staff and are maintained until discharge of the infants. Infected infants are removed from the cohort and placed in isolation.
2. Enforcement of infection control techniques, such as gowning, limited access to the unit, and thorough hand-washing before and after handling each patient.
3. Use of antimicrobial agents. Topical antimicrobial therapy may be used for minor skin infections (pustules); parenteral antistaphylococcal therapy should be used for systemic staphylococcal diseases.
4. Initiation of routine bathing with antistaphylococcal cleaning agents such as 3% hexachlorophene (diluted 1:2 to 1:5) or application of triple dye to the umbilicus of all new admissions to the nursery.
5. If all else fails, closing of the nursery to further admissions until the problem either has been solved or spontaneously disappears.

After an outbreak is controlled, it is sometimes helpful to monitor the activity of staphylococci for a limited period of time by routine culturing of umbilical stumps and noses of infants on discharge from the nursery. Surveillance for clinical infections after discharge by sending postcards to families of affected infants is also helpful.

Bacterial Diarrhea

Any nursery infant with diarrhea should be suspected of having a potentially communicable disease and be treated accordingly. Hand-washing and other routine infection control procedures should be strongly enforced, and bacterial stool cultures should be obtained. If a bacterial pathogen is isolated, the baby in whom it is found should be moved to a special isolation area, if one is available, and given appropriate antimicrobial therapy. If watery stools develop in other infants, they should be cultured, placed in the same isolation room as the index infant, and appropriately treated. Culturing of asymptomatic babies and personnel is not always indicated but is appropriate if it is clear that simple isolation and treatment of symptomatic cases is not controlling an outbreak. Tracing nosocomial transmission of gram-negative infections has been facilitated by molecular characterization of the organisms involved (Alos et al, 1993; Verweij et al, 1993).

Group A Streptococcal Infection

Group A beta-hemolytic *streptococcus* was a common cause of puerperal and neonatal sepsis in the 1930s and early 1940s. With the advent of penicillin and its frequent use in maternity and nursery units, neonatal infections caused by this organism have become relatively uncommon. The primary source of group A streptococci in nursery outbreaks is either an attendant (nurse or physician) working in the unit or the mother. Once group A streptococci are introduced into a nursery, many infants become colonized but few develop clinical disease. The most common clinical manifestation is a low-grade, granulating omphalitis that fails to heal despite the administration of therapy. However, more significant disease may occur, including extensive cellulitis, septicemia, and meningitis.

Identification of one newborn with group A streptococcal infection is enough to warrant epidemiologic investigations of the nursery. All infants in close contact with the index case, a random sampling of other infants, and all nursery personnel should be cultured. Nasopharyngeal and umbilical cultures from infants and nasopharyngeal and rectal cultures from personnel should be obtained. Because nursery and maternity personnel are frequently interchangeable, the epidemiologic work-up should be coordinated with the obstetric service in the hospital.

Infants with streptococcal disease should be given aqueous or procaine penicillin G. During nosocomial outbreaks, all asymptomatic infants colonized with group A streptococci should receive penicillin. The prophylactic use of penicillin for all new admissions to the nursery may also be indicated. Benzathine penicillin G has been used effectively as prophylaxis against group A streptococcal infection in several nursery outbreaks.

Gram-Negative Infections

Since the early 1970s, a number of nursery outbreaks caused by specific gram-negative bacteria have been described, and virtually all have occurred in long-stay intensive care nurseries. Among the causative organisms were *K. pneumoniae, Flavobacterium meningosepticum, P. aeru-* *ginosa, Proteus mirabilis, Serratia marcescens,* and *E. coli.* A common feature of these outbreaks is that the majority of colonized infants are asymptomatic; those in whom disease develops usually have pneumonia, septicemia, or meningitis (Alos et al, 1993; Pegues et al, 1994; Verweij et al, 1993).

Infected fomites represent a common source of nursery outbreaks caused by gram-negative bacteria. Contaminated faucet aerators, sink traps and drains, suction equipment, bottled distilled water, cleansing solutions, humidification apparatus, and incubators have been incriminated (Javett et al, 1956). In addition, healthy colonized infants or nursery personnel may act as a source of infection because the organism is transmitted among infants by way of the hands or gowns of personnel. During epidemics, asymptomatic colonization of infants with the specific pathogen is variable, ranging from 0% to 90%.

The general approach to nursery outbreaks caused by gram-negative organisms is similar to that for epidemics of *S. aureus*. It is often helpful to use selective antibiotic-containing media for isolation of the organisms involved from carriers. In addition to the steps outlined in the discussion of staphylococcal outbreaks, the limitation or even prohibition of certain broad-spectrum antibiotics can contribute to long-term control of the problem.

REFERENCES

Abbott GD: Neonatal bacteriuria: A prospective study in 1,460 infants. BMJ 1:267, 1972.

ACOG: Group B streptococcal infections in pregnancy. Washington, DC: ACOG Technical Bulletin (No. 170), 1992.

Albritton WL, Wiggins GL, Feeley JC: Neonatal listeriosis: Distribution of serotypes in relation to age at onset of disease. J Pediatr 88:481, 1976.

Alexander JB, Giacoia GP: Early onset non-enterococcal group D streptococcal infection in the newborn infant. J Pediatr 92:489, 1978.

Alos JI, Lambert T, Courvalin P: Comparison of two molecular methods for tracing nosocomial transmission of *Escherichia coli* K1 in a neonatal unit. J Clin Microbiol 31:1704, 1993.

American Academy of Pediatrics: Guidelines for prevention of group B streptococcal infection by chemoprophylaxis. Pediatr 90:775, 1992.

American Academy of Pediatrics: *Escherichia coli* and other bacilli: Septicemia and meningitis in neonates. *In* Peter G (Ed): 1994 *Red Book: Report of the Committee on Infectious Diseases,* 23rd ed. Elk Grove Village, IL: American Academy of Pediatrics, 1994, p 184.

Anders JB, Lauer BA, Paisley JW: Campylobacter gastroenteritis in neonates. Am J Dis Child 135:900, 1981.

Anthony B, Giuliano D, Oh W: Nursery outbreak of staphylococcal scalded skin syndrome. Am J Dis Child 124:41, 1972.

Ashwal S, Perkin RM, Thompson JR, et al: Bacterial meningitis in children: Current concepts of neurologic management. Curr Prob Pediatr 24:267, 1994.

Asmar BI: Osteomyelitis in the neonate. Infect Dis Clin North Am 6:117, 1992.

Back NA, Linnemann CC Jr, Pfaller MA, et al: Recurrent epidemics caused by a single strain of erythromycin-resistant *Staphylococcus aureus*. The importance of molecular epidemiology. JAMA 270:1329, 1993.

Baker CJ: Group B streptococcal infection in newborns: Prevention at last? N Engl J Med 314:1702, 1986.

Baker CJ: Vaccine prevention of group B streptococcal disease. Pediatr Ann 22:711, 1993.

Baker CJ, Barrett FF: Transmission of group B streptococci to parturient women and their neonates. J Pediatr 83:919, 1973.

Baker CJ, Kasper DL: Correlation of maternal antibody deficiency with susceptibility to neonatal group B streptococcal infection. N Engl J Med 294:753, 1976.

Bartzokas CA, Paton JH, Gibson MF, et al: Control and eradication of methicillin-resistant *staphylococcus aureus* on a surgical unit. N Engl J Med 311:1422, 1984.

Battisti O, Mitchson R, Davies PA: Changing blood culture isolates in a referral neonatal intensive care unit. Arch Dis Child 56:775, 1981.

Bell AH, Brown D, Halliday HL, et al: Meningitis in the newborn—A 14 year review. Arch Dis Child 64:873, 1989.

Bell TA, Grayston JT, Krohn MA, Kronmal RA: Randomized trial of silver nitrate, erythromycin, and no eye prophylaxis for the prevention of conjunctivitis among newborns not at risk for gonococcal ophthalmitis. Pediatrics 92:755, 1993.

Bennhagen R, Svenningsen NW, Biekiassy AN: Changing pattern of neonatal meningitis in Sweden. A comparative study 1976 vs. 1983. Scand J Infect Dis 19:587, 1987.

Bergstrom T, Larson J, Lincoln K, Winberg J: Studies of urinary tract infections in infancy and childhood. J Pediatr 80:858, 1972.

Berman S: Otitis media in children. N Engl J Med 332:1560, 1995.

Bialkowska-Hobrzanska H, Jaskot D, Hammerberg O: Molecular characterization of the coagulase-negative staphylococcal surface flora of premature neonates. J Gen Microbiol 139:2939, 1993.

Bingen E, Denamur E, Lambert-Zechovsky N, et al: Mother-to-infant vertical transmission and cross-colonization of *Streptococcus pyogenes* confirmed by DNA restriction fragment length polymorphism analysis. J Infect Dis 165:147, 1992.

Blackmon LR, Alger LS, Crenshaw C Jr: Fetal and neonatal outcomes associated with premature rupture of the membranes. Clin Obstet Gynecol 29:779, 1986.

Bland RD: Otitis media in the first six weeks of life: Diagnosis, bacteriology and management. Pediatrics 49:187, 1972.

Blom NA, Vreede WB: Infected cephalhematomas associated with osteomyelitis, sepsis and meningitis. Pediatr Infect Dis J 12:1015, 1993.

Bonadio WA: Acute bacterial meningitis. Cerebrospinal fluid differential count. Clin Pediatr 27:445, 1988.

Borderon E, Desroches A, Tescher M, et al: Value of examination of the gastric aspirate for the diagnosis of neonatal infection. Biol Neonate 65:353, 1994.

Boyer KM, Gotoff SP: Prevention of early-onset neonatal group B streptococcal disease with selective intrapartum chemoprophylaxis. N Engl J Med 314:1665, 1986.

Brook I: The aerobic and anaerobic microbiology of neonatal breast abscess. Pediatr Infect Dis J 10:785, 1991.

Broughton RA, Krafka R, Baker CJ: Non-group D alpha-hemolytic streptococci, new neonatal pathogens. Pediatrics 99:450, 1981.

Bryant RE: Endocarditis and valve-ring abscess caused by *Staphylococcus epidermidis*—an opportunistic pathogen keeping pace with progress. Medical Grand Rounds 1:245, 1982.

Burton DM, Seid AB, Kearns DB, Pransky SM: Neonatal otitis media. An update. Arch Otolaryngol Head Neck Surg 119:672, 1993.

Busby MJ, Rodin AE: Relative contributions of Holmes and Semmelweis to the understanding of the etiology of puerperal fever. Tex Rep Biol Med 34:2, 1976.

Cairo MS: Cotokines: A new immunotherapy. Clin Perinatol 18:343, 1991.

Campognone P, Singer DB: Neonatal sepsis due to nontypeable *Haemophilus influenza*. Am J Dis Child 140:117, 1986.

Carlos CC, Ringertz S, Rylander M, et al: Nosocomial *Staphylococcus epidermidis* septicaemia among very low birth weight neonates in an intensive care unit. J Hosp Infect 19:201, 1991.

Casselbrant ML: Epidemiology of otitis media in infants and preschool children. Pediatr Infect Dis J 8:510, 1989.

Cates KL, Goetz C, Rosenberg N, et al: Longitudinal development of specific and functional antibody in very low birth weight premature infants. Pediatr Res 23:14, 1988.

Centers for Disease Control: Update: Foodborne listeriosis—United States, 1988–1990. MMWR Morb Mortal Wkly Rep 41:250, 1992.

Cherubin CE, Appleman MD, Heseltine PN, et al: Epidemiological spectrum and current treatment of listeriosis. Rev Infect Dis 13:1108, 1991.

Chow AW, Leake RD, Yamauchi T, et al: The significance of anaerobes in neonatal bacteremia, analysis of 23 cases and review of the literature. Pediatrics 54:736, 1974.

Christie C, Hammond J, Reising S, Evans-Patterson J: Clinical and molecular epidemiology of enterococcal bacteremia in a pediatric teaching hospital. J Pediatr 125:392, 1994.

Cohen MB: Etiology and mechanisms of acute infectious diarrhea in infants in the United States. J Pediatr 118:34, 1991.

Daucher JN, Mandell J, Lebowitz RL: Urinary tract infection in infants in spite of prenatal diagnosis of hydronephrosis. Pediatr Radiol 22:401, 1992.

Davies HD, Jones EL, Sheng RY, et al: Nosocomial urinary tract infections at a pediatric hospital. Pediatr Infect Dis J 11:349, 1992.

Derkay CS, Bluestone CD, Thompson AE, Katzdatske D: Otitis media in the pediatric intensive care unit: A prospective study. Otolaryngol Head Neck Surg 100:292, 1989.

de Toledo AR, Chandler JW: Conjunctivitis of the newborn. Infect Dis Clin North Am 6:807, 1992.

Dillon HC: Group A streptococcal infection in a newborn nursery. Am Dis Child 112:177, 1966.

Dodge PR: Neurological sequelae of acute bacterial meningitis. Pediatr Ann 23:101, 1994.

Eavey RD: Abnormalities of the neonatal ear: Otoscopic observations, histologic observations, and a model for contamination of the middle ear by cellular contents of amniotic fluid. Laryngoscope 103:1, 1993.

Edelman R: Prevention and treatment of infectious diarrhea. Speculations on the next 10 years. Am J Med 78:99, 1985.

Edwards MS, Rench MA, Haffar AAM, et al: Long-term sequelae of group B streptococcal meningitis in infants. J Pediatr 106:717, 1985.

Edwards MS, Kasper DL, Jennings JH, et al: Capsular sialic acid prevents activation of the alternative complement pathway by Type III, group B streptococci. J Immunol 128:1278, 1982.

Eisenfeld L, Etamocilla R, Wirtschafter D, et al: Systemic bacterial infections in neonatal deaths. Am J Dis Child 137:645, 1983.

el-Dahr SS, Lewy JE: Urinary tract obstruction and infection in the neonate. Clin Perinatol 19:213, 1992.

Escobar GJ, Zukin T, Usatin MS, et al: Early discontinuation of antibiotic treatment in newborns admitted to rule out sepsis: A decision rule. Pediatr Infect Dis J 13:860, 1994.

Evans ME, Schaffner W, Federspiel CF, et al: Sensitivity, specificity, and pediatric value of body surface cultures in a neonatal intensive care unit. JAMA 259:748, 1988.

Fang FC, McClelland M, Guiney DG, et al: Value of molecular epidemiologic analysis in a nosocomial methicillin-resistant *Staphylococcus aureus* outbreak. JAMA 270:1323, 1993.

Feigin RD, McCracken GH, Klein JO: Diagnosis and management of meningitis. Pediatr Infect Dis J 11:785, 1992.

Foster A, Klauss V: Ophthalmia neonatorum in developing countries. N Engl J Med 332:601 1995.

Franciosi RA, Knostman JD, Zimmerman RA: Group B streptococcal neonatal and infant infections. J Pediatr 83:707, 1973.

Franco SM, Cornelius VE, Andrews BF: Long-term outcome of neonatal meningitis. Am J Dis Child 146:567, 1992.

Frederiksen B, Christiansen P, Knudsen FU: Acute osteomyelitis and septic arthritis in the neonate, risk factors and outcome. Eur J Pediatr 152:577, 1993.

Frommell GT, Rothenberg R, Wang SP, McIntosh K: Chlamydial infections of mothers and infants. J Pediatr 95:28, 1979.

Garite TJ, Freeman RK: Chorioamnionitis in the preterm gestation. Obstet Gynecol 59:539, 1982.

Garner JS, Jarvis WR, Emori TG, et al: CDC definitions for nosocomial infections, 1988. Am J Infect Control 16:128, 1988.

Gaynes RP, Martone WJ, Culver DH, et al: Comparison of rates of nosocomial infections in neonatal intensive care units in the United States. National Nosocomial Infections Surveillance System. Am J Med 91:192, 1991.

Gellert GA, Ewert DP, Bendana N, et al: A cluster of coagulase-negative staphylococcal bacteremias associated with peripheral vascular catheter colonization in a neonatal intensive care unit. Am J Infect Control 21:16, 1993.

Gibbs RS, Romero R, Hillier SL, et al: A review of premature birth and subclinical infection. Am J Obstet Gynecol 166:1515, 1992.

Giebink GS: The microbiology of otitis media. Pediatr Infect Dis J 8:518, 1989.

Giebink GS, Canafax DM, Kempthorne J: Antimicrobial treatment of acute otitis media. J Pediatr 119:495, 1991.

Givner LB, Abramson JS, Wasilauskas B: Apparent increase in the incidence of invasive group A beta-hemolytic streptococcal disease in children. J Pediatrics 118:341, 1991.

Glass RI, Lew JF, Gangarosa RE, et al: Estimates of morbidity and mortality rates for diarrheal disease in American children. J Pediatr 118:27, 1991.

Goldmann DA, Durbin WA Jr, Freeman J: Nosocomial infections in a neonatal intensive care unit. J Infect Dis 144:449, 1981.

Goldmann DA, Freeman J, Durbin WA Jr: Nosocomial infection and death in a neonatal intensive care unit. J Infect Dis 147:635, 1983.

Goldmann DA, Leclair J, Macone, A: Bacterial colonization of neonates admitted to an intensive care environment. J Pediatr 93:288, 1978.

Goossens H, Kremp L, Boury R, et al: Nosocomial outbreak of *Campylobacter jejuni* meningitis in newborn infants. Lancet 2:146, 1986.

Gorbach SL: Bacterial diarrhoea and its treatment. Lancet 2:1378, 1987.

Gordon RC, Barrett FF, Clark DJ: Influence of several antibiotics, singly and in combination, on the growth of *Listeria monocytogenes*. J Pediatr 80:667, 1972.

Green PA, Singh KV, Murray BE, Baker CJ: Recurrent group B streptococcal infections in infants: Clinical and microbiologic aspects. J Pediatr 125:931, 1994.

Greenberg HB, Clark HF, Offit PA: Rotavirus pathology and pathophysiology. Curr Top Microbiol Immunol 185:255, 1994.

Grundmann H, Kropec A, Hartung D, et al: *Pseudomonas aeruginosa* in a neonatal intensive care unit: Reservoirs and ecology of the nosocomial pathogen. J Infect Dis 168:943, 1993.

Gruskay JA, Abbasi S, Anday E, et al: *Staphylococcus epidermidis*–associated enterocolitis. J Pediatr 109:520, 1986.

Gruskay J, Harris MC, Costarino AT, et al: Neonatal *Staphylococcus epidermidis* meningitis with unremarkable CSF examination results. Am J Dis Child 143:580, 1989.

Guerrant RL, Lohr JA, Williams EK: Acute infectious diarrhea. I. Epidemiology, etiology and pathogenesis. Pediatr Infect Dis 5:353, 1986.

Haffejee IE: Neonatal rotavirus infections. Rev Infect Dis 13:957, 1991.

Hammerschlag MR: Neonatal ocular prophylaxis. Pediatr Infect Dis J 7:81, 1988.

Hamoudi AC, Marcon MJ, Cannon HJ, McClead RE: Comparison of three major antigen detection methods for the diagnosis of group B streptococcal sepsis in neonates. Pediatr Infect Dis 2:432, 1983.

Han VKM, Sayed H, Chance GW, et al: An outbreak of *Clostridium difficile* necrotizing enterocolitis: A case for oral vancomycin therapy? Pediatrics 71:935, 1983.

Hargiss C, Larson E: The epidemiology of *Staphylococcus aureus* in a newborn nursery from 1970 through 1976. Pediatrics 61:348, 1978.

Harma P, Pericia M, Kuusela AL: Morbidity of very young infants with and without acute otitis media. Acta Otolaryngol 107:460, 1989.

Hemming VG, Overall JC Jr, Britt MR: Nosocomial infections in a newborn intensive-care unit: Results of forty-one months of surveillance. N Engl J Med 294:1310, 1976.

Hertelendy F, Romero R, Molnar M, et al: Cytokine-initiated signal transduction in human myometrial cells. Am J Repro Immunol 30:49, 1993.

Holbrook KF, Nottebart VF, Hameed SR, Platt R: Automated postdischarge surveillance for post partum and neonatal nosocomial infections. Am J Med 91:125, 1991.

Hristeva L, Bowler I, Booy R, et al: Value of cerebrospinal fluid examination in the diagnosis of meningitis in the newborn. Arch Dis Child 69:514, 1993.

Hudak AP, Lee SH, Issekutz AC, Bortolussi R: Comparison of three serological methods—enzyme-linked immunosorbent assay, complement fixation, and microagglutination—in the diagnosis of human perinatal *Listeria monocytogenes* infection. Clin Invest Med 7:349, 1984.

Huebner J, Pier GB, Maslow JN, et al: Endemic nosocomial transmission of *Staphylococcus epidermidis* bacteremia isolates in a neonatal intensive care unit over 10 years. J Infect Dis 169:526, 1994.

Isenberg SJ, Apt L, Wood M: A controlled trial of povidone-iodine as prophylaxis against ophthalmia neonatorum. N Engl J Med 332:562, 1995.

Ish-Horowicz MR, McIntyre P, Nade S: Bone and joint infections caused by multiply resistant *Staphylococcus aureus* in a neonatal intensive care unit. Pediatr Infect Dis J 11:82, 1992.

Issekutz TB, Evans J, Bortolussi R: The immune response of human neonates to *Listeria monocytogenes* infection. Clin Invest Med 7:281, 1984.

Jafari HS, McCracken GH Jr: Dexamethasone therapy in bacterial meningitis. Pediatr Ann 23:82, 1994.

Javett SN, Heymann S, Mundel B, et al: Myocarditis in the newborn infant. J Pediatr 48:1, 1956

Johnson GM, Lee DA, Regelmann WE, et al: Interference with granulocyte function by *Staphylococcus epidermidis* slime. Infect Immunol 54:12, 1986.

Jones EM, McCulloch SY, Reeves DS, MacGowan AP: A 10 year survey of the epidemiology and clinical aspects of listeriosis in a provincial English city. J Infect 29:91, 1994.

Kaijser B: *E. coli* O and K Antigens and Protective Antibodies in Relation to Urinary Tract Infection. Goteborg, Sweden, University of Goteborg Press, 1972.

Kaplan C: The placenta and viral infections. Semin Diag Pathol 10:232, 1993.

Karmali JA, Norrish B, Lior H, et al: *Campylobacter* enterocolitis in a neonatal nursery. J Infect Dis 149:874, 1984.

Kinney JS, Robertsen CM, Johnson KM, et al: Seasonal respiratory viral infections. Impact on infants with chronic lung disease following discharge from the neonatal intensive care unit. Arch Pediatr Adolesc Med 149:81, 1995.

Klein JO: Current concepts of infectious diseases in the newborn infant. Curr Probl Pediatr 31:405, 1984.

Klein JO, Feigin RD, McCracken GH: Report of the Task Force on Diagnosis and Management of Meningitis. Pediatr 78(Suppl):959, 1986.

Klein JO: Antimicrobial treatment and prevention of meningitis. Pediatr Ann 23:76, 1994.

Kozinn PJ, Taschdjian CL, Wiener H, et al: Neonatal candidiasis. Pediatr Clin North Am 5:803, 1958.

Krasinski K, Perkin R, Rutlege J: Gray baby syndrome revisited. Clin Pediatr 21:571, 1982.

Kumar SP, Delivoria-Papadopoulos M: Infections in newborn infants in a special care unit. A changing pattern of infection. Ann Clin Lab Sci 15:351, 1985.

Laga J, Plummer FA, Piot P, et al: Prophylaxis of gonococcal and chlamydial ophthalmia neonatorum. A comparison of silver nitrate and tetracycline. N Engl J Med 318:653, 1988.

Landau D, Turner ME, Brennan J, Majd M: The value of urinalysis in differentiating acute pyelonephritis from lower urinary tract infection in febrile infants. Pediatr Infect Dis J 13:777, 1994.

Lassiter HA, Wilson JL, Feldhoff RC, et al: Supplemental complement component C9 enhances the capacity of neonatal serum to kill multiple isolates of pathogenic *Escherichia coli*. Pediatr Res 35:389, 1994.

Lee EL, Robinson MJ, Thopng ML, et al: Intraventricular chemotherapy in neonatal meningitis. J Pediatr 91:991, 1977.

Lee SM, Knoppel E, van de Ven C, Cairo MS: Transcriptional rates of granulocyte-macrophage colony-stimulating factor, granulocyte colony-stimulating factor, interleukin-3, and macrophage colony-stimulating factor genes in activated cord versus adult mononuclear cells: Alteration in cytokine expression may be secondary to posttranscriptional instability. Pediatr Res 34:560, 1993.

Madoff LC, Paoletti LC, Tai JY, Kasper DL: Maternal immunization of mice with group B streptococcal type III polysaccharide-beta C protein conjugate elicits protective antibody to multiple serotypes. J Clin Invest 94:286, 1994.

Maisels MJ, Kring E: Risk of sepsis in newborns with severe hyperbilirubinemia. Pediatrics 90:741, 1992.

Manroe BL, Weinberg AG, Rosenfeld CR, Browne R: The neonatal blood count in health and disease. I. Reference values for neutrophilic cells. J Pediatr 95(1):89, 1979.

Marrie TJ, Costerton JW: Scanning and transmission electron microscopy of in situ bacterial colonization of intravenous and intraarterial catheters. J Clin Microbiol 19:687, 1984.

McCracken GH: Current management of bacterial meningitis in infants and children. Pediatr Infect Dis J 11:169, 1992.

McCracken GH, Mize SG: A controlled study of intrathecal antibiotic therapy in gram-negative enteric meningitis of infancy. Report of the Neonatal Meningitis Cooperative Study Group. J Pediatr 89:66, 1976.

McCracken, GH, Sarff LD, Glode, MP, et al: Relation between *Escherichia coli* K1 capsular polysaccharide antigen and clinical outcome of neonatal meningitis. Lancet 2:246, 1974.

McCracken GH Jr, Mize SG, Threlkeld N: Intraventricular gentamicin therapy in gram-negative bacillary meningitis of infancy: Report of the Second Neonatal Meningitis Cooperative Study Group. Lancet 1:787, 1980.

McCracken GH, Mustafa MM, Ramilo O, et al: Cerebrospinal fluid interleukin 1–beta and tumor necrosis factor concentrations and outcome from neonatal gram-negative enteric bacillary meningitis. Pediatr Infect Dis J 8:155, 1989.

Melish M, Glasgow L: Staphylococcus scalded skin syndrome: The expanded clinical syndrome. J Pediatr 78:958, 1971.

Melish M, Glasgow L, Turner M: The staphylococcal scalded-skin syndrome: Isolation and partial characterization of the exfoliatin toxin. J Infect Dis 125:129, 1972.

Milliken J, Tait GA, Ford-Jones L, et al: Nosocomial infections in a pediatric intensive care unit. Crit Care Med 16:233, 1988.

Mohle-Boetani JC, Schuchat A, Plikaytis BD, et al: Comparison of prevention strategies for neonatal group B streptococcal infection. A population-based economic analysis. JAMA 270:1442, 1993.

Mok PM, Reilly BJ, Ash JM: Osteomyelitis in the neonate. Clinical aspects and the role of radiography and scintigraphy in diagnosis and management. Radiology 145:677, 1982.

Molitt DL, Tepas JJ, Talbert JL: The role of coagulase-negative *Staphylococcus* in neonatal necrotizing enterocolitis. J Pediatr Surg 23:60, 1988.

Morrissy RT: Bone and joint infection in the neonate. Pediatr Ann 18:33, 1989.

Mustafa MM, Mertsola J, Ramko O, et al: Increased endotoxin and interleukin-1–beta concentrations in cerebrospinal fluid of infants with coliform meningitis and ventriculitis associated with intraventricular gentamicin therapy. J Infect Dis 160:891, 1989.

Myers JP, Linnemann CC: Bacteremia due to methicillin-resistant *Staphylococcus aureus*. J Infect Dis 145:532, 1982.

Nelson J: Antibiotic concentrations in septic joint effusions. N Engl J Med 284:349, 1971a.

Nelson JD: Duration of neomycin therapy for enteropathogenic *Escherichia coli* diarrheal disease. Pediatrics 48:248, 1971b.

Noel GJ, Kreiswirth BN, Edelson PJ, et al: Multiple methicillin-resistant *Staphylococcus aureus* strains as a cause for a single outbreak of severe disease in hospitalized neonates. Pediatr Infect Dis J 11:184, 1992.

Noya FJD, Baker CJ: Prevention of group B streptococcal infection. Pediatr Infect 6:41, 1992.

Ogden JA, Lister G: The pathology of neonatal osteomyelitis. Pediatrics 55:474, 1975.

O'Hara MA: Ophthalmia neonatorum. Pediatr Clin North Am 40:715, 1993.

Odio CM, Faingezicht I, Paris M, et al: The beneficial effects of early dexamethasone administration in infants and children with bacterial meningitis. N Engl J Med 324:1525, 1991.

Ohman L, Tullus K, Katouli M, et al: Correlation between susceptibility of infants to infections and interaction with neutrophils of *Escherichia coli* strains causing neonatal and infantile septicemia. J Infect Dis 171:128, 1995.

Paisley JW, Lauer BA: Pediatric blood cultures. Clin Lab Med 14:17, 1994.

Panaro NR, Lutwick LI, Chapnick EK: Intrapartum transmission of group A streptococcus. Clin Infect Dis 17:79, 1993.

Patrick CH, John JF, Levkoff AH, Atkins LM: Relatedness of strains of methicillin-resistant coagulase-negative *Staphylococcus* colonizing hospital personnel and producing bacteremias in a neonatal intensive care unit. Pediatr Infect Dis J 11:935, 1992.

Pegues DA, Arathoon EG, Samayoa B, et al: Epidemic gram-negative bacteremia in a neonatal intensive care unit in Guatemala. Am J Infect Control 22:163, 1994.

Peter G, Nelson JS: Factors affecting neonatal *E. coli* K1 rectal colonization. J Pediatr 93:866, 1978.

Peters W, Irving J, Letts M: Long-term effects of neonatal bone and joint infection on adjacent growth plates. J Pediatr Orthop 12:806, 1992.

Philip AGS: Decreased use of antibiotics using a neonatal sepsis screening technique. J Pediatr 98:795, 1981.

Philip AGS, Hewitt JR: Early diagnosis of neonatal sepsis. Pediatrics 65:1036, 1980.

Polin RA, St Geme JW III: Neonatal sepsis. Adv Pediatr Infect Dis 7:25, 1992.

Polk DB, Steele RW: Bacterial meningitis progressing with normal cerebrospinal fluid. Pediatr Infect Dis J 6:1040, 1987.

Pourcyrous M, Bada HS, Korones SB, et al: Significance of serial C-reactive protein responses in neonatal infection and other disorders. Pediatrics 92:431, 1993.

Reboli AC, John JF Jr, Levkoff AH: Epidemic methicillin-gentamicin-resistant *Staphylococcus aureus* in a neonatal intensive care unit. Am J Dis Child 143:34, 1989.

Rench MA, Baker CJ: Neonatal sepsis caused by a new group B streptococcal serotype. J Pediatr 122:638, 1993.

Rennels MB, Levine MM: Classical bacterial diarrhea: Perspectives and update—*Salmonella*, *Shigella*, *Escherichia coli*, *Aeromonas*, and *Pseudomonas*. Pediatr Infect Dis J (1 Suppl):S91, 1986.

Rhodes KH, Henry NK: Antibiotic therapy for severe infections in infants and children. Mayo Clin Proc 67:59, 1992.

Robbins JB, McCracken GH, Gotschlich EC, et al: *Escherichia coli* K1 capsular polysaccharide associated with neonatal meningitis. N Engl J Med 290:1216, 1974.

Robins-Browne RM: Traditional enteropathogenic *Escherichia coli* of infantile diarrhea. Rev Infect Dis 9:28, 1987.

Rodwell RL, Leslie AL, Tudehope DI: Early diagnosis of neonatal sepsis using a hematologic scoring system. J Pediatr 112:176, 1988.

Romero R, Yoon BH, Kenny JS, et al: Amniotic fluid interleukin-6 determinations are of diagnostic and prognostic value in preterm labor. Am J Repro Immunol 30:167, 1993.

Romero R, Sibai B, Caritis S, et al: Antibiotic treatment of preterm labor with intact membranes: A multicenter, randomized, double-blinded, placebo-controlled trial. Am J Obstet Gynecol 169:764, 1993b.

Romero R, Gomez R, Glasso M, et al: Macrophage inflammatory protein-1 alpha in term and preterm parturition: Effect of microbial invasion of this amniotic cavity. Am J Repro Immunol 32:108, 1994a.

Romero R, Mazor M, Munoz H, et al: The preterm labor syndrome. Ann N Y Acad Sci 734:414, 1994b.

Roos KL, Scheld WM: The management of fulminant meningitis in the intensive care unit. Infect Dis Clin North Am 3:137, 1989.

Rubin RH, Weinstein L: Salmonellosis, Microbiologic, Pathologic and Clinical Features. New York, Stratton Intercontinental Medical Book, 1977.

Rudoy RC, Nelson JD: Breast abscess during the neonatal period: A review. Am J Dis Child 129:1931, 1975.

Saez-Llorens X, Jafari HS, Severien C, et al: Enhanced attenuation of meningeal inflammation and brain edema by concomitant administration of anti-CD18 monoclonal antibodies and dexamethasone in experimental *Haemophilus meningitis*. J Clin Invest 88:2003, 1991.

Saez-Llorens X, McCracken GH Jr: Sepals syndrome and septic shock in pediatrics: Current concepts of terminology, pathophysiology, and management. J Pediatr 123:497, 1993.

Sandstrom KI, Bell TA, Chandler JW, et al: Microbial causes of neonatal conjunctivitis. J Pediatr 105:706, 1984.

Saravolatz LD, Markowitz N, Arking L: Methicillin-resistant *Staphylococcus aureus*. Epidemiologic observations during a community-acquired outbreak. Ann Intern Med 96:11, 1982.

Sarff LD, McCracken GH, Schiffer MS, et al: Epidemiology of *Escherichia coli* K1 in healthy and diseased newborns. Lancet 1:1099, 1975.

Sartor O, Anday E: *Campylobacter jejuni* enteritis in a premature neonate. South Med J 80:1593, 1987.

Schaad UB, McCracken GH Jr, Nelson JD: Clinical pharmacology and efficacy of vancomycin in pediatric patients. J Pediatr 96:119, 1980.

Schibler KR, Liechty KW, White WL, Christensen RD: Production of granulocyte colony-stimulating factor in vitro by monocytes from preterm and term neonates. Blood 82:2478, 1993.

Schlech WF III, Lavigne PM, Bortolussi RA, et al: Epidemic listeriosis—Evidence for transmission by food. N Engl J Med 308:202, 1982.

Shaio MF, Yang KD, Bohnsack JF, Hill HR: Effect of immune globulin intravenous on opsonization of bacterial by classic and alternative complement pathways in premature sepsis. Pediatr Res 25:634, 1989.

Shattuck KE, Chonmaitree T: The changing spectrum of neonatal meningitis over a fifteen-year period. Clin Pediatr 31:130, 1992.

Siegel JD, McCracken GH Jr: Group D streptococcal infections. J Pediatr 93:542, 1978.

Siegel JD, McCracken GH Jr: Sepsis neonatorum. N Engl J Med 304:642, 1981.

Siegel JD, McCracken GH Jr, Threlkeld N, et al: Single-dose penicillin prophylaxis against neonatal group B streptococcal infections: A controlled trial in 18,738 newborn infants. N Engl J Med 303:769, 1980.

Siitonen A, Takala A, Ratiner YA, et al: Invasive *Escherichia coli* infections in children: Bacterial characteristics in different age groups and clinical entities. Pediatr Infect Dis J 12:606, 1993.

Smellie JM, Edwards D, Normand ICS, et al: Effect of VUR on renal growth in children with urinary tract infection. Arch Dis Child 56:593, 1981.

Snowe R, Wilfert C: Epidemic reappearance of gonococcal ophthalmia neonatorum. Pediatrics 51:110, 1973.

Spigelblatt L, Saintonge J, Chicoine R, Laverdiere M: Changing pattern of neonatal streptococcal septicemia. Pediatr Infect Dis 4:56, 1985.

Sprunt K: Practical use of surveillance for prevention of nosocomial infection. Semin Perinatol 9:47, 1985.

Squire EN Jr, Reich HM, Merenstein GB, et al: Criteria for the discontinuation of antibiotic therapy during presumptive treatment of suspected neonatal infection. Pediatr Infect Dis 1:85, 1982.

St Geme JW: Nontypeable *Haemophilus influenzae* disease: Epidemiology, pathogenesis, and prospects for prevention. Infect Agents Dis 2:1, 1993.

St Geme JW, Harris MC: Coagulase-negative staphylococcal infection in the neonate. Clin Perinatol 18:281, 1991.

Storch GA, Rajagopalan L: Methicillin-resistant *Staphylococcus auerus* bacteremia in children. Pediatr Infect Dis 5:59, 1986.

Sutherland J: Comment. Pediatrics 51(suppl):351, 1973.

Synnott MB, Morse DL, Hall SM: Neonatal meningitis in England and Wales: A review of routine national data. Arch Dis Child 71:75, 1994.

Talley AR, Garcia-Ferrer F, Laycock KA, et al: Comparative diagnosis of neonatal chlamydial conjunctivitis by polymerase chain reaction and McCoy cell culture. Am J Ophthalmol 117:50, 1994.

Tan TQ, Mason EO Jr, Ou CN, Kaplan SL: Use of intravenous rifampin in neonates with persistent staphylococcal bacteria. Antimicrob Agents Chemother 37:2401, 1993.

Tan TQ, Musser JM, Shulman RJ, et al: Molecular epidemiology of coagulase-negative *Staphylococcus* blood isolates from neonates with persistent bacteremia and children with central venous catheter infections. J Infect Dis 169:1393, 1994.

Taylor DN, Echeverria P: Diarrhoeal disease: Current concepts and future challenges. Molecular biological approaches to the epidemiology of diarrhoeal diseases in developing countries. Trans R Soc Trop Med Hyg 87:3, 1993.

Teberg AJ, Yonekura ML, Salminen C, Pavlova I: Clinical manifestations of epidemic neonatal listeriosis. Pediatr Infect Dis J 6:817, 1987.

Thompson PJ, Greenough A, Hird MF, et al: Nosocomial bacterial infections in very low birth weight infants. Eur J Pediatr 151:451, 1992.

Thompson RL, Wenzel RP: International recognition of methicillin-resistant strains of *Staphylococcus aureus*. Ann Intern Med 97:925, 1982.

Torphy DE, Bond WW: *Campylobacter fetus* infections in children. Pediatrics 64:898, 1979.

Tullus K, Burman LG: Ecological impact of ampicillin and cefuroxime in neonatal units. Lancet 1:1405, 1989.

Unhanand M, Mustafa MM, McCracken GH Jr, Nelson JD: Gram-negative enteric bacillary meningitis: A twenty-one–year experience. J Pediatr 122:15, 1993.

Velasco S, Tarlo M, Olsen K, et al: Temperature-dependent modulation of lipopolysaccharide-induced interleukin-1 beta and tumor necrosis factor alpha expression in cultured human astroglial cells by dexamethasone and indomethacin. J Clin Invest 87:1674, 1991.

Verweij PE, Geven WB, van Belkum A, Meis JF: Cross-infection with *Pseudomonas aeruginosa* in a neonatal intensive care unit characterized by polymerase chain reaction fingerprinting. Pediatr Infect Dis J 12:1027, 1993.

Visintine AM, Oleske JM, Nahmias AJ: *Listeria monocytogenes* infection in infants and children. Am J Dis Child 131:393, 1977.

Wallace RJ, Baker CJ, Quinones FJ, et al: Non-typeable *Haemophilus influenzae* (Biotype 4) as a neonatal, maternal, and genital pathogen. Rev Infect Dis 5:123, 1983.

Wanger AR, Morris SL, Ericsson C, et al: Latex agglutination-negative methicillin-resistant *Staphylococcus aureus* recovered from neonates: Epidemiologic features and comparison of typing methods. J Clin Microbiol 30:2583, 1992.

Warren WS, Stool SE: Otitis media in low-birth-weight infants. J Pediatr 79:740, 1971.

Weissberg ED, Smith AL, Smith DH: Clinical features of neonatal osteomyelitis. Pediatrics 53:505, 1974.

Wheeler MC, Roe MH, Kaplan EL, et al: Outbreak of group A streptococcus septicemia in children. Clinical, epidemiologic and microbiological correlates. JAMA 266:533, 1991.

Williams EK, Lohr JA, Guerrant RL: Acute infectious diarrhea. II. Diagnosis, treatment and prevention. Pediatr Infect Dis 5:458, 1986.

Williams PA, Bohnsack JF, Augustine NH, et al: Production of tumor necrosis factor by human cells in vitro and in vivo, induced by group B streptococci. J Pediatr 123:292, 1993.

Wilson HD, Haltalin K: Acute necrotizing fasciitis in childhood. Am J Dis Child 125:591, 1973.

Wiswell TE, Roscelli JD: Corroborative evidence for the decreased incidence of urinary tract infections in circumcised male infants. Pediatrics 78:96, 1986.

Wooldridge WE: Managing skin infections in children. Postgrad Med 89:109, 1991.

Yagupsky P, Menegus MA, Powell KR: The changing spectrum of group B streptococcal disease in infants: An eleven-year experience in a tertiary care hospital. Pediatr Infect Dis J 10:801, 1991.

Yow MD, Mason ED, Leeds LJ, et al: Ampicillin prevents intrapartum transmission of group B streptococci. JAMA 241:1245, 1979.

Zangwill KM, Schuchat A, Wenger JD, et al: Group B streptococcal disease in the United States, 1990; Report from a multistate active surveillance system. MMWR Morb Mortal Wkly Rep 41:25, 1992.

CHAPTER 44

Other Specific Bacterial Infections

F. Sessions Cole

The bacterial infections discussed in this chapter have been chosen chiefly because their manifestations in the neonatal period differ in some respects from those of later life.

TUBERCULOSIS

In 1925, Debre and LeLong demonstrated convincingly that tuberculosis is, in most instances, not inherited but is acquired by contact. They separated newborn infants from their tuberculous mothers immediately and, in a large series, found that none of the offspring had been infected. Similarly, Ratner and coworkers (1951), carefully reviewing 260 infants born to mothers with tuberculosis, found not one case of congenital tuberculosis, even though 39 of the mothers died of the disease shortly after delivery. There are nevertheless several examples of newborns dying of tuberculosis so early that intrauterine infection must be accepted as the only possible mode of origin. In others, in whom evidence of illness became manifest somewhat later, even though mother and child had been separated promptly after delivery, it appears likely that infection was acquired during birth by inhalation of infected amniotic fluid or vaginal secretions.

Incidence

Because of a 41% increase in the number of cases of tuberculosis among women of child-bearing age in the United States between 1985 and 1992, the risk of congenital tuberculosis has increased during the 1990s (Cantwell et al, 1994; Margono et al, 1994; Vallejo and Starke, 1992). The human immunodeficiency virus (HIV) epidemic among reproductive age women has contributed to this increased risk (Barnes et al, 1991; Jones et al, 1992). The staggering magnitude of the global tuberculosis problem (in 1990, tuberculosis developed in an estimated 8 million people, and 2.6 to 2.9 million people died) coupled with increasing travel, international adoption, and denial of non-emergency medical treatment to undocumented or illegal aliens has further increased the risk of congenital tuberculosis (Iseman and Starke, 1995; Johnson et al, 1992; McKenna et al, 1995; Sudre et al, 1992). In the English language literature between 1985 and 1994, 29 cases of congenital tuberculosis were reported, with the most recent cases in the United States occurring in 1982 and then again in 1994 (Cantwell et al, 1994). Before this review, Hageman and coworkers (1980) reviewed 26 cases of neonatal tuberculosis acquired either in utero or perinatally, all dating from after the time when isoniazid was first introduced. Beitzke (1948) laid down certain criteria for congenital tuberculosis infection, which have recently been revised (Cantwell et al, 1994). These revised criteria for the diagnosis of congenital tuberculosis include proved tuberculous

lesions and at least one of the following: (1) lesions in the first week of life, (2) a primary hepatic complex or caseating hepatic granulomas, (3) tuberculous infection of the placenta or the maternal genital tract, or (4) exclusion of the possibility of postnatal transmission by a thorough investigation of contacts, including the infant's hospital attendants, and by adherence to existing recommendations for treatment for infants exposed to tuberculosis (Cantwell et al, 1994).

Pathology

Hematogenous infection is manifested by enlargement and caseation of the glands at the porta hepatis plus disseminated tubercles throughout the liver, comprising the primary complex. In addition, tubercles are scattered through the lungs and spleen and other viscera; the serous surfaces often are studded with them, and their cavities contain clear yellow fluid. Brain and meninges may be similarly involved. When lesions are most prominent in the lungs and a primary complex cannot be found in and about the liver, it is possible that the disease originated from inhalation of infected amniotic fluid or vaginal secretions at or shortly before delivery. Aspiration of infected material accounts for approximately 50% of the reported cases of congenital tuberculosis, and hematogenous spread accounts for the remaining 50% (Cantwell et al, 1994). The tubercles belong to the Rich category of soft tubercles showing local necrosis with little cellular reaction, indicating overwhelming infection with little host resistance. Almost 50% of the placentae of tuberculous mothers contain acid-fast bacilli, while congenital (i.e., antenatal) infection is rare (Bate et al, 1986).

Diagnosis

Suspicion and recognition are imperative in this disease: more than 50% of cases of progressive primary and acute miliary tuberculosis in infants without proper treatment are fatal (Raucher and Gribetz, 1986). Infants whose disease was acquired in utero may be ill at birth or may develop normally until fever, lethargy, hepatomegaly, and other signs or symptoms occur at several days to several weeks of life. The infection may be sudden and overwhelming or insidious and prolonged. Symptoms are typically nonspecific: poor feeding, listlessness, fever, hepatosplenomegaly, lymphadenopathy, and later, respiratory distress, with a median age at presentation of 24 days (range 1 to 84) (Cantwell et al, 1994). Because the liver is the primary site of bacterial replication, the chest radiograph is often normal until late in the disease course at which time the pattern of involvement is often miliary. Skin lesions (erythematous papules) may be seen.

To determine the specific diagnosis, one must find organisms either in biopsy tissue—liver, lymph nodes, bone marrow (usually not skin lesions)—or in tracheal or gastric aspirates. Acid-fast stains of such materials, even of gastric aspirates, are helpful. The cerebrospinal fluid, although often abnormal, infrequently yields organisms on culture. The presence of granulomas in microscopic sections of biopsy material is also a useful finding, but they are also seen in other neonatal diseases, such as listeriosis. The tuberculin test is rarely positive early in the disease, but may become so later. Presence of demonstrated infection and disease in the mother is often the clue that leads to the correct diagnosis of tuberculosis in the child.

Management

Modern management of neonatal tuberculosis must begin with identification and treatment of the pregnant woman with tuberculosis (Raucher and Gribetz, 1986). The first priority must be prevention of transmission to the fetus and newborn. First, all pregnant women with a history of tuberculosis or with a positive tuberculin skin test should be thoroughly evaluated. In addition, all regular household contacts should be evaluated. The evaluation should include history of exposure to tuberculosis, results of previous skin tests and chest radiographs, previous antituberculous chemotherapy (including agents used, dosage, and duration), prior vaccination with bacille Calmette-Guérin (BCG), results of a recent intradermal Mantoux test, a recent chest radiograph (taken with proper shielding), and results of sputum or gastric aspirate with acid-fast stains and cultures (Raucher and Gribetz, 1986).

The Pregnant Woman with Tuberculous Disease

Once cultures have been obtained, the pregnant woman with active tuberculosis should be started immediately on antituberculous chemotherapy, regardless of stage of pregnancy (Raucher and Gribetz, 1986). The agents to be considered include isoniazid (INH), rifampin, and ethambutol. Although concern about fetal effects of the drugs restricted their use during pregnancy in the past, considerable experience currently suggests their safety. Women with adequately treated tuberculosis are unlikely to infect their infants; however, any clinical suggestion of active disease should prompt acquisition of smears and cultures and reinstitution of therapy. The infant should have a Mantoux test at 2 and 6 months of age.

Conversion of skin reactivity from negative to positive within the past 2 years should prompt initiation of chemotherapy. If the chest radiograph is normal, unchanged, or shows a healed primary complex, INH can be used alone. If the radiograph is abnormal or progressive disease is evident, INH plus ethambutol or rifampin should be started.

Women whose skin tests were positive in the distant past and who are younger than 35 years of age, are asymptomatic, and have never received antituberculous therapy should be given INH before delivery (Raucher and Gribetz, 1986). Regardless of age, women who have a positive skin test, an abnormal chest radiograph (other than a healed Ghon complex or calcifications), or who have close contact with individuals who have active tuberculosis should receive INH preventive therapy.

Congenital Tuberculosis

If the mother has *miliary* disease, untreated in the last part of pregnancy, the infant is at greatest risk of having congenital tuberculosis. The mortality rate among infants with congenital tuberculosis is estimated at 38% overall and 22% among infants who received chemotherapy (Cantwell et al, 1994). Such an infant deserves careful clinical evaluation, including a chest film, smear and culture of gastric washings and urine, examination and culture of the spinal fluid, and drug sensitivities determined on any organism recovered (Bate et al, 1986). The tuberculin test may not become positive for approximately 3 to 5 weeks or longer in such an infant, so reliance on a negative test is unwarranted. The necessity of separating the infant from the mother, who would be hospitalized, is obvious, and institution of INH, 10 mg/kg per day, is appropriate in the absence of manifest disease. The infant with manifest disease should receive INH (10 to 15 mg/kg per day), rifampin (10 to 20 mg/kg per day), pyrazinamide (15 to 30 mg/kg per day), and either streptomycin (20 to 30 mg/kg per day) or ethambutol (15 to 25 mg/kg per day) for the first 2 months, followed by INH and rifampin for 4 to 10 months depending on the severity of disease (Cantwell et al, 1994). If less than 4% of endemic *Mycobacterium tuberculosis* are resistant to INH, three-drug regimens are acceptable as initial treatment (Cantwell et al, 1994). Rifampin appears to have no unusual toxicities in this age group other than the well-recognized occasional problems of hepatotoxicity and allergy.

A study by Escobar and associates (1975) from Cali, Colombia, demonstrates the efficacy of prednisone at 1 mg/kg per day in infants with tuberculous meningitis for the first 30 days of illness. Prednisone therapy should not be initiated until adequate blood levels of antituberculous drugs are achieved, presumably after approximately 48 hours of initiating treatment.

Infant of a Mother on Therapy for Pulmonary Tuberculosis

If the mother is sputum-positive for tuberculosis, the risk to the infant is greater than if the mother was on treatment for at least 2 weeks and is sputum-negative. It seems reasonable to separate the infant from the mother and other family contacts with active tuberculosis as long as they remain sputum-positive. Once the mother's sputum and sputum of family contacts have converted to negative and all are known to be taking medication regularly, separation from the infant is not necessary. Such an infant remains at greater risk than normal, in part because of the likelihood of other unidentified cases of tuberculosis in the environment. The infant should be given prophylactic treatment with INH for 3 months after a chest radiograph and Mantoux test. If the results of the infant's skin test are negative at 3 months of age, therapy may be discontinued.

When compliance with INH administration and follow-up appointments is uncertain, BCG vaccine should be given to the infant (Raucher and Gribetz, 1986). Because of the low frequency of INH-resistant strains in the United States and the concern that INH may decrease efficacy of standard BCG vaccines, separation of the infant from infected family members is recommended until the infant's Mantoux test becomes positive. In hyperendemic areas of developing countries, BCG vaccination is a reasonable intervention. Breast-feeding may be initiated when the need for isolation has passed.

Infant of a Mother with Treated Tuberculosis

The possibility of relapse in the mother is greatest if her disease was arrested for less than 5 years. Since the risk to the infant of a mother with inactive tuberculosis depends on her likelihood of reactivation, careful and frequent examinations of the mother are essential. Indeed, a tuberculin test in all women during pregnancy and at the time of delivery is desirable. A postpartum chest film, one at 3 months, and another at 6 months are indicated in tuberculin-positive mothers. The infant should have a tuberculin test with 5 T.U. (0.1 mL intermediate PPD, or 0.0001 mg) at birth and a chest radiograph. The infant should receive INH prophylaxis until the Mantoux test is negative at 3 months of age and there are no clinical signs of disease (Nakajo et al, 1989). Two drugs (INH and rifampin) should be used if active disease is observed in the infant.

Role of Bacille Calmette-Guérin Vaccine

The arguments for using BCG vaccine are based in part on the experience gained from its wide use in many countries with a very low incidence of subsequent tuberculosis and minimal complications (Centers for Disease Control and Prevention, 1988). One study relevant to its role in newborns from tuberculosis households included 231 vaccinated by multiple puncture techniques and 220 control infants studied over a period of 19 years (Rosenthal et al, 1961). The infants were returned to their respective homes only if the source case was "closed." Even so, the infectivity rate in the nonvaccinated controls was 36.5% at 1 year, suggesting that the state of infectiousness of an adult cannot always be ascertained with accuracy. The results of the Rosenthal study showed that there were three cases of tuberculosis among the 231 vaccinated infants, and 11 cases among the 220 control subjects. The control subjects included four deaths and four cases of miliary disease or meningitis; no deaths or disseminated disease occurred among the vaccinated. More studies in Thailand and Canada have confirmed the benefits of BCG immunization (Chavalittamrong et al, 1986; Young and Hershfield, 1986). The strongest argument for BCG vaccination is the advantage gained from its being given at one time instead of daily, as with chemoprophylaxis. However, because protection against tuberculous infection after BCG immunization requires development of delayed hypersensitivity over approximately 6 weeks, separation from individuals with active disease has been advocated (Raucher and Gribetz, 1986). Kendig and Chernick (1977) advocate the two-site method of BCG immunization, giving the material in two sites of the deltoid at the same time.

Not all trials have demonstrated the protective effect found in Rosenthal's study, and there are many who doubt the usefulness of BCG (CDC, 1996). Its efficacy varies in part because of different potencies of the antigen and variations in the physiologic state of the host, especially perinatal nutritional state and feeding method (formula versus breast) (Grindulis et al, 1984; Ormerod and Garnett, 1988; Pabst et al, 1989). The problem of differing reactions to the vaccine has been lessened by the development of freeze-dried preparation (manufactured by Glaxo Laboratories, Ltd., Middlesex, England, and distributed by Eli Lilly and Co., Indianapolis, IN), which has been found to be comparable to the liquid Danish vaccine in testing on newborns (Griffiths and Gaisford, 1956). The immunizing dose is 0.1 mL by intradermal injection. A small red papule appears at the site of injection within 7 to 10 days and may increase in size over the next few weeks (Cundall et al, 1988). It leaves a smooth or pitted white scar in approximately 6 months. A tuberculin test should be performed in 2 or 3 months, and the immunization repeated if it is negative. Occasionally, local granulomas and regional adenitis ensue. Another problem is the possibility that vaccination with BCG could negate the value of subsequent tuberculin testing. The reaction becomes small 1 year after BCG immunization, and thus an increase in reactivity or a large reaction indicates *M. tuberculosis* infection. Individual differences in tuberculin sensitivity, however, make this distinction often unreliable.

The vaccine should not be given to HIV-infected infants in the United States (CDC, 1996).

Nursery Exposure to Tuberculosis

Experiences with controlling the possible spread of infection from nursery personnel to infants led Light and co-workers (1974) to propose 3 months of oral INH prophylaxis for all exposed infants. The argument is that the acquisition of fulminant disease may occur rapidly and in the absence of a tuberculin conversion. The time lag before effective immunity can be achieved with BCG vaccine makes this form of protection less desirable.

DIPHTHERIA

The virtual disappearance of diphtheria from the scene in many metropolitan areas inevitably decreases the consideration that this disease receives in differential diagnosis. In view of the recent resurgence of other presumed eliminated infections, experienced physicians must be careful lest a new generation of physicians who have had no experience with it forget its characteristics and its hazards.

Incidence

In 1921, more than 200,000 cases of diphtheria were reported in the United States (Centers for Disease Control and Prevention, 1985). Approximately 5% to 10% of the cases were fatal. From 1980 to 1983, 15 cases of respiratory diphtheria were reported, 11 of which occurred in persons

20 years of age or older. In Massachusetts between 1981 and 1991, the incidence of bacteriologically confirmed cases was reported to be 104.5 per 100,000 person-years in infants 1 month old or younger, 12.9 per 100,000 in persons 11 to 19 years old, and 0.56 in persons older than 20 years old (Marchant et al, 1994).

Etiology and Epidemiology

Corynebacterium diphtheriae, generally of the gravis type, is the responsible organism. Its soluble toxin produces antitoxin in the host during the course of natural infection and may be used, modified to toxoid, as a potent antigen to stimulate the formation of antitoxin in inoculated persons. The antitoxic titer from either source persists for a variable number of years and is capable of being boosted by reinfection or by subsequent doses of toxoid. Many newborns receive no antitoxin from a mother whose natural or artificial antitoxin titer had diminished to the vanishing point over the course of years devoid of re-exposure either to *C. diphtheriae* or to stimulating injections. These infants are susceptible to diphtheria, and contact with an infected person or a healthy carrier may cause the disease. Prevention continues to be the best treatment: an exposed or unimmunized pregnant woman should receive two properly spaced disks of tetanus and diphtheria toxoids, preferably during the last two trimesters (CDC, 1994a).

Diagnosis

The diagnosis of diphtheria in the newborn differs in no respect from that in the older child. Faucial diphtheria is recognized by the characteristic membrane, nasal diphtheria by persistent discharge (often sanguineous), and the laryngeal form by slowly progressive hoarseness and aphonia and laryngotracheal obstruction. All are without sharp constitutional reaction. In all forms, diagnosis depends on bacteriologic identification of *C. diphtheriae*. Serodiagnosis by single serum antipertussis toxin antibody enzyme-linked immunosorbent assay has also been useful, but, in the neonatal period, concurrent assessment of maternal serologic status must be obtained (Marchant et al, 1994). Complications, chiefly myocarditis and postdiphtheritic paralysis, have been similarly encountered in the newborn.

Treatment

Diphtheria antitoxin must be given intravenously, when the condition appears serious, or intramuscularly, if the situation is less urgent. Doses of 20,000 to 50,000 units on 2 or 3 successive days is sufficient. Preliminary testing for sensitivity must be carried out. Because penicillin has a bactericidal effect on *C. diphtheriae*, it should be given in doses approximating 300,000 units every 8 to 12 hours. Erythromycin is also effective in the event of penicillin sensitivity. Treatment of complications is carried out as for that in older infants. As discussed in Chapter 40, preterm infants should be immunized on the basis of their chronologic age.

TETANUS NEONATORUM

If public health interventions that emphasize hygiene and immunization were provided in developing countries, neonatal tetanus would decrease worldwide as it has in the United States (CDC, 1994b). During the period 1989–1990, only 1 of 117 cases of tetanus reported in the United States represented a case of neonatal tetanus (Prevots et al, 1992). In contrast, a referral hospital in Plateau State, Nigeria, reported 61 cases in a 4-year period, an overall incidence of 21.8/1000, and a mortality rate of 8.2% (Okuonghae and Airede, 1992). If the incubation period is less than 7 days, greater than 90% mortality has been reported (Dowell, 1984). Hypothermia and bronchopneumonia are the most common events that lead to death (Salimpour, 1977).

Etiology and Pathogenesis

The causative agent is the bacterium *Clostridium tetani*. This gram-positive, anaerobic spore bearer produces a protein neurotoxin (tetanospasmin) that is responsible for this paralysis (Dowell, 1984). This protoplasmic protein is released after the cells of *C. tetani* autolyze. This protein is encoded within a plasmid not directly related to a bacteriophage (Laird et al, 1980). Like the botulinal toxins, tetanospasmin acts at myoneural junctions by inhibiting the release of acetylcholine. Competition experiments have suggested that tetanospasmin and botulinal toxin are bound to different sites. *C. tetani* usually gains entrance into the newborn's body by way of the stump of the umbilical cord that is cut by an unsterile instrument or covered with an unclean dressing. Rarely, a vaccination wound produced by an unclean instrument or by contaminated skin imperfectly cleansed constitutes a portal of entry. The organism is long-lived by virtue of its spore formation, is a normal inhabitant of the intestinal tract of many domestic animals, and hence abounds in the soil of many localities.

Immunity to tetanus depends on the presence in the blood of an adequate concentration of antibody to the toxin. Antibody is efficiently stimulated by immunization with toxoid. The blood of the newborn contains roughly the amount of tetanus antitoxin that is present in the mother's blood. Peterson and colleagues (1955) believe that concentrations as low as 0.01 antitoxin unit/mL may be protective against the disease, and levels higher than this may persist for years in actively immunized persons. Transplacental immunization of the fetus has been effective in achieving long-lasting (up to 5 years) immunologic protection (Insel et al, 1994).

Diagnosis

Signs appear between the 6th and 14th days after birth, most often at the beginning of the 2nd week. Restlessness, irritability, and difficulty in sucking are followed within a day or two by fever, muscle stiffness, and finally, convulsions. The temperature often elevates to between 40° C and 41° C (104° F and 106° F). Physical examination at this stage shows the characteristic trismus and risus sardonicus and the tenseness and rigidity of all muscles, including those of the abdomen. The fists are held tightly clenched and the toes rigidly fanned. Characteristic are the opisthotonic spasms plus clonic jerkings that follow sudden stimulation by touch or by loud noise.

Laboratory investigations are best held to a minimum, because any manipulation produces painful spasms. Diagnosis is clear from the clinical evidence alone, and studies of blood, urine, and cerebrospinal fluid, in all respects normal, add nothing of value. Attempts should be made to cultivate the organism from the presumed portal of entry.

Tetany of the newborn should never be confused with tetanus. Infants with tetany appear well between their convulsive episodes. The infant who is hypertonic from hypoxic-ischemic injury has usually shown evidence of brain injury from birth, before the first sign of tetanus could possibly appear. Extraocular palsies commonly are present and abdominal rigidity absent. Response to stimulation is depressed rather than increased.

Course

The infant may die within a week after onset from respiratory arrest during a convulsive episode. If not, improvement becomes manifest within 3 to 7 days by gradual decline of temperature, decrease in the number of episodes of spasm, and slow resolution of rigidity. Complete disappearance of all signs of illness may take as long as 6 weeks.

Treatment

The first requirement is for tetanus antitoxin to neutralize the circulating toxin not already bound to nerve tissue. Tetanus immune globulin (human) should be given intramuscularly, in a dose of 500 units (McCracken et al, 1971). If this is not available, 10,000 units of equine or bovine tetanus antitoxin should be given intramuscularly. In addition, débridement of the infection site to remove devitalized tissue is imperative (Dowell, 1984). Penicillin, which kills the vegetative form of the bacterium, should be given in a dose of 100,000 to 200,000 units/kg every 12 hours. Tetracycline may be of value as an alternative drug. Treatment with antibiotics and antitoxin should also be considered for infants whose umbilical cords have been cut with or exposed to surfaces that might bear *C. tetani.*

Every known sedative has been used to control spasm, and there is no general agreement as to which one should be chosen. Diazepam (Valium) has become the mainstay of treatment of older children with tetanus, and it is probably also of great value in newborns (1 to 2 mg/kg per day in divided doses). The ideal result is to control spasm without depressing respiration. Drug administration is important. When intensive care and respirators are available, neuromuscular blockade with pancuronium bromide (Pavulon), 0.05 to 0.1 mg/kg administered every 2 to 3 hours for the duration of the spasms (up to 6 weeks), has proved successful (Adams et al, 1979). Endotracheal tubes have largely replaced tracheostomy under these circumstances (Bleck, 1991).

Fluids are best given through an indwelling intravenous catheter at first, later through an indwelling gastric tube. The infant should be under close observation in a darkened room and disturbed and stimulated as infrequently as possible. Active immunization with alum-precipitated or fluid toxoid should be begun as soon as the infant improves, because the disease itself immunizes poorly, if at all.

INFANT BOTULISM

Although *Clostridium botulinum* is widely distributed in soil and water, reports of infant botulism were rare before 1976, when Pickett and coworkers described an outbreak in California. The incidence is unknown. Recent case reports and reviews suggest that this disease is widely distributed in the United States (Hurst and Marsh, 1993; Schreiner et al, 1991; Thilo et al, 1993).

Etiology

Seven types (A, B, C, D, E, F, G) of *C. botulinum,* a heterologous group of obligatory anaerobic, spore-forming, gram-positive, rod-shaped bacteria are distinguished by antigenically distinct toxins (Dowell, 1984). Investigation of 81 cases by the Centers for Disease Control identified a potential source in opened jars of honey that had been added to baby food or used to coat pacifiers. Vacuum cleaner dust was found to contain spores of *C. botulinum* in the household of one infected infant. In the study from Utah (Thompson et al, 1980), it was noted that digging or construction was common in the neighborhoods in which cases were reported. However, food exposures accounted for only a minority of the 68 infant botulism cases reviewed, and pre-existing host factors, especially those related to intestinal flora, may be the most important risk indicators (Spika et al, 1989). Of the 121 cases reported to the Centers for Disease Control from 1975 to 1979, 65 (54%) involved *C. botulinum* type A, 55 (45%) type B, and one, type F. Three of the patients died (Dowell, 1984). The frequency of infant botulism in the United States contrasts with the experience in the United Kingdom where a single case was reported in 1986 (Lancet Editorial, 1986).

Clinical Course

Infant botulism has been described in patients as young as 1 week of age, but the peak incidence occurs at the usual time of weaning, from 6 weeks to 6 months of age. The infants have usually been born at term and described as normal. Constipation is frequently noted. The infants may seem lethargic and slow to feed. Some have a more acute onset of feeding difficulties, pooling of secretions, diminished gag reflex, loss of head control, and generalized weakness. If the diagnosis is not made and appropriate supportive treatment initiated, death from respiratory arrest may occur. Some infants diagnosed as victims of sudden infant death syndrome may have died from unrecognized botulism (Sonnabend et al, 1985).

Diagnosis

The diagnosis depends on recovery of *C. botulinum* with or without its toxin from the stool in the presence of a compatible clinical picture (Dowell, 1984). Stool and serum specimens should be sent to a laboratory equipped to identify the organism and its toxin. Electromyography has been helpful in the clinical diagnosis. Brief small-amplitude motor reaction potentials have been described. Both *C. botulinum* and toxin have been found in the stools of normal infants (Thompson et al, 1980).

Treatment

Botulinal antitoxin has not been useful in infant botulism, perhaps because of the absence of demonstrable toxin in the serum. Ampicillin has been used, although its value in eliminating the organism is uncertain. Aminoglycoside antibiotics are contraindicated because of possible potentiation of neuromuscular weakness (L'Hommedieu et al, 1979).

TYPHOID FEVER

J. P. Crozer Griffith before the beginning of the twentieth century recognized not only that infants could acquire typhoid fever after birth but also that babies born of mothers suffering from the disease acquired the infection in utero.

Incidence

Typhoid fever attained epidemic proportions in the summer and fall of every year throughout most of the United States until the end of the 1920s. By 1902, Griffith was able to report in some detail on 18 patients younger than 2 1/2 years of age whom he had observed personally and on 325 certain cases plus 92 somewhat doubtful ones that he had collected from the literature. Since the early 1920s, typhoid fever among infants has declined in frequency. Griffith and Ostheimer (1902) found 23 examples of congenital typhoid fever among their collected cases. I have not seen one in a pediatric experience that dates from 1923. However, in other countries where *Salmonella typhi* strains are endemic, asymptomatic excretion and life-threatening illness are two forms of the infection that have been observed (Reed and Klugman, 1994; Naqvi et al, 1992). In areas of the world where political conflict leads to warfare and economic devastation (e.g., Iraq after the Gulf War), typhoid fever among infants is observed with increased frequency (The Harvard Study Team, 1991).

Diagnosis

The following case history, first reported by Weech and Chen in 1929, illustrates the course and diagnosis of an infant with typhoid fever.

CASE STUDY 1

A male infant was born prematurely after an uncomplicated pregnancy. Five days postpartum, his mother had fever that proved later to be severe typhoid. The infant became febrile at the age of 26 days, but fever dropped to normal after 24 hours. The spleen was enlarged. White blood cell count was 11,000/mm³. Culture of the blood revealed *B. typhosus (Salmonella typhi* in modern terminology). The next day a bright-red papular eruption appeared over the entire body and lasted 2 days. The white cell count was now 17,000, of which 37% were polymorphonuclears. He had no more fever for 3 weeks, and then low-grade elevation reappeared for a few days. Blood culture was still positive. Two weeks later it was negative. The only other symptom or sign was failure to gain. All other cultures, from stool and urine, remained consistently negative. Eleven Widal tests were performed throughout the course, and none was positive.

Comment

The authors note the extreme youth of their patient, the mildness of the disease and the lack of gastrointestinal symptoms, the generalized exanthem that bore no resemblance to rose spots, the leukocytosis so unlike the leukopenic response of older persons, and the total failure of agglutinins to develop.

Treatment

First chloramphenicol, then ampicillin, was found to be highly effective against *S. typhi*. In the first weeks of the infant's life; ampicillin is the preferred antibiotic.

Schaffer (unpublished data) observed an epidemic of typhoid in northern Mexico in the early 1970s that was caused by a strain of *S. typhi* that was refractory to both chloramphenicol and ampicillin. Presumably, this strain developed because of the availability of these antibiotics without prescriptions. In a recent review of multidrug-resistant typhoid in 58 children, ceftriaxone was more effective than cefotaxime with a significantly lower relapse rate (Naqvi et al, 1992). However, the high cost and problems of parenteral administration of these drugs in rural sites make the development of safe, effective oral therapy a high priority.

Prognosis

Nineteen of the 23 infants with congenital cases collected by Griffith and Ostheimer in 1902 died, 3 recovered, and the fate of 1 was not stated. More recently, all three infants in a small series given parenteral antibiotics (ampicillin, chloramphenicol, or trimethoprim) survived (Chin et al, 1986).

REFERENCES

Adams JM, Kenny JD, Rudolph AJ: Modern management of tetanus neonatorum. Pediatrics 64:472, 1979.
Bailey WC, Albert RK, Davidson PT, et al: Treatment of tuberculosis and other mycobacterial diseases. Am Rev Respir Dis 127:790–796, 1983.
Barnes PF, Bloch AB, Davidson PT, Snider DE Jr: Tuberculosis in patients with human immunodeficiency virus infection. N Engl J Med 324:1644, 1991.
Bate TWP, Sinclair RE, Robinson MJ: Neonatal tuberculosis. Arch Dis Child 61:512–514, 1986.
Beitzke H, cited by Harris EA, McCullough GC, Stone JJ, et al: Congeni-

tal tuberculosis: A review of the disease with report of a case. J Pediatr 32:311, 1948.

Bleck TP: Tetanus: Pathophysiology, management, and prophylaxis. Dis Mon 37:545, 1991.

Cantwell MF, Shehab ZM, Costello AM, et al: Brief report: Congenital tuberculosis. N Engl J Med 330:1051, 1994.

Centers for Disease Control and Prevention: Immunization Practices Advisory Committee statement on diptheria, tetanus, and pertussis. MMWR Morb Mortal Wkly Rep 34:405, 1985.

Centers for Disease Control and Prevention: General recommendations on immunization: Recommendations of the Advisory Committee on Immunization Practices (ACIP). MMWR Morb Mortal Wkly Rep 43:1, 1994a.

Centers for Disease Control and Prevention: Progress towards the global elimination of neonatal tetanus. MMWR Morb Mortal Wkly Rep 43:885, 1994b.

Centers for Disease Control and Prevention: The role of BCG vaccine in the prevention and control of tuberculosis in the United States. MMWR Morb Mortal Wkly Rep 45:RR-4, April 26, 1996.

Chavalittamrong B, Chearskul S, Tuchinda M: Protective value of BCG vaccination in children in Bangkok, Thailand. Pediatr Pulmonol 2:202, 1986.

Chin KC, Simmonds EJ, Tarlow MJ: Neonatal typhoid fever. Arch Dis Child 61:1228–1230, 1986.

Cundall DB, Ashelford DJ, Pearson SB: BCG immunisation of infants by percutaneous multiple puncture. BMJ 297:1173, 1988.

Debre R, LeLong M: The infant born of tuberculous parents, separated before contamination: Its growth and resistance to disease. Ann Med 18:317, 1925.

de Pape AJ: Multiple pseudocystic tuberculosis of bone. J Bone Joint Surg 36B:637, 1954.

Dowell VR Jr: Botulism and tetanus: Selected epidemiologic and microbiologic aspects. Rev Infect Dis 6:S202–S207, 1984.

Editorial: Infant Botulism. Lancet 2:1256–1257, 1986.

Escobar JA, Belsey MA, Duenas A, et al: Mortality from tuberculous meningitis reduced by steroid therapy. Pediatrics 56:1050, 1975.

Griffith JPC, Ostheimer M: Typhoid fever in children under two and a half years of age. Am J Med Sci 124:868, 1902.

Griffiths MI, Gaisford W: Freeze-dried BCG. Vaccination of newborn infants with a British vaccine. BMJ 2:565, 1956.

Grindulis H, Baynham MID, Scott PH, et al: Tuberculin response two years after BCG vaccination at birth. Arch Dis Child 59:614–619, 1984.

Hageman J, Shulman S, Schreiber M, et al: Congenital tuberculosis: Critical reappraisal of clinical findings and diagnostic procedures. Pediatrics 66:980, 1980.

The Harvard Study Team: The effect of the Gulf crisis on the children of Iraq. N Engl J Med 325:977, 1991.

Hurst DL, Marsh WW: Early severe infantile botulism. J Pediatr 122:909, 1993.

Insel RA, Amstey M, Woodin K, Pichichero M: Maternal immunization to prevent infectious disease in the neonate or infant. Int J Tech Assess Health Care 10:143, 1994.

Inselman LS, Kendig EL: Tuberculosis. *In* Chernick V (Ed): Kendig's Disorders of the Respiratory Tract in Children. 5th ed. Philadelphia, WB Saunders, 1990.

Iseman MD, Starke J: Immigrants and tuberculosis control. N Engl J Med 332:1094, 1995.

Johnson DE, Miller LC, Iverson S, et al: The health of children adopted from Romania. JAMA 268:3446, 1992.

Jones DS, Malecki JM, Bigler WJ, et al: Pediatric tuberculosis and human immunodeficiency virus infection in Palm Beach County, Florida. Am J Dis Child 146:1166, 1992.

Laird WJ, Aaronson W, Silver RP, et al: Plasmid-associated toxigenicity in *Clostridium tetani*. J Infect Dis 142:623, 1980.

L'Hommedieu L, Stough R, Brown L, et al: Potentiation of neuromuscular weakness in infant botulism by aminoglycosides. J Pediatr 95:1065, 1979.

Light IJ, Saideman M, Sutherland JM: Management of newborns after nursery exposure to tuberculosis. Am Rev Respir Dis 109:415, 1974.

Marchant CD, Loughlin AM, Lett SM, et al: Pertussis in Massachusetts, 1981–1991: Incidence, serologic diagnosis, and vaccine effectiveness. J Infect Dis 169:1297, 1994.

Margono F, Mroueh J, Garely A, et al: Resurgence of active tuberculosis among pregnant women. Obstet Gynecol 83:911, 1994.

McCracken GH Jr, Dowell DL, Marshall FN: Double-blind trial of equine antitoxin and human immune globulin in tetanus neonatorum. Lancet 1:1146, 1971.

McKenna MT, McCray E, Ontorato I: The epidemiology of tuberculosis among foreign-born persons in the United States, 1986 to 1993. N Engl J Med 332:1071, 1995.

Nakajo MM, Rao M, Steiner P: Incidence of hepatotoxicity in children receiving isoniazid chemoprophylaxis. Pediatr Infect Dis J 8:649, 1989.

Naqvi SH, Bhutta ZA, Farooqui BJ: Therapy of multidrug resistant typhoid in 58 children. Scand J Infect Dis 24:175, 1992.

Okuonghae HO, Airede AI: Neonatal tetanus: Incidence and improved outcome with diazepam. Dev Med Child Neuro 34:448, 1992.

Ormerod LP, Garnett JM: Tuberculin response after neonatal BCG vaccination. Arch Dis Child 63:1491, 1988.

Pabst HF, Godel J, Grace M, et al: Effect of breast-feeding on immune response to BCG vaccination. Lancet 1:295–297, 1989.

Peterson JC, Christie A, Williams WC: Tetanus immunization. XI. Study of the duration of primary immunity and the response to late stimulating doses of tetanus toxoid. Am J Dis Child 89:295, 1955.

Pickett J, Berg B, Chaplin E, et al: Syndrome of botulism in infancy: Clinical and electrophysiologic study. N Engl J Med 295:770, 1976.

Prevots R, Sutter RW, Strebel PM, et al: Tetanus surveillance—United States, 1989–1990. MMWR Morb Mortal Wkly Rep CDC Surveill Summ 41:1, 1992.

Ratner B, Rostler AE, Salgado PS: Care, feeding and fate of premature and full-term infants born of tuberculosis mothers. Am J Dis Child 81:471, 1951.

Raucher HS, Gribetz I: Care of the pregnant woman with tuberculosis and her newborn infant: A pediatrician's perspective. Mt Sinai J Med 53:70–76, 1986.

Reed RP, Klugman KP: Neonatal typhoid fever. Pediatr Infect Dis J 13:774, 1994.

Rosenthal SR, Loewinsohn E, Graham ML, et al: BCG vaccination against tuberculosis in Chicago. Pediatrics 28:622, 1961.

Salimpour R: Cause of death in tetanus neonatorum: Study of 233 cases with 54 necropsies. Arch Dis Child 52:587–594, 1977.

Schreiner MS, Field E, Ruddy R: Infant botulism: A review of 12 years' experience at the Children's Hospital of Philadelphia. Pediatrics 87:159, 1991.

Snider DE, Bacille Calmette-Guérin vaccinations and tuberculin skin tests. JAMA 253:3438, 1985.

Sonnabend OAR, Sonnabend WFF, Krech U, et al: Continuous microbiological and pathological study of 70 sudden and unexpected infant deaths: Toxigenic intestinal *Clostridium botulinum* infection in 9 cases of sudden infant death syndrome. Lancet 2:237–241, 1985.

Spika JS, Shaffer N, Hargrett-Bean N, et al: Risk factors for infant botulism in the United States. Am J Dis Child 143:828–832, 1989.

Sudre P, ten Dam G, Kochi A: Tuberculosis: A global overview of the situation today. Bull World Health Organ 70:149, 1992.

Thilo EH, Townsend SF, Deacon J: Infant botulism at 1 week of age: Report of two cases. Pediatrics 92:151, 1993.

Thompson JA, Glasgow LA, Warpinski JR, et al: Infant botulism: Clinical spectrum and epidemiology. Pediatrics 66:936, 1980.

Vallejo JG, Starke JR: Tuberculosis and pregnancy. Clin Chest Med 13:693, 1992.

Weech AA, Chen KT: Typhoid fever: Report of a case in an infant less than one month of age. Am J Dis Child 38:1044, 1929.

Weinstein L: Current concepts: Tetanus. N Engl J Med 289:1293, 1973.

Young TK, Hershfield ES: A case-controlled study to evaluate the effectiveness of mass neonatal BCG vaccination among Canadian Indians. Am J Public Health 76:783, 1986.

Zalma VM, Older JJ, Brooks GF: The Austin, Texas, diphtheria outbreak: Clinical and epidemiological aspects. JAMA 211:2125, 1970.

CHAPTER 45

Fungal Infections

F. Sessions Cole[*]

COCCIDIOIDOMYCOSIS

Coccidioidomycosis is rare in newborns but it has been reported, especially from endemic areas of the southwestern United States and northern Mexico (Stevens, 1995). *Coccidioides immitis* is a dimorphic soil fungus that causes a mild, self-limiting respiratory illness in immunocompetent children and adults. In infants and newborns, however, the untreated disease is devastating and usually lethal (Child et al, 1985). Transplacental spread has been suggested (Peterson et al, 1993; Shafai, 1978; Spark, 1981). An increasing number of patients were reported during the 1980s (Child et al, 1985; Shehab et al, 1988), and a recent epidemic in California suggested the association of this infection with concurrent human immunodeficiency virus (HIV) infection (Centers for Disease Control and Prevention, 1994). In 1964, Ziering and Rockas described a 3-month-old infant whose initial symptoms appeared within the 1st month of life. In addition to adult-to-infant transmission of coccidioidomycosis, it appears that infants can be infected by porous fomites brought from an endemic area to one in which the disease is rare (Rothman et al, 1962). This following summary of a case described by Townsend and McKey (1953) illustrates the problems of diagnosis and treatment.

CASE STUDY 1

A 3-week-old white female infant had been well until 2 days before admission. The only pertinent fact in the family history was that the father had lived in the San Joaquin Valley for 12 years. The infant exhibited high fever, irritability, and anorexia. She was acutely ill, with a temperature of 104° F, respirations 132/minute. She was pale, and her neck was slightly stiff. Her fontanel was full but not tense. Hemoglobin was 12.3 g/dL and decreased to 8.2 g/dL after 1 week. White blood cells numbered 71,800 cells/mm^3 and decreased gradually to 19,800 with normal differential counts. Cerebrospinal fluid showed 700 cells/mm^3, 80% polymorphonuclear, 195 mg/dL of protein, and 15 mg/dL of sugar on admission. Cell count within the next month varied from 5 to 98, protein from 46 to 64 mg, and sugar from 34 to 49 mg. Cerebrospinal fluid cultures, negative on four occasions, finally became positive for *C. immitis* 1 month after admission. The organism never could be grown from urine, blood, bone marrow, or gastric washings. Complement fixation was positive for *C. immitis* in the first dilution.

The patient appeared better 5 days after multiple antibiotic therapy was started, but then her temperature began to spike. Radiographs showed patchy infiltration of both lungs. The spleen gradually became larger; infiltration of lungs spread. Isoniazid, streptomycin, and para-aminosalicylic acid were given. Despite this therapy, the cervical nodes and spleen grew larger, a papular rash appeared over the trunk, and the infant grew steadily weaker and died 2 months after admission. Autopsy showed disseminated coccidioidomycosis.

Interesting is the fact that repeated coccidioidin skin test results never were positive.

Comment

This 3-week-old infant did not live in but was exposed to a father who had lived in the circumscribed desert region in the U.S. Southwest in which coccidioidomycosis is endemic. The infection manifested itself first as meningoencephalitis, followed by progressive pneumonitis and disseminated lesions, producing splenomegaly, glandular enlargement, and an exanthem. No thrombocytopenia or purpura ever appeared. The skin test result was never positive. Cerebrospinal fluid cultures did not become positive for the fungus until 1 month after the onset. The complement fixation test gave the earliest confirmation of the diagnosis.

In another case, Ziering and Rockas (1964) achieved a notable success in treating their very ill patient, who had extensive pulmonary lesions plus subcutaneous abscesses, osteitis, periostitis, and iridocyclitis. The infant was given courses of amphotericin B over a period of 18 months without toxic effects. His complement fixation titer diminished, and his skin test became positive, indications of marked improvement.

The first report of maternal-infant transmission was a fatal case found by Bernstein and coworkers in 1981. Their patient, born at 36 to 37 weeks' gestation to a mother who had cervical coccidioidomycosis and membranes that had been ruptured for 24 hours, was febrile at 5 days of age and had extensive pneumonia by the 6th day of life. The organisms were seen on Gram stain of the tracheal aspirate and confirmed in postmortem cultures. The course was fulminant, with death at 10 days of age.

Treatment

Before the introduction of amphotericin B, coccidioidomycosis was a uniformly fatal disease (Drutz and Catanzaro, 1978). Mortality has decreased with the availability of am-

---

[*]This chapter includes some contributions from the previous authors, Drs. Arnold Smith and Kenneth McIntosh.

photericin B and, more recently, imidazole therapy (ketoconazole and miconazole), but significant morbidity is still associated with the disease and its treatments (Harrison et al, 1983; Shehab et al, 1988; Stevens, 1995). Amphotericin B is administered intravenously (test dose: 0.1 mg/kg; if tolerated, 0.75 to 1.0 mg/kg per day up to 30 to 50 mg/kg total dose). Imidazole therapy has been shown to be useful as a single agent in coccidioidal meningitis (Shehab et al, 1988). Oral ketoconazole (14 to 23 mg/kg per day as a single daily dose) as well as intraventricular miconazole (3 to 5 mg diluted in 1 mL of 5% dextrose in water or normal saline daily, then once weekly for 2 to 6 months) have been shown to sterilize cerebrospinal fluid within 1 month of therapy (Shehab et al, 1988). It is important to note that imidazole therapy may require prolonged and repeated treatment courses. Although no relapses up to 10 months of therapy were reported in one study (Shehab et al, 1988), systemic infection may recur up to 10 years after initial presentation (Kafka and Catanzaro, 1981; Westley, 1982). Duration of initial therapy ranges from 30 to 90 months. Ketoconazole suppresses adrenal steroid production of both cortisol and aldosterone by partially blocking the 11-beta-hydroxylase step of steroid hormone synthesis (Britton et al, 1988). Although no studies are available in infants, none of 10 prepubertal children required adrenal steroid replacement therapy during acute illness or surgery (Britton et al, 1988).

CRYPTOCOCCOSIS

Cryptococcosis is caused by infection with *Cryptococcus neoformans* (former name, *Torula histolytica*) and is important in the newborn because it invades the central nervous system, where it sets up a meningoencephalitis that closely resembles that produced by *Toxoplasma* and cytomegalovirus. Some of the earliest examples were reported by Neuhauser and Tucker in 1948. Emanuel and colleagues (1961) were able to find 23 affected children reported in the literature. Three definite and three almost certain cases involved illness within the 1st month of life. The increasing frequency of HIV infection among pregnant women will lead to increasing exposure of fetuses and newborns to this pathogen, as a case report suggests (Kida et al, 1989).

Pathogenesis

Cryptococcus is an occasional inhabitant of the female genital tract, and the infant probably acquires infection during passage through the birth canal. Symptoms begin so promptly after birth in some cases that transplacental transmission of infection should be considered. Strains of *C. neoformans* that are pathogenic for humans have been isolated from cow's milk, with or without concomitant bovine mastitis (Emmons, 1953; Pounder et al, 1952).

Diagnosis

The diagnosis and course of three patients with cryptococcosis who were reported by Neuhauser and Tucker (1948) are illustrated in the following case histories.

CASE STUDY 2

A 7-week-old male infant was admitted to the hospital. He had experienced a precipitous delivery and was cyanotic after birth, requiring resuscitation. Twitchings and rigidity followed on the 2nd day and did not entirely disappear for several weeks. He never ate well and, despite tube-feeding, did not gain weight. Upon admission he was emaciated and chronically ill. The head was a bit large, there were cataracts in both eyes, and the spleen and liver were large. Opisthotonos, ankle clonus, and positive Babinski reflex marked his neurologic examination. Cerebrospinal and subdural fluid contained an excess of protein and many red blood cells. Blood cell count was unremarkable, but no mention was made of platelets. He died suddenly after having been in the hospital for 3 weeks. In this case, it is difficult to date the onset, since many of the early symptoms might easily have stemmed from intracranial damage sustained at the time of birth.

CASE STUDY 3

In the second patient, the reason for admission on the 19th day of life was persistent, severe jaundice from birth. Abdominal enlargement was noted at 1 week; the urine was dark, and the stools were light. The spleen and liver were huge. Temperature never exceeded 100° F. He died 4 days after admission. No cause other than the patient's cryptococcal infection was found for the jaundice. Platelets were not mentioned. In this example, infection before birth should be considered.

CASE STUDY 4

The third case differed from the other two in mode of onset. The infant began to have convulsions and incessant crying at 2 weeks of age and was admitted to the hospital 4 days later. He was well at birth and until he was 2 weeks old. The head, heart, and lungs seemed normal on examination. The liver and spleen were very large. Neurologic examinations showed only hyperactive reflexes. The platelets numbered only 66,000/mm³. Otherwise, the blood was normal, as was the urine. On the 9th hospital day, the infant had gross hematuria. Death occurred the following day.

Comment

Radiographs of the skull in all three cases showed spotty calcifications within the substance of the brain. In Case 4, interstitial pneumonitis, focal atelectasis, and a large granulomatous lesion in the right upper lobe were noted on the chest radiograph. Two infants showed chorioretinitis, and two showed physical signs of central nervous system involvement. All had hepatosplenomegaly. Fever was almost nonexistent in all, and all showed hydrocephalus and diffuse areas of focal degeneration throughout their brains.

Cases 2 and 4 are virtually indistinguishable from toxoplasmosis in early life on the basis of history and physical findings alone, whereas Case 3, with the principal involvement in the liver, is highly suggestive of either cytomegalic inclusion disease or viral hepatitis. Diagnosis depends on (1) exclusion of toxoplasmosis by the Sabin dye test and complement fixation studies, (2) exclusion of cytomegalic inclusion disease by the inability to demonstrate inclusion bodies in the cells of urinary sediment or of gastric washings and by virus culture, (3) exclusion of congenital infection with rubella virus or *Treponema pallidum* by appropriate serologic tests. *Cryptococcus* has been seen in and cultivated from the cerebrospinal fluid of newborns five times, twice antemortem and three times postmortem.

Treatment

Untreated infants have died within days to weeks of onset of disease. Amphotericin B in a total intravenous dose of 30 mg/kg over a 3-week period may be adequate therapy for disseminated disease with meningoencephalitis. In treating serious systemic fungal diseases in infants and children, a test dose of amphotericin B (0.1 mg/kg) may be given intravenously over 30 minutes. If this is tolerated without rash, fever, or decrease in blood pressure over the next 3 hours, the maintenance dose is immediately begun (0.75 to 1.0 mg/kg per day in a single infusion over several hours intravenously). Gradually increasing the dose by increments over several days has not been necessary. In cases that progressively deteriorate or relapse, intrathecal therapy, in addition to the intravenous route, often produces a cure, particularly in the absence of underlying disease (Edwards et al, 1970; Sarosi et al, 1969). Because intrathecal therapy is often necessary over a protracted course, an intraventricular reservoir can facilitate this route if used with knowledge of the potential hazards (Diamond and Bennett, 1972). 5-Fluorocytosine (5-FC) should not be used alone, because the emergence of 5-FC–resistant strains has been a major cause of treatment failure with this drug (Block et al, 1973). This drug has a role when used with amphotericin B because the combination is synergistic in vitro and in vivo (Medoff et al, 1971). Although clinical trials with this combination are not available in adults or in children, successful treatment of a preterm infant with a different disseminated fungal infection (candidiasis) has been reported with a dose of 25 mg/kg (Hill et al, 1974).

DISSEMINATED HISTOPLASMOSIS

Approximately 67 cases of disseminated histoplasmosis in children younger than 2 years of age were reported by Leggiadro and associates (1988). The mean age at the time of presentation was 6 months. The increasing frequency of pregnant women with HIV infection will increase the number of infants exposed to opportunistic pathogens (McGregor et al, 1986).

Incidence

The disease is widespread in the United States and elsewhere, but certain areas seem to be heavily contaminated and their populations infected in large numbers. In a recent review of two large urban outbreaks, an estimated 100,000 individuals were infected, but fewer than 0.5% presented with clinical infections (Wheat et al, 1984). Cases are by no means confined to the broad central belt of high infection rate of which Tennessee appears to be the center. In the eastern United States, the shore counties of Maryland are the source of an appreciable number of histoplasmosis cases. Children younger than 2 years of age seem to be highly susceptible, and when they become infected, they almost always have the disseminated form. Cases developing within the 1st month of life are extremely uncommon, but many examples have been reported in the 3rd month and later.

Etiology

The invading organism is a fungus, *Histoplasma capsulatum*. Depending on environmental conditions, the fungus may grow in a yeastlike phase or in a mycelial phase. It is found in the soil in the mycelial phase, and it is from the soil that most human infection appears to be derived (Leggiadro et al, 1988).

Diagnosis

Infected infants become ill with fever that often spikes to high temperature once a day accompanied by rapid enlargement of the spleen and liver, bronchopneumonic pulmonary infiltrations of a nonspecific nature, and progressive pancytopenia (Leggiadro et al, 1988). The disease resembles disseminated tuberculosis in some respects but differs from it in that histoplasmosis is associated with a greater degree of hepatosplenomegaly, has no miliary pulmonary involvement, and fails to invade the meninges. Its later appearance, the usual but not invariable absence of jaundice, and again its lack of tropism for the central nervous system distinguish it from cytomegalic inclusion disease and toxoplasmosis. Differentiation from coccidioidomycosis and cryptococcosis, which make their appearance toward the end of the 1st month of life or later, may be impossible on clinical grounds alone. The diagnosis is influenced somewhat by geographic and epidemiologic considerations, but the final diagnosis depends on laboratory investigations.

A positive histoplasmin skin test is of little use, because the result may be negative in as many as half the early acute cases as well as in those patients who are severely ill with the disease. Histoplasmin reactions are frequently positive when other fungi are the responsible etiologic agents. By far the most reliable laboratory indication of the disease is growth of *H. capsulatum* from peripheral blood, liver biopsy, or bone marrow samples, especially the latter. However, in adults, individuals with known cavitary pulmonary disease may have negative cultures in up to 40% of cases (Wheat et al, 1984). The chief objection to this test is the length of time it takes to obtain a result. Quick and reliable confirmation can be obtained from the demonstration of specific histoplasmosis (H) and mycelia (M) precipitin bands by the Ouchterlony immunodiffusion technique (Holland and Holland, 1966; Wheat et al, 1984). Even though serologic tests are 95% sensitive and specific, these tests cannot differentiate disseminated from focal infection and can be positive in patients with chronic pulmonary infection caused by other fungi (Wheat et al, 1984). Immunoregulatory lymphocyte populations have been shown to be quantitatively and functionally abnormal in a 1-month-old child with disseminated histoplasmosis, but additional immunoregulatory data in infants are lacking (Clapp et al, 1987).

Treatment

Amphotericin B is the only effective therapy. Little and coworkers (1959) reported four cures in children, three of whom were 3, 5, and 8 months of age at the time treatment was begun. The drug is given intravenously, in a daily dosage of 0.25 to 1.0 mg/kg, dissolved in 5% dextrose to a concentration not exceeding 1.0 mg/10 mL of infusate. The infusion must be given slowly over a period of several hours. Infusions are continued for 4 to 8 weeks, daily at first, then every alternate day. A standard treatment course for infants with disseminated histoplasmosis is approximately 35 mg/kg over 6 weeks (Leggiadro et al, 1988). Vomiting and, in some babies, anaphylactoid reactions are not uncommon side effects, but they need not contraindicate continuation of therapy. The author achieved a notable success by this method in a nearly moribund 4-month-old baby. Triple sulfonamide and sulfadiazine have also been used successfully (Leggiadro et al, 1988).

DISSEMINATED CANDIDIASIS

This once rare disease has become a common problem in many nurseries as a result of the intensive use of broad-spectrum antibiotics in premature (and more vulnerable) infants, and the increased use of intravascular catheters for hyperalimentation. Two recent observations suggest mechanisms that mediate increased susceptibility of infants to systemic candida infections. First, epithelial adhesion of invasive *Candida* species is mediated by integrin analogues that recognize ligands present at the surface of the epithelial cell (Bendel and Hostetter, 1993). Because epithelial adhesion is a necessary step in bloodstream or tissue invasion, this mechanism suggests pharmacologic strategies for blocking recognition of ligands to reduce risk of invasive candida infection. Second, Marodi and coworkers (1994) have extended previous observations concerning macrophage activation in newborn infants. They have observed that neonatal macrophages are less responsive to interferon-gamma than adult macrophages. Because macrophage activation is critical for candidacidal defense, this mechanism contributes significantly to enhanced biologic susceptibility in infants.

While compulsive attention must be given to aseptic technique in the management of vascular catheters, it is not clear from currently available data whether these catheters cause infection, whether fluids administered through them (notably hyperalimentation fluid) causes infection, or whether they represent a marker for infants with increased susceptibility to candidiasis (Eppes et al, 1989; Knox et al, 1987; Lacey et al, 1988; Sherertz et al, 1992). *Candida albicans* grows in all alimentation solutions in use, but the rate depends on the composition and temperature (Goldmann and Maki, 1973). The organisms can reach densities of approximately 100,000/mL, and yet the solution appears clear to the eye; further infection from contaminated intravenous fluids produces an insidious infection. Several *Candida* species are known to cause disease in humans (Table 45–1), and Odds (1987) has identified virulence determinants in different species (Table 45–2). Recent work by Hostetter suggests that the most important of these virulence factors mediate epithelial adhesion of invasive *Candida* species through integrin analogues (Bendel and Hostetter, 1993). Specifically, the integrin analogue in invasive *Candida* species shares antigenic, structural, and functional homologies with the beta 2-integrin subunits alpha M and alpha X. Recognition of distinct RGD ligands at the epithelial cell surface by the integrin analogue mediates adhesion and thus virulence. A description of a typical case, reported by Hill and coworkers (1974), follows.

CASE STUDY 5

The patient was a 1928-g infant born to a 33-year-old primigravida at approximately 32 weeks' gestation. The infant, who was delivered by cesarean section because of placenta previa, required intubation and resuscitation in the delivery room. Because of persistent respiratory distress and periods of apnea, the patient was transferred to the University of Minnesota Neonatal Intensive Care Unit at approximately 12 hours of age. Severe hyaline membrane disease necessitated the use of respiratory therapy, and an umbilical artery catheter was inserted to monitor blood gases.

On the 5th hospital day, apnea, acidosis, and questionable pneumatosis intestinalis observed on an abdominal radiograph prompted the institution and continuance of penicillin and kanamycin therapy, although blood, urine, and cerebrospinal fluid cultures remained sterile. Hyperalimentation through the umbilical arterial catheter was started on the 6th hospital day. On the 9th hospital day, a recurrence of apnea and acidosis prompted repeat cultures, and the antibiotic therapy was changed to ampicillin and gentamicin. The patient improved clinically, but after 4 days *Candida albicans* grew out of the blood culture drawn on the 9th day. The catheter in the umbilical artery was removed and replaced 12 hours later with an internal jugular venous catheter, and amphotericin B therapy was initiated. Four days later, after three negative blood cultures and a negative cerebrospinal fluid culture were obtained, the amphotericin B was discontinued. Urine cultures continued to yield 7000 to 50,000 colonies of *C. albicans*/mL. On the 26th hospital day, 17 days after the initial positive blood cultures, edema of the feet, ankles, and knees was observed. This was considered to have a vascular etiology, and the extremities were elevated.

On the 29th hospital day, bilateral knee and ankle effusions developed and were accompanied by warmth and erythema. Synovial fluid contained numerous

TABLE 45–1

Candida Species Associated with Human Disease and the Sites Involved in Candidiasis

Species	Mouth	Vagina	Endocardium	Nervous System	Bone and Joint	Multiorgan Involvement
C. albicans	+ + +	+ + +	+ + +	+ + +	+ + +	+ + +
C. glabrata	+	+	+	+	–	+ +
C. guilliermondi	+	+	+ +	–	+ + +	+ +
C. krusei	+	+	+ +	–	+	+
C. parapsilosis	+	+	+ + +	+	+	+ +
C. tropicalis	+	+	+ +	+ + +	+ + +	+ + +

+ + +, major cause; + +, cause; +, rare cause; –, no cases known.

Reprinted with permission from Odds FC: Candida infections: An overview. CRC Crit Rev Microbiol 15:1, 1987. Copyright CRC Press, Inc., Boca Raton, FL.

polymorphonuclear leukocytes (PMLs), but no organisms were seen on direct examination. *C. albicans* subsequently grew from fluid obtained from both knees and the left ankle. Repeat urine cultures yielded 100,000 colonies of *C. albicans*/mL, although blood cultures remained sterile. A cerebrospinal fluid specimen obtained on the 29th hospital day contained 6 PMNs and 22 monocytes with a glucose of 29 mg/dL and protein of 84 mg/dL. This specimen also yielded *C. albicans* on culture.

Comment

This case illustrates several important principles in the diagnosis of disseminated candidiasis. The infection is septicemic, with blood cultures yielding the organism and the urine containing the organisms cleared by the kidney. Blood cultures obtained through the hyperalimentation catheter sample infected thrombi adjacent to the tip but do not aid in differentiating between diseases that will resolve after catheter removal (Ellis and Spivack, 1967) and life-threatening illness. Peripheral blood cultures obtained by venipuncture are a more reliable indicator of ongoing candidemia. In overwhelming infections, the organisms can be seen in stained smears of buffy coat prepa-

rations (Silverman et al, 1973). Skin lesions can be seen (Bodey and Luna, 1974) that yield the organism on aspiration. Candidal ophthalmitis is an occasional complication of candidemia (Fishman et al, 1972) and can serve as a focus for continued candidemia (Haring et al, 1973). Every infant in whom the diagnosis of candidal sepsis is suspected should have indirect funduscopic examination (McDonnell et al, 1985). Among common presenting symptoms, usually at 1 to 2 months of age, are respiratory deterioration, hyperglycemia, and temperature instability (Baley et al, 1984). Fungal colonization represents a significant risk factor in infants weighing less than 1500 g (Baley et al, 1986). A substantial proportion of infants with persistent signs and symptoms of infection has central nervous system involvement (Faix, 1984). Other manifestations of candidal sepsis in newborn infants are osteomyelitis (Adler et al, 1972; Freeman et al, 1974; Klein et al, 1972), meningitis, endocarditis (Joshi and Wang, 1973; Shapira et al, 1974), and arthritis.

Because of the importance of host factors, the course of disseminated candidiasis is unpredictable, making therapeutic generalizations impossible. If the infection is catheter related, careful consideration should be given to removing the catheter (Eppes et al, 1989; Knox et al, 1987; Lacey et al, 1988). In most instances, amphotericin B is administered until it is clear that there are no occult foci. In patients with meningitis or progressive clinical deteriora-

TABLE 45–2

Possible Virulence Determinants of *Candida* Species

Species*	Able to Form True Hyphae	Able to Resist Phagocytosis	Able to Adhere to Host Surfaces	Able to Secrete Proteinase
C. albicans	+ +	+ +	+ +	+ +
C. tropicalis	±	+ +	+	+
C. parapsilosis	–	+	+	±
C. pseudotropicalis	–	+	±	–
C. krusei	–	+	–	–
C. guilliermondi	–	–	–	–
C. glabrata	–	–	–	–

*Species are listed in their known rank order of pathogenicity.

+ +, Strong/high ability; +, able; ±, little ability; –, very weak or no ability.

Reprinted with permission from Odds FC: Candida infections: An overview. CRC Crit Rev Microbiol 15:1, 1987. Copyright CRC Press, Inc., Boca Raton, FL.

tion, 5-FC is used in combination with amphotericin B (Lilien et al, 1978). Fluconazole (5 to 6 mg/kg every 2 to 3 days) has also been shown to be safe and effective (Fasano et al, 1994; Presterl and Graninger, 1994; Saxen et al, 1993).

Congenital Candidiasis

Many examples of candidal infection acquired in utero have been reported. Dvorak and Gavaller's patient, reported in 1966, had a diffuse macular rash and respiratory distress at birth and died at 34 hours of age. Autopsy showed extensive bronchopneumonia, the sections filled with hyphae and spores. The placenta was also heavily infected with the fungus.

In these instances, ascending infection produces chorioamnionitis with dissemination to the fetus, which can lead to spontaneous abortion (Ho and Aterman, 1970). In most instances, the severity of disseminated candidiasis acquired in utero is such that the infant dies before therapy can be considered (Schirar et al, 1974).

On the one hand, cutaneous candidiasis, evident at the time of birth, can be seen in the absence of systemic involvement (Aterman, 1968; Chapel et al, 1982; Rhatigan, 1968; Wolach et al, 1991). Adverse outcome may also be avoided by accurate prenatal diagnostic procedures and prompt antifungal therapy in the neonatal period (Mazor et al, 1993). On the other hand, cases of systemic candidiasis, probably acquired in utero, have been described in the absence of rash (Johnson et al, 1981; Mamlok et al, 1985; Whyte et al, 1982). The rash, when it does occur, evolves from maculopapular to vesicular to pustular.

It thus appears that *Candida*, like bacteria, may infect the fetus by hematogenous dissemination from the umbilical vessels, leading to systemic infection, or may be limited to cutaneous candidiasis.

Pneumonia Complicating Oral Candidiasis

Adams (1944) reported that five of eight infants who had thrush showed respiratory distress, cyanosis, and leukocytosis. They all had signs of pneumonitis. In one who died, *Candida* had invaded the pulmonary parenchyma, and the author believed this to have been an example of true thrush pneumonitis. Winter (1955) cannot accept Adams' autopsied case as one of mycotic pneumonia but believes that this complication has been demonstrated beyond doubt in a 1 year old and in several older persons.

Mycotic pneumonia has also been reported as an unexpected finding at autopsies of newborns (Koenig, 1971). The course was not always fulminant, and there is little specificity to the roentgenographic picture. Infants with thrush and pneumonia should be suspected of having *Candida* as the infecting agent, particularly if they have been pretreated with broad-spectrum antibiotics. Isolation of *C. albicans* from the blood of such infants is strongly suggestive of bronchopulmonary candidiasis, but demonstration of hyphae in tracheal aspirates obtained at bronchoscopy or pulmonary tissue obtained by open lung biopsy is the best evidence of infection. Although these procedures are hazardous, the possibility of identifying a potentially treatable disease should be strongly considered.

Beckmann and Navarro (1955) recorded the following case history.

CASE STUDY 6

A 2125-g infant was discharged from the nursery on the 10th day of life, well except for thick deposits of thrush upon the tongue. Gentian violet and 2% ferric chloride solution were used locally, but the lesion became ulcerative and spread to involve all the oral and buccal mucous membranes. Cyanosis during feeding appeared, and rales were heard throughout both lungs. At 3 months of age, the infant was admitted to the hospital, weighing 2435 g. His temperature was 98.6° F, and never elevated during his stay. He was malnourished, cyanotic, and critically ill. There were mucopurulent nasal and oral discharges. Radiographs showed patches of pneumonia, atelectasis, and emphysema. Attempted feedings caused choking and cyanosis. Intravenous fluid therapy, transfusion, penicillin, and Gantrisin failed to improve his condition. Mycostatin, 175,000 units orally every 6 hours, was begun, and within 48 hours his mouth was practically healed. The respiratory difficulty improved more slowly and was not gone until the 2nd week of treatment.

Comment

The authors concede that the diagnosis of *C. albicans* pneumonitis was far from proved but believe that the response to the fungicidal antibiotic was striking enough to be highly suggestive.

Thrush Esophagitis

Several cases have been reported in which oral candidiasis has advanced to involve the nasopharynx and esophagus. When this occurs, swallowing becomes almost impossible, and during the attempts to swallow, much liquid appears to be aspirated into the tracheobronchial tree. Choking spells with cyanosis result.

Wolff and coworkers (1955) reported two examples from Birmingham, England. The first is described in the following case history.

CASE STUDY 7

A female infant weighed 2720 g at birth and seemed well until her 16th day, when anorexia and vomiting began. When she was admitted the next day, her general condition seemed good, but the tongue and buccal mucous membranes were covered with a white membrane from which *C. albicans* was identified by smear. After 3 days of treatment with 1% gentian violet locally and 0.01% solution (4 mL, three times a day orally), there was no improvement. It did not respond to sulfonamide or, later, to penicillin. Profuse viscid discharge from the mouth and nose appeared. At this stage the infant could not swallow, and attempts led to repeated bouts of cyanosis. On the 8th day, hydroxystilbamidine was begun, 15 mg (5 mg/kg) in 0.75 mL of water injected slowly into the intravenous infusion tubing. This was repeated every 12 hours. A coagulase-positive *Staphylococcus* was grown from the blood. Streptomycin was given in addition to the other drug. Improvement began while the infant was on hydroxystilbamidine alone. After 6 days, the intravenous drip was removed, and oral feedings were started. On the 18th day, barium swallow showed that incoordination of swallowing was still present, with much iodized oil entering the trachea during the act of deglutition. Gavage feedings were begun again and were able to be discontinued 1 week later.

Comment

Such contiguous spread should be suspected in infants with thrush when swallowing becomes difficult and aspiration seems to be taking place. The contiguous spread can be more anterior and produce signs and symptoms of congenital stridor (Perrone, 1970).

Enteric Candidiasis

Kozinn and Taschdjian (1962) advise against the tendency to forget the possibility of enteric candidiasis in the differential diagnosis of diarrhea in the young infant. The gastrointestinal tract is believed to be the principal habitat of commensal *Candida* species (Odds, 1987). They stress that it is a not uncommon complication of thrush and that it may lead to systemic invasion and death.

The diagnosis should be suspected whenever diarrhea complicates thrush or cutaneous candidiasis, especially if the infant has been on antimicrobial therapy. Direct examination of stools reveals in many cases the mycelial form of the fungus, a finding that is much more significant than visualization of yeast forms. A recently recognized complication of enteric candidiasis is focal gastrointestinal perforation in very-low-birth-weight infants (Meyer et al, 1991; Mintz and Appelbaum, 1993). Bluish discoloration of the abdomen is usually seen in these infants, and no pathologic evidence of necrotizing enterocolitis is detectable. Postoperative treatment with antifungal agents is critical in improving outcomes of these extremely ill infants.

Good clinical response and disappearance of the organisms can be attained with nystatin in 80% of cases. Amphotericin B may be helpful in severe cases.

REFERENCES

Adams JM: A reevaluation of the pneumonias of infancy. J Pediatr 25:369, 1944.

Adler S, Randall J, Plotkin SA: Candidal osteomyelitis and arthritis in a neonate. Am J Dis Child 123:595, 1972.

Ashcraft KW, Leape LL: Candida sepsis complicating parenteral feeding. JAMA 212:454, 1970.

Aterman K: Pathology of candida infection of the umbilical cord. Am J Clin Pathol 49:798, 1968. .

Baley JE, Kliegman RM, Fanaroff AA: Disseminated fungal infections in very low-birth-weight infants: Clinical manifestations and epidemiology. Pediatrics 73:144, 1984.

Baley JE, Kliegman RM, Boxerbaum B, et al: Fungal colonization in the very low birth weight infant. Pediatrics 78:225, 1986.

Beckmann AJ, Navarro JE: Pneumonia complicating oral thrush treated with mycostatin, a new antifungal antibiotic. J Pediatr 46:587, 1955.

Bendel CM, Hostetter MK: Distinct mechanisms of epithelial adhesion for Candida albicans and Candida tropicalis. Identification of the participating ligands and development of inhibitory peptides. J Clin Invest 92:1840, 1993.

Bernstein DI, Tipton JR, Schott SF, et al: Coccidioidomycosis in a neonate: Maternal-infant transmission. J Pediatr 99:752, 1981.

Block ER, Jennings AE, Bennett JE: 5-Fluorocytosine resistance in Cryptococcus neoformans. Antimicrob Agents Chemother 3:649, 1973.

Bodey GP, Luna M: Skin lesions associated with disseminated candidiasis. JAMA 229:1466, 1974.

Britton H, Shehab Z, Lightner E, et al: Adrenal response in children receiving high doses of ketoconazole for systemic coccidioidomycosis. J Pediatr 112:488, 1988.

Burry AF: Hydrocephalus after intrauterine fungal infection. Arch Dis Child 32:161, 1957.

Centers for Disease Control and Prevention: Update—Coccidioidomycosis—California, 1991–1993. MMWR Morb Mortal Wkly Rep 43:421, 1994.

Chapel TA, Gagliardi C, Nichols W: Congenital cutaneous candidiasis. J Am Acad Dermatol 6:926, 1982.

Child DD, Newell JD, Bjelland JC, et al: Radiographic findings of pulmonary coccidioidomycosis in neonates and infants. Am J Radiol 145:216, 1985.

Clapp DW, Kleiman MB, Brahmi Z: Immunoregulatory lymphocyte populations in disseminated histoplasmosis of infancy. J Infect Dis 156:687, 1987.

Diamond RD, Bennett JE: A subcutaneous reservoir for intrathecal therapy of fungal meningitis. N Engl J Med 288:186, 1972.

Drutz DJ, Catanzaro D: Coccidioidomycosis. Am Rev Respir Dis 117:559, 727, 1978.

Dvorak AM, Gavaller B: Congenital systemic candidiasis: Report of a case. N Engl J Med 274:540, 1966.

Edwards VE, Sutherland JM, Tyner JH: Cryptococcosis of the central nervous system. J Neurol Neurosurg Psychiatry 33:415, 1970.

Ellis CA, Spivack ML: The significance of candidemia. Ann Intern Med 67:511, 1967.

Emanuel B, Ching E, Lieberman AD, et al: Cryptococcus meningitis in a child successfully treated with amphotericin B, with a review of the literature. J Pediatr 59:577, 1961.

Emmons CW: Cryptococcus neoformans, strains from an outbreak of bovine mastitis. Mycolpathol Mycol Appl 6:231, 1953.

Eppes SC, Troutman JL, Gutman LT: Outcome of treatment of candidemia in children whose central catheters were removed or retained. Pediatr Infect Dis 8:99, 1989.

Faix RG: Systemic Candida infections in infants in intensive care nurseries: High incidence of central nervous system involvement. J Pediatr 105:616, 1984.

Fasano C, O'Keeffe J, Gibbs D: Fluconazole treatment of neonates and infants with severe fungal infections not treatable with conventional agents. Eur J Clin Microbiol Infect Dis 13:351, 1994.

Fishman LS, Griffin JR, Sapico FL: Hematogenous candida endophthalmitis: A complication of candidemia. N Engl J Med 286:675, 1972.

Freeman JB, Weinke JW, Soper RT: Candida osteomyelitis associated with intravenous alimentation. J Pediatr Surg 9:783, 1974.

Goldmann DA, Maki DG: Infection control in total parenteral nutrition. JAMA 223:1360, 1973.

Haring H, Johnston R, Touloukian R: Successfully treated candida endophthalmitis. Pediatrics 51:1027, 1973.

Harrison HR, Galgiani JN, Reynolds AF, et al: Amphotericin B and imidazole therapy for coccidioidal meningitis in children. Pediatr Infect Dis 2:216, 1983.

Heiner DC: Diagnosis of histoplasmosis. Pediatrics 22:616, 1958.

Henderson JL: Infection in the newborn. Edinburgh Med J 50:535, 1943.

Hill HR, Mitchell TG, Matsen JM, et al: Recovery from disseminated candidiasis in a premature neonate. Pediatrics 53:748, 1974.

Ho CY, Aterman K: Infection of the fetus by candida in a spontaneous abortion. Am J Obstet Gynecol 106:705, 1970.

Holland P, Holland NH: Histoplasmosis in early infancy: Hematologic, histochemical and immunologic observations. Am J Dis Child 112:412, 1966.

Johnson DE, Thompson TR, Ferrieri P: Congenital candidiasis. Am J Dis Child 135:273, 1981.

Joshi W, Wang NS: Repeated pulmonary embolism in an infant with subacute candida endocarditis of the right side of the heart. Am J Dis Child 125:257, 1973.

Kafka JA, Catanzaro P: Disseminated coccidioidomycosis in children. J Pediatr 98:355, 1981.

Kida M, Abromowsky CR, Santoscoy C: Cryptococcosis of the placenta in a woman with acquired immunodeficiency syndrome. Hum Pathol 20:920, 1989.

Klein JD, Yamauchi T, Horlick SP: Neonatal candidiasis meningitis and arthritis: Observations and review of literature. J Pediatr 81:31, 1972.

Knox WF, Hooton VN, Barson AJ: Pulmonary vascular candidiasis and use of central venous catheters in neonates. J Clin Pathol 40:559, 1987.

Koenig ND: Candida pneumonia in newborn infants. Dtsch Med Wochenschr 96:818, 1971.

Kozinn P, Taschdjian CL: Enteric candidiasis: Diagnosis and clinical considerations. Pediatrics 30:71, 1962.

Lacey SR, Zaritsky AL, Azizkhan RG: Successful treatment of candida-infected caval thrombosis in critically ill infants by low-dose streptokinase infusion. J Pediatr Surg 23:1204, 1988.

Leggiadro RJ, Barrett FF, Hughes WT: Disseminated histoplasmosis of infancy. Pediatr Infect Dis 7:799, 1988.

Lilien LD, Ramamurhy RS, Pildes RS: *Candida albicans* meningitis in a premature neonate successfully treated with 5-fluorocytosine and amphotericin B: A case report and review of the literature. Pediatrics 61:57, 1978.

Little J, Bruce J, Andrews H, et al: Treatment of disseminated infantile histoplasmosis with amphotericin B. Pediatrics 24:1, 1959.

Mamlock RJ, Richardson CJ, Mamlok V, et al: A case of intrauterine pulmonary candidiasis. Pediatr Infect Dis 4:692, 1985.

Marodi L, Kaposzta R, Campbell DE, et al: Candidacidal mechanisms in the human neonate. Impaired IFN-gamma activation of macrophages in newborn infants. J Immunol 153:5642, 1994.

Mazor M, Chiam W, Shinwell ES, Glezerman M: Asymptomatic amniotic fluid invasion with *Candida albicans* in preterm premature rupture of membranes. Implications for obstetric and neonatal management. Acta Obstet Gynecol Scand 72:52, 1993.

McDonnell PJ, McDonnell JM, Brown RH, et al: Ocular involvement in patients with fungal infections. Ophthalmology 92:706, 1985.

McGregor JA, Kleinschmidt-DeMasters BK, Ogle J: Meningoencephalitis caused by *Histoplasma capsulatum* complicating pregnancy. Am J Obstet Gynecol 154:925, 1986.

Medoff F, Comfort M, Kobayoshi GS: Synergistic action of amphotericin B and 5-fluorocytosine against yeast-like organisms. Proc Soc Exp Biol Med 138:571, 1971.

Meyer CL, Payne NR, Roback SA: Spontaneous, isolated intestinal perforations in neonates with birth weight less than 1,000 g not associated with necrotizing enterocolitis. J Pediatr Surg 26:714, 1991.

Mintz AC, Applebaum H: Focal gastrointestinal perforations not associated with necrotizing enterocolitis in very low birth weight neonates. J Pediatr Surg 28:857, 1993.

Neuhauser EBD, Tucker A: The roentgen changes produced by diffuse torulosis in the newborn. AJR Am J Roentgenol 59:805, 1948.

Odds FC: Candida infections: An overview. CRC Crit Rev Microbiol 15:1, 1987.

Perrone JA: Laryngeal obstruction due to *Monilia albicans* in a newborn. Laryngoscope 80:288, 1970.

Peterson CM, Schuppert K, Kelly PC, Pappagianis D: Coccidioidomycosis and pregnancy. Obstet Gynecol Surv 48:149, 1993.

Peterson JC, Christie A: Histoplasmosis. Pediatr Clin North Am 2:127, 1955.

Pounder WD, Amberson JM, Jaeger RF: A severe mastitis problem associated with *Cryptococcus neoformans* in a large dairy herd. Am J Vet Res 13:121, 1952.

Presterl E, Graninger W: Efficacy and safety of fluconazole in the treatment of systemic fungal infections in pediatric patients. Multicentre Study Group. Eur J Clin Microbiol Infect Dis 13:347, 1994.

Rhatigan RM: Congenital cutaneous candidiasis. Am J Dis Child 116:545, 1968.

Rothman PE, Graw RG, Harria JC: Coccidioidomycosis—Possible fomite transmission. Am J Dis Child 118:792, 1962.

Sarosi GA, Parker JD, Doto IL, et al: Amphotericin B in cryptococcal meningitis. Ann Intern Med 71:1079, 1969.

Saxen H, Hoppu K, Pohjavuori M: Pharmacokinetics of fluconazole in very low birth weight infants during the first two weeks of life. Clin Pharmacol Ther 54:269, 1993.

Schirar A, Rendu C, Vielk JP, et al: Congenital mycosis (*Candida albicans*). Biol Neonate 24:273, 1974.

Shapira Y, Drucker M, Russell A, et al: Candida endocarditis and encephalitis in an infant. Clin Pediatr 13:542, 1974.

Shafai T: Neonatal coccidioidomycosis in premature twins. Am J Dis Child 132:634, 1978.

Shehab ZM, Britton H, Dunn JH: Imidazole therapy of coccidioidal meningitis in children. Pediatr Infect Dis 7:40, 1988.

Sherertz RJ, Geldhill KS, Hampton KD, et al: Outbreak of Candida bloodstream infections associated with retrograde medication administration in a neonatal intensive care unit. J Pediatr 120:455, 1992.

Silverman EM, Norman LF, Goldman RT: Diagnosis of systemic candidiasis in smears of venous blood stained with Wright's stain. Am J Clin Pathol 60:473, 1973.

Slotkowsky EL: Formation of mucous membrane lesions secondary to prolonged use of one per cent aqueous gentian violet. J Pediatr 51:652, 1957.

Spark RP: Does transplacental spread of coccidioidomycosis occur? Arch Pathol Lab Med 105:347, 1981.

Stevens DA: Coccidioidomycosis. N Engl J Med 332:1077, 1995.

Townsend TE, McKey RW: Coccidioidomycosis in infants. Am J Dis Child 86:51, 1953.

Westley CR: Disseminated coccidioidomycosis in children. J Pediatr 101:154, 1982.

Wheat LJ, French MCV, Kohler RB, et al: The diagnostic laboratory tests for histoplasmosis: Analysis of experience in a large urban outbreak. Ann Intern Med 97:680, 1982.

Wheat LJ, Wass J, Norton J, et al: Cavitary histoplasmosis occurring during two large urban outbreaks. Medicine 63:201, 1984.

Whyte RK, Hussain Z, deSa D: Antenatal infections with *Candida* species. Arch Dis Child 57:258, 1982.

Winter WG Jr: *Candida (Monilia)* infections in children. Pediatr Clin North Am 2:151, 1955.

Wolach B, Bogger-Goren S, Whyte R: Perinatal hematological profile of newborn infants with candida antenatal infections. Biol Neonate 59:5, 1991.

Wolff OH, Petty BW, Astley R, et al: Thrush oesophagitis with pharyngeal incoordination treated with hydroxystilbamidine. Lancet 1:991, 1955.

Ziering WH, Rockas HR: Coccidioidomycosis: Long-term treatment with amphotericin B of disseminated disease in a three-month-old baby. Am J Dis Child 108:454, 1964.

CHAPTER 46

Protozoal Infections: Congenital Toxoplasmosis and Malaria

F. Sessions Cole[*]

CONGENITAL TOXOPLASMOSIS

One of the organisms that causes congenital infection of the human fetus, often presenting in the newborn period as a local or generalized disease, is *Toxoplasma gondii*. It is obscure why this agent, so different in its biologic make-up from cytomegalovirus, rubella, and *Treponema pallidum*, should present so similar a clinical picture. Differentiation from these other syndromes on clinical and laboratory grounds is essential to treatment and prognosis and depends on the extensive knowledge of its epidemiology, clinical behavior, and microbiology gained since the 1960s.

Incidence

Inapparent infection with the protozoan is widespread throughout the world. Population samples indicate that the percentage of adults with antibody is increased at lower geographic latitudes. Feldman (1953) found approximately 10% of his sample positive by complement fixation test in Iceland, 30% in New Orleans, and 65% in Tahiti. However, latitude is by no means the only determining factor. The number of positive reactors in Paris, for instance, is unusually high at 2.3% of all pregnant women who undergo seroconversion during pregnancy; this number has been attributed to Parisians' fondness for raw or undercooked meat. With regard to congenital toxoplasmosis, Hohlfeld and coworkers (1994) recently identified 194 congenitally infected infants and Guerina and associates (1994) 52 such infants, observations that suggest the disease cannot be considered rare.

Serum specimens from 22,845 pregnant women in the Collaborative Perinatal Project were studied by Sever (1988) for evidence of infection with *Toxoplasma*, and 38% of the women showed evidence of toxoplasmosis (detectable antibody at titers of ≥32) at some time in the past. Five infants among the group had confirmed congenital toxoplasmosis. The most recent estimates of frequency of congenital infection in the United States range from 1 to 8 per 1000 livebirths (Wong and Remington, 1994). A study from Malmö, Sweden, revealed that the incidence of primary maternal infection in that city is 4 to 6 per 1000 deliveries (Ahlfors et al, 1989).

Guerina and coworkers (1994) recently reported the results of neonatal screening programs in Massachusetts and New Hampshire for detection of congenital toxoplasmosis. Nineteen of 48 infants identified in this study had abnormalities of either the central nervous system or retina.

After treatment, only 1 of 46 children had a clinically detectable neurologic deficit, and 4 had eye lesions (1 with a macular lesion and 3 with minor retinal scars). McAuley and colleagues (1994) from Chicago have also reported improved outcomes after early treatment. These observations suggest that early diagnosis and treatment may reduce the risk of significant neurologic deficits in infected infants and children.

Etiology

The disease is caused by infestation with a protozoan, *Toxoplasma gondii*, so named because it was first isolated in 1909 from a North African rodent called the "gondi." In addition to the large number of human beings who are infected, many domestic and wild animals and birds harbor the organism. The domestic cat is the only definitive host and is the reservoir of the infective oocysts that are passed in the feces. Maternal toxoplasma infection results primarily from ingestion of undercooked or raw meat, which contains tissue cysts, or ingestion of water or foodstuffs contaminated by oocysts that have been excreted in feces of infected cats (Wong and Remington, 1994). Congenital toxoplasmosis is caused by invasion of the fetal bloodstream by parasites during a stage of maternal parasitemia. It is likely that the parasitemia occurs only with initial infection and often in the absence of any maternal symptoms. Mothers whose infections become chronic and inapparent do not transmit the disease to subsequent fetuses. Desmonts and Couvreur describe infection of the fetus in 33% of all maternal infections. This figure should be considered only an estimate because many mothers in the study received treatment. Data from the Collaborative Perinatal Project (5 of 15 infants, or 33%), and from Sweden (6 of 29 infants, or 21%) indicate that this estimate is reasonable (Ahlfors et al, 1989; Sever et al, 1988). In addition, risk of congenital toxoplasmosis varies considerably with gestational age at the time of maternal infection. In a recently reported series of 2632 primarily infected pregnant women, 194 infected fetuses (7.4%) were identified (Hohlfeld et al, 1994). However, among 100 fetuses in whose mothers infection developed during the first 2 weeks of gestation, none was infected. Among 38 fetuses whose mothers were infected between 27 and 34 weeks' gestation, 11 (28.9%) became infected. Severe neonatal disease is usually seen with first and second trimester infections.

Postnatal infections also occur in children, but the youngest patient was a 7-month-old infant who became ill with diarrhea at 3 months of age. The disease occurred 1 month after the institution of unpasteurized goat's milk feeding and was almost surely the result of that form of alimentation (Riemann et al, 1975).

---

[*]This chapter includes some contributions from the previous authors, Drs. Arnold Smith and Kenneth McIntosh.

Pathology

The *Toxoplasma* is a crescent-shaped organism, 4 to 7 μm long, with a single, approximately central nucleus. In tissues it is intracellular, and small or large agglomerates are often seen. In later stages, the organism is often seen lying within a cystic space, especially in the brain and skeletal and heart muscle.

In the newborn, the principal locus of infection is the central nervous system. Lesions consist of areas of necrosis in which calcium is ultimately deposited and throughout which cysts or the naked parasite may be sparsely scattered. Similar lesions are less abundant in the liver, lungs, myocardium, skeletal muscle, spleen, and other tissues. There is little cellular inflammatory reaction, consisting mostly of lymphocytes, monocytes, and plasma cells. The pathologic picture is not specific unless organisms or cysts can be demonstrated.

Diagnosis

Most of the infants with congenital toxoplasmosis (approximately 85%) have no symptoms or apparent abnormalities at birth (Wong and Remington, 1994). In Desmonts and Couvreur's series, there were two subclinical cases for each clinical one. In such infants, however, disease usually develops as they grow older. The natural history of the disease described by these authors may be different in the 1990s because of antenatal diagnosis, treatment, and the increasing proportion of reproductive-age range women with human immunodeficiency virus (HIV) infection or acquired immunodeficiency syndrome (AIDS). This latter group of women and fetuses/infants presents a unique set of biologic and therapeutic questions (Wong and Remington, 1994). Although data are not yet available to define the risk of congenital toxoplasmosis in HIV-infected mothers, preliminary data suggest a markedly higher rate of transmission (Wong and Remington, 1994). Whether these congenital infections represent reactivation of prior *Toxoplasma* infections or newly acquired infections has not been determined. Coinfection of the fetus with both HIV and *T. gondii* has also been observed. Recent reviews of the natural history of infants who are congenitally infected suggest that prenatal treatment and postnatal treatment for at least 1 year can significantly improve outcome, even in the presence of central nervous system calcifications or retinal changes (Guerina et al, 1994; McAuley et al, 1994).

The so-called classic triad of congenital toxoplasmosis is present in only a small proportion of symptomatic cases. Chorioretinitis, hydrocephalus, and intracranial calcifications were present in 86%, 20%, and 37%, respectively, of the large series of Eichenwald (1957). Fever, hepatosplenomegaly, and jaundice are frequent signs, even in the absence of central nervous system or ocular findings. Rash and pneumonitis occasionally occur. The spinal fluid is often abnormal. Anemia is frequent, and thrombocytopenia and eosinophilia are occasionally seen. Cataracts, microphthalmia, and glaucoma, so common in rubella, are rare. Microcephaly is less common than hydrocephalus. Diarrhea is occasionally a prominent symptom. More recent data from a study of 210 congenitally infected infants by Couvreur and associates (1984) adapted by Remington and

Desmonts (1990) indicate lower frequencies for these signs and symptoms (Table 46–1). These differences may be due to antenatal therapy or to detection of primary maternal infections and subsequent termination of pregnancy.

Neurologic and ocular involvement frequently appear later if they are absent at birth. Convulsions, mental retardation, and spasticity are all common sequelae. A morphologically characteristic relapsing chorioretinitis is the most common sequela of congenital toxoplasmosis, although involvement of the anterior uveal tract also occurs (O'Connor, 1974). It is also clear that most, if not all cases of *Toxoplasma* chorioretinitis represent the sequelae of congenital infection. Treatment has significantly improved the rather grim prognosis of congenital disease.

Although some infants are highly symptomatic at birth, the disease may also be insidious in onset.

In 1953, Beckett and Flynn reported two infants with toxoplasmosis. The first is described in the following case history.

CASE STUDY 1

An infant born at term seemed normal until the 5th day, when ptosis of one lid was noted. In the 4th week, vomiting and pallor developed; in the 5th week, high-pitched cry, enlargement of the head, and opisthotonos were noted. Examination at 6 weeks showed dehydration, pallor, sluggishness, hydrocephalus, bulging fontanel, separated sutures, and right facial nerve palsy. The liver and spleen were not large, purpura was absent, and platelets were normal. Cerebrospinal fluid was grossly abnormal and xanthochromic, containing 200 red blood cells/mm^3 and 2900 mg of protein/dL. Skull radiographs showed fine scattered calcifications.

The epidemiology in this example was noteworthy. The antibody titer of the mother against *Toxoplasma* registered 1:4906, whereas that of a pet dachshund that had had "brain fever" with residual paralysis of one leg at the time of the infant's conception was 1:256.

Other more bizarre forms of the disease have been described. Silver and Dixon's case (1954), described in the following paragraph, is one of the more remarkable ones, demonstrating how protean the manifestations of congenital toxoplasmosis can be.

CASE STUDY 2

This infant's course was one of increasing lethargy, poor appetite, and bleeding manifestations until hospital admission in his 6th week of life. Facial nerve palsy, hepatosplenomegaly, lethargy, pupillary membranes, and cataracts were found. Cerebrospinal fluid was xanthochromic and contained a few white and red blood cells and 1000 mg of protein/dL. Radiographs of the skull showed flaky calcific densities. This patient's

TABLE 46–1

Prospective Study of Infants Born to Women Who Acquired *Toxoplasma* Infection During Pregnancy: Signs and Symptoms in 210 Infants with Proved Congenital Infection

Finding		Number Examined	Number Positive (%)
Prematurity	Birth weight below 2500 g	210	8 (3.8)
	Birth weight of 2500–3000 g		5 (7.1)
Dysmaturity (intrauterine growth retardation)			13 (6.2)
Postmaturity		108	9 (8.3)
Icterus		201	20 (10)
Hepatosplenomegaly		210	9 (4.2)
Thrombocytopenic purpura		210	3 (1.4)
Abnormal blood count (anemia, eosinophilia)		102	9 (4.4)
Microcephaly		210	11 (5.2)
Hydrocephalus		210	8 (3.8)
Hypotonia		210	2 (5.7)
Convulsions		210	8 (3.8)
Psychomotor retardation		210	11 (5.2)
Intracranial calcifications on x-ray examination		210	24 (11.4)
Abnormal ultrasound examination		49	5 (10)
Abnormal computer tomographic scan of brain		13	11 (84)
Abnormal electroencephalographic result		191	16 (8.3)
Abnormal cerebrospinal fluid		163	56 (34.2)
Microphthalmia		210	6 (2.8)
Strabismus		210	11 (5.2)
Chorioretinitis	Unilateral	210	34 (16.1)
	Bilateral		12 (5.7)

Adapted from Remington JS, Desmonts G: Toxoplasmosis. *In* Remington JS, Klein JO (Eds): Infectious Diseases of the Fetus and Newborn Infant. Philadelphia, WB Saunders, 1990, p 132.

course in the hospital was characterized by hypothermia, persistent hypernatremia, and inability to concentrate urine except when treated with posterior pituitary extract. He also showed eosinophilia of the peripheral blood (30%) and of the bone marrow.

Laboratory Findings

Because culture of the organism is tedious and expensive, laboratory diagnosis depends heavily on interpretation of various serologic tests. There are several valuable tests for antibody to *T. gondii*. Although the Sabin-Feldman dye test (lysis of *Toxoplasma* organisms by various dilutions of maternal or infant serum after incubation for 1 hour at 37° C) used to be the standard method, several newer tests easier to perform and of equal reliability have supplanted it in many laboratories, particularly the indirect fluorescent antibody (IFA) test and the enzyme-linked immunosorbent assay (ELISA). Both tests can be adapted to measure IgM antibody. As with other congenital infections, false-positive IgM antibody titers may be caused by rheumatoid factor. Complement fixation and indirect hemagglutination tests may also be performed but are somewhat more difficult to interpret. Detection of IgA antibodies against P30, a major surface protein of *T. gondii*, has recently been reported to be more sensitive than detection of anti-P30 IgM antibodies in identification of congenitally infected infants (DeCoster et al, 1988). All eight congenitally infected infants from 26 mothers infected during pregnancy were identified by

the presence of anti-P30 IgA antibodies, and anti-P30 IgM antibodies were found in three of the eight infected infants.

Antibody develops during acute infection in the mother and remains high or decreases slowly over a year's time. A single high antibody titer implies, but does not prove, recent infection. A serologic diagnosis of acute infection requires an increase in antibody titer in serial samples obtained at least 3 weeks apart and tested in parallel in the same laboratory (Wong and Remington, 1994). In the infant, the titer at birth equals or exceeds the mother's, regardless of whether the baby is congenitally infected. Over the 1st year in the uninfected infant, the titer decreases with a half-life of approximately 30 days. In the infected infant, although the titer may decrease somewhat for the first few months, it increases again to a high level by the first birthday. IgM anti-*Toxoplasma* antibody may be present at birth or at any time for the next few months. A negative *Toxoplasma* antibody titer in the infant's serum at 6 months to 1 year of age essentially excludes the diagnosis.

When symptomatic or serologic evidence of *Toxoplasma* infection is detected during pregnancy, fetal infection can be diagnosed (Hohlfeld et al, 1994; Wong and Remington, 1994). Specific fetal diagnosis is predicated on detection of IgM anti-*Toxoplasma* antibodies and on isolation (by mouse inoculation) of the parasite from fetal blood or amniotic fluid obtained between 20 and 26 weeks of gestation. In the study by Daffos and colleagues (1988), fetal *Toxoplasma* infection was documented by parasite isolation from fetal blood or amniotic fluid in 34 of 746 pregnancies. An additional five pregnancies had serologic fetal biochemical and ultrasonographic evidence of fetal *Toxoplasma* infection. *Toxoplasma*-specific IgM antibodies were identified in fetal blood in only nine cases. Ultrasound examination was helpful in antenatal diagnosis by detecting ascites in two cases and ventricular dilation in 17 cases. Important to note is that 10 of the 17 cases of ventricular dilation were noted in the third trimester after positive results were obtained by blood or amniotic fluid sampling. Ultrasound findings consistent with *Toxoplasma* infection in the context of maternal seroconversion permits consideration of maternal treatment before availability of culture results and findings with which to monitor fetal progress (Daffos et al, 1988). Finally, besides the 34 infected fetuses, an additional three pregnancies resulted in congenital infection. These infections occurred despite antenatal maternal therapy and most likely represent parasite transmission to the fetus after the time of fetal blood sampling (Daffos et al, 1988). When maternal infection is documented during pregnancy, fetal infection before 20 weeks' gestation has been difficult to determine because of the lack of fetal immunologic response (IgM and IgA) (Wong and Remington, 1994). The recent report of the usefulness of polymerase chain reaction, which targets the *B1* gene of *T. gondii*, may permit accurate diagnosis of fetal infection before 20 weeks' gestation (Hohlfeld et al, 1994). These investigators amplified *Toxoplasma*-specific sequences in amniotic fluid and used a positive internal control fragment that competed with the *B1* gene sequences for primer template binding and amplification. Further study of the kinetics of appearance of these sequences in amniotic fluid after maternal infection will be important to evaluate the significance of a negative result.

Antenatal ultrasonography has also been useful in identifying fetuses who are infected. Approximately 36% of fetuses have abnormalities noted, the most common of which is bilateral, symmetric ventricular dilatation (Wong and Remington, 1994). Other prenatally detected abnormalities include intracranial calcifications, increased placental thickness, hepatomegaly, and ascites.

Treatment

Maternal treatment for women who acquire *Toxoplasma* infection during pregnancy reduces the likelihood of congenital transmission by as much as 70% (Daffos et al, 1988; McCabe and Remington, 1988). Because 85% to 95% of women of child-bearing age in the United States are at risk and only 10% of immunocompetent women are symptomatic if infected, serologic screening as described by Daffos and coworkers (1988) before or early in pregnancy should be strongly considered to identify women at risk for infection. Seroconversion should prompt institution of maternal therapy (spiramycin, 3 g per day). This treatment should be continued throughout pregnancy. If fetal infection is diagnosed, 3 weeks of spiramycin therapy should be alternated with 3 weeks of pyrimethamine, 50 mg per day, and sulfadiazine, 3 g per day after the 24th week of gestation (Daffos et al, 1988). Careful hematologic monitoring should be performed along with concurrent treatment with folinic acid. Because of the lack of data, it is currently impossible to estimate the teratogenic and toxic risks to the fetus from antenatal therapy with pyrimethamine and

sulfadiazine. Before initiation of therapy, fetal diagnosis should be attempted to permit evaluation of risk and benefit of these drugs.

Treatment is recommended for all cases of congenital toxoplasmosis or congenital *Toxoplasma* infection. Guidelines for treatment are given in Table 46–2. Future treatment may involve more direct fetal therapy by intra-amniotic infusion of drugs (Matsui, 1994).

After confirmation of fetal infection, therapeutic abortion is a treatment option that needs to be considered. At Stanford University, Wong and Remington (1994) have reported that 53 of 241 pregnant women (22%) diagnosed serologically with *Toxoplasma* infection between 1988 and 1993 elected to terminate their pregnancies. Even though fetal diagnosis may be facilitated considerably by use of molecular methods such as polymerase chain reaction, each woman's decision must be predicated on her understanding of the risks of infection, the benefits of treatment, and the risks of the procedure. In the United States, routine serologic screening, patient education concerning prevention of *Toxoplasma* infection, and regional or national data concerning the incidence or outcome of toxoplasma infection are lacking (Wong and Remington, 1994; Stray-Pedersen, 1993).

Prognosis

It has been known for some time that the prognosis in untreated infants with overt disease at birth is poor (Eichenwald, 1960). Cerebral calcifications were thought to be a particularly ominous finding. Prospective follow-up studies in the 1960s and 1970s of congenitally infected infants asymptomatic at birth have shown that, even in this group, chorioretinitis is frequent and central nervous system involvement is not uncommon. In 1980, Wilson and coworkers found that, in 11 of 13 such infants, chorioretinitis developed and that, in one, seizures and severe psychomotor retardation also developed. In the same study, 11 other children were identified and followed up because they presented with symptoms. All 11 had been asymptomatic at birth. In this group, major neurologic sequelae developed in three, five were blind in both eyes, and three were blind in one eye. Ocular involvement may not begin until the end of the first decade.

More recently, the impact of antenatal diagnosis, antenatal treatment, and treatment during infancy has decreased the frequency of major neurologic sequelae (Daffos et al, 1988; Hohlfeld et al, 1989; McAuley et al, 1994). The overall risk of fetal infection in symptomatic or asymptomatic women who become seropositive is dependent on the time in gestation when maternal infection occurs: the later the stage in gestation, the more likely the transmission of parasites (Hohlfeld et al, 1989). The overall risk of fetal infection in Hohlfeld's study was 7%, most likely a reflection of antenatal spiramycin treatment. Fifty-four infants from this study have been followed up for periods from 6 months to 4 years. The infants' condition at birth is indicated in Table 46–3. Forty-seven of the 54 infants followed up received treatment consisting of pyrimethamine and sulfonamides alternating with spiramycin. The overall rate of subclinical infections was 76%. Fifty-three infants had normal development and neurologic status at follow-up.

TABLE 46–2

Guidelines for the Treatment of Congenital Toxoplasmosis*

Drugs

1. *Pyrimethamine + sulfadiazine:*
   Pyrimethamine: 15 mg/m² per day or 1 mg/kg per day (maximum daily dose is 25 mg) by the oral route. Although the half-life of the drug is 4 to 5 days, it should be given on a daily basis unless breaking of the tablets is grossly inaccurate during preparation of the smaller doses. In such cases, as for very small infants (e.g., when a daily dose of 3 mg is indicated), breaking of a tablet may result in a slightly higher dose, which could be administered every 2 days.
   Sulfadiazine or trisulfapyrimidines: 85 mg/kg per day by the oral route in two divided doses daily.
2. *Spiramycin†:* 100 mg/kg per day by the oral route in two divided doses.
3. *Corticosteroids:* (prednisone or methylprednisolone): 1.5 mg/kg per day by the oral route in two divided doses daily. The drug is continued until the inflammatory process (e.g., high level of cerebrospinal fluid protein [≥100 mg/dL before the age of 1 month], chorioretinitis) has subsided; dosage should then be tapered progressively and discontinued.
4. *Folinic acid:* 5 mg every 3 days (intramuscularly in young infants) during treatment with pyrimethamine. If bone marrow toxicity occurs at this dose, increase to 10 mg every 3 days. If bone marrow toxicity is severe, discontinue pyrimethamine until the abnormality is corrected and then begin pyrimethamine again using 10 mg folinic acid every 3 days. In some infants, it may be necessary to administer folinic acid more frequently.

Indications

1. *Overt congenital toxoplasmosis:* The course of treatment is for 1 year in all cases. For infants in whom clinical signs of the infection are present, treatment during the first 6 months is with pyrimethamine + sulfadiazine. During the following 6 months, 1 month of pyrimethamine + sulfadiazine is alternated with 1 month of spiramycin. Folinic acid should be started as soon as possible. No treatment is usually given after 12 months of age except when there is evidence of evolution of the infection, such as a flare-up of chorioretinitis.
2. *Overt congenital toxoplasmosis with evidence of inflammatory process* (chorioretinitis, high level of cerebrospinal fluid protein, generalized infection, jaundice): as in no. 1 above + corticosteroids.
3. *Subclinical congenital Toxoplasma infection:* Pyrimethamine + sulfadiazine for 6 weeks; thereafter, alternate with spiramycin. Spiramycin is given for 6 weeks and alternated with 4 weeks of pyrimethamine + sulfadiazine to complete a treatment course of 1 year.
4. *Healthy newborn in whom serologic testing has not provided definitive results but maternal infection was proved to have been acquired during pregnancy:* One course of pyrimethamine + sulfadiazine for 1 month. Obtain consultation with appropriate authority to determine necessity for continued therapy and drug and dosage regimen. This decision must be made on an individual basis and depends on multiple factors, including serologic test titers, immune load and clinical findings in the infant.
5. *Healthy newborn born to a mother with high Sabin-Feldman dye test titer—date of maternal infection undetermined:* Spiramycin for 1 month. Then as in no. 4 above. It must be borne in mind that in certain cases the indication for treatment is difficult to define because of a lack of information about the pregnancy and lack of isolation attempts from the corresponding placenta.

*Recommendations of Dr. Jacques Couvreur, Laboratoire de Sérologie Néonatale et de Recherche sur la Toxoplasmose, Institut de Puériculture, Paris.
†Available in the United States only by request to the U.S. Food and Drug Administration.
From Remington JS, Desmonts G: Toxoplasmosis. *In* Remington JS, Klein JO (Eds): Infectious Diseases of the Fetus and Newborn Infant. Philadelphia, WB Saunders, 1990.

Five of the 53 had peripheral chorioretinitis, as demonstrated by a scar noted between 5 and 17 months of life. In one infant who did not receive prenatal treatment because of a false-negative prenatal diagnosis, bilateral chorioretinitis and ventricular dilation developed necessitating a ventriculoperitoneal shunt at 1 month of age. The improving outcome of infants with congenital *Toxoplasma* infection are indicated in Table 46–4.

CONGENITAL MALARIA

Despite the high prevalence of malaria in many parts of the world, congenital malaria, that is, malaria acquired either in utero or in the perinatal period, is a relatively uncommon disease. Maternal parasitemia is presumably frequent, but transmission to the fetus appears to be effectively prevented in most instances by the placental barrier. Disease acquired in utero is, consequently, rare. Transmission at the time of birth is somewhat more common and is probably a consequence of placental leak of infected erythrocytes during delivery combined with inadequate immunity at the time of transmission (Randall and Seidel, 1985).

Etiology and Incidence

The incidence of malaria in the United States and North America increased during the 1980s and 1990s because of increasing overseas travel, immigration, and the spread of drug-resistant parasites (Centers for Disease Control and Prevention, 1989; Lackritz et al, 1991; Lynk and Gold, 1989; Subramanian et al, 1992). Infections have involved all four species of *Plasmodium* infecting humans. The incidence in endemic areas has been estimated to be 0.3%, with disease more likely when a mother acquires malaria for the first time during pregnancy and in primigravidas

TABLE 46–3

Condition of Live Neonates and Positive Findings at Birth

Observations	Number	Percent
Subclinical infection	44/54	81
Multiple cranial calcifications	5/54	9
Single intracranial calcification	2/54	4
Chorioretinitis scar	3/54	6
Abnormal lumbar puncture	1/54	2
Positive findings on inoculation of placenta	23/46	50
Positive cord blood IgM	8/53	15

From Hohlfeld P, Daggos F, Thulliez P, et al: Fetal toxoplasmosis: Outcome of pregnancy and infant follow-up after in utero treatment. J Pediatr 115:765, 1989.

(Miller et al, 1994; Randall and Seidel, 1985). The risk of transfusion-acquired malaria in the United States from 1972 to 1981 was 0.25 per million donor units (Guerro et al, 1983). Transfusion has been infrequently associated with malaria infection in neonatal intensive care units (Bove, 1986; Piccoli et al, 1983; Randall and Seidel, 1985; Shulman et al, 1984).

Diagnosis

The mother may or may not have symptomatic malaria during pregnancy, and cases have been described in which maternal disease was acquired not in an endemic area but through intravenous drug use or transfusion. In most instances, however, the history of exposure to malaria is clear. The child is usually normal at birth. Symptoms appear at 3 to 12 weeks of age. Fever is followed by hepatosplenomegaly, loss of appetite, listlessness, progressive hemolytic anemia, diarrhea, and jaundice.

The diagnosis is normally confirmed by demonstration of characteristic parasites on a thin or thick blood smear, and the particular species is determined by the morphologic appearance of the stained forms. Serologic studies can be used to confirm the diagnosis. If intrauterine transmission occurred, IgM antibody may be present in cord blood (Hindi and Azimi, 1980; Thomas and Chit, 1980). A rapid diagnostic test based on acridine orange staining of

centrifuged parasites in a microhematocrit tube has been reported by Rickman and associates (1989). Although it is not a substitute for the thick blood smear, it may provide easy, prompt diagnosis.

Treatment and Prognosis

Congenital malaria, like transfusion-acquired malaria, has no exoerythrocytic (liver) stage. When the organism is chloroquine sensitive, therefore, chloroquine alone (5 mg/kg of the base by mouth or gavage daily for 5 days) is adequate for treatment, and primaquine is not required. Chloroquine pharmacokinetics has been studied in children, and the drug can be used in infants who do not tolerate enteral treatment. Parenteral chloroquine (0.83 mg of base per kg per hour for 30 hours intravenously, or 3.5 mg/kg every 6 hours by intramuscular or subcutaneous injection) provided there is an acceptable therapeutic ratio (White et al, 1988). When chloroquine resistance is suspected, multiple drugs may be necessary, including parenteral quinidine gluconate or alternatively, exchange transfusion (Miller et al, 1989).

Not every child of every mother with malaria requires treatment at birth, because most will not acquire the disease. When maternal malaria is recognized at parturition, the infant should be followed up carefully, and treatment instituted, if necessary. Blood transfusion is frequently necessary in affected children, and, in areas with a high frequency of HIV infection, these transfusions put congenitally infected children at increased risk for HIV infection (Greenberg et al, 1988). In a recent comparison of 260 children born to HIV-seropositive women with 327 children born to seronegative mothers over a 13-month period, there was no evidence that malaria was more frequent or more severe in children with progressive HIV infection, and malaria did not appear to accelerate the progression of HIV disease (Greenberg et al, 1991).

Follow-up blood smears should confirm that treatment has been successful. In such instances, the prognosis is excellent.

Prevention of malaria during pregnancy represents a high priority for travelers from nonendemic areas as well as women from endemic areas. Even though no chemoprophylactic regimen is completely effective because of differ-

TABLE 46–4

Comparison of Different Outcomes of Liveborn Infants with Congenital *Toxoplasma* Infection

	Trimester											
	First				**Second**				**Third**			
	1972–1981		1982–1988		1972–1981		1982–1988		1972–1981		1982–1988	
Outcome	No.	%	No.	%	No.	%	No.	%	No.	%	No.	
Subclinical	1	10	6	67	23	37	33	77	74	68	2	
Benign	5	50	2	22	28	45	10	23	31	29	0	
Severe	4	40	1	11	11	18	0		3	3	0	
TOTAL	10		9		62		43		108		2	

From Hohlfeld P, Daggos F, Thulliez P, et al: Fetal toxoplasmosis: Outcome of pregnancy and infant follow-up after in utero treatment. J Pediatr 115:765, 1989.

ences in drug resistance, timing of infection during pregnancy, and other currently incompletely understood factors, chloroquine is a safe, well-tolerated, and effective drug for chemoprophylaxis (Garner and Brabin, 1994; Nyirjesy et al, 1993). Travel to areas in which chloroquine-resistant *Plasmodium falciparum* malaria is endemic should be avoided. A recent study of 339 pregnant women who live in an area of multidrug-resistant malaria suggested that mefloquine is safe and effective for antimalarial prophylaxis in the second half of pregnancy (Nosten et al, 1994).

REFERENCES

Ahlfors K, Borjeson M, Huldt G, et al: Incidence of toxoplasmosis in pregnant women in the city of Malmö. Scand J Infect Dis 21:315, 1989.

Beckett RS, Flynn FJ Jr: Toxoplasmosis: Report of two new cases with a classification and with a demonstration of the organisms in the human placenta. N Engl J Med 249:345, 1953.

Bove JR: Transfusion transmitted diseases: Current problems and challenges. Prog Hematol 14:123, 1986.

Centers for Disease Control: Summary of notifiable diseases, United States, 1989. MMWR Morb Mortal Wkly Rep 38:54, 1989.

Couvreur J, Desmonts G, Tournier G, et al: A homogeneous series of 20 cases of congenital toxoplasmosis in 0 to 11 month old infants detected prospectively. Ann Pediatr 31:815, 1984.

Daffos F, Forestier F, Capola-Pavlovsky M, et al: Prenatal management of 746 pregnancies at risk for congenital toxoplasmosis. N Engl J Med 318:271, 1988.

Decoster A, Darcy F, Caron A, et al: IgA antibodies against P30 as markers of congenital acute toxoplasmosis. Lancet 2:1104, 1988.

Desmonts G, Couvreur J: Cerebral toxoplasmosis, a prospective study of 378 pregnancies. N Engl J Med 270:1110, 1974.

Eichenwald H: Congenital toxoplasmosis. A study of one hundred fifty cases. Am J Dis Child 94:411, 1957.

Eichenwald H: A study of congenital toxoplasmosis. *In* Slim JD (Ed): Human Toxoplasmosis. Copenhagen, Munksgaard, 1960.

Feldman HA: The clinical manifestations and laboratory diagnosis of toxoplasmosis. Am J Trop Med 2:420, 1953.

Feldman HA: Toxoplasmosis. N Engl J Med 279:1370, 1431, 1968.

Garner P, Brabin B: A review of randomized controlled trials of routine antimalarial drug prophylaxis during pregnancy in endemic malarious areas. Bull World Health Organ 72:89, 1994.

Greenberg AE, Nguyen-Dinh P, Mann JM, et al: The association between malaria, blood transfusions, and HIV seropositivity in a pediatric population in Kinshasa, Zaire. JAMA 259:545, 1988.

Greenberg AE, Nsa W, Ryder RW, et al: *Plasmodium falciparum* malaria and perinatally acquired human immunodeficiency virus type 1 infection in Kinshasa, Zaire. A prospective, longitudinal cohort study of 587 children. N Engl J Med 325:105, 1991.

Guerina NG, Hsu HW, Meissner HC, et al: Neonatal serologic screening and early treatment for congenital *Toxoplasma gondii* infection. The New England Regional Toxoplasma Working Group. N Engl J Med 330:1858, 1994.

Guero IC, Weniger BC, Schultz MG: Transfusion malaria in the United States, 1972–1981. Ann Intern Med 99:21, 1983.

Hindi RD, Azimi PH: Congenital malaria due to *Plasmodium falciparum*. Pediatrics 66:977, 1980.

Hohlfeld P, Daffos F, Costa JM, et al: Prenatal diagnosis of congenital toxoplasmosis with a polymerase-chain-reaction test on amniotic fluid. N Engl J Med 331:695, 1994.

Hohlfeld P, Daffos F, Thulliez P, et al: Fetal toxoplasmosis: Outcome of pregnancy and infant follow-up after in utero treatment. J Pediatr 115:765, 1989.

Lackritz EM, Lobel HO, Howell BJ, et al: Imported *Plasmodium falciparum* malaria in American travelers to Africa: Implications for prevention strategies. JAMA 265:383, 1991.

Lynk A, Gold R: Review of 40 children with imported malaria. Pediatr Infect Dis J 8:745, 1989.

Matusi D: Prevention, diagnosis, and treatment of fetal toxoplasmosis. Clin Perinatol 21:675, 1994.

McAuley J, Boyer KM, Patel D, et al: Early and longitudinal evaluations of treated infants and children and untreated historical patients with congenital toxoplasmosis: The Chicago Collaborative Treatment Trial. Clin Infect Dis 18:38, 1994.

McCabe R, Remington JS: Toxoplasmosis: The time has come. N Engl J Med 318:313, 1988.

Miller KD, Greenberg AE, Campbell CC: Treatment of severe malaria in the United States with a continuous infusion of quinidine gluconate and exchange transfusion. N Engl J Med 321:65, 1989.

Miller LH, Good MF, Milon G: Malaria pathogenesis. Science 264:1878, 1994.

Nosten F, ter Kuile F, Maelankiri L, et al: Mefloquine prophylaxis prevents malaria during pregnancy: A double-blind, placebo-controlled study. J Infect Dis 169:595, 1994.

Nyirjesy P, Kavasya T, Axelrod P, Fischer PR: Malaria during pregnancy: Neonatal morbidity and mortality and the efficacy of chloroquine chemoprophylaxis. Clin Infect Dis 16:127, 1993.

O'Connor GR: Manifestations and management of ocular toxoplasmosis. Bull NY Acad Med 50:192, 1974.

Piccoli DA, Perlman S, Ephros M: Transfusion-acquired *Plasmodium malariae* infection in two premature infants. Pediatrics 72:560, 1983.

Randall G, Seidel JS: Malaria. Pediatr Clin North Am 32:893, 1985.

Remington JS, Desmonts G: Toxoplasmosis. *In* Remington JS, Klein JO (Eds): Infectious Diseases of the Fetus and Newborn Infant. Philadelphia, WB Saunders, 1990, pp 89–195.

Rickman LS, Long GW, Oberst R, et al: Rapid diagnosis of malaria by acridine orange staining of centrifuged parasites. Lancet 1:68, 1989.

Riemann HP, Meyer ME, Theis JH, et al: Toxoplasmosis in an infant fed unpasteurized goat milk. J Pediatr 87:573, 1975.

Sabin AB, Feldman HA: Dyes as microchemical indicators of a new immunity phenomenon affecting a protozoon parasite (*Toxoplasma*). Science 108:660, 1948.

Sever JL, Ellenberg JH, Ley AC, et al: Toxoplasmosis: Maternal and pediatric findings in 23,000 pregnancies. Pediatrics 82:181, 1988.

Shabin B, Papadopoulou ZL, Jenis H: Congenital nephrotic syndrome associated with congenital toxoplasmosis. J Pediatr 85:366, 1974.

Shulman IA, Saxena S, Nelson JM, et al: Neonatal exchange transfusions complicated by transfusion-induced malaria. Pediatrics 73:330, 1984.

Silver HK, Dixon MS Jr: Congenital toxoplasmosis: Report of case with cataract, "atypical" vasopressin-sensitive diabetes insipidus, and marked eosinophilia. J Dis Child 88:84, 1954.

Stray-Pedersen B: Toxoplasmosis in pregnancy. Baillieres Clin Obstet Gynecol 7:107, 1993.

Subramanian D, Moise KJ Jr, White AC Jr: Imported malaria in pregnancy: Report of four cases and review of management. Clin Infect Dis 15:408, 1992.

Thomas V, Chit CW: A case of congenital malaria in Malaysia with IgM malaria antibodies. Trans R Soc Trop Med Hyg 74:73, 1980.

White NJ, Miller KD, Churchill FC, et al: Choroquine treatment of severe malaria in children. Pharmacokinetics, toxicity, and new dosage recommendations. N Engl J Med 319:1493, 1988.

Wilson CB, Remington JS, Stagno S, et al: Development of adverse sequelae in children born with subclinical congenital *Toxoplasma* infection. Pediatrics 66:767, 1980.

Wong SY, Remington JS: Toxoplasmosis in pregnancy. Clin Infect Dis 18:853, 1994.

CHAPTER 47

Infections with Spirochetal and Parasitic Organisms

F. Sessions Cole

CONGENITAL SYPHILIS

Before 1945, a chapter on congenital syphilis in a textbook devoted to diseases of the newborn would have been the most important one in the infectious disease section because of the great number of newborns affected and the broad variety of clinical syndromes produced. If this chapter had been omitted in the 1950s and 1960s, it would have been scarcely missed. In many parts of the United States, a young pediatrician might have completed 3 years of residency in a large urban hospital without ever having encountered one case, but the situation has changed, and a new syphilis epidemic has developed during the late 1980s and 1990s (Berry and Dajani, 1992).

Incidence

During the 1930s and 1940s, in the congenital syphilis clinic of the Harriet Lane Home in Baltimore, Maryland, 60 to 80 infants and children attended each week for arsenical therapy. Many more were lost to follow up before completing their 2- to 3-year course of treatment. It was unusual if less than three or four new examples were discovered in the general outpatient department in the course of 1 week. Then for several decades the frequency of the disease declined. The curve of incidence has been increasing since the 1970s, however (Fig. 47–1). From 1980 to 1986, the number of cases of congenital syphilis increased from 111 cases to 365 cases per year in the United States. More than 600 cases were reported in 1989. In 48% of cases there was inadequate or no prenatal care, and treatment failed in 19% of total cases and 35% of women who had prenatal care) (Centers for Disease Control and Prevention, 1986). During the 1990s, the epidemic has not been restricted to a single region of the country: the south (178%), the midwest (244%), and the west (777%) have all experienced dramatic increases in incidence of congenital syphilis (Dunn et al, 1993). Although part of this increase has resulted from revisions in surveillance case definition in 1988 and 1989, a true increase in incidence is the major factor in these changes.

Etiology and Pathogenesis

The organism responsible for syphilis is *Treponema pallidum*. This delicate, corkscrew-shaped, flagellated, highly motile spirochete is almost identical in appearance to *Treponema pertenue*, which causes yaws. These two diseases, like smallpox and cowpox, produce a cross-immunity for one another. This fact was established for Alexander Schaffer, the first editor of this textbook, when, after having spent 2 years on yaws-infested Fiji without encountering one case of syphilis, he was transferred to yaws-free India, where syphilis became one of his main medical preoccupations.

Syphilis can be acquired by introduction of *Treponema* through an abrasion in the skin or mucous membrane or by transplacental transmission. Whereas adults and some children become infected percutaneously, young infants almost invariably receive the organism from their mothers via the placenta and the umbilical vein. Transplacental transmission may take place at any time during gestation but ordinarily occurs during the second half of pregnancy. Fetuses infected early may die in utero or are at high risk for significant neurodevelopmental morbidity. The impact of the current epidemic on potentially preventable fetal deaths has not been evaluated. The usual outcome of a third-trimester infection is the birth of an apparently normal infant who becomes ill within the first few weeks of life. Whereas virtually all infants born to women with primary or secondary infection have congenital infection, only 50% are clinically symptomatic. Because of increasing pressure from managed care organizations for early discharge of new mothers, which has occurred during the current epidemic, identification of congenitally infected, asymptomatic infants whose maternal infections occurred late in the third trimester and whose syphilis serologic tests are not yet positive at the time of delivery has presented an unusually difficult problem for tracking and treatment (Dorfman and Glaser, 1990). It is critical that all infants undergo serologic testing for syphilis at the time of delivery and have a source of primary health care capable of tracking both maternal and infant syphilis status (Chhabra et al, 1993; Zenker and Berman, 1991). Early latent infection results in a 40% infant infection rate, and late latent infection results in a 6% to 14% infant infection rate (Wendel, 1988).

Pathology

Because *Treponema* enters the fetal bloodstream directly, the primary stage of infection is completely bypassed. There is no chancre and no local lymphadenopathy. Instead, the liver, the immediate target of the invasion, is flooded with organisms, which then penetrate all the other organs and tissues of the body to a lesser degree. Exactly where they take root and arouse local pathologic response, which in turn produces the presenting signs and symptoms, is unpredictable. Principal sites of predilection are the liver, skin, mucous membranes of the lips and anus, bones, and the central nervous system. If fetal invasion has taken place early, the lungs may be heavily involved in a characteristic *pneumonia alba*, but this condition is seldom compatible with life. *Treponema* may be found in almost any other organ or tissue of the body but seldom causes inflammatory and destructive changes in loci other than the ones named previously.

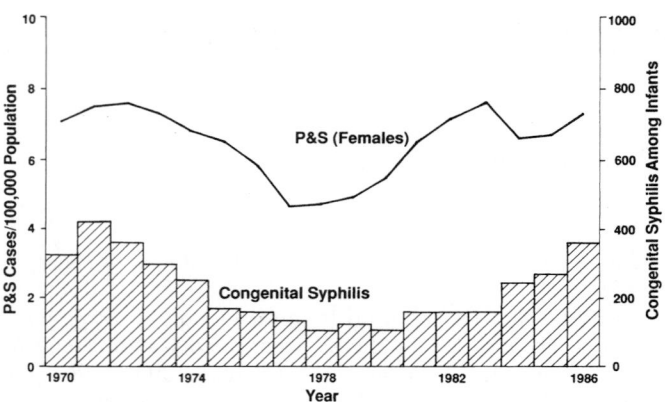

FIGURE 47–1. Case rates of primary and secondary (P&S) syphilis among females and congenital syphilis among infants less than 1 year of age in the United States, 1970 to 1986. Unpublished observations, Statistical Branch, Sexually Transmitted Diseases, Centers for Disease Control and Prevention. (From Ingall D, Dobson SRM, Musher D: Syphilis. *In* Remington JS, Klein JO [eds]: Infectious Diseases of the Fetus and Newborn Infant. Philadelphia, WB Saunders, 1990, pp 367–394.)

Under the microscope, the tissue alterations consist of nonspecific interstitial fibrosis with or without evidence of low-grade inflammatory response in the form of round cell inflammation. Necrosis follows fairly regularly in bone but only rarely in other tissues. Localization and gumma formation are not common in the neonate. Noteworthy is extensive extramedullary hematopoiesis in the liver, spleen, kidneys, and other organs.

Diagnosis

The most common signs and symptoms of congenital infection in the neonatal period are listed in Table 47–1. Additional diagnoses associated with congenital syphilis are nonimmune hydrops, nephrosis, and myocarditis (Wendel, 1988). The earliest sign of congenital syphilis may be snuffles. The nose becomes obstructed and begins to discharge clear fluid at first, then purulent or even sanguineous material later.

TABLE 47–1

Clinical Features of Early Congenital Syphilis

Feature	Age <4 Weeks (%)	Age >4 Weeks (%)
Hepatosplenomegaly	91	87
Joint swellings	3	34
Skin rash	31	55
Anemia	64	89
Jaundice	49	7
Snuffles	12	50
Metaphyseal dystrophy	95	91
Periostitis	37	80
Cerebrospinal fluid changes	44	37

From Hira SK, Bhat GJ, Patel JB, et al: Early congenital syphilis: Clinicoradiologic features in 202 patients. Sex Transm Dis 12:177, 1985.

Cutaneous lesions appear at any time from the 2nd week on. They are sparse or numerous and are copper-colored, round, oval, iris-shaped, circinate, or desquamative. Even more characteristic than their appearance is their distribution, which most frequently includes perioral, perinasal, and diaper regions. Palms and soles are also involved, but the rash is soon replaced there by diffuse reddening, thickening, and wrinkling. In heavily infected infants, the rash may become generalized. Mucocutaneous junctions become involved in typical fashion. The lips become thickened and roughened and tend to weep. Radial cracks appear that traverse the vermilion zone up to and a bit beyond the mucocutaneous margins of the lips. These are the beginnings of the radiating scars that may persist for many years as rhagades. Similar mucocutaneous lesions involve the anus and vulva, but in these locations, the white, flat, moist, raised plaques known as "condylomata" are also encountered, although less frequently.

Radiographs of the bones reveal characteristic osteochondritis and periostitis in 80% to 90% of infants with symptomatic congenital syphilis. In most, the bone lesions are asymptomatic, but in a few, they are severe enough to lead to subepiphyseal fracture and epiphyseal dislocation, extremely painful pseudoparalysis of one or more extremities may supervene. In a recent study by Brion et al. (1991), 12 of 59 asymptomatic, congenitally infected infants had metaphyseal changes consistent with congenital syphilis. Radiographic alterations include an unusually dense band at the epiphyseal ends, below which is a band of translucency whose margins are at first sharp but which later become serrated, jagged, and irregular. The shafts become generally more opaque, but spotty areas of translucency throughout them may give them a moth-eaten look. The periosteum of the long bones becomes more and more thickened. Epiphyses separate because the dense end plate breaks away from the shaft by fracture through the subepiphyseal zone of decalcification. This is exactly what happens in the pseudoparalysis of scurvy, although the reason for the weakening of the subepiphyseal bone is different. In syphilis, pseudoparalysis appears within the first 3 months of life; in scurvy, it seldom presents before 5 months of life.

Signs of visceral involvement include hepatomegaly, splenomegaly, and general glandular enlargement. Palpable epitrochlear nodes are not pathognomonic but are highly suggestive of congenital syphilis. The liver may be greatly enlarged, firm, and nontender. Associated with this may be jaundice, which appears in the 2nd or 3rd week of life, is seldom intense, and does not persist for many days. Anemia, probably indicative of bone marrow infection and hematopoietic suppression, may become severe. Lesions in the gastrointestinal tract and pancreas may occur and produce distention and delay in passage of meconium.

Clinical signs of central nervous system involvement seldom appear in the newborn infant, even though one third to one half of those infected suffer such involvement. This is demonstrated by cerebrospinal fluid changes of increased protein content, by a mononuclear pleocytosis of up to 200 or 300 cells/mm³, or by positive Venereal Disease Research Laboratories (VDRL) test (Table 47–2).

Diagnosis is confirmed by dark-field visualization of *Treponema* in scrapings from any lesion or from any body

TABLE 47–2

Cerebrospinal Fluid Findings in 108 Patients with Congenital Syphilis*

| | % of Total No. of Infants in Age Group for Infants Aged | | | Cerebrospinal Fluid | | |
	91–180 Days (47)†	181–365 Days (31)	366–731 Days (30)	Cells/mL	Protein (mg/100 mL)	VDRL Titer
Asymptomatic (normal)	28	45	63	0–5	15–30	Negative
Minimal involvement	30	32	27	5–30	30–75	Negative
Intermediate involvement	36	20	10	0–100	Moderate increase	Positive
Paretic formula	6	3	0	10–200	50–200	Positive

*Infants with congenital syphilis are defined by clinical status, repeated serologic testing, or dark-field microscopic examination.
†Figures in parentheses refer to number of infants in each age group.
Modified from Moore JF: The Modern Treatment of Syphilis, 2nd ed. Springfield, IL, Charles C Thomas, 1943. Courtesy of Charles C Thomas, Publisher, Springfield, IL, and Platou RV. Adv Pediatr 4:35, 1949.

fluid, by characteristic bone changes on radiographs, and by positive serologic tests for syphilis. These tests must be interpreted with caution, however. Because the IgG portion of reagin is transmitted across the placenta, its finding in the baby's serum means no more than that the mother has or has had syphilis. She may have been cured during pregnancy and yet still have quantities of reagin in her blood or she may not have received treatment at all and still not have passed the disease on to her fetus. A higher titer in the infant's blood than in the mother's is not evidence of fetal infection, nor is an elevated concentration of total IgM in the cord serum.

The most helpful specific test is a positive finding in the newborn's blood of IgM antibody against *T. pallidum*, IgM-FTA-ABS (fluorescent treponemal antibody absorption) (Lewis, 1992; Stoll et al, 1993). This is fluorescent *Treponema* antibody from which antibodies from treponemes other than *T. pallidum* have been removed by absorption. If positive, this finding is usually an indicator of congenital syphilis, although in the presence of rheumatoid factor, false-positive tests are occasionally seen. However, this test is not always positive at first, even when infection is present in the infant, possibly because, if the infection is acquired late in pregnancy, specific antibodies do not have time to form.

Thus, when an infant's blood VDRL is positive at birth, the diagnosis of congenital syphilis is not justified unless pathognomonic signs are also present. If they are not, serial determinations of reagin titer must be performed. If antibodies are passively acquired, the titer decreases to zero within 4 to 12 weeks; it increases if the disease is actually present. If the IgM-FTA-ABS test is also positive at birth, treatment may be initiated. If the test is negative, however, it should be repeated several times at 3- or 4-week intervals.

Treatment

Treatment is recommended for all pregnant women regardless of the stage of pregnancy (Table 47–3). Recent recommendations from the Centers for Disease Control (1988) for treatment of symptomatic or asymptomatic infants are listed in Table 47–4. Long-term follow-up recommendations are outlined in Table 47–5.

Hardy and coworkers (1970) reported a rare case of a male infant who died of congenital syphilis. His mother had received penicillin G 10 days before delivery, and he was given massive doses for 17 days after birth. Even so, *T. pallidum* was recovered from the infant's eyes after his death.

LEPTOSPIROSIS

Lindsay and Luke (1949) reported the first of five cases of congenital leptospirosis (Weil syndrome) on record (Shaked et al, 1993). It is briefly abstracted here because of its similarity to several of the other transplacentally transmitted infections.

CASE STUDY **1**

A male infant's mother had been a waitress in a restaurant known to be infested with rats, but she had never become ill. The infant was born at term, weighing 3540 g; vernix and amniotic fluid were brown, but the infant seemed well. Icterus appeared at 34 hours, and listlessness, cyanosis, dyspnea, and convulsions followed rapidly. The liver enlarged slightly. The blood was essentially normal, although platelets were not counted or mentioned. The urine contained bile. Cerebrospinal fluid was normal. The infant died at 48 hours of life.

Autopsy revealed heavy lungs with bloody, frothy fluid in the trachea and bronchi. There were numerous subpleural hemorrhages, and the parenchyma was congested, edematous, and hemorrhagic, but there was no inflammatory reaction. The enlarged liver showed extensive degenerative and necrotic changes with no evidence of bile stasis or regeneration. There were equally striking degenerative alterations of renal tubular epithelium, with protein and cellular casts within the tubules. Rare leptospirae were seen scattered throughout the liver sections prepared with Dieterle and Levaditi stains. The mother's blood showed a high titer of agglutinins to *Leptospira icterohaemorrhagiae* and *Leptospira canicola*, which disappeared after a few months.

TABLE 47–3

Recommended Treatment of Pregnant Patients with Syphilis

Stages of Syphilis	Drug	Dose
Early (<1 yr duration)	*Recommended*	
Primary, secondary, or early latent		
HIV antibody negative	Benzathine penicillin G	2.4 million units IM single dose; possibly repeat in 1 week
	Procaine penicillin G	600,000 units IM daily × 10–15 days
HIV antibody positive	Procaine penicillin G	1.2 million units IM daily × 15 days
	Aqueous penicillin G	4 million units every 4 hr × 15 days
	Alternative	
	Erythromycin	500 mg qid × 15 days orally
	Penicillin desensitization†	
Latent (>1 yr duration)	*Recommended*	
	Benzathine penicillin G	2.4 million units IM weekly × 3 weeks
	Procaine penicillin G	600,000 units IM daily × 15 days
	Alternative	
	Erythromycin‡	500 mg qid × 30 days orally
	Penicillin desensitization†	

°Use currently discouraged: offspring should be given penicillin.
†For details, see Centers for Disease Control and Prevention: Guidelines for the prevention and control of congenital syphilis. MMWR Morb Mortal Wkly Rep 37:S1, 1988.
‡After neurosyphilis is excluded.
HIV, human immunodeficiency virus; IM, intramuscularly.
From Ingall D, Dobson RM, Musher D: Syphilis. *In* Remington JS, Klein JO (Eds): Infectious Diseases of the Fetus and Newborn Infant. Philadelphia, WB Saunders, 1990, p 387.

TABLE 47–4

Recommended Treatment of the Newborn with Syphilis

Maternal Rx	Clinical Findings	Drug (Penicillin G)	Dose (50,000 units/kg)
None or inadequate	Present or absent	Aqueous	IM or IV daily × 10 days in 2 divided doses
		or	
		procaine	IM daily × 10 days
Adequate	Absent	Benzathine (only if follow-up cannot be ensured)	IM single dose

IM, intramuscularly; IV, intravenously.
From Ingall D, Dobson SRM, Musher D. Syphilis. *In* Remington JS, Klein JO (Eds): Infectious Diseases of the Fetus and Newborn Infant. Philadelphia, WB Saunders, 1990, p 388.

TABLE 47–5

Follow-Up after Treatment or Prophylaxis for Congenital Syphilis

Patient Category	Follow-Up Procedures
Patients receiving diagnosis of congenital syphilis	1. Reagin testing every 3 months for the first 15 months, then every 6 months until negative or stable at low titer 2. Treponemal antibody test after 15 months of age 3. Repeat cerebrospinal fluid evaluation 12 months after treatment if patient received treatment for or showed any signs of central nervous system disease 4. Careful developmental evaluation, vision testing, and hearing testing before 3 years of age or at time of diagnosis
Patients receiving treatment in utero or at birth because of maternal syphilis	1. Reagin testing at birth and then every 3 months until at least 6 months of age and test is negative 2. Treponemal antibody test after 15 months of age
Women receiving treatment for syphilis during pregnancy	1. Reagin testing monthly until delivery, then every 3 months until negative 2. Retreatment anytime there is a fourfold increase in reagin titer

Modified from Rathbun KC: Congenital syphilis: A proposal for improved surveillance, diagnosis and treatment. Sex Transm Dis 10:102, 1983.

Comment

Weil syndrome is contracted through contact with feces of infected rats. The mother doubtless acquired infection in this way but the disease remained asymptomatic. Leptospirae crossed the placenta and produced disease in the fetus that became apparent on the 2nd day of extrauterine life and quickly caused death. Such transplacental transmission has been observed in animals. Among the 15 recently reported women with leptospirosis in pregnancy, 8 had spontaneous abortions, 2 delivered healthy infants, 1 was lost to follow-up, and 4 delivered infants with signs of active leptospirosis (Shaked et al, 1993).

Another case suggested human-to-human transmission through breast milk (Boli and Koellner, 1988). The breast-fed infant became ill at 21 days of age. The infant's mother, a veterinarian, had performed an autopsy on a pregnant cow infected with *Leptospira interrogans* serovar *Hardjo*. The same organism was cultured from the infant's urine. The infant was given high-dose intravenous penicillin for 3 days and subsequently a 10-day course of oral amoxicillin. A Jarisch-Herxheimer reaction was noted after antibiotic therapy was begun.

NEONATAL HELMINTHIASIS*
Hookworm
Definition

Hookworm is a common infection in tropical and subtropical areas. It is caused by *Ancylostoma duodenale* or *Necator americanus*. These nematodes live in the human intestine, feed on blood, and expel ova into the feces.

Epidemiology

It is estimated that perhaps as many as 1 billion people are infected with hookworm, particularly in the developing world, including several tens of millions of children who are likely to suffer developmental consequences from infection (Chan et al, 1994). The most common mode of larval transmission is through penetration of the skin, often the soles of the feet, with the larvae entering the venulas from which they are delivered by the circulation into the lungs and gastrointestinal tract. In some regions of China, the practice of putting sand in diapers to absorb urine has led to infection in infancy.

Other modes of transmission include infection of the infant via colostrum and breast milk (Brabin and Brabin, 1992). The evidence for this is convincing in animals but is indirect in humans because soiled bedding and infant clothing may also be sources of infective larvae. Transplacental infection is probably rare; however, lactogenic transfer can be fatal.

Natural History

With heavy infection, pulmonary lesions may be evident, and cough and dyspnea may occur. The affected child suffers mostly from the consequence of intestinal blood loss, which leads to iron deficiency anemia and hypoalbuminemia.

The diagnosis depends on demonstration of ova in fecal smears. Occult blood in stools is also common.

Treatment

Mebendazole is effective for hookworm disease, ascariasis, enterobiasis, and trichuriasis. The experience with this drug is extensive in children but not in newborns.

Prevention

If a mother is known to have hookworm disease, she should be given treatment, and breast-feeding should be deferred until maternal disease is eradicated. The wisdom of this depends on individual circumstances, because the risk of lactogenic infection is not known. Meticulous attention to personal hygiene is essential in a mother who may be shedding ova in the stool.

Ascaris

Ascariasis is a significant contributor to childhood malnutrition and can be contained by attention to sanitation (Cifuentes et al, 1991, 1992; Hlaing, 1993). Chu and coworkers (1972) encountered an infant of 8 months' gestational age, delivered by cesarean section because of prolonged labor and fetal distress, whose mother vaginally passed a mature worm. The infant was well on the 2nd day but rectally passed a 30-cm mature *Ascaris lumbricoides* and another on the 6th day. The worms almost certainly had penetrated the fetus' intestinal tract after migration into the uterus and across the placenta.

The authors pointed out that similar migrations have been reported for *Schistosoma (Bilharzia)*, *Taenia*, and *Enterobius* helminths.

AMERICAN TRYPANOSOMIASIS

Infection with *Trypanosoma cruzi* (Chagas disease) affects several million individuals in Central and South America. Although 226 of 2651 pregnant women recently surveyed in Brazil were seropositive, and 28.3% had parasitemia, congenital infections occur in only 1% to 4% of women with serologic evidence of having Chagas disease (Bittencourt, 1976; Bittencourt et al, 1985). In Bolivia, nonvectorial transmission through blood transfusion, increased fertility, early age of motherhood, and migration from endemic areas have contributed significantly to persistence of disease in an urban setting (Azogue, 1993). The congenital transmission rate in this study of 910 mothers was 9.5%. Infected infants are usually of low birth weight (Azogue et al, 1985) and may present at birth or during the first weeks of life with jaundice, anemia, petechiae, hepatosplenomegaly, cardiomegaly, and congestive heart failure. Of congenitally infected infants, 57.8% die before 2 years of age. The diagnosis can be made by examining the placenta or with thin and thick blood smears. Serologic tests are also available (Arvin and Yeager, 1990; Bruckner, 1985). Recently, both polymerase chain reaction based detection of *T. cruzi*

___
*This section was written by Mary Ellen Avery.

and detection of antibodies that neutralize trans-sialidase, an enzyme that transfers sialic acid among macromolecules and that has been implicated in invasion of host cells by *T. cruzi*, have been reported (Leguizamon et al, 1994; Russomando et al, 1992). Treatment has been attempted with nitrofurans, 8-aminoquinones, and metronidazole with some success in controlling blood-borne infection (Arvin and Yeager, 1990). Nifurtimox has also been used, but no experience is available in congenitally infected infants. Information concerning treatment should be sought from the Parasitic Disease Drug Service, Centers for Disease Control, Atlanta, Georgia.

REFERENCES

Alford CA, Polt SS, Cassady GE, et al: Gamma-M-fluorescent treponemal antibody in the diagnosis of congenital syphilis. N Engl J Med 280:1086, 1969.

Arvin AM, Yeager AS: Other viral infections of the fetus and newborn. *In* Remington JS, Klein JO (Eds): Infectious Diseases of the Fetus and Newborn Infant. Philadelphia, WB Saunders, 1990, pp 516–527.

Azogue E: Women and congenital Chagas' disease in Santa Cruz, Bolivia: Epidemiological and sociocultural aspects. Soc Sci Med 37:503, 1993.

Azogue E, LaFuente C, Darras C: Congenital Chagas' disease in Bolivia: Epidemiological aspects and pathological findings. Trans R Soc Trop Med Hyg 79:176, 1985.

Berry MC, Dajani AS: Resurgence of congenital syphilis. Infect Dis Clin North Am 6:19, 1992.

Bittencourt AL: Congenital Chagas' disease. Am J Dis Child 130:97, 1976.

Bittencourt AL, Mota E, Filho RR, et al: Incidence of congenital Chagas' disease in Bahaia, Brazil. J Trop Pediatr 31:242, 1985.

Boli CA, Koellner P: Human-to-human transmission of *Leptospira interrogans* by milk. J Infect Dis 158:246, 1988.

Brabin L, Brabin BJ: Parasitic infections in women and their consequences. Adv Parasitol 31:1, 1992.

Brion LP, Manuli M, Rai B, et al: Long-bone radiographic abnormalities as a sign of active congenital syphilis in asymptomatic newborns. Pediatrics 88:1037, 1991.

Bruckner DA: Serologic and intradermal tests for parasitic infections. Pediatr Clin North Am 32:1063, 1985.

Centers for Disease Control and Prevention: Congenital syphilis, United States, 1983–1985. MMWR Morb Mortal Wkly Rep 35:625, 1986.

Centers for Disease Control and Prevention: Guidelines for the prevention and control of congenital syphilis. MMWR Morb Mortal Wkly Rep 37:S1, 1988.

Centers for Disease Control and Prevention: Summary of notifiable diseases, United States, 1989. MMWR Morb Mortal Wkly Rep 38(54), 1989.

Chan MS, Medley GF, Jamison D, Bundy DA: The evaluation of potential global morbidity attributable to intestinal nematode infections. Parasitology 109:373, 1994.

Cheng-I, W: Parasitic diarrhoeas in China. Parasitology Today 4:284, 1988.

Chhabra RS, Brion LP, Castro M, et al: Comparison of maternal sera, cord blood, and neonatal sera for detecting presumptive congenital syphilis: Relationship with maternal treatment. Pediatrics 91:88, 1993.

Chu W-G, Chen P-M, Huang LC, et al: Neonatal ascariasis. J Pediatr 81:783, 1972.

Cifuentes E, Blumenthal U, Ruiz-Palacios G, Bennett S: Health impact evaluation of wastewater use in Mexico. Public Health Rev 19:243, 1991–1992.

Dorfman DH, Glaser JH: Congenital syphilis presenting in infants after the newborn period. N Engl J Med 323:1299, 1990.

Dunn RA, Webster LA, Nakashima AK, Sylvester GC: Surveillance for geographic and secular trends in congenital syphilis—United States, 1983–1991. MMWR Morb Mortal Wkly Rep 42:59, 1993.

Hardy JB, Hardy PH, et al: Failure of penicillin in a newborn with congenital syphilis. JAMA 212:1345, 1970.

Hlaing T: Ascariasis and childhood malnutrition. Parasitology 107:125, 1993.

Hotez PJ: Hookworm disease in children. Pediatr Infect Dis J 8:516, 1989.

Ingall D, Dobson SRM, Musher D: Syphilis. *In* Remington, JS, Klein JO (Eds): Infectious Diseases of the Fetus and Newborn Infant. Philadelphia, WB Saunders, 1990, pp 367–394.

Leguizamon MS, Campetella O, Russomando G, et al: Antibodies inhibiting *Trypanosoma cruzi* trans-sialidase activity in sera from human infections. J Infect Dis 170:1570, 1994.

Lewis LL: Congenital syphilis. Serologic diagnosis in the young infant. Infect Dis Clin North Am 6:31, 1992.

Lindsay S, Luke JW: Fatal leptospirosis (Weil's disease) in a newborn infant. J Pediatr 34:90, 1949.

McCracken GH, Kaplan M: Penicillin treatment for congenital syphilis: A critical reappraisal. JAMA 228:855, 1974.

Nelson NA, Struve VR: Prevention of congenital syphilis by treatment of syphilis in pregnancy. JAMA 161:869, 1956.

Oppenheimer EH, Hardy JBH: Congenital syphilis in the newborn: Clinical and pathological observations in recent cases. Johns Hopkins Med J 129:63, 1971.

Rosen EU, Richardson NJ: A reappraisal of the value of the IgM fluorescent treponemal antibody absorption test in the diagnosis of congenital syphilis. J Pediatr 87:38, 1975.

Russomando G, Figueredo A, Almiron M, et al: Polymerase chain reaction-based detection of *Trypanosoma cruzi* DNA in serum. J Clin Microbiol 30:2864, 1992.

Scotti AT, Logan L: A specific IgM antibody test in neonatal congenital syphilis. J Pediatr 73:242, 1968.

Shaked Y, Shpilberg O, Samra D, Samra Y: Leptospirosis in pregnancy and its effect on the fetus: Case report and review. Clin Infect Dis 17:241, 1993.

Stoll BJ, Lee FK, Larsen S, et al: Clinical and serologic evaluation of neonates for congenital syphilis: A continuing diagnostic dilemma. J Infect Dis 167:1093, 1993.

Wendel GD: Gestational and congenital syphilis. Clin Perinatol 15:287, 1988.

Wilkinson RH, Heller RH: Congenital syphilis: Resurgence of an old problem. Pediatrics 47:27, 1971.

Zenker PN, Berman SM: Congenital syphilis: Trends and recommendations for evaluation and management. Pediatr Infect Dis J 10:516, 1991.

Zimmerman HM: Fatal hookworm disease in infancy and children on Guam. Am J Pathol 22:1081, 1946.

CHAPTER 48

Lung Development and Function

Thomas Hansen and Anthony Corbet

LUNG DEVELOPMENT

The primordial lung bud appears on day 26 of gestation as a ventral epithelial outgrowth from the foregut, with progressive caudal penetration of the primitive lung mesenchyme by continuous dichotomous branching. The mesenchyme exerts an inductive interaction with the epithelium. Lung development may be divided into the following five phases (Langston et al, 1984).

Embryonic Period: Formation of Proximal Airways (4 to 6 weeks)

The right and left main bronchi appear at 4 weeks, the five lobar bronchi at 5 weeks, and the 10 segmental bronchi on each side at 6 weeks.

Glandular Period: Formation of Conducting Airways (7 to 16 weeks)

By the end of the glandular phase a total of about 20 generations of conducting airways have developed, the last eight generations being called *bronchioles*, because they are not destined to develop cartilage like the preceding bronchi. These conducting airways, lined by columnar epithelium, are nourished by capillaries from the bronchial circulation. Cartilage appears at 7 weeks in the trachea and develops peripherally, reaching the last bronchi at term. The pleural membranes and pulmonary lymphatics develop between 8 and 10 weeks.

Canalicular Period: Formation of Acini (17 to 27 weeks)

At 17 weeks the first intra-acinar respiratory bronchioles develop by dichotomous branching from the terminal bronchioles; there are perhaps two or three generations of respiratory bronchioles, marking the birth of the acinus or gas exchange unit of the lung. An increasing number of capillaries appear in the prominent mesoderm and connect with the pulmonary rather than the bronchial arteries. It is the appearance of these capillaries that gives this period the name *canalicular*. From 18 weeks, multiple saccules arise from the last generation of respiratory bronchioles. The saccule is a wide channel with sparsely cellular mesoderm and a double-capillary network. As the acini grow, the saccules elongate, and the distance between the terminal bronchiole and the pleura increases. Initially, the saccules

have a smooth contour and are lined by cuboidal epithelium (Fig. 48–1) (Weibel, 1984). Granular pneumocytes, the sites of synthesis of the pulmonary surfactant, are usually distinguished at 20 weeks by the appearance of lamellar inclusions, but mature lamellar bodies may not be seen until later (Spear et al, 1969). Flattened membranous pneumocytes first appear at 24 weeks. This occurrence, and a progressive decrease of mesoderm with the development of more saccules within each acinus, allows the capillaries to approach closely and bulge into the lumen, at which point the saccules assume a more irregular contour. Gas exchange requires close proximity of capillaries and air

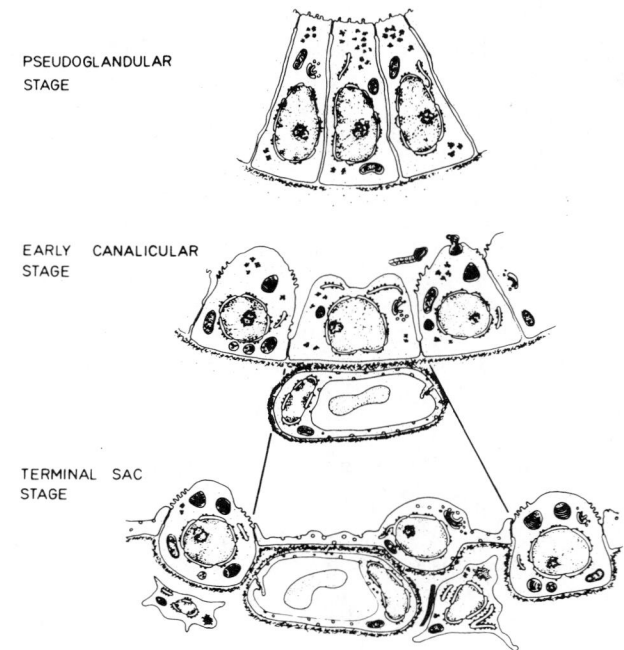

FIGURE 48–1. Epithelial transformation in a developing lung, from a high columnar epithelium of uniform cell population in the glandular phase, to a cuboidal epithelium with two distinct cell types in the canalicular phase. In the late canalicular period and in the saccular phase the prospective lining cells (Type 1) become flattened and broadened so that a thin gas exchange barrier with the endothelial cell of the capillary is formed. Note that secretory Type II cells with lamellar bodies occur in the canalicular phase. (From Burri PH, Weibel ER: Ultrastructure and morphometry of the developing lung. *In* Hodson WA [Ed]: Development of the Lung. New York, Marcel Dekker, 1977, p 215.)

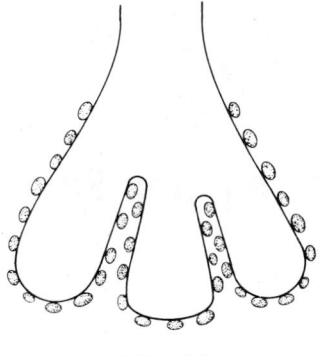
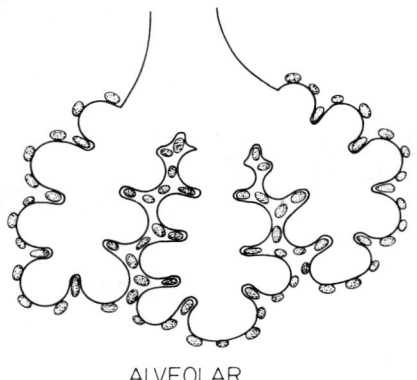

SACCULAR   ALVEOLAR

FIGURE 48–2. Simplified model to show how a saccular lung is transformed postnatally into an alveolar lung. (From Weibel ER: The Pathway for Oxygen: Structure and Function in the Mammalian Respiratory System. Cambridge, Harvard University Press, 1984.)

space. At 19 to 20 weeks, apposition of the capillary endothelial cells and the alveolar-lining epithelial cells occurs, with sporadic points of fusion of their respective basement membranes. From that time, the total area of the alveolar-blood barrier increases exponentially. This structural development is one of the factors that determines preterm viability (DiMaio et al, 1989). Clinical observations are consistent with an insufficient alveolar-blood barrier before 23 to 24 weeks or even later in some infants.

Saccular Period (subsaccular period): Expansion of the Gas-Exchange Sites (28 to 35 weeks)

Beginning at about 28 weeks there is an important change. The appearance of secondary crests begins the division of primary saccules into subsaccules or primitive alveoli, which have a flattened epithelium and a double-capillary network. The interstitium becomes noticeably less prominent, and saccular and subsaccular development accelerates greatly with an exponential increase of lung volume and surface area. In the opinion of the authors, the saccular period is misnamed—the primary saccules appear during the canalicular period; at 28 weeks it is the subsaccules or primitive alveoli that make their appearance and multiply exponentially. Therefore, this period should be called the *subsaccular period.*

Alveolar Period: Expansion of Surface Area (36 weeks to 3 years post-term)

Starting as early as 30 weeks, but nearly always before 36 weeks, the subsaccules become alveoli. Alveolation is accomplished by further thinning of the interstitium and the appearance of a single capillary network, in which one capillary bulges into both the alveoli with which it is associated. The mature alveolus has a very thin wall, a very thin interstitium, and a single capillary network, and it is polyhedral rather than rounded in contour. The process of alveolation starts distally in the subsaccules and proceeds proximally. At term gestation about 50 million alveoli are present, comprising most terminal air spaces. After birth there is a comparative slowing in the development of alveoli during the first 3 months. But later, there is a rapid increase in alveolar number during the first year of life, reaching approximately the adult number of 300 million alveoli by 3 years of age (Fig. 48–2) (Weibel, 1984).

Lung Liquid

The potential airways of the fetus are in contact with amniotic fluid when the glottis is open. The possibility that the lung could contribute to amniotic fluid was first proposed by Jost and Policard (1948), when they demonstrated an increase in lung volume in the rabbit fetus after ligation of the trachea. Secretions from the nasopharyngeal and buccal cavities as well as the lung itself contribute to the tracheal effluent. Rarely does amniotic fluid itself enter the developing lung, except in circumstances of fetal distress. When the fetus is stimulated to gasp, sufficient pressure is applied across the lung to allow entry of amniotic fluid and sometimes its squamous debris and even meconium. The rapid, irregular respiratory movements described as fetal breathing do not, in effect, move much fluid, since fluid is approximately 100 times as viscous as air, and the rapid, small respiratory movements of the fetus are not associated with high transpulmonary pressures.

The lung liquid that fills the potential air spaces of the lung (20 to 30 mL/kg of body weight) is quite distinct from amniotic fluid or plasma (Table 48–1) (Adams et al, 1963; Adamson et al, 1969; Humphreys et al, 1967). Evidence for active secretion of lung liquid was provided by Strang (1977), who measured the ratios of cations and anions between lung liquid and plasma. He and coworkers demonstrated that lung liquid required active transport of chloride ions from plasma in excess of the bicarbonate movement in the opposite direction (Olver and Strang, 1974). This liquid contains large amounts of chloride, relatively small

TABLE 48–1

Interstitial Fluid Estimated from Measurements in Lung Lymph

Component	Lung Liquid	Interstitial Fluid	Plasma	Amniotic Fluid
Sodium (mEq/L)	150	147	150	113
Potassium (mEq/L)	6.3	4.8	4.8	7.6
Chloride (mEq/L)	157	107	107	87
Bicarbonate (mEq/L)	3	25	24	19
pH	6.27	7.31	7.34	7.02
Protein (g/dL)	0.03	3.27	4.09	0.10

Data from Adams 1963; Adamson 1968; Bland 1983; Humphreys 1967.

amounts of bicarbonate, and almost no protein. Its potassium concentration is similar to that of plasma until near term, when it increases in response to surfactant secretion. Fetal lung liquid is secreted by the lung at approximately 4 to 6 mL/kg per hour along an electrochemical gradient that is produced by the active pumping of chloride from the interstitium into the air space. Although the site of the "chloride pump" is unknown, it can be inhibited by a variety of mediators that include beta-agonists, arginine vasopressin, and prostaglandin E$_2$ (Bland, 1988; Walters and Olver, 1978).

For the fetus to complete the transition from intrauterine to extrauterine life, the lung must clear this liquid soon after birth. The process of clearing liquid from the lung actually begins 2 to 3 days prior to birth with a decrease in the rate of secretion of fetal lung liquid. However, lung liquid begins to clear in earnest only with the onset of labor. Data obtained from experiments using fetal lambs show that nearly two thirds of the total clearance of liquid that occurs during the transition from intrauterine to extrauterine life occurs during labor (Bland, 1983, 1988; Bland et al, 1982). With the onset of labor, the pulmonary epithelium changes from a chloride-secreting membrane to a sodium-absorbing membrane with reversal of the direction of flow of lung liquid. This change is an active metabolic process involving increased sodium-potassium adenosine triphosphatase activity in the epithelial cells and serves to drive liquid from the lung lumen into the interstitium. In addition, since lung liquid contains very little protein, oncotic pressure also favors the movement of water from the air space back into the interstitium, and from there into the vascular compartment. (Berthiaume et al, 1987; Bland, 1988; Bland and Nielson, 1992).

When the lungs expand after birth, water moves rapidly from the air spaces to the loose connective tissue of the extra-alveolar interstitium. It is then gradually removed from the lung by lymphatics and pulmonary blood vessels (Bland et al, 1982; Humphreys et al, 1967). The concomitant increase in pulmonary blood flow that occurs with air breathing facilitates water reabsorption into the vascular compartment. In the past, physicians believed that some of the reduction in lung water at birth was caused by vaginal compression of the chest that expelled liquid from the lung. Recent data show, however, that although lung water content in fetal rabbits delivered vaginally with labor is less than the lung water of rabbits delivered by cesarean section without labor, the lung water content in fetal rabbits delivered by cesarean section during labor is not different (Bland et al, 1979). These data suggest that any mechanical effects on the clearance of fetal lung liquid are minimal.

Fetal Breathing

After many years of controversy, it is now established that the fetus breathes (Dawes, 1973). This breathing activity, which is essentially diaphragmatic, is present for 30% to 35% of the time in mothers examined with a real-time ultrasonic scanner (Patrick et al, 1978). It is irregular in rate and amplitude; recorded rates in the human fetus range between 30 to 70 breaths/min. The tidal volume of lung liquid is small, quite insufficient to clear the dead space. Owing to active lung liquid secretion, the net flow

is out of the lung. Periods of apnea may last as long as 1 hour in the normal human fetus. In the lamb, breathing occurs during active sleep, associated with low-voltage electrocortical activity, and is inhibited during quiet sleep, associated with high-voltage electrocortical activity. There appears to be a circadian rhythm, breathing activity being lowest in the early morning and rising during the afternoon to peak in the early evening (Dawes, 1974). Fetal breathing has been detected as early as 10 weeks' gestation. However, it is suppressed as labor approaches, probably owing to a progressive rise of plasma prostaglandins (Kitterman et al, 1983), and remains suppressed during active labor (Boylan and Lewis, 1980).

Fetal breathing is increased by drugs that stimulate the central nervous system, such as caffeine and isoproterenol, and it is inhibited by anesthetics, narcotics, barbiturates, ethanol, and smoking (Manning, 1977). Hypoglycemia or maternal fasting is associated with decreased fetal breathing, whereas it is stimulated after maternal meals and by hyperglycemia. Mild fetal hypoxemia severely depresses fetal breathing, by acting at a midbrain inhibitor (see later), but more severe fetal hypoxemia induces primitive deep gasping by a direct action on the medulla. It is believed that the hypoxia-sensitive carotid body chemoreceptors are active in the fetus and provide a constant stimulus to breathing (Murai et al, 1985), but their effect on the central respiratory neurons is easily overridden by high-voltage electrocortical activity acting through the midbrain inhibitor, or under certain conditions, by endogenous depressants such as prostaglandins, endorphins, or adenosine, which may be present at high levels in the bloodstream (Jansen and Chernick, 1988). The inhibitory effect of maternal ethanol ingestion is mediated by prostaglandins (Smith et al, 1990). Adenosine may be released under conditions of hypoxia, and adenosine antagonists such as theophylline have been found to decrease the depressant effect of hypoxia on ventilatory drive (Darnall, 1985; Runold et al, 1989). The hypoxic response with depression of fetal breathing may be blocked with dopamine antagonists (Lagercrantz, 1992), which suggests that a dopaminergic pathway may connect the midbrain inhibitor with the respiratory centers in the medulla. Hypercarbia has a rapid stimulatory effect on fetal breathing, this effect being exerted by increased hydrogen ion concentration at central chemoreceptors on the surface of the medulla; CO$_2$ diffuses rapidly into the cerebrospinal fluid surrounding these chemoreceptors. A similar stimulation occurs with the production of metabolic acidemia, but only after a latent interval to allow diffusion of organic acids into the cerebrospinal fluid (Harding, 1984). The purpose of fetal breathing appears to be at least twofold. To many physiologists, it is inconceivable that efficient postnatal breathing could be accomplished without prenatal practice. In addition, it appears that growth and development of the lungs (Wigglesworth and Desai, 1982), including the surfactant system (Higuchi et al, 1991), is highly dependent on the distensive forces produced by fetal breathing.

Onset of Continuous Breathing at Birth

Prior to birth, fetal breathing is episodic and dependent on the low-voltage electrocortical state, but after birth, breathing becomes continuous and independent of the electrocortical state. Experimentally in fetal lambs, breathing becomes continuous and independent of electrocortical state when the brain stem is sectioned just below the midbrain level (Dawes et al, 1983). Continuous breathing after birth may be due to suppression of this midbrain inhibitor. Brain sections in this region result in the abolition of the ventilatory depressive response to hypoxia and in the institution of continuous breathing in fetal lambs (Gluckman and Johnston, 1987; Martin-Boddy and Johnston, 1988).

The somatic sensory stimulation associated with delivery can be a powerful stimulus to continuous breathing (Condorelli and Scarpelli, 1975). Similarly, cooling the skin without change of core temperature has been shown to stimulate continuous breathing in fetuses with normal blood gas levels (Gluckman et al, 1983). It is believed that these multiple stimuli, by increasing neuronal traffic in the brain stem, may suppress the midbrain inhibition of breathing during the high-voltage electrocortical state.

Before birth, mild fetal asphyxia with both hypoxemia and hypercarbia, produced by clamping the umbilical cord, always induces continuous fetal breathing, and it does this without cooling or somatic sensory stimulation (Adamson et al, 1987). Mild fetal hypoxemia by itself produces depression of fetal breathing, through the midbrain inhibitor, so breathing stimulated by mild fetal asphyxia is probably due to hypercarbia. After birth, the arterial Po_2 is much higher than before birth, increasing from 30 to 70 mm Hg, and the arterial Pco_2 decreases from 45 mm Hg in the fetus to 35 mm Hg in the newborn. So on first examination, it would seem likely that neither hypoxemia nor hypercarbia could be responsible for continuous breathing after birth. However, it is believed that continuous postnatal breathing must be associated with a resetting of the threshold for both peripheral and central chemoreceptors, so they are stimulated at the new levels for arterial Po_2 and Pco_2. Because the onset of breathing is not abolished by carotid body denervation (Jansen et al, 1981), it seems unlikely that hypoxemia is important in the onset of breathing. Furthermore, it is known that the peripheral chemoreceptors are inactive for several days after birth, both in the lamb (Blanco et al, 1984) and in the human (Hertzberg and Lagercrantz, 1987), presumably because the resetting to a higher Po_2 is delayed. On the other hand, although hypercarbia by itself, induced with CO_2 breathing by the mother, is a powerful stimulus to fetal breathing (Dawes et al, 1982), this is not true during the high-voltage electrocortical state. If hypercarbia is given the prime responsibility for continuous breathing at birth, as seems most likely, there must still be a rapid downward adjustment in the central chemoreceptor threshold for CO_2, about which little is known, and there must still be a reversal of the midbrain inhibition produced by the high-voltage electrocortical state, perhaps induced by increased brain stem neuronal traffic. In addition, clamping the umbilical cord at birth may cut off the supply of a placental inhibitor, and this may facilitate the onset of breathing. It has been demonstrated in the fetal lamb, in which breathing has been stimulated by a cord clamp, that when the cord is unclamped, breathing is soon inhibited (Adamson et al, 1987). The conclusion must be that no single factor is responsible for the onset of continuous breathing at birth (Jansen and Chernick, 1988). In summary, hypoxemia does not play a role for several days after birth; hypercarbia is probably most important, but there must be a very rapid resetting of the central chemoreceptor threshold for Pco_2; and the action of the midbrain inhibitor during the high-voltage electrocortical state must be abolished by increased neuronal traffic in the brain stem; and there must be removal of a placental inhibitor.

SURFACTANT

Composition

Preparations of lung surfactant have been derived from lung lavage fluid; surfactant from mature animals has the composition indicated in Table 48–2. The single most important component is saturated phosphatidylcholine, the backbone of which is the three-carbon glycerol molecule. At the first two carbon positions fatty acid tails are added, while at the head of the molecule, a phosphocholine moiety is added in the third carbon position. During fetal life phosphatidylinositol predominates over phosphatidylglycerol, which replaces it during late gestation and after birth (Hallman and Gluck, 1977).

Function

The insoluble phospholipids of the alveolar lining layer have at least four major functions: (1) to stabilize the lung during deflation; (2) to prevent high surface tension pulmonary edema; (3) to protect the lung against epithelial and endothelial injury; and (4) to provide a defense against infection.

Because they have a hydrophilic head and a hydrophobic fatty acid tail, phospholipid molecules aggregate at the surface of the alveolar lining liquid, thereby displacing water molecules and reducing the surface tension (Possmayer, 1982). As the fatty acid chains in saturated phosphatidylcholine are straight, rather than bent at each unsaturated bond, more molecules of disaturated phosphatidylcholine can be packed into the surface, displacing more water molecules and reducing the surface tension to much lower levels. The surface tension of water is 72

TABLE 48–2

Composition of Surfactant in Mature Animals

Component	Percentage	
Lipid	90	
Saturated phosphatidylcholine		45
Unsaturated phosphatidylcholine		25
Phosphatidylglycerol		5
Other phospholipids		5
Neutral lipids		10
Protein	8	
Carbohydrate	2	

From King RJ: Pulmonary surface active material: Basic concepts. *In* Bloom RS, Sinclair JC, Warshaw JB (Eds): The Surfactant and the Neonatal Lung. Evansville, IN, Mead Johnson, 1979.

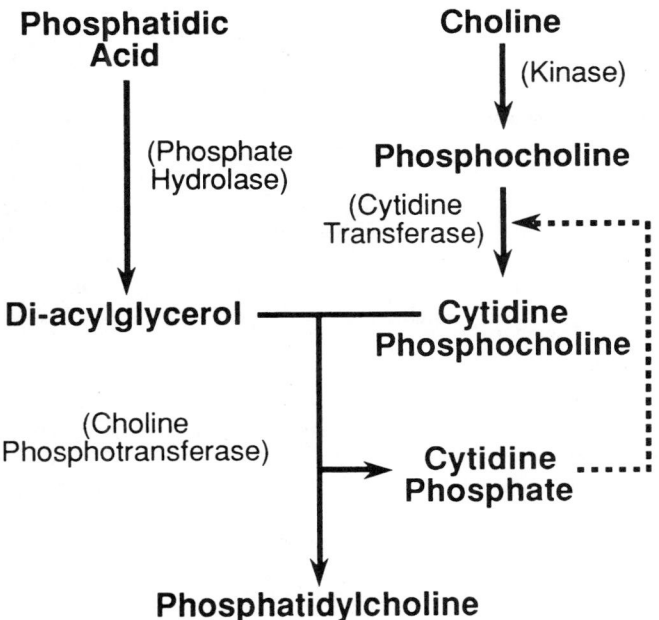

FIGURE 48–3. The synthesis of surfactant phosphatidylcholine by the choline incorporation pathway, using phosphatidic acid as the substrate.

dynes/cm. If the surface is occupied by saturated phosphatidylcholine molecules, packed side by side, the surface tension falls to an equilibrium value of about 25 dynes/cm. If the phospholipid film is compressed, as happens during lung deflation, more water molecules are excluded and the surface tension falls to near zero (Notter and Morrow, 1975). On expansion of the film, as happens during lung inflation, respreading may be too slow, allowing too many water molecules to re-enter the surface. Respreading may be facilitated by the addition of unsaturated phosphatidylcholine (Hawko et al, 1981) and phosphatidylglycerol (Bangham et al, 1979), which make the mixture more fluid.

The pressure required to prevent collapse of spherical airspaces is given by the Laplace equation:

$$P = 2 \cdot \gamma \cdot 10/r$$

where P = pressure in cm H_2O, γ = surface tension in dynes/cm, r = radius in micrometers, and the factor 10 corrects for the units. At the end of deflation the transpulmonary pressure may be as low as 2 cm H_2O. If γ is as high as 10 dynes/cm, airspaces larger than 100-μm radius will remain open, but those that are smaller will collapse at a pressure of 2 cm H_2O. On the other hand, if the surface tension is 1 dyne/cm, then only units smaller than 10 μm radius will collapse at a pressure of 2 cm H_2O. By reducing surface tension to near zero, surfactant guarantees the stability of even the smallest airspaces. This maximizes the surface area at the end of expiration and, thus, the gas-exchange capabilities of the lung.

Synthesis

Surfactant phospholipids are synthesized in the smooth endoplasmic reticulum of granular pneumocytes (VanGolde et al, 1988), cells that line the air spaces and constitute

about 10% of the internal surface area of the lung. The glucose substrate may be derived from glycogen stores or directly from the plasma. In addition, fatty acids may be derived from the plasma pool, from triglycerides following the action of lipoprotein lipase, or from glucose metabolism. The initial phase involves the synthesis of phosphatidic acid, which is similar to phosphatidylcholine, but without the choline head. The major pathway for the synthesis of phosphatidylcholine is the choline incorporation pathway for phosphatidic acid (Fig. 48–3). Most phosphatidylcholine produced is initially unsaturated at the second carbon position. By a process involving phospholipase and acyltransferase enzymes, the unsaturated fatty acid is removed and replaced with saturated palmitic acid, thus remodeling phosphatidylcholine to produce a more surface active molecule (Engle et al, 1980). Other surfactant phospholipids are also produced from phosphatidic acid (Fig. 48–4).

Synthesis, Packaging, Transport, Secretion, Reutilization, and Clearance

After synthesis in the endoplasmic reticulum of granular pneumocytes, surfactant phospholipids are packaged for export in the Golgi apparatus (VanGolde et al, 1988). They emerge as small lamellar bodies coalescing into mature lamellar bodies, which are stored near the apical plasma membrane prior to secretion by exocytosis. Once in the alveolar lining liquid, lamellar bodies are converted into tubular myelin, a specialized form of surfactant that rapidly donates a phospholipid monolayer to the surface (Goerke, 1974) (Fig. 48–5). As a result of breathing and repeated cycles of compression and decompression in the surface monolayer, many surfactant vesicular structures appear in the alveolar liquid. Surfactant phospholipid is taken back into the granular pneumocytes by endocytosis, forming multivesicular bodies, which are rapidly incorporated into lamellar bodies before being secreted again (VanGolde et al, 1988). Thus, there is constant cycling of lamellar bodies, tubular myelin, surfactant vesicles, and multivesicular bodies (Fig. 48–6). Some of the multivesicular bodies are processed by lysosomes, in which case the degradation

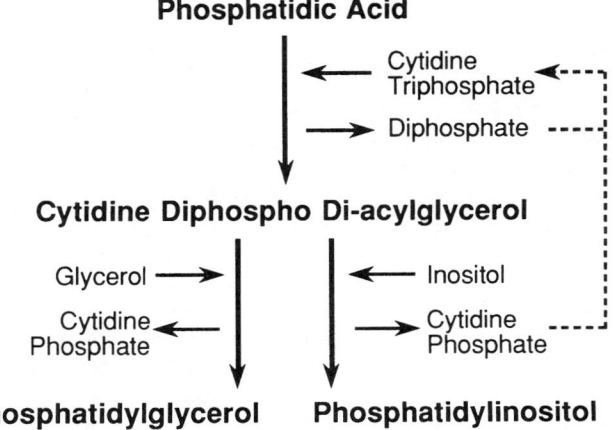

FIGURE 48–4. The synthesis of surfactant phosphatidylglycerol and phosphatidylinositol, using phosphatidic acid as the substrate.

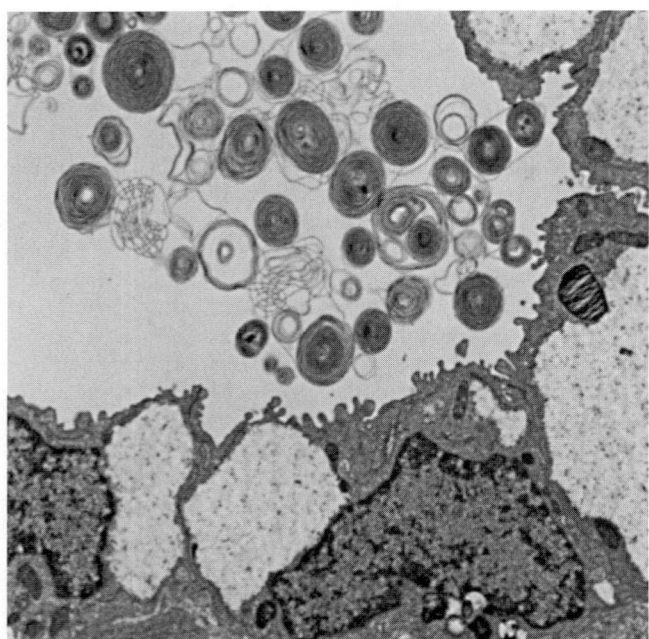

FIGURE 48–5. Fetal rat lung (low magnification), day 20 (term day 22), showing developing Type 2 cells, stored glycogen (pale areas), secreted lamellar bodies, and tubular myelin. (Courtesy of Mary Williams, MD, University of California, San Francisco.)

products may be used for surfactant synthesis or they may be cleared into the plasma. A turnover time of 10 hours has been estimated in the newborn rabbit (Jacobs et al, 1982); this means that in the resting state about 10% of the alveolar storage pool is secreted every hour (Fig. 48–7). In the newborn infant, the process of reutilization is so efficient that 95% of secreted surfactant is recycled and only about 5% of secreted surfactant is cleared from the lung every hour (Jobe and Rider, 1992). It is not known why the surfactant is recycled so efficiently, but one suggestion is that tubular myelin is highly unstable and must be constantly renewed to continue rapidly replenishing the surface monolayer; the process of reutilization prevents the synthetic mechanisms from being overwhelmed by the rapid consumption of monolayer surfactant during breathing.

Surfactant Development

During the glandular phase of lung development epithelial cells are columnar, but during the canalicular phase, they become cuboidal in shape. At about 24 weeks' gestation in the human, many cuboidal cells differentiate into granular pneumocytes, developing an abundant apparatus for synthesis, packaging, and storage of surfactant. Saturated phosphatidylcholine is present early in whole lung extracts and increases after about 24 weeks (Ballard, 1989). Based on the analysis of amniotic fluid samples, the appearance of surfactant in the alveolar fluid is considerably delayed in relation to its appearance in the tissue (Fig. 48–8); but it is clear in the human that if labor, delivery, and breathing occur, the appearance of surfactant in the airspaces may be greatly accelerated, and it is this phenomenon that makes survival after premature birth possible.

Control of Synthesis

The synthesis of the fully developed surfactant package is under control of genetic material in the chromosomes. The information is transcribed from encoded DNA to messenger RNA and translated at the polyribosomes of rough endoplasmic reticulum, where proteins controlling the process are synthesized; these proteins include enzymes, receptors, and transporters. Corticosteroid (Rooney et al, 1979) and thyroid (Ballard et al, 1980) hormones have a well-established regulatory role in accelerating the development of mature surfactant packages, as well as having an effect on lung structure. There is evidence that some glucocorticoid effects may be mediated by fibroblast-pneumocyte factor, synthesized by fibroblasts in the lung interstitium (Smith, 1984). Glucocorticoid and thyroid hormones first bind to their receptors, and the hormone-receptor complexes, after binding to specific regulator sites on the chromosomes, then exert their effects on specific genes in the DNA material. The amount of gene expression is also regulated by catecholamines and cyclic adenosine monophosphate (AMP) (Mettler et al, 1981), which facilitate the transcription process (Martin, 1981).

Control of Secretion

In mature animals a single deep breath completely replenishes the exhausted alveolar surfactant pool (Hildebran et al, 1981); the onset of lung distension after birth is accompanied by brisk surfactant secretion (Gilfillan et al, 1980). Secretion is preceded by an increased intracellular calcium level (Sano et al, 1987), and elemental calcium antagonists inhibit surfactant secretion stimulated by lung inflation in newborn rabbits (Corbet et al, 1991). Catecholamines and cyclic AMP play an important role (Mettler et al, 1981). During labor and at birth, the levels of circulating catecholamines increase enormously and stimulate surfactant secretion (Marino and Rooney, 1981). Other agents that increase cyclic AMP stimulate secretion (such as thyroxine, thyrotropin-releasing hormone, adrenocorticotropic hormone, and prostaglandin E) (Hollingsworth and Gilfillan, 1984). Drugs, such as theophylline, that decrease the degradation of cyclic AMP, increase surfactant secretion (Corbet et al, 1978). During the latter part of gestation, there is an increase in lung adrenergic receptors (Cheng et al, 1980), which increase the response to catecholamines. The density of adrenergic receptors is increased by corticosteroids, thyroid hormone, and estrogen, presumably by their regulation of protein synthesis. In addition, surfactant secretion is regulated by protein kinase C (Sano et al, 1985) and by stimulation of purine receptors with adenosine triphosphate (Rice and Singleton, 1986). There is some evidence that surfactant secretion may be inhibited by extracellular surfactant, in particular by saturated phosphatidylcholine (Suwabe et al, 1991), a phenomenon that may represent a form of feedback control. Secretion may also be inhibited by surfactant proteins (SPs).

Surfactant Clearance

Although surfactant is reutilized continuously by granular pneumocytes, the conservation is not complete. Surfactant,

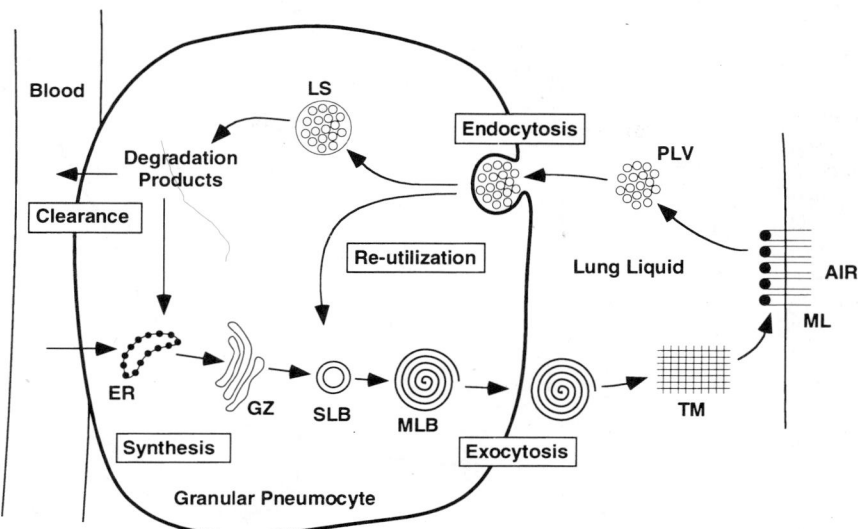

FIGURE 48–6. Possible pathways for synthesis, packaging, transport, secretion by exocytosis, reuptake by endocytosis, reutilization, and clearance of surfactant. ER, endoplasmic reticulum; GZ, Golgi zone; SLB, small lamellar body; MLB, mature lamellar body; TM, tubular myelin figure; ML, monolayer at air-liquid interface; PLV, phospholipid vesicles; LS, lysosomes. After phospholipid vesicles (PLV) are taken back into the granular pneumocyte, they may form multivesicular bodies and enter the reutilization pathway, or they may be degraded by lysosomes, and the degradation products may be either used again in the endoplasmic reticulum or cleared into the blood stream. Another possible pathway for surfactant clearance (not shown) is through alveolar macrophages in the airspaces. In the newborn, the recycling/reutilization process is efficient and clearance is minor; however, in the adult, clearance is more pronounced and recycling/reutilization is less efficient. (Adapted from Jobe AH, Ikegami M: Surfactant metabolism. Clin Perinatol 20:683, 1993.)

excluded from the monolayer during deflation, forms heaps on the air side and micelles or vesicles on the liquid side of the monolayer. The heaps may be consumed by alveolar macrophages and cleared from the lung; the surfactant vesicles may be recycled or cleared from the lung by the granular pneumocytes (Wright and Clements, 1987). Once the surfactant vesicles enter the granular pneumocytes in the form of multivesicular bodies, the lipids may be processed by lamellar bodies and enter the secretion pathway again, they may be processed by lysosomes and enter the synthesis pathway again, or they may be cleared into the

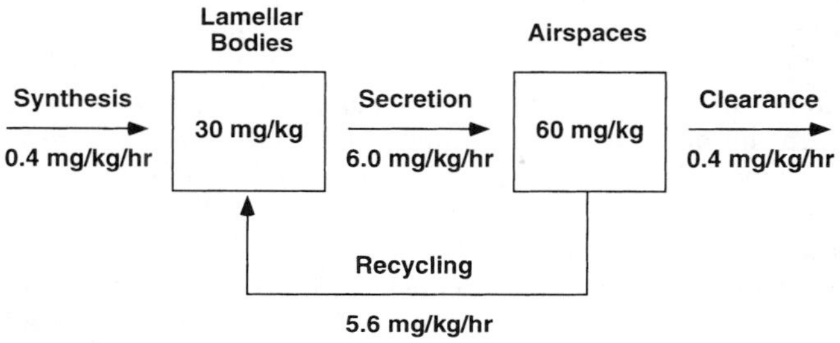

circulation (see Fig. 48–6). If the metabolic pool is to remain constant, the cleared surfactant must be replaced by synthesis of new surfactant (see Fig. 48–7).

Surfactant Protein

There are at least four types of surfactant protein recognized: SP-A, SP-B, SP-C, and SP-D. SP-A is hydrophilic; it has a relative molecular weight of 28,000 but is glycosylated to about 35,000 and then linked by disulfide bonds to form large oligomers greater than 300,000 (Phelps et al, 1986; Whitsett et al, 1985). Each monomeric molecule has a collagen-like domain and a lectin-like domain; the latter is responsible for binding mannose-rich carbohydrate molecules by a calcium-dependent mechanism. SP-A is synthesized in the alveolar Type 2 cell and secreted with phospholipid in lamellar bodies. It forms an integral part of tubular myelin, and although it inhibits surfactant secretion, it stimulates the reutilization process in isolated cells (Wright et al, 1987). SP-A binds to a specific cell surface receptor on the granular pneumocyte (Strayer, 1991) and on the alveolar macrophage, and by influencing both secretion and uptake, as well as clearance, it may be important in determining the surfactant pool size. SP-A binds to phospholipids in a calcium-independent fashion, but both SP-A and calcium, and SP-B, are necessary for the conversion of lamellar bodies to tubular myelin (Hawgood and Poulain, 1995). Moya and associates (1994) have reviewed the evidence that some SP-A may be secreted indepen-

FIGURE 48–7. Surfactant phosphatidylcholine pool sizes and fluxes in mature newborn rabbits. The size of the lamellar body pool and the alveolar surfactant pool is large compared with the rates of surfactant synthesis or clearance, but the rate of surfactant recycling/reutilization is large, about 95% of the secretion rate. (Adapted from Jobe AH, Ikegami M: Surfactant metabolism. Clin Perinatol 20:683, 1993.)

	Lamellar Bodies		Airspaces	
Synthesis →	30 mg/kg	Secretion →	60 mg/kg	Clearance →
0.4 mg/kg/hr		6.0 mg/kg/hr		0.4 mg/kg/hr

Recycling

5.6 mg/kg/hr

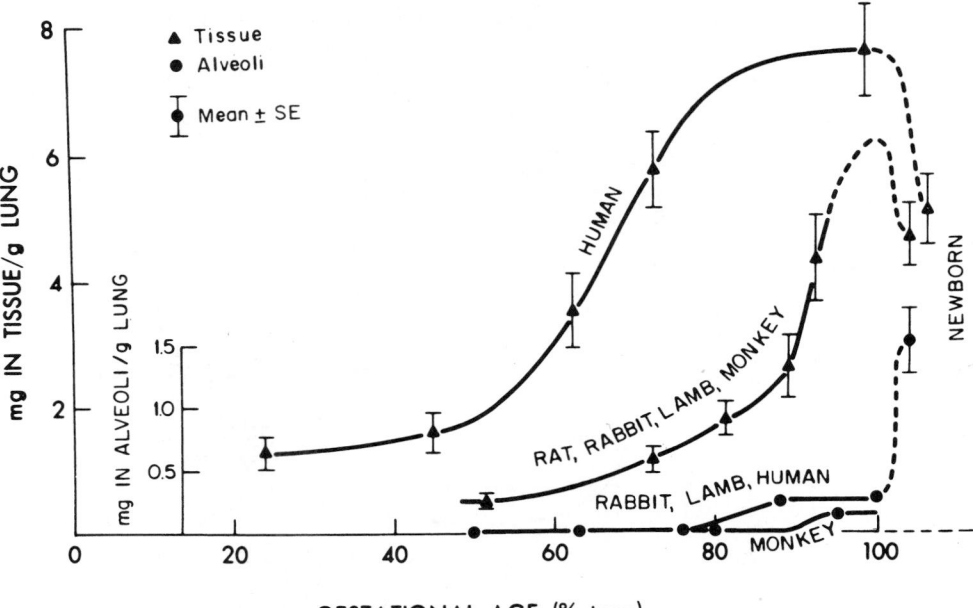

FIGURE 48–8. Concentration of saturated phosphatidylcholine (PC) in lung tissue and alveoli plotted against relative gestational age. Saturated PC appears in the tissues long before it appears in the airspaces. Therefore, respiratory distress syndrome may not be due to a problem with saturated PC synthesis, but rather to a problem with the development of the secretory pathways. (From Clements JA, Tooley WH: Kinetics of surface active material in the fetal lung. *In* Hodson WA [Ed]: Development of the Lung. New York, Marcel Dekker, 1977.)

dently of phospholipid by a constitutive pathway; this SP-A has undergone less post-translational processing, which is necessary for directing SP-A into lamellar bodies. Less is known about SP-D, but it is believed to structurally resemble SP-A, and like SP-A, it binds to carbohydrate molecules (Persson et al, 1990); it is believed that SP-A and SP-D bind to bacteria that bear surface carbohydrates and that they therefore facilitate the process of phagocytosis by alveolar macrophages.

SP-B and SP-C are smaller, with relative molecular weights of 8000 and 5000, respectively; they are both derived by proteolytic processing of larger precursor proproteins (Hawgood, 1991); they appear very early in fetal life, long before the differentiation of Type 2 epithelial cells. These small surfactant proteins are hydrophobic and greatly accelerate the adsorption of phospholipid to the air-liquid interface (Curstedt et al, 1987; Phelps et al, 1987; Suzuki et al, 1986); however, by themselves, these two proteins are not sufficient for full function (Schurch et al, 1992), and SP-A acts cooperatively to further increase their ability to reduce surface tension rapidly (Hawgood, 1991). SP-B is important in the formation of mature lamellar bodies (Hawgood and Poulain, 1995), and it is necessary for the formation of tubular myelin (Williams et al, 1991). SP-B, and SP-C also, are synthesized in Type 2 cells, as well as in Clara cells (Phelps and Harding, 1987).

The genes for SP-A and SP-D are located on chromosome 10, for SP-B on chromosome 2, and for SP-C on chromosome 8. Glucocorticoids increase the synthesis of SP-A, SP-B, and SP-C in cultured lung, and cyclic AMP stimulates SP-A and SP-B production. Other hormones, insulin and transforming growth factor, are reported to inhibit the production of SP-A (Ballard, 1989). In human amniotic fluid, secreted SP-A first appears at 19 weeks' gestation, and secreted SP-B first appears at 31 weeks; then both increase continuously as gestation advances (Pryhuber et al, 1991).

PULMONARY CIRCULATION

The lung has a dual circulation: pulmonary and bronchial. The pulmonary circulation transports poorly oxygenated systemic venous blood to the lung via a branching network of pulmonary arteries. These arteries may be conventional arteries that course through the interstitium and branch with major airways, or they may be supernumerary arteries that branch independently of the airways and supply peribronchial alveolar regions. Both types of arteries ultimately enter the acinus (the gas-exchanging unit of the lung) and branch into a meshwork of capillaries within the alveolar septa. The converging capillaries form venules and pulmonary veins that course through the intralobular and intersegmental septa and then return oxygenated blood to the left atrium (Hoffman, 1975).

The bronchial arteries arise from the systemic circulation. They branch with airways and deliver oxygenated blood to the airways, pulmonary blood vessels, visceral pleura, and connective tissue. Two thirds of this blood returns to the pulmonary veins, while one third returns via the bronchial veins to the azygous vein (Hoffman, 1975).

The pulmonary arteries arise from the sixth branchial arch during the 5th week of gestation. They branch along with the developing airways until the 16th week. After the 16th week, preacinar arteries increase only in diameter and length rather than in number (Hislop and Reid, 1972). Intra-acinar development, however, continues such that the total number of arteries increases tenfold from 20 to 40 weeks' gestation (Levin et al, 1976). During this period capillaries also proliferate in the acinus. The alveolar-capillary membrane thins, and the lung becomes capable of gas exchange with the circulation.

The large fetal pulmonary arteries (>1700 μm in diameter) are elastic and resemble the aorta. Arteries measuring between 180 and 1700 μm in diameter are muscular, whereas those measuring between 100 and 180 μm are surrounded only by a spiral coat of muscle. Arteries measuring less than 100 μm in diameter are nonmuscular (Rabinovitch, 1985). For any given diameter of muscular artery, wall thickness as a percentage of diameter is greater in the fetus than in the adult (Hislop and Reid, 1972). For any given vessel diameter, however, the percentage of wall thickness remains constant throughout the second half of gestation (Levin et al, 1976).

Pulmonary veins grow from the atrium with the airways as far as the secondary bronchi and then course through the connective tissue between pulmonary segments. The pulmonary veins of the fetus are less muscular than those of the adult (Hislop and Reid, 1973). Bronchial arteries develop from the first segmental dorsal aortic arch between the 9th and 12th weeks of gestation.

In the fetus, blood is diverted from the lungs by the relatively high pulmonary vascular resistance and is shunted across the patent ductus arteriosus to the placenta, where gas exchange occurs (Rudolph and Heymann, 1974; Teitel, 1988). Because pulmonary blood flow (hence, venous return) to the left atrium is low, left atrial pressure is less than right atrial pressure, and oxygenated umbilical venous blood is shunted across the foramen ovale to the left ventricle and to the coronary and cerebral circulations. Midway through gestation, the lung receives only 3.5% of the combined ventricular output. Late in gestation, blood flow to the lung increases out of proportion to lung mass and constitutes 7% of the combined ventricular output. This increase can be best accounted for by the marked increase in the number of pulmonary arteries that occurs during the same interval. Recent data show that during this period of increased vascularization, the pulmonary arteries of the fetus begin to constrict in response to their relatively hypoxic milieu. If this increase in vascular tone did not occur, pulmonary blood flow would increase even more during this period (Morin et al, 1988).

With air breathing at birth, pulmonary vascular resistance decreases dramatically and the systemic resistance increases. As a result, the gradient favoring right-to-left shunting of blood at the ductus arteriosus is reversed, and the pulmonary blood flow increases. In fact, a small left-to-right shunt may occur across the ductus arteriosus until ductal closure occurs. In addition, pulmonary venous return increases, left atrial pressure increases, and the right-to-left shunt at the foramen ovale ceases. The net result of these circulatory changes is that the lung replaces the placenta as the organ of gas exchange.

The decrease in pulmonary vascular resistance that occurs with air breathing results from mechanical distention of the lung and from an increase in alveolar oxygen tension (Teitel, 1988). Some of this decrease is the direct result of lung inflation and distention of pulmonary vessels. However, the largest portion is the result of increased secretion of chemical mediators. Both prostacyclin (Leffler et al, 1984) and endothelin-1 (Wong et al, 1994) appear to play some role in the postnatal fall in pulmonary vascular resistance. However, the most important mediator in this process appears to be nitric oxide (NO). Recent data have shown that exogenous administration of NO dramatically reduces pulmonary vascular resistance in the fetus (Kinsella et al, 1992) and that inhibition of NO synthesis markedly attenuates the fall in pulmonary vascular resistance induced

by ventilation and oxygenation of the fetus (Cornfield et al, 1992; Moore et al, 1992).

Postnatal lung development is characterized by remodeling of pulmonary arteries with a thinning of the medial musculature and a further reduction in pulmonary vascular resistance. Arterioles continue to proliferate in the acinus, and the muscularization extends into the acinus so that by adulthood, muscular arteries can be found at the level of the alveolus (Rabinovitch, 1985). Alveoli and alveolar capillaries continue to develop until approximately 3 years of age.

REFERENCES

Adams FH, Fujiwara T, Rowshan G: The nature and origin of the fluid in the fetal lamb lung. J Pediatr 63:881, 1963.

Adamson SL, Richardson BS, Homan J: Initiation of pulmonary gas exchange by fetal sheep in utero. J Appl Physiol 62:989, 1987.

Adamson TM, Boyd RDH, Platt HS, et al: Composition of alveolar liquid in the foetal lamb. J Physiol 204:159, 1969.

Ballard PL: Hormonal regulation of pulmonary surfactant. Endocrinol Rev 10:165, 1989.

Ballard PL, Benson BJ, Brehier A, et al: Transplacental stimulation of lung development in the fetal rabbit by 3,5-dimethyl-3-isopropyl-L-thyronine. J Clin Invest 65:1407, 1980.

Bangham AD, Morley CJ, Phillips MC: The physical properties of an effective lung surfactant. Biochim Biophys Acta 573:552, 1979.

Berthiaume Y, Staub NC, Matthay MA: Beta-adrenergic agonists increase lung liquid clearance in anesthetized sheep. J Clin Invest 79:335, 1987.

Blanco CE, Dawes GS, Hanson MA, McCooke HB: The response to hypoxia of arterial chemoreceptors in fetal sheep and newborn lambs. J Physiol (Lond) 351:25, 1984.

Bland RD: Dynamics of pulmonary water before and after birth. Acta Paediatr Scand 305(Suppl):12, 1983.

Bland RD: Lung liquid clearance before and after birth. Semin Perinatol 12:124, 1988.

Bland RD, Bressack MA, McMillan DD: Labor decreases the lung water content of newborn rabbits. Am J Obstet Gynecol 35:364, 1979.

Bland RD, Hansen TN, Haberkern CM, et al: Lung fluid balance in lambs before and after birth. J Appl Physiol 53:992, 1982.

Bland RD, Nielson DW: Developmental changes in lung epithelial ion transport and liquid movement. Ann Rev Physiol 54:373–394, 1992.

Boylan P, Lewis PJ: Fetal breathing in labor. Obstet Gynecol 56:35, 1980.

Cheng JB, Goldfein A, Ballard PL, et al: Glucocorticoids increase pulmonary beta-adrenergic receptors in fetal rabbit. Endocrinology 107:1646, 1980.

Clements JA, Tooley WH: Kinetics of surface active material in the fetal lung. *In* Hodson WA (Ed): Development of the Lung. New York, Marcel Dekker, 1977, p 349.

Condorelli S, Scarpelli EM: Somatic-respiratory reflex and onset of regular breathing movements in the lamb fetus in utero. Pediatr Res 9:879, 1975.

Corbet AJS, Flax P, Alston C, et al: Effect of aminophyllin and dexamethasone on secretion of pulmonary surfactant in fetal rabbits. Pediatr Res 12:797, 1978.

Corbet A, Voelker R, Murphy F, Owens M: Effect of calcium and calcium antagonists on phospholipid secretion induced by lung inflation in newborn rabbits. Am J Med Sci 301:102, 1991.

Cornfield DN, Chatfield BA, McQueston JA, et al: Effects of birth-related stimuli on L-arginine–dependent pulmonary vasodilation in ovine fetus. Am J Physiol 262:H1474, 1992.

Curstedt T, Jornvall H, Robertson B, et al: Two hydrophobic low-molecular-mass protein fractions of pulmonary surfactant: Characterization and biophysical activity. Eur J Biochem 168:255, 1987.

Darnall RA: Aminophylline reduces hypoxic ventilatory depression: Possible role of adenosine. Pediatr Res 19:706, 1985.

Dawes GS: Revolutions and cyclical rhythms in prenatal life: Fetal respiratory movements rediscovered. Pediatrics 51:965, 1973.

Dawes GS: Breathing before birth in animals and man. N Engl J Med 290:557, 1974.

Dawes GS, Gardner WN, Johnston BM, et al: Effects of hypercapnia on tracheal pressure, diaphragm, and intercostal electromyograms in unanesthetized sheep. J Physiol (Lond) 326:461, 1982.

Dawes GS, Gardner WN, Johnston BM, et al: Breathing in fetal lambs: The effect of brainstem section. J Physiol (Lond) 335:535, 1983.

DiMaio M, Gil J, Ciurea D, et al: Structural maturation of the human fetal lung: A morphometric study of the development of air-blood barriers. Pediatr Res 26:88, 1989.

Engle MJ, Sanders RL, Longmore WJ: Evidence for the synthesis of lung surfactant dipalmitoyl phosphatidylcholine by a "remodelling" mechanism. Biochem Biophys Res Commun 94:23, 1980.

Gilfillan AM, Harkes A, Hollingsworth M: Secretion of lung surfactant following delivery by uterine section. J Dev Physiol 2:101, 1980.

Gluck L, Kulovich MV: Lecithin-sphingomyelin ratios in amniotic fluid in normal and abnormal pregnancy. Am J Obstet Gynecol 115:539, 1973.

Gluckman PD, Gunn TR, Johnston BM: The effect of cooling on breathing and shivering in unanesthetized fetal lambs in utero. J Physiol (Lond) 343:495, 1983.

Gluckman PD, Johnston BM: Lesions in the upper lateral pons abolish the hypoxic depression of breathing in unanesthetized fetal lambs in utero. J Physiol (Lond) 382:373, 1987.

Goerke J: Lung surfactant. Biochim Biophys Acta 344:241, 1974.

Hallman M, Gluck L: Development of the fetal lung. J Perinatol Med 5:3, 1977.

Harding R: Fetal breathing. *In* Beard RW, Nathanielsz PW (Eds): Fetal Physiology and Medicine. New York, Marcel Dekker, 1984, pp 255.

Hawgood S: Structures and properties of the surfactant associated proteins. Annu Rev Physiol 53:375, 1991.

Hawgood S, Poulain FR: Functions of the surfactant proteins: A perspective. Pediatr Pulmonol 19:99, 1995.

Hawko MW, Davis PJ, Keough KMW: Lipid fluidity in lung surfactant: Monolayers of saturated and unsaturated lecithins. J Appl Physiol 51:509, 1981.

Hertzberg T, Lagercrantz H: Postnatal sensitivity of the peripheral chemoreceptors in newborn infants. Arch Dis Child 62:1238, 1987.

Higuchi M, Hirano H, Gotoh K, et al: Relationship of fetal breathing movement pattern to surfactant phospholipid levels in amniotic fluid and postnatal respiratory complications. Gynecol Obstet Invest 31:217, 1991.

Hildebran JN, Goerke J, Clements JA: Surfactant release in excised rat lung is stimulated by air inflation. J Appl Physiol 51:905, 1981.

Hislop A, Reid L: Intrapulmonary arterial development during fetal life—branching pattern and structure. J Anat 113:35, 1972.

Hislop A, Reid L: Fetal and childhood development of the intrapulmonary veins in man—branching pattern and structure. Thorax 28:313, 1973.

Hislop A, Reid L: Development of the acinus in the human lung. Thorax 29:90, 1974.

Hoffman JIE: The normal pulmonary circulation. *In* Scarpelli EM (Ed): Pulmonary Physiology of the Fetus and Newborn and Child. Philadelphia, Lea & Febiger, 1975, p 258.

Hollingsworth M, Gilfillan AM: The pharmacology of lung surfactant secretion. Pharmacol Rev 36:69, 1984.

Humphreys PW, Normand ICS, Reynolds EOR, et al: Pulmonary lymph flow and the uptake of liquid from the lungs of the lamb at the start of breathing. J Physiol 193:1, 1967.

Jacobs H, Jobe A, Ikegami M, et al: Surfactant phosphatidylcholine source, fluxes, and turnover times in 3-day-old, 10-day-old, and adult rabbits. J Biol Chem 257:1805, 1982.

Jansen AH, Chernick V: Onset of breathing and control of respiration. Semin Perinatol 12:104, 1988.

Jansen AH, Ioffe S, Russell BJ, et al: Effect of carotid chemoreceptor denervation on breathing in utero and after birth. J Appl Physiol 51:630, 1981.

Jobe AH, Rider ED: Catabolism and recycling of surfactant *In* Robertson B, VanGolde LMG, Batenburg JJ (Eds): Pulmonary Surfactant: From Molecular Biology to Clinical Practice. Amsterdam, Elsevier, 1992, pp 313–337.

Jost A, Policard A: Contribution expérimentale a l'étude du développement du poumon chez le lapin. Arch Anat Microsc 37:323, 1948.

King RJ: Pulmonary surface-active material: Basic concepts. *In* Bloom RS, Sinclair JC, Warshaw JB (Eds): The Surfactant and the Neonatal Lung. Evansville, IN, Mead Johnson, 1979, p 3.

Kinsella JP, McQueston JA, Rosenberg AA, et al: Hemodynamic effects of oxygenous nitric oxide in ovine transitional pulmonary circulation. Am J Physiol 263:H875, 1992.

Kitterman JA, Liggins GC, Fewell JE, et al: Inhibition of breathing movements in fetal sheep by prostaglandins. J Appl Physiol 54:687, 1983.

Lagercrantz H: What does the preterm infant breathe for? Controversies on apnea of prematurity. Acta Paediatr 81:733, 1992.

Langston C, Kida K, Reed M, Thurlbeck WM: Human lung growth in late gestation and in the neonate. Am Rev Respir Dis 129:607, 1984.

Leffler CW, Hessler JR, Green RS: The onset of breathing at birth stimulates pulmonary vascular prostacyclin synthesis. Pediatr Res 18:938, 1984.

Levin DL, Rudolph AM, Heymann MA, et al: Morphological development of the pulmonary vascular bed in fetal lambs. Circulation 53:144, 1976.

Manning FA: Fetal breathing movements as a reflection of fetal status. Postgrad Med 61:116, 1977.

Marino PA, Rooney SA: The effect of labor on surfactant secretion in newborn rabbit lung slices. Biochim Biophys Acta 664:389, 1981.

Martin DW: Regulation of gene expression. *In* Martin DW, Mayes PA, Rodwell VW (Eds): Harper's Review of Biochemistry. Los Altos, CA, Lange Medical Publications, 1981, pp 402–411.

Martin-Boddy RL, Johnston BM: Central origin of the hypoxic depression of breathing in the newborn. Respir Physiol 71:25, 1988.

Mettler NR, Gray ME, Schuffman S, et al: Beta-adrenergic induced synthesis and secretion of phosphatidylcholine by isolated alveolar type 2 cells. Lab Invest 45:575, 1981.

Moore P, Velvis H, Fineman JR, et al: EDRF inhibition attenuates the increase in pulmonary blood flow due to oxygen ventilation in fetal lambs. J Appl Physiol 73:2151, 1992.

Morin FC III, Egan EA, Ferguson W, et al: Development of pulmonary vascular response to oxygen. Am J Physiol 254:H542, 1988.

Moya FR, Montes JF, Thomas VL, et al: Surfactant protein A and saturated phosphatidylcholine in respiratory distress syndrome. Am J Respir Crit Care Med 150:1672, 1994.

Murai DT, Lee CH, Wallen LD, et al: Denervation of peripheral chemoreceptors decreases breathing movements in fetal sheep. J Appl Physiol 59:575, 1985.

Notter RH, Morrow PE: Pulmonary surfactant: A surface chemistry viewpoint. Ann Biomed Eng 3:119, 1975.

Olver RE, Strang LB: Ion fluxes across the pulmonary epithelium and secretion of lung liquid in the foetal lamb. J Physiol 241:327, 1974.

Patrick J, Fetherston W, Vick H, et al: Human fetal breathing movements at weeks 34 to 35 of gestation. Am J Obstet Gynecol 130:693, 1978.

Persson A, Chang D, Crouch E: Surfactant protein D is a divalent cation–dependent carbohydrate binding protein. J Biol Chem 265:5755, 1990.

Phelps DS, Floros J, Taeusch HW: Post-translational modification of the major surfactant–associated proteins. Biochem J 237:373, 1986.

Phelps DS, Harding H: Immunohistochemical localization of a low-molecular-weight surfactant-associated protein in human lung. J Histochem Cytochem 35:1139, 1987.

Phelps DS, Smith LW, Taeusch HW: Characterization and partial amino acid sequence of a low-molecular-weight surfactant protein. Am Rev Resp Dis 135:1112, 1987.

Possmayer F: The perinatal lung. *In* Jones CT (Ed): Biochemical Development of the Fetus and Neonate. New York, Elsevier, 1982, p 337.

Pryhuber GS, Hull WM, Fink I, et al: Ontogeny of surfactant proteins A and B in human amniotic fluid as indices of fetal lung maturity. Pediatr Res 30:597, 1991.

Rabinovitch M: Morphology of the developing pulmonary bed: Pharmacologic implications. Pediatr Pharmacol 5:31, 1985.

Rice WR, Singleton FM: P_2 purinoceptors regulate surfactant secretion from rat-isolated alveolar type 2 cells. Br J Pharmacol 89:485, 1986.

Rooney SA, Gobran LI, Marino PA, et al: Effects of betamethasone on phospholipid content, composition, and biosynthesis in the fetal rabbit lung. Biochim Biophys Acta 572:64, 1979.

Rudolph AM, Heymann MA: Fetal and neonatal circulation and respiration. Ann Rev Physiol 36:187, 1974.

Runold M, Lagercrantz H, Prabhakar NR, et al: Role of adenosine in hypoxic ventilatory depression. J Appl Physiol 67:541, 1989.

Sano K, Voelker DR, Mason RJ: Involvement of protein kinase C in pulmonary surfactant secretion from alveolar type 2 cells. J Biol Chem 260:12725, 1985.

Sano K, Voelker DR, Mason RJ: Effect of secretagogues on cytoplasmic free calcium in alveolar type 2 epithelial cells. Am J Physiol 253:C679, 1987.

Schurch S, Possmayer J, Cheng S, et al: Pulmonary SP-A enhances adsorption and appears to induce surface sorting of lipid extract surfactant. Am J Physiol 263:L210, 1992.

Smith BT: Pulmonary surfactant during fetal development and neonatal adaptation: Hormonal control. *In* Robertson B, VanGolde LMG, Batenburg JJ (Eds): Pulmonary Surfactant. Amsterdam, Elsevier, 1984, pp 357–381.

Smith GN, Brien JF, Homan J, et al: Indomethacin reversal of ethanol-induced suppression of ovine fetal breathing movements and relationship to prostaglandin E_2. J Dev Physiol 14:29, 1990.

Spear GS, Vaeusorn O, Avery ME, et al: Inclusions in terminal air spaces of fetal and neonatal lung. Biol Neonate 14:344, 1969.

Strang LB: Fetal lung liquid. *In* Neonatal Respiration: Physiological and Clinical Studies. Oxford, Blackwell Scientific Publications, 1977, pp 20–46.

Strayer DS: Identification of a cell membrane protein that binds alveolar surfactant. Am J Pathol 138:1085, 1991.

Suwabe A, Mason RJ, Voelker D: Pulmonary surfactant secretion is regulated by the physical state of extracellular phosphatidylcholine. Am Rev Respir Dis 143:A313, 1991.

Suzuki Y, Curstedt T, Grossman G, et al: The role of the low-molecular-weight apoproteins of pulmonary surfactant. Eur J Respir Dis 69:336, 1986.

Teitel DF: Circulatory adjustments to postnatal life. Semin Perinatol 12:96, 1988.

VanGolde LMG, Batenburg JJ, Robertson B: The pulmonary surfactant system: Biochemical aspects and functional significance. Physiol Rev 68:374, 1988.

Walters DV, Olver RW: The role of catecholamines in lung liquid absorption at birth. Pediatr Res 12:239, 1978.

Weibel ER: The Pathway for Oxygen: Structure and Function in the Mammalian Respiratory System. Cambridge, Harvard University Press, 1984.

Whitsett JA, Hull W, Ross G, et al: Characteristics of human surfactant–associated glycoproteins A. Pediatr Res 19:501, 1985.

Wigglesworth JS, Desai R: Is fetal respiratory function a major determinant of perinatal survival? Lancet 1:264, 1982.

Williams MC, Hawgood S, Hamilton RL: Changes in lipid structure produced by surfactant proteins SP-A, SP-B, and SP-C. Am J Respir Cell Mol Biol 5:41, 1991.

Wong J, Fineman JR, Heymann MA: The role of endothelin and endothelin receptor subtypes in regulation of fetal pulmonary vascular tone. Pediatr Res 35:664–669, 1994.

Wright JR, Clements JA: Metabolism and turnover of lung surfactant. Am Rev Resp Dis 135:426, 1987.

Wright JR, Wager RE, Hawgood S, et al: Surfactant apoprotein 26000–36000 enhances uptake of liposomes by type 2 cells. J Biol Chem 262:2888, 1987.

CHAPTER 49

Control of Breathing

Thomas Hansen and Anthony Corbet

Rhythmic breathing is maintained by alternating discharges of inspiratory and expiratory neurons, located diffusely in the medulla oblongata, and is activated by nonspecific neuronal traffic in the brain stem. One concept is that expiratory neurons discharge continuously under the influence of the reticular activating system, but rhythmic breathing is produced by the central inspiratory activator, which intermittently discharges and temporarily inhibits expiratory neurons (Cohen, 1979). Some of the inspiratory neurons are organized into the nucleus paragigantocellularis lateralis, thought to be the central inspiratory activator, and located close to the central chemoreceptors on the ventral surface of the medulla (Von Euler, 1983).

In adults, inspiration is active, and expiration is passive. Expiration is divided into two phases. In the first phase, a group of inspiratory neurons apply postinspiratory "braking" to slow exhalation. In the second phase, exhalation continues passively, or it is accelerated by contraction of expiratory muscles. The main inspiratory muscles are the diaphragm, intercostals, and upper airway abductors. The main expiratory muscles are intercostal and abdominal groups, which accelerate expiration, and upper airway adductors, which retard expiration by narrowing the larynx.

Inspiration is controlled by an "off-switch" (Fig. 49–1). During inspiration, the augmenting discharge of the central inspiratory activator to inspiratory motor neurons and specialized R_b neurons suddenly causes the off-switch neurons to discharge, transiently inhibiting the central inspiratory activator and allowing passive exhalation. The off-switch is also controlled by the pulmonary volume sensors and the rostral pontine pneumotaxic center, which together decrease the depth and increase the rate of breathing (Kosch et al, 1986). The threshold of the off-switch, and thus the depth and rate of breathing, is modulated up or down from a number of sources—peripheral chemoreceptors, central chemoreceptors, chest wall propriosensors, hypothalamus, and cerebral cortex (Von Euler, 1983). The respiratory control mechanisms develop progressively throughout gestation and infancy, so the system does not attain maturity until late in the 1st year of life. During quiet sleep, modulation of breathing is metabolic, through central and peripheral chemoreceptors, which sense P_{CO_2} and P_{O_2}. During active sleep and wakefulness, there are additional behavioral controls (e.g., crying, sucking, and gross body motions) (Schulte, 1977; Thach et al, 1978).

DEPRESSION OF BREATHING BY HYPOXIA

Before birth, mild hypoxia inhibits breathing, owing to stimulation of a midbrain inhibitor, and this remains true after birth for a variable period of time. Barcroft found continuous breathing in fetal sheep after brain stem transection above the pons, and the same phenomenon occurs under hypoxic conditions after birth (Martin-Boddy and Johnston, 1988). Lagercrantz (1992) reported that dopamine antagonists abolish the hypoxic depression of ventilation and suggested that the midbrain inhibitor may be connected to the respiratory neurons by dopaminergic nerves. In addition to the midbrain inhibitor, adenosine, released by hypoxia, may also depress ventilation (Koos and Matsuda, 1990).

CONTROL OF BREATHING IN THE PREMATURE INFANT

The sensitivity of the central chemoreceptor to CO_2 is reduced in premature infants and increases progressively with gestational age to adult levels by term (Rigatto, 1977). Higher oxygen concentrations increase sensitivity and hypoxemia decreases sensitivity to CO_2. In small premature

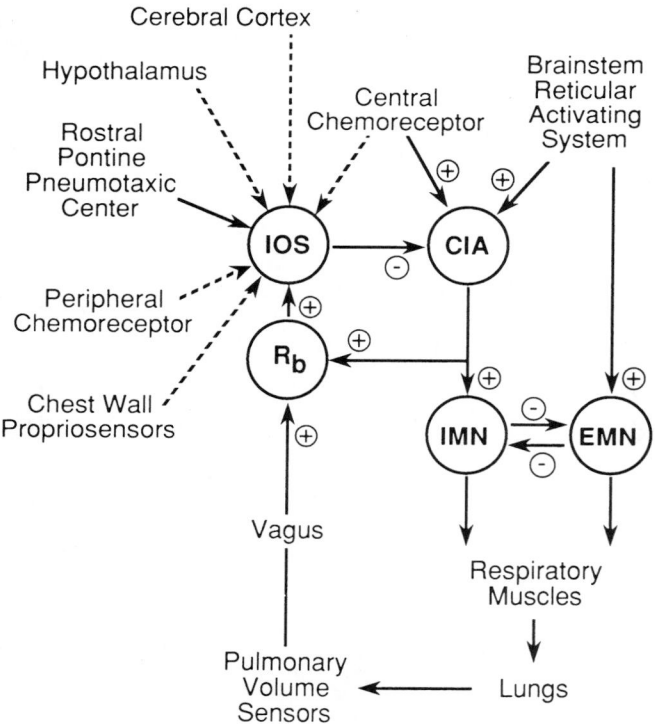

FIGURE 49–1. Possible functional organization of the central respiratory pattern generator. CIA, central inspiratory activator; IOS, inspiratory "off-switch"; IMN, inspiratory motor neurons; EMN, expiratory motor neurons. Solid arrows indicate direct effects. Interrupted arrows indicate modulatory effects. Effects are stimulatory (+) or inhibitory (−). (From Von Euler C: On the central pattern generator for the basic breathing rhythmicity. J Appl Physiol 55:1647, 1983.)

infants, adult levels of sensitivity are reached by 4 weeks' postnatal age (Fig. 49–2).

The term newborn infant responds to decreased oxygen by a transient hyperpnea, followed by a relative ventilatory depression of variable magnitude (Brady and Ceruti, 1966). This phenomenon suggests rapid exhaustion of the peripheral chemoreceptor in the face of moderate hypoxic respiratory center depression produced by the midbrain inhibitor. In small preterm infants, there is no initial hyperpnea, only a sustained decrease in ventilatory activity in response to hypoxia (Alvaro et al, 1992); this means poor peripheral chemoreceptor function.

If the term infant at age 2 to 6 hours is given 100% oxygen to breathe, there is no change in ventilation; the absence of transient depression suggests that the peripheral chemoreceptor is not functional and has not undergone upward resetting of the threshold from the low level in the fetus (Hertzberg and Lagercrantz, 1987). If the term infant, older than a few days, is given 100% oxygen to breathe, there is a transient depression of ventilation (Rigatto and Brady, 1972); this suggests that normal expected activity of the peripheral chemoreceptor appears by 2 days of age. In small preterm infants given 100% oxygen, the peripheral chemoreceptor response is initially absent, but it improves with time, and by 2 weeks of postnatal age the response is as good or better than that seen in term infants (Lagercrantz, 1992). Thus, the main problem in premature infants may be that the peripheral chemoreceptor function is relatively weak, at least in the first few weeks of life. The central hypoxic depression of ventilation, mediated by the midbrain inhibitor, also disappears about 2 to 3 weeks after birth, when the mature response of sustained hypoxic stimulation of ventilation becomes dominant (Rigatto et al, 1975a).

Evidence for the presence of a Hering-Breuer reflex has been obtained, and the strength of the reflex increases with gestational age until term (Gerhardt and Bancalari, 1981) but declines after birth (Bodegard et al, 1969). The Hering-Breuer reflex is mediated by stretch and irritant receptors. The function of stretch receptors is to increase inspiratory flow and tidal volume without changing inspiration time (Haddad and Mellins, 1977). This means that stretch receptors increase the output of the respiratory center. The function of irritant receptors is to shorten inspiration and expiration time and to reduce tidal volume without changing inspiratory flow. These receptors must operate the off-switch neurons (see Fig. 49–1) but have no effect on respiratory center output. The combined activity of stretch and irritant receptors, the volume sensor, shortens both inspiration and expiration, reduces tidal volume, and increases the inspiratory flow. Thus, the increasing activity of the Hering-Breuer reflex throughout gestation is consistent with a maturational increase of respiratory drive induced by the stretch receptors.

PERIODIC BREATHING

A periodic breathing pattern consists of breathing for 10 to 15 seconds, followed by apnea for 5 to 10 seconds, without change of heart rate or skin color. The net effect may be hypoventilation (Rigatto and Brady, 1972). This pattern is common at high altitude and is abolished by supplemental oxygen (Graham et al, 1950) and by continuous positive airway pressure (CPAP). The more premature the infant, the more frequent its occurrence, but to a lesser extent, it persists in term infants and during early infancy (Hoppenbrouwers et al, 1977). Periodic breathing does not occur during the first 2 days of life (Barrington and Finer, 1990) and is more frequent during active sleep. The prognosis is excellent, so no treatment is required. Although it was initially thought that periodic breathing was associated with a high risk for apnea of prematurity (Daily et al, 1969), this concept has been questioned (Barrington and Finer, 1990); these investigators found that periodic breathing does not immediately precede significant apnea spells in preterm infants.

Theoretical models suggest that periodic breathing is due to an imbalance between the peripheral and the central chemoreceptor effect on ventilatory drive (Khoo et al, 1982). Investigators have shown that periodic breathing in

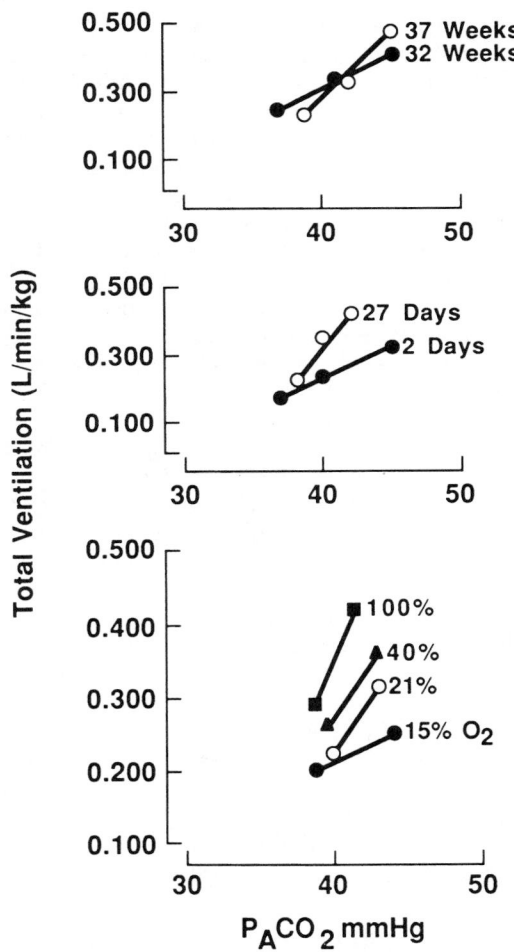

FIGURE 49–2. The relationship between ventilatory sensitivity to carbon dioxide and gestational age, postnatal age, and the concentration of inspired oxygen. (From Rigatto H, Brady J, Verduzco RT: Chemoreceptor reflexes in preterm infants: The effect of gestational and postnatal age on the ventilatory response to inhaled carbon dioxide. Pediatrics 55:614, 1975; and Rigatto H, Verduzco RT, Cates DB: Effects of O_2 on the ventilatory response to CO_2 in preterm infants. J Appl Physiol 39:896, 1975.)

newborn guinea pigs can be induced by suppression of the central chemoreceptor and then abolished by restoration of the balance with suppression of the peripheral chemoreceptor (Wennergren and Wennergren, 1983). In humans at high altitude, with spontaneous periodic breathing owing to hypoxic stimulation of the peripheral chemoreceptor, stimulation of the central chemoreceptor with acetazolamide abolished periodic breathing, whereas further stimulation of the peripheral chemoreceptor with almitrine increased periodic breathing (Hackett et al, 1987). The hypothesis of Barrington and Finer (1990) is that periodic breathing in premature infants is often due to excessive stimulation by the peripheral chemoreceptor, promoting an imbalance; this is consistent with their observation that periodic breathing is not observed in the first 2 days of life when the peripheral chemoreceptor is inactive but is common thereafter when the peripheral chemoreceptor is reset and again functional.

APNEA OF PREMATURITY

Apneic spells usually seen in infants are episodic and random (Daily et al, 1969). Episodes prolonged for 20 seconds or more or those accompanied by bradycardia or color change are considered significant. Perlman and Volpe (1985) have described the cerebral ischemia that accompanies severe bradycardia with heart rate less than 80 beats/min. Infants with significant apnea of prematurity do not perform as well on neurodevelopmental follow-up as similar premature infants without recurrent apneas (Tudehope et al, 1986). The diagnosis of apnea of prematurity can be made only after exclusion of all other causes of recurrent apnea. The incidence of apneic spells is inversely related to gestational age (Henderson-Smart, 1981). Although commonly stated otherwise, apneic episodes frequently start on the 1st day of life (Barrington and Finer, 1991; Henderson-Smart, 1981). In some infants, only bradycardia is recognized, but polygraphic recordings indicate that bradycardia is nearly always preceded by apnea (Dransfield et al, 1983). It is thought that 40% of the episodes are central or diaphragmatic, 10% are obstructive, and 50% are mixed, which may indicate either obstructive followed by central apnea (Martin et al, 1986) or central followed by obstructive apnea (Butcher-Puech et al, 1985). In an individual infant, one type tends to dominate. Central apneas tend to be shorter, whereas obstruction tends to prolong the episode and accelerate the onset of bradycardia. Obstructive apneas are particularly common on the 1st day of life in premature infants (Barrington and Finer, 1991).

It was once thought that bradycardia was not related to hypoxemia (Hiatt et al, 1981) but rather had a central brain stem origin (Schulte, 1977) or was a reflex response to the cessation of lung inflation (Gabriel and Albani, 1976). Henderson-Smart and colleagues (1986), however, concluded that episodes of bradycardia were associated with oxygen desaturation, and Poets and colleagues (1993) have confirmed this. In 80 premature infants just before discharge from the hospital, 193 episodes of bradycardia were recorded; 83% were associated with apnea episodes, and 86% were associated with oxygen desaturations; when all three occurred together, the sequence of events was apnea, followed by desaturation, followed by bradycardia. The

median interval between the onset of apnea and the onset of desaturation was 1 second and between the onset of apnea and the onset of bradycardia was 5 seconds. Although the bradycardia could be due to a direct effect on the heart, the short time interval suggests that the bradycardia is a peripheral chemoreceptor response to hypoxemia, as suggested by earlier workers (Storrs, 1977). There was no evidence that the onset of apnea and bradycardia was simultaneous, as would be expected in a lung or brain stem reflex.

Pathogenesis

The cause is unknown, but a number of theories have been considered for central, diaphragmatic, and obstructive apnea. The neurons of the central pattern generator are poorly myelinated and have a reduced number of dendrites and synaptic connections, thus impairing the capability for sustained ventilatory drive. Prolonged auditory conduction times have been demonstrated in infants with apnea, a problem assumed to reflect the function of the medulla in general (Henderson-Smart et al, 1983). Along similar lines, because infants with apnea of prematurity have a deficiency of catecholamine excretion in the urine, others have suggested a neurotransmitter deficiency (Kattwinkel et al, 1976b). Infants with apnea of prematurity have a decreased ventilatory response to CO_2 inhalation in comparison with premature infants of the same gestation without apnea of prematurity (Gerhardt and Bancalari, 1984a).

The chest wall of premature infants is highly compliant, so considerably more work is performed to generate adequate tidal ventilation. This results in substrate depletion and diaphragmatic failure from fatigue. Evidence for fatigue has been shown by examination of the diaphragmatic electromyogram (Muller et al, 1979).

There is some evidence that the diaphragm may activate before the upper airway abductors, which would predispose to upper airway closure during inspiration. The same problem may occur if abductor activation is insufficient (Mathew, 1985). Because airway obstruction imposes a load on the inspiratory muscles, the ability to load-compensate is important. It has been shown that load compensation is poor in small premature infants and increases as term is approached (Gerhardt and Bancalari, 1982). The poor load compensation is due to the highly compliant chest wall and the presence of an intercostal phrenic inhibitory reflex, which is activated by chest distortion and which shortens the duration of inspiration (Gerhardt and Bancalari, 1984b). This problem predisposes to obstructive apnea, especially under conditions of excessive neck flexion, when the upper airway tends to narrow, and in the supine position, when the tongue falls backward.

Relation to Sleep State

Most apneas occur during active sleep (Schulte, 1977) and are less common during states of quiet sleep or wakefulness. During active sleep, there is a low-voltage electrocortical state, decreased arousal from sleep, decreased muscular tone, absence of upper airway adductor activity, decreased respiratory drive, irregular breathing, and inspiratory chest wall distortion. The loss of chest wall muscle tone and airway adductor activity causes a 30% reduction in lung volume and a decreased arterial Po_2 (Henderson-Smart and Read, 1979). Reduced ventilatory drive causes a slight elevation in arterial Pco_2. The ventilatory response to hypoxia is depressed during active sleep, much more than in quiet sleep. The ventilatory sensitivity to CO_2 is also thought to be more depressed in active sleep (Rigatto, 1982). The newborn and premature infant is asleep 80% of the time, compared with the adult who is asleep for 30% of the time. More than 50% of sleep is active in the small premature infant, and the mature amount of 20% is not reached until 6 months of age (Bryan and Bryan, 1986).

Treatment

All infants at risk for apnea should have a heart rate monitor, which should be continued until the infant is at least 34 weeks' postconceptional age or after that time until the infant has been free of bradycardia for 1 week. Heart rate monitors are preferred because apnea without bradycardia is not significant apnea, obstructive apnea with bradycardia is detected reliably, and false alarms are infrequent. Most monitors in the neonatal intensive care unit also include an apnea monitor; the principal objections to the apnea monitor alone are that it misses obstructive apnea and may confuse bradycardia with breathing. It has become common to monitor with pulse oximetry because of the importance of both oxygen desaturation and heart rate.

Because respiratory center output is dependent on general neuronal traffic, cutaneous stimulation is effective (Kattwinkel et al, 1975). The use of oscillation water beds has been helpful sometimes (Korner et al, 1975). It is reasonable to maintain the patient in the prone position (Kurlak et al, 1994) because in this position there is a significant reduction in the duration of episodes of desaturation and bradycardia. Even in larger premature infants near hospital discharge, there may be advantages to the prone position in the form of improved oxygenation and a better ventilatory response to hypercarbia (Martin et al, 1995). Because diaphragmatic fatigue has been implicated, it is essential to maintain the circulation and a general state of good nutrition; the infusion of amino acids may increase the ventilatory response to hypoxia and hypercarbia (Soliz et al, 1994).

If the patient is hypoxemic, oxygen supplementation is essential, but there is no evidence that significant apnea is reduced if the patient is hyperoxygenated, and harm to the immature retina may be inflicted with such a strategy. Upton and colleagues (1991), using pulse oximetry, found that if the baseline oxygen saturation was higher, the desaturation produced by apnea tended to be less severe, and it was less likely that bradycardia would result. In apneas without bradycardia, the median baseline oxygen saturation was 95% and the median reduction was 5%, whereas the median baseline oxygen saturation was 92% and the median reduction was 9% for those apneas with bradycardia. Upton and colleagues concluded that it is important to keep the premature infant with recurrent apneas relatively well oxygenated. Pulse oximeters vary in their ability to detect hyperoxemia (arterial Po_2 > 90 mm Hg), but in one commonly used instrument, Adams and coworkers (1994)

found that setting the upper limit at 95% detected nearly all instances of hyperoxemia. If the infant must be given occasional bag-mask ventilation, it is important to insure that the oxygen concentration remains stable and is not increased. Because an oxygen hood interferes with access to the infant, many centers prefer to use nasal cannulas to administer oxygen, usually at a flow of 1 to 2 L per minute and with blended oxygen to maintain the pulse oximeter reading in the range of 92% to 96% saturation. Some evidence suggests that nasal cannula therapy may cause improvement in chest wall distortion, less asynchrony between chest and abdomen, and therefore a more efficient breathing strategy (Locke et al, 1993), perhaps by producing a small amount of continuous distending pressure in the nasopharynx; although this pressure may seem unregulated, pulmonary air leak complications have never been reported with this simple technique.

Most infants are treated with methylxanthines, which have been demonstrated to be effective in controlled trials (Murat et al, 1981). Because caffeine produces less tachycardia, has a more favorable therapeutic index, and produces less erratic blood level fluctuations, it may be preferred over theophylline (Aranda and Turmen, 1979). There is some evidence that theophylline, but not caffeine, decreases cerebral blood flow in premature infants (Pryds and Schneider, 1991; Saliba et al, 1989); theophylline may increase the metabolic rate and retard weight gain, and a significant fraction of theophylline is methylated to caffeine in premature infants (Aranda and Turmen, 1979). In a significant number of patients who do not respond to theophylline, a good response is obtained with caffeine (Davis et al, 1987). In a comparative trial, Larsen and colleagues (1995) found caffeine to be equally effective but associated with less tachycardia and less feeding intolerance than theophylline. Either drug may be given for 2 weeks and then stopped to observe whether apnea has ceased, or it may be continued until 32 to 34 weeks' postconceptional age, by which time the problem of apnea has frequently resolved. Infants should not be discharged before caffeine or theophylline has been eliminated because there is evidence that theophylline is effective at quite low levels. Methylxanthines may increase CO_2 sensitivity, decrease diaphragmatic fatigue, and improve load compensation (Gerhardt et al, 1983). Methylxanthines reduce the ventilatory depression following hypoxia by blocking adenosine receptors (Lopes et al, 1994). Others have suggested that theophylline increases the activity of the peripheral chemoreceptors in term infants (Cattarossi et al, 1993), which is consistent with experimental evidence in peripheral chemoreceptor denervated lambs (Blanchard et al, 1986).

The other mainstay of treatment is nasal CPAP (Kattwinkel et al, 1975). Although the effect of 5 cm H_2O should be tried, frequently as much as 8 to 10 cm H_2O is necessary for satisfactory control; this may be because many of these infants have chest cage insufficiency and a low lung volume. Infants may be fed by continuous gastric infusion during this procedure. The chest radiograph should be reviewed periodically to avoid overdistending the lungs. It has been postulated that CPAP provides increased ventilatory drive by directly stimulating the pulmonary stretch receptors (DiMarco et al, 1981; Speidel and Dunn, 1976), but this hypothesis could not be confirmed in premature infants by measurements of the rate of inspiratory flow (Krauss et al, 1986). Also, Krauss and colleagues could not find any improvement in the ventilatory response to inhaled CO_2. Others consider that obstructive and mixed apneas are selectively relieved by CPAP (Miller et al, 1985), which suggests that CPAP may work by supporting the pharynx. In addition, CPAP prevents chest wall distortion during inspiration (Locke et al, 1991), which may improve the efficiency of ventilation and suppress the intercostal phrenic inhibitory reflex; improved load compensation in small premature infants on CPAP has been demonstrated (Martin et al, 1977).

Another drug that has proved useful is doxapram (Barrington et al, 1987). At low doses, it stimulates the peripheral chemoreceptors, whereas at higher doses it stimulates the respiratory center directly. In the United States, the preparation contains 0.9% benzyl alcohol as preservative, but at a dose of 0.5 mg/kg per hour, the amount of benzyl alcohol administered is only 5.4 mg/kg per day, which is far below the levels associated with toxicity in premature infants (Barrington and Finer, 1986). Doxapram should be reserved for infants failing to respond to optimal xanthine and CPAP therapy, in whom mechanical ventilation would be the next step; methylxanthine therapy should be continued during doxapram infusion (Eyal et al, 1985). In addition, doxapram should not be used in the 1st week of life or if the serum bilirubin is high because an association with intraventricular hemorrhage and kernicterus has been reported (Jardine and Rogers, 1988). The drug may be started at 1.0 mg/kg per hour for a few hours to load the patient but then may be decreased to 0.5 mg/kg per hour. Higher doses are not recommended and may be associated with side effects, such as abdominal distention, increased gastric residuals, irritability, hyperglycemia, and mild hypertension (Hayakawa et al, 1986).

Movement-Related Apnea Episodes

Mathew and associates (1991) observed a high incidence of apneas during squirming motions associated especially with arousal from sleep; they suggested that as many as one third of apneas in premature infants may be of this type. Using esophageal pressure measurements, Abu-Osba and coworkers (1982) showed that these motions were associated with increased abdominal expiratory muscle activity against a closed glottis (i.e., Valsalva maneuvers); they also observed some obstructed inspiratory breaths during squirming motions (i.e., Müller maneuvers). These episodes may be associated with greatly reduced minute ventilation and severe oxygen desaturation and bradycardia. These spells are unlikely to respond to methylxanthine therapy, and they may occur in infants on slow rate mechanical ventilation.

Cyanotic Spells Without Apnea in Preterm Infants (V/Q Spells)

In the study by Poets and colleagues (1993), about 15% of premature infants had episodes of bradycardia, which were associated with appropriate nasal air flow but significant oxygen desaturation. The rate at which oxygen desaturation

developed was even more rapid with these spells than during apnea (Samuels et al, 1992). Poets and colleagues (1992) considered the likely causes of this phenomenon and concluded that there is sudden V/Q mismatching secondary to peripheral airway dysfunction. The latter may respond to CPAP therapy or increased positive end-expiratory pressure (PEEP) if the infant is on a ventilator, but this is not proven. Poets and colleagues (1995) have also described episodes of severe oxygen desaturation without bradycardia, without apnea, and without squirming motions, but they were not sure of the cause; they suggested that premature infants less than 32 weeks' gestation should be monitored with pulse oximeters until at least 36 weeks' postconceptional age; this is because of the frequency of these episodes and because of the inability of apnea and heart rate monitors to detect them reliably. Upton and coworkers (1991) also described many episodes of desaturation without bradycardia in premature infants and suggested that pulse oximetry may be the best way to monitor premature infants; it is more important to detect the effect of apnea on heart rate and oxygen saturation than it is to detect the apnea itself.

Bolivar and coworkers (1995) described episodes of oxygen desaturation in premature infants on mechanical ventilation; these episodes were preceded by increased esophageal pressure as a result of active expiratory efforts, produced, it was thought, during efforts at crying. The presence of an endotracheal tube prevented the larynx from closing and allowed the lung volume to decrease suddenly, causing a decrease in lung compliance and an increase in airways resistance; then continued mechanical ventilation or spontaneous breathing was relatively ineffective during a period of severe oxygen desaturation. Bolivar and coworkers suggested that increased PEEP might be effective, that further sedation might prevent the attempts at crying, or that extubation would allow the larynx to function properly to maintain the lung volume.

SYMPTOMATIC RECURRENT APNEA

Apnea is a frequent manifestation of general problems in newborn and premature infants (Kattwinkel, 1977). The more common ones are as follows: (1) local infection such as a scalp abscess; (2) bacteremia or septicemia; (3) necrotizing enterocolitis; (4) hypoxic-ischemic encephalopathy; (5) intracranial hemorrhage, posthemorrhagic hydrocephalus, and periventricular leukomalacia; (6) patent ductus arteriosus with a large left-to-right shunt; (7) gastroesophageal reflux; (8) hypoglycemia; (9) hypocalcemia; (10) anemia; (11) drugs or anesthesia; (12) environmental overheating; (13) any condition causing hypoxemia or hypovolemia; and (14) upper airway obstructions such as nasal stenosis, choanal atresia, or vocal cord paralysis. These should be excluded and appropriately treated before a diagnosis of apnea of prematurity is made.

Apnea Associated with Infection

Small premature infants commonly have systemic infections, and the initial sign is frequently an increased frequency of apnea episodes. Examples include *Staphylococcus epidermidis* bacteremia associated with venous catheters, *Candida* fungal sepsis associated with vaginal delivery and dexamethasone administration, and respiratory syncytial virus pneumonia associated with bronchopulmonary dysplasia and nosocomial spread. It is imperative that infections must be thoroughly excluded or treated in all cases of recurrent apnea.

Apnea Associated with Gastroesophageal Reflux

It has been established that visible postfeeding regurgitation of formula into the pharynx is associated with an increased incidence of apnea in premature infants (Menon et al, 1985); the explanation for this is considered to be an activation of the laryngeal chemoreflex by gastric fluids. This phenomenon has suggested that covert gastroesophageal reflux, which is common in small premature infants, may be associated with recurrent apnea; treatment with theophylline may exacerbate the reflux and make the situation worse. Several polygraphic studies in premature infants have failed to demonstrate a temporal relationship between episodes of apnea and episodes of acid reflux into the esophagus (Ajuriaguerra et al, 1991; Newell et al, 1989; Walsh et al, 1981). Newell and colleagues (1989), however, showed in a subgroup of infants with xanthine-resistant apnea of prematurity that effective control of gastroesophageal reflux with a thickened formula and a more upright position was associated with a significant reduction in the number of apneic spells; this reduction was not immediate but delayed by 1 to 2 days. It has been suggested that the decreased number of apneas was due to the resolution of esophagitis (Booth, 1992). It has become common practice in many centers to treat xanthine-resistant apnea of prematurity with metoclopramide, cisapride, and other antireflux measures, although no controlled trials have established the efficacy of these drugs in preventing apnea.

Apnea Associated with Anemia of Prematurity

There is no agreement on the problem of anemia of prematurity and its relationship to recurrent apnea. In many centers, it is policy to transfuse premature infants with an hematocrit of less than 30% and if the infant has signs of anemia, such as tachycardia, tachypnea, or episodes of apnea or bradycardia. Keyes and associates (1989) found no relationship between hematocrits of 19% to 64% and any of these signs and found no consistent changes after transfusion. Joshi and colleagues (1987) found a significant reduction in the incidence of brief and intermediate apneas and in the incidence of bradycardias after transfusion. Others have had similar results (DeMaio et al, 1989). Ross and coworkers (1989) conducted a controlled trial of blood transfusion in a group of infants who all met the above-mentioned criteria for transfusion. After transfusion there was a significant reduction in the heart rate, in the number of apnea and bradycardia episodes, and in the blood lactate levels in comparison with the group not transfused. Stute and coworkers (1995) found a significant reduction in the number of apneas and the number of bradycardias during the 3 days after transfusion in small premature infants.

Apnea Associated with Anesthesia

Premature infants who have surgery with general anesthesia frequently have major recurrent apnea episodes for a few days after the procedure; the most common case is bilateral inguinal hernia repair. This susceptibility to apnea may persist until 50 to 60 weeks' postconceptional age, so older premature infants must be appropriately observed and treated for apnea following anesthesia (Scherer, 1991).

FEEDING HYPOXEMIA

Feeding hypoxemia is frequent in premature infants given nipple feeds too soon but sometimes occurs in term infants (Rosen et al, 1984). While sucking and swallowing, ventilation is severely interrupted (Shivpuri et al, 1983). The rapid onset of bradycardia is thought to be reflex in origin, whereas the delayed onset of bradycardia is due to oxygen desaturation. Feeding hypoxemia resolves with maturation, usually by 44 weeks' postconceptional age but occasionally as late as 54 weeks' postconceptional age. Infants are treated by frequent interruptions during a feed, by supplemental oxygen while feeding, and in extreme cases by gavage. Sometimes, atropine before feeds may be helpful for the rapid onset of reflex bradycardia (Kattwinkel et al, 1976a).

CONGENITAL HYPOVENTILATION SYNDROME

Although this uncommon condition is more frequently described in older infants (Brouillette et al, 1990), the severe form occurs in newborns and may need attention in the delivery room or the newborn nursery. These infants have significant hypoventilation with small tidal volumes and prolonged apneas while asleep but tend to have more normal ventilation while awake. There is little evidence of a response to asphyxia, so severe oxygen desaturation and hypercarbia develop without signs of an increased effort to breathe. Because the arousal responses may be present but the ventilatory responses to hypoxia and hypercarbia are absent, it is thought that this condition is caused by a failure to integrate signals from the central and peripheral chemoreceptors into the respiratory centers (Marcus et al, 1991). The head sonogram, the head computed tomography scan, and the head magnetic resonance imaging scan are usually normal (Weese-Mayer et al, 1988); the auditory brain stem responses may be abnormal. No respiratory stimulant drugs have been found effective (Oren et al, 1986), at least in the severe newborn type, and most infants must be treated by prolonged home mechanical ventilation with a tracheostomy. Phrenic nerve pacemakers may be useful sometimes (Brouillette et al, 1983), but because the upper airway muscles are not activated by the phrenic nerve, a tracheostomy is still necessary. Initially the ventilator may be needed for much of the day, but there may be some improvement at about the age of 6 months, after which the infant may need the ventilator only at night while sleeping (Oren et al, 1987). Some of these infants may have Hirschsprung disease (O'Dell et al, 1987), a dysautonomia syndrome, or a neuroblastoma, suggesting a more widespread problem. Seizure disorder, mild cerebral atrophy, and developmental delay may occur, possibly as a result of multiple asphyxial episodes. Many families cope with these children surprisingly well, and some of the children may even go to school (Marcus et al, 1991).

Acquired forms of this condition may be associated with the Arnold-Chiari malformation, hypoxic-ischemic encephalopathy, meningitis, brain tumor, and metabolic brain disease. Examples of the obesity hypoventilation syndrome have not been reported in the newborn.

APNEA OF INFANCY

Isolated apneas of 5 to 15 seconds, with or without periodic breathing, occur commonly in term infants during the first 6 months of life (Richards et al, 1984). There is no associated bradycardia or color change, and the episodes resolve spontaneously. Certain infants have significant apneas, usually more than 20 seconds' duration but sometimes shorter and associated with bradycardia or color change. These too usually resolve spontaneously. The diagnosis of apnea of infancy is reserved for those with onset after 38 weeks' gestation, to distinguish them from infants with apnea of prematurity persisting until 42 weeks' postconceptional age (Consensus Statement, 1987).

Usually after discharge from the nursery, some infants with apnea of infancy have an acute life-threatening event (ALTE), requiring resuscitation by vigorous stimulation or positive-pressure ventilation (Consensus Statement, 1987). Apnea of infancy is just one cause of an ALTE, perhaps representing 50% of the cases. Other causes include (1) gastroesophageal reflux, (2) pharyngeal incoordination, (3) convulsions, (4) infection, (5) heart disease, (6) breath-holding spells, (7) central hypoventilation syndrome, (8) central nervous system abnormality, and (9) accidental or intentional smothering by the mother. Many infants with an ALTE, after appropriate investigation to exclude other causes, are considered to have *near-miss sudden infant death syndrome (SIDS)*. Investigation of these infants, by a 24-hour recording of their breathing, reveals that they have an increased incidence of periodic breathing, brief apneas and prolonged apneas, when compared with control infants (Guilleminault et al, 1979). It is not clear if the infants had the same abnormalities before their ALTE. Nevertheless, a significant number of these infants later die suddenly.

SUDDEN INFANT DEATH SYNDROME

SIDS describes the sudden death of an infant, which is unexplained by history, by a thorough death scene investigation, and by an adequate autopsy (Consensus Statement, 1987). Death occurs during sleep, most commonly during the night. The incidence in the United States is generally 2 per 1000 live births. It is a major cause of infant mortality, with a peak incidence between 2 to 4 months. One hypothesis has been that these infants die from obstructive apnea and that they have apnea of infancy before their demise.

In fact, infants with apnea of infancy, diagnosed by pneumogram, have only a slightly increased risk of SIDS over that in the general population, except if they experience an ALTE, when the risk increases to 4%. If they have several ALTEs, the risk is enormous. Only 7% of infants with SIDS, however, have a preceding ALTE. Nonselected infants destined to die of SIDS do not have a breathing pattern, based on 24-hour recordings, that is significantly different from the breathing pattern of closely matched infants who do not die of SIDS (Southall et al, 1986). Infants with SIDS seldom have a prior diagnosis of apnea of infancy or persistent apnea of prematurity. It seems reasonable to conclude that the apnea hypothesis for SIDS remains unproved and that SIDS and apnea of infancy should be considered separate problems.

HOME APNEA MONITORING PROGRAMS

There remains some controversy about whether some infants should have apnea monitoring at home. Parents must be skilled in the use of the monitor, in the interpretation of frequent false alarms, and in cardiopulmonary resuscitation. There is no evidence that home apnea monitoring reduces the number of deaths, and the incidence of SIDS remains unchanged despite the use of home monitors.

The pneumogram performed in premature infants at the time of discharge appears to be of no help in deciding who to monitor for SIDS and should not be used for this purpose (Consensus Statement, 1987). In one British study, 4% of 1157 premature infants discharged from the hospital had unrecognized prolonged apneas by pneumogram. None of the infants with later SIDS had prolonged apneas at discharge, and none with prolonged apneas at discharge had SIDS (Southall et al, 1982). Barrington and associates (1996) performed a pneumogram on small premature infants believed to be ready for discharge from intensive care. In a few with worrisome apneas, discharge was delayed until the recordings improved, but in the end most infants had less worrisome apneas recorded just prior to discharge, and all infants were sent home without a home apnea monitor. During 6 months follow-up, only 3 of 176 infants had an ALTE, and the predischarge pneumogram could not distinguish these 3 from the others without an ALTE. The only justification for the predischarge pneumogram is that it may detect undiagnosed apneas; however, the significance of such apneas is currently unknown.

Nevertheless, some institutions still perform a pneumogram on most small premature infants before discharge, especially if there is a history of recurrent apneas. If persistent apnea of prematurity is found, depending on the severity of the apneas, infants may be kept in the hospital longer, they may be discharged home without a monitor, or they may be discharged home on a monitor with the apparent hope of preventing an ALTE. A national survey showed that the home apnea monitor is not the standard of care (Meadows et al, 1992), and there is no evidence that the home apnea monitor strategy prevents any deaths; it may, however, be cost-effective in comparison with continued hospitalization, and it may be unwise to alienate an anxious and insistent family.

PRONE SLEEPING POSITION

There is suggestive evidence that the prone sleeping position is associated with an increased incidence of SIDS. An American Academy of Pediatrics Task Force on sleeping position and SIDS recommended that infants should sleep in the supine or lateral position (Kattwinkel et al, 1992).

The relative risk of SIDS in the prone position ranges from 3.5 to 9.3 in seven reported studies; no study has reported a relative risk of less than 1.0 (Guntheroth and Spiers, 1992). Critical review of reports from several countries has shown that previously observed large reductions in the SIDS rate with supine or lateral positioning were sustained over time and that further reductions in the incidence of prone positioning were accompanied by further reductions in the incidence of SIDS (CDC, 1996; Hunt, 1994). It was concluded that the supine position was not associated with an increase in complications such as upper airway obstruction or aspiration pneumonia, as had been suggested previously (Hunt and Shannon, 1992).

The decreased incidence of SIDS may be more marked with supine than with lateral positioning (Wigfield et al, 1992); while asleep, the infant placed in the side position may roll into the prone position. It is emphasized that the American Academy of Pediatrics recommendations do not apply to premature infants, to those with significant gastro-esophageal reflux, or to those with craniofacial abnormalities such as the Pierre Robin syndrome or laryngomalacia.

Infants in the normal newborn nursery should be placed in the supine or lateral position. Premature infants should be encouraged into this position before being discharged, unless they are still having significant apnea of prematurity. Mothers should be appropriately advised of the advantages of the supine position.

No consensus on the cause of the problem with prone positioning has been developed. Chiodini and Thach (1993) showed that the prone position may be associated with rebreathing and hypoxia; this is especially true when the infant assumes a persistent face-down position, a not uncommon occurrence, and when the infant sleeps on soft bedding rather than on a firm mattress; the same authors could find little evidence for the development of any airway obstruction, however. Kahn and coworkers (1993) demonstrated that the prone position was associated with a longer duration of sleep, a larger amount of deep sleep, and significantly fewer and shorter arousals from sleep; it seems possible that arousal from sleep may be an important protective mechanism against SIDS, which always occurs during sleep.

REFERENCES

Abu-Osba YK, Brouillette RE, Wilson SL, Thach BT: Breathing pattern and transcutaneous oxygen tension during motor activity in preterm infants. Am Rev Respir Dis 125:382, 1982.

Adams JM, Murfin K, Mort J, et al: Detection of hyperoxemia in neonates by a new pulse oximeter. Neonat Intensive Care 7:42, 1994.

Ajuriaguerra MD, Radvanyi-Bouvet MF, Huon C, Moriette G: Gastroesophageal reflux and apnea in prematurely born infants during wakefulness and sleep. Am J Dis Child 145:1132, 1991.

Alvaro R, Alvarez J, Kwiatkowski K, et al: Small preterm infants (<1500 g) have only a sustained decrease in ventilation in response to hypoxia. Pediatr Res 32:403, 1992.

Aranda JV, Turmen T: Methylxanthines in apnea of prematurity. Clin Perinatol 6:87, 1979.

Barrington K, Finer N: The natural history of the appearance of apnea of prematurity. Pediatr Res 29:372, 1991.

Barrington KJ, Finer NN: Doxapram for apnea of prematurity (Letter). J Pediatr 109:563, 1986.

Barrington KJ, Finer NN: Periodic breathing and apnea in preterm infants. Pediatr Res 27:118, 1990.

Barrington KJ, Finer NN, Li D: Predischarge respiratory recordings in very-low-birth-weight newborn infants. J Pediatr 129:934, 1996.

Barrington KJ, Finer NN, Torok-Both G, et al: Dose-response relationship of doxapram in the therapy for refractory idiopathic apnea of prematurity. Pediatrics 80:22, 1987.

Blanchard PW, Cote A, Hobbs S, et al: Abolition of ventilatory response to caffeine in chemodenervated lambs. J Physiol 61:133, 1986.

Bodegard G, Schweiler GH, Skoglund S, et al: Control of respiration in newborn babies: The development of the Hering-Breuer inflation reflex. Acta Paediatr Scand 58:567, 1969.

Bolivar JM, Gerhardt T, Gonzalez A, et al: Mechanisms for episodes of hypoxemia in preterm infants undergoing mechanical ventilation. J Pediatr 127:767, 1995.

Booth IW: Silent gastro-esophageal reflux: How much do we miss? Arch Dis Child 67:1325, 1992.

Brady JP, Ceruti E: Chemoreceptor reflexes in the newborn infant: Effects of varying degrees of hypoxia on heart rate and ventilation in a warm environment. J Physiol (Lond) 184:631, 1966.

Brouillette RT, Ilbawi MN, Hunt CE: Phrenic nerve pacing in infants and children: A review of experience and report on the usefulness of phrenic nerve stimulation studies. J Pediatr 102:32, 1983.

Brouillette RT, Weese-Mayer DE, Hunt CE: Breathing control disorders in infants and children. Hosp Pract 25:82, 1990.

Bryan AC, Bryan MH: Control of respiration in the newborn. In Thibeault DW, Gregory GA (Eds): Neonatal Pulmonary Care. Norwalk, CT, Appleton-Century-Crofts, 1986.

Butcher-Puech MC, Henderson-Smart DJ, Holley D, et al: Relation between apnea duration and type and neurological status of preterm infants. Arch Dis Child 60:953, 1985.

Cattarossi L, Rubini S, Macagno F: Aminophylline and increased activity of peripheral chemoreceptors in newborn infants. Arch Dis Child 69:52, 1993.

CDC: Sudden infant death syndrome, United States, 1983–1994. MMWR 45:859, 1996.

Chiodini BA, Thach BT: Impaired ventilation in infants sleeping facedown: Potential significance for sudden infant death syndrome. J Pediatr 123:686, 1993.

Cohen MI: Neurogenesis of respiratory rhythm in the mammal. Physiol Rev 59:1105, 1979.

Consensus Statement: National Institutes of Health Consensus Development Conference on Infantile Apnea and Home Monitoring. Pediatrics 79:292, 1987.

Daily WJR, Klaus M, Meyer HB: Apnea in premature infants: Monitoring, incidence, heart rate changes and an effect of environmental temperature. Pediatrics 43:510, 1969.

Davis JM, Spitzer AR, Stefano JL, et al: Use of caffeine in infants unresponsive to theophylline in apnea of prematurity. Pediatr Pulmonol 3:90, 1987.

DeMaio JG, Harris MC, Deuber C, Spitzer AR: Effect of blood transfusion on apnea frequency in growing premature infants. J Pediatr 114:1039, 1989.

DiMarco AF, Von Euler C, Romaniuk JR, Yamamoto Y: Positive feedback facilitation of external intercostal and phrenic inspiratory activity by pulmonary stretch receptors. Acta Physiol Scand 113:375, 1981.

Dransfield DA, Spitzer AR, Fox WW: Episodic airway obstruction in premature infants. Am J Dis Child 137:441, 1983.

Eyal F, Alpan G, Sagi E, et al: Aminophylline versus doxapram in idiopathic apnea of prematurity: A double blind controlled trial. Pediatrics 75:709, 1985.

Gabriel M, Albani M: Cardiac slowing and respiratory arrest in preterm infants. Eur J Pediatr 122:257, 1976.

Gerhardt T, Bancalari E: Maturational changes of reflexes influencing inspiratory timing in newborns. J Appl Physiol 50:1282, 1981.

Gerhardt T, Bancalari E: Components of effective elastance and their maturational changes in human newborns. J Appl Physiol 53:766, 1982.

Gerhardt T, Bancalari E: Apnea of prematurity: I. Lung function and regulation of breathing. Pediatrics 74:58, 1984a.

Gerhardt T, Bancalari E: Apnea of prematurity: II. Respiratory reflexes. Pediatrics 74:63, 1984b.

Gerhardt T, McCarthy J, Bancalari E: Effects of aminophylline on respiratory center and reflex activity in premature infants with apnea. Pediatr Res 17:188, 1983.

Graham BD, Reardon HS, Wilson JL, et al: Physiologic and chemical response of premature infants to oxygen enriched atmosphere. Pediatrics 6:55, 1950.

Guilleminault C, Ariagno R, Korobkin R, et al: Mixed and obstructive sleep apnea and near-miss for sudden infant death syndrome: 2. Comparison of near-miss and normal control infants by age. Pediatrics 64:882, 1979.

Guntheroth WG, Spiers PS: Sleeping prone and the risk of sudden infant death syndrome. JAMA 267:2359, 1992.

Hackett PH, Roach RC, Harrison GL, et al: Respiratory stimulants and sleep periodic breathing at high altitude: Almitrine versus acetazolamide. Am Rev Respir Dis 135:896, 1987.

Haddad GG, Mellins RB: The role of airway receptors in the control of respiration in infants: A review. J Pediatr 91:281, 1977.

Hayakawa F, Hakamada S, Kuno K, et al: Doxapram in the treatment of idiopathic apnea of prematurity: Desirable dosage and serum concentrations. J Pediatr 109:138, 1986.

Henderson-Smart DJ: The effects of gestational age on the incidence and duration of recurrent apnea in newborn babies. Aust Pediatr J 17:273, 1981.

Henderson-Smart DJ, Butcher-Puech MC, Edwards DA: Incidence and mechanism of bradycardia during apnea in preterm infants. Arch Dis Child 61:227, 1986.

Henderson-Smart DJ, Pettigrew AG, Campbell DJ: Clinical apnea and brain-stem neural function in preterm infants. N Engl J Med 308:353, 1983.

Henderson-Smart DJ, Read DJC: Reduced lung volume during behavioral active sleep in the newborn. J Appl Physiol 46:1081, 1979.

Hertzberg T, Lagercrantz H: Postnatal sensitivity of the peripheral chemoreceptors in newborn infants. Arch Dis Child 62:1238, 1987.

Hiatt IM, Hegyi T, Indyk L, et al: Continuous monitoring of PO_2 during apnea of prematurity. J Pediatr 98:288, 1981.

Hoppenbrouwers T, Hodgman JE, Harper RM, et al: Polygraphic studies of normal infants during the first six months of life: III. Incidence of apnea and periodic breathing. Pediatrics 60:418, 1977.

Hunt CE: Infant sleep position and sudden infant death syndrome risk: A time for change. Pediatrics 94:105, 1994.

Hunt CE, Brouillette RT: Sudden infant death syndrome: 1987 perspective. J Pediatr 110:669, 1987.

Hunt CE, Shannon DC: Sudden infant death syndrome and sleeping position. Pediatrics 90:115, 1992.

Jardine DS, Rogers K: Relationship of benzyl alcohol to kernicterus, intraventricular hemorrhage, and mortality in premature infants. Pediatrics 83:721, 1988.

Joshi A, Gerhardt T, Shandloff P, Bancalari E: Blood transfusion effect on the respiratory pattern of preterm infants. Pediatrics 80:79, 1987.

Kahn A, Groswasser J, Sottiaux M, et al: Prone or supine position and sleep characteristics in infants. Pediatrics 91:1112, 1993.

Kattwinkel J: Neonatal apnea: Pathogenesis and therapy. J Pediatr 90:342, 1977.

Kattwinkel J, Brooks J, Myerberg D: Positioning and SIDS: AAP task force on infant positioning and SIDS. Pediatrics 89:1120, 1992.

Kattwinkel J, Fanaroff AA, Klaus MH: Bradycardia in preterm infants: Indications and hazards of atropine therapy. Pediatrics 58:494, 1976a.

Kattwinkel J, Mars H, Fanaroff A, et al: Urinary biogenic amines in idiopathic apnea of prematurity. J Pediatr 88:1003, 1976b.

Kattwinkel J, Nearman HS, Fanaroff AA, et al: Apnea of prematurity: Comparative therapeutic effects of cutaneous stimulation and nasal continuous positive airway pressure. J Pediatr 86:588, 1975.

Keyes WG, Donohue PK, Spivak JL, et al: Assessing the need for transfusion of premature infants and role of hematocrit, clinical signs, and erythropoietin level. Pediatrics 84:412, 1989.

Khoo MCK, Kronauer RE, Srohl KP, Slutsky AS: Factors influencing periodic breathing in humans: A general model. J Appl Physiol 53:644, 1982.

Koos BJ, Matsuda K: Fetal breathing, sleep state and cardiovascular responses to adenosine in sheep. J Appl Physiol 68:489, 1990.

Korner AF, Kraemer HC, Hoffner ME, et al: Effects of waterbed flotation on premature infants: A pilot study. Pediatrics 56:361, 1975.

Kosch PC, Davenport PW, Wozniak JA, et al: Reflex control of inspiratory duration in breathing. J Appl Physiol 60:2007, 1986.

Krauss AN, Goldstein RF, Alfero V, et al: Effect of endotracheal continuous positive airway pressure on sensitivity to carbon dioxide and on respiratory timing in preterm infants. Pediatr Pulmonol 2:103, 1986.

Kurlak LO, Ruggins NR, Stephenson TJ: Effect of nursing position on incidence, type, and duration of clinically significant apnoea in preterm infants. Arch Dis Child 71:F16, 1994.

Lagercrantz H: What does the preterm infant breathe for? Controversies on apnea of prematurity. Acta Paediatr 81:733, 1992.

Larsen PB, Brendstrup L, Skov L, Flachs H: Aminophylline versus caffeine citrate for apnea and bradycardia prophylaxis in premature infants. Acta Paediatr 84:360, 1995.

Locke R, Greenspan JS, Shaffer TH, et al: Effect of nasal CPAP on thoraco-abdominal motion in neonates with respiratory insufficiency. Pediatr Pulmonol 11:259, 1991.

Locke RG, Wolfson MR, Shaffer TH, et al: Inadvertent administration of positive end distending pressure during nasal cannula flow. Pediatrics 91:135, 1993.

Lopes JM, Davis GM, Mullahoo K, Aranda JV: Role of adenosine in the hypoxic ventilatory response of the newborn piglet. Pediatr Pulmonol 17:50, 1994.

Marcus CL, Bautista DB, Amihyia A, et al: Hypercapnic arousal responses in children with congenital central hypoventilation syndrome. Pediatrics 88:993, 1991.

Marcus CL, Jansen MT, Poulsen MK, et al: Medical and psychosocial outcome of children with congenital central hypoventilation syndrome. J Pediatr 119:888, 1991.

Martin-Boddy RL, Johnston BM: Central origin of the hypoxic depression of breathing in the newborn. Respir Physiol 71:25, 1988.

Martin RJ, DiFiore JM, Korenke CB, et al: Vulnerability of respiratory control in healthy preterm infants placed supine. J Pediatr 127:609, 1995.

Martin RJ, Miller MJ, Carlo WA: Pathogenesis of apnea in preterm infants. J Pediatr 109:733, 1986.

Martin RJ, Nearman HS, Katona PG, et al: The effect of a low continuous positive airway pressure on the reflex control of respiration in the preterm infant. J Pediatr 90:976, 1977.

Mathew OP: Maintenance of upper airway patency. J Pediatr 106:863, 1985.

Mathew OP, Thoppil CK, Belan M: Motor activity and apnea in preterm infants. Am Rev Respir Dis 144:842, 1991.

Meadows W, Mendez D, Lantos J, et al: What is the legal standard of medical care when there is no standard of medical care? A survey of the use of home apnea monitoring for graduates of neonatal intensive care units. Neonat Intensive Care 5:43, 1992.

Menon AP, Schefft GL, Thach BT: Apnea associated with regurgitation in infants. J Pediatr 106:625, 1985.

Miller MJ, Carlo WA, Martin RJ: Continuous positive airway pressure selectively reduces obstructive apnea in preterm infants. J Pediatr 106:91, 1985.

Muller N, Volgyesi G, Eng P, et al: The consequences of diaphragmatic muscle fatigue in the newborn infant. J Pediatr 95:793, 1979.

Murat I, Morriette G, Blin MC, et al: The efficacy of caffeine in the treatment of recurrent idiopathic apnea in premature infants. J Pediatr 99:984, 1981.

Newell SJ, Booth IW, Morgan MEI, et al: Gastro-esophageal reflux in preterm infants. Arch Dis Child 64:780, 1989.

O'Dell K, Staren E, Bassuk A: Total colonic aganglionosis (Zuelzer-Wilson syndrome) and congenital failure of autonomic control of ventilation (Ondines curse). J Pediatr Surg 22:1019, 1987.

Oren J, Kelly DH, Shannon DC: Long term follow-up of children with congenital central hypoventilation syndrome. Pediatrics 80:375, 1987.

Oren J, Newth CJL, Hunt CE, et al: Ventilatory effects of almitrine bismesylate in congenital central hypoventilation syndrome. Am Rev Respir Dis 134:917, 1986.

Perlman JM, Volpe JJ: Episodes of apnea and bradycardia in the preterm newborn: Impact on cerebral circulation. Pediatrics 76:333, 1985.

Poets CF, Stebbens VA, Richard D, Southall DP: Prolonged episodes of hypoxemia in preterm infants undetected by cardiorespiratory monitors. Pediatrics 95:860, 1995.

Poets CF, Samuels MP, Southall DP: Potential role of intrapulmonary shunting in the genesis of hypoxemic episodes in infants and young children. Pediatrics 90:385, 1992.

Poets CF, Stebbens VA, Samuels MP, Southall DP: The relationship between bradycardia, apnea, and hypoxemia in preterm infants. Pediatr Res 34:144, 1993.

Pryds O, Schneider S: Aminophylline reduces cerebral blood flow in stable preterm infants without affecting the visual evoked potential. Eur J Pediatr 150:366, 1991.

Richards JM, Alexander JR, Shinebourne EA, et al: Sequential 22-hour profiles of breathing patterns and heart rate in 110 full-term infants during their first 6 months of life. Pediatrics 74:763, 1984.

Rigatto H: Ventilatory response to hypercapnia. Semin Perinatol 1:363, 1977.

Rigatto H: Apnea. Pediatr Clin North Am 29:1105, 1982.

Rigatto H, Brady JP: Periodic breathing and apnea in preterm infants: Evidence for hypoventilation possibly due to central respiratory depression. Pediatrics 50:202, 1972.

Rigatto H, Brady JP, Verduzco RT: Chemoreceptor reflexes in preterm infants: The effect of gestational and postnatal age on the ventilatory response to inhalation of 100% and 15% oxygen. Pediatrics 55:604, 1975a.

Rigatto H, Brady J, Verduzco RT: Chemoreceptor reflexes in preterm infants: The effect of gestational and postnatal age on the ventilatory response to inhaled carbon dioxide. Pediatrics 55:614, 1975b.

Rigatto H, Verduzco RT, Cates DB: Effects of O_2 on the ventilatory response to CO_2 in preterm infants. J Appl Physiol 39:896, 1975c.

Rosen CL, Glaze DG, Frost JD: Hypoxemia associated with feeding in the preterm infant and full-term neonate. Am J Dis Child 138:623, 1984.

Ross MP, Christensen RD, Rothstein G, et al: A randomized trial to develop criteria for administering erythrocyte transfusions to anemic preterm infants 1–3 months of age. J Perinatol 9:246, 1989.

Saliba E, Autret E, Gold F, et al: Effect of caffeine on cerebral blood flow velocity in preterm infants. Biol Neonate 56:198, 1989.

Samuels MP, Poets CF, Stebbens VA, et al: Oxygen saturation and breathing patterns in preterm infants with cyanotic episodes. Acta Paediatr 81:875, 1992.

Scherer LR: Surgical management. *In* Jones MD, Gleason CA, Lipstein SU (Eds): Hospital Care of the Recovering NICU Infant. Baltimore, Williams & Wilkins, 1991.

Schulte FJ: Apnea. Clin Perinatol 4:65, 1977.

Shivpuri CR, Martin RJ, Carlo WA, Fanaroff AA: Decreased ventilation in preterm infants during an oral feed. J Pediatr 103:285, 1983.

Soliz A, Suguihara C, Huang J, et al: Effect of amino acid infusion on the ventilatory response to hypoxia in protein deprived neonatal piglets. Pediatr Res 35:316, 1994.

Southall DP, Richards JM, Rhoden KJ, et al: Prolonged apnea and cardiac arrhythmias in infants discharged from neonatal intensive care units: Failure to predict an increased risk for sudden infant death syndrome. Pediatrics 70:844, 1982.

Southall DP, Richards JM, Stebbens V, et al: Cardiorespiratory function in 16 full-term infants with sudden infant death syndrome. Pediatrics 78:787, 1986.

Speidel BD, Dunn PM: Use of nasal continuous positive airway pressure to treat severe recurrent apnea in very preterm infants. Lancet 2:658, 1976.

Storrs CN: Cardiovascular effects of apnea in preterm infants. Arch Dis Child 52:534, 1977.

Stute H, Greiner B, Linderkamp O: Effect of blood transfusion on cardiorespiratory abnormalities in preterm infants. Arch Dis Child 72:F194, 1995.

Thach BT, Frantz ID, Adler S, et al: Maturation of reflexes influencing inspiratory duration in human infants. J Appl Physiol 45:203, 1978.

Tudehope DI, Rogers YM, Burns YR, et al: Apnea in very low birth weight infants: Outcome at 2 years. Aust Paediatr J 22:131, 1986.

Upton CJ, Milner AD, Stokes GM: Apnoea, bradycardia, and oxygen saturation in preterm infants. Arch Dis Child 66:381, 1991.

Von Euler C: On the central pattern generator for the basic breathing rhythmicity. J Appl Physiol 55:1647, 1983.

Walsh JK, Farrell MK, Keenan WJ, et al: Gastro-esophageal reflux in infants: Relation to apnea. J Pediatr 99:197, 1981.

Weese-Mayer DE, Brouillette RT, Naidich TP, et al: Magnetic resonance imaging and computerized tomography in central hypoventilation. Am Rev Respir Dis 137:393, 1988.

Wennergren G, Wennergren M: Neonatal breathing control mediated by the central chemoreceptors. Acta Physiol Scand 119:139, 1983.

Wigfield RE, Fleming PJ, Berry PJ, et al: Can the fall in Avons sudden infant death rate be explained by changes in sleeping position? BMJ 304:282, 1992.

CHAPTER 50

Pulmonary Physiology of the Newborn

Thomas Hansen and Anthony Corbet

LUNG MECHANICS AND LUNG VOLUMES

The lungs possess physical, or mechanical, properties that resist inflation, such as elastic recoil, resistance, and inertance. The dynamic interaction between these properties determines the effort that must be exerted during spontaneous breathing and the resting and extreme values for the volume of gas in the lung.

Elastic Recoil

The lung contains elastic tissues that must be stretched for lung inflation to occur. Hooke's law requires that the pressure needed to inflate the lung must be proportional to the volume of inflation (Fig. 50–1). Conventionally, volume of inflation is plotted on the y-axis, and the distending pressure is plotted on the x-axis. In this way, the constant of proportionality is volume divided by pressure, or *lung compliance*. Throughout the range of tidal ventilation, the relationship between pressure and volume is linear. At higher lung volumes, as the lung reaches its elastic limit (*total lung capacity*), this relationship plateaus.

The lungs and the chest wall function as a unit (the respiratory system) coupled by the interface between the parietal and visceral pleura. The tendency for the lung to collapse at rest is balanced by the outward recoil of the chest wall resulting in a negative (subatmospheric) intrapleural pressure. In the infant, the chest wall is almost infinitely compliant so that pleural pressure is only slightly subatmospheric. The volume at which this balance occurs is the functional residual capacity (FRC). Deflation below FRC requires an active expiratory maneuver.

Residual volume (RV) is defined as the volume of air that cannot be expired with a forced deflation. Inflation of the respiratory system above FRC requires a positive distending pressure that, at higher lung volumes, must overcome the elastic recoil of both the lung and the chest wall.

As depicted in Figure 50–1, the relative compliance of the lung of the newborn is similar to that of the adult (Krieger, 1963); however, the infant's chest wall compliance (Table 50–1) is greater than the adult's (see Fig. 50–1). Measurements of lung and chest wall compliance suggest that the newborn should have a lower percent RV and a lower percent FRC than the adult. In fact, the percent FRC in the newborn is equal to the adult's, and the infant's percent RV is slightly greater. This seeming paradox exists because FRC and RV are measured while the infant is breathing, and predictions from the pressure volume curves assume that there is no air movement and passive relaxation of all respiratory muscles (Bryan and England, 1984). Data suggest two mechanisms by which the new-

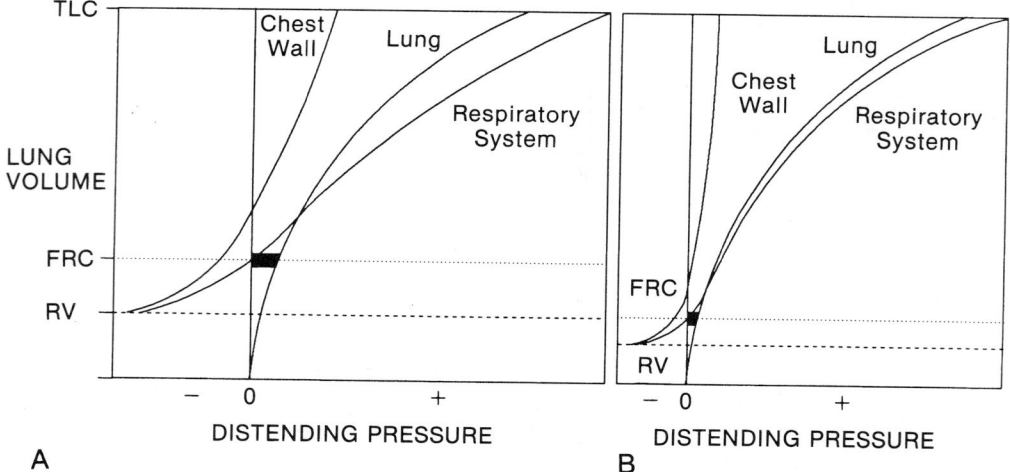

FIGURE 50–1. This is an idealized plot of volume as a function of distending pressure for the lung, chest wall, and respiratory system (lung plus chest wall) of an adult *(A)* and an infant *(B)*. These curves are derived by instilling or removing a measured volume of gas, allowing the respiratory system to come to rest, then measuring the distending pressure for the lung (airway pressure − intrapleural pressure), for the chest wall (intrapleural pressure − atmospheric pressure), and for the respiratory system (airway pressure − atmospheric pressure). Compliance is the change in volume divided by the change in distending pressure. The shaded area is the resting intrapleural pressure at functional residual capacity (FRC). Lung volumes depicted include residual volume (RV), FRC, and total lung capacity (TLC).

TABLE 50–1

Lung Volumes and Mechanics in the Normal Newborn

Lung Volumes	mL/kg
Total lung capacity	63
Functional residual capacity	30
Residual volume	23
Tidal volume	6

Compliance	mL/cm H₂O
Total respiratory system	3
Chest wall	20
Lung	4

Resistance	cm H₂O/mL/sec
Total pulmonary resistance	0.03–0.04

Data from Cook et al, 1957; Gerhardt and Bancalari, 1980; Polgar and Promadhat, 1971; Polgar and String, 1966; Reynolds and Etsten, 1966.

born can maintain a normal FRC during spontaneous breathing: (1) by maintaining inspiratory muscle activity throughout expiration and splinting the chest wall or (2) by increasing expiratory resistance by glottic narrowing. The reason for the elevated RV is not entirely clear, but it could result from airway closure during an active expiration as part of a crying vital capacity maneuver.

Resistance

Resistance to gas flow arises because of friction between gas molecules and the walls of airways (*airway resistance*) and because of friction between the tissues of the lung and the chest wall (*viscous tissue resistance*). Airway resistance represents approximately 80% of the total resistance of the respiratory system (Polgar and String, 1966). In the newborn, nasal resistance represents nearly half the total airway resistance; in the adult, it accounts for about 65% of the airway resistance (Polgar and Kong, 1965).

Gas flows only in response to a pressure gradient (Fig. 50–2). During laminar flow, the pressure difference needed to force gas through the airway is directly related to the flow rate times a constant—airway resistance. During turbulent flow, however, this pressure is directly proportional to a constant times the flow rate squared. Gas flow becomes turbulent at branch points in airways, at sites of obstruction, and at high flow rates. Turbulence occurs whenever flow increases to a point that Reynold's number exceeds 2000. This dimensionless number is directly proportional to the volumetric flow rate and gas density, and it is inversely proportional to the radius of the tube and gas viscosity. Obviously, turbulent flow is most likely to occur in the central airways where volumetric flow is high, rather than in lung periphery where flow is distributed across a large number of airways. Both types of flow exist in the lung, so the net pressure drop is calculated as follows (Pedley et al, 1977):

$$\Delta P = (K_1 \times \dot{V}) + (K_2 \times \dot{V}^2) \qquad (1)$$

It is possible to take advantage of the differences between laminar and turbulent flow to determine the site of airway obstruction in the lung. If obstruction to gas flow is in the central airways, turbulent flow is affected the most. Because turbulent gas flow is density dependent, allowing the patient to breathe a less dense gas (such as helium mixed with oxygen) reduces the resistance to gas flow. If the site of obstruction is peripheral, the mixture of helium and oxygen does not appreciably affect resistance.

Inflation of the lung increases the length of airways and might therefore be expected to increase airway resistance. Lung inflation also increases airway diameter, however. Because airway resistance varies with the fourth to fifth power of the radius of the airway, the effects of changes in airway diameter dominate, and resistance is inversely proportional to lung volume (Rodarte and Rehder, 1986). Thus, airway resistance is lower during inspiration than during expiration because of the effects of changes in intrapleural pressure on airway diameter. During inspiration, pleural pressure becomes negative, and a distending pressure is applied across the lung. This distending pressure increases airway diameter as well as alveolar diameter

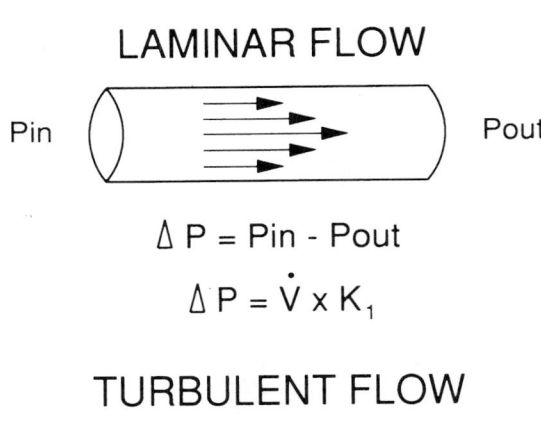

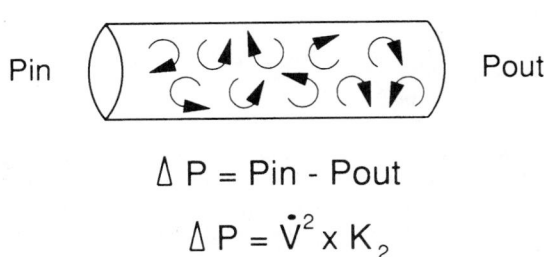

FIGURE 50–2. Gas flow (V̇) through tubular structures occurs only in the presence of a pressure gradient (Pin > Pout). For laminar flow, P is directly proportional to V.

$$\Delta P = \dot{V} \times (8 \times L \times \mu)/(\pi \times r^4)$$

In this case, the constant of proportionality (K_1) is directly related to the length of the airway (L) and the viscosity of the gas (μ) and indirectly proportional to the fourth power of the radius of the airway (r). For turbulent flow, ΔP is proportional to $\dot{V}^2$. The calculation of the constant or proportionality (K_2) is much more complicated. K_2 is directly proportional to the length of the airway, the *density* of the gas, and the fourth root of the Reynold's number and inversely proportional to the *fifth* power of the radius of the airway.

and decreases the resistance to gas flow. During expiration, pleural pressure increases and airways are compressed. Collapse of airways is opposed by their cartilaginous support and by the pressure exerted by gas in their lumina. During passive expiration, these defenses are sufficient to prevent airway closure. When intrapleural pressure is high during active expiration, airways may collapse, and gas may be trapped in the lung. This problem may be accentuated in the small preterm infant with poorly supported central airways.

Inertance

Gas and tissues in the respiratory system also resist accelerations in flow. Inertance is a property that is negligible during quiet breathing and physiologically significant only at rapid respiratory rates.

Dynamic Interaction

Compliance, resistance, and inertance all interact during spontaneous breathing (Fig. 50–3). This interaction is described by the equation of motion for the respiratory system:

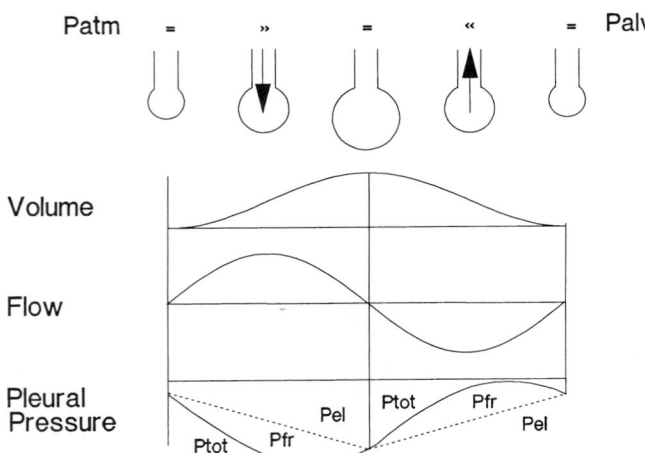

FIGURE 50–3. Gas flows from the atmosphere into the lung only if atmospheric pressure (Patm) is greater than alveolar pressure (Palv). At end exhalation, when Patm equals Palv, there is no gas movement in or out of the lung. During a spontaneous inspiration, the diaphragm contracts, the chest wall expands, and the volume in the intrathoracic space increases. As a result, pleural pressure (Ppl) decreases relative to Patm, and a gradient is created between Ppl and Palv, distending the lung, increasing alveolar volume, and decreasing Palv. A gradient is created between Patm and Palv, and gas flows from the atmosphere into the alveolar space. The rate of gas flow increases rapidly, reaches a maximum (peak flow), then decreases as the alveolus fills with gas and Palv approaches Patm. At peak inspiration, Palv equals Patm, and lung volume is at its maximum, as is Ppl. The curved solid line connecting end expiration to end inspiration is the total driving pressure for inspiration (Ptot). The dotted line represents the pressure needed to overcome elastic forces alone (Pel). The difference between the two lines is the pressure dissipated overcoming flow resistive forces (Pfr). During exhalation, this cycle is reversed.

$$P(t) = (V[t] \times 1/C) + (\dot{V}[t] \times R) + (\ddot{V}[t] \times I) \quad (2)$$

where $P(t)$ is the driving pressure at time, t, $V[t]$ is the lung volume above FRC, C is the respiratory system compliance, $\dot{V}[t]$ is the rate of gas flow, R is the resistance of the respiratory system, $\ddot{V}[t]$ is the rate of acceleration of gas in the airways, and I is the inertance of the respiratory system. If I is neglected, the equation simplifies to:

$$P(t) = (V[t] \times 1/C) + (\dot{V}[t] \times R) \quad (3)$$

At times of zero gas flow (end expiration and end inspiration), the equation further simplifies to:

$$P(t) = (V[t] \times 1/C) \text{ and } C = V(t)/P(t) \quad (4)$$

This series of equations and Figure 50–3 demonstrate that at points of no gas flow (end expiration and end inspiration), only elastic forces are operating on the lung. During inflation or deflation of the lung, however, both elastic and resistive forces are important.

Although the solution to the equation of motion for the respiratory system is beyond the scope of this discussion, the behavior of the respiratory system during passive exhalation is a special situation for which a solution can be obtained relatively easily (Lesouef et al, 1984; McIlroy et al, 1963). Before a passive exhalation maneuver, the infant is given a positive-pressure breath, and the airway is occluded—invoking the Hering-Breuer reflex and a brief apnea. Airway pressure is measured, and the occlusion is released. Expired gas flow is measured using a pneumotachometer and integrated to volume; flow is then plotted as a function of volume (Fig. 50–4A). During a passive exhalation, there are no external forces acting on the respiratory system (P[t] = 0), so the equation of motion simplifies to:

$$(V[t] \times 1/C) + (\dot{V}[t] \times R) = 0$$

Rearranging: $\dot{V}(t) = (-1/[RC]) \times V(t) \quad (5)$

This equation states that during passive exhalation, flow plotted against volume is a straight line with slope $-1/(RC)$. The quantity RC has the units of time and is termed the *respiratory time constant (Trs)*. Trs defines the rate at which the lung deflates during a passive exhalation (see Fig. 50–4). Time constants affect the rate of lung inflation in the same manner that they affect lung deflation (see Chapter 51).

Measurements of Lung Mechanics

A true measurement of static lung compliance requires instilling a known volume of gas into the lung then measuring airway pressure at equilibrium in the absence of respiratory muscle activity (see Fig. 50–1) (McCann et al, 1987). This technique is used to measure compliance during the passive exhalation maneuver described previously (see Fig. 50–4). Another technique for measuring compliance takes advantage of the fact that gas flow is transiently equal to zero at end inspiration and end expiration (see Fig. 50–3). Compliance is calculated by dividing the change in volume between these two points by the concomitant change in

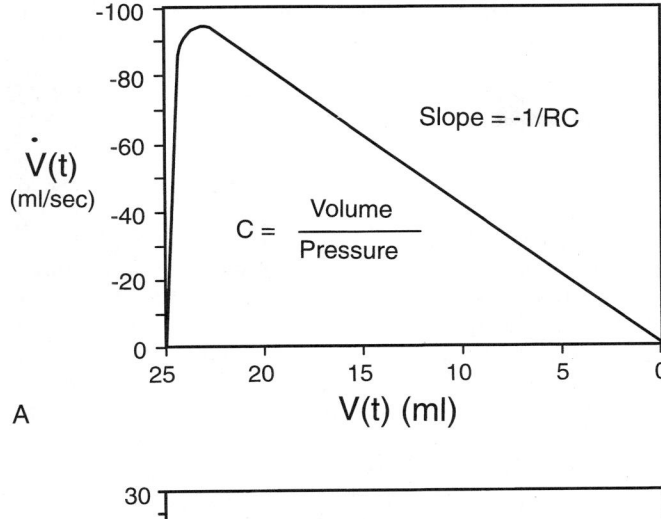

A

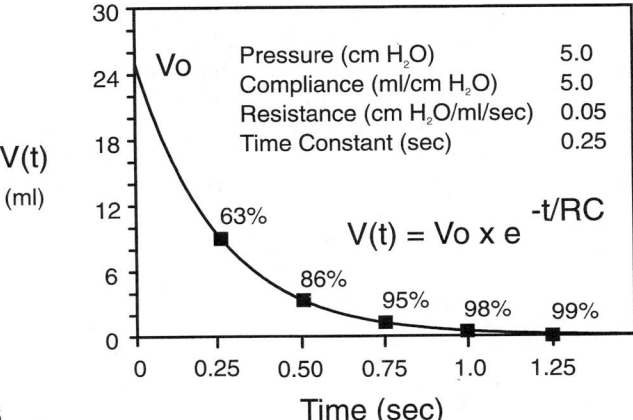

B

FIGURE 50–4. *A,* Plot of flow of gas out of the lung $\dot{V}(t)$ versus volume of gas remaining in the lung $\dot{V}(t)$ for a passive exhalation. Flow of gas out of the lung is negative by convention. After an initial sharp increase, flow decreases linearly as the lung empties. Static compliance of the respiratory system is obtained by dividing the exhaled volume by the airway pressure at the beginning of the passive exhalation. Resistance is calculated from the slope of the flow volume plot ($-1/RC$) and the compliance. This technique has the advantage of not requiring measurements of pleural pressure and being relatively unaffected by chest wall distortion. *B,* $\dot{V}(t)$ is plotted as a function of time for a passive exhalation. The graph is an exponential with the equation:

$$\dot{V}(t) = Vo \times e^{-t (R \times C)}$$

is the starting volume, and *e* is mathematical constant (roughly 2.72). For this example, the time constant is roughly 0.25 second. Calculations show that when exhalation persists for a time equal to one time constant (t = 0.25 sec = 1 × Trs), 63% of the gas in the lung is exhaled. For t = 2Trs, 86% of the gas is exhaled; for 3Trs, 95%; for 4Trs, 98%; and for 5Trs, 99%. If expiration is interrupted before a time t = 3Trs, gas is trapped in the lung.

distending pressure. Because the measurement is made while the infant is breathing, it is termed *dynamic compliance*. In the normal infant, dynamic compliance should be equal to static compliance.

As was alluded to earlier, measurements of compliance are affected by lung size. For example, if a 5 cm H_2O distending pressure results in a 25-mL increase in lung volume in a newborn, calculated lung compliance is 5 mL/ cm H_2O. In an adult, the same 5 cm H_2O distending pressure increases the lung volume by roughly 500 mL, and calculated compliance is 100 mL/cm H_2O. Although the calculated lung compliances are different, the forces needed to carry out tidal ventilation are similar (i.e., lung function is normal in both circumstances). This example points out that if lung compliances are to be compared, they must be corrected for size. This is usually done by dividing compliance by resting lung volume to get *specific compliance*. For the newborn, resting lung volume is roughly 100 mL, so specific compliance is 0.05 mL/cm H_2O/mL lung volume. For the adult, resting lung volume is nearly 2000 mL, so specific compliance is 0.05 mL/cm H_2O/mL lung volume—identical to that of the newborn.

Lung compliance changes with volume history, meaning that it decreases with fixed tidal volumes and increases after deep breaths that recruit air spaces that may have been poorly ventilated or atelectatic. The periodic sigh in spontaneous breathing is associated with an increase in lung compliance and in oxygenation.

Many respiratory disorders result in nonhomogeneous increases in small-airway resistance in the lung. Therefore, if lung compliance remains relatively uniform, the product of resistance and compliance (Trs) varies throughout the lung. During lung inflation, units with normal resistance have the lowest Trs and fill rapidly. Units with high resistance have a longer Trs and fill more slowly. At rapid respiratory rates when the duration of inspiration is short, only those lung units with a short Trs are ventilated. In effect, the ventilated lung becomes smaller. As discussed earlier, as the lung becomes smaller, its measured compliance decreases. Therefore, in infants with ventilation inhomogeneities, dynamic lung compliance decreases as respiratory rate increases. This decrease in lung compliance with increasing respiratory rate is termed *frequency dependence of compliance*, and it is suggestive of inhomogeneous small-airway obstruction.

Resistance of the total respiratory system can be measured using the passive exhalation technique described previously (see Fig. 50–4), or it can be calculated from measurements of distending pressure, volume, and flow (see Fig. 50–3). Points of equal volume are chosen during inspiration and expiration. The gas flow and the distending pressure are measured at each point. The pressure needed to overcome elastic forces should be the same for inspiration and expiration and therefore cancel out. Total resistance, consequently, is equal to distending pressure at the inspiratory point minus distending pressure at the expiratory point, divided by the sum of the respective inspiratory and expiratory point gas flows. Investigators have calculated compliance and resistance by measuring distending pressure, gas flow, and volume (see Fig. 50–3), then fitting these measurements to the equation of motion (see Equation (3)), using multiple linear regression techniques, and solving for the coefficients 1/C and R (Bhutani et al, 1988).

FRC is measured by inert gas dilution techniques (helium dilution) or inert gas displacement (nitrogen washout) (Fig. 50–5). Both of these techniques measure gas that communicates with the airways. The total volume of gas in the thorax at end expiration (thoracic gas volume [TGV]) can be measured using a body plethysmograph and

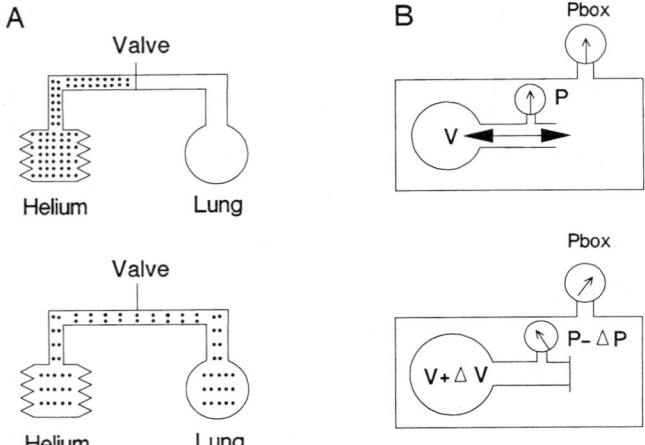

FIGURE 50–5. *A,* Measurement of functional residual capacity (FRC) by helium dilution. At end exhalation, the infant breathes from a bag containing a known volume (V_{bag}) and concentration of helium (He_i) in oxygen. The gas in the infant's lungs dilutes the helium-oxygen mixture to a new concentration (He_f): FRC = Bag volume × (He_i − He_f)/He_f. *B,* Measurement of thoracic gas volume (TGV) using a plethysmograph. The infant breathes spontaneously in a sealed body plethysmograph. At end exhalation, the airway is closed with a shutter. As the infant attempts to inspire against the shutter, the volume of the thorax increases and airway pressure decreases. The increase in volume of the thorax can be measured from the change in the pressure inside of the plethysmograph (Pbox). By Boyle's law: P × TGV = (P − ΔP) × (TGV + ΔV), where *P* is atmospheric pressure, *(P − ΔP)* is airway pressure during occlusion, and *(TGV + ΔV)* is thoracic volume during occlusion. Therefore, TGV = (P − ΔP) × ΔV/ΔP. Because ΔP is small compared with P, this can be simplified to: TGV = P × ΔV/ΔP.

applying Boyle's law. This technique measures all gas in the thorax—even trapped gas that is not in contact with the airways. Obviously, FRC measured by inert gas dilution is less than TGV if significant volumes of trapped gas are present.

ALVEOLAR VENTILATION

The tissues of the body continuously consume O_2 and produce CO_2 (Fig. 50–6). The primary function of the circulation is to pick up O_2 from the lungs and deliver it to the tissues, then to pick up CO_2 from the tissues and deliver it to the lungs. The exchange of O_2 and CO_2 with the blood occurs within the alveolar volume of the lungs. The alveolar volume acts as a "large sink" from which O_2 is continuously extracted by the blood and to which CO_2 is continuously added. This mechanism for acquiring O_2 from the atmosphere and excreting CO_2 into the atmosphere is the *alveolar ventilation* (Slonim and Hamilton, 1987).

The alveolar volume of the lung includes all lung units capable of exchanging gas with mixed venous blood: respiratory bronchioles, alveolar ducts, and alveoli. Because the conducting airways do not participate in gas exchange, they constitute the *anatomic dead space* (V_D). At end exhalation, the FRC is the sum of the volume of gas in the alveolar volume and in the anatomic dead space. During normal breathing, the amount of gas entering and leaving the lung

with each breath is the tidal volume (V_T): V_T × respiratory rate (RR) = minute ventilation ($\dot{V}$). Part of each V_T is wasted ventilation because it moves gas in and out of the V_D. Therefore, alveolar ventilation ($\dot{V}_A$) can be expressed as:

$$\dot{V}_A = (V_T - V_D) \times RR \qquad (6)$$

Alveolar ventilation is an intermittent process, whereas gas exchange between the alveolar space and the blood occurs continuously. Because arterial O_2 and CO_2 tensions (Pa_{O_2} and Pa_{CO_2}) are roughly equal to the O_2 and CO_2 tensions within the alveolar space, these fluctuations in breathing could result in intermittent hypoxemia and hypercarbia. Fortunately the lung has a large buffer—the FRC. The FRC is four to five times as large as the V_T; therefore, only a fraction of the total gas in the lung is exchanged during normal breathing. This large buffer continues to supply O_2 to the blood during expiration and acts as a sump to accept CO_2 from the blood, so alveolar O_2 and CO_2 tensions (Pa_{O_2} and Pa_{CO_2}) change little throughout the ventilatory cycle.

Alveolar ventilation is linked tightly to metabolism. When alveolar ventilation is uncoupled from the body's metabolic rate, hypoventilation or hyperventilation results. During hypoventilation, less O_2 is added to the alveolar space than is removed by the blood, and less CO_2 is

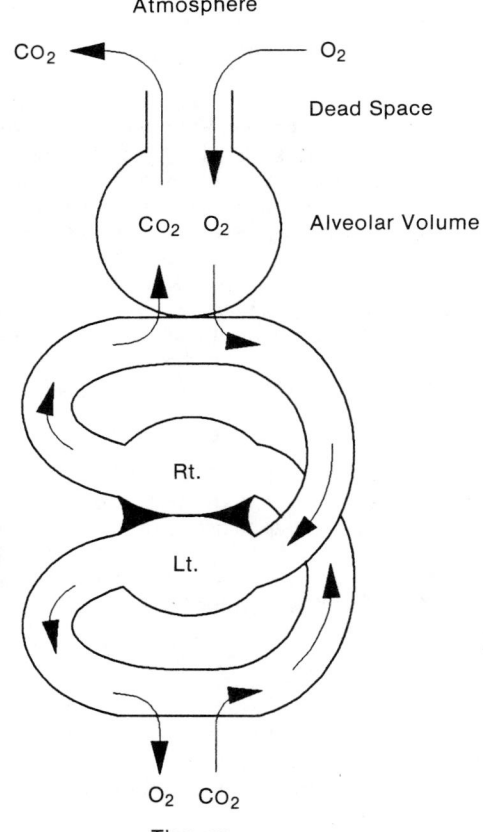

FIGURE 50–6. Schematic showing coupling of alveolar ventilation to tissue oxygen consumption.

removed from the alveolar space than is added by the blood. As a result, P_{AO_2} decreases and P_{ACO_2} increases. The net result of hypoventilation is hypoxemia and hypercapnia. Administering supplemental O_2 increases the quantity of O_2 in each breath delivered to the alveolar space, and it may prevent arterial hypoxemia. For example, suppose a 1-kg male infant has a V_T of 6 mL, an anatomic V_D of 2 mL, and a respiratory rate of 40 breaths/min. His alveolar ventilation is 160 mL per minute ([6 mL − 2 mL] × 40/min). If he breathes room air (21% O_2), he delivers 33.6 mL of O_2 to the alveolar space every minute (160 mL/min × 0.21). If he maintains the same V_T but breathes only 20 times per minute, his alveolar ventilation decreases to 80 mL per minute, only 16.8 mL of O_2 (80 mL/min × 0.21) is delivered to the alveolar space each minute, and his P_{AO_2} and P_{aO_2} decrease. If he is allowed to breathe 50% O_2, O_2 delivery to the alveolar space increases to 40 mL per minute (80 mL/min × 0.50), and both his P_{AO_2} and P_{aO_2} increase. Because O_2 administration has no effect on the accumulation of CO_2, it does not prevent hypercapnia.

Hyperventilation delivers more O_2 to the alveolar space than can be removed by the blood and removes more CO_2 than can be added by the blood. As a result, P_{AO_2} increases and P_{ACO_2} decreases.

Measurements of alveolar ventilation and anatomic V_D in the infant rely on the relationship between CO_2 production ($\dot{V}_{CO_2}$), $\dot{V}_A$, and P_{ACO_2}. The mathematical expression of this relationship states (Cook et al, 1955):

$$F_{ACO_2} = \dot{V}_{CO_2} / \dot{V}_A \tag{7}$$

F_ACO_2 is the ratio of CO_2 to total alveolar gas, or

$$F_{ACO_2} = P_{ACO_2} / (P_B - 47) \tag{8}$$

P_B is the barometric pressure, and 47 mm Hg is the vapor pressure of water at body temperature. Therefore,

$$\dot{V}_A = (\dot{V}_{CO_2} \times [P_B - 47]) / P_{ACO_2} \tag{9}$$

If minute ventilation ($\dot{V}$) is measured, V_D ventilation ($\dot{V}_D$) is calculated as:

$$\dot{V}_D = \dot{V} - \dot{V}_A \tag{10}$$

V_D volume is calculated by dividing by the respiratory rate. This method measures the anatomic V_D in the lung. As seen in the next section, portions of some gas exchanging units in the lung can also function as V_D; therefore, the total V_D, or the physiologic V_D, may be greater than the anatomic V_D. Physiologic V_D is calculated by substituting P_{aCO_2} into Equation (9). When $P_{ACO_2} = P_{aCO_2}$, all the V_D is anatomic V_D, and the gas exchanging units are all functioning normally. As physiologic V_D increases, however, P_{aCO_2} increases relative to P_{ACO_2}. Therefore, the difference between P_{aCO_2} and P_{ACO_2} (the aA.DCO_2) is a measure of efficiency of gas exchange in the lung.

For clinical purposes, $\dot{V}_{CO_2}$ in Equation (9) is assumed to be a constant so that $\dot{V}_A$ is proportional to $1/P_{aCO_2}$. Thus, increased P_{aCO_2} means that alveolar ventilation has decreased; decreased P_{aCO_2} means that alveolar ventilation has increased.

VENTILATION-PERFUSION RELATIONSHIPS

Under ideal circumstances, ventilation and perfusion of the lung are evenly matched ($\dot{V}/\dot{Q} = 1$), both in the lung as a whole and in each individual air space. The air spaces receive O_2 from the inspired gas and CO_2 from the blood. O_2 is transported into the blood, while CO_2 is transported to the atmosphere. Even though $\dot{V}/\dot{Q}$ is 1, CO_2 and O_2 are exchanged in the lung at the same ratio at which they are exchanged in the tissues: A little less CO_2 is transported out than O_2 is transported in, so the respiratory exchange ratio R equals 0.8. If there is no diffusion defect, the gas composition of the air spaces and the blood comes into equilibrium. N_2 makes up the balance of dry gas. The sum of partial pressures of all gases in the air spaces is equal to the atmospheric pressure. The ideal alveolar gas composition is: $PO_2 = 100$, $PCO_2 = 40$, $P_{N_2} = 573$, and $P_{H_2O} = 47$ mm Hg at an atmospheric pressure of 760 mm Hg. The ideal arterial blood composition is the same. Therefore, differences between alveolar and arterial gas composition under ideal circumstances are all zero. Knowing the values for P_{ACO_2} and inspired gas, ideal alveolar gas composition can be calculated from the alveolar gas equations (Farhi, 1966):

$$P_{AO_2} = P_{IO_2} - P_{ACO_2} \times (F_{IO_2} + [1 - F_{IO_2}] / R) \tag{11}$$

$$P_{AN_2} = F_{IN_2} \times (P_{ACO_2} \times [1 - R] / R + [P_B - P_{H_2O}]) \tag{12}$$

Under normal circumstances and certainly in the presence of lung disease, this ideal situation is not the case; some air spaces receive more ventilation than perfusion, and others receive more perfusion than ventilation. A reduction of ventilation may occur because of atelectasis, alveolar fluid, or airway narrowing. Reduced ventilation in one part of the lung may cause increased ventilation elsewhere. A reduction of perfusion may occur if air spaces are collapsed or overdistended or because of gravitational effects, and increased perfusion may occur in congenital heart disease. As with ventilation, reduced perfusion in one part of the lung may cause increased perfusion in other regions. If an air space is relatively overventilated (high $\dot{V}/\dot{Q}$), its gas composition tends toward that of inspired gas, which in the case of room air is $PO_2 = 150$ and $PCO_2 = 0$ mm Hg. If an air space is relatively underventilated (low $\dot{V}/\dot{Q}$), its gas composition tends toward that of mixed venous blood, which is $PO_2 = 40$ and $PCO_2 = 46$ mm Hg. What counts is the $\dot{V}/\dot{Q}$ ratio, not absolute values of $\dot{V}$ or $\dot{Q}$ (West, 1986).

To understand $\dot{V}/\dot{Q}$ imbalance, it is common to view the lung as a three-compartment model (Fig. 50–7): $\dot{V}/\dot{Q} = 0$ (Fig. 50–7A), $\dot{V}/\dot{Q} = 1$ (Fig. 50–7B), and $\dot{V}/\dot{Q} = $ infinity (Fig. 50–7C). The O_2 saturation of blood in each compartment depends on the PO_2 and the O_2 dissociation curve. For illustrative purposes, in a badly diseased lung, 50% of ventilation goes to $\dot{V}/\dot{Q} = 1$ and 50% to $\dot{V}/\dot{Q} = $ infinity, whereas 50% of perfusion goes to $\dot{V}/\dot{Q} = 1$ and 50% to $\dot{V}/\dot{Q} = 0$. Perfusion of $\dot{V}/\dot{Q} = 0$ causes venous admixture, whereas ventilation of $\dot{V}/\dot{Q} = $ infinity causes alveolar V_D. The mixed alveolar gas composition is easily calculated as the mean. For mixed arterial blood, the PO_2 must be read from the O_2 dissociation curve, but because the CO_2

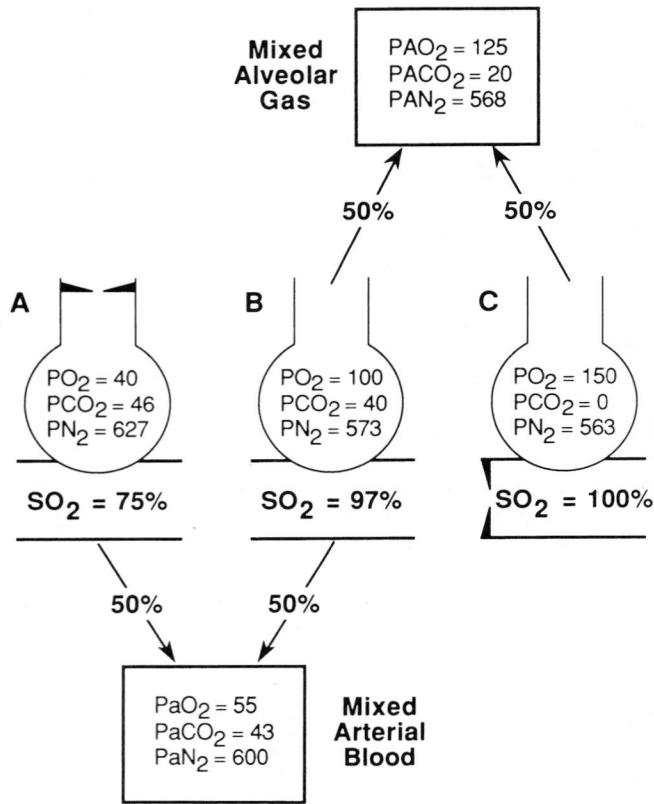

FIGURE 50–7. Three-compartment model of the lung with $\dot{V}/\dot{Q}$ = 0 (A), $\dot{V}/\dot{Q}$ = 1 (B), and $\dot{V}/\dot{Q}$ = infinity (C). The inspired gas is room air, and B is the ideal compartment. The sum of alveolar gas partial pressures is always 713 mm Hg. SO_2 is oxygen saturation in capillary blood. PaO_2 is read from the oxygen dissociation curve for a saturation of 86%. By calculated differences, $Aa.DO_2$ is 70 mm Hg, $aA.DCO_2$ is 23 mm Hg, and $aA.DN_2$ is 32 mm Hg.

dissociation curve is fairly linear, the values for CO_2 are easily calculated as the mean. The abnormalities in distribution of $\dot{V}$ and $\dot{Q}$ have created an $Aa.DO_2 = 70$, $aA.DCO_2 = 23$, and $aA.DN_2 = 32$ mm Hg (see Fig. 50–7). The $Aa.DO_2$ is greater than the sum of the other two because the O_2 dissociation curve is not linear. Of course, the situation in most lungs is not as extreme as the one illustrated. From this illustration, however, it can be seen that:

1. Open low $\dot{V}/\dot{Q}$ units produce increased $Aa.DO_2$, significant hypoxemia, and increased $aA.DN_2$, but because they are poorly ventilated and have a PCO_2 close to the ideal value, they do not change the $aA.DCO_2$ significantly.
2. High $\dot{V}/\dot{Q}$ units produce increased $Aa.DO_2$ without hypoxemia and increased $aA.DCO_2$, but because they are poorly perfused and have a PN_2 close to the ideal value, they do not change the $aA.DN_2$ significantly.

For the calculation of $Aa.DO_2$ and $aA.DN_2$, it is customary to calculate the ideal alveolar gas composition for O_2 and N_2 from the alveolar gas equations and use these values with those measured for arterial PO_2 and PN_2. This emphasizes that part of the $Aa.DO_2$ and $aA.DN_2$ responsible

for hypoxemia. For $aA.DCO_2$, both an arterial and mixed alveolar sample are required.

In the newborn, a fourth compartment in the model is important. A significant part of the venous return may be shunted from right to left at the foramen ovale, ductus arteriosus, pulmonary arteriovenous vessels, or lung mesenchyme without airway development, thus adding mixed venous to mixed arterial blood. This substantially increases the $Aa.DO_2$ but has little effect on $aA.DCO_2$ and no effect on $aA.DN_2$. The last-mentioned is because there is no significant exchange of N_2 in the body, so venous and arterial PN_2 are the same. The effect on $aA.DCO_2$ is small because venous PCO_2 is only slightly higher than arterial. From this analysis, it can be seen that hypoxemia is produced by a true right-to-left shunt and open low $\dot{V}/\dot{Q}$ units. Diffusional problems are not thought to be important in the newborn. Hypoxemia may be modeled as a venous admixture, the part of mixed venous blood, expressed as a fraction of cardiac output, that when added to blood equilibrated with an ideal lung would produce the measured arterial oxygen saturation. It is calculated as follows:

$$\dot{Q}va / \dot{Q}t = C\dot{c}O_2 - CaO_2 / C\dot{c}O_2 - C\bar{v}O_2 \quad (13)$$

where $\dot{Q}va/\dot{Q}t$ = venous admixture, CO_2 = oxygen content, $\dot{c}$ = pulmonary capillary, a = arterial, and $\bar{v}$ = mixed venous blood. For practical application, $C\bar{v}O_2$ is calculated from a constant $a\bar{v}.O_2$ difference, which does introduce an error.

If an infant breathes 100% O_2 for 15 minutes, most N_2 is washed out of the lung, and the PO_2 in open low $\dot{V}/\dot{Q}$ units becomes so high that associated blood is 100% saturated with O_2. The remaining venous admixture is attributed to true right-to-left shunt ($\dot{Q}s/\dot{Q}t$). If an infant has the total venous admixture ($\dot{Q}va/\dot{Q}t$) measured while breathing room air, then true shunt ($\dot{Q}s/\dot{Q}t$) measured while breathing 100% O_2, the venous admixture owing to open low $\dot{V}/\dot{Q}$ units ($\dot{Q}o/\dot{Q}t$) can be calculated as the difference. The venous admixture owing to open low $\dot{V}/\dot{Q}$ units can also be calculated from the $aA.DN_2$ (Markello et al, 1972):

$$\dot{Q}o/\dot{Q}t = PaN_2 - PAN_2 / PoN_2 - PAN_2 \quad (14)$$

where PoN_2 is the PN_2 in the $\dot{V}/\dot{Q}$-0 units (see Fig. 50–7), and PaN_2 is measured and PAN_2 is the ideal value calculated from the alveolar gas equation. In newborns with a significant value for true shunt, this value really represents venous admixture as a fraction of effective pulmonary blood flow ($\dot{Q}o/\dot{Q}c$). A better estimate for $\dot{Q}o/\dot{Q}t$ can be obtained from simple arithmetic (Corbet et al, 1974):

$$\dot{Q}o / \dot{Q}t = \dot{Q}o / \dot{Q}c \cdot (1 - \dot{Q}va / \dot{Q}t) / (1 - \dot{Q}o / \dot{Q}c) \quad (15)$$

The true right-to-left shunt can then be estimated without 100% O_2 breathing using the equation:

$$\dot{Q}s / \dot{Q}t = \dot{Q}va / \dot{Q}t - \dot{Q}o / \dot{Q}t \quad (16)$$

The normal values for the various indices of ventilation-perfusion imbalance in normal newborn infants are shown in Table 50–2.

TABLE 50-2

Indices of Ventilation-Perfusion Imbalance in the Normal Newborn Breathing Room Air

	Aa.Do$_2$ mm Hg	Qva/Qt	aA.Dn$_2$ mm Hg	Qo/Qt	Qs/Qt	aA.Dco$_2$ mm Hg
Newborn	25	0.25	10	0.10	0.15	1
Adult	10	0.07	7	0.05	0.02	1

Adapted from Nelson NM: Respiration and circulation after birth. *In* Smith CA, Nelson NM (Eds): The Physiology of the Newborn Infant. Springfield, IL, Charles C Thomas, 1976.

HEART-LUNG INTERACTION
Effects of the Lung on the Heart

There exists considerable potential for the lung to affect the heart. Because they share the thoracic cavity, changes in intrathoracic pressure accompanying lung inflation are transmitted directly to the heart. In addition, all of the blood leaving the right ventricle must traverse the pulmonary vascular bed, so changes in pulmonary vascular resistance may greatly affect right ventricular function.

Effects of Changes in Intrathoracic Pressure on the Heart

Negative Intrathoracic Pressure

During spontaneous inspiratory efforts, the chest wall and diaphragm move outward, intrathoracic volume increases, and intrathoracic pressure decreases (Fig. 50-8A). The heart also resides within the thoracic cavity and is subject to the same negative intrathoracic pressure during inspiration. With a decrease in intrathoracic pressure, the heart in-

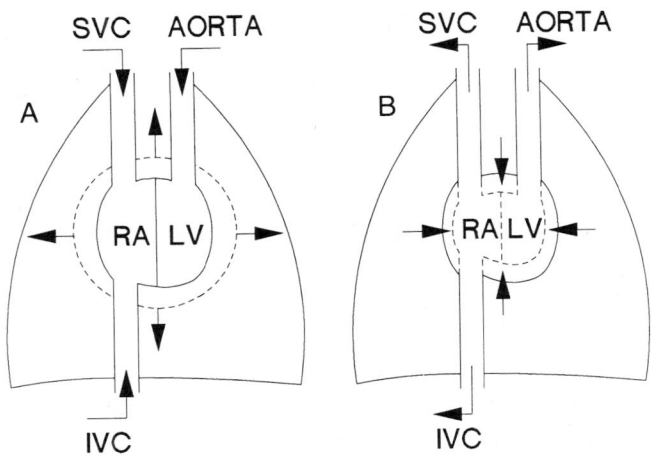

FIGURE 50-8. *A,* Negative intrathoracic pressure increases the volume of the heart and decreases the pressure within the chambers. This facilitates return of blood from the superior vena cava (SVC) and inferior vena cava (IVC) to the right atrium (RA) and impedes ejection of blood from the left ventricle (LV) into the extrathoracic aorta. *B,* Positive intrathoracic pressure decreases the volume of the heart and increases pressure within its chambers. This impedes blood return to the right atrium and augments ejection of blood from the left ventricle.

creases in volume, and the pressure within its chambers decreases relative to atmospheric pressure. Analogous to the lung, when the pressure within the heart decreases, blood is literally sucked back into the heart from systemic veins and arteries. On the right side of the heart, the phenomenon serves to increase the flow of blood from systemic veins into the right atrium, increasing right ventricular preload and ventricular output. On the left side of the heart, ventricular ejection is impaired. During systole, the left ventricle must overcome not only the load imposed by the systemic vascular resistance, but also it must overcome the additional load imposed by the negative intrathoracic pressure (McGregor, 1979).

In infants with normal lungs, spontaneous respiratory efforts result in relatively small swings in pleural pressure (−2 to −3 torr) that have little effect on the pressure within the heart. With airway obstruction or parenchymal lung disease, however, swings in pleural pressure can be much greater (−5 to −20 torr), and systemic arterial pressure may fluctuate as much as 5 to 20 torr depending on where in the respiratory cycle ventricular systole occurs. In older children with asthma or some other form of airway obstruction, these fluctuations in blood pressure constitute pulsus paradoxus and are indicative of severe airway obstruction.

Positive Intrathoracic Pressure

During positive-pressure ventilation, the lung inflates and pushes the chest wall and diaphragm outward (Fig. 50-8B). This outward push generates a pressure in the thoracic space that is greater than atmospheric pressure. The magnitude of the increase (relative transmission of airway pressure to the pleural space) is determined by the volume of lung inflation (which, in turn, is determined by the airway pressure and lung compliance) and by the compliance of the chest wall and diaphragm. If the lung is compliant and the chest wall rigid, little airway pressure is lost inflating the lung, but considerable pressure is generated in the thoracic cavity as the lung attempts to push the rigid chest wall outward. In this instance, intrathoracic pressure (intrapleural pressure) is much greater than atmospheric and in fact nearly equal to airway pressure. If the lung is poorly compliant and the chest wall highly compliant, most of the airway pressure is dissipated trying to inflate the lungs, and little is transmitted to the thoracic cavity.

The effects of positive intrathoracic pressure on the heart are opposite to those of negative intrathoracic pressure. The heart is compressed by the lungs and chest wall, and blood is squeezed out of the heart and the thoracic cavity. Return of blood from systemic veins is impaired, and right ventricular preload and output decrease. If the increase in intrathoracic pressure coincides with ventricular systole, the effect is to augment left ventricular ejection and reduce the load on the left ventricle.

In the infant undergoing positive-pressure ventilation, the degree to which lung inflation compromises venous return is related to the relative compliances of the lung and chest wall. If the infant's lung is poorly compliant and the chest wall is compliant, as in hyaline membrane disease, there is little effect of lung inflation on venous return. If the infant's lung is normally compliant but tight abdominal distention prevents descent of the diaphragm, intrathoracic pressure increases dramatically during positive-pressure ventilation, and venous return and cardiac output can be impaired. This mechanism may help explain the circulatory instability of infants after repair of gastroschisis or omphalocele. A similar situation may arise in the preterm infant with pulmonary interstitial emphysema and massive lung overinflation. In these infants, the heart is tightly compressed between the hyperinflated lungs, the other structures of the mediastinum, and the diaphragm. Venous return may be severely limited and venous pressures so increased that massive peripheral edema often accompanies the reduction in cardiac output.

Although the effects of increased pleural pressure on the right atrium are detrimental, the effects on the left ventricle may be extremely beneficial (Niemann et al, 1980). During cardiopulmonary resuscitation, the chest wall is compressed against the lung, and intrathoracic pressure increases. Because the left ventricle is in the thorax, left ventricular pressure increases as well. A gradient is created favoring flow of blood out of the ventricle and thorax and into the extrathoracic systemic circulation. Between chest compressions, elastic recoil causes the chest wall to pull away from the lung and heart, decreasing pleural pressure and favoring return of venous blood and priming the heart for the next chest compression. A similar phenomenon may result in augmentation of systemic pressure when ventilator breaths coincide with ventricular systole.

Effect of Lung Inflation on Pulmonary Vascular Resistance

The pulmonary interstitium comprises three different interconnected connective tissue compartments, each containing a different element of the pulmonary circulation (Fishman, 1986). The first—the perivascular cuffs—consists of a sheath of fibers that contain the preacinar pulmonary arteries, lymphatics, and bronchi. The second consists of the intersegmental and interlobular septa and contains pulmonary veins and additional lymphatics. The third connects these two within the alveolar septa and contains the majority of the pulmonary capillaries. The first and second compartments represent the extra-alveolar interstitium, whereas the third represents the alveolar interstitium. The perivascular cuffs are surrounded by alveoli and expand during lung inflation (Fig. 50–9A). As a result, pressure within each cuff decreases, distending extra-alveolar blood vessels and decreasing their resistance to blood flow. The alveolar interstitium lies between adjacent alveoli and contains the majority of gas-exchanging vessels in the lung. These vessels are exposed to alveolar pressure on both sides and during lung inflation (Fig. 50–9B) are compressed so that their resistance to blood flow increases.

Therefore, during lung inflation (Fig. 50–9C), the resistance in extra-alveolar vessels (dotted line) decreases, while resistance in alveolar vessels (dashed line) increases. As a result, the overall pulmonary vascular resistance (solid line) decreases initially, with lung inflation reaching its nadir at FRC, and then increases with further inflation.

If transition from intrauterine life to extrauterine life is to be successful, after birth all of the right ventricular

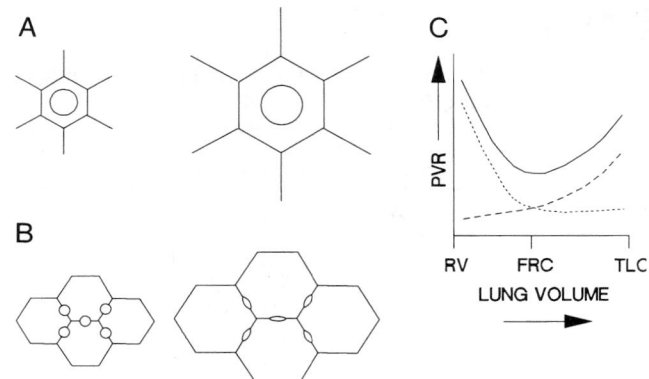

FIGURE 50–9. *A,* Effects of lung inflation on extra-alveolar vessels. *B,* Effects of lung inflation on alveolar vessels. *C,* Effect of lung volume on pulmonary vascular resistance (PVR) (solid line). Inflation is from residual volume (RV) to functional residual capacity (FRC) to total lung capacity (TLC). Dashed line represents alveolar vessels; dotted line represents extra-alveolar vessels.

output must traverse the pulmonary vascular bed. To some extent, this adaptation is facilitated by a reduction in pulmonary vascular resistance that occurs with inflation of the lungs (see Fig. 50–9) to a stable FRC. Inflation of the lung beyond FRC increases pulmonary vascular resistance. If care is not taken during positive-pressure ventilation, it is possible to inflate the lung to the point that alveolar vessels close and blood flow through the lung is impaired. When this occurs, either cardiac output decreases or the blood bypasses the lung via the foramen ovale or ductus arteriosus. Clinically, this is manifest as circulatory insufficiency from impaired right ventricular output or hypoxemia from right-to-left shunting of blood, or both.

Effects of the Heart on the Lung
Pulmonary Edema

Pulmonary edema is the abnormal accumulation of water and solute in the interstitial and alveolar spaces of the lung (Bland and Hansen, 1985; Staub, 1974). In the lung, fluid is filtered from capillaries in the alveolar septa into the alveolar interstitium (Fig. 50–10A) and then siphoned into the lower-pressure extra-alveolar interstitium. The extra-alveolar interstitium contains the pulmonary lymphatics, and under normal conditions, they remove fluid from the lung so that there is no net accumulation in the interstitium. Pulmonary edema results only when the rate of fluid filtration exceeds the rate of lymphatic removal. There are only three mechanisms by which this can occur (Fig. 50–10B): (1) the driving pressure for fluid filtration (filtration pressure) increases, (2) the permeability of the vascular bed (hence, the filtration coefficient K_f) increases, or (3) lymphatic drainage decreases.

Increased Driving Pressure

Filtration pressure can be increased by increased intravascular hydrostatic pressure, decreased interstitial hydrostatic pressure, decreased intravascular oncotic pressure, or increased interstitial oncotic pressure (Fig. 50–10C and D).

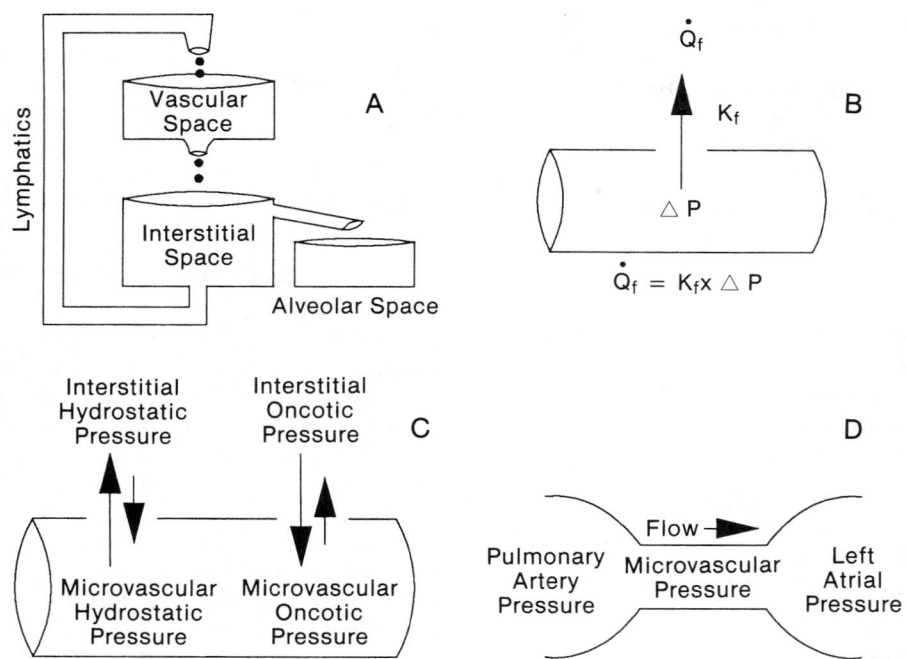

FIGURE 50–10. *A,* In the lung, fluid is continuously filtered out of vessels in the microcirculation into the interstitium and then returned to the intravascular compartment by the lymphatics. Only when the rate of filtration exceeds the rate of lymphatic removal can fluid accumulate in the interstitium. Spillover of fluid into the alveolar space occurs only when the interstitial space fills or when the alveolar membrane is damaged. *B,* Fluid flows out of vessels at a flow rate ($\dot{Q}_f$) that is equal to the driving pressure for fluid flow (ΔP) times the filtration coefficient (K_f): $\dot{Q}_f = K_f \times \Delta P$. K_f can be thought of as the relative permeability of the vascular bed to fluid flux. K_f in the normal lung is a small number so that despite a driving pressure of roughly 5 torr, the net rate of fluid filtration is approximately 1 to 2 mL/kg per hour. *C,* The driving pressure for fluid flow out of the microvascular bed represents a balance of two sets of pressures. Within the blood vessel, hydrostatic pressure tends to push fluid out of the vessel into the interstitium. This pressure is partially opposed by a smaller hydrostatic pressure within the interstitium pushing fluid back into the blood vessel. Within the blood vessel, there also exists a discrete oncotic pressure that results predominantly from intravascular albumin that tends to draw fluid from the interstitium back into the blood vessel. This pressure is opposed by an interstitial oncotic pressure tending to draw fluid from the blood vessel into the interstitium. *D,* The intravascular hydrostatic pressure must be less than pulmonary artery pressure (Ppa) for blood to flow into the microvascular bed and greater than left atrial pressure (Pla) for blood to flow out. Intravascular pressure is roughly equal to 0.4 (Ppa − Pla) + Pla. The interstitial hydrostatic pressure is roughly equal to alveolar pressure. The intravascular oncotic pressure can be calculated from the plasma albumin concentration. The interstitial oncotic pressure is roughly two thirds of the intravascular oncotic pressure. The balance of these pressures favors filtration out of the vessel (in the normal lamb this pressure equals 5 torr).

By far the most common cause of increased filtration pressure is increased intravascular hydrostatic pressure (Table 50–3). In the newborn, intravascular hydrostatic pressure increases with increased left atrial pressure from volume overload or a number of congenital and acquired heart defects. In the preterm and term newborn, evidence suggests that alterations in pulmonary blood flow that are independent of any change in left atrial pressure may also influence fluid filtration in the lung. Preterm infants with patent ductus arteriosus and left-to-right shunts exhibit signs of respiratory insufficiency before they develop any evidence of heart failure, and experiments performed in newborn lambs show that fluid filtration in the lung can be increased by increasing pulmonary blood flow without increasing left atrial pressure (Feltes and Hansen, 1986).

In the newborn with a reduced pulmonary vascular bed, either from lung injury or from hypoplasia, cardiac output appropriate for body size may represent a relative overperfusion to the lung and can result in increased fluid filtration. This phenomenon has been invoked to explain the lung edema that often complicates the course of the infant with bronchopulmonary dysplasia.

The exact cause of pulmonary edema that accompanies severe hypoxia or asphyxia in the newborn is still a controversial issue. Data suggest that it is the result of increased filtration pressure and not the result of any alteration in permeability. Heart failure accounts for some of the increased filtration pressure following severe asphyxia. In addition, there may be some element of pulmonary venous constriction. Finally, there is evidence that hypoxia and

TABLE 50-3

Increased Intravascular Hydrostatic Pressure

Increased Left Atrial Pressure

Intravascular volume overload
   Overzealous fluid administration
   Overtransfusion
   Renal insufficiency
Heart failure
   Left-sided obstructive lesions
   Left-to-right shunts
   Myocardiopathies

Increased Pulmonary Blood Flow

Normal pulmonary vascular bed
   Patent ductus arteriosus
   Increased cardiac output
Reduced pulmonary vascular bed
   Bronchopulmonary dysplasia
   Pulmonary hypoplasia

---

acidosis may redistribute pulmonary blood flow to a smaller portion of the lung and result in relative overperfusion and edema, similar to that seen with anatomic loss of vascular bed (Hansen et al, 1984).

Several investigators have suggested that upper airway obstruction may cause pulmonary edema by decreasing interstitial hydrostatic pressure relative to intravascular hydrostatic pressure. Other data suggest, however, that with airway obstruction vascular pressures decrease with intrapleural pressure in such a way that filtration pressure remains unchanged (Hansen et al, 1985).

Hypoproteinemia in infants results in a decrease in intravascular oncotic pressure. Its effects on filtration pressure, however, are blunted by the simultaneous decrease in protein concentration in the interstitial space of the lung. As a result, edema is unlikely to occur unless hydrostatic pressure also increases (Hazinski et al, 1986).

Increased Permeability

Another possible mechanism for increased fluid filtration in the lung is a change in the permeability of the microvascular membrane to protein—high permeability pulmonary edema. In this form of edema, the sieving properties of the microvascular endothelium are altered so that K_f increases and patients may develop pulmonary edema despite relatively normal vascular pressures (Albertine, 1985). Furthermore, even small changes in vascular pressures can result in a dramatic worsening of pulmonary status. High permeability pulmonary edema usually implies either direct or indirect injury to the capillary endothelium of the lung. Direct injuries result from local effects of an inhaled toxin such as oxygen. Indirect injuries imply that the initial insult occurs elsewhere in the body and that the lung injury occurs secondarily. An example of indirect lung injury is sepsis: Neutrophils activated by bacterial toxins attack endothelial cells in the lung and increase permeability to water and protein (Brigham et al, 1974). Indirect injuries usually involve blood-borne mediators, such as leukocytes, leukotrienes, histamine, or bradykinin. Alveolar overdisten-

tion can also cause high permeability pulmonary edema presumably by direct injury of the pulmonary vascular bed. This type of vascular injury probably accounts for some of the edema that accompanies diseases such as hyaline membrane disease and bronchopulmonary dysplasia, in which maldistribution of ventilation results in areas of alveolar overdistention (Carlton et al, 1990).

Decreased Lymphatic Drainage

In the normal lung, the rate of lung lymph flow is equal to the net rate of fluid filtration, and as long as lymphatic function can keep up with the rate of fluid filtration, water does not accumulate in the lung. Although lymphatics can actively pump fluid against a pressure gradient, studies show that this ability is limited and that lung lymph flow varies inversely with the outflow pressure (pressure in the superior vena cava). Several groups of investigators have demonstrated that, in the presence of an increased rate of transvascular fluid filtration, the rate of fluid accumulation in the lung is substantially greater if systemic venous pressure is increased (Drake et al, 1985). This theory explains why pulmonary edema often complicates the course of infants with bronchopulmonary dysplasia and cor pulmonale and explains the particular problem of edema with pleural effusions complicating the course of superior vena cava syndrome.

Congenital Pulmonary Lymphangiectasis

Congenital pulmonary lymphangiectasis is a rare form of pulmonary lymphatic dysfunction that can be characterized into two groups: (1) cases associated with congenital heart disease and (2) cases not associated with congenital heart disease. The cardiac anomalies may include hypoplastic left heart syndrome, total anomalous pulmonary venous drainage, and pulmonary stenosis, including Noonan syndrome (France and Brown, 1971). The group that does not include associated cardiac anomalies may be of early or late onset and has a wide spectrum of severity. In some individuals, the lesion is asymptomatic, whereas in others it can lead to severe respiratory failure, usually in the first hours after birth but sometimes during the first weeks or months of life. Most infants with this condition die early in the neonatal period. Pulmonary lymphangiectasis has been reported twice as often in males and has been seen in families (Scott-Emaukpor et al, 1981).

Usually the radiologist is the first to suggest the diagnosis after observing dilated lymphatic vessels and sometimes small accumulations of pleural fluid on the chest radiograph. The older infant may have no symptoms or mild to moderate tachypnea with various degrees of hypoxemia. If pleural fluid has accumulated, examination of the fluid is important. If the infant has received milk feedings, pleural fluid is chylous, and if not, there is an elevation in mononuclear cells and moderate protein of up to about 4%. These findings in the absence of fever or other signs of systemic illness are diagnostic of impaired lymphatic drainage.

Lung biopsy is probably not indicated and can be hazardous because once the distended lymphatic channels are severed, they can leak fluid for weeks. Only if the diagnosis is in doubt is open lung biopsy appropriate.

In noncardiac-associated diffuse lymphangiectasis, only supportive treatment is available. The long-term prognosis depends on the severity of the lesion, but this form of pulmonary lymphangiectasis is compatible with asymptomatic life as an adult (Wohl, 1989).

Symptoms

As discussed previously, fluid filtered into the alveolar interstitium ordinarily moves rapidly along pressure gradients into the extra-alveolar interstitium where it is removed by the lymphatics. A delay in this process at birth can result in clinical transient respiratory distress (see Chapter 53). The extra-alveolar interstitium has a large storage capacity. Fluid does not begin to spill over into the alveoli and airways until total lung water is increased more than 50%, unless the alveolar membrane is damaged. Therefore, the first signs and symptoms of pulmonary edema are related to the presence of extra fluid in the interstitial cuffs of tissue that surround airways. As fluid builds up in these cuffs, airways are compressed, and the infants develop signs of obstructive lung disease. The chest may appear hyperinflated, and auscultation reveals rales, rhonchi, and a prolonged expiration. Early in the course, chest radiographs reveal lung overinflation and an accumulation of fluid in the extra-alveolar interstitium—linear densities of fluid that extend from the hilum to the periphery of the lung (the so-called sunburst appearance) and fluid in the fissures. With more severe edema, fluffy densities appear throughout the lung as alveoli fill with fluid (Fig. 50–11). Heart size may be increased in infants with edema from increased intravascular pressure. Initially, infants present with increased $PaCO_2$ secondary to impaired ventilation. Later PaO_2 decreases secondary to ventilation-perfusion mismatching and alveolar flooding. In adults, a ratio of protein concentration in tracheal aspirate to that in plasma greater than 0.5 may help to differentiate permeability pulmonary edema from high-pressure pulmonary edema (Fein et al, 1979).

Treatment

Treatment of pulmonary edema is directed at relieving hypoxemia and lowering vascular pressures. Hypoxemia should be treated with the administration of oxygen and, if necessary, positive-pressure ventilation. Positive end-expiratory pressure frequently improves oxygenation in individuals with pulmonary edema by improving ventilation-perfusion matching within the lung. Available evidence suggests that positive-pressure ventilation *does not* reduce the rate of transvascular fluid filtration in the lung (Woolverton et al, 1978). Optimal treatment of pulmonary edema requires correction of the underlying cause. In infants with patent ductus arteriosus (see Fig. 50–11) or other heart disease amenable to surgery, this is often easily accomplished. In cases of permeability edema or edema from nonsurgical heart defects, correction of the underlying cause may not be possible. In these instances, the only remaining option is to lower vascular pressures (even in permeability edema, lowering vascular pressures lowers the rate of fluid filtration). This can be accomplished by lowering circulating blood volume by use of diuretics and fluid restriction, by improving myocardial function with the use of digitalis or other inotropic agents, or in severe cases by using a drug such as nitroprusside to reduce afterload and lower vascular pressures directly. Whether theophylline reduces airway obstruction in infants with pulmonary edema is not known.

Pulmonary Hemorrhage

Landing (1957) described pulmonary hemorrhage in 68% of lungs of 125 consecutive infants who died in the 1st week of life; massive pulmonary hemorrhage was found in 17.8% of neonatal autopsies at the Johns Hopkins Hospital (Rowe and Avery, 1966). Fedrick and Butler (1971) judged massive pulmonary hemorrhage to be the principal cause of death in about 9% of neonatal autopsies.

Etiology and Pathogenesis

Pulmonary hemorrhage usually occurs between the 2nd and 4th days of life in infants who are being treated with

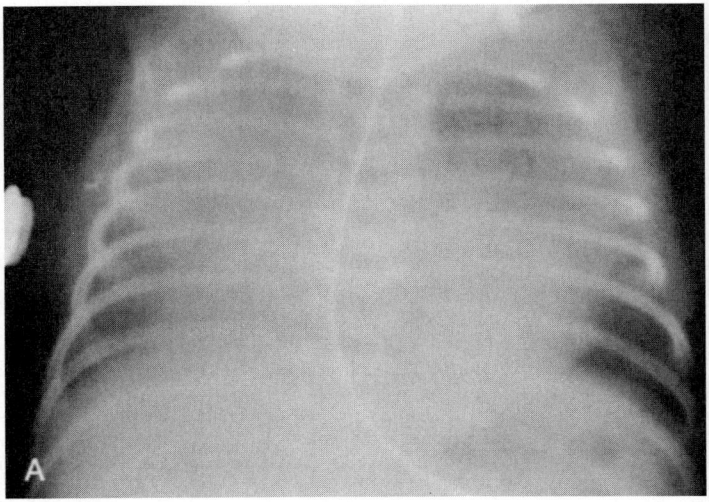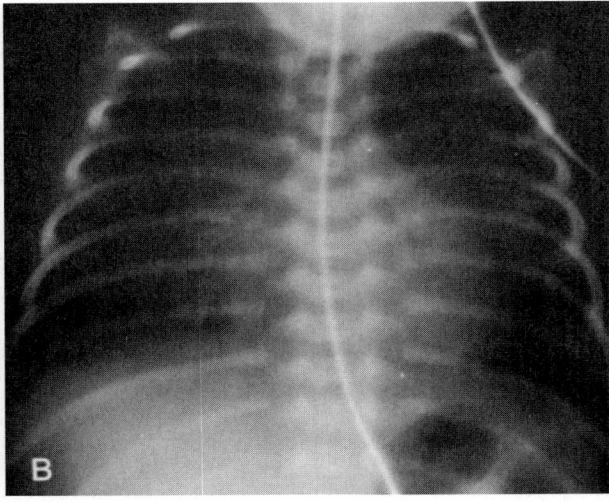

FIGURE 50–11. Preterm infant with a large patent ductus arteriosus and pulmonary edema *(A)*. The same infant 24 hours after the ductus arteriosus was closed by administration of indomethacin *(B)*.

mechanical ventilation. It has been associated with a wide variety of predisposing factors, including prematurity, asphyxia, overwhelming sepsis, intrauterine growth retardation, massive aspiration, severe hypothermia, severe Rh-hemolytic disease, congenital heart disease, and coagulopathies. It is often associated with central nervous system injury, such as asphyxia or intracranial hemorrhage. Cole and associates (1973) studied a group of infants with pulmonary hemorrhage to determine the clinical circumstances under which the illness occurred as well as the hematocrit and protein composition of fluid obtained from lung effluent and arterial or venous blood. Their results indicated that the lung effluent was, in most cases, hemorrhagic edema fluid and not whole blood (i.e., as indicated by hematocrit values significantly lower than those of whole blood). In addition, they did not find that coagulation disorders initiated the condition but probably served to exacerbate it in some cases. They postulated that the important precipitating factor was acute left ventricular failure caused by asphyxia or other events that might increase the filtration pressure and so injure the capillary endothelium of the lung. Thus, pulmonary hemorrhage may be considered as the extreme form of high permeability pulmonary edema.

Pulmonary edema following central nervous system injury probably results from increased hydrostatic pressure and some increase in vascular permeability (Malik, 1985). With the massive sympathetic discharge that accompanies central nervous system injury, left atrial pressure increases, and pulmonary arteries and veins constrict. As a result, microvascular pressure increases dramatically and causes dramatic damage to the microvascular endothelium, increasing its permeability to proteins and red blood cells. In infants with overwhelming sepsis and endotoxin production, increased microvascular permeability is apparent in the pulmonary circulation as well, undoubtedly contributing to the massive pulmonary hemorrhage sometimes seen in this group of infants. Pulmonary hemorrhage also has been described occasionally in the presence of a large patent ductus arteriosus, with a left-to-right shunt that results in high flow and high pressure injurious to the vascular bed.

Pulmonary hemorrhage is also associated with surfactant replacement therapy. Presumably the hemorrhage results from the rapid increase in pulmonary blood flow that accompanies improved lung function after surfactant therapy. The contribution of the patent ductus arteriosus to this increased blood flow remains to be determined. A meta-analysis suggests that surfactant replacement may be associated with an increased risk of pulmonary hemorrhage. This risk, however, is still extremely small compared to the known benefits of surfactant replacement (Pappin et al, 1994; Raju and Langenberg, 1993).

Diagnosis

Infants with any of the conditions mentioned previously should be observed carefully for possible pulmonary hemorrhage. Particular note should be made of any occurrence of blood-stained fluid from endotracheal tube aspirates, especially if repeated suctioning shows an increase in the amount of hemorrhagic fluid. The infant's chest radiograph may show the fluffy appearance of pulmonary edema in addition to the underlying pathology, and the infant may have increased respiratory distress. Frank pulmonary hemorrhage, when it occurs, is an acute emergency, and the fluid has the appearance of fresh blood being pumped directly from the vascular system, although hematocrit values of the fluid are at least 15 to 20 points lower than the hematocrit of circulating blood, in keeping with hemorrhagic pulmonary edema.

Treatment

Effective treatment of pulmonary hemorrhage requires (1) clearing the airway of blood to allow ventilation; (2) use of adequate mean airway pressure, particularly end-expiratory pressure; (3) resisting the temptation to administer large volumes of blood because in most cases the infant has not had a large loss of volume, and thus, administration of excessive volume exacerbates the increase in left atrial pressure and hemorrhagic pulmonary edema; rather red cell replacement should be done as a slow administration of packed cells after the infant's pulmonary status has been stabilized; and (4) evaluation of the possibility of coagulopathy and administration of vitamin K and platelets, if appropriate.

REFERENCES

Albertine KH: Ultrastructural abnormalities in increased-permeability pulmonary edema. Clin Chest Med 6:345, 1985.

Bhutani VK, Sivieri EM, Abbasi S, Shaffer TH: Evaluation of neonatal pulmonary mechanics and energetics: A two factor least mean square analysis. Pediatr Pulmonol 4:150, 1988.

Bland RD, Hansen TN: Neonatal lung edema. *In* Said SI (Ed): The Pulmonary Circulation and Acute Lung Injury. Mount Kisco, NY, Futura Publishing, 1985, p 225.

Brigham KL, Woolverton W, Blake L, et al: Increased sheep lung vascular permeability caused by *Pseudomonas* bacteremia. J Clin Invest 54:792, 1974.

Bryan AC, England SJ: Maintenance of an elevated FRC in the newborn: Paradox of REM sleep. Am Rev Respir Dis 129:209, 1984.

Carlton DP, Cummings JJ, Scheerer RG, et al: Lung overexpansion increases pulmonary microvascular protein permeability in young lambs. J Appl Physiol 69:577, 1990.

Cole VA, Normand ICS, Reynolds EOR, et al: Pathogenesis of hemorrhagic pulmonary edema and massive pulmonary hemorrhage in the newborn. Pediatrics 51:175, 1973.

Cook CD, Cherry RB, O'Brien D, et al: Studies of respiratory physiology in the newborn infant: I. Observations on normal premature and full-term infants. J Clin Invest 34:975, 1955.

Cook CD, Sutherland JM, Segal S, et al: Studies of respiratory physiology in the newborn infant: III. Measurements of mechanics of respiration. J Clin Invest 36:440, 1957.

Corbet AJS, Ross JA, Beaudry PH, et al: Ventilation-perfusion relationships as assessed by aADN$_2$ in hyaline membrane disease. J Appl Physiol 36:74, 1974.

Drake R, Giesler M, Laine G, et al: Effect of outflow pressure on lung lymph flow in unanesthetized sheep. J Appl Physiol 58:70, 1985.

Farhi LE: Ventilation-perfusion relationship and its role in alveolar gas exchange. *In* Caro CG (Ed): Advances in Respiratory Physiology. Baltimore, Williams & Wilkins, 1966.

Fedrick J, Butler NR: Certain causes of neonatal death: IV. Massive pulmonary hemorrhage. Biol Neonate 18:243, 1971.

Fein A, Grossman RF, Jones JG, et al: The value of edema fluid protein measurement in patients with pulmonary edema. Am J Med 67:32, 1979.

Feltes TF, Hansen TN: Effects of a large aorticopulmonary shunt on lung fluid balance in newborn lambs. Pediatr Res 20:368A, 1986.

Fishman AP: Pulmonary circulation. *In* Fishman AP, Fisher AB, Geiger

SR (Eds): Handbook of Physiology. Bethesda, MD, American Physiological Society, 1986, p 131.

France NE, Brown RJK: Congenital pulmonary lymphangiectasis: Report of 11 examples with special reference to cardiovascular findings. Arch Dis Child 46:528, 1971.

Gardner TW, Domm AC, Brock CE, et al: Congenital pulmonary lymphangiectasis. Clin Pediatr 22:75, 1983.

Gerhardt T, Bancalari E: Chestwall compliance in full-term and premature infants. Acta Paediatr Scand 69:359, 1980.

Hansen TN, Gest AL, Landers S: Inspiratory airway obstruction does not affect lung fluid balance in lambs. J Appl Physiol 58:1314, 1985.

Hansen TN, Hazinski TA, Bland R: Effects of asphyxia on lung fluid balance in baby lambs. J Clin Invest 741:370, 1984.

Hazinski TA, Bland RD, Hansen TN, et al: Effect of hypoproteinemia on lung fluid balance in awake newborn lambs. J Appl Physiol 61:1139, 1986.

Krieger I: Studies on mechanics of respiration in infancy. Am J Dis Child 105:439, 1963.

Landing BH: Pulmonary lesions in newborn infants: A statistical study. Pediatrics 19:217, 1957.

Lesouef PN, England SJ, Bryan AC: Passive respiratory mechanics in newborns and children. Am Rev Respir Dis 129:552, 1984.

Malik AB: Mechanisms of neurogenic pulmonary edema. Circ Res 57:1, 1985.

Markello R, Winter P, Olszowka A: Assessment of ventilation-perfusion inequalities by arterial-alveolar nitrogen differences in intensive care patients. Anesthesiology 37:4, 1972.

McCann EM, Goldman SL, Brady JP: Pulmonary function in the sick newborn infant. Pediatr Res 21:313, 1987.

McGregor M: Pulsus paradoxus. N Engl J Med 301:480, 1979.

McIlroy MB, Tierney DF, Nadel JA: A new method for measurement of compliance and resistance of lungs and thorax. J Appl Physiol 18:424, 1963.

Nelson NM: Neonatal pulmonary function. Pediatr Clin North Am 13:769, 1966.

Nelson NM: Respiration and circulation after birth. *In* Smith CA, Nelson NM (Eds): The Physiology of the Newborn Infant. Springfield, IL, Charles C Thomas, 1976.

Nelson NM, Prod'hom LS, Cherry RB, et al: Pulmonary function in the newborn infant: V. Trapped gas in the normal infant's lung. J Clin Invest 42:1850, 1963.

Niemann JT, Rosborough J, Hausknect M, et al: Documentation of systemic perfusion in man and in an experimental model: A "window" to the mechanism of blood flow in external CPR. Crit Care Med 8:141, 1980.

Pappin A, Shenker N, Hack M, et al: Extensive intraalveolar pulmonary hemorrhage in infants dying after surfactant therapy. J Pediatr 124:621, 1994.

Pedley TJ, Sudlow MF, Schroter RC: Gas flow and mixing in the airways. *In* West JB (Ed): Bioengineering Aspects of the Lung. New York, Marcel Dekker, 1977, p 163.

Perlman J, Thach B: Respiratory origin of fluctuations in arterial blood pressure in premature infants with respiratory distress syndrome. Pediatrics 81:399, 1988.

Polgar G, Kong GP: The nasal resistance of newborn infants. J Pediatr 67:557, 1965.

Polgar G, Promadhat V: Pulmonary Function Testing in Children: Techniques and Standards. Philadelphia, WB Saunders, 1971, p 273.

Polgar G, String ST: The viscous resistance of the lung tissues in newborn infants. J Pediatr 69:787, 1966.

Raju TNK, Langenberg P: Pulmonary hemorrhage and exogenous surfactant therapy: A metaanalysis. J Pediatr 123:603, 1993

Reynolds RN, Etsten BE: Mechanics of respiration in apneic anesthetized infants. Anesthesiology 27:13, 1966.

Rodarte JR, Rehder K: Dynamics of respiration. *In* Fishman AP, Macklem PT, Mead J, Geiger SR (Eds): Handbook of Physiology, Vol III. Bethesda, MD, American Physiological Society, 1986, p 131.

Rowe S, Avery ME: Massive pulmonary hemorrhage in the newborn: II. Clinical considerations. J Pediatr 69:12, 1966.

Scott-Emaukpor AB, Warren ST, Kapur S, et al: Familial occurrence of congenital pulmonary lymphangiectasis: Genetic implications. Am J Dis Child 135:532, 1981.

Scully RE, Mark EJ, McNeely WF, et al: Case records of the Massachusetts General Hospital. N Engl J Med 321:309, 1989.

Slonim NB, Hamilton LH: Respiratory Physiology, 5th ed. St. Louis, CV Mosby, 1987, p 52.

Staub NC: Pulmonary edema. Physiol Rev 54:678, 1974.

West JB: Ventilation: Blood Flow and Gas Exchange, 4th ed. St. Louis, CV Mosby, 1986.

Wohl MEB: Case records of Massachusetts General Hospital. N Engl J Med 321:309, 1989.

Woolverton NC, Brigham KL, Staub NC: Effect of positive pressure breathing on lung lymph flow and water content in sheep. Circ Res 42:550, 1978.

CHAPTER 51

Principles of Respiratory Monitoring and Therapy

Michael Gomez, Thomas Hansen and Anthony Corbet

OXYGEN THERAPY

In an emergency, high concentrations of oxygen may be administered by face mask, head hood, or endotracheal tube for the relief of cyanosis. If oxygen must be continued beyond the emergency, it should be warmed, humidified, and delivered by a flow proportioner connected to compressed sources of air and oxygen. The concentration of oxygen should be analyzed continuously or at least every hour, using an oxygen analyzer that is calibrated with air and oxygen every 8 hours. The use of oxygen therapy beyond the emergency period should be monitored by means of regular estimates of arterial oxygen pressure, with continuous analysis of transcutaneous Po_2, or with continuous analysis of oxygen saturation by pulse oximetry. When this is not possible, oxygen should be given in a concentration just sufficient to abolish central cyanosis; within a few hours, arrangements should be made for appropriate measurements. It has become common to administer oxygen by nasal cannula, with adjustments to either the flow or the concentration, according to the results of pulse oximetry.

Monitoring Oxygen Therapy
Arterial Catheters

In infants with significant respiratory distress, it is common to monitor oxygen therapy during the first few days of life using an umbilical arterial catheter. In most infants, the arterial oxygen pressure should be maintained between 50 and 70 mm Hg, but in some patients with labile pulmonary hypertension, it is frequently recommended to keep the arterial oxygen pressure as high as 80 to 100 mm Hg. In infants requiring high ventilator pressures, however, levels between 30 and 40 mm Hg may be accepted, provided that the circulatory status is well maintained and metabolic acidosis does not occur.

The reported complications of umbilical arterial catheters include perforation, vasospasm, thrombosis, embolism, and infection. The most obvious sign of vasospasm is ischemia to the ipsilateral leg, and if this persists after a brief period of warming the contralateral leg, the catheter should be removed. During a difficult insertion procedure, it is possible (although this rarely occurs) to perforate the umbilical artery and enter the peritoneum, with consequent hemoperitoneum and hemorrhagic shock. By far, the most frequently feared complication is thrombosis, and small thrombi, as documented by contrast aortography, may develop around the catheter in up to 95% of infants (Neal et al, 1972). Minute emboli may explain transient episodes of ischemia that later result in bluish discoloration of the toes. Clinical evidence of obstruction to a mesenteric, renal, pelvic, or femoral artery or to the aorta itself is comparatively uncommon but has been found in 13% of autopsy cases (Cochran, 1976). Suggestive evidence was found serendipitously by Jackson and coworkers (1987) that aortic thrombosis, detected by ultrasound, is more common after 11 days than after 4 days of catheterization. Infants with thrombosis can usually be managed conservatively with removal of the catheter and supportive care. Renovascular hypertension may occur and require antihypertensive therapy. The condition usually resolves in time (Caplan et al, 1989). Another significant complication of umbilical arterial catheterization is infection, with sepsis occurring in 5% of cases (Moise et al, 1986). The incidence, however, is clearly higher (13%) if the catheter remains in place more than 14 days.

The problem for clinicians is that the umbilical arterial catheter has become the easiest and most reliable way to monitor oxygen therapy. The need for arterial access should always be weighed against the inherent risks of an indwelling line when a decision is made to leave a catheter in place for more than a few days.

As an alternative to the umbilical arterial catheter, short catheters inserted percutaneously or by the cut-down procedure into the radial, posterior tibial, or dorsalis pedis arteries are now widely used. These catheters sometimes last only a few days to a week, but the rates of infection and other complications are quite low.

Intermittent Arterial Puncture

Arterial samples for blood gas analysis may be obtained by percutaneous needle aspiration of brachial, radial, or temporal arteries. The problem with this procedure is that unless the sample is obtained immediately on penetration or with the use of effective local anesthesia, the infant is disturbed, and this changes the actual oxygen tension, usually in a downward direction. Spasm or thrombosis with local ischemia is, however, comparatively rare.

Noninvasive Monitors

The first noninvasive technique to gain widespread clinical acceptance was the skin-surface oxygen (Pso_2) electrode (Huch et al, 1976; Landers and Hansen, 1994) (Fig. 51–1). The Pso_2 electrode does not measure Pao_2 directly; it simply measures the Po_2 on the surface of the skin. If certain conditions are met—an appropriate electrode temperature for a given skin thickness (Fig. 51–2) and normal circulation—the two measurements are highly related, and the Pso_2 provides a reasonable estimate of the Pao_2 for values between 15 and 150 torr.

Problems arise when the Pso_2 differs from the Pao_2 (Table 51–1). Skin thickness, skin blood flow, oxygen consumption, and electrode temperature all affect the correlation (see Fig. 51–2). The Pso_2 electrode itself may also interfere with the correlation between Pso_2 and Pao_2. The

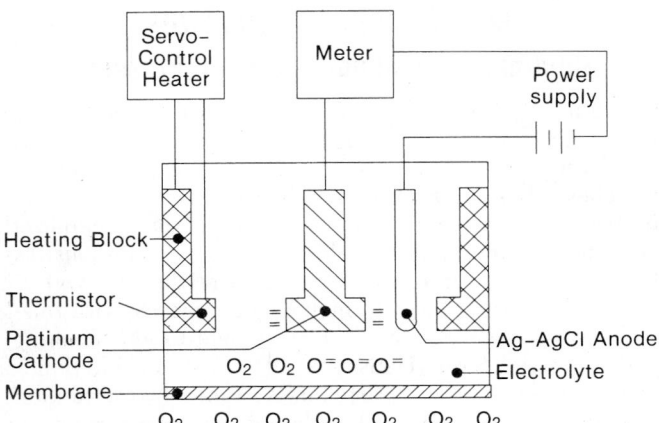

FIGURE 51–1. The PsO$_2$ electrode consists of a servo-controlled heater, a platinum cathode, and a silver–silver chloride anode that is immersed in an electrolyte solution and covered with semipermeable membrane. An external voltage maintains the cathode negative with respect to the anode. Oxygen diffuses across the membrane to the negatively charged cathode, and because it is extremely electrophilic, it readily accepts electrons from the cathode. The reduced oxygen species react with KCl in the electrolyte to form KOH, and liberated Cl $-$ ions are deposited on the anode. As electrons are removed from the cathode, electrons flow from the anode and generate an electrical current that can be measured in the external circuit. This current is proportional to the rate of diffusion of oxygen molecules across the membrane into the electrode. The rate of diffusion, in turn, is proportional to the PsO$_2$ and the permeability of the membrane to oxygen. Oxygen electrodes must be *zeroed* to compensate for the current produced by the external voltage, and a gain must be set to adjust the output for a given membrane permeability.

electrode consumes oxygen at a rate limited by the membrane permeability. If membrane permeability increases, oxygen consumption by the electrode can lower the PsO$_2$. Because an infinite supply of oxygen exists at the time of calibration, the electrode calibrates normally.

The skin surface carbon dioxide (PsCO$_2$) electrode is a glass pH electrode modified so that it can be heated and mounted on the skin (Brunstler et al, 1982; Hansen and Tooley, 1979). CO$_2$ diffuses into the electrode and produces a change in pH. The PsCO$_2$ electrode measures the concentration of CO$_2$ on the surface of the skin and is little affected by skin thickness or membrane permeability. It is affected by blood flow to the skin and must be heated to 42° to 44°C to produce vasodilation. Heating increases PsCO$_2$ relative to PaCO$_2$, and correction factors must be incorporated into the calibration procedure so that the digital or graphic readout of PsCO$_2$ equals PaCO$_2$ (see Fig. 51–2).

Continuous noninvasive estimates of arterial oxygen saturation (SaO$_2$) by pulse oximetry represent an innovative noninvasive monitoring technique (Fig. 51–3) (Pologe, 1987; Wukitsch, 1987). In the red region of the spectrum, reduced hemoglobin absorbs more light than oxyhemoglobin. In the infrared region, oxyhemoglobin absorbs more light than reduced hemoglobin. Total light absorption (at any wavelength) is the sum of the independent absorptions. For whole blood, the ratio of absorption in the red region to that in the infrared region decreases as SaO$_2$ increases.

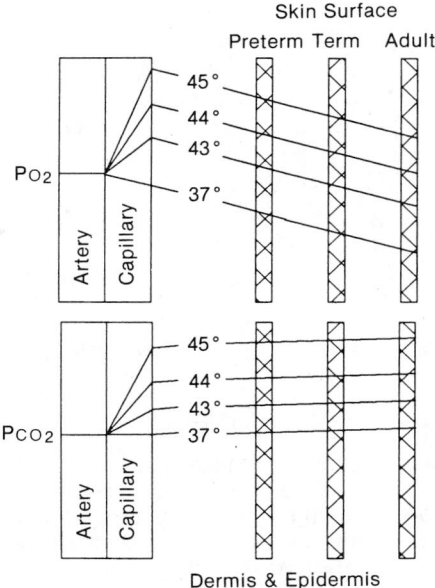

FIGURE 51–2. In unheated skin, as oxygen diffuses from the capillary bed across the dermis and epidermis, PO$_2$ decreases relative to PaO$_2$ because of skin consumption of oxygen (top). As skin thickness increases (preterm infant versus term infant versus adult), this discrepancy increases. To counteract this effect, PsO$_2$ electrodes are heated. Heating increases capillary and tissue PO$_2$ by producing vasodilation, thereby increasing oxygen delivery to the skin, and by shifting the oxygen hemoglobin dissociation curve to the right. The subsequent fall in PO$_2$ as oxygen diffuses to the skin surface counterbalances the effect of heating and lowers PO$_2$ at the skin surface to a value approaching PaO$_2$. Optimal correlation between PaO$_2$ and PsO$_2$ requires that electrode temperature be appropriate for skin thickness. Because of local carbon dioxide production, the PsCO$_2$ of even unheated skin is greater than PaCO$_2$ (bottom). Heating the electrode increases PsCO$_2$ further. The effect of electrode temperature on PsCO$_2$ is constant and predictable so that correction factors can be built into the calibration procedure.

The pulse oximeter is not affected by skin thickness, but it is affected by the circulatory status of the patient. The AC signal detected by the pulse oximeter is only 1% of the DC level, so if changes in tissue perfusion reduce arterial pulsations further, the pulse oximeter cannot function. Al-

TABLE 51–1

Factors Affecting Skin Surface O$_2$ and CO$_2$ Tensions

Increase PsO$_2$	*Increase PsCO$_2$*
Increased PaO$_2$	Increased PaCO$_2$
Increased temperature	Increased temperature
	Increased skin CO$_2$ production
Decrease PsO$_2$	Decreased perfusion
Decreased PaO$_2$	
Decreased skin perfusion	*Decrease PsCO$_2$*
Increased skin thickness	Decreased PaCO$_2$
(age-related)	Decreased temperature
Edema	
Damaged membrane	

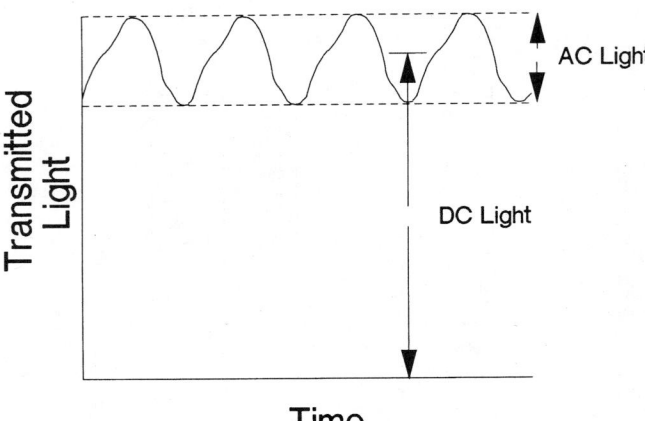

FIGURE 51–3. The pulse oximeter uses light-emitting diodes (LEDs) to send pulses of light of two different wavelengths through tissue containing a peripheral artery. A photodiode located opposite from the LEDs measures the intensity of the transmitted light. At each wavelength, the light transmitted to the diode consists of two components: (1) an AC component, in which the intensity of transmitted light changes with the volume of blood (light absorber) in the artery, and (2) a DC or constant component that results from light being transmitted through the tissues without being absorbed or scattered. The pulse oximeter measures the intensity of transmitted light as it illuminates one LED, then the other, and then switches both off. With both LEDs off, the oximeter can measure and correct for the effects of external light incident on the photodiode. These cycles occur 480 times/second. The pulse oximeter focuses on the pulse added component of the transmitted light by dividing the AC component by the DC component at each wavelength and creating the ratio: R = [ACRED/DCRED]/[ACIR/DCIR]. In this way, it ignores absorbances of venous blood, tissue, and pigmentation.

though the pulse oximeter assumes that there are only two types of hemoglobin present in arterial blood, a consistent effect of fetal hemoglobin on the relationship has not been demonstrated (Jennis and Peabody, 1987; Ramanathan et al, 1987).

Each of these techniques allows continuous noninvasive monitoring of arterial blood gas tensions. The pulse oximeter's advantages are (1) it does not require heat, (2) it has a rapid response time, and (3) it is not affected by skin thickness. This last property makes the pulse oximeter useful in assessing oxygenation in older infants with chronic lung disease. The PsO_2 electrode must be heated and may result in burns to the skin—especially in preterm infants. Therefore, it must be moved to a new site at least every 4 hours. In addition, it is more affected by changes in skin thickness and skin blood flow. The advantages of the PsO_2 electrode are that it estimates PaO_2, rather than SaO_2, and is not subject to wide swings with minor changes in the infant. Although PaO_2 can be roughly calculated from SaO_2, particularly at higher ranges of saturation, the range of PaO_2 values for any given confidence interval of saturations can be broad. As a result, each center should generate acceptable ranges for SaO_2 for given clinical conditions. For example, if the goal is to keep PaO_2 between 50 and 80 torr in a small preterm infant, ranges for SaO_2 must be developed that maintain the PaO_2 within this range (Adams et al, 1994).

MECHANICAL VENTILATION
Continuous Distending Airway Pressure

Continuous distending airway pressure may be applied with positive pressure through nasal prongs or an endotracheal tube or by continuous negative pressure applied to the chest. By stabilizing the poorly supported small airways of the premature infant and preventing the generalized atelectasis of the surfactant-deficient lung, continuous distending pressure improves ventilation in the low $\dot{V}/\dot{Q}$ air spaces, converting them to high $\dot{V}/\dot{Q}$ air spaces, with relief of local vasoconstriction, decreased right-to-left shunting, and improved SaO_2 (Hansen et al, 1979). In addition, a new, open low $\dot{V}/\dot{Q}$ compartment is formed by recruitment of collapsed air spaces. The physiologic consequences of continuous positive airway pressure (CPAP) in hyaline membrane disease (HMD) may include decreased tidal volume (V_T); decreased minute ventilation; increased lung volume; reduced lung compliance; increased work of breathing; increased arterial oxygen pressure; decreased $Aa.DO_2$, $aA.DN_2$, and $aA.DO_2$; and reduced true right-to-left shunt (Corbet et al, 1975).

Intermittent Positive-Pressure Ventilation

Advances in techniques for intermittent positive-pressure ventilation have dramatically altered the outcomes of infants with a variety of lung diseases. To use these techniques effectively, one must have a thorough understanding of how the various components of intermittent positive-pressure ventilation affect the lung of the newborn.

Positive-Pressure Inflation of the Lung

During a positive-pressure breath, gas flows into the lung because airway pressure is greater than alveolar pressure. The volume of gas entering the lung over time is a function of the peak inflation pressure (PIP), duration of inspiration (Ti), and respiratory system compliance (Crs) and resistance (Rrs) (Figs. 51–4 and 51–5). For purposes of this discussion, exhalation is considered to be passive (see Chapter 50).

Most ventilators that are currently in use in neonatal intensive care units are time cycled and pressure limited (Fig. 51–6). PIP, positive end-expiratory pressure (PEEP), Ti, and expiratory time (Te) are adjusted independently (Table 51–2). The rate is altered by changing Ti or Te or both. Mean airway pressure (MAP) is the average pressure at the proximal airway over time. If the inspiratory pressure waveform resembles a square wave (see Fig. 51–6), then:

$$MAP = (PIP - PEEP) \times (Ti/[Ti + Te]) + PEEP$$

Effects of Positive-Pressure Ventilation on Gas Exchange

In infants with parenchymal lung disease, hypoxemia is related to the presence of open but severely underventilated lung units (see Chapter 50). In these units, alveolar ventilation is not sufficient to maintain the alveolar oxygen tension (PAO_2) much above mixed venous PO_2. These lung

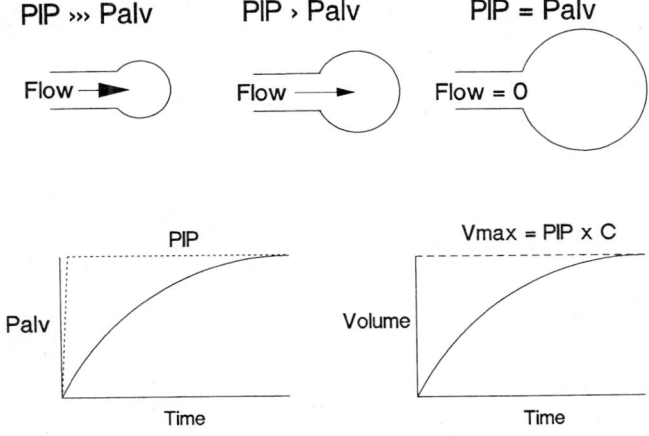

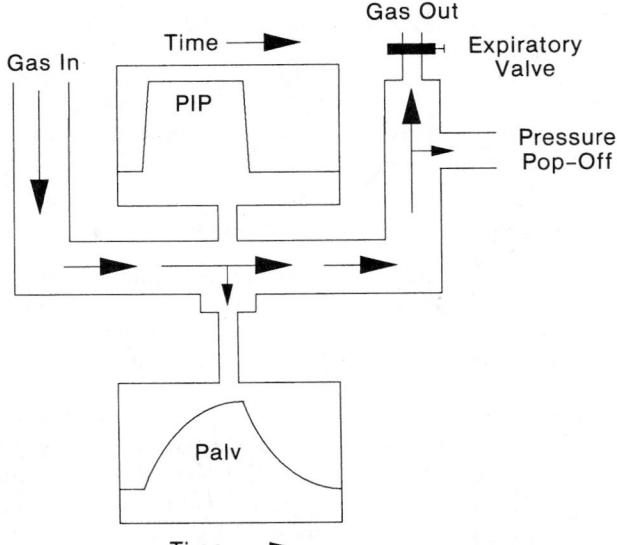

FIGURE 51-4. Positive pressure inflation of the lung. In this example, airway pressure increases rapidly to a plateau (peak inflation pressure [PIP]) (dashed line). Initially, alveolar pressure (Palv) is equal to atmospheric pressure and is much less than airway pressure (PIP >>> Palv). As a result of this large driving pressure, gas flows into the lung, and the volume of gas in the lung increases as a function of time. Obviously, because Palv is directly related to lung volume (Palv = volume/compliance), it also increases as a function of time. Therefore, the driving pressure for gas flow, PIP − Palv, and the rate of gas flow into the lung both decrease over time. Ultimately, Palv becomes equal to PIP, and flow ceases. Therefore, the maximal volume of gas that can enter the lung (Vmax) during any positive-pressure breath is ultimately determined by PIP and compliance (C) (Vmax = PIP × C).

FIGURE 51-6. Time-cycled, pressure-limited ventilator. Gas flows continuously through the ventilator circuit while a flow resistor on the exhalation limb of the circuit provides positive end-expiratory pressure. During inspiration, the expiratory valve is closed, and pressure builds up in the circuit for a preset time (Ti). The rate of the pressure buildup is determined to a large extent by the system flow. In this example, flow is high, and the pressure waveform is a square wave. PIP is limited by venting excessive pressure to the atmosphere. Airway pressure increases rapidly and is held at a plateau. Alveolar pressure increases gradually as gas flows into the lung from the ventilator. The rate of gas flow to the patient is determined by the driving pressure (PIP − Palv) and the resistance (R)—flow = (PIP − Palv)/R—not by the rate of gas flow through the ventilator circuit.

units can cause arterial hypoxemia by two different mechanisms.

Ventilation-Perfusion Mismatch

In term infants with meconium aspiration pneumonia or older infants with bronchopulmonary dysplasia, blood continues to flow past the poorly ventilated lung units and

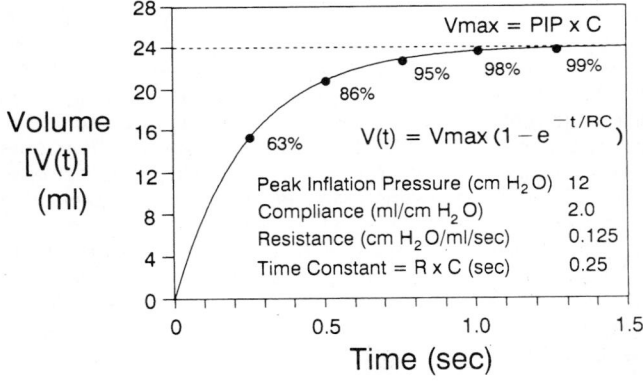

FIGURE 51-5. Lung inflation over time. As in Figure 51-4, airway pressure is rapidly increased to 25 cm H_2O and then maintained at a plateau. The volume of gas in the lung [V(t)] increases over time according to the relationship: $V(t) = Vmax \times (1 - e^{-t/RC})$, where R is the resistance of the respiratory system and C is the compliance. The maximal volume of gas that can flow into the lung (Vmax) is limited by the peak airway pressure (PIP) and C (i.e., Vmax = PIP × C). The rate of lung inflation, similar to the rate of deflation, is described by an exponential equation involving the respiratory time constant (Trs). As described in Chapter 50, Trs = RC. For an inspiratory time equal to one time constant (Ti = 1 × Trs), the lung inflates to 63% of its maximal volume (Vmax). For Ti = 2 × Trs, it reaches 86% of Vmax; for 3 × Trs, 95%; for 4 × Trs, 98%; and for 5 × Trs, 99%. Therefore, the volume of gas entering the lung during a positive-pressure breath is determined by the peak inflation pressure (PIP), the duration of inspiration (Ti), and respiratory system compliance (Crs) and resistance (Rrs).

TABLE 51-2		
Initial and Subsequent Settings for Mechanical Ventilation		
Initial Settings		
F_{IO_2}	As indicated	
System flow	10 L/min	
Rate	60 breaths/min	
Ti/Te	1/4	
PIP	Good breath sounds	
PEEP	5 cm H_2O	
Subsequent Settings	**PEEP**	**PIP**
Low PaO_2, low $PaCO_2$	Increase	
Low PaO_2, high $PaCO_2$		Increase
High PaO_2, high $PaCO_2$	Decrease	
High PaO_2, low $PaCO_2$		Decrease

remains poorly oxygenated. When it mixes with the remainder of the pulmonary venous return, it decreases overall systemic oxygen saturation. The severity of the resultant hypoxemia is directly related to the severity of the hypoxia in the poorly ventilated lung units and to the quantity of blood flowing past them.

Right-to-Left Shunt

In infants with HMD, the cause of hypoxemia is right-to-left shunt. In these infants, intense vasoconstriction occurs in blood vessels supplying severely underventilated lung units causing blood to be directed away from these lung units through intrapulmonary and extrapulmonary shunts (Hansen et al, 1979). The magnitude of the right-to-left shunt, hence the severity of the arterial hypoxemia, is related to the severity of the hypoxia in the open underventilated lung units and to the number of these units present in the lung. Therefore, regardless of the underlying parenchymal disease, the degree of arterial hypoxemia is determined by the PaO_2 in open but severely underventilated units of the lung; the only way to increase arterial oxygen tension (PaO_2) is to increase the PaO_2 in these lung units.

Several studies have shown that increasing the MAP increases PaO_2 in infants with lung disease, suggesting that increases in MAP must somehow increase the PaO_2 in poorly ventilated units of the lung (Herman and Reynolds, 1973; Stewart et al, 1981). As discussed previously, MAP is really a function of PIP, PEEP, and Ti. Increasing MAP by increasing PIP increases the driving pressure for gas flow into poorly ventilated lung units (Fig. 51–7). Increasing MAP by increasing Ti allows more time for gas to distribute to these units. Finally, increasing MAP by increasing PEEP splints small airways open, decreases airway resistance, decreases the time constant for inspiration, and allows more gas to enter the lung unit for any given PIP or Ti. All three techniques improve ventilation to the poorly ventilated lung units and increase their PaO_2. For a given increase in MAP, increasing PEEP or PIP results in a greater increase in PaO_2 than increasing Ti (Stewart et al, 1981). The reason for this discrepancy lies in the effects of mechanical ventilation on the normal parts of the lung.

None of the parenchymal lung diseases, including HMD, are homogeneous (Richardson et al, 1992). Relatively normal lung units coexist with severely underventilated lung units. Because all are connected, however, all are exposed to the same airway pressures during mechanical ventilation. Relatively normal units may have a low airway resistance and high compliance and may be subject to overdistention with increases in MAP. The risk of overdistention is greatest when MAP is increased by increasing Ti, less with increases in PIP, and least with increases in PEEP (see Fig. 51–7). As discussed in Chapter 50, overdistended lung units compress intra-alveolar vessels and redirect blood flow past poorly ventilated lung units or through shunt pathways (Landers et al, 1986). This increase in ventilation-perfusion mismatching tends to offset any increase in PaO_2 that occurs because of increased oxygenation in poorly ventilated lung units. This phenomenon probably explains why PaO_2 increases less when MAP is increased by increasing Ti than when it is increased by increasing PEEP or PIP.

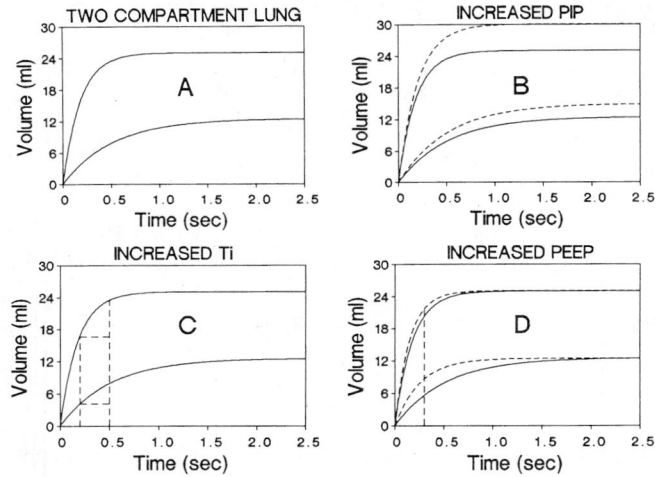

FIGURE 51–7. Effects of ventilatory manipulations on each compartment of a two-compartment lung. *A,* Plot of lung volume over time during a positive pressure inflation of the lung (PIP = 25 cm H_2O). The top curve represents normal lung units (compliance = 1 mL/cm H_2O, resistance = 0.150 cm H_2O/mL/second, and time constant = 0.15 second). These lung units inflate to a greater maximal volume (Vmax = PIP × C = 25 mL) and reach Vmax quickly (5 time constants = 0.75 second). The lower curve represents poorly ventilated lung units (compliance = 0.5 mL/cm H_2O, resistance = 1.0 cm H_2O/mL/second, and time constant = 0.5 second). Obviously, these units have a lower Vmax (12.5 mL) and take longer to reach Vmax (5 time constants = 2.5 seconds). As stated previously, unless there is poor pulmonary blood flow, which can be corrected, the only ventilatory way to increase the patient's PaO_2 is to increase the volume of gas entering poorly ventilated lung units. *B,* Increasing peak inflation pressure (dashed curves) increases the volume of gas entering each group of lung units. The increase is greater in normal lung units than in poorly ventilated lung units for any value of Ti. The net result is overdistention of normal parts of the lung in an attempt to ventilate the poorly ventilated lung units. *C,* Increasing inspiratory time (Ti) from 0.2 to 0.5 second increases the volume of gas entering each group of lung units. As in *B,* the increase, hence tendency for overdistention, is much more pronounced in the normal parts of the lung. *D,* Increasing positive end-expiratory pressure (PEEP) decreases the time constant in each group of lung units. The net effect is to allow more gas to enter each part of the lung for any given PIP or Ti. In this case, the effect is more pronounced in the poorly ventilated lung units. As a result, the likelihood of overdistention of normal lung units is less.

Besides its effects on oxygenation, alveolar overdistention carries the risk of alveolar rupture and pulmonary interstitial emphysema (see Chapter 54). The propensity for increases in Ti to result in alveolar overdistention is supported by its high association with pulmonary air leaks in one study that explored the antecedents of alveolar rupture (Primhak, 1983). It is also supported by the results of two controlled trials showing a higher incidence of pneumothorax in infants ventilated with a long Ti than in those ventilated with a short Ti (Heicher et al, 1981; Oxford Region Controlled Trial, 1991).

The other important function of mechanical ventilation is to ventilate adequately, and the $PaCO_2$ is an indication of this. $PaCO_2$ is equal to the rate of CO_2 production divided by the alveolar ventilation ($\dot{V}A$). The latter is represented by the equation $\dot{V}_A = (V_T - V_D) \times RR$, where V_T is tidal volume, V_D is dead space volume, and RR is respiratory rate. If V_D and CO_2 production are relatively constant, Pa_{CO_2} is proportional to $1 \div (RR \times V_T)$. Pa_{CO_2} decreases if either RR or V_T is increased and Pa_{CO_2} increases if RR or V_T is decreased. On a pressure-limited respirator at a constant inspiratory time, the V_T is determined by the lung compliance and by PIP and PEEP (Fig. 51–8). (If Ti is less than three time constants, increasing Ti increases V_T but at the expense of overdistention of more normal lung units.) Pa_{CO_2} can be decreased by increasing RR, by increasing PIP, or by decreasing PEEP. Conversely, Pa_{CO_2} can be increased by decreasing RR, by decreasing PIP, or by increasing PEEP.

Although it is attractive to try to lower the Pa_{CO_2} by increasing the respirator rate, rather than by adjusting ventilatory pressures, data suggest that this approach may not be entirely without risk. As the respirator rate increases, the absolute time allotted for expiration decreases. If expiratory time decreases to less than three time constants for expiration, gas trapping and alveolar overdistention may occur (Kano et al, 1993).

Applications

Because tiny premature infants characteristically have structurally immature lungs and weak chest walls, many centers have a standard practice of providing some form of respiratory support (i.e., nasal CPAP or mechanical ventilation) for all infants who weigh less than 1250 g. For all infants who weigh between 1250 and 1500 g and have HMD, ventilatory assistance is also necessary, as well as for larger infants with apneic episodes or those who cannot maintain a Pa_{O_2} of more than 50 torr on a continuous distending pressure of 10 to 12 cm H_2O and 100% oxygen. Infants usually are intubated orally with an endotracheal

tube that allows an audible air leak to prevent later development of subglottic stenosis. A 2.5-mm internal diameter (ID) tube is appropriate for infants weighing less than 1 kg, 3.0 mm for those weighing between 1 and 2 kg, and 3.5 mm for those weighing more than 2 kg. For standard use, orotracheal intubation is preferred over nasotracheal because nasotracheal intubation has been found to cause nasal deformities (McMillan et al, 1986).

During intubation, infants often require a fractional inspired oxygen (F_{IO_2}) that is 10% greater than they were receiving before the initiation of mechanical ventilation. It is always valuable to hand-ventilate an infant initially to determine the minimal PIP necessary to achieve good chest wall excursion and good bilateral breath sounds. A rate of 60 breaths/min (which approximates the normal rate for a premature infant) and PEEP of 5 are used. In general, oxygenation can be improved by increasing MAP by increasing PEEP or PIP (see Table 51–1). Ti should rarely be prolonged because of the risk of alveolar overdistention. Hypercarbia is treated by increasing PIP or decreasing PEEP. To allow sufficient time for exhalation, the respirator rate should not ordinarily exceed 80 breaths/min. The entire cardiopulmonary status of the infant must be kept in mind. Data have suggested that attempts to control Pa_{CO_2} rigorously may result in worsened lung injury. Therefore, the authors often allow the Pa_{CO_2} to increase to 50 torr or above in infants with severe respiratory distress (Kraybill et al, 1989). An infant with poor pulmonary blood flow because of hypotension, hypovolemia, cardiac failure, or high pulmonary vascular resistance may also have a low Pa_{O_2}, and treatment should be directed to improving blood pressure and volume and cardiac output.

Weaning can be accomplished, as shown in Table 51–2. For larger infants, weaning to endotracheal CPAP may begin when PIP has been stable at less than 25 cm H_2O and F_{IO_2} is less than 0.40, and then to an oxygen hood when the infants require less than 5 cm H_2O of end-expiratory pressure. For infants weighing less than 1750 g, when PIP is less than 20 cm H_2O and F_{IO_2} is less than 0.30, it is possible to decrease gradually the respiratory rate to 15 to 20 breaths/min and then to wean directly to nasal CPAP (Wung et al, 1975). For this group of infants, the resistance of the endotracheal tube is such that periods of endotracheal CPAP or ventilatory rates less than 15 breaths/min cannot be tolerated (Lesouef et al, 1984). For infants who cannot be weaned from the ventilator because of apnea or chronic lung disease, a respiratory rate of 20 to 30 breaths/min and a slightly prolonged Ti allow the best distribution of ventilation through damaged airways (Chan et al, 1994b).

Ventilator gas should be warmed to 34° to 37°C and humidified to 80% to 90% to prevent excessive water loss from the respiratory tract and injury to the lung from exposure to cold dry air (Chatburn, 1989; Hanssler et al, 1992; Tarnow-Mordi et al, 1989). This warming is most easily accomplished by using a heated nebulizer with heated ventilator circuits to prevent condensation of water in the ventilator tubing. Tracheal suctioning and chest physiotherapy should be minimized in the infant with HMD in the first few days after birth because their secretions are scant, and there is little evidence that suctioning and chest physiotherapy are of benefit. Concern has been

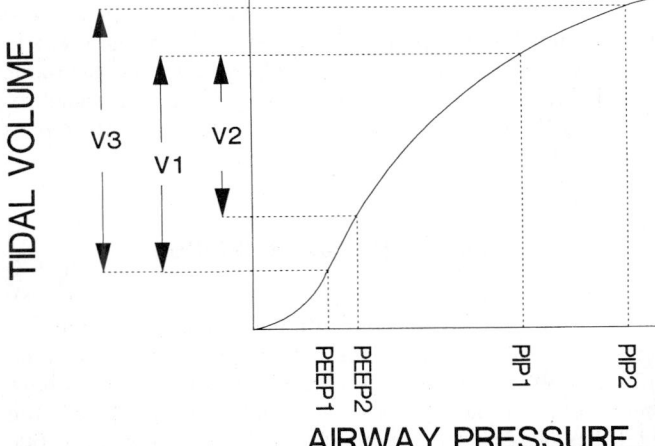

FIGURE 51–8. Determinants of tidal volume. Lung volume is plotted as a function of inflation pressure. As the ventilator cycles between positive end-expiratory pressure (PEEP1) and peak inflation pressure (PIP1), the lung volume changes, generating tidal volume (V1). Increasing PEEP to PEEP2 forces the ventilator to cycle between PEEP2 and PIP1 and results in a lower tidal volume, V2. Leaving PEEP at PEEP1 and increasing peak inflation pressure to PIP2 increases the tidal volume to V3.

expressed that these interventions might increase the risk of intracranial hemorrhage (Greisen et al, 1985). Infants with secretions (e.g., meconium aspiration or pneumonia) and older infants with HMD may require suctioning of the trachea as often as every 2 to 4 hours. Even then, suctioning is often associated with acute side effects of hypoxia, hypertension, and bradycardia (Simbruner et al, 1981) and, with deep suctioning, the risk of airway injury (Miller et al, 1981). If hand ventilation accompanies suctioning, a manometer must be attached to the bag to prevent delivery of excessive PIP.

The use of neuromuscular blockade to facilitate mechanical ventilation in the newborn remains controversial. Paralysis may result in decreased dynamic lung compliance and increased airway resistance and removes any contribution of the infant's own respiratory effort from tidal breathing (Bhutani et al, 1988). Therefore, it is often necessary to increase ventilator pressures after initiation of neuromuscular blockade. Venous return is also impaired by lack of movement and decreased muscle tone; therefore, generalized edema develops with this treatment.

Complications of Therapy

Prolonged orotracheal intubation may cause palatal grooving and may interfere with dentition (Duke et al, 1976; Moylan et al, 1980), whereas nasotracheal intubation may result in cosmetic deformities of the nose (Jung and Thomas, 1974) and even nasal obstruction (see Chapter 57). Subglottic stenosis, although rare, can be a disastrous complication of intubation. A too snugly fitting endotracheal tube, duration of intubation, and number of reintubations all correlate with subsequent subglottic stenosis (Sherman et al, 1986). Some infants have required tracheostomy.

Necrotizing tracheobronchitis (Pietsch et al, 1985) is a necrotic inflammatory process involving the trachea and mainstem bronchi that has been described in newborns requiring mechanical ventilation. Sloughing of the tracheal epithelium results in occlusion of the distal trachea. Infants present with acute respiratory deterioration with symptoms of airway obstruction, hyperexpansion on chest radiograph, and poor chest movement. Emergency bronchoscopy may be necessary to relieve airway obstruction. The lesion is thought to result from drying of the tracheal mucosa secondary to inadequate humidification in the presence of high rates of gas flow and high concentrations of oxygen.

Atelectasis occasionally occurs after extubation from mechanical ventilation, with the right upper lobe most commonly affected. In some instances, atelectasis may reflect injury to the bronchi from suction catheters. In small preterm infants, postextubation atelectasis may result from chest wall instability and may be prevented by weaning to nasal CPAP.

Patient-Triggered Ventilation

Many hospitals use modifications of conventional mechanical ventilation in which the patient is able to initiate ventilator breaths; this is accomplished in different systems by the detection of various types of signal associated with inspiration, such as abdominal motion, chest wall imped-

ance, or airway flow. This technology achieves a greater degree of synchrony between the infant's breathing and the ventilator, and this may improve oxygenation if the infant's breathing was previously asynchronous. Patient-triggered ventilation (PTV) is used in two modes: (1) In synchronized intermittent mandatory ventilation (SIMV), a single triggered breath is given in equal windows of time, with the other patient breaths in each window not assisted; this means that the rate can be slowly reduced with all assisted breaths well synchronized. (2) In assist/control mode (A/C), all breaths are triggered, so the patient controls the ventilator rate, and weaning is accomplished by reducing the PIP. A number of different advantages to these systems have been suggested, but perhaps the most promising is a reduction in cerebral blood flow variability (Rennie et al, 1987), which may help decrease the incidence of intraventricular hemorrhage; this, however, has not been proven in the case of PTV.

The clinical trials that have been performed have used the A/C mode. Visveshwara and colleagues (1991) found that flow-volume curves were more reproducible with PTV than with conventional ventilation and that in a nonrandomized clinical trial small premature infants required a significantly shorter time on the ventilator. They did not show any important reductions in the incidence of pneumothorax, intraventricular hemorrhage, bronchopulmonary dysplasia, or death. These results have been confirmed in true randomized, controlled trials (Chan and Greenough, 1993a; Donn et al, 1994), but there were no reductions in death or complications. Thus, the major benefit of PTV is that weaning from the ventilator is facilitated. In another controlled trial that compared PTV with conventional ventilation at high rates, it was concluded that PTV was less satisfactory (Hird and Greenough, 1991). There seems agreement that this technology can be used only with difficulty in infants weighing less than 1000 g because they may not trigger the ventilator well (Chan et al, 1994b). A comparison between A/C and SIMV showed no difference in the length of the weaning process (Chan and Greenough, 1994a). In a crossover trial, Cleary and coworkers (1995) demonstrated improved oxygenation in infants on SIMV, compared with infants who breathed asynchronously with the ventilator, but they showed no differences for any clinical outcome measures.

High-Frequency Ventilation

Respiratory rates on the ventilator between 60 and 80 breaths/min represent conventional ventilation; high-frequency ventilation (HFV) refers to respirator rates between 150 and 3000 breaths/min. Three types of ventilators have been used for HFV in the newborn (Slutsky, 1988): the high-frequency jet ventilator (HFJV) with rates up to 600 breaths/min, the high-frequency flow interrupter (HFIV) with rates up to 1200 breaths/min, and the high-frequency oscillator (HFOV) with rates up to 3000 breaths/min.

The HFJV delivers a high-pressure puff of gas through a small-bore cannula usually positioned in the airway at the proximal end of the endotracheal tube. The actual volume of gas delivered cannot be known because the volume delivered by the jet may be augmented by gas from the auxiliary circuit that is dragged along with the high-pressure puff. Exhalation is passive.

The HFIV uses a circuit similar to a conventional ventilator. Gas flow through the circuit is interrupted by a motorized rotating ball to produce oscillations. Constant end-expiratory pressure is adjusted by a valve on the expiratory limb of the circuit. As it is for the HFJV, exhalation is passive.

The HFOV uses a piston or moving diaphragm to pump gas in and out of the lung actively. The oscillator uses small tidal volumes (usually less than VD) and relies on a bias flow of gas to flush CO_2 out of the system and maintain a supply of fresh gas at the proximal end of the endotracheal tube.

Mechanisms of Gas Exchange

The mechanism responsible for oxygenation with HFV is the same as for conventional ventilation—it depends on increasing the P_{AO_2} in the poorly ventilated part of the lung (Froese and Bryan, 1987; Slutsky, 1988). Similar to the conventional ventilator, the high-frequency ventilator accomplishes this by increasing MAP. Whether or not HFV results in comparable levels of oxygenation with lower MAPs is still controversial.

The difference between HFV and conventional ventilation lies in the methods of removing CO_2. HFV seemingly defies conventional pulmonary physiology by removing CO_2 by rapid ventilation of the lung with VTs less than the anatomic VD. There are five mechanisms by which HFV might accomplish CO_2 removal:

1. Some alveoli are located near enough to central airways that bulk convection of gas can play a role in CO_2 exchange.
2. Similar to conventional ventilation, HFV relies on molecular diffusion for gas exchange within the terminal lung units.
3. At the high frequencies employed with HFV, gas exchange between lung units with uneven time constants (pendelluft) can set up circulating currents that enhance gas mixing in the lung and CO_2 exchange.
4. The velocity profile of gas in the airways is asymmetric (i.e., in the center of the parabolic gas stream, forward transport is slightly greater than backward transport of gas, and at the edge of the stream, backward transport is greater than forward). At high frequencies, this results in a net forward flow of fresh gas down the center of the airway and a net backward flow of alveolar-airway gas up the airway.
5. At high frequencies, a form of facilitated diffusion occurs secondary to enhanced dispersion of both turbulent and laminar streams of gas flow (Taylor dispersion). During HFV, these mechanisms combine so that the rate of CO_2 elimination is proportional to the respiratory frequency × the VT squared.

Potential Problems

One of the major problems associated with HFV is related to humidification of inspired gas. This is a particular problem with the HFJV, in which inadequate humidification combined with the high-pressure pulses of gas has resulted in cases of necrotizing tracheitis. It is much less of a problem with the HFIV and HFOV, in which the bias flow can be adequately humidified. The other concern with the use of HFV is that of gas trapping. At high frequencies, expiration may be shortened to the point that Te is less than three time constants and gas trapping may occur. This may be a particular problem with ventilators that use a fixed Ti:Te of 1:1.

Clinical Experience

HFJV has been used for short periods of time in infants with HMD (Carlo et al, 1984). In these patients, HFJV provides adequate oxygenation with low MAP and PIP. A single study in which HFJV was used for longer periods of time in infants with intractable respiratory failure suggested that HFJV may be useful in managing patients with air leaks or diaphragmatic hernia (Boros et al, 1985). In infants with pulmonary hypertension, HFJV results in a reduction in arterial P_{CO_2} and required ventilatory pressures, but it has no effect on ultimate outcome (Carlo et al, 1989). One study comparing HFJV to conventional ventilation in an experimental model of meconium aspiration pneumonia found HFJV to be superior, whereas another found conventional ventilation to be superior (Mammel et al, 1983; Trindade et al, 1985). HFIV was used in a controlled trial in preterm infants with respiratory distress syndrome (RDS); the results were not different from those with conventional mechanical ventilation (Pardou et al, 1993).

High-Frequency Ventilation as Rescue Treatment Before Extracorporeal Membrane Oxygenation

Descriptive reports suggest that HFOV or HFJV may be useful in the management of newborn infants with severe respiratory failure, who are on maximal ventilatory support and are being considered for treatment with extracorporeal membrane oxygenation (ECMO) (Baumgart et al, 1992; Carter et al 1990; Cornish et al, 1987). Clark and associates (1994) randomized 19 such patients to conventional mechanical ventilation and 27 to HFOV in a crossover trial with prospectively defined failure criteria; all infants met institutional criteria for ECMO at the time of enrollment. After all patients had been treated with one or both forms of ventilation, as necessary, it was found that the chance of success for HFOV was 51%, compared with only 21% for conventional ventilation. This study supports a trial of HFOV before ECMO; it also suggests that HFOV for this indication should be used only in hospitals that can also provide ECMO because patients who fail HFOV must be managed with conventional ventilation for the purpose of transportation. Additional experience has suggested that HFOV is most successful in cases of RDS and pneumonia and somewhat less successful in cases of meconium aspiration pneumonia (Carter et al, 1990); the experience with HFJV has been the same (Baumgart et al, 1992). There is agreement that in all patients a 6-hour trial of HFOV or HFJV is worthwhile and sufficient to predict success or failure and the likelihood of needing ECMO (Baumgart et al, 1992; Chan et al, 1994a; Paranka et al, 1995).

High-Frequency Ventilation in the Management of Air Leak Problems

In two uncontrolled trials, HFIV appeared to provide some benefit in the management of low-birth-weight infants with pulmonary interstitial emphysema (Frantz et al, 1983; Gaylord et al, 1987). Keszler and colleagues (1991) reported the results of a large multicentered controlled trial in the management of premature infants with pulmonary interstitial emphysema, comparing HFJV with conventional ventilation at rapid rates; the success criteria were prospectively defined, and provision was made for crossover as necessary. Overall, 61% of those who started on HFJV and only 31% of those who started on conventional ventilation were successfully managed, a significantly improved result with HFJV. More patients starting on conventional ventilation had to be crossed over to HFJV. When patients were crossed over to HFJV, the success rate was much higher (45%) than when patients were crossed over to conventional ventilation (9%). Radiographic improvement was clearly more rapid with HFJV. After excluding crossover, the mortality of those starting on HFJV was 35%, compared with 53% in those who started on conventional ventilation. In this study of pulmonary interstitial emphysema, a low volume strategy was pursued, with encouragement of the lung to de-recruit; such a strategy can be followed with other forms of HFV in the management of pulmonary interstitial emphysema.

High-Frequency Ventilation for the Management of Respiratory Distress Syndrome

There have been four controlled trials of HFV as primary management of premature infants with RDS:

1. The HIFI Study Group (1989) conducted a randomized, multicenter trial of HFOV in preterm infants with RDS; 346 infants were assigned to HFOV and 327 infants were assigned to conventional ventilation. There was no difference in the incidence of pulmonary air leaks (PAL), 28-day mortality rate, or 28-day incidence of bronchopulmonary dysplasia. There was a significant increase in the incidence of severe intraventricular hemorrhage and periventricular leukomalacia in those assigned to HFOV, and, as might be expected, at the age of 12 months there were fewer infants with normal neurologic status in the HFOV group (HIFI Study Group, 1990). In addition, in a study of lung mechanics, there was no evidence for reduced lung injury with HFOV (Abbasi et al, 1991). This trial was widely criticized (Bryan and Froese, 1991). All infants were initially on conventional ventilation for a period up to 12 hours before randomization; because of the crossover design, some infants assigned to one group were treated with the other mode of ventilation for a longer period of time; and many centers pursued a low volume strategy without adequate recruitment of the air spaces, and, as is now recognized, this may be injurious to the lungs (Dreyfuss and Saumon, 1994). However, the issue of brain injury raised by this trial remains a serious problem. In a recently published report of a controlled trial for the management of RDS (Wiswell et al, 1996), HFJV was associated with a significantly increased incidence of periventricular leukomalacia.

2. Clark and coworkers (1992) performed a randomized trial comparing three groups of patients with RDS: 26 patients were assigned to conventional ventilation only, 27 patients were assigned to HFOV for 72 hours followed by conventional ventilation, and 30 patients were assigned to HFOV only, until extubation. There were no differences for the 30-day mortality or for the incidence of intraventricular hemorrhage or PAL between any of the three groups. The incidence of bronchopulmonary dysplasia was highest in the conventional ventilation–only group, intermediate in the HFOV and conventional ventilation group, and lowest in the HFOV-only group, and the difference was significant. Survival without bronchopulmonary dysplasia at 36 weeks' postconceptional age was significantly increased by HFOV. This important study suggests that HFOV might be less injurious to the lung, but it was conducted before the advent of surfactant therapy.

3. The HIFO Study Group (1993) performed a randomized trial in patients with RDS: 86 infants were treated with conventional ventilation and 90 were treated with HFOV. There was no change in the neonatal mortality rate and no change in the incidence of bronchopulmonary dysplasia assessed at age 28 days, but the incidence of PAL was significantly reduced in the HFOV group; again, this study was conducted before the advent of surfactant therapy.

4. Ogawa and colleagues (1993) reported a controlled trial of HFOV and conventional ventilation in RDS patients who were also treated with bovine exogenous surfactant; they enrolled 46 infants in each group at the age of 2 hours and were not able to show any advantage with HFOV. This trial casts some doubt on the hypothesis that HFOV may improve the results in RDS patients treated with exogenous surfactant.

After consideration of these four trials, it seems reasonable to conclude that HFOV should not be used for the initial treatment of RDS in premature infants managed with exogenous surfactant; there is no conclusive evidence that HFV reduces the incidence of PAL or bronchopulmonary dysplasia, and there is certainly no evidence that it affects the mortality of infants with RDS. Should conventional ventilation and surfactant fail, however, HFOV is a reasonable form of rescue therapy (Chan et al, 1994a). This conclusion may have to be changed in the future. Frantz (1990) found at his institution during the HIFI trial that HFOV reduced the incidence of bronchopulmonary dysplasia from 50% to 16%. In a recently published report (Gerstmann et al, 1996), a controlled trial of HFOV, initiated early for RDS in surfactant-treated premature infants, showed that the incidence of bronchopulmonary dysplasia was significantly reduced by the use of HFOV compared with conventional ventilation; there was no change in the incidence of IVH or death. These results are consistent with evidence in premature monkeys, in which Jackson and colleagues (1994) demonstrated significantly reduced lung injury when exogenous surfactant is combined with the early use of HFOV.

The usual recommendation for HFOV in the management of severe respiratory failure is to start at a MAP of 2 to 3 cm H_2O above the MAP for conventional ventilation, at a rate of 10 Hz, at an I:E of 1:2, and at a Δ pressure that moves the chest visibly. Chan and Greenough (1993b) recommended a rate of 10 Hz and a MAP of 5 cm H_2O above the MAP on conventional ventilation. In general, oxygenation is controlled with MAP, and ventilation is controlled with Δ pressure. Few changes are made in the rate, but if hypercarbia dictates a larger VT at the same Δ pressure, this can be accomplished by a reduction of the rate to 9 or 8 Hz, and if pulmonary interstitial emphysema dictates a smaller VT at the same Δ pressure, this can be accomplished by an increase in the rate as high as 15 Hz. The MAP may be increased to 25 cm H_2O or higher, but depression of the circulation becomes an important factor and volume support may be needed. When oxygenation is improved, it is usual to wean oxygen first and favor the continued use of high MAP. When the MAP has been weaned to 9 to 12 cm H_2O, it is usual to change the patient back to conventional ventilation at a level of MAP 2 to 3 cm H_2O lower.

SURFACTANT REPLACEMENT THERAPY

Exogenous surfactant therapy has assumed an important place in neonatal intensive care. Most of the clinical studies so far have been concerned with small premature infants and the treatment of RDS; there are few publications concerning other conditions. Because there are so many large controlled trials, it seems reasonable to emphasize these and the meta-analyses that have been performed.

Early Studies

The earliest attempts to provide surfactant replacement therapy were not successful (Chu et al, 1967; Robillard et al, 1964). There were several reasons for this: (1) The preparations consisted only of saturated phosphatidylcholine, which reduces surface tension to low levels but only very slowly; (2) the dose was too small and did not take into account destruction and inactivation of surfactant in the upper airways; and (3) the method of administration was by nebulization, which has not proved to be effective even with better preparations today. Enhorning and colleagues (1973) presented the idea of administering surfactant as a bolus in the upper airway and allowing it to spread peripherally in the lung; they devised an exogenous surfactant by concentrating the lipids in lung lavage fluid from adult rabbits and demonstrated beneficial effects in newborn rabbits subjected at birth to tracheostomy and tracheal deposition of surfactant; later, they showed that the surfactant film in the lung terminal air spaces could be completely reconstituted by pharyngeal deposition of surfactant (Robertson and Enhorning, 1974). Since that time, a vast literature on surfactant replacement therapy in animals has accumulated, confirming its efficacy (Jobe, 1993).

Human Trials

The first successful human clinical trials were conducted in Japan by Fujiwara and coworkers (1980); they prepared exogenous surfactant from a lipid extract of bovine lungs and enriched it by the addition of saturated phosphatidylcholine and other lipids. A single instillation down the endotracheal tube of 10 premature infants with RDS produced a marked improvement in oxygenation. Following this publication, multiple small controlled trials in premature infants were performed with different surfactant preparations: variations of the material used by Fujiwara, a lipid extract of surfactant obtained from bovine lung lavage fluid, surfactant prepared by centrifugation of human amniotic fluid, and synthetic surfactant. Most of these trials suggested that surfactant replacement was a promising new treatment.

Several different types of exogenous surfactant are presently available in the United States: (1) bovine lung mince lipid extract enriched with synthetic lipids (Survanta), (2) bovine lung lavage lipid extract (Infasurf), and (3) a mixture of synthetic lipids (Exosurf). The two bovine surfactants contain SP-B and SP-C but do not contain SP-A; Infasurf contains much more SP-B and SP-C than Survanta; the synthetic surfactant contains no protein, but hexadecanol is intended to accelerate surfactant adsorption to the surface. Large controlled trials have established that these preparations greatly reduce the mortality of preterm infants (Corbet et al, 1991a, 1991b; Hoekstra et al, 1991; Liechty et al, 1991; Long et al, 1991a, 1991b). Two broad clinical strategies were used: (1) prophylaxis within 30 minutes of birth in small premature infants at high risk for HMD and (2) rescue treatment a few hours after birth for infants with a reasonably certain diagnosis of HMD. In Europe, other surfactants are available: (1) porcine lung mince lipid extract enriched by chromatography (Curosurf), (2) another bovine lung lavage lipid extract (Alveofact), and (3) another synthetic surfactant (Pneumactant). These surfactants have proved equally efficacious in large controlled trials (Bevilacqua et al, 1993; Collaborative European Multicentre Study Group, 1988; Gortner et al, 1990, 1992; Morley et al, 1988; Speer et al, 1992; Ten Center Study Group, 1987).

Exogenous surfactants are administered by direct instillation into the endotracheal tube, either with a catheter passed to the distal end or through a ported adapter at the proximal end. Administration may be complicated by arterial oxygen desaturation, airway obstruction and loss of chest wall motion, and reflux of surfactant into the pharynx; these problems can be easily overcome by slowing the rate of administration and by increasing the inspiratory pressure for a short time; in addition, it may be necessary to increase the inspired oxygen for a short time. The use of a catheter requires that infants be removed from mechanical ventilation and given bag-tube ventilation. Trials have shown that it does not matter whether surfactant is given by catheter or through a port, although the port method was associated with less oxygen desaturation and more reflux of the dose up the endotracheal tube. Also, it does not matter if the dose is divided into 2 or 4 aliquots (Zola et al, 1993). Although recommended, it may not be necessary to move the infant into different positions during instillation because exogenous surfactant has remarkable spreading properties. The trachea is usually suctioned just before administration and is not suctioned for 2 to 3 hours afterward, to avoid the removal of any surfactant.

Outcome in Surfactant Clinical Trials

When used at birth, exogenous surfactants reduce the incidence of RDS; the single exception is Exosurf, with which, surprisingly, there was no change in the incidence of RDS. All exogenous surfactants reduce the severity of RDS; they reduce the mortality of RDS by 40% to 60%; and they significantly reduce the overall mortality of premature infants at risk for RDS. The early changes in mortality are reflected in impressive reductions of infant mortality at the age of 1 year (Corbet et al, 1991a, 1991b; Long et al, 1991b). In addition, exogenous surfactants reduce the incidence of pulmonary air leaks by about 50%. This effect is possibly more marked with bovine surfactants (Mercier and Soll, 1993), although this is likely to depend on the ventilation strategy used.

Despite earlier promise, it is now accepted by many observers that surfactants do not reduce the overall incidence of chronic lung disease, perhaps because some of the additional survivors with surfactant have bronchopulmonary dysplasia (Jobe, 1993). In general, the incidence of survival without bronchopulmonary dysplasia is significantly increased (Pramanik et al, 1993), and in the rescue trials of Exosurf, the incidence of bronchopulmonary dysplasia appeared to be significantly reduced (Corbet, 1993; Jobe, 1993).

After analysis of many trials, most observers have concluded that surfactant treatment is not associated with an important change in the incidence of intraventricular hemorrhage, patent ductus arteriosus, or retinopathy of prematurity; however, in more mature infants with birth weight more than 1250 g, the incidence of intraventricular hemorrhage and patent ductus arteriosus was significantly reduced (Long et al, 1991a). In a trial of bovine surfactant, in which early intraventricular hemorrhage was excluded at the time of enrollment, there was a definite reduction in the incidence of subsequent intraventricular hemorrhage in the surfactant-treated group (Fujiwara et al, 1990).

The benefits of surfactant were more limited in infants of 500 to 700 g birth weight enrolled in a large trial of Exosurf (Stevenson et al, 1992), probably because of the limits imposed by the extreme immaturity of all organ systems. Ferrara and coworkers (1991) reported the results in certain selected centers taking part in large Survanta trials; mortality was significantly reduced and the outcome of survivors was improved in surfactant-treated infants with birth weights of 600 to 750 g. In addition, the mortality of this group of tiny infants has improved remarkably in some centers since the introduction of bovine surfactant (Hoekstra et al, 1994). Horbar and associates (1993b) in the NICHD Neonatal Research Network have evaluated the effect of surfactant (mostly Survanta but some Exosurf) on large populations over time and estimated the mortality reduction in various weight groups between 601 and 1300 g before and after the introduction of surfactant. The overall proportionate mortality reduction was 28%, and the mortality reductions were as good in the smaller infants (600 to 700 g) as in the larger infants.

Dose of Surfactant and Its Distribution

Replacement surfactant should be given under conditions of adequate mechanical ventilation and PEEP, to insure optimal distribution to poorly ventilated regions of the lung, and the dose should be 75 to 100 mg/kg, high enough to overcome destruction by macrophages and inhibition by plasma proteins. It has been shown that 60 mg/kg of bovine surfactant does not produce as good results as 120 mg/kg (Konishi et al, 1988) and that 50 mg/kg does not produce as good results as 100 mg/kg (Gortner et al, 1994). Also, it was shown that 100 mg/kg of porcine surfactant produced results as good as 200 mg/kg (Halliday et al, 1993). In animal experiments, the distribution of surfactant to the various regions of the lung has been surprisingly uniform (Davis et al, 1992); this may depend on the dose volume being relatively large (van der Bleek et al, 1993) and on the dose being instilled at a relatively rapid rate (Segerer et al, 1993). The peripheral migration of surfactant may be delayed if HFOV is used after the dose is administered (Heldt et al, 1992). This may be because the bulk flow of inspired gas with HFOV is down the center of the airways, whereas exhaled gas flows out close to the mucosa where surfactant may be deposited; so for patients on HFOV, surfactant administration should be followed by a period of bag-tube ventilation to facilitate distribution.

Number, Interval, and Schedule of Surfactant Doses

It is apparent that the effect of exogenous surfactant is often short-lived, presumably owing to inhibition by plasma proteins in pulmonary edema fluid; multiple doses of surfactant are clearly more effective than a single dose (Corbet et al, 1995b; Dunn et al, 1990; Speer et al, 1992). It has not been firmly established how many doses are best. A large prophylaxis trial using synthetic surfactant showed that three doses at 12-hour intervals were significantly more effective than one dose (Corbet et al, 1995b), but this did not distinguish the effects of two from three doses. Another prophylaxis trial did not show any improvement comparing six doses with three doses, so there is no advantage to more than three doses (Corbet, 1993). It seems reasonable to conclude that prophylaxis should be carried out with either two or three doses. For the rescue approach, several trials have established that there is no advantage to more than two doses of synthetic surfactant (Corbet, 1993; OSIRIS Collaborative Group, 1992). In the case of Survanta, the trials suggested that up to four doses may be necessary in a few patients, although no direct comparisons were performed, and it is not possible to determine if the additional doses actually made a difference to the outcome.

The appropriate interval between doses has not been established; most trials of both synthetic and mammalian surfactants used an interval of 12 hours, but the 6-hour interval used in the Survanta trials was effective (Hoekstra et al, 1991; Liechty et al, 1991). A trial of Exosurf comparing two doses at a 12-hour interval with four doses at shorter intervals as in the Survanta trials found no difference in the response or outcome (Corbet, 1993).

It is not established whether surfactant should be given according to a rigid schedule; the trials of both synthetic surfactants and porcine surfactant were conducted according to rigid schedules, with doses given every 12 hours, whereas the Survanta trials were conducted with more flexible schedules, with doses given as frequently as every 6 hours. The objection to a rigid schedule is that dose administration may be more difficult if ventilator rates and pressures have been reduced to low levels; the surfactant may obstruct the airways and cause a temporary deterioration in gas exchange. In the Survanta trials, further dosing was omitted if the inspired oxygen requirement was less than 30%, and this appears more reasonable to many observers (Jobe, 1993).

Type of Surfactant to Be Used

Direct comparisons in individual large clinical trials have not suggested any major outcome differences between the mammalian and synthetic preparations of exogenous surfactant (Horbar et al, 1993b; Hudak et al, 1994; Tarnow-Mordi and Soll, 1994; Vermont-Oxford Neonatal Network, 1996), but there is a trend toward reduced mortality with mammalian surfactants in most of the trials. Halliday (1995a) has performed a meta-analysis of multiple trials and confirmed that there is, proportionately, a statistically significant improvement in mortality of 20% with mammalian surfactants compared with Exosurf. In addition, the meta-analysis suggested that the incidence of pulmonary air leaks was reduced significantly in the mammalian surfactant groups.

The physiologic response to mammalian surfactant was definitely more rapid, and the lower inspired oxygen levels with mammalian surfactant persisted for 3 days. The latter findings are supported by several other observations. Bovine surfactant produces a more rapid improvement in lung volume and in arterial oxygenation over 2 hours, whereas synthetic surfactant produces a similar, but significantly slower, improvement in these parameters over 6 hours (Cotton et al, 1993). Stenson and colleagues (1994) found a rapid improvement in static lung compliance over 3 hours with Curosurf and no change in static lung compliance over 12 hours with Exosurf. In a comparison of Exosurf with Curosurf, the porcine surfactant produced a rapid improvement in static lung compliance over 6 hours, whereas Exosurf showed no improvement over 6 hours and then a lesser improvement over 24 hours (Choukroun et al, 1994).

In a small comparative trial with Curosurf and Exosurf, the porcine surfactant produced a much more rapid decline in oxygen needs, such that oxygen therapy was necessary for only 10 days compared with 17 days for Exosurf (Rollins et al, 1993). For these reasons, most clinicians now prefer to use a mammalian surfactant; nevertheless, the reduced mortality with a single dose of Exosurf may be impressive (Corbet et al, 1991b), and it may be further improved with two additional doses (Corbet et al, 1995b). In a comparative trial with Curosurf and Survanta (Speer et al, 1995), no significant differences were seen. The slower onset of action of synthetic surfactant may be explained by the relative inefficiency of the lipid additive in speeding adsorption of saturated phosphatidylcholine to the surface, when compared with the SP-B and SP-C present in the mammalian preparations.

In the case of bovine and porcine surfactants, there has been concern about problems of potential antibody production. Chida and colleagues (1991) demonstrated antibodies to surfactant proteins using an enzyme-linked immunosorbent assay technique in serum samples from infants with RDS, but it did not matter whether or not exogenous surfactant was used, suggesting that the antibodies were developed against endogenous surfactant that leaked out of the lung compartment into the circulation. Strayer and associates (1995) demonstrated SP-A/anti SP-A immune complexes in the serum of infants with RDS; it did not matter whether infants received exogenous surfactant, again suggesting that the antibodies were produced against endogenous surfactant in the circulation. In a small proportion of more mature patients treated with Alveofact, antibodies to surfactant proteins have been demonstrated (Bartmann et al, 1991); in a small proportion of patients treated with Curosurf, antibodies were found by a technique using serum samples to immunostain porcine lung (Bambang Oetomo et al, 1993). The significance of these findings is not clear. In other larger mammalian surfactant trials, no evidence of antibody formation has been found (Collaborative European Multicentre Study Group, 1992; Whitsett et al, 1991).

Prophylactic Versus Rescue Strategy

The prophylactic approach in small premature infants produces clearly better results than a late rescue strategy, in which infants are treated at age 6 to 12 hours (Kattwinkel et al, 1993; Kendig et al, 1991; Konishi et al, 1992). Although an early rescue strategy with treatment at age 2 to 3 hours may produce results that are as good as prophylaxis (Dunn et al, 1991; Merritt et al, 1991), a large controlled trial has shown that the results are improved if the treatment is started before the age of 2 hours (OSIRIS Collaborative Group, 1992). An early rescue approach is widely favored so as to minimize the number of patients treated and reduce the costs, but many centers continue the prophylactic strategy in all infants with a birth weight less than 1000 g, in whom the risk for RDS is high (Egberts et al, 1993; European Exosurf Study Group, 1992). Although suggested by some authors, it is not necessary that surfactant be administered immediately at birth, before the first breath; it is far more important to stabilize the infant adequately first. The early rescue strategy would be greatly facilitated by a rapid and reliable bedside test for lung maturity so that occurrence of RDS could be predicted.

Relation of Surfactant to Antenatal Corticosteroid Administration

There is evidence in animal models that surfactant replacement is more effective in those treated with antenatal glucocorticoids (Ikegami et al, 1989; Seidner et al, 1988) and excellent clinical evidence in premature infants to support this position (Farrell et al, 1989; Jobe et al, 1993). The success of surfactant replacement is not reason for obstetricians to abandon antenatal glucocorticoid treatment. It is important to recognize that corticosteroids have a significant effect on the structural and functional maturity of the lung, in addition to their effect on the surfactant system; the development of the ion pumps responsible for lung water clearance and the development of the tight intercellular junctions responsible for decreased permeability to protein are accelerated by antenatal corticosteroid therapy (Jobe, 1991, 1992). In addition, steroids may have beneficial effects on other organ systems, such as the brain, the bowel, and the cardiovascular system. In a prospective controlled trial of prenatal dexamethasone for half the mothers and surfactant for all infants when necessary, Kari and associates (1994) found a significant reduction in the incidence of RDS, less severe RDS, much less intraventricular hemorrhage and periventricular leukomalacia, a more stable blood pressure, and increased survival without bronchopulmonary dysplasia in those treated with prenatal steroids.

Physiologic Effects of Surfactant

The most obvious effect of surfactant is an improvement in oxygenation, frequently within minutes, and the inspired oxygen can be reduced within 1 hour. Improved oxygenation is well correlated with improved lung volume (Alexander and Milner, 1995; Cotton et al, 1993; Svenningsen et al, 1992) and improved static lung compliance (Baraldi et al, 1993; Choukroun et al, 1994; Kelly et al, 1993), both of which occur rapidly and both of which mean increased recruitment of air spaces. The rapid increase in static lung compliance is reflected in the reductions of MAP, which can be made within a few hours of surfactant administration. From multiple measurements made in succession, however, Edberg and colleagues (1990) and Cotton (1994) made the observation that before these improvements in compliance occurred, there was a transient decrease in compliance. This was explained by early stabilization of air spaces that were open with inspiration but closed with expiration; after surfactant, these unstable air spaces were stabilized and remained open during expiration, so the V_T and compliance were transiently reduced. After this early change, more collapsed air spaces were recruited, and compliance increased. In another study of static lung compliance, it was emphasized that even though compliance improved rapidly, the improvement in oxygenation was even more rapid (de Winter et al, 1994); de Winter and colleagues speculated that improved oxygenation was initially due to better ventilation in open but poorly ventilated regions of the lung and that this would not immediately improve lung compliance. Pfenninger and coworkers (1992) found improved static lung compliance 12 hours after administration of Exosurf and a strong correlation between improved oxygenation and improved compliance.

In many studies that examined dynamic lung compliance in mechanically ventilated infants, no change was found after the administration of surfactant (Alexander and Milner, 1995; Armsby et al, 1992; Bhat et al, 1990; Bhutani et al, 1992; Couser et al, 1990; Kelly et al, 1993), which was puzzling. In another study, it was found that increased dynamic lung compliance occurred rapidly after surfactant administration if spontaneous breaths were evaluated (Davis et al, 1988), but increased dynamic lung compliance with ventilator breaths was delayed for 24 hours after surfactant, probably because ventilator breaths commonly produce alveolar overdistention (Bhutani et al, 1992).

Billman and colleagues (1994) have demonstrated a reduction of the $aA.D_{CO_2}$ with Exosurf, which indicates a smaller high V/Q compartment and better V/Q distribution with improved perfusion of normally ventilated alveoli. Bowen and colleagues (1994), however, were unable to demonstrate a reduction in the $aA.D_{N_2}$ with surfactant, which indicates that ultimately the main effect of exogenous surfactant is not in optimizing the distribution of ventilation and perfusion in open air spaces but in the recruitment of new, previously collapsed air spaces.

Adverse Effects of Surfactant

A transient reduction of mean blood pressure and cerebral blood flow has been described with surfactant administration (Cowan et al, 1991; Rey et al, 1994), and this may be followed by increased cerebral blood flow (van de Bor et al, 1991), probably related to an elevated arterial P_{CO_2} (Saliba et al, 1994). These changes may be accentuated by larger doses of surfactant or by a more rapid instillation rate. Others have described a brief but alarming cerebroelectric depression with surfactant administration (Hellstrom-Westas et al, 1992); this coincides with a sharp reduction of brain oxyhemoglobin, as assessed by near infrared spectroscopy (Skov et al, 1992). Others have described a reduced brain oxyhemoglobin, an increased brain deoxyhemoglobin, and an increased brain blood volume during surfactant administration (Fahnenstich et al, 1991). These phenomena may predispose treated infants to intraventricular hemorrhage. Surprisingly, however, there is no evidence for this in the results of multiple clinical trials (Gunkel and Banks, 1993; Pramanik et al, 1993), although in some trials the incidence of intraventricular hemorrhage was increased (Horbar et al, 1990), and in others it was decreased by surfactant (Fujiwara et al, 1990). It has been suggested that because RDS and intraventricular hemorrhage are associated, exogenous surfactant should reduce the incidence of intraventricular hemorrhage, but this has not been the case because of the above-mentioned problems during surfactant administration.

There appears to be an increased incidence of clinical pulmonary hemorrhage associated with surfactant replacement therapy (Raju and Langenberg, 1993), possibly as a result of increased left-to-right shunt flow at an open ductus arteriosus (Clyman et al, 1982). This has been confirmed in echocardiographic studies of premature infants (Seppanen et al, 1994). This effect must be only transient because in the longer term exogenous surfactant therapy is neither associated with an increased incidence of patent ductus arteriosus demonstrated by echocardiography (Reller et al, 1993) nor associated with an increased incidence of symptomatic patent ductus arteriosus requiring treatment (Corbet, 1993; Mercier and Soll, 1993). A study in which clinical pulmonary hemorrhage was strictly defined as bloody tracheal aspirate in the presence of new radiographic densities and increased ventilator requirements found a definite association with patent ductus arteriosus (Garland et al, 1994). It may be that the transient increase in left-to-right shunt flow is sufficient to precipitate a pulmonary hemorrhage in infants with capillary injury. Treatment with exogenous surfactant does not seem to help the capillary injury present in RDS (Jeffries et al, 1993). It remains to be seen whether prophylactic treatment with indomethacin for closure of the patent ductus arteriosus can reduce the incidence of clinical pulmonary hemorrhage after exogenous surfactant.

Poor Responses to Exogenous Surfactant

The data of Fujiwara and colleagues (1988) and Charon and coworkers (1989) indicated that about 65% of infants with RDS have a sustained improvement with exogenous surfactant, about 20% have a transient improvement followed by a relapse requiring further surfactant treatment, and about 15% do not have a significant response. It was not thought that uneven distribution of surfactant during instillation was an important problem. Good responses to surfactant are an index of survival (Hamvas et al, 1993; Kuint et al, 1994); in the case of Survanta, a poor response and the need for a fourth dose has been associated with the development of bronchopulmonary dysplasia (Sobel and Carroll, 1994).

There are several possible reasons for a poor response: (1) The patient may not have RDS; it may be necessary to consider another diagnosis, such as persistent pulmonary hypertension of the newborn, lung hypoplasia, bacterial pneumonia, or congenital heart disease, in those who do not respond to surfactant (Halliday, 1995b). (2) The patient may have RDS, but a severe complication in another organ may cause clinical deterioration, in particular, intraventricular hemorrhage (Easa et al, 1992). (3) The patient may have RDS, but there is an additional problem in the lung, such as pneumonia, interstitial emphysema, or pulmonary edema owing to patent ductus arteriosus or excessive fluid intake (Hallman, 1991). Kobayashi and associates (1991) demonstrated the importance of pulmonary edema in the inhibition of exogenous surfactant and the part played by plasma proteins that leak into the injured lung. Poor responders, before treatment, may have a higher airways resistance than good responders (Wallenbrock et al, 1992); this may reflect the general level of lung injury and lung edema. (4) The RDS may be so severe that the dose is insufficient; some have found poor responses to be associated with higher oxygen and pressure requirements during mechanical ventilation (Collaborative European Multicentre Study Group, 1991; Segerer et al, 1991). (5) It is possible that the ventilator settings may not be optimal. Hallman and colleagues (1993) thought that some clinicians used insufficient levels of PEEP. Schurch (1993) found that Exosurf needed to be cycled at 50 cpm for surface tension to reach zero in a captive bubble surfactometer and suggested that this preparation would function better at higher ventilator rates. (6) The surfactant preparation chosen may not be optimal. Ikegami and coworkers (1993) observed that exogenous surfactants were greatly improved, or activated, if they were first instilled in lamb lungs and then recovered and purified for testing in preterm rabbits; this was presumably due to the addition of endogenous surfactant proteins to the recovered exogenous surfactant (Holm, 1993).

Seeger and colleagues (1993) developed evidence that Curosurf and Survanta are more easily inhibited by plasma proteins in vitro than Infasurf and Alveofact; this may be related to the fact that the latter preparations contain significantly more SP-B and SP-C. In addition, SP-A is of particular importance in protecting surfactant lipids from inhibition by plasma proteins (Yukitake et al, 1995), and none of the presently available exogenous surfactants contain SP-A. When SP-A was added to Infasurf, there was a significant reduction in the sensitivity to inhibition by plasma proteins (Cockshutt et al, 1990). The supplementation of Survanta with SP-B isolated from sheep lungs greatly improves the function of Survanta in rabbit models (Mizuno et al, 1995). In the future, it seems likely that synthetic surfactants containing surfactant proteins or peptides will be developed with a view to minimizing inactivation and improving function.

Follow-Up Evaluation

Extensive and blinded developmental evaluation of treated and control infants enrolled in the trials of Exosurf indicated that there were no differences in the two groups at the age of 1 and 2 years (Corbet, 1993). The indices of general health; the measurements of growth; and the occurrence rates for mental retardation, cerebral palsy, blindness, and deafness were similar in the two groups; this was true whether the infants were treated in the prophylactic or in the rescue mode (Corbet et al, 1995a; Courtney et al, 1995). Most important, despite an increase in the number of survivors in the surfactant-treated group, there was not an absolute increase in the number of handicapped children; there was no evidence that surfactant replacement therapy would place an additional load on community services for handicapped children. The findings in other large-scale trials of other surfactants reached similar conclusions (Collaborative European Multicentre Study Group, 1992; Survanta Multidose Study Group, 1994).

Some patients have had lung mechanics evaluated at follow-up. Abbasi and coworkers (1993) found that infants treated with Exosurf had lower airways resistance and higher forced expiratory flow, indicating there was less injury to the conducting airways with surfactant treatment, but these findings were not confirmed in the Curosurf trials (Walti et al, 1992). In the Survanta trials, no improvements in treated children were found at 2 to 3 years of age.

Economic Analysis

Blinded prospective evaluations of hospital and physician charges were performed during the trials of Exosurf, but all the data are not yet available. For rescue treatment of infants with birth weight 700 to 1350 g (Mauskopf et al, 1995), hospital and physician charges for the 1st year of life were the same, normalized for 100 treated infants versus 100 control infants ($10.07 million versus $10.05 million), but there were 14 more survivors in the treated group. For rescue treatment of infants with birth weight more than 1250 g (Backhouse et al, 1994), hospital and physician charges for the 1st year of life were much lower, normalized per 100 treated infants versus 100 control infants ($4.98 million versus $6.27 million), and there were 3 more survivors in the treated group. If it is assumed that charges bear a constant relationship to costs, it can be stated that costs depend on the mix of smaller versus larger infants; hospitals with more larger infants have lower costs, and those with more smaller infants have similar costs with the introduction of exogenous surfactant therapy.

For prophylactic Exosurf treatment of infants with birth weight 700 to 1100 g, hospital and physician charges for the 1st year of life were increased, normalized for 100 treated infants versus 100 control infants ($14.68 million versus $12.82 million), but there were 11 more survivors in the treated group.

Egberts (1992) has estimated that for infants under 30 weeks' gestation, the optimal strategy is the combination of antenatal steroids followed by prophylactic surfactant. This strategy produces the greatest number of survivors and the lowest number of days in the hospital for each patient; this is the way a clinician should look at the problem. Mugford and associates (1991) estimated that if it were policy for all infants under 31 weeks' gestation to receive antenatal steroids and prophylactic surfactant, the cost per survivor would be reduced by 5% to 16%, but the increased survival as a result of the policy would cause the total cost to the British Health Service to increase by 7% to 32%; this is the way an economist might look at the problem.

Use of Exogenous Surfactant in Conditions Other than Respiratory Distress Syndrome

Surfactant therapy has been used with apparent success in neonatal bacterial pneumonia (Fetter et al, 1995), in meconium aspiration pneumonia (Auten et al, 1991), in congenital diaphragmatic hernia (Bos et al, 1991), and in acquired RDS affecting term infants (Gortner et al, 1994). None of the reports indicate whether surfactant therapy made a difference to the outcome, but in all there was improvement in the level of arterial oxygenation. In a well-designed controlled trial of infants on mechanical ventilation for meconium aspiration pneumonia, three doses of Survanta (each 150 mg/kg) resulted in a sustained reduction in oxygen and MAP requirements after the second dose of surfactant (Findlay et al, 1996). There were significant reductions in the incidence of air leak complications, in the need for ECMO, and in the length of oxygen and ventilator therapy in the treated infants, but the incidence of death and chronic bronchopulmonary dysplasia was not changed.

In congenital diaphragmatic hernia, there are data suggesting that a developmental deficiency of surfactant is present (Wilcox et al, 1994). In bacterial pneumonia, it is possible that RDS is also present at the same time. In addition, it is possible that inflammatory exudate may inactivate surfactant (Fetter et al, 1995). In meconium aspiration pneumonia, there is good evidence that meconium is responsible for surfactant inactivation (Clark et al, 1987; Moses et al, 1991); this is supported by the results in the above-mentioned controlled trial, in which the benefits were not apparent until the second dose was administered (Findlay et al, 1996). Because surfactant dysfunction is only part of the problem, however, it is doubtful that surfactant therapy will achieve the same success in improving the outcome of these disorders as it has in the treatment of RDS.

REFERENCES

Abbasi S, Bhutani VK, Gerdes JS: Long term pulmonary consequences of respiratory distress syndrome in preterm infants treated with exogenous surfactant. J Pediatr 122:446, 1993.

Abbasi S, Bhutani VK, Spitzer AR, Fox WW: Pulmonary mechanics in preterm neonates with respiratory failure treated with high frequency oscillatory ventilation compared with conventional mechanical ventilation. Pediatrics 87:487, 1991.

Adams JM, Murfin K, Mort J, et al: Detection of hyperoxemia in neonates by a new pulse oximeter. Neonat Intensive Care 7:42, 1994.

Alexander J, Milner AD: Lung volume and pulmonary blood flow measurements following exogenous surfactant. Eur J Pediatr 154:392, 1995.

Armsby DH, Bellon G, Carlisle K, et al: Delayed compliance increase in infants with respiratory distress syndrome following synthetic surfactant. Pediatr Pulmonol 14:206, 1992.

Auten RL, Notter RH, Kendig JW, et al: Surfactant treatment of full term newborns with respiratory failure. Pediatrics 87:101, 1991.

Backhouse ME, Mauskopf JA, Jones D, et al: Economic outcomes of colfosceril palmitate rescue therapy in infants weighing 1250 grams or more with respiratory distress syndrome. Pharmacoeconomics 6:358, 1994.

Bambang Oetomo S, Bos F, de Lei L, et al: Immune responses after surfactant treatment of newborn infants with respiratory distress syndrome. Biol Neonate 64:341, 1993.

Baraldi E, Pettenazzo A, Filippone M, et al: Rapid improvement of static compliance after surfactant treatment in preterm infants with respiratory distress syndrome. Pediatr Pulmonol 15:157, 1993.

Bartmann P, Jorch G, Pohlandt F, et al: Antibody response to bovine surfactant in preterm infants. Pediatr Res 29:203A, 1991.

Baumgart S, Hirschl RB, Butler SZ, et al: Diagnosis-related criteria in the consideration of extracorporeal membrane oxygenation in neonates previously treated with high-frequency jet ventilation. Pediatrics 89(3):491, 1992.

Bevilacqua G, Halliday H, Parmigiani S, Robertson B: Randomized multicentre trial of treatment with porcine natural surfactant for moderately severe neonatal respiratory distress syndrome. J Perinat Med 21:329, 1993.

Bhat R, Dziedzic K, Bhutani VK, et al: Effect of single dose surfactant on pulmonary function. Crit Care Med 18:590, 1990.

Bhutani VK, Abbasi S, Long WA, Gerdes JS: Pulmonary mechanics and energetics in preterm infants who had respiratory distress syndrome treated with synthetic surfactant. J Pediatr 120:S18, 1992.

Bhutani VK, Abbasi S, Silvieri EM: Continuous skeletal muscle paralysis: Effect on neonatal pulmonary mechanics. Pediatrics 81:419, 1988.

Billman D, Nicks J, Schumacher R: Exosurf rescue surfactant improves high ventilation perfusion mismatch in respiratory distress syndrome. Pediatr Pulmonol 18:279, 1994.

Bland RD, Kim MH, Light MJ, et al: High-frequency mechanical ventilation in severe hyaline membrane disease. Crit Care Med 8:275, 1980.

Boros SJ, Mammel MD, Coleman JM: Neonatal high-frequency jet ventilation: Four years' experience. Pediatrics 75:657, 1985.

Boros SJ, Matalon SV, Ewald R, et al: The effect of independent variations in inspiratory-expiratory ratio and end-expiratory pressure during mechanical ventilation in hyaline membrane disease: The significance of mean airway pressure. J Pediatr 91:794, 1977.

Bos AP, Tibboel D, Hazebroek FWJ, et al: Surfactant replacement in high risk congenital diaphragmatic hernia. Lancet 2:1297, 1991.

Bowen W, Martin CR, Krauss AN, et al: Ventilation perfusion relationships in preterm infants after surfactant treatment. Pediatr Pulmonol 18:155, 1994.

Bryan AC, Froese AB: Reflections on the HIFI trial. Pediatrics 87:565, 1991.

Brunstler I, Enders A, Versmold HT: Skin surface PCO2 monitoring in newborn infants in shock: Effect of hypotension and electrode temperature. J Pediatr 100:454, 1982.

Caplan MS, Cohn RA, Langman CB, et al: Favorable outcome of neonatal aortic thrombosis and renovascular hypertension. Pediatrics 115:291, 1989.

Carlo WA, Beoglos A, Chatburn RL, et al: High frequency jet ventilation in neonatal pulmonary hypertension. Am J Dis Child 143:233, 1989.

Carlo WA, Chatburn RL, Martin RJ, et al: Decrease in airway pressure during high frequency jet ventilation in infants with respiratory distress syndrome. J Pediatr 104:11, 1984.

Carter JM, Gerstmann DR, Clark RH, et al: High frequency oscillatory ventilation and extracorporeal membrane oxygenation for the treatment of acute neonatal respiratory failure. Pediatrics 85:159, 1990.

Chan V, Greenough A: Randomized controlled trial of weaning by patient triggered ventilation or conventional ventilation. Eur J Pediatr 152:51, 1993a.

Chan V, Greenough A: Determinants of oxygenation during high frequency oscillation. Eur J Pediatr 152:350, 1993b.

Chan V, Greenough A: Comparison of weaning by patient triggered ventilation or synchronous intermittent ventilation in preterm infants. Acta Paediatr 83:335, 1994a.

Chan V, Greenough A: Inspiratory and expiratory times for infants ventilator-dependent beyond the first week. Acta Paediatr 83:1022, 1994b.

Chan V, Greenough A, Gamsu HR: High frequency oscillation for preterm infants with severe respiratory failure. Arch Dis Child 70:F44, 1994a.

Chan V, Greenough A, Muramatsu K: Influence of lung function and reflex activity on the success of patient triggered ventilation. Early Hum Dev 37:9, 1994b.

Charon A, Taeusch HW, Fitzgibbon C, et al: Factors associated with surfactant treatment response in infants with severe respiratory distress syndrome. Pediatrics 83:348, 1989.

Chatburn RL: Physiologic and methodologic issues regarding humidity therapy. J Pediatr 114:416, 1989.

Chida S, Phelps DS, Soll RF, Taeusch HW: Surfactant proteins and anti-surfactant antibodies in sera from infants with respiratory distress syndrome with and without surfactant treatment. Pediatrics 88:84, 1991.

Choukroun ML, Llanas B, Apere H, et al: Pulmonary mechanics in ventilated preterm infants with respiratory distress syndrome after exogenous surfactant: A comparison between two surfactant preparations. Pediatr Pulmonol 18:273, 1994.

Chu J, Clements JA, Cotton EK, et al: Neonatal pulmonary ischemia: Clinical and physiological studies. Pediatrics 40(suppl):709, 1967.

Clark DA, Nieman GF, Thompson JE, et al: Surfactant displacement by meconium free fatty acids: An alternative explanation for atelectasis in meconium aspiration pneumonia. J Pediatr 110:765, 1987.

Clark RH, Gerstmann DR, Null DM, DeLemos RA: Prospective randomized comparison of high frequency oscillatory and conventional ventilation in respiratory distress syndrome. Pediatrics 89:5, 1992.

Clark RH, Yoder BA, Sell MS: Prospective randomized comparison of high frequency oscillation and conventional ventilation in candidates for extracorporeal membrane oxygenation. J Pediatr 124:447, 1994.

Cleary JP, Bernstein G, Mannino FL, Heldt GP: Improved oxygenation during synchronized intermittent mandatory ventilation in neonates with respiratory distress syndrome: A randomized crossover trial. J Pediatr 126:407, 1995.

Clyman RI, Jobe A, Heymann M, et al: Increased shunt through the patent ductus arteriosus after surfactant replacement therapy. J Pediatr 100:101, 1982.

Cochran WD: Umbilical artery catheterization. *In* Moore TD (Ed): Iatrogenic Problems in Neonatal Intensive Care. Proceedings of the 69th Ross Conference on Pediatric Research. Columbus, OH, Ross Laboratories, 1976, p 28.

Cockshutt AM, Weitz J, Possmeyer F: Pulmonary surfactant associated protein A enhances the surface activity of lipid extract surfactant and reverses inhibition by blood proteins in vitro. Biochemistry 36:8424, 1990.

Collaborative European Multicentre Study Group: Surfactant replacement therapy for severe neonatal respiratory distress syndrome: An international randomized clinical trial. Pediatrics 82:683, 1988.

Collaborative European Multicentre Study Group: Factors influencing the clinical response to surfactant replacement therapy in babies with severe respiratory distress syndrome. Eur J Pediatr 150:433, 1991.

Collaborative European Multicentre Study Group: A 2 year follow up of babies enrolled in a European multicentre trial of porcine surfactant replacement for severe neonatal respiratory distress syndrome. Eur J Pediatr 151:372, 1992.

Corbet A: Clinical trials of synthetic surfactant in the respiratory distress syndrome of premature infants. Clin Perinatol 20:737, 1993.

Corbet A, Bose C, Long W, et al: Double blind developmental evaluation at 1 year corrected age of 597 premature infants with birth weights 500–1350 grams enrolled in 3 placebo controlled trials of prophylactic surfactant. J Pediatr 126:S5, 1995a.

Corbet A, Bucciarelli R, Goldman S, et al: Decreased mortality rate among small premature infants treated at birth with a single dose of synthetic surfactant: A multicenter controlled trial. J Pediatr 118:277, 1991a.

Corbet A, Gerdes J, Long W, et al: Double blind randomized trial of one versus three prophylactic doses of synthetic surfactant in 826 700–1100 gram infants: Effects on mortality. J Pediatr 126:969, 1995b.

Corbet AJ, Long WA, Murphy DJ, et al: Reduced mortality in small premature infants treated at birth with a single dose of synthetic surfactant. J Pediatr Child Health 27:245, 1991b.

Corbet AJS, Ross JA, Beaudry PH, Stern L: Effect of positive pressure breathing on aA.DN2 in hyaline membrane disease. J Appl Physiol 38:33, 1975.

Cornish JD, Gertsmann DR, Clark RH, et al: Extracorporeal membrane oxygenation and high-frequency oscillatory ventilation: Potential therapeutic relationships. Crit Care Med 15(9):831, 1987.

Cotton RB: A model of the effect of surfactant treatment on gas exchange in hyaline membrane disease. Semin Perinatol 18:19, 1994.

Cotton RB, Olsson T, Law AB, et al: The physiologic effects of surfactant treatment on gas exchange in newborn premature infants with hyaline membrane disease. Pediatr Res 34:495, 1993.

Courtney SE, Long WA, McMillan D, et al: Double blind 1 year follow-up in 1540 infants with respiratory distress syndrome randomized to rescue treatment with 2 doses of synthetic surfactant or air in four clinical trials. J Pediatr 126:S43, 1995.

Couser RJ, Ferrara TB, Ebert J, et al: Effects of exogenous surfactant therapy on dynamic compliance during mechanical breathing in preterm infants with hyaline membrane disease. J Pediatr 116:119, 1990.

Cowan F, Whitelaw A, Wertheim D, Silverman M: Cerebral blood flow velocity changes after rapid administration of surfactant. Arch Dis Child 66:1105, 1991.

Cvetnic WG, Cunningham MD, Sills JH, Gluck L: Re-introduction of continuous negative pressure ventilation in neonates: Two year experience. Pediatr Pulmonol 8:245, 1990.

Davis JM, Russ GA, Metlay L, et al: Short term distribution kinetics of intratracheally administered exogenous lung surfactant. Pediatr Res 31:445, 1992.

Davis JM, Veness-Meehan K, Notter RH, et al: Changes in pulmonary mechanics after administration of surfactant to infants with respiratory distress syndrome. N Engl J Med 319:476, 1988.

de Winter JP, Merth IT, van Bel F, et al: Changes of respiratory system mechanics in ventilated lungs of preterm infants with two different schedules of surfactant treatment. Pediatr Res 35:541, 1994.

Donn SM, Nicks JJ, Becker MA: Flow synchronized ventilation of preterm infants with respiratory distress syndrome. J Perinatol 14:90, 1994.

Dreyfuss D, Saumon G: Should the lung be rested or recruited? The Charybdis and Scylla of ventilator management. Am J Respir Crit Care Med 149:1066, 1994.

Duke PM, Coulson JD, Santos JI, et al: Cleft palate associated with prolonged orotracheal intubation in infancy. J Pediatr 89:990, 1976.

Dunn MS, Shennan AT, Possmayer F: Single versus multiple dose surfactant replacement therapy in neonates of 30–36 weeks gestation with respiratory distress syndrome. Pediatrics 86:564, 1990.

Dunn MS, Shennan AT, Zayack D, et al: Bovine surfactant replacement therapy in neonates of less than 30 weeks gestation: A randomized controlled trial of prophylaxis versus treatment. Pediatrics 87:377, 1991.

Easa D, Pelke S, Nakamura KT, et al: Exosurf treatment investigational new drug phase: Effect of an individualized third dose in infants with respiratory distress syndrome. Pediatr Pulmonol 14:16, 1992.

Edberg KE, Ekstrom-Jodal B, Hallman M, et al: Immediate effects on lung function of instilled human surfactant in mechanically ventilated newborn infants with IRDS. Acta Paediatr Scand 79:750, 1990.

Egberts J: Estimated costs of different treatments of the respiratory distress syndrome in a large cohort of preterm infants of less than 30 weeks gestation. Biol Neonate 61(suppl 1):59, 1992.

Egberts J, deWinter JP, Sedin G, et al: Comparison of prophylaxis and rescue treatment with Curosurf in neonates less than 30 weeks gestation: A randomized trial. Pediatrics 92:768, 1993.

Emmrich P, Stechele U, Duc G, et al: Transcutaneous PO2 monitoring in routine management of infants and children with cardiorespiratory problems. Pediatrics 57:681, 1976.

Enhorning G, Grossman G, Robertson B: Tracheal deposition of surfactant before the first breath. Am Rev Respir Dis 107:921, 1973.

European Exosurf Study Group: Early or selective surfactant for intubated babies at 26–29 weeks gestation: A European double blind trial with sequential analysis. On-line J Curr Clin Trials Doc #28, 1992.

Fahnenstich H, Schmidt S, Spaniol S, et al: Relative changes in oxyhemoglobin, de-oxyhemoglobin and intracranial blood volume during surfactant replacement therapy in infants with respiratory distress syndrome. Dev Pharmacol Ther 17:150, 1991.

Farrell EE, Silver RK, Kimberlin LV, et al: Impact of antenatal dexamethasone administration on respiratory distress syndrome in surfactant treated infants. Am J Obstet Gynecol 161:628, 1989.

Feihl F, Perret C: Permissive hypercapnia: How permissive should we be? Am J Respir Crit Care Med 150:1722, 1994.

Ferrara TB, Hoekstra RE, Couser RJ, et al: Effects of surfactant therapy on outcome of infants with birth weights of 600–750 grams. J Pediatr 119:455, 1991.

Fetter WPF, Baerts W, Bos AP, van Lingen RA: Surfactant replacement therapy in neonates with respiratory failure due to bacterial sepsis. Acta Paediatr 84:14, 1995.

Findlay RD, Taeusch HW, Walther FJ: Surfactant replacement therapy for meconium aspiration syndrome. Pediatrics 97:48, 1996.

Frantz ID: Newer methods for treatment of respiratory distress. *In* Cowett RM, Hay WW (Eds): The Micropremie: The Next Frontier. Report of the 99th Ross Conference on Pediatric Research. Columbus, OH, Ross Laboratories, 1990, p 29.

Frantz ID, Werthammer J, Stark AR: High frequency ventilation in premature infants with lung disease: Adequate gas exchange at low tracheal pressure. Pediatrics 71:483, 1983.

Fredberg JJ, Glass GM, Boynton BR, et al: Factors influencing mechanical performances of neonatal high-frequency ventilators. J Appl Physiol 62:2485, 1987.

Froese AB, Bryan AD: High-frequency ventilation. Am Rev Respir Dis 135:1363, 1987.

Fujiwara T, Konishi M, Chida S, et al: Surfactant replacement therapy with a single postventilatory dose of a reconstituted bovine surfactant in preterm neonates with respiratory distress syndrome: Final analysis of a multicenter double blind randomized trial and comparison with similar trials. Pediatrics 86:753, 1990.

Fujiwara T, Konishi M, Chida S, Maeta H: Factors affecting the response to a postnatal single dose of a reconstituted bovine surfactant. *In* Lachmann B (Ed): Surfactant Replacement Therapy in Neonatal and Adult Respiratory Distress Syndrome. Berlin, Springer Verlag, 1988, p 91.

Fujiwara T, Maeta H, Chida S, et al: Artificial surfactant therapy in hyaline membrane disease. Lancet 1:55, 1980.

Garland J, Buck R, Weinberg M: Pulmonary hemorrhage risk in infants with a clinically diagnosed patent ductus arteriosus: A retrospective cohort study. Pediatrics 94:719, 1994.

Gaylord MS, Quissell BJ, Lair ME: High-frequency ventilation in the treatment of infants weighing less than 1,500 grams with pulmonary interstitial emphysema: A pilot study. Pediatrics 79:915, 1987.

Gertsmann DR, Minton SD, Stoddard RA, et al: The Provo Multicenter Early High-Frequency Oscillatory Ventilation Trial: Improved pulmonary and clinical outcome in respiratory distress syndrome. Pediatrics 98:1044, 1996.

Gortner L, Bartmann P, Pohlandt F, et al: Early treatment of respiratory distress syndrome with bovine surfactant in very preterm infants: A multicenter controlled clinical trial. Pediatr Pulmonol 14:4, 1992.

Gortner L, Bernsau U, Hellwege HH, et al: A multicenter randomized controlled trial of bovine surfactant for prevention of respiratory distress syndrome. Lung 168(suppl):864, 1990.

Gortner L, Pohlandt F, Bartmann P, et al: High dose versus low dose bovine surfactant treatment in very premature infants. Acta Paediatr 83:135, 1994.

Greisen G, Frederiksen PS, Hertel J, et al: Catecholamine response to chest physiotherapy and endotracheal suctioning in preterm infants. Acta Paediatr Scand 74:525, 1985.

Gunkel JH, Banks PLC: Surfactant therapy and intracranial hemorrhage: Review of the literature and results of new analyses. Pediatrics 92:775, 1993.

Halliday HL: Overview of clinical trials comparing natural and synthetic surfactants. Biol Neonate 67(suppl 1):32, 1995a.

Halliday HL: Surfactant replacement therapy. Pediatr Pulmonol 11:96, 1995b.

Halliday HL, Tarnow-Mordi WO, Corcoran JD, Patterson CC: Multicenter randomized trial comparing high and low dose surfactant regimens for the treatment of respiratory distress syndrome. Arch Dis Child 69:276, 1993.

Hallman M: Lung surfactant in respiratory distress syndrome. Acta Anaesthesiol Scand 35(suppl 95):15, 1991.

Hallman M, Merritt TA, Bry K, et al: Association between neonatal care practices and efficacy of exogenous human surfactant: Results of a bicenter randomized trial. Pediatrics 91:552, 1993.

Hamvas A, Devine T, Cole FS: Surfactant therapy failure identifies infants at risk for pulmonary mortality. Am J Dis Child 147:665, 1993.

Hansen TN, Corbet AJS, Kenny JD, et al: Effects of oxygen and constant positive pressure breathing on aA.DCO2 in hyaline membrane disease. Pediatr Res 13:1167, 1979.

Hansen TN, Tooley WH: Skin surface carbon dioxide tension in sick infants. Pediatrics 64:942, 1979.

Hanssler L, Tennhoff W, Roll C: Membrane humidification—a new method for humidification of respiratory gases in ventilator treatment of neonates. Arch Dis Child 67:1182, 1992.

Heicher DA, Kasting DS, Harrod JR: Prospective clinical comparison of two methods for mechanical ventilation of neonates: Rapid rate and short inspiratory time versus slow rate and long inspiratory time. J Pediatr 98:957, 1981.

Heldt GP, Merritt TA, Golembeski D, et al: Distribution of surfactant, lung compliance, and aeration of preterm rabbit lungs after surfactant therapy and conventional and high frequency oscillatory ventilation. Pediatr Res 31:270, 1992.

Hellstrom-Westas L, Bell AH, Skov L, et al: Cerebro-electric depression following surfactant treatment in preterm neonates. Pediatrics 89:643, 1992.

Herman S, Reynolds EOR: Methods for improving oxygenation in infants mechanically ventilated for severe hyaline membrane disease. Arch Dis Child 48:612, 1973.

HIFI Study Group: High frequency oscillatory ventilation compared with conventional mechanical ventilation in the treatment of respiratory failure in preterm infants. N Engl J Med 320:88, 1989.

HIFI Study Group: High frequency oscillatory ventilation compared with conventional intermittent mechanical ventilation in the treatment of respiratory failure in preterm infants: Neurodevelopmental status at 16–24 months of post term age. J Pediatr 117:939, 1990.

HIFO Study Group: Randomized study of high frequency oscillatory ventilation in infants with severe respiratory distress syndrome. J Pediatr 122:609, 1993.

Hird MF, Greenough A: Randomized trial of patient triggered ventilation versus high frequency positive ventilation in acute respiratory distress. J Perinat Med 19:379, 1991.

Hoekstra RE, Ferrara TB, Payne NR: Effects of surfactant therapy on outcome of extremely premature infants. Eur J Pediatr 153:S12, 1994.

Hoekstra RE, Jackson JC, Myers TF, et al: Improved neonatal survival following multiple doses of bovine surfactant in very premature neonates at risk for respiratory distress syndrome. Pediatrics 88:10, 1991.

Holm BA: Surfactant replacement therapy: New levels of understanding. Am Rev Respir Dis 148:834, 1993.

Horbar JD, Soll RF, Schachinger H, et al: A European multicenter randomized controlled trial of single dose surfactant therapy for idiopathic respiratory distress syndrome. Eur J Pediatr 149:416, 1990.

Horbar JD, Wright EC, Onstad L, et al: Decreasing mortality associated with the introduction of surfactant therapy: An observational study of neonates weighing 601–1300 grams at birth. Pediatrics 92:191, 1993a.

Horbar JD, Wright LL, Soll RF, et al: A multicenter randomized trial comparing two surfactants for the treatment of neonatal respiratory distress syndrome. J Pediatr 123:757, 1993b.

Huch R, Huch A, Albani M, et al: Transcutaneous Po₂ monitoring in routine management of infants and children with cardiorespiratory problems. Pediatrics 57(5):681, 1976.

Hudak ML, Matteson EJ, Baus JA, et al: Infasurf versus Exosurf for the treatment of RDS: A 21 center randomized double masked comparison trial (Abstract). Pediatr Res 35:231A, 1994.

Ikegami M, Jobe AH, Seidner S, Yamada T: Gestational effects of corticosteroids and surfactant in ventilated rabbits. Pediatr Res 25:32, 1989.

Ikegami M, Ueda T, Absolom D, et al: Changes in exogenous surfactant in ventilated preterm lamb lungs. Am Rev Respir Dis 148:837, 1993.

Jackson JC, Truog WE, Standaert TA, et al: Reduction in lung injury after combined surfactant and high frequency ventilation. Am J Respir Crit Care Med 150:534, 1994.

Jackson JC, Truog WE, Watchko JF, et al: Efficacy of thromboresistant umbilical artery catheters in reducing aortic thrombosis and related complications. J Pediatr 110:102, 1987.

Jeffries AL, Dunn MS, Possmayer F, Tai KFY: Radio-active Tc-DTPA clearance in preterm lambs: Effect of surfactant therapy and ventilation. Am Rev Respir Dis 148:845, 1993.

Jennis MS, Peabody JL: Pulse oximetry: An alternative method for the assessment of oxygenation in newborn infants. Pediatrics 79:524, 1987.

Jobe A: Pathogenesis of respiratory failure in the preterm infant. Ann Med 23:687, 1991.

Jobe A: Pulmonary surfactant therapy. N Engl J Med 328:861, 1993.

Jobe AH: Surfactant in the perinatal period. Early Hum Dev 29:57, 1992.

Jobe AH, Mitchell BR, Gunkel JH, et al: Beneficial effects of the combined use of prenatal steroids and postnatal surfactant on preterm infants. Am J Obstet Gynecol 168:508, 1993.

Jonzon A, Oberg PA, Sedin G, et al: High-frequency positive-pressure ventilation by endotracheal insufflation. Acta Anaesthesiol Belg 43(suppl):1, 1971.

Jung AL, Thomas GK: Stricture of the nasal vestibule: A complication of nasotracheal intubation in newborn infants. J Pediatr 85:412, 1974.

Kano S, Lanteri CJ, Pemberton PJ, et al: Fast versus slow ventilation for neonates. Am Rev Respir Dis 148:578, 1993.

Kari MA, Hallman M, Eronen M, et al: Prenatal dexamethasone treatment in conjunction with rescue therapy of human surfactant: A randomized placebo controlled multicenter study. Pediatrics 93:730, 1994.

Kattwinkel J, Bloom BT, Delmore P, et al: Prophylactic administration of calf lung surfactant extract is more effective than early treatment of respiratory distress syndrome in newborns of 29 through 32 weeks gestation. Pediatrics 92:90, 1993.

Kelly E, Bryan H, Possmayer F, et al: Compliance of the respiratory system in newborn infants pre and post surfactant replacement therapy. Pediatr Pulmonol 15:225, 1993.

Kendig JW, Notter RH, Cox C, et al: A comparison of surfactant as immediate prophylaxis and as rescue therapy in newborns of less than 30 weeks gestation. N Engl J Med 324:865, 1991.

Keszler M, Donn SM, Bucciarelli RL, et al: Multicenter controlled trial comparing high frequency jet ventilation and conventional mechanical ventilation in newborn infants with pulmonary interstitial emphysema. J Pediatr 119:85, 1991.

Kobayashi T, Nitta K, Ganzuka M, et al: Inactivation of exogenous surfactant by pulmonary edema fluid. Pediatr Res 29:353, 1991.

Konishi M, Fujiwara T, Chida S, et al: A prospective randomized trial of early versus late administration of a single dose of surfactant TA. Early Hum Dev 29:275, 1992.

Konishi M, Fujiwara T, Naito T, et al: Surfactant replacement therapy in neonatal respiratory distress syndrome: A multicenter randomized clinical trial: Comparison of high versus low doses of surfactant TA. Eur J Pediatr 147:20, 1988.

Kraybill EN, Runyan DK, Bose CL, Khan JH: Risk factors for chronic lung disease in infants with birth weights 751 to 1000 grams. J Pediatr 115:115, 1989.

Kuint J, Reichman B, Neumann L, et al: Prognostic value of the immediate response to surfactant. Arch Dis Child 71:F170, 1994.

Landers S, Hansen TN: Skin surface oxygen monitoring. Perinatol Neonatol 8:39, 1994.

Landers S, Hansen TN, Corbet AJS, et al: Optimal constant positive airway pressure assessed by aADCO2 in hyaline membrane disease. Pediatr Res 20:884, 1986.

Lesouef PN, England SJ, Bryan AC: Total resistance of the respiratory system in preterm infants with and without an endotracheal tube. J Pediatr 104:108, 1984.

Liechty EA, Donovan E, Purohit D, et al: Reduction of neonatal mortality after multiple doses of bovine surfactant in low birth weight neonates with respiratory distress syndrome. Pediatrics 88:19, 1991.

Long WA, Corbet A, Cotton R, et al: A controlled trial of synthetic surfactant in infants weighing 1250 grams or more with respiratory distress syndrome. N Engl J Med 325:1696, 1991a.

Long WA, Thompson T, Sundell H, et al: Effects of two doses of a synthetic surfactant on mortality rate and survival without bronchopulmonary dysplasia in 700–1350 gram infants with respiratory distress syndrome. J Pediatr 118:595, 1991b.

Mammel MC, Gordon MJ, Connett JE, et al: Comparison of high-frequency jet ventilation and conventional mechanical ventilation in a meconium aspiration model. J Pediatr 103:630, 1983.

Mauskopf JA, Backhouse ME, Jones D, et al: Synthetic surfactant for rescue treatment of respiratory distress syndrome in premature infants weighing from 700–1350 grams: Impact on hospital resource use and charges. J Pediatr 126:94, 1995.

McMillan DD, Rademaker AW, Buchan KA, et al: Benefits of orotracheal and nasotracheal intubation in neonates requiring ventilatory assistance. Pediatrics 77:39, 1986.

Mercier CE, Soll RF: Clinical trials of natural surfactant extract in respiratory distress syndrome. Clin Perinatol 20:711, 1993.

Merritt TA, Hallman M , Berry C, et al: Randomized placebo controlled trial of human surfactant given at birth versus rescue administration in very low birth weight infants with lung immaturity. J Pediatr 118:581, 1991.

Miller KE, Edwards DK, Hilton S, et al: Acquired lobar emphysema in premature infants with bronchopulmonary dysplasia: An iatrogenic disease? Pediatr Radiol 138:589, 1981.

Mizuno K, Ikegami M, Chen CM, et al: Surfactant protein B supplementation improves in vivo function of a modified natural surfactant. Pediatr Res 37:271, 1995.

Moise A, Landers S, Fraley K: Colonization and infection of umbilical catheters in newborn infants. Pediatr Res 20:400A, 1986.

Morley CJ, Greenough A, Miller NG, et al: Randomized Trial of Artificial Surfactant (ALEC) given at birth to babies from 23 to 34 weeks' gestation. Early Hum Dev 17(1):41, 1988.

Moses D, Holm BA, Spitale P, et al: Inhibition of pulmonary surfactant function by meconium. Am J Obstet Gynecol 164:477, 1991.

Moylan FMB, Seldin EB, Shannon DC, et al: Defective primary dentition in survivors of neonatal mechanical ventilation. J Pediatr 96:106, 1980.

Mugford M, Piercy J, Chalmers I: Cost implications of different approaches to the prevention of respiratory distress syndrome. Arch Dis Child 66:757, 1991.

Neal WA, Reynolds JW, Jarvis CW, et al: Umbilical artery catheterization: Demonstration of arterial thrombosis by aortography. Pediatrics 50:6, 1972.

Norsted T, Jonzon A, Sedin G: Pancuronium bromide does not lower airway pressures during intermittent positive pressure ventilation in young cats. Acta Anaesthesiol Scand 33:21, 1985.

Ogawa Y, Miyasaka K, Kawano T, et al: A multicenter randomized trial of high frequency oscillatory ventilation as compared with conventional mechanical ventilation in preterm infants with respiratory failure. Early Hum Dev 32:1, 1993.

OSIRIS Collaborative Group: Early versus delayed neonatal administration of a synthetic surfactant: The judgement of OSIRIS. Lancet 340:1363, 1992.

Oxford Region Controlled Trial of Artificial Ventilation Study Group: Multicentre randomised controlled trial of high against low frequency positive pressure ventilation. Arch Dis Child 66:770, 1991.

Paranka MS, Clark RH, Yoder BA, et al: Predictors of failure of high frequency oscillatory ventilation in term infants with severe respiratory failure. Pediatrics 95:400, 1995.

Pardou A, Vermeylen D, Muller MF, Detemmerman D: High frequency ventilation and conventional mechanical ventilation in newborn babies with respiratory distress syndrome: A prospective randomized trial. Intensive Care Med 19:406, 1993.

Pfenninger J, Aebi C, Bachmann D, Wagner BP: Lung mechanics and gas exchange in ventilated preterm infants during treatment of hyaline membrane disease with multiple doses of artificial surfactant (Exosurf). Pediatr Pulmonol 14:10, 1992.

Pietsch JG, Nagaraj HS, Groff DB, et al: Necrotizing tracheobronchitis: A new indication for emergency bronchoscopy in the neonate. J Pediatr Surg 20:391, 1985.

Pologe JA: Pulse oximetry: Technical aspects of machine design. Int Anesthesiol Clin 25:137, 1987.

Pramanik AK, Holtzman RB, Merritt TA: Surfactant replacement therapy for pulmonary diseases. Pediatr Clin North Am 40:913, 1993.

Primhak RA: Factors associated with pulmonary air leak in premature infants receiving mechanical ventilation. J Pediatr 102:764, 1983.

Raju TNK, Langenberg P: Pulmonary hemorrhage and exogenous surfactant therapy: A meta-analysis. J Pediatr 123:603, 1993.

Ramanathan R, Durand M, Larazabal C: Pulse oximetry in very low birthweight infants with acute and chronic lung disease. Pediatrics 79:612, 1987.

Reller MD, Rice MJ, McDonald RW: Review of studies evaluating ductal patency in the premature infant. J Pediatr 122:S59, 1993.

Rennie JM, South M, Morley CJ: Cerebral blood flow velocity in infants receiving assisted ventilation. Arch Dis Child 62:1247, 1987.

Rey M, Segerer H, Kiessling C, et al: Surfactant bolus instillation: Effects of different doses on blood pressure and cerebral blood flow velocities. Biol Neonate 66:16, 1994.

Richardson P, Pace WR, Valdes E, et al: Time dependence of lung mechanics in preterm lambs. Pediatr Res 31:276, 1992.

Robertson B, Enhorning G: The alveolar lining of the premature newborn rabbit after pharyngeal deposition of surfactant. Lab Invest 31:54, 1974.

Robillard E, Alarie Y, Dagenais-Perusse P, et al: Micro-aerosol administration of synthetic di-palmitoyl lecithin in the respiratory distress syndrome: A preliminary report. Can Med Assoc J 90:55, 1964.

Rollins M, Jenkins J, Tubman R, et al: Comparison of clinical responses to natural and synthetic surfactants. J Perinat Med 21:341, 1993.

Saliba E, Nashashibi M, Vaillant MC, et al: Instillation rate effects of Exosurf on cerebral and cardiovascular hemodynamics in preterm neonates. Arch Dis Child 71:F174, 1994.

Schurch S: Surface tension properties of surfactant. Clin Perinatol 20:669, 1993.

Seeger W, Grube C, Gunther A, Schmidt R: Surfactant inhibition by plasma proteins: Differential sensitivity of various surfactant preparations. Eur Respir J 6:971, 1993.

Segerer H, Stevens P, Schadow B, et al: Surfactant substitution in ventilated very low birth weight infants: Factors related to response types. Pediatr Res 30:591, 1991.

Segerer H, van Gelder W, Angenent FWM, et al: Pulmonary distribution and efficacy of exogenous surfactant in lung lavaged rabbits are influenced by the instillation technique. Pediatr Res 34:490, 1993.

Seidner S, Pettenazzo A, Ikegami M, Jobe AH: Corticosteroid potentiation of surfactant dose response in preterm rabbits. J Appl Physiol 64:2366, 1988.

Seppanen M, Kaapa P, Kero P: Acute effects of synthetic surfactant replacement on pulmonary blood flow in neonatal respiratory distress syndrome. Am J Perinatol 11:382, 1994.

Sherman JM, Lowitt S, Stephenson C, et al: Factors influencing acquired subglottic stenosis in infants. J Pediatr 109:322, 1986.

Simbruner G: Inadvertent positive end-expiratory pressure in mechanically ventilated newborn infants: Detection and effect on lung mechanics and gas exchange. J Pediatr 108:589, 1986.

Simbruner G, Coradello H, Fodor M, et al: Effect of tracheal suction on oxygenation, circulation, and lung mechanics in newborn infants. Arch Dis Child 56:326, 1981.

Skov L, Hellstrom-Westas L, Jacobsen T, et al: Acute changes in cerebral oxygenation and cerebral blood volume in preterm infants during surfactant treatment. Neuropediatrics 23:126, 1992.

Slutsky AS: Nonconventional methods of ventilation. Am Rev Respir Dis 138:175, 1988.

Sobel DB, Carroll A: Post surfactant slump: Early prediction of neonatal chronic lung disease. J Perinatol 14:268, 1994.

Speer CP, Gefeller O, Groneck P, et al: Randomized clinical trial of two treatment regimens of natural surfactant preparations in neonatal respiratory distress syndrome. Arch Dis Child 72:F8, 1995.

Speer CP, Robertson B, Curstedt T, et al: Randomized European multicenter trial of surfactant replacement therapy for severe neonatal respiratory distress syndrome: Single versus multiple doses of Curosurf. Pediatrics 89:13, 1992.

Stenson BJ, Glover RM, Parry GJ, et al: Static respiratory compliance in the newborn: 3. Early changes after exogenous surfactant treatment. Arch Dis Child 70:F19, 1994.

Stevenson D, Walther F, Long W, et al: Controlled trial of a single dose of synthetic surfactant at birth in premature infants weighing 500–699 grams. J Pediatr 120:S3, 1992.

Stewart AR, Finer NN, Peters KL: Effects of alteration of inspiratory and expiratory pressures and inspiratory/expiratory ratios on mean airway pressure, blood gases, and intracranial pressure. Pediatrics 67:474, 1981.

Strayer DS, Merritt TA, Hallman M: Levels of SP-A/anti SP-A immune complexes in neonatal respiratory distress syndrome correlate with subsequent development of bronchopulmonary dysplasia. Acta Paediatr 84:128, 1995.

Survanta Multidose Study Group: Two year followup of infants treated for neonatal respiratory distress syndrome with bovine surfactant. J Pediatr 124:962, 1994.

Svenningsen NW, Bjorklund L, Vilstrup C, et al: Lung mechanics (FRC and static pressure volume diagram) after endotracheal surfactant instillation: Preliminary observations. Biol Neonate 61(suppl 1):44, 1992.

Tarnow-Mordi WO, Griffiths ERP, Wilkinson AR: Low inspired gas temperature and respiratory complications in very low birth weight infants. J Pediatr 114:438, 1989.

Tarnow-Mordi WO, Soll RF: Artificial versus natural surfactant: Can we base clinical practice on a firm scientific foundation? Eur J Pediatr 153:S17, 1994.

Ten Center Study Group: Ten center trial of artificial surfactant (ALEC) in premature babies. BMJ 294:991, 1987.

Trindade W, Goldberg RN, Bancalari E, et al: Conventional versus high frequency jet ventilation in a piglet model of meconium aspiration: Comparison of pulmonary and hemodynamic effects. Pediatrics 107:115, 1985.

van de Bor M, Ma EJ, Walther FJ: Cerebral blood flow velocity after surfactant instillation in preterm infants. J Pediatr 118:285, 1991.

van der Bleek J, Plotz FB, van Overbeek FM, et al: Distribution of exogenous surfactant in rabbits with severe respiratory failure: The effect of volume. Pediatr Res 34:154, 1993.

Vermont-Oxford Neonatal Network: A multicenter randomized trial comparing synthetic surfactant with modified bovine surfactant extract in the treatment of neonatal respiratory distress syndrome. Pediatrics 97:1, 1996.

Visveshwara N, Freeman B, Peck M, et al: Patient triggered synchronized assisted ventilation of newborns: Report of a preliminary study and 3 years experience. J Perinatol 11:347, 1991.

Wallenbrock MA, Sekar KC, Toubas PL: Prediction of the acute response to surfactant therapy by pulmonary function. Pediatr Pulmonol 13:11, 1992.

Walti H, Boule M, Moriette G, Relier JP: Pulmonary functional outcome at one year of age in infants treated with natural porcine surfactant at birth. Biol Neonate 61(suppl 1):48, 1992.

Whitsett JA, Hull WM, Luse S, et al: Failure to detect surfactant protein specific antibodies in sera of premature infants treated with Survanta, a modified bovine surfactant. Pediatrics 87:505, 1991.

Wilcox DT, Glick PL, Karamanoukian H, et al: Pathophysiology of congenital diaphragmatic hernia: 5. Effect of exogenous surfactant therapy on gas exchange and lung mechanics in the lamb congenital diaphragmatic hernia model. J Pediatr 124:289, 1994.

Wiswell TE, Graziani LJ, Kornhauser MS, et al: High frequency jet ventilation in the early management of respiratory distress syndrome is associated with a greater risk for adverse outcomes. Pediatrics 98:1035, 1996.

Wukitsch MW: Pulse oximetry: Historical review and Ohmeda functional analysis. Int J Clin Monit Comput 4:161, 1987.

Wung JT, Driscoll JM, Epstein RA, et al: A new device for CPAP by nasal route. Crit Care Med 3:76, 1975.

Yukitake K, Brown CL, Schlueter MA, et al: Surfactant apoprotein A modifies the inhibitory effect of plasma proteins on surfactant activity in vivo. Pediatr Res 37:21, 1995.

Zola EM, Gunkel JH, Chan RK, et al: Comparison of three dosing procedures for administration of bovine surfactant to neonates with respiratory distress syndrome. J Pediatr 122:453, 1993.

CHAPTER 52

Therapies for Intractable Respiratory Failure

Michael Gomez, Thomas Hansen and Anthony Corbet

Although remarkable improvement has occurred in the ability to provide care for infants with respiratory failure using mechanical ventilation, a number of additional approaches to care of the infants with intractable respiratory failure are being developed. The most used (but not the best studied) of these is extracorporeal membrane oxygenation (ECMO). Additional areas of current investigation include the use of inhaled nitric oxide (iNO) and liquid ventilation with perfluorocarbon.

EXTRACORPOREAL MEMBRANE OXYGENATION

A group of infants with severe lung disease, progressive respiratory failure, and life-threatening hypoxemia, who do not respond to maximal ventilatory support, may be considered for ECMO as a treatment of last resort. This is a highly invasive procedure and should not be started without good reason. Physicians using ECMO should review their own experience and determine appropriate criteria for selecting infants with at least an 80% risk of death from their condition. Most centers report that about 80% of such infants survive when treated with ECMO.

Conduct of Extracorporeal Membrane Oxygenation

The system consists of a venous pressure control module, a roller pump, a countercurrent membrane oxygenator, and a heat exchanger, connected in series and primed with heparinized buffered blood (Short and Pearson, 1986) (Fig. 52–1). A catheter (14 French) is inserted in the right internal jugular vein with its tip in the right atrium, and another catheter (8 to 12 French) is inserted in the right common carotid artery with its tip in the arch of the aorta. The infant is given a bolus dose of heparin (50 units/kg) and connected to the system, with venous blood drained by gravity from the right atrium and fully oxygenated blood infused at the aorta. The heart and lungs, to a variable extent, are bypassed. The venous control module regulates the operation of the pump, insuring that the venous drainage from the patient and the pump output to the patient are balanced. Over 30 minutes, the flow is slowly increased to about 120 to 150 mL/kg per minute, after which the mechanical ventilator can be reduced to benign settings, 25% to 30% oxygen, 15 to 20 cm H_2O peak pressure, positive end-expiratory pressure (PEEP) 5 cm H_2O, and a rate of 10 breaths/min (Bartlett et al, 1985), designed to allow the lung comparative rest. Keszler and coworkers (1992) demonstrated that use of a higher PEEP was associated with more rapid recovery of the lung. The arterial oxygen pressure can be maintained between 50 and 70 mm Hg by adjusting the ECMO flow. The venous oxygen saturation may be used to assess the overall level of oxygen-

ation, values below 70% suggesting that the cardiac output may not be sufficient. Heparinization is continued by an adjustable infusion, starting at 40 units/kg per hour, to maintain the activated clotting time at 180 to 220 seconds, up to two times longer than normal. In addition, packed red blood cells are transfused to maintain the hematocrit above 40%, platelets are transfused to maintain the platelet count above 100,000/mm³, and fresh frozen plasma is transfused to maintain the fibrinogen level above 200 mg/dL.

The ECMO flow can usually be weaned to about 90 to 100 mL/kg per minute on the 1st day. An improvement of lung function may be recognized by periodic bag-tube ventilation with increased lung compliance and increased pulse oximeter saturation. After 4 to 5 days, the ECMO flow is further reduced, and the ventilator settings are again increased to assume responsibility for gas exchange. Ideally the settings should be comparatively benign, such as 40% to 50% oxygen, rate 40 to 60 breaths/min, PEEP 5 to 7 cm H_2O, and peak inflation pressure 20 to 25 cm H_2O. After a brief period at a low ECMO flow (30 mL/kg per minute), to ensure adequate pulmonary function, the infant can be decannulated and the vessels ligated; it is usual to place a Broviac central venous line in the right external jugular vein at this time for the purpose of continued parenteral nutrition.

Patient Selection

Patients with meconium aspiration pneumonia, respiratory distress syndrome, neonatal pneumonia, congenital dia-

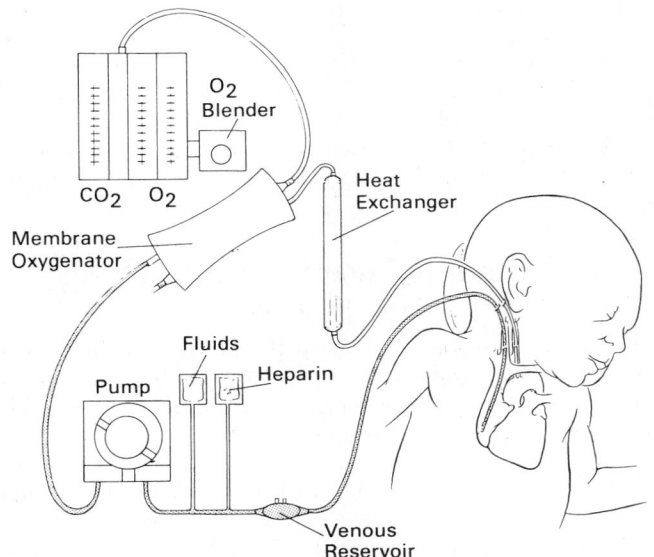

FIGURE 52–1. Extracorporeal membrane oxygenation (ECMO) system. (From Short BL, Miller MK, Anderson KD: Extracorporeal membrane oxygenation in the management of respiratory failure in the newborn. Clin Perinatol 14:737, 1987.)

phragmatic hernia, and persistent pulmonary hypertension of the newborn are prime candidates for this therapy. Because of systemic heparinization, infants weighing less than 2000 g and less than 34 weeks' gestation have a high incidence of cerebral hemorrhage (Cilley et al, 1986) and should be excluded, as should larger infants if they already have evidence for cerebral hemorrhage or cerebral infarction. All patients should have a head ultrasound examination before starting ECMO. Those who are older than 7 days and have been exposed to prolonged mechanical ventilation with oxygen are not good candidates because their lung disease may not be reversible; some centers, however, try ECMO in infants ventilated as long as 10 days. Infants with severe malformations should be excluded. A thorough search for congenital heart disease should be made with echocardiography before ECMO (Palmisano et al, 1992), and occasionally it is necessary to have an emergency chromosome analysis performed in patients with dysmorphic features.

The definition of life-threatening hypoxemia, sufficient to justify ECMO, is highly controversial among neonatal centers. A stringent criterion is that the arterial/alveolar oxygen ratio must be less than 0.04 (Ortega et al, 1988), which corresponds to an arterial PO_2 of less than 30 torr on maximal ventilator support. Other centers prefer to use the less stringent oxygenation index, the product of three factors: (1) the percent oxygen, (2) the mean airway pressure, and (3) the reciprocal of arterial PO_2 (Keszler et al, 1992). Values of 40 or more for 3 hours are considered reliable indications for ECMO, but many infants meeting this criterion may have an arterial PO_2 greater than 50 torr. Another criterion frequently used is an alveolar/arterial oxygen difference of 610 torr, but many infants may have an arterial PO_2 greater than 50 torr, especially if the arterial PCO_2 is low. In the authors' current practice, most patients who are placed on ECMO have an arterial PO_2 that is less than 40 torr. When the arterial oxygen tension is this low, despite intensive medical therapy, there is an increased risk that anaerobic metabolism may result in severe metabolic acidosis, and this increases the likelihood of either death or significant morbidity. Patients with an arterial PO_2 of more than 40 torr have a normal acid-base status and no evidence of anaerobic metabolism (Torrance and Wittnich, 1992) showed that metabolic acidemia did not develop in newborn piglets until the arterial PO_2 was reduced significantly below 40 torr.

Alternatives to Extracorporeal Membrane Oxygenation

The ability to manage infants with severe pulmonary disease has been significantly improved in the past few years using conventional mechanical ventilation (Wung et al, 1985); it is inherent in this approach that arterial PO_2 levels of 40 to 49 torr are often accepted. Dworetz and co-workers (1989) reviewed the experience at Yale with infants who met oxygen index criteria for ECMO; they found that in 1980–1981 only 1 of every 6 such infants survived, whereas in 1986–1988 9 out of 10 such infants survived in their center. This raises serious concerns about the appropriateness of ECMO criteria devised in earlier times. There is suggestive evidence that iNO may reduce the

need for ECMO by about one third in those newborn infants with echocardiographic evidence of persistent pulmonary hypertension (see later). At present, it appears that at least 50% of patients meeting oxygen index criteria for ECMO can be effectively treated with high-frequency oscillator ventilation or high-frequency jet ventilation; this is especially true for infants with respiratory distress syndrome or neonatal pneumonia. It seems prudent that high-frequency ventilation for ECMO candidates should be used only in ECMO centers because it may be difficult to transport patients failing high-frequency ventilation in a non-ECMO center (Walsh-Sukys et al, 1994); unfortunately, this recommendation is widely ignored. In addition to high-frequency ventilation, there is some evidence that conventional mechanical ventilation with lung distention achieved by constant negative pressure around the chest may also be an effective rescue procedure before ECMO (Cvetnic et al, 1990). In the near future, partial liquid ventilation with perfluorocarbons may become a practical alternative to ECMO.

Efficacy of Extracorporeal Membrane Oxygenation

The efficacy of ECMO was assessed in a randomized, controlled trial in adult patients and was found not to be superior to conventional therapy (Zapol et al, 1979). There have been two North American attempts to conduct a randomized, controlled trial of ECMO in newborn infants. In the first (Bartlett et al, 1985), an unusual trial design resulted in a small control group, only one patient, so the results in favor of ECMO were widely discounted. In the second controlled trial (O'Rourke et al, 1989), more appropriately randomized, 6 of 10 infants survived with conventional mechanical ventilation, and 9 of 9 infants survived with ECMO. Although this difference was not significant, further enrollment into the ECMO group suggested superior results with ECMO. Both these trials reflected the bias of investigators in favor of ECMO. In the second trial, the mortality in controls was much lower than the 80% expected. It is now unlikely that a good randomized, controlled trial will be conducted in North America, where ECMO has become almost universally accepted. A controlled trial in Britain demonstrated better survival in infants with intractable respiratory failure with the use of ECMO (UK Collaborative ECMO Trial Group, 1996). Of 93 patients allocated randomly to ECMO, 3 improved and did not need ECMO, 5 were excluded (most for congenital heart disease), 7 died before ECMO could be started, and 78 were treated with ECMO. There were 30 deaths in these 93 patients (32% mortality), compared with 54 deaths among 92 control subjects who were not allocated to ECMO (59% mortality), a significantly better result. The improvement was most noticeable among those with idiopathic persistent pulmonary hypertension, but it was significant in those with meconium-aspiration pneumonia, and even in those with congenital diaphragmatic hernia. The economic analysis of ECMO indicates that although daily charges are higher in ECMO patients than in comparable patients not treated with ECMO, nevertheless overall costs are reduced with ECMO because, taking into account both survivors and nonsurvivors, the length of stay is reduced from 37 days to 21 days (Pearson and Short, 1986).

Outcome in Extracorporeal Membrane Oxygenation

There has been much concern about the long-term outcome of these infants. Schumacher (1993) reviewed multiple reports and found that 81% of 643 patients followed were considered to be normal, 7% had borderline abnormalities, and 12% had serious disabilities. These results are considered to be as good as, and possibly better than, the results in infants with the same conditions treated without ECMO (Klein and Whittlesey, 1994; Schumacher, 1993).

Problems with Extracorporeal Membrane Oxygenation

Because ECMO is an invasive procedure and because contact of blood with a plastic surface sets off a massive release of potent mediators, there are a large number of associated problems, some of which are discussed briefly:

1. The circuit must be constantly observed for large air bubbles and clots, which, if present on the arterial side of the circuit, may embolize into the patient's systemic circulation with potentially disastrous results. Some centers use a trap on the patient's side of the circuit. In addition, an unnoticed disconnection anywhere in the circuit may rapidly cause hemorrhagic shock, so constant vigilance is necessary.

2. If the patient is given too much heparin, there may be hemorrhagic complications, such as bleeding at the operative site, bleeding into the brain, bleeding into the peritoneal or pleural space, or gastrointestinal bleeding. The use of cautery and fibrin glue at the surgical site or the use of systemic aminocaproic acid (Amicar) may help lessen the incidence of hemorrhage. In some cases, the patient may develop excessive consumption of coagulation factors, as the plastic surface of the circuit becomes coated with multiple fibrin thrombus layers; this may become so serious that decannulation or a change of the circuit may be necessary. The level of fibrin split products should remain less than 10 μg/mL during routine ECMO.

3. The patient may develop a low cardiac output, which does not increase when ECMO flow is reduced and which may prolong the length of time on ECMO; this condition is known as the *cardiac stun syndrome* (Hirschl et al, 1992). The reason for this problem may be twofold: that coronary perfusion is dependent on poorly oxygenated left ventricular blood (Kinsella et al, 1992a) and that retrograde flow from the aortic catheter may increase the afterload resistance to left ventricular ejection. This condition should not be confused with the universal reduction of cardiac output and myocardial contractility that occurs because the heart is unloaded in venoarterial ECMO (Kimball et al, 1991).

4. Within a few hours of starting ECMO, the lungs frequently develop a diffuse dense opacification and further loss of compliance; this is thought to be caused by high-permeability pulmonary edema, possibly secondary to activated complement fragments and increased leukotriene production. This pulmonary edema improves within a few days, especially if high PEEP levels are maintained (Keszler et al, 1992). Because surfactant may be inactivated by pulmonary edema fluid, exogenous surfactant therapy may be helpful (Lotze et al, 1993).

5. The urine output often decreases dramatically on ECMO, and the patient may become edematous. As in the case of the lungs, the edema is probably caused by capillary injury from activated complement fragments and increased leukotriene production. This injury cascade leads to hypotension and frequent infusions of colloid to raise the blood pressure; these infusions are in addition to those given to maintain the hematocrit, platelet, and fibrinogen levels. As the capillary injury improves after a few days, the edema may be treated with loop diuretics, but sometimes hemofiltration becomes necessary, especially if pulmonary edema fails to resolve.

6. The use of the carotid artery for cannulation and its ligation at the time of decannulation have raised much concern about the circulation to the brain and the possibility of brain injury. Schumacher and colleagues (1988) reported an increased incidence of right-sided ischemic lesions of the brain, and Mendoza and coworkers (1991) reported more ischemic lesions on the right side and more hemorrhagic lesions on the left side of the brain, but other data do not support these findings (Campbell et al, 1988). In some centers, the carotid artery is reconstructed at the time of decannulation, and this can be accomplished without increasing the risk for brain injury (Taylor et al, 1992). Baumgart and colleagues (1994) found using color-coded Doppler imaging that the brain blood flow profile was improved with this procedure, but head computed tomography scans before discharge and neurodevelopmental status at age 1 year did not suggest any improvement in the outcome. Some centers use a second catheter placed in the cephalad segment of the internal jugular vein to improve the venous drainage of the brain; this improves the total ECMO flow, but the procedure has not been shown to change the outcome.

7. Some patients develop systemic hypertension on ECMO; this may be related to circulation overload and may respond to diuresis or hemofiltration. Because the heart and lungs are bypassed, there may be a deficiency of epinephrine degradation; because renal blood flow is nonpulsatile, there may be high levels of plasma renin; and because the right atrium is decompressed, there may be high levels of arginine vasopressin. Hypertension may predispose to cerebral hemorrhage, so treatment with hydralazine or enalapril may be necessary.

8. A few patients develop excessive hemolysis, related to high pressures in the circuit (>300 torr); this problem may be monitored by measurements of plasma free hemoglobin, which should remain below 40 mg/100 mL.

9. After ECMO, many patients have problems with feeding; the reason for this is not understood, but because the vascular catheters lie near the vagus nerve, there may be temporary injury causing esophageal dysfunction and gastroesophageal reflux. Some of these patients may also develop a superior vena cava syndrome (Zreik et al, 1995) or a chylothorax, and some may have transient vocal cord paralysis, again related to the catheters.

Venovenous Extracorporeal Membrane Oxygenation

The usual type of ECMO is venoarterial, but there has been considerable use of venovenous ECMO, especially with a single dual-lumen catheter placed in the right atrium. The catheter must be carefully placed so that well-oxygenated blood is directed toward the tricuspid valve, to minimize recirculation into the venous drainage.

The major advantage of this technique is that the carotid artery does not have to be sacrificed. In addition, because the pulmonary and coronary circulations receive well-oxygenated blood, there may be significant improvements in pulmonary hypertension and myocardial function. Because of the recirculation problem, often 20% to 40%, the capacity to deliver oxygen is less than in venoarterial ECMO; the ECMO flow must usually be higher, frequently in the range of 120 to 140 mL/kg per minute, and lower levels of arterial PO_2, in the range of 40 to 60 torr, must sometimes be accepted. If the circulation and hemoglobin levels are well maintained and if the patient's acid-base status and blood lactate levels remain normal, it is unlikely that a state of oxygen deficiency exists. Also, because of the recirculation problem, the central venous oxygen saturation cannot be used as an assessment of overall oxygenation. Commonly a cephalad venous catheter is used to monitor cerebral venous oxygen saturation; values less than 60% are considered evidence for oxygen deficiency.

Despite the use of dopamine to maintain the circulation, some patients, perhaps 10%, must be changed to venoarterial ECMO. Nevertheless, Cornish and associates (1993) found that most patients referred to an ECMO center could be managed effectively with venovenous ECMO; myocardial function usually improved, and dopamine could be weaned. The neurodevelopmental outcome of patients after venovenous ECMO is similar to that after venoarterial ECMO (van Meurs et al, 1994).

INHALED NITRIC OXIDE THERAPY

It has long been postulated that vascular tone is an intrinsic property of the blood vessels. The observation that this was true only when the endothelium remained intact (Furchgott and Zawadzki, 1980) led to the suggestion that an endothelial-derived relaxing factor existed. In experiments done by Ignarro and colleagues (1986), it was shown that the endothelial-derived relaxing factor was identical with NO, a gas that could be delivered to the lung by inhalation. NO is produced in the endothelial cell by NO synthase, which catalyzes the conversion of arginine and oxygen to citrulline and NO (Palmer et al, 1988); the NO diffuses to the smooth muscle cell and activates guanyl cyclase, which converts guanosine triphosphate (GTP) into cyclic guanosine monophosphate (GMP) and produces smooth muscle relaxation.

Clinical Experience

There are several reports of using iNO in laboratory animal models to produce a specific decrease in pulmonary artery pressure (Frostell et al, 1991). There was no similar effect on the systemic circulation because on entering the pulmonary bloodstream, NO was rapidly inactivated by combination with hemoglobin, forming first nitroso-hemoglobin and then methemoglobin. This discovery culminated in simultaneous reports by Roberts and colleagues (1992) and Kinsella and associates (1992b), which showed that low-dose inhaled NO (between 5 and 80 ppm) could produce a fall in pulmonary artery pressure, with improved systemic oxygenation, in newborn infants with severe respiratory failure owing to persistent pulmonary hypertension of the newborn. NO did this without decreasing systemic blood pressure or producing other toxic side effects.

This targeted delivery of dilator therapy to the pulmonary vasculature with improved oxygenation had tremendous clinical appeal. There were further reports of improved oxygenation in persistent pulmonary hypertension of the newborn (Kinsella et al, 1993), in congenital heart disease (Roberts et al, 1993), and in acquired respiratory distress syndrome in children (Abman et al, 1994) and in adults (Zapol and Hurfor, 1993). There was wide variability in the effect at various dosage ranges in pulmonary hypertension associated with respiratory distress syndrome (Abman et al, 1993) and with respiratory failure in term infants considered for ECMO (Finer et al, 1994); sometimes a paradoxic deterioration of the patient occurred (Oriot et al, 1993). Finer and co-workers (1994) found that most responding patients had a satisfactory response at levels of less than 20 ppm and that higher doses did not produce any improvement in the response. Buhrer and colleagues (1995) found optimal doses of 8 to 16 ppm, but they noted that it varied with time in the same patient and that the concentration needed frequent adjustment. Even though NO may improve pulmonary vascular resistance, it may have little effect if the lungs are not adequately recruited, if myocardial function is severely impaired, or if systemic circulatory insufficiency is present.

Inhaled Nitric Oxide in Congenital Diaphragmatic Hernia

The use of NO in congenital diaphragmatic hernia is discussed in Chapter 60. In the lamb congenital diaphragmatic hernia model, NO was not effective until exogenous surfactant was given; this emphasizes the importance of adequate recruitment and ventilation. In patients considered for ECMO, NO was not effective before ECMO, but in the same patients after ECMO, NO was often effective in increasing the level of oxygenation.

Inhaled Nitric Oxide in Respiratory Distress Syndrome

Kinsella and associates (1994) showed that NO had a beneficial effect on oxygenation in lambs with respiratory distress syndrome and concluded that there was relief of vasoconstriction in the pulmonary circuit and improvement in V/Q balance. Roze and colleagues (1994), using Doppler echocardiography, distinguished the response of infants with severe hypoxemia, persistent pulmonary hypertension of the newborn, and extrapulmonary shunts from premature infants with severe hypoxemia as a result of respiratory distress syndrome but no extrapulmonary shunts. The infants with persistent pulmonary hypertension of the newborn responded to NO with a large increase in oxygenation, a large increase in pulmonary blood flow, and reduced shunts, whereas those with respiratory distress syndrome responded with a modest increase in oxygenation and no change in pulmonary blood flow. Roze and colleagues' interpretation was that infants with respiratory distress syndrome responded with improved ventilation/perfusion matching rather than increased pulmonary blood flow. The findings in adult respiratory distress syndrome were the same. The successful use of NO in small premature infants with respiratory distress syndrome and suspected lung hypoplasia has been reported (Peliowski et al, 1995). It is emphasized that NO works best in severe respiratory distress syndrome if the terminal air spaces are adequately recruited with exogenous surfactant and mechanical ventilation with adequate levels of PEEP.

Toxicity of Nitric Oxide

With the exception of anesthesia, the use of inhaled gas therapy in medicine is rare. There are concerns about the possible toxicity of NO. When exposed to oxygen, NO is slowly converted to NO_2 (Bouchet et al, 1993). The Centers for Disease Control recommendation is that NO_2 levels not exceed 5 ppm. The higher the oxygen concentration, the higher is the rate of conversion of NO to NO_2; an NO of 20 ppm exposed to 95% oxygen achieves an NO_2 level of 5 ppm after 5 minutes. Higher levels of NO_2 may be associated with high-permeability pulmonary edema and chronic airway inflammation after prolonged exposure (Gaston et al, 1994). In addition, when exposed to superoxide radicals in the lung lining liquid, NO is converted to peroxynitrite, which generates hydroxyl radicals and may produce significant injury to surfactant lipids and proteins (Haddad et al, 1993). There is no evidence that NO treatment is associated with an increased incidence of bronchopulmonary dysplasia. Another concern is that NO may inhibit platelet function or prolong bleeding time and be associated with hemorrhagic complications (Edwards, 1995).

Clinical Protocol

The inherent reactivity of NO and oxygen meant that new techniques needed to be developed to ensure safety. NO, from a mixture in nitrogen, is fed through Teflon tubing into the inspiration line of the ventilator distal to the humidifier, so its exposure to oxygen is as short as possible before inhalation. Exhaled gas is collected by a hood at the PEEP valve and exhausted into the wall suction system of the hospital. The concentrations of NO and NO_2, sampled at the patient manifold, are measured constantly by electrochemical sensors; other detectors using chemolumines-

cence have not proven as satisfactory (Kinsella et al, 1995). The level of methemoglobin in blood does not usually exceed 2%, and the level of NO_2 in the inspired gas does not usually exceed 2 ppm, but they both must be watched closely. Because of the low inspired concentrations of NO, new delivery systems and new detection devices may be developed and tested under different conditions. The NO concentration should be weaned to the minimal effective level, but the weaning should be slow because rapid weaning may be accompanied by severe hypoxemia (Zapol et al, 1994). Despite its potential for toxicity (Stavert and Lehnert, 1990), inhaled NO therapy has proven safe for short-term use (Abman and Kinsella, 1995). Determination of its long-term effects requires further investigation.

Clinical Trials

There have been several large multicenter, multinational trials of iNO therapy. Although there was considerable variation among the trials with regards to entry criteria, prior treatments, randomization, blinding, placebo, dose ranges, and therapeutic outcomes, on the whole, these trials represent a determined attempt to delineate the role that iNO therapy has in the treatment of neonatal respiratory failure (Abman and Kinsella, 1995). Two controlled trials of iNO have demonstrated an important improvement. In the NINOS trial (Neonatal Inhaled Nitric Oxide Study Group, 1997), the mortality in 121 controls and 114 treated infants was the same, but the need for ECMO was reduced from 64% in control subjects to 46% in those given iNO treatment. Similarly, in a smaller trial reported by Roberts and associates (1997), although mortality was unchanged, the need for ECMO was reduced from 71% in control subjects to 40% in treated infants. In a third controlled trial, with a more liberal use of iNO, the need for ECMO was reduced from 34% in control subjects to 22% in the treatment group (Davidson et al, 1997). It seems reasonable to conclude that iNO may reduce the need for ECMO by about one third. It is anticipated that the Food and Drug Administration will release iNO for clinical treatment of the newborn with pulmonary hypertension.

LIQUID VENTILATION

During the past 20 years, investigations have been pursing the possibility of treating ventilatory failure with liquid rather than gaseous ventilation (Shaffer et al, 1984; Wolfson et al, 1996). The discovery of a class of compounds known as fluorocarbons has led to significant advances because they are chemically and physiologically inert. Perfluorocarbon, the compound being used in both animal experimentation and human clinical studies, has a greater solubility for respiratory gases than blood. It has some of the properties of surfactant with a low surface tension. When instilled into the lung, this radiopaque compound gradually recruits alveoli without barotrauma and because of its low vapor pressure is rapidly eliminated by vaporization. Early studies (Greenspan et al, 1990; Leach et al, 1996) in humans suggest that liquid ventilation is tolerated and may be effective in improving compliance and reducing lung injury in humans, but clinical trials are necessary.

REFERENCES

Abman SH, Kinsella JP: Inhaled NO for persistent pulmonary hypertension of the newborn: The physiology matters! Pediatrics 96:1153, 1995.

Abman SH, Griebel JL, Parker DK, et al: Acute effects of inhaled nitric oxide in children with severe hypoxemic respiratory failure. J Pediatr 124(6):881, 1994.

Abman SH, Kinsella JP, Schaffer MS, Wilkening RB: Inhaled NO in the management of a preterm newborn with severe respiratory distress and pulmonary hypertension. Pediatrics 92:606, 1993.

Bartlett RH, Roloff DW, Cornell RG, et al: Extracorporeal circulation in neonatal respiratory failure: A prospective randomized study. Pediatrics 76:479, 1985.

Baumgart S, Hirschl RB, Butler SZ, et al: Diagnosis related criteria in the consideration of extracorporeal membrane oxygenation in neonates previously treated with high frequency jet ventilation. Pediatrics 89:491, 1992.

Baumgart S, Streletz LJ, Needleman L, et al: Right common carotid artery reconstruction after extracorporeal membrane oxygenation: Vascular imaging, cerebral circulation, electro-encephalographic, and neurodevelopmental correlates to recovery. J Pediatr 125:295, 1994.

Bouchet M, Renaudin MH, Raveau C, et al: Safety requirements for use of inhaled NO in neonates. Lancet 341:968, 1993.

Buhrer C, Merker G, Falke K, et al: Dose response to inhaled NO in acute hypoxemic respiratory failure of newborn infants: A preliminary report. Pediatr Pulmonol 19:291, 1995.

Campbell LR, Bunyapen C, Holmes GL, et al: Right common carotid artery ligation in extracorporeal membrane oxygenation. J Pediatr 113:110, 1988.

Cilley RE, Zwischenberger JB, Andrews AF, et al: Intracranial hemorrhage during extracorporeal membrane oxygenation in neonates. Pediatrics 78:699, 1986.

Cornish JD, Gerstmann DR, Clark RH, et al: Extracorporeal membrane oxygenation and high frequency oscillatory ventilation: Potential therapeutic relationships. Crit Care Med 15:831, 1987.

Cornish JD, Heiss KF, Clark RH, et al: Efficacy of venovenous extracorporeal membrane oxygenation for neonates with respiratory and circulatory compromise. J Pediatr 122:105, 1993.

Cvetinic WG, Cunningham MD, Sills JH, et al: Reintroduction of continuous negative pressure ventilation in neonates: Two-year experience. Pediatric Pulmonol 8(4):245, 1990.

Davidson D, Barefield ES, Kattwinkel J, et al: A double-masked, randomized, placebo-controlled dose response study of inhaled nitric oxide for the treatment of persistent pulmonary hypertension of the newborn [abstract]. Pediatr Res 41:144A, 1997.

Dworetz AR, Moya FR, Sabo B, et al: Survival of infants with persistent pulmonary hypertension without extracorporeal membrane oxygenation. Pediatrics 84:1, 1989.

Edwards AD: The pharmacology of inhaled NO. Arch Dis Child 72:F127, 1995.

Finer NN, Etches PC, Kamstra BJ, et al: Inhaled NO in infants referred for extracorporeal membrane oxygenation: Dose response. J Pediatr 124:302, 1994.

Frostell C, Fratacci MD, Wain J, et al: Inhaled NO: A selective pulmonary vasodilator reversing hypoxic pulmonary vasoconstriction. Circulation 83:2038, 1991.

Fuhrman BP, Paczan PR, DeFrancisis M: Perfluorocarbon-associated gas exchange. Crit Care Med 19:712, 1991.

Furchgott RF, Zawadzki JV: The obligatory role of endothelial cells in the relaxation of arterial smooth muscle by acetylcholine. Nature 327:524, 1980.

Gaston B, Drazen JM, Loscalzo J, Stamler JS: The biology of nitrogen oxides in the airways. Am Rev Respir Dis 149:538, 1994.

Glass P, Miller M, Short B: Morbidity for survivors of ECMO: Neurodevelopmental outcome at one year of age. Pediatrics 83:72, 1989.

Greenspan JS, Wolfson MR, Rubenstein D, Shaffer TH: Liquid ventilation of human preterm neonates. J Pediatr 117:106, 1990.

Haddad IY, Ischiropoulos H, Holm BA, et al: Mechanisms of peroxynitrite-induced injury to pulmonary surfactants. Am J Physiol 265(6Pt1):L555, 1993.

Hirschl RB, Heiss KF, Bartlett RH: Severe myocardial dysfunction during extracorporeal membrane oxygenation. J Pediatr Surg 27:48, 1992.

Hirschl RB, Parent A, Tooley R, et al: Liquid ventilation improves pulmonary function, gas exchange, and lung injury in a model of respiratory failure. Ann Surg 221:79, 1995.

Ignarro LJ, Byrns RE, Wood KS: Pharmacological and biochemical properties of endothelial derived relaxing factor (EDRF): Evidence that EDRF is closely related to NO (NO) radical (Abstract). Circulation 74(suppl 2):287, 1986.

Keszler M, Ryckman FC, McDonald JV, et al: A prospective multicenter randomized study of high versus low end expiratory pressure during extracorporeal membrane oxygenation. J Pediatr 120:107, 1992.

Kimball TR, Daniels SR, Weiss RG, et al: Changes in cardiac function during extracorporeal membrane oxygenation for persistent pulmonary hypertension in the newborn infant. J Pediatr 118:431, 1991.

Kinsella JP, Gerstmann DR, Rosenberg AA: The effect of extracorporeal membrane oxygenation on coronary perfusion and regional blood flow. Pediatr Res 31:80, 1992a.

Kinsella JP, Ivy DD, Abman SH: Inhaled NO improves gas exchange and lowers pulmonary vascular resistance in severe experimental hyaline membrane disease. Pediatr Res 36:402, 1994.

Kinsella JP, Neish SR, Ivy DD, et al: Clinical responses to prolonged treatment of persistent pulmonary hypertension of the newborn with low doses of inhaled NO. J Pediatr 123:103, 1993.

Kinsella JP, Neish SR, Shaffer E, Abman SH: Low dose inhalational NO in persistent pulmonary hypertension of the newborn. Lancet 340:818, 1992b.

Kinsella JP, Schmidt JM, Griebel J, Abman SH: Inhaled NO treatment for stabilization and emergency medical transport of critically ill newborns and infants. Pediatrics 96:773, 1995.

Klein MD, Whittlesey GC: Extracorporeal membrane oxygenation. Pediatr Clin North Am 41:365, 1994.

Leach CL, Fuhrman BP, Morin FC III, Rath MG: Perfluorocarbon-associated gas exchange (partial liquid ventilation) in respiratory distress syndrome: A prospective, randomized, controlled study. Crit Care Med 21:1270, 1993.

Leach CL, Greenspan JS, Rubenstein SD, et al, for the LiquiVent Study Group: Partial liquid ventilation with perflubron in premature infants with severe respiratory distress syndrome. N Engl J Med 335:761, 1996.

Leach CL, Holm B, Morin FC III, et al: Partial liquid ventilation in preterm lambs and compatibility with exogenous surfactant. J Pediatr 126(3):412, 1995.

Lotze A, Knight GR, Martin GR, et al: Improved pulmonary outcome after exogenous surfactant therapy for respiratory failure in term infants requiring extracorporeal membrane oxygenation. J Pediatr 122:261, 1993.

Mendoza JC, Shearer LL, Cook LN: Lateralization of brain lesions following extracorporeal membrane oxygenation. Pediatrics 88:1004, 1991.

Neonatal Inhaled Nitric Oxide Study Group: Inhaled NO in full-term and nearly full-term infants with hypoxic respiratory failure. N Engl J Med 336:597, 1997.

Oriot D, Boussemart T, Berthier M, et al: Paradoxical effect of inhaled NO in a newborn with pulmonary hypertension. Lancet 342:364, 1993.

O'Rourke PP, Crone RK, Vacanti JP, et al: Extracorporeal membrane oxygenation and conventional medical therapy in neonates with persistent pulmonary hypertension of the newborn: A prospective randomized study. Pediatrics 84:957, 1989.

Ortega M, Ramos AD, Platzker ACG, et al: Early prediction of ultimate outcome in newborn infants with severe respiratory failure. J Pediatr 113:744, 1988.

Palmer RM, Ashton DS, Moncada S: Vascular endothelial cells synthesize NO from L-arginine. Nature 333:664, 1988.

Palmisano JM, Moler FW, Custer JR, et al: Unsuspected congenital heart disease in neonates receiving extracorporeal life support: A review of 95 cases from the ELSO registry. J Pediatr 121:115, 1992.

Pearson GD, Short BL: An economic analysis of extracorporeal membrane oxygenation. J Intensive Care Med 2:116, 1986.

Peliowski A, Finer NN, Etches PC, et al: Inhaled NO for premature infants after prolonged rupture of membranes. J Pediatr 126:450, 1995.

Roberts JD, Fineman JR, Morin FC III, et al: Inhaled NO and persistent pulmonary hypertension of the newborn. N Engl J Med 336:605, 1997.

Roberts JD, Lang P, Bigatello LM, et al: Inhaled NO in congenital heart disease. Circulation 87:447, 1993.

Roberts JD, Polaner DM, Lang P, et al: Inhaled NO in persistent pulmonary hypertension of the newborn. Lancet 340:818, 1992.

Roze JC, Storme L, Zupan V, et al: Echocardiographic investigation of inhaled nitric oxide in newborn babies with severe hypoxaemia. Lancet 334(8918):303, 1994.

Schumacher RE: Extracorporeal membrane oxygenation: Will this therapy continue to be as efficacious in the future? Pediatr Clin North Am 40:1005, 1993.

Schumacher RE, Barks JDE, Johnston MV, et al: Right sided brain lesions in infants following extracorporeal membrane oxygenation. Pediatrics 92:155, 1988.

Schwieler GH, Robertson B: Liquid ventilation in immature newborn rabbits. Biol Neonate 29:343, 1976.

Shaffer TH, Lowe CA, Bhutani VK, Douglas PR: Liquid ventilation: Effects on pulmonary function in distressed meconium-stained lambs. Pediatr Res 18:47, 1984.

Short BL, Pearson GD: Neonatal extracorporeal membrane oxygenation: A review. J Intensive Care Med 1:47, 1986.

Stavert DM, Lehnert BE: Nitrogen oxides and nitrogen dioxide as inducers of acute pulmonary injury when inhaled at relatively high concentrations for brief periods. Inhalat Toxicol 2:53, 1990.

Taylor BJ, Seibert JJ, Glasier CM, et al: Evaluation of the reconstructed carotid artery following extracorporeal membrane oxygenation. Pediatrics 90:568, 1992.

Torrance SM, Wittnich C: The effect of varying arterial oxygen tension on neonatal acid-base balance. Pediatr Res 31(2):112, 1992.

UK Collaborative ECMO Trial Group: UK collaborative randomised trial of neonatal extracorporeal membrane oxygenation. Lancet 348:75, 1996.

van Meurs KP, Nguyen HT, Rhine WD, et al: Intracranial abnormalities and neurodevelopmental status after venovenous extracorporeal membrane oxygenation. J Pediatr 125:304, 1994.

Walsh-Sukys M, Stork EK, Martin RJ: Neonatal ECMO: Iron lung of the 1990s? J Pediatr 124:427, 1994.

Wilcox DT, Glick PL, Karamanoukian HL, et al: Perfluorocarbon associated gas exchange (PAGE) and NO in the lamb congenital diaphragmatic hernia model. Crit Care Med 23:1858, 1995.

Wolfson MR, Greenspan JS, Shaffer TH: Pulmonary administration of vasoactive substances by perfluorochemical ventilation. Pediatrics 97:449, 1996.

Wung JT, James LS, Kilchevesky E, et al: Management of infants with severe respiratory failure and persistence of fetal circulation, without hyperventilation. Pediatrics 76(4):488, 1985.

Zapol W, Hurfor W: Inhaled NO in adult respiratory distress syndrome and other lung diseases. New Horizons 1:638, 1993.

Zapol WM, Rimar S, Gillis N, et al: NHLBI workshop summary: Nitric oxide and the lung. Am J Respir Crit Care Med 149:1375, 1994.

Zapol WM, Snider MT, Hill DJ, et al: Extracorporeal membrane oxygenation in severe respiratory failure: A randomized prospective study. JAMA 242:2193, 1979.

Zreik H, Bengur AR, Meliones JN, et al: Superior vena cava obstruction after extracorporeal membrane oxygenation. J Pediatr 127:314, 1995.

CHAPTER 53

Disorders of the Transition

Thomas Hansen and Anthony Corbet

HYALINE MEMBRANE DISEASE

Hyaline membrane disease (HMD), frequently referred to as *respiratory distress syndrome* (RDS), occurs after the onset of breathing in infants with insufficiency of the pulmonary surfactant system.

Epidemiology

There are an estimated 40,000 cases of HMD annually in the United States (Farrell and Wood, 1976), about 14% of all low-birth-weight infants (Farrell and Avery, 1975). The incidence is 60% at 29 weeks' gestation but declines with maturation to near 0 by 39 weeks. The condition is more common in male than in female infants (Miller and Futra-kul, 1968); it is more common in white than in nonwhite infants (Richardson and Torday, 1994). At each level of gestational age, RDS is less common in black infants, and this phenomenon is not explained by other factors that may influence lung maturity (Hulsey et al, 1993). At any given gestational age, the incidence is higher for cesarean section without labor than for vaginal delivery (Fedrick and Butler, 1972). There is a significantly increased risk if elective cesarean section is performed before completion of 39 weeks' gestation (Morrison et al, 1995).

When corrected for the important effect of gestational age, the occurrence of HMD is significantly increased in gestational diabetes and in insulin-dependent mothers without vascular disease (Robert et al, 1976). Most such infants of diabetic mothers are large for gestational age, and similar overnourished infants in the absence of maternal diabetes are also at increased risk (Naeye et al, 1974). Evidence suggests that the incidence of RDS in infants of diabetic mothers is now much less, almost certainly because of improved medical control of diabetes (Kjos et al, 1990).

Early reports in comparatively large infants suggested that the risk is decreased in infants who are small for gestational age (Gluck and Kulovich, 1973); however, in much less mature infants seen, comparisons of appropriate-for-gestational-age and small-for-gestational-age infants, both weight matched and gestation matched, suggest that immature small-for-gestational-age infants do not have this advantage (Pena et al, 1988). In fact, there is some evidence that the risk of RDS at constant gestational age may be increased in small-for-gestational-age infants and that the mortality may be higher (Thompson et al, 1992; Tyson et al, 1995). Maternal conditions that compromise fetal growth and may produce decreased risk include pregnancy-induced hypertension, chronic hypertension, subacute placental abruption, narcotic addiction, and maternal smoking. Tubman and colleagues (1991) found an increased risk for RDS in infants of hypertensive mothers; this was because

of the high incidence of cesarean section delivery without benefit of labor.

Suggestions that birth asphyxia predisposes to HMD (Table 53–1) are based on lower Apgar scores in human infants with RDS (James, 1975) and some experimental evidence in lambs (Orzalesi et al, 1965). In an examination of umbilical artery blood at birth, however, it was found that infants with RDS are not more acidemic at birth (Kenny et al, 1976) and that lower Apgar scores associated with RDS are better explained by relative immaturity and defective lung function.

Pathology

The gross findings at autopsy in infants dying without mechanical ventilation include diffuse lung atelectasis, congestion, and edema. If the lungs are inflated at postmortem examination, distensibility is greatly reduced, and the lungs collapse more readily with deflation. On histologic examination, the peripheral air spaces are collapsed, but more proximal respiratory bronchioles, lined with necrotic epithelium and hyaline membranes, have an overdistended appearance (Finlay-Jones et al, 1974) (Figs. 53–1 and 53–2). There is obvious pulmonary edema with congested capillaries, and the lymphatic and interstitial spaces are distended with fluid. The epithelial damage appears within 30 minutes of the onset of breathing, and the hyaline membranes, composed of plasma exudation products and associated with damaged capillaries, appear within 3 hours of birth (Gandy et al, 1970). In experimental animals, the bronchiolar lesions may be completely prevented (Nilsson et al, 1978) and the leakage of protein may be considerably reduced (Ikegami et al, 1992) by the administration of exogenous surfactant at birth. This finding has led to the conclusion that the bronchiolar lesions are secondary to atelectasis in terminal air spaces and to disruptive overdistention of more proximal airways.

Pathophysiology

In HMD, the respiratory rate is elevated, so despite a reduction in each tidal volume, the minute ventilation initially is increased. The functional residual capacity, analyzed by nitrogen washout, is reduced; the greater the need for oxygen, the smaller is the measured value for functional residual capacity (Richardson et al, 1986). In keeping with the reduced static lung compliance found at autopsy, the static lung compliance measured by multiple airway occlusions during exhalation is also markedly reduced, the average value being only 0.5 mL/cm H_2O/kg (Dreizzen et al, 1988). As a result, the work of breathing is greatly increased. Measurements of airway resistance suggest values in the normal range, but there is a tendency toward an

TABLE 53–1

Hyaline Membrane Disease

Epidemiology

Worldwide
Prematurity predisposes
Cesarean section without labor predisposes
Perinatal asphyxia predisposes
Male > female
White > black
Second-born twin at greater risk
PROM spares
IUGR spares
Maternal stress spares
Maternal diabetes predisposes if <37 weeks
Maternal hemorrhage predisposes

Clinical Signs

Onset near the time of birth
Retractions and tachypnea
Expiratory grunt
Cyanosis
Systemic hypotension
Characteristic chest film
Course to death or improvement 3–5 days
Fine inspiratory rales
Hypothermia
Peripheral edema
Pulmonary edema

Pathophysiology

Reduced lung compliance
Reduced FRC
Poor lung distensibility
Poor alveolar stability
Right-to-left shunts
Reduced effective pulmonary blood flow
If hypotensive and hypoxic, poor peripheral perfusion, poor renal
  perfusion, myocardial malfunction
Patent ductus arteriosus contributes

Pathobiochemistry

Respiratory acidosis
Decreased saturated phospholipids
Low AF L/S ratio
Low surfactant-associated proteins
Decreased total serum proteins
Decreased fibrinolysis
Low thyroxine levels

Pathology

Atelectasis
Injury to epithelial cells, edema
Membrane contains fibrin and cellular products
No tubular myelin
Osmiophilic lamellar bodies decreased early, increased later

Etiology

Surfactant deficiency during disease
Probable inadequate hormonal (corticoid) stimulus in utero
DPL synthesis impaired and/or destruction increased
Autonomic dysfunction

Prevention

Prenatal glucocorticoids for >24 hours
Surfactant replacement before 1–2 hours

PROM, prolonged rupture of membranes (>16 hours); IUGR, intrauterine growth retardation; FRC, functional residual capacity; AF, amniotic fluid; L/S, lecithin/sphingomyelin; DPL, dipalmitoyl lecithin.

increase. In one study, the average value was 69 cm $H_2O/$ L per second compared with a reference value of 42 cm H_2O/L per second (Hjalmarson and Olsson, 1974). Edberg and coworkers (1991) found decreased compliance, increased resistance, decreased lung volume, and reduced gas mixing efficiency in very-low-birth-weight infants with RDS. From these data, it can be approximated that the overall time constant in HMD would be less than 0.05 second (see Chapter 50). Because the patency of small peripheral airways depends on proximal spread of surfactant (Macklem et al, 1970), in some regions of lung the local time constants may be more prolonged. The curvature of nitrogen washout traces is better represented by a two-space mathematical model than by a one-space assumption (Richardson and Jung, 1978). The postulated *slow* space may represent parts of the lung with more prolonged time constants.

The Aa.Do₂ and right-to-left shunt while breathing 100% oxygen are greatly increased, many infants having values for shunt in the range of 50% to 90% of cardiac output (Strang and MacLeish, 1961). Because there is no evidence for a diffusion limitation (Krauss et al, 1976), it is commonly stated that large shunts at the foramen ovale and ductus arteriosus and in atelectatic lung constitute the only cause of severe hypoxemia in HMD. If this were true and the shunt were 50%, it can be seen from Figure 53–3 that changing inspired oxygen would have little effect on arterial oxygen pressure, and oxygen therapy would be relatively ineffective. In fact, precipitous changes of arterial oxygen tension and calculated venous admixture occur if inspired oxygen is reduced. This phenomenon indicates the presence of an open, poorly ventilated lung compartment with extremely low V̇/Q̇, representing a significant portion of the lung and producing variable hypoxic vasoconstriction and alterations in right-to-left shunt as the inspired oxygen changes (Corbet et al, 1974). Therefore, in infants with HMD, the severity of arterial hypoxemia is directly related to the size of the open, poorly ventilated compartment. The relationship among V̇/Q̇, alveolar oxygen tension, and changing inspired oxygen (Fig. 53–4) indicates how oxygen

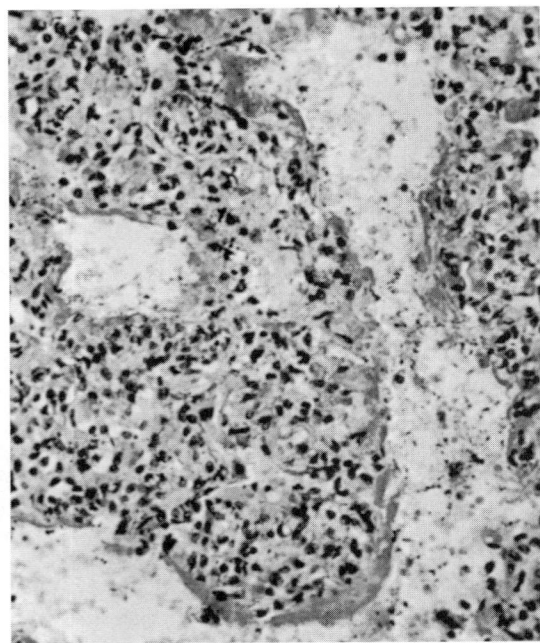

FIGURE 53–1. Photomicrograph of section of lung of an infant born in the 32nd week of gestation weighing 1640 g. He seemed well for 1 hour; then dyspnea appeared and gradually increased with deepening sternal and costal retraction. He died at 22 hours of age. Unexpanded lung, with dilated air spaces lined with thick, homogeneously staining membrane, can be seen.

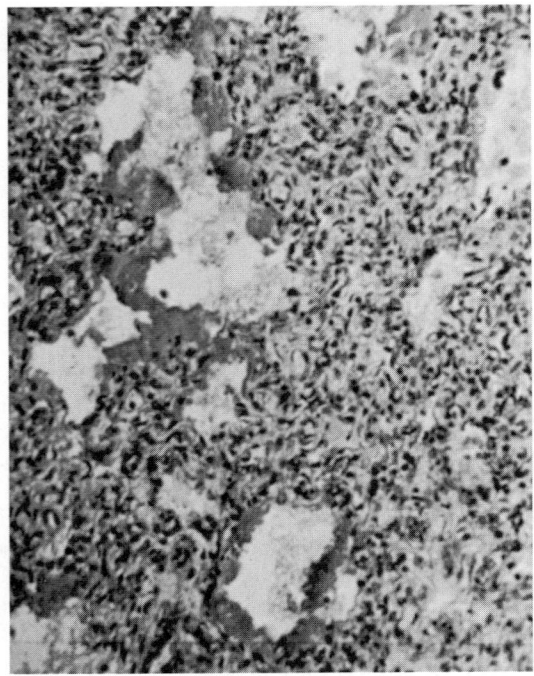

FIGURE 53–2. Photomicrograph of section of lung of a premature infant weighing 2270 g at birth whose dyspnea was first noticed at 8 hours and who died after steadily increasing respiratory difficulty at 27 hours. The appearance of the section of lung is in all respects similar to that in Figure 53–1. The pattern of aeration and atelectasis has been described as Swiss cheese–like in contrast to lace-like aeration.

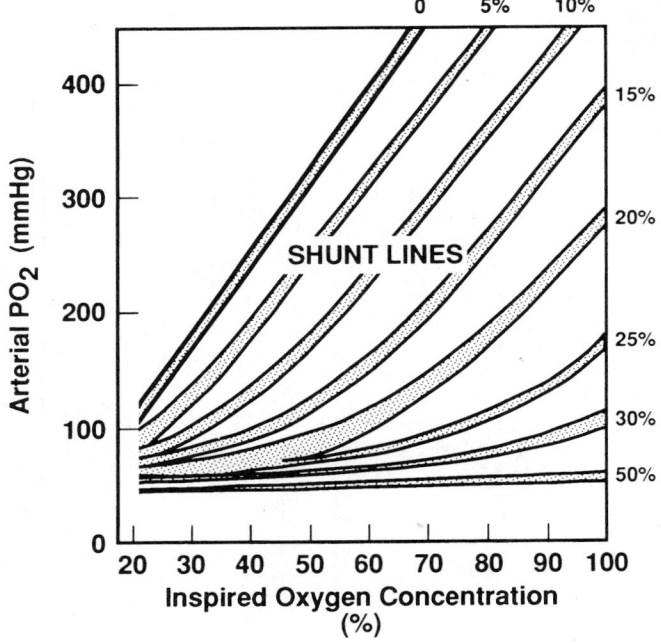

FIGURE 53–3. The relationship between inspired oxygen concentration and arterial P_{O_2} as it is affected by true right-to-left shunting. The assumptions are hemoglobin, 10 to 14 g/dL; arterial P_{CO_2}, 25 to 40 mm Hg; and av-O_2 difference, 5 mL/100 mL. (From Benatar SR, Hewlett AM, Nunn JF: The use of iso-shunt lines for control of oxygen therapy. Br J Anaesthesiol 45:711, 1973.)

as high as 90% is required before the oxygen pressure in low $\dot{V}/\dot{Q}$ units rises significantly (West, 1969) (see also Chapter 50). Because perfusion of the open, extremely low $\dot{V}/\dot{Q}$ compartment is greatly reduced by hypoxic vasoconstriction, it makes only a small contribution to cardiac output, and measurements of aA.D$_{N_2}$ are not greatly increased in HMD (Corbet et al, 1974). It should not be overlooked that this lung compartment makes a significant contribution to the oxygenation defect in HMD.

Measurements of aA.D$_{CO_2}$ and alveolar dead space are markedly increased in HMD (Nelson et al, 1962). Although minute ventilation is increased, the alveolar ventilation is actually decreased, as reflected by the elevated values for arterial CO_2 tension. Because a large part of the lung is collapsed or poorly ventilated, most alveolar ventilation is diverted to a relatively small part of the lung, represented by the reduced functional residual capacity. Because this compartment is small, it is relatively overventilated, so the $\dot{V}/\dot{Q}$ and the measured aA.D$_{CO_2}$ are high (Hansen et al, 1979). Measurements of pulmonary blood flow, using the disappearance of gases that enter ventilated parts of the lung, confirm that perfusion of ventilated lung is low (Chu et al, 1967). Based on the foregoing considerations, an idealized model of the lung in HMD is shown in Figure 53–5 representing the three lung compartments: shunt, open low $\dot{V}/\dot{Q}$, and high $\dot{V}/\dot{Q}$. Under conditions of changed inspired oxygen and changed levels of continuous positive airway pressure (CPAP), there is a close correspondence between predicted and measured values for aA.D$_{CO_2}$, suggesting the validity of this model (Hansen et al, 1979; Landers et al, 1986).

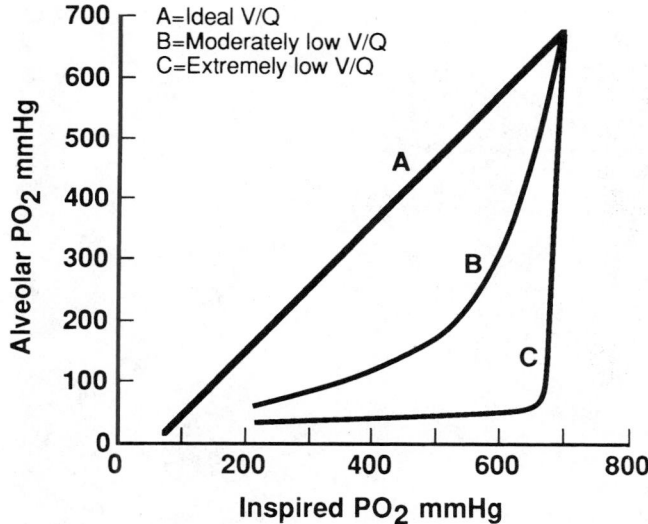

FIGURE 53–4. The relationship between inspired P_{O_2} and alveolar P_{O_2}. In an open lung compartment with extremely low $\dot{V}/\dot{Q}$, the alveolar P_{O_2} rises slowly until greater than 90% oxygen is reached, when it rises rapidly. This phenomenon accounts for the often dramatic changes of arterial P_{O_2} with small changes in inspired O_2, especially reductions of inspired O_2, seen in patients with respiratory distress syndrome. (From West JB: Ventilation perfusion inequality and overall gas exchange in computer models of the lung. Respir Physiol 7:88, 1969.)

In infants with RDS undergoing treatment in a neonatal intensive care unit, the pulmonary artery pressure declines more slowly after birth than in preterm infants without RDS (Seppanen et al, 1994). The systemic artery pressure is maintained similar to that in controls and tends to rise slowly with time; by 24 hours, the systemic artery pressure is well above the pulmonary artery pressure. Extrapulmonary right-to-left shunting at the foramen ovale or the ductus arteriosus disappears by 24 hours (Seppanen et al, 1994), and left-to-right shunting at the ductus arteriosus is

	V/Q>1	V/Q<<1	V/Q=O
Ventilation	0.999	0.001	0.000
Perfusion	0.330	0.030	0.640
	V/Q=3	Qo/Qt	Qs/Qt

FIGURE 53–5. Three-compartment model of hyaline membrane disease (high $\dot{V}/\dot{Q}$, open low $\dot{V}/\dot{Q}$, and shunt; the shunt includes shunt at the ductus, at the foramen, and at collapsed air spaces). The high $\dot{V}/\dot{Q}$ compartment receives nearly all the ventilation. From the measured value for arterial P_{O_2}, the calculated venous admixture is 0.67 of cardiac output. Thus, perfusion of the high $\dot{V}/\dot{Q}$ compartment is 0.33 of cardiac output, and the value for $\dot{V}/\dot{Q}$ is 3. From the latter value, a predicted value of $aA.D_{CO_2}$ can be calculated and compared with the measured value. If a value of 0.03 is assumed for Qo/Qt, the calculated value for Qs/Qt is 0.64. (From Hansen TN, Corbet AJS, Kenny JD, et al: Effects of oxygen and constant positive pressure breathing on $aA.D_{CO_2}$ in hyaline membrane disease. Pediatr Res 13:1167, 1979.)

common by age 24 hours (Dudell and Gersony, 1984). In experimental animals, it is not thought that this early left-to-right ductal shunt makes an important contribution to the overall lung dysfunction of RDS (Morrow et al, 1995), but as the pulmonary artery pressure continues to fall with time, the ductal shunt assumes much greater importance. In preterm infants without RDS, the ductus arteriosus tends to close within 4 days of birth (Reller et al, 1988), whereas in RDS the ductus tends to remain open (Reller et al, 1993) and may become a significant problem by 3 to 4 days of age (Corbet, 1996). (See also Chapter 61.)

Clinical Diagnosis

The infant with HMD is almost always premature and is cyanotic in room air. There is rapid or labored breathing, beginning at or immediately after birth. The severity of respiratory distress can be represented by the Silverman score (Fig. 53–6). Infants usually have a characteristic grunt during expiration, caused by closure of the glottis, the effect of which is to maintain lung volume and gas exchange during exhalation. Frequently the unventilated infant requires 40% to 50% oxygen after birth for relief of central cyanosis but then develops an increasing oxygen requirement over 24 to 48 hours; this may reach as high as 100%. In other infants, the oxygen requirement transiently decreases as acidosis or hypothermia is corrected or fetal lung fluid is cleared; the oxygen requirement begins to increase only after 3 to 6 hours. More severely affected infants have an immediate high oxygen requirement that progresses rapidly to 100%; without mechanical ventilation, they may die within 24 hours. Another group of larger infants needs less oxygen initially and manifests a slowly progressive course of generalized atelectasis over 48 to 72 hours. The urine output is low for the first 24 to 48 hours, but soon after this time a diuresis ensues. If HMD is uncomplicated, recovery starts after 48 hours. The decline in oxygen requirement is relatively rapid after 72 hours, and usually oxygen can be discontinued after 1 week. The very-low-birth-weight infant (<1500 g) usually requires mechanical ventilation and has a more prolonged course. A few infants with RDS also appear to have persistent pulmonary hypertension of the newborn (PPHN); they are easy to ventilate, especially after exogenous surfactant, but

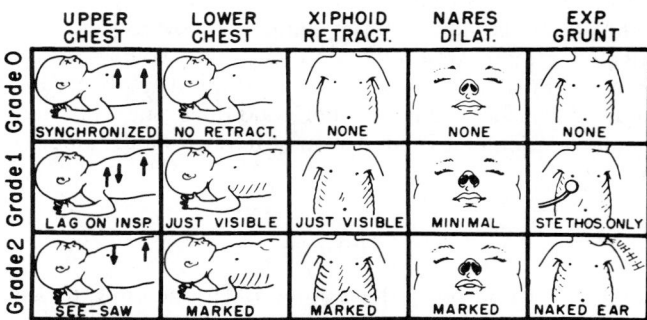

FIGURE 53–6. The Silverman score for assessing the magnitude of respiratory distress. (From Avery ME, Fletcher BD: The Lung and Its Disorders in the Newborn. Philadelphia, WB Saunders, 1974. Courtesy of WA Silverman.)

are difficult to oxygenate, and they have severe pulmonary hypertension as evaluated by echocardiographic criteria (Abman et al, 1993; Chan et al, 1994; Golan et al, 1995; Walther et al, 1992).

Laboratory Diagnosis

Based on arterial blood gas values, infants with HMD have a moderate to severe oxygenation defect, significant hypercarbia, and a mild metabolic acidosis with elevation of blood lactate (Sinclair, 1973). The lecithin/sphingomyelin (L/S) ratio and phosphatidylglycerol (PG) remain low in serial tracheal aspirate samples for 48 hours, then increase with recovery; the saturated phosphatidylcholine (PC) levels remain low in RDS and reach normal levels after 4 to 7 days; the surfactant protein A (SP-A)/saturated PC (SPC) ratio is low in RDS and is even lower in infants destined to develop bronchopulmonary dysplasia (BPD) (Hallman et al, 1991). Stevens and colleagues (1992) showed that SP-A in tracheal aspirate samples was low in infants with RDS, remained low for 3 to 4 days, and then rose in survivors but remained low in nonsurvivors. Moya and colleagues (1994) also found a low SP-A/SPC ratio in infants with RDS, but they detected increasing SP-A in tracheal aspirate samples as early as 12 to 24 hours. Gerdes and colleagues (1992) found that SP-A in tracheal aspirate samples increased after Exosurf administration; because Exosurf does not contain surfactant protein, they attributed this phenomenon to increased lung expansion and therefore increased secretion of endogenous surfactant and SP-A. Another study found that the SP-A/albumin ratio in tracheal aspirate samples was low in RDS; it rose into the normal range at 48 to 72 hours of age but was not changed by the administration of bovine surfactant (Eguchi et al, 1991). Because all of the surfactant proteins are developmentally regulated, it is likely that infants with HMD are also deficient in SP-B and SP-C.

Radiographic Diagnosis

Diffuse, fine granular densities that develop during the first 6 hours of life are seen on the chest radiograph (Fig. 53–7); these densities are influenced by size of the infant, severity of disease, and degree of ventilatory support. The appearance may be more marked at the lung bases than at the apices. The lung volume may appear normal early, especially if the infant is strong enough to overdistend less affected regions, but ultimately the lung volume is decreased. Positive airway pressure frequently obliterates these diagnostic findings. Other conditions, such as pneumonia or pulmonary edema, may have a similar appearance.

Etiology

HMD is primarily a developmental deficiency in the amount of surface-active material at the air-liquid interface of the lung, as demonstrated by pressure-volume curves with air and saline in infants who died from HMD (Avery and Fletcher, 1974). Saline extracts of minced lung have higher surface tension than do controls (Avery and Mead,

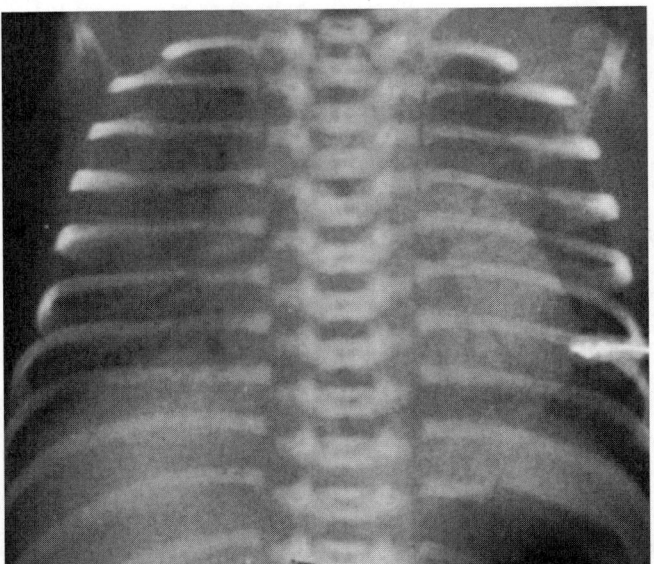

FIGURE 53–7. Typical chest radiograph from an infant with hyaline membrane disease.

1959); this is associated with lower levels of total tissue phospholipid (Brumley et al, 1967) and SPC (Adams et al, 1970). Although based on theoretical considerations of the amount required there appears to be a more than adequate amount of phospholipid present in total lung (Clements and Tooley, 1977), only a small proportion of lung phospholipid is surface-active material (Rieutort et al, 1986). Infants with HMD may synthesize adequate amounts of SPC but cannot package and export it to the alveolar surface in a way that makes it function as surfactant. In infants who die, deMello and associates (1987) has demonstrated the complete absence of tubular myelin and a modest deficiency of lamellar bodies in Type 2 cells in comparison with controls.

deMello and associates (1993) have demonstrated that infants who die with RDS have a deficiency of immunostained SP-A in the endoplasmic reticulum and lamellar bodies of the Type 2 cells. It is not established that infants with RDS have a deficiency of SP-B, but experimentally a specific deficiency of SP-B causes severe respiratory distress (Robertson et al, 1991). Infants with genetic SP-B deficiency have a severe RDS, however, which differs from classic RDS in that it is accompanied by alveolar proteinosis (see later).

It has been suggested that surfactant function in infants with HMD is inhibited by plasma proteins (Ikegami et al, 1986), which leak into the respiratory bronchioles at the sites of overdistention and epithelial damage. In particular, a plasma protein of relative molecular weight 110,000 has been implicated. Fibrinogen, hemoglobin, and albumin are potent inhibitors of surfactant (Seeger et al, 1993). It is of critical importance to the lungs to have adequate surfactant at the gas-liquid interface from the earliest possible moment after birth; otherwise, acute lung injury and surfactant inhibition supervene rapidly and contribute to a cycle of worsening disease (Nilsson et al, 1978). Thus, RDS is due to a developmental deficiency of surfactant at birth, but associated lung injury results in surfactant dysfunction as well.

Based on the results of animal experiments, it is estimated that the air spaces of the newborn infant at term contain about 75 mg/kg of SPC; this compares with only 10 to 15 mg/kg in adults and only 1 to 10 mg/kg in premature infants with RDS (Ikegami et al, 1993). As premature infants recover from RDS, the alveolar pool size approaches that in the term infant. This suggests that newborn infants need more surfactant than adults for adequate function, which may mean that more surfactant is present in an inactive form and that more surfactant is inhibited by excessive fluid and protein in the neonatal lung.

Prevention

Because HMD is a problem of insufficient lung maturity, the best way to prevent it is to prevent premature birth; for this purpose, the effective strategies are thought to be cervical cerclage, discovery and treatment of bacteriuria, and liberal use of tocolytics. At present, however, the two major approaches to the problem are (1) prediction of the risk for HMD by antenatal testing of amniotic fluid samples and (2) antenatal treatment of women in preterm labor with glucocorticoid hormones to accelerate fetal lung maturation. In addition, the prophylactic administration of exogenous surfactant at birth is designed to prevent RDS, and this strategy has been quite successful.

Prenatal Prediction

Before birth, the surfactant system can be assessed in amniotic fluid because some fetal lung fluid enters the amniotic cavity. The most common material measured is lecithin or PC, in particular, SPC. Because changes in amniotic fluid volume may alter the concentration of SPC, it is standardized to the concentration of sphingomyelin, which remains relatively constant throughout gestation; it is expressed as the L/S ratio.

In normal pregnancy, the L/S ratio displays a remarkably stable pattern, increasing slowly to 1 at 32 weeks, rising more rapidly to 2 at 35 weeks, and accelerating rapidly thereafter (Gluck and Kulovich, 1973) (Fig. 53–8). In abnormal pregnancy, there is much wider scatter, reflecting conditions that accelerate or decelerate lung maturation. The ratio may reach 2 as early as 28 weeks or remain at 1 until close to term. The incidence of HMD is only 0.5% for an L/S ratio of 2 or more but 100% for an L/S ratio less than 1; between 1 and 2, the risk of HMD decreases progressively. Elective cesarean section delivery of infants having an unrecognized low L/S ratio carries an unnecessary risk of HMD (Hack et al, 1976).

Phosphatidylinositol (PI) in amniotic fluid progressively increases until 36 weeks and then decreases (Hallman et al, 1976). At about this time, PG appears and increases until term (Fig. 53–9). The appearance time of PG may be accelerated or delayed in the same way as the L/S ratio. Thin-layer chromatography is sensitive, so values for PG of less than 1% of total phospholipid, by reflective densitometry on the chromatographic plate, should be considered negative; this correlates better with the less sensitive but

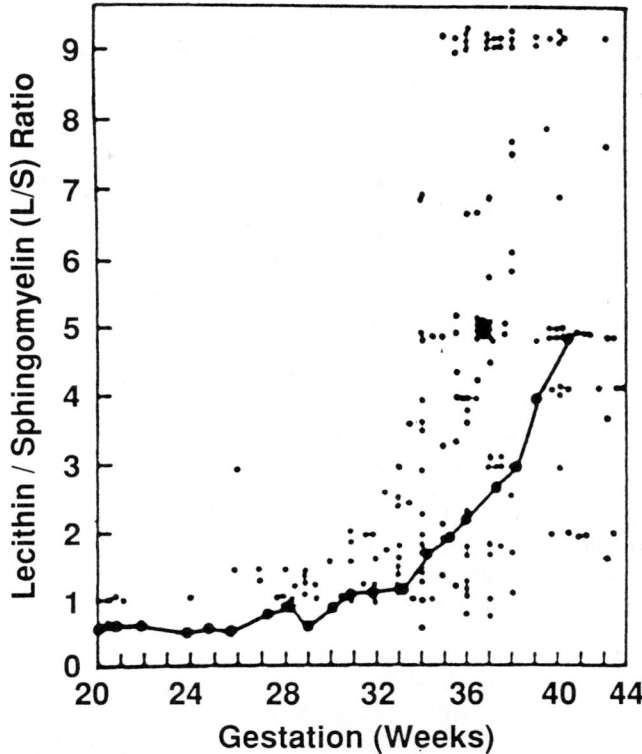

FIGURE 53–8. The L/S ratio in normal and abnormal pregnancies, indicating wide biologic scatter. (From Gluck L, Kulovich MV: The evaluation of functional maturity in the human fetus. *In* Gluck L (Ed): Modern Perinatal Medicine. Chicago, Year Book Medical Publishers, 1974.)

much faster immunologic detection methods for PG, such as the AmnioStat-FLM, which has detection limits of 0.05 μg/mL (Towers and Garite, 1989). The presence of PG at 1% of total phospholipid indicates a remarkably low risk

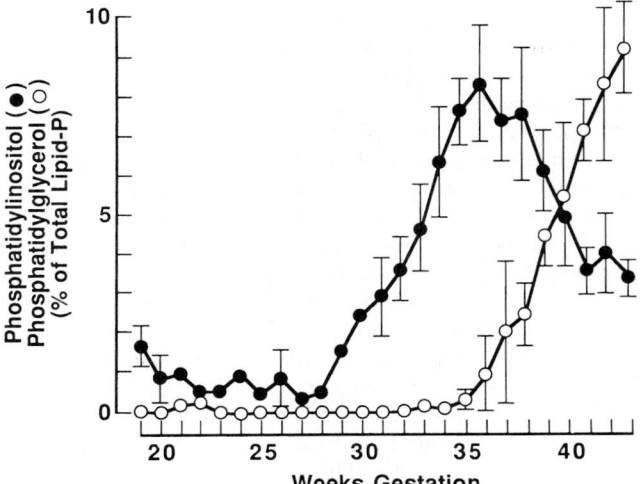

FIGURE 53–9. Changes in the content of phosphatidylglycerol and phosphatidylinositol in amniotic fluid, plotted against gestational age. (From Hallman M, Kulovich MV, Kirkpatrick E, et al: Phosphatidylinositol and phosphatidylglycerol in amniotic fluid: Indices of lung maturity. Am J Obstet Gynecol 125:613, 1976.)

for HMD, less than 0.5%. If a patient has both an L/S ratio of less than 2 and a PG of less than 1%, the risk for HMD is greater than 80% (Hallman and Teramo, 1981). Besides an L/S ratio below 1, this combination is the best predictor of HMD available to the clinician. In certain pregnancies characterized by diabetes and Rh isoimmunization, the L/S ratio has proved less reliable, the risk of HMD at a value between 2 and 3 still being approximately 13%. In those with both an L/S ratio above 2 and PG of 1% or more, however, the risk has been reduced to 0. There are other factors to be considered in the interpretation of the L/S ratio: A low L/S ratio carries a much smaller risk at a more advanced gestation, and in black infants the risk of RDS is low with an L/S ratio of more than 1.2 (Richardson and Torday, 1994).

The measurement of SP-A and SP-B by enzyme-linked immunosorbent assay has been made in amniotic fluid samples for the purpose of predicting the occurrence of RDS (Dilger et al, 1994). Although SP-A and SP-B increased with advancing gestation, the excellent predictive value of the L/S ratio and PG was not improved by the additional measurement of surfactant proteins (Pryhuber et al, 1991).

A rapid test for the evaluation of amniotic fluid samples is the foam stability test, in which samples of variable dilution are shaken with 95% alcohol and the tubes examined for stable foam (Clements et al, 1972); it has not been found entirely satisfactory but may be used in conjunction with other tests. A modification of this shake test is the stable microbubble test, in which stable bubbles are counted under the microscope; fewer than 5 stable microbubbles/mm^2 is considered positive for RDS (Chida et al, 1993). This test has been found to have a positive test predictive value of 95% to 100% and a negative test predictive value of 85% to 90%. This test is rapid and inexpensive and may be adapted to tracheal aspirate samples after birth.

The TDx-FLM assay depends on fluorescence polarization after the introduction of a fluorescent probe into the sample under standardized conditions; in the commercially available application, the polarization values are converted to read the results in mg surfactant/g albumin. In their assessment of this test, Herbert and colleagues (1993) found that values of less than 30 mg/g indicate immaturity and a positive test; the positive test predictive accuracy is 61% and the negative test predictive accuracy is 100%. If the sample has both an immature TDx-FLM and an immature foam stability test, the positive test predictive accuracy is 83%. Herbert and colleagues described their sequential approach to diagnostic testing, using a simple test first and progressively more complex testing next; they were best satisfied with results for the combination of TDx-FLM first, followed by the foam stability test. Tait and coworkers (1987), evaluating the receiver operating curves for TDx-FLM and L/S ratio without PG on a large prospective set of samples, found the TDx-FLM to be slightly better than the L/S ratio without PG. This rapid automated test shows great promise.

Early Postnatal Prediction

The L/S ratio may be used on tracheal aspirate samples to predict RDS, but the threshold level of 2.0 must be raised to 3.0 (Harker et al, 1992). The measurement of PG on tracheal aspirate samples is also useful, and the combination of low L/S ratio and absent PG on tracheal aspirate samples gives a positive test predictive value of 89%. Skelton and Jeffery (1994) have obtained good results with the click test, another modification of the shake test, in tracheal aspirate samples from preterm infants. After shaking a 0.2-mL sample of tracheal aspirate with an equal volume of 95% ethanol, the bubbles, suspended in airless water, are examined under the microscope; if the bubbles increase and decrease in size, this means an active surfactant and therefore a negative test. The positive test predictive accuracy is 100% and the negative test predictive accuracy is 93% for tracheal aspirate samples from preterm infants. This test, or the stable microbubble test described previously, may be used in tracheal aspirate samples of small premature infants at birth for predicting the presence of RDS; in turn, the result may be used in deciding on the use of early surfactant therapy. The measurement of static lung compliance is also useful for this purpose; if the measurement is less than 1.8 mL/cm H$_2$O/m body length, the positive test predictive value is 100%, and if the measurement is more than 1.8, the negative test predictive value is 92% (Wilkie et al, 1994). This test, however, is complex and expensive.

Prophylaxis with Antenatal Glucocorticoid Hormones

A vast literature on the effect of corticosteroid hormones on lung and surfactant maturation in animal and tissue culture models has accumulated (Ballard, 1986). Since 1972, when Liggins and Howie described decreased mortality, decreased incidence of RDS, and less severe RDS in a prospective blinded study done in New Zealand, more than 23 studies have been published worldwide. Not all of these studies have been of appropriate size, and not all have been of sufficient quality to exclude the problems of bias and error; this has resulted in widespread misinterpretation of the results and a regrettable underuse of glucocorticoid therapy (Ryan and Finer, 1995).

The National Perinatal Epidemiology Unit at Oxford published the results of a meta-analysis of 12 randomized, controlled trials (Crowley et al, 1990). To be included, the trials had to meet rigorous standards. Crowley and associates concluded that maternal steroid therapy significantly reduced the incidence of RDS, intraventricular hemorrhage, necrotizing enterocolitis, and neonatal death; in addition, they concluded that the duration and costs of hospital care for the newborn infant were greatly decreased. The benefits applied to all infants at a gestational age of 24 to 34 weeks, and this was not affected by race or gender or by the presence of prelabor rupture of amniotic membranes (Crowley, 1992).

The National Institutes of Health (NIH) reported the conclusions of a panel of experts; the NIH commissioned an updated meta-analysis, a neonatal registry review, and a cost-benefit analysis and evaluated the scientific literature according to the rigorous standards of the U.S. Preventive Services Task Force (NIH Consensus Development Conference Statement, 1995; NIH Consensus Development Panel, 1995). The NIH concluded that the incidence of

RDS, intraventricular hemorrhage, and neonatal death was significantly reduced (odds ratios 0.5, 0.5, and 0.6), and it regarded the evidence as compelling. The benefits were not affected by race or gender or by the presence of premature rupture of membranes, and, most important, the benefits were still apparent in infants in whom exposure was less than 24 hours. In infants of 24 to 28 weeks, the evidence for a reduced incidence of RDS was less certain, but the severity of RDS and the incidence of severe intraventricular hemorrhage were significantly decreased.

There is no reasonable evidence that the incidence of infection is increased in either the mother or the infant. The results of long-term follow-up studies have shown no problems with general health or neurodevelopment that could be attributed to the use of hormone therapy (Ballard, 1986). The NIH panel estimated that if the use of prenatal steroids could be increased from the current level of 15% in preterm infants at 24 to 34 weeks' gestation to a more reasonable level of 60%, the cost savings for initial hospital care alone would be $157 million each year in the United States.

The recommendations of the NIH panel are as follows: (1) All fetuses between 24 and 34 weeks' gestation are candidates for this therapy; (2) the decision should not be influenced by race, gender, premature rupture of membranes, or anticipated surfactant therapy; (3) all patients eligible for tocolytic therapy should receive steroids; (4) because therapy for less than 24 hours is effective, all patients should be treated unless immediate delivery is anticipated; (5) patients of less than 30 weeks' gestation should be treated because of the reduction in intraventricular hemorrhage; (6) treatment may be withheld in the presence of overt amnionitis; (7) treatment consists of betamethasone 12 mg every 24 hours for two doses or dexamethasone 6 mg every 12 hours for four doses.

Liggins and Howie (1972) reported a higher incidence of RDS in infants delivered more than 7 days after maternal steroid treatment, which means that the beneficial effect is reversible. Routine retreatment after 7 days is not recommended, however, unless the mother is still in active labor and imminent delivery before 34 weeks is still a likely possibility (Ballard and Ballard, 1995).

A number of studies have examined the question of the very immature infant, a problem that has been of great concern to many obstetricians. To examine the question of treatment before 30 weeks' gestation, Kattner and colleagues (1992) carried out a meta-analysis with more than 250 infants and found a significant reduction in the incidence of RDS with maternal steroid treatment. Then in a prospective study, they enrolled 135 mothers in a trial of prenatal steroids and found a significant increase in survival in the treated infants. Garite and coworkers (1992) performed a small randomized, controlled trial of prenatal corticosteroids in mothers without premature rupture of membranes at gestational age 24 to 28 weeks; they found no reduction in the incidence of RDS, but they found a dramatic reduction in the incidence of severe intraventricular hemorrhage. The data obtained for the March of Dimes–sponsored Prematurity Prevention Program were analyzed for the effect of prenatal steroids; major reductions in the incidence of RDS, intraventricular hemorrhage, and death were found in infants between 26 and 31 weeks'

gestation and treated with prenatal steroids (Maher et al, 1994). The data for a controlled trial of indomethacin were examined for the effect of antenatal steroids; in infants between 600 and 1250 g birth weight, a large decrease in the incidence of intraventricular hemorrhage was found with antenatal steroid treatment (Ment et al, 1995).

Prenatal glucocorticoids appear to have several other beneficial effects in the small preterm infant (Ballard, 1986). Clyman and associates (1981) demonstrated a significant reduction in the incidence of clinically significant patent ductus arteriosus with prenatal betamethasone therapy. Van Marter and colleagues (1990) reported data indicating that the incidence of BPD is reduced in preterm infants exposed to prenatal corticosteroids; this appears logical in view of the evidence relating RDS, especially severe RDS, to the occurrence of BPD. Other effects observed in animal models include decreased pulmonary protein leaks (Rider et al, 1989), induction of rat lung antioxidant enzymes (Frank et al, 1985), and acceleration of renal function in the fetal lamb (Scholle and Braunlich, 1989; Stonestreet et al, 1983)

The results for prenatal steroid therapy can be further improved; the effects of prenatal steroid and exogenous surfactant therapy proved to be additive in several initial small trials (Jobe et al, 1993). The effect of prenatal steroids has been retrospectively analyzed in the large number of infants enrolled in the many large controlled trials of exogenous surfactant performed in the last 10 years. The beneficial effects of steroids are still clearly apparent (Table 53–2) (Wright et al, 1995), even in populations that have

TABLE 53–2

Risk-Versus-Benefit Analysis of Prenatal Glucocorticoid Therapy

Risks

Possible increased risk of infection in mothers with prolonged rupture of membranes
Disturbs glucose homeostasis in diabetic mothers
Possible impact on T-cell development (with postnatal treatment)
Questionable effect on visual perception in boys

No Difference

Infection in infants
Growth: Height, weight, head circumference; neurologic development; cognitive development
Development of very-low-birth-weight infants
Lung mechanics and growth
Retrolental fibroplasia or vision

Benefit

Improved survival
Decreased incidence of RDS
Decreased severity of RDS
Decreased incidence of significant patent ductus arteriosus
Decreased incidence of intracranial hemorrhage
Decreased incidence of necrotizing enterocolitis
Decreased hospital costs
Decreased hospital stay

RDS, respiratory distress syndrome.

also benefited from the use of exogenous surfactant therapy.

Several other hormones, particularly thyroid hormone, are known to have a positive effect on lung development in tissue culture and animal models; because thyroid hormone does not cross the placenta, thyrotropin-releasing hormone (TRH) has been used instead. Randomized, controlled trials of prenatal TRH, in addition to corticosteroids, have demonstrated further improvements in outcome, related to controls treated with steroids alone. Ballard and colleagues (1992) reported a significant reduction in death and BPD at a postconceptional age of 36 weeks, and Knight and associates (1994) reported a New Zealand trial in which significant reductions in RDS incidence, RDS severity, BPD, and death were found. An Australian controlled trial of TRH, which used a smaller dose of TRH and a longer dosage interval, found a slightly increased risk for RDS occurring in infants born more than 10 days after treatment (ACTOBAT Study Group, 1995). Pierce and coworkers (1992) found decreased survival in oxygen-exposed newborn rats given TRH alone prenatally. This treatment therefore is still regarded as experimental (Ballard et al, 1995; Chiswick, 1995). A large multicenter trial in North America enrolled 1000 women under 30 weeks' gestation and found no significant benefit in decreasing lung disease (Ballard et al, 1997).

Treatment

Resuscitation

The mortality among all infants, including those with HMD, is increased by asphyxia. Therefore, the presence of a skilled resuscitation team at delivery of high-risk infants can reduce the morbidity and mortality of the disease (see Chapter 30).

Lung Expansion

Because secretion of surfactant is impaired by inadequate expansion of the lungs at birth (Lawson et al, 1979), many believe that it is appropriate to intubate all infants weighing less than 1000 g at birth and to initiate mechanical ventilation with positive end-expiratory pressure (PEEP) in the delivery room. Similar treatment may be used for larger premature infants if they have respiratory distress or are not vigorous in the delivery room. For infants less than 1000 g birth weight, the administration of artificial replacement surfactant in the delivery room or soon thereafter may prevent the condition from developing or greatly improve the course of the disease (see Surfactant Replacement).

Surfactant Replacement

Infants less than 1000 g birth weight should be treated prophylactically with exogenous surfactant within 15 to 30 minutes of birth but only after adequate stabilization. Larger infants should be treated as early as possible, preferably before the age of 2 hours and certainly before the age of 6 hours. A mammalian surfactant is currently preferred. The dose should be 100 mg/kg, the interval between doses

should be 12 hours, and two to three doses should be given but omitted when the inspired oxygen decreases below 30%. The dose should be given as rapidly as possible followed by bag-tube ventilation to insure even distribution, but it should not be given so rapidly as to obstruct the airways and promote hypercarbia; the number of aliquots for each dose does not matter, 2 aliquots being as good as 4 aliquots. Although widely practiced, there is little evidence to support rotation and tilting of the patient during the procedure (Broadbent et al, 1995). After surfactant instillation, it is customary to maintain the patient on conventional mechanical ventilation, but Verder and coworkers (1994) have demonstrated that larger infants may be extubated to nasal CPAP and the need for endotracheal intubation and conventional mechanical ventilation reduced. (See further discussion of surfactant replacement in Chapter 51.)

Thermal Neutrality

Infants should be nursed in a warm environment so that oxygen consumption is maintained at minimal levels. This usually means servo-controlling the anterior abdominal skin temperature at 36.5°C, but small premature infants may need to be servo-controlled at 36.9°C to maintain the rectal temperature at 37°C. The measured energy expenditure is 55 calories/kg per day during the first 4 days (Samiec et al, 1994); the caloric intake is usually only 25 calories/kg per day, so it is important to minimize increased caloric expenditure.

Blood Gas Monitoring

Infants with HMD require monitoring of blood pressure, blood gases, electrolytes, calcium, and glucose. Blood samples may be obtained from an umbilical arterial catheter (see Chapter 51).

Oxygen

As previously discussed (see Chapter 50), oxygen therapy is beneficial, despite the presence of large right-to-left shunts. Increased inspired oxygen produces (1) a rise of alveolar oxygen pressure in open low $\dot{V}/\dot{Q}$ units (see Fig. 53–4), (2) relief of regional hypoxic vasoconstriction in this compartment, (3) a reduction in true right-to-left shunt, and (4) an increase of arterial oxygen saturation (Hansen et al, 1979).

Fluid Restriction and Attention to Serum Electrolytes

Because HMD is characterized by high surface tension pulmonary edema (Boughton et al, 1970) and high permeability pulmonary edema (Jefferies et al, 1984), fluid restriction to 50 mL/kg per day is indicated for many infants with HMD for the first 48 hours or until the onset of diuresis. A controlled trial of this kind of fluid restriction, compared with a modest increase in the fluid intake, showed a significant reduction in the incidence of BPD at the age of 1 month and at a postconceptional age near term (Tammela et al, 1992). Close attention should be paid to fluid intake, urine output, urine concentration, and serum electrolytes. Premature infants have an excess of extracellular fluid and are expected to lose at least 10% of body weight by the end of the 1st week of life. It is not necessary or beneficial to administer sodium in the first few days of life (Costarino et al, 1992). Potassium should also be restricted because hyperkalemia may be troublesome (Stefano et al, 1993). In the very immature infant (24 to 26 weeks' gestation) with extremely permeable skin, there may be excessive evaporative losses, and much higher amounts of fluid may be required (see Chapter 34). If the serum sodium rises sharply, especially if it approaches 150 mEq/L, it can be assumed that insensible water losses through the skin are excessive, and the fluid intake should be liberalized accordingly. To minimize insensible water losses, it is useful to manage the infant in a humidified incubator; alternatively, if the infant is on an open warmer, it is useful to place a transparent plastic cover across the infant and across the sides of the bassinet and to run a gentle flow of heated mist into the infant's microenvironment.

Minimal Stimulation

Manipulations, such as heel sticks, tracheal suctioning, diaper changes, and even weighing, should be kept to a minimum because these procedures have been shown to reduce arterial oxygen tension (Lucey, 1981); they probably also increase oxygen consumption and may contribute to the genesis of cerebral hemorrhage by rapidly raising arterial blood pressure to excessive levels. It is not appropriate to give enteral feedings to infants with HMD because this condition is usually accompanied by poor intestinal motility. Many centers now insert an umbilical vein catheter as well as an arterial catheter and use the venous catheter to infuse glucose and the arterial catheter to infuse saline. The major reason for this is that a source of glucose-free blood is needed to monitor glucose tolerance adequately without the use of heel sticks, which are painful to the infant and disturbing. The umbilical vein catheter should be positioned with its tip at the junction of the inferior vena cava and the right atrium. This catheter is well tolerated; it provides for better nutrition; and, contrary to older reports, it is not associated with increased infection or late thrombotic complications (Pereira et al, 1992).

Blood Pressure Support

Premature infants with RDS frequently have a low arterial blood pressure in the first 12 hours of life, as defined by normative data (Versmold et al, 1981). Many extremely-low-birth-weight infants with RDS probably have a low blood pressure for many days after birth, and this may predispose them to brain injury (Kopelman, 1990). In small premature infants without intraventricular hemorrhage, the normal mean blood pressure is more than 30 mm Hg during the 1st week of life (Shortland et al, 1988). Intraventricular hemorrhage is more common in those who have a mean blood pressure less than 30 mm Hg (Miall-Allen et al, 1987), and a mean blood pressure less than 30 mm Hg is more common in those who develop an intraventricular hemorrhage (Puccio et al, 1994).

Adequate oxygenation may be difficult in the presence of hypotension and reduced pulmonary blood flow. In infants with a low hematocrit, poor peripheral perfusion, and metabolic acidosis, the hypotension is often due to hypovolemia and responds to a cautious infusion of 10 or 20 mL/kg of saline, human plasma protein fraction (Plasmanate), or blood. Only a few infants have obvious signs of hypovolemia, however, and echocardiographic studies in small premature infants have shown that many have decreased cardiac contractility, which is reflected in a poor cardiac output and significant hypotension (Gill and Weindling, 1993a). If there are no signs of hypovolemia, the infusion of dopamine at 5 to 10 µg/kg per minute is usually effective at increasing the mean blood pressure. A randomized, controlled trial of Plasmanate versus dopamine in hypotensive preterm infants showed that only 45% responded to Plasmanate, whereas 89% responded to dopamine (Gill and Weindling, 1993b). Others have suggested that dopamine is superior to dobutamine for the correction of hypotension in small premature infants (Christophe Roze et al, 1993); this was confirmed in a controlled trial (Klarr et al, 1994) in which dopamine was successful in elevating the mean blood pressure in 97% of infants, compared to dobutamine, which was successful in 67% of infants. Serial echocardiographic data have shown dopamine dose-dependent increases in cardiac output and stroke volume, without significant changes in heart rate or systemic vascular resistance (Padbury et al, 1986).

Helbock and colleagues (1993) presented evidence that many small preterm infants with RDS have low cortisol levels, and their hypotension is corrected with hydrocortisone; others have found that small premature infants with RDS needing inotrope support have lower cortisol levels than small premature infants with RDS not needing inotrope support (Scott and Watterberger, 1995). Other centers have found that dexamethasone often corrects the low blood pressure in these infants after an interval of 6 to 12 hours (Fauser et al, 1993). Fauser and coworkers suggested that the mechanism involved protein induction of adrenergic receptors. One of the many benefits of prenatal corticosteroid therapy is that the mean blood pressure is higher in treated infants (Kari et al, 1994; Moise, 1995). Evans and Iyer (1993) found that the mean blood pressure increased after successful closure of the ductus arteriosus with indomethacin, but the effect was small. Adequate attention to the blood pressure is important in the management of RDS.

Alkali Therapy

Severe metabolic acidosis may increase pulmonary vascular resistance, impair surfactant synthesis, reduce cardiac output, and ultimately reduce ventilation. An early trial showed that continuous infusion of glucose-bicarbonate solutions reduced the mortality of HMD (Usher, 1963). With the introduction of better methods for oxygenating infants, however, bicarbonate therapy no longer appears to have much benefit (Corbet et al, 1977), and it may be harmful in infants who are not being ventilated adequately and have a high arterial P_{CO_2}.

Continuous Positive Airway Pressure

CPAP may be administered by endotracheal tube, endopharyngeal tube, nasal prongs, face mask, or head box, or it may be administered by negative pressure applied around the body with the airway at atmospheric pressure. Since it was first described (Gregory et al, 1971), CPAP has been shown to reduce mortality in infants who weigh more than 1500 g (Rhodes and Hall, 1973) and to reduce the requirements for oxygen and mechanical ventilation in all infants with RDS (Fanaroff et al, 1973).

Nasal prong CPAP of 5 cm H_2O may be started early for any signs of RDS; this approach is used in many hospitals, even for the tiniest infants (Jacobsen et al, 1993; Kamper et al, 1993; Wung, 1993; Wung et al, 1975), with the expectation that some infants avoid intubation, mechanical ventilation, lung injury, and perhaps chronic lung disease. There may be some evidence for this approach, in that these hospitals may have a lower incidence of BPD than other hospitals (Avery et al, 1987). It may be possible to improve this strategy; some centers that use nasal CPAP in this way have suggested that in larger infants it is reasonable to intubate for surfactant administration and to mechanically ventilate briefly, while surfactant distribution is completed, and then to extubate the infant and continue with nasal CPAP (Verder et al, 1994). In a controlled trial, it was shown that the subsequent requirement for intubation and mechanical ventilation was significantly reduced with the addition of exogenous surfactant to the early nasal CPAP strategy.

In the traditional approach to the use of CPAP support, endotracheal CPAP is frequently used in larger infants (>1500 g) in the hope that mechanical ventilation will not be necessary; it should be started when the oxygen requirement reaches 50%. Many believe that endotracheal CPAP alone is not likely to be successful in smaller infants (<1500 g) and proceed directly to mechanical ventilation. In the larger infants, the initial level of endotracheal CPAP used is 5 cm H_2O at an oxygen requirement of 50%, and the pressure is increased in 1 cm H_2O steps for each 10% increase in the oxygen requirement. The incidence of pulmonary air leak with this regimen is no higher than the spontaneous rate for RDS (Corbet and Adams, 1978). Infants who require an oxygen concentration of more than 80% with endotracheal CPAP of 8 to 10 cm H_2O usually need mechanical ventilation. With the advent of surfactant therapy, it is now common to omit the initial CPAP step, to start surfactant administration and mechanical ventilation when the oxygen requirement is 40% to 50% or less, and to use CPAP only later when the infant is near clinical recovery and extubation. Another possible strategy in larger infants is intubation and mechanical ventilation for surfactant administration and then endotracheal CPAP.

Because CPAP may overdistend the lung and impair the pulmonary circulation, attempts have been made to identify optimal levels. As CPAP is increased and approaches optimum, the aA.D_{CO_2} falls significantly, but as the optimal level is exceeded, both the aA.D_{CO_2} and the arterial P_{CO_2} rise significantly (Landers et al, 1986). Under clinical conditions, increased hypercarbia may indicate excessive CPAP, which should be recognized and corrected before oxygenation deteriorates.

Mechanical Ventilation

Infants with HMD who weigh less than 1500 g and infants treated with exogenous surfactant usually require mechanical ventilation. Otherwise the standard indications are (1) significant apnea, (2) hypercarbia with pH less than 7.20, and (3) arterial oxygen pressure under 50 mm Hg in 80% to 100% oxygen (see Chapter 51). There is no agreement on the settings for rate, peak pressure, inspiratory time, or PEEP, but the principles should not be in doubt. The aim is to correct the blood gas abnormalities with as little lung injury and circulatory compromise as possible. Because the time constant in RDS is short, long inspiration times are not necessary and may be associated with pulmonary air leaks. Oxygenation is dependent on the level of mean airway pressure; in a condition characterized by low lung volume and low lung compliance, it is efficient to use generous levels of PEEP. Many clinicians allow modest hypercarbia to avoid excessive peak pressures and tidal volumes; it is high tidal volumes that injure the lung, not high peak pressures. Under isocarbic conditions, smaller tidal volumes can be used if the rate is higher. Two controlled trials have shown that there is an advantage to ventilating at a rate of 60 breaths/min with a short inspiratory time compared with 30 breaths/min; in each case, there was a significant reduction in the incidence of lung injury with pneumothorax (Heicher et al, 1981; OCTAVE Study Group, 1991). To prevent gas trapping, sufficient time must be allowed for expiration, so there is a limit on how high the rate can be increased; most infants can be managed at a rate of 60 breaths/min initially. If the infant's breathing is asynchronous, especially if the blood pressure is low, it is common to find that the blood pressure wave fluctuates (Perlman and Thach, 1988), a phenomenon associated with an increased incidence of intraventricular hemorrhage (Perlman et al, 1983). Asynchrony is also associated with an increased incidence of pneumothorax. Sometimes an increase in the rate to 70 or 80 breaths/min may promote adequate synchrony (Greenough et al, 1987), or breathing can be suppressed with narcotics (Goldstein and Brazy, 1991). If narcotics are given, expiratory braking may be impaired, so it is again important to use generous levels of PEEP to promote the maintenance of lung volume (Miller et al, 1994). Despite optimal settings, a few infants fail conventional mechanical ventilation and must be rescued with high-frequency oscillator ventilation or extracorporeal membrane oxygenation.

Closure of the Patent Ductus Arteriosus

Especially in infants less than 1000 g birth weight, a patent ductus arteriosus may contribute significantly to the overall problem during recovery from RDS and may predispose the infant to the development of BPD. If the ductus is demonstrated to be patent at the age of 3 to 4 days by two-dimensional echocardiography and pulsed Doppler ultrasonography, the evidence suggests that it is unlikely to close spontaneously within a reasonable time (Dudell and Gersony, 1984), and therefore it should be closed, either with indomethacin therapy or with surgery (see Chapter 61). In infants greater than 1000 g birth weight, in whom the risk for BPD is much less, it is reasonable to close the patent ductus arteriosus later, if signs of a significant left-to-right shunt develop, usually at the age of 5 to 10 days.

Corticosteroids

There has been considerable interest in the use of dexamethasone in the treatment of RDS, with the emphasis being on the prevention of BPD in very small infants. Silverman (1994) has reviewed the evidence that inflammation in RDS begins on the 1st day of life, presumably as a response to lung injury, and this occurs in the absence of infection. (See Chapter 55.)

Prognosis

The chances of survival in HMD are directly related to birth weight and gestational age and are affected by prenatal treatment with glucocorticoids, by surfactant replacement therapy, and by the severity and complications of the disease. (See Chapters 38 and 55.)

TRANSIENT TACHYPNEA OF THE NEWBORN

Transient tachypnea of the newborn (TTN) is also known as *delayed clearance of fetal lung fluid*. In 1966, Avery and coworkers reported on eight near-term infants with early onset of respiratory distress whose chest radiographs showed hyperaeration of the lungs, prominent pulmonary vascular markings, and mild cardiomegaly (Fig. 53–10).

The respiratory symptoms were transient and relatively mild, and most infants improved within 2 to 5 days. The investigators named the disorder *transient tachypnea of the newborn* and speculated that it was the result of delayed clearance of fetal lung liquid.

Pathophysiology

Most authors agree with Avery and coworkers that TTN represents a transient pulmonary edema resulting from delayed clearance of fetal lung liquid. Clearance of the fetal lung liquid actually begins before birth (during the last few days of gestation and during labor). During the first step of this process, secretion of lung liquid is inhibited by increased concentrations of catecholamines and other hormones. Then reabsorption occurs: passively, secondary to differences in oncotic pressure between the air spaces, the interstitium, and blood vessels, and actively, secondary to active transport of sodium out of the air space. Infants born prematurely or those born without labor do not have the opportunity for early lung liquid clearance, and they begin their extrauterine life with excess water in the lungs. After birth, water in the air spaces moves rapidly to the extra-alveolar interstitium, where it pools in perivascular cuffs of tissue and in the interlobar fissures. It is then

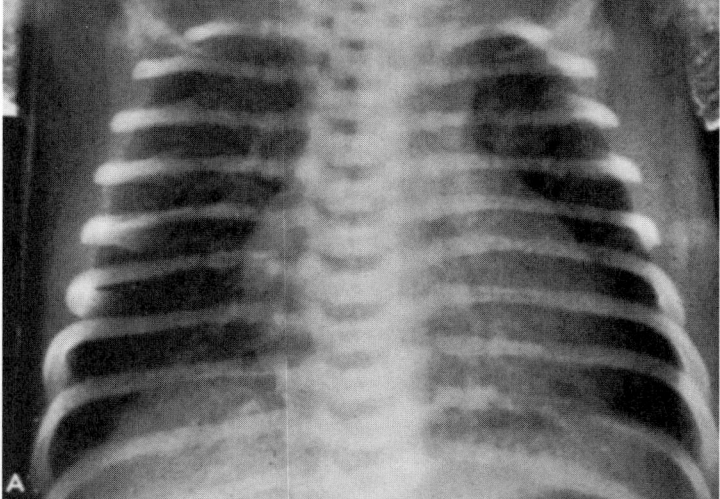
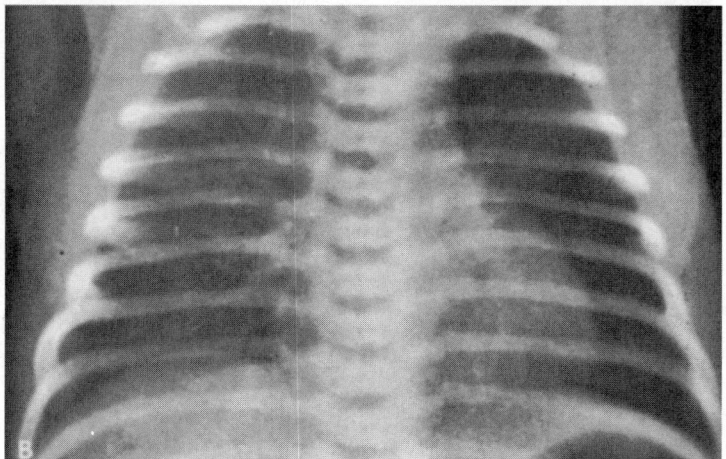

FIGURE 53–10. The large cardiovascular silhouette, air bronchogram, and streaky lung fields were seen at 2 hours of age (*A*) but had cleared by 24 hours of age *(B),* typical of transient tachypnea of the newborn or delayed clearance of lung liquid.

cleared gradually from the lung by the lymphatics or by absorption directly into the small blood vessels (Bland and Nielson, 1992). Infants with TTN, however, are often hypoproteinemic, and decreased plasma oncotic pressure may delay the direct absorption of water into the blood vessels (Cummings et al, 1993). In addition, these infants can have elevated pulmonary vascular pressures and ventricular dysfunction (Halliday et al, 1981), which increase central venous pressure and impair thoracic duct function and the removal of interstitial water by the lymphatics. This is especially true in infants who receive a large transfusion of blood from the placenta as a result of delayed cord clamping or milking of the cord (Saigal et al, 1977).

The symptoms of TTN result from compression of the compliant airways by water that has accumulated in the perivascular cuffs of the extra-alveolar interstitium. This compression results in airway obstruction and hyperaeration of the lungs secondary to gas trapping. Hypoxia results from the continued perfusion of poorly ventilated lung units; hypercarbia results from mechanical interference with alveolar ventilation and from central nervous system depression. Lung function measurements in infants with TTN are compatible with airway obstruction and gas trapping. The functional residual capacity measured by gas dilution is normal or reduced, whereas measurements of thoracic gas volume by plethysmography are increased, suggesting that some of the gas in the lungs is not in communication with the airways (Krauss and Auld, 1971).

Clinical Signs

It was initially thought that TTN was limited to term or larger preterm infants, but it is now clear that very small infants also may present with pulmonary edema from retained fetal lung liquid; this may complicate their surfactant deficiency and account for some of their need for supplemental oxygen and ventilation. There is often a history of heavy maternal sedation, maternal diabetes, or delivery by elective cesarean section. Affected infants may be mildly depressed at birth, and this may mask many of their early symptoms. They are often tachypneic with respiratory rates ranging from 60 to 120 breaths/min and may have hyperinflation with grunting, chest wall retractions, and nasal flaring.

Arterial blood gas tensions often reveal a respiratory acidosis, which resolves within 8 to 24 hours, and mild to moderate hypoxemia. These infants seldom require more than 40% oxygen to maintain an adequate PaO_2 and usually are in room air by 24 hours of age. They have no evidence to indicate right-to-left shunting of blood at the ductus arteriosus or foramen ovale.

Chest radiographs reveal hyperaeration, which is often accompanied by mild cardiomegaly (Fig. 53–11). Water contained in the perivascular cuffs produces prominent vascular markings in a *sunburst pattern* emanating from the hilum. The interlobar fissures are widened, and pleural effusions may be present. Occasionally, coarse, fluffy densities may be present, indicating alveolar edema. The radiographic abnormalities resolve over the first 2 to 3 days after birth.

Clinical Course and Treatment

As its name implies, TTN is a benign, self-limited disease. The infant's need for supplemental oxygen is usually highest at the onset of the disease then progressively decreases. Infants with uncomplicated disease usually recover rapidly without any residual pulmonary disability. Although the

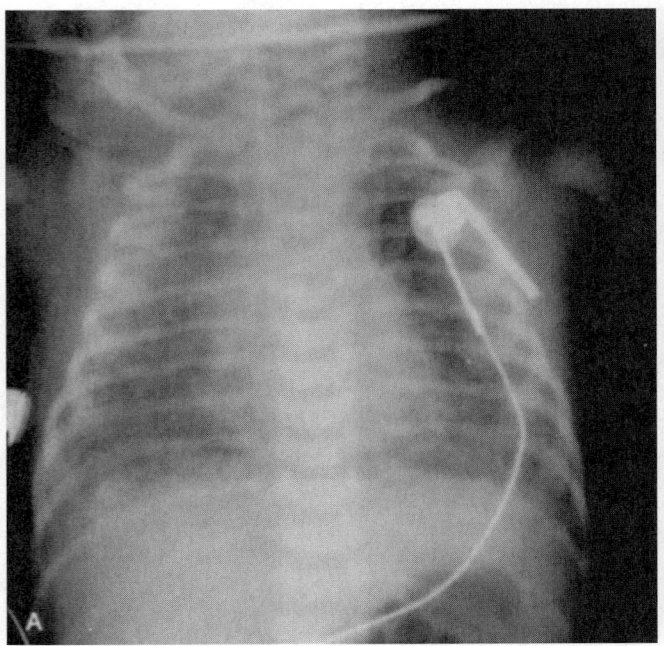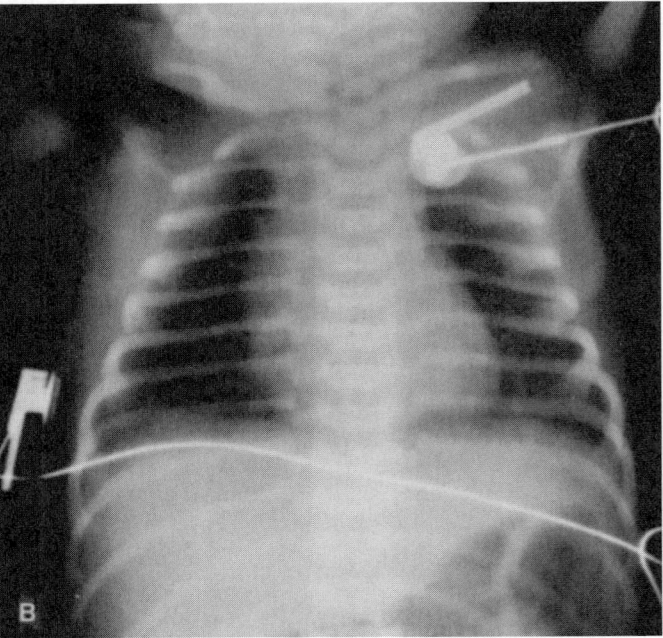

FIGURE 53–11. Chest radiographs from an infant with transient tachypnea of the newborn. Initially the radiograph is compatible with massive interstitial and alveolar edema *(A)*. The radiograph is clear 48 hours later *(B)*.

symptoms of TTN relate to pulmonary edema, one controlled trial that assessed therapy with diuretics found no evidence for their efficacy (Wiswell et al, 1985); however, many infants respond to nasal CPAP.

PERSISTENT PULMONARY HYPERTENSION OF THE NEWBORN

Gersony and coworkers (1969) described a group of term infants without structural heart disease who became cyanotic shortly after birth and had only mild respiratory distress. These infants all had suprasystemic pulmonary arterial pressures and evidence of right-to-left shunting of blood across persistent fetal pathways (the foramen ovale and ductus arteriosus). The nature of these shunts led to the name *persistence of the fetal circulation*. Subsequently the name was changed to *persistent pulmonary hypertension of the newborn* to describe the pathophysiology of the disorder more accurately.

Pathogenesis

Successful transition from intrauterine to extrauterine life requires that the pulmonary vascular resistance decrease precipitously at birth. In infants with PPHN, this decrease does not occur: Pulmonary arterial pressure remains elevated, and blood is shunted right to left across the ductus arteriosus and foramen ovale. In addition, the persistently high pulmonary vascular resistance increases right ventricular afterload and oxygen demand and impairs oxygen delivery to the right ventricle, the posterior wall of the left ventricle, and the subendocardial regions of the right ventricle. Ischemic damage resulting from this reduction in oxygen delivery may cause both right and left ventricular failure, papillary muscle necrosis, and tricuspid insufficiency (Setzer et al, 1980). Finally, increased right ventricular afterload results in displacement of the septum into the left ventricle, impaired left ventricular filling, and reduced cardiac output.

In some instances, pulmonary vascular resistance remains only transiently elevated at birth (Table 53–3) and decreases rapidly once the underlying condition is corrected. There are also a number of other conditions, however, in which the pulmonary vascular resistance remains persistently elevated either because of active constriction of pulmonary vessels or because of some anatomic abnormality.

Active constriction of pulmonary vessels can complicate the course of bacterial sepsis or pneumonia in the newborn (Shankaran et al, 1982). Experiments in animals show that this increase in pulmonary vascular resistance is temporally related to increased plasma thromboxane concentrations (Hammerman et al, 1988); it can be blocked by the administration of inhibitors of prostaglandin synthesis (Rojas et al, 1983). Active constriction of pulmonary vessels can also complicate the course of meconium aspiration pneumonia. Some studies suggest that vasoactive substances present in meconium or amniotic fluid diffuse through the lung and either constrict pulmonary vessels directly or induce platelet aggregation in the microcirculation with the subsequent release of thromboxane. Clinical data support this hypothe-

TABLE 53–3

Causes of Persistent Pulmonary Hypertension

Transient Pulmonary Hypertension

Hypoxia with or without acidosis
Hypothermia
Hypoglycemia
Polycythemia

Persistent Pulmonary Hypertension

Active vasoconstriction
  Bacterial sepsis and/or pneumonia
  Perinatal aspiration syndromes
Underdevelopment of the lung
  Diaphragmatic hernia
  Potter syndrome
  Other causes of pulmonary hypoplasia
Maldevelopment of pulmonary vessels
  Idiopathic
  Chronic intrauterine asphyxia
  Meconium aspiration pneumonitis
  Premature closure of the fetal ductus arteriosus

sis and show an association among perinatal aspiration syndromes, transient thrombocytopenia, and PPHN (Segall et al, 1980). Moreover, pathologic data demonstrate platelet plugging in the microcirculation of the lung of infants dying of PPHN associated with meconium aspiration pneumonia (Levin et al, 1983). Alternatively, in utero hypoxia may lead both to changes in the pulmonary vessels and to passage of meconium, and some infants born through meconium *without* aspiration have PPHN (see later).

Anatomic abnormalities of the pulmonary vascular bed fall into two general categories: those associated with underdevelopment of the lung and those that result from maldevelopment of the vessels. In the case of pulmonary hypoplasia, lung mass is reduced, yet cardiac output is appropriate for body size. As a result, the volume of blood flowing through the existing pulmonary vessels is relatively high, pulmonary arterial pressures are high, and relative pulmonary vascular resistance is increased. In addition to this anatomic impediment to flow, infants with pulmonary hypoplasia are likely to have maldevelopment of the pulmonary vessels and an increased pulmonary vascular resistance from anatomic obstruction of existing vessels (Geggel et al, 1986; Naeye et al, 1976).

Maldevelopment of pulmonary vessels refers predominantly to abnormalities of vascular smooth muscle found in lungs of infants dying from PPHN (Murphy et al, 1981) (Fig. 53–12). In these infants, pulmonary arterial smooth muscle hypertrophies and extends from preacinar arteries into normally nonmuscular intra-acinar arteries, even to the level of the alveolus (Fig. 53–13). This thickened muscle encroaches on the vessel lumen and results in mechanical obstruction to blood flow. In extreme cases, vascular maldevelopment can cause a reduction in number of arteries per cross-sectional area of the lung. A review of the associated clinical entities and the available data from experiments in animals suggests that this vascular maldevelopment is the result of sustained pulmonary hypertension in utero. PPHN is strongly associated with low-grade chronic intrauterine

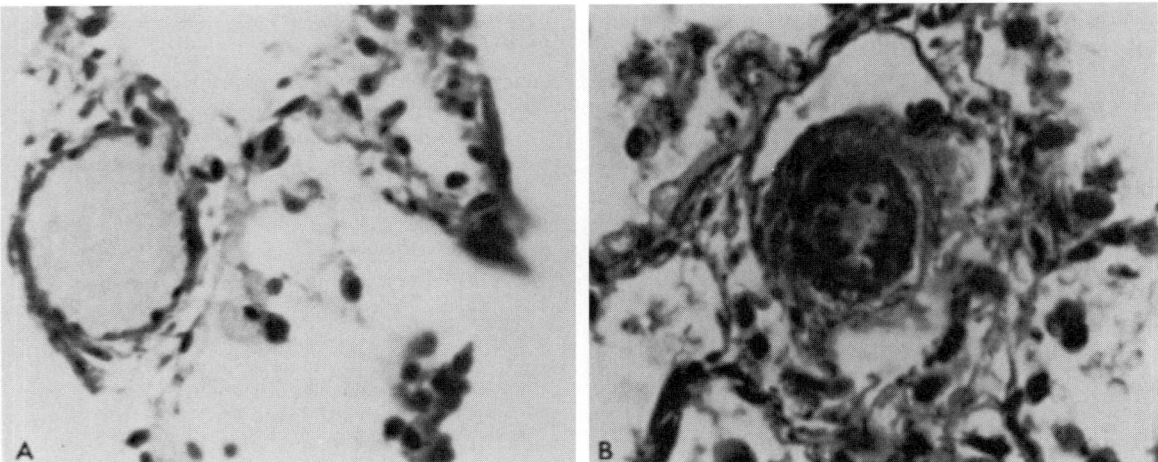

FIGURE 53–12. Photomicrographs of alveolar wall arteries distended with the barium gelatin suspension from a 3-day-old infant with normal lungs *(A)* and a 3-day-old infant with persistent hypertension *(B)*. The normal artery *(A)* is nonmuscular with a single endothelial cell lining surrounded by a thin layer of connective tissue. In *B,* the artery wall is composed of smooth muscle (darkly stained) two-cell-layers thick surrounded by a thick connective tissue sheath enclosing a dilated lymphatic (located superiorly). (Elastin-van Gieson stain ×250.) (Courtesy of Dr. John Murphy.)

hypoxia. In fact, it is likely that unrecognized asphyxia or ductal closure may account for a large proportion of cases labeled as *idiopathic*. In chronically asphyxiated fetuses, pulmonary arterial pressure can be increased by active constriction of pulmonary arterioles secondary to hypoxia.

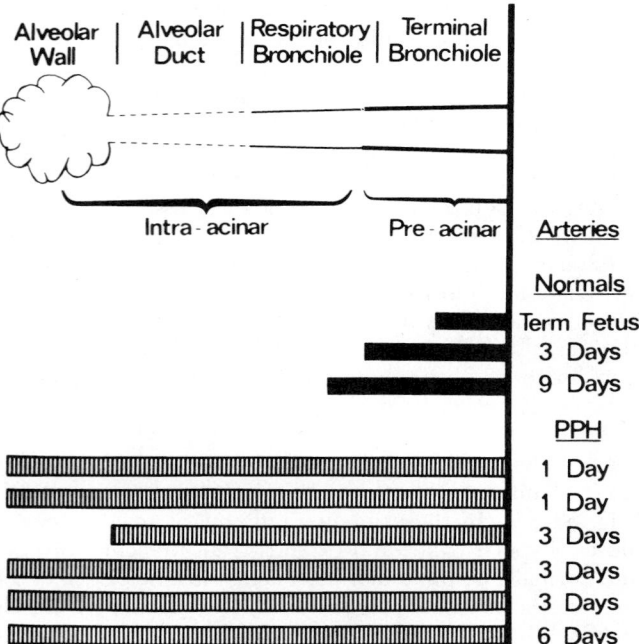

FIGURE 53–13. Vascular maldevelopment in infants with persistent pulmonary hypertension of the newborn. In normal infants, no muscular arteries are found within the acinus. All patients with pulmonary hypertension had extension of muscle into intraacinar arteries. (From Murphy JD, Rabinovitch M, Goldstein JD, Reid LM: The structural basis of persistent pulmonary hypertension of the newborn infant. J Pediatr 98:962, 1981.)

Because the pulmonary circulation is parallel to the systemic circulation, it also can be increased secondary to asphyxia-induced increases in systemic arterial pressure. Experimental data from fetal rats and lambs support both these hypotheses (Soifer et al, 1987); however, although systemic hypertension (even by itself) consistently results in vascular maldevelopment (Levin et al, 1978b), intrauterine hypoxia does not consistently result in vascular maldevelopment (Geggel et al, 1986).

Premature closure of the ductus arteriosus secondary to maternal ingestion of inhibitors of prostaglandin synthesis has been associated with PPHN. In two groups of infants with idiopathic PPHN, those without ductal level shunting had higher salicylate levels than those with ductal level shunting (Perkin et al, 1980). Experiments in animals show that premature closure of the ductus (Morin, 1989; Wild et al, 1989) results in maldevelopment of pulmonary vessels, presumably by forcing a greater portion of the combined ventricular output through the lungs at a significantly higher pressure (Levin et al, 1978a). The association between meconium aspiration pneumonia and vascular maldevelopment is interesting. Of 11 infants dying of meconium aspiration pneumonia, 10 were found to have significant vascular smooth muscle hypertrophy with extension of muscle into intra-acinar arteries (Murphy et al, 1984). This maldevelopment could be secondary to chronic intrauterine asphyxia, the release of vasoactive substances by meconium in the trachea, or a circulating intestinal peptide stimulating both pulmonary vasoconstriction and intestinal motility. Finally, because disorders associated with underdevelopment of the lung also result in intrauterine pulmonary hypertension, it is not too surprising that they also frequently are associated with maldevelopment of existing vessels. This is particularly true in infants with congenital diaphragmatic hernia and accounts for much of the respiratory instability of these infants (see Chapter 60).

It has become apparent that these anatomically abnormal vessels also exhibit certain functional abnormalities (Morin and Stenmark, 1995). One of the more important functions of the vascular endothelium is to produce the vasodilator nitric oxide (NO). NO is produced in endothelial cells from L-arginine by the enzyme NO synthase. It diffuses rapidly into smooth muscle cells where it stimulates production of cyclic guanosine monophosphate (GMP) and smooth muscle relaxation. NO production by endothelial cells is responsible for the vasodilation that occurs in response to substances such as acetylcholine and bradykinin. As a result, these mediators are called *endothelial cell–dependent vasodilators.* Because NO is such a potent pulmonary vasodilator, it is tempting to speculate that impaired NO synthesis contributes to PPHN. In support of this speculation, investigators have shown that infants with PPHN have lower urinary nitrite and nitrate concentrations than do infants without pulmonary disease, suggesting that their ability to produce NO may be impaired (Dollberg et al, 1995). Adults with pulmonary hypertension have reduced expression of NO synthase in their lungs (Giaid and Saleh, 1995), and chronic inhibition of NO production in the fetal lamb results in PPHN (Fineman et al, 1995). Data show that endothelial cell–dependent vasodilation is impaired in fetal lambs with pulmonary hypertension secondary to early closure of the ductus arteriosus (McQueston et al, 1995). How much of this impairment is at the level of NO synthase versus guanylate cyclase remains to be determined (Steinhorn et al, 1995).

In addition to production of the vasodilator NO, endothelial cells also produce endothelin 1, which may act as a pulmonary vasoconstrictor in the newborn. Infants with PPHN have increased concentrations of endothelin 1 in arterial blood. These concentrations correlate with the severity of the pulmonary hypertension (Rosenberg et al, 1993).

Alveolar capillary dysplasia is a rare cause of persistent pulmonary hypertension. This disorder is characterized by failure of formation and ingrowth of alveolar capillaries, medial muscle hypertrophy of pulmonary arteries, and anomalously located pulmonary veins running along with pulmonary arteries. Fewer than 20 such cases have been reported to date, including two reports of affected siblings (Boggs et al, 1994). These patients present with symptoms similar to idiopathic PPHN. This disorder should be considered in patients with idiopathic PPHN who fail to improve (i.e., fail to wean from extracorporeal membrane oxygenation).

Clinical Manifestations

Affected infants are usually delivered at term or post-term and frequently are born through meconium-stained fluid. They are often thought to be normal after brief distress at birth. Then within the first 12 hours after birth, they are recognized as having cyanosis and tachypnea without apnea and retractions or grunting. They frequently have a cardiac murmur that is compatible with tricuspid insufficiency, but systemic blood pressure is normal. Hypoglycemia frequently complicates many of the associated conditions, such as sepsis and meconium aspiration; hypocalcemia also occurs often. Arterial blood gas tensions reveal severe arterial oxygen desaturation with relatively normal CO_2 tensions. In infants with significant ductal level shunting, the oxygen saturation measured from the right brachial or radial artery is greater than that obtained from the umbilical artery. Chest radiographs may reveal cardiomegaly. For infants with idiopathic PPHN, the lung fields are clear and appear undervascularized (Fig. 53–14). For the remainder of the associated entities, chest radiographs reflect the underlying parenchymal disease. Electrocardiograms reveal ventricular hypertrophy appropriate for age; in more severe cases, they also reveal S-T segment depression in the precordial leads, suggestive of ischemia. All infants suspected of having PPHN should undergo ultrasound examination of the heart to rule out cyanotic congenital heart disease, to document right-to-left shunting of blood at the foramen ovale and ductus arteriosus, and to measure systolic time intervals. Prolonged systolic time intervals support a diagnosis of pulmonary hypertension, but they are not definitive because they also can be prolonged by right ventricular dysfunction. Infants in whom cyanotic congenital heart disease cannot be ruled out by echocardiogram should undergo cardiac catheterization. At some point in the course of the disease, most infants with PPHN increase SaO_2, at least transiently, in response to some therapeutic intervention. Infants who can never be oxygenated should be considered for cardiac catheterization.

Therapy

The objectives for therapy for infants with PPHN are to lower the pulmonary vascular resistance, to maintain the systemic blood pressure, to reverse the right-to-left shunts, and to improve arterial oxygen saturation and oxygen delivery to the tissues. Based on results from several centers suggesting that conservative medical management of infants with PPHN may reduce the need for extracorporeal membrane oxygenation and improve outcome (Dworetz et al, 1989; Wung et al, 1985), the authors have adopted an

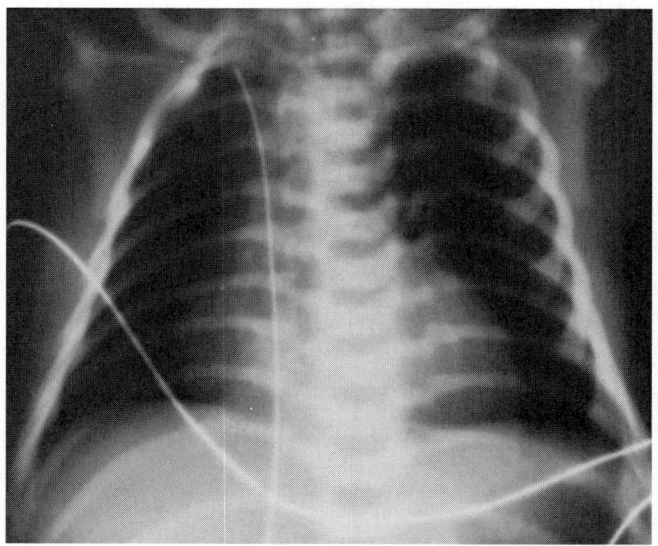

FIGURE 53–14. Chest radiograph from infant with idiopathic persistent pulmonary hypertension of the newborn. Lung fields appear hyperlucent with decreased vascularity.

approach to therapy that seeks to reduce oxygen demand while maximizing oxygen delivery.

All of these infants should be nursed in a neutral thermal environment. Cold stress raises the metabolic rate, increases oxygen consumption, and causes the infant to release norepinephrine, which is a pulmonary vasoconstrictor. Fluids should be restricted and hypoglycemia and hypocalcemia corrected. Systemic hypotension and acidosis should be corrected by judicious use of blood and alkali. Calcium, blood products, and hyperosmolar solutions are potentially vasoactive and should be infused with caution in this group of infants. Infusion of dopamine at low doses (2 to 10 $\mu g/kg/min$) may increase cardiac output without affecting systemic or pulmonary vascular resistance. At higher doses, dopamine exhibits considerable α-adrenergic activity and may result in systemic vasoconstriction and increased blood pressure along with an actual reduction in cardiac output (Feltes et al, 1987). In addition, higher doses of dopamine can constrict pulmonary as well as systemic vessels. If the central hematocrit is greater than 60% to 65%, a partial exchange transfusion should be performed to lower the hematocrit and to reduce the effects of hyperviscosity on the pulmonary artery pressure.

In infants with PPHN, the pulmonary circulation seems to be exceptionally sensitive to changes in oxygen tension. Therefore, it is advisable to try to maintain the PaO_2 between 80 and 100 torr if possible. There is no evidence to suggest that maintaining PaO_2 in excess of 100 torr improves the outcome of the infant with PPHN, and prolonged exposure to excessively high PaO_2 can injure other organs, such as the brain and the eye (Hansen and Gest, 1984). Furthermore, in patients with severe PPHN, attempts to maintain PaO_2 between 80 and 100 torr may result in unacceptable complications of therapy. Therefore, many centers now tolerate much lower values for PaO_2 (≥ 40 torr) in infants with severe PPHN (Wung et al, 1985) and use repeated measurements of blood lactate and pH to provide insurance of adequate tissue oxygenation.

Oxygen should be given by hood, up to 100% if necessary. If oxygen alone does not lower the pulmonary vascular resistance and improve arterial oxygen saturation, the next step is to induce alkalosis. Although several studies in animals have shown that both respiratory and metabolic alkalosis effectively lower pulmonary vascular resistance (Fike and Hansen, 1989; Schreiber et al, 1986), only respiratory alkalosis has been studied in infants (Drummond et al, 1981). The use of neuromuscular blockers such as pancuronium bromide in these infants is controversial and should probably be reserved for infants requiring extremely high inspiratory pressures. Because these infants are extremely sensitive to external stimuli, they should be sedated with either morphine or fentanyl and handled as little as possible. To avoid alveolar overdistention, the inspiratory time is kept short (0.15 to 0.20 second). The lungs of infants with PPHN frequently have normal to prolonged expiratory time constants, so expiratory time must be kept relatively long to prevent gas trapping. Therefore, the respirator rate is set at 60 to 80 breaths/min. Inspiratory pressure is adjusted to control the $PaCO_2$. PEEP is useful only in patients with parenchymal lung disease. If the pulmonary hypertension is severe, however, the infant frequently develops surfactant deficiency and pulmonary

edema and consequently may respond to end-expiratory pressure later in the course of the disease.

After 3 days of ventilation with high concentrations of oxygen and high airway pressures, infants with PPHN develop pulmonary parenchymal abnormalities that are characterized by decreased lung compliance and infiltrates on chest radiograph compatible with pulmonary edema (Sosulski and Fox, 1985). At this point, the pulmonary vascular bed is no longer sensitive to changes in pH and much less sensitive to changes in FIO_2. This probably is in part the result of vascular remodeling that occurs in these infants (Kourembanas et al, 1993; Stenmark et al, 1993).

High-Frequency Ventilation

Both high-frequency jet ventilation and high-frequency oscillator ventilation are highly effective in controlling $PaCO_2$. As a result, several groups have postulated that these ventilatory modalities may be effective in improving oxygenation in infants with PPHN when associated with parenchymal disease. High-frequency jet ventilation results in a reduction in both $PaCO_2$ and ventilator pressures in infants with PPHN but has no effect on ultimate outcome (Carlo et al, 1989). In a single randomized trial, high-frequency oscillator ventilation was more successful than conventional ventilation in reducing the need for extracorporeal membrane oxygenation in this patient population (Clark et al, 1994). (See Chapter 51.)

Surfactant Replacement

Data suggest that surfactant deficiency may play a role in several of the diseases associated with PPHN. Meconium aspiration pneumonia (Sun et al, 1993b) and bacterial pneumonia are both associated with surfactant inactivation, and surfactant replacement therapy appears to improve gas exchange in these infants (Al-Mateen et al, 1994; Auten et al, 1991; Khammash et al, 1993). Infants with congenital diaphragmatic hernia appear to have delayed maturation of the pathways for surfactant synthesis (Suen et al, 1993). Preliminary data from studies in lambs with diaphragmatic hernia suggest that administration of exogenous surfactant may improve outcome (Wilcox et al, 1994). Although these results are promising, surfactant replacement therapy for infants with PPHN must still be considered experimental. For the infant in whom ventilation with oxygen does not result in an acceptable PaO_2, the only other alternative is to try to lower the pulmonary vascular resistance by pharmacologic means.

Nitric Oxide

Several studies have shown that inhalation of NO in concentrations ranging from 5 to 80 ppm selectively dilates pulmonary vessels and improves oxygenation in infants with PPHN (Kinsella et al, 1992; Roberts et al, 1997). As discussed previously, NO is an important regulator of vascular tone, and an inability to generate NO or respond to NO may underly some of the conditions associated with PPHN. (See Chapter 52.)

Tolazoline

Tolazoline was at one time the drug most commonly used to try to dilate the pulmonary vascular bed (Drummond et al, 1981). It is an α-adrenergic blocker with some mild cholinergic properties and is also a potent releaser of histamine, which, in the newborn, is a pulmonary vasodilator. Its effects are not specific for the lung. In most studies, the effects of tolazoline on the systemic circulation are at least as great as those on the pulmonary circulation. In one review of 314 patients, 59% improved after receiving tolazoline, whereas only 54% survived. Complications referable to tolazoline therapy occurred in 70% of the patients: 42% had increased gastrointestinal secretions, 31% had gastrointestinal bleeding, 32% developed hypotension, and 36% became oliguric (Peckham, 1982). *As a result, tolazoline is seldom used to treat infants with PPHN.* If it is to be used, it is administered as a 1 mg/kg bolus over 1 to 2 minutes occasionally followed by 0.15 to 0.30 mg/kg per hour infused through a scalp vein. Tolazoline has a plasma half-life of between 2 and 8 hours and is excreted mostly in the urine. If urine output is less than 1 mL/kg per minute, excretion is reduced markedly (Ward et al, 1986). Its use usually requires circulatory support with volume expansion or the use of pressors. One study showed that endotracheal administration of tolazoline to lambs resulted in more specific pulmonary vasodilation (Curtis et al, 1993), but there are no data in human infants with PPHN to support this route of administration.

Magnesium

Magnesium is a known vasodilator and there have been two uncontrolled trials suggesting that infusion of magnesium may lower pulmonary vascular resistance and improve oxygenation in patients with PPHN (Abu-Osba et al, 1992; Wu et al, 1995). In studies in neonatal piglets with pulmonary hypertension secondary to hypoxia, magnesium did not act as a selective pulmonary vasodilator and had significant effects on the systemic circulation (Ryan et al, 1995).

ATP-MgCl$_2$ and Other Medical Therapy

ATP-MgCl$_2$ is a selective pulmonary vasodilator in the newborn lamb with drug-induced pulmonary hypertension (Fineman et al, 1990). In children with pulmonary hypertension secondary to congenital heart disease, ATP-MgCl$_2$ lowers pulmonary vascular resistance without changing systemic artery pressure (Brook et al, 1994). Although these results are promising, clinical use must await trials in human infants with PPHN.

Despite their early promise, other pharmacologic agents, such as prostacyclin and prostaglandin D$_2$, have not been proven to be efficacious in the treatment of PPHN (Kaapa et al, 1985; Soifer et al, 1982).

Infants that do not respond to medical therapy are now considered candidates for extracorporeal membrane oxygenation in most centers (see Chapter 52).

Outcome

In the past, the mortality for infants with PPHN ranged from 20% to 40%, and the incidence of neurologic handicap ranged from 12% to 25% (Ballard and Leonard, 1984). Sell and coworkers (1985), however, found that only 40% of 40 infants with PPHN in their institution were developmentally normal at 1 to 4 years: 32% had an abnormal or suspect neurologic examination, and 20% had neurosensory hearing loss. A report described 34 infants managed conservatively without induced alkalosis (Marron et al, 1992). All 34 survived. Of the 27 who returned for follow-up, 4 had severe neurologic deficits, 5 had minor abnormalities, and none had any evidence of sensorineural hearing loss.

In most centers, extracorporeal membrane oxygenation has further reduced mortality from severe PPHN. Data from the ECMO Registry shows that for infants requiring extracorporeal membrane oxygenation because of meconium aspiration pneumonia, sepsis, or idiopathic PPHN, the survival rates are now 93%, 76%, and 83%. The improvement for infants with diaphragmatic hernia has not been as dramatic, and survival is still only 58% for those that require extracorporeal membrane oxygenation. Overall, neurologic morbidity for infants with PPHN requiring extracorporeal membrane oxygenation remains high, nearly 20% (Kanto, 1994).

MECONIUM ASPIRATION PNEUMONIA

Meconium, an odorless, thick, blackish green material, is first demonstrable in the fetal intestine during the 3rd month of gestation. It is an accumulation of debris that consists of desquamated cells from the alimentary tract and skin, lanugo hairs, fatty material from the vernix caseosa, amniotic fluid, and various intestinal secretions. Meconium is biochemically composed of a mucopolysaccharide of high blood group specificity, a small amount of lipid, and a small amount of protein that decreases throughout gestation. Its blackish green color is the result of bile pigments.

Pathogenesis

Meconium staining of amniotic fluid (MSAF) occurs in roughly 10% to 26% of all deliveries (Nathan et al, 1994). The risk of MSAF is strongly correlated with gestational age. Before 37 weeks of gestation, the risk of MSAF is less than 2%, whereas the risk after 42 weeks of gestation is nearly 44%.

The cause of MSAF is controversial. At one time, the passage of meconium in utero was thought to be synonymous with fetal asphyxia. At present, however, the relationship between MSAF and fetal asphyxia is unclear. A number of studies have failed to show any consistent effects of MSAF on Apgar score, fetal scalp pH, or incidence of fetal heart rate abnormalities (Abramovici et al, 1974; Baker et al, 1992; Fenton and Steer, 1962; Miller et al, 1975). These studies led to speculation that asphyxial episodes too brief to decrease pH or Apgar scores may cause the passage of meconium in utero. These conclusions were supported by a study showing that there was no correlation between the consistency of meconium and markers of fetal asphyxia (Trimmer and Gilstrap, 1991). Several studies have suggested that the presence of meconium (Nathan et al, 1994), especially thick meconium (Berkus et al, 1994), increases the risk of fetal acidosis and an adverse neonatal outcome. Moreover, one study found that although MSAF correlated poorly with markers of acute intrauterine asphyxia (pH, lactate, and hypoxanthine concentrations), it correlated well with blood erythropoietin concentration (a marker of chronic intrauterine asphyxia). The strong correlation between MSAF and gestational age supports two additional theories: (1) It is possible that the passage of meconium in utero is the result of transient parasympathetic stimulation from cord compression in a neurologically mature fetus. (2) Passage of meconium in utero is a natural phenomenon that reflects the maturity of the gastrointestinal tract. Despite these theories, most physicians agree that MSAF in connection with fetal heart rate abnormalities is a marker for fetal distress and is associated with an increased perinatal morbidity.

Meconium may enter the trachea and airways in utero. In one study, meconium was recovered from the tracheas of 56% of meconium-stained infants in the delivery room (Gregory et al, 1970). Another study (Davis et al, 1985) described 12 infants who died with meconium aspiration pneumonia (MAP), even though their tracheas were suctioned vigorously in the delivery room. These findings suggest that in some instances, particularly with distressed infants who are gasping, considerable peripheral migration of meconium can occur while the fetus is still in utero. Autopsy data that show meconium in the terminal airways of stillborn fetuses support this theory (Brown and Gleicher, 1981). It is highly unlikely, however, that significant intrauterine aspiration of meconium is the result of normal fetal breathing because the rate of production of fetal lung fluid is such that the net movement of fluid is out of the lung. It is more likely that meconium is aspirated into the tracheobronchial tree when the fetus begins to gasp deeply in response to hypoxia and acidosis. Data showing that cord arterial pH is lower in meconium-stained infants with meconium in their tracheas at delivery supports this hypothesis (Yeomans et al, 1989). It is unknown whether the reduced rate of production of fetal lung fluid that accompanies labor contributes to the movement of meconium into the trachea or to its migration peripherally.

If meconium is not removed from the trachea after delivery, with the onset of respiration it migrates from the central airways to the periphery of the lung. Initially, particles of meconium produce mechanical obstruction of the small airways that results in hyperinflation with patchy atelectasis. Later, small airway obstruction is the result of chemical pneumonitis and interstitial edema. During this later stage, hyperinflation persists, and areas of atelectasis become more extensive. In addition, there is infiltration of the alveolar septa by neutrophils, necrosis of alveolar and airway epithelia, and accumulation of proteinaceous debris within the alveolus.

Infants who die of MAP complicated by pulmonary hypertension frequently have evidence of injury to the vascular bed of the lung. In these infants, vascular smooth muscle extends into the walls of normally nonmuscular intra-acinar arterioles and reduces their luminal diameter, which subsequently interferes with the normal postnatal drop in pulmonary vascular resistance. In addition, these infants may demonstrate plugs of platelets in their small vessels that reduce the overall cross-sectional area of the pulmonary vascular bed (Levin et al, 1983).

Airway resistance is increased in newborn infants and experimental animals with MAP (Tran et al, 1980; Yeh et al, 1982). In addition, dynamic lung compliance is reduced while static lung compliance is unchanged, suggesting that airway obstruction is patchy and located in peripheral airways. Functional residual capacity is increased in animals with MAP but not in humans. The effects of meconium on surfactant function have been studied in a number of animal models of meconium aspiration. Although early data suggested that meconium did not impair surfactant function (Tran et al, 1980), more recent data suggest that meconium does inactivate surfactant (Davey et al, 1993; Moses et al 1991; Sun et al, 1993a). Furthermore, several investigators have shown that surfactant replacement may improve gas exchange in animals with MAP (Ohama et al, 1994; Paranka et al, 1992; Sun et al, 1993b). Gas exchange is inevitably altered in MAP. In the absence of persistent pulmonary hypertension, hypoxia is the result of continued perfusion of poorly ventilated lung units, whereas hypercarbia is the result of a decrease in minute ventilation and increase in respiratory dead space. Some infants with MAP have elevated pulmonary arterial pressures with shunting of blood right to left across the foramen ovale and ductus arteriosus (see discussion of pulmonary hypertension).

Clinical Manifestations

Infants with MAP are often postmature and have visible meconium staining of the nails, the skin, and the umbilical cord. Many infants with MAP have been asphyxiated, and much of the early distress may relate more to asphyxia and retained fetal lung fluid complicated by elevated pulmonary vascular resistance than to the presence of meconium in the airways. Infants with MAP have clinical evidence of lung overinflation, with a barrel chest. Auscultation of the chest reveals diffuse rales and rhonchi. The chest radiograph shows patchy areas of atelectasis and areas of overinflation (Fig. 53–15). Pneumothorax and pneumomediastinum are common. The clinical symptoms progress over 12 to 24 hours as meconium migrates to the periphery of the lung. Because meconium must ultimately be removed by phagocytes, respiratory distress and requirements for supplemental oxygen may persist for days or even weeks after birth. Infants who present with a shorter course and with rapid resolution of symptoms are more likely to have had retained fetal lung fluid than MAP.

Therapy

Symptomatic infants with meconium suctioned from their tracheas should be given chest physiotherapy and warmed humidified oxygen to breathe. Lung lavage may result in deterioration of lung function. Because of the high incidence of air leaks, positive-pressure ventilation should be avoided, if possible. Judicious use of nasal or endotracheal CPAP (4 to 7 cm H_2O) may improve oxygenation in the patient who is unresponsive to oxygen administration alone. This improvement in oxygenation is achieved presumably by stabilizing the small airways and improving the ventilation of poorly ventilated lung units. High airway pressures may impair oxygenation by impeding blood flow to well-ventilated lung units. Mechanical ventilation should be reserved for infants with apnea from birth asphyxia or for

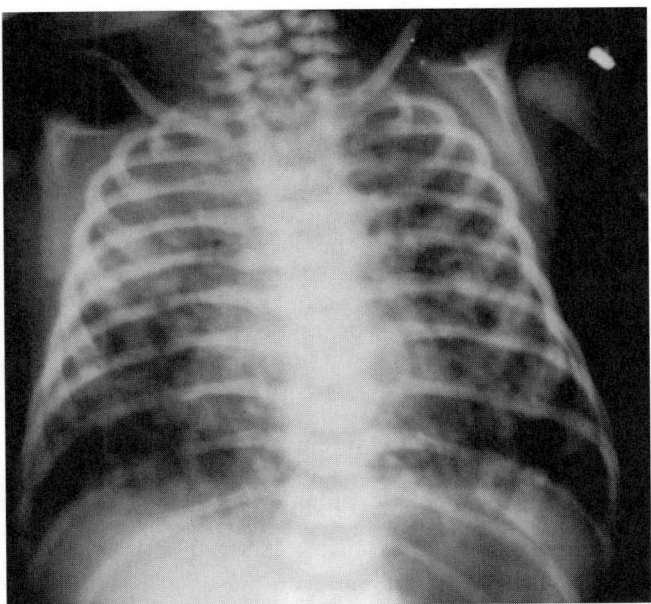

FIGURE 53–15. Chest radiograph of an infant with meconium aspiration pneumonia.

those who cannot maintain their PaO₂ greater than 50 mm Hg in 100% oxygen. These infants are often large and vigorous and tend to fight mechanical ventilation, which makes oxygenation difficult and increases the chances of air leak. If this occurs, the patient may require neuromuscular blockade. Because MAP is an obstructive lung disease, the time constant for expiration is prolonged in severely involved areas of the lung. Careful attention must be paid to expiratory time (ventilatory rate) to prevent inadvertent PEEP, further gas trapping, and alveolar rupture.

The role of antibiotics in the treatment of MAP is controversial. Meconium enhances bacterial growth by reducing host resistance, and the risk of intra-amniotic infection is increased in the presence of MSAF (Romero et al, 1991; Wen et al, 1995). No studies have shown that infection plays a role in the pathogenesis of MAP. Because of the difficulty in distinguishing MAP from bacterial pneumonia, the authors routinely treat infants with presumed MAP with antibiotics pending negative cultures.

The use of corticosteroids for treatment of MAP is not recommended. The time to weaning to room air is prolonged by corticosteroids in infants with MAP (Yeh et al, 1977), and the mortality of rabbits with experimental MAP is increased by treatment with corticosteroids (Frantz et al, 1975).

As discussed earlier, there is some evidence that infants with MAP have surfactant inactivation. A recent controlled trial studied the effects of surfactant replacement (up to 4 doses of 150 mg/kg of beractant every 6 hours) on infants that were being mechanically ventilated for MAP (Findlay et al, 1996). They found that surfactant replacement therapy, if started within 6 hours after birth, improved oxygenation and reduced the incidence of air leaks, severity of pulmonary morbidity, and duration of hospitalization. Other therapies for the infant with MAP and PPHN, including the use of high-frequency ventilation, NO, and

extracorporeal membrane oxygenation, are covered in the section on PPHN and in Chapter 52.

Outcome

The outcome for infants with MAP has improved dramatically. In the past, MAP carried a risk of pneumothorax and pneumomediastinum of between 10% and 20% (Peterson and Pendleton, 1989). This risk increased to as high as 50% if the infant required mechanical ventilation. Now with improved approaches to the management of PPHN and the availability of extracorporeal membrane oxygenation, the mortality for meconium-stained infants is roughly 0.15% (Nathan et al, 1994). The mortality for infants with MAP requiring extracorporeal membrane oxygenation is less than 7% in most centers and approaches 0 is some units.

Prevention

Several older studies have shown that by clearing the airway of meconium at the time of birth, MAP can be virtually eliminated (Carson et al, 1976; Gregory et al, 1970; Ting and Brady, 1975). Based on these results, the American Heart Association and the American Academy of Pediatrics have recommended a combined obstetric and pediatric approach to the infant with MSAF (Bloom and Cropley, 1995). For infants born through thin watery meconium, no special management is necessary. For infants born through thick particulate or *pea soup* meconium, they recommend the following steps:

1. When the infant's head is delivered, the mouth, pharynx, and nose should be thoroughly suctioned by the obstetrician using a 10 French or larger suction catheter.
2. As soon as the infant has been placed on the radiant warmer and before drying, the hypopharynx should be visualized and residual meconium removed by suctioning. Then the trachea should be intubated and meconium suctioned from the lower airway. Tracheal suctioning should be performed using an appropriately sized endotracheal tube and a large-bore meconium aspirator. In the presence of severe asphyxia, it may not be possible to clear the trachea of all meconium, and clinical judgment must be used to determine the amount of suctioning. Intubation and suction is required even when meconium is not visible in the posterior pharynx. Studies have found that 7% to 10% of meconium-stained infants had meconium in their tracheas even when there was not any meconium visible at the vocal cords. A free flow of oxygen should be provided via oxygen tubing to minimize hypoxia during suctioning. After tracheal suctioning, the stomach should be emptied to prevent aspiration of swallowed meconium.

A more recent study questioned the need for intubation and suctioning of *nondistressed* term infants that were meconium stained. This study suggested that in the absence of asphyxia these infants were unlikely to have significant amounts of meconium in their tracheas and that the complications of intubation outweighed any benefit (Linder et al, 1988). This study has led several authors to recommend that direct endotracheal suctioning be reserved for infants born through thick meconium who are depressed and require positive-pressure ventilation (Cunningham et al, 1990; Yoder, 1994). This selective approach to the management of the meconium-stained infant has not received universal support (Kresch et al, 1991; Wiswell and Henley, 1992). In fact, a large retrospective study noted that a number of meconium-stained infants who developed MAP did not require resuscitation at birth and that infants who developed MAP after not having been suctioned may be at increased risk for adverse sequelae (Wiswell and Henley, 1992). As a result of this controversy, the American Heart Association and the American Academy of Pediatrics have added the following statement to their recommendations: "If an infant has passed thick meconium, yet is very active and crying vigorously, a judgment must be made whether the difficulty of intubating a vigorous infant outweighs the advantages of full meconium removal. However, many experienced individuals believe that meconium removal may be of primary importance to prevent the sequelae of meconium aspiration" (Bloom and Cropley, 1995).

A number of investigators have tried to prevent meconium aspiration by infusing saline into the amniotic cavity of mothers with thick MSAF. Several randomized trials have shown that amnioinfusion decreases the risk of meconium below the vocal cords, and a meta-analysis of five controlled trials found that amnioinfusion decreased the risk of meconium below the vocal cords and the risk of MAP (Dye et al, 1994). One large retrospective study (Usta et al, 1995) and a randomized, controlled trial (Spong et al, 1994) found no benefit to a policy of routine amnioinfusion. Furthermore, in the controlled trial, the risk of endometritis-chorioamnionitis was increased in the amnioinfusion group. As a result, the role of amnioinfusion in the prevention of MAP is still controversial.

RESPIRATORY DISTRESS SYNDROME IN TERM INFANTS

It is apparent that a small but significant number of infants have a severe lung disease, which cannot be described under any of the preceding conditions discussed. It is likely that they represent a heterogeneous group, but they all appear to have a condition characterized by the radiologic appearance of pulmonary edema, they may or may not have experienced clinical asphyxia during the delivery process, and they may or may not have evidence of myocardial failure. Because of the last-mentioned, these conditions may be described under names that emphasize the heart as the primary problem (Talner et al, 1992). The infants are usually full-term infants of 38 weeks or more, they may have severe respiratory failure, and they are sometimes candidates for high-frequency oscillator ventilation or extracorporeal membrane oxygenation; there is no evidence for tracheal aspiration of meconium, and bacterial cultures are invariably negative. It is often not possible to be sure of the diagnosis, and clinicians may differ in the diagnosis they assign, but the following conditions represent some of the possibilities.

Postasphyxial Pulmonary Edema

Pulmonary edema in newborn lambs following asphyxia from umbilical cord occlusion was described by Adamson and colleagues (1970). The lambs showed transudation of fluid from the circulation into the lungs in the presence of elevated lung capillary pressures. Infants with this condition are often depressed in the delivery room and require mechanical ventilation immediately or soon after birth (Corbet, 1990). In other infants breathing unassisted, there may be severe respiratory distress because of pulmonary edema, transient cardiomegaly, and cerebral irritation; Strang (1977) called this condition *postasphyxial lung edema*. In many infants, there is postnatal evidence of neurologic depression, and there may be seizures, consistent with a background of intrapartum asphyxia (Prod'hom, 1971). The radiologic appearance of the lungs is that of pulmonary congestion or pulmonary edema with diffuse coarse densities, and in some reports this may be called pneumonia. The heart may be enlarged on the chest radiograph with evidence of mitral or tricuspid valve insufficiency, hypotension, hepatomegaly, poor perfusion, and reduced urine output (Cabal and Siassi, 1988). On the echocardiogram, there may be evidence of poor myocardial contractability and low cardiac output (Walther et al, 1985). Some infants have ischemic changes on the electrocardiogram (Talner et al, 1992), and they may have elevated creatine phosphokinase and liver transaminase levels in the blood. Thibeault and colleagues (1984) described 65 infants with a low pH at birth, who required mechanical ventilation in the first few hours of life and improved soon after the age of 24 hours; they described these infants as having postasphyxial lung disease.

Infants with postasphyxial pulmonary edema do not usually have physical evidence for prematurity as in the case of RDS, or tracheal evidence for meconium aspiration, or bacterial evidence for neonatal pneumonia; instead they have evidence of asphyxia, heart failure, ventricular dysfunction, pulmonary edema, and often pulmonary hypertension. Some of these infants develop clinical pulmonary hemorrhage, which is now known to be hemorrhagic pulmonary edema, the most severe form of postasphyxial pulmonary edema. Treatment consists of oxygen, mechanical ventilation, base infusion, and circulation support, until spontaneous recovery occurs in a few days. Packed red cell transfusion to improve the hematocrit should be cautious. Sometimes these infants fail high-frequency oscillator ventilation and are considered for extracorporeal membrane oxygenation but may be excluded because of ultrasonic evidence for cerebral infarction or hemorrhage, a direct consequence of the asphyxia.

Acquired Respiratory Distress Syndrome

These term infants develop severe RDS soon after birth; the radiologic appearance is that of RDS with the same reticulogranular pattern of diffuse fine densities seen in the premature infant. They have clinical evidence for a low lung volume and reduced lung compliance. There may be a history of asphyxia at birth, as in postasphyxial pulmonary edema, but the radiologic picture is not the same, and the reports have not emphasized any problem with myocardial contractability secondary to asphyxia. It is inherent in this diagnosis that the infants do not have a developmental surfactant deficiency but instead an acquired problem owing to inactivation of normal amounts of surfactant. None of the reports have described lung maturity tests in late amniotic fluid samples or in early tracheal aspirate samples. It is not always clear from the reports why this diagnosis was assigned except that the infants were considered to be mature and to have RDS.

Faix and colleagues (1989) described a set of term infants with RDS who responded to mechanical ventilation with increased PEEP. A similar set of infants was described by Pfenninger and coworkers (1991); these too needed high levels of PEEP. Some of these infants may also respond to exogenous surfactant therapy (Davis et al, 1992; Gortner et al, 1994) or may require high-frequency ventilation or extracorporeal membrane oxygenation.

Congenital Alveolar Proteinosis Owing to SP-B Deficiency

Several families have been described in which full-term infants developed prolonged and eventually fatal RDS; detailed tissue analysis suggested that they had congenital alveolar proteinosis and SP-B deficiency (deMello et al, 1994a). Other families have since been described. The parents give no history of neonatal RDS, and many siblings are not affected; the mode of inheritance is autosomal recessive (Chetcuti and Ball, 1995). The condition is now known to be due to mutations in the SP-B gene; the most commonly described mutation (121 ins 2) involves a 2 base-pair insertion at position 375 in codon 121 of the cDNA (Nogee et al, 1994); the additional two bases produce a frameshift signal for termination of translation after codon 214. There is no detectable mRNA for SP-B.

The chest radiograph shows the granular pattern characteristic of HMD in preterm infants, and hence these infants may initially resemble other term infants with RDS. There is frequently evidence for severe pulmonary hypertension. The alveolar spaces are packed with a proteinaceous material rich in SP-A and SP-C but poor in surfactant phospholipids; there is no normal tubular myelin because of the SP-B deficiency, and surfactant function assessed by pulsating surfactometer is abnormal. The lamellar bodies in granular pneumocytes are poorly formed, and there may be basal, rather than apical, secretion, indicating defective transport protein signaling within the Type 2 epithelial cells (deMello et al, 1994b).

Oxygen, mechanical ventilation, repeated administrations of bovine surfactant containing relatively high levels of SP-B, and eventually extracorporeal membrane oxygenation have not been successful in changing the outcome. A few infants have survived for several months on mechanical ventilation. More recently, several infants have undergone lung transplantation with apparent success.

Prenatal amniotic fluid profiles have shown an L/S ratio of less than 2 and the absence of PG and SP-B at full-term gestation (Hamvas et al, 1994). To establish the diagnosis in newborn infants, tracheal aspirates or lung lavage aspirates should be examined for SP-B by either the enzyme-linked immunosorbent assay or by the Western blot procedure; the presence of any SP-B makes the diagnosis unlikely

(Nogee, 1995). It may be possible to test the infant or the parents for the gene mutation in a DNA diagnostic laboratory. Biopsy or autopsy samples of the affected infant's lung may be examined for surfactant proteins by immunostaining.

Ballard and colleagues (1995) have described a term newborn infant with partial SP-B deficiency, who needed extracorporeal membrane oxygenation and remained on mechanical ventilation until death at 9 months of age. The mother had the previously described point mutation in exon 4, and the father had a new point mutation at codon 236 in exon 7, which resulted in a single amino acid substitution. The infant's surfactant contained low levels of SP-B, more precursor than mature protein, and near-normal levels of mRNA for SP-B; this suggested a defect in translation or in post-translational processing. Other mutations have been reported, frequently occurring in conjunction with the 121 ins 2 mutation.

REFERENCES

Abman SH, Kinsella JP, Schaffer MS, et al: Inhaled nitric oxide in the management of a premature newborn with severe respiratory distress syndrome and pulmonary hypertension. Pediatrics 92:606, 1993.

Abramovici J, Brandes JM, Fuchs K, Timor-Tritsch I: Meconium during delivery: A sign of compensated fetal distress. Am J Obstet Gynecol 118:251, 1974.

Abu-Osba YK, Galal O, Manasra K, et al: Treatment of severe persistent pulmonary hypertension of the newborn with magnesium sulfate. Arch Dis Child 67:31, 1992.

ACTOBAT Study Group: Australian collaborative trial of antenatal thyrotropin releasing hormone (ACTOBAT) for prevention of neonatal respiratory disease. Lancet 345:877, 1995.

Adams FH, Fujiwara T, Emmanouilides GC, Raiha N: Lung phospholipids of human fetuses and infants with and without hyaline membrane disease. Pediatrics 77:833, 1970.

Adamson TM, Boyd RDH, Hill JR, et al: Effect of asphyxia due to umbilical cord occlusion in the foetal lamb on leakage of liquid from the circulation and on permeability of lung capillaries to albumin. J Physiol 207:493, 1970.

Al-Mateen KB, Dailey K, Grimes MM, et al: Improved oxygenation with exogenous surfactant administration in experimental meconium aspiration syndrome. Pediatr Pulmonol 17:75, 1994.

Auten RL, Notter RH, Kendig JW, et al: Surfactant treatment of full-term newborns with respiratory failure. Pediatr 87:101, 1991.

Avery ME, Fletcher BD: The Lung and Its Disorders in the Newborn Infant. Philadelphia, WB Saunders, 1974.

Avery ME, Gatewood OB, Brumley G: Transient tachypnea of newborn: Possible delayed resorption of fluid at birth. Am J Dis Child 111:380, 1966.

Avery ME, Mead J: Surface properties in relation to atelectasis and hyaline membrane disease. Am J Dis Child 97:517, 1959.

Avery ME, Tooley WH, Keller JB, et al: Is chronic lung disease in low-birth-weight infants preventable? A survey of eight centers. Pediatrics 79:26, 1987.

Baker PN, Kilby MD, Murray H: An assessment of the use of meconium alone as an indication for fetal blood sampling. Obstet Gynecol 80:792, 1992.

Ballard PL: Hormones and Lung Maturation. New York, Springer-Verlag, 1986.

Ballard PL, Ballard RA: Scientific basis and therapeutic regimens for use of antenatal glucocorticoids. Am J Obstet Gynecol 173:254, 1995.

Ballard PL, Nogee LM, Beers MF, et al: Partial deficiency of surfactant protein B in an infant with chronic lung disease. Pediatrics 96:1046, 1995.

Ballard RA, Ballard PL, Boardman C, et al, the TRH Collaborative Group: Antenatal thyrotropin releasing hormone (TRH) for the prevention of chronic lung disease (CLD) in the preterm infant. Pediatr Res 41:246A, 1997.

Ballard RA, Ballard PL, Cnaan A, Pinto-Martin J: Thyrotrophin releasing hormone for prevention of neonatal respiratory disease (Letter). Lancet 345:1572, 1995.

Ballard RA, Ballard PL, Creasy R, et al: Respiratory disease in very low birth weight infants after prenatal thyrotropin releasing hormone and glucocorticoid. Lancet 339:510, 1992.

Ballard RA, Leonard CH: Development follow-up of infants with persistent pulmonary hypertension of the newborn. Clin Perinatol 11:737, 1984.

Bancalari E, Garcia OL, Jesse MJ: Effects of continuous negative pressure on lung mechanics in idiopathic respiratory distress syndrome. Pediatrics 51:485, 1973.

Bauer CR, Morrison JC, Poole WK, et al: Decreased incidence of necrotizing enterocolitis after prenatal glucocorticoid therapy. Pediatrics 73:682, 1984.

Benatar SR, Hewlett AM, Nunn JF: The use of iso-shunt lines for control of oxygen therapy. Br J Anaesthesiol 45:711, 1973.

Benitz WE, Malachowski N, Cohen RS, et al: Use of sodium nitroprusside in neonates: Efficacy and safety. J Pediatr 106:102, 1985.

Berkus MD, Langer O, Samueloff A, et al: Meconium-stained amniotic fluid: Increased risk for adverse neonatal outcome. Obstet Gynecol 84:115, 1994.

Bland RD, Nielson DW: Developmental changes in lung epithelial ion transport and liquid movement. Ann Rev Physiol 54:373, 1992.

Bloom RS, Cropley C: Lesson 2: Initial steps. *In* AHA/AAP Neonatal Resuscitation Steering Committee (Eds): Textbook of Neonatal Resuscitation, 2nd ed. Elk Grove Village, IL, American Heart Association/Academy of Pediatrics, 1995, pp 2-3–2-36.

Boggs S, Harris MC, Hoffman DJ, et al: Misalignment of pulmonary veins with alveolar capillary dysplasia: Affected siblings and variable phenotypic expression. J Pediatr 124:125, 1994.

Bolton DPG, Cross KW: Further observations on cost of preventing retrolental fibroplasia. Lancet 1:445, 1974.

Boughton K, Gandy G, Gairdner D: Hyaline membrane disease: II. Lung lecithin. Arch Dis Child 45:311, 1970.

Broadbent R, Fok TF, Dolovich M, et al: Chest position and pulmonary deposition of surfactant in surfactant depleted rabbits. Arch Dis Child 72:F84, 1995.

Brook MM, Fineman JR, Bolinger AM, et al: Use of ATP-MgCl2 in the evaluation and treatment of children with pulmonary hypertension secondary to congenital heart defects. Circulation 90:1287, 1994.

Brown BL, Gleicher N: Intrauterine meconium aspiration. Obstet Gynecol 57:26, 1981.

Brumley GW, Hodson WA, Avery ME: Lung phospholipids and surface tension correlations in infants with and without hyaline membrane disease. Pediatrics 40:13, 1967.

Cabal LA, Siassi B: Shock in the newborn infant. *In* Emmanouilides GC, Baylen BG (Eds): Neonatal Cardiopulmonary Distress. Chicago, Year Book Medical Publishers, 1988, p 290.

Carlo WA, Beoglos A, Chatburn RL, et al: High-frequency jet ventilation in neonatal pulmonary hypertension. Am J Dis Child 143:233, 1989.

Carson BS, Losey RW, Bowes WA, Simmons MA: Combined obstetric and pediatric approach to prevent meconium aspiration syndrome. Am J Obstet Gynecol 126:712, 1976.

Chan V, Greenough A, Gamsu HR: High frequency oscillation for preterm infants with severe respiratory failure. Arch Dis Child 70:F44, 1994.

Chetcuti PAJ, Ball RJ: Surfactant apoprotein B deficiency. Arch Dis Child 73:F125, 1995.

Chida S, Fujiwara T, Konishi M, et al: Stable microbubble test for predicting the risk of respiratory distress syndrome: Prospective evaluation of the test on amniotic fluid and gastric aspirate. Eur J Pediatr 152:152, 1993.

Chiswick M: Antenatal TRH. Lancet 345:872, 1995.

Christophe Roze J, Tohier C, Maingueneau C, et al: Response to dobutamine and dopamine in the hypotensive very preterm infant. Arch Dis Child 69:59, 1993.

Chu J, Clements JA, Cotton EK, et al: Neonatal pulmonary ischemia: Clinical and physiological studies. Pediatrics 40:709, 1967.

Clark RH, Yoder BA, Sell MS: Prospective, randomized comparison of high-frequency oscillation and conventional ventilation in candidates for extracorporeal membrane oxygenation. J Pediatr 124:447, 1994.

Clements JA, Platzker ACG, Tierney DF, et al: Assessment of the risk of respiratory distress syndrome by a rapid test for surfactant in amniotic fluid. N Engl J Med 286:1077, 1972.

Clements JA, Tooley WH: Kinetics of surface active material in the fetal lung. *In* Hodson WA (Ed): Development of the Lung. New York, Marcel Dekker, 1977.

Clyman RI, Ballard PL, Sniderman S, et al: Prenatal administration of betamethasone for prevention of patent ductus arteriosus. J Pediatr 98:123, 1981.

Collaborative Group on Antenatal Steroid Treatment: Effect of antenatal dexamethasone administration on the prevention of respiratory distress syndrome. Am J Obstet Gynecol 141:276, 1981.

Corbet A: Respiratory disorders in the newborn. *In* Chernick V, Kendig EL (Eds): Disorders of the Respiratory Tract in Children. Philadelphia, WB Saunders, 1990, p 288.

Corbet A: Clinical trials of synthetic surfactant in the respiratory distress syndrome of premature infants. Clin Perinatol 20:737, 1993.

Corbet A: Medical manipulation of the ductus arteriosus. *In* Garson A, Bricker JT, Fisher DJ, Neish SR (Eds): The Science and Practice of Pediatric Cardiology. Philadelphia, Lea & Febiger, 1996.

Corbet A, Adams J: Current therapy in hyaline membrane disease. Clin Perinatol 5:299, 1978.

Corbet AJS, Adams JM, Kenny JD, et al: Controlled trial of bicarbonate therapy in high risk premature newborn infants. J Pediatr 91:771, 1977.

Corbet AJS, Ross JA, Beaudry PH, Stern L: Ventilation perfusion relationships as assessed by aA.DN2 in hyaline membrane disease. J Appl Physiol 36:74, 1974.

Corbet AJS, Ross JA, Beaudry PH, Stern L: Effect of positive pressure breathing on aA.DN2 in hyaline membrane disease. J Appl Physiol 38:33, 1975.

Costarino AT, Gruskay JA, Corcoran L, et al: Sodium restriction versus daily maintenance replacement in very low birth weight premature neonates: A randomized blind therapeutic trial. J Pediatr 120:99, 1992.

Crowley MR, Fineman JR, Soifer SJ: Effects of vasoactive drugs on thromboxane A2 mimetic-induced pulmonary hypertension in newborn lambs. Pediatr Res 29:167, 1991.

Crowley P: Corticosteroids after preterm premature rupture of membranes. Obstet Gynecol Clin North Am 19:317, 1992.

Crowley P, Chalmers I, Keirse MJNC: The effects of corticosteroid administration before preterm delivery: An overview of the evidence from controlled trials. Br J Obstet Gynaecol 97:11, 1990.

Cummings JJ, Carlton DP, Poulain FR, et al: Hypoproteinemia slows lung liquid clearance in young lambs. J Appl Physiol 74:153, 1993.

Cunningham AS, Lawson EE, Martin RJ, et al: Tracheal suction and meconium: A proposed standard of care. J Pediatr 116:153, 1990.

Curtis J, O'Neill T, Pettett G: Endotracheal administration of tolazoline in hypoxia-induced pulmonary hypertension. Pediatrics 92:403, 1993.

Davey AM, Becker JD, Davis JM: Meconium aspiration syndrome: Physiological and inflammatory changes in a newborn piglet model. Pediatr Pulmonol 16:101, 1993.

Davis JM, Richter SE, Kendig JW, Notter RH: High frequency jet ventilation and surfactant treatment of newborns with severe respiratory failure. Pediatr Pulmonol 13:108, 1992.

Davis RO, Philips JB, Harris BA, et al: Fetal meconium-aspiration syndrome occurring despite airway management considered appropriate. Am J Obstet Gynecol 151:731, 1985.

deMello DE, Chi EY, Doo E, Lagunoff D: Absence of tubular myelin in lungs of infants dying with hyaline membrane disease. Am J Pathol 127:131, 1987.

deMello DE, Heyman S, Phelps DS, Floros J: Immunogold localization of SP-A in lungs of infants dying of respiratory distress syndrome. Am J Pathol 142:1631, 1993.

deMello DE, Heyman S, Phelps DS, et al: Ultrastructure of lung in surfactant protein B deficiency. Am J Respir Cell Mol Biol 11:230, 1994a.

deMello DE, Nogee LM, Heyman S, et al: Molecular and phenotypic variability in the congenital alveolar proteinosis syndrome associated with inherited surfactant protein B deficiency. J Pediatr 125:43, 1994b.

Dilger I, Schwedler G, Dudenhausen JW: Determination of the pulmonary surfactant associated protein SP-B in amniotic fluid with a competition ELISA. Gynecol Obstet Invest 38:24, 1994.

Dollberg S, Warner BW, Myatt L: Urinary nitrite and nitrate concentrations in patients with idiopathic persistent pulmonary hypertension of the newborn and effect of extracorporeal membrane oxygenation. Pediatr Res 37:31, 1995.

Dreizzen E, Migdal M, Praud JP, et al: Passive compliance of total respiratory system in preterm newborn infants with respiratory distress syndrome. J Pediatr 112:778, 1988.

Drew JH: Immediate intubation at birth of the very low birthweight infant. Am J Dis Child 136:207, 1982.

Drummond WH, Gregory GA, Heymann MA, Phibbs RH: The independent effects of hyperventilation, tolazoline and dopamine on infants with persistent pulmonary hypertension. J Pediatr 98:603, 1981.

Dudell GG, Gersony WM: Patent ductus arteriosus in neonates with severe respiratory disease. J Pediatr 104:915, 1984.

Dworetz AR, Moya FR, Sabo B, et al: Survival of infants with persistent pulmonary hypertension without extracorporeal membrane oxygenation. Pediatrics 84:1, 1989.

Dye T, Aubry R, Gross S, et al: Amnioinfusion and the intrauterine prevention of meconium aspiration. Am J Obstet Gynecol 171:1601, 1994.

Edberg KE, Sandberg K, Silberberg A, et al: Lung volume, gas mixing, and mechanics of breathing in mechanically ventilated very low birth weight infants with idiopathic respiratory distress syndrome. Pediatr Res 30:496, 1991.

Eguchi H, Koyama N, Tanaka T, et al: Surfactant apoprotein A (SP-A) in tracheal aspirates of newborn infants with RDS. Acta Paediatr Jpn 33:649, 1991.

Enhorning G, Shennan A, Possmayer F, et al: Prevention of neonatal respiratory distress syndrome by tracheal instillation of surfactant: A randomized clinical trial. Pediatrics 76:145, 1985.

Evans N, Iyer P: Change in blood pressure after treatment of patent ductus arteriosus with indomethacin. Arch Dis Child 68:584, 1993.

Faix RG, Viscardi RM, DiPietro MA, Nicks JJ: Adult respiratory distress syndrome in full term infants. Pediatrics 83:971, 1989.

Fanaroff AA, Cha CC, Sosa R, et al: Controlled trial of continuous negative external pressure in the treatment of severe respiratory distress syndrome. J Pediatr 82:921, 1973.

Farrell PM, Avery ME: State of the art: Hyaline membrane disease. Am Rev Respir Dis 111:657, 1975.

Farrell PM, Wood RE: Epidemiology of hyaline membrane disease in the United States: Analysis of national mortality statistics. Pediatrics 58:167, 1976.

Fauser A, Pohlandt F, Bartmann P, Gortner L: Rapid increase of blood pressure in extremely low birth weight infants after a single dose of dexamethasone. Eur J Pediatr 152:354, 1993.

Fedrick J, Butler NR: Hyaline membrane disease. Lancet 2:768, 1972.

Feltes TF, Hansen TN, Martin CG, et al: The effects of dopamine infusion on regional blood flow in newborn lambs. Pediatr Res 21:131, 1987.

Fenton AN, Steer CM: Fetal distress. Am J Obstet Gynecol 83:354, 1962.

Fike C, Hansen TN: Effects of alkalosis on hypoxic pulmonary vasoconstriction in newborn rabbit lungs. Pediatr Res 25:383, 1989.

Findlay RD, Taeusch HW, Walther FJ: Surfactant replacement therapy for meconium-aspiration syndrome. Pediatrics 97:48, 1996.

Fineman JR, Crowley MR, Soifer SJ: Selective pulmonary vasodilation with ATM-MgCl2 during pulmonary hypertension in lambs. J Appl Physiol 69:1836, 1990.

Fineman JR, Wong J, Morin FCI, et al: Chronic nitric oxide inhibition in utero produces persistent pulmonary hypertension in newborn lambs. J Clin Invest 93:2675, 1995.

Finer NN, Etches PC, Kamstra BJ, et al: Inhaled nitric oxide in infants referred for extracorporeal membrane oxygenation: Dose response. J Pediatr 124:302, 1994.

Finlay-Jones JM, Papadimitriou JM, Barter RA: Pulmonary hyaline membrane: Light and electron microscopic study of the early stage. J Pathol 112:117, 1974.

Frank L, Lewis PL, Sosenko IRS: Dexamethasone-stimulated fetal rat lung antioxidant enzyme activity in parallel with surfactant stimulation. Pediatrics 75:569, 1985.

Frantz ID, Wang NS, Thach BT: Experimental meconium aspiration: Effects of glucocorticoid treatment. J Pediatr 86:438, 1975.

Gandy G, Jacobson W, Gairdner D: Hyaline membrane disease: Cellular changes. Arch Dis Child 45:289, 1970.

Garite TJ, Rumney PJ, Briggs GG, et al: A randomized placebo controlled trial of betamethasone for the prevention of respiratory distress syndrome at 24–28 weeks gestation. Am J Obstet Gynecol 166:646, 1992.

Geggel RL, Aronovitz MJ, Reid LM: Effects of chronic in utero hypoxemia on rat neonatal pulmonary arterial structure. J Pediatr 108:756, 1986.

Gerdes J, Whitsett J, Long W: Elastase activity and surfactant protein concentration in tracheal aspirates from neonates receiving synthetic surfactant. J Pediatr 120:S34, 1992.

Gersony WM, Duc GV, Sinclair JC: "PFC" syndrome (persistence of the fetal circulation). Circulation 39(suppl):III-87, 1969.

Giaid A, Saleh D: Reduced expression of endothelial nitric oxide synthase in the lungs of patients with pulmonary hypertension. N Engl J Med 333:214, 1995.

Gill AB, Weindling AM: Echocardiographic assessment of cardiac function in shocked very low birth weight infants. Arch Dis Child 68:17, 1993a.

Gill AB, Weindling AM: Randomised controlled trial of plasma protein fraction versus dopamine in hypotensive very low birth weight infants. Arch Dis Child 69:284, 1993b.

Gluck L, Kulovich MV: Lecithin-sphingomyelin ratios in amniotic fluid in normal and abnormal pregnancy. Am J Obstet Gynecol 115:539, 1973.

Gluck L, Kulovich MV: The evaluation of functional maturity in the human fetus. In Gluck L (Ed): Modern Perinatal Medicine. Chicago, Year Book Medical Publishers, 1974.

Golan A, Zalzstein E, Zmora E, et al: Pulmonary hypertension in respiratory distress syndrome. Pediatr Pulmonol 19:221, 1995.

Goldstein RF, Brazy JE: Narcotic sedation stabilizes arterial blood pressure fluctuations in sick premature infants. J Perinatol 11:365, 1991.

Gortner L, Pohlandt F, Bartmann P: Bovine surfactant in full term neonates with adult respiratory distress syndrome-like disorders (Letter). Pediatrics 93:538, 1994.

Greenough A, Greenall F, Gamsu H: Synchronous respiration: Which ventilator rate is best? Acta Paediatr Scand 76:713, 1987.

Gregory GA, Gooding CA, Phibbs RH, Tooley WH: Meconium aspiration in infants—a prospective study. J Pediatr 85:848, 1970.

Gregory GA, Kitterman JA, Phibbs RH, et al: Treatment of idiopathic respiratory distress syndrome with continuous positive airway pressure. N Engl J Med 284:1333, 1971.

Gribetz I, Frank NR, Avery ME: Static volume pressure relations of excised lungs of infants with hyaline membrane disease, newborn and stillborn infants. J Clin Invest 38:2168, 1959.

Hack M, Fanaroff A, Klaus M: Neonatal respiratory distress following elective delivery: A preventable disease? Am J Obstet Gynecol 126:43, 1976.

Hageman JR, Conley M, Francis K, et al: Delivery room management of meconium staining of the amniotic fluid and the development of meconium aspiration syndrome. J Perinatol 8:127, 1988.

Halliday HL, McClure G, McCreid M: Transient tachypnea of the newborn: Two distinct clinical entities? Arch Dis Child 56:322, 1981.

Hallman M, Kulovich MV, Kirkpatrick E, et al: Phosphatidylinositol and phosphatidylglycerol in amniotic fluid: Indices of lung maturity. Am J Obstet Gynecol 125:613, 1976.

Hallman M, Merritt TA, Akino T, Bry K: Surfactant protein A, phosphatidylcholine, and surfactant inhibitors in epithelial lining fluid. Am Rev Respir Dis 144:1376, 1991.

Hallman M, Merritt TA, Jarvenpaa AL, et al: Exogenous human surfactant for treatment of severe respiratory distress syndrome: A randomized prospective clinical trial. J Pediatr 106:963, 1985.

Hallman M, Teramo K: Measurement of the lecithin sphingomyelin ratio and phosphatidylglycerol in amniotic fluid: An accurate method for the assessment of fetal lung maturity. Br J Obstet Gynaecol 88:806, 1981.

Hammerman C, Komar K, Abu-Khudair H: Hypoxic vs septic pulmonary hypertension. Am J Dis Child 142:319, 1988.

Hamvas A, Cole FS, deMello DE, et al: Surfactant protein B deficiency: Antenatal diagnosis and prospective treatment with surfactant replacement. J Pediatr 125:356, 1994.

Hansen TN, Corbet AJS, Kenny JD, et al: Effects of oxygen and constant positive pressure breathing on aADCO$_2$ in hyaline membrane disease. Pediatr Res 13:1167, 1979.

Hansen TN, Gest AL: Oxygen toxicity and other ventilatory complications of treatment of infants with persistent pulmonary hypertension. Clin Perinatol 11:653, 1984.

Harker LC, Merritt TA, Edwards DK: Improving the prediction of surfactant deficiency in very low birth weight infants with respiratory distress. J Perinatol 12:129, 1992.

Heicher DA, Kasting DS, Harrod JR: Prospective clinical comparison of two methods for mechanical ventilation of neonates: Rapid rate and short inspiratory time versus slow rate and long inspiratory time. J Pediatr 98:957, 1981.

Helbock HJ, Insoft RM, Conte FA: Glucocorticoid responsive hypotension in extremely low birth weight newborns. Pediatrics 92:715, 1993.

Herbert WNP, Chapman JF, Schnoor MM: Role of the TDx FLM assay in fetal lung maturity. Am J Obstet Gynecol 168:808, 1993.

Hjalmarson O, Olsson T: Mechanical and ventilatory parameters in healthy and diseased newborn infants. Acta Paediatr Scand 247(suppl):26, 1974.

Horbar JD, Sutherland J, Philip AGS, et al: Multicenter trial of single dose surfactant-TA for treatment of respiratory distress syndrome (Abstract). Pediatr Res 23:410A, 1988.

Howie RN: Pharmacological acceleration of lung maturation. *In* Raivio KO, Hallman N, Kouvalainen K, Valimaki I (Eds): Respiratory Distress Syndrome. New York, Academic Press, 1984, pp 385–396.

Hulsey TC, Alexander GR, Robillard PY, et al: Hyaline membrane disease: The role of ethnicity and maternal risk factors. Am J Obstet Gynecol 168:572, 1993.

Ikegami M, Jobe A, Berry D: A protein that inhibits surfactant in respiratory distress syndrome. Biol Neonate 50:121, 1986.

Ikegami M, Jobe AH, Tabor BL, et al: Lung albumin recovery in surfactant treated preterm ventilated lambs. Am Rev Respir Dis 145:1005, 1992.

Ikegami M, Ueda T, Absolom D, et al: Changes in exogenous surfactant in ventilated preterm lamb lungs. Am Rev Respir Dis 148:837, 1993.

Jacob J, Gluck L, DiSessa T, et al: The contribution of PDA in the neonate with severe RDS. J Pediatr 96:79, 1980.

Jacobsen T, Gronvall J, Petersen S, Andersen GE: Minitouch treatment of very low birth weight infants. Acta Paediatr 82:934, 1993.

James LS: Perinatal events and respiratory distress syndrome. N Engl J Med 292:1291, 1975.

Jefferies AL, Coates AL, O'Brodovich H: Pulmonary epithelial permeability in hyaline membrane disease. N Engl J Med 311:1075, 1984.

Jobe A: Pulmonary surfactant therapy. N Engl J Med 328:861, 1993.

Jobe AH, Mitchell BR, Gunkel JH: Beneficial effects of the combined use of prenatal corticosteroids and postnatal surfactant on preterm infants. Am J Obstet Gynecol 168:508, 1993.

Kaapa P, Koivisto M, Ylikorkala O, Koiuvalainen K: Prostacyclin in the treatment of neonatal pulmonary hypertension. J Pediatr 107:951, 1985.

Kamper J, Wulff K, Larsen C, Lindequist S: Early treatment with nasal continuous positive airway pressure in very low birth weight infants. Acta Paediatr 82:193, 1993.

Kanto WP: A decade of experience with neonatal extracorporeal membrane oxygenation. J Pediatr 24:335, 1994.

Kari MA, Hallman, M, Eronen M, et al: Prenatal dexamethasone therapy in conjunction with rescue therapy of human surfactant: A randomized placebo controlled multicenter study. Pediatrics 93:730, 1994.

Kattner E, Metze B, Waib E, Obladen M: Accelerated lung maturation following maternal steroid treatment in infants born before 30 weeks gestation. J Perinat Med 20:449, 1992.

Kenny JD, Adams JM, Corbet AJS, Rudolph AJ: The role of acidosis at birth in the development of hyaline membrane disease. Pediatrics 58:184, 1976.

Khammash H, Perlman M, Wojtulewicz J, et al: Surfactant therapy in full-term neonates with severe respiratory failure. Pediatrics 92:135, 1993.

Kinsella JP, Neish SR, Shaffer E, et al: Low-dose inhalational nitric oxide in persistent pulmonary hypertension of the newborn. Lancet 340:819, 1992.

Kjos SL, Walther FJ, Montoro M, et al: Prevalence and etiology of respiratory distress syndrome in infants of diabetic mothers: Predictive values of fetal lung maturation tests. Am J Obstet Gynecol 163:898, 1990.

Klarr JM, Faix RG, Pryce CJE, et al: Randomized blind trial of dopamine versus dobutamine in preterm infants with respiratory distress syndrome. J Pediatr 125:117, 1994.

Knight DB, Liggins GC, Wealthall SR: A randomized controlled trial of antepartum thyrotropin releasing hormone and betamethasone in the prevention of respiratory disease in preterm infants. Am J Obstet Gynecol 171:11, 1994.

Kopelman AE: Blood pressure and cerebral ischemia in very low birth weight infants. J Pediatr 116:1000, 1990.

Kourembanas S, McQuillan LP, Leung GK, Faller DV: Nitric oxide regulates the expression of vasoconstrictors and growth factors by vascular endothelium under both normoxia and hypoxia. J Clin Invest 92:99, 1993.

Krauss AN, Auld PAM: Pulmonary gas trapping in premature infants. Pediatr Res 5:10, 1971.

Krauss AN, Klain DB, Auld PAM: Carbon monoxide diffusing capacity in newborn infants. Pediatr Res 10:771, 1976.

Kresch MJ, Brion LP, Fleischman AR: Delivery room management of meconium-stained neonates. J Perinatol 11:46, 1991.

Landers S, Hansen TN, Corbet AJS, et al: Optimal constant positive airway pressure assessed by arterial alveolar difference for CO_2 in hyaline membrane disease. Pediatr Res 20:884, 1986.

Lawson EE, Birdwell RL, Huang PS, Taeusch HW: Augmentation of pulmonary surfactant secretion by lung expansion at birth. Pediatr Res 13:611, 1979.

Levin DL, Fixler DE, Morriss FC, Tyson J: Morphologic analysis of the pulmonary vascular bed in infants exposed in utero to prostaglandin synthetase inhibitors. J Pediatr 92:478, 1978a.

Levin DL, Heymann MA, Kitterman JA, et al: Persistent pulmonary hypertension of the newborn infant. J Pediatr 89:626, 1976.

Levin DL, Hyman AI, Heymann MA, Rudolph AM: Fetal hypertension and the development of increased pulmonary vascular smooth muscle: A possible mechanism for persistent pulmonary hypertension of the newborn infant. J Pediatr 92:265, 1978b.

Levin DL, Weinberg AG, Perkin RM: Pulmonary microthrombi syndrome in newborn infants with unresponsive persistent pulmonary hypertension. J Pediatr 102:299, 1983.

Liggins GC, Howie RN: A controlled trial of antepartum glucocorticoid treatment for prevention of the respiratory distress syndrome in premature infants. Pediatrics 50:515, 1972.

Linder N, Aranda JV, Tsur M, et al: Need for endotracheal intubation and suction in meconium-stained neonates. J Pediatr 112:613, 1988.

Lucey JF: Clinical uses of transcutaneous oxygen monitoring. Adv Pediatr 28:27, 1981.

MacArthur BA, Howie RN, Dezoete JA, Elkins J: School progress and cognitive development of 6 year old children whose mothers were treated antenatally with betamethasone. Pediatrics 70:99, 1982.

Macklem PT, Proctor DF, Hogg JC: The stability of peripheral airways. Respir Physiol 8:191, 1970.

Maher JE, Cliver SP, Goldenberg RL, et al: The effect of corticosteroid therapy in the very premature infant. Am J Obstet Gynecol 170:869, 1994.

Marron MJ, Crisafi MA, Driscoll JM Jr, et al: Hearing and neurodevelopmental outcome in survivors of persistent pulmonary hypertension of the newborn. Pediatrics 90:392, 1992.

McQueston JA, Kinsella JP, Ivy DD, et al: Chronic pulmonary hypertension in utero impairs endothelium-dependent vasodilatation. Am J Physiol 268:H288, 1995.

Ment LR, Oh W, Ehrenkranz RA, et al: Antenatal steroids, delivery mode, and intraventricuolar hemorrhage in preterm infants. Am J Obstet Gynecol 172:795, 1995.

Merritt TA, Harris JP, Roghmann K, et al: Early closure of the patent ductus arteriosus in very low birth weight infants: A controlled trial. J Pediatr 99:281, 1981.

Miall-Allen VM, DeVries LS, Whitelaw AGL: Mean arterial blood pressure and neonatal cerebral lesions. Arch Dis Child 62:1068, 1987.

Miller FC, Read JA: Intrapartum assessment of the postdate fetus. Am J Obstet Gynecol 141:516, 1981.

Miller HC, Futrakul P: Birth weight, gestational age, and sex as determining factors in the incidence of respiratory distress syndrome of prematurely born infants. J Pediatr 72:628, 1968.

Miller FC, Sacks DA, Yeh SY, Paul RH, Schifrin BS, Martin CB, Hon EH: Significance of meconium during labor. Am J Obstet Gynecol 122:573, 1975.

Miller J, Law AB, Parker RA, et al: Effects of morphine and pancuronium on lung volume and oxygenation in premature infants with hyaline membrane disease. J Pediatr 125:97, 1994.

Moise AA, Wearden ME, Kozinetz CA, et al: Antenatal steroids are associated with less need for blood pressure support in extremely premature infants. Pediatrics 95:845, 1995.

Morales WJ, Diebel D, Lazar AJ, et al: The effect of antenatal dexamethasone administration on the prevention of respiratory distress syndrome in preterm gestations with premature rupture of membranes. Am J Obstet Gynecol 154:591, 1986.

Morin FC III: Ligating the ductus arteriosus before birth causes persistent pulmonary hypertension in the newborn lamb. Pediatr Res 25:245, 1989.

Morin FC, Stenmark KR: Persistent pulmonary hypertension of the newborn. Am J Respir Crit Care Med 151:2010, 1995.

Morrison JJ, Rennie JM, Milton PJ: Neonatal respiratory morbidity and mode of delivery at term: Influence of timing of elective cesarian section. Br J Obstet Gynaecol 102:101, 1995.

Morrow RW, Taylor AF, Kinsella JP, et al: Effect of ductal patency on organ blood flow and pulmonary function in the preterm baboon with hyaline membrane disease. Crit Care Med 23:179, 1995.

Moses D, Holm BA, Spitale P, et al: Inhibition of pulmonary surfactant function by meconium. Am J Obstet Gynecol 164:477, 1991.

Moya RM, Montes HF, Thomas VL, et al: Surfactant protein A and saturated phosphatidylcholine in respiratory distress syndrome. Am J Respir Crit Care Med 150:1672, 1994.

Murphy JD, Rabinovitch M, Goldstein JD, Reid LM: The structural basis of persistent pulmonary hypertension of the newborn infant. J Pediatr 98:962, 1981.

Murphy JD, Vawter GF, Reid LM: Pulmonary vascular disease in fetal meconium aspiration. J Pediatr 104:758, 1984.

Naeye RL, Freeman RK, Blanc WA: Nutrition, sex, and fetal lung maturation. Pediatr Res 8:200, 1974.

Naeye RL, Schochat SJ, Whitman V, Maisels MJ: Unsuspected pulmonary vascular abnormalities associated with diaphragmaic hernia. Pediatrics 58:902, 1976.

Nathan L, Leveno KJ, Carmody TJ III, et al: Meconium: A 1990s perspective on an old obstetric hazard. Obstet Gynecol 83:329, 1994.

Nelson NM, Prod'hom LS, Cherry RB, et al: Pulmonary function in the newborn infant: Perfusion, estimation by analysis of the arterial-alveolar carbon dioxide difference. Pediatrics 30:975, 1962.

NIH Consensus Development Conference Statement: Effect of corticosteroids for fetal maturation on perinatal outcomes, 1994. Am J Obstet Gynecol 173:246, 1995.

NIH Consensus Development Panel: Effect of corticosteroids for fetal maturation of perinatal outcomes. JAMA 273:413, 1995.

Nilsson R, Grossman G, Robertson B: Lung surfactant and the pathogenesis of neonatal bronchiolar lesions induced by artificial ventilation. Pediatr Res 12:249, 1978.

Nogee LM: Clinical significance of surfactant protein B deficiency. Neonatal Respir Dis 5:1, 1995.

Nogee LM, Garnier G, Dietz HC, et al: A mutation in the surfactant protein B gene responsible for fatal neonatal respiratory disease in multiple kindreds. J Clin Invest 93:1860, 1994.

Ohama Y, Itakura Y, Koyama N, et al: Effect of surfactant lavage in a rabbit model of meconium aspiration syndrome. Acta Paediatr Jpn 36:236, 1994.

Orzalesi MM, Motoyama EK, Jacobson HN, et al: The development of the lungs of lambs. Pediatrics 35:373, 1965.

Oxford Region Controlled Trial of Artificial Ventilation Group: Multicentre randomised controlled trial of high- against low-frequency positive pressure ventilation. Arch Dis Child 66:770, 1991.

Padbury JF, Agata Y, Baylen BG, et al: Dopamine pharmacokinetics in critically ill newborn infants. J Pediatr 110:293, 1986.

Papageorgiou AN, Colle E, Farri-Kostopoulos E, Gelfand MM: Incidence of respiratory distress syndrome following antenatal betamethasone: Role of sex, type of delivery and prolonged rupture of membranes. Pediatrics 67:614, 1981.

Papageorgiou AN, Doray J-L, Ardilia R, et al: Reduction of mortality, morbidity and respiratory distress syndrome in infants weighing less than 1,000 grams by treatment with betamethasone and ritodrine. Pediatrics 83:493, 1989.

Paranka MS, Walsh WF, Stancombe BB: Surfactant lavage in a piglet model of meconium-aspiration syndrome. Pediatr Res 31:625, 1992.

Peckham GJ: Risk-benefit relationships of current therapeutic approaches. Proceedings of the 83rd Ross Conference on Cardiovascular Sequelae of Asphyxia in the Newborn, 1982, p 110.

Pena IC, Teberg AJ, Finella KM: The premature small for gestational age infant during the first year of life: Comparison by birth weight and gestational age. J Pediatr 113:1066, 1988.

Pereira GR, Lim BK, Ing C, Medeiros HF: Umbilical versus peripheral vein catheterization for parenteral nutrition in sick premature infants. Yonsei Med J 33:224, 1992.

Perkin RM, Levin DL, Clark R: Serum salicylate levels and right-to-left ductus shunts in newborn infants with persistent pulmonary hypertension. J Pediatr 96:721, 1980.

Perlman J, Thach BT: Respiratory origin of fluctuations in arterial blood pressure in premature infants with respiratory distress syndrome. Pediatrics 81:399, 1988.

Perlman JM, McMenamin JB, Volpe JJ: Fluctuating cerebral blood flow velocity in respiratory distress syndrome: Relation to the development of intraventricular hemorrhage. N Engl J Med 309:204, 1983.

Peterson HG, Pendleton ME: Contrasting roentgenographic pulmonary patterns of the hyaline membrane and fetal-aspiration syndromes. Am J Roentgenol 73:800, 1989.

Pfenninger J, Tschaeppeler H, Wagner P, et al: Paradox of adult respiratory distress syndrome in neonates. Pediatr Pulmonol 10:18, 1991.

Pierce MR, Sosenko IRS, Frank L: Prenatal thyroid releasing hormone and thyroid releasing hormone plus dexamethasone lessen the survival of newborn rats during prolonged high O_2 exposure. Pediatr Res 32:407, 1992.

Prod'hom LS: The paediatric aspect of foetal asphyxia: The post asphyxia syndrome. *In* Proceedings of the 2nd European Congress on Perinatal Medicine. Basel, Karger, 1971, p 131.

Pryhuber GS, Hull WM, Fink I, et al: Ontogeny of surfactant proteins A and B in human amniotic fluid as indices of fetal lung maturation. Pediatr Res 30:597, 1991.

Puccio VF, Nahum L, Massone ML, et al: Arterial blood pressure and cerebral hemorrhage in the critically ill premature infants. J Perinat Med 22(suppl 1):93, 1994.

Reller MD, Ziegler ML, Rice MJ, et al: Duration of ductal shunting in healthy preterm infants: An echocardiographic color flow Doppler study. J Pediatr 112:441, 1988.

Reller MD, Rice MJ, McDonald RW: Review of studies evaluating ductal patency in the premature infant. J Pediatr 122:S59, 1993.

Rhodes PG, Hall RT: Continuous positive airway pressure delivered by face mask in infants with the idiopathic respiratory distress syndrome: A controlled study. Pediatrics 52:1, 1973.

Richardson CP, Jung AL: Effects of continuous positive airway pressure on pulmonary function and blood gases of infants with respiratory distress syndrome. Pediatr Res 12:771, 1978.

Richardson DK, Torday JS: Racial differences in predictive value of the lecithin/sphingomyelin ratio. Am J Obstet Gynecol 170:1273, 1994.

Richardson P, Bose CL, Carlstrom JR: The functional residual capacity of infants with respiratory distress syndrome. Acta Paediatr Scand 75:267, 1986.

Rider E, Jobe A, Ikegami M, et al: Effects of maternal corticosteroid dose on surfactant pool sizes, protein leaks and SPC precursor incorporation in preterm rabbits. Clin Res 37:207A, 1989.

Rieutort M, Farrell PM, Engle MJ, et al: Changes in surfactant phospholipids in fetal rat lungs from normal and diabetic pregnancies. Pediatr Res 20:650, 1986.

Robert MF, Neff RK, Hubbell JP, et al: Association between maternal diabetes and the respiratory distress syndrome in the newborn. N Engl J Med 294:357, 1976.

Roberts JD, Fineman JR, Morin FC III, et al: Inhaled nitric oxide and persistent pulmonary hypertension of the newborn. N Engl J Med 336:605, 1997.

Roberts JD, Polaner DM, Lang P, et al: Inhaled nitric oxide in persistent pulmonary hypertension of the newborn. Lancet 340:818, 1992.

Robertson B, Kobayashi T, Ganzuka M, et al: Experimental neonatal respiratory failure induced by a monoclonal antibody to the hydrophobic surfactant associated protein SP-B. Pediatr Res 30:239, 1991.

Rojas J, Larsson LE, Ogletree ML, et al: Effects of cyclooxygenase inhibition on the response to group B streptococcal toxin in sheep. Pediatr Res 17:107, 1983.

Romero R, Hanoaka S, Mazor M, et al: Meconium-stained amniotic fluid: A risk factor for microbial invasion of the amniotic cavity. Am J Obstet Gynecol 164:859, 1991.

Rosenberg AA, Kennaugh J, Koppenhafer SL, et al: Elevated immunoreactive endothelin-1 levels in newborn infants with persistent pulmonary hypertension. J Pediatr 123:109, 1993.

Ryan CA, Finer NN: Antenatal corticosteroid therapy to prevent respiratory distress syndrome. J Pediatr 126:317, 1995.

Ryan CA, Finer NN, Barrington KJ: Effects of magnesium sulphate and nitric oxide in pulmonary hypertension induced by hypoxia in newborn piglets. Arch Dis Child 71:F151, 1995.

Saigal S, Wilson R, Usher R: Radiological findings in symptomatic neonatal plethora resulting from placental transfusion. Radiology 125:1851, 1977.

Samiec TD, Radmacher P, Hill T, Adamkin DH: Measured energy expenditure in mechanically ventilated very low birth weight infants. Am J Med Sci 307:182, 1994.

Scholle S, Braunlich H: Effects of prenatally administered thyroid hormones or glucocorticoids on maturation of kidney function in newborn rats. Dev Pharmacol Ther 112:162, 1989.

Schreiber ME, Heymann MA, Soifer SJ: Increased arterial pH, not decreased $PACO_2$, attenuates hypoxia-induced pulmonary vasoconstriction in newborn lambs. Pediatr Res 20:113, 1986.

Scott SM, Watterberger KL: Effect of gestational age, postnatal age, and illness on plasma cortisol concentrations in premature infants. Pediatr Res 37:112, 1995.

Seeger W, Grube C, Gunther A, Schmidt R: Surfactant inhibition by plasma proteins: Differential sensitivity of various surfactant proteins. Eur Respir J 6:971, 1993.

Segall ML, Goetzman BW, Schick JB: Thrombocytopenia and pulmonary hypertension in the perinatal aspiration syndromes. J Pediatr 96:727, 1980.

Sell EJ, Gaines JA, Gluckman C, Williams E: Persistent fetal circulation. Am J Dis Child 139:25, 1985.

Seppanen MP, Kaapa PO, Kiro PO, Saraste M: Doppler derived systolic pulmonary artery pressure in acute neonatal respiratory distress syndrome. Pediatrics 93:769, 1994.

Setzer E, Ermocilla R, Tonkin I, et al: Papillary muscle necrosis in a neonatal autopsy population: Incidence and associated clinical manifestations. J Pediatr 96:289, 1980.

Shankaran S, Farooki Q, Desai R: Beta-hemolytic streptococcal infection appearing as persistent fetal circulation. Am J Dis Child 136:725, 1982.

Shortland DB, Evans DH, Levene MI: Blood pressure measurements in very low birth weight infants over the first week of life. J Perinat Med 16:93, 1988.

Silverman M: Chronic lung disease of prematurity: Are we too cautious with steroids? Eur J Pediatr 153(suppl 2):S30, 1994.

Sinclair JC: Pathophysiology of hyaline membrane disease. *In* Winter RW (Ed): The Body Fluids in Pediatrics. Boston, Little, Brown, 1973.

Sinclair JC, Engel K, Silverman WA: Early correction of hypoxemia and acidemia in infants of low birthweight: A controlled trial of oxygen breathing, rapid alkali infusion and assisted ventilation. Pediatrics 42:565, 1968.

Skelton R, Jeffery H: Click test: Rapid diagnosis of the respiratory distress syndrome. Pediatr Pulmonol 17:383, 1994.

Soifer SJ, Kaslow D, Roman C, Heymann MA: Umbilical cord compression produces pulmonary hypertension in newborn lambs: A model to study the pathophysiology of persistent pulmonary hypertension in the newborn. J Dev Physiol 9:239, 1987.

Soifer SJ, Morin FC III, Heymann MA: Prostaglandin D_2 reverses induced pulmonary hypertension in the newborn lamb. J Pediatr 100:458, 1982.

Sosulski R, Fox WW: Transition phase during hyperventilation therapy for persistent pulmonary hypertension of the neonate. Crit Care Med 13:715, 1985.

Spong CY, Ogundipe OA, Ross MG: Prophylactic amnioinfusion for meconium-stained amniotic fluid. Am J Obstet Gynecol 171:931, 1994.

Stefano JL, Norman ME, Morales MC, et al: Decreased erythrocyte sodium-potassium-ATPase activity associated with cellular potassium loss in extremely low birth weight infants with non-oliguric hyperkalemia. J Pediatr 122:276, 1993.

Steinhorn RH, Russell JA, Morin FCI: Disruption of cGMP production in pulmonary arteries isolated from fetal lambs with pulmonary hypertension. Am J Physiol 268:H1483, 1995.

Stenmark KR, Dempsey EC, Badesch DB, et al: Regulation of pulmonary vascular wall cell growth: Developmental and site-specific heterogeneity. Eur Respir Rev 3:629, 1993.

Stevens PA, Schadow B, Bartholain S, et al: Surfactant protein A in the course of respiratory distress syndrome. Eur J Pediatr 151:596, 1992.

Stonestreet BS, Hansen MB, Laptock AR, et al: Glucocorticoids accelerate renal function maturation in fetal lambs. Early Hum Dev 8:331, 1983.

Strang LB: Neonatal lung oedema. *In* Neonatal Respiration: Physiological and Clinical Studies. Oxford, Blackwell Scientific Publications, 1977, p 251.

Strang LB, MacLeish MH: Ventilatory failure and right to left shunt in newborn infants with respiratory distress. Pediatrics 28:17, 1961.

Suen H, Catlin EA, Ryan DP, et al: Biochemical immaturity of lungs in congenital diaphragmatic hernia. J Pediatr Surg 28:471, 1993.

Sun B, Curstedt T, Robertson B: Surfactant inhibition in experimental meconium aspiration. Acta Paediatr Scand 82:182, 1993a.

Sun B, Curstedt T, Song GW, et al: Surfactant improves lung function and morphology in newborn rabbits with meconium aspiration. Biol Neonate 63:96, 1993b.

Sundell H, Garrott J, Blankenship WJ, et al: Studies on infants with type II respiratory distress syndrome. J Pediatr 78:754, 1971.

Tait JF, Foerder CA, Ashwood ER, Benedetti TJ: Prospective clinical evaluation of an improved fluorescence polarization assay for predicting fetal lung maturity. Clin Chem 33:554, 1987.

Talner NS, Lister G, Fahey JT: Effect of asphyxia on the myocardium of the fetus and newborn. *In* Polin RA, Fox WW (Eds): Fetal and Neonatal Physiology. Philadelphia, WB Saunders, 1992.

Tammela KT, Lanning FP, Koivisto ME: The relationship of fluid restriction during the first month of life and the occurrence and severity of bronchopulmonary dysplasia in low birth weight infants: A 1 year radiological follow up. Eur J Pediatr 151:367, 1992.

Thibeault DW, Hall FK, Sheehan MB, Hall RT: Postasphyxial lung disease in newborn infants with severe perinatal acidosis. Am J Obstet Gynecol 150:393, 1984.

Thompson PJ, Greenough A, Gamsu HR, Nicolaides KH: Ventilatory requirements for respiratory distress syndrome in small for gestational age infants. Eur J Pediatr 151:528, 1992.

Ting P, Brady JP: Tracheal suction in meconium aspiration. Am J Obstet Gynecol 122:767, 1975.

Towers CV, Garite TJ: Evaluation of the new AmnioStat-FLM test for the detection of phosphatidylglycerol in contaminated fluids. Am J Obstet Gynecol 160:298, 1989.

Tran N, Lowe C, Sivieri EM, Shaffer TH: Sequential effects of acute meconium obstruction on pulmonary function. Pediatr Res 14:34, 1980.

Trimmer KJ, Gilstrap LC: "Meconiumcrit" and birth asphyxia. Am J Obstet Gynecol 165:1010, 1991.

Tubman TRJ, Rollins MD, Patterson C, Halliday HL: Increased incidence of respiratory distress syndrome in babies of hypertensive mothers. Arch Dis Child 66:52, 1991.

Tyson JE, Kennedy K, Broyles S, Rosenfeld CA: The small for gestational age infant: Accelerated or delayed pulmonary maturation? Increased or decreased survival? Pediatrics 95:534, 1995.

Usher R: Reduction in mortality from respiratory distress syndrome with early administration of intravenous glucose and sodium bicarbonate. Pediatrics 32:966, 1963.

Usta IM, Mercer BM, Aswad NK, et al: The impact of a policy of amnioinfusion for meconium-stained amniotic fluid. Obstet Gynecol 85:237, 1995.

Van Marter LJ, Leviton A, Kuban KCK, et al: Maternal glucocorticoid therapy and reduced risk of bronchopulmonary dysplasia. Pediatrics 86:331, 1990.

Verder H, Robertson B, Greisen G, et al: Surfactant therapy and nasal continuous positive airway pressure for newborns with respiratory distress syndrome. N Engl J Med 331:1051, 1994.

Versmold HT, Kitterman JA, Phibbs RH, et al: Aortic blood pressure during the first 12 hours of life in infants with birthweight 610–4220 grams. Pediatrics 67:607, 1981.

Walther FJ, Benders MJ, Leighton JO: Persistent pulmonary hypertension in premature neonates with severe respiratory distress syndrome. Pediatrics 90:899, 1992.

Walther FJ, Siassi B, Ramadan NA, et al: Cardiac output in infants with transient myocardial dysfunction. J Pediatr 107:781, 1985.

Ward RM, Daniel CH, Kendig JW, Wood MA: Oliguria and tolazoline pharmacokinetics in the newborn. Pediatrics 77:307, 1986.

Wen TS, Eriksen NL, Blanco JD, et al: Association of clinical intra-amniotic infection and meconium. Am J Perinatol 10:438, 1995.

West JB: Ventilation perfusion inequality and overall gas exchange in computer models of the lung. Respir Physiol 7:88, 1969.

Wilcox DT, Glick PL, Karamanoukian H, et al: Pathophysiology of congenital diaphragmatic hernia: V. Effect of exogenous surfactant therapy on gas exchange and lung mechanics in the lamb congenital diaphragmatic hernia model. J Pediatr 124:289, 1994.

Wild LM, Nickerson PA, Morin FC III: Ligating the ductus arteriosus before birth remodels the pulmonary vasculature of the lamb. Pediatr Res 25:251, 1989.

Wilkie RA, Bryan MH, Tarnow-Mordi WO: Static respiratory compliance in the newborn: 2. Its potential for selection of infants for early surfactant treatment. Arch Dis Child 70:F16, 1994.

Wiswell TE, Henley MA: Intratracheal suctioning, systemic infection, and the meconium aspiration syndrome. Pediatrics 89:203, 1992.

Wiswell TE, Rawlings JS, Smith FR, Goo ED: Effect of furosemide on the clinical course of transient tachypnea of the newborn. Pediatrics 75:908, 1985.

Wright LL, Horbar JD, Gunkel H, et al: Evidence from multicenter networks on the current use and effectiveness of antenatal corticosteroids in low birth weight infants. Am J Obstet Gynecol 173:263, 1995.

Wu T, Ru-Jeng T, Yau KT: Persistent pulmonary hypertension of the newborn treated with magnesium sulfate in premature neonates. Pediatrics 96:472, 1995.

Wung JT: Respiratory management for low birth weight infants. Crit Care Med 21(suppl):S364, 1993.

Wung JT, Driscoll JM, Epstein RA, Hyman AI: A new device for CPAP by nasal route. Crit Care Med 3:76, 1975.

Wung J-T, James LS, Kichevsky E, James E: Management of infants with severe respiratory failure and persistence of the fetal circulation, without hyperventilation. Pediatrics 76:488, 1985.

Yeh TF, Lilien LD, Aiyanadar B, Pildes RS: Lung volume, dynamic lung compliance, and blood gases during the first 3 days of postnatal life in infants with meconium aspiration syndrome. Crit Care Med 10:588, 1982.

Yeh TF, Scrinivasan G, Harris V, Pildes RS: Hydrocortisone therapy in meconium aspiration syndrome: A controlled study. J Pediatr 90:140, 1977.

Yeomans ER, Gilstrap LC III, Leveno KJ, et al: Meconium in the amniotic fluid and fetal acid-base status. Obstet Gynecol 73:175, 1989.

Yoder BA: Meconium-stained amniotic fluid and respiratory complications: Impact of selective tracheal suction. Obstet Gynecol 83:77, 1994.

Yoder PR, Gibbs RS, Blanco JD, et al: A prospective controlled study of maternal and perinatal outcome after intra-amniotic infection at term. Am J Obstet Gynecol 145:695, 1983.

Zachman RD: The NIH multicenter study and miscellaneous clinical trials of antenatal corticosteroid administration. *In* Farrell PM (Ed): Lung Development: Biological and Clinical Perspectives: II. Neonatal Respiratory Distress. New York, Academic Press, 1982.

CHAPTER 54

Air Block Syndromes

Thomas Hansen and Anthony Corbet

Pulmonary interstitial emphysema (PIE), pneumomediastinum, subcutaneous emphysema, pneumothorax, pneumopericardium, pneumoperitoneum, and intravascular air are all manifestations of air block syndrome, and all begin with some degree of PIE (Kirkpatrick et al, 1974; Macklin and Macklin, 1944).

PULMONARY INTERSTITIAL EMPHYSEMA
Pathophysiology

PIE is the result of alveolar rupture from overdistention of alveoli abutting against nonalveolar structures and marginal alveoli (Figs. 54–1 and 54–2) (Caldwell et al, 1970; Hansen and Gest, 1984). It occurs most commonly in preterm or term infants undergoing mechanical ventilation for some form of parenchymal lung disease. In these infants, distribution of inspired gas is nonuniform, with the bulk of each breath being distributed to the more normal lung units. As a result, these lung units may become overdistended and rupture. Gas trapping from an insufficient expiratory time can also result in alveolar overdistention and rupture. Once alveolar rupture occurs, air is forced from the alveolus into the loose connective tissue sheaths surrounding airways and pulmonary arterioles and into the interlobular septa containing pulmonary veins. The air follows a track along these sheaths to the hilum of the lung, producing the characteristic radiographic appearance of PIE (Fig. 54–3).

PIE increases the volume of gas within the lung parenchyma and splints the lung in full inflation, thereby decreasing lung compliance. Air trapped within the interstitial cuffs compresses airways and increases airway resistance.

In addition, air in the interstitial space impairs lymphatic function, allowing fluid to accumulate in the interstitial cuffs and in alveoli (Leonidas et al, 1979). $PaCO_2$ increases, and PaO_2 decreases. The increase in $PaCO_2$ occurs early and is the result of increased respiratory dead space and reduced minute ventilation. The decrease in PaO_2 results in part from reduction in alveolar ventilation and in part from ventilation-perfusion mismatch secondary to mechanical obstruction of airways by interstitial air and edema fluid. It also results from compression of pulmonary arterioles by air in the perivascular cuffs with increased pulmonary vascular resistance (Brazy and Blackmon, 1977) and right-to-left shunting of blood.

Once interstitial air reaches the hilum of the lung, it coalesces to form large hilar blebs, or it tracks beneath the visceral pleura to form large subpleural pockets of air. In both instances, these accumulations of air can be large enough to compress normal lung and impair ventilation or cause circulatory embarrassment by encroaching on mediastinal structures (Plenat et al, 1978).

Prevention

The cause of PIE is alveolar overdistention and rupture. Therefore, ventilatory techniques that minimize alveolar overdistention would be expected to reduce the risk of PIE. Previous data have shown that increases in inspiratory time are associated with pulmonary air leaks (Primhak, 1983), and two controlled trials have shown that techniques for ventilation that rely on shorter inspiratory times decrease the incidence of PIE (Heicher, 1981; OCTAVE, 1991).

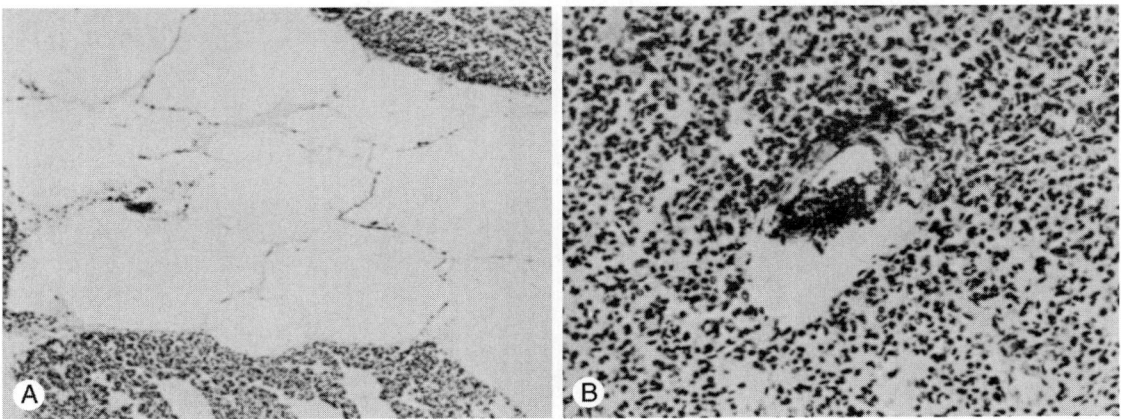

FIGURE 54–1. *A,* Photomicrograph of the lung of an infant who died of emphysema and bilateral pneumothorax. The alveoli in the center show much distention, their septa thinned. Some of the septa have ruptured. In the periphery, the lung is atelectatic. *B,* Higher-power view showing a blood vessel in cross-section. The vessel is compressed by a surrounding collar of air that has filled and ballooned the perivascular space.

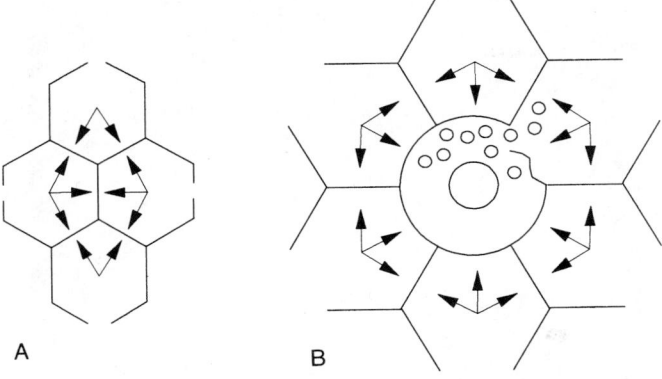

FIGURE 54–2. Mechanism of alveolar rupture. Partitional alveoli *(A)* have their bases lying against other alveoli, whereas marginal alveoli *(B)* abut against bronchi, blood vessels, or pleura. During lung inflation, these two different types of alveoli behave quite differently. Partitional alveoli are free to expand equally in all directions because they abut on the equally distensible walls of adjacent alveoli. In addition, the pressure within each alveolus is balanced by an equal pressure inside surrounding alveoli so no unbalanced forces across the alveolar wall occur. Marginal alveoli, especially those surrounding blood vessels, are tethered at the base to a less distensible structure and are not as free to expand in all directions. During lung inflation, the connective tissue sheaths surrounding pulmonary blood vessels attempt to expand with the alveoli, whereas the vessels themselves increase in size only slightly. As a result, unbalanced forces develop across the wall at the base of the alveolus, and air ruptures into the adjacent connective tissue sheath.

Treatment

Because the site of the air leak behaves like a check valve, gas trapping occurs and results in further alveolar overdistention and rupture. Therefore, the first step in treatment must be to interrupt this cycle by putting the more severely involved areas in the lung to rest. If PIE is unilateral, this can be done by positioning the infant with the involved side down (Swingle et al, 1984) or by selectively intubating the main stem bronchus on the uninvolved side (Brooks et al, 1977). If PIE is bilateral, the involved areas can be put to rest by taking advantage of regional differences in time constants in the lung. Areas with PIE have airway compression and long time constants for inspiration and expiration. Mechanical ventilation using short inspiratory times (0.1 second), low inflation pressures, and small tidal volumes are ineffective in inflating these areas of the lung and should not contribute to further gas trapping (Meadow and Cheromcha, 1985). Over time, these areas deflate and collapse. It may be difficult to maintain oxygenation and ventilation while selectively underventilating the areas of the lung with PIE. If this happens, it may be necessary to increase the respirator rate to 80 to 100 breaths/min. The advantage of rapid-rate ventilation is that it makes maximal use of the less severely involved lung units and may compensate for the respiratory deterioration associated with selective underventilation of areas with extensive PIE. A multicenter controlled trial (Keszler et al, 1991) found that high-frequency jet ventilation allowed the use of lower peak and mean airway pressures in the treatment of infants with PIE than did rapid-rate conventional ventilation. Furthermore, high-frequency jet ventilation led to more frequent and rapid improvement in PIE than did rapid-rate conventional ventilation.

Prognoses

PIE is a serious complication of mechanical ventilation. Infants who develop PIE have a significantly increased mortality and risk of developing chronic lung disease (Gaylord et al, 1985; Powers and Clemens, 1993). In fact, for infants who develop PIE on days 0 or 1 after birth, the gestational age–adjusted odds ratio for risk of dying is nearly 10 to 1 and for developing chronic lung disease is 3 to 1 (Powers and Clemens, 1993).

PNEUMOMEDIASTINUM AND PNEUMOTHORAX
Epidemiology

The incidence of spontaneous pneumomediastinum and pneumothorax in term infants is 1% to 2%, presumably because high transpulmonary pressures exerted at birth, when coupled with some degree of ventilation inhomogeneity, result in alveolar overdistention and rupture (Chernick and Avery, 1963; Lubchenco, 1959). In the presence of underlying lung disease, the incidence of pneumothorax increases dramatically. Ten percent of infants with retained fetal lung fluid develop pneumothorax, as do 5% to 10% of spontaneously breathing infants with hyaline membrane disease. Continuous positive airway pressure does not appear to increase the incidence of pneumothorax in infants with hyaline membrane disease, but positive-pressure ventilation does produce an increase (incidence between 20% and 50% of ventilated infants). Positive-pressure ventilation

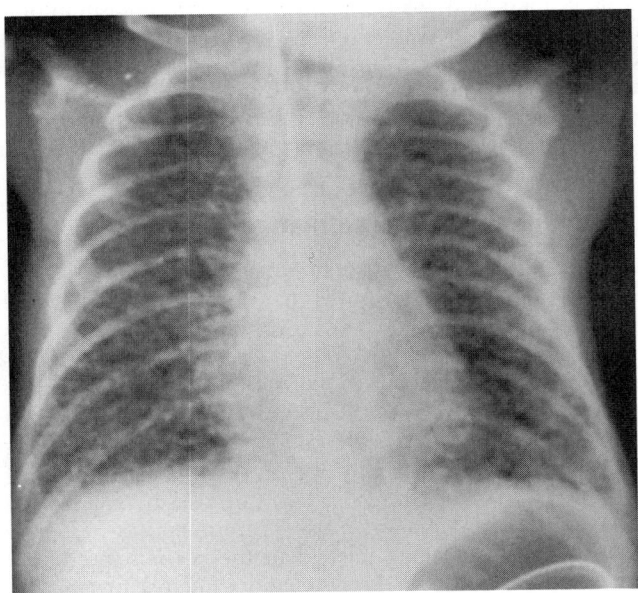

FIGURE 54–3. Pulmonary interstitial emphysema. The lung is grossly hyperinflated with coarse radiolucencies extending from the pleura to the hilum. These radiolucencies represent bubbles of air in the perivascular and peribronchial interstitial cuffs.

of term infants with meconium aspiration pneumonia or persistent pulmonary hypertension is associated with an incidence of pneumothorax of roughly 40%.

Natural History

Pneumomediastinum occurs when air that has tracked through the perivascular and peribronchial cuffs to the hilum ruptures into the mediastinum. From there air can rupture through the mediastinum into the pleural space and produce tension pneumothorax. Available evidence suggests that air in the mediastinum seldom achieves enough tension to cause circulatory embarrassment because as the tension increases, air can dissect into the soft tissues of the neck to produce subcutaneous emphysema or rupture into the intrapleural space. Tension pneumothorax can result in high pressures within the pleural space, collapsing the lung on the involved side and resulting in immediate hypoxia and hypercapnia. In addition, by compressing mediastinal structures and impeding venous return, pneumothorax may result in circulatory collapse.

Diagnosis

Pneumomediastinum is usually asymptomatic or associated with mild tachypnea. In the spontaneously breathing infant, however, pneumothorax usually results in clinically significant tachypnea, grunting, irritability, pallor, and cyanosis. The cardiac point of maximal impulse may be shifted away from the pneumothorax, and often the affected hemithorax appears to bulge. Differential breath sounds are unreliable markers of pneumothorax in the infant. Arterial pressure tracings may reveal a reduction in pulse pressure. In the infant on the mechanical ventilator, signs may be more dramatic with sudden onset of hypoxemia and cardiovascular collapse (Ogata et al, 1976). Transillumination of the chest is increased over the affected side. Pneumothorax should be confirmed by chest radiograph (Fig. 54–4), if at all possible. Needle aspiration of the chest to diagnose pneumothorax relieves acute distress but should be discouraged. If needle aspiration is performed, it should ordinarily be followed by tube thoracostomy.

Treatment

Asymptomatic or mildly symptomatic spontaneously breathing infants may simply be observed closely until spontaneous resolution occurs. Although allowing infants to breathe 100% oxygen hastens reabsorption of intrapleural air (Chernick and Avery, 1963), the risk associated with prolonged hyperoxia limits usefulness of this therapy in preterm infants. Infants with moderate to severe symptoms and all infants receiving positive-pressure ventilation must be treated with tube thoracostomy. Because most mechanically ventilated infants are nursed supine and because gas rises, the tube is usually placed in the second intercostal space in the midclavicular line and directed toward the diaphragm so that the tip lies between the lung and the anterior chest wall (Allen et al, 1981). Alternatively the tube may be inserted at the midaxillary line and directed anteriorly. When placing the tube, one must take care to

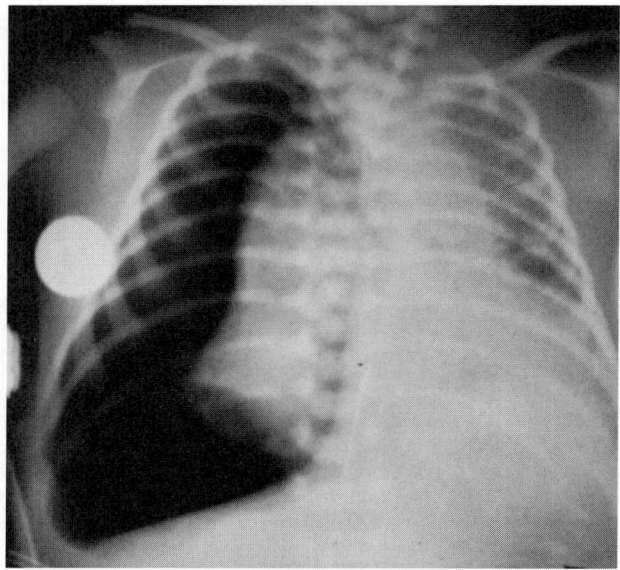

FIGURE 54–4. Tension pneumothorax. The lung on the involved side is collapsed, and the mediastinum is shifted to the opposite side. Pleura can be seen bulging into the intercostal spaces.

avoid impaling the lung, especially if a trocar is used to direct the tube rather than curved hemostats. Care must also be taken to avoid placing the tube too far into the chest and compressing mediastinal structures (Gooding et al, 1981). The thoracostomy tube usually is connected to water seal with 10 to 20 cm H$_2$O negative pressure and is left in place until it ceases to drain. The negative pressure should be discontinued, and the tube should be left under the water seal for 12 to 24 hours before removal. Infant chest tubes should never be clamped.

PNEUMOPERICARDIUM

Pneumopericardium results from direct tracking of interstitial air along the great vessels into the pericardial sac (Varano and Maisels, 1974). Gas under tension in the pericardium impairs atrial and ventricular filling, decreases stroke volume, and ultimately decreases cardiac output and systemic blood pressure. Infants present with increasing cyanosis, muffled heart sounds, and decreased systemic blood pressure. The chest radiograph is diagnostic (Fig. 54–5). Needle aspiration alleviates the acute symptoms, but because recurrence rate is high (53%), continuous tube drainage is frequently necessary (Reppert et al, 1977). The mortality rate associated with pneumopericardium has been reported to be as high as 75%.

PNEUMOPERITONEUM

Pneumoperitoneum results from dissection of air from the mediastinum along the sheaths of the aorta and vena cava, with subsequent rupture into the peritoneal cavity. Infants with this condition present with sudden abdominal distention and a typical abdominal radiograph. Occasionally the pneumoperitoneum may be large enough to cause respiratory embarrassment by compromising descent of the dia-

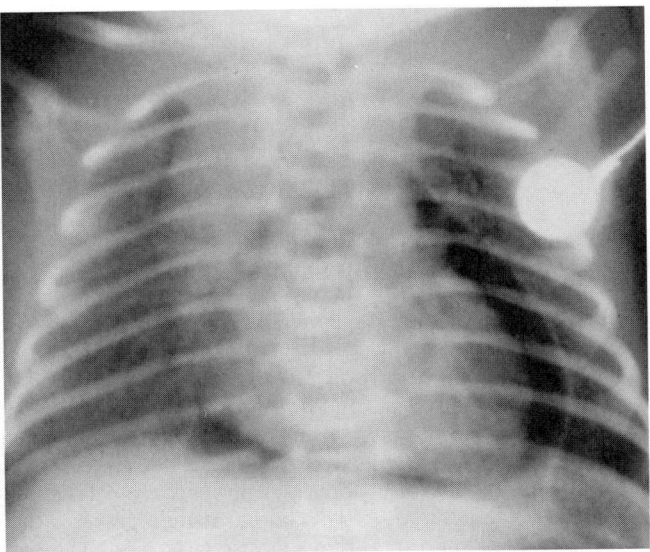

FIGURE 54–5. Pneumopericardium. A thin rim of pericardium is visible and clearly separated from the heart by air within the pericardial sac.

phragm and may require drainage. A more common problem, however, is the difficulty of distinguishing this cause of peritoneal air from a primary gastrointestinal catastrophe, such as perforated ulcer or necrotizing enterocolitis (Knight and Abdenour, 1981). Obtaining more than 0.5 mL of green or brown fluid on paracentesis is suggestive of primary bowel disease, especially if bacteria are present on Gram stain. Measurement of the Po_2 of the gas aspirated from the abdomen may also be of some help because it is likely to be high if the gas is of pulmonary origin. Finally, a careful upper gastrointestinal series performed with water-soluble contrast material may be of use in distinguishing the cause of intraperitoneal air (Cohen et al, 1982).

INTRAVASCULAR AIR

Intravascular air results from air being pumped directly into the pulmonary venous system and occurs only when airway pressure is extremely high (70 cm H_2O). It results in immediate cardiovascular collapse and is often diagnosed when air is withdrawn from the umbilical arterial catheter. Although intravascular air is usually fatal, placing the infant head down on the left side may favor displacement of cerebral emboli.

REFERENCES

Allen RW, Jung AL, Lester PD: Effectiveness of chest tube evacuation of pneumothorax in neonates. J Pediatr 99:629, 1981.

Brazy JE, Blackmon LR: Hypotension and bradycardia associated with airblock in the neonate. J Pediatr 90:796, 1977.

Brooks JG, Bustamante SA, Koops BL, et al: Selective bronchial intubation for the treatment of severe localized pulmonary interstitial emphysema in newborn infants. Pediatrics 91:648, 1977.

Caldwell EJ, Powell RD, Mullooly JP: Interstitial emphysema: A study of physiologic factors involved in experimental induction of the lesion. Am Rev Respir Dis 102:516, 1970.

Chernick V, Avery ME: Spontaneous alveolar rupture at birth. Pediatrics 32:816, 1963.

Cohen MD, Schreiner R, Lemons J: Neonatal pneumoperitoneum without significant adventitious pulmonary air: Use of metrizamide to rule out perforation of the bowel. Pediatrics 69:587, 1982.

Gaylord MS, Thieme RE, Woodall DL, Quissell BJ: Predicting mortality in low-birth-weight infants with pulmonary interstitial emphysema. Pediatrics 76:219, 1985.

Gooding CA, Kerlan RK, Brasch RC: Partial aortic obstruction produced by a thoracostomy tube. J Pediatr 98:471, 1981.

Hansen TN, Gest AL: Oxygen toxicity and other ventilatory complications of treatment of infants with persistent pulmonary hypertension. Clin Perinatol 11:653, 1984.

Heicher DA, Kasting DS, Harrod JR: Prospective clinical comparison of two methods for mechanical ventilation of neonates: Rapid rate and short inspiratory time versus slow rate and long inspiratory time. J Pediatr 98:957, 1981.

Keszler M, Donn SM, Bucciarelli RL, et al: Multicenter controlled trial comparing high-frequency jet ventilation and conventional mechanical ventilation in newborn infants with pulmonary interstitial emphysema. J Pediatr 119:85, 1991.

Kirkpatrick BV, Felman AH, Eitzman DV: Complications of ventilator therapy in respiratory distress syndrome. Am J Dis Child 128:496, 1974.

Knight PJ, Abdenour G: Pneumoperitoneum in the ventilated neonate: Respiratory or gastrointestinal origin? J Pediatr 98:972, 1981.

Leonidas JC, Bhan I, McCauley GK: Persistent localized pulmonary interstitial emphysema and lymphangiectasia: A causal relationship? Pediatrics 64:165, 1979.

Lubchenco LO: Recognition of spontaneous pneumothorax in premature infants. Pediatrics 24:996, 1959.

Macklin MT, Macklin CC: Malignant interstitial emphysema of the lungs and mediastinum as an important occult complication in many respiratory diseases and other conditions: An interpretation of the clinical literature in the light of laboratory experiment. Medicine 23:281, 1944.

Meadow WL, Cheromcha D: Successful therapy of unilateral pulmonary emphysema: Mechanical ventilation with extremely short inspiratory time. Am J Perinatol 2:194, 1985.

Ogata E, Gregory GA, Kitterman JA, et al: Pneumothorax in respiratory distress syndrome: Incidence and effect on vital signs, blood gases and pH. Pediatrics 58:177, 1976.

Oxford Region Controlled Trial of Artificial Ventilation Study Group (OCTAVE): Multicentre randomised controlled trial of high against low frequency positive pressure ventilation. Arch Dis Child 66:770, 1991.

Plenat F, Vert P, Didier F, Andre M: Pulmonary interstitial emphysema. Clin Perinatol 5:351, 1978.

Powers WF, Clemens JD: Prognostic implications of age at detection of air leak in very low birth weight infants requiring ventilatory support. J Pediatr 123:611, 1993.

Primhak RA: Factors associated with pulmonary air leak in premature infants receiving mechanical ventilation. J Pediatr 102:764, 1983.

Reppert SM, Ment LR, Todres ID: The treatment of pneumopericardium in the newborn infant. J Pediatr 905:115, 1977.

Swingle HM, Eggert LD, Bucciarelli RL: New approach to management of unilateral tension pulmonary interstitial emphysema in premature infants. Pediatrics 74:354, 1984.

Varano LA, Maisels MJ: Pneumopericardium in the newborn: Diagnosis and pathogenesis. Pediatrics 53:941, 1974.

Yuksel B, Greenough A: Persistence of respiratory symptoms into the second year of life: Predictive factors in infants born preterm. Acta Paediatr Scand 81:832, 1992.

CHAPTER 55

Chronic Lung Disease

Thomas Hansen and Anthony Corbet

BRONCHOPULMONARY DYSPLASIA

Definition

Bronchopulmonary dysplasia (BPD) was first described by Northway and associates in 1967 in a report on 32 infants. They described the severe chronic lung disease (CLD) that occurs in very sick, small infants with severe hyaline membrane disease who require treatment with mechanical ventilation and oxygen. They suggested it might result from several different causes, such as pulmonary healing, a residual toxic effect of oxygen itself, barotrauma of intermittent positive-pressure ventilation, the problems of endotracheal intubation, or a combination of these factors.

Since then, much has been learned about BPD, and an appreciation has emerged that CLD may also occur in a group of infants who have not previously had hyaline membrane disease. Consequently, the spectrum of patients affected by CLD includes tiny preterm infants who require ventilatory support because of pulmonary structural immaturity as well as infants with severe initial surfactant deficiency. For purposes of uniform reporting, however, the definition of CLD has been changed to *respiratory sequelae in an infant requiring oxygen at more than 28 days after birth.* Many physicians have questioned this definition, however, because it includes such a wide range of infants, that is, from those who ultimately appear to have no residual problems at one extreme to those with severe BPD, as described by Northway and associates (1967), at the other. A proposed, more practical definition would be *respiratory sequelae in an infant who reaches 36 weeks postmenstrual age but cannot be discharged from the hospital because of continued oxygen or mechanical ventilatory requirement, or an infant who is discharged home on oxygen or ventilatory support.*

Incidence

Merritt and coworkers (1988) have reviewed the epidemiology of BPD. The incidence is clearly highest in very-low-birth-weight (VLBW) infants who require mechanical ventilation for severe respiratory distress. The incidence is inversely related to birth weight (75% for survivors weighing 700 to 800 g and 13% for those weighing 1250 to 1500 g) (Avery et al, 1987). Based on expected survival and estimating that full resolution takes 3 years, one would expect that there are at least 3000 infants with BPD in the United States at any given time.

With the survival of an increasing number of infants of 24 to 26 weeks' gestation, the number of infants with significant BPD has also risen markedly (Zimmerman and Farrell, 1994) and is probably at least 7000.

Pathologic Stages

There are four distinctive clinical and pathologic stages to BPD, as described by Northway and associates (1967). Although therapeutic approaches since 1967 have modified some of their findings, the original descriptions remain useful. Postmortem examination of the lung during Stage 1 (at 1 to 3 days of age) reveals marked alveolar and interstitial edema with hyaline membranes, atelectasis, and necrosis of bronchial mucosa. The chest radiograph is consistent with hyaline membrane disease (Fig. 55–1A).

During Stage 2 (at 4 to 10 days of age), atelectasis becomes more extensive, alternating with areas of emphysema. There is widespread necrosis and repair of bronchial mucosa. Cellular debris fills the airways. On chest radiograph study, the lung fields are opaque with air bronchograms (Fig. 55–1B). Interstitial air is commonly evident.

During Stage 3 (at 11 to 30 days of age), extensive bronchial and bronchiolar metaplasia and hyperplasia evolve. Areas of emphysema are surrounded by areas of atelectasis, accompanied by massive interstitial edema with thickening of the basement membranes. On chest radiographic study, the lung now appears cystic with areas of hyperinflation and areas of atelectasis (Fig. 55–1C).

During Stage 4 (after 30 days of age), there is massive fibrosis of the lung with destruction of alveoli and airways. In addition, there is hypertrophy of bronchial smooth muscle and metaplasia of airway mucosa. Finally, there is actual loss of pulmonary arterioles and capillaries and medial muscular hypertrophy of remaining vessels. The chest radiographic study reveals massive fibrosis and edema with areas of consolidation and areas of overinflation (Fig. 55–1D).

Etiology and Pathogenesis

Current theories on the cause of BPD include those originally suggested by Northway and coworkers (1967) expanded by further knowledge that suggests additional causal components. Most workers in the field believe that the cause is multifactorial. Probable contributing factors are discussed in the following sections.

Genetic Predisposition

Even for infants of early gestational age, there is clearly a difference in the maturational level of the lung in infants of certain families compared with those of others. It is also clear that a familial history of asthma and reactive airway disease puts the infant at an additional disadvantage (Bertrand et al, 1985; Nickerson and Taussig, 1980).

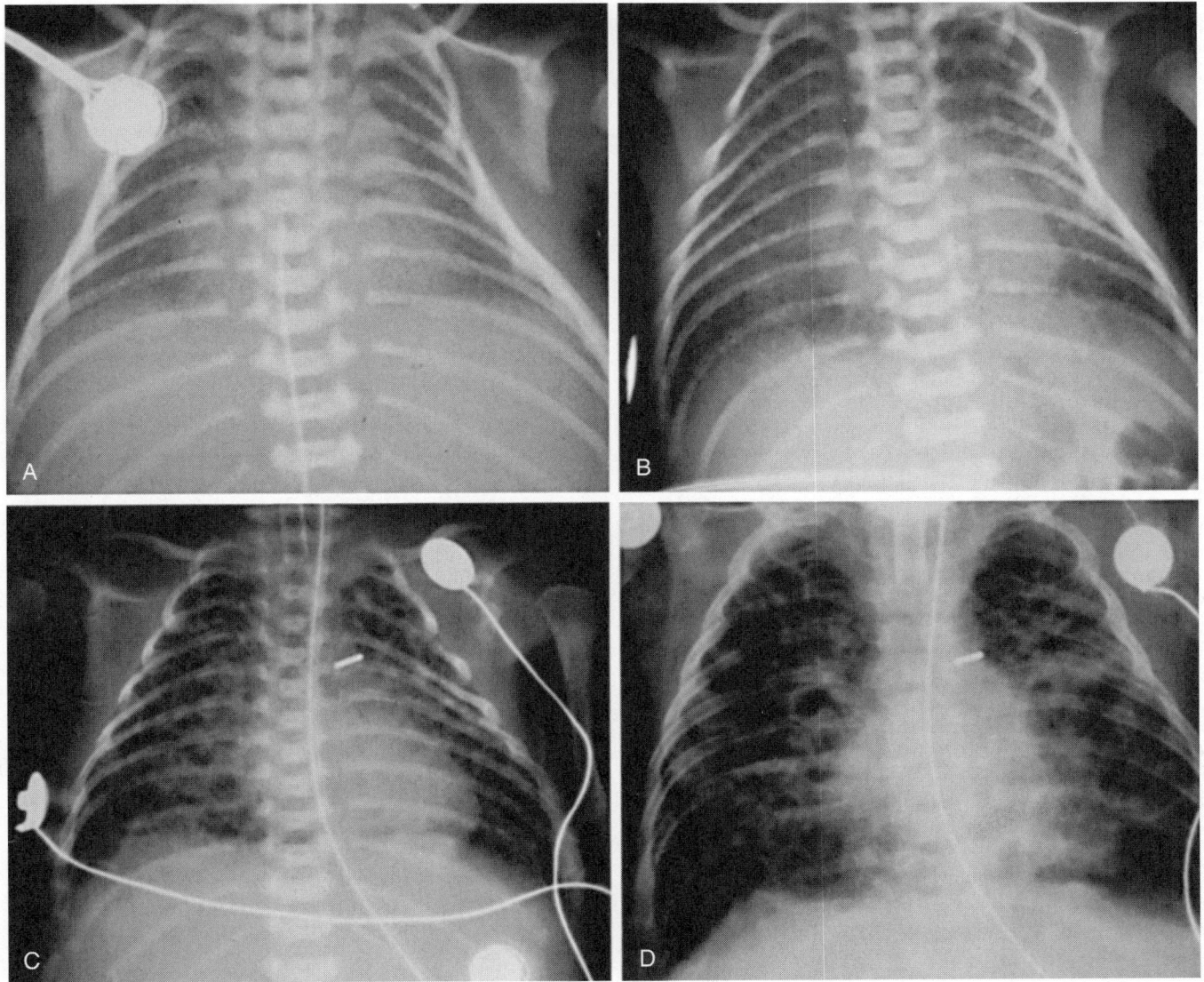

FIGURE 55–1. *A* to *D*, Radiographs illustrating the four stages of bronchopulmonary dysplasia.

Immaturity of the Lung

As demonstrated by the high incidence (70% to 75%) of BPD in very-premature infants (<26 weeks), immaturity is clearly a major etiologic factor, whether it is surfactant deficiency that leads to severe hyaline membrane disease or immaturity of the parenchymal structure of the lung or chest wall that contributes to chronic pulmonary insufficiency of prematurity.

Oxygen Toxicity

Although the cause of BPD is not known, there is a strong clinical association between BPD and exposure to high concentrations of oxygen (Hansen and Gest, 1984). BPD was first described as a form of CLD that occurred only in survivors of hyaline membrane disease who were ventilated with 80% to 100% oxygen for more than 150 hours. Subsequent reports have continued to show an association between oxygen exposure and lung damage in ventilated and nonventilated infants and, in fact, have suggested that even prolonged exposure to 60% oxygen can be toxic to the lungs of newborn infants (Philip, 1975).

Data obtained from experiments in animals and human volunteers and information gleaned from reports of patients inadvertently exposed to high concentrations of oxygen provide support for the theory that oxygen is a causative agent in BPD (Deneke and Fanburg, 1980); also in ventilated animals, oxygen damages the lung independent of the ventilator (DeLemos et al, 1988). In experimental animals, oxygen toxicity follows a course similar to BPD and has similar postmortem findings. Oxygen toxicity has an initial exudative phase that lasts up to 7 days, which is characterized by damage to airway and alveolar epithelium and capillary endothelium. With loss of endothelial and epithelial integrity, there is massive interstitial and alveolar edema with formation of hyaline membranes. Finally, there is a marked infiltration of the lung by neutrophils, the significance of which is still unclear. Animals surviving this phase enter the proliferative phase, which is characterized by proliferation of alveolar Type 2 cells and interstitial fibrosis. The amount of fibrosis is related to the length of the exposure to oxygen in the proliferative phase.

Experimental and clinical data have shown that humans are also susceptible to oxygen toxicity and that the course is similar to that seen in experimental animals (Philip, 1975). Short-term exposure to high concentrations of oxygen results in tracheitis and damage to airway epithelium, impaired mucociliary clearance, atelectasis, and eventually a significant alveolar-capillary leak. Long-term exposure results in pulmonary edema and impaired gas exchange.

Damage to the lung during oxygen toxicity appears to be mediated by reactive oxygen species produced during the univalent reduction of molecular oxygen. These species include superoxide anion (O_2^-), hydrogen peroxide (H_2O_2), and hydroxyl radical (OH^-). O_2^- is generated by the transfer of a single electron to molecular oxygen and the rate of O_2^- generation is increased by exposure to increased concentrations of oxygen. O_2^- is rapidly converted to H_2O_2 by one of several superoxide dismutases (SODs). O_2^- and H_2O_2 are both capable of causing tissue injury but are considered weak oxidants. Their real importance, however, relates to their ability to react with iron to generate the highly reactive OH^- radical. These reactive oxygen species damage the lung by initiating lipid peroxidation, inactivating sulfhydryl enzymes and damaging nucleic acids (Warner and Wispe, 1992). Superoxide also reacts with endogenous nitric oxide at a rapid rate (three times faster than its reaction with SOD) to form peroxynitrite ($ONOO^-$). This highly volatile molecule is known to cause lipid peroxidation and is likely to be responsible for some of the oxidant damage in BPD (Banks et al, 1996).

The lung is equipped with antioxidant enzymes to protect it from injury by reactive oxygen. SODs, located in the mitochondria (Mn SOD), cytosol (Cu Zn SOD), and outside the cells (extracellular SOD), catalyze the conversion of superoxide anion to hydrogen peroxide (Tsan, 1993). H_2O_2 concentrations are kept low by catalase, located in the peroxisomes, and by glutathione peroxidase, located in the cytosol and the mitochondria. Glutathione peroxidase converts H_2O_2 to water in a reaction with glutathione, and is the predominant mitochondrial defense against H_2O_2 (Smith, 1992). In this reaction, glutathione (GSH) acts as a donor of hydrogen atoms in the detoxification of hydrogen peroxide and is converted to the disulfide (GSSG). GSSG is converted back to GSH in a reaction with nicotinamide adenine dinucleotide phosphate, reduced form (NADPH) catalyzed by glutathione reductase. NADPH is supplied by the pentose shunt. Finally, because of its lipid solubility and ability to donate hydrogen atoms, vitamin E is important in stopping the chain reaction of lipid peroxidation in cell membranes. These defense mechanisms develop roughly in parallel with the surfactant system and may be inadequate at birth in preterm infants, especially those with hyaline membrane disease (Frank, 1985). In particular, recent data suggest that preterm infants may be glutathione deficient at birth and more susceptible to injury by reactive oxygen, even in relatively low oxygen environments (Smith et al, 1993). The glutathione content of lung epithelial cells is up to 100 times greater than in the plasma, and this is reflected in high levels in alveolar epithelial lining fluid (Cantin et al, 1987); this may represent the first line of defense against oxygen. On the first day of life, premature infants destined to develop BPD may have lower levels of glutathione in bronchoalveolar lavage fluid than infants not destined to develop BPD (Grigg et al, 1993).

Augmentation of the lung antioxidants by inducing the enzyme systems, or by direct supplementation, may offer some protection from oxygen toxicity (Freeman et al, 1985). Transgenic mice that overexpress Mn SOD are resistant to oxygen-induced lung injury (Wispe et al, 1992). A single study suggested that administration of SOD to preterm infants reduced the incidence of BPD; however, the effect was small, and SOD supplementation has not subsequently gained clinical acceptance (Rosenfeld et al, 1984). Vitamin E supplementation is discussed later in the section on prevention.

Barotrauma (Volutrauma)

BPD is a disease that made its appearance only after the introduction of positive-pressure mechanical ventilation for premature infants with RDS. Prior to that, CLD was reported only occasionally in infants treated with high oxygen concentrations without positive-pressure ventilation. But this condition, known as *pulmonary fibroplasia*, was not the same as BPD; there was radiologic evidence of parenchymal fibrosis without the evidence of airway involvement so typical of BPD, and the condition was much milder in its clinical course (Shepard et al, 1968). In their analysis of the histology of infants dying with BPD, Taghizadeh and Reynolds (1976) concluded that BPD was due to overdistension of terminal airways by high inflation pressures at a time when the terminal airspaces could not be inflated easily because of surfactant deficiency. Follow-up studies of some of the early survivors with CLD have suggested that persistently increased airway resistance seems to be related only to whether or not infants were mechanically ventilated with positive pressure rather than to the duration of oxygen exposure (Stocks, 1979).

It is now clear from numerous experimental studies that barotrauma, particularly that associated with high inspiratory pressures, is a major factor in the evolution of lung injury, independent of any injury produced by oxygen (Carlton et al, 1990; Kolobow et al, 1987; Parker et al, 1993); it is characterized by epithelial disruption in the conducting airways and increased capillary permeability to proteinaceous fluid. It is not high pressure alone that causes lung injury but rather high tidal volumes associated with overdistension; for when chest expansion is physically restricted during mechanical ventilation in experimental animals, the inflation pressures remain high, but lung injury is remarkably reduced or absent (Hernandez et al, 1989). It would be more correct to speak of *volutrauma* (Dreyfuss and Saumon, 1994; Hernandez et al, 1989). Several clinical studies have found an association between hypocarbia and an increased incidence of BPD (Garland et al, 1995; Kraybill et al, 1989), suggesting that the peak inflation pressure was too high in relation to the lung compliance. There is a strong association between the occurrence of pneumothorax and pulmonary interstitial emphysema, always associated with lung overdistension, and an increased incidence of BPD. In a multivariate analysis of autopsy data, Gorenflo and colleagues (1995) found a strong association between the occurrence of pulmonary interstitial emphysema in the first week of life and the occurrence of interstitial cell proliferation/lung fibrosis in BPD infants surviving more than 28 days.

Currently, there is no evidence that appropriate levels of PEEP contribute to BPD. In their animal model of lung overdistension and lung injury, Webb and Tierney (1974) found that increased positive end-expiratory pressure (PEEP) was protective against lung injury caused by high inflation pressures. Others have confirmed this finding (Jarriel et al, 1989; Johnson et al, 1989). In a comparison of three Harvard-affiliated neonatal intensive care units (NICUs) with different rates of BPD, Van Marter and associates (1992) also found that increased PEEP was protective against BPD. Dreyfuss and Saumon (1994) have discussed the lung injury that occurs when the airspaces are allowed to collapse during expiration and must be re-recruited with each breath by high inflation pressures; the use of generous levels of PEEP prevents this phenomenon.

Stern (1979) pointed out that infants treated with negative-pressure respirators between 1965 and 1975 never developed BPD, despite exposure to 100% oxygen for remarkably long periods. The negative-pressure respirator was a highly inefficient ventilator, and despite usual rates of 60 breaths/min, it seldom corrected the arterial PCO_2 to under 45 mm Hg, and therefore seldom overdistended the lung; moreover, it oxygenated infants only if high levels of expiratory distending pressure were used, which may have been protective against lung injury. Despite these deficiencies, the results for the negative-pressure respirator in infants over 1500 g were generally good (Ballard et al, 1973; Stern et al, 1970), and BPD in some of these patients would have been expected, especially on the basis of prolonged oxygen therapy.

Inflammation

In response to a primary form of injury, oxygen toxicity or volutrauma, there is an inflammatory response (Ogden et al, 1984; Pierce and Bancalari, 1995), which is reflected in increased numbers of neutrophils in the bronchial lavage samples as early as the second day of life (Arnon et al, 1993; Ogden et al, 1984). The bronchial lavage sample neutrophil count peaks on the fourth day of life and then declines rapidly to normal by the end of the first week in those who recover from respiratory distress syndrome (RDS) but declines much more slowly and persists in those who go on to develop BPD (Figs. 55–2 and 55–3). The neutrophils are of neonatal, not maternal, origin (Grigg et al, 1993), and surfactant therapy does not induce any change in the neutrophil profile during the first week of life (Arnon et al, 1993; Merritt et al, 1986).

More specifically, there is the appearance of increasing high levels of neutrophil elastase during the first few days of life in RDS (Merritt et al, 1983; Speer et al, 1993). The neutrophil elastase levels follow the same course as the neutrophils, peaking at 4 days, declining to normal by 1 week in those who recover, and persisting in those who go on to develop BPD. In the bronchial lavage samples during the first week, there are also elevated levels of mediators and cytokines, such as leukotrienes, platelet-activating factor, fibronectin, fibroblast-activating factors, and others (Silverman, 1994); there are elevated levels of interleukins and adhesion molecules (Kotecha et al, 1995); and in one of the earliest responses to injury, there are markedly elevated levels of interleukin-6 in bronchial lavage samples on the first day of life in those destined to develop BPD (Bagchi et al, 1994).

In patients with RDS who recover without BPD, there is a compensatory increase in proteinase inhibitor in the bronchial lavage samples, whereas in RDS which progresses to BPD, there is no such change, and the ratio of

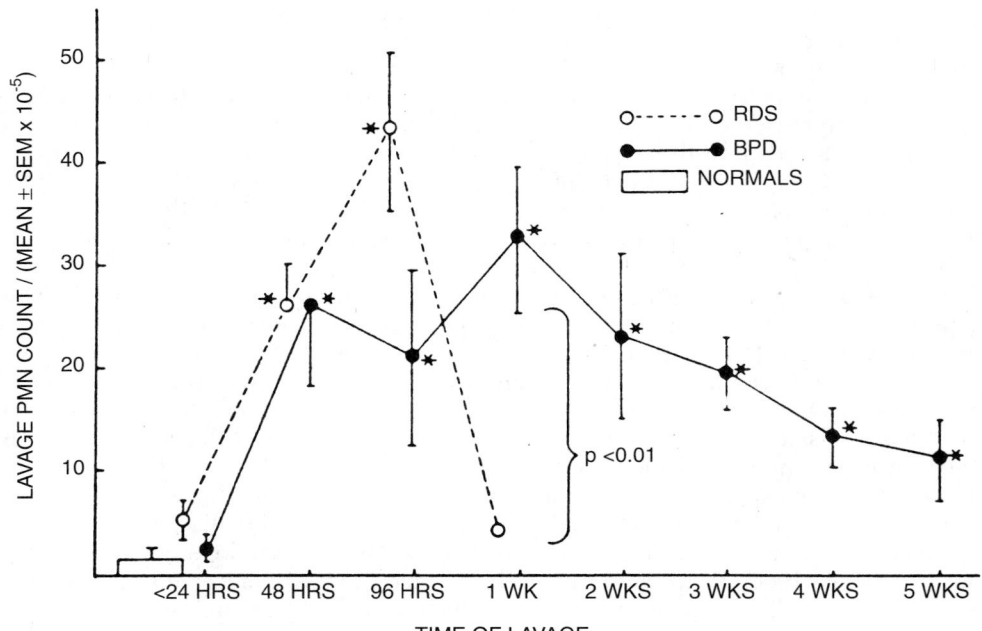

FIGURE 55–2. Bronchial lavage sample neutrophil counts in premature infants with respiratory distress syndrome (RDS) followed by recovery (open circles) and in premature infants with RDS followed by the development of bronchopulmonary dysplasia (closed circles). The profile for neutrophil elastase was similar. (From Ogden BE, Murphy SA, Saunders GC, et al: Neonatal lung neutrophils and elastase/proteinase inhibitor imbalance. Am Rev Respir Dis 130:817, 1984.)

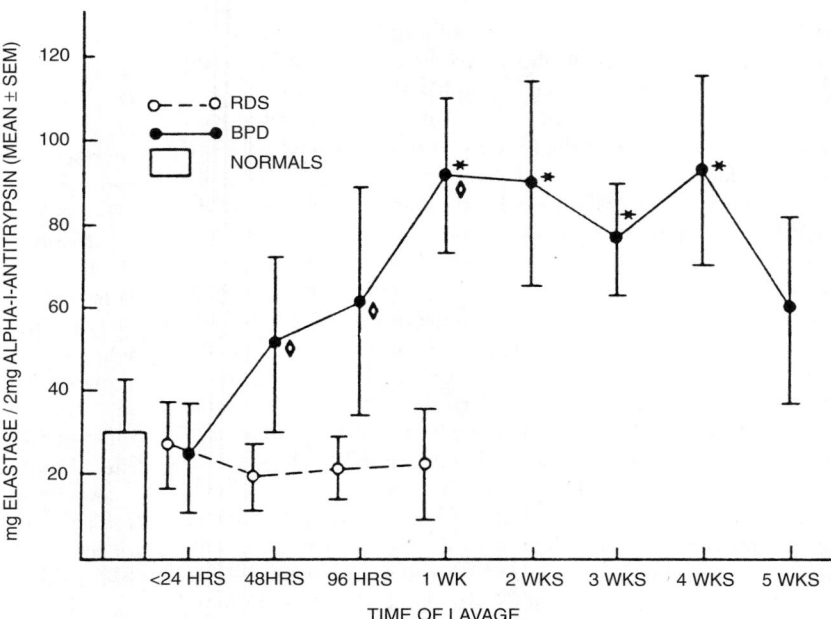

FIGURE 55–3. The ratio of neutrophil elastase/ proteinase inhibitor from bronchial lavage samples in control infants (open bar), in premature infants with respiratory distress syndrome (RDS) followed by recovery (open circles), and in premature infants with RDS followed by the development of bronchopulmonary dysplasia (closed circles). This illustrates the potential for an elastolytic destruction of lung tissue in bronchopulmonary dysplasia (BPD). (From Ogden BE, Murphy SA, Saunders GC, et al: Neonatal lung neutrophils and elastase/proteinase inhibitor imbalance. Am Rev Respir Dis 130:817, 1984.)

elastase to proteinase inhibitor becomes, and continues to be, unfavorable (Watterberg et al, 1994). It is believed that the lung is subjected to elastase (Bruce et al, 1992) and mediator attacks (Silverman, 1994) and that this further injury plays an important role in the genesis of BPD. The urinary levels of desmosine, an elastin degradation product, were demonstrated to be elevated at the age of 1 week in infants who later developed BPD, compared with infants who did not develop BPD (Bruce et al, 1985). If the plasma levels of proteinase inhibitor are low, this makes the lung particularly susceptible to further injury and the development of BPD (Merritt et al, 1983); the plasma levels of proteinase inhibitor are known to be low in RDS. In addition, there may be present inactivators of proteinase inhibitors (Bruce et al, 1982), which may further upset the balance in favor of proteolytic injury and the development of BPD. In infants who do not develop BPD, the neutrophils undergo programmed cell death (apoptosis) and are ingested by macrophages without releasing their elastase or other destructive enzymes (Grigg et al, 1991); this process may be disturbed in those who develop BPD.

Later, between 1 and 4 weeks of age, the bronchial lavage samples contain increased levels of additional factors, such as fibronectin, platelet-derived growth factor, tumor necrosis factor, histamine, and others (Silverman, 1994); this is the time when BPD is developing and there is persistent inflammation and persistent high permeability pulmonary edema (Jeffries et al, 1984), aggravated by mediators, chemoattractants, and cytokines. Premature infants with early BPD have higher levels of neutrophils, complement fragments, leukotrienes, and interleukins in the bronchial lavage samples, and increased levels of albumin, which reflect the capillary injury typical of BPD (Groneck et al, 1994). In addition, the levels of fibronectin in tracheal aspirate samples are elevated in infants with early BPD (Gerdes et al, 1986; Watts and Bruce, 1992), and this would favor the development of pulmonary fibrosis, seen in the later stages of BPD.

Pulmonary Edema and Patent Ductus Arteriosus

Some studies have stressed the importance of pulmonary edema, due to excessive fluid administration, in the genesis of BPD (Brown et al, 1978; Van Marter et al, 1990). A controlled trial of fluid restriction in the management of RDS has established that reduced fluid administration is associated with a decreased incidence of BPD (Tammela et al, 1992); there was a significant reduction in the number of deaths and in the incidence of BPD by radiologic criteria in the fluid-restricted group. In the analysis of three Harvard NICUs referred to earlier, it was concluded that the major cause of BPD was excessive fluid and colloid administration (Van Marter et al, 1992).

Patent ductus arteriosus (PDA) makes a major contribution to the genesis of BPD by favoring the development of pulmonary edema. Dudell and Gersony (1984) showed, in a population of small premature infants with RDS, that if the ductus closed spontaneously at the age of 3 days, then the incidence of BPD was low (22%), but if it remained open at the age of 3 days, the incidence of BPD was significantly higher (68%). However, for therapeutic closure of the PDA, the data are not so convincing. If the ductus was surgically closed at the age of about 1 week, the duration of intubation and hospitalization was greatly shortened (Cotton et al, 1978). Although there was no documentation that the incidence of BPD was reduced, this study has been widely interpreted to mean that it was. Some studies, in which the ductus was closed with indomethacin given at the age of 3 days, have suggested that the incidence of BPD was reduced (Merritt et al, 1981), but not all studies have confirmed this (Hammerman et al, 1986). In a study of tracheal aspirate samples, Varsila and coworkers (1995) found that neutrophil myeloperoxidase levels were elevated in small premature infants with PDA and that indomethacin treatment caused a significant reduction; it was believed that closure of the ductus or treatment with indomethacin might reduce lung injury due to neutrophils and, hence, reduce the incidence of BPD.

Eronen and associates (1994) reported that antenatal treatment with indomethacin for preterm labor was associated with an increased incidence of BPD, perhaps because of postnatal oliguria and fluid retention (Norton et al, 1993). Increased BPD has not been reported in trials of postnatal administration of indomethacin for intraventricular hemorrhage prevention or PDA treatment, but fluid retention is frequently observed, and this may contribute to the difficulties in demonstrating a possible reduced incidence of BPD with early closure of the PDA.

Infection

During the past 10 years, reports have appeared (Holtzman et al, 1989; Sanchez and Regan, 1988; Wang et al, 1988) suggesting that organisms such as *Ureaplasma, Chlamydia,* or cytomegalovirus may produce chronic infection and thereby contribute to the pathogenesis of BPD. Cassell and colleagues (1988) have claimed that *Ureaplasma* pneumonia is responsible for many cases of BPD, but other studies have not supported this hypothesis (Heggie et al, 1994). Alfa and associates (1995) found placental cultures positive for *Ureaplasma* in 20% to 25% of mothers, regardless of gestational age at delivery; throat cultures on the first day of life were positive in 19% of VLBW infants, in 6% of larger preterm infants, and in 1% of term infants, indicating that small, premature infants are most susceptible to acquisition of *Ureaplasma*. Among VLBW infants, BPD developed in all those with *Ureaplasma* colonization but in only one third of those without *Ureaplasma* colonization. It is not clear that affected infants must develop *Ureaplasma* pneumonia before developing BPD. A recent meta-analysis of multiple studies of this problem has suggested that colonization alone with *Ureaplasma* may nearly double the risk for developing BPD (Wang et al, 1995). This controversy can be settled only by large prospective therapeutic trials with effective antibiotics.

Other Factors

Nutritional factors may well play a role in the development of BPD (Frank and Sosenko, 1988); undernourished animals are vulnerable to lung injury. After experiments in rats, it was suggested that a diet high in polyunsaturated fatty acids may protect against oxygen toxicity (Sosenko et al, 1988), but a randomized, controlled trial of early administration of intravenous lipids to small premature infants failed to find any benefit and demonstrated some harm (Sosenko et al, 1993). Hammerman and Aramburo (1988) reported a controlled trial of intravenous lipids in small premature infants and concluded that the incidence of BPD was increased. This finding may be the result of the high level of hydroperoxides in lipid preparations exposed to light (Neuzil et al, 1995).

After initially promising studies, it is now clear that vitamin E does not prevent lung injury in hyperoxic lambs (Hansen et al, 1982) and that vitamin E deficiency is not associated with an increased incidence of BPD (Ehrenkranz et al, 1979).

There is some evidence that premature infants are deficient in vitamin A as a result of too early delivery, that vitamin A is important in the process of epithelial repair in the injured lung, that infants with BPD have more evidence of vitamin A deficiency than infants without BPD, and that attempts to supplement vitamin A are hampered by vitamin A degradation in the intravenous tubing used for parenteral nutrition (Shenai et al, 1990; Stahlman et al, 1988). In a controlled trial of vitamin A supplementation, Shenai and colleagues (1987) found a significant reduction in the incidence of BPD in the treated infants. But these results could not be confirmed; in a second controlled trial of vitamin A supplementation with intramuscular injections, in infants weighing 700 to 1100 g, no benefit was demonstrated (Pearson et al, 1992); this may have been because the control subjects had adequate levels of vitamin A from routine vitamin supplementation (Pearson et al, 1994).

Another factor under consideration is that premature infants may be deficient in selenium, with low levels of selenium-dependent glutathione peroxidase in red blood cells and possibly in the lung (Friel et al, 1993; Sluis et al, 1992). Darlow and associates (1995) found a significant inverse relationship between plasma selenium levels at the age of 28 days and the number of days of oxygen therapy in premature infants, but they could not discern whether this was cause or effect. No trials of selenium supplementation in premature infants have appeared at this time.

In summary, BPD is a multifactorial disease in which inflammation, following oxygen toxicity, volutrauma, or infection, and possibly other factors such as excessive hydration and nutritional insufficiency, may play a role. Using a multivariate logistic regression analysis, Corcoran and coworkers (1993) have devised a scoring system to assess the probability of BPD at the age of 1 week. The independent variables were (1) gestational age; (2) birth weight; (3) gender; (4) age at intubation; (5) duration of inspired oxygen more than 60%; (6) duration of peak inflation pressure more than 25 cm H_2O; and (7) diagnosis of RDS. Using a probability of less than 25% as low risk, and a probability of more than 25% as high risk, the sensitivity was 83% and the specificity was 85%. This indicates a good level of predictability based on these factors alone. They observed a declining incidence in the condition over the passage of time, mostly based on the systematic use of lower pressures and less oxygen in managing this condition.

Clinical Course

Stage 4 BPD is a type of chronic obstructive lung disease. The infants have a barrel chest, prolonged expiration time, expiratory wheezing, and evidence of lung overinflation on chest radiograph (Merritt and Boynton, 1988) (see Fig. 55–1). Pulmonary function tests demonstrate increased airway resistance and functional residual capacity and decreased tidal volume (Heldt, 1988a). Increased airway resistance is in part the result of damage and destruction of airways, in part the result of increased airway reactivity, and in part a manifestation of the interstitial edema that invariably accompanies BPD. Infants with BPD have bronchial smooth muscle hypertrophy, and cold air provocation tests and trials of bronchodilators have demonstrated that bronchospasm may contribute to their increased airway resistance (Greenspan et al, 1989), even when they are as young as 14 days. In addition, infants with BPD have radiographic and clinical evidence of pulmonary edema. Presumably, the loss of arterioles and capillaries in the lung along with some vascular remodeling results in increased blood flow through remaining vessels and increased filtration of fluid from these vessels. In infants with cor pulmonale, systemic venous pressure is high and the ability of the lymphatics to clear this filtered fluid is impaired. Fluid in perivascular cuffs compresses airways and increases airway resistance.

In infants with BPD, static lung compliance is usually decreased but may be increased if damage to the lung is sufficient to result in loss of elastic recoil. Dynamic compliance is invariably decreased and nitrogen washout is delayed, indicating a severe maldistribution of ventilation. Maldistribution of ventilation results in mismatch of ventilation and perfusion, which leads to hypoxemia. Although the respiratory rate is usually increased, physiologic dead space is also increased so that alveolar ventilation is decreased and arterial PCO_2 is increased.

Obliteration of arterioles and capillaries results in a reduction in available surface area for gas exchange and may contribute to arterial hypoxemia, especially during exercise. The loss of vessels, coupled with smooth muscle hypertrophy from chronic alveolar hypoxia, may also result in pulmonary hypertension and cor pulmonale. With cor pulmonale, cardiac output falls and oxygen delivery may be impaired.

Treatment

Nutrition

Since infants with BPD usually outgrow their CLD, a major aim of therapy is provision of adequate nutritional support for growth and prevention of complications. Nutritional support is complicated by an increased resting metabolic rate (Kurzner et al, 1988; Weinstein and Oh, 1981; Yeh et al, 1989), with a caloric need for as much as 140 to 160 kcal/kg per day in the face of a relative inability to tolerate fluid loads. Thus, these infants must often be fed high-caloric-density formulas supplemented with calcium and potassium to replace losses resulting from concomitant diuretic therapy.

Oxygen Therapy

Supplemental oxygen should be administered to maintain the infant's arterial PO_2 between 55 and 70 mm Hg and the pulse oximeter reading above 95% to prevent alveolar hypoxia. Reduced alveolar oxygen levels may cause airway constriction (Tay-Uyboco et al, 1989) and pulmonary hypertension (Abman et al, 1985); oxygen must be given in sufficient amounts to prevent cor pulmonale. This approach may require prolonged mechanical ventilation initially, but eventually patients can be managed with administration of oxygen by nasal continuous positive airway pressure (CPAP), Oxy-Hood, or nasal cannula. In the past, chronic oxygen administration usually required prolonged hospitalization; however, several neonatal programs have reported successful management of these infants at home (Goldberg

and Monahan, 1989; Hudak et al, 1989; Pinney and Cotton, 1976). It is important that infants remain well oxygenated during and after feeds (Singer et al, 1992), during sleep (Harris and Sullivan, 1995), and during other activities.

Blood Transfusion

Booster transfusions of blood to maintain the hematocrit above 40% have been shown to reduce resting oxygen consumption and to increase systemic oxygen transport in infants with BPD (Alverson et al, 1988) and some programs also administer erythropoietin and iron to minimize transfusion.

Fluid Restriction and Diuretic Therapy

Fluid restriction may reduce interstitial edema in the lung and improve pulmonary function; therefore, these infants are usually fed with concentrated formulas. It has been shown in a controlled trial that furosemide facilitates extubation from mechanical ventilation in BPD (McCann et al, 1985). Furosemide alone (Engelhardt et al, 1986; Kao et al, 1983), and chlorothiazide in combination with spironolactone (Kao et al, 1984), has been shown to be effective in improving lung mechanics and gas exchange, thus reducing the oxygen requirements in infants with BPD; however, the effects last only so long as the drugs are continued. Chronic diuretic therapy may result in excessive urinary losses of calcium, potassium, sodium, and chloride. Calcium loss may compromise bone mineralization and exacerbate osteopenia of prematurity. In addition, prolonged administration of furosemide has been associated with nephrocalcinosis in infants with BPD (Ezzedeen et al, 1988; Hufnagle et al, 1982) and also with cholelithiasis (Callahan et al, 1982). Although it has been suggested that substitution of chlorothiazide for furosemide may reduce calcium wasting, a recent study has questioned this effect (Atkinson et al, 1988); and Engelhardt and associates (1989) were unable to demonstrate improvement in lung mechanics with chlorothiazide-spironolactone treatment. In addition, chloride loss can result in metabolic alkalosis, decreased ventilatory drive, and hypercarbia; this may contribute to an erroneous conclusion that furosemide therapy is ineffective (Hazinski, 1985). These infants must be supplemented with potassium chloride and occasionally sodium chloride to prevent the bicarbonate concentration from reaching 30 mEq/L. Alternate-day furosemide therapy has proved effective while minimizing the electrolyte disturbances (Rush et al, 1990).

Kao and coworkers (1984) have reported the results of a controlled trial comparing chlorothiazide-spironolactone with placebo; all infants were eligible to receive furosemide when needed, and the trial was continued until oxygen supplementation could be discontinued. The placebo group needed significantly more furosemide therapy. Patients were scored on the basis of respiratory rate, chest retractions, inspired oxygen, and arterial PCO_2; infants in the chlorothiazide-spironolactone group had significantly improved clinical scores, but there was no difference in the length of oxygen supplementation, and side effects such as nephrocalcinosis and deafness were not reduced in the chlorothiazide-spironolactone group. According to Rush and Hazinski (1992), furosemide therapy may be initiated in the following situations: (1) in 1-week-old ventilator-dependent patients with early BPD; (2) in infants with stable BPD who suddenly deteriorate from excessive fluids; (3) in infants with chronic BPD that is not improving; and (4) in infants in whom there is a need for increased volume and calorie intake. The clinician should continue diuretics if improvement occurs when they are given, or deterioration occurs when they are stopped. The use of diuretics has decreased since the advent of steroid therapy. In general, furosemide may be continued 2 to 3 days a week until oxygen is no longer required.

Bronchodilators

Infants with BPD often have a family history of asthma (Nickerson and Taussig, 1980) and frequently have very high levels of urinary leukotrienes, comparable to those seen in asthma (Davidson et al, 1995). Episodes of acute deterioration in infants with BPD resemble acute asthmatic attacks and are often attributed to bronchospasm. Furthermore, increased airway resistance secondary to broncho-constriction is believed to play a role in prolonging ventilator requirements in this population of infants. Multiple authors have shown that administration of a variety of beta-adrenergic agents to infants with BPD results in improvements in lung compliance, airway resistance, and gas exchange (Cabal et al, 1987; Denjean et al, 1992; Jarriel et al, 1993; Rotschild et al, 1989; Sosulski et al, 1986).

Management of acute episodes of bronchoconstriction is best accomplished by the use of beta-adrenergic agents. For ventilated infants, albuterol may be delivered by metered-dose inhaler, using a spacer placed between the ventilator circuit connector and endotracheal tube connector (Rozycki et al, 1991). This technique allows more precise control of the delivered dose than techniques of in-line nebulization. In one study a dose of 100 μg of albuterol by metered-dose inhaler significantly increased respiratory system compliance and decreased resistance in 65% of patients, and 200 μg was effective in the remainder (Denjean et al, 1992). These changes lasted 3 hours and were accompanied by increased oxygen saturation by pulse oximetry and an increased heart rate. Beta-adrenergic agents may also be administered by nebulization into the ventilator circuit or into a face mask. The usual medication is albuterol (1 mg/kg) repeated every 4 to 6 hours (Kao et al, 1988); the large dose is a reflection of the inefficiency of this method of administration. In some instances it may be useful to assess the response to a single dose of terbutaline (5 to 10 μg/kg) administered subcutaneously (Jarriel et al, 1993; Sosulski et al, 1986) and then to continue bronchodilator therapy only if a significant improvement in lung function is observed. Both terbutaline and albuterol produce some tachycardia, which is well tolerated, and in some patients there is hyperglycemia, hypertension, or tremor. In rare situations terbutaline may be administered as a continuous intravenous infusion (0.25 to 0.50 μg/kg per minute) in very ill ventilator-dependent patients with evidence of severe bronchoconstriction.

Inhaled beta-adrenergic agents are also useful in the chronic management of infants with BPD and increased airway reactivity. In addition, administration of theophylline has been shown to relieve bronchoconstriction (Rooklin et al, 1979) and in some centers is used in combination with a selective beta$_2$-adrenergic agonist. As it is very poorly absorbed from the respiratory tract, it does not produce significant systemic effects. One further medication, which works differently, is cromolyn sodium; it is a mast cell stabilizer and inhibits the release of histamine and leukotrienes, which may play a role in producing bronchoconstriction (Davis et al, 1990). It has been tried in infants with severe BPD and may be effective.

Although there are multiple studies of the short-term effects of these drugs (Clarke et al, 1993), there are no long-term studies, so we do not know if the length of mechanical ventilation, oxygen therapy, or hospitalization is decreased, or if the incidence of BPD is reduced, or if survival is improved.

Systemic Corticosteroids

A number of clinical trials have suggested that dexamethasone is valuable in shortening the time to extubation and the length of time the patient remained on mechanical ventilation (Ariagno, 1988; Avery et al, 1985; Cummings et al, 1989; Harkavy et al, 1989; Kazzi et al, 1990; Mammel et al, 1983). Watterberg and Scott (1995) have suggested a possible basis for steroid therapy. They found that 1-week-old premature infants destined to develop BPD had a poor cortisol response to corticotropin when compared with control infants not destined to develop BPD. This may mean that such infants are not able to adequately suppress the inflammatory response to lung injury and need appropriate therapeutic intervention. Ballard and associates (1996), however, found that levels of cortisol were elevated in infants with RDS compared with those without lung disease and that there was no difference in cortisol levels in infants who went on to develop BPD versus those who did not.

The Collaborative Dexamethasone Trial Group (1991) in Europe performed a large controlled trial of corticosteroids in ventilator-dependent premature infants with BPD enrolled at the age of 30 days and found that a 7-day course of dexamethasone, repeated in some cases, significantly reduced the time to extubation from a median of 18 days in the control group to a median of 11 days in the treated group. The median time on oxygen was decreased by 19 days, but the length of hospitalization was not shortened by dexamethasone treatment. This trial also showed some benefits in extubated infants on oxygen therapy. In another important trial, it was shown that a 3-day dexamethasone course, at the age of 30 days in infants with BPD, significantly reduced the oxygen requirements, significantly increased the static lung compliance, and significantly reduced neutrophils, neutrophil elastase, fibronectin, and albumin in tracheal aspirate samples (Yoder et al, 1991). These authors concluded that steroids suppressed lung inflammation and improved the permeability of lung capillaries and that dexamethasone exerted its favorable effects within 3 days. Papile and colleagues (1996) found no difference in outcome for early (14-day) versus late (28-day) administration of steroids in preterm infants with early CLD.

Brundage and coworkers (1992) gave 30-day-old infants

with BPD a 7-day course of dexamethasone and found major improvements in lung mechanics: static lung compliance was increased by 77% and airway resistance was reduced by 33%. They believed that a critical level of improved lung compliance was important for the success of extubation. Durand and associates (1995) demonstrated, in a controlled trial of surfactant-treated premature infants aged 7 to 14 days, that a 3-day course of dexamethasone, tapered over 4 additional days, produced dramatic improvements in the treated group. There was a significant increase in static lung compliance; oxygen and ventilator requirements were greatly reduced; the median time on mechanical ventilation was reduced from 35 to 20 days; the incidence of BPD at 28 days was reduced from 68% to 32%; the incidence of BPD at 36 weeks' postconceptional age was reduced from 47% to 10%; and survival without BPD was increased from 45% to 83%. Brozanski and colleagues (1995) showed in a controlled trial that a 3-day course of dexamethasone, starting at 7 days of age and repeated every 10 days, also produced improved results in the treated group. At 36 weeks' postconceptional age, there was a significant decrease in the incidence of BPD from 77% in control subjects to 54% in treated infants, and there was a significant increase in survival without BPD from 20% in control subjects to 40% in treated infants.

The side effects of dexamethasone include hyperglycemia, hypertension, neutrophilia, infection, and reduced growth and in the animal model disturbed myelinization and neurodevelopment. Some infants have developed concentric hypertrophic cardiomyopathy, especially with prolonged treatment, which resolves with time after discontinuation of the drug (Sicard and Werner, 1992). Other infants treated with dexamethasone have developed systemic candidiasis, which is a worrisome complication associated also with extreme prematurity and vaginal delivery (Rowen et al, 1995). Schwarze and Bartmann (1994) showed that dexamethasone suppresses the lymphocyte proliferative response to mitogen stimulation in whole blood cultures of newborn infants. Although long courses of dexamethasone may suppress adrenal function (Ng et al, 1989), it does not appear that a 5- to 7-day course of dexamethasone at 0.5 mg/kg per day significantly suppresses function of the adrenal gland (Brundage et al, 1992; Wilson et al, 1988). The dose of 0.5 mg/kg is a pharmacologic dose, however, and there is evidence (Durand et al, 1995) that a more physiologic dose (0.25 mg/kg), twice the amount necessary to saturate the glucocorticoid receptors (Ballard et al, 1995), would be adequate to mimic the physiologic stress level produced in sick infants with RDS. The mechanism of action of dexamethasone is probably a suppression of lung inflammation (Watts and Bruce, 1992; Yoder et al, 1991) or a suppression of lung collagen synthesis (Co et al, 1993); however, others have suggested reduced protein leakage resulting in decreased surfactant inhibition (Kari et al, 1994) and reduced pulmonary edema following enhanced diuresis (Gladstone et al, 1989).

Despite the current enthusiasm for steroid treatment of BPD, the 3-year follow-up evaluation of infants in the Collaborative Dexamethasone Trial (1991) did not suggest any long-term outcome advantage for those treated with steroids (Jones et al, 1995), and indeed Yeh and associates (1997) found an increase in neurodevelopmental abnormal-

ities at 2 years of age in infants with respiratory failure treated beginning at 12 hours of life (with a tapered 28-day course beginning with 0.25 mg/kg). The evidence to date suggests that the benefits are short term. It may be that the full beneficial effect can be obtained with a low-dose short course of steroids with a reduction in concerns about potential long-term deleterious effects. These trials are underway and caution is advised.

Inhaled Corticosteroids

There have been few studies of inhaled steroids in the treatment of this condition. In a controlled trial, LaForce and Brudno (1993) found that beclomethasone by metered-dose inhaler produced improved airway resistance and improved dynamic lung compliance after treatment for 2 weeks in comparison with controls. In a small controlled trial of nebulized flunisolide for 28 days in ventilator dependent infants with BPD, improvements were found in oxygen requirements, lung mechanics, and time to extubation in comparison with control groups (Pokriefka et al, 1993). Konig and coworkers (1992) have described the use of nebulized flunisolide in older infants with BPD. In another small controlled trial of nebulized dexamethasone for 10 days in ventilator-dependent preterm infants, the dynamic lung compliance was markedly improved and airway resistance was modestly improved, whereas no such improvements occurred in the control subjects (Pappagallo et al, 1991). Rozycki and associates (1991) have described an excellent method for administering medication using a metered-dose inhaler with a spacer and a ventilation bag.

Vasodilators

The most severe complication of BPD is cor pulmonale with pulmonary hypertension associated with a very high mortality rate. Infants whose disease has reached this stage may require cardiac catheterization to determine their response to increased oxygen or to agents that might reduce pulmonary vascular resistance. No agents have yet been established as useful, although early trials of inhaled nitric oxide show some promise (Banks et al, 1997).

Prevention

Prevention of preterm birth is, of course, the most effective means of preventing BPD; if we could recognize premature labor and delay delivery until 30 weeks' gestation, more than 75% of BPD cases would not occur (Rush and Hazinski, 1992). Short of that possibility, acceleration of lung maturation with prenatal glucocorticoid treatment (see Chapters 49 and 53) is the optimal approach (Van Marter et al, 1990); it is known that prenatal steroids induce the development of antioxidant enzymes in the lung, as well as surfactant synthesis enzymes (Frank et al, 1985), and have a beneficial effect as lung structure as well. There is some evidence that the addition of thyrotropin-releasing hormone to betamethasone for antenatal prophylaxis against RDS may be effective in further reducing the incidence of BPD (Ballard et al, 1992).

Preventive management of the newborn now includes administration of exogenous surfactant at birth, but only in the case of rescue treatment with synthetic surfactant is there any evidence for reduced BPD (Corbet, 1993; Jobe, 1993), and the effect is small. In institutions that routinely use nasal CPAP initially after birth, there may be a reduced use of mechanical ventilation and a reduced incidence of BPD (Avery et al, 1987); however, there are no controlled trials to confirm this idea. Maintenance of low inspired oxygen concentrations is believed to be important in preventing oxygen toxicity; it is recommended that the arterial P_{O_2} be maintained at 50 to 70 mm Hg and not higher. Reduced inspired oxygen can be accomplished to some degree by the use of continuous distending pressure. Mechanical ventilation with a strategy of reduced inflation pressures and acceptance of relatively high levels of arterial P_{CO_2} may reduce the incidence of BPD (Rhodes et al, 1983); but again, this hypothesis for permissive hypercarbia has never been adequately tested in clinical trials. Clark and colleagues (1992) have presented evidence from controlled trials that high-frequency oscillatory ventilation may reduce the incidence of BPD in comparison with infants treated with conventional mechanical ventilation. Cleary and colleagues (1995) also found some evidence of decreased BPD with use of synchronized intermittent mandatory ventilation.

Although a number of therapies including vitamin E, vitamin A, inositol supplementation, SOD, and treatment of potential infection with *Ureaplasma* have been tried, no clear benefit for any of these has been demonstrated.

In an attempt to suppress the inflammation that follows lung injury, there has been wide interest in the early use of steroids on the first day of life; this strategy may be considered either as treatment for RDS or as prevention for BPD. Yeh and coworkers (1990) have published evidence that dexamethasone administration on the first day of life may prevent the development of BPD in many infants. Sanders and associates (1994) showed that the administration of two doses of dexamethasone to high-risk infants under 30 weeks' gestation, during the first 24 to 30 hours after birth, significantly improved lung function and decreased ventilatory requirements. Another potential approach to reducing lung injury is the use of liquid ventilation with perfluorocarbon. Animal studies suggest beneficial effects, and clinical trials in severe respiratory distress are underway (see also Chapter 53).

Outcome

The mortality rate among infants with BPD after discharge from the hospital is roughly 10%. Survivors have an increased incidence of lower respiratory tract infections and of increased airway reactivity in the first year after discharge (Smyth et al, 1981). Later, although pulmonary function studies may indicate increased small airway resistance among children with BPD, the exercise tolerance of these children is comparable to that of their normal peers (Bader et al, 1987; Heldt et al, 1980). Growth may be delayed initially, but catch-up growth occurs with resolution of the pulmonary abnormalities.

Neurodevelopmental Outcome

In general, when discharged to a good home, and when provided with appropriate nutrition and oxygen supple-

mentation, these infants achieve a reasonable neurodevelopmental status if they have not sustained a significant intracranial insult (Leonard et al, 1994). Gray and colleagues (1995) examined a large cohort of premature infants at the age of 2 years and compared infants with BPD and birth-weight matched control subjects. They found an increased incidence of neurodevelopmental disabilities in those with BPD, but the problems were related to periventricular hemorrhage, cerebral ventricular dilation, and sepsis; BPD was not an independent risk factor for neurologic disability. However, Campbell and coworkers (1988) have recently reported a progressive neurologic syndrome in some infants with BPD and have raised concerns that this syndrome may be caused by some of the therapies being used in the clinical management of these infants.

CHRONIC PULMONARY INSUFFICIENCY OF PREMATURITY

Chronic pulmonary insufficiency of prematurity (CPIP), which occurs usually in premature infants weighing less than 1200 g at birth, is also known as *late-onset respiratory distress* and is characterized by the development of serious respiratory difficulty and recurrent apnea after the first few days of life. During the first month, these infants exhibit a substantially reduced lung volume that is manifested clinically by an oxygen requirement of 25% to 40%, the presence of modest hypercarbia, and poorly defined, diffuse lung densities without cystic changes on the chest radiograph. The AaD_{O_2}, aAD_{CO_2}, and aAD_{N_2} all are increased (Krauss et al, 1975) (see Chapter 50 for definition of terms).

The very compliant chest wall of these infants probably contributes to the atelectasis associated with this condition; small premature infants have more flexible ribs and less intercostal muscle mass than larger more mature infants. Heldt (1988a) has measured the volume displacement of the diaphragm during inspiration in small premature infants and related it to the volume of each breath; he found that the volume displacement of the diaphragm was much greater than the lung volume change in small infants and attributed the difference to chest wall distortion or collapse during inspiration; the difference decreased with increasing maturity, as the chest wall became less compliant and chest wall distortion decreased. This phenomenon is believed to be almost universal in small premature infants but is likely more prominent in those who develop the signs of CPIP. It means that the diaphragm is less effective in producing a normal lung minute volume and that diaphragmatic work is greatly increased.

Apnea and bradycardia spells are common, but the relationship between apnea and CPIP is not firmly established; most authors believe that apnea of prematurity is related to deficiencies in respiratory drive, but diaphragmatic fatigue related to chest wall distortion may also be important. Both conditions appear to respond well to prolonged management with low concentrations of oxygen administered by nasal CPAP or by nasal cannula therapy. Clinical recovery in CPIP generally occurs during the second month of life (Krauss et al, 1975), but apnea and bradycardia may persist in some infants for a longer period. The best interpretation of the data is that CPIP aggravates apnea of prematurity by producing diaphragmatic fatigue.

WILSON-MIKITY SYNDROME

Wilson-Mikity syndrome is an eponym for a form of late-developing respiratory distress in small premature infants, which was described in 1960 by Wilson and Mikity. It may, in fact, represent one end of the spectrum of CPIP. It is characterized by the onset of tachypnea, chest retractions, and cyanosis at 1 to 4 weeks of age in infants who were free of RDS at birth. Some of these infants have mechanical ventilation for other reasons, such as apnea, but they need low pressures and low oxygen concentrations. Their respiratory distress progresses for about 2 months and then slowly regresses until recovery is achieved over a period of 1 to 2 years. As the condition develops, the chest radiograph shows that the lung has a "bubbly" appearance, with diffuse streaks of infiltrate and widespread cystic change; during the recovery phase, hyperinflation is present at the lung bases, with flattening of the diaphragm, and streaky atelectasis at the apices.

The cause of Wilson-Mikity syndrome is unknown. The airways of premature infants are extremely compliant (Burnard, 1966), and if compliance values are unevenly distributed, this might cause airway closure and gas trapping in certain regions of the lung, and adjacent compression atelectasis in other regions. In Burnard's experience, this condition was rarely diagnosed following the advent of CPAP treatment; it is possible that higher mean airway pressures stabilized the peripheral airways and prevented widespread closure.

REFERENCES

Abman SH, Wolfe, RR, Accurso, FJ, et al: Pulmonary vascular response to oxygen in infants with severe bronchopulmonary dysplasia. Pediatrics 75:90, 1985.

Alfa MJ, Embree JE, Degagne P, et al: Transmission of *Ureaplasma urealyticum* from mothers to full and preterm infants. Pediatr Infect Dis J 14:341, 1995.

Alverson DC, Isken VH, Cohen RS: Effect of booster blood transfusions on oxygen utilization in infants with bronchopulmonary dysplasia. J Pediatr 113:722, 1988.

Ariagno RL: Use of steroids. *In* Merritt TA, Northway WH, Boynton BR (Eds): Bronchopulmonary Dysplasia. Boston, Blackwell Scientific Publications, 1988.

Arnon S, Grigg J, Silverman M: Pulmonary inflammatory cells in ventilated preterm infants: Effect of surfactant treatment. Arch Dis Child 69:44, 1993.

Atkinson SA, Shah JK, McGee C, et al: Mineral excretion in premature infants receiving various diuretic therapies. J Pediatr 113:540, 1988.

Avery GB, Fletcher AB, Kaplan M, et al: Controlled trial of dexamethasone in respirator-dependent infants with bronchopulmonary dysplasia. Pediatrics 75:106, 1985.

Avery ME, Tooley WH, Keller JB, et al: Is chronic lung disease in low-birth-weight infants preventable? A survey of eight centers. Pediatrics 79:26, 1987.

Bader D, Ramos AD, Lew CD, et al: Childhood sequelae of infant lung disease: Exercise and pulmonary function abnormalities after bronchopulmonary dysplasia. J Pediatr 110:693, 1987.

Bagchi A, Viscardi RM, Tacia KV, et al: Increased activity of interleukin-6 but not tumor necrosis factor in lung lavage of premature infants is associated with the development of bronchopulmonary dysplasia. Pediatr Res 36:244, 1994.

Ballard RA, Kraybill E, Blankenship W: Idiopathic respiratory distress syndrome: Treatment with continuous negative pressure ventilation. Am J Dis Child 125:676, 1973.

Ballard RA, Ballard PL, Creasy R, et al: Respiratory disease in very-low-birth-weight infants after prenatal thyrotropin-releasing hormone and glucocorticoid. Lancet 339:510, 1992.

Ballard PL, Ballard RA: Scientific basis and therapeutic regimens for use of antenatal glucocorticoids. Am J Obstet Gynecol 173:254, 1995.

Ballard PL, Ballard RA, Planer BC, et al: Plasma cortisol concentrations in premature infants. Pediatr Res 39:325A, 1996.

Banks BA, McClelland M, Ischiropoulos H, et al: Plasma nitrotyrosine as an indicator of nitric oxide–derived oxidant stress in infants with bronchopulmonary dysplasia. Pediatr Res 39:325A, 1996.

Banks BA, Seri I, McClelland MM, et al: Plasma nitrotyrosine (PNT) in full-term infants treated with inhaled nitric oxide (iNO) for persistent pulmonary hypertension of the newborn (PPHN). Pediatr Res 41:138A, 1997.

Banks BA, Seri I, Ischiropoulos H, et al: Inhaled nitric oxide (iNO) in infants with severe ventilator dependent bronchopulmonary dysplasia (BPD). Pediatr Res 41:246A, 1997.

Berman W Jr, Katz R, Yabek SM, et al: Long-term follow-up of bronchopulmonary dysplasia. J Pediatr 109:45, 1986.

Bertrand JM, Riley SP, Popkin J, et al: The long-term pulmonary sequelae of prematurity: The role of familial airway hyperreactivity and the respiratory distress syndrome. N Engl J Med 312:742, 1985.

Brown ER, Stark A, Sosenko I, et al: Bronchopulmonary dysplasia: Possible relationship to pulmonary edema. Pediatrics 92:982, 1978.

Brozanski BS, Jones JG, Gilmour CH, et al: Effect of pulse dexamethasone therapy on the incidence and severity of chronic lung disease in the very-low-birth-weight infant. J Pediatr 126:769, 1995.

Bruce MC, Boat TF, Martin RJ, et al: Proteinase inhibitors and inhibitor inactivation in neonatal airways secretions. Chest 81(suppl):44S, 1982.

Bruce MC, Wedig K, Jentoft N, et al: Altered urinary excretion of elastin crosslinks in premature infants who developed bronchopulmonary dysplasia. Am Rev Respir Dis 131:568, 1985.

Bruce MC, Schuyler M, Martin RJ, et al: Risk factors for the degradation of lung elastic fibers in the ventilated neonate: Implications for impaired lung development in bronchopulmonary dysplasia. Am Rev Respir Dis 146:204, 1992.

Brundage KL, Mohsini KG, Froese AB, et al: Dexamethasone therapy for bronchopulmonary dysplasia: Improved respiratory mechanics without adrenal suppression. Pediatr Pulmonol 12:162, 1992.

Burnard ED: The pulmonary syndrome of Wilson and Mikity, and respiratory function in very small premature infants. Pediatr Clin North Am 13:999, 1966.

Cabal LA, Larrazabalo C, Ramanathan R, et al: Effects of metaproterenol on pulmonary mechanics, oxygenation, and ventilation in infants with chronic lung disease. J Pediatr 110:116, 1987.

Callahan J, Haller JO, Cacciarelli AA, et al: Cholelithiasis in infants: Association with total parenteral nutrition and furosemide. Radiology 143:437, 1982.

Campbell RL, McAlister W, Volpe JJ: Neurologic aspects of bronchopulmonary dysplasia. Clin Pediatr 27:7, 1988.

Cantin A, North SL, Hubbard RC, Crystal RG: Normal alveolar epithelial lining fluid contains high levels of glutathione. J Appl Physiol 63:152, 1987.

Carlton DP, Cummings JJ, Scheerer RG, et al: Lung overexpansion increases pulmonary microvascular permeability in young lambs. J Appl Physiol 69:577, 1990.

Cassell GH, Waites KB, Crouse DT, et al: Association of *Ureaplasma urealyticum* infection of the lower respiratory tract with chronic lung disease and death in very-low-birth-weight infants. Lancet 2:240, 1988.

Clark RH, Gerstmann DR, Null DM, DeLemos RA: Prospective randomized comparison of high-frequency oscillatory and conventional ventilation in respiratory distress syndrome. Pediatrics 89:5, 1992.

Clarke JR, Aston H, Silverman M: Delivery of salbutamol by metered-dose inhaler and valved spacer to wheezy infants: Effect on bronchial responsiveness. Arch Dis Child 69:125, 1993.

Cleary JP, Bernstein G, Mannino FL, Heldt GP: Improved oxygenation during synchronized intermittent mandatory ventilation in neonates with respiratory distress syndrome: A randomized crossover trial. J Pediatr 126:407, 1995.

Clement A, Chadelat K, Sardet A, et al: Alveolar macrophage status in bronchopulmonary dysplasia. Pediatr Res 23:470, 1988.

Co E, Chari G, McCulloch K, Vidyasagar D: Dexamethasone treatment suppresses collagen synthesis in infants with bronchopulmonary dysplasia. Pediatr Pulmonol 16:36, 1993.

Collaborative Dexamethasone Trial Group: Dexamethasone therapy in neonatal chronic lung disease: An international placebo, controlled trial. Pediatrics 88:421, 1991.

Cotton RB, Stahlman MT, Bender HW, et al: Randomized trial of early closure of symptomatic patent ductus arteriosus in small preterm infants. J Pediatr 93:647, 1978.

Corbet A: Clinical trials of synthetic surfactant in the respiratory distress syndrome of premature infants. Clin Perinatol 20:737, 1993.

Corcoran JD, Patterson CC, Thomas PS, Halliday HL: Reduction in the risk of bronchopulmonary dysplasia from 1980–1990: Results of a multivariate logistic regression analysis. Eur J Pediatr 152:677, 1993.

Cummings JJ, D'Eugenio DB, Gross SJ: A controlled trial of dexamethasone in preterm infants at high risk for bronchopulmonary dysplasia. N Engl J Med 320:1505, 1989.

Darlow BA, Inder TE, Graham PJ, et al: The relationship of selenium status to respiratory outcome in the very-low-birth-weight infant. Pediatrics 96:314, 1995.

Davidson D, Drafta D, Wilkens BA: Elevated urinary leukotriene E_4 in chronic lung disease of extreme prematurity. Am J Respir Crit Care Med 151:841, 1995.

Davis JM, Sinkin RA, Aranda JV: Drug therapy of bronchopulmonary dysplasia. Pediatr Pulmonol 8:117, 1990.

DeLemos, RA, Coalson JJ, Gerstmann DR, et al: Oxygen toxicity in the premature baboon with hyaline membrane disease. Am Rev Respir Dis 136:677, 1988.

Deneke SM, Fanburg BL: Normobaric oxygen toxicity of the lung. N Engl J Med 303:76, 1980.

Denjean, A, Guimaraes H, Migdal M, et al: Dose-related bronchodilator response to aerosolized salbutamol (albuterol) in ventilator-dependent premature infants. J Pediatr 120:974, 1992.

Dreyfuss D, Saumon G: Should the lung be rested or recruited? The Charybdis and Scylla of ventilator management. Am J Respir Crit Care Med 149:1066, 1994.

Dudell GG, Gersony WM: Patent ductus arteriosus in neonates with severe respiratory disease. J Pediatr 104:915, 1984.

Durand M, Sardesai S, McEvovy C: Effects of early dexamethasone therapy on pulmonary mechanics and chronic lung disease in very-low-birth-weight infants: A randomized, controlled trial. Pediatrics 95:584, 1995.

Ehrenkranz RA, Ablow RC, Warshaw JB: Prevention of bronchopulmonary dysplasia with vitamin E administration during the acute stages of respiratory distress syndrome. J Pediatr 85(suppl):873, 1979.

Engelhardt B, Blalock WA, Donlevy S, et al: Effect of spironolactone-hydrochlorothiazide on lung function in infants with chronic bronchopulmonary dysplasia. J Pediatr 114:619, 1989.

Engelhardt B, Elliott S, Hazinski TA: Short- and long-term effects of furosemide on lung function in infants with bronchopulmonary dysplasia. J Pediatr 109:1034, 1986.

Eronen M, Peesonen E, Kurki T, et al: Increased incidence of bronchopulmonary dysplasia after antenatal administration of indomethacin to prevent preterm labor. J Pediatr 124:782, 1994.

Ezzedeen R, Adelman RD, Ahlfors CE: Renal calcification in preterm infants: Pathophysiology and long-term sequelae. J Pediatr 113:532, 1988.

Fiascone JM, Rhodes RG, Grandgeorge SR, et al: Bronchopulmonary dysplasia: A review for the pediatrician. Curr Prob Pediatr 19:169, 1989.

Frank L: Effects of oxygen on the newborn. Fed Proc 44:2328, 1985.

Frank L, Lewis PL, Sosenko IRS: Dexamethasone stimulation of fetal rat lung antioxidant enzyme activity in parallel with surfactant stimulation. Pediatrics 75:569, 1985.

Frank L, Sosenko IR: Undernutrition as a major contributing factor in the pathogenesis of bronchopulmonary dysplasia. Am Rev Respir Dis 138:725, 1988.

Freeman BA, Turrens JF, Mirza Z, et al: Modulation of oxidant lung injury by using liposome-entrapped superoxide dismutase and catalase. Fed Proc 44:2591, 1985.

Friel JK, Andrews WL, Long DR, et al: Selenium status of very-low-birth-weight infants. Pediatr Res 34:293, 1993.

Garland JS, Buck RK, Allred EN, Leviton A: Hypocarbia before surfactant therapy appears to increase bronchopulmonary dysplasia risk in infants with respiratory distress syndrome. Arch Pediatr 149:617, 1995.

Gerdes JS, Yoder MC, Douglas SD, et al: Tracheal lavage and plasma fibronectin: Relationship to respiratory distress syndrome and development of bronchopulmonary dysplasia. J Pediatr 108:601, 1986.

Gerdes JS, Harris MC, Polin RA: Effects of dexamethasone and indo-

methacin on elastase, α_1-proteinase inhibitor, and fibronectin in bronchoalveolar lavage fluid from neonates. J Pediatr 113:727, 1988.

Gerhardt T, Hehre D, Feller R, et al: Serial determination of pulmonary function in infants with chronic lung disease. J Pediatr 110:446, 1987.

Gladstone IM, Ehrenkrantz RA, Jacobs HC: Pulmonary function tests and fluid balance in neonates with chronic lung disease during dexamethasone treatment. Pediatrics 84:1072, 1989.

Goldberg AI, Monahan CA: Home health care for children assisted by mechanical ventilation: The physician's perspective. J Pediatr 114:378, 1989.

Goodman G, Perkin RM, Anas NG, et al: Pulmonary hypertension in infants with bronchopulmonary dysplasia. J Pediatr 112:67, 1988.

Gorenflo M, Vogel M, Herbst L, et al: Influence of clinical and ventilatory parameters on morphology of bronchopulmonary dysplasia. Pediatr Pulmonol 19:214, 1995.

Gray PH, Burns YR, Mohay HA, et al: Neurodevelopmental outcome of preterm infants with bronchopulmonary dysplasia. Arch Dis Child 73:F128, 1995.

Greenspan JS, DeGiulio PA, Bhutani VK: Airway reactivity as determined by a cold air challenge in infants with bronchopulmonary dysplasia. J Pediatr 114:452, 1989.

Grigg J, Barber A, Silverman M: Bronchoalveolar lavage fluid glutathione in intubated premature infants. Arch Dis Child 69:49, 1993.

Grigg JM, Savill JS, Sarraf C, et al: Neutrophil apoptosis and clearance from neonatal lungs. Lancet 338:720, 1991.

Grigg J, Arnon S, Chase A, Silverman M: Inflammatory cells in the lungs of premature infants on the first day of life: Perinatal risk factors and origin of cells. Arch Dis Child 69:40, 1993.

Groneck P, Gotze-Speer B, Oppermann M, et al: Association of pulmonary inflammation and increased microvascular permeability during the development of bronchopulmonary dysplasia: A sequential analysis of inflammatory mediators in respiratory fluids of high-risk preterm neonates. Pediatrics 93:712, 1994.

Hallman M, Bry K, Hoppu K, et al: Inositol supplementation in premature infants with respiratory distress syndrome. N Engl J Med 326:1233, 1992.

Hammerman C, Aramburo MJ: Decreased lipid intake reduces morbidity in sick premature neonates. J Pediatr 113:1083, 1988.

Hammerman C, Strates E, Valaitis S: The silent ductus: Its precursors and its aftermath. Pediatr Cardiol 7:121, 1986.

Hansen TN, Gest AL: Oxygen toxicity and other ventilatory complications of treatment of infants with persistent pulmonary hypertension. Clin Perinatol 11:6653, 1984.

Hansen TN, Hazinski TA, Bland RD: Vitamin E does not prevent oxygen induced lung injury in newborn lambs. Pediatr Res 16:583, 1982.

Harkavy KL, Scanlon JW, Chowdhry PK, Grylack LJ: Dexamethasone therapy for chronic lung disease in ventilator-dependent and oxygen-dependent infants: A controlled trial. J Pediatr 115:979, 1989.

Harris MA, Sullivan CE: Sleep pattern and supplementary oxygen requirements in infants with chronic neonatal lung disease. Lancet 345:831, 1995.

Hazinski TA: Furosemide decreases ventilation in young rabbits. J Pediatr 106:81, 1985.

Heggie AD, Facobs MR, Butler VT, et al: Frequency and significance of isolation of *Ureaplasma urealyticum* and *Mycoplasma hominis* from cerebrospinal fluid and tracheal aspirate specimens from low-birth-weight infants. J Pediatr 124:956, 1994.

Heldt GP: Development of stability of the respiratory system in preterm infants. J Appl Physiol 65:441, 1988a.

Heldt GP: Pulmonary status of infants and children with bronchopulmonary dysplasia. *In* Merritt TA, Northway WJ, Boynton BR (Eds): Bronchopulmonary Dysplasia. Boston, Blackwell Scientific Publications, 1988b, p 421.

Heldt GP, McIlroy MB, Hansen TN, et al: Exercise performance of the survivors of hyaline membrane disease. Pediatrics 96:995, 1980.

Hernandez LA, Peevy KJ, Moise AA, Parker JC: Chest wall restriction limits high airway pressure–induced lung injury in young rabbits. J Appl Physiol 66:2364, 1989.

Holtzman RB, Hageman JR, Yogev R: Role of *Ureaplasma urealyticum* in bronchopulmonary dysplasia. J Pediatr 114:1061, 1989.

Hudak BB, Allen MD, Hudak ML, et al: Home oxygen therapy for chronic lung disease in extremely low-birth-weight infants. Am J Dis Child 143:357, 1989.

Hufnagle KG, Khan SN, Penn D, et al: Renal calcifications: A complication of long-term furosemide therapy in preterm infants. Pediatrics 70:360, 1982.

Jarriel, S, Richardson, P, Pace, R, et al: Positive end-expiratory pressure (PEEP) reduces ventilation inhomogeneities in hyaline membrane disease in lambs. Pediatr Res 25:314A, 1989.

Jarriel WS, Richardson P, Knapp RD, Hansen TN: A nonlinear regression analysis of nonlinear, passive-deflation flow-volume plots. Pediatr Pulmonol 15:175, 1993.

Jefferies AL, Coates G, O'Brodovich HM: Pulmonary epithelial permeability in hyaline membrane disease. N Engl J Med 311:1075, 1984.

Jobe A: Pulmonary surfactant therapy. N Engl J Med 328:861, 1993.

John E, Ermocilla R, Golden J, et al: Effects of gas temperature and particulate water on rabbit lungs during ventilation. Pediatr Res 14:1186, 1980.

Johnson WH Jr, Young JA, Hernandes LA, et al: Positive end-expiratory pressure (PEEP) prevents barotrauma-induced microvascular injury due to high peak inspiratory pressure (PIP). Pediatr Res 25:369A, 1989.

Jones R, Wincott E, Elbourne D, et al: Controlled trial of dexamethasone in neonatal chronic lung disease: A 3-year follow-up. Pediatrics 96:897, 1995.

Kao LC, Warburton D, Cheng MH, et al: Effect of oral diuretics on pulmonary mechanics in infants with chronic bronchopulmonary dysplasia: Results of a double-blind crossover sequential trial. Pediatrics 74:37, 1984.

Kao LC, Warburton D, Sargent CS, et al: Furosemide acutely decreases airways resistance in chronic pulmonary dysplasia. J Pediatr 103:624, 1983.

Kao LC, Durand DJ, Nickerson BG: Improving pulmonary function does not decrease oxygen consumption in infants with bronchopulmonary dysplasia. J Pediatr 112:616, 1988.

Kari MA, Raivio KO, Venge P, Hallman M: Dexamethasone treatment of infants at risk for chronic lung disease: Surfactant components and inflammatory parameters in airway specimens. Pediatr Res 36:387, 1994.

Kazzi NJ, Brans YW, Poland RL: Dexamethasone effects on the hospital course of infants with bronchopulmonary dysplasia who are dependent on artificial ventilation. Pediatrics 86:722, 1990.

Kitajima H, Nakayama M, Miyano A, et al: Significance of chorioamnionitis. Early Hum Dev 29:125, 1992.

Kolobow T, Moretti MP, Fumagalli R, et al: Severe impairment in lung function induced by high peak airway pressure during mechanical ventilation: An experimental study. Am Rev Respir Dis 135:312, 1987.

Konig P, Shatley M, Levine C, Mawhinney TP: Clinical observations of nebulized flunisolide in infants and young children with asthma and bronchopulmonary dysplasia. Pediatr Pulmonol 13:209, 1992.

Kotecha S, Chan B, Azam N, et al: Increase in interleukin-8 and soluble intercellular adhesion molecule-1 in bronchoalveolar lavage fluid from premature infants who develop chronic lung disease. Arch Dis Child 72:F90, 1995.

Krauss AN, Klain DB, Auld PAM: Chronic pulmonary insufficiency of prematurity (CPIP). Pediatrics 55:55, 1975.

Kraybill EN, Runyan DK, Bose CL, et al: Risk factors for chronic lung disease in infants with birth weights of 751 to 1000 grams. J Pediatr 115:115, 1989.

Kurzner SI, Garg M, Bautista DB, et al: Growth failure in bronchopulmonary dysplasia: Elevated metabolic rates and pulmonary mechanics. J Pediatr 112:73, 1988.

LaForce WR, Brudno DS: Controlled trial of beclomethasone diproprionate by nebulization in oxygen- and ventilator-dependent infants. J Pediatr 122:285, 1993.

Leonard C, Piecuch R, Ballard RA: Outcome of very-low-birth-weight infants: Multiple gestation versus singletons. Pediatrics 93:611, 1994.

Mammel MC, Green TP, Johnson DE, Thompson TR: Controlled trial of dexamethasone therapy in infants with bronchopulmonary dysplasia. Lancet 1:1356, 1983.

McCann EM, Lewis K, Deming DD, et al: Controlled trial of jurosemide therapy in infants with chronic lung disease. J Pediatr 106:957, 1985.

Merritt TA, Hallman M, Holcomb K, et al: Human surfactant treatment of severe respiratory distress syndrome: Pulmonary effluent indicators of lung inflammation. J Pediatr 108:741, 1986.

Merritt TA, Harris JP, Toghmann K, et al: Early closure of the patent ductus arteriosus in very-low-birth-weight infants: A controlled trial. J Pediatr 99:281, 1981.

Merritt TA, Boynton BR: Clinical presentation of bronchopulmonary dysplasia. In Merritt, TA, Northway, WH, Jr, Boynton, BR (Eds): Contemporary Issues in Fetal and Neonatal Medicine. Vol. 4, Bron-

chopulmonary Dysplasia. Boston, Blackwell Scientific Publications, 1988, p. 179.

Merritt TA, Cochrane CG, Holcomb K, et al: Elastase and alfa 1-proteinase inhibitor activity in tracheal aspirates during respiratory distress syndrome: role of inflammation in the pathogenesis of bronchopulmonary dysplasia. J Clin Invest 72:656, 1983.

Moshini, K, Tanswell, K.: Resolution of acquired lobar emphysema with dexamethasone therapy. J Pediatr 11:901, 1987.

Neuzil J, Darlow BA, Inder TE, et al: Oxidation of parenteral lipid emulsion by ambient light and phototherapy lights: potential toxicity of routine parenteral feeding. J Pediatr 126:785, 1995.

Ng PC, Blackburn ME, Brownlee KG, et al: Adrenal response in very low birth weight babies after dexamethasone treatment for bronchopulmonary dysplasia. Arch Dis Child 64:1721, 1989.

Nickerson BG, Taussig LM.: Family history of asthma in infants with bronchopulmonary dysplasia. Pediatrics 65:1140, 1980.

Northway WH, Rosan RC, Porter DY: Pulmonary disease following therapy of hyaline membrane disease. N Engl J Med 276:357. 1967.

Norton ME, Merrill J, Cooper BAB, et al: Neonatal complications after the administration of indomethacin for preterm labor. N Engl J Med 629:1602, 1993.

O'Brodovich HM, Mellins RB.: Bronchopulmonary dysplasia— unresolved neonatal acute lung injury. Am Rev Respir Dis 132:694, 1985.

Ogden BE, Murphy SA, Saunders GC, et al: Neonatal lung neutrophils and elastase/protease inhibitor imbalance. Am Rev Respir Dis 130:817, 1984.

Papile LA, Stoll B, Donovan E, et al for the NICHD Neonatal Research Network: Dexamethasone therapy in infants at risk for chronic lung disease (CLD): A multi-center, randomized, double-masked trial. Pediatr Res 39(4):236A, 1996.

Pappagallo M, Bhutani VK, Abbasi S: Nebulized steroid trial in ventilator dependent preterm infants (abstract). Pediatr Res 29:327A, 1991.

Parker JC, Hernandez LA, Peevy KJ: Mechanisms of ventilator induced injury. Crit Care Med 21:131, 1993.

Pearson E, Bose C, Snidow T, et al: Trial of vitamin A supplementation in very low birth weight infants at risk for bronchopulmonary dysplasia. J Pediatr 121:420, 1992.

Pearson E, Stiles A, Bose C: Vitamin A and bronchopulmonary dysplasia (letter). J Pediatr 124:328, 1994.

Philip, AGS.: Oxygen plus pressure plus time: The etiology of bronchopulmonary dysplasia. Pediatrics 55:44, 1975.

Pierce MR, Bancalari E: The role of inflammation in the pathogenesis of bronchopulmonary dysplasia. Pediatr Pulmonol 19:371, 1995.

Pinney, MA, Cotton, EK.: Home management of bronchopulmonary dysplasia. Pediatrics 58:856, 1976.

Pokriefka EM, Mehdizadeh B, Rabbani A: Inhaled flunisolide in bronchopulmonary dysplasia (abstract). Pediatr Res 33:341A, 1993.

Rhodes, PG, Graves, GR, Patel, DM, et al: Minimizing pneumothorax and bronchopulmonary dysplasia in ventilated infants with hyaline membrane disease. J Pediatr 103:634, 1983.

Rooklin AR, Moomjian AS, Shutack JG, et al: Theophylline therapy in bronchopulmonary dysplasia. J Pediatr 95(suppl):882, 1979.

Rosenfeld, W, Evans, H, Concepcion, L, et al: Prevention of bronchopulmonary dysplasia by administration of bovine superoxide dismutase in preterm infants with respiratory distress syndrome: J Pediatr 105:781–785, 1984.

Rotschild A, Solimano A, Puterman M, et al: Increased compliance in response to salbutamol in premature infants with developing bronchopulmonary dysplasia. J Pediatr 115:984, 1989.

Rowen JL, Atkins JT, Levy ML, et al: Invasive fungal dermatitis in the under 1000 gram neonate. Pediatrics 95:682, 1995.

Rozycki HJ, Byron PR, Dailey K, Gutcher GR: Evaluation of a system for the delivery of inhaled beclomethasone dipropionate to intubated neonates. Dev Pharmacol Ther 16:65, 1991.

Rush MG, Hazinski TA: Current therapy of bronchopulmonary dysplasia. Clin Perinatol 19:563, 1992.

Rush MG, Engelhardt B, Parker RA, et al: Double blind placebo controlled trial of alternate day furosemide therapy in infants with chronic bronchopulmonary dysplasia. J Pediatr 117:112, 1990.

Sanchez, PJ, Regan, UA.: *Ureaplasma urealyticum* colonization and chronic lung disease in low-birth weight infants. Pediatr Infect Dis 7:542, 1988.

Sanders RJ, Cox C, Phelps DL, Sinkin RA: Two doses of early intravenous dexamethasone for the prevention of bronchopulmonary dysplasia in babies with respiratory distress syndrome: Pediatr Res 36:122–128, 1994.

Sauve RS, Singhai N: Long-term morbidity of infants with bronchopulmonary dysplasia. Pediatrics 76:725, 1985.

Schwarze J, Bartmann P: Influence of dexamethasone on lymphocyte proliferation in whole blood cultures of neonates. Biol Neonate 65:295, 1994.

Shenai JP, Rush MB, Stahlman MT, et al: Plasma retinol-binding protein response to vitamin A administration in infants susceptible to bronchopulmonary dysplasia. J Pediatr 116:607, 1990.

Shenai JP, Kennedy KA, Chytil F, Stahlman MT: Clinical trial of vitamin A supplementation in infants susceptible to bronchopulmonary dysplasia. J Pediatr 111:269, 1987.

Shepard FM, Johnston RB, Klatte EC, et al: Residual pulmonary findings in clinical hyaline membrane disease. N Engl J Med 279:1063, 1968.

Sicard RE, Werner JC: Dexamethasone induces a transient relative cardiomegaly in neonatal rats. Pediatr Res 31:359, 1992.

Silverman M: Chronic lung disease of prematurity: Are we too cautious with steroids? Eur J Pediatr 153 (suppl 2):S30, 1994.

Singer L, Martin RJ, Hawkins SW, et al: Oxygen desaturation complicates feeding in infants with bronchopulmonary dysplasia after discharge. Pediatrics 90:380, 1992.

Sluis KB, Darlow BA, George PM, et al: Selenium and glutathione peroxidase levels in premature infants in a low selenium community (Christchurch, NZ). Pediatr Res 32:189, 1992.

Smith CV: Free radical mechanisms of tissue injury. *In* Moslen MT, Smith CV (Eds): Free radical mechanisms of tissue injury. Boca Raton: CRC Press, 1992, p. 1–22.

Smith CV, Hansen TN, Martin NE, McMicken HW, Elliott SJ: Oxidant stress responses in premature infants during exposure to hyperoxia: Pediatr Res 34:360–365, 1993.

Smyth JA, Tabachnik E, Duncan WJ, et al: Pulmonary function and bronchial hyperreactivity in long-term survivors of bronchopulmonary dysplasia. Pediatrics 68:336, 1981.

Sosenko IR, Innis SM, Frank L: Polyunsaturated fatty acids and protection of newborn rats from oxygen toxicity. J Pediatr 112:630, 1988.

Sosenko IRS, Pierce MR, Bancalari E: Effect of early initiation of intravenous lipid administration on the incidence and severity of chronic lung disease in premature infants. J Pediatr 123:975, 1993.

Sosulski R, Abbasi S, Bhutani VK, Fox WW: Physiologic effects of terbutaline on pulmonary function of infants with bronchopulmonary dysplasia. Pediatr Pulmonol 2:269, 1986.

Speer CP, Ruess D, Harms K, et al: Neutrophil elastase and acute pulmonary damage in neonates with severe respiratory distress syndrome. Pediatrics 91:794, 1993.

Stahlman MT, Gray ME, Chytil F, et al: Effect of retinol on fetal lamb tracheal epithelium with and without epidermal growth factor. Lab Invest 59:25, 1988.

Stern L (Ed): The respiratory system in the newborn. Clin Perinatol 14:3, 1987.

Stern L: The role of respirators in the etiology and pathogenesis of bronchopulmonary dysplasia. J Pediatr 85 (suppl):867, 1979.

Stern L, Ramos A, Outerbridge EW, Beaudry P: Negative pressure artificial respiration: Use and treatment of respiratory failure of the newborn. Can Med Assoc J 102:595, 1970.

Stocks J, Godfrey S, Reynolds EOR: Airway resistance in infants after various treatments for hyaline membrane disease: Special emphasis on prolonged high levels of inspired oxygen. Pediatrics 61:178, 1979.

Taghizadeh A, Reynolds EOR: Pathogenesis of bronchopulmonary dysplasia following hyaline membrane disease. Am J Pathol 82:241, 1976.

Tammela KT, Lanning FP, Koivisto ME: The relationship of fluid restriction during the first month of life to the occurrence and severity of bronchopulmonary dysplasia in low birth weight infants: A one-year radiological follow up. Eur J Pediatr 151:367, 1992.

Tay-Uyboco JS, Kwiatkowski K, Cates DB, et al: Hypoxic airway constriction in infants of very low birth weight recovering from moderate to severe bronchopulmonary dysplasia. J Pediatr 115:456, 1989.

Tsan M-F: Superoxide dismutase and pulmonary oxygen toxicity: Proc Soc Exp Biol Med 203:286–290, 1993.

U.S. Congress, Office of Technology Assessment: Technology-Dependent Children: Hospital v. Home Care. Washington, DC.: U.S. Government Printing Office, OTA-TM-H–38, May 1987.

Van Marter LJ, Leviton A, Kuban KCK, et al: Maternal glucocorticoid therapy and reduced risk of bronchopulmonary dysplasia. Pediatrics 86:331, 1990.

Van Marter LJ, Pagano M, Allred EN, et al: Rate of bronchopulmonary dysplasia as a function of neonatal intensive care practices. J Pediatr 120:938, 1992.

Van Marter LJ, Leviton A, Allred EN, et al: Hydration during the first days of life and the risk of bronchopulmonary dysplasia in low birth weight infants. J Pediatr 116:942, 1990.

Varsila E, Hallman M, Venge P, Andersson S: Closure of patent ductus arteriosus decreases pulmonary myeloperoxidase in premature infants with respiratory distress syndrome. Biol Neonate 67:167, 1995.

Wang EEL, Frayha H, Watts J, et al: Role of Ureaplasma urealyticum and other pathogens in the development of CLD of prematurity. Pediatr Infect Dis 7:547, 1988.

Wang EEL, Ohlsson A, Kellner JD: Association of *Ureaplasma urealyticum* colonization with chronic lung disease of prematurity: Results of a meta-analysis. J Pediatr 127:640, 1995.

Warner BB, Wispe JR: Free radical-mediated diseases in pediatrics: Semin Perinatol 16:47–57, 1992.

Watterberg KL, Carmichael DF, Gerdes JS, et al: Secretory leukocyte protease inhibitor and lung inflammation in developing bronchopulmonary dysplasia. J Pediatr 125:264, 1994.

Watterberg KL, Scott SM: Evidence of early adrenal insufficiency in babies who develop bronchopulmonary dysplasia. Pediatrics 95:120, 1995.

Watts CL, Bruce MC: Effect of dexamethasone therapy on fibronectin and albumin levels in lung secretions of infants with bronchopulmonary dysplasia. J Pediatr 121:597, 1992.

Webb HH, Tierney DF: Experimental pulmonary edema due to intermittent positive pressure ventilation with high inflation pressures: Protection by positive end expiratory pressure. Am Rev Respir Dis 110:556, 1974.

Weinstein MR, Oh W: Oxygen consumption in infants with bronchopulmonary dysplasia. Pediatrics 99:958, 1981.

Wilson MG, Mikity VC: A new form of respiratory disease in premature infants. Am J Dis Child 99:489, 1960.

Wilson DM, Baldwin RB, Ariagno RL: A randomized placebo controlled trial of effects of dexamethasone on hypothalamic pituitary adrenal axis in preterm infants. J Pediatr 113:764, 1988.

Wispe JR, Warner BB, Clark JC, et al: Human Mn-superoxide dismutase in pulmonary epithelial cells of transgenic mice confers protection from oxygen injury. J Biol Chem 267:23937, 1992.

Yeh TF, Lin YJ, Lin CH, et al: Early postnatal (<12 hours) dexamethasone (D) therapy for prevention of BPD in preterm infants with RDS—a two-year follow-up study. Pediatr Res 41:188A, 1997.

Yeh TF, McClenan DA, Ajayl OA: Metabolic rate and energy balance in infants with bronchopulmonary dysplasia. J Pediatr 114:448, 1989.

Yeh TF, Torre JA, Rastogi A, et al: Early postnatal dexamethasone therapy in premature infants with severe respiratory distress syndrome: A double blind controlled study. J Pediatr 117:273, 1990.

Yoder MC, Chua R, Tepper R: Effect of dexamethasone on pulmonary inflammation and pulmonary function of ventilator dependent infants with bronchopulmonary dysplasia. Am Rev Respir Dis 143:1044, 1991.

Zimmerman JJ, Farrell PM: Advances and issues in bronchopulmonary dysplasia. Curr Prob Pediatr 24:159–170, 1994.

CHAPTER 56

Neonatal Pneumonias

Thomas Hansen and Anthony Corbet

PNEUMONIA ACQUIRED FROM THE MOTHER

Most pneumonias acquired from the mother have an onset of clinical signs within the first 3 days after birth. It is estimated that the incidence of early-onset pneumonia is 0.5% of all live births. Two types of pneumonia appear to be acquired from the mother: (1) *congenital or intrauterine pneumonia* and (2) *transnatal pneumonia*. In transnatal pneumonias, however, the onset may be delayed well beyond 3 days with certain types of pathogens, such as *Chlamydia*.

Congenital Pneumonia

Infections with onset in the fetus present as either transplacental or postamnionitis pneumonia.

Transplacental Pneumonia

In transplacental pneumonia, bacteria cross the placenta and invade the fetal lungs by the hematogenous route, as in congenital syphilis and in some cases of listeriosis with maternal septicemia. Pneumonia may be well established in utero, causing fetal death or immediate severe disease at birth. Most cases of transplacental pneumonia have evidence of preceding maternal infection with inflammatory lesions of the placenta, as in the case of syphilis or listeriosis.

Postamnionitis Pneumonia

Amnionitis can be explained by invasion of bacteria (Lauweryns et al, 1973) or other infective agents, such as viruses, mycoplasmas, or fungi. This is believed to be an ascending infection, arising from vaginal flora and beginning in the amnion at the cervical os, then spreading by the membranes to the chorionic plate (Blanc, 1961) (Fig. 56–1). For aspiration into the lung, significant fetal asphyxia with deep continuous gasping is thought to be necessary. This is evidenced by the presence of aspirated amniotic squames in the lungs.

Most cases of amnionitis, however, are not associated with pneumonia in the newborn. In some infants, aspiration of infected amniotic fluid occurs, but the lung parenchyma is not invaded by pathogens. As a result, neutrophils of maternal origin are confined to the air spaces, fetal neutrophils do not infiltrate the septal walls, and fibrinous exudate does not occur. Blood culture in these infants is negative, and the clinical picture is that of fetal asphyxia, with or without postasphyxial pulmonary edema. In the presence of amnionitis, a true pneumonia is frequently absent for two reasons: (1) There may be no significant fetal asphyxia (i.e., gasping does not occur), and (2) some bacteria may not produce lung inflammation even if aspira-

tion does occur; this may be partly due to the anti-infective properties of surface-active material.

When an active postamnionitis pneumonia does occur, the usual organisms are group B streptococcus; *Escherichia coli*; and, sometimes, enterococcus, *Haemophilus influenzae*, *Streptococcus viridans*, *Listeria*, or anaerobes. These cases are characterized by lung inflammation, fetal neutrophils in both the septal walls and the saccules, fibrinous exudate into the air spaces, and usually a positive blood culture.

Factors Predisposing to Amnionitis and Pneumonia

The conditions associated with amniotic fluid infection are

1. Premature labor
2. Rupture of membranes before the onset of labor
3. Prolonged membrane rupture ($\geq$24 hours) before delivery
4. Prolonged active labor with cervical dilation
5. Frequent obstetric digital examinations

The strong association of amnionitis with premature birth may be due to a developmental deficiency of bacteriostatic factors in amniotic fluid (Schlievert et al, 1975) or to the infection per se as the precipitating factor for preterm labor. With an increasing latent interval between rupture of membranes and labor, the incidence of clinical amnionitis also increases (Burchell, 1964) as well as the frequency of bacteremia in cord blood samples collected at birth (Tyler and Albers, 1966). If gestational age is adequately controlled, however, there is no evidence for increased perinatal mortality in premature infants with ruptured membranes (Daikoku et al, 1981; Schutte et al, 1983). A prolonged interval between rupture of membranes and the onset of labor is a significant independent factor favoring an increased incidence of amnionitis only for gestations of 37 weeks or more (Johnson et al, 1981). In preterm gestations, a prolonged interval between membrane rupture and the onset of labor does not necessarily increase the risk of amnionitis because preterm gestations are more prone to amnionitis for reasons independent of membrane rupture. In fact, infection may be one of the *causes* of premature labor because amnionitis often occurs in the presence of intact membranes (Naeye and Peters, 1978). Thus, in assessing the risk of neonatal infection in premature infants, the important thing to consider is not the length of membrane rupture but whether or not preterm labor occurred and whether or not amnionitis was present.

Active labor with cervical dilation has a considerable effect on the incidence of amnionitis. As the duration of labor increases, more women have bacteria in the amniotic fluid. The absence of labor and delivery by cesarean section are associated with a greatly reduced risk of amnionitis and of congenital pneumonia (Avery, 1984). Data also suggest

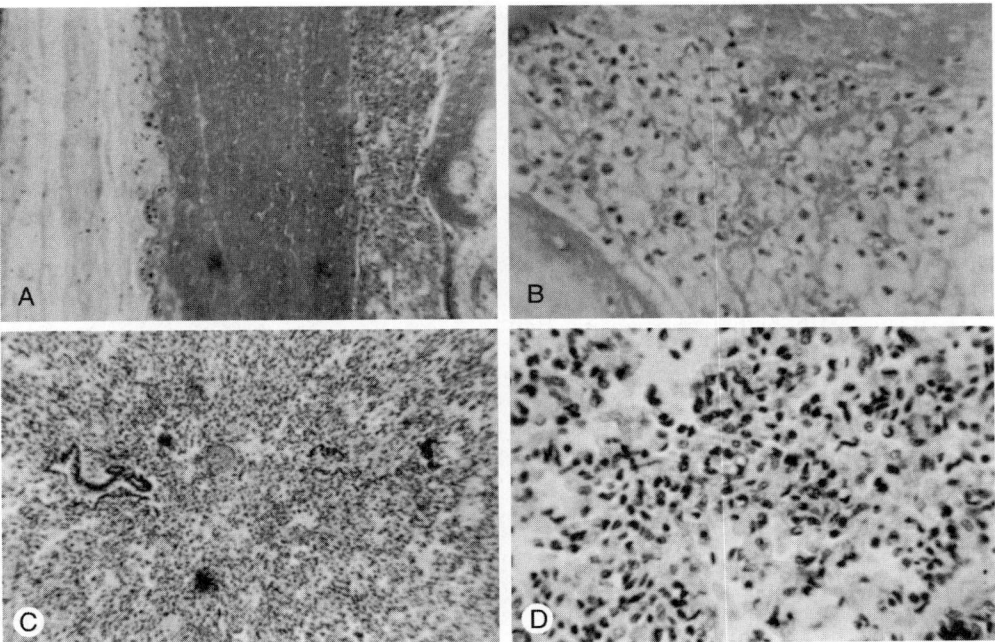

FIGURE 56–1. *A,* Microscopic section of placenta showing leukocyte infiltration and ascending fetal infection, which lead to a congenital or intrauterine infection, in this case postamnionitis pneumonia. *B,* High-power view of the subchorionic region showing leukocyte infiltration. *C,* Low-power view of section of lung showing dense homogeneous exudation and leukocytic infiltration. No amniotic debris is visible. *D,* Higher-power view of the same. The mother's labor was induced, because of Rh incompatibility, 2 weeks before term. Manual stripping of the membranes did not succeed on one day and was repeated the following day. The infant was promptly exchange transfused but died for unknown reasons in the midst of the procedure. The findings of placentitis and pneumonitis were unexpected but may have been related to the membrane stripping procedures done to induce labor. (This case was presented by Dr. Peter Gruenwald at a Johns Hopkins Fetal Mortality Clinic. The photographs are reprinted with his kind permission.)

that obstetric digital examinations after rupture of membranes significantly increase the chance of amniotic infection (Schutte et al, 1983). Amnionitis is more common in undernourished populations, perhaps because bacteriostatic factors may be lacking in the amniotic fluid (Naeye and Blanc, 1970). There appears to be a racial predisposition to amnionitis; at comparable levels of family income, amnionitis is more frequent among black than among white women. Infants of mothers with active urinary tract infection in the 2 weeks before birth are at increased risk for amnionitis (Naeye, 1979a).

Yoder and associates (1983) have estimated that in the presence of amnionitis, term infants are subject to an 8% risk of infection with a positive blood culture and a 4% risk of congenital pneumonia. Other estimates for term infants have been lower (Koh et al, 1979), but the risk of infection is clearly greater in premature infants.

Transnatal Pneumonia

In transnatal pneumonia, there is no evidence of either preceding amnionitis or maternal infection, although the infant is believed to aspirate vaginal bacteria during the birth process. The onset of clinical signs of pneumonia is delayed for a few hours or days or even longer. A true inflammatory process in the lung is always present. Many

cases of group B streptococcal pneumonia represent cases of transnatal pneumonia; there may be no evidence for a preceding amnionitis in the mother.

Early-Onset Pneumonia

Diagnosis

Clinical Findings

Some infants have a history of fetal tachycardia and loss of beat-to-beat variability. It is not uncommon for the Apgar score to be low and the first breath delayed or for the cord pH to reflect significant fetal asphyxia. The usual clinical picture is that of respiratory distress with onset at or soon after birth. Sometimes, however, the onset of respiratory distress is delayed, preceded by increasing tachypnea during the 1st day of life. Infants with infection often have poor peripheral perfusion and tachycardia. Larger infants who are not on mechanical ventilation may have brief or prolonged apneas with bradycardia, significant lethargy, and poor feeding. Other signs are abdominal distention, temperature instability, unexplained metabolic acidosis, or excessive jaundice. Some infants progress to a state of septic shock, with or without pulmonary hypertension. Pulmonary hemorrhage may occur, and there may be disseminated intravascular coagulation.

Laboratory Findings

Analysis of the *gastric aspirate*, collected at or soon after birth, is a useful screening test (Ramos and Stern, 1969). The presence of white cells of maternal origin can be interpreted as indicating inflammation of the amnion and therefore an increased risk of pneumonia in the infant, but it does not mean the infant has pneumonia. The presence of bacteria on Gram stain reflects swallowed vaginal flora and may reflect heavy colonization and increased risk for infection. If the bacteria are identified as group B streptococci or *E. coli*, organisms with high pathogenicity, the level of suspicion for pneumonia should be high, especially in the face of prematurity or asphyxia (Figs. 56–2 and 56–3). The positive gastric aspirate is not diagnostic of pneumonia; it indicates only increased risk.

Culture and Gram stain of *tracheal aspirate*, collected within 8 hours of delivery, is also helpful (Sherman et al, 1984) because the trachea is normally sterile and, it is hoped, colonization after intubation has not occurred. The presence of bacteria on Gram stain has a 47% positive test predictive accuracy (Sherman et al, 1980) and a 79% negative test predictive accuracy. Brook and coworkers (1980), worried about the high number of false-positive tests, tested tracheal aspirate samples for white cells by Wright stain and found white cells present only in cases of proven pneumonia. Patients with both bacteria and white cells in early tracheal aspirate samples are highly likely to have pneumonia.

Blood culture should be done in all cases of suspected pneumonia as well as *cerebrospinal fluid analysis* because meningitis may also be present. Lumbar puncture may be postponed if the infant's condition is extremely unstable. *Surface cultures* are of little value because they indicate

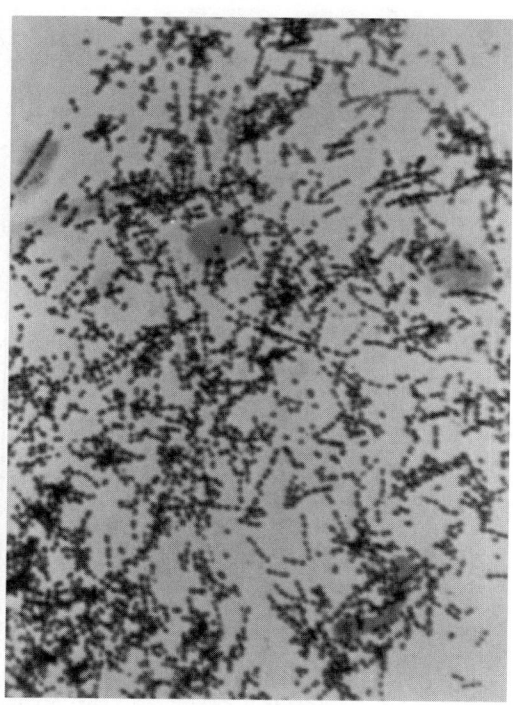

FIGURE 56–3. Gram stain of gastric aspirate from an infant with congenital pneumonia. Note the myriad of streptococci evident on this smear. This finding suggests heavy maternal colonization with group B streptococci, which in an infant with signs of pneumonia and infection strongly suggests the bacterial diagnosis and the appropriate antibiotic therapy. (Courtesy of Dr. William Cochran, Boston Hospital for Women.)

only the state of colonization and are never diagnostic of bacterial infection (Evans et al, 1988).

Radiographic Findings

In the most severe cases of congenital pneumonia, the chest radiograph shows diffuse homogeneous density (Figs. 56–4 and 56–5). In other cases, the picture is one of diffuse reticulogranular density similar to that in hyaline membrane disease, or it may have a somewhat more coarse reticulonodular density. Occasionally the picture is more like that expected in older infants, with linear radiating densities similar to those found in bronchopneumonia (Fig. 56–6) or, less commonly, lobar consolidation. Pleural effusions may be present. Sometimes the radiograph initially is normal, but later films show abnormalities developing over the first few days; this course is suggestive of a transnatal pneumonia (Fig. 56–7). The diffuse pattern is consistent with intrauterine acquisition, whereas the bronchopneumonia pattern suggests infection by aspiration at birth.

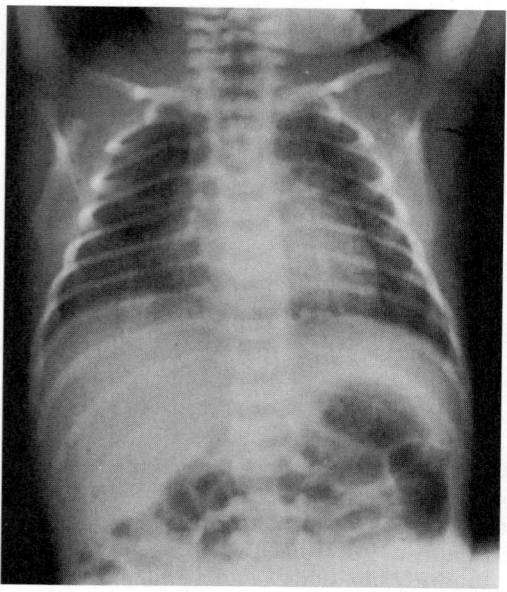

FIGURE 56–2. Radiograph of an infant, age 4 hours, with moderate tachypnea, born to a mother with group B streptococcal urinary tract infection. Although the infiltrates appear only moderate, the infant died of septicemia and pneumonia at 20 hours of age.

Treatment

Antibiotic treatment with a broad-spectrum penicillin and an aminoglycoside is indicated, pending culture results. Without cerebrospinal fluid findings, it is usual to double the customary dose of ampicillin to ensure adequate cerebrospinal fluid levels. Plasma aminoglycoside levels should

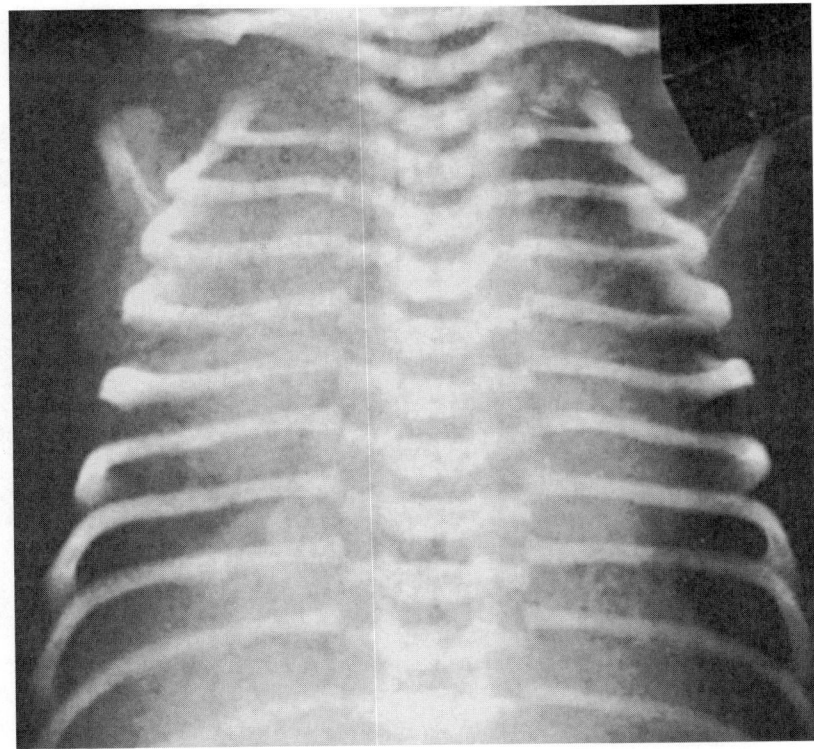

FIGURE 56–4. Congenital pneumonia. Anteroposterior view of chest taken at 16 hours of age. The lungs appear to be almost completely consolidated, the periphery of the left lung and the extreme right base alone containing air. The opacification is homogeneous and dense.

be monitored because of unpredictable and prolonged elimination half-life. When the results of appropriate cultures are available, treatment with the single most effective antibiotic may be the treatment of choice for gram-positive bacterial infections. It is often wise to repeat the blood culture at 48 to 72 hours to document effectiveness of the antibiotic regimen. Regardless of the antibiotic used, treatment should be continued for 10 to 14 days.

Specific Pneumonias Acquired from the Mother

Group B Streptococcal Pneumonia of Early Onset

Pneumonia caused by group B streptococcal infections may be either of the postamnionitis or of the transnatal form.

Epidemiology

Group B streptococcal disease with onset before 3 days of life is manifested by (1) septicemia without diagnosed pneumonia in 30% of the cases, (2) pneumonia with bacteremia in 40%, and (3) septicemia or pneumonia with meningitis in 30% (Baker, 1979). The distribution of bacterial strains causing disease is the same as that in vaginal flora. Mothers are reported to have vaginal colonization rates as high as 28%, and similar rates of colonization are seen in the newborn (Paredes et al, 1977). The attack rate is estimated to be 3 per 1000 live births but is higher with preterm delivery and with evidence of maternal amnionitis.

Diagnosis

More than 80% of infants with pneumonia develop respiratory distress at birth or within a few hours. *Blood and cerebrospinal fluid cultures* are most important for determining the diagnosis. In addition, the *rapid latex agglutination test* for capsular polysaccharide antigen performed

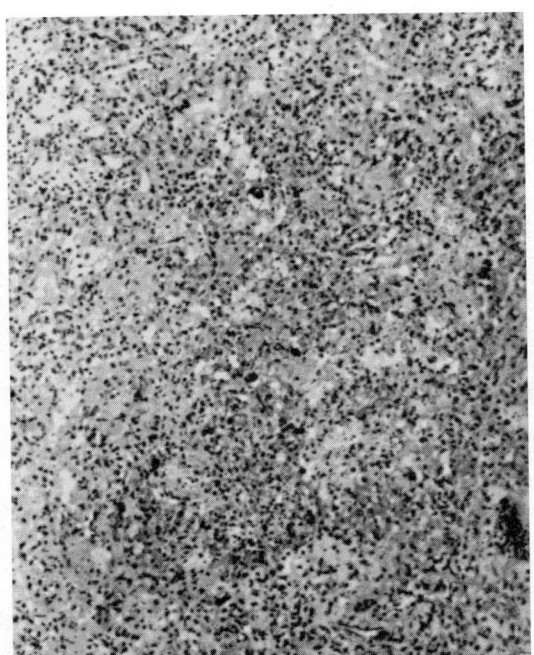

FIGURE 56–5. Congenital pneumonia. Microscopic section of lung from the same patient as in Figure 56–4 shows widespread homogeneous exudation and leukocytic infiltration. Alveoli, bronchi, and interstitial tissue are all equally involved.

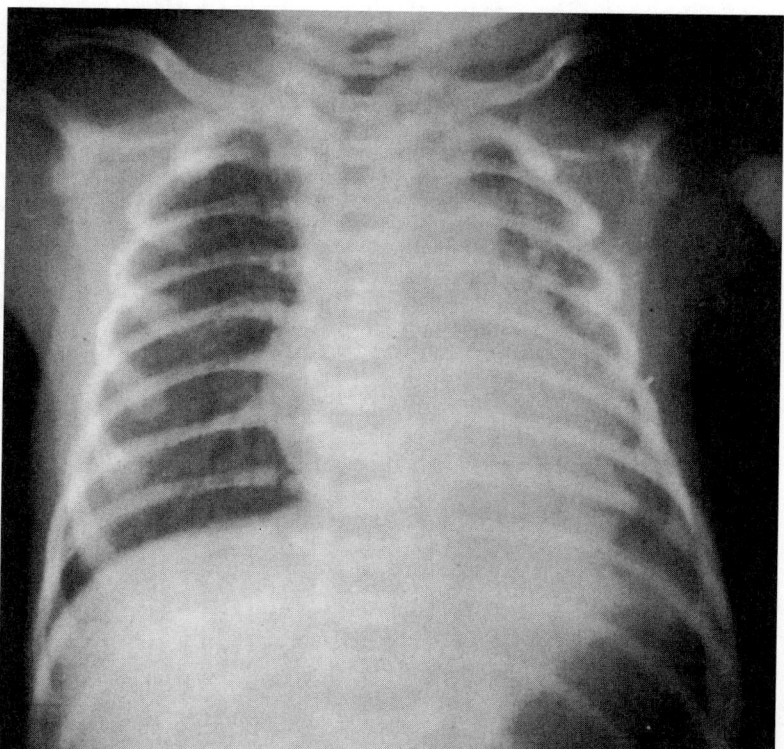

FIGURE 56–6. There is soft linear infiltration spreading outward fanwise from the right hilus. The left lung is almost entirely opacified by confluent areas of homogeneous density. This infant, whose weight was 1956 g, was born 11.5 hours after membranes had been ruptured. Amniotic fluid was meconium stained; Apgar score was 2 at 1 minute. Tachypnea and dyspnea were followed by apneic spells then convulsions; the infant died at 25 hours of age.

on heated concentrated urine has proved useful (Hamoudi et al, 1983). It is frequently performed on urine collected by bag, after thorough cleansing of the perineum to remove colonizing bacteria. False-positive results may occur from heavy colonization (Sanchez et al, 1990) or intestinal absorption of antigen (Ascher et al, 1991). When the test is properly performed, the negative test-predictive accuracy is 100%, and the positive test-predictive accuracy is 80%. This test also diagnoses infection after antibiotics have been given to the mother or infant, but the data for predictive accuracy were obtained in infants with signs of illness, not in apparently healthy newborns.

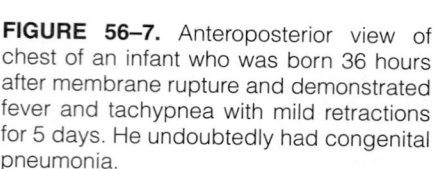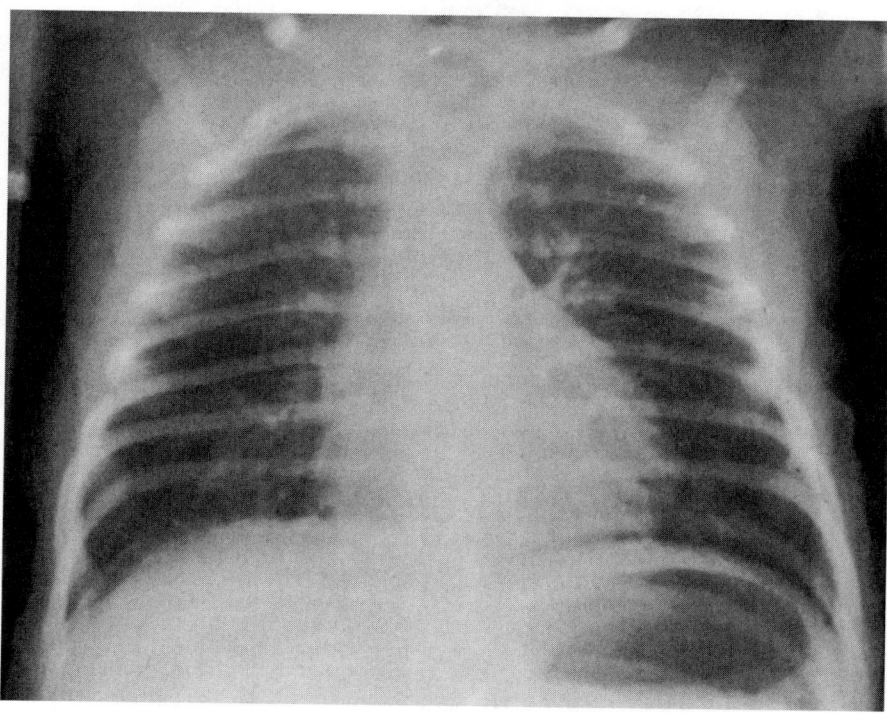

FIGURE 56–7. Anteroposterior view of chest of an infant who was born 36 hours after membrane rupture and demonstrated fever and tachypnea with mild retractions for 5 days. He undoubtedly had congenital pneumonia.

Treatment

The synergistic combination of ampicillin and gentamicin is recommended for 3 days, followed by ampicillin or penicillin alone for a total of 10 to 14 days. The antibiotic dose should be higher than usually recommended because the minimal inhibitory concentration is high, and recurrence has been reported after the use of lower doses (Baker, 1979).

Prevention

All pregnant women should have vaginal and rectal cultures performed at 26 weeks' gestation (Gibbs et al, 1992) or as soon as possible thereafter. Among those who are positive at 26 weeks' gestation, 75% remain positive at term, whereas in those who are negative, only 6% become positive by term (Gotoff, 1988). Women with positive cultures should have ampicillin prophylaxis, with an initial dose of 2 g during labor, if they have any of the following: (1) gestation less than 37 weeks, (2) rupture of membranes exceeding 12 hours, (3) amnionitis or fever, (4) a history of group B streptococcal urinary infection, or (5) a history of infection in a previous newborn (Gibbs et al, 1992). If the mother does not have a culture available, ampicillin should be given if she has any of the above-mentioned risk factors (Gibbs et al, 1992). Many centers omit the screening procedure and during labor treat all mothers with the risk factors. After delivery, term infants without signs of illness do not need treatment, provided that the mother received a 2-g dose of ampicillin at least 1 hour before delivery (Baker, 1990). Antigen detection tests are not useful in infants without signs of illness (AAP Committee, 1992). Apparently well term infants of colonized mothers should remain under observation in the hospital for 48 hours or longer. Term infants with signs of illness and all preterm infants (<2000 g) with or without signs of illness should have a complete blood count and blood culture, and then be treated with antibiotics for at least 48 hours and longer if the blood culture is positive or signs of illness, such as tachypnea, poor perfusion, or neutropenia, persist (AAP Committee, 1992).

There have been some recent changes in this recommended approach. The 26-week culture is often neither practical nor completely reliable. About 25% to 30% of newborn cases of group B streptococcal infection do not have maternal risk factors (Baker and Edwards, 1995), and so may not receive maternal prophylaxis. Instead, it has been recommended that a maternal culture be done at 36 weeks' gestation (AAP Committee, 1997); this is believed to predict the culture status at term more reliably than the 26-week culture. Mothers with positive cultures at 36 weeks' gestation should receive prophylaxis in labor even if the risk factors are absent. Penicillin may be preferred by some authorities because it is more specific and antibiotic resistance is less likely to develop, but others still favor ampicillin because enteric bacteria may also cause infection in the newborn (Gotoff and Boyer, 1997). Because the time for which prophylactic antibiotics are administered to the mother may be important, term infants without signs of illness should be treated with antibiotics for at least 48 hours if the mother was culture positive and did not receive antibiotics for 4 hours prior to delivery (AAP Committee, 1997).

Pneumonia Caused by *Listeria Monocytogenes*

Listeria monocytogenes is a gram-positive, beta-hemolytic bacillus, sometimes confused with diphtheroids. It may cause a febrile illness in the mother, but asymptomatic rectal and vaginal colonization is common. The pneumonia occurring in infants infected with *L. monocytogenes* may be transplacental, postamnionitis, or transnatal in type. In transplacental pneumonia, granulomatous disease of the placenta is present. The amniotic fluid in *Listeria* amnionitis has a greenish or chocolate-brown appearance. The chest radiograph shows a diffuse reticulonodular pattern of pneumonia if the onset is intrauterine. In transnatal pneumonia, the chest radiograph shows a bronchopneumonia pattern. These infants should have a lumbar puncture because meningitis may accompany the pneumonia.

The recommended treatment for *L. monocytogenes* pneumonia is ampicillin and gentamicin for 3 days, followed by ampicillin alone for a total of 10 to 14 days (Gordon et al, 1970). The earlier the onset, the worse the prognosis; the mortality rate is close to 100% in transplacental pneumonia, despite adequate antibiotic therapy, but quite low in transnatal pneumonia.

Pneumonia Alba Caused by Syphilis

Pneumonia alba, a classic transplacental pneumonia, occurs in infants of mothers with syphilis. This diagnosis should be suspected when infants with congenital pneumonia have other signs of congenital syphilis, such as desquamation of the palms and soles, macular rash, hepatosplenomegaly, metaphysitis, thrombocytopenia, obstructive hepatitis, hydrops, or meningoencephalitis (Mascola et al, 1985). A patient was described with congenital pneumonia, hepatosplenomegaly, periostitis, and growth retardation (Edell et al, 1993). The treatment of choice is crystalline penicillin for 10 days.

Herpes Simplex Pneumonia

Herpes simplex pneumonia is acquired by aspiration of the virus from the vaginal canal secretions during delivery, and thus this condition is a typical transnatal pneumonia. The infection is disseminated in about a third of the cases, and pneumonia is present in most of these; pneumonia is not present in the more usual localized forms of herpes infection of the skin, eyes, or brain. In 30% of all cases of herpes infection, a maternal genital lesion has been documented, but in most cases shedding of the virus is asymptomatic (Whitley et al, 1980). The onset of disseminated disease with herpes pneumonia in the newborn infant typically occurs at 5 to 7 days after birth, and the mortality rate is at least 85%. Infected infants manifest respiratory distress and poor perfusion similar to that with bacterial septicemia. Diffuse densities and lobar consolidation are apparent on the chest radiograph. Often the diagnosis can be confirmed within 1 to 3 days by viral growth in tissue cultures of tracheal aspirate samples. Controlled trials have shown that treatment with acyclovir (30 mg/kg per day) for

10 to 14 days is superior to vidarabine therapy (Whitley et al, 1986). Prevention consists of delivery by cesarean section if virus shedding can be identified in the mother; however, for most infants with this disease, the mothers are apparently asymptomatic.

Varicella Pneumonia

An infant, delivered vaginally, whose mother develops chickenpox within 5 days before delivery or within 2 days after delivery is at risk for transnatal pneumonia as a result of aspiration of infected secretions from the vaginal canal, and these newborn infants should receive herpes zoster immune globulin (125 units) as soon as possible. The onset for varicella pneumonia is between 5 and 10 days after birth. The disease is severe, with pneumonia, skin rash, coagulopathy, and liver disease, and it is associated with a mortality rate of 30% (Meyers, 1974). Infants born more than 5 days after the onset of maternal rash receive adequate antibody protection and have less severe disease. The recommended treatment for varicella pneumonia is intravenous vidarabine (15 mg/kg per day) for 10 to 14 days.

Systemic Candidiasis with Pneumonia

About 25% of infants weighing less than 1500 g at birth are colonized by *Candida*, probably during the birth process. This colonization is usually evident by 1 week of age, but it may take 2 to 3 weeks before multiplication is sufficient for cultures to be positive (Baley et al, 1986). The common sites for colonization are the rectum, groin, and throat, but systemic disease occurs only in infants who are colonized. About 70% of infants with systemic candidiasis have pneumonia. These infants are usually small premature infants, about 1 month of age, who have required mechanical ventilation, prolonged use of intravascular catheters, and multiple courses of antibiotics. The signs resemble those of bacterial septicemia. There may be respiratory deterioration with increased oxygen or ventilator requirements, apnea and bradycardia, temperature instability, glucose intolerance, hypotension, thrombocytopenia, or feeding intolerance and abdominal distention. Recovery of *Candida* from the tracheal aspirate cannot differentiate colonization from infection, and the only way to prove pneumonia is by open lung biopsy. If the fungus can be recovered from the blood, cerebrospinal fluid, urine, or other body fluids, however, or if eye disease is present, infection of the lung is likely. The radiographic signs of *Candida* pneumonia are nonspecific against the usual background of chronic lung disease. The recommended treatment is amphotericin (1 mg/kg per day) for 30 days (Butler and Baker, 1988).

Chlamydial Pneumonia

Although the onset of pneumonia caused by *Chlamydia trachomatis* is usually delayed until 1 to 3 months of age, it is considered to be a transnatal pneumonia, the pathogen being acquired from the mother's vagina at delivery (Gilbert, 1986). About 2% to 10% of pregnant women have vaginal colonization with *Chlamydia*; in a San Francisco

study, the rate was 4.7% (Schachter et al, 1986). In infants of colonized mothers, about 35% develop conjunctivitis, and 20% may develop pneumonia (Schachter et al, 1979). The eye condition is largely prevented by the widespread use of antibiotic ointment at birth. The majority of cases of pneumonia are mild, and Schachter and colleagues (1979) noted that 25% of infants at home required hospitalization.

The pneumonia is characterized by insidious respiratory distress, cough, wheezing, absence of fever, and bilateral diffuse densities and hyperinflation on the chest radiograph (Harrison et al, 1978). Significant eosinophilia and elevated serum immunoglobulin M (IgM) levels are frequently observed.

Infants with chronic lung disease are said to be particularly susceptible (Stagno et al, 1981); however, in a prospective study in a London intensive care unit, only one case of *Chlamydia* pneumonia was identified among 280 infants (Rudd and Carrington, 1984), and that infant also had conjunctivitis. Sollecito and coworkers (1992) described a group of premature infants who had respiratory distress syndrome initially and who developed pneumonia while being weaned from the ventilator. These infants had severe apnea spells and underexpansion of the lungs; some had eosinophilia.

To confirm the diagnosis, nasopharyngeal or tracheal secretions should be plated in specific tissue culture cells (Harrison et al, 1978); after 48 to 72 hours, the monolayers are Giemsa stained and examined for inclusions. This test is commercially available. Alternatively, secretions should be examined for antigen, using rapid direct slide immunofluorescence with monoclonal antibodies (Bell et al, 1984). An enzyme-linked immunosorbent assay test is not considered suitable for use with respiratory secretions because of many false-positive tests (Preece et al, 1989). The recommended treatment is oral erythromycin (10 mg/kg every 6 hours) for 14 days.

Pneumonia Caused by *Ureaplasma* and *Mycoplasma*

There have been isolated reports of congenital pneumonia caused by *Ureaplasma urealyticum* (Brus et al, 1991; Panero et al, 1995; Quinn et al, 1985; Ursi et al, 1995; Waites et al, 1989) and *Mycoplasma hominis* (Ursi et al, 1995). Mycoplasmas and ureaplasmas are commonly associated with amnionitis in the mother; the pneumonia has an early onset, but the specific diagnosis may be made comparatively late in the clinical course. The organisms are cultured only with special media after a period of 3 to 5 days, but DNA tests for the urease gene using polymerase chain reaction (PCR) can indicate the organism's presence within 24 hours (Blanchard et al, 1993). Commonly used antibiotics are not effective in treatment. Therefore, this diagnosis should be considered, among other diagnoses, in any infants appearing to have infection with pneumonia but not responding to antibiotic therapy. The appropriate treatment is intravenous erythromycin lactobionate (10 mg/kg every 12 hours) for 14 days.

Some clinicians have claimed that untreated *Ureaplasma* pneumonia is a common cause of bronchopulmonary dysplasia (Cassell et al, 1988; Horowitz et al, 1992). Crouse and associates (1993) found that a positive tracheal aspirate culture was significantly more often associated with radiologic evidence of pneumonia in premature infants with birth weight less than 2500 g, but the evidence in those with birth weight less than 1250 g, in whom pneumonia is more common, was less conclusive. Ohlsson and colleagues (1993) reviewed the evidence that the white cell count was elevated in cases of pneumonia, but it was not clear from the report which cases had pneumonia. Thureen and colleagues (1993) identified prospectively a group of neonatal intensive care unit infants who were thought to have late-onset pneumonia and compared them with a group of controls not suspected of pneumonia; they found *Ureaplasma* in tracheal aspirate samples in equal numbers in each group and strongly questioned whether *Ureaplasma* was responsible for disease in these infants. Other studies have found that tracheal aspirate samples positive for *Ureaplasma* are not associated with an increased incidence of chronic lung disease (Heggie et al, 1994; Saxen et al, 1993). Sanchez and Regan (1990) showed that rates of mucosal colonization were high and that the rates were much higher in infants with birth weights less than 1000 g (89%) than in larger premature infants (54%); this may be the reason why some have found a higher incidence of bronchopulmonary dysplasia in colonized infants. This controversy can be settled only with large prospective studies.

NOSOCOMIAL PNEUMONIA
Pathogenesis

Although hospital-acquired pneumonia is a problem for all newborn and premature infants, it has become a particular problem for those requiring mechanical ventilatory support. These infections are a major determinant of late morbidity and mortality.

Endotracheal intubation is the single most important factor predisposing to nosocomial pneumonia. The risk for intubated patients is about four times higher than in nonintubated patients (Cross and Roup, 1981) and even higher with tracheostomy. The endotracheal tube eliminates the upper airway as a bacterial filter, tracheal mucosal damage encourages colonization, and ventilator equipment may be contaminated.

Predisposing factors in the occurrence of nosocomial infection are

1. Birth weight less than 1500 g
2. Prolonged hospitalization
3. Severe underlying disease
4. Multiple invasive procedures
5. Overcrowding
6. Low nurse/patient ratio
7. Contaminated ventilator equipment
8. Insufficiently washed hands of health care personnel (Hemming et al, 1976)

The nose, throat, and rectum are colonized with bacteria during the first 3 days of life. Normally the predominant bacteria in the nose are *Staphylococcus aureus*, in the throat hemolytic streptococci, and in the rectum *E. coli* and *Lactobacillus*.

Colonization is somewhat delayed in those admitted to the neonatal intensive care unit immediately after birth, especially those treated with antibiotics. The colonizing bacteria are often different (e.g., *S. aureus, Staphylococcus epidermidis,* or *Klebsiella* in the throat or *Klebsiella, Enterobacter,* or *Citrobacter* in the rectum) presumably a reflection of exposure to antibiotics. It is thought that colonization with so-called normal flora provides protection against infection but that colonization with unusual flora is associated with an increased risk of infection (Sprunt et al, 1978).

The trachea and bronchi are normally sterile, despite heavy colonization in the nose and throat. Placement of an endotracheal tube, however, soon leads to colonization of the trachea (Harris et al, 1976). This is especially true if the patient is intubated after 12 hours of age, for more than 72 hours, or more than once. The presence of colonization in the trachea and bronchi does not mean infection in the absence of clinical signs, but it substantially increases the risk (Johanson et al, 1972). Nosocomial pneumonia may also result from the inhalation of aerosols containing bacteria (Simmons and Wong, 1982); this requires routine daily decontamination procedures and periodic surveillance cultures of respiratory therapy equipment.

Diagnosis

The clinical diagnosis of nosocomial pneumonia depends on the appearance of new infiltrates on the chest radiograph, increased oxygen and ventilator requirements, an abnormal white cell count, and the finding of purulent tracheal secretions. Bacteriologic diagnosis depends on culture results from blood, tracheal aspirate, and pleural fluid, if available.

In an early study, a good correlation was shown between tracheal aspirate bacteria and bacteria grown from blood in cases of bacterial pneumonia in adult patients (Schwartz et al, 1984). Tracheal aspirates, as performed in the neonatal intensive care unit, are subject to contamination from the throat. It has been suggested that this problem can be overcome by passing a long sterile catheter with a stylet through the endotracheal tube into a peripheral bronchus and aspirating a sample for culture after brief saline lavage (Frankel et al, 1988). Investigators have found the standard tracheal aspirate sample not to be useful in the diagnosis of nosocomial pneumonia in premature infants. Webber and coworkers (1990) observed 41 cases of nosocomial pneumonia in an Oxford neonatal intensive care unit; most were preterm infants on mechanical ventilation. In only seven was the blood culture positive, but in only one of these seven was the tracheal sample positive for the same organism. They suggested that antibiotic choice should be made on the basis of past experience in the neonatal intensive care unit, rather than on the results of tracheal aspirate culture. In a similar experience with positive blood cultures in nosocomial infection of neonatal intensive care unit infants, Slagle and associates (1989) found that the tracheal aspirate sample identified the correct organism in the blood in only 19% of cases.

Thureen and colleagues (1993) published excellent data further questioning the results for tracheal aspirate specimens. They identified infants prospectively in the neonatal intensive care unit who were suspected of having a lung infection on the basis of increased oxygen or ventilation requirements, then they selected a contemporary control infant who was stable for the prior week; they performed a standard set of tests with predefined abnormal results in both groups. The chest radiograph and the white blood count were abnormal in the study group significantly more often than in the controls. The tracheal aspirate culture was positive in 35% of both groups and was of no help in distinguishing the two groups. In adult patients with endotracheal tubes in place, it has been known for a long time that there is little correlation between tracheal aspirate samples and samples collected from small bronchi with a catheter wedged in the peripheral lung (Matthew et al, 1977); the latter samples are much more often correct.

Treatment

The choice of antibiotics depends on the recent history of infection in the neonatal intensive care unit. In the past, ampicillin and gentamicin have frequently been chosen, but in view of the prevalence of staphylococcal species, in many hospitals the appropriate choices now are vancomycin and gentamicin. During an outbreak of *Pseudomonas* infection, the proper choice may be ceftazidime and tobramycin. If sensitivities become known, this choice can be changed for the individual patient.

Specific Nosocomial Pneumonias

Staphylococcus Aureus Pneumonia

S. aureus colonize the nose frequently but may also colonize the throat and trachea of debilitated infants. The chest radiograph suggests a nonspecific bronchopneumonia, frequently superimposed over chronic lung disease. In more severe cases, ultimately leading to death, there are multiple small lung abscesses. These infants have lethargy, poor circulation, increased oxygen and ventilator requirements, and changes in the white blood cell count. The treatment of choice is vancomycin in most cases, but in a few cases methicillin for 14 days is appropriate.

Pneumonia from *Staphylococcus Epidermidis*

A normal inhabitant of the skin, *S. epidermidis* may also colonize the throat and trachea of small debilitated infants. Although it more frequently causes a generalized infection, about one fifth of the cases have lung involvement, with the chest radiograph suggesting a nonspecific bronchopneumonia (LaGamma et al, 1983). Because infection is usually resistant to methicillin, the treatment is vancomycin for 14 days, with monitoring of plasma levels.

Pseudomonas Pneumonia

Pseudomonas is not part of the normal flora at any site, and its isolation from throat or tracheal aspirate is cause for considerable concern. It is sometimes isolated from moist equipment, such as nebulizers, humidifiers, incubators, and faucets, and disinfectant and respiratory therapy solutions, which act as dangerous sources of infection. The signs are nonspecific, but necrotic skin ulcerations are characteristic, if present. The chest radiograph suggests

bronchopneumonia. Small premature infants with a tracheal tube in place are susceptible (Barson, 1971). The mortality is high because of antibiotic resistance. Treatment consists of an anti-*Pseudomonas* penicillin, such as ticarcillin, and an aminoglycoside, such as gentamicin, tobramycin, or amikacin. Synergistic activity is thought to be important. Ceftazidime may be the best treatment, in combination with an aminoglycoside.

Klebsiella Pneumonia

Klebsiella is not part of the normal flora at any site, and its isolation from the throat, tracheal aspirate, or rectum is cause for alarm. Its transmission is usually by the hands of attendants from one infant to another. On the chest radiograph, there is a nonspecific bronchopneumonia, but because this is a necrotizing pneumonia, lung abscesses and pneumatoceles may also be evident (Papageorgiou et al, 1973). The mortality is high. Because *Klebsiella* is frequently ampicillin resistant, the treatment is currently cefotaxime and amikacin for 14 days.

Cytomegalovirus Pneumonia

Small premature infants may acquire cytomegalovirus infection around the age of 1 to 3 months. About one third of such infants have pneumonia, which may contribute to the development of bronchopulmonary dysplasia (Sawyer et al, 1987) or otherwise complicate its course (Ballard et al, 1979). Characteristically, there is increased respiratory distress, greater oxygen or ventilator requirements, hepatosplenomegaly, a peculiar gray color suggestive of sepsis, thrombocytopenia, and both an atypical and absolute lymphocytosis. It is thought that most of these infants acquire this infection from multiple seropositive blood transfusions, although it may be acquired perinatally from a cytomegalovirus-positive mother. The lung infection lasts about 2 weeks, but some cases are more prolonged. Deaths have generally been related to systemic infection beyond the lungs. The diagnosis is made by identifying cytomegalovirus in tissue culture by plating urine, throat washings, or tracheal secretions. Although the culture is frequently positive within 7 days, it may take up to 4 weeks. Preventive measures include limiting the number of blood transfusions, limiting the number of blood donors, or using only seronegative blood. Because seronegative blood may become scarce, an alternative is to use filtered leukocyte-depleted blood (Lane et al, 1992).

Respiratory Syncytial Virus Pneumonia

The respiratory syncytial virus causes bronchiolitis and pneumonia with respiratory distress in infants and frequently lethargy and apnea as well and has been seen in small premature infants, usually those with chronic lung disease, especially during the winter months. It may be acquired in the community after discharge but is frequently acquired from visitors or health care personnel in the hospital. Adults and older children who are infected have signs of an upper respiratory infection; they constitute a major threat to the susceptible host and, where possible, should be excluded from attendance or visitation. Infection may also be spread from patient to patient. The virus is transmitted by direct contact with infected secretions, which remain infectious for hours on environmental hard and soft surfaces and are then carried by the hands of attendants to the mucous membranes of susceptible hosts. Adequate hand-washing diminishes noscomial spread, and infected patients should be cohorted and isolated with gown, glove, and mask precautions. The characteristic finding on the chest radiograph is hyperinflation, with or without lobar densities suggesting pneumonia. Identification of the virus in tissue culture takes 3 to 8 days or longer. The most rapid method of diagnosis is antigen detection by enzyme-linked immunosorbent assay or the direct fluorescent antibody test performed on tracheal aspirate secretions. The sensitivity of these rapid tests in comparison with culture methods is in the range of 80% to 90%.

The treatment recommended is aerosol administration of the antiviral drug ribavirin (Taber et al, 1983) by hood, mask, or ventilator for 3 to 7 days. Although controlled trials showed that ribavirin-treated infants recovered faster than untreated infants and had significantly improved arterial oxygenation (Hall et al, 1983), there is some evidence that ribavirin may be toxic, especially as a teratogen (Rodriguez et al, 1987); as a result, many centers do not use this therapy. Special precautions must be taken with ventilators to prevent obstruction of mechanical valves (Outwater et al, 1988). A large controlled trial showed that ribavirin provided considerable benefit to infants who needed ventilatory support (Smith et al, 1991); the duration of mechanical ventilation, oxygen therapy, and hospital stay was significantly reduced, and hospital costs were decreased. Another controlled trial examined the results for the standard dose given continuously over 18 hours per day versus a high dose given intermittently for 2 hours three times a day (Englund et al, 1994); the hospital course and clinical scores were the same, but with the high-dose regimen, access to the patient for nurses and family was much improved, and environmental contamination with the high-dose regimen by hood was markedly reduced. The AAP Committee on Infectious Diseases (1996) has changed its recommendation for ribavirin and now states that it should only be considered in the treatment of this infection. Some evidence, not published yet, suggests that this therapy may not be efficacious and that it may prolong the course of mechanical ventilation in sicker patients. This area of therapeutics suffers badly from lack of truly large well-controlled trials. A specific high-titer immunoglobulin preparation, given at monthly intervals to high-risk infants, has shown promise for passive immunoprophylaxis against this condition (Groothuis et al, 1993).

Pneumocystis Carinii Pneumonia

Pneumocystis carinii pneumonia has been seen in epidemic form in European premature nurseries but has been identified only sporadically in North America in immunocompetent infants under 3 months of age (Stagno et al, 1980) as well as in older immunocompromised patients. It may have been overlooked in the past. The parasite causes a diffuse interstitial mononuclear pneumonia without fever. In small prematures, the onset is insidious during the 3rd month of

life, with tachypnea, retractions, cyanosis, crepitant rales, cough, eosinophilia, and a diffuse granular infiltrate on the chest radiograph. Epidemics represent infant-to-infant spread and can be terminated by isolation techniques. The diagnosis may be made by examination of tracheal secretions for the encapsulated cyst or may require lung aspirate, using a Gomori methenamine silver stain. Alternatively the antigen may be detected by counterimmunoelectrophoresis (Pifer, 1983). The treatment is administration of trimethoprim-sulfamethoxazole for 14 days.

ASPIRATION PNEUMONIA IN THE NEWBORN INFANT
Aspiration During the Birth Process

It is sometimes difficult to understand what clinicians mean when they refer to the diagnosis of aspiration pneumonia in a newborn infant. The most common situation is the aspiration of meconium, which results in meconium aspiration pneumonia, as discussed in Chapter 53.

Another situation is the aspiration of large volumes of amniotic fluid (Schaffer and Avery, 1971), in which case the infant experiences severe fetal asphyxia to initiate deep continuous gasping and presents after birth with signs of postasphyxial pulmonary edema or a related condition. It remains unclear whether aspiration of amniotic fluid alone causes a problem because the fetal lung is normally filled with clear liquid. Because the amniotic fluid is filled with squamous epithelial cells, these cells may obstruct the peripheral airways, and such a picture is commonly seen at autopsy in stillborn infants (Fig. 56–8). Jose and colleagues (1981) instilled large amounts of amniotic fluid with squamous cells into the lungs of adult rabbits and found no adverse effects, compared with the instillation of clear fluid. It is now thought unlikely that clear amniotic fluid causes respiratory distress.

Another possibility is the aspiration of blood, most likely from the mother, but there have been no unique descriptions of this condition. In view of the lung liquid in the airways before birth, it is unlikely that blood would cause a problem for the newborn infant.

Finally, the infant may aspirate infected amniotic fluid, and in the few instances in which the organisms are invasive, this may cause a postamnionitis pneumonia, as previously discussed. In most cases, the organisms are not invasive, so the clinical picture is that of postasphyxial pulmonary edema or a related condition.

Aspiration After Birth

Under certain circumstances after birth, the infant may aspirate gastric contents, either acidic gastric secretions or milk formula, or both. This may occur in esophageal atresia, with or without a fistula, in cases of laryngotracheoesophageal cleft, in conditions associated with pharyngeal incoordination such as birth asphyxia, and in conditions associated with gastroesophageal reflux such as marked prematurity or severe bronchopulmonary dysplasia. The typical aspiration pneumonia with esophageal atresia involves the right upper and lower lobes of the lung and sometimes the left perihilar region; there is a loss of lung

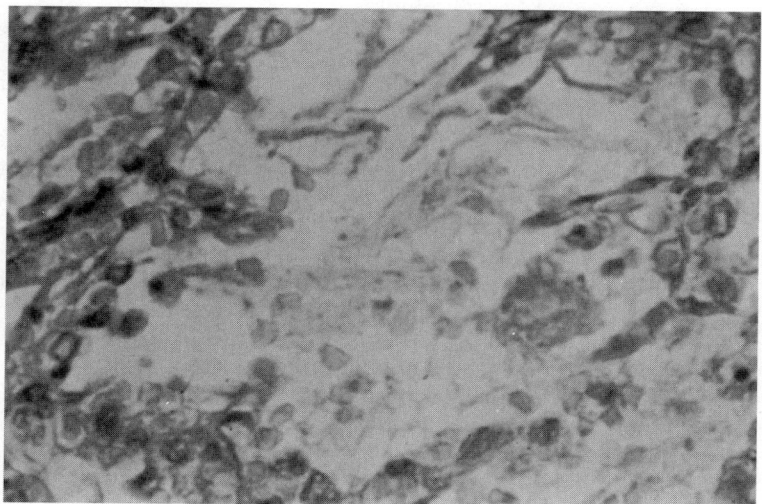

FIGURE 56–8. Section of lung of a full-term infant weighing 3400 g, who died 15 minutes after birth, having gasped only a few times. Prolonged labor, uterine inertia, stimulation of labor by oxytocin (Pitocin), and, finally, midforceps extraction characterized his delivery. The microscopic section shows much fluid and debris and many squames within dilated terminal air spaces. Virtually every section from both lungs looked like this one.

compliance owing to edema, hemorrhage, and atelectasis, and there may be a secondary infection for which antibiotics are usually prescribed.

Although postnatal aspiration pneumonia is greatly feared, it is comparatively uncommon under modern neonatal intensive care unit conditions, even in tiny premature infants. The larynx is richly endowed with a variety of mechanoreceptors and chemoreceptors, which initiate laryngeal closure and prolonged apnea when stimulated by unusual fluids at the laryngeal opening (Bartlett, 1985); this reflex is powerful in the newborn, especially in small premature infants, and diminishes with development as the cough reflex becomes more active. Most infants become apneic when the opening to the larynx is bathed in gastric fluid (Perkett and Vaughan, 1982; Pickens et al, 1989), and apnea prevents the aspiration of gastric material into the lungs. Infants who are appropriately resuscitated after an apneic episode frequently have formula suctioned from the pharynx or larynx, but the chest radiograph done later rarely shows evidence of a true aspiration pneumonia.

Because of the possible danger of aspiration pneumonia if there is unrecognized esophageal atresia or another problem, it is common practice for the first feed to be glucose water. This may not be a logical practice, however, because glucose water is just as irritating to the lungs as milk formula (Olson, 1970), and so many clinicians think that water is preferred for the first feeding. Also because of the possible danger, it was once recommended that feedings for premature infants be delayed for several days after birth, but this recommendation has survived only for the smallest of premature infants. The American Academy of Pediatrics has recommended that normal term infants be placed supine, or on the side, after feeds; this has accompanied the acceptance that postnatal aspiration pneumonia in such infants, when placed supine, has never been described.

Infants on long-term mechanical ventilation and formula feedings may develop evidence of aspiration into the lungs and aspiration pneumonia. The diagnosis is made by finding lipid-laden macrophages in the tracheal aspirate samples (Nickerson, 1987), an occurrence that reflects gastroesophageal reflux, tracheal aspiration, and interference with the normal tracheal clearance mechanisms by the indwelling endotracheal tube. Others have confirmed this phenomenon by using a blue dye in the formula and recovering this dye in the tracheal aspirate samples.

REFERENCES

AAP Committee on Infectious Diseases: Reassessment of the indications for ribavirin therapy in respiratory syncytial virus infections. Pediatrics 97:137, 1996.

AAP Committee on Infectious Diseases and on Fetus and Newborn: Guidelines for prevention of group B streptococcal infection by chemoprophylaxis. Pediatrics 90:775, 1992.

AAP Committee on Infectious Diseases and on Fetus and Newborn: Revised guidelines for prevention of early-onset group B streptococcal infection. Pediatrics 99:489, 1997.

Ascher DP, Wilson S, Mendiola J, Fischer GW: Group B streptococcal latex agglutination testing in neonates. J Pediatr 119:458, 1991.

Avery ME: Pneumonia. *In* Avery ME, Taeusch HW (Eds): Diseases of the Newborn, 5th ed. Philadelphia, WB Saunders, 1984.

Baker CJ: Group B streptococcal infections in neonates. Pediatr Rev 1:5, 1979.

Baker CJ: Antibiotic therapy in neonates whose mothers have received intrapartum group B streptococcal chemoprophylaxis. Pediatr Infect Dis J 9:149, 1990.

Baker CJ, Edwards MS: Group B streptococcal infections. *In* Remington J, Klein JO (Eds): Infectious Diseases of the Fetus and Newborn Infant. Philadelphia, WB Saunders, 1995, p 980.

Baker CJ, Webb BJ, Jackson CV, et al: Countercurrent electrophoresis in the evaluation of infants with group B streptococcal disease. Pediatrics 65:1110, 1980.

Baley JE, Kliegman RM, Boxerbaum B, et al: Fungal colonization in the very low birth weight infant. Pediatrics 78:225, 1986.

Ballard RA, Drew L, Hufnagle KG, et al: Acquired cytomegalovirus infection in preterm infants. Am J Dis Child 133:482, 1979.

Barson AJ: Fatal *Pseudomonas aeruginosa* bronchopneumonia in a children's hospital. Arch Dis Child 46:55, 1971.

Bartlett D: Ventilatory and protective mechanisms of the infant larynx. Am Rev Respir Dis 131(suppl):S49, 1985.

Bell TA, Kuo C, Stamm WE, et al: Direct fluorescent monoclonal antibody stain for rapid detection of infant *Chlamydia trachomatis* infections. Pediatrics 74:224, 1984.

Blanc WA: Pathways of fetal and early neonatal infection. J Pediatr 59:473, 1961.

Blanchard A, Hentschel J, Duffy L, et al: Detection of *Ureaplasma urealyticum* by polymerase chain reaction in the urogenital tract of adults in amniotic fluid, and in the respiratory tract of newborns. Clin Infect Dis 17(suppl 1):S148, 1993.

Brook I, Martin WJ, Finegold SM: Bacteriology of tracheal aspirates in intubated newborn. Chest 78:875, 1980.

Brus F, van Waarde WM, Schoots C, Oetomo SB: Fatal ureaplasmal pneumonia and sepsis in a newborn infant. Eur J Pediatr 150:782, 1991.

Burchell RC: Premature spontaneous rupture of the membranes. Am J Obstet Gynecol 88:251, 1964.

Butler KM, Baker CJ: *Candida:* An increasingly important pathogen in the nursery. Pediatr Clin North Am 35:543, 1988.

Cassell GH, Waites KB, Crouse DT, et al: Association of *Ureaplasma urealyticum* infection of the lower respiratory tract with chronic lung disease and death in very low birth weight infants. Lancet 2:240, 1988.

Cross AS, Roup B: Role of respiratory assistance devices in endemic nosocomial pneumonia. Am J Med 70:681, 1981.

Crouse DT, Odrezin GT, Cutter GR, et al: Radiographic changes associated with tracheal isolation of *Ureaplasma urealyticum* from neonates. Clin Infect Dis 17(suppl 1):S122, 1993.

Daikoku NH, Kaltreider DF, Johnson TRB, et al: Premature rupture of membranes and preterm labor: Neonatal infection and perinatal mortality risks. Obstet Gynecol 58:417, 1981.

Edell DS, Davidson JJ, Mulvihill DM, et al: A common presentation of an uncommon cause of neonatal respiratory distress syndrome: Pneumonia. Pediatr Pulmonol 15:376, 1993.

Englund JA, Piedra PA, Ahn YM, et al: High dose short duration ribavirin aerosol therapy compared with standard ribavirin therapy in children with suspected respiratory syncytial virus infection. J Pediatr 125:635, 1994.

Evans ME, Schaffner W, Federspiel CF, et al: Sensitivity, specificity, and predictive value of body surface cultures in a neonatal intensive care unit. JAMA 259:248, 1988.

Frankel LR, Smith DW, Lewiston NJ: Bronchoalveolar lavage for diagnosis of pneumonia in the immunocompromised child. Pediatrics 81:785, 1988.

Gibbs RS, Hall RT, Yow MD, et al: Consensus: Perinatal prophylaxis for group B streptococcal infection. Pediatr Infect Dis J 11:179, 1992.

Gilbert GL: Chlamydial infections in infancy. Aust Paediatr J 22:13, 1986.

Goldmann DA, Leclair J, Macone A: Bacterial colonization of neonates admitted to an intensive care environment. J Pediatr 93:288, 1978.

Gordon RC, Barrett FF, Yow MD: Ampicillin treatment of listeriosis. J Pediatr 77:1067, 1970.

Gotoff SP: Prophylaxis for early onset group B streptococcus. Contemp Obstet Gynecol 33:25, 1988.

Gotoff SP, Boyer KM: Prevention of early-onset neonatal group B streptococcal disase. Pediatrics 99:866, 1997.

Groothuis JR, Simoes EAF, Levin MJ, et al: Prophylactic administration of respiratory syncytial virus immune globulin to high risk infants and young children. N Engl J Med 329:1524, 1993.

Hall CB, McBride JT, Walsh EE, et al: Aerosolized ribavirin treatment of infants with respiratory syncytial viral infection. N Engl J Med 308:1443, 1983.

Hamoudi AC, Marcon MJ, Cannon HJ, et al: Comparison of three major antigen detection methods for the diagnosis of group B streptococci in a newborn nursery. Pediatrics 58:679, 1983.

Harris H, Wirtschafter D, Cassady G: Endotracheal intubation and its relationship to bacterial colonization and systemic infection of newborn infants. Pediatrics 58:816, 1976.

Harrison HR, English MG, Lee CK, et al: *Chlamydia trachomatis* infant pneumonitis. N Engl J Med 298:702, 1978.

Heggie AD, Facobs MR, Butler VT, et al: Frequency and significance of isolation of *Ureaplasma urealyticum* and *Mycoplasma hominis* from cerebrospinal fluid and tracheal aspirate specimens from low birth weight infants. J Pediatr 124:956, 1994.

Hemming VG, Overall JC, Britt MR: Nosocomial infections in a newborn intensive-care unit. N Engl J Med 294:1310, 1976.

Horowitz S, Landau D, Shinwell ES, et al: Respiratory tract colonization with *Ureaplasma urealyticum* and bronchopulmonary dysplasia in neonates in southern Israel. Pediatr Infect Dis J 11:847, 1992.

Johanson WG, Pierce AK, Sanford JP: Nosocomial respiratory infections with gram-negative bacilli. Ann Intern Med 77:701, 1972.

Johnson JWC, Daikoku NH, Neibyl JR, et al: Premature rupture of the membranes and prolonged latency. Obstet Gynecol 57:547, 1981.

Jose J, Schreiner R, Mirkin L, et al: Non-association of cell content with respiratory distress in adult rabbits aspirating human amniotic fluid (abstract). Pediatr Res 15:1672, 1981.

Koh KS, Chan FH, Monfared AH, et al: The changing perinatal and maternal outcome in chorioamnionitis. Obstet Gynecol 53:730, 1979.

LaGamma EF, Drusin LM, Mackles AW, et al: Neonatal infections: An important determinant of late NICU mortality in infants less than 1000 g at birth. Am J Dis Child 137:838, 1983.

Lane TA, Anderson KC, Goodnough LT, et al: Leukocyte reduction in blood component therapy. Ann Intern Med 117:151, 1992.

Lauweryns J, Bernat R, Lerut A, et al: Intrauterine pneumonia. Biol Neonate 22:301, 1973.

Maki DG, Alvarado CJ, Hassemer CA, et al: Relation of the inanimate hospital environment to endemic nosocomial infection. N Engl J Med 307:1562, 1982.

Mascola L, Pelosi R, Blount JH, et al: Congenital syphilis revisited. Am J Dis Child 139:575, 1985.

Matthew EB, Holstrom FMG, Kaspar RL: A simple method for diagnosing pneumonia in intubated or tracheostomized patients. Crit Care Med 5:76, 1977.

Meyers JD: Congenital varicella in term infants: Risk reconsidered. J Infect Dis 129:215, 1974.

Naeye RL: Causes of the excessive rates of perinatal mortality and prematurity in pregnancies complicated by maternal urinary-tract infections. N Engl J Med 300:819, 1979a.

Naeye RL: Coitus and associated amniotic-fluid infections. N Engl J Med 301:1198, 1979b.

Naeye RL, Blanc WA: Relation of poverty and race to antenatal infection. N Engl J Med 283:555, 1970.

Naeye RL, Peters EC: Amniotic fluid infections with intact membranes leading to perinatal death: A prospective study. Pediatrics 61:171, 1978.

Nickerson BG: A test for recurrent aspiration in children. Pediatr Pulmonol 3:65, 1987.

Ohlsson A, Wang E, Vearncombe M: Leukocyte counts and colonization with *Ureaplasma urealyticum* in preterm neonates. Clin Infect Dis 17(suppl 1):S144, 1993.

Olson M: The benign effects on rabbits lungs of the aspiration of water compared with 5% glucose and milk. Pediatrics 46:538, 1970.

Outwater KM, Meissner HC, Peterson MB: Ribavirin administration to infants receiving mechanical ventilation. Am J Dis Child 142:512, 1988.

Panero A, Pacifico L, Rossi N, et al: *Ureaplasma urealyticum* as a cause of pneumonia in preterm infants: Analysis of the white cell response. Arch Dis Child 73:F37, 1995.

Papageorgiou A, Bauer CR, Fletcher BD, et al: *Klebsiella* pneumonia with pneumatocele formation in a newborn infant. Can Med Assoc J 109:1217, 1973.

Paredes A, Wong P, Mason EO, et al: Nosocomial transmission of group B streptococci in a newborn nursery. Pediatrics 59:679, 1977.

Pennington JE: Community-acquired and hospital-acquired pneumonia in adults. *In* Simmons DH (Ed): Current Pulmonology, Vol 7. Chicago, Year Book Medical Publishers, 1986.

Perkett EA, Vaughan RL: Evidence for a laryngeal chemoreflex in some human preterm infants. Acta Paediatr Scand 71:969, 1982.

Phillip AGS, Hewitt JR: Early diagnosis of neonatal sepsis. Pediatrics 65:1036, 1980.

Pickens DL, Schefft GL, Thach BT: Pharyngeal fluid clearance and aspiration preventive mechanisms in sleeping infants. J Appl Physiol 66:1164, 1989.

Pierce AK, Sanford JP: Bacterial contamination of aerosols. Arch Intern Med 131:156, 1973.

Pifer LL: *Pneumocystis carinii:* A diagnostic dilemma. Pediatr Infect Dis 2:177, 1983.

Preece PM, Anderson JM, Thompson RG: Chlamydia trachomatis infection in infants: A prospective study. Arch Dis Child 64:525, 1989.

Quinn PA, Gillan JE, Markestad T, et al: Intrauterine infection with ureaplasma urealyticum as a cause of fatal neonatal pneumonia. Pediatr Infect Dis J 4:538, 1985.

Ramos A, Stern L: Relationship of premature rupture of the membranes to gastric fluid aspirate in the newborn. Am J Obstet Gynecol 105:1247, 1969.

Rodriguez WJ, Dang Bui RH, Connor JD, et al: Environmental exposure of primary care personnel to ribavirin aerosol when supervising treatment of infant with respiratory syncytial virus infections. Antimicrob Agents Chemother 31:1143, 1987.

Rudd PT, Carrington DA: A prospective study of chlamydial, mycoplasmal, and viral infections in a neonatal intensive care unit. Arch Dis Child 59:120, 1984.

Sanchez PJ, Regan JA: Vertical transmission of Ureaplasma urealyticum from mothers to preterm infants. Pediatr Infect Dis J 9:398, 1990.

Sanchez PJ, Siegel JD, Cushion NB, et al: Significance of a positive urine group B streptococcal latex agglutination test in neonates. J Pediatr 116:601, 1990.

Sawyer MH, Edwards DK, Spector SA: Cytomegalovirus infection and bronchopulmonary dysplasia in premature infants. Am J Dis Child 141:303, 1988.

Saxen H, Hakkarainen K, Pohjavuori M, Miettinen A: Chronic lung disease of preterm infants in Finland is not associated with *Ureaplasma urealyticum* colonization. Acta Paediatr 82:198, 1993.

Schachter J, Grossman M, Sweet RL, et al: Prospective study of perinatal transmission of chlamydia trachomatis. JAMA 255:3374, 1986.

Schachter J, Holt J, Goodner E, et al: Prospective study of chlamydial infection in neonates. Lancet 2:377, 1979.

Schaffer AJ, Avery ME: Aspiration syndromes. *In* Diseases of the Newborn. Philadelphia, WB Saunders, 1971.

Schlievert P, Larsen B, Johnson W, et al: Bacterial growth inhibition by amniotic fluid. Am J Obstet Gynecol 122:809, 1975.

Schutte MF, Treffers PE, Kloosterman GJ, et al: Management of premature rupture of membranes: The risk of vaginal examination to the infant. Am J Obstet Gynecol 146:395, 1983.

Schwartz DB, Oslon DE, Kauffman CA: The utility of pharyngeal and tracheal cultures during endotracheal intubation. Chest 86:335, 1984.

Selden R, Lee S, Wang WLL, et al: Nosocomial *Klebsiella* infections: Intestinal colonization as a reservoir. Ann Intern Med 74:657, 1971.

Sherman MP, Chance KH, Goetzman BW: Gram's stains of tracheal secretions predict neonatal bacteremia. Am J Dis Child 138:848, 1984.

Sherman MP, Goetzman BW, Ahlfors CE, et al: Tracheal aspiration and its clinical correlates in the diagnosis of congenital pneumonia. Pediatrics 65:258, 1980.

Shurin PA, Alpert S, Rosner B, et al: Chorioamnionitis and colonization of the newborn infant with genital mycoplasmas. N Engl J Med 293:5, 1975.

Simmons BP, Wong ES: Guidelines for prevention of nosocomial pneumonia. Infect Control 3:327, 1982.

Slagle TA, Bifano EM, Wolf JW, Gross SJ: Routine endotracheal cultures for the prediction of sepsis in ventilated babies. Arch Dis Child 64:34, 1989.

Smith DW, Frankel LR, Mathers LH, et al: A controlled trial of aerosolized ribavirin in infants receiving mechanical ventilation for severe respiratory syncytial virus infection. N Engl J Med 325:24, 1991.

Sollecito D, Midulla M, Bavastrelli M, et al: *Chlamydia trachomatis* in neonatal respiratory distress of very preterm babies: Biphasic clinical picture. Acta Paediatr Scand 81:788, 1992.

Sprunt K, Leidy G, Redman W: Abnormal colonization of neonates in an intensive care unit: Means of identifying neonates at risk of infection. Pediatr Res 12:998, 1978.

Stagno S, Brasfield DM, Brown MB, et al: Infant pneumonitis associated with cytomegalovirus, *Chlamydia, Pneumocystis* and *Ureaplasma*: A prospective study. Pediatrics 68:322, 1981.

Stagno S, Pifer LL, Hughes WT, et al: *Pneumocystis carinii* pneumonitis in young immunocompetent infants. Pediatrics 66:56, 1980.

Taber LH, Knight V, Gilbert BE, et al: Ribavirin aerosol treatment of bronchiolitis associated with respiratory syncytial virus infection in infants. Pediatrics 72:613, 1983.

Thureen PJ, Moreland S, Rodden DJ, et al: Failure of tracheal aspirate cultures to define the cause of respiratory deteriorations in neonates. Pediatr Infect Dis J 12:560, 1993.

Tyler CW, Albers WH: Obstetric factors related to bacteremia in the newborn infant. Am J Obstet Gynecol 94:970, 1966.

Ursi D, Ursi JP, Ieven M, et al: Congenital pneumonia due to *Mycoplasma* pneumonia. Arch Dis Child 72:F118, 1995.

Waites KB, Crouse DT, Philips JB, et al: Ureaplasmal pneumonia and sepsis associated with persistent pulmonary hypertension of the newborn. Pediatrics 83:84, 1989.

Webber S, Wilkinson AR, Lindsell D, et al: Neonatal pneumonia. Arch Dis Child 65:207, 1990.

Whitley RJ, Alford CA, Hirsch MS, et al: Vidarabine versus acyclovir therapy in herpes simplex encephalitis. N Engl J Med 314:144, 1986.

Whitley RJ, Nahmias AJ, Visintine AM, et al: The natural history of herpes simplex virus infection of mother and newborn. Pediatrics 66:489, 1980.

Yoder PR, Gibbs RS, Blanco JD, et al: A prospective controlled study of maternal and perinatal outcome after intra-amniotic infection at term. Am J Obstet Gynecol 145:695, 1983.

CHAPTER 57

Diseases of the Airways

Thomas Hansen and Anthony Corbet

Respiratory distress as a result of partial or complete obstruction of the nares or upper airway may present as a serious, life-threatening event shortly after birth. Infants who have no apparent respiratory distress when crying but who develop cyanosis and severe retractions when quiet or attempting to feed should be evaluated immediately for choanal atresia. The diagnosis may be more complex in the infant with inspiratory stridor or expiratory wheezing.

NASAL STENOSIS

With birth trauma, the nasal septum may become buckled or, less commonly, dislocated. Most cases respond to decongestant and steroid nasal drops, but dislocations require surgical manipulation (Presscott, 1995). In nasal piriform aperture stenosis, there is excessive bone formation in the nasal processes of the maxillary bone; there is severe obstruction and difficulty in passing a catheter. The obstruction is best demonstrated by computed tomography (CT) scan (Truong and Oudjhane, 1994). In most cases, the problem is resolved with nasal drops, but in more severe cases surgery to remove excessive bone and nasal stenting are required.

CHOANAL ATRESIA
Epidemiology

This malformation, caused by persistence of the bucconasal membrane, occurs in 1 per 10,000 births and has a significant female preponderance. About half the occurrences are bilateral, in which case there may be an immediate neonatal emergency. Associated anomalies are present in 50% of the cases (Hall, 1979), including the Treacher Collins syndrome. The most common collection of anomalies is called the *CHARGE association*, consisting of some combination of *c*olobomas of the eyes, congenital *h*eart disease, choanal *a*tresia, *r*etardation of physical and mental *g*rowth, and *e*ar anomalies associated with deafness (Pagon et al, 1981).

Diagnosis

Because newborns are preferential nose breathers for the first 2 to 3 weeks of life, bilateral choanal atresia is associated with chest retractions and severe cyanosis, particularly during feedings, and relieved only when the mouth is opened to cry. A catheter cannot be passed through the nose, and nasal instillation of radiopaque dye demonstrates obstruction. CT scan is the method of choice in making a definitive diagnosis.

Treatment

Emergency prophylaxis consists of endotracheal intubation. Although 90% of cases are bony, rather than membranous, in some the bone is soft and easily penetrated. Correction can be accomplished using the transnasal approach with either Hegar dilators (Stahl and Jurkiewicz, 1985) or a carbon dioxide surgical laser (Healy et al, 1978). After creating the appropriate airway, polyvinyl tubes are sutured in place to prevent subsequent closure. The tubes are lavaged with saline and suctioned, and after 6 weeks, they can be removed. This procedure is often definitive, or it can be followed by a transpalatal operation when the infant is much larger. If CT scan demonstrates a thick bony component, transpalatal surgery during the newborn period is probably the best method of correction.

PHARYNGEAL DEFORMITIES
Pierre Robin Syndrome

The Pierre Robin syndrome has an incidence of 1 per 2000 births. The major feature is micrognathia with posterior displacement of the tongue into the pharynx, but 60% of the patients also have a cleft palate. Hereditary transmission may be through a dominant gene with variable expressivity. Because the pharyngeal airway is narrowed, obstructive respiratory distress and cyanosis are common during the newborn period; these episodes may progress to dangerous spells of apnea (Cozzi and Pierro, 1985). Obstruction is common when the infant is in the supine position, during feeding, and in active sleep, when pharyngeal muscle tone is absent. Excessive air swallowing, followed by gastric distention, vomiting, and tracheal aspiration are frequent problems. The pharyngeal obstruction is maintained by the generation of large negative pressures in the lower pharynx during inspiration and swallowing (Fletcher et al, 1969). Chronic obstruction leads to carbon dioxide retention, failure to thrive, and development of pulmonary hypertension with right ventricular failure (Johnson and Todd, 1980).

In an emergency, tracheal intubation should be performed. It is now customary to pass a 3.5-mm tube through the nose and into the hypopharynx (Heaf et al, 1982). This prevents the generation of negative pressure and greatly relieves the respiratory difficulty. The nasopharyngeal tube may be left in place for weeks or even months with adequate lavage and suctioning. The infant should be placed in the prone position to prevent the tongue from falling backward. If a nasopharyngeal tube does not adequately relieve the obstruction, tracheotomy is indicated to prevent progression to cor pulmonale. Nutrition can be maintained with a hypercaloric formula fed by nasogastric tube or gastrostomy. With the passage of time, the problem becomes less threatening, especially after a few months, when the infant gains better control of the tongue (Mallory and Paradise, 1979). Oral feedings can be introduced, usually with a long lamb's nipple to help hold the tongue forward.

With adequate nutrition and growth of the mandible, the problem usually resolves by 6 to 12 months of age.

Glossoptosis-Apnea Syndrome

The Pierre Robin syndrome is not the only condition characterized by the tongue obstructing the airway. Infants with unilateral choanal atresia, choanal stenosis, or swelling of the nasal mucosa may generate large negative pressures in the pharynx and, in the absence of adequate muscular control over the tongue, may develop pharyngeal obstruction that causes respiratory distress, cyanosis, and severe episodes of apnea (Cozzi and Pierro, 1985).

Pharyngeal Incoordination

Pharyngeal incoordination causes choking and cyanosis with feedings and may be complicated by aspiration pneumonia (Avery and Fletcher, 1974). It may be seen in infants with severe hypoxic-ischemic encephalopathy and pseudobulbar palsy, in infants with Arnold-Chiari malformation, and in infants with Möbius syndrome. Although some infants may gradually improve, the long-term management includes tube feedings or even gastrostomy.

LARYNGEAL DEFORMITIES
Congenital Laryngeal Stridor

A relatively common condition, congenital laryngeal stridor (laryngomalacia) is due to the prolapse of poorly supported supraglottic structures, the arytenoids, aryepiglottic folds, and the epiglottis, into the airway during inspiration. Despite loud inspiratory stridor and significant chest retractions, usually from birth or the 1st month of life, the infant seldom has cyanosis, hypercarbia, notable feeding difficulty or growth failure, or abnormal cry (Richardson and Cotton, 1984). Congenital stridor is worse in the supine position with the neck flexed and better in the prone position with the neck extended (Cotton and Richardson, 1981). Obstruction is worse during episodes of agitation and better when the infant is calmed. Radiographic demonstration of prolapse of the aryepiglottic folds supports the diagnosis; ultrafast cine CT scan is effective at demonstrating the abnormalities without disturbance to the airway structures (Galvin et al, 1994). Confirmation may be obtained at laryngoscopy, but care must be taken not to fixate the supraglottic tissues with the instrument. Some practitioners prefer to pass a flexible fiberoptic bronchoscope through the nose. In some cases, gastroesophageal reflux or episodes of obstructive apnea may be associated with this condition (Belmont and Grundfast, 1984). About 18% of infants with a congenital lesion of the airway have a second lesion of some kind. Thus, the evaluation of stridor must include the examination of the entire upper aerodigestive tract (Friedman et al, 1984). The treatment is conservative, tracheostomy rarely being required, and the condition spontaneously improves over about 18 months (Smith and Catlin, 1984).

Vocal Cord Paralysis

Unilateral cord paralysis is usually left-sided; stridor and retractions are not marked, and the voice is weak and hoarse. The infant may cough and choke during feedings. The condition is due to a lesion involving the recurrent laryngeal nerve, perhaps caused by excessive stretching of the neck during delivery. Other possible causes include trauma from ligation of a patent ductus arteriosus (Davis et al, 1988). Right-sided vocal cord paralysis has been reported as a complication of extracorporeal membrane oxygenation (Schumacher et al, 1989), presumably as a result of the surgical dissection for insertion of the catheters. Stridor may be less if the infant lies on the paralyzed side, when the affected cord can fall away from the midline (Cotton and Richardson, 1981). The condition often tends to improve over a period of several weeks or months.

Bilateral cord paralysis is a much more serious condition, accompanied by serious inspiratory stridor. Frequently, however, the cry is normal. The diagnosis may be suspected at laryngoscopy and then confirmed with flexible fiberoptic bronchoscopy in the neonatal intensive care unit, rigid bronchoscopy in the operating room, or ultrafast cine CT scan in the radiology department. Associated problems may include pharyngeal incoordination with swallowing difficulty, recurrent apnea, and tracheal aspiration. Usually, severe central nervous system problems are also present, such as hypoxic-ischemic encephalopathy, cerebral hemorrhage, Arnold-Chiari malformation, hydrocephalus, or brain stem dysgenesis. The stridor may improve slowly if brain swelling subsides after birth. Tracheostomy is frequently required (Smith and Catlin, 1984), and the prognosis is usually poor.

Congenital Laryngeal Stenosis

The larynx may be partially obstructed by a web or cyst that causes inspiratory stridor from birth and a hoarse cry. The diagnosis of congenital laryngeal stenosis is made by laryngoscopy. Treatment consists of endoscopic lysis with microlaryngeal surgery or a carbon dioxide laser (Smith and Catlin, 1984). Usually, one application is sufficient to correct this difficulty, and the prognosis is excellent.

Laryngeal Atresia

In laryngeal atresia, the larynx may be completely obstructed by a web, seen in the delivery room during attempts to intubate the cyanotic infant. An endotracheal tube can sometimes be forced beyond the obstruction into the trachea. Otherwise a large-bore needle should be inserted percutaneously into the trachea to maintain marginal gas exchange while preparations for emergency tracheostomy are made. Most infants with laryngeal atresia have other lethal malformations (Smith and Catlin, 1984).

Congenital Subglottic Stenosis

Congenital subglottic stenosis is secondary to malformation of the cricoid cartilage. In severe cases, stridor is present from birth, and respiratory distress is obvious. In milder cases, excessive *croup* in an older infant may indicate the presence of this malformation (Healy et al, 1988; McGill, 1984).

Subglottic Hemangioma

Subglottic hemangioma, often in association with cutaneous hemangioma, may cause inspiratory stridor and expiratory wheezing, which progress with slow enlargement of the tumor (Cotton and Richardson, 1981). Although some have advocated high-dose corticosteroid therapy (Brown et al, 1972), intubation or tracheostomy is usually required. Results of removal by carbon dioxide laser have been encouraging (Healy and McGill, 1984) and have enabled treatment without tracheostomy in many cases.

Acquired Subglottic Stenosis

Extubation after prolonged endotracheal intubation is sometimes followed by inspiratory stridor and expiratory wheezing, produced by subglottic edema and fibrosis. The risk is greatest in infants who have had tightly fitting endotracheal tubes, frequent intubations, and prolonged intubation and mechanical ventilation (Downing and Kilbride, 1995; Sherman et al, 1986). The initial evaluation of these patients may be performed with a flexible bronchoscope after extubation in the neonatal intensive care unit.

For management of this condition, adequate humidification of inspired gas; nebulization of racemic epinephrine; and systemic, nebulized, or topical dexamethasone have proved useful. In cases with no response to these measures, reintubation with a smaller endotracheal tube for a short period, while growth occurs, may be helpful. Couser and associates (1992) reported the results of a controlled trial in which three doses of dexamethasone were given, starting 4 hours before extubation, to premature infants at high risk for subglottic edema; the incidence of stridor in the treated group was greatly reduced.

Difficult cases should be evaluated by rigid bronchoscopy and in some cases by ultrafast cine CT scan. In some infants, an anterior cricoid split procedure may be successful (Seid and Canty, 1985). In this operation, a vertical incision is made in the cricoid and first two tracheal cartilages, after which the airway is stented open with a larger endotracheal tube, which prevents the cut ends of the cartilage from abutting. The tube is maintained in place for 7 to 14 days, with the help of heavy sedation, and then removed under cover of steroid treatment (Tavin et al, 1994). More severely affected infants may require tracheostomy, followed by a formal surgical procedure with rib grafts to reconstruct the subglottic space later in life (Rowe et al, 1991).

Laryngotracheoesophageal Cleft

In laryngotracheoesophageal cleft, a longitudinal communication is present between the airway and esophagus, stretching from the larynx into the upper trachea or sometimes as far as the carina. Such infants have respiratory distress and cyanosis, associated with tracheal aspiration of saliva and feedings. The chest radiograph may show evidence of aspiration pneumonia, and the cine esophagogram shows contrast material spilling into the trachea. The airway must be adequately secured with an endotracheal tube or tracheostomy (Richardson and Cotton, 1984); an esophagostomy diverts saliva, and feedings should be accomplished by gastric division and gastrostomy. Attempts at operative repair through a lateral pharyngotomy, and thoracotomy if necessary, have been successful in a few infants (Burroughs and Leape, 1974; Cotton and Schreiber, 1981).

TRACHEAL DEFORMITIES
Tracheal Agenesis Syndrome

In this rare condition, the trachea is atretic just below the vocal cords, or it is absent all the way down to the carina (Altman et al, 1972). These infants usually have a tracheoesophageal fistula as well as severe cardiac malformations. Despite the presence of a larynx, intubation cannot be accomplished; however, if the tracheal tube is positioned in the esophagus and connected to a mechanical ventilator, reasonable gas exchange can be obtained through the tracheoesophageal fistula. When the atresia is high, a tracheostomy can be done. If survival seems possible, gastric division and a gastrostomy for feeding should be performed. Reconstructive surgery is not likely to be successful, however, and the prognosis is extremely poor.

Congenital Tracheal Stenosis

In congenital tracheal stenosis, a segment of the trachea is narrowed, usually starting in the subglottic region and producing inspiratory stridor, expiratory wheezing, and often cyanotic episodes. The segment may be short or long; occasionally the entire trachea is hypoplastic, and the bronchi may be involved. The narrowing is caused by complete or nearly complete tracheal cartilage rings. Mild inflammation and small mucus plugs may cause life-threatening deterioration. In many cases, other congenital malformations are also present, such as vascular ring anomalies, congenital heart defects, tracheoesophageal fistula, especially the H type, and hemivertebrae (Benjamin et al, 1981); there is also an association with pulmonary agenesis (Voland et al, 1986). A series of cases without accompanying defects has been reported in premature infants, who presented with difficulties at tracheal intubation (Hauft et al, 1988).

Patients with this deformity can usually be intubated, but the endotracheal tube cannot be advanced and should not be forced; mechanical ventilation with generous levels of positive end-expiratory pressure may be helpful to stabilize the infant. Tracheostomy is not indicated and interferes with making the diagnosis (Nakayama et al, 1982). Sometimes the diagnosis can be made by chest radiographs, with air as the contrast medium, with inspiration and expiration films, and with high-kilovolt techniques, the so-called lateral airways xeroradiogram (Benjamin, 1980), and fluoroscopy is often useful (Lobe et al, 1987); flexible fiberoptic bronchoscopy in the neonatal intensive care unit or rigid bronchoscopy in the operating room is usually required. Because it is important to examine the lower limits of the stenosis, it is necessary to proceed with tracheobronchography, but this may sometimes cause acute decompensation (Loeff et al, 1988). As an alternative, ultrafast cine CT scan has been developed as a useful diagnostic technique to define the lower limits of stenosis (Galvin et al, 1994).

In most cases, the stenosis requires treatment of some kind in the operating room: simple balloon dilation at rigid bronchoscopy for short stenoses and segmental excision or tracheoplasty for longer stenoses. Balloon dilation is not likely to be successful in the case of a complete tracheal cartilage ring because cartilage cannot be stretched, but forcible balloon dilation and tracheal splitting through a bronchoscope has been accomplished (Messineo et al, 1992). Longaker and colleagues (1990) described segmental resection of the stenosis with end-to-end anastomosis, followed by serial balloon dilations through a rigid bronchoscope; they resected nearly two thirds of the tracheal length and claimed that the residual stenosis would grow without restenosis. Sasaki and coworkers (1992) described the use of esophagus for tracheoplasty in patients with a long tracheal stenosis and believed that collapse of this tissue into the tracheal lumen was not a large problem. Lobe and colleagues (1987) described the successful use of cartilage grafts for tracheoplasty; they used ingenious anesthesia techniques for operating on the major airway, and they described the use of an endotracheal tube as an internal stent for 3 weeks postoperatively.

The use of cardiopulmonary bypass has improved treatment in many cases and may avert the need for complex anesthesiology techniques (Loeff et al, 1988). After resection or tracheoplasty, the patient may need fixation in a brace for at least 6 weeks to maintain neck flexion and prevent tension on the anastomosis suture line (Nakayama et al, 1982).

RUPTURE OF THE TRACHEA

This uncommon lesion may occur just below the cords as a result of severe traction with a difficult delivery; the infant presents with pneumomediastinum, pneumothorax, or subcutaneous emphysema, accompanied by other signs of birth trauma such as vocal cord, brachial, or phrenic palsy (Hogason et al, 1992). Tracheal intubation may be difficult because the trachea bends at the site of injury. At flexible fiberoptic bronchoscopy, the endotracheal tube can be positioned past the rupture and maintained in position using a total body brace for 10 to 14 days to ensure adequate healing. If tracheal stenosis occurs, this can later be resected with end-to-end anastomosis, making use of cardiopulmonary bypass if necessary.

ACQUIRED TRACHEOBRONCHIAL STENOSIS

Lesions of of the trachea and main bronchi are being increasingly recognized as acquired complications of prolonged intubation of infants in the neonatal intensive care unit. These lesions are thought to be inflammatory, related to movement of the endotracheal tube and suction catheter. To prevent these problems, the endotracheal tube should be adequately fixed in position, and it is recommended that in routine suctioning the catheter should not be pushed past the end of the endotracheal tube (Bailey et al, 1988). These cases may be suspected in infants with recurrent lobar atelectasis, emphysema, or both, especially of the right lower lobe; with difficulties after extubation; or with a resistance noted during use of the suction catheter (Friedberg and Forte, 1987). Most of these lesions are just

above or below the carina. The usual time of diagnosis is about 4 weeks of age.

The initial diagnostic approach may be with flexible fiberoptic bronchoscopy in the neonatal intensive care unit or rigid bronchoscopy in the operating room, but these infants are often in poor condition, and the best way to establish the length of the stenosis is by contrast tracheobronchography performed in the neonatal intensive care unit. This procedure has been described by Betremieux and coworkers (1995). A fine catheter filled with water-soluble contrast material is positioned with its tip precisely at the end of the endotracheal tube; 0.2 mL contrast material is injected rapidly followed by 5 mL of air, then two plain films are taken with 30 seconds of bag tube ventilation in between; the contrast material is suctioned, and mechanical ventilation is resumed. In a significant number of infants, the findings suggest mucus plug obstruction, which responds to chest physical therapy, and further investigation can be avoided.

Mild inflammatory stenoses may respond to topical or inhaled steroids or racemic epinephrine, and systemic steroids may be used (Elkerbout et al, 1993). In some cases, granuloma tissue has been biopsy excised through the rigid bronchoscope (Miller et al, 1987) or subjected to electroresection (Greenholz et al, 1987). In those with a mature stenosis, balloon dilation may be undertaken with rigid bronchoscopy in the operating room; several operative sessions may be needed. The success rate is only 50%, however, and the mortality rate is as high as 33% (Betremieux et al, 1995). Alternatively, dilations may be accomplished with bougies through a rigid bronchoscope, which may allow a better feel for the operator (Albert, 1995). These infants are small and premature and have frequent complications, such as bronchopulmonary dysplasia and infection; a greatly feared risk is airway rupture by the dilation procedure. The use of alternative strategies, such as carbon dioxide laser, operative stenting, and surgical resection with grafting, is limited by the small size and severe illness of these infants. If the stenosis is short, however, as is often the case, resection with end-to-end anastomosis can be accomplished with skilled anesthesiology techniques (Albert, 1995). As a last resort, cadaver tracheal transplantation or live donor heart-lung transplantation may be considered in larger and older infants.

Tracheobronchomalacia

Rarely, development of tracheal cartilage support may be delayed, resulting in tracheobronchomalacia, a condition characterized by expiratory wheezing and respiratory distress. The chest radiograph shows diffuse overinflation. The abnormalities of the trachea can be well demonstrated with ultrafast cine CT scan (Galvin et al, 1994; Kimura et al, 1990); in particular, a good idea of the peripheral extent of the lesion can be obtained. At bronchoscopy, the anterior and posterior walls of the trachea are approximated during expiration (Salzberg, 1983). The bronchoscope may support the walls of the trachea, so the respiratory distress may be alleviated by passage of the bronchoscope to the carina, but this may disguise the extent of the abnormalities.

Many affected infants with tracheomalacia improve by 6 to 12 months of age. Severe cases may benefit from tracheostomy and treatment with continuous positive airway pressure, which prevents tracheal collapse. Prolonged treatment for 1 to 2 years may be required (Wiseman et al, 1985). Prolonged tracheostomy by itself may be useful, with the tube acting as a stent for the compliant trachea (Cogbill et al, 1983), but this is less useful when the bronchi are also involved. In some cases, a special long tracheostomy tube has been successful, even with bronchial involvement (Zinman, 1995).

A strong association with tracheoesophageal fistula has been reported (Benjamin et al, 1976), but tracheomalacia does not occur in patients with esophageal atresia without a fistulous connection to the trachea (Rideout et al, 1991). Filler and associates (1992) have reported a large series of infants in which the flaccid trachea was compressed between the aorta anteriorly and the dilated esophagus posteriorly; most of these patients responded to aortopexy, fixation of the aorta to the sternum, which has the effect of supporting the attached trachea. An alternative is tracheopexy, in which the trachea is fixed directly to the sternum (Benjamin et al, 1976).

Tracheomalacia has been seen in respirator-dependent infants with bronchopulmonary dysplasia (Sotomayor et al, 1986), who present with severe cyanotic episodes (bronchopulmonary dysplasia spells). Many of these patients also have gastroesophageal reflux (Jacobs et al, 1994). Penn and colleagues (1988) have described the effect of prolonged mechanical ventilation in lamb tracheas and demonstrated increased collapse and increased flow resistance correlated with deformation of the trachea. The trachea of premature infants is compliant and may be excessively stretched during mechanical ventilation; because the tracheal compliance decreases with maturity, it is the very immature infant who is prone to tracheomalacia. Some premature infants have greatly enlarged tracheas or tracheomegaly after mechanical ventilation (Bhutani et al, 1986). Downing and Kilbride (1995) found that the factors associated with the development of tracheomalacia were immaturity, higher mean airway pressure, and prolonged mechanical ventilation. Infants with bronchopulmonary dysplasia and tracheomalacia may have significant dynamic compression of the trachea from reactive lower airway disease with forceful expiration and thus gain some improvement from bronchodilator therapy. Increased smooth muscle tone may help support the trachea during expiration, so bronchodilator therapy may sometimes make the situation worse (McCubbin et al, 1989).

Flexible bronchoscopy in the neonatal intensive care unit, with the patient still intubated and breathing spontaneously, is an excellent way to evaluate the problem (Wood, 1985); in the case of rigid bronchoscopy in the operating room, collapse of the trachea may be abolished by positive pressure from the ventilator, and dynamic compression of the trachea may be abolished by general anesthesia (Jacobs et al, 1994). Ultrafast cine CT scan has also proved invaluable to help establish this diagnosis if the infant can go to the radiology department.

The usual treatment is continued tracheal intubation with high levels of continuous positive airway pressure or positive end-expiratory pressure with mechanical ventilation and empiric attempts to wean as the infant grows older (Jacobs et al, 1994). Many of these patients must have a tracheostomy to avoid laryngeal complications. McCoy and colleagues (1992) described a group of infants with bronchopulmonary dysplasia and severe cyanotic spells during episodes of agitation; they observed tracheal collapse at flexible bronchoscopy, initiated by agitation and relieved by soothing the patient or by sedation; thus, adequate sedation is an important part of management in patients with bronchopulmonary dysplasia spells. Many of the most severely affected patients respond well to aortopexy (McCoy et al, 1992).

Malignant Lobar Hyperexpansion in Bronchopulmonary Dysplasia

Azizkhan and colleagues (1992) have described a condition they called *acquired lobar hyperinflation* in infants with bronchopulmonary dysplasia; this condition was due to bronchomalacia with diffuse involvement but more severe involvement in the affected lung lobe. These patients were evaluated by ultrathin flexible videobronchoscopy, performed during mechanical ventilation. Selective intubation of the less involved lung provided only transient benefit. These patients can sometimes be managed medically, but many benefit immediately from surgical lobectomy; a few infants are operated on under emergency circumstances, with malignant hyperexpansion of the affected lobe and compression of surrounding lung. In general, the results of surgery may be good, although some patients eventually die from underlying bronchopulmonary dysplasia and its complications.

VASCULAR RINGS

The trachea may be compressed by (1) a double aortic arch, (2) a right aortic arch, (3) left-sided origin of the innominate artery or right-sided origin of the left common carotid artery, or (4) an anomalous origin of the left pulmonary artery from the right pulmonary artery (Hendren and Kim, 1978). With a right aortic arch, the trachea is compressed by the main pulmonary trunk, aortic arch, and ligamentum arteriosus. The anomalous innominate or carotid arteries form a tight crotch, which impinges on the anterior trachea. The anomalous left pulmonary artery returns to the left by passing between the esophagus and trachea, compressing the trachea between the right and left pulmonary arteries. Infants with tracheal compression have inspiratory stridor and expiratory wheezing. The onset of symptoms is usually later in the neonatal period. These infants often lie with the head and neck hyperextended to stretch the trachea and make it less compressible. If the esophagus is compressed, feeding is associated with regurgitation. The chest radiograph may show mild overinflation; a right-sided aorta; and, with appropriate technique, evidence of tracheal narrowing. A barium swallow examination may show indentation of the esophagus. Magnetic resonance imaging has proved to be accurate in defining most vascular malformations compressing the airway. Bronchoscopy should reveal a pulsatile mass at the carina, and echocardiography confirms the diagnosis. After surgical relief, the respiratory distress may persist for weeks or longer because of localized tracheal deformity, either stenosis or tracheomalacia, and in some cases a second operation may be required to repair the trachea further.

TRACHEAL COMPRESSION BY EXTRINSIC MASSES

The trachea may be compressed by a bronchogenic cyst, an enteric or duplication cyst, or a neurogenic tumor or teratoma (Benjamin, 1980). These may be demonstrated by anterior and lateral chest films and especially well by CT scan. They may also compress the esophagus and be demonstrated with a barium swallow.

BRONCHOSCOPY AND BRONCHOGRAPHY

Albert (1995) has described the advantages and disadvantages of the methods used in the diagnostic approach to tracheobronchial obstructions. The instillation of nonionic contrast material for tracheobronchography does not seem to cause serious bronchospasm and, despite the iodine, does not seem to affect thyroid function seriously in premature infants. The lower trachea and main bronchi beyond the stenosis are well demonstrated. The technique does not differentiate a soft stenosis with granulation tissue from a hard stenosis owing to fibrosis, and because it is two-dimensional, it does not identify a complete tracheal ring in congenital stenosis. An advantage is that it can be performed in the neonatal intensive care unit (Betremieux et al, 1995).

Flexible fiberoptic bronchoscopy can also be performed in the neonatal intensive care unit, usually after a period of hyperoxygenation to prevent oxygen desaturation. The instrument may be passed for short intervals through the endotracheal tube during mechanical ventilation (Dab et al, 1993); the smallest available flexible bronchoscope is 2.2-mm outside diameter; it does not have a suction channel; however, it does have the capacity for distal angulation, and it can be passed through a 3.0-mm internal diameter endotracheal tube for brief periods of time. Flexible bronchoscopy can differentiate soft from hard stenoses, in contrast to tracheobronchography, and the instrument may sometimes penetrate easily beyond the stenosis; the image is of lower quality than that with a rigid bronchoscope, however, and continued ventilation is not always easily accomplished. Two other ultrathin flexible bronchoscopes are also available (1.8-mm and 2.3-mm outside diameter), but they do not have a suction channel (Wood, 1985), although they do now have the capacity for modest distal angulation. These instruments can be passed through a small 2.5-mm internal diameter endotracheal tube during mechanical ventilation to evaluate the lower trachea and the main bronchi of very small infants; they can be advanced and withdrawn repeatedly to assist in the maintenance of adequate ventilation; they may be most useful to evaluate obstruction from granulation tissue or tracheobronchomalacia in infants with bronchopulmonary dysplasia. A 2.7-mm outside diameter flexible bronchoscope with capacity for better distal angulation is also available (Wood, 1985); this can be passed through a 3.5-mm internal diameter endotracheal tube to examine the lower trachea, main bronchi, and segmental bronchi of larger infants, but there

is no suction channel. The standard pediatric flexible bronchoscope is 3.5-mm outside diameter, and it has a 1.2-mm suction channel for removal of mucus plugs. All flexible bronchoscopes can be used with reasonable quality video recording, so the examinations can be played back later (Wood, 1985).

The rigid bronchoscope with a glass rod telescope requires transfer to the operating room, extubation, and general anesthesia. It, however, gives a better image, anesthesia and ventilation are easily maintained through the bronchoscope, suction is available, biopsies can be performed, solutions can be injected, and it can be used for balloon or bougie dilation procedures. The smallest available rigid bronchoscope is 2.5-mm outside diameter.

REFERENCES

Albert D: Management of suspected tracheobronchial stenosis in ventilated neonates. Arch Dis Child 72:F1, 1995.

Altman RP, Randolph JG, Shearin RB: Tracheal agenesis: Recognition and management. J Pediatr Surg 7:112, 1972.

Avery ME, Fletcher BD: The Lung and Its Disorders in the Newborn Infant. Philadelphia, WB Saunders, 1974.

Azizkhan RG, Grimmer DL, Askin FB, et al: Acquired lobar emphysema (overinflation): Clinical and pathological evaluation of infants requiring lobectomy. J Pediatr Surg 27:1145, 1992.

Bailey C, Kattwinkel J, Teja K, Buckley T: Shallow versus deep endotracheal suctioning in young rabbits: Pathologic effects on the tracheobronchial wall. Pediatrics 82:746, 1988.

Belmont JR, Grundfast K: Congenital laryngeal stridor (laryngomalacia): Etiologic factors and associated disorders. Ann Otol Rhinol Laryngol 93:430, 1984.

Benjamin B: Endoscopy in congenital tracheal anomalies. J Pediatr Surg 15:164, 1980.

Benjamin B, Cohen D, Glasson M: Tracheomalacia in association with congenital tracheo-esophageal fistula. Surgery 79:504, 1976.

Benjamin B, Pitkin J, Cohen D: Congenital tracheal stenosis. Ann Otol Rhinol Laryngol 90:364, 1981.

Betremieux P, Treguier C, Pladys P, et al: Tracheobronchography and balloon dilatation in acquired neonatal tracheal stenosis. Arch Dis Child 72:F3, 1995.

Bhutani VK, Ritchie WG, Shaffer TH: Acquired tracheomegaly in very preterm infants. Am J Dis Child 140:449, 1986.

Brown SH, Neerhout RC, Fonkalsrud EW: Prednisone therapy in the management of large hemangiomas in infants and children. Surgery 71:168, 1972.

Burroughs N, Leape LL: Laryngotracheoesophageal cleft: Report of a case successfully treated and review of the literature. Pediatrics 53:516, 1974.

Cogbill TH, Moore FA, Accurso FJ, et al: Primary tracheomalacia. Ann Thorac Surg 35:538, 1983.

Cohn RC, Kercsmar C, Dearborn D: Safety and flexibility of flexible endoscopy in children with bronchopulmonary dysplasia. Am J Dis Child 142:1225, 1988.

Cotton RT, Richardson MA: Congenital laryngeal anomalies. Otolaryngol Clin North Am 14:203, 1981.

Cotton RT, Schreiber JH: Management of laryngotracheoesophageal cleft. Ann Otol 90:401, 1981.

Couser RJ, Ferrara TB, Falde B, et al: Effectiveness of dexamethasone in preventing extubation failure in preterm infants at increased risk for airway edema. J Pediatr 121:591, 1992.

Cozzi F, Pierro A: Glossoptosis-apnea syndrome in infancy. Pediatrics 75:836, 1985.

Crockett DM, Healy GB, McGill TJ, et al: Computed tomography in the evaluation of choanal atresia in infants and children. Laryngoscope 97:174, 1987.

Dab I, Malfroot A, Goosens A: Therapeutic bronchoscopy in ventilated neonates. Arch Dis Child 69:533, 1993.

Davis JT, Baciewicz FA, Suriyapa S, et al: Vocal cord paralysis in premature infants undergoing ductal closure. Ann Thorac Surg 46:214, 1988.

Douglas B: The treatment of micrognathia associated with obstruction by a plastic procedure. Plast Reconstr Surg 1:300, 1946.

Downing GJ, Kilbride HW: Evaluation of airway complications in high risk preterm infants: Application of flexible fiberoptic airway endoscopy. Pediatrics 95:567, 1995.

Elkerbout SC, van Lingen RA, Gerritsen J, Roorda RJ: Endoscopic balloon dilatation of acquired airway stenosis in newborn infants: A promising treatment. Arch Dis Child 68:37, 1993.

Filler RM, Messineo A, Vinograd I: Severe tracheomalacia associated with esophageal atresia: Results of surgical treatment. J Pediatr Surg 27:1136, 1992.

Fletcher MM, Blum SL, Blanchard CL: Pierre-Robin syndrome: Pathophysiology of obstructive episodes. Laryngoscope 79:547, 1969.

Friedberg J, Forte V: Acquired bronchial injury in neonates. Int J Pediatr Otorhinolaryngol 14:223, 1987.

Friedman EM, Williams M, Healy GB, et al: Pediatric endoscopy: A review of 616 cases. Ann Otol 93:517, 1984.

Friedman EM, Vastola AD, McGill TJ, et al: Chronic pediatric stridor: Etiology and outcome. Laryngoscope 100:277, 1990.

Galvin JR, Gingrich RD, Hoffman E, et al: Ultrafast computed tomography of the chest. Radiol Clin North Am 32:775, 1994.

Greenholz SK, Hall RJ, Lilly JR, Shikes RH: Surgical implications of bronchopulmonary dysplasia. J Pediatr Surg 22:1132, 1987.

Hall BD: Choanal atresia and associated multiple anomalies. J Pediatr 95:395, 1979.

Hauft SM, Perlman JM, Siegel MJ, et al: Tracheal stenosis in the sick premature infant: Clinical and radiologic features. Am J Dis Child 142:206, 1988.

Heaf DP, Helms PJ, Dimwiddie R, et al: Nasopharyngeal airways in Pierre Robin syndrome. J. Pediatr 100:698, 1982.

Healy GB: Subglottic stenosis. Otolaryngol Clin North Am 22:599, 1989.

Healy GB, McGill T: CO₂ laser in subglottic hemangioma—an update. Ann Otol Rhinol Laryngol 93:270, 1984.

Healy GB, McGill T, Jako GJ, et al: Management of choanal atresia with the carbon-dioxide laser. Ann Otol Rhinol Laryngol 87:658, 1978.

Healy GB, Schuster SR, Jonas RA, et al: Correction of segmental tracheal stenosis in children. Ann Otol Rhinol Laryngol 97:444, 1988.

Hendren WH, Kim SH: Pediatric thoracic surgery. *In* Scarpelli EM, Auld PAM, Goldman HS (Eds): Pulmonary Disease of the Fetus and Newborn and Child. Philadelphia, Lea & Febiger, 1978, p 166.

Hogason AKM, Boe G, Finne PH: Rupture of the trachea: An unusual complication of delivery. Acta Paediatr 81:944, 1992.

Jacobs IN, Wetmore RF, Tom LWC, et al: Tracheobronchomalacia in children. Arch Otolaryngol Head Neck Surg 120:154, 1994.

Johnson GM, Todd DW: Cor pulmonale in severe Pierre Robin syndrome. Pediatrics 65:152, 1980.

Kimura K, Soper RT, Kao SCS, et al: Aortosternopexy for tracheomalacia following repair of esophageal atresia: Evaluation by cine CT and technical refinement. J Pediatr Surg 25:769, 1990.

Lobe tracheoesophageal, Hayden CK, Nicolas D, Richardson CJ: Successful management of congenital tracheal stenosis in infancy. J Pediatr Surg 22:1137, 1987.

Loeff DS, Filler RM, Vinograd I, et al: Congenital tracheal stenosis: A review of 22 patients from 1965 to 1987. J Pediatr Surg 23:744, 1988.

Longaker MT, Harrison MR, Adzick NS: Testing the limits of neonatal tracheal resection. J Pediatr Surg 25:790, 1990.

Mallory SF, Paradise JL: Glossoptosis revisited: On the development and resolution of airway obstruction in the Pierre Robin syndrome. Pediatrics 64:946, 1979.

McCoy KS, Bagwell CE, Wagner M, et al: Spirometric and endoscopic evaluation of airway collapse in infants with bronchopulmonary dysplasia. Pediatr Pulmonol 14:23, 1992.

McCubbin M, Frey EE, Wagener JS, et al: Large airway collapse in bronchopulmonary dysplasia. J Pediatr 114:304, 1989.

McGill T: Congenital diseases of the larynx. Otolaryngol Clin North Am 17:57, 1984.

McGovern FH: Bilateral choanal atresia: A new method of management. Laryngoscope 71:480, 1961.

Messineo A, Forte V, Joseph T, et al: The balloon posterior tracheal split: A technique for managing tracheal stenosis in the premature infant. J Pediatr Surg 27:1142, 1992.

Miller RW, Woo P, Kellman RK, Slagle TS: Tracheobronchial abnormalities in infants with bronchopulmonary dysplasia. J Pediatr 111:779, 1987.

Nakayama DK, Harrison MR, deLorimier AA, et al: Reconstructive surgery of obstructing lesions of the intrathoracic trachea in infants and small children. J Pediatr Surg 17:854, 1982.

Pagon RA, Graham JM, Zonana J, et al: Coloboma, congenital heart disease, and choanal atresia with multiple anomalies: CHARGE association. J Pediatr 99:223, 1981.

Penn RB, Wolfson MR, Shaffer TH: Effect of ventilation on mechanical properties and pressure flow relationships of immature airways. Pediatr Res 23:519, 1988.

Presscott CAJ: Nasal obstruction in infancy. Arch Dis Child 72:287, 1995.

Richardson MA, Cotton RT: Anatomic abnormalities of the pediatric airway. Pediatr Clin North Am 31:821, 1984.

Rideout DT, Hayashi AH, Gillis DA, et al: The absence of clinically tracheomalacia in patients having esophageal atresia without tracheoesophageal fistula. J Pediatr Surg 26:1303, 1991.

Rowe RW, Betts J, Free E: Peri-operative management of laryngotracheal reconstruction. Anesth Analg 73:483, 1991.

Saltzberg AM: Congenital malformations of the lower respiratory tract. *In* Kendig EL, Chernick V (Eds): Disorders of the Respiratory Tract in Children. Philadelphia, WB Saunders, 1983, p 169.

Sasaki S, Hara F, Ohwa T, et al: Esophageal tracheoplasty for congenital tracheal stenosis. J Pediatr Surg 27:645, 1992.

Schumacher RE, Weinfeld IJ, Bartlett RH: Neonatal vocal cord paralysis following extracorporeal membrane oxygenation. Pediatrics 84:793, 1989.

Seid AB, Canty TG: The anterior cricoid split procedure for the management of subglottic stenosis in infants and children. J Pediatr Surg 20:388, 1985.

Sherman JM, Lowitt S, Stephenson C, et al: Factors influencing acquired subglottic stenosis in infants. J Pediatr 109:322, 1986.

Smith RJH, Catlin FI: Congenital anomalies of the larynx. Am J Dis Child 138:35, 1984.

Sotomayor JL, Godinez RI, Borden S, et al: Large airway collapse due to acquired tracheobronchomalacia in infancy. Am J Dis Child 140:367, 1986.

Stahl RS, Jurkiewicz MJ: Congenital posterior choanal atresia. Pediatrics 76:429, 1985.

Stern LM, Fonkalsrud EW, Hassakis P, et al: Management of Pierre Robin syndrome in infancy by prolonged naso-esophageal intubation. Am J Dis Child 124:79, 1972.

Tavin E, Singer L, Bassila M: Problems in postoperative management after anterior cricoid split. Arch Otolaryngol Head Neck Surg 120:823, 1994.

Truong DT, Oudjhane K: Anterior nasal stenosis as a cause of neonatal nasal airway obstruction. Arch Pediatr Adolesc Med 148:279, 1994.

Voland JR, Benirschke K, Saunders B: Congenital tracheal stenosis with associated cardiopulmonary anomalies: Report of 2 cases with a review of the literature. Pediatr Pulmonol 2:247, 1986.

Wiseman NE, Duncan PG, Cameron CB: Management of tracheobronchomalacia with continuous positive airway pressure. J Pediatr Surg 20:489, 1985.

Wood RE: Clinical applications of ultrathin flexible bronchoscopes. Pediatr Pulmonol 1:244, 1985.

Zinman R: Tracheal stenting improves airway mechanics in infants with tracheobronchomalacia. Pediatr Pulmonol 19:275, 1995.

CHAPTER 58

Malformations of the Mediastinum and Lung Parenchyma

Thomas Hansen, Anthony Corbet and Mary Ellen Avery

CONGENITAL PULMONARY CYSTS

Most pulmonary cysts in the newborn are pneumatoceles, acquired after pneumonia or during the course of pulmonary interstitial emphysema or bronchopulmonary dysplasia. Congenital cysts are much less common; they may be single or multiple but are always confined to one lobe of the lung; and other organs are not affected by cystic changes. Although acquired cysts tend to disappear with time, congenital cysts are persistent. All cysts have a communication with the peripheral airways, and for this reason they are filled with air except at birth, when they may be filled with fluid for several hours after birth.

Diagnosis

Newborns who develop signs of cystic disease of the lungs usually manifest the effects of rapid expansion of the cysts. The most common presentation is with air trapping, tension cyst, pneumothorax, and severe respiratory distress that requires lobectomy (Gwinn et al, 1970). Tachypnea or respiratory distress may begin at birth or any time thereafter and progress rapidly or slowly; the infant's condition may become critical within hours or remain static for weeks or months. In a few cases, older infants may present with recurrent episodes of pneumonia; it may then be difficult to decide whether the cyst is congenital or acquired (Figs. 58–1 through 58–3).

Radiographic Findings

Large balloon cysts filled with air under tension are often mistaken for a tension pneumothorax. One hemithorax is overfilled, the diaphragm is flattened or even concave, and the mediastinum and heart are pushed to the contralateral side. Points that may distinguish balloon cysts from a pneumothorax are (1) a delicate linear pattern within the translucent area denoting the cyst's fine trabeculation, which is not present in the case of a pneumothorax; (2) the presence of compressed lung at the apex and at the costophrenic and cardiohepatic angles, often demarcated from the cyst by a curving line visible in one or another projection; and (3) the absence of all hilar shadows. In pneumothorax, the collapsed lung is often visible as a dense shadow projecting from the hilar region or upward from the diaphragm. It may be difficult to distinguish between congenital pulmonary cyst and congenital lobar emphysema; a chest com-

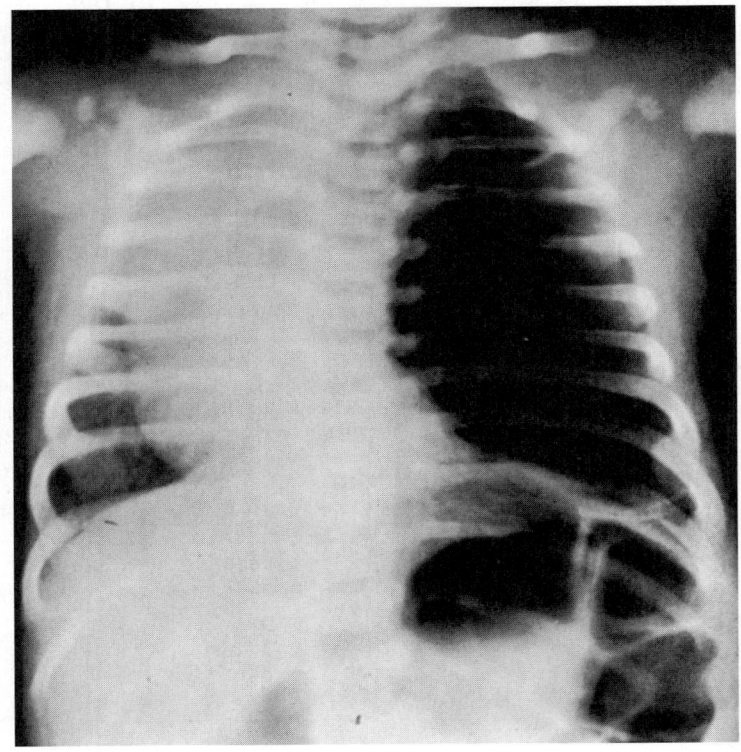

FIGURE 58–1. Anteroposterior chest film made at 8 weeks of age. Note the shift of heart and mediastinum far to the right, herniation of left lung into right hemithorax, and deviation of trachea to the right. The overfilled, overaerated left hemithorax suggests the appearance of tension cyst rather than pneumothorax because the left hilus is empty and the lower border is curved. No collapsed lung can be seen. (From Hill LF: Conference at Raymond Blank Memorial Hospital for Children, Des Moines, Iowa. J Pediatr 38:511, 1951.)

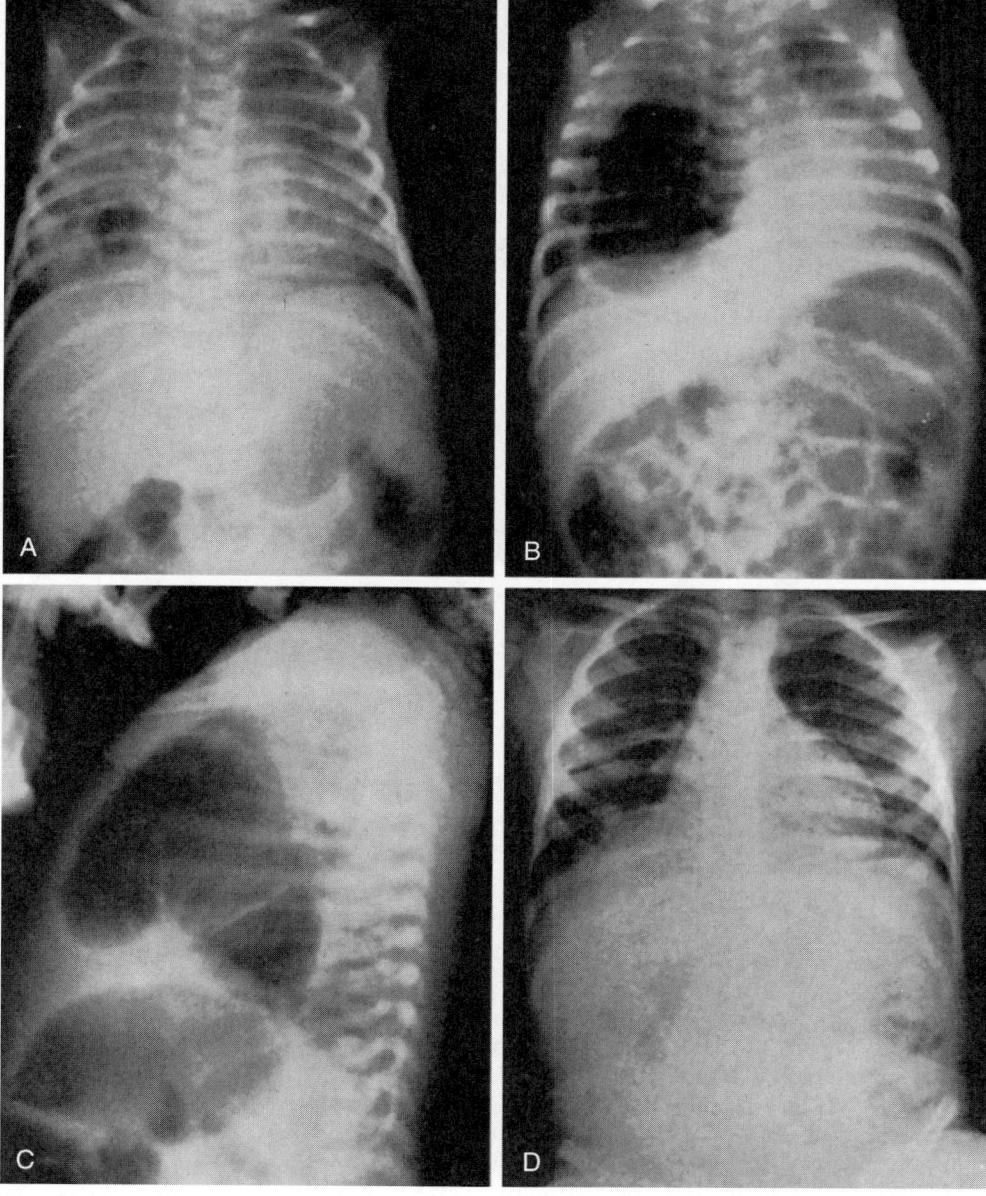

FIGURE 58–2. *A*, Anteroposterior view of the chest taken on the 21st day of life. An air-filled cyst can be seen in the right lower part of the chest. *B* and *C*, Thirty days later, showing great increase in size of cyst and dislocation of heart toward the left axilla. *D*, Anteroposterior view at the age of 3 years. The lungs appear essentially normal. (From Swan H, Aragon GE: Surgical treatment of pulmonary cysts in infancy. Pediatrics 14:651, 1954.)

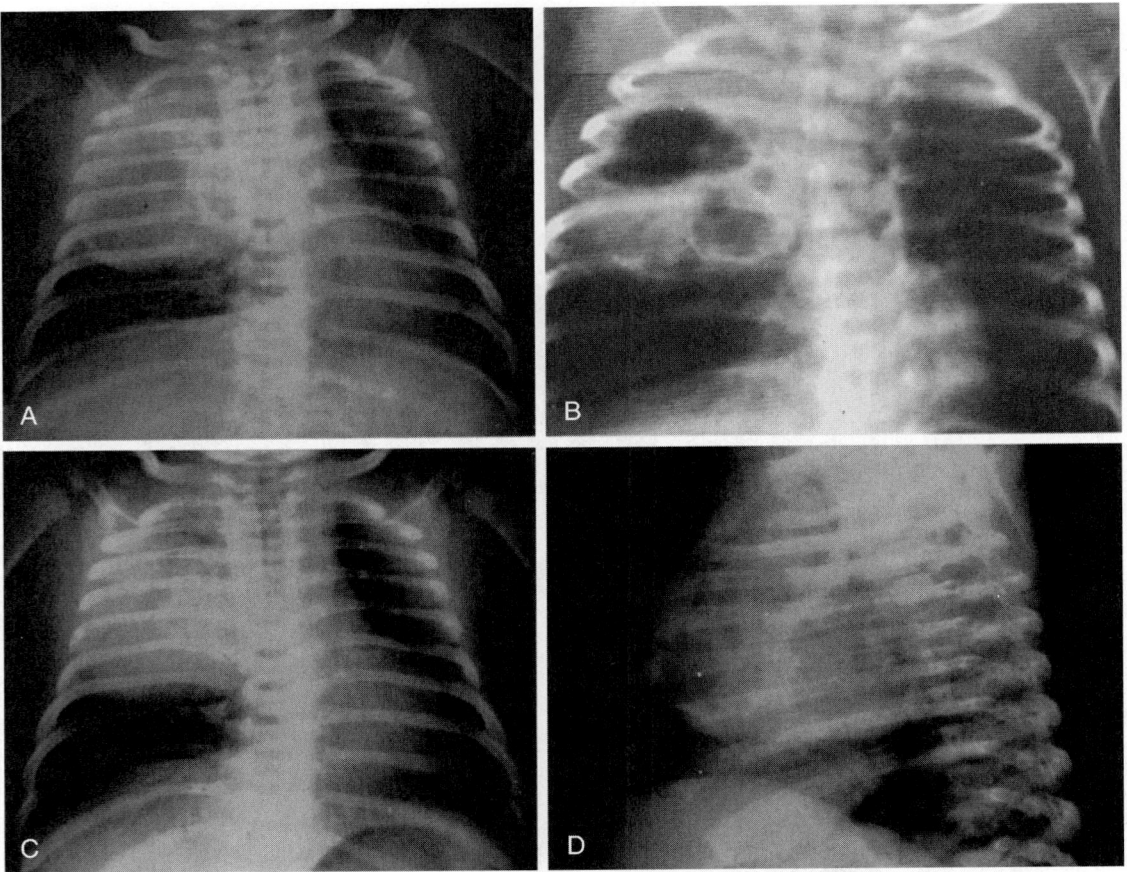

FIGURE 58–3. *A* to *C*, Anteroposterior views of the chest of an infant at different times showing the great variability in appearance of the same cystic lung. Differences in appearance depend on whether one or all of the component cysts are air filled or fluid filled at that particular time. *D*, Lateral view made on the same day that *C* was taken.

puted tomography (CT) scan often demonstrates the cystic nature of the former lesion (Kravitz, 1994).

Treatment

The absolute indication for immediate surgical treatment is increasing air tension within the cyst. Repeated aspirations of air by needle and syringe or constant suction through a catheter introduced into the cyst may be necessary in an emergency situation, but these maneuvers provide only temporary relief. Operation should then consist of removal of as small a portion of the lung as possible, either a segment of a lobe or the entire lobe. If the older patient has recurrent bouts of infection, associated with a congenital cyst, lobectomy is again indicated.

Prenatal Management

Large fluid-filled cysts, producing mass effects, polyhydramnios, and fetal hydrops, have been treated with thoracoamniotic catheters, with resolution of both the cyst and the hydrops condition (Revillon et al, 1993).

CONGENITAL CYSTIC ADENOMATOID MALFORMATION

This condition may affect any single lobe of the lung, causing a great increase in mass from multiple cystic proliferation (Merenstein, 1969), and this may result in lung compression and significant pulmonary hypoplasia. The lesion is a type of hamartoma with cystic structures. Many of the infants are stillborn or premature or both. Associated malformations are present in about 20% of affected infants; there may be renal agenesis, jejunal atresia, diaphragmatic hernia, hydrocephalus, and skeletal anomalies. In the case of congenital heart disease, the lesion is frequently truncus arteriosus or tetralogy of Fallot (Morin et al, 1994). Owing to its great mass, this malformation displaces the mediastinum and impedes venous return to the heart, accounting for a 50% incidence of hydrops fetalis. Another complication is polyhydramnios, which may be due to esophageal compression with impaired fetal swallowing (Revillon et al, 1993). In addition, polyhydramnios may occur because the cysts communicate with the airways and secrete fluid actively. After birth, because they are connected to the airways, the multiple cysts fill with air and produce further compression of the adjacent lung. If born alive, these infants have an early onset of respiratory distress, and the diagnosis is made by the chest radiograph (Fig. 58–4). This condition may be confused with congenital diaphragmatic hernia, but in cystic adenomatoid malformation, the abdominal gas pattern is normal, and a feeding catheter follows the normal path.

Natural Course

There are two major pathologic types. In the macrocystic type, the cysts are more than 5 mm in diameter, the cysts are visible on fetal ultrasonography, and the prognosis is better. In the microcystic type, the cysts are less than 5 mm in diameter, the mass has a solid appearance, and the prognosis is worse, more commonly associated with large size, mediastinal shift, polyhydramnios, pulmonary hypoplasia, and hydrops fetalis. In a large series diagnosed prenatally, Thorpe-Beeston and Nicolaides (1994) reported that 51% were on the left side, 35% were on the right, and 14% were bilateral. In this series, 59% were macrocystic and 41% were microcystic. In 33%, there was an elective termination of pregnancy; in 5%, there was intrauterine death; 43% developed hydrops fetalis; 62% were liveborn; and in 26%, there was a neonatal death. It was considered that survival was better if the mass was macrocystic and if there was no hydrops or polyhydramnios. Spontaneous regression with normal lungs at birth has been described in several series; in one series, 13 out of 32 cases showed

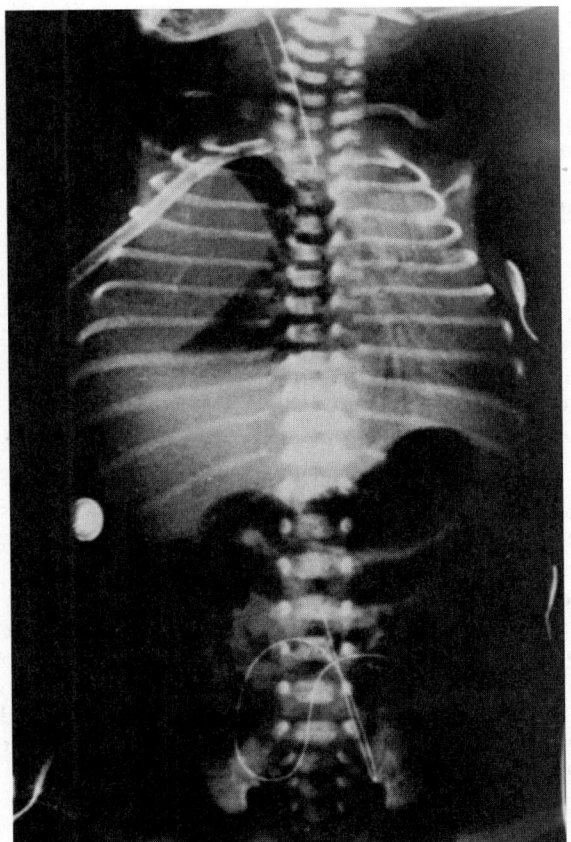

FIGURE 58–4. Cystic adenomatoid malformation of the lung, with chest tube on the right.

regression before birth (Revillon et al, 1993). Masses that disappear are usually the microcystic type, and this phenomenon does not occur in those with hydrops fetalis (Morin et al, 1994).

Prenatal Diagnosis

In prenatal diagnosis, there may be confusion with bronchopulmonary sequestration, in which case color flow Doppler should be used to distinguish the systemic blood supply to the sequestration (Morin et al, 1994). Chromosome analysis and fetal echocardiography should be performed, and the fetus should be followed for increasing mass size and signs of hydrops fetalis.

Prenatal Management

Those fetal patients at 32 weeks or more should have betamethasone prophylaxis against respiratory distress syndrome if necessary and then delivery as soon as possible. Those fetal patients at less than 32 weeks should be considered for fetal surgery if there are signs of hydrops (see also discussion in Chapter 60). In the case of large cysts, it is possible to perform fetal thoracentesis, perhaps on a repeated basis, to drain the fluid from the mass and allow the remaining lung to develop normally (Obwegeser et al, 1993). Others have placed a catheter from the cystic mass to the amniotic cavity, to provide a more prolonged decompression of the mass (Bernaschek et al, 1994). Adzick and colleagues (1993) reported three cases that had placement of a thoracoamniotic shunt; two infants survived, but they had pulmonary hypoplasia and needed high-frequency oscillatory ventilation and extracorporeal membrane oxygenation. Surgeons have performed lobectomy on fetuses with large cystic adenomatoid malformations producing mass effects, with mediastinal shift, lung hypoplasia, vena caval compression, and hydrops fetalis. Adzick and colleagues (1993) reported a series of six cases with microcystic disease and hydrops; the first fetus died of premature delivery and pulmonary hypoplasia soon after operation, four fetuses survived with resolution of hydrops and good lung development, and the last was a fetal death for unknown reasons in the postoperative phase. Harrison and coworkers (1990) reported one additional fetus with early hydrops successfully operated at 23 weeks. Others have claimed that many cases improve spontaneously during the last trimester (Revillon et al, 1993), but in a large series the chance of this occurring was considered to be only 6% (MacGillivray et al, 1993). Hydrops, the usual indication for surgery, is not known to resolve spontaneously and always signifies a poor outcome.

Postnatal Management

Prenatal diagnosis may also allow plans to be made for resection of the tumor immediately after delivery (Adzick et al, 1985). If there is severe gas trapping, selective bronchial intubation and either needle or tube thoracostomy may give temporary relief, but the treatment of choice is lobectomy as soon as possible after delivery (Morin et al, 1994). Rescorla and colleagues (1990) reported a case in which lobectomy was complicated by pulmonary hypertension secondary to lung hypoplasia, and the patient survived after extracorporeal membrane oxygenation.

INTRATHORACIC TUMORS AND FLUID-FILLED CYSTS

A large variety of solid tumors and fluid-filled cysts, in addition to the air-filled cysts just described, are encountered in the thoraces of adults. Many of these have already been observed in newborns, and others will no doubt be recorded. Those that result from congenital maldevelopment, such as intrathoracic cysts of gastrointestinal origin and dermoid cysts or teratomatous tumors, are more common in the neonatal period than are neoplasms and lymphomas. This last group, which in adults accounts for up to 40% of most series of mediastinal tumors, is of small numerical importance in the young infant. Too few neonatal cases have accumulated up to the present to warrant detailed classification.

Hope and Koop (1959) put forth the concept that intrathoracic mass lesions are best subdivided into those that arise in the posterior, middle, and anterior mediastinal spaces. A few others arise within the substance of the lung itself. In the posterior space, neurogenic tumors, duplications of the foregut, and neurenteric and bronchogenic cysts are most commonly encountered in the newborn. The middle mediastinum is the site almost exclusively of vascular lesions, whereas enlarged thymus and teratomas are masses most often seen in the anterior mediastinal space.

Thymus

The thymus occupies the upper anterior mediastinum, and it is more prominent in the newborn period than at any time of life. It may be so large as to reach the diaphragm or obscure both cardiac borders on radiographs. The normal thymus can be distinguished from an abnormal mass by the absence of tracheal deviation or compression. It changes in position with respiration and is less prominent with deep inspiration. It also involutes with stress as well as with corticosteroid therapy. Absence of the thymic shadow in an infant should alert one to the possibility of thymic agenesis and subacute combined immunodeficiency.

The cardiothymic/thoracic ratio provides an index of thymic size. Fletcher and associates (1979) as well as Gewolb and colleagues (1979) noted that a large ratio is present on the 1st day in infants at risk for hyaline membrane disease, presumably because of less than normal levels of glucocorticoids before birth. Thymic cysts have been reported in infants but rarely in newborns. Thompson and Love (1972) described a persistent cervical thymoma in a newborn infant that presented as an outpouch in the sternal notch with crying.

Mediastinal Neuroblastoma

Neuroblastoma, the most common solid tumor in the mediastinum of infants, arises from neural tissue, either intercostal or sympathetic nerves for the most part. Because it typically lies in the thoracic gutter, it is almost always posterior in location, and it may involve superior, middle, or inferior mediastinum. From here it may extend to either side and invade one or both lungs. Extension through a vertebral foramen may result in neurologic manifestations.

Diagnosis

Diagnosis is suggested by the discovery of an intrathoracic mass. It may follow radiography of the chest because of lower respiratory tract infection. Such infections afflict these infants more commonly than others because the growing tumor compresses bronchi. Alternatively, radiographs may be taken because of increasing dyspnea coupled with the physical signs of a solid intrathoracic mass.

Differentiation from other posterior mediastinal masses may be impossible before exploration. Neuroblastoma is not likely to be so sharply demarcated or to have so smooth and round a lower border as does a mediastinal cyst. Invasion of neighboring lung parenchyma strongly supports a diagnosis of neuroblastoma. Elevated urinary vanillylmandelic acid may be present. Its absence does not rule out neuroblastoma (Figs. 58–5 and 58–6).

Treatment

Exploration is indicated for any intrathoracic mass. If the tumor proves to be neuroblastoma, as much of it should be excised as is feasible surgically. The tumor should be staged according to the system of Evans and colleagues (1971), and subsequent therapy should be dictated by the stage.

Prognosis

The outlook for neuroblastomas in extra-adrenal locations is better than that for their suprarenal counterparts (Young et al, 1970). If the lesion can be completely removed and if no distant metastases are present, the probable survival rate is better than 75%.

Bronchogenic Cysts

Fluid-filled cysts of tracheobronchogenous origin are distinguished with difficulty from those of gastroenterogenous origin.

Incidence

In several series of cases of neoplasms and cysts of the mediastinum among patients of all ages reported from various clinics, bronchogenic cysts outnumber those of gastric or enteric derivation. Most observers comment on the fact that the distribution differs in young infants and children, so that gastroenterogenous and enterogenous ones outnumber the bronchogenic. In a 20-year experience and review of the literature, de Paredes and associates (1970) found 68 cases and added 12 of their own. In the newborn, bronchogenic cysts are encountered infrequently.

Pathology

Bronchogenic cysts seldom attain large size. They contain clear fluid and are lined with columnar, cuboidal, or pseu-

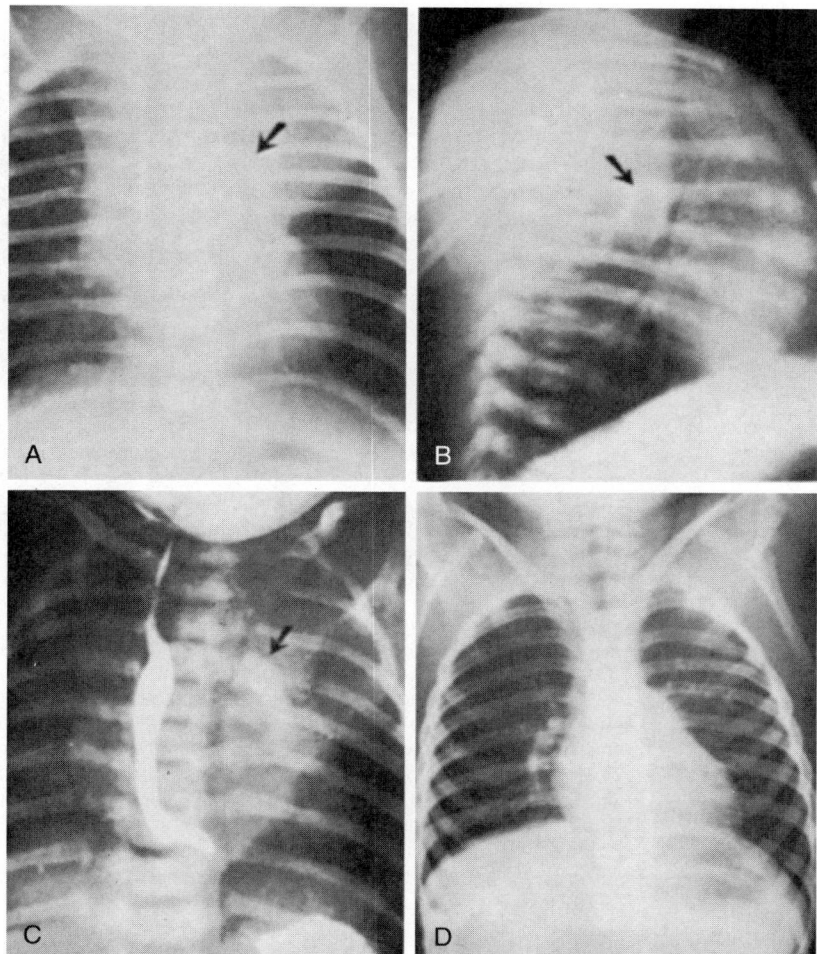

FIGURE 58–5. Neuroblastoma. A 7-week-old male infant entered the hospital for repair of an inguinal hernia and was found to have an enlarged lymph node in the left cervical region. This finding prompted a radiographic examination of the chest. *A,* Anteroposterior radiograph showing a large area of density in the left upper hemithorax. Within the homogeneous density, a curvilinear calcification is present (arrow). *B,* Lateral radiograph showing the mass lesion to be in the posterior mediastinum with some anterior deviation of the trachea. The calcification appears to be in the shape of a horseshoe (arrow). *C,* Anteroposterior view of barium-filled esophagus showing the large size of the mass lesion more graphically. The calcification is more clearly visualized (arrow). At operation, the lesion proved to be a neuroblastoma. It was entirely excised. *D,* Posteroanterior radiograph 5 years later showing a normal chest. (From Hope JW, Koop CE: Differential diagnosis of mediastinal masses. Pediatr Clin North Am 6:379, 1959.)

dostratified epithelium, and their walls generally contain smooth muscle and cartilage. They may, but do not always, communicate with the tracheobronchial tree. They tend to lie in the posterior mediastinum, but some have been found in the anterior space.

Diagnosis

Lying as they do, near the carina, these cysts commonly produce signs of respiratory embarrassment from birth or soon after. Generally their size is not such that they can be discovered by percussion or auscultation, but physical signs are likely to reveal their secondary effects, emphysema or atelectasis, rather than the tumor itself. Opsahl and Berman (1962) reported a case that showed emphysema on the left, followed by clearing, then equally notable emphysema on the right.

Radiographic examination often shows a mass projecting forward from the superior mediastinal shadow, not large and not necessarily rounded (Figs. 58–7 and 58–8). Ultrasonography can help localize the lesion. Barium swallow test may reveal indentation of the esophagus from an anterior direction. Bronchoscopy reveals compression of the trachea and often of one major bronchus.

Treatment

Immediate excision should be performed.

ESOPHAGEAL, GASTROGENIC, AND ENTEROGENOUS CYSTS

Three varieties of intrathoracic fluid-filled cysts are discussed together because they are indistinguishable on clinical grounds. Esophageal, gastrogenic, and enterogenous cysts may also be called *neurenteric cysts* or *duplication cysts.* Together they constitute a large group of mediastinal masses found in the neonatal period. Although they are not encountered frequently, they are far from uncommon. These cysts are duplicated segments of the foregut that have become partially or completely detached from the parent viscus. They lie in or near the posterior mediastinum but with increasing size may project far into one or the other hemithorax. Their walls are composed of a mucosal layer, characteristic of that of their site of origin, and of one or more muscular layers. They contain fluid that is also similar to the secretion normally manufactured in their parent locus; the material within gastrogenic cysts contains pepsin and hydrochloric acid in roughly the same concentrations as are present in gastric juice.

The foregut becomes duplicated in the course of embryonic development by failure of complete resorption of occluding epithelium, resulting in the formation of a supernumerary wall. The high percentage of vertebral malformations associated with gastroenterogenous cysts led Veeneklaas (1952) to suggest that the primary embryonic defect

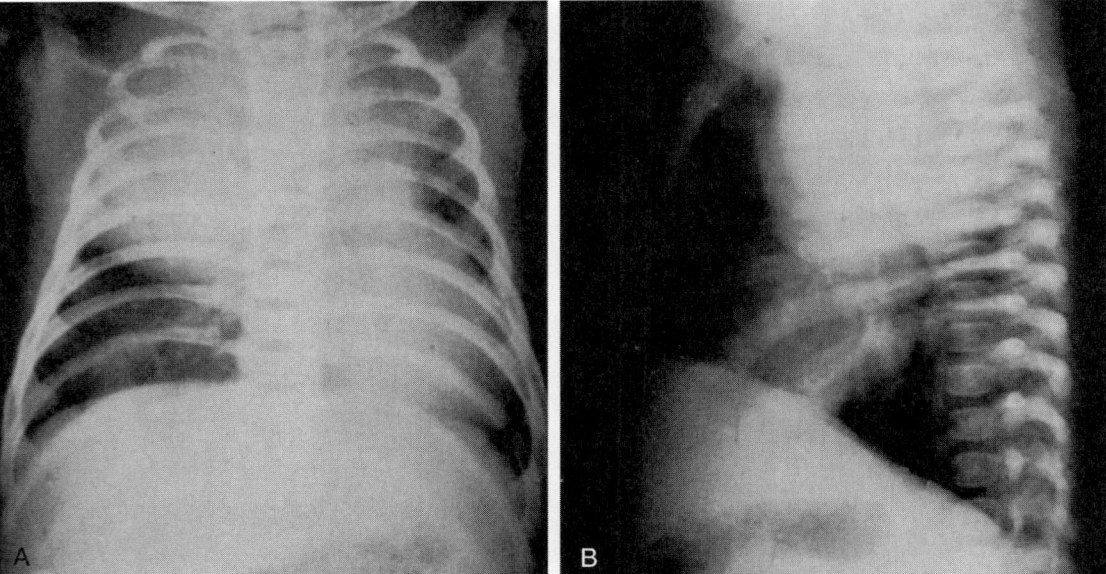

FIGURE 58–6. Neuroblastoma. *A*, Anteroposterior view of the chest of a 7-week-old infant admitted because of a severe respiratory infection. An opacity is seen filling the upper half of the right hemithorax and extending beyond the midline halfway to the left axilla. Its lower and left borders are rounded. The heart is displaced to the left and downward. The opacity gives the appearance of a solid tumor. *B*, Lateral view shows an opaque mass jutting forward from the posterior chest wall from the clavicle halfway down the chest to abut on the heart. Its outline is round. At operation, a tumor was seen in the mediastinum that invaded all adjacent structures, including the left upper lobe. Biopsy revealed neuroblastoma. No excision was attempted. Radiotherapy was ineffective. Aminopterin was begun 2 months later and was followed by rapid improvement. Two years later, the patient appeared perfectly well, and no tumor was visualized on x-ray films. (Case 7 of Dr. Gladys Boyd, abstracted with her kind permission.)

lies in abnormal persistence of the primitive adherence of the foregut to the notochord at the site of the duplication. When the foregut descends from its early position in the neck, this adhesion causes anomalies in the vertebral bodies derived from the notochord. This adhesion also breaks off the duplicated portion of the foregut and prevents its complete descent into the thorax and abdomen along with the mature foregut.

Diagnosis

Clinical signs depend on the size and location of the duplication cyst. Because the cysts are all posterior and lie close to the trachea, esophagus, and great vessels, they are seldom present without signs of abnormality. Cyanosis, tachypnea, and dyspnea are often present from birth. Swallowing difficulty and vomiting are less frequent. Recurrent lower respiratory tract infections characterize a few. Hemorrhage, from either the mouth or nose, from lungs or stomach, or in the form of melena, is not at all uncommon. In most instances, hemorrhage indicates that the cyst is of gastrogenic origin because the fluid within these cysts contains pepsin and is capable of eroding through the cyst wall to enter surrounding organs, such as the trachea or esophagus. Technetium scans are useful in delineating cysts lined with gastric mucosa. Radiographs of the chest show abnormal shadows that are often difficult to distinguish from unusual cardiac contours (Fig. 58–9). Lateral and oblique films may be needed to make the differentiation with certainty. In one or another projection, the rounded border of the cyst contiguous to the heart should be able to be visualized. Barium swallow test commonly shows displacement of the esophagus. Gastroenterogenous cysts may either partially or totally compress the bronchus, with consequent lung overdistention or atelectasis. Sometimes the symptoms are intermittent as the cyst enlarges or empties. Bronchoscopy and esophagoscopy are not ordinarily required to confirm the diagnosis, but when performed, they may show compression of one or both structures from without. Cyst puncture should not be performed. Superina and colleagues (1984) reviewed 25 years' experience with neurenteric cysts at the Hospital for Sick Children in Toronto and noted that a spinal component may accompany the mediastinal cyst in as many as 20% of the children. They recommended careful radiographic evaluation of the spinal canal with CT scan and then excision of the intraspinal cyst, if possible, before the onset of neurologic signs in later childhood.

Treatment

Operation is indicated as soon as the diagnosis of mediastinal mass is made. It is neither necessary nor wise to delay exploration until a specific diagnosis has been made.

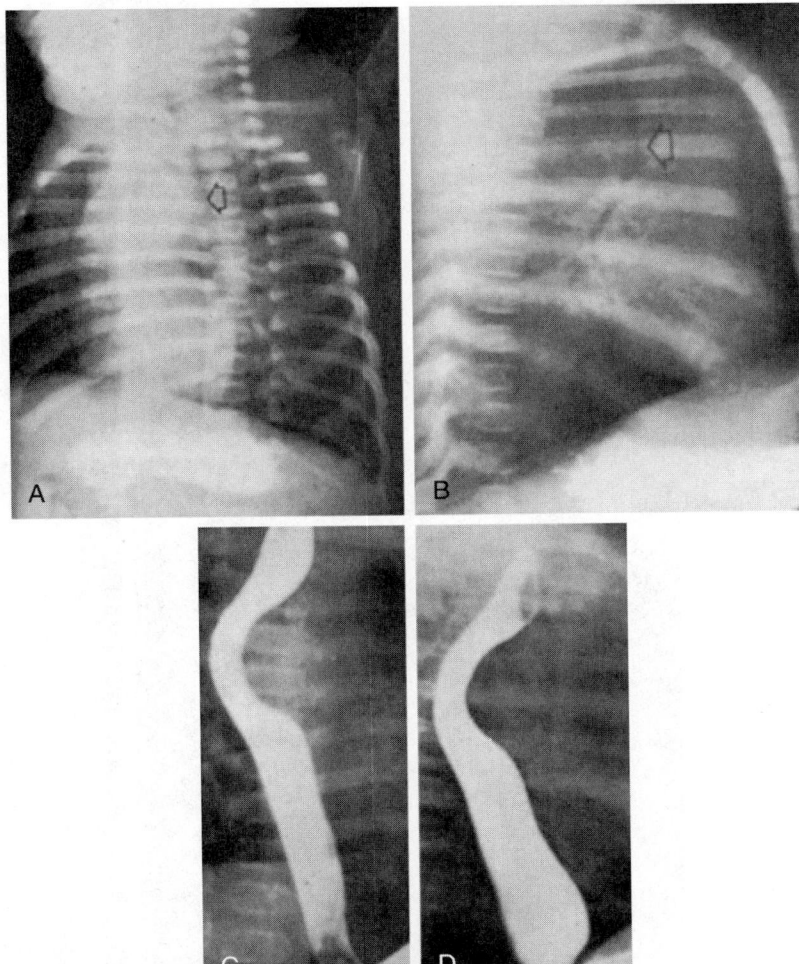

FIGURE 58–7. Bronchogenic cyst. A 10-week-old male infant with dyspnea since birth. *A,* Left anterior oblique radiograph showing a mass lesion just above the carina (arrow). *B,* Lateral radiograph showing anterior deviation of the trachea (arrow). *C,* Anteroposterior view of barium-filled esophagus showing extreme deviation of the esophagus to the right just above the level of the carina. *D,* Lateral view of barium-filled esophagus showing posterior deviation of the esophagus just above the level of the carina. A bronchogenic cyst was removed at operation. (From Hope JW, Koop CE: Differential diagnosis of mediastinal masses. Pediatr Clin North Am 6:379, 1959.)

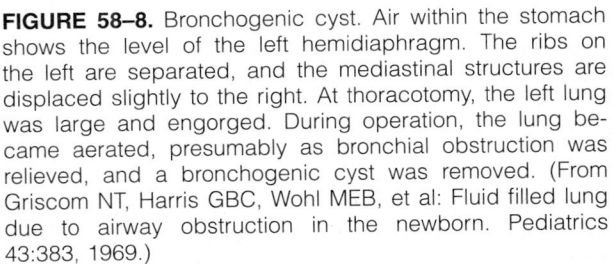

FIGURE 58–8. Bronchogenic cyst. Air within the stomach shows the level of the left hemidiaphragm. The ribs on the left are separated, and the mediastinal structures are displaced slightly to the right. At thoracotomy, the left lung was large and engorged. During operation, the lung became aerated, presumably as bronchial obstruction was relieved, and a bronchogenic cyst was removed. (From Griscom NT, Harris GBC, Wohl MEB, et al: Fluid filled lung due to airway obstruction in the newborn. Pediatrics 43:383, 1969.)

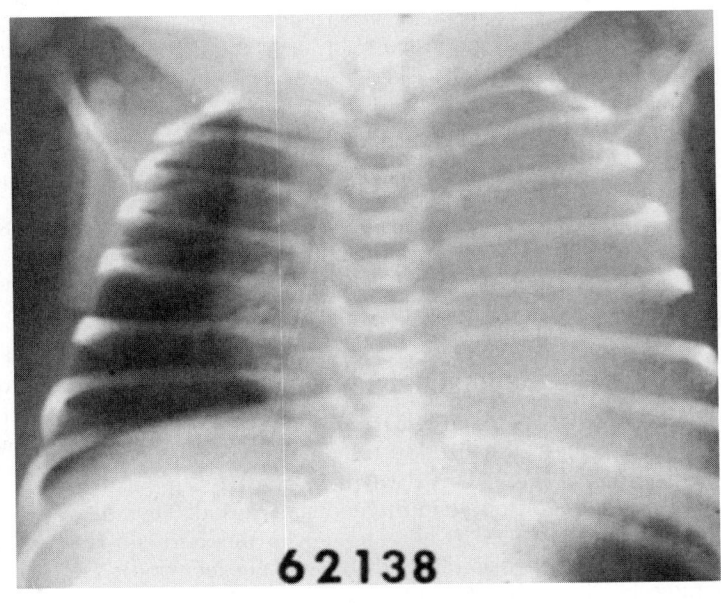

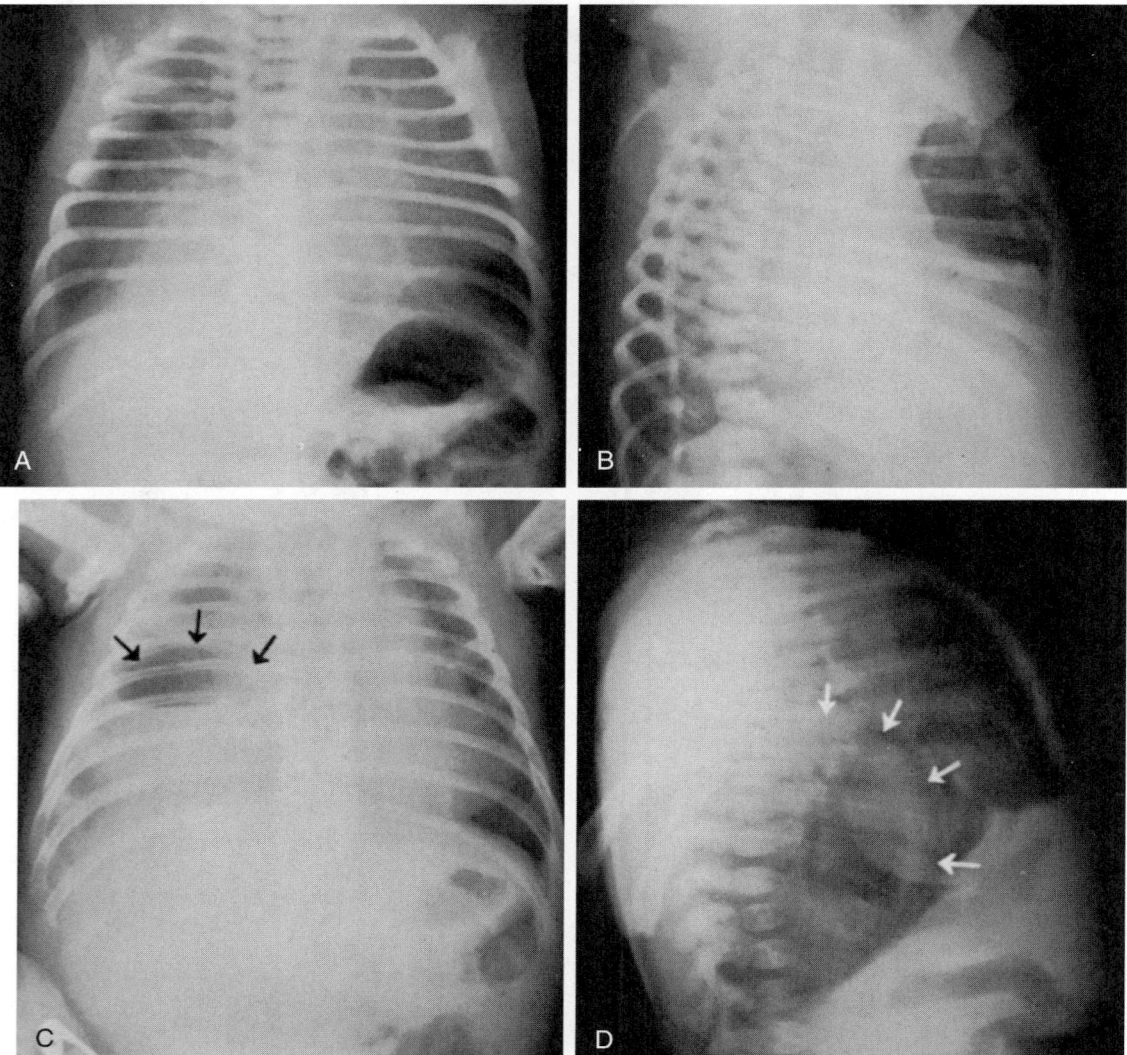

FIGURE 58–9. Enterogenous cyst. *A,* Anteroposterior view of the chest taken within the 1st week of life, interpreted as showing atelectasis of right upper and lower lobes. The left border of the heart almost touches the left axillary wall, whereas the right border appears to be almost as far in the right hemithorax. It is difficult to tell whether this shadow is that of a hugely enlarged heart or whether it is composed of more than one element. *B,* Lateral view showing the opacity filling the lower half of the chest, which is also difficult to diagnose, but it almost surely is not all heart. *C,* Anteroposterior view taken 4 weeks later. In the interim, fluid had been withdrawn six times, and in the process air had been introduced into the right hemithorax. Now one can see a mass in the right middle and lower hemithorax containing a bubble of air that delineates its rounded upper border. Removal of fluid has permitted the heart to return to a position more nearly normal. *D,* Lateral view, same day. Here the rounded margin of almost the entire cyst can be visualized. (From Leahy LJ, Butsch WL: Surgical management of respiratory emergencies during the first few weeks of life. Arch Surg 59:466, 1949. Copyright 1949, American Medical Association.)

Mediastinal Teratomas

The shadow of the enlarged thymus is the most common radiopaque mass visualized in the anterior mediastinum of the newborn. The enlarged thymus, however, appears to cause little if any trouble in the neonatal period. Thymoma has not been reported. When an anterior mediastinal mass is associated with respiratory distress in the newborn, the strong likelihood is that the lesion is a teratoma (Fig. 58–10). Seibert and coworkers (1976) reported one infant

with tracheal compression from a teratoma. Normal thymus should not compress the trachea or great vessels. All other anterior masses (e.g., lymphomas, lymphangiomas, substernal thyroids) occur infrequently in this age period.

Fibrosarcoma of the Lung

An unusual solid tumor of the lung in a newborn was reported to one of the authors in a personal communication

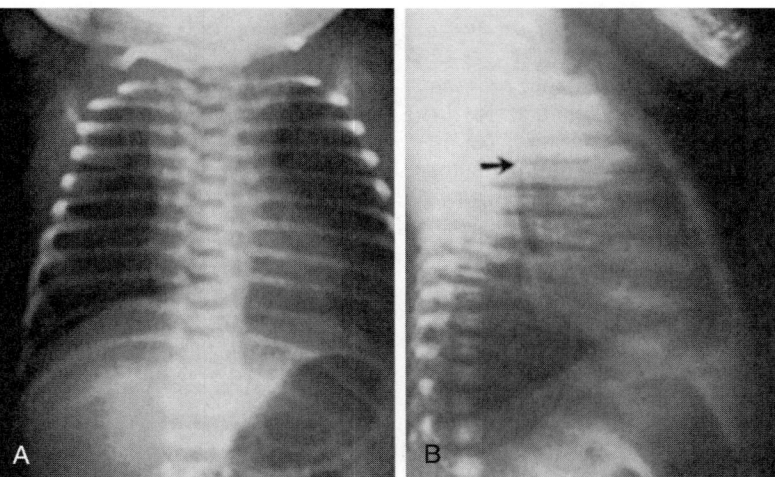

FIGURE 58–10. Mediastinal teratoma. An 11-day-old male infant with severe respiratory distress and cyanosis since 2 days of age. *A,* Anteroposterior radiograph showing extreme hyperaeration of both lung fields and a wide superior mediastinum. *B,* Lateral radiograph showing extreme hyperaeration of the lungs and a mass filling the anterior mediastinum, producing posterior deviation and compression of the trachea (arrow). The tumor was excised and proved to be a benign teratoma lying behind a normal thymus gland and in front of the trachea. (From Hope JW, Koop CE: Differential diagnosis of mediastinal masses. Pediatr Clin North Am 6:379, 1959.)

(Robb D, Auckland, New Zealand). As far as the authors can determine, this is the only fibrosarcoma of the lung thus far identified in a newborn.

Hamartoma of Lung

Hamartoma is not a true neoplasm. It is a mass composed of the normal elements that make up an organ, combined in an abnormal manner. In the lung, it is usually encapsulated and firm and ordinarily does not attain a great size. Under the microscope, varying amounts of mesenchymal and epithelial elements are seen, often surrounding bits of cartilage.

BRONCHOPULMONARY SEQUESTRATION

More than 300 cases of bronchopulmonary sequestration have been reported in the literature; these were reviewed by Carter in 1969 and by Landing in 1979. They have only rarely produced symptoms in newborn infants and have usually been detected on chest radiographs taken for other reasons; more commonly, a sequestered lobe manifests itself in children or young adults by repeated infections in a fluid-filled lung cyst. The lesion should be suspected in infants with cystic lesions, especially in the lower lobes (Fig. 58–11). The malformation is slightly more common in males and is distinctly more likely on the left side;

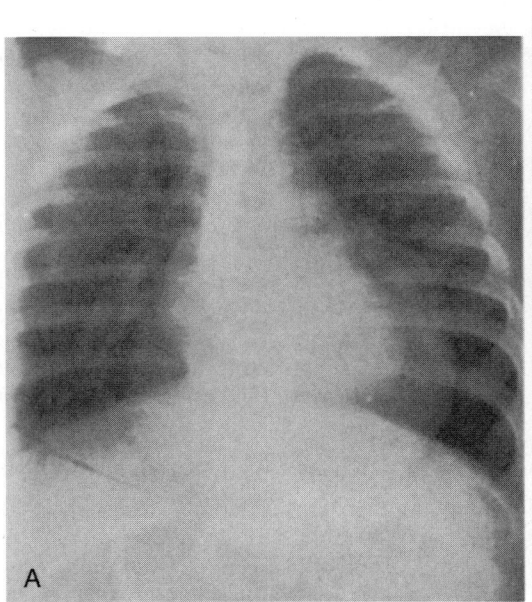
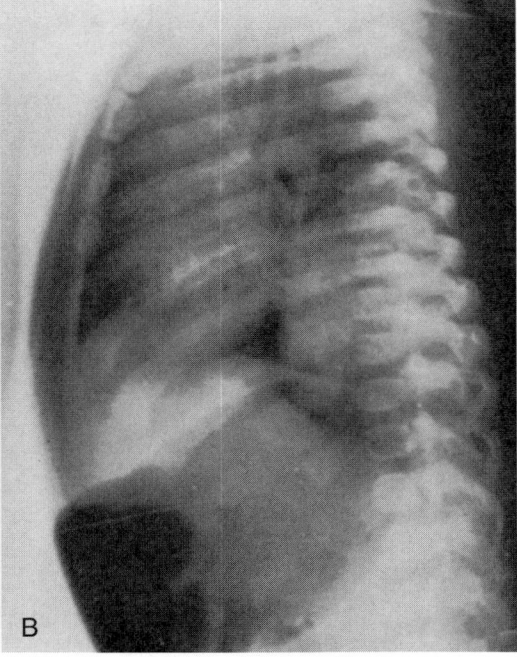

FIGURE 58–11. Accessory lung lobe. *A,* Anteroposterior view shows a homogeneous circular shadow surrounding the heart shadow. The heart appears normal and the lungs clear. *B,* In the lateral view, the disc-shaped mass lies in the posterior mediastinum and proved to be an accessory lobe, a variant of pulmonary sequestration that derives its blood supply from the pulmonary, instead of the systemic, system.

approximately two thirds of the cases involve the left lower lobe.

Sequestration is a term for nonfunctioning lung tissue that does not communicate with the tracheobronchial tree and that derives its blood supply from the aorta. There may be a single large anomalous vessel, but sometimes multiple small anomalous arteries from above or below the diaphragm supply the sequestered lobe. The venous drainage may be pulmonary or systemic; the latter may be into the inferior vena cava, the azygous vein, or the portal vein; in the case of pulmonary venous return, there may be a large left-to-right shunt and possible congestive heart failure. In greater than 80% of the cases, a communication with the foregut can be demonstrated by contrast studies (Heithoff et al, 1976); the usual location is the lower esophagus or gastric fundus. The affected lung is highly abnormal, consisting of atelectatic areas interspersed with fluid-filled cysts. There is an increased incidence of associated malformations (e.g., diaphragmatic hernia, congenital heart disease, eventration of the diaphragm, enterogenous cysts, and vertebral or rib anomalies).

Bronchopulmonary sequestration is thought to be caused by an accessory lung bud originating lower down in the primitive foregut. If the bud originates early, the normal and sequestered lung have a common pleural covering, in which case the sequestration is considered to be intralobar, whereas if the supernumerary bud originates later, the sequestered lung has its own pleura and is considered to be extralobar; in some cases, an extralobar sequestration may be subdiaphragmatic in location. About 75% of cases are intralobar sequestrations, but in cases presenting in the newborn period, extralobar sequestrations are more common. If the sequestered lobe is found to obtain its blood supply from the pulmonary system, rather than from the systemic system, it may be called an *accessory lung lobe*. Other malformations occur in 60% of extralobar sequestrations and in 10% of intralobar sequestrations.

Prenatal Diagnosis

The diagnosis of bronchopulmonary sequestration may be made in the fetus, but in some cases solid chest masses have been known to resolve by the time of delivery (Mac-Gillivray et al, 1993). A sequestration is a solid, highly echogenic chest mass, and the systemic blood supply may be demonstrated by color-coded Doppler ultrasonography (Dolkart et al, 1992). In some cases, the lesions have been associated with mediastinal shift, polyhydramnios, and hydrops fetalis, in which case the prognosis is poor, and stillbirth or early neonatal death is common. There may be unilateral or bilateral pleural effusions (see also Chapter 59).

Postnatal Diagnosis

Most infants with bronchopulmonary sequestration are not symptomatic in the neonatal period, but if the sequestration is sufficiently large, there may be persistent cyanosis and respiratory distress (Pearl, 1972), with or without lung hypoplasia. Some cases may present with a large unilateral hydrothorax, possibly secondary to lymphatic obstruction in the sequestration (Boyer et al, 1996; Hernanz-Schulman

et al, 1991). Brus and colleagues (1993) reported an infant with nonimmune hydrops fetalis, bilateral hydrothoraces, and severe pulmonary hypoplasia secondary to an extralobar pulmonary sequestration. Infants with a large left-to-right shunt through the sequestration may present with congestive heart failure in the newborn period, especially if born prematurely (Kolls et al, 1992). Later in infancy, frequent bouts of pneumonia may occur. On the chest radiograph, the classic appearance consists of a triangular or oval-shaped basal lung mass on one side of the chest, usually the left side. Ultrasound examination confirms the presence of a thoracic mass (Schlesinger et al, 1994); the chest CT scan is also helpful (Boyer et al, 1996). The definitive diagnosis is made with angiography, which delineates the feeding vessels to the sequestration; the usual study is contrast aortography (Kravitz, 1994), but other less invasive techniques, such as magnetic resonance angiography (Doyle, 1992) and color-coded Doppler ultrasonography (Eisenberg et al, 1992; Smart and Hendry, 1991), have been used successfully. The barium swallow test frequently demonstrates contrast material entering the sequestered lung.

Management

If a large hydrothorax is discovered before birth, this may be drained by insertion of a thoracoamniotic shunt to allow further lung development (Hernanz-Schulman et al, 1991). Depending on the degree of associated lung hypoplasia, the newborn infant may need no mechanical ventilation, only conventional ventilation, or high-frequency oscillatory ventilation and extracorporeal membrane oxygenation (Morin et al, 1994). Large pleural effusions present at birth should be treated with immediate tube thoracostomy. Further treatment consists of surgical resection in all cases; this is true even if there are no signs of respiratory distress because repeated lung infections in the future are the rule. It is helpful to have an angiographic study preoperatively to alert the surgeon to the position of the anomalous vessels from the aorta and to the position of the venous drainage system. The arterial vessels may bleed postoperatively if not found and ligated, and the venous drainage may represent the sole venous drainage of the ipsilateral lung. If the lesion disappears before birth, the residual lesion should be sought with chest CT scans or chest magnetic resonance imaging scans; if found, these lesions should be resected because of the risks for infection, hemorrhage, and malignant transformation. Although lung resection is recommended, resection of an intralobar sequestration may make the management of pulmonary hypoplasia more difficult.

CONGENITAL LOBAR EMPHYSEMA

Congenital lobar emphysema describes a condition with respiratory distress caused by overinflation of one lobe of the lung, usually the left upper, right upper, or right middle lobe. There is no emphysematous destruction of lung tissue, as the name might imply. The onset may be any time in the first 6 months of life, but 50% of cases present in the newborn period. The respiratory distress may be severe, but in many cases it is mild, without cyanosis in room air. The chest radiograph shows overdistention of one lobe, compression of the adjacent lung, herniation across the mediastinum, and diaphragmatic depression. The chest CT scan shows decreased vessels owing to compression in the involved lung and increased vessels owing to overperfusion on the opposite side. About 15% of the cases are associated with congenital heart disease, usually patent ductus arteriosus or ventricular septal defect, and other cases may be associated with rib anomalies and cystic renal lesions (Kravitz, 1994). Before making this diagnosis, a mucus plug obstruction should be excluded by vigorous physical therapy or suction applied at rigid bronchoscopy.

Some authors contend that most cases are caused by local bronchial cartilage deficiency, with airway closure and gas trapping in exhalation (Campbell, 1969). Other causes have been suggested (e.g., redundant bronchial mucosal fold, stenosis of the bronchial wall, or external compression by an anomalous pulmonary artery or mediastinal mass). It is possible for a lobe to be rotated on its pedicle with resultant obstruction (Hislop and Reid, 1971).

Sometimes the condition represents a polyalveolar lobe in which, despite a normal number of airways, there is a fivefold increase in the number of alveoli in each acinus (Hislop and Reid, 1970). Infants with this condition tend to have prolonged retention of fetal lung liquid in the affected lobe after birth and to have early signs of respiratory distress on the 1st day of life (Cleveland and Weber, 1993).

Most cases can be evaluated with the chest radiograph, especially if films are taken in both inspiration and expiration. The chest CT scan is useful for defining a mediastinal mass or a vascular ring and in the evaluation of possible bronchial stenosis (Stigers et al, 1992). The ventilation/perfusion study is useful in assessing lung function, which may be surprisingly good in many cases.

In those with congenital lobar emphysema and severe respiratory distress, the treatment is surgical lobectomy, the results of which have been excellent. In infants with mild tachypnea and no significant oxygen requirement, the treatment may be expectant (Shannon et al, 1977). The mild symptoms frequently subside by the age of 1 year. Stigers and coworkers (1992) managed five of their eight cases without surgery. Whether treated medically or surgically, at age 10 most such children have evidence of mild airway obstruction, suggesting a more generalized abnormality of the airways (McBride et al, 1980).

UNILATERAL PULMONARY AGENESIS

This condition may be a unilateral lung agenesis without main bronchus development on one side and therefore without a carina, or it may be a unilateral lung aplasia with a carina and a main stem bronchial pouch as evidence of arrested bronchial development. Left-sided lung agenesis is slightly more common and is sometimes associated with severe congenital heart disease, such as tetralogy of Fallot; cases have been described in asymptomatic adults. Right-sided lung agenesis may cause more problems from mediastinal shift and obstruction of major vessels and airways and is more frequently associated with congenital heart disease, such as ventricular septal defect and coarctation of the aorta. The contralateral lung may be enlarged and hypertrophied, it may be overdistended and overperfused,

and it may herniate into the opposite hemithorax, usually through the anterior mediastinum; this means that there may be no obvious evidence for asymmetry of the chest in the newborn, and asymmetry may only develop with further growth during later infancy. For this reason, breath sounds may be heard on the involved side, but not posteriorly.

Some patients with this condition may die in the delivery room, and others may have severe respiratory distress syndrome that does not respond to mechanical ventilation; this may lead to consideration for extracorporeal membrane oxygenation. Some patients may have only modest and transient respiratory distress at birth, and it is also possible for there to be no signs of illness in the newborn. The clinical presentation may be with congenital heart disease, frequently with cyanosis. In lung agenesis, the ipsilateral pulmonary artery is absent, so cyanosis cannot be attributed to perfusion of airless lung mesenchyme. There may be other anomalies, such as esophageal atresia and polycystic kidneys, and hemivertebrae are particularly common.

The chest radiograph shows homogeneous density in place of the lung, the ribs may appear closer together on the involved side, and there is mediastinal shift and tracheal deviation. A chest CT scan may be necessary to confirm the absence of lung tissue on one side (Kravitz, 1994). Bronchoscopy shows the absence of the ipsilateral main stem bronchus, and this may be confirmed by bronchography. The echocardiogram demonstrates the absence of the ipsilateral pulmonary artery and any associated congenital heart defects. If there is confusion with dextrocardia, an electrocardiogram may be useful.

If they survive the neonatal period, these infants may develop recurrent pneumonia and reactive airways disease, but the reason for this is not clear. One suggestion is that in the case of lung aplasia, the remnant bronchial pouch allows the accumulation of stagnant secretions and therefore predisposes to infection in the normal lung (Borja et al, 1970).

PULMONARY HYPOPLASIA

Pulmonary hypoplasia is a pathologic condition in which the combined lung weight is less than 1.2% of body weight, the standardized autopsy lung volume is less than 60% of predicted lung volume, lung DNA is less than 100 mg/kg of body weight, or the radial alveolar count is less than 4 (Langston and Thurlbeck, 1986). The incidence at autopsy is approximately 10% of newborns, and the overall incidence is thought to be approximately 2 per 1000 live births (Knox and Barson, 1986). Infants with pulmonary hypoplasia present usually with respiratory distress and cyanosis in room air. On the chest radiograph, the lungs appear small and clear unless another condition is superimposed, the diaphragms are elevated, and the thorax may appear bell shaped. These infants have significant hypercarbia, which responds poorly to mechanical ventilation, and the risk of pneumothorax is high. They often have persistent pulmonary hypertension, as a result of a reduced vascular bed and secondary arterial muscle hypertrophy (Hislop et al, 1979). In addition, the hypoplastic lung may also have an immature surfactant profile, so some infants also have respiratory distress syndrome (Nakamura et al, 1988; Wigglesworth et al, 1981).

Normal lung growth depends on lung distention (Wigglesworth and Desai, 1982), which, in turn, depends on space to occupy and expansion caused by lung fluid secretion and fetal breathing. Conditions causing oligohydramnios and fetal thoracic compression are associated with pulmonary hypoplasia, owing to increased loss of lung fluid into the amniotic cavity; it is possible that in oligohydramnios the amniotic fluid pressure is low, so when the larynx is opened, excessive lung fluid is expelled. Conditions associated with oligohydramnios include renal agenesis, renal dysplasia, obstructive uropathy (Thomas and Smith, 1974), and chronic amnion rupture (Thibeault et al, 1985). Lung compression may also be due to congenital diaphragmatic hernia, cystic lung disease, eventration of the diaphragm, ascites, or pleural effusion, all of which may cause pulmonary hypoplasia. Effective fetal breathing may be impaired by chest cage insufficiency as in congenital thoracic dystrophy, by neuromuscular problems such as motor neuron disease or myotonic dystrophy, and by brain malformations that affect the brain stem such as iniencephaly. Patients with giant omphalocele may have pulmonary hypoplasia because the lower chest cage is not adequately supported by abdominal contents (Hershenson et al, 1985). Finally, in a significant number of infants, no cause for primary pulmonary hypoplasia can be found (Swischuk et al, 1979), although suppression of fetal breathing caused by maternal use of tobacco, barbiturates, or ethanol may be implicated (Collins et al, 1985).

In many cases of hypoplasia, the number of bronchial generations is reduced, suggesting an insult occurring between 10 and 14 weeks' gestation, as in diaphragmatic hernia or renal dysplasia. Although the total number of acini is reduced, the number of alveoli per acinus is relatively well preserved (Hislop et al, 1979). In many cases of chronic amnion rupture, the onset is much later, the bronchial number is normal, and the number of alveoli per acinus is reduced.

CHRONIC AMNION RUPTURE

In chronic amnion rupture, Nimrod and colleagues (1984) concluded that serious lung hypoplasia was unlikely to occur if the membranes ruptured after 26 weeks' gestation, apparently because a sufficient number of air spaces may have developed by then. This is in agreement with the data of Moessinger and associates (1986), who found in a guinea pig model that hypoplasia was most likely if amnion rupture occurred in the canalicular stage of lung development and was not significant if amnion rupture occurred in the terminal sac (saccular) stage of lung development. McIntosh and Harrison (1994) found that the minimal duration of rupture for the development of lung hypoplasia was 2 weeks for survivors and 3 weeks for those who died. In addition, the median length of rupture for those with compression deformities of the face and limbs was 28 days, and for those with pulmonary hypoplasia it was 31 days, indicating the close relationship of pulmonary hypoplasia with the fetal compression syndrome. Although fetal breathing movements may disappear in oligohydramnios, thoracic compression and loss of lung fluid are the cause of lung

hypoplasia in chronic amnion rupture (Adzick et al, 1984). Blott and associates (1987), however, found that the presence of sustained fetal breathing movements may protect against the development of pulmonary hypoplasia.

The possibilities for treatment are limited. A major objective of fetal surgery today is the relief of fetal lung compression, such as that caused by diaphragmatic hernia. Lobar lung transplantation for pulmonary hypoplasia may become possible in the future.

Kitterman (1993) has warned that many infants with severe respiratory distress syndrome and born in situations that might suggest pulmonary hypoplasia in fact do not have this condition and make a good recovery; he suggests that clinicians be skeptical of this diagnosis in infants who survive. McIntosh (1988) described three infants with prolonged amnion rupture, small lungs, and compression deformities, who required high pressures with mechanical ventilation on the 1st day of life but who markedly improved on the 2nd day of life and recovered in room air.

PULMONARY HEMANGIOMATOSIS

Pulmonary hemangiomatosis is a proliferation of small blood vessels that may be peribronchovascular, septal, or pleural in location. If the lesions also involve the airways, hemoptysis may occur.

Natural History

Pulmonary hemangiomatosis may be a part of a disseminated hemangiomatosis that can involve the liver, gastrointestinal tract, central nervous system, and skin. Cutaneous lesions may be present at birth or develop within the first few weeks of life. In some instances, the hemangiomas may be confined to the lung and remain asymptomatic until childhood. Because the flow through the hemangiomas in the lung is right to left, there is significant venous admixture and associated clubbing of all digits. In some instances, clubbing may take place even in the absence of arterial desaturation. The major symptom is dyspnea, which is progressive. The most likely cause of death is from bleeding or in adults from pulmonary hypertension.

Diagnosis

The diagnosis is suggested by the chest radiograph, which may resemble an interstitial infiltrate or thickened fissures. Pulmonary angiography and magnetic resonance imaging are useful in diagnosis.

Treatment

In at least one instance, a 12-year-old boy had a good response to treatment with interferon alfa-2a administered subcutaneously. He received daily interferon therapy for 14 months during which his dyspnea remitted, his digital clubbing resolved, and his pulmonary function tests were restored to normal. Abnormal vessels were still evident in the angiogram, but their density had been substantially reduced (White et al, 1989). This therapy seems to be less toxic than long-term corticosteroids or cyclophosphamides, which have been used in the past.

Prognosis

Experience with interferon is too recent to know whether all visceral hemangiomas respond.

PULMONARY ARTERIOVENOUS MALFORMATIONS

Although rare, pulmonary arteriovenous fistula or angioma is characterized by persistent cyanosis in the newborn, but unless the fistula is large and compresses the surrounding lung, it does not cause respiratory distress (Hodgson et al, 1959). Lesions may be single or multiple and aneurysmal or microscopic in size. About 50% of the cases are associated with hereditary hemorrhagic telangiectasia (Rendu-Osler-Weber syndrome). The chest radiograph most commonly shows a small mass lesion, usually in the lower lobes; the electrocardiogram may suggest unusual left ventricular dominance. The diagnosis can be made at cardiac catheterization, in which a selective cine-angiogram of the pulmonary artery shows the lesion in the lung (Mitchell and Austin, 1993). Alternatively the diagnosis may be made with a radionuclide perfusion study or digital subtraction angiography. The best treatment is conservative surgical excision with lobectomy or segmentectomy as necessary. For large lesions, embolotherapy may be useful. Multiple hemangiomas may respond to glucocorticoid therapy or newer inhibitors of angiogenesis. The mortality and morbidity in untreated cases is considerable (Dines et al, 1983). Most cases are diagnosed in adults; fewer than 10% are diagnosed in infancy.

REFERENCES

Abell MR: Mediastinal cysts. AMA Arch Pathol 61:360, 1956.

Adzick NS, Harrison MR, Flake AW, et al: Fetal surgery for cystic adenomatoid malformation of the lung. J Pediatr Surg 28:806, 1993.

Adzick NS, Harrison MR, Glick PC: Fetal cystic adenomatoid malformation: Prenatal diagnosis and natural history. J Pediatr Surg 20:483, 1985.

Adzick NS, Harrison MR, Glick PL, at al: Experimental pulmonary hypoplasia and oligohydramnios: Relative contributions of lung fluid and fetal breathing movements. J Pediatr Surg 19:658, 1984.

Anspach WE, Wolman IJ: Large pulmonary air cysts of infancy, with special reference to pathogenesis and diagnosis. Surg Gynecol Obstet 56:634, 1933.

Bates M: Total unilateral pulmonary sequestration. Thorax 23:311, 1968.

Bernaschek G, Deutinger J, Hansmann M, et al: Feto-amniotic shunting: Report of the experience of four European centres. Prenat Diagn 14:821, 1994.

Blott M, Greenough A, Nicolaides KH, et al: Fetal breaking movements as predictor of favorable pregnancy outcome after oligohydramnios due to membrane rupture in second trimester. Lancet 2:129, 1987.

Borja AR, Ransdell HT, Villa S: Congenital developmental arrest of the lung. Ann Thorac Surg 10:317, 1970.

Boyd GL: Solid intrathoracic masses in children. Pediatrics 19:142, 1957.

Boyer J, Dozor A, Brudnicki A, et al: Extralobar pulmonary sequestration masquerading as a congenital pleural effusion. Pediatrics 97:115, 1996.

Brooks JW: Tumors of the chest. *In* Kendig EL, Chernick V (Eds): Disorders of the Respiratory Tract in Children. Philadelphia, WB Saunders, 1983.

Brus F, Nikkels PGJ, van Loon AJ, Okken A: Non-immune hydrops fetalis and bilateral pulmonary hypoplasia in a newborn infant with extralobar pulmonary sequestration. Acta Paediatr 82:416, 1993.

Buntain WL, Isaacs H, Payne VC, et al: Lobar emphysema, cystic adenomatoid malformation, pulmonary sequestration and bronchogenic cyst in infancy and childhood: A clinical group. J Pediatr Surg 9:85, 1974.

Burnett WE, Caswell HT: Lobectomy for pulmonary cysts in a fifteen-day-old infant with recovery. Surgery 23:84, 1948.

Caffey J: On the natural regression of pulmonary cysts during early infancy. Pediatrics 11:48, 1953.

Campbell PE: Congenital lobar emphysema: Etiological studies. Aust Paediatr J 5:226, 1969.

Carter R: Pulmonary sequestration—collective review. Ann Thorac Surg 7:68, 1969.

Clark NS, Nairn RC, Gowar FJS: Cystic disease of the lung in the newborn treated by pneumonectomy. Arch Dis Child 31:358, 1956.

Cleveland RH, Weber B: Retained fetal lung liquid in congenital lobar emphysema: A possible predictor of polyalveolar lobe. Pediatr Radiol 23:291, 1993.

Collins MD, Moessinger AC, Kleinerman J, et al: Fetal lung hypoplasia associated with maternal smoking: A morphometric analysis. Pediatr Res 19:408, 1985.

Cooke FN, Blades BB: Cystic disease of the lungs. J Thorac Surg 23:546, 1952.

de Paredes CG, Pierce WS, Johnson DG, et al: Pulmonary sequestration in infants and children: A 20-year experience and review of the literature. J Pediatr Surg 5:136, 1970.

Dines DE, Seward JB, Bernatz PE, et al: Pulmonary arteriovenous fistulas. Mayo Clin Proc 58:176, 1983.

Dolkart LA, Reimers FT, Helmuth WV, et al: Antenatal diagnosis of pulmonary sequestration: A review. Obstet Gynecol Surv 47:515, 1992.

Doyle AJ: Demonstration of blood supply to pulmonary sequestration by MR angiography. AJR Am J Roentgenol 158:989, 1992.

Eisenberg P, Cohen HL, Coren C: Color Doppler in pulmonary sequestration diagnosis. J Ultrasound Med 11:175, 1992.

Ellis FH Jr, Kirklin JW, Hodgson CH, et al: Surgical implications of the mediastinal shadow in thoracic roentgenograms of infants and children. Surg Gynecol Obstet 100:532, 1955.

Erkalis AJ, Griscom NT, McGovern JB: Bronchogenic cyst of the mediastinum. N Engl J Med 281:1150, 1969.

Evans AE, D'Angio GJ, Randolph J: A proposed staging for children with neuroblastoma. Cancer 27:324, 1971.

Ferguson CC, Young LN, Sutherland JB, et al: Intrathoracic gastrogenic cyst—preoperative diagnosis by technetium pertechnetate scan. J Pediatr Surg 8:827, 1973.

Fischer CC, Tropea F Jr, Bailey CP: Congenital pulmonary cysts: Report of an infant treated by lobectomy with recovery. J Pediatr 23:219, 1943.

Fletcher BD, Masson M, Lisbona A, et al: Thymic response to endogenous and exogenous steroids in premature infants. J Pediatr 95:111, 1979.

France NE, Brown RJK: Congenital pulmonary lymphangiectasis: Report of 11 examples with special reference to cardiovascular findings. Arch Dis Child 46:528, 1971.

Gerle RD, Jaretski A, Ashley CA, et al: Congenital bronchopulmonary foregut malformation: Pulmonary sequestration communicating with the gastrointestinal tract. N Engl J Med 278:1413, 1968.

Gewolb IH, Lebowitz RL, Taeusch HW: Thymic size and its relationship to the respiratory distress syndrome. J Pediatr 95:108, 1979.

Goodwin SR, Graven SA, Haberkern CM: Aspiration in intubated premature infants. Pediatrics 75:85, 1985.

Gottschalk W, Abramson D: Placental edema and fetal hydrops. Obstet Gynecol 10:626, 1957.

Graham GG, Singleton JW: Diffuse hamartoma of the upper lobe in an infant: Report of successful surgical removal. AMA J Dis Child 89:609, 1955.

Gross RE: Congenital cystic lung: Successful pneumonectomy in a three-week-old baby. Ann Surg 123:229, 1946.

Gwinn JL, Lee FA, Rao PS: Radiological case of the month. Am J Dis Child 119:341, 1970.

Harrison MR, Adzick NS, Jennings RW, et al: Antenatal intervention for congenital cystic adenomatoid malformation. Lancet 336:965, 1990.

Heitoff KB, Sane SM, Williams HJ, et al: Bronchopulmonary foregut malformations: A unifying etiological concept. AJR Am J Roentgenol 126:46, 1976.

Hernanz-Schulman M, Stein SM, Neblett WW, et al: Pulmonary sequestration: Diagnosis with color Doppler sonography and a new theory of associated hydrothorax. Radiology 180:817, 1991.

Hershenson MB, Brouillette RT, Klemka L, et al: Respiratory insufficiency in newborns with abdominal wall defects. J Pediatr Surg 20:348, 1985.

Hill LF: Conference at Raymond Blank Memorial Hospital for Children, Des Moines, Iowa. J Pediatr 38:511, 1951.

Hislop A, Hey E, Reid L: The lungs in congenital bilateral renal agenesis and dysplasia. Arch Dis Child 54:32, 1979.

Hislop A, Reid L: New pathological findings in emphysema of childhood: Polyalveolar lobe with emphysema. Thorax 25:682, 1970.

Hislop A, Reid L: New pathological findings in emphysema of childhood: Overinflation of a normal lobe. Thorax 26:190, 1971.

Hodgson CH, Burchell HB, Good CA, et al: Hereditary hemorrhagic telangiectasia and pulmonary arteriovenous fistula. N Engl J Med 261:625, 1959.

Holder TM, Christy MG: Cystic adenomatoid malformation of the lung. J Thorac Cardiovasc Surg 47:590, 1964.

Hope JW, Koop CE: Differential diagnosis of mediastinal masses. Pediatr Clin North Am 6:379, 1959.

Izzo C, Rickham PP: Neonatal pulmonary hamartoma. J Pediatr Surg 3:77, 1968.

Kafka V, Beco V: Simultaneous intra- and extrapulmonary sequestration. Arch Dis Child 35:51, 1960.

Kitterman JA: Transient severe respiratory distress mimicking pulmonary hypoplasia in preterm infants. J Pediatr 123:969, 1993.

Knox WF, Barson AJ: Pulmonary hypoplasia in a regional perinatal unit. Early Hum Dev 14:33, 1986.

Kolls JK, Kiernan MP, Ascuitto RJ, et al: Intralobar pulmonary sequestration presenting as congestive heart failure in a neonate. Chest 102:974, 1992.

Kravitz RM: Congenital malformations of the lung. Pediatr Clin North Am 41:453, 1994.

Kwittken J, Reiner L: Congenital cystic adenomatoid malformation of the lung. Pediatrics 30:759, 1962.

Landing BH: Congenital malformations and genetic disorders of the respiratory tract (larynx, trachea, bronchi and lungs). Am Rev Respir Dis 120:151, 1979.

Langston C, Thurlbeck WM: Conditions altering normal lung growth and development. *In* Thibeault DW, Gregory GS (Eds): Neonatal Pulmonary Care. Norwalk, CT, Appleton-Century-Crofts, 1986.

Leahy LJ, Butsch WL: Surgical management of respiratory emergencies during the first few weeks of life. Arch Surg 59:466, 1949.

MacGillivray TE, Adzick NS, Harrison MR, et al: Disappearing fetal lung lesions. J Pediatr Surg 28:1321, 1993.

McBride JT, Wohl MEB, Strieder DJ, et al: Lung growth and airway function after lobectomy in infancy for congenital lobar emphysema. J Clin Invest 66:962, 1980.

McIntosh N: Dry lung syndrome after oligohydramnios. Arch Dis Child 63:190, 1988.

McIntosh N, Harrison A: Prolonged premature rupture of membranes in the preterm infant: A seven year study. Eur J Obstet Gynecol Reprod Biol 57:1, 1994.

Merenstein GB: Congenital cystic adenomatoid malformation of the lung. Am J Dis Child 118:772, 1969.

Mitchell RO, Austin EH: Pulmonary arteriovenous malformation in the neonate. J Pediatr Surg 28:1536, 1993.

Moessinger AC, Collins MH, Blanc WA, et al: Oligohydramnios-induced lung hypoplasia: The influence of timing and duration in gestation. Pediatr Res 20:951, 1986.

Morin L, Crombleholme TM, D'Alton ME: Prenatal diagnosis and management of fetal thoracic lesions. Semin Perinatol 18:228, 1994.

Nakamura Y, Yamamoto I, Funatsu Y, et al: Decreased surfactant level in the lung with oligohydramnios: A morphometric and biochemical study. J Pediatr 112:471, 1988.

Nimrod C, Varela-Gittings F, Machin G, et al: The effect of very prolonged membrane rupture on fetal development. Am J Obstet Gynecol 148:540, 1984.

Nishibayashi SW, Andrassy RJ, Woolley MM: Congenital cystic adeno-

matoid malformation: A 30-year experience. J Pediatr Surg 16:704, 1981.

Obwegeser R, Deutinger J, Bernaschek G: Fetal pulmonary cyst treated by repeated thoracentesis. Am J Obstet Gynecol 169:1622, 1993.

Opsahl T, Berman EJ: Bronchogenic mediastinal cysts in infants: Case report and review of the literature. Pediatrics 30:372, 1962.

Pearl M: Sequestration of the lung. Am J Dis Child 124:706, 1972.

Rescorla FJ, West KW, Vane DW, et al: Pulmonary hypertension in neonatal cystic lung disease: Survival following lobectomy and extracorporeal membrane oxygenation in two cases. J Pediatr Surg 25:1054, 1990.

Revillon Y, Jan D, Plattner V, et al: Congenital cystic adenomatoid malformation of the lung: Prenatal management and prognosis. J Pediatr Surg 28:1009, 1993.

Sabiston DC Jr, Scott HW Jr: Primary neoplasms and cysts of the mediastinum. Ann Surg 136:777, 1952.

Schlesinger AE, DiPietro MA, Statter MB, Lally KP: Utility of sonography in the diagnosis of bronchopulmonary sequestration. J Pediatr Surg 29:52, 1994.

Seibert JJ, Marvin WJ, Schieker RM: Mediastinal teratoma: A rare cause of severe respiratory distress in the newborn. J Pediatr Surg 11:253, 1976.

Shannon DC, Todres ID, Moylan FMB: Infantile lobar hyperinflation: Expectant treatment. Pediatrics 59:1012, 1977.

Smart LM, Hendry GMA: Imaging of neonatal pulmonary sequestration including Doppler ultrasound. Br J Radiol 64:324, 1991.

Spock A, Schneider S, Baylin GJ: Mediastinal gastric cysts: A case report and review of the English literature. Am Rev Respir Dis 94:97, 1966.

Stigers KB, Woodring JH, Kanga JF: The clinical and imaging spectrum of findings in patients with congenital lobar emphysema. Pediatr Pulmonol 14:160, 1992.

Stocker JT, Drake RM, Madewell JE: Cystic and congenital lung disease in the newborn. Perspect Pediatr Pathol 4:93, 1978.

Superina RA, Ein SH, Humphreys R: Cystic duplications of the esophagus and neuroenteric cysts. J Pediatr Surg 19:527, 1984.

Swan H, Aragon GE: Surgical treatment of pulmonary cysts in infancy. Pediatrics 14:651, 1954.

Swischuk LE, Richarson CJ, Nichols MM, et al: Primary pulmonary hypoplasia in the neonate. J Pediatr 95:573, 1979.

Thibeault DW, Beatty EC, Hall RT, et al: Neonatal pulmonary hypoplasia with premature rupture of fetal membranes and oligohydramnios. J Pediatr 107:273, 1985.

Thomas IT, Smith,DW: Oligohydramnios, cause of the non-renal features of Potter's syndrome, including pulmonary hypoplasia. J Pediatr 84:811, 1974.

Thompson RE, Love WG: Persistent cervical thymoma, apparent with crying. Am J Dis Child 124:761, 1972.

Thorpe-Beeston JG, Nicolaides KH: Cystic adenomatoid malformation of the lung: Prenatal diagnosis and outcome. Prenat Diagn 14:677, 1994.

Veeneklaas GMH: Pathogenesis of intrathoracic gastrogenic cysts. Am J Dis Child 83:500, 1952.

Wexler HA, Valdes-Dapena M: Congenital cystic adenomatoid malformation: A report of three unusual cases. Radiology 126:737, 1978.

White CW: Treatment of hemangiomatosis with recombinant interferon alpha. Semin Hematol 27:15, 1990.

White CW, Sondheimer HM, Crough EC, et al: Treatment of pulmonary hemangiomatosis with recombinant interferon alfa-2a. N Engl J Med 320:1197, 1989.

Wigglesworth JS, Desai R: Is fetal respiratory function a major determinant of perinatal survival? Lancet 1:264, 1982.

Wigglesworth JS, Desai R, Guerrini P: Fetal lung hypoplasia: Biochemical and structural variations and their possible significance. Arch Dis Child 56:606, 1981.

Young LW, Rubin P, Hanson RE: The extra-adrenal neuroblastoma: High radiocurability and diagnostic accuracy. AJR Am J Roentgenol 108:75, 1970.

CHAPTER 59

Accumulation of Fluid in the Pleural Space

Thomas Hansen and Anthony Corbet

PLEURAL EFFUSION

The pleural space exists between the parietal pleura of the chest wall and the visceral pleura of the lung. Each pleural surface is comprised of a mesothelial layer that covers a layer of connective tissue containing lymphatics, blood vessels, and nerves. In the parietal pleura, lymphatic channels communicate with the pleural space to provide a direct pathway for fluid and protein reabsorption. It was initially believed that the blood supply to the parietal pleura emanated from the systemic circulation and that the blood supply to the visceral pleura emanated from the pulmonary circulation. The capillary hydrostatic pressure in the visceral pleura was believed to be correspondingly low leading to the assumption that fluid was filtered out of the parietal pleura and reabsorbed by the visceral pleura. Data now show, however, that the blood supply to the visceral pleura emanates from the bronchial circulation: Both pleural surfaces filter fluid into the pleural space, and the lymphatics are responsible for most of the fluid reabsorption (Wiener-Kronish et al, 1985).

Fluid accumulates in the pleural space only if the rate of filtration increases or if the rate of lymphatic clearance decreases (or if both of these processes occur). The rate of fluid filtration can be increased by increasing the filtration pressure. The parietal pleura is drained by the systemic veins, and the visceral pleura is drained by the pulmonary veins. Therefore, filtration pressure increases with increases in either systemic or pulmonary venous pressure. Raised venous pressure (along with hypoproteinemia) is the most likely cause for pleural effusions that complicate heart failure as well as for effusions that occur with hydrops fetalis. The rate of fluid filtration into the pleural space also increases if the permeability of the pleura to water and protein increases (e.g., with infection).

Any impairment of lymphatic function from direct mechanical obstruction or from raised central venous pressure has marked effects on the rate of clearance of pleural fluid (Mellins et al, 1970). Raised venous pressure contributes substantially to the problem of effusions complicating heart failure or hydrops fetalis and accounts for the massive pleural effusions that accompany superior vena cava thrombosis (Dhande et al, 1983).

Pleural effusions should be suspected in any infant with respiratory difficulty who is hydropic or who has been receiving intravenous nutrition. Infants who receive central venous alimentation should have the glucose content of the pleural fluid checked immediately to make sure that the catheter has not perforated into the pleural space. Differential breath sounds are valuable in localizing unilateral effusions. The chest radiograph is diagnostic (Fig. 59–1). Thoracentesis is useful to identify effusions secondary to infections and to distinguish chylothorax from other causes of pleural effusions.

Infants with hydrops fetalis can occasionally have effusions that are large enough to impair ventilation and require drainage in the delivery room. Once the underlying abnormality is corrected, most effusions resolve without further need for drainage. Effusions that accompany superior vena cava syndrome can persist and require interventions similar to those described for persistent chylothorax.

CHYLOTHORAX

Accumulations of chyle in the pleural space may be congenital or acquired. Congenital chylothorax is probably one part of the spectrum of anomalies that result from intrauterine obstruction of the thoracic duct (Chervenak et al, 1983; Smeltzer et al, 1986). It may occur alone or in combination with other lymphatic anomalies. Presumably, lymph flow obstruction results in the development of fistulas between the thoracic duct and the pleural space or in rupture of the thoracic duct. Congenital chylothorax occurs more commonly in males than in females (2:1), and it occurs more commonly on the right side (right, 53%; left, 35%; bilateral, 12%) (Chernick and Reed, 1970). Acquired chylothorax results from damage to the thoracic duct. It has been reported as a surgical complication of the repair of diaphragmatic hernia, tracheoesophageal fistula, and a variety of congenital heart disorders.

Acquired chylothorax is usually diagnosed by a chest radiograph obtained because of a change in respiratory

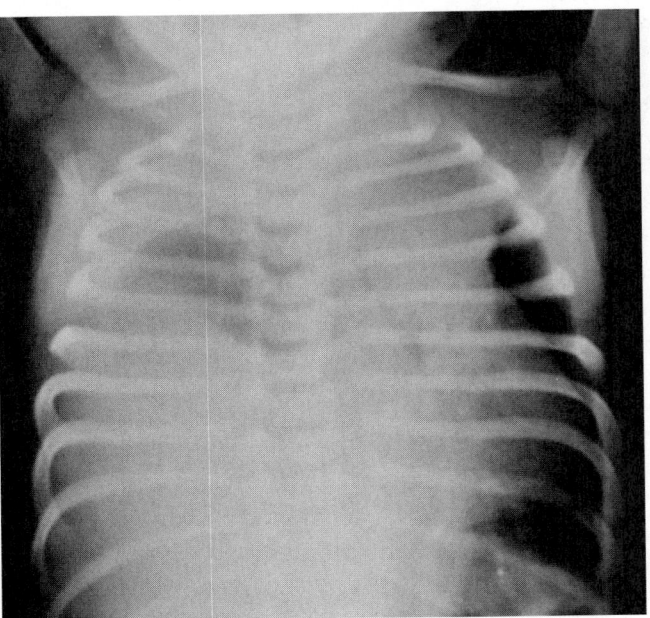

FIGURE 59–1. Chest radiograph of an infant with a right-sided chylothorax.

TABLE 59–1

Composition of Chyle

Measurement	Units	Mean	Range
Total protein	g/dL	3.56	1.89–6.17
Albumin	g/dL	2.24	1.26–3.0
Total lipids	mg/dL	1180	56–3500
Cholesterol	mg/dL	81	48–200
Triglycerides	mg/dL	197	123–234
White blood cells	/mm³	15,200	0–29,000
Lymphocytes	%	90	70–100
pH	—	7.5	7.4–7.8
Specific gravity	—	1.013	1.008–1.027

From Brodman RF: Congenital chylothorax: Recommendation for treatment. NY State J Med 75:553, 1975.

status. Congenital chylothorax has been diagnosed in utero by ultrasonography. Bilateral chylothoraces should be considered in the differential diagnosis of any infant who cannot be ventilated in the delivery room. Thoracentesis is required for a definitive diagnosis. Chyle can be distinguished from transudates by its high protein and lipid content; it can be distinguished from exudates by its high lipid content, the characteristic preponderance of lymphocytes, and its slightly alkalotic pH (Table 59–1).

Treatment of chylothorax may require repeated thoracenteses or even thoracostomy tube drainage to prevent respiratory failure (Brodman, 1975). Drainage has been performed in the fetus to try to prevent compression of the lungs and pulmonary hypoplasia (Rodeck et al, 1988; Schmidt et al, 1985). Once drainage is accomplished, these infants are placed on formulas containing medium-chain triglycerides, rather than long-chain fats, to reduce thoracic duct lymph flow and the rate of reaccumulation of chyle. Oral intake of protein and water also stimulates thoracic duct lymph flow, however, so often the infant is not allowed anything by mouth, and nutritional support must be provided intravenously.

A variety of approaches have been used with some success to treat the infant with persistent chylothorax, including direct attempts at repair, patching with fibrin glue (Stenzl et al, 1983), and obliteration of the pleural space with sclerosing agents. Chylothorax has also been managed successfully using a pleuroperitoneal shunt (Azizkhan et al, 1983). Finally, some reports suggest that ligation of the thoracic duct below the area of leakage is highly effective in stopping reaccumulation (Stringel et al, 1984). Thoracic duct ligation appears to be well tolerated without accumulations of fluid in the peripheral tissues or in the peritoneum.

The prognosis for infants with chylothorax is good. In a review of 34 cases, two thirds of the infants with chylothorax responded to thoracentesis alone, and only 5 infants died (15%). The complications reported in this review included weight loss from malnutrition, hypoproteinemia, and lymphopenia (Brodman, 1975).

REFERENCES

Azizkhan RG, Canfield J, Alford BA, et al: Pleuroperitoneal shunts in the management of neonatal chylothorax. J Pediatr Surg 18:842, 1983.

Brodman RF: Congenital chylothorax: Recommendations for treatment. N Y State J Med 75:553, 1975.

Chernick V, Reed MH: Pneumothorax and chylothorax in the neonatal period. J Pediatr 76:624, 1970.

Chervenak FA, Isaacson G, Blakemore KJ, et al: Fetal cystic hygroma: Cause and natural history. N Engl J Med 309:822, 1983.

Dhande V, Kattwinkel J, Alford B: Recurrent bilateral pleural effusions secondary to superior vena cava obstruction as a complication of central venous catheterization. Pediatrics 72:109, 1983.

Mellins RB, Levine OR, Fishman AP: Effect of systemic and pulmonary venous hypertension on pleural and pericardial fluid accumulation. J Appl Physiol 29:564, 1970.

Rodeck CH, Fisk NM, Fraser DI, et al: Long-term in utero drainage of fetal hydrothorax. N Engl J Med 319:1135, 1988.

Schmidt W, Harms E, Wolf D: Successful prenatal treatment of nonimmune hydrops fetalis due to congenital chylothorax: Case report. Br J Obstet Gynaecol 92:685, 1985.

Smeltzer DM, Stickler GB, Fleming RE: Primary lymphatic dysplasia in children: Chylothorax, chylous ascites, and generalized lymphatic dysplasia. Eur J Pediatr 145:286, 1986.

Stenzl W, Rigler B, Tscheliessnigg KH, et al: Treatment of postsurgical chylothorax with fibrin glue. Thorac Cardiovasc Surg 31:35, 1983.

Stringel G, Mercer S, Bass J: Surgical management of persistent postoperative chylothorax in children. Can J Surg 27:543, 1984.

Wiener-Kronish JP, Berthiaume Y, Albertine KH: Pleural effusions and pulmonary edema. Clin Chest Med 6:509, 1985.

CHAPTER 60

Disorders of the Chest Wall and Diaphragm

Thomas Hansen, Anthony Corbet and Roberta A. Ballard

DISORDERS OF THE CHEST WALL

Abnormalities of the bone and muscle of the chest wall may be a mechanical hindrance to ventilation. Although bony abnormalities are rare, they may be recognized immediately and are sometimes amenable to operative correction.

Defects in fusion of the sternum are uncommon. *Complete separation of the sternum* allows protrusion of cardiovascular structures, a condition known as *ectopia cordis*. Lethal malformations of the heart are commonly associated with this condition. *Upper sternal clefts* are more common. Early operation is advised to shield the underlying structures from injury and because of the greater ease of approximating the separated parts in the first days of life, compared with later.

The most common of the sternal defects is *pectus excavatum*, sometimes associated with the Pierre Robin syndrome and Marfan syndrome. Rarely is it a fixed or severe deformity until several months of postnatal age. A family history of some type of anterior thoracic deformity was found in 37% of patients, according to Welch (1980). The indications for operative correction are debatable. In the authors' opinion, correction should not be undertaken until several years of age and then only in those few children in whom the deformity appears to be progressing. Serial photographs are the best way to document changes in pectus excavatum. Periodic evaluation of cardiovascular status with ultrasonography and electrocardiogram and assessment of pulmonary function are appropriate in the presence of progressive deformity. Results of operative correction are excellent in more than 80% of patients and almost always lead to improvement. Recurrences are possible during later active growth.

A rare deformity of the thoracic cage, *asphyxiating thoracic dystrophy*, is part of a serious generalized chondrodystrophy (Fig. 60–1). It was first described by Jeune and coworkers in 1954. The ribs are broad and short, and the thorax is rigid. Some degree of lung hypoplasia may be present. Renal cystic dysplasia may be present and lead to hypertension and renal failure. About 60 cases have been reported. Oberkaid and coworkers (1977) studied 10 of them and noted that only two patients were alive at the time of the report. One of the two was in excellent health at 15 years of age. The more severely affected infants had respiratory distress from birth. Three patients have been described in one family; the expectation is occurrence in one of four siblings. No parent-child occurrence has been described. The disorder is familial and is inherited as an autosomal recessive trait. Attempts at operative correction have not been successful. Prenatal diagnosis with ultrasonography is possible.

Severe underdevelopment of the thoracic rib cage, accompanied usually by lethal pulmonary hypoplasia, may be seen in other conditions, such as the *thanatophoric dwarfism syndrome*, the *short rib–polydactyly syndrome*, and the *camptomelic dwarfism syndrome*. These infants do not survive for long after birth.

Deficiency of pectoral muscles on one side (Poland syndrome) may be associated with abnormal ribs (two to four) and hypoplasia of the breast. Breathing may be paradoxic and the cardiac impulse easily observed through the soft tissues. No operative intervention is required in infancy, although mammoplasty may later be desirable in affected girls after puberty.

Other causes of thoracic dysfunction are diseases of the muscles, including myasthenia gravis, poliomyelitis, amyotonia congenita, congenital muscular dystrophy, glycogen storage disease, and spinal cord injury or tumor. Such conditions are usually recognized in the context of the associated systemic muscular weakness or paralysis. They should be suspected in any infant in whom hypoventilation is present when the chest radiograph shows normal heart and lungs.

DISORDERS OF THE DIAPHRAGM
Congenital Diaphragmatic Hernia

Most infants with congenital diaphragmatic hernia (CDH) are mature, two thirds are male, and in 90% the hernia is left-sided. Incidence has been reported in between 1 in 2000 and 1 in 10,000 live births (Langham et al, 1996). In the newborn, nearly all hernias pass through the posterolateral foramen of Bochdalek. The pathophysiology of CDH has been reviewed by Glick and colleagues (1996).

Pathogenesis

The diaphragm develops anteriorly as a septum between the heart and liver and progresses backward to close last at the left Bochdalek foramen around 8 to 10 weeks' gestation. The bowel migrates from the yolk sac at about 10 weeks, and if it arrives before the foramen has closed, a hernia results. Lung compression from an early age is associated with pulmonary hypoplasia, most severe on the ipsilateral side but also present on the contralateral side. There is a marked reduction in the number of bronchial generations and a less marked reduction in the number of alveoli per acinus. The number of arterial vessels is proportionally reduced (Bohn et al, 1987), and there is a modest increase in the medial muscle of pulmonary arterioles, together with abnormal extension of muscle into arterioles at the acinar level (Geggel et al, 1985). In many cases, herniation occurs comparatively late in gestation, or the hernia is small, in which case the lung hypoplasia is less marked (Adzick et al, 1985).

After birth when the hernia fills with air, compression

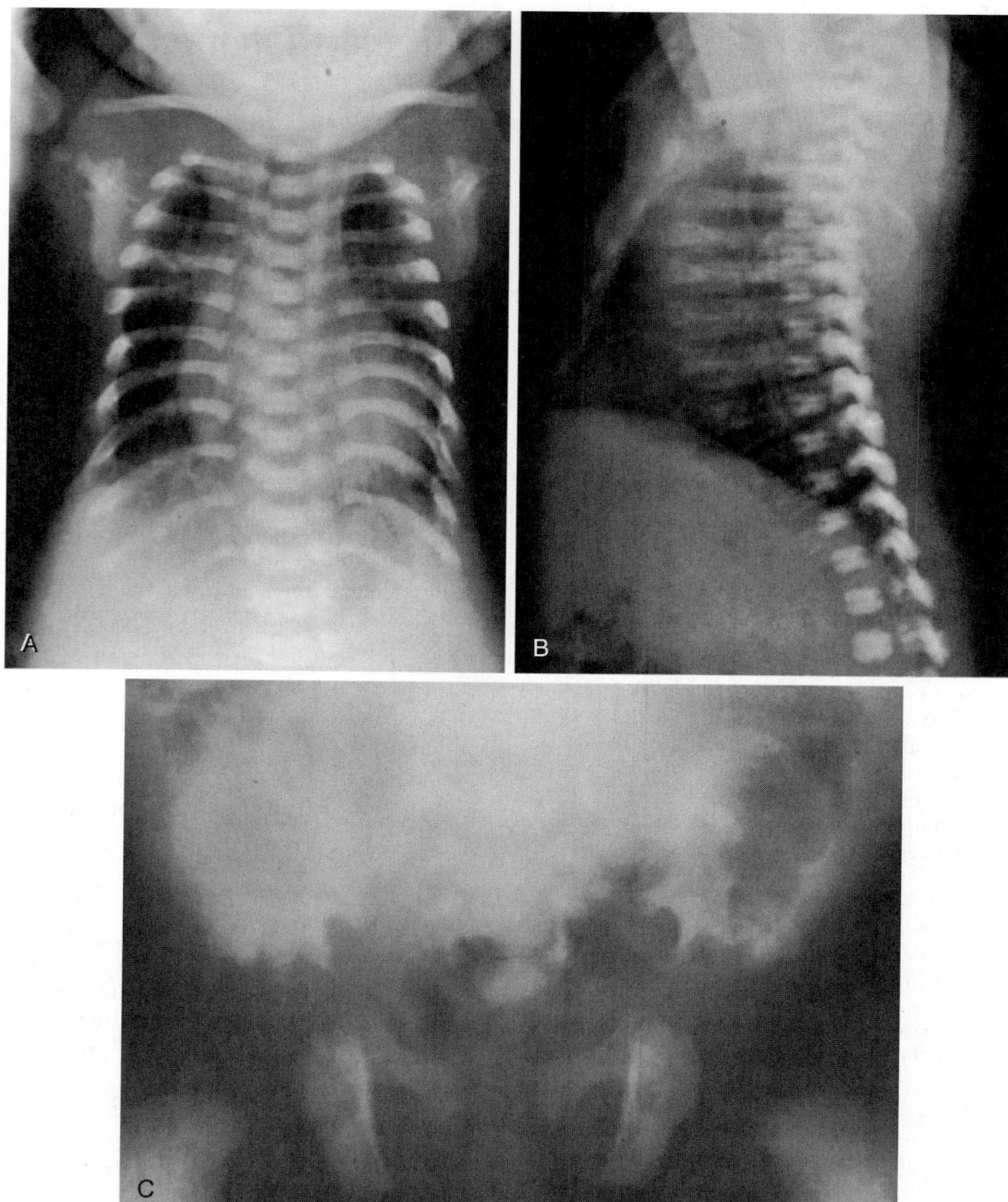

FIGURE 60–1. *A,* Anteroposterior radiograph of infant with asphyxiating thoracic dystrophy. The thoracic circumference is reduced as compared with the abdominal circumference, and the liver and spleen are displaced downward. *B,* Lateral projection of the same infant further demonstrates the reduced thoracic volume. (*A* and *B* courtesy of Dr. John Kirkpatrick.) *C,* Radiograph of the pelvis shows flaring of the iliac crest and irregular calcification of the triradiate cartilage with typical bony protrusions. (*C* from Avery ME, Fletcher BD, Williams RG: The Lung and Its Disorders in the Newborn Infant, 4th ed. Philadelphia, WB Saunders, 1981.)

of the lungs is increased, thus superimposing atelectasis on pulmonary hypoplasia. The prognosis depends on the degree of pulmonary hypoplasia (Nguyen et al, 1983), with its associated reduction in alveolar and vascular surface area. There may be severe hypercarbia and hypoxemia with persistent pulmonary hypertension and large right-to-left shunts at the atrial and ductal levels. The pulmonary hyper-

tension has a fixed element because of anatomic changes and a reactive vasoconstrictive element, which is responsive to clinical conditions. Kobayashi and Puri (1994) have shown in this condition that pulmonary hypertension is accompanied by markedly elevated levels of endothelin in the plasma and markedly increased expression of endothelin immunoreactivity in lung endothelial cells.

Diagnosis

An increasing percentage of diaphragmatic hernias are now diagnosed antenatally by ultrasonography. Antenatal diagnosis allows evaluation of the fetus for possible additional anomalies as well as counseling of the family as to possible treatment approaches and prognosis. It is still unclear, however, what factors are the most accurate for predicting eventual outcome (Wilcox et al, 1996a) (see discussion later). For those not diagnosed in utero, the onset of symptoms is usually with respiratory distress in the first few hours or days of life. Patients with the most severe symptoms present in the delivery room with a difficult resuscitation and have a high incidence of pneumothorax in the more common left-sided hernias. Breath sounds are absent on the left side, the chest is barrel shaped, the abdomen is scaphoid, and the heart beat is displaced to the right. The diagnosis is made easily with a chest radiograph, aided by a feeding tube placed in the stomach. The left hemithorax is filled with a mass, usually incorporating air-filled bowel loops, and the stomach tube enters the chest. The heart is displaced to the right, and the abdomen is remarkably devoid of gas patterns (Fig. 60–2).

Associated Anomalies

Fauza and Wilson (1994) reviewed 166 cases of CDH and found that 39% had associated anomalies and 61% were isolated; many of the listed anomalies may not be clinically evident, but many have an adverse effect on the outcome. About two thirds of the anomalies were cardiac, including hypoplastic left heart syndrome, atrial septal defect, ven-

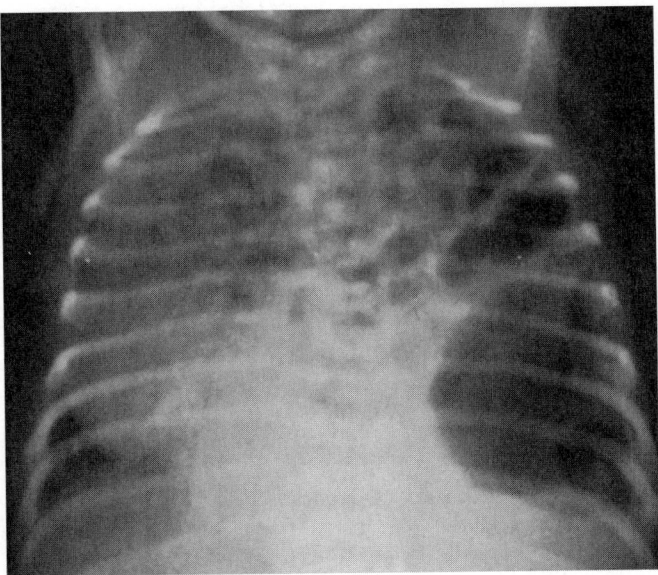

FIGURE 60–2. Left-sided diaphragmatic hernia. Anteroposterior view of the chest taken on the 2nd day of life. The chest is overexpanded and barrel shaped. Round translucencies of varying size fill the left hemithorax and part of the right. The heart occupies the lower lateral corner of the right hemithorax. Both diaphragms are depressed, the left more than the right. The translucency in the left lower hemithorax resembles stomach, slightly above it looks like large bowel, and the remainder appear to be loops of small bowel.

tricular septal defect, coarctation of the aorta, and Ebstein anomaly. Other anomalies in this series included esophageal atresia, trisomy 18, hydronephrosis, hydrocephalus, and omphalocele. It is important to assess these patients by echocardiography, but the study is often technically difficult because of the malposition of the heart (Ryan et al, 1994). It has been reported that left ventricular mass is reduced in CDH and that this may adversely affect the outcome (Schwartz et al, 1994); it is not clear why this problem occurs, but one suggestion is that fetal venous return across the foramen ovale to the left side of the heart may be reduced by displacement of the heart within the chest, and the change in flow dynamics might cause underdevelopment of the left ventricle (Allan et al, 1996).

Prediction of Outcome

In an early study, it was found that in those diagnosed during the first 6 hours of life the mortality was 68%, in those diagnosed at 6 to 24 hours of age the mortality was 59%, and in those diagnosed after 24 hours of age the mortality was 22% (Raphaely and Downes, 1973). In a more recent study, however, which may reflect improvements in care over time, it was found that in those needing treatment in the first 6 hours of life, the mortality was 44%, and in those needing treatment after 6 hours, the mortality was close to 0% (Marshall and Sumner, 1982). These data imply that if the lungs are good enough to bridge the first 6 hours of life, the results of treatment are likely to be good.

Others believe that the prognosis is best assessed by the arterial PCO_2 and the intensity of conventional mechanical ventilation required, as a reflection of the degree of pulmonary hypoplasia. Bohn and coworkers (1987) assessed the mortality in terms of a critical arterial PCO_2 of 40 mm Hg and a critical ventilation index of 1000 (where ventilation index = mean airway pressure × ventilator rate). Their data were accumulated before the availability of extracorporeal membrane oxygenation (ECMO). Wung and colleagues (1995), however, have reported excellent outcome in infants who have been managed with gentle ventilation and permissive hypercarbia. This approach makes the predictive value of $PaCO_2$ less important.

Wilson and colleagues (1991) and others (O'Rourke et al, 1988) have found that a postductal PaO_2 of greater than 100 mm Hg was associated with much better survival (91%) than that of infants who never experienced a honeymoon period. Obviously, if this PaO_2 is associated with a normal $PaCO_2$ without vigorous ventilation, this combination is most promising.

Hasegawa and coworkers (1994) also demonstrated the predictive value of the ratio of the left and right pulmonary artery dimensions, as measured by ultrasound. If the left artery was smaller than the right artery, severe pulmonary hypoplasia and severe pulmonary hypertension were more likely to be present.

Treatment

In infants with a prenatal diagnosis or as soon as the diagnosis is suspected, a double-lumen orogastric tube should be passed and suctioned continuously to reduce the amount of air in the hernia and decrease compression of the lung. The infant should not be ventilated by bag and mask but instead immediately intubated and ventilated using a low peak pressure (<30 cm H_2O) if possible. Because the danger of pneumothorax is high and substantially increases mortality (Hansen et al, 1984), paralysis with pancuronium and sedation with morphine are indicated; paralysis provides the additional benefit that swallowing air is abolished, which helps keep the hernia decompressed. Surfactant should be administered because there is accumulating evidence that the lungs in infants with severe diaphragmatic hernias are immature in addition to hypoplastic (Bohn et al, 1996; Glick et al 1992a, 1992b; Suen et al, 1993; Wilcox et al, 1994, 1995b, 1996b). Administration of surfactant (prophylactically when possible) may not only treat surfactant deficiency and improve compliance, but also may lower pulmonary vascular resistance and improve pulmonary blood flow (O'Toole et al, 1996b) (see discussion later).

The infant should have an umbilical arterial catheter inserted and, if possible, an umbilical venous catheter with its tip at the junction of the inferior vena cava and right atrium. In forms of CDH with the liver in the chest, the catheter does not go through the ductus venous and should not be left in place. Right-to-left shunting can be followed by the use of pulse oximeters above and below the ductus. Blood pressure support should be given in the form of colloid and continuous dopamine infusion if hypotension is present. It is prudent to restrict the volume of crystalloid administered because pulmonary edema may cause deterioration. Alkalosis may be produced by administration of sodium bicarbonate or tris(hydroxymethyl)aminomethane (Tham). Although the definitive treatment is surgical reduction of the hernia, there is no evidence that this is an emergency, and time should be spent in adequately stabilizing the infant (Bohn et al, 1996; Charlton et al, 1992; Goh et al, 1992).

Other Treatment Approaches

High-Frequency Ventilation

Tamura and colleagues (1988) reported two infants with high-risk CDH treated successfully with high-frequency oscillatory ventilation; the major advantage was improved control of the arterial P_{CO_2}. For infants with severe respiratory failure on maximal conventional mechanical ventilation and approaching ECMO inclusion criteria, the success rate for high-frequency jet ventilation in avoiding ECMO has been reported as 33% (Baumgart et al, 1992), and the success rate for high-frequency oscillatory ventilation in avoiding ECMO has been reported as 22% (Paranka et al, 1995). A trial of up to 6 hours of high-frequency ventilation is considered worthwhile, but most responsive patients improve within 1 hour, so the trial need not be prolonged and ECMO need not be unduly delayed. High-frequency ventilation may also be used in patients with less severe pulmonary hypoplasia. Although there is no evidence that high-frequency ventilation is superior to conventional ventilation, it may be a good choice if the patient develops a pneumothorax on conventional ventilation.

Inhaled Nitric Oxide

Inhaled nitric oxide has been used successfully in the treatment of persistent pulmonary hypertension of the newborn (see Chapter 53), and several investigators have tried this therapy in infants with persistent pulmonary hypertension of the newborn complicating the course of CDH (Bohn et al, 1996; Dillon et al, 1995; Finer et al, 1992; Henneberg et al, 1995). Karamanoukian and associates (1994) treated CDH infants with nitric oxide and found that before ECMO there was little response, but about 1 week later, after ECMO, the same patients responded to nitric oxide treatment with sustained improvements in oxygenation. In the lamb model of CDH, there was a good response to nitric oxide but in this case only after the animals had received exogenous surfactant treatment (Karamanoukian et al, 1995). It is not yet clear whether this is true for the human infant.

Extracorporeal Membrane Oxygenation

There have been no randomized controlled trials that specifically examined the efficacy of ECMO in the management of CDH. Many centers using ECMO have not seen an improvement in the survival of patients with CDH, but this may be because of a change in the referral pattern to these centers, with more severe cases being sent for treatment. Atkinson and coworkers (1991) compared infants with an oxygenation index of 40 or more; before ECMO, the mortality was 95%, and after the introduction of ECMO, the mortality was 31%. Infants who presented with respiratory distress in the first 6 hours of life were analyzed before and after the introduction of ECMO in the Netherlands (vanden Staak et al, 1995). Patients without exclusion criteria, who were suitable candidates for ECMO, were classified according to whether or not they met ECMO inclusion criteria. Before the availability of ECMO, in those who met ECMO inclusion criteria, the mortality was 100%, whereas after the introduction of ECMO, in those who met ECMO inclusion criteria, the mortality was 39%, a highly significant improvement.

At present, the standard criteria for ECMO are used in CDH patients, but in general the results have not been as good as in other conditions, such as meconium aspiration pneumonia. Attempts have been made to decrease the number of infants subjected to ECMO and to improve the results for ECMO treatment of CDH by changing the inclusion criteria. Some centers require that the patient show evidence of the so-called honeymoon period, in which the postductal arterial P_{O_2} should be at least 100 mm Hg on at least one occasion (O'Rourke et al, 1988; Stolar et al, 1988); otherwise the patient is considered to have severe pulmonary hypoplasia and not to be a candidate for ECMO. Steimie and associates (1994) considered a honeymoon period to be represented by any arterial P_{O_2} above 50 mm Hg. When they included infants who never had an arterial P_{O_2} above 50 mm Hg, the results overall were worse; they found that survival of the additional patients without a honeymoon period was only 27%. They considered lack of a honeymoon period, as they defined it, to be a relative contraindication for ECMO.

Others have wanted to use ECMO in more cases. They

have argued that the overall results for survival in CDH patients might be improved if infants with CDH were started on ECMO earlier, at a higher level of arterial Po_2, to take into account that the arterial Pco_2 is often elevated in CDH (vanden Staak et al, 1993). There has been no confirmation of this idea.

In the final analysis, the degree of lung hypoplasia along with the severity of pulmonary vascular disease determines the outcome with ECMO. The aim of ECMO is to have the patient survive long enough for reactive pulmonary hypertension to resolve, which may take up to 2 to 3 weeks, but if there is severe lung hypoplasia, death becomes inevitable. Antunes and coworkers (1995) evaluated the prognosis with preoperative measurements of lung volume by the helium dilution method; there were clear differences for those who survived without ECMO (16 mL/kg), those who survived with ECMO (12 mL/kg), and those who died despite ECMO (5 mL/kg). A lung volume of less than 9 mL/kg delineated infants with such severe lung hypoplasia that they were unlikely to survive, even after prolonged ECMO for up to 4 weeks.

The presence of congenital heart disease is a relative contraindication to ECMO but only if the lesion is known to be untreatable (Ryan et al, 1994), as in the case of hypoplastic left heart syndrome. Overall the mortality is doubled by the presence of congenital heart disease (Cunnif et al, 1990). In infants with other anomalies, it is important to assess the chromosome status as rapidly as possible to avoid using ECMO in infants with severe genetic problems, but this may be difficult in an emergency situation.

Surgery

For many years, it was considered imperative to reduce the hernia surgically as soon as possible after birth. Cartlidge and associates (1986) reported a markedly improved survival when surgery, instead of being done immediately, was delayed for a period of 4 to 16 hours of stabilization; they recommended that surgery not be performed until the pH was at least 7.20. To explore why early surgery may be harmful, Sakai and colleagues (1987) measured the static respiratory system compliance before and after surgery in infants who presented in the first 6 hours of life and were operated immediately. The surgical technique included, when considered necessary, the use of abdominal muscle flaps for diaphragm repair and nonclosure of abdominal muscle to avoid overfilling the abdominal cavity. These authors found no improvement in compliance after surgery, and most patients had major reductions in compliance, suggesting that surgery had made matters worse. This was thought to be due mostly to tension in the chest wall generated by the repaired diaphragm and to tension generated by the abdominal wall after closure of the muscle layers, rather than to reduced compliance in the lung itself.

In a prospective controlled trial, Nakayama and coworkers (1991) compared a group of infants who had early emergency repair at about 11 hours of age with a group who had delayed repair, many of them after a period of ECMO, at about 5 to 6 days of age. They confirmed that respiratory system compliance was not improved after surgery and was usually decreased, and this was true

whether or not they had early or delayed surgery. Before surgery, the delayed surgery group had a significant improvement in respiratory system compliance, which may ultimately have been helpful. The mortality in the early surgery group was 54%, whereas in the delayed surgery group the mortality was only 11%. Although the delayed surgery group was thought to have more severe disease initially, the results for delayed surgery looked better; however, this study, similar to others before it, may have been misleading because it was not properly randomized.

Nio and colleagues (1994) have reported the results of a randomized, controlled trial of early versus delayed surgical repair of CDH in 32 infants, who presented with respiratory distress within 12 hours of birth. All patients were treated with ECMO according to standard criteria. The early group had surgery at about 10 hours of age, and the delayed group had surgery at about the age of 1 week. There was no difference in the need for ECMO or in the mortality between the two groups. The authors concluded that if the patient could be adequately stabilized with mechanical ventilation, early surgery was suitable, but if the patient could not be stabilized, preoperative ECMO and delayed surgery was a more reasonable course.

Surgical Management. Some surgeons recommend placement of a thoracostomy tube to protect against the catastrophic development of tension pneumothorax, but the underwater seal should be at atmospheric pressure and not placed to suction. Others believe that no chest tube should be placed and air in the pleural cavity not removed, so as to discourage overdistention of the contralateral lung (Cloutier et al, 1983). They believe that overdistention may be sufficient to compress pulmonary capillaries and reduce pulmonary blood flow; Ramenofsky (1979) used a dog model of CDH to show that suction to the ipsilateral pleural space caused overdistention and deterioration of gas exchange, which could be reversed by instillation of air back into the ipsilateral pleural space. No matter what is done concerning the chest tube, every attempt should be made to keep the mediastinum in the midline and not to overdistend the contralateral lung. Wung and colleagues (1995) have reported excellent results emphasizing delayed surgery, avoidance of lung overdistention, and no chest tube.

Postoperatively, patients often require quite large volumes of colloid to overcome the effects of third-space fluid losses on systemic perfusion. All too commonly, the course is complicated by the development of pulmonary hypertension. If the systemic arterial pressure is not well maintained with inotropics, there may be increased right-to-left shunting at the ductus arteriosus and foramen ovale. There is no evidence that hyperventilation is helpful in these infants, but Wung and colleagues (1995) have been successful using permissive hypercarbia. Attempts to increase pulmonary blood flow with tolazoline, nitroprusside, and other drugs have only occasionally been successful and if they reduce systemic arterial pressure may instead be harmful.

The left lung may take only a few days to expand and fully occupy the hemithorax, which means that atelectasis predominated over hypoplasia. Otherwise the space, initially filled with air, becomes filled with fluid. The lung may slowly increase in size over the next few weeks, but in the most severe cases, growth may take several months. Histologically, there is growth in the number of alveoli and a reduction in the muscle mass of pulmonary arteries, but these improvements are more marked on the contralateral side (Beals et al, 1992), and the time course is such that it is at least a week before improvement occurs.

Surgery On or Off Extracorporeal Membrane Oxygenation. Although delayed surgery has become common, some centers have performed surgery while the patient is still on ECMO (Breaux et al, 1991), and some centers wait until the patient can be taken off ECMO (Adolph et al, 1995). The technique of surgery on ECMO calls for the use of topical thrombin powder or fibrin glue, the use of less heparin with acceptance of shorter activated clotting times (180 to 200 seconds), and the use of antifibrinolytic agents (Wilson et al, 1994a). In the experience of many, the incidence of hemorrhagic complications is greater; surgical site hemorrhage needing transfusion occurred in 38%, 18%, and 6% of those repaired on, before, and after ECMO (Vasquez and Cheu, 1994). These complications may contribute to a worse outcome (Lally et al, 1992).

The major reason for performing surgical repair on ECMO is the fear of rebound pulmonary hypertension after decannulation. In a large Canadian experience, however, Sigalet and colleagues (1995) have not found rebound pulmonary hypertension to be a problem in following their strategy of initial stabilization, ECMO if necessary, and delayed surgical repair after decannulation. Some centers find it useful to monitor the patient with serial echocardiography and to operate only after the pulmonary artery pressure reaches 30 to 50 mm Hg or a left-to-right shunt appears (Haugen et al, 1991). Some centers offer a second course of ECMO, and this may be quite useful in the case of CDH (Lally and Breaux, 1995); surgical reinsertion of the catheters has usually been possible.

Mortality

For those presenting in the first 6 hours of life, Adzick and colleagues (1985) found no difference in mortality for left-sided versus right-sided hernias, but all infants with bilateral hernias died. The mortality for associated polyhydramnios was 89% compared with 45% for those without associated polyhydramnios. Prematurity was associated with a higher mortality rate, as expected. The mode of delivery, whether vaginal or abdominal, and immediate surgery after birth made no difference to the outcome. Those with a prenatal diagnosis and planned delivery have better resuscitation at birth, as reflected in the 5-minute Apgar score, but there is no evidence that this has improved the survival rate. Langman and coworkers (1996) reviewed the epidemiology and outcome for these infants.

Complications

It is common for infants with CDH to have evidence of esophageal dilation, esophageal dysfunction, and gastroesophageal reflux (Stolar et al, 1990), and some of these infants require a Nissen fundoplication in the predischarge phase (Kieffer et al, 1995; Koot et al, 1993; Nagaya et al, 1994; Sigalet et al, 1994). Esophageal dilation and dysfunc-

tion are more common in infants who had polyhydramnios before birth. There is often a minimal or absent left diaphragmatic crus, and it may be necessary to refashion this at the time of hernia repair (Sigalet et al, 1994). It is possible that a tight primary repair of the diaphragm may apply excessive tension to the diaphragm at the gastroesophageal junction and that a synthetic patch should be used more often (Kieffer et al, 1995).

Some infants may develop intestinal obstruction related to volvulus and adhesions and require a laparotomy. In a few instances repaired with a synthetic patch, a recurrent diaphragmatic hernia has developed, sometimes within a few months but often at about the age of 18 months, and the diaphragmatic patch may need to be repaired (Atkinson and Poon, 1992). Other infants have complications associated with the development of bronchopulmonary dysplasia. Of course, these infants may have the usual complications related to the use of ECMO, other invasive procedures, and indwelling venous catheters; the most notable have been extra-axial fluid collections in the brain, pleural effusions owing to chylothorax, and superior vena cava syndromes.

Outcome of Survivors

D'Agostino and coworkers (1995) provided data for the 1st year of life in 16 surviving patients who were treated with ECMO during the years 1990–1992 in Philadelphia. Before discharge from the hospital, 13 infants had gastroesophageal reflux; 11 infants were poor oral feeders and needed tube feedings; and 10 infants had bronchopulmonary dysplasia, some of mild severity. At the age of 1 year, 11 infants had symmetric hypotonia. In addition, three infants still needed ventilatory support for bronchopulmonary dysplasia. On the Bayley Scales of Infant Development, the mean mental score was 87, which was considered to be average, and the mean psychomotor score was 75, indicating a significant level of motor impairment in some infants. The scores were worse in those who needed a synthetic patch for repair of the diaphragm and were better in those who did not need a patch (an indicator of severity). The authors considered that seven infants had normal cognitive and motor function. Only 1 out of 14 infants had a significant hearing loss.

Lund and colleagues (1994) followed 33 patients with CDH for a period of 2 to 3 years; 20 of these patients were treated with ECMO. They found deafness needing amplification in 7 infants, seizure disorder that resolved by 12 months of age in 4 infants, developmental delays without evidence of cerebral palsy in 15 infants, and evidence of growth failure in many infants. Abnormal head computed tomography scans were found in 10 infants, usually with bifrontal brain atrophy or ventriculomegaly, both of uncertain significance. Six infants needed surgery for bowel obstruction, and six infants needed fundoplication for gastroesophageal reflux. Chest wall deformities were seen in one third of infants, usually pectus excavatum, presumably the result of chronic respiratory distress, and scoliosis developed in four infants, possibly the result of tight diaphragmatic repairs. In older children, although the chest radiograph may appear normal, lung volumes are slightly reduced, and there is persistent evidence of a reduced vascular bed in the left lung (Reid and Hutcherson, 1976; Wohl et al, 1977).

Prenatal Diagnosis and Possible Fetal Surgery

There has been controversy over how to assess the results of therapy for CDH, especially whether the denominator should be all fetuses with the condition or all those infants referred for surgical treatment. It is important to know the mortality with conventional therapy when assessing the suitability of other therapies.

Harrison and colleagues (Adzick et al, 1985, 1989; Harrison et al, 1994) at the University of California, San Francisco, have produced evidence that there is a large hidden mortality in this condition, which is not reflected in the results reported from ECMO referral centers. A significant number of infants have associated lethal malformations, some are stillborn, some are either electively not resuscitated in the delivery room or cannot be resuscitated despite the best efforts of clinicians, and some are not transported to an appropriate center for surgery and ECMO. These authors concluded that when the diagnosis is made before birth, the true mortality is about 60% for those without lethal malformations and about 80% for the total population; this contrasts with the results from ECMO referral centers, which report mortalities of 20% to 40%. Two other groups, however, have failed to find a relevant difference in mortality for those diagnosed before birth versus those diagnosed after birth; they found that most of the difference was explained by a higher incidence of lethal malformations in those with a prenatal diagnosis (Sharland et al, 1992; Wilson et al, 1994b). It is doubtful that prenatal diagnosis alone indicates a higher mortality, but it may be that prenatal diagnosis is precipitated by an event such as polyhydramnios that may be associated with a poor prognosis.

It is an appealing notion that the earlier in gestation the hernia occurs and the larger the hernia, the more severe the degree of pulmonary hypoplasia and the worse the outcome. To improve the results, Harrison and coworkers (1993a, 1993b) suggested surgical reduction of the hernia before 30 weeks' gestation, and for this to be a viable alternative form of therapy, they needed to identify the fetus at greatest risk. In a group who all had antenatal diagnosis, Adzick and colleagues (1989) found evidence that diagnosis before 24 weeks' gestation and the development of polyhydramnios, usually after 24 weeks' gestation, were poor prognostic signs. This finding has not been absolutely confirmed. After exclusion of malformations, Sharland and associates (1992) reported a 72% mortality for those diagnosed before 25 weeks' gestation and a 52% mortality for those diagnosed later in gestation. Wilson and colleagues (1994b) indicated a similar trend in their subpopulation of infants with prenatal diagnosis.

Harrison and coworkers (1994) found in a homogeneous group of infants, all of whom had prenatal diagnosis before 24 weeks' gestation, that the true mortality, after excluding malformations, was 58%, compared with a 37% mortality, if only infants reaching an ECMO center were considered. Thus, in those with a prenatal diagnosis and without associated malformations, the evidence suggests that diagnosis before 24 weeks' gestation may be associated with a worse

outcome; this may justify consideration for fetal surgery. Other data have suggested that the presence of polyhydramnios (Adzick et al, 1985), the presence of stomach in the hernia (Burge et al, 1989; Hatch et al, 1992), a reduced lung/thorax area ratio (Kamata et al, 1992), or a reduced left ventricular mass (Crawford et al, 1989; Sharland et al, 1992), all possibly reflections of a large hernia, may also predict a bad outcome and be useful in selecting suitable candidates for fetal surgery.

Prevention of Surfactant Deficiency

It has been shown that the alveolar lavage fluid of lambs with a surgically induced diaphragmatic hernia is deficient in surfactant phospholipids and that exogenous surfactant produces marked improvement in the blood gases and lung mechanics of these lambs (Wilcox et al, 1994). Also, in a rat model of CDH, insufficiency of surfactant development has been demonstrated, and lung surfactant maturation can be accelerated with antenatal betamethasone treatment or thyrotropin-releasing hormone (Suen et al, 1993, 1994b). Both in humans and in the lamb model, however, there is no evidence that the lecithin/sphingomyelin ratio and phosphatidylglycerol profile in amniotic fluid samples accurately indicate lung surfactant immaturity (Sullivan et al, 1994; Wilcox et al, 1995b). It is possible that only the ipsilateral lung is immature (George et al, 1987), and this is hidden by the contribution of both lungs to the amniotic fluid samples. Lotze and coworkers (1994) gave repeated doses of bovine surfactant to nine infants on ECMO and compared them with eight air-treated controls; they could find no advantage to surfactant treatment. Surfactant may need to be administered prophylactically to be effective, however. Glick and colleagues (1992a) reported three infants, two of them premature, who were diagnosed prenatally and treated in the delivery room with a bovine surfactant. Although they were all high risk by ultrasound criteria, they all survived without ECMO, and despite there being no controls, the authors considered that exogenous surfactant had played an important part in the outcome. Many clinicians currently administer antenatal betamethasone in addition to prophylactic surfactant.

Fetal Surgery

The group at University of California, San Francisco, performed fetal surgical repair of CDH before 30 weeks' gestation in highly selected cases. One of the many difficulties of fetal surgery is in removal of the liver from the chest without compromising the umbilical circulation (Harrison et al, 1993a). In their first summary, Harrison and colleagues reported that they operated on 6 cases chosen from a total of 45 cases; 3 were operative deaths, 1 died at birth, and 2 were late neonatal deaths. In their second summary, Harrison and colleagues (1993b) reported that they operated on 14 new cases chosen from a total of 61 further cases; 5 died during operation, 3 were fetal deaths within 48 hours after operation, 2 died of prematurity, and 4 were survivors, none of whom needed ECMO. In a situation in which they expected 40% survival, they obtained only a 30% survival. Furthermore, not all clinicians agree with the criteria used for selection; the prenatal identification of patients with the most severe lung hypoplasia, those most likely to fail after ECMO, remains a significant problem (Weinstein and Stolar, 1993). In addition, postsurgical premature labor with premature birth is a constant threat to the success of this approach (Longaker et al, 1991). This approach has now been abandoned.

Several other approaches to fetal surgery have been suggested. DiFiore and coworkers (1994) and Hedrick and colleagues (1994) found that tracheal ligation in the lamb CDH model caused the lungs to enlarge with lung fluid, resulting in reduction of the hernia and excellent lung growth. Bealer and colleagues (1995) have used translaryngeal insertion of a hydrophilic plug to obstruct the trachea of fetal lambs and achieve the same result; the plug can be removed at birth. Ongoing clinical trials of this technique have not yet produced definitive results (Mychaliska et al, 1996).

Liquid Ventilation

Observations on the use of perflurocarbon to distend the lung and provide gas exchange (see Chapter 52) have led to current trials of partial liquid ventilation in infants with CDH, both before and during treatment with ECMO (Pranikoff et al, 1996). Animal studies have been promising (Wilcox et al, 1995a).

Unilateral Agenesis of the Diaphragm

Among 31 newborns with CDH presenting in the first 6 hours of life, Muràskas and coworkers (1993) reported eight cases of unilateral diaphragmatic agenesis, in which no remnant of skeletal muscle could be found at the subcostal margin. A prenatal diagnosis was more common in agenesis of the diaphragm. Others have found lower Apgar scores and a longer period of preoperative stabilization in this condition (Tsang et al, 1995). These infants have more severe gas exchange problems and more severe bilateral pulmonary hypoplasia than even fatal cases of CDH. Despite repair with a synthetic patch and despite the use of ECMO, the outcome is frequently fatal, and the long-term survival is reported as less than 30%. This condition has been observed more often in recent years, presumably because of antenatal diagnosis and the improved ability to resuscitate infants and transport them to referral centers. This group of infants should be considered separately in assessing the results for CDH.

Right-Sided Diaphragmatic Hernia of Delayed Onset

This condition should not be confused with a right-sided hernia that is present at birth, as discussed earlier. Because the liver is a large organ, herniation into the thorax may be a slow process and may occur after birth only with the onset of breathing. The lung problem reflects compression atelectasis rather than hypoplasia, and the right basal mass may present a confusing appearance on the chest radiograph of the newborn infant (Fig. 60–3). The right leaf of the diaphragm may appear elevated as in eventration or paralysis of the diaphragm. Alternatively the clinician may

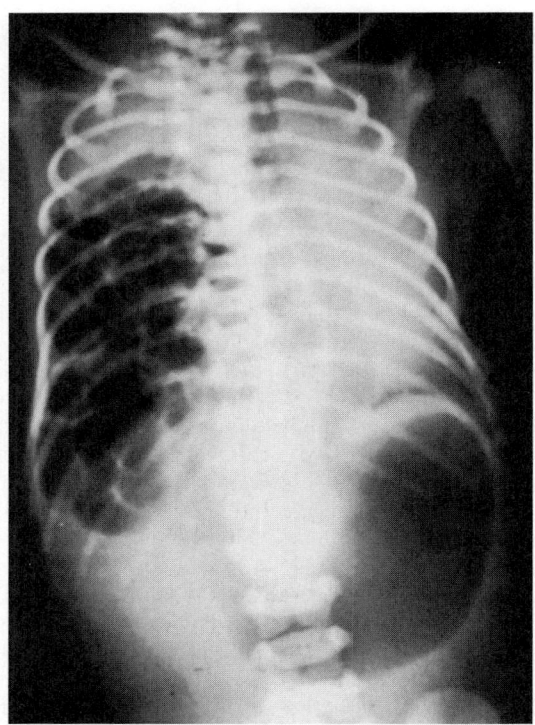

FIGURE 60–3. Right-sided diaphragmatic hernia. This infant was resuscitated by mask and bag without intubation. The consequence was disastrous overdistention of stomach and bowel. When lungs resist insufflation, intubation is mandatory to prevent this kind of complication.

think the patient has a right basal pneumonia or a pleural effusion; some patients have had a chest tube placed, which may injure the liver. The abdominal gas pattern on the right side may appear higher than usual and the lower edge of the liver more horizontal. Ultrasonography or a radionuclide liver scan usually indicates that the liver is excessively high. There has been an unexplained association of this condition with group B streptococcal sepsis (Handa et al, 1992); it may be that increased negative pleural pressures and increased positive abdominal pressures encourage herniation into the chest.

Eventration of the Diaphragm

Eventration of the diaphragm results from insufficient muscle development or absence of phrenic nerves, so that the diaphragm is replaced by a fibrous sheet. An eventration may be localized or diffuse, and most of the latter are unilateral, frequently on the left side. Many, especially those that are localized, produce no clinical signs. When severe, however, newborns have significant respiratory distress. There may be lung hypoplasia on the affected side and, if the mediastinum is shifted, even hypoplasia on the contralateral side. In addition, basal lung compression may cause atelectasis, poor drainage, and complicating bronchopneumonia. The diagnosis is suspected from undue elevation of the diaphragm in frontal and lateral chest radiographs and may be confirmed by fluoroscopy or ultrasound examination (Figs. 60–4 and 60–5). The major cause of

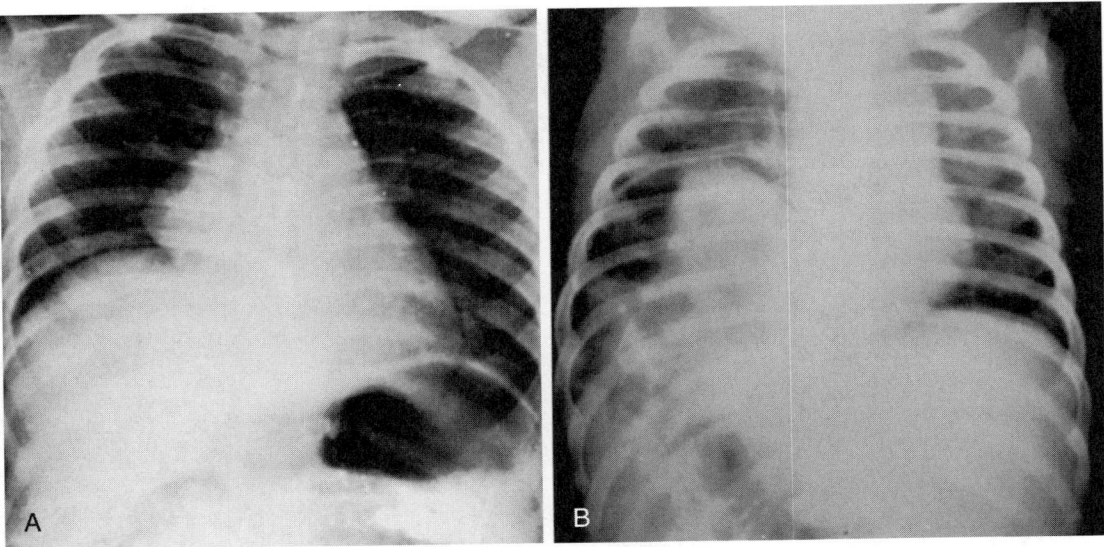

FIGURE 60–4. Eventration of diaphragm. *A,* Anteroposterior view of the chest showing a moderately elevated right diaphragm. This case history is not summarized in the text because the infant was completely asymptomatic, the radiograph having been taken because a sibling had tuberculosis. There had been no difficulty in labor and no respiratory trouble in the newborn. The probable diagnosis is eventration of the diaphragm. *B,* Diaphragmatic paralysis has the same appearance. On fluoroscopy, paradoxic diaphragmatic movement would indicate paralysis.

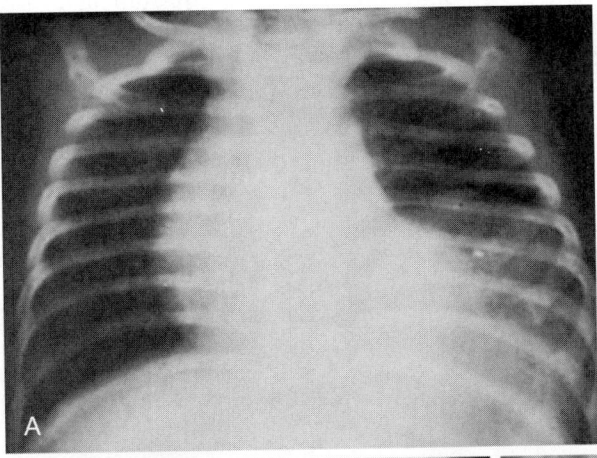

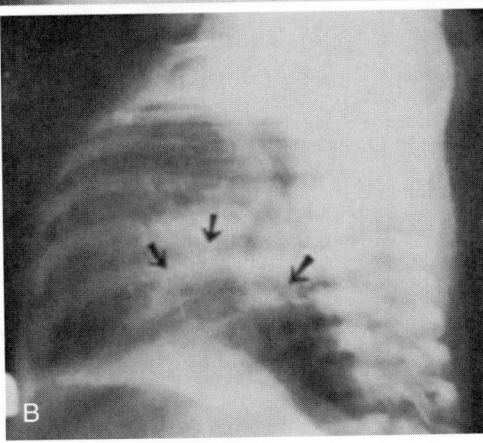

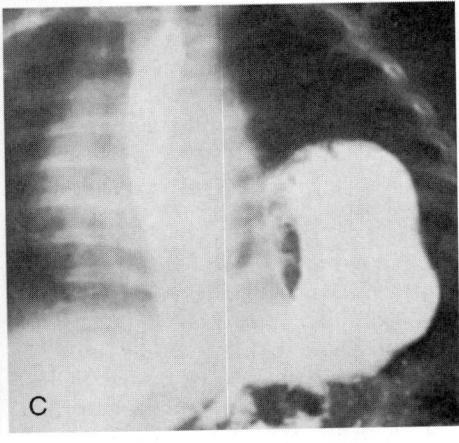

FIGURE 60–5. Eventration of diaphragm. *A,* Anteroposterior view of the chest made at 3.5 months of age. The left diaphragm is elevated to the level of the fourth rib. The heart is displaced a little to the right. *B,* Lateral view on same date. The left diaphragm can be seen considerably higher in the chest than the right. Arrows point to the domed diaphragm. *C,* With barium in the esophagus and stomach, the stomach can be seen to lie largely within the thorax. It is inverted. The esophagus is displaced toward the right.

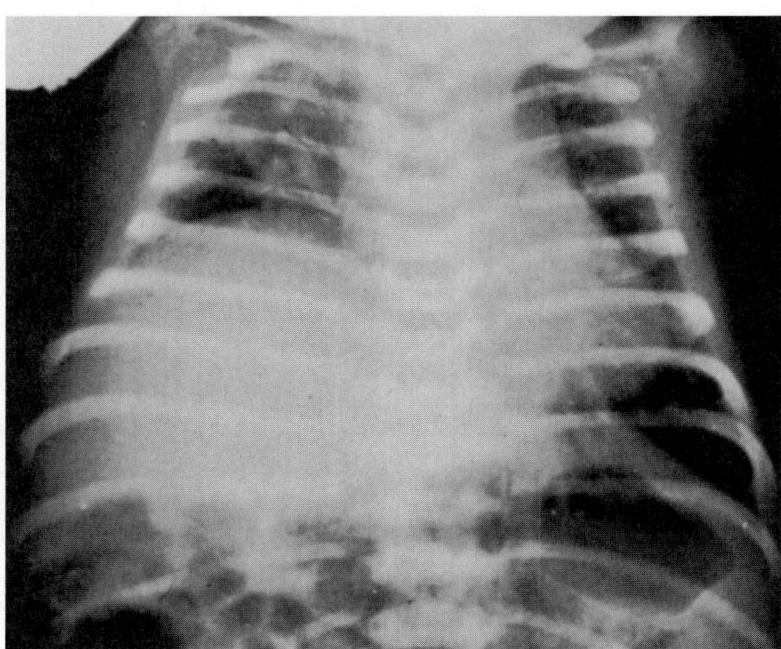

FIGURE 60–6. Paralysis of diaphragm. Anteroposterior view of the chest made when patient was 3 weeks old. Labor had been difficult and prolonged because of shoulder dystocia; delivery was completed by forceps extraction. Right-sided Erb palsy, tachypnea, and dyspnea were noted, and there was one severe bout of pneumonitis at 4 weeks. All finally cleared at 2.5 months of age. The right diaphragm is elevated to the level of the fourth rib. The right lung contains patches of increased density. The heart is displaced a little toward the left. The left lung is moderately emphysematous, its diaphragm flattened and depressed.

confusion is a paralyzed diaphragm, but evidence for birth trauma or thoracotomy is absent in eventration. The diaphragm may show minimal motion while breathing, or the motion may be paradoxic, rising with inspiration and falling with expiration. In those cases in which signs are persistent, the treatment of choice is surgical plication (Goldstein and Reid, 1980; Wayne et al, 1974). Follow-up of patients with plicated diaphragms suggests that the functional outcome is good in nearly all cases (Kizilcan et al, 1993).

Paralysis of the Diaphragm

There are two clinical situations in which diaphragmatic paralysis may occur, after birth trauma or after thoracotomy.

Birth Trauma

Although sometimes bilateral, most cases of diaphragmatic paralysis are unilateral on the right side. The usual presentation is with respiratory distress, produced largely by overactivity of the normal hemidiaphragm. In cases of bilateral paralysis, however, there is cyanosis and poor breathing effort that requires mechanical ventilation. The infants are usually large and have other signs of birth trauma. There is excessive stretching of the C3 to C5 nerve roots in the neck. The diaphragm is an especially important respiratory muscle in the newborn. Furthermore, during active sleep, the intercostals are inhibited, the supine position of the newborn pushes the paralyzed diaphragm upward, and the newborn is especially prone to muscle fatigue. The diagnosis is suggested on the chest radiograph if the right hemidiaphragm is two intercostal spaces higher than the left or if the left hemidiaphragm is one intercostal space higher than the right (Fig. 60–6). On fluoroscopy or ultrasound examination, the involved diaphragm shows either limited or paradoxic motion (Ambler et al, 1985). There may be

associated basal atelectasis, which explains why some infants are markedly improved by nasal continuous positive airway pressure. When both hemidiaphragms are paralyzed, these infants require prolonged mechanical ventilation (Aldrich et al, 1980). Although many improve over 2 weeks, further improvement is possible over a period of 2 months. Once it is believed no further improvement will occur, and the patient cannot be weaned from ventilatory support, surgical plication of the diaphragm should be performed.

Post-Thoracotomy

Diaphragmatic paralysis from phrenic nerve trauma is a known reason for failure to wean from mechanical ventilation after a thoracic operation, such as ligation of patent ductus arteriosus, creation of a systemic pulmonary shunt, or repair of a tracheoesophageal fistula. Management is similar to that for paralysis after birth trauma.

REFERENCES

Adolph V, Flageole H, Perreault T, et al: Repair of congenital diaphragmatic hernia after weaning from extracorporeal membrane oxygenation. J Pediatr Surg 30:349, 1995.

Adzick NS: On the horizon: Neonatal lung transplantation. Arch Dis Child 67:455, 1992.

Adzick NS, Harrison MR, Glick PL, et al: Diaphragmatic hernia in the fetus: Prenatal detection and outcome in 94 cases. J Pediatr Surg 20:357, 1985.

Adzick NS, Vacanti JP, Lillehei CW, et al: Fetal diaphragmatic hernia: Ultrasound diagnosis and clinical outcome in 38 cases. J Pediatr Surg 24:654, 1989.

Aldrich TK, Herman JH, Rochester DF: Bilateral diaphragmatic paralysis in the newborn infant. J Pediatr 97:988, 1980.

Allan LD, Irish MS, Glick PL: The fetal heart in diaphragmatic hernia. Clin Perinatol 23:795, 1996.

Ambler R, Gruenewald S, John E: Ultrasound monitoring of diaphragm activity in bilateral diaphragmatic paralysis. Arch Dis Child 60:170, 1985.

Antunes MJ, Greenspan JS, Cullen JA, et al: Prognosis with pre-operative pulmonary function and lung volume assessment in infants with congenital diaphragmatic hernia. Pediatrics 96:1117, 1995.

Atkinson JB, Ford EG, Humphries B, et al: The impact of extracorporeal membrane support in the treatment of congenital diaphragmatic hernia. J Pediatr Surg 26:791, 1991.

Atkinson JB, Poon MW: ECMO and the management of congenital diaphragmatic hernia with large diaphragmatic defects requiring a prosthetic patch. J Pediatr Surg 27:754, 1992.

Baumgart S, Hirschl R, Butler SZ, et al: Diagnosis related criteria in the consideration of extracorporeal membrane oxygenation in neonates previously treated with high frequency jet ventilation. Pediatrics 89:491, 1992.

Bealer JF, Skarsgard ED, Hedrick MH, et al: The PLUG Odyssey: Adventures in experimental fetal tracheal occlusion. J Pediatr Surg 30:361, 1995.

Beals DA, Schloo BL, Vacanti JP, et al: Pulmonary growth and remodelling in infants with high risk congenital diaphragmatic hernia. J Pediatr Surg 27:997, 1992.

Bohn DJ, Pearl R, Irish MS, Glick PL: Postnatal management of congenital diaphragmatic hernia. Clin Perinatol 23:843, 1996.

Bohn D, Tamura M, Perrin D, et al: Ventilatory predictors of pulmonary hypoplasia in congenital diaphragmatic hernia, confirmed by morphologic assessment. J Pediatr 111:423, 1987.

Breaux CW, Rouse TM, Cain WS, Georgeson KE: Improvement in survival of patients with congenital diaphragmatic hernia utilizing a strategy of delayed repair after medical and/or extracorporeal membrane oxygenation stabilization. J Pediatr Surg 26:333, 1991.

Burge DM, Atwell JD, Freeman NV: Could the stomach site help predict outcome in babies with left sided congenital diaphragmatic hernia diagnoses antenatally. J Pediatr Surg 24:567, 1989.

Cartlidge PHT, Mann NP, Kapila L: Pre-operative stabilisation in congenital diaphragmatic hernia. Arch Dis Child 61:1226, 1986.

Charlton AJ, Bruce J, Davenport M: Timing of surgery in congenital diaphragmatic hernia: Low mortality after pre-operative stabilization. Anaesthesia 46:820, 1992.

Cloutier R, Fournier L, Levasseur L: Reversion to fetal circulation in congenital diaphragmatic hernia: A preventable postoperative complication. J Pediatr Surg 18:551, 1983.

Crawford DC, Wright VM, Drake DP, Allan LD: Fetal diaphragmatic hernia: The value of fetal echocardiography in the prediction of postnatal outcome. Br J Obstet Gynaecol 96:705, 1989.

Cunniff C, Jones KL, Jones MC: Patterns of malformation in children with congenital diaphragmatic defects. J Pediatr 116:258, 1990.

D'Agostino JA, Bernbaum JC, Gerdes M, et al: Outcome for infants with congenital diaphragmatic hernia requiring extracorporeal membrane oxygenation: The first years. J Pediatr Surg 30:10, 1995.

DiFiore JW, Fauza DO, Slavin R, et al: Experimental fetal tracheal ligation reverses the structural and physiological effects of pulmonary hypoplasia in congenital diaphragmatic hernia. J Pediatr Surg 29:248, 1994.

Dillon PW, Cilley RE, Hudome SM, et al: Nitric oxide reversal of recurrent pulmonary hypertension and respiratory failure in an infant with CDH after successful ECMO therapy. J Pediatr Surg 30:743, 1995.

Fauza DO, Wilson JM: Congenital diaphragmatic hernia and associated anomalies: Their incidence, identification, and impact on prognosis. J Pediatr Surg 29:1113, 1994.

Finer NN, Tierney AL, Hallgren R, et al: Neonatal congenital diaphragmatic hernia and extracorporeal membrane oxygenation. Can Med Assoc J 146:501, 1992.

Geggel RL, Murphy JD, Langleben D, et al: Congenital diaphragmatic hernia: Arterial structural changes and persistent pulmonary hypertension after surgical repair. J Pediatr 107:457, 1985.

George K, Cooney TP, Chiu BK, Thurlbeck WM: Hypoplasia and immaturity of the terminal lung unit (acinus) in congenital diaphragmatic hernia. Am Rev Respir Dis 136:947, 1987.

Glick PL, Irish MS, Holm BA (Eds): New Insights into the Pathophysiology of Congenital Diaphragmatic Hernia. Clinics in Perinatology, Vol 23. Philadelphia, WB Saunders, 1996.

Glick PL, Leach CL, Besner GE, et al: Pathophysiology of congenital diaphragmatic hernia: III. Exogenous surfactant therapy for the high risk neonate with CDH. J Pediatr Surg 27:866, 1992a.

Glick PL, Stannard VA, Leach CL, et al: Pathophysiology of congenital diaphragmatic hernia: II. The fetal lamb model is surfactant deficient. J Pediatr Surg 27:382, 1992b.

Goh DW, Drake DP, Brereton RJ, et al: Delayed surgery for congenital diaphragmatic hernia. Br J Surg 79:644, 1992.

Goldstein JD, Reid LM: Pulmonary hypoplasia resulting from phrenic nerve agenesis and diaphragmatic amyoplasia. J Pediatr 97:282, 1980.

Gyllesward A: Pectus excavatum: A clinical study with long-term postoperative follow-up. Acta Pediatr Scand 255(suppl):1, 1975.

Handa N, Suita S, Shono T, Kukita J: Right sided diaphragmatic hernia following group B streptococcal pneumonia and sepsis. J Pediatr Surg 27:764, 1992.

Hansen J, James S, Burrington J, Whitfield J: The decreasing incidence of pneumothorax and improving survival of infants with congenital diaphragmatic hernia. J Pediatr Surg 19:385, 1984.

Harrison MR, Adzick NS, Estes JM, Howell LJ: A prospective study of the outcome for fetuses with diaphragmatic hernia. JAMA 271:382, 1994.

Harrison MR, Adzick NS, Flake AW, Jennings RW: The CDH two-step: A dance of necessity. J Pediatr Surg 28:813, 1993a.

Harrison MR, Adzick NS, Flake AW, et al: Correction of congenital diaphragmatic hernia in utero: VI. Hard earned lessons. J Pediatr Surg 28:1411, 1993b.

Harrison MR, Adzick NS, Longaker MT, et al: Successful repair in utero of a fetal diaphragmatic hernia after removal of herniated viscera from the left chest. N Engl J Med 322:1582, 1990.

Hasegawa S, Kohno S, Sugiyama T, et al: Usefulness of echocardiographic measurement of bilateral pulmonary artery dimensions in congenital diaphragmatic hernia. J Pediatr Surg 29:622, 1994.

Hatch EI, Kendall J, Blumhagen J: Stomach position as an in utero predictor of neonatal outcome in left sided diaphragmatic hernia. J Pediatr Surg 27:778, 1992.

Haugen SE, Linker D, Eik-Nes S, et al: Congenital diaphragmatic hernia: Determination of the optimal time for operation by echocardiographic monitoring of the pulmonary arterial pressure. J Pediatr Surg 26:560, 1991.

Hedrick MH, Estes JM, Sullivan KM, et al: Plug the lung until it grows (PLUG): A new method to treat congenital diaphragmatic hernia in utero. J Pediatr Surg 29:612, 1994.

Henneberg SW, Jepsen S, Andersen PK, Pedersen SA: Inhalation of nitric oxide as a treatment of pulmonary hypertension in congenital diaphragmatic hernia. J Pediatr Surg 30:853, 1995.

Jeune N, Cararon R, Berand C, et al: Polychondrodystrophie avec blocage thoracique d'évolution fatale. Pediatrie 9:390, 1954.

Kamata S, Hasegawa T, Ishikawa S, et al: Prenatal diagnosis of congenital diaphragmatic hernia and perinatal care: Assessment of lung hypoplasia. Early Hum Dev 29:375, 1992.

Karamanoukian HL, Glick PL, Wilcox DT, et al: Pathophysiology of congenital diaphragmatic hernia: VIII. Inhaled nitric oxide requires exogenous surfactant therapy in the lamb model of congenital diaphragmatic hernia. J Pediatr Surg 30:1, 1995.

Karamanoukian HL, Glick PL, Zayek M, et al: Inhaled nitric oxide in congenital hypoplasia of the lungs due to diaphragmatic hernia or oligohydramnios. Pediatrics 94:715, 1994.

Kieffer J, Sapin E, Berg A, et al: Gastro-esophageal reflux after repair of congenital diaphragmatic hernia. J Pediatr Surg 30:1330, 1995.

Kizilcan F, Tanyel FC, Hicsonmez A, et al: The long term results of diaphragmatic plication. J Pediatr Surg 28:42, 1993.

Kobayashi H, Puri P: Plasma endothelin levels in congenital diaphragmatic hernia. J Pediatr Surg 29:1258, 1994.

Kohler E, Babbitt DP: Dystrophic thoraces and infantile asphyxia. Radiology 94:55, 1970.

Koot VCM, Bergmeijer JH, Bos AP, Molenaar JC: Incidence and management of gastro-esophageal reflux after repair of congenital diaphragmatic hernia. J Pediatr Surg 28:48, 1993.

Lally KP, Breaux CW: A second course of extracorporeal membrane oxygenation in the neonate—is there a benefit? Surgery 117:175, 1995.

Lally KP, Paranka MS, Roden J, et al: Congenital diaphragmatic hernia: Stabilization and repair on ECMO. Ann Surg 216:569, 1992.

Langer JC, Filler RM, Bohn DJ, et al: Timing of surgery for congenital diaphragmatic hernia: Is emergency operation necessary? J Pediatr Surg 23:731, 1988.

Langham MR, Kays DW, Ledbetter DJ, et al: Congenital diaphragmatic hernia—epidemiology and outcome. Clin Perinatol 23:671, 1996.

Longaker MT, Golbus MS, Filly RA, et al: Maternal outcome after fetal surgery: A review of the first 17 human cases. JAMA 265:737, 1991.

Lotze A, Knight GR, Andersen KD, et al: Surfactant (beractant) therapy for infants with congenital diaphragmatic hernia on ECMO: Evidence of persistent surfactant deficiency. J Pediatr Surg 29:407, 1994.

Lund DP, Mitchell J, Kharasch V, et al: Congenital diaphragmatic hernia: The hidden morbidity. J Pediatr Surg 29:258, 1994.

Maier HC, Bortone F: Complete failure of sternal fusion with herniation of pericardium. J Thorac Surg 18:851, 1949.

Marshall A, Sumner E: Improved prognosis in congenital diaphragmatic hernia: Experience of 62 cases over 2 year period. J R Soc Med 75:607, 1982.

Michalevicz D, Chaimoff C: Use of a silastic sheet for widening the abdominal cavity in the surgical treatment of diaphragmatic hernia. J Pediatr Surg 24:265, 1989.

Muraskas JK, Husain A, Myers TF, et al: An association of pulmonary hypoplasia with unilateral agenesis of the diaphragm. J Pediatr Surg 28:999, 1993.

Mychaliska GB, Bullard KM, Harrison MR: In utero management of congenital diaphragmatic hernia. Clin Perinatol 23:823, 1996.

Nagaya M, Akatsuka H, Kato J: Gastro-esophageal reflux occurring after repair of congenital diaphragmatic hernia. J Pediatr Surg 29:1447, 1994.

Nakayama DK, Motoyama EK, Tagge EM: Effect of pre-operative stabilization on respiratory system compliance and outcome in newborn infants with congenital diaphragmatic hernia. J Pediatr 118:793, 1991.

Newman BM, Jewett TC, Lewis A, et al: Prosthetic materials and muscle flaps in the repair of extensive diaphragmatic defects: An experimental study. J Pediatr Surg 20:362, 1985.

Newman KD, Anderson KC, Van Meurs K, et al: Extracorporeal membrane oxygenation and congenital diaphragmatic hernia: Should any infant be excluded? J Pediatr Surg 25:1048, 1990.

Nguyen L, Guttman FM, DeChadarevian JP, et al: The mortality of congenital diaphragmatic hernia: Is total pulmonary mass inadequate, no matter what? Ann Surg 198:766, 1983.

Nio M, Haase G, Kennaugh J, et al: A prospective randomized trial of delayed versus immediate repair of congenital diaphragmatic hernia. J Pediatr Surg 29:618, 1994.

Oberkaid F, Danks DM, Mayne V, et al: Asphyxiating thoracic dysplasia: Clinical, radiological and pathological information on 10 patients. Arch Dis Child 52:758, 1977.

O'Rourke PP, Vacanti JP, Crone RK, et al: Use of the postductal PaO_2 as a predictor of pulmonary vascular hypoplasia in infants with congenital diaphragmatic hernia. J Pediatr Surg 23:904, 1988.

O'Toole SJ, Irish MS, Holm BA, Glick PL: Pulmonary vascular abnormalities in congenital diaphragmatic hernia. Clin Perinatol 23:781, 1996a.

O'Toole SJ, Karamanoukian HL, Morin FC III, et al: Surfactant decreases pulmonary vascular resistance and increases pulmonary blood flow in the fetal lamb model of CDH. J Pediatr Surg 31:507, 1996b.

Paranka MS, Clark RH, Yoder BA, Null DM: Predictors of failure of high frequency oscillatory ventilation in term infants with severe respiratory failure. Pediatrics 95:400, 1995.

Pranikoff T, Gauger PH, Hirschl RB: Partial liquid ventilation in newborn patients with congenital diaphragmatic hernia. J Pediatr Surg 31:613, 1996.

Ramenofsky ML: The effects of intrapleural pressure on respiratory insufficiency. J Pediatr Surg 14:750, 1979.

Raphaely RC, Downes JJ: Congenital diaphragmatic hernia: Prediction of survival. J Pediatr Surg 8:815, 1973.

Ravitch MM: Congenital Deformities of the Chest Wall and Their Operative Correction. Philadelphia, WB Saunders, 1977.

Reid IS, Hutcherson RJ: Long-term follow-up of patients with congenital diaphragmatic hernia. J Pediatr Surg 11:939, 1976.

Ryan CA, Perreault T, Johnston-Hodgson A, Finer NN: Extracorporeal membrane oxygenation in infants with congenital diaphragmatic hernia and cardiac malformations. J Pediatr Surg 29:878, 1994.

Sabiston DC: The surgical management of congenital bifid sternum with partial ectopia cordis. J Thorac Surg 35:118, 1958.

Sakai H, Tamura M, Hosokawa Y, et al: Effect of surgical repair on respiratory mechanics in congenital diaphragmatic hernia. J Pediatr 111:432, 1987.

Schnitzer JJ, Kikiros CS, Short BL, et al: Experience with abdominal wall closure for patients with congenital diaphragmatic hernia repaired on ECMO. J Pediatr Surg 30:19, 1995.

Schumacher RE, Farrell PM: Congenital diaphragmatic hernia: A major remaining challenge in neonatal respiratory care. Perinatol Neonatol 9:29, 1985.

Schwartz SM, Vermilion RP, Hirschl RB: Evaluation of left ventricular mass in children with left sided congenital diaphragmatic hernia. J Pediatr 125:447, 1994.

Sharland GK, Lockhart SM, Heward AJ, Allan LD: Prognosis in fetal diaphragmatic hernia. Am J Obstet Gynecol 166:9, 1992.

Sigalet DL, Nguyen LT, Adolph V, et al: Gastro-esophageal reflux associated with large diaphragmatic hernias. J Pediatr Surg 29:1262, 1994.

Sigalet DL, Tierney A, Adolph V, et al: Timing of repair of congenital diaphragmatic hernia requiring extracorporeal membrane oxygenation support. J Pediatr Surg 30:1183, 1995.

Steimie CN, Meric F, Hirschl RB, et al: Effect of extracorporeal life support on survival when applied to all patients with congenital diaphragmatic hernia. J Pediatr Surg 29:997, 1994.

Stolar C, Dillon P, Reyes C: Selective use of extracorporeal membrane oxygenation in the management of congenital diaphragmatic hernia. J Pediatr Surg 23:207, 1988.

Stolar CJH, Levy JP, Dillon PW, et al: Anatomic and functional abnormalities of the esophagus in infants surviving congenital diaphragmatic hernia. Am J Surg 159:204, 1990.

Suen HC, Bloch KD, Donahue PK: Antenatal glucocorticoid corrects pulmonary immaturity in experimentally induced congenital diaphragmatic hernia in rats. Pediatr Res 35:523, 1994a.

Suen HC, Catlin EA, Ryan DP, et al: Biochemical immaturity of lungs in congenital diaphragmatic hernia. J Pediatr Surg 28:471, 1993.

Suen H, Losty P, Donahue P, et al: Combined antenatal thyrotrophin-releasing hormone and low-dose glucocorticoid therapy improves the pulmonary biochemical immaturity in congenital diaphragmatic hernia. J Pediatr Surg 29:359, 1994b.

Sullivan KM, Hawgood S, Flake AW, et al: Amniotic fluid phospholipid analysis in the fetus with congenital diaphragmatic hernia. J Pediatr Surg 29:1020, 1994.

Tamura M, Tsuchida Y, Kawano T, et al: Piston pump type high frequency oscillatory ventilation for neonates with congenital diaphragmatic hernia: A new protocol. J Pediatr Surg 23:478, 1988.

Tsang TM, Tam PKH, Dudley NE, Stevens J: Diaphragmatic agenesis as a distinct clinical entity. J Pediatr Surg 30:16, 1995.

vanden Staak FHJM, De Haan AFJ, Geven WB, et al: Improving survival for patients with high risk congenital diaphragmatic hernia by using extracorporeal membrane oxygenation. J Pediatr Surg 30:1463, 1995.

vanden Staak FHJ, Thiesbrummel A, de Haan AFJ, et al: Do we use the right entry criteria for extracorporeal membrane oxygenation in congenital diaphragmatic hernia? J Pediatr Surg 28:1003, 1993.

Van Meurs KP, Rhine WD, Benitz WE, et al: Lobar lung transplantation as a treatment for congenital diaphragmatic hernia. J Pediatr Surg 29:1557, 1994.

Vasquez WD, Cheu HW: Hemorrhagic complications and repair of congenital diaphragmatic hernias: Does timing of the repair make a difference? Data from the Extracorporeal Life Support Organization. J Pediatr Surg 29:1002, 1994.

Wayne ER, Campbell JB, Burrington JD, et al: Eventration of the diaphragm. J Pediatr Surg 9:643, 1974.

Weinstein S, Stolar CJH: Newborn surgical emergencies: Congenital diaphragmatic hernia and extracorporeal membrane oxygenation. Pediatr Clin North Am 40:1315, 1993.

Welch KJ: Chest wall deformities. *In* Holder TM, Ashcraft KW (Eds): Pediatric Surgery. Philadelphia, WB Saunders, 1980, p 162.

Wilcox DT, Glick PL, Karamanoukian H, et al: Pathophysiology of congenital diaphragmatic hernia: V. Effect of exogenous surfactant therapy on gas exchange and lung mechanics in the lamb congenital diaphragmatic hernia model. J Pediatr 124:289, 1994.

Wilcox D, Glick P, Karamanoukian H, et al: Perflubron associated gas exchange improves pulmonary mechanics, oxygenation, ventilation and allows nitric oxide delivery in the hypoplastic lung congenital diaphragmatic hernia lamb model. Crit Care Med 23:1858, 1995a.

Wilcox DT, Glick PL, Karamanoukian H, et al: Pathophysiology of congenital diaphragmatic hernia: XII. Amniotic fluid lecithin/sphingomyelin ratio and phosphatidylglycerol concentrations do not predict surfactant status in congenital diaphragmatic hernia. J Pediatr Surg 30:410, 1995b.

Wilcox DT, Irish MS, Holm BA, Glick PL: Prenatal diagnosis of congenital diaphragmatic hernia with predictors of mortality. Clin Perinatol 23:701, 1996a.

Wilcox DT, Irish MS, Holm BA, Glick PL: Pulmonary parenchymal abnormalities in congenital diaphragmatic hernia. Clin Perinatol 23:771, 1996b.

Wilson JM, Bower LK, Lund DP: Evolution of the technique of congenital diaphragmatic hernia repair on ECMO. J Pediatr Surg 29:1109, 1994a.

Wilson JM, Fauza DO, Lund DP, et al: Antenatal diagnosis of isolated congenital diaphragmatic hernia is not an indicator of outcome. J Pediatr Surg 29:815, 1994b.

Wilson JM, Lund DP, Lillehei CW, Vacanti JP: Congenital diaphragmatic hernia: Predictors of severity in the ECMO era. J Pediatr Surg 26:1028, 1991.

Wohl MEB, Griscou NT, Strieder DJ, et al: The lung following repair of congenital diaphragmatic hernia. J Pediatr 90:405, 1977.

Wung JT, Sahni R, Moffitt ST, et al: Congenital diaphragmatic hernia: Survival treated with very delayed surgery, spontaneous respiration, and no chest tube. J Pediatr Surg 30:406, 1995.

PART IX
CARDIOVASCULAR SYSTEM

CHAPTER 61

Patent Ductus Arteriosus in the Premature Infant

Ronald I. Clyman

The ductus arteriosus represents a persistence of the terminal portion of the left pulmonary or sixth branchial arch. More muscular than the elastic pulmonary artery and aorta at either end, the ductus arteriosus also has a looser structure with increased amounts of acid mucopolysaccharide in the muscle media. During fetal life, it serves to divert blood away from the fluid-filled lungs toward the descending aorta and placenta. Obliteration of the ductus arteriosus takes place after birth. In the full-term animal or human neonate, the ductus begins to constrict rapidly after delivery with initiation of air breathing. In addition to both circumferential and longitudinal vasoconstriction, the media indents into the lumen and the intima increases in size, forming intimal mounds that help to occlude the lumen.

REGULATION OF DUCTUS ARTERIOSUS PATENCY

Since the initial studies of Kennedy and Clark (1942), many investigators have demonstrated that oxygen is responsible for constricting the ductus arteriosus after birth. However, the biochemical basis for the oxygen response has never been fully explained (Coceani et al, 1984; Fay and Jobsis, 1972). Although neural and hormonal factors possibly contribute to ductus closure under physiologic conditions, they do not mediate oxygen-induced vessel closure. A cytochrome P450 hemoprotein, which is located in the plasma membrane of the vascular smooth muscle cells, appears to act as a receptor for the oxygen-induced events in the ductus (Coceani et al, 1989b, 1994). Oxygen causes membrane depolarization, which, in turn, is associated with an increase in smooth muscle intracellular calcium (Nakanishi et al, 1993) and formation of the potent vasoconstrictor, endothelin-1 (Coceani et al, 1989a).

The ductus also produces several vasodilators that oppose the ability of oxygen to constrict the vessel. The postnatal increase in Po_2 stimulates the release of prostaglandin E_2 (PGE_2) from cells in the muscle media and adventitia. There is some evidence to suggest that the PGE_2 produced by the ductus may be stimulated by reactive oxygen metabolites (Clyman et al, 1989). A nitric oxide (NO)-like vasodilator is also produced by the ductus arteriosus after birth. Therefore, closure of the ductus at birth occurs through a process that alters the balance between dilating and contracting factors.

Oxygen has a greater constrictor effect in the ductus from near-term versus immature fetuses. The increased effectiveness of oxygen in the mature ductus arteriosus is due to a developmental alteration in the sensitivity of the vessel to locally produced vasodilators. Isolated ductus arteriosus, from preterm animals, is much more sensitive to the dilating action of PGE_2 and NO than are those from animals near term (Clyman, 1987). In addition to being much more sensitive to the vasodilators PGE_2 and NO, the ductus from extremely immature fetuses (< 0.7 gestation) also has decreased contractile capacity. These factors probably account for the higher incidence of persistent patent ductus arteriosus in preterm infants. Inhibitors of prostaglandin production such as indomethacin, ibuprofen, and mefenamic acid have proven themselves to be effective agents in promoting ductus closure. It follows that drugs interfering with NO synthesis or function also could become useful adjuncts, especially in situations in which indomethacin has proven to be ineffective. The factors that alter the sensitivity of the ductus to locally produced PGE_2 are unknown. Elevated cortisol concentrations in the fetus have been found to decrease the sensitivity of the ductus to PGE_2 (Clyman et al, 1981b); consistent with these findings, prenatal administration of glucocorticoids causes a significant reduction in the incidence of patent ductus arteriosus (PDA) in premature human and animal infants (Clyman et al, 1981a, 1981b; Collaborative Group on Antenatal Steroid Therapy, 1985; Momma et al, 1981; Thibeault et al, 1978; Waffarn et al, 1983).

In normal full-term animals, loss of responsiveness to PGE_2 shortly after birth prevents the ductus arteriosus from reopening once it has constricted. Loss of ductus arteriosus responsiveness is directly related to the degree of prior ductus arteriosus constriction because constriction causes loss of luminal blood flow and ischemia of the inner vessel wall. This appears to be the first step in permanent closure of the ductus. In contrast to full-term infants, premature infants are more likely to have a ductus arteriosus that continues to dilate in response to PGE_2 and NO. This occurs even after complete obliteration of ductus luminal blood flow. Consequently, once the ductus arteriosus has closed in the premature infant (either spontaneously or as a result of indomethacin), it may reopen at a later date, with recurrence of the left-to-right shunt (Mellander et al, 1984). The incidence of ductus arteriosus reopening is inversely related to gestational age: in 33% of infants delivered before 26 weeks' gestation, the ductus arteriosus reopens after initial closure (demonstrated by echocardiography), whereas in only 5% of infants delivered after 26 weeks' gestation, the ductus arteriosus reopens (Weiss et al, 1995). When the ductus arteriosus reopens after initial successful closure, it is most frequently due to the effects of endogenous PGE$_2$. As a result, 70% of those ductus arteriosus that reopen can be closed again with a second treatment course of indomethacin. The factors that maintain ductus arteriosus responsiveness to PGE$_2$ after postnatal constriction in immature newborns are unknown. The oxygen consumption of the near-term ductus arteriosus is normally greater than that of other vascular smooth muscles (Fay, 1971). In contrast, the O$_2$ consumption of the premature ductus arteriosus appears to be much lower than that of animals near term. This might be due to the low circulating concentrations of thyroid hormones in immature fetuses and neonates. Because O$_2$ consumption is reduced in the preterm ductus arteriosus, the preterm vessel is more resistant to ischemic damage during postnatal constriction. Consistent with this hypothesis is the observation that premature infants with low concentrations of thyroid hormones have an increased incidence of PDA compared with those with normal concentrations.

In full-term infants, once the ductus arteriosus constricts, rapid histologic changes ultimately lead to obliteration of the lumen of the vessel and prevent reopening at a later date. As the fetus approaches term, there is intimal thickening and fragmentation of the internal elastic lamina. After birth, the intima of the ductus arteriosus increases in size, forming mounds that ultimately occlude the lumen. The rapid increase in intimal thickening is due to extensive constriction and shortening of the vessel, in addition to migration of smooth muscle cells from the muscle media, proliferation of luminal endothelial cells, and accumulation of hyaluronan in the subendothelial region (de Reeder et al, 1988; Toda et al, 1980). Shortly after birth, cells in the inner part of the muscle media appear to disintegrate. This may be due to anoxia in the region of the wall that is normally nourished by diffusion from the ductal lumen. Over the next number of weeks, the muscle fibers of the inner media ultimately atrophy and are replaced by connective tissue. The outer media of the ductus is supplied by vasa vasorum, which transiently become hyperemic and increase in density after birth. In the full-term infant, anatomic closure is complete within 1 to 3 months after birth. In contrast, in the preterm infant, this pattern of closure frequently does not occur. The vessel is fetal in appearance with diminished intimal mounds, an intact internal elastic lamina, absent cytolytic necrosis, and absent vasa vasorum (Gittenberger-de-Groot et al, 1980). As a result, there is potential in preterm infants for their ductus to reopen late in the hospital course. For an in-depth discussion, see Gluckman and Heymann, 1993.

HEMODYNAMIC AND PULMONARY ALTERATIONS

Virtually all shunting through the ductus in the preterm infant is left-to-right. Only in larger infants with persistent pulmonary hypertension does right-to-left shunting become a problem (see Chapter 53). The pathophysiologic features of a PDA depend both on the magnitude of the left-to-right shunt and on the cardiac and pulmonary responses to the shunt. There are important differences between immature and mature infants in the ability of the heart to handle a volume load. Immature infants have less cardiac

sympathetic innervation. Before term, the myocardium has more water and less contractile mass. Therefore, in the immature fetus the ventricles are less distensible than at term and also generate less force per gram of myocardium (even though they have the same ability to generate force per sarcomere as those in more mature infants) (Friedman, 1972). The relative lack of left ventricular distensibility in immature infants is more a function of the ventricle tissue constituents than of poor muscle function. As a result, left ventricular distention secondary to a large left-to-right PDA shunt may produce a higher left ventricular end-diastolic pressure at smaller ventricular volumes in the immature than in the mature infant. Elevations in left ventricular end-diastolic pressures, which increase pulmonary venous pressures and cause pulmonary congestion, occur with smaller left-to-right shunts in immature than in mature infants.

In preterm lamb and human newborns (Clyman et al, 1987; Shimada et al, 1994) with a PDA, left ventricular output can be increased to maintain their "effective" systemic blood flow as long as the left-to-right shunt is less than or equal to 50% of left ventricular output. With shunts greater than 50% of left ventricular output, "effective" systemic blood flow declines, despite increases in left ventricular output. The increase in left ventricular output associated with a PDA is accomplished not by an increase in heart rate, but by an increase in stroke volume (Clyman et al, 1987; Shimada et al, 1994). Stroke volume increases primarily as a result of the simultaneous decrease in afterload resistance on the heart and the increase in left ventricular preload. Despite the ability of the left ventricle to increase its output with increasing amounts of ductus shunt, blood flow distribution is significantly rearranged. This redistribution of systemic blood flow occurs even with small shunts (Clyman et al, 1987). Blood flow to the skin, bone, and skeletal muscle is most likely to be affected by the left-to-right ductus shunt. The next most likely organs to be affected are the gastrointestinal tract and kidneys. These organs receive decreased blood flow resulting from a combination of decreased perfusion pressure (related to a decrease in diastolic pressure) and localized vasoconstriction. These organs may experience significant hypoperfusion before there are any signs of left ventricular compromise. This decrease in organ perfusion may explain some of the pathophysiologic manifestations of a PDA in preterm infants.

Very-low-birth-weight infants with a PDA have been found to have increased flow in the ascending aorta and decreased flow in the descending aorta, with an associated metabolic acidosis (Johnson et al, 1978). Such alterations in cardiac output distribution have been implicated in the high incidence of intracranial hemorrhage (Martin et al, 1982; Perlman et al, 1981) and necrotizing enterocolitis (Cotton et al, 1978; Kitterman, 1975) associated with PDA. Significant aortic backflow has been observed over large distances in some infants with PDA, consistent with a "diastolic steal" of blood from the abdominal organs to the pulmonary artery (Spach et al, 1980). The continuous distention of the pulmonary vessels during diastole may be important in the production of pulmonary vascular disease and bronchopulmonary dysplasia.

The decreased ability of the preterm infant to maintain

active pulmonary vasoconstriction (Lewis et al, 1976) may be responsible in part for the earlier presentation of a "large" left-to-right PDA shunt in the most immature infants (Gersony et al, 1983; Jacob et al, 1980). In addition, therapeutic maneuvers (e.g., surfactant replacement) that lead to decreased pulmonary vascular resistance can exacerbate the amount of left-to-right shunt in preterm infants with respiratory distress syndrome (RDS) (Clyman et al, 1982; Fujiwara et al, 1980). Two recent meta-analyses of the surfactant therapy trials have demonstrated an increased incidence of both clinically symptomatic PDAs and pulmonary hemorrhages in the infants receiving prophylactic surfactant (Alpan and Clyman, 1995; Raju and Langenberg, 1993).

The factors responsible for preventing fluid and proteins from moving from the plasma to the lung interstitium (microvascular barrier) and from the interstitium to the air spaces (alveolar barrier) have been described previously in detail (Staub, 1980). Several groups have observed an improvement in lung compliance in preterm infants with a PDA of several days' duration following ligation of the PDA (Gerhardt and Bancalari, 1980; Johnson et al, 1978; Naulty et al, 1978). With a wide-open PDA, the pulmonary vasculature is exposed to systemic blood pressure and increased pulmonary blood flow. Because the premature infant with RDS frequently has a low plasma oncotic pressure and may have increased capillary permeability, increases in microvascular perfusion pressure that result from PDA may increase interstitial and alveolar lung fluid. Leakage of plasma proteins into the alveolar space may inhibit surfactant function and increase surface tension in the immature air sacs, which are already compromised by surfactant deficiency (Ikegami et al, 1983). The increased FIO_2 and mean airway pressures required to overcome these early changes in compliance caused by PDA may be important factors in the association of PDA with chronic lung disease (Brown, 1979; Cotton et al, 1978). However, these changes in pulmonary mechanics only occur after several days of exposure to a PDA.

Even though preterm animals with a PDA have increased fluid and protein clearance into the lung interstitium, a simultaneous increase in lung lymph flow appears to eliminate the excess fluid and protein from the lung. This compensatory increase in lung lymph flow acts as an "edema safety factor," inhibiting fluid accumulation in the lungs. As a result, there is no net increase in water or protein accumulation in the lung, or change in pulmonary mechanics during the first 24 to 72 hours after delivery (Alpan et al, 1989; Krauss et al, 1989; Pérez Fontán et al, 1987; Shimada et al, 1989). This delicate balance between PDA-induced fluid filtration and lymphatic reabsorption is consistent with the observation made in human infants that closure of the ductus arteriosus within the first 24 hours after birth has no effect on the course of the newborn's respiratory disease. However, if a symptomatic left-to-right shunt persists beyond the first 24 to 72 hours or if lung lymphatic drainage is impaired, as it is in the presence of pulmonary interstitial emphysema or fibrosis, the likelihood of edema increases dramatically. After several days of lung disease and mechanical ventilation, the residual functioning lymphatics are more easily overwhelmed by the same size PDA shunt that could be accommodated on the first day

after delivery. As a result, it is most common for a "hemodynamically significant shunt" with pulmonary edema and alterations in pulmonary mechanics to develop in infants with a persistent PDA at 7 to 10 days after birth. In these infants, improvement in lung compliance occurs following closure of the PDA.

DIAGNOSIS

Studies designed to determine how a PDA contributes to an infant's morbidity or when a PDA becomes a persistent PDA have been hampered by the lack of consistent diagnostic criteria for defining the condition. A PDA can be defined by echocardiographic or clinical criteria. Echocardiographic signs are the most sensitive and accurate means of diagnosing the presence of a PDA; on the other hand, clinical signs have the highest correlation with the development of long-term, PDA-related morbidity.

The combination of two-dimensional echocardiographic visualization of the ductus with either pulsed, continuous wave, or color Doppler measurements appears to be not only very sensitive but also specific for identifying ductus patency (Drayton and Skidmore, 1987; Gentile et al, 1981; Huhta et al, 1984; Mellander et al, 1987; Stevenson et al, 1980). This combination may also be useful in determining pressure gradients across the ductus (Musewe et al, 1987). Determining the size of the lumen of the ductus arteriosus and the magnitude of the Doppler signal from the shunt give only qualitative measures of the size of the shunt. M-mode measurements of LA:Ao ratio (diameter of the left atrium to that of the aortic root) greater than 1.4 (Johnson et al, 1983), Doppler-derived measurements of cardiac output (Walther et al, 1989), or evidence of diastolic retrograde flow in the descending aorta helps to determine when moderate-to-large PDA shunts are present (Ellison et al, 1983; Evans and Iyer, 1994; Iyer and Evans, 1994; Mellander et al, 1987; Serwer et al, 1982).

Although the magnitude of shunt flow plays a significant role in creating neonatal morbidity, equally important factors are the duration of exposure to the shunt and the infant's ability to compensate for the shunt. For example, the same magnitude left-to-right PDA shunt may be clinically "silent" when present within the first 24 hours after delivery, whereas it may be associated with signs of congestive failure if it persists for 7 to 10 days. Even though echocardiographic findings can predict in which infants clinical symptoms eventually will develop (Mellander et al, 1987; Walther et al, 1989), it does not automatically follow that treatment of the PDA should begin when these signs are first present (see *Treatment*).

Clinical signs of a PDA usually appear later than echocardiographic signs but have a higher correlation with the development of PDA-associated neonatal morbidity. Ellison and coworkers (1983) attempted to evaluate several commonly used criteria for diagnosing a large left-to-right shunt through the ductus arteriosus by noting the occurrence of each sign both before and 36 to 48 hours after surgical ligation (Fig. 61–1). No single criterion alone sufficed as an indicator of PDA. Certain signs, such as continuous murmur or hyperactive left ventricular impulse, were specific for a PDA, but lacked sensitivity; conversely, ventilatory support criteria were very sensitive, but lacked speci-

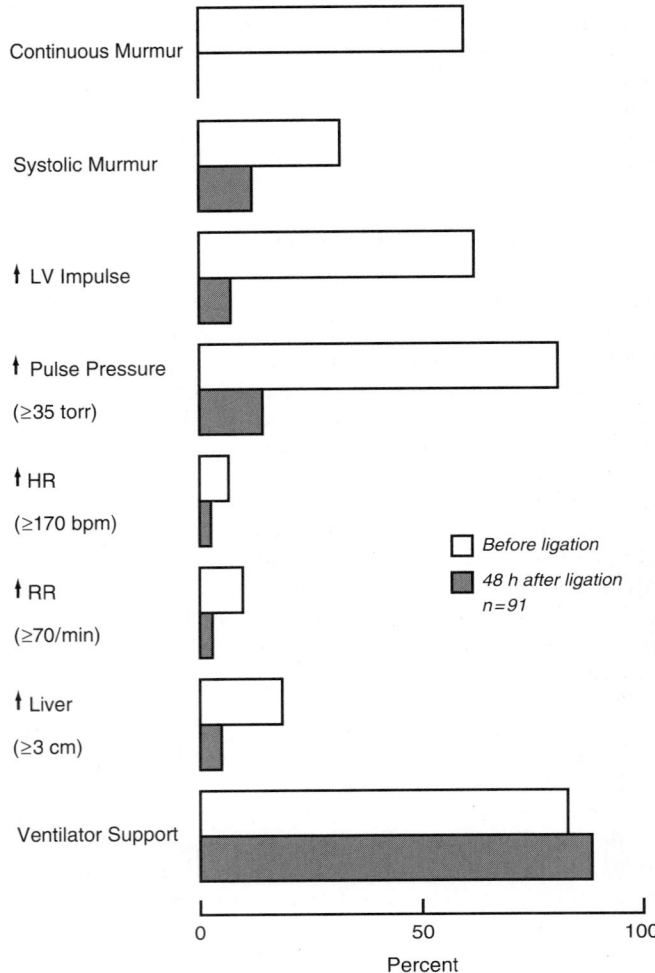

FIGURE 61–1. Clinical signs associated with a patent ductus arteriosus. (Data from Ellison RC, Peckham GJ, Lang P, et al: Evaluation of the preterm infant for patent ductus arteriosus. Reproduced by Permission of PEDIATRICS, Vol 71, Pages 364–372, Copyright 1983.)

ficity. On the other hand, the appearance of three or more of these clinical signs (systolic murmur, hyperdynamic precordial impulse, full pulses, widened pulse pressure, or worsening respiratory status) correlates well with the subsequent development of PDA-related morbidity (see *Treatment*). Therefore, when considering the relative merits of using clinical or echocardiographic methods for determining the presence of a PDA, not only the accuracy of the method must be considered but also which method identifies the PDA that will lead to other neonatal morbidities.

INCIDENCE

Pulsed Doppler echocardiographic assessments of full-term infants indicate that functional closure of the ductus has occurred in almost 50% of all full-term newborns by 24 hours, in 90% by 48 hours, and in all by 72 hours (Gentile et al, 1981). The rate of ductus closure is delayed in preterm infants; however, essentially all healthy preterm infants of 30 weeks' gestation or greater will have a closed

ductus by the 4th day after birth (Reller et al, 1993) (Table 61–1). RDS also delays ductus closure; however, in most infants who are 30 weeks' gestation or greater, the actual impact of RDS on ductal shunting may be less than commonly assumed (see Table 61–1). On the other hand, preterm infants of less than 30 weeks' gestation with severe respiratory distress have a high incidence of persistent PDA (Dudell and Gersony, 1984; Hammerman et al, 1986) (see Table 61–1).

Clinical symptoms do not develop in all infants with echocardiographic or Doppler-demonstrable ductus patency; the more mature the infant, the less the likelihood that ductus patency within the first 48 hours after delivery will require subsequent therapeutic intervention (Dudell and Gersony, 1984; Mellander et al, 1987). On the other hand, infants with RDS (Thibeault et al, 1975), perinatal asphyxia (Cotton et al, 1981), or excessive fluid administration during the first days of life (Bell et al, 1980; Green et al, 1980) are more susceptible to development of clinically symptomatic PDA.

The recent introduction of exogenous surfactant therapy has altered both the incidence and the presentation of the PDA. Although surfactant has no effect on the contractile behavior of the ductus, its effects on pulmonary vascular resistance lead to an earlier clinical presentation of the left-to-right shunt in preterm animals (Clyman et al, 1982; Shimada et al, 1989) and infants (Kaapa et al, 1993; Reller et al, 1991, 1993); it also causes a greater perceived need by physicians to treat the PDA (Heldt et al, 1989). A recent meta-analysis of the surfactant trials has found that there is an increased risk for development of a clinically symptomatic PDA following surfactant therapy; this risk is highest among infants who have received prophylactic treatment with surfactant (Alpan and Clyman, 1995).

TREATMENT

Unless there is a primary defect of the ductus wall, constriction and permanent anatomic closure should occur spontaneously. To forestall the use of therapeutic interventions to close the PDA (indomethacin or surgical ligation), other conservative measures have been advocated (e.g., fluid restriction, diuretics, and digitalis). Although excessive fluid administration has been associated with an increased incidence of PDA (Bell et al, 1980), fluid restriction is unlikely to cause ductus closure (Green et al, 1980). In addition, the combination of fluid restriction and diuretics frequently leads to electrolyte abnormalities, dehydration, and, most important, caloric deprivation. Furthermore, furosemide, the most commonly used diuretic, has been associated with an increased incidence of PDA in one study (Green et al, 1983). Digitalis would not be expected to be very useful because myocardial contractility is increased rather than reduced in infants with PDA. One controlled study by McGrath failed to show any effect of digoxin (McGrath, 1978). Finally, there may be an interaction between digoxin and indomethacin that increases the patient's susceptibility to the toxic effects of digoxin (Berman et al, 1978; Koren et al, 1984; Wilkerson and Glenn, 1977).

The addition of positive end-expiratory pressure has been found useful in managing infants with a PDA. When end-expiratory pressure is added, the amount of left-to-

TABLE 61–1

Incidence of Patent Ductus Arteriosus (%)

Gestation (wk)	Postnatal Age (hours)							
	0–24		24–48		48–72		72–96	
	Healthy	RDS	Healthy	RDS	Healthy	RDS	Healthy	RDS
>40	55		0		0		0	
38–40	85		50		5		0	
34–37	96		42		12		4	
30–33	87	87	31	56	13	25	0	11
≤29	80	88	40	84	20	77	7	65

RDS, respiratory distress syndrome.
Data from Dudell and Gersony, 1984; Gentile, et al, 1981; Hammerman, et al, 1986; Reller et al, 1993.

right shunt through the ductus arteriosus decreases; as a result, effective systemic blood flow increases (Cotton et al, 1980). A low hematocrit has been shown to aggravate left-to-right shunting by lowering the resistance to blood flow through the pulmonary vascular bed (Lister et al, 1982). Higher hematocrits diminish excessive shunting through the PDA and help ensure systemic oxygen delivery when perfusion is limited. Similarly, demands on left ventricular output should be minimized in infants with PDA by maintaining adequate oxygenation and by keeping the patient in a neutral thermal environment. Nevertheless, such therapies usually only delay, rather than prevent, the ultimate need for PDA closure. Cotton and colleagues (1978) demonstrated that failure to close the ductus after significant clinical symptoms of cardiovascular compromise have developed (approximately 7 to 10 days after birth) significantly increases neonatal morbidity. Ligation of a symptomatic PDA in premature infants can be done in the neonatal intensive care unit with low mortality and morbidity (Mikhail et al, 1982; Wagner et al, 1984).

Indomethacin appears to be an effective alternative to surgery for treatment of a PDA (Gersony et al, 1983). Its efficacy and toxicity have been explored extensively, and it appears comparable to surgical ligation in preventing the complications associated with a PDA: bronchopulmonary dysplasia (BPD), necrotizing enterocolitis (NEC), intracranial hemorrhage (ICH), and intolerance of enteral feedings (Gersony et al, 1983). In most intensive care nurseries, indomethacin has replaced surgery as the preferred therapy for a persistent PDA, probably because the most frequently occurring risks associated with ligation (increased incidence of cicatricial retinopathy of prematurity and need for thoracotomy) seem more serious than those associated with indomethacin (decreased urine output and increased bleeding other than ICH) (Gersony et al, 1983). Even though there may be general consensus on the efficacy of indomethacin for treatment of a PDA, questions about proper dosage, treatment duration, and optimal timing of treatment remain controversial.

Dose

Many variations in dosage regimens have been reported in the literature. When giving treatment to 8- to 10-day-old infants with left-to-right shunts that are causing cardiovascular compromise, the response of the ductus to indomethacin depends on the size of the dose as well as on the number of doses administered (Yeh et al, 1983, 1989). In most instances, a single dose has not resulted in persistent constriction of the ductus arteriosus. I recommend an initial dose of 0.2 mg/kg of lyophilized indomethacin, by intravenous (never intra-arterial) administration over 20 to 30 minutes when treating a clinically symptomatic PDA in infants weighing more than 1250 g or older than 7 days. A second and third dose of 0.2 mg/kg are given 12 and 36 hours after the first dose. Infants who weigh less than 1250 g at birth are given only 0.1 mg/kg for the second and third dose (unless they are older than 7 days). Plasma clearance of indomethacin depends on postnatal age (Brash et al, 1981; Smith et al, 1984; Thalji et al, 1980; Yaffe et al, 1980; Yeh et al, 1989). Therefore, a dosage regimen recommended for infants at the end of the 1st week (when the half-life of the drug is 21 hours) (Yaffe et al, 1980; Yeh et al, 1989) may lead to elevated and prolonged plasma concentrations when used in infants on day 1 (when the half-life is 71 hours) (Smith et al, 1984). Conversely, a single loading dose of indomethacin (0.2 mg/kg), without subsequent maintenance doses, can be effective in preventing clinical symptoms associated with a PDA when administered within the first 24 hours after delivery (Krueger et al, 1987).

Duration

Prostaglandin production is only transiently suppressed following indomethacin therapy. Within 6 to 7 days after completion of therapy, circulating PGE_2 concentrations return to the normal range (Seyberth et al, 1982). This interval may not allow enough time for anatomic remodeling of the ductus in the most immature infants. A prolonged maintenance course of low-dose indomethacin (0.1 mg/kg every 24 hours for 5 to 7 days) appears to both increase the success of the initial closure rate and decrease the relapse rate when compared with a shorter course (2–3 doses over 24 hours) (Hammerman and Aranburo, 1990; Rennie and Cooke, 1991; Rhodes et al, 1988). This dosage regimen still needs further evaluation because, in some reports (Rennie and Cooke, 1991; Rhodes et al, 1988), a higher mortality rate was observed in the infants receiving prolonged maintenance indomethacin.

In addition to its effects on the ductus, indomethacin also is associated with vasoconstriction of other vascular beds (e.g., cerebral, mesenteric, renal). Prolonging the rate of indomethacin infusion (20–30 min) alleviates some of the decrease in organ blood flow (Colditz et al, 1989); a continuous indomethacin infusion, of the same total daily dose, appears to decrease the detrimental effects of indomethacin even further (Hammerman et al, 1995).

Timing

The postnatal age at which indomethacin is administered plays an important role in determining its effectiveness. Several investigators have suggested that the relative ineffectiveness of indomethacin in treating conditions in infants of advanced postnatal age may be due to rapid drug clearance with a resultant inability to maintain "desired" plasma concentrations (Brash et al, 1981; Thalji et al, 1980). However, even when indomethacin concentrations have been maintained in the "desired" range, the ability of the drug to produce ductus closure remains inversely proportional to the postnatal age at the time of treatment (Achanti et al, 1986; Rennie et al, 1986; Rheuban et al, 1987). With advancing postnatal age, dilator prostaglandins play less of a role in maintaining ductus patency (Clyman et al, 1983). As a result, indomethacin becomes less effective in producing PDA closure (Achanti et al, 1986). It appears that in some situations, prostaglandins may not be the dominant factor maintaining ductus patency (Cotton et al, 1991).

A second type of indomethacin treatment failure is found in patients whose ductus initially constricts when treated with indomethacin only to reopen several days later. Recurrence of a symptomatic PDA after initial successful treatment is independent of initial plasma indomethacin concentrations (Brash et al, 1981; Gersony et al, 1983; Ramsey et al, 1987). The rate of reopening, which is greatest among the most immature infants, appears to be related to the timing of treatment with indomethacin and the completeness of initial ductus closure after treatment (Weiss et al, 1995). Infants whose ductus is closed with indomethacin during the first 2 days after delivery (Kaapa et al, 1983; Mahony et al, 1982, 1985) appear to have a lower incidence of reopening when compared with those receiving treatment after the first week (Brash et al, 1981; Gersony et al, 1983; Hammerman et al, 1986; Ivey et al, 1979; Mellander et al, 1984; Ramsey et al, 1987; Rudd et al, 1983). Because of the lower incidence of indomethacin failure and ductus reopening when indomethacin is administered within the first 48 hours, there is less need for surgical ligation than when it is given after the 1st week.

Indomethacin treatment may be most effective in the first 24 to 48 hours after delivery, but is that necessarily the best time to administer it? Ninety percent of infants with severe respiratory distress have echocardiographic evidence of a PDA during the first 24 hours; however, in only 40% do symptoms subsequently develop of a hemodynamically large left-to-right shunt that will require intervention with indomethacin or surgery. In addition, in most infants, symptoms of cardiovascular compromise do not develop before 7 days (Alpert et al, 1979; Cotton et al, 1978;

Gersony et al, 1983). Therefore, treatment given within the first 24 to 48 hours implies that, in approximately 60% of such infants, symptoms of cardiovascular compromise would never have developed. Because indomethacin has been associated with several frequent as well as infrequent complications (Alpan et al, 1985; Appleton et al, 1986; Friedman et al, 1978; Gersony et al, 1983; Krueger et al, 1987; Rennie et al, 1986; Yeh et al, 1989; Yeh et al, 1982a), such an aggressive approach to therapy can be justified only if early treatment can be demonstrated to significantly alter outcome in these infants.

A recently reported meta-analysis of more than 25 randomized, controlled trials examined the relative merits of the different timing strategies that have been used to treat the PDA (Clyman, 1996). In each of the trials, a backup treatment (either indomethacin or surgical ligation) was included to close the PDA, if the initial study treatment failed. As was demonstrated previously, clinical signs of a PDA frequently develop in premature infants within the first 2 to 3 days of life (early symptomatic PDA) (Cotton et al, 1978); however, it may not be until 7 to 10 days after birth that signs of congestive failure develop (late symptomatic PDA) (Cotton et al, 1978). The initial treatment trials (*Late Symptomatic Rx Versus Later Backup Rx*) were designed to evaluate the effectiveness of indomethacin in closing the late symptomatic PDA (Table 61–2). Infants were randomized to receive indomethacin or no additional therapy when signs of congestive failure developed (age 7 to 10 days). If the infant's condition did not improve within 2 to 6 days after initial randomization, then backup treatment was started. The *Early Symptomatic Rx Versus Late Symptomatic Rx* trials were designed to evaluate whether the early treatment of a symptomatic PDA, when clinical signs first appeared (age 1–3 days), would decrease PDA-related morbidity below that of a backup treatment strategy that was not initiated until signs of congestive failure appeared (age 7–12 days). The *Prophylactic Rx Versus Early Symptomatic Rx* trials were designed to evaluate whether administration of indomethacin, before the appearance of any PDA clinical signs (usually within the first 24 hours after birth), would reduce morbidity to less than that associated with a strategy wherein no treatment was given until signs of an early symptomatic PDA appeared (age 3–4 days). All three treatment strategies prevented either the development or the need for backup treatment of a symptomatic PDA (Clyman, 1996).

Surgical Ligation

The studies listed in Table 61–3 reserved surgical ligation for infants who either failed backup therapy with indomethacin or in whom contraindications to its use developed at the time it was needed. The prophylactic treatment strategy significantly reduced the need for surgical ligation when compared with a strategy that is not initiated until early symptoms appear. Early symptomatic treatment of the PDA, although not as effective as prophylactic treatment, does reduce the need for surgical ligation when compared with a late symptomatic treatment strategy. However, if indomethacin treatment has not been given before the late symptomatic stage, differences in timing no

---

TABLE 61–2

Characteristics of Strategies Used to Evaluate Timing of Treatment for Patent Ductus Arteriosus

Study Design	Trials (N)	Patients (N)	Birth Weight g	Gestation (weeks)	HMD (%)	Postnatal Age Study Rx (days)	Postnatal Age Backup Rx (days)	Backup Treatment Needed for Control Patients (%)
Late symptomatic treatment vs. later symptomatic treatment	5	428	1216 ±108	30 ±1	90 ±11	8.9 ±1.5	12.8 ±4.5	58 ±22
Early symptomatic treatment vs. late symptomatic treatment	8	264	1255 ±442	29 ±2	94 ±10	2.0 ±0.9	8.3 ±3.0	63 ±20
Prophylactic treatment vs. early symptomatic treatment	17	1580	1001 ±123	28 ±1	83 ±13	0.7 ±0.5	3.4 ±0.5	38 ±15

°Values are mean ± SD.
HMD, hyaline membrane disease.
Adapted from Clyman RI: Commentary: Recommendations for the postnatal use of indomethacin. An analysis of four separate treatment strategies. J Pediatr 128:601–607, 1996.

Pulmonary Morbidity

Infants who receive late symptomatic treatment of their PDA, when signs of congestive failure are present, have significant improvement in pulmonary compliance (Stefano et al, 1991; Yeh et al, 1981). Once late symptoms of a PDA appear (age 8–10 days), a brief delay (48 hours) (Gersony et al, 1983) before initiating indomethacin does not appear to increase the risks of long-term pulmonary morbidity; however, failure to close the ductus at this junction is associated with significant pulmonary morbidity and long-term ventilator requirements (Cotton et al, 1978).

If infants are given indomethacin when early PDA symptoms appear, they have less long-term pulmonary morbidity than if treatment is delayed until late symptoms develop (usually an additional 5–10 days). Two thirds of the control patients in the *Early Symptomatic PDA Treatment* trials ultimately needed backup treatment of their PDA. The patients who received the early symptomatic treatment had both a significant reduction in BPD and a significant reduction in the duration of mechanical ventila-

tion when compared with those who received late symptomatic treatment.

In contrast, infants who are prophylactically given indomethacin (before the onset of symptoms) do not have any further decrease in long-term pulmonary morbidity when compared with those receiving early symptomatic treatment. In these trials, backup therapy was started for early symptoms (age 3–4 days), long before late symptoms of congestive failure occurred. As a result, the patients in the prophylactic treatment trials had been exposed to a left-to-right PDA shunt only during the period when their pulmonary lymphatics were capable of rapidly eliminating the extra fluid entering the lung interstitium (see *Hemodynamic and Pulmonary Alterations*). In addition, a symptomatic PDA that required backup therapy ultimately developed in less than 40% of the control patients in the prophylactic treatment trials.

Necrotizing Enterocolitis

A large left-to-right shunt through a PDA decreases mesenteric blood flow in premature animals (Meyers et al, 1991) and infants (Shimada et al, 1994). In a randomized, controlled trial of early versus late surgical ligation of a PDA,

---

TABLE 61–3

Neonatal Morbidity Associated with Different Patent Ductus Arteriosus Treatment Strategies

	Symptomatic PDA	Surgical Ligation	Pulmonary Morbidity	NEC	Pulmonary Hemorrhage	ICH	ROP	Death	Renal Toxicity
Late symptomatic treatment vs. later symptomatic treatment	↓	—	—	—			—	—	↑
Early symptomatic treatment vs. late symptomatic treatment	↓	↓	↓	↓		—	—	—	↑
Prophylactic treatment vs. early symptomatic treatment	↓	↓	—	—	↓	↓	—	—	↑

↓, significant reduction in morbidity ($P < 0.05$); ↑, significant increase in morbidity ($P < 0.05$); —, no difference in morbidity; ICH, intracranial hemorrhage; NEC, necrotizing enterocolitis; ROP, retinopathy of prematurity.
Adapted from Clyman RI: Commentary: Recommendations for the postnatal use of indomethacin. An analysis of four separate treatment strategies. J Pediatr 128:601–607, 1996.

surgical closure of the ductus, within 5 days of birth and before initiating feedings, significantly lowered the incidence of NEC among preterm infants with similar feeding histories (Cassady et al, 1989). This study suggests that a symptomatic PDA probably does contribute to the development of NEC. Indomethacin also decreases mesenteric blood flow (Meyers et al, 1991) and has been associated with sporadic cases of intestinal perforation (Alpan et al, 1985). This has raised appropriate concern about its overzealous use. However, a meta-analysis of the multiple indomethacin trials supports the view that indomethacin may be as effective as surgical ligation in decreasing the incidence of NEC (Clyman, 1996). Just as was observed in the early surgical ligation study, early treatment of a symptomatic PDA with indomethacin is associated with a significantly decreased incidence of NEC. Prophylactic treatment with indomethacin offers no additional advantage (see Table 61–3).

Pulmonary Hemorrhage

Concerns about transient, rapid increases in pulmonary blood flow following surfactant administration have existed since the first accounts of pulmonary hemorrhage were reported in 1990 (Bose et al, 1990). A meta-analysis of the surfactant trials found that the rate of pulmonary hemorrhage was significantly increased when surfactant therapy was used (Raju and Langenberg, 1993). Although the mechanisms responsible for pulmonary hemorrhage following surfactant therapy are uncertain, a recent retrospective cohort study found that a clinically detectable PDA was significantly associated with the onset of the hemorrhage (Garland et al, 1994). More than 90% of pulmonary hemorrhages occur during the first 72 hours after birth (Garland et al, 1994). Although no data are available from the early symptomatic and the late symptomatic treatment trials, it might be anticipated that these two strategies, which initiate treatment after symptoms of a PDA appear (after 48 hours), would be ineffectual in altering the incidence of pulmonary hemorrhage. In contrast, prophylactic treatment with indomethacin significantly reduces the incidence of pulmonary hemorrhage (Clyman, 1996).

Intracranial Hemorrhage

Previous studies have shown that indomethacin decreases cerebral blood flow, decreases reactive postasphyxial cerebral hyperemia, accelerates maturation of the germinal matrix microvasculature, and decreases the incidence of ICH in experimental animals (Dahlgren et al, 1981; Ment et al, 1983, 1992). The effects of indomethacin on ICH do not appear to be due to its effects on ductus patency (Ment et al, 1985, 1988). Because most ICHs occur within the first 3 days after birth, beneficial effects would be expected only when indomethacin is given in a prophylactic strategy (within the first 8–24 hours after birth). When prophylactic indomethacin is given to infants with normal echoencephalograms, there is a significant reduction in both the incidence of all grades (I–IV) as well as the most severe grades (III, IV) of ICH (Clyman, 1996). The dramatic effects of prophylactic indomethacin in this group of infants with known, normal echoencephalograms is somewhat tem-

pered when prophylactic indomethacin is administered to populations in which the prior ICH status is unknown. Between 30% and 50% of infants in whom an ICH ultimately develops have evidence of an ICH on their screening preindomethacin echoencephalogram. When indomethacin is administered prophylactically, without knowledge of prior ICH status, there is no longer a difference in the overall incidence of ICH; however, there is still a significant reduction in the incidence of severe (Grade III, IV) ICH (Clyman, 1996).

The beneficial effects of prophylactic indomethacin may not apply to all preterm infants. In studies wherein the effects of indomethacin have been examined by weight group (i.e., <1000 g versus ≥1000 g), the most beneficial effects have been found in the larger infants. Prophylactic indomethacin does not appear to alter the incidence of ICH in infants with birth weights less than 1000 g (Clyman, 1996).

Centers that experience a higher incidence of Grades III and IV ICH also appear to benefit the most from prophylactic indomethacin. In centers where the incidence of Grades III and IV ICH in the control population is greater than 10%, indomethacin produces a significant reduction in severe ICH. In contrast, in centers where the incidence is less than 10%, indomethacin does not have the same significant effect (Clyman, 1996).

The long-term effects of prophylactic indomethacin on cerebral function have not been fully evaluated. The preliminary findings show that, if anything, there is a decreased incidence of both periventricular leukomalacia (Ment et al, 1994a, 1994b; Setzer-Bandstra et al, 1988) and later motor abnormalities (Setzer-Bandstra et al, 1987) in the infants who receive prophylactic indomethacin (see Chapters 68 and 69).

Retinopathy of Prematurity and Death

None of the three indomethacin treatment strategies (prophylactic, early symptomatic, and late symptomatic) altered the incidence of retinopathy of prematurity or death.

Renal Toxicity

All three treatment strategies (prophylactic, early symptomatic, and late symptomatic) are associated with significant transient reductions in urine output and elevations in serum creatinine concentration.

CONTRAINDICATIONS TO USE OF INDOMETHACIN

Most contraindications are relative, and few are beyond dispute.

Poor Renal Function

Many centers do not use indomethacin if serum creatinine is more than 1.7 mg/dL, or if urine output is less than 1 mL/kg per hour. The reasoning behind this is that indomethacin may decrease urine output further and cause significant water and electrolyte problems. Whether giving indomethacin to a patient with moderate renal failure damages the kidney is uncertain; nevertheless, it is prudent to withhold indomethacin in infants who have significant renal failure. In some infants, indomethacin administration is followed by a markedly decreased urine output, which must be allowed for when replacing fluid and electrolyte losses. Early reports suggested that furosemide or dopamine might minimize the renal side effects (Seri et al, 1984; Yeh et al, 1982b), but subsequent studies have not corroborated these earlier findings (Fajardo et al, 1992).

Bleeding Disorders and Low Platelets

Frank renal or gastrointestinal bleeding is a contraindication to the use of indomethacin. ICH, however, is not a contraindication to the use of indomethacin (Ment et al, 1994a). As discussed previously, indomethacin may actually decrease the incidence of ICH.

Indomethacin impairs platelet function for 7 to 9 days (Friedman et al, 1978). Usually, this has not been clinically relevant; however, it is customary to withhold indomethacin if platelets are less than 50,000/mm³, even in the absence of overt bleeding.

Necrotizing Enterocolitis

If infants have signs of early NEC, indomethacin is usually contraindicated, partly because NEC may be due to bowel ischemia secondary to the ductus arteriosus, and indomethacin may further decrease blood flow to the bowel. A more important reason is that, if closing the ductus arteriosus prevents the progression of NEC, as many neonatologists believe, then surgical ligation is a more certain and rapid way of achieving ductus closure. Indomethacin may take 36 hours to close the PDA, and such a delay may not preserve bowel viability.

Sepsis

Indomethacin should not be used if sepsis is strongly suspected, because it impairs white blood cell motility.

SUMMARY

A PDA is an important problem in the small preterm infant. The clinical consequences of a PDA are related to the degree of left-to-right shunt with its associated increase in blood flow to the lungs and decrease to the kidneys and intestines. Treatment with indomethacin has been demonstrated in many studies to be effective in closing a PDA, particularly when given within the first few days after birth.

The current use of exogenous surfactant has caused the symptomatic PDA to present earlier than it did during the presurfactant era. The presence of a large, symptomatic PDA that persists through the end of the first week after birth increases the likelihood of pulmonary morbidity, pulmonary hemorrhage, NEC, and the ultimate need for surgical ligation. Early treatment of a clinically symptomatic PDA, in the first days after delivery, reduces the risk of development of these morbidities if the group of infants receiving treatment has a high chance (>50%) of developing a persistent PDA. Several centers have noted that very-low-birth-weight infants in whom a murmur develops, even without other signs of a ductus, are at high risk (80%) for development of persistent, large PDA shunts (Mahony et al, 1982, 1985). It seems appropriate to apply treatment in these very-low-birth-weight infants when their PDA first becomes apparent and before signs of a large shunt are evident.

Although prophylactic indomethacin reduces the chances of development of a symptomatic PDA, this approach does not appear to offer any additional advantage in reducing pulmonary morbidity or NEC when compared with early symptomatic treatment. This finding is not surprising in that less than 40% of the placebo-treated infants in the prophylactic trials ever had a symptomatic PDA that required treatment. On the other hand, prophylactic indomethacin may be the most appropriate strategy to follow when populations of infants can be identified in whom either the incidence of Grade III, IV ICH (>10%) or severe pulmonary hemorrhage (>10%) is high, or in whom indomethacin failure and the need for surgical ligation is frequent (>30%).

REFERENCES

Achanti B, Yeh TF, Pildes RS: Indomethacin therapy in infants with advanced postnatal age and patent ductus arteriosus. Clin Invest Med 9:250–253, 1986.

Alpan G, Clyman RI: Cardiovascular effects of surfactant replacement with special reference to the patent ductus arteriosus. *In* Robertson B, Taeusch HW (Eds): Surfactant Therapy for Lung Disease: Lung Biology in Health and Disease. Vol 84. New York, Marcel Dekker, 1995, pp 531–545.

Alpan G, Mauray F, Clyman RI: Effect of patent ductus arteriosus on water accumulation and protein permeability in the premature lungs of mechanically ventilated premature lambs. Pediatr Res 26:570–575, 1989.

Alpan GM, Eyal F, Vinograd I, et al: Localized intestinal perforations after enteral administration of indomethacin in premature infants. J Pediatr 106:277–281, 1985.

Alpert BS, Lewins MJ, Rowland DW, et al: Plasma indomethacin levels in preterm newborn infants with symptomatic patent ductus arteriosus—Clinical and echocardiographic assessments of response. J Pediatr 95:578–582, 1979.

Appleton RS, Graham TP, Cotton RB, et al: Abnormal diastolic cardiac function following indomethacin therapy of patent ductus arteriosus. Pediatr Res 20:167A, 1986.

Bell EF, Warburton D, Stonestreet B, Oh W: Effect of fluid administration on the development of symptomatic patent ductus arteriosus and congestive heart failure in premature infants. N Engl J Med 302:598–604, 1980.

Berman W Jr, Dubynsky O, Whitman V, et al: Digoxin therapy in low-birth-weight infants with patent ductus arteriosus. J Pediatr 93:652–655, 1978.

Bose C, Corbet A, Bose G, et al: Improved outcome at 28 days of age for very low birth weight infants treated with a single dose of a synthetic surfactant. J Pediatr 117:947–953, 1990.

Brash AR, Hickey DE, Graham TP, et al: Pharmacokinetics of indomethacin in the neonate. N Engl J Med 305:67–72, 1981.

Brown E: Increased risk of bronchopulmonary dysplasia in infants with patent ductus arteriosus. J Pediatr 95:865–866, 1979.

Cassady G, Crouse DT, Kirklin JW, et al: A randomized, controlled trial of very early prophylactic ligation of the ductus arteriosus in babies who weighed 1000 g or less at birth. N Engl J Med 320:1511–1516, 1989.

Clyman RI: Commentary: Recommendations for the postnatal use of indomethacin. An analysis of four separate treatment strategies. J Pediatr 128:601–607, 1996.

Clyman RI: Ductus arteriosus: Current theories of prenatal and postnatal regulation. Semin Perinatol 11:64–71, 1987.

Clyman RI, Ballard PL, Sniderman S, et al: Prenatal administration of betamethasone for prevention of patent ductus arteriosus. J Pediatr 98:123–126, 1981a.

Clyman RI, Jobe A, Heymann MA, et al: Increased shunt through the patent ductus arteriosus after surfactant replacement therapy. J Pediatr 100:101–107, 1982.

Clyman RI, Mauray F, Heymann MA, Roman C: Cardiovascular effects of a patent ductus arteriosus in preterm lambs with respiratory distress. J Pediatr 111:579–587, 1987.

Clyman RI, Mauray F, Roman C, et al: Effects of antenatal glucocorticoid administration on the ductus arteriosus of preterm lambs. Am J Physiol 241:H415–H420, 1981b.

Clyman RI, Mauray F, Roman C, et al: Factors determining the loss of ductus arteriosus responsiveness to prostaglandin E_2. Circulation 68:433–436, 1983.

Clyman RI, Saugstad OD, Mauray F: Reactive oxygen metabolites relax the lamb ductus arteriosus by stimulating prostaglandin production. Circ Res 64:1–8, 1989.

Coceani F, Armstrong C, Kelsey L: Endothelin is a potent constrictor of the lamb ductus arteriosus. Can J Physiol Pharmacol 67:902–904, 1989a.

Coceani F, Hamilton NC, Labuc J, Olley PM: Cytochrome P 450 linked monooxygenase: Involvement in the lamb ductus arteriosus. Am J Physiol 246:H640–H643, 1984.

Coceani F, Kelsey L, Ackerley C, et al: Cytochrome P450 during ontogenic development: Occurrence in the ductus arteriosus and other tissues. Can J Physiol Pharmacol 72:217–226, 1994.

Coceani F, Wright J, Breen C: Ductus arteriosus: Involvement of a sarcolemmal cytochrome P-450 in O_2 constriction? Can J Physiol Pharmacol 67:1448–1450, 1989b.

Colditz P, Murphy D, Rolfe P, Wilkinson AR: Effect of infusion rate of indomethacin on cerebrovascular responses in preterm neonates. Arch Dis Child 64:8–12, 1989.

Collaborative Group on Antenatal Steroid Therapy: Prevention of respiratory distress syndrome: Effect of antenatal dexamethasone administration. Publication No 85–2695, National Institutes of Health, 1985, p 44.

Cotton RB, Haywood JL, FitzGerald GA: Symptomatic patent ductus arteriosus following prophylactic indomethacin. A clinical and biochemical appraisal. Biol Neonate 60:273–282, 1991.

Cotton RB, Lindstrom DP, Kanarek KS, et al: Effect of positive-end-expiratory-pressure on right ventricular output in lambs with hyaline membrane disease. Acta Paediatr Scand 69:603–606, 1980.

Cotton RB, Lindstrom DP, Stahlman MT: Early prediction of symptomatic patent ductus arteriosus from perinatal risk factors: Discriminant analysis. Acta Paediatr Scand 70:723–727, 1981.

Cotton RB, Stahlman MT, Berder HW, et al: Randomized trial of early closure of symptomatic patent ductus arteriosus in small preterm infants. J Pediatr 93:647–651, 1978.

Dahlgren N, Nilsson B, Sakabe T, Siesjo BK: The effect of indomethacin on cerebral blood flow and oxygen consumption in the rat at normal and increased carbon dioxide tensions. Acta Physiol Scand 111:475–485, 1981.

de Reeder EG, Girard N, Poelmann RE, et al: Hyaluronic acid accumulation and endothelial cell detachment in intimal thickening of the vessel wall. The normal and genetically defective ductus arteriosus. Am J Pathol 132:574–585, 1988.

Drayton MR, Skidmore R: Ductus arteriosus blood flow during first 48 hours of life. Arch Dis Child 62:1030–1034, 1987.

Dudell GG, Gersony WM: Patent ductus arteriosus in neonates with severe respiratory disease. J Pediatr 104:915–920, 1984.

Ellison RC, Peckham GJ, Lang P, et al: Evaluation of the preterm infant for patent ductus arteriosus. Pediatrics 71:364–372, 1983.

Evans N, Iyer P: Assessment of ductus arteriosus shunt in preterm infants supported by mechanical ventilation: Effect of interatrial shunting. J Pediatr 125:778–785, 1994.

Fajardo CA, Whyte RK, Steele BT: Effect of dopamine on failure of indomethacin to close the patent ductus arteriosus. J Pediatr 121:771–775, 1992.

Fay FS: Guinea pig ductus arteriosus. I. Cellular and metabolic basis for oxygen sensitivity. Am J Physiol 221:470–479, 1971.

Fay FS, Jobsis FF: Guinea pig ductus arteriosus. III. Light absorption changes during response to O_2 Am J Physiol 223:588–595, 1972.

Friedman WF: The intrinsic physiologic properties of the developing heart. *In* Friedman WF, Lesch M, Sonnenblick EH (Eds): Neonatal Heart Disease. New York, Grune and Stratton, 1972, pp 21–49.

Friedman Z, Whitman V, Maisels MJ, et al: Indomethacin disposition and indomethacin induced platelet dysfunction in premature infants. J Clin Pharmacol 18:272–279, 1978.

Fujiwara T, Maeta H, Chida S, et al: Artificial surfactant therapy in hyaline-membrane disease. Lancet 1:55–59, 1980.

Garland J, Buck R, Weinberg M: Pulmonary hemorrhage risk in infants with a clinically diagnosed patent ductus arteriosus: A retrospective cohort study. Pediatrics 94:719–723, 1994.

Gentile R, Stevenson GM, Dooley T, et al: Pulsed Doppler echocardiographic determination of time of ductal closure in normal newborn infants. J Pediatr 98:443–448, 1981.

Gerhardt T, Bancalari E: Lung compliance in newborns with patent ductus arteriosus before and after surgical ligation. Biol Neonate 38:96–105, 1980.

Gersony WM, Peckham GJ, Ellison RC, et al: Effects of indomethacin in premature infants with patent ductus arteriosus: Results of a national collaborative study. J Pediatr 102:895–906, 1983.

Gittenberger-de-Groot AC, Van Ertbruggen I, Moulaert AJMG, Harinck E: The ductus arteriosus in the preterm infant: Histologic and clinical observations. J Pediatr 96:88–93, 1980.

Gluckman PD, Heymann MA: Perinatal and Pediatric Pathophysiology: A Clinical Perspective, 1st ed. London, Edward Arnold, 1993.

Green TP, Thompson TR, Johnson D, Lock JE: Fluid administration and the development of patent ductus arteriosus. N Engl J Med 303:337–338, 1980.

Green TP, Thompson TR, Johnson DE, Lock JE: Furosemide promotes patent ductus arteriosus in premature infants with the respiratory distress syndrome. N Engl J Med 308:743–748, 1983.

Hammerman C, Aranburo MJ: Prolonged indomethacin therapy for the prevention of recurrences of patent ductus arteriosus. J Pediatr 117:771–776, 1990.

Hammerman C, Glaser J, Schimmel MS, et al: Continuous versus multiple rapid infusions of indomethacin: Effects on cerebral blood flow velocity. Pediatrics 95:244–248, 1995.

Hammerman C, Strates C, Valaitis S: The silent ductus: Its precursors and its aftermath. Pediatr Cardiol 7:121–127, 1986.

Heldt GP, Pesonen E, Merritt TA, et al: Closure of the ductus arteriosus and mechanics of breathing in preterm infants after surfactant replacement therapy. Pediatr Res 25:305–310, 1989.

Huhta JC, Cohen M, Gutgesell HP: Patency of the ductus arteriosus in normal neonates: Two dimensional echocardiography vs Doppler assessment. J Am Coll Cardiol 4:561–564, 1984.

Ikegami M, Jacobs H, Jobe A: Surfactant function in respiratory distress syndrome. J Pediatr 102:443–447, 1983.

Ivey HH, Kattwinkel J, Park TS, Krovetz LJ: Failure of indomethacin to close patent ductus arteriosus in infants weighing under 1000 g. Br Heart J 41:304–307, 1979.

Iyer P, Evans N: Re-evaluation of the left atrial to aortic root ratio as a marker of patent ductus arteriosus. Arch Dis Child 70:F112–F117, 1994.

Jacob J, Gluck G, DiSessa T, et al: The contribution of PDA in the neonate with severe RDS. J Pediatr 96:79–87, 1980.

Johnson DS, Rogers JH, Null DM, DeLemos RA: The physiologic consequences of the ductus arteriosus in the extremely immature newborn. Clin Res 26:826A, 1978.

Johnson GL, Breart GL, Gewitz MH, et al: Echocardiographic characteristics of premature infants with patent ductus arteriosus. Pediatrics 72:864–871, 1983.

Kaapa P, Lanning P, Koivisto M: Early closure of patent ductus arteriosus with indomethacin in preterm infants with idiopathic respiratory distress syndrome. Acta Paediatr Scand 72:179–184, 1983.

Kaapa P, Seppanen M, Kero P, Saraste M: Pulmonary hemodynamics after synthetic surfactant replacement in neonatal respiratory distress syndrome. J Pediatr 123:115–119, 1993.

Kennedy JA, Clark SL: Observations on the physiological reactions of the ductus arteriosus. Am J Physiol 136:140–147, 1942.

Kitterman JA: Effects of intestinal ischemia in necrotizing enterocolitis in the newborn infant. *In* Moore TD (Ed): Report of the 68th Ross Conference of Pediatric Research. Columbus, OH, Ross Laboratories, 1975, pp 38–42.

Koren G, Zarfin Y, Perlman M, MacLeod SM: Effects of indomethacin on digoxin pharmacokinetics in preterm infants. Pediatr Pharmacol 4:25–30, 1984.

Krauss AN, Fatica N, Lewis BS, et al: Pulmonary function in preterm infants following treatment with intravenous indomethacin. Am J Dis Child 143:78–81, 1989.

Krueger E, Mellander M, Bratton D, Cotton R: Prevention of symptomatic patent ductus arteriosus with a single dose of indomethacin. J Pediatr 111:749–754, 1987.

Lewis AB, Heymann MA, Rudolph AM: Gestational changes in pulmonary vascular responses in fetal lambs in utero. Circ Res 39:536–541, 1976.

Lister G, Hellenbrand WE, Kleinman CS, Talner NS: Physiologic effects of increasing hemoglobin concentration in left-to-right shunting in infants with ventricular septal defects. N Engl J Med 306:502–506, 1982.

Mahony L, Caldwell RL, Girod DA, et al: Indomethacin therapy on the first day of life in infants with very low birth weight. J Pediatr 106:801–805, 1985.

Mahony L, Carnero V, Brett C, et al: Prophylactic indomethacin therapy for patent ductus arteriosus in very-low-birth-weight infants. N Engl J Med 306:506–510, 1982.

Martin CG, Snider AR, Katz SM, et al: Abnormal cerebral blood flow patterns in preterm infants with a large patent ductus arteriosus. J Pediatr 101:587–593, 1982.

McGrath RL: General discussion. Session III: Persistent patency of ductus arteriosus in premature infants. Report of the 75th Ross Conference on Pediatric Research. Columbus, Ohio, Ross Laboratories, 1978, p 92.

Mellander M, Larsson LE, Ekström-Jodal B, Sabel KG: Prediction of symptomatic patent ductus arteriosus in preterm infants using Doppler and M-mode echocardiography. Acta Paediatr Scand 76:553–559, 1987.

Mellander M, Leheup B, Lindstrom DP, et al: Recurrence of symptomatic patent ductus arteriosus in extremely premature infants, treated with indomethacin. J Pediatr 105:138–143, 1984.

Ment LR, Duncan CC, Ehrenkranz RA, et al: Randomized indomethacin trial for prevention of intraventricular hemorrhage in very low birth weight infants. J Pediatr 107:937–943, 1985.

Ment LR, Duncan CC, Ehrenkranz RA, et al: Randomized low-dose indomethacin trial for prevention of intraventricular hemorrhage in very low birth weight neonates. J Pediatr 112:948–955, 1988.

Ment LR, Oh W, Ehrenkranz RA, et al: Low-dose indomethacin and prevention of intraventricular hemorrhage: A multicenter randomized trial. Pediatrics 93:543–550, 1994a.

Ment LR, Oh W, Ehrenkranz RA, et al: Low-dose indomethacin therapy and extension of intraventricular hemorrhage: A multicenter randomized trial. J Pediatr 124:951–955, 1994b.

Ment LR, Stewart WB, Ardito TA, et al: Indomethacin promotes germinal matrix microvessel maturation in the newborn beagle pup. Stroke 23:1132–1137, 1992.

Ment LR, Stewart WB, Scott DT, Duncan CC: Beagle puppy model of intraventricular hemorrhage: Randomized indomethacin prevention trial. Neurology 33:179–184, 1983.

Meyers RL, Alpan G, Lin E, Clyman RI: Patent ductus arteriosus, indomethacin, and intestinal distension: Effects on intestinal blood flow and oxygen consumption. Pediatr Res 29:569–574, 1991.

Mikhail M, Lei W, Toews W, et al: Surgical and medical experience with 734 premature infants with patent ductus arteriosus. J Thorac Cardiovasc Surg 83:349–357, 1982.

Momma K, Mishihara S, Ota Y: Constriction of the fetal ductus arteriosus by glucocorticoid hormones. Pediatr Res 15:19–21, 1981.

Musewe NN, Smallhorn JF, Benson LN, et al: Validation of Doppler derived pulmonary arterial pressure in patients with ductus arteriosus under different hemodynamic states. Circulation 76:1081–1091, 1987.

Nakanishi T, Gu H, Hagiwara N, Momma K: Mechanisms of oxygen-induced contraction of ductus arteriosus isolated from the fetal rabbit. Circ Res 72:1218–1228, 1993.

Naulty CM, Horn S, Conry J, Avery GB: Improved lung compliance after ligation of patent ductus arteriosus in hyaline membrane disease. J Pediatr 93:682–684, 1978.

Pérez Fontán JJ, Clyman RI, Mauray F, et al: Respiratory effects of a patent ductus arteriosus in premature newborn lambs. J Appl Physiol 63:2315–2324, 1987.

Perlman JM, Hill A, Volpe JJ: The effect of patent ductus arteriosus on flow velocity in the anterior cerebral arteries: Ductal steal in the premature newborn infant. J Pediatr 99:767–771, 1981.

Raju TNK, Langenberg P: Pulmonary hemorrhage and exogenous surfactant therapy—A metaanalysis. J Pediatr 123:603–610, 1993.

Ramsey JM, Murphy DJ, Vick GW III, et al: Response of the patent ductus arteriosus to indomethacin treatment. Am J Dis Child 141:294–297, 1987.

Reller MD, Buffkin DC, Colasurdo MA, et al: Ductal patency in neonates with respiratory distress syndrome. A randomized surfactant trial. Am J Dis Child 145:1017–1020, 1991.

Reller MD, Rice MJ, McDonald RW: Review of studies evaluating ductal patency in the premature infant. J Pediatr 122:S59–S62, 1993.

Rennie JM, Cooke RWI: Prolonged low dose indomethacin for persistent ductus arteriosus of prematurity. Arch Dis Child 66:55–58, 1991.

Rennie JM, Doyle J, Cooke RWI: Early administration of indomethacin to preterm infants. Arch Dis Child 61:233–238, 1986.

Rheuban KS, Everett AD, Zellers TM, et al: Ductus arteriosus closure rates and indomethacin levels in premature infants. Pediatr Res 21:387A, 1987.

Rhodes PG, Ferguson MG, Reddy NS, et al: Effects of prolonged versus acute indomethacin therapy in very low birth weight infants with patent ductus arteriosus. Eur J Pediatr 147:481–484, 1988.

Rudd P, Montanez P, Hallidie-Smith K, Silverman M: Indomethacin treatment for patent ductus arteriosus in very low birthweight infants: Double blind trial. Arch Dis Child 58:267–270, 1983.

Seri I, Tulassay T, Kiszel J, Csomor S: The use of dopamine for the prevention of the renal side effects of indomethacin in premature infants with patent ductus arteriosus. Int J Pediatr Nephrol 5:209–214, 1984.

Serwer GA, Armstrong BE, Anderson PA: Continuous wave Doppler ultrasonographic quantitation of patent ductus arteriosus flow. J Pediatr 100:297–299, 1982.

Setzer-Bandstra E, Duenas ML, Rodriguez I, et al: Prophylactic indomethacin for prevention of intraventricular hemorrhage (IVH): Neurodevelopmental follow-up. Pediatr Res 21:391A, 1987.

Setzer-Bandstra E, Montalvo BM, Goldberg R, et al: Prophylactic indomethacin for prevention of intraventricular hemorrhage in premature infants. Pediatrics 82:533–542, 1988.

Seyberth HW, Müller H, Wille L, et al: Recovery of prostaglandin production associated with reopening of the ductus arteriosus after indomethacin treatment in preterm infants with respiratory distress syndrome. Pediatr Pharmacol 2:127–141, 1982.

Shimada S, Kasai T, Konishi M, Fujiwara T: Effects of patent ductus arteriosus on left ventricular output and organ blood flows in preterm infants with respiratory distress syndrome treated with surfactant. J Pediatr 125:270–277, 1994.

Shimada S, Raju TNK, Bhat R, et al: Treatment of patent ductus arteriosus after exogenous surfactant in baboons with hyaline membrane disease. Pediatr Res 26:565–569, 1989.

Smith M, Setzer ES, Garg DC, Goldberg RN: Pharmacokinetics of prophylactic indomethacin in very low birthweight premature infants. Pediatr Res 18:161A, 1984.

Spach MS, Serwer GA, Anderson PAW, et al: Pulsatile aortopulmonary pressure flow dynamics of patent ductus arteriosus in patients with various hemodynamic states. Circulation 61:110–122, 1980.

Staub NC: Pathogenesis of pulmonary edema. Prog Cardiovasc Dis 23:53–80, 1980.

Stefano JL, Abbasi S, Pearlman SA, et al: Closure of the ductus arteriosus with indomethacin in ventilated neonates with respiratory distress syndrome. Effects of pulmonary compliance and ventilation. Am Rev Respir Dis 143:236–239, 1991.

Stevenson JG, Kawabori I, Guntheroth WG: Pulsed Doppler echocardiographic diagnosis of patent ductus arteriosus: Sensitivity, limitations and technical features. Cath Cardiovasc Diagn 6:255–263, 1980.

Thalji AA, Carr I, Yeh TF, et al: Pharmacokinetics of intravenously administered indomethacin in premature infants. J Pediatr 97:995–1000, 1980.

Thibeault DW, Emmanouilides GC, Dodge ME: Pulmonary and circulatory function in preterm lambs treated with hydrocortisone in utero. Biol Neonate 34:238–247, 1978.

Thibeault DW, Emmanouilides GC, Nelson RJ, et al: Patent ductus arteriosus complicating the respiratory distress syndrome in preterm infants. J Pediatr 86:120–126, 1975.

Toda T, Tsuda N, Takagi T, et al: Ultrastructure of developing human ductus arteriosus. J Anat 131:25–37, 1980.

Waffarn F, Siassi B, Cabal L, Schmidt PL: Effect of antenatal glucocorticoids on clinical closure of the ductus arteriosus. Am J Dis Child 137:336–338, 1983.

Wagner HR, Ellison RC, Zierler S, et al: Surgical closure of patent ductus arteriosus in 268 preterm infants. J Thorac Cardiovasc Surg 87:870–875, 1984.

Walther FJ, Kim DH, Ebrahimi M, Siassi B: Pulsed Doppler measurement of left ventricular output as early predictor of symptomatic patent ductus arteriosus in very preterm infants. Biol Neonate 56:121–128, 1989.

Weiss H, Cooper B, Brook M, et al: Factors determining reopening of the ductus arteriosus after successful clinical closure with indomethacin. J Pediatr 127:466–471, 1995.

Wilkerson RD, Glenn TM: Influence of nonsteroidal anti-inflammatory drugs on ouabain toxicity. Am Heart J 94:454–459, 1977.

Yaffe SJ, Friedman WF, Rogers D, et al: The disposition of indomethacin in premature babies. J Pediatr 97:1001–1006, 1980.

Yeh TF, Achanti B, Jain R, et al: Indomethacin therapy in premature infants with PDA—Determination of therapeutic plasma levels. Dev Pharmacol Ther 12:169–178, 1989.

Yeh TF, Luken JA, Raval D, et al: Indomethacin treatment in small vs large premature infants with ductus arteriosus—Comparison of plasma indomethacin concentration and clinical response. Br Heart J 50:27–30, 1983.

Yeh TF, Raval D, Lilien LD, et al: Decreased plasma glucose following indomethacin therapy in premature infants with patent ductus arteriosus. Pediatr Pharmacol 2:171–177, 1982a.

Yeh TF, Thalji A, Luken L, et al: Improved lung compliance following indomethacin therapy in premature infants with persistent ductus arteriosus. Chest 80:698–700, 1981.

Yeh TF, Wilks A, Betkerur M, et al: Furosemide prevents the renal side effects of indomethacin therapy in premature infants with patent ductus arteriosus. J Pediatr 101:433–437, 1982b.

Evaluation of Newborns with Possible Cardiac Problems

Walker A. Long, Elman G. Frantz, G. William Henry, Michael D. Freed
and Michael Brook

Accurate, timely diagnosis is the foundation of effective treatment in all areas of medicine. Accuracy and timeliness in diagnosis are especially important in symptomatic newborn infants, whether premature or term, because dramatic changes in gas exchange and circulation begin at the moment of birth. Many serious pulmonary and cardiac disorders that affect newborns become obvious or are exacerbated as the normal postnatal cardiopulmonary adaptations unfold.

At birth, the fetus must begin its transition from the hypoxic, warm, dark, secure, and water-filled caverns of fetal life to the oxygen-rich, cold, bright, uncertain, and gas-filled world of respiring mammals. The most dramatic changes are the cessation of perfusion of the placenta and the emptying of fluid from the lungs, both of which normally occur within a few minutes of birth. Of equal importance, but occurring over hours rather than minutes, is the transition from a parallel circulation, with high pulmonary vascular resistance and consequent right-to-left shunting at the foramen ovale and ductus arteriosus, to a serial circulation, in which blood must traverse the pulmonary vascular bed, now greatly reduced in resistance, to reach the body (Long, 1990a; Rudolph, 1970).

This metamorphosis, roughly equivalent to turning from a tadpole into a frog, is obviously remarkably successful in the great majority of cases but does result in problems in three circumstances. First, malfunctions or delays in the transition from placental to pulmonary gas exchange, or from parallel to serial circulation, can cause symptoms in apparently otherwise healthy term infants. Two well-known examples are transient tachypnea of the newborn, which results from delayed resorption of fetal lung fluid, and idiopathic persistent pulmonary hypertension of the newborn syndrome (PPHNS), which results from delayed postnatal reduction in pulmonary vascular resistance (Long, 1990b). Second, successful normal transition to air breathing and serial circulation precipitates symptoms when the underlying pulmonary or cardiovascular systems have abnormalities that did not threaten fetal survival but do threaten postnatal survival. This problem also largely affects term infants; examples include diaphragmatic hernia and pulmonary atresia. Third, premature delivery or delayed maturity (as seen in infants of diabetic mothers) may complicate the normal transition to air breathing and serial circulation. Immaturity of the lungs and the ductus in premature infants or infants of diabetic mothers often results in both impaired gas exchange from respiratory distress syndrome (RDS) and lung overperfusion with consequent pulmonary edema from left-to-right ductal shunt (Clyman, 1990; Corbet, 1996; Long et al, 1996). The net result in such infants, despite the advent of surfactant (Fujiwara et al, 1980; Long et al, 1996), is still too often

chronic lung disease from the high oxygen concentrations and ventilator pressures required to maintain gas exchange.

Early diagnosis remains the key to minimizing morbidity and mortality among symptomatic newborn infants, whether term or preterm. Separating cardiovascular from pulmonary problems in symptomatic newborns can be difficult for even experienced diagnosticians. Further, not infrequently cardiovascular and pulmonary problems coexist, even in premature infants (Huhta, 1990b). In fact, in virtually every infant with RDS, patent ductus arteriosus (PDA) is also present because maturations of the surfactant system and ductal tissue are both incomplete. Left-to-right ductal shunts in infants with RDS compromise pulmonary compliance (Balsan et al, 1991; Corbet, 1996; Griffin et al, 1972; Heldt et al, 1989; Long, 1992; Long et al, 1996; Stefano et al, 1991; Yeh et al, 1991). Serial evaluation is equally important in the management of symptomatic newborn infants. Serial evaluation is essential in confirming initial diagnoses, in assessing the stage and progress of the normal postnatal respiratory and circulatory transition to air breathing and serial circulation, and in assessing the impact of therapeutic interventions.

DIAGNOSTIC APPROACHES

In evaluating the symptomatic newborn, at least two issues must be addressed simultaneously. The most important issue is how sick the infant is now and how much sicker the infant is likely to become without intervention over the next few hours. This assessment can be difficult if it has to be made over the telephone, particularly when the only information available is provided by relatively inexperienced health care professionals in distant hospitals. The judgment of how sick the infant is now and how much sicker the infant is likely to become in the next few hours drives decisions about the urgency of possible transport to a tertiary center, about the performance of further diagnostic testing at the local hospital (such as arterial blood gases, blood cultures, chest radiographs, or echocardiograms), and about the possibly immediate institution of therapeutic measures. Such measures, which might include supplemental oxygen, endotracheal intubation, antibiotics, pressors, transfusion, surfactant, or prostaglandin E_1 (PGE_1) (depending on the working diagnosis), must sometimes be instituted even before the arrival of a team for neonatal stabilization and transport. Although better than 9 times out of 10 a single diagnosis accounts for all symptoms in a given newborn, it is obviously important not to overlook a second diagnosis when two diseases are present. For example, failure to recognize underlying transposition of the great vessels (TGV) in the small-for-dates infant with obvious meconium aspiration pneumonia can be calamitous.

The second major issue is the distinction between heart disease and lung or systemic disease. Accurately making this fundamental distinction is useful in stabilizing symptomatic newborns. Infants with virtually any form of congenital heart disease that causes symptoms in the first 48 hours after birth can be stabilized by initiation of PGE$_1$. Mechanical ventilation and antibiotics can at least temporarily stabilize the great majority of infants with respiratory failure or sepsis (or both). In reaching the preliminary clinical judgment as to whether heart or lungs or systemic problems are causing symptoms, all information available from the history, physical examinations, laboratory tests, and any therapeutic trials (such as supplemental oxygen) must be considered quickly but carefully.

History

As in all areas of medicine, the patient's history contributes a great deal to the differential diagnosis of symptomatic newborn infants. In the case of newborns, the history is obtained from the maternal obstetric records, the records of birth, the records of postnatal care including records of transport, and interviews of the parents as well as health care providers. Any of these sources of information may provide the essential clue to either the criticality of illness or the preliminary distinction between heart and lung or systemic illness.

Pregnancy

Much useful information can be garnered from the history of the pregnancy. Length of pregnancy is the single most important fact available from the maternal history because typically quite different diseases afflict term and premature infants. Symptomatic term infants suffer from a wide spectrum of heart, lung, and systemic diseases, whereas symptomatic premature infants typically have lung disease complicated by left-to-right ductal shunting. Other important information includes (1) the presence or absence of maternal or gestational diabetes because the incidences of RDS, congenital heart disease, cardiomyopathy, and hypoglycemia are all higher in diabetic pregnancies; (2) results of amniocentesis and fetal ultrasonography because the incidence of congenital heart disease is high in chromosomal disorders (Noonan, 1990a) and in a variety of syndromes that can be diagnosed prenatally, such as VACTERL (*v*ertebral, *a*nal, *c*ardiac, *t*racheal, *e*sophageal, *r*enal, and *l*imb) syndrome (Noonan, 1990b); (3) the length of rupture of membranes because the incidence of infection increases with the duration of rupture and because prolonged leakage of amniotic fluid is strongly associated with pulmonary hypoplasia; (4) evidence of maternal infection, including fever, uterine tenderness, or purulent vaginal discharge, any of which raises the risk of fetal/neonatal infection; (5) maternal use of over-the-counter or prescription medications, such as ibuprofen (which can close the ductus in utero and cause postnatal pulmonary hypertension), phenytoin (Dilantin) (associated with fetal Dilantin syndrome,

characterized by cleft palate, muscular ventricular septal defect [VSD], and hypoplastic nails), and lithium (associated with Ebstein anomaly) (Long and Willis, 1984); and (6) identification of fetal dysrhythmias, such as complete heart block or supraventricular tachycardia.

Labor

The events of labor are also important in the assessment of the symptomatic newborn. Infants delivered before the spontaneous onset of labor are at higher risk of RDS. Infants born with meconium staining are at risk for meconium aspiration pneumonia. Infants born after fetal distress are at risk for the consequences of asphyxia, such as shock lung and myocardial dysfunction.

Delivery

Information on the delivery of the infant can also be useful. A history of shoulder dystocia or nuchal cord can be a clue to underlying asphyxia despite seemingly normal Apgar scores. Delivery by cesarean section is associated with transient tachypnea of the newborn in term and near-term infants. Apgar scores at 1 and 5 minutes provide insight into the infant's uteroplacental reserve during labor and delivery.

Postnatal Course

Information on the infant's postnatal course can provide crucial insight into both the criticality of illness and the preliminary distinction between heart and lung disease. The single most important piece of information is the presence or absence of a symptom-free interval after birth. Infants who are symptomatic from birth almost always have parenchymal lung disease of one kind or another. Infants with parenchymal lung disease severe enough to require mechanical ventilation are obviously critically ill and are at risk for sudden death from complications such as pneumothorax or pneumopericardium.

Symptom-Free Interval

Infants who appear to have an uncomplicated initial postnatal adaptation and later become symptomatic may also have lung disease, but systemic or cardiac diseases are also common. The postnatal age at which the infant first develops symptoms and the presence or absence of prior feeding can be helpful.

Age at Presentation—Less than 4 Hours

Infants who appear to be well at birth but develop symptoms within the first 4 hours may still have lung disease, but lung disease becomes less likely with each passing hour. Infants with ductal dependent congenital heart disease who develop symptoms within 4 hours of birth are far more likely to have inadequate pulmonary blood flow from hypoplasia of the right heart than inadequate systemic blood flow from hypoplasia of the left heart. Infants with obstruction to pulmonary blood flow usually develop obvious cyanosis within 4 hours of birth as a result of closure of the ductus. Infants with TGV also usually develop obvious cyanosis within 4 hours of birth, unless VSD or other factors complicate the transposition. Ductal closure in infants with TGV worsens cyanosis by reducing mixing of the two circulations.

Age at Presentation—Greater than 4 Hours

Infants who first develop symptoms after 4 hours of age seldom have intrinsic lung disease. The presence of a symptom-free interval after birth, however, offers no protection from the possibility of immediately life-threatening illness. Infants with symptom-free intervals exceeding 4 hours usually have systemic disorders, such as sepsis or inborn errors of metabolism; disorders that can affect the lungs, such as tracheoesophageal fistula; or ductal dependent congenital heart disease. Infants with these disorders, like infants with intrinsic lung disease, can obviously become critically ill in a short time. Infants with inborn errors of metabolism can become critically ill rapidly after milk feedings. Similarly, infants with late-onset, group B streptococcal sepsis can become critically ill rapidly and die unless the condition is recognized and antibiotics are started. Infants who have ductal dependent congenital heart disease also die unless the condition is recognized and the ductus is reopened.

Ductal Dependent Congenital Heart Disease

Infants with ductal dependent congenital heart disease usually present in one of three patterns: cyanosis, shock with congestive heart failure, or shock without congestive heart failure (Table 62–1). Further, each pattern has a typical age of presentation.

Cyanosis—Less than 4 Hours

Infants whose lives depend on ductal patency for pulmonary blood flow (e.g., pulmonary atresia, critical pulmonary stenosis, severe tetralogy of Fallot [TOF], some forms of tricuspid atresia) present in the first few hours of life (almost always before 4 hours of age) with cyanosis despite good air exchange. Even modest constriction of the pulmonary end of the ductus precipitates worsening cyanosis in

TABLE 62–1

Presentations of Ductal Dependent Congenital Heart Disease

Cyanosis	Shock with Congestive Heart Failure	Shock Without Congestive Heart Failure
Pulmonary atresia	Aortic atresia	Coarctation
Critical pulmonary stenosis	Mitral atresia	Interrupted arch
Tetralogy of Fallot		
Tricuspid atresia		
Transposition of the great vessels		

such infants, and constriction of the pulmonary end of the ductus normally begins shortly after birth. Such infants can be cyanotic in the delivery room, and sometimes they end up intubated and mechanically ventilated as a result. More frequently, infants with pulmonary atresia and the like are assigned Apgar scores of 9 and 9 (one off for color) and are sent to the normal nursery initially. There progressive cyanosis and tachypnea result in transfer to intensive care. In the neonatal intensive care unit, administration of oxygen has no effect on the cyanosis, and the possibility of congenital heart disease arises. Reopening the pulmonary end of the ductus with PGE$_1$ in deeply cyanotic infants with hypoplasia of the right heart is a lifesaving measure.

Infants with TGV and intact ventricular septum are also made more cyanotic by ductal closure, but in such infants ductal closure reduces mixing of the two circulations rather than pulmonary blood flow. Similar to infants with hypoplasia of the right heart, infants with uncomplicated TGV also present by 4 hours of age in the great majority of cases.

Shock—Greater than 4 Hours

Infants whose lives depend on ductal patency for systemic blood flow (e.g., interrupted aortic arch, hypoplastic left heart syndrome [HLHS], critical aortic coarctation) almost always present after 4 hours of age with poor perfusion and hyperpnea. Cyanosis is not part of the presentation. Time of presentation, cause of hyperpnea, and presence or absence of congestive heart failure usually vary with underlying cardiovascular anatomy.

Shock with Congestive Heart Failure—4 to 24 Hours

When the entire systemic cardiac output is dependent on ductal patency (e.g., aortic or mitral atresia), affected infants usually present early (4 to 24 hours of age) with pulmonary congestion, decreased lung compliance, and signs of shock. In such infants, normal postnatal ductal constriction of the pulmonary end of the ductus compromises coronary blood flow as well as lower body blood flow, impairs ventricular function, and also forces more blood flow into the lungs. The end result is typical left-sided congestive heart failure characterized by pulmonary edema, reduced lung compliance, and poor systemic perfusion. The progressive impairment of cardiac function caused by ductal closure in such infants culminates in obvious shock with cool, gray extremities; hypotension; tachycardia; and metabolic acidosis.

Shock Without Congestive Heart Failure—8 Hours to 14 Days

In contrast, when only perfusion of the lower body is dependent on ductal patency (e.g., interrupted aortic arch, critical aortic coarctation), coronary flow is supplied normally from antegrade flow through the aorta, and constriction of the pulmonary end of the ductus does not result in myocardial infarction or excessive pulmonary blood flow. As a result, affected infants tolerate closure of the pulmonary end of the ductus better and usually present later than infants in whom all of systemic perfusion is compromised by ductal closure. Infants in whom only perfusion of the lower body is compromised by ductal closure usually present after 8 hours of age with progressive acidosis. Pulmonary congestion is not prominent in such infants, unless systemic acidosis is severe enough to compromise cardiac function.

Infants in whom lower body perfusion is ductal dependent thus usually present with what appears to be a metabolic problem or sepsis rather than congestive heart failure. Typical findings include Kussmaul type of hyperpnea, mottling, but unimpaired gas exchange. Decreased lung compliance and pulmonary edema are not present in most such infants until late in their courses, when progressive metabolic acidosis impairs cardiac function. Metabolic acidosis and azotemia progressively worsen from lack of perfusion of the kidneys and lower body, and eventually shock ensues from acidosis-induced cardiac compromise. Pulmonary congestion, however, is not a prominent feature of the symptoms of infants in whom only lower body perfusion is dependent on ductal patency; instead, listlessness, pallor, cool lower extremities, and poor feeding are usually the presenting symptoms.

Physical Examination

Systematic physical examination of the newborn provides much useful information about the criticality of illness and the preliminary distinction between lung disease and heart or systemic disease. The general physical examination of the infant often provides more important information than the cardiovascular or pulmonary examinations. Serial physical examinations are critically important in symptomatic newborns to determine (1) how symptomatic infants tolerate any required procedures or diagnostic tests, (2) whether attempted therapeutic interventions are in fact effective, and (3) when treatments that do prove to be effective need adjustments.

General Appearance

A great deal of useful information can usually be obtained by taking a few moments to inspect the infant who may have heart disease. The first question to be answered by inspection is whether the infant is too large, too small, or just right in size. Several neonatal cardiovascular problems are associated with excessive intrauterine somatic growth. Infants who are large for gestational age (typically >4 kg) may be products of diabetic pregnancies, and maternal diabetes is associated with increased risk of congenital heart disease, hypertrophic cardiomyopathy, and hypoglycemia among offspring. When maternal hyperglycemia results in profound fetal hyperinsulinemia, severe cardiac dysfunction can occur postnatally from either hypertrophic cardiomyopathy or hypoglycemia. Infants who have Beckwith-Wiedemann syndrome are also typically large for gestational age, and the associated postnatal hypoglycemia can also result in profound cardiac dysfunction. For unexplained reasons, infants with TGV are also apt to be large for gestational age.

Similarly, infants who are too small are also at increased risk of difficulties during postnatal adaptation. Infants who are small because they are premature obviously are at high risk of RDS and persistent ductal patency. Infants who

are small because of intrauterine growth retardation have increased risk of polycythemia, a disorder that can result in severe cardiopulmonary compromise, particularly when central hematocrit exceeds 70%. Infants with a variety of chromosomal abnormalities that have high incidences of congenital heart disease are also often small for gestational age; trisomies 13 and 18 are the most common such abnormalities.

The second question to be answered by inspection is whether the newborn infant who may have heart disease is acutely ill or not. Newborn infants who are acutely ill look the part. Early during evolution of acute illness, sick newborns look worried and appear to be frightened. Later in the course of acute illness, sick newborns appear to retreat from interaction with the outside world and focus intently on the illness they are battling. In the final stages of acute illness, newborns become progressively less responsive; moribund newborns are unresponsive. Even during the late stages of acute illness, prompt reversal of the illness is often possible if the right diagnosis is recognized and appropriate therapy is provided.

The third question to be answered from general inspection of the symptomatic newborn infant is whether multiple congenital anomalies are present. Infants who have more than two externally visible anomalies are highly likely to exhibit associated internal anomalies, even if the three or more external anomalies identified are relatively minor. For example, a newborn with findings as simple as a sacral dimple, extra digit, and single umbilical artery is also likely to have renal or cardiac anomalies. Certain anomalies commonly occur in association with specific chromosomal abnormalities that are accompanied by cardiac malformations; for example, cleft lip and palate are frequently present in infants with trisomy 13, and scalp defects are often present in infants with trisomy 18 (Noonan, 1990a).

The fourth question to be answered from general inspection of the symptomatic newborn infant is whether the infant has an obvious syndrome that could account for symptoms (Noonan, 1990b). Such syndromes might have a chromosomal basis and characteristic cardiac defects (e.g., Turner syndrome/coarctation), an unknown basis and typical cardiac defects (e.g., VACTERL syndrome/VSD), or an unknown basis and no cardiac defects (e.g., Potter syndrome/pulmonary hypoplasia).

Vital Signs

The second step in physical examination of the newborn who may have heart disease is evaluation of vital signs. Newborns who are febrile or hypothermic, hypotensive or hypertensive, bradycardic or tachycardic, or apneic or tachypneic need immediate diagnostic and therapeutic interventions. Changes in vital signs are always present in acutely ill newborn infants, and observed changes correlate with the acuity of the illness.

Each of the vital signs can contribute information critical to the initial assessment of the acuity of illness, to the preliminary distinction between heart and lung disease, and on occasion to the final diagnosis. Serial comparisons of the vital signs are invaluable in determining (1) whether attempted therapeutic interventions are in fact effective and (2) when treatments that do prove to be effective need adjustments.

Measurement of *temperature* is an important step. Infants who are either hypothermic or febrile are sick, whether or not they also have underlying heart or lung disease. Fever is not a common finding in sick newborn infants, but when present, it is highly significant. Fever can complicate administration of PGE_1, but more commonly fever signifies serious infections in newborns. Such infections may be accompanied by cardiac involvement. Cardiac involvement in systemic neonatal infections ranges from structural abnormalities such as pulmonary stenosis and PDA seen in congenital rubella to endotoxin-induced pulmonary vasospasm and cardiac dysfunction seen in group B streptococcal sepsis. Hypothermia, which occurs far more commonly than fever in newborns, is both a marker for and a cause of serious compromise. Energy stores are not large in the term newborn and scant to nonexistent in the premature newborn. Thermogenesis requires a great deal of energy and oxygen, and sick newborns are frequently unable to maintain normal body temperature without external thermal support, such as radiant heat or use of an incubator.

Measurement of *blood pressure* also provides information critical to assessment of the newborn infant who may have cardiovascular problems. For any recorded or reported blood pressure measurement, the first question to be asked is where the measurement was obtained. Because of variations in the origin of the arteries arising from the aortic arch and in the location of aortic interruption and coarctation, obstruction to blood flow can exist between (1) the right arm and the rest of the body, (2) the left arm and the rest of the body, (3) both arms and the rest of the body, or even (4) the head and the rest of the body (with arteries to both arms arising distal to the interruption or coarctation). The last-mentioned can be quite difficult to recognize. In any case, the net result is that what appears to be systemic hypotension at first glance in the sick term infant can sometimes be a sign of aortic obstruction instead.

Thus, the second question to be asked in evaluating the blood pressure of the newborn infant who may have cardiovascular problems is what the blood pressures are in the (other three) extremities. The key to accurate assessment of blood pressure in the newborn is measurement of blood pressures *in all four extremities*. Identification of the fact that systemic arterial pressure is normal in all four extremities at a given point in time provides substantial, albeit fleeting, reassurance that the infant does not at that time have compromised systemic perfusion. Recognition of isolated upper extremity hypertension is virtually diagnostic of aortic obstruction, and prompt initiation of PGE_1 in such infants can prevent subsequent rapid evolution of an apparently stable infant into a critically ill infant.

The normal range for blood pressure varies with both gestational age and postnatal age. In the term infant, systolic pressures less than 50 and greater than 90 mm Hg and diastolic pressures less than 30 and greater than 60 mm Hg are clearly abnormal and merit investigation. In the premature infant, ready access to normograms is important in assessing blood pressure measurements. Abnormal blood pressures can either be the cause of observed symptoms (e.g., pulmonary edema from idiopathic neonatal systemic hypertension) or simply reflect the severity of the underlying illness from which the infant suffers (e.g., hypotension from severe neonatal sepsis).

Infants who are hypotensive are inherently unstable and may quickly become acutely ill. The identification of hypotension in a newborn calls for rapid assessment and rapid institution of appropriate countermeasures. Hypotension may herald a wide variety of disorders that quickly kill the inaccurately or too slowly diagnosed newborn infant. Disorders that can present as hypotension include pneumothorax, pneumopericardium (Long, 1990c), HLHS, critical aortic stenosis, interrupted aortic arch, critical coarctation, hypoglycemia, and sepsis. Shock associated with interrupted aortic arch and critical coarctation can usually be reversed rapidly if PGE_1 is initiated.

Assessment of *heart rate* can also provide information critical to the assessment of the acuity of illness, to the preliminary distinction between heart and lung disease, and to the final diagnosis. Similar to abnormal blood pressures, abnormal heart rates can either be the cause of observed symptoms (e.g., congenital complete heart block and paroxysmal atrial [supraventricular] tachycardia) or simply reflect the severity of the underlying illness from which the infant suffers.

Similar to blood pressure, the normal range for heart rate also varies with gestational age and postnatal age. In the newborn infant, sustained heart rates in excess of 180 beats/min are always abnormal and should prompt rapid inquiry. Similarly, persistent heart rates of less than 100 beats/min are seldom seen in newborns except in healthy term infants, in whom heart rates approaching 60 beats/min during deep sleep can be observed. As a general rule, heart rate increases proportionally with the acuity of illness, but when death approaches, bradycardia supervenes.

The first question to be answered in the evaluation of *tachycardias* is whether the rhythm is sinus or not. In times of stress, the sinus node can accelerate up to 230 beats/min in the newborn. Heart rates above 230 beats/min are rarely due to sinus tachycardias; episodes of atrial flutter or paroxysmal atrial tachycardias are usually responsible. Recording of a 12-lead electrocardiogram is essential in evaluation of rapid tachycardias; sometimes placement of an esophageal lead is necessary for identification of atrial flutter.

When the tachycardia is sinus but less than 200 beats/min, little information about the acuity of illness, the preliminary distinction between heart and lung disease, or the final diagnosis can be surmised. The affected infant may or may not have a serious underlying illness and may or may not have lung or heart disease. When the tachycardia is sinus, sustained, and greater than 200 beats/min, the newborn is virtually always seriously ill and needs rapid evaluation and treatment.

Measurement of *respiratory rate* also provides useful information. Tachypnea is a reliable sign of serious illness in both term and premature newborns. Sustained respiratory rates of greater than 80 breaths/min are virtually always abnormal in newborns, even when the respirations are shallow. Sustained respiratory rates less than 20 breaths/min represent hypoventilation and require immediate evaluation. In addition to respiratory rate, it is also useful to observe both the *pattern of breathing* and the *work of breathing*. Periodic breathing is commonplace in premature infants and does occur in some healthy term infants; unless the periods of hypopnea during periodic breathing result in bradycardias of less than 60 beats/min, periodic breathing is usually benign. Hyperpnea, or deep breathing, even at relatively slow rates, is always abnormal and usually reflects systemic acidosis. Hyperpnea is a hallmark of infants with HLHS. Hyperpnea can also reflect injury to the respiratory control center in the pons, an unusual injury in newborn infants except in bleeding diatheses (e.g., idiopathic thrombocytopenic purpura).

Observing how much work is required for each breath is also useful (Table 62–2). In cyanotic congenital heart diseases with *decreased pulmonary blood flow*, such as pulmonary atresia, TOF, and some forms of tricuspid atresia, tachypnea is present, but work of breathing is normal because lung compliance is normal (Bancalari et al, 1977). Such infants have what appears to be effortless tachypnea. If the proper diagnosis is not recognized, however, systemic acidosis from hypoxemia eventually supervenes, and dyspnea occurs.

In cyanotic congenital heart diseases with *increased pulmonary blood flow* (such as total anomalous pulmonary venous drainage [TAPVD], truncus arteriosus, and other forms of tricuspid atresia), pulmonary congestion results in decreased lung compliance and increased work of breathing (Bancalari et al, 1977). The diminution in compliance is inversely related to pulmonary arterial pressure, not magnitude of shunt. Thus, infants with increased pulmonary blood flow have not only tachypnea, but also dyspnea and increased work of breathing.

In addition, infants with *left-to-right shunts*, such as VSD, atrioventricular septal defect (AVSD), PDA, and arteriovenous malformation (AVM) also have reduced lung compliance (Bancalari et al, 1977). As in cyanotic heart diseases with increased pulmonary blood flow, the diminution in lung compliance observed in infants with uncomplicated left-to-right shunts is inversely related to pulmonary arterial pressure, not size of the shunt. Pulmonary hypertension (stiff lung vessels) can certainly cause stiff airways on a mechanical basis because tense pulmonary arterial vessels resist the motion of chest inflation. Elevations in pulmonary arterial pressure, however, also cause reduced lung compliance by exacerbating pulmonary edema, a known inhibitor of the surfactant system (Kobayashi et al, 1991). Infants with large shunts typically manifest dyspnea and increased work of breathing. In the premature infant, left-to-right shunt from PDA is a common cause of dyspnea and increased work of breathing.

Similarly, in congenital heart diseases characterized by *pulmonary venous congestion* (such as aortic and mitral atresia), pulmonary venous hypertension decreases lung compliance and causes increased work of breathing. Increased work of breathing is identified by flaring of the alae nasae, intercostal retractions, subcostal retractions, and, in the premature infant, sternal retractions. Infradiaphragmatic TAPVD is an important cause of pulmonary venous congestion in symptomatic newborn infants. In addition, left ventricular dysfunction from any cause also causes pulmonary venous hypertension by elevating left atrial pressure. The net result of pulmonary venous hypertension is reduced pulmonary compliance from consequent pulmonary arterial hypertension and from pulmonary edema. In the term infant, the most common myopathic causes of left ventricular dysfunction include asphyxia, congenital myocarditis, and hypoglycemia. Endocardial fibroelastosis is not seen frequently today.

Gestational Age and Height, Weight, Head Circumference

Formal estimates of gestational age (e.g., Dubowitz) provide useful information, as do plots of measurements of height, weight, and head circumference on the appropriate growth charts. In acutely ill newborns, however, such efforts are best deferred until stabilization and more important diagnostic evaluations are complete. In most cases, important disparities in fetal development, such as severe intrauterine growth retardation or macrosomia, are obvious from simple inspection. For example, the growth-retarded 1000-g infant who is really 42 weeks' gestation and the 2500-g infant of a diabetic mother who is really only 32 weeks' gestation are obvious from the observed (versus expected) thickness of their skins (i.e., degree of translucency) as well as their accompanying postures and muscle tones.

Skin

Examination of the skin (and nails) can provide much useful information about the newborn. The skin and nails should be inspected visually. Yellowish staining of the nails indicates passage of meconium in utero long before delivery and the occurrence of some prenatal insult or stress. Hypoplasia of the nails is associated with Dilantin syndrome. The skin should be inspected to determine its integrity and color, pressed to observe capillary refill, palpated to determine consistency, and lightly pinched to examine turgor.

Inspection of the Skin

Small holes in the skin are typical of trisomy 13; these usually are 1 to 3 mm in diameter and most commonly

---

TABLE 62–2

Work of Breathing and Congenital Heart Disease

Normal Work of Breathing	Increased Work of Breathing
Cyanotic CHD with decreased pulmonary blood flow: pulmonary atresia, PS, tricuspid atresia (+ small VSD/or PS)	Cyanotic CHD with increased pulmonary blood flow: TAPVD, truncus arteriosus, tricuspid atresia (+ large VSD, no PS) Shunts: PDA, VSD, AVSD, AVM
Cyanotic CHD with inadequate mixing: TGV	Pulmonary venous congestion: HLHS, asphyxia, hypoglycemia, EFE, cardiomyopathy

CHD, congenital heart disease; VSD, ventricular septal defect; PS, pulmonary stenosis; TGV, transposition of the great vessels; TAPVD, total anomalous pulmonary venous drainage; PDA, patent ductus arteriosus; AVSD, atrioventricular septal defect; HLHS, hypoplastic left heart syndrome; EFE, endocardial fibroelastosis; AVM, arteriovenous malformation.

occur over the scalp. The *color* of the skin depends on a number of factors, including gestational age, presence or absence of meconium staining, vasomotor tone, concentration of hemoglobin, oxygen saturation, pH, level of bilirubin, and cardiac output. The epidermis and dermis are virtually translucent in extremely immature infants (<26 weeks), and the skin appears gelatinous. *Acrocyanosis*, which usually occurs in healthy term infants, is often said to be a function of peripheral vasomotor instability. Acrocyanosis is probably instead a vestigial remnant of the vasomotor mechanisms that drive the fetus's adaptive response to hypoxemia. Acrocyanosis is characterized by cyanosis limited to the peripheral circulation, usually the hands and feet. Occasionally acrocyanosis occurs in the entire left or right side of the body (harlequin response). The lips and tongue always remain pink in acrocyanosis, and affected infants are asymptomatic. Acrocyanosis does not cause *differential cyanosis*, which is defined as cyanosis limited to the left arm, the left arm and head, the upper body, or the lower body.

Differential cyanosis is an important physical finding that *always* indicates a major cardiovascular problem in the newborn (Table 62–3). Right-to-left ductal shunting causes differential cyanosis (Long, 1984). Right-to-left ductal shunting can occur only when the ductus is patent and the pulmonary arterial pressure exceeds systemic pressure. Such right-to-left ductal shunts, one of several criteria diagnostic of PPHNS, can result from a wide variety of disorders, including many forms of congenital heart disease (Long, 1984, 1990b; Long et al, 1984b, 1984c). Whether the cyanosis in differential cyanosis occurs in the upper body or lower body is determined by underlying cardiac anatomy.

When the cyanosis in *differential cyanosis* is present in the *lower body* (both legs, both legs and right arm, or both legs and right arm and head), right-to-left ductal shunt of deoxygenated blood from the pulmonary artery to the lower extremities accounts for the visibly lower oxygen content in the lower body. Differential cyanosis with cyanosis in the lower body is far more common than differential cyanosis with cyanosis in the upper body. Meconium aspiration (with associated persistent pulmonary hypertension) is the single most common cause of differential cyanosis, but congenital heart disease must be excluded in every case (Long, 1984, 1990b).

When the cyanosis in *differential cyanosis* is present in the *upper body* (left arm, left arm and head, or entire upper body), either TGV or supracardiac TAPVD must be present (with or without other forms of congenital heart disease). In both disorders, the most highly oxygenated blood in the body is in the pulmonary artery rather than ascending aorta. When the highly oxygenated blood from the pulmonary artery crosses the ductus right to left, the lower body and legs have visibly higher oxygen. In infants with TGV, oxygen content in the pulmonary artery is higher than the aorta because the pulmonary artery arises from the left ventricle, and the left ventricle receives oxygenated pulmonary venous return from the left atrium.

In infants with supracardiac TAPVD, oxygen content is higher in the pulmonary artery than aorta because pulmonary venous return enters the heart from the superior vena cava. It is well understood that during fetal life and in the immediate newborn period, the superior vena caval flow streams into the right ventricle and goes out to the pulmonary artery and that the inferior vena caval flow streams across the foramen ovale into the left heart and goes out to the aorta. The net result in supracardiac TAPVD is that highly oxygenated pulmonary venous blood, mixed with systemic venous blood from the superior vena cava, goes into the right ventricle and out the pulmonary artery. Right-to-left ductal shunt in afflicted infants results in good oxygenation of the lower extremities and cyanosis of the upper extremities.

Pallor

Infants who are pale may have anemia or shock. Congenital heart disease does not cause anemia, but congenital heart disease is an important cause of shock. Infants who are in shock generally are pale but have a grayish appearance, and the skin is cool to touch. In the late stages of shock when death is near, the skin takes on a splotchy appearance that resembles livido reticularis in the normal newborn except that the splotches are blue rather than red.

Capillary Refill

In normal infants, refill of the capillaries after gentle pressure of the skin with the thumb for 5 seconds takes 1 to 2 seconds both in the extremities (palms and soles) and in the central circulation (forehead and central chest). Delayed capillary refill is a sign of inadequate cardiac output. Capillary refill that takes more than 3 to 4 seconds indicates moderate impairment of cardiac output; capillary refill that takes more than 5 to 6 seconds indicates severe impairment of cardiac output. As in other parts of the physical examination, serial assessments of capillary refill can be valuable in determining whether attempted therapeutic interventions are effective and when adjustments to effective treatments are needed. Because the newborn has remarkable peripheral vasomotor control and can shut down perfusion to the extremities in times of stress (e.g., cold, infection, hypoglycemia, cardiac compromise), the best places to follow capillary refill serially in infants who are compromised are the forehead and central chest.

TABLE 62–3

Differential Cyanosis and Congenital Heart Disease

Lower Body Cyanosis	Upper Body Cyanosis
Left atrial hypertension: IAA, coarctation, aortic stenosis, mitral stenosis	TAPVD above the diaphragm TGV
Cardiomyopathy: EFE, hypoglycemia	
Infradiaphragmatic TAPVD	

IAA, interrupted aortic arch; TAPVD, total anomalous pulmonary venous drainage; EFE, endocardial fibroelastosis; TGV, transposition of the great vessels.

Skin Resilience

Thickness of the skin varies with gestational age and nutritional well-being. The normal skin is flexible and instantly resumes its flat, smooth shape when lifted into a fold. The skin of infants who are dehydrated requires 1 to several seconds to resume its normal shape after being lifted into a fold. Infants who are moribund develop *doughy* skin that cannot be lifted into a fold; this phenomenon is termed *sclerema*.

Head

Measurements of head circumference and plots on percentile charts are not needed to identify macrocephaly and microcephaly; both are, with experience, obvious from inspection. In sick newborns, macrocephaly suggests congenital hypothyroidism, and microcephaly suggests congenital infection (e.g., rubella or cytomegalovirus). The anterior fontanel is an important window on the brain. The brain swells and bulges through the fontanel in hydrocephalus, encephalitis, meningitis, and severe asphyxia. In congenital cerebral arteriovenous malformation of the brain, a bruit can be heard over the anterior fontanel.

Neck

In general, examination of the neck does not provide much useful information. The necks of most newborns are short and fat, and changes in cervical vascular pulsations are not usually detectable. One exception to this rule is among infants with cerebral arteriovenous malformation, many of whom demonstrate bounding pulsations in the neck from the large volumes of blood coursing through the carotid arteries and jugular veins. Loose skin at the base of the neck suggests Turner syndrome.

Chest Inspection

The importance of observing the rate, pattern, and depth of breathing has already been described. Another important item to note during inspection of the chest in any acutely ill newborn is the residual volume (anterior-posterior diameter) of the chest. Infants with reduced anterior-posterior diameters have reduced lung compliance; in the great majority of cases, pulmonary immaturity and surfactant deficiency are responsible. In infants with increased anterior-posterior diameters of the chest, air trapping is present. The most common cause of air trapping in term newborns is meconium aspiration; in premature newborn infants, air trapping usually represents excessive mechanical ventilation, tension pneumothorax, or, later in their neonatal course, chronic lung disease.

Auscultation of the Chest

Auscultation of the chest also provides important information. The most important observation to make in auscultation of the chest in acutely ill newborn infants is symmetry of chest inflation and symmetry of breath sounds. Asymmetric chest motion and asymmetric air movement virtually always indicate a potentially life-threatening difficulty, such as pneumothorax, intubation of a main stem bronchus instead of the trachea, or chylothorax.

Rales

The character of the breath sounds is also important. Infants with disorders that cause atelectasis, such as RDS and congenital pneumonia, exhibit rales that are clearly audible even during mechanical ventilation. Term infants seldom have RDS, unless they are either delivered by elective cesarean section before spontaneous labor or are products of a diabetic pregnancy. Premature infants of 32 weeks' gestation or less are at substantial risk of RDS, unless a course of maternal steroid treatment has been completed before delivery. Similarly, infants with disorders that cause pulmonary venous congestion, such as cardiomyopathy, aortic atresia, and mitral atresia, also exhibit rales. In contrast, wheezing is distinctly uncommon in newborn infants; unilateral wheezing suggests congenital bronchial stenosis.

Examination of the Heart

Osler taught that examination of the heart consisted of five parts: inspection, palpation, percussion, auscultation, and contemplation. In evaluating acutely ill newborn infants who might or might not have cardiac disease, consistently performing all five parts of the physical examination of the heart, as taught by Osler, is worthwhile.

Cardiac Inspection

Visual assessment of precordial cardiac motion should determine three things: (1) whether the heart is in the left or right chest, (2) whether the heart is enlarged (or displaced laterally), and (3) whether the heart is volume-loaded or not. In symptomatic newborns, dextrocardia virtually always means complex congenital heart disease, and cardiomegaly virtually always means that cardiac compromise is contributing to the observed symptoms. Volume-loaded hearts exhibit dynamic precordial motion that can be identified easily from across the room. The most common example of volume loading of the heart in neonatal intensive care units is observed among premature infants ventilated for RDS; dynamic precordial activity in such infants virtually always indicates substantial left-to-right ductal shunts, even in the absence of murmurs and bounding pulses. In term infants, dynamic precordial activity usually indicates significant tricuspid regurgitation, which is most commonly associated with either birth asphyxia or PPHNS.

Cardiac Auscultation

Listening to the heart provides information useful in the differential diagnosis and management of symptomatic newborns. The first matter to establish is where the heart sounds are loudest. Even in the absence of visible or palpable precordial impulses, the presence of dextrocardia should be readily divined by comparing the intensity of the heart sounds over the left and right chests. The second matter to be determined is whether both components of the second heart sound are present. If so, the aortic valve

TABLE 62–4

Differential Diagnosis of Systolic Murmurs by Location in Acyanotic Infants

Apex	Tricuspid/Septal Area	Pulmonary Area	Aortic Area
Mitral regurgitation	Tricuspid regurgitation VSD	Pulmonary stenosis PDA Coarctation ASD	Aortic stenosis Subaortic stenosis

VSD, ventricular septal defect; PDA, patent ductus arteriosus; ASD, atrial septal defect.

and the pulmonary valve are both present. If not, either one could be missing, or TGV could be present. At the rapid heart rates many newborns exhibit, confirming splitting of the second sound can be a challenge at times even for experienced clinicians.

The third matter to be accomplished is to localize systolic and diastolic murmurs to one of the four cardinal areas of the heart: the mitral area (apex), tricuspid/septal area (lower left sternal border), pulmonary area (upper left sternal border), or aortic area (upper right sternal border). Placing murmurs anatomically over a structure in the heart is useful in differential diagnosis (Table 62–4). Fourth, it is important to listen for radiation of systolic murmurs to the axillae and back. Murmurs that radiate well to both axillae mean either bilateral peripheral pulmonary stenosis (common in premature infants) or pathology in the pulmonary outflow tract. Murmurs that radiate only to the left axilla often represent mitral regurgitation but can represent isolated left peripheral pulmonary stenosis as well as pulmonary stenosis (the systolic jet in pulmonary stenosis tends to be directed into the left pulmonary artery). Murmurs that radiate well to the back suggest coarctation. Finally, in infants with heart failure, it is important to listen over the anterior fontanel and liver for a bruit because AVMs of the brain and liver are important causes of high-output congestive heart failure in newborn infants.

As with other parts of the physical examination, serial auscultation of the heart can be quite useful in assessing whether attempted therapeutic interventions are in fact effective and when treatments that do prove to be effective need adjustments. For example, appearance of a systolic or continuous murmur over the pulmonary area after initiation of PGE$_1$ in an infant with pulmonary atresia indicates reopening of the ductus. Similarly, diminution of a systolic murmur over the lower left sternal border (i.e., diminution of tricuspid regurgitation) after initiation of nitric oxide in an infant with PPHNS indicates reduction in pulmonary arterial pressure.

Age at Which Murmur Is First Heard

The age at which a murmur is first heard has diagnostic significance. Murmurs heard in the delivery room are always due either to stenosis (such as aortic or pulmonary stenosis) or to regurgitation (such as tricuspid or mitral

regurgitation) and are never due to shunts. Shunts are not heard in the delivery room because vascular resistances in lungs and body are equal at birth, and left-to-right shunts do not occur in the absence of resistance (pressure) gradients. Thus, it is irrelevant whether only the normal communications between the systemic and pulmonary circulations present at birth (foramen ovale and ductus arteriosus) are patent, or other abnormal communications between the left and right heart (such as atrial septal defect [ASD] or VSD) are also present at birth; all such lesions are inaudible in the delivery room because pulmonary and systemic vascular resistances are equal.

Typically, murmurs from uncomplicated VSDs are not audible until the second or third day after birth, and murmurs from uncomplicated ASDs are not audible until several weeks of life (Table 62–5).

Abdominal Examination

Much can also be learned from a careful examination of the abdomen. As with other parts of the physical examination, it is important to look carefully at the abdomen before feeling it. Abdomens that are missing either part (omphalocele) or all (prune belly) of the abdominal wall are obvious, and the incidence of congenital heart disease is increased. Abdomens that are intact and distended are distended by fluid (ascites or blood), gas (pneumoperitoneum, intestinal perforation, tracheoesophageal fistula), tissue (hepatomegaly, splenomegaly, or tumor), or luminal obstruction (necrotizing enterocolitis, Hirschsprung disease, duodenal atresia). Abdomens that are intact but appear to be empty usually are empty because the abdominal contents are in the chest (diaphragmatic hernia).

Palpation of the abdomen also yields much useful information. The presence of crepitus indicates dissection of subcutaneous air leak down from the chest. In the normal newborn infant, the edge of the liver is usually palpable 1 cm below the right costal margin in the right upper quadrant. Liver distention or displacement is present if the liver

TABLE 62–5

Causes of Congestive Heart Failure During the 2nd Through 4th Weeks of Life

Acyanotic (PaO$_2$ > 150 mm Hg in 100% O$_2$)
    Coarctation of the aorta
    Aortic stenosis
    Myocarditis
    Endocardial fibroelastosis
    Patent ductus arteriosus
    Aortopulmonary window
    Arteriovenous fistula
    Ventricular septal defect
    Atrioventricular septal defects
    Hypoplastic left heart syndrome
Cyanotic (PaO$_2$ < 150 mm Hg in 100% O$_2$)
    Total anomalous pulmonary venous connection
    Truncus arteriosus
    Transposition and ventricular septal defect
    Tricuspid atresia and ventricular septal defect
    Single ventricle

edge is more than 2 cm below the right costal margin. In situs inversus totalis and in some forms of heterotaxia, the liver is on the left side, rather than on the right side. In situs ambiguus, the liver can be felt on both sides of the abdomen. If the edge of the liver is pulsatile, tricuspid regurgitation is present (Courvoisier's sign). If the liver has a bruit over it, hepatic arteriovenous malformation is present.

Serial examination of the edge of the liver is a useful tool in assessing the adequacy of volume replacement in critically ill infants because the liver readily distends and shrinks in response to changes in vascular volume. The size of the liver is a rough indicator of central venous pressure.

Extremities

Examination of the extremities should focus on the presence or absence of deformities as well as on the character of the peripheral pulses, peripheral capillary refill, and presence or absence of edema. Deformities of the upper extremities (and face) are associated with cardiac malformations; embryologically the upper extremities and heart form at about the same time. Peripheral edema is observed in newborn infants with hydrops fetalis, a topic discussed elsewhere. The presence or absence of peripheral cyanosis is not useful in assessing symptomatic newborns because normal newborns frequently have acrocyanosis.

Peripheral Arterial Pulses

Confirmation of symmetric peripheral arterial pulsations is essential in any symptomatic newborn infant. Bilateral diminution or absence of lower extremity arterial pulses in the presence of a strong right or left upper extremity pulse is virtually pathognomonic of coarctation or interrupted aortic arch. Pulses in all four extremities must be carefully palpated and compared. If the right subclavian artery arises aberrantly from the descending aorta distal to the site of coarctation or interruption, only the pulse in the left arm may be hypertensive. Further, umbilical arterial catheterization not infrequently causes reduced femoral arterial and distal pedal pulsations on the ipsilateral side. What can initially appear to be diminished arterial pressures in the lower extremities is far more frequently unilateral femoral arterial vasospasm from umbilical arterial catheterization.

Laboratory Studies

Many diagnoses can be strongly suspected from the history and physical examination, but final diagnoses virtually always require laboratory confirmation. Further, serial laboratory studies are useful in assessing responses to treatment. For example, the septic-appearing newborn infant born to a febrile mother with uterine tenderness and purulent discharge quite likely has bacterial sepsis, but blood cultures are essential to confirm the diagnosis of bacterial sepsis, to optimize antibiotic choices and doses, and to confirm that the antibiotics are effective in vivo. Laboratory studies performed in evaluating symptomatic newborns can be divided into two categories, *general screening laboratory studies* and *laboratory studies for cardiac diagnosis* (Table 62–6).

TABLE 62–6

Laboratory Studies in Symptomatic Infants Who May Have Congenital Heart Disease

General Screening Laboratory Tests	Laboratory Studies for Cardiac Diagnosis
Hematocrit	Hyperoxia test
Glucose	12-lead electrocardiogram
Blood culture	Echocardiography
Arterial blood gas	Cardiac catheterization
Chest radiograph	

General Screening Laboratory Tests

Several general screening laboratory studies are essential in evaluating any symptomatic newborn and should be immediately available in any hospital that has an obstetric service. Every sick newborn infant should have an immediate blood culture, hematocrit, blood glucose, arterial blood gas, and chest radiograph. Polycythemia and hypoglycemia are readily reversible causes of respiratory distress and cardiac dysfunction that should never be missed. Arterial pH is the single best laboratory measurement of the symptomatic newborn's clinical status. A chest radiograph should also be performed at once in any infant who develops respiratory distress or cyanosis because a large variety of life-threatening disorders can be quickly diagnosed by chest radiography. A number of such disorders can either be immediately reversed (e.g., thoracostomy for tension pneumothorax) or at least stabilized for later definitive treatment (e.g., placement of a nasogastric tube to remove gastrointestinal air in congenital diaphragmatic hernia) if the correct diagnosis is recognized on the chest radiograph. The chest radiograph provides useful information not only about the chest and its contents, but also about the abdomen.

Arterial Blood Gases

Measurements of arterial blood gases provide important insight into both cardiopulmonary function and cardiopulmonary reserve in symptomatic newborns. The most important determination provided by an arterial blood gas measurement is pH. Arterial pH is an excellent barometer of the adequacy of both cardiac and pulmonary function. If arterial pH is in the normal range, the symptomatic newborn remains compensated and is not in danger of immediate collapse. If acidosis is present, the symptomatic newborn is unstable and at high risk for rapid deterioration.

The second most important determination provided by an arterial blood gas measurement is arterial P_{CO_2}. The arterial P_{CO_2} level provides insight as to the cause of acidosis: Normal or low levels of P_{CO_2} in the presence of acidosis indicate metabolic acidosis; elevated levels of P_{CO_2} in the presence of acidosis indicate respiratory failure. The most common cause of metabolic acidosis observed in the neonatal intensive care unit is fetal asphyxia. The most common postnatal cause of metabolic acidosis in the neonatal intensive care unit is septic shock, but HLHS and inborn errors of metabolism are also important causes. During mechanical ventilation of newborn infants, serial measurements of P_{CO_2} are the main criteria by which minute ventilation is adjusted (although chest motion and radiographic determinations of lung inflation are also important guides).

Information important in the diagnosis and management of symptomatic newborns can also be provided by determinations of arterial P_{O_2}, but in general too much focus is placed on arterial P_{O_2} measurements in interpreting blood gases. As stated earlier, pH and P_{CO_2} measurements are far more important than arterial P_{O_2} measurements. The eye is a fair oximeter and can certainly determine whether an infant is hypoxemic. During fetal life, P_{O_2} measurements in the high 20s were normal, and the fetus adapted to hypoxia by having fetal hemoglobin, polycythemia, and elevated levels of 2,3-diphosphoglycerate. Those adaptations do not disappear at birth. For these reasons, a P_{O_2} measurement in the 40s is certainly not a medical emergency in the newborn as long as pH and P_{CO_2} are normal. In fact, at normal pH, newborns are 80% saturated at a P_{O_2} of 40 mm Hg. Many dangerous interventions and much consequent iatrogenic damage are perpetrated in both term and premature newborns because of largely unwarranted efforts to get or maintain arterial P_{O_2} measurements above 70 mm Hg. P_{O_2} measurements above 50 mm Hg are a far better target when lung disease accounts for symptoms. In cyanotic heart disease, depending on the lesion, a saturation of 70% may be perfectly acceptable.

Those caveats notwithstanding, arterial P_{O_2} measurements can provide useful information in the diagnosis and management of symptomatic newborns (Long, 1984, 1990b; Long et al, 1984a). The most important role of arterial P_{O_2} measurements is to determine when hyperoxia is present. Hyperoxia is mostly irrelevant in term infants but is a medical emergency in premature infants at risk of retinopathy of prematurity (<32 weeks' gestation). Hyperoxia cannot be detected by the human eye, in contrast to hypoxemia.

The first question to be asked when evaluating any arterial P_{O_2} measurement is what concentration of oxygen was the infant breathing? The second question to be asked is from what artery was the sample drawn? These two questions are critical because arterial P_{O_2} varies significantly with inspired oxygen concentrations, underlying cardiac anatomy, ductal patency, and the balance of pulmonary and systemic vascular resistance. The important issue is the P_{O_2} of the blood being supplied to the brain and coronary arteries, not the lower body. If the infant is not cyanotic, the P_{O_2} of the blood going to the brain and coronaries is probably fine. A blood gas measurement is not necessary to determine this fact. The clinician should not adjust inspired oxygen concentrations and ventilator settings in response to low P_{O_2} measurements obtained from the umbilical artery without first confirming that the P_{O_2} in the right radial artery is also low. Every sick newborn, term or premature, has the capacity and propensity for right-to-left ductal shunting (Chu et al, 1967; Long, 1990b, 1992). The possibility of right-to-left ductal shunting of unoxygenated pulmonary arterial blood into the descending aorta causing falsely low umbilical arterial P_{O_2} measurements should be considered on every umbilical arterial blood gas. The most practical way to minimize chances of being misled by unsuspected right-to-left ductal shunts (which typically vary considerably with ventilator changes, suctioning, and stimulation) is to compare simultaneous right radial and umbilical arterial P_{O_2} measurements as well as right arm and leg transcutaneous oxygen saturations frequently.

Differential Oximetry

Positive Arterial P_{O_2} Gradients Between the Right Arm and Descending Aorta. Right-to-left ductal shunting, one of the diagnostic criteria for PPHNS (Long, 1984, 1990b), occurs when the ductus is patent and the pulmonary arterial pressure exceeds systemic pressure. Such right-to-left ductal shunts can cause large differences between arterial P_{O_2} measurements obtained from the upper body and lower body. A difference in P_{O_2} of 10 mm Hg or more between the right arm and umbilical arterial catheter is diagnostic of PPHNS. Sometimes P_{O_2} differences of better than 200 mm Hg between the right arm and descending aorta are observed in afflicted infants.

In better than 99 out of 100 instances of right-to-left ductal shunting, the P_{O_2} is higher in the right arm than in the umbilical artery. These positive gradients in P_{O_2} between the right arm and umbilical artery are caused by right-to-left ductal shunting of unoxygenated pulmonary arterial blood into the descending aorta. Such positive P_{O_2} gradients between the right arm and umbilical artery have many causes, including most commonly various forms of lung disease (e.g., meconium aspiration, pneumonia, RDS). Several forms of congenital heart disease also cause right-to-left ductal shunting and positive P_{O_2} gradients between the right arm and umbilical artery (e.g., interrupted aortic arch, critical coarctation, aortic stenosis, endocardial fibroelastosis, infradiaphragmatic TAPVD, AVSD, arteriovenous malformation) (Long, 1990b; Long et al, 1984a, 1984c).

Negative Arterial P_{O_2} Gradients Between the Right Arm and Descending Aorta. In two forms of congenital heart disease, the most highly oxygenated blood is in the pulmonary artery rather than the ascending aorta: TGV and supracardiac TAPVD. When right-to-left ductal shunting occurs in infants with TGV and supracardiac TAPVD, highly oxygenated blood is shunted from the pulmonary artery into the descending aorta. The net result is higher P_{O_2} measurements in the descending aorta than in the right arm or negative P_{O_2} gradients between the right arm and umbilical artery. Negative P_{O_2} gradients, admittedly rare, are nevertheless diagnostic of what is termed *transposition physiology* and always mean either TGV or supracardiac TAPVD.

Chest Radiography

The chest radiograph is the single most useful general screening test in making the preliminary distinction between lung disease and heart or systemic disease in symptomatic newborns. The chest radiograph is also useful in the preliminary assessment of how sick the infant is or is likely to become. As in other components of the evaluation of symptomatic newborns, serial chest radiographs can be useful in confirming initial diagnoses, in assessing whether attempted therapeutic interventions are effective, and in making adjustments to treatments that are effective.

In the newborn, the standard chest radiograph is taken with the infant flat on his or her back, and the field imaged includes the abdomen. All information captured on the chest radiograph, including the identifying information, bony structures, soft tissues, abdominal contents, lungs, and heart, should be examined systematically because information of clinical importance can lie anywhere.

Identifying Information. It is imperative to confirm that the chest radiograph hanging on the view box and presented for review (1) does in fact belong to the patient in question and (2) is the one most pertinent to the question at hand. It is also important to determine where the presented film fits in the sequence of chest radiographs likely to already have been taken of that patient. Clinicians experienced in the evaluation of sick newborns seldom make the mistake of examining a chest radiograph in isolation when other chest radiographs exist. Usually with a little persistence and ingenuity, any other films taken of the infant can be identified, located, and assembled for simultaneous review. All available chest radiographs should be arranged in chronologic order. The name of the patient, unit number of the patient, date and time of the radiograph, and the right and left orientation of each film (as labeled by the technician) should be carefully noted, and any inconsistencies among the radiographs should be resolved.

Most patients admitted to neonatal intensive care units are admitted before first names given by the parents reach patient registration. The initials usually assigned, BB and BG, do not provide much differentiation of patients with the same last name in the same neonatal intensive care unit. This problem becomes more difficult when same-sex twins, triplets, or greater are admitted. Thus, attention to the medical record number is essential in identification of the patient.

Even the medical record number cannot be relied on for patient identification because mistakes in numerical entry and transcription do occur. If the chest radiographs look as if they are from different patients, even though the names and unit numbers match, it is best to presume that the chest radiographs are from different patients until careful investigation proves otherwise. Until the multimedia electronic medical record with a universal patient identifier arrives, the best protection against the iatrogenic error of acting clinically on information contained in a chest radiograph actually from a different patient is vigilance. Applying treatments to the wrong patient is one of the most serious errors in medicine.

Errors in the labeling of *right* and *left* on the chest radiograph also occur. These errors typically occur when the technician shoots the film with right and left properly labeled but notes what appears to be the heart on the wrong side of the chest when the film is developed. Too often the next step by the technician is to conclude that he or she mislabeled right and left and then to compound that mistake by relabeling the exposed film to make the heart appear to be normally placed on the left side of the chest. Failure to recognize dextrocardia because of this sequence of errors can prove to be a costly mistake. Prompt

cardiologic evaluation is important in infants with dextrocardia and symptoms because complex congenital heart disease is usually present. After confirming the identity of the patient, the chronologic sequence of the films, and the proper right/left orientation, the next step is systematic survey of the contents of each film.

Bony Structures. Careful examination of all bony structures visible on the chest radiograph provides much useful information. For example, the skeleton provides information about gestational age. Accurate assessment of gestational age can add to the judgment about the likelihood of RDS versus other lung or heart diseases accounting for respiratory distress in larger premature infants. The absence of femoral head calcifications means that the infant is less than 36 weeks. The presence of humeral head calcifications means that the infant is at least 38 weeks.

The number of ribs should be counted on each infant; the presence of only 11 ribs suggests underlying trisomy 21. Trisomy 21 is associated with acyanotic (typically VSDs and AVSDs) but sometimes cyanotic (typically TOF) congenital heart disease. Infants with trisomy 21 also sometimes exhibit slow postnatal relaxation of pulmonary vascular tone (e.g., PPHNS), particularly when they also have AVSDs. Such infants can be quite blue for several days after birth (without pulmonary stenosis or right ventricular outflow obstruction) just from right-to-left intracardiac shunting secondary to pulmonary hypertension. Usually only supplemental oxygen is indicated; after several days, pulmonary vascular resistance eventually falls, and these infants begin to develop large left-to-right intracardiac shunts. In contrast, the presence of 13 ribs suggests underlying trisomy 13, a chromosomal disorder typically associated with severe and complex congenital heart disease.

The presence of hemivertebrae is suggestive of VACTERL syndrome, a syndrome usually accompanied by congenital heart disease (Noonan, 1990b). Congenital scoliosis is frequently associated with other congenital anomalies, including congenital heart disease (Noonan, 1990b).

Soft Tissues. The chest radiograph also provides a snapshot of the soft tissues of the neck and of the lateral thorax and abdomen. In infants with hydrops fetalis, edema of the soft tissues of the chest and abdomen is usually obvious from the thickness of the skin. Leakage of extrapulmonary air from the pleural space into the lateral subcutaneous spaces along the chest wall and abdomen and from the mediastinum into the neck can be readily identified by examination of the soft tissues captured on the chest radiograph. Extrapulmonary air is most commonly observed in premature infants mechanically ventilated for RDS, but term infants with meconium aspiration also commonly develop extrapulmonary air, as do term infants hyperventilated for PPHNS. It is also not uncommon to see subcutaneous air after chest tubes are removed during recovery from surgery for congenital heart disease.

Catheter and Tube Positions. A common reason for obtaining chest radiographs in symptomatic newborns is to determine the positions of inserted catheters and tubes. Distinguishing the course of an umbilical arterial catheter (down from the central abdomen into the pelvis, then up along the left side of the vertebral column) from an umbilical venous catheter (up from the central abdomen along the right side of the vertebral column) is important. Early diagnosis of infradiaphragmatic TAPVD can be missed when what is thought to be umbilical arterial blood is drawn out of what is really an umbilical venous catheter. Highly oxygenated blood (pulmonary venous return) courses through the umbilical vein in infradiaphragmatic TAPVD (Long et al, 1984b).

It is also important to notice when catheters in the umbilical vein have really passed across the foramen ovale into the left atrium because emboli of air or clot released into the left atrium are especially hazardous. In fact, umbilical venous catheters are most safely positioned at the junction of the inferior vena cava and right atrium. This position minimizes risks of perforation and of inadvertent migration across the foramen ovale into the left atrium. On the anteroposterior radiograph, the key to recognizing left atrial position of an umbilical venous catheter is a slight leftward tilt of the tip of the catheter toward the midline. On the lateral radiograph, left atrial placement of an umbilical venous catheter is obvious from the posterior course of the catheter across the foramen ovale into the left atrium. Left atrial placement of an umbilical venous catheter is sometimes done on purpose when no other access to arterial blood is available but should never be permitted to happen by accident.

The course of umbilical arterial catheters inserted high enough to cross the diaphragm can lead to recognition of a right-sided aortic arch. Normally, high umbilical catheters always stay to the left of the vertebral column. If an umbilical catheter crosses the vertebral column above the diaphragm and ascends on the right, right-sided aortic arch is present. Right-sided aortic arch is strongly associated with TOF and truncus arteriosus.

Another common reason for obtaining a chest radiograph is to check placement of a newly inserted endotracheal tube. Less commonly, chest radiographs are obtained to check the positions of percutaneously inserted silastic central lines and attempted duodenal tube placements. Chest radiographs obtained for any reason should be used in serial assessment of cardiopulmonary function because changes in lung inflation, lung perfusion, and heart size over time can provide information critical to both diagnosis and management.

Abdomen. Information useful in diagnostic assessment of symptomatic newborns is frequently found on the abdominal portion of chest radiographs. Air has to be in the gastrointestinal tract, however, to extract useful information for cardiovascular diagnosis and assessment—although the absence of air in the gastrointestinal tract is in itself useful information. When air is present and one can therefore see the position of the abdominal contents, the first question to be addressed is the location of the liver and stomach. Problems with heterotaxia are virtually always accompanied by complex congenital heart disease. Complete situs inversus, with the heart in the right chest, the stomach on the right, and the liver on the left, is almost always benign from a cardiac point of view. Discordance between thoracic and abdominal situs, however, is always associated with major cardiovascular malformations (Table 62–7).

The second question to be addressed in evaluating the abdominal findings on a chest radiograph is the size of the liver. The liver in newborn infants is readily distensible, and it expands and contracts quickly with changes in blood volume and right atrial pressure. Thus, the size of the liver on serial radiographs can be useful in following adequacy of volume replacement, of diuresis, and of treatment for pulmonary hypertension.

The third question to be addressed in evaluating the abdominal findings on a chest radiograph is whether or not free air is present. Recognition of the *football sign* from free air making the hepatic ligament visible can be the only clue to perforation of the gut or peritoneal dissection of extrapulmonary air.

The fourth question to be addressed in evaluating the abdominal findings on a chest radiograph is whether ascites is present. Ascites is most commonly seen in term newborns as part of hydrops fetalis, a disorder with many causes, including fetal arrhythmias. In premature newborns, ascites is more often seen as a manifestation of hyperalimentation-induced hepatic dysfunction or necrotizing enterocolitis.

Lungs. The status of the lungs is the single most important piece of information available on the chest radiograph. In evaluating the lungs, it is important to assess (1) lung inflation, (2) lung density and homogeneity, and (3) lung vascularity. In addition, the presence of pleural fluid can be an important diagnostic key (Long et al, 1984a). The most common disorder associated with pleural effusion in newborns is meconium aspiration, but group B streptococcal pneumonia and congenital heart disease are also associated with pleural fluid. Pleural effusion is so uncommon

TABLE 62–7

Thoracoabdominal Discordance and Congenital Heart Disease

Heart	Stomach	Liver	Spleen	Diagnosis	Heart Disease
Left	Left	Right	Left	Normal	None
Left	Right	Left	Right	Thoracoabdominal discordance	Complex
Left	Midline	Midline	Absent	Asplenia	Complex
Left	Midline	Midline	Present	Polysplenia	Complex
Right	Right	Left	Right	Situs inversus totalis	None
Right	Left	Right	Left	Thoracoabdominal discordance	Complex
Right	Midline	Midline	Absent	Asplenia	Complex
Right	Midline	Midline	Present	Polysplenia	Complex

in infants with RDS that its presence should suggest an alternative diagnosis, such as pneumonia or infradiaphragmatic TAPVD.

Lung Inflation. One useful technique in assessing lung inflation is to count the number of posterior ribs visible on the right side of the chest above the diaphragm. In general, when fewer than eight posterior ribs are visible above the diaphragm, the lungs are hypoinflated, and when more than 10 posterior ribs are visible above the diaphragm, the lungs are hyperinflated. Comparing the magnitude of inflation in serial chest films is critical to serial assessments of heart size because changes in lung inflation can mask or exaggerate apparent changes in heart size.

Hypoinflation can be an important clue to the correct underlying diagnosis (e.g., RDS, pulmonary hypoplasia) in symptomatic infants. Hypoinflation also makes interpretation of lung density, lung vascularity, and heart size far more difficult. In mechanically ventilated infants, hypoinflation can also reflect low lung compliance (*stiff lungs*) as well as inadequate inspiratory or end-expiratory pressure. Similarly, hyperinflation can be a clue to the correct underlying diagnosis (e.g., chronic lung disease, meconium aspiration) in symptomatic infants or reflect excessive inspiratory or end expiratory pressure during mechanical ventilation.

Lung Density and Homogeneity. The second assessment to make in radiographic evaluation of the lungs in symptomatic newborns is whether the parenchymal lung fields are normal or opacified and, if opacified, whether the opacifications are homogeneous or asymmetric. Vigorous positive pressure ventilation can cause what would otherwise be a diffusely atelectatic lung to appear to be normally inflated and to have normal-appearing parenchyma. In any case, the presence of normal inflation and normal parenchymal lung fields in spontaneously ventilating, symptomatic infants rules out structural problems of the lung (e.g., diaphragmatic hernia, pulmonary hypoplasia, pneumothorax, congenital lobar emphysema) and parenchymal diseases of the lung (e.g., RDS, congenital group B streptococcal pneumonia, meconium aspiration) as possible causes. In such infants, the likelihood of a systemic illness or congenital heart disease accounting for symptoms is high.

When parenchymal opacities are present on the chest radiograph, an important question is whether those opacities are *homogeneous* or *asymmetric*. Homogeneous densities usually represent RDS or congenital pneumonia, but adult respiratory distress syndrome does occur in newborn infants (Faix et al, 1989). Cardiogenic pulmonary edema can also be seen as a result of cardiac dysfunction from asphyxia as well as of structural congenital heart diseases that cause left atrial hypertension. Asymmetric densities, if bilateral, are most commonly seen in meconium aspiration in term infants and in chronic lung disease in premature infants. Meconium aspiration is the most common cause of PPHNS, but every infant with PPHNS, including those with meconium aspiration, requires careful cardiovascular evaluation to rule out the many known cardiac causes of pulmonary hypertension (Long, 1984, 1990b). Similarly, every premature infant with chronic lung disease requires

careful cardiovascular evaluation to ferret out the possible contribution of silent PDA to the lung dysfunction (Long et al, 1996). Unilateral parenchymal densities can represent localized pneumonias, aspiration, atelectasis, and congenital anomalies.

Lung Vascularity. The third assessment to make in radiographic evaluation of the lungs in symptomatic newborns is whether the pulmonary vascularity is normal, decreased, or increased. Certainly in some cases separating vascular changes from parenchymal changes can be difficult. Nevertheless, attempting to distinguish whether pulmonary vascularity is normal, decreased (Fig. 62–1), or increased (Fig. 62–2) and following changes in pulmonary vascularity serially on subsequent chest radiographs can be useful in differential diagnosis (Table 62–8) and management. The distinction between pulmonary venous engorgement from left atrial hypertension (or pulmonary venous obstruction) and pulmonary arterial engorgement from left-to-right shunt is more difficult in sick newborn infants than in older children and adults, at least in part because chest radiographs are taken supine in newborn infants. One useful marker for pulmonary venous congestion is the presence of pleural fluid (Long et al, 1984a).

One important radiographic appearance to recognize is the picture of *congestive heart failure with a small heart* (Fig. 62–3), a pattern typical of infradiaphragmatic TAPVD (Long, 1984, 1990b; Long et al, 1984b). A similar pattern can be observed in some infants with retained amniotic fluid, however. In infants with various forms of hypoplasia of the right heart and inadequate pulmonary blood flow,

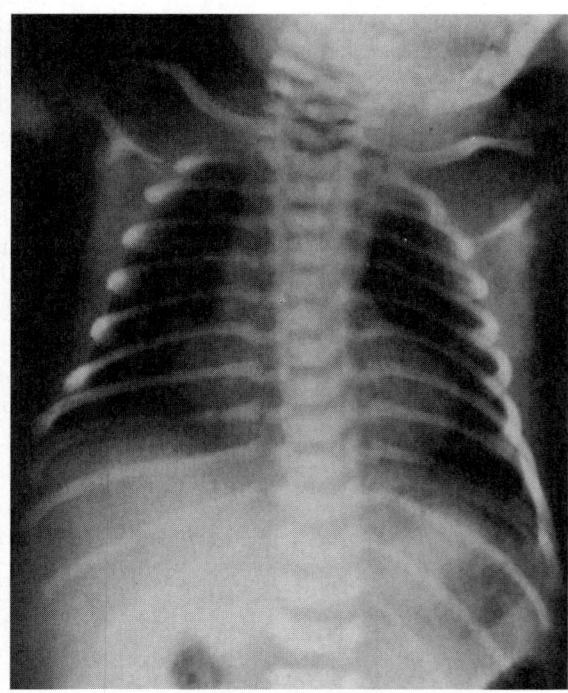

FIGURE 62–1. Chest radiograph in a newborn infant with pulmonary atresia and ventricular septal defect. The pulmonary vascularity is diminished, and the heart size is normal. (From Long WA [Ed]: Fetal and Neonatal Cardiology. Philadelphia, WB Saunders, 1990.)

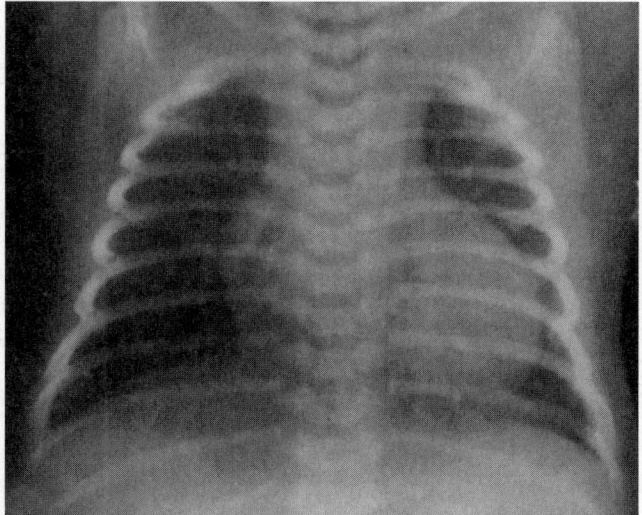

FIGURE 62–2. Chest radiograph in a 2-week-old infant with atrioventricular septal defect. The pulmonary vascularity is increased. Pulmonary edema is not present. The heart is mildly enlarged. (From Long WA [Ed]: Fetal and Neonatal Cardiology. Philadelphia, WB Saunders, 1990.)

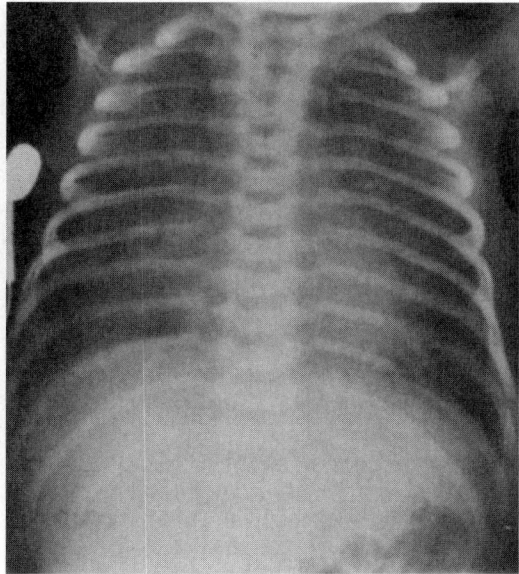

FIGURE 62–3. Chest radiograph in a newborn infant with obstructed total anomalous pulmonary venous drainage to the portal vein. The pulmonary vascularity is increased. Pulmonary edema is present. The heart size is normal. This pattern represents *congestive heart failure with a small heart.* (From Long WA [Ed]: Fetal and Neonatal Cardiology. Philadelphia, WB Saunders, 1990.)

reduction in pulmonary oligemia in response to infusion of PGE$_1$ (and reopening of the ductus) is usually readily evident on serial chest radiographs. Similarly, increased pulmonary vascularity is usually readily evident at least on the side of the shunt on postoperative chest radiographs after surgical placement of modified Blalock-Taussig shunts.

Heart and Great Vessels. A great deal of useful information about the heart and great vessels can be obtained from the chest radiograph. Systematic review of the chest radiograph should enable the clinician to determine (1) whether the heart *position* is normal or whether dextrocardia (Fig. 62–4) or mesocardia is present, (2) whether the heart *size* is normal or abnormal, and (3) whether the heart *contour* is normal or abnormal. In addition, the chest radiograph should enable the clinician to determine whether the pulmonary artery is normal or not. These assessments provide useful insights into differential diagnosis (Table 62–9), but the value of the radiographic appearance of the heart is far greater when it is considered in conjunction with the status of the pulmonary vascularity

(see Table 62–8) and the entire clinical picture of the patient.

On the chest radiograph of the normal heart, the right border is formed by the right atrium, and most of the left heart border is formed by the left ventricle. The most characteristic feature of normal cardiac contour is the *bump* at the upper left margin of the heart derived from the normal size and position of the pulmonary artery.

Right atrial enlargement is readily evident on chest radiograph from extension of the right heart border into the right chest because the right atrium makes up the right heart border. The rest of the contour of the heart is unchanged by right atrial enlargement. Right atrial enlargement is characteristic of critical pulmonary stenosis, Ebstein anomaly (Fig. 62–5), and in utero closure of the ductus secondary to maternal ingestion of over-the-counter inhibitors of cyclo-oxygenase (such as aspirin, ibuprofen). The right atrium also enlarges in ASD but not in the newborn period.

TABLE 62–8

Differential Diagnosis of Sick Newborn Infants: Pulmonary Vascularity

Normal Vascularity	Decreased Vascularity	Increased Vascularity
Lung diseases	Idiopathic PPHNS	Cyanotic CHD (ITAPVD, truncus arteriosus, tricuspid atresia)
Systemic diseases	Tetralogy of Fallot	CHF (HLHS, critical aortic stenosis, critical coarctation, interrupted aortic arch)
Incidental CHD	Pulmonary atresia	Shunts (PDA, VSD, AVSD, AVM)

PPHNS, persistent pulmonary hypertension of the newborn syndrome; CHD, congenital heart disease; ITAPVD, infradiaphragmatic total anomalous pulmonary venous drainage; CHF, congestive heart failure; HLHS, hypoplastic left heart syndrome; PDA, patent ductus arteriosus; VSD, ventricular septal defect; AVSD, atrioventricular septal defect; AVM, arteriovenous malformation.

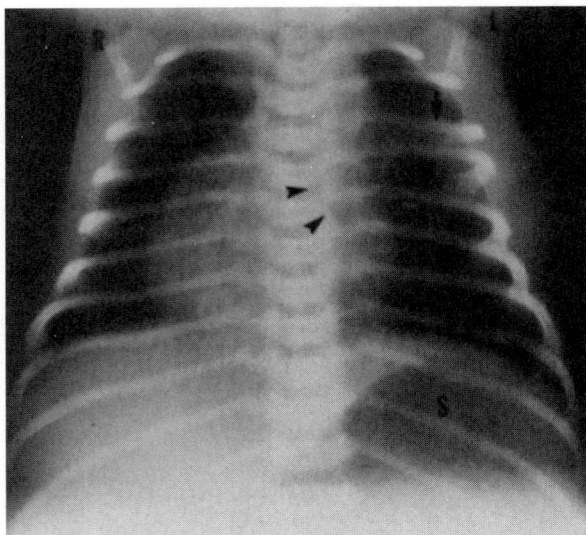

FIGURE 62–4. Dextrocardia in a cyanotic 7-day-old infant status post left Blalock-Taussig shunt for pulmonary atresia/transposition of the great vessels. The stomach (S) is on the left, and the liver is on the right. The arrowheads indicate the longer bronchus on the left side; the arrows indicate the rib deformity from the shunt. This infant demonstrates thoracoabdominal discordance with the heart reversed but the abdominal organs in the normal position (see Table 62–9). (From Long WA [Ed]: Fetal and Neonatal Cardiology. Philadelphia, WB Saunders, 1990.)

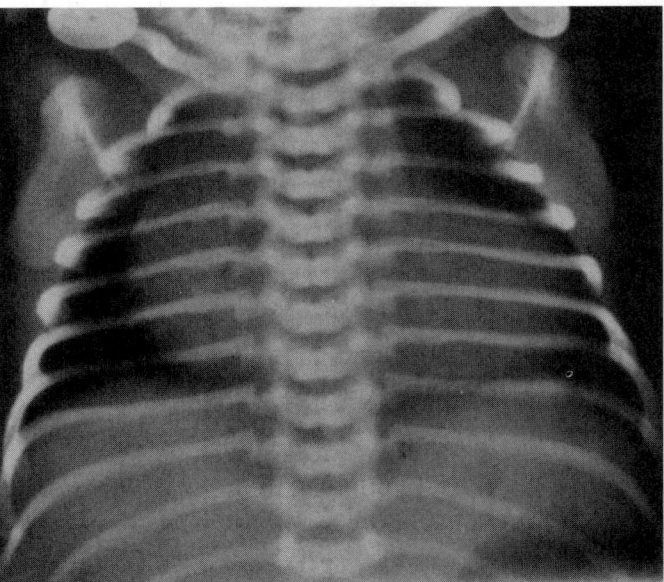

FIGURE 62–5. Chest radiograph in a 1-day-old infant with severe cyanosis secondary to Ebstein's anomaly. The extension of the heart into the right chest is due to right atrial enlargement. The pulmonary vascularity is diminished from right-to-left atrial shunt. (From Long WA [Ed]: Fetal and Neonatal Cardiology. Philadelphia, WB Saunders, 1990.)

When the pulmonary artery is transposed, absent, or diminutive, the cardiac silhouette appears abnormal because the bump created by the normal pulmonary artery is not present. If the pulmonary artery is absent (pulmonary atresia) or hypoplastic (TOF, most forms of tricuspid atresia), absence of the normal shadow of the pulmonary artery usually makes the heart appear to be boot-shaped (*coeur en sabot*) (see Fig. 62–15). If the pulmonary artery is transposed (TGV), the abnormal position of the pulmonary artery creates an *egg-on-side* appearance to the cardiac silhouette (Fig. 62–6; see Table 62–9).

Left atrial enlargement is more difficult to detect on a chest radiograph than right atrial enlargement because the left atrium lies behind the heart in the anteroposterior projection. Left atrial enlargement can be recognized from (1) a double density behind the heart just to the right of the vertebral column and (2) splaying of the main stem bronchi from the usual angulation of 45 degrees to near 90 degrees. The latter finding occurs because left atrial enlargement can elevate the left main stem bronchus. When shunt vascularity is evident, the presence of left atrial enlargement means that the atrial septum is intact and that the shunt must be at the ventricular or ductal level.

Laboratory Studies for Cardiac Diagnosis

The three most important laboratory tests in diagnosis of neonatal cardiac disorders are electrocardiography, echo-

TABLE 62–9

Differential Diagnosis from Heart Position, Size, and Shape in Symptomatic Newborn Infants

Position	Size	Contour/Shape	Pulmonary Artery	Diagnosis
Normal	Normal	Normal	Normal	Lung/systemic disease
Normal	Normal	Snowman	Normal	Supracardiac TAPVD
Normal	Normal	Egg on side	Not seen	TGV
Normal	Normal	Boot-shaped	Not seen	Pulmonary atresia, TOF, tricuspid atresia
Normal	Increased	Right atrial enlargement	Normal	Critical pulmonary stenosis/Ebstein anomaly, ASD, AVSD
Normal	Increased	Left atrial enlargement	Normal	IAA, critical coarctation/aortic stenosis, EFE, cardiomyopathy, VSD, PDA
Normal	Decreased	Normal	Normal	ITAPVD
Right chest	Any	Any	Any	Complex CHD

TAPVD, total anomalous pulmonary venous drainage; TGV, transposition of the great vessels; TOF, tetralogy of Fallot; IAA, interrupted aortic arch; EFE, endocardial fibroelastosis; VSD, ventricular septal defect; PDA, patent ductus arteriosus; ITAPVD, infradiaphragmatic total anomalous pulmonary venous drainage; CHD, congenital heart disease; ASD, atrial septal defect; AVSD, atrioventricular septal defect.

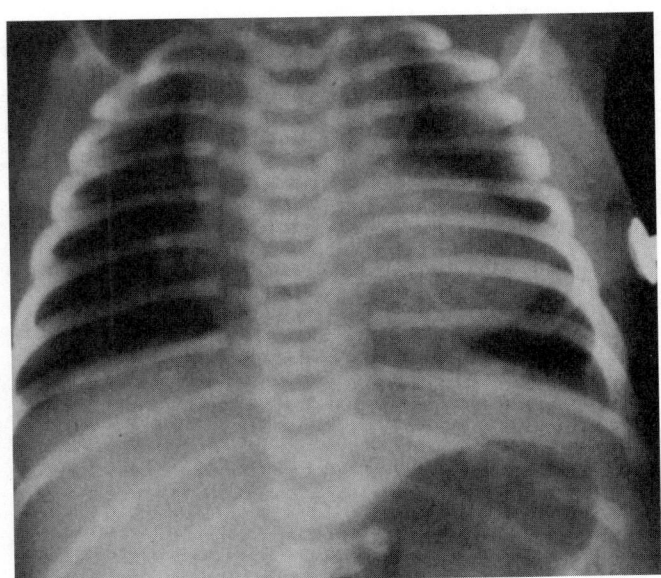

FIGURE 62–6. Chest radiograph in an infant with transposition of the great vessels and intact ventricular septum. The heart size is normal, but the abnormal position of the pulmonary artery makes the apex of the heart appear to be upturned, and causes the *egg on side* appearance. (From Long WA [Ed]: Fetal and Neonatal Cardiology. Philadelphia, WB Saunders, 1990.)

cardiography, and cardiac catheterization. The hyperoxia test is a well-known maneuver designed to distinguish infants with congenital heart disease from those with lung disease, but it lacks both specificity and sensitivity and is therefore more misleading than useful. Electrocardiography is mainly useful in sorting out disorders of cardiac rate and rhythm. Echocardiography is by far the most valuable diagnostic tool in evaluating newborns with possible cardiac disease because it can provide the fine details of cardiovascular structure and function noninvasively. Cardiac catheterization, once the gold standard of neonatal cardiovascular diagnosis, is largely a therapeutic procedure today. Diagnostic cardiac catheterization is still performed in certain circumstances, however. Diagnostic cardiac catheterization is still required occasionally in newborns in whom more precise anatomic definition is required for (1) the coronary circulation (e.g., possible anomalous left coronary artery), (2) the pulmonary venous connections (e.g., partial or complete anomalous pulmonary venous return in the setting of complex congenital heart disease), (3) the pulmonary arterial tree (e.g., pulmonary atresia with hypoplasia of the branch pulmonary arteries), and (4) the aortic arch (e.g., assessment of probable coarctation in the setting of PDA).

Hyperoxia Test

In the hyperoxia test, an infant with suspected or possible congenital heart disease is placed on 100% oxygen (or in other iterations, 100% oxygen plus constant positive airway pressure). If arterial PO_2 does not rise above some magical level (100 mm Hg in some hands, 50 mm Hg in others), the infant is supposed to have cyanotic congenital heart disease. If the PO_2 rises above 200 mm Hg, congenital

heart disease is supposed to be ruled out. The problem with this test is that it does not work (Long, 1990b). All that a PO_2 less than 50 mm Hg on 100% oxygen really means is that the infant has either a large intracardiac or a large intrapulmonary right-to-left shunt—if the arterial sample in question really reflects the oxygen content being ejected from the systemic ventricle (a false assumption in many cases). For example, many infants with severe RDS have a PO_2 less than 50 mm Hg on 100% oxygen before the administration of surfactant or institution of positive airway pressure. A persistent PO_2 in the 30s in the absence of respiratory distress and in the absence of radiographic abnormalities in the lungs does suggest cyanotic heart disease, however.

Similarly, all that a PO_2 greater than 200 mm Hg really means is that highly oxygenated blood is reaching the artery from which the sample was drawn; it does not mean that highly oxygenated blood is being ejected from the systemic ventricle. For example, arterial PO_2 measurements greater than 200 mm Hg can be found in the descending aorta (umbilical arterial catheter) in TGV when the ductus is patent and pulmonary vascular resistance exceeds systemic resistance. Arterial PO_2 measurements on 100% oxygen greater than 200 mm Hg that are derived from blood ejected from the systemic ventricle can be seen in many forms of life-threatening congenital heart disease, including HLHS, infradiaphragmatic TAPVD, interrupted aortic arch, critical aortic stenosis, and critical coarctation (Long, 1984, 1990b).

For these reasons, the hyperoxia test should be abandoned as a test for congenital heart disease. It has no value in discriminating congenital heart disease from lung disease. In fact, the hyperoxia test is dangerous in that it can provide a false indication to unsuspecting clinicians that heart disease is present and, more importantly, false reassurance that it is absent. The fact that the hyperoxia test should be abandoned as a putative discriminator between heart and lung disease should not be taken to mean that there is no value in knowing that hypoxemia persists despite 100% oxygen. Failure of PO_2 to rise above 100 mm Hg in 100% oxygen does mean that a large right-to-left shunt is present and that the infant has a serious problem that merits rapid investigation.

Electrocardiography

The 12-lead electrocardiogram is not particularly helpful in evaluation of symptomatic newborn infants except in two circumstances. First, the 12-lead electrocardiogram is essential in diagnosing disorders of cardiac rate and rhythm. Rhythm strips from bedside monitors are not useful in identifying disorders of rhythm and should not be relied on. Typical disorders of rate and rhythm seen in newborns include supraventricular tachycardia (SVT), also known as *paroxysmal atrial tachycardia*, and complete heart block. Complete heart block is usually well tolerated if the resting ventricular rate is greater than 55 beats/min and the heart is structurally normal. Complete congenital heart block is now typically diagnosed prenatally, although occasional infants with complete congenital heart block are still delivered by emergency cesarean section for fetal bradycardia presumed to be secondary to fetal distress.

SVT is now frequently first diagnosed prenatally, particularly when the SVT is persistent enough to cause hydrops fetalis. In most newborns with SVT, good control can be achieved with digoxin alone; less commonly the combination of digoxin and propranolol is required. Recording a 12-lead electrocardiogram is indicated after abolition of SVT to look for underlying Wolff-Parkinson-White syndrome. Infants with SVT who have underlying Wolff-Parkinson-White syndrome are more likely to have recurrences and are more likely to have SVT that is difficult to suppress pharmacologically. A single normal 12-lead electrocardiogram does not exclude Wolff-Parkinson-White syndrome because the bypass tract can come and go from the surface electrocardiogram.

Multifocal atrial tachycardia has the poorest prognosis of neonatal tachyarrhythmias but is rare. Neonatal atrial flutter can be difficult to recognize, but injections of adenosine (to abolish presumed SVT) usually induce brief periods of higher degrees of block that permit recognition of flutter.

Second, determination of axis with the 12-lead electrocardiogram is also useful. In the most common form of congenital heart disease associated with trisomy 21, left axis deviation is almost always present (Fig. 62–7). Absence of left axis deviation virtually excludes the diagnosis of AVSD in infants with trisomy 21. In the absence of readily available cardiologic consultation, a screening 12-lead electrocardiogram in infants with trisomy 21 to exclude left

axis deviation can provide reassurance to the pediatrician or neonatologist (and parents) that the most commonly encountered form of congenital heart disease is not present. Shunt murmurs in infants with trisomy 21 and AVSD are frequently not present for several days after birth, given the often dilatory postnatal relaxation of pulmonary vascular resistance commonly observed in infants with trisomy 21. In cyanotic infants, mild left axis deviation suggests pulmonary atresia, and extreme left axis deviation suggests tricuspid atresia.

Echocardiography

The single most useful diagnostic test in the evaluation of symptomatic infants who may have congenital heart disease is echocardiography because it can provide detailed noninvasive assessment of cardiovascular structure and function. Comprehensive summaries of neonatal echocardiography are available elsewhere (Sanders, 1990). Although neonatal echocardiography can be a highly accurate diagnostic tool, similar to all diagnostic tools, neonatal echocardiography has limitations. The purposes of this brief summary are to (1) highlight the limitations of neonatal echocardiography and (2) suggest ways in which neonatologists can assist in improving the diagnostic information derived from neonatal echocardiography.

Limitations. The information provided by neonatal echocardiography in detection of cardiovascular problems in symptomatic newborns is unmatched by any other diagnostic approach. Nevertheless, neonatal echocardiography has several limitations. The most important limitation of neonatal echocardiography is that its accuracy depends on the experience and skill of the person performing the test. An echocardiogram performed by inexperienced personnel is usually better than no echocardiogram at all—as long as both the clinician ordering the test and the person performing it are aware of the limitations of the information garnered. Far more valuable information can be obtained if the person performing the echocardiogram is either a full-time pediatric cardiac ultrasonographer or an experienced pediatric cardiologist. In general, cardiac ultrasonographers who spend the great majority of their time with adult patients and adult cardiologists are uncomfortable performing and interpreting neonatal echocardiograms because they seldom use the two most important views for accurate cardiac assessment of newborns: the subxiphoid view and the arch view. Technicians and cardiologists trained for adult echocardiography are not familiar with these views because they are not possible in most adult patients.

A second limitation of neonatal echocardiography is that it provides only a snapshot of cardiac anatomy and function at a given point in time. This fact reduces both the sensitivity and the specificity of neonatal echocardiography because of the many changes in cardiovascular structure and function normally taking place in the first hours, days, and weeks after birth. Depending on when echocardiography is performed, these ongoing changes in cardiovascular structure and function can obscure both the presence and the absence of several important forms of congenital heart disease. Some infants are underdiagnosed or overdiagnosed

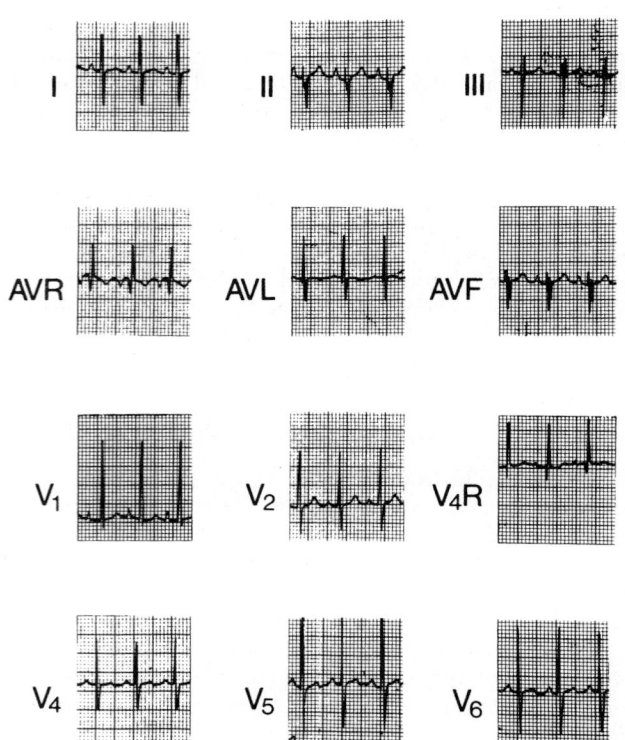

FIGURE 62–7. Twelve-lead electrocardiogram demonstrating left axis deviation in atrioventricular septal defect, with negative deflection in AVF. In an immediate newborn infant, the upright T in V1 and the S wave in V6 would be normal, but otherwise right ventricular hypertrophy is present. (From Long WA (Ed): Fetal and Neonatal Cardiology. Philadelphia, WB Saunders, 1990.)

by neonatal echocardiography when echocardiography is performed too soon after birth.

Several disorders can be missed (i.e., neonatal echocardiography lacks sensitivity, or causes false-negative diagnoses) when echocardiography is performed too soon after birth and not repeated later. The most important (and most difficult to diagnose) example of a diagnosis that is commonly missed because echocardiography is performed too soon after birth is coarctation. As long as the aortic end of the ductus is patent, many infants who have coarctation are not diagnosable by either echocardiography or cardiac catheterization. Normally the aortic end of the ductus does not close until after 10 days of age, although the pulmonary end usually shuts by the end of the first day of life in term infants. It is only closure of the aortic end of the ductus that precipitates significant obstruction in many infants with coarctation. Coarctation cannot be excluded until the aortic end of the ductus closes.

A second example of a malformation that can be missed when echocardiograms are performed shortly after birth is a small or moderate VSD. Such defects are usually identified by color flow Doppler–detected left-to-right shunts, rather than by direct visualization of ventricular septal dropout. Yet left-to-right shunts in VSDs cannot occur until pulmonary vascular resistance falls below systemic resistance, a development that occurs slowly in some infants.

A third example of a malformation that can be missed when echocardiograms are performed too soon (or too infrequently) after birth is failure to demonstrate ductal patency in premature infants who have chronic lung disease. Silent PDA in infants with chronic lung disease is the most common diagnosis missed by neonatal echocardiography. In infants with chronic lung disease, pulmonary vascular resistance is usually not only high, but also highly variable. Infants with chronic lung disease who have not had the ductus ligated almost always have intermittent left-to-right ductal shunts that wax and wane over periods of minutes in response to changes in pulmonary vascular resistance. Thus, absence of left-to-right ductal shunting at a single point in time by echocardiography in infants with chronic lung disease provides little reassurance that ductal patency is not contributing to pulmonary compromise.

Two disorders that are commonly overdiagnosed by neonatal echocardiography (i.e., disorders in which neonatal echocardiography lacks specificity, or yields false-positive diagnoses) when the study is performed too soon after birth are PDA and ASD. In the case of PDA, the ductus is obviously normally patent at birth. In term infants, the pulmonary end of the ductus often does not fully constrict until 24 hours after birth. In premature infants, the ductus is not likely to shut for quite some time. As a result, any infant who has an echocardiogram performed in the first 24 hours after birth is highly likely to exhibit ductal patency. If the affected infant is term and is otherwise normal, this phenomenon is normal and needs no further follow-up unless a murmur persists. In the premature infant, the ductus is unlikely to close permanently until the age at which the infant would have reached full term had the infant remained in utero and not been born prematurely.

Similarly the foramen ovale is normally patent at birth and typically remains patent in up to 90% of infants for the first year of life. Distinguishing left-to-right atrial shunt across a patent foramen ovale from left-to-right shunt across a small or even moderate ASD is usually impossible in the first days and often first months after birth. Sometimes the final assessment of what is a patent foramen ovale versus ASD cannot be made until the end of the first year of life.

A third limitation of echocardiography is that sound waves do not travel as well in air as in tissue or fluid. The net result is that the resolution of echocardiography is worst in some cases in which it is most needed—infants with what appears to be severe lung disease in whom underlying congenital heart disease must be excluded (e.g., infants with PPHNS, meconium aspiration). The resolution of echocardiography is poor in infants who have air trapping. Air trapping is typical in infants hyperventilated for PPHNS or any other reason, in infants with meconium aspiration, in premature infants with chronic lung disease, and in infants with air leaks (pulmonary interstitial emphysema). The heart cannot be visualized if anterior pneumothorax is present or if pneumopericardium is present (Long, 1990c).

A fourth limitation of echocardiography is that it can create images of only what is present, and a lot of congenital heart disease is concerned with what may be missing. Determining whether anatomic structures that are not well visualized are truly absent sometimes requires persistent scanning as well as other diagnostic approaches. For example, failure to demonstrate pulmonary venous drainage to the left atrium could represent (1) technical problems with the image (not too uncommon in sick, hyperventilated infants), (2) severe reductions in pulmonary blood flow from PPHNS, (3) anomalous pulmonary venous drainage elsewhere, or (4) atresia of the pulmonary veins (worst case). Pulmonary angiography is still required occasionally to sort these four possibilities out.

Finally, another limitation of neonatal echocardiography is that its resolution, although improving virtually every year, is not perfect. With current equipment, it is not possible in all infants to (1) determine with certainty the origins and branching of the coronary arteries, (2) identify the connection of all four pulmonary veins, (3) delineate hypoplastic branch and peripheral pulmonary arteries, and (4) diagnose coarctation before the aortic end of the ductus closes except in severe cases.

Improving Utility of Neonatal Echocardiography. Practices differ in different hospitals, but in many hospitals today neonatal echocardiograms are ordered by a variety of specialists and subspecialists, including general pediatricians, neonatologists, family practitioners, intensivists, and congenital heart surgeons. In some instances, what is needed is consultation by a pediatric cardiologist, rather than an echocardiogram. In others, all that may be needed is a targeted echocardiogram; examples include ventilated premature infants with RDS with documented PDA in whom the neonatologist wants to know whether indomethacin has closed the ductus. In yet others, what is needed is a thorough clinical evaluation by an experienced pediatric cardiologist, including a comprehensive echocardiogram; examples include term infants in shock or respiratory failure.

The utility of neonatal echocardiography can be improved in several ways. Most importantly the physician with primary responsibility for the patient and the consulting pediatric cardiologist need to communicate directly. It is helpful for the pediatric cardiologist to know what the primary physician is looking for or worried about. For any problems other than routine ones, a phone call to the consulting pediatric cardiologist to describe the problem and ask for help is probably the most effective first step. Understanding what the clinical question or issue is enables the pediatric cardiologist to assist in decisions about laboratory tests and to give special scrutiny to the areas that are most pertinent during both clinical examination and, if necessary, echocardiography.

Other more specific measures can improve the diagnostic accuracy of echocardiography in particular clinical situations. For example, the sensitivity of echocardiographic detection of left-to-right ductal shunt is increased among premature infants with chronic lung disease when afflicted infants are sedated with fentanyl. Fentanyl relaxes afflicted infants, drops pulmonary vascular resistance, and brings out previously occult left-to-right ductal shunts. Similarly, during runs of extracorporeal membrane oxygenation for severe respiratory failure or for postoperative support after surgery for congenital heart disease, reducing extracorporeal membrane oxygenation transiently so that more blood is pumped by the heart permits much better visualization of cardiac structure and function.

Diagnostic Cardiac Catheterization

Indications. With the advent and refinement of echocardiographic and Doppler ultrasound techniques over the past two decades, the role of cardiac catheterization and angiocardiography in the diagnosis of neonatal congenital heart disease has diminished. In many cases, cardiac catheterization may be entirely unnecessary or may be tailored to provide limited anatomic information that complements the echocardiographic diagnosis. In practice, the utilization of cardiac catheterization for the diagnosis of congenital heart disease in the newborn varies widely from center to center, depending on the quality of echocardiographic support, the type of surgery planned, and the preferences of the attending cardiologist and surgeon. The overriding principle determining the indications for cardiac catheterization in an individual patient should be whether or not all important anatomic and physiologic questions have been answered sufficiently to guide proper treatment. The decision about diagnostic catheterization should not be influenced by whether the patient has a congenital heart anomaly that is typically diagnosed only by echocardiography.

Facility, Equipment, and Technique. Cardiac catheterization of newborns should be undertaken only in a hospital facility with an appropriately equipped catheterization suite staffed by technical personnel who are skilled and experienced in managing newborns. These qualifications generally correlate with a minimal volume of procedures, as recognized by an American Academy of Pediatrics position statement (American Academy of Pediatrics, 1991). In addition to skilled personnel in the catheterization laboratory, an entire hospital-based team, including particularly neona-

tal intensivists and a cardiovascular surgeon experienced in managing congenital heart disease, is essential.

Performing neonatal cardiac catheterization safely begins with transporting the often critically ill patient between the intensive care unit and the catheterization laboratory before and after the procedure. The same skilled nursing and respiratory therapy personnel who staff the hospital-to-hospital neonatal transport team along with the patient's nurse in the intensive care unit can be used. Because of the newborn's high body surface area-to-volume ratio and attendant susceptibility to hypothermia, a regulated thermal environment is important. The authors position the patient on the table on top of a continuous warm-air flow mattress (Warmtouch, Mallinckrodt Medical, Inc., St. Louis, MO). Attention must be paid to positioning of essential support equipment (e.g., ventilator, intravenous pump stands) to allow access to the patient and positioning of the x-ray cameras. Continuous pulse oximetric monitoring and monitoring of systemic blood pressure by existing arterial line or automated cuff sphygmomanometry are employed. Critically ill newborns usually require sedation in the intensive care unit before the procedure (e.g., continuous fentanyl infusion), and this infusion is maintained during the procedure. Minimally symptomatic infants often require only a pacifier, but supplemental small doses of a narcotic (e.g., 0.5 to 1.0 μg/kg of fentanyl) may be used as needed.

The technique of neonatal cardiac catheterization varies widely from center to center, depending on the preferences of the operator. These preferences affect the chosen route of vascular access, the selection of catheters and other equipment, and many other technical aspects. For most diagnostic right heart studies, the authors prefer a percutaneous approach to a femoral vein for ease of catheter manipulations and exchanges, although the authors have occasionally used the umbilical vein. (The authors prefer the umbilical vein approach for bedside Rashkind atrioseptostomy, discussed further in Chapter 64.) For retrograde left heart studies, the umbilical artery is frequently available and ideal, obviating risk of femoral arterial injury. With improvements in catheter and introducer sheath design, a 3, or at most 4, French system is sufficient for diagnostic studies and is minimally traumatic when used after percutaneous entry into a femoral artery. In selected circumstances, unusual access sites may be used, such as the right radial artery when the aortic arch is interrupted, the right subclavian artery is not aberrant, and a left ventricular angiogram does not opacify the ascending segment. Isolation and cannulation of vessels by a cutdown technique is an option but is rarely necessary. Planned interventional procedures may dictate particular access routes and are discussed in Chapter 65.

A dizzying array of diagnostic catheters and wires are available commercially. This wide selection allows the operator to select an instrument that is well tailored to the task at hand. For most diagnostic purposes, a soft, 5 French, balloon-tipped, flow-directed, angiographic or wedge catheter is used for right heart and transforaminal left heart studies, minimizing the risk of perforation or myocardial staining during angiography. Occasionally a more torque-directed catheter is necessary to aid certain catheter courses (e.g., crossing a restrictive atrial defect or critically stenotic pulmonary valve) or to facilitate selective ventriculography of a hypoplastic chamber. Retrograde left heart studies are most often performed using a 3 or 4 French pigtail catheter after exchanging over a wire through a standard umbilical artery catheter or after placing a femoral arterial hemostatic sheath. A 4 French multipurpose catheter is sometimes more maneuverable and is often adequate for hand angiographic injections, particularly when cardiac output is low.

Catheter Course. The course of the cardiac catheter through the vascular system is usually routine, but common variations occur. These variations are diagnostically useful and are important for the operator to recognize to limit injudicious catheter manipulations. In newborns, the venous catheter can almost invariably be passed across an interatrial defect to the left heart, sometimes obviating the need for a retrograde study. When the cardiac situs is abnormal, the venous catheter may pass to the left of the spine (in the inferior vena cava with situs inversus) or posterior to the heart (in the azygos or hemiazygos vein with situs ambiguus and interruption of the inferior vena cava). When a left superior vena cava persists, the catheter may pass into it via the enlarged ostium of the coronary sinus. When the pulmonary venous connections are anomalous, the catheter may pass into the pulmonary veins directly from the right atrium or superior vena cava or from the innominate vein via a left vertical vein. When the ventriculoarterial connections are abnormal, the catheter may pass from the right ventricle to the aorta (directly or via a VSD). When the ductus arteriosus is patent, it may be crossed antegrade with the venous catheter or retrograde with the arterial catheter. The retrograde arterial catheter may enter aortic collateral vessels, aberrant subclavian arteries, normal brachiocephalic or coronary vessels, or the right ventricle from the aorta (when the ventriculoarterial connections are abnormal).

Hemodynamic Data Collection. The diagnostic information obtained at cardiac catheterization includes oximetric data, intravascular and intracardiac pressures, and angiography. Although routinely collected, oximetric data suffer from numerous confounding variables that limit their utility, particularly in newborns. Sampling error owing to streaming and incomplete admixture owing to multiple levels of intracardiac shunting (especially at the ductal level) may be more prevalent and problematic in newborns with heart disease than in older children. The influences of assisted ventilation, supplemental oxygen administration, vasotonic agents, sedatives and paralytics, and unknown oxygen consumption make Fick method calculations of blood flow less reliable. Vascular resistances and blood flows, particularly pulmonary, may be quite labile throughout the course of the procedure in a critically ill newborn.

Despite these limitations, qualitative interpretation of measured oxygen saturations at different sites may be helpful in some instances. Low oxygen saturation ($< 50\%$) in the systemic veins suggests impaired systemic blood flow (except when profound systemic arterial hypoxemia or anemia is present). High (usually $> 90\%$) oxygen saturation in the systemic veins suggests anomalous pulmonary venous drainage or an arteriovenous malformation. A significant increase ($> 10\%$) in oxygen saturation from the systemic veins to the right atrium usually indicates a left-to-right atrial shunt (as in critical left heart obstructions), anomalous pulmonary venous drainage to the right atrium, or atrioventricular valve insufficiency into the right atrium from a ventricle containing highly saturated blood. A significant increase in oxygen saturation from the right atrium to the ventricular level indicates a left-to-right shunt through a VSD or venous admixture in a single ventricle. A significant increase in oxygen saturation from the right ventricle to the pulmonary artery indicates a left-to-right shunt through the ductus or an aortopulmonary window, collateral vessel, or surgically placed shunt. A significant decrease in oxygen saturation from the pulmonary veins to the left atrium indicates an atrial level right-to-left shunt (as in critical right heart obstructions) or anomalous systemic venous drainage. A significant decrease in oxygen saturation from the left atrium to the left ventricle indicates a ventricular level right-to-left shunt (as in pulmonary outflow obstruction with a VSD). A significant decrease in oxygen saturation from the left ventricle to the aorta usually occurs when the aorta is partially related to the right ventricle (as in TOF, truncus arteriosus, and double-outlet right ventricle). A significant difference in oxygen saturation between ascending and descending aorta indicates a right-to-left ductal shunt, the ascending aortic value being higher with normally related great vessels and the descending aortic value being higher with transposed great vessels. Low systemic arterial oxygen saturation suggests critically impaired pulmonary blood flow (e.g., pulmonary atresia) or inadequate intracardiac mixing with TGV.

Many intravascular and intracardiac pressures can be predicted by Doppler ultrasound techniques. Atrial and ventricular end-diastolic pressures, however, require direct measurement. Dominant atrial A waves are seen with ipsilateral atrioventricular valve atresia. Dominant V waves reflect significant atrioventricular valve regurgitation. A large pressure difference between the atria denotes a restrictive interatrial defect with tricuspid or mitral atresia and may indicate the need for atrial septostomy or septectomy. Elevated ventricular end-diastolic pressures occur with critical ventricular outflow obstruction, volume overload, or primary myocardial dysfunction. Pulmonary arterial pressure is elevated, often to systemic levels, in the first weeks of life, particularly when pulmonary blood flow is increased or the ductus is widely patent. Pressure gradients across stenotic valves or vessels may not accurately indicate the severity of obstruction when, as is often true of neonatal ductus dependent obstructions, blood flow through the stenotic area is low.

In a few particular clinical scenarios, pressure data obtained at cardiac catheterization are of special interest and diagnostic value. Occasionally the infant with transposition of the great arteries and intact ventricular septum presents late (> 2 weeks of age), and the preparedness of the left ventricle to perform against high systemic afterload following a planned arterial switch repair is uncertain. Although some surgical groups have reported equally favorable outcomes in patients up to 1 month of age regardless of hemodynamic findings (Idriss et al, 1988; Mee, 1991), others rely on direct measurement of left ventricular pressure at cardiac catheterization to guide selection of patients

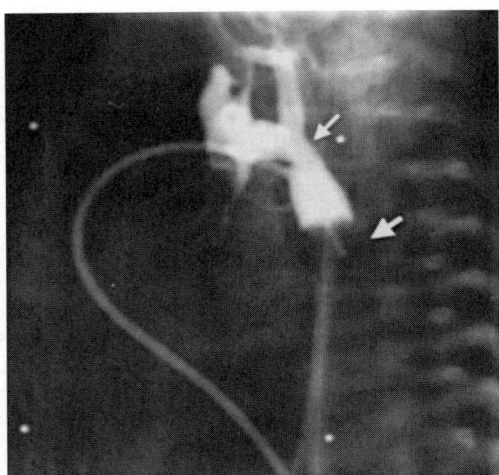

FIGURE 62–8. Lateral-view aortogram using the balloon occlusion technique in a newborn infant suspected of having aortic coarctation based on clinical and echocardiographic findings. The balloon-tipped catheter with multiple side-holes proximal to the balloon is passed antegrade through the ductus to the descending thoracic aorta, and the contrast injection is performed with the balloon (large arrow) occluding flow causing reflux of contrast material into the isthmus and tranverse aortic arch showing no discrete coarctation (small arrow).

for primary repair or staged repair after preparatory banding of the pulmonary artery (Jonas et al, 1989). In infants with pulmonary atresia and intact ventricular septum, measurement of markedly suprasystemic right ventricular pressure may be associated with coronary sinusoids and a right ventricular dependent coronary circulation and may guide the therapeutic approach (Hanley et al, 1993). In newborns with a single ventricle and a bulboventricular foramen supplying aortic blood flow, simultaneous measurement of ventricular and aortic systolic pressure identifies a restrictive bulboventricular foramen (although absence of a gradient does not exclude obstruction when systemic output is low). Also, in double-inlet left ventricle, measurement of left atrial pressure and the interatrial pressure gradient in the setting of an intact or restrictive atrial septum can identify or exclude mitral inflow obstruction.

Angiography. Of all the diagnostic information obtained at cardiac catheterization in newborns, angiographic demonstration of the anatomy is of primary importance and may be tailored to supplement well-documented echocardiographic anatomy. In most instances, a thorough understanding of the cardiovascular anatomy coupled with the clinical setting allows the physiology to be deduced. Selected circumstances in which angiographic definition of the anatomy is especially helpful or in which use of less common techniques is especially helpful are discussed here.

The common acyanotic forms of congenital heart disease with left-to-right shunts *dependent* on low pulmonary vascular resistance (Rudolph, 1970) rarely require diagnostic angiographic assessment in the neonatal period. Critical obstructions (i.e., pulmonary and aortic stenosis) are studied in the setting of a therapeutic intervention and are

discussed later. Coarctation of the aorta may be challenging to diagnose or exclude, particularly in patients with major intracardiac defects and a large ductus arteriosus. A retrograde juxtaductal or transverse aortogram or an antegrade balloon occlusion descending thoracic aortogram (Keane et al, 1985) demonstrates the intraluminal filling defect and extent of proximal aortic hypoplasia (Fig. 62–8). Occasionally angiography is necessary to distinguish between coarctation and interruption of the aortic arch. Rarely in interrupted aortic arch, contrast material injected into the left ventricle does not sufficiently opacify the aortic arch, and hand injection of contrast material via a right radial artery intravenous catheter is diagnostic (if the right subclavian artery does not arise aberrantly from the descending aorta).

Cyanotic congenital heart disease in newborns is generally diagnosed echocardiographically, but frequently specific anatomic details are delineated angiographically. In transposition of the great arteries, coronary artery anomalies are common and may be demonstrated by aortography. The *laid-back* view, obtained by an antegrade aortic root injection filmed with extreme caudal angulation of the x-ray beam, provides a look down the barrel of the ascending aorta and is especially valuable for visualizing the coronary origins and course (Mandell et al, 1990) (Fig. 62–9).

TOF occurs in its classic form with right ventricular outflow obstruction and in a more complex form with complete pulmonary atresia. Newborns with pulmonary atresia usually have more severe and variable associated vascular abnormalities, such as extreme hypoplasia, nonconfluence, or abnormal arborization of the native pulmonary arteries and major aortopulmonary collateral arteries, and benefit from angiographic assessment. When the ductus arteriosus is widely patent, a juxtaductal aortogram allows visualization of the pulmonary arterial anatomy. When an infant presents after ductal closure, pulmonary venous wedge angiography by hand injection of contrast material fills the native pulmonary arteries retrograde via the pulmonary capillary bed (Nihill et al, 1978) (Fig. 62–

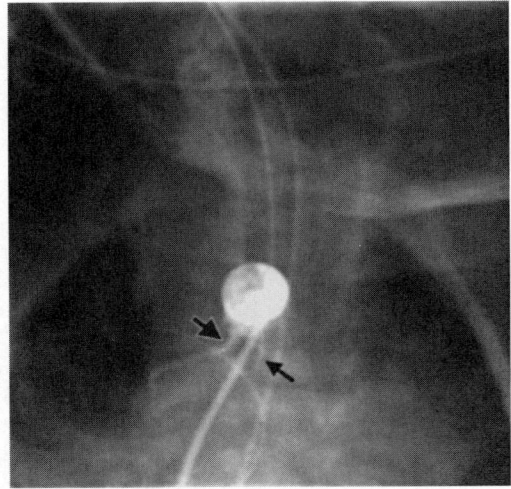

FIGURE 62–9. Anteroposterior aortogram with extreme caudal angulation of the x-ray beam performed via the venous catheter in a newborn infant with transposition of the great arteries. The right (large arrow) and left (small arrow) coronary arteries are seen.

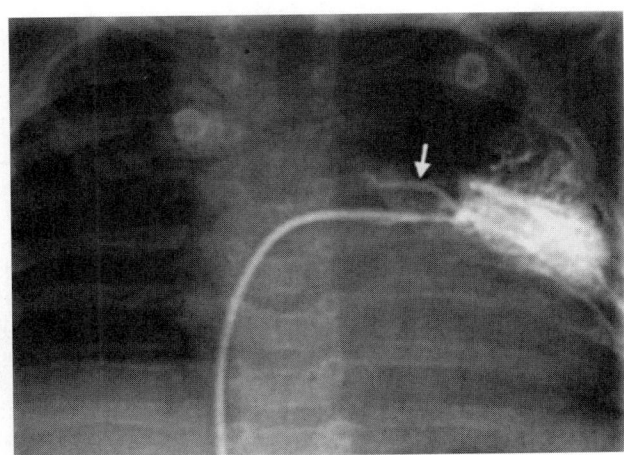

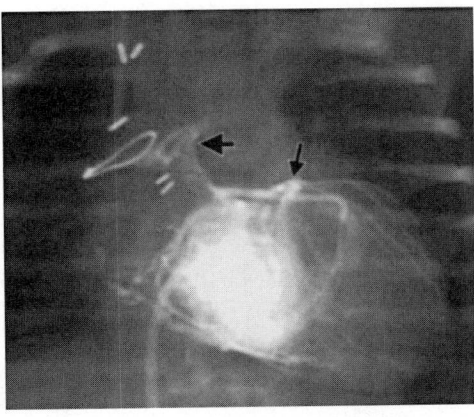

FIGURE 62–10. Pulmonary venous wedge angiogram using an end-hole catheter opacifies a severely hypoplastic left pulmonary artery (arrow) in a patient with pulmonary atresia, ventricular septal defect, and small aortopulmonary collateral vessels.

FIGURE 62–12. Anteroposterior right ventricular angiogram in a newborn with pulmonary atresia, intact ventricular septum, and suprasystemic right ventricular pressure demonstrates retrograde filling of the coronary arteries (small arrow) and ascending aorta (large arrow) from sinusoidal connections with the right ventricular cavity.

10). Selective contrast injections into aortopulmonary collateral vessels often fill the native pulmonary arteries and aid in identifying arborization abnormalities (Fig. 62–11). Although some operators prefer selective coronary arteriography to detect coronary anomalies even in newborns (Takahashi et al, 1983), aortography or left ventriculography is generally sufficient to diagnose or exclude anomalous origin of the anterior descending coronary from the right coronary artery (the most prevalent variation associated with TOF).

Pulmonary atresia with an intact ventricular septum presents an entirely different set of diagnostic considerations that guide angiographic assessment. Right ventriculography allows quantitation of the degree of hypoplasia of the chamber and tricuspid valve annulus, determination of whether the chamber is tripartite or not, and proximity

of the outflow tract to the pulmonary trunk (the position of which may be identified by simultaneous placement of a retrograde catheter via the ductus). Right ventriculography also identifies sinusoidal connections to the coronary arteries and may fill the ascending aorta (Fig. 62–12). Aortic root angiography should opacify both coronary artery beds, or the coronary circulation may be dependent on suprasystemic right ventricular perfusion pressure.

Total anomalous pulmonary venous drainage is usually associated with pulmonary venous obstruction when it requires angiographic assessment in the newborn. A pulmonary arteriogram generally allows visualization of the anomalous site of drainage except when pulmonary blood flow is critically reduced because of the venous obstruction. Alternatively the venous catheter may be passed to the common pulmonary venous chamber for selective angiography, although this may be most difficult when it is most necessary (i.e., the obstruction is severe). Occasionally selective bilateral branch pulmonary arteriography improves angiographic identification of mixed sites of drainage (supradiaphragmatic and infradiaphragmatic in the same patient).

Truncus arteriosus may be associated with truncal valve dysfunction, branch pulmonary artery stenosis, interrupted aortic arch, or coronary artery anomalies. A large-volume, rapidly injected, truncal root angiogram, usually with the antegrade catheter, can demonstrate most, if not all, of these features in a single injection.

Tricuspid atresia may occur with transposed or normally related great arteries, a large or small VSD, and varying degrees of pulmonary stenosis and pulmonary arterial hypoplasia. A large-volume, rapidly injected, left ventriculogram, with the venous catheter, can demonstrate most, if not all, of these features in a single injection. In newborns with ductus-derived pulmonary blood flow, a juxtaductal aortogram visualizes the pulmonary artery anatomy.

Several other complex cyanotic congenital heart malformations may require angiographic assessment. In double inlet left ventricle with transposed great arteries, ventriculography may aid in the evaluation of the bulboventricular

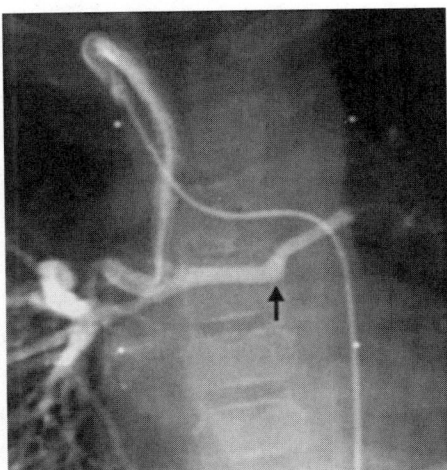

FIGURE 62–11. Selective angiogram in an aortopulmonary collateral vessel opacifies confluent hypoplastic *gull-wing* central pulmonary arteries (arrow) in a patient with pulmonary atresia, ventricular septal defect, and multiple aortopulmonary collateral vessels.

foramen and its egress to the aorta. In the heterotaxia syndromes (asplenia/polysplenia), anomalous systemic and pulmonary venous drainage and pulmonary atresia with associated pulmonary arterial hypoplasia are common, and angiography is particularly valuable in their assessment. Finally, postoperative patients occasionally require angiography to evaluate residual intracardiac shunts, obstructions, or the patency of a surgically placed aortopulmonary shunt.

Complications. As with all medical decisions or interventions, the benefits or diagnostic value of cardiac catheterization must be weighed against the attendant risks of complications related to the procedure. Neonatal cardiac catheterization is generally considered to have a higher risk of serious complications than is cardiac catheterization of older infants and children, and early surveys supported this impression. Mortality directly attributable to the procedure was 1% to 1.75% in newborns and infants under 1 year of age but less than 0.5% in older children (Kennedy et al, 1982; Stanger et al, 1974). A more recent survey (Cassidy et al, 1992) found a mortality rate of 0.2%, and the incidence of potentially serious complications (perforation, sepsis, bleeding requiring transfusion, serious arrhythmias, hypercyanotic spells, or embolism) was 2.4%. In reviewing continuous quality improvement statistics from 1989 through 1996 at the authors' hospital, 2 out of nearly 1300 patients died as a result of the procedure (unpublished data). One of these deaths was in a patient with deep baseline cyanosis who became agitated after attempted sedation and suffered cardiopulmonary arrest before obtaining vascular access. No procedural mortality was observed in newborns.

This improved safety record is observed despite a greater frequency of interventional procedures and more patients undergoing diagnostic procedures after surviving surgery with complex disease. The lower complication rate is likely attributable to many factors, including more refined equipment, the increased collective experience of technical staff and operator, improved preprocedure stabilization with PGE_1, and improved patient selection owing to the use of echocardiography. Although the potential diagnostic value of cardiac catheterization must be carefully considered in each individual newborn, the risk of morbidity and mortality from the procedure should not be a contraindication.

COMMON PRESENTATIONS AND SPECIFIC CARDIAC PROBLEMS

The range of developmental abnormalities and problems with pregnancy, labor, and delivery that can result in postnatal symptoms is quite broad. Nevertheless, the great majority of infants with serious or life-threatening problems present in one of eight different ways (Table 62–10). Familiarity with the common cardiovascular causes of these eight presentations can provide earlier insight into the correct diagnosis and management for better than 9 out of 10 infants with potentially serious cardiovascular problems.

Complete Transposition of the Great Arteries

In transposition of the great arteries, the position of the great arteries is reversed; that is, the aorta arises anteriorly

from the right ventricle and the pulmonary artery posteriorly from the left ventricle. The pulmonary and systemic circulations are therefore arranged in parallel rather than in series, with the systemic venous blood passing through the right heart chambers then back out to the body, and pulmonary venous blood traversing the left heart and returning to the lungs. Survival after birth depends on mixing between the circuits.

Transposition of the great arteries in the newborn is often an isolated defect, but other associated malformations involving defects of the atrial or ventricular septum, stenosis or atresia of the pulmonic valve, and anomalies of the atrioventricular valves are not uncommon and may alter the physiology considerably. Interestingly, extracardiac anomalies are unusual in newborns with transposition of the great arteries. Transposition of the great arteries occurs in slightly more than 1 per 4500 live births. There is a strong sex predilection in transposition of the great arteries, with males outnumbering females by almost 2:1.

The pulmonary and systemic circulations are arranged in parallel rather than in series, with the aorta arising from the right ventricle and the pulmonary artery from the left. In utero, there is little disruption in fetal hemodynamics (Fig. 62–13) because blood returning from the systemic and pulmonary veins passes unimpeded into the atrium and ventricles in the normal fashion. Blood from the right ventricle is pumped into the ascending aorta then to the systemic arteries and placenta. Blood from the left ventricle passes into the pulmonary artery, then, because of the high pulmonary resistance, most is diverted into the ductus arteriosus and descending aorta. The only variation from the normal fetal circulation is that the slightly less saturated blood from the superior vena cava is preferentially shunted to the head vessels rather than through the ductus arteriosus, and the more saturated blood from the inferior vena cava is shunted to the lungs rather than to the cerebral circulation. Despite these differences, in utero development appears normal, and thus far no major extrauterine abnormalities have been identified.

After birth, newborns completely depend on mixing between pulmonary and systemic circulations for survival. For a while the fetal pathways, the ductus arteriosus and foramen ovale, suffice. By a few hours of age, the pulmonary resistance is significantly lower than the systemic, so shunting of hypoxemic blood from the aorta to the pulmonary artery is facilitated. Because the pulmonary circuit cannot be overloaded, obligatory shunting of pulmonary venous return from left atrium to right atrium occurs. This bidirectional shunting from aorta to pulmonary artery and left atrium to right atrium improves mixing and prevents severe cyanosis. As the ductus arteriosus closes, however, the obligatory shunting is eliminated, and the only site of mixing is the foramen ovale. Although some bidirectional shunting may occur allowing deoxygenated blood to get to the lungs and oxygenated blood to the systemic circulation, this is usually inadequate, and severe systemic hypoxemia (Po_2, 15 to 40 mm Hg; O_2 saturation, 30 to 60) results.

The physical examination is usually unrewarding except for generalized cyanosis. Although peripheral pulses may be somewhat bounding and the right ventricular impulse slightly hyperactive, the heart sounds are usually normal, with physiologic splitting of the second sound present

TABLE 62–10

Eight Commonly Occurring Presentations of Infants Needing Cardiovascular Evaluation

Presentation	Lung Diseases	Heart/Systemic Diseases	Differentiating Points
Respiratory distress	RDS, pneumonia, ARDS, meconium aspiration, TTNB, diaphragmatic hernia, PPHNS (pulmonary causes), congenital lobar emphysema	CHF (any cause), absent pulmonary valve, PPHNS (cardiac causes)	Cardiomegaly is not present in pulmonary causes but is common in cardiac causes
Cyanosis	Idiopathic PPHNS	Cyanotic CHD, with either increased (TGV, truncus, TAPVD, TA) or decreased (TOF, PA, critical PS, Ebstein anomaly) pulmonary blood flow	Idiopathic PPHNS: normal cardiac contour, clear lungs/ decreased pulmonary vessels Cyanotic CHD: either increased pulmonary vessels or abnormal cardiac contour
Shock	Pulmonary hemorrhage, tension pneumothorax	IAA, coarctation, AS, HLHS, cardiomyopathy, pneumopericardium, pericardial tamponade, sepsis	Hematocrit of secretions from endotracheal tube: > 30% in pulmonary hemorrhage, < 10% in pulmonary edema from cardiac dysfunction Heart size is normal in pulmonary hemorrhage and increased in cardiac dysfunction and pericardial tamponade
Murmur	None	PDA, PPS, PS, AS, TR, VSD, MR, AVSD, coarctation	Location and radiation of murmur point to correct diagnosis
Multiple congenital anomalies	Choanal atresia, tracheoesophageal fistula, esophageal atresia (causing aspiration), tracheomalacia	Type of heart disease varies widely, depending on other anomalies/ underlying syndrome, chromosomes	Failed passage of nasal tube to stomach is diagnostic of choanal atresia, esophageal atresia, and most types of tracheoesophageal fistula
Prematurity	RDS, pneumonia	PDA	Active precordium, murmur, left atrial enlargement on echo, color flow detected shunt in PDA visualization of ductal shunt
Asphyxia	ARDS	Ischemic cardiomyopathy with pulmonary edema	Cardiomegaly, left ventricular dysfunction, and elevated cardiac enzymes present in ischemic cardiomyopathy

RDS, respiratory distress syndrome; ARDS, adult respiratory distress syndrome; TTNB, transient tachypnea of the newborn; PPHNS, persistent pulmonary hypertension of the newborn syndrome; CHF, congestive heart failure; CHD, congenital heart disease; TGV, transposition of the great vessels; TAPVD, total anomalous pulmonary venous drainage; TA, tricuspid atresia; TOF, tetralogy of Fallot; PA, pulmonary atresia; PS, pulmonary stenosis; IAA, interrupted aortic arch; AS, aortic stenosis; HLHS, hypoplastic left heart syndrome; PDA, patent ductus arteriosus; PPS, peripheral pulmonary stenosis; TR, tricuspid regurgitation; VSD, ventricular septal defect; MR, mitral regurgitation; AVSD, atrioventricular septal defect.

about half the time. Prominent heart murmurs are uncommon, although there may be a short grade 2/6 systolic murmur along the left sternal border. A loud murmur should alert one to the possibility of associated heart disease (e.g., a VSD). Signs of congestive failure are usually absent, although tachypnea may be present, probably as a compensatory mechanism for the hypoxemia.

Because there is little disturbance in the intrauterine blood flow, the electrocardiogram is usually normal showing right axis deviation and right ventricular hypertrophy that is within the normal limits for age. The chest radiography is also usually normal for a newborn, although the relative

anteroposterior position of the great vessels and the usual (although unexplained) absence of a thymic shadow give the narrow appearance of the superior mediastinum frequently described as an *egg-on-side* appearance. The pulmonary blood flow is rarely increased in the first few days of life, although it may be increased in infants who present later.

Transposition of the great arteries should be strongly suspected in any cyanotic newborn showing normal-to-increased pulmonary blood flow on the radiograph and right ventricular hypertrophy on the electrocardiogram. A severely hypoxemic infant breathing comfortably with a

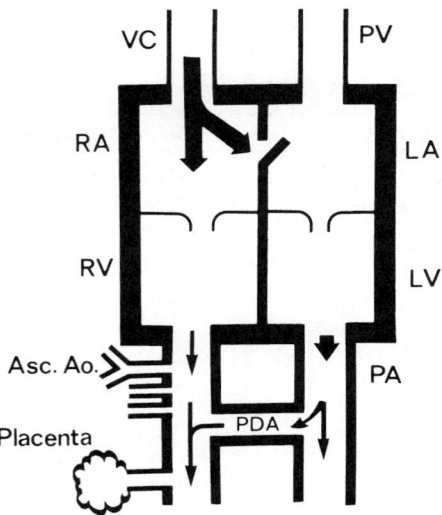

FIGURE 62–13. Schematic diagram of the fetal circulation in transposition of the great arteries. Venous blood returning to the heart via the vena cava passes either into the right atrium, right ventricle, and aorta or through the foramen ovale to the left atrium, left ventricle, and pulmonary artery. As in the normal fetus, most of the blood entering the main pulmonary artery is diverted through the ductus arteriosus into the descending aorta and placenta because of the high pulmonary vascular resistance. Asc Ao, ascending aorta; LA, left atrium; LV, left ventricle; PA, pulmonary artery; PDA, patent ductus arteriosus; PV, pulmonary vein; RA, right atrium; RV, right ventricle; VC, vena cava.

Tetralogy of Fallot

In 1888, Fallot described a series of cyanotic patients with a VSD, pulmonary stenosis, right ventricular hypertrophy, and an aorta that appeared to be over the ventricular septum. For many years, it has been appreciated that the last two manifestations are secondary to the first two lesions.

The VSD location is predictably high in the ventricular septum; additional defects are present in 15% of the patients. The degree of pulmonic obstruction at the infundibulum (subvalvular) or secondarily at the pulmonary valve or peripheral pulmonary arteries is variable, ranging from mild stenosis to complete atresia, and accounts for the variability of presentation. Associated anomalies include ASDs, right aortic arch (25%), and anomalies of the coronary arteries (5%). TOF occurs slightly less frequently than transpositions (1 of every 5000 live births) and accounts for 9% of infants presenting in the 1st week of life.

In utero there does not seem to be any major hemodynamic disturbance, and consequently, newborns with TOF are well developed at birth. During fetal life, the aorta carries an increased percentage of combined ventricular output with the exact proportion a function of the degree of pulmonic stenosis (Fig. 62–14). The ductus arteriosus is smaller than normal because its flow is diminished, and it may be quite tortuous. Because there is no volume or pressure overload within the heart, the ventricles and atrioventricular valves usually develop normally.

After birth, the degree of shunting depends on the

normal physical examination, chest radiograph, and electrocardiogram almost invariably has transposition. All other types of cyanotic congenital heart disease are associated with diminished or congested pulmonary vascular markings on the radiograph and a single second heart sound. Persistent fetal circulation can usually be distinguished by echocardiography.

Untreated transposition of the great arteries in infants is associated with a dismal prognosis; 30% die in the 1st week, and 50% die in the first months of life. The management involves three phases: rapid correction of metabolic derangements, palliation, and later correction. If the infant is acidotic with a pH of less than 7.25 when first seen, sodium bicarbonate should be given to correct the base deficit. In those who are severely acidotic or in whom further palliation must be delayed, PGE_1 is used to open the ductus arteriosus and improve mixing and oxygenation.

Surgical correction historically has involved rerouting the blood at the atrial level (Senning or Mustard procedures). More recently, most centers have performed an arterial switch including coronary relocation as a primary operation in the perinatal period. Surgical mortality has been reduced to about 5% to 10% in most centers, with excellent medium-term survival (up to 10 to 15 years) (Casteñeda et al, 1994).

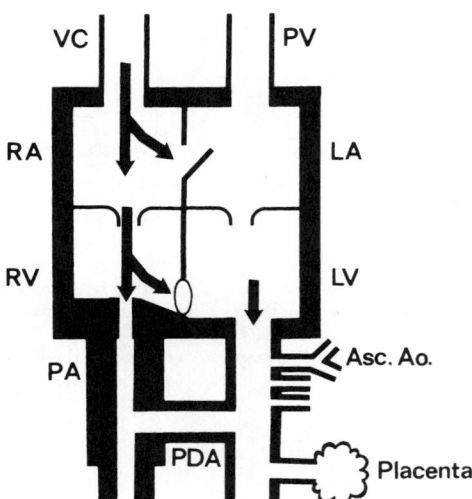

FIGURE 62–14. Schematic diagram of the circulation in the fetus with tetralogy of Fallot. Because of the right ventricular outflow obstruction, some of the right ventricular output passes across the ventricular septal defect into the left ventricle and out the aorta. If the pulmonary stenosis is severe, pulmonary blood flow may be augmented by blood from the aorta passing through the ductus arteriosus. Blood flow to the placenta is unimpeded. The abbreviations in this diagram are the same as those used in Figure 62–13.

severity of the pulmonary stenosis and the relative pulmonary and systemic arteriolar resistance. In the newborn with severe pulmonary stenosis, the resistance to blood passing out the right ventricular outflow tract is high, and desaturated venous blood preferentially passes through the VSD into the aorta, resulting in arterial hypoxemia and cyanosis. If the pulmonary stenosis is mild, there may be little resistance to blood passing out the pulmonary artery; infants with this condition may behave similar to those with a VSD, with increasing left-to-right shunt and heart failure as the pulmonary arteriolar resistance drops over the first weeks of life. The usual hallmarks of TOF, arterial hypoxemia and cyanosis, may be completely absent in this group at first. Occasionally, mild-to-moderate pulmonary stenosis may occur in a balanced situation in which pulmonary and systemic resistances are equal and little shunt in either direction occurs; often these infants shunt right-to-left with crying.

The presentation of infants with tetralogy is a function of the degree of pulmonary stenosis. Those with severe obstruction usually present in the first days with extreme cyanosis as the ductus arteriosus closes. Those with lesser degrees of pulmonary stenosis may be only mildly cyanotic and present with a systolic ejection murmur along the left sternal border in the delivery room or in the nursery. The pulmonary component of the second heart sound is diminished or inaudible. Signs of congestive heart failure are absent except in a small group with an absent pulmonary valve who present with a to-and-fro murmur at the left upper sternal border owing to pulmonary stenosis and regurgitation. Tetralogy *spells*, which are attacks of paroxysmal dyspnea associated with irritability, extreme cyanosis, and loss of the systolic murmur, are an emergency because cerebral hypoxemia may lead to convulsions, coma, and death. Spells are unusual in the first months of life.

Because the right ventricle receives normal flow in utero, the electrocardiogram of the newborn with TOF is normal, showing right axis deviation and right ventricular hypertrophy. The heart size on the chest radiograph is usually normal because neither the atria nor the ventricles are exposed to a volume overload. In those who are hypoxemic, the pulmonary blood flow is decreased because venous blood is being diverted away from the lungs to the systemic circuit. The main pulmonary artery segment is often diminished, giving the classic *coeur-en-sabot* appearance (Fig. 62–15). A right aortic arch is present in one fourth of the cases.

The cyanotic infant with decreased pulmonary blood flow and a normal heart size on the chest radiograph, right axis deviation and right ventricular hypertrophy on the electrocardiogram, and a systolic ejection murmur on examination usually has TOF. Infants with a systolic murmur without cyanosis may be confused with patients with isolated valvular pulmonary stenosis or even those with a VSD. More complicated lesions with a physiology similar to that of TOF, ventricular defect, and pulmonary stenosis must be differentiated by echocardiography or angiocardiography. Examples are double-outlet ventricle with pulmonary stenosis, single ventricle with pulmonary stenosis, and transposition.

Historically, the approach to TOF has been either early palliation with an aortopulmonary shunt or corrective surgery. Most centers now reserve palliative surgery for those younger than 1 year, but an increasing number of surgeons are doing corrective operations at the time of presentation. Surgery involves closing the VSD, usually through a right ventriculotomy; resecting infundibular muscle; and if the infundibular muscle, pulmonary valve, and main pulmonary artery are hypoplastic, using a pericardial patch to open the narrowed area. Failure to close the VSD is unusual, although some degree of residual right ventricular outflow tract obstruction is common. When the patch crosses the pulmonary annulus, the children are left with pulmonary regurgitation. Recently, long-term (30-year) follow-up studies have become available, with an actuarial survival of more than 86% at 30 years for those repaired during childhood (Murphy et al, 1993).

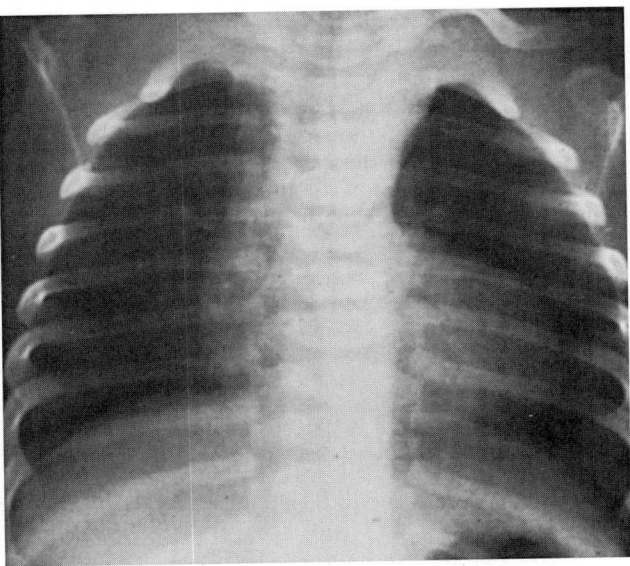

FIGURE 62–15. Plain anteroposterior roentgenogram from a newborn with tetralogy of Fallot. Note the absent main pulmonary artery segment and uplifted apex (coeur-en-sabot). The pulmonary blood flow is decreased.

Tetralogy of Fallot with Pulmonary Atresia

TOF with pulmonary atresia is the severest form of TOF, with the deviated parietal band of the infundibulum completely occluding the right ventricular outflow tract. Because there is no antegrade flow through the pulmonic valve, development of the pulmonary arteries depends on flow from the ductus arteriosus and embryologic intersegmental or bronchial arteries. If the flow into the pulmonary arteries is proximal, the mediastinal portion of the right and left pulmonary arteries may be of good size. If, however, the collaterals insert well within the hilum of the lungs, the mediastinal portions may be hypoplastic or even atretic. Even when central pulmonary arteries are present, there may be incomplete arborization of the pulmonary arteries with some or most of the lung parenchyma supplied via the collateral systemic arteries rather than the mediastinal pulmonary arteries.

A cyanotic infant showing decreased pulmonary blood flow on the radiograph, right ventricular hypertrophy on the electrocardiogram, and no murmur or a continuous murmur usually has TOF with pulmonary atresia. Newborns with transposition and an intact ventricular septum have no murmurs and may be just as cyanotic but have normal or increased pulmonary blood flow visible on chest radiographs. Infants with total anomalous pulmonary venous return usually show a pulmonary venous congestion pattern on the chest radiographs. More complicated lesions simulating TOF with pulmonary atresia must be distinguished by two-dimensional echocardiogram or angiography.

Those infants with large collaterals and congestive heart failure can usually be distinguished from infants with a VSD, PDA, or aortopulmonary window on the basis of their arterial hypoxemia as well as from those with truncus arteriosus and transposition with a VSD on the basis of the continuous murmurs.

Since there is no forward pulmonary blood flow, these infants frequently become very sick when the ductus arteriosus closes. For those who present with severe hypoxemia and acidosis, PGE_1 is usually sufficient to give temporary improvement. Reparative surgery is more problematic than in infants with a pulmonary stenosis because of the common accompaniment of hypoplasia or even discontinuity of pulmonary arteries.

Some centers use a palliative systemic-to-pulmonary artery shunt in the perinatal period with later repair. Other centers have been doing primary repair in those with an adequate pulmonary tree by closing the VSD and using an external conduit (usually aortic homograft) between the right ventricle and pulmonary artery. Surgery is necessary later in childhood because of the fixed size of the conduit, which becomes relatively smaller with somatic growth. For children with hypoplastic or discontinuous pulmonary arteries, a staged procedure is frequently necessary involving palliative surgical operations (unifocalization) and catheterization laboratory intervention to dilate or stent the hypoplastic pulmonary arteries (Castañeda et al, 1994).

Pulmonary Atresia with an Intact Ventricular Septum

In pulmonary atresia with an intact ventricular septum (approximately 1/14,000 births), the pulmonary valve is an imperforate membrane. In more than 80% of the newborn patients, the right ventricle is moderately or severely hypoplastic, often having a volume of only 1 or 2 mL at birth. The tricuspid valve annulus is also hypoplastic, corresponding to the size of the right ventricle, and the valve may be stenotic owing to fusion of the chordae. The right atrium is invariably enlarged and hypertrophied and may be enormous in infants with severe tricuspid regurgitation. The high pressure within the right ventricular cavity causes dilation of the normal myocardial sinusoids, and connections are often present between the sinusoids and coronary arteries, with flow going from right ventricle to ascending aorta. Obstructions in the coronary arteries are not uncommon in this group with sinusoids, and myocardial perfusion may be via the right ventricle, the aorta, or both. In contrast to patients with TOF associated with pulmonary atresia, the infants with pulmonary atresia and an intact ventric-

ular septum almost invariably have normal pulmonary arteries.

Prenatally, egress of blood from the right ventricle is prevented by the pulmonary atresia (Fig. 62–16). All the venous blood returning to the right atrium must pass through the foramen ovale to the left atrium, left ventricle, and ascending aorta; these chambers are dilated compared with those in the normal fetus. Conversely, because flow to the right ventricle is minimal, this chamber is usually hypoplastic. The pulmonary blood flow in utero is derived entirely from the aorta via a small, usually tortuous, ductus arteriosus. This physiologic arrangement does not disrupt the normal growth and development during fetal life. After birth, there is a continuation of the fetal pattern; the pulmonary blood flow continues to be totally dependent on the small ductus arteriosus. As this closes in the first hours or days of life, the minimal pulmonary blood flow diminishes further, and severe hypoxemia and acidosis follow.

Infants with pulmonary atresia are mildly cyanotic soon after birth but are often intensely cyanotic by 24 hours of age as the ductus arteriosus constricts. On physical examination, the second heart sound is single. A continuous murmur, from left-to-right shunting through the ductus arteriosus, or a systolic regurgitant murmur along the left sternal border, secondary to tricuspid regurgitation, may be heard; however, in about 20% of infants, no murmur is audible. The liver is enlarged if tricuspid regurgitation is severe and the foramen ovale is restrictive.

On chest radiographs, the cardiothoracic ratio is increased because of dilation of the right atrium and left ventricle, and the pulmonary vascular markings are invariably reduced. The aortic arch is to the left of the trachea in almost all infants. The electrocardiogram is characteristic and extremely helpful in the differential diagnosis (Fig.

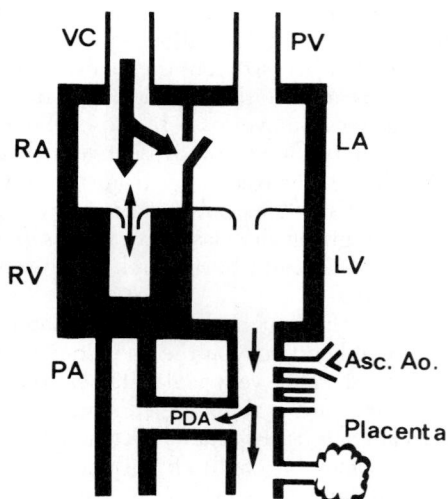

FIGURE 62–16. Schematic diagram of the circulation in the fetus with pulmonary atresia and an intact ventricular septum. All the systemic venous return from the vena cava passes across the foramen ovale into the left atrium. Pulmonary blood flow before and after birth is derived from the aorta via the ductus arteriosus. Because right ventricular flow is minimal, the chamber remains quite small. The abbreviations in this diagram are the same as those used in Figure 62–13.

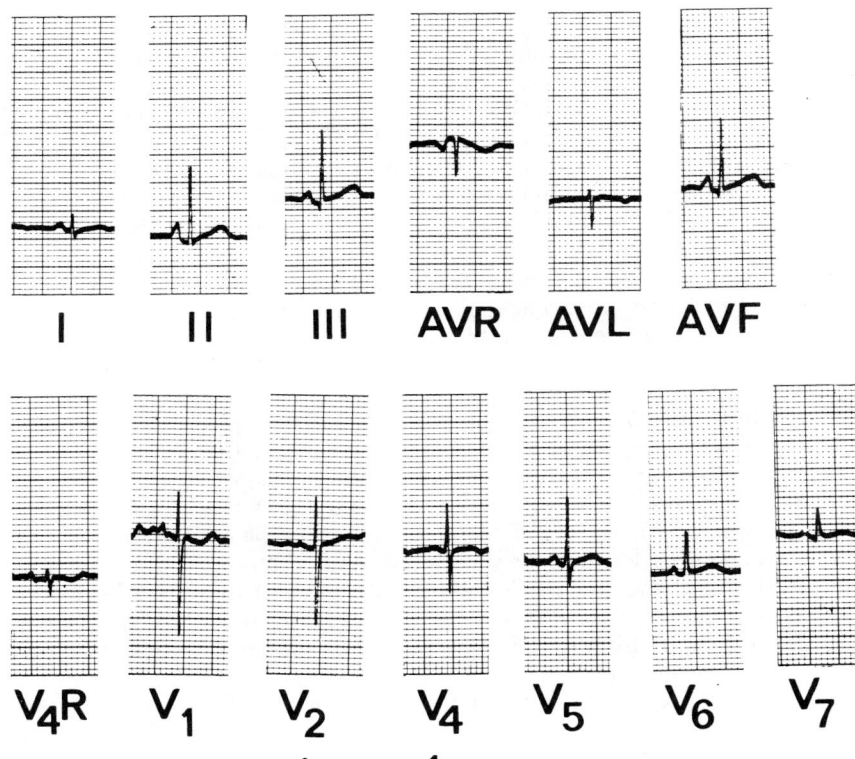

FIGURE 62–17. Electrocardiogram from a 3-day-old newborn with pulmonary atresia and an intact ventricular septum. Note the leftward QRS axis (+ 75 degrees) and the left ventricular predominance for age. The P waves are tall and peaked in II, suggesting right atrial hypertrophy.

I   II   III   AVR   AVL   AVF

V₄R   V₁   V₂   V₄   V₅   V₆   V₇
              ½   ½

62–17). Because of the right ventricular hypoplasia and low volume of blood in the right ventricle and large left ventricle in utero, there is a left ventricular predominance in the precordial leads, with a QRS axis of + 30 to + 120 degrees. Right atrial hypertrophy is also often seen.

A cyanotic newborn with pulmonary atresia and an intact ventricular septum can usually be distinguished from an infant with transposition of the great arteries with an intact ventricular septum because the latter child has a split second heart sound, increased pulmonary flow on the radiograph, right ventricular hypertrophy on the electrocardiogram, and a characteristic echocardiogram. Infants with tricuspid atresia and a hypoplastic right ventricle show decreased pulmonary flow on the radiograph and left ventricular predominance on electrocardiogram, but they almost invariably have a QRS axis of − 30 to − 90 degrees on the electrocardiogram, whereas infants with pulmonary atresia have a QRS axis of + 30 to + 120 degrees. Infants with pulmonary stenosis and a hypoplastic right ventricle may be difficult to distinguish from those with pulmonary atresia before angiography but usually have a pulmonary ejection murmur rather than a regurgitant murmur and a valve that can be seen on two-dimensional echocardiography.

The initial treatment must be directed at correcting the metabolic acidosis with oxygen and bicarbonate. The value of PGE₁ to dilate the ductus arteriosus, increase pulmonary blood flow, and improve oxygenation has been well demonstrated (Freed et al, 1981). PGE₁ is useful in allowing time for stabilization of the infants before initiation of surgery.

The surgical therapy of pulmonary atresia with an intact ventricular septum depends on the degree of hypoplasia of the right ventricle and tricuspid valve (Hanley FL et al, 1993). When near normal in size, a pulmonary valvulotomy or right ventricular outflow tract patch may suffice. If the right ventricle and tricuspid valve are intermediate in size, a right ventricular outflow tract patch and palliative aortopulmonary shunt are frequently performed in the perinatal period. If the right ventricle and tricuspid valve grow, the palliative shunt can be closed either in the interventional catheterization laboratory or surgically. If there is no significant growth, a Fontan operation is required, directing systemic venous blood to the pulmonary artery, bypassing the right ventricle. For children with extreme hypoplasia of the right ventricle and tricuspid valve, frequently with sinusoidal connections and right-to-left shunting between the right ventricle and the coronary arteries, the long-term approach should be directed toward the Fontan, although a palliative aortopulmonary shunt must be done in the perinatal period since the Fontan will not work with the elevated pulmonary vascular resistance of the perinatal period.

Pulmonary Stenosis with an Intact Ventricular Septum

In this lesion (1/14,000 live births), the pulmonary valve has a narrowed orifice that is usually due to fusion of the three pulmonary commissures. The size of the right ventricular cavity can be normal but is usually somewhat hypoplastic in those infants who present with cyanosis in the 1st month of life. The size of the chamber is rarely, if ever, as small as that seen in infants with pulmonary atresia and an intact ventricular septum, and abnormalities of the tricuspid valve and right ventricular sinusoidal–coronary artery fistulas are less common. The main and peripheral pulmonary arteries are usually normal.

In utero the obstruction at the pulmonary valve results in hypertrophy as well as a loss of compliance of the right ventricle. This leads to diversion of an increased proportion of venous return through the foramen ovale to the left side of the heart and ascending aorta. If the stenosis appears early in gestation and is severe, significant hypoplasia of the right ventricle with corresponding enlargement of the left ventricle occurs, resembling that seen in pulmonary atresia and an intact ventricular septum. If the stenosis is milder and occurs later in gestation, the right ventricle can be normal or near normal in size.

After birth, the degree of right-to-left shunting at the atrial level and thus arterial hypoxemia depends on the degree of pulmonary stenosis and right ventricular hypoplasia. If the stenosis is severe, right-to-left shunting at the atrial level may be massive and adequate pulmonary blood flow dependent on left-to-right shunting through the ductus arteriosus. If the stenosis is milder, with most of the pulmonary blood flow through the pulmonary valve, there may be little effect from ductal closure. As the pulmonary arteriolar resistance (in series with the pulmonary valve resistance) decreases over the first few weeks of life, the right-to-left shunt at the atrial level and, thus, the systemic hypoxemia may decrease.

In mild pulmonary stenosis, a loud systolic ejection murmur at the left upper sternal border may be the only finding. In moderate or severe stenosis, the murmur is less prominent, but cyanosis is present, increasing as the ductus arteriosus constricts. There is a prominent *a* wave in the jugular venous pulse reflecting reduced right ventricular compliance, and the liver is often enlarged and may even be pulsatile. The pulmonary component of the second heart sound is delayed and diminished and may be inaudible.

On chest radiograph, there is mild cardiomegaly owing to an enlarged right atrium and diminished pulmonary blood flow. Poststenotic dilation in the main pulmonary artery in the newborn is unusual. The electrocardiogram is normal if the pulmonary stenosis is mild or moderate. With severe pulmonary stenosis and a diminutive right ventricle, the electrocardiogram usually demonstrates right atrial enlargement and left ventricular predominance with a QRS axis of $+30$ to $+120$ degrees, similar to that seen in pulmonary atresia with an intact ventricular septum.

With severe obstruction and right ventricular hypoplasia, pulmonary stenosis can be confused with pulmonary atresia with an intact ventricular septum. Usually an ejection rather than regurgitant murmur at the left upper sternal border allows one to differentiate these conditions, but occasionally echocardiography, angiography, or even surgical inspection is necessary to make the diagnosis with certainty. Newborns with tricuspid atresia usually have a superior axis (-90 to -30 degrees) on the electrocardiogram, and those with transposition rarely have a loud murmur and have normal or increased flow on the chest radiograph. If the right ventricle is not diminutive, the electrocardiogram has right ventricular predominance, and it may be difficult to differentiate pulmonary stenosis with an intact ventricular septum from pulmonary stenosis with

a VSD (TOF). Echocardiography usually detects the latter because of the overriding aorta and absence of echoes in the area of the ventricular septum. The murmur of mild valvular pulmonary stenosis can be confused with the murmur of a VSD, ASD, or peripheral pulmonary stenosis.

The treatment of the cyanotic newborn with critical pulmonary stenosis is surgical intervention or balloon dilation (Caspi J et al, 1990). For the severely hypoxemic neonate, oxygen and PGE$_1$ are the initial therapy, with bicarbonate added if metabolic acidosis is present. While the gold standard used to be surgical valvotomy, balloon valvuloplasty has replaced surgical therapy as a first approach at most centers. The procedure can be done at low risk and a very high likelihood of long-term palliation.

Tricuspid Atresia

In tricuspid atresia (1/20,000 live births), there is a failure of development of the right atrioventricular valve; therefore an intra-atrial communication, usually a patent foramen ovale, is necessary for survival. There is usually a VSD connecting a large left ventricular cavity with a hypoplastic chamber that represents the infundibulum or outflow portion of the right ventricle. The great arteries may be either normally related (Type I) or transposed (Type II), and there may be pulmonary atresia (a), pulmonary stenosis (b), or no pulmonary stenosis (c). About 70% of infants with tricuspid atresia have Type I, with three fourths of these having pulmonary stenosis (b). In contrast, of the 30% who have Type II (transposition), more than three fourths have no pulmonary stenosis (c). The presentation of newborns with tricuspid atresia depends on the anatomy. Those with severe pulmonary stenosis or atresia present with cyanosis in the first few days of life. Infants with a large VSD and no pulmonary stenosis present with congestive heart failure, usually late in the 1st or during the 2nd month as the pulmonary vascular resistance falls.

The presence of tricuspid atresia in utero must be compatible with a relatively normal intrauterine circulation because growth and development proceed normally. Because the tricuspid valve is atretic, all systemic venous return is diverted across the foramen ovale into left atrium and left ventricle (Fig. 62–18). If the great arteries are normally related and the ventricular septum is intact or if the pulmonary valve is atretic, all the left ventricular output passes through the aorta, and pulmonary blood flow is via the ductus arteriosus. If the VSD is large, some of the left ventricular output passes through the VSD into the hypoplastic right ventricle, exiting the pulmonary artery if the vessels are normally related and exiting the aorta if transposition is present. Either way, there is antegrade flow through the pulmonary artery and ductus arteriosus.

After birth, there is little change in the circulation, but the normal postnatal alterations impose significant handicaps. The newborns with pulmonary atresia or severe pulmonary stenosis continue to depend on the ductus arteriosus for pulmonary blood flow. When the ductus begins to close, severe hypoxemia, acidosis, and eventually death follow.

Infants with pulmonary stenosis or atresia (a,b) are usually cyanotic soon after birth, with the cyanosis increasing as the ductus arteriosus closes. Those with pulmonary ste-

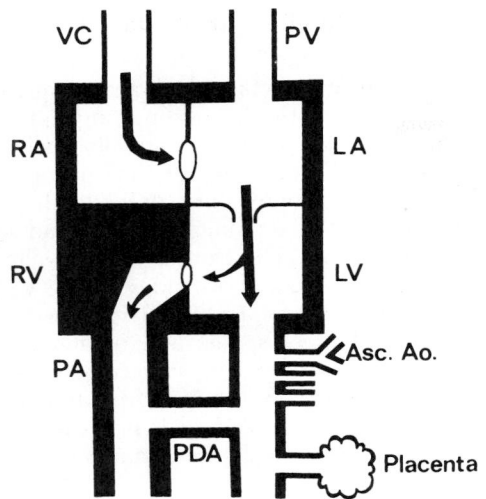

FIGURE 62–18. Schematic diagram of the circulation in the fetus with tricuspid atresia. All the venous return from the vena cava passes across the atrial septum into the left atrium and ventricle. Pulmonary blood flow before (and after) birth is via a ventricular septal defect or through the ductus arteriosus. Blood flow to the placenta for oxygenation is unimpeded. The abbreviations in this diagram are the same as those used in Figure 62–13.

nosis usually have a loud systolic ejection murmur along the left sternal border; those with pulmonary atresia may have no murmur at all or a continuous murmur from the ductus arteriosus. Infants with type c (no pulmonary stenosis) may have minimal cyanosis with an ejection murmur and heart failure as the major manifestations of heart disease. The heart size and the pulmonary blood flow visible on the radiographs are determined by the degree of pulmonary stenosis. Infants with pulmonary atresia or stenosis have a small heart with decreased pulmonary blood flow; those without pulmonary stenosis have a large heart with increased pulmonary flow. A right aortic arch is occasionally present.

The electrocardiogram is usually helpful. Because of the right ventricular hypoplasia and increased left ventricular flow in utero, left ventricular predominance with diminished right ventricular forces is almost universal. The QRS axis is almost always superior (0 to −90 degrees) in Type I, probably in large part owing to early origin of the left bundle of the conducting system and the resultant abnormal depolarization sequence. Right atrial hypertrophy is frequently present.

In the cyanotic infant, tricuspid atresia can be differentiated from transposition, TOF, and Ebstein disease of the tricuspid valve by the demonstration of left ventricular predominance on the electrocardiogram and from pulmonary atresia or stenosis with a diminutive right ventricle on the basis of the superior QRS axis. In the minimally cyanotic infant, tricuspid atresia can be differentiated from the atrioventricular canal type of VSD by electrocardiography or echocardiography and from the more complicated types of acyanotic heart disease by the presence of arterial hypoxemia, which is especially evident while the infant is crying.

In the severely hypoxic infant, the primary treatment is oxygen, bicarbonate, and PGE$_1$, followed by a systemic-to-pulmonary artery shunt. For those with a large enough VSD sufficient to provide adequate pulmonary blood flow, no palliation may be necessary in the perinatal period. For those with a large, nonrestrictive VSD and no pulmonary stenosis, the increased pulmonary blood flow may lead to congestive heart failure and require a palliative banding procedure. The Fontan operation (right atrium–to–pulmonary artery connection) provides palliation for children with tricuspid atresia. This cannot be done in the perinatal period because of increased pulmonary vascular resistance and is usually performed somewhere between 6 months and 3 years of age. It has provided good long-term palliation with a complication rate (arrhythmias, stroke, protein-losing enteropathy, or atrial arrhythmias) of about 1% per year (Cetta et al, 1996).

Ebstein Anomaly of the Tricuspid Valve

In 1866, Ebstein described the heart of a 19-year-old man with cyanosis and palpitations who died of heart failure with an anomaly of the tricuspid valve. The lesion (1/80,000 live births), now known as Ebstein anomaly of the tricuspid valve, is due to redundancy and dysplasia of the tricuspid valve with adherence of a variable portion of the septal and, often, posterior leaflets to the right ventricular wall so that the free portion of the leaflets is displaced downward, away from the normal atrioventricular ring. Thus, the atrium and ventricle are divided in three segments: a normal right atrium, a portion of the atrium above the displaced valve that is partly ventricular myocardium, and the true right ventricle. The tricuspid valve is usually regurgitant and, at least in the newborn, stenotic. The right atrium is often large, in part owing to the muscularized segment but primarily because of the tricuspid stenosis and regurgitation; the right ventricle is correspondingly small. An ASD (or patent foramen ovale) is almost always present in the newborn, and pulmonary stenosis and atresia are not uncommon. Other associated lesions such as VSDs, coarctation, and transposition are rarely seen.

In utero the incompetent or stenotic tricuspid valve diverts systemic venous return through the foramen ovale into the left side of the heart, resulting in increased left atrial and ventricular flow. The tricuspid regurgitation into the right atrium leads to severe right atrial dilation and hypertrophy before birth and may cause in utero heart failure with edema or anasarca.

After birth, the degree of hypoxemia is a function of the right-to-left shunting at the atrial level. This depends on the degree of difficulty with which blood passes through the right ventricle and pulmonary artery into the lungs. With high pulmonary vascular resistance of the newborn increasing right ventricular afterload, the tricuspid regurgitation may be exacerbated and the right-to-left shunting at the atrial level massive. These severely hypoxic infants may depend on the ductus arteriosus for most of their pulmonary blood flow, and when the ductus closes, the hypoxemia may be severe, and acidosis may develop. If the foramen ovale is restrictive, preventing decompensation of the right atrium, right-sided heart failure with hepatomegaly may be prominent.

If the tricuspid stenosis and regurgitation are less severe, right-to-left shunting and, therefore, cyanosis may be less prominent. In either case, as the pulmonary vascular resistance drops over the first few days and weeks of life, reducing right ventricular afterload and tricuspid regurgitation, dramatic improvements in arterial saturation and congestive heart failure may be seen.

The infants with Ebstein anomaly who present during the neonatal period are almost invariably cyanotic. Right-sided congestive heart failure with hepatomegaly owing to severe tricuspid regurgitation is frequently present. On auscultation, there may be a quadruple rhythm composed of a loud first sound, single second sound, and loud third and fourth sounds. A pansystolic murmur of tricuspid regurgitation is often audible.

On chest radiographs, the cardiac silhouette is usually enlarged because of massive dilation of the right atrium. The largest hearts in infants with congenital disease are seen in this condition. Often it is difficult for one to see enough lung field to note the diminished pulmonary flow.

The P waves on the electrocardiogram are often tall and peaked, suggesting right atrial hypertrophy. Right ventricular conduction abnormalities prolonging the QRS duration are common, although they are not seen as frequently in the newborn as in the older child. Wolff-Parkinson-White syndrome with a short P-R interval and a delta wave may be seen in as many as 20% of children, and atrial tachycardias and flutter are not uncommon.

On chest radiographs, the hearts of children with Ebstein disease are large. In the minimally distressed infant with cyanosis, a murmur along the left sternal border, right ventricular hypertrophy on the electrocardiogram, and massive cardiomegaly, the diagnosis is almost certain.

Patients with pulmonary atresia with an intact ventricular septum or tricuspid atresia may have cyanosis and cardiac enlargement, but they usually have left rather than right ventricular hypertrophy on the electrocardiogram, and the tricuspid valve is hypoplastic or atretic on echocardiogram rather than large and redundant as in Ebstein disease. Infants with transposition of the great arteries or TOF may be just as cyanotic, but the former have increased pulmonary vascularity, and the latter rarely show cardiac enlargement on chest radiographs.

The treatment of Ebstein anomaly in the newborn period is based on two premises: (1) many infants improve markedly over the first weeks of life as the pulmonary resistance drops, and (2) surgical approaches to treating these critically ill newborns have been problematic. PGE$_1$ may be helpful in improving oxygenation in a severely cyanotic infant by maintaining patency of the ductus arteriosus until the pulmonary resistance falls. In older children, tricuspid annuloplasty or valve replacement may be successful in those with significant congestive heart failure or hypoxemia (Danielson et al, 1992). Pharmacologic therapy or ablation is useful for those with atrial arrhythmias. In those with minimal symptoms, a conservative, nonsurgical approach is probably preferable. Attempts to close the tricuspid valve transforming Ebstein disease to a single ventricle physiology and then performing a Fontan operation (right atrium–to–pulmonary artery anastomosis) has been tried with mixed results.

Truncus Arteriosus

Truncus arteriosus (about 1/33,000 live births) has been defined as the cardiac defect in which a single great artery arises from the base of the heart supplying the coronary, pulmonary, and systemic arteries. Embryologically, truncus probably results from atresia (rather than hypoplasia as is seen in TOF) of the subpulmonary infundibulum, partial or complete absence of the pulmonary valve, and an aortopulmonary septal defect. The truncal valve usually resembles a normal aortic valve and overrides a large VSD.

In utero the main consequence of truncus arteriosus is complete mixing of the systemic and pulmonary venous return above the truncal valve. The truncus is usually large, and the ductus arteriosus arising from the pulmonary arteries may be smaller than normal. Because blood flow through the heart is normal, the atrium and ventricles develop normally.

After birth, the flow to the pulmonary arteries and systemic arteries is a function of the relative resistances in the two circuits. Initially the pulmonary resistance is high, and pulmonary flow equals or slightly exceeds systemic flow. Over the first hours or days of life, however, the pulmonary arteriolar resistance decreases, and pulmonary blood flow increases. As the pulmonary venous return increases, the left ventricle must eject an increasing volume load, which eventually leads to congestive failure. Because there is common mixing of systemic and pulmonary venous blood above the truncal valve, the degree of hypoxemia decreases as the pulmonary flow increases so that these infants are only mildly cyanotic until left heart failure and pulmonary edema interfere with oxygen exchange, and pulmonary venous desaturation ensues. In some infants, the pulmonary arteries are hypoplastic or stenotic at their origin; in these patients, the pulmonary blood flow is restricted, and cyanosis rather than congestive failure may be the presenting symptom.

Children with truncus arteriosus usually present in the 1st month (and often in the 1st week) with predominantly left-sided heart failure. Tachypnea, poor feeding, increased perspiration, and intermittent cyanosis are usually prominent, and hepatomegaly is occasionally present. On physical examination, the cardiac impulse is hyperactive, and the pulses are usually bounding secondary to the diastolic run-off from the aorta. On auscultation, the second heart sound is single, although the phonocardiogram can often detect multiple components, presumably from the abnormal truncal valve cusps. Commonly a systolic ejection click is audible. Although a continuous murmur is often thought to be characteristic of truncus, it is actually unusual because pulmonary hypertension is the rule. Systolic ejection murmurs of moderate intensity (grade 2 or 3/6) as a result of relative truncal stenosis are common, and a mid-diastolic flow rumble across the mitral valve is often present.

The heart is enlarged on the chest radiograph because of dilation of the left atrium and ventricle. The pulmonary vascular markings are increased, and pulmonary venous congestion is frequently seen. A right aortic arch is present in about one fourth of cases. The QRS axis is usually normal, with biventricular hypertrophy present in about 60% of infants, left ventricular hypertrophy in 20% and pure right ventricular hypertrophy in the remainder.

A newborn with mild cyanosis, congestive heart failure, and bounding pulses probably has truncus arteriosus. Infants with a VSD, PDA, aortopulmonary window, arteriovenous fistula, or coarctation of the aorta are not cyanotic, and infants with TOF and pulmonary atresia and large collaterals who may have cyanosis and heart failure have loud continuous murmurs. In infants with tricuspid atresia and a large VSD, the electrocardiogram shows a superior axis and left ventricular hypertrophy, and infants with transposition and a large VSD do not usually have bounding pulses.

For the newborn with congestive heart failure, digoxin and diuretics may be tried but rarely suffice. Surgical repair, closing the VSD so that left ventricular blood is diverted exclusively through the truncal valve, dividing the pulmonary artery, removing it from the site of the aorta, and connecting the right ventricle to the distal pulmonary artery using a conduit (usually aortic homograft) is the procedure of choice by age 3 months to prevent pulmonary vascular disease. This approach continues to carry a significant risk but has been done in many centers with survival in the 80% to 90% range. Inevitably, surgery to replace the conduit as the children grow is necessary.

Total Anomalous Pulmonary Venous Connection

In this anomaly (1/17,000 live births), the pulmonary veins have no connection with the left atrium and drain either directly or, more commonly, indirectly into the right atrium via one of the normal embryonic channels. The embryologic defect seems to be a failure of development of the common pulmonary vein normally connecting the developing pulmonary venous plexus with the posterior aspect of the left atrium. As a consequence, one or more of the normal anastomotic channels between the pulmonary venous plexus of the lung buds and the cardinal or umbilicovitelline vein persists, allowing drainage of the pulmonary blood flow into the systemic venous atrium. If the connection to the left common cardinal system persists, postnatal drainage is to the left innominate vein (35% of cases) or to the coronary sinus (19%). Other pathways that may persist include the right common cardinal system (drainage to right superior vena cava or azygos, 11% of cases) and the umbilicovitelline system (ductus venosus or portal system, 21%). Alternatively the pulmonary veins may drain directly into the right atrium (4%). The presence of an interatrial communication, either a patent foramen ovale or a true ASD, is necessary to sustain life after birth.

The postnatal presentation depends on the degree of obstruction to pulmonary venous drainage. If obstruction is severe (almost invariable with drainage into the umbilicovitelline system and frequent with drainage into the right superior vena cava or innominate vein), the children present within the 1st week of life. If obstruction is mild or absent, presentation is usually during the second half of the 1st year or later.

In utero there is little hemodynamic disruption from total anomalous pulmonary venous connection because before birth the pulmonary blood flow represents only 5% to 10% of combined ventricular output, an amount that can be handled by the anomalous systemic venous connection

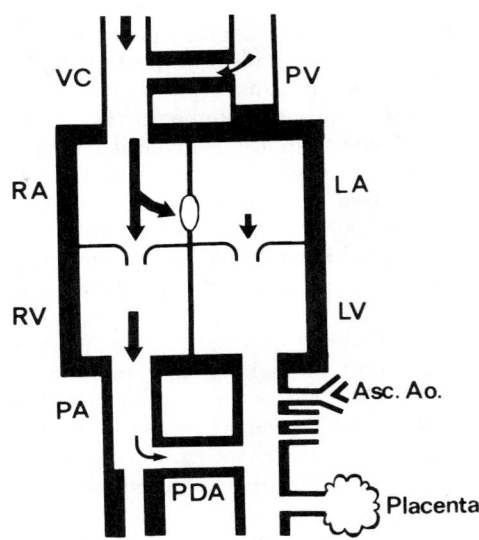

FIGURE 62–19. Schematic diagram of the circulation in a fetus with total anomalous pulmonary venous connection. The intracardiac circulation is normal. Pulmonary venous connection is to the anomalous channel connecting with one of the systemic veins. In utero, there is no hemodynamic embarrassment because pulmonary blood flow is minimal. After birth, if the anomalous channel restricts egress of blood from the pulmonary veins, pulmonary venous hypertension and pulmonary edema follow. The abbreviations are the same as those used in Figure 62–13.

(Fig. 62–19). The drainage of pulmonary venous blood to the right side of the heart rather than the left causes no apparent sequelae; the newborns are normal in size and development.

After birth, the fetal pathways persist. The pulmonary venous return continues to drain to the right atrium via one of the systemic venous channels, where it mixes with the normal systemic venous return. A portion of the totally mixed pulmonary and systemic venous return passes into the left atrium, left ventricle, and aorta, and the rest passes into the right ventricle and pulmonary artery. As the pulmonary arteriolar resistance drops, the pulmonary blood flow increases, and if there is obstruction to the increased pulmonary venous flow, pulmonary edema follows.

The pulmonary venous obstruction increases the pulmonary vascular resistance above systemic, diverting blood from the pulmonary artery into the descending aorta as long as the ductus arteriosus remains open. When the ductus begins to close, the increased pulmonary resistance elevates right ventricular and right atrial pressure and leads to increasing right-to-left shunting at the atrial level. The increased pulmonary resistance secondary to the obstruction reduces pulmonary flow, and the pulmonary edema reduces the oxygen content of the blood that is not obstructed, resulting in arterial hypoxemia and, eventually, acidosis and death.

In infants with severe pulmonary venous obstruction, the predominant finding is cyanosis. The heart is not hyperactive, and other than experiencing tachypnea, the infant is usually comfortable, at least initially. The second heart sound is single or narrowly split and accentuated. Often no murmurs are audible.

In newborns with lesser degrees of pulmonary venous obstruction, cyanosis may be less impressive, and the signs and symptoms of heart failure—tachypnea, dyspnea, and feeding difficulties—may predominate. In these infants, the right ventricular impulse is hyperdynamic, and the second heart sound is widely split, with the pulmonary component increased. A systolic ejection murmur at the left upper sternal border and a mid-diastolic murmur at the left lower sternal border secondary to increased blood flow across the pulmonary and tricuspid valves may be audible.

In infants with severe obstruction, the heart is normal in size on the chest radiograph, and pulmonary venous congestion is obvious. Those with milder obstruction have right ventricular dilation and increased pulmonary blood flow. Occasionally the dilated accessory venous channels to the left or right superior vena cava can be seen on the anteroposterior projection.

The electrocardiogram almost invariably shows right axis deviation and right ventricular hypertrophy. In the 1st week, this may be difficult to distinguish from normal, but in those who present in the 2nd week, the right ventricular hypertrophy becomes more obvious and may be associated with right atrial hypertrophy. Angiocardiography, either in the common pulmonary vein entered from the systemic venous connection or in the pulmonary artery with usual long filming, outlines the site or sites of pulmonary venous drainage except when the obstruction is almost complete (Fig. 62–20).

In the infant with severe cyanosis that is unresponsive to oxygen and a small heart and pulmonary venous congestion visible on the radiographs, the diagnosis is usually clear. It is occasionally difficult to distinguish infants with total anomalous pulmonary venous return from those with persistent fetal circulation with or without primary lung disease because (1) both groups of patients demonstrate tachypnea, dyspnea, and cyanosis on physical examination as well as haziness of the lung fields on radiographs, and (2) both may transiently improve with 100% oxygen because a perfusion imbalance may occur in either condition. In preterm infants, lung disease is more common, but in the term infant, the index of suspicion must be high for total anomalous pulmonary venous return. Echocardiography or even catheterization may occasionally be necessary to distinguish the two with certainty. HLHS may also be associated with pulmonary edema on radiographs, but there is usually extreme cardiac enlargement with increased pulmonary blood flow visible on the films and severe circulatory collapse.

The treatment of TAPVC with obstruction is surgical. The horizontal common pulmonary vein posterior to the heart is connected to the back wall of the left atrium and the anomalous systemic venous channel is ligated. Initially, surgical mortality was high, although repair can now be accomplished in more than 85% of children (Cobanoglu and Menashe, 1993). Long-term results have usually been quite good, with a small incidence of residual stenosis at the anastomotic site present in some.

Asplenia

Asplenia is one of the heterotaxia syndromes (1/12,000 live births) that are characterized by positional abnormalities of

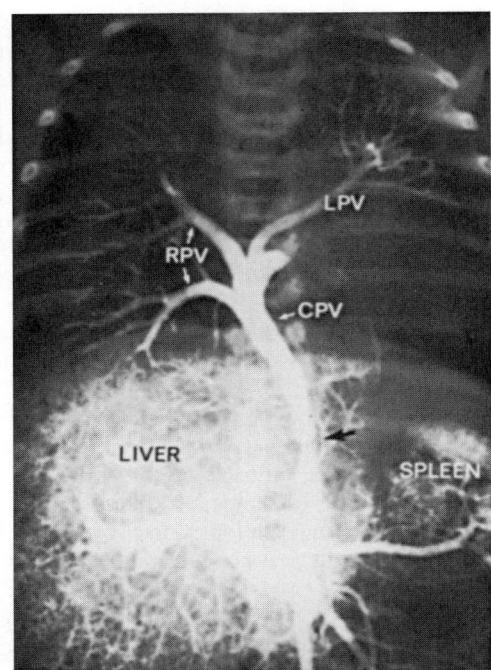

FIGURE 62–20. A postmortem angiogram in a newborn who died with total anomalous pulmonary venous connection into the portal system. The right and left pulmonary veins drain into a common trunk that descends below the diaphragm to join the portal system. Note the discrete narrowing in the pulmonary vein (arrow) that probably occurs as it pierces the diaphragm. CPV, common pulmonary vein; LPV, left pulmonary vein; RPV, right pulmonary vein.

the abdominal viscera (midline liver, stomach on the right, malrotation of the gut); splenic abnormalities (absence of spleen or multiple tiny splenules); and complex, usually cyanotic, congenital heart disease. For convenience, heterotaxia syndromes have been classified as asplenia and polysplenia, although the disease associated with asplenia may be present with a normal spleen, and polysplenia heart disease may exist with no spleen, many splenules, or a normal spleen.

In asplenia, there is *bilateral right-sidedness*. The liver tends to be midline, with right and left lobes equal in size. Both lungs are trilobed with epiarterial bronchi (bronchus over the pulmonary artery) similar to the bronchus seen in the normal right lung. There is often no rotation or reverse rotation of the midgut loop, with abnormal mesenteric attachments. Often the entire small bowel is on one side of the abdomen and the large intestine on the other. Cardiac malformations usually include bilateral superior vena cava, inferior vena cava either to the right or left of the spine, common atrium, complete atrioventricular canal, single ventricle, and total anomalous pulmonary venous return. Transposition of the great arteries is common, and severe pulmonary stenosis or atresia is almost invariably present. A helpful pathognomonic feature of asplenia, demonstrable by echocardiography, catheter passage, or angiocardiography, is the finding of the abdominal aorta and inferior vena cava on the same side of the spine.

The infants are usually normal at birth, a finding that

suggests relatively normal intrauterine development. This is not surprising because virtual common mixing of systemic venous and pulmonary venous blood normally occurs before birth, and the pulmonary stenosis or atresia and TAPVD are less important in utero because pulmonary blood flow is minimal.

After birth, the presentation is usually similar to that of newborns with a large VSD and severe pulmonary stenosis or atresia—profound cyanosis, especially as the ductus arteriosus closes.

Cyanosis is usually the presenting symptom. If the infant has pulmonary stenosis rather than atresia, a systolic murmur is audible along the left sternal border. The second heart sound is single. The asplenia syndrome may be diagnosed by the plain chest radiograph. The liver is midline and symmetric, and the stomach is found in the midline or on the right or left side of the abdomen. If the chest film is of good quality, the bilateral epiarterial bronchi are visible. The heart may be in the right chest (dextrocardia), midline (mesocardia), or in the left chest (levocardia) and is usually normal in size with reduced pulmonary vascularity. The electrocardiogram is variable. There is often a superior QRS axis (0 to − 120 degrees) with a counterclockwise loop in the frontal plane typical of an endocardial cushion defect. The configuration of the QRS complex depends on the position of the heart in the chest and the presence or absence of a ventricular septum. The P-wave axis is usually inferior and anterior with a normal P-R interval.

Infants with asplenia must be differentiated from those with large VSD and pulmonary stenosis or atresia (TOF). The characteristic picture of abdominal heterotaxia with bilateral epiarterial bronchi on chest radiographs should alert one to the probability of the asplenia syndrome. Finding the inferior vena cava and abdominal aorta on the same side of the spine seems to be pathognomonic. The finding of Howell-Jolly and Heinz bodies in red cell smears is presumptive evidence of asplenia, and the absence of spleen on ultrasound or radionuclide scan is confirmatory.

It is often more difficult to differentiate between asplenia and polysplenia. In general, the heart disease is more complex with asplenia; the lungs are trilobed, the bronchi are epiarterial, the P-wave axis is normal, and the inferior vena cava is present on the same side as the abdominal aorta. In the polysplenia syndrome, the lungs are bilobed, the bronchi hyparterial (bronchus beneath the pulmonary artery), the inferior vena cava absent, and the P-wave axis superior. Severe pulmonary stenosis is frequent in infants with asplenia and less common in polysplenia.

Temporary infusion of PGE$_1$ helps those who depend on the ductus arteriosus for pulmonary blood flow. Occasionally, the increased pulmonary blood flow may unmask latent pulmonary venous obstruction from total anomalous pulmonary venous connection that is frequently present. Palliation in the form of a systemic-to-pulmonary artery shunt has been successful in most. The Fontan operation directly connecting the systemic venous return to the pulmonary artery, leaving the single ventricle to pump pulmonary venous blood to the body, has been attempted with increasing success. The surgical mortality should be less than 15%, with the long-term complications rate (arrhythmias, strokes, protein-losing enteropathy, and congestive heart failure) approximately 1% per year.

Because children without spleens have a high risk of sepsis and, at least in the authors' experience, a higher rate of mortality from sepsis than from heart disease, the authors believe that pneumococcal vaccine and prophylactic antibiotics should be administered to all asplenic patients who survive beyond the neonatal period.

Polysplenia

In polysplenia, there is *bilateral left-sidedness*. Multiple splenules are usually present, with the mass of splenic tissue approximating that in the normal spleen. The lungs are usually bilobed, with bilateral hyparterial bronchi (bronchus beneath the pulmonary artery) present in about two thirds of the cases. The liver is often midline, and, in most infants, the stomach is on the right side. The heart disease may be as complex as that in the infants with asplenia but often is limited to abnormalities of pulmonary venous and systemic venous return. Absence of the renal-to-hepatic portion of the inferior vena cava is common, with the hepatic veins draining directly into the right atrium and the lower inferior vena cava into the right or left superior vena cava via an azygos or hemiazygos connection. The superior vena cava is frequently bilateral, and the pulmonary veins often enter separately into both atria, with the right and left veins draining into the ipsilateral atrium. Large ASDs are common, and a common atrium is not unusual. Other cardiac anomalies less frequently seen include pulmonary stenosis, double outlet right ventricle, and endocardial cushion defects. Infants with transposition of the great arteries and single ventricle are uncommon.

The prenatal and postnatal hemodynamics depend on the lesions present. If only abnormalities of pulmonary venous and systemic venous return are present, newborns are rarely symptomatic. If an endocardial cushion type of VSD without pulmonary stenosis is present, congestive failure may occur as the pulmonary vascular resistance drops. Less commonly the pulmonary stenosis is severe, and cyanosis from a right-to-left shunt predominates.

The clinical findings depend on the associated lesions present. Cyanosis may be present if there is pulmonary stenosis or atresia; congestive failure predominates if there is an endocardial cushion defect without pulmonary obstruction.

The most distinctive feature of the electrocardiogram is the superior P-wave axis, usually known as a *coronary sinus rhythm*, with a negative P wave in leads II, III, and AVF. If an endocardial cushion defect is present, the QRS axis is almost always superior (0 to −90 degrees) with a counterclockwise loop in the frontal plane. The chest radiograph is also often distinctive, with a transverse midline liver, right-sided stomach, and absence of the inferior vena cava shadow above the diaphragm in the lateral projection. If the technique is optimal, the bilateral hyparterial bronchi can often be seen.

The precise defect present determines the treatment. Those with exclusively atrial anomalies rarely require treatment in the perinatal period. For those with more complex anatomy, corrective operations are usually possible. Those without pulmonary stenosis require a palliative pulmonary artery banding operation to reduce congestive heart failure, and those with severe pulmonary stenosis require a palliative aortopulmonary shunt. The prognosis depends on the lesions present but is usually better than that associated with asplenia, since the heart disease is rarely as complex.

Coarctation of the Aorta

The sine qua non of this anomaly (1/7000 live births) is the presence of a constriction in the aorta distal to the left subclavian artery, usually at the site of insertion of the ductus arteriosus. There may be, in addition, tubular hypoplasia of the aortic arch and intracardiac anomalies. Because there is normally little flow across the aortic isthmus in utero, the tubular hypoplasia of the arch does not affect fetal growth and development. In the presence of a posterior shelf, there is also no significant hemodynamic difficulty because the flow is small and the large ductus arteriosus allows ample room for it to bypass the narrowing (Fig. 62–21).

After birth, the constriction in the aorta increases left ventricular afterload. In the presence of a VSD, this increased systemic resistance leads to a large left-to-right shunt. As the pulmonary vascular resistance falls, the left-to-right shunt increases, resulting in a volume as well as a pressure overload of the left ventricle. In addition to congestive heart failure, there is failure of the blood to pass from ascending to descending aorta if the coarctation is severe. The results are tissue hypoxia, lactic acidosis, and eventual death after the ductus arteriosus closes.

Those infants with a juxtaductal coarctation but no associated anomalies have a slightly different hemodynamic picture. In these newborns, closure of the ductus arteriosus leads to an acute increase in afterload to the left ventricle because blood must be pumped through the narrowed

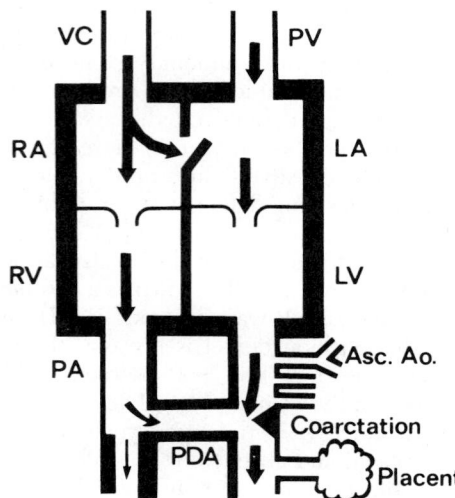

FIGURE 62–21. Schematic representation of the circulation in a fetus with coarctation of the aorta. The intracardiac blood flow is relatively normal. In utero, the constriction in the aorta is of no physiologic significance because the open ductus arteriosus allows blood to go around the obstruction. After birth, when the ductus closes, the narrowing is exhibited. The abbreviations are the same as those used in Figure 62–13.

segment. Because no obstruction was present in utero, no collateral vessels have developed. Owing in part to a reduced number of sympathetic receptors, the neonatal myocardium is not able to respond to increased work as well as the left ventricle of an older child or adult can. Consequently, congestive heart failure, with elevation of left ventricular end-diastolic, left atrial, and pulmonary venous pressures follows. Occasionally the acute left atrial dilation causes the septum secundum to become incompetent, resulting in an atrial left-to-right shunt. If the coarctation is not too severe, congestive failure may be mild, and there may be time for compensatory mechanisms (e.g., left ventricular hypertrophy or collateral vessels that bypass the obstruction) to develop.

The newborn with coarctation of the aorta presents with the usual signs and symptoms of congestive heart failure: dyspnea, tachypnea, tachycardia, hepatomegaly, poor feeding, and increased perspiration. A careful examination of the peripheral pulses demonstrates that pulses and blood pressure (by Doppler or flush method) in the legs are diminished compared with those in the arms. Blood pressure in both arms must be measured because it may be diminished in the left arm if the coarctation involves the origin of the left subclavian artery, and it may be decreased in the right arm in the rare situation in which the right subclavian arises anomalously below the coarctation as the last vessel of the aortic arch rather than as the first branch of the innominate. Occasionally the pulses in the legs *wax and wane* as the ductus arteriosus opens and closes. In the newborn with an isolated juxtaductal coarctation, there may be no murmur or, occasionally, a short systolic ejection murmur in the axilla or back. In newborns with tubular hypoplasia and a VSD, there is usually a harsh pansystolic murmur at the left lower sternal border, but its absence does not rule out a ventricular defect.

In the absence of complex intracardiac anomalies, there is right axis deviation and right ventricular hypertrophy on the electrocardiogram reflecting normal intrauterine blood flow. On the chest radiograph, the heart is enlarged with the pulmonary vascularity congested, and if a left-to-right shunt is present from a stretched foramen ovale, the heart is actively engorged. Poststenotic dilation in the descending aorta and rib notching, usually present in older children with coarctation, are not seen in newborns.

The diagnosis of coarctation of the aorta (Fig. 62–22) is obvious if there is a marked discrepancy in blood pressure between the arms and legs. As already mentioned, however, in some newborns the pulses wax and wane, presumably as the ductus arteriosus closes. Therefore, one must check the pulses and blood pressure more than once if there is any possibility of coarctation.

Coarctation of the aorta must be differentiated from other causes of congestive heart failure in the 1st or 2nd week of life. HLHS usually causes a symmetric decrease in pulses with equal blood pressures in the arms and legs and severe right ventricular hypertrophy on the electrocardiogram. Aortic stenosis also causes a symmetric decrease in pulses but is usually associated with left ventricular hypertrophy and ST-T changes on the electrocardiogram. Echocardiography or catheterization may be necessary to differentiate these lesions if no difference in pulses or blood pressure is apparent.

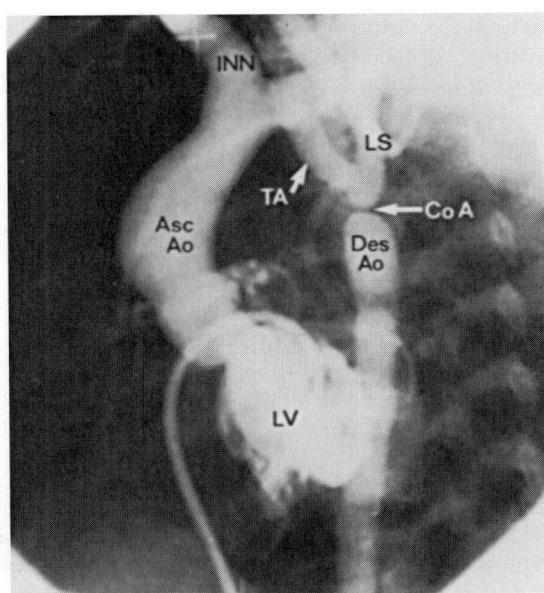

FIGURE 62–22. Lateral left ventricular angiogram in a newborn with coarctation of the aorta without a ventricular septal defect. There is a discrete narrowing in the aorta just distal to the origin of the left subclavian artery. The transverse aortic arch between the innominate artery and the left subclavian is moderately hypoplastic. Asc Ao, ascending aorta; CoA, coarctation of the aorta; Des Ao, descending aorta; INN, innominate artery; LS, left subclavian artery; LV, left ventricle; TA, transverse aortic arch.

The medical treatment of a newborn with congestive heart failure from coarctation of the aorta includes digitalis and diuretics and, if acidosis or low output is present, PGE₁, to dilate the ductus arteriosus. Those with a juxtaductal coarctation without associated heart disease are usually repaired sugically by excision of the narrowed segment and end-to-end anastomosis (Zehr et al, 1995). Some centers with an active, aggressive, interventional catheterization laboratory have performed balloon dilation in the perinatal period. This may have to be repeated in the first year of life because of recurrence, but it has become the procedure of choice in some centers.

For those with complex intracardiac anomalies (usually with tubular hypoplasia of the aortic arch), palliative or corrective operations for the underlying heart disease are frequently necessary in addition to surgical or balloon therapy of coarctation of the aorta.

Interrupted Aortic Arch

Infants with an interrupted aortic arch (1/50,000 live births) have a discontinuity between the ascending and descending aorta. Almost any cardiac anomaly can be associated with interrupted aortic arch, but a PDA and a VSD are almost invariably present, and aortic stenosis, double outlet right ventricle, truncus arteriosus, and single ventricle are not uncommon. The embryologic defect in interrupted aortic arch is not known. More than two thirds of the newborns with interrupted aortic arch have been found to have Di-George syndrome (Van Mierop and Kutsche, 1986), now

known to be due to a deletion in the 22 chromosome (22q11).

In the normal fetus, the left ventricle supplies the ascending aorta and the right ventricle supplies the descending aorta through the ductus arteriosus, with only 10% of combined ventricular output passing through the arch of the aorta from ascending to descending aorta. In the fetus with an interrupted aortic arch, no blood passes through the aortic isthmus, but this results in no major observable hemodynamic abnormalities (Fig. 62–23). After birth, however, the descending aorta continues to depend on the ductus arteriosus to provide systemic output. When the ductus begins to close, flow to the descending aorta diminishes, and tissue hypoxia, acidosis, and death follow. Rarely the ductus arteriosus remains open. In these infants, congestive heart failure occurs as the pulmonary vascular resistance falls over the first weeks of life and pulmonary blood flow increases.

The clinical presentations of the various types of interruption are similar. As the pulmonary vascular resistance falls, the newborns develop the signs and symptoms of congestive heart failure: respiratory distress, tachypnea, tachycardia, hepatomegaly, poor feeding, and increased perspiration. As the ductus arteriosus closes, the pulses and perfusion in the lower body diminish and mottling appears. Although differential cyanosis should be observable, because the upper body receives fully saturated blood from the left ventricle and the lower body receives desaturated venous blood from the pulmonary artery, it is rarely clinically apparent because a large left-to-right shunt through a VSD tends to increase the pulmonary artery oxygen saturation, and pulmonary venous desaturation from pulmonary edema lowers the aortic saturation, making the differences

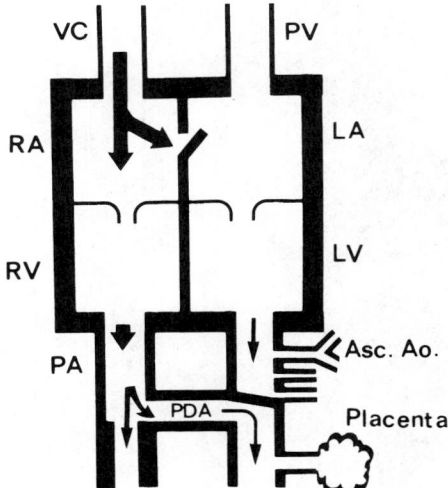

FIGURE 62–23. Schematic diagram of the circulation in a fetus with an interrupted aortic arch. The intracardiac flow is normal. Blood from the right atrium passes through the right ventricle, pulmonary artery, and ductus arteriosus to the descending aorta and placenta. Flow to the ascending aorta is derived from blood passing through the foramen ovale and left heart chambers. No blood crosses from ascending to descending aorta. After birth, when the ductus arteriosus constricts, blood supply to the lower half of the body is compromised. The abbreviations are the same as those used in Figure 62–13.

minimal and not clinically visible, even to the experienced observer. The presence of strong pulses in the left carotid but not in the left subclavian artery or in the right carotid but not left carotid artery can often localize the site of the interruption. Heart murmurs are rarely impressive in these infants, but a systolic murmur can sometimes be heard along the left sternal border, presumably from the VSD. The second sound is usually loud and single.

Because intrauterine flows are normal, the electrocardiogram is rarely helpful at birth; there is usually right axis deviation and right ventricular hypertrophy that is normal for age. No specific anomalies are present on the chest radiograph other than generalized cardiac enlargement and increased pulmonary vascular markings often associated with pulmonary venous congestion.

The diagnosis of an interrupted aortic arch (Fig. 62–24) is difficult but should be suspected in any newborn with early congestive heart failure. The finding of differential blood pressures between the arms and legs suggests either coarctation of the aorta or interruption: differences in the pulse between the right and left carotid arteries make the latter condition more probable. Other acyanotic heart diseases in the newborn in which congestive heart failure occurs (e.g., aortic stenosis and HLHS) can usually be excluded by the differential pulses in interrupted aortic arch or by the electrocardiographic finding of left ventricular hypertrophy and strain in aortic stenosis and the echocardiographic demonstration of a small ascending aorta in HLHS.

The initial treatment of newborns with interrupted aortic arch should be aimed to reopen the ductus with PGE$_1$ and treat the congestive heart failure and acidosis. After stabilization, the interrupted aortic arch can usually be repaired by direct anastomosis between the proximal and distal ends of the aortic arch. Since virtually all infants have a VSD, the operation is usually done under cardiopulmonary bypass with closure of the VSD at the same time. Perinatal survival is now above 75% (Norwood et al, 1983), with long-term prognosis usually quite good, although balloon dilation of the anastomotic site is frequently required later in childhood.

Aortic Stenosis

Although left ventricular outflow obstruction in childhood may occur below or above the valve, for all practical purposes only valvular aortic stenosis (1/16,000 live births) causes severe symptoms in the neonatal period. The valve is usually unicommissural and unicuspid, and the tissue is thickened, nodular, and severely deformed. The myocardium is always hypertrophied, but the left ventricular cavity varies in size. It may be dilated, normal, or hypoplastic; when small, the defect gradually becomes a part of HLHS. In many infants, the left ventricular endocardium is thickened and covered with a gray layer of fibrous and elastic tissue that may involve the papillary muscles, resulting in mitral regurgitation. This *endocardial fibroelastosis* is probably secondary to myocardial hypoxia from the thick myocardium, which, in the presence of high intracavitary pressures, cannot be adequately perfused in the endocardial layers. Associated lesions, such as coarctation of the aorta, VSD, and ASD, are occasionally seen.

In utero the presence of left ventricular outflow obstruction imposes a pressure load on the left ventricle. If the stenosis occurs early in gestation and is severe, the afterload reduces flow through the ventricle, and left ventricular hypoplasia and HLHS may result. If the stenosis is less severe, the left ventricular size is normal, but the myocardium is hypertrophied, and fibroelastosis from inadequate endocardial perfusion may be present.

After birth, the left ventricular output normally must increase by about 50% with the switch from a parallel to an in-series circulation. In the presence of severe aortic obstruction, the marginally compensated left ventricle may be unable to handle increased volume load. If the foramen ovale is closed, the left atrial pressure rapidly increases, leading to pulmonary edema. Occasionally, left atrial dilation makes the septum primum incompetent, allowing the left atrium to decompress through the foramen ovale. This left-to-right shunt at the atrial level may exacerbate the congestive heart failure.

The infant with critical aortic stenosis is usually normal at birth. A systolic murmur is invariably audible along the left sternal border with radiation to the right upper sternal border but may be only grade 2 or 3/6. The symptoms of congestive heart failure—respiratory distress, poor feeding, and tachypnea—may be delayed by hours to weeks; however, once symptoms occur, they may progress rapidly, leading to a low output state with cool, mottled extremities; diminished pulses; and a murmur that is barely audible. The murmur is rarely associated with a thrill, even when output is adequate, but a systolic ejection click at the apex may be present. In stark contrast with its radiographically

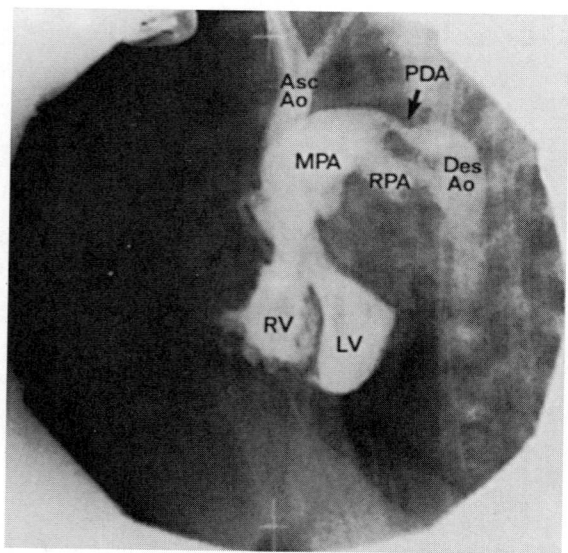

FIGURE 62–24. Lateral left ventricular angiogram of a newborn with an interrupted aortic arch. There is no connection between the ascending and descending aorta; blood flow to the descending aorta is derived from the pulmonary artery through a closing ductus arteriosus. A ventricular septal defect connecting the right and left ventricle is present. Asc Ao, ascending aorta; Des Ao, descending aorta; LV, left ventricle; MPA, main pulmonary artery; PDA, patent ductus arteriosus; RPA, right pulmonary artery; RV, right ventricle.

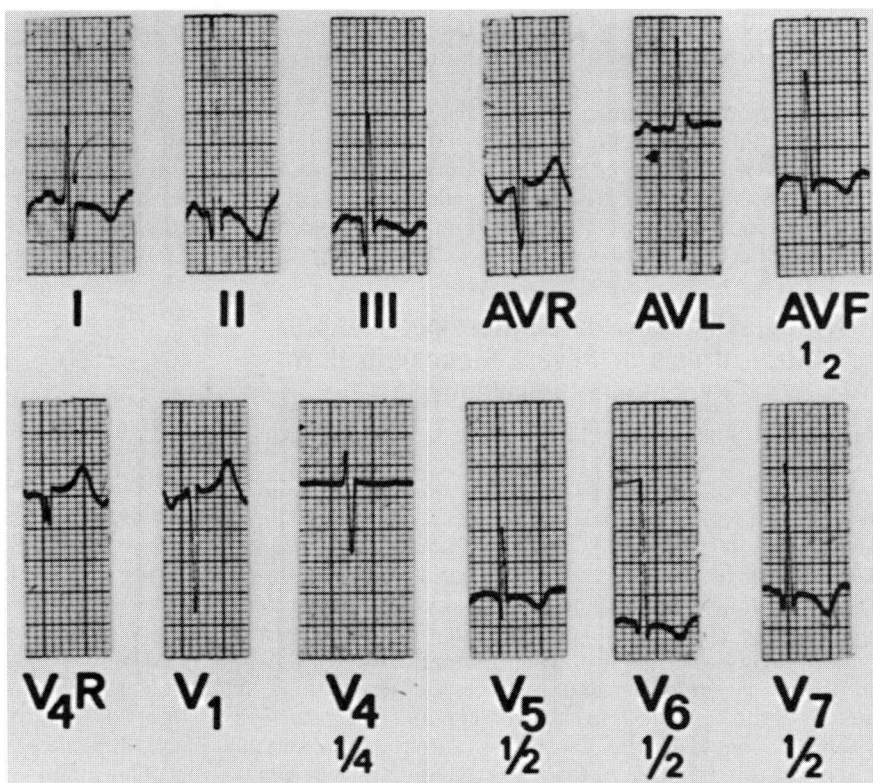

FIGURE 62–25. Electrocardiogram in a newborn with aortic stenosis. There is left ventricular hypertrophy for age. The inverted T waves in the left precordium suggest left ventricular strain (ischemia).

visible enlargement, the heart is rarely hyperactive on palpation.

The most frequent electrocardiographic pattern is left ventricular hypertrophy with inverted T waves over the left precordium, suggesting left ventricular ischemia (Fig. 62–25). Occasionally, right ventricular hypertrophy may be seen, but in our experience, this is associated with at least some hypoplasia of the left ventricle. Even in those with right ventricular predominance, inverted T waves over the left precordium are common.

In infants with congestive heart failure, the heart is invariably enlarged on chest radiographs and may be massive. The pulmonary vessels are indistinct owing to pulmonary venous congestion and may also be actively engorged if there is a large left-to-right shunt at the atrial level from a stretched foramen ovale. Using a long-axis view of the left ventricular outflow tract, two-dimensional echocardiography shows severe immobility of the aortic valve with little or no systolic opening, left ventricular hypertrophy, left atrial dilation, and poststenotic dilation in the ascending aorta. Evaluation of the ascending aorta with Doppler technique shows increased velocity of blood flow, allowing estimation of the gradient.

At cardiac catheterization, the left ventricle can usually be approached through the foramen ovale, but occasionally a retrograde study across the aortic valve or even a transatrial septal puncture may be necessary. There is usually a pressure gradient of greater than 40 mm Hg between the left ventricle and ascending aorta, with the left ventricular systolic pressure exceeding 120 mm Hg, but occasionally in infants with severe congestive heart failure, the left ventricle cannot generate such a high pressure, and the

gradient may be less. The left ventricular end-diastolic pressure is invariably elevated and has been observed to be as high as 35 mm Hg. If the foramen ovale is incompetent, a left-to-right shunt at the atrial level may be present, with the pulmonary flow–to–systemic flow ratio occasionally exceeding 3:1. A left ventricular angiocardiogram in the left anterior oblique projection outlines the domed, thickened aortic valve.

Aortic stenosis must be differentiated from other causes of heart failure in the 1st month of life. With aortic atresia and HLHS, there is congestive failure but no left ventricular hypertrophy on the electrocardiogram. In coarctation of the aorta with or without a VSD, the pulses are weak or absent in the legs but are usually palpable in the arms and carotids, and left ventricular strain on the electrocardiogram is usually not present. The murmur of aortic stenosis is loudest at the right or left upper sternal borders, whereas in infants with coarctation the murmur is louder at the lower left sternal border or into the axilla. Finally, aortic stenosis is associated with an ejection click that is rarely present in the newborn with coarctation of the aorta. With acyanotic lesions causing congestive heart failure, such as VSDs, AVCDs, and PDA, there is usually a hyperactive precordium associated with the large left-to-right shunts. In tricuspid atresia, truncus arteriosus, and single ventricle, there is usually cyanosis with crying.

These infants are usually very sick when first seen, and the usual medical management with digoxin, diuretics, and correction of the acidosis must be accomplished without delay. Aortic valvotomy under inflow occlusion or a cardiopulmonary bypass has been the procedure of choice. More recently, many interventional catheterization laboratories have attempted balloon dilation of the aortic valve with success that approaches that of the surgical procedure (Zeevi et al, 1989). The long-term prognosis is fair, with repeat dilation of the valve commonly necessary later in childhood. Valve replacement either with a prosthetic valve or, more recently, a pulmonary autograft has been necessary in some infants surviving initial palliation and is likely to be necessary for most patients later in childhood or as an adult.

Hypoplastic Left Heart Syndrome: Aortic or Mitral Atresia or Severe Stenosis with a Hypoplastic Left Ventricle

On gross pathologic examination, the hearts of children with HLHS (1/6000 live births) are all similar, with severe hypoplasia of the left ventricle and ascending aorta and a dilated right ventricle and pulmonary artery. The aortic valve may be atretic with a complete absence of any recognizable valve tissue or may be fused and domed with an eccentric pinhole orifice. The mitral valve is atretic in one fourth of the cases and hypoplastic in the rest. The left ventricle may be slitlike if both mitral and aortic valves are atretic but somewhat more developed when there is some flow through the mitral valve. The ascending aorta is hypoplastic between the coronaries and the innominate artery, and a coarctation of the aorta may be present. VSDs are uncommon.

In a fetus with a hypoplastic left heart, the right ventricle must support the entire circulation (Fig. 62–26). Almost all the systemic venous return that enters the right atrium

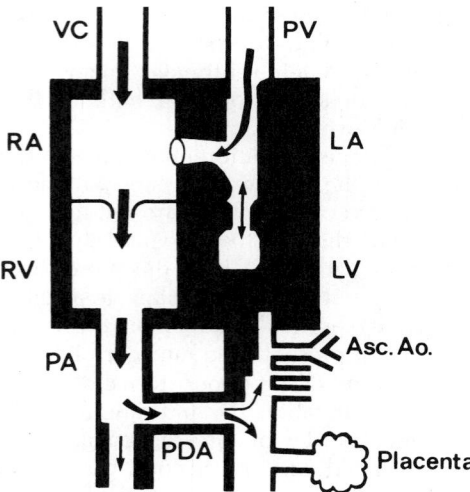

FIGURE 62–26. Schematic diagram of the circulation in a fetus with hypoplastic left heart syndrome. There is aortic atresia and hypoplasia of the left ventricle, left atrium, and mitral valve. The systemic venous return from the vena cava passes through the right heart chambers into the ductus arteriosus then to the descending aorta and placenta as well as the ascending aorta. The pulmonary venous return goes through a foramen ovale into the right atrium. After birth, the foramen may be obstructive as pulmonary flow increases. When the ductus arteriosus constricts, flow to the systemic circulation is reduced, and low-output shock and death follow. The abbreviations are the same as those used in Figure 62–13.

passes into the right ventricle and is ejected into the pulmonary artery. A small portion of blood may pass through the foramen ovale, but with mitral or aortic atresia this is minimal. Because the pulmonary resistance is high, virtually all the blood entering the pulmonary artery is diverted through the ductus arteriosus into the aorta rather than passing into the lungs. Most blood flow is retrograde into the aortic arch and ascending aorta. Flow to the subclavian, carotid, and coronary arteries is therefore also retrograde. The ascending aorta is small because the coronary arteries are the only continuation after the takeoff of the innominate artery.

After birth, the pulmonary vascular resistance falls, and the systemic resistance increases so that an increasing proportion of blood from the single pulmonary trunk goes to the lungs rather than through the ductus arteriosus. The increased pulmonary blood flow leads to an increase in pulmonary venous return that cannot freely exit from the left atrium because of hypoplasia of the left atrium and foramen ovale. Pulmonary venous hypertension and pulmonary edema result. As the ductus arteriosus begins to close at 12 to 48 hours of age, the perfusion to the systemic circulation is reduced, resulting in systemic and coronary ischemia. Newborns with this disease are the sickest patients seen by the pediatric cardiologist, with the median age of death 4.5 days in untreated infants.

The infants are usually normal at birth, but tachypnea and dyspnea soon develop as the pulmonary blood flow increases. Cyanosis is rarely prominent, despite the total mixing of the systemic and pulmonary circulations, because the pulmonary blood flow is so increased. Congestive heart failure with tachypnea, hepatomegaly, and poor feeding is usually present by 24 to 48 hours of age. Finally, as the ductus arteriosus begins to close, the signs of low output—mottling, grayness of the skin, and markedly diminished pulses—follow. One third are in vascular collapse by the time they reach the physician, with blood pressures of 40 mm Hg or less, and they are hypothermic, hypoglycemic, and ashen in color. Auscultation is rarely helpful because prominent murmurs are unusual, and the second heart sound is single.

The electrocardiogram reflects the intrauterine circulation, showing right axis deviation and right ventricular predominance that may be normal for age. Occasionally, diminished left-sided forces owing to left ventricular hypoplasia can be appreciated. Right atrial hypertrophy is seen in about two thirds of the infants. Coronary ischemia frequently results in ST-T wave changes. A marked sinus tachycardia is usually present. The heart is markedly enlarged on chest radiographs, with both increased pulmonary blood flow and pulmonary venous congestion prominent. Angiography demonstrates severe hypoplasia of the ascending aorta (Fig. 62–27).

Infants with HLHS must be differentiated from those with other causes of respiratory distress in the 1st month of life. In the early stages, the tachypnea may suggest lung disease, but the appearance of congestive heart failure with tachycardia, hepatomegaly, and cardiac enlargement on radiographs should allow the two to be differentiated. Nonstructural heart diseases, myocarditis, transient myocardial ischemia, and intrauterine supraventricular tachycardia

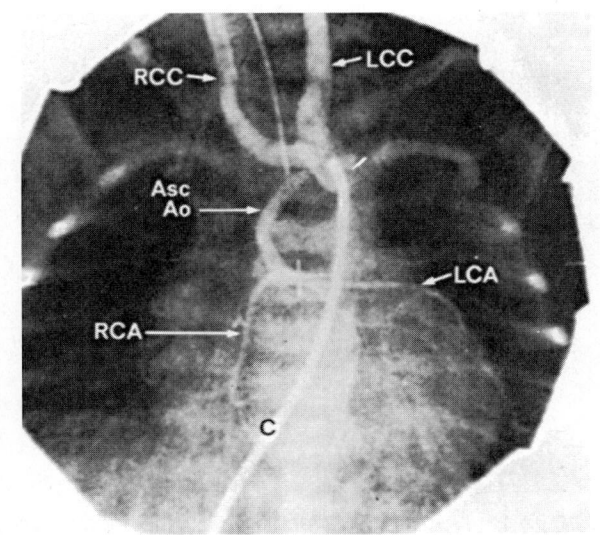

FIGURE 62–27. Angiogram in the aorta in a child with the hypoplastic left heart syndrome with aortic atresia. There is no antegrade flow through the aortic valve. Blood flow to the hypoplastic ascending aorta is retrograde from the ductus arteriosus. Asc Ao, ascending aorta; C, catheter; LCA, left coronary artery; LCC, left common carotid artery; RCA, right coronary artery; RCC, right common carotid artery.

must be ruled out as must other causes of vascular collapse, such as sepsis.

After the onset of congestive heart failure, HLHS must be differentiated from the two other common structural causes of failure early in the 1st week of life: aortic stenosis and the coarctation syndrome. There is usually left ventricular hypertrophy on the electrocardiogram in the former, and a difference in pulses and blood pressure between the upper and lower extremities is normally present in the latter.

Since the hypoplastic left heart syndrome has been uniformly fatal, treatment was initially terminated at the time of definitive diagnosis and comfort care given. More recently, centers have tried a more aggressive approach, either with staged surgical repair or cardiac transplantation. If either of the latter procedures are considered, congestive heart failure should be treated with digoxin, and diuretics and PGE_1 should be given to dilate the ductus arteriosus to improve systemic perfusion. Bicarbonate should be given to treat the metabolic acidosis.

The staged surgical procedure involves turning the defect into a single ventricle that can later be repaired by a modified Fontan procedure. The first stage in the perinatal period involves dividing the pulmonary artery connecting the proximal portion to the aorta so that the right ventricle becomes the systemic pump. Pulmonary blood flow is provided via an aortopulmonary shunt. An atrial septal defect is created to decompress the hypertensive left atrium. A second stage involves dividing the aortopulmonary shunt and directly connecting the systemic venous return to the pulmonary artery (Fontan).

Other centers have gone directly to neonatal cardiac transplantation. Since the availability of hearts is limited in the perinatal period, approximately 25% of children have died on the transplant list.

The most recent data would suggest an initial mortality of 25% to 35% with either the staged surgical approach or transplantation, including those who die on the transplant waiting list. Survival to the age of eight years is about 65% and is almost identical with either staged surgical repair or transplantation. Further data will be necessary to decide which of these two surgical approaches is preferable (Bove and Lloyd, 1996; Razzouk et al, 1996).

Ventricular Septal Defects

VSDs (1/3000 live births) may be isolated, part of a more complex cardiac anomaly such as TOF, or associated with other congenital cardiac defects such as coarctation of the aorta. In this section, only the isolated defect is considered; the more complicated types are discussed elsewhere in this chapter. Ventricular defects have been classified according to their location in the ventricular septum. The most common site is the membranous portion of the septum that lies between the crista supraventricularis and the papillary muscle of the conus when the heart is viewed from the right ventricular side. Less common sites are the area above the crista (subpulmonary), the muscular portion of the septum below the tricuspid valve (atrioventricular septal defect), and the anterior trabecular portion of the ventricular septum near the apex of the right ventricle. The size of VSDs varies: They can be as small as a pinhole or large enough to make the ventricular septum almost completely absent. In about 10% of infants, multiple defects are present.

Because the right and left sides of the heart are arranged in parallel before birth, the presence of a large communication at the ventricular level in addition to the normal ductus connection at the great vessel level does not significantly alter the fetal circulation. After birth, the hemodynamics depend on the size of the defect and the pulmonary and systemic vascular resistances. If the defect is large (> 1 cm^2/m^2 body size or equal to at least half the size of the aortic valve), it offers no resistance to flow. The systolic pressures in both ventricles and both great vessels are approximately equal, and the degree of intracardiac shunting is determined by the systemic and pulmonary vascular resistances. For the first few hours of life, the resistances are about equal, and little shunting (left-to-right or right-to-left) occurs. Over the following hours, days, and weeks, the pulmonary vascular resistance gradually falls, increasing the proportion of blood ejected by the left ventricle that goes through the VSD into the pulmonary artery. When the pulmonary blood flow is about three times greater than the systemic flow, the left ventricle can no longer accommodate the volume load, and signs and symptoms of congestive heart failure develop. In full-term infants with an isolated ventricular defect, this usually occurs late in the 1st or during the 2nd month of life, but failure is occasionally seen earlier, sometimes in the 1st week, presumably owing to a more rapid fall in the pulmonary vascular resistance. The left-to-right shunting at the ventricular level results in increased flow in the pulmonary artery, pulmonary veins, left atrium, and left ventricle, with the latter chamber ejecting blood directly into the pulmonary artery. The right atrium and right ventricle are not volume overloaded, but in the presence of a large defect the right ventricle must generate pressures equal to those of the left ventricle, so there is usually right ventricular hypertrophy without significant dilation.

If the ventricular defect is small, it does offer resistance to flow, and the pressures in the two ventricles may differ. These infants are a heterogeneous group, with the hemodynamics depending on the size of the hole rather than the pulmonary vascular resistance. If the defect is small, the right ventricular and pulmonary artery pressures may be normal and the pulmonary blood flow less than twice the systemic flow. These infants are rarely symptomatic, and a murmur is usually the sole indication of heart disease. If the defect is larger, the right heart pressures may be close to systemic pressures, with flow ratios exceeding 3:1. These infants may have congestive heart failure.

Newborns with a small VSD have a grade 2 or 3/6 high-pitched, pansystolic murmur along the left sternal border and are asymptomatic. Even if the defect is large, the elevated pulmonary resistance prevents significant shunting in the first few days and weeks of life, so heart failure is unusual. Later, as the left-to-right shunt increases, signs and symptoms of congestive failure—tachypnea, tiring with feeding, poor weight gain, diaphoresis, and hepatomegaly—develop.

On physical examination, the cardiac impulse is usually hyperactive, and the apex is displaced laterally. A systolic thrill and grade 4/6 pansystolic murmur can be appreciated along the left sternal border. If the left-to-right shunt is large, a mid-diastolic rumble is audible at the apex from the increased flow across a structurally normal mitral valve. If the pulmonary artery pressure is increased, the pulmonary component of the second heart sound is single or narrowly split and accentuated.

Although the electrocardiogram is usually an accurate tool for assessing the hemodynamics in older children with a VSD, it is less valuable in the newborn because the normal pattern of right ventricular predominance masks the typical changes. A normal progression from right to left ventricular predominance over the 1st month is usual for a small VSD, and an increase in both right and left ventricular forces over the 1st month of life is typical of a large ventricular defect with pulmonary hypertension.

The chest film is a better tool than the electrocardiogram in the evaluation of a newborn with a ventricular defect. If the heart is normal in size and the pulmonary vascular markings are normal, the left-to-right shunt is small. With large shunts, the cardiac silhouette is enlarged, and the pulmonary vascular markings are increased and, if there is an elevated pulmonary venous pressure, indistinct. The two-dimensional echocardiogram can usually allow visualization of defects that are larger than 2 mm and rule out associated cardiac anomalies. Doppler assessment of the flow through the defect gives an estimate of the interventricular gradient and may be helpful to estimate the size. Color Doppler can frequently pick up small defects that cannot be imaged otherwise. VSDs also can be visualized with angiography (Fig. 62–28).

An infant who has congestive heart failure and a systolic murmur in the first 2 weeks of life is not likely to have an isolated ventricular defect. If cyanosis is absent, coarctation (with or without a ventricular defect), critical aortic stenosis, or HLHS is more likely. They can usually be differenti-

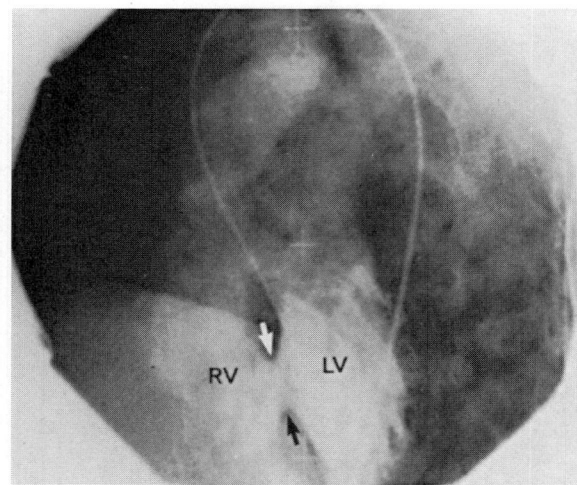

FIGURE 62–28. Left ventricular angiogram in the hepatoclavicular *four-chamber* projection using 40 degrees of left anterior obliquity and 40 degrees of cranial angulation. A large midmuscular ventricular septal defect is outlined by the arrows. LV, left ventricle; RV, right ventricle.

ated by the absence of femoral pulses in coarctation, the presence of left ventricular hypertrophy with strain on the electrocardiogram in aortic stenosis, and the appearance of a shocklike picture in HLHS. If cyanosis is present, truncus arteriosus, tricuspid atresia, or TOF must be considered. In the asymptomatic newborn with a murmur, mild aortic stenosis, valvular or peripheral pulmonary stenosis, and TOF can be confused, especially if the lesions are mild.

One must treat newborns with a VSD with the knowledge that many, if not most, small defects close spontaneously and that up to 20% of large defects also get much smaller or close. Newborns with a small or moderate size VSD often require no treatment. For those with mild heart failure, digoxin and diuretics and the usual anticongestive measures often suffice. Occasionally a child with a large defect responds poorly to anticongestive measures with continued severe heart failure and poor weight gain despite maximal medical management. For these infants, reparative surgery is necessary.

Surgery can be done at a very low risk (<5%) with a very high probability of a surgical cure. For those with multiple muscular defects, pulmonary artery banding is sometimes performed in the hope that some or most of the defects will close spontaneously, making later surgical repair easier.

Atrioventricular Septal Defects

The atrioventricular canal portion of the heart is formed from the endocardial cushions, a mass of embryonic mesenchymal tissue that forms the structures in the middle portion of the heart: the lower portion of the atrial septum, the upper portion of the ventricular septum, and the septal portions of the mitral and tricuspid valves. Any one or all of the components may be abnormal in an endocardial cushion defect, the modern term for which is AVSD. The spectrum of abnormalities in AVSD range from an isolated cleft in the mitral or tricuspid valve to a complete atrioventricular canal with a huge deficiency of the atrial and ventricular septum and a common atrioventricular valve. A variety of classifications have been proposed, but the tremendous spectrum of variations makes sharp distinctions difficult, and a description of the anomalies is preferable: atrial septal defect of the ostium primum type, ventricular septal defect of the atrioventricular canal type, clefts of the mitral or tricuspid valve, single atrioventricular valve, and complete atrioventricular septal defect. Atrioventricular septal defects are the most common type of heart disease present in Down syndrome. Up to 45% of infants with atrioventricular septal defects have trisomy 21. Other cardiac anomalies are often present in association with AVSDs. Heterotaxia syndromes, single ventricle, double outlet right ventricle, transposition, and pulmonary stenosis are the most common.

The hemodynamics of AVSDs are complex. Shunting in these infants may be dependent or obligatory. Dependent shunting through either an ASD or VSD is a function of the pulmonary and systemic vascular resistance. In the newborn period, when the pulmonary vascular resistance is high, little left-to-right shunt may be present. As the pulmonary resistance drops over the first days and weeks of life, the pulmonary blood flow increases, eventually leading to congestive heart failure as the left ventricle becomes overloaded. Obligatory shunting occurs from a high pressure chamber to a low pressure chamber, usually from ventricle to atrium, and is independent of resistance. In AVSDs, obligatory shunting is usually from left ventricle through the mitral portion of the atrioventricular valve into the left atrium and across the atrial defect into the right atrium or, less frequently, directly into the right atrium. This left-to-right shunt caused by atrioventricular valve regurgitation is independent of the status of the pulmonary vasculature and may occur even with the high pulmonary vascular resistance seen in the newborn period.

The degree of intracardiac shunting at any given time is the result of a complex interplay between the pulmonary and systemic resistances affecting the dependent shunting and the obligatory shunting. In the first weeks of life, however, when the pulmonary vascular resistance tends to be high, the newborns who present with congestive failure tend to have obligatory shunts owing to atrioventricular valve regurgitation.

When there is only an ostium primum atrial defect present, infants with AVSD rarely, if ever, are seen in the neonatal period. Infants with AVSD who have an isolated ventricular defect present similarly to the previously described newborns with membranous or muscular ventricular defects. The age at presentation of infants with a complete AVSD is related to the presence of atrioventricular valve regurgitation; if it is severe, the infants may present in the first 1 or 2 weeks of life with the usual manifestations of heart failure, tachycardia, tachypnea, feeding difficulties, and sweating. If the atrioventricular valves are competent, infants present later in the 1st month or even in the 2nd month of life. The precordium is usually hyperactive on palpation, with the maximal impulse displaced laterally and inferiorly. A thrill at the lower left sternal border may be present. If there is significant atrial shunting, the first heart sound is accentuated. In the usual case with pulmonary

hypertension, the pulmonary component of the second heart sound is loud. Heart murmurs may be quite variable, but usually there is a loud pansystolic murmur at the lower left sternal border and a flow rumble across the mitral valve best heard at the apex. In the presence of mitral regurgitation, a pansystolic murmur at the apex is audible, but it may be hard to distinguish from the murmur of the VSD.

The electrocardiographic features in infants with AVSDs are characteristic. Because of posterior displacement of the atrioventricular node, His bundle, and distal left bundle as well as hypoplasia of the anterior portion of the left fascicle and an early origin of the left bundle, there is a characteristic superior QRS axis (0 to −150 degrees) on electrocardiogram. These children also have a prolonged P-R interval, biatrial hypertrophy, and biventricular hypertrophy (Fig. 62–29).

The heart is almost invariably enlarged on the chest radiograph, and the pulmonary blood flow is increased and often congested (see Fig. 62–2). The size of the cardiac silhouette is often out of proportion with the increased pulmonary blood flow, presumably owing to the atrioventricular valve regurgitation.

AVSDs should be considered in all infants who show congestive heart failure, a left-to-right shunt, and a superior axis on the electrocardiogram. Infants with tricuspid atresia without significant pulmonary stenosis may also demonstrate a large heart with increased pulmonary blood flow on the radiograph and a superior axis on the electrocardiogram, but they are desaturated and almost invariably have pure left ventricular hypertrophy on the electrocardiogram, as opposed to the right or biventricular hypertrophy seen in infants with atrioventricular canal defects. Echocardiography can resolve any remaining questions. When congestive failure is present, the usual medical management consisting of digoxin, diuretics, and high-calorie formula should be started. In some infants, this suffices for many months, but frequently surgery is required because of persistent congestive heart failure and failure to thrive.

Surgical repair involves dividing the common atrioventricular valve and closing the ASD and VSD using either one patch or two, attaching the mitral portion of the atrioventricular valve on the left side of the patch and the tricuspid portion on the right side of the patch. Hospital mortality following correction of a complete atrioventricular canal in infancy ranges from 3% to 10%. The development of significant atrioventricular valve regurgitation or subaortic stenosis is occasionally encountered, but a 10-year survival is now expected to be in the 85% to 90% range (Bando et al, 1995).

Arteriovenous Fistulas

Arteriovenous fistulas (1/100,000 live births) are a rare cause of congestive heart failure in the newborn. There are two types of fistulous connections: a direct communication between an artery and vein bypassing the capillary bed and, less commonly in the newborn, an angioma with multiple arterial and venous supply. Although arteriovenous fistulas causing heart failure have been described in the subclavian, internal mammary, and vertebral arteries and hemangiomas may be found in the skin, pelvis, and coro-

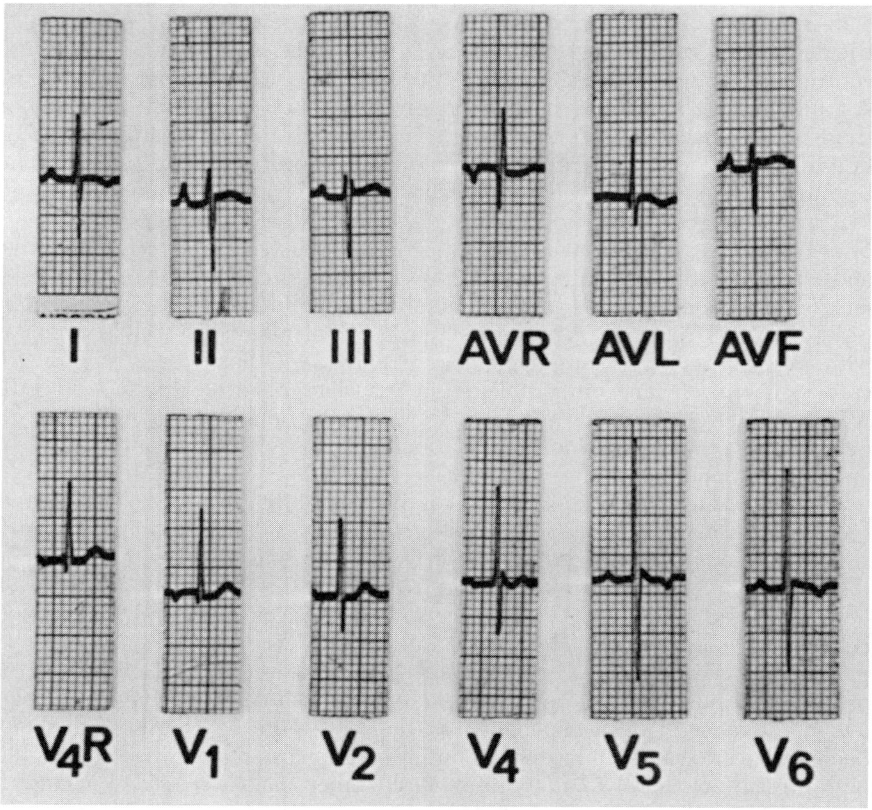

FIGURE 62–29. Electrocardiogram of a 1-week-old newborn with a complete atrioventricular septal defect. The QRS axis is −90 degrees with a predominant negative deflection in leads II, III, and AVF. The tall peaked P wave in lead II reflects right atrial hypertrophy, and the upright T waves in V_4R and V_1 suggest right ventricular hypertrophy. There is also first-degree heart block with a P-R interval of 0.17 second.

nary arteries, most of the newborns with heart failure have either a cerebral arteriovenous fistula or a hemangioma of the liver.

Arteriovenous fistulas are present in utero but do not seem to cause significant hemodynamic embarrassment. At birth, infants are well developed without evidence of heart failure, but profound heart failure may develop within a few hours. This dramatic change is a result of the shift from the parallel to the in-series circulation after birth. In utero, the systemic venous return including the arteriovenous fistula is divided into two streams. Part of the venous return goes through the right heart chambers into the pulmonary artery, and the rest goes through the foramen ovale to the left-sided heart chambers. After birth, the entire systemic return, including return from the fistula, must pass through the right heart as well as the pulmonary arteries and then to the left heart and aorta. In addition, the removal of the low resistance placenta circuit after birth increases the systemic resistance and forces more blood through the arteriovenous fistula. These changes occurring with the transitional circulation suddenly impart a large volume overload to the right and left sides of the heart. The neonatal heart is unable to tolerate the increased systemic venous return, and heart failure and circulatory collapse result.

Congestive heart failure with tachypnea, dyspnea, and feeding difficulties is usually present within the first few days of life. Cyanosis is occasionally seen secondary to pulmonary venous desaturation and to right-to-left shunting at the atrial or ductal levels. The peripheral pulses are generally diminished but may be increased in the

arteries feeding the fistula. Infants with a cerebral arteriovenous fistula may have dilated veins in the neck. Cardiac enlargement with a hyperdynamic cardiac impulse is present on palpation, and a soft systolic ejection murmur over the semilunar valves or a diastolic flow murmur across the atrioventricular valves may be audible on auscultation. Occasionally a continuous bruit may be heard over the fistula.

Right axis deviation, right ventricular hypertrophy, and ST-T wave changes are usually present on the electrocardiogram. On the chest radiograph, there is generalized cardiac enlargement with increased pulmonary blood flow and pulmonary venous congestion. In infants with a cerebral arteriovenous fistula, the superior mediastinum is often widened because of dilation of the ascending aorta, carotid arteries, jugular vein, and superior vena cava.

The presence of vascular collapse and congestive heart failure in the 1st week of life suggests myocarditis or a left-sided obstructive lesion, such as HLHS, coarctation of the aorta, or aortic stenosis. If there is a bruit over the head with normal or brisk pulses in the head vessels and dilated veins in the neck, a fistula is likely. Occasionally the clinical diagnosis remains unclear, and echocardiography or catheterization is necessary.

For the newborn with circulatory collapse, the usual treatment of congestive heart failure is correction of acidosis and administration of digoxin and diuretics followed by diagnostic study. For newborns with a cerebral or hepatic arteriovenous fistula, coiling of the feeding vessels has occasionally been successful. For those with smaller fistulas, successful therapy has been possible; for the majority of infants with large arteriovenous fistulas with multiple feeding vessels, the prognosis is guarded. Interferon has been tried with limited success.

TRANSIENT MYOCARDIAL ISCHEMIA

A number of newborns suffer a form of myocardial ischemia that frequently is transient but that may be associated with significant cardiovascular symptoms and even death. In some of these infants, the signs of respiratory distress and congestive heart failure or shock are predominant; in others, myocardial dysfunction and tricuspid regurgitation are the presenting symptoms.

The infants are usually born at term by a delivery complicated by hypoxic stress that occurs before or during birth. Fetal scalp pH measurement is in the range of 6.9 to 7.1. The Apgar score is usually less than 3 at 1 minute. Respiratory distress and cyanosis are frequently present soon after birth, with affected infants developing the signs and symptoms of congestive heart failure (tachypnea, tachycardia, hepatomegaly, and a gallop rhythm) within a few hours. Some develop hypotension and cardiovascular collapse and shock. About half the newborns have systolic heart murmurs. In most, the murmur is at the left lower sternal border and suggests tricuspid regurgitation, but in a few the murmur is loudest at the apex and sounds like mitral regurgitation.

The chest radiograph invariably shows cardiomegaly. There is usually a diffuse haziness with pulmonary venous congestion in those with predominantly left-sided heart failure. In those with right-sided heart failure, pulmonary congestion may be absent and pulmonary blood flow may be diminished by right-to-left atrial shunting. The electrocardiogram shows right ventricular predominance that is normal for age and right atrial hypertrophy in the majority. Diffuse ST-T changes are usually present, with the most common pattern being ST depression in the midprecordium and persistent T-wave inversion over the left precordium.

Transient myocardial ischemia should be suspected in all newborns who experience birth asphyxia and who have respiratory distress, cyanosis, or signs of congestive failure soon after birth. Echocardiography is helpful in distinguishing infants who have tricuspid regurgitation associated with transient ischemia from those who have tricuspid regurgitation caused by Ebstein disease of the tricuspid valve or critical pulmonary stenosis or pulmonary atresia with an intact ventricular septum.

The treatment is symptomatic. Digitalis and diuretics should be given for congestive heart failure and metabolic abnormalities of hypoglycemia, and acidosis should be corrected promptly. Those with severe respiratory distress may need intubation and assisted ventilation. Those with cardiovascular collapse may benefit from ionotropic support with dopamine or dolbutamine. Afterload reduction with nitroprusside should be reserved for those most severely affected. For those who are first seen with severe acidosis and cardiogenic shock, the prognosis remains grim, with death likely occurring from heart failure, low cardiac output, or failure of a necessary organ system.

Myocarditis

Myocarditis (1/80,000 live births) occurs in all age groups, but there is higher frequency in the 1st month than in any other period of life. It is a well-recognized entity with a clinical pattern sufficiently distinctive for one to make an antemortem diagnosis. Although often a fulminant disease, it is not invariably fatal, and early recognition and prompt treatment may alter the outcome. Any infective agent can cause myocarditis, although the enteroviruses, particularly coxsackie B and ECHO viruses, are the most common.

On gross examination, the heart is enlarged and dilated. The cardiac muscle feels flabby and is often pale or nutmeg-like in color. Microscopic examination reveals a multicellular infiltration of the myocardium. Lymphocytes, large mononuclear cells, eosinophils, and polymorphonuclear leukocytes are present in varying numbers with either patchy or diffuse distribution. Necrosis and fragmentation of muscle fibers may be present. Although rare in patients with primary myocarditis, involvement of the endocardium and pericardium may occur. When the coxsackie virus is the causative agent, involvement of other organs, particularly the central nervous system, is common. Involvement of multiple organs is even more common with rubella and herpesviruses.

Most serious coxsackie virus infections occur in the first 10 days of life. The clinical course of young infants with myocarditis is variable. The initial symptoms may be mild and include lethargy, failure to feed, vomiting, or diarrhea. Jaundice may be present, and evidence of a mild upper respiratory tract infection is sometimes noted. In the milder forms of the disease, clinical manifestations may be limited to slight tachypnea, tachycardia, and poor heart sounds. Frequently there are no premonitory symptoms. The infant becomes seriously ill suddenly. Respirations increase, become labored, and are often accompanied by a grunt. The infant appears restless and anxious. The skin is pale, mottled, and mildly cyanotic. The temperature may be slightly or greatly elevated or subnormal. The pulse rate is usually rapid, between 150 and 200, and weak. Occasionally bradycardia is present. The percussion note over the chest may be normal or hyper-resonant. Dullness is uncommon. The breath sounds are usually harsh, and rales may be heard at the bases. Although there is always some degree of cardiac enlargement, it is often difficult to detect clinically. The heart sounds are mushy, particularly the first sound, and a gallop rhythm may be present. The liver is almost invariably enlarged. Edema is an uncommon finding, and venous engorgement is almost never detected. There may be signs referable to central nervous system involvement, including lethargy, seizures, or coma with occasional focal signs suggesting meningoencephalitis.

Chest radiographs show generalized cardiac enlargement as well as haziness of the lung fields. At times, it is not possible to make the distinction between congestion and pneumonia. Electrocardiograms often show abnormalities. Low-voltage QRS complexes and low, isoelectric, or inverted T waves are the most frequent findings. There may also be significant disturbances in conduction, such as heart block, extrasystoles, and ventricular or atrial tachycardia. The electrocardiographic abnormalities are frequently transient. Elevations of aspartate transaminase, lactic dehydrogenase, and cardiac creatine phosphokinase are variably present with levels dependent on the extent of tissue damage.

The diagnosis of myocarditis should be suspected in any newborn with congestive heart failure in whom structural heart disease has been excluded by two-dimensional echocardiogram. The suspicion should be heightened if there is a known respiratory infection in the mother or proven viral illness in other nursery infants. The acute form of myocarditis is commonly mistaken for overwhelming *sepsis* or a severe *lower respiratory tract infection*. This is especially true for the latter because cyanosis and respiratory distress may initially suggest pneumonia. Myocarditis should be suspected if there are tachycardia, poor heart sounds with or without gallop rhythm, a degree of dyspnea disproportionate with the pulmonary findings, and radiographic evidence of cardiac enlargement. Myocarditis must also be differentiated from other cardiac conditions that may occur in the neonatal period, such as congenital heart disease with congestive failure precipitated by infection, the acute form of endocardial fibroelastosis, and paroxysmal tachycardia. Coarctation of the aorta, a not uncommon cause of heart failure in the newborn, must always be excluded by careful evaluation of the pulses and blood pressures in the arms and legs.

Endocardial fibroelastosis is usually associated with left ventricular hypertrophy indicated in electrocardiographic tracings by high-voltage R waves in precordial leads taken over the left side of the heart. The left ventricular pattern may not be as striking in the first few days or weeks of life. In myocarditis, low-voltage complexes are characteristic and are the result of severe disturbances in myocardial function. Occasionally, infants with endocardial fibroelastosis in severe heart failure may have low voltage temporarily.

Congestive heart failure is frequently present with paroxysmal tachycardia, but in this condition the heart rate is usually much more rapid than in myocarditis. Almost invariably the rate is greater than 220 beats/min if the tachycardia itself is severe enough to cause heart failure. Mild forms of myocarditis are particularly difficult to recognize. Signs of heart failure may not be prominent or may be absent entirely. The clinical manifestations may include pallor, slight increase in the respiratory rate, tachycardia, and poor heart sounds. Such findings in an infant who has signs of infection and who appears to have a disproportionate degree of cardiac embarrassment should suggest the possibility of myocarditis. Although electrocardiographic studies may aid in the diagnosis, there is no specific pattern, and a normal tracing does not rule out the disorder.

Young infants with myocarditis may become critically ill with such rapidity that treatment should be instituted as soon as the diagnosis is suspected. Oxygen therapy and digitalis should be started at once with the usual anticongestive measures. Afterload reduction with nitroprusside may be helpful for those who are not hypotensive. A clinical trial is underway to test the efficacy of intravenous gamma globulin, but data are not yet available to know if this is effective. For those most severely involved, cardiac transplantation may be the most reasonable option, although the availability of neonatal hearts on short notice remains highly problematic.

Endocardial Fibroelastosis

Endocardial fibroelastosis (approximately 1/70,000 live births) may occur as an isolated or primary condition or in association with a variety of congenital and acquired cardiac lesions. In the latter groups, the clinical entity is that of the underlying cardiac disease, and the fibroelastosis is a secondary finding on postmortem examination. The description that follows is limited mainly to infants with the primary or isolated form of endocardial fibroelastosis.

Gross enlargement of the heart is a constant finding. The weight is increased, and there are hypertrophy and dilation of one or more chambers. This is especially true of the left ventricle, which is the most frequent site of endocardial thickening. Involvement of the left atrium is fairly common, but less than half have an additional lesion of the right ventricle and right atrium. Fibroelastosis confined to the right side of the heart is rare. On gross examination, the endocardium is diffusely thickened and smooth and has a porcelain-white appearance (Fig. 62–30). About half the cases show involvement of one or more valves, the mitral more commonly than the others. In contrast to the usual pattern of congenital abnormalities, there is a striking absence of other malformations. Microscopic examination shows an increase in the fibrous and elastic tissue within the endocardium with some extension into the myocardium. When the valves are involved, the picture is similar to that of the endocardium. There is no evidence of inflammation in the heart. Pneumonia and signs of congestive heart failure are commonly associated autopsy findings.

On auscultation, the heart sounds may be normal or muffled, and a third heart sound is frequently present. Heart murmurs may be present in more than 50% of patients, usually a Grade I to Grade II pansystolic murmur at the apex from mitral regurgitation secondary to papillary muscle dysfunction. Diastolic murmurs are uncommon.

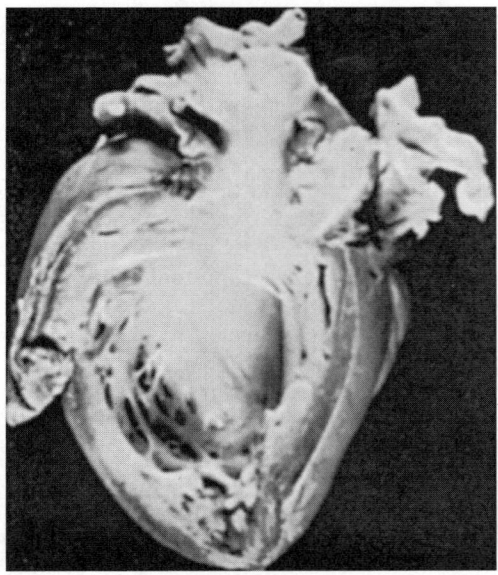

FIGURE 62–30. Endocardial fibroelastosis in an infant who died at the age of 9 days. The endocardium of both ventricles is thickened and porcelain-white in appearance.

Chest radiographs invariably show cardiac enlargement that is usually significant, with increased pulmonary vascularity secondary to pulmonary venous congestion. Left atrial enlargement is common. The electrocardiogram almost invariably reveals left ventricular hypertrophy with tall R waves over the left precordium, frequently associated with prominent Q waves and T-wave inversion. Supraventricular or nodal tachycardia, complete heart block, or other arrhythmias may occasionally be seen.

Endocardial fibroelastosis should be suspected in the newborn if abnormalities of cardiac rhythm (e.g., heart block, atrial tachycardia) are present. In the most acute form, diagnosis is difficult. These infants often resemble patients with sepsis or pneumonia. The presence of tachycardia, cardiomegaly, and hepatomegaly should lead to the suspicion of heart failure owing to primary heart disease. Differentiation from primary myocarditis may be particularly difficult. The findings in both conditions are remarkably similar. One distinguishing feature is the strikingly low voltage noted on the electrocardiogram in severe myocarditis, but low voltage may occasionally occur in endocardial fibroelastosis. The left ventricular pattern commonly found in endocardial fibroelastosis may be slight or absent in the patient less than 1 week old with an acute case. The diagnosis should be suspected in any young infant with an enlarged heart, particularly when there is little or no cyanosis and no audible heart murmurs. Absence of the latter signs should exclude most other forms of congenital heart disease. The presence of palpable femoral pulsations eliminates coarctation of the aorta. Infants with anomalous origin of the left coronary artery may have a similar clinical and radiographic picture. The electrocardiogram in this condition is often distinctive, however, and shows a pattern of coronary insufficiency with inverted T waves in leads I and II plus a prominent Q wave in lead I. Glycogen storage disease of the heart is a rare cause of cardiac enlargement in infancy. Here the enlargement is usually globular, without specific chamber enlargement. The electrocardiographic pattern is more bizarre in glycogen storage disease, and a short P-R interval is often present. A specific diagnosis can be made by analysis of the glycogen content of skeletal muscle.

Treatment is symptomatic. Transplantation may be necessary for those most seriously affected.

Cardiomyopathy of the Infant of the Diabetic Mother

Many large-for-gestational-age infants born to diabetic mothers have an asymmetric hypertrophic cardiomyopathy involving primarily the ventricular septum. Fetal hyperinsulinemia contributes directly to septal hypertrophy. Microscopic examination has demonstrated hypertrophy of the fibers with areas of cellular disarray. The exact mechanism of the cardiac hypertrophy and the reason that the hypertrophy primarily affects the ventricular septum remain a matter of conjecture.

Affected infants, who are usually puffy and plethoric, may present with the signs and symptoms of congestive heart failure: tachypnea, tachycardia, and hepatomegaly. They usually have respiratory distress and frequently cyanosis from birth. Systolic ejection murmurs are common and,

at least according to one study, seem to be correlated with the degree of obstruction to left ventricular ejection by the septal hypertrophy. Cardiac enlargement on the chest radiograph is almost universal, and pulmonary venous congestion is seen in most symptomatic patients. These abnormalities, however, do not correlate with the echocardiographic findings of wall or septal thickness. On echocardiographic evaluation of symptomatic infants, the right ventricular anterior wall, the ventricular septum, and the left ventricular posterior wall are thickened, but the septal wall is disproportionately hypertrophied so that the septal wall–to–left ventricular posterior wall ratio is increased above normal in about one half of infants (Gutgesell et al, 1980). The internal dimensions of the right and left ventricle were normal, as was the percentage of dimensional change, a measure of cardiac function. In 5 of the 24 infants, there was evidence of left ventricular outflow tract obstruction owing to apposition of the anterior leaflet of the mitral valve to the hypertrophied interventricular septum during systole. The echocardiogram is diagnostic and should be performed on all infants of diabetic mothers with signs or symptoms of respiratory distress or congestive heart failure. Other forms of heart disease must be excluded because the incidence of congenital heart disease in infants of diabetic mothers is five times that of the normal population.

The treatment is symptomatic. Hypoglycemia, hypocalcemia, and hypomagnesemia and polycythemia should be corrected, and maintenance fluid should be provided intravenously if oral intake is not possible. Occasional increasing respiratory distress requires intubation and assisted ventilation. Unless severely depressed myocardial contractility can be demonstrated on echocardiogram, digitalis and other ionotropic agents are contraindicated since they may lead to increasing left ventricular outflow tract obstruction.

The prognosis in this group of newborns is excellent. Of 11 symptomatic infants reported by Way and colleagues in 1975, all were asymptomatic by 1 month of age, with the radiograph in all and the electrocardiogram in 10 returning to normal. Echocardiograms showed regression of septal thickness in all the patients, and repeat cardiac catheterizations in 2 of the 11 have shown normal hemodynamics with elimination of gradients of 30 and 74 mm Hg between the left ventricle and the aorta. The findings of Gutgesell and co-workers are similar.

Glycogen Storage Disease of the Heart

Glycogen storage disease is a rare condition that may produce symptoms from birth. There are at least 22 types of which only 3 affect the heart. The most common is Pompe disease, usually classified as Type IIa. It is transmitted through a single recessive autosomal gene. The defect is due to the congenital absence of alpha-1,4-glycosidase (lysosomal acid maltose) from intracellular lysosomes. This results in the accumulation of normal glycogen in lysosomal sacs of virtually all tissues, where it cannot be degraded by glycolytic enzymes.

The heart is always enlarged, often to enormous proportions. The walls of both ventricles are thick, but the atria are normal. Microscopic examination shows infiltration of the muscle fibers with large vacuoles of glycogen. Varying amounts of glycogen deposition are also found in the skeletal muscles, liver, kidneys, and central nervous system. Frequently the infant appears normal at birth but goes on to have a history of poor feeding, lassitude, a feeble cry, protruding tongue, and failure to gain weight. Hypotonia may be striking, and the tongue may appear thick. Cardiac enlargement is the rule. A systolic heart murmur may be noted, but it is often soft and variable. The liver is not usually enlarged.

The usual parameters for glycogen metabolism are normal, including glucose tolerance and response to epinephrine and glucagon. These infants do not suffer from hypoglycemia. Radiologic examination shows gross generalized cardiomegaly, although the heart need not be enlarged at birth. The electrocardiogram may show abnormalities at birth or after a period of some weeks: The presence of a short P-R interval, huge precordial voltages, and evidence of left ventricular hypertrophy is universal. T-wave inversion, ST-T elevation, and deep Q waves are frequently seen. On echocardiogram, thickening of the left ventricular free wall disproportionate to the thickness of the interventricular septum is seen. Cardiac catheterization and angiography are rarely indicated.

The diagnosis is rarely made in the neonatal period unless there is a family history of the disease. The early symptoms are ill defined and, with the exception of intermittent episodes of dyspnea, do not suggest a cardiac abnormality. The patient is more likely to be several weeks or months old before the cardiac enlargement is detected. The diagnosis should be suspected in any infant with an enlarged heart in the absence of structural heart disease, especially if the enlargement is great. Muscle weakness is an important additional clue. Macroglossia is often present and may be confused with cretinism or Down syndrome.

Tumors of the Heart

Cardiac tumors are rare but when present the manifestations of heart disease may appear infrequently in the neonatal period. Several types of tumors have been described—rhabdomyomas are the most common and are frequently associated with tuberous sclerosis. Most commonly the tumors are multiple, but occasionally only one is found (Fig. 62–31). They are situated in the walls of the right or left ventricle or occasionally in the interventricular septum and, on occasion, project into the lumen and obstruct one of the valves or the outflow tract of the right or left ventricle. Histologically they consist of numerous nodular areas with vacuoles that contain glycogen. On electron microscopy the glycogen is seen in the cytoplasm and in the mitochondria. Fibromas, solitary tumors in the septal or parietal wall of the left ventricle, are usually not encapsulated with tissue mixing with the myocardial cells in the wall. They have been described in the neonatal period and occasionally cause problems by compressing the anterior descending coronary artery, interfering with the conduction system, or obstructing right or left ventricular outflow. Other tumors, including teratoma, lipoma, hemangioma, hamartoma, and sarcoma, are considerably less common, especially in the perinatal period.

The clinical picture is extremely variable. Many infants, especially those with multiple intramural rhabdomyomas,

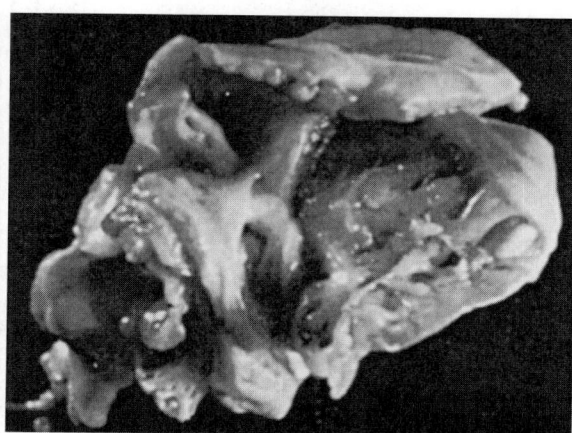

FIGURE 62–31. Age 1 month. Multiple rhabdomyomas. Gross specimen of the opened heart shows numerous nodular masses within the walls of the ventricle that protrude into the chamber of the heart.

are asymptomatic and are identified on two-dimensional echocardiogram performed because minor obstructions lead to turbulence and murmurs. Occasionally, newborns present with arrhythmias, including atrial flutter or fibrillation or ventricular tachycardia, or complete heart block because of interference with the conduction system. Heart murmurs are usually not present unless the tumor projects into the cardiac cavity and obstructs blood flow. Changes in the cardiac examination depend on the location and severity of the intracavitary obstruction to flow. The electrocardiographic findings are variable, with right, left, and combined ventricular hypertrophy being reported, although occasionally the electrocardiogram is normal. Often there is evidence of abnormal repolarization with inverted T waves. On chest radiographic studies, the heart is usually normal in the absence of significant hemodynamic disruption, although in children with large fibromas the tumor may distort the cardiac contour. Two-dimensional echocardiogram is now the best tool to evaluate the size, location, number, and hemodynamic severity of the tumor or tumors (Fig. 62–32).

Most rhabdomyomas and fibromas need no therapy. The natural history has not been determined conclusively because these tumors are so uncommon. Most of the intramural lesions do not progress and enlarge, however, and some may become relatively smaller with time.

Cardiac Dysrhythmias

Cardiac dysrhythmias are not uncommon in the newborn, accompanying the significant changes in circulatory hemodynamics and gas exchange that occur with the switch from the in utero to extrauterine circulations. In a review of more than 3000 apparently normal newborns (Southall et al, 1981), about 1% revealed dysrhythmias on a routine 10-second electrocardiogram before discharge. The vast majority of these dysrhythmias were of little significance, but life-threatening arrhythmias may occur on rare occasions (Ferrer, 1983).

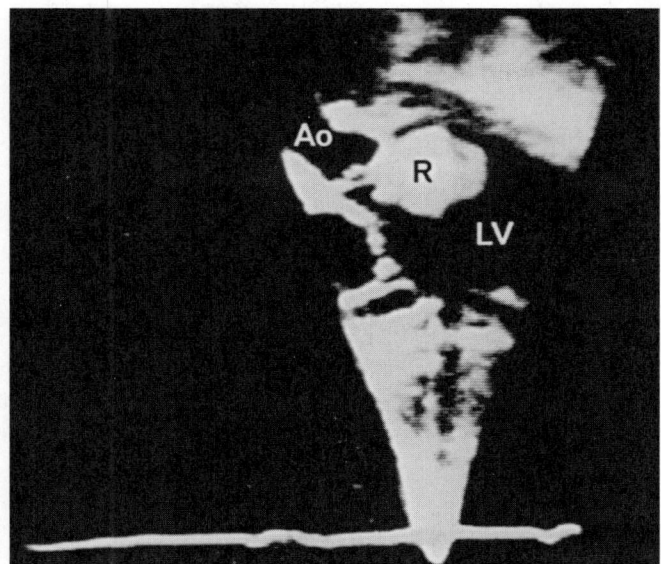

FIGURE 62–32. A subxiphoid view on two-dimensional echocardiogram of the left ventricle (LV) and aorta (Ao) in a 1-week-old infant with tuberous sclerosis. Note the rhabdomyoma (R) that is arising just below the aortic valve and that projects into the lumen of the left ventricle, causing subaortic stenosis. (Courtesy of Roberta G. Williams, M.D.)

Sinus Arrhythmia, Sinus Tachycardia, and Sinus Bradycardia

Sinus arrhythmia is a phasic variation of the sinus node discharge that may occur either in cycle with respiration or independent of it. It is quite common and, as far as can be determined, is of no clinical significance. On electrocardiogram, the P-P interval is irregular and the P wave, P-Q interval, and QRS complexes are normal.

Sinus tachycardia can be defined as a heart rate that exceeds the upper range of normal, usually 175 to 190 beats/min in a full-term infant and 195 beats/min in a premature infant. The P-P interval is short, but the P wave, P-Q interval, and QRS complexes are normal. It is usually a manifestation of increased adrenergic activity that may be the result of crying, feeding, or blood letting, but it may also be secondary to congestive heart failure, shock, anemia, or fever. No treatment is necessary if the significant secondary causes of the tachycardia can be ruled out.

Sinus bradycardia is a heart rate that falls below what is generally accepted as normal (i.e., below 90 to 100 beats/ min), with a normal P wave preceding each QRS. Occasionally the sinus mechanism is so depressed that the junctional tissue depolarizes first, resulting in a junctional escape rhythm. Sinus bradycardia has been associated with defecation, hiccupping, yawning, and nasopharyngeal stimulation, probably as a result of parasympathetic stimulation, and is frequently seen with prolonged apnea. Also, it may be seen with severe systemic disease, particularly that associated with acidosis, hypoxemia, or increased intracranial pressure. Occasionally, otherwise normal infants have a sinus bradycardia of 80 to 90 beats/min in the absence of other findings, probably because of immaturity of the autonomic nervous system and increased vagal tone. In deep sleep, healthy newborn infants can occasionally exhibit heart rates as low as 60 beats per minute. If systemic and primary cardiac disease can be excluded, no treatment is necessary.

Ectopic Beats: Supraventricular and Ventricular

Although during routine predischarge screening in one series the incidence of ectopic beats was less than 1% (Southall et al, 1981), continuous monitoring of healthy newborns shows that the incidence of ectopic beats is much greater, as high as 13%. Supraventricular ectopic beats are usually preceded by a P wave with an abnormal contour, have a normal-appearing QRS, and are followed by an incomplete compensatory pause before the next P wave. Ventricular ectopic beats usually have a wide abnormal QRS, a tall T wave in the opposite direction from the QRS, and a full compensatory pause. These arrhythmias may be seen with metabolic abnormalities, hypoxia, or digoxin toxicity or after cardiac surgery, but they are also frequently seen in otherwise normal newborns. Treatment includes correction of the predisposing factors when possible; in otherwise normal infants, no treatment is necessary unless couplets or atrial or ventricular tachycardia is present because the prognosis is excellent, with ectopy usually disappearing within the 1st month of life.

Paroxysmal Supraventricular Tachycardia

Paroxysmal SVT is one of the most common serious dysrhythmias occurring in the fetus and newborn. Although precise incidence data are not available, the generally accepted frequency is approximately 1 of every 25,000 children. Although usually relatively benign in the older child, the dysrhythmias may be life-threatening in the fetus or newborn, who generally has a higher ventricular rate and is less able to rely on other mechanisms for support of a failing circulation. On electrocardiogram there is a rapid regular rhythm, usually 230 to 320 beats/min, that originates in the atria or junctional region with normal, abnormal, or inapparent P waves; a normal or slightly widened QRS; and ST segments that are normal or slightly depressed (Fig. 62–33). Several mechanisms play a part in the genesis of SVTs, but a rapid ectopic pacemaker or a circus type of re-entry secondary to different refractory periods of adjacent conducting bundles is the most common. Wolff-Parkinson-White syndrome, in which there is a direct muscular connection between the atrium and ventricle that allows re-entry, is recognizable on the electrocardiogram by a short P-Q interval and slow initial ventricular depolarization (delta wave) and is present in about 50% of the cases (Fig. 62–34).

SVT may occur in the fetus. It may not cause symptoms before birth, but occasionally the rapid rate may lead to in utero congestive failure with fetal edema or hydrops and fetal death. Rarely the fetal SVT is intermittent, and the authors have observed infants with hydrops born with normal electrocardiograms who subsequently demonstrate recurrent SVT.

The newborn with SVT presents with signs and symptoms of low cardiac output and congestive heart failure; fussiness, refusal to feed, vomiting, tachypnea, and hepatomegaly are common. At first, the infants have some duski-

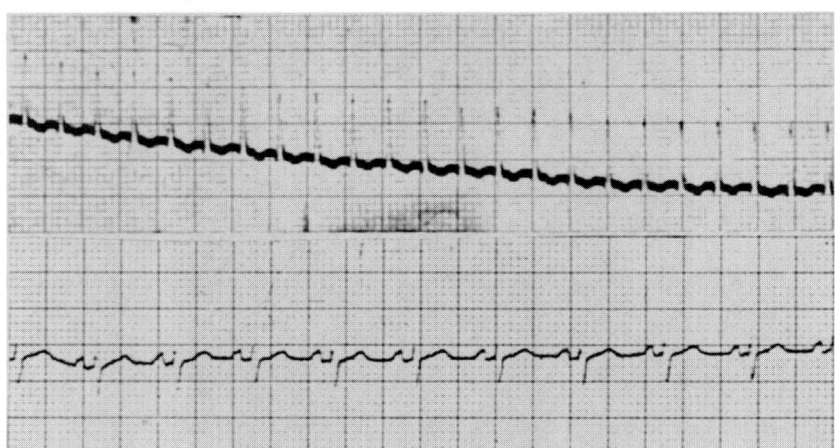

FIGURE 62–33. The upper tracing is lead III in a 7-day-old infant during a paroxysm of supraventricular tachycardia. The lower tracing (lead I) is in the same infant after the attack.

ness or cyanosis of the skin, but later their skin turns ashen gray, and their extremities become cool owing to extreme peripheral vasoconstriction. Cardiac examination usually reveals no problem other than tachycardia. Underlying heart disease may be difficult to detect, even if present, because of the rapid heart rate. At first, the chest radiograph may be normal, but, by the time symptoms occur, there is usually cardiac enlargement, often with pulmonary venous congestion. The echocardiogram is helpful in ruling out associated heart disease.

SVT is diagnosed electrocardiographically. Occasionally, normal newborns with increased adrenergic activity may have heart rates exceeding 200 beats/min, but these infants do not have congestive failure, and the rate slows down when they are quiet. Sometimes, however, it may be difficult to distinguish newborns with a tachycardia associated with severe congestive failure caused by myocarditis or congenital heart disease from those with SVT. Rates of 220 beats/min or more in the newborn are rarely, if ever, of sinus origin and thus require treatment. Rates of 220 beats/min or less in the newborn usually represent sinus rhythm. The presence of heart failure with a rate of 200 to 220 beats/min suggests underlying heart disease because this rate alone is rarely rapid enough to cause significant congestive heart failure in the newborn. Another helpful electrocardiographic sign is that SVT is almost always regular, with variation in heart rate of more than 1 to 2 beats/min being an unusual occurrence. Therefore, any variation in

rate with crying or feeding is likely to signify a sinus mechanism. Rarely a therapeutic trial of adenosine may be necessary to sort out the underlying mechanism.

SVT in a newborn represents an emergency, and treatment should not be delayed. Vagal stimulation, including gagging, carotid sinus massage, or ice compresses to the head, is rarely effective. Adenosine is approved for intravenous use for paroxysmal SVTs in adults and children. It has now become the first-line treatment for paroxysmal atrial tachycardia. Adenosine is given as an intravenous bolus starting at 0.05 mg/kg and increased by 0.05 mg/kg until tachycardia resolves (usually within seconds). Adenosine is a remarkably safe and effective agent for treating both term and preterm infants with SVT (Paret et al, 1996). It acts by inducing complete atrioventricular block transiently. By this mechanism, the re-entry circuit is interrupted. Half-life of adenosine in the blood after injection is only seconds. Adenosine is ineffective in treatment of other tachycardias; therefore a response is diagnostic as well as therapeutic. Older treatments include digoxin with half the total intravenous digitalizing dose of 0.02 mg/kg in term infants (0.015 mg/kg in premature infants) given immediately and the rest in divided doses over the next 12 to 18 hours. Other regimens that have been used include overdrive atrial pacing DC cardioversion (0.25 to 1 joule/kg) synchronized to the peak of the QRS complex to avoid the vulnerable period of the T wave, propranolol (0.01 to 0.1 mg/kg intravenously), phenylephrine (0.005 to 0.02 mg/kg

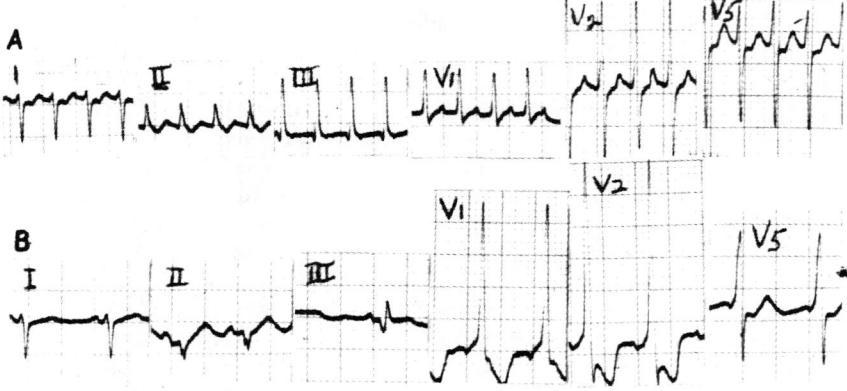

FIGURE 62–34. Electrocardiogram in a 4-day-old infant. *A*, Supraventricular tachycardia. *B*, Tracing after the tachycardia stopped shows a typical Wolff-Parkinson-White pattern with a short P-R interval and a wide QRS. The delta waves can be seen just before the upstroke of the R waves in the precordial leads.

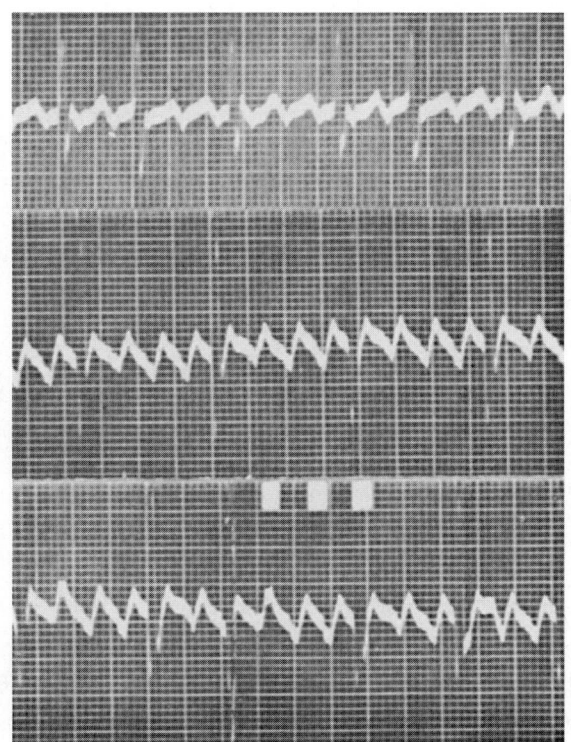

FIGURE 62–35. Standard limb leads during an attack of atrial flutter.

intravenously), or edrophonium (0.2 mg/kg intravenously). Calcium channel blockers should be avoided in neonates, because they can cause cardiovascular collapse.

Atrial Flutter

Atrial flutter is a relatively rare dysrhythmia in the neonatal period. The atrial rate ranges between 360 and 480 beats/min, with the ventricular response one half or, less com-

monly, one third of that. The atrial activity is best seen as a saw-toothed pattern of the P waves in leads II and V_{4R} to V_2. Newborns with atrial flutter may have congestive heart failure from the tachycardia, but more commonly the 2:1 or 3:1 block reduces the ventricular rate so that the dysrhythmia is well tolerated (Fig. 62–35).

The treatment involves digitalization and, if this fails to revert the rhythm to sinus, cardioversion. The prognosis is not as favorable as with atrial tachycardia because recurrences are more common, but most infants without associated structural heart disease usually do well. Ongoing treatment with digoxin is usually successful in preventing recurrences. If this approach is not successful, propranolol or quinidine can be added.

Ventricular Tachycardia

Ventricular tachycardia (three or more premature complexes in a row) in the newborn is uncommon. When it does occur, it is usually in association with structural heart disease and is triggered by cardiac catheterization, surgery, anesthesia, metabolic abnormalities, or digitalis toxicity. The QRS complexes are wide and tall, and the T waves are directed opposite to the QRS complex. The rate is usually less than 200 beats/min, but higher rates have been reported. The initial treatment should be lidocaine (1 mg/kg intravenously) or cardioversion. Other drugs that may occasionally be useful include phenytoin (diphenylhydantoin), procainamide, quinidine, and propranolol. In the idiopathic variety, echocardiography and angiocardiography should be performed to rule out the possibility that a resectable tumor is the source of the tachycardia. Treatment must be individualized, with the long-term prognosis depending primarily on the underlying cardiac problem.

Atrioventricular Block
First-Degree and Second-Degree Heart Block

First-degree heart block is a prolongation of the P-R interval beyond the normal limits, 0.164 seconds on the first

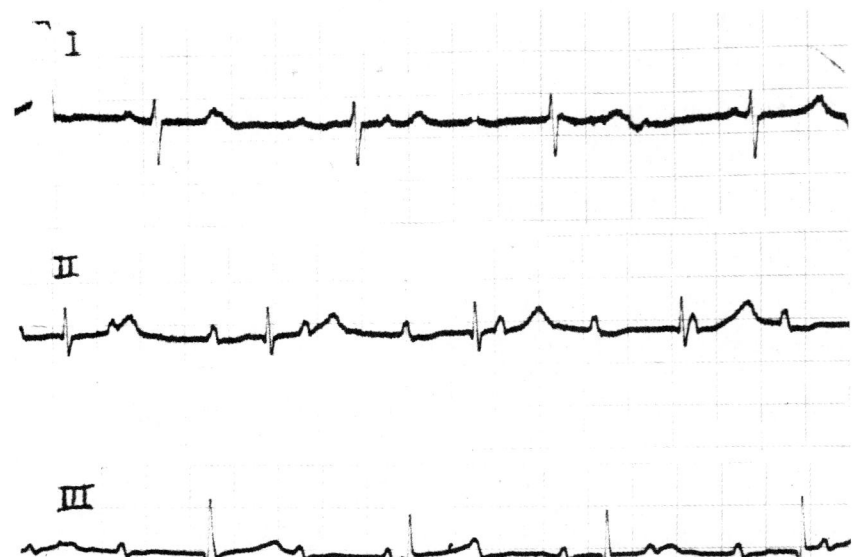

FIGURE 62–36. Age 4 days. Standard limb leads. Complete heart block is present. The ventricular rate is 90, the atrial rate 120.

day of life, and 0.14 seconds for the rest of the neonatal period. It is of no hemodynamic significance by itself and requires no treatment. In second-degree heart block, there is an intermittent failure of impulse transmission from atria to ventricles. It may be exhibited as a progressive prolongation of the P-R interval in successive cycles followed by an unconducted atrial impulse (Wenckebach or Mobitz Type I) or failure of atrial impulse transmission with dropped ventricular beats and no progressive prolongation of the P-R interval (Mobitz Type II). Both Type I and Type II may be manifestations of infection or digitalis toxicity. Neither type needs treatment, but both should be watched carefully because either may lead to third-degree or complete heart block.

Third-Degree Heart Block

In complete heart block, there is complete failure of the atrial impulse to lead to a ventricular response; the atria and ventricles beat independently, with the latter having a slower rate. On the surface electrocardiogram, there is no fixed relationship between the P waves and the QRS complex (Fig. 62–36). Complete heart block is a relatively common problem in the newborn, occurring in 1 of every 15,000 to 20,000 live births. Histologically there may be an absence of a connection between the atrial conduction tissue and the atrioventricular node, absence or degeneration of the connection between the atrioventricular node tissue and the distal conducting tissue, or a lesion beyond the atrioventricular node that interrupts the bundle of His.

REFERENCES

American Academy of Pediatrics: Section on Cardiology: Guidelines for pediatric diagnostic and treatment centers. Pediatrics 87:576, 1991.

Balsan MJ, Jones JG, Guthrie RD: Effects of a clinically detectable PDA on pulmonary mechanics measures in VLBW infants with RDS. Pediatr Pulmonol 111:161, 1991.

Bancalari E, Jesse MJ, Gelband H, Garcia O: Lung mechanics in congenital heart disease with increased and decreased pulmonary blood flow. J Pediatr 90:192, 1977.

Bando K, Turrentine MW, Sun K, et al: Surgical management of complete atrioventricular septal defects: A twenty-year experience. J Thorac Cardiovasc Surg 110:1543–1552, 1995.

Bove EL, Lloyd TR: Staged reconstruction for hypoplastic left heart syndrome: Contemporary results. Ann Surg 224:387–394, 1996.

Burnard ED: The cardiac murmur in relation to symptoms of the newborn. BMJ 1:134, 1939.

Caspi J, Coles JG, Benson LN, et al: Management of neonatal critical pulmonic stenosis in the balloon valvotomy era. Ann Thorac Surg 49:273–278, 1990.

Cassidy SC, Schmidt KG, van Hare GF, et al: Complications of pediatric cardiac catheterization: A three-year study. J Am Coll Cardiol 19:1285, 1992.

Castañeda AR, Jonas RA, Mayer JE Jr, Hanley FL: Cardiac Surgery of the Neonate and Infant. Philadelphia, WB Saunders, 1994.

Cetta F, Feldt RH, O'Leary PW, et al: Improved early morbidity and mortality after Fontan operation: The Mayo Clinic experience, 1987 to 1992. J Am Coll Cardiol 28:480–486, 1996.

Chu J, Clements JA, Cotton EK, et al: Neonatal pulmonary ischemia: Part 1. Clinical and physiological studies. Pediatrics 40:709, 1967.

Clyman RI: Medical treatment of patent ductus arteriosus in premature infants. In Long WA (Ed): Fetal and Neonatal Cardiology. Philadelphia, WB Saunders, 1990, pp 682–690.

Clyman RI, Jobe A, Heymann M, et al: Increased shunt through the patent ductus arteriosus after surfactant replacement therapy. J Pediatr 100:101, 1982.

Cobanoglu A, Menashe VD: Total anomalous pulmonary venous connec-

tion in neonates and young infants: Repair in the current era [see comments]. Ann Thorac Surg 55:43–48, 1993.

Corbet A: Medical manipulation of the ductus arteriosus. In Garson A, Bricker JT, Fisher DJ, Neish SR (Eds): The Science and Practice of Pediatric Cardiology. Philadelphia, Williams & Wilkins, 1998, pp 2489–2513.

Danielson GK, Driscoll DJ, Mair DD, et al: Operative treatment of Ebstein's anomaly. J Thorac Cardiovasc Surg 104:1195–1202, 1992.

Dudell GG, Gersony WM: Patent ductus arteriosus in neonates with severe respiratory disease. J Pediatr 104:915, 1984.

Faix RG, Viscardi RM, DiPietro MA, Nicks JJ: Adult respiratory distress syndrome in full term infants. Pediatrics 83:971, 1989.

Ferrer PL: Arrhythmias in the neonate. In Roberts NK, Gelband H (Eds): Cardiac Arrhythmias in the Neonate, Infant, and Child. New York, Appleton-Century-Crofts, 1997.

Freed MD, Heymann MA, Lewis AB, et al: Prostaglandin E₁ in infants with ductus arteriosus dependent congenital heart disease. Circulation 64:899, 1981.

Fujiwara T, Maeta H, Chida S, et al: Artificial surfactant therapy in hyaline membrane disease. Lancet 1:55, 1980.

Griffin AJ, Ferrara JD, Lax JO, Cassels DE: Pulmonary compliance: An index of cardiovascular status in infancy. Am J Dis Child 123:89, 1972.

Gutgesell HP, Speer ME, Rosenberg HS: Characterization of the cardiomyopathy in infants of diabetic mothers. Circulation 61:441, 1980.

Hanley FL, Sade RM, Blackstone EH, et al: Outcomes in neonatal pulmonary atresia with intact ventricular septum: A multi-institutional study. J Thorac Cardiovasc Surg 105:406, 1993.

Heldt GP, Pesonen E, Merritt TA, et al: Closure of the ductus arteriosus and mechanics of breathing in preterm infants after surfactant replacement therapy. Pediatr Res 25:305, 1989.

Huhta J: Patent ductus arteriosus in the preterm neonate. In Long WA (Ed): Fetal and Neonatal Cardiology. Philadelphia, WB Saunders, 1990a, pp 389–400.

Huhta J: Structural heart disease in the low birth weight neonate. In Long WA (Ed): Fetal and Neonatal Cardiology. Philadelphia, WB Saunders, 1990b, pp 419–424.

Idriss FS, Ilbawi MN, Delean SY, et al: Transposition of the great arteries with intact ventricular septum: Arterial switch in the first month of life. J Thorac Cardiovasc Surg 95:255, 1988.

Jonas RA, Giglia TM, Sanders SP, et al: Rapid, two-stage arterial switch for transposition of the great arteries and intact ventricular septum beyond the neonatal period. Circulation 80(suppl I):I-203, 1989.

Keane JF, McFaul R, Fellows K, Lock J: Balloon occlusion angiography in infancy: Methods, uses, and limitations. Am J Cardiol 56:495, 1985.

Kennedy JW and the Registry Committee of the Society for Cardiac Angiography: Complications associated with cardiac catheterization and angiography: Symposium on catheterization complications. Cathet Cardiovasc Diagn 8:5, 1982.

Kinsella JP, Neish SR, Shaffer E, Abman AH: Low dose inhalational nitric oxide in persistent pulmonary hypertension of the newborn. Lancet 340:819, 1992.

Kitterman JA, Edmunds LH, Gregory GA, et al: Patent ductus arteriosus in premature infants: Incidence relation to pulmonary disease and management. N Engl J Med 287:473, 1973.

Kobayashi T, Mitta K, Ganzuka M, et al: Inactivation of exogenous surfactant by pulmonary edema fluid. Pediatr Res 29:353, 1991.

Long WA, Structural cardiovascular abnormalities presenting as persistent pulmonary hypertension of the newborn. Clin Perinatol 11:601, 1984.

Long WA: Developmental pulmonary circulatory physiology. In Long WA (Ed): Fetal and Neonatal Cardiology. Philadelphia, WB Saunders, 1990a, pp 76–96.

Long WA: Persistent pulmonary hypertension of the newborn syndrome (PPHNS). In Long WA (Ed): Fetal and Neonatal Cardiology. Philadelphia, WB Saunders, 1990b, pp 627–655.

Long WA: Pneumopericardium. In Long WA (Ed): Fetal and Neonatal Cardiology. Philadelphia, WB Saunders, 1990c, pp 377–388.

Long WA: The changing natural history of patent ductus arteriosus in respiratory distress syndrome: Impact of surfactant replacement. In Long WA, Tilson HH (Eds): Proceedings of the Exosurf Neonatal Treatment IND Investigators' Meeting. Langhorne, PA, Adis Publishing, 1992, pp 89–94.

Long WA, Henry GW: Central neural and autonomic regulation of fetal cardiovascular function. In Polin RA, Fox WW (Eds): Neonatal and Fetal Medicine: Physiology and Pathophysiology. Philadelphia, WB Saunders, 1992, pp 629–645.

Long WA, Willis PW IV: Maternal lithium and neonatal Ebstein's anomaly: Evaluation with cross-sectional echocardiography. Am J Perinatol 1:182, 1984.

Long WA, Lawson EE, Harned HS Jr, Kraybill EN: Pleural effusion in the first days of life: A prospective study. Am J Perinatol 1:190, 1984a.

Long WA, Lawson EE, Henry GW, Harned HS Jr: Infradiaphragmatic total anomalous pulmonary venous drainage: New diagnostic, physiologic, and surgical considerations. Am J Perinatol 1:227, 1984b.

Long WA, Schall SA, Henry GW: Cerebral arteriovenous malformation presenting as persistent fetal circulation: Diagnosis by cross-sectional echo. Am J Perinatol 1:236, 1984c.

Long WA, Zeng G, Henry GW: Pharmacologic adjuncts: II. Exogenous surfactants. *In* Goldsmith JP, Korotkin EH (Eds): Assisted Ventilation of the Neonate, 3rd ed. Philadelphia, WB Saunders, 1996, pp 305–325.

Long WA, Zeng G, Henry GW: New drugs for perinatal practice: The role of industry-sponsored clinical trials. Semin Perinatol 19:132, 1995a.

Long WA, Zucker J, Kraybill EN (Eds): Symposium on Synthetic Surfactant: II. Health and Developmental Outcomes at One Year. J Pediatr 125:S1–S102, 1995b.

Mandell VS, Lock JE, Mayer JE, et al: The "laid-back" aortogram: An improved angiographic view for demonstration of coronary arteries in transposition of the great arteries. Am J Cardiol 65:1379, 1990.

Mee RBB: Results of the arterial switch procedure for complete transposition with intact ventricular septum. Cardiol Young 1:97, 1991.

Murphy JG, Gersh BJ, Mair DD, et al: Long-term outcome in patients undergoing surgical repair of tetralogy of Fallot [see comments]. N Engl J Med 329:593–599, 1993.

Naulty CM, Horn S, Conry J, Avery GB: Improved lung compliance after ligation of patent ductus arteriosus in hyaline membrane disease. J Pediatr 93:682, 1978.

Neghme RA, O'Connor TZ, Lister G, Bracken M: Patent ductus arteriosus. *In* Sinclair JC, Bracken MB (Eds): Effective Care of the Newborn Infant. Oxford, Oxford University Press, 1992, pp 281–324.

Nihill MR, Mullins CE, McNamara DG: Visualization of the pulmonary arteries in pseudotruncus by pulmonary vein wedge angiography. Circulation 58:140, 1978.

Noonan J: Chromosomal abnormalities. *In* Long WA (Ed): Fetal and Neonatal Cardiology. Philadelphia, WB Saunders, 1990a, pp 578–594.

Noonan J: Syndromes. *In* Long WA (Ed): Fetal and Neonatal Cardiology. Philadelphia, WB Saunders, 1990b, pp 604–626.

Norwood WI, Lang P, Castañeda AR, Hougen TJ: Reparative operations for interrupted aortic arch with ventricular septal defect. J Thorac Cardiovasc Surg 86:832–837, 1983.

Paret G, Steinmetz D, Kuint J, et al: Adenosine for the treatment of paroxysmal supraventricular tachycardia in full-term and preterm newborn infants. Am J Perinatol 13:343, 1996.

Podrid PJ, Kowey PR (Eds): Cardiac Arrhythmias: Mechanisms, Diagnosis, and Management. Baltimore, Williams & Wilkins, 1995.

Rassouk AJ, Chinnock RE, Gundry SR, et al: Transplantation as a primary treatment for hypoplastic left heart syndrome: Intermediate-term results. Ann Thorac Surg 62:1–7, 1996.

Rudolph AM: The changes in the circulation after birth: Their importance in congenital heart disease. The Lewis A. Conner Memorial Lecture, Dallas, Texas, 1969. Circulation 41:343, 1970.

Sanders S: Echocardiography. *In* Long WA (Ed): Fetal and Neonatal Cardiology. Philadelphia, WB Saunders, 1990, pp 310–329.

Southall DP, Johnson AM, Shinebourne EA, et al: Frequency and outcome of disorders of cardiac rhythm and conduction in a population of newborn infants. Pediatrics 68:58, 1981.

Stanger P, Heymann M, Tarnoff H, et al: Complications of cardiac catheterization of neonates, infants, and children: A three-year study. Circulation 50:595, 1974.

Stefano JL, Abbasi S, Perlman SA, et al: Closure of the ductus arteriosus with indomethacin in ventilated neonates with respiratory distress syndrome. Am Rev Respir Dis 143:236, 1991.

Takahashi M, Schieber RA, Wishner SH, et al: Selective coronary arteriography in infants and children. Circulation 68:1021, 1983.

Taylor PV, Taylor KF, Norman A, et al: Prevalence of maternal R_o (SSA) and L_a (SSB) autoantibodies in relation to complete heart block. Br J Rheumatol 27:128, 1988.

Van Mierop LHS, Kutsche L: Cardiovascular anomalies in DiGeorge syndrome and importance of neural crest as a possible pathogenic factor. Am J Cardiol 58:133, 1986.

Way GL, Wolfe RR, Pettet G, et al: Echocardiographic assessments of ventricular dimensions and myocardial function in infants of diabetic mothers. Pediatr Res 9:273, 1975.

Yeh TF, Thalji A, Luken L, et al: Improved lung compliance following indomethacin therapy in premature infants with patent ductus arteriosus. Chest 80:698, 1991.

Zeevi B, Keane JF, Castañeda AR, et al: Neonatal critical valvular aortic stenosis: A comparison of surgical and balloon dilation therapy [see comments]. Circulation 80:831–839, 1989.

Zehr KJ, Gillinov AM, Redmond JM, et al: Repair of coarctation of the aorta in neonates and infants: A thirty-year experience. Ann Thorac Surg 59:33–41, 1995.

Zeng G, Henry GW, Long WA: Persistent pulmonary hypertension of the newborn syndrome and myocardial ischemia of the newborn. *In* Anderson RH (Ed): Paediatric Cardiology, 2nd ed. London, Churchill Livingstone, in press.

CHAPTER 63

Preoperative and Postoperative Care of the Newborn with Congenital Heart Disease

Lela W. Brink

STABILIZATION AND TRANSPORT
Identification of the Infant at Risk

Early identification of the neonate with congenital heart disease is important. In the first 24 hours of life, cyanosis is the most common presenting symptom. Many more cyanotic neonates have respiratory disease than primary cardiac anomalies. The difficulty, therefore, is differentiating the infant with congenital heart disease from the infant with pulmonary disease. The common cyanotic lesions that may present in the 1st day of life include truncus arteriosus, total anomalous pulmonary venous return, transposition of the great vessels, tricuspid atresia, tetralogy of Fallot, and pulmonary atresia (Perloff, 1978) (Table 63–1).

Neonates with congenital heart disease may present with central cyanosis but few signs or symptoms of respiratory distress. Because the cause of the cyanosis is usually intracardiac right-to-left shunting, there is little change when the infant is placed in oxygen with a fraction of inspired oxygen (FIO_2) of 1.0. Further evaluation of the cyanosis may include endotracheal intubation and the delivery of positive end-expiratory pressure. Infants with primary pulmonary disease will generally show significant improvement in oxygenation with these maneuvers, whereas infants with cyanotic congenital heart disease will have little improvement. A more difficult differential diagnosis is presented by the infant with persistent pulmonary hypertension resulting in right-to-left shunting. Echocardiographic evaluation of the infant with severe refractory hypoxemia permits identification of cyanotic congenital heart disease and persistent pulmonary hypertension (Meyer, 1995).

Evaluation of the chest radiograph may help in the differential diagnosis. The presence of cyanosis and decreased pulmonary blood flow on chest radiograph almost always is either cyanotic congenital heart disease or persistent pumonary hypertension. It is more difficult to distinguish lung disease from heart disease if the chest radiograph demonstrates pulmonary congestion or opacification. In the first days of life, total anomalous pulmonary venous connection (TAPVC) with obstruction is characterized by opacification of the lung fields and can mimic respiratory distress syndrome. At the time of ductal closure, severe left-sided obstructive lesions, critical aortic stenosis, aortic atresia, or hypoplastic left heart syndrome may also present with significant pulmonary opacification on chest radiograph (Kelley et al, 1982).

A group of essentially asymptomatic newborns presents with an abnormal physical examination in the newborn period. The presence of a significant murmur can lead to identification of congenital heart disease before symptoms develop. Occasionally an infant is identified because of diminished femoral pulses at the time of discharge from the newborn nursery or on an early follow-up examination. Other infants are identified because congenital heart disease is a significant component of a more complex syndrome (e.g., Down syndrome).

Although several congenital cardiac lesions typically present within the first 24 hours of life with cyanosis, others may not present until several days of age or even the 2nd week of postnatal life. Typical presentations after the 1st day of life include shock or congestive heart failure (Artman and Graham, 1982). The differential diagnosis includes blood loss, anemia, sepsis, and congenital metabolic abnormalities but also other causes of shock as well as congenital heart disease. Resuscitation is initiated to reverse the signs and symptoms of respiratory failure and shock (Bloom et al, 1990). Treatment for sepsis is generally instituted early. If the child fails to respond to the usual resuscitative measures, therapy with prostaglandin E_1 (PGE_1) should be considered pending a complete cardiac evaluation (Elliot et al, 1975).

Infants with acyanotic congenital heart disease that is not ductal dependent rarely experience symptoms in the neonatal period. Infants with ductal-dependent left-sided obstructive lesions, such as coarctation of the aorta, critical aortic stenosis, and hypoplastic left heart syndrome, experience symptoms at the time of ductal closure and present in the early neonatal period. The signs and symptoms are those of shock and respiratory failure. Most often, these patients are initially thought to have neonatal sepsis. Pulmonary congestion may be significant. Secondary organ system injury will occur from inadequate end-organ delivery of oxygen secondary to ductal closure. In the majority of the patients with ductal-dependent left-sided obstructive lesions, tachypnea and pallor are the presenting symptoms. Metabolic acidemia is frequently present. Because of the luxuriant pulmonary blood flow that results from ductal closure in the presence of left-sided outflow obstruction, the acidemia is often accompanied by a surprisingly high partial pressure of arterial oxygen (PaO_2). Later as the circulatory failure progresses, hydrostatic pulmonary edema impairs gas exchange and PaO_2 falls.

Stabilization of the Neonate with Possible Congenital Heart Disease

When a neonate or infant presents with respiratory failure or shock, the initial approach to stabilization is determined by the symptoms at presentation. The differential diagnosis for any sick infant must include congenital heart disease. After the initial evaluation and stabilization, consideration should be given to starting PGE_1, unless the infant is

TABLE 63–1

Common Congenital Heart Lesions

Cyanotic	Acyanotic
Decreased Pulmonary Blood Flow	Atrial septal defect
	Ventricular septal defect
Pulmonary atresia	Patent ductus arteriosus
Tricuspid atresia	Left-sided obstructive lesions
Tetralogy of Fallot	Coarctation of the aorta
Transposition of the great vessels	Aortic stenosis (atresia)
Increased Pulmonary Blood Flow	Mitral stenosis (atresia)
Total anomalous pulmonary venous return	Hypoplastic left heart syndrome

responding rapidly to more routine measures. Reopening of the ductus should be a priority in infants who are not improving rapidly, particularly if immediate cardiac evaluation is not available. Failure to reopen the ductus arteriosus in infants who are critically ill with ductal-dependent congenital heart disease is often fatal. Giving PGE_1 to an infant who later proves to have sepsis or an inborn error of metabolism seldom causes harm.

Airway and Ventilation. Primary respiratory failure is the most common cause of cyanosis and arrest in infants. Patency of the airway, adequacy of ventilation, and secure delivery of oxygen are the primary goals during the initial resuscitation and stabilization. After opening the airway, bag-valve-mask ventilation should be initiated if spontaneous ventilation does not return. If continued ventilatory support is required, an endotracheal tube should be placed. If significant circulatory compromise, poor perfusion, diminished pulses, or reduced blood pressure is present, myocardial depressant drugs should be avoided and the circulation supported when pharmacologic agents are chosen to facilitate endotracheal intubation. Once the airway is secured, the initial support should be with an FIO_2 of 1.0 and adequate ventilation.

Circulation. Initial attention should be focused on the systemic circulation, with an evaluation of perfusion, peripheral pulses, and the adequacy of intravascular volume. The physical examination should include an evaluation of color, pulses (and blood pressure) in all four extremities, signs of pulmonary congestion, and a complete cardiac evaluation. Hepatomegaly may be an important sign of right-sided heart failure or a marker of the adequacy of intravascular volume replacement. The chest radiograph also may give clues as to the extent of cardiac failure or the adequacy of pulmonary blood flow.

One of the initial issues in the resuscitation of neonates is obtaining adequate vascular access for administration of intravenous fluid administration or assessment of intravascular pressures. Peripheral intravenous catheters can be placed for the initial resuscitation. In the immediate newborn, central vascular catheters can be placed via the umbilical vein or umbilical artery. These can be used for the measurement of intravascular pressures or for the infusions of fluids or medications. In older infants, central venous catheters can be placed by experienced clinicians in the

internal jugular, subclavian, or femoral routes. Peripheral arterial catheters can be placed in the radial, posterior tibial, and dorsalis pedis arteries. Care should be taken in the placement of such cannulas. In patients with critical coarctation, the right radial artery is the only site for the measurement of preductal pressures and blood gases. Often the surgeon prefers to place this cannula. Alternatively, the most experienced intensivist or neonatologist should attempt placement. Interpretation of blood gases and pressures may vary with the location of the catheter, whether preductal or postductal, and the type of cardiac anomaly.

The initial fluid resuscitation is focused on adequate volume replacement with an isotonic fluid (normal saline, Ringer's lactate, or 5% albumin). If there is clinical evidence of cardiac failure, small aliquots of volume should be used: 3 to 5 mL/kg rather than the larger 10 to 20 mL/kg dose frequently recommended. Volume infusion should be discontinued if there is evidence of progression of circulatory failure or clinical evidence of adequate intravascular volume replacement. If the circulatory failure does not reverse with volume replacement, consideration should be given to beginning inotropic support.

The decision to initiate inotropic support and the selection of pharmacologic agents depend on the age of the child, cardiac disease, and physiologic stability. Extensive reviews of the individual agents and the use of vasoactive agents in pediatrics are published (Zaritsky and Chernow, 1984) (Table 63–2).

If with the usual resuscitation and evaluation it becomes clear that there is (1) potential for inadequate pulmonary blood flow secondary to a right-sided obstructive lesion or (2) evidence of inadequate systemic blood flow secondary to a potential left-sided obstructive lesion, consideration should be given to beginning therapy with PGE_1. PGE_1 is used to reopen and then maintain the patency of the ductus arteriosus in neonates with congenital heart disease. Reopening the ductus stabilizes infants with ductal-dependent congenital heart disease until a definitive evaluation or palliative or corrective surgery can be accomplished. The usual dose of PGE_1 is 0.05 to 0.1 μg/kg/min. In small infants and at higher doses, there is a significant incidence of apnea. Mechanical ventilation may be required in up to 10% of the infants receiving PGE_1.

Transport of the Neonate with Congenital Heart Disease

Infants with congenital heart disease are generally cared for at regional tertiary referral centers. It is important to establish lines of referral, consultation, and communication about the transport of these high-risk patients. Transport by a specially trained neonatal or pediatric transport team with experience in the care of infants with congenital heart disease is ideal. Serial assessments and adjustments in management are usually required throughout transport in infants with symptomatic congenital heart disease.

Transport Personnel. The actual configuration of the transport team may vary among institutions. Expertise in neonatal and pediatric nursing is essential. Expertise in intubation, airway management, and mechanical ventilation may be provided by registered nurses (RNs), respiratory

TABLE 63–2

Vasoactive Agents

Medication	Dose	Pharmacologic Action
Catecholamines		
Dopamine	1–20 µg/kg/min	1. Low dose, 1–3 µg/kg/min, dopaminergic action primarily dilates renal vascular bed 2. Five to 10 µg/kg/min beta-adrenergic dosing with primarily inotropic effects 3. Ten to 20 µg/kg/min beta-adrenergic dosing with inotropic, chronotropic, and vasoconstrictive effects Dopamine is a naturally occurring catecholamine. Clinical inotropic and chronotropic effects require the release of endogenous stores of catecholamines, epinephrine, and norepinephrine.
Dobutamine	2–20 µg/kg/min	Synthetic catecholamine with selective beta-adrenergic effects. Dominantly inotropic with varying effect on blood pressure depending on its effect on peripheral vascular resistance. Variable degree of tachycardia may be noted.
Epinephrine	0.01–1 µg/kg/min	Epinephrine is a naturally occurring "endogenous" catecholamine that acts directly on the adrenergic receptor sites. The response to epinephrine is dose related. At relatively low dose, the effects are primarily beta-adrenergic chronotropic and inotropic. At higher doses (>0.3 µg/kg/min), the vasoconstrictive effects (vasopressor effects) of epinephrine are more predictable.
Phosphodiesterase Inhibitors		
Amrinone	5–10 µg/kg/min	Amrinone, a bipyridine, possesses positive inotropic characteristics and is a potent pulmonary and systemic vasodilator. Effect on blood pressure depends on the relative effects of the increase in inotropy, the effective preload, and relative fall in peripheral vascular resistance. Long-term administration has been associated with thrombocytopenia. Because of the relatively long half-life, a loading dose is often given to facilitate achieving steady-state kinetics. Doses of 0.75 to 3 mg/kg have been used.
Milrinone	0.5–1.0 µg/kg/min	A bipyridine, 10 to 30 times more potent then amrinone, the intravenous formulation of milrinone reportedly is associated with less thrombocytopenia than amrinone. The inotropic, chronotropic, and vasodilatory effects of the two agents are similar in equipotent dosing. Bolus doses of 50 µg/kg have been used in neonates with congenital heart disease. Loading doses are used in the order of 0.
Vasodilators		
Nitroprusside	0.5–5 µg/kg/min	Nitroprusside is a systemic and pulmonary vasodilator used in the management of hypertensive crises or for afterload reduction to improve cardiac output in patients with ventricular failure. It causes peripheral vasodilation by direct action on venous and arteriolar smooth muscle.
Nitroglycerin	0.5–5 µg/kg/min	Nitroglycerin is a vasodilator that affects the systemic, pulmonary, and coronary vessels. It reduces cardiac oxygen demand by decreasing left ventricular pressure and systemic vascular resistance. It improves coronary flow and improves collateral flow through ischemic areas.

therapists (RTs), physician extenders, or physicians. The most common configurations for neonatal transport are RN-RN or RN-RT. Medical direction for transport should be provided by pediatric intensivists or neonatologists based at the receiving hospital. The availability of continual communication between the transport personnel and the physician directing transport is optimal. Standards for the training of personnel for neonatal and pediatric transport have been developed by national organizations.

Transport Equipment. Provision of a neutral thermal environment minimizes the physiologic stress on a neonates with congenital heart disease. A transport isolette is ideal for provision of thermoneutrality; isolettes can be configured with appropriate cardiorespiratory monitors, (electrocardiogram [ECG], respiratory, blood pressure, pulse oximetry) as well as a ventilator to facilitate the movement of the infant from the referring hospital to the receiving hospital, regardless of the vehicle and mode of transport. Intravenous infusion pumps capable of accurate infusions of low volumes of fluids are essential. Dedicated equipment bags for airway, vascular access, and medications are also useful; the contents vary to support the protocols and procedures of the individual transport teams.

Transport Vehicle. The mode of transport and the vehicle chosen will depend on the distance traveled, the physiologic stability of the infant, the availability of equipment, and the weather. Infants with congenital heart disease can be safely transported by experienced personnel in medically equipped vehicles by ground, rotor wing, or fixed wing.

During transport to the receiving institution, serial assessments and modifications of therapy are necessities for unstable patients. For this reason, there must be ready access to equipment, medications, the patient, and medical support from the receiving institution.

PREOPERATIVE CARE
General Principles

Many infants identified in the neonatal period with congenital heart disease will not require surgery before discharge from the nursery. The preterm infant with patent ductus arteriosus and significant cardiac failure secondary to left-to-right shunting may require surgical intervention if medical management fails. The care of these infants preoperatively is focused on the management of the pulmonary disease and prematurity.

In infants requiring surgical palliation or repair in the neonatal period, the goal of preoperative care is maintenance of cardiorespiratory stability. The timing of surgery will depend on the anatomic and physiologic characteristics of the cardiac lesion, gestational age, and complicating problems in the neonate (Castaneda et al, 1989). In the preterm neonate with congenital heart disease, supportive care, including long-term maintenance on PGE_1, may be required. PGE_1 administration is associated with an increased incidence of apnea. Many infants who are about to be transported are intubated with the initiation of PGE_1 therapy to avoid apnea in a closed isolette aboard a helicopter or airplane. If there is no pulmonary reason for intubation, the dose of prostaglandin can generally be decreased once ductal patency is established and early extubation of these infants is considered. Supportive care appropriate for any other infant of similar gestational age is essential.

Care of Infants with Ductal-Dependent Pulmonary Flow: The Patient with a Critical Right-Sided Obstructive Lesion or Transposition of the Great Vessels

Infants with suspected right-sided obstructive lesions resulting in decreased pulmonary blood flow require maintenance of ductal patency with PGE_1 until a complete assessment of the cardiac lesion has been performed. Many term neonates with cyanotic congenital heart disease secondary to right-sided obstructive lesions are candidates for definitive repair. Palliation with systemic-to-pulmonary artery shunt may be the option selected in small infants or in those with very small or poorly developed pulmonary arteries.

Before palliation or definitive repair, stabilization on PGE_1 is required. The goals for support should be to minimize invasive therapies, minimize infectious risks, maximize caloric intake, and maximize the infant-parental contact. PGE_1 therapy is initiated to re-establish or to maintain ductal patency, thereby ensuring adequate pulmonary blood flow. The determinants of pulmonary blood flow include the size of the ductus arteriosus (or shunt) and the pressure gradient across the ductus. The concentration of FIO_2 and the magnitude of ventilatory support can affect pulmonary vascular resistance and pulmonary pressure. Intravascular volume, inotropic state and level of vasomotor tone can affect systemic pressure. The optimal pulmonary-systemic blood flow (Q_s) ratio (Q_p-Q_s) is 1:1. The best noninvasive gauge of pulmonary blood flow is systemic oxygenation. A systemic oxygen saturation of 75% to 85% usually reflects good mixing and adequate pulmonary blood flow. Pulmonary blood flow will also increase with the physiologic fall in pulmonary vascular resistance that occurs in the 1st week of life in the otherwise normal term neonate. A similar fall in pulmonary vascular resistance will occur with the resolution of pulmonary parenchymal disease. Throughout this period of stabilization, the ability to provide adequate nutrition for growth may be limited.

In addition to therapy with PGE_1, infants with transposition of the great arteries, especially those with intact ventricular septum, may require balloon atrial septostomy to ensure adequate mixing. Again monitoring of peripheral arterial saturations is a good marker of adequate mixing. Many factors affect the timing of definitive repair with the arterial switch operation. Early repair should be timed to allow the natural fall in pulmonary vascular resistance to begin. If surgical intervention is delayed significantly, the anatomic smooth-walled left ventricle may begin involution in response to the decrease in stroke work that results from pumping to the low-pressure pulmonary bed.

Care of the Infant with Ductal-Dependent Systemic Flow: The Patient with a Critical Left-Sided Obstructive Lesion

Infants with critical left-sided obstructive lesions may be identified early while relatively asymptomatic or may present later with severe circulatory failure at the time of functional ductal closure. Some infants present early in life with tachypnea, respiratory distress, or a murmur. Respiratory symptoms occur secondary to increased pulmonary congestion but may be relatively mild until the ductus arteriosus begins to close. When the ductus arteriosus closes, differences in blood pressure or pulses in the upper and lower extremities may be evident. Echocardiography is the best technique to identify a significant left-sided obstructive lesion (mitral or aortic stenosis, coarctation of the aorta, or other lesion in the spectrum of hypoplastic left heart syndrome). However, the echocardiographic diagnosis of coarctation of the aorta may be very difficult in the neonate if the aortic end of the ductus arteriosus is widely patent at the time of examination (Rychik et al, 1991).

Infants often do not become symptomatic with left-sided obstructive lesions until ductal closure occurs after 4 hours of age. Some infants present later, at 2 to 3 weeks of age. These infants present to their pediatricians or the emergency room acutely ill. Often their color is poor and is described as gray. A septic work-up is generally performed. A chest radiograph may show increased markings compatible with pulmonary edema or pneumonia. Often the child is intubated and begun on antibiotics before the referral call. In the process of data collection, an arterial blood gas may be obtained. Often the initial arterial blood gas demonstrates a PaO_2 significantly higher than the referring physician would anticipate based on the chest radiogram and the infant's color. The pH often demonstrates a significant metabolic acidemia resulting from the decrease in systemic perfusion secondary to ductal closure. After initial stabilization and beginning PGE_1, transport to a referral center is essential. Many of these infants will have evidence of significant end-organ dysfunction that can delay or prevent later surgical palliation or correction (Norwood and Pigott, 1989).

Stabilization of the neonate with ductal-dependent systemic flow is aimed at providing adequate organ perfusion. To achieve adequate systemic flow, a pressure gradient must exist that drives flow from the pulmonary through the ductus to the systemic arterial bed. The first and most critical parameter is to ensure ductal patency. Once ductal patency is established, the pulmonary vascular resistance must be increased to the extent that pulmonary artery pressure exceeds systemic pressure (Morray et al, 1986). The most potent pulmonary vasoconstrictor we have is hypoxia. Weaning of FIO_2 to room air or the lowest possible FIO_2 to sustain adequate end-organ delivery of oxygen is imperative. After the acute resuscitation, inotropic agents, if required, should minimize systemic vasoconstriction (to decrease the resistance to systemic flow). For this reason dobutamine is usually preferable to either high-dose dopamine or epinephrine. If a further increase in pulmonary vascular resistance is required to increase the pulmonary pressure and provide an adequate pressure gradient for systemic flow, several options are available: (1) endotracheal intubation and paralysis with intentional hypoventilation to allow partial pressure of arterial carbon dioxide to rise and pH to fall, (2) spontaneous rebreathing or breathing of a mixture of gases that includes inspired carbon dioxide, or (3) spontaneous breathing hypoxic gas mixture. Combinations of these techniques have been used successfully (Norwood and Pigott, 1989).

Assessment of the adequacy of systemic organ perfusion in patients with ductal-dependent systemic flow may be difficult using the usual clinical parameters. Serial measurements of systemic arterial saturations are useful in evaluation of systemic perfusion. Excessive increases in pulmonary flow result in increases in systemic saturations in excess of 90%. In contrast, excessive reductions in pulmonary flow are represented by systemic saturations of less than 70%. In such cases, hypoxemia may compromise end-organ oxygen delivery despite increased systemic perfusion. Adequate systemic blood flow is usually present in infants with ductal-dependent systemic circulation, if systemic saturation is between 75% and 85% on PGE_1. Near-normal systemic arterial blood pressures for age should also result. Although a bit counterintuitive, vasopressor agents may decrease right-to-left flow through the ductus and therefore decrease end-organ perfusion. Adequate systemic oxygen delivery may require the maintenance of relatively elevated oxygen-carrying capacity to compensate for the hypoxemia and compromise in cardiac output. The hematocrit should usually be maintained in the range of 40% to 55%.

Infants with ductal-dependent systemic perfusion can usually be stabilized on PGE_1 but not indefinitely. Planning for definitive therapy, when possible, or palliation should begin with the identification of the anatomic and physiologic abnormalities.

The Patient with TAPVC

Neonates with partially or completely obstructed total anomalous pulmonary venous return present with significant pulmonary congestion and respiratory failure. Echocardiography is essential in term infants with hypoxemia, respiratory distress, and diffuse interstitial edema on chest radiograph to differentiate TAPVC from diffuse pulmonary disease. Stabilization of these patients is focused on achieving adequate gas exchange and supporting cardiac function. Once obstructed TAPVC has been identified, surgical intervention is emergent (Sano et al, 1989).

Infants with unobstructed TAPVC or partial anomalous pulmonary venous connection have increased pulmonary blood flow and can experience cardiac failure. The treatment in neonates would include inotropic support when indicated and diuresis. In patients unresponsive to pharmacologic therapies alone, consideration should be given to endotracheal intubation and mechanical ventilation until surgical intervention can be performed. However, most infants with unobstructed total or partial anomalous venous return can be managed medically for several months.

The Neonate with Cardiac Failure Secondary to Increased Pulmonary Blood Flow from Intracardiac Left-to-Right Shunting

Few term neonates experience failure secondary to increased pulmonary blood flow from atrial or ventricular shunts in the immediate newborn period unless the left-to-right shunt is complicated by other lesions such as coarctation of the aorta. The increase in pulmonary vascular resistance that is present at birth prevents a large volume of left-to-right shunting in most term infants for several weeks. Identification of newborn infants with structural heart disease at risk for early congestive heart failure is important and may be difficult. One such problem is patency of the aortic end of the ductus arteriosus, delaying presentation and diagnosis of coarctation of the aorta in an infant who otherwise appears to have an uncomplicated ventricular septal defect.

Transport of the Neonate to and from the Operating Room

Ideally, the critically ill neonate will be stabilized in the intensive care unit (ICU) before transport to the operating room. Depending on the severity of illness of the infant, endotracheal intubation, mechanical ventilation, continuous monitoring of gas exchange, continuous infusions of one or multiple vasoactive agents, including PGE_1, and continuous measurement of intravascular pressures may be required. Maintaining this level of support during transport to and from the operating room requires the same organization and teamwork similar to that of interhospital transport.

Communication. The most important element is a careful and complete report between the physicians and the nursing staff caring for the child in the ICU unit to those caring for the child in the operating room and vice versa. An initial report should be requested from the operating room as the patient comes off by-pass, usually about 1 hour before transport. This preliminary report from the operating room nurse to the ICU nurse should identify the key issues of support, including mechanical ventilation, pressure monitoring catheters (arterial, central venous, left atrial, pulmonary artery), tubes (nasogastric, Foley, chest tubes), and vasoactive agents. In addition, information on the length of time on cardiopulmonary by-pass, cross-clamp time, circulatory arrest time, and any operative problems such as bleeding or arrhythmias is essential to understanding the intraoperative stresses affecting the postoperative patient. A brief update should be called to the ICU as the operating room team prepares to leave the operating room. This update should include information about any additional catheters or vasoactive infusions and any subsequent events.

POSTOPERATIVE MANAGEMENT
Transfer from the Operating Room

The bed space is prepared to include an overbed warmer, appropriate intravenous infusion pumps, syringe pumps, suction, appropriate monitoring cables, including ECG, respiratory, pulse oximetry, and the correct pressure cables and transducers. Medications commonly used during resuscitation are left at the bedside either in their original containers or drawn up in unit dose syringes according to a precalculated and posted list. A standard set of postoperative laboratory measurements are obtained on the open heart patients shortly after arrival in the ICU. The appropriate blood drawing tubes and requisitions are prepared in advance so that these can be sent to the laboratory in a timely manner. The usual postoperative laboratory studies include a complete blood count, prothrombin time and partial thromboplastin time, chemistry panel, and an arterial blood gas with plasma electrolytes, ionized calcium, glucose, and hemoglobin. The appropriate ventilator and ventilation monitors, if any, are set up at the bedside before the patient's arrival.

The attending physician and resident anesthesiologist as well as members of the surgical team accompany the patient to the ICU. The primary nurse is responsible for the assessment of the child, the transfer of the child from the transport monitor to the ICU monitor, the transfer of pressure catheters, and the receiving of the clinical report. As the transfer of the patient to the ICU monitor is occurring, the anesthesiologist generally (1) communicates the updated clinical status to the ICU nurse and physician, (2) establishes the baseline ventilator settings, (3) communicates any problems related to ventilation to the clinical care team and respiratory therapists, and (4) continues the clinical management of the patient, including administration of medications and fluid or blood products until report is given.

Approximately 15 minutes after the child has been placed on the ventilator (unless the patient is unstable and requires baseline studies sooner), the initial laboratory work should be drawn and sent to the laboratory. The nurse should identify the earliest appropriate time for the postoperative ECG and chest radiograph.

General Principles of Postoperative Management: The Neonate After Open Heart Surgery

Respiratory. Identification of any intraoperative problems with ventilation must be made at the time of transfer. Identification of patients and lesions at risk for concomitant pulmonary hypertension is important, because modes of ventilation and oxygen administered may require adjustment. An understanding of whether the surgery has been corrective or palliative and the level of systemic oxygenation to be anticipated is imperative. If a child's chest is left open, an option frequently chosen for neonates after complex open heart surgery, ventilation should be adjusted accordingly because the chest wall resistance and elastic recoil will be minimal. In patients with an "open chest" or in those with hemodynamic instability, main-

taining an adequate level of sedation and neuromuscular blockade will facilitate accurate assessment of both the hemodynamic and respiratory status of the patient early during recovery from anesthesia and cardiopulmonary bypass.

During bypass the ventilator is turned off and the lungs are collapsed. The bypass procedure and the process of lung collapse may lead to pulmonary capillary membrane injury, surfactant deficiency, pulmonary microemboli, contusion, or hemorrhage. Rerecruitment of the lung may be incomplete, and areas of atelectasis or pooling of secretions can result in alterations of pulmonary vascular resistance and pulmonary blood flow. A thorough understanding of the pathophysiology that results from bypass and of the hemodynamic changes resulting from the surgical procedure as well as the underlying congenital heart lesion are necessary to optimize ventilation, oxygenation, and perfusion (Kern, 1995).

In many postoperative neonates, the risk of pulmonary hypertension is considerable (Hickey and Hansen, 1989). Pulmonary hypertensive crises can be precipitated by many stimuli, including particularly changes in inspired oxygen and suctioning. To avoid pulmonary hypertensive crises, many institutions advocate the maintenance of deep sedation and a near-anesthetic level of narcotic for the first 24 hours of the postoperative course. Fentanyl, 5 to 20 μg/kg/hr, has been given to minimize the risks of pulmonary hypertensive crises (Hickey and Hansen, 1985). Care with manual ventilation and suctioning procedures is required. In patients at high risk for pulmonary hypertension, the level of inspired oxygen is weaned slowly, and the same FIO_2 as the ventilator (or in some institutions an FIO_2 5% to 10% above that of the ventilator) is used during manual ventilation required for suctioning to prevent significant alterations in alveolar oxygen (Hoffman et al, 1981). Suctioning is done for brief periods of time by two caregivers to ensure the briefest discontinuation of ventilation and supplemental oxygen.

In most patients who return to the ICU with an open chest, neuromuscular blockade is continued until the chest is closed because the absence of chest wall resistance and recoil make spontaneous respiratory efforts useless and confusing.

Fluid and Electrolytes. After cardiopulmonary bypass, most neonates have excess total body water; as a result restriction of fluids is usually instituted. At times, fluid restriction is difficult because of the numerous support medications that are required. In general, an attempt is made to minimize crystalloid infusions to one half to two thirds of maintenance (50 to 66 mL/kg/day) in patients who have undergone cardiopulmonary bypass. This is often impossible because of the number of vasoactive infusions and medications the child is receiving and the number of intravascular pressure monitoring catheters that must be maintained. In general, pressure catheters are transduced with either normal saline or 0.5 normal saline; therefore, no additional sodium is added to the other fluids administered to infants.

Glucose. Maintenance intravenous fluid is generally begun with 10% dextrose in water. Careful monitoring of serum glucose is required to ensure that hypoglycemia does not occur, because the paralyzed sedated neonate will not demonstrate typical symptoms. Serum glucose is monitored with the arterial blood gas every 1 to 2 hours until stable. It is not unusual in the initial postoperative laboratory to see a relatively high serum glucose. Many anesthesiologists, surgeons, and perfusionists use high doses of steroids before the initiation of cardiopulmonary bypass.

Potassium. This is an intracellular cation, and serum or plasma determinations do not reflect total body potassium stores. During cardiopulmonary bypass, large amounts of potassium may be administered or released, or both, by the transfusion of blood products, hemolysis, and acidemia. Renal dysfunction will increase the incidence of hyperkalemia, which is much more toxic than hypokalemia. For these reasons, potassium should not be added to the initial postoperative fluids. If serum potassium is less than 3.0 mEq/L, cautious replacement with infusion of potassium chloride, 0.25 mEq/kg over 1 to 2 hours, should be given. If serum potassium concentration exceeds 6 mEq/L, treatment for hyperkalemia should be initiated. The usual protocols for treatment of hyperkalemia include (1) the removal of potassium from all intravenous fluids, (2) measure to move potassium into the intracellular spaces, alkalinization with sodium bicarbonate, 1 to 2 mEq/kg, or an infusion of glucose and insulin (dextrose 25% to deliver 1 g/kg of glucose and insulin 0.5–1 U/g of glucose), (3) stabilization of the cardiac cell membrane with an infusion of calcium chloride ($CaCl_2$) (10–20 mg/kg), (4) removal of potassium by diuresis with furosemide (Lasix) (1 mg/kg) or sodium polystyrene sulfonate (Kayexalate) (1.0 to 1.5 g/kg) per rectum.

Calcium. The initial laboratory data obtained postoperatively should include a measurement of ionized calcium. Hypocalcemia is a frequent problem in the postoperative cardiac patient. Infusions of blood products, alterations in arterial acid base status, and ongoing tissue injury all alter the level of ionized calcium. Neonates with congenital heart disease may have an abnormal requirement for calcium as a result of concomitant DiGeorge syndrome.

The inotropic state of the heart may be very dependent on levels of ionized calcium. Maintenance of an ionized calcium of greater than 4 (normal, 3.5–5.5 mg/dL) is generally beneficial. In general, low levels of ionized calcium are treated with $CaCl_2$, 10 to 20 mg/kg as a slow intravenous infusion through a central catheter. Because of the many medications usually required in the postoperative period, constant infusions of calcium are difficult to maintain. In addition, the usual preparations of calcium gluconate or gluceptate for constant infusion in intravenous fluid may not be effective because of the relative inefficiency of hepatic function in the postoperative period (Nakanishi, 1987).

Magnesium. Post-bypass patients may have significant hypomagnesemia. Restoration of a normal serum magnesium may facilitate maintenance of normal calcium. Normalization of serum magnesium may also be important in ensuring a stable cardiac rhythm.

Fluids. Minimizing maintenance intravenous fluids in the postoperative period should not limit the fluids given to replace losses in intravascular volume. Significant intravascular losses of volume in the first several postoperative hours may be related to bleeding, chest tube drainage, alterations in vasomotor tone, or alterations in inotropic state. The choice of volume to be infused should be made with great care. If oxygen-carrying capacity is needed, blood loss has occurred, or is anticipated or if capillary leak is a problem, red cells should be infused as needed. If the patient is coagulopathic, the fresh frozen plasma or cryoprecipate may be the volume infusion of choice. In general, during the first postoperative night, careful infusion of small amounts of colloid are required to maintain intravascular volume.

Throughout the postoperative period, careful monitoring of urine output and renal function is required. Postbypass acute renal failure is not uncommon (Hilberman, 1979). Episodic hypotension or renal hypoperfusion may increase the frequency of renal dysfunction (Kron, 1985). Many institutions use "renal-dose dopamine" to attempt to maintain preferential blood flow to the kidneys in the postoperative period (Girardin et al, 1989). In the presence of stable hemodynamics, a diuresis may be initiated or maintained with a dose of furosemide (0.5–1 mg/kg) even on the 1st postoperative day. If a single dose of diuretic does result in urine output, occult renal hypoperfusion or renal damage should be suspected.

Cardiovascular. Myocardial dysfunction is a common problem after neonatal heart surgery. The duration of cardiopulmonary bypass, length of cross-clamp time or total circulatory time, as well as the type and method of cardioplegia all affect the degree of myocardial edema and ischemia (Kern et al, 1995). Other factors affecting myocardial function and recovery include the type of cardiac lesion and whether a ventriculotomy was performed. Cardiac compromise may be suspected if difficulty is encountered coming off cardiopulmonary bypass, if large doses of vasopressors are required in the initial postoperative period, or if metabolic acidemia occurs or worsens in the first several hours postoperatively. Myocardial dysfunction peaks at 4 to 12 hours after surgery. Careful monitoring may permit early identification and intervention during this time, minimizing secondary injury and the attendent sequelae (Wernovsky et al, 1992).

Maintenance of cardiac rate and sinus rhythm, assurance of adequate preload, and optimization of myocardial function and control of vasomotor tone are essential to maintaining adequate cardiac output (Humes et al, 1989). Tachycardias and bradycardias may compromise cardiac output. Although bradydysrhythmias, especially heart block, may indicate severe myocardial dysfunction, cardiac output can be maintained with cardiac pacing. Most patients will have temporary transthoracic pacing wires placed on both the atria and ventricles after complex cardiac repairs. With contemporary pacing technology, atrioventricular sequential pacing can usually be established, thereby controlling heart rate and optimizing ventricular filling by ensuring that atrial contraction precedes ventricular contraction. Tachydysrhythmias, especially junctional tachycardia, can also indicate severe myocardial dysfunction as well as compromise cardiac output. Atrial tachycardia (supraventricular tachycardia [SVT] or atrial flutter) associated with significant hemodynamic collapse should be treated with cardioversion. Alternatively, atrial override pacing can be attempted if wires are in place. An atrial electrogram (recording from the atrial wires) can help determine the actual atrial rate and regularity and assist in diagnosis of the rhythm disturbance (Yabek et al, 1980). If SVT is noted and the hemodynamic state is relatively stable, a rapid intravenous infusion of adenosine, 50 to 100 μg/kg, can be used to break the rhythm abnormality (Rossi et al, 1992). Digoxin should be used with extreme caution in the immediate postoperative period. Junctional tachycardia can be very difficult to control and will not respond to the therapeutic measures described for atrial tachycardia. In general, the best way to control junctional tachycardia is to lower body temperature. To monitor core temperature effectively, an esophageal temperature probe (which will reflect cardiac temperature) should be placed. Temperature is initially lowered by removal of heat sources and topical cooling using fans cool clothes and ice packs. Usually lowering the core temperature to approximately 35° C will slow the ventricular rate. Deliberate hypothermia has risks, including adverse effects on the immune system and white cell function. Small reduction in the infusion rates of catecholamines can be helpful in slowing or abolishing tachyarrhythmias. Noncatecholamine inotropes should be used if tolerated when malignant tachydysrhythmias remain a significant problem. The bipyridines, amrinone and milrinone, have been used, but the vasodilator effects sometimes result in an intrinsic tachycardia (Alousi and Johnson, 1986; Robinson et al, 1993).

Significant myocardial dysfunction in neonates often can be overcome with the use of inotropic agents. The choice of inotropic agent is often empiric. Dobutamine should be considered as a first-line drug, but its use may result in significant vasodilation and adversely affect blood pressure as well as coronary perfusion in some patients. Dopamine has less effect on stable vasomotor tone but is effective only in the presence of endogenous catecholamines (Bohn et al, 1980). If neither of these agents improves cardiac output, consideration should be given to the use of epinephrine. Epinephrine may be effective in very low doses (0.03–0.05 μg/kg/min) in chronically stressed neonates, but higher pharmacologic doses of vasopressor may be required (Anand et al, 1990; Port et al, 1990). Vasodilator drugs have been used to augment cardiac output by decreasing afterload in patients with low cardiac output (Artman and Graham, 1987). Nitroprusside and nitroglycerin have been used in the postoperative period to decrease systemic and pulmonary vascular resistance and improve ventricular function (Benitz et al, 1985; Benson et al, 1979). Infusions of vasoactive agents should be titrated to maintain adequate end-organ perfusion rather than normalization of blood pressure. Serial assessment of urine output and plasma acid load are the best markers of end-organ perfusion in the sick neonate.

In the initial postoperative period, many neonates will demonstrate significant reactivity of the pulmonary vascular bed. Acute elevations in pulmonary artery pressure may result in life-threatening right-sided heart failure. If significant pulmonary hypertension occurs, pulmonary vasodilators such as nitroglycerin or PGE₁ should be adminis-

tered. Recently, significant attention has been given to the use of more specific pulmonary vasodilators such as prostacyclin (PGI_2) or inhaled nitric oxide in the postoperative cardiac patient (Ignarro et al, 1987; Palmer et al, 1987; Kinsella et al, 1992; Roberts et al, 1993).

Careful administration of volume may be required to optimize intravascular volume and improve cardiac output. Serial monitoring of right and left atrial pressures and central venous saturation can be useful in monitoring filling volume and cardiac output, respectively. The choice of volume agent is often determined by other physiologic needs, such as the need to optimize oxygen-carrying capacity (blood), the need for correction of coagulopathy (fresh frozen plasma or platelets), and the need to normalize oncotic pressure (albumin).

During the initial postoperative period, optimizing cardiac output and minimizing the adverse effects of the pharmacologic agents required to support cardiac function are the primary goals. Later, during the recovery phase, the goal changes to decreasing tissue edema, including myocardial edema, through diuresis while maintaining intravascular volume.

Closure of the chest is generally best delayed until the infant is stable and significant diuresis has begun. Usually, by the time chest closure is indicated, the infant is also ready for the discontinuation of neuromuscular blockade, reduction in sedation, and weaning of vasoactive agents and respiratory support. However, after chest closure, it is wise to reassess the needs for respiratory and cardiovascular support before beginning significant weaning.

Central Nervous System. One of the most devastating sequelae of neonatal cardiac surgery is neurologic disability. Neurologic injury may be related to acute complications such as stroke from micro- or macroembolic phenomenon or air, ischemia, or inadequate cerebral preservation during total circulatory arrest (Greeley et al, 1989; Ferry, 1990; Wright et al, 1979). Persistent low cardiac output in the postoperative period may also result in progression of hypoxic ischemic injury. At present, no accurate or reliable methods of monitoring cerebral perfusion and substrate delivery are available. In addition, anesthetic agents and high doses of sedatives and neuromuscular blocking agents mask the presence of significant neurologic injury.

Postoperative Care of the Neonate After Palliative Shunt

Most neonates who have inadequate pulmonary blood flow from disorders such as tetralogy of Fallot or pulmonary atresia and who are not candidates for complete repair undergo palliative shunting with or without accompanying pulmonary valvotomy. Such infants frequently go to the operating room on PGE₁ to maintain pulmonary blood flow. The anesthetic, thoracotomy, lung deflation, and hemodynamic changes caused by the placement of a surgical shunt all may significantly affect hemodynamics and gas exchange postoperatively.

Respiratory. The goals of ventilatory support in the postoperative period after palliative shunts are to maintain recruitment of the alveolar-capillary membrane and prevent overdistention, thereby minimizing pulmonary vascular resistance and increasing flow through the shunt. The initial FIO$_2$ is maintained at 1.0 until the initial postoperative evaluation is complete. The pulmonary vasodilator effects of oxygen are used to increase pulmonary blood flow. Once the initial evaluation is complete, the FIO$_2$ can be weaned to maintain systemic oxygen saturation in the 75% to 85% range, usually indicative of a Q$_p$-Q$_s$ of 1:1. Maximal pulmonary blood flow is achieved with spontaneous ventilation and the generation of a negative intrathoracic pressure.

Fluids and Electrolytes. In the infant with cyanotic congenital heart disease and a new systemic to pulmonary artery shunt, maintenance of adequate intravascular volume is important. Total fluids can be infused at 66% to 100% maintenance. Boluses of blood, fresh frozen plasma, colloid, or crystalloid may be required as the pulmonary vascular bed dilates in response to recovery from anesthesia and surgery and in response to the normal drop in pulmonary vascular resistance associated with postnatal development. Hematocrit should be maintained in the 40% to 55% range. The choice of colloid or crystalloid is generally not based on specific criteria. In the immediate postoperative period, more efficient volume expansion can be achieved with colloid than an equal volume of crystalloid.

Once the pulmonary vascular bed dilates or pulmonary vascular resistance falls, or both, pulmonary edema may become a significant problem. Fluid restriction, inotropic support, or diuresis, or a combination, may be required.

Circulatory. To maintain adequate shunt flow, a pressure gradient must be maintained between the systemic and pulmonary circulations. Measures that lower pulmonary vascular resistance or increase systemic arterial pressure will increase flow through the shunt. Dopamine can be used to raise systemic arterial pressure. Occasionally, a more potent vasoconstrictor is needed to ensure adequate pulmonary blood flow into the relatively high pulmonary vascular resistance of the neonatal lung. Either epinephrine or phenylephrine can be used as a more powerful systemic arterial vasoconstrictor. Both vasopressors should be given through a secure catheter into the central circulation. Epinephrine is a potent inotrope as well as a vasoconstrictor. If inotropy is not required, phenylephrine is a very specific alpha-adrenergic agonist. In the neonate, higher doses of phenylephrine are required to achieve arterial vasoconstriction; doses of 1 to 2 μg/kg/min (or higher) may be required in the early postoperative period to maintain shunt flow and systemic arterial systolic pressure greater than 85 mm Hg in a term infant.

After the initial assessment, shunt flow should be monitored by measurements of heart rate, respiratory rate, and systemic oxygenation as well as by assessment of perfusion, liver size, and shunt murmur. Excessive shunt flow is detected by signs of congestive heart failure and hyperkinetic circulation. Occlusion of a shunt should be suspected when there is compromise in systemic oxygenation and the absence of a shunt murmur. Occlusion of a shunt is a surgical emergency, and shunt flow should be documented by echocardiography as soon as possible.

REFERENCES

Alousi A, Johnson D: Pharmacology of the bipyridines: Amrinone and milrinone. Circulation 73:10, 1986.

Anand KJS, Phil D, Hansen DD, Hickey PR: Hormonal-metabolic stress responses in neonates undergoing cardiac surgery. Anesthesiology 73:661, 1990.

Artman M, Graham TP Jr: Congestive heart failure in infancy recognition and management. Am Heart J 103:1040, 1982.

Artman M, Graham TP Jr: Guidelines for vasodilator therapy of congestive heart failure in infants and children. Am Heart J 113:994, 1987.

Benitz WE, Malachowski N, Cohen RS, et al: Use of sodium nitroprusside in neonates: Efficacy and safety. J Pediatr 106:102, 1985.

Benson LN, Bohn D, Edmonds JP: Nitroglycerine therapy in children with low cardiac index after heart surgery. Cardiovasc Med 4:207, 1979.

Benzing G, Helmsworth JA, Schrieber JT: Nitroprusside and epinephrine for the treatment of low output in children after open heart surgery. Ann Thorac Surg 27:523, 1979.

Bloom RS, Cropley L, Chameides L (Eds): Textbook of Neonatal Resuscitation. Elk Grove Village, IL, American Academy of Pediatrics, 1990.

Bohn DJ, Poirier CS, Edmonds JF, Barker GA: Hemodynamic effects of dobutamine after cardiopulmonary bypass in children. Crit Care Med 8:367, 1980.

Bush A, Busst C, Booth K: Does prostacyclin enhance the selective pulmonary vasodilator effect of oxygen in children with congenital heart disease? Circulation 74:135, 1986.

Bush A, Busst C, Knight WB, Shinebourne EA: Modification of pulmonary hypertension secondary to congenital heart disease by prostacyclin therapy. Am Rev Respir Dis 136:767, 1987.

Castaneda AR, Mayer JE Jr, Jonas RA, et al: The neonate with critical congenital heart disease: Repair—A surgical challenge. J Thorac Cardiovasc Surg 98:869, 1989.

Cohen M, Fuster V, Steele PM, et al: Coarctation of the aorta. Circulation 80:840, 1989.

Drummond WH, Lock JE: Neonatal "pulmonary vasodilator" drugs: Current status. Dev Pharmacol Ther 7:1, 1984.

Elliot RB, Starling MB, Neutz JM: Medical manipulation of the ductus arteriosus. Lancet 1:140, 1975.

Ferry PC: Neurologic sequelae of open-heart surgery in children: An "irritating question." Am J Dis Child 144:369, 1990.

Girardin E, Berner M, Rouge JC, et al: Effect of low dose dopamine on hemodynamic and renal function in children. Pediatr Res 26:200, 1989.

Gold JP, Jonas RA, Lang P, et al: Transthoracic intracardiac monitoring lines in pediatric surgical patients: A ten-year experience. Ann Thorac Surg 42:185, 1986.

Greeley W, Ungerleider RM, Smith LR, Reves JG: The effects of deep hypothermic cardiopulmonary bypass and total circulatory arrest on cerebral blood flow in infants and children. J Thorac Cardiovasc Surg 97:737, 1989.

Hickey PR, Hansen DD: Pulmonary hypertension in infants: Postoperative management. *In* Yacoub M (Ed): Annals of Cardiac Surgery. London, Current Science, 1989, pp 16–22.

Hickey PR, Hansen DD, Wessel DL, et al: Blunting of stress responses in the pulmonary circulation of infants by fentanyl. Anesth Analg 64:1137, 1985.

Hilberman M, Derby G, Spencer RJ, Stinson EB: Sequential pathophysiological changes characterizing the progression from renal dysfunction to acute renal failure following cardiac operation. J Thorac Cardiovasc Surg 79:838, 1979.

Hoffman JIE, Rudoph AM, Heymann MA: Pulmonary vascular disease with congenital heart lesions: Pathologic features and causes. Circulation 64:873, 1981.

Humes RA, Porter CJ, Puga FJ, et al: Utility of temporary atrial epicardial electrodes in postoperative pediatric cardiac patients. Mayo Clin Proc 64:516, 1989.

Ignarro L, Buga G, Woods K, et al: Endothelium derived relaxing factor produced and released from artery and vein is nitric oxide. Proc Natl Acad Sci U S A 84:9265, 1987.

Kelley MJ, Jaffe CC, Kleinman CS: The chest radiograph. *In* Kelley MJ, Jaffe CC, Kleinman CS (Eds): Cardiac Imaging in Infants and Children. Philadelphia, WB Saunders, 1982, pp 7–89.

Kern FH, Greeley WJ, Ungerleider RM: Cardiopulmonary bypass. *In*

Nichols DG, Cameron DE, Greeley WJ, et al (Eds): Critical Heart Disease in Infants and Children. St. Louis, MO, Mosby-Yearbook, 1995, pp 497–529.

Kinsella JP, Neish SR, Shaffer E, Abman SH: Low dose inhalational nitric oxide in persistent pulmonary hypertension of the newborn. Lancet 340:819, 1992.

Kron IL, Joob AW, Van Meter C: Acute renal failure in the cardiovascular surgical patient. Ann Thorac Surg 39:590, 1985.

Meyer RA: Echocardiography. *In* Emmanouilides GC, Riemenschneider TA, Allen HD, Gutgesell HP (Eds): Heart Disease in Infants, Children and Adolescents, 5th ed. Baltimore, MD, Williams and Wilkins, 1995, pp 241–293.

Morray JP, Lynn AM, Kahana M: The effect of pH and pCO_2 on pulmonary and systemic hemodynamics following surgery in children with congenital heart disease and pulmonary hypertension. Anesthesiology 65:A451, 1986.

Nakanishi T, Seguchi M, Takao A: Intracellular calcium concentration in newborn myocardium. Circulation 76:IV-455, 1987.

Norwood WI, Pigott JD: Hypoplastic left sided heart syndrome. *In* Grillo HC, Austen WG, Wilkins EW Jr, et al (Eds): Current Therapy in Cardiothoracic Surgery. Toronto: BC Decker, 1989, pp 473–480.

Palmer RMJ, Ferrige AG, Moncada S: Nitric oxide release accounts for the biologic activity of endothelium-derived relaxing factor. Nature 327:524, 1987.

Park JK, Dell RB, Ellis K, Gersony WM: Surgical management of the infant with coarctation of the aorta and ventricular septal defect. J Am Coll Cardiol 20:176, 1992.

Perloff JK: Introduction: Formulation of the problem. *In* Perloff JK (Ed): The Clinical Recognition of Congenital Heart Disease, 2nd ed. Philadelphia, WB Saunders, 1978, pp 1–7.

Port JD, Gilbert EM, Larrabee P: Neurotransmitter depletion compromises the ability of indirect acting amines to provide inotropic support in the failing human heart. Circulation 81:929, 1990.

Roberts JD Jr, Lang P, Bigatello LM, et al: Inhaled nitric oxide in congenital heart disease. Circulation 87:447, 1993.

Robinson BW, Gelband H, Mas MS: Selective pulmonary and systemic vasodilator effects of amrinone in children: New therapeutic implications. J Am Coll Cardiol 21:1461, 1993.

Rossi AF, Steinberg LG, Kipel G, et al: Use of adenosine in the management of perioperative arrythmias in the pediatric cardiac intensive care unit. Crit Care Med 20:1107, 1992.

Rubis LJ, Stephenson LW, Johnston MR, et al: Comparison of effects of prostaglandin E_1 and nitroprusside on pulmonary vascular resistance after open heart surgery. Ann Thorac Surg 32:563, 1981.

Rychik J, Murdison KA, Chin AJ, Norwood WI: Surgical management of severe aortic outflow obstruction in lesions other than the hypoplastic left heart syndrome: Use of a pulmonary artery to aorta anastomosis. J Am Coll Cardiol 18:809, 1991.

Sano S, Brawn WJ, Mee RBB: Total anomalous pulmonary venous drainage. J Thorac Cardiovasc Surg 97:886, 1989.

Wernovsky G, Jonas RA, Newburger JW: The Boston circulatory arrest study: Hemodynamics and hospital course after the arterial switch operation (abstract). Circulation 86(suppl 1):237A, 1992.

Wright JS, Hicks RG, Newman DC: Deep hypothermic arrest: Observations on later development in children. J Thorac Cardiovasc Surg 77:466, 1979.

Yabek SM, Aki BF, Berman W JR, et al: Use of atrial epicardial electrodes to diagnose and treat postoperative arrythmias in children. Am J Cardiol 46:285, 1980.

Zaritsky A, Chernow B: Use of catecholamines in pediatrics. J Pediatr 105:341, 1984.

CHAPTER 64

Therapeutic Cardiac Catheterization

Elman G. Frantz

The mainstay of treatment for most major congenital heart malformations in the neonate is surgery. However, the modern era of improved survival for infants with congenital heart disease, largely due to the development of cardiopulmonary bypass techniques allowing extensive reconstructive surgery, was advanced by the pioneering application of a therapeutic catheter-based technique. In 1966, Rashkind and Miller described the balloon atrioseptostomy technique for palliation of infants with transposition of the great arteries (Rashkind and Miller, 1966). Over the past decade, other therapeutic catheterization procedures, routinely used in older children, have been increasingly and successfully applied to neonates and are often preferred over surgical alternatives.

BALLOON ATRIOSEPTOSTOMY

Prior to the introduction of the Rashkind balloon atrioseptostomy procedure, the mortality rate for infants with transposition of the great arteries and intact ventricular septum was about 90% by 2 months of age. With routine application of balloon atrioseptostomy, the presurgical mortality fell to about 10% at 2 months of age (Paul and Wernovsky, 1995). When combined with a surgical atrial baffle repair (Mustard, 1964; Senning, 1959), balloon atrioseptostomy helped to transform transposition of the great arteries from a uniformly lethal congenital anomaly into one with a generally excellent functional outcome in the majority of patients.

Indications

In the era of prostaglandin E_1 and the arterial switch repair of transposition of the great arteries, balloon atrioseptostomy has become less essential as life-saving palliation but remains important for the preoperative stabilization effort. We and others prefer to perform a balloon atrioseptostomy procedure for newborns with transposition of the great arteries if surgery is not planned within 12 to 24 hours or if the patient is clinically unstable. Balloon atrioseptostomy may also be indicated in some infants with critical right or left heart obstructions and obligatory atrial level shunts.

Technique

Several manufacturers market balloon catheters intended for atrioseptostomy. We prefer the American-Edwards "Fogarty" catheter. This 5 French catheter has an angled tip to facilitate entry into the left atrium and its 1.8 cc balloon volume results in a 15 mm diameter balloon (Fisher and Paul, 1970). Much larger balloon volumes result in small increases in diameter as a sphere's volume is proportional to the cube of its radius.

The septostomy catheter may be passed under fluoroscopic guidance through a 7, or over-sized 6, French introducer sheath after percutaneous entry into a femoral vein as a component of a diagnostic cardiac catheterization. Preferably, if invasive hemodynamics and angiography are not deemed necessary, the balloon septostomy may be performed at the bedside in the intensive care unit under echocardiographic guidance. In the latter instance, the catheter is usually introduced directly into the umbilical vein without a sheath. Again, the angled tip on the catheter aids passage through the ductus venosus to the inferior vena cava and into the left atrium. If the umbilical vein or ductus venosus are not patent, the femoral vein may be entered percutaneously at the bedside. With either approach, the bedside procedure is brief, avoids the potential risks of transport to and from the catheterization laboratory, and allows superior monitoring of the balloon position relative to vital structures with immediate assessment of efficacy by two-dimensional and Doppler echocardiography (Fig. 64–1).

Once the catheter tip is in the left atrium, the balloon is inflated to its maximum capacity with saline (echocardiographically-guided) or dilute contrast material (fluoroscopically-guided) and "locked" to maintain full inflation. After confirming that the balloon is free from the pulmonary veins and mitral orifice, the catheter is jerked, rapidly and forcefully, yet with a short, controlled excursion, across the atrial septum. The balloon is then rapidly deflated so as not to impede venous return. It is important to use the maximum balloon size on the first pullback in order to tear, and not simply stretch, the floor of the oval fossa. The catheter is then replaced into the left atrium and a total of three to five pullbacks are performed, although the first is generally effective. Substantial resistance is usually felt on the first pullback and minimal resistance thereafter.

Results

The immediate hemodynamic effects of balloon atrioseptostomy are salutary and gratifying, producing a rise in systemic arterial oxygen saturation and abolition of any interatrial pressure gradient. With appropriate, widespread use of prostaglandin E_1 prior to definitive diagnosis, the rise in systemic arterial oxygen saturation may not be dramatic if ductus-derived intercirculatory mixing was good before the procedure. Over the ensuing hours, the improvement in systemic oxygen delivery should promote resolution of metabolic acidosis, if present. If surgery is delayed for days, balloon atrioseptostomy will allow discontinuance of the prostaglandin E_1 infusion, thereby minimizing pulmonary overcirculation, excessive aortopulmonary run-off, and sometimes, the need for prolonged assisted ventilation, improving the preoperative condition of the

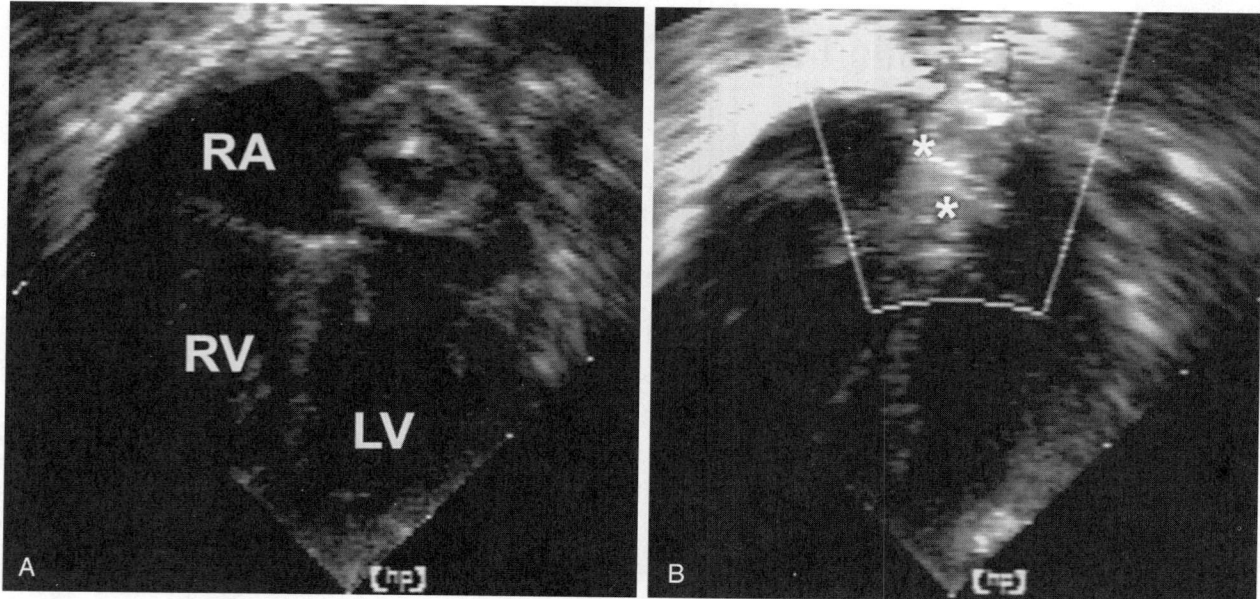

FIGURE 64–1. *A,* A Rashkind balloon atrioseptostomy catheter has been passed from the umbilical vein to the left atrium in a newborn with transposition of the great arteries. The inflated balloon occupies most of the left atrium but is free of the mitral valve leaflets that are open in this diastolic frame. LV, left ventricle; RA, right atrium; RV, right ventricle. *B,* The atrial defect created by the Rashkind procedure is evident by color flow Doppler. The margins of the defect are demarcated by the asterisks.

patient. However, when an atrial defect is the only site of intercirculatory mixing in transposition of the great arteries, particularly if pulmonary vascular resistance remains elevated, systemic arterial saturations may remain uncomfortably low. Prior to routine early operation, successful balloon atrioseptostomy resulted in resting systemic arterial oxygen saturations in the 55% to 60% range in the majority of infants with an intact ventricular septum (Fisher and Paul, 1970; Tynan, 1972). This condition was followed expectantly with greater comfort prior to the use of continuous pulse oximetric monitoring. Most of these infants did well and subsequently underwent an atrial baffle surgical repair.

BALLOON PULMONARY VALVULOPLASTY

The application of the balloon valvuloplasty technique to older children with congenital pulmonary stenosis was reported by Kan et al in 1982 (Kan et al, 1982). Soon thereafter, the procedure was extended to newborns with critical pulmonary valve obstruction (Zeevi et al, 1988). More recently, the technique has been used in an effort to palliate infants with tetralogy of Fallot (Qureshi et al, 1988). In the past several years, balloon pulmonary valvuloplasty has been performed on newborns with pulmonary atresia and intact ventricular septum (Latson, 1991; Rosenthal et al, 1993; Rosenthal et al, 1993).

Indications

Although older infants and children with valvar pulmonary stenosis are selected for balloon pulmonary valvuloplasty based primarily on the transvalvar pressure gradient, the procedure is generally deferred until an older age in asymptomatic newborns with normal systemic arterial oxy-

gen saturations and normal right ventricular function even when the gradient is large. However, when a neonate presents with ductus-dependent pulmonary blood flow, hypoxemia due to right-to-left atrial shunt, right ventricular dysfunction, or evidence of suprasystemic right ventricular pressure, the procedure may be undertaken urgently. A subset of newborns with tetralogy of Fallot may be considered less-than-ideal candidates for primary surgical repair, and balloon pulmonary valvuloplasty may be performed as a first-stage palliation to improve pulmonary blood flow, relieve hypoxemia, and encourage growth of the pulmonary valve annulus, thereby minimizing the need for transannular right ventricular outflow tract patching during subsequent surgical repair (Sluysmans et al, 1995). However, many of the reported infants with tetralogy of Fallot who have undergone this procedure may have been managed by primary repair in some centers (Reddy et al, 1995). The rare neonate with membranous pulmonary atresia and intact ventricular septum who has a nearly normal-sized right ventricle may be treated with perforation of the atretic membrane and balloon pulmonary valvuloplasty alone, whereas those newborns with more significant right ventricular hypoplasia may be treated with balloon valvuloplasty and a surgical shunt.

Technique

In most patients requiring balloon pulmonary valvuloplasty in the neonatal period, maintaining ductal patency with prostaglandin E_1 will lessen the risk and aid some technical aspects of the procedure. After routine diagnostic cardiac catheterization with right ventriculography (Fig. 64–2A), the pulmonary valve annulus is measured, and a balloon dilatation catheter with a diameter 1.2 to 1.4 times greater than the measured annulus diameter is chosen for eventual definitive valvuloplasty. An end-hole catheter is passed across the stenotic valve to the pulmonary artery. Often, the catheter tip must be positioned below the valve, and a floppy-tipped 0.014- to 0.018-inch wire advanced out the tip to the pulmonary artery. A Judkins curve right coronary catheter with the tip pointing posteriorly works well for this maneuver. Usually, the wire will pass across the ductus to the descending aorta, providing a secure wire position with the stiff, trackable portion of the wire crossing the stenotic valve enabling smooth catheter exchanges (Fig. 64–2B). Alternatively, the wire may be positioned in a distal branch pulmonary artery, preferably the left. A 4-, 5-, or 6-mm diameter balloon catheter is passed over the wire and used to "predilate" a critically stenotic valve allowing subsequent passage of the larger definitive balloon. A circumferential indentation or "waist" on the balloon is usually seen at low inflation pressure, which disappears at higher inflation pressures. Incomplete abolition of the waist implies a dysplastic valve and/or annular hypoplasia. Follow-up hemodynamics and right ventriculography are performed. Once the patient is settled in the intensive care unit after the procedure, the prostaglandin E_1 infusion is discontinued.

In hypoxemic infants with tetralogy of Fallot, the technique is essentially the same. Because these infants generally have significant pulmonary annular and arterial hypoplasia, the diameter of the final balloon chosen is often smaller than the final balloon used for infants with isolated, typical, valvar stenosis. Although hypercyanotic spells precipitated by the procedure are unusual, the operator must be prepared to manage such spells with oxygen, morphine, propranolol, and/or phenylephrine, and a surgeon should be available to perform an emergency shunt. When possible, ductus-derived pulmonary blood flow should be maintained with an infusion of prostaglandin E_1.

In newborns with pulmonary atresia, intact ventricular septum, and close proximity of the right ventricular outflow tract to the pulmonary trunk, balloon pulmonary valvuloplasty may be performed after initial perforation of the "membrane" (Fig. 64–3A). We and others have used the stiff end of an 0.014 in coronary angioplasty wire (Latson, 1991), whereas some operators have used a radiofrequency catheter (Rosenthal, 1993) or laser-tipped probe (Rosenthal, 1993) to perforate the atretic segment. It is helpful to place a catheter retrograde through the ductus against the pulmonary arterial aspect of the atretic membrane as a marker (Fig. 64–3B). An end-hole catheter is positioned in the right ventricular outflow tract and seated against the atretic membrane pointing posteriorly toward the pulmonary trunk. The stiff end of the wire may be hand-shaped near the tip so that it will follow the curve of the catheter, avoiding an anterior course and perforation of the free wall of the right ventricle. After perforating the membrane and advancing the wire a short distance, the catheter may be advanced over the wire or, if it will not advance, the wire may be removed and reversed and the floppy tip advanced across the perforation and across the ductus to the descending aorta. "Predilation" followed by serially larger balloons may then progress as for typical pulmonary stenosis.

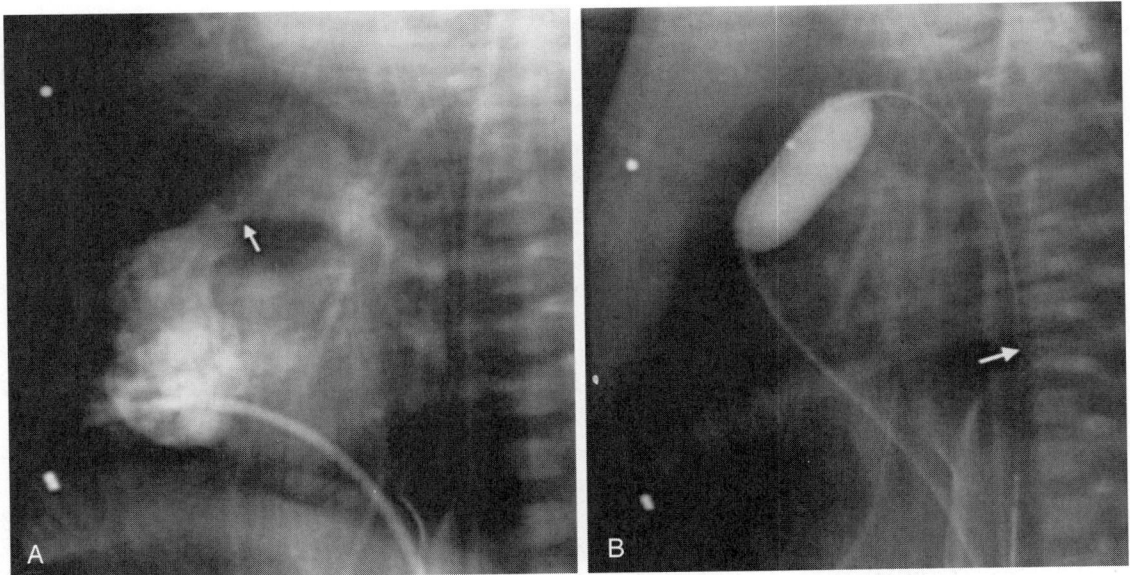

FIGURE 64–2. *A,* A lateral right ventriculogram in a newborn with critical pulmonary stenosis showing a faintly opacified narrow jet of contrast material passing through the stenotic valve orifice *(arrow).* The pulmonary valve annulus measured 6.8 mm in diameter. Severe tricuspid insufficiency opacifies the right atrium. *B,* The fully inflated 8 mm diameter balloon catheter in the same patient has lost its "waist," indicating an effective valvuloplasty. The arrow indicates the guidewire positioned in the descending aorta via the ductus facilitating balloon catheter exchanges. This patient's right ventricular pressure fell from 93 to 65 mm Hg; the valve gradient fell from 38 to 5 mm Hg. At 1-year-follow-up the Doppler-estimated gradient is <15 mm Hg with complete resolution of tricuspid insufficiency.

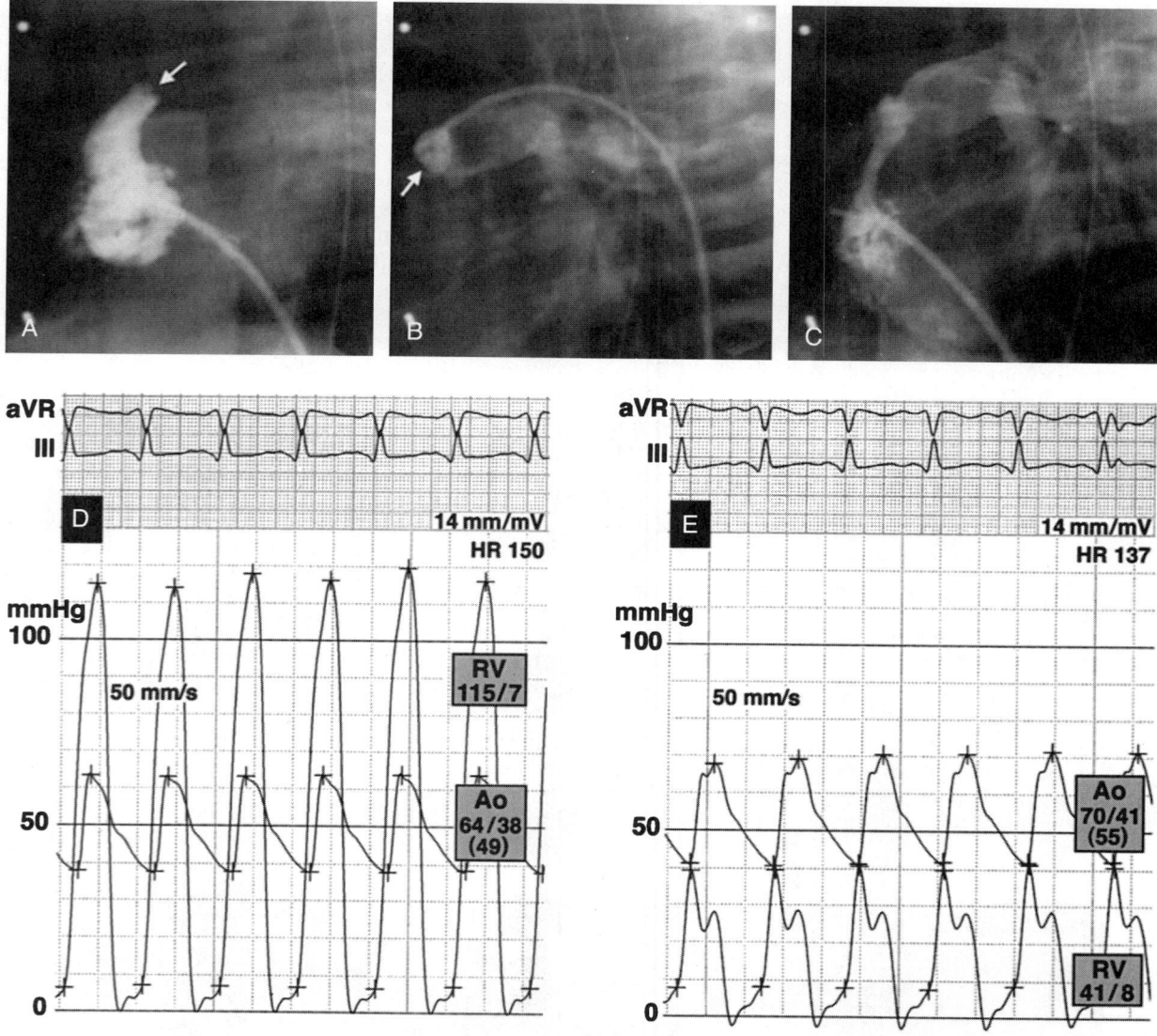

FIGURE 64–3. *A,* A lateral right ventriculogram in a newborn with pulmonary atresia and intact ventricular septum. The right ventricle is moderately hypoplastic. The arrow indicates the level of the atretic "membrane." *B,* A retrograde catheter passed via the ductus demarcates the pulmonary arterial aspect of the "membrane" *(arrow).* This catheter is left in place during perforation of the "membrane" to guide proper positioning of the tip of the right ventricular catheter. *C,* The lateral right ventriculogram following valvuloplasty with a 6 mm diameter balloon shows significant antegrade output filling the pulmonary arteries. *D,* Simultaneous right ventricular (RV) and aortic (Ao) pressures in the same patient prior to valvuloplasty showing markedly supra-systemic RV pressure. *E,* Simultaneous RV and Ao pressures in the same patient after valvuloplasty showing striking reduction in RV pressure. This patient underwent an adjunctive modified Blalock-Taussig shunt and is awaiting re-evaluation of right ventricular growth.

Results

The immediate effects of balloon pulmonary valvuloplasty are evident as a reduction in right ventricular pressure with an improvement in antegrade right ventricular output and a decrease in tricuspid insufficiency angiographically. Right-to-left atrial shunting diminishes, and systemic arterial oxygen saturation rises. However, some degree of residual right-to-left shunt and systemic arterial hypoxemia may

persist after an efficacious balloon valvuloplasty if the right ventricle is somewhat hypoplastic or poorly compliant. Accurate assessment of the residual right ventricular outflow gradient must be deferred until after ductal closure with its associated fall in pulmonary arterial pressure and may be obtained by Doppler echocardiography.

The ability to accomplish a technically successful balloon valvuloplasty in neonates with critical pulmonary valve stenosis has varied widely from center to center (Caspi et al,

1990) but appears to be improving with more widespread application of interventional techniques. The long-term functional and hemodynamic outcome in these infants is generally excellent unless significant right ventricular hypoplasia is present. In one series, 94% of infants in whom the procedure was successfully accomplished required no surgical intervention, although 10% required repeat valvuloplasty. Ninety percent of these patients had pulmonary valve gradients of less than 30 mmHg 3 years later (Colli et al, 1995). In the largest single-institution series, including some patients with pulmonary atresia, the procedure was accomplished in 84% of attempts with short-term success in 95%. Thirteen percent of patients required a surgical shunt and 26% required eventual right ventricular surgery during a 9.7 year follow-up period (Gournay et al, 1995). Several authors have reported the value of indices of hypoplasia of the pulmonary annulus, tricuspid annulus, or right ventricular cavity for predicting the need for subsequent repeat valvuloplasty or early adjunctive interventions such as an aortopulmonary shunt or transannular right ventricular outflow tract patch (Fedderly et al, 1995; Hanley et al, 1993).

The success of balloon pulmonary valvuloplasty in infants with tetralogy of Fallot depends greatly on the relative contributions of valvar obstruction compared to subvalvar or supravalvar obstruction. Most hypoxemic newborns with tetralogy of Fallot have significant anterior deviation of the infundibular septum as a predominant component of their pulmonary outflow obstruction. However, when the procedure is effective, systemic arterial oxygen saturation increases immediately. Approximately one third of patients do not derive lasting benefit and require palliative surgery in short order. Approximately two thirds of patients can have surgical intervention deferred for at least several months and can then undergo primary repair (Sreeram et al, 1991). A subset of these patients undergo primary repair without transannular right ventricular outflow tract enlargement due to growth of the pulmonary valve annulus in the interval between the catheterization procedure and the surgical procedure (Reddy et al, 1995). Avoidance of a transannular patch at repair is beneficial because it minimizes the severity of pulmonary insufficiency and its long-term deleterious effects on right ventricular function and arrhythmogenic potential.

The outcome of balloon pulmonary valvuloplasty in neonates with pulmonary atresia is dependent on the degree of associated right ventricular hypoplasia and dysfunction (Fedderly et al, 1995). Often, perforation and balloon dilation of an atretic membrane provides effective relief of right ventricular hypertension (see Fig. 64–3D and E) and allows some antegrade pulmonary blood flow (see Fig. 64–3C). However, balloon (or surgical) valvotomy alone is rarely sufficient because pulmonary blood flow frequently remains ductus-dependent. An adjunctive surgical shunt (e.g., modified Blalock-Taussig) may then be performed, allowing a longer interval for right ventricular growth and recovery which, if it occurs, allows subsequent transcatheter occlusion of the shunt.

BALLOON AORTIC VALVULOPLASTY

Critical congenital aortic stenosis remains one of the most challenging and difficult forms of neonatal heart disease to treat successfully. Associated left ventricular, aortic, and mitral hypoplasia and dysfunction are often severe and limit therapeutic options and outcomes. Surgical valvotomy results in significant early mortality of 30% to 35%. Balloon aortic valvuloplasty offers an opportunity to accomplish an effective valvotomy with a lower immediate mortality of about 10% in selected patients (Egito et al, 1997).

Indications

Careful selection is crucial to identify newborns who are good candidates for balloon valvuloplasty and to recognize infants who are better served by a single-ventricle/Norwood approach because of the severity of associated left heart abnormalities. An echocardiographic score using indexed measurements of aortic root size, mitral area, and the long axis of the left ventricle predicts failure of an attempted "two-ventricle" approach, guiding referral for an early Norwood approach (Rhodes et al, 1991). Attempted valvuloplasty in this group of infants, even with low procedural mortality, in order to "give the left ventricle a chance" has resulted in an unusually high surgical mortality at later Norwood operation and should be avoided.

Newborns with congenital aortic stenosis requiring intervention in the neonatal period generally manifest findings of congestive heart failure, if not cardiogenic shock, and are usually dependent on the ductus arteriosus for adequate systemic blood flow. Rarely, an infant may be selected for balloon valvuloplasty owing to the echocardiographic severity of aortic stenosis and left ventricular dysfunction despite the paucity of symptomatology. The transvalvular pressure gradient, obtained by Doppler techniques or direct catheter measurement, is not a reliable indicator of the severity of obstruction because of reduced left ventricular stroke output.

Technique

Because of the fragile condition of most infants with critical aortic stenosis, the catheterization procedure is usually undertaken with the support of a continuous prostaglandin E_1 infusion and assisted ventilation. A retrograde aortic approach is preferred by most operators, from the umbilical artery or, percutaneously, from the femoral artery. The umbilical arterial approach minimizes vascular complications but catheter/wire manipulations to cross the stenotic valve and subsequent catheter exchanges are sometimes difficult. When the femoral arterial route is used, balloon dilatation catheters up to 8 mm in diameter may be passed through a 5 French hemostatic sheath. Some operators prefer an antegrade route (Hausdorf et al, 1993) or a surgical cutdown approach to the carotid (Fischer et al, 1990) or subscapular (Alekyan et al, 1995) arteries.

From the retrograde approach, a 3 French pigtail catheter is passed, uncoiled over a straight, floppy-tipped, 0.018-inch wire, around the aortic arch to the aortic root. The direction of the leading wire tip is aimed at the site of the anticipated aortic orifice and is advanced and withdrawn, slightly altering the amount of wire out of the pigtail, until the wire is seen passing into the left ventricle. Care must be taken to avoid trauma to the coronary ostia and to avoid perforating a valve cusp (rather than traversing the orifice).

Ventricular ectopy usually heralds entry into the left ventricle, but ectopy may be absent if endocardial fibroelastosis is prominent. The pigtail catheter is advanced into the left ventricle, and pressures and an angiogram are obtained. If left ventricular dysfunction is severe, the ventriculogram may be deferred, and balloon selection may be based on echocardiographic measurements of annulus diameter. The dilating balloon is chosen to have a diameter of 0.9 times the aortic annular diameter in an effort to achieve acceptable relief of stenosis while producing a minimum of aortic insufficiency. A standard J-tipped 0.018-inch wire with a hand-formed apical loop or a nitinol wire (Microvena Corp., White Bear Lake, MN) with a short flexible tip may be used as an exchange wire and is positioned in the left ventricular cavity via the pigtail catheter. The pigtail catheter is removed and the balloon dilating catheter is advanced over the wire to the aortic annulus and is inflated several times until the "waist" on the balloon disappears (Fig. 64–4). A catheter is then replaced over the wire for pressure measurements and an aortogram to assess the severity of any aortic insufficiency. The patient is then returned to the intensive care unit and the prostaglandin E₁ infusion is discontinued. If left ventricular function is severely impaired, continuous infusion of inotropic agents may be continued for several days.

Results

The immediate hemodynamic effects of balloon aortic valvuloplasty are an improvement in left ventricular output and function associated with a reduction in transvalvar pressure gradient. The peak systolic pressure gradient was reduced by 54% in one large series, and left ventricular end-diastolic pressure fell by 20% (Egito et al, 1997). The accompanying fall in left atrial pressure diminishes the severity of pulmonary edema and the symptoms of congestive heart failure. Mitral insufficiency, if present, usually decreases in severity.

However, the catheter-determined gradient obtained immediately after balloon valvuloplasty often underrepresents the severity of the eventual residual obstruction once left ventricular function normalizes and cardiac output increases with somatic growth. About one third of patients require repeat valvuloplasty within 4 months (Egito et al, 1997).

Medium-term results at about 4 years after the procedure are notable for 88% survival and 83% of survivors are asymptomatic. Recurrent aortic stenosis is common, and aortic insufficiency is audible in 24% and moderately severe in 11%. Associated congenital heart defects, mostly mitral stenosis or coarctation of the aorta, become more important in follow-up of about one third of the patients (Egito et al, 1997).

In appropriately selected neonates with critical aortic stenosis, balloon valvuloplasty has become the favored initial therapeutic approach in most centers, yielding outcomes similar to surgical valvotomy with lower procedural mortality risk.

BALLOON COARCTATION ANGIOPLASTY

In general, balloon angioplasty of native, or previously unoperated, aortic coarctation remains controversial because of concerns about incomplete relief of obstruction and the development of aneurysms at the site of angioplasty (Tynan et al, 1990). However, as experience with the procedure increases, the hemodynamic outcome in most infants over 6 months of age is good, and the incidence of true aneurysms is low and probably no greater for angioplasty of native obstructions than it is for angioplasty of postoperative restenosis. Despite these encouraging results in older infants and children, restenosis is the rule rather than the exception in neonates so that primary surgical repair is favored in most centers (Fletcher et al, 1995; Rao et al, 1996).

Indications

When aortic coarctation is diagnosed in the neonate, it is usually juxtaductal and results in severe obstruction to

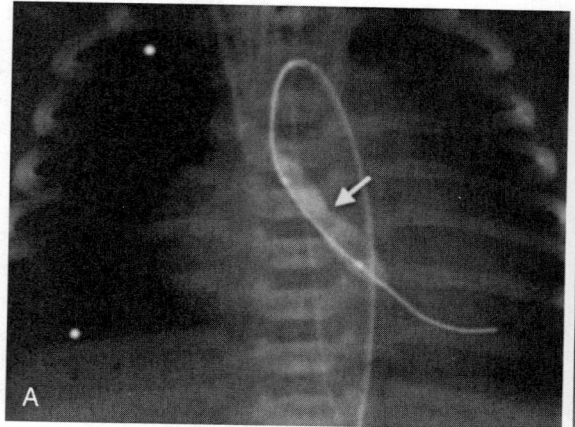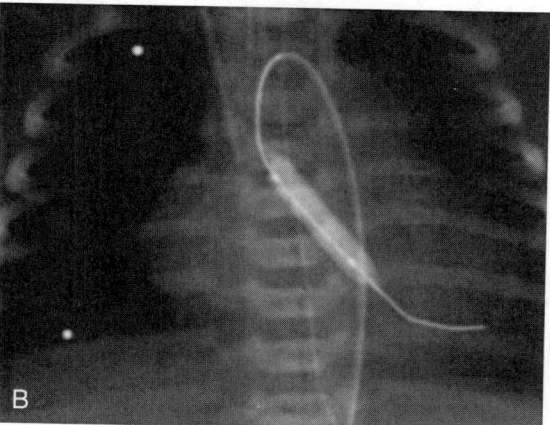

FIGURE 64–4. *A,* A 6-mm diameter balloon catheter has been passed over an exchange wire from the umbilical artery in a newborn with critical aortic valve stenosis and a valve annulus of 6.5 mm. The arrow indicates the "waist" formed on the balloon by the stenotic valve at an early phase of balloon inflation. *B,* The fully inflated balloon in the same patient shows complete loss of the waist.

systemic blood flow as the ductus constricts. Symptoms of congestive heart failure or cardiogenic shock with metabolic acidosis are common, and the indications for intervention, usually surgical, are clear. However, if the patient is considered a poor operative candidate, balloon coarctation angioplasty may be undertaken as a palliative step to allow eventual surgical repair under more favorable conditions. Extreme prematurity is an example of a clinical state that may make operative intervention less appealing, and balloon angioplasty can be performed via umbilical arterial access to avoid vascular complications. We have encountered three neonates with coarctation of the aorta, all weighing between 900 and 1000 g, in the past several years. Two of them underwent balloon coarctation angioplasty from an umbilical arterial approach and the third was managed with a low-dose chronic prostaglandin infusion owing to lack of umbilical arterial access after late presentation (Fig. 64–5).

Technique

In the premature infant, preventing hypothermia during the procedure and intra-hospital transport is especially important. An umbilical arterial catheter often will have been placed prior to the diagnosis for standard neonatal monitoring. If not, the umbilical artery may be cannulated directly at the stump or by a cutdown on the anterior abdominal wall below the stump. A 0.014-inch coronary angioplasty exchange wire or nitinol wire with a straight floppy tip is passed through the existing catheter and across the site of coarctation to the ascending aorta. Care must be taken to confirm that the wire has passed to the aorta and not through a persistent ductus to the pulmonary trunk. A cutoff 3 French pigtail catheter is passed over the wire to the site of coarctation, the wire is removed, and an aortogram is performed. For a premature infant, a coronary angioplasty

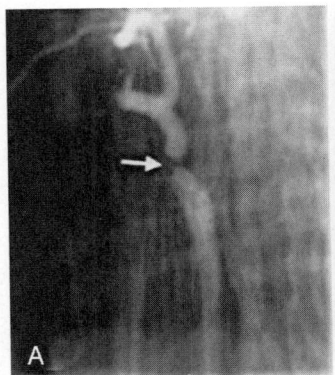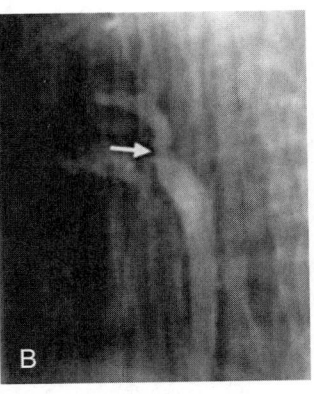

FIGURE 64–5. *A,* A lateral aortogram in a 32-week gestation, small-for-gestational age, 950-g, premature infant showing near-complete obstruction due to a juxtaductal aortic coarctation *(arrow)*. *B,* The lateral aortogram in the same patient following angioplasty of the coarctation with a 3-mm diameter coronary angioplasty balloon shows enlargement of the diameter of the coarctation site to approximately the caliber of the aortic isthmus *(arrow)* and slight reopening of the ductus. The systolic pressure gradient across the coarctation fell from 58 to 12 mm Hg. This patient developed restenosis several months later and underwent uncomplicated surgical repair at a weight of about 3 kg.

balloon catheter with a 3.0- to 4.0-mm diameter balloon is chosen to approximate the diameter of the isthmus of the aorta and is exchanged for the pigtail catheter over the wire. A term neonate may require a balloon diameter of 4.0 to 6.0 mm. The balloon is inflated several times for 10 to 20 seconds per inflation in the site of the coarctation at a pressure sufficient to completely abolish the "waist." The pigtail catheter is then replaced for final pressure measurements and aortography. Close clinical and echo-Doppler reassessment is important to recognize and quantify restenosis and to time referral for surgical repair.

Results

The immediate results of balloon coarctation angioplasty of native coarctation of the aorta are appealing with a dramatic reduction in coarctation pressure gradient, an increase in angiographic coarctation diameter, and amelioration of symptoms of congestive heart failure, if present. However, in the largest single-center experience, 88% of infants older than 7 months remained free of repeat intervention at 3 years of follow-up, whereas 77% of neonates required further intervention within about 6 months. Hypoplasia of the aortic isthmus was strongly associated with a high incidence of early restenosis (Fletcher et al, 1995). Other authors have reported similar high rates of restenosis in neonates related to smaller isthmic diameter (Rao and Koscik, 1995; Redington et al, 1990). Small, nonprogressive aneurysms developed at the site of angioplasty in less than 2% of patients (Fletcher et al, 1995).

It is clear that balloon coarctation angioplasty is a palliative procedure in the majority of neonates. Nonetheless, in selected patients who, for a variety of reasons, are considered unfavorable surgical candidates, balloon angioplasty of aortic coarctation can have an important adjunctive role in the overall therapeutic plan by allowing surgical repair under optimal circumstances.

EMBOLIZATION THERAPY

Systemic arteriovenous malformations (cerebral vein of Galen, hepatic, or others) may present with intractable congestive heart failure in the neonatal period. The prognosis for neurologically intact survival for infants with large vein of Galen malformations is quite poor regardless of the mode of therapy. Transcatheter embolization with Gianturco coils is possible, but outcomes remain as unfavorable as with surgical therapy (Friedman et al, 1991). Embolization with the liquid adhesive, n-butyl-cyanoacrylate, resulted in more favorable survival and neurologic outcomes in a small number of infants (Verma et al, 1993).

Pulmonary arteriovenous malformations rarely present with severe cyanosis in infancy except when a single large fistula connects the pulmonary artery and left atrium. A case report of successful transcatheter closure using a clamshell septal occluder device has been published (Preminger et al, 1995). Gianturco coils have been used to embolize the multiple smaller malformations associated with hereditary hemorrhagic telangiectasia in older patients, but this is rarely, if ever necessary, in the neonatal period.

Embolization of aortopulmonary collateral vessels associated with pulmonary atresia with ventricular septal defect and hypoplastic true pulmonary arteries using Gianturco coils is a frequently used adjunct in the overall management scheme of these infants in order to control pulmonary blood flow and allow for growth of the central pulmonary arteries (Perry et al, 1989). Again, this transcatheter intervention is rarely performed in the neonate.

FUTURE DIRECTIONS OF INTERVENTIONAL MANAGEMENT OF THE DUCTUS ARTERIOSUS

Persistent patency of the ductus arteriosus may be a hemodynamic asset or a liability in the neonatal period depending on the clinical setting (see Chapter 61). Premature infants frequently require medical or surgical intervention to close the ductus in order to prevent morbid complications such as intracranial hemorrhage, necrotizing enterocolitis, and chronic lung disease. Neonates with ductus-dependent congenital heart disease occasionally require long-term maintenance of ductal patency prior to surgical intervention. Transcatheter interventions to manage ductal patency are not generally applicable to neonates, particularly premature ones, but several recent reports illustrate the potential for future applicability.

Transcatheter closure of the smaller ductus arteriosus in asymptomatic infants and children using Gianturco coils has become a well-accepted, highly successful procedure (Lloyd et al, 1993; Moore et al, 1994). However, constraints of equipment size and the caliber of the symptomatic neonatal ductus relative to nearby vital vascular channels (i.e., the aorta and left pulmonary artery), limit the feasability of this approach in newborns. An intriguing modification of this technique, using a specially designed detachable coil delivered antegrade through a 3 French catheter, has shown promising results in neonatal piglets weighing about 1500 to 2000 grams (Grabitz et al, 1996). A case of successful ductal occlusion in a 4.3 kg, 2-month-old infant, using a newly developed vascular occlusion device ("coils in a bag"), has been reported (Grifka et al, 1996). As currently constructed, this device is delivered through an 8 French sheath, but its design is appealing and could potentially be miniaturized.

The first-stage surgical interventions for certain ductus-dependent forms of congenital heart disease are palliative. Several reports of the use of coronary artery stents to maintain ductal patency and palliate newborns with pulmonary atresia and hypoplastic left heart syndrome (Gibbs et al, 1992, 1993; Slack et al, 1994) have been published. Although the outcomes in these few cases have been mostly poor, deaths were not directly attributable to the stent placement.

It is likely that refinements in catheterization equipment design and technical expertise will result in increased applicability and availability of therapeutic catheter-based interventions to manage patency of the ductus arteriosus in the neonatal period, possibly even in premature infants.

REFERENCES

Alekyan BG, Petrosyar YS, Coulson JD, et al: Right subscapular artery catheterization for balloon valvuloplasty of critical aortic stenosis in infants. Am J Cardiol 76:1049–1052, 1995.

Caspi J, Coles JG, Benson LN, et al: Management of neonatal critical pulmonic stenosis in the balloon valvotomy era. Ann Thorac Surg 49:273–278, 1990.

Colli AM, Perry SB, Lock JE, Keane JF: Balloon dilation of critical pulmonary stenosis in the first month of life. Cathet Cardiovasc Diagn 34:23–28, 1995.

Egito EST, Moore P, O'Sullivan JO, et al: Transvascular balloon dilation for neonatal critical aortic stenosis: Early and mid-term results. J Am Coll Cardiol 29:442–447, 1997.

Fedderly RT, Lloyd TR, Mendelsohn AM, Beekman RH: Determinants of successful balloon valvotomy in infants with critical pulmonary stenosis or membranous pulmonary atresia with intact ventricular septum. J Am Coll Cardiol 25:460–465, 1995.

Fischer DR, Ettedgui JA, Park SC, et al: Carotid artery approach for balloon dilation of aortic valve stenosis in the neonate: A preliminary report. Am J Cardiol 15:1633–1636, 1990.

Fisher E, Paul MH: Transposition of the great arteries: Recognition and management. *In* Downing DF (Ed): Cardiovascular Clinics, vol 2. Philadelphia, F.A. Davis, 1970, p 211.

Fletcher SE, Nihill MR, Grifka RG, et al: Balloon angioplasty of native coarctation of the aorta: Midterm follow-up and prognostic factors. J Am Coll Cardiol 25:730–734, 1995.

Friedman DM, Madrid M, Berenstein A, et al: Neonatal vein of Galen malformations: Experience in developing a multidisciplinary approach using an embolization treatment protocol. Clin Pediatr (Phila) 30:621–629, 1991.

Gibbs JL, Rothman MT, Rees MR, et al: Stenting of the arterial duct: A new approach to palliation for pulmonary atresia. Br Heart J 67:211–212, 1992.

Gibbs JL, Wren C, Watterson KG, et al: Stenting of the arterial duct combined with banding of the pulmonary arteries and atrial septectomy or septostomy: A new approach to palliation for the hypoplastic left heart syndrome. Br Heart J 69:551–555, 1993.

Gournay V, Piechaud JF, Delogu A, et al: Balloon valvotomy for critical stenosis or atresia of the pulmonary valve in newborns. J Am Coll Cardiol 26:1725–1731, 1995.

Grabitz RG, Neuss MB, Coe JY, et al: A small interventional device to occlude persistently patent ductus arteriosus in neonates: Evaluation in piglets. J Am Coll Cardiol 28:1024–1030, 1996.

Grifka RG, Vincent JA, Nihill MR, et al: Transcatheter patent ductus arteriosus closure in an infant using the Gianturco-Grifka vascular occlusion device. Am J Cardiol 78:721–723, 1996.

Hanley FL, Sade RM, Freedom RM, et al, and the Congenital Heart Surgeons Society: Outcomes in critically ill neonates with pulmonary stenosis and intact ventricular septum: A multi-institutional study. J Am Coll Cardiol 22:183–192, 1993.

Hausdorf G, Schneider M, Schirmer KR, et al: Anterograde balloon valvuloplasty of aortic stenosis in children. Am J Cardiol 71:460–462, 1993.

Kan JS, White RJ Jr, Mitchell SE: Percutaneous balloon valvuloplasty: A new method for treatment of congenital pulmonary stenosis. N Engl J Med 307:540–542, 1982.

Latson LA: Nonsurgical treatment of a neonate with pulmonary atresia and intact ventricular septum by transcatheter puncture and balloon dilation of the atretic valve membrane. Am J Cardiol 68:277–279, 1991.

Lloyd TR, Fedderly R, Mendelsohn AM, et al: Transcatheter occlusion of patent ductus arteriosus with Gianturco coils. Circulation 88:1412–1420, 1993.

Moore JW, George L, Kirkpatrick SE, et al: Percutaneous closure of the small patent ductus arteriosus using occluding spring coils. J Am Coll Cardiol 23:759–765, 1994.

Mustard WT: Successful two-stage correction of transposition of the great vessels. Surgery 55:469–472, 1964.

Paul MH, Wernovsky G: Transposition of the great arteries. *In* Emmanouilides GC, Allen HD, Riemenschneider TA, Gutgesell HP (Eds): Heart Disease in Infants, Children, and Adolescents, 5th ed. Baltimore, Williams & Wilkins Co, 1995, p 1154.

Perry SB, Radtke W, Fellows KE, et al: Coil embolization to occlude aortopulmonary collateral vessels and shunts in patients with congenital heart disease. J Am Coll Cardiol 13:100–108, 1989.

Preminger TJ, Perry SB, Burrows PE: Vascular anomalies. *In* Emmanouilides GC, Allen HD, Riemenschneider TA, Gutgesell HP (Eds): Heart Disease in Infants, Children, and Adolescents, 5th ed. Baltimore, Williams & Wilkins, 1995, p 804.

Qureshi SA, Kirk CR, Lamb RK, et al: Balloon dilatation of the pulmonary valve in the first year of life in patients with tetralogy of Fallot: A preliminary study. Br Heart J 60:232–235, 1988.

Rao PS, Galal O, Smith PA, Wilson AD: Five- to nine-year follow-up results of balloon angioplasty of native aortic coarctation in infants and children. J Am Coll Cardiol 27:462–470, 1996.

Rao PS, Koscik R: Validation of risk factors in predicting recoarctation after initially successful balloon angioplasty for native aortic coarctation. Am Heart J 130:116–121, 1995.

Rashkind WJ, Miller WW: Creation of an atrial septal defect without thoracotomy: A palliative approach to complete transposition of the great arteries. JAMA 196:991–992, 1966.

Reddy VM, Liddicoat JR, McElhinney DB, et al: Routine primary repair of tetralogy of Fallot in neonates and infants less than three months of age. Ann Thorac Surg 60:S592–S596, 1995.

Redington AN, Booth P, Shore DF, Rigby ML: Primary balloon dilatation of coarctation of the aorta in neonates. Br Heart J 64:277–281, 1990.

Rhodes LA, Colan SD, Perry SB, et al: Predictors of survival in neonates with critical aortic stenosis. Circulation 84:2325–2335, 1991.

Rosenthal E, Qureshi SA, Chan KC, et al: Radiofrequency-assisted balloon dilatation in patients with pulmonary atresia and an intact ventricular septum. Br Heart J 69:347–351, 1993.

Rosenthal E, Qureshi SA, Kakadekar AP, et al: Technique of percutaneous laser-assisted valve dilatation for valvar atresia in congenital heart disease. Br Heart J 69:556–562, 1993.

Senning A: Surgical correction of transposition of the great vessels. Surgery 45:966–980, 1959.

Slack MC, Kirby WC, Towbin JA, et al: Stenting of the ductus arteriosus in hypoplastic left heart syndrome as an ambulatory bridge to cardiac transplantation. Am J Cardiol 74:636–637, 1994.

Sluysmans T, Neven B, Rubay J, et al: Early balloon dilatation of the pulmonary valve in infants with tetralogy of Fallot: Risks and benefits. Circulation 91:1506–1511, 1995.

Sreeram N, Saleem M, Jackson M, et al: Results of balloon pulmonary valvuloplasty as a palliative procedure in tetralogy of Fallot. J Am Coll Cardiol 18:159–165, 1991.

Tynan M: Haemodynamic effects of balloon atrial septostomy in infants with transposition of the great arteries. Br Heart J 34:791–794, 1972.

Tynan M, Finley JP, Fontes V, et al: Balloon angioplasty for the treatment of native coarctation: Results of the valvuloplasty and angioplasty of congenital anomalies registry. Am J Cardiol 65:790–792, 1990.

Verma R, Friedman DM, Madrid M, et al: Recent improvement in outcome using transcatheter embolization techniques for neonatal aneurysmal malformations of the vein of Galen. Pediatrics 91:583–586, 1993.

Zeevi B, Keane JF, Fellows KE, et al: Balloon dilation of critical pulmonary stenosis in the first week of life. J Am Coll Cardiol 11:821–824, 1988.

CHAPTER 65

Fetal Cardiology/Telemedicine

John L. Cotton, James P. Loehr and Walker A. Long

Newborn cardiology, similar to the rest of medicine, has changed remarkably over the last 15 years and continues to change at an accelerating rate. Technical advances such as two-dimensional echocardiography and color flow Doppler, indomethacin, prostaglandin E_1, balloon valvuloplasty, coil occlusions, and surfactant have improved the outcomes of sick newborn infants remarkably and are likely to continue as long as a public support for basic research is maintained. The most important improvement of the last 15 years, however, has been in the expertise of the physicians and other health care professionals caring for newborns with cardiac problems. This chapter reviews two developments that have the potential to enhance early and appropriate access for sick newborn infants who may have cardiac problems: fetal cardiology and telemedicine.

FETAL CARDIOLOGY
Anatomic Assessments in the Fetus

Fetal echocardiography has evolved from the use of simple M-mode scanning to modern techniques of two-dimensional real-time imaging, pulsed and continuous-wave spectral Doppler, and Doppler color flow mapping. These new methods have allowed the pediatric cardiologist to evaluate fetal cardiac structure and function and to monitor therapeutic interventions used to treat fetal cardiac disease.

Indications

There are multiple indications for a referral for fetal echocardiography. These can be broadly categorized as familial risk factors, fetal risk factors, and maternal risk factors (Friedman et al, 1993). The most common reason for referral for fetal echocardiography is an abnormal four-chamber view on routine screening ultrasonography (Cooper et al, 1995). Other fetal risk factors found on screening ultrasound scans include fetal arrhythmias (Meijboom et al, 1994), nonimmune hydrops (Smythe et al, 1992), polyhydramnios (Callan et al, 1991), and major fetal noncardiac anomalies. Chromosomal abnormalities found by amniocentesis, including trisomy 21, trisomy 13, trisomy 18, and Turner syndrome, are associated with a high incidence of congenital heart disease and should lead to fetal echocardiography. A history of congenital heart disease in one family member increases the risk of congenital heart disease in the fetus from 0.8% to 3% to 4%, with a possibly higher risk in families with a history of left ventricular outflow tract obstruction (Fyler et al, 1980; Nora and Nora, 1978) (Fig. 65–1). Maternal risk factors include diseases such as Type I diabetes (Friedman et al, 1993), which is associated with hypertrophic cardiomyopathy and transposition of the great vessels; connective tissue disorders, which have an increased incidence of complete heart block; hyperthyroid-

ism, which causes fetal tachyarrhythmias; and other illnesses including metabolic diseases and pheochromocytoma. Certain maternal viral infections, such as rubella, coxsackievirus, and toxoplasmosis, are also associated with structural heart disease. Finally, exposure to certain teratogens, including alcohol, lithium, phenytoin (Dilantin), retinoic acid, and warfarin (Coumadin), increases the risk of congenital heart disease.

Only about 10% of congenital heart disease is detected prenatally (Simpson and Marx, 1994; Tegnander et al, 1995). Fetal echocardiography allows the precise definition of fetal cardiac anatomy as early as 10 weeks' gestation (Dolkart and Reimers, 1991). High-resolution two-dimensional scanning can determine cardiac position and allows visualization of the cardiac chambers, valves, and arterial and venous connections. The velocity of arterial and venous blood flow and incidence and amount of valvular regurgitation and stenoses can be quantitated with spectral and color Doppler (Sharland et al, 1990). M-mode scanning is used to determine chamber size and function and for delineation of fetal arrhythmias. Many complex congenital heart malformations require prostaglandin E_1 to maintain ductal patency after birth to supply either pulmonary blood flow (i.e., pulmonary atresia) or systemic perfusion (i.e., interrupted aortic arch). If ductal dependent congenital heart disease is known prenatally, appropriate obstetric plans can be made for delivery at a tertiary care center equipped with facilities capable of managing such infants. Therapy with prostaglandin E_1 can then be instituted soon after birth to avoid ductal closure and prevent ischemic organ damage. Prenatal counseling can also be offered to the parents to help them prepare for the infant's postnatal course. Prenatal diagnosis allows the option of in utero therapies or early delivery for management of certain fetal problems. Finally, in certain instances of severe congenital heart disease, the option of termination of the pregnancy may also be offered.

Technique

Fetal echocardiography is an excellent tool for noninvasive evaluation of cardiac anatomy. The most optimal time to perform the examination is at 16 to 22 weeks' gestation (Fyfe and Kline, 1990; Simpson and Marx, 1994), although some forms of congenital heart disease may not become evident until later in gestation (Allan, 1988). The method of scanning a fetal heart is systematic so that all cardiac structures are seen in multiple views. Initially, fetal orientation within the uterus is determined, and the cardiac position within the chest is resolved (Comstock, 1987; Cordes et al, 1994). The position of the aorta and inferior vena cava in relation to the spine is used to determine visceroatrial situs. Once visceroatrial situs is established, the major cardiac structures are determined through the following

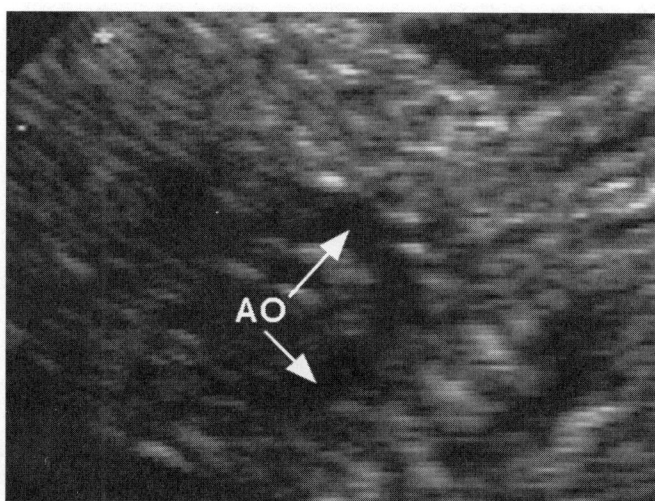

FIGURE 65–1. Fetal echocardiogram demonstrating a normal aortic arch. Note the visualization of arch vessels. The fetus had an older sibling with aortic stenosis. AO, aorta.

two-dimensional echocardiographic views: (1) standard four chamber, (2) superior vena cava–right atrium–inferior vena cava, (3) right ventricular long axis from apex to pulmonary valve, (4) left ventricular long axis from apex to aortic valve, (5) short axis of the ventricles, (6) ductal arch from main pulmonary artery to descending aorta, (7) aortic arch, and (8) short axis of the great vessels. The specific techniques have been reviewed (McCurdy and Reed, 1993). These techniques significantly augment the information obtained from the four-chamber view, which screens for cardiac chamber malformations but does not assess the connections to the great vessels, abnormalities of systemic and pulmonary venous return, and valvular dysfunction. The sensitivity for detecting congenital heart disease from the four-chamber view ranges from 15% to 68% (Achiron et al, 1992; Bromely et al, 1992; Ott, 1995). This sensitivity contrasts with focused fetal echocardiography, which has much better sensitivity and good specificity. The sensitivity of focused fetal echocardiography ranges from 51% to 95%, and specificity has been reported between 95% and 99% (Buskens et al, 1996; Martin and Ruckman, 1990; Rustico et al, 1990). Factors that limit the accuracy of the evaluation include maternal obesity, multiple gestation, abnormal amounts of amniotic fluid, distortion of the thoracic contents by other masses, or an unfavorable fetal position (Chang et al, 1991). Atrial septal defects, small ventricular septal defects, anomalies of pulmonary venous return, and coarctation of the aorta remain difficult to define in the fetus (Sharland et al, 1994). These limitations are fully discussed with the parents at the time of the study.

After the two-dimensional anatomy has been evaluated, pulsed and color Doppler flow mapping is then performed. Blood flow velocity across the valves can be quantitated, as can direction and magnitude of flow across the foramen ovale. Both ductal and aortic arch flow can be seen with Doppler scanning. Reversal of blood flow across the ductus arteriosus or foramen ovale has been associated with severe congenital heart disease (Berning et al, 1996). If any cardiac arrhythmias are noted, further investigation can be done to determine the exact rhythm, including M-mode through the atria and ventricles or pulse Doppler of the left ventricular inflow and outflow signals (Steinfeld et al, 1986). Pulse Doppler of the umbilical vessels adds useful information about placental function and congestive heart failure (Al-Gazali et al, 1987). Finally, any effusions in the pericardial, pleural, or abdominal cavities should be noted because structural cardiac abnormalities have been associated with hydrops fetalis. The presence of hydrops has dire prognostic significance for the survival of the fetus (Silverman et al, 1985).

Normal data have been established for the measurement of various cardiac chambers and vessels throughout the second and third trimesters (Devore et al, 1985; Dolkart and Reimers, 1991; Rane et al, 1990) (see Chapter 62). Using these data in conjunction with gestational age (derived either from dates or biophysical profile), estimation of chamber volumes can be made (Silverman and Schmidt, 1990). The end-diastolic volumes of the fetal left and right ventricle increase exponentially from 18 weeks until term. Initially the right ventricle is dominant in size, but this imbalance becomes less significant late in gestation. An ejection fraction of approximately 67% is usually maintained (Schmidt et al, 1995).

Findings in Disease States

Prenatal diagnoses of tricuspid valve dysplasia (Sharland et al, 1991a), tricuspid atresia (Devore et al, 1987), pulmonary stenosis (Rice et al, 1993), atrioventricular septal defects (Machado et al, 1988) (Fig. 65–2), tetralogy of Fallot (Callan and Kan, 1991; Devore et al, 1988) (Fig. 65–3), critical aortic stenosis (Huhta et al, 1987; Robertson et al, 1989), hypoplastic left heart syndrome (Blake et al, 1991), subaortic stenosis (Chang et al, 1991), left ventricular aneurysm (Jacobsen et al, 1991), hypoplastic aortic arch (Sharland et al, 1994), hypertrophic cardiomyopathy (Gandi et al, 1995), asymmetric septal hypertrophy (Cooper et al, 1992), and cardiac tumors (Holley et al, 1995) have all been described.

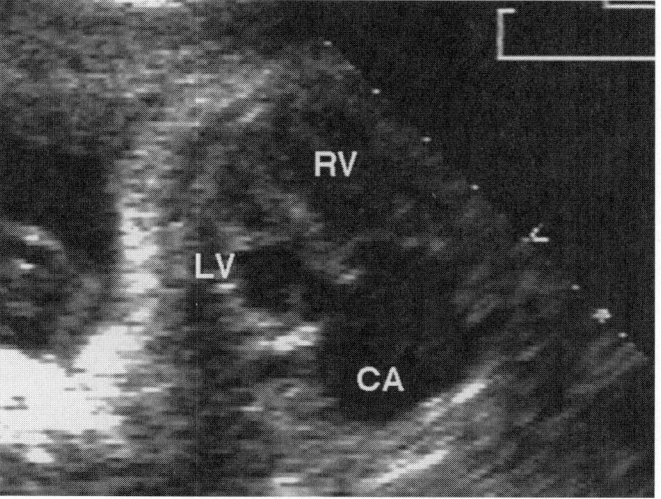

FIGURE 65–2. Common atrium in a fetus, later confirmed postnatally. This is one of the forms of atrioventricular septal defect. LV, left ventricle; RV, right ventricle; CA, common atrium.

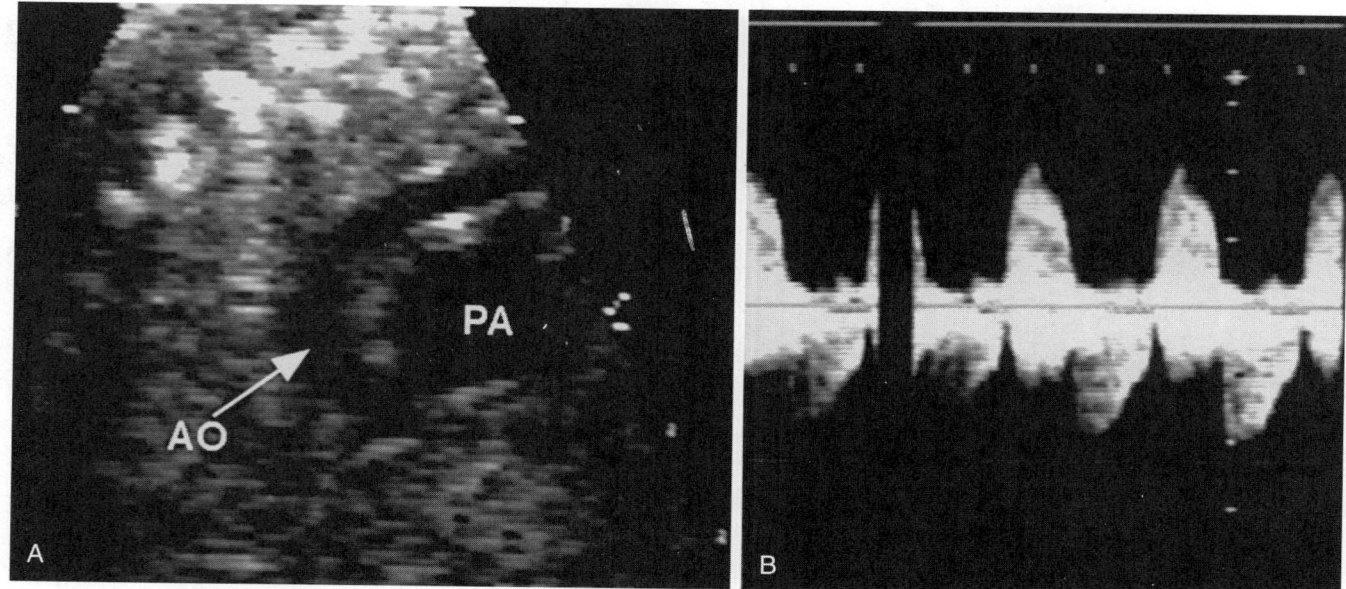

FIGURE 65–3. Tetralogy of Fallot with absent pulmonary valve. Marked dilation of the pulmonary artery is seen in *A*, and severe pulmonary stenosis and insufficiency are documented by continuous-wave Doppler in *B*. The infant died of respiratory insufficiency soon after birth. AO, aorta; PA, pulmonary artery.

Cardiac malposition as well as abnormalities of visceroatrial situs has been associated with severe congenital heart disease. Left atrial isomerism is commonly found in conjunction with complete atrioventricular septal defects as well as other more complex forms of the heterotaxia syndromes. The frequency of left atrial isomerism prenatally appears to exceed the incidence of right atrial isomerism, a relationship that is reversed postnatally. The association of left atrial isomerism with complete atrioventricular block has an extremely poor prognosis (Phoon et al, 1996) (Fig. 65–4).

The identification of severe abnormalities of the tricuspid valve prenatally also carries a poor prognosis. Tricuspid regurgitation is found in about 7% of fetuses but is trivial in 80% of these (Respondek et al, 1995). It is often difficult to distinguish correctly Ebstein anomaly of the tricuspid valve from tricuspid valvar dysplasia. Right atrial enlargement is usually associated with severe tricuspid regurgitation. When found in conjunction with right ventricular outflow tract obstruction, both lesions have a similarly poor outcome. Right ventricular outflow tract stenosis or atresia may develop late in gestation, necessitating repeat echocardiography later in the pregnancy. Severe tricuspid valve abnormalities are found more rarely postnatally than prenatally, indicative of fetal wastage (Hornberger et al, 1991; Oberhoffer et al, 1992; Sharland et al, 1991a). A partial reason for the fetal wastage may be the high frequency of hydrops seen in fetuses with severe tricuspid regurgitation; additionally, severe cardiomegaly, defined as a cardiothoracic ratio greater than 0.6, is associated with lethal pulmonary hypoplasia (Chaoui et al, 1994). One study reported the perinatal mortality of tricuspid regurgitation in the presence of anatomic heart disease of 83%, despite prenatal anticipation of the abnormality (Fig. 65–5). Half of the autopsies performed demonstrated pulmonary hypoplasia (Hornberger et al, 1991).

Right ventricular outflow tract obstructions such as pulmonary stenosis can progress to pulmonary atresia. These may also be associated with tricuspid regurgitation and severe right atrial enlargement (Todros et al, 1988). Fetuses with tetralogy of Fallot can have significant variability in the size of the pulmonary arteries, from diminutive in the case of severe right ventricular outflow tract obstruction to the extreme enlargement seen in tetralogy of Fallot with absence of the pulmonary valve (see Fig. 65–3). In the former case, hypoplasia of the pulmonary vessels may develop gradually during gestation as a result of inadequate pulmonary flow. The possibility of the development of pulmonary atresia should prompt repeat echocardiography closer to term (Hornberger et al, 1995b). Anomalous right ventricular muscle bundles in association with a ventricular septal defect have been identified in utero (Leandro et al, 1994).

The assessment of left ventricular disease in the fetus centers on the size of the left ventricle as well as the size and patency of the mitral and aortic valves. Poor growth of the left ventricle and mitral and aortic valves during gestation has been documented (Allan et al, 1989; Sharland et al, 1991b). The mechanism of this progression is unknown, but it may be related to diminished blood flow through the left ventricle during a crucial time in myocardial development. Although some have speculated that premature closure or restriction of the foramen ovale can cause this lesion, others maintain that early closure of the foramen is the result rather than the cause of left ventricular hypoplasia, citing occasional occurrence of reverse (left-to-right) shunting at the atrial level in these fetuses (Hornberger et al, 1995b; Kleinman and Copel, 1992; Sharland et al, 1991b). With severe left ventricular outflow tract obstruction, the ductus arteriosus is usually enlarged. Coarctation of the aorta is extremely hard to identify in this setting, but the associated finding of distal aortic arch hypoplasia is

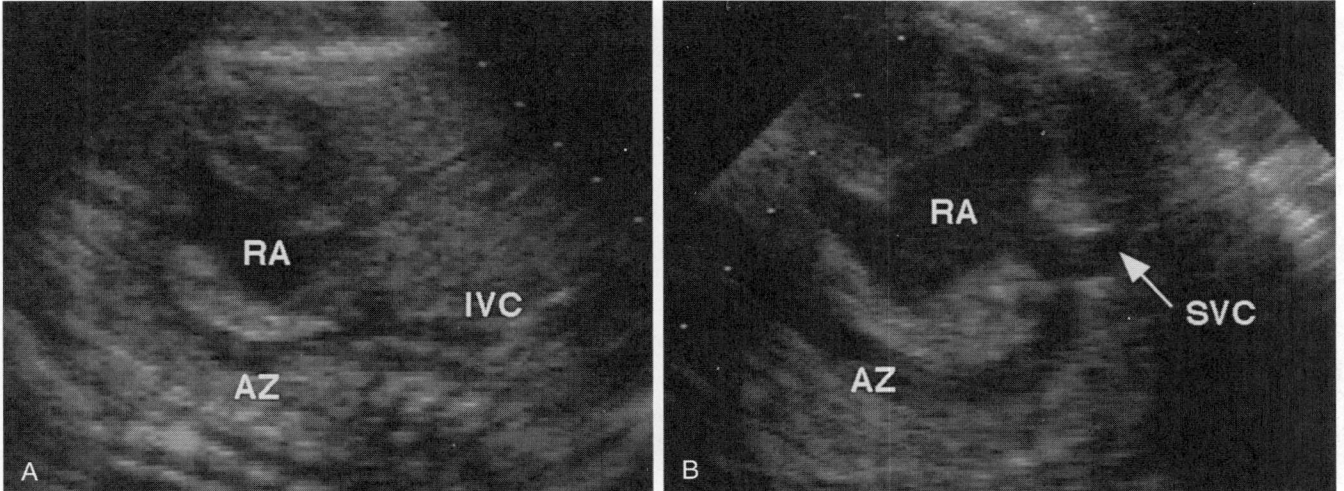

FIGURE 65–4. Left atrial isomerism in a fetus. Interruption of the inferior vena cava is seen in *A*, and azygos vein continuation to the superior vena cava is demonstrated in *B*. The infant had complex structural heart disease and complete atrioventricular block and eventually died of complications of biliary atresia. RA, right atrium; IVC, inferior vena cava; AZ, azygos vein; SVC, superior vena cava.

suggestive of the diagnosis (Hornberger et al, 1994; Sharland et al, 1994). Prenatal knowledge of severe hypoplasia of the left ventricle may not alter the poor postnatal prognosis to any great extent (Chang et al, 1991).

In addition to diagnosis of structural heart disease, fetal echocardiography has been used to diagnose fetal arrhythmias and to document efficacy of medical therapy (Allan et al, 1983; Strasburger et al, 1986). The more common arrhythmias that have been reported include complete heart block, sinus bradycardia, supraventricular tachycardia, atrial flutter, and isolated premature atrial and ventricular beats. Once the cause of a particular fetal arrhythmia

has been determined, the decision to treat can be made using structural information, gestational age, and the presence or absence of hydrops.

During certain medical therapeutic measures for the mother, fetal echocardiography has an important role in monitoring the health of the fetus. Specifically, the use of indomethacin for preterm labor or polyhydramnios has been shown to cause multiple abnormalities in the fetus (Mohen et al, 1992; Takahashi et al, 1996). Constriction of the ductus arteriosus or tricuspid regurgitation has been found in up to 10% of fetuses of mothers receiving indomethacin. The effect appears to be greatest in fetuses

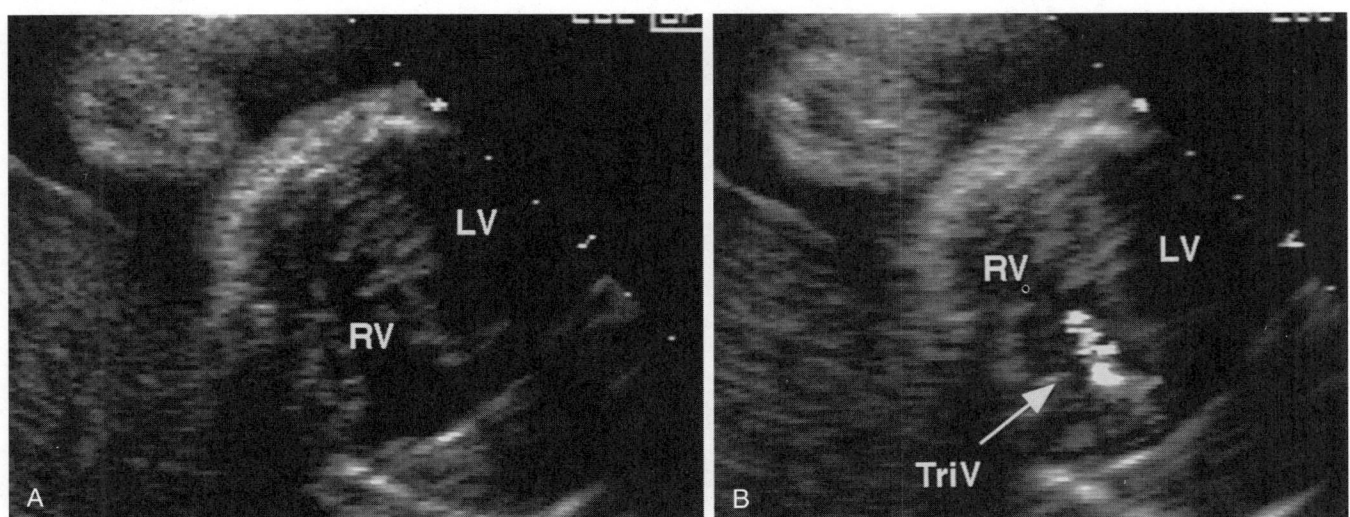

FIGURE 65–5. Tricuspid regurgitation in a fetus with a cardiomyopathy. *A* shows markedly abnormal myocardium, and the tricuspid regurgitation is shown by color flow Doppler in *B*. The infant died in the 1st year of life awaiting cardiac transplantation. LV, left ventricle; RV, right ventricle; TriV, tricuspid valve.

greater than 34 weeks' gestation. The amount of constriction can be quantified by pulse Doppler evaluation of the flow through the ductus, and therapy can be adjusted if a significant gradient across the ductus is found (Respondek et al, 1995). Pulmonary hypertension has resulted from surgical constriction of the fetal lamb ductus (Abman et al, 1989); the risk of postnatal pulmonary hypertension may mandate early delivery if ductal constriction is persistent (Fig. 65–6).

Perinatal Bradyarrhythmias

The normal fetal heart rate is 100 beats/min or more by 6 weeks' gestation (Doubilet and Benson, 1995). Fetal bradycardia is defined as a heart rate of less than 100 beats/min (Ito et al, 1994). The two major causes of fetal bradycardia are atrial extrasystoles with atrioventricular block and congenital complete atrioventricular block (CCAVB). During profound bradycardia caused by CCAVB, abnormalities in umbilical venous flow and increases in biventricular size are observed (Indik et al, 1991; Veille and Covitz, 1994). Decreases in right ventricular function may occur with severe bradycardia, and this change has been shown to be accompanied by the development of hydrops (Veille and Covitz, 1994) (Fig. 65–7). As noted previously, hydrops can also be seen in instances of structural heart disease and CCAVB.

CCAVB occurs in about 1 in 20,000 births. About 25% to 30% have CCAVB in association with congenital heart disease (Ross, 1990), which worsens the prognosis generally and increases the likelihood of nonimmune hydrops in the fetus (Gembruch et al, 1989). One of the most lethal forms of congenital heart disease associated with CCAVB is left atrial isomerism. In these hearts, there is anatomic discontinuity between the atrioventricular node and the His-Purkinje system (Ho et al, 1992). The prognosis of CCAVB with L-transposition of the great vessels, if uncomplicated by other major lesions, is generally favorable, although pacemaker placement may be necessary.

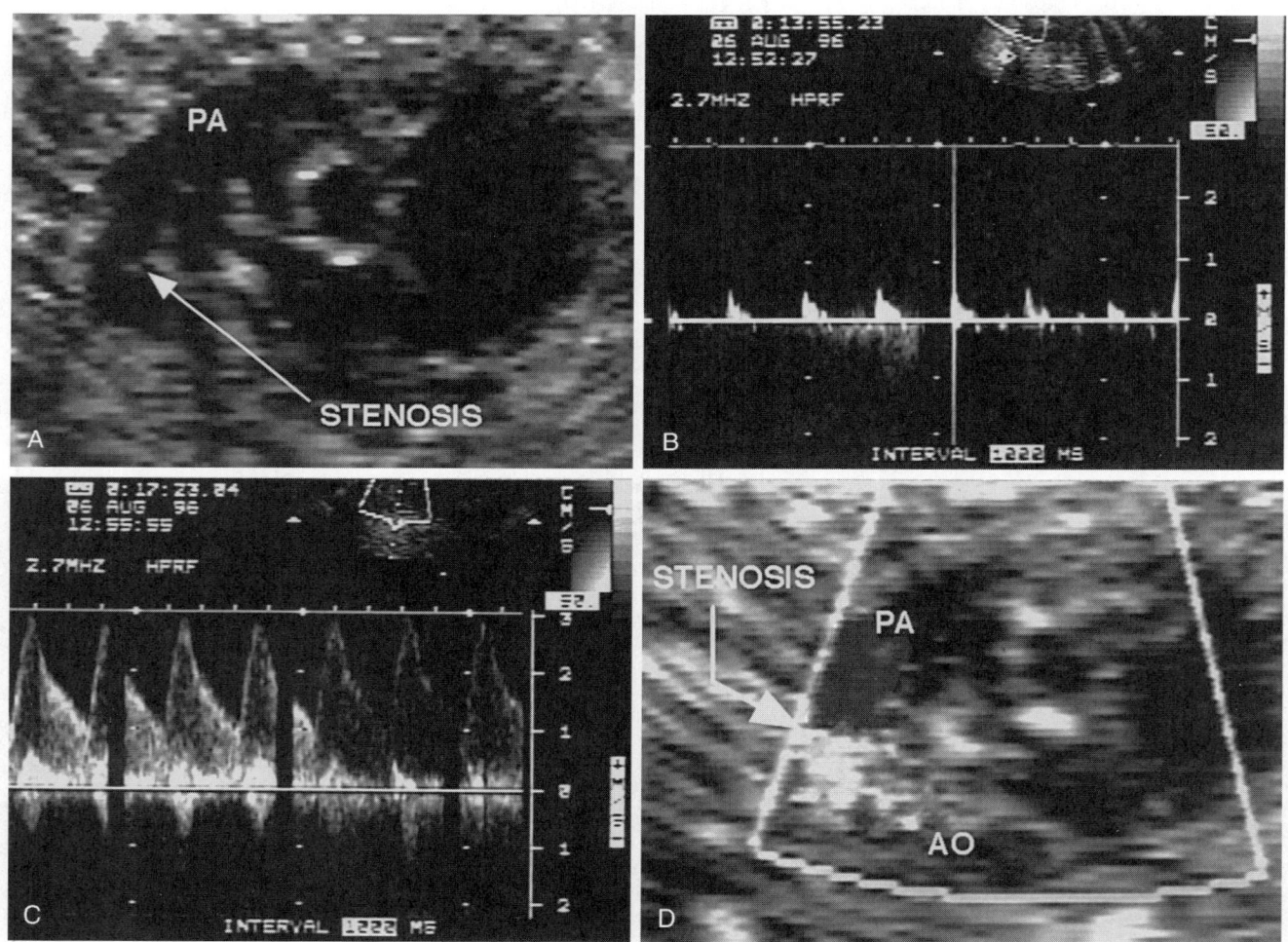

FIGURE 65–6. Constriction of the ductus arteriosus. The constriction is visible in *A*. Low-velocity flow in the pulmonary artery is documented by spectral Doppler in *B*, with high velocity and continuous flow detected distal to the site of obstruction in *C*. The flow disturbance is again demonstrated by color flow imaging in *D*. The fetus also had mild tricuspid regurgitation. The mother was not receiving indomethacin, and the child underwent planned early delivery without incident.

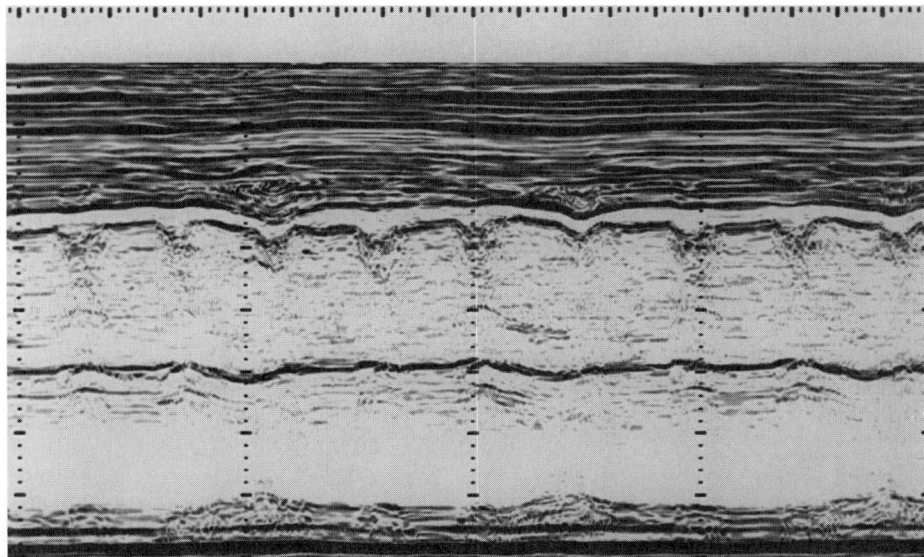

FIGURE 65–7. M-mode of complete atrioventricular block in a fetus. Note the faster atrial contractions than ventricular contractions. There is also a small pericardial effusion seen as a clear band on the tracing.

Diagnostic Considerations

CCAVB in the absence of structural heart disease is highly associated with maternal connective tissue disease. The atrioventricular block is probably caused by deposition of immunoglobulin in fetal cardiac tissue (Litsey et al, 1985), resulting in replacement of the atrial-nodal junction areas with fibrous tissue (Ho et al, 1992). The mother of an affected fetus is frequently asymptomatic but carries immunoglobulin G (IgG) antibodies against the small nuclear and cytoplasmic riobonucleoproteins Ro (SS-A) and La (SS-B) (Silver et al, 1992; Waltuck and Buyon, 1994). The Ro particle consists of 60 and 52 kDa polypeptides in association with small RNA known as hY1-5; at least a portion of the Ro particle is associated with the 48-kDa La polypeptide (Silverman et al, 1991). Symptomatic mothers usually have systemic lupus erythematosus, Sjögren syndrome, or an undifferentiated collagen vascular disease. Asymptomatic mothers have about a 50% likelihood of developing disease within a few years of birth of an affected child, but many remain asymptomatic for life. CCAVB usually occurs at 16 to 24 weeks' gestation, coincident with increased transfer of maternal IgG into the fetal circulation (Waltuck and Buyon, 1994). Historically the anti-Ro autoantibody was first associated with lupus-related CCAVB; however, the anti-La antibody cross-reacts with laminin, a major component of the cardiac sarcolemmal membrane, and has been shown to bind to cardiac myocytes, in distinction to anti-Ro (Li et al, 1995). In one study, fetal death was more strongly associated with anti-La than anti-Ro, although the difference was not statistically significant (Waltuck and Buyon, 1994). Another study demonstrated the strongest association of CCAVB with a combination of anti 48-kD La and anti 52-kDa Ro autoantibodies, with mothers also demonstrating antibodies to a 60-kDa Ro particle (Buyon et al, 1989). In addition to the effects of these and probably other autoantibodies on the conduction system, the lupus anticoagulant and antiphospholipid antibodies (anticardiolipin) have been associated with placental decidual plate thromboses resulting in fetal death (Silver et al, 1992).

Mothers with lupus should be followed for fetal bradycardia throughout pregnancy starting at 14 weeks' gestation (Fabbri and Hamner, 1992; Fyfe et al, 1993). Screening for autoantibodies should include coagulation studies, anticardiolipin antibody, and anti-Ro and anti-La (Silver et al, 1992). The risk of CCAVB in a child of a mother with known systemic lupus erythematosus is 1% to 2%, but the recurrence risk in a sibling is about 20% (Strasburger, 1990). The risk of CCAVB increases to about 5% in mothers with lupus who carry the anti-Ro antibody (Ramsey-Goldman et al, 1986), but high titers of anti-Ro antibody are not more predictive (Lockshin et al, 1988). Although the risk of CCAVB is clearly higher in the presence of both the anti-Ro and anti-La autoantibodies, some exposed infants have only cutaneous signs of lupus, complicating assertions that prophylactic treatment should be employed (Silverman et al, 1991). Transplacental passage of antibody is not in itself sufficient for the development of neonatal lupus, as the occurrence of disease in one twin has been reported (Callen et al, 1985). The antibodies are detectable in the newborn only for the first several months, consistent with transplacental passage of antibody (Scott et al, 1983).

Intrauterine Therapy

Some fetuses with CCAVB go on to develop poor myocardial function with hydrops, considerably increasing the risk of a demise (Veille and Covitz, 1994). Treatment of the mother during pregnancy should be considered if myocardial dysfunction occurs in a previable fetus (Silverman et al, 1991). Maternal therapies to attenuate or prevent the effect of maternal connective tissue disease are difficult to evaluate because of the lack of prospective studies and the multiple therapies used. Fetuses with CCAVB do not increase their heart rate in response to maternal atropine or beta agonists (Carpenter et al, 1986; Martin et al, 1988), and at least one hydropic fetus has failed to respond to intra-abdominal isoproterenol (Martin et al, 1988). In one report of dexamethasone use after the development of CCAVB, one of the five fetuses that had 2:1 atrioventricular block did not progress to complete block. Dexamethasone was used because of its ability to cross the placenta, and additional stress doses were given at the time of delivery (Copel et al, 1995). Plasmapheresis has also been employed in hydrops associated with CCAVB, with continuation of poor myocardial function but resolution of pleural and pericardial effusions (Carpenter et al, 1986). There are reports of women with a particularly poor history of fetal wastage undergoing plasmapheresis and prednisolone therapy before the development of block, with a consequent decrease in the titer of anti-Ro antibodies and subsequent delivery of a normal infant (Barclay et al, 1987). Prophylactic treatment of other fetuses with oral steroids, in one instance combined with acetylsalicylic acid, however, failed to prevent CCAVB (Carreira et al, 1993; Waltuck and Buyon, 1994). Fetuses with hydrops have been treated with maternal digoxin (Carpenter et al, 1986) and repeated paracentesis in an attempt to prevent pulmonary hypoplasia (Martin et al, 1988).

Intrauterine pacing has been accomplished in fetal lambs (Assad et al, 1994; Scagliotti et al, 1987), as has fetal transcatheter ablation of the atrioventricular node to produce atrioventricular block experimentally (Assad et al, 1995). Intrauterine transvenous pacing has been performed via the inferior vena cava in a 24-week gestation fetus with hydrops, but the fetus died during attempts to replace a dislodged pacing lead. This approach may become more feasible with improvements in pacing lead and ultrasound visualization capability (Walkinshaw et al, 1994). A direct transcutaneous approach to the right ventricle with a pacing electrode has also been performed, but pacing was successful only for a few hours (Carpenter et al, 1986). Whether intrauterine pacing would be more successful if applied before the development of hydrops is not known, but there are obvious ethical issues about employing intrauterine pacing in a fetus without congestive heart failure who might otherwise progress to term without intervention.

Fetuses with CCAVB without hydrops can be delivered vaginally, with monitoring of the fetal atrial rate either by Doppler ultrasound or by scalp electrocardiogram after rupture of membranes. Cesarean sections should be performed in fetuses with hydrops when otherwise appropriate from the perinatal standpoint because of the risk of sudden deterioration in the condition of the fetus (Ross, 1990). Early delivery of fetuses with hydrops has been performed by cesarean section or vaginally (Simpson and Marx, 1994; Veille and Covitz, 1994). Fetuses with CCAVB and severe structural heart disease are usually not considered for early delivery because the postnatal survival of these infants is poor (Gembruch et al, 1989; Simpson and Marx, 1994).

Postnatal Management

Infants with CCAVB are followed closely after birth for the development of congestive heart failure or complications of low cardiac output. Permanent pacemakers have been placed in infants as small as 1.3 kg (Gillette et al, 1992) and as early as 29 weeks' gestation (Ohmi et al, 1992). Pacing through exteriorized wires has been reported in a 1.2-kg premature infant (Martin et al, 1988). The pulse generator is placed in a variety of locations, from intra-abdominally with the use of a Gore-Tex pocket (Ohmi et

al, 1992), in the retroperitoneum (Sosa et al, 1988), and by a transvenous approach in infants in the 2.6- to 2.8-kg range (Stojanov et al, 1994; Till et al, 1990). The retroperitoneal route may allow for the placement of larger pulse generators, allowing for earlier institution of dual-chamber pacing (Sosa et al, 1988). There is no question, however, that the smaller the infant, the greater are the technical problems, including skin erosion over the generator site (Shearin and Fleming, 1978) and perforation of the right ventricle with temporary transvenous pacing. Emergency pacing may be necessary in the delivery room (Ohmi et al, 1992). Pacing is performed in the asymptomatic newborn with an average heart rate of less than 55 beats/min because of the risk of death in infants with slow heart rates (Michaelsson and Engle, 1972; Pinsky et al, 1982). Use of digoxin has been advocated to treat congestive heart failure, but administration of digoxin is probably safer after pacemaker implantation (Michaelsson and Engle, 1972). Other risk factors that pertain to the issue of pacemaker implantation include the presence of junctional exit block, ventricular ectopy, or the lack of change in heart rate with physical activity (Dewey et al, 1987).

Perinatal Tachyarrhythmias

Fetal arrhythmias occur in about 2% of pregnancies. Indications for referral to a cardiac specialist include a sustained heart rate of greater than 180 beats/min, repetitive irregular beats, or unexplained hydrops. Proper diagnosis of the arrhythmia is performed by using M-mode techniques to define the relationship of atrial and ventricular contraction and Doppler methods to evaluate flow across atrioventricular valves (Fyfe et al, 1993). The evaluation should include a complete echocardiographic evaluation for structural defects, with particular attention to abnormalities of the tricuspid valve (Hansmann et al, 1991). Signs of hydrops should be sought.

Diagnostic Considerations

The most frequent tachyarrhythmia seen in the fetus is premature atrial extrasystoles, followed by supraventricular tachycardia (SVT) and atrial flutter (Koehler et al, 1995). Premature atrial contractions (PACs) usually resolve spontaneously before or shortly after birth. It is important to distinguish blocked PACs from sinus bradycardia because suspicion of the latter can prompt emergency delivery for fetal distress. About 1% of patients with PACs develop SVT. Aneurysmal bulging of the atrial septum may be associated with PACs (Fyfe et al, 1993; Rice et al, 1988). Sinus tachycardia can occur with hyperthyroidism (Ito et al, 1994). In atrial flutter, atrial rates can approach 500 beats/min, and the rhythm is irregular owing to variable atrioventricular block. Atrial flutter and SVT can coexist in the same fetus. Junctional and ventricular tachycardia and atrial fibrillation are quite rare in the fetus (Fyfe et al, 1993; Ito et al, 1994; Strasburger, 1990).

Fetal cardiac function during arrhythmias is evaluated echocardiographically. Postextrasystolic potentiation of fractional shortening has been observed after an isolated premature beat, indicating a functioning Frank-Starling mechanism as early as 21 to 24 weeks' gestation (Reed et al, 1987). Flow reversal is observed in the inferior vena cava during PACs, SVT, and atrial flutter (Reed et al, 1990). Sustained SVT, defined as persistence of the tachycardia greater than 50% of the time (Ito et al, 1994), results in diminished mean velocity across all cardiac valves. Cardiac function improves on conversion of the dysrhythmia (Kleinman and Copel, 1992; Reed et al, 1987).

Supraventricular Tachycardia

SVT is the most common sustained tachyarrhythmia in the fetus (Fyfe et al, 1993). Postnatal transesophageal echocardiography reveals that hydropic infants are similar to infants diagnosed postnatally in the mechanism of the tachycardia (orthodromic reciprocating tachycardia) and in the frequency of pre-excitation (about 33%). The only significant difference is a slightly slower heart rate in hydropic fetuses, perhaps indicating that hydrops results from prolonged duration of a slightly slower tachycardia than in those diagnosed postnatally (Zales et al, 1988).

Sustained tachyarrhythmias should be treated because of their propensity to lead to fetal hydrops (Hansmann et al, 1991; Ito et al, 1994; van Engelen et al, 1994). Drug therapy is more difficult once hydrops occurs because of poor placental transmission of drugs in the hydropic state (Hansmann et al, 1991; Kleinman and Copel, 1991a). The traditional treatment of fetal SVT is maternal digoxin (Table 65–1). Usually a loading dose of 0.5 to 1.25 mg is given over 24 hours, with maintenance doses of 0.25 to 0.75 mg per day. The regimen may be more effective if the two loading doses of 0.25 to 0.5 mg are given intravenously. Maternal digoxin levels are followed to achieve levels in the high therapeutic range. Digoxin slows conduction through the atrioventricular node and increases its refractoriness, thus terminating the tachycardia. It also has a positive inotropic effect. Digoxin can decrease the refractoriness of accessory electrophysiologic connections; however, the hazards of this property pertain to the possible rapid ventricular response in the presence of atrial fibrillation, which is vanishingly rare in the fetus. Digoxin is incompletely transferred to the fetus by the placenta; the presence of digoxin-like immunoreactive substances also complicates the interpretation of digoxin levels in the fetus (Ito et al, 1994). Maternal digoxin therapy can be successful in the presence of hydrops (Gough et al, 1986).

Considerable institutional variability exists in the treatment of the fetus in SVT resistant to conversion with maternal digoxin. Maternal digoxin therapy may also be limited because of maternal side effects (Hansmann et al, 1991). Some practitioners are hesitant to add a second agent in the absence of hydrops (Kleinman and Copel, 1991a). Hydropic fetuses take a longer time to achieve control and require more drugs for control than nonhydropic fetuses (van Engelen et al, 1994). The chance of successful conversion of SVT with combination drug therapy is about 80%; drugs such as quinidine, verapamil, propafenone, and amiodarone significantly alter digoxin clearance, making it necessary to decrease the digoxin dose (Ito et al, 1994). Combinations of digoxin with verapamil (Hansmann et al, 1991), quinidine, and flecainide have been successfully used. Quinidine monotherapy is usually avoided because of its propensity to increase the ventricular response in atrial flutter or fibrillation. Flecainide has also shown effectiveness as a single agent, but it does have

---

TABLE 65–1

Maternal Drug Administration for Fetal Arrhythmias

Drug	Loading Dose	Maintenance Dose	Feto/Maternal Ratio	Drug Interactions	Major Toxicities
Digoxin	0.25–0.5 mg IV × 2–3	0.25–0.75 mg/d	0.2–1.15	Quinidine, amiodarone, verapamil, flecainide	GI, CNS, and proarrhythmia
Procainamide	100 mg IV q 5 min; max 1 g	2–6 mg/min IV	Proc 0.3–1.3 NAPA 0.9–1.2	Amiodarone, propranolol	Hypotension, GI, CNS, proarrhythmia
Quinidine		200–300 mg po tid/qid	0.24–0.94	Digoxin, verapamil, amiodarone	GI, CNS, proarrhythmia
Flecainide		300–600 mg/d divided bid/tid	0.5–0.8	Digoxin, amiodarone, propranolol	CNS, proarrhythmia
Propafenone		150–300 mg po q 8 h	0.2	Digoxin, quinidine, amiodarone	Asthma, hypotension, CNS, GI, proarrhythmia
Propranolol	1–3 mg IV	30–320 mg/d divided tid/qid	0.3–1.3 (less protein binding in fetus)	Quinidine	Effects of beta blockade
Amiodarone	800–1200 mg/d	400–800 mg/d	0.1–0.5	Digoxin, quinidine, procainamide, flecainide	Abnormal thyroid function, ocular, hepatic
Verapamil	5–10 mg IV	240–480 mg/d divided tid/qid	0.1–0.2	Digoxin, flecainide	Death in newborns, CNS, GI, proarrhythmia

NAPA, N-acetyl procainamide; Proc, procainamide; CNS, central nervous system; GI, gastrointestinal.
Data from Hansmann et al, 1991; Ito et al, 1994; Kleinman and Copel, 1991b; Simpson and Marx, 1994; van Engelen et al, 1994.

proarrhythmic effects, including the slowing of atrial flutter leading to a possibly higher ventricular rate (Ito et al, 1994).

Alternatively, direct therapy of the fetus via the umbilical vein can be considered. The direct administration of adenosine to the fetus serves as both a diagnostic and therapeutic maneuver (Kleinman and Copel, 1991a, 1991b); SVT should terminate abruptly with 1:1 atrioventricular conduction. The short half-life of adenosine necessitates its rapid delivery intravenously and makes it useless as a transplacental agent. In atrial flutter, the degreee of atrioventricular block is transiently increased by adenosine, making flutter contractions somewhat easier to visualize and failing to terminate the tachycardia. If the response to adenosine is consistent with the diagnosis of SVT, direct administration of digoxin to the fetus has been advocated. If fetal and maternal digoxin levels are already in the high therapeutic range (1.5 to 2.0 ng/mL) or if digoxin has been ineffective, intravenous procainamide can be administered (Kleinman and Copel, 1991a). Intravenous flecainide, propafenone, and amiodarone have also been employed; sudden cardiac arrest during direct administration of amiodarone has been reported (Hansmann et al, 1991), and its long half-life, although allowing infrequent direct dosing to the fetus, also makes termination of therapy owing to fetal toxicity problematic (Kleinman and Copel, 1991b). Amiodarone is transmitted poorly across the placenta. Fetal deaths have been reported after the direct administration of verapamil (Hansmann et al, 1991); the dangers of administering this drug to newborns are well known, and this mode of therapy should probably not be used. Outpatient use and monitoring of these newer modes of therapy is unwise (Kleinman and Copel, 1991a). Although drug can be applied directly to the fetus with this technique, drug can also be passed back to the mother, who acts as a large reservoir for drug clearance (Ito et al, 1994).

Atrial Flutter

Atrial flutter is generally more difficult to control than SVT (van Engelen et al, 1994). Digoxin is the principal drug used to treat atrial flutter; by increasing the degree of atrioventricular block, digoxin lowers the ventricular rate. If the rhythm fails to convert or if the ventricular response is unacceptably rapid, coadministration of procainamide (Simpson and Marx, 1994) or quinidine has been advocated (Hansmann et al, 1991; Kleinman and Copel, 1991b; Strasburger 1990). Quinidine introduces problems of proarrhythmia, and it alters digoxin pharmacokinetics, mandating a 50% decrease in the digoxin dose. Administration of amiodarone to the mother or directly to the fetus can be considered if the combination of digoxin and quinidine fails to succeed (Hansmann et al, 1991; Kleinman and Copel, 1991a).

Ventricular Tachycardia

Ventricular tachycardia is rare in the fetus. Newborns are usually stable if the ventricular rate is not excessive (van Engelen et al, 1994); treatment of this dysrhythmia in the fetus has been recommended only if the heart rate is greater than 200 beats/min or if hydrops is present. There is not sufficient experience with this arrhythmia to describe a proven mode of therapy, but direct treatment of the fetus with lidocaine or maternal treatment with mexiletine could be considered. Digoxin and verapamil should be avoided (Kleinman and Copel, 1991a, 1991b).

Postnatal Therapy

The postnatal therapy of newborns with SVT has been reviewed (Kugler and Danford, 1996). After initial stabilization of the infant, which may include ventilatory support and attention to acid-base status, an electrocardiogram should be performed to document the arrhythmia. Immediate conversion of SVT is desirable and can be accomplished with either cardioversion or the use of intravenous adenosine, starting at 100 μg/kg and increasing the dose to a maximum of 250 μg/kg. It is the authors' and others' experience that the most frequent cause of failure to convert SVT with adenosine is that the bolus of medication was not delivered rapidly. After conversion of the rhythm, long-term therapy is usually begun with digoxin unless the infant is shown to have Wolff-Parkinson-White syndrome; in this circumstance, other agents are employed with the assistance of a pediatric cardiologist.

The goal of therapy in the newborn with atrial flutter is not only to control the ventricular rate, but also to convert the tachycardia. The most effective mode of therapy is DC cardioversion. Digoxin is usually satisfactory for long-term management. Management of ventricular tachycardia depends on symptoms and on the presence or absence of underlying cardiac disease.

Interventions to Alter Fetal Anatomy

Surgical or transcatheter intervention in the fetus remains in its infancy but may hold great promise in the future as a method to prevent or attenuate the effects of congenital cardiac malformations. Fetal thoracic surgery in animals has advanced significantly. Tracheal ligation improves the pulmonary hypoplasia seen in experimental diaphragmatic hernia, and fetoscopic procedures may make it possible to plug the trachea via that technique (DiFiore et al, 1994; Hedrick et al, 1994). Pulmonary artery banding has been performed in fetal sheep, with demonstrable changes in biventricular performance as a result (Reller et al, 1992; Sandhu et al, 1994).

Thoracic surgery has been successfully performed in the human fetus for the treatment of diaphragmatic hernia and cystic adenomatoid malformations (Adzick et al, 1993). The greatest problem appears to be uterine irritability and subsequent preterm labor (Flake and Harrison, 1995). Experimental work suggests that removal of abdominal contents from the thorax can result in less lung hypoplasia if delivery does not occur soon after the procedure. The most optimal time to perform surgery from the standpoint of avoiding premature labor appears to be between 24 and 30 weeks' gestation (Harrison et al, 1990). Methods of fetal cardiac bypass are currently in development in experimental animals; these techniques hold great promise for intrauterine cardiac surgery if the problems of premature labor and hazard to the mother can be surmounted (Hawkins et al, 1994; Reddy et al, 1996).

Candidates for fetal cardiac intervention in the future might include fetuses with congenital complete atrioventricular block or ventricular outflow tract obstruction (Flake and Harrison, 1995). Interventions in any form of fetal heart disease in which there is massive cardiomegaly might result in improved pulmonary function simply by reducing the size of the heart before birth (Kleinman and Copel, 1992). More needs to be known about the natural history of these lesions in the fetus, and the risk of any intervention needs to be weighed against the risk to the fetus and to the mother (Flake and Harrison, 1995). Fetal transesophageal echocardiography has been performed in animals and might provide improved visualization of the fetal heart during invasive procedures (Kohl et al, 1996). It has been postulated that balloon dilation of the stenotic right ventricular outflow tract in early gestation might result in improved growth of the pulmonary arteries by increasing flow (Hornberger et al, 1995b; Kleinman and Copel, 1992). Severe obstruction to left ventricular outflow has a particularly dismal prognosis after birth, prompting efforts at fetal intervention. Opening of the atrial septum in the fetus with a restrictve foramen ovale is not likely to be of value (Allan et al, 1989). Balloon dilation of the aortic valve has been performed successfully by passing a catheter transabdominally through the left ventricular apex (Allan et al, 1995), but failures have occurred as well, perhaps in part owing to extremely poor left ventricular function at the time of the procedure (Maxwell et al, 1991). It is not clear whether early dilation of the aortic valve would result in improved left ventricular function and growth (Allan et al, 1989; Hornberger et al, 1995a; Sharland et al, 1991b). Advances in this important area of investigation depend on close cooperation between the fetal echocardiographer, interventional pediatric cardiologist, and pediatric cardiac surgeon.

TELEMEDICINE

Few technologies share the potential of advanced telecommunications to change the practice of medicine. Telemedicine has the potential to dash all of the traditional barriers to the practice of medicine, including historical patterns of referral, time, distance, and state and national borders. Telemedicine also has the potential to bring the best in medical expertise to any bedside, regardless of geography. Telemedicine will improve access, reduce cost, and increase quality in several highly specialized areas of medicine, including fetal and newborn cardiology.

Telemedicine is defined as the care of individual patients over distances using advanced telecommunications equipment.

In its initial phases, telemedicine has largely been based on relatively expensive, room-based, broad-band technology designed for interaction of small groups of people at fixed locations. This approach can be near ideal for specific uses, such as administrative meetings, didactic teaching, and technical demonstrations.

Telemedicine has recently moved from dedicated rooms to desk tops. Desk-top telemedicine puts the technology in front of people where they work in the laboratories, intensive care units, and clinics and permits telemedicine to become a seamless and routine tool in daily practice. Desk-top telemedicine is currently practiced using high-speed telephone lines such as ISDN (integrated serial digital network) over which transmissions cost a small fraction of transmissions over fiber optic or ATM (asynchronous transfer mode) connections. Each ISDN line carries 128 kilobytes per second, whereas a standard telephone line (POTS, plain old telephone service) now carries up to 56 kilobytes per second with the latest modem. Broad-band technology such as ATM typically provides up to 155 megabytes per second. ATM may be critical for sharing large patient databases or information systems between or among hospitals but is not necessary for high-quality video conferencing or transmissions of echocardiograms today. Commercial television broadcasts and cardiac ultrasound scanners record at 30 frames per second; even the best human eye cannot perceive individual frames at frame rates greater than 22 frames per second. Low-cost, off-the-shelf, desk-top video conferencing equipment such C-Phone (C-Phone Incorporated, Wilmington, NC) can now digitize and transmit 30 frame-per-second analogue video signals at 384 kilobytes per second using three ISDN lines. Within 4 years, technical advances will permit the same transmissions over the internet for pennies.

The net result of telemedicine in newborn cardiology is that nurseries in need of help in diagnosing or managing a potential cardiac problem (whether because the local expert is out of town, across town, or does not exist) are now getting it immediately without having to transfer the patient or wait for a consultant to arrive (Fisher et al, 1996; Rendina et al, in press). Using desk-top video conferencing, it is possible to provide a virtual pediatric cardiology service to any nursery. Desk-top video conferencing is being used to guide acquisition of echocardiograms as well as provide echocardiographic interpretations, radiographic consultations, physician-to-physician consultations, and conferences with parents in distant hospitals. Similarly, obstetricians and perinatologists are beginning to use desk-top video conferencing for reviews of fetal scans and fetal echocardiograms and consultations with distant colleagues.

The distinction between telemedicine and other forms of medicine is likely to blur as hospitals begin to (1) use digital technology internally for information storage and transfer and (2) move to electronic, multimedia medical records. Transferring an electronic medical record with an attached clip of an echocardiogram to the building next door over an intranet is ultimately not different from transferring the same data across town or across an ocean over ISDN lines today or the internet tomorrow. The obvious implication of the advent of the digital age in medicine is consolidation of health care delivery, as the distinction as to what is internal (in our hospital) and what is external (in their hospital) begins to disappear. The good news from the digital transformation of the health care system will be reductions in errors, reductions in costs, improvements in quality, and improvements in access. The bad news will be heightened competition and progressive consolidation.

REFERENCES

Abman S, Shanley PF, Accurso FJ: Failure of postnatal adaptation of the pulmonary circulation after chronic intrauterine pulmonary hypertension in fetal lambs. J Clin Invest 83:1849, 1989.

Achiron R, Glaser J, Gelernter I, et al: Extended fetal echocardiographic examination for detecting cardiac malformations in low risk pregnancies. BMJ 304:671, 1992.

Adzick N, Harrison MR, Flake AW, et al: Fetal surgery for cystic adenomatoid malformation of the lung. J Pediatr Surg 6:806, 1993.

Al-Gazali W, Chapman MG, Chita SK, et al: Doppler assessment of umbilical artery blood flow for the prediction of outcome in fetal cardiac abnormality. Br J Obstet Gynaecol 94:742, 1987.

Allan LD: Development of congenital lesions in mid or late gestation. Int J Cardiol 19:361, 1988.

Allan LD, Anderson RH, Sullivan ID, et al: Evaluation of fetal arrhythmias by echocardiography. Br Heart J 50:240, 1983.

Allan LD, Crawford DC, Sheridan R: Aetiology of non-immune hydrops: The value of echocardiography. Br J Obstet Gynaecol 93:223, 1986.

Allan LD, Maxwell DJ, Carminati M, et al: Survival after fetal aortic balloon valvuloplasty. Ultrasound Obstet Gynecol 5:90, 1995.

Allan LD, Sharland GK, Chita SK, et al: Chromosomal anomalies in fetal congenital heart disease. Ultrasound Obstet Gynecol 1:8, 1991.

Allan LD, Sharland GK, Tynan MJ: The natural history of hypoplastic left heart syndrome. Int J Cardiol 25:341, 1989.

Assad R, Aiello VD, Jatene MB, et al: Cryosurgical ablation of fetal atrioventricular node: New model to treat fetal malignant tachyarrhythmias. Ann Thorac Surg 60:S629, 1995.

Assad R, Jatene MB, Moreira LFP, et al: Fetal heart block: A new experimental model to assess fetal pacing. Pacing Clin Electrophysiol 17:1256, 1994.

Barclay CS, French MAH, Ross LD, et al: Successful pregnancy following steroid therapy and plasma exchange in a woman with anti-Ro (SS-A) antibodies: Case report. Br J Obstet Gynaecol 94:369, 1987.

Berning RA, Silverman NH, Villegas M, et al: Reversed shunting across the ductus arteriosus or atrial septum in utero heralds severe congenital heart disease. J Am Coll Cardiol 27:481, 1996.

Blake DM, Copel JA, Kleinman CS: Hypoplastic left heart syndrome: Prenatal diagnosis, clinical profile and management. Am J Obstet Gynecol 165:529, 1991.

Bromely B, Estroff JA, Sanders SP, et al: Fetal echocardiography: Accuracy and limitations in a population at high and low risk for heart defects. Am J Obstet Gynecol 166:1473, 1992.

Buskens E, Stewart PA, Hess J, et al: Efficacy of fetal echocardiography and yield by risk category. Obstet Gynecol 87:423, 1996.

Buyon JP, Ben-Chetrit E, Karp S, et al: Acquired congenital heart block: Pattern of maternal antibody response to biochemically defined antigens of the SSA/Ro-SSB/La system in neonatal lupus. J Clin Invest 84:627, 1989.

Callan NA, Kan JS: Prenatal diagnosis of tetralogy of Fallot with absent pulmonary valve. Am J Perinatol 8:15, 1991.

Callan NA, Maggio M, Steger S, et al: Fetal echocardiography: Indications for referral, prenatal diagnosis, and outcomes. Am J Perinatol 8:390, 1991.

Callen J, Fowler JF, Kulick KB, et al: Neonatal lupus erythematosus occurring in one fraternal twin. Arthritis Rheum 28:271, 1985.

Carpenter R, Strasburger JF, Garson A, et al: Fetal ventricular pacing for hydrops secondary to complete atrioventricular block. J Am Coll Cardiol 8:1434, 1986.

Carreira P, Gutierrez-Larraya F, Gomez-Reino JJ: Successful intrauterine therapy with dexamethasone for fetal myocarditis and heart block in a woman with systemic lupus erythematosus. J Rheumatol 20:1204, 1993.

Chang AC, Huhta JC, Yoon GY, et al: Diagnosis, transport, and outcome in fetuses with left ventricular outflow obstruction. J Thorac Cardiovasc Surg 102:841, 1991.

Chaoui R, Bollmann R, Goldner B, et al: Fetal cardiomegaly: Echocardiographic findings and outcome in 19 cases. Fetal Diagn Ther 9:92, 1994.

Comstock CH: Normal fetal heart axis and position. Obstet Gynecol 70:255, 1987.

Cooper MJ, Enderlein MA, Dyson DC, et al: Fetal echocardiography: Retrospective review of clinical experience and in evaluation of indications. Obstet Gynecol 86(4 pt 1):577, 1995.

Cooper MJ, Enderlein MA, Tarnoff H, et al: Asymmetric septal hypertrophy in infants of diabetic mothers: Fetal echocardiography and the impact of maternal diabetic control. Am J Dis Child 146:226, 1992.

Copel J, Buyon JP, Kleinman CS: Successful in utero therapy of fetal heart block. Am J Obstet Gynecol 173:1384, 1995.

Cordes TM, O'Leary PW, Seward JB, et al: Distinguishing right from left: A standardized technique for fetal echocardiography. J Am Soc Echocardiogr 7:47, 1994.

De Lia J, Emery MG, Sheafor SA, et al: Twin transfusion syndrome: Successful in utero treatment with digoxin. Int J Gynaecol Obstet 23:197, 1985.

Devore GR, Siassi B, Platt LD: Fetal echocardiography: V. M-mode measurements of the aortic root and aortic valve in the second and third trimester normal fetus. Am J Obstet Gynecol 152:543, 1985.

Devore GR, Siassi B, Platt LD: Fetal echocardiography: The prenatal diagnosis of tricuspid atresia (type Ic) during the second trimester of pregnancy. J Clin Ultrasound 15:317, 1987.

Devore GR, Siassi B, Platt LD: Fetal echocardiography: VIII. Aortic root dilatation—a marker for tetralogy of Fallot. Am J Obstet Gynecol 159:129, 1988.

Dewey R, Capeless MA, Levy AM: Use of ambulatory electrocardiographic monitoring to identify high-risk patients with congenital complete heart block. N Engl J Med 316:835, 1987.

DiFiore J, Fauza DO, Slavin R, et al: Experimental fetal tracheal ligation reverses the structural and physiological effects of pulmonary hypoplasia in congenital diaphragmatic hernia. J Pediatr Surg 29:612, 1994.

Dolkart LA, Reimers FT: Transvaginal fetal echocardiography in early pregnancy: Normative data. Am J Obstet Gynecol 165:688, 1991.

Doubilet P, Benson CB: Embryonic heart rate in the early first trimester: What rate is normal? J Ultrasound Med 14:431, 1995.

Fabbri E, Hamner LH: Congenital complete heart block associated with maternal anti-Ro antibody: A case report. J Perinatol 12:225, 1992.

Fisher JB, Albotiras ET, Berdusis K, et al: Rapid identification of congenital heart disease by transmission of echocardiograms. Am Heart J 131:1225, 1996.

Flake A, Harrison MR: Fetal surgery. Ann Rev Med 46:67, 1995.

Friedman AH, Copel JA, Kleinman CS: Fetal echocardiography and fetal cardiology: Indications, diagnosis, and management. Semin Perinatol 17:76, 1993.

Fyfe DA, Kline CH: Fetal echocardiographic diagnosis of congenital heart disease. Pediatr Clin North Am 37:45, 1990.

Fyfe D, Meyer KB, Case CL: Sonographic assessment of fetal cardiac arrhythmias. Semin Ultrasound CT MR 14:286, 1993.

Fyler DC, Buckley LP, Hellenbrand WE, et al: Report of the New England Regional Infant Cardiac Program. Pediatrics 65(2 suppl):376, 1980.

Gandi JA, Zhang XY, Maidman JE: Fetal cardiac hypertrophy and cardiac function in diabetic pregnancies. Am J Obstet Gynecol 173:1132, 1995.

Gembruch U, Hansmann M, Redel DA, et al: Fetal complete heart block: Antenatal diagnosis, significance, and management. Eur J Obstet Gynecol Rep Biol 31:9, 1989.

Gillette P, Ziegler VL, Winslow AT, et al: Cardiac pacing in neonates, infants, and preschool children. Pacing Clin Electrophysiol 15(pt 2):2046, 1992.

Gough JD, Keeling JW, Castle B, et al: The obstetric management of non-immunological hydrops. Br J Obstet Gynaecol 93:226, 1986.

Hansmann M, Gembruch U, Bald R, et al: Fetal tachyarrhythmias: Transplacental and direct treatment of the fetus—a report of 60 cases. Ultrasound Obstet Gynecol 1:162, 1991.

Harrison M, Langer JC, Adzick NS, et al: Correction of congenital diaphragmatic hernia in utero: V. Initial clinical experience. J Pediatr Surg 25:47, 1990.

Hawkins J, Clark SM, Shaddy RE, et al: Fetal cardiac bypass: Improved placental function with moderately high flow rates. Ann Thorac Surg 57:293, 1994.

Hedrick M, Estes JM, Sullivan KM, et al: Plug the lung until it grows (PLUG): A new method to treat congenital diaphragmatic hernia in utero. J Pediatr Surg 29:612, 1994.

Ho S, Anderson RH, Allan L: Disposition of the atrioventricular conduction tissues in the heart with isomerism of the atrial appendages: Its relation to congenital complete heart block. J Am Coll Cardiol 20:904, 1992.

Holley DG, Martin GR, Brenner JI, et al: Diagnosis and management of fetal cardiac tumors: A multicenter experience and review of published reports. J Am Coll Cardiol 26:516, 1995.

Holzgreve W, Holzgreve B, Curry CJR: Nonimmune hydrops fetalis: Diagnosis and management. Semin Perinatol 9:52, 1985.

Hornberger LK, Sahn DJ, Kleinman CS, et al: Antenatal diagnosis of coarctation of the aorta: A multicenter experience. J Am Coll Cardiol 23:417, 1994.

Hornberger LK, Sahn DJ, Kleinman CS, et al: Tricuspid valve disease with significant tricuspid insufficiency in the fetus: Diagnosis and outcome. J Am Coll Cardiol 17:167, 1991.

Hornberger LK, Sanders SP, Rein A, et al: Left heart obstructive lesions and left ventricular growth in the midtrimester fetus: A longitudinal study. J Am Coll Cardiol 92:1531, 1995a.

Hornberger LK, Sanders SP, Sahn DJ, et al: In utero pulmonary artery and aortic growth and potential for progression of pulmonary outflow tract obstruction in tetralogy of Fallot. J Am Coll Cardiol 25:739, 1995b.

Huhta JC, Carpenter RJ, Moise KJ, et al: Prenatal diagnosis and postnatal management of critical aortic stenosis. Circulation 75:573, 1987.

Indik J, Chen V, Reed KL: Association of umbilical venous with inferior vena cava blood flow velocities. Obstet Gynecol 77:551, 1991.

Ito S, Magee L, Smallhorn J: Drug therapy for fetal arrhythmias. Clin Perinatol 21:543, 1994.

Jacobson RL, Perez A, Meyer RA, et al: Prenatal diagnosis of fetal left ventricular aneurysm: A case report and review. Obstet Gynecol 78:535, 1991.

Kleinman CS, Copel JA: Direct fetal therapy for cardiac arrhythmias: Who, what, when, where, why and how? Ultrasound Obstet Gynecol 1:158, 1991a.

Kleinman CS, Copel JA: Electrophysiological principles and fetal antiarrhythmic therapy. Ultrasound Obstet Gynecol 1:286, 1991b.

Kleinman CS, Copel JA: Fetal cardiovascular physiology and therapy. Fetal Diagn Ther 7:147, 1992.

Kleinman CS, Donnerstein RL, Jaffe CC, et al: Fetal echocardiography: A tool for evaluation of in utero cardiac arrhythmias and monitoring of in utero therapy: Analysis of 71 patients. Am J Cardiol 51:237, 1983.

Koehler D, Meyer KB, Kline CH, et al: Fetal echocardiography: A review of 1,028 consecutive examinations. J S C Med Assoc 91:333, 1995.

Kohl T, Szabo Z, VanderWall KJ, et al: Experimental fetal transesophageal and intracardiac echocardiography utilizing intravascular ultrasound technology. Am J Cardiol 77:899, 1996.

Kugler J, Danford DA: Management of infants, children, and adolescents with paroxysmal supraventricular tachycardia. J Pediatr 129:324, 1996.

Leandro J, Dyck JD, Smallhorn JF: Intra-utero diagnosis of anomalous right ventricular muscle bundles in association with a ventricular septal defect: A case report. Pediatr Cardiol 15:246, 1994.

Li J-M, Horsfall AC, Maini RN: Anti-La (SS-B) but not anti Ro52 (SS-A) antibodies cross-react with laminin-a role in the pathogenesis of congenital heart block? Clin Exp Immunol 99:316, 1995.

Litsey S, Noonan JA, O'Connor WN, et al: Maternal connective tissue disease and congenital heart block: Demonstration of immunoglobulin in cardiac tissue. N Engl J Med 312:98, 1985.

Lockshin M, Bonfa E, Elkon K, et al: Neonatal lupus risk to newborns of mothers with systemic lupus erythematosus. Arthritis Rheum 31:697, 1988.

Machado MV, Crawford DC, Anderson RH, et al: Atrioventricular septal defect in prenatal life. Br Heart J 59:352, 1988.

Martin GR, Ruckman RN: Fetal echocardiography: A large clinical experience and follow-up. J Am Soc Echocardiogr 3:4, 1990.

Martin T, Arias F, Olander DS, et al: Successful management of congenital atrioventricular block associated with hydrops fetalis. J Pediatr 112:984, 1988.

Maxwell D, Allan L, Tynan MJ: Balloon dilatation of the aortic valve in the fetus: A report of two cases. Br Heart J 65:256, 1991.

McCurdy CM, Reed KL: Basic technique of fetal echocardiography. Semin Ultrasound CT MR 14:267, 1993.

Meijboom EJ, van Englen AD, van de Beek EW, et al: Fetal arrhythmias. Curr Opin Cardiol 9:97, 1994.

Michaelsson M, Engle MA: Congenital complete heart block: An international study of the natural history. Cardiovasc Clin 4:85, 1972.

Mohen D, Newnham JP, D'Orsogna L: Indomethacin for the treatment of polyhydramnios: A case of constriction of the ductus arteriosus. Aust N Z J Obstet Gynaecol 32:243, 1992.

Nicolaides KH, Rodeck CH, Watson LJ, et al: Fetoscopy in the assessment of unexplained fetal hydrops. Br J Obstet Gynaecol 92:671, 1985.

Nora JJ, Nora AH: The evolution of specific genetic and environmental counseling in congenital heart disease. Circulation 57:205, 1978.

Oberhoffer R, Cook AC, Lang D, et al: Correlation between echocardiographic and morphological investigations of lesions of the tricuspid valve diagnosed during fetal life. Br Heart J 68:580, 1992.

Ohmi M, Tofukuji M, Sato K, et al: Permanent pacemaker implantation in premature infants less than 2,000 grams of body weight. Ann Thorac Surg 54:1223, 1992.

Okamura K, Murotsuki J, Kobayashi M, et al: Umbilical venous pressure and Doppler flow patterns of inferior vena cava in the fetus. Am J Perinatol 11:255, 1994.

Ott WJ: The accuracy of antenatal fetal echocardiography screening in high and low risk patients. Am J Obstet Gynecol 172:1741, 1995.

Phoon CK, Villegas MD, Ursell PC, et al: Left atrial isomerism detected in fetal life. Am J Cardiol 77:1083, 1996.

Pinsky W, Gillette PC, Garson A, et al: Diagnosis, management, and long-term results of patients with congenital complete atrioventricular block. Pediatrics 69:728, 1982.

Porreco RP, Barton SM, Haverkamp AD: Occlusion of umbilical artery in acardiac, acephalic twin. Lancet 337:326, 1991.

Ramsey-Goldman R, Hom D, Deng JS, et al: Anti-SS-A antibodies and fetal outcome in maternal systemic lupus erythematosus. Arthritis Rheum 29:1269, 1986.

Rane HS, Purandare HM, Chakravarty A, et al: Fetal echocardiography—norms for M-mode measurements. Ind Heart J 42:351, 1990.

Reddy V, Liddicoat JR, Klein JR, et al: Long-term fetal outcome after fetal cardiac bypass: Fetal survival to full term and organ abnormalities. J Thorac Cardiovasc Surg 111:536, 1996.

Reed K, Appleton CP, Anderson CF, et al: Doppler studies of vena cava flows in human fetuses: Insights into normal and abnormal cardiac physiology. Circulation 81:498, 1990.

Reed K, Sahn DJ, Marx GR, et al: Cardiac doppler flows during fetal arrhythmias: Physiologic consequences. Obstet Gynecol 70:1, 1987.

Reller M, Morton MJ, Giraud GD, et al: Severe right ventricular pressure loading in fetal sheep augments global myocardial blood flow to submaximal levels. Circulation 86:581, 1992.

Rendina M, Long WA, deBliek R, Henry GW: Effect size and experimental power analysis of a pediatric cardiology telemedicine system. J Telemed Telecare (in press).

Respondek M, Weil SR, Huhta JC: Fetal echocardiography during indomethacin treatment. Ultrasound Obstet Gynecol 5:86, 1995.

Rice MJ, McDonald RW, Reller MD: Fetal atrial septal aneurysm: A cause of fetal atrial arrhythmias. J Am Coll Cardiol 12:1292, 1988.

Rice MJ, McDonald RW, Reller MD: Progressive pulmonary stenosis in the fetus: Two case reports. Am J Perinatol 10:424, 1993.

Robertson MA, Byrne PJ, Penkoske PA: Perinatal management of critical aortic valve stenosis diagnosed by fetal echocardiography. Br Heart J 61:365, 1989.

Ross B: Congenital complete atrioventricular block. Pediatr Clin North Am 37:69, 1990.

Rustico MA, Benettoni A, D'Ottavio G, et al: Fetal echocardiography: The role of the screening procedure. Eur J Obstet Gynecol Reprod Biol 36:19, 1990.

Sandhu S, Heckman JL, Balsara R, et al: Chronic alterations in cardiac mechanics after fetal closed heart operation. Ann Thorac Surg 57:1409, 1994.

Scagliotti D, Shimokochi DD, Pringle KC: Permanent cardiac pacemaker implant in the fetal lamb. Pacing Clin Electrophysiol 10:1253, 1987.

Schmidt KG, Silverman NG, Harrison MR, et al: High-output cardiac failure in fetuses with large sacrococcygeal teratoma: Diagnosis by echocardiography and Doppler ultrasound. J Pediatr 114:1023, 1989.

Schmidt KG, Silverman NH, Hoffman J: Determination of ventricular volumes in human fetal hearts by two-dimensional echocardiography. Am J Cardiol 76:1313, 1995.

Scott J, Maddison PJ, Taylor PV, et al: Connective tissue disease, antibodies to ribonucleoprotein, and congenital heart block. N Engl J Med 309:209, 1983.

Sharland GK, Chan KY, Allan LD: Coarctation of the aorta: Difficulties in prenatal diagnosis. Br Heart J 71:70, 1994.

Sharland GK, Chita SK, Allan LD: The use of color Doppler in fetal echocardiography. Int J Cardiol 28:229, 1990.

Sharland GK, Chita SK, Allan LD: Tricuspid valve dysplasia or displacement in intrauterine life. J Am Coll Cardiol 17:944, 1991a.

Sharland GK, Chita SK, Fagg NLK, et al: Left ventricular dysfunction in the fetus: Relation to aortic valve anomalies and endocardial fibroelastosis. Br Heart J 66:419, 1991b.

Shearin R, Fleming WH: Fourteen years of implanted pacemakers in children. Ann Thorac Surg 25:144, 1978.

Silver M, Laxer RM, Laskin CA, et al: Association of fetal heart block and massive placental infarction due to maternal autoantibodies. Pediatr Pathol 12:131, 1992.

Silverman E, Mamula M, Hardin JA, et al: Importance of the immune response to the Ro/La particle in the development of congenital heart block and neonatal lupus erythematosus. J Rheumatol 18:120, 1991.

Silverman NH, Kleinman CK, Rudolph AM, et al: Fetal atrioventricular valve insufficiency associated with nonimmune hydrops: A two-dimensional echocardiographic and pulsed Doppler ultrasound study. Circulation 72:825, 1985.

Silverman NH, Schmidt KG: Ventricular volume overload in the human fetus: Observations from fetal echocardiography. J Am Soc Echocardiogr 3:20, 1990.

Simpson LL, Marx GR: Diagnosis and treatment of structural fetal cardiac abnormality and dysrhythmia. Semin Perinatol 18:215, 1994.

Smythe JF, Copel JA, Kleinman CS: Outcome of prenatally detected cardiac malformations. Am J Cardiol 69:1471, 1992.

Sosa E, Van Doesburg N, Kratz C, et al: Implantation of a permanent pacemaker in a premature infant. Tex Heart Inst J 15:128, 1988.

Steinfeld L, Rappaport HL, Rosebach HC, et al: Diagnosis of fetal arrhythmias using echocardiographic and Doppler techniques. J Am Coll Cardiol 8:1425, 1986.

Stojanov P, Hrnjak V, Nedeljkovic V, et al: Transvenous permanent pacing in a one-day-old infant. Pacing Clin Electrophysiol 17:1811, 1994.

Strasburger J: Fetal arrhythmias. *In* Garson A, Bricker JT, McNamara DG (Eds): The Science and Practice of Pediatric Cardiology. Philadelphia, Lea & Febiger, 1990, pp 1905–1911.

Strasburger JF, Huhta JC, Carpenter RJ, et al: Doppler echocardiography in the diagnosis and management of persistent fetal arrhythmias. J Am Coll Cardiol 7:1386, 1986.

Takahashi Y, Harada K, Ishida A, et al: Doppler echocardiographic findings of indomethacin-induced occlusion of the fetal patent ductus arteriosus. Am J Perinatol 13:15, 1996.

Tegnander E, Eik-Nes SH, Johansen OJ, et al: Prenatal detection of heart defects at the routine fetal examination at 18 weeks in a non-selected population. Ultrasound Obstet Gynecol 5:372, 1995.

Till J, Jonmes S, Rowland E, et al: Endocardial pacing in infants and children 15 kg or less in weight: Medium-term follow-up. Pacing Clin Electrophysiol 13:1385, 1990.

Todros T, Presbitero P, Gaglioti P, et al: Pulmonary stenosis with intact ventricular septum: Documentation of the development of the lesion echocardiographically during fetal life. Int J Cardiol 19:355, 1988.

van Engelen A, Weijtens O, Brenner JI, et al: Management outcome and follow-up of fetal tachycardia. J Am Coll Cardiol 24:1371, 1994.

Veille J, Covitz W: Fetal cardiovascular hemodynamics in the presence of complete atrioventricular block. Am J Obstet Gynecol 170:1258, 1994.

Walkinshaw SA, Welch CR, McCormack J, et al: In utero pacing for fetal congenital heart block. Fetal Diagn Ther 9:183, 1994.

Waltuck J, Buyon JP: Autoantibody-associated congenital heart block: Outcome in mothers and children. Ann Intern Med 120:544, 1994.

Zales V, Dunnigan A, Benson DW: Clinical and electrophysiologic features of fetal and neonatal paroxysmal atrial tachycardia resulting in congestive heart failure. Am J Cardiol 62:225, 1988.

PART X

NEUROLOGIC SYSTEM

CHAPTER 66

Introduction and Overview of Antenatal Central Nervous System Insults

Jan Goddard-Finegold

Neonatal neurology has become a vital subspecialty as neonatal medical care has become more successful. With the survival of many extremely low-birth-weight infants now a certainty, attention to the status of the nervous system and to the quality of life of such infants has become a priority. The newborn brain has some degree of equipotentiality, so that the functions of damaged areas can be subserved by other parts of the still developing brain (Vargha-Khadem et al, 1994). In fact, some infants with what appear to be extensive lesions show only minimal deficit (Fawer et al, 1983). This is not absolute, however, and it is becoming apparent that if one function is taken over by another part of the brain, there can be sacrifice of at least some of that part's original functions (Vargha-Khadem et al, 1994). It is also becoming clear that damage to the developing brain early on may cause compromise of integrated developmental processes and can lead to increasing deficits with age, as the central nervous system's functional requirements become more complex (Banich et al, 1990). Focal lesions in the adult usually lead to specific, neuroanatomically defined deficits, whereas what appear to be focal or at least unilateral lesions in newborns and young infants often lead to global developmental deficits (Vargha-Khadem et al, 1994).

It is extremely difficult to make predictions of outcome in most newborns with such lesions; furthermore, it is not always possible to define accurately the full extent of the lesions. It is known, for instance, that unilateral intraventricular hemorrhage can be associated with severe depression of cerebral blood flow and possible secondary injury in regions of the hemisphere not directly contiguous to the lesion (Volpe et al, 1983). Confounding the problem for the clinician is the fact that premature newborns may be completing from 8 to 14 or more weeks of what should have been intrauterine brain growth and development in the not always optimal extrauterine environment. Even with the best of circumstances and without specifically identified adverse neonatal events (specifically, with no hypoxia or hypotension), such infants still show major neurologic abnormality in 8% of cases (Low et al, 1993). Thus, it is important to have a basic understanding of the processes of normal brain development, some of the common congenital central nervous system abnormalities, and some mechanisms that might underlie acquired injuries and the reactions of the immature nervous system to such injuries. It is also imperative to plan for continued neurodevelopmental assessment and intervention, when necessary, for all surviving very-low-birth-weight infants.

Chapters 66 through 69 discuss the development, physiology, and pathology of the central nervous system for three distinct epochs: the intrauterine state, during birth, and the neonatal period. The problems that are unique to each period and the adaptations and responses of the nervous system at each period are detailed and compared.

CHROMOSOME ABNORMALITIES

From 30% to 60% of all human conceptuses do not complete intrauterine development. Most of these failures occur early in embryonic development and are associated with chromosome aneuploidy and polyploidy (Tyson and Kalousek, 1992). Chromosome abnormalities are identified in 5% to 10% of cases of fetal death occurring after 20 weeks of gestation (Kalousek et al, 1990). Chromosome defects occur in about 0.5% of infants born alive (Hall, 1987). Consistent data have been derived from perinatal autopsies; in those cases, 5% to 6% have had chromosome abnormalities (Machin and Crolla, 1974; Sutherland et al, 1978). Thirteen percent of infants in those series with lethal multisystemic malformations have had abnormal karyotypes (Machin and Crolla, 1974; Sutherland et al, 1978).

Although most isolated central nervous system malformations do not have an associated identifiable chromosome abnormality, 40% of deaths occurring in the first postnatal year are due to central nervous system malformations that occur prenatally, and 25% of all conceptuses have developmental disturbances that involve the central nervous system (these contribute significantly to the 30% to 60% of conceptuses that are not maintained) (Evrard, 1989; Sutherland et al, 1978). Of infants born alive, 1 in 200 has an abnormality of the central nervous system (Young, 1988). Thus, central nervous system malformations contribute to significant prenatal mortality and postnatal mortality and morbidity, whether there is multisystem involvement or an isolated central nervous system defect.

INFECTIONS

Infection in utero is not uncommon and can result in fetal loss at all stages of gestation as well as fetal malformations, intrauterine growth failure, premature delivery, and the consequences of continued postnatal infection (Klein and Remington, 1995). The incidence of infection with several agents is known. There are about 4.1 million live births in the United States annually, of which 1% excrete cytomegalovirus (10% of these infants are symptomatic, and 5% are severely symptomatic). Up to 15% are infected with *Chlamydia trachomatis* (Klein and Remington, 1995; Wegman, 1992). Herpes simplex virus, *Toxoplasma gondii*, and varicella zoster virus each infect 1 per 1000 liveborn infants. Human immunodeficiency virus (HIV) infects 13% to 40% of infants born alive to mothers who have the virus (Connor and McSherry, 1994; Klein and Remington, 1995). About 1.5 per 1000 child-bearing women are infected with HIV, and data have shown that the rate of vertical transmission to the neonate can be decreased by treatment of the mother during pregnancy with zidovudine (Conner et al, 1994; Gwinn et al, 1991). Other in utero infections include bacterial infections and those due to syphilis, rubella virus, enteroviruses, parvovirus B19, and *Borrelia burgdorferi* (Fanaroff et al, 1994; Klein and Remington, 1995).

Congenital infections that frequently affect the developing central nervous system include *Toxoplasmosis*, cytomegalovirus, rubella, syphilis, varicella zoster, herpes simplex, and HIV (Bale, 1994). Knowledge of the effects of these agents on the developing nervous system, current means of diagnosis, and treatment options may decrease damage to the central nervous system. As an example, when diagnosed in utero, *Toxoplasmosis* can be treated with various regimens, depending on the gestational age; if infected late in gestation, the infected infant can be treated throughout the first postnatal year (Swisher et al, 1994). Both of these strategies have significantly enhanced cognitive and motor development in treated infected infants compared to non-treated infected babies (Swisher et al, 1994). Two regimens using ganciclovir for infants diagnosed postnatally with symptomatic cytomegalovirus infection also showed promise for improving the neurologic status of some infants (Nigro et al, 1994).

DRUGS AND THE INTRAUTERINE NERVOUS SYSTEM

Prenatal illicit drug exposure contributes to adverse pregnancy outcomes and notable effects on the developing nervous system. Current estimates are that 375,000 of the 4 million infants born each year in the United States are exposed to illicit drugs prenatally (Alexander, 1992). From 10% to 50% of women in different hospital populations test positively for such drugs at delivery, and the most common drug used is cocaine (Alexander, 1992). Alcohol use during pregnancy is frequent enough to cause an incidence of fetal alcohol syndrome of 1% in high-risk populations (Alexander, 1992). Fetal alcohol syndrome is now recognized as the most common known cause of mental retardation (Abel and Sokol, 1987).

Drugs of abuse are not the only problems for the developing nervous system, however. From 0.3% to 0.6% of pregnant women have epilepsy (Bjerkedal and Bahna, 1973), and both seizures and the anticonvulsants used to control them can have effects on the fetus and the fetal central nervous system. Furthermore, pregnancy can alter the dosage requirements for anticonvulsants. Dosage requirements during pregnancy increase for phenytoin, phenobarbital, carbamazepine, primidone, and ethosuximide (Lander et al, 1977). In addition, some anticonvulsants are teratogenic, possibly related to folate antagonism or to the induction of chromosome abnormalities (Aminoff, 1994).

Up to 11% of infants exposed in utero to phenytoin develop the fetal hydantoin syndrome with the features of intrauterine and postnatal growth retardation, microcephaly, dysmorphic facies, and variable degrees of mental retardation (Hanson et al, 1976). Up to 33% of exposed infants have milder forms of dysmorphism or disability (Hanson et al, 1976). Similar problems have been described in infants exposed in utero to phenobarbital, carbamazepine, and, as mentioned previously, alcohol (Aminoff, 1994). Facial dysmorphism and neural tube defects have been associated with prenatal exposure to sodium valproate or valproic acid (DiLiberti et al, 1984; Nosel and Klein, 1992). Postnatal syndromes in infants associated with withdrawal from various agents, including opiates, benzodiazepines, barbiturates, amphetamines, cocaine, phencyclidine, glutethimide (Doriden), ethchlorvynol (Placidyl), and pentazocine (Talwin), are well documented (Bean, 1991; Desmond and Wilson, 1975).

INTRAUTERINE TRAUMATIC INJURY

Trauma occurs in 1 of every 12 pregnancies (ACOG, 1993). Most often the trauma is due to motor vehicle accidents, but falls and direct assaults to the abdomen are next in incidence (ACOG, 1993). In inner-city populations, the incidence of battering during pregnancy is as high as the incidence of overall trauma during pregnancy in lower-risk populations (Helton et al, 1987). When the trauma is minor, abruptio placentae occurs 1% to 5% of the time; when the injury is major, abruptio placentae occurs 40% to 50% of the time (Goodwin and Breen, 1990; Pearlman et al, 1990; Rothenberger et al, 1978). Uterine rupture occurs in 0.6% of injuries during pregnancy and usually happens after significant, direct abdominal impact (ACOG, 1993). Although direct fetal injury is unusual after blunt trauma, when it does occur, it usually involves the fetal skull and brain (ACOG, 1993). Such injury is most likely to happen when there is trauma to the maternal pelvis when the fetal head is already engaged. Penetrating trauma, such as that due to gunshot wounds to the uterus, affects the fetus two thirds of the time (Buchsbaum, 1979). Perinatal mortality in these cases ranges from 41% to 71% (Buchsbaum, 1979). Maternal mortality in these cases is approximately 5%.

INTRAUTERINE GROWTH RESTRICTION

Intrauterine growth restriction is one term used to describe the growth-impaired infant. Other terms used for this same problem include *pseudomature, small for dates, dysmature, fetal malnourished, chronic fetal distress, intrauterine growth retardation*, and *small for gestational age* (Crouse and Cassady, 1994). Four percent to 8% of all infants born in developed countries have intrauterine growth restriction, which is usually defined clinically in an infant when weight is below the 10th percentile for gestational age and clinical features of growth restriction are present (Creasy and Resnick, 1994). Lubchenco and colleagues (1966) also include infants at the 10th percentile, whereas some clinicians prefer to use the 3rd percentile for this cut-off, and others use greater than 2 standard deviations below the mean (Crouse and Cassady, 1994).

Many clinicians believe, however, that using these lower cut-off values leaves out a group of infants who, although not as growth restricted, are still at risk for intrauterine and perinatal complications. In addition, uncritical use of the 10th percentile cut-off criterion can be problematic in some cases because infants whose growth is restricted, who would have been large infants, may show all of the physical signs of intrauterine growth restriction and yet be above the 10th percentile for weight or length (Crouse and Cassady, 1994). Thus, most clinicians look for clinical signs of intrauterine growth restriction and do not go solely on weight for the clinical diagnosis. Clinical signs include asymmetric growth, loss of soft tissue, decreased skin-fold thickness, decreased breast tissue, and reduced thigh circumference (Crouse and Cassady, 1994). Indicators of longer-term growth failure include widened cranial sutures; reduced foot, femoral, and crown-heel lengths; and delayed epiphyseal development. In severely growth-restricted infants, head circumference may be decreased.

In asymmetric growth restriction (usually intrauterine growth restriction occurring late in pregnancy), the weight is decreased, but length and head size are not. In symmetric growth restriction all growth indices, including head size, are decreased. These definitions can be problematic, however, and asymmetric growth restriction can also be said to be present when weight and length are reduced, but head size is not. The division into two classifications of growth restriction may be simply a way of acknowledging the duration and severity of the underlying problem (Brar and Rutherford, 1988). Symmetric growth restriction is usually caused by events that are present early on in the pregnancy, such as early intrauterine infection (5% to 10% of cases) or chromosome abnormalities (5% to 15% of cases)(Creasy and Resnick, 1994). Asymmetric growth restriction is usually due to deficiencies that occur during the latter part of pregnancy, including problems such as the effects of multiple gestations ($\leq$ 3% of cases) and various causes of placental insufficiency (25% to 30% of cases). Neonatal mortality is increased 10-fold when the infant is below the 2.5 percentile; intrauterine growth-restricted infants weighing 1500 to 2500 g at 38 to 42 weeks' gestation have a 5 to 30 times increase in mortality compared to infants in the 10th to 50th percentiles, and infants who weigh less than 1500 g at term have a 70-fold to 100-fold increase in mortality (Creasy and Resnick, 1994; Williams et al, 1982).

Only a decade ago, fewer than one third of all intrauterine growth-restricted infants were recognized before delivery, whereas today the majority of such infants are identified before delivery (Fanaroff et al, 1994). Thirty percent to 60% of the perinatal deaths of intrauterine growth-restricted infants are due to congenital anomalies. Other problems causing intrauterine growth restriction include maternal antiphospholipid antibody syndrome and maternal cigarette smoking, alcohol use, cocaine use, and other drug use. Metabolic problems such as maternal homozygous phenylketonuria (PKU), hypothyroidism, and diabetes with vascular disease can all cause intrauterine growth

restriction (Creasy and Resnick, 1994). Maternal malnutrition can cause intrauterine growth restriction during any part of the pregnancy (Brasel and Winick, 1972).

The intrauterine growth-restricted fetus is at risk for central nervous system damage because of the increased risk of intrapartum asphyxia, meconium aspiration, and acidosis at delivery (especially in cases of placental insufficiency) (Fanaroff et al, 1994; Gregory et al, 1974). Intrauterine growth-restricted infants are also at risk for postnatal hypoglycemia because of reduced substrate stores, other metabolic problems, and polycythemia secondary to chronic subacute hypoxia. In one study, 50% of children with intrauterine growth restriction had learning deficits when tested at 9 to 11 years (Low et al, 1992). As a population, intrauterine growth-restricted infants also have an increased risk of cerebral palsy when born after 33 weeks' gestational age (Blair and Stanley, 1990).

METABOLIC DISEASE IN THE FETUS OR MOTHER

Prenatal diagnosis of inherited metabolic disease is now possible in a large number of diseases, many of which are likely to become apparent in the newborn period (Clarke et al, 1992). In addition, it has become possible for affected mothers to survive and reproduce; well-known examples include mothers with PKU and mothers heterozygous for ornithine transcarbamylase deficiency (OTC)(Clarke et al, 1992). Untreated mothers with PKU have given birth to infants with microcephaly, mental retardation, low birth weight, and congenital heart disease. Intrauterine brain damage can also occur in male fetuses carried by mothers heterozygous for OTC deficiency (Clarke et al, 1992).

For further discussion, see Chapters 21, 22, 24, and 25.

HYPOXIA AND ISCHEMIA

It has been apparent for some time now that only about 8% to 22% of cases of cerebral palsy in the population can be attributed to peripartum events (Blair and Stanley, 1988; Torfs et al, 1990). This means that most cases of static encephalopathy are due to prenatal factors or genetic factors, and a smaller proportion is due to more easily identifiable postnatal factors. The use of prenatal ultrasound monitoring has made it possible to detect some brain lesions prenatally; in addition, it has been possible to relate the onset of brain damage to some known adverse circumstances (de Vries et al, 1987). Particular attention has been paid to severe maternal conditions, such as anaphylaxis, respiratory or cardiac failure, seizures, trauma, carbon monoxide poisoning, and coagulopathy. Conditions of the fetus that have led to prenatal brain injury include multiple pregnancy, embolization of cerebral vessels from placental or fetal veins, fetal thrombocytopenia, and disturbances in fetal cerebral circulation that lead to prenatal germinal matrix hemorrhage—intraventricular hemorrhage (present in 5% of stillborns) (Cocker et al, 1965; Courville, 1959; D'Alton et al, 1984; Dudley and D'Alton, 1986; Larroche, 1986; Leech and Kohnen, 1974; Naidu et al, 1983; Zalneraitis et al, 1979). Problems of the placenta and cord can also lead to fetal brain injury; most commonly cited reasons include placental abruption, true knots in the cord, tight nuchal cord, and placental insufficiency leading to severe intrauterine growth restriction with chronic effects on brain growth (de Vries et al, 1987). Routine intrauterine and early postnatal imaging, especially in cases of postnatal encephalopathy, makes timing of intrauterine lesions more accurate and their relationship to postnatal symptoms better defined.

REFERENCES

Abel EL, Sokol RJ: Incidence of fetal alcohol syndrome and economic impact of FAS-related anomalies. Drug Alcohol Depend 19:51, 1987.

Alexander D: Introduction. *In* Zagon IS, Slotkin TA (Eds): Maternal Substance Abuse and the Developing Nervous System. New York, Academic Press, 1992, pp 1–3.

American College of Obstetricians and Gynecologists (ACOG): ACOG Technical Bulletin No. 161: Trauma During Pregnancy. Int J Gynecol Obstet 40:165, 1993.

Aminoff MJ: Neurologic disorders. *In* Creasy RK, Resnick R (Eds): Maternal-Fetal Medicine: Principles and Practice. Philadelphia, WB Saunders, 1994, pp 1071–1101.

Bale JF (Ed): Congenital infections of the central nervous system. Semin Pediatr Neurol 1:1, 1994.

Banich MT, Levine SC, Kim H, et al: The effects of developmental factors on IQ in hemiplegic children. Neuropsychologia 28:35, 1990.

Bean X: Maternal substance abuse. *In* Taeusch HW, Ballard RA, Avery ME (Eds): Schaffer and Avery's Diseases of the Newborn, 6th ed. Philadelphia, WB Saunders, 1991, pp 243–253.

Beaudet AL, Scriver CR, Sly WS, Valle D: Genetics and biochemistry of variant human phenotypes. *In* Scriver CR, Beaudet AL, Sly WS, Valle D (Eds): The Metabolic Basis of Inherited Disease, 6th ed. New York, McGraw-Hill, 1989, pp 3–165.

Bjerkedal T, Bahna SL: The course and outcome of pregnancy in women with epilepsy. Acta Obstet Gynecol Scand 52:245, 1973.

Blair E, Stanley FJ: Intrapartum asphyxia: A rare cause of cerebral palsy. J Pediatr 112:515, 1988.

Blair E, Stanley F: Intrauterine growth and spastic cerebral palsy: I. Association with birth weight for gestational age. Am J Obstet Gynecol 162:229, 1990.

Brar HS, Rutherford SP: Classification of intrauterine growth retardation. Semin Perinatol 12:2, 1988.

Brasel JA, Winick M: Maternal nutrition and prenatal growth: Experimental studies of effects of maternal undernutrition on fetal and placental growth. Arch Dis Child 47:479, 1972.

Buchsbaum HJ: Penetrating injury of the abdomen. *In* Buchsbaum HJ (Ed): Trauma in Pregnancy. Philadelphia, WB Saunders, 1979, pp 82–100.

Clarke LA, Dimmick JE, Applegarth DA: Pathology of inherited metabolic diseases. *In* Dimmick JE, Kalousek DK (Eds): Developmental Pathology of the Embryo and Fetus. Philadelphia, JB Lippincott, 1992, pp 199–234.

Cocker J, George SW, Yates PO: Perinatal occlusion of the middle cerebral artery. Dev Med Child Neurol 7:235, 1965.

Conner EM, Sperling RS, Gelber R, et al: Reduction of maternal-infant transmission of human immunodeficiency virus with zidovudine treatment: Pediatric AIDS Clinical Trials Group Protocol 076 Study Group. N Engl J Med 331:1173, 1994.

Connor E, McSherry G: Treatment of HIV infection in infancy. Clin Perinatol 21:163, 1994.

Courville CB: Antenatal and paranatal circulatory disorders as a cause of cerebral damage in early life. J Neuropathol Exp Neurol 18:115, 1959.

Creasy RK, Resnick R: Intrauterine growth restriction. *In* Creasy RK, Resnick R (Eds): Maternal-Fetal Medicine: Principles and Practice. Philadelphia, WB Saunders, 1994, pp 558–574.

Crouse DT, Cassady G: The small-for-gestational-age infant. *In* Avery GB, Fletcher MA, MacDonald MG (Eds): Neonatology: Pathophysiology and Management of the Newborn, 4th ed. Philadelphia, JB Lippincott, 1994, pp 369–398.

D'Alton ME, Newton ER, Cetrulo CL: Intrauterine fetal demise in multiple gestation. Acta Genet Med Gemellol 33:43, 1984.

Desmond MM, Wilson GS: Neonatal abstinence syndrome: Recognition and diagnosis. Addict Dis 2:113, 1975.

de Vries JIP, Visser GHA, Mulder EJH, et al: Diurnal and other variations in fetal movement and heart rate patterns at 20–22 weeks. Early Hum Dev 15:333, 1987.

DiLiberti JH, Farndon PA, Dennis NR, et al: The fetal valproate syndrome. Am J Med Genet 19:473, 1984.

Dudley DKL, D'Alton ME: Single fetal death in twin gestation. Semin Perinatol 10:65, 1986.

Evrard P: Preface. *In* Evrard P, Minkowski A (Eds): Developmental Neurobiology. New York, Raven Press, 1989, pp V–VI.

Fanaroff AA, Martin RJ, Miller MJ: Identification and management of high-risk problems in the neonate. *In* Creasy RK, Resnick R (Eds): Maternal-Fetal Medicine: Principles and Practice. Philadelphia, WB Saunders, 1994, pp 1135–1172.

Fawer C-L, Levene MI, Dubowitz LMS: Intraventricular hemorrhage in a preterm neonate: Discordance between clinical course and ultrasound scan. Neuropediatrics 14:242, 1983.

Goodwin TM, Breen MT: Pregnancy outcome and fetomaternal hemorrhage after noncatastrophic trauma. Am J Obstet Gynecol 162:665, 1990.

Gregory GA, Gooding CA, Phibbs RH, et al: Meconium aspiration in infants—a prospective study. J Pediatr 85:848, 1974.

Gwinn M, Pappaioanou M, George R, et al: Prevalence of HIV infection in childbearing women in the United States: Surveillance using newborn blood samples. JAMA 265:1704, 1991.

Hall BD: Nonchromosome malformations and syndromes associated with stillbirth. Clin Obstet Gynecol 30:278, 1987.

Hanson JW, Myrianthopoulos NC, Harvey MAS, et al: Risks to the offspring of women treated with hydantoin anticonvulsants, with emphasis on the fetal hydantoin syndrome. J Pediatr 89:662, 1976.

Helton AS, McFarlane J, Anderson ET: Battered and pregnant: A prevalence study. Am J Public Health 77:1337, 1987.

Kalousek DK, Fitch N, Paradice B: Pathology of the Embryo and Fetus. New York, Springer-Verlag, 1990.

Klein JO, Remington JS: Current concepts of infections of the fetus and newborn infant. *In* Remington JS, Klein JO (Eds): Infectious Diseases of the Fetus and Newborn Infant. Philadelphia, WB Saunders, 1995, pp 1–19.

Lander CM, Edwards VE, Eadie MJ, et al: Plasma anticonvulsant concentrations during pregnancy. Neurology 27:128, 1977.

Larroche J-C: Fetal encephalopathies of circulatory origin. Biol Neonate 50:61, 1986.

Leech RW, Kohnen P: Subependymal and intraventricular hemorrhages in the newborn. Am J Pathol 77:465, 1974.

Low JA, Froese AB, Galbraith RS, et al: The association between preterm newborn hypotension and hypoxemia and outcome during the first year. Acta Paediatr 82:433, 1993.

Low JA, Handley-Derry MH, Burke SO, et al: Association of intrauterine fetal growth retardation and learning deficits at age 9 to 11 years. Am J Obstet Gynecol 167:1499, 1992.

Lubchenco LO, Hansman C, Boyd E: Intrauterine growth in length and head circumference as estimated from live births at gestational ages from 26 to 42 weeks. Pediatrics 37:403, 1966.

Machin GA, Crolla JA: Chromosomal constitution of 500 infants dying during the perinatal period. Humangenetik 23:183, 1974.

Naidu S, Messmore H, Caserta V, et al: Central nervous system lesions in neonatal isoimmune thrombocytopenia. Arch Neurol 40:552, 1983.

Nigro G, Scholz H, Bartmann U: Ganciclovir therapy for symptomatic congenital cytomegalovirus infection in infants: A 2-regimen experience. J Pediatr 124:318, 1994.

Nosel PG, Klein NW: Methionine decreases the embryotoxicity of sodium valproate in the rat: In vivo and in vitro observations. Teratology 46:499, 1992.

Pearlman MD, Tintinalli JE, Lorenz RP: A prospective controlled study of outcome after trauma during pregnancy. Am J Obstet Gynecol 162:1502, 1990.

Rothenberger D, Quattlebaum FW, Perry JF Jr, et al: Blunt maternal trauma: A review of 103 cases. J Trauma 18:173, 1978.

Seashore MR, Rinaldo P: Metabolic disease of the neonate and young infant. Semin Perinatol 17:318, 1993.

Sutherland GR, Carter RF, Bauld R, et al: Chromosome studies at the paediatric necropsy. Ann Hum Genet 42:173, 1978.

Swisher CN, Boyer K, McLeod R, and the other members of the Toxoplasmosis Study Group: Congenital toxoplasmosis. Semin Pediatr Neurol 1:4, 1994.

Torfs CP, van den Berg BJ, Oechsli FW, et al: Prenatal and perinatal factors in the etiology of cerebral palsy. J Pediatr 116:615, 1990.

Tyson RW, Kalousek DK: Chromosomal abnormalities in stillbirth and neonatal death. *In* Dimmick JE, Kalousek DK (Eds): Developmental Pathology of the Embryo and Fetus. Philadelphia, JB Lippincott, 1992, pp 83–142.

Vargha-Khadem F, Isaacs E, Muter V: A review of cognitive outcome after unilateral lesions sustained during childhood. J Child Neurol 9(suppl 2):2S67, 1994.

Volpe JJ, Herscovitch P, Perlman JM, et al: Positron emission tomography in the newborn: Extensive impairment of regional cerebral blood flow with intraventricular hemorrhage and hemorrhagic intracerebral involvement. Pediatrics 72:589, 1983.

Wegman ME: Annual summary of vital statistics—1991. Pediatrics 90:835, 1992.

Williams Rl, Creasy RK, Cunningham GC, et al: Fetal growth and perinatal viability in California. Obstet Gynecol 59:624, 1982.

Young ID: Genetics of neurodevelopmental abnormalities. *In* Levene MI, Bennett MJ, Punt J (Eds): Fetal and Neonatal Neurology and Neurosurgery. Edinburgh, Churchill Livingstone, 1988, pp 249–257.

Zalneraitis EL, Young RSK, Krishnamoorthy KS: Intracranial hemorrhage in utero as a complication of iso-immune thrombocytopenia. J Pediatr 95:611, 1979.

CHAPTER 67

The Intrauterine Nervous System

Jan Goddard-Finegold

CENTRAL NERVOUS SYSTEM DEVELOPMENT

Adverse events occurring during the early phases of development can have dramatic effects on the nervous system of the newborn and usually occur before the pregnancy is discovered. This section presents an overview of central nervous system (CNS) development. In the following section, CNS malformations and their relationships to developmental processes are discussed.

Early Events

The earliest developmental stages include the one-celled embryo, the cleaving embryo, the blastocyst, the process of implantation and development of the amniotic cavity and umbilical vesicle, the formation of chorionic villi, and the formation of axial features (right and left sides, rostral and caudal ends). All of these events occur during the first 14 postconceptual days. At 16 days, the site of the future neural plate can be defined by autoradiographic means, and at about 18 days, the neural groove can be seen (England, 1988; O'Rahilly and Muller, 1994).

Neurulation

At 18 days, neurulation begins, when the embryo's crown-rump length is about 1.0 to 1.5 mm. An area of thickened neuroectoderm, the neural plate, is formed after induction by the underlying notochord and mesoderm. The neural plate gives rise to the brain and spinal cord. At 20 to 21 days, the neural groove forms in the midline with a neural fold on either side. Areas that become the forebrain, midbrain, and hindbrain can be identified at this early stage. By day 22, the neural folds are beginning to fuse to form the neural tube and central canal (England, 1988; O'Rahilly and Muller, 1994) (Fig. 67–1).

Neural Crest Migration

As the rostral parts of the neural folds fuse, the neural crest is formed from ectodermal cells on both sides of the neural tube. The neural crest cells migrate shortly after neural tube closure. They become sensory, sympathetic, and parasympathetic ganglia; chromaffin cells of the adrenal medulla; skin melanocytes; enteric neurons in the gastrointestinal tract; and facial connective tissue (O'Rahilly and Muller, 1994).

Neural Tube Closure

The neural folds fuse first in what will be the occipitocervical region. Experimental data suggest that fusion may occur in multiple sites simultaneously (Golden and Chernoff,

1995). By days 24 to 25, fusion has occurred cephalically to the level of the colliculi, and fusion continues rostrally and caudally until only the most rostral neuropore and most caudal neuropore are open. By day 24, the rostral neuropore has closed; by day 26, the caudal neuropore has closed at the site corresponding to S2 (O'Rahilly and Muller, 1994) (Fig. 67–2).

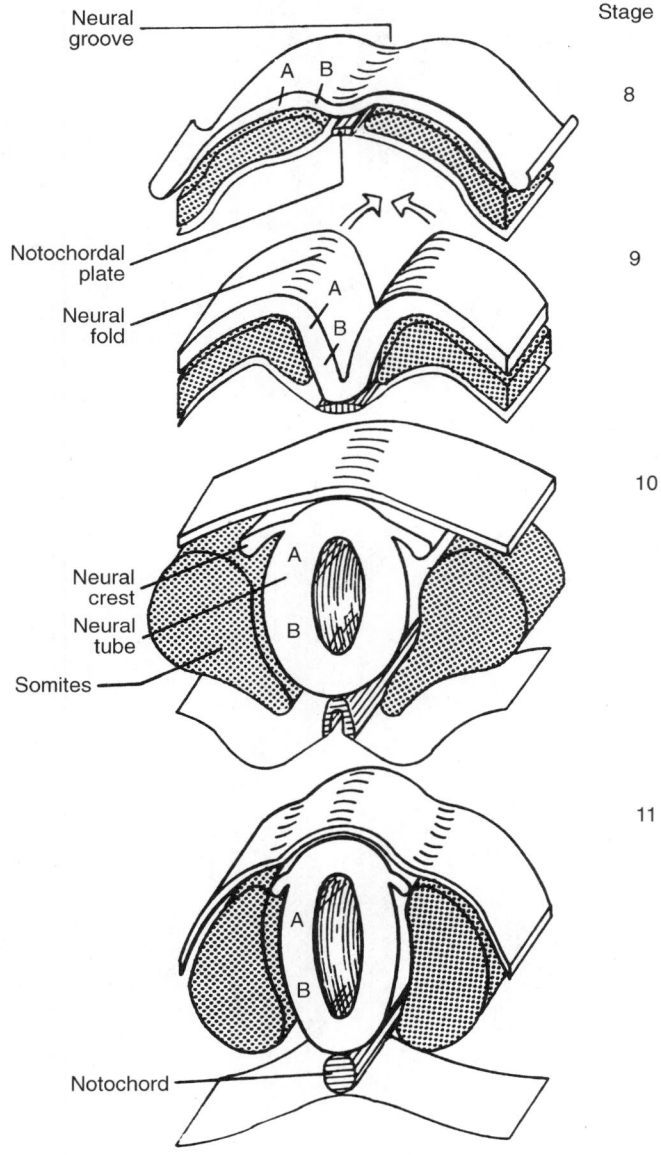

FIGURE 67–1. Formation of the neural tube. (From O'Rahilly R, Muller F: The Embryonic Human Brain. New York, Wiley-Liss, 1994, p 41.)

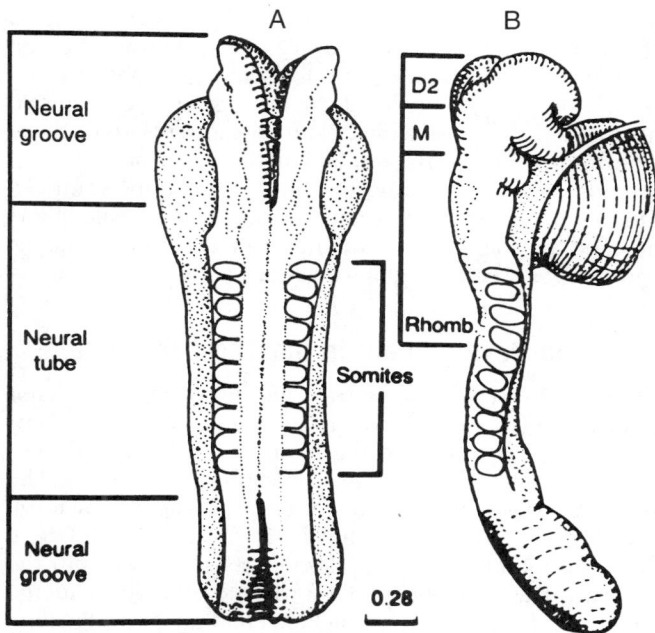

FIGURE 67–2. Positions of anterior and posterior neuropores. (From O'Rahilly R, Muller F: The Embryonic Human Brain. New York, Wiley-Liss, 1994, p 45.)

Secondary Neural Tube Formation

A process of secondary neural tube formation also occurs during postconceptual days 30 to 50, in which vacuoles form in a caudal cell mass that surrounds the lower neural tube. The vacuoles join together and connect with the central canal of the already present neural tube (England, 1988; O'Rahilly and Muller, 1994).

Caudal Regression

At postconceptual days 41 to 51, the caudalmost part of the neural tube and central canal begins to regress as the tail of the embryo disappears. Atrophy of the caudal neural tube results in formation of a fibrous strand called the *filum terminale*, which is present throughout life. As the vertebral bodies grow, the end of the central canal (the conus medullaris) becomes placed higher in the vertebral column, eventually reaching the L1-2 level (usually by 2 weeks postnatally). This may be due to proportionately greater lengthening of the spinal vertebrae compared to the spinal cord (England, 1988; O'Rahilly and Muller, 1994).

Morphogenesis After Neural Tube Closure

As the rostral neuropore is closing, the optic vesicles are being formed. When the embryo has reached a length of about 5 mm, both neuropores have closed, thus isolating the developing ventricular system from the amniotic fluid. At this time, the choroid plexuses have not yet formed, parts of the neural crest are still appearing, the retinal and lens placodes are developing, and the indentation for the adenohypophysis is present. Also at this stage, the cerebellum begins to form as well as some somatic and visceral

efferent nuclei, the common afferent tract, and the ganglia for most of the cranial nerves.

At about 32 days, when the embryo is 5 to 7 mm long, the cerebral hemispheres become identifiable. Specific areas, such as the hypothalamic, amygdaloid, hippocampal, and olfactory regions, can be defined. The cerebellum is more recognizable, and some blood vessels are now present. Various tracts and cranial nerve nuclei are formed, and by the next day, the diencephalon and its regions and the epithalamus, subthalamus, and hypothalamus are evident. Vertebrae can now be seen clearly. By day 37, the components of the circle of Willis are present (O'Rahilly and Muller, 1994).

At about 44 days, the optic fibers are forming but not yet entering the chiasmatic plate. The red nucleus can be recognized, and the substantia nigra is forming. Choroid plexuses are developing, and the production of cerebrospinal fluid within the ventricles begins. Frontal and temporal poles of the cerebral hemispheres can be seen, and the pontine flexure is deep. Tracts present at stage 18 (44 days, 13 to 17 mm length) include the stria medullaris thalami, mamillothalamic tract, medial and lateral tectobulbar tracts, dentatorubral tract, and tractus solitarius. By 48 days, the optic nerves have arrived at the chiasm. The globus pallidus has developed, and the habenula is well formed. Connections from the cerebellum are increasing. During stages 18 and 19, electrical activity can be detected in the brain stem (England, 1988; O'Rahilly and Muller, 1994).

At 51 days, the optic commissure is present, and numerous other fiber connections are forming. Notably, those of the olfactory system can be identified. It is at this stage that intrinsic neocortical vascularization begins, and fibers from the cuneate and gracilis nuclei are decussating (England, 1988; O'Rahilly and Muller, 1994).

Appearance of the Cortical Plate

When the embryo is about 22 to 24 mm, at about 52 days, the cortical plate appears. The cortical plate develops as neurons migrate between the marginal and intermediate zones and gives rise to the neurons of layers II–VI. At this point, it is also possible to define subpial and subplate layers–these become layer I and white matter (O'Rahilly and Muller, 1994). At this stage, glial cells and Schwann cells can be identified between the fibers of the cranial nerves.

At stage 21, the tentorium cerebelli is present, and by stage 22 (54 days), the internal capsule and olfactory tracts are seen. Thalamocortical fibers are present at stage 21 before corticothalamic fibers can be seen in the internal capsule. By stage 22, the cortical plate has expanded to cover half of the hemispheric surface. The role of the cortical plate and subplate neurons in the formation of the six-layered cortex are discussed in the next section in more detail.

By the end of the embryonic period, at about 57 days, or 8 postovulatory weeks, most of the major elements of the brain can be recognized (Fig. 67–3). The optic tract reaches the lateral geniculate body, and the external germinal layer of the cerebellum has begun to spread. The ventricular layer is present in all brain regions, and the

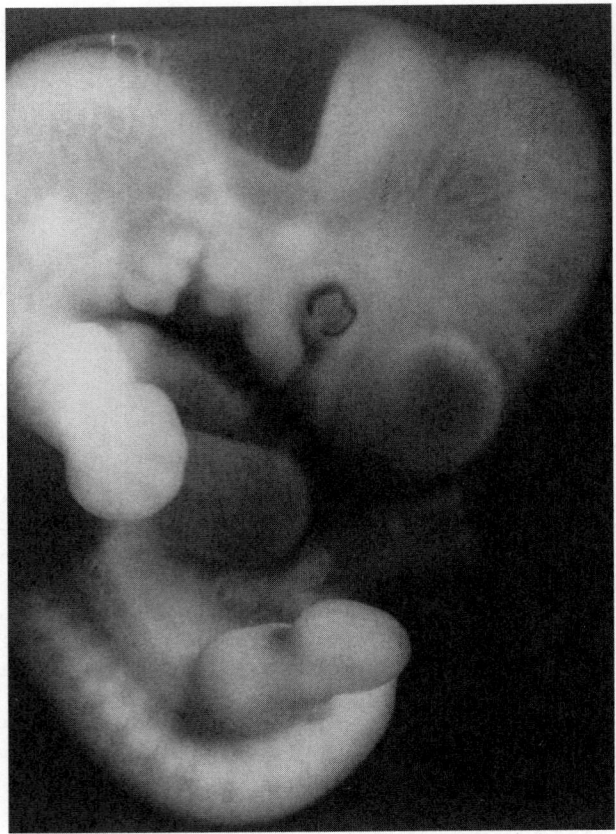

FIGURE 67–3. The human brain at the end of the embryonic period. (From O'Rahilly R, Muller F: The Embryonic Human Brain. New York, Wiley-Liss, 1994, p 115.)

cortical plate covers almost the entire neocortical surface. The pyramidal decussation can now be identified, and the insula has become indented (O'Rahilly and Muller, 1994).

Brain Development in the Postembryonic Period

The fetal period is characterized by numerous external events, including increasing definition of parts of the brain; enlargement of the cerebral hemispheres; union of the cerebellar halves and demarcation of the vermis; appearance of sulci; and disappearance of the embryonic cervical, pontine, and mesencephalic flexures. Internally the growth of the corpus callosum occurs noticeably.

In the early fetal period (first trimester, *early postembryonic phase*), there is controversy as to exactly when fusion of the medial walls of the cerebral hemispheres occurs, and the mechanisms of formation of the cavum septi pellucidi have not been completely determined. Nevertheless, the diencephalic nuclei are present, and the globus pallidus is clearly identifiable. The inferior olivary nucleus and its subdivisions can be seen, and projections to the cerebellum have formed. In the early postembryonic period, the cortical plate extends to the occipital pole, and the external capsule, the hippocampal sulcus, and the third ventricular choroid plexus are apparent (O'Rahilly and Muller, 1994).

The ventricular germinal eminences are expanding dramatically at this stage; their blood supply comes from striatal arteries through a capillary plexus. During the first trimester, the dorsal and ventral thalamic regions are well delineated, and the nuclei of the basal ganglia, the choroid fissure, and the internal and external capsules are distinct.

After the fetus is 100 mm in length, the corpus callosum extends caudally, covering the roof of the third ventricle. During the second trimester, the internal capsule fibers descend, passing between the putamen and caudate nuclei and then between the globus pallidus and the thalamus.

Brain Development in the Third Trimester

At about 28 weeks, the fetus is 265 mm long. The major sulci and gyri are present at this time, and the corpus callosum is composed of the rostrum, genu, central part, and splenium. The septum pellucidum is present. The subplate region of the visual cortex has dissipated by term, whereas the prefrontal subplate is present for up to 6 postnatal months. The subplate neurons relocate into the cortical plate, become part of white matter, or undergo cell death. Postnatal events include continuing myelination, growth of corticocortical and association fibers, dendritic arborization and pruning as well as continued synaptogenesis and synapse elimination. These events are discussed further in the following sections (O'Rahilly and Muller, 1994).

Neurotransmitter Systems

The brain stem is more mature than the rest of the brain at the end of the embryonic period and already contains monoamine-synthesizing neurons at that time. By the middle of gestation, the spinal cord, cerebellum, and forebrain have almost the adult distribution of monoamine-synthesizing neurons. Norepinephrine-synthesizing neurons are present in various parts of the medulla, in the locus caeruleus, and in the nucleus subcaeruleus. Dopamine neurons are present in the substantia nigra (pars compacta), in the midbrain tegmentum and rostral pons, and in the arcuate nucleus of the hypothalamus. Serotonin-synthesizing neurons are present in part of the reticular formation of the midbrain, in the rostral pons, and in the raphe of the pons and medulla (England, 1988).

Histogenesis

Cells that give rise to the neurons and glia of the nervous system are initially the neuroepithelial cells that line the neural tube. These germinal cells pass through a cycle of DNA synthesis and mitosis, and, as this occurs, their nuclei change position. Metaphase nuclei remain close to the neural tube lumen (or ventricle later in development), whereas telophase and interphase nuclei become positioned further from the lumen or ventricle. Late interphase and prophase nuclei approach the lumen as they progress toward metaphase and mitosis. Until metaphase, cell processes are attached at the internal and external limiting membranes. At metaphase, the external attachment is lost. Postmitotic cells migrate away from the germinal zone and undergo further differentiation in the mantle layer. Both neurons and glia arise from the germinal neuroepithelial cells and differ in their proliferative potentials. Some of the neuroepithelial and neuroglial cells can be stimulated to re-enter the mitotic cycle, some neuroglial cells temporarily leave the cycle, and all postmitotic neurons permanently leave the mitotic cycle. The phenomenon of movement of the neuroepithelial cell nucleus during mitosis has not been fully explained and is not unique to neuroepithelium (Jacobson, 1991).

Different Cell Types

There are differences in timetables for production of different types of neurons and of glial cells in the germinal zone. Large neurons are produced before intermediate-sized neurons, and intermediate-sized neurons are produced before small neurons. Motor nuclei usually complete their cell populations before sensory nuclei. Although most neurons are produced before birth in mammals, some neurons are produced postnatally. This may have meaningful consequences for infants who have postnatal CNS insults. The areas best known for postnatal neurogenesis include the olfactory bulb, hippocampus, brain stem nuclei, and cerebellar cortex. Glial cells are still being produced in the neuraxis after neuronal production is completed (Jacobson, 1991; Wilkinson et al, 1990).

Cortical Plate and Subplate Neurons

Four transient tangential layers form during the process of cerebral cortical development. These (from the ventricle to the brain surface) are the ventricular, subventricular, intermediate, and marginal zones. The earliest cell proliferation occurs in the ventricular zone; later cell proliferation occurs in the subventricular zone. The intermediate zone becomes the white matter, and the marginal zone becomes layer I (the outermost layer) of the cortex. The cortical plate, which develops as neurons migrate between the marginal and intermediate zones, becomes layers II–VI. In addition, it has become clear that the cortical plate develops within a preplate. The preplate consists of the earliest generated neurons and a plexus of nerve fibers. The preplate has also been divided into a superplate and a deep subplate. Both of these contain the earliest generated neurons.

It is now known that in the second trimester, two subcortical afferent systems are present in the subplate. These are thalamocortical fibers and basal forebrain fibers, and they seem to wait in the subcortical region for some time before their fibers penetrate the cortical plate. It has been known for some time that the neurons of layer IV in the cortex receive their predominant ascending inputs from the thalamus. Interestingly, however, the thalamic axons are present in the cortex long before the layer IV neurons have reached the cortical plate. Apparently the axons wait in the subplate for a period of weeks; at the same time the axons are in the subplate region, they are in proximity to postmitotic neurons. These neurons mature early but undergo cell death after the thalamic axons have grown into the cortical plate. The hypothesis that these subplate neurons interact with the thalamic axons and play a role in thalamocortical development has been substantiated by studies that have shown that deletion of the early subplate neurons prevents the thalamic axons from innervating the cortex. Thus, it seems that the transient subplate *pioneer* neurons play an important role in target selection by the thalamocortical axons (Ghosh et al, 1990; Jacobson, 1991; O'Rahilly and Muller, 1994).

Formation of Cortical Layers

The first neurons migrate outward to layer I. Neurons in the subsequent layers are pushed to deeper levels by the neurons arriving from below. Thus, older neurons are actually deeper in the cortex (i.e., away from the pial surface) except for layer I neurons. The II–VI layers are formed in an *inside-out* sequence. Variations of this process occur in the hippocampus and cerebellum. Notably, nonspecific thalamocortical fibers are first recognized in layers VI–V, specific thalamocortical fibers in layers V–IV, callosal fibers in layer III, and corticocortical fibers in layer II. The major processes involved in formation of the cortical layers are occurring from between 7 and 11 weeks' gestation to term (Jacobson, 1991).

Rakic and Sidman (1969) presented evidence for the existence of a later migration period for neurons reaching the pulvinar. They studied human fetal brains using the rapid Golgi method and showed that from 18 to 34 weeks of gestation, germinal cells from the ganglionic eminence (the portion of the telencephalon composed of immature cells that lies above the corpus striatum and protrudes into the lateral ventricle) migrate away from it, crossing beneath the sulcus terminalis to enter the diencephalon and form a layer that they described as the *corpus gangliothalamicus*. This structure is part of the developing pulvinar. As the ganglionic eminence (also called the *germinal matrix*) regresses in size, the pulvinar becomes larger. Rakic and Sidman thus hypothesized that cells from the ganglionic eminence migrate into the pulvinar during the 5th to 8th months of gestation. It is not difficult to extrapolate from this information that this particular process may be going on during the time that many preterm infants are incurring germinal matrix and intraventricular hemorrhages and other forms of brain pathology that are likely to have direct impact on this region of the brain. Further neuropathologic, neuroimaging, and follow-up studies are necessary to determine if specific neurodevelopmental deficits can be correlated with damage in the region of the ganglionic eminence or with loss of volume in the pulvinar.

Migration of Neurons

Early migration of neurons seems to be either by unaligned movement or along neuroepithelial cells. Later on, however, neurons in the cortex, hippocampus, and cerebellum are guided by radial glial cells. The radial glial cell can be identified histochemically by glial fibrillary acidic protein staining and does not divide during the period of neuronal migration. After that period, the radial glia become astrocytes. In the spinal cord, radial glia also become oligodendroglia. The neuron advancing along a radial glial process is thought to move at 4 μm per hour in vivo. The migration of neurons along radial glial guides leads to the columnar functional organization of the cortex. A model of abnormal neuronal migration, in which neurons do not reach their usual position in the cortex, is found in the reeler mouse. Also, a severe depletion of radial glial fibers has been shown to be present in holoprosencephaly. Other CNS malformations and syndromes that have abnormalities of neuronal migration include fetal alcohol syndrome, microcephaly vera, lissencephalies, pachygyria and agyria, cerebrohepatorenal syndrome (Zellweger), HARD + E syndrome (*h*ydrocephalus, *a*gyria, retinal *d*ysplasia, and *en*cephalocele), various types of heterotopias, and polymicrogyria (Gadisseux et al, 1990; Herschkowitz, 1988; Jacobson, 1991; Marin-Padilla, 1988; Rakic, 1988; Rorke, 1994).

Morphogenetic or Naturally Occurring Cell Death

Naturally occurring cell death, or apoptosis, occurs in the nervous system as well as in other tissues during development. Cell death occurs when transient embryonic tissues undergo dissolution; when tissues undergo processes such as separation, fusion, folding, bending, or cavitation; or when tissues are remodeled and cell numbers are adjusted after initial overproduction. Specific genes seem to be involved in the control of morphogenetic cell death, and hormones also seem to play an important role in the process. Certain growth factors may reduce cell death. For example, cell death in the superior cervical ganglion is retarded by treatment with nerve growth factor. The removal of target sites induces neuronal cell death, and the provision of extra postsynaptic targets reduces the incidence of neuronal cell death in numerous experimental paradigms. It may be that growth factors necessary for neuronal survival can be supplied only in certain quantities via postsynaptic targets. Thus, many neurons, in essence, probably must compete for their survival. Insufficient programmed cell death has been suggested as a possible cause of the defects in a frontoethmoidal encephalocele. Insufficient cell death in the region of the rostral neuropore is also thought to cause too many surviving cells that may form heterotopias, such as nasal gliomas. In animal models, overabundant cell death, such as that produced by the administration of retinoic acid, has resulted in caudal regression syndromes, spina bifida, and spinal dysraphism (Alles and Sulik, 1990; Jacobson, 1991; O'Rahilly and Muller, 1994).

Axonal Growth and Targeting

Knowledge of the structure of axons has increased remarkably during the past two decades. The cytoskeletal network of the axon has been described, and the transport of materials in axons and dendrites has been shown by cinematography, videomicroscopy, and electron microscopy and by using radioactive tracers. Both anterograde and retrograde transport have been documented, with anterograde transport shown at both slow and fast rates, whereas retrograde transport occurs only at fast rates (Bisby, 1982).

Slow transport carries cytoskeletal proteins and proteins of the axoplasmic matrix; fast transport carries membrane proteins, acetylcholinesterase, parts of mitochondria, other organelles, vesicles, and neurotropic viruses. Fast transport

occurs at 50 to 400 mm/day (Black and Lasek, 1980). The materials transported in axons are used in various ways. Some are used to build new structures for the axon, some are recirculated, some are metabolized, and some are released at the axon terminals.

Elongation of axons and of dendrites occurs at their growth cones, which are present at their tips when growth is occurring. The extension and movement of the growth cone are the means by which the axon finds direction, a pathway, and, ultimately, a target. Growth cone morphology and motility can be regulated by free intracellular calcium ions. Growth cones are also known to adhere to the extracellular matrix and then to break those adhesions by releasing proteases and other substances that activate proteolytic enzymes. Growth cones are also directly affected by nerve growth factor.

Critical processes involving neuronal connections during neural development include (1) axon growth and pathway determination; (2) dendrite growth and development; (3) axonal target selection; (4) synaptic, axonal, dendritic, and neuronal elimination to avoid redundancy and mismatching; and (5) synaptic functional refinement (Jacobson, 1991).

Dendritic and Synaptic Development

Dendrite outgrowth usually occurs after the extension of the axon and may be delayed for some time after the migration of the neuron. Branching of dendrites substantially increases the dendritic surface area, which ultimately forms 90% of the postsynaptic surface of the neuron. Different neurons have different, and characteristic, dendritic sizes, shapes, and patterns. Dendrites differ from axons in having ribosomes, rough and smooth endoplasmic reticulum, and Golgi structures (axons do not). Axons are frequently myelinated, and dendrites are only rarely myelinated (notably in the olfactory system). During development, the morphology of dendrites may change; in human infants, the dendrites of the superior cervical ganglion neurons are long, but they become shorter with age. A period also exists during which there is an outgrowth of an excessive number of dendritic branches followed by a *pruning* phase, in which there is loss of extra dendrites.

Dendritic growth in the cortex has been shown to be impaired by malnutrition, phenylketonuria, radiation injury, and certain hormone deficiencies or excesses (especially thyroid); dendritic morphology has been shown to be abnormal in some cases of mental retardation (Cordero et al, 1986; Huttenlocher, 1991; Lacey, 1984; Rami et al, 1986; Schade and Caviness, 1968). In Down syndrome, dendritic arborization has been shown to be increased in the infantile period but reduced in the juvenile period, and the number of dendritic spines has been shown to be reduced in children with Down syndrome who are older than 4 months of age (Becker et al, 1986; Takashima et al, 1981). Some studies have shown that the number of afferent inputs is important for the determination of the size and complexity of dendritic trees. In addition, the development of dendrites and axodendritic and dendrodendritic synapses goes together. Dendrites have the highest metabolic rate of all parts of the neuron, and this metabolic activity peaks during synaptogenesis. Similar to dendrites, synapses are formed in excess in many regions of the nervous system and then undergo a process of selective elimination. Many questions still have not been answered about the basic processes involved in dendritic and synaptic development and organization; the answers to these questions are especially pertinent for infants born prematurely and whose brains are developing for a major part of the last trimester in the extrauterine environment. At least one study has shown that immature infants dying in the neonatal period have smaller visual cortical neurons with shorter basilar dendrites than postconceptional age–matched mature controls, suggesting that their cortical development may be delayed (Jacobson, 1991; Takashima et al, 1982).

Myelination

Schwann cells myelinate axons in the periphery, and oligodendroglia myelinate central axons. Schwann cells are derived from the neural crest and migrate to the peripheral nerves. They require interaction with neurons to differentiate completely, and they produce galactocerebroside and myelin basic protein only when they are actively myelinating axons. Myelination is not necessary for axons to function, however, and impulse conduction is present before myelination has commenced during development. Myelination serves to increase the conduction velocity of the nerve impulse.

Schwann cells are still able to divide after finding their way into peripheral nerves, and, in fact, most Schwann cell proliferation seems to occur after contact with axons. In the periphery, one Schwann cell myelinates one axon, whereas in the CNS, one oligodendroglial cell can myelinate many axons. There is a period of intense proliferation of oligodendrocytes prior to myelination; this has been termed *myelination gliosis* and is also associated with an increase in vascularization. Compared to other events in the development of the nervous system, myelination begins late and lasts a long time, well into the first decade in humans (myelination is actually not totally complete until the 20s). Phylogenetically older parts of the nervous system are myelinated before phylogenetically newer parts, and large neurons with long axons are myelinated before small neurons with short axons. Because myelination covers such a long period of time, and because it involves a continuous process of degradation and synthesis throughout the lifetime of the individual, it is especially vulnerable to environmental influences (Jacobson, 1991; Kinney et al, 1988).

Specific Issues in Vascular Development

The earliest parts of the nervous system are essentially avascular. Blood vessels form as a meshwork in the meninges before growing into the CNS from the pial surface in a caudal-rostral progression. The blood-brain barrier is essentially a function of capillary endothelial cell tight junctions and develops under the influence of astrocytes. Brain blood vessel formation and blood-brain barrier capacities are present early in the CNS, but maximal capillary sprouting occurs during the period of dendritic growth and glial cell proliferation.

The vascular development in the periventricular areas of the developing brain is particularly clinically relevant because the immature infant is susceptible to ischemic injury in the white matter around the ventricles and to hemorrhage in the germinal eminence region (part of the ventricular zone) (Takashima and Tanaka, 1978a, 1978b). The periventricular white matter may be particularly susceptible to ischemia or to reduced substrate supply because for a period of time it has a decreased density of blood vessels at the junction of penetrating vessels that extend downward from the cortex and deep white matter vessels that branch upward. This is also true for the subcortical vessels at the depths of the sulci in the more mature infant. The conditions of periventricular leukomalacia and subcortical leukomalacia are well-known pathologic entities (Takashima and Tanaka, 1978a; Takashima et al, 1978).

The germinal eminence is supplied by striatal arteries through a dense capillary network that is particularly susceptible to hemorrhage in the preterm infant. The hemodynamics of this region and the biology of the maturation of its vessels are current research areas that continue to hold promise for prevention of intraventricular hemorrhage. Information suggests that maturation of vessels of the germinal eminence can be influenced by the postnatal environment and by agents such as indomethacin (Ment et al, 1991). Studies of the ultrastructural features of the blood-brain barrier in this region in an animal model have also suggested that postnatal endothelial basal lamina deposition occurs before tight junction formation and glial investiture and that basal lamina induction influences the latter two processes (Ment et al, 1995). In the human preterm infant less than 34 weeks' gestational age, the period of risk for germinal matrix and intraventricular hemorrhage is the first 3 to 4 postnatal days, regardless of gestational age (Ment et al, 1995). This suggests that postnatal induction of vascular maturation may occur at the same rate and over the same period of time in these infants.

Neuromuscular Development

Skeletal muscles arise from somites that form from mesoderm, the muscles for the trunk originating from the myotomes that line the neural tube (Figarella-Branger and Pellissier, 1995). Muscle precursor cells for the limbs and ventral part of the body wall migrate from the dermomyotomes and differentiate into myoblasts after they are in their respective locations. Axial and limb muscles develop from at least two different cell lineages; the lateral parts of the somites form the limb and ventral body wall musculature, and the axial muscles originate from the dorsomedial parts of the somites. The remaining part of the dorsomedial somite, or dermomyotome, becomes dermis (Ordahl and LeDouarin, 1992). The part of the somite called the *sclerotome* gives rise to the vertebral column and ribs.

Myoblasts proliferate and then fuse to form primary myotubes. The ultrastructure of the myotube has recognizable components of the mature muscle system. After a period of time, secondary myoblasts line up under the basal lamina of the primary myotubes and fuse to form secondary myotubes. These then separate from the primary myotubes to form a new generation of myotubes. Neural cell adhesion molecule (NCAM) seems to be involved in the myoblast fusion process and in myotube formation (Knudsen et al, 1990). Cell-substrate adhesion molecules (integrins) and certain growth factors also seem to play a role in myoblast fusion (Sue-Menko and Boettiger, 1987). Cell adhesion molecules also play a role in the secondary phase of myogenesis, the alignment of myoblasts along myotubes to make the secondary myotubes.

In postnatal life, the nuclei of myofibers, the fiber diameter, and the length of myofibers increase. The maturation of the muscle involves a number of processes, including the development of the contractile apparatus, its positioning in the muscle sarcomere, and the development of the sarcotubular system and the transverse tubules (Schiaffino and Margreth, 1969). Innervation of muscle is completed after birth. Other parts of the muscular system, including the muscle spindles, Golgi tendon organs, and pacinian corpuscles, take time to mature (Landon, 1982).

Mature muscle consists of four recognized types: I, IIA, IIB, and IIC, each of which has monosynaptic innervation. Mature muscle fibers are innervated by motor neurons, with large fibers (type alpha) innervating fast motor units and type beta fibers innervating slow motor units and some intrafusal fibers. A progression of events occurs to complete the motor innervation of muscle, including the processes of nerve bundling and branching, growth and spread of nerves into muscle, and matching of a specific neuromuscular junction to an appropriate muscle target (Figarella-Branger and Pellissier, 1995).

NCAM seems to play a particularly important role in innervation and seems to be distributed on developing myotube membranes corresponding to acetylcholine receptor sites (Rieger et al, 1985). NCAM expression changes as innervation proceeds, and mature fibers do not express the molecule. It is re-expressed, however, on denervated fibers (Cashman et al, 1987; Covault et al, 1986; Moore and Walsh, 1985).

Muscle fiber type specialization corresponds to motor neuron specialization, as one motor neuron type innervates muscle fibers of the same type. Fiber diversity seems to occur early in development and may reflect myoblast diversity. Thus, there seems to be some sort of recognition between motor neuron types and different types of muscle fibers, so that specific developing motor neurons selectively innervate muscle fibers of a single type (Condon et al, 1989). All of these developmental processes require genetic control, including regulatory and structural gene input.

In humans, myoblast proliferation occurs until the 7th week of gestation, after which myotube formation begins. Between 8 and 12 weeks, primitive nerves and neuromuscular contacts can be seen (Juntunen and Teravainen, 1972). Secondary myoblasts are seen between 12 and 14 weeks, and tertiary myotubes are seen at 16 to 17 weeks. Fiber type diversity can be seen as early as 14 weeks with sensitive techniques, and by 20 weeks' gestation, the adenosine triphosphatase technique can be used to detect fiber diversity. During the later parts of gestation, adult slow and fast myosin heavy chains are discernible in the secondary and tertiary myotubes (Pons et al, 1986). At 25 weeks' gestation, the multiple sites of acetylcholinesterase staining are no longer present, and NCAM expression disappears after 30 weeks. This probably reflects the elimination of synapses and organization of monosynaptic innervation (Figarella-Branger and Pellissier, 1995; Toop, 1975).

Critical Periods, Central Nervous System Plasticity, and Selective Vulnerability

This brief review of development of the nervous system does not include discussion of its molecular biology and genetics. Nevertheless, processes that are important in the developing nervous system are being studied at the molecular genetics level to understand their basic mechanisms. Some of those processes underly the phenomena of critical periods, CNS plasticity, and selective vulnerability, all of which are important for the outcome of the newborn brain. When a specific condition is required for a developmental event to occur, and that condition must be present over a specific time period, that condition and that period are *critical* (Jacobson, 1991). Usually, critical periods are times that are extremely sensitive to external events–that is, they are the singular times at which a developmental event can occur and occur optimally; interference with that event cannot be corrected later. Such processes as neurogenesis have been considered to be critical events; however, Bayer and colleagues (1995) have stressed that in human development, the periods of neurogenesis, neuronal migration, and neuronal differentiation are overlapping rather than distinct epochs (Fig. 67–4). Nevertheless, the concept of

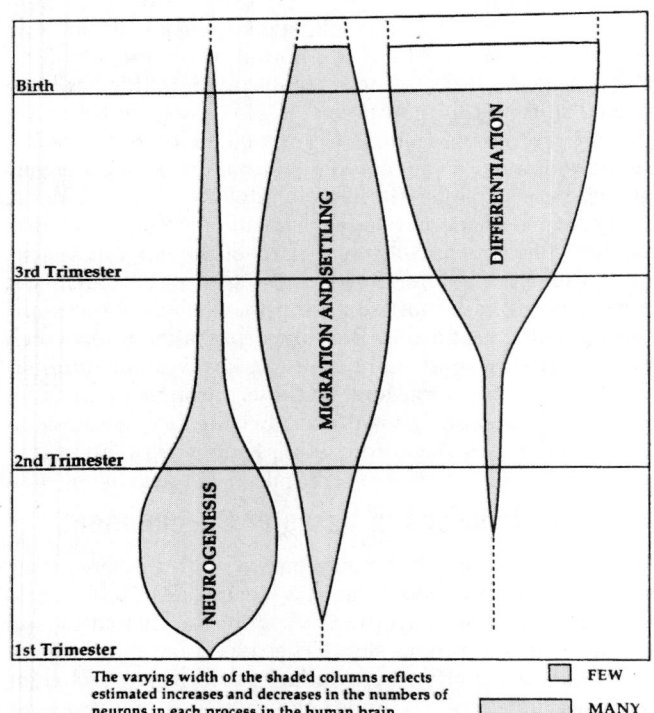

THE TIME COURSE OF DEVELOPMENTAL PROCESSES BETWEEN NEURONAL POPULATIONS

FIGURE 67–4. A diagrammatic representation of the extensive overlay between neurogenesis, migration, and cytodifferentiation during central nervous system development. (From Bayer SA, Altman J, Russo RJ, Zhang X: Embryology. *In* Duckett S [Ed]: Pediatric Neuropathology. Baltimore, Williams & Wilkins, 1995, p 101.)

critical events is important and is in contradistinction to CNS plasticity, which implies that there is a certain amount of flexibility in the young nervous system, so that adaptability is possible when injury to the developing nervous system occurs. It is probably more accurate to use the term *plasticity* to refer to *limited* homeostatic mechanisms that allow the nervous system to function normally even though there have been changes in either the external or the internal milieu (Jacobson, 1991). The concept of plasticity has been oversimplified in clinical usage and should not be used to assume that the young infant brain can recover after any degree of injury.

Selective vulnerability implies that there is a hierarchy of likelihood of injury to various parts of the nervous system or to its cellular components after defined insults. Such vulnerability depends on factors such as the intrinsic vulnerability of a particular cell type, the age of the individual, the blood supply to the region involved, and the nature and duration of the insult (Armstrong, 1995). Mechanisms behind differing vulnerabilities are currently being defined, and the complexities of selective vulnerabilities are becoming more apparent. For instance, in the newborn brain, some neurons are more vulnerable than others to hypoxia, and this vulnerability seems in part to be related to the absence of certain intracellular enzymes, such as reduced nicotinamide-adenine dinucleotide diaphorase (nitric oxide synthase) (Ferriero et al, 1988). The absence of a particular enzyme or substrate may make a cell more susceptible to peroxidant injury, to excitatory amino acid–mediated injury, to calcium-mediated events, or to other critical effects.

CENTRAL NERVOUS SYSTEM MALFORMATIONS

A true malformation results when a disruption occurs in an intrinsic developmental process; acquired defects occur when an already normally formed brain is injured by a secondary process, such as vascular compromise, hypoxia-ischemia, infection, a teratogen (i.e., environmental poison, toxin, or medication), or physical compression or disruption. The type of defect resulting from such agents depends on the stage of development at which the injury occurs, the type and duration of the insult, and other factors. The lesions resulting from such injuries are usually *encephaloclastic* in nature, meaning that destruction of already present brain tissue occurs, but they can look much like primary developmental lesions in some cases (Roessmann, 1995). In this section, the emphasis is on primary malformations of the CNS; however, primary malformations can have multifactorial origins.

Timing of Specific Lesions: Overview

O'Rahilly and Muller (1994) have detailed some neuroteratologic conditions and have correlated their timing with that of normal processes. A summary of their findings is presented followed by clinicopathologic descriptions of representative abnormalities. It should be stressed that these abnormalities may be multifactorial in origin, caused by problems such as chromosomal defects, external teratogenetic influences, developmental dysgeneses, or acquired prenatal or postnatal insults.

Abnormalities of the nervous system that can have their beginning at stage 8, or around 18 postconceptual days, include those arising from mesenchymal disturbances. Such disturbances can cause abnormal elevation of the neural folds and abnormal formation of facial structures, optic precursors, and cerebrum. These malformations are variable in their presentation but are termed *holoprosencephalies* because many are associated with failure of formation of two hemispheres from the prosencephalon. The initial mesenchymal defect can lead to problems that occur during the first 4 to 5 postconceptual weeks. Abnormal division of the hemispheres can also be associated with failure of formation of two optic evaginations, leading to a single eye, or *cyclopia* or *synophthalmia*, occurring at around 20 days, when the ocular structures remain paired but are within a single globe. The earliest phase of development of anencephaly also occurs at this period, with failure of closure of the rostral neural groove.

By 22 days, production of the neural crest is occurring, and abnormalities of the neural crest at this stage can cause a reduction in the size of cranial nerve ganglia as well as incomplete formation of the cranium. Because the optic primordia are developing at this stage, it is thought that when anophthalmos occurs, either in conjunction with anencephaly or as an isolated defect, the optic primordia have failed to form normally. Other abnormalities that are also influenced by malformations of the rhombencephalic or mesencephalic crest include holoprosencephaly, encephalomeningocele, and facial abnormalities seen in fetal alcohol syndrome.

At or around 24 days, the rostral neuropore closes, and the progression of abnormalities causing anencephaly may continue. At this stage, the nasal discs begin to form. Thus, abnormalities at this stage may lead to arhinencephaly, with or without holoprosencephaly.

At stage 12, 26 days, occipital encephaloceles may form as a result of absent basal mesenchyme usually present at this time. At 28 to 30 days, cases of anencephaly have been documented in which the neural tube was open over the midbrain and forebrain, although fusion at the rostral neuropores had occurred. At this stage and slightly before, cerebellar agenesis can arise, as the first part of the body of the cerebellum is forming. Most of the motor nuclei of the cranial nerves are also beginning to develop at this time, thus leading to the supposition that the underlying defect in Möbius syndrome (absent nuclei of cranial nerves six and seven) occurs at this stage.

At 32 days, many basal areas of the forebrain are developing. These regions are frequently absent in holoprosencephaly, suggesting again that the defect is a much earlier inductive event and is not due primarily to failure of cleavage of the hemispheres.

The Dandy-Walker malformation is composed of vermal dysgenesis, cystic dilation of the fourth ventricle, a high tentorium, and usually hydrocephalus. This is usually associated with lack of perforation of the foramen in the roof of the fourth ventricle. The time of origin of this complex is thought to be at 6 to 8 fetal weeks.

Other abnormalities occur predominantly in the fetal period, including agenesis of the corpus callosum, lissencephaly, polymicrogyria, microcephaly vera, pachygyria and agyria, heterotopias, aqueductal stenosis, and other defects. These are discussed further in subsequent sections.

Central Nervous System Malformations in Chromosomal Disorders

In Down syndrome (trisomy 21), the brain is small (about three fourths normal weight) and short in the anterior-posterior dimensions (Fig. 67–5). There are small frontal lobes, slanted orbital gyri, and flattened occipital lobes. The superior temporal gyrus is small (Norman, 1992). Dendritic atrophy has been shown to be present in children by 1 to 2 years of age in Down syndrome, associated with defective cortical layering (Becker et al, 1986; Takashima et al, 1981).

Trisomy 13 is associated with holoprosencephaly in about one third of cases, and the other cases usually show either abnormalities of the forebrain or no specific abnormalities in a small brain. When holoprosencephaly or arhinencephaly is present, the brain usually has cerebellar heterotopias as well (Norman, 1992).

Trisomy 18 has variable brain abnormalities, including abnormal gyri, hippocampal and olivary dysplasias, cerebellar heterotopias, agenesis of the corpus callosum, various forms of neural tube defect, and holoprosencephaly (Norman, 1992).

Miller-Dieker syndrome (Fig. 67–6) is characterized by Type I or four-layered lissencephaly and is due to a microdeletion of the short arm of chromosome 17 (Dobyns et al, 1984; Ledbetter et al, 1992). Another term for lissencephaly is *agyria* (Friede, 1989). Other findings in this syndrome include microcephaly; large fontanels; bitemporal hollowing; extra soft tissue over the metopic ridge; short nose with upturned nares; ear anomalies; prominent occiput; micrognathia; and neurologic abnormalities, including severe mental retardation, seizures, and abnormal tone (frequently decerebrate posturing) (Encha-Razavi, 1995). Type I lissencephaly has a thickened cortex with a reduced white matter volume. The thickened cortex has only four horizontal layers that do not display normal cellular organization; in addition, the periventricular white matter that is present usually contains nodular heterotopias.

Heterotopias are usually found in the inferior olivary nuclei as well (Encha-Razavi, 1995; Friede, 1989).

Neural Tube Defects

Neural tube defects, encompassing craniorachischisis totalis, anencephaly, myeloschisis, encephaloceles, and meningomyeloceles (and Arnold-Chiari malformation), were, until recently, one of the most frequent congenital malformations encountered in newborns, occuring in about 3 in 1000 births on the East Coast of the United States, in about 1 in 1000 births on the West Coast of the United States, and at a higher rate in various regions of the United Kingdom. In 1970, the occurrence rate for England and Wales was 4.5 in 1000 births; in 1991, this rate had dropped to 0.18 in 1000 (Seller, 1994). For the most part, the lower occurrence rates reflect two major interventions: in utero diagnosis with termination of affected pregnancies and maternal periconceptional folate therapy (which is estimated to prevent 60% of neural tube defects) (Czeizel and Dudas, 1992; MRC Vitamin Study Research Group, 1992; Oakley et al, 1994; Smithells et al, 1981). A decline in numbers of infants with neural tube defects has also been noted in the Republic of Ireland, however, where neither prenatal diagnosis nor termination of pregnancy is practiced (Seller, 1994).

The development of the neural tube is a critical process in the formation of the nervous system. As mentioned earlier, the neural groove and folds begin to appear by day 18. Closure of the neural tube begins a few days later, with anterior neuropore closure on day 24 and caudal neuropore closure by day 26. Animal studies are providing new insights into this process and suggest that, instead of the zipper concept of closure, there are multiple closure sites, with the head being most complex. Inbred strains of mice show differences in the timing of the various closure sites and in the exact locations and sequences of closure, all of which are dependent on different, specific genes (Golden and Chernoff, 1993; Seller, 1994; Van Allen et al, 1993). A study of the sites of human anterior neural tube defects supports the hypothesis that there are multiple locations of

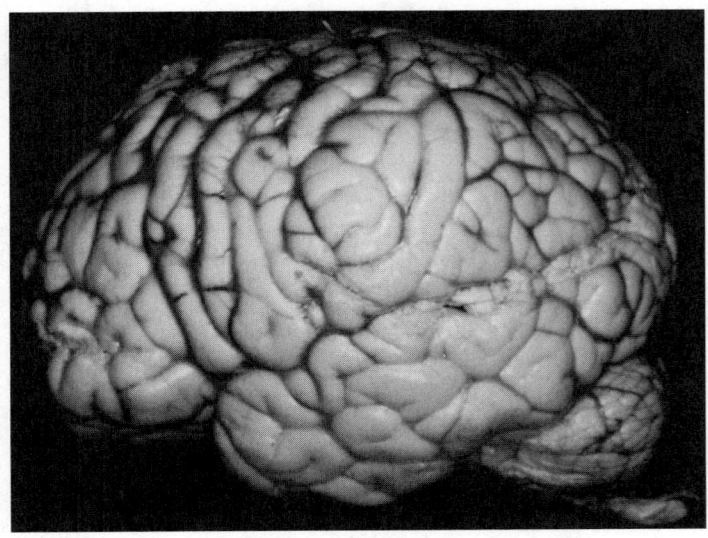

FIGURE 67–5. The brain of a child with Down syndrome. Note box-like shape and narrow superior temporal gyrus. (Courtesy of Dr. Dawna L. Armstrong, Department of Pathology, Texas Children's Hospital.)

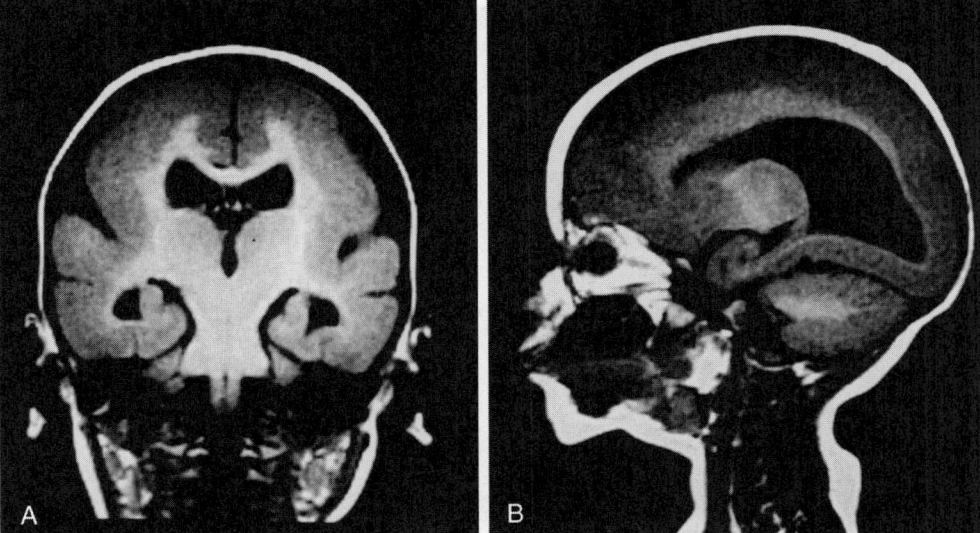

FIGURE 67–6. T1-weighted magnetic resonance images of the brain of a child with type I lissencephaly (characteristic of Miller-Dieker syndrome). *A*, Coronal view. *B*, Sagittal view. (Courtesy of Dr. C. McCluggage, Department of Radiology, Texas Children's Hospital.)

anterior neural tube closure; furthermore, there seem to be two mechanisms involved in the formation of the defect—failure of closure to occur at one or more of the sites and failure of two closures to meet (Golden and Chernoff, 1995). The role of folate in this process is not certain, but it is known that folate is a cofactor for some of the enzymes involved in DNA synthesis; it is also involved in methylation, and some of the developmental genes operate by means of methylation (Adams et al, 1992; Seller, 1994).

Further complexity is apparent in the evidence for multifactorial influences involved in the production of neural tube defects. A particular mouse model of neural tube defects, the curly tail variant with the responsible *ct* gene localized to distal chromosome 4, has at least three modifier loci that influence the incidence of the neural tube defects (Neumann et al, 1994).

Anencephaly and Encephaloceles

The defects referred to as *neural tube defects* are those that result from abnormalities of neural tube closure or from splitting of the neural tube (schisis) (Roessmann, 1995). Failure of closure of the anterior neuropore is thought to be the mechanism for anencephaly and cranial encephalocele. It is thought that anencephaly represents an early neurulation defect and that encephalocele represents a postneurulation event. Anencephaly is a lethal malformation in which the calvaria is absent and the intracranial contents are replaced by vascularized, disorganized glial tissue (area cerebrovasculosa) (Menkes, 1991; Roessmann, 1995). The hypothalamus and cerebellum are usually malformed, the anterior lobe of the pituitary is present, and the internal carotid arteries are hypoplastic, which may be secondary to abnormal brain formation. Because the anencephalic infant has a period of exencephaly, in which the brain tissue extrudes through the unformed calvaria and then is degraded by exposure to the amniotic fluid, some investigators have hypothesized that the primary defect is the abnormal skull formation. There are some cases in which remnants of calvarial bones are present, with

normal brain under the protective bones (Roessmann, 1995).

Anencephaly can be diagnosed by fetal ultrasound examination and by measuring alpha-fetoprotein (AFP) in maternal serum. AFP is the major serum protein in the early embryo and is fetus specific. It normally passes from the fetal serum into fetal urine and then into amniotic fluid; in the amniotic fluid, it is swallowed by the fetus and catabolized in the fetal gastrointestinal tract (Brock, 1976). In anencephaly, open spina bifida, and open encephalocele, there is leakage of fetal serum directly into the amniotic fluid, and amniotic fluid AFP levels as well as maternal serum levels are elevated. When a neural tube defect is closed (i.e., covered by intact skin), however, the AFP level is not elevated; this occurs in about 5% of neural tube defects (Milunsky et al, 1980).

Figure 67–7 shows an anencephalic infant. Cranium bifidum occurs when there is failure of fusion of the midline of the skull; when meningeal tissue or meninges plus glial tissue protrude through the defect, this is termed *cranial meningocele*. Protrusion of brain tissue through cranial defects is more common, and such lesions are termed *encephaloceles* or *cephaloceles*. Sixty percent to 80% of encephaloceles occur in the occipital region, with the remainder in the parietal, frontonasal, intranasal, or nasopharyngeal regions. Up to 50% of cases have hydrocephalus (Diebler and Dulac, 1987; Menkes, 1991; Volpe, 1995a).

A study of a series of children with encephaloceles reported overall mortality at 29% (45% in infants with posterior defects; 0 in infants with anterior defects). About one half of infants with encephaloceles had other major congenital anomalies, including cleft lip or palate, craniosynostosis, myelomeningocele, hydrocephalus, agenesis of the corpus callosum, anophthalmia, porencephaly, arhinencephaly, complex congenital heart disease, and other systemic abnormalities (Brown and Sheridan-Pereira, 1992). Neurologic deficits were severe in 33% of survivors with anterior defects and in 33% of survivors with posterior defects (fewer with posterior defects survived); mild neurologic deficits were found in 17% of survivors of anterior

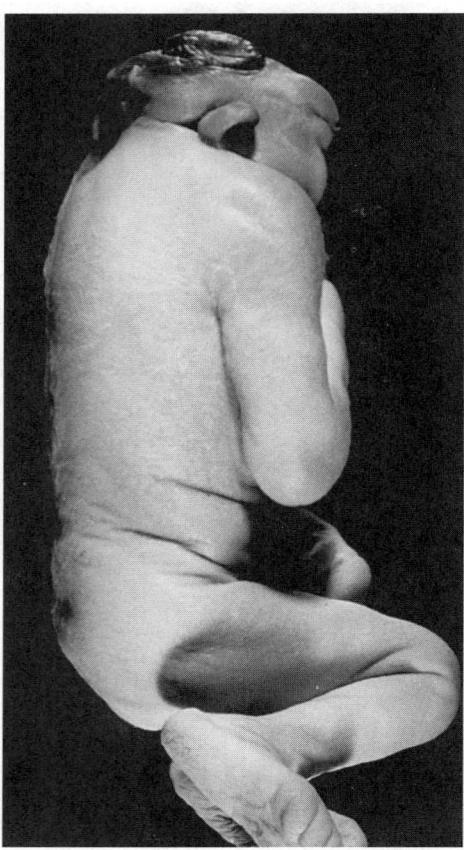

FIGURE 67–7. An anencephalic infant. (Courtesy of Dr. Dawna L. Armstrong, Department of Pathology, Texas Children's Hospital.)

defects and in 50% of survivors of posterior defects (Brown and Sheridan-Pereira, 1992). Both anencephaly and cranium bifidum with occipital encephaloceles affect girls more than boys.

Figure 67–8 shows an infant with large occipital encephalocele. Examination of the infant with occipital and pari-

etal encephaloceles can be aided by transillumination, skull radiographs, ultrasound examination, computed tomography scans, and magnetic resonance imaging (MRI). Decisions about which modality to use depend on the individual cases and whether other cerebral anomalies or hydrocephalus is suspected. Frontonasal encephaloceles pulse or bulge with brief bilateral jugular vein compression, indicating communication with the subarachnoid space. Nasal *gliomas*, dermoids, and teratomas can all occur in the same region. Intranasal encephalocele should be suspected when an intranasal mass is found in a child with a broad nasal bridge and widely spaced eyes. Some of these children may also present with recurrent meningitis (Menkes, 1991). Basal encephaloceles are not usually diagnosed until childhood and can be located in the nasopharynx, sphenoid sinus, or posterior orbit. Treatment of encephaloceles, when possible, is surgical removal, early in life.

Meningocele, Meningomyelocele, and Lipomeningomyelocele

In spina bifida occulta, there is usually no neurologic deficit early in postnatal life, and the malformation consists of a defect in the vertebral arches, in some cases with a split spinal cord that resembles the neural plate but contains all of the necessary components (Roessmann, 1995). Symptoms can develop later on, however, especially when there are associated spinal cord abnormalities. The defect is usually located at L5 or S1 and may show localized dermal sinuses or dimples (35%), lipoid tumors (29%), or abnormalities of the filum terminale (24%) (Anderson, 1975; Menkes, 1991). Spina bifida occulta occurs in about 5% of the normal population (James and Lassman, 1972).

When there is herniation of the meninges or the meninges and spinal cord through the spinal defect, the lesion is referred to as *spina bifida cystica*; 80% of these lesions are meningomyeloceles, and 20% are meningoceles (Friede, 1989; Menkes, 1991). The lesion most often occurs in the lumbar or lumbosacral region (69% of cases), and 95% of children with lumbar or lumbosacral meningomyelocele have the brain abnormalities referred to as the Arnold-Chiari II malformation (Fig. 67–9). The incidence of men-

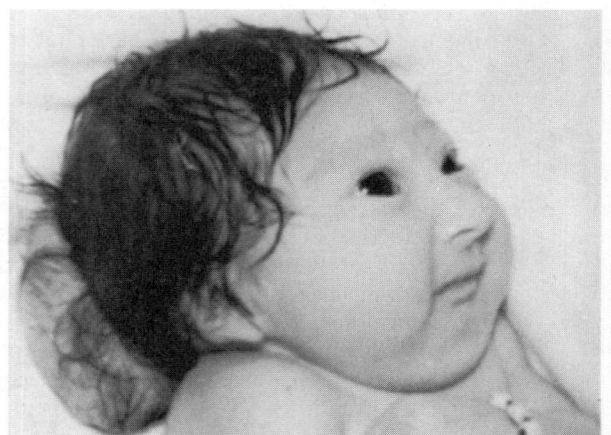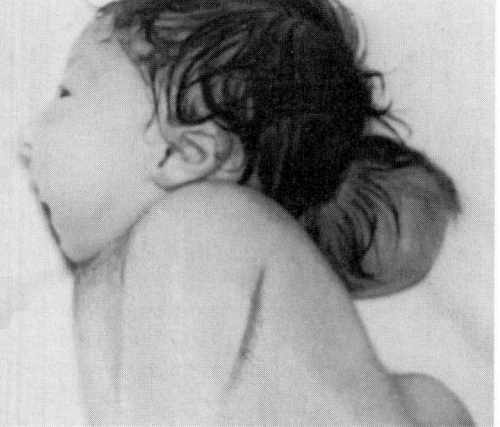

FIGURE 67–8. Occipital meningoencephalocele. The sloping forehead and small head circumference are evident, although progressive ventricular enlargement often subsequently occurs in such children.

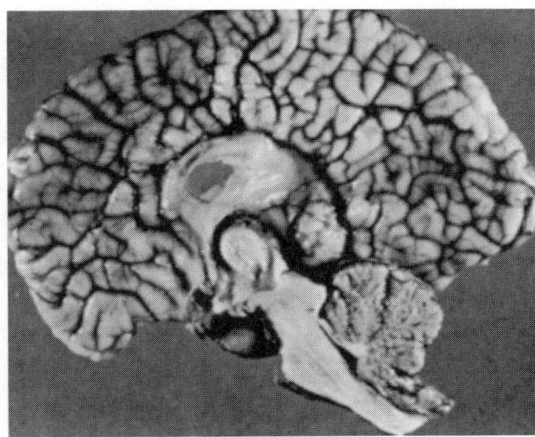

FIGURE 67–9. Arnold-Chiari malformation. Child with a thoraco-lumbar meningomyelocele. The Arnold-Chiari malformation consists of elongation of the lower brain stem with downward displacement of the inferior part of the vermis of the cerebellum. The tectal plate is beaked, and the massa intermedia is enlarged. Polymicrogyria is present.

ingomyelocele in the United States is now about 0.2 to 0.4 per 1000 live births (Yen et al, 1992).

When the lesion is a meningocele, it is usually skin covered, and neurologic function is usually normal (sometimes there are other abnormalities of spinal cord or brain). Meningomyeloceles are usually not skin covered unless a lipoma overlies the defect, forming a lipomeningomyelocele (Menkes, 1991) (Fig. 67–10).

Arnold-Chiari Malformation

The Arnold-Chiari malformation was first described in 1883 by Cleland. Chiari documented the malformations in

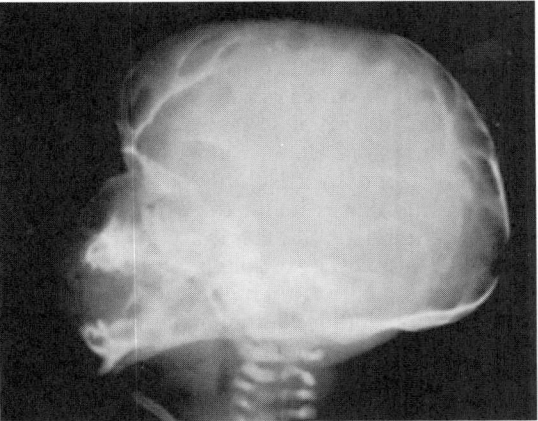

FIGURE 67–11. Lückenschädel, or craniolacunia. Honeycombed pattern of the skull in newborn infant with meningomyelocele, usually associated with hydrocephalus.

detail in 1891 and 1896, and Arnold added a description in a patient with myelomeningocele and sacral defects (1894). Chiari described three lesions: Type I, herniation of the cerebellar tonsils; Type II, the Arnold-Chiari prototype; and Type III, cervical spina bifida with cerebellar encephalocele. Later, Chiari included cerebellar hypoplasia as Type IV (Friede, 1989).

The pathology of the Arnold-Chiari malformation includes lückenschädel, or craniolacunia (in 43% of 120 patients with spina bifida) (Friede, 1989) (Fig. 67–11); a short, fenestrated falx; a shallow posterior fossa with enlarged foramen magnum, sometimes with only a rudimentary tentorium; anomalies of the cervical spine (21 of 30 cases); and tightly crowded brain stem and cerebellum with

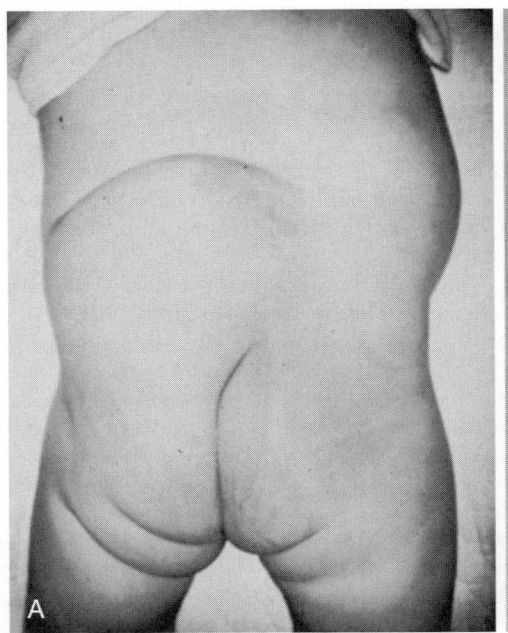 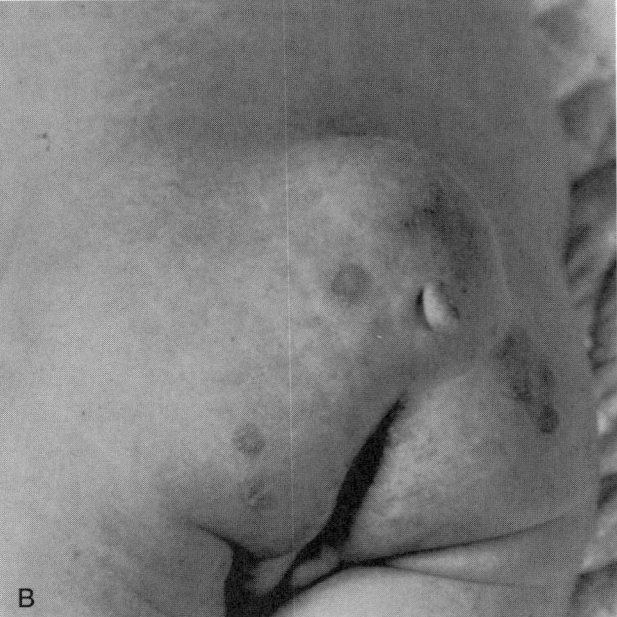

FIGURE 67–10. *A* and *B,* Two examples of lipomeningocele. Each presented in the left buttock as a firm, well-circumscribed, lobulated tumor that became tense when the infant cried. Over the surface of *B* are some macular erosions and a congenital skin tag and dimple. This last feature may be a pilonidal dimple displaced by the tumor.

caudal displacement (Blaauw, 1971). The fourth ventricle is compressed, and herniated cerebellar tissue extends into the cervical spinal canal. The caudal displacement of the brain stem causes the roots of the cranial nerves to project rostrally and be elongated (Friede, 1989; Naidich et al, 1980). The brain stem shows caudal displacement of the dorsal medulla, the fourth ventricle, and the choroid plexus. The tissue that is below the fourth ventricle forms a mass that compresses the cervical cord (this appears Z-shaped in median sagittal sections).

There are frequently other abnormalities in posterior fossa structures, including flattening and asymmetry of the cerebellar hemispheres and incomplete separation of the cerebellar hemispheres. There is also beaking of the midbrain at the level of the quadrigeminal plate, and the cervical spinal nerve roots project cranially to their foramina (instead of showing a lateral or descending course). Abnormalities of the spinal cord, including hydromyelia, syringomyelia, and diastematomyelia, can also be seen in this malformation. Almost all patients with meningomyelocele (Fig. 67–12) have the Arnold-Chiari malformation. Hypotheses about the origins of the Arnold-Chiari malformation are numerous and include the following, as summarized by Friede (1989): (1) traction from below, (2) pressure from above, (3) primary malformation of the

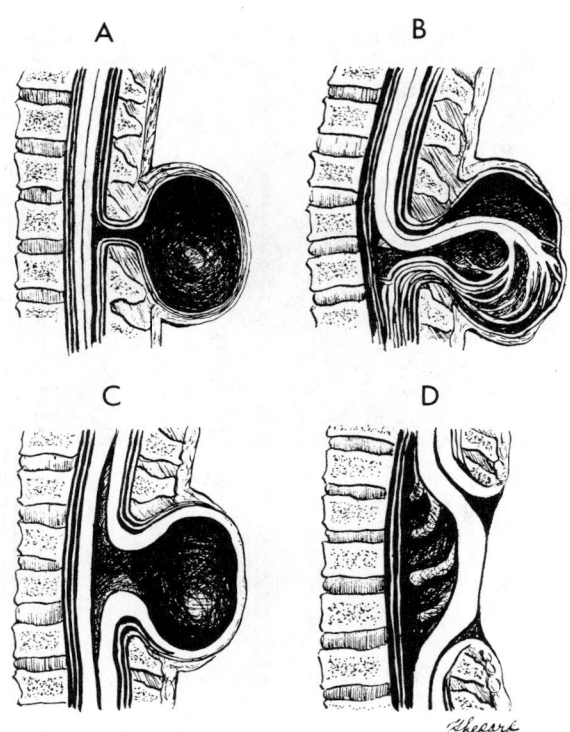

FIGURE 67–13. Diagram of meningoceles. *A*, Meningocele: Through the bony defect (spina bifida), the meninges herniate and form a cystic sac filled with spinal fluid. The spinal cord does not participate in the herniation and may or may not be abnormal. *B*, Myelomeningocele: Spina bifida with myelomeningocele; the spinal cord is herniated into the sac and ends there or may continue in an abnormal way further downward. *C*, Myelocystocele or syringomyelocele: The spinal cord shows hydromyelia; the posterior wall of the spinal cord is attached to the ectoderm and undifferentiated. *D*, Myelocele: The spinal cord is araphic; a cystic cavity is in front of the anterior wall of the spinal cord. (From Benda CE: Developmental Disorders of Mentation and Cerebral Palsies. New York, Grune & Stratton, 1952.)

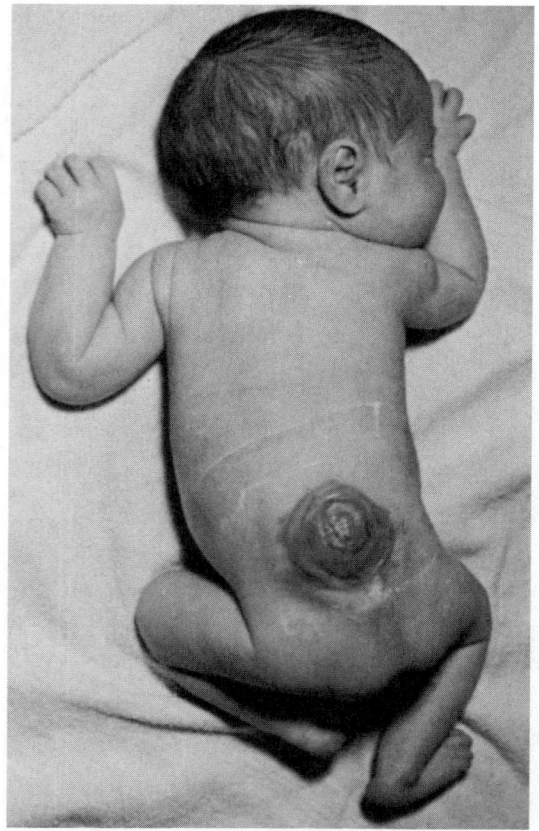

FIGURE 67–12. Lumbar meningomyelocele in a 3-day-old infant. There is moderate weakness of the proximal muscle groups and more extensive weakness of the distal musculature in the lower extremities. The lesion was flat at birth but began to elevate in the next 2 days.

hindbrain, or (4) primary malformation of the basicranium. The most compatible theory to date is primary malformation of the basicranium, causing a disproportion between the hypoplastic posterior fossa and the relatively rapid but late growth of the cerebellum (Marin-Padilla and Marin-Padilla, 1981; Muller and O'Rahilly, 1980). It is thought that the hydrocephalus that usually accompanies the Arnold-Chiari malformation is due to the obstruction at the foramen magnum and compression of the fourth ventricle, preventing any communication between the fourth ventricular compartment and the cranial subarachnoid space. In addition, 40% to 75% of patients with the Arnold-Chiari malformation have associated aqueductal stenosis, and 10% have aqueductal atresia (Gilbert et al, 1986; Peach, 1965; Stein and Schut, 1979).

Nevertheless, hydrocephalus is not universal, and its development in patients with meningomyeloceles can be correlated with the site of the lesion (Fig. 67–13). Sixty percent of patients with occipital, cervical, thoracic, or sacral lesions develop hydrocephalus, whereas 90% of those with thoracolumbar, lumbar, or lumbosacral lesions do so

(Lorber, 1961). Increased intracranial pressure is present in about 15% of newborns with meningomyelocele; in some infants, there are no signs of increased pressure because of decompression owing to cerebrospinal fluid leakage through the meningomyelocele (Stein and Schut, 1979). In these infants, hydrocephalus and increased pressure can become evident after surgical closure of the meningomyelocele. Most infants with hydrocephalus develop abnormal increases in head size within a month after birth (Stein and Schut, 1979).

As in anencephaly, fetal diagnosis of open meningomyelocele is made by quantitating maternal serum AFP and by ultrasound or MRI of the fetus in cases in which the protein is elevated. Another marker, amniotic fluid acetylcholinesterase, is also used to diagnose neural tube defects in utero, along with amniotic AFP levels, increasing the sensitivity of the screening when the maternal serum AFP level is questionable or high (Cuckle, 1994). Maternal serum AFP is elevated when there has been fetal blood contamination of the amniotic fluid, in cases of esophageal and duodenal atresia or annular pancreas, omphalocele, gastroschisis, congenital nephrosis, polycystic kidneys, renal agenesis, or fetal demise. It can also be elevated in multiple gestations (Brock, 1976; Volpe, 1995a). The best time for determination in maternal serum is 16 to 18 weeks of gestation and in amniotic fluid 14 to 16 weeks of gestation. Ultrasound or MRI is done routinely in many centers now, certainly in any questionable case or in any case in which there is an affected sibling. The risk of recurrence for neural tube defects in general is 2% to 5% when there has been one affected previous child; the risk increases when there have been more than one affected sibling (from 5% to 12% when there have been two) (Laurence, 1981). These values reflect differences in recurrence rates in different places and populations, recurrence rates in the United States being at the lower end of the ranges and lower than those in Great Britain or Quebec but similar to recurrence rates in British Columbia (Crowe et al, 1985; Janerich and Piper, 1978).

Occult Dysraphisms

Occult dysraphic states are the result of defects in caudal neural tube formation (i.e., canalization and caudal regression). The lesions include myelocystocele; diastematomyelia-diplomyelia; meningocele-lipomeningocele; lipoma, teratoma, and other tumors; dermal sinus with or without dermoid or epidermoid cyst formation; and tethered cord (Towfighi and Housman, 1991). More severe lesions include neurenteric cyst, anterior meningocele, and the findings of the caudal regression syndrome (dysraphia of sacrum and coccyx, atrophy of muscles and bones of the legs, fusion of spinal nerves and sensory ganglia, or agenesis of the distal spinal cord) (Towfighi and Housman, 1991). Infants of diabetic mothers are at increased risk for these lesions as well as for more severe neural tube defects (Becerra et al, 1990). It is important to examine newborns for evidence of occult dysraphisms by looking for midline skin findings—hair, hemangiomas, pigmented spots, skin tags, aplasia cutis congenita, cutaneous dimples or tracts, or any subcutaneous mass (Albright et al, 1989; Hall et al, 1981; Scatliff et al, 1989). Problems occurring in infancy

and childhood related to these lesions include delay in walking, delay in sphincter control, anatomic abnormalities of the feet or legs, and pain in the back or legs. Gait and spincter abnormalities, foot deformities, and scoliosis occur in older patients.

Clinical Management

Clinical management of the newborn with a neural tube defect has to be individualized. In the past, selective aggressive treatment was instituted for infants thought to have a chance for the best outcome; this approach did not always result in a good outcome. At present, aggressive surgical therapy is advocated for most infants; to date, this has resulted in patients with increased cognitive abilities, increased ambulation, a lower incidence of incontinence, and lower mortality (Hunt and Holmes, 1975; McLone et al, 1985; Stein et al, 1974, 1975).

Patients with occult dysraphisms require radiographs of the spine to diagnose the bony defect. Computed tomography, myelography, MRI, and real-time ultrasonography are used to visualize the anatomy, the tissue–cerebrospinal fluid relationships, and mobility of the cord. Because rapid, sometimes irreversible, neurologic deterioration can occur, surgery is performed in some infants to prevent neurologic deficits (Gower et al, 1988; Scatliff et al, 1989).

Disorders of the Prosencephalon
Holoprosencephaly

Failure of formation of the two telencephalic vesicles and the subsequent cerebral hemispheres results in holoprosencephaly or holotelencephaly (Fig. 67–14). This lesion can be varied, with some affected brains displaying partially formed hemispheres (lobar holoprosencephaly). Most severe cases are characterized by absence of the interhemispheric fissure and presence of a single anterior ventricle. The third ventricle is usually fused, and the basal ganglia are a single mass (Roessmann, 1995). Facial defects may be associated with holoprosencephaly and may vary from

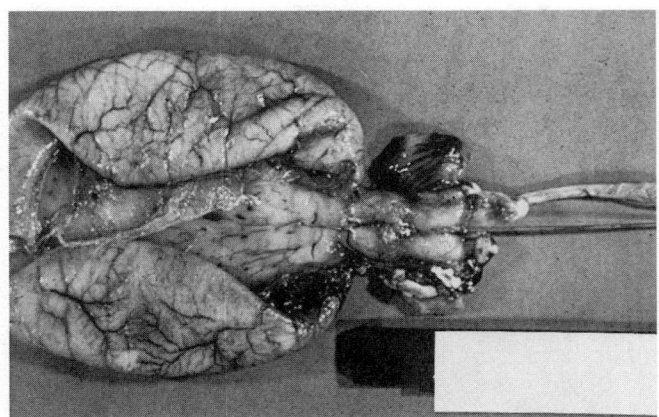

FIGURE 67–14. Holoprosencephaly. This brain has one central ventricular cavity with no division of the hemispheres. (Courtesy of Dr. Dawna L. Armstrong, Department of Pathology, Texas Children's Hospital.)

hypotelorism to cebocephaly (a flattened single nostril situated centrally between the eyes) to cyclopia. Infants with trisomy 13 frequently have holoprosencephaly, but infants with isolated holoprosencephaly do not have chromosomal abnormalities. Most infants with severe lesions are stillborn or die shortly after birth; those who survive have motor and cognitive impairment. Infants who survive may have diabetes insipidus or inappropriate secretion of antidiuretic hormone, or both (Hasegawa et al, 1990).

Arhinencephaly

Arhinencephaly, absence of the olfactory bulbs and tracts, always accompanies holoprosencephaly but can exist as an isolated lesion. It is usually found incidentally at autopsy. Leech and Shuman have hypothesized that a single mechanism operating to disrupt midline structures at different stages of development could lead to arhinencephaly, holoprosencephaly, septo-optic dysplasia, and agenesis of the corpus callosum (Roessman, 1995; Leech and Shuman, 1986).

Agenesis of the Corpus Callosum

Agenesis of the corpus callosum is shown in Figure 67–15. Although sometimes found at autopsy as an incidental finding in otherwise normal individuals, this lesion is frequently associated with other defects that lead to symptoms. Two hypotheses have been tendered for its causation: (1) a disturbance of the cells that form the lamina terminalis, which is the medial portion of the anterior telencephalon, and (2) interference with the glial sling that bridges the developing hemispheres, across which axons are led to form the corpus callosum (Roessmann, 1995; Silver et al, 1982). When there is agenesis of the corpus callosum, the medial portion of each hemisphere has abnormal gyration with absence of the cingulate gyrus and sulcation that is perpendicular to the long axis of the hemisphere. The lateral angles of the ventricles point upward, toward the vertex, and fornices are widely separated. Bundles run parallel to the ventricle carrying callosal fibers in an ante-rior-posterior direction; these are referred to as *Probst bundles*. Agenesis of the corpus callosum can be total or partial; when partial, the splenium is involved, and the genu remains intact (Roessmann, 1995; Schaefer, 1991). Agenesis of the corpus callosum is frequently found in abnormalities of chromosomes 8, 11, 13 to 15, and 18 (Jeret et al, 1987). Four syndromes are characterized by agenesis of the corpus callosum: Aicardi, acrocallosal, Andermann, and Shapiro syndromes (Jeret et al, 1987). Agenesis of the corpus callosum is also variably found in fetal alcohol syndrome, Dandy-Walker syndrome, Leigh disease, and in association with the Arnold-Chiari II malformation. Other CNS lesions are common (29% to 80%) in patients with agenesis of the corpus callosum (Jeret et al, 1987; Parrish et al, 1979).

Agenesis of the Septum Pellucidum: Septo-Optic Dysplasia

Agenesis of the septum pellucidum frequently acompanies optic nerve hypoplasia and agenesis or thinning of the corpus callosum (Williams et al, 1993). This triad, known as *septo-optic dysplasia*, is clinically associated with pituitary dwarfism and other forms of hypothalamic-pituitary dysfunction. (It should be noted that although agenesis of the septum pellucidum is never an isolated finding, optic nerve hypoplasia can occur unilaterally or bilaterally without other associated lesions) (Barkovich and Norman, 1989; Ouvrier and Billson, 1986; Zeki et al, 1992). Frequently, other cerebral abnormalities are present, including schizencephaly and absence of the pituitary infundibulum. Children with septo-optic dysplasia are blind or have reduced vision and nystagmus. Their neurodevelopmental prognosis has been controversial. In earlier studies, cerebral palsy was found in 57%, mental retardation in 71%, epilepsy in 37%, and behavior problems in 20% of children with septo-optic dysplasia (Acers, 1981; Margalith et al, 1984). A more recent neurodevelopmental study of seven children with unilateral or bilateral optic nerve hypoplasia, whose only other documentable CNS abnormality was absence of the septum pellucidum, found normal cognitive development, intact neurologic status, normal language development, and age-appropriate behavior in six of the seven (Williams et al, 1993). Thus, the abnormalities found in many patients with septo-optic dysplasia are probably due to other associated brain lesions.

The cavum septi pellucidi is an opening formed by the separation of the lamellae of the septum pellucidum; the lamellae fuse as the fetal brain matures (Mott et al, 1992). The cavum septi pellucidi may persist into extrauterine life, especially in preterm infants. Mott and associates (1992) have documented the presence of a cavum septi pellucidi in all infants less than 36 weeks' gestation routinely studied by cranial sonographic examination. A cavum septi pellucidi was present in 36% of term newborns in Mott's series.

Migration Disorders
Agyria and Pachygyria

Agyria and *lissencephaly* are synonymous terms for a brain with no gyri. Agyria and pachygyria differ in severity;

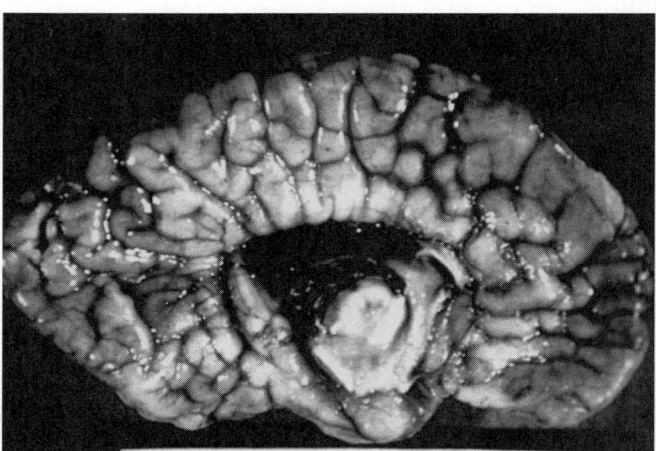

FIGURE 67–15. Agenesis of the corpus callosum. (Courtesy of Dr. Dawna L. Armstrong, Department of Pathology, Texas Children's Hospital.)

pachygyria describes a brain with a reduced number of coarse, broadened gyri (Friede, 1989). Agyric brains are most commonly classified as lissencephaly Type I and lissencephaly Type II (Evrard et al, 1989). In Type I, the earliest generated neurons, which would normally end up in layers VI and V, instead keep a more superficial position. Neurons produced later also settle in the depth of the cerebral mantle and do not continue to migrate. The end product is a four-layered cortex. This defect seems to occur between 12 and 16 weeks' gestation in the human; heterotopia of the inferior olivary nucleus is also part of this disorder. Type I lissencephaly or agyria is part of the Miller-Dieker syndrome (see Fig. 67–7).

Type II lissencephaly differs in involving the cerebral hemispheres and the cerebellum. The cortex is penetrated by vessels and glial septa, causing it to be divided into coarse masses (Evrard et al, 1989). The cerebellar cortex is microgyric. The brain in Type II lissencephaly also has hydrocephalus and neuronal heterotopias. It has been suggested that this pathologic picture may result from a destructive process during and after the second trimester of gestation (Evrard et al, 1989). Syndromes in which Type II lissencephaly occurs include Walker-Warburg syndrome and Fukuyama congenital muscular dystrophy (Fukuyama et al, 1984; Roessmann, 1995; Warburg, 1987). These syndromes are similar pathologically and also have eye and skeletal muscle defects (Pagon and Chandler, 1978). Type III lissencephaly is a variant that has been associated with micrencephaly (Encha-Razavi, 1995).

Polymicrogyria

The cortical surface in polymicrogyria has been compared to Moroccan leather (Friede, 1989). On cut surface, there is an abnormally thick cortex resulting from the piling of many small gyri with fused surfaces (Friede, 1989); this can resemble pachygyria on computed tomography or MRI images. There may be associated heterotopias of the white matter. The microscopic features usually include (1) an abnormal cell layer arrangement and intracortical fibers, (2) excessive folding of various layers, and (3) fusion of gyri (Friede, 1989). The cortex is usually four layers, consisting of a molecular layer, an upper dense layer, a middle layer of low density, and a deep cell layer next to the white matter. The neurons are smaller than usual and appear immature. There are usually abnormally dense myelinated fibers running tangentially in the molecular layer. The leptomeninges may be abnormally vascularized. Polymicrogyria probably represents a developmental defect occurring at around 5 to 6 months of gestation, which is when cortical gyration begins.

Heterotopias

Nodular heterotopias are masses of gray matter usually close to the ventricular walls (Friede, 1989). They are irregular nodules that are separated from each other by bands of myelinated fibers. Most often they are found at the corners of the lateral ventricles or at the edges of the temporal horns of the lateral ventricles. They consist of neurons and glial tissue in a disorganized fashion. Nodular heterotopias may coexist with other forms of cortical dysplasia and with other malformations. In rats, x-irradiation late in gestation produces heterotopias; heterotopias have been associated in humans with fever sustained between 4 and 14 weeks of gestation and with methylmercury poisoning (Choi et al, 1978; Pleet et al, 1981).

Neurocristopathies

The neural crests form during weeks 3 to 4 of gestation. As the neural tube closes, the neural crest cells become isolated between the neural tube and the posterior ectoderm (Reznik and Pierard, 1995). This layer differentiates into cephalic and truncal neural crests. The cephalic neural crest form the trigeminal neural crest, the facial-auditory neural crest, and the glossopharyngeal and vagal neural crest. These give rise to the cranial nerves and their sensory ganglia as well as to parts of the branchial arcs (Reznik and Pierard, 1995). The truncal neural crest becomes fragmented along with the truncal somites. After the neural crest anlage are formed, neural crest cells migrate throughout the entire embryo. Migration is rostrocaudal, along the medial axis of the embryo (LeDouarin, 1982). After migration is accomplished, the neural crest cells are located in four areas: (1) nervous system—meningioblasts and Schwann cells and ganglion and paraganglion cells (including enteric ganglion cells of the digestive tract); (2) endocrine system—chromaffin cells of the adrenal medulla and several types of endocrine and paraendocrine cells; (3) pigmented system—melanoblasts in all tissues except the retina; and (4) skeletal system of the head, face, and neck. Abnormalities thus can arise in the migration or differentiation of the neural crest cells, or neural crest derivatives may develop tumors (Jacobson, 1991; Reznik and Pierard, 1995).

Disorders thought to arise from abnormalities of neural crest formation, migration, proliferation, or differentiation include the LEOPARD syndrome; multiple lentigines syndrome; NAME syndrome; LAMB syndrome; and the Peutz-Jeghers-Touraine syndrome (Table 67–1). Tumors derived from neural crest cells include those arising from Schwann cells, perineural cells, or fibrocytes; from neural sense organs; from ganglionic or neuroendocrine cells; or from melanogenic cells (Reznik and Pierard, 1995). Some neurocutaneous syndromes, such as neurofibromatosis, hypomelanosis of Ito, and neurocutaneous melanosis, as well as other entities, such as multiple schwannoma syndrome (without neurofibromatosis), multiple mucosal neuromas, multiple hamartomas syndrome, cutaneous meningiomas, and multiple endocrine neoplasia, are all thought to involve neural crest cells in some way. The derivation of neurocutaneous syndromes, however, is not clearly, always, or only from neural crest cells, and thus the term *neurocristopathy* is no longer used to describe those diseases. In fact, many of the diseases previously classified as neurocutaneous syndromes are now being called *hereditary tumor syndromes of the nervous system*, with more definition of their pathogenesis becoming available through molecular genetic studies (Louis and von Deimling, 1995).

Hirschsprung disease is a disorder of neural crest development and occurs in 1 in 5000 births (Edery et al, 1994; Romeo et al, 1994). It is characterized by absence of hindgut intramural ganglion cells, which causes intestinal

TABLE 67–1

Disorders of Neural Crest Formation, Migration, Proliferation, or Differentiation

LEOPARD	Multiple Lentigines	Electrocardiographic defects	Ocular hypertelorism	Pulmonary stenosis	Genital Abnormalities	Growth Retardation	Sensorineural Deafness
Multiple Lentigines	Cutaneous pigmented macules	Obstructive cardiomyopathy	Genital abnormalities	Delayed puberty	Sensorineural hearing loss	Hypertelorism and skeletal abnormalities	Growth retardation
NAME	Cutaneous Nevi	Atrial myxoma	Myxoid neurofibromas	Ephelides			
LAMB	Lentigines	Atrial myxoma	Mucocutaneous myxoma	Blue nevi			
Peutz-Jeghers-Touraine	Mucocutaneous lentigines	Gastrointestinal polyposis	Schwannoma of the gut; acoustic neurinomas	Increased risk of malignancies			

obstruction in the neonatal period. A gene associated with some cases of Hirschsprung disease has been mapped to chromosome 10 and localized to the *RET* proto-oncogene (Edery et al, 1994; Romeo et al, 1994; Yin et al, 1994). Mutations that affect the RET protein seem also to be present in patients with multiple endocrine neoplasia Type 2A (Donis-Keller et al, 1993; Mulligan et al, 1993).

Neuroblastoma is a neuroectodermal tumor that occurs mostly in children. It usually arises from the adrenal gland but can arise from sympathetic ganglia, the neuroendocrine system, or the ovary (Reznik and Pierard, 1995). It is sometimes seen in association with neurofibromatosis. Cutaneous metastases from neuroblastoma can occur as multiple skin nodules and have been seen in the newborn.

Möbius Syndrome

Möbius syndrome typically consists of bilateral facial and abducens palsies caused by absence or hypoplasia of the cranial nerve nuclei. In some cases, there is involvement of other cranial nerves. Associated features, such as mental retardation, dextrocardia, and endocrine and muscular abnormalities, have been described (Costa and Hauw, 1995). It is not known whether Möbius syndrome is a result of abnormal differentiation of either mesodermal or ectodermal structures, an abnormality of cellular migration, or proliferation or programmed cell death or whether it is an effect of early regression of parts of the brain stem arterial supply (Bavinck and Weaver, 1986; Volpe, 1995b). Clinical features of Möbius syndrome have been compiled by Volpe (1995b) and include severe facial diplegia (100%), bilateral abducens palsy (82%), total external ophthalmoplegia (25%), oculomotor palsy (21%), bilateral ptosis (10%), tongue weakness (30%), talipes equinovarus (31%), hand or arm malformation (21%), and pectoralis hypoplasia (13%).

Proliferation Disorders

Micrencephaly

Micrencephaly is a condition in which smallness of the brain or of the cerebral hemispheres is the only lesion; microcephaly is used to describe a small cranial vault induced either by micrencephaly or by acquired atrophic lesions (e.g., multicystic encephalopathy, hydranencephaly, diffuse cortical atrophy) (Friede, 1989). The pathogenesis of micrencephaly has been better defined, and two subgroups have been postulated (Evrard et al, 1989; Rakic, 1988): *radial microbrain* and *micrencephaly vera*. The first entity is thought to be due to a reduced number of proliferative units; the second is thought to be due to reduced size of proliferative units (Evrard et al, 1989; Rakic, 1988). Radial microbrains, as described in seven cases by Evrard and colleagues (1989), have normal gyri and cortical lamination but have abnormal numbers of cortical neuronal columns. The number of cells per column is normal, however. This implies that the abnormality occurs at the time of stem cell division.

Micrencephaly vera is the term used to describe small brains that are usually well formed (although usually not as small as radial microbrains) with simple gyral patterns (Evrard et al, 1989). In these brains, the number of cortical

neuronal columns is normal, but the cell number in each column is reduced. Evrard and colleagues (1989) have shown the absence of residual germinal matrix in one such brain at 26 weeks' gestation. This abnormality would most likely occur between 6 and 18 weeks' gestation, when the later proliferative events are occurring. Both of these forms of micrencephaly may be caused by genetic abnormalities, teratogenic influences, or sporadically. Autosomal dominant, autosomal recessive, and X-linked recessive types have been described (Robain and Lyon, 1972; Warkany et al, 1981). Irradiation before 18 weeks' gestation is a well-known teratogenic agent that can produce micrencephaly, and use of alcohol and cocaine during this time in pregnancy can also result in micrencephaly. Maternal hyperphenylalanine has also been associated with these defects in nonphenylketonuric offspring (Lenke and Levy, 1980; Waisbren and Levy, 1990).

Many dysgenetic syndromes have microcephaly as a component. The genetic bases of some of the syndromes are becoming clearer, and some of the syndromes are associated with deficiencies of myelin or reduced white matter, with or without associated micrencephaly (Friede, 1989).

Macrencephaly

Just as micrencephaly implies a small brain, macrencephaly describes a large brain that is generally well formed (Friede, 1989). It is distinguished from macrocephaly, which defines a large head from a number of causes. It has been hypothesized that macrencephaly is due to abnormalities that cause increased cellular proliferation, but quantitative studies are lacking. A number of syndromes are associated with macrencephaly. Those that include generalized growth disturbances are listed in the following section; others include familial macrencephaly (autosomal dominant or autosomal recessive), sporadic macrencephaly, macrencephaly associated with neurocutaneous syndromes, macrencephaly associated with known chromosomal disorders (fragile X syndrome and Klinefelter syndrome), and unilateral macrencephaly (hemimegalencephaly) (Volpe, 1995c). In some cases of familial macrencephaly, brain imaging studies show prominent extracerebral subarachnoid spaces in addition to the large brain. During the first few postnatal years in these infants, the size of the extracerebral spaces diminishes, although the brain remains large. Clinical features of familial macrencephaly include head size at birth greater than the 90th percentile, rapid postnatal head growth, normal intelligence in 60%, and mental retardation in 10% (DeMyer, 1972). Almost all of such infants have a parent with macrencephaly (Volpe, 1995c). When macrencephaly is autosomal recessive, other neurologic deficits are more likely to be present (Warkany et al, 1981).

Macrencephaly and Growth Disorders

Macrencephaly can also be associated with generalized growth disorders, including Beckwith-Wiedemann syndrome (high birth weight, exomphalos, large tongue, renal and pancreatic hyperplasia, fetal adrenal cytomegaly, hemihypertrophy, Wilms tumor, eventration of the diaphragm, hypoglycemia, grooves on the ear lobes), cerebral gigantism, and achondroplasia (DeMyer, 1972; Dodge et al, 1983). Although macrencephaly and other features of these syndromes are likely to be present in the newborn, neurologic abnormalities (except those associated with hypoglycemia in Beckwith-Wiedemann syndrome) are usually not common in the newborn.

Neurocutaneous Syndromes

Neurocutaneous syndromes that can be diagnosed in the newborn in some cases include neurofibromatosis I, Sturge-Weber disease, and tuberous sclerosis. The gene for neurofibromatosis I, on chromosome 17, is involved in the regulation of cell proliferation through the *ras* proto-oncogene (Gutmann and Collins, 1992). Neurofibromas usually contain a mixed population of cells, including Schwann cells, perineurial cells, and mast cells (Reznik and Pierard, 1995). Forty percent of infants with neurofibromatosis have five cafe-au-lait lesions greater than 5 cm in size at birth, and 20% to 40% of these infants have macrocephaly eventually (Fois et al, 1993; Listernick and Charrow, 1990). Occasionally, optic nerve glioma and plexiform neuroma of the eyelid are seen in the newborn with neurofibromatosis (Listernick and Charrow, 1990).

Sturge-Weber disease, a sporadic disease of mesoblastic origin also known as *encephalofacial angiomatosis*, is characterized by a cutaneous nevus or port-wine stain in the areas of the sensory branches of the trigeminal nerve as well as a vascular malformation that involves the leptomeninges, choroid, and cortex homolaterally (Reznik and Pierard, 1995). The port-wine stain is evident at birth, and cerebral atrophy can be present at birth (Reznik and Pierard, 1995). Glaucoma is sometimes present at birth, and all children with Sturge-Weber disease should be followed for development of glaucoma. Cerebral calcifications can sometimes be seen on neuroimaging in the newborn with Sturge-Weber disease but are usually not manifest until 6 months of age or later (Kitahara and Maki, 1978; Nelhaus et al, 1967; Volpe, 1995c).

Tuberous sclerosis is characterized by abnormal proliferations of both neurons and glial cells as well as hamartomas in other organs (Yoshimura et al, 1990). The genetics are complicated with two genes now identified for this disease, one on chromosome 16 and the other on chromosome 9 (Green et al, 1994). The typical cutaneous hypopigmented spots are frequently present in the neonatal period, and seizures may occur in the newborn with tuberous sclerosis (Sugita et al, 1985). Infants with tuberous sclerosis at several months of age may manifest infantile spasms (Roth and Epstein, 1971). Subependymal nodules and cortical tubers can sometimes be diagnosed by computed tomography, ultrasound, or MRI in the newborn period (Bell et al, 1991).

Incontinentia pigmenti is a rare disorder with a predilection for females. In eight families with hereditary incontinentia pigmenti, genetic linkage analysis has shown a gene locus at Xq28. Other families have shown X/autosomal translocations with the same phenotype, however. The disease is manifest by well-described dermatologic features that pass through four stages (Cohen, 1987; Rosman, 1992; Wettke-Schafer, 1983; Wiley and Frias, 1974). Lesions seen during the neonatal period in 90% of cases are macular,

papular, vesicular, erythematous, and bullous; may be pustular; and are characterized by the presence of eosinophils (Rosman, 1992). Half of the cases show skin lesions at birth. These early-phase lesions usually are present for several months (and may be present for several years). In the second stage, the skin lesions have been described as lichenoid or keratotic, verrucous, or pustular. This stage usually occurs at 2 to 6 weeks of age but may be present at birth if the first stage was present in utero. In the third stage, the lesions become pigmented, occurring usually between 3 and 6 months of age (but they may be delayed). The pigmentation is usually tan, brownish, or grayish and can be in streaks, whorls, flecks, or other configurations. These lesions, too, can be seen at birth, suggesting that the other lesions have been present in utero. The pigmented lesions usually last for decades. When the fourth stage occurs, it consists of fading of the pigmented lesions followed by the appearance of atrophic scars (Cohen, 1987).

Other findings in incontinentia pigmenti include eye, bone, dental, and nail abnormalities as well as CNS involvement in 30% to 50% of cases (Simmons et al, 1986; Simmonsson, 1972; Wettke-Schafer, 1983). The most common CNS abnormalities are psychomotor retardation, seizures, spastic paralyses, and microcephaly. Most children with incontinentia pigmenti have more than one neurologic abnormality.

Cerebellar Malformations

The malformations of the cerebellum are usually classified by involvement of either the neocerebellum or the paleocerebellum. Because the development of the vermis occurs before that of the cerebellar hemispheres, the flocculi of the hemispheres and the vermis are called *paleocerebellum*, and the remaining cerebellar hemispheres are called *neocerebellum*.

The Dandy-Walker malformation and related disorders are primarily associated with aplasia or hypoplasia of the vermis of the cerebellum (Costa and Hauw, 1995; Friede, 1989). The Dandy-Walker malformation consists of complete or partial agenesis of the vermis; cystic dilation of the fourth ventricle; and enlargement of the posterior fossa with upward displacement of the lateral sinuses, tentorium, and torcular (D'Agostino, 1963; Friede, 1989; Hart et al, 1972). Dandy and Blackfan, then Taggart and Walker originally described the syndrome and ascribed its components to nonpatency of the foramina of Luschka and Magendie. Others have pointed out that atresia of the foramina does not have to be present to have the syndrome (Benda, 1954). More than 80% of those with the Dandy-Walker malformation develop signs of hydrocephalus during the first postnatal year; some have hydrocephalus at birth. Those diagnosed after 12 months of age usually have delayed developmental milestones, with or without increased head size (Costa and Hauw, 1995; Hart et al, 1972). Neurologic signs may include cranial nerve palsies, apnea, nystagmus, and truncal ataxia. The diagnosis can be made by ultrasonography in utero or by computed tomography or MRI scan postnatally. Treatment usually requires ventricular and posterior fossa shunting.

The Dandy-Walker variant consists of hypoplasia of the cerebellar vermis and hemispheres without enlargement of the posterior fossa. In other variants, there is enlargement of the posterior fossa and the cisterna magna, without vermian hypoplasia (Altman et al, 1992). Atresia of the foramina of Luschka and Magendie may occur in the Dandy-Walker syndrome, but atresia does not have to be present for the other features to be present. Isolated atresias of the foramina may occur without associated aplasia of the vermis or cystic dilation of the fourth ventricle.

Abnormalities of the cerebellum are also found in Joubert syndrome, which is thought to be autosomal recessive and is characterized by abnormal eye movements, ataxia, mental retardation, and periods of hyperpnea alternating with periods of apnea (Joubert et al, 1969). This syndrome may also have other malformations, such as occipital meningoencephaloceles, microcephaly, low-set ears, polydactyly, and retinal dysplasia (Egger et al, 1982; Friede and Boltshauser, 1978). The cerebellar lesion is usually complete or partial agenesis of the vermis, but there can also be dysplasia of the dentate nucleus, cerebellar heterotopias, anomalies of brain stem nuclei, and absence of decussation of the pyramidal tracts (Curatolo et al, 1980). Patients with this syndrome usually die before 3 years of age (Curatolo et al, 1980).

Other rare defects associated with cerebellar vermian hypoplasia, some of which can be diagnosed in the newborn period, include the COACH syndrome (*c*erebellar vermis hypoplasia or aplasia, *o*ligophrenia, congenital nonprogressive *a*taxia, *c*oloboma, and *h*epatic fibrosis), tectocerebellar dysraphia (occipital encephalocele containing cerebellar tissue with malformation of the tectum), and rhombencephalosynapsis (aplasia of the vermis with fused, small cerebellar hemispheres) (Verloes and Lambotte, 1989). Other abnormalities of the nervous system may be present with rhombencephalosynapsis, including septooptic dysplasia, arhinencephaly, and fused cerebellar peduncles (Michaud et al, 1982).

Aplasia and hypoplasia of the cerebellar hemispheres are usually associated with other brain malformations. Complete absence of the cerebellum has been reported in several siblings but is extremely rare (Riccardi and Marcus, 1978). Absence of one cerebellar hemisphere is not as rare and may be asymptomatic (Costa and Hauw, 1995). In reported cases of bilateral cerebellar hemispheric aplasia, there has been atrophy of the basis pontis as well and severe neurologic symptoms, including microcephaly, mental retardation, and spasticity, with death before 1 year of age (Norman and Urich, 1958). It should be noted that pontoneocerebellar hypoplasia has been reported in association with prenatal exposure to phenytoin (Gadisseux et al, 1984).

Other malformations of the cerebellum may play a role in juvenile-onset cerebellar signs and symptoms; two such malformations include absence or thinning of the superficial granular layer and cerebellar heterotopias (Friede, 1989; Jervis, 1950). These are not likely to be recognized as causes of neurologic problems in the newborn but may be found at autopsy.

Arteriovenous Malformation of the Vein of Galen

An arteriovenous malformation (AVM) of the vein of Galen frequently causes symptoms in the newborn period. This malformation consists of a meshwork of arteries extending from the vertebrobasilar system that feeds, sometimes along with branches of the anterior and middle cerebral arteries, into the vein of Galen. Because of the large shunt of blood through the malformation, the newborn usually presents with cardiomegaly and heart failure. Infants presenting with heart failure with this lesion in the newborn period usually have a large AVM with a poorer prognosis than infants presenting later. The preferential steal (diversion) of blood through the malformation can also cause infarction of brain tissue (Norman, 1992). A review of seven newborns with vein of Galen AVMs showed that six of the seven presented with heart failure (Norman and Becker, 1974). Two of the newborns had antenatal brain infarcts, five had periventricular leukomalacia, and three had hemorrhagic infarcts (all infants died, and the brains were examined at autopsy). It has been suggested that, despite the poor prognosis, surgery can be helpful for some infants by slowing or arresting the otherwise progessive deterioration associated with the lesion (Phillips et al, 1986). Other types of vascular malformations occur in the brains of infants and children, but they are not as likely to present in the newborn period as AVM of the vein of Galen.

Choroid Plexus Cysts

Choroid cysts are mentioned briefly here because the association has been made between them and trisomy 18 (Fitzsimmons et al, 1989; Norman, 1992). Cysts can now be seen on ultrasound examinations in fetuses, and it has been suggested that when they are present before 20 to 22 weeks' gestation, amniocentesis should be done for chromosome analysis (Fitzsimmons et al, 1989). This practice is controversial, however, and the risk of amniocentesis may outweigh the number of infants identified with trisomy (Benacerraf et al, 1990). Choroid plexus cysts in general are thought not to be significant without other systemic or CNS malformations (Norman, 1992).

Arachnoid Cysts

Arachnoid cysts are pockets within the arachnoid filled with fluid that is similar to cerebrospinal fluid. They usually do not communicate with other parts of the subarachnoid space, and common locations are the sylvian fissure, the interhemispheric fissure, and the cisterna magna (Hanieh et al, 1988). It is not clear why the cysts form, but children with these lesions can present with increased intracranial pressure or large heads. Decompression of arachnoid cysts can be accomplished surgically.

DESTRUCTIVE LESIONS IN UTERO

Varying degrees of destruction of the brain can occur in utero related to events that cause brain necrosis and cavitation (Norman, 1992). Such lesions include a range of defects from isolated cysts to hydranencephaly. Similar lesions have been produced in experimental models by trauma, arterial vascular obstruction, infection, hyperthermia, and endotoxin (Norman, 1978). Usually it is not possible to define the exact cause of such lesions.

Aqueductal Stenosis

Although aqueductal obstruction can be the result of several types of pathology, including stenosis, forking, atresia, or septum formation, when due to gliosis, it has been classified as postinflammatory (Russell, 1949). A form of stenosis without evidence of gliosis is apparently sex linked and is also associated with other malformations, including abnormal thumbs, agenesis of the corpus callosum, and agenesis of the corticospinal tracts (Norman, 1992; Roessmann, 1995). Because the fetal brain before 17 to 20 weeks' gestation does not show gliosis as a result of aquired damage, it is not always possible to tell if an aqueductal lesion is a true malformation or is secondary to intrauterine infection or other insult (Roessmann, 1995).

Hydrocephalus

The term *hydrocephalus* implies an increased amount of cerebrospinal fluid within the ventricles, under pressure, as a result of an obstruction to the outflow of cerebrospinal fluid or an overproduction of cerebrospinal fluid. Obstruction to outflow can be at the foramen of Monro, in a ventricle, at the aqueduct, at the foramina of Luschka and Magendie, in one or more cisterns, or at the places of absorption in the arachnoid villi (Shaw and Alvord, 1995). Hydrocephalus as a result of overproduction of cerebrospinal fluid can occur with choroid plexus papillomas, carcinomas, or hyperplasia. Choroid plexus papillomas can be seen as congenital brain tumors, and hydrocephalus associated with choroid plexus papilloma may be a combination of obstruction to outflow by the papilloma and overproduction of cerebrospinal fluid (Shaw and Alvord, 1995). The term *communicating hydrocephalus* is used to define cases in which the ventricular system and cisterns communicate. In *noncommunicating hydrocephalus*, there is obstruction at some point within the ventricular system or between the cisterns (Shaw and Alvord, 1995).

Hydrocephalus is frequently associated with developmental anomalies of the brain, including the Dandy-Walker malformation and variants, Chiari malformations, lissencephalies and cerebro-ocular muscular syndromes, holoprosencephaly, and other defects with maldevelopment or loss of cerebral tissue. Hydrocephalus can also be a consequence of aqueductal occlusion (see earlier), tumors or cysts that obstruct various parts of the ventricular system, or postinflammatory states (postmeningitic, posthemorrhagic). Surgical treatment of hydrocephalus, most commonly by ventriculoperitoneal shunting, has increased survival of affected infants dramatically with improved cognitive outcome.

Hypoxic-Ischemic Lesions

Intrauterine hypoxic-ischemic lesions are usually manifest as complete or incomplete necrosis or hemorrhage in either or both white and gray matter (Encha-Razavi, 1995). Fetal brains are particularly prone to rarefaction or cavitary lesions of white matter, especially in the periventricular regions, centrum semiovale, and subcortical white matter (Encha-Razavi, 1995). The cerebellum may also be affected. The areas most likely to be infarcted are those that correspond to areas of poor vascularization between dorsal and basal penetrating arteries (Takashima and Tanaka, 1978a). Such lesions are also found frequently in premature infants who die after having sustained prenatal or postnatal hypoxia-ischemia. When lesions with necrosis, cavitation, and mineral deposits are apparent by ultrasound scanning at birth, they are due to intrauterine injury because these findings take days to weeks to develop (Encha-Razavi, 1995; Friede, 1989).

Gray matter lesions are more likely to be found in term infants. They may be found as parasagittal lesions, as laminar cortical necrosis, as pontosubicular necrosis, and as necrosis of the basal ganglia. Experimental studies in primates have suggested that total asphyxial injury results in brain stem damage; partial asphyxia with acidosis results in cerebral cortical injury with edema; partial asphyxia without acidosis results in white matter injury; and a combination of partial and total asphyxia results in basal ganglia injury plus lesions of the neocortex (the more severe the total asphyxia, the more brain stem injury also occurs) (Painter, 1995). Human newborns also show cerebellar lesions after significant hypoxia-ischemia. These designations are helpful but not universal because there are significant physiologic, anatomic, and developmental differences between primates and humans that have to be considered.

Hydranencephaly

One of the most devastating intrauterine encephaloclastic lesions is hydranencephaly, which is loss of tissue in the territories supplied by the internal carotid arteries (Encha-Razavi, 1995). The brain stem is usually intact, but the hemispheres are usually replaced by fluid-filled cavities surrounded by a leptomeningeal membrane with remnants of the damaged cortex (Encha-Razavi, 1995).

Hemorrhagic Lesions

Fresh hemorrhage, especially petechial hemorrhages and subependymal germinal matrix hemorrhages, occurs in fetal brains; choroid plexus hemorrhage also occurs (Encha-Razavi, 1995). Periventricular and subcortical infarctions can also be hemorrhagic.

Lesions Caused by Infections

Aqueductal stenosis has already been mentioned as a postinfectious or postinflammatory sequela; it has been documented in particular after mumps infection in utero (Norman, 1992). Rubella, cytomegalovirus, *Listeria monocytogenes*, and *Toxoplasma gondii* are agents known to affect the developing nervous system. They can cause meningitis, choroiditis, and multicystic encephalopathy with resulting microcephaly or hydrocephalus (Encha-Razavi, 1995). Varicella zoster and herpes simplex type 2 infection can affect the fetus, although herpes type 2 more commonly affects the fetus at birth. When varicella zoster infection occurs in utero, a congenital defects syndrome can occur with damage to sensory nerves and cutaneous manifestations, ophthalmic involvement, encephalitis, and damage to the spinal cord (Grose, 1994). Intrauterine infection with herpes simplex virus type 2 involves the skin, eyes, and CNS. Infection with human immunodeficiency virus is thought to occur in utero in a minority of cases, and neuropathology in the fetus is not yet well documented.

Lesions Associated with Metabolic Disease

Metabolic disease in the mother or the fetus can result in neuropathology in the fetus. Abnormalities in infants of untreated phenylketonuric mothers and of mothers heterozygous for ornithine transcarbamylase deficiency were mentioned in Chapters 24 and 25. Diabetes mellitus in the mother has been associated with neural tube defects in the offspring (Norman, 1992). Infants dying of metabolic disease in the fetal or neonatal period may show secondary findings of hypoxia-ischemia; in lipid storage diseases, they may show characteristic cells containing abnormal by-products (such as cerebroside in Gaucher disease) (Norman, 1992).

DEVELOPMENTAL PHARMACOLOGY

Antenatal use of alcohol, nicotine, marijuana, cocaine, and opioids continues to be a hazard for the developing nervous system (Alexander, 1992). In addition, environmental contamination and inadvertant exposure to agents such as lead and mercury can affect the intrauterine nervous system. A number of antiepileptic drugs have fetal CNS effects, as does isotretinoin, a vitamin A analogue, which is now prescribed for severe acne and is a known teratogen with severe effects on the CNS and other systems (Fernhoff and Lammer, 1984; Rosa, 1983). This section covers the effects of alcohol, isotretinoin, the hydantoins, and cocaine as well as the environmental toxins, mercury and polychlorinated biphenyls (PCBs), on the developing nervous system.

Drugs and the Developing Nervous System
Alcohol

The fetal alcohol syndrome, a combination of CNS and systemic effects of chronic fetal exposure to alcohol, is now considered the most common *known* cause of mental retardation worldwide (Alexander, 1992). The worldwide incidence is thought to be 1.9 per 1000 live births, and the overall incidence in the United States is approximately 0.33 per 1000 live births (Committee on Substance Abuse, 1993). Less obvious dysmorphic, cognitive, and behavioral consequences of in utero exposure to alcohol are called *fetal alcohol effects* and occur more frequently than fetal alcohol syndrome.

The syndrome consists of prenatal and postnatal growth retardation, with length affected more than weight initially (Jones et al, 1973). Nearly all affected infants have microcephaly with neurodevelopmental delay and intelligence quotients ranging generally from 65 to 85. A particular abnormality has been noted on the electroencephalogram of some infants (Ioffe and Chernick, 1988). The dysmorphic features of the syndrome consist of short palpebral fissures, epicanthal folds, midfacial hypoplasia, short upturned nose, hypoplastic long or smooth philtrum, thin

upper lip vermilion, abnormal palmar creases, joint abnormalities, ear anomalies, abnormalities of the external genitalia, and cutaneous hemangiomas (Jones et al, 1973). About 50% of infants have congenital heart defects.

CNS abnormalities usually include micrencephaly with abnormalities of neuronal and glial migration (Ferrer and Galofre, 1987; Jones, 1975; Peiffer et al, 1979) that are seen as heterotopias and abnormalities of brain stem and cerebellar development. Schizencephaly and polymicrogyria have been reported, as have agenesis of the corpus callosum, septo-optic dysplasia, forms of holoprosencephaly, neural tube defects, arhinencephaly, and abnormal dendritic formation (Ferrer and Galofre, 1987; Jones, 1975). A number of neurodevelopmental events are affected by alcohol, and the precise mechanism of action is not known, although several hypotheses are being studied in experimental models. What is known is that the occurrence of the syndrome and the severity are directly related to the amount and timing of the consumption of alcohol by the mother. Notably, mothers consuming more than 2 ounces of absolute alcohol per day at the time of and shortly after conception delivered infants with fetal alcohol syndrome in 19% of cases (Hanson et al, 1978).

Retinoic Acid

Retinoic acid is a vitamin A metabolite that plays a role in many developmental processes. Alcohol may act on the fetus through this compound because ethanol competitively antagonizes the enzyme that converts vitamin A to retinol, which then is converted to retinoic acid (Duester, 1991; Keir, 1991). As mentioned previously, retinoic acid may play a role in the genesis of neural tube defects (Alles and Sulik, 1990).

In addition, and extremely important from a public health standpoint, is the fact that the vitamin A analogue isotretinoin is a teratogen itself, causing craniofacial abnormalities with cleft palate, ear defects, CNS defects, and heart lesions (DeLaCruz et al, 1984; Fernhhoff and Lammer, 1984; Lott et al, 1984; Rizzo et al, 1991; Rosa, 1983). The ears can be small and malformed or absent with abnormal ear canals. The CNS abnormalities include aqueductal stenosis, migrational defects, micrencephaly, vermian atresia, and migration abnormalities of the brain stem and cerebellum.

Because isotretinoin is prescribed for acne in women in the early child-bearing years, the potential for this embryopathy must be kept in mind. This drug should not be prescribed casually, and careful attention to the sexual histories of the patients using this drug and to their use of contraception is extremely important before its use. The patients should be counseled about the teratogenic effects of isotretinoin.

Hydantoins

The fetal hydantoin syndrome is a constellation of findings that may occur with several of the anticonvulsant drugs when they are taken during pregnancy (Albengres and Tillement, 1983; Hanson and Buehler, 1982; Hill et al, 1974; Speidel and Meadow, 1972). The syndrome consists of growth disturbance, characteristic facies, cranial abnormalities, hypoplastic nails and distal phalanges, and neuro-developmental delay (Hill, 1976; Monson et al, 1973). Similar findings may be present after intrauterine exposure to barbiturates, primidone, and carbamazepine (Jones et al, 1989; Krauss et al, 1984; Myhre and Williams, 1981; Seip, 1976). Usually these infants have small heads with enlarged fontanels (approximately 30% are microcephalic), ocular hypertelorism, a broad nasal bridge, and hypoplasia of the nails and distal phalanges. Other findings, such as cleft lip and palate, heart anomalies, gingival hypertrophy, wide-set nipples, bilateral inguinal hernias, simian creases, digital thumbs, and pilonidal sinuses, have been reported to lesser, varying extents (Hill et al, 1974). The brain pathology of this syndrome is not defined. It is now thought that a genetic predisposition must be present for the syndrome to occur; the syndrome has occurred in one, but not the other, of heteropaternal dizygotic twins (Phelan et al, 1982). Because the antiepileptic drugs that cause this syndrome are metabolized to a toxic epoxide that is then detoxified by an epoxide hydrolase, it has been hypothesized that fetuses with low levels of epoxide hydrolase are at greater risk of being affected (Buehler et al, 1990; Finnell et al, 1992).

Cocaine

Cocaine use is widespread in the United States; in one New York City hospital, records showed that 13% of the infants born there had been exposed to cocaine in utero (Fox, 1994). Cocaine has many physiologic effects, including CNS stimulation by antagonism of catecholamine uptake at nerve endings. Reactions include dilation of the pupils, increased heart rate and blood pressure, tachycardia, and exaggerated reflexes. The cocaine user may be agitated, may be anorectic, may have cardiac arrhythmias, and may have seizures (Fox, 1994). Use in pregnancy can lead to preterm labor, preeclampsia, acute pulmonary edema, and abruptio placentae (Fox, 1994; Jones, 1991). It has been hypothesized that other fetal effects can result from vascular compromise in utero, leading to decreased fetal, uterine, and placental blood flow (Jones, 1991). CNS defects in exposed infants include cerebellar necrosis, hydranencephaly, multicystic encephalomalacia, intracranial hemorrhage, Möbius syndrome, optic nerve abnormalities, hydrocephalus, microcephaly, spinal cord transection, and other abnormalities (Gieron-Korthals et al, 1994; Ryan et al, 1987). A current suggestion is that these malformations may be due to a combination of in utero insults in this population of infants and that they are probably not due to the effects of cocaine alone. Transient dystonia in the neonatal period has been associated with prenatal cocaine exposure (Beltran and Coker, 1995).

The later behavioral and cognitive effects of cocaine exposure in utero have not been clearly determined, and there is controversy as to whether early abnormal responses to environmental stimuli in cocaine-exposed infants have meaning for later neurodevelopmental outcome. Cocaine metabolites can be detected noninvasively in urine, meconium, and hair; the detection period for urine is up to 4 days before sample collection. Analysis of meconium detects the metabolites after use up to 6 weeks before birth. The metabolites can be detected in hair for up to the entire pregnancy, depending on the length of the strands used for analysis (Fox, 1994). There are still problems in interpreting results in hair, but it seems a promising means of detection for the future.

Environmental Toxins: Mercury and Polychlorinated Biphenyls

Knowledge of the effects of exposure to toxins such as mercury and PCBs has come from industrial accidents, in which pregnant women have ingested badly contaminated foods or water (Amin-Zaki, 1979; Chen and Hsu, 1994; Harada, 1978; Kuratsune et al, 1972). After the mercury poisoning of the water and fish of Minamata Bay, Minamata, Japan, many fetuses were affected (Harada, 1978). Infants showed multiple neurologic defects, including spastic cerebral palsy with ataxia, mental retardation, dysarthria, and hypersalivation (Harada, 1978).

PCB poisoning has occurred in both the United States and Japan. Infants with in utero exposure have had intrauterine growth restriction, brown coloration of the skin and mucous membranes, widely open fontanels, abnormal calcifications in the skull, teeth present at birth, and neuro-developmental delay (Harada, 1978; Rogan et al, 1988). Long-term follow-up of PCB-exposed children has been carried out by Chen and Hsu (1994), with assessments of intelligence, somatosensory evoked potentials, and pattern visual evoked potentials. Their findings have suggested that prenatal exposure to PCBs affects higher cortical functions.

NEUROLOGICALLY COMPROMISED FETUS*

Not all neurologic problems can be diagnosed before birth or even some time after birth, and sometimes the causes of neurologic abnormalities cannot be determined with certainty. The prevalence of some abnormalities and their risk of recurrence, however, can be estimated. It is known, for instance, that genetic chromosomal, monogenic, and multifactorial abnormalities are present in 5.3% of individuals under the age of 25 (many of the abnormalities leading to early death would not be counted in this statistic), and many involve the nervous system (Beaudet et al, 1995). One well-known multifactorial neurologic abnormality, neural tube defect, seems to differ in frequency or prevalence depending on geographic factors, ethnic or racial background, the season during which conception occurs, maternal age and parity, and socioeconomic factors (Phillips and Elias, 1989). In the past, the prevalence of neural tube defects was 1.6 in 1000 in whites, 0.9 in 1000 in blacks, and 2.5 in 1000 in Puerto Ricans in the United States (Phillips and Elias, 1989). These rates have all decreased substantially (see the section on CNS malformations).

It is not always known why individuals have static encephalopathy (cerebral palsy); however, the most common causes are prenatal in origin (usually quoted as at least 50% of the total number) (Miller, 1992; Sunshine, 1989). In fact, fewer than 10% of cases can be shown to have

---

*Parts of this section have been published previously in Goddard-Finegold J: The neurologically compromised fetus. Semin Perinatol 17:304–311, 1993.

originated solely in the intrapartum period and only 10% to 18% in the postnatal period (Miller, 1992). Importantly, most children who ultimately show the signs and symptoms of cerebral palsy become symptomatic only as the first year of postnatal life progresses; they are not symptomatic during the neonatal period, and neurophysiologic or sonographic studies may show evidence of brain injury dating from the fetal period (Scher et al, 1991). Survivors in the group of infants who do have neonatal encephalopathy and other signs indicative of intrapartaum asphyxia have an average 25% incidence of permanent neuromotor or neuropsychologic deficits (Vannucci, 1990).

The issues of intrauterine infection and drug exposure have been discussed earlier. Clearly, enhancing diagnostic and treatment capabilities for prenatal problems such as these will reduce the burden of neurologic morbidity in offspring, and increasing public awareness of the problems related to drug and alcohol intake during pregnancy will certainly prevent many infants from suffering unnecessary CNS damage.

Assessment of Fetal Neurologic Status

Fetal Imaging

One of the most effective ways to assess fetal well-being is by ultrasound imaging. Fetal size, the presence of some fetal anomalies, the quantity of amniotic fluid, and the quantity and quality of fetal movements can be determined using ultrasound imaging.

Fetal Size. The intrauterine growth-retarded fetus, defined as the fetus whose weight is below the 10th percentile for gestational age, can be detected. Intrauterine growth retardation occurs in association with numerous pregnancy-associated problems that affect the nutrient or blood supply to the fetus; growth retardation can also be seen in fetuses with intrinsic problems, such as chromosomal abnormalities. Whenever there is decreased intervillous placental perfusion, such as with multiple gestations and serious placental pathology (abruptio, infarction, and placenta previa), there is likely to be a growth-retarded infant (Besinger et al, 1989; Hardwick et al, 1992). Various measurements, including the biparietal diameter, estimations of the amount of amniotic fluid present, abdominal circumference, and umbilical artery flow velocities, have increased the sensitivity and specificity of intrauterine diagnosis of the intrauterine growth-retarded infant (Besinger et al, 1989).

Both the growth-retarded fetus and the macrosomic fetus are at risk for neurologic complications, especially from hypoxia, before and during delivery. The postdates infant, infant of a diabetic mother, and infant of an obese mother are especially likely to be macrosomic (birth weight greater than 4500 g) (Thomas et al, 1989). These infants are at especially increased risk of complications at delivery, including shoulder dystocia (frequently leading to Erb palsy), meconium aspiration, and asphyxia (Thomas et al, 1989).

Fetal Central Nervous System Anomalies: Hydrocephalus and Neural Tube Defects. Fetal hydrocephalus oc-

curs in from 0.12 to 2.5 per 1000 births and can be diagnosed by ultrasound examination (Chervenak, 1989; Hardwick et al, 1992). A total of 124 cases of fetal hydrocephalus were reviewed by Evrard and colleagues (1989). Most of the cases were due to acquired obstructions of cerebrospinal fluid flow, usually as a result of prenatal infection or hemorrhage (Evrard et al, 1989). Prenatal primary hydrocephalus owing to nonperforation of the foramen of Luschka or Magendie or to abnormalities of subarachnoid cerebrospinal fluid reabsorption was rare. Fetal hydrocephalus can be diagnosed by prenatal ultrasound with measurement of biparietal diameter and ventricular size. The ratio of the diameter of the lateral ventricle and the cerebral mantle thickness can be used, but Evrard and colleagues (1989) stress that care must be taken to differentiate hydrocephalus from other CNS malformations, such as partial agenesis of the corpus callosum, cystic dilation of the choroid plexus, choroid plexus papillomas, and holoprosencephalies. Usually the diagnosis is made at around 30.5 weeks of gestation. Because ventricular size can be somewhat variable, when antenatal hydrocephalus is suspected earlier in gestation, it is advisable to repeat the ventricular measurements on successive sonograms (Chervenak, 1989; Evrard et al, 1989). It is also advisable to look carefully for other anomalies when fetal hydrocephalus is diagnosed; in a study of 53 cases of fetal hydrocephalus, major malformations were present in 83% (Chervenak, 1989).

Fetal ultrasonography and maternal serum AFP determinations are the most frequently used aids for diagnosing neural tube defects (Crane, 1992). Anencephaly can be diagnosed as early as 10 to 12 weeks' gestational age by fetal ultrasound; however, sonographic detection of open spina bifida is not as reliable (Crane, 1992). Amniotic fluid AFP and acetylcholinesterase determinations are also used when the ultrasound examination does not show a clear-cut lesion and the serum AFP is high (Crane, 1992).

Determination of Fetal Movement. The assessment of the quantity and quality of fetal movements as well as fetal position by ultrasonography has added useful information to that usually gained by asking about the mother's perceptions of her infant's movements. Specific types of fetal movements have been categorized, the timing of their appearance during gestation has been determined, and changes in frequency with increasing gestation have also been observed (Prechtl, 1989; Rayburn, 1989). Movements of certain types of abnormal fetuses have been characterized, and correlations with heart rate patterns and with fetal states have been made (Prechtl, 1989; Rayburn, 1989). In addition, comparisons have been made of monitored fetal movements to those reported by the mother (Gellinger et al, 1978).

Some neurologically compromised fetuses have extremely abnormal movements (or lack of movement). Anencephalic fetuses exhibit disturbed motor behavior (Prechtl, 1989). Excessive bursts of activity have been documented in these fetuses, and the movements have been described as jerky, causing large uterine shifts (Prechtl, 1989). Growth-retarded fetuses have been shown by Bekedam and coworkers (1985) to have slow, undynamic, monotonous movements, and fetuses with known chromosomal abnormalities have shown persistence of immature movement patterns (i.e., jerky movements and twitches usually seen at 13 to 14 weeks of gestation in normal fetuses have been shown still to be predominant at 19 to 20 weeks) (Boue and Vignal, 1982). When Gellinger and colleagues (1978) compared ultrasound quantitations with subjective maternal assessments of fetal movements, there was no correlation when maternal assessments were consistently of low fetal movement. Fetal movements have also been correlated with fetal heart rate patterns. By 20 to 22 weeks, there are diurnal variations for both fetal movements and heart rate patterns, with decreased movements, heart rate, and variation in the morning and increased movements, heart rate, and variation at night (deVries et al, 1988). Most important, and confirming clinical impressions that have been held for some time, was the finding that there is a significant association between abnormal fetal movements and stillbirth or poor neonatal condition (Leader et al, 1981). Abnormal fetal movements have been defined variously, including a day of no fetal movement or 2 consecutive days with fewer than 10 fetal movements or as the mother reporting fewer fetal movements than 3 per 12 hours or complete cessation of fetal movement for the same time period (Horimoto et al, 1993; Thomas et al, 1989).

Fetal Stress and Nonstress Tests

The concept that CNS function has measurable effects on fetal heart rate patterns is the basis for both the fetal nonstress and fetal stress tests (Hon and Quilligan, 1968; Smith and Phelan, 1989). Initial studies of fetal heart rate during labor indicated that abnormal fetal heart rate patterns (especially repeated late decelerations) were associated with greater incidence of fetal morbidity (Hon and Quilligan, 1968). Two tests have been developed based on these observations: (1) assessment of fetal heart rate patterns during contractions induced by oxytocin before the onset of labor (contraction stress test), and (2) the assessment of fetal heart rate patterns during fetal movements (the nonstress test)(Smith and Phelan, 1989). The nonstress test is considered *reactive* (indicating fetal well-being and the presence of an intact CNS) when fetal heart rate accelerates as fetal movements occur. Problems can be predicted when there is no heart rate reaction to fetal movement or when the nonstress test shows significant variable decelerations in heart rate (Smith and Phelan, 1989). Significant variable decelerations have been associated with umbilical cord compression.

The nonstress test is now used routinely to assess fetuses in many high-risk pregnancies. In a study by Devoe (1982), infants with abnormal contraction stress tests after nonreactive nonstress testing had a higher incidence of depressed Apgar scores at 5 minutes, intrauterine growth retardation, birth by primary cesarean section, and greater mortality incidence. There is also increased risk of fetal morbidity and mortality in fetuses with persistent nonreactive nonstress tests (Brown and Patrick, 1981). If the nonstress test is performed in very preterm infants (<26 to 28 weeks of gestation), however, immaturity of the nervous system may itself cause there to be a *nonreactive* result (Castillo et al, 1989).

Fetal Vibroacoustic Stimulation

Another method to assess fetal neurologic well-being is the application of a vibratory sound stimulus to the maternal abdomen to induce a startle response in the fetus and gain an objective idea of neurologic integrity (Divon et al, 1985). Movement and cardiac responses to sound stimuli have been compared, showing that between 37 and 40 weeks of gestation, cardiac responses are greater than movement responses, and that the amplitude of the cardiac response is increased when there is concomitant movement. The responses depend on the state of the fetus, with high variability heart rate patterns occurring when there are active periods and low variability heart rate patterns during sleep (Lecanuet et al, 1986). When there are repeated sound stimuli, the fetal responses decrease. This is called *habituation* and implies a normally functioning nervous system. Habituation has been shown to be abnormal in cases of anencephaly, in some intrauterine growth-retarded infants, in some meconium-stained infants, and in some fetuses with abnormal biparietal diameters (Leader et al, 1982). The safety of vibroacoustic stimulation has been questioned, and thus this procedure is not widely used.

Fetal Biophysical Profile

Independent variables such as fetal breathing movements, fetal body movements, fetal tone, amniotic fluid volume, and the fetal nonstress test have been used to assess fetal well-being. These individual tests have high false-positivity rates, however, sometimes 50% or more. Combining the tests has resulted in more accurate differentiation of an abnormal fetus; the combined data also correlate more closely with mortality outcome. Thus, a biophysical profile is obtained when the five variables listed are all measured during the same observation period. When all five variables are considered, the false-positive rate is considerably reduced, and the incidence of fetal distress increases as more of the tests in the profile become abnormal (Manning et al, 1980).

Fetal Doppler Blood Flow Studies

In addition to fetal movement evaluations, heart rate correlations, and vibroacoustic stimulation, it is also possible to assess blood flow velocity waveforms of the umbilical arteries and of the middle cerebral arteries using Doppler methodology (Weiss et al, 1992). Reduction, absence, or reversal of end-diastolic flow velocities in the umbilical arteries implies moderate to extreme increases in placental vascular resistance. In one study, 29 of 37 surviving infants with absent or reversed end-diastolic flow velocities in the umbilical arteries showed intrauterine growth retardation (Weiss et al, 1992); 11 of 37 had abnormal neurologic examinations at discharge, and 17 of 37 had evidence of abnormal resistance of the middle cerebral arteries on Doppler examination. At present, the value of Doppler flow velocity studies for long-term neurologic prognosis is not yet clear.

Near-Infrared Spectroscopy

Near-infrared spectroscopy is a newly available method for noninvasive monitoring of cerebral oxygenation, blood volume, and blood flow (Rea et al, 1985). Light in the near-infrared spectrum is produced by laser diodes and is passed through the brain. Light in certain near-infrared wavelengths is absorbed by the iron in hemoglobin and the copper in cytochrome aa_3 (part of the mitochondrial electron transport chain). Iron and copper absorb different wavelengths depending on their oxidation or reduction status. Using algorithms derived for scatter of infrared light through newborn brain, interoptrode distances, and other physical properties affecting the infrared light, the amount of oxidized or reduced hemoglobin can be quantitated, and the oxidation status of cytochrome aa_3 can be determined. In addition, by instituting a transient change in F_{IO_2}, the immediate change in amount of oxygenated hemoglobin can be used as a *tracer* for estimating cerebral blood flow (Edwards et al, 1988). Currently, techniques for using near-infrared spectroscopy technology on the fetal head during labor are being perfected (Rolfe et al, 1991).

Special Problems of Fetal Assessment
Akinetic Fetus

Fetuses with abnormalities of the nervous system, nerve innervation, or muscle; with defective skin or connective tissue; or with structural limitations of movement (e.g., oligohydramnios, extrauterine pregnancy, bicornuate uterus) may show lack or diminution of fetal movements and may have other manifestations of the *fetal akinesia deformation sequence* (Hall, 1986, 1992; Jones, 1988). Fetal akinesia can result in pulmonary hypoplasia, polyhydramnios, contractures of fetal joints (arthrogryposis), a short umbilical cord, short gut, and dysmorphic features (Jones, 1988). Fetal akinesia has been associated with certain syndromes, including cerebro-oculofacioskeletal syndrome, chromosomal abnormalities, Freeman-Sheldon syndrome, cerebroarthrodigital syndrome, and the multiple pterygium syndrome. The fetal akinesia sequence has also been called the *Pena-Shokeir phenotype* (Hall, 1986; Jones, 1988). Infants with fetal and neonatal neuromuscular weakness (e.g., anterior horn cell disease, congenital muscular dystrophy, congenital hypomyelination neuropathy) may also show reduced fetal movement and, if severe enough, part or all of the Pena-Shokeir phenotype.

Intrauterine Fetal Brain Death

When prenatal evaluation shows a fixed heart rate pattern, intrauterine fetal brain death should be suspected (Zimmer et al, 1992). Although fetal brain death has already occurred, in some instances fetal systemic growth and development are not affected. Fetal body and breathing movements are usually decreased or absent. Usually when fixed fetal heart rates are detected and fetal movement has ceased, further studies, such as fetal movement and heart rate correlations, vibroacoustic stimulation, and ultrasound imaging of the fetal head, show evidence of severe brain injury. If other causes of a fixed heart rate have been excluded (such as anencephaly, prolonged fetal deep sleep state, other developmental CNS anomalies, and effects of drugs or hypoxia), these findings most likely represent fetal brain death (Zimmer et al, 1992). It is also possible that

some fetal tachyarrhythmias may exceed the capability of the monitoring system to respond appropriately electronically and should be considered in the differential diagnosis.

Antenatal Central Nervous System Damage and Cerebral Palsy

The potential for highly specific diagnostic capabilities, preventive measures, and therapies seems great for high-risk fetuses in the future. As more effective postnatal, neuronal and glial protection agents, and prevention strategies for hypoxic-ischemic injury become available, their application to the fetus will not lag far behind. Thus, the accurate assessment of the neurologic status of the fetus will become even more important, and the timing of the onset of neurologic insult will be more feasible. This will also be important for elucidating the relative roles of prenatal, perinatal, and postnatal factors with respect to neurologic outcome. Currently, it is thought that primary antepartum events account for about 20% of cases of neonatal hypoxic-ischemic encephalopathy; primary intrapartum events are thought to account for 35% of cases, and both antepartum and intrapartum factors are thought to play a role in an additional 35%. Only about 10% of infants have hypoxic-ischemic encephalopathy due solely to postnatal events. These figures relate only to the incidence of neonatal encephalopathy and not to neurologic outcome. Data on term infants from the National Collaborative Study indicate that only 37% of patients with cerebral palsy came from the group with the greatest number of risk factors; furthermore, 97% of the infants with the highest risk did not develop cerebral palsy. In studies of patients with cerebral palsy, it has become clear that in only about 8% can the cerebral palsy be attributed to perinatal hypoxic-ischemic events. This implies that there are a number of prenatal factors that play a role in the genesis of cerebral palsy that have yet to be identified both in individual cases and in populations of patients.

REFERENCES

Acers TE: Optic nerve hypoplasia: Septo-optic-pituitary dysplasia syndrome. Trans Am Ophthalmol Soc 79:425, 1981.

Adams B, Dorfler P, Aguzzi A, et al: pax-5 encodes the transcription factor BSAP and is expressed in B lymphocytes, the developing CNS, and adult testes. Genes Dev 6:1589, 1992.

Albengres E, Tillement JP: Phenytoin in pregnancy: A review of the reported risks. Bil Res Preg 4:71, 1983.

Albright AL, Gartner JC, Wiener ES: Lumbar cutaneous hemangiomas as indicators of tethered spinal cords. Pediatrics 83:977, 1989.

Alexander D: Introduction. *In* Zagon IS, Slotkin TA (Eds): Maternal Substance Abuse and the Developing Nervous System. New York, Academic Press, 1992, pp 1–3.

Alles AJ, Sulik KK: Retinoic acid-induced spina bifida: Evidence for a pathogenetic mechanism. Development 108:73, 1990.

Altman NR, Naidich TP, Braffman BH: Posterior fossa malformations. AJNR Am J Neuroradiol 13:691, 1992.

Amin-Zaki L: Prenatal methyl mercury poisoning: Clinical observations over five years. Am J Dis Child 133:172, 1979.

Anderson FM: Occult spinal dysraphism: A series of 73 cases. Pediatrics 55:826, 1975.

Armstrong DD: Neonatal encephalopathies. *In* Duckett S (Ed): Pediatric Neuropathology. Baltimore, Williams & Wilkins, 1995, pp 334–352.

Barkovich AJ, Norman D: Absence of the septum pellucidum: A useful sign in the diagnosis of congenital brain malformations. Am J Radiol 152:353, 1989.

Bavinck JN, Weaver DD: Subclavian artery supply disruption sequence: Hypothesis of a vascular origin for Poland, Klippel-Feil, and Moebius anomalies. Am J Med Genet 23:903, 1986.

Bayer SA, Altman J, Russo RJ, et al: Embryology. *In* Duckett S (Ed): Pediatric Neuropathology. Baltimore, Williams & Wilkins, 1995, pp 54–108.

Beaudet AL, Scriver CR, Sly WS, et al: Genetics, biochemistry, and molecular basis of variant human phenotypes. *In* Scriver CR, Beaudet AL, Sly WS, Valle D (Eds): The Metabolic and Molecular Bases of Inherited Disease, 7th ed. New York, McGraw-Hill, 1995, pp 53–229.

Becerra JE, Khoury MJ, Cordero JF, et al: Diabetes mellitus during pregnancy and the risks for specific birth defects: A population-based case-control study. Pediatrics 85:1, 1990.

Becker LE, Armstrong DL, Chan F: Dendritic atrophy in children with Down syndrome. Ann Neurol 20:520, 1986.

Bekedam DJ, Visser GHA, DeVries JJ, et al: Motor behaviour in the growth retarded fetus. Early Human Dev 12:155, 1985.

Bell DG, King BF, Hattery RR, et al: Imaging characteristics of tuberous sclerosis. AJR Am J Roentgenol 156:1081, 1991.

Beltran RS, Coker SB: Transient dystonia of infancy, a result of intrauterine cocaine exposure? Pediatr Neurol 12:354, 1995.

Benacerraf BR, Harlow B, Frigoletto FD Jr: Are choroid plexus cysts an indication for second-trimester amniocentesis? Am J Obstet Gynecol 162:1001, 1990.

Benda CE: The Dandy-Walker syndrome or the so-called atresia of the foramen of Magendie. J Neuropathol Exp Neurol 13:14, 1954.

Besinger RE, Repke JT, Ferguson JE: Preterm labor and intrauterine growth retardation: Complex obstetrical problems with low birth weight infants. *In* Stevenson DK, Sunshine P (Eds): Fetal and Neonatal Brain Injury: Mechanisms, Management, and the Risks of Practice. Philadelphia, BC Decker, 1989, pp 11–33.

Bisby MA: Functions of retrograde transport. Fed Proc 41:2307, 1982.

Blaauw G: Defect in posterior arch of atlas in myelomeningocele. Dev Med Child Neurol 13(suppl 25):113, 1971.

Black MM, Lasek RJ: Slow components of axonal transport: Two cytoskeletal networks. J Cell Biol 86:616, 1980.

Boue J, Vignal P: Ultrasound movement patterns of fetuses with chromosome abnormalities. Prenat Diagn 2:61, 1982.

Brock DJ: Mechanisms by which amniotic-fluid alpha-feto-protein may be increased in fetal abnormalities. Lancet 2:345, 1976.

Brown MS, Sheridan-Pereira M: Outlook for the child with a cephalocele. Pediatrics 90:914, 1992.

Brown R, Patrick J: The nonstress test: How long is enough? Am J Obstet Gynecol 141:646, 1981.

Buehler BA, Delimont D, Van Waes M, et al: Prenatal prediction of risk of the fetal hydantoin syndrome. N Engl J Med 322:1567, 1990.

Cashman N, Covault J, Wollman R, et al: Neural cell adhesion molecule in normal, denervated, and myopathic human muscle. Ann Neurol 21:481, 1987.

Castillo RA, Devoe LD, Arthur M, et al: The preterm nonstress test: Effects of gestational age and length of study. Am J Obstet 160:172, 1989.

Chen Y-J, Hsu C-C: Effects of prenatal exposure to PCBs on the neurological function of children: A neuropsychological and neurophysiological study. Dev Med Child Neurol 36:312, 1994.

Chervenak FA: Current perspectives on the diagnosis, prognosis, and management of fetal hydrocephalus. *In* Hill A, Volpe JJ (Eds): Fetal Neurology. New York, Raven Press, 1989, pp 231–253.

Choi BH, Lapham LW, Amin-Zaki L, et al: Abnormal neuronal migration, deranged cerebral cortical organization, and diffuse white matter astrocytosis of human fetal brain: A major effect of methylmercury poisoning in utero. J Neuropathol Exp Neurol 37:719, 1978.

Cohen BA: Incontinentia pigmenti. Neurol Clin North Am 5:361, 1987.

Committee on Substance Abuse and Committee on Children with Disabilities: Fetal alcohol syndrome and fetal alcohol effects. Pediatrics 91:1004, 1993.

Condon KW, Soileau LC, Silberstein L, et al: Development and innervation of muscle fiber types in the rat hindbrain. *In* Landmesser LT (Ed): The Assembly of the Nervous System. New York, Alan R. Liss, 1989, pp 51–65.

Cordero ME, Trejo M, Carcia E, et al: Dendritic development in the neocortex of adult rats following a maintained prenatal and/or early postnatal life undernutrition. Early Hum Dev 14:245, 1986.

Costa C, Hauw JJ: Pathology of the cerebellum, brainstem, and spinal cord. *In* Duckett S (Ed): Pediatric Neuropathology. Baltimore, Williams & Wilkins, 1995, pp 217–239.

Covault J, Merlie JP, Goridis C, et al: Molecular forms of NCAM and its RNA in developing and denervated skeletal muscle. J Cell Biol 102:731, 1986.

Crane JP: Sonographic detection of neural tube defects. *In* Elias S, Simpson JL (Eds): Maternal Serum Screening for Fetal Genetic Disorders. New York, Churchill-Livingstone, 1992, pp 59–74.

Crowe CA, Heuther CA, Oppenheimer SG, et al: The epidemiology of spina bifida in south-western Ohio—1970–1979. Dev Med Child Neurol 27:176, 1985.

Cuckle HS: Screening for neural tube defects. *In* Bock G, Marsh J (Eds): Neural Tube Defects: Ciba Foundation Symposium 181. Chicester, John Wiley & Sons, 1994, pp 253–267.

Curatolo P, Mercuri S, Cotroneo E: Joubert syndrome: A case confirmed by computerized tomography. Dev Med Child Neurol 22:362, 1980.

Czeizel AE, Dudas I: Prevention of the first occurrence of neural tube defects by periconceptional vitamin supplementation. N Engl J Med 317:1832, 1992.

D'Agostino AN, Kernohan JW, Brown JR: Dandy-Walker syndrome. J Neuropathol Exp Neurol 22:450, 1963.

DeLaCruz E, Sun S, Vangvanichyzkorn K, et al: Multiple congenital malformations associated with maternal isotretinoin therapy. Pediatrics 74:428, 1984.

DeMyer W: Megalencephaly in children: Clinical syndromes, genetic patterns, and differential diagnosis from other causes of megalocephaly. Neurology 22:634, 1972.

Devoe LD: Antepartum FHR testing in preterm pregnancy. Obstet Gynecol 50:431, 1982.

deVries LS, Larroche J-C, Levene MI: Fetal encephalopathy of circulatory origin. *In* Levene MI, Bennett MJ, Punt J (Eds): Fetal and Neonatal Neurology and Neurosurgery. Edinburgh, Churchill-Livingstone, 1988, pp 339–346.

Diebler C, Dulac O: Pediatric Neurology and Neuroradiology. Berlin, Springer-Verlag, 1987, pp 51–57.

Divon MY, Platt LD, Cantrell CJ, et al: Evoked fetal startle response: A possible intrauterine neurological examination. Am J Obstet Gynecol 153:454, 1985.

Dobyns WB, Stratton RF, Greenberg F: Syndromes with lissencephaly: I. Miller-Dieker and Norman-Roberts syndromes and isolated lissencephaly. Am J Med Genet 18:509, 1984.

Dodge PR, Holmes SJ, Sotos JF: Cerebral gigantism. Dev Med Child Neurol 25:248, 1983.

Donis-Keller H, Dou S, Chi D, et al: Mutations in the RET proto-oncogene are associated with MEN 2A and FMTC. Hum Mol Genet 2:851, 1993.

Duester G: A hypothetical mechanism for fetal alcohol syndrome involving ethanol inhibition of retinoic acid synthesis at the alcohol dehydrogenase step. Alcohol Clin Exp Res 15:568, 1991.

Edery P, Lyonnet S, Mulligan LM, et al: Mutations of the RET proto-oncogene in Hirschsprung's disease. Nature 367:378, 1994.

Edwards AD, Wyatt JS, Richardson C, et al: Cotside measurement of cerebral blod flow by near infrared spectroscopy. Lancet 2:770, 1988.

Egger J, Bellman MM, Ross EM, et al: Joubert-Boltshauser syndrome with polydactyly in siblings. J Neurol Neurosurg Psychiatry 45:737, 1982.

Encha-Razavi F: Fetal neuropathology. *In* Duckett S (Ed): Pediatric Neuropathology. Baltimore, Williams & Wilkins, 1995, pp 108–123.

England MA: Normal development of the central nervous system. *In* Levene MI, Bennett MJ, Punt J (Eds): Fetal and Neonatal Neurology and Neurosurgery. Edinburgh, Churchill-Livingstone, 1988, pp 3–31.

Evrard P, Kadhim HJ, de Saint-Georges P, et al: Abnormal development and destructive processes of the human brain during the second half of gestation. *In* Evrard P, Minkowski A (Eds): Developmental Neurobiology. Nestle Nutrition Workshop Series, 12. New York, Raven Press, 1989, pp 1–12.

Fernhoff PM, Lammer EJ: Craniofacial features of isotretinoin embryopathy. J Pediatr 105:595, 1984.

Ferrer I, Galofre E: Dendritic spine anomalies in fetal alcohol syndrome. Neuropediatrics 18:161, 1987.

Ferriero DM, Arcavi LJ, Sagar SM, et al: Selective sparing of NADPH-diaphorase neurons in neonatal hypoxia-ischemia. Ann Neurol 24:670, 1988.

Figarella-Branger D, Pellissier JF: Pathologic changes in muscle development. *In* Duckett S (Ed): Pediatric Neuropathology. Baltimore, Williams & Willkins, 1995, pp 785–822.

Finnell RH, Buehler BA, Kerr BM, et al: Clinical and experimental studies linking oxidative metabolism to phenytoin-induced teratogenesis. Neurology 42(suppl 5):25, 1992.

Fitzsimmons J, Wilson D, Pascoe-Mason J, et al: Choroid plexus cysts in fetuses with trisomy 18. Obstet Gynecol 73:257, 1989.

Fois A, Calistri L, Balestri P, et al: Relationship between café-au-lait spots as the only symptom and peripheral neurofibromatosis (NF-1)—a follow-up study. Eur J Pediatr 152:500–504, 1993.

Fox CH: Cocaine use in pregnancy. J Am Board Fam Pract 7:225, 1994.

Friede RL: Developmental Neuropathology, 2nd ed. New York, Springer-Verlag, 1989.

Friede RL, Boltshauser E: Uncommon syndromes of cerebellar vermis aplasia: I. Joubert syndrome. Dev Med Child Neurol 20:758, 1978.

Fukuyama YM, Ohsawa M, Suzuki H: Congenital progressive muscular dystrophy of the Fukuyama type: Clinical genetic and pathologic considerations. Brain Dev 3:1, 1984.

Gadisseux JF, Kadhim HJ, van den Bosch de Aguilar P, et al: Neuron migration within the radial glial fiber system of the developing murine cerebrum: An electron microscopic autoradiographic analysis. Dev Brain Res 52:39, 1990.

Gadisseux JF, Rodriguez J, Lyon G: Pontoneocerebellar hypoplasia—a probable consequence of prenatal destruction of the pontine nuclei and a possible role of phenytoin intoxication. Clin Neuropathol 3:160, 1984.

Gettinger A, Roberts AB, Campbell S: Comparison between subjective and ultrasound assessments of fetal movement. Br Med J 2:88–90, 1978.

Ghosh A, Antonini A, McConnell SK, et al: Requirement for subplate neurons in the formation of thalamocortical connections. Nature 347:179, 1990.

Gieron-Korthals MA, Helal A, Martinez CR: Expanding spectrum of cocaine induced central nervous system malformations. Brain Dev (Netherlands) 16:253, 1994.

Gilbert JN, Jones KL, Rorke LB, et al: Central nervous system anomalies associated with meningomyelocele, hydrocephalus, and the Arnold-Chiari malformation: Reappraisal of theories regarding the pathogenesis of posterior neural tube closure defects. Neurosurgery 18:559, 1986.

Golden JA, Chernoff GF: Intermittent pattern of neural tube closure in two strains of mice. Teratology 47:73, 1993.

Golden JA, Chernoff GF: Multiple sites of anterior neural tube closure in humans: Evidence from anterior neural tube defects (anencephaly). Pediatrics 95:506, 1995.

Gower DJ, Del Curling O, Kelly DLJ, et al: Diastematomyelia—a 40-year experience. Pediatr Neurosci 14:90, 1988.

Green AJ, Johnson PH, Yates JR: The tuberous sclerosis gene on chromosome 9q34 acts as a growth suppressor. J Hum Mol Genet 3:1833, 1994.

Grose C: Congenital infections caused by varicella zoster virus and herpes simplex virus. Semin Pediatr Neurol 1:43, 1994.

Gutmann DH, Collins FS: Recent progress toward understanding the molecular biology of von Recklinghausen neurofibromatosis. Ann Neurol 31:555, 1992.

Hall DE, Udvarhelyi GB, Altman J: Lumbosacral skin lesions as markers of occult spinal dysraphism. JAMA 246:2606, 1981.

Hall JG: Invited editorial comment: Analysis of Pena-Shokeir phenotype. Am J Med Genet 25:99, 1986.

Hall JG: Developmental defects in stillborn and newborn infants. *In* Dimmick JE, Kalousek DK (Eds): Developmental Pathology of the Embryo and Fetus. Philadelphia, JB Lippincott, 1992, pp 111–142.

Hanieh A, Simpson DA, Worth JB: Arachnoid cyst: A critical survey of 41 cases. Childs Nerv Syst 4:92, 1988.

Hanson JW, Buehler BA: Fetal hydantoin syndrome: Current status. J Pediatr 101:816, 1982.

Hanson JW, Streissguth AP, Smith DW: The effects of moderate alcohol consumption during pregnancy on fetal growth and morphogenesis. J Pediatr 92:457, 1978.

Harada M: Congenital minamata disease: Intrauterine and methyl mercury poisoning. Teratology 18:285, 1978.

Hardwick DF, Dimmick JE, Kalousek DK, et al: Concepts of intrauterine development and embryofetal pathology. *In* Dimmick JE, Kalousek DK (Eds): Developmental Pathology of the Embryo and Fetus. Philadelphia, JB Lippincott, 1992, pp 26–54.

Hart MN, Malamud N, Ellis WG: The Dandy-Walker syndrome: A clinico-pathological study based on 28 cases. Neurology 22:771, 1972.

Hasegawa Y, Hasegawa T, Yokoyama T, et al: Holoprosencephaly associ-

ated with diabetes insipidus and syndrome of inappropriate secretion of antidiuretic hormone. J Pediatr 117:756, 1990.

Herschkowitz N: Brain development in the fetus, neonate, and infant. Biol Neonate 54:1, 1988.

Hill RM: Fetal malformations and antiepileptic drugs. Am J Dis Child 130:923, 1976.

Hill RM, Verniaud WM, Horning MG, et al: Infants exposed in utero to antiepileptic drugs. Am J Dis Child 127:645, 1974.

Hon EH, Quilligan EJ: Electronic evaluation of the fetal heart rate. Clin Obstet Gynecol 11:145, 1968.

Horimoto N, Koyanagi T, Maeda H, et al: Can brain impairment be detected by in utero behavioural patterns? Arch Dis Child 69:3, 1993.

Hunt GM, Holmes AE: Some factors relating to intelligence in treated children with spina bifida cystica. Dev Med Child Neurol 17(suppl):65, 1975.

Huttenlocher PR: Dendritic and synaptic pathology in mental retardation. Pediatr Neurol 7:79, 1991.

Ioffe S, Chernick V: Development of the EEG between 30 and 40 weeks gestation in normal and alcohol-exposed infants. Dev Med Child Neurol 30:797, 1988.

Jacobson M: Developmental Neurobiology. New York, Plenum Press, 1991.

James CCM, Lassman LP: Spinal Dysraphism: Spina Bifida Occulta. London, Butterworth, 1972.

Janerich DT, Piper J: Shifting genetic patterns in anencephaly and spina bifida. J Med Genet 15:101, 1978.

Jeret JS, Serur D, Wisniewski KE, et al: Clinicopathological findings associated with agenesis of the corpus callosum. Brain Dev 9:255, 1987.

Jervis GA: Early familial cerebellar degeneration (report of three cases in one family). J Nerv Ment Dis 111:398, 1950.

Jones KL: Aberrant neuronal migration in the fetal alcohol syndrome. Birth Def 7:131, 1975.

Jones KL: Pena-Shokeir phenotype (fetal akinesia/hypokinesia sequence). *In* Jones KL (Ed): Smith's Recognizable Patterns of Human Malformation, 4th ed. Philadelphia, WB Saunders, 1988, pp 144–146.

Jones KL: Developmental pathogenesis of defects associated with prenatal cocaine exposure: Fetal vascular disruption. Clin Perinatol 18:139, 1991.

Jones KL, Lacro RV, Johnson KA, et al: Pattern or malformations in the children of women treated with carbamazepine during pregnancy. N Engl J Med 320:1661, 1989.

Jones KL, Smith DW, Ulleland CN, et al: Pattern of malformation in offspring of chronic alcoholic mothers. Lancet 1:1267, 1973.

Joubert M, Eisenring JJ, Robb JP, Andermann F: Familial agenesis of the cerebellar vermis: A syndrome of episodic hyperpnea, abnormal eye movements, ataxia, and retardation. Neurology 19:813, 1969.

Juntunen J, Teravainen H: Structural development of myoneural junctions in the human embryo. Histochemistry 32:107, 1972.

Keir WJ: Inhibition of retinoic acid synthesis and its implications in fetal alcohol syndrome. Alcohol Clin Exp Res 15:560, 1991.

Kinney HC, Brody BA, Kloman AS, et al: Sequence of central nervous system myelination in human infancy. J Neuropathol Exp Neurol 47:217, 1988.

Kitahara T, Maki Y: A case of Sturge-Weber disease with epilepsy and intracranial calcifications at the neonatal period. Eur Neurol 17:8, 1978.

Knudsen K, McElwee SA, Myers L: A role for the neural cell adhesion molecule NCAM in myoblast interaction during myogenesis. Dev Biol 138:159, 1990.

Krauss CM, Holmes LB, Vanlang QN, et al: Four siblings with similar malformations after exposure to phenytoin and primidone. J Pediatr 105:750, 1984.

Kuratsune M, Yoshimura T, Matsuzaka J: Yusho, a poisoning caused by rice oil contaminated with chlorinated biphenyls. Environ Health Perspect 1:119, 1972.

Lacey DJ: Hippocampal dendritic abnormalities in a rat model of phenylketonuria. Ann Neurol 16:577, 1984.

Landon DN: Skeletal muscle, normal morphology, development and innervation. *In* Mastaglia FL, Walton J (Eds): Skeletal Muscle Pathology. New York, Churchill-Livingstone, 1982, pp 1–87.

Laurence KM: Recurrence risk of neural tube defects (letter). J Med Genet 18:322, 1981.

Leader LR, Baillie P, Martin B, et al: Fetal habituation in high-risk pregnancies. Br J Obstet Gynaecol 89:441, 1982.

Leader LR, Baillie P, Van Schalkwyk DJ: Fetal movements and fetal outcome: A prospective study. Obstet Gynecol 57:431, 1981.

Lecanuet J-P, Granier-Deferre C, Cohen H, et al: Fetal responses to acoustic stimulation depend on heart rate variability pattern, stimulus intensity, and repetition. Early Hum Dev 13:269, 1986.

Ledbetter SA, Kuwano A, Dobyns WB, et al: Microdeletions of chromosome 17p13 as a cause of isolated lissencephaly. Am J Hum Genet 50:182, 1992.

LeDouarin NM: The Neural Crest. New York, Cambridge University Press, 1982.

Leech RW, Shuman RM: Holoprosencephaly and related midline cerebral anomalies: A review. J Child Neurol 1:3, 1986.

Lenke RR, Levy HL: Maternal phenylketonuria and hyperphenylalanemia: An international survey of the outcome of untreated and treated pregnancies. N Engl J Med 303:1202, 1980.

Listernick R, Charrow J: Neurofibromatosis type 1 in childhood. J Pediatr 116:845, 1990.

Lorber J: Systematic ventriculographic studies in infants born with meningomyelocele and encephalocele. Arch Dis Child 36:381, 1961.

Lott IT, Bocian M, Bribram HW, et al: Fetal hydrocephalus and ear anomalies associated with maternal use of isotretinoin. J Pediatr 105:597, 1984.

Louis DN, von Deimling A: Hereditary tumor syndromes of the nervous system: Overview and rare syndromes. Brain Pathol 5:145, 1995.

Manning FA, Platt LD, Sipos L: Antepartum fetal evaluation: Development of a fetal biophysical profile. Am J Obstet Gynecol 136:787, 1980.

Margalith D, Jan JE, McCormick AQ, et al: Clinical spectrum of congenital optic nerve hypoplasia: A review of 51 patients. Dev Med Child Neurol 26:311, 1984.

Marin-Padilla M: Early ontogenesis of the human cerebral cortex. *In* Peters A, Jones EG (Eds): Cerebral Cortex: Vol 7. Development and Maturation of Cerebral Cortex. New York, Plenum Press, 1988, pp 1–30.

Marin-Padilla M, Marin-Padilla TM: Morphogenesis of experimentally induced Arnold-Chiari malformation. J Neurol Sci 50:29, 1981.

McLone DG, Dias L, Kaplan WE, et al: Concepts in the management of spina bifida. *In* Marlin AE (Ed): Concepts in Pediatric Neurosurgery, Vol 5. Basel, Karger, 1985, pp 97–106.

McLone DG: Continuing concepts in the management of spina bifida. Pediatr Neurosurg 18:254, 1992.

Menkes JH: Malformations of the central nervous system. *In* Taeusch HW, Ballard RA, Avery ME (Eds): Diseases of the Newborn, 6th ed. Philadelphia, WB Saunders, 1991, pp 426–445.

Ment LR, Stewart WB, Ardito TA, et al: Beagle pup germinal matrix maturation studies. Stroke 2:390, 1991.

Ment LR, Stewart WB, Ardito TA, et al: Germinal matrix microvascular maturation correlates inversely with the risk period for neonatal intraventricular hemorrhage. Dev Brain Res 84:142, 1995.

Michaud J, Mizrahi EM, Urich H: Agenesis of the vermis with fusion of the cerebellar hemispheres, septo-optic dysplasia, and associated anomalies: Report of a case. Acta Neuropathol (Berlin) 56:161, 1982.

Miller G: Cerebral palsies. *In* Miller G, Ramer JC (Eds): Static Encephalopathies of Infancy and Childhood. New York, Raven Press, 1992, pp 11–27.

Milunsky A, Alpert E, Neff RK, et al: Prenatal diagnosis of neural tube defects: IV. Maternal serum alpha-fetoprotein screening. Obstet Gynecol 55:60, 1980.

Monson RR, Rosenberg L, Hartz SC, et al: Diphenylhydantoin and selected congenital malformations. N Engl J Med 289:1049, 1973.

Moore SE, Walsh FS: Specific regulation of NCAM cell adhesion molecule during muscle development. EMBO J 4:623, 1985.

Mott SH, Bodensteiner JB, Allen WC: The cavum septi pellucidi in term and preterm newborn infants. J Child Neurol 7:35, 1992.

MRC Vitamin Study Research Group: Prevention of neural tube defects: Results of the MRC vitamin study. Lancet 338:132, 1992.

Muller F, O'Rahilly R: The human chondrocranium at the end of the embryonic period proper, with particular reference to the nervous system. Am J Anat 159:33–58, 1980.

Mulligan LM, Kwok JB, Healey CS, et al: Germ-line mutations of the RET proto-oncogene in multiple endocrine neoplasia type 2A. Nature 363:458, 1993.

Myhre SA, Williams R: Teratogenic effects associated with maternal primidone therapy. J Pediatr 99:160, 1981.

Naidich TP, Pudlowshi RM, Naidich JB: Computed tomographic signs of Chiari II malformation: II. Midbrain and cerebellum. Radiology 134:391, 1980.

Nelhaus G, Haberland C, Hill BJ: Sturge-Weber disease with bilateral intracranial calcifications at birth and unusual pathologic findings. Acta Neurol Scand 43:314, 1967.

Neumann PE, Frankel WN, Letts VA, et al: Multifactorial inheritance of neural tube defects: Localization of the major gene and recognition of modifiers in *ct* mutant mice. Nat Genet 6:357, 1994.

Norman MG: Perinatal brain damage. Perspect Pediatr Pathol 4:41, 1978.

Norman MG: Central nervous system. *In* Dimmick JE, Kalousek DK (Eds): Developmental Pathology of the Embryo and Fetus. Philadelphia, JB Lippincott, 1992, pp 341–383.

Norman MG, Becker LE: Cerebral damage in neonates resulting from arteriovenous malformation in the vein of Galen. J Neurol Neurosurg Psychiatry 37:252, 1974.

Norman RM, Urich H: Cerebellar hypoplasia associated with systemic degeneration in early life. J Neurol Neurosurg Psychiatry 21:159, 1958.

Oakley GP, Erickson JD, James LM, et al: Prevention of folic acid–preventable spina bifida and anencephaly. *In* Bock G, Marsh J (Eds): Neural Tube Defects: CIBA Foundation Symposium 181. Chicester, John Wiley & Sons, 1994, pp 212–231.

O'Rahilly R, Muller F: The Embryonic Human Brain: An Atlas of Developmental Stages. New York, Wiley-Liss, 1994.

Ordahl CP, LeDouarin N: Two myogenic lineages within the developing somite. Development 114:339, 1992.

Ouvrier R, Billson F: Optic nerve hypoplasia: A review. J Child Neurol 1:181, 1986.

Pagon RA, Chandler JW: Hydrocephalus, agyria, retinal dysplasia, encephalocele (HARD +E) syndrome: An autosomal recessive condition. Birth Def 14:233, 1978.

Painter MJ: Animal models of perinatal asphyxia: Contributions, contradictions, clinical relevance. Semin Pediatr Neurol 2:37, 1995.

Parrish ML, Roessmann U, Levinsohn MW: Agenesis of the corpus callosum: A study of the frequency of associated malformations. Ann Neurol 6:349, 1979.

Peach B: Arnold-Chiari malformation: Anatomic features in 20 cases. Arch Neurol 12:613, 1965.

Peiffer J, Majewski F, Fischbach H: Alcohol embryo and fetopathy: Neuropathology of 3 children and 3 fetuses. J Neurol Sci 41:125, 1979.

Phelan MC, Pellock JM, Nance WE: Discordant expression of fetal hydantoin syndrome in heteropaternal dizygotic twins. N Engl J Med 307:99, 1982.

Phillips OP, Elias S: Genetics and epidemiology of neural tube defects. *In* Elias S, Simpson JL (Eds): Maternal Serum Screening for Fetal Genetic Disorders. New York, Churchill-Livingstone, 1989, pp 1–23.

Phillips SJ, Dooley JM, Camfield PR: Vein of Galen malformation with cerebral calcification: A reversible cause of neurodegenerative disease. Can J Neurol Sci 13:103, 1986.

Pleet H, Graham JM Jr, Smith DW: Central nervous system and facial defects associated with maternal hyperthermia at four to 14 weeks' gestation. Pediatrics 67:785, 1981.

Pons F, Leger JOC, Chevallay M, et al: Immunocytochemical analysis of myosin heavy chains in human fetal skeletal muscles. J Neurol Sci 76:151, 1986.

Prechtl H: The Neurological Examination of the Full Term Newborn Infant, 2nd ed. London, Spastics International Medical Publications, 1977.

Prechtl HFR: Fetal behavior. *In* Hill A, Volpe JJ (Eds): Fetal Neurology. New York, Raven Press, 1989, pp 1–16.

Rakic P: Defects of neuronal migration and the pathogenesis of cortical malformations. Prog Brain Res 73:15, 1988.

Rakic P, Sidman RL: Telencephalic origin of pulvinar neurons in the fetal human brain. Z Anat Entwickl Gesch 129:53, 1969.

Rami A, Patel AJ, Rabie A: Thyroid hormone and development of the rat hippocampus: Morphological alterations in granule and pyramidal cells. J Neurosci 19:1217, 1986.

Rayburn WF: Antepartum fetal monitoring: Fetal movement. *In* Hill A, Volpe JJ (Eds): Fetal Neurology. New York, Raven Press, 1989, pp 17–36.

Rea PA, Crowe J, Wickramasinghe Y, et al: Non-invasive optical methods for the study of cerebral metabolism in the human newborn: A technique for the future? J Med Eng Technol 9:160, 1985.

Reznik M, Pierard GE: Neurophakomatoses and allied disorders. *In* Duckett S (Ed): Pediatric Neuropathology. Baltimore, Williams & Wilkins, 1995, pp 734–755.

Riccardi VM, Marcus ES: Congenital hydrocephalus and cerebellar agenesis. Clin Genet 13:443, 1978.

Rieger F, Grumet M, Edelman GM: NCAM at the vertebrate neuromuscular junction. J Cell Biol 101:285, 1985.

Rizzo R, Lammer EJ, Parano E, et al: Limb reduction defects in humans associated with prenatal isotretinoin exposure. Teratology 44:599, 1991.

Robain O, Lyon G: Familial microcephalies due to cerebral malformation: Anatomical and clinical study. Acta Neuropathol 20:96, 1972.

Roessmann U: Congenital malformations. *In* Duckett S (Ed): Pediatric Neuropathology. Baltimore, Williams & Wilkins, 1995, pp 123–149.

Rogan WJ, Galden BC, Hung KL, et al: Congenital poisoning by polychlorinated biphenyls and their contaminants in Taiwan. Science 241:334, 1988.

Rolfe P, Wickramasinghe Y, Thorniley MS: The potential of near infrared spectroscopy for detection of fetal cerebral hypoxia. Eur J Obstet Gynecol 42:S24, 1991.

Romeo G, Ronchetto P, Luo Y, et al: Point mutations affecting the tyrosine kinase domain of the RET proto-oncogene in Hirschsprung's disease. Nature 367:377, 1994.

Rorke LB: A perspective: The role of disordered genetic control of neurogenesis in the pathogenesis of migration disorders. J Neuropathol Exp Neurol 53:105, 1994.

Rosa FW: Teratogenicity of isotretinoin. Lancet 2:513, 1983.

Rosman NP: Incontinentia pigmenti: Presentations, pathology, pathogenesis, and prognosis. *In* Fukuyama Y, Suzuki Y, Kamoshita S, Casaer P (Eds): Fetal and Perinatal Neurology. Basel, Karger, 1992, pp 174–186.

Roth JC, Epstein CJ: Infantile spasms and hypopigmented macules: Early manifestations of tuberous sclerosis. Arch Neurol 25:547, 1971.

Russell DS: Observations on the Pathology of Hydrocephalus. London, Her Majesty's Stationery Office, 1949.

Ryan L, Ehrlich S, Finnegan L: Cocaine abuse in pregnancy: Effects on the fetus and newborn. Neurotoxicol Teratol 9:295, 1987.

Scatliff JH, Kendall BE, Kingsley DP, et al: Closed spinal dysraphism: Analysis of clinical, radiological, and surgical findings in 104 consecutive patients. ANJR Am J Neuroradiol 10:269, 1989.

Schade JP, Caviness VF: Pathogenesis of X-irradiation effects in the monkey cerebral cortex: IV. Alterations in dendritic organization. Brain Res 7:59, 1968.

Schaefer GB: Partial agenesis of the corpus callosum: Correlation between appearance, imaging, and neuropathology. Pediatr Neurol 7:39, 1991.

Scher MS, Belfar H, Martin J, et al: Destructive brain lesions of presumed fetal onset: Antepartum causes of cerebral palsy. Pediatrics 88:898, 1991.

Schiaffino S, Margreth A: Coordinated development of the sarcoplasmic reticulum and a system during post-natal differentiation of rat skeletal muscle. J Cell Biol 41:855, 1969.

Seip M: Growth retardation, dysmorphic facies and minor malformations following massive exposure to phenobarbitone in utero. Acta Paediatr Scand 65:617, 1976.

Seller MJ: Risks in spina bifida. Dev Med Child Neurol 36:1021, 1994.

Shaw CM, Alvord EC: Hydrocephalus. *In* Duckett S (Ed): Pediatric Neuropathology. Baltimore, Williams & Wilkins, 1995, pp 149–211.

Silver J, Lorenz SE, Wahlsten D, et al: Axonal guidance during development of the great cerebral commissures: Descriptive and experimental studies, in vivo, on the role of preformed glial pathways. J Comp Neurol 210:10, 1982.

Simmons DA, Kegel MF, Scher RK, et al: Subungual tumors in incontinentia pigmenti. Arch Dermatol 122:1431, 1986.

Simmonsson H: Incontinentia pigmenti: Bloch-Sulzberger syndrome associated with infantile spasms. Acta Paediatr Scand 61:612, 1972.

Smith CV, Phelan JP: Antepartum fetal assessment: The nonstress test. *In* Hill A, Volpe JJ (Eds): Fetal Neurology. New York, Raven Press, 1989, pp 61–74.

Smithells RW, Sheppard S, Schorah CJ, et al: Apparent prevention of neural tube defects by periconceptional vitamin supplementation. Arch Dis Child 56:911, 1981.

Speidel BD, Meadow SR: Maternal epilepsy and abnormalities of the fetus and newborn. Lancet 2:839, 1972.

Stein SC, Schut L: Hydrocephalus in myelomeningocele. Childs Brain 5:413, 1979.

Stein SC, Schut L, Ames MD: Selection for early treatment in myelomeningocele: A retrospective analysis of various selection procedures. Pediatrics 54:553, 1974.

Stein SC, Schut L, Ames MD: Selection of early treatment of myelomen-

ingocele: A retrospective analysis of selection procedures. Dev Med Child Neurol 17:311, 1975.

Sue-Menko A, Boettiger D: Occupation of the extra-cellular matrix receptor, integrin, is a control point for myogenic differentiation. Cell 51:51, 1987.

Sugita K, Itoh K, Tabeuchi Y, et al: Tuberous sclerosis: Report of two cases studied by computer-assisted cranial tomography within one week after birth. Brain Dev 7:433, 1985.

Sunshine P: Epidemiology of perinatal asphyxia. *In* Stevenson DK, Sunshine P (Eds): Fetal and Neonatal Brain Injury: Mechanisms, Management, and the Risks of Practice. Philadelphia, BC Decker, 1989, pp 2–11.

Takashima S, Armstrong D, Becker LE: Subcortical leukomalacia: Relationship to development of cerebral sulcus and its vascular supply. Arch Neurol 35:470, 1978.

Takashima S, Becker LE, Armstrong DL, et al: Abnormal neuronal development in the visual cortex of the human fetus and infant with Down syndrome: A quantitative and qualitative Golgi study. Brain Res 225:1, 1981.

Takashima S, Becker LE, Chan F-W: Retardation of neuronal maturation in premature infants compared with term infants of the same postconceptional age. Pediatrics 69:33, 1982.

Takashima S, Tanaka K: Development of cerebral architecture and its relationship to periventricular leukomalacia. Arch Neurol 35:11, 1978a.

Takashima J, Tanaka K: Microangiography and vascular permeability of the subependymal matrix in the premature infant. Can J Neurol Sci 5:45, 1978b.

Thomas RL, Ferguson JE, Repke JT: Complications of labor and delivery: Selected medical and surgical considerations. *In* Stevenson DK, Sunshine P (Eds): Fetal and Neonatal Brain Injury: Mechanisms, Management, and the Risks of Practice. Philadelphia, BC Decker, 1989, pp 34–45.

Toop J: The histochemical development of human skeletal muscle and its motor innervation. *In* Bradley WG, Gardner-Medwin D, Walton JN (Eds): Recent Advances in Myology. Amsterdam, Excerpta Medica, 1975, pp 322–329.

Towfighi J, Housman C: Spinal cord abnormalities in caudal regression syndrome. Acta Neuropathol (Berlin) 81:458, 1991.

Van Allen MI, Kalousek DK, Chernoff GF, et al: Evidence for multi-site closure of the neural tube in humans. Am J Med Genet 47:723, 1993.

Vannucci RC: Current and potentially new management strategies for perinatal hypoxic-ischemic encephalopathy. Pediatrics 85:961, 1990.

Verloes A, Lambotte C: Further delineation of a syndrome of cerebellar hypo/aplasia, oligophrenia, congenital ataxia, coloboma, and hepatic fibrosis. Am J Med Genet 32:227, 1989.

Volpe JJ: Neural tube formation and prosencephalic development. *In* Volpe JJ: Neurology of the Newborn, 3rd ed. Philadelphia, WB Saunders, 1995a, pp 3–42.

Volpe JJ: Neuromuscular disorders: Muscle involvement and restricted disorders. *In* Volpe JJ: Neurology of the Newborn, 3rd ed. Philadelphia, WB Saunders, 1995b, pp 634–671.

Volpe JJ: Neuronal proliferation, migration, organization, and myelination. *In* Volpe JJ: Neurology of the Newborn, 3rd ed. Philadelphia, WB Saunders, 1995c, pp 43–92.

Waisbren SE, Levy HL: Effects of untreated maternal hyperphenylalanemia on the fetus: Further study of families identified by routine cord blood screening. J Pediatr 116:926, 1990.

Warburg M: Ocular malformations and lissencephaly. Eur J Pediatr 146:450, 1987.

Warkany U, Lemire RJ, Cohen MM Jr: Mental Retardation and Congenital Malformations of the Nervous System. Chicago, Year Book Medical Publishers, 1981.

Weiss E, Ulrich S, Berle P: Blood flow velocity waveforms of the middle cerebral artery and abnormal neurological evaluations in live-born fetuses with absent or reversed end-diastolic flow velocities of the umbilical arteries. Eur J Obstet Gynecol Reprod Biol 45:93, 1992.

Wettke-Schafer RG: X-linked dominant inherited diseases with lethality in hemizygous males. Hum Kantner Genet 64:1, 1983.

Wiley HE, Frias JL: Depigmented lesions in incontinential pigmenti: A useful diagnostic sign. Am J Dis Child 128:546, 1974.

Wilkinson M, Hume R, Strange R, et al: Glial and neuronal differentiation in the human fetal brain 9–23 weeks of gestation. Neuropathol Appl Neurobiol 16:193, 1990.

Williams J, Brodsky MC, Griebel M, et al: Septo-optic dysplasia: The clinical insignificance of an absent septum pellucidum. Dev Med Child Neurol 35:490, 1993.

Yen IH, Khoury MJ, Erickson JD, et al: The changing epidemiology of neural tube defects—United States, 1968–1989. Am J Dis Child 146:857, 1992.

Yin L, Barone V, Seri M, et al: Heterogeneity and low detection rate of RET mutations in Hirschsprung disease. Eur J Hum Genet 2:272, 1994.

Yoshimura K, Hayashi Y, Nakal Y, et al: Brain and cardiac tumors with neonatal tuberous sclerosis. Brain Dev 12:358, 1990.

Zeki SM, Hollman AS, Dutton GN: Neuroradiological features of patients with optic nerve hypoplasia. J Pediatr Ophthalmol Strabismus 29:107, 1992.

Zimmer EZ, Jakobi P, Goldstein I, et al: Cardiotopographic and sonographic findings in two cases of antenatally diagnosed intrauterine fetal brain death. Prenat Diagn 12:271, 1992.

CHAPTER 68

The Nervous System During Birth

Jan Goddard-Finegold

NEUROPHYSIOLOGY OF BIRTH

Just as the cardiovascular system is undergoing transitions during and after the birth process, so too is the cerebrovascular system. Knowledge that a significant proportion of cerebral injury occurs in utero, and probably before any labor has occurred, makes it imperative that clinicians understand as much about fetal cerebral physiologic reactions as possible. Ideally, the intrauterine human brain should be monitored in a noninvasive way, to avoid inducing labor, infection, bleeding, or other problems. Some monitoring has been possible using Doppler ultrasound techniques, but information gained regarding blood flow velocities from this method is not exact (Martin et al, 1990). Studies of intrauterine near-infrared spectroscopy are current research protocols. Long-term monitoring can be done in fetal sheep and nonhuman primates, and the information gained from such studies is valuable, although not always completely applicable because of species differences. Thus, there is much still to learn in the area of fetal-neonatal cerebral physiology and changes that occur before and during the birth process. Probably the most important issues studied to date include fetal cerebrovascular responses to hypoxia, changes in perfusion pressure, increased intracranial pressure, and changes in pH and carbon dioxide (Jones and Hudak, 1992).

Labor and Vaginal Delivery

The contractions of the uterus during normal labor cause reductions in maternal blood flow to the placenta (Borell et al, 1965; Marsal and Lindblad, 1992). During normal labor, this is compensated by an increase in blood flow that occurs during the relaxation phases (Lees et al, 1971). In addition, the maternal circulation compensates by increasing blood pressure and cardiac output (Hendricks and Quilligan, 1956; Ueland and Hansen, 1969). Short-term changes in maternal placental blood flow during contractions do not adversely affect the fetus; however, when uteroplacental blood flow is decreased significantly during a problematic labor, fetal hypoxemia can develop. This can ultimately lead to changes in fetal heart rate, blood pressure, and organ blood flow (Dawes, 1968). Fetal cerebral blood flow velocity in the anterior cerebral arteries has been estimated using Doppler ultrasound during labor. Mean velocities do not seem to change during normal labor, and there is conflicting evidence regarding the effect of labor on diastolic velocities. One study has shown that head compression during contractions results in increased cerebrovascular resistance with decreased diastolic flow velocities (Lang et al, 1988).

Anesthesia and the Fetal Brain

Anesthesia used in the mother is rapidly transported to the fetus (Marsal and Lindblad, 1992). Placental blood flow does not seem to be altered by epidural anesthesia, and the fetal circulatory responses with epidural anesthesia do not seem to differ from those without epidural anesthesia. The main problem with epidural anesthesia is the systemic hypotension that sometimes results from the sympathetic blockade (Albright, 1989). In those cases in which maternal systolic blood pressure falls below 80 mm Hg or in which there is marginal uteroplacental blood supply from the outset, the fetus will have bradycardia and may require more rapid delivery (Albright, 1989).

Other types of anesthesia can lower placental blood flow as well as aortic blood flow in the fetus, including the local anesthetics used in paracervical blocks (Albright, 1985; Willdeck-Lund et al, 1979). There are also isolated reports of misplaced paracervical anesthetics being injected directly into the fetal brain. Lowered aortic blood flow may be a significant problem for the fetus with insufficient cerebral autoregulatory capacities, leading potentially to cerebral ischemia. General anesthetics are known to have effects on cerebral blood flow in adults (Lassen and Shapiro, 1981). Thiopental can reduce cerebral blood flow as much as 50%; most of the other agents, with the exception of ketamine, also decrease cerebral blood flow to some extent (Lassen and Shapiro, 1981). Ketamine increases cerebral blood flow and is not likely to be used for maternal anesthesia; it is especially not used in patients with increased intracranial pressure.

The main problem with general anesthesia in the pregnant woman is the risk of hypoxia and the effect of hypoxia on the fetal brain (Albright, 1989). The increased metabolic needs and decreased respiratory reserve of the pregnant woman make it especially important to preoxygenate the patient before administering general anesthesia (Albright, 1989).

Effects of general anesthetic agents, local anesthetics, and sedative drugs can all be seen in the term newborn but are not usually problematic unless the infant is asphyxiated. Hypoxia and acidosis lower the infant's ability to tolerate the depressant effects of lidocaine or mepivacaine (Albright, 1985; Morishima et al, 1972). Premature newborns are more susceptible to drug effects and may show respiratory and central nervous system depression at delivery and require resuscitation after relatively low maternal doses. Thus, when possible, anesthetics that undergo rapid enzymatic breakdown are used in mothers of preterm infants (Albright, 1989).

Mechanical Events and Central Nervous System Trauma

Significant birth trauma is responsible for about 2% of stillbirths and neonatal deaths in the United States and occurs to some extent in 6 to 8 of every 1000 live births

(Robertson et al, 1990; Schullinger, 1993). Notably, statistics indicate that midforceps deliveries are associated with admission of the newborn to the intensive care unit in 9.2% of cases, whereas cesarean section deliveries are associated with intensive care unit admission only 2.3% of the time (Lucas, 1994). In the same study, successful vacuum extraction deliveries resulted in no admissions to the neonatal intensive care unit, but unsuccessful vacuum extractions usually lead to either forceps or cesarean section deliveries. Approximately half of the injuries in the midforceps group were attributable directly to the instrument, resulting in skull fractures, seventh nerve palsies, and dural thrombosis. Problems that have been reported after vacuum extraction include bruising, scalp trauma, retinal hemorrhages, cephalohematomas, subaponeurotic hemorrhages (subgaleal hemorrhages), and intracranial hemorrhages (intraventricular, intracerebral, subdural) (Lucas, 1994).

In general, trauma in the newborn is most often manifest as skull fracture (Ward, 1993). Neurosurgical intervention is usually not necessary when the fracture is linear but may be indicated when the fracture is depressed (especially if depressed more than 0.5 cm) (Ward, 1993) (Fig. 68–1). Elevation of a depressed fracture is always indicated if there is neurologic deficit. Subperiosteal and subgaleal hemorrhages can also occur in the absence of vacuum extractor or forceps use. Subgaleal hematomas can be quite large and may cause a significant decrease in hematocrit with resulting hyperbilirubinemia; they cross sutures and are not usually associated with skull fractures (Ward, 1993). Subperiosteal hematomas (cephalohematomas) do not cross sutures and may be associated with skull fracture. *Caput succedaneum* refers to edema below the scalp but can include subgaleal hemorrhage (Fig. 68–2). Other types of hemorrhages that can occur during delivery include subarachnoid, subdural, extradural, and intraparenchymal

hemorrhages (Ward, 1993). Other types of traumatic birth injuries, including spinal cord, plexus, cranial nerve, and peripheral nerve injuries, are discussed in Chapter 69.

Fetal Brain Responses to Asphyxia

Fetal brain and cerebrovascular responses to asphyxia are not completely understood. In addition, such responses are complicated, involving reactions to multiple stresses that are part of or accompany asphyxia, including hypoxia, acidosis, hypercarbia, in some cases hypoglycemia, and hypotension. Studies in fetal animals have been done to determine normal autoregulatory capacity, cerebral blood flow responses to hypovolemic hypotension and to intrauterine asphyxia, cardiovascular and cerebral blood flow responses to hypoxemia and acidemia, and fetal cerebral blood flow responses to changes in cephalic pressure.

Jones and colleagues (1978) have shown that fetal lamb cerebral blood flow increases more during hypoxia than in juvenile lamb or adult sheep. Baseline cerebral blood flow is higher in the lamb fetus, however, making this a relative, rather than an absolute, difference. Ashwal and colleagues (1980) also showed that fetal lambs respond to hypoxia by increasing cerebral blood flow as much as 92% and that they maintain increased cerebral blood flow of 50% above control values 60 minutes after fetal oxygenation is restored. Apparently, fetal cerebral oxygen transport is high when compared to fetal cerebral oxygen consumption, probably as a result of higher oxyhemoglobin affinity in the fetus (Jones and Traystman, 1984). Adult hemoglobin has lower oxygen affinity, resulting in greater oxygen extraction by the brain; transfusion of the fetal lamb with adult blood results in lowering of both baseline cerebral blood flow in the fetus and the cerebral blood flow response to hypoxia (Koehler et al, 1982). These studies have shown that arte-

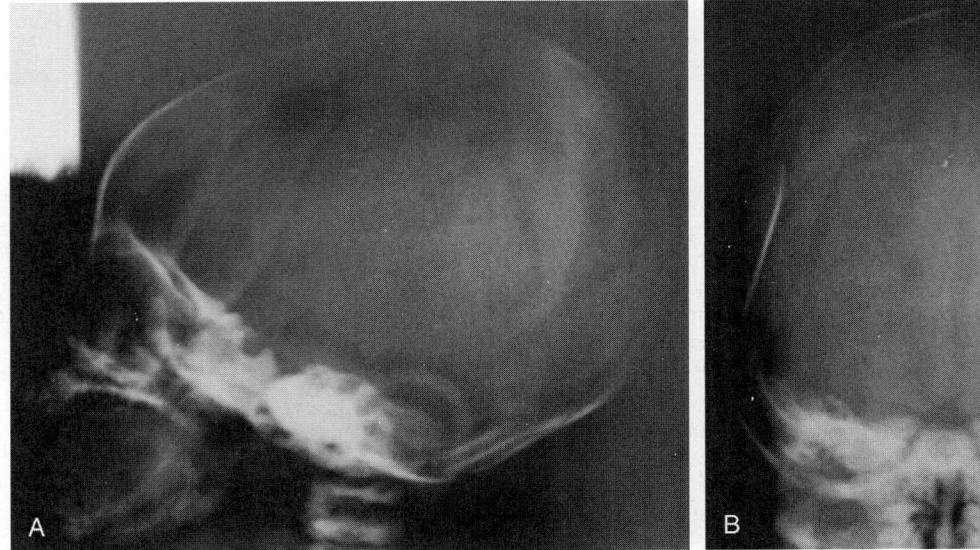
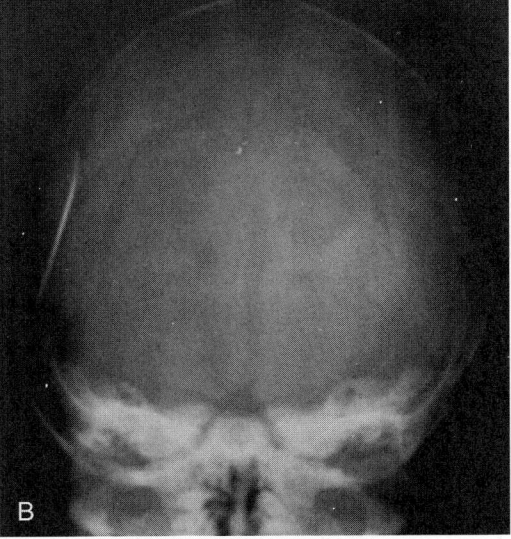

FIGURE 68–1. *A* and *B*, Lateral and anteroposterior skull x-ray films of a 1-day-old infant. Depressed skull injury is visualized clearly on the anteroposterior view as a linear streak of increased density. Such injuries are the result of inward buckling of the poorly mineralized skull of the newborn. The actual break in the continuity of the bone is present over a short distance only.

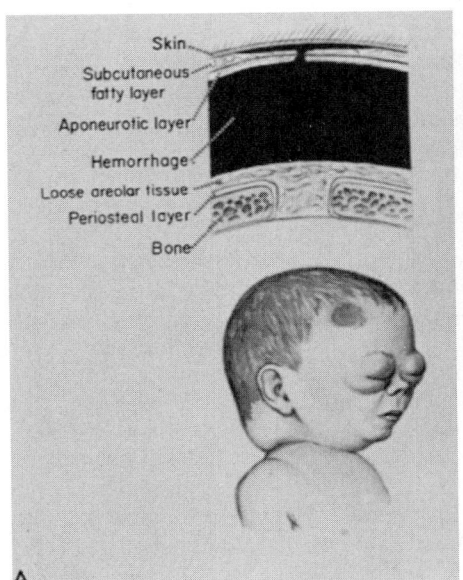
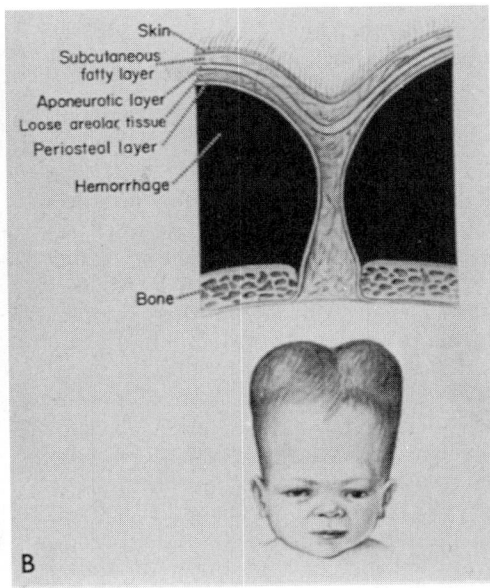
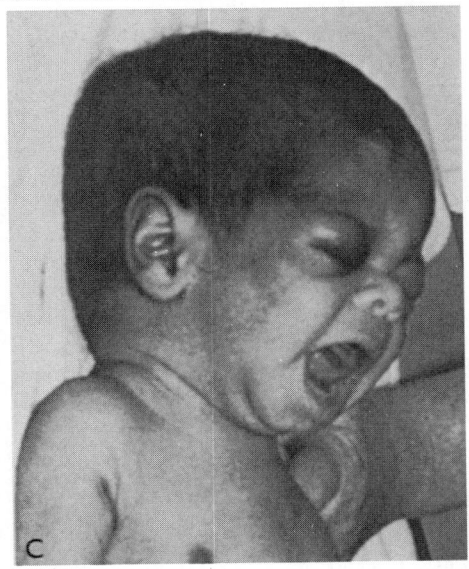

FIGURE 68–2. *A,* Location of edema and hemorrhage in caput succedaneum. *B,* Location of hemorrhage in cephalhematoma. *C,* Patient with massive hemorrhagic caput succedaneum, whose hemoglobin level fell to 2.2 g/dL by the age of 48 hours. (Courtesy of Daniel J. Pachman, M.D., of the University of Illinois Pediatric Department. The photograph, but not the sketches, appeared in Pediatrics 29:907, 1962.)

rial oxygen content and oxyhemoglobin affinity are the most important factors for brain tissue oxygenation; tissue oxygenation decreases as arterial oxygen content decreases, but the degree of decrease is determined by the oxyhemoglobin affinity (Jones and Traystman, 1984). Similar to hypoxemia, anemia also causes fetal cerebral blood flow to increase, but this response may be related more to decreased blood viscosity than to changes in tissue oxygen (Fumia et al, 1984).

Fetal autoregulation, or the capacity to maintain cerebral blood flow at a constant level despite changes in cerebral perfusion pressure over a defined range, has been studied in the fetal lamb (Papile et al, 1985). The fetal lamb's autoregulatory range seems to be between about 45 and 80 mm Hg with fetal aortic blood pressure averaging 55 mm Hg at 80% of term gestation (Arnold et al, 1991; Papile et al, 1985). Interestingly, Arnold and coworkers (1991) found that this autoregulatory range remained constant over the first 2 postnatal weeks in the lamb, although the mean arterial blood pressure rose from 55 mm Hg to 73 mm Hg over that time period. These findings suggest that the mean aortic blood pressure of the fetus is nearer to the lower limit of autoregulation, whereas the mean aortic blood pressure of the infant lamb is nearer to the upper limit. This suggests that although the fetus may be more susceptible to ischemic brain injury, the newborn may be more susceptible to hyperemic injury. The ability of the fetus to maintain autoregulatory capacities in the face of physiologic stresses remains unclear, although one study in fetal lambs suggested that autoregulation is lost after asphyxia induced by umbilical cord clamping (Lou et al, 1979).

The vasodilatory effects of hypercapnia are less pronounced in immature brains than in adult brains, but the effects of hypercapnia on autoregulation in the fetus are not known. Hypercapnia in mature brains is known to abolish autoregulation when P_{CO_2} is greater than 70 mm Hg (Harper, 1966).

Labor and vaginal delivery result in pressure on the fetal skull. Descent of the fetal head during labor has been known to result in episodic fetal bradycardia, and in fetal lambs, pressure applied to the fetal head by head cuff inflation at 200 mm Hg results in initial bradycardia followed by tachycardia and return to normal after cuff deflation (O'Brien et al, 1984). During the cuff inflation, mean aortic blood pressure increases. Cerebral blood flow to all brain regions decreases significantly during inflation, falling by 95% overall (O'Brien et al, 1984). Relative distribution of cerebral blood flow changes during the increased cephalic pressure, with the percentage of total cerebral blood flow going to the cortex decreasing from 65% to 56% and the percentage of flow going to the brain stem increasing from 5.6% to 12.5%, despite the reductions in absolute flow (O'Brien et al, 1984). Responses to cephalic pressure may be altered by the presence of other physiologic stresses, such as asphyxia. These findings suggest that there is relative sparing of the brain stem when cerebral blood flow is reduced during cephalic pressure, but it should be noted that in these studies blood flow still decreased by 88% to the brain stem and by 96% to the cortex. *Sparing*, thus, is a relative term.

Brain Stem and Autonomic Influences

Brain stem mechanisms are important for the fetal and neonatal ventilatory responses to hypoxia (Noble, 1991). The late-gestation fetus responds to hypoxemia with a cessation of fetal breathing movements (Boddy et al, 1974). The newborn response differs in having an initial increase in ventilation followed by decreased ventilatory effort (Rigatto, 1984). The effect of hypoxia on fetal breathing can be prevented in fetal lambs by transection of the brain stem at the level of the colliculi (Dawes et al, 1983). In newborn rabbits and rats, transection at the level of the rostral pons can abolish the decrease in ventilation that follows the initial increase (Hanson and Williams, 1989; Martin-Body and Johnston, 1988). Neurons in this pontine region are sensitive to hypoxia in the fetus and newborn and respond differently than in the adult. In the adult, the main ventilatory response to hypoxia is hyperpnea, whereas in the late-gestation fetus, the initial response is apnea, offering an explanation for the respiratory depression present in the newborn delivered after intrauterine asphyxia.

Carotid arterial chemoreceptors and baroreceptors are active in the 90-day lamb fetus (term is 147 days); however, their sensitivity is less than that of the adult to hypoxia (Blanco et al, 1984). Conversely the carotid baroreceptors have greater sensitivity to arterial blood pressure changes in earlier gestation fetal lambs (88 to 113 days) compared to later gestation fetuses (131 to 144 days). Sensitivity, however, increases again postnatally in the lamb (Blanco et al, 1988). This change in sensitivity seems to correlate with the increase in blood pressure that occurs postnatally. Cardiovascular efferent reflexes also change with gestational age. Fetuses near term respond to hypoxia with bradycardia and an increase in arterial blood pressure; this response is not present earlier in gestation (i.e., up to 120 days) (Boddy et al, 1974; Iwamoto et al, 1989; Walker et al, 1979). The bradycardia is reflex in origin and can be prevented by vagotomy (Boddy et al, 1974) or by atropine

(Martin, 1985). Experimental studies in near-term lambs showed that hypoxia causes increases in cerebral, myocardial, and adrenal blood flow with decreases in pulmonary, skin, and skeletal muscle flow (Rudolph, 1985). Notably, denervation of chemoreceptors by vagotomy does not alter the vasodilation that occurs in the brain during hypoxia in the near-term fetal lamb or the postnatal lamb (Miyabe et al, 1989).

The effects of hypoxia on the fetal adrenal medulla have been reviewed, with the conclusion that the sympathetic responses are not fully developed by the time of birth in the lamb (Jones and Wei, 1985). Nevertheless, there is a rise in plasma catecholamines after hypoxia; after the initial decrease in heart rate, if the hypoxia is not too severe, there follows a return of heart rate to the prehypoxia level (Jones et al, 1988). It is thought that this is due to an increase in both maternal and fetal catecholamine levels. In younger fetuses, hypoxia may be met with an increase in heart rate initially (Boddy et al, 1974; Iwamoto et al, 1989).

Asphyxia implies the presence of both hypoxia and hypercarbia, with resulting acidosis, and usually occurs when there is a decrease in placental perfusion for some reason. Studies indicate that reductions of uterine blood flow up to 50% are actually well tolerated acutely by term fetal sheep when oxygenation is considered (Skillman et al, 1985); however, carbon dioxide transport is affected more quickly. Chronically the hypoxemia becomes much more severe. As in hypoxia alone, late-gestation fetal lambs respond to asphyxia from decreased perfusion with a fall in heart rate, and, if the cord is compressed, with an increase in arterial pressure. The increase in arterial pressure has been shown to correlate with gradual decreases in uterine blood flow (Yaffe et al, 1987). Chronically hypoxic or asphyxiated lamb fetuses can show heart rate and blood pressure patterns that return to normal but also seem to respond differently when acidosis or growth retardation is present. In particular, growth-retarded hypoxic fetuses have been noted to have significantly lower fetal heart rates (Bocking et al, 1988, 1989; Walker et al, 1990).

ANTENATAL BRAIN PROTECTION

The majority of cases of static encephalopathy (cerebral palsy) are due to intrauterine brain injury or to unknown genetic or other factors, with only a modest percentage due to intrapartum asphyxia (Blair and Stanley, 1988; Torfs et al, 1990). It is also well known that preterm infants are more likely to have neurologic injury, probably owing to prenatal and postnatal hypoxia and ischemia as well as to the adverse physiologic factors affecting the immature brain in the extrauterine environment.

Clearly, one way of decreasing neurologic abnormalities associated with adverse intrauterine and perinatal stresses would be to (1) identify actual and potential adverse events and (2) protect the brain while the fetus is still in utero. Ways of doing the latter include enhancing normal structural and physiologic maturation of the fetus, so that preterm delivery can be met with term physiologic responses, or counteracting the injurious stresses and their effects directly in term or preterm infants. Corticosteroids are known to enhance fetal maturation, and their antenatal use has been studied for more than 20 years (see also Chapter

4). Agents thought to affect cellular responses to hypoxia, for example, *N*-methyl-D-aspartate receptor antagonists and antioxidants, are being tested experimentally in animals but are not yet available for use in humans. Some agents thought to have effects on autoregulation (phenobarbital, indomethacin), postnatal circulatory adaptation (corticosteroids), or bleeding tendencies (vitamin K) are given prenatally or postnatally in attempts to prevent intracerebral ischemia, hyperemia, or hemorrhage.

Stimulation of Maturation in the Preterm Fetus

Administration of corticosteroids to mothers delivering preterm was initiated in 1972 to increase fetal lung maturity. It has since become apparent that treatment of women with corticosteroids before delivery of a preterm infant is associated with large reductions in the incidence of early neonatal death, respiratory distress syndrome, intraventricular hemorrhage, and necrotizing enterocolitis (Report of Consensus Development Conference, 1994). Unfortunately, information from approximately 500 perinatal centers indicates that, to date, only 18% or fewer eligible women are treated with antenatal corticosteroids.

Data from large meta-analyses indicate that the effect of antenatal corticosteroids in decreasing intraventricular hemorrhage is independent of the effect on lung disease, suggesting that there is a separate effect on the vulnerable brain regions or blood vessels (Crowley, 1994; Crowley et al, 1990). A distinct mechanism for the protective action of prenatal corticosteroids against intraventricular hemorrhage has yet to be shown. The accumulated positive information regarding the use of corticosteroids for fetal maturation has led a recent National Institutes of Health consensus panel to conclude that their antenatal use, even for a short period of time before preterm delivery, is advantageous (Report of Consensus Development Conference, 1994).

Pharmacologic Strategies

Other pharmacologic strategies have been used antenatally to reduce the incidence of postnatal brain injury. Treatments aimed at decreasing the incidence of both hypoxic-ischemic injury and intraventricular hemorrhage have included prenatal administration of phenobarbital, vitamin K, and both agents together (Morales, 1991). The degree of reduction in the incidence of intraventricular hemorrhage after antenatal treatment with these agents has not been as great as that produced by use of antenatal corticosteroids.

REFERENCES

Albright GA: What is the place of bupivacaine in obstetric epidural analgesia? Can Anaesth Soc J 32:392, 1985.

Albright GA: Effects of anesthesia on the fetus and neonate. *In* Stevenson DK, Sunshine P (Eds): Fetal and Neonatal Brain Injury: Mechanisms, Management, and the Risks of Practice. Philadelphia, BC Decker, 1989, pp 46–56.

Arnold BW, Martin CG, Alexander BJ, et al: Autoregulation of brain blood flow during hypotension and hypertension in infant lambs. Pediatr Res 29:110, 1991.

Ashwal S, Majcher JS, Vain N, et al: Patterns of fetal lamb regional cerebral blood flow during and after prolonged hypoxia. Pediatr Res 18:1104, 1980.

Blair E, Stanley JF: Intrapartum asphyxia: A rare cause of cerebral palsy. J Pediatr 112:515, 1988.

Blanco CE, Dawes GS, Hanson MA, et al: The response to hypoxia of arterial chemoreceptors in fetal sheep and new-born lambs. J Physiol 351:25, 1984.

Blanco CE, Dawes GS, Hanson MA, et al: Carotid baroreceptors in fetal and newborn sheep. Pediatr Res 24:342, 1988.

Bocking AD, Gagnon R, White SE, et al: Circulatory responses to prolonged hypoxemia in fetal sheep. Am J Obstet Gynecol 159:1418, 1988.

Bocking AD, White S, Gagnon R, et al: Effect of prolonged hypoxemia on fetal heart rate accelerations and decelerations in sheep. Am J Obstet Gynecol 161:722, 1989.

Boddy K, Dawes GS, Fisher R, et al: Foetal respiratory movements, electrical and cardiovascular responses to hypoxaemia and hypercapnia in sheep. J Physiol 243:599, 1974.

Borell U, Fernstrom I, Ohlson L, et al: Influence of uterine contractions on the uteroplacental blood flow at term. Am J Obstet Gynecol 93:44, 1965.

Crowley P: Update of the antenatal steroid meta-analysis: Current knowledge and future research needs. *In* Report of the Consensus Development Conference on the Effect of Corticosteroids for Fetal Maturation on Perinatal Outcomes. NIH Pub No. 95–3784. Bethesda, MD, National Institutes of Health, 1994, pp 93–95.

Crowley P, Chalmers I, Keirse MJNC: The effects of corticosteroid administration before preterm delivery: An overview of the evidence from controlled studies. Br J Obstet Gynaecol 97:11, 1990.

Dawes GS: Fetal and Neonatal Physiology. Chicago, Year Book Medical Publishers, 1968.

Dawes GS, Gardner WN, Johnston BM, et al: Breathing in fetal lambs: The effect of brainstem section. J Physiol 335:535, 1983.

Fumia FD, Eledstone DI, Holzmann IR: Blood flow and oxygen delivery to fetal organs and oxygen delivery as functions of fetal hematocrit. Am J Obstet Gynecol 150:274, 1984.

Hanson MA, Williams BA: The effect of decerebration and brain-stem transection on the ventilatory response to acute hypoxia in normoxic and chronically hypoxic newborn rats. J Physiol 414:25, 1989.

Harper AM: Autoregulation of cerebral blood flow: Influence of the arterial blood pressure on the blood flow through the cerebral cortex. J Neurol Neurosurg Psychiatry 29:398, 1966.

Hendricks CH, Quilligan EJ: Cardiac output during labor. Am J Obstet Gynecol 71:953, 1956.

Iwamoto HS, Kaufman T, Keil LC, et al: Responses to acute hypoxemia in fetal sheep at 0.6–0.7 gestation. Am J Physiol 256:H613, 1989.

Jones CT, Roebuck MM, Walker DW, et al: The role of the adrenal medulla and peripheral sympathetic nerves in the physiological responses of the fetal sheep to hypoxia. J Dev Physiol 10:17, 1988.

Jones CT, Wei G: Adrenal-medullary activity and cardiovascular control in the fetal sheep. *In* Kunzel W (Ed): Fetal Heart Rate Monitoring. Berlin, Springer-Verlag, 1985, pp 127–135.

Jones MD, Hudak ML: Regulation of the fetal cerebral circulation. *In* Polin RA, Fox WW (Eds): Fetal and Neonatal Physiology. Philadelphia, WB Saunders, 1992, pp 682–690.

Jones MD Jr, Sheldon RE, Peeters LL, et al: Regulation of cerebral blood flow in the ovine fetus. Am J Physiol 235:H162, 1978.

Jones MD Jr, Traystman RJ: Cerebral oxygenation of the fetus, newborn and adult. Semin Perinatol 8:205, 1984.

Koehler RC, Traystman RJ, Jones MD Jr: Comparison of cerebrovascular response to hypoxic and carbon monoxide hypoxia. Am J Physiol 251:H756, 1982.

Lang GD, Levene MI, Dougall A, et al: Direct measurements of fetal cerebral blood-flow velocity with duplex Doppler ultrasound. Eur J Obstet Gynecol Reprod Biol 29:15, 1988.

Lassen NA, Shapiro HM: Anaesthesia and cerebral blood flow. *In* Gordon E (Ed): A Basis and Practice of Neuroanaesthesia. New York, Excerpta Medica, 1981, pp 139–172.

Lees MH, Hill JD, Ochsner AJ III, et al: Maternal placental and myometrial blood flow of the rhesus monkey during uterine contractions. Am J Obstet Gynecol 110:68, 1971.

Lou HC, Lassen NA, Tweed WA, et al: Pressure passive cerebral blood flow and breakdown of the blood-brain barrier in experimental fetal asphyxia. Acta Paediatr Scand 68:57, 1979.

Lucas MJ: The role of vacuum extraction in modern obstetrics. Clin Obstet Gynecol 37:794, 1994.

Marsal K, Lindblad A: Fetal and placental circulation during labor. *In* Polin RA, Fox WW (Eds): Fetal and Neonatal Physiology. Philadelphia, WB Saunders, 1992, pp 703–710.

Martin CB: Pharmacological aspects of fetal heart rate regulation during hypoxia. *In* Kunzel W (Ed): Fetal Heart Rate Monitoring. Berlin, Springer-Verlag, 1985, pp 170–184.

Martin CG, Hansen TN, Goddard-Finegold J, et al: Prediction of brain blood flow using pulsed Doppler ultrasonography in newborn lambs. J Clin Ultrasound 18:487, 1990.

Martin-Body RL, Johnston BM: Central origin of the hypoxic depression of breathing in the newborn. Respir Physiol 71:25, 1988.

Miyabe M, Jones JD Jr, Koehler RC, et al: Chemodenervation does not alter cerebrovascular response to hypoxic hypoxia. Am J Physiol 257:H1413, 1989.

Morales WJ: Antenatal therapy to minimize neonatal intraventricular hemorrhage. Clin Obstet Gynecol 34:328, 1991.

Morishima HO, Heymann MA, Rudolph AM, et al: Toxicity of lidocaine in the fetal and newborn lamb and its relationship to asphyxia. Am J Obstet Gynecol 112:72, 1972.

Noble R: Brain stem mechanisms mediating the neonatal ventilatory response to hypoxia. *In* Hanson MA (Ed): The Fetal and Neonatal Brain Stem. New York, Cambridge University Press, 1991, pp 48–59.

O'Brien WF, Davis SE, Grissom MP, et al: Effect of cephalic pressure on fetal cerebral blood flow. Am J Perinatol 1:223, 1984.

Papile LA, Rudolph AM, Heymann MA, et al: Autoregulation of cerebral blood flow in the preterm fetal lamb. Pediatr Res 19:159, 1985.

Report of the Consensus Development Conference on the Effect of Corticosteroids for Fetal Maturation on Perinatal Outcomes. NIH Pub No. 95-3784. Bethesda, MD, National Institutes of Health, 1994.

Rigatto H: Control of ventilation in the newborn. Ann Rev Physiol 46:661, 1984.

Robertson PA, Laros RK Jr, Zhan BL: Neonatal and maternal outcome in low-pelvic and midpelvic operative deliveries. Am J Obstet Gynecol 162:1436, 1990.

Rudolph AM: Distribution and regulation of blood flow in the fetal and neonatal lamb. Circ Res 57:811, 1985.

Schullinger JN: Birth trauma. Pediatr Clin North Am 40:1351, 1993.

Skillman CA, Plessinger MA, Woods JR, et al: Effect of graded reductions in uteroplacental blood flow on the fetal lamb. Am J Physiol 249:H1098, 1985.

Torfs CP, van den Berg BJ, Oechsli FW, et al: Prenatal and perinatal factors in the etiology of cerebral palsy. J Pediatr 116:615, 1990.

Ueland K, Hansen JM: Maternal cardiovascular dynamics: II. Posture and uterine contractions. Am J Obstet Gynecol 103:1, 1969.

Walker AM, Cannata JP, Dowling MH, et al: Age-dependent pattern of autonomic heart rate control during hypoxia in fetal and newborn lambs. Biol Neonate 35:198, 1979.

Walker AM, de Preu NP, Horne RSC, et al: Autonomic control of heart rate differs with electrocortical activity and chronic hypoxaemia in fetal lambs. J Dev Physiol 14:43, 1990.

Ward JD: Central nervous system trauma. *In* Pellock JM, Myer EC (Eds): Neurologic Emergencies in Infancy and Childhood. Boston, Butterworth-Heinemann, 1993, pp 91–102.

Willdeck-Lund G, Lindmark G, Nilsson BA: Effect of segmental epidural analgesia upon the uterine activity with special reference to the use of different local anaesthetic agents. Acta Anaesth Scand 23:519, 1979.

Yaffe H, Parer JT, Block BS, et al: Cardiorespiratory responses to graded reductions of uterine blood flow in the sheep. J Dev Physiol 9:325, 1987.

CHAPTER 69

The Newborn Nervous System

Jan Goddard-Finegold, Eli M. Mizrahi and Rita T. Lee

PERINATAL DEPRESSION AND THE BRAIN
Definition of Perinatal Depression

Depression or distress in the newborn is defined as decreased or ineffective respiration resulting in poor air exchange, in many cases associated with bradycardia and frequently associated with poor tone, poor color, and poor reflex irritability (the basis of the Apgar score for term infants) (Benitz et al, 1989). The causes of perinatal depression are numerous, and the presence of neonatal depression by itself does not imply the presence of central nervous system (CNS) damage. The presence of neonatal depression indicates the need for prompt initiation of effective ventilation; in most cases, there is an immediate positive response to resuscitation. The very premature infant may not have the neurologic integrity to meet the tone, irritability, and respiratory requirements for the Apgar score.

Resuscitation and the Brain

The brain requires an adequate supply of oxygen and glucose. During asphyxia, both of these substrates are reduced or absent, and the by-products of anaerobic metabolism accumulate. Experimental data indicate that irreversible injury to vulnerable parts of the brain in newborn primate and lamb models occurs after 30 minutes of severe, incomplete asphyxia and after about 12 minutes of total asphyxia (Brann and Myers, 1975; Myers, 1969; Williams et al, 1992). These time periods are longer than those required for injury in adult brains.

The first route to supplying these substrates is through effective ventilation. Whether this is accomplished simply by supplying additional oxygen, by mask ventilation, or by intubation and mechanical ventilation depends on the severity of the respiratory depression and the underlying problem. After a severe asphyxial episode before or during birth, newborns can have respiratory depression, hypotonia, and a suppressed electroencephalogram (EEG) (Williams et al, 1992). The neurologic depression may occur because of accumulation of inhibitory neuromodulators in the brain (Mallard et al, 1993). Prolonged suppression of the EEG in fetal lambs indicates a poor outcome, and prolonged neurologic depression in postasphyxial newborn human infants also predicts poor outcome (Sarnat and Sarnat, 1976).

There is current debate about the effects of hyperglycemia and hypoglycemia on the neonatal brain during and after hypoxic-ischemic insult. In adults, neurologic outcome is worse after hypoxic-ischemic or traumatic brain injury when glucose levels are high and tissue lactate accumulates. Glucose transport into the brain is reduced and lactate buildup is less, however, in the newborn. Thus, the consequences of low serum glucose—hypoglycemia and low brain glucose—are deleterious at this stage (Duffy et al, 1975; Holowach-Thurston et al, 1974; Moore et al, 1971). Therefore, glucose supplementation is important because the newborn no longer has a placental glucose supply. This supplementation is especially important for preterm and growth-restricted infants because their glycogen stores are usually minimal. Glucose consumption is also increased by infection, hypoxia, hypothermia, and hyperthermia, leading often to hypoglycemia (Benitz et al, 1989).

Improved cardiac output and tissue perfusion can also be gained through correction of acidemia. Infants with respiratory depression as the result of an event late in delivery usually have only respiratory acidosis. Infants with longer-lived intrauterine distress with inadequate substrate delivery to tissues have metabolic acidosis. Some of the causes of persistent metabolic acidosis include decreased cardiac output, severe anemia, hypoxia (sepsis, severe asphyxia), tissue infarction (necrotizing enterocolitis, intraventricular hemorrhage, pulmonary hemorrhage), and inborn metabolic errors (Benitz et al, 1989). Bicarbonate may be administered for severe acidosis, but this must be done judiciously and not before ensuring adequate ventilation. There are many side effects of the use of bicarbonate; current debate, in fact, has shown little to recommend the routine practice of infusing bicarbonate in the acidotic newborn (Hein, 1993). Thus, when possible, the best therapy for correction of acidemia is correction of the underlying problem.

Evidence suggests that brain temperature affects the extent of brain injury after experimental hypoxic-ischemic insults in animal models. Notably, modest hypothermia has been associated with a significant decrease in mortality and in the extent of histologic brain injury when instituted before or after the hypoxic-ischemic insult in adult and newborn animal models (Buchan and Pulsinelli, 1990; Busto et al, 1987; Yager et al, 1993). The thermoneutral environment has been taught as ideal for the newborn infant to maintain hydration, reduce shivering and energy loss, and reduce metabolic requirements (Glatzl-Hawlik and Bell, 1992). In light of the experimental information suggesting that a lower temperature may protect the brain, it is advisable not to render newborns hyperthermic during resuscitation.

Associated Clinical Findings After Intrauterine Asphyxia

When the cause of neonatal depression is intrauterine asphyxia (failure of delivery of oxygen and failure of removal of metabolic waste, usually associated with impaired tissue perfusion), there are usually other associated findings. Meconium staining may be present, although meconium is present in 8% to 20% of all deliveries, and light meconium is usually not associated with symptoms. Acidosis is usually present, but the degree of acidosis does not correlate with the degree of depression of the Apgar score in term infants unless the acidosis is quite severe (pH ≤7.05). More importantly, significant asphyxia causing CNS damage in the intrapartum period is associated with neonatal encephalopathy and, frequently, with evidence of dysfunction of one or more systemic organs. When depression and signs suggesting some asphyxia at delivery occur but no neurologic syndrome, there is not likely to be neurologic damage resulting from that episode of asphyxia (Sunshine, 1989). Levene and colleagues (1985) found that severe encephalopathy was present in 2.1 births per 1000.

POSTNATAL NEUROLOGIC ADAPTATION
Newborn Central Nervous System Metabolic Adaptation

Brain oxidative metabolism, glucose utilization, and blood flows have been studied in both fetal and neonatal animals. Oxidative metabolism in the brain is higher in the newborn lamb than in the fetus at late gestation (Jones et al, 1982; Rosenberg et al, 1982). During the perinatal period itself, no changes have been seen in cerebral oxidative metabolism (Richardson et al, 1989). During the last 2 months of gestation, glucose metabolism increases about threefold, and during the first few postnatal days, there is further increase (Abrams et al, 1984). Analysis of regional glucose metabolism has shown that there are large increases in the brain stem and subcortical regions as the lamb nears term.

Cerebral blood flow also increases during the last half of gestation, paralleling the fall in oxygen content as the fetus nears term (Iwamoto et al, 1989; Jones et al, 1978, 1981; Rudolph and Heymann, 1970). When the changes in arterial oxygen content are taken into account, there is still a significant increase in cerebral blood flow as the fetal lamb matures. The increase in global cerebral blood flow is also coupled with a change in the hierarchy of flow; instead of the brain stem predominance seen in the fetus, blood flow to the cortex seems to be greater in the newborn lamb (Richardson et al, 1989).

Glucose metabolism in human newborns has been evaluated using positron emission tomography (PET). Chugani and Phelps (1986) have shown that glucose metabolism is highest in the sensorimotor cortex, thalamus, brain stem, and vermis of the cerebellum in infants younger than 5 weeks' postnatal age. Studies in other species, notably dog and monkey, have shown different results, indicating that interspecies differences exist in the timing and extent of postnatal metabolic changes. In general, however, the rule is that metabolic activity increases at birth and in the early postnatal period. Importantly, although peak growth and development of the brain occur in utero, there is continued rapid growth during the perinatal period and beyond, and the increases in metabolic activity parallel this continued maturation and requirement for energy expenditure. In comparison to prenatal brain developers (guinea pig) and postnatal brain developers (dog and rat), the human is a *perinatal brain developer* (Richardson, 1991). These definitions reflect the fact that the guinea pig brain is quite mature at birth, the dog and rat brains are quite immature,

and, in comparison, the human brain is somewhere in the middle. These variations in brain maturation at birth can be documented in electrocortical patterns at birth as well as by behavioral and metabolic indices (Roffwarg et al, 1966; Szeto et al, 1985).

Importantly the shifts in oxidative and glucose metabolism as well as cerebral blood flow that occur over the fetal to newborn period may play an important role in determining different brain vulnerabilities to intrauterine, intrapartum, and postpartum hypoxia-ischemia.

Newborn Cerebrovascular Adaptation

In the previous section, it was stated that cerebral blood flow increases from the fetal to the newborn period. The autoregulatory capacity in lambs does not seem to change from the late fetal to the newborn period, however, despite increases in blood pressure over that time period (Arnold et al, 1991). In human infants, Doppler flow velocities have been estimated in the pericallosal artery postnatally and have shown that the upper limit of autoregulation increases as gestational age increases, from 45 to 60 mm Hg to 85 to 100 mm Hg from 33 to 50 weeks' gestational age (Raemakers et al, 1990; Wallen, 1992). A study conducted within 72 hours of birth has also shown that very preterm infants (24 to 31 weeks' gestational age) have a range of autoregulation that is narrow, over about 31 to 40 mm Hg (Van De Bor and Walther, 1991).

Cerebral blood flow reactivity to changes in blood pressure and to PCO_2 has also been studied using xenon-133 clearance in preterm infants and correlated with the development of cerebral lesions (Pryds et al, 1989). Pryds and colleagues showed that cerebral blood flow, $PaCO_2$, and mean arterial blood pressures all increased with age. Cerebral blood flow and $PaCO_2$ reactivities were depressed in 1-day-old infants but not in infants from 24 to 48 hours of postnatal age. In infants without intracranial hemorrhages, cerebral blood flows increased modestly with increasing mean arterial blood pressure; the changes in cerebral blood flow were not significant and were not interpreted as representing pressure-passive reactivity. The infants who subsequently suffered severe intracranial hemorrhages had significant changes in cerebral blood flow associated with changes in mean arterial blood pressure (4.0% change in blood flow per mm Hg change in mean arterial blood pressure, $P<.02$) (Pryds et al, 1989). Similar studies done by the same investigators in severely asphyxiated newborn infants showed that the most severely affected infants had high cerebral blood flows with absent reactivity to changes in carbon dioxide or blood pressure (Pryds et al, 1990b). These studies suggest that the normal very-low-birth-weight preterm infant has cerebral vascular reactivity to PCO_2 and modest cerebral blood flow changes in response to blood pressure changes. The infant at risk for brain injury seems to have either pressure-passive or unreactive cerebral circulation.

More mature infants (33 to 50 weeks' gestational age) show increases in autoregulatory limits as mean arterial blood pressure increases, and Low and coworkers (1991) have shown that stable preterm infants increase their systemic blood pressures and decrease their heart rates during the days following delivery (Raemakers et al, 1990). Mean arterial blood pressures in infants less than 1500 g birth weight increase from 38 to 45 mm Hg during the first 4 postnatal days, and in infants of greater than 1500 g birth weight, pressures increase from 43 to 54 mm Hg. Heart rates in the same two groups decrease over the first 4 postnatal days from means of 159 to 144 beats/min and from 154 to 136 beats/min.

POSTNATAL BRAIN PROTECTION

Minimal Stimulation Protocols for the Preterm Infant

Because of the narrow range of autoregulation in the preterm infant, and the possibility that infants of varying gestational ages may lose autoregulatory capacities after even moderate asphyxia, efforts to reduce dramatic fluctuations in systemic blood pressure (thereby hypothetically reducing fluctuations in cerebral blood flow) have been instituted in most neonatal intensive care units. These efforts consist mainly of *minimal stimulation* protocols, in which the amount of handling of infants and the number and types of procedures are held to a minimum. In addition, the lights in the immediate environment are dimmed, and noise levels are kept as low as possible. In some cases, very preterm infants are also paralyzed during mechanical ventilation to prevent breathing efforts that interfere with the ventilator and affect blood pressure and blood flow (Perlman et al, 1983, 1985). These efforts reduce blood pressure fluctuations, and it is hypothesized that some of the decreased incidence in intraventricular hemorrhage relates in part to the adoption of such protocols. Because of other parallel changes in neonatal intensive care, including changes in ventilatory practices, however, it has not been possible to prove unequivocally the effectiveness of minimal stimulation in this regard (Szymonowicz et al, 1986).

Pharmacologic Strategies

Prenatal and postnatal pharmacologic strategies are being studied for reducing both hypoxic-ischemic and hemorrhagic brain injury. Presently, pharmacologic therapies aimed at reducing the incidence of intraventricular hemorrhage include (1) prenatal corticosteroid administration, (2) prenatal or postnatal vitamin K administration, (3) prenatal or postnatal administration of phenobarbital, and (4) postnatal administration of indomethacin (Bedard et al, 1984; Crowley, 1994; Donn et al, 1981; Kaempf et al, 1990; Kuban et al, 1986; Ment et al, 1994a, 1994b; Morales and Koerton, 1986; Morales et al, 1988; Shankaran et al, 1986; Whitelaw et al, 1983). Vitamin E has also been administered in attempts to prevent both retinopathy of prematurity and intraventricular hemorrhage (Speer et al, 1984). Other strategies being considered for protection against hypoxic-ischemic injury, but not yet part of the pharmacologic armamentarium, include use of antioxidant agents, *N*-methyl-D-aspartate (NMDA) receptor antagonists, calcium channel blockers, and nonglucocorticosteroids (lazaroids).

NEUROLOGIC, MATURATIONAL, AND BEHAVIORAL ASSESSMENTS

Initial Observations: Behavioral States and Mental Status

The purpose of the neurologic examination of the newborn is to assess the integrity of the nervous system through the behaviors and reflex responses of the newborn. This also means paying attention to any findings from the general physical examination that might give clues to problems in the nervous system. The head should be examined carefully. The fronto-occipital circumference should be measured and charted, and the sutures should be palpated. Any suspected craniosynostosis should be followed up with appropriate radiologic studies. A port-wine stain in the trigeminal nerve branch distributions may be associated with abnormalities in the retinal choroid or in the meningeal vasculature (Sturge-Weber syndrome). Midline defects (hair whorls, tufts, dimples, cysts, or encephaloceles) should be noted so that appropriate neuroimaging and neurosurgical consultation can be obtained. The eyes and skin should be examined for evidence of diseases that also affect the brain (e.g., neurofibromatosis, Sturge-Weber syndrome, incontinentia pigmenti, tuberous sclerosis).

The quality and intensity of neonatal neurologic responses depend on the behavioral state of the infant—defined as quiet sleep, rapid-eye-movement (REM) sleep, quiet alertness, active alertness, or crying (Prechtl, 1977). A depressed infant may be stuporous or comatose—examples of abnormal states of consciousness. Abnormal states of consciousness can be determined by assessing the responses of the infant to gentle shaking, to a light shining in the eyes, or to sound (arousal maneuvers) as well as by assessing the infant's quality and quantity of spontaneous and reflex movements (Volpe, 1995a). It is imperative to note the infant's state for each examination. It is also important to note the quality and intensity of all newborn responses: Are they sustained or easily diminished, can they be elicited over and over, or does the infant lessen (habituate) the response? Neurologically normal newborns do not have overactive responses and usually habituate most responses to some extent on repetitive testing.

Although the neurologic examination is recorded in a sequential standardized format, the order in which the examination is done does not necessarily correlate with that format. It is essential that the tests of neurologic function be gestational age specific. Because the neurologic status of an infant can depend on behavioral state, and because some findings are more easily elicited in certain states, it is imperative to carry out repeated examinations when findings are not definite on one examination.

The mental status of the infant corresponds closely to behavioral state. It is especially important to recognize the infant with variations such as nervous system irritability or depression, however, because both indicate possible nervous system dysfunction. Irritability may be manifest by the following: hyperalertness, restlessness, jitteriness or persistent tremor, hypertonus, or hyper-reflexia. The irritable infant usually has a high-pitched, unpleasant cry. Depression manifests as decreased respiratory effort, abnor-

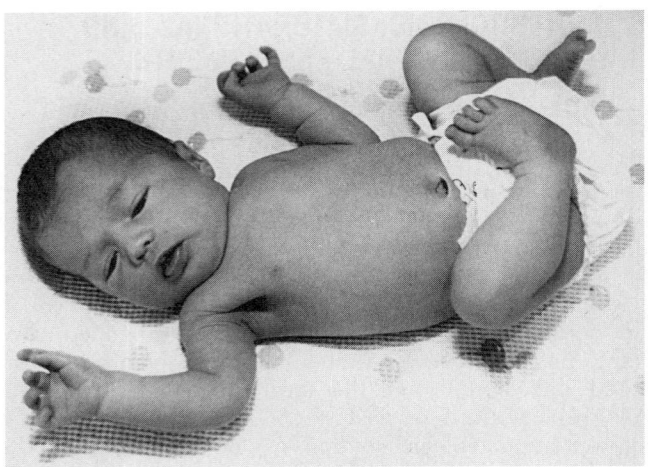

FIGURE 69–1. Normal tone and posture of a term infant in the supine position. (Photo by Jan Goddard-Finegold of Anneliese Moise Gest, at 40 weeks' corrected gestational age; printed with permission of her parents.)

mal eye movements, decreased alertness (lethargy, stupor, or coma), poorly sustained or absent cry, and depressed reflexes. The depressed infant may be hypotonic; the comatose infant may show flaccidity (this can also be present when there is neuromuscular disease, myopathy, or spinal cord injury). The irritable infant and the depressed infant can both exhibit seizures, and the irritable infant may show exaggerated athetoid movements (Prechtl, 1977). Some tremor and athetoid movements are normal in full-term infants, however, during the first few postnatal days.

Posture, Tone, and Spontaneous Activity

Tone is best assessed in the awake, alert state by passive movement of the limbs, neck, and trunk. Tone is particularly dependent on maturation; flexor tone becomes noticeable in the lower extremities at about 28 weeks' gestation. The term infant holds a posture that is predominantly flexor in both the upper and the lower extremities (Figs. 69–1 and 69–2). The progression of development of tone from 28 to 40 weeks' gestational age is shown in Figure

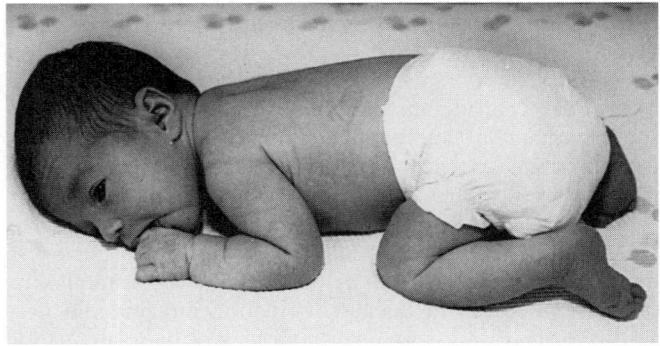

FIGURE 69–2. Normal tone and posture of a term infant in the prone position. (Photo by Jan Goddard-Finegold of Anneliese Moise Gest, at 40 weeks' corrected gestational age; printed with permission of her parents.)

69–3. If the infant is in the *asymmetric tonic neck posture*, tone is more extensor on the side to which the head is turned and more flexor on the opposite side. Thus, it is important to keep the infant's head in neutral position during the examination of posture and tone.

The traction response consists of the infant's actively maintaining the head briefly in line with the trunk, when the examiner gently pulls the infant from the supine position by the hands. During this response, the palmar grasp is stimulated, the elbows flex, and the flexor muscles of the neck raise the head briefly. Abnormalities of the traction response can be seen in infants who are hypotonic (head lag) as well as in infants who are hypertonic (head usually hyperextended).

Maturational Indices

Assessment of neurologic maturity includes assessment of tone and several gestational age–dependent reflexes (Amiel-Tison, 1968). The most frequently used reflexes include (1) pupillary reaction to light (develops between 29 and 31 weeks' gestation), (2) glabellar reflex (32 to 34 weeks), (3) neck-righting reflex (34 to 37 weeks), (4) traction response (>33 weeks), and (5) head turning to diffuse light (32 to 36 weeks) (Amiel-Tison, 1968; Menkes, 1991a). Other signs that appear and disappear with age are listed in Table 69–1 (Paine and Oppe, 1966).

Cranial Nerve Examination

The pupillary reactions to light can be tested by shading one eye at a time with the examiner's hand and then removing the hand. The pupils should be equal and round, and the newborn should have conjugate eye movements from time to time. Some newborns have strabismus, which is not abnormal at this time unless it is constant. Although transient horizontal nystagmus may be seen in normal newborns, sustained nystagmus is pathologic (Menkes, 1991a; Prechtl, 1977). Following is inconsistent at this stage, but some term infants fix for fairly long periods of time. Usually the doll's eye test is strongly positive in newborns during the first couple of postnatal weeks; the best way to test for doll's eyes is to turn the head slowly in each direction, watching the position of the eyes. The head should be kept to the right and to the left for several seconds. When testing for facial strength, it should be noted that some infants have failure of depression of one corner of the mouth on crying. This is due to congenital absence of the depressor anguli oris muscle and does not indicate facial nerve injury (Fenichel, 1994).

Motor Examination

The motor examination at this stage primarily consists of assessment of power of active movement and range of movement. Resistance to passive movement is also assessed. This examination is best done when the infant is alert, quiet or active. In the prone position, the newborn full-term infant keeps the legs partially flexed and adducted. The infant can rotate the head from side to side and can momentarily lift it off of the mattress. Supine, the

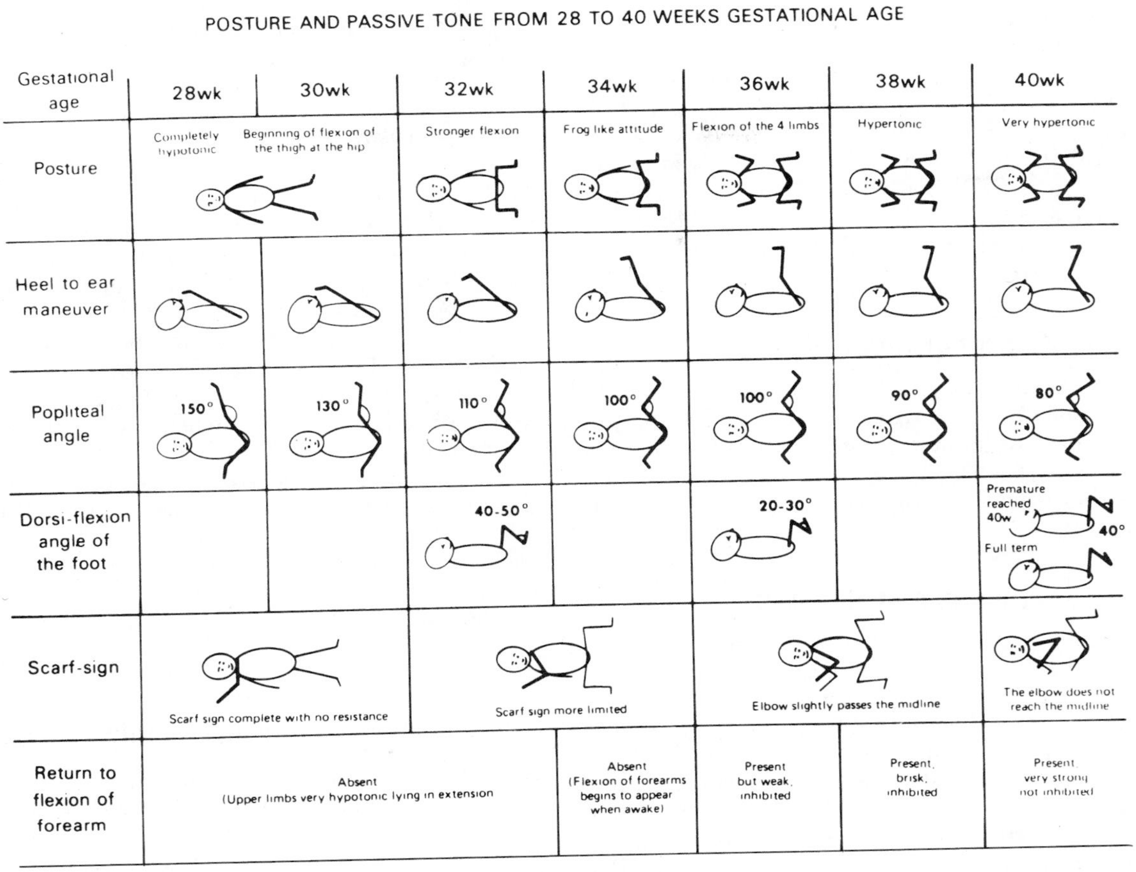

POSTURE AND PASSIVE TONE FROM 28 TO 40 WEEKS GESTATIONAL AGE

FIGURE 69–3. Posture and passive tone from 28 to 40 weeks' gestation, indicating increasing muscle tone in upper and lower extremities, which develops with increasing gestational age. (Adapted from Amiel-Tison C, David SW: Newborn neurologic examination. *In* Rudolph AM, Hoffman JIE [Eds]: Pediatrics, 19th ed. Norwalk, CT, Appleton & Lange, 1991.)

infant has poorly coordinated limb movements on both sides. Some of these movements appear to be *athetoid.* Asymmetry of movement, when one or both limbs on one side do not move or move less than the limbs on the other side, may indicate weakness.

Tone is assessed by the infant's resistance to passive movement as well as by the scarf sign and the traction response. For the scarf sign, the infant is held with one of the examiner's hands supporting his or her back; with the other hand, the examiner takes the infant's hand on one side and pulls the arm across the chest to the opposite shoulder. The position of the elbow with respect to the midline is noted. If the elbow passes the midline, hypotonia is present. The degree of hypotonia in the scarf sign de-

TABLE 69–1

Reflexes of Value in Assessing Gestational Age*

Reflex	Stimulus	Positive Response	Gestation (weeks) if Reflex Is:	
			Absent	**Present**
Pupil reaction	Light	Pupil contraction	<31	≥29
Traction	Pull up by wrists from supine	Flexion of neck or arms	<36	≥33
Glabellar tap	Tap on glabella	Blink	<34	≥32
Neck righting	Rotation of head	Trunk follows	<37	≥34
Head turning	Diffuse light from one side	Head turning to light	Doubtful	≥32

*Note: 24 weeks means 203 days after the first day of the last menstrual period. If there is a conflict between two results, the reflex placed higher in the table is more likely to give the true gestational age.

(From Robinson, RJ: Assessment of gestational age by neurological examination. Arch Dis Child 41:437, 1966.)

creases as an immature infant approaches term (see Table 69–1). Hypotonia is a common motor abnormality found in newborns with neurologic abnormalities and is usually associated with some degree of weakness (Volpe, 1995a). It is important to distinguish the patterns of weakness associated with CNS disease; spinal cord disorders; and abnormalities of lower motoneurons, nerve roots, peripheral nerves, neuromuscular junctions, or muscles. These disorders are discussed in some detail in the section on Neuromuscular Disorders.

Sensory Examination

The sensory examination can be carried out by using a sharp object, such as the broken end of a wooden Q-tip, to see if the infant withdraws and grimaces. When there is a level of motor dysfunction, suggesting spinal cord injury, the level below which sensory loss is absent should be determined.

Examination of Reflexes

Several primitive reflexes have already been mentioned (glabellar, tonic neck, neck righting, traction). Other primitive reflexes include respiratory reflexes, cardiovascular reflexes, coughing reflex, sneezing reflex, swallowing reflex, and rooting and sucking reflexes (Menkes, 1991a). Palmar and plantar grasp responses are primitive reflexes, as are reflex placing and stepping and the Landau reflex (in which the infant is suspended prone on one of the examiner's hands—the infant then shows a reflex extension of the trunk, causing an upward curvature of the spine with lifting of the head). These reflexes decrease in intensity as higher cortical functions become manifest.

Tendon reflexes can also be tested in the newborn (these are tests of phasic tone) (Fenichel, 1994). They are best tested with the head in the midline, so as not to elicit the tonic neck reflex. The patellar reflex is the most easily elicited in the perinatal period.

The plantar response (or Babinski reflex) is a response elicited by stroking the foot from heel to toe along the lateral aspect (Bodensteiner, 1992). The reflex is mediated by the L5-S2 spinal roots and consists of plantar flexion of the toes. When there is hyperactivity particularly of the S1 spinal segment, this stimulus also recruits the extensor hallucis longus, causing extension (dorsiflexion) of the big toe (the Babinski sign). In the newborn, elicitation of the extensor response seems to depend on the nature of the nociceptive stimulus used. When there is a subthreshold stimulus, the flexor response may be present; when the stimulus is sufficiently noxious, the extensor response occurs (Bodensteiner, 1992). By the end of the 1st year, in most infants, the plantar response becomes uniformly flexor, even with a sufficiently noxious stimulus. The Babinski sign in the infant younger than 1 year of age is not considered pathologic; when it is present in older children and adults, it is a sign of upper motor neuron dysfunction.

Postural reflexes include the tonic neck reflex, the Moro reflex, and the withdrawal reflex. The asymmetric tonic neck reflex is tested by slowly turning the head in one direction, allowing the ipsilateral arm to extend and the contralateral arm to flex. Leg extension on the side to which the head is turned is less consistent. When the tonic neck reflex is overly strong and sustained, it is said to be *obligatory*. When there is an obligatory tonic neck response in one direction, there is an abnormality in the contralateral hemisphere (Fenichel, 1994).

The Moro reflex is a startle reaction that occurs when the head is allowed to fall backward a few centimeters with the child supported in the supine position. There are phases to the Moro response: initial movements in which the arms are spread out and the hands are opened, followed by arm adduction and flexion over the chest with closing of the fists, finalized in some cases with a cry. Exaggerated Moro responses may occur when there is CNS irritability, as in infants after severe asphyxia; asymmetric Moro responses may occur when there is paralysis owing to brachial plexus injury.

The withdrawal reflex is a spinal reflex that is present from 28 weeks' gestation (Fenichel, 1994). Touching the sole of the foot with the broken tip of a wooden Q-tip elicits the response, which can be variable. Flexion of the pricked leg usually occurs with extension of the contralateral leg; however, the contralateral limb may show flexion or incomplete extension.

Assessment of Autonomic Function

It has been known for some time that the newborn heart does not have full sympathetic innervation and, therefore, is more sensitive to exogenous catechols (Friedman, 1973). Parasympathetic innervation is more complete at birth, and thus vagal reflexes are strongly operational (Phillips et al, 1964). Bradycardia may follow head or umbilical cord compression in utero or may occur after sneezing, hiccoughing, or yawning in newborns (Hellman et al, 1961; Phillips et al, 1964). As term is approached, there is an increase in baroreflex sensitivity (Gootman et al, 1972), and tests of blood pressure changes during postural variations have been tried in newborns. An upright tilt has led to increased systolic blood pressure followed by a drop, then by a return to steady-state values (Moss et al, 1963). The response to tilting seems to depend on the degree and duration of tilt, however. Other vasomotor responses have been recorded during exchange transfusions in newborn infants: With blood removal, pressure falls, and when an equal volume of blood is returned, blood pressure rises above control values (Wallgren et al, 1964). It has been suggested that a simulated Valsalva maneuver can be used to test baroreceptor function by observing blood pressure changes—however, the authors do not suggest invoking Valsalva maneuvers for this purpose, and the authors do not suggest tilting for testing purposes. It is useful to monitor blood pressure in newborns when possible and to observe spontaneous changes that occur with procedures, postural changes, and naturally occurring events.

Evaluation of Vision and Hearing

Evaluation for vision includes tests of visual following and opticokinetic nystagmus. The range of eye movements is assessed as well as the optic fundi. Visual following may be delayed in some full-term infants without implying an abnormality of the subcortical or cortical visual systems. Any suspected abnormalities, however, must be followed up carefully; high-risk infants are at greater risk of visual impairment usually in conjunction with cognitive impairment (Miranda et al, 1977; Miranda and Hack, 1979).

Infants with hearing impairment may have abnormal startle patterns: Either they do not startle appropriately, or they may startle excessively to visual stimuli (Volpe, 1995a). It is vital for language development to recognize hearing loss early, and the use of brain stem auditory evoked potentials is extremely important for diagnosis. If the hearing loss is a progressive disorder, occurring over the first months of life, however, the neonatal brain stem–evoked responses may not be abnormal (Kennedy, 1992; Stapells and Kurtzberg, 1991; Volpe, 1995a). Notably, in one study of congenital cytomegalovirus infection, 10.4% of infected infants (the incidence of infection in the study population was 1.3%) had evidence of sensorineural hearing loss (1.1 per 1000 live births) (Hicks et al, 1993). Another study of infants with otherwise asymptomatic cytomegalovirus infection showed that 8 of 59 infected infants had sensorineural hearing loss; 6 of the 8 infants had further deterioration of their hearing with time, and a ninth infant in the study developed sensorineural hearing loss during the 1st postnatal year (Williamson et al, 1992). Infants with persistent pulmonary hypertension of the newborn have been known in the past to be at risk for hearing loss (Hendricks-Munoz and Walton, 1988); however, this appears to be related to treatment modalities and not as much to the underlying problem. Marron and associates (1992) reported prospective follow-up data on 27 of 34 infants with persistent pulmonary hypertension of the newborn who survived after conservative therapy (no paralysis and no hyperventilation to induce alkalosis). None of the children had sensorineural hearing loss. It is important to obtain family histories also because hereditary forms of deafness account for a significant proportion of cases (Barton et al, 1962; Konigsmark, 1969).

Neurobiologic Risk Assessment

Prediction of long-term neurodevelopmental outcome from nursery neurologic evaluations is difficult. Brazy and colleagues (1991) attempted to address the problem of long-term predictions by devising a neurobiologic risk score that is based primarily on indices that might reflect brain injury. These investigators weighted 13 different items that they thought reflected possible causes of neural cell injury (hypoxemia, ischemia, inadequate metabolic substrate, or direct injury). At 2 weeks of age, or when the infants were ready for discharge, the items were assessed by chart review. The infants also underwent neurodevelopmental assessments at 6, 15, and 24 months' corrected ages. When the Neurobiologic Risk Score (NBRS) was applied to 68 infants of less than 1500 g birth weight, seven of the indices accounted for most of the variation in neurodevelopmental outcome: pH, ventilation, infection, seizures, intraventricular hemorrhage, periventricular leukomalacia, and hypoglycemia. The use of these seven items for the NBRS had great sensitivity at both the 6-month and the 24-month assessments. If an infant had a revised NBRS of 5 or more at 2 weeks or 6 or more at discharge, the infant was significantly more likely to have one or more neurodevelopmental abnormalities at all of the follow-up periods. This type of risk assessment may be useful; however, clinicians are cautioned to use it in conjunction with careful follow-up and prospective neurodevelopmental testing.

Diagnostic Tests

Major techniques for imaging the nervous system (ultrasound, computed tomography [CT], magnetic resonance imaging [MRI]), electroencephalography, and other electrophysiologic tests are discussed in subsequent sections. Cerebrospinal fluid (CSF) examination (lumbar puncture), which is frequently helpful in the neurologic assessment of the newborn, is considered here.

Cerebrospinal Fluid Examination

CSF is obtained for examination most frequently in newborns by lumbar puncture. Lumbar puncture is usually done to rule out meningitis and can be carried out in the lateral decubitus or the sitting position. Pressure readings are more accurate from the lateral decubitus position, but the midline may be more easily defined in the sitting position. To prevent the intraspinal introduction of tissue, a styletted needle is recommended (Shaywitz, 1972); however, in the newborn, it is sometimes advantageous to use a nonstyletted butterfly needle. When the butterfly tubing is held vertically, the CSF rises in the tubing, and pressure can be estimated. In addition, when there is a traumatic tap, sometimes uncontaminated CSF can still be obtained by cutting off the butterfly tubing containing the clear fluid (Fishman, 1992; Greenshear et al, 1971).

CSF pressure is lower in infants than in children and adults. CSF pressures obtained in newborns ranged from 10 to 20 cm H_2O in one study and averaged 27 cm H_2O in another (Minns, 1984; Welch, 1980). Composition of the CSF in newborns has been reported in several studies. Naidoo (1968) found that healthy term infants, from birth to 24 hours' postnatal age, had 0 to 70 polymorphonuclear leukocytes, 0 to 20 monocytes, 32 to 240 mg/dL protein, and 32 to 78 mg/dL glucose, with 0 to 1070 red blood cells in nontraumatic taps.

Pinheiro and coworkers (1993) reported the effect of local anesthesia on the success rate of lumbar puncture in the newborn. In their study, newborns were held in a modified lateral recumbent position without the neck flexed, and struggling was scored. Forty-eight infants were subcutaneously injected with 0.2 to 0.5 mL of 1% lidocaine before the procedure; 52 infants were not. Struggling increased during the injection of the lidocaine, but the struggling response to the lumbar puncture was significantly reduced. The success rate of the lumbar punctures in the two groups was the same, however, with the number of traumatic taps and repeated punctures virtually the same in both groups. The authors concluded that the use of the injected local anesthesia did not make performing the lumbar puncture more difficult and did not alter the success rate of the procedure; however, they did not assess the use of topically applied anesthetic.

NEUROPHYSIOLOGIC ASSESSMENT
Electroencephalography
General Considerations

The EEG has an important role in the diagnosis and management of neurologic disorders in newborns. It can provide useful information concerning brain function, in contrast to techniques that assess brain structure. Neonatal electroencephalography is most valuable when it is correlated with the infant's medical history, when a plan or recording is based on history and clinical findings, when there is careful patient observation and appropriate stimulation during the recording, when EEG findings are considered in relation to the infant's state of alertness and to relevant laboratory data, and when there is direct consultation between the clinical neurophysiologist and the physicians requesting the EEG.

This section describes the clinical circumstances in which electroencephalography may be helpful in the care of newborns. This is not intended to be a comprehensive review of neonatal electroencephalography but rather is designed to provide the clinician with an understanding of the ways in which the EEG can be applied to clinical diagnosis and management of the newborn. A number of other current discussions of neonatal electroencephalography provide further details of recording techniques, normal and abnormal EEG features, and methods of analysis (Hrachovy et al, 1990; Lombroso, 1982; Scher, 1989; Tharp, 1980; Torres and Anderson, 1985).

Technical Considerations

The American Electroencephalographic Society (1994) has provided guidelines for the recording of the neonatal EEG. Some of the basic technical requirements for obtaining optimal recordings of the EEG in older children and adults apply to recording in newborns. There are, however, some significant differences: (1) fewer scalp electrodes are needed in newborns, although electrodes placed in the midline are critical; (2) in addition to the EEG, other measures must be recorded simultaneously to allow for adequate wake/sleep cycle assessment, including electrocardiogram (ECG), movements of respirations, electrooculogram, and surface electromyography (EMG) of various muscle groups; (3) typically, one selection of an array of electrode channels (a montage) is recorded throughout the recording; (4) recordings must be long enough in duration to allow for sleep to be sampled; and (5) the recording of the neonatal EEG requires technologists specially trained in this technique, in the handling of newborns, and in the understanding of neonatal clinical problems.

Considerations in Electroencephalogram Interpretation

Interpretation of the neonatal EEG is based on several principles, some of which are unique to this age group. The normal EEG undergoes rapid changes as a consequence of rapid brain development in the perinatal period. Abnormalities may be characterized by altered developmental characteristics as well as by specific patterns or waveforms. Patterns and waveforms that are normal at one age may be abnormal at another. Although many aspects of the neonatal EEG have been determined by careful clinical investigation to be either normal or abnormal, there are other aspects that are of uncertain significance (Hrachovy et al, 1990). Finally, certain abnormal EEG findings in the immediate neonatal period may be present only transiently and may change to less abnormal findings within a few hours or days, as the infant's condition stabilizes or improves. Thus, the prognostic significance of these findings is best established only in relationship to their persistence or change over time (Tharp et al, 1981).

Brain Development and the Electroencephalogram

Brain growth and differentiation are reflected in rapidly changing electrographic findings in the newborn. These changes have been characterized from 27 weeks' conceptional age to the end of the neonatal period (44 weeks' conceptional age). They have been categorized into changes of continuity, development of age-specific waveforms, hemispheric synchrony, and development of wake/sleep cycles. During this period, the EEG gradually changes from a discontinuous pattern of bursts of activity between periods of electrical quiescence to a continuous pattern. Waveforms with specific character and location over the scalp appear and disappear in an orderly progression during this period. After an initial early period in which activity is synchronous over the two hemispheres, the EEG becomes relatively asynchronous, then gradually the degree of synchrony increases with age. Finally, early in development, there are no EEG changes that are specifically correlated with the wake/sleep cycle. With increasing age, clearly defined EEG patterns are correlated with the various stages of sleep and with wakefulness (Dreyfus-Brisac and Monod, 1964; Ellingson and Peters, 1980).

Application of Electroencephalography to Clinical Care of the Newborn

The newborn EEG is most valuable when performed to answer a specific clinical question. The neonatal EEG can be helpful in considering several clinical questions.

What Is the Conceptional Age of the Infant? The physical examination and the maternal history may not provide information specific enough to make an accurate determination of age. In addition, there may be instances in which history and physical examination may provide conflicting estimates of the infant's age. Because the neonatal EEG has developmental features that appear during specific developmental epochs, the EEG can be helpful in assessing conceptional age.

Has the Infant Suffered a Diffuse Central Nervous System Injury? This question is generally prompted by the finding of an abnormal state of alertness or the clinical suspicion that the infant may have had a seizure. The EEG may be abnormal, with either diffuse or focal features, or both, indicating CNS dysfunction. The most frequent EEG characterizations of diffuse CNS injury are the following: depressed and undifferentiated background activity, a suppression-burst pattern, the presence of multifocal sharp waves, electrocerebral silence, or dyschronism (dysmaturity of the EEG). These should be viewed as descriptions of the disordering of brain function and not as representative of a specific pathologic process. A generalized disturbance of brain function as evidenced by the EEG may be the result of hypoxia-ischemia, metabolic disorders, infection, or, at times, intracranial hemorrhage. Therefore, EEG findings consistent with cerebral dysfunction require detailed evaluation as to cause.

Is There Evidence of Focal Central Nervous System Injury? The EEG may be helpful in evaluation of some infants with certain types of focal lesions. Persistent asymmetry of voltage has statistically been associated with focal structural or space-occupying lesions, such as intracerebral hemorrhage, subdural hemorrhage, subdural effusion, focal ischemia or infarction, cystic lesions, or congenital malformations. The finding of focal depression or persistent voltage asymmetry requires further evaluation with available imaging techniques.

There has been considerable discussion in the literature concerning the specificity of the finding of positive rolandic sharp waves in the diagnosis of intraventricular hemorrhage. Early reports suggested that the finding of positive rolandic sharp waves was diagnostic of intraventricular hemorrhage; however, more recent studies indicate that positive rolandic sharp waves are most specific for periventricular leukomalacia, which may result from or be associated with several different types of injury, including intraventricular hemorrhage (Blume and Dreyfus-Brisac, 1982; Clancy and Tharp, 1984; Novotny et al, 1987).

When Did Central Nervous System Injury Occur? In the immediate neonatal period, the finding of EEG features indicating delayed maturational development may suggest that a CNS injury may have occurred in utero (Hrachovy et al, 1990). Thus, the finding of immature EEG features in relation to gestational age (dyschronism) suggests that the insult may have been prenatal.

What Is the Prognosis? The EEG may be helpful in the determination of the prognosis of a newborn with suspected cerebral injury. It is generally thought that the greater the EEG abnormality, the more grave the prognosis. In making this correlation, however, it is critical to determine the timing of the EEG to the suspected time of injury and the rate of resolution of the EEG abnormalities over time. The ideal time to record the EEG is within 24 hours of suspected injury. The EEG should be repeated within 24 hours, then, depending on the findings, further studies should be planned. Although the initial EEG may be severely abnormal, the accuracy of prognosis is based on the evolution (degree and rate of resolution) of the abnormality. A normal initial EEG (within 24 hours of birth) reliably suggests a good prognosis (Hrachovy et al, 1990).

Is There Evidence of Brain Death? Brain death is a clinical diagnosis in the newborn. The finding of electrocerebral silence in the newborn indicates the destruction of the neocortex. Brain stem function, however, may still be present. Some infants have survived for several years, even though electrocerebral silence had been noted in the neonatal period (Mizrahi et al, 1985). The diagnosis of brain death in the newborn cannot be based on electrographic findings alone.

Is the Infant Experiencing Seizures? As discussed in the section on Seizures and Other Paroxysmal Disorders, not all behaviors currently considered to be neonatal seizures are accompanied by EEG seizure activity (Kellaway and Mizrahi, 1990; Mizrahi and Kellaway, 1987). Focal clonic seizures have a close, consistent relationship to EEG seizure activity. In addition, a limited range of so-called subtle seizures (focal tonic seizures) and some myoclonic seizures may also occur in close relationship to EEG seizure activity. Generalized tonic, almost all subtle (best characterized as *motor automatisms*), and most myoclonic seizures, however, do not have a close relationship to EEG seizure activity and may occur in the absence of any electrical seizure discharges. As discussed subsequently, these clinical events may not be of epileptic origin and may be primitive reflex behavior. The recording of the EEG during clinical events suspected of being seizures provides a basis for considering their pathophysiology.

In addition to EEG seizure activity occurring in association with clinical seizure activity, electrical seizure activity may also occur in the absence of any clinical activity. This activity may occur if the infant is pharmacologically paralyzed, if the infant has suffered severe brain injury, or if the infant had originally experienced clinical seizures associated with electrical seizure activity and then had been treated with antiepileptic drugs (AEDs). In untreated infants with focal clonic seizures, the EEG seizure activity is closely associated with the clinical seizure. When AED therapy is initiated, the clinical event may be controlled, but the electrical seizure activity may persist. Thus, the clinical seizure becomes *decoupled* from the electrical seizure (Mizrahi and Kellaway, 1987). When clinical seizures are controlled by AEDs, further EEG monitoring is necessary to detect persistent electrical seizure activity.

Electroencephalography is essential in the evaluation of newborns suspected of having seizures. Equally critical, however, is careful observation of the newborn during recording to insure accurate clinical correlation with EEG findings.

Electroencephalography and Video Monitoring

The simultaneous recording of the EEG with a video image of infants, children, and adults has become routine in neurophysiology laboratories. The technique has been important in both clinical management and clinical research providing the basis for detection, characterization, and quantification of seizure activity and its differentiation from other paroxysmal clinical events. The EEG/video monitoring of newborns has specific problems that have limited its widespread application: Recordings must be performed at the bedside in the busy environment of a critical care unit; technologists, instrumentation, and neurophysiologists must be continuously available to capture suspected clinical events; special expertise is required; specialized instrumentation is needed; and recording protocols must be established and rigorously followed (Mizrahi, 1994). Despite the difficulties of EEG/video monitoring in newborns, the technique has provided important information concerning neonatal seizures (see the section on Seizures and Other Paroxysmal Disorders) and, at centers where monitoring is available, has become a powerful tool for diagnosis and management in the nursery.

The technical basis of monitoring is the simultaneous recording of EEG; video; and a number of other measures of movement, respirations, and heart rate, which all can be used to characterize paroxysmal clinical events. Depending on instrumentation capabilities, the following measures can be recorded with EEG and video: thoracic and abdominal respiratory effort, airway flow, ECG, EMG of various muscle groups, electro-oculogram, blood pressure, pulse oximetry, and end-expiratory carbon dioxide.

The correlation of EEG findings with any changes in these measures or with the infant's behavior helps the neurophysiologist assess the type of events recorded and determine their pathophysiologic mechanisms. The most important clinical questions addressed by monitoring relate to neonatal seizures: Is the infant experiencing seizures; what type of seizures; what are the clinical components of the seizures; and what is the response to therapy? As in monitoring of older children and adults, the finding that paroxysmal clinical events are not seizures of epileptic origin is just as important as the confirmation of that finding. Thus, monitoring may demonstrate clinical events such as apnea (obstructive or central), paroxysmal changes in heart rate or blood pressure (not related to electrical seizure activity), nonepileptic seizures (see the section on Seizures and Other Paroxysmal Disorders), jitteriness of the newborn, and normal behaviors or movements of the newborn initially thought to be abnormal.

Electromyography and Nerve Conduction Studies

The application of EMG and nerve conduction studies in the newborn requires specialized expertise, an understanding of the type of information that can be obtained, and the knowledge of when EMG should be attempted in the course of the evaluation of possible neuromuscular disorders (Fenichel, 1990b; Jones, 1993).

Electromyography

The goals of EMG application are to determine the presence of neuromuscular dysfunction, and, if present, to localize the abnormality to a specific level of the motor unit (Jones, 1993). Normally, contraction is represented as a motor unit potential, which is characterized by amplitude, duration, number, and morphology. Based on the electrical features of the muscle at rest and during contraction, neuromuscular abnormalities can be characterized as disorders of anterior horn cells, peripheral nerve, or muscle. In addition, the response to repetitive stimulation may identify disorders of the neuromuscular junction.

Most often, EMG is used in the newborn to evaluate hypotonia, including the confirmation of physical signs, the characterization of the disorder, and the localization within the motor unit of the dysfunction (Fenichel, 1990a, 1990b). This information can then be applied to the determination of cause, prognosis, and therapy. The sequence of evaluation of these infants is important. Laboratory studies such as creatine phosphokinase assay should be performed before EMG, which, because of manipulation of the muscle by the needle examination, may falsely elevate the enzyme. Muscle biopsy should be performed in muscles not examined by EMG to avoid sampling muscle disrupted by needle penetration. Above all, the need for EMG should be considered in relation to the timing of the study (i.e., the potential yield of the study may increase with the age of the newborn, and the delay of the study may lessen the need for its repeat and provide more definite clinical information).

Nerve Conduction Studies

Motor and sensory nerve conduction velocities may be determined by electrical stimulation to assess the presence of peripheral nerve dysfunction. Nerve conduction velocities increase with increasing age. Therefore, age-dependent normal values are required for accurate assessment (Dubowitz et al, 1968; Miller et al, 1983). Evaluation by nerve conduction studies may be helpful in newborns suspected of having neuropathy, most often clinically manifested by hypotonia (Khater-Boidin and Duron, 1992).

Sensory Evoked Potentials

Sensory stimulation usually results in an electrical response that can be recorded using scalp electrodes. These responses are, however, for the most part, lower in amplitude and shorter in latency when compared to the spontaneous electrical activity of the brain. Instrumentation has been developed to record the response to repeated sensory stimulation, to average these responses, and to reduce the appearance of the spontaneous electrical cerebral activity. As a consequence, electrical potentials produced by repetitive auditory, visual, or tactile (somatosensory) stimulation can be enhanced, and the spontaneous background EEG activity is diminished in appearance. This allows for the measure of the amplitude and latency of specific waveforms, which characterize brain stem auditory evoked potentials (BAEPs), visual evoked potentials (VEPs), and somatosensory evoked potentials (SEPs).

Each is designed to test the transit time of the modality-specific sensory pathway from the site of stimulation to the most rostral generators within the brain. Thus, evoked potentials depend on both peripheral nervous system and CNS pathways. This aspect represents both a strength and a limitation of the application of evoked potentials to neonatal neurologic evaluation. The response allows the characterization of various components of a single sensory system pathway. Depending on the specific modality used, the site of dysfunction within specific pathways can be precisely localized, but at times this may be difficult. Because propagation of the response is a manifestation of peripheral nervous system and CNS conduction, the transit time (i.e., the latency of the response) depends on the degree of myelination of conducting fibers. Although these different modalities of evoked potential studies have been employed in diverse clinical settings in the evaluation of older children and adults, their application is relatively limited in newborns. They can be of value, however, when specifically applied (Fenichel, 1990a).

Brain Stem Auditory Evoked Potentials

BAEPs are responses recorded at the scalp that are generated by repetitive clicks delivered by headphones. The response is a series of waveforms that typically occur within 10 msec after the click is delivered. The peaks of the waves are generated by specific regions within the auditory pathways—from auditory nerve through midbrain. The absolute latency of the responses and the difference in latency between waveforms (the interpeak latencies) are measured. Amplitudes of response are also measured. Delays in latency (absolute or interpeak) and, at times, diminution of latency indicate abnormalities of the auditory conduction pathways.

In the nursery, BAEPs can be helpful in the assessment of hearing and, in the presence of abnormalities, allow the differentiation of conductive and sensorineural hearing loss. The BAEP may also indicate the presence of brain stem dysfunction, by virtue of the delay of waveforms generated within the brain stem itself. This type of interpretation is made difficult, however, by the dependency of normal conduction times on the degree of myelination of fibers.

Visual Evoked Potentials

VEPs are produced in response to flashing light presented to each eye. A single waveform is typically generated, which is analyzed for morphology, amplitude, and latency. In addition, the response generated by each eye is compared to the other (interocular differences), and the representation of the responses recorded on the two sides of the scalp are also compared (interhemispheric differences). The most clear abnormality is the absence of a response. Because of the variability of responses with flash stimulation in newborns, abnormality of VEPs based on latency and amplitude measures is not consistently reliable.

In newborns, flash VEPs have been used to assess the integrity of the visual pathways in hopes of estimating visual perception or acuity. In addition, because the visual pathways traverse subcortical and cortical structures, VEPs have been used to assess the functional integrity of adjacent structures. In the assessment of vision, however, VEPs only can indicate the relative intactness of the pathways but cannot provide information as to whether the infant actually can see or appreciate images. Other techniques, including imaging and EEG, may provide more specific information concerning the presence of structural abnormalities in the neonatal brain.

Somatosensory Evoked Potentials

SEPs are produced by electrical stimulation of nerves of distal limbs and recording at specific anatomic points along the pathway; the electrical impulse travels to the cortex. Upper extremity SEPs are typically produced by stimulation of the median nerves at the wrist and recorded at sites that include the elbow, Erb point, posterior cervical region at the neck, and scalp over the motor cortex contralateral to the stimulated limb. Lower extremity SEPs are typically produced by stimulation of the common peroneal nerve at the knee or posterior tibial nerve at the ankle and recorded at the lumbar spine region and the scalp. Each site is recorded on a separate channel; the absolute and interpeak latencies and amplitudes of the individual waveforms are measured. Abnormalities can localize the site of dysfunction through a relatively long pathway, which includes peripheral nerve, spinal cord dorsal columns, brain stem, and cortex. The application of these tests in the newborn is limited, however, by the degree of peripheral nervous system and CNS myelination, and thus, their use is, for the most part, reserved for older infants.

NEUROIMAGING

Neuroimaging of the newborn has entered an era of increasing sophistication, encompassing both structural and functional imaging. Transillumination is the simplest and least expensive method and one that should still be used. Ultrasonography, CT, MRI, and near-infrared spectroscopy (NIRS) can all be used to assess the newborn brain in various ways (for structure, blood flow velocity, oxygenation, blood volume changes, and estimates of volume of blood flow). Functional MRI, near-infrared time-of-flight analysis (for structural and physiologic imaging), nuclear magnetic resonance spectroscopy (MRS) (for biochemical monitoring), and positron emission tomography (for quantitative autoradiography in vivo) all continue to be used mainly in experimental realms, but the goal for the next decade is to make them less expensive, more accessible, more accurate, and without hazard. This section presents an overview of the primary modalities of neuroimaging in the newborn period.

Transillumination

Transillumination of the head is done by shining a high-intensity light over the infant's skull; close contact with the scalp is maintained by having a rubber collar at the end of the light source (this can be a specially designed transilluminator, the *Chun gun*, or it can be a large flashlight). Transillumination is best accomplished in a totally darkened room. Transillumination is increased when the infant is light skinned; has sparse, light hair; has a thin skull; and has a fluid collection in or under the scalp. Transillumination is decreased when the infant is dark-skinned with dark hair, has a thick skull or increased bone marrow, or has blood underneath the scalp, such as subgaleal hematoma (Volpe, 1995b). When the above-mentioned moderators are taken into account, and the normal findings on transillumination are considered for each gestational age (infants have been studied from 26 to 42 weeks' gestational age) (Vyhmeister et al, 1977), transillumination is abnormal when ventriculomegaly, fluid collections in the subdural or subarachnoid spaces, or decreased cerebral cortical mantle is present. Abnormal fluid collections or tissue loss in either the anterior or posterior compartments can be shown by transillumination. Transillumination is followed by other neuroimaging techniques for verification of suspected abnormalities.

Ultrasonography

Ultrasonography has become the imaging modality of choice in the neonatal intensive care unit because of its noninvasiveness and bedside applicability. A-mode echoencephalography was introduced in the mid-1950s as a means of determining midline cerebral shifts (Elliott, 1984). Two-dimensional, B-mode echoencephalography was introduced in the 1960s for imaging ventricular anatomy but was superseded by CT in adult neurology. With improvement of the imaging capabilities of the method, its portability, its lack of radiation hazard, and real-time function, however, it has become the first-line imaging procedure at the bedside in the nursery, especially for infants weighing less than 1500 g who are at risk for intraventricular and parenchymal hemorrhage, periventricular white matter lesions, and ventriculomegaly (Babcock and Han, 1981; Bejar et al, 1980; Elliott, 1984). CT offers advantages for detection of subarachnoid, cerebellar, and subdural hemorrhages. Ultrasonography uses pulsed sound waves to generate images; to date, there has been no association of the use of ultrasound imaging with any adverse biologic effects.

Images are obtained by changing the angle of the ultrasound beam through the fontanels and sutures. In this way, various sagittal and coronal *slices* can be visualized of the neonatal brain. This imaging technique is excellent, in particular, for visualization of the ventricular system and the periventricular regions. When further detail of brain is required, CT or MRI is preferable.

Skull Radiographs

Skull radiographs are still useful in neonatal neurology. Most often, they are obtained to determine the presence of skull fractures or the presence and definition of craniosynostosis, occipital osteodiastasis (usually after traumatic breech delivery), abnormal bone characteristics (e.g., thinning, thickening, lacunar skull), and abnormalities of the spine and craniocervical junction.

Computed Tomography

CT is an x-ray technique with high-resolution computerized image reconstruction. CT is used in the newborn, when more detail is needed than ultrasonography can provide, especially for subdural and subarachnoid hemorrhage as well as lesions in the posterior fossa and for brain calcifications. The value of MRI as a superior imaging modality is becoming evident, however, and CT is being used less frequently when MRI is available. Both CT and MRI require sedation of newborns; both can be accomplished in ventilated infants.

Magnetic Resonance Imaging

MRI, which requires no ionizing radiation, can detect lesions that are missed by CT. Notably, MRI is particularly excellent for imaging morphologic detail, myelination indices, developmental disorders (e.g., myelination and migration defects, partial agenesis of the corpus callosum), early and late cerebral ischemic lesions (cortical and white mat-

ter), hemorrhagic lesions, venous thromboses, and lesions of the posterior fossa and spinal cord (Volpe, 1995b).

MRI is based on the fact that the atomic nuclei of certain elements (such as hydrogen or phosphorus) behave as spinning magnets when exposed to a magnetic field (Martin et al, 1991). The alignment of the atomic nuclei in the magnetic field can be altered by brief pulses of radio waves; when the radio waves are discontinued, the atomic nuclei return to their original positions, and energy is given off (the atomic nuclei return to a lower energy state). Return of atomic nuclei to a lower energy state is called *relaxation*. The frequency of radio waves released is specific for specific atomic nuclei and is determined by the strength of the surrounding magnetic field and other environmental factors. Using computer techniques, images can be constructed that depict either the distribution of atomic nuclei with a particular relaxation time in a slice of tissue or the concentration of particular atomic nuclei (Martin et al, 1991).

NEUROMETABOLIC AND PHYSIOLOGIC ASSESSMENTS
Magnetic Resonance Spectroscopy

As in MRI, the basis for nuclear MRS is the measurement of the absorption of specific radiofrequencies by atomic nuclei with magnetic moments in a magnetic field (Chance et al, 1989). The elements most commonly used for medical purposes include phosphorus, hydrogen, carbon, sodium, and fluorine. Thus, measurements can be made noninvasively of metabolites important for energy metabolism, such as adenosine triphosphate (ATP), phosphocreatine (PCr), and the product of their breakdown, inorganic phosphate (Pi). Extrapolation can be made from the measurements of these compounds for the concentration of adenosine diphosphate (ADP), and intracellular pH can be estimated. MRS has been used to study brain metabolism in newborn infants; although the infant must be in a strong magnetic field for the MRS study, the infant can be monitored and ventilated, if necessary. Spectra are obtained as *peaks* for specific signal intensities. Concentrations of the metabolites are proportional to the areas under the peaks. This noninvasive technology is especially useful for evaluating the brain after hypoxia-ischemia or other metabolic insults that newborn infants may experience. The PCr/Pi ratio appears to be particularly helpful for prognostic purposes in such infants. In a study by Hamilton and colleagues (1986), PCr/Pi ratios were correlated with ultrasound findings and outcome. Fifteen of 27 infants with ultrasound scans suggestive of hypoxic-ischemic injury had PCr/Pi ratios below the range for normal infants; 9 of these 15 infants died, and the other 6 developed cerebral atrophy. Twelve infants whose PCr/Pi ratios were within the normal range survived; three who had ratios at the lower end of normal also developed atrophy (Chance et al, 1989; Hamilton et al, 1986).

Near-Infrared Spectroscopy

NIRS is a noninvasive technique for the detection of changes in concentrations of brain oxyhemoglobin, deoxyhemoglobin, and oxidized cytochrome aa_3, based on the absorption of near-infrared light by the iron and copper atoms in hemoglobin and cytochrome aa_3 (Jobsis, 1977; Rea et al, 1985; von Siebenthal et al, 1992; Wyatt et al, 1989). When a brief change in oxygen saturation is used as a tracer, cerebral blood flow can be estimated using a modification of the Fick principle (Edwards et al, 1988). When a gradual change in oxygen saturation is instituted, cerebral blood volume can be estimated using NIRS (Wyatt et al, 1989). Because cytochrome aa_3 is a critical component of the respiratory electron transport chain, its oxidation-reduction status is an indication of intracellular oxygenation. Infrared light can penetrate tissues up to 8 cm in depth, thereby making it realistic for assessing the newborn brain. The metabolic and hemodynamic information that can be gained by NIRS, along with studies that show that blood flow estimations obtained with NIRS compare favorably with those obtained in animals using invasive, time-honored methods, and its non-invasive bedside applicability make it a realistic candidate to be a long-awaited *cerebral function monitor* (Goddard-Finegold et al, 1994; Newton et al, 1995).

Doppler Cerebral Blood Flow Velocity Estimation

Doppler ultrasound makes use of the fact that frequency shifts occur when sound waves are reflected from a moving object; the frequency shift is proportional to the velocity of the object. When Doppler is used to assess blood flow velocity, the sound waves are reflected by moving red blood cells. Doppler ultrasound has been used to quantitate blood flow velocity in umbilical vessels and cerebral vessels in the fetus as well as blood flow velocity in cerebral vessels in newborn preterm and term infants. Flow velocities and resistance indices have been quantitated to estimate the status of the newborn cerebral circulation (Bada et al, 1979; Raju, 1991).

Positron Emission Tomography

PET is a way of performing quantitative autoradiography in the living human (Sokoloff, 1985). When a chemical reaction occurs, one type of molecule is converted to another. The rate of this reaction can be determined by measuring the rate of decrease of one type of molecule and the rate of appearance of the product. In general, this entails labeling of one of the reactants and measuring the rate of accumulation of the labeled product (Sokoloff, 1985). In PET, a radioactive label that undergoes chemical change by decaying with the emission of positrons is used; its distribution in the tissue of interest is measured by the radiation emitted over a period of time (Ter-Pogossian, 1985). The radionuclides ^{11}C, ^{13}N, ^{15}O, and ^{18}F are used to label selected compounds, which can be injected systemically and whose reaction products are known (e.g., oxygen, glucose, amino acids, fatty acids). Particularly important for human studies is the fact that all of these nuclides have extremely short half-lives (2 to 110 minutes), which enables their use in larger quantities and in repeated studies with much less radiation exposure. Methods for the detection and collimation of positron-emitting radionuclides led to the development of PET (Ter-Pogossian, 1985).

To date, PET has been used to measure cerebral blood flow, cerebral blood volume, and cerebral metabolism. One study using PET in six newborns with intraventricular hemorrhage and periventricular infarction used ^{15}O-labeled water to measure regional cerebral blood flow (Volpe et al, 1983). In these six infants, periventricular blood flow was considerably reduced in the areas of hemorrhagic infarction; in addition, blood flow was markedly reduced in the parietal-occipital white matter of the same hemisphere (Volpe et al, 1983). PET showed that impairment of blood flow was much more extensive than anticipated by the extent of the lesion.

NEUROLOGIC INJURY IN THE NEWBORN
Brain Depression and Recovery; Injury and Repair

The brain cellular responses to asphyxia are at least partly explained by experimental studies of hypoxia-ischemia. Apparently the earliest neuronal responses to oxygen lack include the release of adenosine and the opening of potassium channels (Rothman, 1992). This sequence causes the neuronal membrane to hyperpolarize, reducing the ability of the cell to produce action potentials. Calcium currents are also depressed, decreasing the release of synaptic neurotransmitters. Intracellular calcium increases moderately, however, activating calcium-dependent potassium channels and increasing the membrane hyperpolarization. Another potassium channel is opened when ATP concentrations decrease, further limiting the excitability of the neuron. These early events probably spare energy during periods of oxygen lack; they appear to be easily reversible when perfusion and oxygenation return to normal. Studies have shown that hypoxia-ischemia has a deleterious effect on an enzyme necessary for glucose metabolism, altering the binding characteristics of hexokinase, so that it is less available for glucose that is present (Gray et al, 1994). This biochemical change is not immediately reversible, lasting for some hours into reoxygenation and reperfusion (Gray et al, 1994). When tissue deoxygenation persists, other mechanisms come into play. Especially notable are those associated with (1) release of the amino acid glutamate, (2) production of neuronal and vascular nitric oxide, and (3) release of oxygen free radicals (Faraci and Brian, 1994; Rothman, 1992; Vannucci, 1990b).

There is now ample evidence to suggest that glutamate is a neurotransmitter (Monaghan et al, 1983; Rothman, 1992). There are four receptor types for glutamate, with the most avid being NMDA (Rothman, 1992). The NMDA receptor is one of the most physiologically active, and the channels that are activated by it depolarize neurons, are voltage dependent, and have a high permeability to calcium (Mayer et al, 1984, 1987; Rothman, 1992). When glutamate is present and neurons depolarize, their NMDA channels open. This is followed by more depolarization and intracellular accumulation of calcium. Under normal conditions, glutamate is intracellular and does not affect NMDA receptors. When synaptically released glutamate is present extracellularly, it is rapidly transported back across the cell membrane by pump mechanisms. When there is continued hypoxia-ischemia, however, the pump and transport mechanisms fail, and glutamate that is leaked from neurons is not transported out of the extracellular space. When this happens, levels of glutamate that are toxic to neurons accumulate. The glutamate-mediated toxicity is thought to be secondary to increased intracellular calcium concentrations. Areas of the brain with high concentrations of NMDA receptors seem to be most sensitive to hypoxic-ischemic injury. Also, the concentrations of NMDA receptors in various parts of the brain change with development, perhaps offering one reason for changing *selective vulnerabilities* with age.

Glutamate receptor antagonists such as MK-801 have been used experimentally to decrease neuronal damage from hypoxia-ischemia; however, the therapeutic window for the use of such agents has yet to be determined. In addition, drugs that block glutamate receptors have their own toxicities clinically, and it is not clear whether it is necessary to block all of the major receptors to achieve clinical effectiveness. Other strategies include finding ways to block endogenous glutamate release during hypoxia-ischemia; for instance, adenosine blocks glutamate release and synaptic activity (Goldberg et al, 1988; Swan et al, 1987).

Other mechanisms also play a role in hypoxic-ischemic brain injury. Glutamate release does not have the same deleterious effects on glial cells that it has on neurons, and neurons containing NADPH-diaphorase (nitric oxide synthase) seem to be more resistant to hypoxia-mediated cell death, for reasons that are not completely clear (Ferriero et al, 1988). Nitric oxide is a potent vasodilator (previously named *endothelium-derived relaxing factor*) that is produced by a number of cell types, including neurons, glia, and endothelial cells. Nitric oxide synthase converts L-arginine to nitric oxide and citrulline (Faraci and Brian, 1994). Importantly, when L-arginine is present, nitric oxide is preferentially made by nitric oxide synthase. When L-arginine is not present, however, nitric oxide synthase in the brain generates superoxide and hydrogen peroxide (Manzoni et al, 1992; Pou et al, 1992). When nitric oxide combines with superoxide, a toxic peroxynitrite is formed. Thus, it has been hypothesized that nitric oxide can be both helpful and detrimental during hypoxia: Nitric oxide can cause vasodilation and increased blood flow, and nitric oxide also blocks NMDA receptors (Faraci and Brian, 1994). Excessive production of nitric oxide can activate NMDA receptors and increase the likelihood of free radical formation (peroxynitrite), both of which can contribute to neuronal damage (Faraci and Brian, 1994).

Although hypoxic-ischemic brain injury is frequent enough to warrant much study of its pathogenesis, other types of injury to the brain do occur, and other factors also complicate hypoxic-ischemic brain injury. For instance, brain injury also occurs after prolonged hypoglycemia, with significant and prolonged hyperammonemia and with severe hyperbilirubinemia as well as with other metabolic insults. Traumatic brain injury can result in cerebral contusion, axonal tearing, and brain hemorrhage. It is well known that hemorrhage can occur with many types of brain injury. It is now thought that hemorrhage can further complicate brain injury by adding toxic free radical species. For example, it has been shown experimentally that xanthine oxidase is produced during ischemia/reperfusion insults. When this occurs, hydrogen peroxide is generated, which can then react with ferrous iron to form toxic hydroxy radicals. In an experimental animal model of ischemia/reperfusion, animals with low iron diets had less brain injury than animals with normal diets (Patt et al, 1990). An extrapolation from this work is that tissue with increased iron from heme products could also provide iron to interact with hydrogen peroxide to produce hydroxy radicals. If unchecked by antioxidant mechanisms, these radicals could then initiate lipid peroxidation, causing disruption of cellular membranes (Halliwell and Gutteridge, 1984).

Brain injury frequently consists of damage to neurons, axons, glia, and vascular elements, and thus adequate brain repair must include restoration of all of these elements to normal. Different strategies, including pharmacologic means of brain protection (e.g., calcium channel antagonists, NMDA receptor antagonists, free radical scavengers, nitric oxide synthase inhibitors, and monosialoganglioside GM_1) and postinsult treatments (e.g., hypothermia, control of glucose, use of nonglucocorticoid steroids, reduction of edema, and other secondary injury), are being assessed in various ways. Such protective strategies against hypoxic-ischemic brain injury are being studied in fetal and newborn animal models. A study in chronically instrumented fetal sheep examined the effect of pretreatment with monosialoganglioside GM_1 on brain injury after 30 minutes of severe cerebral ischemia (Tan et al, 1993). GM_1 has been shown to protect neurons against excitotoxicity and to have a direct membrane stabilization effect, probably through direct incorporation into plasma membranes (Tan et al, 1993). The fetal sheep pretreated with GM_1 before ischemic insult showed improved recovery of primary edema, reduced duration of epileptiform activity, and reduced brain histologic damage without any effects on blood pressure or metabolic status (Tan et al, 1993). Further studies should give information about the therapeutic window and any potential toxicities of GM_1.

In addition, some techniques have been employed to attempt either reconstitution of neurotransmitter systems (transplantation of embryonic neurons into the damaged brain) or stimulation of regeneration of central axons (by use of peripheral nerve grafts) (Bjorklund et al, 1980; David and Aguayo, 1981). At present, both of these strategies are experimental; they have not been attempted in newborns.

Clinical Encephalopathies

Postasphyxial (Hypoxic-Ischemic) Encephalopathy

Whether imposed by lack of oxygen in the blood or lack of blood reaching the brain, hypoxia is the main insult causing hypoxic-ischemic encephalopathy. Asphyxia implies hypoxia caused by respiratory insufficiency of one type or another, with the added component of some degree of carbon dioxide retention. During ischemia, metabolic by-products build up in the tissues, and during reperfusion, the reintroduction of oxygen can lead to the buildup of toxic oxygen radical species, which then lead to membrane lipid peroxidation. Metabolic changes occur immediately in the brain during hypoxia-ischemia (and asphyxia), leading to suppression of electrical activity, cortical depression, and stupor or coma. As discussed in the previous section, these events have been associated with changes in many cellular parameters, and the amount of recovery from such insults depends on a number of factors, not least of which are the degree of asphyxia or hypoxia-ischemia and the duration. Other factors, such as temperature, glucose availability, gestational age, and previous insults, all play roles in determining the amount of resulting brain compromise and ultimate injury.

Metabolic Encephalopathy

Metabolic encephalopathies occur when either vital substrates are withdrawn (such as glucose) or when there is accumulation of a metabolite that is toxic in concentrations that are higher than normal (ammonia, branched-chain amino acids and ketoacids, phenylalanine, glycine, valine, methionine, and others). Other acids that are well known to accumulate are those associated with disorders of *organic acid metabolism*. Such disorders have been recognized for propionate and methylmalonate metabolism, pyruvate and mitochondrial metabolism, defects of medium-chain acyl-coenzyme A (CoA) dehydrogenase, glutaric acidemia, glutathione synthetase deficiency, molybdenum cofactor deficiency, and defects of carbohydrate metabolism (galactosemia, glycogen storage disease type I, fructose-1,6-diphosphatase deficiency, and phosphoenolpyruvate carboxykinase deficiency, among others).

Glucose is the primary metabolic fuel for the brain, is transported to the brain via the blood, and is produced primarily in the liver. Brain transport of glucose depends on specific proteins that carry glucose across the blood-brain barrier. Glucose transporter protein deficiencies lead to seizures, microcephaly, and cognitive deficits in affected infants (DeVivo et al, 1991). Such infants have low CSF glucose with normal serum glucose values. A current treatment is the ketogenic diet. The normal newborn can rapidly use fuels other than glucose, such as ketones, for brain energy. Ketones in the newborn brain are readily delivered from the blood by carrier-mediated transport. Studies in hypoglycemic infants, however, have shown that ketone bodies are not present in the amounts necessary to provide sufficient energy in newborn infants; ketones do not increase during fasting in newborns (as they do in older infants and children); and ketones do not increase during hypoglycemia in the newborn (Stanley et al, 1979). The lack of ketones is probably due to limitations of hepatic ketone synthesis during the newborn period.

Hypoglycemia is defined as a plasma glucose level less than 40 mg/dL, regardless of gestational age (despite the lack of knowledge about acceptable glucose levels in very preterm infants) (Ogata, 1994). Plasma levels of glucose this low, although defined as hypoglycemia, do not necessarily correlate with symptoms.

The mechanisms underlying cellular injury that occurs during hypoglycemia are still being elucidated. Significant hypoglycemic injury causes selective neuronal necrosis, especially in superficial cortical areas and in the spinal cord (Anderson et al, 1967). The injury is probably not totally due to lack of energy, however, because ATP levels are much higher in the brain after hypoglycemia than after hypoxia-ischemia (Mayman and Tijerina, 1971). Current data suggest that damage during hypoglycemia may be due to the release of excitotoxins, as in hypoxia-ischemia (Auer, 1986; Wieloch, 1985).

Hepatic encephalopathy is probably the most frequent clinical symptom complex associated with hyperammonemia. In the newborn, however, there are possible inborn errors of urea cycle metabolism that cause hyperammonemia and encephalopathy. Infants with such disorders are usually affected in the perinatal period with the introduction of protein into the diet through milk. Symptoms include irritability, lethargy, poor feeding, seizures, coma, and death. The enzyme deficiencies include carbamylphosphate synthetase deficiency, ornithine transcarbamylase deficiency, arginosuccinate deficiency, arginosuccinase deficiency, and arginase deficiencey (Lockwood, 1985). Neuropathologic changes have been particularly apparent in astrocytes after hyperammonemic states. In addition, the ammonia ion can substitute for sodium and potassium, with effects on membrane electrical properties, the chloride pump, and postsynaptic inhibitory mechanisms (Lockwood, 1985). Almost all metabolic functions of the nervous system are affected by hyperammonemia.

Toxic or Abstinence Encephalopathy

Effects of maternal anesthesia can be recognized as neurologic depression in some newborns, especially newborns who are already compromised and acidotic (Albright, 1989). When local anesthetics are transferred to an asphyxiated fetus, significant bradycardia can occur (Morishima et al, 1972). When local anesthetic is accidentally injected into the fetal scalp, the outcome can be fetal death (Sinclair et al, 1965).

Other drugs that usually cause symptoms in the neonatal period include those of recreational use or abuse. In addition to direct fetal effects, these agents also cause addiction of the fetus in utero and withdrawal symptoms after birth. Narcotic addiction is characterized by a withdrawal syndrome of persistent wakefulness, irritability, jitteriness, crying, hyperactivity, hyperreflexia, hyperthermia and sweating, excessive but inefficient sucking, diarrhea and vomiting, rhinorrhea, tachypnea, hiccups, poor weight gain, and infrequently seizures (Cohen et al, 1989).

Cocaine is a nervous system stimulant and a vasoconstrictor (Cohen et al, 1989). The vasoconstriction can be especially prominent in the placenta, and placental abruption has been associated with cocaine use. Cerebral infarcts have occurred in infants exposed to cocaine in utero (Chasnoff et al, 1986). Symptoms and signs seen in cocaine-exposed infants in the perinatal period include poor feeding; sleeplessness; tremors; irritability; and decreased birth weight, length, and head circumference (Oro and Dixon, 1987).

Bilirubin

Studies of bilirubin in the 1960s showed that when dissociated from albumin in the circulation, it could enter the CNS no matter how mature the animal (Diamond and Schmid, 1966), and that its toxicity is probably most dependent on its rate of clearance from the interstitial fluid and CSF because poisons that increase the concentration of bilirubin in the CSF cause the yellow staining of brain nuclei (Ernster et al, 1957). Because the extracellular space of the CNS in the newborn is greater than in the adult, its solutes are cleared less rapidly; in addition, the rate of formation and turnover of CSF is less in the newborn (Aprison and Segar, 1963; Bass and Lundborg, 1973; Davson et al, 1962). These facts and the supposition that the space between any capillary ultrafiltrate and susceptible neurons may be much smaller than in the adult brain provide some postulated reasons for the vulnerability of the neonatal nervous system to bilirubin encephalopathy (Odell and Schutta, 1985; Rapaport, 1976). Adults with unconjugated hyperbilirubinemia can exhibit bilirubin encephalopathy and *kernicterus* at autopsy; however, the chance of an adult's having unconjugated bilirubin in concentrations greater than the concentrations of circulating albumin is far less likely than that of a newborn (Odell and Schutta, 1985).

Bilirubin is toxic to the brain in several ways. In brain slices, bilirubin has been shown to depress oxygen consumption (Day, 1954). Bilirubin at high concentrations uncouples oxidative phosphorylation in mitochondria in vitro, and inclusion of albumin in the incubation medium could protect the mitochondria from the effects of the bilirubin (Mustafa et al, 1969). Bilirubin has also been shown to affect water and sodium transport across the toad bladder membrane (Brem et al, 1985), and in cultured ascites cell lines, bilirubin inhibits potassium transport and increases sodium and water retention (Corchs et al, 1982). Neuronal swelling is found in kernicteric brains and may result from similar physiologic effects of bilirubin. Neuronal transport and enzyme systems are affected by bilirubin. Notably, bilirubin inhibits the activation of protein kinase and decreases the phosphorylation of synapsin I in synaptic vesicles (Hansen et al, 1988). In cultured neuroblastoma cell lines, bilirubin impairs mitochondrial action, impairs the activity of sodium, potassium-ATPase, causes decreased thymidine uptake, and causes decreased incorporation of methionine (Amit et al, 1989). Physiologic studies have shown that bilirubin impairs nerve conduction; action potentials are decreased by bilirubin in hippocampal brain slices (Hansen et al, 1988). Unconjugated bilirubin has been shown in adult brains to lower cortical EEG amplitudes and, in some cases, to abolish the EEG tracing (Wennberg and Hance, 1986). Bilirubin also reduces the transport of tyrosine and the synthesis of dopamine, especially at high concentrations (Cashore, 1989). These effects all provide some reasons for the encephalopathic effects of bilirubin.

The clinical condition of bilirubin encephalopathy has been well described, and its autopsy correlative findings, or kernicterus, have been known since 1903 (Schmorl, 1903). The clinical manifestations of full-blown kernicterus are usually recognized as lethargy (developing after the first 48 postnatal hours), an incomplete Moro response, and often opisthotonic posturing after abrupt postural changes (Odell and Schutta, 1985). The infant's suck is ineffective, and the cry is cerebral (high pitched). The infant may have abnormal eye movements, characterized by persistent downward gaze and rotary nystagmus, and episodes of

hypothermia and hyperthermia. At the end stage of the disease, decerebrate posturing occurs. Bilirubin pigment is found at autopsy, along with swelling and vacuolization of neurons, in numerous nuclei and structures, but not usually in the cerebral cortex (Schutta et al, 1970; Vaughan et al, 1950). Areas usually affected include the basal ganglia, cerebellum, hippocampus, medulla oblongata, subthalamic nuclei, thalamus, corpus striatum, fourth ventricle, dentate nucleus, olivary nuclei, nuclei in the floor of the fourth ventricle, lentiform nucleus, midbrain, spinal cord, globus pallidus, ependyma, the pons, the mamillary bodies, the caudate nucleus, and the cerebral cortex, in descending order of frequency (Claireaux, 1961).

Current guidelines for treatment of hyperbilirubinemia in the newborn have been published by the American Academy of Pediatrics (Provisional Committee for Quality Improvement and Subcommittee on Hyperbilirubinemia, 1994). Infants with jaundice before 24 hours' postnatal age are considered to have *pathologic* jaundice and to require further work-up and possible phototherapy or exchange transfusion early in the course of the hyperbilirubinemia. Otherwise healthy term infants whose jaundice becomes apparent after the first 24 hours are treated with phototherapy when total serum bilirubin is greater than 15 mg/dL (μmol/L) in the first 25 to 48 hours and with exchange transfusion if the bilirubin is 20 mg/dL or greater in the first 25 to 48 hours (after failure of intensive phototherapy). More detailed guidelines for persisting jaundice are given in the American Academy of Pediatrics report.

Infectious Encephalopathy

Most pediatricians are familiar with infants who are encephalopathic because of CNS infection. Viral encephalitides are, in particular, associated with neurochemical abnormalities and cellular dysfunction in the brain, characterized by direct cytolysis, impairment of synaptic transmission, alteration of metabolism of neurotransmitters, and fusion of cell membranes (Rammohan et al, 1985). Brain findings in viral encephalitis include mononuclear perivascular inflammatory infiltrates and degeneration of neurons. Hemorrhage occurs commonly into areas of necrosis in herpesvirus infections. A number of viral infections are characterized by intracellular inclusion bodies (herpesvirus, cytomegalovirus, measles, subacute sclerosing panencephalitis, polio, and rabies) (Fishman, 1992). In infants and children, encephalitides are clinically characterized by alterations of consciousness, headache, neurologic abnormalities, and fever (Fishman, 1992). Viral encephalitis is recognized in newborns by alterations in consciousness, neurologic signs, hypothermia or hyperthermia, and seizures and is especially likely to be due to herpesvirus type 2. In recent years, infants with human immunodeficiency virus (HIV) have been recognized with progressive encephalopathies developing between 2 months and 5 years of age, after infection during the prenatal or perinatal period. Subacute encephalopathies associated with viral infections are characterized by cellular dysfunction and demyelination (subacute sclerosing panencephalitis, postinfectious encephalomyelitis syndromes), but these are not diagnosed in the newborn period. Newborn infants, especially preterm infants, are at particular risk for bacterial or spirochetal infections of the nervous system and in some cases for fungal or for parasitic infections (such as *Toxoplasmosis*) (see the section on Infections of the Newborn Nervous System).

Asphyxial and Hypoxic-Ischemic Injury
Clinical Diagnosis

The well-taken history and review of the pregnancy course give clues to antenatal factors that might have caused hypoxia-ischemia. Review of fetal monitoring studies and ultrasound examinations and any fetal acid-base determinations is always helpful. Infants who are depressed at birth with low Apgar scores, acidosis, and the need for ventilatory assistance should be admitted to the intensive care unit. Infants with signs of neonatal depression, who are resuscitated immediately and have no subsequent signs of encephalopathy, have usually had only transient, late, depressive events without likely sequelae. These infants should be watched carefully and monitored, if necessary, during the 1st or 2nd postnatal day; it should be remembered, however, that the presence of depression at birth is not necessarily synonymous with the occurrence of perinatal asphyxia or neonatal encephalopathy—the majority of infants with neonatal depression do not have neonatal encephalopathy. Infants with low Apgar scores may have causes other than asphyxia, such as CNS congenital abnormalities, drug effects, vagal responses to head compression or oropharyngeal suctioning, or antenatal neurologic damage (Badawi et al, 1996; O'Brien et al, 1984). Infants with severe acidosis (mixed or metabolic) have usually had longer standing depression. When an infant has low Apgar scores (0 to 3) that persist longer than 5 minutes, severe acidosis (pH ≤7.0), neonatal encephalopathy, and some degree of systemic organ injury, the infant can be diagnosed as having had perinatal asphyxia significant enough possibly to cause neurologic sequelae (ACOG, 1993).

Grades of Severity

Neonatal encephalopathy is recognized as mild, moderate, or severe and can be graded in various ways. The grading scheme of Sarnat and Sarnat has been in use since 1976 (Sarnat and Sarnat, 1976); this scheme has been modified by Volpe (1995c) and others (Novotny, 1989). In general, mild encephalopathy is characterized by alternating levels of consciousness—including periods of lethargy, irritability, and hyperalertness (Novotny, 1989). The infants are jittery, feed poorly, and do not have normal sleep cycles. The cranial nerve examination is normal, muscle tone may be increased, and deep tendon reflexes are frequently increased. Some autonomic signs are present, such as pupillary dilation and tachycardia. Most of the primitive reflexes are normal, with the exception of the Moro, which may be increased. Infants with mild encephalopathy do not have seizures.

The infant with moderate encephalopathy is more lethargic with poor feeding and hypotonia. Clonus is usually present, and the gag reflex is usually depressed. There may be abnormal movements, including spontaneous myoclonus or extrapyramidal dysfunction. The pupils are usually con-

stricted, and the infant may have bradycardia. Seizures frequently occur within the first 24 hours.

The severely encephalopathic infant is comatose and flaccid with absent reflexes. The pupils often are fixed or sluggishly reactive, and the doll's eye reflex is absent. The infant may be bradycardic and frequently has apnea and hypotension.

The neurologic sequelae in infants with hypoxic-ischemic encephalopathy are related to the degree of the encephalopathy; infants with low Apgar scores, delayed respirations, meconium staining, or problems of fetal heart rate patterns, who do not show signs of encephalopathy, are not likely to show neurologic sequelae unless intrauterine brain damage is already present (Nelson and Ellenberg, 1987; Robertson and Finer, 1985). In fact, studies indicate that most cases of spastic cerebral palsy do not result from intrapartum asphyxia. Blair and Stanley (1988) showed that in only 15 of 183 patients with spastic cerebral palsy (8%) could the condition be attributed to intrapartum asphyxia. Other studies have also confirmed that birth asphyxia is a relatively rare cause of later static encephalopathy (Torfs et al, 1990). It is becoming clearer that antepartum events and genetic factors play significant roles in the pathogenesis of cerebral palsy (Scher et al, 1991).

Pathogenesis

Significant hypoxemia is caused in the peripartum and neonatal period by several kinds of problems. Chief among these is asphyxia with inadequate placental gas exchange, usually accompanied by insufficient respiratory function in the infant at birth with hypoxia, hypercarbia, acidosis, and sometimes hypoglycemia and coagulopathy (Armstrong, 1995). After birth, hypoxia is associated with severe respiratory distress syndrome or apneic spells or with desaturation owing to cardiac disease or pulmonary hypertension owing to persistent fetal circulation. When there is circulatory insufficiency and systemic hypotension associated with any of the above-mentioned in the infant, especially when there is compromise of cerebral autoregulation, cerebral ischemia may occur along with hypoxemia.

The pathogeneses of brain injury during insults such as those listed here are frequently multifactorial but relate, in general, to vascular and metabolic factors, distribution of excitatory amino acid receptors, and effectiveness of cerebral circulatory control (Adams et al, 1966; Armstrong et al, 1987; Brann and Myers, 1975; Bredt and Snyder, 1992; DeReuck, 1984; De Reuck et al, 1972; D'Souza et al, 1992; Ferriero et al, 1988; Greenamyre et al, 1987; Greisen, 1992; Livera et al, 1991; McDonald and Johnston, 1990; Miall-Allen et al, 1987; Myers, 1975; Nelson and Silverstein, 1994; Oka et al, 1993; Pape and Wigglesworth, 1979; Pryds et al, 1990a, 1990b; Rorke, 1992; Rosenberg, 1988; Takashima and Tanaka, 1978; Takashima et al, 1978; Volpe, 1995d). These factors are discussed subsequently with relation to the sites and types of lesions produced by hypoxic-ischemic insults.

Sites and Types of Lesions

Sites commonly injured by hypoxia-ischemia vary to some extent in the preterm and term brain. Neuronal injury is particularly common in the cerebral cortex, CA1 region of the hippocampus, Purkinje cells of the cerebellum, and anterior horn cells of the spinal cord in the term newborn. Neuronal injury is seen in the basal ganglia and thalamus and in the cranial nerve nuclei of the brain stem equally in term and preterm infants, and neuronal injury is particularly common in the subiculum of the hippocampus, the ventral pons, the inferior olivary nuclei, the cerebellar internal granule cells, and more diffusely in the spinal cord in preterm infants (Armstrong, 1995).

Differences in susceptibility of cortical neurons to injury in the term and preterm infant relate probably to differences in vascular distributions and in neuronal differentiation. Cortical vascular anastomoses are more abundant in the preterm infant, whereas term infants have more injury in areas where anastomoses have diminished, leaving *border zones* between major arterial territories. Parasagittal cerebral injury in the term infant, with involvement of both gray and white matter, is an example of this type of injury; parasagittal injury tends to be greatest in the posterior cerebrum, in the border zone region for all three major cerebral vessels. Cellular injury in term infants tends to affect more highly differentiated cells (cortical neurons in the calcarine cortex, Purkinje cells in the cerebellum). Basal ganglia and thalamic injury from hypoxia-ischemia occurs less frequently than the other types of injury in both term and preterm infants. It is characterized by necrosis (sometimes hemorrhagic), followed by capillary proliferation, neuronal loss, gliosis, and hypermyelination (Rorke, 1982). The hypermyelination is an abnormal myelination of astrocytic processes and gives the affected areas in the basal ganglia (especially the putamen) a marbled appearance (Friede, 1989). Thus, this entity has been called *status marmoratus* or *état marbré* (Vogt and Vogt, 1926).

The brain stem is affected frequently in newborns with hypoxic-ischemic damage, both in term and in preterm newborns, as is the cerebellum. Cranial nerve nuclei are particularly susceptible in the term newborn. In the preterm newborn, brain stem injury is more global.

Cellular susceptibilities to injury seem to depend on maturational factors, metabolic factors (sparing of neurons with NADPH diaphorase-nitric oxide synthase, sparing of dopamine-synthesizing neurons), metabolic rate, and presence and density of glutamate receptor types. Glutamate receptors seem to be highly concentrated in the basal ganglia in the perinatal period (Greenamyre et al, 1987), and the glutamate receptor subtype most clearly related to neuronal death in the striatum is the receptor subtype of greatest density in that region in the perinatal period (McDonald et al, 1990).

Periventricular leukomalacia (white matter injury) occurs in both term and preterm infants but is particularly prevalent in the preterm infant (Armstrong and Norman, 1974; Banker and Larroche, 1962) (Fig. 69–4). The incidence of cystic periventricular leukomalacia in one study was 3.2% of infants weighing less than 1500 g at birth (Perlman et al, 1996). The two most common sites of occurrence of this lesion are at the level of the occipital radiation at the trigone of the lateral ventricles and at the level of the cerebral white matter around the foramen of Monro (Shuman and Selednik, 1980; Volpe, 1995d), two regions that are particularly prominent border zones be-

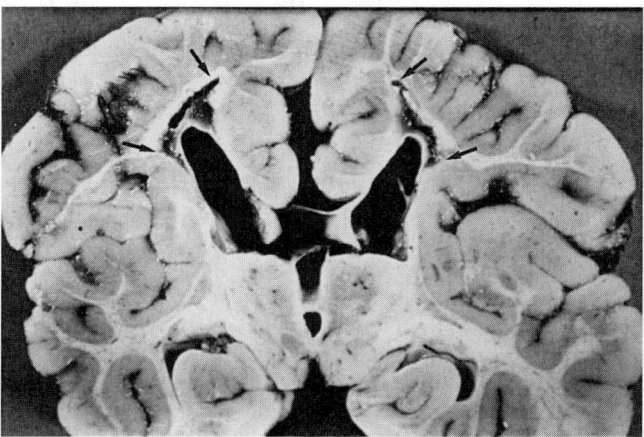

FIGURE 69–4. Periventricular leukomalacia; the extent of the bilateral lesions is shown by the arrows. (Photo courtesy of Dr. Dawna L. Armstrong, Department of Pathology, Texas Children's Hospital.)

tween penetrating branches of major arteries in the preterm brain. The cellular response in periventricular leukomalacia consists of necrosis of the cellular elements and processes (resulting in axonal swellings and periodic acid–Schiff reaction positive staining of cells). Oligodendrocytes are especially vulnerable to injury in these regions. There is infiltration by macrophages and astrocytic activation. The end result is frequently multiple cysts or a large cavitary lesion; there may be hemorrhage into the area of necrosis (25% at autopsy) (Armstrong and Norman, 1974). Although cavitation may be apparent in 1 to 3 weeks, it is also possible for gliosis to occur over a period of time, with subsequent loss of cavities. The constriction of the white matter may lead to secondary enlargement of the ventricles. Cavitation occurs as a consequence of necrosis in the immature brain more frequently than in the mature brain probably because of the high water content, low myelin component, and relatively limited glial response in the immature brain.

Periventricular leukomalacia may be a sequela in premature infants who are subject to episodes of ischemia. A correlation has been shown between the occurrence of hypocarbic alkalosis in the first 24 postnatal hours in very-low-birth-weight infants and subsequent development of periventricular leukomalacia (Fujimoto et al, 1994). Hypocarbic alkalosis may cause considerable cerebral vasoconstriction. Episodes of apnea and bradycardia have also been shown to reduce cerebral perfusion in the preterm newborn and are associated with an increased risk for cerebral palsy (McDonald, 1967; Perlman and Volpe, 1985a). The presence of periventricular leukomalacia, cystic periventricular leukomalacia in particular, is associated with an increased risk for cerebral palsy (Fazzi et al, 1992, 1994; Jongmans et al, 1993; Pidcock et al, 1990).

The border zone concept implies that blood supply is lost first, when perfusion pressure falls, at the places where arterial sources do not penetrate fully. Cerebral perfusion pressure in the preterm newborn is particularly likely to fall when systemic blood pressure falls. This may be because the range of autoregulation (the range of blood pressures over which cerebral blood flow remains constant) is narrower than in the infant, child, or adult, or it may be because under certain conditions autoregulation fails. Autoregulation fails in all species studied when significant hypoxia is induced. Ranges of autoregulation seem to vary with development and species, and autoregulation can be affected by pharmacologic agents (Louis et al, 1994; Yamashita et al, 1993).

It is apparent, however, that other factors also probably play roles in the genesis of periventricular leukomalacia, including susceptibility of myelination glia to hypoxia, acidosis, hypoglycemia, and other metabolic insults; cerebrovascular instability and ischemia/reperfusion injury; presence of prenatal white matter injury or prenatal infection (herpes simplex, cytomegalovirus, or bacterial infections); and effects of cytokines (Adinolfi, 1993). Periventricular leukomalacia has been documented prenatally in a number of cases (Iida et al, 1993; Rettwitz-Volk et al, 1993). A study of a large cohort has shown that preterm infants born to mothers with premature rupture of membranes or chorioamnionitis are at increased risk for periventricular leukomalacia (Perlman et al, 1996). Earlier experimental studies in an animal model showed that endotoxemia could be associated with white matter lesions (Gilles et al, 1976).

Other types of injuries that lead to cavitation or loss of brain tissue include ischemic infarctions (Volpe, 1995d). These may be focal or multifocal and occur with occlusions, loss of blood flow, or hemorrhage involving specific cerebral vessels with resulting brain necrosis in the respective vascular territories. Thus, these lesions are thought to be the result of ischemic or hemorrhagic injuries with tissue hypoxia; the infant may or may not have systemic hypoxia or hypotension. Correlations of lesion types with the time of insult have shown that second-trimester ischemic insults often cause porencephalies and hydranencephalies, whereas third-trimester ischemic insults more often cause multicystic encephalomalacia (Amato et al, 1991; Fernandez et al, 1986; Larroche, 1986; Scher et al, 1991). Case histories associated with these injuries have included maternal cardiac failure, attempted suicide (gas inhalation), trauma, and anaphylaxis; placental and cord catastrophes; and vascular accidents in the fetus associated with vascular malformations (Stewart et al, 1978; Volpe, 1995d). Focal infarctions can be due to vessel occlusion or maldevelopment, both of which can be difficult to verify. Multifocal lesions can occur with thromboemboli (especially with twin gestations and placental vascular anastomoses) as well as with hypercoagulable states (antiphospholipid antibodies, deficiencies of protein C or protein S, or antithrombin III) (Clouse and Comp, 1986; Devilat et al, 1993; Hess, 1992; Pegelow et al, 1992). Other problems of coagulation, including disseminated intravascular coagulation, hypernatremia and dehydration, and polycythemia, can all be associated with thrombosis. Vasculitis associated with bacterial meningitis can also cause arterial or venous thromboses, infarction being more common with arterial thrombosis (Volpe, 1995d). In utero hemorrhagic lesions can occur secondary to isoimmune thrombocytopenia in the fetus and can result in later cystic cavitations (Naidu et al, 1983; Zalneraitis et al, 1979).

Timing of Lesions

Acute and chronic lesions of both gray and white matter are discussed in this section. Lesions of the sulcul cortex are termed *ulegyria* and are usually microscopic when acute. There is diffuse pallor in the cortex at the depth of the involved sulci, with vacuolization of the tissue. These areas also show cellular changes, including nuclear pyknosis, chromatolysis, and loss of neurons (Friede, 1989). Later stages of ulegyria can vary in extent, with less severe lesions consisting of multiple patches of neuron loss and gliosis at the depths of the sulci (the crowns are spared). The gliosis is frequently intermixed with abnormal myelinated fibers, called *fibromyelinic plaques*, which are similar to those seen in status marmoratus of the basal ganglia (Friede, 1989). When the cortical sulcal injury is more severe, more of the cortex is destroyed, and the gyri have a crown of more normal tissue on a base of glial scar. There may be areas of cavitation as well as evidence of cortical laminar necrosis (usually layer three of the cortex) (Friede, 1989). Ulegyria usually occurs in arterial border zones, frequently between the anterior and middle cerebral arterial territories or between the middle and posterior cerebral arterial zones. Such lesions are frequently bilateral, but they can be unilateral (Friede, 1989) (Fig. 69–5).

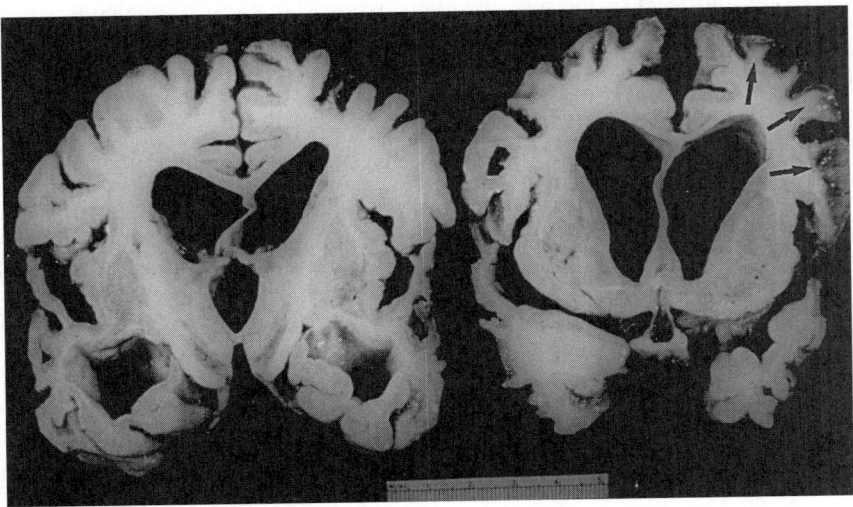

FIGURE 69–5. Ulegyria; crowns of gyral tissue above glial scars are marked by arrows. (Photo courtesy of Dr. Marvin A. Fishman, Division of Pediatric Neurology, Texas Children's Hospital.)

Although the injury to the basal ganglia occurs during the hypoxic-ischemic episode, the resulting status marmoratus is not visible until myelination is underway. Glial scars are already present when the abnormal myelination patterns start to form—at about 6 months of age. Late lesions of status marmoratus are characterized by pale streaks in the basal ganglia or thalamus. Microscopically there is neuronal loss and glial scarring (Friede, 1989).

Early lesions of periventricular leukomalacia are termed *coagulation necrosis*. The white matter becomes vacuolated and periodic acid–Schiff reaction positive. A few days into the lesion, glia become activated and proliferate, microglia are activated, and macrophages move into the region. Axons become swollen. Over the course of the ensuing weeks, cavitation develops. Late lesions show cavitary lesions with gliotic walls; the axonal swellings can become calcified and persist for long periods of time (Friede, 1989). Periventricular leukomalacia frequently accompanies other lesions of prematurity, including germinal matrix and intraventricular hemorrhages (Armstrong et al, 1987).

Treatment

Diagnostic and treatment regimens for hypoxic-ischemic encephalopathy are not standardized, as shown by answers to a questionnaire sent by Donn and coworkers (1988) to major institutions. Diagnostic tests performed frequently in newborns thought to have been asphyxiated included electroencephalography, cranial sonography, arterial blood gases, and serum calcium determinations (Donn et al, 1988). Brain stem auditory evoked response testing was used less frequently than the EEG but was used relatively frequently because the results have been shown to have some prognostic significance (Hecox and Cone, 1981; Kileny and Connelly, 1980).

Widely used therapies included fluid restriction and phenobarbital for treatment of seizures. Lumbar puncture was usually done by 38% of respondents and sometimes done by 40%; creatine kinase enzymes were usually ascertained by 28% and sometimes by 33% (Donn et al, 1988). Serum lactate, pyruvate, and osmolality were determined to variable extents. Rarely used therapies included mannitol, glycerol, hypothermia, hyperglycemia, and pentobarbital coma. More commonly used therapies, in addition to fluid restriction and seizure therapy, included hyperventilation, sedation, and phenobarbital as prophylaxis; furosemide; paralysis; and corticosteroids.

In general, the treatment of the infant with hypoxic-ischemic encephalopathy is supportive: ventilatory therapy when necessary; fluid restriction to lessen the degree of cerebral edema and effects of inappropriate secretion of antidiuretic hormone; maintenance of normal glucose and calcium levels, acid-base and electrolyte balance, and serum osmolality; provision of calories; and treatment of seizures. Many infants with hypoxic-ischemic encephalopathy have elevated ammonia levels as well as elevated serum glutamic oxaloacetic transaminase values, probably secondary to impaired liver function and increased protein breakdown. Brain-specific creatine kinase (CK-BB) seems to be an indicator of brain injury when measured in spinal fluid early in the course of hypoxic-ischemic encephalopathy (DePraeter et al, 1991).

Lumbar puncture is helpful for diagnosis of subarachnoid or intraventricular hemorrhage; to rule out meningitis in certain cases; and for determination of CSF pressure, lactate, hydroxybutyrate dehydrogenase, or CK-BB. Ultrasound and CT scans are useful for determining if structural brain injury is present early in the course of the encephalopathy (sometimes suggesting intrauterine brain injury) and for determining the progression of CNS lesions, such as hemorrhage, hydrocephalus, periventricular leukomalacia, atrophy, and multicystic encephalomalacia. Although ultrasound scans are useful and probably sensitive in the early postnatal period for changes in brain water content, in general they lack both sensitivity and specificity and should be followed by CT or MRI scans.

The EEG is useful and can correlate with specific types of brain injury. Burst suppression, voltage suppression, or an isoelectric tracing can be seen with diffuse cortical necrosis; rolandic sharp waves are frequently present in infants with periventricular leukomalacia or periventricular hemorrhagic infarction (Bejar et al, 1986; Marret et al, 1986; Novotny et al, 1987; Tharp et al, 1989). Localized periodic lateralized epileptiform discharges imply the presence of focal cerebral infarction (Scher and Beggarly, 1989).

At present, glutamate receptor antagonists, inhibitors of nitric oxide synthesis, calcium channel blockers, free radical scavengers and inhibitors, monosialogangliosides, hypothermia, and higher dose barbiturates are being used only experimentally, mainly in animal studies (Gunn et al, 1994; Hamada et al, 1994; Hill, 1991; Miller, 1993; Tan et al, 1993; Vannucci, 1990a). Their risk/benefit ratios are still uncertain (Hill, 1991).

Relationship of Lesions to Neurologic Sequelae

As mentioned in previous sections, the major types of brain injury resulting from hypoxia-ischemia include varying degrees of neuronal loss (cortex, hippocampus, thalamus, basal ganglia, brain stem, cerebellum, and spinal cord), periventricular white matter injury, and gray and white matter injury in areas of infarction. Cortical neuronal necrosis can be associated with cognitive deficits, vision loss, or seizure disorders in survivors, and cognitive deficits may also be related to injury in association areas. Injury to the thalamus is associated with intellectual deficit as well as with spastic quadriparesis (Malamud, 1950). Basal ganglia injury is associated with movement disorders (dystonia, choreoathetosis), and periventricular white matter injury is associated with spastic pareses of varying severity, spastic diplegia being the most common. Hypotonia may be a consequence of cerebral injury or of injury to the anterior horn cells of the spinal cord. Newborns with parasagittal cerebral injury can show proximal limb weakness, greater in the upper than the lower extremities. This presentation contrasts with spastic diplegia caused by periventricular leukomalacia, in which lower extremity weakness is usually greater than that of the upper extremities.

Brain stem injury is often manifest as difficulty with sucking, swallowing, and facial movement, but similar difficulties can also be related to damage of cerebral origin (pseudobulbar palsy). Hearing loss secondary to hypoxic injury to brain stem dorsal cochlear nuclei or to the cochlea can be present. Sexual precocity may occur in infants with injury to the hypothalamus. Infants with unilateral cerebral infarctions (especially of the middle cerebral artery territory) usually have some degree of hemiparesis.

Although most patients who have neurologic sequelae exhibit what is termed *static encephalopathy* after hypoxic-ischemic insults, implying that the brain injury is not progressive, some of the manifestations of the injuries are not apparent early in the child's life. For instance, movement disorders usually become apparent during the preschool years (up to age 4 to 5 years). Not all newborns with hypoxic-ischemic encephalopathy have neurologic sequelae, however. The infant who recovers quickly in the neonatal period and is asymptomatic by the end of the first postnatal week has a high likelihood of being normal at long-term follow-up (Robertson and Finer, 1985; Sarnat and Sarnat, 1976). Infants with moderate encephalopathy have relatively low mortality (5%), and neurologic sequelae occur in about 20% of survivors. Conversely, infants with severe neonatal encephalopathy have a high likelihood of dying (75%), and likelihood of neurologic sequelae is almost certain in survivors (Robertson and Finer, 1985).

Prognostication can sometimes be aided by neuroimaging and by the EEG. In particular, CT scan findings can be helpful because term infants with normal scans in the neonatal period are usually normal on follow-up, and infants with marked decreased density on CT in the neonatal period are usually abnormal on follow-up (Adsett et al, 1985; Fitzhardinge et al, 1981). In preterm infants, documentation of hypodensity on CT scan may be more difficult, and the ultrasound scan is more frequently used in the neonatal period. Ultrasonography is especially useful for documenting periventricular echolucenies (tissue loss and cysts) and ventricular dilation, and these lesions in preterm infants correlate with neurologic deficits on follow-up in 60% to 90% of the infants. Notably, mild echodensities and small periventricular cysts are not necessarily associated with abnormal outcomes (Pidcock et al, 1990). If cystic brain lesions are already present on scans done early in the 1st postnatal week, intrauterine injury has occurred.

Intraventricular Hemorrhage

Intraventricular hemorrhage is mainly a lesion of the premature brain (Fig. 69–6). Fifteen years ago, intraventricular hemorrhage was diagnosed in close to 40% of infants with birth weights less than 1501 g (Ahmann et al, 1980; Goddard-Finegold and Mizrahi, 1987; Papile et al, 1978a; Shinnar et al, 1982). Current incidence rates average close to 25%, with and without various preventive treatment modalities (Batton et al, 1994; Garland et al, 1995; O'Shea et al, 1992; Philip et al, 1989), but higher incidences are found in the lowest-birth-weight infants (Amato et al, 1993). The outlook for the very-low-birth-weight infant with intraventricular hemorrhage remains an important issue because the incidence of problems such as hydrocephalus, seizures, static encephalopathy, blindness, mental retardation, and learning disabilities is higher in those with symptomatic hemorrhages (Kitchen et al, 1986; Papile et al, 1983; Skouteli et al, 1985; Williamson et al, 1982; Yu et al, 1986). The severity of neurologic sequelae is not always due just to intraventricular hemorrhage, however, because additional lesions are frequently found at autopsy in infants who succumb (Armstrong et al, 1987; Skullerud and Wes-

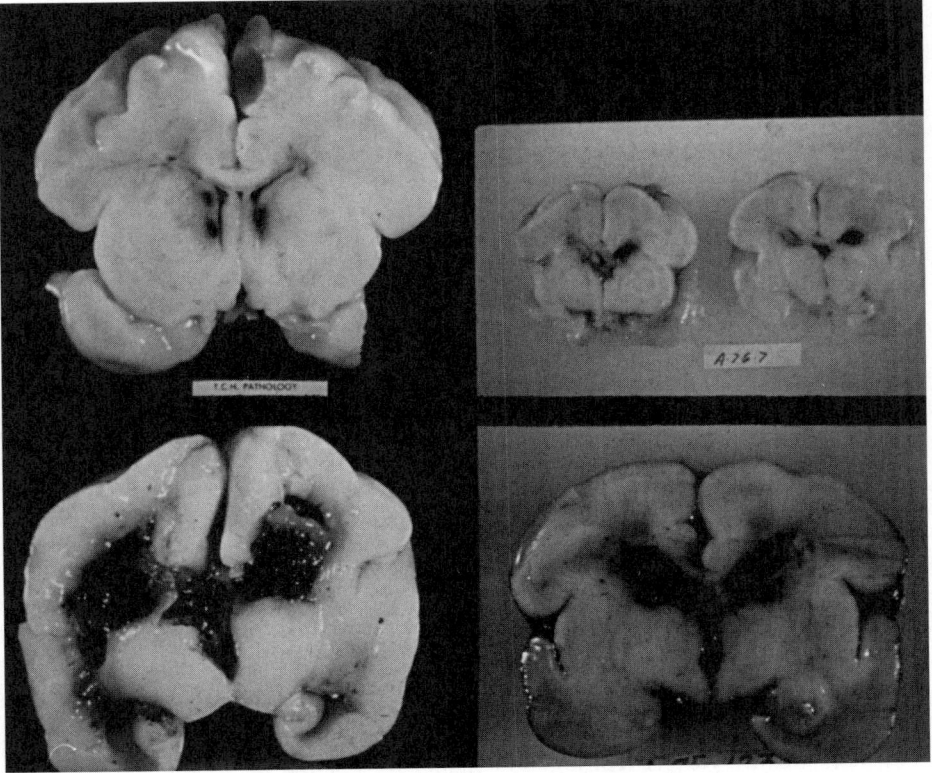

FIGURE 69–6. Intraventricular hemorrhage; lesions of Grade I to Grade IV severity (see text). (Photos courtesy of Dr. Dawna L. Armstrong, Department of Pathology, Texas Children's Hospital.)

tre, 1986). Other lesions often associated with intraventricular hemorrhage are periventricular infarction and pontosubicular necrosis; both of these can be associated with debilitating neurologic sequelae (Armstrong et al, 1987; Leech et al, 1979; Skullerud and Westre, 1986). Intraventricular hemorrhage occurs rarely in term infants but has been reported in a number of circumstances (Cartwright et al, 1979; Donat et al, 1978; Fenichel et al, 1984; Heafner et al, 1985; Lacey and Terplan, 1982; Mitchell and O'Tuama, 1980; Palma et al, 1979; Scher et al, 1982; Wehberg et al, 1992).

Clinical Diagnosis

Intraventricular hemorrhage is usually diagnosed during the first 72 postnatal hours in very preterm infants and is infrequently diagnosed later in the 1st postnatal week (Ahmann et al, 1980; Papile et al, 1978a; Shinnar et al, 1982). Most affected infants are less than 32 weeks' gestational age, are mechanically ventilated, and have had some degree of asphyxia or hemodynamic instability (or both) (Goddard-Finegold and Mizrahi, 1987; Volpe, 1995e). Although about 25% of newborns with intraventricular hemorrhage are asymptomatic, the other 75% can have symptoms of varying degrees (Papile et al, 1978a; Volpe, 1995e). The classic, but infrequent, presentation is one of sudden deterioration with a bulging fontanel, decrease in blood pressure, drop in hematocrit, and seizure activity. Neurologic manifestations in these infants include flaccidity, loss of pupillary reactions, loss of extraocular movements, respiratory abnormalities, and coma. Some infants manifest a more protracted course, however, that is often described as *saltatory* because symptoms wax and wane over a period of time. These infants usually show a change from alertness to irritability or stupor, with a decrease in activity, hypotonia, and other neurologic abnormalities. They may recover for periods of time, only to become symptomatic again later. It is thought that this course reflects episodes of intermittant bleeding. Metabolic problems may also herald the onset of intraventricular hemorrhage: Some infants become hypoglycemic or hypothermic (or both). Decreased CSF glucose is frequently associated with intraventricular hemorrhage (hypoglycorrhachia) (Mathew and Volpe, 1980), and diabetes insipidus has been reported after intraventricular hemorrhage (Adams et al, 1976).

Concepts of Pathogenesis

Information from autopsy studies has shown that intraventricular hemorrhage in preterm infants originates in most cases from the subventricular germinal matrix layer (GML) (Larroche, 1974; Leech and Kohnen, 1974). This zone is highly cellular and gives rise to neurons and glia during gestation (Gressens et al, 1992). Preterm infants less than 32 weeks' gestational age have persisting germinal matrix with cellularity becoming scant by term. The germinal matrix is also a vascular region, with vascularity decreasing as term approaches. Both the characteristics of the vessels themselves and their distribution seem to be important in the pathogenesis of hemorrhage. The vessels are histologically immature, with less collagen support and less elastin than more mature vessels (Haruda and Blanc, 1981; Pinar

et al, 1985). Trommer and colleagues (1987) showed that the vessels of the GML in newborn puppies are larger in size, have thinner walls, and lack support from surrounding neuropil compared to vessels elsewhere in the cerebrum. Another study in newborn puppies showed that GML vessels undergo basement membrane maturation during the first 4 postnatal days (Ment et al, 1991).

A study of human preterm brain showed that large periventricular channels in the GML do not stain with alkaline phosphatase (arteries, arterioles, and capillaries stain with alkaline phosphatase) (Moody et al, 1994). This study suggested that most hemorrhage in the GML was perivenous in origin. Earlier autopsy studies of Towbin (1968) had suggested that hemorrhages originated from stasis and rupture of terminal veins. Hambleton and Wigglesworth (1976), who injected barium solutions into the carotid arteries of preterm newborns at autopsy, showed disruption of the capillary plexus in the GML at pressures of greater than 80 mm Hg, without disruption of the terminal veins (it should be mentioned, however, that the meaning of a postmortem injection pressure is not clear). When barium solution was injected into the jugular vein, GML leaks occurred in one instance, leading these investigators to suggest that increases in arterial or venous pressures could be transmitted to the capillary plexus, causing hemorrhage from the capillaries, the capillary-arteriolar junctions, or the capillary-venule junctions. Takashima and Tanaka (1978) studied the vascular permeability of the GML with microangiography and benzidine stains. Their findings suggested that the GML is an end zone or border zone between cerebral arteries and the collecting zone of the deep cerebral veins. Using fluorescein isothiocyanate–dextran in rabbits, they showed that permeability was increased in the vessels of this region by hypoxia and by hypoxia associated with increased venous pressure (Takashima and Tanaka, 1978). Other studies in both animals and humans (Brown et al, 1994; Funato et al, 1992; Goddard et al, 1978, 1980a, 1980b; Gronlund et al, 1994) have shown a relationship between GML hemorrhage and increases in systemic blood pressure. The increases in systemic blood pressures have also been linked to increases in cerebral blood flow (Goddard-Finegold et al, 1990; Pasternak et al, 1983).

Intraventricular hemorrhage has also been produced experimentally after hypovolemia and hypotension followed by reperfusion (Goddard-Finegold et al, 1982; Ment et al, 1982), and intraventricular hemorrhage has been documented in infants who remain hypotensive for periods of time (Miall-Allen et al, 1987). All of these possible hemodynamic pathogeneses make sense because hypoxia and hypotension could cause injury to the endothelium of GML vessels with hemorrhage resulting in reperfusion, and acute increases in blood flow (associated with hypertension) could cause vessel rupture independently or in association with previous vessel injury.

The role of blood pressure changes in the genesis of intraventricular hemorrhage has interested numerous investigators, leading to studies of the reactions of the cerebral vasculature in the newborn. Major questions have revolved around the ability of the preterm newborn to *autoregulate*, or to maintain constant cerebral blood flow in the face of changes in blood pressure over a defined range. The infant with absent or limited autoregulatory capacities is likely to translate systemic arterial pressures directly to cerebral perfusion pressures. Such a *pressure-passive* state could be reflected in the especially vulnerable GML vessels.

Numerous studies have indicated that immature infants are at risk for having pressure-passive cerebral circulations, especially after even modest asphyxial events (Lou et al, 1979; Milligan, 1980; Pryds et al, 1989). A pressure-passive cerebral circulation is thought to be a particular problem when arterial blood pressures fluctuate widely. Perlman and coworkers (1983) showed that infants with fluctuating cerebral blood flow velocities, which correlated with fluctuating blood pressures and ventilator pressures, were at high risk of developing intraventricular hemorrhage. In addition, when the same population of infants was paralyzed so that cerebral blood flow velocities and systemic arterial pressures did not fluctuate, the incidence of intraventricular hemorrhage diminished (Perlman et al, 1985b). Fujimura and colleagues (1979) reported that infants with intraventricular hemorrhage were more likely than those without to have had an early period of hypotension followed by an increase in systemic blood pressure.

Interestingly, several clinical situations have been shown to be associated with increases in blood pressure in at-risk newborns. Wimberley and colleagues (1979) showed that crying, feeding, and stimulation caused increased blood pressure. Hypertension has been reported during seizures (Perlman and Volpe, 1985b) and during procedures such as intubation and suctioning (Ninan et al, 1986). Brazy and Lewis (1986) showed increases in systemic blood pressure in preterm infants during movements, with coughing, and with breath holding.

Other means of increasing cerebral blood flow include rapid volume expansion and vasodilation caused by hypercapnia. Papile and associates (1978b) confirmed a relationship between intraventricular hemorrhage and rapid volume infusion, and Wallin and colleagues (1990) showed a relationship between severe hypercarbia and intraventricular hemorrhage. Other factors are associated with increases in cerebral blood flow, with or without associated increases in systemic blood pressure. Two such factors are anemia and hypoglycemia, but a direct role for them in causing intraventricular hemorrhage has not been shown (Pryds et al, 1990a).

Additional factors thought to be important in the pathogenesis of intraventricular hemorrhage include increased venous pressure (which can occur during labor and delivery; during asphyxia; and during mechanical ventilation, pneumothorax, and other abnormal respiratory states), cerebral ischemia (which can occur during hypotension from multiple causes or during severe hypocapnia), and hypocoagulable states. Drugs that impair hemostasis (aspirin, heparin) have been shown to increase the risk of intraventricular hemorrhage (Lesko et al, 1986; Rumack et al, 1981). Conflicting reports have been published about the role of cocaine exposure in increasing the risk for intraventricular hemorrhage. Singer and colleagues (1994) showed that cocaine-exposed preterm infants of birth weights less than 1500 g had a higher incidence of Grades I and II intraventricular hemorrhage. Another prospective study has not shown this association (Dusick et al, 1993).

Timing of Hemorrhages

Studies in the 1980s showed that intraventricular hemorrhage could occur early in the postnatal period, could extend further during the following days and weeks, but rarely occurred primarily after 72 postnatal hours (Dolfin et al, 1983; Van de Bor et al, 1986). A prospective study showed that 90% of hemorrhages were diagnosed by 72 hours and 100% by 108 hours after birth (Van De Bor et al, 1986). Bejar and coworkers (1980) showed the presence of hemorrhages as early as the 1st postnatal hour in low-birth-weight infants studied with real-time ultrasound scans. Dolfin and associates (1983) prospectively studied 64 infants from 2 to 72 hours' postnatal age. The total incidence of intraventricular and subependymal hemorrhages in this study was 31%, with 19% of the infants having severe hemorrhages. All hemorrhages occurred within the first 62 postnatal hours, and extension of hemorrhages after 72 hours occurred in three cases (Dolfin et al, 1983).

In a more recent prospective study, 229 newborns from 600 to 1250 g birth weight were prospectively evaluated using real-time ultrasonography within the first 11 postnatal hours (Ment et al, 1992). Forty-three of the 229 infants had germinal matrix or intraventricular hemorrhage (18 germinal matrix hemorrhages, 21 Grade II hemorrhages, 1 Grade III hemorrhage, and 3 Grade IV hemorrhages). The infants in this study with early intraventricular hemorrhage had more vertex, vaginal deliveries than the infants without hemorrhages and less maternal tocolytic therapy (Ment et al, 1992). Of 61 infants with low-grade hemorrhage diagnosed in the first 6 to 11 postnatal hours, 21 had increase in size of the hemorrhage during the first 5 postnatal days (Ment et al, 1994a, 1994b).

Funato and coworkers (1992) performed prospective ultrasound scans on 33 very-low-birth-weight infants during the first 48 postnatal hours. Sixteen of the infants developed intraventricular hemorrhage, and in four infants the hemorrhage occurred during the ultrasound scanning. Clinical events occurring at the time of the hemorrhages in three of the infants included (1) manual ventilation in an infant with primary pulmonary hypertension, (2) infusion of calcium gluconate and sodium bicarbonate for correction of hyperkalemia, and (3) administration of surfactant for respiratory failure secondary to pulmonary hemorrhage. In the fourth infant, the presence of hypertension (relative to the admission blood pressure) was noted at the time of the hemorrhage, and compared to the blood pressures of infants without hemorrhages, the other three infants also had persistent or rapid increases in blood pressure at the time of the intraventricular hemorrhage (after previous hypotension) (Funato et al, 1992). Several studies have documented that the lower an infant's birth weight, the greater the likelihood that intraventricular hemorrhage will occur during the 1st postnatal day (Leviton et al, 1991; Paneth et al, 1993; Perlman and Volpe, 1986).

Sites and Grades of Hemorrhage

Intracerebral hemorrhages in the preterm infant usually originate in the subependymal germinal matrix region with extension into the ventricular system and from there into the aqueduct, cisterns, and subarachnoid spaces. Armstrong and colleagues (1987) have shown that extension into surrounding white matter does not occur unless white matter damage is already present. It has been suggested that periventricular hemorrhagic infarction occurs after substantial intraventricular hemorrhage has occluded periventricular venous return (Volpe, 1989a).

The germinal matrix is most pronounced at the head of the caudate near the foramen of Monro between 28 and 32 weeks' gestation. At and after 28 weeks' gestation, hemorrhage is usually found at this site; before 28 weeks' gestation, hemorrhage seems to localize over the body of the caudate nucleus (Larroche, 1974; Leech and Kohnen, 1974). In the autopsy studies by Armstrong and colleagues (1987), the choroid plexus was a site of hemorrhage in addition to the germinal matrix in 50% of preterm infants with intraventricular hemorrhage. In term infants with intraventricular hemorrhage, the choroid plexus is usually the site of origin of hemorrhage (Armstrong et al, 1987).

Periventricular and intraventricular hemorrhages have been graded by extent and location by Papile and colleagues (1978a). This grading system is used most frequently, and grading of hemorrhages can be accomplished by either ultrasound visualization or by CT scan. Grade I is a subependymal hemorrhage only; Grade II is intraventricular hemorrhage without ventricular dilation; Grade III is intraventricular hemorrhage with ventricular dilation; and Grade IV is intraventricular hemorrhage and the presence of intraparenchymal blood (Papile et al, 1978a). It should be cautioned that ventricular dilation described for Grade III hemorrhage in the original study reflected obstructive hydrocephalus secondary to intraventricular blood; it may be difficult to distinguish between this situation and that of intraventricular hemorrhage with pre-existing cerebral atrophy and ventriculomegaly. Also, although Grade IV hemorrhage indicates the presence of parenchymal blood, the blood does not have to be adjacent to the ventricles. Knowledge gained since 1978 has shown that most parenchymal blood is not caused by extravasation of blood from the ventricles; rather, it is caused by a separate but related process, usually in the white matter.

Associations with Hemorrhage

Hypoglycorrhachia

Low CSF glucose (hypoglycorrhachia) has been described in association with intraventricular hemorrhage as well as with other neurologic disease states, including bacterial meningitis, meningeal carcinomatosis, hypoglycemia, glucose transporter protein deficiency, and subarachnoid hemorrhage (DeVivo et al, 1991; Mathew et al, 1979; Mathew and Volpe, 1980). Fifteen preterm infants with intracranial hemorrhage were evaluated by Mathew and colleagues (1979), and 14 survived. Sequential lumbar punctures were performed to determine the course of the hypoglycorrhachia. All of the infants had CSF xanthochromia, elevated CSF protein, CSF pleocytosis, and hemosiderin-containing macrophages in the CSF (Mathew et al, 1979). The number of cells in the CSF and the protein concentrations returned to normal before resolution of the hypoglycorrhachia in this study. Hypoglycorrhachia was present as long

as 33 days after the hemorrhage in one case, and all infants developed low CSF glucoses between 1 and several days after the hemorrhage.

Mathew and Volpe (1980) have also shown that CSF lactate is high immediately after hemorrhage but returns to near normal by the time hypoglycorrhachia is present; similarly the CSF cell count is usually low by the time hypoglycorrhachia is present. This has led to the hypothesis that the hypoglycorrhachia is caused by damage to or inhibition of the glucose transporter system by blood breakdown products. It is not known if the hypoglycorrhachia following intraventricular hemorrhage is deleterious to the brain; however, congenital glucose transporter deficiency states are known to be associated with seizures, microcephaly, and mental retardation (DeVivo et al, 1991). Infants with hypoglycorrhachia as a result of intracranial hemorrhage may continue to have low CSF/blood glucose ratios for a period of time. This may be found when lumbar punctures are done to relieve posthemorrhagic hydrocephalus and, without other findings, should not be thought to indicate infection (Green and Shaw, 1994).

Hemispheric Metabolic Depression

Infants with Grade IV intraventricular hemorrhage have always been at greatest risk for severe neurologic sequelae. Autopsy studies have suggested that when there is parenchymal hemorrhage, this occurs because underlying brain tissue is already compromised (Armstrong et al, 1987). Metabolic studies using PET have shown that cerebral blood flow is depressed in areas of hemorrhagic cerebral involvement (Volpe et al, 1983). These studies have also shown that there is a twofold to fourfold reduction in cerebral blood flow throughout the entire affected hemisphere, encompassing an area extending a considerable distance from the actual hematoma. Autopsies in the infants who have succumbed after being studied with PET have shown extensive damage of the entire hemisphere (Volpe et al, 1983). Thus, the PET studies have provided functional clues to the extent of brain injury present in the preterm infants evaluated. These studies have confirmed that infants with intracranial hemorrhages are at risk for damage in other brain regions that may not be visible on ultrasound scans and may take time to become apparent on CT.

Periventricular Venous Infarction

Periventricular venous infarction is destruction of white matter, frequently hemorrhagic, that is thought to be a consequence of obstruction of venous return owing to pressure on veins in the floor of the ventricle by homolateral intraventricular clot (Volpe, 1989a). This situation is probably made worse when the periventricular region has already been compromised by hypoxia/ischemia, the antecedent for periventricular leukomalacia (Armstrong et al, 1987). Survivors may show loss of brain tissue in the region with ventricular enlargement. Severe neurologic sequelae are associated with this lesion.

Periventricular Leukomalacia

Periventricular leukomalacia is frequently found at autopsy in conjunction with intraventricular hemorrhage. Armstrong and associates (1987) reported the association in 75% of infants who came to autopsy after surviving at least 1 week after the diagnosis of intraventricular hemorrhage. The pathology of periventricular leukomalacia has been discussed in a previous section. Periventricular leukomalacia may be due to multiple factors (e.g., hypoxia/ischemia, endotoxemia, hypoglycemia, effects of glutamate release on glia and axons). Periventricular leukomalacia can be hemorrhagic, and it seems reasonable to propose that periventricular venous infarction is a severe form of periventricular leukomalacia because in both the end result is destruction of white matter. It is not clear what role venous obstruction plays in less severe forms of periventricular leukomalacia, just as it is not clear if previously existing periventricular leukomalacia is essential for the genesis of periventricular venous infarction.

Posthemorrhagic Hydrocephalus

Hydrocephalus is defined as ventriculomegaly with CSF under increased pressure because of an imbalance in CSF production, CSF flow, or CSF absorption. What used to be termed *hydrocephalus ex vacuo* is now called *ventriculomegaly with cerebral atrophy* and does not imply that CSF is under increased pressure, unless hydrocephalus is also present. Over the years, it has become clear that infants with intraventricular hemorrhage can have normal ventricles, posthemorrhagic hydrocephalus, hydrocephalus that resolves, or ventriculomegaly with cerebral atrophy. A small percentage have hydrocephalus and atrophy. In the series by Albright and Fellows (1981), hydrocephalus followed intracerebral hemorrhage (intraventricular or intraparenchymal) in 32% of infants. Allan and colleagues (1984) reported 26 infants with ventriculomegaly, in 12 of whom hydrocephalus was eventually diagnosed. These represented 13% of the infants with intraventricular hemorrhages. Ventriculomegaly was defined as dilation of the ventricles that either stabilized or reversed in infants with head circumferences that increased less than 2 cm per week and had no signs or symptoms of increased intracranial pressure. Posthemorrhagic hydrocephalus was defined as progressive dilation of the ventricles (by scan) associated with an increase in head circumference greater than 2 cm per week and with symptoms of increased pressure (apnea with bradycardia, stupor, vomiting, or brain stem ocular signs) (Allan et al, 1984). Infants with ventriculomegaly were observed carefully but had no intervention. Infants with posthemorrhagic hydrocephalus underwent either serial lumbar punctures for relief of pressure or external ventricular drainage. Serial lumbar punctures or external drainage were discontinued in those who had three successive weekly scans with stable ventricular size. Those who had recurrence of hydrocephalus or unremitting increase in ventricular size underwent ventricular shunt placement when their weights were 2000 g or greater. Of 12 infants with posthemorrhagic hydrocephalus, only 3 required permanent shunts. All 14 infants with ventriculomegaly as defined here had normal head growth, although 2 of these infants had developmental delay or spastic diplegia (Allan et al, 1984).

Although it has been reported that infants with moderate to marked intraventricular hemorrhage are those most likely to incur posthemorrhagic hydrocephalus, Fishman and coworkers (1984) reported 11 premature infants who had moderate to marked degrees of ventricular enlargement after minor subependymal or intraventricular hemorrhages. Six of the 11 continued to have ventricular dilation after 1 month of age, with head growth either normal (in 3) or excessive (in 3). Four of the six infants had only subependymal hemorrhage on ultrasound scan. This study made clear (1) the necessity to watch for hydrocephalus in infants with (apparently) only minor degrees of hemorrhage, (2) the fact that ventriculomegaly could progress beyond 1 month of age, and (3) that increases in ventricular size could occur without increases in head circumference or signs of increased intracranial pressure. Increases in ventricular size without increases in fronto-occipital circumference may occur because of the ease of compressibility of the immature white matter and because of the presence of a relatively large subarachnoid space in the premature infant.

In a prospective study of infants with progressive posthemorrhagic hydrocephalus, 13% of infants with intraventricular hemorrhage (53 of 409) developed hydrocephalus that was arrested in 35 and became severe in 18 (Dykes et al, 1989). Furthermore, a study of infants with and without ventriculomegaly showed a significantly higher incidence of neurologic deficits and developmental delay in the group with ventriculomegaly (Shankaran et al, 1989). Most notably, infants who required shunts but did not respond to shunting with ventricular decompression had worse neurologic outcomes. This implies that these infants had some degree of cerebral atrophy before shunting (Shankaran et al, 1989).

Posthemorrhagic hydrocephalus can occur acutely or over a period of time, probably as a result of impairment of CSF egress or absorption. Acute hydrocephalus is usually due to obstruction of CSF outflow by clot; subacute hydrocephalus is thought to be due to an obliterative arachnoiditis that occurs downstream from the fourth ventricular outflow and in the arachnoid villi. Hydrocephalus can be apparent by ultrasound scan within the first few days after intraventricular hemorrhage or several weeks later. In cases in which there is evidence of only minimal hemorrhage on ultrasound scan, it is worthwhile to remember that blood may still reach the subarachnoid spaces and not be seen on the scan; therefore, it is reasonable to monitor ventricular size in these infants at monthly intervals until discharge.

Treatment

Numerous prophylactic regimens, including prenatal administration of vitamin K, phenobarbital, and corticosteroids, have been shown to have some beneficial effects on the incidence of postnatal intraventricular hemorrhage (Crowley et al, 1990; Kaempf et al, 1990; Leviton et al, 1993; Morales and Koerton, 1986; Morales et al, 1988; Shankaran et al, 1986). Of all the prenatal regimens, antenatal corticosteroids have had the most consistently positive effects (NIH Consensus Statement, 1994). Postnatal regimens have included various strategies for administration of phenobarbital, indomethacin, paralysis, ethamsylate, fresh frozen plasma, vitamin E, and minimal stimulation protocols (Bedard et al, 1984; Beverley et al, 1985; Donn et al,

1981; Goddard-Finegold and Mizrahi, 1987; Ment et al, 1994a; Perlman and Volpe, 1985; Speer et al, 1984). Each of these prevention strategies has supporting and detracting data in the literature. General prevention measures also include avoidance of bolus infusions, continuous monitoring of blood pressure and avoidance of hypotension or hypertension; prevention and rapid treatment of pneumothorax; careful regulation of intake of sodium and glucose; avoidance of hyperosmolar states; and careful management of the open ductus arteriosus (Goddard-Finegold and Mizrahi, 1987). For the most part, however, treatment of infants once intraventricular hemorrhage has occurred has been supportive, with control of ventilation, seizures, metabolic and fluid status, temperature, and nutritional state. Attention is also paid to coagulation status to reduce the likelihood of extension of bleeding (all infants in the United States receive prophylactic vitamin K at birth). Minimal stimulation protocols are continued because hemodynamic instability may be even more severe after intraventricular hemorrhage has occurred.

Once hydrocephalus is diagnosed, medical therapy to reduce production of CSF by the choroid plexus can be instituted by using isosorbide or glycerol or acetazolamide (Diamox) (Laurent et al, 1985; Salfield et al, 1981; Shinnar et al, 1985). If the infant is symptomatic because of increased intracranial pressure, mannitol can be given acutely, followed by decompression of the ventricles by lumbar puncture or by insertion of an external ventricular drain. In such infants, with open fontanels, lumbar puncture has not been associated with herniation. Serial lumbar punctures have been used to remove CSF, to gain time before inserting a permanent shunt, or to determine if an infant's hydrocephalus will ultimately resolve.

Serial lumbar punctures have also been performed in infants after intraventricular hemorrhage in attempts to prevent the onset of hydrocephalus. The goal has been the removal of blood and protein thought to be responsible for the arachnoiditis. Although some studies initially raised hopes, the current consensus is that serial lumbar punctures have not been successful when used for this purpose (Anwar et al, 1985; Mantovani et al, 1980; Papile et al, 1980). Currently, investigators are looking into ways to dissolve clots and remove fibrin products from the ventricular system immediately after intraventricular hemorrhage to prevent posthemorrhagic hydrocephalus (Todo et al, 1991; Whitelaw et al, 1992).

Relationship of Hemorrhagic Lesions to Neurologic Sequelae

Low and colleagues (1993) have shown that very-low-birthweight infants with no apparent hypoxia, hypotension, or hemorrhage are still at some risk for neurologic disability. The mechanisms of injury underlying such disability are not known, but one could suppose that even in the best of circumstances, the immature brain may not develop optimally in the extrauterine environment. Thus, one might speculate that infants with neurologic sequelae who have only had subependymal hemorrhages or isolated intraventricular hemorrhage may have either areas of previously unsuspected brain injury or functional disorders of brain development that are not currently detectable by neuro-

imaging. What is known is that infants with documented intraparenchymal hemorrhage, periventricular venous infarction, or periventricular leukomalacia have much higher incidences of neurologic sequelae (Guzzetta et al, 1986). A compilation of current information has shown that when periventricular injury is extensive, mortality is high (81%), major motor deficits are universal (100%), and cognitive deficits are common (85%). When periventricular lesions are smaller and localized, mortality is less (37%), major motor deficits are common but not universal (80%), cognitive deficits are less frequent (53%), and some infants are normal (10%) (Volpe, 1995d).

Superficial Cranial Traumatic Injury

A frequent superficial cranial traumatic injury is hemorrhagic edema of the scalp (Abroms and Rosen, 1993). This is termed *caput succedaneum* and usually resolves quickly. It is frequently associated with molding of the head and overriding sutures as a result of pressure during delivery (Menkes, 1991b). Subgaleal hemorrhage, occurring under the scalp aponeurosis but external to the periosteum, can be more severe, with extensive bleeding sometimes necessitating a blood transfusion. A cephalohematoma occurs under the periosteum of a skull bone and does not cross suture lines. Large cephalohematomas may calcify and persist for a period of time, giving the skull an asymmetric appearance (Abroms and Rosen, 1993). It is useful to obtain radiologic studies in some cases to determine if a skull fracture is present, especially if there appears to be a skull depression in association with the cephalohematoma. Compound depressed fractures require surgical reduction; simple depressed fractures may be elevated in some cases by nonsurgical means (Menkes, 1991b).

Traumatic Brain Injury

Traumatic brain injury is often associated with traumatic hemorrhages. One of the most dangerous situations occurs when there is injury to the middle meningeal artery or to a major vein or sinus (Abroms and Rosen, 1993). Middle meningeal artery injury usually occurs with a linear skull fracture and results in an epidural hematoma, which can cause mass effect, increased intracranial pressure, and death within a few hours of occurrence. Prompt surgical attention is required to evacuate the blood and occlude the middle meningeal artery.

Subdural hemorrhages can also occur after traumatic injury. Because the bleeding is less rapid, however, the symptoms may be delayed for several hours. Posterior fossa subdural hemorrhages can be particularly ominous because of brain stem compression. Symptoms associated with posterior fossa subdural hemorrhage can also be delayed up to several days and can include lethargy, bulging fontanel, seizures, eye deviation, facial weakness, trunk and limb hypotonia, and respiratory abnormalities (Abroms and Rosen, 1993). This is a critical situation.

When subdural hemorrhage is present over the convexities, there may be minimal symptoms or signs such as hemiparesis, eye deviation, and pupillary abnormalities (Volpe, 1995f). Subdural hematomas may become chronic, with subacute symptoms becoming apparent as the infant exhibits seizures, developmental delay, and anemia (sometimes severe enough to cause heart failure) (Menkes, 1991b). Detection of subdural hematomas is accomplished best by using CT scanning; ultrasound is not reliable for the diagnosis of subdural hemorrhage.

Traumatic Spinal Cord Injury

Traumatic injuries to the spinal cord are not common but can be devastating when they do occur. Lesions can occur from stretching, compression, or transection of the cord; from hemorrhage into or around the cord; and from infarction of the cord (Abroms and Rosen, 1993; Menkes, 1991b). Infants are especially at risk of spinal cord injury during difficult breech deliveries (Stem and Rand, 1959), and in about 20% of such cases of spinal cord injury, there is also injury to the brachial plexus or to the lower brain stem (or both) (Menkes, 1991b). When injury is extensive, death occurs soon after delivery. Less severe injury can result in respiratory compromise and hypotonia or flaccid paraplegia (Bucher et al, 1979; Menkes, 1991b). These are usually associated with urinary retention; abdominal distention; paradoxic respirations; and absence of deep tendon reflexes, sweating, and sensation below the level of the injury. After a period of time, the infant with cord transection shows reflex withdrawal movements and other isolated spinal reflexes, eventually exhibiting spasticity (Menkes, 1991b). In addition to injuries directly from hyperextension and traction, injury to the cord can occur from spinal epidural hematomas (especially with trauma to the neck), after vertebral artery injury (can lead to upper cervical cord infarction and death of the newborn), from traumatic cervical cord hemorrhage (hematomyelia), or from spinal artery occlusion (can follow umbilical artery catheterization or air embolus from a peripheral vein) (Abroms and Rosen, 1993).

Traumatic Nerve Injuries

Facial Nerve Injury

Damage to peripheral nerves can also occur during labor and delivery, with the facial nerve, brachial plexus, and phrenic and laryngeal nerves noted in descending frequency (Abroms and Rosen, 1993; Levine et al, 1984). Facial nerve injury is the most common peripheral nerve injury in the newborn, with incidences of between 2 and 8 per 1000 births (Falco and Eriksson, 1990; Levine et al, 1984). Most cases of facial nerve injury resolve spontaneously. The clinical findings of complete facial nerve injury include drooping of the mouth, flattening of the nasolabial fold, and widening of the palpebral fissure on the side of the injury; there is also paucity of movement of the side of the face and inability to wrinkle the forehead or to close the eye (lower motor neuron lesion) (Abroms and Rosen, 1993). The injury can occur to varying degrees, with some cases involving only weakness in a small group of muscles (Menkes, 1991b). When there is difficulty in closing the eye, the eye of the newborn should be protected with artificial tears and covered. If the facial palsy does not begin to resolve within a few weeks, the infant should be referred to a pediatric neurologist.

Levine and coworkers (1984) have reported a decreasing incidence of facial nerve injuries with a decrease in the use of forceps during delivery. The injury also occurs in infants delivered without forceps, however, probably because the nerve can be injured when the face is pressed against the sacral promontory or against the ischial spines in utero (Hepner, 1952).

Congenital unilateral facial paralysis can also be due to a developmental hypoplasia or absence of the facial nerve (Shapiro et al, 1996). In such cases, the paralysis does not resolve, and electroneurography reveals diminished or no responses from homolateral facial muscles. In cases of traumatic facial nerve injury, electroneurography usually shows normal facial nerve function within 48 hours of injury, despite traumatic compression or transection injury (the distal portions of the nerve can still function early in the course of the injury) (Shapiro et al, 1996). The degree of decrease in facial nerve function that occurs for a period of time after traumatic injury is predictive of eventual recovery; however, in congenital developmental defects of the facial nerve, recovery of function does not occur.

When one corner of the mouth fails to move downward and outward during crying but all other facial movements are normal, the infant has congenital hypoplasia or absence of the angularis oris muscle. About 20% of infants with this minor anomaly have other associated congenital anomalies, with cardiac anomalies the most frequent association (Franco and Tunnessen, 1996).

Brachial Plexus Injury

Injury to the brachial plexus has great social and practical implications, and thus, pediatricians should have knowledge of its natural history and treatment. At the present time, surgical repair is available for infants whose injuries do not heal spontaneously. Brachial plexus injury consists of weakness or paralysis of upper extremity muscles innervated by the cervical nerve roots C5 to C8 and thoracic root T1 (i.e., the roots supplying the brachial plexus). The reported incidence of brachial plexus birth injuries varies greatly, from 0.3 to 2 per 1000 live births (Greenwald et al, 1984; Painter and Bergman, 1982; Specht, 1975). The true incidence has to be derived from delivery room data because many infants are "cured" of subtle and transient deficits before being seen by consultants.

Sever (1916) postulated that traumatic delivery caused stretch damage to the brachial plexus, with injury occurring in descending order from the suprascapular nerve through C5, C6, and C7. The brachial plexus, with its roots anchored to the cervical cord, is thought to be damaged by severe lateral traction during delivery. The upper roots are most vulnerable to injury, but with greater degrees of traction, the lower roots of the plexus are more likely to undergo avulsion (spinal cord–nerve rootlet disconnection) resulting in total paralysis.

Sharpe (1916), Gordon and coworkers (1973), and Zancolli (1981) described the obstetric and fetal factors that may lead to brachial plexus injury, including multiparous mothers, prolonged or augmented labors, abnormal presentations, shoulder dystocia, increased birth weight, and signs of fetal distress with low Apgar scores. Brachial plexus injury has been seen with premature births as well as with cesarean section births (Hardy, 1981).

Lesions may occur at any point from the spinal canal where nerve rootlets leave the spinal cord, to nerve roots, trunks, and divisions and cords of the brachial plexus and its peripheral nerves. The most common form of brachial plexus injury is that involving Erb point—the point where C5 and C6 join to form the upper trunk of the brachial plexus—resulting in the typical upper plexus lesion known as *Erb palsy*. A lesion at the juncture of C8 and T1, as they form the lower trunk of the brachial plexus, produces weakness of the distal upper extremity known as *Klumpke palsy*.

The least severe injuries, neuropraxic lesions, produce nerve conduction blocks via hemorrhage and edema involving the neural sheath but resolve rapidly and completely. Axonotmesis, disruption of internal neural elements with nerve sheaths remaining intact, produces an intermediate injury, which may allow regeneration of axons (and recovery of function) using the remaining nerve sheath as a guide for growth. Complete rupture of the nerve root, neurotmesis, implies disruption of both neural and sheath elements. A neuroma, a mass of fibrous tissue and disorganized regenerating neural elements, usually forms; recovery is most often unsatisfactory. The most severe injury is avulsion, in which nerve rootlets are torn from the spinal cord proximal to the formation of a mixed nerve root. Avulsed rootlets do not recover their function.

Although most newborns with birth-related brachial plexus injury present with flaccid arms (Laurent and Lee, 1994), a predominant lesion is established in 2 to 6 weeks. The large majority, 71% to 90% of cases, involve the upper extremity, presenting as an Erb palsy (Eng, 1971; Gordon et al, 1973; Laurent et al, 1990), with a smaller number presenting as a combined lesion (C5-T1). A pure Klumpke paralysis is rare. In typical Erb palsy, the arm is extended, the shoulder is internally rotated and adducted, the forearm is pronated, and the wrist and fingers are flexed, placing the extremity in the typical *waiter's tip* position. In Klumpke palsy, the arm is flexed, the forearm is supinated with the shoulder in a normal position, and the wrist and fingers are flaccid.

Horner syndrome is often present in lesions involving the entire plexus (and in the unusual pure lower plexus lesion). This manifests in the newborn as ipsilateral miosis and ptosis as a result of interruption of sympathetic innervation from T1.

If C4 is involved, the loss of phrenic nerve function may lead to diaphragmatic paralysis. Deep tendon reflexes are usually absent at biceps, triceps, and brachioradialis. The Moro reflex is diminished or absent because of shoulder involvement, and the palmar grasp reflex may also be decreased or absent. Other traumatic lesions, such as fractures of the clavicle or humerus, cervical cord injury, or facial palsy, may be seen (Al-Rajeh et al, 1990; Eng, 1971). Sensory deficits may be subtle and difficult to assess in the newborn because of inconsistent responses and overlapping of dermatomes. Sensory loss at C5 (over the lateral aspect of the shoulder) is most common, with diffuse sensory loss seen in more severe, combined brachial plexus injuries.

Most important for determination of appropriate treatment is repeated meticulous examination for degree of injury, associated traumatic lesions, and evidence of spontaneous recovery. Although EMG studies have not been useful as independent predictors or recovery in some series (Laurent and Lee, 1994), others regard EMG as having an important confirmative and predictive value (Eng, 1996; Terzis et al, 1987). Definition of diaphragmatic paralysis can be made with fluoroscopy or with real-time ultrasonography (Ambler et al, 1985). CT myelography and MRI may provide information as to presence of avulsions but are best performed before contemplated surgery (Hunt, 1988; Laurent and Lee, 1994; Laurent et al, 1990; Urabe et al, 1991).

Prognosis depends on the severity of the injury. As a general rule, the faster the recovery, the more complete the functional return (Gilbert and Tassin, 1987). The Collaborative Perinatal Study reported complete functional return in 93% of infants with brachial plexus injury, with 88% recovering by 4 months of age (Gordon et al, 1973). Laurent and colleagues (1993) have summarized 16 reported series involving more than 1000 infants with brachial plexus injury; most authors observed beginning improvement at 6 months or less for patients who would have good return of muscle function. Michelow and coworkers (1994) published a series in which a multimuscle scoring system applied at 3 months of age allowed correct prediction of eventual outcome in 95% of cases.

For the 1st week, when there is likely to be pain associated with the acute injury, the limb should be gently immobilized across the chest. The *statue of liberty* point is no longer used because of its propensity for causing contractures at the shoulder and elbow. Therapy should begin after the 1st week, with regular passive range of motion exercises and hand and wrist splinting when appropriate. For the small group of infants who do not show beginning muscle recovery by 5 to 6 months, evaluation for surgical repair is appropriate (see the section on Brachial Plexus Injuries under Conditions Amenable to Neurosurgical Intervention) (Hunt, 1988; Laurent et al, 1990; Laurent and Lee, 1994).

Phrenic and Laryngeal Nerve Injuries

Phrenic nerve injury (causing paralysis of the ipsilateral diaphragm) and laryngeal nerve injury (causing vocal cord paralysis) are rare injuries as a result of birth trauma (Abroms and Rosen, 1993). Phrenic nerve injury can occur in conjunction with brachial plexus injury, the forces for both being excessive lateral traction on the neck and arm. Symptomatic infants show tachypnea and respiratory distress, sometimes with cyanosis; fluoroscopy shows paradoxic movements of the diaphragms (when the paralysis is unilateral, as is most often the case). Again, most cases resolve spontaneously after some supportive care (which may include intubation and positive-pressure ventilation). Those that do not resolve may require surgical plication of the affected diaphragm (Abroms and Rosen, 1993). Laryngeal nerve injury also occurs infrequently, probably as a result of head rotation and compression of the thyroid cartilage against the hyoid bone (Abroms and Rosen, 1993).

Metabolic and Degenerative Diseases and the Newborn Nervous System

Recognition of metabolic and degenerative diseases in the newborn is sometimes difficult but important: difficult because the signs and symptoms can seem nonspecific and can be confounded by the presence of drugs, infection, or hypoxia, but important because although a number of metabolic diseases cannot be treated effectively, some can be, and the window of time during which neurologic injury can be averted may be narrow. (See also Chapter 25.)

Saudubray and Carpentier (1995) have divided the categories of metabolic diseases that present in the newborn period into five major types with typical presentations. This scheme is a helpful approach to diagnosis and is presented in an abbreviated form here:

Type I, neurologic distress: intoxication, with ketosis. The cardinal disease represented here is maple syrup urine disease, in which a newborn becomes symptomatic with feeding difficulties and encephalopathy leading to coma after an initial symptom-free period.

Type II, neurologic distress: intoxication, with ketoacidosis and hyperammonemia. These disorders have an earlier onset than Type I, with symptoms beginning frequently during the 1st postnatal day. The infants are acutely ill and may develop coma within hours. Many of the organic acidurias are included in Type II, and many of these disorders also have marked hyperammonemia (Saudubray and Carpentier, 1995). Organic acidurias frequently diagnosed include methylmalonic, propionic, and isovaleric acidemia; less frequently diagnosed are glutaric aciduria type II (multiple acyl-CoA dehydrogenase deficiency) and hydroxymethylglutaryl-CoA lyase deficiency (in these, ketosis is absent, and hypoglycemia is frequent).

Type III: energy deficiency. This category is different from the previous two in that the infants are not as acutely ill, although they are acidotic and may have lactic acidosis. Biotin-responsive multiple carboxylase deficiency can present with lactic acidosis, and thus Saudubray and Carpentier (1995) urge physicians to treat all patients with lactic acidosis of unknown cause with biotin after blood and urine samples have been obtained for studies. Diseases grouped in this category include pyruvate carboxylase deficieny, pyruvate dehydrogenase deficiency, respiratory chain disorders, and multiple carboxylase deficiency (Saudubray and Carpentier, 1995).

Type IVa: neurologic distress, intoxication, with hyperammonemia but without ketoacidosis. This category is represented by the urea cycle defects, and infants with such defects usually have a short symptom-free interval followed by rapid development of neurologic symptoms and coma. Blood ammonia is extremely high, and respiratory alkalosis and moderate lactic acidemia may be present. There is no ketonuria, which is an important diagnostic distinction between this class of diseases and the organic acidurias with hyperammonemia. The two main urea cycle disorders are ornithine transcarbamylase deficiency (sex-linked) and carbamyl phosphate synthetase deficiency. These two diseases cannot be diagnosed by amino acid analyses, and liver biopsy is required for enzyme diagnosis. Other urea cycle defects (citrullinemia, argininosuccinic aciduria, and argininemia) can be diagnosed by amino acid analyses, which show elevated concentrations of citrulline, argininosuccinate, and arginine. Significant hyperammonemia can also be seen in some of the fatty acid oxidation disorders in the neonatal period (Saudubray and Carpentier, 1995). Ammonia determinations should be done in any infant with the rapid onset of neurologic symptoms because delay can mean permanent neurologic sequelae or death, and rapid treatment can mean reversal of some or all symptoms.

Type IVb, neurologic distress: energy deficiency, no ketoacidosis and no hyperammonemia. This group is characterized by nonketotic hyperglycinemia. Infants with this disorder present at birth or within a few hours with hypotonia, myoclonic jerks, and coma and have a burst-suppression pattern on the EEG (Mises et al, 1982). This disorder is diagnosed by finding elevated plasma glycine levels and elevated CSF/plasma glycine ratio. Other disorders in this spectrum of disease include sulfite oxidase deficiency and sulfite and xanthine oxidase deficiencies, which present with hypotonia, seizures, myoclonic jerks, dysmorphic features, and microcephaly (Saudubray and Carpentier, 1995; Wadman et al, 1983). These deficiencies are also present in molybdenum cofactor deficiency (see earlier). Saudubray and Carpentier (1995) also include the peroxisomal disorders, Zellweger syndrome and neonatal adrenoleukodystrophy, in this category because they also have no symptom-free interval, presenting with dysmorphic features, hypotonia, and early-onset seizures. Pyridoxine-dependent seizures are also listed in this category; these seizures are resistant to anticonvulsants, and improvement in the EEG tracing can be seen as pyridoxine (vitamin B_6) is administered.

Type IVc: storage disorders without metabolic disturbances. Storage disorders that have been diagnosed during the newborn period include GM_1 gangliosidosis, Gaucher disease, mucopolysaccharidosis Type VII, sialidosis, galactosialidosis, sialuria, and Niemann-Pick disease type C. Two other degenerative diseases that are not as well understood, neuronal ceroid lipofuscinosis and neuroaxonal dystrophy, are discussed subsequently.

Type V: hypoglycemia with hepatomegaly and liver dysfunction. The diseases in this category that present with hypoglycemia (often with hypoglycemic seizures), hepatomegaly, ketosis, and lactic acidosis include glucose-6-phosphatase deficiency (Type I glycogen storage disease), glycogenosis Type III, and fructose-1,6-diphosphatase deficiency. Other disorders in this category present mainly with hepatic dysfunction and jaundice (hypoglycemia may be present but usually not marked). The disorders in this group include tyrosinemia Type I, galactosemia, hereditary fructose intolerance when the diet contains frucose, alpha$_1$-antitrypsin deficiency, Wilson disease, and neonatal hemochromatosis (Saudubray and Carpentier, 1995).

Neuronal Ceroid Lipofuscinosis

During the past few years, some disorders that are usually diagnosed in older patients have been described in newborns because diagnostic acumen and capabilities have increased. The case history of a term infant with microcephaly, status epilepticus, and death at 36 postnatal hours was reported (Barohn et al, 1992). Autopsy of this infant revealed changes in the brain consistent with neuronal ceroid lipofuscinosis. The usual patient with ceroid lipofuscinosis is normal at birth but has subsequent deterioration of cognitive function, vision, and motor abilities, often with seizures, in the infantile form (Haltia-Santavuori), the late infantile form (Jansky-Bielschowsky), the juvenile form (Spielmeyer-Vogt or Batten), or the adult form (Kufs) (Swick, 1989). Nevertheless, three other patients have been reported with neonatal ceroid lipofuscinosis, suggesting that it should be part of the differential diagnosis for intractable neonatal seizures or microcephaly (Edathodu et al, 1984; Garbarg et al, 1987; Humphreys et al, 1985). Vacuolated lymphocytes are present in neuronal ceroid lipofuscinosis (Bennett and Berry, 1995).

Infantile Neuroaxonal Dystrophy

Infantile neuroaxonal dystrophy is characterized pathologically by spheroid bodies in axons and, in some cases, mineralization of neurons in the basal ganglia and thalamus (Venkatesh et al, 1994). It has been suggested that infantile neuroaxonal dystrophy (also called *Seitelberger disease*) and Hallervorden-Spatz disease have features in common (Gilman and Barrett, 1973). Several cases of infantile neuroaxonal dystrophy presenting at birth have been reported; Venkatesh and coworkers (1994) have reported a case presenting within several hours of birth with extreme hypertonicity, with axonal spheroids and mineralization of the basal ganglia at autopsy. Most usually, this disorder presents at the end of the 1st postnatal year with progressive cognitive and motor deterioration, bilateral pyramidal tract signs, hypotonia, and early visual problems, without seizures (Venkatesh et al, 1994). The storage product and gene defect in this disease are not known.

Gaucher Disease

Gaucher disease has also been diagnosed in the newborn in a form similar to a mouse model of the disease (Sidransky et al, 1992). Gaucher disease is caused by deficiency of the lysosomal enzyme glucocerebrosidase. One newborn in whom Gaucher disease was identified presented with hepatosplenomegaly, hypertonia, hyperreflexia, neck hyperextension, and poor sucking and swallowing; the infant died at 2 months of age (Sidransky et al, 1992). A second infant, also diagnosed with Gaucher disease, had absent fetal movements, polyhydramnios, and thickened skin and after birth had no spontaneous movements or respiratory efforts (Sidransky et al, 1992). Fifteen additional infants diagnosed with Gaucher disease in the neonatal period have been reported, and some of these cases have had collodion skin. These infants resembled a transgenic mouse model of Gaucher disease (Lipson et al, 1991; Sidransky et al, 1992). Other metabolic diseases that affect the nervous system are discussed in Chapter 25.

Infections of the Newborn Nervous System

Infections of the newborn nervous system are covered in Part VII (Chapters 40 to 47).

CONDITIONS AMENABLE TO NEUROSURGICAL INTERVENTION
Dysraphic States

The term *dysraphism* is used to denote all of the conditions associated with abnormal fusion of the posterior neuropore and that are usually associated with spina bifida. The conditions presenting to the neurosurgeon include meningocele, myelomeningocele, neural plaque, myelocystocele, lipomeningocele, lipomyelomeningocele, lipomyeloschisis, lipomyelolipoma, anterior meningocele, rachischisis, and Chiari II malformation (see Chapter 67) (Reigel and Rotenstein, 1994). Spina bifida occulta is considered a dysraphism, not usually requiring surgical intervention but associated with an increased incidence of occult intraspinal lesions (Reigel and Rotenstein, 1994). Except for spina bifida occulta, most of these lesions are diagnosed in the immediate newborn period, and surgical repair is undertaken shortly after diagnosis.

The clinical manifestations and pathology of the dysraphic lesions listed are detailed in previous sections. Repair of dysraphic lesions begins with an initial physical and neurologic examination, determination of extent of the lesion(s) and neurologic deficit, and maintenance of the infant's homeostasis (maintenance of temperature, calorie, and fluid and electrolyte status; treatment of infection; and protection of the lesion). The presence of any orthopedic deformities should be determined. Bladder function should be assessed, and when neurogenic bladder is present, the appropriate maneuvers must be initiated to empty the bladder intermittently (Credé maneuver or intermittent catheterization). Bowel incontinence is usually associated with bladder incontinence (Reigel and Rotenstein, 1994).

Neurosurgical repair of myelomeningocele consists of reconvolution of the spinal cord within the spinal canal; restoration of the continuity of the dural sac surrounding the reconstituted spinal cord; primary spinal osteotomy for kyphosis (when present); and meticulous, five-layer closure of the lesion (Reigel and Rotenstein, 1994). When hydrocephalus is present at birth, a ventriculoperitoneal shunt is placed before closure of the myelomeningocele; this is done because it has been noted that hydrocephalus can be worsened (or its onset hastened) by closure of the back lesion (Reigel and Rotenstein, 1994). Infants without early signs of hydrocephalus should be followed closely with fronto-occipital circumference measurements, ultrasonography, and, when necessary, CT or MRI scans because 80% to 90% of those with myelomeningocele develop hydrocephalus, frequently within the 1st postnatal month.

Current statistics show that 90% of infants born with myelomeningocele survive, at least 80% have normal intelligence, and 85% ambulate (with or without aids) (McLone, 1992). Eighty percent of patients with myelomeningocele are able to be socially continent with pharmacologic therapy and intermittent catheterization (McLone, 1992). Current care in most centers involves a multidisciplinary team of physicians (neurosurgeons, orthopedists, urologists, and pediatricians) as well as nurses, social workers, and physical therapists. Surgery in some cases is done within 24 hours of birth; when surgery is delayed, the surface of the lesion is serially cultured to determine if infection has occurred.

Surgery is not performed until sterilization of the lesion and CSF is ensured (Reigel and Rotenstein, 1994).

Postsurgical care includes normal positioning and handling by the nurses and parents, with careful attention to status of the wound for cellulitis, CSF leakage, or wound breakdown. Wound infection is treated with appropriate drainage, cleansing, and use of systemic antibiotics. When ventriculitis is present, a ventricular drainage device often must be inserted for instillation of intrathecal antibiotics.

Intellectual outcome of infants with myelomeningocele, without the complications of intracerebral hemorrhage or ventriculitis, is usually good, with intelligence quotients within normal ranges (McLone, 1992). Intelligence can be considerably impaired after CSF shunt infections, however, and other problems, such as difficulties with hand use, dominance, and coordination as well as memory, have been reported in children with myelomeningocele (Reigel and Rotenstein, 1994).

Hydrocephalus

A number of temporizing measures can be used to postpone the placement of a shunt device for the correction of hydrocephalus in newborns. These have been discussed in the section on Intraventricular Hemorrhage because this is the most common cause of hydrocephalus in the neonatal period. For infants whose hydrocephalus is progressive, however, the placement of a shunt device is necessary. The success of surgical shunting procedures for control of hydrocephalus and resulting increased intracranial pressure has largely been due to the development of pressure-activated shunt valves, siphon control devices, and Silastic shunt tubing (Rekate, 1994).

Shunt devices today consist of a catheter, which is placed proximal to the site of obstruction of CSF, usually in the lateral ventricle, positioned where the ventricles are most enlarged (Sainte-Rose et al, 1991–1992); a reservoir and a valve system (which may be separate or combined); and a distal catheter that is usually placed into the peritoneal cavity (Rekate, 1994). Slit valves are placed in some distal tubing to add resistance, and the main shunt valves used today can be pressure activated by one mechanism or another, to prevent too rapid or unnecessary CSF drainage. In addition, an antisiphoning device is often built into the system to prevent a gravity-induced pressure differential that can lead to rapid drainage, negative intracranial pressure, and collapse of the ventricular system (Rekate, 1994). Overdrainage is a serious problem that can result in fatal subdural hematomas when ventricular decompression results in rapid brain shrinkage and tearing of bridging veins.

The surgical placement of a shunt is not without complications, and the patient with a shunt requires careful attention and follow-up. Equipment failure, disconnection, migration, and shunt infections can all occur. Abdominal complications, including small bowel obstruction; ureter obstruction; omental cysts; and perforations of bladder, bowel, or gallbladder, are infrequent complications. Neurologic complications in shunted children include slit-ventricle syndrome (episodic signs and symptoms of increased intracranial pressure in patients with slit-like ventricular systems), seizures, neuro-ophthalmologic problems, subdural collections, craniosynostosis, and the possibility of

spread of primary brain tumors through a shunt system (reported in primitive neuroectodermal tumor, astrocytoma, glioblastoma, germinoma, and endodermal sinus tumors) (Marlin and Gaskill, 1994). Despite these potential problems, the outlook for shunted children who have good follow-up is generally good, with cognitive outcome in cases without shunt infections dependent primarily on the cause of the hydrocephalus.

Hematomas and Fluid Collections

Hematomas occur in the newborn brain under several circumstances, and some require rapid surgical evacuation. Intraventricular hemorrhages of the premature infant have been discussed earlier. Convexity subdural and cerebellar hemorrhages (parenchymal and subdural) are considered here.

Whenever hemorrhage occurs in a term or preterm newborn, the coagulation status of the infant must be assessed. Infants with disseminated intravascular coagulation, coagulopathy secondary to a large cutaneous angioma, vitamin K deficiency (especially in newborns with chronic gastrointestinal disorders), drug-related coagulopathies, platelet disorders, or forms of hemophilia can have cerebral hemorrhages with or without hemorrhages in other organs. Mechanical trauma during birth can also cause hemorrhages, in particular, subdural hematomas over the cerebral convexities, cerebellar hematomas, or posterior fossa subdural hematomas (Aronyk, 1994). When cerebellar hemorrhages occur in preterm infants, surgical evacuation is often necessary. Sometimes such hemorrhages in term infants can be managed with temporary CSF drainage or medically. Acute posterior fossa subdural hematoma in any newborn (particularly in the preterm infant), however, can lead to rapid brain stem compression and death. Symptoms include lethargy, irritability, bulging anterior fontanel, nuchal rigidity, hypertonicity, respiratory abnormalities, lower cranial nerve palsies, and ultimately respiratory arrest (Aronyk, 1994, Serfontein et al, 1980). Posterior fossa subdural hematomas are not diagnosable by ultrasonography, and thus coronal CT scans or MRI must be done to diagnose this lesion neuroradiologically.

Convexity subdural hematomas may be silent but can also present with focal neurologic abnormalities, seizures, or both. Most can be managed with subdural taps; some may require craniotomy. Chronic subdural collections may occur when subdural hematomas are not completely evacuated in newborns; however, in young infants and children, the presence of chronic subdural collections should alert the physician to look carefully for evidence of trauma other than birth trauma (in particular, child abuse).

Brachial Plexus Injuries

Modern neurosurgical techniques and the widespread acceptance of brachial plexus repair in adults have stimulated interest in surgical management for infants. Operative intervention may take the form of neurolysis, excision of neuromas, sural nerve grafting, or neurotization of avulsed nerves using intact donor roots, depending on findings at surgery (Laurent et al, 1993).

Recovery of antigravity function in 80% to 90% of surgically treated patients with upper brachial plexus lesions (C5-C7) has been reported (Laurent et al, 1990, 1993; Gilbert et al, 1991). More severe lesions involving C5-T1 innervated muscles have a poorer operative prognosis (Gilbert et al, 1991; Laurent and Lee, 1994). Orthopedic procedures as well as muscle and tendon transfers to augment the function of muscles still lacking antigravity function during early childhood have been well described.

Congenital Brain Tumors

Brain tumors diagnosed within the 1st postnatal year are considered to be congenital in origin, and current neuroimaging techniques have made earlier diagnoses of such lesions possible. In a series from Japan, 26 (11.3%) of 231 such tumors were diagnosed in the neonatal period, and of the neonatal tumors, teratomas were the most common, accounting for nine cases (Oi et al, 1990). A series of 45 cases of neonatal brain tumors from the United States included 12 teratomas; 12 primitive neuroectodermal tumors; 9 astrocytomas (Grades I through III); 4 cases of glioblastoma multiforme; 3 choroid plexus papillomas; and single cases each of ependymoma, medulloepithelioma, germinoma, angioblastic meningioma, and ganglioglioma (Buetow et al, 1990). Another series of cases occurring before 1 year of age included 22 children: 7 with astrocytomas, 6 with primitive neuroectodermal tumors, 3 with papilloma or carcinoma of the choroid plexus, 2 with malignant teratomas, 2 with dermoid tumors, and 1 each with embryonal rhabdomyosarcoma and chloroma. Fifteen of the 22 tumors were supratentorial in location (Haddad et al, 1991).

Neurosurgical resection is the treatment of choice for most of these lesions, with best results for choroid plexus tumors, dermoids, and astrocytomas. Radiation therapy and chemotherapy are used selectively in cases of congenital brain tumors. In general, the outcome is poor; in the series reported from Japan, total or subtotal resections were achieved in only 59% of the infants and in 74% of the newborns (Oi et al, 1990). Seventy-six percent of the newborns with tumors and 73% of the infants had mental retardation on follow-up. Diagnosis of brain tumors in utero by ultrasound examination in two cases at 31 and 33 weeks' gestation has also been reported (Alvarez et al, 1987).

Vascular Malformations

The vein of Galen aneurysm has been previously mentioned as a relatively rare vascular malformation that may cause congestive heart failure in the newborn, with high morbidity and mortality (Moriarity and Steinberg, 1995). In both vein of Galen malformations and other vascular malformations, endovascular obliteration can be accomplished by embolizing particulate material into the feeding vessels of the malformation; in other cases, staged embolization and resections can be done (Humphreys, 1994). A series of 28 patients in whom embolizations of vein of Galen malformations were done has been reported (Lylyk et al, 1993). In this series, 39% of the patients were newborns. Of patients, 54% had congestive heart failure, 21% had seizures, 14% had hydrocephalus, and 11% had intra-

ventricular hemorrhage. In 46% of the patients, the embolization procedures resulted in complete obliteration of the malformation, and in 82% improvement in clinical status was achieved. There was an 18% mortality in this series (Lylyk et al, 1993).

At least two cases of arteriovenous malformations in full-term newborns presenting with intraventricular hemorrhage have been reported (Heafner et al, 1985; Schum et al, 1979). In one case, the vascular malformation was defined by arteriography on the roof of the third ventricle; it was removed surgically, and the infant recovered (Heafner et al, 1985).

Craniosynostoses

Craniosynostosis (premature closure of the sutures) is relatively common, occurring in 0.4 per 1000 infants (Chadduck, 1994). Sagittal synostosis is familial in 2% of cases, and coronal synostosis is familial in 8% (Hunter and Rudd, 1976, 1977). When premature fusion of one or more sutures occurs, brain growth forces other parts of the cranium to enlarge, leading to cranial deformities. When the sagittal suture closes prematurely, scaphocephaly or dolichocephaly occurs (Fig. 69–7); coronal synostosis results in brachycephaly or plagiocephaly. Metopic synostosis causes trigonocephaly. Other, more complicated forms of craniosynostosis can also occur. Sagittal synostosis is the most common form. Certain teratogens have been associated with craniosynostoses (phenytoin, valproic acid, aminopterin, methotrexate, retinoic acids, and oxymetazoline) (Chadduck, 1994). Numerous syndromes, including Crouzon disease and Apert disease, have craniosynostosis as one of a number of abnormalities. It is important to document other problems that might be associated with craniosynostosis, such as midfacial retrusion, septo-optic dysplasia, or ventriculomegaly, before surgery is initiated.

Three-dimensional reconstructions after neuroimaging studies are often helpful in planning surgery for complicated craniofacial abnormalities. In sagittal craniosynostosis, various procedures have been used, including removal of the fused suture followed by parasagittal craniectomies, with and without placement of some form of plastic to prevent reanastomosis of the bony edges. Experience with these patients has led to the conclusion that surgery should be carried out relatively early—within the first few postnatal weeks—to ensure a good cosmetic result (Chadduck, 1994).

Intracranial and Epidural Abscesses

Brain abscess does not occur frequently in newborns, although the incidence may be increasing because of the survival of susceptible very-low-birth-weight infants (Davies, 1988). Abscesses seem to occur either during meningitis or as a result of sepsis or contiguous bone infection (cranial osteomyelitis).

In the past, diagnosis of brain abscesses was usually made late, and as a result, therapy was not always effective. Current neuroimaging techniques have made it possible to diagnose brain abscesses much earlier. The organisms usually involved include *E. coli*, *Proteus* species, and *Citrobacter* species. *Staphylococcus aureus*, *Mycoplasma hom-*

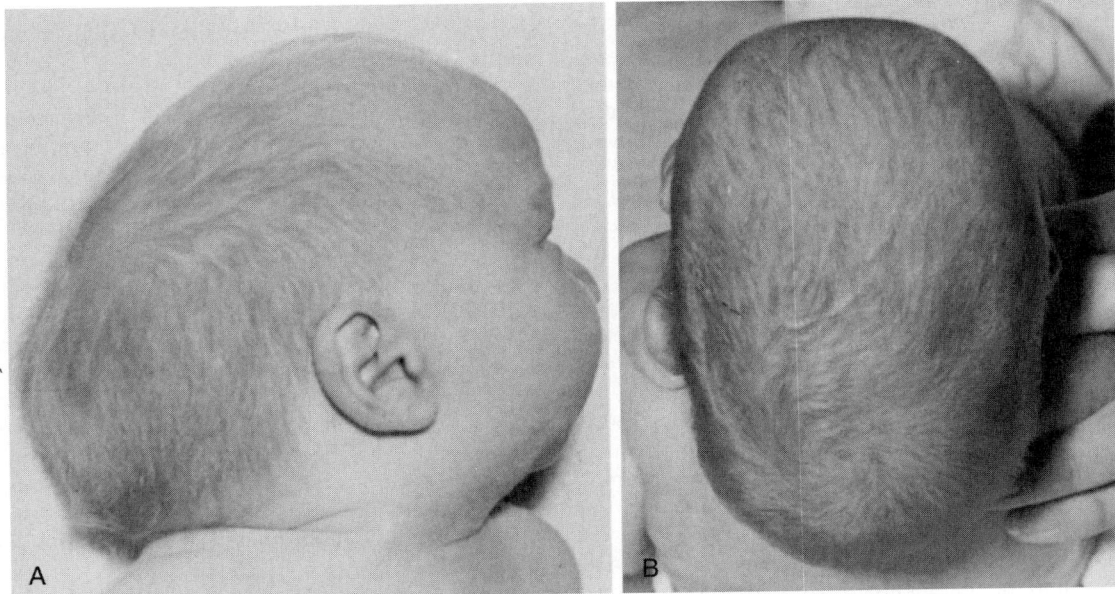

FIGURE 69–7. Three-week-old infant with sagittal craniosynostosis. *A*, Lateral view demonstrates the elongated head shape with tapering in the occipital region. Except for the abnormal configuration of the head, the child is developmentally normal for age. *B*, Vertex view reveals the characteristic long, narrow shape of the calvaria with premature closure of the sagittal suture.

inis, and group B streptococci have also been isolated from abscesses in newborns (Baker and Edwards, 1983; Fischer et al, 1981). As mentioned in the section on Infections of the Newborn Nervous System, *Candida* species can also cause brain abscesses. Treatment usually consists of antibiotic therapy and, if necessary, aspiration or surgical excision of the lesion(s).

Spinal epidural abscess is rare in newborns but has been reported after repeated lumbar punctures during a course of meningitis and in an infant with paralysis of the left arm at birth (Bergman et al, 1983; Davies, 1988; Miller and Hesch, 1962). Antibiotic therapy, surgical aspiration of the abscess, and, in some cases, decompression laminectomies are required.

SEIZURES AND OTHER PAROXYSMAL DISORDERS
Clinical Significance

Seizure occurrence is significant for several reasons. Seizures may be the most frequent clinical sign of CNS dysfunction in the newborn; their presence requires a thorough investigation for potentially treatable causes of the underlying CNS disorder. Depending on type, duration, recurrence, and severity, the seizures themselves may require treatment with AEDs.

The reported incidence of neonatal seizures has varied, owing to definitions and methods of seizure identification and surveillance. Early studies reported that seizures occurred in 0.15% to 0.5% of all live births (Eriksson and Zetterstrom, 1979; Holden et al, 1982; Spellacy et al, 1987). More recent studies suggested a higher incidence in higher-risk groups: 1.5% in premature newborns older than

30 weeks' conceptional age and 3.9% in those less than 30 weeks' conceptional age (Scher et al, 1993). Lanska and colleagues (1995) determined an overall risk of seizures to be 4.4 per 1000 live births, varying inversely with birth weight (57.5 per 1000 live births with birth weights <1500 g; 4.4 per 1000 live births, 1500 to 2499 g; 2.8 per 1000 live births, 2500 to 3999 g; and 2.0 per 1000 live births, ≥4000 g).

Despite their clinical significant and incidence, there are a number of problems in diagnosis and management, underscoring the dynamic nature of the field of study of neonatal seizures. As these problems continue to be addressed, current tenets of clinical practice may be refined or changed. It may be difficult to identify clinical seizures accurately, to designate seizure pathophysiology (i.e., epileptic or nonepileptic) accurately, to know the natural history of acute seizures, or to determine the specific relationship between seizure occurrence and risk or etiologic factors (Kellaway and Mizrahi, 1990; Mizrahi, 1987; Mizrahi and Kellaway, 1987). The utilization of AED therapy has been re-examined, and the clinical efficacy of some agents has been called into question (Mizrahi, 1989; Moshe, 1987; Painter et al, in press). The effect of seizures on the developing brain is also being closely examined, and outcome has been linked more closely to the underlying etiologic factors rather than to the occurrence of the seizures themselves.

Characterization

The clinical manifestations of seizures in the newborn differ from those of older infants or children primarily because of the rapid rate of brain development near term and the types and number of etiologic factors that may be responsible for brain injury during the neonatal period. Early investigators characterized neonatal seizures as stereotypic motor activity (Dreyfus-Brisac and Monod, 1964); anarchic or atypical behaviors, such as ocular movements, orobuccolingual movements, and limb and body movements of progression (Dreyfus-Brisac and Monod, 1964; Minkowski and Sainte Anne-Dargassies, 1956); or phenomena thought secondary to activation of the autonomic nervous system, such as changes in heart rate, changes in respirations, changes in systemic blood pressure, and vasomotor changes (e.g., flushing, pupillary dilation, and excessive salivation) (Cadilhac et al, 1959; Fenichel et al, 1980; Goldberg et al, 1982; Lou and Friis-Hansen, 1979; Schulte, 1966). Volpe (1973) designated a group of some of these behaviors and clinical signs as *subtle* seizures. This group included ocular signs, orobuccolingual movements, progression movements (rowing, stepping, and pedaling limb movements), and some signs referable to autonomic nervous system activation.

All of the clinical types of motor and behavioral seizures were recorded and further characterized in studies using time-synchronized, EEG/polygraphic/video monitoring of newborns (Kellaway and Mizrahi, 1990; Mizrahi and Kellaway, 1987). Clonic seizures were observed to be unifocal, multifocal, alternating, migratory, or hemiconvulsive. Tonic seizures were observed to be either generalized or focal. Generalized seizures were observed to be either symmetric or asymmetric. Ocular signs were characterized as either random movements or sustained tonic deviation. Movements of progression included stepping or pedaling of the legs and swimming or rowing movements of the arms. Myoclonic seizures were described as generalized, focal, or fragmentary (multifocal). Clinical events resembling generalized spasms were also noted.

The findings of these EEG/video monitoring clinical investigations suggested that not all of these clinical events were of epileptic origin. Some types of spontaneous clinical events could be provoked by stimulation of the infant, could be suppressed by light restraint of the infant, and did not consistently occur with simultaneously recorded EEG seizure activity. Other seizure types could not be provoked by stimulation, could not be suppressed by restraint, and occurred with a consistent electrocortical signature. These findings lead to the consideration that not all clinical events currently considered to be neonatal seizures were engendered by the same pathophysiologic mechanism: Clinical seizures eventually were characterized and classified as seizures of either epileptic or nonepileptic origin.

This is the most controversial aspect of the terminology of neonatal seizures: the application of the terms *epileptic* and *nonepileptic*. The term *seizure* may be used to designate an abnormal paroxysmal clinical event. Some types of clinical events may be generated by paroxysmal, hypersynchronous neuronal discharges characteristic of epileptogenesis. These can be referred to as *epileptic seizures* and include focal and multifocal clonic, focal and asymmetric tonic, and some myoclonic seizures. Other clinical seizures may be generated and propagated by nonepileptic mechanisms. These can be referred to as *nonepileptic seizures* and include generalized symmetric tonic posturing; some myoclonic events; and the motor automatisms of progres-

sion movements, ocular signs, and orobuccolingual movements.

Another important distinction in the characterization of neonatal seizures is to differentiate them accurately from nonepileptic paroxysmal events, which may be either normal or abnormal. Jitteriness may be regional or generalized and can be suppressed by restraint of the limbs. Some infants may experience myoclonus during sleep only, which is a normal phenomenon. Episodic apnea or periodic breathing are rarely manifestations of seizures in isolation, without other motor signs of seizures. Although there has been much interest in sudden changes in heart rate and systemic blood pressure as manifestations of neonatal seizures, again, their finding as signs of clinical seizures without other motor changes is rare. Because orobuccolingual movements have been characterized as seizures, sucking movements of newborns prompt significant concern at the bedside. Random, infrequent, and not well-sustained sucking, particularly in intubated infants, is not likely to be a seizure.

Pathophysiology

In clinical investigations, some events are designated as *epileptic* in origin because of their precise and consistent relationship to electrical seizure activity on an EEG recorded simultaneously with the videotaped clinical seizures. The epileptic discharge is defined by the hypersynchronous firing of an aggregate of cortical neurons. Discharges may be confined to specific regions or spread rapidly to other regions. Thus, epileptic seizures tend to be manifested as unifocal or multifocal events, with irregular rather than sequential spread over cortical regions.

The suggestion that other types of events are generated by *nonepileptic* mechanisms is based on EEG/video monitoring and clinical data and their correlation with animal studies. First, these clinical events are not consistently accompanied by EEG seizure activity and most often occur in the absence of any electrical seizure activity. Second, the spontaneously occurring clinical events can be suppressed by restraint or repositioning of the infant. For example, generalized tonic posturing can be arrested by repositioning of the infant's head and neck. In addition, clinical events identical to the spontaneously occurring events can be provoked by tactile stimulation. For example, stroking the infant's back or rubbing the infant's limb can provoke posturing or motor automatisms. Finally, increasing intensity or sites of tactile stimuli result in increasing the degree of paroxysmal movements, and stimulation at one site can provoke paroxysmal movements at another site. These clinical features of suppression of movement, evocation of clinical events, temporal and spatial summation, and irradiation of the response are not suggestive of an epileptic process but rather are characteristic of reflex physiology (Sherrington et al, 1932; Starzl et al, 1951).

Animal models of reflex physiology can be used to explain how nonepileptic seizures can be engendered. Normally, brain stem structures facilitate the primitive movements of progression (such as stepping, pedaling, or swimming) and posture (such as truncal and limb extension or flexion). In the immature animal, these primitive movements may occur reflexively. Eventually, however, the forebrain develops and inhibits brain stem facilitory centers, allowing the cortex to *override* primitive reflex behaviors. This allows more voluntary movements to become manifest as development progresses. If the forebrain is depressed, removed, or disconnected, the facilitory brain stem centers are allowed to mediate reflex behaviors without rostral inhibition. These unchecked reflex behaviors can be characterized by suppression and evocation of clinical events, spatial and temporal summation, and irradiation of the response and may occur because of rich extrapyramidal sensory input to the brain stem (Sherrington et al, 1932; Sprague and Chambers, 1954; Starzl et al, 1951).

All of these features are characteristic of generalized tonic posturing and many of the types of so-called subtle seizures (swimming and pedaling movements and some orobuccolingual movements). Because of this putative pathophysiologic mechanism of disinhibition of brain stem facilitatory centers, these clinical events in infants have been referred to as *brain stem release phenomena* and as *motor automatisms* (Kellaway and Hrachovy, 1983; Mizrahi and Kellaway, 1984, 1987).

Classification

The most widely used classification system is one initially proposed and revised by Volpe (1973, 1989b). The latest revision allows for the possibility that some seizure types may occur in the absence of simultaneous EEG seizure activity and expands the categories of clinical seizures. Another classification system has been proposed by Mizrahi and Kellaway (1984, 1987; Kellaway and Mizrahi, 1990; Mizrahi, 1994), which has been developed from findings of their EEG/video monitoring studies (Table 69–2). This system recognizes the possibility that not all neonatal seizures may be initiated or generated by an epileptic process.

Regardless of the system used, each has some limitations. There is a lack of specific data concerning paroxysmal changes in heart rate, respirations, and systemic blood pressure. The issue of whether apnea alone can be a manifestation of neonatal seizures has not been completely resolved. Some early studies suggested that apnea may be a sole seizure manifestation; others have not found apnea as a seizure phenomenon unless accompanied by other signs, such as clonic or tonic seizures (Mizrahi and Kellaway, 1987). Similarly, it has also not yet been firmly established whether paroxysmal tachycardia, hypertension, or tachypnea may exist as sole features of clinical seizures or coexist with other clinical manifestations. The classification systems emphasize the clinical manifestations of seizures. Electrical seizure activity, however, may occur in the absence of any clinical signs, representing an important electroclinical entity that can, obviously, be appreciated only by recording the EEG.

In many instances, it may be possible to identify and classify seizures at the bedside according to their presumed pathophysiology (Table 69–3). Epileptic seizures cannot be suppressed by restraint and, typically, cannot be provoked. Clinical events that can be suppressed and evoked most likely can be classified as nonepileptic in origin. In addition to these characteristics, epileptic and nonepileptic neonatal seizures may have other constellations of clinical characteristics.

TABLE 69–2

Clinical Characteristics of Neonatal Seizures

Designation	Characterization
Focal clonic	Repetitive, rhythmic contractions of muscle groups of the limbs, face, or trunk
	May be unilateral or multifocal
	May appear synchronously or asynchronously in various body regions
	Cannot be suppressed by restraint
Focal tonic	Sustained posturing of single limbs
	Sustained asymmetric posturing of the trunk
	Sustained eye deviation
	Cannot be provoked by stimulation or suppressed by restraint
Myoclonic	Arrhythmic contractions of muscle groups of the limbs, face, or trunk
	Typically not repetitive or may recur at a slow rate
	May be generalized, focal, or fragmentary
	May be provoked by stimulation
Generalized tonic	Sustained symmetric posturing of limbs, trunk, and neck
	May be flexor, extensor, or mixed extensor/flexor
	May be provoked by stimulation
	May be suppressed by restraint or repositioning
Ocular signs	Random and roving eye movements or nystagmus
	Distinct from tonic eye deviation
Orobuccolingual movements	Sucking, chewing, tongue protrusions
	May be provoked by stimulation
Progression movements	Rowing or swimming movements of the arms
	Pedaling or bicycling movements of the legs
	May be provoked by stimulation
	May be suppressed by restraint or respositioning

From Mizrahi EM: Neonatal seizures. *In* Shinnar S, Amir N, Branski D (Eds): Pediatric and Adolescent Medicine, Vol 6, Childhood Seizures. New York, Karger, 1995. Reproduced with permission of S. Karger AG, Basel.

The overall appropriate approach to seizure recognition, characterization, and classification includes (1) observation of the spontaneous events, (2) attempts to restrain or suppress the events, (3) attempts to provoke similar events by tactile stimulation, and (4) documentation of these findings. Detailed description, rather than initial classification, is critical. Classification of seizures can eventually be based on the description of the witnessed clinical events.

Etiology

Although some of the previous discussion of neonatal seizures has emphasized seizure type and pathophysiology, this discussion of etiology applies to all seizure types regardless of pathophysiology. The occurrence of neonatal seizures indicates the presence of CNS dysfunction and should prompt an orderly, thorough clinical and laboratory investigation of the underlying cause. Major etiologic factors are hypoxic-ischemic encephalopathy, meningitis, en-

TABLE 69-3

Classification of Neonatal Seizures Based on Electroclinical Findings and Presumed Pathophysiology

Clinical Seizures with a Consistent Electrocortical Signature, Pathophysiology—Epileptic

    Focal clonic
        Unifocal
        Multifocal
        Hemiconvulsive
        Axial
    Focal tonic
        Asymmetric trunk posturing
        Limb posturing
        Sustained eye deviation
    Myoclonic
        Generalized
        Focal

Clinical Seizures Without a Consistent Electrocortical Signature, Pathophysiology—Presumed Nonepileptic

    Myoclonic
        Generalized
        Focal
        Fragmentary
    Generalized tonic
    Motor automatisms
        Orobuccolingual movements
        Ocular signs
        Progression movements

Electrical Seizures Without Clinical Seizure Activity, Pathophysiology—Epileptic

cephalitis, intracranial hemorrhage (intraventricular, intracerebral, subarachnoid), cerebral infarction, congenital anomalies of the brain, metabolic disorders (hypoglycemia, hypomagnesemia, hypocalcemia), inborn errors of metabolism, and genetic disorders. For some infants, however, despite a thorough evaluation, no specific cause for the seizures or associated risk factors are be identified.

Attention has been focused on some specific etiologic factors. The clinical signs and laboratory findings traditionally associated with the diagnosis of hypoxic-ischemic encephalopathy are currently considered, by a number of investigators, to lack specificity and not consistently to predict long-term neurologic outcome (Nelson and Leviton, 1991; Paneth, 1993). Thus, specific criteria for this diagnosis are currently being re-evaluated and may eventually require a review of conclusions drawn from investigations using less precise diagnostic criteria.

There has also been renewed interest in two syndromes of benign neonatal convulsions: benign familial neonatal convulsions and benign neonatal convulsions. Benign familial neonatal convulsions are thought to have a pattern of autosomal dominant transmission based on a locus on chromosome 20 (Leppert et al, 1989; Quattlebaum, 1979), although reports suggest some genetic heterogeneity (Lewis et al, 1993). The disorder is considered to be benign because initial clinical descriptions reported no neurologic sequelae in affected infants. More recent studies suggest, however, that not all infants with benign familial neonatal

convulsions experience normal long-term outcome (Ronen et al, 1993).

Benign neonatal convulsions occur in infants with no family history of neonatal seizures. The infants are typically full-term and the products of normal pregnancies and deliveries. The seizures are usually brief, often clonic, and typically occur between the 4th and 6th day of postnatal life. No cause can be identified. The infants are neurologically normal before, between, and after the seizures.

Evidence suggests that specific seizure types may be associated with various etiologic factors, depending on their resulting degree and severity of brain injury (Kellaway and Mizrahi, 1990; Mizrahi and Kellaway, 1987). The presumed nonepileptic seizures of generalized tonic posturing and motor automatisms have been most often associated with diffuse brain injury caused by factors such as hypoxia-ischemia, severe meningitis or encephalitis, and infarction or hemorrhage that may involve both cerebral hemispheres. Seizures of epileptic origin, such as focal clonic or focal tonic seizures, have been most often associated with etiologic factors that tend to produce focal brain injury, such as localized infarction or hemorrhage, or some metabolic disorders, such as hypocalcemia, hypoglycemia, and hypomagnesemia. Although these generalizations may be helpful in initial bedside clinical assessment, they cannot be used to exclude specific causes because some infants with diffuse brain injury can experience epileptic seizures with or without nonepileptic events.

Prognosis

Early investigations reported mortality ranging from 20% to 42% and morbidity from 3% to 27% in newborns with seizures (Burke, 1954; Cadilhac et al, 1959; Craig, 1960; Harris and Tizard, 1960). Later, when outcome was analyzed in relation to cause, certain risk factors were associated with varying degrees of neurologic abnormalities and developmental delay. Normal outcomes occurred with increasing frequency in association with each of the following etiologic factors: hypoxia-ischemia, CNS infection, cerebral hemorrhage, hypoglycemia, and hypocalcemia (Bergman et al, 1983; Clancy et al, 1985; Kellaway and Mizrahi, 1990; Lombroso, 1983; Mannino and Trauner, 1983; McInerny and Schubert, 1969; Rose and Lombroso, 1970). Clancy and colleagues (1985) indicated that the incidence of epilepsy was as high as 56% in children who had seizures in the newborn period. Risk factors that increased the probability of newborns with seizures developing subsequent epilepsy included coma and significant background EEG abnormalities during the neonatal period, eventual development of cerebral palsy or mental retardation, and spikes and sharp and slow wave activity on postnatal follow-up EEGs.

There is still no clear consensus as to whether there are long-term neurologic or cognitive sequelae of neonatal seizures per se (Holmes, 1991). It does appear, however, that the most important determinant of outcome is the degree of brain injury associated with seizure occurrence. The factors that caused the seizures and concomitant brain disturbance are the most likely factors that determine long-term outcome rather than the seizures themselves (Bergman et al, 1983; Holden et al, 1982; Kellaway and Mizrahi, 1990).

Treatment

Objectives in the therapy of neonatal seizures include maintenance of systemic homeostasis, treatment of etiologic factors underlying the seizures, and cessation of seizures with AEDs. Despite these clear goals, their achievement may be difficult: Causative factors are not always identifiable, and their precise relationship to the seizures themselves may not be readily apparent. Some clinical seizure types may not warrant AED therapy, and when given, AEDs may incompletely control seizures.

Several factors should ideally be considered in the development of a plan of therapy for neonatal seizures: cause or associated risk factors, characterization and classification of seizure type, determination of pathophysiology, assessment of duration and severity of the seizures, understanding of the natural history of the seizure disorder, and assessment of the expected effects of the seizures and AEDs on the developing brain. Information concerning all of these factors, however, may not be complete. Despite this lack of complete data, consideration of each factor may provide the basis for rational management decisions at the bedside.

Three phases of therapy can be individualized to each infant: (1) initial medical management, (2) cause-specific therapy, and (3) AED therapy. Adequate ventilation and circulatory perfusion should be ensured because changes in respirations, heart rate, and blood pressure may occur in association with seizures, as a consequence of causative factors, or in association with AED therapy. The therapy of identified specific causative factors is essential. Treatable causes include CNS and systemic infections and metabolic factors, such as hypocalcemia, hypomagnesemia, and hypoglycemia. Pyridoxine deficiency is often cited as a treatable cause of medically refractory neonatal seizures, although it is exceedingly rare.

The AEDs traditionally used for neonatal seizures are phenobarbital, phenytoin, and diazepam in the following dosages: phenobarbital 20 mg/kg as a loading dose, followed by additional dosages of 10 mg/kg to achieve serum levels between 20 and 40 μg/mL; phenytoin 20 mg/kg as a loading dose to achieve serum levels between 15 and 20 μg/mL; diazepam 0.1 to 0.3 mg/kg in repeated dosages. Lorazepam has been reported to be safe and efficacious (Maytal et al, 1991; Painter and Alvin, 1990). Other agents used and reported to be useful include carbamazepine, primidone, paraldehyde (now unavailable in the United States), and lidocaine (Hellstrom-Westas et al, 1992; Painter and Alvin, 1990). These agents have been used as additional therapy when first-line AEDs have failed to control seizures.

The decision to initiate AED therapy is based on seizure type, pathophysiology, duration, and severity; natural history of the seizure disorder; and anticipated effects of both the seizures and the selected AEDs on the infant. At some centers, EEG or EEG/video monitoring may be available to assist in diagnosis and management.

When initiation of AED therapy is based on features of the clinical seizure alone, without benefit of electroencephalography, four situations may be encountered:

1. *Focal clonic or focal tonic seizures that are prolonged and recurrent.* Focal clonic seizures are repetitive and rhythmic muscle contractions that cannot be arrested by restraint or repositioning. Focal tonic seizures, such as sustained posturing of a limb, also cannot be altered by these maneuvers. Focal tonic seizure eye deviation can be differentiated from the random eye movements of nonepileptic motor automatisms because the epileptic tonic eye deviation is sustained and cannot be evoked by stimulation. These seizure types are considered epileptic in origin. Following the determination of pathophysiology, duration and severity must be considered. When seizures are sustained and prolonged, they are treated with AEDs.

2. *Focal clonic or focal tonic seizures that are brief and infrequent.* The clinical characteristics of these seizures are the same as those described earlier, but duration is shorter and frequency less, and their natural history may be brief. Although AEDs may be used in attempts to control the seizures, their use is being re-evaluated. This is based on the following ideas: Epileptic seizures may be a response to a transient, underlying brain disorder; in some infants, after an initial injury, seizures may resolve spontaneously; and potential adverse effects of AEDs may outweigh the potential risk of brief, infrequent seizures on the developing brain (Moshe, 1987). Despite these developing concepts, specific criteria for what constitutes brief, infrequent seizures have not been established, and issues of whether AEDs and seizures adversely affect the immature brain have not yet been resolved.

3. *Generalized tonic posturing and motor automatisms that are unresponsive to stimulation and can be suppressed with restraint.* Generalized tonic posturing and motor automatisms (including ocular signs, orobuccolingual movements, and movements of progression) may be presumed to be of nonepileptic origin, based on the characterization of the events and their response to clinical maneuvers: The spontaneous events can be suppressed by restraint or repositioning of the limbs or trunk, and events similar to spontaneous events can be evoked by tactile stimulation. Traditionally, these clinical events have been treated with AEDs. Although their frequency and severity may be reduced by AEDs, this is more likely due to CNS depressant effects of these drugs rather than to their antiepileptic properties. Overall, if generalized tonic posturing and motor automatisms demonstrate characteristic clinical features, they can be presumed to be of nonepileptic origin and do not require AED therapy (Mizrahi, 1989; Mizrahi and Kellaway, 1987). Although the clinical events may be initially quite dramatic, their natural course is one of gradual spontaneous resolution without AED therapy.

4. *Generalized tonic posturing and motor automatisms that may not be responsive to stimulation or restraint.* For some infants, generalized tonic posturing and motor automatisms are typical of nonepileptic events, but clinical maneuvers or restraint, repositioning, and stimulation do not result in characteristic responses.

In these instances, the infants may be treated with AEDs with the understanding that clinical observation and maneuvers alone cannot provide data to indicate underlying pathophysiology.

If the initiation of AED therapy is based on EEG or EEG/video monitoring, two additional clinical circumstances may be encountered that determine whether AED therapy should be initiated:

1. *Clinical seizures that are present in the absence of EEG seizure activity.* These clinical seizure types include generalized tonic posturing and motor automatisms. The clinical features suggest they are nonepileptic in origin, and the lack of EEG seizure activity at the time of the clinical seizures further supports this idea. These clinical events are not treated with AEDs when they occur in the absence of electrical seizure activity.

2. *EEG seizure activity that is present in the absence of any clinical seizures.* Electrical seizure activity occurring in the absence of any clinical seizure activity is treated with AEDs. These electrical seizures, however, may be highly resistant to therapy despite high doses of several AEDs.

At the onset of treatment, the end point of AED therapy must be defined as either the cessation of clinical seizures or cessation of electrical seizure activity (if EEG is available). Clinical seizures of epileptic origin may be controlled with AED therapy, but the electrical seizure activity that initially accompanied the clinical seizures may persist (referred to as *decoupling* of the clinical from the electrical seizure) (Mizrahi and Kellaway, 1987, 1992). Further AED therapy may be used in attempts to eliminate electrical seizure activity, but this may be difficult or, more often, may not be accomplished (Painter et al, in press). These attempts may lead to high doses of multiple AEDs; may not successfully control EEG seizure activity; and may be associated with the clinical problems of CNS depression, systemic hypotension, and respiratory depression. In this circumstance, the clinician must weigh the potential risks of vigorous AEDs against the potential benefits and likelihood of success of therapy. Therapeutic strategies may be devised to strike an even balance, such as attaining high therapeutic levels of phenobarbital and phenytoin, then using individual doses of a benzodiazepine in attempts to reduce or eliminate electrical seizure discharges.

Following acute therapy, infants are typically placed on regimens of maintenance AEDs. Typically, this is in the form of phenobarbital alone or with phenytoin if it had been required during acute management (maintenance dosage of each is 3 to 4 mg/kg/day).

No specific practice guidelines have been established to assist in the decision to discontinue AEDs after a period of clinical seizure control. Thus, in clinical practice, this is highly individualized. The probable natural history of the treated disorder should be the most significant factor in this clinical decision, although it has not been well characterized. If seizures represent a short-lived phenomenon produced in reaction to an acute injury, long-term AED therapy might be maintained for a period beyond which seizures might have resolved. Reported maintenance schedules range from 1 week up to 12 months after the last seizure, although specific clinical and EEG predictors of recurrent seizures after AED withdrawal have not been identified (Brod et al, 1988; Gal et al, 1984). There has been increasing clinical interest in short-term therapy, however, with AED withdrawal 2 weeks after the infant's last clinical seizure.

A final consideration of AED therapy is the risk/benefit ratio. Although under intensive investigation, there is no clear consensus as to whether epileptic seizures adversely affect the developing brain (Holmes, 1991). In addition, there are no detailed clinical studies of the adverse systemic effects of seizures, although infants with prolonged seizures may experience changes in respirations, heart rate, or blood pressure and may have an increased level of energy utilization. These may be unwelcome clinical findings in an infant who may already be medically compromised. There is an equal lack of consensus concerning the possible adverse effects of AEDs on the developing brain. Experimental data suggest alteration in cell growth and energy substrate utilization (Bergey et al, 1981; Diaz and Schain, 1978; Neale et al, 1985), although the applicability of these findings to human newborns has been called into question. There have been few studies of adverse effects of acute AED therapy, although vigorous treatment may result in CNS depression, hypotension, bradycardia, and respiratory depression (Goldberg et al, 1986). There are few studies of the effect of long-term therapy on newborns and young infants.

Overall, a regimen that may minimize perceived risk and maximize therapeutic benefit includes acute therapy to eliminate clinical seizures, maintenance therapy after seizure control is attained, and withdrawal of AEDs 2 weeks after the last clinical seizure. Additional basic science and clinical investigations are needed, however, to establish firmly the rational basis for this or other management schemes.

Electroencephalography and Electroencephalography/Video Monitoring

EEG and EEG/video monitoring have been discussed in detail in the section on Neurophysiologic Assessment and are mentioned here to reiterate their usefulness. As stated previously, the EEG plays an important role in the assessment of neonatal seizures. In addition, the EEG is a useful tool for determining conceptional age; whether an infant has suffered a diffuse or focal CNS injury; timing of CNS injury in some cases; and, when degree and rate of resolution of CNS injury can be determined by sequential EEGs, prognosis (Hrachovy et al, 1990). The EEG can be used in the substantiation of brain death and to determine if an infant is having epileptic seizure activity. EEG/video monitoring is an especially helpful adjunct for correlating clinical and electrographic seizure activity, for determining when behaviors are probably not epileptic in origin, and for helping to identify clinical events that may be important (such as apnea) but that are not related to seizure activity.

Nonseizure Paroxysmal Events

Repetitive nonepileptic events have been described throughout this section; however, one specific diagnosis should be mentioned. Neonatal sleep myoclonus is a benign disorder that should not be confused with epileptic seizures or with brain stem release phenomena. Characterized by repetitive myoclonic jerks that occur only during sleep, benign neonatal sleep myoclonus is not associated with EEG abnormalities. Noise, motion (particularly rocking motion), and certain drugs (benzodiazepines) may trigger or exacerbate the myoclonus, and the myoclonus does not stop with restraint (Alfonso et al, 1995). Benign neonatal sleep myoclonus requires no treatment and is usually not apparent after 6 months of age (Alfonso et al, 1995; Daoust-Roy and Seshia, 1992).

NEUROMUSCULAR DISORDERS

Neuromuscular disorders can involve any of the components of the motor unit, including the anterior horn cell, its axon or myelin sheath, nerve root, the neuromuscular junction, or the muscle fibers. The brain can be involved in some neuromuscular disorders, and abnormalities of tone and strength can, of course, also be due to disorders or injuries involving the brain or parts of the spinal cord.

Central Hypotonia

Hypotonia is a frequent symptom in newborns that may reflect an abnormality of the CNS; a systemic toxic, metabolic, infectious, or degenerative disease; a disorder of ligaments or connective tissue; or a neuromuscular disorder. Hypotonia implies decreased resistance to passive muscle stretch and decreased resting tone, and it may or may not be associated with muscle weakness.

It is useful to determine if the hypotonic newborn has a central disorder that is responsible. In these cases, there may be other neurologic signs, but usually hypotonia is greater than the degree of muscle weakness. Examples include hypoxic-ischemic encephalopathy, cerebral hemorrhage, systemic infection, toxic encephalopathy, hypothyroidism, Down syndrome, Prader-Willi syndrome, degenerative or metabolic diseases, endocrine diseases, or connective tissue diseases (DeVivo and Hays, 1986). Spinal cord injury or malformation can be associated early in the course with hypotonia and severe muscle weakness. Normal preterm infants are hypotonic at birth and develop increasing tone with maturity. The most common causes of central hypotonia in newborns are hypoxic-ischemic encephalopathy and dysgenetic syndromes.

Motoneuron Diseases

Spinal muscular atrophy (SMA) (anterior horn cell disease) is the most common form of neurogenic hypotonia in early infancy and is second only to the muscular dystrophies as a cause of neuromuscular disease in childhood (Houston et al, 1994). Autosomal recessive in inheritance, the gene locus has been mapped to the long arm of chromosome 5 (Soares et al, 1993). SMA occurs in about 8 per 100,000 live births, with SMA I (Werdnig-Hoffmann disease) symptomatic before 6 months of age, not infrequently in utero or in the newborn period (Dubowitz, 1995; Mostacciuolo et al, 1992; Russman and Schwartz, 1993). Infants with

SMA I do not sit independently and have a life expectancy of 2 years or less. SMA II and III are less severe forms of SMA with longer life expectancies.

It is not clear if the basic defect in SMA is degeneration or failure of development of anterior horn cells in the spinal cord and motor nuclei in the lower brain stem (Russman and Schwartz, 1993). Nevertheless, the presentation and course of the disease in newborns are well known and predictable. The mother may have noted decreased fetal movements during the last part of the infant's gestation. After birth, the clinical picture is of an infant with symmetric severe weakness and flaccidity that is greater in the lower limbs than in the upper and is greater proximally than distally. Head control is poor in both the prone and the supine positions. Respiration is impaired because of weakness of the intercostal muscles; relative sparing of the diaphragm causes abdominal breathing, resulting in a bell-shaped appearance to the chest. The bulbar muscles are weak causing poor cry, weak suck and swallow, pooling of secretions, and aspiration; tongue fasciculations are frequently present (although sometimes difficult to distinguish from tremor of the tongue in very young infants). Because upper cranial nerves are spared, however, the infant usually has an alert expression and normal eye movements. There may be spontaneous movements of the ankles, toes, hand, and fingers, but there is no ability to raise the limbs against gravity. Cardiac muscle is not affected, and the infants do not have arthrogryposis (multiple congenital contractures of limbs); deep tendon reflexes are absent (Dubowitz, 1995).

Nerve conduction studies show normal or slightly decreased motor nerve conduction velocities with normal sensory nerve potentials. There is abnormal spontaneous activity on EMG with fibrillations and sharp waves as well as increased mean duration and amplitude of motor unit action potentials. Some motor unit potentials are polyphasic (Miller, 1997). Creatine kinase activity in the serum may be mildly elevated, and muscle biopsy shows atrophy of both Type 1 and Type 2 muscle fibers. These are rounded and are in large groups between fascicles of enlarged Type 1 fibers (which are thought to be fibers that have been reinnervated). Degeneration of muscle fibers is not seen in severe SMA (Dubowitz, 1995). In the newborn, only the pattern of atrophy may be apparent. The infant presenting as a newborn with severe SMA rarely survives the 1st postnatal year.

Other motoneuron disorders presenting in the newborn period seem to be more heterogeneous diseases, often with involvement of anterior horn cells and the CNS, and frequently having arthrogryposis as an associated clinical finding. One example is infantile neuronal degeneration, in which there is SMA, joint deformity (arthrogryposis), abnormalities in the thalamus and cerebellum, and absent or decreased sensory nerve action potentials (Steiman et al, 1980). Other forms of neurogenic arthrogryposis can occur rarely and can be sporadic, autosomal recessive, or X-linked (Greenberg et al, 1988).

Axonal Diseases

At least one hereditary motor and sensory neuropathy (hereditary motor and sensory neuropathy type III) has been described as presenting in very early infancy (Dyck, 1975). In addition, hypomyelinating neuropathies are an ill-defined group of diseases that present in the neonatal period or in early infancy (Dubowitz, 1995). The affected newborn is hypotonic and weak, without deep tendon reflexes. Distal weakness is prominent, and the infant usually has difficulty with feeding and respiration. Extraocular movements are usually spared, although facial weakness may be present. Diagnostic studies show reduced motor nerve conduction velocities and elevated CSF protein. Some cases have shown absence of peripheral myelin with increased numbers of Schwann cells (Charnas et al, 1988; Karch and Urich, 1975; Miller, 1997). Sensory nerves can also be affected (although this is difficult to detect clinically). Hypomyelinating neuropathies are variable in their presentation and prognosis. In some cases, there can be improvement in strength as time passes. These disorders appear to be similar to Charcot-Marie-Tooth disease Type 1A, a demyelinating hereditary motor and sensory neuropathy that presents later in life (caused by a duplication at 17p11.2) (Patel and Lupski, 1994).

Other neuropathies can involve peripheral sensory and autonomic neurons. One example is familial dysautonomia (Riley-Day syndrome), which is characterized by pale, blotchy skin; hypotonia; feeding difficulties; poor suck and swallow; vomiting; abdominal distention; loose bowel movements; irritability; temperature and blood pressure instability; absent corneal reflexes; decreased or absent deep tendon reflexes; absent fungiform papillae on the tongue; and general failure to thrive (Ouvrier et al, 1990). The gene for this autosomal recessive disorder is located at 9q31-q33 (Blumenfeld et al, 1993). Other findings in this syndrome include absence of the axon reflex flare and pupillary denervation hypersensitivity: injection of 0.1 mL 1:10,000 histamine sulfate intradermally causes a wheal but not a flare, and placing dilute (0.0625%) pilocarpine into the conjunctival sac causes miosis. Conjunctival installation of pilocarpine causes no change in the normal pupil (Axelrod et al, 1987).

Diseases of the Neuromuscular Junction

Diseases of the neuromuscular junction can be acquired or congenital, transient or lifelong. Transient acquired neonatal myasthenia gravis occurs in 10% to 15% of infants born to mothers with myasthenia gravis, either active or in remission (Elias et al, 1979; Papazian, 1992). Transient neonatal myasthenia is characterized by weakness and hypotonia that is apparent within the first 3 postnatal days. The infant often has feeding and respiratory difficulties and may require mechanical ventilation. Diagnosis can be supported by a positive response to intramuscular or subcutaneous injection of an anticholinesterase agent, usually edrophonium chloride (Tensilon) (intravenously 0.03 mg/kg) (Dubowitz, 1995). Edrophonium has more rapid onset of action and shorter duration of action than neostigmine. Repetitive nerve stimulation at 10 to 50 Hz causes transmission fatigue in infants with myasthenia and can also be used to aid in the diagnosis.

In most cases, the infant with transient myasthenia gravis has antibodies directed against the nicotinic acetylcholine receptor that have been transferred from the affected mother. These antibodies cause a postsynaptic failure of neuromuscular transmission (Lindstorm et al, 1988). Most infants require treatment with an anticholinesterase drug, with recovery within several weeks. Treatment with anticholinesterase agents must be carefully monitored because side effects include diarrhea, increased secretions, muscle fasciculations, and cholinergic weakness (Miller, 1997). Treatment is discontinued by gradually decreasing the dose of the anticholinesterase as the infant improves.

The congenital myasthenic syndromes are only rarely diagnosed in the newborn period and, in contrast to transient neonatal myasthenia, are not characterized by the presence of acetylcholine receptor antibodies. A number of defects of the neuromuscular junction can cause a myasthenia-like picture, and they may present with fluctuating hypotonia and weakness. They frequently also present with ptosis, ophthalmoplegia, and bulbar and respiratory weakness (including apnea). The response to anticholinesterase drugs is not always positive; some forms of congenital myasthenia may be worsened by anticholinesterases (slow-channel syndrome, acetylcholinesterase deficiency) (Dubowitz, 1995). The diagnostic features of these diseases on EMG are more complicated than those of transient neonatal myasthenia; the reader is referred to Engel (1994).

Toxic Myasthenic Syndromes

Certain drugs can exacerbate already existing myasthenia and should be avoided, including muscle relaxants (curare, gallamine triethiodide, decamethonium, succinylcholine) and drugs that increase neuromuscular blockade (quinine, quinidine, neomycin, procaine) (Dubowitz, 1995). Other drugs can depress respirations (morphines, benzodiazepines), and their effects may be potentiated by the anticholinesterases (morphines). Magnesium at toxic levels and frequently used aminoglycoside antibiotics can cause neuromuscular junction failure in newborns (Wright and McWuillen, 1971).

Infantile Botulism

Infantile botulism is usually seen between 2 weeks and 6 months of age; thus, infants may be readmitted to the intensive care nursery with this disorder. It is seen in infants who ingest *Clostridium botulinum*. Some honeys have been shown to contain *C. botulinum*, and most pediatricians discourage giving honey to young infants (Arnon et al, 1979). The bacteria colonize the infant intestine and produce botulinum toxin, which then causes presynaptic cholinergic blockade of skeletal and smooth muscle as well as autonomic function (Thompson et al, 1980). The symptoms can be mild (hypotonia and constipation) or severe (sudden death). Classically the disease presents with constipation and poor feeding followed by progressive weakness and hypotonia and loss of deep tendon reflexes (Miller, 1997). There is usually paralysis of the pupillary muscles and ptosis. The disease may last 1 to 2 months and can relapse (Glauser et al, 1990). Diagnosis can be made by repetitive nerve stimulation and EMG as well as by isolation of the organism from the stool.

Neonatal Tetanus

Also a clostridial infection, tetanus is caused by infection of the umbilical stump. It is not uncommon in underdeveloped countries but is only rarely seen in the United States in home-delivered infants (Adams et al, 1979; Menkes, 1991c). Tetanus toxin inhibits the release of gamma-aminobutyric acid (GABA) and glycine from the presynaptic inhibitory nerve terminals surrounding motoneurons. This causes uncontrolled firing of the motoneurons resulting in muscle spasms. Symptoms of neonatal tetanus develop between the 5th and 10th postnatal days and consist of irritability, trismus, and poor suck followed by opisthotonos and generalized spasms (Menkes, 1991c). Spasms may be accompanied by apnea; they may be spontaneous or appear with stimulation. Treatment is difficult and consists of paralysis and mechanical ventilation, penicillin, and tetanus antiserum (intravenously and into the umbilical stump) (Adams et al, 1979). Symptoms last from 25 to 45 days.

Diseases of Muscle

Diseases that are characterized by specific structural abnormalities of muscle that are present from birth are called *congenital myopathies*. These disorders do not include muscular dystrophies, inflammatory myopathies, or disorders caused by known metabolic abnormalities or inborn errors of metabolism (Dubowitz, 1995; Miller, 1997). A number of congenital myopathies have been described during the past few decades. They are listed, along with characteristic findings, in Table 69–4. Not all present in the neonatal period, however, and when manifest in the newborn, most cause nonspecific symptoms of weakness and hypotonia. Congenital myopathies that have been diagnosed in the newborn include the following: (1) Nemaline myopathy can be severe, with generalized weakness and hypotonia involving the facial, bulbar, and respiratory muscles and sparing the eye muscles. (2) Central core disease is mild in the newborn, with muscle weakness and hypotonia, proximal greater than distal; congenital hip dislocation is common. (3) Multicore/minicore myopathy causes mild proximal weakness in the newborn. (4) Myotubular myopathy consists of two genetic subtypes—X-linked recessive and autosomal dominant. The X-linked form presents at birth with severe weakness and hypotonia; facial weakness and ophthalmoplegia can be present, and respiratory failure is common. (5) Congenital fiber type disproportion is characterized by generalized weakness including the face and deformational features (Dubowitz, 1995; Miller, 1997).

Other rarer myopathies may also present in the neonatal period (Dubowitz, 1995; Miller, 1997). Muscle biopsy is required for diagnosis of specific congenital myopathies. Some have been linked to specific gene loci (the gene for X-linked myotubular myopathy is located on chromosome Xq28) (Leichti-Gallati et al, 1993).

Muscular Dystrophies

The muscular dystrophies are defined as inherited disorders with progressive degeneration of skeletal muscle (Du-

TABLE 69–4

Congenital Myopathies

Disease	Inheritance	Course	Histology	Laboratory Studies
Central core	Dominant or sporadic	Nonprogressive proximal weakness; muscle cramps; malignant hyperthermia	Fiber size variation; slight atrophy; central cores in type 1 fibers	CK normal; EMG nonspecific changes
Multicore/minicore disease	Autosomal recessive	Variable weakness; face and diaphragm involved	Variation in fiber size; internal nuclei; minicores in type 1 fibers	CK normal; EMG nonspecific changes
Nemaline myopathy	Dominant or recessive	Usually nonprogressive; nocturnal hypoventilation; dysmorphisms present; some cases have a severe neonatal course with fatal outcome	Rod bodies on Gomori trichrome stain	EMG may show a denervation pattern
Myotubular myopathy (centronuclear)	X-linked (Xq28); autosomal dominant; or uncertain	Severe neonatal course (fatal) in some with X-linked form; otherwise, variable weakness; ptosis and eye muscle weakness	Central nuclei; may show Type 1 fiber atrophy	Mixed myopathic/denervation pattern
Congenital fiber type disproportion	?Dominant or recessive	Floppy newborns; contractures; dislocated hip; static or improves with time; respiratory infections during the first year of life	Type 1 fibers smaller than Type 2 fibers (Type 2 fibers are normal sized or enlarged)	

CK, creatine kinase; EMG, electromyography.

bowitz, 1995). Increasing knowledge of the genetics and pathophysiology of some of these disorders has complicated the picture because similar clinical phenotypes may have different modes of inheritance and different gene loci and products. In addition, some forms of congenital muscular dystrophy also have associated brain malformations. Severe X-linked dystrophinopathy (Duchenne) only rarely presents in the newborn period and is characterized by high serum creatine kinase levels, absence of arthrogryposis, and regeneration and degeneration in the muscle biopsy specimen (Miller, 1997). The gene locus for Duchenne muscular dystrophy is Xp21. Other dystrophies that present in the newborn include pure congenital muscular dystrophies (with or without merosin° deficiency), congenital muscular dystrophy with brain malformations or mental retardation (Fukuyama type, muscle-eye-brain disease [the muscle-eye-brain disease has also been referred to as *cerebro-ocular dysplasia muscular dystrophy syndrome* (see Chapter 67)], Walker-Warburg syndrome), congenital muscular dystrophy with cerebellar atrophy and hypoplasia, and congenital muscular dystrophy with occipital agyria (Miller, 1997).

Fukuyama congenital muscular dystrophy is autosomal recessive with a defect in chromosome 9q31-33 (Toda et al, 1993). This syndrome includes congenital muscular dystrophy as well as cerebral neuronal migration defects. The brain has abnormal gyral patterns (pachygyria and polymicrogyria), and eye defects are minor in this disease. The newborn with Fukuyama congenital muscular dystrophy has generalized weakness, hypotonia, muscle contractures, facial and bulbar involvement, seizures, and mental retardation, with survival into the teens (Miller, 1997). This syndrome has mainly been diagnosed in Japan, where it was first described.

Muscle-eye-brain disease and Walker-Warburg syndrome have similar findings, but infants with Walker-Warburg syndrome are more severely affected. This syndrome is characterized by muscular dystrophy with severe brain and eye malformations, including retinal detachment or dysplasia (or both); optic nerve hypoplasia; microphthalmia; colobomas; anterior chamber abnormalities, including glaucoma, buphthalmos, cataracts, and cloudy corneas; and other abnormalities (Towfighi et al, 1984). The brain in the Walker-Warburg syndrome has a cobblestone cortex, lissencephaly, white matter cystic changes, ventriculomegaly, and brain stem and cerebellar hypoplasia (Towfighi et al, 1984). Infants with Walker-Warburg syndrome rarely survive more than a few months. Infants with Walker-Warburg syndrome and with muscle-eye-brain disease present with hypotonia, weakness, feeding difficulties, respiratory difficulties, poor vision, and apathy. Mental retardation and seizures are present in both disorders.

The pure congenital muscular dystrophies with or without merosin are relatively nonprogressive dystrophies that can present in the neonatal period. Infants with merosin deficiency are more severely affected, with severe weakness, hypotonia, respiratory difficulties, and multiple contractures, at the outset. Those without merosin deficiency have less respiratory involvement and fewer contractures and appear to do better later on.

Myotonic dystrophy is a multisystem disorder inherited as an autosomal dominant disease with variable expression, characterized in part by muscular dystrophy and myotonia. In adults, the disease also affects the heart, brain, eye, endocrine system, and gastrointestinal system. Myotonia is a failure of the muscle to relax after contraction and can sometimes be seen in infants whose eyes have a delay in opening after a period of closure with crying (Dubowitz, 1995). Myotonia in affected adults can be elicited by percussion of a muscle. On EMG, myotonia has a characteristic pattern of a prolonged series of rhythmic activity of high amplitude and high frequency that wanes and slows with time (Dubowitz, 1995). Myotonic dystrophy is the most common muscular dystrophy in adults (5 per 100,000). The congenital form is inherited from the mother and can be particularly severe in the neonatal period. The newborn presents with hypotonia, difficulty with sucking and swallowing, respiratory failure, and deformities such as talipes equinovarus (Dubowitz, 1995). Fetal movements may have been decreased, and hydramnios is usually noted. Preterm delivery is not infrequent. The infants have evident facial diplegia, a *tent-shaped* mouth, and inability to close the eyes completely. Myotonia is not usually seen in the newborn.

The infant with myotonic dystrophy who survives the neonatal period improves with time, although milestones are delayed. Myotonia becomes apparent after 2 to 3 years, and mental retardation of varying degrees is part of the disorder in the congenital form. Creatine kinase is usually normal, and EMG may be myopathic in the newborn. Muscle biopsy in the newborn shows maturational delay of the muscle with some atrophy of Type 1 fibers; in older patients, muscle biopsy shows variation in muscle fiber size, proliferation of internal nuclei, ring fibers, and varying degrees of muscle degeneration as well as increases in amounts of connective and adipose tissue (Dubowitz, 1995).

The genetics of myotonic dystrophy are interesting, as the gene has been localized to chromosome 19q13.3, and within that region a variable trinucleotide repeat insert consisting of 50 to several thousand CTG repeats has been discovered (Aslandis et al, 1992; Buxton et al, 1992; Harley et al, 1992). The region involved affects a protein kinase gene that has been named *myotonin protein kinase* (Brook et al, 1992). A progressive increase in the size of the trinucleotide repeat from generation to generation is associated with progressively earlier onset and increased severity of the disease; this phenomenon, *anticipation*, occurs in other neurologic diseases, including spinocerebellar ataxia I, fragile X syndrome, Huntington chorea, and X-linked spinobulbar muscular atrophy. It is still not clear, however, why the congenital form of myotonic dystophy is inherited from affected mothers and not from affected fathers.

Genetic Diseases That Involve Muscle

The subtitle to this section is probably a misnomer because many of the neuromuscular diseases in the first part of this section are now known to be due to specific genetic errors.

°Merosin is part of the extracellular protein laminin. It links with dystrophin-associated glycoproteins, which then link with the cytoskeletal protein dystrophin. Patients with Duchenne dystrophy are dystrophin deficient.

There are some inherited storage and endocrine diseases, however, that involve multiple organ systems including muscle. Several of these that present in the neonatal period are described here.

Glycogenoses

The glycogenoses include nine enzyme defects that involve muscle; two of the glycogenoses are frequently symptomatic in the newborn period (Types II and III, Pompe disease, and Forbes or Cori disease) (Dubowitz, 1995). *Pompe disease* (acid maltase deficiency—this prevents intralysosomal degradation of glycogen) is a multisystem disease involving heart, muscle, CNS, liver, kidneys, and leukocytes. Infants may be hypotonic at birth or may present with cardiac or respiratory failure. In some cases, there is a normal period of several weeks, followed by decompensation. Infants with Pompe disease clinically resemble those with SMA I. The diaphragm is not spared in Pompe disease, facial weakness is usually present, and the tongue may be enlarged owing to increased lysosomal storage of glycogen. Severely affected infants with Pompe disease usually die during infancy. A milder form of acid maltase deficiency has been reported in patients who present later with features resembling limb-girdle dystrophy, with or without cardiac involvement, and sometimes with glycogen deposition in the CNS (Courtecuisse et al, 1965; Isch et al, 1966; Smith et al, 1966; Zellweger et al, 1965). The ECG in affected infants shows huge QRS complexes with short P-R intervals (Dubowitz, 1995). EMG may show either a myopathic or a denervation pattern but in addition shows pseudomyotonic bursts that are characteristic of Type II glycogenosis. The muscle biopsy specimen shows excess glycogen with a vacuolar myopathy and distortion of the normal muscle pattern. The abnormal enzyme activity can be demonstrated in lymphocytes (Dubowitz, 1995).

Type III glycogenosis, also known as Forbes or Cori disease and debrancher enzyme deficiency, affects skeletal muscle modestly and can present in the neonatal period as hypotonia and weakness. Type III glycogenosis involves liver and cardiac muscle and is associated with a longer survival period than Pompe disease. Type III glycogenosis may cause an elevated creatine kinase; EMG may be normal or show varying degrees of myopathic or denervation patterns. Motor nerve conduction may be slowed. Excess storage of the abnormal glycogen in the muscle is intrasarcoplasmic and subsarcolemmal (not lysosomal). Enzyme analysis for amylo-1,6-glucosidase (debrancher enzyme) can be done in leukocytes (Dubowitz, 1995).

Phosphorylase Deficiency

McArdle disease (muscle phosphorylase deficiency) is restricted to striated muscle and usually is diagnosed in older children or adults who present with muscle fatigability, cramps on exertion, weakness, and sometimes myoglobinuria (Dubowitz, 1995). There have been at least two reports of phosphorylase deficiency presenting in the newborn period. One infant was symptomatic at 4 weeks of age with progressive generalized weakness and respiratory failure and died at 3 months of age (DiMauro and Hartlage, 1978). Another infant with phosphorylase deficiency was

weak and flaccid at birth with contractures and died at 16 days (Milstein et al, 1989).

Phosphofructokinase Deficiency

Phosphofructokinase deficiency (Type VII glycogen storage disease), which usually presents with myoglobinuria and cramps on exercise, also has been diagnosed as a severe infantile form. Again the presentation is a hypotonic infant with progressive weakness; some infants have had seizures, cortical blindness, and mental retardation (Amit et al, 1992).

Lipid Storage Diseases

Other systemic disorders that can affect muscle include lipid storage diseases and mitochondrial disorders. Defects of lipid metabolism that affect muscle include carnitine deficiency (myopathic), systemic carnitine deficiency (lipid storage myopathy as well as hepatic encephalopathy), and carnitine palmityltransferase deficiency (Dubowitz, 1995). Carnitine is necessary for transfer of medium-chain and long-chain fatty acids into the mitochondrion for beta-oxidation. Patients with these disorders are not usually symptomatic in the newborn period but have weakness that becomes evident in childhood; the encephalopathic form of systemic carnitine deficiency presents as recurrent episodes of nausea, vomiting, confusion, or coma, with or without hypoglycemia and lactic acidosis (DiMauro et al, 1980).

Other lipid disorders that may be symptomatic in the newborn period or in early infancy include medium-chain acyl-CoA dehydrogenase deficiency, which can present early with hypoglycemic episodes or sudden infant death or later with exercise-induced muscle cramps; long-chain acyl-CoA dehydrogenase deficiency, which can present in the first 6 months with cardiac muscle involvement or later with coma on fasting or with later-onset muscle pain; glutaric aciduria Type II, in which one subset of patients with this disease presented with muscle weakness in early infancy; and long-chain 3-hydroxyacyl-CoA dehydrogenase deficiency, with onset from 3 days to 3 years with nonketotic hypoglycemia, sudden infant death, cardiomyopathy, and myopathy (Hale et al, 1990; Jackson et al, 1991; Stanley et al, 1983; Turnbull et al, 1984).

Mitochondrial Myopathies

Mitochrondrial myopathies in the newborn are usually due to defects of the electron transport (respiratory) chain (DeVivo, 1993). Other abnormalities of mitochondrial metabolism usually cause progressive encephalopathy (pyruvate carboxylase and pyruvate dehydrogenase complex deficiencies) (see Chapter 25). *Cytochrome-c oxidase deficiency* is the most likely respiratory chain disorder to present as a myopathy during the neonatal period (Nagai et al, 1993). The disorder is characterized by severe generalized weakness, hypotonia, hyporeflexia, poor feeding, respiratory difficulty, and lactic acidosis. When hepatomegaly, cardiomyopathy, and renal tubular defects are present, the disorder is called the *De Toni-Fanconi-Debré syndrome*. Some infants may also have macroglossia. Although a reversible form of cytochrome-*c* oxidase deficiency also occurs, in the severe, progressive form, the infant usually dies before 6 months of age (Tritschler et al, 1991).

Peroxisomal Diseases

Peroxisomal diseases can present in the neonatal period with severe hypotonia and weakness along with other findings (including dysmorphic facial features in Zellweger syndrome), hepatomegaly, cataracts, retinopathy, epiphyseal stippling, and, in some cases, rhizomelia (Brown et al, 1993; Miller, 1997).

Diseases of the Peripheral Nerve

Peripheral neuropathies are rare in infants. Undoubtedly, as more genetic defects underlying neuromuscular disorders are discovered, clinicians will be able to identify affected infants in families known to have herditary motor and sensory or sensory and autonomic neuropathies before symptoms are apparent.

Other infantile neuropathies that cause weakness and hypotonia in infants and children include metachromatic leukodystrophy, globoid cell leukodystrophy (Krabbe disease), infantile neuroaxonal dystrophy, giant axonal neuropathy, neonatal adrenoleukodystrophy, hypertrophic interstitial polyneuropathy, and peroneal muscular atrophy (DeVivo and Hays, 1986). Neonatal adrenoleukodystrophy is a peroxisomal disorder that is recessively inherited characterized by hypotonia, seizures, and developmental delay. Peripheral neuropathy is present in this disorder in 30% to 50% of cases (Ouvrier et al, 1990).

REFERENCES

Abrams RM, Ito J, Frisinger JE, et al: Local cerebral glucose utilization in fetal and neonatal sheep. Am J Physiol 246:R608, 1984.

Abroms IF, Rosen BA: Neurologic trauma in newborn infants. Semin Neurol 13:100, 1993.

Adams JH, Brierley JB, Connor RC, et al: The effects of systemic hypotension upon the human brain: Clinical and neuropathological observations in 11 cases. Brain 89:235, 1966.

Adams JM, Kenny JD, Rudolph AJ: Central diabetes insipidus following intraventricular hemorrhage. J Pediatr 88:292, 1976.

Adams JM, Kenny JD, Rudolph AJ: Modern management of tetanus neonatorum. Pediatrics 64:472, 1979.

Adinolfi M: Infectious diseases in pregnancy, cytokines and neurological impairment: An hypothesis. Dev Med Child Neurol 35:549, 1993.

Adsett DB, Fitz CR, Hill A: Hypoxic-ischaemic cerebral injury in the term newborn: Correlation of CT findings with neurological outcome. Dev Med Child Neurol 27:155, 1985.

Ahmann PA, Lazzara A, Dykes FD, et al: Intraventricular hemorrhage in the high-risk preterm infant: Incidence and outcome. Ann Neurol 7:118, 1980.

Albright GA: Effects of anesthesia on the fetus and newborn. In Stevenson DK, Sunshine P (Eds): Fetal and Neonatal Brain Injury: Mechanisms, Management, and the Risks of Practice. Philadelphia, BC Decker, 1989, pp 46–56.

Albright L, Fellows R: Sequential CT scanning after neonatal intracerebral hemorrhage. AJR Am J Roentgenol 136:949, 1981.

Alfonso I, Papazian O, Jeffries HE: A simple maneuver to provoke benign neonatal sleep myoclonus. Pediatrics 96:1161, 1995.

Allan WC, Dransfield DA, Tito AM: Ventricular dilation following periventricular-intraventricular hemorrhage: Outcome at age 1 year. Pediatrics 73:158, 1984.

Al-Rajeh S, Corea JR, Al-Sibai MH, et al: Congenital brachial palsy in the eastern province of Saudi Arabia. J Child Neurol 5:35, 1990.

Alvarez M, Chitkara U, Lynch L, et al: Prenatal diagnosis of fetal brain tumors. Fetal Ther 2:203, 1987.

Amato M, Huppi P, Herschkowitz N, et al: Prenatal stroke suggested by intrauterine ultrasound and confirmed by magnetic resonance imaging. Neuropediatrics 22:100, 1991.

Amato M, Konrad D, Huppi P, et al: Impact of prematurity and intrauterine growth retardation on neonatal hemorrhagic and ischemic brain damage. Eur Neurol 33:299, 1993.

Ambler R, Gruenewald S, John E: Ultrasound monitoring of diaphragm activity in bilateral diaphragmatic paralysis. Arch Dis Child 60:170, 1985.

American College of Obstetricians and Gynecologists (ACOG): Fetal and neonatal neurologic injury. ACOG Technical Bulletin Number 163. Int J Gynecol Obstet 41:97, 1993.

American Electroencephalographic Society (AEEGS): Minimum technical standards for pediatric electroencephalography. J Clin Neurophysiol 11:6, 1994.

Amiel-Tison C: Neurological evaluation of the maturity of newborn infants. Arch Dis Child 43:89, 1968.

Amit R, Bashan N, Abarbanel JM, et al: Fatal familial infantile glycogen storage disease—multisystem phosphofructokinase deficiency. Muscle Nerve 15:455, 1992.

Amit Y, Chan G, Fedunec S, et al: Bilirubin toxicity in a neuroblastoma cell line N-115: I: Effects on Na^+,K^+-ATP_{ase}, (^3H)-thymidine uptake, L-(^{35}S)-methionine incorporation, and mitochondrial function. Pediatr Res 25:364, 1989.

Anderson JM, Milner RDG, Stritch SJ: Effects of neonatal hypoglycaemia on the nervous system: A pathological study. J Neurol Neurosurg Psychiatry 30:295, 1967.

Anwar M, Kadam S, Hiatt IM, et al: Serial lumbar punctures in prevention of post-hemorrhagic hydrocephalus in preterm infants. J Pediatr 107:446, 1985.

Aprison MH, Segar WE: Electrolyte distribution and water content in six discrete areas of the developing mammalian brain. Rec Adv Biol Psychol 5:279, 1963.

Armstrong D, Norman MG: Periventricular leucomalacia in newborns: Complications and sequelae. Arch Dis Child 49:367, 1974.

Armstrong DD: Neonatal encephalopathies. In Duckett S (Ed): Pediatric Neuropathology. Baltimore, Williams & Wilkins, 1995, pp 334–352.

Armstrong DL, Sauls CD, Goddard-Finegold J: Neuropathologic findings in short-term survivors of intraventricular hemorrhage. Am J Dis Child 141:617, 1987.

Arnold BW, Martin CG, Alexander BJ, et al: Autoregulation of brain blood flow during hypotension and hypertension in infant lambs. Pediatr Res 29:110, 1991.

Arnon SS, Midura TF, Damus K, et al: Honey and other environmental risk factors for infant botulism. J Pediatr 94:331, 1979.

Aronyk KE: Post-traumatic hematomas. In Cheek WR (Ed): Pediatric Neurosurgery: Surgery of the Developing Nervous System. Philadelphia, WB Saunders, 1994, pp 279–296.

Aslandis C, Jansen G, Amemiya C, et al: Cloning of the essential myotonic dystrophy region and mapping of the putative defect. Nature 355:548, 1992.

Auer RN: Progress review: Hypoglycemic brain damage. Stroke 17:699, 1986.

Axelrod FB, Porges RF, Sein ME: Neonatal recognition of familial dysautonomia. J Pediatr 110:946, 1987.

Babcock DS, Han BK: The accuracy of high resolution real-time ultrasonography of the head in infancy. Radiology 139:665, 1981.

Bada HS, Hajjar W, Chua C, et al: Noninvasive diagnosis of neonatal asphyxia and intraventricular hemorrhage by Doppler ultrasound. J Pediatr 95:775, 1979.

Badawi N, Kurinszuk J, Blair E, et al: Early prediction of the development of microcephaly after hypoxic-ischemic encephalopathy in the newborn (letter to the editor). Pediatrics 97:151, 1996.

Baker CJ, Edwards MS: Group B streptococcal infections. In Remington JS, Klein JO (Eds): Infectious Diseases of the Fetus and Newborn Infant. Philadelphia, WB Saunders, 1983, pp 820–881.

Banker BQ, Larroche J-C: Periventricular leukomalacia of infancy: A form of neonatal anoxic encephalopathy. Arch Neurol 7:386, 1962.

Barohn RJ, Dowd DC, Kagan-Hallet KS: Congenital ceroid-lipofuscinosis. Pediatr Neurol 8:54, 1992.

Barton ME, Court SD, Walker W: Causes of severe deafness in school children in Northumberland and Durham. BMJ 1:351, 1962.

Bass NH, Lundborg P: Postnatal development of bulk flow in the cerebrospinal fluid system of the albino rat: Clearance of carboxyl (^{14}C) insulin after intrathecal infusion. Brain 52:323, 1973.

Batton DG, Holtrop P, DeWitte D, et al: Current gestational age-related incidence of major intraventricular hemorrhage. J Pediatr 125:623, 1994.

Bedard MP, Shankaran S, Slovis TL, et al: Effect of prophylactic phenobarbital on intraventricular hemorrhage in high-risk infants. Pediatrics 73:435, 1984.

Bejar R, Coen RW, Merritt TA, et al: Focal necrosis of the white matter (periventricular leukomalacia): Sonographic, pathologic, and electroencephalographic features. AJNR Am J Neuroradiol 7:1073, 1986.

Bejar R, Curbelo V, Coen RW, et al: Diagnosis and follow-up of intraventricular and intracerebral hemorrhages by ultrasound studies of the infant's brain through the fontanelles and sutures. Pediatrics 66:661, 1980.

Benitz WE, Frankel LR, Stevenson DK: Immediate management. *In* Stevenson DK, Sunshine P (Eds): Fetal and Neonatal Brain Injury: Mechanisms, Management, and the Risks of Practice. Philadelphia, BC Decker, 1989, pp 94–104.

Bennett MJ, Berry GT: Use of the clinical laboratory for evaluating metabolic disease. *In* Duckett S (Ed): Pediatric Neuropathology. Baltimore, Williams & Wilkins, 1995, pp 823–829.

Bergey GK, Swaiman KF, Schrier BK, et al: Adverse effects of phenobarbital on morphological and biochemical development of fetal mouse spinal cord neurons in culture. Ann Neurol 9:584, 1981.

Bergman I, Painter MJ, Hirsch RP, et al: Outcome in newborns with convulsions treated in an intensive care unit. Ann Neurol 14:642, 1983.

Beverley DW, Pitts-Tucker TJ, Congdon PJ, et al: Prevention of intraventricular haemorrhage by fresh frozen plasma. Arch Dis Child 60:710, 1985.

Bjorklund A, Dunnett SB, Stenevi U, et al: Reinnervation of the denervated striatum by substantia nigra transplants: Functional consequences as revealed by pharmacological and sensorimotor testing. Brain Res 199:307, 1980.

Blair E, Stanley JF: Intrapartum asphyxia: A rare cause of cerebral palsy. J Pediatr 112:515, 1988.

Blume WT, Dreyfus-Brisac C: Positive Rolandic sharp waves in neonatal EEG: Types and significance. Electroencephalogr Clin Neurophysiol 53:277, 1982.

Blumenfield A, Slaugenhaupt SA, Axelrod FB, et al: Localization of the gene for familial dysautonomia on chromosome 9 and definition of DNA markers for genetic diagnosis. Nat Genet 4:160, 1993.

Bodensteiner JB: Plantar responses in infants. J Child Neurol 7:311, 1992.

Brann AW, Myers RE: Central nervous system findings in the newborn monkey following severe in utero partial asphyxia. Neurology 25:327, 1975.

Brazy JE, Eckerman CO, Oehler JM, et al: Nursery neurobiologic risk score: Important factors in predicting outcome in very low birth weight infants. J Pediatr 118:783, 1991.

Brazy JE, Lewis DV: Changes in cerebral blood volume and cytochrome aa_3 during hypertensive peaks in preterm infants. J Pediatr 108:983, 1986.

Bredt DS, Snyder SH: Nitric oxide, a novel neuronal messenger. Neuron 8:3, 1992.

Brem AS, Cashore WJ, Pacholski M, et al: Effects of bilirubin on transepithelial transport of sodium, water, and urea. Kidney Int 27:51, 1985.

Brierley JB, Excell BJ: The effects of profound systemic hypotension upon the brain of M. rhesus: Physiological and pathological observations. Brain 89:269, 1966.

Brod SA, Ment LR, Enrenkranz RA, et al: Predictors of success for drug discontinuation following neonatal seizures. Pediatr Neurol 4:13, 1988.

Brook JD, McCurrach ME, Harley HG, et al: Molecular basis of myotonic dystrophy: Expansion of a trinucleotide (CTG) repeat at the 3' end of a transcript encoding a protein kinase family member. Cell 68:799, 1992.

Brown FR, Voigt R, Singh AK, et al: Peroxisomal disorders: Neurodevelopmental and biochemical aspects. Am J Dis Child 147:617, 1993.

Brown WD, Gerfen GW, Vachon LA, et al: Real-time ultrasonography of arterial intraventricular hemorrhage in preterm infants. Pediatr Neurol 11:325, 1994.

Buchan A, Pulsinelli WA: Hypothermia but not the N-methyl-D-aspartate antagonist, MK-801, attenuates neuronal damage in gerbils subjected to transient global ischemia. J Neurosci 10:311, 1990.

Bucher HU, Boltshauser E, Friderich J, et al: Birth injury to the spinal cord. Helv Paediatr Acta 34:517, 1979.

Buetow PC, Smirniotopoulos JG, Done S: Congenital brain tumors: A review of 45 cases. AJNR Am J Neuroradiol 11:793, 1990.

Burke JB: Prognostic significance of neonatal convulsions. Arch Dis Child 29:342, 1954.

Busto R, Dietrich W, Mordecai G, et al: Small differences in intraischemic brain temperature critically determine the extent of neuronal injury. J Cereb Blood Flow Metab 7:729, 1987.

Buxton J, Shelbourne P, Davies J, et al: Detection of an unstable fragment of DNA specific to individuals with myotonic dystrophy. Nature 355:547, 1992.

Cadilhac J, Passouant P, Ribstein M: Convulsions in the newborn: EEG and clinical aspects. Electroencephalogr Clin Neurophysiol 11:604, 1959.

Cartwright GW, Culbertson K, Schreiner RL, et al: Changes in clinical presentation of term infants with intracranial hemorrhage. Dev Med Child Neurol 21:730, 1979.

Cashore WJ: Effects of bilirubin and albumin on dopamine synthesis in striatal synaptosomes. Pediatr Res 25:210A, 1989.

Chadduck WM: Craniosynostosis. *In* Cheek WR (Ed): Pediatric Neurosurgery: Surgery of the Developing Nervous System. Philadelphia, WB Saunders, 1994, pp 111–123.

Chance B, Smith DS, Delivoria-Papadopoulos M, et al: New techniques for evaluating metabolic brain injury in newborn infants. Crit Care Med 17:465, 1989.

Charnas L, Trapp B, Griffin J: Congenital absence of peripheral myelin: Abnormal Schwann cell development causes lethal arthrogryposis multiplex congenita. Neurology 38:966, 1988.

Chasnoff IF, Bussey ME, Savich R, et al: Perinatal cerebral infarction and maternal cocaine use. J Pediatr 108:456, 1986.

Chugani HT, Phelps ME: Maturational changes in cerebral function in infants determined by ^{18}FDG positron emission tomography. Science 231:840, 1986.

Claireaux AE: Pathology of human kernicterus. *In* Sass-Kortsak A (Ed): Kernicterus. Toronto, University of Toronto Press, 1961, p 140.

Clancy R, Malin S, Laraque D, et al: Focal motor seizures heralding stroke in full-term newborns. Am J Dis Child 139:601, 1985.

Clancy RR, Tharp BR: Positive Rolandic sharp waves in the electroencephalograms of premature newborns with intraventricular hemorrhage. Electroencephalogr Clin Neurophysiol 57:395, 1984.

Clouse LH, Comp PC: The regulation of hemostasis: The protein C system. N Engl J Med 314:1298, 1986.

Cohen RS, Benitz WE, Stevenson DK: Fetal injury from drug abuse in pregnancy: Alcohol, narcotic, cocaine, and phencyclidine. *In* Stevenson DK, Sunshine P (Eds): Fetal and Neonatal Brain Injury: Mechanisms, Management, and the Risks of Practice. Philadelphia, BC Decker, 1989, pp 57–64.

Committee on Infectious Diseases, American Academy of Pediatrics (Eds): Report of the Committee on Infectious Diseases, 22nd ed. Elk Grove Village, IL, American Academy of Pediatrics, 1991.

Corchs JL, Serrani RE, Venera G, et al: Inhibition of K$^+$ influx in Ehrlich ascites cells by bilirubin and ouabain. Experientia 38:1069, 1982.

Courtecuisse V, Royer P, Habib R, et al: Glycogenose musculaire par deficit d'alpha,4-glucosidase simulant une dystrophie musculaire progressive. Arch Francaises de Pediatrie 22:1153, 1965.

Craig WS: Convulsive movements occurring in the first ten days of life. Arch Dis Child 35:336, 1960.

Crowley P: Update of the antenatal steroid meta-analysis: Current knowledge and future research needs. Report of the Consensus Development Conference on the Effect of Corticosteroids for Fetal Maturation on Perinatal Outcomes. NIH Pub No. 95–3784. Bethesda, US Department of Health and Human Services, 1994, pp 93–95.

Crowley P, Chalmers I, Keirse MJNC: The effects of corticosteroid administration before preterm delivery: An overview of the evidence from controlled studies. Br J Obstet Gynaecol 97:11, 1990.

Daoust-Roy J, Seshia SS: Benign neonatal sleep myoclonus: A differential diagnosis of neonatal seizures. Am J Dis Child 146:1236, 1992.

David S, Aguayo AJ: Axonal elongation into peripheral nervous system "bridges" after central nervous system injury in adult rats. Science 214:931, 1981.

Davies PA: Bacterial and fungal infections. *In* Levene MI, Bennett MJ, Punt J (Eds): Fetal and Neonatal Neurology and Neurosurgery. Edinburgh, Churchill Livingstone, 1988, pp 427–449.

Davson H, Kleeman CR, Levin E: Quantitative studies of the passage of different substances out of the cerebrospinal fluid. J Physiol 161:126, 1962.

Day R: Inhibition of brain respiration in vitro by bilirubin: Reversal of inhibition by various means. Proc Soc Exp Biol Med 85:261, 1954.

DePraeter C, Vanhaesebrouck P, Govaert P, et al: Creatine kinase isoenzyme BB concentrations in the cerebrospinal fluid of newborns: Relationship to short-term outcome. Pediatrics 88:1204, 1991.

DeReuck JL: Cerebral angioarchitecture and perinatal brain lesions in premature and full-term infants. Acta Neurol Scand 70:391, 1984.

DeReuck JL, Chattha AS, Richardson EP Jr: Pathogenesis and evolution of periventricular leukomalacia in infancy. Arch Neurol 27:229, 1972.

Devilat M, Toso M, Morales M: Childhood stroke associated with protein C or S deficiency and primary antiphospholipid syndrome. Pediatr Neurol 9:67, 1993.

DeVivo D, Trifiletti RR, Jacobson RI, et al: Defective glucose transport across the blood-brain barrier as a cause of persistent hypoglychorrhachia, seizures, and developmental delay. N Engl J Med 325:703, 1991.

DeVivo DC: The expanding clinical spectrum of mitochondrial diseases. Brain Dev 15:1, 1993.

DeVivo DC, Hays AP: Disorders of the neuromuscular system. In Fishman MA (Ed): Pediatric Neurology. New York, Grune & Stratton, 1986, pp 111–135.

Diamond I, Schmid R: Experimental bilirubin encephalopathy: The mode of entry of bilirubin-14C into the central nervous system. J Clin Invest 45:678, 1966.

Diaz J, Schain RJ: Phenobarbital: Effects of long-term administration on behavior and brain of artificially reared rats. Science 199:90, 1978.

DiMauro S, Hartlage PL: Fatal infantile form of muscle phosphorylase deficiency. Neurology 28:1124, 1978.

DiMauro S, Lombes A, Nakase H, et al: Cytochrome c oxidase deficiency. Pediatr Res 28:536, 1980.

Dolfin T, Skidmore MB, Fong KW, et al: Incidence, severity, and timing of subependymal and intraventricular hemorrhages in preterm infants born in a perinatal unit as detected by serial real-time ultrasound. Pediatrics 71:541, 1983.

Donat JF, Okazaki H, Kleinberg F, et al: Intraventricular hemorrhages in full-term and premature infants. Mayo Clin Proc 53:437, 1978.

Donn SM, Goldstein GW, Schork MA: Neonatal hypoxic-ischemic encephalopathy: Current management practices. J Perinatol 3:49, 1988.

Donn SM, Roloff DW, Goldstein GW: Prevention of intraventricular haemorrhage in preterm infants by phenobarbitone—a controlled trial. Lancet 2:215, 1981.

Dreyfus-Brisac C: The electroencephalogram of the premature infant and full-term newborn: Normal and abnormal development of waking and sleeping patterns. In Kellaway P, Petersen J (Eds): Neurological and Electroencephalographic Correlative Studies in Infancy. New York, Grune & Stratton, 1964, pp 186–206.

Dreyfus-Brisac C, Monod N: Electroclinical studies of status epilepticus and convulsions in the newborn. In Kellaway P, Petersen I (Eds): Neurological and Electroencephalographic Correlative Studies in Infancy. New York, Grune & Stratton, 1964, pp 250–272.

D'Souza SW, McConnell SE, Slater P, et al: N-methyl-D-aspartate binding sites in neonatal and adult brain. Lancet 339:1240, 1992.

Dubowitz V: Muscle Disorders in Childhood, 2nd ed. Philadelphia, WB Saunders, 1995.

Dubowitz V, Whittaker GF, Brown BH, et al: Nerve conduction velocity: An index of neurological maturity of the newborn infant. Dev Med Child Neurol 10:741, 1968.

Duffy TE, Kohle SJ, Vannucci RC: Carbohydrate and energy metabolism in perinatal rat brain: Relation to survival in anoxia. J Neurochem 24:271, 1975.

Dusick AM, Covert RF, Schreiber MD, et al: Risk of intracranial hemorrhage and other adverse outcomes after cocaine exposure in a cohort of 323 very low birth weight infants. J Pediatr 122:438, 1993.

Dyck PJ: Inherited neuronal degeneration and atrophy affecting peripheral motor, sensory, and autonomic neurons. In Dyck PJ, Thomas PK, Lambert EH (Eds): Peripheral Neuropathy, Vol 2. Philadephia, WB Saunders, 1975, pp 825–867.

Dykes FD, Dunbar B, Lazarra A, et al: Posthemorrhagic hydrocephalus in high-risk preterm infants: Natural history, management, and long-term outcome. J Pediatr 114:611, 1989.

Edathodu Ak, Dyken PR, Trefz JI, et al: Two new forms of neuronal ceroid-lipofuscinoses: Expanded clinical, morphologic, and biochemical classification. Neurology 34:150, 1984.

Edwards AD, Wyatt JS, Richardson C, et al: Cotside measurement of cerebral blood flow by near infrared spectroscopy. Lancet 2:770, 1988.

Elias SB, Butler I, Appel SH: Neonatal myasthenia gravis in the infant of a myasthenic mother in remission. Ann Neurol 6:72, 1979.

Ellingson RJ, Peters JF: Development of EEG and daytime sleep patterns in full-term infants during the first 3 months of life: Longitudinal observations. Electroencephalogr Clin Neurophysiol 49:112, 1980.

Elliott D: Ultrasonography of the neonatal brain. In Sarnat HB (Ed): Topics in Neonatal Neurology. New York, Grune & Stratton, 1984, pp 233–256.

Eng GD: Brachial plexus palsy in newborn infants. Pediatrics 48:18, 1971.

Eng GD: Obstetrical brachial plexs palsy (OBPP): Outcome with conservative management. Muscle Nerve 19:884, 1996.

Engel AG: Congenital myasthenic syndromes. Neurol Clin North Am 12:401, 1994.

Epstein LG, Sharer LR, Joshi VV, et al: Progressive encephalopathy in children with acquired immune deficiency syndrome. Ann Neurol 17:488, 1985.

Eriksson M, Zetterstrom R: Neonatal convulsions: Incidence and causes in the Stockholm area. Acta Paediatr Scand 68:807, 1979.

Ernster L, Herlin L, Zetterstrom R: Experimental studies on the pathogenesis of kernicterus. Pediatrics 20:647, 1957.

Falco NA, Eriksson E: Facial nerve palsy in the newborn: Incidence and outcome. Plast Reconstr Surg 85:1, 1990.

Faraci FM, Brian JE: Nitric oxide and the cerebral circulation. Stroke 25:692, 1994.

Fazzi E, Lanzi G, Gerardo A, et al: Neurodevelopmental outcome in very-low-birth-weight infants with or without periventricular haemorrhage and/or leukomalacia. Acta Paediatr 81:808, 1992.

Fazzi E, Orcesi S, Caffi L, et al: Neurodevelopmental outcome at 5–7 years in preterm infants with periventricular leukomalacia. Neuropediatrics 25:134, 1994.

Fenichel GM: Electroencephalography and evoked potentials. In Fenichel GM: Neonatal Neurology, New York, Churchill Livingstone, 1990a, pp 225–253.

Fenichel GM: Hypotonia, arthrogryposis, and rigidity. In Fenichel GM: Neonatal Neurology, New York, Churchill Livingstone, 1990b, pp 35–63.

Fenichel GM: Neurological examination of the newborn. Int Pediatr 9:77, 1994.

Fenichel GM, Olson BJ, Fitzpatrick JE: Heart rate changes in convulsive and nonconvulsive neonatal apnea. Ann Neurol 7:577, 1980.

Fenichel GM, Webster DL, Wong WKT: Intracranial hemorrhage in the term newborn. Arch Neurol 41:30, 1984.

Fernandez F, Perez-Higueras A, Hernandez R, et al: Hydranencephaly after maternal butane gas intoxication during pregnancy. Dev Med Child Neurol 28:361, 1986.

Ferriero DM, Arcavi LJ, Sagar SM, et al: Selective sparing of NADPH-diaphorase neurons in neonatal hypoxia-ischemia. Ann Neurol 24:670, 1988.

Fischer EG, McLennan JE, Suzuki Y: Cerebral abscess in children. Am J Dis Child 135:746, 1981.

Fishman MA: Infectious diseases. In David RB (Ed): Pediatric Neurology for the Clinician. Norwalk, CT, Appleton & Lange, 1992, pp 249–268.

Fishman MA, Dutton RV, Okumura S: Progressive ventriculomegaly following minor intracranial hemorrhage in premature infants. Dev Med Child Neurol 26:725, 1984.

Fishman RA: Cerebrospinal Fluid in Diseases of the Nervous System, 2nd ed. Philadelphia, WB Saunders, 1992, pp 160–161.

Fitzhardinge PM, Flodmark O, Fitz CR, et al: The prognostic value of computed tomography as an adjunct to assessment of the term infant with postasphyxial encephalopathy. J Pediatr 99:777, 1981.

Franco SM, Tunnessen WW: Picture of the month: Congenital hypoplasia of the depressor anguli oris muscle. Arch Pediatr Adolesc Med 150:325, 1996.

Friede RL: Developmental Neuropathology, 2nd ed. New York, Springer-Verlag, 1989.

Friedman WF: The intrinsic physiologic properties of the developing heart. In Friedman WF (Ed): Neonatal Heart Disease. New York, Grune & Stratton, 1973, pp 21–49.

Fujimoto S, Togari H, Yamaguchi N, et al: Hypocarbia and cystic periventricular leukomalacia in premature infants. Arch Dis Child 71:F107, 1994.

Fujimura M, Salisbury DM, Robinson RO, et al: Clinical events relating to intraventricular hemorrhage in the newborn. Arch Dis Child 54:409, 1979.

Funato M, Tamai H, Noma K, et al: Clinical events in association with timing of intraventricular hemorrhage in preterm infants. J Pediatr 121:614, 1992.

Gal P, Sharpless MK, Boer HR: Outcome in newborns with seizures: Are chronic anticonvulsants necessary? Ann Neurol 15:610, 1984.

Garbarg I, Torvik A, Hals J, et al: Congenital neuronal ceroid-lipofuscinosis: A case report. Acta Pathol Microbiol Immunol Scand 95:119, 1987.

Garland JS, Buck R, Leviton A: Effect of maternal glucocorticoid exposure on risk of severe intraventricular hemorrhage in surfactant-treated preterm infants. J Pediatr 126:272, 1995.

Gilbert A, Brockman R, Carlioz H: Surgical treatment of brachial plexus birth palsy. Clin Orthop 264:39, 1991.

Gilbert A, Tassin JL: Obstetrical palsy: A clinical, pathological, and surgical overview. *In* Terzis J (Ed): Microreconstruction of Nerve Injuries. Philadelphia, WB Saunders, 1987, pp 529–553.

Gilles FH, Leviton A, Kerr CS: Endotoxin leucoencephalopathy in the telencephalon of the newborn kitten. J Neurol Sci 27:183, 1976.

Gilman S, Barrett RE: Hallervorden-Spatz disease and infantile neuroaxonal dystrophy: Clinical characteristics and nosological considerations. J Neurol Sci 19:189, 1973.

Glatzl-Hawlik M-A, Bell EF: Environmental temperature control. *In* Polin RA, Fox WW (Eds): Fetal and Neonatal Physiology. Philadelphia, WB Saunders, 1992, pp 515–527.

Glauser TA, Maguire HC, Sladky JT: Relapse of infant botulism. Ann Neurol 28:187, 1990.

Goddard J, Lewis RM, Alcala H, Zeller RS: Intraventricular hemorrhage: An animal model (abstract). Ann Neurol 13:488, 1978.

Goddard J, Lewis RM, Alcala H, Zeller RS: Intraventricular hemorrhage: An animal model. Biol Neonate 37:39, 1980a.

Goddard J, Lewis RM, Armstrong DL, Zeller RS: Moderate, rapidly induced hypertension as a cause of intraventricular hemorrhage in the newborn beagle model. J Pediatr 96:1057, 1980b.

Goddard-Finegold J, Armstrong DL, Zeller RS: Intraventricular hemorrhage following volume expansion after hypovolemic hypotension in the newborn beagle. J Pediatr 100:796, 1982.

Goddard-Finegold J, Donley DK, Adham BI, et al: Phenobarbital and cerebral blood flow during hypertension in the newborn beagle. Pediatrics 86:501, 1990.

Goddard-Finegold J, Louis PT, Rodriguez DL, et al: Near infrared spectroscopic (NIRS) estimations of cerebral blood flow (CBF) in newborn piglets. Ann Neurol 36:496, 1994.

Goddard-Finegold J, Mizrahi EM: Understanding and preventing perinatal, intracerebral, peri- and intraventricular hemorrhage. J Child Neurol 2:170, 1987.

Goldberg MP, Monyer H, Weiss JH, et al: Adenosine reduces cortical neuronal injury induced by oxygen or glucose deprivation in vitro. Neurosci Lett 89:323, 1988.

Goldberg RN, Goldman SL, Ramsay RE, et al: Detection of seizure activity in the paralyzed newborn using continuous monitoring. Pediatrics 69:583, 1982.

Goldberg RN, Moscoso P, Bauer CR, et al: Use of barbiturate therapy in severe perinatal asphyxia: A randomized controlled trial. J Pediatr 109:851, 1986.

Gootman N, Gootman PM, Buckley NM, et al: Central vasomotor regulation in the newborn piglet *Sus scrofa*. Am J Physiol 222:994, 1972.

Gordon M, Rich H, Deutschberger J, et al: The immediate and long term outcome of obstetric birth trauma. Am J Obstet Gynecol 117:51, 1973.

Gray SM, Adams V, Yamashita Y, et al: Hexokinase binding in ischemic and reperfused piglet brain. Biochem Med Metab Biol 53:145, 1994.

Green KA, Shaw NJ: Is a low cerebrospinal fluid blood glucose ratio indicative of infection in patients with post haemorrhagic hydrocephalus? Early Hum Dev 36:187, 1994.

Greenamyre T, Penney JB, Young AB, et al: Evidence for transient perinatal glutamatergic innervation of globus pallidus. J Neurosci 7:1022, 1987.

Greenberg F, Genolio KR, Kejtmancik F, et al: X-linked infantile spinal muscular atrophy. Am J Dis Child 142:217, 1988.

Greenshear J, Mofenson HC, Borafsky LG, et al: Lumbar puncture in the neonate: A simplified technique. J Pediatr 78:1034, 1971.

Greenwald AG, Schute PC, Shiveley JL: Brachial plexus birth palsy. J Pediatr Orthop 4:689, 1984.

Greisen G: Effect of cerebral blood flow and cerebrovascular autoregulation on the distribution, type, and extent of cerebral injury. Brain Pathol 2:223, 1992.

Gressens P, Richelme C, Kadhim HJ, et al: The germinative zone produces the most cortical astrocytes after neuronal migration in the developing mammalian brain. Biol Neonate 61:4, 1992.

Gronlund JU, Korvenranta H, Kero P, et al: Elevated arterial blood pressure is associated with peri-intraventricular haemorrhage. Eur J Pediatr 153:836, 1994.

Grose C: Congenital infections caused by varicella zoster virus and herpes simplex virus. Semin Pediatr Neurol 1:43, 1994.

Gunn AJ, Williams CE, Mallard C, et al: Flunarizine, a calcium channel antagonist, is partially prophylactically neuroprotective in hypoxic-ischemic encephalopathy in the fetal sheep. Pediatr Res 35:657, 1994.

Guzzetta F, Shackelford GD, Volpe S, et al: Periventricular intraparenchymal echodensities in the premature newborn: Critical determinant of neurologic outcome. Pediatrics 78:995, 1986.

Haddad SF, Menezes AH, Bell WE, et al: Brain tumors occurring before 1 year of age: A retrospective review of 22 cases in an 11 year period (1977–1987). Neurosurgery 29:8, 1991.

Hale DE, Stanley CA, Coates PM: The long-chain acyl-CoA dehydrogenase deficiency. *In* Tanaka K, Coates PM (Eds): Fatty Acid Oxidation: Clinical, Biochemical and Molecular Aspects. New York, Alan R. Liss, 1990, pp 303–311.

Halliwell B, Gutteridge JMC: Oxygen toxicity, oxygen radicals, transition metals, and disease. J Biochem 219:1, 1984.

Hamada Y, Hayakawa T, Hattori H, et al: Inhibitor of nitric oxide synthesis reduces hypoxic-ischemic brain damage in the neonatal rat. Pediatr Res 35:10, 1994.

Hambleton G, Wigglesworth JS: Origin of intraventricular hemorrhage in the preterm infant. Arch Dis Child 51:651, 1976.

Hamilton PA, Hope PL, Cady EB, et al: Impaired energy metabolism in brains of newborn infants with increased cerebral echodensities. Lancet 1:1242, 1986.

Hansen TWR, Paulsen O, Gjerstad L, et al: Short-term exposure to bilirubin reduces synaptic activation in rat transverse hippocampal slices. Pediatr Res 23:453, 1988.

Hardy AE: Birth injuries of the brachial plexus. J Bone Joint Surg (Am) 63:98, 1981.

Harley HG, Brook JD, Rundle SA, et al: Expansion of an unstable DNA region and phenotypic variation in myotonic dystrophy. Nature 355:545, 1992.

Harris R, Tizard JPM: The electroencephalogram in neonatal convulsions. J Pediatr 57:501, 1960.

Haruda F, Blanc WA: The structure of intracerebral arteries in premature infants and the autoregulation of cerebral blood flow (abstract). Ann Neurol 10:303, 1981.

Heafner MD, Duncan CC, Kier EL, et al: Intraventricular hemorrhage in a term newborn secondary to a third ventricular AVM. J Neurosurg 63:640, 1985.

Hecox KE, Cone B: Prognostic importance of brain stem auditory evoked responses after asphyxia. Neurology 31:1429, 1981.

Hein HA: The use of sodium bicarbonate in neonatal resuscitation: Help or harm? Pediatrics 91:496, 1993.

Hellman LM, Johnson HL, Tolles WE, et al: Some factors affecting the fetal heart rate. Am J Obstet Gynecol 82:1055, 1961.

Hellstrom-Westas L, Svenningse NW, Westgren U, et al: Lidocaine for treatment of severe seizures in newborn infants: II. Blood concentrations of lidocaine and metabolites during intravenous infusion. Acta Paediatr Scand 81:35, 1992.

Hendricks-Munoz KD, Walton JP: Hearing loss in infants with persistent fetal circulation. Pediatrics 81:650, 1988.

Hepner WR Jr: Some observations on facial paresis in the newborn infant: Etiology and incidence. Pediatrics 8:494, 1952.

Hess DC: Stroke associated with antiphospholipid antibodies. Stroke 23:23, 1992.

Hicks T, Fowler K, Richardson M, et al: Congenital cytomegalovirus infection and neonatal auditory screening. J Pediatr 123:779, 1993.

Hill A: Current concepts of hypoxic-ischemic cerebral injury in the term newborn. Pediatr Neurol 7:317, 1991.

Holden KR, Mellits ED, Freeman JM: Neonatal seizures: I. Correlation of prenatal and perinatal events with outcomes. Pediatrics 70:165, 1982.

Holmes GL: Do seizures cause brain damage? Epilepsia 32(suppl 5):S14, 1991.

Holowach-Thurston J, Hauhart RE, Jones EM: Anoxia in mice: Reduced glucose in brain with normal or elevated glucose in plasma and increased survival after glucose treatment. Pediatr Res 8:238, 1974.

Houston K, Buschange PH, Iannaccone St, et al: Craniofacial morphology of spinal muscular atrophy. Pediatr Res 36:265, 1994.

Hrachovy RA, Mizrahi EM, Kellaway P: Electroencephalography of the newborn. *In* Daly DD, Pedley TA (Eds): Current Practice of Clinical

Electroencephalography, 2nd ed. New York, Raven Press, 1990, pp 201–242.

Humphreys RP: Vascular malformations of the brain. *In* Cheek WR (Ed): Pediatric Neurosurgery: Surgery of the Developing Nervous System. Philadelphia, WB Saunders, 1994, pp 524–532.

Humphreys S, Lake BD, Schulz CL: Congenital amaurotic idiocy—a pathological, histochemical, biochemical, and ultrastructural study. Neuropathol Appl Neurobiol 11:475, 1985.

Hunt D: Surgical management of brachial plexus birth injuries. Dev Med Child 30:824, 1988.

Hunter AGW, Rudd NL: Craniosynostosis: I. Sagittal synostosis: Its genetics and associated clinical findings in 214 patients who lacked involvement of the coronal suture(s). Teratology 14:185, 1976.

Hunter AGW, Rudd NL: Craniosynostosis: II. Coronal synostosis: Its familial characteristics and associated clinical findings in 109 patients lacking bilateral polysyndactyly or syndactyly. Teratology 15:301, 1977.

Iida K, Takashima S, Taeuchi Y, et al: Neuropathologic study of newborns with prenatal-onset leukomalacia. Pediatr Neurol 9:45, 1993.

Isch F, Juif JG, Sacrez R, et al: Glycogenose musculaire a forme myopathique pare deficit en maltase acid. Pediatrie 21:71, 1966.

Iwamoto HS, Kaufman T, Keil LC, et al: Responses to acute hypoxemia in fetal sheep at 0.6–0.7 gestation. Am J Physiol 256:H613, 1989.

Jackson S, Bartlett K, Land J, et al: Long-chain 3-hydroxyacyl-CoA dehydrogenase deficiency. Pediatr Res 29:406, 1991.

Jobsis JJ: Non-invasive, infra-red monitoring of cerebral and myocardial oxygen sufficiency and circulatory parameters. Science 198:1264, 1977.

Jones HR: Pediatric electromyography. *In* Brown WF, Bolton DF (Eds): Clinical Electromyography. Boston, Butterworth-Heineman, 1993.

Jones MD, Rosenberg AA, Simmons MA, et al: Oxygen delivery to the brain before and after birth. Science 216:324, 1982.

Jones MD, Traystman RJ, Simmons MA, et al: Effects of changes in arterial O_2 content on cerebral blood flow in the lamb. Am J Physiol 240:H209, 1981.

Jones MD Jr, Sheldon RE, Peeters LL, et al: Regulation of cerebral blood flow in the ovine fetus. Am J Physiol 235:H162, 1978.

Jongmans M, Henderson S, deVries L, et al: Duration of periventricular densities in preterm infants and neurological outcome at 6 years of age. Arch Dis Child 69:9, 1993.

Kaempf JW, Porreco R, Molina R, et al: Antenatal phenobarbital for the prevention of periventricular and intraventricular hemorrhage: A double-blind, randomized, placebo-controlled multi-hospital trial. J Pediatr 117:933, 1990.

Karch SB, Urich H: Infantile polyneuropathy with defective myelination: An autopsy study. Dev Med Child Neurol 17:504, 1975.

Kellaway P, Hrachovy RA: Status epilepticus in newborns: A perspective on neonatal seizures. *In* Delgado-Escueta AV, Wasterlain CG, Treiman DM, Porter RJ (Eds): Advances in Neurology, vol 34: Status Epilepticus. New York, Raven Press, 1983, pp 93–99.

Kellaway P, Mizrahi EM: Clinical electroencephalographic, therapeutic, and pathophysiological studies of neonatal seizures. *In* Wasterlain C, Vert P (Eds): Neonatal Seizures. New York, Raven Press, 1990, pp 1–14.

Kennedy CR: The assessment of hearing and brain stem function. *In* Eyre JA (Ed): The Neurophysiological Examination of the Newborn Infant. New York, MacKeith Press, 1992.

Khater-Boidin J, Duron B: Nerve conduction. Clin Dev Med 120:155, 1992.

Kileny P, Connelly C: Auditory brain stem responses in perinatal asphyxia. Int J Pediatr Otorhinol 2:147, 1980.

Kitchen WH, Rickards AL, Ryan MM, et al: Improved outcome to two years of very low-birthweight infants: Fact or artifact? Dev Med Child Neurol 28:479, 1986.

Konigsmark BW: Hereditary deafness in man. N Engl J Med 281:774, 1969.

Kuban KC, Leviton A, Krishnamoorthy KS, et al: Neonatal intracranial hemorrhage and phenobarbital. Pediatrics 77:443, 1986.

Lacey DJ, Terplan K: Intraventricular hemorrhage in full-term newborns. Dev Med Child Neurol 24:332, 1982.

Lanska MJ, Lanska DJ, Baumann RJ, et al: A population-based study of neonatal seizures in Fayette county, Kentucky. Neurology 45:724, 1995.

Larroche J-C: Hemorrhagies cerebrales intraventriculares chez le premature: I. Anatomie et physiopathologie. Biol Neonate 7:36, 1974.

Larroche J-C: Fetal encephalopathies of circulatory origin. Biol Neonate 50:61, 1986.

Laurent JP, El-Hibri H, Okumura S, et al: Glycerol's effect on cerebrospinal fluid formation. Concept Pediatr Neurosurg 5:84, 1985.

Laurent JP, Lee RT: Birth-related upper brachial plexus injuries in infants: Operative and nonoperative approaches. J Child Neurol 9:111, 1994.

Laurent JP, Shenaq S, Lee R, et al: Upper brachial plexus birth injuries: A neurosurgical approach. Concepts Pediatr Neurosurg 10:156, 1990.

Laurent JP, Shenaq S, Lee RT, et al: Neurosurgical correction of upper brachial plexus birth injuries. J Neurosurg 79:197, 1993.

Leech RW, Kohnen P: Subependymal and intraventricular hemorrhages in the newborn. Am J Pathol 77:465, 1974.

Leech RW, Olson MI, Alvord EC: Neuropathologic features of idiopathic respiratory distress syndrome. Arch Pathol Lab Med 103:341, 1979.

Leichti-Gallati S, Wolff G, Ketelson U-P, et al: Prenatal diagnosis of X-linked centronuclear myopathy by linkage analysis. Pediatr Res 33:201, 1993.

Leppert M, Anderson VE, Quattlebaum TG, et al: Benign familial neonatal convulsions linked to genetic markers on chromosome 20. Nature 337:647, 1989.

Lesko SM, Mitchell AA, Epstein MF, et al: Heparin use as a risk factor for intraventricular hemorrhage in low-birth-weight infants. N Engl J Med 314:1156, 1986.

Levene HL, Kornberg J, Williams THC: The incidence and severity of post-asphyxial encephalopathy in full-term infants. Early Hum Dev 11:21, 1985.

Levine MG, Holroyde J, Woods JR, et al: Birth trauma: Incidence and predisposing factors. Obstet Gynecol 63:792, 1984.

Leviton A, Kuban KC, Pagano M, et al: Antenatal corticosteroids appear to reduce the risk of postnatal germinal matrix hemorrhage in intubated low birth weight newborns. Pediatrics 91:1083, 1993.

Leviton A, Pagano M, Kuban KC, et al: The epidemiology of germinal matrix hemorrhage during the first half-day of life. Dev Med Child Neurol 33:138, 1991.

Lewis TB, Leach RJ, Ward K, et al: Genetic heterogeneity in benign familial neonatal convulsions: Identification of a new locus on chromosome 8q. Am J Hum Genet 53:670, 1993.

Lindstrom J, Shelton D, Fujii Y: Myasthenia gravis. Adv Immunol 42:233, 1988.

Lipson AH, Rogers M, Berry A: Collodion babies with Gaucher's disease: A further case. Arch Dis Child 66:667, 1991.

Livera LN, Spencer SA, Thorniley MS, et al: Effects of hypoxaemia and bradycardia on neonatal cerebral haemodynamics. Arch Dis Child 66:376, 1991.

Lockwood AH: Ammonia-induced encephalopathy. *In* McCandless DW (Ed): Cerebral Energy Metabolism and Metabolic Encephalopathy. New York, Plenum Press, 1985, pp 203–222.

Lombroso CT: Neonatal electroencephalography: *In:* Niedermeyer E, Lopes deSilva F (Eds): Electroencephalography: Basic Principles, Clinical Applications, and Related Fields. Baltimore, Urban & Schwarzenberg, 1982, pp 599–637.

Lombroso CT: Prognosis in neonatal seizures. Adv Neurol 34:101, 1983.

Lou HC, Friis-Hansen B: Arterial blood pressure elevations during motor activity and epileptic seizures in the newborn. Acta Paediatr Scand 68:803, 1979.

Lou HC, Lassen NA, Friis-Hansen B: Impaired autoregulation of cerebral blood flow in the distressed newborn infant. J Pediatr 94:118, 1979.

Louis PT, Yamashita Y, Del Toro J, et al: Brain blood flow responses to indomethacin during hemorrhagic hypotension in newborn piglets. Biol Neonate 66:359, 1994.

Low JA, Froese AB, Galbraith RS, et al: The association between preterm newborn hypotension and hypoxemia and outcome during the first year. Acta Paediatr 82:433, 1993.

Low JA, Froese AB, Smith JT, et al: Blood pressure and heart rate of the preterm newborn following delivery. Clin Invest Med 14:183, 1991.

Lylyk P, Vinuela F, Dion JE, et al: Therapeutic alternatives for vein of Galen vascular malformations. J Neurosurg 78:438, 1993.

Malamud N: Status marmoratus: A form of cerebral palsy following either birth injury or inflammation of the central nervous system. J Pediatr 37:610, 1950.

Mallard EC, Williams CE, Gunn AJ, et al: Frequent episodes of brief ischemia sensitize the fetal sheep brain to neuronal loss and induce striatal injury. Pediatr Res 33:61, 1993.

Mannino FL, Trauner DA: Stroke in newborns. J Pediatr 102:605, 1983.

Mantovani JF, Pasternak JF, Mathew OP, et al: Failure of daily lumbar punctures to prevent the development of hydrocephalus following intraventricular hemorrhage. J Pediatr 97:278, 1980.

Manzoni O, Prezeau L, Marin P, et al: Nitric oxide-induced blockade of NMDA receptors. Neuron 8:653, 1992.

Marlin AE, Gaskill SJ: Cerebrospinal fluid shunts: Complications and results. *In* Cheek WR (Ed): Pediatric Neurosurgery: Surgery of the Developing Nervous System. Philadelphia, WB Saunders, 1994, pp 221–233.

Marret S, Parain D, Samson-Dollfus D, et al: Positive rolandic sharp waves and periventricular leukomalacia in the newborn. Neuropediatrics 17:199, 1986.

Marron M-J, Crisafi MA, Driscoll JM Jr, et al: Hearing and neurodevelopmental outcome in survivors of persistent pulmonary hypertension of the newborn. Pediatrics 90:392, 1992.

Martin JH, Brust JCM, Hilal S: Imaging the living brain. *In* Kandel ER, Schwartz JD, Jessell TM (Eds): Principles of Neural Science, 3rd ed. New York, Elsevier Press, 1991, pp 309–324.

Mathew OP, Bland HE, Pickens JM, et al: Hypoglychorrhachia in the survivors of neonatal intracranial hemorrhage. Pediatrics 63:851, 1979.

Mathew OP, Volpe JJ: Neonatal intraventricular hemorrhage: Hypoglycorrhachia and its relationship to CSF lactate levels. J Pediatr 97:292, 1980.

Mayer ML, MacDermott AB, Westbrook GL, et al: Agonist- and voltage-gated calcium entry in cultured mouse spinal cord neurons under voltage clamp measured using arsenazo III. J Neurosci 7:3230, 1987.

Mayer ML, Westbrook GL, Guthrie PB: Voltage-dependent block by Mg^{2+} of NMDA responses in spinal cord neurons. Nature 309:261, 1984.

Mayman CI, Tijerina ML: The effect of hypoglycemia on energy reserves in adult and newborn brain. Clin Dev Med 39/40:242, 1971.

Maytal J, Novak GP, King K: Lorazepam in the treatment of refractory neonatal seizures. J Child Neurol 6:319, 1991.

McDonald A: Children of Very Low Birthweight: M.E.I.U. Research Monograph No. 1. London, Spastics Society and Heineman Press, 1967.

McDonald JW, Johnston MV, Young AB: Differential ontogenic development of three receptors comprising the NMDA receptor/channel complex in the rat hippocampus. Exp Neurol 110:237, 1990.

McInerny TK, Schubert WK: Prognosis of neonatal seizures. Am J Dis Child 117:261, 1969.

McLone DG: Continuing concepts in the management of spina bifida. Pediatr Neurosurg 18:254, 1992.

McLone DG, Dias L, Kaplan WE, et al: Concepts in the management of spina bifida. *In* Marlin AE (Ed): Concepts in Pediatric Neurosurgery, Vol 5. Basel, Karger, 1985, pp 97–106.

Menkes J: Neurologic evaluation of the newborn infant. *In* Taeusch HW, Ballard RA, Avery ME (Eds): Diseases of the Newborn, 6th ed. Philadelphia, WB Saunders, 1991a, pp 395–405.

Menkes JH: Perinatal central nervous system asphyxia and trauma. *In* Taeusch HW, Ballard RA, Avery ME (Eds): Diseases of the Newborn, 6th ed. Philadelphia, WB Saunders, 1991b, pp 406–422.

Menkes JH: Diseases of the motor unit. *In* Taeusch HW, Ballard RA, Avery ME (Eds): Diseases of the Newborn, 6th ed. Philadelphia, WB Saunders, 1991c, pp 450–455.

Ment LR, Oh W, Ehrenkrantz RA, et al: Low-dose indomethacin and prevention of intraventricular hemorrhage: A multicenter randomized trial. Pediatrics 93:543, 1994a.

Ment LR, Oh W, Ehrenkranz RA, et al: Low-dose indomethacin therapy and extension of intraventricular hemorrhage: A multicenter randomized trial. J Pediatr 124:951, 1994b.

Ment LR, Oh W, Philip AGS, et al: Risk factors for early intraventricular hemorrhage in low birth weight infants. J Pediatr 121:776, 1992.

Ment LR, Stewart WB, Ardito TA, et al: Beagle pup germinal matrix maturation studies. Stroke 2:390, 1991.

Ment LR, Stewart WB, Duncan CC, et al: Beagle puppy model of intraventricular hemorrhage. J Neurosurg 57:219, 1982.

Miall-Allen VM, de Vries LS, Whitelaw AG: Mean arterial blood pressure and neonatal cerebral lesions. Arch Dis Child 62:1068, 1987.

Michelow BJ, Clarke HM, Curtis DG, et al: The natural history of obstetrical brachial plexus palsy. Plast Reconstr Surg 93:675, 1994.

Miller G: Hypotonia and neuromuscular disease. *In* Fanaroff AJ, Martin RC (Eds): Diseases of the Fetus and Newborn. St. Louis, Mosby, 1997, pp 911–924.

Miller GA, Heckmatt JZ, Dubowitz LM, et al: Use of nerve conduction velocity to determine gestational age in infants at risk and in very-low-birth-weight infants. J Pediatr 103:109, 1983.

Miller VS: Pharmacologic management of neonatal cerebral ischemia and hemorrhage: Old and new directions. J Child Neurol 8:7, 1993.

Miller WH, Hesch JA: Nontuberculosis spinal epidural abscess: Report of a case in a 5-week-old infant. Am J Dis Child 104:269, 1962.

Milligan DW: Failure of autoregulation and intraventricular haemorrhage in preterm infants. Lancet 1:896, 1980.

Milstein JM, Herron TM, Haas JE: Fatal infantile phosphorylase deficiency. J Child Neurol 4:186, 1989.

Minkowski A, Sainte-Anne-Dargassies S: Les convulsions du nouveau-né. Evolut Psychiatr 1:279, 1956.

Minns RA: Intracranial pressure monitoring. Arch Dis Child 59:486, 1984.

Miranda SB, Hack M: The predictive value of neonatal visual-perceptual behaviors. *In* Field TM (Ed): Infants Born at Risk: Behavior and Development. New York, SP, 1979.

Miranda SB, Hack M, Fantz RL, et al: Neonatal pattern vision: A predictor of future mental performance? J Pediatr 91:642, 1977.

Mises J, Moussalli-Salefranque F, Laroque ML, et al: EEG findings as an aid to the diagnosis of neonatal non ketotic hyperglycinemia. J Inherit Metab Dis 5(suppl 2):117, 1982.

Mitchell W, O'Tuama L: Cerebral intraventricular hemorrhages in infants: A widening age spectrum. Pediatrics 65:35, 1980.

Mizrahi EM: Neonatal seizures: Problems in diagnosis and classification. Epilepsia 28(suppl 1):S46, 1987.

Mizrahi EM: Consensus and controversy in the clinical management of neonatal seizures. Clin Perinatol 16:485, 1989.

Mizrahi EM: Electroencephalographic-video monitoring in newborns, infants, and children. J Child Neurol 9(suppl):S46, 1994.

Mizrahi EM, Kellaway P: Characterization of seizures in newborns and young infants by time-synchronized electroencephalographic/polygraphic/video monitoring. Ann Neurol 16:383, 1984.

Mizrahi EM, Kellaway P: Characterization and classification of neonatal seizures. Neurology 37:1837, 1987.

Mizrahi EM, Kellaway P: The response of electroclinical neonatal seizures to antiepileptic drug therapy. Epilepsia 33(suppl 3):S114, 1992.

Mizrahi EM, Pollack MA, Kellaway P: Neocortical death in infants: Behavioral, neurologic, and electroencephalographic characteristics. Pediatr Neurol 1:302, 1985.

Monaghan DT, Holets VR, Toy DW, et al: Anatomical distribution of four pharmacologically distinct 3H-L glutamate binding sites. Nature 306:176, 1983.

Moody DM, Brown WR, Challa VR, et al: Alkaline phosphatase histochemical staining in the study of germinal matrix hemorrhage and brain vascular morphology in a very-low-birth-weight newborn. Pediatr Res 35:424, 1994.

Moore TJ, Lione AP, Regan DM, et al: Brain glucose metabolism in the newborn rat. Am J Physiol 221:1746, 1971.

Morales WJ, Angel JL, O'Brien WF, et al: The use of antenatal vitamin K in the prevention of early neonatal intraventricular hemorrhage. Am J Obstet Gynecol 159:774, 1988.

Morales WJ, Koerton J: Prevention of intraventricular hemorrhage in very low birth weight infants by maternally administered phenobarbital. Obstet Gynecol 68:295, 1986.

Moriarity JL, Steinberg GK: Surgical obliteration for vein of Galen malformation: A case report. Surg Neurol 44:365, 1995.

Morishima HO, Heymann MA, Rudolph AM, et al: Toxicity of lidocaine in the fetal and newborn lamb and its relationship to asphyxia. Am J Obstet Gynecol 112:72, 1972.

Moshe SL: Epileptogenesis and the immature brain. Epilepsia 28(suppl 1):S3, 1987.

Moss AJ, Duffie ER, Emmanouilides GC: Blood pressure and vasomotor reflexes in the newborn infant. Pediatrics 32:175, 1963.

Mostacciuolo ML, Danieli GA, Trevisan C, et al: Epidemiology of spinal muscular atrophies in a sample of the Italian population. Neuroepidemiology 11:34, 1992.

Mustafa MG, Cowger ML, King TE: Effects of bilirubin on mitochondrial reactions. J Biol Chem 244:6403, 1969.

Myers RE: Atrophic cortical sclerosis associated with status marmoratus in a perinatally damaged monkey. Neurology 19:1177, 1969.

Myers RE: Four patterns of perinatal brain damage and their conditions of occurrence in primates. Adv Neurol 10:223, 1975.

Nagai T, Tuchiyz Y, Taguchi Y, et al: Fatal infantile mitochondrial encephalomyopathy with complex I and IV deficiencies. Pediatr Neurol 9:151, 1993.

Naidoo BT: The cerebrospinal fluid in the healthy newborn infant. S Afr Med J 42:933, 1968.

Naidu S, Messmore H, Caserta V, et al: CNS lesions in neonatal isoimmune thrombocytopenia. Arch Neurol 40:552, 1983.

Neale EA, Sher PK, Braubard BI, et al: Differential toxicity of chronic exposure to phenytoin, phenobarbital, or carbamazepine in cerebral cortical cell cultures. Pediatr Neurol 1:143, 1985.

Nelson C, Silverstein FS: Acute disruption of cytochrome oxidase activity in brain in a perinatal rat stroke model. Pediatr Res 36:12, 1994.

Nelson KB, Ellenberg JH: The asymptomatic newborn and risk of cerebral palsy. Am J Dis Child 141:1333, 1987.

Nelson KB, Leviton A: How much of neonatal encephalopathy is due to birth asphyxia? Am J Dis Child 145:1325, 1991.

NIH Consensus Statement: Effect of Corticosteroids for Fetal Maturation on Perinatal Outcomes. Vol. 12, No. 2, 1994.

Ninan A, O'Donnell N, Hamilton K, et al: Physiologic changes induced by endotracheal installation and suctioning in critically ill preterm infants with and without sedation. Am J Perinatol 3:94, 1986.

Novotny EJ: Hypoxic-ischemic encephalopathy. *In* Stevenson PK, Sunshine P (Eds): Fetal and Neonatal Brain Injury: Mechanisms, Management, and the Risks of Practice. Philadelphia, BC Decker, 1989, pp 113–122.

Novotny EJ Jr, Tharp BR, Coen RW, et al: Positive Rolandic sharp waves in the EEG of the premature infant. Neurology 37:1481, 1987.

O'Brien WF, Davis SE, Grissom MP, et al: Effect of cephalic pressure on fetal cerebral blood flow. Am J Perinatol 1:223, 1984.

Odell GB, Schutta HS: Bilirubin encephalopathy. *In* McCandless DW (Ed): Cerebral Energy Metabolism and Metabolic Encephalopathy. New York, Plenum Press, 1985, pp 229–261.

Ogata ES: Carbohydrate homeostasis. *In* Avery GB, Fletcher MA, MacDonald MG (Eds): Neonatology: Pathophysiology and Management of the Newborn, 4th ed. Philadelphia, JB Lippincott, 1994, pp 568–584.

Oi S, Kokunai T, Matsumoto S: Congenital brain tumors in Japan (ISPN Cooperative Study): Specific clinical features in newborns. Childs Nerv Syst 6:86, 1990.

Oka A, Belliveau MJ, Rosenberg PA, et al: Vulnerability of oligodendroglia to glutamate: Pharmacology, mechanisms, and prevention. J Neurosci 13:1441, 1993.

Oro AS, Dixon SD: Perinatal cocaine and methampetamine exposure: Maternal and neonatal correlates. J Pediatr 111:571, 1987.

O'Shea TM, Savitz DA, Hage ML, et al: Prenatal events and the risk of sub-ependymal/intraventricular hemorrhage in very low birth weight newborns. Paediatr Perinat Epidemiol 6:352, 1992.

Ouvrier R, Billson F: Optic nerve hypoplasia: A review. J Child Neurol 1:181, 1986.

Ouvrier RA, McCleod JG, Pollard JD: Peripheral Neuropathies in Childhood. New York, Raven Press, 1990, pp 131–133.

Paine RS, Oppe TE: Neurologic examination of children. Clin Dev Med 20/21, 1966.

Painter MJ, Alvin J: Choice of anticonvulsants in the treatment of neonatal seizures. *In* Wasterlain CG, Vert P (Eds): Neonatal Seizures. New York, Raven Press, 1990, pp 243–256.

Painter MJ, Bergman I: Obstetrical trauma to the neonatal central and peripheral nervous system. Semin Perinatol 6:89, 1982.

Painter MJ, Scher MS, Paneth NS, et al: Randomized trial of phenobarbital v. phenytoin treatment of neonatal seizures. Pediatr Res (in press).

Palma PA, Miner ME, Morriss FH, et al: Intraventricular hemorrhage in the newborn born at term. Am J Dis Child 133:941, 1979.

Paneth N: The causes of cerebral palsy: Recent evidence. Clin Invest Med 16:95, 1993.

Paneth N, Pinto-Martin J, Gardiner J, et al: Incidence and timing of germinal matrix/intraventricular hemorrhage in low birth weight infants. Am J Epidemiol 137:1167, 1993.

Papasian CJ, Parker JC: Bacterial and fungal infections. *In* Duckett S (Ed): Pediatric Neuropathology. Baltimore, Williams & Wilkins, 1995, pp 352–373.

Pape KE, Wigglesworth JS: Haemorrhage, Ischaemia and the Perinatal Brain. Philadelphia, JB Lippincott, 1979.

Papile LA, Burstein J, Burstein R, et al: Incidence and evolution of subependymal and intraventricular hemorrhage: A study of infants with birth weights less than 1,500 gm. J Pediatr 92:529, 1978a.

Papile LA, Burstein J, Burstein R, et al: Relationship of intravenous sodium bicarbonate infusions and cerebral intraventricular hemorrhage. J Pediatr 93:834, 1978b.

Papile LA, Burstein J, Burstein R, et al: Posthemorrhagic hydrocephalus in low-birth-weight infants: Treatment by serial lumbar punctures. J Pediatr 97:273, 1980.

Papile LA, Munsick-Bruno G, Schaefer A: The relationship of cerebral intraventricular hemorrhage and early childhood neurologic handicaps. J Pediatr 103:273, 1983.

Pasternak JF, Groothuis DR, Fischer JM, et al: Regional cerebral blood flow in the beagle model of neonatal intraventricular hemorrhage: Studies during systemic hypertension. Neurology 33:559, 1983.

Patel PI, Lupski JR: Charcot-Marie-Tooth disease: A new paradigm for the mechanism of inherited disease. Trends Genet 10:128, 1994.

Patt A, Horesh IR, Berger EM, et al: Iron depletion or chelation reduces ischemia/reperfusion-induced edema in gerbil brains. J Pediatr Surg 25:224, 1990.

Pegelow CH, Ledford M, Young JN, et al: Severe protein S deficiency in a newborn. Pediatrics 89:674, 1992.

Perlman JM, Goodman S, Kreusser KL, et al: Reduction in intraventricular hemorrhage by elimination of fluctuating cerebral blood flow velocity in preterm infants with respiratory distress syndrome. N Engl J Med 312:1353, 1985.

Perlman JM, McMenamin JB, Volpe JJ: Fluctuating cerebral blood flow velocity in respiratory distress syndrome. N Engl J Med 309:204, 1983.

Perlman JM, Risser R, Broyles RS: Bilateral cystic periventricular leukomalacia in the premature infant: Associated risk factors. Pediatrics 97:822, 1996.

Perlman JM, Volpe JJ: Episodes of apnea and bradycardia in the preterm newborn: Impact on cerebral circulation. Pediatrics 76:333, 1985a.

Perlman JM, Volpe JJ: Seizures in the preterm infant: Effects on cerebral blood flow velocity, intracranial pressure, and arterial blood pressure. J Pediatr 102:288, 1985b.

Perlman JM, Volpe JJ: Intraventricular hemorrhage in extremely small premature infants. Am J Dis Child 140:1122, 1986.

Philip AG, Allan WC, Tito AM, et al: Intraventricular hemorrhage in preterm infants: Declining incidence in the 1980's. Pediatrics 84:797, 1989.

Phillips SJ, Agafe FJ, Silverman WA, et al: Autonomic cardiac reactivity in premature infants. Biol Neonate 6:225, 1964.

Pidcock FS, Graziani LJ, Stanley C, et al: Neurosonographic features of periventricular echodensities associated with cerebral palsy in preterm infants. J Pediatr 116:417, 1990.

Pinar MH, Edwards WH, Fratkin J, et al: A transmission electron microscopy study of human cerebral cortical and germinal matrix (GM) blood vessels in premature newborns (abstract). Pediatr Res 19:394, 1985.

Pinheiro JMB, Furdon S, Ochoa LF: Role of local anesthesia during lumbar puncture in newborns. Pediatrics 91:379, 1993.

Pou S, Pou WS, Bredt DS, et al: Generation of superoxide by purified brain nitric oxide synthase. J Biol Chem 267:24173, 1992.

Prechtl H: The Neurological Examination of the Full Term Newborn Infant, 2nd ed. London, Spastics International Medical Publications, 1977.

Provisional Committee for Quality Improvement and Subcommittee on Hyperbilirubinemia, American Academy of Pediatrics: Practice parameter: Management of hyperbilirubinemia in the healthy term newborn. Pediatrics 94:558, 1994.

Pryds O, Christensen NJ, Friis-Hansen B: Increased cerebral blood flow and plasma epinephrine in hypoglycemic, preterm newborns. Pediatrics 85:172, 1990a.

Pryds O, Greisen G, Lou H, et al: Heterogeneity of cerebral vasoreactivity in preterm infants supported by mechanical ventilation. J Pediatr 115:638, 1989.

Pryds O, Greisen G, Lou H, et al: Vasoparalysis associated with brain damage in asphyxiated term infants. J Pediatr 117:119, 1990b.

Quattlebaum TG: Benign familial convulsions in the neonatal period and early infancy. J Pediatr 95:257, 1979.

Raemakers VT, Casaer P, Daniels H, et al: Upper limits of brain blood flow autoregulation in stable infants of various conceptional age. Early Hum Dev 24:249, 1990.

Raju TN: Cerebral Doppler studies in the fetus and newborn infant. J Pediatr 119:165, 1991.

Rammohan KW, Farooqui AA, Horrocks LA: Neurochemical effects of viral infections in the central nervous system. *In* McCandless DW (Ed): Cerebral Energy Metabolism and Metabolic Encephalopathy. New York, Plenum Press, 1985, pp 433–445.

Rapaport SI: Blood-Brain Barrier in Physiology and Medicine. New York, Raven Press, 1976.

Rea PA, Crowe J, Wickramasinghe Y, et al: Non-invasive optical methods for the study of cerebral metabolism in the human newborn: A technique for the future? J Med Eng Technol 9:160, 1985.

Reigel DH, Rotenstein D: Spina bifida. *In* Cheek WR (Ed): Pediatric Neurosurgery: Surgery of the Developing Nervous System. Philadelphia, WB Saunders, 1994, pp 51–76.

Rekate HL: Treatment of hydrocephalus. *In* Cheek WR (Ed): Pediatric Neurosurgery: Surgery of the Developing Nervous System. Philadelphia, WB Saunders, 1994, pp 202–220.

Rettwitz-Volk W, Fiedler A, Horn M: Intrauterine tachycardia and periventricular leukomalacia. Am J Perinatol 10:212, 1993.

Richardson BS: Metabolism of the fetal brain: Biological and pathological development. *In* Hanson MA (Ed): The Fetal and Neonatal Brain Stem. New York, Cambridge University Press, 1991, pp 87–105.

Richardson BS, Carmichael L, Homan J, et al: Regional blood flow change in the lamb during the perinatal period. Am J Obstet Gynecol 160:919, 1989.

Robertson C, Finer N: Term infants with hypoxic-ischemic encephalopathy: Outcome at 3.5 years. Dev Med Child Neurol 27:473, 1985.

Roffwarg HP, Muzio JN, Dement WC: Ontogenetic development of the human sleep-dream cycle. Science 152:604, 1966.

Ronen GM, Rosales TO, Connolly M, et al: Seizure characteristics in chromosome 20 benign familial neonatal convulsions. Neurology 43:1355, 1993.

Rorke LB: Pathology of Perinatal Brain Injury. New York, Raven Press, 1982.

Rorke LB: Anatomical features of the developing brain implicated in pathogenesis of hypoxic-ischemic injury. Brain Pathol 2:211, 1992.

Rose AL, Lombroso CT: Neonatal seizure states. Pediatrics 45:404, 1970.

Rosenberg AA: Regulation of cerebral blood flow after asphyxia in neonatal lambs. Stroke 19:239, 1988.

Rosenberg AA, Jones MD, Traystman RJ, et al: Response of cerebral blood flow to changes in pCO$_2$ in fetal, newborn, and adult sheep. Am J Physiol 242:H862, 1982.

Rothman SM: Biochemistry of hypoxic-ischemic brain injury. *In* Polin RA, Fox WW (Eds): Fetal and Neonatal Physiology. Philadelphia, WB Saunders, 1992, pp 1608–1613.

Rudolph AM, Heymann MA: Circulatory changes during growth in the fetal lamb. Cir Res 26:289, 1970.

Rumack CM, Guggenheim MA, Rumack BH, et al: Neonatal intracranial hemorrhage and maternal use of aspirin. Obstet Gynecol 58:52S, 1981.

Russman BS, Schwartz RC: Neuromuscular diseases of childhood. Curr Opin Pediatr 5:669, 1993.

Sainte-Rose C, Piatt JH, Pierre-Kahn A, et al: Mechanical complications in shunts. Pediatr Neurosurg 17:2, 1991–1992.

Salfield AW, Lorber J, Lonton T: Isosorbide in the management of infantile hydrocephalus. Arch Dis Child 56:806, 1981.

Sarnat H, Sarnat M: Neonatal encephalopathy following fetal distress. Arch Neurol 33:696, 1976.

Saudubray J-M, Carpentier C: Clinical phenotypes: Diagnosis/algorithms. *In* Scriver CR, Beaudet AL, Sly WS, Valle D (Eds): The Metabolic and Molecular Bases of Inherited Disease, Vol I, 7th ed. New York, McGraw-Hill, 1995, pp 327–400.

Scher MS: Pediatric electroencephalography and evoked potentials. *In* Swaiman KF (Ed): Pediatric Neurology: Principles and Practices. St. Louis, CV Mosby, 1989, pp 67–103.

Scher MS, Aso K, Beggarly ME, et al: Electrographic seizures in preterm and full-term newborns: Clinical correlates, associated brain lesions, and risk for neurologic sequelae. Pediatrics 91:128, 1993.

Scher MS, Beggarly M: Clinical significance of focal periodic discharges in newborns. J Child Neurol 4:175, 1989.

Scher MS, Belfar H, Martin J, et al: Destructive brain lesions of presumed fetal onset: Antepartum causes of cerebral palsy. Pediatrics 88:898, 1991.

Scher MS, Wright FS, Lockman LA, et al: Intraventricular hemorrhage in the full-term newborn. Arch Neurol 39:769, 1982.

Schmorl G: Zur Kenntnis des Ikterus neonatorum, insbesondere der dabei auf tretenden Gehirnveraenderungen. Verh D Detsch Pathol Ges 6:109, 1903.

Schulte FJ: Neonatal convulsions and their relation to epilepsy in early childhood. Dev Med Child Neurol 8:381, 1966.

Schum TR, Meyer GA, Grausz JP, et al: Neonatal intraventricular hemorrhage due to an intracranial arteriovenous malformation: A case report. Pediatrics 64:242, 1979.

Schutta HS, Johnson L, Neville HE: Mitochondrial abnormalities in bilirubin encephalopathy. J Neuropathol Neurol 29:296, 1970.

Serfontein GL, Rom S, Stein S: Posterior fossa subdural hemorrhage in the newborn. Pediatrics 65:40, 1980.

Sever JWL: Obstetric paralysis. Am J Dis Child 12:541, 1916.

Shankaran S, Cepeda E, Ilagan N, et al: Antenatal phenobarbital for the prevention of neonatal intracerebral hemorrhage. Am J Obstet Gynecol 154:53, 1986.

Shankaran S, Koepke T, Woldt E, et al: Outcome after posthemorrhagic ventriculomegaly in comparison with mild hemorrhage without ventriculomegaly. J Pediatr 114:109, 1989.

Shapiro NL, Cunningham MJ, Parikh SR, et al: Congenital unilateral facial paralysis. Pediatrics 97:261, 1996.

Sharpe W: The operative treatment of brachial plexus paralysis. JAMA 66:876, 1916.

Shaywitz BA: Epidermoid spinal cord tumors and previous lumbar puncture. J Pediatr 80:638, 1972.

Sherrington CS, Creed RS, Denny-Brown DE, et al: Reflex Activity of the Spinal Cord. London, Oxford University Press, 1932.

Shinnar S, Gammon K, Bergman EW, et al: Management of hydrocephalus in infancy: Use of acetazolamide and furosemide to avoid cerebrospinal fluid shunts. J Pediatr 107:31, 1985.

Shinnar S, Molteni RA, Gammon K, et al: Intraventricular hemorrhage in the preterm infant: A changing outlook. N Engl J Med 306:1464, 1982.

Shuman RM, Selednik LJ: Periventricular leukomalacia: A one-year autopsy study. Arch Neurol 37:231, 1980.

Sidransky E, Sherer DM, Ginns EI: Gaucher disease in the newborn: A distinct Gaucher phenotype is analogous to a mouse model created by targeted disruption of the glucocerebrosidase gene. Pediatr Res 32:494, 1992.

Sinclair JC, Fox HJ, Lentz JF: Intoxication of the fetus by a local anesthetic: A newly recognized complication of maternal and caudal anesthesia. N Engl J Med 273:1173, 1965.

Singer LT, Yamashita TS, Hawkins S, et al: Increased incidence of intraventricular hemorrhage and developmental delay in cocaine-exposed, very low birth weight infants. J Pediatr 124:765, 1994.

Skouteli HN, Dubowitz LMS, Levene MI, et al: Predictors for survival and normal neurodevelopmental outcome of infants weighing less than 1001 grams at birth. Dev Med Child Neurol 27:588, 1985.

Skullerud K, Westra B: Frequency and prognostic significance of germinal matrix hemorrhage, periventricular leukomalacia, and pontosubicular necrosis in preterm newborns. Acta Neuropathol 70:257, 1986.

Smith HL, Amick LD, Sidbury JB Jr: Type II glycogenosis: Report of a case with four-year survival and absence of acid maltase associated with an abnormal glycogen. Am J Dis Child 111:475, 1966.

Soares VM, Brzustowicz LM, Kleyn PW, et al: Refinement of the spinal muscular atrophy locus to the interval between D55435 and MAP1B. Genomics 15:365, 1993.

Sokoloff L: Application of quantitative autoradiography to the measurement of biochemical processes in vivo. *In* Reivich M, Alavi A (Eds): Positron Emission Tomography. New York, Alan R. Liss, 1985, pp 1–42.

Specht EE: Brachial plexus injury in the newborn. Clin Orthop 110:32, 1975.

Speer ME, Blifeld C, Rudolph AJ, et al: Intraventricular hemorrhage and vitamin E in the very low birth weight infant: Evidence for efficacy of early intramuscular vitamin E administration. Pediatrics 74:1107, 1984.

Spellacy WN, Peterson PQ, Winegar A, et al: Neonatal seizures after cesarean delivery: Higher risk with labor. Am J Obstet Gynecol 157:377, 1987.

Sprague JM, Chambers WW: Control of posture by reticular formation and cerebellum in intact, anesthetized and unanesthetized, and in decerebrated cat. Am J Physiol 176:52, 1954.

Stanley CA, Anday EK, Baker L, et al: Metabolic fuel and hormone responses to fasting in newborn infants. Pediatrics 64:613, 1979.

Stapells DR, Kurtzberg D: Evoked potential assessment of auditory system integrity in infants. Clin Perinatol 18:497, 1991.

Starzl TE, Taylor CW, Magoun HW: Collateral afferent excitation of reticular formation of the brain stem. J Neurophysiol 14:479, 1951.

Steiman GS, Rorke LB, Brown MJ: Infantile neuronal degeneration masquerading as Werdnig-Hoffman disease. Ann Neurol 8:317, 1980.

Stem WE, Rand RW: Birth injuries to the spinal cord. Am J Obstet Gynecol 78:498, 1959.

Stewart RM, Williams RS, Lukl P, et al: Ventral porencephaly: A cerebral defect associated with multiple congenital anomalies. Acta Neuropathol (Berl) 42:231, 1978.

Sunshine P: Epidemiology of perinatal asphyxia. *In* Stevenson DK, Sunshine P (Eds): Fetal and Neonatal Brain Injury: Mechanisms, Management, and the Risks of Practice. Philadelphia, BC Decker, 1989, pp 2–11.

Swan JH, Evans MC, Meldrum BS: Ischaemic brain damage: Protection by 2-chloroadenosine, a modulator of excitatory neurotransmission. J Cereb Blood Flow Metab 7(suppl):S145, 1987.

Swick HM: Diseases of gray matter. *In* Swaiman KF (ed): Pediatric Neurology: Principles and Practice. St. Louis, CV Mosby, 1989, pp 777–781.

Szeto HH, Vo TDH, Dwyer G, et al: The ontogeny of fetal lamb electrocortical activity: A power spectral analysis. Am J Obstet Gynecol 153:462, 1985.

Szymonowicz W, Yu VYH, Walker A, et al: Reduction in periventricular haemorrhage in preterm infants. Arch Dis Child 61:661, 1986.

Takashima J, Tanaka K: Microangiography and vascular permeability of the subependymal matrix in the premature infant. Can J Neurol Sci 5:45, 1978.

Takashima S, Armstrong D, Becker LE: Subcortical leukomalacia: Relationship to development of cerebral sulcus and its vascular supply. Arch Neurol 35:470, 1978.

Tan WKM, Williams CE, Gunn AJ, et al: Pretreatment with monosialoganglioside GM1 protects the brain of fetal sheep against hypoxic-ischemic injury without causing systemic compromise. Pediatr Res 34:18, 1993.

Ter-Pogossian MM: Positron emission tomography instrumentation. *In* Reivich M, Alavi A (Eds): Positron Emission Tomography. New York, Alan R. Liss, 1985, pp 43–61.

Terzis JK, Liberson WT, Levine R: Our experience in obstetrical brachial plexus palsy. *In* Terzis J (Ed): Microreconstruction of Nerve Injuries. Philadelphia, WB Saunders, 1987, pp 513–528.

Tharp BR: Neonatal and pediatric electroencephalography. *In* Aminoff MJ (Ed): Electrodiagnosis in Clinical Neurology. New York, Churchill-Livingstone, 1980, pp 67–117.

Tharp BR, Cukier F, Monod N: The prognostic value of the electroencephalogram in premature infants. Electroencephalogr Clin Neurophysiol 51:219, 1981.

Tharp BR, Scher MS, Clancy RR: Serial EEGs in normal and abnormal infants with birth weights less than 1200 grams—a prospective study with long term follow-up. Neuropediatrics 20:64, 1989.

Thompson JA, Glasgow LA, Warpinski JR, et al: Infant botulism: Clinical spectrum and epidemiology. Pediatrics 66:936, 1980.

Toda T, Segawa M, Nomura Y, et al: Localization of a gene for Fukuyama type congenital muscular dystrophy to chromosome 9q31-33. Nat Genet 5:283, 1993.

Todo T, Usui M, Takakura K: Treatment of severe intraventricular hemorrhage by intraventricular infusion of urokinase. J Neurosurg 74:81, 1991.

Torfs CP, van den Berg BJ, Oechsli FW, et al: Prenatal and perinatal factors in the etiology of cerebral palsy. J Pediatr 116:615, 1990.

Torres F, Anderson C: The normal EEG of the human newborn. J Clin Neurophysiol 2:89, 1985.

Towbin A: Cerebral intraventricular hemorrhage and subependymal matrix infarction in the fetus and premature newborn. Am J Pathol 52:121, 1968.

Towfighi J, Sassani JW, Suzuki K, et al: Cerebro-ocular-dysplasia–muscular dystrophy (COD-MD) syndrome. Acta Neuropathol 65:110, 1984.

Tritschler JH, Bonilla E, Lombes A, et al: Differential diagnosis of fatal and benign cytochrome c oxidase-deficient myopathies of infancy. Neurology 41:300, 1991.

Trommer BL, Groothuis DR, Pasternak JF: Quantitative analysis of cerebral vessels in the newborn puppy: The structure of germinal matrix vessels may predispose to hemorrhage. Pediatr Res 22:23, 1987.

Turnbull DM, Bartlett K, Stevens DL, et al: Short-chain acyl-CoA dehydrogenase deficiency associated with a lipid-storage myopathy and secondary carnitine deficiency. N Engl J Med 311:1232, 1984.

Urabe F, Matsuishi T, Kojima K, et al: MR imaging of birth brachial palsy in a two-month-old infant. Brain Dev 13:130, 1991.

Van De Bor M, Van Bel F, Lineman R, et al: Perinatal factors and periventricular-intraventricular hemorrhage in preterm infants. Am J Dis Child 140:1125, 1986.

Van De Bor M, Walther FJ: Cerebral blood flow velocity regulation in preterm infants. Biol Neonate 59:329, 1991.

Vannucci RC: Current and potentially new management strategies for perinatal hypoxic-ischemic encephalopathy. Pediatrics 85:961, 1990a.

Vannucci RC: Experimental biology of cerebral hypoxia-ischemia: Relation to perinatal brain damage. Pediatr Res 27:317, 1990b.

Vaughan VC III, Allen FH Jr, Diamond LK: Erythroblastosis fetalis: IV. Further observations on kernicterus. Pediatrics 6:706, 1950.

Venkatesh S, Coulter DL, Kemper TD: Neuroaxonal dystrophy at birth with hypertonicity and basal ganglia mineralization. J Child Neurol 9:74, 1994.

Vogt C, Vogt O: Die nosologische Stellung des Status marmoratus des Striatum. Psychiatr Neurol Wochenschr (Halle) 28:85, 1926.

Volpe JJ: Neonatal seizures. N Engl J Med 289:413, 1973.

Volpe JJ: Intraventricular hemorrhage and brain injury in the premature infant: Neuropathology and pathogenesis. Clin Perinatol 16:361, 1989a.

Volpe JJ: Neonatal seizures. Pediatrics 84:422, 1989b.

Volpe JJ: The neurological examination: Normal and abnormal features. *In* Volpe JJ: Neurology of the Newborn, 3rd ed. Philadelphia, WB Saunders, 1995a, pp 95–124.

Volpe JJ: Specialized studies in the neurological evaluation. *In* Volpe JJ: Neurology of the Newborn, 3rd ed. Philadelphia, WB Saunders, 1995b, pp 125–171.

Volpe JJ: Hypoxic-ischemic encephalopathy: Clinical aspects. *In* Volpe JJ: Neurology of the Newborn, 3rd ed. Philadelphia, WB Saunders, 1995c, pp 314–372.

Volpe JJ: Hypoxic-ischemic encephalopathy: Neuropathology and pathogenesis. *In* Volpe JJ: Neurology of the Newborn, 3rd ed. Philadelphia, WB Saunders, 1995d, pp 279–313.

Volpe JJ: Intracranial hemorrhage: Germinal matrix—intraventricular hemorrhage of the premature infant. *In* Volpe JJ: Neurology of the Newborn, 3rd ed. Philadelphia, WB Saunders, 1995e, pp 403–463.

Volpe JJ: Intracranial hemorrhage. *In* Volpe JJ: Neurology of the Newborn, 3rd ed. Philadelphia, WB Saunders, 1995f, pp 373–402.

Volpe JJ, Herscovitch P, Perlman JM, et al: Positron emission tomography in the newborn: Extensive impairment of regional cerebral blood flow with intraventricular hemorrhage and hemorrhagic intracerebral involvement. Pediatrics 72:589, 1983.

von Siebenthal K, Bernert G, Casaer P: Near-infrared spectroscopy in newborn infants. Brain Dev 14:135, 1992.

Vyhmeister N, Schneider S, Cha C: Cranial transillumination norms of the premature infant. J Pediatr 91:980, 1977.

Wadman SK, Duran M, Breemer FA, et al: Absence of hepatic molybdenum cofactor: An inborn error of metabolism leading to a combined deficiency of sulphite oxidase and xanthine dehydrogenase. J Inherit Metab Dis 6:78, 1983.

Wallen LD: Developmental physiology of the fetus and newborn and physiologic changes related to birth, cerebral adaptation, and apnea. Curr Opin Pediatr 4:200, 1992.

Wallgren G, Baur M, Rudhe U: Hemodynamic studies of induced hypo- and hypervolemia in the newborn infant. Acta Paediatr 53:1, 1964.

Wallin LA, Rosenfeld CR, Laptook AR, et al: Neonatal intracranial hemorrhage: II. Risk factor analysis in an inborn population. Early Hum Dev 23:129, 1990.

Wehberg K, Vincent M, Garrison B, et al: Intraventricular hemorrhage in the full-term newborn associated with abdominal compression. Pediatrics 89:327, 1992.

Welch K: The intracranial pressure in infants. J Neurosurg 52:693, 1980.

Wennberg RP, Hance AJ: Experimental bilirubin encephalopathy: Importance of total protein, protein binding, and blood brain barrier. Pediatr Res 20:789, 1986.

Whitelaw A, Placzek M, Dubowitz L, et al: Phenobarbitone for prevention of periventricular haemorrhage in very low birth weight infants: A randomized, double-blind, trial. Lancet 2:1168, 1983.

Whitelaw A, Rivers RP, Creighton L, et al: Low dose intraventricular fibrinolytic treatment to prevent posthaemorrhagic hydrocephalus. Arch Dis Child 67:12, 1992.

Wieloch T: Hypoglycemia-induced neuronal damage prevented by an N-methyl-D-aspartate antagonist. Science 230:681, 1985.

Williams CE, Gunn AJ, Mallard EC, et al: Outcome after ischemia in the developing sheep brain: An electroencephalographic and histological study. Ann Neurol 31:14, 1992.

Williamson W, Demmler G, Percy A, et al: Progressive hearing loss in infants with asymptomatic congenital cytomegalovirus infection. Pediatrics 90:862, 1992.

Williamson WD, Desmond MM, Wilson GW, et al: Early neurodevelopmental outcome of low birth weight infants surviving neonatal intraventricular hemorrhage. J Perinat Med 10:34, 1982.

Wimberley PD, Lou HC, Pedersen H, et al: Hypertensive peaks in the pathogenesis of intraventricular hemorrhage in the newborn: Abolition by phenobarbitone sedation. Acta Paediatr Scand 71:537, 1979.

Wright EA, McWuillen MP: Antibiotic induced neuromuscular blockade. Ann NY Acad Sci 183:358, 1971.

Wyatt JS, Edwards AD, Azzopardi D, et al: Magnetic resonance and near infrared spectroscopy for investigation of perinatal hypoxic-ischaemic brain injury. Arch Dis Child 64:953, 1989.

Yager J, Towfighi J, Vannucci RC: Influence of mild hypothermia on hypoxic-ischemic brain damage in the immature rat. Pediatr Res 34:525, 1993.

Yamashita Y, Goddard-Finegold J, Contant CF, et al: Phenobarbital and cerebral blood flow during hypotension in newborn pigs. Pediatr Res 33:598, 1993.

Yu VYH, Downe L, Astbury J, Bajuk B: Perinatal factors and adverse outcome in extremely low birthweight infants. Arch Dis Child 61:554, 1986.

Zalneraitis EL, Young RSK, Krishnamoorthy KS: Intracranial hemorrhage in utero as a complication of iso-immune thrombocytopenia. J Pediatr 95:611, 1979.

Zancolli EA: Classification and management of the shoulder in birth palsy. Orthop Clin North Am 12:433, 1981.

Zellweger H, Illingworth-Brown B, McCormick WF, et al: A mild form of muscular glycogenosis in two brothers with alpha 1,4-glucosidase deficiency. Ann Paediatr (Basel) 205:413, 1965.

PART XI

GASTROINTESTINAL AND NUTRITIONAL CONDITIONS

CHAPTER 70

Developmental Anatomy and Physiology of the Gastrointestinal Tract

Carol Lynn Berseth

DEVELOPMENTAL PHYSIOLOGY

The gastrointestinal tract is formed as a result of invagination and folding of the embryo as early as the 4th week of gestation. When the buccopharyngeal and cloacal membranes rupture, complete continuity is established between the primitive gastrointestinal tract and the exterior environment. A series of evaginations, elongations, and dilations results in the ultimate formation of the esophagus, stomach, duodenum, liver, and pancreas from the foregut; the jejunum, ileum, and ascending and transverse colon from the midgut; and the descending and rectosigmoid colon from the hindgut. As the gut rapidly elongates during the first trimester, it herniates into the umbilical cord. It re-enters the abdominal cavity and rotates counterclockwise around the superior mesenteric artery and achieves its final position by 20 weeks' gestation (Fig. 70–1). All of the anatomic structures of the gastrointestinal tract are recognizable and well formed by the second trimester. Functional maturation of these structures, however, occurs well after anatomic maturation. Many functions are still immature at birth in the term infant and are not established until 2 to 4 years of age (Table 70–1).

Maturation and growth of the gastrointestinal tract are regulated by genetic endowment, the biologic clock, endogenous events such as the release of hormones, and exposure to exogenous factors such as amniotic fluid or enteral feedings (Lebenthal and Lee, 1983). As a result of continuity of the gastrointestinal tract to the intrauterine environment, the fetal gut is bathed in amniotic fluid as early as 4 weeks' postconceptual age. By 20 weeks, 15 mL of amniotic fluid traverses the fetal gut; this volume rapidly increases to 400 to 500 mL by term. Amniotic fluid contains nutrients as well as hormones and growth factors that may provide stimulation for maturation. Functional maturation occurs along axes directed proximodistally and aborally. Concurrently, vascular and neural structures migrate with similar axes to support and regulate intestinal function. Vascular supply is provided by the celiac, superior mesenteric, and inferior mesenteric arteries. Enteric neurons are derived from neuroblasts that originate in the vagal region of the neural crest and migrate along the gastrointestinal tract with the descending fibers of the vagus nerve. Because structural development appears to develop asynchronously with functional development, a brief review of structural development precedes a description of functional development.

Oropharynx and Esophagus

Non-nutritive sucking begins at approximately 20 weeks' gestation (Herbst, 1983). It is characterized by mouthing movements that may or may not be coordinated with swallowing. Nutritive sucking, which does not appear until 32 to 34 weeks' gestation, consists of prolonged bursts of sucking that contain swallows. Superficial glands are present in the pharyngeal and esophageal mucosa by 20 weeks and squamous cells by 28 weeks. Mucous and lingual lipase are also secreted. The upper esophageal sphincter is present by 32 weeks. The neuroblasts and circular muscle throughout the body of the esophagus appear by the end of the first trimester, and esophageal peristalsis is present in the preterm infant. More immature infants, however, display nonperistalic tertiary peristalsis, which gradually decreases with postnatal age.

The lower esophageal sphincter, which is responsible for preventing reflux of gastric content, is a 0.6- to 1-cm area of increased muscular tone located in the distal esophageus. Its tone is regulated by vagal and sympathetic nerves. Lower esophageal sphincter basal pressures range from 20 to 40 mm Hg in term infants and as low as 5 mm Hg in infants born at 27 weeks' gestation (Newell et al, 1988).

Stomach

The structure of the stomach is well established by 6 weeks; the circular and longitudinal muscles appear by 9 weeks; and the endocrine, chief, mucus, and parietal cells appear by 12 weeks. By 16 weeks, all of these latter cells are secreting hydrochloric acid, intrinsic factor, pepsin, gastrin, and mucus. Although acid secretion is present shortly after birth in preterm and term infants, it is approximately 10% of that seen in adults. Adult values are achieved by 3 months' postnatal age. Acid secretion is less in preterm infants compared to term infants (Fig. 70–2). Gastric emptying is slower in preterm infants compared to term infants (Cavell, 1979). The method of feeding may also alter gastric emptying in preterm infants. Moreover gastric emptying may be delayed by the presence of some nutrients such as casein, medium-chain triglycerides, or diluted formula.

Pancreas

The rotation and fusion of the dorsal and ventral buds of the pancreas are complete by 7 weeks. Differentiation of

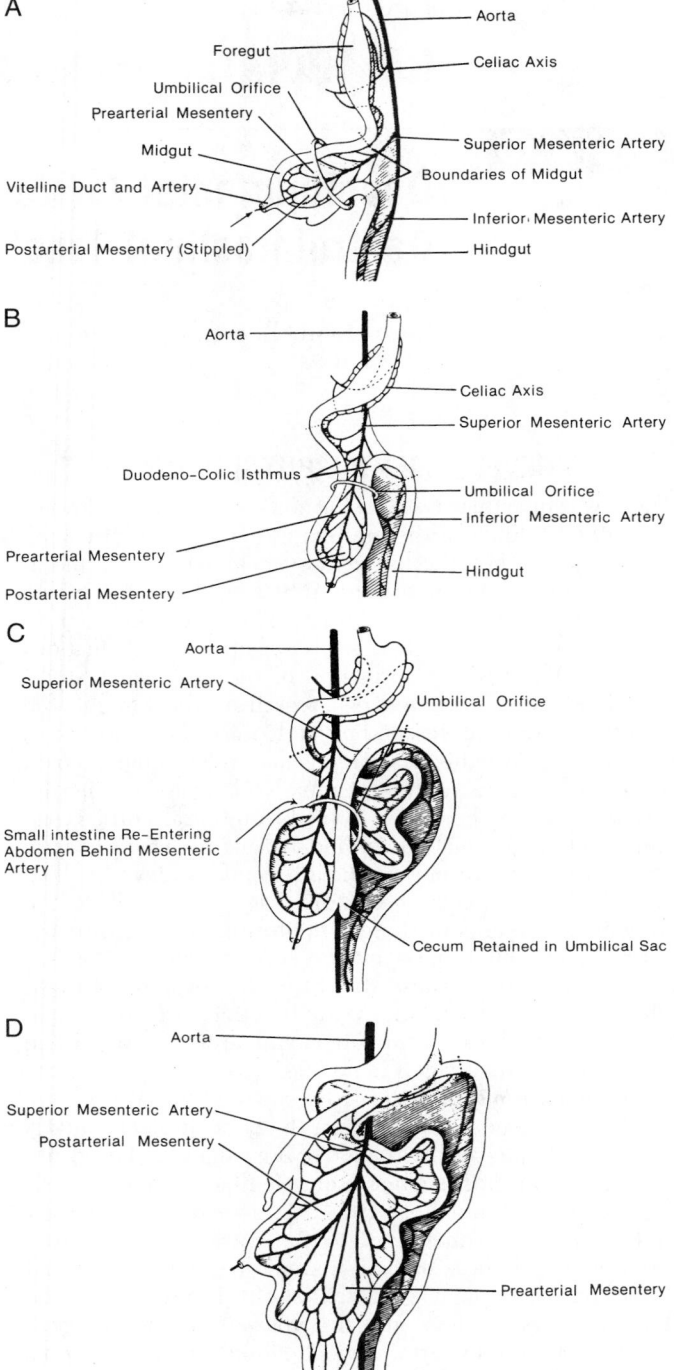

FIGURE 70–1. Diagram showing normal rotation of alimentary tract. *A*, Fifth week of intrauterine life (lateral view). The foregut, midgut, and hindgut are shown with their individual blood supply supported by the common dorsal mesentery in the sagittal plane. The midgut loop has been extruded into the umbilical cord. *B*, Eighth week of intrauterine life (anterioposterior view). The first stage of rotation is being completed. Note the narrow duodeno-colic isthmus from which the midgut loop depends and the right-sided position of the small intestine and left-sided position of the colon. Maintenance of this position within the abdomen after birth is termed *nonrotation*. *C*, About the 10th week of intrauterine life, during the second stage of rotation (anterior-posterior view). The bowel in the temporary umbilical hernia is in the process of reduction; the most proximal part of the prearterial segment entering the abdomen to the right of the superior mesenteric artery is held forward close to the cecum and ascending colon, permitting the bowel to pass under it. As the coils of small intestine collect within the abdomen, the hindgut is displaced to the left and upward. *D*, Eleventh week of intrauterine life at the end of the second stage of rotation. From its original sagittal position, the midgut has rotated 270 degrees in a counterclockwise direction about the origin of the superior mesenteric artery. The essentials of the permanent disposition of the viscera have been attained. (*A* to *D* from Gardner CE Jr, Hart D: Arch Surg 29:942, 1934. Copyright 1934, American Medical Association.)

the endocrine and exocrine structure is present by 14 weeks. Pancreatic zymogen granules are detected in the acini by 14 weeks, as is immunoreactive insulin. By 16 weeks, amylase is present. Trypsin, lipase, and amylase are secreted into the duodenum by 31 weeks (Zoppi et al, 1972). Concentrations of these enzymes are lower in preterm than term infants and, in turn, are significantly lower in term infants than children (Fig. 70–3). Postnatally, trypsin increases in concentration, followed by chymotrypsin, carboxypeptidase, lipase, and amylase (Lebenthal and Lee,

1980). Postprandial release of these enzymes is initially blunted at birth and cannot be stimulated by specific nutrients. For example, high-protein diets can increase trypsin and lipase secretion, but a high-fat diet does not stimulate lipase secretion (Zoppi et al, 1972).

Liver

The liver is derived as an outbudding from the duodenum. The cranial portion of the bud differentiates into hepatic

TABLE 70–1

Anatomic and Functional Maturation of the Gastrointestinal Tract

			Postconceptual Age, weeks			
10	**15**	**20**	**25**	**30**	**35**	**40**
Mouth	Salivary glands	Swallow		Lingual lipase	*Sucking*	
Esophagus	Muscle layers present	Striated epithelium present		*Poor lower esophageal sphincter tone*		
Stomach	Gastric glands present	G cells appear		*Gastric secretions present*	*Slow gastric emptying*	°
Pancreas	Exocrine and endocrine tissue differentiate	Zymogen present		*Reduced trypsin, lipase*		°
Liver	Lobules form	*Bile secreted*		*Fatty acids absorbed*		°
Intestine	Crypt and villus form	*Glucose transport present*		*Dipeptidase, sucrase, and maltase active*	*Lactase active*	
Colon		Crypts and villi recede			*Meconium passed*	

°Full functional maturation occurs postnatally.
Italics = Functional maturation.

parenchyma and the caudal portion the gallbladder. Lobules and bile canaliculi are present by 6 weeks; bile acids are synthesized by 12 to 14 weeks, and they are actively secreted by 22 weeks. There are qualitative and quantitative differences in bile acid synthesis in preterm infants. First, bile acid synthesis is decreased in the preterm infant compared to the term infant. Synthesis in the term infant, in turn, is approximately half of that seen in adults (Watkins et al, 1975) (Fig. 70–4). Similarly, bile acid pool size in preterm infants is approximately one third that seen in term infants. Pool size in term infants, in turn, is approximately one half that seen in adults. Hepatic hydroxylation is not fully developed in the fetus, and there is a decreased cholic acid:deoxycholic acid ratio. It has also been noted

that atypical bile acids are present in the fetus; these are formed using fetal biosynthesis pathways. These compounds are not typically seen in adults and represent only a small percentage of bile acids by term (Nakagawa and Setchell, 1990). Thus, it has been suggested that measurement of monohydroxyl bile acids in amniotic fluid may be used as an index of maturity (DeLeze et al, 1978). Degradation of bile salts also differs in preterm infants, in that preterm and term infants rely on taurine conjugation rather than glycine conjugation as in the adult.

Although in vitro studies have previously suggested that the active ileal transport mechanism of bile salts is absent (deBelle et al, 1979), in vivo kinetic studies using isotopes suggest that the transport mechanism is present but immature (Heubi and Balistreri, 1980). Because hepatic uptake, secretion, and transport are impaired in the newborn, serum bile acid concentrations are elevated. These elevated levels persist for 6 to 8 weeks postnatally and slowly decline to adult values by 6 months (Suchy et al, 1981). Because there is immaturity of the hepatic processing of bile salts at multiple sites, newborns are prone to develop cholestasis in response to stresses such as sepsis, mildly hepatotoxic drugs, or exposure to parenteral nutrition.

Small Intestine

By the time the intestine elongates, rotates, and returns to the abdominal cavity, the mucosal and muscular structures are well developed. The crypt and villi structure is present throughout. Because of rapid proliferation of epithelial tissue, the duodenum is transiently obstructed, but it is fully patent by 12 weeks. During the second trimester, the glycocalyx has appeared, and the brush border is structurally well defined. Endocrine cells are well established, and granules containing gastrin, secretin, cholecystokinin, motilin, serotonin, somatostatin, and substance P are present by 12 to 18 weeks. Gastrin, secretin, motilin, and

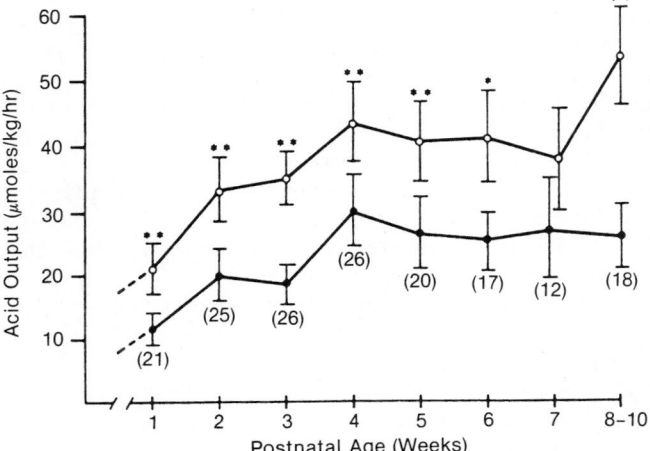

FIGURE 70–2. Basal acid output (●) and pentagastrin-stimulated acid output (○) in preterm infants. Number of subjects studied at each age is given in parentheses. *$P < .05$. **$P < .01$. (From Hyman PE, Clarke DD, Everett SL: Gastric acid secretory function in preterm infants. J Pediatr 106:468, 1985.)

gastrin inhibitory polypeptide are localized to duodenum and jejunum, whereas enteroglucagon, neurotensin, somatostatin, and vasoactive intestinal polypeptide are distributed throughout the intestines. Brush-border membrane function, however, is immature. Although alpha-glucosidases, dipeptidases, and sucrase are functional by the end of the second trimester, lactase does not appear until 32 to 34 weeks' gestation. By 13 to 20 weeks' gestation, sucrase and maltase activities are 50% to 75% of those found in term infants and adults.

Lactase activity is present by 9 weeks (Fig. 70–5). By 24 weeks, however, its activity is still less than 25% of that found in term infants (Antonowicz et al, 1974; Auricchio et al, 1965). The abrupt rise in lactase activity that is noted to occur from 32 to 34 weeks' gestation coincides with

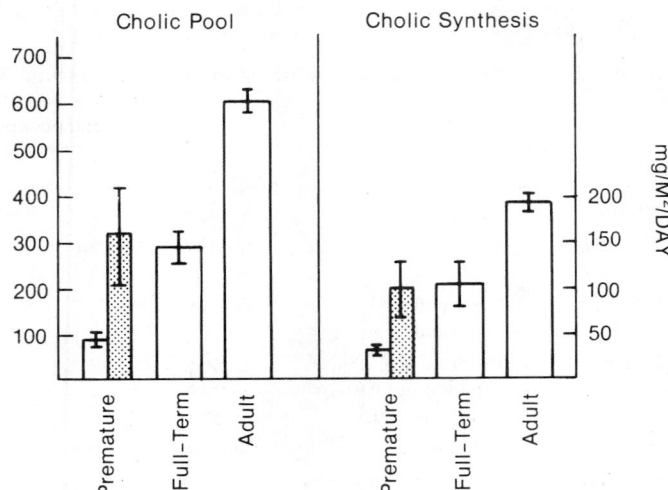

FIGURE 70–4. Comparison of bile acid pool size and synthesis rate in premature infants, full-term infants, and adults, corrected for body surface area. Shaded bars refer to premature infants whose mothers had received prenatal treatment with dexamethasone or phenobarbital. Data are mean ± SE. (Courtesy of Dr. John B. Watkins, Children's Hospital, Philadelphia, PA.) Values for premature infants are from Watkins JB, Szczepanik P, Gould JB, et al: Bile salt metabolism in the premature infant: Preliminary observations of pool size and synthesis rate following prenatal administration of dexamethasone and phenobarbital. Gastroenterology 69:706, 1975; those for term infants are from Watkins JB, Ingall D, Szczepanik P, et al: Bile-salt metabolism in the newborn: Measurement of pool size and synthesis by stable isotope technique. N Engl J Med 288:431, 1973; and those for adults are from Vlahcevic et al, 1971.

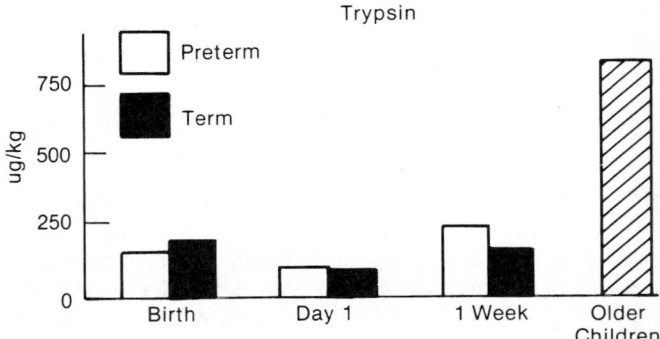

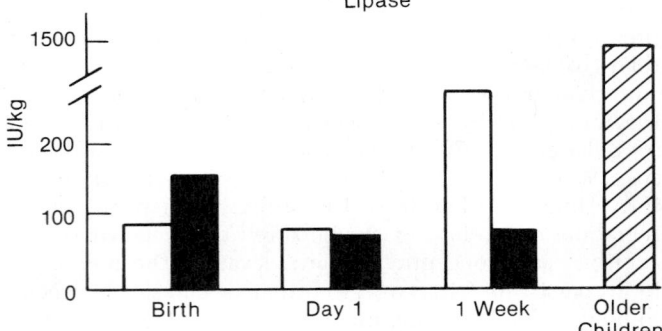

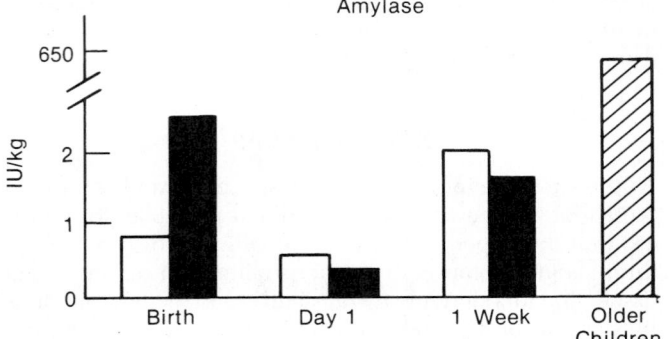

FIGURE 70–3. Pancreatic enzyme activity in preterm (32 to 34 weeks' gestational age) and full-term infants fed a balanced formula. (Data from Zoppi G, Andreotti G, Pajno-Ferrara F, et al: Exocrine pancreas function in premature and term infants. Pediatr Res 6:880, 1972; they represent mean values.)

an increase in lactase mRNA, implying that its delay in appearance is due to transcriptional control (Villa et al, 1992). When lactase first appears, its activity is distributed throughout the small intestine in a uniform manner. Shortly thereafter, a proximal gradient is established (Lacroix et al, 1984). Thus, lactase has been observed to be present in the colon at 13 to 20 weeks' gestation (Ménard and Pothier, 1987).

Sucrase and maltase also are present by 9 weeks' gestation. The activities of these enzymes achieve levels as high as 75% of those found in term infants by the end of the second trimester. Sucrase-isomaltase exists in a single high-molecular-weight form (Triadoru and Zweibaum, 1985). Glucoamylase, which is responsible for absorption of starches and glucose polymers, is present by the end of the second trimester with activities approximately half that found at term (Antonowicz et al, 1974).

There are numerous brush-border peptidases, including alpha-glutamyl transpeptidase, aminopeptidase, oligoaminopeptidase, dipeptidylaminopeptidase IV, and carboxypeptidase. All are present by the end of the second trimester.

Colon

The cecal dilation that forms the hindgut appears by 4 weeks, and by 12 weeks haustra and taeniae appear. When the rotation of the midgut is completed at 12 weeks, the

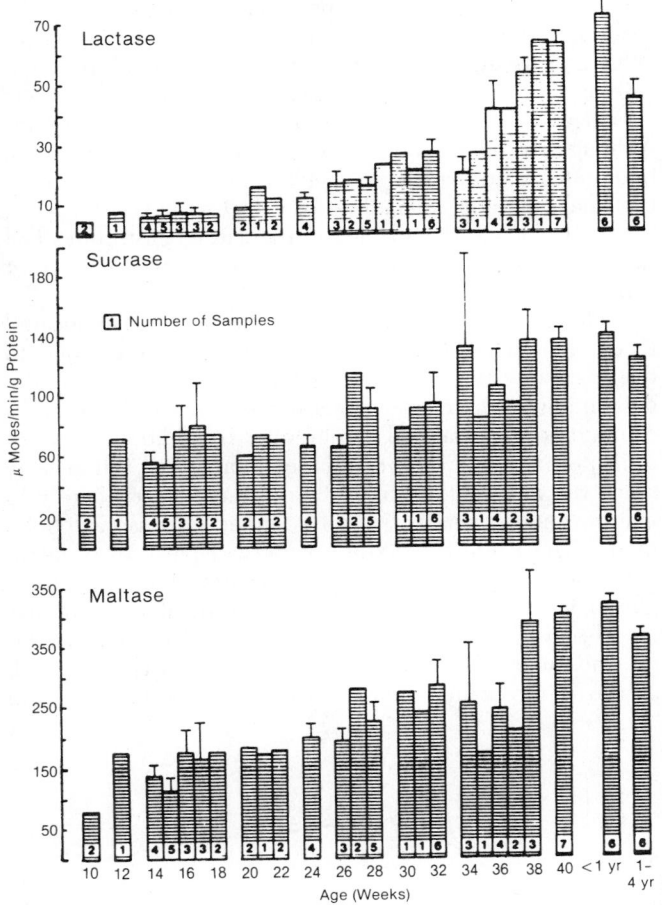

FIGURE 70–5. Developmental patterns of jejunal disaccharidase activities in human fetuses. (From Antonowicz I, Lebenthal E: Developmental pattern of small intestinal enterokinase and disaccharidase activities in the human fetus. Gastroenterology 72:1301, 1977.)

cecum descends into the right iliac fossa. The rectum forms by 8 weeks, and formation of complete muscle layers and neural migration of ganglia cells are accomplished by 24 weeks. Morphologically the premature colon contains villi and crypts and possesses disaccharidase activities until 22 weeks' gestation. Although the villi and disaccharidase activities decrease to disappear by term, sucrase and glucoamylase activities may be present as late as 28 to 32 weeks' gestation (Raul et al, 1986).

Vascularization

Development of the mesenteric circulatory system parallels that of the intestine. Arterial supply occurs as a series of unpaired ventral outbuddings of vessels from the aorta to form the celiac axis, superior mesenteric artery, and inferior mesenteric artery. The celiac trunk originates at the level of T12–L1; passes next to the median arcuate ligament of the diaphragm; and splits to form the splenic, left gastric, and hepatic arteries. Branches of the left gastric artery supply the lesser and greater curvature of the stomach. Vessels from the hepatic artery supply the pancreas and

duodenum. The superior mesenteric artery arises at L1 just caudal to the celiac trunk and supplies flow to the jejunum and ileum. Smaller branches form a series of arcades before entering the wall of the intestine. Therefore, there is considerable collateral flow, and there are additional anastomoses with branches from the inferior mesenteric artery. The inferior mesenteric artery originates at L3 and supplies branches to the colon and rectum. Although there are rich collaterals throughout the gastrointestinal tract, watershed areas of marginal supply exist as in the areas of the distal transverse colon and the upper rectum. In addition, the mucosa has the greatest need for vascular supply because of its high metabolic activity. Thus, it is the layer most sensitive to impairment of blood supply.

There are two points of regulation of mesenteric blood flow, the arteriole and the precapillary sphincter, and there are two levels of control, intrinsic and extrinsic. Intrinsic control by local factors regulates blood flow in response to changes in arterial pressure tissue oxygenation. Vasodilation, for example, occurs in response to occlusion (reactive hyperemia) or feeding (functional hyperemia) and involves tonic changes at both the arteriolar and the precapillary level. Extrinsic regulation is mediated by the splanchnic nerves by sympathetic input. In addition, circulating endogenous and exogenous factors, such as hormones, histamine, and prostaglandins, may modulate vascular tone. There is also present a phenomenon called the *autoregulatory escape* (Shepherd and Granger, 1973). When gut blood flow is decreased by stimulating periarterial mesenteric nerves (i.e., the extrinsic system) or by infusion of norepinephrine, it is restored within minutes by the intrinsic regulation (Shepherd et al, 1973). This escape mechanism is present in newborn swine (Nowicki et al, 1991), as is functional hyperemia (Crissinger and Burney, 1992), and both are presumed to be present in human newborns.

Gastrointestinal Hormones and Peptides

Numerous regulatory gut peptides are produced in the gastrointestinal tract. Several function as true hormones, including gastrin, cholecystokinin, motilin, pancreatic polypeptide, and somatostatin. Others have paracrine or neurocrine function, including gastric inhibitory polypeptide, bombesin, vasoactive intestinal polypeptide, neurotensin, enteroglucagon, and peptide YY. All of these peptides are identified to be present in the fetal intestine by the end of the first trimester. Adult distribution of these peptides may not be established until the end of the third trimester. All of these peptides are present in the plasma of preterm and term infants (Lucas et al, 1980). Of special note is the occurrence of transient hypergastrinemia described in term newborns during the 1st postnatal week (Lucas et al, 1980). It has been postulated that this phenomenon occurs as a result of poor gastric acid secretion (which provides negative feedback on gastrin release), immaturity of the G cell in storing gastrin, and immaturity of systemic inhibitory feedback mechanisms.

In addition to its function in regulating acid secretion, gastrin is a potent trophic factor for the stomach (Lichtenberger and Johnson, 1974). Thus, it has been speculated that neonatal hypergastrinemia serves to promote growth and maturation in the immature stomach. The presence of neonatal hypergastrinemia has not been confirmed by other investigators, however, and there have been no studies in human infants to confirm that gastrin in fact plays a role in regulating gastrointestinal growth. More recently, plasma concentrations of motilin, gastric inhibitory polypeptide, and peptide YY have all been shown to be increased in preterm infants compared to term infants (Berseth, 1992). All of these previous studies have evaluated the plasma concentrations of peptides in the fasting state. Because several of these peptides function as true hormones, more recent studies have evaluated whether these peptides are released in response to feeding. It appears that these hormones are released in response to feeding; however, their releases are limited in the newborn compared to the adult (Fig. 70–6) (Berseth et al, 1992; Lucas et al, 1980). With routine enteral feedings, releases of these peptides become brisker and more intense over the first postnatal month (Berseth, 1992; Lucas et al, 1980).

Neural Regulation

Control of gastrointestinal functions is provided primarily by the enteric nervous system (ENS). The ENS is a subsystem of the autonomic nervous system and is composed of complex neural circuits located within the gut wall. The basic unit of the ENS is the nerve cell, which functions by releasing neurotransmitters to other neurons or to effector cells (i.e., striated or smooth muscle). In general, the neurotransmitter acetylcholine is involved in excitatory synaptic events and norepinephrine in inhibitory synaptic events. Although the central nervous system and the ENS function in an integrated manner to regulate gastrointestinal events, the final common regulation for effectors is via the ENS. Thus, the ENS is capable of regulating gastrointestinal function independent of the central nervous system or spinal nerves.

Enteric neurons originate from the neuroblasts located in the neural crest in the vagal region. They migrate to the gastrointestinal tract along the same pathways as the descending fibers of the vagus nerve. During this process of migration, neural cells proliferate. In addition, they are multipotential and express catecholamines. When they reach the gut wall late in gestation, they differentiate into mature enteric neurons that no longer express catecholamines. The ENS consists of a variety of plexuses of nerve cell bodies and interneuronal circuits. The myenteric plexus is located between the longitudinal and circular muscle layers. The submucosal plexus is located between the muscularis mucosa and the circular muscle layer. All of the differentiated neurons express serotoninergic and

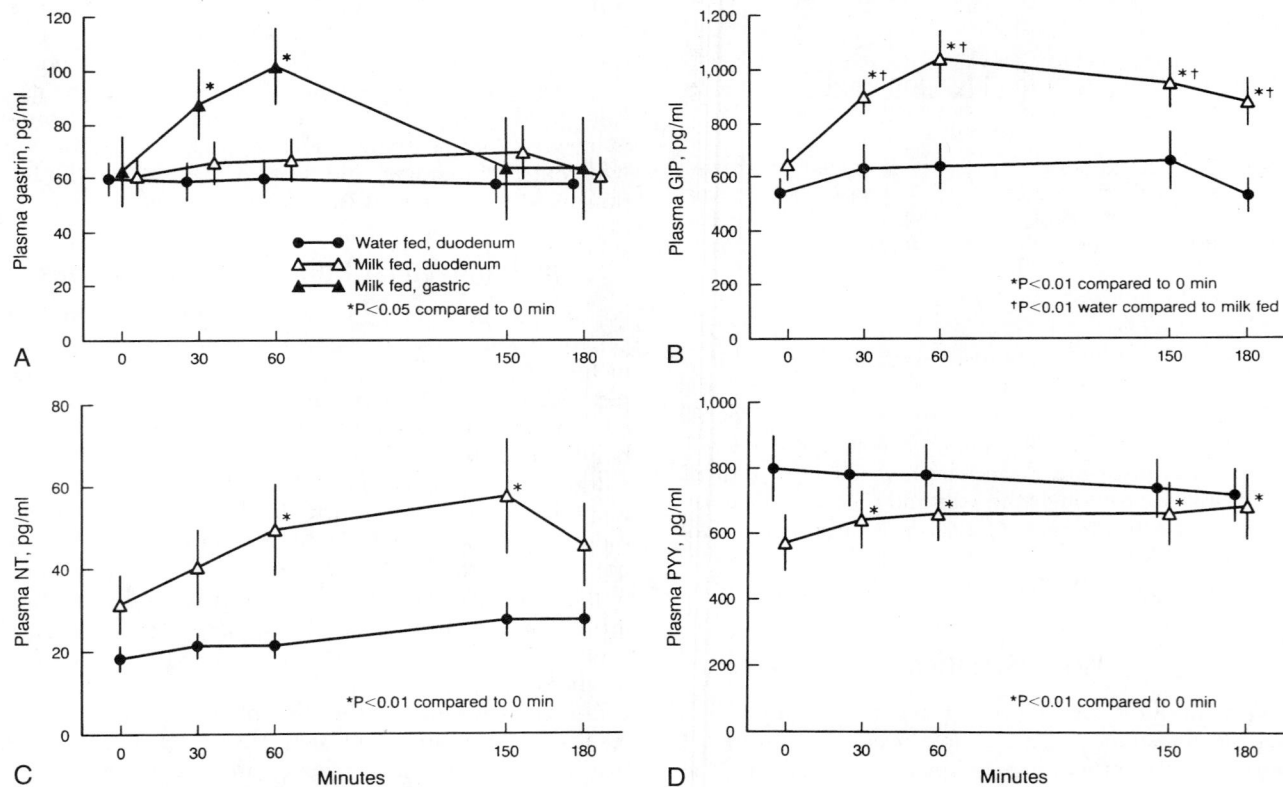

FIGURE 70–6. Plasma concentrations of four gastrointestinal peptides in response to a 2-hour slow infusion feeding. Values for infants fed water intraduodenally (●) and values for infants fed formula intraduodenally △. Plasma concentrations of gastrin *(A)*, gastric inhibitory polypeptide (GIP) *(B)*, neurotensin (NT) *(C)*, and peptide YY (PYY) *(D)* are similar during fasting and postprandial sampling. When infants were fed milk, plasma concentrations of gastrin did not increase with intraduodenal feeding. When feedings were given intragastrically, shown in *A* ▲, plasma gastric concentrations increased significantly over fasting values. (Data summarized in Berseth CL: Responses of gastrointestinal peptides and motor activity to milk and water feedings in preterm and term neonates. Pediatr Res 31:587, 1992.)

peptidergic neurotransmitters, such as serotonin, substance P, and neuropeptide Y. Neurotransmitters are present by immunohistochemical staining by 24 weeks. The adult distribution along the length of the intestine of the transmitters may not be achieved until close to term.

Abnormalities in neural migration are reflected in clinical disease. Neural structures are abnormal in patients with Chagas disease, achalasia, chronic intestinal pseudoobstruction, and Hirschsprung disease (Cohen, 1974; Schuffler and Jonah, 1982). Chemical ablation of myenteric neurons in rats results in hypertrophy of the longitudinal and circular muscle and, subsequently, myoelectric activity (Holle and Forth, 1990). In fetal sheep who have had artificial exteriorization of the bowel in utero to stimulate gastroschisis, profound disruption of the myenteric plexus occurs concurrently with the presence of highly disturbed motility (Holle and Forth, 1990). More recently, an absence of nitric oxide has been demonstrated among infants who have pyloric stenosis and Hirschsprung disease. Nitric oxide is thought to provide inhibitory input to the ENS as a nonadrenergic, noncholinergic neurotransmitter. Hence, its absence results in increased muscle tone.

Host Defenses

Because the gut is in continuity with the neonatal environment, it is constantly exposed to antigens and bacteria. The newborn has a complex series of host defenses that are immune and nonimmune in nature. Many potential antigens and organisms never reach the intestinal mucosa because of the presence of nonimmune host defenses. First, gastric acid and gastric and pancreatic proteases process proteins to form smaller, less allergenic peptides. Second, gastric emptying and intestinal peristalsis prevent stasis of intraluminal materials and actually propel and expel potentially harmful contents. Third, mucus forms a physical barrier and traps glycoproteins, which bind toxins and pathogens, making them unavailable to bind to the intestinal mucosa.

The immune system of host defense is composed of cellular components and secretory components. T cells, B cells, and macrophages are present in the fetal intestine by 20 weeks' gestation. Lymphocytes proliferate in response to a mitogen as early as 12 weeks, and M cells that specialize in the antigenic processing of macromolecules are present by 17 weeks. Antigenic stimulation of lymphoid tissues, however, cannot be demonstrated until 46 weeks. This deficiency is most concerning because the preterm gut absorbs macromolecules directly by pinocytosis. Although plasma immunoglobulin A (IgA) is relatively low in the newborn, secretory IgA is present by 22 weeks' gestation. The newborn intestine has few IgA-producing plasma cells, however, and when preterm infants are fed exogenous protein they are unable to form antibodies (Rieger and Rothberg, 1985).

When an antigen stimulates the host defense system, a variety of soluble proteins regulate growth and differentiation of lymphocytes. These are called *cytokines* and include the interleukins, tumor necrosis factors, interferon, and platelet-activating factor.

Motor Activity

Motor activity is responsible for the forward movement of nutrients throughout the alimentary tract. To feed successfully, there must be coordinated sucking and swallowing, an ability to empty the stomach, coordinated propagation of nutrients through the intestine, and expulsion of waste products from the colon. All of these tasks are achieved by motor activity, which requires intact function of muscle, the nerves that regulate them, and the hormones that modulate their activity.

The muscle layers of the alimentary tract are present by 14 weeks and the nerves and endocrine components by 20 to 24 weeks. Muscle mass is less in the preterm infant than in the term infant, however, and thus forcefulness of contraction is less. This is reflected in lower esophageal sphincter tone in the preterm infant and diminished amplitude of muscle contraction in stomach and duodenum (Berseth, 1992; Ittman et al, 1992). Coordinated activity is also absent, suggestive of an immaturity in neural regulation of motor activity. The sucking mechanism does not appear until 32 to 34 weeks, esophageal peristalsis is diminished before term, gastric emptying is delayed in preterm infants, and migrating activity is often absent in preterm infants. Although most gastrointestinal hormones and peptides are present in the very preterm infant, receptors may not be. For example, gastrin regulation of lower esophageal sphincter tone appears to be impaired (Cohen, 1974), and normal cyclical variation of the hormone motilin does not appear to initiate intestinal migrating activity in the term infant (Jadcherla et al, 1997).

Motor activity in the preterm stomach and intestine has been extensively studied. Gastric emptying requires that antral motor activity and duodenal motor activity be adequate and that their actions be coordinated. Antral motor activity is similar in the 24-week preterm infant and the term infant (Ittman et al, 1992). Duodenal motor activity as well as its coordination with antral activity, however, differs in preterm and term infants. The absence of coordination of antral and duodenal motor activity thus appears to reflect immaturity of duodenal function rather than antral function. In the adult, motor activity cycles through three patterns every 60 to 90 minutes. Often the muscle is still or quiescent for 10 to 20 minutes. This quiescence is then replaced by irregular contractions, which, in turn, are replaced by an episode of intense regular contractions that migrate distally through the bowel. This entire sequence of patterns is called the *interdigestive cycle* (Fig. 70–7). Complete interdigestive cycles are present in term infants (Amarnath et al, 1989). They are rarely seen in preterm infants, however. In extremely premature infants (24 to 28 weeks gestation), unorganized irregular contractions are seen, and little quiescence is present (Berseth, 1992) (Fig. 70–8). In older preterm infants (28 to 32 weeks), motor quiescence begins to appear, and motor activity is organized into short bursts of phasic activity called *clusters* (Baker and Berseth, 1995). In more mature preterm infants (32 to 36 weeks), motor patterns become increasingly more organized, episodes of motor quiescence as well as clusters lengthen (Baker and Berseth, 1995), and migrating activity is occasionally seen (Berseth, 1992).

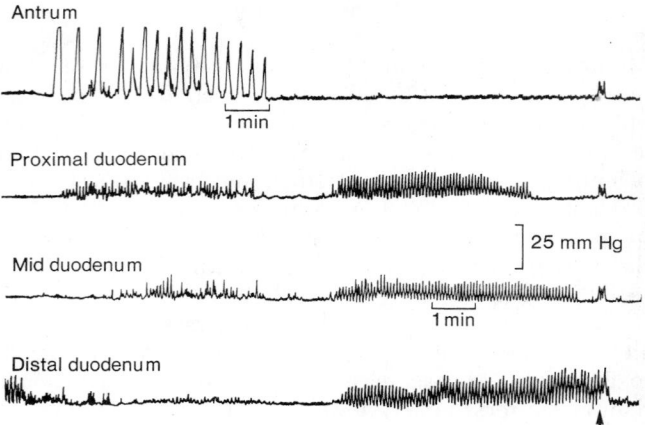

FIGURE 70–7. Migrating motor complex in a term infant. The uppermost line of tracing displays motor contractions recorded from the antrum, and the lower three lines display motor contractions recorded from the duodenum. Phasic activity present in the antrum is temporally associated with the appearance of intense phasic activity that migrates distally to the three duodenal leads. (From Ittman PI, Amarnath R, Berseth CL: Maturation of antroduodenal motor activity in preterm and term infants. Dig Dis Sci 37:14, 1992.)

Gut Flora

The gut is sterile in utero, but colonization begins at birth. The pattern of bacterial growth reflects the maternal and neonatal environment, and enteric bacteria colonize the human infant in an oral-to-anal direction (Rotimi and Duerden, 1981). In healthy infants, aerobic organisms appear within a few hours. Anaerobic organisms are present by 24 hours and increase in number over the first 3 weeks (Cooperstock and Zedd, 1983). Because the route of access of organisms to the intestine is by ingestion, stools of breast milk–fed infants have a predominance of *Bifidobacterium*, whereas stools of formula-fed infants have a predominance of *Bacteroides* and *Clostridium* (Simhon et al, 1982). These organisms are capable of metabolizing bile acids as well as nonabsorbed proteins, lipids, and carbohydrates and thus may potentially play an important role in further processing of nutrients in the preterm newborn. Thus, alterations in gut flora by use of drugs or by shortened bowel length may result in profound intestinal dysfunction.

FUNCTIONAL MATURATION
Digestion of Carbohydrates

Carbohydrates contribute approximately 40% of the caloric intake in healthy term infants. Lactose present in breast milk and formulas is the predominant source of carbohydrate. Some preterm formulas also contain glucose polymers. Although preterm infants have relatively low levels of lactase activity, preterm infants display normal growth with little diarrhea when they are fed lactose-containing milk and formula (MacLean and Fink, 1980). It is speculated that the relative absence of lactase activity is compensated for by the conversion of malabsorbed lactose by colonic bacteria to volatile organic acids, which are subse-

quently absorbed. It is not unusual, however, for stools of breast-fed preterm infants to contain disaccharides. Glucose polymers require amylase for hydrolysis. Because pancreatic amylase levels are quite low, these polymers are likely hydrolyzed by salivary amylase or absorbed directly at the mucosal level via mucosal glucoamylase, which has its maximal activity against polymers with chain lengths of five to nine units (Kerzner et al, 1991). Once lactose and polycose are hydrolyzed to glucose, active glucose transport occurs by 17 weeks via two systems: a low-affinity, high-capacity sodium-glucose cotransport system found along the entire length of the intestines and a low-affinity, high-

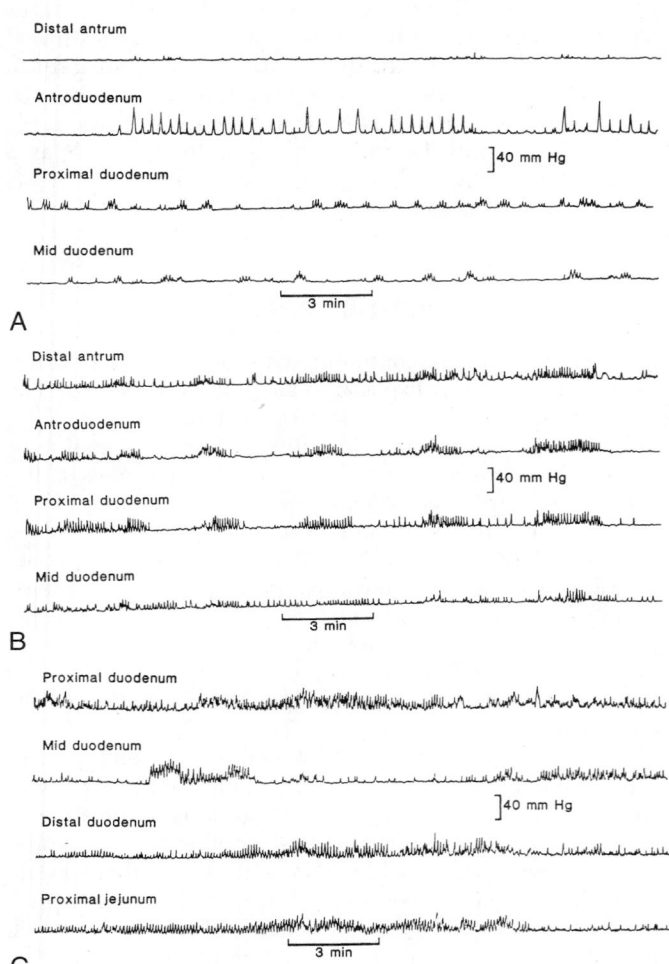

FIGURE 70–8. Serial gastrointestinal manometric tracings from an individual infant at birth (32 weeks) *(A)*, 2 weeks postnatal age (34 weeks) *(B)*, and 4 weeks postnatal age (36 weeks) *(C)*. In *A*, clusters of phasic contractions occur in the two duodenal leads. Clusters are of short duration (approximately 0.75 minutes), have low amplitude (approximately 12 mm Hg), and recur frequently. Two weeks later in the same infant, clusters are present in all leads *(B)*. Individual clusters have a longer duration (approximately 2.5 minutes), have a higher amplitude (approximately 20 mm Hg), and recur less often. At 4 weeks of age in *C*, only one cluster can be displayed because its duration is now prolonged. (From Berseth CL: Gestational evolution of small intestinal motility in preterm and term infants. J Pediatr 115:649, 1989.)

capacity system localized to the proximal small intestine (Malo, 1988).

Digestion of Lipids

Fat provides 50% of the caloric intake of the newborn. Fat absorption is important not only for the utilization in structural growth and cell membrane integrity, but also in facilitating the absorption of fat-soluble vitamins. There are two components of fat processing—that which occurs in the lumen of the intestine and that which occurs at the level of the mucosa. In the lumen, fats must be emulsified and hydrolyzed to form free fatty acids and monoglycerides. This process is achieved by bile acids and lipases, both of which are limited in presence or function (or both) in the preterm infant. Alternate mechanisms for fat hydrolysis appear to be present in the newborn. Lingual lipases and gastric lipases are present by 26 weeks' gestation. Lingual lipases are produced by serous glands located in the posterior third of the tongue, and non-nutritive sucking is a mechanism for its release. Lingual lipase tolerates the low gastric pH 3.5 to 5.5. Gastric lipase, secreted by gastric glands, also contributes to luminal hydrolysis of fats in newborns (Cohen et al, 1971). Additional lipases are also present in breast milk. The major breast milk lipase is bile salt–stimulated lipase. In contrast to endogenous lipases, this lipase is capable of hydrolyzing all three ester bonds of triglycerides. A second lipase that resembles lipoprotein lipase has also been described to be present in breast milk. Thus, it appears that these lipases substitute for the absence of pancreatic lipase. Furthermore, in contrast to pancreatic lipases, these three lipases function well in an environment that has low bile salt concentration, as is the case in the preterm infant. Because of decreased bile acid synthesis, preterm infant intraluminal bile acid concentration is 1 to 2 mmol/L (Katz and Hamilton, 1977), or approximately half of the critical micellar concentration required for adequate fat absorption. Thus, these alternate lipases appear to be well adapted for function in the immature environment of the preterm infant.

There is also a relationship between intraluminal Ca^{++} concentration and fat absorption. In newborns, a high intake of Ca^{++} impairs fat absorption, and for this reason the high Ca^{++} content in cow's milk can cause malabsorption of fats (Hanna et al, 1970). Conversely, high fat intake may also impair Ca^{++} absorption. Therefore the optimal relationship of dietary fat and Ca^{++} has not yet been identified for the preterm infant.

The source of dietary fat also influences absorption. Preterm infants digest and absorb fats better if they are derived from human milk than formula (Foman et al, 1970). Vegetable fats are absorbed better than animal fats. Unsaturated fats are absorbed better than saturated fats. Medium-chain and short-chain triglycerides are absorbed better than long-chain triglycerides (Roy et al, 1975).

Once the luminal phase of fat processing is completed, the mucosal phase of absorption must occur. The mucosal phase involves the passage of mixed micelles through the unstirred water layer at the mucosal cell surface. Monoglycerides and free fatty acids diffuse directly into the cells. Both of these processes appear to be well developed in the preterm infant. Thus, the inefficiency of fat absorption in the preterm infant, which ranges from 40% to 90%, largely reflects immaturity of intraluminal processing.

Digestion of Proteins

Although proteins contribute less than 10% of ingested calories, they provide important bricks for the structure of somatic growth. Initial digestion of protein begins in the stomach, where dietary protein is denatured by gastric acid and cleaved to large polypeptides by pepsin. Because acid secretion is significantly lower in the preterm infant, it is not known how efficient this initial processing is. Gastric contents then are expelled into the upper intestine, where pancreatic proteases are capable of fairly efficient splitting of the peptides to oligopeptides and amino acids. As detailed previously, most of the brush borders and cytosolic peptidases are well developed in the preterm infant, and the peptide transport system is efficient. In addition, there appears to be an alternate method for protein uptake in the intestine. Macromolecules can be actively taken up by pinocytosis by the neonatal intestine (Walker, 1978). In fact, preterm infants have been demonstrated to absorb intact lactoferrin of maternal origin (Hutchens et al, 1991).

Electrolytes, Minerals, Vitamins, and Metals
Electrolytes

Animal studies suggest that newborns may have unique fluid and electrolyte fluxes. Rat pups initially show a net secretion of water in the small intestine, which is reversible by the addition of glucose (Younoszai et al, 1978). Compared with 7-week-old rats, intraluminal osmotic loads in 2-week-old pups cause a greater increase in water, sodium, and chloride secretion by the small intestine, and other data show similar findings in humans.

Vitamin Absorption

Limited data are available regarding vitamin absorption in the newborn. The capacity to absorb folate is lower than that found in adults, and in addition, the reduced secretion of intrinsic factor by the stomachs of term and preterm infants may affect the absorption of vitamin B_{12}. Intrinsic factor is secreted by 3 months of age in term infants in amounts similar to those in adults. Stores at birth last almost 12 months.

Calcium

Calcium is absorbed primarily in the duodenum by an active transport process (Koo and Tsang, 1988). Early studies suggested that the amount of calcium absorbed was dependent on gestational age and postnatal age and independent of the source (i.e., cow's milk versus human milk) (Shaw, 1976); however, more recent data in the preterm infant show that up to 90% of calcium in breast milk may be absorbed (Chappell et al, 1986; Ehrenkranz et al, 1985).

Phosphorus

Phosphorus is absorbed principally in the jejunum by simple diffusion and an active transport process that is vitamin

D dependent. In preterm infants fed human milk with low phosphorus content, phosphorus absorption approaches 90% of intake (Senterre et al, 1983). The process does not appear to be affected by vitamin D intake. The percentage of phosphorus absorbed in infants decreases as phosphorus intake increases. Excessive amounts of either calcium or phosphorus decrease the absorption of the other because of the precipitation of insoluble calcium phosphate (see Chapter 78).

Magnesium

Magnesium absorption occurs throughout the entire gastrointestinal tract at a similar rate and does not appear to vary with either gestational age or postnatal age (Tantibhedhyakul and Hashim, 1978). Magnesium absorption is 43% to 73% when intake is normal (Greer and Tsang, 1985). Isolated deficiencies of magnesium absorption have also been described.

Copper

Copper is absorbed in the duodenum. Ehrenkranz and coworkers (1989) demonstrated that 53% of copper was absorbed in formula-fed preterm infants. This increased to 72% when preterm infants were fed human milk.

Zinc

Zinc is absorbed in the duodenum and proximal jejunum. In newborns, absorption rates vary from 32% with cow's milk to 52% with human milk. Voyer and colleagues (1982) showed that in preterm infants of 30 to 32 weeks' gestation, zinc absorption could be enhanced by the addition of medium-chain triglycerides to formula or breast milk, suggesting that the process is linked to fat absorption. Higashi and associates (1988) studied zinc balance in premature infants given the minimum dietary zinc requirement and showed that zinc balance changes from negative to positive at about 36 weeks. They suggested that oral zinc supplementation in preterm infants of less than 36 weeks' gestation may lead to an increase in fecal extraction and that intravenous supplementation seems necessary to obtain a zinc retention rate similar to the fetal rate.

Iron

Iron for the newborn is provided as iron salts of nonheme iron. Absorption of the small amount of iron in breast milk approaches 50%, even in the preterm infant. Because iron absorption is only 4% from both fortified and nonfortified formulas, iron supplementation is necessary (Rios et al, 1975).

Motility of the Digestive System

The major limitations to enteral alimentation do not appear to be digestion or absorption but the propulsion of chyme along the gastrointestinal tract. The human fetus can swallow as early at 17 weeks' gestation, and swallowing appears to play an important role in the regulation of amniotic fluid volume. For example, hydramnios is often seen in pregnancies in which fetal swallowing is impaired, such as when esophageal atresia or upper intestinal atresia is present. Exposure to factors in amniotic fluid appears to be important for gastrointestinal development. Mucosal maturation in the stomach is delayed in rabbits if the esophagus is ligated, and maturation returns to normal if the esophagus is exposed to amniotic fluid or epidermal growth factor.

In both premature and term infants younger than 12 hours of age, peristalsis in the body of the esophagus is poorly coordinated in response to swallowing. Simultaneous nonperistaltic contractions are often present along the entire length of the esophagus. Lower esophageal sphincter pressure is frequently decreased. Gastric emptying in the premature and young newborn is slow, compared with emptying in older children. Cavell (1979) showed that the emptying pattern for breast milk in healthy preterm infants was more rapid than for formula and was biphasic in nature. The emptying pattern for infant formula, however, was linear. As in adults, meal composition also affects gastric emptying, with delay occurring as caloric density increases. Emptying is also delayed more with glucose or lactose than with glucose polymers and with long-chain triglycerides than with medium-chain triglycerides (Siegal et al, 1985). This last finding, however, has not been documented in preterm infants of fewer than 32 weeks' gestation.

McLain (1963), in one of the earliest studies of small bowel motility in human newborns, suggested that motility increases with advancing gestational age. Until 30 weeks, contrast material did not progress through the small intestine of the fetus; however, at 32 weeks, contrast material passed through the small bowel to the colon in 9 hours, compared with a transit time of 4.5 to 7 hours in term infants. Migrating motor complexes, first seen around 33 weeks' gestation, are an interdigestive phenomenon that functions to sweep gut contents over long segments of

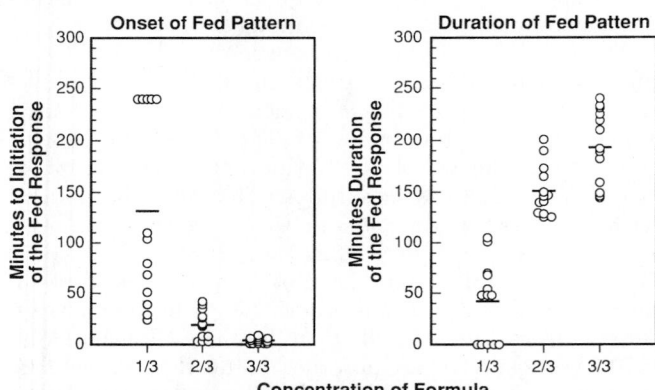

FIGURE 70–9. Motor activity responses to feeding formula diluted to ⅓ strength, ⅔ strength, and ⅗ strength. In the left panel, there is an increasing delay of the onset of the fed response as progressively more diluted formula is given (r = −.62; P <.01). In the right panel, the duration of the fed response is sustained progressively longer as more concentrated formula is given (r = .49; P <.01). (From Koenig WJ, Amarnath RP, Hench V, Berseth CL: Manometrics for preterm and term infants: A new tool for old questions. Pediatrics 95:203, 1995. Reproduced by Permission of PEDIATRICS, Vol 95 Page 203 Copyright 1995.)

intestine between meals. This pattern is inhibited by eating, which initiates postprandial mixing-type contractions. In the term infant, the time between migrating motor complexes is 44 minutes, or about half the time observed in older children. The propagation rate, however, is 3.1 cm per minute in term infants, compared with 8.2 cm per minute for older children, and the duration time is 10.9 minutes in infants, compared with 7.2 minutes for older children. Berseth (1992) has suggested that early feeding may be important in hastening the maturation of motility in preterm infants. In addition, she has also shown that the composition of feeding may alter motor responses. For example, duodenal motor activity normally increases in response to feeding. When the preterm infant is fed diluted formula, motor responses are delayed in onset and are less intense (Fig. 70–9).

Meconium is the thick black material that collects in the distal portion of the small intestine and colon of the fetus and consists of intestinal secretions, bile, desquamated cellular debris, and amniotic fluid. Ninety-four percent of newborns pass a meconium stool within 24 hours after birth. In premature infants, rectal sphincteric reflexes may be absent or impaired, and fecal passage is therefore delayed. Other bases for the failure of meconium passage have also been suggested (i.e., the absence of colonic bulk movement or of giant migrating complexes), but no data have been reported to clarify what causes failure to stool.

REFERENCES

Amarnath RP, Berseth CL, Malagelada J-R, et al: Postnatal maturation of small intestinal motility in preterm neonates. J Gastrointest Motil 1:138, 1989.

Antonowicz I, Chang SK, Grand RJ: Development and distribution of liposomal enzymes and disaccharidases in human fetal intestine. Gastroenterology 67:51, 1974.

Auricchio S, Rubino A, Mürset G: Intestinal glycosidase activities in the human embryo, fetus, and newborn. Pediatrics 3S:944, 1965.

Back P, Walter K: Developmental pattern of bile acid metabolism as revealed by bile acid analysis of meconium. Gastroenterology 78:671, 1980.

Baker J, Berseth CL: Postnatal change in inhibitory regulation of intestinal motor activity in human and canine neonates. Pediatr Res 38:133, 1995.

Berseth CL: Effect of early feeding on maturation of the preterm infant's small intestine. J Pediatr 120:947, 1992.

Berseth CL, Nordyke CK, Valdes MG, et al: Responses of gastrointestinal peptides and motor activity to milk and water feedings in preterm and term neonates. Pediatr Res 31:587, 1992.

Bisset WM, Watt JB, Rivers RPA, et al: Ontogeny of fasting small intestinal motility in human infant. Gut 29:483, 1988.

Bryant MG, Buchan AM, Gregor M, et al: Development of intestinal regulatory peptides in the human fetus. Gastroenterology 83:47, 1982.

Cavell B: Gastric emptying in preterm infants. Acta Paediatr Scand 68:725, 1979.

Chappell JE, Clandinen MT, Kearney-Volpe C: Fatty acid balance studies in premature infants fed human milk or formula: Effect of calcium supplementation. J Pediatr 108:439, 1986.

Cohen M, Morgan GRH, Hofmann AF: Lipolytic activity of human gastric and duodenal juice against medium and long chain triglycerides. Gastroenterology 60:1, 1971.

Cohen S: Developmental characteristics of lower esophageal sphincter function: A possible mechanism for infantile cholasia. Gastroenterology 67:252, 1974.

Cohen S: Motor disorders of the esophagus. N Engl J Med 301:184, 1979.

Cooperstock MS, Zedd AJ: Intestinal flora of infants. In Hentgis D (Ed): Human Intestinal Microflora in Health and Disease. New York, Academic Press, 1983, p 79.

Crissinger KD, Burney DL: Influence of luminal nutrient composition on hemodynamics and oxygenation in developing piglet intestine. Pediatr Res 31:106A, 1992.

deBelle RC, Vaupshas V, Vitullo BB, et al: Intestinal absorption of bile salts: Immature development in the neonate. J Pediatr 94:472, 1979.

DeLeze G, Paumgartner G, Karlaganis G, et al: Bile acid pattern in human amniotic fluid. Eur J Clin Invest 8:41, 1978.

Ehrenkranz RA, Ackerman BA, Nelli CM, et al: Absorption of calcium in premature infants as measured with a stable isotope [46]Ca extrinsic tag. Pediatr Res 19:178, 1985.

Ehrenkranz RA, Gettner PA, Nelli CM: Nutrient balance studies in premature infants fed premature formula or fortified human milk. J Pediatr Gastroenterol Nutr 8:58, 1989.

Foman SJ, Ziegler EE, Thomas LN, et al: Excretion of fat by normal full-term infants fed various milks and formulas. Am J Clin Nutr 23:1299, 1970.

Greer FR, Tsang RC: Calcium, phosphorus, magnesium and vitamin D requirements for the preterm infant. In Tsang RC (Ed): Vitamin and Mineral Requirements in Preterm Infants. New York, Marcel Dekker, 1985, pp 99–136.

Hamosh M: Lingual and breast milk lipases. Adv Pediatr 29:33, 1982.

Hanna FM, Navarete DH, Hsu FA: Calcium-fatty acid absorption in term infants fed human milk and prepared formulas simulating human milk. Pediatrics 45:216, 1970.

Herbst JJ: Development of suck and swallow. J Pediatr Gastroenterol Nutr 2:S131, 1983.

Heubi JE, Balistreri WF: Bile salt metabolism in infants and children after protracted diarrhea. Pediatr Res 14:943, 1980.

Heubi JE, Fondacaro JD, Balistreri WF: Bile salt absorption in neonates. J Pediatr 95:1085, 1979.

Higashi A, Ikeda T, Iribe K, Matsuda I: Zinc balance in premature infants given the minimal dietary zinc requirement. J Pediatr 112:262, 1988.

Holle GE, Forth W: Myoelectric activity of small intestine after chemical ablation of myenteric neurons. Am J Physiol 258:G519, 1990.

Hutchens TW, Henry JF, Yip TT, et al: Origin of intact lactoferrin and its DNA-binding fragments found in the urine of human milk fed preterm infants: Evaluation by stable isotope enrichment. Pediatr Res 29:243, 1991.

Ittman PI, Amarnath R, Berseth CL: Maturation of antroduodenal motor activity in preterm and term infants. Dig Dis Sci 37:14, 1992.

Jadcherla SR, Klee G, Berseth CL: Regulation of migrating motor complexes by motilin and pancreatic polypeptide in human neonates. Pediatr Res 1997, in press.

Katz L, Hamilton JR: Fat absorption in infants of birthweight less than 1300 gm. J Pediatr 90:431, 1977.

Kerzner B, Sloan HR, Haase GL, et al: The jejunal absorption of glucose oligomers in the absence of pancreatic enzymes. Pediatr Res 15:250, 1981.

Koo WWK, Tsang RC: Calcium, magnesium and phosphorous in nutrition during infancy. In Tsang RC, Nichols BS (Eds): Nutrition During Infancy. Philadelphia, Hanley & Belfus, 1988, pp 175–189.

Lacroix B, Kedinger M, Simon-Assman P, Haffen K: Early organogenesis of human small intestine: Scanning electron microscopy and brush border enzymology. Gut 25:925, 1984.

Lebenthal E, Lee PC: Development of functional responses in human exocrine pancreas. Pediatrics 66:556, 1980.

Lebenthal E, Lee PC: Interactions of determinants in the ontogeny of the gastrointestinal tract: A unified concept. Pediatr Res 17:19, 1983.

Lichtenberger LM, Johnson LR: Gastrin in the ontogenic development of the small intestine. Am J Physiol 227:390, 1974.

Lucas A, Bloom SR, Aynsley-Green A: Development of gut hormone responses to feeding in neonates. Arch Dis Child 55:678, 1980.

Lucas A, Bloom SR, Aynsley-Green A: Postnatal surges in plasma gut hormones in term and preterm infants. Biol Neonate 41:63, 1982.

MacLean WC, Fink BB: Lactase malabsorption by premature infants: Magnitude and clinical significance. J Pediatr 97:383, 1980.

Malo C: Kinetic evidence for heterogeneity in Na + -D-glucose co-transport systems in the normal human fetal small intestine. Biochem Biophys Acta 938:181, 1988.

McLain CR Jr: Amniography studies of the gastrointestinal motility of the human fetus. Am J Obstet Gynecol 86:1079, 1963.

Ménard D, Pothier P: Differential distribution of digestive enzymes in isolated epithelial cells from developing human fetal small intestine and colon. J Pediatr Gastroenterol Nutr 6:509, 1987.

Motil KJ: Development of the gastrointestinal tract. In Wyllie R, Hyanes JS (Eds): Pediatric Gastrointestinal Disease. Philadelphia, WB Saunders, 1993.

Nakagawa M, Setchell KDR: Bile acid metabolism in early life: Studies of amniotic fluid. J Lipid Res 31:1089, 1990.

Newell SJ, Sarkar PK, Durbin GM, et al: Maturation of the lower esophageal sphincter in the preterm baby. Gut 29:167, 1988.

Nowicki P, Miller C, Hayes J: Effect of sustained mesenteric nerve stimulation on intrinsic vascular oxygenation in developing swine. Am J Physiol 260:G333, 1991.

Raul F, Lacroix B, Aprahamian M: Longitudinal distribution of brush border hydrolases and morphological maturation in the intestine of the preterm infant. Early Hum Dev 13:225, 1986.

Rieger CHL, Rothberg RM: Development of the capacity to produce specific antibody to an ingested food antigen in the premature infant. J Pediatr 87:515, 1985.

Rios E, Hunter RE, Cook J: The absorption of iron as supplements in infant cereal and infant formulas. Pediatrics 55:686, 1975.

Rotimi VO, Duerden BI: The bacterial flora in normal neonates. J Med Microbiol 14:51, 1981.

Roy CC, Ste-Marie M, Chartrand L, et al: Correction of the malabsorption of the preterm infant with a medium chain triglyceride formula. Pediatrics 86:446, 1975.

Ruger CHL, Rothberg RM: Development of the capacity to produce specific antibody to an ingested food antigen in the premature infant. J Pediatr 87:515, 1975.

Schuffler MD, Jonah A: Chronic idiopathic intestinal pseudo-obstruction caused by degenerative disorder of the myenteric plexus: The use of Smith's method to define neuropathy. Gastroenterology 82:476, 1982.

Senterre J, Putet G, Salle B, et al: Effects of vitamin D and phosphorous supplementation on calcium retention in preterm infants fed banked human milk. J Pediatr 103:305, 1983.

Shaw JCL: Evidence of the defective skeletal mineralization in low birth weight infants: The absorption of calcium and fat. Pediatrics 57:16, 1976.

Shepherd A, Granger J: Autoregulatory escape in the gut: A systems analysis. Gastroenterology 65:77, 1973.

Shepherd A, Mailman D, Burks T, et al: Effects of norepinephrine and sympathetic stimulation on extraction of oxygen and Rb in perfused canine small bowel. Circ Res 33:166, 1973.

Siegal M, Krantz B, Lebenthal E: Effect of fat and carbohydrate composition on the gastric emptying of isocaloric feedings in premature infants. Gastroenterology 89:785, 1985.

Simhon A, Douglas JR, Drasar BS, et al: Effect of feeding on infant's fecal flora. Arch Dis Child 57:54, 1982.

Strawczynski H, Beck IT, McKenna RD, et al: The behavior of the lower esophageal sphincter in infants and its relationship to gastroesophageal reflux. J Pediatr 64:17, 1964.

Suchy FJ, Balistreri WF, Heubi JE, et al: Physiologic cholestasis: Elevation of the primary serum bile acid concentrations in normal infants. Gastroenterology 80:1037, 1981.

Tantibhedhyangkal P, Hashim SA: Medium-chain triglyceride feeding in premature infants: Effects on calcium and magnesium absorption. Pediatrics 61:537, 1978.

Triadoru N, Zweibaum A: Maturation of sucrase-isomaltase complex in human fetal small and large intestine during gestation. Pediatr Res 19:136, 1985.

Villa M, Ménard D, Semenza G, Mantei N: Expression of the lactase enzymatic activity and mRNA in human fetal jejunum. FEBS Lett 301:202, 1992.

Voyer M, Davikis M, Artener I, et al: Zinc balances in preterm infants. Biol Neonate 42:87, 1982.

Walker WA: Antigen handling by the gut. Arch Dis Child 53:527, 1978.

Watkins JB, Szczepanik P, Gould JB, et al: Bile metabolism in the premature infant: Preliminary observations of pool size and synthesis rate following prenatal administration of dexamethasone and phenobarbital. Gastroenterology 69:706, 1975.

Worniak ER, Fenton TR, Milla PJ: The development of fasting small intestinal motility in human neonates. *In* Roman C (Ed): Gastrointestinal Motility. London, Lancaster Press, 1983, pp 265–270.

Younoszai MK, Sapario RS, Laughlin M, et al: Maturation of jejunum and ileum in rats: Water and electrolyte transport during in vivo perfusion of hypertonic solutions. J Clin Invest 62:271, 1978.

Zoppi G, Andreotti G, Pajno-Ferrara F, et al: Exocrine pancreas function in premature and term infants. Pediatr Res 6:880, 1972.

CHAPTER 71

Disorders of the Teeth, Mouth, and Neck

Carol Lynn Berseth

TEETH

Infants may be born with one or more erupted teeth. These are usually lower incisors, which are called *natal teeth*, to differentiate them from neonatal teeth, which erupt during the 1st month. Natal teeth should be extracted because their roots are poorly formed and they present a danger of aspiration when they loosen.

MOUTH

Tiny cystic lesions may be visible in the mouths of 80% of newborns. Those located on the hard palate on either side of the raphe are called *Epstein pearls*, and those located on the mandibular and maxillary alveolar ridges are called *Bohn nodules*. A ranula is a retention cyst of the sublingual salivary gland that presents as a pea-sized mass on the anterior floor of the mouth. Most cysts disappear within 1 month, but larger ones that interfere with feeding may require surgical excision.

Tumors of the mouth are rare in the newborn; however, when they are present, careful evaluation with computed tomography is necessary to define the anatomy and to determine if a connection with the central nervous system is present. An *epignathus* is any type of growth that arises from the upper jaw or palate and projects from the mouth (Fig. 71–1). Although most of these tumors are polyps, dermoids, or teratomas, they often cause respiratory or feeding difficulty. The definitive treatment is surgical removal.

Congenital epulis is a misnamed tumor that arises from the upper or lower jaw and projects into the mouth and impairs normal sucking. These tumors are covered with squamous epithelium and contain vascular connective tissue, large polyhedral round cells, and spindle-shaped cells (Langley and Davson, 1950), and they are considered to be benign. Histochemical staining of these tumors demonstrates that these tumor cells represent early mesodermal cells that express pericytic and myofibroblastic features (Damm et al, 1993).

Salivary gland lesions are rare in the newborn. Tumors or infection of the salivary gland (sialadenitis) may arise anywhere salivary gland tissue is present, including the floor of the mouth and the parotid regions. Hemangiomas are the most common tumors found in this region and lymphangiomas the second most common (Welch and Trump, 1979). Both of these benign lesions are typically confined to the intracapsular portion of the gland, although surface sentinel lesions may be present. Treatment consists of confirming a histologic diagnosis via open biopsy and long-term observation of the lesion. Juxtaparotid lymphangiomas that invade the gland should be locally excised. Suppurative parotitis may present during the 1st month of life and involve one or both parotid glands. Pus may be expressed from the Stensen duct by putting gentle pressure on the gland. The infant may become septic; extension to the submaxillary gland is not uncommon. The offending organism is usually *Staphylococcus aureus* or *Escherichia coli*, but broad-spectrum antibiotic coverage is necessary until the organism has been identified and sensitivities established.

TONGUE

Aglossia congenita, or congenital absence of the tongue, has been described. Taste sensation is present, and these children can learn to speak. Ankyloglossia inferior (tongue-tie) is common in newborns. The frenulum of the newborn is normally short, but this does not interfere with sucking and swallowing. Because the frenulum lengthens with postnatal age, it should not be cut.

Ankyloglossia superior, attachment of the tongue to the roof of the mouth, is a rare anomaly that must be recognized at birth because respiratory obstruction may occur. Other lesions, such as micrognathia, macroglossia, and cleft palate, are frequently associated with this anomaly (Spivack and Bennett, 1968).

True macroglossia, or enlargement of the tongue, results in continuous protrusion of the tongue from the mouth making feeding difficult and respiration noisy. Macroglossia is often present in infants who have Down syndrome or Beckwith-Wiedemann syndrome. Lymphangioma and idiopathic muscular hypertrophy are additional common causes of macroglossia. Characteristically the gross appearance of a lymphangioma is that of a raised firm mass in the tongue, which has a warty-looking surface. The treatment for lymphangioma is surgical removal, if possible, or reduction of the tumor bulk with reshaping of the tongue. Infants with idiopathic muscular hypertrophy should be treated conservatively because the relative size of the tongue often becomes smaller as the mandible grows postnatally.

Thyroid tissue may persist as a solid or cystic mass in the posterior midline of the tongue or under it. Because the presence of this mass represents a failure of migration of normal thyroid tissue, no other thyroid tissue may exist. A thyroid scan should be performed when one is evaluating midline lingual tumors.

NASOPHARYNX

Nasopharyngeal tumors are rare and are polyps, dermoids, or teratomas. Often these lesions are on a stalk and project into the mouth. Those not projecting externally may be palpated as movable, sausage-shaped masses in the pharynx. These lesions should be removed urgently because acute respiratory distress may occur if the nasopharynx is obstructed.

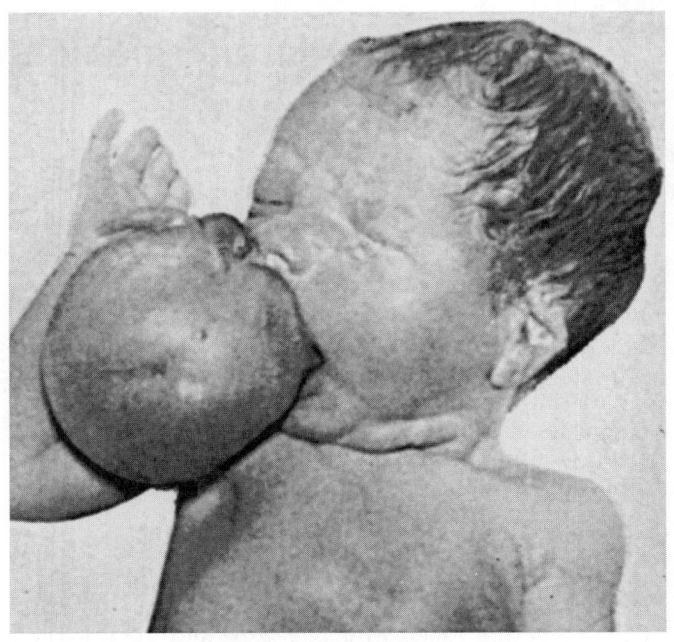

FIGURE 71–1. Infant with epignathus: The orange-sized mass attached to the maxilla protrudes grotesquely from the mouth. (From Wynn SK, Waxman S, Ritchie G, Askofsky M: Am J Dis Child 91:495, 1956. Copyright 1956, American Medical Association.)

NECK

Cystic hygroma is the most common lateral neck mass in the newborn (Fig. 71–2). Derived from lymphatic tissue, these multilobular, multicystic masses may rapidly enlarge and cause respiratory compromise. Thus, excision is the treatment of choice.

Branchial cleft anomalies may present as skin tags, pits, sinuses, fistulas, or cysts in the preauricular and lateral cervical region. Most are remnants of the second branchial cleft and pouch, and 10% to 15% occur bilaterally (Bill and Vadheim, 1955). Sinuses and fistulas may be discovered during the newborn period, but cysts require time to fill

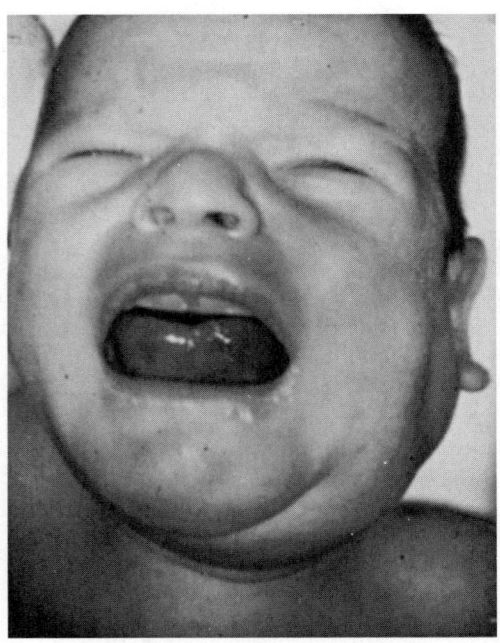

FIGURE 71–2. Hygroma of the neck and tongue.

and are usually not recognized until childhood. Ultrasound or computed tomography scan of the neck may be useful to define anatomic relationships, and surgical removal is the treatment of choice.

Sternomastoid tumor can be seen and palpated within the body of the sternocleidomastoid muscle as a hard, smooth oval mass. By histopathology, these lesions are caused by endomysial fibrosis and deposition of collagen and fibroblasts around individual muscle fibers that subsequently undergo atrophy. The cause is unknown, but the incidence is seven times higher following breech delivery (Ling and Low, 1973) and among infants who have had specific fetal positioning in utero (Rosegger and Steinwendner, 1992). Torticollis is not always present; instead there may be rotation of the head to the side opposite the tumor. Cranial and facial asymmetry may also occur. In most infants, the lesion resolves within 6 to 12 months. Surgical splitting of the muscle is indicated if severe hemihypoplasia develops (Wirth et al, 1992).

Midline neck masses in newborns include cystic hygromas, hemangiomas, teratomas, goiter, ectopic thyroid tissue, and ectopic thymic tissue (Fig. 71–3). Goiters may be visible at birth and may be associated with the presence of hypothyroidism, hyperthyroidism, or euthyroidism. The second most common location for ectopic thyroid tissue is the anterior midline of the neck, just at or below the hyoid bone (Meyerowitz and Buchholz, 1969). Although this tissue may be easily mistaken for a thyroglossal duct cyst, thyroglossal duct cysts are rarely present in the newborn. Before removal of ectopic thyroid tissue, it must be determined if this tissue is the infant's only functioning thyroid tissue.

Thymic tissue arises high in the cervical region of the embryo as two lateral buds. The buds migrate caudad and join in the anterior mediastinum. Abnormal migration results in ectopic location or cyst formation (or both), which may present as a lateral or midline neck mass (Thompson and Love, 1972) and requires surgical removal.

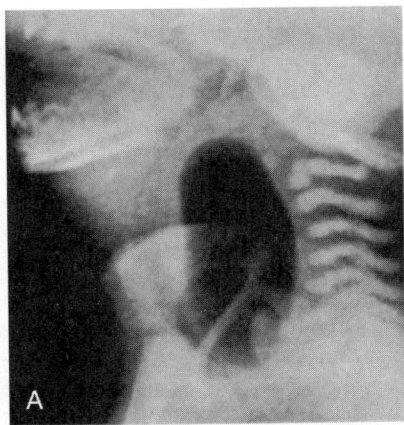

FIGURE 71–3. *A,* Lateral radiograph of the neck shows an air-containing cyst displacing the air passages and esophagus forward. *B,* Lateral view of the neck with patient quiet, demonstrating straight, unobstructed tracheal air column. *C,* Lateral view of the neck with patient crying demonstrates mass lesion between the manubrium and the trachea, displacing the lower cervical trachea backward and moderately narrowing this portion of the trachea. (From Thompson, RE, Love WG: Persistent cervical thymoma apparent with crying. Am J Dis Child 124:761, 1972. Copyright 1972, American Medical Association.)

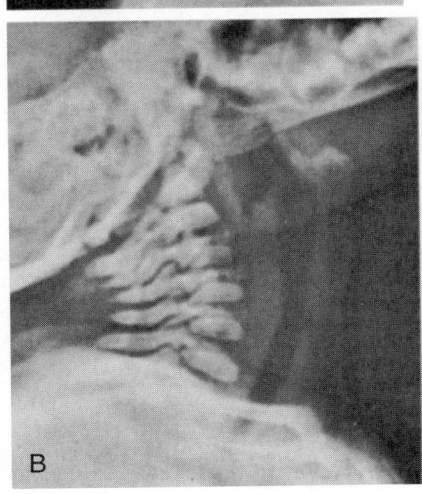

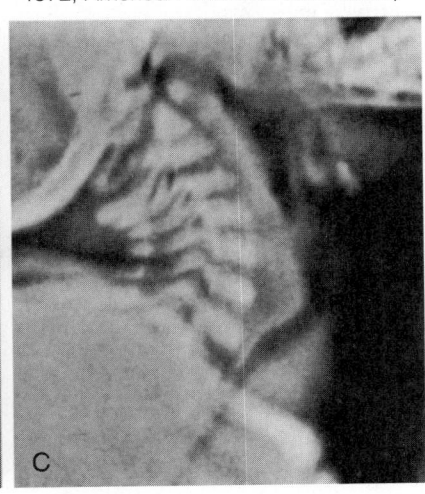

REFERENCES

Badami JP, Athey PA: Sonography in the diagnosis of branchial cysts. Am J Radiol 137:1245, 1981.

Beckwith JB: Macroglossia, omphalocele, adrenal cytomegaly, gigantism and hyperplastic visceromegaly. Birth Def 5:188, 1969.

Bill AH, Vadheim JL: Cysts, sinuses and fistulas of the neck arising from the first and second branchial clefts. Am Surg 142:904, 1955.

Chappuis JP: Current aspects of cystic lymphangioma in the neck. Arch Pediatr 1:186, 1994.

Damm DD, Cibull ML, Geissler RH, et al: Investigation into the histogenesis of congenital epulis of the newborn. Oral Surg Oral Med Oral Pathol 76:205, 1993.

Grosfield JL, Skinner MA, Rescorla FJ, et al: Mediastinal tumors in children: Experience with 196 cases. Ann Surg Oncol 1:121, 1994.

Langley FA, Davson J: Epulis in the newborn. Arch Dis Child 25:89, 1950.

Ling CM, Low YS: Sternomastoid tumor and muscular torticollis. J Bone Joint Surg 55:236, 1973.

Meyerowitz BR, Buchholz RB: Midline cervical ectopic thyroid tissue. Surgery 65:358, 1969.

Orlian AI, Perl C: Treating multiple congenital epulides in a newborn. J Am Dent Assoc 126:647, 1995.

Rosegger H, Steinwendner G: Transverse fetal position syndrome—a combination of congenital skeletal deformities in the newborn infant. Padiatrie und Padolog 27:125, 1992.

Spivack J, Bennett JE: Glossopalatine ankylosis. Plast Reconstr Surg 42:129, 1968.

Thompson RE, Love WG: Persistent cervical thymoma apparent with crying. Am J Dis Child 124:761, 1972.

Warden PJ: Ankyloglossia: A review of the literature. Gen Dentistry 39:252, 1991.

Welch KJ, Trump DS: The oropharynx and jaws. *In* Ravitch MM (Ed): Pediatric Surgery. Chicago, Year Book Medical Publishers, 1979, p 308.

Wirth CJ, Hagena FW, Wuelker N, Siebert WE: Bi-terminal tenotomy for the treatment of congenital muscular torticollis. J Bone Joint Surg (Am) 74:427, 1992.

CHAPTER 72

Disorders of the Esophagus

Carol Lynn Berseth

ESOPHAGEAL ATRESIA WITH TRACHEOESOPHAGEAL FISTULA

Definition. Esophageal atresia and tracheoesophageal fistula may occur as separate congenital defects, but more frequently they are seen together as a compound defect (Fig. 72–1). Esophageal atresia with distal tracheoesophageal fistula is by far the most common form, accounting for 85% of the cases.

Epidemiology. The incidence of esophageal atresia with tracheoesophageal fistula varies from 1 per 3000 to 1 per 4000 live births (Meyers, 1974; Raffensperger, 1990). Most series show a slight male predominance and an increased incidence in premature infants (Reckham, 1981). The role genetic factors play is unclear; however, this anomaly has been described in siblings as well as identical twins (Hausmann et al, 1957; Woolley et al, 1961). In addition, two kindreds with autosomal dominant transmission have been reported (Pletcher et al, 1991).

Etiology. The anomaly occurs before the 8th week of gestation, but the exact mechanism is unknown. The foregut divides into a ventral and a dorsal tube when the lateral walls invaginate, giving rise to the trachea and esophagus. When this process of division is abnormal or when there is compression of these primitive tubes by an extrinsic structure, such as an anomalous blood vessel, esophageal atresia or tracheoesophageal fissure (or both) may result. Other anomalies may occur in as many as 40% of infants with tracheoesophageal atresias. These anomalies are usually gastrointestinal (anal atresia, pyloric stenosis, duodenal obstruction, and malrotation) or cardiovascular (Greenwood and Rosenthal, 1976). One cluster of congenital anomalies seen often among infants of diabetic mothers has been named the VATER association (Vertebral anomalies, Anal anomalies, Tracheoesophageal fistula with Esophageal atresia, and Radial limb dysplasia and renal anomalies) (Quan and Smith, 1973). An extension of this is the VACTERAL association, which includes Cardiac and Limb anomalies.

Diagnosis. Polyhydramnios is present in approximately one third of mothers bearing infants with esophageal atresia because the fetus is unable to swallow amniotic fluid. Within hours after birth, these infants accumulate large amounts of oral secretions, which may precipitate coughing, choking, and respiratory distress. The infants vomit when they are fed, and if the infant has a distal tracheoesophageal connection, abdominal distention may ensue as the intestine fills with air. The presence of a flat or gasless abdomen should suggest an esophageal atresia without tracheoesophageal fistula (see Fig. 72–1B). Fourteen percent of patients with a gasless abdomen, however, may have a tracheoesophageal fistula that is partially obliterated and still requires surgical repair (Goh et al, 1991). The most dramatic presentation of tracheoesophageal fistula occurs in those infants who have a tracheoesophageal fistula proximal to the esophageal atresia (see Fig. 72–1D, E, G). These infants develop life-threatening respiratory failure from aspiration almost immediately after birth.

Infants with the H-type tracheoesophageal fistula (see Fig. 72–1F) do not usually develop symptoms in the newborn period. Instead, these infants usually present with a history (over months to years in duration) of mild respiratory distress related to feeding or recurrent pneumonias.

If a diagnosis of esophageal atresia is suspected, a soft 5 or 8 French feeding tube can be passed into the esophagus until it meets an obstruction. On occasion, the tube coils in a blind pouch, creating the false impression that the esophagus is patent. A plain film confirms the position of the tube and frequently demonstrates the presence of an air-filled upper esophageal pouch (Fig. 72–2). The presence of gas in the abdomen suggests that a distal tracheoesophageal fistula is present.

Treatment. Preoperative care of esophageal atresia includes the insertion of a sump suction catheter into the proximal esophageal pouch for the continuous evacuation of secretions. The infant should also be placed in the upright position to decrease the reflux of gastric secretions through the fistula and into the lungs. Hydration is maintained by intravenous fluids, and surgical repair is undertaken when the infant's general condition permits. Thus, surgical repair in preterm infants may be delayed postnatally until the infant is clinically stable enough for surgery.

At surgery, an extrapleural or transpleural approach is used, the fistula is divided, and an anastomosis between the proximal and distal esophageal segments is achieved using an end-to-end or end-to-side anastomosis. Usually a gastrostomy is also placed.

Postoperative care consists of respiratory support, antibiotics, and intravenous nutritional support. Enteral feedings via a gastrostomy or a transpyloric tube may be started on the 3rd or 4th postoperative day. These are initially given by continuous infusion. Bolus feedings may be introduced once full enteral alimentation is achieved. Small amounts of oral feedings may be started 7 to 10 days postoperatively after confirmation by radiographic contrast study that there are no esophageal anastomotic leaks.

Prognosis. The overall survival rate in term infants without respiratory complications preoperatively approaches 95% (Holder and Ashcraft, 1970). Among premature infants or those with moderate to severe respiratory disease, survival is 85%. Infants with multiple anomalies or those with severe respiratory disease have a 75% survival rate. Leakage postoperatively from the anastomotic site may cause mediastinitis, sepsis, and thoracic empyema. These

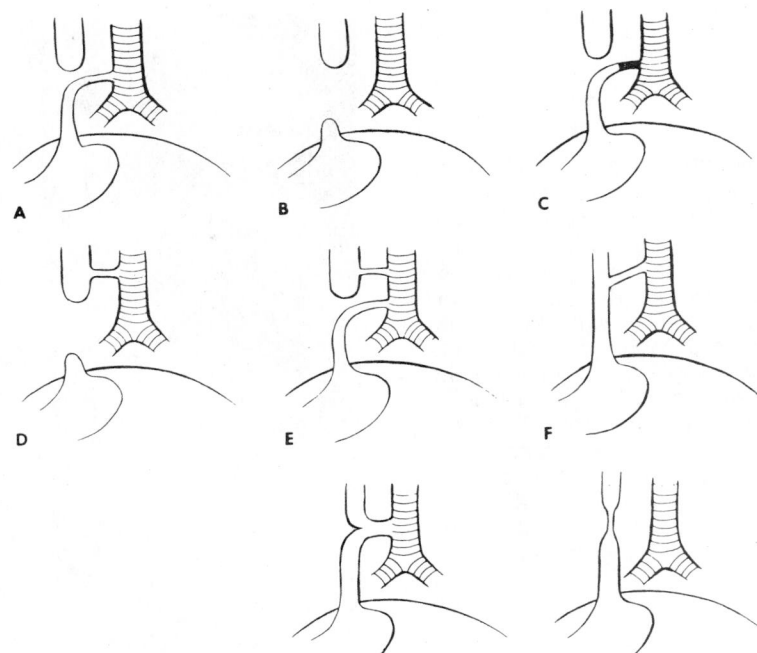

FIGURE 72–1. Types of tracheoesophageal fistulas: *A* is overwhelmingly the most common, accounting for 85% of esophageal malformations. *B* is next most common and can be distinguished from *A* by the absence of air in the intestinal tract on roentgenogram. All the other types have been noted sporadically. (From Avery ME, et al: The Lung and Its Disorders in the Newborn Infant, 4th ed. Philadelphia, WB Saunders, 1981.)

self-contained minor leaks form small pseudodiverticula, which resolve spontaneously or form an esophagocutaneous fistula. If the lung remains inflated, these close spontaneously.

Virtually all infants with esophageal atresia have residual problems with strictures and abnormal esophageal motility and swallowing. Esophageal stricture at the anastamotic site should be suspected if feeding difficulty develops, particularly after the 3rd week. Repeated dilation may be necessary to relieve the stricture.

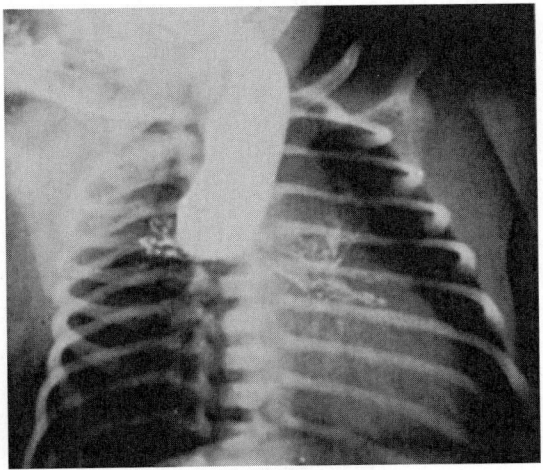

FIGURE 72–2. Anteroposterior view of the chest made on the second day of life, after an iodized oil (Lipiodol) swallow. A large dilated upper esophageal pouch ending blindly in the midchest can be seen. There is no air in the abdomen, a fact suggesting either that there is no fistula or that, if one is present, it is an upper one. Some dye has seeped into the lungs and an outline of a broad fistula tract coursing to the left of the lower end of the pouch is visible.

Gastroesophageal reflux occurs in 70% of patients after tracheoesophageal fistula repair (Roberts et al, 1980), owing to lower esophageal sphincter incompetence or abnormal motility in the body of the esophagus (Whitington et al, 1977). Medical therapy may be successful initially, but most patients require antireflux surgery.

TRACHEOESOPHAGEAL FISTULA WITHOUT ESOPHAGEAL ATRESIA

Tracheoesophageal fistula without esophageal atresia is rare. Only 5% of tracheoesophageal fistulas occur in the absence of esophageal atresia. Most of these fistulas are located superior to the second thoracic vertebra and can be repaired via a neck incision. A few also occur at the carina. Symptoms include coughing and cyanosis with feeding and recurrent episodes of pneumonia. If the diagnosis of tracheoesophageal fistula is suspected, oral feedings should be withheld and replaced by gavage feedings. A thick barium upper gastrointestinal series should be done to demonstrate the lesion (Figs. 72–3 and 72–4). If this is unsuccessful, simultaneous endoscopic examination of the trachea and esophagus may be done; the injection of a small amount of methylene blue into the trachea and its subsequent appearance in the esophagus may be diagnostic. The treatment is surgical ligation of the fistula.

LARYNGOTRACHEOESOPHAGEAL CLEFT

Laryngotracheoesophageal cleft is a communication of the larynx and trachea with the esophagus. The defect varies in length, with the shortest being the length of the arytenoid cartilages and the longest extending the entire length of the trachea (Fig. 72–5). These clefts form between the 5th and 7th weeks of gestation when there is a failure of the

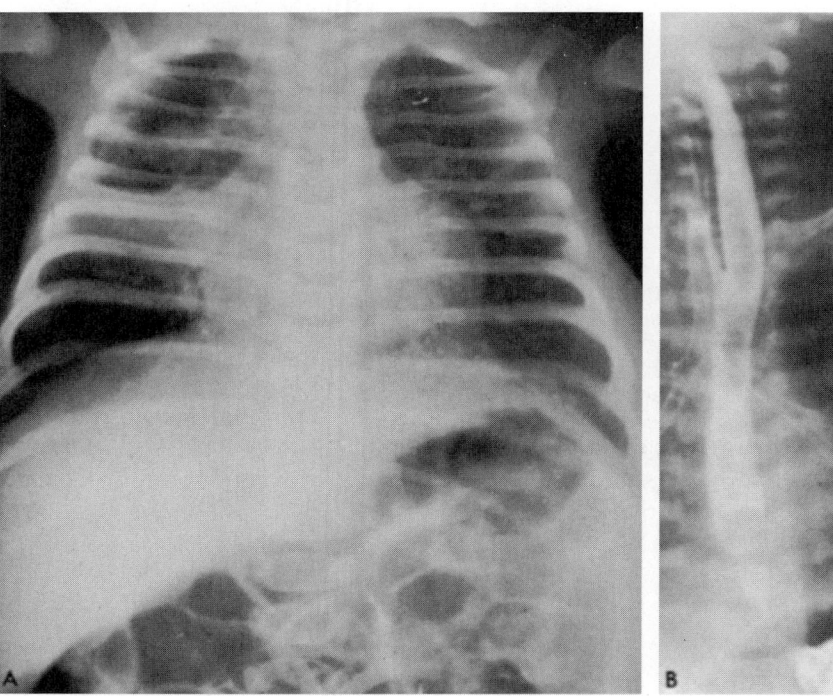

FIGURE 72–3. *A,* Anteroposterior view of chest of an infant 6 months old. There is atelectasis of the right middle lobe, hyperinflation of the right lower lobe, and some patchy opacification elsewhere. *B,* Spot film taken after barium swallow outlines the esophagus and a fistula of large caliber coursing from it upward toward the trachea. A faint bronchogram is visible. There is no atresia or stenosis of the esophagus. A tracheoesophageal fistula without esophageal atresia was found at autopsy. (Courtesy of Dr. Thomas D. Michael, Baltimore.)

rostral advance and fusion of the lateral ridges of the laryngotracheal groove. One fifth of the clefts are associated with esophageal atresia and tracheoesophageal fistula. Clinical presentation occurs early in the newborn period and is similar to that for esophageal atresia with tracheoesophageal fistula except that stridor may also be present. A carefully done esophageal dye study should establish the diagnosis. Tracheal spillover, however, may be misinter-

preted to be due to the presence of a high H-type fistula or the presence of incoordination of the swallowing mechanism. Patients with clefts should undergo bronchoscopic examination with immediate surgical repair. A temporary

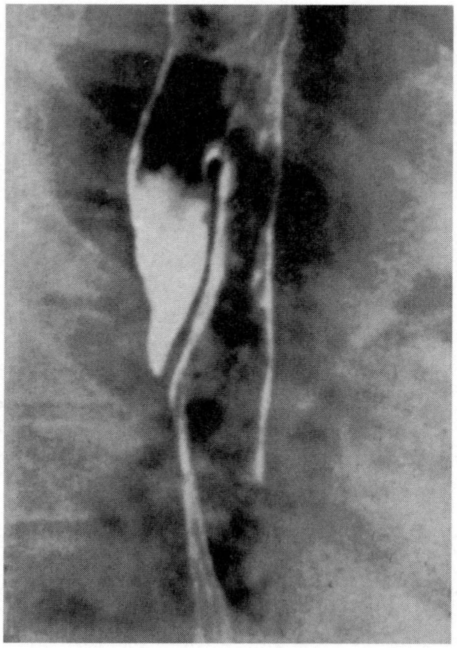

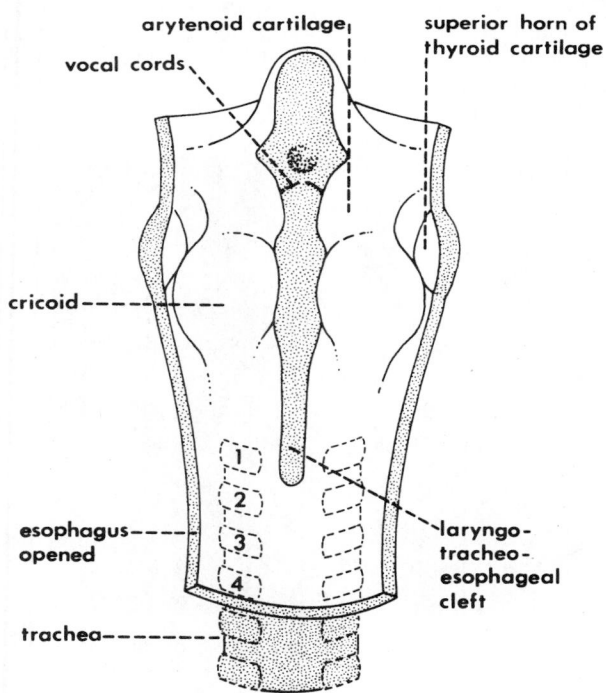

FIGURE 72–5. Illustration of the anatomy of a laryngotracheoesophageal cleft. (From Burroughs N, Leape LL: Laryngotracheoesophageal cleft: Report of a case successfully treated and review of the literature. Pediatrics 53:517, 1974. Reproduced by permission of Pediatrics.)

FIGURE 72–4. Roentgenogram after barium swallow, showing diverticulum before operation. The fistula is not demonstrated. (Robb D: Aust NZ J Surg 22:120, 1952.)

tracheostomy is often placed because breakdown of the closure is common.

ESOPHAGEAL STENOSIS

The lumen of the esophagus may be narrowed because of congenital stenosis, webs, external pressure, or acquired strictures.

CONGENITAL STENOSIS

There are two forms of congenital stenosis. In the first form, the stenosis is associated with the presence of abnormal tissue in the esophageal wall, such as respiratory tissue including cartilage and ciliated epithelium (Ohkawa et al, 1975). This lesion is usually located in the distal third of the esophagus. Most of these infants are asymptomatic until solids are introduced into the diet. Vomiting and discomfort are then noted during or shortly after feeding. The diagnosis is made by a radiographic contrast study. The treatment, surgical resection of the short affected segment with primary anastomosis, has generally been successful.

The second type of stenosis is, in fact, a variant of esophageal atresia. In this form of stenosis, the two segments of the esophagus are juxtaposed but separated by either a full thickness of esophageal wall or a thin diaphragm of mucous membrane. The diaphragm or web does not completely occlude the lumen, and vomiting, particularly after taking solid foods, is the presenting complaint. The diagnosis can be made using a barium study of the esophagus. A thin membrane may respond to dilation, but in some cases surgical resection may be necessary.

ESOPHAGEAL DUPLICATIONS

Esophageal duplications represent 10% to 15% of all gastrointestinal duplications. Vacuoles are formed during the early developmental obliteration of the esophageal lumen. If these vacuoles coalesce during recanalization, duplications are formed. The cysts are usually small and take on a spherical configuration, but they may also be tubular extending along the entire length of the esophagus. Sixty percent are located in the distal esophagus. Dysphagia or vomiting is the usual presenting manifestation, unless the cyst is large, in which case respiratory symptoms may occur. These lesions seldom present in the neonatal period.

HIATAL HERNIA

Etiology. Hiatal hernia refers to a defect in which at least 15% to 20% of the stomach is located in the chest (Fig. 72–6). In the newborn, hiatal hernia is due to either abnormal development of the diaphragm or a failure of the esophagus to elongate to permit the stomach to migrate caudally. The result is a short esophagus with the stomach completely or partially trapped above the diaphragm. Although the cause is not known, there is a familial occurrence of hiatal hernia (DiBella et al, 1991; Thomas and Carre, 1991).

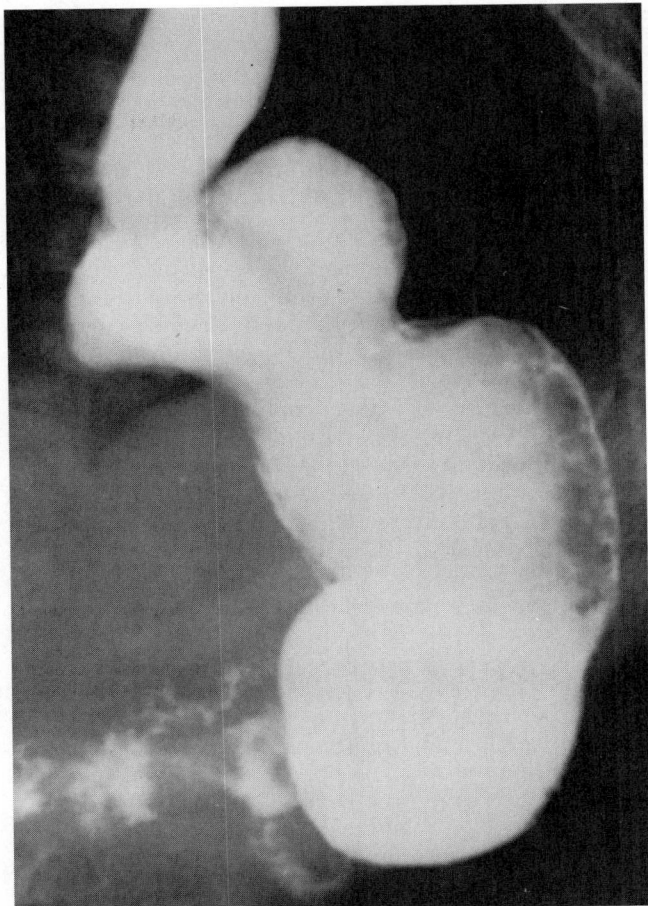

FIGURE 72–6. Upper gastrointestinal series from a 1-month-old newborn showing a large hiatus hernia and gastroesophageal reflux. The infant presented with massive vomiting following feeding. (Courtesy of Dr. Hoosang Taybi, Children's Hospital, Oakland, CA.)

Diagnosis. The primary symptom is vomiting, although its frequency and volume may vary with the size of the defect. The diagnosis may be made on an upper gastrointestinal series (see Fig. 72–6).

Treatment and Prognosis. Large defects require surgical closure of the diaphragmatic defect and the performance of a Nissan fundoplication (Johnson, 1986).

ACHALASIA

Achalasia is an idiopathic primary motility disorder of the esophagus characterized by (1) an increased lower esophageal sphincter pressure, (2) failure of the lower esophageal sphincter to relax, and (3) a loss of effective peristalsis in the body of the esophagus. Fewer than 20 infants with this disorder have been described (Asch et al, 1974). Presenting symptoms include vomiting and recurrent aspiration pneumonia. The diagnosis can be made from an upper gastrointestinal series, which shows a symmetric beak-like narrowing at the gastroesophageal junction, with moderate to advanced dilation above this stenotic point. Esophageal manometry is necessary to confirm the diagnosis. In infants, the treatment of choice is the Heller myotomy. The major complication following surgery is reflux, and an antireflux procedure at the time of the myotomy has been proposed (Lemmer et al, 1985).

CRICOPHARYNGEAL DYSFUNCTION

Some newborns aspirate at times despite having what appears to be a normal sucking and swallowing mechanism. If the problem is persistent, evaluation with a cineradiographic swallowing study is indicated. Diagnostic considerations include cricopharyngeal achalasia, familial dysautonomia, or myasthenia gravis. Blank and Silbiger (1972) described a newborn with cricopharyngeal achalasia. On barium swallow, a transverse submucosal bar was seen that was indistinguishable from the cricopharyngeus muscle. Treatment consisted of repeated bougienage. Linde and Westover (1962) noted that infants with familial dysautonomia may have pharyngeal dysfunction at birth that causes chronic aspiration. In addition, poor esophageal peristalsis delays esophageal emptying.

DIFFUSE ESOPHAGEAL SPASM

Diffuse esophageal spasm is an exceedingly rare problem in newborns. This esophageal motility disorder is characterized by tertiary esophageal peristaltic waves of increased amplitude and duration. It presents with symptoms of extreme agitation and vomiting during feeding. The diagnosis can be made by a barium study of the esophagus or by esophageal manometry. Extensive experience from adult series reports success using nitroglycerin or calcium channel blocking agents (Short and Thomas, 1992).

RUPTURE OF THE ESOPHAGUS

Esophageal perforation occurs in premature infants secondary to malpositioned endotracheal tubes as well as stiff nasogastric tubes (Krasna et al, 1987). Five newborns have been described with spontaneous rupture of the esophagus. In one instance, the rupture occurred just proximal to a stenosing web, but in the other four, the ruptures were unexplained. Hematemesis, hydropneumothorax, or both are the presenting manifestations. An esophagram can confirm the diagnosis, and emergent surgical repair is necessary.

REFERENCES

Asch MJ, Liebman W, Lachman RS, et al: Esophageal achalasia: Diagnosis and cardiomyotomy in a newborn infant. J Pediatr Surg 9:911, 1974.

Blank RH, Silbiger M: Cricopharyngeal achalasia as a cause of respiratory distress in infancy. J Pediatr 81:95, 1972.

Botha GSM: The gastro-esophageal region in infants: Observations in anatomy with special reference to the closing mechanism and partial thoracic stomach arch. Dis Child 33:78, 1958.

Burroughs N, Leape LL: Laryngotracheoesophageal cleft: Report of a case successfully treated and review of the literature. Pediatrics 53:516, 1974.

Carre LJ: The natural history of the partial thoracic stomach ("hiatal hernia") in children. Arch Dis Child 34:344, 1959.

DiBella D, Meli C, DiFedes GF, Mollica F: Genetic role in hernia of the esophageal hiatus: Description of the disease in 2 brothers. Pediatr Med Chir 13:209, 1991.

Fontan JP, Heldt GP, Heyman MB, et al: Esophageal spasm associated with apnea and bradycardia in an infant. Pediatrics 73:5255, 1984.

Goh DW, Brereton RJ, Spitz L: Esophageal atresia with obstructed tracheoesophageal fistula and gasless abdomen. J Pediatr Surg 26:160, 1991.

Greenwood RD, Rosenthal A: Cardiovascular malformations associated with tracheoesophageal fistula and esophageal atresia. Pediatrics 57:87, 1976.

Grunwald P: Asphyxia, trauma and shock at birth. Arch Pediatr 67:103, 1950.

Hausmann PF, Close AS, Williams LP: Occurrence of tracheoesophageal fistula in three consecutive siblings. Surgery 41:542, 1957.

Herbst JJ: Gastroesophageal reflux. J Pediatr 98:859, 1981.

Herbst JJ, Minton SD, Book LS: Gastroesophageal reflux causing respiratory distress and apnea in newborn infants. J Pediatr 95:763, 1979.

Hillemeier AC, Gnil BB, McCallum R, et al: Esophageal and gastric motor abnormalities in gastroesophageal reflux during infancy. Gastroenterology 84:741, 1983.

Hohf RP, Kimball ER, Ballenger JJ: Rupture of the esophagus in the neonate. JAMA 181:939, 1962.

Holder TM, Ashcraft KW: Esophageal atresia and tracheoesophageal fistula (collective review). Ann Thorac Surg 9:445, 1970.

Johnson DG: The Nissan fundoplication. *In* Ashcraft KW, Holder TM (Eds): Pediatric Esophageal Surgery. Orlando, Grune & Stratton, 1986, pp 193–208.

Krasna IH, Rosenfeld D, Benjamin BG, et al: Esophageal perforation in the neonate: An emerging problem in the nursery. J Pediatr Surg 22:784, 1987.

Kutiyanawa M, Wyse AK, Brereton RJ, et al: CHARGE and esophageal atresia. J Pediatr Surg 27:558, 1992.

Lemmer JH, Coran AG, Wesley JR, et al: Achalasia in children: Treatment by anterior esophageal myotomy (modified Heller operation). J Pediatr Surg 20:333, 1985.

Linde LM, Westover JL: Esophageal and gastric abnormalities in dysautonomia. Pediatrics 29:303, 1962.

Merriam JC Jr, Benirschke K: Esophageal erosions in the newborn. Lab Invest 8:39, 1959.

Meyers NA: Oesophageal atresia: The epitome of modern surgery. Ann R Coll Surg Engl 54:312, 1974.

Ohkawa H, Takahashi H, Hoshino Y, et al: Lower esophageal stenosis in association with tracheobronchial remnants. J Pediatr Surg 10:453, 1975.

Orenstein SR, Magill HL, Brooks P: Thickening of infant feedings for therapy of gastroesophageal reflux. J Pediatr 110:181, 1987.

Oski FA: Iron-fortified formulas and gastrointestinal symptoms in infants: A controlled study. Pediatrics 66:168, 1980.

Pletcher BA, Friedes JS, Greg WR, Toulonkian RJ: Familial occurrence of esophageal atresia with and without tracheoesophageal fistula: Report of two unusual kindreds. Am J Med Genet 39:380, 1991.

Quan L, Smith DW: The VATER association: Vertebral defects, anal atresia, T-fistula with esophageal atresia, radial and renal dysplasia: A spectrum of associated defects. J Pediatr 104:7, 1973.

Raffensperger JG: Esophageal atresia and tracheoesophageal stenosis. *In* Raffensperger JG (Ed): Swenson's Pediatric Surgery, 5th ed. Norwalk, CT, Appleton & Lange, 1990, pp 697–717.

Randolph JG, Lilly JR, Anderson KD: Surgical treatment of gastroesophageal reflux in infants. Ann Surg 180:479, 1974.

Reckham PP: Infants with esophageal atresia weighing under 3 pounds. J Pediatr Surg 16:595, 1981.

Roberts CC, Herbst JJ, Jolley SG, et al: Evaluation of tests for gastroesophageal reflux in patients operated on for tracheoesophageal fistula. Pediatr Res 14:509, 1980.

Short TP, Thomas E: An overview of the role of calcium antagonists in the treatment of achalasia and diffuse esophageal spasm. Drugs 43:177, 1992.

Skinner MA, Shorter NA: Primary neonatal cricopharyngeal achalasia: A case report and review of the literature. J Pediatr Surg 27:1509, 1992.

Spitzer AR, Boyle JT, Tuchman DN, et al: Awake apnea associated with gastroesophageal reflux: A specific clinical syndrome. J Pediatr 104:200, 1984.

Thomas PS, Carre IJ: Findings on barium swallow in younger siblings of children with hiatal hernia (partial thoracic stomach). J Pediatr Gastroenterol Nutr 12:174, 1991.

Vandenplas T, Sacre-Smits L: Seventeen-hour continuous esophageal pH monitoring in the newborn: Evaluation of the influence of position in asymptomatic and symptomatic babies. J Pediatr Gastroenterol Nutr 4:356, 1985.

Walsh JK, Farrell MK, Keenan WJ, et al: Gastroesophageal reflux in infants: Relation to apnea. J Pediatr 99:197, 1981.

Werlin SL, Dodds WJ, Hogan WJ, et al: Mechanisms of gastroesophageal reflux in children. Pediatrics 97:244, 1980.

Whitington PF, Shermeta DW, Eto DSY, et al: Role of lower esophageal sphincter incompetence in recurrent pneumonia after·repair of esophageal atresia. J Pediatr 91:550, 1977.

Woolley MM, Chinnock RF, Paul RH: Premature twins with esophageal atresia and tracheoesophageal fistula. Acta Paediatr 50:423, 1961.

CHAPTER 73

Disorders of the Stomach

Carol Lynn Berseth

HYPOPLASIA OF THE STOMACH

Hypoplasia of the stomach (congenital microgastria) is an exceedingly rare lesion in which fetal rotation of the stomach does not occur. Tissues fail to differentiate into a distinct fundus, body, antrum, and pyloric canal. The gastroesophageal junction is incompetent, and food may be stored in the distal esophagus. Therefore, vomiting is the major clinical presentation. Survival is possible (Blank and Chisholm, 1973), but additional gastrointestinal anomalies may be present.

GASTRIC DUPLICATION

Gastric duplications are spherical or hollow-tubular structures that (1) are lined by a mucosal layer composed of gastric, small bowel, or colonic epithelium; (2) contain a smooth muscle coat contiguous with the muscle of the stomach; and (3) are contiguous with the stomach wall. Most do not communicate with the gastric lumen and are located along the greater curvature. Embryologically the lesion arises during the 4th week of gestation when normally the embryonic notochordal plates and endoderm separate. A band between them may cause a traction diverticulum leading to gut cyst formation (McLetchie et al, 1954). In addition, associated anomalies occur in 50% of these patients; the most common are esophageal duplication and vertebral abnormalities. The treatment is complete surgical excision of the cyst.

PYLORIC ATRESIA

Pyloric atresia is rare, and it often is accompanied by a history of polyhydramnios. Pyloric atresia may be due to vascular compromise that occurs early in gestation, similar to that which occurs to cause intestinal and colonic atresias. The presence of a gasless abdomen on a plain film and the failure of contrast material to leave the stomach on an upper gastrointestinal series are suggestive of the diagnosis and warrant urgent operative intervention. Simple excision of the diaphragm may be adequate, but some patients may require gastroduodenostomy or gastrojejunostomy.

ANTRAL WEB OR DIAPHRAGM

Antral webs or diaphragms are usually incomplete or contain an orifice and therefore produce a partial gastric outlet obstruction. Of 44 cases in pediatric patients, 60% were diagnosed before 3 months of age (Bell et al, 1977). Nonbilious vomiting is the most common presenting symptom. A careful upper gastrointestinal series (Fig. 73–1) may demonstrate the web, but upper gastrointestinal endoscopy may be necessary for diagnosis in some cases. Surgical

intervention usually consists of excision of the web and pyloroplasty.

PYLORIC STENOSIS

Definition and Epidemiology. Hypertrophy of the pyloric muscle in early infancy results in partial gastric outlet obstruction. The incidence is 1 to 3 per 1000 live births, and males are affected four times more often than females. First-borns account for half of the cases. Whites are at greater risk than blacks (Laron and Horne, 1957). Premature infants are affected with the same frequency as term infants.

Etiology. The exact cause of pyloric stenosis is unknown. Hereditary factors may play a role because there is a 7% incidence of pyloric stenosis among the siblings of affected patients.

Diagnosis. Vomiting is the primary presenting symptom. It may occur from birth to 12 weeks, but most often the onset occurs between the 3rd and 5th weeks. In premature infants, the onset follows the same pattern postnatally, regardless of the postconceptual age. At first, vomiting may occur infrequently. With time, the frequency and volume of the emesis increases, and projectile vomiting develops. Weight loss, dehydration, and metabolic alkalosis may occur as a consequence of the vomiting. Gastric peristaltic waves may be seen passing obliquely from the left upper quadrant across the midline when the infant is fed. Jaundice may occasionally occur, but indirect hyperbilirubinemia recedes 5 to 10 days after pyloromyotomy. In most instances of pyloric stenosis, a definite tumor, or "olive," can be felt either in the epigastric area or just to the right of the midline in the right upper quadrant. When the clinical presentation is atypical, the lesion can be demonstrated on an upper gastrointestinal series. The most significant radiographic sign is curvature, elongation, and narrowing of the pyloric channel, the *string sign* (Fig. 73–2). More recently, ultrasound has been used to make the diagnosis (Fig. 73–3) (Hallam et al, 1995; Neilson and Hollman, 1994).

Treatment. The stomach should be decompressed, and dehydration and metabolic alkalosis should be corrected with intravenous fluids before surgery. Pyloromyotomy (Fredet-Ramstedt operation) involves splitting the hypertrophied pyloric muscle. Feedings may be resumed 8 to 12 hours after surgery and quickly advanced so that by 24 hours the infant is ingesting formula or breast milk.

Prognosis. Overall the mortality from this operation is less than 0.5% (Scharli et al, 1969). Perforation of the

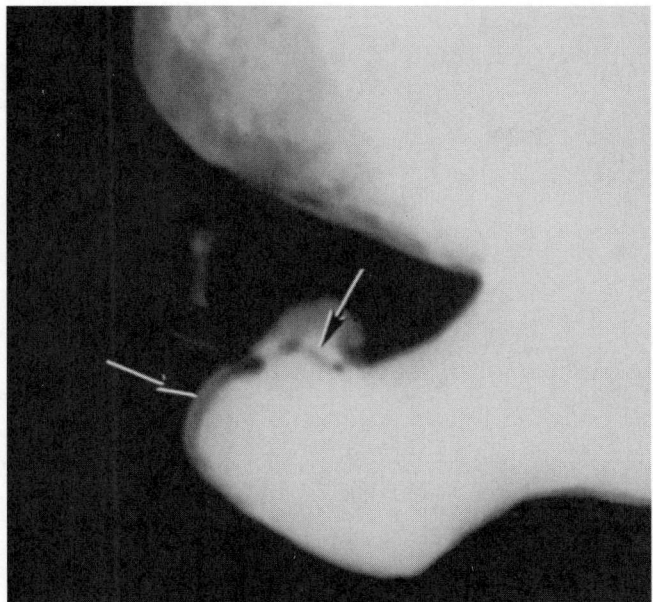

FIGURE 73–1. The arrows point to a thin antral diaphragm, the orifice of which can be seen. This infant began vomiting at 2 weeks of age. The film was taken at 2 months of age. (Courtesy of Dr. Paul Nancarrow, Children's Hospital, Oakland, CA.)

stomach at the time of surgery is seen in less than 2%. These are recognized and closed at the time of surgery. Incomplete pyloromyotomy is rare.

PYLOROSPASM

The diagnosis of infantile pylorospasm is made by radiographic evaluation, and it must be differentiated from pylo-

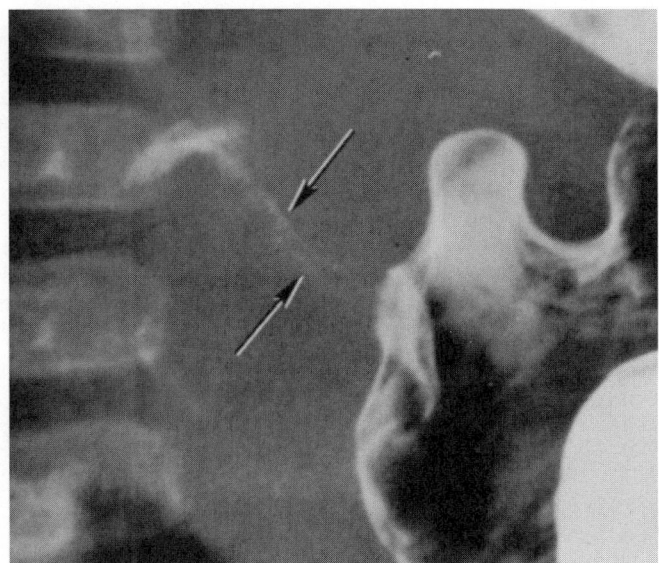

FIGURE 73–2. Upper gastrointestinal series illustrating the "string sign" (arrows) diagnostic for pyloric stenosis. This 2-month-old infant began vomiting at 3 weeks of age. (Courtesy of Dr. Paul Nancarrow, Children's Hospital, Oakland, CA.)

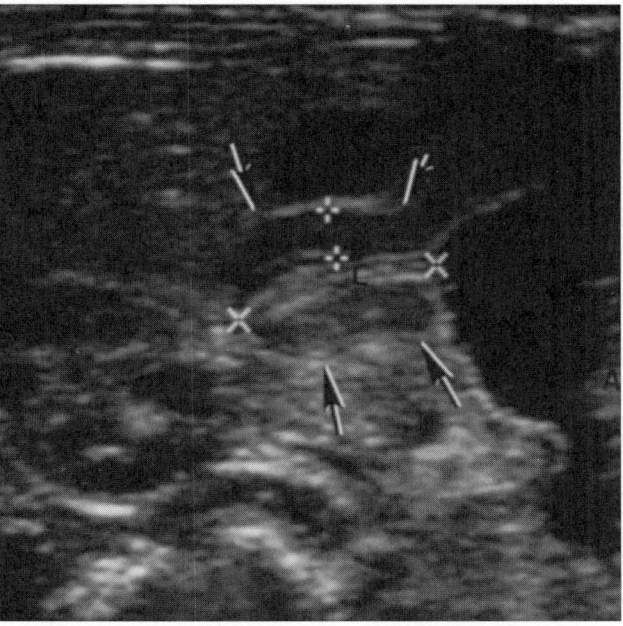

FIGURE 73–3. Ultrasonographic study of the right upper quadrant in a 1-month-old infant with a 1-week history of vomiting. The length (+) of the pylorus is 18.4 mm (normal up to 16 mm) and wall thickness (×) is 4.5 mm (normal is up to 4.0 mm). The arrows outline the muscular wall and point to the lumen (L). A is the antral lumen. (Courtesy of Dr. Ronald M. Cohen, Children's Hospital, Oakland, CA.)

ric stenosis. Radiographically, infants with pylorospasm show a narrow distal antrum, but in contrast to pyloric stenosis, the caliber of the channels intermittently narrows and widens. Peristalsis is present in the affected area, and there are no features of muscular hypertrophy, as seen with pyloric stenosis. During the examination, an initial delay in the passage of barium may be followed by a sudden emptying of the stomach. The cause of pylorospasm is unknown. Conservative medical management consisting of atropine sulfate 0.04 mg/kg/d intravenously given in eight doses 10 to 15 minutes before each meal may be more successful than metoclopramide in relieving the spasm. Pylorospasm is usually transient, and it resolves within 1 to 2 weeks.

PEPTIC ULCER DISEASE

Definition and Epidemiology. Ulceration of the gastric or duodenal mucosa is rare in the newborn. Peptic ulcers may be classified as primary if they occur in otherwise healthy individuals or secondary if they are seen in association with underlying systemic disorders. In the newborn, most ulcers are secondary and are found in the duodenum (Bell et al, 1981).

Etiology. The cause of peptic ulcer disease is unknown but is probably multifactorial even in patients with secondary ulcers (Byrne, 1985). Genetic factors, emotional factors, dietary and environmental factors, the amount of hydrochloric acid, and local tissue resistance factors contribute to ulcer formation in the older child and adolescent. In the newborn, a breakdown of local tissue resistance plays the

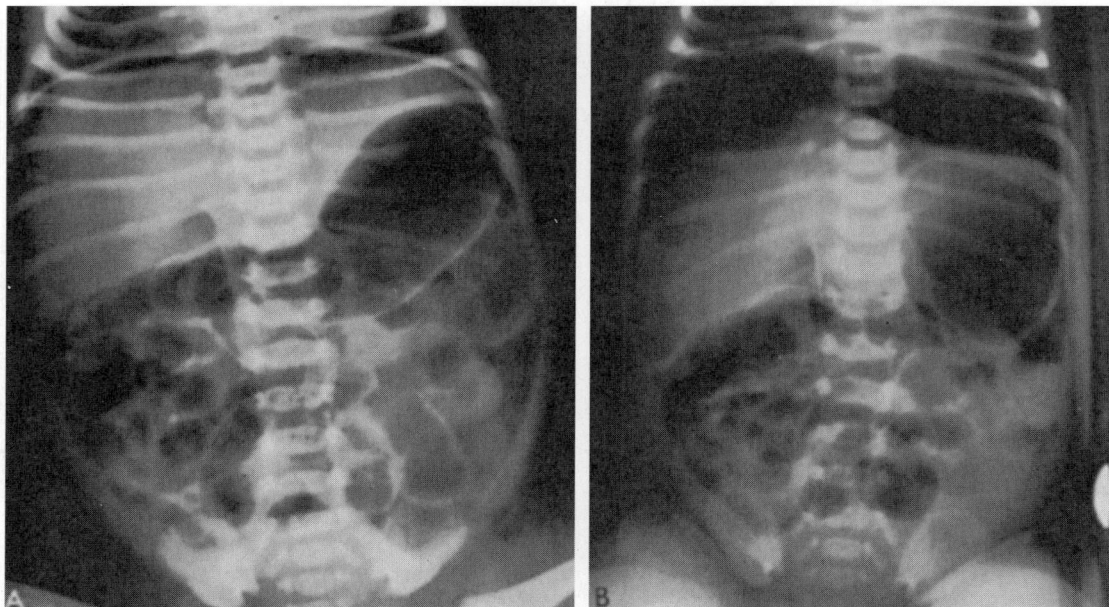

FIGURE 73–4. *A,* Anteroposterior view of abdomen taken in the erect position at 72 hours of age. There is air in the stomach and intestine, and one gets the distinct impression that some of the air is outside of the lumen of the bowel. A layer of air is clearly visible above the liver and below the diaphragm. *B,* Ten hours later. By now, there is a huge accumulation of air between the diaphragm and the liver.

major role. Normally the mucosal cell is protected by a complex barrier, which includes gastric mucus, the secretion of bicarbonate by the mucosal cell, the *alkaline tide*, mucosal blood flow, and prostaglandins. Drugs, such as indomethacin, that block prostaglandin synthesis or acidosis and shock, which affect blood flow and bicarbonate production, precipitate events that disrupt this barrier and thus permit mucosal cell destruction, inflammation, and ulcer formation to occur.

Diagnosis. In the newborn, hematemesis, hematochezia, and perforation of the stomach or duodenum are presenting clinical manifestations. At times, the loss of blood may be considerable, causing a rapid drop in the hematocrit and the development of shock. At other times, bleeding may be gradual and recognized only by the presence of "coffee grounds" or a Hemoccult-positive stool. In general, radiographic studies in the newborn are not useful in demonstrating the presence of ulceration or gastritis. Upper gastrointestinal fiberoptic endoscopy can be done in the smallest of infants. For suspected peptic ulcer disease, endoscopy is the procedure of choice.

Treatment. Blood loss into the gastrointestinal tract requires prompt and adequate replacement. A nasogastric tube should be passed and the stomach lavaged with room-temperature saline (Andrus and Ponsky, 1987). Antacid therapy 1 mL/kg every 2 hours and/or H₂ blockers 1.5 to 2 mg/kg every 6 hours is then begun. If there is no further bleeding after 24 hours, feedings may be resumed. The antacids should be continued at the same dose and given 1 hour after each feeding for 6 to 8 weeks.

GASTRIC PERFORATION

Spontaneous perforation of the stomach in the newborn occurs most often during the first 5 days of life (Fig. 73–4) (Bell, 1985). Perinatal stress leading to localized ischemia appears to be the causative mechanism in 80% of the cases. In 20% of the cases, however, no cause can be identified. Potential causes include rapid overdistention, trauma from passage of a nasogastric tube, and spontaneous rupture of weak points in the gastric wall along the greater curvature where muscle is deficient. Shaw and coworkers (1965) showed that the stomach of a normal infant, when sufficiently distended with air to raise intragastric pressure to a critical level, would rupture.

Symptoms that typically occur by the 2nd to 5th day include refusal to suck, vomiting, and abdominal distention. Plain films of the abdomen show the presence of free air. Immediate decompression, fluid resuscitation, and broad-spectrum antibiotic administration should be followed by immediate surgical intervention to close the tear. Early recognition and treatment result in an overall survival rate of 90% (Bell, 1985).

REFERENCES

Andrus CH, Ponsky JL: The effects of irrigant temperature in upper gastrointestinal hemorrhage: A requiem for iced saline lavage. Am J Gastroenterol 82:1062, 1987.
Bell JJ: Perforation of the gastrointestinal tract and peritonitis in the neonate. Surg Gynecol Obstet 160:20, 1985.
Bell MJ, Keating JP, Ternberg JL, et al: Perforated stress ulcers in infants. J Pediatr Surg 16:998, 1981.
Bell MJ, Ternberg JL, McAlister W, et al: Antral diaphragm—a cause of gastric outlet obstruction in infants and children. J Pediatr 90:196, 1977.

Blank E, Chisholm AJ: Congenital microgastria: A case report with 26-year follow-up. Pediatrics 51:1037, 1973.

Byrne WJ: Diagnosis and treatment of peptic ulcer disease in children. Pediatr Rev 7:182, 1985.

Hallam D, Hansen B, Bodner B, et al: Pyloric size in normal infants and infants suspected of having hypertropic pyloric stenosis. Acta Radiol 36:261, 1995.

Laron Z, Horne LM: The incidence of infantile pyloric stenosis. Am J Dis Child 94:151, 1957.

McLetchie NGB, Purves JK, Saunders RL: The genesis of gastric and certain intestinal diverticula and enterogenous cysts. Surg Gynecol Obstet 9:135, 1954.

Neilson D, Hollman AS: The ultrasonic diagnosis of infantile hypertrophic pyloric stenosis: Technique and accuracy. Clin Radiol 49:246, 1994.

Scharli A, Sieber WK, Kiesewetter WB: Hypertrophic pyloric stenosis at the Children's Hospital of Pittsburgh from 1912 to 1967. J Pediatr Surg 4:108, 1969.

Shaw A, Blanc WA, Santulli TV, et al: Spontaneous rupture of the stomach: A clinical and experimental study. Surgery 58:561, 1965.

Wieczorek RL, Seidman I, Ranson JHC, et al: Congenital duplication of the stomach: Case report and review of the English literature. Am J Gastroenterol 79:597, 1984.

CHAPTER 74

Disorders of the Intestine and Pancreas

Carol Lynn Berseth

MECHANICAL OBSTRUCTION

Complete or partial obstruction of the small bowel or colon is not unusual in the newborn. A variety of lesions, intrinsic or extrinsic, may be responsible (Table 74–1). Success or failure in terms of morbidity and mortality depends not so much on pinpointing the exact location of the lesion as it does on correctly diagnosing obstruction as the cause of the clinical symptoms and then instituting prompt operative intervention.

Vomiting, particularly of bile-stained material, with abdominal distention or the failure to pass meconium are symptoms highly suggestive of the presence of intestinal obstruction. If the obstruction is high or complete, symptoms start soon after birth. Vomiting of bile suggests that the lesion is located distal to the ampulla of Vater, whereas sporadic vomiting may be seen in patients with partial obstruction caused by malrotation, duplications, or annular pancreas. Abdominal distention may be present soon after birth, reaching a peak at 24 to 48 hours with visible peristaltic waves. Failure to pass meconium within 24 hours after birth suggests the presence of a colonic lesion. Infants with high obstruction or even those with obstruction as low as the ileum pass meconium, so this finding by itself does not exclude obstruction. Prenatal diagnosis of gastrointestinal obstruction has been successful and is becoming more common (Langer et al, 1989).

Palpation of the abdomen may reveal a solid or cystic mass. Occasionally, hard masses are palpable throughout the abdomen, a finding consistent with meconium ileus.

The initial radiographic studies obtained should be plain films in the supine and left lateral position. Normally, air fills the stomach immediately after birth, the small bowel within 12 hours, and the colon within 24 hours. When obstruction exists, the air pattern stops abruptly at that point, leaving the remainder of the bowel airless. Obstruction at the pylorus produces one large bubble outlining the dilated stomach, whereas duodenal obstructions produce a "double-bubble" appearance (Fig. 74–1). Distal obstructions show a series of dilated, air- and fluid-filled loops of intestine. Obstruction resulting from meconium ileus is an exception in that air–fluid levels usually are not seen. In an incomplete obstruction, gas may be seen distal to dilated loops of bowel.

If the diagnosis is in doubt or a meconium plug is suspected, a contrast enema can be done. The finding of a microcolon is suggestive of small bowel atresia or meconium ileus. An upper gastrointestinal series is done only if the plain film and enema are nondiagnostic (see also Chapter 80).

Intrinsic Obstruction

Atresias

Definition and Etiology

Atresia, complete obstruction of the lumen of the bowel, should be distinguished from stenosis, which is a narrowing of the lumen. Atresias account for one third of all intestinal obstructions in the newborn, occurring in 1 of every 1500 live births. Sites of occurrence, in order of frequency, are jejunoileal, duodenal, and colonic. Failure of the gut to recanalize during the 8th to 10th weeks of gestation seems to be the most likely cause for duodenal atresia. In the jejunum, ileum, and colon, vascular compromise early in gestation may be responsible for bowel atresias (Louw, 1966). Other potential causes in utero include incarceration of the physiologic umbilical hernia, localized volvulus, intussusception, focal peritonitis, and peritoneal band formation.

Duodenal Atresia

Thirty percent of all atresias occur in the duodenum and most are distal to the ampulla. Approximately 70% of infants with duodenal atresia also have other associated anomalies including, in order of frequency, Down syndrome, annular pancreas, cardiovascular malformations, malrotation, esophageal atresia, small bowel lesions, and anorectal lesions (Young and Wilkinson, 1968). Anatomically, duodenal atresia may occur in several forms (Fig. 74–2). Bile-stained vomiting on the 1st day of life and a

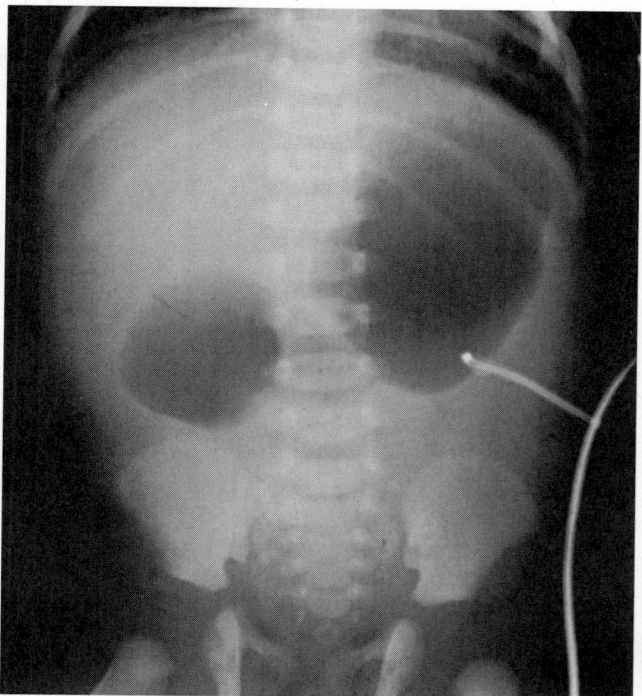

FIGURE 74–1. Abdominal film from a 12-hour-old infant with vomiting. A "double-bubble" sign is present. At laparotomy duodenal atresia was found. (Courtesy of Dr. Ronald M. Cohen, Children's Hospital, Oakland, CA.)

TABLE 74-1

Causes of Intestinal Obstruction in the Newborn

Mechanical		Functional
Congenital	**Acquired**	
Intrinsic	Necrotizing	Hirschsprung disease
Atresias	enterocolitis	Meconium plug
Stenoses	Intussusception	syndrome
Meconium ileus	Peritoneal	Ileus
Anorectal malformations	adhesions	Peritonitis
Enteric duplications		
Extrinsic		Intestinal pseudo-
Volvulus		obstruction
Peritoneal bands		syndrome
Annular pancreas		
Cysts and tumors		
Incarcerated hernias		

history of polyhydramnios are common presenting symptoms. Abdominal distention is usually absent. Dehydration with a metabolic alkalosis rapidly ensues. The diagnosis may be made on plain abdominal films with the appearance of the double-bubble sign (see Fig. 74–1). Medical therapy consists of the passage of a nasogastric tube and correction of dehydration and electrolyte abnormalities. Urgent surgical intervention is necessary. Because of the high incidence of multiple atresias (15%), inspection of the entire bowel is carried out before constructing a duodenojejunostomy or, more recently, a duodenoduodenostomy (Weber et al, 1986) (see also Chapter 80). The mortality rate following surgery is less than 10% (Mooney et al, 1987). Most deaths that now occur are due to related major anomalies.

Jejunoileal Atresia

Fifty-five percent of intestinal atresias occur in the jejunum or ileum. Of these, 31% occur in the proximal jejunum, 20% in the distal jejunum, 13% in the proximal ileum, and 36% in the distal ileum (De Lorimier et al, 1969). Associated extraintestinal anomalies are infrequent (7%), and unlike in duodenal atresia, Down syndrome is uncommon (1%). A useful classification is shown in Figure 74–3 (Martin and Zerella, 1976). Signs and symptoms of jejunoileal atresia include maternal polyhydramnios, bilious vomiting, abdominal distention, which may not become obvious until the 2nd or 3rd day of life, failure to pass meconium, and jaundice. On a plain film, dilated loops of bowel with no gas in the rectum are seen (Fig. 74–4). Contrast enema using Gastrografin or barium may not reach the obstruction, but the appearance of a microcolon in the normal anatomic position is strong evidence that other lesions, such as malrotation, colonic atresia, and aganglionosis are unlikely. Meconium ileus can also be excluded. The type of surgical operation depends on the lesion, but the procedure of choice is primary closure with end-to-end anastomosis. Survival rate, with the availability of postoperative intravenous nutritional support, exceeds 90%.

Colonic Atresia

Less than 10% of atresias occur in the colon, and stenosis is even less common. Seventy-five percent of the atresias

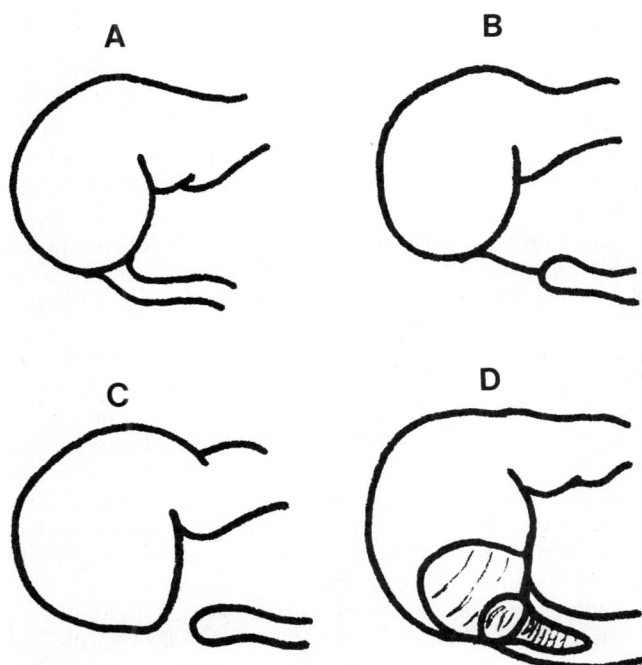

FIGURE 74–2. Forms of intrinsic duodenal obstruction. *A,* Duodenal atresia with continuity of the bowel wall. *B,* Duodenal atresia with a fibrous cord joining segments. *C,* Complete atresia with two separate segments. *D,* Wind sock deformity.

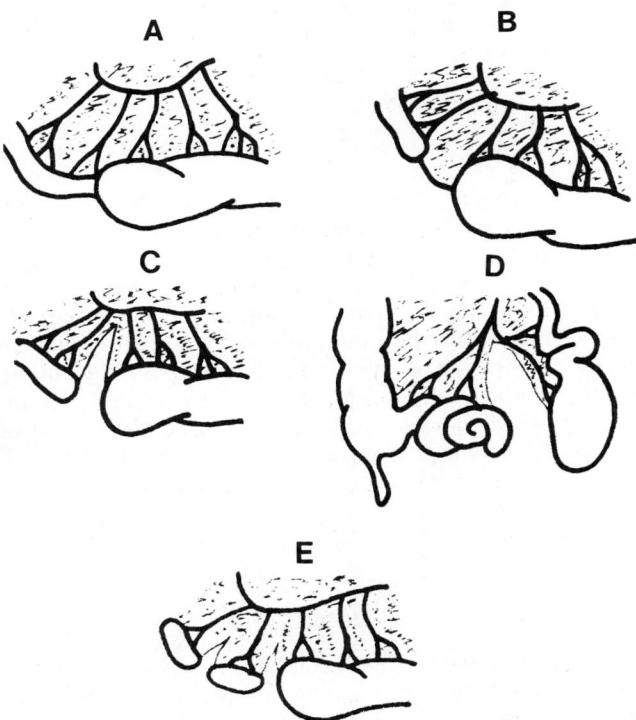

FIGURE 74–3. Classification of intestinal atresias. *A,* Mucosal atresia with intact bowel wall and mesentery. *B,* Blind ends joined by a fibrous cord. *C,* Blind ends separated by a mesenteric defect. *D,* Blind ends with the "apple-peel" atresia. *E,* Multiple atresias.

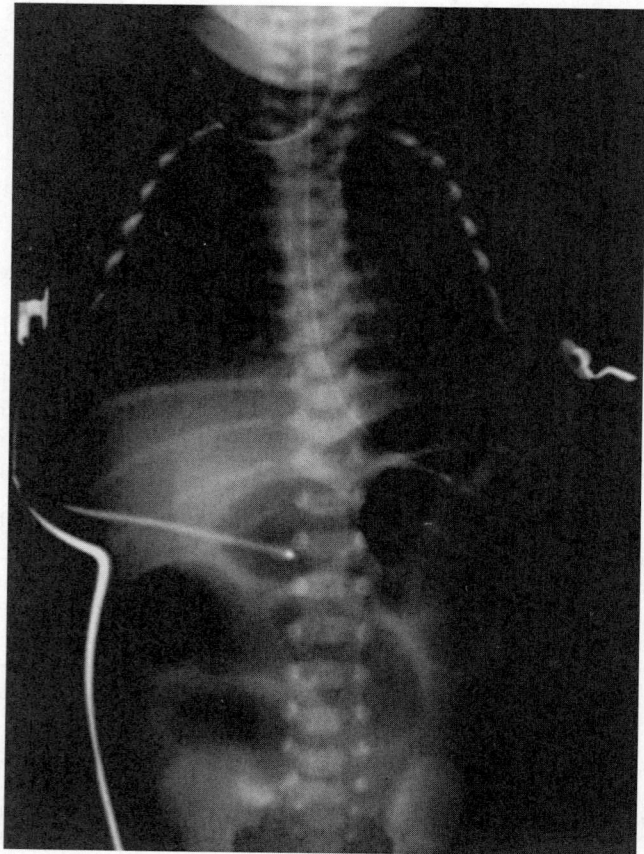

FIGURE 74–4. Plain abdominal film in a 24-hour-old infant with vomiting and abdominal distention. Multiple dilated bowel loops are present. No gas is seen in the rectum. At surgery proximal ileal atresia was found. (Courtesy of Dr. Ronald M. Cohen, Children's Hospital, Oakland, CA.)

are found proximal to the splenic flexure, usually in the ascending colon (Sturim and Ternberg, 1966), with a significant amount of colon missing in most infants. Associated anomalies of the gastrointestinal wall may occur in one third of the infants. Clinical symptoms of colonic atresia include abdominal distention and vomiting beginning on the 2nd or 3rd day of life and failure to pass meconium. On plain radiographs, dilated loops of bowel are present, but a contrast enema is essential to make the definitive diagnosis. One surgical approach involves primary anastomosis, whereas another involves initial colostomy or ileostomy with subsequent anastomosis. Survival with the second approach is greater than 90% (Boles et al, 1976).

Stenosis

Duodenal stenosis may be secondary to an intrinsic defect (see Fig. 74–3) or the result of compression by extrinsic lesions. These include annular pancreas, peritoneal bands, aberrant superior mesenteric artery, or a preduodenal portal vein. Depending on the degree of obstruction, vomiting may begin at any time after birth. Because most lesions involve the second or third portion of the duodenum, the vomiting is bilious. Plain films are usually not diagnostic,

but on upper gastrointestinal series the area of stenosis can be delineated; differentiation of the cause may not be possible before surgery.

Meconium Ileus

Definition and Etiology

Meconium ileus refers to an intraluminal intestinal obstruction produced by thick inspissated meconium. Ninety percent of patients with meconium ileus have cystic fibrosis (CF). Indeed, 10% to 15% of CF patients present with meconium ileus. Recently, DNA markers for the CF gene have been identified and localized on chromosome 7 (Rommens et al, 1989). Mornet and coworkers (1988) showed different haplotypic variants for CF chromosomes in families with meconium ileus as compared with families with no meconium ileus. To explain this finding they suggested there were different mutations at the same locus: one for CF and one for meconium ileus. However, Kerem and colleagues (1989a) were unable to verify this observation.

Severe pancreatic involvement is not a consistent finding in CF patients presenting with meconium ileus (Waters et al, 1990). In utero, some CF fetuses produce exceptionally viscid secretions from the mucous glands of the small intestine. The meconium formed is dry and contains higher than usual concentrations of protein, including albumin (Schwachmann and Antonowicz, 1981). The abnormal meconium adheres firmly to the mucosal surface of the distal small bowel creating an intraluminal obstruction. Histologically, the goblet cells and mucous glands are prominent and distended with an eosinophilic material that merges with the intraluminal meconium for a cast of the crypts and villi. Proximal to the obstruction there may be intestinal muscular hypertrophy.

Diagnosis

Prenatal diagnosis of CF is possible (Lemna et al, 1990). A family history of CF should alert the clinician to the possibility of meconium ileus. In the simple form in which obstruction occurs in the middle and distal ileum without perforation and peritonitis, signs of obstruction appear within the first 48 hours in an otherwise healthy infant. Abdominal distention is noticed between 12 and 24 hours, after which vomiting occurs. No meconium is passed. Physical examinations may reveal hard palpable masses throughout the abdomen that are freely movable in any direction. Meconium ileus complicated by volvulus, atresias, meconium peritonitis, or pseudocyst formation is found in one third of the patients. Newborns with these complications present earlier than those with simple meconium ileus, usually within the first 24 hours of life. They appear sicker, with severe vomiting, signs of neonatal sepsis, and more marked distention causing respiratory distress.

Radiographic examination with the infant in the erect position shows dilated loops of bowel. Fluid levels are inconspicuous because of the viscous nature of the meconium, which produces a coarse granular, or ground-glass, appearance. The abdominal film may show, in addition to the distended gas-filled loops, intra-abdominal calcification indicative of meconium peritonitis (Fig. 74–5). A cross-

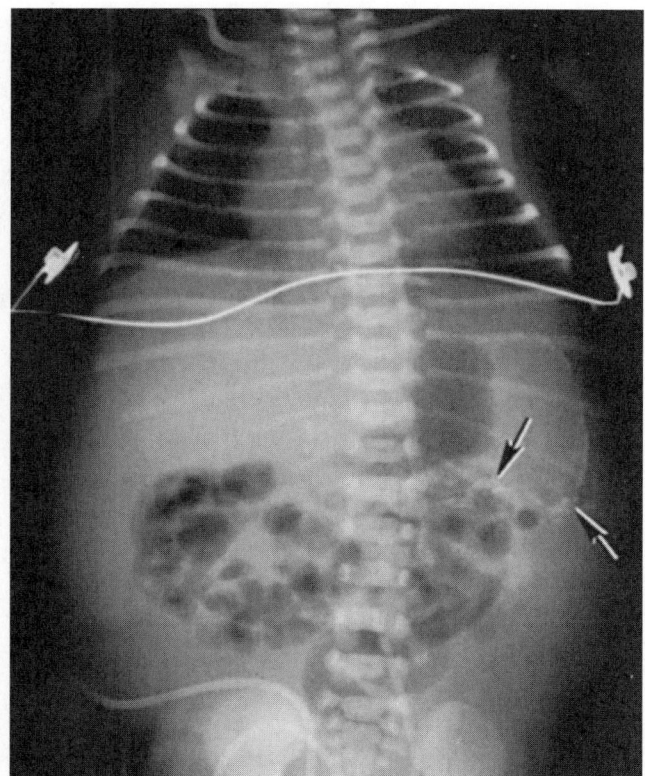

FIGURE 74–5. Ten-hour-old infant with ascites and abdominal calcification (arrows) secondary to meconium peritonitis. No gas is present in the rectum. The infant had ileal atresia and a subsequent sweat chloride test was positive. (Courtesy of Dr. Ronald M. Cohen, Children's Hospital, Oakland, CA.)

intervention, not another enema. If the enema is successful, meconium passage continues for 24 to 48 hours. Acetylcysteine, 5 mL every 6 hours for 5 days, is given via a nasogastric tube. Broad-spectrum antibiotics should also be given.

Surgical intervention in simple meconium ileus may consist of enterotomy with irrigation and immediate closure, resection of the ileum with irrigation and primary anastomosis, or, in the past, resection of the ileum and construction of a Mikulicz-type ileostomy or a Bishop Koop ileostomy. More recently, the need for an ileostomy has been questioned (Nguyen et al, 1986). Complicated meconium ileus always requires surgical intervention. The operative procedure depends on the pathologic findings.

Prognosis

Operative mortality is well under 20% for simple meconium ileus. The severity of pulmonary involvement affects eventual outcome.

Anorectal Malformations
Definition and Epidemiology

Anorectal anomalies occur in 1 of every 5000 births and are slightly more common in males (deVries and Cox, 1985). Associated anomalies occur in more than half of these infants and are more frequent in cases in which the rectal pouch lies above the puborectalis sling. Vertebral malformations are the most common, followed by genitourinary malformations (28%) and gastrointestinal malformations (13%) (Kiesewetter and Chang, 1977).

Etiology

The proctoderm comprises the anus and a canal that extends cephalad a short distance to meet the blind end of the hindgut, which has simultaneously moved caudad. Around the 7th to 8th week of gestation these should make contact, separated only by an anal membrane. At the same time, the lower urinary tract develops alongside the lower intestinal tract, separated by the urorectal membrane. Anal malformations arise locally from maldevelopment within the proctoderm. Atresias, stenoses, and fistulas arise from imperfect resolution of the anorectal membrane with or without concomitant failure of the urorectal membrane to separate completely the rectal and genitourinary anlagen.

Diagnosis and Treatment

Inspection of the perianal area will reveal abnormal anatomy in cases of anorectal anomaly. Table 74–2 lists the various types and relative frequencies of anorectal anomalies.

Anal Stenosis

Anal stenosis accounts for approximately 8% of anorectal anomalies. The lesion represents a narrowing of a normally formed anorectum at its lower most extremity. The onset of symptoms varies depending on the size of the opening.

table lateral film with the baby in the prone position helps establish whether air is in the rectum. The presence of air–fluid levels suggests the presence of jejunal or ileal atresia. The presence of a single grossly distended loop of bowel suggests the presence of postnatal volvulus. Perforations after birth result in free intraperitoneal air.

All newborns with meconium ileus should be evaluated for CF. Boat and coworkers (1989) have reviewed the clinical, physiologic, and genetic aspects of CF. The identification and cloning of the primary CF gene and the ability to identify mutations causing CF have advanced the clinician's ability to provide accurate diagnosis as well as counseling (Kerem et al, 1989b; Lemna et al, 1990; Rommens et al, 1989).

Treatment

In simple meconium ileus, approximately 60% of the infants have their obstructions successfully relieved by a hyperosmolar enema (Noblett, 1969). Before the hyperosmolar enema is given, other complications, such as perforation, volvulus, or atresia, must be excluded. The hypertonic enema draws water into the intestinal tract, dislodging and breaking up the meconium. Because of rapid fluid shifts, great care must be taken to maintain fluid and electrolyte balance. Failure of the infant to pass meconium within several hours after the enema is an indication for surgical

TABLE 74–2

Anatomic Classification of Anorectal Malformations

Lesion		Frequency (%)			Survival (%)
		Overall	Male	Female	
Low (below the levator)	Anal stenosis	8			100
	Imperforate anal membrane	6			95
	Anal agenesis	36			84
	No fistula	7	7	0	
	Fistula	29	8	21	
	Anovulvar		1	14	
	Anoperineal		8	7	
High (above the levator)	Rectal agenesis	47			72
	No fistula	13	11	2	
	Fistula	31	21	10	
	Rectourethral		24		
	Rectovesical		1		
	Rectovaginal			8	
	Rectocloacal			3	
	Rectal atresia	3	1	2	57
Overall					80

Data from Kiesewetter WB, Chang JHT: Imperforate anus: A five to thirty year follow-up perspective. Prog Pediatr Surg 10:81–90, 1977.

Defecation is difficult and the stools may be ribbon-like. Treatment consists of dilation but in some cases it may be necessary to excise the fibrous tissue and mobilize the rectum, suturing it to the lower part of the anal canal. The prognosis is good in as much as the anorectal region is basically normal.

Imperforate Anal Membrane

An imperforate anal membrane accounts for 6% of all anorectal anomalies. The newborn fails to pass meconium. On inspection of the perineum, a greenish bulging membrane of epithelium is seen overlying the anal orifice. Excision of the membrane relieves the problem, and sphincter function is usually normal.

Anal Agenesis

Anal agenesis without fistulas accounts for 7% of the lesions and is seen almost exclusively in males. Normal bowel descends through the levator sling, but because of abnormal anal development, only an anteriorly placed dimple is present externally. These infants fail to pass meconium. Anoplasty is the procedure of choice.

Anal agenesis with "fistula" formation occurs in 29% of patients. The fistulas are ectopic openings of the anus. In males, the fistula is almost always to the perineum but rarely to the urethra. In females, it may be either to the vulva (63%) or to the perineum (37%). Any opening or presence of a spot of meconium in the vulva, or along the perineal raphe in a male, should suggest this lesion. There are a number of anoplasty techniques to move the anus to its normal anatomic location.

Rectal Agenesis

Rectal agenesis lesions make up 47% of anorectal anomalies. In the female, these high supralevator lesions occur both with and without fistula. Meconium is either not passed at all or is passed through the fistula, which is not visible on the perineum. The fistula opens either into the vagina or into the urogenital sinus, which is a common passageway for the urethra and vagina. Males may also have rectal agenesis with or without fistula formation. Fistulas in the male are rectourethral or rectovesical and can be detected by examining the urine for meconium in an infant who fails to pass meconium rectally. Patients with high anomalies are treated initially with diverting colostomy, followed by a pull-through procedure performed when the patient is between 1 and 2 years of age.

Rectal Atresias

Rectal atresias are rare lesions that present as a bowel obstruction with the failure to pass meconium. The obstructing membrane lies just above the levator sling. This lesion is managed surgically in a manner similar to rectal agenesis.

Prognosis

Early survival figures given in Table 74–2 are dependent primarily on the absence of associated anomalies. From the same series, with a follow-up period of 5 to 30 years, continence was achieved in 75% of patients (Kiesewetter and Chang, 1977). In another 14%, soiling occasionally occurred, but the patient had a socially acceptable degree of continence. Ditesheim and Templeton (1987) reported continence rates of 65% to 70% in their 25-year follow-up of patients operated on for high imperforate anus. In this series quality of life correlated closely with the establishment of continence. Iwai and coworkers (1988), using electromyography and anal manometry, stated that problems with continence following repair of high imperforate anus were due to external anal sphincter dysfunction. Posterior sagittal anorectoplasty promises to revolutionize the surgical approach and outcome for imperforate anus (Pena, 1985).

Enteric Duplications

Duplications of the gastrointestinal tract are relatively rare. Sixty-five percent are located in the small bowel with more than half of these occurring in the ileum (Favara et al, 1971). Thirty percent of instances are associated with other anomalies, the most common being intestinal atresias. Spherical duplications are more common than tubular ones. Duplications are generally located on the mesenteric side of the lumen, are lined by intestinal mucosa, and share a common wall and mesenteric blood supply with the adjacent intestine, but usually do not communicate with the gut lumen. The diagnosis is made in at least half of the patients in the neonatal period (Grosfeld et al, 1970). Presenting symptoms include vomiting and signs of obstruction with the presence of a palpable mass. Plain films of the abdomen may show displacement of adjacent viscera by a mass. Upper gastrointestinal series and barium enema demonstrate a filling defect or, rarely, may show a communication between the cyst and normal bowel. Treatment is surgical excision with primary anastomosis.

Extrinsic Obstruction

Malrotation with Volvulus

Definition, Epidemiology, and Etiology

Anomalies of intestinal rotation occur in 1 per 6000 live births. Malrotation of the gut occurs between the 8th and 10th week of gestation when the elongating intestine returns to the abdominal cavity. If the mesenteric attachments do not develop properly, the midgut lies free, attached to the posterior abdominal wall at only two points: the duodenum and the proximal colon. It may therefore twist in either direction, but when volvulus occurs it is usually in the clockwise direction. The twisting may make several complete turns, resulting in obstruction of the duodenojejunal junction. Compromise of the circulation of the twisted bowel leads to the rapid development of gangrene.

Diagnosis

Of symptomatic patients, 80% are seen with evidence of high intestinal obstruction during the 1st month of life. Bilious vomiting, once it begins, occurs after each meal. Because the obstruction is often incomplete, all gradations of distention are seen. Interruption of blood flow leads to peritonitis, sepsis, and shock. Plain film of the abdomen may show dilated stomach and duodenum with little air in the distal bowel. An upper gastrointestinal series should be done initially. If the diagnosis is unclear, a barium enema is indicated (Fig. 74–6).

Treatment

Immediate operation is imperative to prevent irreversible ischemic damage to the gut. The volvulus is reduced by counterclockwise rotation, and the Ladd bands are divided. Nonviable bowel can be resected, but in the absence of perforation, many pediatric surgeons wait to resect bowel at a second procedure 24 to 36 hours after the initial operation. During this interval the infant is given volume expanders and broad-spectrum antibiotics.

Prognosis

The operative mortality rate is less than 15% and depends on the infant's clinical condition at the time of surgery.

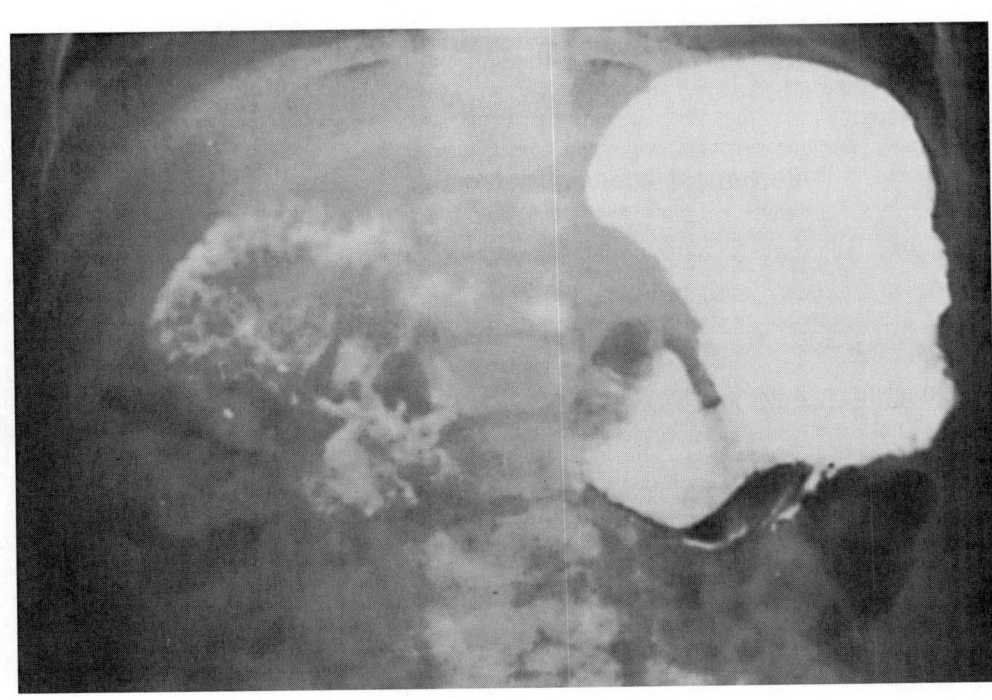

FIGURE 74–6. Unequivocal malrotation, proved by the presence of the cecum and appendix in the left lower quadrant; the lower end of the midgut mesentery is therefore improperly located. There is also barium in the stomach, but the duodenum and ligament of Treitz are not shown.

Morbidity depends on the amount of bowel resected and the need for long-term parenteral nutrition.

Annular Pancreas

Annular pancreas is an uncommon lesion that arises from a persistence of the dorsal pancreatic bud, which develops into its own lobe, grows around the left side of the duodenum, and then entraps the duodenum when it fuses to the bilobate ventral pancreatic bud. In 10% to 20% of cases, there are associated anomalies including duodenal atresia, malrotation, duodenal diaphragm, and Down syndrome (Kiernan et al, 1980). Most cases, however, are not diagnosed until adulthood. Symptoms in the newborn are those of partial obstruction (i.e., vomiting and abdominal distention). Treatment is surgical. The procedure of choice is duodenoduodenostomy or duodenojejunostomy. No attempt should be made at operative dissection or division of the pancreatic annulus.

Intussusception

Intussusception is the invagination of one loop of bowel into a loop distal to it. Although intussusception is a relatively common cause of intestinal obstruction in infants 6 to 18 months old, it is extremely rare in the 1st month of life. Talwalker (1962) reviewed the case histories of 24 newborns with intussusception (Table 74–3). Eight arose in the jejunum, which resulted in an unusually high proportion of jejunal to ileocecal intussusceptions. Vomiting and blood in the stools were almost always present. Unlike in the older infants, pain and a palpable mass were rare. Plain films show dilated loops above the obstruction with an almost gasless abdomen distally. Barium enema shows the column ending in a meniscus with a coiled-spring pattern extending proximally. The passage of blood or blood-stained mucus, with signs of obstruction clinically and on plain films, warrants the performance of a proctoscopic examination and barium enema. In older infants a barium enema is not only diagnostic but in 81% of the patients is also therapeutic (Gierup et al, 1972). Hydrostatic reduction in the newborn has been successful in only 40%, and surgical reduction is therefore usually necessary.

Peritoneal Adhesions

Obstruction may follow the development of adhesions between one hollow viscus and another as a result of healed peritonitis. The initial inflammation may have taken place weeks to months before. Causes include bacterial infection, chemical irritation, such as that occurring with bile peritonitis, or mechanical irritation from a previous laparotomy.

Mesenteric Thrombosis

Thrombosis may occur in either the veins or the arteries of the mesenteric vessels of the newborn. The venous form is almost always secondary to abdominal inflammatory disease and is accompanied by dehydration, shock, and increased blood viscosity. The arterial form is due to emboli, either septic or nonseptic. In the past decade, this syndrome has been associated with umbilical artery catheterization, sepsis, and shock. Infants of poorly controlled diabetic mothers are susceptible to thromboses in many organs, one of which is the mesentery (Oppenheimer and Avery, 1968).

Prevention and Treatment

Mesenteric thrombosis has probably become rare because of vigorous initial stabilization of blood pressure and attention to hydration. Better control of diabetes in pregnancy has been associated with fewer complications, including venous thromboses.

Once the lesion is suspected, correction of hemoconcentration is mandatory, and consultation with a pediatric surgeon is appropriate to discuss the necessity for and timing of surgical exploration.

FUNCTIONAL OBSTRUCTION
Hirschsprung Disease
Definition and Epidemiology

Hirschsprung disease is a lower intestinal obstruction caused by agenesis of ganglion cells in the Auerbach and Meissner plexuses. The lesion originates in the rectum and extends proximally over a variable distance. In 80% to 90% of the patients, involvement does not extend more proximally than the sigmoid colon. With involvement limited to the rectosigmoid, males predominate 4:1. Both sexes are equally affected in long-segment disease. Aganglionic megacolon occurs in 1 in 5000 live births and accounts for 5% of neonatal intestinal obstructions. It is uncommon in low-birth-weight infants and not infrequently associated with Down syndrome (up to 15%) and other chromosome disorders. Occasionally it may coexist with Ondine's curse.

There appears to be a relatively rare autosomal dominant form of Hirschsprung disease that has been ascribed to mutations in tyrosine kinase receptor gene mapping of the region called the RET proto-oncogene (Angrist). There is also a large kindred in which there is an association of Waardenburg syndrome and Hirschsprung disease as well as multiple endocrine neoplasia and Hirschsprung disease. Future attempts to map and characterize the gene that regulates the migration and differentiation of the autonomic regulation of the colon will likely help to clarify the origin of this disorder.

TABLE 74–3

Intussusception in the Newborn

| Type | Number | Methods of Treatment | | |
		Reduction	Resection	None
Ileocecal	12	6	3	3
Jejunal	8	2	6	—
Ileal	3	2	1	—
Colonic	1	—	1	—

Adapted from Talwalker VC: Intussusception in the newborn. Arch Dis Child 37:203–208, 1962.

Diagnosis

Delay in the passage of meconium beyond 24 hours occurs in 95% of newborns with this disease. Other clinical findings include evidence of lower intestinal obstruction (abdominal distention and vomiting), obstipation, and failure to thrive. The development of enterocolitis may lead to diarrhea, dehydration, and shock. In some patients, the disease resembles the meconium plug syndrome, initially responding to an enema with the passage of meconium. However, within a few days the symptoms of constipation recur.

A barium enema may not be diagnostic in the newborn. Only rarely is the characteristic narrowed rectosigmoid segment distal to a dilated sigmoid segment seen. The typical caliber differential does not become apparent until the infant is 3 or 4 weeks of age. However, the persistence of barium in the rectum and sigmoid for more than 24 hours after the examination is highly suggestive of Hirschsprung disease.

The definitive diagnosis may be made on rectal suction biopsy (Campbell and Noblett, 1969). If ganglion cells are not present in three specimens of sufficient depth after serial sectioning, a full-thickness biopsy can be done before diverting colostomy.

Treatment

Definitive treatment for Hirschsprung disease is operative. Most pediatric surgeons defer definitive repair until the patient is 8 to 12 months of age, temporizing by performing a colostomy. A number of definitive procedures are available, including the Swenson pull-through, the Duhamel operation, and the Soave endorectal pull-through (Joseph and Sim, 1988; Vane and Grosfeld, 1986). All have their proponents, and the choice depends on the experience of the surgeon.

Prognosis

The mortality rate for enterocolitis is 20%. Prompt diagnosis and therapy should improve this figure. The operative mortality rate is less than 5%, and a good surgical outcome in terms of continence can be expected in 80%.

Meconium Plug Syndrome

Meconium plug syndrome was initially described as an intestinal obstruction in the newborn that is relieved by the passage of an inspissated gray plug of meconium from the distal colon (Ellis and Clatworthy, 1966). It was initially thought that the meconium itself was abnormal. However, this syndrome has come to be considered a form of colonic dysmotility without an abnormality of intramural ganglion cells.

Infants pass no meconium for the first 24 to 48 hours of life and eventually symptoms of distal intestinal obstruction develop. Contrast enema may be both diagnostic and therapeutic. Because Hirschsprung disease is diagnosed in half of these patients eventually, careful follow-up is necessary.

Pseudo-Obstruction Syndrome

The chronic idiopathic intestinal pseudo-obstruction syndrome comprises a group of motility disorders of both muscular and neurogenic origin. Patients may become symptomatic at any time, including during the neonatal period (Anuras et al, 1986; Byrne et al, 1977). Symptoms include abdominal distention and vomiting. With onset in the newborn period, there is unlikely to be a "resolution" of the obstruction, as is seen in older patients. Pharmacologic agents such as metoclopramide, cisapride, bethanechol chloride, prostaglandins, cholecystokinin, pentagastrin, ceruletide, and acetylcholine have been tried without success (Golladay and Byrne, 1981). Surgical intervention is usually not successful and should be avoided. Treatment consists of long-term parenteral nutritional support.

A variant of pseudo-obstruction is the megacystismicrocolon-intestinal hypoperistalsis syndrome, as described by Berdon and associates (1981) and reviewed by Vintzileos and coworkers (1986). Rarely seen in males, this disorder presents in the newborn period with signs of a bowel obstruction. In addition, bilateral flank masses (hydronephrotic kidneys) and a single large midline abdominal mass (megacystis) suggest an obstructive uropathy. Ultrasound, voiding cystourethrogram, and barium enema are diagnostic. Surgical exploration usually reveals a massively dilated bladder and a short, malfixed small intestine with a microcolon. Adequate peristalsis never returns, so that long-term parenteral nutrition is necessary.

DISORDERS OF THE PANCREAS
Cystic Fibrosis

The usual presentation of CF in the newborn period is meconium ileus. However, this diagnosis should be considered in the young infant with failure to thrive and hypoalbuminemia, even in the absence of respiratory disease. Incidence figures for whites vary from 1 in 600 to 1 in 2500 and for American blacks, 1 in 17,000. CF is an autosomal recessive disorder. (See the discussion of genetic diagnosis with meconium ileus.) In addition to being concerned about failure to thrive and hypoalbuminemia, parents may complain that the infant is constipated or passes large, malodorous stools. The diagnosis can be made on a sweat test. Nutritional therapy is directed at providing adequate calories for growth and improving protein digestion and absorption. Predigested formulas with a significant percentage of their fat as medium-chain triglycerides often accomplish this goal. If the infant is fed regular formula or breast milk, enzyme supplementation is necessary. Even with more elemental formulas, enzymes may increase absorption by 50%. Half of a capsule with feedings is usually sufficient. Fat-soluble vitamin supplementation is not usually necessary in these infants but vitamin levels should be followed up at 4- to 6-month intervals.

Shwachman Syndrome

Shwachman syndrome is characterized by pancreatic insufficiency and bone marrow dysfunction (Aggett et al, 1980). The defect appears to be with enzyme secretion and acinar function, not bicarbonate secretion and duct function (Hill et al, 1982). Microscopically, there is an absence of acinar tissue with preservation of the islets and ducts. The hematologic defect is primarily a severe neutropenia, although mild anemia and thrombocytopenia may be present. The cause of Shwachman syndrome is genetic, but the mode of inheritance is unknown. Clinically, the infants present with neutropenia and failure to thrive. Pancreatic enzyme replacement improves nutrition, but the mortality rate during childhood remains high (30%) because of recurrent infections and the associated development of leukemia (Woods et al, 1981).

Pancreatic Agenesis

Several forms of insulin-requiring diabetes have been described in the newborn period. One form of pancreatic agenesis also includes exocrine pancreatic insufficiency (Howard et al, 1980). In addition to diabetes, the clinical presentation includes edema, hypoproteinemia, and failure to thrive. Steatorrhea can be documented. Therapy includes enzyme replacement and insulin. Survival is possible.

Isolated Enzyme Defects

Isolated deficiencies of trypsinogen (Townes et al, 1967) and lipase have been reported. Trypsinogen deficiency presents with hypoproteinemia, edema, and failure to thrive. With lipase deficiency, steatorrhea and poor growth are the presenting manifestations.

Nesidioblastosis

Nesidioblastosis is a relatively rare cause of severe neonatal hypoglycemia. The cause is unknown, but histologically there is diffuse proliferation of nesidioblasts, the immature pancreatic cells that differentiate to form the pancreatic islets (Laidlaw, 1938). There is a genetic predisposition of the disease in as much as an autosomal recessive pattern of appearance has been described, but not all patients have a familial history. Hyperinsulinemic hypoglycemia typically presents early postnatally. Aggressive glucose administration is required to maintain normoglycemia (Aynsley-Green et al, 1981). The diagnosis is made by confirming the presence of hyperinsulinemia when hypoglycemia is present. Although the treatment in the past has been resection of 75% to 90% of the pancreas, long-term follow up of such patients demonstrates that insulin secretion in children undergoing treatment in this manner 6 to 21 years later is abnormal and frank diabetes developed in many patients in puberty (Leibowitz et al, 1995). Thus, an attempt should be made to manage these infants with diazoxide and the long-acting somatostatin analogue, octreotide (Tauber et al, 1994) to avoid the use of subtotal pancreatectomy. Infants given long-term pharmacologic therapy with these agents still demonstrate defects in beta-cell function but have a lower incidence of diabetes as adolescents (Liebowitz et al, 1995).

REFERENCES

Aggett PJ, Cavanaugh NPC, Matthew DJ: Shwachman's syndrome. Arch Dis Child 55:331–347, 1980.

Angrist M, Bolk S, Thiel B, et al: Mutation analysis of the RET receptor kinase in Hirschsprung disease. Hum Mol Genet 4:821–830, 1995.

Anuras S, Metros FA, Soper RT, et al: Chronic intestinal pseudo obstruction in young children. Gastroenterology 91:62–70, 1986.

Aynsley-Green A, Polak JM, Bloom SR, et al: Nesidioblastosis of the pancreas: Definition of the syndrome and management of the severe neonatal hyperinsulinemic hypoglycemia. Arch Dis Child 56:496–508, 1981.

Berdon WE, Baker DN, Blank WA, et al: Megacystis-microcolon intestinal hypoperistalsis syndrome: A new cause of intestinal obstruction in the newborn. Report of radiologic findings in five newborn girls. AJR Am J Roentgenol 137:749–755, 1981.

Boat TF, Welsh MJ, Beaudet AL, et al: Cystic fibrosis. *In* Scriver CR, Beaudet AL, Sly WS, et al (Eds): The Metabolic Basis of Inherited Disease, 6th ed. New York, McGraw-Hill, 1989, pp 2649–2680.

Boles ET, Vassy LE, Ralston M: Atresia of the colon. J Pediatr Surg 11:69, 1976.

Byrne WJ, Cipil L, Ruler AR, et al: Chronic idiopathic intestinal pseudo-obstruction syndrome in children clinical characteristics and prognosis. J Pediatr 90:585–589, 1977.

Campbell PE, Noblett HR: Experience with rectal suction biopsy in the diagnosis of Hirschsprung's disease. J Pediatr Surg 4:410–415, 1969.

De Lorimier AA, Fonkalsrud EW, Hays DW: Congenital atresia and stenosis of the jejunum and ileum. Surgery 65:819–827, 1969.

deVries PA, Cox KL: Surgery of anorectal anomalies. Surg Clin North Am 65:1139–1169, 1985.

Ditesheim JA, Templeton JM: Short-term versus long-term quality of life in children following repair of high imperforate anus. J Pediatr Surg 22:581–587, 1987.

Dow E, Cross S, Wolgemuth DJ, et al: Second locus for Hirschsprung disease/Waardenberg syndrome in a large Mennonite kindred. Am J Med Genet 53:75–80, 1994.

Ellis DG, Clatworthy HW: The meconium plug syndrome revisited. J Pediatr Surg 1:54–61, 1966.

Favara BE, Franciosi RA, Akers DR: Enteric duplications: 37 cases, a vascular theory of pathogenesis. Am J Dis Child 122:501–506, 1971.

Gierup J, Jonulf H, Levaditis A: Management of intussuscepeon in infants and children: A survey based on 288 consecutive cases. Pediatrics 50:535–540, 1972.

Golladay ES, Byrne WJ: Intestinal pseudo-obstruction. Surg Gynecol Obstet 153:257–273, 1981.

Grosfeld JL, O'Neill JA, Clatworthy HW: Enteric duplications in infancy and childhood: An 18 year review. Ann Surg 172:8390, 1970.

Hill RE, Durie PR, Gaskin KJ: Steatorrhea and pancreatic insufficiency in Shwachman's syndrome. Gastroenterology 83:22–27, 1982.

Howard CP, Go VLW, Infante AJ, et al: Long-term survival in a case of functional pancreatic agenesis. J Pediatr 97:786–789, 1980.

Iwai N, Yanagihara J, Takahasi T: Voluntary anal continence after surgery for anorectal malformations. J Pediatr Surg 23:393–397, 1988.

Joseph VT, Sim CK: Problems and pitfalls in the management of Hirschsprung's disease. J Pediatr Surg 23:398–402, 1988.

Kerem E, Corey M, Levison H: Clinical and genetic comparisons of patients with cystic fibrosis, with or without meconium ileus. J Pediatr 114:767–773, 1989a.

Kerem BS, Rommens JM, Buchanan JA, et al: Identification of the cystic fibrosis gene: Genetic analysis. Science 245:1073, 1989b.

Kiernan PD, ReMine SG, Kiernan PC, et al: Annular pancreas. Arch Surg 115:46–50, 1980.

Kiesewetter WB, Chang JHT: Imperforate anus: A five to thirty year follow-up perspective. Prog Pediatr Surg 10:81–90, 1977.

Laidlaw GF: Nesidioblastoma, the islet cell tumor of the pancreas. Am J Pathol 14:125–134, 1938.

Langer JC, Adzick NS, Filly RA, et al: Gastrointestinal tract obstruction in the fetus. Arch Surg 124:1183–1187, 1989.

Leibowitz G, Glasser B, Higazi AA, et al: Hyperinsulinemic hypoglycemia of infancy (nesioblastosis) in clinical remission: High incidence of diabetes mellitus and persistent beta-cell dysfunction at long-term follow-up. J Clin Endocrinol Metab 80:386–392, 1995.

Lemna WK, Feldman GL, Kerem B, et al: Mutation analysis for heterozygote detection and the prenatal diagnosis of cystic fibrosis. N Engl J Med 322:291–296, 1990.

Louw JH: Jejunoileal atresia and stenosis. J Pediatr Surg 1:8–15, 1966.

Martin LW, Zerella JT: Jejunoileal atresia: A proposed classification. J Pediatr Surg 11:399–406, 1976.

Mata AG, Rosenpart RM: Interobserver variability in the radiographic diagnosis of necrotizing enterocolitis. Pediatrics 66:68–71, 1980.

Mooney D, Lewis JE, Weber TR: Newborn duodenal atresia: An improving outlook. Am J Surg 153:347–349, 1987.

Mornet E, Serre JL, Farrell M: Genetic differences between cystic fibrosis with and without meconium ileus. Lancet 1:376–378, 1988.

Nguyen LT, Youssef S, Guttman FM, et al: Meconium ileus: Is a stoma necessary? J Pediatr Surg 21:766, 1986.

Noblett HR: Treatment of uncomplicated meconium ileus by Gastrografin enema: A preliminary report. J Pediatr Surg 4:190–195, 1969.

Oppenheimer EN, Avery ME: Clinical-pathologic conference. J Pediatr 73:143, 1968.

Park RW, Grand RJ: Gastrointestinal manifestations of cystic fibrosis: A review. Gastroenterology 81:1143–1161, 1981.

Pena A: Surgical treatment of high imperforate anus. World J Surg 9:236–245, 1985.

Ponder BA: The gene causing multiple endocrine neoplasia type 2 (MEN 2). Ann Med 26:199–203, 1994.

Ralston CW, Ament ME, Berquist W, et al: Somatic growth and developmental functioning in children receiving prolonged home total parenteral nutrition. J Pediatr 105:842–847, 1984.

Rommens JM, Zengerling S, Bums J: Identification and regional localization of DNA markers on chromosome 7 for cloning of the cystic fibrosis gene. Am J Hum Genet 43:645–663, 1989.

Rothschild HB, Storch A, Meyers B: Mesenteric occlusion in a newborn infant. J Pediatr 43:569–571, 1953.

Schwachmann H, Antonowivcz I: Studies on meconium. In Lebenthal E. (Ed.): Textbook of Gastroenterology and Nutrition in Infancy. New York, Raven Press 1981.

Seges RA, Kenny A, Bird GW, et al: Pediatric surgical patients with severe anaerobic infection: Report of 16 T-antigen positive cases and possible hazard of blood transfusion. J Pediatr Surg 16:905–910, 1981.

Shaul WL: Clues to the early diagnosis of neonatal appendicitis. J Pediatr 98:473–476, 1981.

Sturim HS, Ternberg JL: Congenital atresia of the colon. Surgery 59:458–465, 1966.

Talwalker VC: Intussusception in the newborn. Arch Dis Child 37:203–208, 1962.

Tauber MT, Harris AG, Rochiccidi P: Clinical use of the long acting somatostatin analogue octreotide in pediatrics. Eur J Pediatr 153:304–310, 1994.

Townes PL, Bryson M, Miller C: Further observations on trypsinogen deficiency disease: Report of a second case. J Pediatr 71:220–224, 1967.

Vane DW, Grosfeld JL: Hirschsprung's disease. Experience with the Duhamel operation in 195 cases. Pediatr Surg Int 1:95–99, 1986.

Vintzileos AM, Eisenfeld LI, Herson VC, et al: Megacystismicrocolon-intestinal hypoperistalsis syndrome. Am J Perinatol 3:297–302, 1986.

Waters DL, Domey SF, Gaskin KJ, et al: Pancreatic function in infants identified as having cystic fibrosis in a neonatal screening program. N Engl J Med 322:303, 1990.

Weber TR, Lewis JE, Mooney D, et al: Duodenal atresia: A comparison of techniques of repair. J Pediatr Surg 21:1133–1136, 1986.

Woods WG, Roloff JS, Lukens JN, et al: The occurrence of leukemia in patients with the Shwachman syndrome. J Pediatr 99:425–428, 1981.

Young DG, Wilkinson AW: Abnormalities associated with neonatal duodenal obstruction. Surgery 63:832–840, 1968.

Zachary RB: Meconium and fecal plugs in the newborn. Arch Dis Child 32:22–27, 1957.

CHAPTER 75

Disorders of the Liver

Carol Lynn Berseth

Cholestasis in the neonate results from extrahepatic or intrahepatic abnormalities. Alagille and coworkers (1975) have suggested that clinical criteria may be useful to discern jaundice caused by extrahepatic from that caused by intrahepatic abnormalities in approximately 80% of cases. Infants with intrahepatic disease tend to exhibit acholic stools intermittently rather than consistently and acholic stools tend to develop later in life (e.g., postnatal week 4 rather than week 2) compared with infants with extrahepatic disease. Infants with intrahepatic disease are less likely than an infant with extrahepatic disease to have a liver with a hard consistency (Alagille et al, 1975). In addition radiographic or nuclear medicine studies and histologic evaluation of biopsy material may be useful in obtaining a more definitive diagnosis. A more detailed discussion of this topic is found in Chapter 86.

In short, extrahepatic causes of cholestasis include biliary atresia, choledochal cysts, and congenital stenosis of the common bile duct. All three entities are rare (biliary atresia is the most common with an incidence of 1 in 8000) and are more commonly seen in peoples of the Pacific or Indian Ocean regions. All require surgical repair. Approximately 2% to 3% of infants with biliary atresia have a surgically correctable defect. In another 20% of infants, the gallbladder and cystic duct are present and patent, and a portocholecystostomy can be performed. The remaining infants usually undergo hepatic portenterostomy, also called a Kasai procedure. In many of these infants, postoperative cholangitis develops, which is manifested by the presence of fever, increasing jaundice, and acholic stools. Most typically these episodes are caused by *Escherichia coli* and are treated with antibiotics for 3 weeks. The long-term prognosis for these patients is fair; in many, end-stage hepatic failure develops and patients require liver transplantation. Intrahepatic disease, most commonly of infectious or metabolic origin, is the more common cause of cholestasis in the newborn.

HEPATITIS

Numerous viral agents cause neonatal hepatitis. At least five major hepatitis viruses have been described and include hepatitis A, hepatitis B, hepatitis C, hepatitis D, and hepatitis E. Other viral causes of hepatitis include infection with cytomegalovirus, Epstein Barr virus, herpes simplex, varicella-zoster, adenovirus, enterovirus, rubella, and arbovirus. If hepatitis presents in the neonatal period with jaundice, hepatomegaly and elevation of serum transaminase concentrations, a thorough evaluation should be undertaken to make a specific diagnosis as outlined in the chapter on hyperbilirubinemia. Serologic studies, liver biopsy, and viral isolation are used to establish the diagnosis. More specific information about hepatitis is reviewed in Chapter 86.

Of the five hepatitis viruses, hepatitis B virus (HBV) causes the most concern for neonatologists. HBV is a 43-nm virion that contains an outer shell, which contains the surface antigen (HBsAg), an inner shell, which contains the core antigen, and the inner contents, which contain the e antigen (HBeAg) and the double-stranded DNA. Temporally, the surface antigen is detected early in the disease, followed by the core antigen and the e antigen. When e antigen is present, DNA is also present in the serum, indicating that active viral replication is occurring. Fewer than 5% of fetuses whose mothers have hepatitis acquire HBV in utero, in as much as 95% have no evidence of HBV at birth. Approximately 60% of these infants, however, acquire HBV perinatally. The rate of perinatal acquisition depends on the presence of the hepatitis B e antigen. If mothers are HBsAg positive but HBeAg negative, the rate of neonatal infection is less than 20%. However, the rate of transmission increases to 90% if the mother is HBeAg positive (Stevens et al, 1979).

Most infants who acquire hepatitis B infection are asymptomatic. Most HBeAg-positive infants exhibit a long period of immune HBV tolerance with high serum HBV DNA but minimally elevated serum alanine transferase levels and minimal histologic changes on liver biopsy. In the third decade of life, however, there is a transition in viral immunity, because serum HBV DNA decreases. By that time, many women may have already delivered infants of their own to whom they have passed along hepatitis infection. At the time of transition, chronic active hepatitis develops in approximately half of the patients. The risk of chronic disease development is inversely related to the age at which infection occurs, such that chronic disease develops in 20% to 50% of persons who are infected in early childhood and in 80% to 90% of those infected in infancy. Of those in whom chronic disease develops, hepatocellular carcinoma will develop in a substantial number of the individuals when they reach their 60s. Chronic HBV is responsible for 80% of all cases of hepatocellular carcinoma. Thus, reduction of perinatal acquisition of HBV is done, not out of concern for the neonatal disease, which is mild, but as a public health measure based on concerns for the high rate of chronic active hepatitis and risk for hepatocellular carcinoma.

Passive immunity against HBV can be provided by hepatitis B immune globulin, which is prepared from humans with high serum concentrations of HBsAg. Although passive prophylaxis prevents perinatal acquisition of HBV, its effect is transient and 20% to 50% of infants can become carriers by 1 year of age. Active prophylaxis using inactivated virus vaccine given three or four times during infancy elicits protective serum concentrations of HB surface antibodies. When passive and active immunization is combined there is 90% efficacy among infants born to mothers who are HBsAg and HBeAg positive. Since 1988, it has been the recommendation by the U.S. Public Health Service that all pregnant women be tested for HBsAg and that immunization be provided to infants of mothers who are found to be positive regardless of their HBeAg status. The doses and schedule of administration of vaccine is detailed in Chapters 43 and 86. Protective levels of HBS antibody can be observed until 5 to 6 years of age, but long-term studies have not yet been published. The breast milk of HBsAg-positive mothers contains HBsAg; however, breast-feeding can be permitted if infants are vaccinated.

Although perinatal transmission of hepatitis C is reportedly rare (Lam et al, 1993), the transmission rate is high among mothers who are human immunodeficiency virus (HIV) positive (Giovannini et al, 1990). Most infants who acquire hepatitis C virus are asymptomatic until early childhood when the use of alpha-2b-interferon has held some promise for treatment (Davis et al, 1989; Ruiz-Moreno et al, 1992).

Hepatitis resulting from syphilis is being seen more frequently. Newborns present with hepatosplenomegaly and jaundice during the 1st month of life. Serum transaminase levels may reach 500 IU. Liver biopsy shows a picture consistent with giant cell hepatitis. Even after penicillin therapy, liver dysfunction may persist for up to 2 months (Long et al, 1984).

Bacterial hepatitis may produce cholestasis by two mechanisms. The first is associated with generalized sepsis with bacterial invasion of the liver and markedly elevated transaminase levels, hepatomegaly, and liver necrosis. Treatment and prognosis are the same as for neonatal sepsis. The second mechanism is a "toxic cholestasis." No direct invasion or destruction of the hepatocytes occurs. Therefore, transaminases are usually seen with severe urinary tract infections caused by *E. coli* or *Proteus* or with pneumonia and generalized sepsis from *Pneumococcus*. The mechanism is thought to be caused by a toxin that inhibits hepatic excretory function. Successful treatment of the infection results in resolution of the cholestasis.

INHERITED AND METABOLIC LIVER DISORDERS

Alpha₁-Antitrypsin Deficiency

Alpha₁-antitrypsin deficiency is caused by accumulation of alpha₁-antitrypsin in the hepatocyte with subsequent hepatocellular necrosis (Morse, 1978; Talamo, 1975). Alpha₁-antitrypsin is an alpha₁-globulin and is a major serum protease inhibitor. It is inherited as an autosomal recessive trait. Although there are several phenotypes, only the homozygous Pi (protease inhibitor) ZZ and, rarely, the MZ types have been associated with liver disease in infancy. The ZZ phenotype occurs in 1 in 2000 live births, but cholestasis develops in only 10% in the neonatal period, typically by 8 to 10 weeks. Of those in whom cholestasis develops, it remains permanent and complete in 50%. However, if spontaneous remission occurs, it characteristically occurs by 6 months of age. Thereafter, the course is highly variable among those who do not have remission, and hepatic failure does develop in some infants who require transplantation. The absence of the alpha₁-globulin fraction seen on serum electrophoresis is highly suggestive of the disorder.

Definitive diagnosis depends on finding a reduced serum alpha₁-antitrypsin level, Pi typing, and liver biopsy that shows periodic acid–Schiff (PAS)-positive cytoplasmic granules with variable degrees of hepatic necrosis and fibrosis. There is no specific treatment.

Cystic Fibrosis

Cholestasis in early infancy can be an initial presentation of cystic fibrosis (Park and Grand, 1981). Half of such infants also have meconium ileus. Liver disease eventually occurs in up to 50% of cystic fibrosis patients. Cirrhosis develops in 5% but only 2% have clinical findings. Liver biopsy in the infants shows evidence of excessive biliary mucus with mild periportal inflammation and fibrosis. Bile duct plugging may also be present. Focal biliary cirrhosis, characterized by inspissated granular eosinophilic material in ductules and bile duct proliferation, develops later and may progress to multilobular biliary cirrhosis.

Galactosemia

Galactosemia is an autosomal recessive disorder of carbohydrate metabolism that results from deficient galactose-1-phosphate uridyltransferase activity. Accumulation of galactose-1-phosphate results in cholestasis, hepatomegaly, hypoglycemia, cataracts, vomiting, and failure to thrive. The diagnosis is made by demonstrating low levels of erythrocyte galactose-1-phosphate uridyltransferase activity. Treatment consists of removing all sources of galactose (lactose) from the diet (see also Chapter 25).

Hereditary Fructose Intolerance

Hereditary fructose intolerance is a congenital deficiency of fructose-1-phosphatase that results in the accumulation of fructose and fructose-1-phosphate in body tissues. Introduction of fructose into the diet results in vomiting, hepatomegaly, and jaundice. Treatment is to eliminate fructose and sucrose from the diet (Odievre et al, 1978) (see also Chapter 25).

Tyrosinemia

Tyrosinemia is a rare autosomal recessive disorder characterized by decreased activity of p-hydroxyphenylpyruvic acid oxidase, methionine-activating enzyme, and cystathionine synthetase. Both acute and chronic forms have been described. The acute form presents with vomiting, failure to thrive, liver failure, and renal tubular dysfunction, usually within the first 3 to 6 weeks of life (Carson et al, 1976). Plasma and urine aminograms reveal elevated levels of tyrosine and its metabolites. Dietary restriction of tyrosine and phenylalanine may slow the progress of the liver disease, but without a liver transplant, most infants die during the 1st year of life (see also Chapter 25).

Lipid Storage Diseases

Niemann-Pick disease, Gaucher disease, Wolman disease, and cholesterol ester storage disease are rare genetic disorders of lipid metabolism. They present with hepatospleno-megaly and varying degrees of liver dysfunction, including cholestasis (see Chapter 25).

Familial Recurrent Cholestasis

Familial recurrent cholestasis (Byler disease) is an autosomal recessive disorder characterized by episodic cholestasis. The initial presentation is within the first 6 months of life. The cholestatic episodes may last weeks to months. Cirrhosis eventually develops. Death from liver failure occurs between 2 and 15 years of age.

Recurrent Cholestasis with Lymphedema

Recurrent cholestasis with lymphedema (Aagenaes syndrome) is a rare genetic disorder characterized by cholestasis and lymphedema of the lower extremities. Cirrhosis develops in some patients.

Cerebrohepatorenal Syndrome

Cerebrohepatorenal (Zellweger) syndrome is one of a group of disorders of peroxisomal dysfunction. Inherited as an autosomal recessive trait, it presents in the neonatal period with cholestasis, hepatomegaly, profound hypotonia, and dysmorphic features (Moser et al, 1984). The diagnosis is made by demonstrating abnormal very-long-chain fatty acid levels in the serum (see Chapter 25).

Paucity of Interlobular Bile Ducts (Alagille Syndrome)

Two forms of this disease occur. Those who have the syndromatic form of the disease have cholestasis, characteristic facial features, vertebral anomalies, cardiac murmurs, and mental retardation (Alagille et al, 1975). There is usually a familial occurrence. Infants who have the nonsyndromatic form do not have the characteristic facies or a family history of the disease. The diagnosis for both forms is made histologically by noting an absence or paucity of interlobular bile ducts. The long-term prognosis for the syndromatic form is fair, because it typically does not regress. However, fibrosis, cirrhosis, or portal hypertension develops in only a few patients. Among infants who have the nonsyndromatic form, cirrhosis and portal hypertension develop in approximately half.

TOTAL PARENTERAL NUTRITION–ASSOCIATED CHOLESTASIS
Definition and Epidemiology

Cholestasis develops in 50% of infants with birth weights less than 1000 g after 2 weeks of parenteral nutrition (Merritt, 1986). In newborns with birth weights between 1000 and 2000 g, the incidence is 15%. The incidence increases with the duration of parenteral nutrition. Cholestasis develops in up to 90% of low-birth-weight infants after 13 weeks of total parenteral nutrition.

No precise cause has been found, but a number of factors appear to be important. These include immaturity of biliary excretion, lack of oral feedings, toxicity of certain amino acid components of the parenteral nutrition solution, and inadequate intake of certain nutrients such as taurine. Lipid infusion does not appear to play a role. The final common pathway may be the accumulation in the serum and bile of toxic bile acids, such as glycolithocholate.

Diagnosis

Serum bile salt concentrations increase before clinical jaundice becomes obvious. After 2 weeks or more on total parenteral nutrition, there is a gradual increase in the conjugated bilirubin with a modest increase in the serum transaminases and alkaline phosphatase (Fig. 75–1). Physical findings are limited to jaundice and hepatomegaly. In some infants the gallbladder becomes hydropic and is palpable. The diagnosis is made by excluding other causes of cholestasis. Histologic changes on liver biopsy are nonspecific and therefore not diagnostic.

Treatment

Treatment consists of the introduction of enteral alimentation and the discontinuation of intravenous nutrition. If total parenteral nutrition must be used, sufficient protein (at least 8% of the total calories) should be provided to prevent hepatic steatosis.

Although this disease was previously treated with phenobarbital, its use has not been shown to be effective (Cleghorn et al, 1986); conversely, its use has been reported to worsen the disease (Nemeth et al, 1990). Therefore, treatment with ursodioxycholate is preferred (Beau et al, 1994). Ursodioxycholate, a naturally occurring dihydroxy bile salt that comprises 1% of the total bile pool, desaturates bile

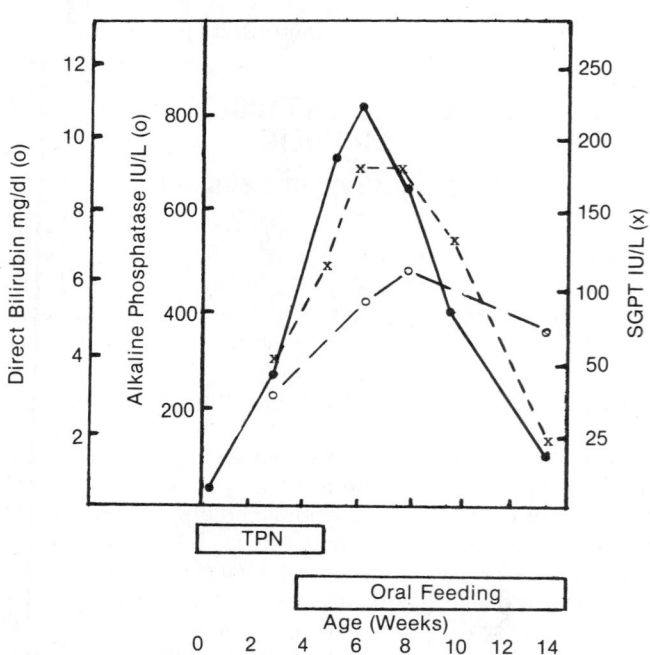

FIGURE 75–1. Typical pattern of liver function tests in a premature infant on total parenteral nutrition.

TABLE 75-1

Hepatic Histologic Changes Observed in Pediatric Patients Receiving Total Parenteral Nutrition

Histologic Lesion	Duration of TPN (Days)			
	0–10	10–30	30–60	>60
Steatosis	+ +	+	+	
Extramedullary Erythropoiesis	+ +	+ +	+	
Periportal Inflammation	+	+	+ +	+ + +
Cholestasis		+ +	+ + +	+ + +
Fibrosis		+	+	+ + +
Ductular proliferation		+	+	+ + +
Cirrhosis			+	+ + + +

TPN, total parenteral nutrition; +, mild or inconsistent finding; + +, consistent finding or generally more than mild when present; + + +, frequently seen and moderate to severe when present.

From Merritt RJ: Cholestasis associated with total parenteral nutrition. J Pediatr Gastroenterol Nutr 5:10, 1986.

and dissolves cholesterol present in gallstones. It can reduce direct hyperbilirubinemia significantly; however; its precise mechanism is unknown. It is thought that it displaces hepatotoxic bile acids from bile to the serum, decreases the actual toxicity of bile acids to the liver, and reduces the immune responses to cholestasis that are thought to aggravate the liver disease seen in total parenteral nutrition–induced cholestasis. Two preliminary studies have also reported improvement of cholestasis in infants given cholecystokinin, a gastrointestinal peptide that increases bile flow, biliary tract motility, and contraction of the sphincter of Oddi (Rintala et al, 1995; Teitelbaum et al, 1995).

Prognosis

After discontinuation of the parenteral nutrition, liver function abnormalities usually resolve after 4 to 12 weeks. Gallbladder hydrops also resolves with the institution of feedings. Gallstones that necessitate cholecystectomy do develop in some infants. Progressive cirrhosis may develop in a small number of infants despite discontinuation of the parenteral nutrition (Table 75–1). Deaths have been reported from liver failure. Liver transplantation may be required.

DRUG-INDUCED CHOLESTASIS

As part of the evaluation of cholestasis in the newborn, each drug that the infant is receiving should be carefully considered as a potential cause or contributing factor. The following is a partial list: erythromycin estolate, ampicillin, oxacillin, diazepam, phenothiazines, and thiazide diuretics. Stricker and Spoelstra (1985) provide a more comprehensive review.

HYPERAMMONEMIA

Hyperammonemia in the first few days of life is caused either by a urea cycle disorder or a transient hyperammo-nemia of the newborn. Later in the neonatal period, fulminant hepatic failure may result in hyperammonemia. See Chapter 25 for complete discussion.

LIVER TRANSPLANTATION

Recent advances in techniques for liver transplantation have made successful treatment of liver failure possible in many infants (Esquivel et al, 1987; Starzl et al, 1989a, 1989b).

REFERENCES

Alagille D, Odievre M, Gautier M, Dommergues JP: Hepatic ductular hypoplasia associated with characteristic facies, vertebral malformations, retarded physical, mental, and sexual development, and cardiac murmur. J Pediatr 86:63–71, 1975.

Beau P, Labat-Labourdette J, Ingrand P, Beauchant M: Is ursodeoxycholic acid an effective therapy for total parenteral nutrition–related liver disease? J Hepatol 20:240–244, 1994.

Carson NAJ, Biggart JD, Bittles AH, et al: Hereditary tyrosinaemia. Clinical, enzymatic and pathological study of an infant with the acute form of the disease. Arch Dis Child 51:106–111, 1976.

Cleghorn EE, Merritt RJ, Subramanian N, et al: Phenobarbital does not prevent total parenteral nutrition–associated cholestasis in noninfected neonates. J Parenter Enteral Nutr 10:282–283, 1986.

Davis GL, Ballart LA, Schiff ER, et al: Treatment of chronic hepatitis C with recombinant interferon alfa: A multicenter randomized, control trial. N Eng J Med 321:1501–1506, 1989.

Esquivel CO, Iwatsuki S, Gordon RD, et al: Indications for pediatric liver transplantation. J Pediatr 111:1039–1045, 1987.

Gordon ER, Shaffer EA, Sass-Kortsak J: Bilirubin secretion and conjugation in the Crigler-Najjar syndrome type II. Gastroenterology 70:761–764, 1976.

Giovannini M, Tagger A, Ribero ML, et al: Maternal-infant transmission of hepatitis C virus and HIV infection: A possible interaction. Lancet 335:1166, 1990.

Krugman S: Viral hepatitis. Pediatr Rev 13:203–245, 1992.

Lam JPH, McOmish F, Burns SM, et al: Infrequent vertical transmission of hepatitis C virus. J Infect Dis 167:572–576, 1993.

Lok ASF: Natural history and control of perinatally acquired hepatitis B virus infection. Dig Dis 10:46–52, 1992.

Long WA, Ulshen MH, Lawson EE: Clinical manifestations of congenital syphilitic hepatitis: Implications for pathogenesis. J Pediatr Gastroenterol Nutr 3:351–355, 1984.

Maisels MJ: Jaundice in the newborn. Pediatr Rev 3:305–319, 1982.

Merritt RJ: Cholestasis associated with total parenteral nutrition. J Pediatr Gastroenterol Nutr 5:9–22, 1986.

Morse JO: Alpha₁-antitrypsin deficiency. N Engl J Med 299:1045–1048, 1099–1105, 1978.

Moser AE, Singh L, Brown FR, et al: The cerebrohepatorenal (Zellweger) syndrome. N Engl J Med 310:1141–1146, 1984.

Nemeth A, Wilkstrom S, Standvik B: Phenobarbital can aggravate a cholestatic bile pattern in infants with obstructive cholangiopathy. J Pediatr Gastroenterol Nutr 10:290–297, 1990.

Odievre M, Genffl C, Gauffer M, et al: Hereditary fructose intolerance in childhood: Diagnosis, management and course in 55 patients. Am J Dis Child 132:605–610, 1978.

Park RW, Grand RJ: Gastrointestinal manifestations of cystic fibrosis: A review. Gastroenterology 81:1143–1161, 1981.

Rintala RJ, Lindahl H, Pohjavouri M: Total parenteral nutrition–associated cholestasis in surgical neonates may be reversed by intravenous cholecystokinin—A preliminary report. J Pediatr Surg 30:827–830, 1995.

Ruiz-Moreno M, Rua MJ, Castillo I, et al: Treatment of children with chronic hepatitis C with recombinant interferon-alpha: A pilot study. Hepatology 16:882–885, 1992.

Starzl TE, Demetris AJ, Thiel DV: Liver transplantation. Part I. N Engl J Med 321:1014, 1989a.

Starzl TE, Demetris AJ, Thiel DV: Liver transplantation. Part II. N Engl J Med 321:1092, 1989b.

Stevens CE, Neurath RA, Beasley RP, et al: HBeAg and anti-HBe detection by radioimmunoassay: Correlation with vertical transmission of hepatitis B virus in Taiwan. J Med Virol 3:237–241, 1979.

Stricker BH, Spoelstra P: Drug-Induced Hepatic Injury. New York, Elsevier, 1985.

Talamo RC: Basic and clinical aspects of alpha$_1$-antitrypsin deficiency. Pediatrics 56:91–99, 1975.

Teitelbaum DH, Han-Markey T, Schumacher RE: Treatment of parenteral nutrition–associated cholestasis with cholecystokinin-Octapeptide. J Pediatr Surg 30:1082–1085, 1995.

Wright TL, Donegan E, Hsu E, et al: Recurrent and acquired hepatitis C virus infection in liver transplant recipients. Gastroenterology 103:317–327, 1992.

Disorders of the Umbilical Cord, Abdominal Wall, Urachus, and Omphalomesenteric Duct

Carol Lynn Berseth

The umbilical region is the site of intricate, complex activity during embryonic life. Early in gestation, there is a widely open communication between the yolk sac and primitive gut. Later the entire midgut passes through this communication to form a large physiologic umbilical hernia that persists in utero for several weeks. Thereafter the gut returns to its position in the abdominal cavity. By the third trimester, the aperture around the vessels, omphalomesenteric (vitelline) duct, and urachus begins to narrow. After birth, the umbilical arteries contract, blood flow ceases, their internal and medial layers undergo aseptic necrosis, and the stump separates. Alterations in this orderly but complex sequence of events result in serious congenital anomalies.

UMBILICAL CORD LESIONS
Noncoiled Umbilical Blood Vessels

The three vessels within the cord are coiled to form a helical structure. The number of twists can differ greatly (from 0 to 40) and, rarely, reach 380 per cord (Lacro et al, 1987). Left-twisted vessels outnumber right-twisted vessels 7 to 1. Absence of any twists occurs in about 4% to 5% of pregnancies (Edmonds, 1954). The helical structure is identifiable by ultrasound by the end of the first trimester. Although it is not established why the vessels have this geometric arrangement, it is known that like a telephone cord, such a configuration is more able to resist external compression stretch or torsion, and it remains flexible (Strong et al, 1993). The absence of coils is associated with increased abnormalities that include single umbilical artery trisomy 21 and coarctation of the aorta. Approximately 10% of infants without coils are stillborn, and the incidence of preterm birth is greater than expected.

Single Umbilical Artery

Normally the umbilical cord is composed of two arteries and a vein. A single umbilical artery occurs in 1% of single births and 7% of twin births. In approximately one third of these infants, gastrointestinal obstructive lesions and urogenital abnormalities are present. Therefore, the presence of a single umbilical artery warrants careful physical examination.

Granuloma of the Umbilicus

If the separation of the umbilical stump is delayed beyond 5 to 8 days after birth, granulation tissue may be produced and delay epithelialization. Granulomas must be differentiated from everted gastric or intestinal mucosa, which permits the entrance of a fine probe. Treatment for both is judicious desiccation with silver nitrate.

Delay in Separation of the Cord

If the umbilical cord fails to separate after more than 14 days, investigation for a possible defect in neutrophil function and chemotaxis should be undertaken.

Umbilical Infection

The presence of serous, purulent, or sanguineous drainage from the umbilicus for a number of days after the cord has separated can be an early clinical presentation of omphalitis. Infection may remain restricted to the cord or may spread to involve the surrounding skin causing erythema and warmth to touch. Treatment consists of parenteral antibiotics including antistaphylococcal coverage.

Septic Umbilical Arteritis

In this relatively uncommon disorder, bacteria may invade or spread along the lumen, the inner necrosing coats, or the mantle of loose connective tissue of the umbilical artery. If the iliac and abdominal ends of the artery are sealed, the infection forms an abscess; if the artery remains patent externally, the umbilicus drains purulent material. If the mantle zone is involved, peritonitis may ensue. Infection may also track along the course of the artery to form abscesses in the scrotum or the thigh. If the iliac end of the umbilical artery is patent, generalized sepsis may occur by vascular spread of bacteria.

ABDOMINAL WALL DEFECTS
Omphalocele
Definition and Epidemiology

Omphalocele refers to a congenital defect in the formation of the umbilical portion of the abdominal wall that is larger than 4 cm in diameter (Table 76–1; Figs. 76–1 and 76–2). The defect occurs in 1 in 6000 to 10,000 live births. Although many are isolated defects, many are part of a constellation of malformations (such as Beckwith-Wiedemann syndrome or trisomy 18), and a few cases are associated with maternal ingestion of valproic acid for seizure control (Boussemart et al, 1995).

Etiology

Early in fetal life, the small intestine lies outside of the abdominal cavity. By the 10th week, the midgut returns to

TABLE 76–1

Characteristics of Gastroschisis and Omphalocele

Defect	Gastroschisis	Omphalocele
Covering sac	Absent	Present, but may be torn
Fascial defect	Small	Small or large
Cord attachment	Onto the abdominal wall	Onto the sac
Herniated bowel	Edematous	Normal
Prematurity (%)	50–60	10–20
Associated anomalies (%)	10–15	45–55
Gastrointestinal	18	37
Cardiac	2	20
Trisomy syndromes	—	30
Necrotizing enterocolitis (%)	18	Only if sac is ruptured
Malabsorption	Common	Only if sac is ruptured

the abdomen, and the somatic layers of the cephalic, caudal, and lateral folds join to close the defect in the abdominal wall. For unknown reasons, this closure may not occur. Two types of omphalocele are recognized (Margulies, 1945). In the first type, the failure of closure occurs in the 3rd week of gestation, and the resulting defect is large. Three subtypes make up this first type. An epigastric omphalocele occurs when there is abnormal closure of the cephalic fold. Because these somites form the lower thoracic wall, failure of closure results in the Cantrell pentalogy, which includes cleft sternum, diaphragmatic defects, pericardial defects, cardiac anomalies, and omphalocele. The classic omphalocele occurs when there is an interruption in lateral fold development resulting in an abdominal wall defect that lies between the epigastric and hypogastric regions. In addition to loops of bowel, liver may also herniate through the abdominal wall defect. The umbilicus arises

from an anterior position on the omphalocele, and the muscular abdominal wall is normal. Failure in closure of the caudal fold results in a hypogastric omphalocele. Associated defects include bladder exstrophy and imperforate anus (Fig. 76–3).

The second type of omphalocele is often called an *umbilical hernia*. By definition, the defect in the abdominal wall is less than 4 cm in diameter, and the exterior ionized sac contains only loops of bowel (Fig. 76–4). This defect arises between the 8th and 10th weeks owing to a failure of closure of the umbilical ring (see next section).

Diagnosis

Alpha-fetoprotein (AFP) is synthesized in the fetal liver and is excreted by the fetal kidneys. It also crosses the placenta and appears in the maternal circulation by 12 weeks' gestation. Maternal plasma levels of AFP are elevated when fetuses have neural tube defects, abdominal wall defects, or atresia of the duodenum or esophagus. Maternal serum AFP is used as a screening test because there is a 40% rate of false-positive results. Analysis of amniotic AFP and acetylcholinesterase-pseudocholinesterase can be sensitive in detecting abdominal wall defects, especially gastroschisis (Saleh et al, 1993; Saller et al, 1994). Human chorionic gonadotropin levels have shown promise in small series to detect abdominal wall defects (Schmidt et al, 1993).

Ultrasound evaluation is not useful during the first trimester because the midgut is normally herniated. Therefore, current recommendations are for its use beyond 14 weeks (Cyr et al, 1986). The combined use of maternal serum AFP and ultrasound at 19 weeks has been shown in a series of 8000 patients to have excellent sensitivity in identifying abdominal wall defects (Luck, 1992). Once an abdominal wall defect has been identified, ultrasound can often distinguish omphalocele from gastroschisis. Because the association of cardiac anomalies and chromosomal disorders is high, fetal echocardiography and amniocentesis should also be performed. Vaginal delivery does not ad-

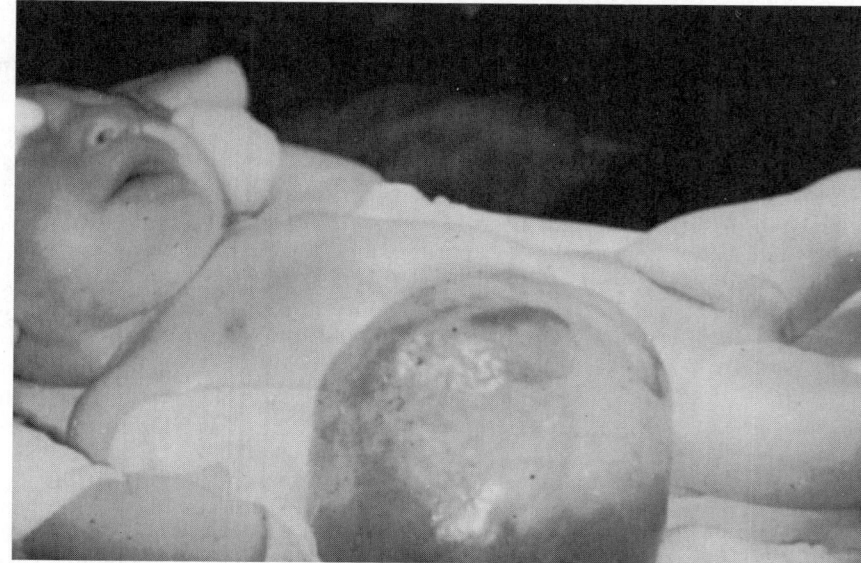

FIGURE 76–1. A mass is seen protruding from the umbilical region. No specific structures can be identified. It is covered by whitish, glistening membrane and is obviously an omphalocele.

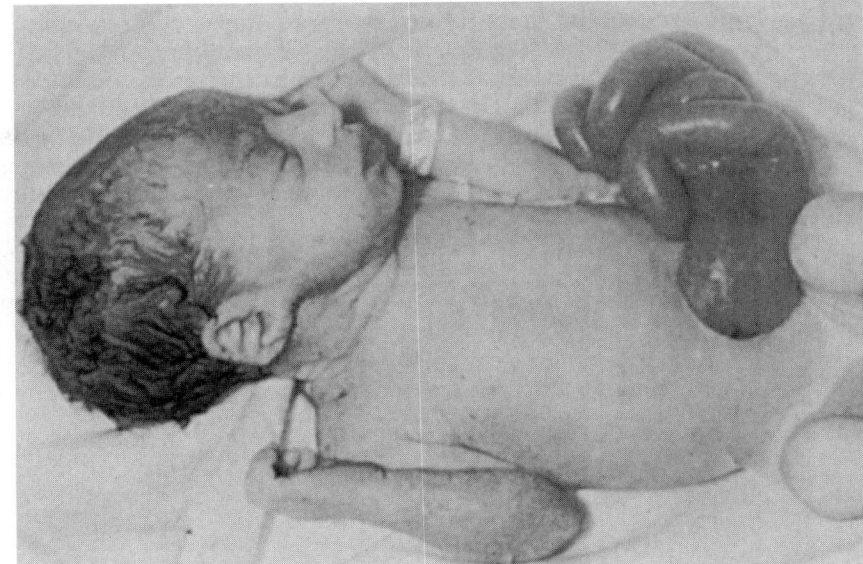

FIGURE 76–2. Omphalocele in which the containing amniotic-peritoneal membrane must have been torn away during delivery. Loops of bowel lie free on the abdominal wall. (Courtesy of Dr. Arnold Tramer, Baltimore, MD.)

versely affect outcome; therefore, the need for cesarean section should be based on obstetric indications alone (Lewis et al, 1990; Sipes et al, 1990). If not discovered prenatally, the diagnosis is obvious at birth. If the sac ruptures, the bowel loops may be edematous and matted together and can mimic gastroschisis.

Treatment

The presence of exteriorized bowel results in heat loss and extravasation of fluid and provides a major portal of entry for bacteria. When the omphalocele is first seen, the sac should be kept moist by wrapping it with gauze sponges that have been soaked in warmed normal saline. A plastic covering is then wrapped around the defect to limit water and heat loss. Care should be taken to place the contents above the abdomen if the patient is prone to prevent kinking of mesenteric vessels. Alternatively the infant can be positioned on the side facing the exteriorized loops of bowel. A nasogastric tube is passed to decrease the accumulation of air in the bowel. The infant should be given 1.5 times maintenance intravenous fluids and broad-

spectrum antibiotics. Thereafter, any inspection and manipulation of the abdominal contents should be done with sterile gloves.

Operative repair should be done as soon as possible. Small defects can be closed with a single-stage repair. For larger defects, primary repair may cause respiratory failure and compression of the vena cava because the abdominal cavity is too small to accommodate the bowel. In these infants, a staged repair using a prosthetic material called a *silo* is used to cover the defect. After the bowel is gradually pushed into the abdominal cavity over 7 to 10 days, finally closure can be achieved (Schuster, 1979).

A third approach has been introduced. In these infants, fascial closure cannot be achieved after the silo has been removed. A tear-shaped patch is used to achieve fascial

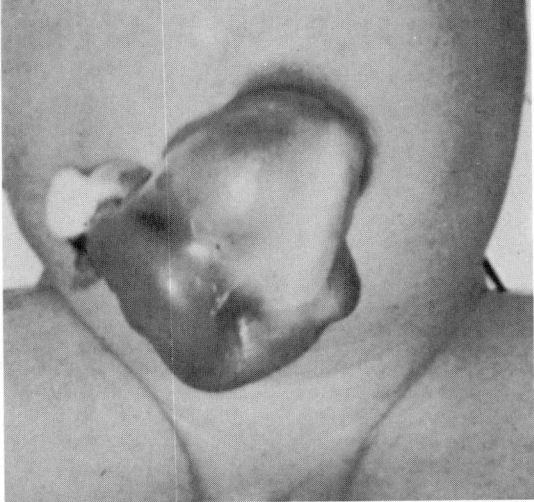

FIGURE 76–4. A comparatively small mass protrudes from the umbilical region, and a loop of bowel can be readily recognized running around its lower margin. The mass is completely covered by shiny transparent membrane—clearly an umbilical cord hernia.

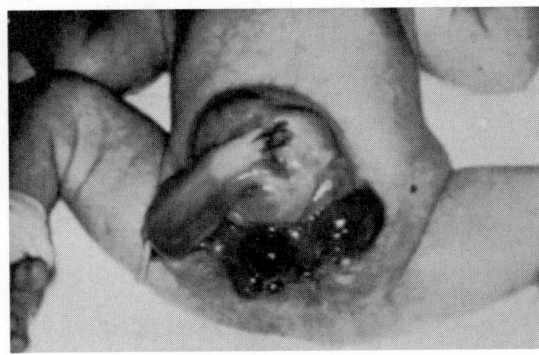

FIGURE 76–3. A combination of omphalocele and ectopia vesicae. The bright structure below the omphalocele is an everted, exstrophic bladder.

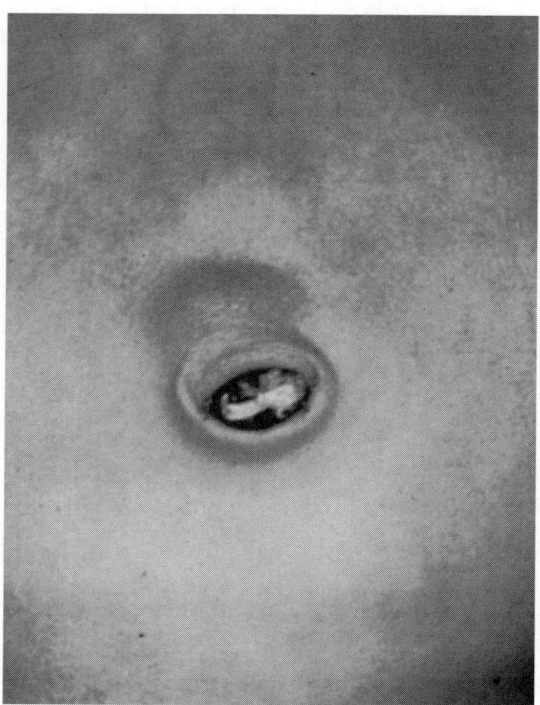

FIGURE 76–5. Two definite bulges are seen cephalad to the umbilicus, one above the other. Two distinct apertures could be felt in the midline. This represents a minor defect of the abdominal wall.

closure. Final fascial repair is done 2 to 5 months later (Krasna, 1995).

Postoperatively, protracted ileus usually necessitates prolonged parenteral nutrition. Attention must also be directed to the diagnosis and management of associated anomalies.

Prognosis

Mortality with associated heart disease is 80%. Without heart disease, 70% survive.

Umbilical Hernia

The umbilical ring is formed when the mesoderm of the muscle and fascia around the umbilical vessels and urachus contract. Umbilical hernia differs from omphalocele in that skin and subcutaneous tissue cover the original defect and separation of the rectus muscle persists. These lesions are found in 30% of black infants and 4% of white infants; there is a high familial incidence. The condition is more common in infants weighing under 1500 g, as 75% may have small hernias. The hernia aperture varies in size from 1 to 4 cm in diameter at the base of the umbilicus. The sac may contain a loop of bowel that may easily be pushed back into the abdomen. Approximately 80% of these hernias close spontaneously by 3 to 4 years, and the risk of incarceration is exceedingly low (Fig. 76–5). Larger hernias, however, may require surgical closure (Lassaletta et al, 1975) (Fig. 76–6).

Gastroschisis
Definition and Epidemiology

Gastroschisis is the herniation of abdominal contents through an abdominal wall defect, usually occurring on the right side of a normally positioned umbilical cord (see Table 76–1). This lesion is approximately one third as common as omphalocele. If associated anomalies are present, they are usually gastrointestinal in origin, including malrotation and atresias. Infants with gastroschisis tend to have intrauterine growth retardation.

Etiology

Although the cause of these lesions is not known, many speculate that they may be of vascular origin. Intrauterine interruption of the omphalomesenteric artery has been proposed, an explanation that accounts for many of the clinically observed differences between this lesion and omphalocele (Hoyme et al, 1981).

Diagnosis and Treatment

As described for an omphalocele, gastroschisis may be correctly diagnosed prenatally. Because the peritoneal sac

FIGURE 76–6. Large triangular herniation of and above the umbilicus. The bulge contained easily reducible bowel. A large aperture could be felt just above the umbilicus and a second, smaller one several centimeters above it. Between them the rectus muscles were diastatic. This is a large defect of the abdominal wall demanding surgical closure.

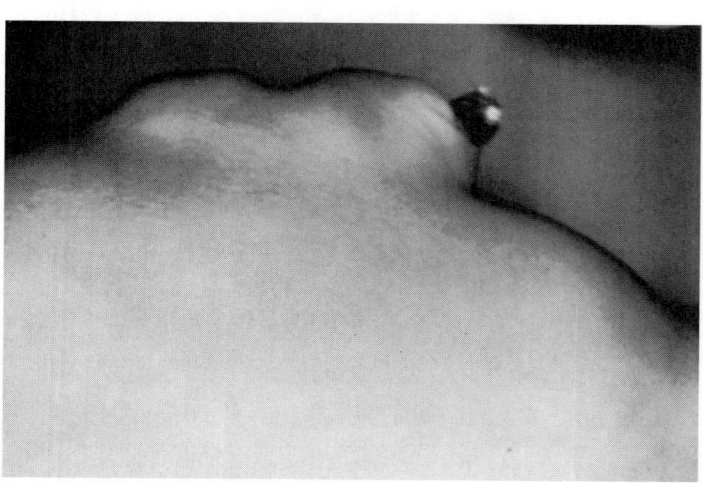

is absent, the fetal bowel is continuously bathed in amniotic fluid, which results in significant intestinal dysmorphia. As with omphalocele, the need for cesarean section should be restricted to obstetric indications only (Langer et al, 1988).

As described for omphalocele, the bowel contents should be kept moist and relatively sterile at birth. A nasogastric tube is passed for decompression, and 1.5 times maintenance intravenous fluids given. Broad-spectrum antibiotics should also be started. Because the abdominal wall defect is often small, vascular compromise occurs more readily, and great care should be taken to position the infant and the exteriorized bowel to prevent kinking of mesenteric vessels. As for omphalocele, primary closure is often possible, but larger defects may require staged repair. Postoperatively, prolonged ileus may occur because of intestinal dysmorphology, which often includes the myenteric plexus. These infants are at increased risk for necrotizing enterocolitis. Prolonged obstruction and malabsorption are frequent complications in the postoperative period.

Prognosis

Reported mortality figures vary from 10% to 30%.

Prune-Belly Syndrome

Prune-belly syndrome refers to a triad of anomalies consisting of a deficiency of abdominal musculature, cryptorchidism, and urinary tract abnormalities. The most common urinary tract anomalies seen in this triad are megaloureter, cystic renal dysplasia, urethral obstruction, and megacystis (Lattimer, 1958). Associated gastrointestinal (malrotation) anomalies occur in 30%, and cardiac anomalies occur in 20%. The syndrome rarely occurs in females, and its exact cause is unknown. One theory proposes that there is a failure in the development of the abdominal wall between the 6th and 8th weeks of gestation. A second theory holds that primary urethral obstruction with early bladder distention gives rise to abdominal distention and other secondary anomalies (Moerman et al, 1984). At birth, the defect is visually obvious. The abdomen is shapeless, and the skin hangs in wrinkled folds. There may be an open patent urachus, which by itself signals a poor prognosis. Of immediate concern is the evaluation and relief of urinary tract obstruction. Approximately 20% of patients with prune-belly syndrome die in the neonatal period from renal dysplasia or pulmonary hypoplasia, but of the 80% who survive, 30% develop renal failure during childhood (Burbige et al, 1987).

Inguinal Hernia

The gonads are formed during the 5th to 12th weeks of gestation. The testes descend through the internal ring at 28 weeks. In the general population, inguinal hernias occur in 1% of all live births. The incidence of inguinal hernia in low-birth-weight and very-low-birth-weight infants is as follows: 500 to 1000 g, 42%; 1000 to 1500 g, 10%; and 1500 to 2000 g, 3% (Peevy et al, 1986). With preterm delivery and the accompanying increase in intra-abdominal pressure, testicular descent and inguinal canal closure do not take place, thus explaining the increased incidence of inguinal hernia.

Additional risk factors for inguinal hernias are the presence of cystic fibrosis, congenital dislocation of the hip, the presence of a ventriculoperitoneal shunt, and the presence of abdominal wall defects. Although many inguinal hernias can be repaired electively, as many as 10% to 30% may become incarcerated or strangulated (Rowe and Clatworthy, 1970). Therefore, repeated examinations may be necessary, particularly if an infant develops instability, a tense fluctuant scrotal mass, or vomiting. Approximately 80% of these incarcerated hernias may be reduced nonoperatively by placing the infant in Trendelenburg position with sedation and an ice pack applied to the inguinal-scrotal area (Scherer and Grosfeld, 1993). The most common complication of operative repair is postoperative apnea (Stewart, 1982).

Diaphragmatic Hernia
Definition and Epidemiology

The incidence of congenital diaphragmatic hernia is 1 in 1000 to 6000 births. Diaphragmatic hernias may be of two types (Fig. 76–7): through a posterolateral defect (foramen of Bochdalek) or through a retrosternal defect (foramen of Morgagni). Ninety-eight percent are of the posterolateral variety, and 90% of these involve the left leaf of the diaphragm. The incidence of diaphragmatic hernia is 1 in 4000 live births. See Chapter 60 for extensive discussion of this entity.

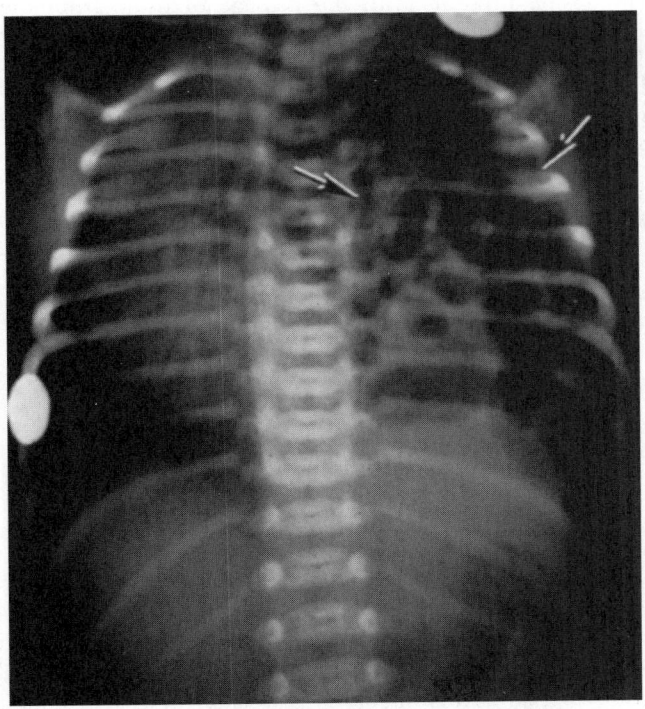

FIGURE 76–7. Plain film of the abdomen and chest of a 2-hour-old infant who developed severe respiratory distress. Loops of bowel are present in the chest with a shifting of the mediastinum to the right (arrows). (Courtesy of Dr. Ronald M. Cohen, Children's Hospital, Oakland, CA.)

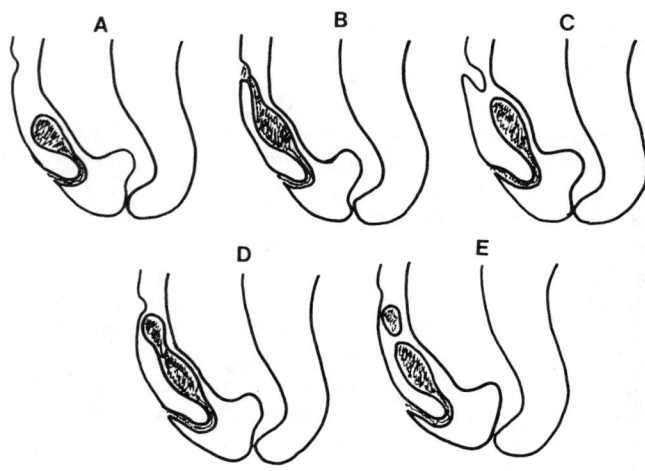

FIGURE 76–8. Urachal anomalies. *A,* Normal anatomy. *B,* Completely patent urachus. *C,* Blind external tract–urachal sinus. *D,* Blind internal tract–bladder diverticulum. *E,* Urachal cyst.

URACHAL LESIONS

The urachus is the remnant of the allantois that extends from the bladder portion of the cloaca to the umbilicus. The urachus may remain completely patent throughout its length or fail to obliterate (Ney and Friedenberg, 1968) (Fig. 76–8). All varieties of this defect are rare.

Completely Patent Urachus

This lesion presents with the passage of urine from the umbilicus. Injection of radiopaque contrast material into the orifice outlines the urachal tract and fills the bladder. Treatment consists of surgical excision of the umbilicus along with the entire urachus and a small portion of the bladder. Results are usually good.

Blind External Type

When only the distal end of the urachus fails to obliterate, a draining sinus results. Drainage of urine begins sometime after the cord separates. Treatment consists of surgical excision of the sinus tract.

Blind Internal Type

Failure of obliteration of the proximal end of the urachus results in a bladder diverticulum. It produces no symptoms and may be coincidentally discovered on cystogram. Nothing needs to be done surgically.

Urachal Cyst

Incomplete obliteration of the midportion of the urachus leads to the development of a urachal cyst. Cysts may present at birth or may grow slowly and become obvious at anytime during infancy or childhood. The cysts frequently become infected. Plain films may show the lesion just beneath the abdominal wall. Surgical excision should be performed.

MALFORMATIONS OF THE OMPHALOMESENTERIC DUCT

In the developing embryo, the omphalomesenteric (vitelline) duct connects the yolk sac to the primitive midgut through the umbilical cord. In the normal course of ontogeny, the duct becomes obliterated and disappears. Under certain circumstances, all or portions of the duct may persist (Fig. 76–9).

Patent Omphalomesenteric Duct

More than 200 cases of patent omphalomesenteric duct (enteroumbilical fistula) have been reported. It presents with the passage of meconium and fecal matter through the umbilicus. This may begin at birth or occur within 1 to 2 weeks. The most significant danger with this lesion is evagination of the small bowel through the umbilical orifice. Mortality increases fivefold when this occurs. Once this lesion is diagnosed, it should be corrected by surgical excision of the umbilicus and the duct.

Omphalomesenteric Sinus

Failure of distal closure of the duct leads to the formation of a sinus. Persistent watery discharge from the umbilical cord is the initial presentation. Examination of the umbilicus reveals a red nodule projecting from the base. Gentle massage results in the extrusion of mucus, which differentiates this lesion from an umbilical granuloma. Injection of radiopaque contrast material outlines the sinus tract. Treatment consists of surgical excision.

Omphalomesenteric Duct Cyst

When the middle portion of the omphalomesenteric duct persists and eventually fills with secretions, a cyst forms.

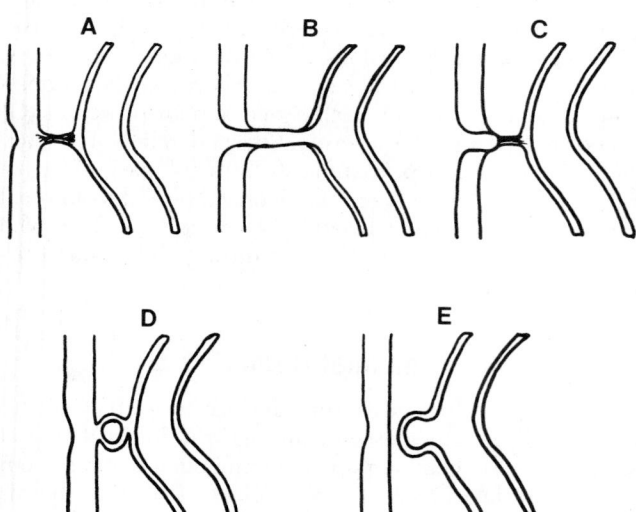

FIGURE 76–9. Omphalomesenteric (vitelline) duct anomalies. *A,* Normal anatomy. *B,* Patent omphalomesenteric duct. *C,* Blind external tract–umbilical sinus. *D,* Omphalomesenteric duct cyst. *E,* Blind internal tract–Meckel diverticulum.

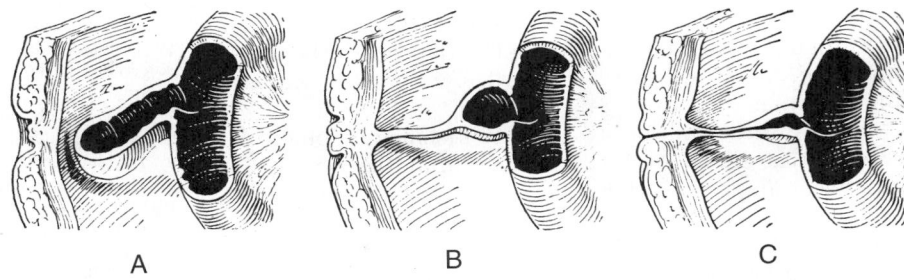

FIGURE 76–10. Meckel diverticulum of the ileum. *A,* Ordinary blind sac. *B,* Diverticulum continued to umbilicus as a cord. *C,* Diverticulum with fistulous opening of umbilicus. (From Arey LB: Developmental Anatomy, rev 7th ed. Philadelphia, WB Saunders, 1974.)

This may be detected as an enlarging umbilical mass. Treatment consists of surgical excision.

Meckel Diverticulum

When the proximal, or intestinal, end of the omphalomesenteric duct fails to become obliterated completely, an outpouching of the ileum persists. The diverticulum may be as short as 2 cm or as long as 90 cm. It is usually tent shaped, but it may be tubular. It may arise from any point of the small intestine as close as 3 cm proximal to the cecum or as far as 100 cm distant from it. The junction usually lies at some point in the ileum, rarely in the jejunum, and exceptionally in the duodenum. It must arise from the antimesenteric side of the bowel, a fact that distinguishes Meckel diverticulum from duplications. Its distal end usually lies free in the peritoneal cavity, but some are attached to the umbilicus by a fibrous cord, and a small minority remain patent to the umbilicus (omphalomesenteric fistula) (Fig. 76–10). Its structure simulates that of small bowel, with well-defined mucosa, submucosa, muscularis, and serosa. In about one fifth of cases, it is the site of ectopic pancreatic or gastric tissue. Aberrant pancreatic tissue is usually present as a small mass in the wall, whereas gastric mucosa replaces or overlies the usual intestinal mucosa at some point or points. A pancreatic mass may act as a leader to produce intussusception. Gastric mucosa may cause peptic ulceration and bleeding; the latter is almost always the presenting sign if Meckel diverticulum becomes symptomatic. The fibrous cord, if present, may produce intestinal obstruction. Rarely, inflammation of the diverticulum may lead to peritonitis.

Incidence

A Meckel diverticulum can be discovered in 1.5% to 2% of all persons. Only a small proportion of these ever become symptomatic, and when they do, this usually happens beyond the age of 4 months. Only exceptionally do they cause illness in the neonatal period. Males outnumber females by 3:1 to 5:1.

Diagnosis

Hemorrhage from the bowel is the definitive sign of Meckel diverticulum. A few cases in older children and adults may produce the signs and symptoms of diverticulitis, but this condition has never been described in young infants. Hemorrhage is often sudden and catastrophic, causing a precipitous fall in the hematocrit level and a shock-like state within a few hours. The first few stools passed may be composed almost entirely of unchanged

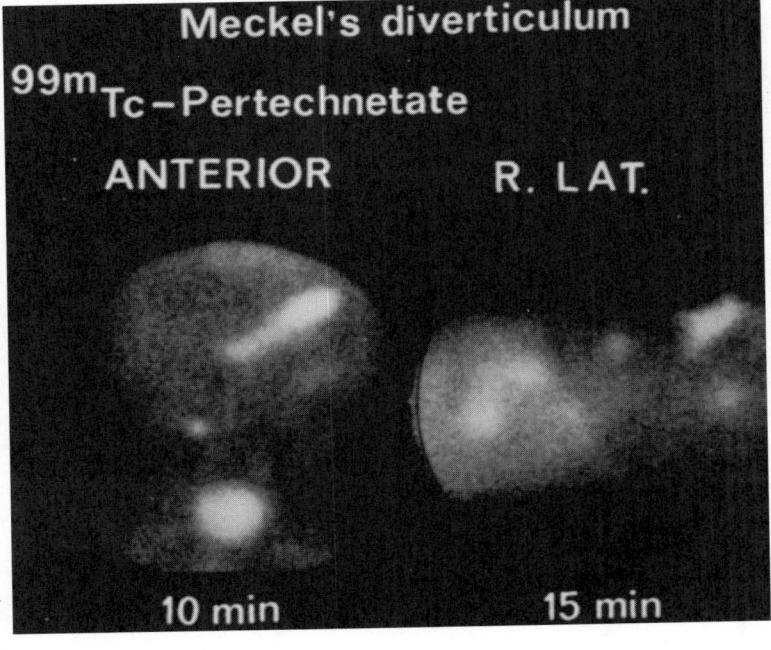

FIGURE 76–11. Anterior gamma camera view of the abdomen of a 2-year-old infant. Note the small well-defined area of increased uptake located in the right lower quadrant. The stomach and bladder are also visualized. On the lateral view, some radioactivity is evident on the diaper as well. (Courtesy of Dr. S. Treves, Children's Hospital, Boston, MA.)

blood; later, they become burgundy colored, then tarry. In other instances, bleeding is constant and occult. About 25% of individuals with Meckel diverticulum present with intussusception.

Meckel diverticulum must be differentiated from other disorders that produce gross bleeding from the bowel: peptic ulcer, duplication, intestinal polyp, intussusception, and intestinal hemangioma. Fissure in ano, proctitis, and ulcerative colitis ordinarily do not lead to gross hemorrhage, blood loss being confined to the passage of bloody mucus or of stools containing a surface accumulation of blood. The most useful differential point is that hematemesis usually coexists with rectal bleeding when peptic ulcer is present, whereas hematemesis rarely occurs with Meckel diverticulum. The mass of duplication is sometimes palpable.

Scans after intravenous injection of technetium-99m pertechnetate are often, but not always, diagnostic of Meckel diverticulum because the technetium is concentrated in gastric mucosa. Pentagastrin or cimetidine is useful in enhancing the image of gastric mucosa on subsequent technetium scans (Fig. 76–11).

Treatment

Blood replacement therapy is the prime treatment regardless of the cause of bleeding. If bleeding ceases, careful observation for recurrence of bleeding is often all that is needed because peptic ulcer rarely recurs. A second episode of bleeding, however, strongly suggests that other diagnostic procedures be explored, including endoscopy and laporatomy. If a diverticulum is discovered, it must be excised.

REFERENCES

Abrahamson J: Repair of inguinal hernias in infants and children. Clin Pediatr 12:617, 1973.

Adzick NS, Vacanti I, Lillehei CW, et al: Fetal hernia: Ultrasound diagnosis and clinical outcome in 38 cases. J Pediatr Surg 24:654, 1989.

Bloss RS, Aranda JV, Beardmore HE: Congenital diaphragmatic hernia: Pathophysiology and pharmacologic support. Surgery 89:518, 1981.

Boussemart T, Bonneau D, Levard G, et al: Omphalocele in a newborn baby exposed to sodium valproate in utero. Eur J Pediatr 154:220, 1995.

Burbige KA, Amodio J, Berdon WE, et al: Prune-belly syndrome: Thirty-five years of experience. J Urol 137:86, 1987.

Cyr DR, Mack LA, Schoenecker SA, et al: Bowel migration in the normal fetus: US detection. Radiology 161:119, 1986.

Edmonds HW: The spiral twist of the normal umbilical cord in twins and singletons. Am J Obstet Gynecol 67:102, 1954.

Goldfine C, Haddow JE, Knight GJ, et al: Amniotic fluid alpha-fetoprotein and acetylcholinesterase measurements in pregnancies associated with gastroschisis. Prenat Diagn 8:697, 1989.

Greenwood RD: Cardiovascular malformation associated with omphalocele. J Pediatr 85:818, 1974.

Harrison MR, Bjordal RL, Langmark F, et al: Congenital diaphragmatic hernia: The hidden mortality. J Pediatr Surg 13:227, 1978.

Hoyme HE, Higginbottom MC, Jones KL: The vascular pathogenesis of gastroschisis: Intrauterine interruption of the omphalomesenteric artery. J Pediatr 98:228, 1981.

Krasna IH: Is early fascial closure necessary for omphalocele and gastroschisis? J Pediatr Surg 30:23, 1995.

Lacro RV, Jones KL, Benirschke K: The umbilical cord twist: Origin, direction, and relevance. Am J Obstet Gynecol 157:833, 1987.

Langer JC, Filler RM, Bohn DJ, et al: Timing of surgery for congenital diaphragmatic hernia: Is emergency operation necessary? J Pediatr Surg 23:731, 1988.

Lassaletta L, Fonkalsrud EW, Tovar JA, et al: Management of umbilical hernias in infancy and childhood. J Pediatr 10:405, 1975.

Lattimer JK: Congenital deficiency of the abdominal musculature and associated genitourinary anomalies: A report of 22 cases. J Urol 79:343, 1958.

Lewis DF, Towers CV, Garita TJ, et al: Fetal gastroschisis and omphalocele: Is cesarean section the best method of delivery? Am J Obstet Gynecol 163:773, 1990.

Luck CA: Value of routine ultrasound scanning at 19 weeks: A four year study of 8849 deliveries. Br Med J 304:1474, 1992.

Margulies L: Omphalocele. Am J Obstet Gynecol 49:695, 1945.

Meguid M, Canty T, Eraklis AJ: Complications of Meckel's diverticulum in infants. Surg Gynecol Obstet 139:541, 1974.

Moerman P, Fryns J, Goddeeris P, et al: Pathogenesis of the prune belly syndrome: A functional urethral obstruction caused by prostatic hypoplasia. Pediatrics 73:470, 1984.

Ney C, Friedenberg RM: Radiographic findings in anomalies of the urachus. J Urol 99:288, 1968.

Paidas MJ, Crombleholme TM, Robertson FM: Prenatal diagnosis and management of the fetus with an abdominal wall defect. Semin Perinatol 18:196, 1994.

Peevy KJ, Speed FA, Hoff CJ: Epidemiology of inguinal hernia in preterm neonates. Pediatrics 77:246, 1986.

Rogers LW, Ostrow PT: The prune belly syndrome. J Pediatr 83:786, 1973.

Rowe MI, Clatworthy HW: Incarcerated and strangulated hernias in children. Arch Surg 101:136, 1970.

Saleh AA, Isada NB, Johnson MP, et al: Amniotic fluid acetylcholinesterase is found in gastroschisis but not omphalocele. Fetal Diagn Ther 8:168, 1993.

Saller DN, Canick JA, Palmoki GE, et al: Second-trimester maternal serum alpha-fetoprotein, unconjugated estriol, and hCG levels in pregnancies with ventral wall hernias. Obstet Gynecol 84:852, 1994.

Scherer LR III, Grosfeld JL: Inguinal and umbilical anomalies. Pediatr Clin North Am 40:1121, 1993.

Schmidt D, Rose E, Greenberg F: An association between fetal abdominal wall defects and elevated levels of human chorionic gonadotropin in mid-trimester. Prenat Diagn 13:9, 1993.

Schuster S: Omphalocele, hernia of the umbilical cord and gastroschisis. *In* Ravitch MM (Ed): Pediatric Surgery. Chicago, Year Book Medical Publishers, 1979, pp 778–900.

Sipes SL, Weiner CP, Sipes DR, et al: Gastroschisis and omphalocele: Does either antenatal diagnosis or route of delivery make a difference in perinatal outcome? Obstet Gynecol 76:195, 1990.

Stewart DJ: Preterm infants are more prone to complications following minor surgery than are term infants. Anesthesiology 56:304, 1982.

Strong TH, Elliott JP, Radin TG: Noncoiled umbilical blood vessels: A new marker for the fetus at risk. Obstet Gynecol 81:409, 1993.

West KN, Bengston K, Rescorla FJ, et al: Delayed surgical repair and ECMO improves survival in congenital diaphragmatic hernia. Am Surg 216:454, 1992.

CHAPTER 77

Ascites and Peritonitis

Carol Lynn Berseth

ASCITES

Generalized abdominal enlargement may be due to intestinal distention, hepatomegaly, tumors, peritonitis, and ascites. Therefore the presence or absence of each of these entities must be determined when evaluating the presence of suspected ascites. The use of imaging techniques such as radiography, ultrasonography, and computed tomography scanning may be useful in determining whether abdominal masses are present and in determining the type of ascites present, as detailed subsequently. In addition, paracenteses to obtain peritoneal fluid for laboratory analysis provides additional clues as to the cause of ascites. Most commonly, ascitic fluid in newborns is analyzed for content of red blood cells, white blood cells, protein, and fat content, but additional analysis as shown in Table 77–1 can be useful.

Ascites may be identified early in fetal life by obstetric ultrasound. Accumulation of fluid in the abdomen of the fetus may be so massive as to necessitate delivery by cesarean section. The presence of ascites may produce respiratory distress after birth (Fig. 77–1). Immediate paracentesis to aspirate ascitic fluid may be diagnostic as well as therapeutic. Ascites may be chylous, urinary, biliary, or pancreatic. It may be secondary to neonatal hydrops or congestive heart failure or caused by the rupture of a large ovarian cyst in the fetus during delivery. Although hyponatremia is found in 70% of these infants, electrolytes are commonly normal at birth because of the presence of the maternal-placental circulation. Postnatally, however, the presence of ascitic fluids containing high concentrations of urea, creatnine, and potassium triggers physiologic equilibration with the extracellular fluid, which may result in dramatic shifts of free water and solutes. Thus, sodium moves from the vascular compartment to the peritoneal cavity and causes hyponatremia. There have been case reports of the use of shunts and modified extracorporeal membrane oxygenation circuits to manage some of these severe cases (Pettitt, 1992; Rector and Whittlesey, 1993).

Chylous Ascites

The most common cause of neonatal ascites is chylous ascites, and it occurs more often in males. In the newborn, chylous ascites is usually due to a congenital failure of the lymphatic channels to communicate (Cochran et al, 1985). The initial paracentesis may yield clear fluid, but after enteral feedings are initiated, subsequent paracenteses yield a milky fluid that is high in triglyceride content. Leukocyte counts may also be elevated, and protein content is variable. Because chylous ascites may accompany intestinal malrotation and incomplete volvulus, appropriate imaging should be done to rule out the presence of intestinal malrotation. Treatment consists of repeated paracentesis to relieve distention and avoid respiratory embar-

rassment. The use of a formula containing medium-chain triglycerides decreases the formation of chyle. If chyle formation persists despite the specialized formula, intravenous alimentation may be necessary. Most patients undergo spontaneous remission, and the outlook for total recovery is good.

Urinary Ascites

Urinary ascites accounts for 25% of all cases of neonatal ascites, and it is due to an obstructive uropathy. The male:female ratio is 5:1. Posterior urethral valves are the most common cause (Mann et al, 1974), but other lesions that can cause urinary ascites include ureteroceles, urethral atresia, bladder neck obstruction, neurogenic bladder, and bladder hematoma. Although the most common cause of disruption of the urinary collecting system is the presence of a tear in the collecting system itself—most often located at the calyceal fornix—perforation of the bladder has also been described.

Paracentesis yields urine. Evaluation should include an abdominal ultrasound study, intravenous pyelogram, and voiding cystourethrogram to characterize the abnormalities in the urinary tract and its collecting system. Surgical decompression of the urinary tract or definitive correction of the lesions should be performed with urgency.

Biliary Ascites

Biliary ascites is caused by spontaneous perforation of the biliary tree. In 68%, the perforation occurs in the main biliary tree. The remainder are located at the junction of the cystic and common ducts or in an accessory bile duct. Two clinical forms are apparent. In the acute form, the infant presents with abdominal distention, vomiting, absent bowel sounds, and unstable vital signs. Clinical jaundice may not be present. In the more chronic form, which occurs in about 80% of reported cases, clinical jaundice appears early, followed by gradual abdominal distention. Paracentesis reveals fluid with a bilirubin content above 4

TABLE 77–1

Laboratory Studies Useful in the Evaluation of Ascites

Routine	Special
Red cell count	Triglycerides
White cell count with differential	Amylase
Specific gravity	Bilirubin
Total protein	
Culture	

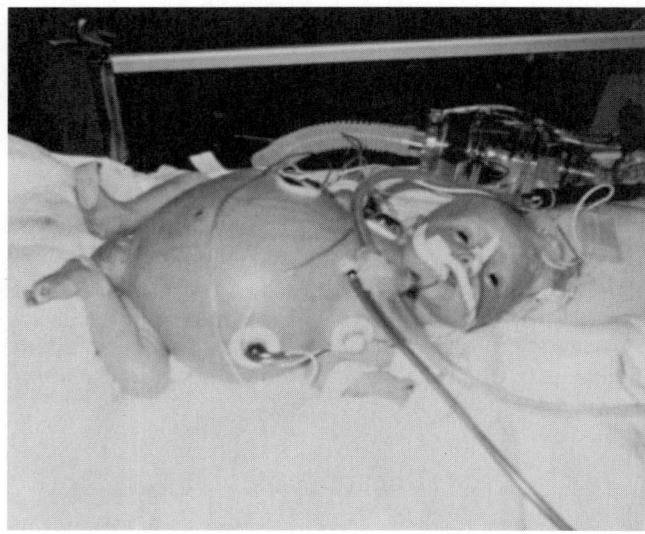

FIGURE 77–1. Full-term infant at 2 hours of age with massive ascites, which subsequently proved to be chylous. The distention was controlled with repeated paracentesis and an elemental diet. By 6 months of age, paracentesis was no longer necessary. At 13 months of age, the infant remains on an elemental diet and is growing and developing normally.

g/dL. Technetium liver scan is confirmatory (So et al, 1983). Laparotomy with a biliary drainage procedure is essential for survival. Survival after surgery is 80%.

Pancreatic Ascites

This extremely rare lesion may be the presenting manifestation of pancreatitis secondary to a pancreatic duct anomaly. Except for the presence of abdominal distention, infants are asymptomatic. The concentrations of amylase, fat, and protein in the ascitic fluid may be elevated. Urine and serum amylase levels may be normal. Most infants require a surgical drainage procedure.

Ruptured Ovarian Cyst

Ahmed (1971) reported this complication in a review of newborns with ovarian cysts. The presenting symptoms at birth included ascites or hemoperitoneum.

PERITONITIS

Peritonitis in the newborn can be classified as either bacterial or chemical (Fonkalsrud et al, 1966). Chemical peritonitis occurs as an inflammatory response to the presence of a caustic material. The two most common forms of chemical peritonitis are due to the presence of meconium or bile as a result of spillage from the intestine or biliary tree.

Meconium peritonitis may result from intestinal perforation that occurs in utero or shortly after birth. Most typically these cases of intestinal perforation are secondary to bowel obstruction; almost half are due to meconium ileus

(Santulli, 1980). At autopsy or surgery, the tear may be obvious or may have healed over. Although uncommon, other causes of meconium peritonitis are intussusception, volvulus, incarcerated internal hernia, imperforate anus, and meconium plugs. It has been speculated that intestinal perforation that occurs in the absence of obstruction may be due to the presence of localized defects or vascular accidents.

Infectious peritonitis may be primary or secondary. Primary peritonitis occurs as a result of hematogenous or lymphatic spread, and secondary peritonitis occurs as a result of a primary abdominal catastrophe, such as necrotizing enterocolitis, appendicitis, biliary tract disease, rupture of a visceral abscess, or infection of indwelling foreign objects. Bacterial peritonitis in newborns is most commonly secondary. Thus, the organisms involved are mixed anaerobic and aerobic (Brook, 1989). The pathogenesis of peritonitis is multifactorial. First, many gut bacteria produce endotoxins, which activate inflammatory mediators such as tumor necrosis factor, interleukins, leukotrienes, and the complement systems, all of which can cause increased vascular permeability and coagulation abnormalities. Anaerobes do not produce endotoxin but instead adhere to epithelial cells and produce exoenzymes, such as hyaluronidase and protease. In addition, anaerobes possess capsules, which reduce the ability of immunoregulatory T cells to contain and compartmentalize infection. Moreover, there is a synergism of anaerobic and aerobic bacteria that is enhanced in the presence of irritants such as hemoglobin or bile. Finally, the exudation of intraperitoneal fluid that is triggered by these infections results in large fluid shifts, mechanical compromise of pulmonary function, and presence of a fibrinous glue, which may result in adherence of peritoneal surfaces and mesentery to result in abscess formation.

A new organism that has emerged as a causal agent of peritonitis is *Candida*, which is present in approximately 10% of cases of bowel perforation. Fungal peritonitis is more likely to occur in those infants who are extremely premature, require prolonged umbilical artery catheterization, have prolonged exposure to antibiotics, and require prolonged intubation (Karlowiez, 1993).

Management includes surgical drainage and antibiotics. Antifungal therapy may also be considered. In addition, aggressive rehydration and correction of electrolyte abnormalities must be provided.

REFERENCES

Ahmed S: Neonatal and childhood ovarian cysts. J Pediatr Surg 6:702, 1971.

Brook I: A 12-year study of aerobic and anaerobic bacteria in intraabdominal and postsurgical abdominal wound infections. Surg Gynecol Obstet 169:387, 1989.

Clarke HS Jr, Mills ME, Parres JA, Kropp KA: The hyponatremia of neonatal urinary ascites: Clinical observations, experimental confirmation and proposed mechanism. J Urol 150:778, 1993.

Cochran WJ, Klish WJ, Brown MR, et al: Chylous ascites in infants and children: A case report and literature review. J Pediatr Gastroenterol Nutr 4:668, 1985.

Fonkalsrud EW, Ellis DG, Clatworthy HW: Neonatal peritonitis. J Pediatr Surg 1:227, 1966.

Griscom NT, Colodny AH, Rosenberg HK: Diagnostic aspects of neonatal ascites: Report of 27 cases. AJR Am J Roentgenol 128:961, 1977.

Kalwinsky D, Frittelli G, Oski FA: Pancreatitis presenting as unexplained ascites. Am J Dis Child 128:734–736, 1974.

Karlowiez MG: Risk factors associated with fungal peritonitis in very low birth weight neonates with severe necrotizing enterocolitis: A case control study. Pediatr Infect Dis J 12:574, 1993.

Mann CM, Leape LL, Holder TM: Neonatal urinary ascites: A report of 2 cases of unusual etiology and a review of the literature. J Urol 111:124, 1974.

Mollitt DL, Tepas JJ, Talbert JL: The microbiology of neonatal peritonitis. Arch Surg 123:176, 1988.

Pettitt B: Use of a modified Denver peritoniovenous shunt in a newborn with intractable ascites. J Pediatr Surg 27:108, 1992.

Prevot J, Rickham PP, Hecker WC: Acute biliary peritonitis. Prog Pediatr Surg 1:196, 1971.

Rector FE, Whittlesey G: Effective control of chylons ascitis: An alternative approach. J Pediatr Surg 28:76, 1993.

Santulli TV: Meconium ileus. *In* Holder TM, Ashcraft KW (Eds): Pediatric Surgery. Philadelphia, WB Saunders, 1980, pp 367–372.

So SKS, Lindahl JA, Sharp HL, et al: Bile ascites during infancy: Diagnosis using Tc-99m sequential antiphotography. Pediatrics 71:402, 1983.

CHAPTER 78

Parenteral and Enteral Nutrition

Richard J. Schanler, Carol Lynn Berseth and Steven A. Abrams

GENERAL CONSIDERATIONS

For infants born at term, the gastrointestinal tract is functionally mature to process enteral nutrients adequately. Although there are deficiencies in a variety of gastrointestinal functions at birth, a rapid transition and maturation occurs over the first few postnatal days. This transition occurs as a result of maturation occurring within the infant as well as maturation triggered by the exposure of the gut to exogenous nutrients. Successful ingestion and processing of nutrients requires that certain inherent behaviors and skills be present in the newborn and that the infant learn new skills. This series of complex interactions results in the patterns of feeding that are observed the first few postnatal days.

Although infants may be placed to breast in the delivery room or offered a bottle feeding within 4 hours of birth, the infant may not demonstrate fully competent sucking and swallowing until the third or fourth feeding. Often oral intake is modest (1 to 2 oz per feeding attempt) the first 1 to 2 days after birth, but it generally improves by 72 hours.

The first stool is passed by 24 to 48 hours (Sherry and Kramer, 1955). In the first 2 days, generally meconium stools are passed. Thereafter, stools may contain part meconium and part fecal material. By the 4th day, stools contain fecal material only. The frequency and consistency of stools are highly variable. A healthy infant may produce 1 to 10 stools per day. In general, the stools of breast-fed infants are more frequent and liquid than those of formula-fed infants. Stools are rarely formed. Rather they are soft or semiliquid and may range in color from yellow, green, or brown.

Infants may vomit blood or blood-stained contents the first day after birth. The most common cause is the presence of blood in the stomach that was swallowed during the birthing process. As little as 3 mL of ingested blood may result in the passage of one or more blood-containing stools the first 24 hours. If larger volumes are ingested, hematochezia may persist for 2 to 3 days.

Although most of these episodes of hematemesis and hematochezia are the result of ingested maternal blood, bleeding may also result from the presence of a stress-induced peptic ulcer, esophagitis, bleeding disorders, or congenital anomalies of the gastrointestinal tract. Therefore, it is important to determine whether the blood present in the vomitus or stool is of maternal or fetal origin. This is done using the Apt test. Fetal hemoglobin is resistant to alkalinization, whereas adult hemoglobin is not. In the laboratory, the pink or red filtrate of the vomitus or stool is mixed with sodium hydroxide. If the hemoglobin present in the sample is maternal in origin, it is denatured and the solution turns from pink or red to yellow. If it is fetal in origin, it is not denatured and its color does not change.

Regurgitation is common among newborns. Regurgitation of the first few feedings is not uncommon. The newborn who vomits, however, should be observed and examined frequently. The nature of the material regurgitated may provide useful clues to the location of obstruction. Pure mucus or a mixture of mucus and saliva alone denotes obstruction proximal to the stomach and suggests esophageal atresia. Unaltered or coagulated milk, unstained with bile, suggests gastroesophageal reflux or obstruction at the pylorus or in the duodenum proximal to the ampulla of Vater. Bile-stained vomitus suggests narrowing or obstruction of the intestinal lumen distal to the ampulla. The presence of bile in vomitus is suggestive, but not absolutely diagnostic, of organic obstruction.

In addition to gastrointestinal lesions, there are numerous other causes of vomiting. Intracranial lesions, chiefly subdural hemorrhage and hydrocephalus, may produce vomiting. Infections of almost any system may present with vomiting, and in some cases, the vomiting may continue until the infection is controlled. Metabolic disorders, such as galactosemia, hereditary fructose intolerance, tyrosinemia, and adrenal cortical hyperplasia, also may cause vomiting.

In some newborns, especially premature infants, *functional* constipation may become a problem. Stools not only are passed at long intervals, but also, when passed, are small, hard, and dry. Constipation in these tiny infants may produce anorexia, distention, and vomiting. Laxative medications in general should be avoided, but a glycerin suppository (usually only a fraction of one is necessary) is permissible and often effective. The exact cause of this type of constipation is not known, but weakness of the intestinal and abdominal musculature may play an important role. Infants of mothers with preeclampsia who have hypermagnesemia may present with lethargy and hypotonia, and their passing of meconium may be delayed.

NUTRITIONAL NEEDS OF THE FULL-TERM INFANT

The goals for nutritional support of the healthy full-term infant are to provide nutrient deposition and body composition to match that of the infant who is breast-fed exclusively. The Recommended Dietary Allowances (RDA) for the first 6 months after birth assume that the breast-fed infant receives 750 mL milk per day (National Academy of Sciences, 1989). In the second 6 months, approximately 600 mL are ingested daily with other foods (Table 78–1). Table 78–2 is included to familiarize the reader with common conversion factors for nutrients discussed in the chapter.

TABLE 78–1

Recommended Dietary Allowances for Full-Term Infants

Component, units/d	0–6 months	6–12 months
Estimated body weight, kg	6	9
Energy, kcal	650	850
Protein, g	13	14
Calcium, mg	400	600
Phosphorus, mg	300	500
Magnesium, mg	40	60
Sodium, mg	120	200
Potassium, mg	500	700
Chloride, mg	180	300
Zinc, μg	5000	5000
Copper, μg	400–600	600–700
Chromium, μg	10–40	20–60
Manganese, μg	300–600	600–1000
Selenium, μg	10	15
Vitamin A, IU	1250	1250
Vitamin D, IU	300	400
Vitamin E, IU	3	4
Vitamin K, μg	5°	10
Thiamine (vitamin B$_1$), μg	300	400
Riboflavin (vitamin B$_2$), μg	400	500
Pyridoxine (vitamin B$_6$), μg	300	600
Niacin, mg	5	6
Biotin, μg	10	15
Pantothenic acid, mg	2	3
Folic acid, μg	25	35
Vitamin B$_{12}$, μg	0.3	0.5
Ascorbic acid, mg	30	35

°Vitamin K, 0.5–1.0 mg, also administered at birth.

Data from National Academy of Science (Ed): Recommended Dietary Allowances, 10th ed. Washington, DC, National Academy Press, 1989.

Breast-Feeding

The Committee on Nutrition of the American Academy of Pediatrics strongly recommends breast-feeding for full-term infants (American Academy of Pediatrics, 1980a; Nutrition Committee of the Canadian Paediatric Society and American Academy of Pediatrics, 1978) because of its ac-

TABLE 78–2

Conversion Factors for Nutrients

Calcium	40 mg = 1 mmol = 2 mEq
Phosphorus	31 mg = 1 mmol
Magnesium	24 mg = 1 mmol = 2 mEq
Sodium	23 mg = 1 mmol = 1 mEq
Potassium	39 mg = 1 mmol = 1 mEq
Chloride	35 mg = 1 mmol = 1 mEq
Vitamin A	1 μg retinol = 3.33 IU vitamin A = 6 μg β-carotene = 1.83 μg retinal palmitate = 1 retinol equivalent (RE)
Vitamin E	1 mg α-tocopherol = 1 IU vitamin E
Vitamin D	1 μg vitamin D (cholecalciferol) = 40 IU vitamin D (cholecalciferol)
Niacin	1 mg niacin = 1 niacin equivalent (NE) = 60 mg tryptophan

knowledged benefits with respect to infant nutrition and host defense. Contraindications are maternal illness, including human immunodeficiency virus (HIV), if alternatives are available (see later section on general considerations in breast-feeding).

Nutritional Aspects

The approximate compositions of mature human milk obtained after 1 month of lactation and commonly used commercial formulas are shown in Appendix 2. The total nitrogen content in human milk declines with postpartum age (Schanler and Oh, 1980), and the protein quality (proportion of whey and casein) of human milk (30% casein and 70% whey) differs from that in bovine milk and milk-based formula (82% casein and 18% whey) (Hambraeus, 1977). The whey fraction provides lower concentrations of phenylalanine, tyrosine, and methionine and higher concentrations of taurine than the casein fraction of milk (Hambraeus, 1977). These differences may be significant because infants have a relative inability to process phenylalanine and methionine and have a relative inability to form taurine compared with adults.

The constituents of the whey fraction differ between human and bovine milks. The human whey proteins include alpha-lactalbumin, which serves as a nutritional protein for the infant, as well as lactoferrin, lysozyme, and secretory immunoglobulin A (sIgA), which serve important roles in host defense (Hambraeus, 1977). These three latter proteins are present only in trace quantities in bovine milk, and the major whey protein in bovine milk, beta-lactoglobulin, is thought to cause milk protein allergy and colic (Jakobsson et al, 1985; Savilahti and Kuitunen, 1992). The whey fraction in human milk also contains nonprotein nitrogen-containing compounds, such as free amino acids, taurine, and urea, which may contribute to nitrogen utilization in the infant (Carlson, 1985; Heine et al, 1986).

Lipids in human milk are comprised of organized milk fat globules, containing fatty acids (high in palmitic 16:0, oleic 18:1, linoleic 18:2n-6, and linolenic 18:3n-3) distributed on the triglyceride molecule (16:0 at the 2-position of the molecule). The mixture of fatty acids in commercial formulas differs from that in human milk (Hamosh, 1987; Innis, 1992; Jensen and Jensen, 1992). Generally, commercial formulas have a greater quantity of medium chain–length fatty acids. Arachidonic acid (20:4n-6) and docosahexaenoic acid (22:6n-3), derivatives of linoleic and linolenic acids, are found in human but not bovine milk (Carlson et al, 1986; Clandinin et al, 1992; Innis et al, 1990; Uauy and Hoffman, 1991). These fatty acids are precursors of prostaglandins as well as components of phospholipids found in brain and red cell membranes. Their presence has been associated with improved cognition, growth, and vision (Carlson et al, 1993; Crawford, 1993; Uauy and Hoffman, 1991). Human milk also contains bile salt–stimulated lipase, which contributes significantly to the digestion of fats present in human milk (Hamosh, 1987; Innis, 1992; Jensen and Jensen, 1992).

Human milk contains approximately 7% lactose. As described in Chapter 70, however, lactase absorption may not be fully present in the newborn. Thus, a softer stool consistency, more nonpathogenic bacterial fecal flora, and improved absorption of minerals have been attributed to the presence of small quantities of unabsorbed lactose from human milk feeding (MacLean and Fink, 1980; Whyte et al, 1978; Ziegler and Fomon, 1983). Oligosaccharides, including the glycoproteins and mucins, are important in the host defense of the infant.

Host Defense

Data from numerous studies suggest that there is decreased morbidity in breast-fed versus formula-fed full-term infants (Cunningham, 1977; Cunningham et al, 1991; Howie et al, 1990). The presence of specific factors such as sIgA, lactoferrin, lysozyme, oligosaccharides, growth factors, and cellular components in human milk may contribute to the improved host defense of the breast-fed infant (Hambraeus, 1977). The enteromammary immune system, summarized in Figure 78–1, is one way the dynamic immune system protects the infant (Kleinman and Walker, 1979). When the mother is exposed to foreign antigens, her gastrointestinal plasma cells produce sIgA antibody, which circulates to mucosal surfaces, one of which is the mammary gland. Thus, specific antibody is present in her milk. When the infant ingests the milk, the infant receives specific passive immunity. This system is active in infants against a variety of antigens. The complex interplay among the immune components results in a reduced incidence of gastrointestinal and respiratory diseases and otitis media among breast-fed infants (Cunningham, 1979; Cunningham et al, 1991; Duncan et al, 1993; Glass et al, 1983; Glass and Stoll, 1989).

General Considerations in Breast-Feeding

Mothers who are breast-feeding may need assistance in establishing skills for nursing. Colostrum and early transition milk may be limited in volume, and mothers need to be reassured that frequent nursing stimulates improvement in human milk production. The infant generally loses weight the first few days as redistribution and excretion of free water occurs. This weight loss may be more dramatic in the breast-feeding infant, whose mother's milk supply has not yet been established. The physician should monitor progress with the mother's nursing skills, the infant's feeding skills, and the infant's weight over this first postnatal week. In the first few weeks after birth, an infant should receive 8 to 12 feedings each day and sleep contentedly between feedings (Freed et al, 1991; Lawrence, 1994). By day 3, breast-fed infants usually have three to four wet diapers and one to two yellow stools. By week 1, there should be six pale yellow diapers per day and a yellow stool with each feeding. By 1 month, the stool frequency may diminish to three per day.

Numerous drugs and viruses may be excreted in human milk. Human milk may contain hepatitis B virus, cytomegalovirus, herpes simplex if lesions are localized to the breast, and HIV. The World Health Organization and the American Academy of Pediatrics currently do not recommend discontinuing breast-feeding for the HBsAg-positive mother. The infant, however, should be given hepatitis B immunoglobulin and hepatitis B vaccine. Although it is common practice in the United States to avoid breast-feeding by HIV-positive mothers, it is not a World Health

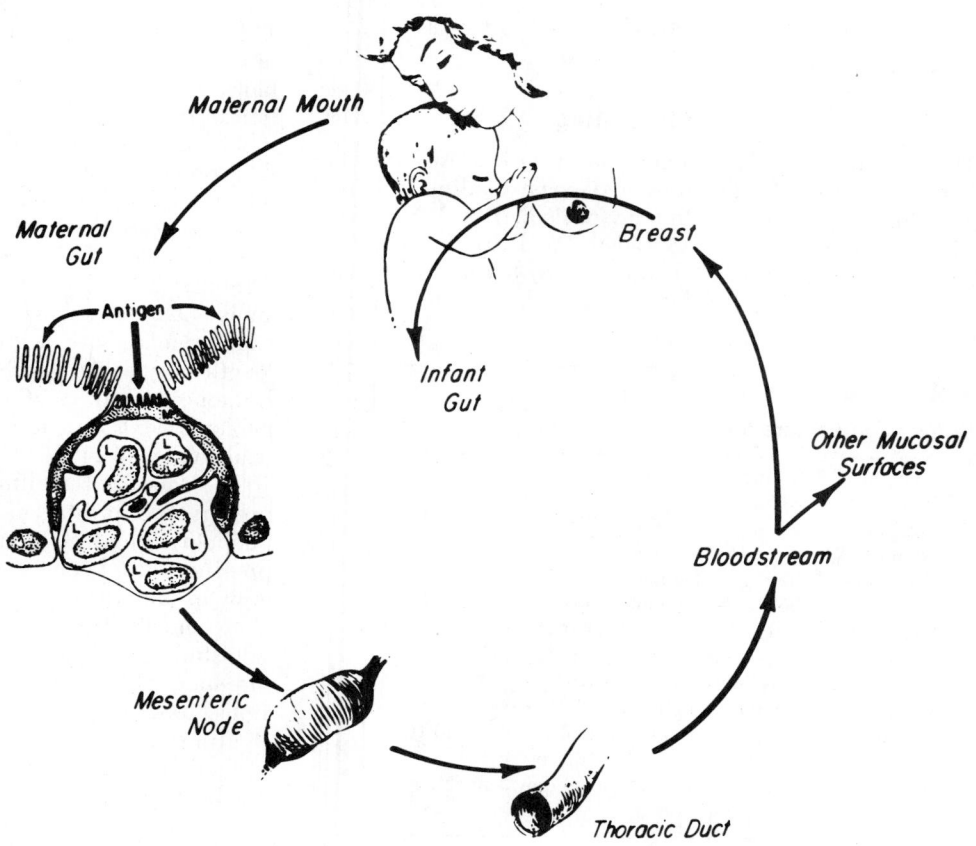

FIGURE 78–1. The enteromammary immune system. Antigen presented to maternal gut is brought into proximity to lymphoid follicles by specialized transport cells (M). The presence of antigen commits the lymphoblasts (L) to specific immunoglobulin A (IgA) production, and they then migrate via mesenteric nodes and thoracic duct into the systemic circulation. During periods of proper hormonal stimulation, these cells populate the breast and secrete sIgA, which is ingested by the infant and functions in the infant gut much as endogenous IgA. T cells, B cells, and macrophages also are extruded into the breast milk and are immunologically active. (From Kleinman RE, Walker WA: The enteromammary immune system. Dig Dis Sci 24:876, 1979.)

Organization policy because of the immune protection it provides. Although most drugs ingested by the mother are excreted in human milk (American Academy of Pediatrics, 1994), interruption of nursing currently is indicated only occasionally (see Appendix 1).

Supplements for Breast-Fed Infants

In general, the healthy, breast-fed, full-term infant receiving adequate sunlight exposure does not require vitamin and mineral supplements (Lawrence, 1994). The breast-fed infant, however, should receive vitamin K at birth. Moreover, the physician should be aware that the vitamin D concentration in human milk may be insufficient to prevent rickets. Although most breast-fed infants do not require vitamin D supplements, those who do not receive sunlight exposure and who also have dark skin pigmentation may need vitamin D supplementation of 400 IU per day. Because the concentration of iron declines during lactation, the breast-fed infant needs an iron supplement by 6 months of age (Lawrence, 1994).

Formulas for Full-Term Infants

The design of infant formulas is based on the composition of human milk. Because of the increased bioavailability of nutrients in human milk, the content of many nutrients in commercial formula must be greater than in human milk to ensure similar rates of nutrient deposition. Cow milk–based formulations are most often used, and soy-based or hydrolysate-based formulas are not indicated under routine circumstances. Soy-based formulations may be used when dietary lactose is contraindicated, such as in galactosemia. Soy-based formulas are often used following gastroenteritis; however, once the brush-border lactase activity is restored, cow milk–based formula can be reintroduced. Hydrolysate-based formulations are used for cow milk–protein allergy, as described later in Chapter 79. Standard vitamin supplements are recommended for infants who are receiving commercial formulas until their daily intake exceeds 1 L.

NUTRITIONAL NEEDS OF THE LOW-BIRTH-WEIGHT INFANT

In the neonatal period, the low-birth-weight (LBW) infant faces significant nutritional challenges. First, LBW infants either are born at the beginning of the third trimester of pregnancy or are products of pregnancies complicated by diminished uterine blood flow. These circumstances result in decreased nutrient deposition in the fetus. Second, the medical conditions of many of these infants result in increased nutrient needs. The daily weight gain of the LBW infant, therefore, when expressed per kilogram body weight, is nearly double that of a full-term infant (Butte et al, 1984; Schanler et al, 1985). Nutrient recommendations for LBW infants have been derived from chemical analyses of fetal cadavers to determine the net deposition or retention of particular nutrients during the last trimester of pregnancy (Widdowson, 1982; Ziegler et al, 1976), and these data have been computed on a daily basis per kilogram body weight (Table 78–3). Although the original data

TABLE 78–3

Estimated Intrauterine Nutrient Accretion Rates*

Nutrient	Unit/kg/d
Calcium (mg)	105
Copper (μg)	50
Magnesium (mg)	2.7
Nitrogen (mg)	325
Phosphorus (mg)	70
Potassium (mg)	66
Sodium (mg)	28
Zinc (μg)	240

*Values averaged from last trimester, adjusted for body weight.

Adapted from (1) Widdowson EM: Importance of nutrition in development, with special reference to feeding low-birth-weight infants. In Sauls HS, Bachhuber WL, Lewis LA (Eds): Meeting Nutritional Goals for Low-Birth-Weight Infants. Used with permission of Ross Products Division, Abbott Laboratories, Columbus, OH 43216 from Second Ross Clinical Research Conference, © 1982 Ross Products Division, Abbott Laboratories; and (2) Ziegler EE, O'Donnell AM, Nelson SE, et al: Body composition of the reference fetus. Growth 40:329, 1976.

were derived from fetal carcass analyses, the data for several minerals have been corroborated by noninvasive neutron activation techniques (Ellis et al, 1993).

To determine the intake needed for a particular nutrient, the factorial approach is used (Ziegler et al, 1981). This method includes a summation of the quantity of the nutrient deposited and an estimate of nutrient losses. For infants receiving total parenteral nutrition (TPN), the advisable intake includes estimates of nutrient deposition, cutaneous and urinary losses, and an additional allowance to account for variability. For enteral nutrition, the factorial approach is amended to account also for the bioavailability of the particular nutrient. The differences between the estimated parenteral and enteral nutrient needs of LBW infants is given in Table 78–4.

Energy Needs

The daily energy needs for the growing LBW infant are summarized in Table 78–5 (Sinclair, 1971). The range in resting energy expenditure ranges from 49 to 60 kcal/kg per day at 8 to 63 days' postnatal age (Sinclair, 1978). Because the parenterally nourished LBW infant has less fecal energy loss, fewer episodes of cold stress, and less activity, the actual energy needs for growth are lower for the preterm infant than for the term infant and range from 80 to 100 kcal/kg per day. In chronic disease, such as bronchopulmonary dysplasia, the resting energy expenditure may rise significantly (Weinstein and Oh, 1981; Yunis and Oh, 1989).

Parenteral Nutrition

Amino Acids

The use of parenteral nutrition containing glucose and amino acids reverses the negative nitrogen balance characteristic of the first days after birth (Anderson et al, 1979; Schanler et al, 1994), increases the serum concentration of

Comparison of Suggested Parenteral and Enteral Fluid, Energy, and Nutrient Intakes for Low-Birth-Weight Infants

Component, units	Parenteral Intake unit/kg/d	Enteral Intake unit/kg/d
Water, mL	150	150
Energy, kcal	80–100	120–130
Protein, g	3.0–3.5	3.5
Fat, g	1.0–4.0	5.0–7.0
Carbohydrate, g	16	12.0–14.0
Calcium, mg	80–120	200–220
Phosphorus, mg	60–90	100–110
Magnesium, mg	9–10	7–10
Sodium, mEq	2.0–4.0	2.0–8.0
Potassium, mEq	2.0–3.0	2.0–3.0
Chloride, mg	2.0–3.0	2.0–3.0
Zinc, μg	350–450	1000–2000
Copper, μg	65	65–300
Chromium, μg	0.4	0.1–0.4
Manganese, μg	10	7.5
Selenium, μg	2.0	1.0–2.0
Vitamin A, IU	500	700–2000
Vitamin D, IU	160	400 IU/d
Vitamin E, IU	2.8	5–25 IU/d
Thiamine (vitamin B_1), μg	350	20–40 μg/d
Riboflavin (vitamin B_2), μg	150	60 μg/d
Pyridoxine (vitamin B_6), μg	180	35–60 μg/d
Niacin, mg	6.8	0.8 mg/d
Folic acid, μg	56	50 μg/d
Vitamin B_{12}, μg	0.3	0.1–0.5 μg/d
Ascorbic acid, mg	32	35 mg/d

°Vitamin K, 0.5–1.0 mg at birth.

Adapted from American Academy of Pediatrics Committee on Nutrition: Pediatrics 75:976, 1985, used with permission of the American Academy of Pediatrics; and Greene HL, Hambidge KM, Schanler R, Tsang RC: Guidelines for the use of vitamins, trace elements, calcium, magnesium, and phosphorus in infants and children receiving total parenteral nutrition: Report of the Subcommittee on Pediatric Parenteral Nutrient Requirements for the Committee on Clinical Practical Issues of The American Society for Clinical Nutrition. Am J Clin Nutr 48:1324, 1988. © Am J Clin Nutr, American Society for Clinical Nutrition.

Partition of Energy Needs for Growing Low-Birth-Weight Infants

Component	kcal/kg/d
Resting energy expenditure	50
Intermittent activity (+30% above resting)	15
Occasional cold stress (thermoregulation)	10
Thermic effect of feeding (synthesis)	8
Fecal loss (10% of intake)	12
Growth allowance (energy storage)	25
Totals	120

From Sinclair JC: Metabolic rate and body size of the newborn. Clin Obstet Gynecol 14:840, 1971.

essential amino acids (Rivera et al, 1989), and increases the rate of protein synthesis (Rivera et al, 1993). Several amino acid solutions are available, and the percentage of essential/total amino acids is variable among them, ranging from 40% to 53% (Table 78–6). Evidence indicates that histidine, tyrosine, cysteine, and taurine may be conditionally essential amino acids (Mitton, 1994). Tyrosine and cysteine are not present in all amino acid preparations, principally because of difficulties in solubility (Mitton, 1994). Taurine and glutamic acid are not present in all solutions, although their need is questioned (Mitton, 1994; Zelikovic et al, 1990).

There is a direct relationship between the quantity of nitrogen (amino acids) provided in TPN and nitrogen balance or retention (Malloy et al, 1984; Zlotkin et al, 1981). In addition, specific amino acids may affect nitrogen balance. The addition of cysteine hydrochloride to TPN increases plasma free and total cyst(e)ine and urinary cyst(e)ine concentrations (Malloy et al, 1983), but increasing cysteine intake does not increase nitrogen balance or weight gain (Zlotkin et al, 1981). Therefore, cysteine hydrochloride is added to TPN solutions to meet presumed cysteine needs and to enhance the solubility of the calcium and phosphorus salts because it can lower the pH of the TPN solution (Schanler et al, 1994).

Nitrogen retention can be increased in infants receiving TPN in one of three ways: by changing the mixture of essential/nonessential amino acids, increasing the nitrogen intake, or increasing the energy intake (Zlotkin et al, 1981). There is a positive relationship between energy intake and nitrogen balance for any given nitrogen intake, in that nitrogen balance (retention) increases as energy intake increases from 50 to 90 kcal/kg per day (Pierro et al, 1988; Zlotkin et al, 1981). Significant positive relationships are also observed between nitrogen retention and intake in long-term studies conducted for 3 weeks using a 2.2% mixture of multiple essential and nonessential amino acids (TrophAmine) and 20% intravenous fat emulsion (Intralipid) (Schanler et al, 1994). Thus, the current recommendation for TPN in LBW infants is that it provide approximately 3 to 3.5 g/kg per day of amino acids (Mitton, 1994; Schanler et al, 1994).

Intravenous Lipid Emulsions

Intravenous lipid emulsions containing soybean oil (with or without safflower oil) with glycerin and egg yolk phospholipid emulsifiers are available in 10% or 20% concentrations to supplement parenteral nutrition regimens (Table 78–7). Intravenous lipid emulsion can be used in sick LBW infants as early as the day of birth without short-term adverse effects (Gilbertson et al, 1991). Early administration of intravenous lipid reverses essential fatty acid deficiency, provides needed energy for tissue healing and growth, and equalizes the distribution of nonprotein calories (Friedman et al, 1976; Gutcher and Farrell, 1991).

Intravenous lipid reportedly protects the lung from oxygen toxicity by increasing the content of polyunsaturated fatty acids in the lung (Sosenko et al, 1991). This finding may be especially important in ventilator-dependent LBW infants. There have been some concerns, however, regarding the worsening of pulmonary function and the potential

TABLE 78–6

Amino Acid Composition of Selected Parenteral Mixtures Adjusted to 1% Dilution (1 g Amino Acid/dL)

Component	Aminosyn-PF (Abbott)	FreAmine III (McGaw)	Novamine (Clintec)	Travasol (Clintec)	TrophAmine (McGaw)
Essential amino acids	(48%)°	(48%)	(44%)	(40%)	(53%)
Isoleucine	76†	69	50	60	82
Leucine	119	91	69	73	140
Lysine	68	73	79	58	82
Methionine	18	53	50	40	34
Phenylalanine	43	56	69	56	48
Threonine	51	40	50	42	42
Tryptophan	18	15	17	18	20
Valine	65	66	64	58	78
Nonessential amino acids	(52%)	(52%)	(56%)	(60%)	(47%)
Alanine	70	71	145	207	54
Arginine	123	95	98	115	122
Histidine	31	28	60	48	48
Proline	81	112	60	68	68
Serine	50	59	39	50	38
Tyrosine	6	—	2.6	4	24
Glycine	39	140	69	103	36
Cysteine	—	<2.4	—	—	<2.3
Aspartic acid	55	—	29	—	32
Glutamic acid	60	—	50	—	50
Taurine	5	—	—	—	2.5

°Percentage of total amino acids listed.
†mg/g amino acid.

for oxidant toxicity as a result of the use of intravenous lipid (Hammerman and Aramburo, 1988; Pitkanen et al, 1991; Sosenko et al, 1993). In vitro studies suggest that hydroperoxides present in lipid emulsions may be deleterious to lung function (Helbock et al, 1993). Clinical studies, however, have not confirmed a risk from the administration of intravenous lipid emulsions. Even when administered

TABLE 78–7

Intravenous Lipid Emulsions for Low-Birth-Weight Infants

	Intralipid (Kabi-Vitrum)	Liposyn (Abbott)
Concentrations	10%, 20%	10%, 20%
Oil source	Soybean 100%	Soybean 50% Safflower 50%
Fatty acids (%)		
Linoleic acid	50	66
Linolenic acid	9	4
Other	41	30
Egg yolk phospholipids (g/dL)	1.2	1.2
Glycerin (g/dL)	2.25	2.5
Energy density (kcal/mL)	1.1, 2.0	1.1, 2.0
Osmolarity (mOsm/L)	260, 260	276, 258

Adapted from Rombeau JL, Caldwell MD (Eds): Clinical Nutrition: Parenteral Nutrition, 2nd ed. Philadelphia, WB Saunders, 1993, pp 310–320; and Heird WC, Kashyap S, Gomez MR: Parenteral alimentation of the neonate. Semin Perinatol 15:493, 1991.

within 12 hours of birth, LBW infants do not experience an increase in oxygen requirement or the development of chronic respiratory disease (Sosenko et al, 1993). Deleterious effects on pulmonary function, however, have been demonstrated in adults who received large doses of intravenous lipid with markedly elevated (339 mg/dL) plasma triglyceride concentrations (Greene et al, 1976). Although the issue has not been settled conclusively, it appears that the benefits of intravenous lipid outweigh the potential risks and that monitoring of serum triglyceride concentrations may be helpful in determining potential toxicity.

The concentration of the lipid emulsion (10% versus 20%) may affect the infant's tolerance of the preparation. For example, LBW infants receiving the 20% solution at the same or even greater lipid intakes had lower serum concentrations of triglycerides, cholesterol, and phospholipids than similar infants receiving the 10% solution (Haumont et al, 1989, 1992). It is postulated that the excess phospholipid, cholesterol, and liposomes contained in the 10% solution accumulate to form lipoprotein X. These lipoprotein X particles then compete with lipoprotein lipase to reduce the clearing of triglycerides (Haumont et al, 1989, 1992; Mitton, 1994). Thus, regardless of the dose of lipid or the age of the infant, most LBW infants should receive the 20% solution.

The method of lipid infusion also is a concern. Intermittent infusion may produce higher serum triglyceride concentrations than continuous infusion of the same dose (Kao et al, 1984). Intermittent infusions and lipid-free intervals do not appear to be justified in routine circumstances (Brans et al, 1986).

Energy Distribution

A balanced distribution between calories derived from glucose and fat is necessary to avoid potential effects on respiratory metabolism (Table 78–8). When the caloric distribution permits a significant surplus of glucose, glucose is converted to fat, which increases the production of carbon dioxide, which, in turn, causes an increase in alveolar minute ventilation and raises the respiratory quotient, resulting in an increase in oxygen consumption (Bresson et al, 1991; Piedboeuf et al, 1991). Daily monitoring of the intakes for all energy sources in TPN is essential to ensure a relatively balanced distribution of calories derived from glucose and fat.

Conditional Nutrients

Several conditionally essential nutrients are being evaluated for inclusion in TPN solutions for newborns, including carnitine, inositol, choline, and glutamine. Data conflict concerning the need for carnitine supplementation of TPN for LBW infants. Supplementation of TPN with L-carnitine (10 mg/kg/day) resulted in greater plasma total carnitine and acylcarnitine concentrations in infants of 29 to 33 weeks' gestation compared with control infants receiving TPN without carnitine (Schmidt-Sommerfeld et al, 1983). Study infants who were supplemented with carnitine also appeared to have greater fatty acid oxidation. Other investigators, however, observed a slower weight gain and an increase in protein oxidation in L-carnitine–supplemented infants (Sulkers et al, 1990). Supplementation of TPN with inositol in the first week after birth has been reported to reduce the incidence of chronic pulmonary disease in LBW infants with respiratory distress syndrome (Hallman et al, 1992). No data exist concerning the inclusion of glutamine in parenteral solutions for LBW infants. The use of choline to prevent hepatic cholestasis also is speculative.

Calcium, Phosphorus, and Magnesium

Bone undermineralization, fractures, and rickets may result from inadequate intakes of calcium and phosphorus (Koo, 1992; MacMahon et al, 1989). Chest wall stability may be reduced and atelectasis may occur if undermineralization progresses (Glasgow and Thomas, 1977). Phosphorus deficiency has been associated with diaphragmatic paralysis and respiratory failure in adults (Aubier et al, 1985). Calcium and phosphorus deficiency may lead to hypercalciuria and, in combination with the use of diuretics, may result in nephrocalcinosis (Atkinson et al, 1988; Stafstrom et al, 1992).

Although there is a direct relationship between intake and net retention, the delivery of optimal intakes is often limited by the lack of solubility of calcium and phosphorus in intravenous solution. Careful attention to pH, amino acid concentration and source, and temperature is necessary so as to provide a recommendation for the appropriate quantity of calcium and phosphorus in TPN (Fitzgerald and MacKay, 1986).

It has been suggested that increased intakes of calcium and phosphorus can be achieved if each is delivered separately (Hoehn et al, 1987). When this alternate-day infusion method was used, however, hypercalciuria and hypercalcemia occurred on the days phosphorus was omitted, and hyperphosphaturia and hyperphosphatemia occurred on the days when calcium was omitted. The two minerals, therefore, must be delivered together for deposition into bone. It is generally agreed that calcium/phosphorus ratios of 1:1 (molar) or greater are appropriate for LBW infants (Greene et al, 1988; Koo, 1992). Calcium/phosphorus ratios less than 1:1 have resulted in elevated urinary phosphorus and serum phosphorus concentrations, suggestive of inadequate phosphorus utilization because of inadequate calcium intake (Prestridge et al, 1993).

The parenteral needs for calcium, phosphorus, and magnesium were derived in a longitudinal study evaluating serial balance studies using TrophAmine 2.2% (130 mL/kg/day) and Intralipid 20% (20 mL/kg/day) (Prestridge et al, 1993; Schanler et al, 1994). Intrauterine accretion rates were most closely approximated in parenteral nutrition solutions containing 80 mg calcium, 80 mg phosphorus, and 7 mg magnesium per 100 mL (Prestridge et al, 1993; Schanler et al, 1994). These quantities of mineral also resulted in increased bone mineral content well beyond the TPN study interval (Prestridge et al, 1993).

Electrolytes

Generally the parenteral needs for sodium and potassium are determined by the infant's clinical circumstance, with a range of intakes recommended (see Table 78–4). The majority of sodium intake is derived from common medications received by the LBW infant (Schanler et al, 1994). Mild acidosis may occur when infants are receiving parenteral nutrition because the LBW infant has decreased renal reabsorption of bicarbonate. Moreover, the use of amino acid solutions with low pH (generally 5.5 to 6.5) and the use of cysteine hydrochloride further reduce the pH (Mitton, 1994). The addition of acetate to the solution, as either the sodium or potassium salt, has been reported to correct the acidosis. The small quantity of acetate, 1 to 2 mEq/kg per day, has not been observed to affect the solubility of the minerals in TPN solutions containing TrophAmine and cysteine hydrochloride (Laine et al, 1991).

Trace Elements

Suggested parenteral intakes of copper and zinc for LBW infants have been evaluated from serial balance studies

---

TABLE 78–8

Distribution of Energy Sources in Parenteral Nutrition Solutions for Low-Birth-Weight Infants

	Unit*	kcal*	% kcal
Glucose (12.5%)	16.3 g	55.3	(51%)
Protein (2.4%)	3.1 g	12.4	(11.5%)
Fat (20%)	4.0 g	40.0	(37%)
Total fluid	150 mL	—	—
Total calories	—	107.7	(100%)

*Per kilogram per day.

conducted during the first 3 weeks postnatally (Schanler et al, 1994). Net retention and urinary excretion did not increase over the 3 weeks of study, suggesting that these elements were used by the infant during the early period of postnatal life. Estimated parenteral intakes of zinc range from 350 to 450 µg/kg per day (Greene et al, 1988; Schanler et al, 1994; Zlotkin and Buchanan, 1983). A greater dose may be indicated in LBW infants with ongoing intestinal losses of zinc. Differences in recommendations for trace elements may arise because of the various sources of amino acids used and medical conditions of the infants studied.

An estimate of zinc status can be obtained from serum zinc concentrations, which range between 70 and 120 µg/dL in adults. Severe zinc deficiency generally is associated with plasma zinc concentrations below 20 to 30 µg/dL (Greene et al, 1988). Copper status is more difficult to define with serum indices (Sutton et al, 1985). Plasma copper and ceruloplasmin concentrations increase with postmenstrual age (Greene et al, 1988). At 30 weeks, plasma copper concentrations are 35 µg/dL and at 40 weeks are between 50 and 60 µg/dL. Copper needs are increased in cases of excess biliary losses and in patients with jejunostomies. It is important to recognize that impaired biliary secretion leads to a buildup of copper. Therefore, it is advised that copper intakes be reduced in patients with impaired biliary excretion, such as that which occurs in TPN cholestasis.

Selenium is a component of glutathione peroxidase, and its absence from long-term parenteral nutrition solutions results in a deficiency of the element (Kien and Ganther, 1983; Lockitch et al, 1989; Van Caillie-Bertrand et al, 1984). Approximately 75% of an absorbed dose is excreted by the kidney, so selenium intake should be reduced in patients with impaired renal function. The recommended intake of 2 mg/kg per day is derived from the selenium intake of the full-term breast-fed infant.

Recommendations for manganese intakes are not clearly defined (Greene et al, 1988). The ratio of manganese to zinc in the available trace element solution used for LBW infants provides a greater intake of manganese than presumed to be needed. Manganese excretion is diminished markedly in cholestatic syndromes. The use of manganese in cholestatic disease should be avoided.

Chromium needs may be associated with insulin activity at the receptor level (Greene et al, 1988). Chromium deficiency, therefore, may result in impaired glucose tolerance. High doses of chromium may accumulate in the body (Bougle et al, 1993). A recommended intake of approximately 0.3 µg/kg per day appears to be appropriate.

Vitamin A

Vitamin A circulates in association with retinol-binding protein, which is synthesized in the liver and bound to the vitamin before secretion (Greene et al, 1986; Zachman, 1989). Estimates of vitamin A needs, therefore, depend on the concentration of retinol-binding protein in circulation. The synthesis of retinol-binding protein is affected by protein and energy intake. In adults and healthy children, there is a positive correlation between vitamin A and retinol-binding protein, both moieties in a molar ratio of 1:1

(Greene et al, 1988). The vitamin A/retinol-binding protein ratio in LBW infants, however, is lower (Greene et al, 1986; Shenai et al, 1990). This may be a result of deficient hepatic stores or intakes of the vitamin (or both).

As much as 70% to 80% of vitamin A is lost in the delivery system because it is adsorbed to plastic and degraded by light exposure (Greene et al, 1986). The addition of vitamin A to intravenous lipid solutions results in greater delivery of the vitamin (Baeckert et al, 1988; Greene et al, 1987). When retinal palmitate is used, the losses in vitamin A delivery are minimized (Greene et al, 1987). The substitution of retinal palmitate for retinol in parenteral nutrition solutions also appears to maintain the greater plasma retinol concentrations that are achieved if retinol is mixed and infused with intravenous lipid (Greene et al, 1987).

An association between deficient vitamin A status and the development of bronchopulmonary dysplasia has been reported (Shenai et al, 1985). High doses of intramuscular vitamin A (averaging 1500 to 2000 IU/kg/day) resulted in greater plasma vitamin A and retinol-binding protein concentrations and a lower incidence of bronchopulmonary dysplasia (Shenai et al, 1985, 1990). The recommended parenteral intakes of vitamin A (Table 78–9) approximate this dose. The probable losses of the vitamin in the intravenous delivery system, however, result in lower plasma concentrations than those achieved in infants receiving the vitamin by the intramuscular route. Thus, a best estimate for vitamin A needs during parenteral nutrition would encourage a higher dose and a change in the formulation so it can be mixed and delivered with intravenous lipid emulsion.

Vitamin E

The need for vitamin E is directly related to the content of polyunsaturated fatty acids (PUFA) in the diet. This is particularly important in parenteral nutrition because the proportion of PUFA in intravenous fat emulsions is high. Vitamin E doses of 2.1 versus 4.6 mg per day have been evaluated during 3 to 4 weeks of parenteral nutrition therapy (Phillips et al, 1987). The higher dose resulted in a large proportion of elevated plasma vitamin E concentrations (>3.5 mg/dL) in infants less than 1000 g birth weight (Phillips et al, 1987). A vitamin E dose of 3.5 mg per day reportedly produced adequate plasma vitamin E concentrations at 7 days' postnatal age in infants 1000 g birth weight or less. In neither study were lipid intakes reported. A dose of 2.8 mg/kg per day administered in intravenous lipid, however, resulted in appropriate plasma vitamin E concentrations (Baeckert et al, 1988).

Water-Soluble Vitamins

Current formulations generally provide more water-soluble vitamins than are needed by LBW infants (see Table 78–9). Plasma ascorbate (vitamin C) and vitamin B_2 (riboflavin) concentrations reportedly were elevated in LBW infants receiving parenteral nutrition (Baeckert et al, 1988; Greene et al, 1991; Moore et al, 1986). The elevated riboflavin concentrations appear paradoxical in view of the known degradation of the vitamin under infusion and nursery lighting conditions. Thus, significantly lower doses of some

TABLE 78–9

Suggested Intakes of Vitamins for Low-Birth-Weight Infants Receiving Total Parenteral Nutrition

Vitamin	Current Suggestion* (unit/kg/d)	Best Estimate for New Formulation (unit/kg/d)	Maximum Not to Exceed Full-Term Infant (unit/d)
Fat-soluble vitamins			
A (μg)	280	500	700
E (mg)	2.8	2.8	7
K (μg)	80	80	200
D (μg)	4	4	10
Water-soluble vitamins			
B_1, thiamine (mg)	0.48	0.35	1.2
B_2, riboflavin (mg)	0.56	0.15	1.4
B_6, pyridoxine (mg)	0.40	0.18	1.0
Niacin (mg)	6.8	6.8	17
Pantothenate (mg)	2	2	5
Biotin (μg)	8	6	20
Folate (μg)	56	56	140
Vitamin B_{12} (μg)	0.40	0.30	1.0
Ascorbic acid (mg)	32	25	80

°Practical approach using 40% of a vial of MVI-Pediatric (Astra Pharmaceutical Products, Westborough, MA) per kg body weight or 2 mL/kg/d.

Adapted from Greene HL, Hambridge KM, Schanler R, Tsang RC: Guidelines for the use of vitamins, trace elements, calcium, magnesium, and phosphorus in infants and children receiving total parenteral nutrition: Report of the Subcommittee on Pediatric Parenteral Nutrient Requirements for the Committee on Clinical Practical Issues of the American Society for Clinical Nutrition. Am J Clin Nutr 48:1324, 1988. © Am J Clin Nutr, American Society for Clinical Nutrition.

water-soluble vitamins are indicated (see Table 78–9). When used in a dose of 2 mL/kg per day (40% of the vial M.V.I. Pediatric), no deficiencies of thiamine or riboflavin were detected, and plasma concentrations of folate and vitamin B_{12} indicated sufficient status (Levy et al, 1992).

Monitoring Parenteral Nutrition

A sample recipe for the preparation of a parenteral nutrition mixture for LBW infants is given in Table 78–10. The lower range of nutrient concentrations is used when TPN is initiated, and the upper range is used if parenteral nutrition is given for more than 2 weeks. LBW infants receiving parenteral nutrition should have biochemical monitoring to avoid excesses or deficiencies of particular nutrients (Table 78–11). Complications related to TPN therapy may occur. There may be extravascular infiltration of the solution resulting in skin slough and localized infection. Systemic infection, emboli, and metabolic complications, such as electrolyte disturbances, hepatic dysfunction, nephrocalcinosis, and osteopenia, also have been recognized.

Enteral Nutrition

Protein

The quality of protein (e.g., the greater proportion of whey to casein) in human milk is particularly suitable for the LBW infant (Schanler and Garza, 1987a). The quantity and quality of protein needed for LBW infants have been investigated longitudinally (Raiha et al, 1976). Infants were fed one of five preparations: formulas that provided protein intakes of 2.25 or 4.50 g/kg per day (containing whey or casein) or pasteurized human milk that provided a protein

intake of 1.6 g/kg per day. LBW infants who received 4.5 g/kg per day and infants given casein-dominant milk had greater plasma amino acid concentrations of phenylalanine, tyrosine, and methionine during the 8-week study (Gaull et al, 1977; Rassin et al, 1977). Infants fed whey-dominant formulas had higher plasma threonine concentrations and improved retention of cyst(e)ine and taurine compared with infants fed casein-dominant formula (Kashyap et al, 1987). Because elevations of particular amino acids may be toxic to brain development, there is a potential concern that feeding LBW infants a high-protein intake, especially of a casein-dominant milk, may be harmful (Moro et al, 1989).

The aforementioned studies also demonstrated that the lowest plasma concentrations of phenylalanine, tyrosine, and methionine were observed in infants fed human milk. Human milk–fed LBW infants also had the lowest protein intakes and the lowest serum albumin concentrations of the five groups studied (Fomon and Ziegler, 1977). Other investigators have now confirmed these findings, suggesting that after the first 2 weeks of feeding, human milk may not provide adequate protein intake for the LBW infant (Polberger et al, 1990; Ronnholm et al, 1982; Schanler and Oh, 1980). Protein intakes of 2.2 and 2.8 g/kg per day result in lower serum indices, weight gain, and nitrogen retention, whereas protein intakes of 3.8 g/kg per day appeared somewhat excessive (Kashyap et al, 1986, 1988). Therefore, it is recommended that preterm infants receive 3.5 g/kg per day protein with energy intakes of 120 kcal/kg per day (Kashyap et al, 1986). Thus, protein intakes from unfortified human milk or full-term infant formulas are inadequate for feeding LBW infants. The protein contents of human milk and various preterm formulas are summarized in Table 78–12.

Although human milk is not adequate for meeting the

TABLE 78–10

Recommended Preparation of Total Parenteral Nutrition Solution for Low-Birth-Weight Infants

Component	Concentration/Additive	Intake
Glucose	12.5%	(Glucose = 16 g/kg/d)
Amino acids°	2.4%	(Amino acids = 3.1 g/kg/d)
Cysteine HCl	30 mg/g amino acids	
NaCl	2.6 mmol	(Na = 3.4 mmol/kg/d)
KCl	0–0.2 mmol	(Total K = 3.1–3.8 mmol/kg/d)
K_2PO_4-$KHPO_4$†	1.5–2.0 mmol P	(P = 2.0–2.6 mmol/kg/d)
Ca gluconate‡	1.5–2.0 mmol Ca	(Ca = 2.0–2.6 mmol/kg/d)
$MgSO_4$	0.25 mmol	(Mg = 0.3 mmol/kg/d)
MVI-Pediatric[R]§	40% of vial	(2 ml/kg/d)
MTE-5‖	0.1 mL/kg/d	(Zn, Cu, Mn, Cr, Se)
$ZnSO_4$	200 μg/kg/d	(Total Zn = 400 μg/kg/d)
		(Cu = 40 μg/kg/d)
		(Mn = 10 μg/kg/d)
		(Cr = 0.4 μg/kg/d)
		(Se = 2 μg/kg/d)
Heparin	1 unit/mL	
Intralipid 20%¶	5–20 mL/kg/d	
Total fluid	150 mL/kg/d	

°TrophAmine (McGaw).

†Monobasic-dibasic phosphate contains 1.4 mmol K/mmol P or 1.3 mmol Na/mmol P, depending on the preparation used. Use the higher P concentration for TPN duration >2 weeks.

‡Use the higher concentration for TPN duration >2 weeks. Add last in the preparation of TPN.

§Astra Pharmaceutical Products (Westborough, MA).

‖Lymphomed (Deerfield, IL).

¶Begin lipid at 1 g/kg/d and increase stepwise to 4 g/kg/d.

protein needs of LBW infants, a variety of methods are available for augmenting the protein intakes of human milk–fed LBW infants, including the use of lyophilized human milk protein and bovine protein sources (Polberger et al, 1990; Ronnholm et al, 1982; Schanler and Garza, 1987a). Plasma amino acid patterns occasionally differ when preterm infants are fed these milks, depending on the protein source used in fortification, but no consistent differences in nitrogen utilization or growth are observed from the use of either human or bovine protein sources.

Fat

Fat is the major energy source for the newborn. As described for the full-term infant, human milk fat digestion and absorption in the preterm infant are facilitated by the complex organization of the human milk fat globule, the pattern of fatty acids, their distribution on the triglyceride molecule, and the presence of bile salt–stimulated lipase (Hamosh, 1987; Innis, 1992; Jensen and Jensen, 1992). A slight but significant increase in fat absorption was reported when LBW infants were fed a mixture containing 40% fresh human milk and 60% formula compared to being fed 100% formula (Alemi et al, 1981).

Manufacturers of infant formulas modify their fat blends to mimic the fat absorption in human milk. Generally, commercial formulations have a greater quantity of medium chain–length fatty acids to compensate for the absence of the lipid system in human milk (Innis, 1992; Jensen and Jensen, 1992). In addition, the saturated fatty acids, especially palmitic acid, may not be absorbed as readily because of the differences in intrinsic packaging of human milk compared with commercial fat preparations. The malabsorbed palmitic acid, therefore, has a greater tendency toward soap formation, which could potentially interfere with mineral absorption.

Research has focused on the respective derivatives of linoleic and linolenic acids, arachidonic acid (20:4n-6), and docosahexaenoic acid (22:6n-3). These very long-chain fatty acids, which are found in human but not bovine milk, are components of phospholipids found in brain and red cell membranes (Carlson et al, 1986). When supplemented with marine oil, formula-fed LBW infants had red blood cell concentrations of 22:6n-3 that parallel those of similar infants fed human milk (Clandinin et al, 1992). Follow-up studies of supplemented infants suggest improvements in visual acuity (Carlson et al, 1993; Uauy and Hoffman,

TABLE 78–11

Biochemical Monitoring for Low-Birth-Weight Infants Receiving Total Parenteral Nutrition

Energy	Urine glucose, serum triglycerides
Protein	Blood urea nitrogen, albumin, prealbumin
Minerals	Ca, P, Mg, Na, K, Cl, alkaline phosphatase activity
Other	Creatinine, conjugated bilirubin, CO_2, alanine aminotransferase, trace element concentrations

TABLE 78–12

Nutrient Composition of Preterm Human Milk, Fortified Human Milk, Preterm Formulas, and Specialized Formulas (see also Appendix 2)

	Preterm Human Milk 1 week	Mature Human Milk (MM) 1 month	EHMF* + MM	SNC† + MM	EPF‡ 24	SSC§ 24	Pregestimil**	Similac 27††	PediaSure‡‡
Volume, mL	100	100	100	100	100	100	100	100	100
Energy, kcal	67	70	84	76	81	81	67	91	100
Protein, g	2.4	1.8	2.5	2.0	2.4	2.2	1.9	2.5	3.0
% Whey/casein	70/30	70/30	70/30	65/35	60/40	60/40	0/100	18/82	18/82
Fat, g	3.8	4.0	4.0	4.2	4.1	4.4	2.7	4.8	4.9
% MCT/LCT	2/98	2/98	2/98	25/75	40/60	40/60	55/45	8/92	20/80
Carbohydrate, g	6.1	7.0	9.7	7.8	9.0	8.6	6.9	9.6	11.2
% Lactose	100	100	72	72	40	50	0%	100%	0%
Calcium, mg	25	22	112	116	134	146	63	82	96
Phosphorus, mg	14	14	59	60	67	73	42	64	79
Magnesium, mg	3.1	2.5	3.5	6.1	5.5	9.7	7.3	6.4	20
Sodium, mg	50	30	37	33	32	35	26	31	38
Potassium, mg	70	60	75	82	83	104	73	120	129
Chloride, mg	90	60	78	63	69	66	58	74	100
Zinc, μg	500	320	1030	770	1215	1215	630	683	1167
Copper, μg	80	60	120	130	100	200	63	82	100
Vitamin A, IU	560	400	1350	475	1013	550	255	273	254
Vitamin D, IU	4	4	214	63	219	122	50	55	50
Vitamin E, mg	1.0	0.3	4.9	1.8	5.1	3.2	2.5	2.7	2.3
Vitamin C, mg	5.4	5.6	17.2	17.8	16	30	7.8	8	10

*Enfamil Human Milk Fortifier (EHMF) (Mead Johnson Nutritionals, Evansville, IN), 4 packets + 100 mL mature milk.
†Similac Natural Care (SNC) 24 (Ross Laboratories, Columbus, OH) diluted 1:1 with mature milk.
‡Enfamil Premature Formula (EPF) 24 (Mead Johnson).
§Similac Special Care (SSC) 24 (Ross Laboratories).
**Mead Johnson.
††Ready To Feed (Ross Laboratories).
‡‡With fiber (Ross Laboratories).
MCT, medium-chain triglyceride; LCT, long-chain triglyceride.
Data from Butte et al, 1984; Gross et al, 1980; Litov and Combs, 1991; Moran et al, 1983; Newman, 1994; Schanler, 1988; Slagle and Gross, 1988.

1991). These data indicate that human milk may be suitable for LBW infants not only for the ability to promote fat absorption in the immature infant, but also because of the profound metabolic functions attributed to this particular pattern of essential fatty acids. Recommendations for the supplementation of preterm formulas with marine oil have been published (Van Aerde and Clandinin, 1993).

The proportion of medium-chain fatty acids, here defined as carbon length 6:0 to 12:0, is below 12% of total fatty acids in human milk but approaches 50% in preterm formulas (see Table 78–12). Previous reports suggested that medium-chain fatty acids were absorbed passively and to a greater extent than long-chain fatty acids and affected growth and mineral absorption positively (Roy et al, 1975; Tantibhedhyangkul and Hashim, 1978). Data comparing LBW infants receiving medium-chain fatty acids at 42% versus 7% of total fatty acids in a crossover design demonstrated no differences in the absorption of fat and weight gain (Hamosh et al, 1989). No differences were observed between medium-chain fatty acids 46% versus 4% in energy digestibility, expenditure and storage, nitrogen retention, or weight gain in LBW infants (Whyte et al, 1986). Other reports also confirm the lack of effect of medium-chain fatty acids on weight gain and mineral absorption compared with exclusive long-chain fatty acid diets (Huston et al, 1983). When used in a high proportion, medium-chain fatty acids may be incompletely oxidized, which contributes to increased urinary dicarboxylic acid excretion and metabolic inefficiency compared with long-chain fatty acids (Borum, 1992; Wu et al, 1986). It appears that the metabolism of medium-chain fatty acids may require carnitine (Rebouche et al, 1990). When added exogenously to milk, medium-chain fatty acids have been reported to adhere to feeding tubes and diminish fat delivery to the infant (Mehta et al, 1988). Thus, there are no compelling data to suggest that a high proportion of medium-chain fatty acids is needed for preterm formulas.

One can capitalize on the variability in the fat content of human milk in feeding the LBW infant. The fat content of human milk varies among women, changes during the day, rises slightly during lactation, and increases dramatically within a single milk expression (Hall, 1979; Neville et al, 1984). The fat content of hindmilk may be 1.5-fold to 3-fold greater than that of foremilk (Valentine et al, 1994). No differences between foremilk and hindmilk are reported for the contents of nitrogen, calcium, phosphorus, sodium, or potassium (Table 78–13). Thus, the use of hindmilk can be recommended for LBW infants whose rate of weight gain is low (<15 g/kg/day) (Valentine et al, 1994).

Because it is not homogenized, on standing, the fat separates out of human milk (Bhatia and Rassin, 1988). The separated fat may adhere to collection containers, feeding tubes, and syringes, instead of being delivered to the infant (Greer et al, 1984). The greatest loss of fat in this manner occurs from continuous milk infusion systems. Care should be taken that continuous milk infusion systems use a short length of tubing. If the system contains a cassette interface, much of the fat is lost when it is discarded (Schanler, 1988a). Milk infusion systems employing a syringe and pump, in which the syringe is oriented upright, allow more complete delivery of fat. Fat loss is

TABLE 78–13

Composition of Foremilk and Hindmilk*

	Foremilk	Hindmilk
Volume (L)	0.30 ± 0.10†	0.44 ± 0.14
Energy (kcal)	629 ± 108	824 ± 77
Total nitrogen (g)	2.1 ± 0.27	2.1 ± 0.32
Fat (g)	28.6 ± 8.1	47.8 ± 8.5
Calcium (mg)	273 ± 40	272 ± 44
Phosphorus (mg)	152 ± 28	157 ± 30
Sodium (mg)	75 ± 23	72 ± 22
Potassium (mg)	432 ± 49	419 ± 43
Zinc (mg)	2.91 ± 0.88	2.75 ± 0.88
Copper (mg)	0.29 ± 0.09	0.27 ± 0.10

*Concentrations in units/L.
†X ± SD.
Data from Valentine CJ, Hurst NM, Schanler RJ: Hindmilk improves weight gain in low-birth-weight infants fed human milk. J Pediatr Gastroenterol Nutr 18:474, 1994.

reduced from 48% to less than 8% with these simple changes in methods of continuous infusion (Schanler, 1988a).

Carbohydrate

Although mucosal lactose levels are low until 32 to 34 weeks' gestation, LBW infants have the capacity to absorb more than 90% of the lactose present in human milk (Atkinson et al, 1981; De Curtis et al, 1986). Artificial formulas for LBW infants contain a mixture, usually 50:50, of lactose and glucose polymers. In general, the replacement of some lactose with glucose polymers reduces the osmolality compared with a formulation based entirely on lactose as the carbohydrate source. No beneficial effect on mineral absorption was reported when a formulation containing a mixture of lactose and glucose polymers was compared with lactose alone (Wirth et al, 1990). Improved mineral absorption was reported when an exclusive lactose-containing formula was used compared with a formula containing sucrose and corn syrup solids (glucose polymers) as the carbohydrate source (Ziegler and Fomon, 1983).

Calcium, Phosphorus, and Magnesium

A linear relationship exists between calcium (or phosphorus) intake and net retention in enterally fed LBW infants (Schanler and Rifka, 1994). LBW infants who are fed unfortified human milk never achieve intrauterine accretion rates for calcium and phosphorus. Intakes of calcium and phosphorus greater than 3.5 and 3.0 mmol/kg per day can be achieved by feeding specialized preterm cow milk–based formulas (see Table 78–12). Full-term infant formulas and specialized formulas, however, provide inadequate quantities of calcium and phosphorus to meet the needs of LBW infants (see Table 78–12).

The reported absorption of calcium averages 60% of intake (Schanler and Rifka, 1994). Phosphorus absorption varies from 90% in human milk-fed to 80% in commercial formula-fed infants (Schanler and Rifka, 1994). Several factors affect the absorption of calcium and phosphorus, including postnatal age; intake of calcium and phosphorus; and content of lactose, fat, and vitamin D of the ingested food. Vitamin D, however, may be responsible for only a small component of calcium absorption in LBW infants (Bronner et al, 1992).

The most optimal times to supply sufficient calcium and phosphorus to LBW infants are during the initial hospitalization with TPN, with the initiation of enteral feeding, and with the beginning of exclusive breast-feeding. Bone mineral content after hospital discharge has been used as an indicator of mineral status in LBW infants fed fortified human milk during hospitalization (Abrams et al, 1989; Chan, 1993). When fortified human milk was discontinued at hospital discharge and commercial cow milk–based formula substituted, LBW infants had rapid increases in bone mineral content and caught up by 6 months' postnatal age to the bone mineralization of the full-term infant (Abrams et al, 1989). When breast-feeding was continued after hospital discharge, LBW infants failed to catch up, such that at 1 year postnatal age their bone mineral content lagged behind the group switched to formula (Abrams et al, 1989). Catch-up bone mineral content in the human milk–fed LBW infant did not occur until 2 years (Schanler et al, 1992). These data imply that if in-hospital calcium and phosphorus retentions meet intrauterine standards, differences in bone mineral content postdischarge may be avoided. Furthermore, the data underscore the need for monitoring mineral status in the follow-up of LBW infants. In the early months post–hospital discharge, LBW infants may benefit from diets enriched in calcium and phosphorus (Bishop et al, 1993). At present, infants who should receive such enriched diets have not been identified definitively.

Preterm human milk contains approximately 20% of the calcium and phosphorus found in artificial formulas designed for LBW infants in the United States (see Table 78–12). In human milk, calcium and phosphorus exist in ionized and complexed forms that are easily absorbed. The salts in commercial formulas, however, are relatively insoluble. Thus, in the design of commercial formulas, greater quantities of these minerals are added to compensate for their poorer bioavailability.

Human milk contains too little calcium and phosphorus to meet the recommended needs of LBW infants (Atkinson et al, 1983; Schanler, 1991; Schanler and Oh, 1980). Prolonged deficiency of these minerals tends to stimulate bone resorption in an attempt to maintain a normal serum calcium concentration. This bone activity often is correlated with elevated serum alkaline phosphatase activity or reduced bone density on radiographs (or both). Thus, skeletal radiographs may reveal poor bone mineralization, rickets, and fractures in the LBW infant fed human milk (Koo et al, 1988). Lucas and colleagues (1989) reported that the majority of LBW infants who had elevated serum alkaline phosphatase activities were those who had been fed human milk. When these infants were re-evaluated 9 and 18 months later, their linear growth was significantly lower than that seen in the group that had the higher serum activity of alkaline phosphatase in the neonatal period (Lucas et al, 1989).

Supplementation of human milk with both calcium and phosphorus improves the net retention of both minerals (Salle et al, 1986). The need for augmented intakes of calcium and phosphorus in LBW infants also is apparent in studies assessing biochemical indicators and bone mineral content (Horsman et al, 1989). Current management of human milk–fed LBW infants emphasizes the need for supplements of both calcium and phosphorus (Salle et al, 1986; Schanler and Garza, 1987b).

Major technical considerations limit the ability to meet guidelines concerning enteral intakes of calcium and phosphorus for LBW infants. Because the bioavailability of calcium and phosphorus is lower in formulas than in human milk, their content in formulas must be greater to achieve recommended intakes. Because formulas that contain high concentrations of calcium and phosphorus have been noted to precipitate and form sediment within the bottle, uniform delivery of calcium and phosphorus, even as fortifiers for human milk, is not ensured (Bhatia and Rassin, 1988). Newer formulations in the United States, however, have obviated some of the solubility issues by using thickeners and stabilizers, such as carrageenan. The effect of these stabilizers on nutrient bioavailability is unknown, and therefore they have not been advocated unanimously. The addition of calcium and phosphorus has been attempted using a variety and combination of sources: calcium lactate, calcium gluconate, monobasic and dibasic phosphates, calcium phosphate tribasic, and calcium glycerophosphate (Schanler, 1991). Calcium lactate provides 13 mg elemental calcium/100 g powder; calcium gluconate (10% solution) provides 9 mg calcium/mL. Calcium glycerophosphate provides 19% calcium and 15% phosphorus. Sodium phosphate dibasic powder is 22% phosphorus and 32% sodium; sodium phosphate monobasic is 26% phosphorus and 19% sodium. Sodium monobasic-dibasic phosphate solution provides 90 mg phosphorus and 4 mEq sodium per mL. Calcium caseinate (1 g of powder) provides 0.9 g protein, 16 mg calcium, and 8 mg phosphorus and may be adequate if whey protein is unavailable.

By providing a more stable suspension of nutrients, commercially available fortifiers for human milk may be beneficial because they favor solubility. In addition, the commercial formulations contain a number of nutrients in one mixture. The potential problem with the use of a multicomponent formulation, however, is that single-nutrient adjustments are not practical. Currently, commercial formulations are available in a powder form (Enfamil Human Milk Fortifier, Mead Johnson Nutritional Division, Evansville, IN) and in a liquid form (Similac Natural Care 24, Ross Laboratories, Columbus, OH). The commercial preparations differ in their composition (see Table 78–12).

The absorption of magnesium is significantly greater in unfortified human milk (73%) compared with formula (48%) (Schanler and Rifka, 1994). Net magnesium retention in human milk–fed LBW infants meets intrauterine estimates. Thus, the data from balance studies and biochemical monitoring suggest that magnesium supplements are not needed for LBW infants fed human milk (Schanler and Abrams, 1995). Similar studies in LBW infants fed preterm formulas indicate that, despite lower absorption compared with human milk, intrauterine estimates for magnesium accretion are surpassed. The effect of this greater magnesium intake and retention is unknown.

Trace Elements

Zinc

LBW infants receiving pooled pasteurized human milk (intakes approximately 0.7 mg/kg/day) were in negative zinc balance for 60 days postnatally and never met the intrauterine accretion rate (Dauncey et al, 1977). In contrast, intakes of 1.8 to 2 mg/kg per day were associated with net retention of zinc that surpassed intrauterine accretion rates (Ehrenkranz et al, 1989; Tyrala, 1986). The absorption and retention of zinc from human milk appears to be significantly greater, especially if postmenstrual age is considered. In more mature human milk–fed LBW infants older than 34 weeks, zinc intakes of 0.7 to 0.8 mg/kg per day were adequate to meet intrauterine accretion rates (Ehrenkranz et al, 1989; Higashi et al, 1988). Reports of symptomatic zinc deficiency in human milk–fed preterm infants are a reminder of the decline in milk zinc concentration as lactation advances (Sievers et al, 1992). The infants reported to be zinc deficient were several months of age (Zimmerman et al, 1982). It appears that a best estimate, however, for zinc intakes is nearer to the 2 mg/kg per day intake.

Copper

LBW infants receiving pooled pasteurized human milk (copper intakes approximately 85 µg/kg/day) were in negative copper balance for 30 days postnatally and never met the intrauterine accretion rate (Dauncey et al, 1977). Copper retention was quite variable from formula providing intakes of 294 µg/kg per day (Tyrala, 1986). Several LBW infants with those intakes, however, did achieve the intrauterine accretion rate. Formulas providing approximately 190 µg/kg per day resulted in net copper retention below intrauterine estimates (Ehrenkranz et al, 1989). Human milk intakes providing 87 and 152 µg/kg per day from unfortified and fortified human milk approached and met intrauterine accretion rates (Ehrenkranz et al, 1989). These data indicate that the needs for copper vary with the type of milk fed. For human milk–fed LBW infants, a supplement of approximately 65 µg/kg per day (total 110 µg/kg/day) would be satisfactory, but for formula-fed LBW infants, an intake of 300 µg/kg per day enables the LBW infant to meet intrauterine needs.

Iron

The concentration of iron in human milk declines through lactation, from approximately 0.6 mg/L at 2 weeks to 0.3 mg/L after 5 months of lactation (Siimes et al, 1979). The absorption of iron is affected adversely by blood transfusion (Dauncey et al, 1978). LBW infants fed human milk were in negative iron balance, which, if untransfused, corrected with iron supplements (Dauncey et al, 1978). Iron absorption also appears to be facilitated by a modest degree of anemia. Thus, the usual recommendations for LBW infants suggest delaying iron supplementation until 2 to 3 months' postnatal age, a time when hemoglobin concentrations are at a nadir (Dallman, 1974; Lundstrom et al, 1977). The provision of small doses of iron at 2 mg/kg per day beginning 2 weeks postnatally, however, has been demonstrated, in the absence of blood transfusions, to prevent the development of iron deficiency at 3 months postnatally (Lundstrom et al, 1977). Experience with the use of recombinant erythropoietin for the treatment of anemia of prematurity indicates that higher doses of iron are needed, in the range of 6 mg/kg per day, to support the more rapid rate of erythropoiesis (Ehrenkranz et al, 1994).

Generally, ferrous sulfate (25 mg/mL, 2 mg/kg/day) drops are used in human milk–fed LBW infants beginning soon after the achievement of complete enteral feedings. Formula-fed LBW infants should receive iron-fortified formula from the onset of milk feeding (Hall et al, 1993).

Sodium and Potassium

A comparison of sodium intakes of 2.9 and 1.6 mmol/kg per day in LBW infants suggested that the former intake provided more appropriate serum sodium concentrations (Roy et al, 1976). Hyponatremia also may result in LBW infants primarily fed human milk because the sodium content of preterm milk continues to decline through lactation. The need for these electrolytes may increase during or after diuretic usage.

Vitamins

Vitamin A and riboflavin concentrations decline in human milk under conditions of light exposure and after passage through feeding tubes (Bates et al, 1985). Ascorbic acid concentrations are lower in infants fed pooled human milk (Heinonen et al, 1986). Supplementary vitamins are provided in human milk fortifiers and in preterm formulas (Schanler, 1988b). Thus, there is no recommendation for additional multivitamin supplements for infants receiving adequate intakes of preterm formulas or fortified human milk. A multivitamin supplement, however, should be added to unfortified human milk or standard term commercial formulas until the infant is consuming 1 L of milk per day (American Academy of Pediatrics, 1980).

Additives for Enteral Feeding

Additives are available to augment the energy (glucose polymers, long-chain and medium-chain triglycerides) and protein (bovine casein or whey) components of the diet. It is important to recognize that additions of energy, without commensurate increases in protein, may dilute the proportion of the protein calories. Furthermore, the addition of nonprotein energy may lead one to ignore needs for minerals and other essential nutrients. Examples of nutrient constituents of three 27 kcal/oz prepared formulas are shown in Table 78–14 to illustrate this point. By reconstituting or using a prepared formula to achieve greater caloric density rather than using additives, a more balanced energy intake can be achieved without the loss of protein and minerals.

Human Milk for Low-Birth-Weight Infants

The benefits of feeding LBW infants human milk are beginning to be recognized. Specific factors such as sIgA, lactoferrin, lysozyme, oligosaccharides (including mucins),

TABLE 78–14

Distribution of Energy and Selected Nutrients in Formulas Containing Additives*

Component	Similac 27 kcal/oz Ready-to-feed	Similac 20 kcal/oz Plus Fat	Similac 20 kcal/oz Plus Carbohydrate
Energy, kcal/dL	90	90	90
Protein, g/dL (% kcal)	2.4 (11%)	1.4 (6%)	1.4 (6%)
Fat, g/dL (% kcal)	4.7 (47%)	6.2 (56%)	3.6 (36%)
Carbohydrate, g/dL (% kcal)	9.5 (42%)	7.2 (32%)	13.0 (58%)
Calcium, mg/dL	81	49	49
Sodium, mg/dL	31	18	18
Zinc, μg/dL	675	500	500
Vitamin A, IU/dL	270	200	200

*Products of Ross Laboratories (Columbus, OH) selected for comparative purposes.
Used with permission of Ross Products Division, Abbott Laboratories, Columbus, OH 43216.

growth factors, and cellular components may affect the host defense of the LBW infant (Goldman et al, 1982; Hambraeus, 1977). The quantity of host defense factors in preterm milk is greater than in term milk (Goldman et al, 1982). Lactoferrin, lysozyme, and sIgA are specific human whey proteins that are particularly resistant to hydrolysis and, as such, line the gastrointestinal tract to play a primary role in host defense (Schanler et al, 1986). The enteromammary immune system (see Fig. 78–1) is the mechanism through which the human milk–fed infant receives a portion of its host protection (Kleinman and Walker, 1979). To what extent the enteromammary immune system functions in the LBW infant–mother dyad is unknown. Protocols that encourage skin-to-skin contact between the LBW infant and mother may affect milk protective antibody concentrations.

A lower incidence of infections in LBW infants fed their mothers' milk partially or exclusively compared with similar infants fed formula exclusively has been reported (Narayanan et al, 1980, 1981). One large, multicenter study observed that either exclusively or partially human milk–fed LBW infants had a significantly lower incidence of necrotizing enterocolitis than similar infants fed formula exclusively (Lucas and Cole, 1990). Although the mechanism for the protective role of human milk in necrotizing enterocolitis is unclear, the protective role of IgA and IgG in feeding LBW infants has been demonstrated (Eibl et al, 1988). The infants fed the immunoglobulin preparation had a significantly higher fecal excretion of IgA, suggesting a local protective effect throughout the gastrointestinal tract. Similar data on the fecal excretion of human milk immune factors have been reported in LBW infants fed fortified human milk (Schanler et al, 1986).

Few studies have evaluated the effect of diet on neurodevelopmental outcomes in LBW infants. Data suggest that children who received human milk during their hospitalization as LBW infants had significantly greater scores on the Weschler Intelligence Scales for Children–Revised (WISC-R) than children who never received human milk as LBW infants (Lucas et al, 1992). There are some corroborating data from a longitudinal assessment of full-term infants that suggest a positive relationship between cognitive abilities and duration of breast-feeding (Rogan and

Gladen, 1993). Thus, a variety of reasons are emerging to encourage either the exclusive or partial use of human milk for LBW infant feeding.

Despite the potential benefits, human milk–fed LBW infants manifest slower growth rates and inadequate intakes of specific nutrients to meet their greater needs (Schanler and Oh, 1980; Atkinson et al, 1981). Inadequate nutrient intakes may result from compositional variability of human milk; losses associated with collection, storage, and feeding procedures; or inherently lower nutrient concentrations than those needed by growing LBW infants (Butte et al, 1988; Gross et al, 1980; Hall, 1979; Schanler, 1988a). Growth and nutritional status may improve in LBW infants by the avoidance of restricted milk intakes; the prevention of fat losses in collection, storage, and preparation of the milk; and the use of hindmilk and nutrient fortifiers (Greer and McCormick, 1988; Narayanan, 1982; Schanler et al, 1985). The composition of the fortifiers is described in Table 78–12 and in specific previous sections.

Collection and Storage of Human Milk

An important property of breast-feeding is its relative freedom from bacterial contamination. Contamination can be a problem, however, when milk is artificially collected and stored. Standards have been published by the Human Milk Banking Association of North America. A variety of bacteria; bacterial toxins; and viruses such as rubella, cytomegalovirus, and hepatitis may be transmitted by breast-feeding. For these reasons, human milk banks processing pooled milk from multiple donors use pasteurization methods to avoid disease transmission. Because maternal T lymphocytes may be absorbed intact through the gastrointestinal tract of newborn infants, there are theoretical concerns about the safety of feeding *fresh* (unfrozen or unheated) human milk from a mother other than the infant's own.

Human milk is microbiologically safe for feeding to the mother's own infant if the mother's hands and collection equipment are properly cleaned before collection. Electric breast pumps are generally more effective than manual pumps or manual expression. Hand pumps of the bicyclehorn variety may cause breast trauma or contamination of milk and should not be used. Glass or hard plastic containers should be used for milk storage. Milk to be fed within 48 hours of collection can be refrigerated without significant bacterial proliferation.

Freezing is the preferred method of storing milk that will not be fed within 48 hours. Single milk expressions should be packaged separately for freezing. In contrast to heat treatment, freezing preserves most of the nutritional and immunologic benefits of human milk. Efforts should be made to collect clean milk with minimal bacterial contamination and to store it in a freezer until it is gently thawed and fed. After milk is thawed, it should not be frozen again.

PRACTICAL FEEDING ISSUES

Once the decision has been made to initiate enteral feedings, the physician must determine what to feed, how much to feed, the route to feed by, and how rapidly to advance the volume of feedings. Although numerous studies have attempted to address these issues, no consensus exists among neonatology caregivers (Churella et al, 1985).

What to Feed

There is a wide diversity of practice concerning the appropriate fluid to use in initiating feeding. Many neonatal intensive care units (NICUs) offer a sterile water feeding first to test the infant's ability to suck and to empty the stomach. For very-low-birth-weight infants, sterile water feedings may be given for 24 to 48 hours. In other NICUs, infants are placed directly to the breast or given milk or formula. Many NICUs choose to feed formula that has been diluted 1:1. Others initiate feedings with 24 kcal/oz formulas, and others begin with 20 kcal/oz formulas. Other NICUs feed 5% dextrose in water solutions. The use of 10% .dextrose in water should be avoided because it is hyperosmolar compared to human milk or formula. One should also be aware that gastric emptying and intestinal transit are slowed when fluids are hyposmolar or hyperosmolar compared with human milk. Thus, an infant who has gastric residuals when fed diluted formula may have improved feeding tolerance when given undiluted formula (Koenig et al, 1995).

Most preterm infants are given unfortified human milk or preterm formula. As the benefits of human milk for the LBW infant are being acknowledged, more NICUs are using human milk exclusively. Once full caloric intake is achieved, the caloric density of these formulas can be enhanced by using fortifiers or 24 kcal/oz cow milk–based formulas. Soy formulas are not recommended for routine use in preterm infants (American Academy of Pediatrics, 1983). Soy formulas have been noted to result in decreased phosphorus absorption in LBW infants, which places the infants at risk for osteopenia. Elemental formulas also are not routinely used to feed healthy preterm infants because mucosal function is adequately mature enough to process regular infant formulas. Both types of formulas also contain lower mineral concentrations than preterm formulas and fortified human milk (see Table 78–12).

Route of Feeding

Infants who have an active suck can ingest milk and formula. Preterm infants, however, do not commonly have a coordinated suck before 32 to 34 weeks' gestation. In addition, mature infants who have suffered asphyxial insults or who have significant tachypnea may not have the skills to suck. Thus, many LBW infants must be fed by tube. Most NICUs provide enteral nutrition by orogastric tubes and transpyloric tubes.

Although verification of tube placement is necessary for transpyloric tubes, the need for repeated radiographic exposure can be limited by using pH testing of tube drainage to document a change from acidic to neutral pH. There are concerns that gastric acid plays a role in inactivating bacterial growth and that the addition of acid to milk instilled into the upper duodenum results in a lower incidence of intestinal infections and necrotizing enterocolitis. Although the presence of milk or formulas in the stomach is required to stimulate the release of the hormone gastrin, transpyloric feedings are often used to overcome delayed gastric emptying in an attempt to avoid reliance on parenteral nutrition.

Rate of Feeding

The two most commonly used feeding rates are slow, continuous feedings and intermittent (bolus) feedings given over 15 minutes every 3 to 4 hours. Although bolus feedings may permit a more powerful physiologic stimulus for the release of gastrointestinal hormones, LBW infants absorb nutrients better and gain weight faster when they are given continuous infusion feedings (Parker et al, 1981). Bolus feedings are temporally associated with apnea, cyanosis, and decreases in pH and PaO_2 in some infants. In some infants, these events may be related to gastroesophageal reflux (Orenstein and Orenstein, 1988). Bolus feedings may also cause gastric distention, increased intra-abdominal pressure, and elevation of the diaphragm among infants with chronic lung disease whose chest compliance and diaphragmatic work may be compromised. Therefore, slow infusion feedings may be useful in older preterm infants who have severe chronic lung disease. Slow infusion feedings elicit a more mature duodenal motor response to feeding and more complete gastric emptying than do bolus feedings (DeVille et al, 1993). In studies among debilitated adults, slow infusion feedings resulted in fewer episodes of gastroesophageal reflux than bolus feeding. Collectively, these data suggest that the very preterm infant may not be physiologically prepared to process bolus feedings as well as slow infusion feedings. A feeding regimen used in studies offers a compromise of these two techniques by alternating 2-hour episodes of slow feeding infusions with 2-hour episodes of fasting. This technique permits one to capitalize on the better weight gain achieved by slow infusion and yet provide adequate stimulus for hormone release (Berseth et al, 1992).

When and How Much to Feed

Enteral nutrition can be used to achieve two goals: the stimulation of growth, integrity, and function of the intestine and the provision of calories. Although the former goal can be achieved using small volumes of feeding, clinical needs often force the clinician to increase volumes to achieve the latter.

Numerous studies in rat, pig, dog, rabbit, and guinea pig have shown that newborn animals maintained on parenteral nutrition alone exhibit better growth and maturation of the gastrointestinal tract when they are given small enteral feedings. In fact, these trophic effects of luminal nutrients on intestinal growth can be achieved when only 15% of daily caloric needs are provided enterally. Studies in preterm infants have shown that infants fed as little as 1% to 12% of their caloric intake for 1 to 2 weeks demonstrate greater intestinal functional maturation than do infants fed nothing or sterile water, as reflected by plasma concentrations of gastrointestinal hormones (Berseth, 1992; Meetze et al, 1992), feeding tolerance, somatic growth (Berseth, 1992; Dunn et al, 1988; Slagle and Gross, 1988), and hepatic function (Slagle and Gross, 1988b). In a parallel manner, motor responses to feeding can be elicited by feeding volumes as small as 24 mL/kg per day (Berseth, 1990). Thus, it appears that there is an emerging consensus that preterm infants benefit from the use of 10 to 24 mL/kg per day to induce the maximal benefit of enhancing intestinal growth.

The use of enteral nutrients to provide the sole source of caloric intake, however, is fraught with risk. The incidence of necrotizing enterocolitis is significantly higher among infants who have been fed compared with those who have not been fed (Stoll, 1994). Although the risk of necrotizing enterocolitis is not higher among infants who are fed early compared with those whose feedings are delayed, none of these studies have evaluated the risk for necrotizing enterocolitis when volumes are advanced beyond the minimal enteral nutrition volumes of 10 to 24 mL/kg per day. In fact, the use of increased volumes may cause changes in vascular flow and oxygen consumption that exceed the capabilities of the preterm intestine. Two retrospective studies have shown that when feeding volumes are increased significantly beyond minimal enteral volumes, the risk of necrotizing enterocolitis significantly increases (McKeown et al, 1992; Owens and Berseth, 1995). Thus, many NICUs maintain minimal enteral nutrition volumes for a prolonged time and thereafter advance feeding volumes slowly (i.e., by 5 to 20 mL/kg every few days). Tolerance to enteral feedings must be monitored vigilantly because necrotizing enterocolitis can occur 3 to 4 months postnatally. Most NICUs recommend monitoring abdominal circumference, the presence of gastric residuals that exceed 25% to 50% of the volume fed, the presence of bilious aspirates from a tube that has been documented radiographically to be positioned in the stomach, and episodes of vomiting. Because many preterm infants exhibit numerous episodes of feeding problems, a measured response to each episode is necessary. Because necrotizing enterocolitis can occur among these infants, however, experienced judgment is required to evaluate each episode.

NUTRITIONAL ASSESSMENT

The nutritional status of the LBW infant is monitored (Table 78–15) by daily assessments of fluid and energy intake and evaluation of the rate of growth in weight, length, and head circumference. Growth parameters are plotted on graph paper or a specific chart for current LBW infants' growth (Shaffer et al, 1987). Because older charts

TABLE 78–15

Nutritional Assessment of the Low-Birth-Weight Infant

Fluid intake (mL/kg/d)	Daily
Parenteral intake	
Enteral intake	
Nutrient intake (unit/kg/d)	Daily
Energy intake (kcal)	
Protein intake (g)	
Specific nutrient (unit)	
Anthropometry	
Body weight (g)	Same time each day
Length (cm)	Weekly
Head circumference (cm)	Weekly
Biochemical monitoring°	
Hemoglobin, hematocrit	Weekly
Reticulocyte count	Weekly
Serum electrolytes	Weekly × 2, then q 2 wk†
Calcium, phosphorus	Weekly × 2, then q 2 wk
Alkaline phosphatase	Weekly × 2, then q 2 wk
Albumin, blood urea nitrogen	Weekly × 2, then q 2 wk‡
Other assessments	
Renal ultrasound§	2 months

°For infants receiving TPN exclusively, see Table 78–13.
†If infant receiving human milk or diuretics.
‡Add prealbumin if abnormal.
§To evaluate for nephrocalcinosis.

did not include sufficient numbers of infants less than 1000 g and nutrition practices have changed dramatically, differences are noted between 1948 and 1988 charts (Dancis et al, 1948; Shaffer et al, 1987). The rates of weight gain and growth milestones, such as the age at which birth weight is regained, 14 versus 31 postnatal days, differ between the 1948 and 1988 charts. The charts are helpful, but equally important is the computation of the weekly rate of growth. The average values for weight, length, and head circumference for LBW infants are 15 g/kg per day, 1.0 cm per week, and 1.0 cm per week (Gross and Eckerman, 1983; Shaffer et al, 1987; Usher and McLean, 1969). Once the infant reaches 2.5 kg, a daily weight gain of 20 to 30 g per day is appropriate.

The nutritional status of the LBW infant also is monitored by serial evaluations of biochemical indices. These assessments include serum calcium, phosphorus, alkaline phosphatase activity, albumin, and blood urea nitrogen. If more specific indices of protein status are needed, the serum prealbumin (transthyretin) is measured. Serum sodium, chloride, and bicarbonate are evaluated in human milk–fed infants or infants receiving diuretics. The hemoglobin and reticulocyte count are monitored to assess anemia. Specific determinations of plasma zinc and copper are not routinely useful, but zinc may be measured in infants with unusual losses, such as after gastrointestinal surgery and from enterostomies. The pattern of changes in biochemical indices may be more reflective of nutritional status than isolated values. A renal ultrasound scan to detect the presence of nephrocalcinosis is useful in LBW infants receiving prolonged courses of parenteral nutrition or diuretics.

DISCHARGE PLANNING

As the LBW infant nears the time of hospital discharge, several concerns regarding the nutritional management of the infant must be considered. If the infant has been fed fortified human milk or preterm formulas, the ability of the infant to consume ad libitum quantities of unfortified human milk or standard formula (20 kcal/oz) and continue to demonstrate appropriate growth must be determined. The infant with slow growth or in whom biochemical abnormalities of nutritional status have been identified may require an enriched milk after hospital discharge. This may be accomplished by adding a standard formula diluted to 24 kcal/oz to alternate with breast-feeding or by using 24 kcal/oz formula exclusively. Follow-up studies of LBW infants are beginning to suggest that growth and bone mineralization will be affected positively by feeding enriched milks after discharge (Bishop et al, 1993; Chan, 1993). Growth and biochemical nutritional status should be monitored after discharge. Further research is needed to identify norms for posthospitalization growth and biochemical indices of LBW infants.

Acknowledgments

This work is a publication of the USDA/ARS Children's Nutrition Research Center, Department of Pediatrics, Baylor College of Medicine and Texas Children's Hospital, Houston, TX. Funding has been provided from the USDA/ARS under Cooperative Agreement No. 58-6250-1-003. The contents of this publication do not necessarily reflect the views or policies of the USDA, and mention of trade names, commercial products, or organizations does not imply endorsement by the U.S. government.

REFERENCES

Abrams SA, Schanler RJ, Tsang RC, Garza C: Bone mineralization in former very low birth weight infants fed either human milk or commercial formula: One year follow-up observation. J Pediatr 114:1041, 1989.

Alemi B, Hamosh M, Scanlon JW, et al: Fat digestion in very low-birthweight infants: Effect of addition of human milk to low birthweight formula. Pediatrics 68:484, 1981.

American Academy of Pediatrics, Committee on Nutrition: Encouraging breast-feeding. Pediatrics 65:657, 1980a.

American Academy of Pediatrics, Committee on Nutrition: Vitamin and mineral supplement needs in normal children in the United States. Pediatrics 66:1015, 1980b.

American Academy of Pediatrics, Committee on Nutrition: Soy-protein formulas: Recommendations for use in infant feeding. Pediatrics 72:359, 1983.

American Academy of Pediatrics, Committee on Nutrition: Nutritional needs of low-birth-weight infants. Pediatrics 75:976, 1985.

American Academy of Pediatrics, Committee on Nutrition: The transfer of drugs and other chemicals into human milk. Pediatrics 93:137, 1994.

Anderson TL, Muttart CR, Bieber MA, et al: A controlled trial of glucose versus glucose and amino acids in premature infants. J Pediatr 94:947, 1979.

Atkinson SA, Bryan MH, Anderson GH: Human milk feeding in premature infants: Protein, fat and carbohydrate balances in the first two weeks of life. J Pediatr 99:617, 1981.

Atkinson SA, Radde IC, Anderson GH: Macromineral balances in premature infants fed their own mothers' milk or formula. J Pediatr 102:99, 1983.

Atkinson SA, Shah JK, McGee C, Steele BT: Mineral excretion in premature infants receiving various diuretic therapies. J Pediatr 113:540, 1988.

Aubier M, Murciano D, Lecocguic Y, et al: Effect of hypophosphatemia on diaphragmatic contractility in patients with acute respiratory failure. N Engl J Med 313:420, 1985.

Baeckert PA, Greene HL, Fritz I, et al: Vitamin concentrations in very low birth weight infants given vitamins intravenously in a lipid emulsion: Measurement of vitamins A, D, E, and riboflavin. J Pediatr 113:1057, 1988.

Bates CJ, Liu DS, Fuller NJ, et al: Susceptibility of riboflavin and vitamin A in breast milk to photodegradation and its implications for the use of banked breast milk in infant feeding. Acta Paediatr Scand 74:40, 1985.

Berseth CL: Neonatal small intestinal motility: Motor responses to feeding in term and preterm infants. J Pediatr 117:777, 1990.

Berseth CL: Effect of early feeding on maturation of the preterm infant's small intestine. J Pediatr 120:947, 1992.

Berseth CL, Nordyke CK, Valdes MG, et al: Responses of gastrointestinal peptides and motor activity to milk and water feedings in preterm and term infants. Pediatr Res 31:587, 1992.

Bhatia J, Rassin DK: Human milk supplementation: Delivery of energy, calcium, phosphorus, magnesium, copper and zinc. Am J Dis Child 142:445, 1988.

Bishop NJ, King FJ, Lucas A: Increased bone mineral content of preterm infants fed with a nutrient enriched formula after discharge from hospital. Arch Dis Child 68:573, 1993.

Borum PR: Medium-chain triglycerides in formula for preterm neonates: Implications for hepatic and extrahepatic metabolism. J Pediatr 120:S139, 1992.

Bougle D, Bureau F, Deschrevel G, et al: Chromium and parenteral nutrition in children. J Pediatr Gastroenterol Nutr 17:72, 1993.

Brans YW, Dutton EB, Andrew DS, et al: Fat emulsion tolerance in very low birth weight neonates: Effect on diffusion of oxygen in the lungs and on blood pH. Pediatrics 78:79, 1986.

Bresson JL, Bader B, Rocchiccioli F, et al: Protein-metabolism kinetics and energy-substrate utilization in infants fed parenteral solutions with different glucose-fat ratios. Am J Clin Nutr 54:370, 1991.

Bronner F, Salle BL, Putet G, et al: Net calcium absorption in premature infants: Results of 103 metabolic balance studies. Am J Clin Nutr 56:1037, 1992.

Butte NF, Garza C, Johnson CA, et al: Longitudinal changes in milk composition of mothers delivering preterm and term infants. Early Hum Dev 9:153, 1984.

Butte NF, Garza C, Smith EO: Variability of macronutrient concentrations in human milk. Eur J Clin Nutr 42:345, 1988.

Butte NF, Garza C, Smith EO, Nichols BL: Human milk intake and growth of exclusively breast-fed infants. J Pediatr 104:187, 1984.

Carlson SE: Human milk nonprotein nitrogen: Occurrence and possible functions. In Barness LA (Ed): Advances in Pediatrics. Chicago, Year Book Medical Publishers, 1985, pp 43–70.

Carlson SE, Rhodes PG, Ferguson M: Docosahexaenoic acid status of LBW infants at birth and following feeding with human milk and formula. Am J Clin Nutr 44:798, 1986.

Carlson SE, Werkman SH, Rhodes PG, et al: Visual-acuity development in healthy preterm infants: Effect of marine-oil supplementation. Am J Clin Nutr 58:35, 1993.

Chan GM: Growth and bone mineral status of discharged very low birth weight infants fed different formulas or human milk. J Pediatr 123:439, 1993.

Churella HR, Bachhuber WL, MacLean WC: Survey: Methods of feeding low-birth-weight infants. Pediatrics 76:243, 1985.

Clandinin MT, Parrott A, Van Aerde JE, et al: Feeding preterm infants a formula containing C20 and C22 fatty acids simulates plasma phospholipid fatty acid composition of infants fed human milk. Early Hum Dev 31:41, 1992.

Crawford MA: The role of essential fatty acids in neural development: Implications for perinatal nutrition. Am J Clin Nutr 57:703S, 1993.

Cunningham AS: Morbidity in breast-fed and artificially fed infants. J Pediatr 90:726, 1977.

Cunningham AS: Morbidity in breast-fed and artificially fed infants: II. J Pediatr 95:685, 1979.

Cunningham AS, Jelliffe DB, Jelliffe EFP: Breast-feeding and health in the 1980s: A global epidemiologic review. J Pediatr 118:659, 1991.

Dallman PR: Iron, vitamin E, and folate in the preterm infant. J Pediatr 85:742, 1974.

Dancis J, O'Connell JR, Holt LE Jr: A grid for recording the weight of premature infants. J Pediatr 33:570, 1948.

Dauncey MJ, Davies CG, Shaw JCL, Urman J: The effect of iron supplements and blood transfusion on iron absorption by low birth weight infants fed pasteurized human breast milk. Pediatr Res 12:899, 1978.

Dauncey MJ, Shaw JCL, Urman J: The absorption and retention of magnesium, zinc, and copper by low birth weight infants fed pasteurized human breast milk. Pediatr Res 11:1033, 1977.

De Curtis M, Senterre J, Rigo J: Estimated and measured energy content of infant formulas. J Pediatr Gastroenterol Nutr 5:746, 1986.

DeVille KT, Shulman RJ, Berseth CL: Slow infusion feeding enhances gastric emptying in preterm infants compared to bolus feeding. Clin Res 41:787A, 1993.

Dickerson RN, Brown RO, White KG: Parenteral nutrition solutions. *In* Rombeau JL, Caldwell MD (Eds): Clinical Nutrition: Parenteral Nutrition, 2nd ed. Philadelphia, WB Saunders, 1993, pp 310–320.

Duncan B, Ey J, Holberg CJ, et al: Exclusive breast-feeding for at least 4 months protects against otitis media. Pediatrics 91:867, 1993.

Dunn L, Hulman S, Weiner J, Kliegman R: Beneficial effects of early hypocaloric enteral feeding on neonatal gastrointestinal function: Preliminary report of a randomized trial. J Pediatr 112:622, 1988.

Ehrenkranz RA, Gettner PA, Nelli CM, et al: Zinc and copper nutritional studies in very low birth weight infants: Comparison of stable isotope extrinsic tag and chemical balance methods. Pediatr Res 26:298, 1989.

Ehrenkranz RA, Sherwonit EA, Nelli CM, Janghorbani M: Recombinant human erythropoietin stimulates incorporation of absorbed iron into RBCs in VLBW infants. Pediatr Res 35:311A, 1994.

Eibl MM, Wolf HM, Furnkranz H, Rosenkranz A: Prevention of necrotizing enterocolitis in low-birth-weight infants by IgA-IgG feeding. N Engl J Med 319:1, 1988.

Ellis KJ, Shypailo RJ, Schanler RJ, Langston C: Body elemental composition of the neonate: New reference data. Am J Hum Biol 5:323, 1993.

Fitzgerald KA, MacKay MW: Calcium and phosphate solubility in neonatal parenteral nutrient solutions containing TrophAmine. Am J Hosp Pharm 43:88, 1986.

Fomon SJ, Ziegler EE: Protein intake of premature infants: Interpretation of data. J Pediatr 90:504, 1977.

Freed GL, Landers S, Schanler RJ: A practical guide to successful breast-feeding management. Am J Dis Child 145:917, 1991.

Friedman Z, Danon A, Stahlman MT, Oates JA: Rapid onset of essential fatty acid deficiency in the newborn. Pediatrics 58:640, 1976.

Gaull GE, Rassin DK, Raiha NCR, Heinonen K: Milk protein quantity and quality in low-birthweight infants: III. Effects on sulfur amino acids in plasma and urine. J Pediatr 90:348, 1977.

Gilbertson N, Kovar IZ, Cox DJ, et al: Introduction of intravenous lipid administration on the first day of life in the very low birth weight neonate. J Pediatr 119:615, 1991.

Glasgow JFT, Thomas PS: Rachitic respiratory distress in small preterm infants. Arch Dis Child 5:268, 1977.

Glass RI, Stoll BJ: The protective effect of human milk against diarrhea. Acta Paediatr Scand 351:131, 1989.

Glass RI, Svennerholm AM, Stoll BJ, et al: Protection against cholera in breast-fed children by antibodies in breast milk. N Engl J Med 308:1389, 1983.

Goldman AS, Garza C, Nichols BL, et al: Effects of prematurity on the immunologic system in human milk. J Pediatr 101:901, 1982.

Greene HL, Courtney Moore ME, Phillips B, et al: Evaluation of a pediatric multiple vitamin preparation for total parenteral nutrition: II. Blood levels of vitamins A, D, and E. Pediatrics 77:539, 1986.

Greene HL, Hambidge KM, Schanler R, Tsang RC: Guidelines for the use of vitamins, trace elements, calcium, magnesium, and phosphorus in infants and children receiving total parenteral nutrition: Report of the Subcommittee on Pediatric Parenteral Nutrient Requirements from the Committee on Clinical Practice Issues of The American Society for Clinical Nutrition. Am J Clin Nutr 48:1324, 1988.

Greene HL, Hazlett D, Demaree R: Relationship between Intralipid-induced hyperlipemia and pulmonary function. Am J Clin Nutr 29:127, 1976.

Greene HL, Phillips BL, Franck L, et al: Persistently low blood retinol levels during and after parenteral feeding of very low birth weight infants: Examination of losses into intravenous administration sets and method of prevention by addition to a lipid emulsion. Pediatrics 79:894, 1987.

Greene HL, Smith R, Pollack P, et al: Intravenous vitamins for very-low-birth-weight infants. J Am Coll Nutr 10:281, 1991.

Greer FR, McCormick A: Improved bone mineralization and growth in premature infants fed fortified own mother's milk. J Pediatr 112:961, 1988.

Greer FR, McCormick A, Loker J: Changes in fat concentration of human milk during delivery by intermittent bolus and continuous mechanical pump infusion. J Pediatr 105:745, 1984.

Gross SE, Eckerman CO: Normative early head growth in low birth weight infants. J Pediatr 104:946, 1983.

Gross SJ, David RJ, Bauman L, Tomarelli RM: Nutritional composition of milk produced by mothers delivering preterm. J Pediatr 96:641, 1980.

Gutcher GR, Farrell PM: Intravenous infusion of lipid for the prevention of essential fatty acid deficiency in premature infants. Am J Clin Nutr 54:1024, 1991.

Hall B: Uniformity of human milk. Am J Clin Nutr 32:304, 1979.

Hall RT, Wheeler RE, Benson J, et al: Feeding iron-fortified premature formula during initial hospitalization to infants less than 1800 grams birth weight. Pediatrics 92:409, 1993.

Hallman M, Bry K, Hoppu K, et al: Inositol supplementation in premature infants with respiratory distress syndrome. N Engl J Med 326:1233, 1992.

Hambraeus L: Proprietary milk versus human breast milk in infant feeding, a critical appraisal from the nutritional point of view. Pediatr Clin North Am 24:17, 1977.

Hammerman C, Aramburo MJ: Decreased lipid intake reduces morbidity in sick premature neonates. J Pediatr 113:1083, 1988.

Hamosh M: Lipid metabolism in premature infants. Biol Neonate 52(suppl 1):50, 1987.

Hamosh M, Bitman J, Liao TH, et al: Gastric lipolysis and fat absorption in preterm infants: Effect of medium-chain triglyceride or long-chain triglyceride-containing formulas. Pediatrics 83:86, 1989.

Haumont D, Deckelbaum RJ, Richelle M, et al: Plasma lipid and plasma lipoprotein concentrations in low birth weight infants given parenteral nutrition with twenty or ten percent lipid emulsion. J Pediatr 115:787, 1989.

Haumont D, Richelle M, Deckelbaum RJ, et al: Effect of liposomal content of lipid emulsions on plasma lipid concentrations in low birth weight infants receiving parenteral nutrition. J Pediatr 121:759, 1992.

Heine W, Tiess M, Wutzke KD: 15N tracer investigations of the physiological availability of urea nitrogen in mother's milk. Acta Paediatr Scand 75:439, 1986.

Heinonen K, Mononen I, Mononen T, et al: Plasma vitamin C levels are low in premature infants fed human milk. Am J Clin Nutr 43:923, 1986.

Heird WC, Kashyap S, Gomez MR: Parenteral alimentation of the neonate. Semin Perinatol 15:493, 1991.

Helbock HJ, Motchnik PA, Ames BN: Toxic hydroperoxides in intravenous lipid emulsions used in preterm infants. Pediatrics 91:83, 1993.

Higashi A, Ikeda T, Iribe K, Matsuda I: Zinc balance in premature infants given the minimal dietary zinc requirement. J Pediatr 112:262, 1988.

Hoehn GJ, Carey DE, Rowe JC, et al: Alternate day infusion of calcium and phosphorus in very low birth weight infants: Wasting of the infused mineral. J Pediatr Gastroenterol Nutr 6:752, 1987.

Horsman A, Ryan SW, Congdon PJ, et al: Bone mineral accretion rate and calcium intake in preterm infants. Arch Dis Child 64:910, 1989.

Howie PW, Forsyth JS, Ogston SA, et al: Protective effect of breast-feeding against infection. BMJ 300:11, 1990.

Huston RK, Reynolds JW, Jensen C, Buist NRM: Nutrient and mineral retention and vitamin D absorption in low-birth-weight infants: Effect of medium-chain triglycerides. Pediatrics 72:44, 1983.

Innis SM: Human milk and formula fatty acids. J Pediatr 120:S56, 1992.

Innis SM, Foote KD, MacKinnon MJ: Plasma and red blood cell fatty acids of low-birth-weight infants fed their mother's expressed breast milk or preterm infant formula. Am J Clin Nutr 51:994, 1990.

Jakobsson I, Lindberg T, Benediktsson B: Dietary bovine β-lactoglobulin is transferred to human milk. Acta Paediatr Scand 74:342, 1985.

Jensen RG, Jensen GL: Specialty lipids for infant nutrition: I. Milks and formulas. J Pediatr Gastroenterol Nutr 15:232, 1992.

Kao LC, Cheng MH, Warburton D: Triglycerides, free fatty acids, free fatty acids/albumin molar ratio, and cholesterol levels in serum of neonates receiving long-term lipid infusions: Controlled trial of continuous and intermittent regimens. J Pediatr 104:429, 1984.

Kashyap S, Forsyth M, Zucker C, et al: Effects of varying protein and energy intakes on growth and metabolic response in low birth weight infants. J Pediatr 108:955, 1986.

Kashyap S, Okamoto E, Kanaya S: Protein quality in feeding low birth weight infants: A comparison of whey-predominant versus casein-predominant formulas. Pediatrics 79:748, 1987.

Kashyap S, Schulze K, Forsyth M, et al: Growth, nutrient retention, and metabolic response in low birth weight infants fed varying intakes of protein and energy. J Pediatr 113:713, 1988.

Kien CL, Ganther HE: Manifestations of chronic selenium deficiency in a child receiving total parenteral nutrition. Am J Clin Nutr 37:319, 1983.

Kleinman RE, Walker WA: The enteromammary immune system. Dig Dis Sci 24:876, 1979.

Koenig WJ, Amarnath RP, Hench V, Berseth CL: Manometrics for preterm and term infants: A new tool for old questions. Pediatrics 95:203, 1995.

Koo WWK: Parenteral nutrition-related bone disease. JPEN J Parenter Enteral Nutr 16:386, 1992.

Koo WWK, Sherman R, Succop P, et al: Sequential bone mineral content in small preterm infants with and without fractures and rickets. J Bone Miner Res 3:193, 1988.

Laine L, Shulman RJ, Pitre D, et al: Cysteine usage increases the need for acetate in neonates who receive total parenteral nutrition. Am J Clin Nutr 54:565, 1991.

Lawrence RA (Ed): Breastfeeding: A Guide for the Medical Profession, 4th ed. St. Louis, Mosby-Year Book, 1994.

Levy R, Herzberg GR, Andrews WL, et al: Thiamine, riboflavin, folate, and vitamin B12 status of low birth weight infants receiving parenteral and enteral nutrition. JPEN J Parenter Enteral Nutr 16:241, 1992.

Litov RE, Combs GF: Selenium in pediatric nutrition. Pediatrics 87:339, 1991.

Lockitch G, Jacobson B, Quigley G, et al: Selenium deficiency in low birth weight neonates: An unrecognized problem. J Pediatr 114:865, 1989.

Lucas A, Brooke OG, Baker BA, et al: High alkaline phosphatase activity and growth in preterm neonates. Arch Dis Child 64:902, 1989.

Lucas A, Cole TJ: Breast milk and neonatal necrotizing enterocolitis. Lancet 336:1519, 1990.

Lucas A, Morley R, Cole TJ: Breast milk and subsequent intelligence quotient in children born preterm. Lancet 339:261, 1992.

Lundstrom U, Siimes MA, Dallman PR: At what age does iron supplementation become necessary in low birthweight infants? J Pediatr 91:878, 1977.

MacLean WC, Fink BB: Lactose malabsorption by premature infants: Magnitude and clinical significance. J Pediatr 97:383, 1980.

MacMahon P, Blair ME, Treweeke P, Kovar IZ: Association of mineral composition of neonatal intravenous feeding solutions and metabolic bone disease of prematurity. Arch Dis Child 64:489, 1989.

Malloy MH, Rassin DK, Richardson CJ: Cyst(e)ine measurements during total parenteral nutrition. Am J Clin Nutr 37:188, 1983.

Malloy MH, Rassin DK, Richardson CJ: Total parenteral nutrition in sick preterm infants: Effects of cysteine supplementation with nitrogen intakes of 240 and 400 mg/kg/day. J Pediatr Gastroenterol Nutr 3:239, 1984.

McKeown RE, Marsh TD, Amarnath U, et al: Role of delayed feeding and of feeding increments in necrotizing enterocolitis. J Pediatr 121:764, 1992.

Meetze WH, Valentine C, McGuigan JE, et al: Gastrointestinal priming prior to full enteral nutrition in very low birth weight infants. J Pediatr Gastroenterol Nutr 15:163, 1992.

Mehta NR, Hamosh M, Bitman J, Wood DL: Adherence of medium-chain fatty acids to feeding tubes during gavage. J Pediatr 112:474, 1988.

Mitton SG: Amino acids and lipid in total parenteral nutrition for the newborn. J Pediatr Gastroenterol Nutr 18:25, 1994.

Moore MC, Greene HL, Phillips B, et al: Evaluation of a pediatrics multiple vitamin preparation for total parenteral nutrition in infants and children: I. Blood levels of water-soluble vitamins. Pediatrics 77:530, 1986.

Moran JR, Vaughan R, Stroop S: Concentrations and total daily output of micronutrients in breast milk of mothers delivering preterm: A longitudinal study. J Pediatr Gastroenterol Nutr 2:629, 1983.

Moro GE, Fulconis F, Minoli IE: Growth and plasma amino acid concentrations in very low birthweight infants fed either human milk protein fortified human milk or whey-predominant formula. Acta Paediatr Scand 78:18, 1989.

Narayanan I: Human milk in the developing world: To bank or not to bank? Indian J Pediatr 19:395, 1982.

Narayanan I, Prakash K, Bala S, et al: Partial supplementation with expressed breast-milk for prevention of infection in low-birth-weight infants. Lancet 2:561, 1980.

Narayanan I, Prakash K, Gujral VV: The value of human milk in the prevention of infection in the high-risk low-birth-weight infant. J Pediatr 99:496, 1981.

National Academy of Sciences (Ed): Recommended Dietary Allowances, 10th ed. Washington, DC, National Academy Press, 1989.

Neville MC, Keller RP, Seacat J, et al: Studies on human lactation: I. Within-feed and between-breast variation in selected components of human milk. Am J Clin Nutr 40:635, 1984.

Newman V: Vitamin A and breast-feeding: A comparison of data from developed and developing countries. Food Nutr Bull 15:161, 1994.

Nutrition Committee of the Canadian Paediatric Society, American Academy of Pediatrics: Breastfeeding. Pediatrics 65:591, 1978.

Orenstein S, Orenstein D: Gastroesophageal reflux and respiratory disease. J Pediatr 112:847, 1988.

Owens L, Berseth CL: Is there a volume threshold for enteral feeding and necrotizing enterocolitis? Pediatr Res 37:315A, 1995.

Parker P, Stroop S, Greene H: A controlled comparison of continuous versus intermittent feeding in the treatment of infants with intestinal disease. J Pediatr 99:360, 1981.

Phillips B, Franck LS, Greene HL: Vitamin E levels in premature infants during and after intravenous multivitamin supplementation. Pediatrics 80:680, 1987.

Piedboeuf B, Chessex P, Hazan J, et al: Total parenteral nutrition in the newborn infant: Energy substrates and respiratory gas exchange. J Pediatr 118:97, 1991.

Pierro A, Carnielli V, Filler RM, et al: Characteristics of protein sparing effect of total parenteral nutrition in the surgical infant. J Pediatr Surg 23:538, 1988.

Pitkanen O, Hallman M, Andersson S: Generation of free radicals in lipid emulsion used in parenteral nutrition. Pediatr Res 29:56, 1991.

Polberger SKT, Axelsson IE, Räihä NCR: Urinary and serum urea as indicators of protein metabolism in very low birthweight infants fed varying human milk protein intakes. Acta Paediatr Scand 79:737, 1990.

Prestridge LL, Schanler RJ, Shulman RJ, et al: Effect of parenteral calcium and phosphorus therapy on mineral retention and bone mineral content in very low birth weight infants. J Pediatr 122:761, 1993.

Raiha NCR, Heinonen K, Rassin DK, Gaull GE: Milk protein quantity and quality in low-birth-weight infants: I. Metabolic responses and effects on growth. Pediatrics 57:659, 1976.

Rassin DK, Gaull GE, Raiha NCR, Heinonen K: Milk protein quantity and quality in low-birth-weight infants: IV. Effects on tyrosine and phenylalanine in plasma and urine. J Pediatr 90:356, 1977.

Rebouche CJ, Panagides DD, Nelson SE: Role of carnitine in utilization of dietary medium-chain triglycerides by term infants. Am J Clin Nutr 52:820, 1990.

Rivera A, Bell EF, Bier DM: Effect of intravenous amino acids on protein metabolism of preterm infants during the first three days of life. Pediatr Res 33:106, 1993.

Rivera A, Bell EF, Stegink LD, Ziegler EE: Plasma amino acid profiles during the first three days of life in infants with respiratory distress syndrome: Effect of parenteral amino acid supplementation. J Pediatr 115:465, 1989.

Rogan WJ, Gladen BC: Breast-feeding and cognitive development. Early Hum Dev 31:181, 1993.

Ronnholm KAR, Sipila I, Siimes MA: Human milk protein supplementation for the prevention of hypoproteinemia without metabolic imbalance in breast milk-fed, very low birth weight infants. J Pediatr 101:243, 1982.

Roy CC, Ste-Marie M, Chartrand L, et al: Correction of the malabsorption of the preterm infant with a medium-chain triglyceride formula. J Pediatr 86:446, 1975.

Roy RN, Chance GW, Radde IC, et al: Late hyponatremia in very low birthweight infants. Pediatr Res 10:526, 1976.

Salle B, Senterre J, Putet G, Rigo J: Effects of calcium and phosphorus supplementation on calcium retention and fat absorption in preterm infants fed pooled human milk. J Pediatr Gastroenterol Nutr 5:638, 1986.

Savilahti E, Kuitunen M: Allergenicity of cow milk proteins. J Pediatr 121:S12, 1992.

Schanler RJ: Special methods in feeding the preterm infant. *In* Tsang RC, Nichols BL (Eds): Nutrition During Infancy. Philadelphia, Hanley & Belfus, 1988a, pp 314–325.

Schanler RJ: Water soluble vitamins: C, B1, B2, B6, niacin, biotin, and pantothenic acid. *In* Tsang RC, Nichols BL (Eds): Nutrition During Infancy. Philadelphia, Hanley & Belfus, 1988b, pp 236–252.

Schanler RJ: Calcium and phosphorus absorption and retention in preterm infants. Excerpta Med 2:24, 1991.

Schanler RJ, Abrams SA: Postnatal attainment of intrauterine macromineral accretion rates in low birth weight infants fed fortified human milk. J Pediatr 126:441, 1995.

Schanler RJ, Burns PA, Abrams SA, Garza C: Bone mineralization outcomes in human milk-fed preterm infants. Pediatr Res 31:583, 1992.

Schanler RJ, Garza C: Plasma amino acid differences in very low birth weight infants fed either human milk or whey-dominant cow milk formula. Pediatr Res 21:301, 1987a.

Schanler RJ, Garza C: Improved mineral balance in very low birth weight infants fed fortified human milk. J Pediatr 112:452, 1987b.

Schanler RJ, Garza C, Nichols BL: Fortified mothers' milk for very low birth weight infants: Results of growth and nutrient balance studies. J Pediatr 107:437, 1985.

Schanler RJ, Goldblum RM, Garza C, Goldman AS: Enhanced fecal excretion of selected immune factors in very low birth weight infants fed fortified human milk. Pediatr Res 20:711, 1986.

Schanler RJ, Oh W: Composition of breast milk obtained from mothers of premature infants as compared to breast milk obtained from donors. J Pediatr 96:679, 1980.

Schanler RJ, Rifka M: Calcium, phosphorus, and magnesium needs for low birth weight infants. Acta Paediatr 83:111, 1994.

Schanler RJ, Shulman RJ, Prestridge LL: Parenteral nutrient needs of very low birth weight infants. J Pediatr 125:961, 1994.

Schmidt-Sommerfeld E, Penn D, Wolf H: Carnitine deficiency in premature infants receiving total parenteral nutrition: Effect of L-carnitine supplementation. J Pediatr 102:931, 1983.

Shaffer SG, Quimiro CL, Anderson JV, Hall RT: Postnatal weight changes in low birth weight infants. Pediatrics 79:702, 1987.

Shenai JP, Chytil F, Stahlman MT: Vitamin A status of neonates with bronchopulmonary dysplasia. Pediatr Res 19:185, 1985.

Shenai JP, Rush MG, Stahlman MT, Chytil F: Plasma retinol-binding protein response to vitamin A administration in infants susceptible to bronchopulmonary dysplasia. J Pediatr 116:607, 1990.

Sherry SN, Kramer I: The time of passage of the first stool and the first urine by the newborn infant. J Pediatr 46:158, 1955.

Sievers E, Oldigs H-D, Daerner K, Schaub J: Longitudinal zinc balances in breast-fed and formula-fed infants. Acta Paediatr 81:1, 1992.

Siimes MA, Vuori E, Kuitunen P: Breast milk iron a declining concentration during the course of lactation. Acta Paediatr Scand 68:29, 1979.

Sinclair JC: Metabolic rate and body size of the newborn. Clin Obstet Gynecol 14:840, 1971.

Sinclair JC: Energy balance of the newborn. *In* Sinclair JC (Ed): Temperature Regulation and Energy Metabolism in the Newborn. New York, Grune & Stratton, 1978, pp 187–204.

Slagle TA, Gross SJ: Vitamin E. *In* Tsang RC, Nichols BL (Eds): Nutrition During Infancy. Philadelphia, Hanley & Belfus, 1988a, pp 277–288.

Slagle TA, Gross SJ: Effect of early low-volume enteral substrate on subsequent feeding tolerance in very low birth weight infants. J Pediatr 113:526, 1988b.

Sosenko IRS, Innis SM, Frank L: Intralipid increases lung polyunsaturated fatty acids and protects newborn rats from oxygen toxicity. Pediatr Res 30:413, 1991.

Sosenko IRS, Rodriguez-Pierce M, Bancalari E: Effect of early initiation of intravenous lipid administration on the incidence and severity of chronic lung disease in premature infants. J Pediatr 123:975, 1993.

Stafstrom CE, Gilmore HE, Kurtin PS: Nephrocalcinosis complicating medical treatment of posthemorrhagic hydrocephalus. Pediatr Neurol 8:179, 1992.

Stoll BJ: Epidemiology of necrotizing enterocolitis. Clin Perinatol 21:205, 1994.

Sulkers EJ, Lafeber HN, Degenhart HJ, et al: Effects of high carnitine supplementation on substrate utilization in low-birth-weight infants receiving total parenteral nutrition. Am J Clin Nutr 52:889, 1990.

Sutton AM, Harvie A, Cockburn F, et al: Copper deficiency in the preterm infant of very low birthweight. Arch Dis Child 60:644, 1985.

Tantibhedhyangkul P, Hashim SA: Medium-chain triglyceride feeding in premature infants: Effects on calcium and magnesium absorption. Pediatrics 61:537, 1978.

Tyrala EE: Zinc and copper balances in preterm infants. Pediatrics 77:513, 1986.

Uauy R, Hoffman DR: Essential fatty acid requirements for normal eye and brain development. Semin Perinatol 15:449, 1991.

Usher R, McLean F: Intrauterine growth of live-born Caucasian infants at sea level: Standards obtained from measurements in 7 dimensions of infants born between 25 and 44 weeks of gestation. Pediatrics 74:901, 1969.

Valentine CJ, Hurst NM, Schanler RJ: Hindmilk improves weight gain in low-birth-weight infants fed human milk. J Pediatr Gastroenterol Nutr 18:474, 1994.

Van Aerde JE, Clandinin MT: Controversy in fatty acid balance. Can J Physiol Pharmacol 71:707, 1993.

Van Caillie-Bertrand MV, Degenhart HJ, Fernandes J: Selenium status of infants on nutritional support. Acta Paediatr Scand 73:816, 1984.

Weinstein MR, Oh W: Oxygen consumption in infants with bronchopulmonary dysplasia. J Pediatr 99:958, 1981.

Whyte RK, Campbell D, Stanhope R, et al: Energy balance in low birth weight infants fed formula of high or low medium-chain triglyceride content. J Pediatr 108:964, 1986.

Whyte RK, Homer R, Pennock CA: Faecal excretion of oligosaccharides and other carbohydrates in normal neonates. Arch Dis Child 53:913, 1978.

Widdowson EM: Importance of nutrition in development, with special reference to feeding low-birth-weight infants. *In* Sauls HS, Bachhuber WL, Lewis LA (Eds): Meeting Nutritional Goals for Low-Birth-Weight Infants: Proceedings of the Second Ross Clinical Research Conference. Columbus, OH, Ross Laboratories, 1982, pp 4–11.

Wirth FH, Numerof B, Pleban P, Neylan MJ: Effect of lactose on mineral absorption in preterm infants. J Pediatr 117:283, 1990.

Wu PYK, Edmond J, Auestad N, et al: Medium-chain triglycerides in infant formulas and their relation to plasma ketone body concentrations. Pediatr Res 20:338, 1986.

Yunis KA, Oh W: Effects of intravenous glucose loading on oxygen consumption, carbon dioxide production, and resting energy expenditure in infants with bronchopulmonary dysplasia. J Pediatr 115:127, 1989.

Zachman RD: Retinol (vitamin A) and the neonate: Special problems of the human premature infant. Am J Clin Nutr 50:413, 1989.

Zelikovic I, Chesney RW, Friedman AL, Ahlfors CE: Taurine depletion in very low birth weight infants receiving prolonged total parenteral nutrition: Role of renal immaturity. J Pediatr 116:301, 1990.

Ziegler EE, Biga RL, Fomon SJ: Nutritional requirements of the premature infant. *In* Suskind RM (Ed): Textbook of Pediatric Nutrition. New York, Raven Press, 1981, pp 29–39.

Ziegler EE, Fomon SJ: Lactose enhances mineral absorption in infancy. J Pediatr Gastroenterol Nutr 2:288, 1983.

Ziegler EE, O'Donnell AM, Nelson SE, Fomon SJ: Body composition of the reference fetus. Growth 40:329, 1976.

Zimmerman AW, Hambidge KM, Lepow ML, et al: Acrodermatitis in breast-fed premature infants: Evidence for a defect in mammary zinc secretion. Pediatrics 69:176, 1982.

Zlotkin SH, Bryan MH, Anderson GH: Intravenous nitrogen and energy intakes required to duplicate in utero nitrogen accretion in prematurely born human infants. J Pediatr 99:115, 1981a.

Zlotkin SH, Bryan MH, Anderson GH: Cysteine supplementation to cysteine-free intravenous feeding regimens in newborn infants. Am J Clin Nutr 34:914, 1981b.

Zlotkin SH, Buchanan BE: Meeting zinc and copper intake requirements in the parenterally fed preterm and fullterm infant. J Pediatr 103:441, 1983.

CHAPTER 79

Special Gastrointestinal Concerns

Carol Lynn Berseth and Steven A. Abrams

NECROTIZING ENTEROCOLITIS

Necrotizing enterocolitis (NEC) is the most commonly occurring gastrointestinal emergency in preterm infants. With the advent of modern neonatology, its incidence has ranged from 10% to 25% over the past 30 years. Approximately one third to one half of all very-low-birth-weight infants develop signs or symptoms suggestive of NEC; approximately one third to one half of those infants are eventually given a diagnosis of NEC. Of those infants who develop NEC, approximately half require surgery. Mortality ranges from 25% to 30%. Of those who survive, approximately 25% experience long-term sequelae.

Epidemiology

The incidence of NEC varies geographically and temporally. It typically occurs in a pattern of clustered cases. Although 10% of all cases of NEC occur in term infants, it is more commonly seen in preterm infants, particularly those with birth weights less than 1000 g. The incidence appears to be similar among male and female infants, but it is more common among black infants (Mizrahi et al, 1965; Wilson et al, 1983).

The age of onset of NEC is inversely related to gestational age, with a mean age of 3 to 4 days for term infants and 3 to 4 weeks for infants born at less than 28 weeks' gestation. NEC is 10 times more common among infants who have been fed compared to those who have not received enteral nutrition, and it occurs more commonly among infants fed formula compared to those fed breast milk. NEC, however, does occur among infants who have never been fed and who have received breast milk feedings.

NEC occurs in epidemics. Most neonatal intensive care units (NICUs) experience a low endemic incidence of NEC that is periodically punctuated by sporadic epidemics. A wide variety of organisms have been associated with these outbreaks, including *Klebsiella pneumoniae, Escherichia coli,* clostridia, coagulase-negative staphylococcus, and rotavirus. Most typically, these outbreaks occur during times of nursery crowding, but it is not clear that NEC is caused by infectious agents. Although a single, clear-cut cause for NEC has not been identified, several contributing risk factors have been identified: bowel ischemia, immaturity of host defense, and enteral feedings.

Bowel Ischemia

The role of ischemia in the pathogenesis of NEC has been supported by reports of increased occurrences of NEC among infants who have low Apgar scores, umbilical vessel catheterization, polycythemia, and reduced aortic blood flow. It has been postulated that when the preterm infant

is stressed by periods of hypoxia or hypotension, blood flow is redistributed via input from the adrenergic system away from the splanchnic bed. More recent evidence, however, suggests that these neurogenic events are transient and are reversed within 1 to 2 minutes by local vascular events called the *autoregulatory escape*, which restores intestinal tissue oxygenation. In fact, case-control studies have failed to confirm that hypoxic events occur any more frequently among infants who develop NEC compared to those who do not (Wilson et al, 1983).

Despite the lack of a direct causal relationship of hypoxia and NEC, regulation of vascular bed flow differs in preterm infants and adults, as described in Chapter 1, and these unique differences may make the preterm intestine more vulnerable to hypoxia during the period of reperfusion that typically follows a period of ischemia. During reperfusion, oxygen free radicals are generated; these free radicals can cause the tissue damage that is typically seen in reperfusion injuries. These free radicals result from the enzymatic breakdown of hypoxanthine that accumulates during ischemia and from activated neutrophils that adhere to the gut microvasculature after ischemic injury.

The high tissue levels of xanthine that result from episodes of ischemia may contribute in part to NEC, but the occurrence of NEC also appears to be related to other vascular events that are related to the use of centrally placed vascular catheters. Vascular access in most preterm infants is achieved by the use of umbilical arterial or venous catheters. NEC is also seen among infants who have had umbilical catheters inserted to perform an exchange transfusion for hyperbilirubinemia or polycythemia. Increases in portal venous pressure that may occur during an exchange transfusion in term infants can result in a decrease in ileal and colonic blood flow (Touloukian et al, 1973). It is not clear that this myogenic vasoconstriction occurs in preterm infants (Crissinger, 1989a). Exchange transfusions, however, are no longer a common procedure in this population.

Umbilical arterial catheters may pose more serious risk to the intestinal vasculature. It has been suggested that embolization of catheters may result in embolization of mesenteric arteries. Infusion of medications such as calcium may cause vasospasm in humans and frank intestinal necrosis in rabbits (Book and Herbst, 1980). Emboli, however, cannot be demonstrated to be present in the intestinal circulation of infants who have NEC (Tyson et al, 1976).

NEC has also been described among infants who have received indomethacin for treatment of a patent ductus arteriosus. It is speculated that indomethacin causes a generalized decrease in splanchnic bed flow that may compromise vascular supply to the distal ileum and colon. NEC also has an increased incidence among infants who are polycythemic (Leake et al, 1975). Polycythemia has been shown to cause a reduction in intestinal perfusion in swine (Nowicki et al, 1984) and intestinal necrosis in puppies

(LeBlanc et al, 1984). It has also been shown that antenatal exposure to cocaine is associated with postnatal development of NEC. Cocaine may cause a generalized fetal hypoxia as a result of impaired uterine blood flow. It can also cause selective intestinal ischemia that is not reversed by the autoregulatory escape mechanism. Thus, cocaine-related NEC may be vascular in origin.

Host Defense Factors

As reviewed in Chapter 70, host defenses in the preterm gastrointestinal tract are either absent or functionally immature. Because of the variety of agents that have been identified with outbreaks of NEC, it is unclear whether these organisms actually cause NEC or represent secondary infections. Although specific bacteria have been reported during some outbreaks of NEC, these same bacteria can frequently be cultured from unaffected infants.

Nevertheless, several immunologically based strategies have been employed to treat or prevent NEC. Several small studies have shown that the administration of oral antibiotics can reduce the incidence of NEC (Egan et al, 1976); however, there are concerns that liberal use of these medications may permit the overgrowth of resistant organisms. Other investigators have shown that the administration of oral immune globulin reduces the occurrence of NEC (Eibl et al, 1988), but this practice has not been validated by additional studies.

Other investigations have assessed whether mediators of inflammation contribute to the tissue damage of NEC. Platelet-activating factor, which is synthesized by white cells, stimulates the release of complement, oxygen radicals, catecholamines, prostaglandins, thromboxane, and leukotrienes. In animal models, the administration of exogenous platelet-activating factor causes neutrophil aggregation, platelet aggregation, systemic hypotension, and ischemic bowel necrosis. During artificially created episodes of ischemia/reperfusion of mesenteric circulation in animals, plasma platelet-activating factor levels increase, and severe bowel necrosis occurs. This sequence of events can be prevented if platelet-activating factor antagonists are administered (Kubes et al, 1990). Plasma platelet-activating factor concentrations are higher among infants who have NEC compared to age-matched control infants (Caplan et al, 1990). Furthermore, providing enteral feedings results in increased levels of platelet-activating factor (MacKendrick et al, 1993). Other mediators that are currently under investigation are tumor necrosis factor, endothelium-1, prostaglandins, and nitric oxide.

Because NEC occurs less frequently among infants fed breast milk, and because breast-feeding appears to protect infants from a number of diseases (Grulee et al, 1935), numerous investigators have attempted to delineate the factors in breast milk that contribute to neonatal host defense. As detailed in Chapter 78, breast milk contains immunoglobulins, leukocytes, and antibacterial agents. When neonatal rats were fed maternal milk, the incidence of NEC was significantly lower than that seen in neonatal rats fed artificial formula (Barlow et al, 1974). For breast milk to confer this protection from NEC, intact leukocytes had to be present in the milk. The protective effects conferred by the ingestion of breast milk were also reproduced

by feeding the immunoglobulin fraction of breast milk alone. In a large prospective trial, infants fed formula had a 2.5-fold greater risk of developing NEC than did infants fed breast milk. Furthermore, infants fed artificial formula supplemented by a preparation of human serum gamma immunoglobulin A (IgA) and IgG experienced a significant reduction in NEC (Eibl et al, 1988). Thus, it appears that host defense conferred by feeding breast milk may provide some protection against the development of NEC. Additional research in this area is still needed, however, to elucidate the component(s) that confer this protection and the mechanism(s) whereby this protection is conferred.

Enteral Feeding

Although NEC occurs in infants who have never been fed, its incidence is much higher among infants who have been fed compared to those who have not. Earlier studies suggested that delaying the onset of the initiation of enteral feeding reduced the incidence of NEC (Lucas and Cole, 1990); however, more recent studies have not confirmed this observation. In fact, several randomized prospective studies have failed to show an increase in the occurrence of NEC among infants fed early (within the first postnatal week) compared to those whose feedings are initiated late (2 to 3 weeks' postnatal age) (Berseth, 1992; Dunn et al, 1988; LaGamma et al, 1985; Meetze et al, 1992). NEC has been linked to the use of hyperosmolar formulas (Abrams et al, 1975), however, and to the rapid advancement of feeding volumes that exceed 25 mL/kg per day (McKeown et al, 1992). It is also important for the clinician to realize that the addition of medications such as theophylline, sodium bicarbonate, and calcium supplements as well as vitamins may significantly raise the osmotic loads of formulas (Ernst et al, 1983).

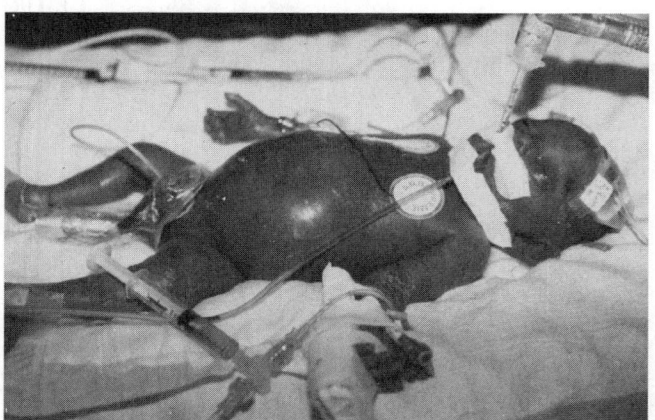

FIGURE 79–1. Clinical presentation of a preterm infant with necrotizing enterocolitis. This infant was born at 28 weeks' gestation and had been receiving enteral feedings for 1 week when he developed acute abdominal distention, hematochezia, and vomiting. Note the discoloration of the skin overlying the abdomen. Also, this infant required endotracheal intubation because of respiratory compromise that occurred as a result of the upward pressure of the abdominal contents on the diaphragm. (Courtesy of Dr. Lalo Cabrera-Meza, Baylor College of Medicine.)

Clinical Presentation

The clinical signs and symptoms of NEC are highly variable. In general, infants demonstrate gastrointestinal dysfunction, as reflected in the presence of abdominal distention, vomiting, bilious drainage from enteral feeding tubes, or hematochezia, and systemic illness, as reflected in temperature instability, apnea, lethargy, or hypotension (Fig. 79–1). The presentation of these signs and symptoms may be acute or insidious. Although a number of infants develop NEC within the 1st week of life, it is also a disease seen in the NICU graduate who has been transferred to the intermediate care nursery. Because the onset of NEC is inversely related to gestational age, clinicians must be exceedingly vigilant in assessing very preterm infants for a protracted postnatal period that may extend to 10 to 12 weeks.

The initial evaluation of an infant who exhibits the signs or symptoms of NEC should include a radiographic examination of the abdomen, collection of body fluids for culture, a metabolic evaluation including electrolytes, and a complete blood count. The intestinal inflammatory process often causes shifts in body fluid distribution resulting in hypotension and acid-base imbalance. In addition, inflammation and swelling of the abdominal contents can cause upward compression against the diaphragm, resulting in respiratory embarrassment. Thus, infants who are acutely ill may also require evaluation of respiratory status by laboratory and radiographic testing.

The severity of NEC is staged using criteria proposed by Bell and colleagues (1978) and later modified by Kliegman and associates (1982). These criteria are based on systemic intestinal signs and radiologic signs. As shown in Table 79–1, radiographic findings must be present to confirm a diagnosis of NEC.

Nonspecific radiographic findings in suspected but unproved NEC are dilated bowel loops, bowel wall thickening, and increased peritoneal fluid. The diagnostic radiographic finding in NEC is the presence of intestinal pneumatosis. This radiographic finding is caused by the presence of hydrogen in the bowel wall as a by-product of bacterial metabolism (Fig. 79–2A). There are two commonly observed radiographic patterns. More typically, there is a linear streak of gas within the bowel wall. This streaking may be visualized in a single discrete portion of the small intestine or may extend throughout the entire small and large intestine. The other pattern seen in NEC is a bubbly pattern that is similar to that seen in newborn infants who retain meconium in the intestine (Fig. 79–2B). Because this pattern can be confused with that of retained meconium, it is less specific for NEC than the linear streaking pattern. If intestinal pneumatosis extends into the portal venous circulation, linear branching areas of radiolucency may appear overlying the liver (Fig. 79–3).

If NEC progresses to bowel perforation, pneumoperitoneum may be identified radiographically. Most typically, free air is visualized on a cross-table lateral or right lateral decubitus film (Fig. 79–4A). Occasionally, free air can be

TABLE 79–1

Modified Bell's Staging Criteria for Necrotizing Enterocolitis

Stage	Systemic Signs	Intestinal Signs	Radiologic Signs	Treatment
I. Suspected				
A	Temperature instability, apnea, bradycardia	Elevated pregavage residuals, mild abdominal distention, occult blood in stool	Normal or mild ileus	NPO, antibiotics × 3 days
B	Same as IA	Same as IA, plus gross blood in stool	Same as IA	Same as IA
II. Definite				
A: Mildly ill	Same as IA	Same as I, plus absent bowel sounds, abdominal tenderness	Ileus, intestinal pneumatosis	NPO, antibiotics × 7–10 days
B: Moderately ill	Same as I, plus mild metabolic acidosis, mild thrombocytopenia	Same as I, plus absent bowel sounds, definite abdominal tenderness, abdominal cellulitis, right lower quadrant mass	Same as IIA, plus portal vein gas, with or without ascites	NPO, antibiotics × 14 days
III. Advanced				
A: Severely ill, bowel intact	Same as IIB, plus hypotension, bradycardia, respiratory acidosis, metabolic acidosis, disseminated intravascular coagulation, neutropenia	Same as I and II, plus signs of generalized peritonitis, marked tenderness, and distention of abdomen	Same as IIB, plus definite ascites	NPO, antibiotics × 14 days, fluid resuscitation, inotropic support, ventilator therapy, paracentesis
B: Severely ill: bowel perforated	Same as IIIA	Same as IIIA	Same as IIB, plus pneumoperitoneum	Same as IIA, plus surgery

NPO, nulla per os (nothing by mouth).
From Walsh MC, Kliegman RM, Fanaroff AA: Necrotizing enterocolitis: A practitioner's perspective. Pediatr Rev 9:225, 1988. Reproduced by permission of Pediatrics.

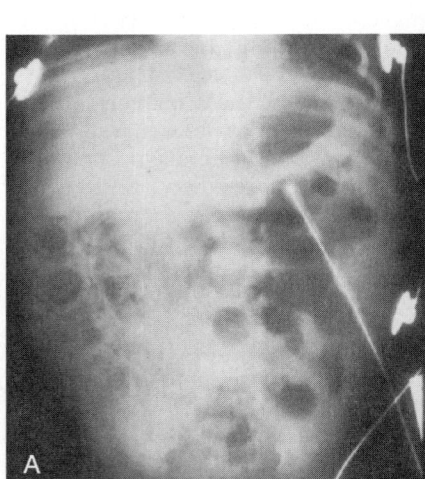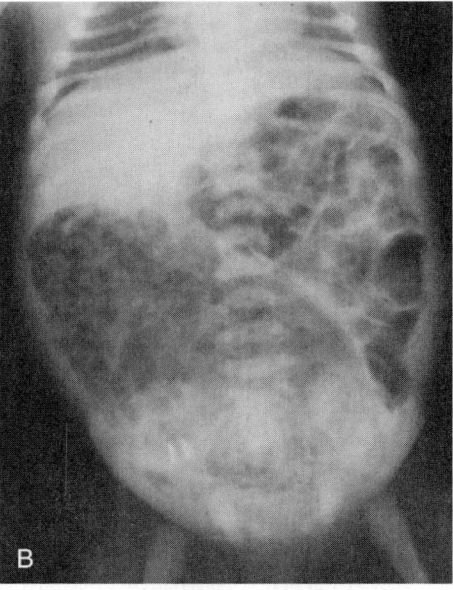

FIGURE 79–2. *A*, This is a typical abdominal radiograph finding of intestinal pneumatosis seen in necrotizing enterocolitis, which appears as dark concentric rings around the bowel loops in the right upper quadrant. *B*, This radiograph displays the *bubbly gas* pattern occasionally seen in necrotizing enterocolitis. (Courtesy of Dr. Lalo Cabrera-Meza, Baylor College of Medicine.)

visualized as a central periumbilical collection on an anteroposterior film (Fig. 79–4*B*).

Medical Management

The medical management of NEC requires attention to acute care as well as long-term care. Acute care is focused on providing aggressive supportive care while attempting

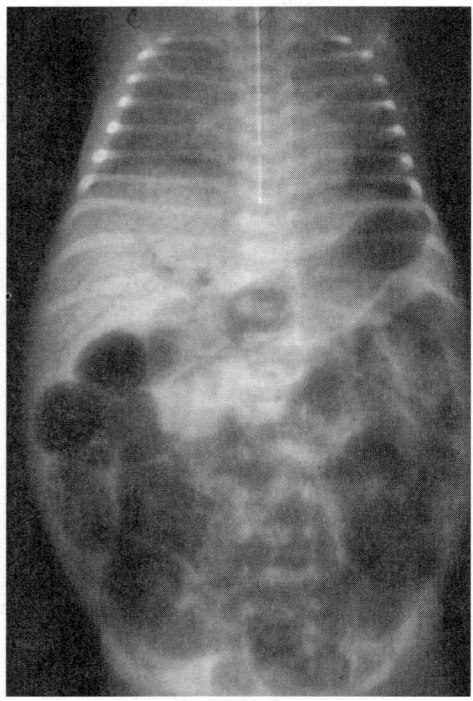

FIGURE 79–3. This radiograph displays the presence of portal gas, which is seen as linear dark streaks within the hepatic density. (Courtesy of Dr. Lalo Cabrera-Meza, Baylor College of Medicine.)

to limit the progression of disease. If the infant is receiving enteral nutrition, feedings should be discontinued and the stomach should be decompressed. Body fluids should be collected for culturing, and broad-spectrum antibiotic therapy should be initiated. Although NICUs may choose specific coverage based on their specific nursery flora, antibiotic coverage usually includes ampicillin or a cephalosporin and an aminoglycoside. In some nurseries, additional antistaphylococcal antibiotics may be given. In the event of bowel perforation, anaerobic coverage may be added by using clindamycin or metronidazole.

Because enteral nutrients are generally discontinued for 10 to 14 days, placement of central vascular lines is often necessary to deliver parenteral nutrition. Because NEC is an inflammatory process that results in substantial third space fluid loss, substantial volume support may be needed during the first 48 to 72 hours of treatment. In addition to the aggressive use of fluids and volume expanders such as albumen, pressor agents, such as dopamine, may be required to maintain the infant's blood pressure and peripheral perfusion. Because many infants with NEC develop apnea or respiratory compromise owing to abdominal distention and upward compression on the diaphragms, many require intubation and ventilatory support. Frequent monitoring of blood gases assists in management decisions concerning ventilator support as well as fluid management.

Radiographic evaluations should be repeated every 6 to 8 hours during the first 48 to 72 hours of the disease to assess whether the disease is progressing or to determine if pneumoperitoneum is present. Approximately one quarter to one half of infants with NEC require surgical intervention (Janik and Ein, 1980; Kosloske, 1985; Kosloske et al, 1980).

The most common indication for surgery is the presence of pneumoperitoneum. Other indications for surgery may be the presence of clinical deterioration despite aggressive medical therapy (Kosloske et al, 1980), the presence of portal vein gas (Cikrit et al, 1985), the presence of a persistently dilated loop of bowel on serial radiographs

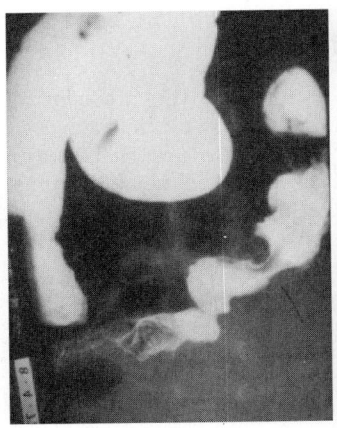

FIGURE 79–4. *A,* This radiograph demonstrates intestinal perforation as displayed by the presence of a gas lucency that lies between the hepatic density and the outer abdominal wall. *B,* This radiograph is from another infant whose bowel is perforated. In *B,* air lies anterior to the loops of intestine as well as along the right abdominal wall, where it is displacing loops of bowel medially. (Courtesy of Dr. Lalo Cabrera-Meza, Baylor College of Medicine.)

(Cikrit et al, 1985; Kosloske et al, 1980; Pokorny and Fowler, 1991), or evidence of peritonitis and gangrenous bowel by paracentesis (Ricketts, 1986). The purposes of surgery are to excise necrotic bowel, to decompress intestine, to remove necrotic material, and to preserve as much bowel length as possible. To this end, a variety of procedures are used and may be modified for use in a specific patient.

The severity of NEC usually subsides in 48 to 72 hours. Thereafter, infants are typically given antibiotics and parenteral nutrition for 10 to 14 days. Then enteral nutrition may be slowly reintroduced.

Long-Term Complications

Approximately 75% of infants who develop NEC survive. Half of surviving infants incur a long-term complication. The two most common complications are intestinal strictures and short bowel syndrome.

Because NEC is an inflammatory process that involves all layers of the bowel, fibrosis commonly forms during the healing phase. Strictures occur in infants who have been managed medically or surgically, with an incidence from 25% to 33%. Although NEC occurs most commonly in the distal ileum, strictures occur most commonly in the large bowel (Fig. 79–5), and 80% are located on the left side (Schwartz et al, 1982). These infants typically develop recurrent abdominal distention 2 to 3 weeks after recovery from NEC. The areas of stricture can be identified by barium enema examination. Surgical resection of the strictured areas is necessary. Because infants who have had surgical resection may develop strictures, contrast studies are routinely performed in these patients before definitive reanastomosis of the bowel is performed so that areas of stricture can be resected at the time of surgery.

Although the bowel may hypertrophy postoperatively

after resection, infants may develop malabsorption owing to shortened bowel length. It is estimated that infants require 25 cm of small intestine if the ileocecal valve is absent and 11 cm if it is present (Dorney et al, 1985). As outlined in the next section, medical and surgical management must address issues related to malabsorption, bacterial overgrowth, and alterations in intestinal transit.

SHORT BOWEL SYNDROME

The normal small intestine length in the term infant is 200 to 300 cm. The most common cause of short gut in the newborn is resection because of the presence of NEC,

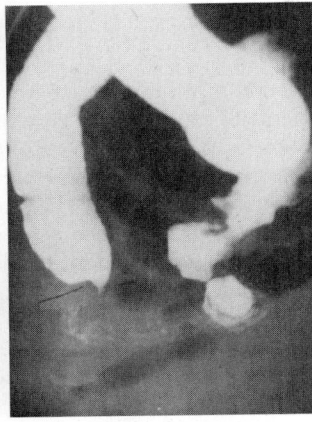

FIGURE 79–5. This barium study was obtained in an infant who had recovered from necrotizing enterocolitis and was experiencing intermittent episodes of abdominal distention when enteral feedings were given. Note that multiple areas of stricture are present. (Courtesy of Dr. Lalo Cabrera-Meza, Baylor College of Medicine.)

midgut volvulus, or congenital anomalies, such as jejunal or ileal atresia and gastroschisis. Thus, newborns most typically have short gut characterized by losses of ileum and ileocecal valve.

Reduction in bowel length results in loss of surface area for absorption of nutrients; thus, malnutrition and fluid electrolyte loss occur. Loss of the ileocecal valve results in greater disease because the absence of the valve permits colonic bacteria to reflux into the distal ileum and colonize it. Thus, outcome from intestinal resection depends on two factors: the length of bowel remaining and whether the ileocecal valve is intact. Although previous studies have indicated that infant patient survival requires the presence of 15 cm of intestine when the ileocecal valve is intact and 38 cm when it is absent (Wilmore, 1972), more recent studies during the era of the use of parenteral nutrition have indicated that newborns can survive with as little as 11 cm of ileum if the ileocecal valve is intact and 25 cm if the ileocecal valve is absent (Dorney et al, 1985). Predictions concerning survival are rarely accurate, however, because newborns have a significant potential for intestine growth and adaptation.

Intestinal adaptation after intestinal resection depends on several factors. First, the remaining bowel dilates and the mucosa hypertrophies. These two responses result in an increased absorption area per unit length of intestine. Second, as the infant grows in body length, the intestine elongates, increasing absorptive area. Third, adaptation occurs differently in ileum and jejunum. Ileal mucosa increases in size and function much more effectively than does jejunal mucosa (Dowling, 1982). Although ileal structures can perform jejunal functions, jejunal structures cannot perform ileal functions. Complete adaptation of all four of these aspects may not be completed for 2 years (Cooper et al, 1984; Grosfeld et al, 1986; Purdam and Kirby, 1991). Therefore, many neonatologists may be responsible for managing the care in only early stages of adaptation in an infant who develops short gut syndrome, and they must exercise restrained patience in caring for infants with this disease.

Treatment

The first priority of treatment must be the provision of adequate calories for growth. This must be first achieved by using parenteral nutrition to establish positive nitrogen balance. Thereafter, clinical care for the newborn must address four issues: (1) malabsorption of nutrients and fluids, (2) gastric hypersecretion, (3) bacterial overgrowth, and (4) encouragement of intestinal adaptation.

Because bile salts and fat-soluble vitamins and trace minerals are absorbed in the distal ileum, infants with short bowel syndrome develop steatorrhea and specific vitamin and mineral deficiencies. Cholestyramine, an ion-exchange resin that binds bile salts, is often used to reduce steatorrhea. Although cholestyramine reduces steatorrhea, it does not reduce fat malabsorption, and attention should still be given to nutritional needs for fat. Fats can be given either parenterally or enterally. Deficiencies of vitamins A, D, E, K, and B_{12} as well as zinc and magnesium have all been described in infants with short gut. Therefore, levels of all

of these substrates should be monitored and supplemented appropriately.

Gastric acid hypersecretion occurs after intestinal resection in adults and children (Clark, 1984). Infants have limited gastric acid secretion, and it has not been confirmed that gastric acid hypersecretion occurs in preterm infants postresection. Cimetidine and rimantadine, however, are commonly used to suppress acid secretion to prevent low pH in the duodenum, which can inactivate pancreatic enzymes or impair micelle formation.

Bacterial overgrowth can occur intermittently as a result of reflux of colonic contents into the distal ileum in the absence of an ileocecal valve. Bacterial overgrowth can also occur as the result of the presence of hypotonic, dilated bowel segments or the presence of fistulas. Bacterial overgrowth can impair fat and vitamin B_{12} absorption and depress mucosal levels of maltase, sucrose, lactase, and enterokinase (Gianella et al, 1974) resulting in malabsorption and profound diarrhea. Patients may require intermittent cyclical treatment with double antibiotic regimens, such as metronidazole and trimethoprim-sulfamethoxazole or oral vancomycin and gentamicin, to suppress episodes of bacterial overgrowth and its attendant complications.

Finally, these patients require adequate long-term nutritional support. Most infants are initially supported by parenteral nutrition supplemented by additional fluid and electrolytes to overcome losses caused by malabsorption and losses via ostomy sites. Enteral feedings are exceedingly important in providing stimulation for intestinal growth and adaptation. The physical presence of luminal nutrients stimulates mucosal growth. In addition, enteral nutrients stimulate the release of hormones and pancreatic biliary secretions, which also stimulate intestinal growth. Enteral nutrients, however, may also cause diarrhea because mucosal hypoplasia may result in inadequate processing of enteral nutrients. Therefore, most infants are initially fed small volumes of elemental formulas that are lactose-free and contain medium-chain triglycerides. As adaptation occurs, more complex standard formulas can be used to stimulate mucosal hyperplasia better (Purdum and Kirby, 1991). Fluid and electrolyte losses via ostomy sites should be replaced, and reinfusion of ostomy losses into discontiguous distal bowel segments prevents bowel atrophy while awaiting reanastomosis (Purdum and Kirby, 1991). The stool pH may be acidic if malabsorption, bacterial overgrowth, or both are present. Because acidic fecal material has a more rapid transit, the addition of sodium bicarbonate to feedings may be needed to maintain the stool pH above 6.

Although most infants can be managed medically until intestinal adaptation occurs, approximately 10% to 15% are dependent on total parenteral nutrition. A variety of surgical techniques have been used in small numbers of patients, including surgically reversing 2.5 to 4 cm of bowel to slow transit, tapering dilated loops of intestine by resection of the antimesenteric border, and performing the Bianchi procedure. Intestinal transplantation may also be an option available for a limited number of patients as transplantation technique and survival improve.

OSTEOPENIA OF PREMATURITY

Osteopenia of prematurity occurs when bone mineral content in an infant is significantly decreased compared to that seen in a fetus or infant of comparable size or gestational age. It may occur in as many as one half of all infants who have birth weights less than 1000 g and are fed human milk or formulas that have not been fortified. The term *osteopenia of prematurity* is used in place of the older term *rickets of prematurity* to identify infants who have evidence of decreased bone mineralization without the presence of classic radiologic signs of rickets (Steichen et al, 1980).

Epidemiology

Although rickets in older children is more commonly due to vitamin D deficiency, most cases of osteopenia in premature infants are due to deficiencies in calcium and phosphorus. Osteopenia occurs more frequently among infants who are born at less than 28 weeks' gestation, who require long-term parenteral nutrition, or who require medications that affect mineral metabolism. These medications can include caffeine, diuretics (especially furosemide), and corticosteroids (Atkinson, 1994). Decreases in bone mineralization also occur in infants born to diabetic mothers and in infants born small for gestational age (Minton et al, 1983; Palacios et al, 1992). High tissue levels of aluminum have also been described in a small number of children and adults with bone mineral abnormalities (Sedman et al, 1985); however, aluminum toxicity is an uncommon cause of osteopenia in preterm infants (Koo et al, 1992).

Etiology

Fetal calcium and phosphorus accretion rates rise exponentially during the third trimester in utero. During the middle of the third trimester, the fetus accretes approximately 100 to 120 mg/kg per day of calcium and 70 mg/kg per day of phosphorus (Greer and Tsang, 1985; Widdowson and Spray, 1951). Upon birth, the infant relies on the ingestion of milk to provide ongoing exogenous sources of calcium and phosphorus. Human milk is relatively low in calcium and phosphorus, however, relative to the in utero accretion rates of these minerals. Although preterm infants absorb minerals well from human milk, their net retentions of calcium and phosphorus are only approximately 20 to 30 mg/kg per day as seen in Table 79–2 (Greer and Tsang,

TABLE 79–2

Approximate Mineral Retention for Premature Infants on Typical Feeding Regimens (at 160 mL/kg/day)

	Calcium Retention (mg/kg/day)	Phosphorus Retention (mg/kg/day)
In utero	100–120	70
Human milk	30	20
Fortified human milk	100	70
Term formula	40	40
Preterm formula	100	90

Modified from Greer and Tsang, 1985; Schanler and Abrams, 1995; and Schanler and Rifka, 1994.

1985). Although these absorption rates are adequate for most term infants, they are far below the in utero accretion rates of these minerals and thus are inadequate for premature infants.

Formulas designed for term infants—including special formulas containing soy-protein and casein—have greater amounts of calcium and phosphorus than human milk. The minerals in these formulas are not absorbed as well as those from human milk, however, and the net retention of these minerals by premature infants remains far below in utero accretion rates (Greer and Tsang, 1985). Thus, bone density lags behind in utero levels when premature infants are fed formulas designed for term infants (Steichen et al, 1980). Therefore, without mineral supplementation, neither human milk nor term-infant formulas can meet the calcium and phosphorus needs of very-low-birth-weight infants.

Currently, several commercial mineral supplements and formulas are marketed for use for premature infants. When preterm infants are fed these products, their net calcium retention is comparable to that achieved in utero (Abrams et al, 1991; Schanler and Abrams, 1995). Because products formulated before 1990 often contained sediment from the precipitation of minerals (Bhatia and Fomon, 1983), currently marketed products now use stabilizers such as carrageenan to improve mineral solubility. Nonetheless, solubility problems as well as attempts to avoid high renal solute load and hyperosmolarity provide practical limits to the amount of minerals that can be added to formula or human milk fortifiers.

Calcium and phosphorus delivery is also impaired in premature infants who receive parenteral nutrition. In a manner similar to that for formulas, parenteral nutrition solutions have also been reformulated to permit greater mineral solubility. Studies have shown that these newly formulated parenteral nutrition sources now provide net retentions of 70 to 80 mg/kg per day of calcium and phosphorus, resulting in increased bone mineralization when compared to solutions containing less minerals (Prestridge et al, 1993).

In general, the provision of 400 IU per day of vitamin D to the orally fed premature infant is adequate to maintain normal vitamin D levels (Cooke et al, 1990). Although lower intakes may suffice, vitamin D intakes that exceed 400 IU per day are unlikely to be beneficial and have the potential to cause vitamin D toxicity. Moreover, it is not currently confirmed that calcium absorption in premature infants is vitamin D dependent. Because infants exhibit similar rates of fractional calcium absorption regardless of the amount of vitamin D ingested, it has been postulated that calcium intake is achieved via a passive, vitamin D–independent pathway (Bronner et al, 1992). Furthermore, plasma 1,25-dihydroxyvitamin D concentrations are not related to calcium absorption in premature infants (Cooke et al, 1990). No evidence of clinical benefit was found by providing 2000 IU of vitamin compared to 400 IU per day to premature infants (Evans et al, 1989).

Differential Diagnosis

Osteopenia of prematurity is generally suspected when an elevated alkaline phosphatase activity or lowered serum phosphorus is documented during regular monitoring of these biochemical parameters. As detailed in Chapter 78, routine monitoring should be performed for infants who are receiving parenteral nutrition or who are receiving feedings that do not provide adequate calcium and phosphorus. Although plasma concentrations of biochemical markers are not highly sensitive and specific for osteopenia of prematurity, values for alkaline phosphatase exceeding 800 IU/L or serum phosphorus values less than 3.5 mg/dL may be indicative of the presence of significant osteopenia. Moderate elevations in alkaline phosphatase (400 to 800 IU/L) are commonly seen in rapidly growing premature infants, and when these elevations are present, treatment should be limited to careful monitoring of mineral intake to insure that it is sufficient.

Although laboratory testing can be useful to suggest that osteopenia is present, biochemical testing is not definitive, and the correlation between radiologic changes and alkaline phosphatase activity is poor (Lyon et al, 1987). Premature infants with normal bone radiographs and normal bone growth can have significant elevations of alkaline phosphatase activity (Walters et al, 1986). A condition in which extremely elevated alkaline phosphatase activity is present without identifiable pathology also has been described (Kraut et al, 1985). In some circumstances, significant osteopenia can exist with normal biochemical values as well.

The presence of osteopenia can be more definitively assessed by direct radiologic or histologic evaluation by using a standard radiograph, a bone mineral densitometer, or a bone biopsy. Bone biopsies are rarely performed in infants. Histologic studies from the ribs of premature infants with clinical diagnoses of rickets, however, have confirmed the presence of both osteomalacia and osteoporosis (Oppenheimer and Snodgrass, 1980). Bone densitometry using single-photon absorptiometry or newer whole-body techniques of bone mineral measurement such as dual-energy x-ray absorptiometry are highly sensitive for small amounts of bone deficiency. Although these techniques are widely used in adults, they are generally reserved for use as research tools for pediatric and neonatal evaluation.

Therefore, most evaluations for bone demineralization in premature infants with biochemical evidence of osteopenia are performed using standard radiographs of the long bones or ribs (Fig. 79–6). Although useful, this technique does not detect mild osteopenia (James et al, 1986). A standard score has been developed to characterize radiographic findings of the wrist in premature infants (Koo, 1983). Decreased lucency of the cortical bone with or without epiphyseal changes is characteristic of significant osteopenia. Although the presence of a fracture can be the presenting sign of osteopenia of prematurity, most infants with decreased bone mineralization, including some with severe rickets, do not have fractures.

Evaluation of vitamin D or parathyroid hormone status is generally not necessary in infants with osteopenia of prematurity. Sophisticated biochemical testing, including measurement of markers of bone formation and resorption, is not widely available.

When infants with chronic pulmonary or cardiac disease are given calcium-wasting diuretics, hypercalciuria and nephrocalcinosis may develop (Venkataraman et al, 1983).

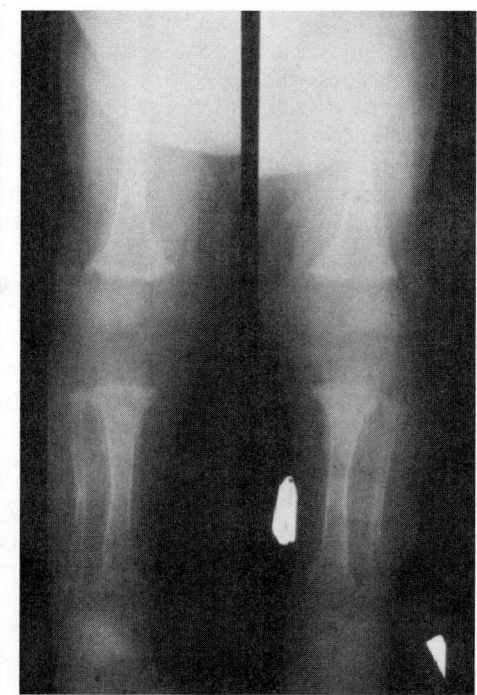

FIGURE 79–6. Radiographs of the lower extremities of a preterm infant with osteopenia. Note the *washed-out* appearance of the bones of the lower extremities and feet because of loss of bone density. In addition, there is *periostitis* present on the left. The distal ends of the lower extremities appear widened and frayed.

A 24-hour urine specimen may be used to demonstrate the presence of hypercalciuria, although urinary calcium excretion is generally greater in premature infants than in older children (Abrams et al, 1994). If nephrocalcinosis is suspected, an abdominal ultrasound scan may demonstrate the presence of nephrocalcinosis.

Management

The mainstay of therapy for osteopenia of prematurity is the provision of adequate calcium and phosphorus to permit mineralization of bone. It is important that supplementation include both calcium and phosphorus. Provision of supplemental calcium without phosphorus may not resolve the mineral deficit and can worsen hypercalciuria or cause hypercalcemia (Rowe and Carey, 1987). For most infants, this goal can be achieved by feeding one of several commercially available high mineral–containing formulas or human milk containing fortification products. For infants who have lactose intolerance or cow milk protein sensitivity, small amounts of supplemental calcium and phosphorus may be added directly to human milk or formula. For infants who are receiving parenteral nutrition, calcium and phosphorus content can be maximized using a variety of techniques to avoid formation of precipitates (Schanler and Rifka, 1994). Although it is suggested that using a non–calcium-losing diuretic such as a thiazide diuretic may improve osteopenia, treatment for hypercalciuria and nephrocalcinosis in premature infants has not been evaluated.

Most premature infants with osteopenia respond to high levels of enteral or parenteral mineral supplementation by demonstrating an improvement in radiographic findings or biochemical markers (or both) over several weeks. Infants with severe cholestasis or other chronic illnesses, however, may need long-term high-dose supplementation of minerals. Rarely an older premature infant with cholestasis or other diseases limiting production of the active forms of vitamin D may also benefit from therapy with 25-hydroxyvitamin D or 1,25-dihydroxyvitamin D.

A conservative orthopedic approach is advocated for premature infants with fractures secondary to osteopenia. A good outcome is generally expected with attention to positioning and use of simple splints (Koo et al, 1989).

Prognosis

The outlook for healing of established osteopenia depends on its cause (i.e., the reason that mineral intake could not be optimized). Osteopenia associated with an extremely elevated alkaline phosphatase activity (>1200 IU/L) has been associated with a deficit in body length at 18 months compared with infants with less elevated alkaline phosphatase activity (Lucas et al, 1989). The potential for catch-up growth beyond 18 months is unknown.

A catch-up phase of mineralization can occur late in the 1st year and 2nd year of life in premature infants such that bone mineralization levels in these infants are comparable to those of term infants (Abrams et al, 1989; Horsman et al, 1989; Schanler et al, 1992). A more rapid catch-up may occur by the use of high mineral–containing formulas after hospital discharge (Chan, 1993). Specific long-term benefit to this approach remains to be identified. The effects of prematurity on adult bone mineralization and the risk of adult osteoporosis are also unknown.

Prevention

Because osteopenia of prematurity is generally caused by poor mineral delivery, its occurrence can be decreased by close attention to the use of these minerals in enteral and parenteral nutrition. Thus, parenteral nutrition should be initiated shortly after birth to provide intakes of 60 to 80 mg/kg per day of calcium and phosphorus. Human milk–fed infants should be supplemented with mineral fortifiers, and formula-fed infants should receive a high mineral–containing formula designed for premature infants.

Although optimal postnatal age to discontinue these increased mineral intakes has not been identified, they are generally used until the preterm infant achieves somatic weights of 1.8 to 2.0 kg. Longer-term use of high mineral–containing formulas and human milk fortification may be considered for infants who have chronic illness or whose birth weight was less than 1000 g.

COW MILK PROTEIN ALLERGY
Definition

Cow milk protein allergy (CMPA) has been defined as an adverse reaction after the ingestion of cow milk owing to immunologic hypersensitivity to milk protein(s) (Hill et al,

1986). Adverse reactions include a wide range of clinical expression, including gastrointestinal symptoms such as colitis and protein-losing enteropathy and more poorly defined symptoms including bronchitis, colic, and atopic dermatitis (Odze et al, 1995; Walther and Kootstra, 1983).

Epidemiology

The frequency of CMPA ranges from 2% to 7% (Host et al, 1988). It occurs more frequently in infants fed cow milk or a cow milk–based formula than in those fed human milk. Nonetheless, it does occur in approximately 0.5% of breast-fed infants (Jacobsson and Lindberg, 1979) as a result of maternal ingestion of cow milk protein and transfer of antigenic proteins to human milk (Jacobsson et al, 1985).

Although the specific cause of CMPA is unknown, it frequently displays a familial incidence. For example, it has been estimated that a child with a first-degree affected relative has a 30% risk of developing CMPA (Gerrard et al, 1967). Acute infectious gastroenteritis has also been identified as a risk factor for developing CMPA (Italian Collaborative Working Study, 1988) because of the increased absorption of macromolecules during an acute infection (Stintzing et al, 1986). Several studies have also suggested that ingestion of cow milk formula in the first weeks of life may increase the incidence of allergic symptoms (Host et al, 1988); however, this effect has not been confirmed by others (Lindfors and Enocksson, 1988).

Differential Diagnosis

Because a large number of symptoms have been attributed to CMPA, clinical evaluation for infectious causes of gastroenteritis or respiratory symptoms may be necessary. The diagnosis of CMPA is confirmed when clinical improvement occurs when a milk-free diet is given and relapse occurs when a milk challenge is given (Goldman et al, 1963). Thus, there are no specific biochemical tests for CMPA. Some investigators have found evaluation of immunoglobulins to be helpful but not diagnostic (Italian Collaborative Working Study, 1988). The presence of cow milk–specific IgE and an index of lymphocyte stimulation with beta-lactoglobulin is the most sensitive (88%) and specific (67%) test for predicting whether a clinical reaction to cow milk protein will occur (Tainio and Savilahti, 1990). Jejunal biopsies are not usually necessary to diagnose CMPA in newborns (Sumithran and Lyngkaran, 1977). If biopsy specimens are obtained, however, they demonstrate partial or total villous atrophy or an increase in the presence of eosinophils in the lamina propria, epithelial mucosa, or muscularis mucosa (Savilahti and Verkasalo, 1984). Biopsies may be useful to demonstrate the absence of parasites, ova, or crypt architectural abnormalities (Odze et al, 1995).

Management

The management of CMPA is the removal of cow milk protein from the diet. Some advocate the use of soy protein–based formulas as an initial therapeutic technique (Businco et al, 1992). As many as 30% of infants who have

CMPA, however, exhibit allergy to soy protein (Kleinman et al, 1992; Powell, 1978). Thus, it is currently recommended that soy-based formulas not be used for treatment of CMPA (American Academy of Pediatrics, 1983).

Hypoallergenic formulas contain hydrolyzed protein to decrease their allergic potentials. Casein hydrolysate formulas are more extensively hydrolyzed and cause less allergic reactions (Businco et al, 1989; Wahn et al, 1992). On rare occasions, infants may remain allergic to these formulas, and an elemental diet consisting of free amino acids as the protein source may be needed (Odze et al, 1995).

Breast-fed infants with CMPA usually improve when dairy products are removed from the mother's diet (Barau and Dupont, 1994). If severe colitis persists in breast-fed infants, however, hypoallergenic or elemental formulas may be necessary. Sensitivity to cow milk protein decreases with age. As many as 28% of children with CMPA are tolerant of milk protein by 2 years of age and 78% by 6 years of age (Bishop et al, 1990).

GASTROESOPHAGEAL REFLUX
Physiology

The lower esophageal sphincter (LES) is a 1- to 2-cm segment of the distal esophagus that is functionally identified as an area of high pressure. Its primary function is to prevent reflux of gastric contents into the distal esophagus. Infants frequently regurgitate, and it would superficially appear that gastrointestinal reflux (GER) is related to poor LES tone. Multiple factors affect LES pressure, however, including the intrinsic muscle tone of the sphincter; gastric distention; acute or chronic brain injury; position of the sphincter; angle of the indentation of the esophagus at entry of the stomach; and factors that alter sphincter circumference, such as edema, increases in intra-abdominal pressure, and delayed gastric emptying.

Three types of decreases in LES tone have been identified to occur in infants: persistently low sphincter tone, episodes of basal tone drift, and acute episodes of transient relaxation of sphincter tone. Basal tone in healthy term infants is lower than that seen in adults. Low basal LES tone, however, is found only in a small number of infants who have GER. Esophageal inflammation has been identified only among infants whose LES tone is less than 5 mm Hg, and low basal LES tone is seen in only 20% of infants who have documented esophagitis (Dodds et al, 1982). Sondheimer (1980) has shown that some episodes of reflux may occur when the basal tone of the LES gradually drifts downward during sleep. The most common event associated with reflux is the transient LES relaxation. Transient LES relaxations occur when the LES relaxes to the level of gastric pressure for 5 to 35 seconds. These episodes occur five to six times hourly in the healthy adult but are increased in occurrence in children and adults who have esophagitis (Cucchiara et al, 1988).

Presentation

In non-newborns, GER is clinically suspected when infants exhibit poor weight gain owing to regurgitation, nonspecific irritability, and apnea. Because newborns cannot verbalize pain, GER may also present as recurrent fussiness, feeding aversion, bradycardia, or cyanotic episodes. There is an increased incidence of GER in infants who have central nervous system abnormalities, bronchopulmonary dysplasia, cystic fibrosis, and esophageal atresia (Bendig et al, 1982; Dudley and Phelan, 1976; Lew et al, 1981). In addition, other NICU therapies may alter normal physiologic regulation and anatomic relationships and predispose an infant to developing GER. Xanthines, used to treat apnea, reduce LES tone and increase gastric acid secretion (Berquist et al, 1984; Vandenplas et al, 1986). The use of orogastric tubes may reduce LES pressure (Berezin et al, 1986). Increasing intra-abdominal pressure by delivering chest physiotherapy may also reduce LES pressure and increase the occurrence of reflux (Newell et al, 1987). There is also an association of GER with respiratory symptoms. GER occurs more commonly among infants with bronchopulmonary dysplasia and who have experienced acute life-threatening events (Gioffre et al, 1987; Veereman-Wauters et al, 1991). Moreover, the instillation of acidic agents into the distal esophagus can induce bronchospasm (Herve et al, 1986). The strong temporal association of GER and respiratory disease, however, has not been shown to be a causal one, and the mechanism for this association has not been delineated.

Evaluation

Controversy currently surrounds issues related to diagnostic testing for GER. Several techniques are available. Because of the lack of agreement concerning diagnostic techniques, their use is generally reserved for infants whose symptoms are relatively severe.

The barium swallow is the first study that should be done to evaluate GER. It is a poor method to demonstrate the presence of GER; rather it is used to confirm the presence of normal esophageal, gastric, and intestinal anatomy because congenital anomalies in any of these structures may cause mild episodes of vomiting. Because this study is not performed under physiologic conditions (i.e., the patient is supine on a cold table, often crying or struggling, and provocative maneuvers such as abdominal compression may be used) and because the patient is monitored fluoroscopically for a brief period (generally <5 minutes), the frequency of GER demonstrated during these evaluations has little relationship with the presence of real reflux disease.

The pH probe is the most commonly used diagnostic test for evaluating GER. Testing is done by positioning a pH probe in the distal esophagus. Placement of the probe is documented fluoroscopically or by estimation, using the Strobel formula (Strobel et al, 1979). Typically, pH is monitored for 20 to 24 hours. The neonatologist should be aware that interpretation of pH probe studies is limited by several factors. First, the ability to detect pH changes may be altered by the anatomic location of the probe. If the probe is located too proximal to the gastroesophageal junction, it may not detect reflux adequately; conversely, if it is located too distally, it inappropriately identifies the presence of acid. Second, the ability to detect acidosis up to 2 hours postprandially in infants is limited because milk buffers any acid contained in refluxate. Thus, many centers feed apple juice (pH 4) to maintain a more accurate ability to detect the presence of acidosis postprandially. Third, variability of infant position may alter variability of pH probe results (Hampton et al, 1990).

Because all healthy individuals have GER, a variety of techniques for scoring pH probe studies have been proposed (Orenstein et al, 1987a; Sondheimer, 1980; Sutphen and Dillard, 1986; Vandenplas and Sacre-Smits, 1987). In general, the number of acid reflux episodes, the average duration of such episodes, and the overall proportion of time that the pH is less than 4 are quantified.

Technetium scintigraphy can be used to monitor for reflux, pulmonary aspiration, or both. Its ability to detect episodes is limited because it is performed during a single feeding for a 2- to 3-hour postprandial period. Endoscopy and esophageal manometry are rarely used in the neonatal age group. Because of the limitations of the diagnostic techniques for newborns, many gastroenterologists proceed to a trial of therapy before extensive diagnostic studies are performed.

Treatment

Conservative treatment for GER includes positioning and dietary changes. A decade ago, infants with GER were positioned upright supine. This position for preterm newborns may place them at risk for airway obstruction if the head drops down on the chest (Orenstein et al, 1983). Therefore, placing infants prone or on their side may be safer and equally effective (Orenstein and Whitington, 1983). In a large controlled study, however, head elevation showed no benefit over the flat prone position (Orenstein, 1990). A supine position improves gastric emptying and decreases aspiration.

Because gastric distention may contribute to the occurrence of GER, infants may experience less GER if they are fed smaller volumes more frequently. Because reflux occurs more typically postprandially, however, there may be an increased risk for GER incurred by this practice. Another dietary manipulation is to add rice cereal to the milk. Although this therapy does not reduce reflux, it does decrease emesis (Bailey et al, 1987; Orenstein et al, 1987b).

Because no pharmacologic agent currently used can reduce the occurrence of transient LES relaxations, prokinetic agents that improve gastric emptying or esophageal sphincter tone have been used to reduce the symptoms of GER. Bethanecol, a cholinergic drug, increases LES basal tone and overall forcefulness of esophageal peristalsis (Sondheimer and Arnold, 1986); however, it has not demonstrated consistent efficacy in clinical trials (Orenstein et al, 1986; Sondheimer et al, 1984), and it has a potential for exacerbating bronchospasm, which limits its use in infants with bronchopulmonary dysplasia. Metoclopramide, a dopamine antagonist, also increases gastric emptying and augments LES basal tone but causes central nervous system side effects, an important limitation for infants recovering from respiratory distress syndrome who are trying to establish normal sucking skills. Cisapride, a noncholinergic non-antidopaminergic agent, has been approved in tablet form by the Food and Drug Adminstration for use in the United States, but liquid suspensions are not approved for outpatient use. Therefore, experience with this new drug is currently limited. Although antacids and histamine receptor antagonists, such as cimetidine and rimantadine, are used in children, gastric acid secretion in preterm newborns is relatively low (Hyman et al, 1985), and these agents may have limited benefit.

Surgical therapy is reserved for infants who have severe GER. The most commonly used procedure is the Nissen fundoplication. Postoperative complications are common (Byrne et al, 1982; Spitz and Kirtane, 1985; Wilkinson et al, 1987) and include failure of the wrap, overtightness of the wrap, and delayed gastric emptying. Because tincture of time provides improvement of GER in most patients, consideration should be given to the use of transpyloric feedings on a temporary basis in this population of infants to obviate the need for surgery.

REFERENCES

Necrotizing Enterocolitis

Abrams CA, Phillips LL, Berkowitz C, et al: Hazards of over-concentrated milk formula. JAMA 232:1136, 1975.

Barlow B, Santulli TV, Heird WC, et al: An experimental study of acute neonatal enterocolitis—the importance of breast milk. J Pediatr Surg 9:587, 1974.

Bell JM, Ternberg JL, Feigin RD, et al: Neonatal necrotizing enterocolitis: Therapeutic decisions based upon clinical staging. Ann Surg 187:1, 1978.

Berseth CL: Early feeding enhances maturation of the preterm small intestine. J Pediatr 120:947, 1992.

Book S, Herbst J: Intra-arterial infusions and intestinal necrosis in the rabbit: Potential hazards of umbilical artery injections of ampicillin, glucose, and sodium bicarbonate. Pediatrics 65:1145, 1980.

Book LS, Herbst JJ, Jung AL: Comparison of fast- and slow-feeding rate schedules to the development of necrotizing enterocolitis. J Pediatr 89:463, 1976.

Caplan MS, Sun XM, Hsueh W, et al: Role of platelet activating factor and tumor necrosis factor-alpha in neonatal necrotizing enterocolitis. J Pediatr 116:960, 1990.

Cashore WJ, Peter G, Lauermann M, et al: Clostridia colonization and clostridial toxin in neonatal necrotizing enterocolitis. J Pediatr 98:308, 1981.

Cikrit D, Mastandrea J, Grosfeld JL, et al: Significance of portal vein in necrotizing enterocolitis: Analysis of 53 cases. J Pediatr Surg 20:425, 1985.

Cone TE: History of the Care and Feeding of the Premature Infant. New York, Little, Brown, 1985.

Crissinger K, Granger D: Mucosal injury induced by ischemia and reperfusion in the piglet intestine: Influences of age and feeding. Gastroenterology 97:920, 1989.

Crissinger K, Grisham J, Granger D: Developmental biology of oxidant-producing enzymes and antioxidants in the piglet intestine. Pediatr Res 25:612, 1989.

Dunn L, Hulman S, Weiner J, et al: Beneficial effects of early hypocaloric enteral feeding on neonatal gastrointestinal function: Preliminary report of a randomized trial. J Pediatr 112:622, 1988.

Egan EA, Mantilla G, Nelson RM, et al: A prospective controlled trial of oral kanamycin in the prevention of neonatal necrotizing enterocolitis. J Pediatr 89:467, 1976.

Eibl M, Wolf HM, Furnkranz H, et al: Prevention of necrotizing enterocolitis in low birth weight infants by IgA-IgG feeding. N Engl J Med 319:1, 1988.

Ernst JA, Williams JM, Glick MR, et al: Osmolality of substances used in the intensive care nursery. Pediatrics 72:347, 1983.

Gastinne H, Wolff M, Delatour F, et al: A controlled trial in intensive care units of selective decontamination of the digestive tract with nonabsorbable antibiotics. N Engl J Med 326:594, 1992.

Goldman HI: Feeding and necrotizing enterocolitis. Am J Dis Child 134:553, 1980.

Grulee CG, Sanford HN, Schwartz H: Breast and artificially fed infants: A study of the age incidence in the morbidity and mortality in twenty thousand cases. JAMA 104:1986, 1935.

Janik JS, Ein SH: Peritoneal drainage under local anesthesia for necrotizing enterocolitis (NEC) perforation: A second look. J Pediatr Surg 15:565, 1980.

Kliegman RM, Hack M, Jones P, et al: Epidemiologic study of necrotizing enterocolitis among low-birth-weight infants: Absence of identifiable risk factors. J Pediatr 100:440, 1982.

Kosloske AM: Surgery of necrotizing enterocolitis. World J Surg 9:277, 1985.

Kosloske AM, Papile L-A, Burstein J: Indications for operation in acute necrotizing enterocolitis of the neonate. Surgery 87:502, 1980.

Kubes P, Ibbotson G, Russell J, et al: Role of platelet-activating factor in ischemia/reperfusion-induced leukocyte adherence. Am J Physiol 259:G300, 1990.

La Gamma EF, Ostertag SG, Birenbaum H: Failure of delayed oral feedings to prevent necrotizing enterocolitis. Am J Dis Child 139:385, 1985.

Leake R, Thanopoulos B, Nielberg R: Hyperviscosity syndrome associated with necrotizing enterocolitis. Am J Dis Child 129:1192, 1975.

LeBlanc M, D'Cruz C, Pate K: Necrotizing enterocolitis can be caused by polycythemic hyperviscosity in the newborn dog. J Pediatr 105:804, 1984.

Lucas A, Cole TJ: Breast milk and neonatal necrotizing enterocolitis. Lancet 336:1519, 1990.

MacKendrick W, Hill N, Hsueh W, et al: Increase in plasma platelet activating factor levels in enterally fed preterm infants. Biol Neonate 64:89, 1993.

McKeown RE, Marsh TD, Amaranth U, et al: Role of delayed feeding and of feeding increments in necrotizing enterocolitis. J Pediatr 121:764, 1992.

Meetze WH, Valentine C, McGuigan JE, et al: Gastrointestinal priming prior to full enteral nutrition in very low birth weight infants. J Pediatr Gastroenterol Nutr 15:163, 1992.

Mizrahi A, Barlow O, Berdon W, et al: Necrotizing enterocolitis in premature infants. J Pediatr 66:697, 1965.

Nowicki P, Oh W, Yao A, et al: Effect of polycythemia on gastrointestinal blood flow and oxygenation in piglets. Am J Physiol 247:G220, 1984.

Pokorny WJ, Fowler CL: Isoperistalic intestinal lengthening for short bowel syndrome. Surg Gynecol Obstet 172:39, 1991.

Ricketts RR: The surgical role of paracentesis in the management of infants with necrotizing enterocolitis. Am Surg 52:61, 1986.

Ricketts RR: Surgical treatment of necrotizing enterocolitis and the short bowel syndrome. Clin Perinatol 21:14, 1994.

Santulli TV, Schullinger JN, Heird WC, et al: Acute necrotizing enterocolitis in infancy: A review of 64 cases. Pediatrics 55:376, 1975.

Schwartz MZ, Hayden CK, Richardson CJ, et al: A prospective evaluation of intestinal stenosis following necrotizing enterocolitis. J Pediatr Surg 17:764, 1982.

Smith MF, Borriello SP, Clayden GS, et al: Clinical and bacteriological findings in necrtizing enterocolitis: A controlled study. J Infect 2:23, 1980.

Touloukian R, Kadar A, Spencer R: The gastrointestinal complications of neonatal umbilical venous exchange transfusion: A clinical and experimental study. Pediatrics 51:36, 1973.

Tyson J, deSa D, Moore S: Thromboatheromatous complications of umbilical arterial catheterization in the newborn period. Arch Dis Child 51:744, 1976.

Walsh MC, Kliegman RM: Necrotizing enterocolitis: Treatment based on staging criteria. Pediatr Clin North Am 33:179, 1986.

Wilson R, delPortillo M, Schmidt E, et al: Risk factors for necrotizing enterocolitis in infants weighing more than 2,000 grams at birth: A case-controlled study. Pediatrics 71:19, 1983.

Short Bowel Syndrome

Bianchi A: Intestinal loop lengthening—a technique of increasing small intestinal length. J Pediatr Surg 15:145, 1980.

Clark JH: Management of short bowel syndrome in the high-risk infant. Clin Perinatol 11:189, 1984.

Cooper A, Floyd TF, Ross AJ III, et al: Morbidity and mortality of short-bowel syndrome acquired in infants: An update. J Pediatr Surg 19:711, 1984.

Dorney SFA, Ament ME, Berquist WE, et al: Improved survival in very short small bowel of infants with use of long-term parenteral nutrition. J Pediatr 107:521, 1985.

Dowling RH: Small bowel adaptation and its regulation. Scand J Gastroenterol 17:53, 1982.

Gianella RA, Rout WR, Toskes PP: Jejunal brush border injury and impaired sugar and amino acid uptake in the blind loop syndrome. Gastroenterology 67:965, 1974.

Grosfeld JL, Rescoria FJ, West KW: Short bowel syndrome in infancy and childhood: Analysis of survival in 60 patients. Am J Surg 151:41, 1986.

Purdum PP III, Kirby DF: Short-bowel syndrome: A review of the role of nutrition support. JPEN J Parenter Enteral Nutr 15:93, 1991.

Wilmore DW: Factors correlating with a successful outcome following extensive intestinal resection in newborn infants. J Pediatr 80:88, 1972.

Osteopenia of Prematurity

Abrams SA, Esteban NV, Vieira NE, Yergey AL: Dual tracer stable isotopic assessment of calcium absorption and endogenous fecal excretion in low birth weight infants. Pediatr Res 29:615, 1991.

Abrams SA, Schanler RJ, Tsang RC, Garza C: Bone mineralization in former very low birth weight infants fed either human milk or commercial formula: One-year follow-up. J Pediatr 114:1041, 1989.

Abrams SA, Yergey AL, Schanler RJ, et al: Hypercalciuria in premature infants receiving high mineral-containing diets. J Pediatr Gastroenterol Nutr 18:20, 1994.

Atkinson SA: Calcium and phosphorus needs of premature infants. Nutrition 10:66, 1994.

Bhatia J, Fomon SJ: Formulas for premature infants: Fate of the calcium and phosphorus. Pediatrics 72:37, 1983.

Bronner F, Salle BL, Putet G, et al: Net calcium absorption in premature infants: Results of 103 metabolic balance studies. Am J Clin Nutr 56:1037, 1992.

Chan GM: Growth and bone mineral status of discharged very low birth weight infants fed different formulas or human milk. J Pediatr 123:439, 1993.

Cooke R, Hollis B, Conner C, et al: Vitamin D and mineral metabolism in the very low birth weight infant receiving 400 IU of vitamin D. J Pediatr 116:423, 1990.

Evans JR, Allen AC, Stinson DA, et al: Effect of high-dose vitamin D supplementation on radiographically detectable bone disease of very low birth weight infants. J Pediatr 115:779, 1989.

Forbes GB: Some remarks on bone mineralization. J Pediatr 113:167, 1988.

Greer FR, Tsang RC: Calcium, phosphorus, magnesium, and vitamin D requirements for the preterm infant. *In* Tsang RC (Ed): Vitamin and Mineral Requirements in Preterm Infants. New York, Marcel Dekker, 1985, pp 99–136.

Horsman A, Ryan SW, Congdon PJ, et al: Bone mineral content and body size 65 to 100 weeks postconception in preterm and full term infants. Arch Dis Child 64:1579, 1989.

James JR, Congdon PJ, Truscott J, et al: Osteopenia of prematurity. Arch Dis Child 61:871, 1986.

Koo WW, Gupta JM, Nayanar VV, et al: Skeletal changes in premature infants. Arch Dis Child 57:447, 1982.

Koo WW, Krug-Wispe SK, Succop P, et al: Sequential serum aluminum and urine aluminum:creatinine ratio and tissue aluminum loading in infants with fractures/rickets. Pediatrics 89:877, 1992.

Koo WW, Sherman R, Succop PM, et al: Fractures and rickets in very low birth weight infants: Conservative management and outcome. J Pediatr Orthop 9:326, 1989.

Kraut JR, Metrick M, Maxwell NR, Kaplan MM: Isoenzyme studies in transient hyperphosphatasemia of infancy: Ten new cases and a review of the literature. Am J Dis Child 139:736, 1985.

Lucas A, Brooke OG, Baker BA, et al: High alkaline phosphatase activity and growth in preterm neonates. Arch Dis Child 64:902, 1989.

Lyon AJ, McIntosh N, Wheeler K, Williams JE: Radiological rickets in extremely low birthweight infants. Pediatr Radiol 17:56, 1987.

Minton SD, Steichen JJ, Tsang RC: Decreased bone mineral content in small-for-gestational-age infants compared with appropriate-for-gestational-age infants: Normal serum 25-hydroxyvitamin D and decreasing parathyroid hormone. Pediatrics 71:383, 1983.

Oppenheimer SJ, Snodgrass GJ: Neonatal rickets: Histopathology and quantitative bone changes. Arch Dis Child 55:945, 1980.

Palacios J, Rodriguez S, Rodriguez JI: Intrauterine long bone growth in small-for-gestational-age infants. Eur J Pediatr 151:304, 1992.

Prestridge LL, Schanler RJ, Shulman RJ, et al: Effect of parenteral calcium and phosphorus therapy on mineral retention and bone mineral content in very low birth weight infants. J Pediatr 122:761, 1993.

Rowe JC, Carey DE: Phosphorus deficiency syndrome in very low birth weight infants. Pediatr Clin North Am 34:997, 1987.

Schanler RJ, Abrams SA: Can we meet intrauterine macromineral accretion rate postnatally in low birth weight infants fed fortified human milk? J Pediatr 126:441, 1995.

Schanler RJ, Burns PA, Abrams SA, Garza C: Bone mineralization outcomes in human milk-fed preterm infants. Pediatr Res 31:583, 1992.

Schanler RJ, Rifka M: Calcium, phosphorus and magnesium needs for the low-birth-weight infant. Acta Paediatr 405(suppl):111, 1994.

Sedman AB, Klein GL, Merritt RJ, et al: Evidence of aluminum loading in infants receiving intravenous therapy. N Engl J Med 312:1337, 1985.

Steichen J, Gratton T, Tsang R: Osteopenia of prematurity: The cause and possible treatment. J Pediatr 96:528, 1980.

Venkataraman PS, Han BK, Tsang RC, et al: Secondary hyperparathyroidism and bone disease in infants receiving long-term furosemide therapy. Am J Dis Child 137:1157, 1983.

Walters EG, Murphy JF, Henry P, et al: Plasma alkaline phosphatase activity and its relation to rickets in pre-term infants. Ann Clin Biochem 23:652, 1986.

Widdowson E, Spray C: Chemical development in utero. Arch Dis Child 26:205, 1951.

Ziegler EE, O'Donnell AM, Nelson SE, Fomon SJ: Body composition of the reference fetus. Growth 40:329, 1976.

Cow Milk Protein Allergy

American Academy of Pediatrics, Committee on Nutrition: Soy-protein formulas: Recommendations for use in infant feeding. Pediatrics 72:359, 1983.

Barau E, Dupont C: Allergy to cow's milk proteins in mother's milk or in hydrolyzed cow's milk infant formulas as assessed by intestinal permeability measurements. Allergy 49:295, 1994.

Bishop JM, Hill DJ, Hosking CS: Natural history of cow milk allergy: Clinical outcome. J Pediatr 116:862, 1990.

Businco L, Bruno G, Biampietro PG, Cantani A: Allergenicity and nutritional adequacy of soy protein formulas. J Pediatr 121:S21, 1992.

Businco L, Cantai A, Lohghi A, Giampietro PG: Anaphylactic reactions to a cow's milk whey protein hydrolysate (Alfa-Ré, Nestlé) in infants with cow's milk allergy. Ann Allergy 62:333, 1989.

Cow's milk allergy in the first year of life: An Italian Collaborative Study. Acta Paediatr Scand Suppl 348:1, 1988.

Gerrard JW, Lubos MC, Hardy LW, et al: Milk allergy: Clinical picture and familial incidence. Can Med Assoc J 97:780, 1967.

Goldman AS, Anderson DW, Sellers WA, et al: Milk allergy: I. Oral challenge with milk and isolated milk proteins in allergic children. Pediatrics 32:425, 1963.

Hill DJ, Firer MA, Shelton MJ, Hosking CS: Manifestations of milk allergy in infancy: Clinical and immunologic findings. J Pediatr 109:270, 1986.

Host A, Husby S, Osterballe O: A prospective study of cow's milk allergy in exclusively breast-fed infants. Acta Paediatr Scand 77:663, 1988.

Jacobsson I, Lindberg T: A prospective study of cow's milk protein intolerance in Swedish infants. Acta Paediatr Scand 68:853, 1979.

Jacobsson I, Lindberg T, Benediktsson B, Hansson BG: Dietary bovine β-lactoglobulin is transferred to human breast milk. Acta Paediatr Scand 76:453, 1985.

Kleinman RE: Cow milk allergy in infancy and hypoallergenic formulas. J Pediatr 121:LS116, 1992.

Lindfors A, Enocksson E: Development of atopic disease after early administration of cow milk formula. Allergy 43:11, 1988.

Odze RD, Wershel BK, Leichtner AM, Antonioli DA: Allergic colitis in infants. J Pediatr 126:163, 1995.

Powell GK: Milk and soy-induced enterocolitis of infancy: Clinical features and standardization of challenge. J Pediatr 98:553, 1978.

Savilahti E, Verkasalo M: Intestinal cow's milk allergy: Pathogenesis and clinical presentation. Clin Rev Allergy 2:7, 1984.

Stintzing G, Johansen K, Magnusson KE, et al: Intestinal permeability in small children during and after rotavirus assessed with different-size polyethyleneglycols (PEG 400 and PEG 1000). Acta Paediatr Scand 75:1005, 1986.

Sumithran E, Lyngkaran N: Is jejunal biopsy really necessary in cow's milk protein intolerance? Lancet 1:1122, 1977.

Tainio VM, Savilahti E: Value of immunologic tests in cow milk allergy. Allergy 45:189, 1990.

Wahn U, Wahl R, Rugo E: Comparison of the residual allergenic activity of six different hydrolyzed protein formulas. J Pediatr 121:S80, 1992.

Walther FJ, Kootstra G: Necrotizing enterocolitis as a result of cow's milk allergy? Z Kinderchir 38:110, 1983.

Gastroesophageal Reflux

Bailey DJ, Andres JM, Danek GD, et al: Lack of efficacy of thickened feeding as treatment for gastroesophageal reflux. J Pediatr 110:187, 1987.

Bendig DW, Seilheimer DK, Wagner ML, et al: Complications of gastroesophageal reflux in patients with cystic fibrosis. J Pediatr 100:536, 1982.

Berezin S, Schwartz SM, Halata MS, et al: Gastroesophageal reflux secondary to gastrostomy tube placement. Am J Dis Child 140:699, 1986.

Berquist WE, Rachelefsky GS, Rowshan N, et al: Quantitative gastroesophageal reflux and pulmonary function in asthmatic children and normal adults receiving placebo, theophylline, and metaproterenol sulfate therapy. J Allergy Clin Immunol 73:253, 1984.

Byrne WJ, Euler AR, Ashcraft E, et al: Gastroesophageal reflux in the severely retarded who vomit: Criteria for and results of surgical intervention in twenty two patients. Surgery 91:95, 1982.

Byrne WJ, Euler AR, Campbell M: Body position and esophageal sphincter pressure in infants. Am J Dis Child 136:523, 1982.

Cucchiara S, Staiano A, DiLorenzo C, et al: Pathophysiology of gastroesophageal reflux and distal esophageal motility in children with gastroesophageal reflux disease. J Pediatr Gastroenterol Nutr 7:830, 1988.

Dodds WJ, Dent J, Hogan WJ, et al: Mechanisms of gastroesophageal reflux in patients with reflux esophagitis. N Engl J Med 307:1547, 1982.

Dudley NE, Phelan PD: Respiratory complications in long-term survivors of esophageal atresia. Arch Dis Child 51:279, 1976.

Gioffre RM, Burin S, Mitchell I: Antereflux surgery in infants with bronchopulmonary dysplasia. Am J Dis Child 141:648, 1987.

Hampton FJ, MacFadyen UM, Simpson H: Reproducibility of 24 hour esophageal pH studies in infants. Arch Dis Child 65:1249, 1990.

Herve P, Denjean A, Jian R, et al: Intraesophageal perfusion of acid increases the bronchomotor response to methacholine and to isocapnic hyperventilation in asthmatic patients. Am Rev Respir Dis 134:986, 1986.

Hyman PE, Clarke DD, Everett SL, et al: Gastric acid secretory function in preterm infants. J Pediatr 106:467, 1985.

Lew C, Keens T, O'Neal M, et al: Gastroesophageal reflux prevents recovery from bronchopulmonary dysplasia. Clin Res 29:149A, 1981.

Newell SJ, Booth IW, Morgan MEI, et al: Gastroesophageal reflux in the pre-term infant. Pediatr Res 22:104, 1987.

Orenstein SR: Prone positioning in infant gastroesophageal reflux: Is elevation of the head worth the trouble? J Pediatr 117:184, 1990.

Orenstein SR, Klein HA, Rosenthal MS: Simultaneous comparison of pH probe and scintigraphy for gastroesophageal reflux (GER). Gastroenterology 92:1561, 1987a.

Orenstein SR, Lofton SW, Orenstein DM: Bethanechol for pediatric gastroesophageal reflux: A prospective, blind, controlled study. J Pediatr Gastroenterol Nutr 5:549, 1986.

Orenstein SR, Magill HL, Borrks P: Thickening of infant feedings for therapy of gastroesophageal reflux. J Pediatr 110:181, 1987b.

Orenstein SR, Whitington PF: Positioning for prevention of infant gastroesophageal reflux. J Pediatr 103:534, 1983.

Orenstein SR, Whitington PF, Orenstein DM: The infant seat as treatment for gastroesophageal reflux. N Engl J Med 309:760, 1983.

Sondheimer J, Arnold G: Early effects of bethanechol on the esophageal motor function of infants with gastroesophageal reflux. J Pediatr Gastroenterol Nutr 5:47, 1986.

Sondheimer JM: Continuous monitoring of distal esophageal pH: A diagnostic test for gastroesophageal reflux in infants. J Pediatr 96:804, 1980.

Sondheimer JM, Hoddes E: Gastroesophageal reflux with drifting onset in infants: A phenomenon unique to sleep. J Pediatr Gastroenterol Nutr 15:418, 1992.

Sondheimer JM, Mintz HL, Michaels M: Bethanechol treatment of gastroesophageal reflux in infants: Effect on continuous esophageal pH records. J Pediatr 104:128, 1984.

Spitz L, Kirtane J: Results and complications of surgery for gastroesophageal reflux. Arch Dis Child 66:743, 1985.

Strobel CT, Byrne WJ, Ament ME, Euler AR: Correlation of esophageal lengths in children with height: Application to the Tuttle test without prior esophageal manometry. J Pediatr 49:81, 1979.

Sutphen JL, Dillard VL: Effects of maturation and gastric acidity on gastroesophageal reflux in infants. Am J Dis Child 140:1062, 1986.

Veereman-Wauters G, Bochner A, VanCaillie-Bertrand M: Gastroesophageal reflux in infants with a history of near miss sudden infant death syndrome. J Pediatr Gastroenterol Nutr 12:319, 1991.

Vandenplas Y, DeWolf D, Sacre L: Influence of xanthines on gastroesophageal reflux in infants at risk for sudden infant death syndrome. Pediatrics 77:807, 1986.

Vandenplas Y, Sacre-Smits L: Continuous 24-hour esophageal pH monitoring in 285 asymptomatic infants 0–15 months old. J Pediatr Gastroenterol Nutr 6:220, 1987.

Wilkinson JD, Dudgeon DL, Sondheimer JM: A comparison of medical and surgical treatment of gastroesophageal reflux in severely retarded children. J Pediatr 99:202, 1987.

CHAPTER 80

Gastrointestinal Surgical Emergencies of the Newborn

Mary L. Brandt

Neonatal surgery became possible in the 1940s and 1950s with the advent of the neonatal intensive care unit and refinement of neonatal anesthesia and perioperative care (Soper and Kimura, 1989). Surgical emergencies of the gastrointestinal tract in the newborn are common and require rapid diagnosis and treatment to ensure optimal outcomes. As many as 25% to 30% of infants admitted to the neonatal intensive care unit require a surgical procedure, many of them for congenital or acquired conditions of the gastrointestinal tract or abdominal wall.

INTESTINAL OBSTRUCTION
Esophageal Obstruction

Esophageal atresia (EA) with or without tracheoesophageal fistula (TEF) occurs in 1 in 3000 to 4000 births (Holder, 1993; Rowe et al, 1995b). The cause remains unknown, although some familial occurrence has been reported (Holder, 1993; Rowe et al, 1995b). The preoperative management of the infant with an EA/TEF consists of three important steps: (1) confirming the diagnosis and type of anomaly, (2) evaluating and controlling the pulmonary complications, and (3) looking for associated anomalies.

The classification of EA and tracheoesophageal fistula is based on the anatomic anomaly. The most common anomaly is EA with distal TEF, which occurs in 86% of patients (Fig. 80–1, *far left*) (Holder, 1993; Rowe et al, 1995b). In this anomaly, the upper esophagus ends in a blind pouch, and the distal esophagus ends in a fistulous tract to the distal, membranous trachea (Holder, 1993; Rowe et al, 1995b). The next most common anomaly is isolated EA, without TEF (5%). The least common anomalies are isolated TEF, without EA (3%); EA with a proximal and distal TEF (3%); and EA with a proximal TEF (1%).

The diagnosis of EA, with or without TEF, may be suspected prenatally or postnatally and is confirmed by physical examination and diagnostic imaging. Prenatal ul-

trasound studies may suggest the diagnosis if there is polyhydramnios, failure to see the fetal stomach, or visualization of a dilated esophageal pouch (Holder, 1993). After birth, infants with EA drool and may exhibit signs of respiratory distress owing to aspiration. This aspiration is either of saliva, which spills over from the proximal esophageal pouch, or of gastric contents, which enter the airway through the TEF. The fistulous connection also allows air to enter the stomach with positive pressure ventilation or crying, creating gastric distention, abdominal distention, or both. This distention can cause further deterioration in the infant's respiratory status by its mechanical effect on the diaphragm and by increasing the risk of reflux into the fistula.

The diagnosis of EA is confirmed by the passage of a 10 to 12 French orogastric tube, which obstructs at 9 to 13 cm from the oropharynx (Holder, 1993). A smaller tube should not be used because it may curl in the esophageal pouch (Holder, 1993). Inadvertent penetration of the posterior oropharynx with the orogastric tube gives the impression of an obstruction at approximately the same level (Blair et al, 1987). A lateral radiograph of the neck and chest is necessary to demonstrate the orogastric tube posterior to the esophagus. Patients with a pharyngeal perforation can usually be treated without surgery, by removing the tube; placing a chest tube, if indicated; and starting appropriate antibiotics (Johnson et al, 1982; Mollitt et al, 1981). After placement of the tube, a radiograph of the chest and abdomen is obtained, which shows the tube in the esophageal pouch and, in the case of a TEF, will also show air in the stomach. Contrast studies to opacify the proximal pouch are rarely indicated and, if ordered, should be done only by a radiologist with considerable experience. A small amount (1 mL) of dilute barium can be gently instilled into the proximal pouch, then rapidly removed, to delineate more accurately the anatomy of the pouch and to determine if a proximal TEF is present. In the case of a suspected isolated TEF (without EA), the most accurate

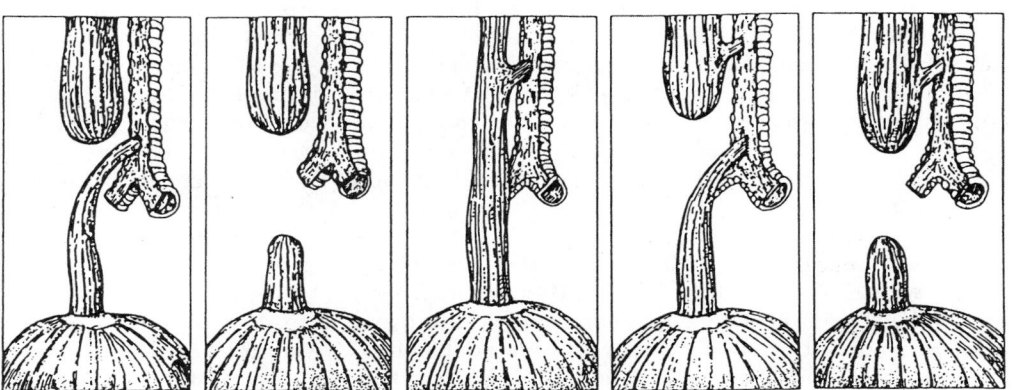

FIGURE 80–1. The five types of esophageal atresia and tracheoesophageal fistula. (From Ashcraft KW: Esophageal atresia/tracheoesophageal fistula. *In* Atlas of Pediatric Surgery. Philadelphia, WB Saunders, 1994, p 38.)

test is a prone, pull-back esophagram (Ein et al, 1983). In this examination, the infant is placed prone with an orogastric tube in the distal esophagus. The tube is slowly withdrawn, instilling a small amount of barium every centimeter or so. With a lateral fluoroscopic view of the mediastinum, a small fistula can be seen with this technique (Ein et al, 1983).

The decision of when to operate and what procedure will likely be performed is based on the following anatomic considerations: (1) Is there a connection from the esophagus to the airway? (2) If so, is it proximal, distal, or both? (3) Is there likely to be a long gap between the proximal and distal portions of the esophagus? Whether or not there is a connection to the airway is established by plain abdominal radiographs, which demonstrate air in the stomach if there is a fistulous communication. Because of the high percentage of patients with EA and distal TEF, this is most likely to be an isolated distal fistula. In stable infants, controlled opacification of the proximal pouch with contrast material or visualization by endoscopy may be necessary to rule out a proximal fistula (Holder, 1993). Long gap EA is almost universal in infants with isolated EA and is usually present in EA with an isolated proximal fistula (Holder, 1993). In infants with a distal TEF associated with EA, there is rarely a long gap (Holder, 1993).

The preoperative pulmonary complications associated with EA/TEF occur because of aspiration of oral contents or reflux of gastric contents into the airway. Evaluation of the pulmonary complications is based on the physical examination, blood gas evidence of respiratory compromise, and appearance of the chest radiograph. The aspiration of saliva can be minimized by placing a Replogle tube with continuous suction into the proximal esophageal pouch. Reflux of gastric contents can be minimized by elevating the infant's head and minimizing any positive pressure ventilation. If gastric distention, with reflux, becomes an important problem in the sick, small infant, a decompressive gastrostomy can be performed with local anesthesia at the bedside (Holder, 1993). If the fistula is large, there may be a significant loss of tidal volume if the infant requires positive pressure ventilation. This volume loss can usually be controlled by placing the gastrostomy to a chest tube system on water seal (Fann et al, 1988). In extreme cases, in which the infant may not tolerate a thoracotomy and definitive procedure, a Fogarty catheter can be passed with a bronchoscope to occlude the fistula (Filston et al, 1982).

Associated anomalies are common, occurring in 50% to 70% of patients with EA/TEF (Holder, 1993; Rowe et al, 1995b). The VACTERL association is present in 25% to 30% of children with EA/TEF (Rowe et al, 1995b). The VACTERL, previously referred to as VATER, association, consists of the association of Vertebral anomalies, Anal agenesis (imperforate anus), Cardiac defects (most commonly patent ductus arteriosus, atrial septal defect, and ventricular septal defect), TE fistula, Renal anomalies, and Limb anomalies (most often radial anomalies) (Corsello et al, 1993; Manning et al, 1986; Quan and Smith, 1973). Infants with EA/TEF and the VACTERL association tend to have higher proximal pouches, more complications, and a higher mortality than infants with isolated EA/TEF (Holder, 1993; Touloukian and Keller, 1988; Weber et al,

1980). Cardiac anomalies occur in 35% of patients and are the leading cause of death in infants who die with a EA/TEF (Holder, 1993; Rowe et al, 1995b). Echocardiography should be performed on all infants with cyanosis, evidence of heart failure, a murmur, or an abnormal cardiac silhouette on chest radiograph, followed by cardiac catheterization, if indicated (Holder, 1993). The cardiac defect may require repair before repair of the EA/TEF, especially in anomalies that are not duct dependent (Spitz, 1993). Gastrointestinal anomalies occur in 15% of patients (Rowe et al, 1995b). Anal atresia is the most common gastrointestinal anomaly seen and requires a diverting colostomy at the time of the first anesthetic (Holder, 1993). Duodenal atresia may also occur (Holder, 1993). Duodenal atresia is particularly difficult to diagnose in infants with isolated EA because there is no air in the gastrointestinal tract to demonstrate the duodenal obstruction on abdominal radiograph. Ultrasound, however, can be used to show the fluid-filled, dilated duodenum and stomach. A prompt gastrostomy, with or without repair of the duodenal atresia, is indicated in these infants to minimize aspiration from the dilated, obstructed stomach. Other, less common, associated anomalies include pyloric stenosis (rare), genitourinary anomalies (5%), neurologic anomalies (5%), and skeletal anomalies (2%) (Holder, 1993).

Following delineation of the anatomy and the search for associated anomalies, the operative strategy for the infant can be developed. If possible, it is always preferable to correct the anomaly with the first anesthetic. In small or very ill infants, however, the outcome will probably be better if the procedure is staged (Alexander et al, 1993). Three classification systems have been established to determine prognosis and to help determine which patients will benefit from a staged procedure (Table 80–1). In general, any size or gestational age infant who does not have significant associated anomalies and who has a reasonably stable pulmonary status should undergo primary repair of the EA and ligation of the TEF. Infants with the lowest probability of survival are likely to benefit from a staged approach. If the infant has significant aspiration at birth, he or she should be ventilated with the minimum positive pressure possible and given antibiotics. In most cases, a primary repair is possible after 2 to 3 days of recuperation from the initial aspiration. For infants with extreme pulmonary compromise or significant associated anomalies, an initial gastrostomy for decompression with later repair of the EA/TEF may be indicated.

The postoperative care of the infant consists of ventilatory support, as indicated, and nutritional support. The infant should be extubated as quickly as is safe to minimize positive pressure on the newly closed fistulous tract. Total parenteral nutrition should be started because the infant will be without enteral nutrition for 7 to 10 days at a minimum. The infant initially needs frequent oral and airway suctioning. The surgeon should have marked a suction catheter during surgery to indicate the distance from the anastomosis to the lips. The suction catheter should not be passed to the level of the anastomosis to avoid disrupting the fresh anastomosis. If no catheter was marked, a distance of 5 to 8 cm should be safe. Some surgeons place the neck in a flexed position to take some of the tension off the esophageal anastomosis. Even if the

TABLE 80–1

Transesophageal Fistula and Esophageal Atresia

Staging System	Best Group (Survival %)	Moderate Group (Survival %)	Worst Group (Survival %)
Waterston (Strodel et al, 1979; Waterston et al, 1962)	A: >2500 g and otherwise well (96–100%)	B: 2000–2500 g and well or >2500 g with moderate associated anomalies (96%)	C: <2000 g or >2000 g with severe associated anomalies (59%)
Holder (Holder, 1993)	"Healthy" (100%)	"Associated problems but relatively stable" (>90%)	"Very ill babies" (severe prematurity with weight <1500 g, <32 weeks usually in this group) (82%)
Spitz (Spitz et al, 1994)	>1500 g, without major cardiac disease (97%)	<1500 g or major cardiac disease (59%)	<1500 g and major cardiac disease (22%)

neck is not placed in flexion, extension of the neck should be avoided in the first week or two after surgery. A chest tube is placed at surgery to control any anastomotic leak that might occur. Antibiotics are usually continued until the chest tube is removed. On the 5th to 7th postoperative day, most surgeons obtain a barium swallow examination to evaluate the anastomosis for a leak. If no leak is demonstrated, the infant is started on oral feeds, and the chest tube is removed a day or two later. If a leak is demonstrated, the chest tube is left in place and the infant is kept nulla per os (nothing by mouth).

Five significant complications can occur after repair of an EA/TEF: esophageal anastomotic leak, esophageal stricture, gastroesophageal reflux, recurrent TEF, and tracheal obstruction. The incidence of anastomotic leak is around 10% to 15% (Rowe et al, 1995b). The diagnosis is usually made by the presence of saliva in the chest tube and is confirmed by a contrast swallow study (Rowe et al, 1995b). The treatment is expectant, with parenteral nutritional support, because most of these leaks close spontaneously (Rowe et al, 1995b). A minor esophageal stricture is almost universal after repair of an EA/TEF. Significant strictures occur in 5% to 10% of infants (Rowe et al, 1995b). The diagnosis is suspected with aspiration, failure to take adequate enteral feeds, or, in older children, esophageal obstruction by food or foreign bodies (Rowe et al, 1995b). The diagnosis is confirmed by barium swallow examination. Treatment is with esophageal dilation, either with Jackson dilators or by balloon dilation (Benjamin et al, 1993; Shah and Berman, 1993). Gastroesophageal reflux, which occurs with high frequency (40% to 70%) in these children, may increase the incidence and recurrence of strictures (Holder, 1993; Pieretii et al, 1974). Although medical management of the gastroesophageal reflux usually will control symptoms, 15% to 45% of these children ultimately require an antireflux procedure (Holder, 1993). Because of the inherent dysmotility of the esophagus in children with EA/TEF, a partial fundoplication (Thal, Boix-Ochoa) may be preferable to a complete wrap (Nissen) (Boix-Ochoa, 1986; Holder, 1993; Rowe et al, 1995b). Clinically significant tracheal obstruction may occur in as many as 25% of children with EA/TEF as a consequence of tracheomalacia (Corbally et al, 1993; Rowe et al, 1995b). The onset of symptoms (cyanosis, bradycardia, and apnea, usually with or immediately after feeding) is usually in the months

following repair of the EA/TEF but may occur in the immediate postoperative period (Holder, 1993). These symptoms may be difficult to distinguish from aspiration due to an esophageal stricture, aspiration owing to poor esophageal motility, recurrent TEF, or simple gastroesophageal reflux. Evaluation of all these possibilities is important. The diagnosis of tracheal obstruction due to tracheomalacia is made by bronchoscopy (Holder, 1993). In the child without significant distress, the treatment is time. Most symptoms improve over the first year or two of life (Holder, 1993). The surgical treatment of severe tracheomalacia is aortopexy, or suspending the aorta (and therefore the anterior trachea) to the posterior surface of the sternum (Corbally et al, 1993; Holder, 1993). Indications for aortopexy include severe apnea, recurrent respiratory distress and infection, worsening stridor, and near-miss sudden infant death syndrome (Corbally et al, 1993). The incidence of recurrent TEF is probably less than 10% (Rowe et al, 1995b). The TEF most likely recurs in the immediate postoperative period, but the diagnosis may not be made for months or years. The symptoms of a recurrent TEF are the same as gastroesophageal reflux, with aspiration, coughing with feeds, and recurrent pulmonary infections. Small fistulas may close spontaneously, but if a fistula persists for longer than 4 weeks, surgical closure is indicated (Rowe et al, 1995b). Most surgeons prefer to wait 3 to 6 months after the initial EA/TEF repair, if possible, to decrease inflammation and edema (Holder, 1993).

Gastric and Duodenal Obstruction

Gastric obstruction is uncommon in newborns and is most commonly due to pyloric atresia (Raffensberger, 1994). In this condition, the infant demonstrates nonbilious vomiting soon after birth. There may be a familial occurrence, with a suspected autosomal recessive inheritance (Raffensberger, 1994). This rare condition may be suspected with the presence of a single bubble rather than the double bubble of duodenal obstruction.

The diagnosis of duodenal obstruction is suspected with the clinical presentation of a vomiting infant and is confirmed by the presence of a double bubble on flat plate radiograph of the abdomen. The vomiting may be either bilious or nonbilious, depending on the level of obstruction. The differential diagnosis of duodenal obstruction in the newborn includes duodenal atresia, malrotation, duodenal stenosis, duodenal web, annular pancreas, and anterior portal vein. Malrotation usually, but not always, has air distal to the duodenum in conjunction with the double bubble. Because of the high association of duodenal atresia with Down syndrome (30% to 40%), the diagnosis may be suspected in infants with the physical manifestations of trisomy 21. Other anomalies associated with duodenal atresia include malrotation (19%), TEF (7%), and congenital heart disease (17%) (Raffensberger, 1994). Biliary atresia has also been associated with annular pancreas (Heij and Niessen, 1987).

The treatment of duodenal obstruction is surgical. A duodenal obstruction is not considered a surgical emergency, however. Because there cannot be a closed loop obstruction, there is little, if any, chance for ischemia of the duodenum. Most surgeons elect to proceed with the surgery within a day or two of diagnosis, allowing time to evaluate the infant for associated anomalies as well as time for stabilization of the infant. A complete duodenal obstruction, however, may be associated with a malrotation (19% of patients), and provisions should be made to operate quickly if there is any clinical deterioration consistent with a volvulus (Raffensberger, 1994). Before surgery, an orogastric tube is placed to decompress the stomach, and the infant is given maintenance fluids (usually 10% dextrose in water with 3 mEq sodium chloride and 2 mEq potassium chloride/100 mL) and replacement fluid for the nasogastric losses (usually 5% dextrose in 0.5 normal saline with 2 mEq potassium chloride/100 mL). The surgical correction of duodenal atresia is based on resecting or bypassing the area of obstruction. This is usually accomplished by anastomosing the duodenum proximal to the obstruction to the duodenum distal to the obstruction (Fig. 80–2). In some cases, when a duodenoduodenostomy is not possible, the proximal jejunum is used to bypass the obstruction. When the obstruction is due to a web, rather than a complete atresia, resection of the web without bypass is sufficient. Postoperatively, there is a significant period of duodenal dyskinesia until the marked dilation of the proximal duodenum begins to resolve. Although some infants are able to eat within 5 to 7 days of surgery, it is not uncommon for it to take several weeks until motility returns to the duodenum. It may be helpful to place a percutaneous central line in infants with duodenal atresia, in anticipation of the need for prolonged parenteral nutrition. Deciding when to start feeds for these infants can be difficult. Because the pylorus is usually rendered incompetent by most of the surgical procedures, there is easy reflux of duodenal contents into the stomach. This reflux results in high outputs of bilious material via the orogastric tube. After a week or so, the author places the orogastric tube to gravity drainage for a day or two, followed by elevation of the tube for an additional day or two, to see if the secretions are tolerated before starting feeds.

Malrotation

To understand malrotation, it is helpful to understand the embryologic events leading to this fascinating but dangerous condition. There are three stages of rotation of the bowel, and, therefore, there are anomalies of rotation associated with each of these stages (Table 80–2). The majority of anomalies occur in stage II, as the bowel returns to the abdomen. The term *malrotation*, as it is used clinically, usually refers to incomplete rotation of the bowel as it returns to the abdomen.

Malrotation, or partial rotation of the bowel, can present with duodenal obstruction, volvulus, or chronic symptoms of obstruction or can be an asymptomatic finding on a contrast study. In the newborn period, the most common presentation is partial or complete duodenal obstruction (Smith, 1986). Because the cecum usually fixes to the right lateral abdominal wall in stage III, bands to the lateral abdominal wall form. However, because the malrotated cecum is abnormally positioned superiorly in the abdomen, these fixating bands (Ladd's bands) cross the duodenum, causing the obstruction. The mesentery of the small bowel is normally fixed in the left upper quadrant, at the ligament of Treitz, and the right lower quadrant, at the cecum. With malrotation, the mesentery lacks this posterior fixation and can easily twist, creating a volvulus. Other presentations of malrotation, more common in older children, include chronic diarrhea and malabsorption from chronic obstruction of the intestinal lymphatics, intermittent vomiting and pain from recurrent partial volvulus, and constipation (Brandt et al, 1985; Smith, 1986).

The diagnosis of malrotation may be suggested on an abdominal radiograph by an abnormal air pattern, the presence of an orogastric tube in a malrotated duodenum, or duodenal obstruction (double bubble) (Smith, 1986). The procedure of choice to diagnose malrotation is a limited upper gastrointestinal contrast study, with just enough contrast material given to visualize the duodenum. Complete

FIGURE 80–2. The proximal duodenum is anastomosed to the duodenum distal to the obstruction, bypassing the area of obstruction. (From Ashcraft KW, Holder TM: Intestinal atresia and stenosis. *In* Ashcraft K, Holder T [Eds]: Pediatric Surgery, 2nd ed. Philadelphia, WB Saunders, 1993, p 315.)

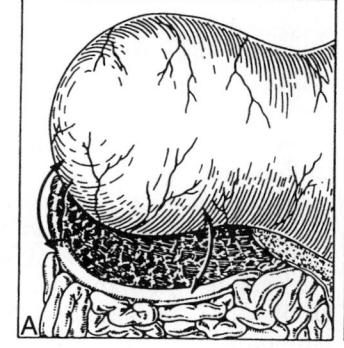
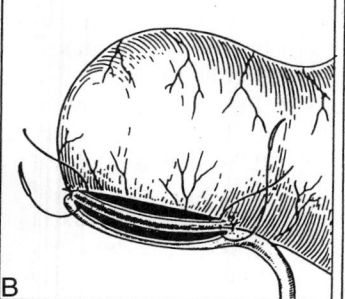
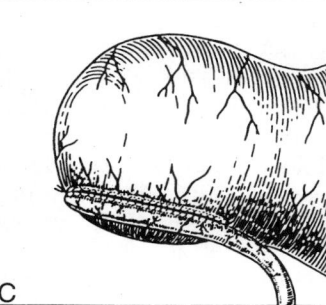

TABLE 80–2

Stages of Intestinal Rotation and Types of Malrotation

Stage	Normal	Abnormal
I	Herniation of the bowel from the abdomen	Duodenum can become prematurely fixed before rotating = isolated duodenal malrotation
II	Return of the bowel to the abdomen with 270-degree counterclockwise rotation	Failure to return = omphalocele
		Failure to completely rotate = nonrotation (90 degrees instead of 270 degrees) = *malrotation (180 degrees instead of 270 degrees)* Reversed rotation (90 degrees of counterclockwise rotation followed by 180 degrees of *clockwise* rotation in stage II) Hyperrotation (>270 degrees rotation) = hyperdescent of the cecum
III	Fixation of the rotated intestine	Undescended cecum (cecum ascends with liver—right colon does not lengthen) Inverted cecum (cecum ascends with liver—right colon lengthens) Mobile cecum Retroperitoneal cecum Lack of fixation of duodenum or colon with internal herniation

duodenal obstruction does not rule out a malrotation because there is an association of duodenal atresia with malrotation. Although a barium enema may show a displaced cecum, because of the variability of cecal fixation and rotation (see Table 80–2), this is not as reliable as assessing the position of the duodenum. In the case of a volvulus, if a barium enema is performed, an obstruction may be identified at the level of the transverse colon (Smith, 1986).

Malrotation should be considered a true surgical emergency. The surgical procedure to correct malrotation not only relieves the duodenal obstruction (if present), but also strives to decrease the risk of future volvulus as well. The Ladd procedure, as currently performed, consists of five steps: (1) Any volvulus is reduced, (2) Ladd's bands are lysed, (3) intrinsic duodenal obstruction is ruled out by passing an orogastric tube into the duodenum, (4) the appendix is removed, and (5) the base of the mesentery is widened to flatten it and decrease the risk of volvulus. Finally, the intestines are left in a position of nonrotation, with the small bowel on the right side of the abdomen and the colon on the left. In patients with the incidental finding of malrotation on contrast studies, most surgeons recommend proceeding with surgery to reduce the risk of future volvulus (Brandt et al, 1985).

Volvulus, or clockwise rotation of the intestine around the superior mesenteric artery, is one of the most devastating surgical conditions of infants and children. Acute volvulus usually presents as a clear intra-abdominal crisis with distention, hematemesis, acidosis, and shock (Smith, 1986). An abdominal radiograph may suggest a volvulus if no distal air can be identified or if the abdomen is gasless (Smith, 1986). Treatment should be instituted in an aggressive manner, with rapid fluid resuscitation and operative exploration. In clear-cut cases, the benefit of obtaining a quick contrast study of the duodenum, to confirm the diagnosis, should be weighed against the time this takes because the goal is to relieve the ischemia as quickly as possible. Unfortunately, in many cases, by the time the infant is ill enough to make the diagnosis, it is already too late to save the intestine.

Small Bowel Obstruction

The most common causes of neonatal small bowel obstructions are small bowel atresia or stenosis, meconium ileus, meconium peritonitis, and incarcerated inguinal hernia. Other, less common, causes include intestinal duplication, incarcerated internal hernia, and intussusception. Small bowel obstruction in the newborn varies in presentation, depending on the level of the obstruction. A proximal jejunal obstruction, similar to a duodenal obstruction, manifests itself with early vomiting or intolerance of feeds but does not have much associated abdominal distention. A more distal obstruction does not become evident until after air is swallowed and usually is associated with significant abdominal distention. Passage of a normal meconium stool after birth does not rule out a distal small bowel obstruction because 20% of infants with a small bowel atresia pass a normal stool (Touloukian, 1993). Jaundice is common, occurring in 40% of infants with a proximal atresia and 20% of infants with a distal small bowel atresia (Touloukian, 1993).

All infants with a suspected bowel obstruction should have intravenous resuscitation, thermal protection, and routine laboratory evaluation (complete blood count, electrolytes). A nasogastric or orogastric tube should be placed to low intermittent suction and the losses replaced with 5% dextrose and 0.45 normal saline with added potassium (assuming the infant has demonstrated normal renal function). In all but the very proximal obstructions, the next step is a water-soluble contrast enema. This serves to confirm the diagnosis by demonstrating a microcolon and may be therapeutic if the infant has a meconium ileus. In addition, a contrast enema rules out the rare but potentially devastating associated colonic atresia (Puri et al, 1981). Although it is important to correct any fluid or electrolyte imbalances in infants with a bowel obstruction, the fundamental concept is that early surgery is the goal, if there is a risk of bowel compromise. The critical issue in bowel obstruction is whether or not there is a closed loop obstruction present. If the bowel can be easily decompressed, as in the case of a duodenal or very proximal jejunal atresia, there is little risk of vascular compromise and little likelihood of severe physiologic imbalances from fluid loss and loss of mucosal integrity. Bowel that cannot be decompressed or decompressed only partially continues to fill with secreted fluid. This distention not only represents a significant third space loss, but also results in venous stasis and finally arterial compromise to the bowel with a loss in mucosal or bowel wall integrity.

Small bowel atresia is the most common congenital cause of intestinal obstruction in the newborn, occurring in 1 in 2700 births (Touloukian, 1993). The cause of small bowel atresia is believed to be prenatal vascular compromise to the affected bowel. The severity of the atresia increases the more proximal the vascular accident. In distal vascular compromise, there may be a stenosis or a web (Type 1) with an intact mesentery (Fig. 80–3). In more proximal vascular compromise, there is a cord-like segment between the segments (Type 2) and, finally, a gap between the two portions of bowel with a mesenteric defect (Type 3). In the most severe form of intestinal atresia, the *apple-peel* or *Christmas tree* atresia (Type 3b), the proximal superior mesenteric artery is occluded in utero and the small bowel receives retrograde flow via the ileocolic artery, the terminal branch of the inferior mesenteric artery. In

this anomaly, the intestine is coiled around the ileocolic artery, which is the sole blood supply for the midgut. Infants with this anomaly are usually premature and may have significant shortening of the small bowel length (Touloukian, 1993). Fewer than 10% of patients with small bowel atresia have associated anomalies (Touloukian, 1993). Infants with small bowel atresia should be evaluated for cystic fibrosis (Touloukian, 1993). In infants with cystic fibrosis, a distended fetal loop of bowel, filled with heavy meconium, twists on itself. The prenatal volvulus then reabsorbs, resulting in a small bowel atresia.

A standard, right supraumbilical transverse incision is used by most surgeons to approach the infant with suspected small bowel atresia. The area of obstruction is identified, and other, more distal, areas of obstruction are ruled out by injecting saline into the lumen of the distal bowel. The ultimate goal of the surgery is to restore intestinal continuity with an anastomosis of the two atretic ends. There are two problems that can make this difficult: (1) the size discrepancy between the distended, proximal segment and the unused, tiny distal segment and (2) the presence of more than one atresia. In most cases, despite the size discrepancy, the two ends can be anastomosed, usually by beveling the smaller bowel to make it fit the larger bowel. Other options include resecting the bulbous, proximal bowel; plicating the proximal bowel; or tapering it to a smaller size (De Lorimer and Harrison, 1983; Grosfeld et al, 1979; Touloukian, 1993). With multiple atresias, most surgeons exteriorize the two ends of the most proximal atresia and repair the distal atresia(s). In this setting, before take-down and closure of the stomas, contrast studies should be performed to confirm that there is no anastomotic stricture.

Postoperatively, adequate intestinal decompression and nutritional support are the cornerstones of therapy. The severely distended proximal bowel has decreased motility for days or weeks. In addition, the transition from a large diameter to small diameter results in altered bowel motility and emptying. The rule, rather than the exception, is a prolonged period until normal bowel function returns. For this reason, placement of a central venous catheter or PIC line at the time of repair of the atresia may be indicated.

Meconium ileus is the cause of obstruction in up to one third of newborns with small bowel obstruction (Andrassy and Nirgiotis, 1993; de Lorimer et al, 1969). Meconium ileus is most commonly associated with cystic fibrosis, although it can rarely occur in patients who do not have cystic fibrosis (Dolan and Touloukian, 1974; Fakhoury et al, 1992). Meconium ileus is the earliest manifestation of cystic fibrosis and occurs in 10% to 20% of patients with cystic fibrosis (Andrassy and Nirgiotis, 1993; Rowe et al, 1995c; Ziegler, 1994). Meconium ileus is classified as either uncomplicated or complicated. Uncomplicated meconium ileus, with inspissated meconium obstructing the distal ileum, occurs in 40% to 80% of patients (Andrassy and Nirgiotis, 1993; Docherty et al, 1992; Lloyd, 1986). Meconium ileus is classified as complicated if there is an associated volvulus, gangrene, prenatal or postnatal perforation, or small bowel atresia. On physical examination, infants with uncomplicated meconium ileus become distended in the first day or two of life. They rarely pass a stool, and their anus appears small, even stenotic (Andrassy and Nir-

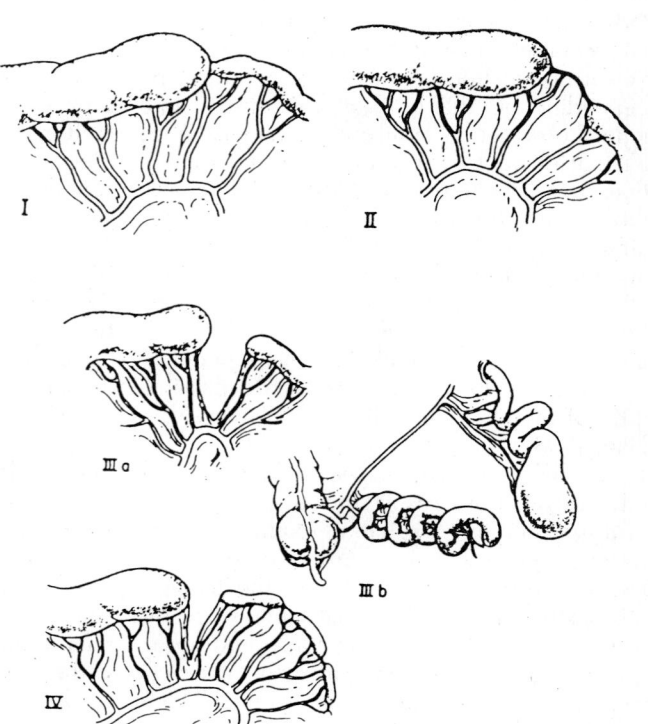

FIGURE 80–3. Classification of intestinal atresias. (From Rowe MI, O'Neill JA Jr, Grosfeld JL, et al: Intestinal atresia and stenosis. *In* Essentials of Pediatric Surgery. St. Louis, Mosby–Year Book, 1995, p 511.)

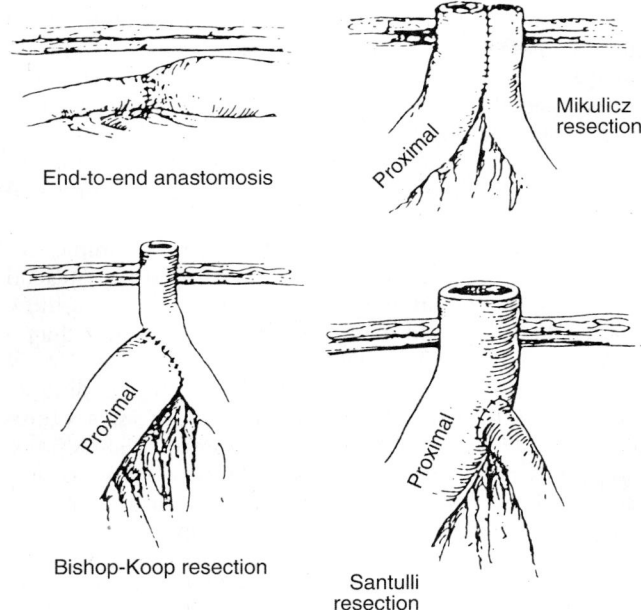

FIGURE 80–4. Surgical options in meconium ileus. (From Rowe MI, O'Neill JA Jr, Grosfeld JL, et al: Colon, rectum, and anus. *In* Essentials of Pediatric Surgery. St. Louis, Mosby–Year Book, 1995, p 612.)

giotis, 1993). Occasionally a large, "doughy" loop of bowel is palpable (Andrassy and Nirgiotis, 1993). Infants with complicated meconium ileus may be much more ill, especially in the presence of a bowel perforation or gangrene (Andrassy and Nirgiotis, 1993).

The diagnosis of meconium ileus can be suspected on plain radiograph of the abdomen and is confirmed by a contrast enema. The flat plate radiograph of the abdomen is abnormal in two thirds of patients with meconium ileus (Andrassy and Nirgiotis, 1993). The bowel loops may be distended, consistent with a small bowel obstruction, but may not demonstrate typical air-fluid levels (Andrassy and Nirgiotis, 1993). The inspissated meconium may give a ground-glass or soap-bubble appearance. If prenatal perforation has occurred, intra-abdominal calcifications may be present. The calcifications occur within a few days of perforation as a result of the saponification induced by the presence of pancreatic enzymes (Rowe et al, 1995c). The contrast enema should be performed with water-soluble contrast material. Diatrizoate meglumine (Gastrografin) has been the traditional contrast material used, but its high osmolality (1900 mOsm) can lead to sequestration of fluid in the small bowel. Many radiologists now recommend 20% to 25% Hypaque, which is still slightly hypertonic (300 to 400 mOsm) with or without a small amount of Tween added as an emulsifier (Kao and Franken, 1995; Parker, 1996). The contrast enema demonstrates a microcolon and pellets of inspissated meconium in the terminal ileum (Rowe et al, 1995c). The differential diagnosis of microcolon with inspissated meconium should also include Hirschsprung disease, hypothyroidism, small left colon syndrome, and meconium plug syndrome (Andrassy and Nirgiotis, 1993).

The obstruction associated with uncomplicated meco-

nium ileus can be relieved by a water-soluble enema in the majority of patients. Surgery is reserved for those patients with uncomplicated meconium ileus who do not respond to the water-soluble contrast enema and for patients with complicated meconium ileus. In uncomplicated meconium ileus, the objective of surgery is to evacuate the inspissated meconium. A second objective, for most surgeons, is to provide access to the distal small bowel and colon to allow further irrigation of the abnormal meconium. The surgery usually consists of a small enterotomy and evacuation of the inspissated meconium. Another strategy is to place a tube enterostomy or T-tube into the bowel, which serves as a temporary irrigation port for the first week or two after surgery (Fitzgerald and Conlon, 1989; Harberg et al, 1981; O'Neill et al, 1970). Once oral feedings and enzyme replacement are started, the T-tube is pulled, avoiding the need for a second surgical procedure. In complicated meconium ileus, a bowel resection may be needed. The two ends may be anastomosed together, brought out as separate stomas, or sewn end-to-side with the distal limb brought out (Bishop-Coop procedure) or the proximal end brought out (Santulli procedure) (Fig. 80–4).

Postoperatively, prophylactic pulmonary toilet should be instituted. To prevent the reoccurrence of the meconium ileus, pancreatic enzymes and *N*-acetylcysteine are started by mouth (Lloyd, 1986). If a distal enterostomy or tube enterostomy is left is place, gentle instillation of *N*-acetylcysteine solution can be started on the first postoperative day (Harberg et al, 1981; Lloyd, 1986).

Colonic Obstruction

Colonic obstruction in the newborn can be due to congenital obstruction, intraluminal occlusion, or functional obstruction. Congenital obstruction of the colon is usually due to an imperforate anus (Figs. 80–5 and 80–6). Other, less common, causes of congenital obstruction of the colon include colonic atresia, colonic duplication, and congenital segmental dilation of the colon (Philippart, 1986). Anorectal malformations represent a wide spectrum of problems, with fascinating anatomy. The Wingspread classification, developed in 1984, classifies these anomalies as high, intermediate, or low (Stephens and Smith, 1984). On physical diagnosis, findings consistent with a low anomaly include a perineal (cutaneous) fistula, a subepithelial tract (usually in the raphe in boys), anal stenosis, an anal membrane, or the *bucket-handle* deformity (Pena, 1993; Templeton and O'Neill, 1986). Physical findings present with a high anomaly include a flat or rocker bottom with missing gluteal folds, absence of contraction of the external sphincters with scratching of the perineum, a vestibular fistula in a girl, the passage of meconium or air from the urethra or vagina, an abnormal hymen, the presence of gas in the bladder on radiographs, cleft scrotum or proximal hypospadias, or the presence of a significant sacral anomaly (Pena, 1993; Rowe et al, 1995a; Templeton and O'Neill, 1986). In 20% of cases, the physical examination is not able to differentiate between a low and high anomaly (Pena, 1993; Templeton and O'Neill, 1986). The Wangensteen and Rice invertogram usually is able to differentiate between high and low anomalies in this case (Templeton and O'Neill, 1986). For this radiograph, performed after at least 16 to 24 hours of

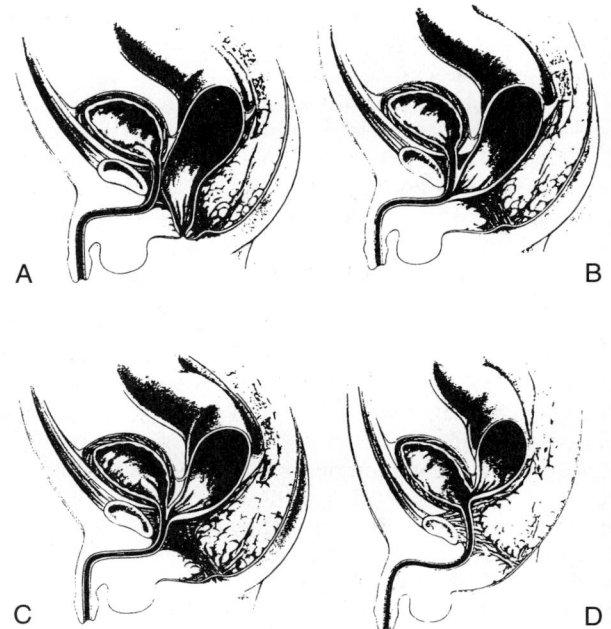

FIGURE 80–5. Examples of the most common male defects. *A,* Low defect with perineal fistula. *B,* Rectourethral bulbar fistula. *C,* Rectourethral prostate fistula. *D,* Rectobladder neck fistula. (From Pena A: Male defects. *In* Atlas of Surgical Management of Anorectal Malformations. New York, Springer-Verlag, 1990, p 26.)

life, the infant is held head down for at least 3 minutes, the perineum is marked with a radiopaque substance, and a true lateral pelvic radiograph is obtained (Templeton and O'Neill, 1986). Alternatively the infant can be placed

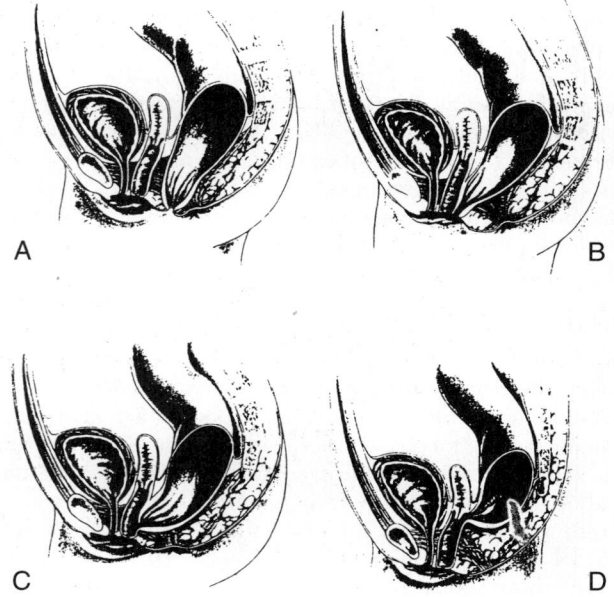

FIGURE 80–6. Examples of the most common female defects. *A,* Perineal (cutaneous) fistula. *B,* Vestibular fistula. *C,* Low rectovaginal fistula. *D,* High rectovaginal fistula. (From Pena A: Female defects. *In* Atlas of Surgical Management of Anorectal Malformations. New York, Springer-Verlag, 1990, p 50.)

prone, with the pelvis elevated, and a cross-table lateral film obtained (Templeton and O'Neill, 1986). A line is drawn between the pubis and the coccyx (*PC line*), and a mark is placed on the ischium (*I point*). If the most distal air is above the PC line, the defect is high. If the most distal air is below the I point, the malformation is low. In between the PC line and the I point, the lesion is termed *intermediate.*

For low lesions, dilation of a fistula, or a simple anoplasty, may be all that is needed. For anteriorly displaced lesions, most surgeons perform a true anal transposition, usually when the child is 6 to 8 months old, rather than a cut-back anoplasty (Templeton and O'Neill, 1986). In all cases, a biopsy is sent to rule out Hirschsprung disease, which is rarely associated with imperforate anus (Templeton and O'Neill, 1986). For high or intermediate lesions, a colostomy is performed. A descending colostomy is preferred over a transverse colostomy for several reasons: (1) There is less distance to the atretic portion of the colon, allowing more accurate imaging; (2) if it is necessary to wash out the distal bowel to decrease the risk of urinary tract infection, this is more easily accomplished; and (3) if there is a urinary fistula, there is less exposure of urine to the colonic mucosa and, therefore, less risk of a hyperchloremic metabolic acidosis (Templeton and O'Neill, 1986). A truly diverting, double-barrel colostomy is preferred by most surgeons, although many perform loop colostomies as well (Pena, 1993; Templeton and O'Neill, 1986).

The formal anoplasty is carried out 4 to 8 weeks after creation of the colostomy. There is evidence that early repair, rather than waiting until the previously recommended 10 kg or 1 year of age, may be beneficial (Freeman et al, 1980; Pena, 1993). The posterior sagittal approach, developed and refined by Pena, is used by the vast majority of surgeons in North America (Pena, 1988, 1993; Pena and de Vries, 1982). With this technique, all anomalies are approached through a posterior, midline incision. The muscle complex of the external and internal sphincters is carefully divided in the midline and, following the pull-through, are carefully reconstructed around the neorectum. Any anterior vaginal or urethral fistula is approached by opening the rectum posteriorly and separating the rectum from the vagina or urethra from within the lumen of the bowel (Pena, 1993). After the anoplasty, antibiotics are given for 72 hours. If urethral dissection was necessary, a Foley catheter is left in place at least 5 days. Daily anal dilations are started 2 weeks after surgery to avoid anal stricture. The colostomy is closed when an adequate anal diameter is demonstrated, usually 6 to 8 weeks later.

The outcome of the surgery is dictated by the functional results and the degree of complications encountered. Mortality is rare after surgery for imperforate anus and usually is the result of associated problems (Rowe et al, 1995a; Templeton and O'Neill, 1986). Mortality rates have been reported as less than 1% for low malformations and as high as 5% to 10% in infants with high lesions (Rowe et al, 1995a). Complications after surgery include wound infection, pelvic sepsis, anal stricture, anal prolapse, and functional obstruction due to unrecognized Hirschsprung disease (Rowe et al, 1995a). Functionally, most patients suffer from some degree of constipation or incontinence (or both) (Pena, 1993). In general, the lower the malformation, the more likely the functional outcome will be good (Pena, 1993). The presence of a significant sacral anomaly (two or more abnormal vertebrae) greatly affects the prognosis because innervation to the rectum will most likely be abnormal (Pena, 1993). Satisfactory continence can be expected in 75% of patients with intermediate anomalies, 65% of patients with high anomalies, and only 20% of girls with complex cloacal anomalies (Rowe et al, 1995a). These patients are primarily handicapped by inadequate sensation at the anal verge and proximally in the rectum. In addition, they have altered rectal motility. Most patients, with a combination of enemas, diet, and pharmacologic management, can achieve acceptable social continence (Pena, 1993). This goal, however, requires a great degree of trial and error on the part of the child's family and physicians.

Colonic atresia is the least common form of intestinal atresia and is an infrequent cause of colonic obstruction (Touloukian, 1993). The incidence is believed to be close to 1 in 20,000 births (Philippart, 1986; Rowe et al, 1995d). Skeletal anomalies, including syndactyly, polydactyly, absent radius, and clubfoot, are frequently associated (Philippart, 1986; Rowe et al, 1995d). Other reported associated anomalies include small bowel atresia, ocular deformities, congenital heart disease, Hirschsprung disease, and abdominal wall defects (Johnson and Dean, 1981; Philippart, 1986). These infants present with the clinical signs and symptoms of a distal bowel obstruction. Radiographs of the abdomen show dilated loops of bowel, with air-fluid levels. Pneumoperitoneum from colonic perforation is common (Philippart, 1986). The diagnosis is confirmed, in the absence of free air, by contrast enema. The site of obstruction is most commonly the transverse colon, with sigmoid colon next in frequency (Rowe et al, 1995d; Touloukian, 1993). Rapid surgery is indicated, after stabilization, to decrease the risk of colonic perforation (Philippart, 1986). At surgery, the abdomen is explored to eliminate any other, more proximal, atresia(s). Most infants require a temporary end colostomy, although a primary anastomosis may be considered in some cases (Philippart, 1986; Touloukian, 1993).

Intraluminal obstruction of the colon is most commonly due to meconium plug syndrome, which is thought to be caused by an imbalance of meconium mass and colonic motility in the prenatal period (Clatworthy et al, 1956; Philippart, 1986). This may occur in conjunction with small left colon syndrome, seen most commonly in infants of diabetic mothers, in Hirschsprung disease, or in the presence of hypermagnesemia (Andrassy and Nirgiotis, 1993; Philippart, 1986; Stewart et al, 1977). Meconium plug may occur as a complication of cystic fibrosis or Hirschsprung disease, warranting both a sweat chloride test and rectal biopsy in all infants with this diagnosis (Andrassy and Nirgiotis, 1993; Lloyd, 1986; Rowe et al, 1995c; Vinograd et al, 1983). As with meconium ileus, a water-soluble contrast enema is usually both diagnostic and therapeutic.

Functional obstruction of the colon is most commonly caused by Hirschsprung disease. Hirschsprung disease occurs in 1 in 5400 to 7200 births (Skinner, 1996). There is a strong male predominance (80%) except in long segment disease (Skinner, 1996). Overall, 22% of infants with Hirschsprung disease have associated anomalies (Skinner, 1996). Down syndrome occurs in 8% of patients with Hirschsprung disease, and in these patients, the incidence

of congenital heart disease approaches 50% (Ryan et al, 1992; Skinner, 1996). The trend has been for earlier diagnosis, with a decrease in the rate of enterocolitis as the presenting symptom (Klein et al, 1984; Rescorla et al, 1992; Skinner, 1996). Currently, approximately 6% of infants present with enterocolitis, with sepsis, fever, diarrhea, abdominal distention, and hematochezia (Klein et al, 1984; Rescorla et al, 1992; Skinner, 1996). Delay in the diagnosis of Hirschsprung disease past 1 week of age or the presence of Down syndrome increases the risk of enterocolitis (Skinner, 1996). In the newborn period, 35% of infants present with the signs and symptoms of a bowel obstruction (abdominal distention, bilious emesis, or gastric drainage). The classic finding of failure to pass meconium in the first day of life may not be as accurate as previously thought, with only 58% of infants with Hirschsprung disease meeting this criterion in one study (Puri, 1993).

The diagnosis of Hirschsprung disease should be considered in any infant who demonstrates the radiographic findings of a distal bowel obstruction. The diagnosis is usually made on contrast enema and is confirmed by rectal biopsy. In the newborn, the first enema should be with water-soluble contrast to rule out (and treat) meconium-related obstruction. A second, barium, enema may be needed for more accurate diagnosis. It is important to avoid any rectal manipulation before the study, which may lead to evacuation of the rectum and masking of the transition zone. The classic transition zone is often difficult to visualize in the newborn period, and the barium enema is positive in only 80% of patients subsequently proven to have Hirschsprung disease (Klein et al, 1984; Skinner, 1996; Taxman et al, 1986). In virtually every patient with total colon Hirschsprung disease, the barium enema is nondiagnostic (De Campo et al, 1984). The diagnosis may be suspected the following day when a plain radiograph of the abdomen may reveal failure to pass the barium. Manometry, which may be helpful in older children, is technically difficult in the newborn and may give misleading results.

Rectal biopsy is the gold standard for the diagnosis of Hirschsprung disease. The biopsy can be done at the bedside with a suction rectal biopsy forcep and should be taken at least 1.5 cm above the dentate line (Aldridge and Campbell, 1968; Andrassy et al, 1981; Noblett, 1969). This is an especially effective biopsy technique in the newborn, with less than 3% of specimens inadequate to make the diagnosis (Andrassy et al, 1981). The specimen is fixed and examined with routine hematoxylin and eosin staining. Frozen sections are not indicated because they are less accurate than permanent sections. The presence of ganglion cells effectively eliminates the diagnosis of Hirschsprung disease. The absence of ganglion cells in the submucosal plexus is highly suggestive but not completely diagnostic of Hirschsprung disease. If hypertrophic nerve fibers are identified, this further supports the diagnosis (Skinner, 1996). Some pathologists believe that the addition of acetylcholinesterase staining increases the diagnostic accuracy of the histologic examination (Skinner, 1996; Wakely and McAdams, 1984). Other studies have shown that acetylcholinesterase staining, because it is so technically difficult, may lead to misleading results in up to 10% of cases (Athow et al, 1990).

After confirmation of the diagnosis, the next step is to

determine the extent of disease. In 75% of patients, the aganglionic segment extends to the rectosigmoid area (Kleinhaus et al, 1979; Skinner, 1996). The distribution for the remaining 25% of patients is approximately 11% in the descending colon, 4% at the splenic flexure, 2% in the transverse colon, 1% in the ascending colon, and 8% involving the entire colon (Kleinhaus et al, 1979).

The initial surgical management of Hirschsprung disease consists of decompression of the intestine until a definitive operation can be achieved. Classically, this has been accomplished by the creation of a colostomy proximal to the aganglionic segment in the newborn period. Rectal irrigations may be an alternative to creation of a colostomy. Rectal irrigations are effective in the vast majority of patients with less than total colonic disease and may allow evaluation and treatment until the definitive procedure can be performed. This nonoperative decompression is accomplished by four to six rectal irrigations a day and is facilitated by feeding the infant breast milk or a predigested formula (Skinner, 1996).

The surgical treatment of Hirschsprung disease began in the late 1940s, when Swenson and Bill elucidated the true pathophysiology of the disease (Skinner, 1996; Swenson and Bill, 1948; Swenson et al, 1949). The definitive operation for Hirschsprung disease consists of removal of the aganglionic segment, combined with pulling down normally innervated bowel to the anus (Table 80–3). Swenson's procedure consists of an intra-abdominal dissection of the rectum to a level just proximal to the dentate line. The bowel is then divided at the transition zone, and the distal

aganglionic segment is everted out the anus. The aganglionic segment is amputated just proximal to the dentate line, and the proximal ganglionic bowel is pulled down and sewn circumferentially to this level. Since Swenson's original procedure was developed, two trends have developed: less dissection, with less tissue damage, and earlier operation. In Duhamel's procedure, the aganglionic segment is left in place, and the ganglionic segment is brought posterior to it, in the presacral space. The two portions of bowel are then anastomosed, usually with a stapler, by creating an opening between the two walls (Duhamel, 1956, 1964). The Soave-Boley procedure, instead of dissecting the outer wall of the rectum, similar to the Swenson, dissects the *inner wall* (the submucosal layer) of the bowel (Boley, 1964; Soave, 1964). In this way, the mucosa is removed to a level just proximal to the dentate line. Similar to the Swenson, the ganglionic bowel is pulled down, in this case, through the retained muscular cuff, and anastomosed to the anus. Georgeson's procedure uses the growing field of laparoscopic surgery to decrease further the extent of dissection necessary (Georgeson et al, 1995). In this procedure, the intra-abdominal rectum is mobilized using laparoscopic instruments. The mucosal sleeve is removed from the aganglionic segment via a transanal dissection. The anastomosis is identical to the Soave-Boley procedure (Georgeson et al, 1995).

Postoperatively, all patients are still at risk for enterocolitis, with an incidence as high as 33% (Blane et al, 1994; Elhalaby et al, 1995). The mean time from surgery to the enterocolitis is 29 months, although it can occur from days

TABLE 80–3

Procedures for Hirschsprung Disease

	Swenson	Duhamel	Soave	Georgeson
Incision	Transabdominal	Transabdominal	Transabdominal	No abdominal incision; laparoscopic technique used for abdominal portion
Distal Aganglionic Bowel	Removal in entirety to just proximal to the dentate line	Distal aganglionic bowel left in place	Muscular wall left in place distal to peritoneal reflection; mucosal removed from aganglionic segment (abdominal approach)	Portion of muscular wall left in place distal to peritoneal reflection; mucosa removed from aganglionic segment (perineal approach)
Anastomosis	Full thickness	Back wall of aganglionic segment anastomosed to front wall of ganglionic bowel	To cut edge of mucosa, just proximal to dentate line	To cut edge of mucosa, just proximal to dentate line
Unique Indications		Total colon disease; may be best procedure for second operation		
Contraindications			More difficult in patients with history of extensive enterocolitis	Long segment disease
Unique Complications	?Increased enterocolitis, potential for parasympathetic nerve damage, anal stricture	Reservoir inertia with constipation	Muscular cuff abscess, ?increased diarrhea and incontinence, anal stricture	Complications of laparoscopy, anal stricture

to years following surgery (Blane et al, 1994). The cause is most likely a persistently hypertonic anal sphincter, although an abnormal intestinal immune system has been implicated as well (Skinner, 1996). Rapid diagnosis and therapy with rectal irrigations, nasogastric suction, and intravenous antibiotics is important in the treatment of enterocolitis (Skinner, 1996). Routine irrigations in the postoperative period may help prevent enterocolitis (Marty et al, 1995). Other postoperative complications include anal stricture, incontinence, constipation, and cuff abscess (see Table 80–3).

Based on historical review, the outcome from these procedures is essentially identical, although adequate data are not yet available to compare Georgeson's procedure with the three traditional procedures (Nixon, 1985; Skinner, 1996). No prospective trial has ever been done to compare procedures for Hirschsprung disease (Skinner, 1996). Mortality is low, and there is no difference based on the procedure performed (Skinner, 1996). There is a slightly higher risk of death with total colon Hirschsprung disease, with a history of enterocolitis, or if associated problems such as Down syndrome are present (Caniano et al, 1990; Rescorla et al, 1992; Skinner, 1996). Functionally, approximately 90% of patients undergoing a pull-through for Hirschsprung disease have a satisfactory outcome (Skinner, 1996). Incontinence (2% to 25% of patients) and constipation (8% to 14% of patients) are the two most significant functional problems reported after a pull-through (Skinner, 1996).

INTESTINAL PERFORATION

Intestinal perforation in the newborn is most commonly caused by necrotizing enterocolitis (50% to 67% of patients) (Foglia, 1995; Steves and Ricketts, 1987). Pneumoperitoneum is the classic, and usually diagnostic, finding in intestinal perforation. On physical examination, the abdomen becomes distended and tympanitic. The infant may develop respiratory distress because of compression of the diaphragm. Pneumoperitoneum may also be diagnosed by the appearance of air in the scrotum in infants with a hernia or patent processus vaginalis (Coppes et al, 1991). On flat radiograph of the abdomen, the findings may be subtle, with air present over the liver, surrounding the falciform ligament, or free in the anterior abdomen (the football sign) (Bayatpour et al, 1979). A left lateral decubitus position allows the air to rise over the liver, where it can be more easily seen. Although pneumoperitoneum in the newborn may be due to necrotizing enterocolitis, the differential diagnosis includes iatrogenic perforation of the stomach or duodenum with a gastric tube, spontaneous rupture of the bowel from a distal functional obstruction owing to Hirschsprung disease, intestinal perforation secondary to meconium-induced obstruction, and mediastinal dissection of air in an infant on positive pressure ventilation (Foglia, 1995). In infants with pneumoperitoneum and associated pneumomediastinum, a paracentesis may eliminate an abdominal source and prevent an unnecessary laparotomy (Steves and Ricketts, 1987).

Neonatal gastric perforation may occur because of iatrogenic injury, inadvertent overinsufflation, obstructions distal to the perforation, or spontaneously (Campbell, 1986).

Spontaneous gastric perforation is most likely due to postnatal overdistention of the stomach, and not, as has been previously suggested, a congenital absence of muscle, increased gastric acidity, or gastric compression during birth (Bayatpour et al, 1979; Campbell, 1986).

Isolated perforation of the colon is unusual in the newborn and should suggest distal obstruction, such as Hirschsprung disease (Ajayi et al, 1969). Perforated appendicitis can also occur in the newborn, even the premature newborn (Schorlemmer and Herbst, 1983). A rectal biopsy should be performed in these infants to rule out Hirschsprung disease. Iatrogenic perforation of the colon can occur with placement of a rectal thermometer or during a contrast enema and should be treated by diverting colostomy with, when possible, primary closure of the perforation (Greenbaum et al, 1969).

NECROTIZING ENTEROCOLITIS

Necrotizing enterocolitis is now the most commonly seen critical condition of the gastrointestinal tract in newborns, occurring in 2% to 2.5% of all infants admitted to a neonatal intensive care unit (Amoury, 1993; Foglia, 1995). The cause remains elusive, although it is clearly a pathology based on insufficient perfusion of immature intestine. The overall outcome after severe necrotizing enterocolitis is improving. Currently the survival after surgical intervention is 70% to 80% (Foglia, 1995). The outcome depends on the amount of bowel resected, the functional status of the remaining intestine, and the presence of associated problems of prematurity.

The diagnosis of necrotizing enterocolitis can be difficult because the initial signs and symptoms are neither specific nor sensitive. Most infants initially are lethargic and develop apnea and bradycardia. They usually develop a feeding intolerance or increased gastric residuals. As the disease progresses, the signs of volume loss and sepsis appear, with tachycardia, hypotension, poor perfusion, temperature instability, and progressive decline. The findings more specific for necrotizing enterocolitis include abdominal distention, palpable loops of bowel, abdominal tenderness, abdominal wall erythema or induration, and blood in the stool.

Infants suspected of having necrotizing enterocolitis should undergo a plain radiograph of the abdomen. Serial radiographs of the abdomen should be ordered, every 6 to 12 hours, with flat and left lateral decubitus films requested. Progression of the degree of bowel wall distention, an increase in intra-abdominal fluid, and diminishing bowel gas with asymmetric loops are all signs of progressive disease (Foglia, 1995). Nonspecific radiographic signs that may be seen in infants with necrotizing enterocolitis include bowel distention, bowel wall edema, and gastric distention (Amoury, 1993; Foglia, 1995). Signs more specific for necrotizing enterocolitis include pneumatosis intestinalis, portal vein gas, intraperitoneal fluid, fixed bowel loops, and pneumoperitoneum (Amoury, 1993; Foglia, 1995). Pneumatosis intestinalis is the classic finding in necrotizing enterocolitis but is seen only in 70% to 80% of infants subsequently proven to have necrotizing enterocolitis (Foglia, 1995; Kosloske, 1979). Pneumatosis occurs first in the submucosa and appears as "bubbles" on radiographs

(Foglia, 1995). As the disease progresses, the gas becomes subserosal and appears linear on radiograph of the abdomen (Foglia, 1995). If pneumatosis is seen in the colon alone, the infant has a better prognosis than if the gas is seen in small bowel and colon (Leonidas and Hall, 1976). Portal venous gas may be a marker for more severe disease because there is a 38% incidence of severe bowel necrosis and mortality rates as high as 70% associated with this finding (Grosfeld et al, 1991). Intraperitoneal fluid is usually a sign of significant loss of integrity of the bowel wall, with impending or recent perforation (Foglia, 1995). Fixed bowel loops are suggestive of ischemic bowel (Foglia, 1995; Leonidas et al, 1976). Half of the patients with fixed bowel loops on abdominal radiograph subsequently need surgery for necrosis (Leonard et al, 1982). There is no indication for any contrast studies in the evaluation of necrotizing enterocolitis, with the exception of a limited upper gastrointestinal series to rule out a malrotation, if that is a concern. Contrast enemas, in particular, are contraindicated because they may lead to a perforation, rather than diagnose it. Ultrasound has been suggested as a more sensitive method to detect pneumatosis intestinalis and portal vein gas (Bomelburg and von Lengerke, 1992; Foglia, 1995). In addition, it may aid in directing paracentesis of free abdominal fluid or in identifying abscess cavities. A report has also suggested that there is decreased flow in the superior mesenteric artery in newborns with necrotizing enterocolitis, which may serve as another diagnostic criterion for necrotizing enterocolitis (Deeg et al, 1993; Foglia, 1995).

The overall treatment of necrotizing enterocolitis is designed to optimize bowel recovery and minimize the risk of systemic sepsis. The role of surgery in meeting this goal is complex. In all infants, the initial treatment is to stop feeds and place the bowel at rest, by placing an orogastric tube to low intermittent suction. Triple antibiotics, to cover gram-positive, gram-negative, and anaerobic enteric organisms, are begun, and the infant's overall homeostasis is protected by temperature control, fluid replacement, and careful monitoring. Overall, 50% to 60% of infants with severe necrotizing enterocolitis need surgery (Amoury, 1993). Surgical interventions should be designed to remove all truly nonviable intestine at an appropriate time, without giving the child a short gut syndrome. Perforation is the only absolute indication for operative intervention. The difficulty lies in being able to assess accurately whether or not perforation has occurred and to time the surgery in such a way as to minimize the risk of systemic sepsis while maximizing bowel recovery. Pneumoperitoneum on plain radiograph is diagnostic of perforation. Other findings strongly suggestive of perforation include a fixed or progressive metabolic acidosis; a fixed intestinal loop on plain radiographs; an abdominal mass on physical examination; abdominal wall erythema or induration; rapidly increasing intra-abdominal fluid; and, most difficult to define, "worsening clinical status despite maximal medical therapy" (Amoury, 1993; Foglia, 1995; Kosloske et al, 1980). Preoperatively, all attempts should be made to correct hypovolemia, anemia, electrolyte imbalances, and coagulopathy (Foglia, 1995).

The choice of procedures is based on the operative findings. In the unstable severely premature infant, simple abdominal drainage, by placing right and left lower quadrant drains, may be the procedure of choice (Ein et al, 1990). Most infants, however, undergo exploratory laparotomy. The findings at surgery can be grouped into three general categories: (1) isolated perforation or localized necrotizing enterocolitis, (2) multiple localized areas of necrosis, and (3) pan-necrosis.

Isolated perforation of the small bowel is most likely caused by an entirely different pathophysiology and should not be considered as necrotizing enterocolitis. In this condition, there is an antimesenteric perforation of the small bowel, usually in the mid to distal ileum. The bowel mucosa is well vascularized, and there is no evidence of necrosis. This entity is easily treated by resection of the perforation with an end-to-end anastomosis (Harberg et al, 1983; Kiesewetter et al, 1979). In rare cases, extremely limited necrotizing enterocolitis, with otherwise healthy-appearing bowel in a relatively stable infant, may also most appropriately be treated with resection and primary anastomosis (Harberg et al, 1983; Kiesewetter et al, 1979). In most cases of isolated necrosis, the area is resected and both ends brought out as stomas. The proximal stoma is usually brought out separate from the wound, and the distal stoma, or mucous fistula, is usually brought out in the corner of the incision (Foglia, 1995).

With multiple areas of necrosis, there are several operative approaches, depending on the overall condition of the infant and the extent of disease. If two or three isolated areas can be resected, the most proximal area of resection can be brought out as two stomas and the distal areas of resection anastomosed (Foglia, 1995). In very ill infants or if the disease is extensive or not yet defined, the options include closure with a planned second look, placement of drains, and resecting all necrotic bowel then closing the intestinal lumen with multiple metal clips (Foglia, 1995; Grosfeld, 1996). Surgical options in the case of pan-necrosis include proximal diversion only; "patch, drain, and wait"; and the placement of drains only (Foglia, 1995; Martin and Neblett, 1981; Moore, 1989). In the case of pan-necrosis, doing nothing may be the most appropriate decision. For these infants, the likelihood of overall survival must be considered, as well as the ethical considerations of survival with short gut syndrome. The only possible option at present, if there is loss of the entire small bowel, is small bowel transplant. If the infant, because of associated problems of prematurity or other reasons, is not a candidate for small bowel transplant, it is not only acceptable, but also compassionate to stop aggressive treatment and control pain.

ABDOMINAL WALL DEFECTS

Omphalocele and gastroschisis are fairly common anomalies, occurring with a combined incidence of approximately 1 in every 4000 live births (Tunell, 1993). Gastroschisis occurs two to three times more frequently than omphalocele and appears to be increasing in incidence (Tunell, 1993).

Omphalocele occurs when there is an arrest of the return of the contents of the abdomen to the abdominal cavity at approximately 12 weeks' gestation (see Table 80-2) (Tunell, 1993). The diagnosis of an omphalocele can be suspected as early as 13 or 14 weeks by prenatal ultrasound studies (Tunell, 1993). In omphalocele, the abdominal wall defect is at the level of the umbilicus, and the umbilical cord is located on the apex of the herniated bowel. In cases of prenatal or perinatal rupture of an omphalocele, it is difficult to distinguish the defect from a gastroschisis without close inspection of the site of insertion of the umbilical cord. In all cases of gastroschisis, the umbilical cord inserts normally, and the defect is lateral to the umbilical cord. In all but the rare case, the defect is to the right of the cord. In most cases, prenatal ultrasound studies are accurate in differentiating an omphalocele from a gastroschisis (Lindfors et al, 1986).

The distinction between an omphalocele and gastroschisis has important prognostic significance. Approximately 33% of children with an omphalocele have an associated chromosomal anomaly, such as trisomy 13, 18, or 21 (Tunell, 1993). Other syndromes associated with omphaloceles include Beckwith-Weidemann syndrome and prune-belly syndrome (Tunell, 1993). There is a high rate of associated anomalies with omphalocele, including cardiac anomalies, which occur in 15% to 25% of infants (Schuster, 1986). Gastroschisis rarely has associated major anomalies. Malrotation, as with omphalocele, is nearly universal. Undescended testes are frequent as well (Tunell, 1993). The most common problems associated with gastroschisis are the result of vascular insufficiency associated with the herniated and exposed bowel. Intestinal anomalies occur in 14% of patients, and two thirds of these anomalies are atresias or stenoses (Gornall, 1989; Pokorny et al, 1981; Schuster, 1986). Postoperatively, necrotizing enterocolitis has been reported to occur in as many as 20% of patients with gastroschisis (Tunell, 1993).

The prenatal diagnosis of an abdominal wall defect by ultrasound allows better planning as well as time to educate the parents. In cases of a large omphalocele, defined by liver herniated into the defect, with multiple associated anomalies, termination of the pregnancy may be offered to the parents. As the fetus grows, the dimensions of the herniated abdominal contents usually proportionally decrease (Tunell, 1993). The decision for the route of delivery is ultimately an obstetric decision, which should be based on the status of the mother and fetus, not on the presence of the abdominal wall defect. In cases in which the liver is included in the herniated abdominal contents, a cesarean section may be indicated (Paidas et al, 1994). Otherwise, numerous studies have shown no benefit to the infant with cesarean versus vaginal delivery (Moretti et al, 1990; Tunell, 1993).

After birth, the preoperative management of infants is directed at preventing fluid and heat loss from the exposed bowel or amnion, preventing injury to the exposed structures, evaluating the infant for any associated anomalies, and otherwise stabilizing and preparing the infant for surgery. One, or preferably two, upper extremity peripheral intravenous lines are started, and a 10% dextrose solution containing sodium chloride and potassium chloride is started. Because of the potential for compression of the inferior vena cava after reduction of the bowel and closure of the abdomen, lower extremity intravenous lines should be avoided. The rate of fluid infusion should take into account the infant's maintenance fluid and the fluid losses incurred because of the exposed amnion or bowel. Most

infants with a gastroschisis require an initial fluid bolus of 20 mL/kg of a colloid solution, followed by 120 to 170 mL/kg/day of crystalloid (Mollitt et al, 1978). The fluid rate is adjusted to maintain good perfusion and a good urine output. An orogastric or nasogastric tube should be placed to low intermittent suction to keep the bowel decompressed. The bowel, or amnion, should be wrapped with Kerlex moistened with warm saline and then covered with a waterproof covering to prevent evaporation. The author places the infant into an adult "bowel bag," cinching the bag around the chest, although some surgeons prefer plastic wrap, such as Saran wrap (Tunell, 1993). The infant should be placed on his or her side, rather than in a supine position. In this position, there is less chance of the herniated bowel falling off the abdomen, with a potential distraction injury to the mesenteric vessels. The infant is allowed several hours for transition, during which time evaluation of associated anomalies and preparation for the operating room can take place.

At the time of surgery, all efforts are made to maximize the space in the abdominal cavity. The gastric tube is used to evacuate the contents of the stomach and small bowel, and enemas can be used to evacuate the colon. The abdominal wall can be physically stretched, which also increases the space available. After examining the bowel, an attempt is made to reduce the herniated contents. Indicators that the infant cannot tolerate a reduction with primary closure include a marked increase in the pressure necessary to ventilate (usually >40 cm H_2O), a decrease in overall perfusion to the skin, marked venous congestion of the lower extremities, or any ischemic discoloration in the bowel (Tunell, 1993). Some venous congestion to the lower extremities is to be expected and usually resolves within 24 to 48 hours by elevating the legs. More objective measures of intra-abdominal pressure have been studied, including intragastric pressure, intravesicular pressure, and differences between the venous pressure in the superior and inferior vena cavae (Gorenstien et al, 1985; Wesley et al, 1981; Yaster et al, 1989). Unfortunately, none of these methods to date have helped in deciding which infants can be closed primarily and which should not. In patients with a gastroschisis, it is often difficult to determine if an intestinal atresia is present at the time of closure of the abdominal wall defect. Whether or not an atresia is clearly identified, no attempt is usually made to repair it at the time of reduction because the inflamed, thickened bowel increases the technical difficulty and risk of postoperative complications. Infants with an associated intestinal atresia are usually returned to the operating room 4 to 6 weeks after the closure of the abdominal wall defect, to allow time for the extensive inflammation to resolve (Schuster, 1986).

The ultimate goal of surgery for abdominal wall defects is reduction of the herniated contents with closure of the defect. In some infants, the abdominal cavity is not large enough to reduce the contents, or a marginal pulmonary or cardiac status may prohibit the resultant increase in intra-abdominal pressure. In these cases, an alternative to primary closure must be used. Gross (1948) described leaving the muscular defect alone, mobilizing the skin, and achieving skin coverage of the herniated contents. This technique creates, in essence, a huge ventral hernia that can be repaired at a later date. Currently, most surgeons prefer the use of a silo for graduated reduction of the herniated contents with secondary closure. In this technique, sheets of plastic (previously Silastic, which is not currently available owing to the legal ramifications of Silastic breast implants) are sewn to the fascial edges of the defect. Alternatively the bottom of a 100 or 250-mL intravenous bag can be removed and the edges of the bag sewn to the fascia of the defect, similar to the plastic bag closure used in adult trauma (Hirshberg et al, 1994). A plastic silo has been designed that has a spring-loaded ring at its base. The ring can be placed inside the abdominal cavity to hold the bag in place, eliminating the need to sew the bag in place (Fischer et al, 1995). Regardless of the type of silo used, the postoperative treatment is the same. On a daily basis, the herniated bowel is gently reduced into the abdomen by squeezing the bag or rolling it down like a toothpaste tube. A row of sutures, a clamp, or sterile safety pins are then placed to keep the bowel from herniating back into the bag. After 7 to 10 days, the patient is returned to the operating room, the silo is removed, and the defect is closed.

The postoperative management of these infants may include massive fluid resuscitation because third space loss into the distended bowel and abdominal cavity is the rule. Antibiotics are usually continued for 3 to 7 days or until closure of the abdominal wall if a silo was placed. After primary reduction of an abdominal wall defect, the infant should be watched closely for any signs of a potential abdominal compartment syndrome. If there is any indication of compromised bowel (bloody discharge, acidosis, sepsis) or of decreased renal or central venous perfusion, the infant should be returned to the operating room and a silo placed.

REFERENCES

Ajayi O, Solanke T, Seriki O, Nohrer S: Hirschsprung's disease in the neonate presenting as cecal perforation. Pediatrics 43:102, 1969.

Aldridge R, Campbell P: Ganglion cell distribution in the normal rectum and anal canal: A basis for the diagnosis of Hirschsprung's disease by anorectal biopsy. J Pediatr Surg 3:475, 1968.

Alexander F, Johanningman J, Martin L: Staged repair improves outcome of high-risk premature infants with esophageal atresia and tracheoesophageal fistula. J Pediatr Surg 28:151, 1993.

Amoury R: Necrotizing enterocolitis. In Ashcraft K, Holder T (Eds): Pediatric Surgery. Philadelphia, WB Saunders, 1993, pp 341–357.

Andrassy R, Isaacs H, Weitzman J: Rectal suction biopsy for the diagnosis of Hirschsprung's disease. Ann Surg 193:419, 1981.

Andrassy R, Nirgiotis J: Meconium disease of infancy: Meconium ileus, meconium plug syndrome and meconium peritonitis. In Ashcraft K, Holder T (Eds): Pediatric Surgery. Philadelphia, WB Saunders, 1993, pp 249–267.

Athow A, Filipe M, Drake D: Problems and advantages of acetylcholinesterase histochemistry of rectal suction biopsies in the diagnosis of Hirschsprung's disease. J Pediatr Surg 25:520, 1990.

Bayatpour M, Bernard L, McCune F, Bariel W: Spontaneous gastric rupture in the newborn. Am J Surg 137:267, 1979.

Benjamin B, Robb P, Glasson M: Esophageal stricture following esophageal atresia repair: Endoscopic assessment and dilatation. Ann Otol Rhinol Laryngol 102:332, 1993.

Blair G, Filler R, Theodorescu D: Neonatal pharyngoesophageal perforation mimicking esophageal atresia: Clues to diagnosis. J Pediatr Surg 22:770, 1987.

Blane C, Elhalaby E, Coran A: Enterocolitis following endorectal pull through in children with Hirschsprung's disease. Pediatr Radiol 24:164, 1994.

Boix-Ochoa J: The physiologic approach to the management of gastric esophageal reflux. J Pediatr Surg 21:1032, 1986.

Boley S: New modification of the surgical treatment of Hirschsprung's disease. Surgery 56:1015, 1964.

Bomelburg T, von Lengerke H: Intrahepatic and portal venous gas detected by ultrasonography. Gastrointest Radiol 17:237, 1992.

Brandt M, Pokorny W, McGill C, Harberg F: Late presentations of malrotation. Am J Surg 150:767, 1985.

Campbell J: Other conditions of the stomach. In Welch K, et al (Eds): Pediatric Surgery. Chicago, Year Book Medical Publishers, 1986, pp 821–828.

Caniano D, Teitelbaum D, Qualman S: Management of Hirschsprung's disease in children with trisomy 21. Am J Surg 159:402, 1990.

Clatworthy H, Howard W, Lloyd J: The meconium plug syndrome. Surgery 39:131, 1956.

Coppes M, Roukema J, Bax N: Scrotal pneumatocele: A rare phenomenon. J Pediatr Surg 26:1428, 1991.

Corbally M, Spitz L, Kiely E, et al: Aortopexy for tracheomalacia in oesophageal anomalies. Eur J Pediatr Surg 3:264, 1993.

Corsello G, Maresi E, Corrao A, et al: VATER/VACTERL association: Clinical variability and expanding phenotype including laryngeal stenosis. Am J Med Genet 44:813, 1993.

De Campo J, Mayne V, Boldt D, et al: Radiological findings in total aganglionosis coli. Pediatr Radiol 14:205, 1984.

Deeg K, Rupprecht T, Schmid E: Doppler sonographic detection of increased flow velocity in the celiac trunk and superior mesenteric artery in infants with necrotizing enterocolitis. Pediatr Radiol 23:578, 1993.

De Lorimer A, Fonkalsrud E, Hays D: Congenital atresia and stenosis of the jejunum and ileum. Surgery 65:819, 1969.

De Lorimer A, Harrison M: Intestinal plication in the treatment of atresia. J Pediatr Surg 18:734, 1983.

Docherty J, Zaki A, Coutts J, et al: Meconium ileus: A review 1972–1990. Br J Surg 79:571, 1992.

Dolan T, Touloukian R: Familial meconium ileus not associated with cystic fibrosis. J Pediatr Surg 9:821, 1974.

Duhamel B: Une nouvelle operation pour le megacolon congenial. Presse Med 64:2249, 1956.

Duhamel B: Retrorectal and transanal pullthrough procedure for the treatment of Hirschsprung's disease. Dis Colon Rect 7:455, 1964.

Ein S, Shandling B, Wesson D, Filler R: A 13 year experience with peritoneal drainage under local anesthesia for necrotizing enterocolitis perforation. J Pediatr Surg 25:1034, 1990.

Ein S, Stringer D, Stephens C, et al: Recurrent tracheoesophageal fistulas: Seventeen year review. J Pediatr Surg 18:436, 1983.

Elhalaby E, Coran A, Blane C, et al: Enterocolitis associated with Hirschsprung's disease: A clinical-radiological characterization based on 168 patients. J Pediatr Surg 30:76, 1995.

Fakhoury K, Durie P, Levison H, Canny G: Meconium ileus in the absence of cystic fibrosis. Arch Dis Child 67:1204, 1992.

Fann J, Hartmann G, Shocat S: "Waterseal" gastrostomy in the management of premature infants with tracheoesophageal fistula and pulmonary insufficiency. J Pediatr Surg 23:29, 1988.

Filston H, Chitwood WJ, Schkolne B, Blackmon L: The Fogarty balloon catheter as an aid to management of the infant with esophageal atresia and tracheoesophageal fistula complicated by severe RDS or pneumonia. J Pediatr Surg 17:149, 1982.

Fischer J, Chun K, Moores D, Andrews H: Gastroschisis: A simple technique for staged silo closure. J Pediatr Surg 30:1169, 1995.

Fitzgerald R, Conlon K: Use of the appendix stump in the treatment of meconium ileus. J Pediatr Surg 24:899, 1989.

Foglia R: Necrotizing enterocolitis. Curr Probl Surg 32:757, 1995.

Freeman N, Burge D, Soar J, et al: Anal evoked potentials. Z Kinderchir 31:22, 1980.

Georgeson K, Fuenfer M, Hardin W: Primary laparoscopic pull-through for Hirschsprung's disease in infants and children. J Pediatr Surg 30:1017, 1995.

Gorenstien A, Goitein K, Schiller M: Simultaneous superior and inferior vena cava pressure recordings in giant omphalocele repair—a possible guideline for prevention of postoperative circulatory complications. Z Kinderchir 40:329, 1985.

Gornall P: Management of intestinal atresia complicating gastroschisis. J Pediatr Surg 24:522, 1989.

Greenbaum E, Carson M, Kincannon W, O'Loughlin B: Rectal thermometer-induced pneumoperitoneum in the newborn: Report of two cases. Pediatrics 44:539, 1969.

Grosfeld J, Ballantine T, Shoemaker R: Operative management of intestinal atresia and stenosis based on pathologic findings. J Pediatr Surg 14:368, 1979.

Grosfeld J, Cheu H, Schletter M: Changing trends in necrotizing enterocolitis. Ann Surg 214:300, 1991.

Gross R: A new method for surgical treatment of large omphaloceles. Surgery 24:277, 1948.

Harberg F, McGill C, Saleem M, et al: Resection with primary anastomosis for necrotizing enterocolitis. J Pediatr Surg 18:743, 1983.

Harberg F, Senekjian E, Pokorny W: Treatment of uncomplicated meconium ileus via T-tube ileostomy. J Pediatr Surg 16:61, 1981.

Heij H, Niessen G: Annular pancreas associated with congenital absence of the gallbladder. J Pediatr Surg 22:1033, 1987.

Hirshberg A, Wall MJ, Mattox K: Planned reoperation for trauma: A two year experience with 124 consecutive patients. J Trauma 37:365, 1994.

Holder T: Esophageal atresia and tracheoesophageal malformations. *In* Ashcraft K, Holder T (Eds): Pediatric Surgery. Philadelphia, WB Saunders, 1993, pp 249–267.

Johnson D, Foker J, Munson D, et al: Management of esophageal and pharyngeal perforation in the newborn infant. Pediatrics 70:592, 1982.

Johnson J, Dean B: Hirschsprung's disease coexisting with colonic atresia. Pediatr Radiol 11:97, 1981.

Kao S, Franken E Jr: Nonoperative treatment of simple meconium ileus: A survey of the Society for Pediatric Radiology. Pediatr Radiol 25:97, 1995.

Kiesewetter W, Taghizadeh F, Bower R: Necrotizing enterocolitis: Is there a place for resection and primary anastomosis? J Pediatr Surg 14:360, 1979.

Klein M, Coran A, Wesley J, Drongowski R: Hirschsprung's disease in the newborn. J Pediatr Surg 19:370, 1984.

Kleinhaus S, Boley S, Sheran M, Sieber W: Hirschsprung's disease: A survey of the members of the surgical section of the American Academy of Pediatrics. J Pediatr Surg 14:588, 1979.

Kosloske A: Necrotizing enterocolitis in the neonate: Collective review. Surg Gynecol Obstet 148:259, 1979.

Kosloske A, Papile L, Burstein J: Indications for operation in acute necrotizing enterocolitis of the neonate. Surgery 87:502, 1980.

Leonard TJ, Johnson J, Pettett P: Critical evaluation of the persistent loop sign in necrotizing enterocolitis. Radiology 142:385, 1982.

Leonidas J, Hall R: Neonatal pneumatosis coli: A mild form of necrotizing enterocolitis. J Pediatr 89:456, 1976.

Leonidas J, Hall R, Amoury R: Critical evaluation of the roentgen signs of neonatal enterocolitis. Ann Radiol 219:123, 1976.

Lindfors K, McGahan J, Walter J: Fetal omphalocele and gastroschisis: Pitfalls in sonographic diagnosis. AJR Am J Roentgenol 147:797, 1986.

Lloyd D: Meconium ileus. *In* Welch K, et al (Eds): Pediatric Surgery. Chicago, Year Book Medical Publishers, 1986, pp 849–858.

Manning P, Morgan R, Coran A, et al: Fifty years' experience with esophageal atresia and transesophageal fistula. Ann Surg 204:446, 1986.

Martin L, Neblett W: Early operation with intestinal diversion for necrotizing enterocolitis. J Pediatr Surg 16:252, 1981.

Marty T, Seo T, Sullivan J, et al: Rectal irrigations for the prevention of postoperative enterocolitis in Hirschsprung's disease. J Pediatr Surg 30:652, 1995.

Mollitt D, Ballantine T, Grosfeld J, et al: A critical assessment of fluid requirements in gastroschisis. J Pediatr Surg 3:217, 1978.

Mollitt D, Schullinger J, Santulli T: Selective management of iatrogenic esophageal perforation in the newborn. J Pediatr Surg 16:989, 1981.

Moore T: The management of necrotizing enterocolitis by "patch, drain, and wait." Pediatr Surg Int 4:110, 1989.

Moretti M, Khoury A, Rodriguez J, et al: The effect of mode of delivery on the perinatal outcome in fetuses with abdominal wall defects. Am J Obstet Gynecol 163:833, 1990.

Nixon H: Hirschsprung's disease: Progress in management and diagnostics. World J Surg 9:189, 1985.

Noblett H: A rectal suction biopsy tube for use in diagnosis of Hirschsprung's disease. J Pediatr Surg 4:406, 1969.

O'Neill J, Grosfeld J, Boles E, et al: Surgical treatment of meconium ileus. Am J Surg 119:99, 1970.

Paidas M, Crombleholme T, Robertson F: Prenatal diagnosis and management of the fetus with an abdominal wall defect. Semin Perinatol 18:196, 1994.

Pena A: Posterior sagittal anoplasty: Results in the management of 332 cases of anorectal malformations. Pediatr Surg Int 3:94, 1988.

Pena A: Imperforate anus and cloacal malformations. *In* Ashcraft K, Holder T (Eds): Pediatric Surgery. Philadelphia, WB Saunders, 1993, pp 372–392.

Pena A, de Vries P: Posterior sagittal anorectoplasty: Important technical considerations and new applications. J Pediatr Surg 17:796, 1982.

Philippart A: Atresia, stenosis, and other obstructions of the colon. *In* Welch K, et al (Eds): Pediatric Surgery. Chicago, Year Book Medical Publishers, 1986, pp 984–988.

Pieretii R, Shandling B, Stephens C: Resistant esophageal stenosis associated with reflux after repair of esophageal atresia. J Pediatr Surg 9:355, 1974.

Pokorny W, Harberg F, McGill C: Gastroschisis complicated by intestinal atresia. J Pediatr Surg 16:261, 1981.

Puri P: Hirschsprung's disease: Clinical and experimental observations. World J Surg 17:374, 1993.

Puri P, Blake N, O'Donnell B, Guiney J: Delayed primary anastomosis following spontaneous growth of esophageal segments in esophageal atresia. J Pediatr Surg 16:180, 1981.

Quan L, Smith D: The VATER association: Vertebral defects, anal atresia, T-E fistula with esophageal atresia, radial and renal dysplasia: A spectrum of associated anomalies. J Pediatr 82:104–107, 1973.

Raffensberger JG: Pyloric and duodenal obstruction. *In* Raffensberger JG (Ed): Swenson's Pediatric Surgery, 5th ed. Norwalk, CT, Appleton & Lange, 1994, pp 509–516.

Rescorla F, Morrison A, Engles D, et al: Hirschsprung's disease: Evaluation of mortality and long-term function in 260 cases. Arch Surg 127:934, 1992.

Rowe M, O'Neill J Jr, Grosfeld J, et al: Anorectal disorders. *In* Essentials of Pediatric Surgery. St. Louis, Mosby-Year Book, 1995a, pp 596–609.

Rowe M, O'Neill J Jr, Grosfeld J, et al: Congenital abnormalities of the esophagus. *In* Essentials of Pediatric Surgery. St. Louis, Mosby-Year Book, 1995b, pp 397–408.

Rowe M, O'Neill J Jr, Grosfeld J, et al: Disorders of the peritoneum and peritoneal cavity. *In* Essentials of Pediatric Surgery. St. Louis, Mosby-Year Book, 1995c, pp 462–467.

Rowe M, O'Neill J Jr, Grosfeld J, et al: Intestinal atresia and stenosis. *In* Essentials of Pediatric Surgery. St. Louis, Mosby-Year Book, 1995d, pp 508–514.

Ryan E, Ecker J, Christakis N, Folkman J: Hirschsprung's disease: Associated anomalies and demographics. J Pediatr Surg 27:76, 1992.

Schorlemmer G, Herbst C Jr: Perforated neonatal appendicitis. South Med J 76:536, 1983.

Schuster S: Omphalocele and gastroschisis. *In* Welch K, et al (Eds): Pediatric Surgery. Chicago, Year Book Medical Publishers, 1986, pp 740–763.

Shah M, Berman W: Endoscopic balloon dilatation of esophageal strictures in children. Gastrointest Endosc 39:153, 1993.

Skinner M: Hirshsprung's disease. Curr Probl Surg 33:389, 1996.

Smith E: Malrotation of the intestine. *In* Welch K, et al (Eds): Pediatric Surgery. Chicago, Year Book Medical Publishers, 1986.

Soave F: A new surgical technique for the treatment of Hirschsprung's disease. Surgery 56:1007, 1964.

Soper R, Kimura K: Overview of neonatal surgery. Clin Perinatol 16:1, 1989.

Spitz L: Esophageal atresia and tracheoesophageal fistula in children. Curr Opin Pediatr 5:347, 1993.

Spitz L, Kiely E, Morecroft J, et al: Oesophageal atresia: At-risk groups for the 1990s. J Pediatr Surg 29:723, 1994.

Stephens F, Smith E: Classification, identification and assessment of surgical treatment of anorectal anomalies. Pediatr Surg Int 1:200, 1984.

Steves M, Ricketts R: Pneumoperitoneum in the newborn infant. Am Surg 53:226, 1987.

Stewart D, Nixon G, Johnson D, et al: Neonatal small left colon syndrome. Ann Surg 186:741, 1977.

Strodel W, Coran A, Kirsh M, et al: Esophageal atresia: A 41 year experience. Arch Surg 114:523, 1979.

Swenson O, Bill A: Resection of the rectum and rectosigmoid with preservation of the sphincter for benign spastic lesions producing megacolon. Surgery 24:212, 1948.

Swenson O, Rheinlander J, Diamond I: Hirschsprung's disease: A new concept in etiology: Operative results in thirty-four patients. N Engl J Med 241:551, 1949.

Taxman T, Yulish B, Rothstein F: How useful is the barium enema in the diagnosis of infantile Hirschsprung's disease? Am J Dis Child 140:881, 1986.

Templeton J, O'Neill J Jr: Anorectal malformations. *In* Welch K, et al (Eds): Pediatric Surgery. Chicago, Year Book Medical Publishers, 1986, pp 1022–1037.

Touloukian R: Intestinal atresia and stenosis. *In* Ashcraft K, Holder T (Eds): Pediatric Surgery. Philadelphia, WB Saunders, 1993, pp 305–319.

Touloukian R, Keller M: High proximal pouch esophageal atresia with vertebral, rib and sternal anomalies: An additional component to the VATER association. J Pediatr Surg 23:76, 1988.

Tunell W: Omphalocele and gastroschisis. *In* Ashcraft K, Holder T (Eds): Pediatric Surgery. Philadelphia, WB Saunders, 1993, pp 341–357.

Vinograd I, Mogle P, Peleg O, et al: Meconium disease in premature infants with very low weight. J Pediatr 103:963, 1983.

Wakely P, McAdams J: Acetylcholinesterase histochemistry and the diagnosis of Hirschsprung's disease: A 3 1/2 year experience. Pediatr Pathol 2:35, 1984.

Waterston D, Bonham-Carter R, Aberdeen E: Oesophageal atresia, tracheoesophagel fistula—a study of survival in 218 infants. Lancet 1:819, 1962.

Weber T, Smith W, Grosfeld J: Surgical experience in infants with the VATER syndrome. J Pediatr Surg 15:849, 1980.

Wesley J, Drongowski R, Coran A: Intragastric pressure measurements: A guide for reduction and closure of the Silastic chimney in omphalocele and gastroschisis. J Pediatr Surg 16:264, 1981.

Yaster M, Scherer T, Stone M, et al: Prediction of successful primary closure of congenital abdominal wall defects using intraoperative measurements. J Pediatr Surg 24:1217, 1989.

Ziegler M: Meconium ileus. Curr Probl Surg 31:731, 1994.

CHAPTER **81**

Bilirubin Metabolism

James R. MacMahon, David K. Stevenson, and Frank A. Oski[*]

HISTORICAL PERSPECTIVE

Although jaundice was known as a sign of disease to both Hippocrates and Galen, the first mention of it with regard to newborns is found in *Ein Regiment der Jungen Kinder*, a "pediatric text" written by Bartholomeus Metlinger in 1473. In North America, the 1652 correspondence of John Winthrop, Jr., governor of Connecticut, included his recommendations about herbal remedies for jaundice in the first months of life, mentioning the use of barberry root, turmeric, and saffron (Cone, 1979). In 1751, John Burton's *An Essay Towards a Complete New System of Midwifery, Theoretical and Practical*, included the following description of neonatal jaundice and proposed intervention:

> The Want of Respiration to squeeze forward the Bile, and the Resistance made to its Entry into the Guts of foetuses by the tough Slime which lines the Intestinal tube make the Effusion of their Bile very slow, and therefore, their Gallbladder is generally full of a green Bile. Hence at birth or soon after, children are observed to have the jaundice, the thick slime produces the same Effect in them, as if Stones or the Gravel obstructed the Neck of the Gallbladder. The Jaundice generally yields to any gentle Purgative, and very often is carried away by any Medicine that increases the Contractions of the Gut.
>
> *Burton, 1751*

Following in this tradition, William Potts Dewees wrote in 1825 that jaundice in the newborn "is but too often fatal, with whatever propriety or energy we may attempt to relieve it." Yet he recommended treating the jaundiced infant with castor oil, "a small teaspoonful every two hours, until it purges freely" (Dewees, 1825).

These examples demonstrate that jaundice was long ago recognized as a sign of illness and was known to be related to hepatic function and intestinal elimination, but it was not understood physiologically. Only with the scientific advances of the latter half of the nineteenth century could understanding of the processes involving bilirubin metabolism and jaundice be furthered, combining pathology, physiology, chemistry, and biology.

In 1847, Virchow observed the accumulation of microscopic yellow crystal formation in bruises, in wound fluid, and in subcutaneous hematomas following phagocytosis of red blood cells (Virchow, 1847). This observation provided the first experimental evidence for a link between bilirubin and heme. Since that time, much effort has been spent exploring the various aspects of this relationship, including mechanisms that control or influence the chemical reactions producing the pigment, bilirubin transport systems, movement of bilirubin across tissue barriers and cell walls, and the conjugation, excretion, elimination, absorption, and clinical consequences associated with the presence of bilirubin in vital organs. In this chapter, the current information pertaining to these issues is reviewed, with attention to persistent questions, controversies, and future areas of inquiry.

FORMATION OF BILIRUBIN

Bilirubin is a yellow-orange crystalline pigment formed by the reduction of biliverdin, a green pigment, which is derived from the catabolism of heme. The rate-limiting reaction in the pathway from heme to bilirubin is the oxidation of heme to form biliverdin, a process controlled by heme oxygenase (HO). The degradation of heme to bilirubin requires the presence of oxygen (O_2) and the reduced form of nicotinamide adenine dinucleotide phosphate (NADPH) and releases carbon monoxide (CO) and iron (Fe^{3+}).

Heme, which is a porphyrin ring surrounding a ferric (Fe^{3+}) ion, is the nonamino acid portion of several hemoproteins including hemoglobin, myoglobin, catalase, peroxidase, NO synthase, and mitochondrial and microsomal cytochromes (Fig. 81–1).

Heme is an essential molecule in all oxygen-dependent metabolism, making every cell a potential source of bilirubin. However, under usual circumstances bilirubin production primarily results from the destruction of hemoglobin contained in erythrocytes.

In newborns, approximately 80% of the bilirubin produced each day is derived from the catabolism of heme derived from the hemoglobin of circulating erythrocytes. The other 20% comes from the breakdown of nonerythropoietic heme, that is, other heme proteins and free heme in the liver, and from the destruction of erythrocyte precursors in the marrow or soon after their release into circulation. Such destruction of red cell precursors or young erythrocytes is termed "ineffective erythropoiesis."

Any process that accelerates the destruction of red blood cells can lead to increases in degradable erythropoietic heme and thus potentially an increase in the bilirubin load.

---

[*]Deceased.

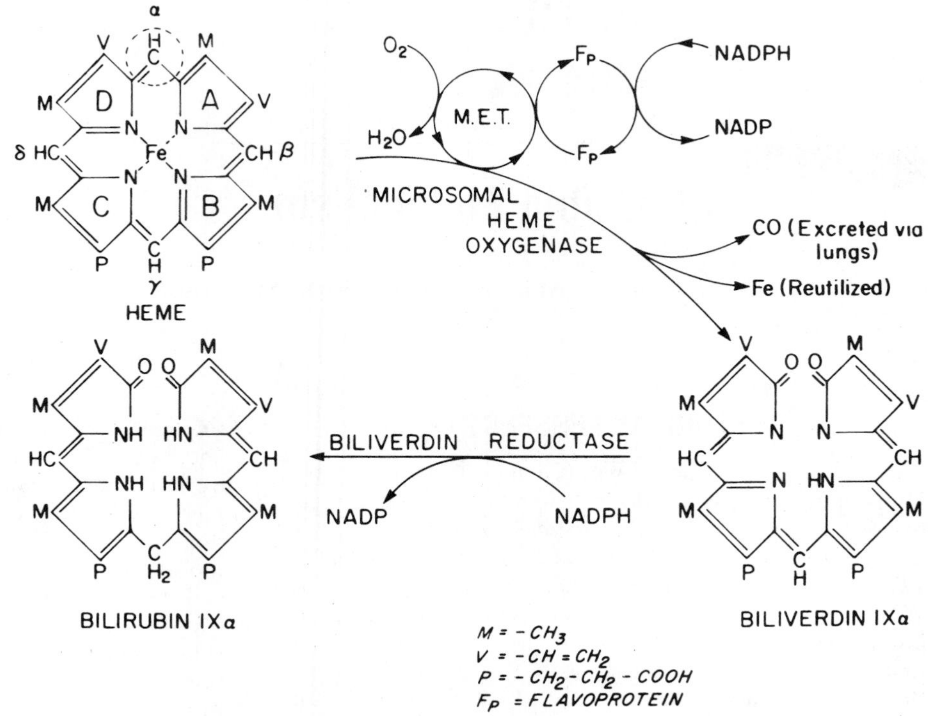

FIGURE 81–1. Catabolism of heme to bilirubin IXα by microsomal heme oxygenase and biliverdin reductase. M.E.T., microsomal electron transport system. (From Berlin NI, Berk PD: Quantitative aspects of bilirubin metabolism for hematologists. Blood 57:983, 1981.)

$$M = -CH_3$$
$$V = -CH = CH_2$$
$$P = -CH_2 - CH_2 - COOH$$
$$F_P = FLAVOPROTEIN$$

BREAKDOWN OF HEME

The first step in the catabolic pathway of the heme molecule is also the rate-limiting step: the creation of biliverdin through the action of the microsomal enzyme, HO. This enzyme opens up the alpha-methene bridge of the heme (see Fig. 81–1), with the alpha-methene carbon quantitatively converted to CO. This opening of the ring allows for the removal of the iron, which can be recycled, the production of CO, which can be removed via ventilation, and the formation of biliverdin, which is immediately reduced by the action of biliverdin reductase.

The enzyme cytochrome P450 reductase (NADPH-cytochrome c [p450] reductase) is an essential cofactor in the breakdown of heme to biliverdin, contributing one electron to reduce heme to the ferrous (Fe^{2+}) state (Yoshida and Kikuchi, 1978). In the ferrous state, heme binds oxygen to begin a lengthy sequence of steps toward auto-oxidation. An intermediary alpha-hydroxy heme is reduced by release of the alpha-methene bridge carbon as CO. With the consumption of several oxygen molecules and electrons, a biliverdin–iron complex is formed and the iron component is then released for recycling. To accomplish the degradation of one mole of heme to bilirubin, it is estimated that 5 to 6 moles of NADPH and 3 molecules of O_2 are required (Maines, 1984; Rodgers and Stevenson, 1990; Tenhunen et al, 1969).

Biliverdin is water soluble and could be readily excreted, as is demonstrated by the normal physiology of birds, reptiles, and amphibians (Stocker et al, 1987). In mammals, however, biliverdin is rapidly converted to bilirubin through the action of biliverdin reductase in another energy-consuming step. Unlike biliverdin, bilirubin is lipophilic and hydrogen binding; it partitions readily into cellular membranes and is virtually insoluble at normal pH. For the body to rid itself of this insoluble end product, therefore, transport and elimination mechanisms are necessary.

BILIRUBIN TRANSPORT

Bilirubin produced in the peripheral regions of the body is transported to the liver, tightly (but reversibly) bound to albumin. Bilirubin formed in the reticuloendothelial system or hepatic parenchymal cells is released into the circulation. Unbound bilirubin cannot be transported in serum or excreted by the liver or kidneys because the solubility of free bilirubin is extremely low, below a pH of 7.8. However, unconjugated bilirubin becomes soluble in aqueous solution when it is attached to proteins with high affinity for nonpolar (hydrophobic) compounds, such as plasma albumin or hepatic ligandin.

Plasma albumin is the most abundant protein in plasma, accounting for 50% of total proteins (Notorianni, 1990). It has the ability to bind endogenous compounds such as bilirubin as well as drugs and metal ions as a result of reactive groups projecting from its tertiary structure. Whereas albumin has an affinity for and can bind unconjugated bilirubin molecules, other compounds may compete for binding sites on the albumin molecule. There is one high-affinity binding site for bilirubin on the albumin molecule. A second site with much less affinity (0.3% as much) is known to exist (Brodersen and Bartels, 1969). Bilirubin can occupy this second site if bilirubin levels are extremely high or when binding to the first site is altered.

Albumin also has a high affinity for acidic drugs such as penicillin and sulfonamide. Because these drugs bind at the predominate binding site for bilirubin, they compete with bilirubin and are capable of displacing the bilirubin molecule from the albumin molecule (Notorianni, 1990).

Other drugs have been shown to displace bilirubin from albumin by reducing the affinity of the albumin for the bilirubin. These drugs include digoxin, gentamicin, furosemide, tolbutamide, and sulfisoxazole. Bilirubin is known to be displaced also by some preservatives used in drug preparations; acetyltryptophan and caprylate, which are used in most albumin preparations, have a displacing effect, which may partially explain the inability of albumin infusions to reduce free bilirubin levels clinically. Bilirubin binding is a dynamic process, with some unbound bilirubin always in equilibrium with that which is bound to the albumin (Table 81–1).

At the average serum albumin concentration of a term neonate, 3.5 to 5.0 mg/dL, there are enough albumin binding sites to carry bilirubin up to a maximum serum bilirubin concentration of 25 to 30 mg/dL (450 μM/L), with a small amount of bilirubin remaining unbound and in equilibrium with the bound bilirubin. However, at higher levels of bilirubin, the albumin binding sites may become saturated and the amount of free (i.e., unbound) bilirubin then increases substantially. The amount of free bilirubin doubles when the total bilirubin level is 15 to 20 mg/dL, quadruples at 25 mg/dL, and increases eightfold at 30 mg/dL (Notorianni, 1990).

Much effort has been expended on tests of serum bilirubin binding capacity. Data suggest that the theoretical "tight" binding capacity of albumin for bilirubin may be diminished in the newborn period. Low pH may have a direct effect on the binding of bilirubin to albumin and is known to increase movement of bilirubin into tissue, altering equilibrium between the bound and the unbound, thereby promoting the dissociation of bilirubin from albumin binding sites (Odell and Cohen, 1960). Such an effect might occur because of the impact of changes in pH in the neonate on the changing solubility of free bilirubin at varying pH values. As pH decreases, the solubility of free bilirubin decreases and bilirubin moves out of solution and enters cells more easily than the bound bilirubin (Bratlid, 1972; Nelson et al, 1974; Wennberg, 1988). Neonates have a lower pH than older infants and adults (Notorianni, 1990) and have a lower concentration of albumin in the first few days of life. Bilirubin binding may be further depressed in premature infants, whose course is frequently complicated by hypoalbuminemia, hypoxia, hypoglycemia, acidosis, hypothermia, hemolysis, and septicemia. The resulting increase in free bilirubin has been implicated in bilirubin neurotoxicity at relatively low serum bilirubin levels in premature infants. (Gartner et al, 1970; Stern and Denton, 1965).

The transport of bilirubin into various cellular compartments, including the skin, is poorly understood but may be of clinical importance with regard to an infant's susceptibility to toxic effects of bilirubin. Body tissues may serve as a reservoir for free bilirubin when serum levels are elevated, partially protecting the brain from the bilirubin entry and deposition.

UPTAKE OF BILIRUBIN AT THE HEPATOCYTE

Bilirubin from the bilirubin–albumin complex is taken up at the surface of the liver parenchymal cells, where the bilirubin is transferred across the cell membrane without the albumin molecule. The hepatocyte plasma membrane may recognize and bind the albumin-bound bilirubin and transfer it directly to a membrane transport system. Immediately after passing through the cell wall, the bilirubin is bound to intracellular proteins. Several proteins manufactured by the hepatocyte bind bilirubin in the cytoplasm. The most important one is ligandin. The exact nature and function of this protein and other binding proteins are still being investigated, although their presence and the intracellular pH are considered important in maintaining the solubility of bilirubin while inside the cells, and the binding of bilirubin inside the cell prevents backflow of bilirubin into the circulation. In addition to enhancing uridine diphosphoglucuronyl transferase (UDPG-T) activity and influencing plasma membrane transport mechanisms, phenobarbital increases the concentration of ligandin, allowing for more binding sites for bilirubin inside the hepatocyte (Potter et al, 1994).

CONJUGATION OF BILIRUBIN

The liver converts bilirubin to an excretable, relatively polar (hence water soluble) conjugate (Fig. 81–2). Conjugation consists of the transfer of one or two glucuronic acid residues from uridine diphosphoglucuronic acid (UDPGA), resulting in a bilirubin monoglucuronide or diglucuronide. Two enzymes participate in the conjugation process. One is UDPG-T, which is associated with the

---

TABLE 81–1

Drugs Capable of Displacing Bilirubin from Albumin*†

Analgesics, antipyretics	Penicillins°°·††
Sodium salicylate	Propicillin
Phenylbutazone	Cloxacillin
Antiseptics, disinfectants	Other
Paraben, methyl-‡	Novabiocin
Paraben, isopropyl	Stabilizers for albumin preparation
Phenyl salicylate	Tryptophan, N-acetyl-D-
Antibiotics, sulfa compounds	Tryptophan, N-acetyl-L-
Sulfaphenazole	Tryptophan, N-acetyl-DL-
Sulfadiazine	Caprylic acid
Sulfadimethoxine	Mendelic acid
Sulfamethizole	X-ray contrast material
Sulfisoxazole	Sodium iodipamide
Sulfamoxole	Meglumine ioglycamate
Sulfamoxazole	Iopanoic acid
Sulfathiazole	Sodium ipodate
Sulfamexazine	
Cephalosporins§	
Ceftriaxone	
Cefoperazone	
Cefonicid	
Cefotetan	
Cefometazole	

° Ability to displace bilirubin may depend on pH, bilirubin concentration, and concentration of drug.
† Reference, except where noted, is Broderson (1978).
§ Broderson and Robertson (1989); Robertson et al (1988).
°° Bratlid, 1976.
‡ Rasmussen et al (1976).
†† Fink et al (1988).

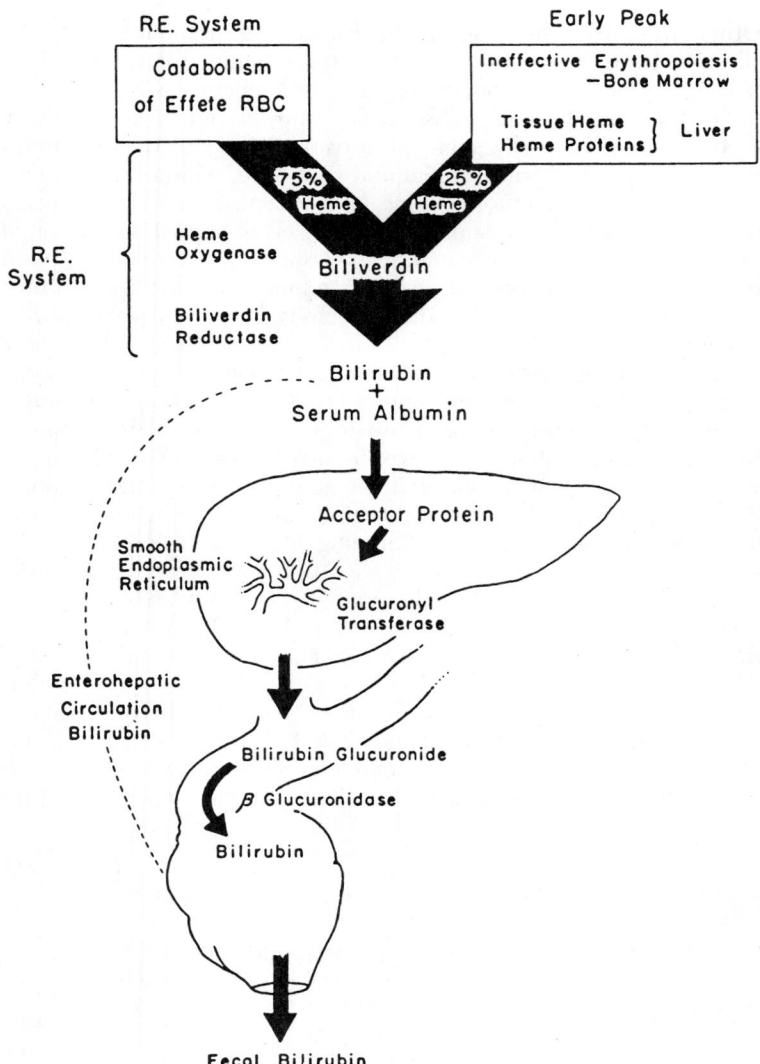

FIGURE 81–2. Bilirubin metabolism in the newborn. (From Maisels MJ: Jaundice in the newborn. Pediatr Res 3:306, 1982. Reproduced by permission of Pediatrics.)

smooth endoplasmic reticulum. This enzyme has been shown to be induced by certain drugs, such as phenobarbital, suggesting a clinical mode for enhancing conjugation and elimination of bilirubin (see Chapter 87.) UDPG-T catalyzes the formation of bilirubin monoglucuronides, which can be excreted or which can be stored and converted to diglucuronides. A second enzyme, located in the plasma membrane of the hepatocyte, is responsible for the addition of the second glucuronide (Schmid, 1978) (Fig. 81–3). In the neonatal period, especially in premature infants, conjugation may be impaired because of reduced transferase activity and possible absence of UDPGA. Indeed, in the first 48 hours of life, conjugated bilirubin is almost all in the form of monoglucuronide; thereafter, diglucuronides dominate.

Cord blood of normal newborns contains little, if any, conjugated bilirubin. However, cord blood of fetuses with intrauterine hemolysis can have both monoglucuronide and diglucuronide forms of conjugated bilirubin, suggesting that the presence of critical amounts of bilirubin can induce conjugation prematurely.

EXCRETION OF BILIRUBIN

Once conjugated, bilirubin is excreted into the bile against a large concentration gradient, an active process dependent on energy expenditure. Transport of conjugated bilirubin from the hepatocyte to the canaliculus is the rate-limiting step in the transhepatic transport of bilirubin. Conjugated bilirubin is not itself reabsorbed once it reaches the intestines. However, unlike adults, newborns have in their stool and intestinal mucosa the enzyme beta-glucuronidase, which can hydrolyze the monoglucuronides and diglucuronides of conjugated bilirubin, returning the bilirubin into the unconjugated state, which can be readily absorbed. Also, unlike in adults, in whom bacteria in the intestinal lumen degrade conjugated bilirubin to a nonabsorbable end product such as stercobilin, the newborn's intestinal lumen is sterile and only gradually colonized in the transition after birth. Thus, the neonate is at risk for enhanced enterohepatic absorption of bilirubin because of two factors, the presence of beta-glucuronidase and the absence of bacteria. Interruption of the enterohepatic circulation of

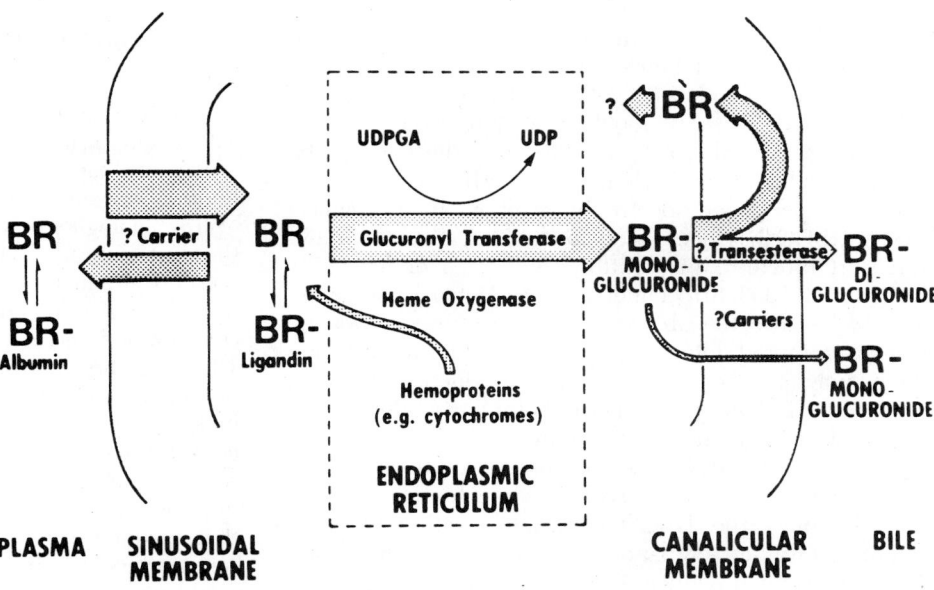

FIGURE 81–3. Bilirubin transport and conjugation in the hepatocyte. Bilirubin (BR) that has been transferred across the sinusoidal membrane is converted to bilirubin monoglucuronide by glucuronyl transferase located in the endoplasmic reticulum. The monoglucuronide is then either excreted into the bile or converted to bilirubin diglucuronide by a glucuronyl transferase believed to be located in the canalicular membrane. (From Schmid R: Bilirubin metabolism: State of the art. Gastroenterology 74:1307, 1978.)

bilirubin has been attempted with some success, using such agents as agar, albumin, and charcoal. These strategies are further discussed in Chapter 87.

FETAL BILIRUBIN METABOLISM

In utero, placental transfer of unconjugated bilirubin directly to the mother allows the fetus to maintain low bilirubin levels, with the fetal liver playing a minor role in bilirubin excretion. Bilirubin UDPG-T is detectable at approximately 20 weeks of gestation, but its quantity remains "low" until after birth. Before 20 weeks' gestation, intestinal contents and the bile of fetuses contain small amounts of unconjugated bilirubin. In later gestation, severe fetal hyperbilirubinemia can induce enzyme production, enhancing the ability of the fetus to conjugate bilirubin.

Bilirubin formed from heme catabolism during fetal life appears to be eliminated by two mechanisms. Bilirubin that enters the placental circulation is cleared across the placenta into the maternal circulation. The concentration of bilirubin in the venous blood returning from the placenta has been found to be lower than the concentration in the umbilical arteries that transport blood to the placenta. Only unconjugated bilirubin is cleared via the placental circulation. Conjugated bilirubin, when formed *in utero*, remains in the fetus and may accumulate in fetal plasma and other tissues. Infants with severe hemolytic disease may be born with increased concentrations of conjugated bilirubin in their blood.

The second route for bilirubin clearance in the fetus is by way of the fetal liver. This excretory pathway is limited in the fetus as a consequence of reduced hepatic blood flow, low levels of hepatocyte ligandin, and limited UDPG-T activity. Conjugated bilirubin that is excreted into the fetal gut is largely hydrolyzed and reabsorbed into the fetal circulation.

Bilirubin can be found in normal amniotic fluid at about 12 weeks of gestation. It usually disappears from the amni-

otic fluid by the 36th to 37th weeks of pregnancy. Increased levels of bilirubin are found in the amniotic fluid of infants with severe hemolytic disease and in association with fetal intestinal obstruction.

The mechanism by which bilirubin gets into the amniotic fluid is still a matter of speculation. It has been suggested that bilirubin reaches the amniotic fluid from tracheobronchial secretions, fetal urine, meconium, diffusion across the umbilical vessels, diffusion from the skin, or direct transfer from the maternal circulation. In rabbits, there is a close relation between the concentration of unconjugated bilirubin in the plasma and that found in tracheal fluid.

In the chapters to follow, various causes of neonatal hyperbilirubinemia are discussed. Jaundice is usually the result of one or more of the following mechanisms:

1. Overproduction of bilirubin
2. Defective uptake and transport of bilirubin within the hepatocyte
3. Impaired conjugation within the hepatic microsomes
4. Defects in bilirubin excretion
5. Increased reabsorption of bilirubin from the intestinal tract

RECENT DEVELOPMENTS IN BILIRUBIN METABOLISM
Measurement of Bilirubin Production

The series of reactions by which heme is degraded to bilirubin results in equimolar production of CO and bilirubin. This fact has proven useful to investigators searching for noninvasive methods to measure heme catabolism and bilirubin production. Gas chromatographic methods have been developed for the accurate detection of CO *in vitro* and *in vivo* (Cavallin-Stahl et al, 1978; Sunderman et al, 1982; Vreman and Stevenson, 1988). These methods have been well correlated with bilirubin production measurements *in vivo* and *in vitro*. Thus in neonates, CO excretion measurements offer a valid and noninvasive index of change in the rate of heme catabolism (Ostrander et al, 1982; Stevenson et al, 1979). The CO diffuses out of the cells, and binds to the hemoglobin of circulating erythrocytes (Rodgers et al, 1994). In this state, the CO can be measured as blood carboxyhemoglobin (HbCO), using CO oximeters, specialized spectrophotometers. In the clinical setting, HbCO has been used to diagnose hemolysis and increased bilirubin production (Necheles et al, 1976; Slusher et al, 1993; Strocchi et al, 1992; Uetani et al, 1989). As well, because the ability of CO to diffuse across the placenta is limited, fetal HbCO may be useful in detecting fetal hemolysis and excessive bilirubin production (Widness et al, 1994). To overcome spectrophotometric interference from fetal hemoglobin and bilirubin itself, newer CO oximeters have been developed to correct for these factors (Vreman and Stevenson, 1994).

In the lung, the HbCO dissociates, with CO being excreted by way of ventilation. The rate of CO production can be determined by measuring the rate of total body CO excretion, or it can be estimated by measuring the CO concentration in end-tidal breath samples.

Through these technologic advances, sensitive noninvasive assays for HO activity, HbCO levels, end tidal breath CO concentrations, and total body CO excretion have been achieved. Estimates of CO production can be correlated with bilirubin production *in vitro* and *in vivo* and used as valid and noninvasive indices of total bilirubin production. Using these methods, total bilirubin production has been shown to be increased in infants such as those with Rh and ABO hemolytic disease and other causes of hemolysis, infants of diabetic mothers, and infants of mothers who smoke tobacco. However, well, breast-fed neonates have demonstrated no such increase in bilirubin production, despite a propensity for jaundice, which is attributed primarily to enhanced enterohepatic circulation (Gartner, 1994; Stevenson et al, 1993).

Instruments capable of measuring bilirubin concentrations transcutaneously have been developed to make noninvasive assessment practical. However, these devices measure either the color of the skin or reflectance at specific wavelengths rather than true bilirubin concentrations. Consistent and clinically useful correlations between the measures and the true serum bilirubin concentration have not been achieved for a variety of reasons, and changes in the skin color may not always reflect directly changes in serum concentration. Transcutaneous measurements of bilirubin have been shown to be inaccurate also because the yellow color of skin is affected by several factors including postnatal age, presence of other pigments, crying, location on the body, and even the amount of light to which the skin is exposed (Amato, 1994; Yamouchi and Yamouchi, 1991a, 1991b, 1991c). These devices have most commonly been used for screening populations, not for specific case management or acute intervention decisions. The nature of the correlation of skin color to serum concentration is such that a given jaundice meter reading can encompass a large range of serum levels. Additionally, dark skinned individuals may not be assessed well by these meters (Brown, 1984). Efforts to standardize the results and to make transcutaneous bilirubinometry practical are continuing.

Efforts to Reduce Bilirubin Production

Efforts are underway to develop safe methods to reduce the production of bilirubin by controlling or blocking the catabolism of heme. Several metalloporphyrin analogues of heme are known to inhibit the enzyme HO, the rate-limiting enzyme in the degradation of heme (Fig. 81–4).

Tin analogues have been the most widely studied of these compounds in humans. Both tin protoporphyrin and mesoporphyrin have been shown to inhibit HO competitively *in vitro* and to reduce bilirubin production *in vivo* (Drummond and Kappas, 1981). The mesoderivative has a 10-fold greater inhibitory effect on HO. Both these compounds are also potential photosensitizers capable of enhancing the photodegradation of bilirubin as well as other compounds (Vreman et al, 1988). Phototoxic reactions would be undesirable side effects in populations experiencing uncontrolled exposure to light. It has been suggested that singlet oxygen production and lipid peroxidation are responsible for tin-protoporphyrin–induced phototoxicity (Dennery et al, 1993; McDonagh and Palma, 1985).

Zinc protoporphyrin has also been extensively studied as a potential HO inhibitor, although its efficacy compared to the tin compounds is somewhat controversial (Drummond and Kappas, 1981; Maines, 1981). The zinc protoporphyrin molecule appears to be less photoreactive than the tin compounds, demonstrating little photosensitizing activity *in vitro* and none *in vivo* (Vreman et al, 1991). Zinc mesoporphyrin and zinc deuteroporphyrin 2,4-bis glycol (ZnBG) have also been studied, the latter being orally absorbable and even more potent than the tin porphyrins for inhibiting HO. The search continues for effective inhibitors of HO that are nonphotosensitizing, biocompatible, and resistant to degradation.

POSSIBLE BENEFITS OF BILIRUBIN

Ever since Virchow described yellow crystal formation at sites of hemolysis, the metabolic link between heme and bilirubin has been explored. So closely are they related that bilirubin formation appears to be essential for regulation of intracellular heme levels. Because the catabolism of heme is the only known source of both bilirubin and CO in humans, speculation has been growing with regard to possible roles that these two by-products play in normal physiology.

Until recently, it has been assumed that bilirubin is merely a useless catabolic waste product. Investigators have come to question this assumption. Hypothesizing that bilirubin formation is uneconomic and (theoretically) unnecessary, investigators have sought to identify a purpose for its production. If reptiles, amphibians, and birds use biliverdin as the end product of heme degradation, why would mammals have evolved the complex energy-requiring system of excretion for bilirubin unless the end product is beneficial?

One theory suggests that the placenta is incapable of transferring polarized molecules such as biliverdin from the fetal to the maternal circulation. Conversion to the nonpolar bilirubin allows placental transfer to occur, avoiding buildup of biliverdin in the fetus. What risk, if any, such a buildup might present is unknown.

A second theory touts bilirubin as a beneficial protective

FIGURE 81–4. Metalloporphyrin complexes and their chemical structures. Substrates and inhibitors of heme oxygenase belong to a large family of metalloporphyrins with varying metal moieties and porphyrin ring substituents. (From Rodgers PA, Stevenson DK: Developmental biology of heme oxygenase. *In* Maisels MJ [Ed]: Clinics in Perinatology. Neonatal Jaundice. Philadelphia, WB Saunders, 1990, p 278.)

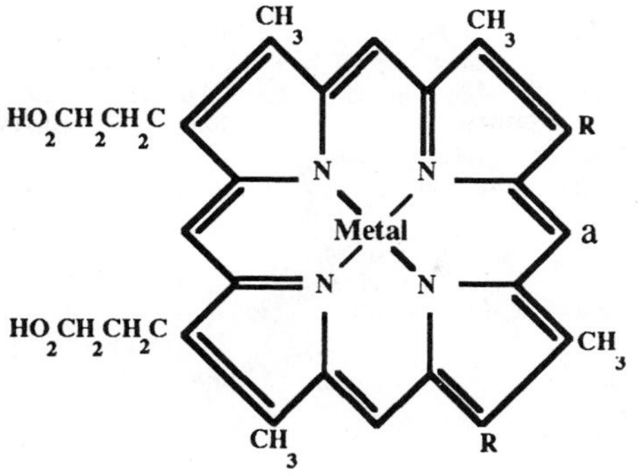

Metals:

1. Fe - Heme
2. Sn - Tin Metalloporphyrin
3. Zn - Zinc Metalloporphyrin
4. Cr - Chromium Metalloporphyrin
5. Mn - Manganese Metalloporphyrin

R-Chemical Group:

1. R=Vinyl (CH_2=CH-) - Protoporphyrin
2. R=Ethyl (CH_3-CH_2-) - Mesoporphyrin
3. R=Deutero (H-) - Deuteroporphyrin
4. R=2,4 Bis Glycol (CH_2OH-CHOH-) - Deuteroporphyrin 2,4 Bis Glycol

antioxidant. Reactive free oxygen radicals are being increasingly implicated as contributing or exacerbating factors in many diseases including cancer, cardiovascular disease, bronchopulmonary dysplasia, emphysema, and aging (Cross et al, 1987). Endogenous defensive antioxidant enzymes such as catalase have been identified. In addition to these enzymes, there are smaller nonprotein, nonenzyme molecules that may play a role in blocking oxidative damage. These include vitamin E, beta-carotene, and ascorbic acid, and recent studies suggest that bilirubin may also be such an endogenous antioxidant (McDonagh, 1990). Consistent with this hypothesis is that, during the newborn period, demand for tissue protection may be especially high and other antioxidants may not be readily available.

Additionally, it has been shown that HO, the enzyme that leads to bilirubin formation, is itself a heat-shock protein that may be induced as a general response to oxidative stress, including hyperthemia (Ewing and Maines, 1993; Ewing et al, 1992; Maines, 1988). Because heme is capable of catalyzing oxygen radical reactions, defense against oxidative damage could occur by stimulating HO to deplete the intracellular heme, or by enhanced production of bilirubin. It seems plausible, then, that bilirubin might play a beneficial role, particularly in the immediate postpartum period when oxidative stresses may occur and when there are depressed levels of endogenous vitamin E and other antioxidant enzymes. Such arguments suggest that bilirubin is more than merely a waste product or a dangerous toxin, but whether it actually plays a significant physiologic or antioxidant role in fetal, infant, or adult life is unknown and awaits further investigation.

Controversy exists regarding the CO by-product of heme catabolism, as well. Considered in the past to be a poison, CO has recently been shown to be used by the brain and vascular tissues as an intercellular messenger in much the same fashion as NO (Morita and Kourembanas, 1995). CO, generated by HO, can diffuse into neighboring cells, stimulating the activity of guanylate cyclase, the enzyme that helps to produce intracellular messenger cyclic guanosine monophosphate. This area of inquiry exposes questions regarding the presence and role of HO in brain tissue in the normal state and regarding its significance locally in times of stress.

REFERENCES

Amato M: Transcutaneous, capillary, and arterial bilirubin levels (letter). J Pediatr 125:332, 1994.

Amato M, Huppi P, Markus D: Assessment of neonatal jaundice in low birth weight infants comparing transcutaneous, capillary and arterial bilirubin levels. Eur J Pediatr 150:59–61, 1990.

Bratlid D: Bilirubin binding by human erythrocytes. Scand J Clin Lab Invest 29:91–94, 1972.

Bratlid D: Pharmacologic aspects of neonatal hyperbilirubinemia. Birth Defects XII:184–191, 1976.

Bratlid D: How bilirubin gets into the brain. Clin Perinatol 17:449–466, 1990.

Brodersen R: Competitive binding of bilirubin and other substances to plasma albumin: Equilibrium studies in vitro. Birth Defects XII:179–183, 1976.

Brodersen R, Bartels P: Enzymatic oxidation of bilirubin. Eur J Biol Chem 10:468–473, 1969.

Brodersen R: Free bilirubin in blood plasma of the newborn: Effects of albumin, fatty acids, pH, displacing drugs and phototherapy. *In* Stern L, Oh W, Friis-Hansen B (Eds): Intensive Care in the Newborn II. New York, Masson, 1978, pp 331–345.

Brodersen R, Robertson A: Ceftriaxone binding to human serum albumin: Competition with bilirubin. Mol Pharmacol 36:478–483, 1989.

Brown AK, Kim MH, Valencia G, et al: Factors affecting transcutaneous measurement of bilirubin: Influence of race, gestational age, phototherapy and albumin binding capacity. *In* Rubaltelli FF, Jori G (Eds): Neonatal Jaundice. New Trends in Phototherapy. New York, Plenum Press, 1984, pp 95–109.

Burton J: An essay towards a complete new system of midwifery, theoretical and practical. London, J Hodges, 1751.

Cavallin-Stahl E, Johnsson GI, Lundh B: A new method for determination of microsomal heme oxygenase based on quantitation of carbon monoxide formation. Scand J Clin Invest 38:69, 1978.

Cone TE: The History of American Pediatrics. Boston, Little, Brown, 1979.

Cross CE, Halliwell B, Borish ET, et al: Oxygen radicals and human disease. Ann Intern Med 107:526–545, 1987.

Dennery PA, Vreman HJ, Rodgers PA, Stevenson DK: Role of lipid peroxidation in metalloporphyrin-mediated phototoxic reactions in neonatal rats. Pediatr Res 33(1):87–91, 1993.

Dewees WP: Treatise on the Physical and Medical Treatment of Children. Philadelphia, HC Carey & I Lea, 1825.

Drummond GS, Kappas A: Prevention of neonatal hyperbilirubinemia by tin-protoporphyrin IX, a potent competitive inhibitor of heme oxidation. Proc Natl Acad Sci U S A 78:6466–6470, 1981.

Ewing JF, Haber SN, Maines MD: Normal and heat-induced patterns of expression of heme-oxygenase-1 (HSP32) in rat brain; hyperthermia causes rapid induction of mRNA and protein. J Neurochem 58(3):1140–1149, 1992.

Ewing JF, Maines MD: Glutathione depletion induces heme oxygenase-1 (HSP32) mRNA and protein in rat brain. J Neurochem 60(4):1512–1519, 1993.

Fink S, Karp W, Robertson A: Effect of penicillins on bilirubin-albumin binding. J Pediatr 113:566–568, 1988.

Gartner LM: Neonatal jaundice. Pediatr Rev 15:422–432, 1994.

Gartner LM, Snyder RN, Chalon RS, Bernstein L: Kernicterus: High incidence in premature infants with low serum bilirubin concentrations. Pediatrics 45:906–908, 1970.

Hintz SR, Vreman HJ, Stevenson DK: Mortality of metalloporphyrin-treated neonatal rats after light exposure. Dev Pharmacol Ther 14:187–192, 1990.

Kappas A, Simionatta CS, Drummond GS, et al: The liver excretes large amounts of heme into bile when heme oxygenase is inhibited competitively by Sn-protoporphyrin. Proc Natl Acad Sci U S A 82:896–900, 1985.

Keino H, Nagae H, Mimura S, et al: Dangerous effects of tin-protoporphyrin plus photoirradiation on neonatal rats. Eur J Pediatr 149:278–279, 1990.

Land EJ, McDonagh AF, McGarvey DJ, Truscott TG: Photophysical studies of tin (IV)-protoporphyrin: Potential phototoxicity of a chemotherapeutic agent proposed for the prevention of neonatal jaundice. Proc Natl Acad Sci U S A 85:5249–5253, 1988.

Langbaum ME, Pomerance JJ, Farber SJ, Rosenthal P: Comparison of arterial and capillary bilirubin values in neonates with arterial lines. J Pediatr 123:794–796, 1993.

Maines MD: Zinc protoporphyrin is a selective inhibitor of heme oxygenase activity in the neonatal rat. Biochem Biophys Acta 673:339–350, 1981.

Maines MD: New developments in the regulation of heme metabolism and their implications. CRC Crit Rev Toxicol 12:241, 1984.

Maines MD: Heme oxygenase: Function, multiplicity, regulatory mechanisms, and clinical applications. FASEB J 2(10):2557–2568, 1988.

McDonagh AF: Is bilirubin good for you? Clin Perinatol 17:359–369, 1990.

McDonagh AF, Palma LA: Tin-protoporphyrin: A potent photosensitizer of bilirubin destruction. Photochem Photobiol 42:261–264, 1985.

Morita T, Kourembanas S: Endothelial cell expression of vasoconstrictors and growth factors is regulated by smooth muscle cell–derived carbon monoxide. J Clin Invest 96:2676–2682, 1995.

Necheles TR, Rai US, Valaes T: The role of haemolysis in neonatal hyperbilirubinemia as reflected in carboxyhemoglobin levels. Acta Paediatr Scand 65:361–367, 1976.

Nelson T, Jacobsen J, Wennberg RP: Effect of pH on the interaction of bilirubin with albumin and tissue culture cells. Pediatr Res 8:963–967, 1974.

Notorianni L: Plasma protein binding of drugs in pregnancy and in neonates. Clin Pharmacokinet 18(1):20–36, 1990.

Odell GB, Cohen S: The effect of pH on the binding of bilirubin. Am J Dis Child 105:525–530, 1960.

Ostrander CR, Cohen RS, Hopper AO, et al: Paired determinations of blood carboxyhemoglobin concentration and carbon monoxide excretion rate in term and preterm infants. J Lab Clin Med 100:745–755, 1982.

Posselt AM, Kwong LK, Vreman HJ, Stevenson DK: Suppression of carbon monoxide excretion rate by tin protoporphyrin. Am J Dis Child 140:147–150, 1986.

Potter BJ, Ni JZ, Wolfe K, Stump D, Berk PD: Induction of a dose related increase in sulfobromophthalein uptake velocity in freshly isolated rat hepatocytes by phenobarbitol. Hepatology 20:1078–1085, 1994.

Qato MK, Maines MD: Prevention of neonatal hyperbilirubinemia in non-human primates by Zn-protoporphyrin. Bio Chem J 226:51–57, 1985.

Rasmussen LF, Ahlfors CE, Wennberg RP: The effect of paraben preservatives on albumin binding of bilirubin. J Pediatr 89(3):475–478, 1976.

Robertson A, Fink S, Karp W: Effect of cephalosporins on bilirubin-albumin binding. J Pediatr 112:291–294, 1988.

Robertson A, Karp W, Bordersen R: Bilirubin displacing effect of drugs used in neonatology. Acta Paediatr Scand 80:1119–1127, 1991.

Rodgers PA, Vreman HJ, Stevenson DK: Heme catabolism in rhesus neonates inhibited by zinc protoporphyrin. Dev Pharmacol Ther 18:449–460, 1989.

Rodgers PA, Stevenson DK: Developmental biology of heme oxygenase. Clin Perinatol 17:275–291, 1990.

Rodgers PA, Vreman HJ, Dennery PA, Stevenson DK: Sources of carbon monoxide (CO) in biological systems and applications of CO detection technologies. Semin Perinatol 18(1):2–10, 1994.

Schmid R: Bilirubin metabolism: State of the art. Gastroenterology 74:1307, 1978.

Slusher TM, Vreman HJ, McLaren DW, et al: Carboxyhemoglobin predicts bilirubin-related morbidity and mortality in infants (abstr). Pediatr Res 33:237A, 1993.

Stern L, Denton RL: Kernicterus in small premature infants. Pediatrics 35:483–485, 1965.

Stevenson DK, Ostrander CR, Cohen RS, et al: Relationship of heme catabolism to jaundice: Bilirubin production in infancy. Perinatol Neonatal 5:35, 1979.

Stevenson DK, Rodgers PA, Vreman HJ: The use of metalloporphyrins for the chemoprevention of neonatal jaundice. Am J Dis Child 143:353–356, 1989.

Stevenson DK, Bartoletti AL, Ostrander CR, Johnson JD: Pulmonary excretion of carbon monoxide in the human infant as an index of bilirubin production. IV. Effects of breast-feeding and caloric intake in the first postnatal week. Pediatrics 65:1170–1172, 1990.

Stevenson DK, Vreman HJ, Oh W, et al: Bilirubin production in breast-fed only or formula-fed only well term infants. Pediatr Res 33:238A, 1993.

Stevenson DK, Vreman HJ, Stevenson DK, et al: Bilirubin production in healthy term infants as measured by carbon monoxide in breath. Clin Chem 40:1934–1939, 1994.

Stocker R, Yamamoto Y, McDonagh AF, et al: Bilirubin is an antioxidant of possible physiologic importance. Science 235:1043–1046, 1987.

Strocchi A, Schwartz S, Ellefson M, et al: A simple carbon monoxide breath test to estimate erythrocyte turnover. J Lab Clin Med 120:392–399, 1992.

Sunderman FW, Downs JR, Reid MC, et al: Gas-chromatographic assay for heme oxygenase activity. Clin Chem 28:2026, 1982.

Tenhunen R, Marver HS, Schmid R: Microsomal heme oxygenase. J Biol Chem 244:1388, 1969.

Uetani Y, Nakamura H, Okamoto O, et al: Carboxyhemoglobin measurements in the diagnosis of ABO hemolytic disease. Acta Paediatr Jpn 31:171–176, 1989.

Virchow R: Die pathologischen pigmenten. Arch Pathol Anat Physiol Klin Med 1:379–486, 1847.

Vreman HJ, Downum KR, Stevenson DK: Generation of CO by tin protoporphyrin as a function of light exposure. Pediatr Res 23:265A, 1988.

Vreman HJ, Lee OK, Stevenson DK: In vitro and in vivo characteristics of a heme oxygenase inhibitor: ZnBG. Am J Med Sci 302:335–341, 1991.

Vreman HJ, Rodgers PA, Gale R, Stevenson DK: Carbon monoxide excretion as an index of bilirubin production in rhesus monkeys. J Med Primatol 18:449–60, 1989.

Vreman HJ, Rodgers PA, Stevenson DK: Zinc protoporphyrin administration for suppression of increased bilirubin production by iatrogenic hemolysis in rhesus neonates. J Pediatr 117:292–297, 1990.

Vreman HJ, Stevenson, DK: Heme oxygenase activity as measured by carbon monoxide production. Anal Biochem 168:31, 1988.

Vreman HJ, Stevenson DK: Metalloporphyrin-enhanced photodegradation of bilirubin in vitro. Am J Dis Child 144:590–594, 1990.

Vreman HJ, Stevenson DK: Carboxyhemoglobin determined in neonatal blood with a CO-oximeter unaffected by fetal oxyhemoglobin. Clin Chem 40(8):1522–1527, 1994.

Vreman HJ, Stevenson DK, Oh W, Fanaroff AA, Wright LL, Lemons JA: Semiportable electrochemical instrument for determining carbon monoxide in breath. Clin Chem 40:1927–33, 1994.

Wennberg RP: The importance of free bilirubin acid salt in bilirubin uptake by erythrocytes and mitochondria. Pediatr Res 23:443–447, 1988.

Widness JA, Lowe LS, Stevenson DK, et al: Direct relationship of fetal carboxyhemoglobin with hemolysis in allo-immunized pregnancies. Pediatr Res 35(6):713–719, 1994.

Yamouchi Y, Yamouchi I: Transcutaneous bilirubinometry: Variability of transcutaneous bilirubin measurements on the forehead with injury. Acta Paediatr Jpn 33:655–657, 1991a.

Yamouchi Y, Yamouchi I: Factors affecting transcutaneous bilirubin measurement: The effect of daylight. Acta Paediatr Jpn 33:658–662, 1991b.

Yamouchi Y, Yamouchi I: Factors affecting transcutaneous bilirubin measurement: Effect of postnatal age. Acta Paediatr Jpn 33:663–667, 1991c.

Yoshida T, Kikuchi G: Features of the reaction of heme degradation catalyzed by the reconstituted microsomal heme oxygenase system. J Biol Chem 253:4230, 1978.

CHAPTER 82

Physiologic Jaundice

James R. MacMahon, David K. Stevenson and Frank A. Oski*

Etymology

- Bile—from Latin *bilis,* but the Latin probably had Celtic origins *(bistlis).*
- Bilirubin and Biliverdin—simply "red bile" and "green bile," latinized.
- Icterus—from Greek *ikteros,* meaning yellow colored, a word applied to a yellow bird as well.
- Jaundice—from Old French *jaundice,* a word rooted in the Latin *galbinus,* meaning greenish yellow, from *galbus.*

Jaundice is the visible manifestation in skin and sclera of elevated serum concentrations of bilirubin. Most adults are jaundiced when serum bilirubin levels exceed 2.0 mg/dL (34 μM/L). Neonates, however, may not appear jaundiced until the serum bilirubin concentration exceeds 5.0 to 7.0 mg/dL (119 μM/L). Each year, some degree of jaundice develops in approximately 60% to 70% of the 4 million babies born in the United States. In babies born prematurely, the incidence is approximately 80%.

Chemical hyperbilirubinemia, defined as a serum total bilirubin level of 2.0 mg/dL (34 μM/L) or more, is virtually universal in newborns during the 1st week of life. Bilirubin concentrations in premature babies are even higher, persist longer, and are more likely to be associated with neurologic injury than those in term neonates (Lockitch, 1994). Debate and controversy remain in efforts to define either normal or physiologic ranges of serum bilirubin concentration in newborns, because the data are influenced by such variables as length of gestation, birth weight, nutritional status, mode of feeding, race, and even geographic location. Even within a single racial group, genetic variation may affect the intensity and duration of physiologic jaundice. At issue is whether the normal range should be determined by rate of increase in serum bilirubin concentration, a level for a specific postpartum age, or the maximum level attained.

An understanding of bilirubin production, extracellular and intracellular transport, conjugation, and elimination, as described in Chapter 81, provides the basis for discussion of what has long been thought of as "physiologic" jaundice of the newborn, a condition considered clinically benign and etiologically nonpathologic.

Traditionally, a distinction has been made between this physiologic jaundice and hyperbilirubinemia, which is either pathologic in origin or severe enough to be considered deserving of further evaluation and intervention. This latter group has been called "nonphysiologic," although frequently no disease is identified as being causative or consequent.

Basing their interpretation of normal ranges of serum bilirubin concentration in neonates on the National Collaborative Perinatal Project, authors of chapters in leading pediatric textbooks have agreed that, if the total serum bilirubin concentration exceeded 5 mg/dL on the 1st day of life in a term neonate, 10 mg/dL on the 2nd day, or 12 to 13 mg/dL thereafter, the bilirubin is, by definition, not physiologic. In recent years, the significance of these numbers has been questioned.

Data from a mixed population of babies weighing more than 2500 g in San Francisco revealed that, using the aforementioned parameters, 13.1% of the babies would be classified as nonphysiologic (10% of whites, 4.4% of blacks, and 23% of Asians) (Newman et al, 1990). The data of Maisels and Gifford (1986) indicate that the 97th percentile of maximal total bilirubin concentration in healthy mature newborns is 12.4 mg/dL if formula fed and 14.8 mg/dL if breast-fed.

The elevation of serum bilirubin concentrations in healthy-appearing babies results from the convergence of several developmental situations specific to the neonate. Gartner and coworkers (1977) divided the clinical course of physiologic jaundice into two phases. Phase I includes the first 5 days of life in term infants and is characterized by a rapid increase in bilirubin levels for 3 or 4 days when the level begins to decline. Phase II is characterized by stable but elevated bilirubin levels lasting about 2 weeks. In preterm infants, phase I lasts 6 to 7 days, and the bilirubin levels reached are higher than in term babies. After phase II, serum bilirubin levels become comparable with adult levels. Data from multiple studies show that physiologic jaundice usually results in peak bilirubin levels between days 3 and 5 of life. In 1981, Maisels proposed criteria that can be used to exclude the diagnosis of physiologic jaundice. Since then, these criteria have been adjusted upward to accommodate conditions related to breast-feeding, state of hydration, and so on. In addition, it must be remembered that absence of these criteria does not guarantee that the jaundice is physiologic (Table 82–1).

Distinctive aspects of normal newborn physiology that contribute to neonatal hyperbilirubinemia include (1) increased bilirubin synthesis, (2) less effective binding and transportation, (3) less efficient hepatic conjugation and excretion, and (4) enhanced absorption of bilirubin via the enterohepatic circulation.

INCREASED BILIRUBIN SYNTHESIS

In neonates, hemoglobin breaks down at twice the adult rate (Maisels et al, 1971), and there is an increased rate of red cell degradation in the marrow even before release. In addition, bilirubin synthesis in healthy neonates results from a greater erythrocyte mass at birth and a shorter half-life of neonatal red blood cells. Normal term newborns

*Deceased.

TABLE 82–1

Criteria that Rule Out the Diagnosis of Physiologic Jaundice

1. Clinical jaundice in the first 24 hours of life.
2. Total serum bilirubin concentration increasing by more than 5 mg/dL (85 μmol/L) per day.
3. Total serum bilirubin concentration exceeding 12.9 mg/dL (221 μmol/L) in a full-term infant or 15 mg/dL (257 μmol/L) in a premature infant.
4. Direct serum bilirubin concentration exceeding 1.5 to 2 mg/dL (26–34 μmol/L).
5. Clinical jaundice persisting for more than 1 week in a full-term infant or 2 weeks in a premature infant.

From Maisels MJ: *In* Avery GB (Ed): Neonatology, 2nd ed. Philadelphia, JB Lippincott, 1981, p 484.

have a hemoglobin level of approximately 19 g/dL, and a hematocrit of approximately 50% to 55%. Polycythemia, defined as a hematocrit greater than 65%, occurs in 1.4% to 1.8% of infants born at sea level and in 4% of those born at altitude.

The life span of erythrocytes is less than 70 days for premature babies. It is estimated to be approximately 70 to 90 days in healthy term infants compared to 120 days in adults.

BINDING AND TRANSPORTATION

The full-term newborn infant has a significantly lower plasma albumin level than an adult and, therefore, correspondingly fewer bilirubin binding sites. The albumin level is dependent on gestational age, and the more premature an infant is, the lower the level. Plasma albumin level increases rapidly over the first few days after birth, resulting in a mean increase over the first 7 days of almost 30%. Adult levels are reached by about 5 months of age (Notorianni, 1990).

Albumin binding of compounds in neonates is similar to that in adults, in that acidic drugs and bilirubin are bound to albumin, but the affinity of the compounds to albumin may be altered. It has been suggested that there are endogenous displacing agents in newborns and that the albumin may be structurally different, attaining adult characteristics at 10 to 12 months of age (Miyoshi et al, 1966).

CONJUGATION AND EXCRETION

During intrauterine life, removal of bilirubin from the fetus is accomplished by way of the placenta and maternal-fetal circulation, and the bilirubin in cord blood is virtually all unconjugated. At birth, blood supply to the right lobe of the liver changes from the high oxygen content of the umbilical vein to portal venous flow. Blood flow through the hepatic arteries develops only in the 1st week of extrauterine life. In addition, the ductus venous may remain partially patent for several days, allowing blood to bypass the liver altogether. All these factors can contribute to a delay in plasma clearance of bilirubin.

The conjugating capacity of normal infants varies greatly; delayed conjugation and excretion may in some cases be related to immaturity of the liver cell itself. The activity of the glucuronyl transferase system in the newborn liver must be induced. Evidence that it can be induced prenatally in cases of severe fetal hemolysis (see Chapter 81) suggests that elevated bilirubin levels may be necessary to induce the conjugating enzymes. Production of glucuronyl transferase has been shown to be enhanced when certain drugs are administered.

Phenobarbital is known to have this effect, and clinical application of this knowledge is discussed in Chapter 81. However, there also are pharmaceutical substances that can inhibit glucuronyl transferase activity. Steroids structurally related to estrogen and progesterone have been shown to have this effect *in vitro* and *in vivo,* as have phenothiazines and the ester proprionate preparation of erythromycin (Hsia et al, 1960).

ENHANCED ENTEROHEPATIC CIRCULATION

Intestinal absorption of bilirubin successfully excreted into the intestines is enhanced by several features of newborn physiology, which thus add to the tendency of newborns to become jaundiced. Conjugated bilirubin, either as the monogluronide or diglucuronide, is unstable and can be spontaneously or enzymatically hydrolyzed to unconjugated bilirubin, which is easily absorbed through the mucosa. In addition, absorption is enhanced by the sterility of the intestinal contents; older children and adults have intestinal flora that can metabolize conjugated bilirubin to break down products, such as urobilin and stercobilin, which are water soluble and relatively easy to excrete. Newborns have no such advantage; instead, the neonatal intestinal mucosa has a greater concentration of beta-glucuronidase than does the adult. This enzyme can deconjugate bilirubin, resulting in more unconjugated bilirubin that can be absorbed via the enterohepatic circulation, adding to the unconjugated bilirubin load. Two other factors accelerating the deconjugation of bilirubin glucuronide in the newborn intestine are the mildly alkaline pH of the proximal intestine, which facilitates nonenzymatic hydrolysis, and the dominance of monoglucuronides as the main excretion form of bilirubin in the first few days of life.

All the aforementioned factors have the effect of increasing the serum bilirubin of the healthy newborn; the premature newborn is even more susceptible to almost all of these influences. Because individual variation in the maturation of any of these systems is great, there is a wide range of serum bilirubin levels in a normal neonatal population. Slight perturbations in any of these processes could result in increased bilirubin levels. For example, through studies of carbon monoxide (CO) production, it has been determined that infants of diabetic mothers have a propensity for jaundice because of both enhanced bilirubin formation and impaired elimination. Any pathologic process that increases bilirubin production or impairs its elimination is superimposed on normally occurring physiologic jaundice in newborns. In the clinical setting, any such pathologic disorder should be identified and treated as necessary. What remains controversial is the danger posed by bilirubin levels encountered in the absence of pathologic disorders, as well as when to pursue investigations to identify or rule out disease.

EPIDEMIOLOGY

Although all babies experience some degree of hyperbilirubinemia in the first few days of life and most have some physiologic jaundice, the extent and the duration of the elevation in serum bilirubin levels vary among populations of different racial compositions or in different geographic distributions. The pattern of physiologic jaundice described previously in this chapter, reaching maximal levels on the 3rd or 4th day of life, is commonly seen in term infants of European or African ancestry. In the United States, black infants have slightly lower peak bilirubin concentrations than other groups. In contrast, Native American infants and infants of Asian ancestry have a different pattern of neonatal jaundice, with a more rapid increase of serum bilirubin concentration in the first few days, a higher peak bilirubin level, and a relatively prolonged course with the peak bilirubin level reaching its maximum several days later. The subsequent return to more normal levels occurs more slowly in these populations as well (Gartner, 1994).

Investigations involving babies in Japan, Asians born in the United States, Navajo, Sioux, Eskimos in Alaska, and Hispanics in Los Angeles (mostly from families in northern Mexico) have consistently shown higher levels of bilirubin in the first few days of life in all these groups. The reasons for such racial or ethnic differences are unclear. Studies assessing CO production suggest that an increased rate of heme catabolism leading to increased synthesis of bilirubin may be an important contributing cause. There is no strong evidence in favor of enhanced intestinal absorption or diminished conjugation or excretion in these populations (Johnson, 1992). However, in larger studies that have assessed the increase in bilirubin synthesis in Asians, it is clear that not all individuals in a population are high producers of bilirubin (Fisher et al, 1988). Whether these populations are at higher risk for toxic effects of hyperbilirubinemia has not been determined. Italian studies looking for specific genetic markers within racial groups suggest that there may be genetic traits involving red cell membrane stability as well as factors involved with bilirubin conjugation that contribute to neonatal jaundice, although environmental as well as genetic factors may play a role (Lucarini et al, 1991).

The knowledge that racial groups differ in the peak bilirubin levels could have important implications for management of these infants. Using criteria for intervention based on Caucasian and African populations might lead to overtreatment of significant numbers of infants from other races.

For several years there has been considerable controversy regarding the influence of breast-feeding on serum bilirubin levels. Most studies indicate that infants who are breast-fed are several times as likely to have serum bilirubin levels greater than 12 mg/dL than formula-fed babies. In addition, breast-fed babies are thought to have higher levels of bilirubin throughout the first several weeks of life. The question has been asked, "Is physiologic jaundice in the newborn exaggerated in breast-fed babies?" Many studies have attempted to answer this question, and results are conflicting. Investigations with data showing no difference between breast-fed and formula-fed babies generate considerable correspondence, indicating the impression of many clinicians that breast-fed babies are more icteric on the 3rd day of life than formula-fed babies (Boggs, 1974). A meta-analysis of a large series of studies showed that nearly 13% of breast-fed babies versus 4% of formula-fed babies had bilirubin levels of 12 mg/dL or higher on days 3 to 6 of life, and 2% of breast-fed infants versus 0.3% of those fed formula exceeded bilirubin levels of 15 mg/dL (Schneider, 1986). The consensus of practitioners and investigators in the past decade is that breast-feeding is indeed associated with statistically significant elevations of serum bilirubin concentrations.

BREAST-FEEDING JAUNDICE

Two separate patterns of jaundice in breast-feeding infants have been described. The first has been termed *breast-feeding associated jaundice,* or simply *breast-feeding jaundice,* a condition that occurs in the 1st week of life; the second is less common and is called *breast milk jaundice* and presents as prolonged hyperbilirubinemia lasting into the 3rd week of life or beyond. Several reports suggesting that the cause of breast-feeding jaundice may be nutritional show that this condition can be prevented by encouraging frequent (e.g., nine times daily) breast-feeding in the first 3 days of life and by avoidance of supplementation with water or glucose solutions (DeCarvalho et al, 1982; Varimo et al, 1986; Yamauchi and Yamauchi, 1990). To explain the phenomenon of breast-feeding jaundice, attention has been given to such factors as dehydration, caloric intake, frequency and volume of feedings, and supplementation. Of these, dehydration has been discredited as a major issue because of normal serum osmolalities and the absence of hematocrit changes consistent with the degree of hyperbilirubinemia. As well, some studies suggest that water supplementation actually leads to further elevation of bilirubin levels. Breast-fed babies pass less stool in the first few days of life, suggesting that increased amounts of bilirubin are absorbed into the enterohepatic circulation. Early and frequent feedings may overcome this by increasing evacuation and decreasing the intestinal transit time. There is also evidence that caloric intake can influence bilirubin levels independently of other factors. In studies of adults and a variety of animals, starvation or general deprivation of calories has been shown to lead to increases in serum bilirubin levels along with changes in liver functions. The mechanisms for this starvation jaundice are not known, but may involve shifts in bilirubin pools, less efficient conjugation, enhanced absorption from the intestines, or a systemic effect modulating cell transport of bilirubin. Consistent with the concept that the increase in bilirubin concentration is related to conjugation and absorption rather than bilirubin production or heme catabolism are studies of CO production showing no difference between breast-fed and formula-fed infants (Stevenson et al, 1994).

Recent evidence suggests that the increase in jaundice in the first few days of life in breast-fed babies is best explained by fewer calories and less frequent feeds. The implications are that better management of breast-feeding could reduce the frequency and severity of jaundice in the 1st week of life. Changes in hospital breast-feeding policies may not only prevent toxicity of hyperbilirubinemia but could also lead to reductions in unnecessary laboratory testing, hospitalization, and medical intervention. Breast-feeding jaundice is an important issue for the practitioner, especially because the incidence of breast-feeding has increased from 33% of babies in the United States in 1975 (Gartner, 1994) to 50% to 60% in recent years (Martinez and Krieger, 1985; Ryan et al, 1991), and the length of routine newborn hospital length of stay has shortened to about 1 day. Breast-feeding jaundice is a diagnosis of exclusion, and, most importantly, increased bilirubin production should be eliminated as a contributing cause.

BREAST MILK JAUNDICE

The second identified pattern of jaundice in some otherwise healthy breast-fed babies has been called breast milk jaundice. Considered by some researchers to be an extension of physiologic hyperbilirubinemia beyond the first 5 or 6 days of life and continuing for weeks, this entity was first described in 1963 (Arias et al, 1963) and was considered to be a disease that occurred in less than 1% to 2% of the breast-feeding population. Epidemiologic studies suggest it is much more frequent, affecting as many as 10% to 30% of the breast-fed infants in the 2nd to 6th week of life, with some experiencing hyperbilirubinemia into the 3rd month (Gartner, 1994; Linn et al, 1985). With the realization that the prolongation of jaundice in breast-fed infants is so common, the view of this condition has changed from that of a disorder to perhaps a normal extension of physiologic jaundice.

One hypothesis regarding this prolonged jaundice associated with breast-feeding suggests that it results from enhanced enterohepatic absorption of unconjugated bilirubin related to the presence of an unidentified factor in human milk. This theory holds that breast-fed infants who do not have the prolonged jaundice either do not respond to this factor in their mother's milk or their mother's milk lacks it. Another possibility is that breast-fed infants are able to metabolize and excrete the resulting increase in bilirubin load, successfully accommodating for the enhanced intestinal absorption of bilirubin. No specific factor has been identified and etiologic theories are still considered speculative.

The cause of this breast milk jaundice has been sought ever since it was first considered a disease state. Several metabolites in breast milk have been considered as etiologic agents, and usually their activity has been described as inhibiting conjugation or enhancing the intestinal absorption of bilirubin through the enterohepatic circulation. Early studies suggested that the prolonged unconjugated hyperbilirubinemia in otherwise healthy breast-fed babies was due to the inhibition of hepatic glucuronyl transferase, the enzyme responsible for conjugating bilirubin in preparation for excretion. Initially an unusual steroid metabolite of progesterone (pregnane-3-alpha, 20-beta-diol) was considered as a likely candidate because it was known to inhibit hepatic glucuronyl transferase *in vitro*. Later studies cast doubt on the relevance of this chemical to breast milk jaundice. Other inhibitors of glucuronyl transferase have

been suggested, including free fatty acids and several lipases (including lipoprotein lipase [serum–stimulated lipase] and bile salt–stimulated lipase). However, studies of the amount and the composition of fat in jaundice-causing milk have resulted in contradictory reports, leading to suggestions that yet another factor (e.g., beta-glucuronidase) might be present that could deconjugate bilirubin in the intestine, allowing for even more intestinal absorption. However, no clear relationship between the levels of this enzyme in breast milk and the level of bilirubin in infant serum has been demonstrated and none of the aforementioned theories has been confirmed. Consideration that breast milk jaundice may be a normal event does nothing to explain its cause, so the search for a true link between breast milk composition and breast milk jaundice will continue.

Over the past 30 years, much investigation has been carried out to explain both breast-feeding jaundice and breast milk jaundice. No single and exclusive cause for either condition has been identified. As the epidemiology of these conditions is better understood, it seems possible that their being perceived as disease states may disappear. Breast-feeding jaundice may simply be related to feeding practices, and breast milk jaundice may simply be an extension of what has commonly been termed physiologic jaundice.

REFERENCES

Arias IM, Gartner LM, Seifter S, Furman M: Neonatal unconjugated hyperbilirubinemia associated with breast feeding and a factor in milk that inhibits glucuronide formation *in vitro*. J Clin Invest 42:913, 1963.

Beazley JM, Alderman B: Neonatal hyperbilirubinemia following the use of oxytocin in labour. Br J Obstet Gynaecol 82:265–271, 1975.

Boggs TR: Serum bilirubin values in first 4 postnatal days of breast-fed and bottle-fed infants. J Pediatr 84:284, 1974.

Cady HM: Serum bilirubin values in first 4 postnatal days of breast-fed and bottle-fed infants. J Pediatr 84:284, 1974.

DeCarvalho M, Hall M, Harvey D: Effects of water supplementation on physiological jaundice in breast-fed babies. Arch Dis Child 56:568–569, 1981.

DeCarvalho M, Klaus MH, Merkatz RB: Frequency of breast feeding and serum bilirubin concentration. Am J Dis Child 136:737–738, 1982.

Fisher AF, Nakamura H, Uetani V, et al: Comparison of bilirubin production in Japanese and Caucasian infants. J Pediatr Gastroenterol Nutr 7:27–29, 1988.

Forsyth JS, Donnet L, Ross PE: A study of the relationship between bile salts, bile salt-stimulated lipase, and free fatty acids in breast milk: Normal infants and those with breast milk jaundice. J Pediatr Gastroenterol Nutr 11:205–210, 1990.

Friedman L, Lewis PJ, Clifton P, Bulpitt CJ: Factors influencing the incidence of neonatal jaundice. BMJ 1:1235–1237, 1978.

Gartner LM: Neonatal jaundice. Pediatr Rev 15:422–432, 1994.

Gartner LM, Auerbach KG: Breast milk and breast feeding jaundice. Adv Pediatr 34:249–274, 1987.

Gartner LM, Lee KS, Auerbach KG: Development of bilirubin transport and metabolism in the newborn rhesus monkey. J Pediatr 90:513, 1977.

Hardy JB, Drage JS, Jackson EC: The first year of life: The collaborative perinatal project of the national institutes of neurological and communicative disorders and stroke. Baltimore, Johns Hopkins University Press, 1979, pp 104.

Hamosh M: Breast milk jaundice (editorial). J Pediatr Gastroenterol Nutr 11:145–146, 1990.

Herrera AJ: Supplemented versus unsupplemented breast feeding. Perinatal Neonatol May/June 70–1, 1984.

Hsia DYY, Dowben RM, Shaw R, Grossman A: Inhibition of glucuronyl transferase by progestational agents from serum of pregnant women. Nature 187:693, 1960.

Jeffares MJ: A multifactorial survey of neonatal jaundice. Br J Obstet Gynaecol 84:452–455, 1977.

Johnson JD: Jaundice in Navajo neonates. Clin Pediatr 31:716–718, 1992.

King S, Novogroder M: Serum bilirubin values in first 4 postnatal days of breast-fed and bottle-fed infants. J Pediatr 84:285, 1974.

Kurinij N, Schiono PH, Rhoads GG: Breast-feeding incidence and duration in black and white women. Pediatrics 81:365–371, 1988.

Linn S, Schoenbaum SC, Monson RR, et al: Epidemiology of neonatal hyperbilirubinemia. Pediatrics 75:770–774, 1985.

Lockitch G: Beyond the umbilical cord: Interpreting laboratory tests in the neonate. Clin Biochem 27:1–6, 1994.

Lucarini N, Gloria-Bottini F, Tucciarone L, et al: The role of a genetic variability in neonatal jaundice. A prospective study on full term, blood group-compatible infants. Experimentia 47:1218–1221, 1991.

Maisels MJ: Neonatal jaundice. *In* Avery GB (Ed): Neonatology. 2nd ed. Philadelphia, JB Lippincott, 1981, p 484.

Maisels MJ, Gifford K: Normal serum bilirubin levels in the newborn and the effect of breast feeding. Pediatrics 78:837–843, 1986.

Maisels MJ, Pathak A, Nelson NM, et al: Endogenous production of carbon monoxide in normal and erythroblastotic newborn infants. J Clin Invest 50:1–8, 1971.

Maisels MJ, Vain N, Acquavita AM, et al: The effect of breast feeding frequency on serum bilirubin levels. Am J Obstet Gynecol 170:880–883, 1994.

Martinez GA, Krieger FW: 1984 Milk feeding patterns in the United States. Pediatrics 76:1004–1008, 1985.

Martinez JC, Maisels MJ, Otheguy C, et al: Hyperbilirubinemia in the breast-fed newborn: A controlled trial of four interventions. Pediatrics 91:470–473, 1993.

Mathew PM, Wharton BA: Investigation and management of neonatal jaundice: A problem oriented case record. Arch Dis Child 56:949–953, 1981.

Miyoshi K, Saijo K, Kotani Y, et al: Characteristic properties of fetal human albumin (alb f) in isomerization equilibrium. Tokushima J Exp Med 13:121–126, 1966.

Newman TB, Easterling E, Goldman ES, Stevenson DK: Laboratory evaluation of jaundice in newborns: Frequency, cost and yield. Am J Dis Child 144:364–368, 1990.

North AF Jr: Serum bilirubin values in first 4 postnatal days of breast-fed and bottle-fed infants. J Pediatr 84:285, 1974.

Notorianni LJ: Plasma protein binding of drugs in pregnancy and in neonates. Clin Pharmacokinet 18:2036, 1990.

Ryan AS, Rush D, Krieger FW, Lewandowski GE: Recent declines in breast-feeding in the United States through 1989. Pediatrics 88(4):719–727, 1991.

Schneider AP: Breast milk jaundice in the newborn. A real entity. JAMA 255:3270–3274, 1986.

Sivasuriya M, Tan KL, Salmon YM, Karim SM: Neonatal serum bilirubin levels in spontaneous and induced labor. Br J Obstet Gynaecol 85:619–623, 1978.

Stern L: Bilirubin metabolism in the newborn: Its mechanisms and relationship to kernicterus. *In* Rubaltelli F, Jori G (Eds): Neonatal Jaundice: New Trends in Phototherapy. New York, Plenum Press, 1983, pp 1–11.

Stevenson DK, Vreman HJ, Oh W, et al: Bilirubin production in healthy term infants as measured by carbon monoxide in breath. Clin Chem 40(10):1934–1939, 1994.

Varimo P, Simila S, Wendt L, Kolvisto M: Frequency of breast feeding and hyperbilirubinemia. Clin Pediatr 25:112, 1986.

Vest MF, Grieder H: Erythrocyte survival in the newborn infant as measured by chromium[51] and its relation to the postnatal serum bilirubin level. J Pediatr 59:194–199, 1961.

Wilson DC, Afrasiabi M, Reid MM: Breast milk beta-glucuronidase and exaggerated jaundice in the early neonatal period. Biol Neonate 61:232–234, 1992.

Yamauchi Y, Yamanouchi I: Breastfeeding frequency during the first 24 hours after birth in full-term neonates. Pediatrics 86:171–175, 1990.

CHAPTER 83

Bilirubin Toxicity, Encephalopathy, and Kernicterus

James R. MacMahon, David K. Stevenson and Frank A. Oski*

Neonatal jaundice can be an entirely benign physiologic process; it can also be the first sign of serious illness with associated toxicity manifested into the nervous system. The terms *bilirubin encephalopathy* and *kernicterus* represent clinical and pathologic observations of bilirubin toxicity in the central nervous system. Often the term kernicterus is used to include an entire spectrum of clinical and pathologic manifestations attributed to bilirubin. However, kernicterus, by strict definition, includes only the neuropathologic changes that are characterized by pigment deposition in specific regions of the brain, especially the basal ganglia, pons, and cerebellum. Of all infants in whom kernicterus develops, 50% die, and the survivors may have choreoathetoid cerebral palsy, high-frequency auditory nerve deafness, and mental retardation. The term *bilirubin encephalopathy* is correctly applied to the clinical manifestations of the effects of bilirubin on the central nervous system: there is a broad spectrum of neurologic signs attributed to bilirubin, ranging from subtle behavioral changes, such as lethargy and irritability to seizures, mental retardation, and death. Because it is not clear under what conditions neurotoxicity develops or at what concentration of serum bilirubin this damage occurs, there is little agreement about what constitutes a "safe level" of bilirubin. The effect of even moderate increases in serum bilirubin levels on early development remains a source of controversy, especially because some clinical manifestations are reversible upon reduction of the serum bilirubin concentration.

Before exchange transfusions were used to control bilirubin levels in isoimmune hemolytic disease, kernicterus was a common postmortem finding in infants dying with severe jaundice. In recent years, kernicterus has been documented in ill, low-birth-weight (mainly premature) infants whose serum bilirubin levels remained much lower than the levels formerly associated with kernicterus. Whether this "low bilirubin" kernicterus is associated with prematurity alone or is necessarily associated with stresses such as hypoxia, acidosis, respiratory distress, and neonatal septicemia is uncertain.

In the following paragraphs, the history of kernicterus is reviewed, clinical findings are described, and current understanding of the processes leading to bilirubin neurotoxicity are discussed. Finally, new approaches to diagnosis, prediction of risk, and prevention are presented.

CLINICAL MANIFESTATIONS OF BILIRUBIN TOXICITY

Bilirubin neuropathy does not usually become overt until high bilirubin levels have been established for several hours. A prodrome of reversible signs has been described

which includes decreased activity, loss of interest in feeding, changes in the infant's cry, lethargy, irritability, and possibly apnea. If the bilirubin level is rapidly decreased (e.g., by way of exchange transfusion), these findings can often be reversed.

If hyperbilirubinemia persists, however, these more subtle findings are followed within a few hours by rigid extension of all four extremities, tight-fisted posturing of arms, crossed extension of the legs, and a high pitched irritable cry. Sometimes these changes are accompanied with opisthotonos or seizure activity. After several months in patients who survive, reduced muscle tone, difficulty feeding, and spastic or choreoathetoid cerebral palsy usually develop, with tremors, fine motor clumsiness, and poor visual tracking or a fixed upward gaze. High-frequency hearing loss and mental retardation are also part of this syndrome. The most common findings later in childhood are choreoathetosis, ocular paralysis, and eighth nerve deafness; severe mental retardation and spastic cerebral palsy occur in a minority. In general, the motor findings are the most obvious abnormalities in long-term survivors.

Classic findings of kernicterus are not often seen in neonatal follow-up clinics for premature and low-birth-weight infants, because most affected infants do not survive into childhood. However, a spectrum of mild neurologic disabilities and subtle developmental delays has been associated with moderate elevation of serum indirect bilirubin concentration. Because developmental delays related to other factors of prematurity, neonatal illness, or environmental situations are commonly associated with neonatal intensive care, there is controversy regarding the reversibility or long-term implications of the subtle neurologic damage attributed to bilirubin in low-birth-weight babies. Debates about the need for aggressive or conservative treatment for mild to moderate hyperbilirubinemia in infants persist.

HISTORY

The relation between the clinical encephalopathy associated with elevated serum bilirubin concentration and the gross pathologic changes seen as yellow staining of specific areas of the central nervous system was observed and described as early as 1875. Orth described bilirubin crystals in the brain of a newborn who died with icterus neonatorum. He hypothesized that there was a primary necrosis of parts of the brain and that these damaged tissues absorbed icteric pigmentation (Orth, 1875). Schmorl, in 1904, coined the term *kernikterus* (sic) for such focal icteric pigmentation in degenerated zones of the brain (*kern*, meaning nucleus or ganglion, and *ikterus* meaning yellow) (Schmorl, 1904). He believed that necrosis resulted from vascular damage caused by some toxin, perhaps bile, or by thrombo-

---

*Deceased.

sis. He observed that the staining of the neural tissue occurred in only a minority of babies having severe jaundice, in that he identified only six instances of kernicterus in 120 cases of jaundice of the newborn that came to autopsy.

In the ensuing 2 decades, numerous accounts of patients with similar clinical courses and anatomic changes were reported (Zimmerman, 1933). During this time, theories concerning the relationship between icterus and staining of the nuclei did not advance from the 1907 discussion by Beneke. He was the first to suggest that septicemia might play an important role in icterus gravis neonatorum, and he theorized that the pigmentation of brain tissue was caused by (1) a peculiar attraction of bile pigments to ganglion cells, leading to their necrosis, (2) damage to ganglion cells by bile salts, which then pigmented, or (3) ischemic or traumatic insult that allowed the cells to become pigmented (Beneke, 1907).

As early as 1915 there were descriptions of children who survived severe neonatal jaundice with resultant mental retardation and neuromuscular dysfunction, with the jaundice being considered the causal agent (Guthrie, 1913; Spiller, 1915).

In their review of the literature regarding kernicterus in 1933, Zimmerman and Yanet observed that all the children appeared normal at birth, although many were premature. The jaundice began early, usually before the 2nd day of life, and evidence of involvement of the central nervous system, including convulsions and spasticity, was frequent; death usually occurred by the 5th day of life.

In 1916, an advance in the understanding of this disease was made possible by the observation of Van Den Bergh and Muller that serum from patients with hemolytic jaundice could be differentiated from serum of patients with obstructive jaundice on the basis of chemical reactions. They observed that the hemolytic serum did not react promptly with diazotized sulfanilic acid except in the presence of alcohol; the other serum reacted in an aqueous solution. They termed these reactions "indirect" and "direct," which has come to be recognized as unconjugated and conjugated, respectively (Van Den Bergh and Muller, 1916).

Diamond and colleagues in 1932 recognized that generalized edema of the fetus (hydrops fetalis), icterus gravis, and congenital anemia of the newborn (until that time considered three unrelated syndromes) were in fact all part of a single condition, which they termed *erythroblastosis fetalis*. This was followed by the demonstration in 1939 of a serologic basis for maternal-fetal blood group incompatibility and the identification of the Rh system of antigens (Landsteiner and Weiner, 1940; Levine and Stetson, 1939). The stage was set for an expansion of progress in understanding hemolytic disease of the newborn and therapeutic interventions.

EXCHANGE TRANSFUSION

Although the first successful exchange transfusion performed on an infant with familial icterus gravis was reported in 1925 (Hart, 1925), this mode of intervention was not accepted until hemolytic disease of the newborn was conceptually understood in the 1940s. Exchange transfu-

sion decreases the risk of bilirubin encephalopathy by reducing the total bilirubin load, increasing the binding sites of plasma albumin, and shifting bilirubin out of tissue into the plasma as well as providing erythrocytes less apt to hemolyze. Early attempts at exchange transfusion involved removing blood from the sagittal sinus or radial artery and infusing blood into the saphenous vein. With the development of polyethylene tubing, Diamond and coworkers in 1946 introduced the technique of alternate removal and administration of blood for each transfusion via umbilical vein catheterization (Diamond et al, 1951).

Before exchange transfusion came into common usage in the 1950s, kernicterus affected 15% of live born infants with erythroblastosis. Seventy percent of patients with kernicterus died within 1 week of birth, and many of the remainder died during the 1st year of life (Hsia et al, 1952). Survivors had permanent neurologic sequelae and were thought to account for 10% of all cases of cerebral palsy. Considering the severe morbidity of this condition, the major contribution provided by exchange transfusion can be appreciated, even though the procedure was recognized as having inherent risks of its own.

By 1950, kernicterus was thought to occur almost entirely as a sequel to erythroblastosis fetalis, and the relationship between the damage and the severity of jaundice was recognized. Even then, only the Rh incompatibility was considered critical. There was debate about whether other blood groups played any role at all; prematurity, sepsis, pulmonary damage, and maternal diabetes were seen as cofactors in the development of clinical or pathologic disease.

In a series of publications between 1950 and 1952, Diamond, Allen, Hsia, and coworkers summarized the contemporary knowledge and state-of-the-art approaches regarding kernicterus, erythroblastosis, and interventions to prevent neurologic damage from high serum concentrations of unconjugated bilirubin (Allen et al, 1950). In concluding the series of articles, they wrote "kernicterus is likely to occur in babies with serum bilirubin above 30 mg. per 100 cc and unlikely to occur when serum bilirubin remains below 20 mg. per 100 cc" (Hsia et al, 1952). Often taken out of context, this sentence has had an enduring effect on decisions regarding clinical intervention, standards of care, hospitalization policies, and even legal concerns. Controversies about appropriate treatment of hyperbilirubinemia to prevent kernicterus continue (see Chapter 87).

With the publication describing congenital familial nonhemolytic jaundice with kernicterus in 1952, Crigler and Najjar not only exposed a new disease or family of diseases (currently understood to be hereditary deficiencies of bilirubin uridinediphosphoglucuronyl transferase) but they also advanced the understanding of kernicterus as a process related more to elevated unconjugated bilirubin levels rather than to specific blood group incompatibilities or even hemolysis.

PHOTOTHERAPY

The next major advances in the management of neonatal jaundice involved prevention of isoimmunization and a simpler method to reduce the peak serum bilirubin concentration—phototherapy. Although Native Americans had long been aware of the beneficial effects of the sun in reducing the yellow color of babies exposed to its light, phototherapy for neonatal hyperbilirubinemia was first proposed in 1958 by Cremer and colleagues in England (Cremer et al, 1958). Subsequently this therapy has been used for the reduction of elevated serum bilirubin levels and for the "prophylactic" prevention of hyperbilirubinemia in premature infants. With the development of Rh-immune globulins to prevent maternal isoimmunization and the introduction of phototherapy, the need for exchange transfusions in healthy term babies was reduced significantly.

The progress in preventing maternal-fetal blood group incompatibility and in reducing bilirubin concentration coincided with the development of neonatology as a specialty and the ability to rescue sick premature babies. Kernicterus was reappearing in the autopsies of sick low-birth-weight infants, particularly in those with severe respiratory distress, acidosis, and sepsis. It was evident in neonates whose serum bilirubin level was never elevated to the extremes reported earlier, suggesting that bilirubin toxicity in low-birth-weight babies might be in some way different from that in full-term infants with erythroblastosis fetalis. Even though kernicterus is mainly seen in premature babies with respiratory distress, acidosis, and moderately elevated bilirubin levels, the same questions are being asked as they were decades earlier. Is bilirubin the cause of the damage or is staining of tissue caused by antecedent injury? Are patients dying with kernicterus or of kernicterus? In some cases, bilirubin encephalopathy is observed before death and the yellow neuronal staining in a classic distribution of kernicterus is the only prominent finding in the central nervous system at autopsy, providing evidence of a real toxicity attributed to bilirubin itself.

BILIRUBIN TOXICITY

To understand neonatal bilirubin toxicity more completely, several factors need further exploration, including how bilirubin enters the brain, what it does to the neurons, what effects are reversible, and whether neurotoxicity can be predicted in time to be prevented (Table 83–1).

Bilirubin into the Brain

The mechanism by which unconjugated bilirubin enters the brain and damages it is unclear. Several hypotheses regarding entrance of bilirubin into the brain have been advanced and are not yet disproven.

One hypothesis involving free bilirubin (i.e., bilirubin that is not bound to albumin) has been widely accepted although never conclusively proven. Recognizing the lipophilic nature of free bilirubin, this hypothesis presumes that free bilirubin, in equilibrium with bound bilirubin, has access to tissues. Thus, any increase in the amount of free bilirubin or reduction in the amount or binding capacity of albumin could increase the level of unbound bilirubin within the brain tissue, saturating membranes and causing precipitation of bilirubin acid within the nerve cell membrane. Consistent with this hypothesis is the knowledge that even during physiologic hyperbilirubinemia some unbound bilirubin crosses the blood–brain barrier freely.

The clinical significance of this passage of free bilirubin into the brain during physiologic jaundice is unclear. Could this be the cause of transient changes in attention, alertness, and motor performance documented during moderate serum bilirubin elevations? This theory raises concern about the duration of jaundice as well as the peak level attained, and suggests that any situation that decreases the affinity or binding capacity of albumin or increases movement of bilirubin into tissue (e.g., acidosis, hypoalbuminemia, and action of competitively bound drugs as discussed in Chapter 81) would thus exacerbate the entry of bilirubin into brain tissue.

A second hypothesis not only involves the binding of bilirubin to albumin but, also, in particular, focuses on the state of the bilrubin available to cross cell membranes. This hypothesis is based on close examination of the chemical nature of bilirubin in solution and seeks to explain the increased risk to acidotic infants. At alkaline pH, bilirubin forms a water-soluble sodium salt, but the solubility of this substance at neutral or lower pH is extremely low. Bilirubin therefore is found in plasma as a dianion bound to albumin after dissociation of two hydrogen ions. However, the amount of bilirubin acid (i.e., bilirubin that has not dissociated the hydrogen ions) may be excessive and tends to precipitate readily from serum only when a lipid membrane is present, suggesting that it is the supersaturated bilirubin acid that precipitates in the tissues of icteric infants (Brodersen and Stern, 1990). In this model, the degree of supersaturation is determined by the concentration of free bilirubin, relative to the solubility at the pH of plasma. However, it is accepted that some bilirubin can pass from albumin to tissues by direct contact of the bilirubin–albumin molecule with a cellular surface. In this theory, the rate of tissue uptake of bilirubin would depend on both the concentration of albumin-bound bilirubin and the pH, with low pH enhancing precipitation and tissue uptake. Any increase in free albumin could reverse the process. This theory provides an explanation for the role that acidosis may play in the development of kernicterus (Gartner et al, 1970; Stern and Denton, 1965). The low albumin levels of premature infants coupled with the acidosis of respiratory distress places these infants at risk for kernicterus in the face of only moderate hyperbilirubinemia. Whether brain bilirubin oxidase can degrade bilirubin rapidly enough to prevent the deposition of bilirubin acid at the cellular level is controversial and variations of this hypothesis have been suggested (Wennberg, 1988). It is still unclear whether bilirubin acid or bilirubin acid salt (monobasic bilirubin) is

---

TABLE 83–1

Factors that Increase Susceptibility to Neurotoxicity Associated with Hyperbilirubinemia

Asphyxia	Caloric deprivation
Hyperthermia	Prolonged hyperbilirubinemia
Septicemia	Low gestational age
Hypoalbuminemia	Low birth weight
Acidosis	Excessive hemolysis

the form of bilirubin involved in the crossing of cell membranes or in tissue binding.

A third theory suggests that bound bilirubin enters the brain mainly through a damaged blood–brain barrier. The importance of a mature and intact blood–brain barrier stems from demonstration that the barrier to albumin and bilirubin can be reversibly opened under conditions of vascular injury, abnormal circulation, or abnormal osmolality (Bratlid, 1991). Hyperthermia and septicemia may have similar effects (Levine, 1983). Such loss of integrity of the blood–brain barrier could make entry of bilirubin into the brain possible at any serum bilirubin concentration. According to this hypothesis, the local toxicity of bilirubin to the central nervous system would still require dissociation of the bilirubin from albumin at the cell membrane or in the cell, because free bilirubin is known to be more toxic than bound bilirubin in in vitro preparations. Even with a damaged blood–brain barrier, however, more bilirubin than albumin enters the brain, suggesting that several mechanisms of bilirubin entry may be operant simultaneously (see Table 83–1).

Bilirubin Toxicity at the Cellular Level

Similar to the controversy regarding the entry of bilirubin into brain tissue is the understanding of how bilirubin actually exerts its toxic effect at the cellular level. Four possible mechanisms have been theorized: interruption of normal neurotransmission, mitochondrial dysfunction, cellular and intracellular membrane impairment, and interference with enzyme activity (Palmer and Smith, 1990).

Neurotransmission has been theorized as an early target of bilirubin toxicity since reversible changes in brain stem auditory evoked responses (BAER) have been recorded at moderate levels of hyperbilirubinemia. Bilirubin has been shown in vitro to inhibit phosphorylation of enzymes (e.g., synapsin I), which are critical in neurotransmitter release. In addition, changes in membrane potential in cells involved in synapse transmission are known to occur in the presence of varying levels of bilirubin.

Mitochondrial function has been believed for many years to be an important part of the pathogenesis of irreversible bilirubin encephalopathy. Even though the molecular mechanisms are still not understood, some researchers have hypothesized that bilirubin acid precipitates in phospholipid membranes, resulting in mitochondrial dysfunction. Other researchers, however, suggest that bilirubin forms reversible complexes with various cellular membranes, thereby explaining the reversal of some clinical signs of bilirubin toxicity in response to exchange transfusions and rapid reduction of bilirubin levels. Further research is necessary to explain more fully the molecular mechanisms. Perhaps the impact of bilirubin on either neurotransmission or on mitochondrial function relates to the effect of bilirubin acid on the ability of ions (e.g., hydrogen, sodium, and potassium) to cross the membranes. As an example supporting this concept, benzyl alcohol, a preservative recently implicated in a kernicterus epidemic, is known to have an impact on such membrane fluidity. Hydrogen ion gradients across cellular and mitochondrial membranes may be important in controlling mitochondrial function and neurotransmitter release at the synapses. Any

changes in the ability of the membranes to maintain hydrogen ion gradients may be critical in bilirubin toxicity, especially because the binding of bilirubin to cells or mitochondria is proportional to the hydrogen concentration in the local environment (Nelson et al, 1974, Odell, 1965; Wennberg, 1988).

A fourth hypothesis to explain intracellular bilirubin toxicity holds that bilirubin acid is capable of binding receptor sites on specific enzymes, rendering the enzymes inoperative, or at least severely diminishing their activities.

The pathogenesis of kernicterus, especially the "low bilirubin" variety, and the exact mechanism of bilirubin toxicity to the central nervous system are still not fully understood. Bilirubin encephalopathy is a multifactorial process that requires a critical level of free bilirubin, access to the brain across the blood–brain barrier, and presence of susceptible nerve cells. The severity and duration of hyperbilirubinemia, the maturity of the structures involved, the binding capability of albumin, the physiologic environment, and the cell membrane composition and metabolic state are probably all critical to the development of neurodysfunction. Decisions based simply on the total or unconjugated serum bilirubin levels seem simplistic; these other factors must be taken into consideration as well.

PREDICTING ENCEPHALOPATHY

From the aforementioned information, it is understandable that controversy remains regarding the toxicity of low and moderate levels of bilirubin in the premature and in the full-term infant. Despite the progress made in clinical management, there is no agreement as to what constitutes a "safe" level of bilirubin. New assessment tools have been sought to identify factors that could be used to predict impending encephalopathy or to identify subtle findings that could be reversed. Various new techniques are being used in this regard (Vohr, 1990).

Because the auditory pathway of the neonate is particularly vulnerable to insult from bilirubin, BAER has been suggested as a tool that could identify or predict early effects of hyperbilirubinemia on the central nervous system. Studies have regularly correlated increased bilirubin concentrations with changes in amplitude and latency of these responses. BAER testing is accurate and noninvasive, and assesses the functional status of the auditory nerve in the brain stem auditory pathway. BAER testing could be used to screen hyperbilirubinemic full-term and premature infants for sensorineural hearing loss and could be incorporated into the assessment of need for exchange transfusions (Nwaesei et al, 1984; Wennberg et al, 1982).

INFANT CRY ANALYSIS

Analysis of characteristics of infant crying, or "cry analysis," has progressed so that alterations in cry characteristics have been documented in several perinatal risk situations including hyperbilirubinemia. Early work in this field involved spectrographic methods, but recent advances in high-speed computer technology have improved the ability to measure cry characteristics efficiently and accurately (Lester, 1987). It has been shown that with moderately elevated bilirubin levels there is interference with neural conduction, as demonstrated by the BAER, and changes in neural function in adjoining pathways, with resultant impacts on vocal cords (increased tension or phonation).

NUCLEAR MAGNETIC RESONANCE

Another advance in the search for a rapid, noninvasive measure of impending or actual brain cell injury in the face of hyperbilirubinemia has been proposed using nuclear magnetic resonance (NMR) techniques, both imaging and spectroscopy (Palmer and Smith, 1990). NMR is a form of spectroscopy using magnetism and radio frequency energy. It is a noninvasive method that could be used to characterize anatomic structural changes in variable metabolic states. Compared with ultrasonography or computerized tomography, magnetic resonance imaging provides superior anatomic detail without exposing the neonate to ionizing radiation. NMR spectroscopy, especially using phosphorus-31 with its ability to measure phosphorus metabolites, is being used to improve understanding of the interaction of hyperbilirubinemia and asphyxia. Phosphorus-31 NMR spectroscopy captures the phosphorus metabolites as levels decline, elevate, and shift in relation to each other to maintain cellular homeostasis in the face of oxygen depletion.

Brain biochemical activity and "energy failure" are detectable by these techniques, allowing for identification and study of the progression from initial to irreversible tissue damage. Using phosphorus-31 NMR spectroscopy, studies involving animal models have demonstrated the cumulative effect of bilirubin and hypoxia being far more significant than either alone in disrupting brain energy metabolism (Ives et al, 1988). Similarly, hyperosmolar blood–brain barrier opening and hyperbilirubinemia have been shown to disturb cortical energy metabolism only when they coexist (Ives et al, 1989). NMR spectroscopic changes have also been reported in a jaundiced newborn rhesus monkey after displacement of bilirubin with a sulfa drug (Ahlfors et al, 1986).

NMR technology has been proposed as a rapid noninvasive measurement of impending or actual brain cell injury during periods of hyperbilirubinemia. It may enable the diagnosis of reversible brain injury in sufficient time to intervene and to determine what is irreversible for timely prognostication. Diffusion-weighted NMR imaging (DWI) applies a special gradient on the water signal to measure its diffusivity, which can be used as an early physiologic marker of neuronal injury. In other models of brain injury, such as neonatal hypoxic-ischemic encephalopathy or stroke, DWI shows significant changes quite early, while still reversible and before the more permanent injury occurs that is normally shown by conventional NMR imaging (Fisher et al, 1995; Rhine et al, 1994). This could have important implications in bilirubin encephalopathy if DWI is shown to demonstrate ongoing, severe neuronal dysfunction in the affected regions of the brain (e.g., basal ganglia) which might prompt intervention such as exchange transfusion. After extreme hyperbilirubinemia, conventional NMR images have been anatomically specific and symmetric, with abnormalities seen having the distribution characteristic of kernicterus (Martich-Kriss et al, 1995; Penn et al, 1994). Further spectroscopic and imaging studies are needed to better characterize kernicterus and to help de-

termine which changes suggestive of neurotoxicity might be found in more moderate hyperbilirubinemia.

CONCLUSION

Despite years of progress in understanding the processes by which excess bilirubin concentration places the newborn at risk and even with the advances in technology that allow measurement of the effects early in the process, the question of what is a critical threshold of bilirubin for the neonate in terms of long-term or permanent morbidity remains unanswered. A safe level of bilirubin concentration and a safe duration of exposure have not been determined, nor have all the factors (e.g., acidosis, hypoxia) that influence the risk of long-term neurodevelopmental handicaps been fully explained. Until these issues are adequately understood, a cautious approach to clinical management must be pursued.

REFERENCES

Ahlfors CE, Bennett SH, Shoemaker CT, et al: Changes in the auditory brainstem response associated with intravenous infusion of unconjugated bilirubin into infant rhesus monkeys. Pediatr Res 20(6):511–515, 1986.

Allen FH Jr, Diamond LK, Vaughan VC III: Erythroblastosis fetalis: VI. Prevention of kernicterus. Am J Dis Child 80:779–791, 1950.

Beneke R: Uber den kernicterus der neugeborenen. Munchen Med Wchnsch 54:2023, 1907.

Benaron DA, Bowen FW: Variation of initial serum bilirubin rise in newborn infants with type of illness. Lancet 338(8759):78–81, 1991.

Bratlid D: How bilirubin gets into the brain. Clin Perinatol 17:449–465, 1990.

Bratlid D: Bilirubin toxicity: Pathophysiology and assessment of risk factors. N Y State J Med 91:489–492, 1991.

Brodersen R, Stern L: Deposition of bilirubin acid in the central nervous system—A hypothesis for the development of kernicterus. Acta Paediatr Scand 79:12–19, 1990.

Cremer RJ, Perryman PW, Richards DH: Influence of light on the hyperbilirubinaemia of infants. Lancet 1:1094–1097, 1958.

Crigler JF Jr, Najjar VA: Congenital familial non-hemolytic jaundice with kernicterus. Pediatrics 10:169–179, 1952.

Diamond LK, Allen FH, Thomas WO Jr: Erythroblastosis fetalis, VII. Treatment with exchange transfusion. N Engl J Med 244:39, 1951.

Diamond LK, Blackfan KD, Baty JM: Erythroblastosis fetalis and its association with universal edema of the fetus, icterus gravis neonatorum, and anemia of the newborn. J Pediatr 1:269, 1932.

Fisher M, Prichard JW, Warach S: New magnetic resonance techniques for acute ischemic stroke. JAMA 274:908–911, 1995.

Gartner L, Snyder RM, Chabon RS, et al: Kernicterus: High incidence in premature infants with low serum bilirubin concentrations. Pediatrics 45:906–917, 1970.

Goperlud JM, Delivoria-Papadopoulos M: Nuclear magnetic resonance imaging and spectroscopy following asphyxia. Clin Perinatol 20(2):345–367, 1993.

Guaran RL, Drew JH, Watkins AM: Jaundice: Clinical practice in 88,000 liveborn infants. Aust N Z J Obstet Gynaecol 32:186–192, 1992.

Guthrie L: Case of kernikterus associated with choreiform movements. Proc R Soc Med 7:86–87, 1913–1914.

Hart AP: Familial icterus gravis of the newborn and its treatment. Can Med Assoc J 15:1008, 1925.

Hsia DY, Allen FH Jr, Geliss, Diamond LK: Erythroblastosis fetalis. VIII. Studies of serum bilirubin in relation to kernicterus. N Engl J Med 247:668–671, 1952.

Ives NK, Bolas NM, Gardiner RM: The effects of bilirubin on brain energy metabolism during hyperosmolar opening of the blood–brain barrier: An in vivo study using 31P nuclear magnetic resonancy spectroscopy. Pediatr Res 26(4):356–361, 1989.

Ives NK, Cox DW, Gardiner RM, et al: The effects of bilirubin on brain energy metabolism during normoxia and hypoxia: An in vitro study using 31P nuclear magnetic resonance spectroscopy. Pediatr Res 23(6):569–573, 1988.

Landsteiner K, Wiener AS: An agglutinable factor in human blood recognizable by immune sera for Rhesus blood. Proc Soc Exp Biol 43:223, 1940.

Lester BM: Developmental outcome prediction from acoustic cry analysis in term and preterm infants. Pediatrics 80:529–534, 1987.

Levine P, Stetson R: An unusual case of intra-group agglutination. JAMA 113:126, 1939.

Levine RL: Bilirubin and the blood brain barriers. *In* Levine RL, Maisels MJ (Eds): Hyperbilirubinemia in the Newborn. Report of the 85th Ross Conference on Pediatric Research. Columbus, Ohio, Ross Laboratories, 1983, pp 125–140.

MacGillivray MH, Crawford JD, Robey JS: Congenital hypothyroidism and prolonged neonatal hyperbilirubinemia. Pediatrics 40:283, 1967.

Martich-Kriss V, Kollias SS, Ball WS Jr: MR findings in kernicterus. Am J Neuroradiol 16(4):819–821, 1995.

Nelson T, Jacobson J, Wennberg RP: Effect of pH on the interaction of bilirubin with albumin and tissue culture cells. Pediatr Res 8:963, 1974.

Nwaesei C, Van Aerde J, Boyden M, et al: Changes in auditory brainstem responses in hyperbilirubinemia infants before and after exchanged transfusions. Pediatrics 74:800–803, 1984.

Odell GB: The influence of pH on distribution of bilirubin between albumin and mitochondria. Proc Soc Exp Biol Med 120:352, 1965.

Orth J: Ueber das vorkommen von bilirubinkrystallen bei neugebornen kindern. Virchows Arch F Anat Pathol 63:447, 1875.

Palmer CC, Smith MB: Assessing the risk of kernicterus using nuclear magnetic resonance. Clin Perinatol 17(2):307–329, 1990.

Penn AA, Enzmann DR, Hahn JS, et al: Kernicterus in a full term infant. Pediatrics 93(6):1003–1006, 1994.

Rhine WD, DeCrespigny A, Pelc LR, et al: Magnetic resonance studies of immature rabbit hypoxic-ischemic encephalopathy. Pediatr Res 35:386A, 1994.

Schmorl G: Zur kenntnis des icterus neonatorum, insbesondere der dabei auftretenden Gehirnveranderungen. Verhandl D Deutsch Path Gesellsch 6:109, 1904.

Spiller WG: Severe jaundice in the newborn child a cause of spastic cerebral diplegia. Am J Med Sci 149:345, 1915.

Stern L, Denton RL: Kernicterus in small premature infants. Pediatrics 10:483–485, 1965.

Van Den Bergh AAH, Muller P: Uber eine direkte und eine indirekte diazoreaktionen auf bilirubin. Biochem Z 77:90, 1916.

Vohr BR: New approaches to assesing the risks of hyperbilirubinemia. Clin Perinatol 17:293–306, 1990.

Wennberg RP: The importance of free bilirubin acid salt in bilirubin uptake by erythrocytes and mitochondria. Pediatr Res 23:443–447, 1988.

Wennberg RP: Cellular basis of bilirubin toxicity. N Y State J Med 91:493–496, 1991.

Wennberg RP, Ahlfors CE, Bickers R, et al: Abnormal auditory brainstem response in a newborn infant with hyperbilirubinemia: Improvement with exchange transfusion. J Pediatr 100:624–626, 1982.

Zimmerman HM, Yannet H: Kernicterus: Jaundice of the nuclear masses of the brain. Am J Dis Child 45:470, 740–753, 1933.

CHAPTER 84

Unconjugated Hyperbilirubinemias

James R. MacMahon, David K. Stevenson and Frank A. Oski[*]

As discussed in Chapter 82, the capacity for removal of bilirubin is limited in infants. Overproduction of bilirubin combined with immature mechanisms for conjugation and enhanced intestinal enterohepatic circulation of bilirubin contribute to the absorption and development of jaundice, which, in most infants, is mild enough to be considered physiologic and nontoxic and which is almost entirely comprised of unconjugated bilirubin. However, when excessive production of bilirubin saturates the immature mechanism for bilirubin uptake and conjugation or when the process of bilirubin uptake and conjugation is defective or deficient, the level of unconjugated bilirubin in the serum can accumulate to toxic concentrations. Accordingly, there is a variety of pathologic conditions that may result in severe or prolonged unconjugated hyperbilirubinemia (Table 84–1). Even though the most prevalent of these involve overproduction of bilirubin, impaired uptake and conjugation and excessive enterohepatic circulation can be responsible for severe clinical disorders. Because most cases of dangerous or extreme hyperbilirubinemia are related to hemolysis, identification of overproduction of bilirubin is useful in the early identification of the increased risk for bilirubin toxicity. Measurement of end-expiratory carbon monoxide (CO) levels or hemoglobin CO (HbCO) levels, discussed in Chapter 81, are techniques that have not yet come into general use yet.

In a recent review of 88,000 live born infants in Melbourne, Australia, from 1971 to 1989, it was determined that 12.4% of all the infants had hyperbilirubinemia, defined as total bilirubin levels over 9 mg/dL (Guaran, 1992). Correlates of jaundice were determined in 32% of the infants. Most often these were prematurity (20%) followed by isoimmunization (7%), with sepsis, bruising, and glucose-6-phosphate dehydrogenose (G6PD) deficiency accounting for less than 2% each. Of the infants defined as having hyperbilirubinemia, the maximum levels exceeded 20 mg/dL in 2% (212 of 10,944), representing 0.25% of all the births. Nearly 60% of these infants had some determined cause of jaundice, with the hemolysis of isoimmunization (54 of 212) being the most common identifiable cause of the severe hyperbilirubinemia. The largest single group with high bilirubin levels, however, comprised babies with no known cause of jaundice (90 of 212).

In the newborn period, unconjugated hyperbilirubinemia is common, multifactoral, and associated with a variety of physiologic and pathologic conditions.

In this chapter, pathologic conditions responsible for un-conjugated hyperbilirubinemia are discussed (see Table 84–1).

---

[*]Deceased.

EXCESSIVE PRODUCTION OF BILIRUBIN (HEMOLYSIS)
Rh Isoimmunization

The most common identified pathologic cause leading to hyperbilirubinemia is hemolytic disease of the newborn. The destruction of red cells in the fetus and newborn most commonly results from Rh and ABO blood group incompatibility with the maternal blood type. The hematologic details of this phenomenon are discussed in Part XIII.

The first understanding of hemolytic disease in the newborn resulted from the studies of erythroblastosis fetalis resulting from presence of Rh antibody. The Rh antibody in the mother is produced in response to the presence of Rh antigen of the fetal red blood cell membrane. Initially, maternal response to this antigenic stimulus is production of IgM antibodies, which do not cross the placenta in significant amounts. Later, IgG antibodies are formed which cross into the fetus and attach to antigenic sites on the red blood cell membrane. Although small volumes of fetal red cells may enter the maternal circulation throughout pregnancy, the major sensitizing event is delivery, during which a greater amount of fetal blood may enter the

TABLE 84–1

Causes of Unconjugated Hyperbilirubinemia

Excessive production of bilirubin (hemolysis)
  Blood group heterospecificity (incompatibility)
    Rh
    ABO
    Minor blood groups
  Red blood cell enzyme abnormalities
    Glucose-6-phosphate dehydrogenase
    Pyruvate kinase
  Sepsis
  Red blood cell membrane defects
    Hereditary spherocytosis, elliptocytosis, poikilocytosis
  Extravascular blood
  Polycythemia
Impaired conjugation or excretion
  Hormonal deficiency
    Hypothyroidism
    Hypopituitarism
  Disorders of bilirubin metabolism
    Crigler-Najjar syndrome: Type I
    Crigler-Najjar syndrome: Type II (Arias disease)
    Gilbert disease
    Lucey-Driscoll syndrome
Enhanced enterohepatic circulation
  Intestinal obstruction, pyloric stenosis
  Ileus, meconium plugs, cystic fibrosis

maternal circulation. For this reason, blood group incompatibility is less likely to cause hemolysis or hyperbilirubinemic complications with the first pregnancy. Mothers are frequently sensitized by transplacental hemorrhage of only 0.5 mL, an amount not uncommon in active labor or during obstetric complications or procedures such as amniocentesis and therapeutic abortions. The development of maternal sensitization can be identified by the **indirect antiglobulin (Coombs') reaction in the mother,** which identifies the presence of IgG antibody in her circulation or from spectrophotometric examination of amniotic fluid. Because the placenta efficiently transports bilirubin to the mother, affected infants do not appear significantly jaundiced at birth, but the hemolysis experienced may result in severe anemia, hydrops, and intrauterine death. After delivery of the infant, the hemolysis resulting from Rh sensitization may result in rapid development of hyperbilirubinemia reaching levels requiring intervention. Presence of the Rh antigen in an infant is identified by blood typing; isoimmunization, which is the attachment of maternal antibody to fetal red blood cells, can be identified with a positive **direct antiglobulin (Coombs') reaction in the infant.** Red cells coated with maternal antibodies are destroyed in the fetal or newborn liver and spleen, resulting in excessive amounts of hemoglobin being catabolized to bilirubin. The severity of the Rh-induced hemolysis depends on several factors including the antigenicity of the fetal erythrocytes (e.g., males in general are more antigenic than females), degree of sensitization, the specific Rh antigen involved, and the amount of maternal-fetal transfusion. Fifteen percent to 20% of Rh-positive infants born to Rh-negative sensitized mothers show no clinical signs of illness, whereas 25% have severe disease with fetal death, hydrops, or severe anemia at birth.

ABO Incompatibility

Hemolytic disease caused by maternal anti-A or anti-B antibodies reacting with fetal A or B antigens on the erythrocyte surface, a process similar to Rh incompatibility, is more common but generally milder than hemolytic disease caused by Rh incompatibility. This condition occurs almost exclusively in type O mothers, in that the relevant antibodies produced by A mothers or B mothers are mostly IgM antibodies that do not cross the placenta. The jaundice of ABO heterospecificity usually appears within the first 24 to 72 hours after birth, later than that of Rh incompatibility.

Minor Blood Group Incompatibility

Traditionally, less than 2% of infants with hemolytic disease have isoimmunization caused by minor blood group antibodies. However, because the cases resulting from Rh incompatibility have dramatically declined since the use of blocking antibodies (RhoGAM) was instituted, there is a higher percentage of contribution from minor blood group incompatibilities.

Red Blood Cell Enzyme Abnormalities

Congenital nonspherocytic hemolytic anemia has been associated with a group of red blood cell enzymopathies that result in chronic spontaneous hemolysis of early onset that persists throughout life. In the newborn period, marked hyperbilirubinemia can occur as a result of the severe hemolysis (Matthay and Mentzer, 1981; Olsen, 1969; Valaes, 1969). The two most studied of these defects, G6PD deficiency and pyruvate kinase (PK) deficiency, may be associated with hemolytic anemia and jaundice even in the absence of a recognized trigger agent or event in the neonatal period.

Glucose-6-Phosphate-Dehydrogenase Deficiency

G6PD deficiency is a sex-linked recessive trait whose occurrence in several forms has a geographic distribution, with increased prevalence in African, Mediterranean, and Asian regions. Some of the clinical manifestations of this condition, such as favism and hemolytic reactions to certain drugs, were well recognized long before the deficiency of the enzyme was recognized. Although severe neonatal jaundice is the most common clinical manifestation of G6PD deficiency, the relationship between hyperbilirubinemia and the hemolytic anemia was recognized only when the enzyme deficiency was identified in the late 1950s (Newton and Frajola, 1958; Zinkham, 1959). Since then, it has become apparent that the situation in the neonatal period is special, because severe jaundice rather than the anemia may predominate in the clinical presentation. Moreover, severe neonatal jaundice develops apparently spontaneously in some G6PD deficient babies. G6PD-deficient red cells cannot activate the pentose phosphate metabolic pathway and therefore they are unable to defend adequately against oxidant stresses. Because of this phenomenon, severe hyperbilirubinemia can result from hemolysis associated with sepsis, exposure to chemicals such as naphtha in mothballs, or administration of pharmaceutical agents (Table 84–2). Even though some of these agents and stresses have received public attention, others represent generally unsuspected dangers, such as the intramuscular injection of vitamin K analogues, or the inhalation of paradichlorobenzene, which is used in many countries in moth repellents, car and carpet fresheners, and bathroom deodorizers (Siegel and Watson, 1986; Valaes, 1994). Exposure of the newborn to a hemolytic agent can occur transplacentally, via breast milk, or directly by inhalation, ingestion, or injection.

Understanding of the processes leading to the clinical manifestations of G6PD deficiency has come from studies examining the intracellular events following exposure of red blood cells to naphthoquinones (Harley and Robin, 1962, 1963; Sass-Kortsak, 1962). In these studies, oxidation of hemoglobin to methemoglobin and Heinz body formation and growth stimulating hormone depletion were described even in normal erythrocytes. All these phenomena are exaggerated in red blood cells deficient in G6PD, because the pentose phosphate pathway is essential to the defense against such oxidative stress. The data in these studies suggest that neonates with G6PD deficiency may be particularly susceptible to the hemolytic action of vitamin K analogues. Experts currently recommend that oral vitamin K_1 be given for prevention of hemorrhagic disease in newborns in populations with a high incidence of G6PD deficiency (Jorgensen et al, 1991; Valaes, 1994).

TABLE 84–2

Agents Producing Hemolysis in Patients with Glucose-6-Phosphate Dehydrogenase Deficiency

Antimalarials	Others
Pamaquine	Ascorbic acid
Pentaquine	Chloramphenicol
Plasmoquine	Chloroquine
Primaquine	Aniline dyes
Quinacrine	Dimercaprol (BAL)
Quinine	Fava beans
Quinocide	Methylene blue
Sulfonamides	Nalidixic acid
Sulfacetamide	Naphthalene° (used in mothballs)
Sulfamethoxazole	Naphthoquinones° (used in
Sulfanilamide	mothballs)
Sulfamethoxypyridazine	Paradichlorbenzenes (moth
Sulfapyridine	repellent, car freshener,
Sulfisoxazole	bathroom deodorizer)
Trisulfapyrimidine	Phenylhydrazene
Sulfones	Probenecid
Nitrofurans	Quinidine
Furaltadone	Tolbutamide
Furazolidone	Vitamin K, water-soluble analogues
Nitrofurantoin	Menadione diphosphate
Nitrofurazone	Menadione sodium disulfate
Thiazolesulfone	
Antipyretics and Analgesics	
Acetophenetidin	
Acetylsalicylic acid	
Aminopyrine	
Antipyrone	
p-Aminosalicylic acid	

°Most severe and numerous hemolytic episodes.
Adapted from Oski FA, Nalman JL: Hematologic Problems in the Newborn, 2nd ed. Philadelphia, WB Saunders, 1972; and Valaes F: Severe neonatal jaundice associated with glucose-6-phosphate dehydrogenase deficiency: Pathogenesis and global epidemiology. Acta Paediatr Suppl 394:58–76, 1994.

Different genetic forms of the enzyme deficiency have characteristic risks, with the Mediterranean region exhibiting a more severe type of deficiency, called Gd^Mediterranean, than the type found in West Africa, termed Gd A−. The initial association between G6PD deficiency and neonatal hyperbilirubinemia and kernicterus was reported from Greece (Doxiadis et al, 1961), and in 1969 it was recognized as a serious public health problem there (Valaes et al, 1969). Reports from other Mediterranean countries followed. A similar relationship between G6PD deficiency and hyperbilirubinemia was reported in neonates in China and in ethnic groups of other east Asian countries (Lie-Injo et al, 1977; Phornphutkul et al, 1969), and it appears that the Asian forms of this condition have a severe reduction in enzyme activity similar to the Mediterranean forms. Reports from Africa associating G6PD deficiency of the Gd A− type with neonatal hyperbilirubinemia and kernicterus in infants in Nigeria, Senegal, Ghana, and South Africa were significant because the earlier reports had suggested that only the Gd^Mediterranean form of the enzyme deficiency was severe enough to cause kernicterus. Early reports suggesting that black infants with G6PD deficiency

exhibit no increased incidence or severity of hemolysis and jaundice have been shown to be incorrect, although their enzyme deficiency, the GD A− form of the disease, is less severe than the others. The susceptibility to hemolysis is not dependent only on the level of enzyme deficiency but also on the amount of oxidant stress or degree of exposure to an offending agent. Normal erythrocytes can be similarly affected if the stress or exposure is severe enough.

Between 200 and 400 million people are estimated to carry the G6PD deficiency gene. In Greece, for example, the prevalence is estimated at 2% to 4% (Valaes, 1994). Even though the distribution of this genetic trait has historically been centered in the tropics where malaria has flourished, several centuries of migration have led to worldwide dissemination of the gene. Therefore, physicians in all countries need to be familiar with the clinical manifestations and risks of G6PD deficiency.

Severe jaundice develops in approximately 5% of Caucasion or Asian infants with this disorder, usually after 24 to 48 hours of life and sometimes only after some trigger event. Maximum bilirubin level is reached between the 3rd and 5th days of life after exposure to a triggering agent or event. A recent report of such a case (Penn et al, 1994) is a reminder to practitioners that the cause may be subtle but the consequences devastating.

Also, red cells deficient in G6PD are unable to reduce methylene blue to leukomethylene blue; therefore, exposure to even normally acceptable levels of methylene blue causes hemolytic anemia and hyperbilirubinemia when the dye accumulates and functions as a hemoglobin oxidizing agent. Thus, severe hyperbilirubinemia, and even kernicterus, have resulted from the use of methylene blue in patients with unsuspected G6PD deficiency.

Pyruvate Kinase Deficiency

Pyruvate kinase (PK) deficiency is an autosomal recessive disorder occurring uncommonly in all ethnic groups. PK is a key enzyme in the production of adenosine triphosphate in red blood cells. Its deficiency leads to shortened red blood cell survival, resulting in excess hemolysis. Unexplained jaundice in a newborn, with no isoimmunization or no sepsis or drug administration, but with evidence of hemolysis (excessive CO production, anemia, reticulocytosis) raises the possibility of this disorder. Although it occurs much less frequently than G6PD deficiency, this disease represents a classic example of a specific enzyme deficiency leading to a series of events resulting in a major effect on overall health of the individual.

Septicemia

Sepsis is one of the important treatable problems associated with bilirubin overproduction. From the earliest studies of septicemia in newborns, it was observed that 25% to 30% had clinical jaundice early in the illness, sometimes reaching extreme levels. The hyperbilirubinemia in septic neonates is thought to be a consequence of rapid hemolysis, although there are several theories regarding the mechanism of occurrence. Neonatal erythrocytes are susceptible to cell injury and Heinz body formation in response to oxidative stress. In addition, heme oxygenase (HO) is known to be induced by oxidants, and its induction could lead to increased catabolism of heme to bilirubin (see Chapter 81). Unstable hemoglobins are known to precipitate to form Heinz bodies when exposed to certain chemicals (e.g. methylene blue), resulting in production of erythrocytes that tend to lyse. It is possible that some aspect of sepsis has similar effects.

Recent data suggest that bilirubin is a protective antioxidant and that initially in infection bilirubin levels may be decreased as a result of its consumption (Benaron and Bowen, 1991). However, the predominant view that sepsis results commonly in hyperbilirubinemia suggests that this protective mechanism is overwhelmed in septicemia, which manifests with increased levels of unconjugated bilirubin.

Red Blood Cell Membrane Defects
Hereditary Spherocytosis

Hereditary spherocytosis is characterized by spherocytic erythrocytes that are abnormally fragile under osmotic stress. This condition is inherited as a mendelian dominant trait, but in 10% to 25% of cases, neither parent is found to have spherocytes (Robinson, 1957).

Jaundice develops in approximately 50% of infants with spherocytes and is usually misdiagnosed as physiologic jaundice. Because isoimmunization is not involved as an etiologic factor, the direct Coombs' test in the infant is negative. The diagnosis is made by examination of a peripheral smear of blood and recognition of the abnormal shape of erythrocytes. Red cell fragility tests are also abnormal.

Hereditary Elliptocytosis

Even less common than hereditary spherocytosis is hereditary elliptocytosis, which usually is found as a red blood cell morphologic abnormality without significant anemia.

However, occasionally in the neonatal period, there is enough hemolysis resulting from increased osmotic fragility to cause hyperbilirubinemia. The peripheral smear in these cases demonstrates many budding erythrocytic forms similar to those seen in pyropoikilocytosis (Austin and Desforges, 1969).

Extravascular Blood

Blood that has been swallowed or that remains entrapped after a hemorrhagic event commonly leads to hyperbilirubinemia because of the excess bilirubin production resulting from the breakdown of hemorrhagic red blood cells. The common sites for such substantial collections of blood in term infants are cephalohematomas and the space beneath the galeal aponeurosis. Intracranial hemorrhages are more frequent in ill premature infants, and they may be more subtle than other sites of blood sequestration.

Polycythemia

Because neonatal erythrocytes have a shorter life span and increased fragility compared to those of older infants and children, any excess in the number or concentration of erythrocytes at birth can be associated with increased heme degradation and bilirubin production. For this reason, any baby who is plethoric or polycythemic runs some risk of development of hyperbilirubinemia. Because polycythemia is regularly associated with newborns with specific clinical entities (e.g., trisomy 21, maternal diabetes), these entities are associated with increased risks of neonatal jaundice.

Infants of diabetic mothers have factors, in addition to polycythemia, that may contribute to their risk for hyperbilirubinemia. For example, hypoglycemia can be associated with high levels of unconjugated bilirubin. In this instance, the cause is not excess bilirubin production, but rather limitation of conjugation. Glucose is a substrate that participates in the synthesis of the bilirubin–glucuronide conjugate; its absence may reduce the capacity to conjugate bilirubin, accentuating jaundice in young infants.

IMPAIRED CONJUGATION OR IMPAIRED EXCRETION OF BILIRUBIN (NONHEMOLYTIC UNCONJUGATED HYPERBILIRUBINEMIA)
Hypothyroidism

Congenital hypothyroidism can be accompanied by prolonged hyperbilirubinemia (unconjugated), presumably on the basis of delay in maturation of the bilirubin conjugating enzymes (MacGillivray et al, 1967). First recognized in 1954, this association has been documented in approximately 10% of all newborns with hypothyroidism. Several mechanisms may be involved in this process because only a portion of hypothyroid patients with jaundice demonstrate rapid resolution of the problem after hormonal therapy. It is unclear whether the protracted jaundice in hypothyroidism is a consequence of delayed maturation of hepatic conjugating capacity, but a similar picture of protracted jaundice, often in association with refractory hypoglycemia, is seen in infants with congenital hypopituitarism.

The exact impact or role of the thyroid hormones on conjugation awaits further study. It appears that the prolonged jaundice associated with congenital hypothyroidism may stem from a delayed maturation of the ability of the liver to conjugate bilirubin because of the hormone-dependent variations in uridine diphosphate UDP-glucuronosyl transferase activity. Recent reports also suggest that the thyroid hormones cause changes in protein expression, rather than enzyme latency, although some coordinated regulation of glucuronidation and levels of cytochrome P450 has also been hypothesized (Goudonnet et al, 1990). Differential actions of thyroid hormones and chemically related compounds on UDP-glucuronosyl transferases and cytochrome P450 isozymes in animal studies suggest that the physiochemical characteristics of the hormones are important in determining the impact of these chemicals (Goudonnet et al, 1990). Clinically a similar picture is seen in infants with congenital hypopituitarism, although this condition is much less common than hypothyroidism.

Inherited Disorders of Bilirubin Metabolism

The entire group of inherited disorders of bilirubin metabolism (nonhemolytic unconjugated hyperbilirubinemia) can be simplistically divided into three major types according to the degree of bilirubin UDP-glucuronosyl transferase activity and response to enzyme-inducing agents such as phenobarbital. The pattern of inheritance is different among these groups as well. The principal features of these three forms of the disorder are listed in Table 84–3.

Crigler-Najjar Syndrome: Type I

In 1952, just when the Rh isoimmunization problems were being clarified and understood as the major cause of kernicterus, a report of congenital familial nonhemolytic jaundice with kernicterus was authored by Crigler and Najjar (see Chapter 83). That report describes a severe, often lethal, unconjugated hyperbilirubinemia afflicting as many as 15 children in one family pedigree with no evidence of blood group incompatibility, hemolysis, or primary biliary obstruction. The bilirubin concentration reached levels of 25 to 35 mg/dL, but other liver function tests were normal. Subsequent reports have documented bilirubin levels as high as 45 mg/dL. Crigler-Najjar syndrome has come to be recognized as the most severe form of a group of inherited disorders of bilirubin metabolism that result from reduction or absence of UDP-glucuronosyl transferases activity. In 1969, Arias and colleagues described a second type of severe nonhemolytic hyperbilirubinemia that is more common. The original condition described by Crigler and Najjar became known as Crigler-Najjar syndrome Type I, and the new condition was called Crigler-Najjar syndrome Type II, or Arias disease (Arias, 1971). The Type I form of this inherited disorder is extremely rare. Family studies of Type I patients have exposed partial deficiencies in glucuronidation of salicylates and menthol among siblings, parents, and grandparents of affected patients (Childs et al, 1959), supporting the view that this is inherited as an autosomal recessive characteristic that results in virtual absence of UDP-glucuronyl transferase activity. The parents of these patients are anicteric heterozygotes. The patients with Type I disease have pale bile containing no bilirubin. Whereas in the past kernicterus resulted early in life, patients with this condition can currently be treated with phototherapy and agents that reduce the enterohepatic circulation of bilirubin, leading the possibility of a normal life.

If Crigler-Najjar syndrome Type I is left untreated, bilirubin production from the breakdown of hemoglobin in erythrocytes and other heme proteins occurs normally, but the unconjugated bilirubin accumulates in plasma and tissues. A new steady state is eventually attained as bilirubin is degraded by other pathways.

The Gunn rat provides an animal model of the Crigler-Najjar Type I disease. This animal produces no UDP-glucuronosyl transferase and experiences severe jaundice. This animal model has served well in the understanding of the biologic processes involving bilirubin metabolism and the genetic defects associated with deficiency of conjugating enzymes.

TABLE 84–3

Congenital Nonhemolytic Unconjugated Hyperbilirubinemia: Clinical Syndromes

Characteristics	Marked (Crigler-Najjar Type I)	Moderate (Arias disease, Crigler-Najjar Type II)	Mild (Gilbert Disease)
Steady-state serum bilirubin	>20 mg/dL	<20 mg/dL	<5 mg/dL
Range of bilirubin values	14–50 mg/dL	5.3–37.6 mg/dL	0.8–10 mg/dL
Total bilirubin in bile	<10 mg/dL (increased with phototherapy)	50–100 mg/dL	Normal
Conjugated bilirubin in bile	Absent	Present (only monoglucuronide)	Present (50% monoglucuronide)
Bilirubin–UDPG-T activity in vitro	None detected	None detected	20%–30% of normal
Bilirubin clearance	Extremely decreased	Markedly decreased	20%–30% of normal
Hepatic bilirubin uptake	Normal	Normal	Reduced
Glucuronide formation with other substrates	Decreased	Decreased	Decreased
Response to phenobarbital			
Plasma bilirubin	Unchanged	Decreased but remains above normal range	Within normal range
Bilirubin–UDPG-T activity	None detected	None detected	Within normal range
Glucuronidation of other substrates	Increased from previous subnormal levels	Increased from previous subnormal levels	Increased
Smooth endoplasmic reticulum	Hypertrophy	Hypertrophy	Hypertrophy
Bilirubin encephalopathy	Usually present	Uncommon. May occur only in the neonatal period	Not present
Genetics	Autosomal recessive. Parents often related, both demonstrate impairment of glucuronidation but have normal bilirubin levels.	Heterogeneity of defect distinctly possible.	Autosomal dominant (heterozygotes). Usually one of the parents demonstrates similar abnormality.

UDPG-T, uridine diphosphate glucuronosyl transferase.
Adapted from Valaes T: Bilirubin metabolism: Review and discussion of inborn errors. Clin Perinatol 3:177, 1976.

Crigler-Najjar Syndrome: Type II (Arias Disease)

Crigler-Najjar syndrome Type II (Arias disease) is more common but more difficult to recognize in the 1st week of life. Children with Type II disease excrete small amounts of bilirubin glucuronide into the bile, which is yellow. The hyperbilirubin experienced by these patients is less severe than in Type I disease, with levels varying from 8 to 25 mg/dL, with less risk of kernicterus. The inheritance of Type II disease is still uncertain. Initially the inheritance was thought to be autosomal dominant, because abnormalities of glucuronidation were found in only one parent of each patient. However, subsequent studies identified mild serum bilirubin elevations and decreased glucuronyl transferase activity in some siblings and other parents (Labrune et al, 1989; Okolicsanyi et al, 1988). Some investigations have suggested that this condition could be a homozygous form of Gilbert disease. Patients with this form of UDP-glucuronosyl transferase deficiency are clinically cured by the use of phenobarbital or other substances known to induce the enzyme activity (see Chapter 87).

This characteristic differentiates the two types of Crigler-Najjar syndrome because Type I patients experience no decrease in serum bilirubin or enhanced conjugation in response to drug therapy (Sinaasappel and Jansen, 1991).

In the more than 40 years since the report by Crigler and Najjar, advances in molecular biology and genetics have led to an understanding of the molecular basis of these defects in glucuronidation. The organizational gene, termed *ugt 1*, that expresses B-UGT (bilirubin 5′ diphosphate-glucuronosyl transferase or bilirubin UDP-glucuronosyl transferase) in humans and rats has been identified and described. It consists of five exons, four of which encode the carboxy-terminal domain of all UGT isoforms, and one encodes the amino-terminal half of each isoform. Because B-UGT is the only physiologically significant form of the enzyme, a mutation in any of the five exons can lead to either Type I or Type II diseases depending on the severity of the impact of the mutation on enzyme activity. Patients with as little as 4% of normal enzyme activity are clinically in the Type II category; they have moderate elevations of bilirubin without ill health or neurotoxicity.

Because all these patients are normal in every regard except for a single gene defect that happens to code for this one enzyme, therapeutic intervention using gene therapy has been proposed. Several modes of gene therapy have been suggested, including transplantation of normal hepatocytes, retrovirus-mediated gene transfer, adenovirus-mediated gene transfer, and noninvasive receptor–mediated delivery of hepatocytes. Until these techniques are tested further, liver transplantation will be the main mode of treatment for the more severely afflicted individuals.

Gilbert Disease

A mild form of UDP-glucuronosyl transferase deficiency was identified before Crigler and Najjar reported their severe family pedigree. Known as Gilbert disease, this condition was initially described in 1901 (Gilbert and Lereboullet, 1901) and later acquired a variety of names including physiologic hyperbilirubinemia, icterus intermittens juvenilis, constitutional hepatic dysfunction, and familial nonhemolytic jaundice (Crigler and Najjar, 1952). Although many patients with this condition have severe neonatal hyperbilirubinemia, the diagnosis is most often made in later adolescence. It is estimated that 2% to 6% of the general population may have this condition, which is characterized by a hereditary, mild chronic or recurrent nonhemolytic jaundice with otherwise normal liver function tests, and no excess pigment in the urine (Odell and Gourlye, 1989). Patients often complain of fatigue and asthenia associated with their jaundice. Because caloric deprivation results in hyperbilirubinemia in the child or adult with this disease, it is possible that many infants with unexplained hyperbilirubinemia are actually demonstrating the earliest manifestations of this disease. Like Criggler-Najjar syndrome Type II, Gilbert disease can be treated with phenobarbital, which induces the necessary enzymes, although no specific treatment is usually necessary. This condition represents a heterogeneous group of disorders that result in at least a 50% decrease in bilirubin glucuronosyl transferase activity (Gourley, 1994).

Lucey-Driscoll Syndrome

The *Lucey-Driscoll syndrome* was originally described in 24 infants born of eight mothers. Kernicterus developed in four of the infants in the original report as a result of their intense hyperbilirubinemia. The sera from the mothers of these infants contained a substance that markedly inhibited the conjugation in vitro of aglycones such as O-aminophenol. This inhibitory material was also detected in the sera of the infants and was postulated to have been transplacentally acquired. The substance eventually disappears from the circulation of both the mother and the infant and is believed to be a gestational hormone. This syndrome should be considered in those circumstances in which siblings experience intense, transient hyperbilirubinemia of unexplained cause.

ENHANCED ENTEROHEPATIC CIRCULATION OF BILIRUBIN

In young infants, unconjugated hyperbilirubinemia has been documented with high intestinal obstruction, especially with hypertrophic pyloric stenosis. Jaundice rapidly disappears after operation. In the past it was thought that this represented one of a number of conditions in which enhanced enterohepatic circulation of bilirubin resulted in unconjugated hyperbilirubinemia. Studies have shown that an essential etiologic feature of jaundice with pyloric stenosis is a markedly reduced activity of UDP-glucuronosyl transferase at the time of corrective surgery. Normal enzyme activity is seen in nonjaundiced infants with pyloric stenosis. Therefore, concerns have been raised that jaundice with pyloric stenosis may represent an early manifestation of Gilbert syndrome exposed by factors related to undernutrition. Other researchers have suggested that this jaundice results from reduced portal and hepatic artery blood flow or simply a delay in maturation of the enzymes needed for conjugation. Until long-term enzyme presence and activity have been assessed after treatment of upper intestinal obstruction, the cause of this jaundice may be unclear.

Other intestinal conditions that are thought to cause

hyperbilirubinemia because of increased enterohepatic circulation include lower intestinal obstruction, hypoperistalsis, paralytic ileus regardless of cause (e.g., drug induced), and meconium plugs. In all these conditions, there is virtually no removal of bilirubin secreted into the intestines, and reabsorption is enhanced by the stasis and the sterility of the intestinal lumen, as discussed in Chapter 82.

CONCLUSION

Unconjugated hyperbilirubinemia is the manifestation of a large and diverse group of clinical entities. To emphasize the pathophysiologic processes involved, this chapter considered the conditions associated with excess bilirubin production separately from those related to impaired conjugation, excretion, or elimination. There is a clinical relevance to this distinction, in that excessive bilirubin production can be identified from the CO production resulting from heme degradation. In addition, the risk of neurotoxicity in the newborn infant is greater in situations associated with increased bilirubin production than in those conditions associated primarily with impaired bilirubin excretion or elimination. The former present earlier in more unstable infants and the latter present later in otherwise well infants.

REFERENCES

Arias M: Inheritable and congenital hyperbilirubinemia; models for the study of drug metabolism. N Engl J Med 285:1416–1421, 1971.

Arias M, Gartner LM, Cohen M, et al: Chronic non-hemolytic unconjugated hyperbilirubinemia with glucuronyl transferase deficiency. Am J Med 44:395–409, 1969.

Arias M, Wolfson S, Lucey JF, et al: Transient familial neonatal hyperbilirubinemia. J Clin Invest 44:1442–1450, 1956.

Austin RF, Deforges JF: Hereditary elliptocytosis: An unusual presentation of hemolysis in the newborn associated with transient morphological abnormalities. Pediatrics 44:196, 1969.

Benaron DA, Bowen FW: Variation in serum bilirubin with illness during the first few days of life: Possible evidence for a free radical scavenging reaction. Lancet 338(8759):78–81, 1991.

Brown AK: Hyperbilirubinemia in black infants, role of glucose-6-phosphate dehydrogenase deficiency. Clin Pediatr 31:712–715, 1992.

Childs B, Sidbury JB, Migeon CJ: Glucuronic acid conjugation by patients with familial non-hemolytic jaundice and their relatives. Pediatrics 23:903–913, 1959.

Crigler JF Jr, Najjar VA: Congenital familial non-hemolytic jaundice with kernicterus. Pediatrics 10:169–179, 1952.

Dawodu Ah, Owa JA, Familusi JB: A prospective study of the role of bacterial infection and glucose-6-phosphate dehydrogenase deficiency in severe neonatal jaundice in Nigeria. Trop Geogr Med 36:127–132, 1984.

Dennery PA, Rhine WD, Stevenson DK: Neonatal jaundice. What now? Clin Pediatr 34:103–107, 1995.

Doxiadis SA, Fessas P, Valaes T: Glucose-6-phosphate dehydrogenase deficiency: A new etiologic factor in severe neonatal jaundice. Lancet 1:297–301, 1961.

Familusi JB, Dawodu AH, Owa JA: Some epidemiological aspects of neonatal hyperbilirubinemia in Nigeria. In Fukuyama Y, Arima M, Mokawa K, Yamaguchi K (Eds): Child Neurology. International Congress Series, Vol 579. Proceedings of the Tokyo Meeting, 1981. Amsterdam: Elsevier, 1983, pp 272–280.

Gibbs WN, Gray R, Lowry M: Glucose-6-phosphate dehydrogenase deficiency and neonatal jaundice in Jamaica. Br J Haematol 43:263–274, 1979.

Gilbert A, Lereboullet P: La cholemie simple familial. Semaine Medicále 21:241–443, 1901.

Goudonnet H, Magdalou J, Mounie J, et al: Differential action of thyroid hormones and chemically related compounds on the activity of UDP-glucuronosyl tranferases and cytochrome P-450 isozymes in rat liver. Biochim Biophys Acta 1035(1):12–19, 1990.

Gourley GR: Disorders of bilirubin metabolism. In Suchy FJ (Ed): Liver Disease in Children. St Louis, Mosby–Year Book, 1994, pp 401–413.

Guaran RL, Drew JH, Watkins AM: Jaundice: Clinical practice in 88,000 liveborn infants. Aust N Z J Obstet Gynaecol 32:186–192, 1992.

Harley JD, Robin H: Haemolytic activity of Vitamin K3: Evidence for a direct effect on cellular enzymes. Nature 193:478–480, 1962.

Harley JD, Robin H: Adaptive mechanisms in erythrocytes exposed to naphthoquinones. Aust J Exp Biol 41:281–292, 1963.

Harper RJ, Yoon JJ: Handbook of Neonatology. Chicago, Year Book, 1987, p 297.

Jorgensen FS, Felding P, Vinther S, Andersen GE: Vitamin K to neonates: Peroral versus intramuscular administration. Acta Paediatr Scand 80:304–307, 1991.

Labrune P, Myava A, Hennion C, et al: Crigler-Najjar Type II disease inheritance: A family study. J Inherit Metab Dis 12:50302–50306, 1989.

Levin SE, Charlton RW, Freiman I: Glucose-6-phosphate dehydrogenase deficiency and neonatal jaundice in South African Bantu infants. J Pediatr 65:757, 1964.

Lie-Injo LE, Virik HK, Lim PW, et al: Red cell metabolism and severe neonatal jaundice in West Malaysia. Acta Haematol 58:152–160, 1977.

MacGillivray MH, Crawford JD, Robey JS: Congenital hypothyroidism and prolonged neonatal hyperbilirubinemia. Pediatrics 40:283, 1967.

Matthay KK, Mentzer WC: Erythrocyte enzymopathies in the newborn. Clin Haematol 10:31–55, 1981.

Newton WA Jr, Frajola WJ: Drug-sensitive chronic hemolytic anemia: Family studies. Clin Res 6:392, 1958.

Odell GB, Gourlye GR: Hereditary hyperbilirubinemia. In Lebenthal E (Ed): The Textbook of Gastroenterology and Nutrition in Infancy, 2nd ed. New York, Raven Press, 1989, pp 949–967.

O'Flynn MED, Hsia DYY: Serum bilirubin levels and glucose-6-phosphate dehydrogenase deficiency in newborn American Negroes. J Pediatr 68:160, 1963.

Okolicsanyi L, Nassauto G, Muraca M, et al: Epidemiology of unconjugated hyperbilirubinemia: Revisited. Semin Liver Dis 8:179–182, 1988.

Olsen JE: Neonatal nonspherocytic hemolytic anemia due to glucose-6-phosphate dehydrogenase deficiency in a Danish infant. Acta Paediatr Scand 58:187–190, 1969.

Owa JA, Dawodu AH, Familusi JB: Kernicterus in Nigerian infants. West Afr J Med 6:11–20, 1987.

Penn AA, Enzmann DR, Hahn JS, Stevenson DK: Kernicterus in a full term infant. Pediatrics 93:1003–1006, 1994.

Phornphutkul C, Whitaker JA, Worathumrong N: Severe hyperbilirubinemia in Thai newborns in association with erythrocyte G6PD deficiency. Clin Pediatr 8:275–278, 1969.

Robinson GC: Hereditary spherocytosis in infancy. J Pediatr 50:447, 1957.

Sass-Kortsak A, Thalme B, Ernster L: Commentary: Haemolytic activity of vitamin K3. Nature 193:480–481, 1962.

Siegel E, Watson S: Mothball toxicity. Pediatr Clin North Am 33:369–374, 1986.

Sinaasappel M, Jansen PL: The differential diagnosis of Crigler-Najjar disease, Type 1 and 2, by bile pigment analysis. Gastroenterology 100:783–789, 1991.

Slusher TM, Vreman HJ, McLaren DW, et al: Glucose-6-phosphate dehydrogenase deficiency and carboxyhemoglobin concentrations associated with bilirubin-related morbidity and death in Nigerian infants. J Pediatr 126:102–108, 1994.

Valaes T: Bilirubin and red cell metabolism in relation to neonatal jaundice. Postgrad Med J 45:86–106, 1969.

Valaes T: Severe neonatal jaundice associated with glucose-6-phosphate dehydrogenase deficiency: Pathogenesis and global epidemiology. Acta Paediatr Suppl 394:58–76, 1994.

Valaes T, Karaklis A, Stravrakakis D, et al: Incidence and mechanism of neonatal jaundice related to glucose-6-phosphate dehydrogenase deficiency. Pediatr Res 3:448–458, 1969.

Vreman HJ, Stevenson DK: Determination of carboxyhemoglobin in neonatal blood with a CO-oximeter unaffected by fetal oxyhemoglobin. Clin Chem 40:1522–1527, 1994.

Vreman HJ, Stevenson DK, Oh W, et al: Semi-portable, electrochemical instrument for determining carbon monoxide in breath. Clin Chem 40:1927–1933, 1994.

Zinkham WH, Lenhard RE: Metabolic abnormalities of erythrocytes from patients with congenital non-spherocytic hemolytic anemia. J Pediatr 55:319–336, 1959.

CHAPTER 85

Obstructive Jaundice due to Biliary Atresia and Neonatal Hepatitis

James R. MacMahon, David K. Stevenson and Frank A. Oski*

In the past 3 decades, there has been a major reorientation in thinking with respect to the entity termed *congenital atresia of the bile ducts*. In the past, clinicians attempted to distinguish hepatitis from atresia by a variety of diagnostic procedures and deferred operative intervention for several months in the hope that patients with hepatitis would improve, while assuming that little or nothing could be done for infants with anatomic abnormalities.

There is a growing consensus that neonatal hepatitis and biliary atresia may be opposite ends of a single spectrum of disease and that the pathologic process observed is dynamic. The pathologic picture observed depends on the time and nature of intrauterine insult and the age at which the infant is examined.

BILIARY ATRESIA
Historical Perspective

Congenital obliteration of the bile ducts was first described in the medical literature when Heschl reported an infant who died at 7 months of age and whose postmortem microscopic examination showed complete absence of large and small ducts within the liver and no trace of hepatic or common bile ducts (Heschl, 1865). A survey of the medical literature in 1891 (Thomson, 1891) and subsequent reviews published in the first half of this century (Benecke, 1907; Dahl-Iversen and Gormsen, 1944; Holmes, 1916; Stolkind, 1939) demonstrated that, among a large number of case studies, the extent of the atresia could vary from a small area of partial stenosis in a single duct to complete absence of all extrahepatic biliary structures (Ahrens et al, 1951). Even though atresia of extrahepatic ducts dominated these case reports, some of the reports made specific comments about absence or paucity of the intrahepatic bile ducts, and in three cases the extrahepatic bile ducts were found to be normal.

During this era, the dominant theory regarding the pathophysiology of biliary atresia held that the condition resulted from a developmental structural anomaly consisting of failure of recanalization of the bile ducts, which in early embryonic stages appear to be occluded by proliferating duct cells.

Competing theories suggested that the cause of biliary atresia is (1) injury to the fetal liver by "toxins" carried across the placenta resulting in fetal hepatitis or cirrhosis followed by descending cholangitis and eventual obliteration of the extrahepatic ducts (Rolleston, 1901), (2) obstruction of a patent bile duct at the papilla of Vater with consequent ascending cholangitis leading to widespread obstruction (Benecke, 1907), or (3) postnatal infection ascending the biliary system from the intestinal lumen.

Despite a century of investigation, the pathophysiology of biliary atresia is still uncertain and continues to spawn competing theories. Nevertheless, surgical interventions in recent decades have provided a more complete understanding of the ductile disease processes and the progression to biliary atresia. Evidence has accumulated to support the concept that these conditions are neither isolated phenomena nor static conditions caused simply by the lack of duct formation or by some structural defect in duct formation, as previously hypothesized. Instead, both extrahepatic biliary atresia and intrahepatic paucity of bile ducts are seen as the result of progressive, destructive, inflammatory cholangiopathies of uncertain origin. Current theory holds that an initial insult leads to inflammation at some level of the hepatobiliary tract, and the end result represents a continuing inflammatory process at the primary site of injury, be that the hepatocytes or the bile ducts. The initial injury, which is thought to occur in utero, and the sustaining mechanisms are still not fully defined. The various presentations and problems seen with neonatal obstructive cholangiopathy represent a continuum in which each entity is simply a particular manifestation of one basic disease process. Intrahepatic ducts may disappear over a period of several months in the presence of complete extrahepatic obstruction. For this reason, surgical intervention must be performed early to be beneficial.

Progress in the surgical management of this condition has been dramatic and unabated over the past 40 years. Based on the assumption that the intrahepatic ducts are usually intact and that the ducts of the right lobe communicate with those of the left, various cholangioenterostomies were proposed and tried in the late 1940s (Gray et al, 1948; Longmire and Sanford, 1949). Accompanied by advances in diagnostic technology allowing more sophisticated preoperative assessment of the location and extent of the duct pathology, the Kasai portoenterostomy became the standard therapy for extrahepatic biliary atresia in the 1970s. Currently, liver transplantation is used when intrahepatic disease or damage is substantial (Ryckman et al, 1992).

Without surgical intervention, the outlook is known to be miserable, with a "spontaneous cure rate" of only approximately 1% (Vacanti et al, 1990). With the advent of liver transplantation, survival rates are reported as high as 90% and an inadequate supply of donor livers has led to the use of portions of livers from related donors (Cox et al, 1991). Currently, extrahepatic biliary atresia represents the most common indication for liver transplantation in children (Lachaux et al, 1995).

---

*Deceased.

Patterns of Disease

Loose and ambiguous use of the term *biliary atresia* has led to confusion concerning the approach to therapy. Only surgical exploration, an operative cholangiogram if a gallbladder is present, a careful dissection of the porta hepati, and microscopic examination of liver tissue can enable the classification of the patient's disease as intrahepatic or extrahepatic biliary obstruction with or without atresia.

With this information, the following diagnostic classification can be made:

1. Complete intrahepatic biliary atresia
   a. Normal extrahepatic biliary system
   b. Hypoplastic extrahepatic biliary system
   c. Complete extrahepatic biliary atresia
2. Complete extrahepatic biliary atresia
   a. Normal number of intrahepatic ducts
   b. Decreased number of intrahepatic ducts
3. Hypoplasia of the extrahepatic biliary trees
   a. Normal number of intrahepatic ducts
   b. Decreased number of intrahepatic ducts

Such classification is essential since infants with functioning intrahepatic ducts have come to be able to benefit from surgical procedures using a variety of anastomotic techniques to promote adequate biliary drainage. However, current discussions of the cause and pathogenesis of biliary atresia still group the various patterns of paucity and fibrosis of bile ducts into the broader categories of *extrahepatic biliary atresia* and *paucity of the interlobular bile ducts*, a term that has largely replaced *intrahepatic biliary atresia*.

EXTRAHEPATIC BILIARY ATRESIA
Pathology

Almost every conceivable pattern of absence or atresia of one or more of the components of the biliary outflow tract has been encountered. All the extrahepatic ducts or, rarely, all the intrahepatic ducts may be absent. The hepatic, cystic, or common duct may be atretic. The gallbladder may be absent or hypoplastic, or it may have no connection with the liver or the duodenum. Stenosis rather than complete atresia may be found.

What has traditionally been called extrahepatic bile duct atresia is currently seen as a disease affecting portions of the biliary tree lying outside the liver as well as the intrahepatic bile ducts (Desmet and Callea, 1990). In the first 2 to 3 months of life, a variable number of bile-draining intrahepatic ducts are patent in nearly all patients. In the presence of progressive fibrosis and obstruction of extrahepatic ducts, the interlobular ducts (intrahepatic) begin to be destroyed and decrease progressively after 8 weeks of age, and the liver itself becomes fibrotic (Desmet, 1994).

In the 1st month after birth, the liver of patients with extrahepatic bile duct atresia demonstrates nonspecific bilirubinostasis and resembles the liver seen in neonatal hepatitis, with bilirubin granules in hepatocytes and intercellular bile plugs (Desmet, 1994). After approximately 4 to 6 weeks, histologic changes characteristic of extrahepatic bile duct atresia are found, with multiplication of pre-existing ductules and progressive periductal fibrosis (Desmet, 1992). Some authors recommend delaying diagnosis by liver biopsy until 6 weeks of age because these findings are more specific than the early histologic changes.

Once periductal fibrosis has occurred, with atrophy of the biliary epithelium, radiographic investigations can demonstrate hypoplasia of the intrahepatic portions of the biliary tree. Because determining this stage of the disease may have prognostic implications, the number and size of the ducts at the porta hepatis are important features to investigate.

The atresia of the intrahepatic bile ducts is usually incomplete but is evident by a reduced ratio of interlobular ducts to the number of portal tracts. Because the development and maturation of the biliary tree are not complete until about 4 weeks beyond the normal gestation period, these ratios may vary according to the maturity of the baby. What is a normal ratio in a premature baby would be considered abnormal in more mature infants (Kahn et al, 1989). The intrahepatic picture may present variable features; thus, a variety of terms describing the findings has emerged, including intrahepatic bile duct atresia, hypoplasia, paucity of intrahepatic bile ducts, and ductopenia. The precise diagnosis of the intrahepatic pathologic conditions requires a sufficiently large liver biopsy specimen which can be obtained by surgical wedge biopsy or by percutaneous needle biopsy if the latter contains at least five portal tracts (Desmet, 1994).

The liver shows all gradations of damage ranging from biliary stasis to advanced biliary cirrhosis, depending on the length of time the particular infant survives. Before the era of surgical treatment and liver transplantation, the natural course of the disease was well described. The spleen enlarges as portal hypertension advances. The bones may become rachitic or osteoporotic because of defective absorption of both vitamin D and calcium. In advanced cases, foci of destruction of skeletal muscle may be discovered after careful search. Weinberg and coworkers (1958) correlated this lesion with prolonged deprivation of vitamin E.

Etiology

There is little evidence that congenital biliary atresia is familial or hereditary. It is presumed to result from some noxious process that adversely affects the development of the bile duct system during gestation. A variety of causes has been proposed, including infectious agents such as congenital rubella, cytomegalovirus (Hart et al, 1991), and reovirus 3 (Morecki et al, 1984), ischemia, immunologic phenomena, and pancreatic reflux. No single pathogenic mechanism is recognized, but extrahepatic biliary atresia is the most common structural anomaly that results in neonatal jaundice, affecting 1 in 15,000 births (Stein and Vacanti, 1994). An antenatal onset of these disease processes is suggested by the fact that 15% of biliary atresia patients have other major anomalies outside the biliary system, such as polysplenism and congenital heart disease (Chandra, 1974). The final pattern evolves from two distinct portions of the liver anlage: the larger cranial part forming parenchyma as well as hepatic and common ducts and the small caudal part eventuating in gallbladder and cystic duct. These two portions must accomplish juncture secondarily.

Congenital defects of many kinds are the end results of imperfections in this complex evolution.

Diagnosis

Clinical Presentation

The typical presentation of a patient with extrahepatic biliary atresia is an apparently well child in whom jaundice gradually develops between 3 and 6 weeks of age. The prime sign of congenital biliary atresia is this increasing and persisting jaundice. Many times, the icterus appears to be a continuation of physiologic icterus of the newborn, and serious trouble is suspected only when the color fails to fade at the expected time. In other cases, jaundice is not seen until 1, 2, or even 3 or more weeks have passed, after which it persists and deepens. A history dating the onset of jaundice after 6 weeks of age is good evidence (after 4 weeks, fair evidence) that the disorder is something other than atresia. Often, jaundice appears variable in intensity, alternately deepening and lightening. Because complete atresia would be expected to give rise to jaundice that steadily increases in intensity, such variability tends to be misleading. A significant delay in diagnosis or treatment can have tragic consequences if jaundice in an infant is erroneously attributed to physiologic hyperbilirubinemia or to breast-feeding. If the conjugated (direct reacting) bilirubin comprises more than 20% of the total bilirubin, cholestasis should be considered in the differential diagnosis (Balistreri, 1985).

The second diagnostic sign is absence of bile in the stools. In some cases, infants pass the typical clay-colored stools from the 4th or 5th day of life. In other instances, confusion arises because stools fail to become absolutely white for several weeks or months or because some are clay-colored yet others contain a tinge of brown or green. The usual phenomenon is that heavily jaundiced intestinal epithelial cells may be sloughed off and incorporated in the bulk of the stool. These two factors, variability in intensity of jaundice and delay and variability in absoluteness of acholia in stools, cause uncertainty regarding the congenital origin and completeness of the obstruction, and not too much weight should be assigned to these "red herrings." Within these limitations, jaundice and acholic stools constitute the pathognomonic signs. Consistent presence of pigmented stools tends to rule out biliary atresia as a diagnosis. A simple yet reliable maneuver to assess bile output is to obtain duodenal fluid to assess the bilirubin content. If bile-stained fluid is collected from the duodenum, biliary atresia is virtually excluded (Greene et al, 1979); in most patients with neonatal hepatitis, bile-stained fluid is present. Jaundice steadily increases to its maximum degree, ultimately imparting to the infant a deep yellow color, from the bilirubin that is mixed with a greenish discoloration from the biliverdin. The liver soon becomes large and extremely firm. In the first few months, the baby does not appear or act as though ill. Venous dilatation appears over the surface of the protuberant abdomen, greatest over its upper half, and ascites develops. The spleen enlarges.

Fat-soluble vitamins are poorly absorbed in the absence of bile salts from the intestine, but deficiencies in vitamins A, D, and K do not become manifest until after the neonatal period. Vitamin E deficiency may be demonstrated by laboratory tests, and the absorption of an orally administered dose of Aquasol E has been proposed as a simple test for distinguishing hepatitis from biliary atresia.

Blood content is normal in the neonatal period. Hemoglobin content and red and white blood cell counts fall within the usual range, and there is no excess of nucleated erythrocytes or reticulocytes. The urine contains bile in large quantities but no urobilinogen. By 4 to 6 weeks of age, most patients are anemic with elevations in their reticulocyte count.

Liver Function Tests

Serum bilirubin becomes elevated by the end of the first several weeks of life and gradually increases to a maximum, where it remains throughout life, with minor fluctuations. Much of the bilirubin is of the direct type.

Liver function tests may indicate liver damage but not until considerably later in life, after cirrhotic alterations have begun to develop.

Blood cholesterol level tends to increase gradually pari passu with increasing liver damage. This never happens as early as the neonatal period.

Several transaminating enzymes have been measured in the sera of infants with persistent jaundice. Values for serum aspartate aminotransferase (AST) in normal adults range from 8 to 40 units (in normal newborns, from 13 to 120 units) per milliliter of serum per minute. From 5 to 35 units of alanine aminotransferase (ALT) are present in adult serum, and in newborn serum there are 12 to 90 units (Kove et al, 1958). In bile duct atresia, the activities of these enzymes may increase to levels ranging from 500 to 700 units, whereas in hepatitis this figure may increase to as high as more than 1000 units. There is a good deal of overlapping in these two conditions. The ratio of serum gamma-glutamyl transpeptidase to AST is elevated in infants with obstructive cholangiopathy. Platt and coworkers (1981) proposed that the measurement of this ratio may be a sensitive means of distinguishing infants with extrahepatic biliary atresia from those with neonatal hepatitis. This distinction may be evident as early as 5 to 14 days of life. The ratio may also be elevated in neonates with alpha$_1$-antitrypsin deficiency who demonstrate bile duct proliferation.

Imaging Studies

Ultrasonography

When biliary obstruction is suspected from the clinical presentation, the first screening study performed is ultrasonography. Although frequently nondiagnostic, ultrasonography is valuable as a noninvasive tool to examine the hepatobiliary structure for the presence and size of a gallbladder, choledochal cysts, cholelithiasis, polysplenia, and relevant vascular anomalies (Cox et al, 1987). Comparing preprandial and postprandial studies may demonstrate changes in the size of the gallbladder and bile ducts, effectively ruling out the diagnosis of extrahepatic biliary atresia, although false-positive tests have been reported (Green and Carroll,

1986; Ikeda et al, 1989). Ductal dilatation is usually not a feature of biliary atresia, but the common duct may not be visualized or portions of it may appear to be of normal size.

Computed tomography and magnetic resonance imaging could provide similar information, but the need for heavy sedation and the absence of intra-abdominal fat for contrast render these techniques less useful than ultrasonography.

Hepatobiliary Scintigraphy

Radionuclide imaging can be used in assessing both the physiology and anatomy of the hepatobiliary system. In the 1970s, the rose bengal ^{131}I excretion test was used to distinguish biliary atresia from hepatitis. Since then, isotopes of technetium-99m (Tc 99m) have come to be used for this purpose. Hepatobiliary imaging is accomplished by the intravenous injection of Tc 99m hepatic 2,6-dimethyl-iminodiacetic acid (HIDA) and its derivatives ("the HIDA scan"). In the normal physiologic state, hepatocytes promptly extract this material from the blood and secrete it into bile canaliculi, from which it is then directed to bile ducts and, eventually, the intestinal lumen. In biliary atresia, hepatocyte function is intact early in the disease, allowing for a fair degree of hepatic extraction to occur. However, the failure of the isotopes to clear the liver and be excreted into the biliary tract or intestine is suggestive of biliary atresia (Cox et al, 1987). By contrast, in neonatal hepatitis, cellular uptake is sluggish or absent, and the lack of a resolvable liver image in small infants is a demonstration of a severe degree of liver cell dysfunction, which is seen almost exclusively in hepatitis.

In an effort to image even small amounts of secretory activity from the dysfunctional hepatocytes involved in hepatitis, pretreatment of patients for 5 days with phenobarbital (5 mg/kg per day) is the usual practice because it enhances the accuracy of hepatobiliary imaging (Majd, 1983).

Radionuclide imaging is no longer commonly performed to detect hepatic space-occupying lesions because there is little sensitivity for lesions smaller than several centimeters in diameter (Keller, 1994).

In an infant with persistent jaundice and apparent biliary obstruction, efforts should be made by 6 to 8 weeks of age to determine the precise cause. In addition to conventional measurements of liver enzymes, diagnostic procedures should include one or more of the following to determine whether obstruction is present: ultrasonography, HIDA scan, duodenal intubation and analysis for bile acids, and needle biopsy of the liver or laparoscopy with biopsy and cholangiogram. If the tests are equivocal or indicate the presence of obstruction, surgery should be performed to establish a precise diagnosis and possibly correct or ameliorate the problem. Surgery should be performed by a surgeon who is familiar with the problem and capable of performing an anastomosis if indicated. At the time of exploratory laparotomy, a cholangiogram as well as a liver biopsy specimen should be obtained.

Liver Biopsy

The percutaneous liver biopsy is the most specific and sensitive method of diagnosing biliary atresia (Ferry et al,

1985; Tolia et al, 1986). This procedure can be performed in even the smallest infants using sedation and local anesthesia. A diagnosis of extrahepatic biliary atresia can be made in 90% to 95% of patients (Brough and Bernstein, 1974; Ferry et al, 1985).

The characteristic features of biliary obstruction include bile ductular proliferation, bile plugs, and portal tract edema and fibrosis. Because these characteristics develop over time, they may not be seen in the first few weeks of life (Suchy, 1994). Inflammatory changes, focal hepatocellular necrosis, cellular swelling, and giant cell transformation of hepatocytes are seen when intrahepatic duct obstruction occurs, along with ductular injury and paucity. These findings contrast with those of neonatal hepatitis, in which hepatocellular damage and inflammation, mostly portal infiltration with mononuclear cells, are the outstanding signs. Giant cell transformation is far from universal in intrahepatic duct obstruction and duct proliferation is only rarely seen (Fig. 85–1).

Prognosis

Death occurs in all cases of extrahepatic biliary atresia that cannot be surgically corrected or in which liver transplantation is impossible. An occasional infant may suddenly and spontaneously be relieved of jaundice after many months. This does not mean that atresia is reversible but indicates that the diagnosis was incorrect. Errors of this sort have been made even after careful exploration at reputable clinics. Therefore, the grave prognosis should be qualified when communicating it to the parents by pointing out that this slim possibility exists. Most deaths are caused by either hepatic failure or the bleeding of portal hypertension and occur between 6 months and 2 years of age. A few children live years longer. Kernicterus does not complicate biliary atresia because much of the accumulated bilirubin is of the direct kind, and dangerous levels of indirect hyperbilirubinemia are not reached.

Surgical Intervention

With the advances in surgical management of extrahepatic biliary atresia, dramatic improvement in survival statistics has occurred. The Kasai portoenterostomy has resulted in relief of biliary obstruction, but its long-term impact is controversial, because the mechanisms of the disease process are still not entirely understood. Liver transplantation is lifesaving for children with liver failure, and 50% to 75% of all children needing liver transplants are given the diagnosis of biliary atresia before the transplantation (Vacanti et al, 1990). Transplantation following portoenterostomy raises questions as to the choice of operative procedure, and because hepatic dysfunction often progresses even after portoenterostomy, the timing of surgery and the procedure used may become problematic. In addition, because the portoenterostomy results in scarring, subsequent transplantation is more difficult than in children with no previous surgery. Dissection is difficult, blood loss is greater, and operating time is longer in patients who have had the portoenterostomy as primary surgical treatment. However, the Kasai portoenterostomy offers significant benefit for many patients by delaying the need for trans-

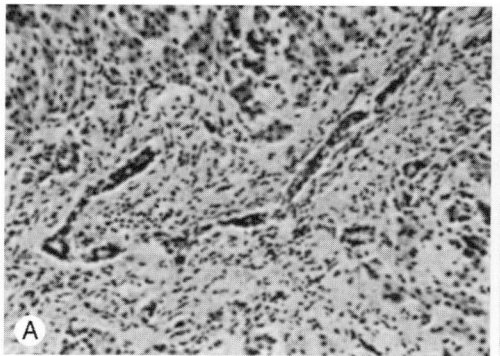
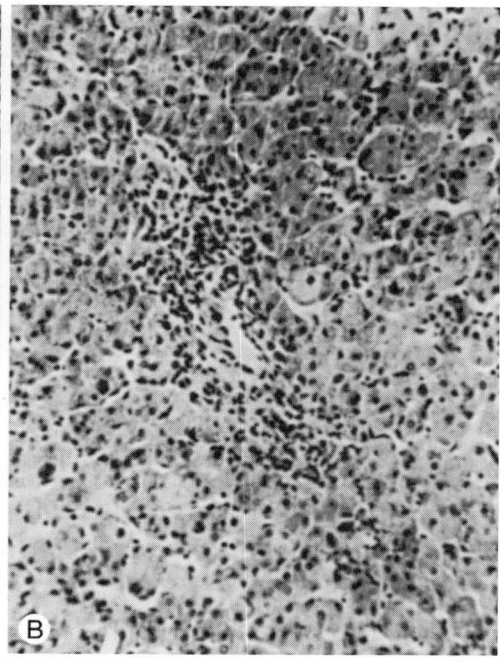

FIGURE 85–1. *A,* Bile duct proliferation and portal fibrosis in an infant with obstruction of the common duct by a plug of inspissated secretion. (Original magnification, ×200.) *B,* Hepatitis with moderate portal inflammation; hepatocellular changes are mild, and multinucleated cells are few. (Original magnification, ×200.) (From Brough AJ, Bernstein J: Liver biopsy in the diagnosis of infantile obstructive jaundice. Pediatrics 43:519, 1969. Reproduced by permission of Pediatrics.)

plantation (Vacanti et al, 1990). A common scenario leading to transplantation is an infant or toddler whose portoenterostomy has failed and in whom recurrent cholangitis has developed with rapidly progressive portal hypertension, malnutrition, mineral and vitamin deficiencies, and liver failure. Early identification of these patients correlates with improved long-term outcome following liver transplantation. Primary transplantation without initial portoenterostomy is not recommended in biliary atresia unless the initial presentation occurs when the child is older than 120 days of age with an enlarged firm liver and biopsy-documented advanced cirrhosis (Kasai et al, 1989; Ryckman et al, 1992). Several factors seen on liver biopsy, including focal necrosis and the presence of giant cells, correlate with failure of the Kasai procedure. Patients older than 8 to 10 weeks of age with this histology should not have the Kasai procedure but should be considered for primary liver transplantation (Filston, 1995).

Until the 1990s, the most important prognostic factor in pediatric liver transplantation was the age and size of the recipient (Starzl et al, 1987). Children weighing less than 10 to 12 kg had a lower survival rate and a frequent complication of hepatic artery thrombosis (Cox et al, 1991). The clinical status before transplantation, especially portal hypertension and nutritional imbalance, also influenced the post-transplantation morbidity and survival rate. However, the availability of donor livers was limited so that a mortality rate of children waiting for a suitable donor was 25% to 46%. Modification in transplantation strategy has improved the outlook considerably. Reduction in size of the donor liver is feasible, donor livers with ABO blood types mismatched with the recipient blood type can be used (Cox et al, 1991), and liver tissue from living related donors (usually the left lobe) has proven satisfactory (Lachaux, 1995). These factors have increased the donor pool size and allowed for better preparation of the patient and timing of

the procedure, resulting in survival rates in excess of 90% even in children weighing less than 10 kg.

PAUCITY OF THE INTERLOBULAR BILE DUCTS

Atresia of the intrahepatic bile ducts, as previously discussed, is usually not complete, but instead consists of a reduced ratio of the number of interlobular bile ducts to the number of portal tracts. For this reason, the term *paucity of the interlobular bile ducts* (PILBD) is used to describe a variety of intrahepatic cholangiopathies, which previously were called intrahepatic biliary atresia ductular hypoplasia, ductular paucity, and ductopenia. This condition may represent an isolated defect, called nonsyndromic PILBD, or it may be associated with specific extrahepatic anomalies, in which case it is termed syndromic PILBD.

Syndromic Paucity of the Interlobular Bile Ducts

Syndromic PILBD, also known as Alagille syndrome and arteriohepatic dysplasia, is a disease with progressive bile duct destruction. It may be the most common of the familial intrahepatic cholestatic syndromes, but it is not as common as extrahepatic biliary atresia (Riely, 1994). This is a multisystem disorder, which includes chronic cholestasis with PILBD on biopsy, congenital heart disease (e.g., peripheral pulmonic stenosis), butterfly vertebrae, eye involvement, and typical facies (Krantz et al, 1997). Not all affected patients have all these findings. Some patients with this syndrome have a deletion or translocation in the short arm of chromosome 20 (Byrne et al, 1986; Legirs et al, 1990; Piccoli et al, 1993).

In patients with Alagille syndrome with severe biliary involvement, jaundice occurs in the first 6 weeks of life, suggesting extrahepatic biliary atresia. Over time, the jaundice improves but pruritus and lichenification of the skin caused by severe persisting cholestasis become problems. Eventually, xanthomata may develop from hypercholesterolemia, rickets, fat malabsorption, growth failure, and neurologic sequelae of vitamin E malabsorption. Despite normalization of calcium, phosphorus, and vitamin D intakes and of blood levels, recurrent or poorly healing long bone fractures are a frequent complication. Some patients eventually require liver transplantation.

Nonsyndromatic Paucity of the Interlobular Bile Ducts

Nonsyndromatic PILBD may be an isolated hepatic abnormality or one component of a more complex systemic process. No one specific etiology has been assigned to this condition and its relationship with extrahepatic bile duct atresia is debated, although both are seen as progressive, destructive, inflammatory cholangiopathies. Unlike syndromic PILBD, nonsyndromic PILBD is not regularly associated with specific extrahepatic anomalies. Although most cases are idiopathic, this condition, like extrahepatic bile duct atresia, has been associated with chromosomal anomalies (e.g., Turner syndrome, trisomy 21), endrocrinopathies (e.g., hypopituitarism), altered bile acid metabolism, and other miscellaneous disorders (Desmet, 1994). Intrauterine infections that have been associated with PILBD include cytomegalovirus, rubella, and hepatitis B. The cholangiopathy appears to proceed to bile duct destruction more rapidly in the nonsyndromic variant of PILBD.

Because nonsyndromic PILBD may coexist with extrahepatic biliary atresia in the same patient and extrahepatic bile duct atresia eventually leads to intrahepatic ductopenia, it is unclear whether these are overlapping clinical syndromes or varying presentations of a single entity, neonatal sclerosing cholangiopathy.

Complete Atresia of the Intrahepatic Bile Ducts

An extraordinary variant of the biliary atresia group, in which no intrahepatic bile ducts are to be found in detailed microscopic examination of liver tissue, was studied carefully and described by Ahrens and colleagues (Ahrens et al, 1951). This condition is thought to be extremely infrequent, and may represent the most extreme form of PILBD. Its clinical course is similar to that of milder PILBD and differs in some particulars from that of atresia of the extrahepatic ducts.

Pathology

The absence of bile ducts of any size within the liver substance is characteristic of PILBD. Bile capillaries are present within each lobule, and these often are dilated and contain plugs of inspissated bile. Extrahepatic ducts are usually absent also, but in 3 of 10 early reported cases the extrahepatic duct system seemed normal. No remnants of compressed, chronically inflamed, or fibrosed ducts are found, and there is no apparent pericholangitis. Fibrosis is

minimal, and cirrhosis develops extremely slowly and seldom reaches the degree it does when atresia is extrahepatic. Ahrens and coworkers (1951) believe that this slow development of cirrhosis stems from the absence of intrahepatic ducts, a condition in which there cannot be liver injury by distention, backflow of bile, and periductal inflammation.

Laboratory Investigations

The blood, stool, and urine findings are initially exactly the same with PILBD as those in extrahepatic atresia. Blood lipid content gradually increases over the course of months or years of biliary obstruction of any type.

Clinical Course

The chief difference between the clinical course of PILBD and that of extrahepatic atresia is that the former disease progresses more slowly than the latter. Jaundice appears at the same time and is equally persistent, but the liver enlarges much more slowly in intrahepatic atresia and does not become so hard and nodular. The patient's nutritional state remains fairly good, and the life span is long. Infants with intrahepatic atresia show a great tendency toward development of cutaneous xanthomatosis. This sign is not seen before 18 months of age, usually later, and it may be more apparent in this group because of the increased life expectancy of the infants. Xanthomas appear and disappear with fluctuations in the serum lipid content.

Treatment

No specific treatment of PILBD is available. Cholestyramine is more likely to lower the bilirubin level and relieve itching in this form of jaundice than in the extrahepatic obstructive variety.

Prognosis

The first reports of long-term follow-up of patients with PILBD (Alagille et al, 1987; Depreterre et al, 1987) suggested survival rates of 75% to 80% with variable morbidity among survivors. Hepatocellular carcinoma, pancreatitis, and liver failure may develop in patients surviving into adulthood (Schwarzenberg et al, 1992). A report of the outcome of patients with Alagille syndrome in whom cholestatic liver disease had developed before 3 months of age was less optimistic, with 50% of patients dying or requiring liver transplantation before 19 years of age (Hoffenberg et al, 1995). For these patients, liver transplantation improves the prognosis for both morbidity and mortality.

The nonsyndromic forms of PILBD have a similar prognosis, long-term course, and eventual need for liver transplantation as patients with Alagille syndrome.

CHOLEDOCHAL CYST

Cystic dilatation of the common duct results from congenital defect of the duct wall or a mucosal valve, or abnormal course of the duct through the duodenal wall. The dilatation is confined to the common duct itself and does not involve the hepatic or cystic ducts or the gallbladder. It may reach the size of an orange or grow even larger.

Incidence

More than 200 cases of choledochal cyst have been reported in all age groups, but it is rare for it to become symptomatic and to be diagnosed within the neonatal period. In Brough and Bernstein's experience (1969), with 39 proven cases of obstructive lesions causing persistent neonatal jaundice, 36 were extrahepatic atresias, 1 was an obstructive bile plug, and 2 were choledochal cysts.

Diagnosis

In older persons, a triad consisting of jaundice, abdominal pain, and upper abdominal tumor strongly suggests the diagnosis. In the neonatal period, the mass is not necessarily large enough to palpate, but it may be huge, filling the entire abdomen. Pain is not prominent or easy to localize. When a cystic mass is felt within the abdomen in the presence of jaundice, the possibility of choledochal cyst must be considered seriously. Wide fluctuations in the depth of the jaundice are highly suggestive. In the final analysis, differential diagnosis can be made only by cholecystography or by direct observation after laparotomy.

Laboratory Investigations

Because jaundice results from blockage by the expanding cyst of entry of bile into the duodenum, the findings are those of obstructive jaundice. Stools become acholic, the urine contains bile but no urobilin, and the serum bilirubin level elevates, with a large percentage of the total bilirubin being direct. Biopsy of the liver reveals a picture indistinguishable from that of extrahepatic atresia.

Treatment

After the cyst has been visualized by cholecystography or by exploratory laparotomy, its walls should be anastomosed to that of the duodenum.

Prognosis

Cholecystoduodenostomy should result in cure. Again, if operative intervention is delayed, irreversible liver damage may occur.

PSEUDOCHOLEDOCHAL CYSTS

Whereas choledochal cyst results from a congenital defect of the common duct, pseudocholedochal cyst is an iatrogenic disorder that follows injury to the common duct at operation.

NEONATAL HEPATITIS

Between one third and one half of infants with persistent obstructive jaundice do not have primary biliary atresia.

Although, as previously indicated, biliary atresia and neonatal hepatitis may be different behaviors of the same disease process, in many instances an entity defined as neonatal hepatitis can be recognized as distinct in its pathologic picture and clinical course. The distinctive pathologic picture is the presence of a cholestatic inflammatory process. Giant cell transformation occurs, but significant bile duct proliferation is absent. Biopsy specimens may demonstrate disorganized lobular architecture, fibrosis, round cell infiltration, and extramedullary hematopoiesis.

Incidence

Neonatal hepatitis cannot be considered rare, because it is observed in two or three patients every year in most large children's hospitals. Milder forms of this entity are much more common and may occur in great numbers during certain viral epidemics such as rubella outbreaks.

Etiology

Neonatal hepatitis has multiple causes. Viral agents recognized to produce the disease include rubella, cytomegalovirus, herpes simplex, Epstein-Barr virus, coxsackievirus, and the hepatitis B virus. Hepatitis may also be observed in infants born with congenital infections resulting from toxoplasmosis and syphilis. In addition, a clinical picture indistinguishable from that observed with infectious agents may be seen in some infants with severe hemolytic disease or galactosemia. In many instances, an etiologic agent is not determined. Familial cases do occur, and in such patients the disease appears to carry a much worse prognosis (see Chapters 42 and 86).

Pathology

The microscopic pictures of the livers of children with neonatal hepatitis have been compared with those of children suffering from congenital extrahepatic duct atresias. In most patients, the distinction can be made by the histologic pattern.

Diagnosis

Jaundice is the primary sign of neonatal hepatitis. It has been observed at birth, but usually it becomes apparent days or weeks after birth. Onset more than 4 weeks after birth (particularly after 6 weeks) makes this diagnosis more likely than that of biliary atresia. Abdominal distention and hepatic enlargement appear with or soon after the jaundice. Later, with advancing cirrhosis, the liver may shrink in size and become hard. At this stage, splenomegaly becomes prominent and ascites may develop. Fever is usually absent. These infants, in contrast to those with biliary atresia, may appear ill, eat poorly, and vomit. Stools become acholic within the first few weeks of the disease process, but this sign may be intermittent. Striking intermittence may strongly, but not absolutely, indicate the absence of congenital atresia. The urine darkens at the same time that color disappears from the stool.

Fletcher and coworkers (1964) reported an extraordinary case of an infant with neonatal hepatitis who was born with massive ascites. He was greatly improved by exchange transfusion and, with excellent supportive care, made a complete recovery after 7 weeks of being very ill.

In many instances, the clinical differentiation of hepatitis from biliary atresia is not possible with absolute certainty.

Laboratory Investigations

Differentiation between obstructive jaundice on the basis of hepatocellular disease caused by neonatal hepatitis and that caused by obstruction of the extrahepatic biliary tree is often difficult. Hepatitis often produces prolonged and essentially complete obstruction of the passage of bile from the liver into the gastrointestinal tract. Certain diagnostic procedures, however, may aid in making a distinction. A gradually increasing serum bilirubin level suggests atresia, whereas an irregularly declining serum bilirubin level suggests hepatitis. The presence of a serum that is positive for alpha-fetoprotein suggests the diagnosis of neonatal hepatitis.

As discussed previously, hepatobiliary imaging using isotopes of Tc 99m can be used in identifying patients with hepatitis and then distinguishing hepatitis from the various forms of biliary atresia. Because the cellular uptake in neonatal hepatitis is impaired, a clear liver image does not develop in patients with hepatitis even though a small percentage of the radioactive material is excreted into the stool.

The fat-soluble vitamin E is poorly absorbed when bile salts do not reach the small intestine. Measurement of vitamin E absorption as described by Lubin and coworkers (1971) or by Melhorn and associates (1972) is a simple procedure that correlates well with the results of isotope imaging and the pathologic picture found at laparotomy.

Administration of phenobarbital or cholestyramine increases the isotope excretion and lowers the serum bilirubin and bile salts in many patients with intrahepatic obstruction.

Recovery of a viral agent or serologic demonstration of an infection with rubella, hepatitis B virus, cytomegalovirus, or toxoplasmosis may suggest the presence of neonatal hepatitis, although these agents have also been associated with presence of a pathologic picture of biliary atresia. Reovirus type 3 is more closely associated with extrahepatic biliary atresia than with hepatitis.

Many infants ultimately require surgical exploration, cholangiography, and liver biopsy so that the cause of the persistent jaundice may be determined. Before such procedures are performed, other diseases that may produce liver diseases must also be excluded. These include alpha$_1$-antitrypsin deficiency, galactosemia, tyrosinemia, and cystic fibrosis.

It has become the consensus that operative diagnosis should not be postponed beyond 2 months of age so that those patients with correctable forms of biliary atresia can be cured.

Prognosis

The prognosis for infants presenting with evidence of hepatitis is largely a function of the cause of the disease. In general, most infants with viral and bacterial causes of hepatitis recover without residual evidence of chronic liver disease of cirrhosis. Rapid resolution of hepatic dysfunction occurs in newborns with galactosemia if diagnosis is promptly established and galactose-containing feeds are removed from the diet. In contrast, hepatitis as a result of cystic fibrosis, alpha$_1$-antitrypsin deficiency, cystic fibrosis, or tyrosinemia often progresses to chronic liver disease. The prognosis for infants with idiopathic forms of neonatal giant cell hepatitis is widely variable. Approximately 20% to 40% of such patients die within the 1st year of life, chronic liver disease develops in another 20% to 40% and the remaining recover entirely.

REFERENCES

Ahrens EH, Harris RC, MacMahon HE: Atresia of the intrahepatic bile ducts. Pediatrics 8:628–646, 1951.

Alagille D, Estrada A, Hadchouel M, et al: Syndromic paucity of interlobular bile ducts (Alagille syndrome or arteriohepatic dysplasia): A view of 80 cases. J Pediatr 110:195–200, 1987.

Alagille D, Odievre M, Gautier M, et al: Hepatic ductular hypoplasia associated with characteristic facies, vertebral malformations, retarded, physical, mental and sexual development, and cardiac murmur. J Pediatr 86:63–71, 1975.

Balistreri WF: Neonatal cholestasis. J Pediatr 106:171–184, 1985.

Benecke R: Die entstehung der kongenitalen atresia der grossen gallengange. Marburg, Universitats Programm, 1907.

Brough AJ, Bernstein J: Liver biopsy in the diagnosis of infantile obstructive jaundice. Pediatrics 43:519, 1969.

Brough AJ, Bernstein J: Conjugated hyperbilirubinemia in early infancy. Human Pathol 5:507, 1974.

Byrne J, Harrod M, Friedman J, et al: del(20p) with manifestations of arteriohepatic dysplasia. Am J Med Genet 24:673–678, 1986.

Chandra RS: Biliary atresia and other structural anomalies in congenital polysplenia syndrome. J Pediatr 85:649–655, 1974.

Cox KL, Nakazato P, Berquist W, et al: Liver transplantation in infants weighing less than 10 kilograms. Trans Proc 23:1579–1580, 1991.

Cox KL, Stadalnik RC, McGahan JP, et al: Hepatobiliary scintigraphy with Technetium-99m disofenin in the evaluation of neonatal cholestasis. J Pediatr Gastroenterol Nutr 6:885–891, 1987.

Dahl-Iversen E, Gormsen H: Sur l'occlusin congenitale des voies biliares. Acta Chir Scand 89:333–338, 1944.

Deprettere A, Portman B, Mowat A: Syndromic paucity of the interlobular bile ducts: Diagnostic difficulty; severe morbidity throughout early childhood. J Pediatr Gastroenterol Nutr 6:865–871, 1987.

Desmet VJ: Pathology of neonatal cholestasis. *In* Lentz M, Riechen J (Eds): Pediatric Cholestasis: Novel Approaches to Treatment. Dordrecht, Kluwer Academic Publishers, 1992, pp 55–74.

Desmet VJ: The cholangiopathies. *In* Suchy FJ (Ed): Liver Disease in Children. St Louis, Mosby-Year Book, 1994, pp 145–165.

Desmet VJ, Callea F: Cholestatic syndromes of infancy and childhood. *In* Zakin D, Boyer TD (Eds): Hepatology. A Textbook of Liver Disease, Vol 2, 2nd ed. Philadelphia, WB Saunders, 1990, pp 1355–1395.

Ferry DG, Selby ML, Udall J, et al: Guide to early diagnosis of biliary obstruction in infancy. Clin Pediatr 24:305–311, 1985.

Filston HC: What's new in pediatric surgery. Pediatrics 96:748–757, 1995.

Fletcher CB, Eakin EL, Rothman PE: Fetal ascites-liver giant-cell transformation. Am J Dis Child 108:554, 1964.

Gray HK, DuShane JW, Henegar GC: Cholecystogastromy for congenital atresia of common bile duct. Professional Staff Meetings, Mayo Clin 23:473–475, 1948.

Green D, Carroll BA: Ultrasonography in the jaundiced infant: A new approach. J Ultrasound Med 5:323–329, 1986.

Greene HL, Helinek GL, Moran R, et al: A diagnostic approach to prolonged obstructive jaundice by 24-hour collection of duodenal fluid. J Pediatr 95:412–414, 1979.

Hart MH, Kaufman SS, Vanderhoof JA, et al: Neonatal hepatitis and extrahepatic biliary atresia associated with cytomegalovirus in two twins. Am J Dis Child 145:302–305, 1991.

Heschl H: Vollstandiger Defekt der Gallenwege, beobachtet an einem 7

Monate alt verstorbene weiblichen Kinde. Wien Med Wochnschr 15:493–498, 1865.

Hoffenberg EJ, Narkewicz MR, Sondheimer JM, et al: Outcome of syndromic paucity of interlobular bile ducts (Alagille syndrome) with onset of cholestasis in infancy. J Pediatr 127:220–224, 1995.

Holmes JB: Congenital obliteration of the bile ducts. Am J Dis Child 11:405–431, 1916.

Ikeda S, Sera Y, Akagi M: Serial ultrasonic examination to differentiate biliary atresia from neonatal hepatitis—Special reference to changes in size of the gallbladder. Eur J Pediatr 148:396–400, 1989.

Kahn E, Markowitz J, Aiges H, et al: Human ontogeny of the bile duct to portal space ratio. Hepatology 10:21–23, 1989.

Kasai M, Mochizuki I, Ohkohchi N, et al: Surgical limitation for biliary atresia: Indication for liver transplantation. J Pediatr Surg 24:851–854, 1989.

Keller MS: Imaging of the liver and biliary tract. *In* Suchy FJ (Ed): Liver Diseases in Children. St Louis, Mosby-Year Book, 1994, pp 309–329.

Kove S, Goldstein S, Wrobleski F: Serum transaminase activity in neonatal period: Valuable aid in differential diagnosis of jaundice in the newborn infant. JAMA 168:860, 1958.

Krantz ID, Piccoli DA, Spinner NB: Alagille syndrome. J Med Genet 34:152–157, 1997.

Lachaux A, Boillot O, Stamm D, et al: Liver transplantation in end-stage biliary cirrhosis in infants weighing less than 12 kilograms. Trans Proc 27:1704–1705, 1995.

Legirs E, Fryns J, Eyshens B, et al: Alagille syndrome (arteriohepatic dysplasia) and del(20)(p11.2). Am J Med Genet 35:532–535, 1990.

Longmire WP, Sanford MC: Intrahepatic cholangiojejunostomy for biliary obstruction. Ann Surg 130:455–458, 1949.

Lubin BH, Baehner RL, Schwartz E, et al: Red cell peroxide hemolysis test in differential diagnosis of obstructive jaundice in the newborn period. Pediatrics 48:562, 1971.

Majd M: (99m)-Tc IDA Scintigraphy in the evaluation of neonatal jaundice. Radiographics 3:88–89, 1983.

Melhorn DK, Gross S, Izant RJ Jr: The red cell hydrogen peroxide hemolysis test and vitamin E absorption in the differential diagnosis of jaundice in infancy. J Pediatr 81:1082, 1972.

Morecki R, Glaser JH, Cho S, et al: Biliary atresia and reovirus type 3 infection. N Engl J Med 310:1610, 1984.

Piccoli D, Moleadam N, Rand E, et al: Phenotype and genetic analysis of syndromic bile duct paucity (Alagille syndrome) (abst 61). Program of the 7th Meeting of the North American Society for Pediatric Gastroenterology and Nutrition. Chicago, November 5–6, 1993.

Platt MS, Potter JL, Boeckman CR, et al: Elevated SGTP/SGOT ratio. An early indicator of infantile obstructive cholangiopathy. Am J Dis Child 135:834, 1981.

Riely CA: Familial intrahepatic cholestasis syndromes. *In* Suchy FJ (Ed): Liver Disease in Children. St Louis, Mosby-Year Book, 1994, pp 443–459.

Rolleston HD, Hayne LB: Case of congenital hepatic cirrhosis with obliterative cholangitis. BMJ 1:758–761, 1901.

Ryckman FC, Fisher RA, Pedersen SH, et al: Liver transplantation in children. Semin Pediatr Surg 1:162–172, 1992.

Ryckman FC, Ziegler MM, Pederson SH, et al: Liver transplantation in children. *In* Suchy FJ (Ed): Liver Disease in Children. St Louis, Mosby-Year Book, 1994, pp 930–950.

Schwarzenberg S, Grothe R, Sharp H, et al: Long-term complications of arteriohepatic dysplasia. Am J Med 93:171–175, 1992.

Starzl TE, Esquivel C, Gordon R, et al: Pediatric liver transplantation. Transplant Proc 19(4):3230–3235, 1987.

Stein JE, Vacanti JP: Biliary atresia and other disorders of the extrahepatic biliary tree. *In* Suchy FJ (Ed): The Disease in Children. St Louis, Mosby-Year Book, 1994, pp 426–442.

Stolkind E: Congenital abnormalities of gallbladder and extrahepatic ducts. Br J Child Dis 36:115–122, 1939.

Suchy FJ: Approach to the infant with cholestasis. *In* Suchy FJ (Ed): Liver Disease in Children, St Louis, Mosby-Year Book, 1994, pp 349–355.

Thomson J: On congenital obliteration of bile ducts. Edinburgh Med J 37:523–530, 1891.

Tolia V, Dubois RS, Kagalwalla A, et al: Comparison of radionuclear scintigraphy and liver biopsy in the evaluation of neonatal cholestasis. J Pediatr Gastroenterol Nutr 5:30–34, 1986.

Vacanti JP, Shamberger RC, Eraklis A, et al: The therapy of biliary atresia combining the Kasai portoenterostomy with liver transplantation: A single center experience. J Pediatr Surg 25:149–152, 1990.

Weinberg T, Gordon HH, Oppenheimer EH, et al: Myopathy in association with tocopherol deficiency in cases of congenital biliary atresia and cystic fibrosis of the pancreas. Am J Pathol 34:565, 1958.

CHAPTER 86

Other Conjugated Hyperbilirubinemias

James R. MacMahon, David K. Stevenson and Frank A. Oski*

Although the clinician commonly associates the accumulation of conjugated bilirubin in the serum of the newborn with the possible presence of either neonatal hepatitis or biliary atresia, it must be appreciated that a large number of heterogeneous disorders are associated with laboratory evidence of conjugated hyperbilirubinemia (Table 86–1).

METABOLIC DEFECTS

Conjugated bilirubin may be retained as a result of an isolated specific defect in hepatic bilirubin transport, as occurs in the Dubin-Johnson and Rotor syndromes, or as a result of a more generalized disturbance in hepatic biliary secretion. This more generalized defect is termed *cholestasis*. Obstruction of a mechanical nature may produce cholestasis, but not all cases of cholestasis result from obstructive jaundice.

Dubin-Johnson syndrome and Rotor syndrome are rarely diagnosed in the neonatal period, although both may initially manifest themselves during this period by the elevation in conjugated ("direct"-reacting) bilirubin. First reported in 1954, the Dubin-Johnson syndrome is caused by a deficiency in the canalicular secretion of conjugated bilirubin and other anions (Dubin, 1958). Intrahepatic storage is normal, resulting in the reflux of conjugated bilirubin back into the circulation. Bile salt secretion occurs normally and affected patients are not pruritic. The most characteristic laboratory feature of this disease is the markedly increased urinary excretion of the type I isomer of coproporphyrin. This metabolic error is inherited as an autosomal recessive trait. Liver biopsy is normal except for the presence of brownish-black granules that have many of the characteristics of melanin. Jaundice in women with the Dubin-Johnson syndrome becomes more intense during the last trimester of pregnancy and when estrogen-containing oral contraceptives have been used before pregnancy. Total bilirubin levels in patients with this condition are usually between 1.5 and 6 mg/dL, although levels as high as 25 mg/dL have been reported (Gustein et al, 1968).

Rotor syndrome was first reported in 1948 and is much less common than Dubin-Johnson syndrome. It is also inherited as an autosomal recessive trait and is characterized by the presence of lifelong mild conjugated hyperbilirubinemia (Rotor et al, 1948). No pigment accumulates in the liver of affected patients, in contrast to the biopsy findings in patients with the Dubin-Johnson syndrome. The defect in this disorder is believed to be the result of a disturbance in the hepatic storage of anions.

Other rare metabolic defects may produce injury to the hepatocytes and often result in the retention of conjugated bilirubin. Alpha₁-antitrypsin deficiency may be the most common of the inherited metabolic defects associated with

liver disease in the newborn period, affecting approximately 1 in 1600 to 2000 live births in North America and northern European populations (Perlmutter, 1994). This autosomal recessive disorder is associated with 85% to 90% reduction in serum concentrations of alpha₁-antitrypsin and is the most common genetic cause of liver disease for which children undergo liver transplantation. Eventually this condition leads to premature development of emphysema, chronic liver disease, and hepatocellular carcinoma, but the presentation in the neonatal period may mimic that of neonatal hepatitis with jaundice, abnormal liver function tests, and bilirubinuria. The homozygous form of the severe deficiency, designated as the PiZZ genotype by protein electrophoresis, is the only mutant form of the disease associated with liver disease in childhood. The alpha₁-antitrypsin deficiency is caused by a defect in transport of alpha₁-antitrypsin, a secretory protein, from endoplasmic reticulum to the Golgi apparatus, resulting in the accumulation of alpha₁-antitrypsin in the endoplasmic reticulum (Mornex et al, 1986). It is this intracellular accumulation of the mutant alpha₁-antitrypsin molecules that results in liver disease. The defect is caused by a single nucleotide substitution resulting in a single amino acid substitution (Jeppsson, 1976). It is estimated that between 10% and 20% of individuals with the PiZZ genotype are seen with conjugated hyperbilirubinemia, cirrhosis, or both during infancy or early childhood. When the disease is symptomatic in the neonatal period, it usually leads to fatal cirrhosis. The finding of little or no alpha₁ globulin on routine protein electrophoresis suggests that the disease is present. The diagnosis can be made by demonstration that serum is deficient in trypsin-inhibitory activity and that the patient possesses a PiZZ type on electrophoresis. It is possible to detect specific alpha₁-antitrypsin variants by amplification of genomic DNA using the polymerase chain reaction (Petersen et al, 1988). This technique is rapid and sensitive, and it may prove useful for confirming the diagnosis or in prenatal assessments. Liver biopsy in affected patients demonstrates hepatocytes containing amorphous clumps of pink-staining material in the cytoplasm of the cell. These granules are positive on periodic acid–Schiff and resistant to diastase digestion. No effective therapy except liver transplantation is available to halt the progress of the disease.

Galactosemia, tyrosinemia, fructosemia, Niemann-Pick disease, Gaucher disease, glycogenosis type IV, and cystic fibrosis are other metabolic disorders in which conjugated hyperbilirubinemia may be observed in the newborn period. In general, other features of the disease dominate the clinical picture, and the patients rarely have a simple problem in the differential diagnosis of conjugated hyperbilirubinemia (Andres, 1996).

Gatzimos and Jowitt (1955) first called attention to the association between jaundice and cystic fibrosis. Many of these infants may have a history of delayed passage of the

°Deceased.

TABLE 86–1

Disorders of the Newborn Associated with Conjugated (Direct-Reacting) Hyperbilirubinemia

I. Obstruction to biliary flow
  1. Extrahepatic biliary atresia
  2. Paucity of intrahepatic ductules (intrahepatic biliary atresia)
  3. Choledochal cyst (bile duct stenosis)
  4. Bile-plug syndrome (inspissated bile syndrome)
  5. Cystic fibrosis
  6. Choledocholithiasis
  7. Tumors
  8. Hepatic hemangioendotheliomas
  9. Lymphadenopathy
II. Hepatic cell injury
  1. Infection
    Bacterial
      Syphilis
      Listeriosis
      Tuberculosis
      Escherichia coli urinary tract infection
    Viral
      Rubella
      Cytomegalovirus
      Herpes
      Coxsackie B
      Hepatitis B
      Hepatitis A
      Reovirus type 3
      Enterovirus (coxsackie, echo)
    Parasitic
      Toxoplasmosis
    Idiopathic
      Neonatal hepatitis (giant cell hepatitis)
  2. Toxic
    Bacterial sepsis (*E. coli, Listeria,* monocytogenes, *Proteus, Pneumococcus*)

    Intravenous alimentation
    Drugs
  3. Metabolic errors
    Galactosemia
    Fructosemia
    Tyrosinemia
    Alpha$_1$-antitrypsin deficiency
    Cystic fibrosis
    Infantile Gaucher disease
    Glycogenosis type IV
    Wolman disease
    Idiopathic neonatal hemochromatosis
    Niemann-Pick disease
    Cerebrohepatorenal syndrome (Zellweger disease)
    Byler disease
    Trihydroxycoprostanic acidemia
    Rotor syndrome
    Dubin-Johnson syndrome
  4. Immunologic neonatal lupus erythematosus
  5. Chromosomal disorders
    Trisomy 17–18
    Trisomy 21
III. Chronic bilirubin overload
  1. Erythroblastosis fetalis
  2. Glucose-6-phosphate dehydrogenase deficiency and other erythrocyte enzyme deficiencies
  3. Spherocytosis, elliptocytosis, pyknocytosis
  4. Congenital erythropoietic porphyria

Adapted from Gartner LM: Disorders of bilirubin metabolism. *In* Nathan DG, Oski FA (Eds): Hematology of Infancy and Childhood, 2nd ed. Philadelphia, WB Saunders, 1981, p 108.

first meconium stool. These infants can be demonstrated to have thick tenacious bile plugging their biliary tree. Needle biopsy of the liver may demonstrate the characteristic eosinophilic plugs in the portal bile ducts, which may be accompanied by hyperplasia. The jaundice usually resolves spontaneously. A diagnosis of cystic fibrosis in the newborn period can be established by demonstrating the increased concentration of sweat chloride.

NEONATAL HEMOCHROMATOSIS

Neonatal hemochromatosis (NH) is a condition that results from liver disease of intrauterine onset, which is associated with extrahepatic deposits of stainable iron (siderosis) sparing the spleen, bone marrow, and lymph nodes. The liver disease is manifested in the first hours or days of extrauterine life. NH presents with hypoglycemia, hypoalbuminemia, and hemorrhagic diathesis, and it leads to hyperbilirubinemia in the first few days of life (Knisely, 1992). NH is etiologically separate from human leukocyte antigen–linked heritable hemochromatosis. The initial manifestations result from inadequate synthesis of albumin and clotting factors caused by hepatic disease. The elevated bilirubin

concentration appears to be caused by both the increased bilirubin load from extravasated blood of a bleeding diathesis and the impaired ability of the liver to synthesize and excrete bilirubin.

The causes of intrauterine liver disease and the mechanisms leading to hemochromatic siderosis in this condition are obscure, and the differential diagnosis includes many causes of hepatic insufficiency (Knisely, 1994). Diagnosis is based on tissue distribution of stainable iron, as established by biopsy or magnetic resonance imaging studies (Hayes et al, 1992), and abnormalities in circulating concentrations of iron and iron-binding proteins (Silver et al, 1987).

Treatment of NH depends on early recognition, support for hepatic insufficiency, and rapid intervention with early liver transplantation if necessary (Knisely et al, 1994). Principal complications are hypoglycemia, hemorrhage, and hypotension. Deferoxamine administration and iron depletion alone do not adequately treat this condition (Jonas, 1987).

SEPSIS

Both generalized sepsis and severe urinary tract infections, particularly with *Escherichia coli*, during the 1st month of life may be accompanied by an increase in the serum concentration of conjugated bilirubin. Bacterial products are believed to produce a toxic injury to the hepatocellular excretory system. Liver biopsy of infected and jaundiced newborns reveals cholestasis, focal liver cell necrosis, and other nonspecific changes. Direct infection of the liver is not evident. Despite the marked increases in the concentration of bilirubin that may accompany infection, the serum values for alkaline phosphatase and the transaminases are either normal or only slightly elevated. Treatment of the infection produces a decline in the bilirubin concentrations without evidence of residual liver damage.

TOXIC HEPATITIS

Although bacterial infections may produce a "toxic" hepatitis, this term is more commonly applied to circumstances in which exposure to exogenous substances produces cholestasis with variable degrees of hepatocellular injury, inflammation, or fibrosis.

The most common cause of toxic hepatitis or cholestatic jaundice observed in neonatal intensive care nurseries is the prolonged use of total parenteral nutrition.

Cholestatic jaundice induced by parenteral nutrition is seen with greatest frequency in the most immature infants. It is estimated that this complication will develop in at least 10% of infants with a gestational age of less than 32 weeks if they receive parenteral nutrition for periods of 3 to 4 weeks. In contrast, cholestatic jaundice develops in only about 1% of infants with gestational ages of more than 36 weeks under similar circumstances.

Bacterial infections appear to contribute to the development of cholestasis.

Liver biopsies in infants in whom cholestatic jaundice develops in association with parenteral nutrition demonstrate both hepatocellular damage and cholestasis. Giant cell transformation may also be observed. The cause of the cholestasis is unclear but may relate to the inhibition of bile flow by amino acid. Evidence of hepatic dysfunction but not clinical jaundice can be demonstrated within 1 week of the initiation of total parenteral nutrition. This effect appears to be independent of the newborn's underlying condition and unrelated to the concomitant use of intravenous lipid. The initial effect of the amino acid infusion appears to be on the canalicular membrane and is reflected by increases in the serum concentrations of gamma glutamyl transpeptidase and 5'-nucleotidase.

Discontinuation of the parenteral nutrition usually produces a disappearance of the hepatic abnormalities, although evidence of hepatocellular damage and fibrosis may persist over several weeks. Newborns receiving total parenteral nutrition should be monitored, at least weekly, with measurement of conjugated bilirubin values and serum bile acids.

THE BILE-PLUG SYNDROME

It has been suspected for many years that obstructive jaundice could be caused by plugs in the extrahepatic bile ducts. Bernstein and coworkers (1977) proved this theory by demonstrating such plugs in two infants, one of whom became jaundiced as early as 6 days and the other as late as 7 weeks of age. The second baby was saved after demonstration by cholangiogram of obstruction in the distal end of the common duct and following the removal of an impacted mass of dark, granular, bile-colored material.

REFERENCES

Andres JM: Neonatal hepatobiliary disorders. Clin Perinatol 23(2):321, 1996.

Bernstein J, Braylan R, Brough AJ: Bile-plug syndrome: A correctable cause of obstructive jaundice in infants. Pediatrics 43:273, 1969.

Bernstein J, Chang CH, Brough AJ, et al: Conjugated hyperbilirubinemia in infants associated with parenteral alimentation. J Pediatr 90:361, 1977.

Brath SV, Davies P, Papadopoulov A, et al: Parenteral nutrition–related cholestasis in postsurgical neonates: Multivariate analysis of risk factors. J Pediatr Surg 31:604, 1996.

Dubin IN: Chronic idiopathic jaundice: A review of fifty cases. Am J Med 24:268–292, 1958.

Escobedo MB, Barton LL: The frequency of jaundice in neonatal bacterial infections. Clin Pediatr 13:656, 1974.

Gatzimos CD, Jowitt RH: Jaundice in mucoviscidosis (fibrocystic disease of the pancreas). J Dis Child 80:182, 1955.

Gustein SL, Alpert L, Arias IM: Studies of hepatic excretory function. IV. Biliary excretion of sulfobromophthalein sodium in a patient with Dubin-Johnson syndrome and a biliary fistula. Isr J Med Sci 4:36–40, 1968.

Hayes AM, Jamarillo D, Levy HM, et al: Neonatal hemochromatosis: Diagnosis with MRI imaging. AJR Am J Roentgenol 159:623–625, 1992.

Jeppsson J-O: Amino acid substitution Glu-Lys in alpha-1-antitrypsin PiZ. FEBS *Lett* 65:195–197, 1976.

Jonas MM, Kaweblum YA, Fojaco R: Neonatal hemochromatosis: Failure of deferoxamine therapy. J Pediatr Gastroenterol Nutr 6:984–988, 1987.

Knisely AS: Neonatal hemochromatosis. Adv Pediatr 39:383–403, 1992.

Knisely AS: Neonatal hemochromatosis. *In* Suchy FJ (Ed): Liver Disease in Children. St Louis, Mosby-Year Book, 1994, pp 783–790.

Mornex J-P, Chytil-Weir A, Martinet Y, et al: Expression of the α_1 antitrypsin gene in mononuclear phagocytes of normal and alpha-1-antitrypsin-deficient individuals. J Clin Invest 77:1952–1961, 1986.

Moss AL, Das JB, Ansari G, et al: Hepatobiliary dysfunction during total parenteral nutrition is caused by infusate, not the route of administration. J Pediatr Surg 28:391, 1993.

Odievre M, Martin JP, et al: Alpha-1-antitrypsin deficiency in liver disease in children: Phenotypes, manifestations, and prognosis. Pediatrics 57:226, 1976.

Pereira GR, Sherman MS, DiGiacomo J, et al: Hyperalimentation-induced cholestasis. Increased incidence and severity in premature infants. Am J Dis Child 135:842, 1981.

Perlmutter DH: α_1 Antitrypsin deficiency. *In* Suchy FJ (Ed): Liver Disease in Children. St Louis, Mosby-Year Book, 1994, pp 686–704.

Petersen KB, Kolvroa S, Bolund L, et al: Detection of alpha-1-antitrypsin genotypes by analysis by amplified DNA sequences. Nucleic Acids Res 16:352, 1988.

Quigley EM, Marsh MN, Shaffer JL, et al: Hepatobiliary complications of total parenteral nutrition. Gastroenterology 104:286, 1993.

Rosenthal P: Neonatal hepatitis and congenital infections. *In* Suchy FJ (Ed): Liver Disease in Children. St. Louis, CV Mosby, 1994, pp 414–425.

Rotor AB, Manahan L, Florentin A: Familial nonhemolytic jaundice with direct van den Bergh reaction. Acta Med Phil 5:37–49, 1948.

Silver MM, Beverly DW, Valberg LS, et al: Perinatal hemochromatosis: Clinical, morphologic, and quantitative iron studies. Am J Pathol 128:538–554, 1987.

Taylor WF, Qaqundah BY: Neonatal jaundice associated with cystic fibrosis. Am J Dis Child 123:161, 1972.

CHAPTER 87

Management of Neonatal Hyperbilirubinemia

James R. MacMahon, David K. Stevenson and Frank A. Oski*

Hyperbilirubinemia remains a common, important, and sometimes pathologic condition of the newborn. Because the risk of jaundice-associated neurotoxicity continues to be a major concern of physicians caring for newborns, management of neonatal hyperbilirubinemia is a subject of considerable discussion and debate. In this chapter, issues affecting management decisions and current recommendations are discussed.

Since the introduction of blood exchange transfusion in the 1950s for the treatment of hyperbilirubinemia associated with hemolytic disease of the newborn and since Rh-negative mothers have routinely received the anti-Rh globulin as a measure to prevent isoimmunization, the occurrence of bilirubin encephalopathy in newborns has been reduced greatly. However, the knowledge that low levels of serum bilirubin can be associated with bilirubin encephalopathy in small premature infants and that hypoxia, acidosis, and sepsis may be associated with higher risk has prevented the emergence of a single reliable criterion for instituting treatment of hyperbilirubinemia. As discussed in Chapter 83, the neurotoxicity of bilirubin is not an all-or-none phenomenon, but ranges from subtle reversible changes in neural function to permanent structural and functional impairment related to discrete cell death and regional yellow staining of brain tissue. Besides the classic signs of kernicterus, neurologic sequelae (e.g., disturbances of visual-motor function and impaired nonverbal intelligence) have been described in surviving premature infants who had hyperbilirubinemia in the neonatal period. However, whether such nonspecific findings may have been related to either the degree or the duration of hyperbilirubinemia or to some other factors is uncertain and will not be ascertained by further analysis of current data. Thus, predictors of bilirubin encephalopathy, besides total serum bilirubin concentration, have been sought, and guidelines for intervention have been fraught with lively controversy. Criteria based entirely on clinical experience and measurement of total serum bilirubin have weaknesses and may result in overtreatment of term infants. In contrast, more liberal criteria may lead to undertreatment of some infants, a situation that could inadvertently contribute to permanent damage in susceptible infants. Understanding susceptibility is key to solving this clinical problem. Some researchers have argued for a case-based approach using not only the determination of total unconjugated serum bilirubin concentrations to develop criteria for treatment plans but also measures of albumin binding capacity, determination of the integrity and maturity of the blood–brain barrier, and an assessment of the conjugating power of the liver. Because the basic mechanisms behind the development of bilirubin toxicity are not completely understood, however, such new treatment criteria have not been systematically or successfully implemented (Bratlid, 1995).

---

* Deceased.

THE TERM INFANT

Because well term neonates present, as a group, less risk for bilirubin encephalopathy compared to premature or sick infants, most authors discussing clinical management of neonatal hyperbilirubinemia frame their discussion in the context of only one of these groups. As medical practice faces increasing economic constraints, the management of hyperbilirubinemia concerns not only which tests to complete and which clues to follow but also the balance of risks of undertreatment with the cost and consequences of overtreatment.

With regard to management of the jaundiced term neonate who is deemed to be "healthy," controversy has characterized the discussions for several decades. In 1959, Mores and associates evaluated 54 full-term infants without evidence of isoimmunization who had total serum bilirubin levels greater than 20 mg/dL and who received no exchange transfusion. Citing normal development in all 54 subjects after 2 years of follow-up, this study concluded that "it is useless to perform an exchange transfusion on full term infants with intensive jaundice without isoimmunization because these infants are neither in danger, nor ill; they are only icteric" (Mores et al, 1959). Since that time, much has been learned about the processes of bilirubin metabolism but not much more about the mechanisms of neurotoxicity. Although many studies confirm the low risk to term infants who do not have excessive hemolysis or rigid elements in serum bilirubin levels, any statement suggesting total absence of risk is viewed as overly simplistic and dangerous.

In response to these controversies, the American Academy of Pediatrics (AAP) published guidelines for the management of the jaundiced neonate (American Academy of Pediatrics, 1994). Intended to apply only to the healthy full-term neonate, these guidelines describe a range of acceptable practices, recognizing that more precise recommendations cannot be formulated from current scientific literature, and with the acknowledgment that (1) "factors influencing bilirubin toxicity to the brain cells of newborn infants are complex and incompletely understood," (2) "It is not known at what bilirubin concentration or under what circumstances significant risk of brain damage occurs or when the risk of brain damage exceeds the risk of treatment," and (3) "Concentrations considered harmful may vary in different ethnic groups, or geographic locations. . . . Reasons for apparent geographic differences in risk for kernicterus are not clear." In addition, these recommendations were presented at a time when the management decisions were increasingly problematic because of mounting pressures for early discharge from the hospital and a greater prevalence of breast-feeding in the American population.

EVALUATION AND DIAGNOSTIC PROCEDURES

The AAP Practice Parameter lists factors to be considered when assessing a jaundiced infant (Table 87–1). Regarding the evaluation of the jaundiced newborn, the AAP recommendations reinforce the fact that because the determination of specific risk factors and the identification of illnesses early are critical to the management of these patients, a careful history and physical examination remain the most important diagnostic procedures.

Of particular significance is a family history of severe unexplained jaundice requiring exchange transfusion, suggesting the possibility of glucose-6-phosphate dehydrogenase (G6PD) deficiency or some other cause of hemolytic disease. When the family history, ethnic or geographic origin, or timing of jaundice suggests such a diagnosis, appropriate laboratory assessment in the infant should be performed.

Maternal prenatal testing routinely should include ABO and Rh typing and a serum screen for unusual isoimmune antibodies. When the mother has not had prenatal blood grouping or is Rh negative, a direct Coombs test and Rh typing on the infant's cord blood are recommended to anticipate and closely monitor an infant at risk of severe hemolysis and to determine the need for the mother to receive Rho(D) antibody (anti Rh globulin).

Serum bilirubin determinations are indicated in all infants who appear jaundiced in the first 24 hours of life, because such an early appearance of jaundice is almost always associated with hemolytic disease or illness. In other infants, serum bilirubin levels are indicated if estimates from sequential observations show that the jaundice is moderate or greater (estimate of serum bilirubin in excess of 12 mg/dL [200 μM/L]).

With increasing pressure to discharge babies from the hospital at 24 hours of age or less, most jaundiced infants will not be diagnosed by nursery personnel. Therefore, 2 to 3 days after discharge (corresponding to the time of the normal transitional peek of hyperbilirubinemia), follow-up should be provided by a health-care professional in an office, clinic, or at home to all newborns discharged less than 48 hours after birth. Because bacterial sepsis is a significant risk factor for bilirubin encephalopathy and may be associated with elevated bilirubin levels caused by hemolysis or inadequate nutrition or hydration, further evaluation of newborns in whom abnormal signs such as feeding difficulty, lethargy, apnea, or temperature instability develop must be initiated to rule out underlying illness or sepsis (see Table 87–1).

Because approximately one third of healthy breast-fed infants have jaundice that persists beyond 2 weeks of age (Linn et al, 1985), breast-feeding need not be routinely interrupted solely for the purpose of establishing a diagnosis of breast milk or breast-feeding jaundice (Gartner, 1994).

Any report of dark urine, light stools, or persistence of jaundice beyond 2 weeks should prompt a measurement of direct (conjugated) serum bilirubin levels. Otherwise, determination of direct bilirubin levels is most often not useful in the healthy neonate. Other data that are useful in evaluating an infant with neonatal jaundice are listed in Table 87–2.

SUSCEPTIBILITY TO BILIRUBIN NEUROTOXICITY

Appreciating the factors that may be associated with increased risk for brain injury associated with increased hyperbilirubinemia is central to determining which patients should be treated and which intervention should be undertaken. Some patients demonstrate a steady and excessive increase in serum bilirubin levels over the first several days of extrauterine life, enabling clinicians to predict bilirubin levels by extrapolation. Other infants exhibit a more sudden change in total serum bilirubin concentration, making prediction of the course of hyperbilirubinemia impossible (e.g., in G6PD-deficient or septic infants).

Specific clinical situations such as sepsis, isoimmunization, and other causes of hemolysis are known to be associated with elevated risks for neurotoxicity, even at serum bilirubin levels otherwise considered moderate or mild. Why this problem occurs is not known with certainty, but increased bilirubin production is a finding common to these situations.

Some experts think that bilirubin production rates may be the critical piece of information distinguishing jaundiced infants at excessive risk of encephalopathy from those who, although equally jaundiced in appearance and having similarly elevated total serum bilirubin concentrations, are at

---

TABLE 87–1

Factors to Be Considered When Assessing a Jaundiced Infant

Factors that suggest the possibility of hemolytic disease
    Family history of significant hemolytic disease
    Onset of jaundice before age 24 hours
    An increase in serum bilirubin levels of more than 0.5 mg/dL per hour
    Pallor, hepatosplenomegaly
    Rapid increase in the TSB level after 24 to 48 hours (consider G6PD deficiency)
    Ethnicity suggestive of inherited disease (e.g., G6PD deficiency)
    Failure of phototherapy to lower the TSB level
Clinical signs suggesting the possibility of other diseases such as sepsis or galactosemia in which jaundice may be one manifestation of the disease
    Vomiting
    Lethargy
    Poor feeding
    Hepatosplenomegaly
    Excessive weight loss
    Apnea
    Temperature instability
    Tachypnea
Signs of cholestatic jaundice suggesting the need to rule out biliary atresia or other causes of cholestasis
    Dark urine or urine positive for bilirubin
    Light-colored stools
    Persistent jaundice for more than 3 weeks

TSB, total serum bilirubin; G6PD, glucose-6-phosphate dehydrogenase.
Used with permission of the American Academy of Pediatrics: Practice parameter: Management of hyperbilirubinemia in the healthy term newborn. Pediatrics 94:559, 1994.

TABLE 87–2

Data Collection in the Diagnosis of Neonatal Jaundice

Information	Significance
Family History	
Parent or sibling with history of jaundice or anemia	Suggests hereditary hemolytic anemia such as hereditary spherocytosis
Previous sibling with neonatal jaundice	Suggests hemolytic disease due to ABO or Rh isoimmunization
History of liver disease in siblings or disorders such as cystic fibrosis, galactosemia, tyrosinemia, hypermethioninemia, Crigler-Najjar syndrome, or alpha₁-antitrypsin deficiency	All associated with neonatal hyperbilirubinemia
Maternal History	
Unexplained illness during pregnancy	Consider congenital infections such as rubella, cytomegalovirus, toxoplasmosis, herpes, syphilis, hepatitis A or B, Epstein-Barr virus
Diabetes mellitus	Increased incidence of jaundice among infants of diabetic mothers
Drug ingestion during pregnancy	Ingestion of sulfonamides, nitrofurantoins, antimalarials may initiate hemolysis in G6PD deficient infant
History of Labor and Delivery	
Vacuum extraction	Increased incidence of cephalhematoma and jaundice
Oxytocin-induced labor	Increased incidence of hyperbilirubinemia
Delayed cord clamping	Increased incidence of hyperbilirubinemia among polycythemic infants
Apgar score	Increased incidence of jaundice in asphyxiated infants
Infant's History	
Delayed passage of meconium or infrequent stools	Increased enterohepatic circulation of bilirubin. Consider intestinal atresia, annular pancreas, Hirschsprung disease, meconium plug, drug-induced ileus (hexamethonium)
Caloric intake	Inadequate caloric intake results in delay in bilirubin conjugation
Vomiting	Suspect sepsis, galactosemia, or pyloric stenosis; all associated with hyperbilirubinemia.
Infant's Physical Examination	
Small for gestational age	Infants frequently polycythemic and jaundiced
Head size	Microcephaly seen with intrauterine infections associated with jaundice
Cephalhematoma	Entrapped hemorrhage associated with hyperbilirubinemia
Plethora	Polycythemia
Pallor	Suspect hemolytic anemia
Petechiae	Suspect congenital infection, overwhelming sepsis, or severe hemolytic disease as cause of jaundice
Appearance of umbilical stump	Omphalitis and sepsis may produce jaundice
Hepatosplenomegaly	Suspect hemolytic anemia or congenital infection
Optic fundi	Chorioretinitis suggests congenital infection as cause of jaundice
Umbilical hernia	Consider hypothyroidism
Congenital anomalies	Jaundice occurs with increased frequency among infants with trisomic conditions

Laboratory Data

Maternal	
Blood group and indirect Coombs' test	Necessary for evaluation of possible ABO or Rh incompatibility
Serology	Rule out congenital syphilis
Infant	
Hemoglobin	Anemia suggests hemolytic disease or large entrapped hemorrhage. Hemoglobin above 22 g/dL associated with increased incidence of jaundice
Reticulocyte count	Elevation suggests hemolytic disease
Red cell morphology	Spherocytes suggest ABO incompatibility or hereditary spherocytosis. Red cell fragmentation seen in disseminated intravascular coagulation
Platelet count	Thrombocytopenia suggests infection
White cell count	Total white cell count less than 5000/mm³ or band/neutrophil ratio >0.2 suggests infection
Sedimentation rate	Values in excess of 5 during the first 48 hours indicate infection or ABO incompatibility
Direct bilirubin	Elevation suggests infection or severe Rh incompatibility
Immunoglobulin M	Elevation indicates infection
Blood group and direct and indirect Coombs' test	Required to rule out hemolytic disease as a result of isoimmunization
Carboxyhemoglobin level	Elevated in infants with hemolytic disease or entrapped hemorrhage
Urinalysis	Presence of reducing substance suggests diagnosis or galactosemia

less risk. Previous discussions (see Chapter 83) alluded to the saturation of the albumin-binding sites and elevated levels of unbound bilirubin as being critical to the neurotoxic effects of bilirubin. In addition to the capacity of albumin to bind bilirubin in the circulation, the total tissue load of bilirubin may be important to consider.

When serum bilirubin concentrations are lower than the level that saturates the bilirubin-binding sites of albumin, the measured "total serum bilirubin" represents all the unconjugated bilirubin in circulation, whether bound to albumin or not. However, this total serum bilirubin concentration does not reflect the tissue load or total body load of bilirubin. This is a critical difference, because a high bilirubin production rate is thought to result in a more rapid transfer of bilirubin to tissue, causing patients with high rates of production to have substantially higher tissue loads than those with low production rates. If the capacity to keep bilirubin in circulation is exceeded more rapidly, a surrogate for this circumstance is the rate of increase of bilirubin in circulation or the postnatal age at which a particular level is reached; for example, a serum concentration of 20 mg/dL at 48 hours of age represents a different risk from that of 20 mg/dL at 7 days of age. When the total serum concentration increases enough to "saturate" the albumin-binding sites and the body load is particularly heavy, the tissue load is already high and any further increase in serum bilirubin represents bilirubin with great potential to enter the brain, which may have been spared until that time. If the tissue load is small, however, further deposition of bilirubin in the body may be possible, relieving the brain of immediate risk. It has been hypothesized that this high tissue load in patients with increased bilirubin production may explain why these patients are vulnerable to brain damage at the same bilirubin levels that do not seem to endanger babies with low rates of bilirubin production. This concept of a total body load or tissue load may also explain why babies with increased bilirubin production (e.g., hemolysis) have a more profound rebound in serum

bilirubin levels after treatment with either exchange transfusion or phototherapy. If this hypothesis is sustained, identifying patients with increased bilirubin production will be extremely useful in determining the level of risk for neurotoxicity and scheduling interventions (see Chapter 83).

Methods of identifying such patients by carbon monoxide measurements in expiratory gas analysis or noninvasive percutaneous measures are also discussed in Chapter 81.

TREATMENT

AAP guidelines for treatment and intervention of hyperbilirubinemia in the healthy term newborn are summarized in Table 87–3 and in Figure 87–1. These guidelines are recommended for infants initially seen with elevated total serum bilirubin levels as well as for infants who have been followed up for clinical jaundice. Because direct bilirubin measurements vary substantially as a function of differences of individual laboratories and their instrumentation, the direct bilirubin measurement should not be subtracted from the total serum bilirubin level in determining management strategy. Infants less than 24 hours of age who are jaundiced are generally considered to have a "pathologic" process and require further evaluation. There is continuing uncertainty about what specific total serum bilirubin levels warrant exchange transfusion, and intensive phototherapy is recommended while preparations are being made for exchange transfusion. This is especially relevant for infants who have a total serum bilirubin concentration in the exchange transfusion range when initially seen (see Table 87–3). Intensive phototherapy is expected to cause a decline in total serum bilirubin level of 1 to 2 mg/dL within 4 to 6 hours (American Academy of Pediatrics, 1994); if no decline occurs, the presence of hemolytic disease or some other pathologic process is suggested and warrants further investigation, and most experts recommend exchange transfusion. Practices vary between ordering sequential individ-

TABLE 87–3

American Academy of Pediatrics Guidelines for the Management of Hyperbilirubinemia in the Healthy Term Newborn

Age (hours)	Total Serum Bilirubin Level, mg/dL (μmol/L)			
	Consider Photherapy°	Phototherapy	Exchange Transfusion if Intensive Phototherapy Fails†	Exchange Transfusion and Intensive Phototherapy
25–48‡	≥12 (170)	≥15 (260)	≥20 (340)	≥25 (430)
49–72	≥15 (260)	≥18 (310)	≥25 (430)	≥30 (510)
>72	≥17 (290)	≥20 (340)	≥25 (430)	≥30 (510)

° Phototherapy at these total serum bilirubin (TSB) levels is a clinical option, meaning that the intervention is available and may be used on the basis of individual clinical judgment.

† Intensive phototherapy should produce a decline of TSB of 1 to 2 mg/dL within 4 to 6 hours, and the TSB level should continue to decline and remain below the threshold level for exchange transfusion. If this does not occur, phototherapy has failed. Intensive phototherapy includes the use of more than one bank of lamps containing "special blue" bulbs, maximizing the surface area illuminated by using a phototherapy blanket or other means, and providing phototherapy on a continuous, noninterrupted schedule.

‡ Term infants who are clinically jaundiced at ≤24 hours old are not considered healthy and require further evaluation.

Used with permission of the American Academy of Pediatrics: Practice parameter: Management of hyperbilirubinemia in the healthy term newborn. Pediatrics 94:560, 1994.

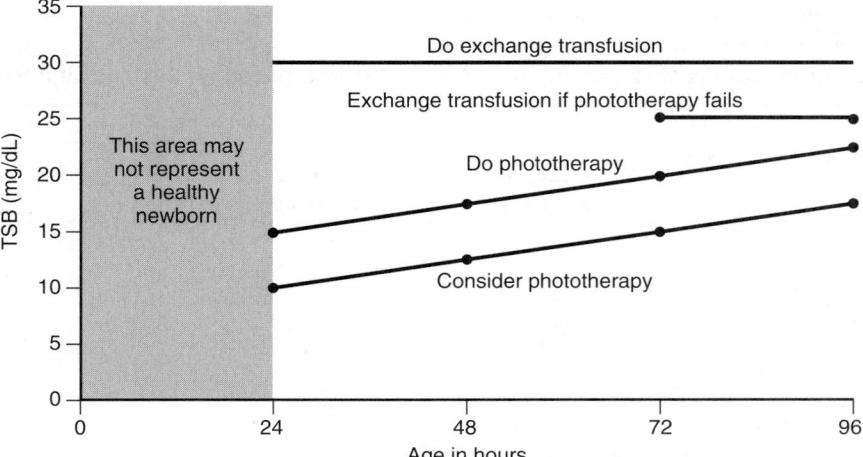

FIGURE 87–1. Guidelines for treatment and intervention of hyperbilirubinemia in the healthy term newborn. (From Gartner LM: Neonatal jaundice. Pediatr Rev 15(11):429, 1994. Reproduced by Permission of *Pediatrics in Review*, Copyright 1994.)

ualized laboratory tests or "batching" them in a "hyperbilirubinemia workup." For example, once a total bilirubin level is obtained and is seen to be elevated, some clinicians obtain a direct Coombs test and blood group type and await the results before proceeding to further tests. Others, to minimize patient inconvenience and to gather more complete information initially, study hemoglobin, reticulocyte count, blood group, direct Coombs test, and blood cell count and differential and inspect a blood film all at once. Consideration of practical and economic issues plays a role in such decisions, and practice variations are expected.

The controversies remaining in the AAP recommendations center on two areas. First, the guidelines are said to apply to infants without signs of illness or apparent hemolytic disease. The bilirubin levels cited by the committee's policy for initiating phototherapy are high enough that increased bilirubin production could well be a contributing cause and it becomes the responsibility of the physician to determine whether such a contributing cause is likely. Assuming the absence of hemolysis when there is a negative Coombs test does not suffice, because this test identifies isoimmunization primarily. Obtaining a direct estimate of bilirubin production, by measuring the carboxyhemoglobin level or the end-tidal carbon monoxide in breath, may be the only reliable way to exclude hemolysis (see Chapter 81). Although the feasibility of these techniques has been demonstrated, they have not been available to most physicians until recently.

The second area of controversy involves the levels of bilirubin cited for initiating phototherapy or considering exchange transfusion. Some experts think that the AAP recommendations are overly simplistic because they do not consider the duration of moderate to severe hyperbilirubinemia and because they belittle the risk of hyperbilirubinemia when the total serum bilirubin level ranges from 25 to 30 mg/dL (425–510 μM/L), especially without knowing the albumin-binding capacity or its affinity for bilirubin.

MANAGEMENT OF THE PRETERM INFANT

The increased intensity and duration of hyperbilirubinemia in the preterm infant as well as the assumed immaturity of the blood–brain barrier lead to concern about greater risks of bilirubin encephalopathy in this patient population. Is the "healthy" preterm infant at greater risk of bilirubin encephalopathy at serum bilirubin concentrations less than 20 mg/dL (340 μM/L)? Or is the premature infant at greater risk because of the greater frequency with which such patients suffer from pathologic conditions such as sepsis, acidosis, hypoxia, shock, and intracranial hemorrhage? Many clinicians use gestational age, birth weight, and health status adjustments to determine the need for phototherapy and exchange transfusion, although controlled trials supporting these policies have not been carried out. The guidelines in Table 87–4 suggest one approach to the implementation of exchange transfusion in premature babies.

Because neurotoxicity has been related to the serum total bilirubin level, this measure has traditionally been the parameter most often used in assessing the severity of hyperbilirubinemia and in decisions regarding management. During the years in which practice guidelines suggested instituting phototherapy to keep the total bilirubin level less than 20 mg/dL (340 μM/L) in term infants, severe bilirubin encephalopathy rarely occurred. In infants weighing less than 1500 g, efforts were usually made to keep total serum bilirubin concentration less than 12 mg/dL (200 μM/L) and less than 14 mg/dL (240 μM/L) in infants weighing 1500 to 2500 g, with similar good results. There is concern, however, that more subtle neurodevelopmental abnormalities may occur at these levels and that prolonged elevations at lower levels may also be damaging, suggesting that the current guidelines for premature or low-birth-weight babies may still not be adequate to eliminate risk.

OTHER FACTORS TO CONSIDER

Other chapters in this book have discussed in detail bilirubin metabolism, stressing the importance of excess bilirubin production (rather than simply hemolysis) as a risk factor for encephalopathy. Excess bilirubin production includes hemolysis resulting from isoimmune reactions, hemolysis from other causes (e.g., G6PD deficiency, erythrocyte membrane disorders), and nonhemolytic processes

TABLE 87–4

Guideline for the Management of Hyperbilirubinemia Based on Gestational Age and Relative Health of the Newborn

| | Total Serum Bilirubin Level mg/dL (μmol/L) | | | |
| | Healthy | | Sick | |
	Phototherapy	Exchange Transfusion	Phototherapy	Exchange Transfusion
Premature				
<1000 g	5–7	Variable	4–6	Variable
1001–1500 g	7–10	Variable	6–8	Variable
1501–2000 g	10–12	Variable	8–10	Variable
2001–2500 g	12–15	Variable	10–12	Variable
Term				
>2500 g	15–18	20–25	12–15	18–20

From Halamek LP, Stevenson DK: Neonatal jaundice. *In* Fanaroff AA, Martin RJ (Eds): Neonatal-Perinatal Medicine. Diseases of the Fetus and Infant, 6th ed. St. Louis, Mosby-Year Book, 1997, p 1371.

leading to excess bilirubin production. A Coombs test is not sufficient to identify all causes of excess bilirubin production and is not a good measure of the degree or intensity of hemolysis.

Research continues to identify parameters that can guide clinicians toward more appropriate intervention than the measures traditionally used. In addition to the factors listed in Table 87–1, the total serum bilirubin concentration has been the critical parameter in developing management guidelines. Other measures are listed in Table 87–5, and some of these hold promise for becoming useful tools in the decision-making process. However, they have not yet been included in standard practice parameters (see Table 87–2).

FREE PLASMA BILIRUBIN

Free plasma bilirubin is the fraction of bilirubin not bound to albumin. This has been considered the critical portion of unconjugated bilirubin because of its ability to cross the blood–brain barrier easily. Although there is a constant dynamic state between bound and unbound bilirubin at the albumin-binding sites, free bilirubin levels are known to increase when plasma albumin levels are diminished or when bilirubin is displaced from the albumin by drugs and chemicals that competitively attach to the albumin-binding

TABLE 87–5

Potential Criteria for Treatment of Neonatal Jaundice

Total serum bilirubin concentration
Unconjugated serum bilirubin concentration
Free plasma bilirubin (not bound to albumin)
Reserve albumin binding capacity
Bilirubin production rates
   Serum carboxyhemoglobin
   End-tidal respiratory carbon monoxide
Neurophysiologic criteria
Visual evoked potentials
Somatosensory potentials
Auditory evoked potentials

sites (see Table 81–1). Encephalopathy is virtually nonexistent if the unbound bilirubin levels are maintained less than 0.8 μg/dL in infants weighing less than 1500 g and less than 0.1 μg/dL in infants weighing 1500 to 2500 g (Bratlid, 1995; Nakamura et al, 1992). Studies using auditory brain stem auditory evoked responses have demonstrated significantly more abnormalities in newborns with unbound bilirubin concentrations equal to or greater than 1.0 μg/dL, suggesting that measuring unbound bilirubin concentrations may be helpful for evaluating bilirubin effects and may predict the risk of bilirubin encephalopathy in full term newborns with hyperbilirubinemia. Until recently, there has been no simple accurate method of determining free bilirubin levels when they are in such low concentrations, but using a commercially available device, unbound bilirubin concentrations have been measured at the bedside by the peroxidase method in academic settings (Nakamura et al, 1992).

RESERVE ALBUMIN-BINDING CAPACITY

Some authors have suggested the use of the reserve albumin-binding capacity to determine how much of a range of safety is available before albumin-binding sites become saturated. The conceptual basis for this proposal is the knowledge that unbound bilirubin accumulates in the brain only after the albumin-binding sites have been saturated, and the theory that the oversaturation by bilirubin allows unbound bilirubin to gain access to the brain. However, the dynamic process involved in attachment of bilirubin to albumin suggests that this parameter might be an unreliable measure of the amount of unbound bilirubin. Even when the binding sites are not fully occupied with bilirubin, there is some unbound bilirubin that can diffuse across the blood–brain barrier. Using the availability of binding sites as a proxy for unbound bilirubin levels could therefore be unreliable, underestimating risks of neurotoxicity. Among the tests currently suggested for estimating albumin-binding capacity are bilirubin titration tests, dye binding tests, and selective binding of tracer ligands. Some of these tests are semiquantitive and most are impractical in the neonatal clinical setting (Bratlid, 1995).

BILIRUBIN PRODUCTION RATES

Because of the inadequacies and ambiguities of the aforementioned parameters suggested for assessing neurotoxic risk of hyperbilirubinemia, some neonatologists postulate that measuring bilirubin production rates may be the best index of potential bilirubin encephalopathy. Unconjugated bilirubin production has traditionally been estimated from the rate of increase in serum total bilirubin concentration during the first 24 to 48 hours after birth. However, the rate of increase in serum bilirubin does not reflect only bilirubin production but also distribution and elimination.

Degradation of heme results in the production of one molecule of carbon monoxide (CO) with each molecule of biliverdin produced. The biliverdin is then reduced to bilirubin. The CO diffuses out of cells and binds to hemoglobin in circulating erythrocytes. It can be measured as carboxyhemoglobin in the blood. The carboxyhemoglobin dissociates in the lungs, releasing measurable CO to the exhaled breath.

Techniques have recently been developed that result in clinically useful measurements of exhaled carbon monoxide or percutaneous measurement of carboxyhemoglobin. These measures correlate well with bilirubin production rates. Monitoring bilirubin production rates as well as total serum bilirubin concentration has been suggested as a guide to initiation of treatment and management for severe neonatal jaundice. Continuous monitoring of these parameters would be ideal, especially in situations of rapid increase in bilirubin concentration, and instruments capable of such measures are becoming available for clinical application using portable electrochemical sensors (Stevenson et al, 1994; Vreman et al, 1994).

MODES OF INTERVENTION TO REDUCE SERUM BILIRUBIN CONCENTRATION

Once the clinician has determined that a neonate's serum bilirubin concentration is elevated enough to present a risk of encephalopathy or is increasing in a way that predicts significant risk, intervention to reduce the bilirubin concentration becomes imperative. Therapeutic intervention decisions must be tempered by clinical judgment based on the history, course, and physical findings. The current accepted modes of intervention and others that are still in various stages of investigation are listed in Table 87–6.

Hydration

There is no evidence that excess fluid administration affects the serum bilirubin concentration. Some infants, especially

---

TABLE 87–6

Treatment Modalities

Hydration
Phototherapy
Exchange transfusion
Drugs to increase conjugation
Inhibiting reabsorption (binding in the gut)
Inhibiting bilirubin production

---

those being breast-fed, may be mildly dehydrated and may need supplemental fluid intake to correct their dehydration. However, the idea that the baby's serum can be diluted to reduce the total bilirubin level is not supported by studies. Reduction in serum bilirubin concentration, which appears to be a response to rehydration, especially with increased oral nutrition, may be related to the correction of dehydration, to more effective intestinal motility (with the increased oral intake leading to elimination of conjugated bilirubin via stool), or to enhanced removal of photoproducts in both urine and stool. Because milk-based formula is less likely to enhance reabsorption of bilirubin by the enterohepatic circulation, it is often recommended for use for oral correction of mild dehydration in hyperbilirubinemic children.

Phototherapy

Since Cremer and associates (1958) first proposed the use of phototherapy as a treatment for hyperbilirubinemia, much has been learned about the mechanism of action and techniques of administering this mode of therapy. Phototherapy has become the most common treatment used for neonatal hyperbilirubinemia (Costarino et al, 1985). Still, there is no standardized method for delivering phototherapy. The phototherapy units vary widely, the types of lamps used differ, the amount of skin exposed to phototherapy often depends on other clinical issues, and the intensity of the light varies according to the lamp power and the distance from the skin. Usually the dose of phototherapy is based on what is convenient to administer, rather than what is most effective.

The efficacy of phototherapy is influenced by the following factors: (1) the spectrum of light delivered, the blue-green region of the visible spectrum being the most effective, (2) the energy output or irradiance of the phototherapy light, measured in $\mu W/cm^2/nm$, and (3) the surface area of the infant exposed to phototherapy (Landry et al, 1985).

The amount of light to which a baby is exposed during phototherapy is minute compared with exposure later in life, even during the 1st year of life. With the light sources currently used, it is impossible to overdose the patient with phototherapy. Conventional phototherapy involves exposing a maximal area of skin to an irradiance of 7 to 10 $\mu W/cm^2/nm$ (Garg et al, 1995).

High-intensity phototherapy involves increasing the irradiance to more than 25 $\mu W/cm^2/nm$ and was first described in 1977 (Tan, 1977). The rationale for high-intensity phototherapy is the demonstration of a dose–response relationship to bilirubin degradation until a saturation dose is reached at about 40 $\mu W/cm^2/nm$ of appropriate light. The use of high-intensity phototherapy has been advocated by investigators who have documented more effective reduction of total bilirubin levels with no long-term complications.

Commonly used phototherapy units contain a number of daylight, cool white, or "special blue" fluorescent tubes. Others use tungsten-halogen lamps. These lamps may be part of a radiant warming device, included as a bank of lights shining on the baby, or included in fiberoptic vests or blankets, which are used to increase the surface area exposed or to aid in continuing phototherapy while a baby is held or fed. Special blue fluorescent tubes make the baby appear blue, occasionally causing discomfort to nursery personnel.

Recommendations to optimize phototherapy include using the most effective spectrum, using the maximum irradiance available, and exposing as much skin as possible to the therapy. Intermittent skin exposure using one continuous light source and rotating the baby to expose different areas of the skin has not been shown to improve the effect of phototherapy. There is no convincing rationale for using intermittent phototherapy, but interrupting phototherapy for feeding or brief parental visits may be tolerated in less severely affected infants. Therefore, the systems that provide a fiberoptic light source in the mattress under the baby and standard lighting above have been recommended. The administration of high-intensity phototherapy using a transparent waterbed has been shown to be significantly more effective at reducing bilirubin than conventional phototherapy (Garg et al, 1995).

Despite its apparent safety and enthusiastic application, the photochemical reactions responsible for the decline in serum bilirubin levels are incompletely understood. Bilirubin is known to undergo photodegradation in vivo and in vitro, resulting in photoproducts that are more polarized and therefore more water soluble and potentially excretable than native bilirubin. The initial and most rapid reactions occurring as a result of phototherapy produce configurational isomers that change the shape of the molecule without changing the structure. These isomers are the most abundant serum photoisomers and may account for up to 20% of total serum bilirubin in babies undergoing phototherapy. The most prominent of these configurational isomers is called 4z,15e bilirubin (native bilirubin being 4z,15z bilirubin). The second most rapid photochemical reaction leads to the formation of structural isomers, the most prominent known as lumirubin. Formation of this compound appears to be irreversible. Although certain phototherapy reactions reach their peak at relatively low levels of irradiance (6–9 μW/cm^2/nm), the production of lumirubin is directly proportional to the energy output on the skin (Garg et al, 1995). High-intensity phototherapy results in greater amounts of lumirubin among the photosomers.

In summary, it appears that the decrease in serum bilirubin resulting from phototherapy is mainly a result of excretion of photoproducts in the bile and subsequent removal in stool. Configurational isomers are maximally produced at conventional levels of irradiance, but structural isomers are more efficiently produced by high-intensity phototherapy and may account for the increased efficacy of high-intensity phototherapy.

Because these photoproducts are not conjugated for excretion but merely rendered more polar, their reabsorption by way of the enterohepatic circulation can diminish the effectiveness of phototherapy.

Rebounding Bilirubin Levels

In the absence of hemolytic disease in healthy term infants, the cessation of phototherapy results in a mild rebound in the level of serum bilirubin concentration. In one small study involving term and preterm infants, the average re-

bound after cessation of phototherapy was less than 1 mg/dL (17 μM/L) (Lazar et al, 1993).

Hospital discharge does not need to be delayed for observation for rebound in such cases. However, in the presence of hemolytic disease or in sick or low-birth-weight babies, such reassurance may not be warranted. Because hemolysis or other processes responsible for increased bilirubin production may continue, the rebound in these cases depends not only on the effectiveness of phototherapy but also on the severity of the bilirubin production.

Exchange Transfusion

With the initiation of exchange transfusion as an intervention for the hyperbilirubinemia of erythroblastosis fetalis, the history of kernicterus in newborns was forever changed. Despite many advances in the understanding of hemolytic and neonatal physiology, exchange transfusion remains the ultimate treatment to prevent neurotoxic damage from hyperbilirubinemia. As discussed previously, the controversies regarding management of hyperbilirubinemia swirl around questions about when to institute certain management techniques, not about the techniques themselves.

Exchange transfusion removes much of the circulating bilirubin and "sensitized" red cells (erythrocytes with maternal antibodies attached), replacing them with red cells compatible with the mother's antibody-rich serum and providing fresh albumin with binding sites for bilirubin. The process is tedious, in that 5 to 10 mL aliquots are removed and replaced sequentially until about twice the volume of the neonate's circulating blood volume has been exchanged. The anticoagulant of choice in the blood being infused is citrate-phosphate-dextrose. Because the citrate chelates calcium ions, there may be a need for calcium gluconate infusion during the course of the exchange. High concentration of glucose in the infusate may stimulate insulin production and increase the risk of severe hypoglycemia (Rubaltelli and Griffith, 1992).

Blood stored for more than 4 days has excessive potassium levels, and such blood requires erythrocyte washing and resuspension in compatible plasma. All these issues, as well as the temperature of the infusate and the environment, lead to possible stress and instability in the infant, especially in one who is ill and of low birth weight. The amount of bilirubin removed by each transfusion is a function of the initial serum bilirubin and the amount of blood exchanged. After an exchange transfusion, low levels of serum bilirubin concentration may increase rapidly for several hours as bilirubin in tissues "migrates" back into the circulation.

Exchange transfusions are not free of risk. Some reports estimate a risk of morbidity resulting from the procedure at 5% with apnea, bradycardia, cyanosis, vasospasm, and hypothermia being the most common problems. Mortality rate estimates run as high as 0.5%.

Inducing Enzymes to Increase Conjugation

Increasing the ability of the body to excrete bilirubin by stimulating the ability of the liver to conjugate it has been attempted since Trolle (1961) observed less hyperbilirubinemia in babies of mothers receiving phenobarbital as anticonvulsant therapy.

Several pharmacologic agents have been identified as liver enzyme inducers, and those inducing uridine diphosphate (UDP)-glucuronosyl transferase have been shown to increase the conjugation and excretion of bilirubin.

Phenobarbital and nicotinamide were the first agents used for prevention and treatment of hyperbilirubinemia in newborns, and phenobarbital continues to be used in Gilbert disease and Crigler-Najjar syndrome Type II (Arias disease). Type I disease does not respond well to this therapy (Rubaltelli and Griffith, 1992).

The effect of phenobarbital (at a dosage of 2.5 mg/kg per day) on serum bilirubin levels begins within a few days of its administration. This characteristic has made it less than optimal in the usual neonatal hyperbilirubinemia, because the serum bilirubin is already high or rapidly increasing in the first few days. Phototherapy has been shown to be more effective in this situation, and adding phenobarbital to phototherapy has not been shown to have any advantage. However, postnatal phenobarbital administration may provide a useful approach to later elevation of bilirubin levels, like that seen in the hyperbilirubinemia in Asians, Native Americans, and other ethnic and genetic subgroups. It has been used with some success in congenital disorders of bilirubin metabolism in which it lowers bilirubin levels for 15 to 20 days after which a new steady state is reached, which is lower than pretreatment levels.

Prenatal administration of phenobarbital in anticipation of hyperbilirubinemia has been suggested in an effort to "prime the pump" of the conjugation process. One untoward side effect of this approach, however, is a decrease in prothrombin levels in the newborn, but this effect can be remedied by vitamin K administration.

Several chemicals used in traditional Chinese medicine have an enzyme-inducing effect similar to that of phenobarbital (Yin et al, 1991). In studies involving rats and rabbits, yin zhi huang at 30 to 60 mg/kg per day has been shown to accelerate the plasma clearance and conjugation of bilirubin even to a greater degree than phenobarbital at 60 mg/kg per day. Both drugs increase glucuronyl transferase activity, but because they have dissimilar effects on other liver enzymes, it appears that their mechanism of action may be different. Yin zhi huang, which is widely used in Asia to treat neonatal hyperbilirubinemia, is a decoction of four plants, *Artemisia, Gardenia, Rheum,* and *Scutellaria baicalensis.* The gardenia portion and phenobarbital have similar inducing effects also on glutathione-s-transferase, an enzyme involved in intracellular bilirubin transport in the liver (Yin et al, 1991b).

Blocking Bilirubin Reabsorption

Neonatal hyperbilirubinemia is exacerbated by, if not caused by, enhanced reabsorption in the enterohepatic circulation. The absence of intestinal flora in neonates prevents the degradation of bilirubin in meconium and stool to products like urobilinogen, which could be excreted. Bilirubin glucuronide arriving in the intestines is readily deconjugated to bilirubin and reabsorbed. Some of the products of phototherapy, especially the configurational isomers of bilirubin, also return to the native bilirubin form

and may be reabsorbed. To counteract this process, various strategies have been used to bind the bilirubin in the intestinal lumen to substances that resist absorption. Seen as an effective low-risk, low-cost therapy, products such as activated charcoal and dried agar (an extract of seaweed) have been used with inconsistent results. A review of the early studies involving agar identified methodologic problems, allowing neither recommendation nor rejection of this approach (Kemper et al, 1988).

More recent studies (Caglayan et al, 1993) using doses of 500 mg/kg of agar every 6 hours suggest that agar therapy can be used to augment the efficacy of phototherapy and perhaps it could be used as therapy by itself (Caglayan et al, 1993). Besides resulting in a more rapid decline in serum bilirubin levels, the use of agar increased stool frequency, suggesting enhanced clearance of intraluminal bilirubin regardless of binding. Cholestyramine was similarly considered but was found to cause hyperchloremic acidosis (Nicolopoulos et al, 1978).

Bilirubin oxidase derived from the fungus *Myrothecium verrucarea* has been suggested as another oral agent, but its effectiveness at interrupting reabsorption is based on its ability to degrade bilirubin to biliverdin and other nontoxic substances enzymatically rather than by binding the pigment in the lumen (Murao and Tanaka, 1981). Studies involving the Gunn rat support this approach, but adequate data in humans are not yet available (Johnson et al, 1988).

Inhibiting Bilirubin Production

Whereas other modes of intervention are directed at disposing of excess bilirubin already produced, attempts to decrease the production of bilirubin have met with moderate success. Studies in vitro and in both animals and humans have shown that certain metalloporphyrins can reduce the production of bilirubin, substantially reducing serum levels. These studies suggest that, in cases of hyperbilirubinemia caused by excess bilirubin production (i.e., catabolism of heme), these metalloporphyrins could be used to prevent the accumulation of dangerous levels of serum bilirubin, thus obviating more expensive, time-consuming, or hazardous interventions such as phototherapy and exchange transfusion. The mechanism of action of these compounds is competitive inhibition of the activity of heme oxygenase, the rate-limiting enzyme in heme catabolism. Tin or zinc protoporphyrin, tin or zinc mesoporphyrin, and other synthetic analogues of the natural metalloporphyrin (ferroporphyrin-heme) are potent competitors of heme oxygenase, the critical enzyme in the catabolism of heme. Their action is based on the fact that the catalytic site of heme oxygenase recognizes metalloporphyrins with central metal ions other than iron (Fig. 87–2). Heme oxygenase actually favors some of these metalloporphyrins over heme as a substrate, sometimes by a large factor (Cornelius and Rodgers, 1984; Valaes et al, 1994; Vreman et al, 1990, 1991).

The potency of metalloporphyrins and their side effects are influenced by the central metal cation and the nature of the side chains. Tin porphyrins are more potent than zinc or cobalt porphyrins. With side chains comprised of ethyl groups, mesoporphyrins are far more potent and stable than the other forms. Currently, tin mesoporphyrin

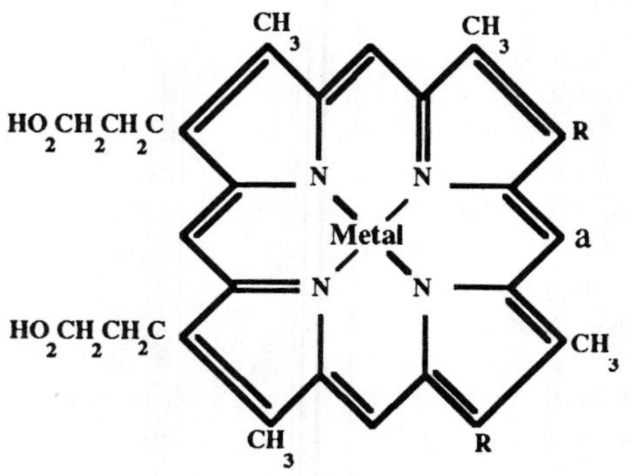

FIGURE 87–2. Metalloporphyrin complexes and their chemical structures. Substrates and inhibitors of heme oxygenase belong to a large family of metalloporphyrins with varying metal moieties and porphyrin ring substituents. (From Rodgers PA, Stevenson DK: Developmental biology of heme oxygenase. *In* Maisels MJ (Ed): Clinics in Perinatology. Neonatal Jaundice. Philadelphia, WB Saunders, 1990, p 278.)

Metals:

1. Fe - Heme
2. Sn - Tin Metalloporphyrin
3. Zn - Zinc Metalloporphyrin
4. Cr - Chromium Metalloporphyrin
5. Mn - Manganese Metalloporphyrin

R-Chemical Group:

1. R=Vinyl (CH_2=CH-) - Protoporphyrin
2. R=Ethyl (CH_3-CH_2-) - Mesoporphyrin
3. R=Deutero (H-) - Deuteroporphyrin
4. R=2,4 Bis Glycol (CH_2OH-CHOH-) - Deuteroporphyrin 2,4 Bis Glycol

is approved for chemical use in the United States. Administered intramuscularly in doses from 1 μmol to 6 μmol/kg, a dose-related moderation in the development of hyperbilirubinemia has been observed with minimal side effects (Valaes et al, 1994).

Because these synthetic metalloporphyrins do not bind molecular oxygen, they are not metabolically degraded by ring rupture and do not add to the body pool of bilirubin. The metalloporphyrins also do not affect the metabolic disposition of preformed bilirubin, but they may have some inhibitory effect on the biliary excretion of bilirubin (Beri and Chandra, 1993).

The potential benefits of this chemopreventive approach to the management of hyperbilirubinemia could be substantial, especially in premature babies in whom threshold levels for the manifestation of bilirubin toxicity are controversial and uncertain. Proponents of metalloporphyrins have demonstrated the effectiveness and apparent innocuousness of these compounds, but research continues in identifying which of the compounds is most effective at reducing bilirubin production without toxic side effects. For example, if phototherapy is to be used in conjunction with metallophorphyrin therapy, the effect of photodegradation on the metalloporphyrin and any ensuing risks would become substantial issues. For example, adults and children with cholestasis have high levels of copper porphyrins that are vulnerable to photo-induced chemical alterations resulting in the formation of brown pigments, made famous by the term the *bronze baby syndrome* (Rubaltelli et al, 1983).

Each metalloporphyrin currently being evaluated has its own characteristics related to efficacy and side effects. These compounds are administered intramuscularly in a dose based on body weight, and their effectiveness appears to be dose related (and compound specific) in all gestational age groups tested. Administration of these compounds also produces a dose-dependent decrease in the proportion of newborns requiring phototherapy. When phototherapy is used as an adjunct to metalloporphyrin administration, a decrease in the duration of phototherapy is seen, especially on days 3 to 7 of life, which is related to metalloporphyrin dose. It is not clear which of these

metalloporphyrins will eventually prove to be most efficacious and safe, and research in their use continues.

INTERRUPTION OF BREAST-FEEDING

Breast-fed babies generally have serum bilirubin concentrations slightly above that of formula-fed babies. Some babies may experience prolonged jaundice, termed *breast-milk jaundice* (see Chapter 82). Interrupting or continuing breast-feeding is a management decision that clinician and mother must decide upon together. Options include continuing breast-feeding with optimal support, supplementing breast-feeding with bottle feeding to guarantee optimal hydration, or discontinuing breast-feeding and relying on formula or parenteral feeding. The choice among these options may depend on the strength and condition of the infant, the availability of the parents, the infant's environment, and the intensity of the treatments prescribed. There is no one certain way, but every attempt to accommodate long-term breast-feeding should be encouraged. The 1994 AAP practice parameter "Managing Hyperbilirubinemia in the Healthy Term Newborn" included a statement discouraging the interruption of breast-feeding in healthy term newborns and encouraging continued and frequent breast-feeding (at least 8–10 times every 24 hours).

CONCLUSION

The management of hyperbilirubinemia presents a complicated scenario to the clinician. The purpose of treatment is to prevent neurotoxic effects of bilirubin and to identify and treat illnesses that can be associated with excess bilirubin production, impaired conjugation, or inadequate elimination of the pigment. Modes of treatment include interfering with bilirubin production; enhancing the transport, binding, or conjugation of bilirubin; or removing bilirubin in urine, feces, and blood. Controversies remain regarding which treatment or combination of therapies is safest and most effective and which criteria should serve as indicators for instituting therapy.

REFERENCES

American Academy of Pediatrics: Practice parameter: Management of hyperbiliburubinemia in the healthy term newborn. Pediatrics 94:558–565, 1994.

Aono S, Yamada Y, Keino H, et al: A new type of defect in the gene for bilirubin uridine 5'-diphosphate-glucuronosyltransferase in a patient with Crigler-Najjar syndrome Type I. Pediatr Res 35(6):629–632, 1994.

Beri R, Chandra R: Chemistry and biology of heme. Effect of metal salts, organometals, and metalloporphyrins on heme synthesis and catabolism, with special reference to clinical implications and interactions with cytochrome P-450. Drug Metab Rev 25(1–2):49–152, 1993.

Bratlid D: How bilirubin gets into the brain. Clin Perinatol 17:449–465, 1990.

Bratlid D: Bilirubin toxicity: Pathophysiology and assessment of risk factors. N Y State J Med 91(11):489–492, 1991.

Bratlid D: Neonatal and congenital hyperbilirubinemias: Evaluation of neonatal jaundice. Presentation at the International Bilirubin Workshop, Trieste, Italy, April 6–8, 1995.

Brodersen R: Prevention of kernicterus, based on recent progress in bilirubin chemistry. Acta Paediatr Scand 66:625–634, 1977.

Caglayan S, Candemir H, Aksit S, et al: Superiority of oral agar and phototherapy combination in the treatment of neonatal hyperbilirubinemia. Pediatrics 92(1):86–89, 1993.

Cashore WJ: Bilirubin binding tests. In Levine RL, Maisels MJ (Eds): Hyperbilirubinemia in the Newborn. Report of the 85th Ross Conference on Pediatric Research. Columbus, OH, 1983, pp 101–110.

Cornelius CE, Rodgers PA: Prevention of neonatal hyperbilirubinemia in rhesus monkeys by tin protoporphyrin. Pediatr Res 18:728–730, 1984.

Costarino AT, Ennever JF, Baumgart S, et al: Bilirubin photoisomerization in premature neonates under low- and high-dose phototherapy. Pediatrics 75(3):519–522, 1985.

Cremer RJ, Perryman PW, Richards DH: Influence of light on the hyperbilirubinaemia of infants. Lancet 1:1094–1097, 1958.

Dobbs RH, Cremer RJ: Phototherapy (looking back). Arch Dis Child 50:833–836, 1975.

Drummond GS, Kappas A: Prevention of neonatal hyperbilirubinemia by tin protoporphyrin IX, a potent competitive inhibitor of heme oxidation. Proc Natl Acad Sci U S A 78:6466–6470, 1981.

Ennever JF: Blue light, green light, white light, more light: Treatment of neonatal jaundice. Clin Perinatol 17(2):467–481, 1990.

Ennever JF, Costarino AT, Polin RA, et al: Rapid clearance of a structural isomer of bilirubin during phototherapy. J Clin Invest 79:1674–1678, 1987.

Ennever JF, McDonagh AF, Speck WT: Phototherapy for neonatal jaundice: Optimal wavelengths of light. J Pediatr 103:295–299, 1983.

Funato M, Tamai H, Shimada S, Nakamura H: Vigintiphobia, unbound bilirubin, and brainstem responses. Pediatrics 93:50–53, 1994.

Garg AK, Prasad RS, AlHifzi I: A controlled trial of high-intensity double-surface phototherapy on a fluid bed versus conventional phototherapy in neonatal jaundice. Pediatrics 95(6):914–916, 1995.

Gartner LM: Neonatal jaundice. Pediatr Rev 15:(11):422–431, 1994.

Johnson L, Dworanczyk R, Abbasi M, Dalin C: Bilirubin oxidase (BOX) feedings significantly decrease serum bilirubin (B) levels in jaundiced infant Gunn rats (abstr). Pediatr Res 22:412A, 1988.

Kappas A, Drummond GS, Henschke C, Valaes T: Direct comparison of sn-mesoporphyrin, an inhibitor of bilirubin production, and phototherapy in controlling hyperbilirubinemia in term and near-term newborns. Pediatrics 95:168–174, 1995.

Kemper K, Horwitz RI, McCarthy P: Decreased neonatal serum bilirubin with plain agar: A meta-analysis. Pediatrics 82(4):631–638, 1988.

Kimura A, Ushijima K, Kage M, et al: Neonatal Dubin-Johnson syndrome with severe cholestasis: Effective phenobarbital therapy. Acta Paediatr Scand 80:381–385, 1991.

Landry RJ, Scheidt PC, Hammond RW: Ambient light and phototherapy conditions of eight neonatal care units: A summary report. Pediatrics 75(Suppl):434–436, 1985.

Lazar L, Litwin A, Nerlob P: Phototherapy for neonatal nonhemolytic hyperbilirubinemia. Analysis of rebound and indications for discontinuing phototherapy. Clin Pediatr 32:264–267, 1993.

Linn S, Shoenbaum SC, Monson RR, et al: Epidemiology of neonatal hyperbilirubinemia. Pediatrics 75:770–774, 1985.

Maisels MJ, Newman TB: Kernicterus occurs in full term, healthy newborns without apparent hemolysis. Pediatr Res 3:239A, 1994.

Mores A, Fargasova I, Minarikova E: The relation of hyperbilirubinemia in newborns without isoimmunization to kernicterus. Acta Pediatr Scand 48:590, 1959.

Murao S, Tanaka N: A new enzyme 'bilirubin oxidase' produced by Myrothecium verrucarea MT-1. Agricult Biolog Chem 45:2383–2385, 1981.

Nakamura H, Yonetani M, Uetani Y, et al: Determination of unbound bilirubin for prediction of kernicterus in low birthweight infants. Acta Paediatr Jpn 34:642–647, 1992.

Newman TB, Maisels MJ: Evaluation and treatment of jaundice in the term newborn: A kinder, gentler approach. Pediatrics 89:809–818, 1992.

Nicolopoulos D, Hadjigeorgiou E, Malamitsi A, et al: Combined treatment of neonatal jaundice with cholestyramine and phototherapy. J Pediatr 93:684–688, 1978.

Penn AA, Enzmann DR, Hahn JS, Stevenson DK: Kernicterus in a full term infant. Pediatrics 93:1003–1006, 1994.

Rhine WD, Benitz WE, Dennery PA, et al: Bilirubin measurements and long term outcome. Pediatrics 94:246, 1994.

Robertson A, Brodersen R: Effect of drug combinations on bilirubin-albumin binding. Dev Pharmacol Ther 17(1–2):95–99, 1991.

Rubaltelli F, Camurri S, Sala M: Treatment of neonatal hyperbilirubinemia. Pediatr Med Chir 12(1):17–23, 1990.

Rubaltelli FF, Griffith PF: Management of neonatal hyperbilirubinaemia and prevention of kernicterus. Drugs 43(6):864–872, 1992.

Rubaltelli FF, Jori G, Reddi E: Bronze baby syndrome: A new porphyrin-related disorder. Pediatr Res 17:327–330, 1983.

Slusher TM, Vreman HJ, McLaren DW, Stevenson DK: Carboxyhemoglobin predicts bilirubin-related morbidity and mortality in infants. Pediatr Res 33:237A, 1993.

Stevenson DK, Vreman HJ, Oh W, et al: Bilirubin production in well term infants with and without hemolysis. Pediatr Res 33:238A, 1993.

Stevenson DK, Vreman HJ, Oh W, et al: Bilirubin production in health term infants as measured by carbon monoxide in breath. Clin Chem 40:1934–1939, 1994.

Tan KL: The nature of the dose-response relationship of phototherapy for neonatal hyperbilirubinemia. J Pediatr 90:448–452, 1977.

Tan KL: Efficacy of fluorescent daylight, blue, and green lamps in the management of nonhemolytic hyperbilirubinemia. J Pediatr 114:132–137, 1989.

Trolle D: Discussion on the advisability of performing exchange transfusion in neonatal jaundice of unknown aetiology. Acta Paediatr Scand 50:392, 1961.

Valaes T, Harvey-Wilkes K: Pharmacologic approaches to the prevention and treatment of neonatal hyperbilirubinemia. Clin Perinatol 17:245–273, 1990.

Valaes T, Petmezaki S, Henschke C, et al: Control of jaundice in preterm newborns by an inhibitor of bilirubin production: Studies with tin-mesoporphyrin. Pediatrics 93(1):1–11, 1994.

Vohr BR: New approaches to assessing the risks of hyperbilirubinemia. Clin Perinatol 17:293–306, 1990.

Vreman HJ, Baxter LM, Stone RR, Stevenson DK: Evaluation of an automated end-tidal carbon monoxide instrument for infant breath analysis. J Clin Invest 43:174A, 1995.

Vreman HJ, Ekstrand BC, Stevenson DK: Selection of metalloporphyrin heme oxygenase inhibitors based on potency and photoreactivity. Pediatr Res 33:195–200, 1993.

Vreman HJ, Oh W, Stevenson DKS: In vitro and in vivo characteristics of a heme oxygenase inhibitor: ZnBG. Am J Med Sci 302:335–341, 1991.

Vreman HJ, Rodgers PA, Stevenson DKS: Zinc protoporphyrin administration for suppression of increased bilirubin production by iatrogenic hemolyses in rhesus neonates. J Pediatr 117:292–297, 1990.

Vreman HJ, Stevenson DK, Oh W, et al: Semiportable electrochemical instrument for determining carbon monoxide in breath. Clin Chem 40:1927–1933, 1994.

Vreman HJ, Stevenson DK, Oh W, et al: Variability of interlaboratory bilirubin measurements. Pediatr Res 37:243A, 1995.

Yamauchi Y, Kasa N, Yamanouchi I: Is it necessary to change babies' position during phototherapy? Early Hum Dev 20:221–227, 1989.

Yeung CY, Lee FT, Wong HN: Effect of a popular Chinese herb on neonatal bilirubin protein binding. Biol Neonate 58:98–103, 1990.

Yin J, Miller M, Wennberg RP: Induction of hepatic bilirubin-metabolizing enzymes by the traditional Chinese medicine yin zhi huang. Dev Pharmacol Ther 16(3):176–184, 1991a.

Yin J, Wennberg RP, Xia YC, et al: Effect of a traditional Chinese medicine, yin zhi huang, on bilirubin clearance and conjugation. Dev Pharmacol Ther 16(1):59–64, 1991b.

CHAPTER **88**

Hemostatic Disorders in Newborns

Maureen Andrew and Lu Ann Brooker

The diagnosis and management of acquired and congenital hemostatic disorders in newborns differ from those of older patients owing to a unique hemostatic system at birth and age-related pathologic conditions. For example, physiologic levels of many coagulation proteins are low, making the diagnosis of some inherited and acquired hemostatic problems difficult. Because the hemostatic system is dynamic and age dependent, multiple reference ranges reflecting both the gestational and postnatal ages of infants are necessary (Andrew, Paes, Johnston, 1990; Andrew, Paes, Milner, 1987, 1988). The index of suspicion for severe congenital deficiencies of components of hemostasis must be increased, because most severe deficiencies present in the neonatal period.

Although the hemostatic system of the young can be considered immature, it must also be considered physiologic because it provides protection from hemorrhagic and thrombotic complications in healthy newborns (Sutor, 1992). However, the immaturity of the hemostatic system in the very young leaves them vulnerable to acquired hemostatic disorders (Hathaway, 1987; Kries et al, 1988).

After confirming the presence of a hemostatic problem, the clinician is faced with the problem of providing safe and effective treatment. Just as for adults, the efficacy and safety of therapeutic interventions require testing in randomized, controlled trials, whenever feasible, whereas alternative study designs can be useful in dealing with rare or consistently life-threatening events. Guidelines for the classification of study design, and therefore the strength of the finds, have been established (Michelson et al, 1995). In this chapter, conclusions from studies with strong designs are given greater weight than are conclusions of studies with weaker designs. The chapter provides a brief review of developmental hemostasis and the diagnosis and management of both bleeding and thromboembolic disorders in newborns.

PHYSIOLOGY OF HEMOSTASIS
Coagulation System

Physiologically, blood is maintained in a fluid phase. In response to a damaged vessel wall, platelets, plasma coagulation proteins, and the damaged vessel contribute to the formation of a hemostatic plug. Figure 88–1 provides a scheme of the current concepts of the coagulation system

discussed in recent reviews (Seguin and Topper, 1995; Vermylen et al, 1987; Vieira et al, 1991). The central purpose of coagulant proteins is to generate thrombin from prothrombin. Thrombin is a serine protease with potent coagulant functions. Thrombin (1) cleaves fibrinopeptides A (FPA) and B (FPB) from fibrinogen, resulting in fibrin formation; (2) it activates factor V (FV), FVIII, and FXI, thereby enhancing its own generation; (3) it promotes fibrin cross-linking by activating FXIII; and (4) it is a potent physiologic activator of platelets.

Coagulant Proteins

Components of the coagulation system do not cross the placenta but are synthesized by the fetus with detectable levels by approximately 10 weeks' gestational age (GA). Plasma concentrations of coagulant proteins in healthy fetuses and newborns are available and are summarized in Table 88–1. Plasma concentrations of most coagulant proteins of newborns differ significantly from those of adults (see Table 88–1). Plasma levels of the vitamin K (VK)-dependent coagulant proteins (FX, FIX, FVII, FII) and the contact factors (FXII, FXI, prekallikrein [PK], and high-molecular-weight kininogen (HMWK)) are approximately 50% of adult values at birth (Andrew, Paes, John-

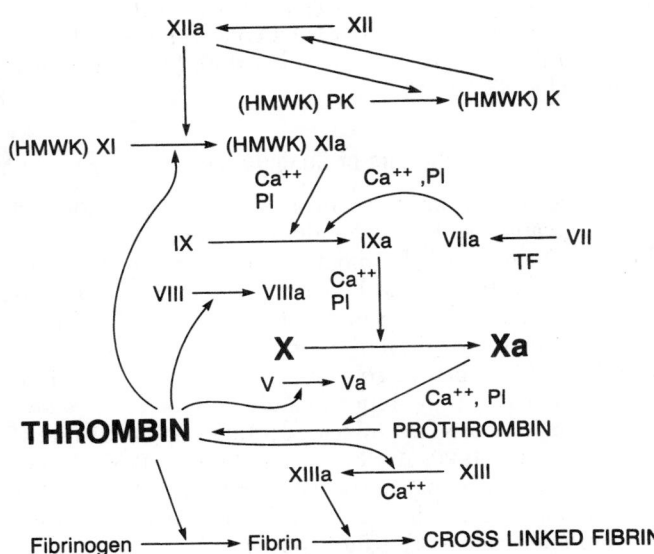

FIGURE 88–1. Physiology of normal hemostasis.

This work was supported by Project 7 from the Medical Research Council of Canada's Group in Development Lung Biology.

Reference Values* for Components of the Coagulation System in Healthy Fetuses (19–27 weeks' GA) and Premature Infants at Birth (28–31 weeks' GA)

| Coagulation Tests | Gestational Age (weeks) | | | |
| | 19–27 | | 28–31 | |
	M	(B)	M	(B)
PT (sec)	—		15.4(14.6–16.9)°°	
APTT (sec)	—		108(80.0–168)°°	
Fibrinogen (g/L)	1.0(±0.43)††		2.56(1.60–5.50)°°	
II (U/mL)	0.12(±0.02)‡		0.31(0.19–0.54)°°	
V (U/mL)	0.41(±0.10)†		0.65(0.43–0.80)°°	
VII (U/mL)	0.28(±0.04)‡		0.37(0.24–0.76)°°	
VIII (U/mL)	0.39(±0.14)†		0.79(0.37–1.26)°°	
vWF (U/mL)	0.64(±0.13)†		1.41(0.83–2.23)°°	
IX (U/mL)	0.10(±0.01)‡		0.18(0.17–0.20)°°	
X (U/mL)	0.21(±0.03)‡		0.36(0.25–0.64)°°	
XI (U/mL)	—		0.23(0.11–0.33)°°	
XII (U/mL)	0.22(±0.03)		0.25(0.05–0.35)°°	
PK (U/mL)	—		0.26(0.15–0.32)°°	
HK (U/mL)	—		0.32(0.19–0.52)°°	
ATIII (U/mL)	0.24(±0.03)§		0.28(0.20–0.38)°°	
HCII (U/mL)	0.27(±0.05)§		—	
Protein C (U/mL)	0.11(±0.03)‡		—	

°All factors except fibrinogen are expressed as units per milliliter (U/mL) where pooled plasma contains 1.0 U/mL. All values are extrapolated from designated references: †(Forestier et al, 1986), ‡(Forestier et al, 1985), §(Toulon et al, 1986), °°(Barnard et al, 1979), ††(Holmberg et al, 1974); they are expressed as a mean (M) followed by the lower and upper boundary (B).

PT, prothrombin time; APTT, activated partial thromboplastin time; II, factor II procoagulant; vWF, von Willebrand factor; PK, prekallikrein; HK, high-molecular-weight kininogen; ATIII, antithrombin ATIII; HCII, heparin cofactor II.

From Andrew M, Paes B, Milner R, et al: Development of the human coagulation system in the full-term infant. Blood 70:165, 1987.

ston, 1990; Andrew, Paes, Milner, 1987, 1988; Andrew, Vegh, Johnston, 1992). In contrast, plasma concentrations of fibrinogen, FVIII, and FV are not decreased at birth or during early childhood (Andrew, Paes, Johnston, 1990; Andrew, Paes, Milner, 1987, 1988; Andrew, Vegh, Johnston, 1992). By 6 months of age plasma concentrations of most coagulant proteins are in the lower part of the adult normal range (Table 88–2).

Inhibitors of Coagulation

There are several proteins involved in the regulation of the coagulation system. The direct plasma inhibitors of thrombin include antithrombin (AT [formerly ATIII]), α_2-macroglobulin (α_2M), and heparin cofactor II (HCII). AT-mediated inhibition of thrombin is potentiated by certain glycosaminoglycans, most important, heparan sulfate and heparin. At birth, plasma concentrations of the direct inhibitors AT and HCII are approximately 50% of adult values, whereas α_2M levels are increased (Table 88–3) (Andrew, Paes, Johnston, 1990; Andrew, Paes, Milner, 1987, 1988). By 6 months of age, plasma concentrations of AT and HCII reach adult levels, whereas α_2M levels are nearly twice those of adult values (see Table 88–3).

The indirect inhibitors of thrombin include protein C,

protein S, and tissue factor pathway inhibitor (TFPI). When thrombin is generated in vivo, it binds to an endothelial cell receptor, thrombomodulin (TM), and can no longer cleave fibrinogen, FV, or FVIII. However, thrombin can activate protein C to its activated form (APC). APC, a VK-dependent serine protease, enzymatically inactivates FVa and FVIIIa by limited proteolytic cleavage. The enzymatic activity of APC is enhanced by another VK-dependent protein, protein S. Plasma concentrations of protein C and S are reduced at birth by 60% and remain low during the first weeks of life (see Table 88–3) (Andrew, Vegh, Johnston, 1992). Protein C circulates in a fetal form that differs from the adult by a twofold increase in single-chain protein C (Manco-Johnson et al, 1991). Protein S, which circulates as both a free (active) and C_4B-bound (inactive) form in adults, circulates only in the free, active form at birth because C_4B-binding protein is absent in newborn plasma (Moalic et al, 1988; Schwarz et al, 1988). In contrast with proteins C and S, plasma concentrations of TM are increased during infancy and early childhood (Andrew, Vegh, Johnston, 1992). Whether this reflects increased endothelial expression of TM in the young is unknown, but it is an interesting speculation.

A second indirect mechanism for regulating thrombin generation is by an inhibitor of the FVIIIa/tissue factor (TF) pathway, called the *TFPI*. TFPI forms a complex with FXa, and the TFPA/FXa complex inhibits FVIIa, thereby inhibiting the generation of thrombin. There is limited information on the influence of age on TFPI. Cord plasma concentrations of TFPI are decreased to 64% of adult values (Warr et al, 1989).

Thrombin Regulation of Plasma

Physiologic differences in plasma concentrations of coagulation proteins at birth significantly influence thrombin regulation, a key step in hemostasis.

Thrombin Generation. Values for the prothrombin time (PT) and the activated partial thromboplastin time (APTT) are prolonged in newborns. More sensitive assays show that thrombin generation is delayed and decreased by approximately 50% in plasmas from newborns compared with adults (Andrew, 1990; Shah et al, 1992; Vieira et al, 1991). By 6 months of age, the capacity to generate thrombin remains approximately 20% less than for adults (Andrew, Paes, Johnston, 1990; Shah et al, 1992; Vieira et al, 1991). The plasma concentration of prothrombin, which is decreased at birth, is critically important to the amount of thrombin generated in newborn plasma (Andrew et al, 1990).

Thrombin Inhibition. The inhibition of ^{125}I-thrombin in newborn plasma is slower than in adult plasma, likely reflecting the low plasma concentrations of AT (Schmidt et al, 1989; Shah et al, 1992). However, the total capacity to inhibit thrombin is similar for newborns and adults owing to the increased binding of thrombin by α_2M (Fischer, 1981). In addition to the increased binding of thrombin to α_2M in newborn plasma, the amount of thrombin complexing to HCII is increased owing to a circulating dermatan sulfate proteoglycan (DSPG) that catalyzes thrombin inhi-

TABLE 88-2

Reference Values* for Coagulation Tests in Healthy Full-Term Infants During the First Six Months of Life

Coagulation Tests	Day 1 M (B)	Day 5 M (B)	Day 30 M (B)	Day 90 M (B)	Day 180 M (B)	Adult M (B)
PT (sec)	13.0(10.1–15.9)°	12.4(10.0–15.3)°	11.8(10.0–14.3)°	11.9(10.0–14.2)°	12.3(10.7–13.9)°	12.4(10.8–13.9)
INR	1.00(0.53–1.62)	0.89(0.53–1.48)	0.79(0.53–1.26)	0.81(0.53–1.26)	0.88(0.61–1.17)	0.89(0.64–1.17)
APTT (sec)	42.9(31.3–54.5)	42.6(25.4–59.8)	40.4(32.0–55.2)	37.1(29.0–50.1)°	35.5(28.1–42.9)°	33.5(26.6–40.3)
TCT (sec)	23.5(19.0–28.3)°	23.1(18.0–29.2)	24.3(19.4–29.2)	25.1(20.5–29.7)°	25.5(19.8–31.2)°	25.0(19.7–30.3)
Fibrinogen (g/L)	2.83(1.67–3.99)°	3.12(1.62–4.62)°	2.70(1.62–3.78)°	2.43(1.50–3.79)°	2.51(1.50–3.87)°	2.78(1.56–4.00)
II (U/mL)	0.48(0.26–0.70)	0.63(0.33–0.93)	0.68(0.34–1.02)	0.75(0.45–1.05)	0.88(0.60–1.16)	1.08(0.70–1.46)
V (U/mL)	0.72(0.34–1.08)	0.95(0.45–1.45)	0.98(0.62–1.34)	0.90(0.45–1.32)	0.91(0.55–1.27)	1.06(0.62–1.50)
VII (U/mL)	0.66(0.28(1.04)	0.89(0.35–1.43)	0.90(0.42–1.38)	0.91(0.39–1.43)	0.87(0.47–1.27)	1.05(0.67–1.43)
VIII (U/mL)	1.00(0.50–1.78)°	0.88(0.50–1.54)°	0.91(0.50–1.57)	0.79(0.50–1.25)°	0.73(0.50–1.09)	0.99(0.50–1.49)
vWF (U/mL)	1.53(0.50–2.87)	1.40(0.50–2.54)	1.28(0.50–2.46)	1.18(0.50–2.06)	1.07(0.50–1.97)	0.92(0.50–1.58)
IX (U/mL)	0.53(0.15–0.91)	0.53(0.15–0.91)	0.51(0.21–0.81)	0.67(0.21–1.13)	0.86(0.36–1.36)	1.09(0.55–1.63)
X (U/mL)	0.40(0.12–0.68)	0.49(0.19–0.79)	0.59(0.31–0.87)	0.71(0.35–1.07)	0.78(0.38–1.18)	1.06(0.70–1.52)
XI (U/mL)	0.38(0.10–0.66)	0.55(0.23–0.87)	0.53(0.27–0.79)	0.69(0.41–0.97)	0.86(0.49–1.34)	0.97(0.67–1.27)
XII (U/mL)	0.53(0.13–0.93)	0.47(0.11–0.83)	0.49(0.17–0.81)	0.67(0.25–1.09)	0.77(0.39–1.15)	1.08(0.52–1.64)
PK (U/mL)	0.37(0.18–0.69)	0.48(0.20–0.76)	0.57(0.23–0.91)	0.73(0.41–1.05)	0.86(0.56–1.16)	1.12(0.62–1.62)
HK (U/mL)	0.54(0.06–1.02)	0.74(0.16–1.32)	0.77(0.33–1.21)	0.82(0.30–1.46)°	0.82(0.36–1.28)°	0.92(0.50–1.36)
XIIIₐ (U/mL)	0.79(0.27–1.31)	0.94(0.44–1.44)°	0.93(0.39–1.47)°	1.04(0.36–1.72)°	1.04(0.46–1.62)°	1.05(0.55–1.55)
XIII_b (U/mL)	0.76(0.30–1.22)	1.06(0.32–1.80)	1.11(0.39–1.73)°	1.16(0.48–1.84)°	1.10(0.50–1.70)	0.97(0.57–1.37)

°Values that do not differ significantly from adult values.

All factors except fibrinogen are expressed as units per milliliter (U/mL) where pooled plasma contains 1.0 U/mL. All values are expressed as mean (M) followed by the lower and upper boundary encompassing 95% of the population (B).

PT, prothrombin time; APTT, activated partial thromboplastin time; TCT, thrombin clotting time; II, factor II procoagulant; vWF, von Willebrand factor; PK, prekallikrein; HK, high-molecular-weight kininogen; INR, international normalized ratio.

From Andrew M, Paes B, Johnston M: Development of the hemostatic system in the neonate and young infant. Am J Pediatr Hematol Oncol 12:95, 1990.

bition by HCII (Andrew, Mitchell, Paes, 1992; Delorme et al, 1993). DSPG is also present in plasmas from pregnant women and is likely released from the placenta (Delorme et al, 1991). The length of time that DSPG circulates in newborns is not known, except that it is still present during the first week of life in sick infants with respiratory distress syndrome (RDS) (Shah et al, 1992).

Conversion of Fibrinogen to Fibrin

Fibrinogen. At birth, plasma concentrations of fibrinogen are similar to adult levels. However, "fetal" fibrinogen has an increased sialic acid content compared with adult fibrinogen (Galanakis and Mosesson, 1976; Hamulyak et al, 1983; Witt et al, 1969). The thrombin clotting time (TCT), if performed without Ca²⁺ in the system, is prolonged in newborns, reflecting the fetal fibrinogen (Gralnick et al, 1978). If sialic acid is removed, fetal fibrinogen appears indistinguishable from adult fibrinogen (Galanakis and Mosesson, 1976; Hamulyak et al, 1983; Witt et al, 1969). The physiologic significance of fetal fibrinogen is unknown. Fetal fibrinogen disappears during early infancy, and plasma concentrations during childhood remain similar to adults.

Fibrin Clots. The capacity of newborn fibrin clots to bind thrombin has been assessed by measuring FPA production by fibrin clots prepared from adult and cord plasma (Patel et al, 1995). Cord plasma clots generate significantly less FPA compared with clots formed in adult plasma owing to decreased concentrations of prothrombin (Patel et al,

1995). Increasing cord plasma concentrations of prothrombin increases FPA production by cord clots. This observation suggests that thrombi in newborns or children with low plasma concentrations of prothrombin may have a decreased propensity of propagate.

Mechanisms Contributing to the Age Dependency of Coagulation

Potential mechanisms responsible for decreased plasma concentrations of coagulation proteins include decreased synthesis, increased clearance or consumption, and the presence of proteins with decreased activity.

Coagulation Factor Synthesis. Evaluation of messenger RNA (mRNA) in fetal and adult hepatocytes shows that transcript levels for several coagulation proteins are similar in size and the nucleotide sequence is identical (Hassan et al, 1990). However, the expression of mRNA is variable, with adult values for some coagulation proteins and decreased expression for others (Hassan et al, 1990; Karpatkin, 1991; Kisker, 1988). Similarly, hepatocyte content of specific coagulation proteins differs and does not necessarily match the mRNA expression (Hassan et al, 1990).

Coagulation Factor Clearance. At least some coagulation proteins are cleared more rapidly in newborns than in adults (Andrew, Mitchell, Berry, 1988). The half-life of fibrinogen is significantly shorter in newborn animals and in infants with RDS compared with adults (Daffos et al, 1984; Feusner et al, 1983). The half-life of AT is shorter

TABLE 88–3

Reference Values* for the Inhibitors of Coagulation in Healthy Infants During the First Six Months of Life

	Full-Term Infants										
	Day 1		**Day 5**		**Day 30**		**Day 90**		**Day 180**		**Adult**
Inhibitor Levels	**M**	**(B)**	**M**	**(B)**	**M**	**(B)**	**M**	**(B)**	**M**	**(B)**	**M** **(B)**
AT (U/mL)	0.63(0.39–0.87)		0.67(0.41–0.93)		0.78(0.48–1.08)		0.97(0.73–1.21)†		1.04(0.84–1.24)†		1.05(0.79–1.31)
α_2M (U/mL)	1.39(0.95–1.83)		1.48(0.98–1.98)		1.50(1.06–1.94)		1.76(1.26–2.26)		1.91(1.49–2.33)		0.86(0.52–1.20)
C₁E-INH (U/mL)	0.72(0.36–1.08)		0.90(0.60–1.20)†		0.89(0.47–1.31)		1.15(0.71–1.59)		1.41(0.89–1.93)		1.01(0.71–1.31)
α_1AT (U/mL)	0.93(0.49–1.37)†		0.89(0.49–1.29)†		0.62(0.36–0.88)		0.72(0.42–1.02)		0.77(0.47–1.07)		0.93(0.55–1.31)
HCII (U/mL)	0.43(0.10–0.93)		0.48(0.00–0.96)		0.47(0.10–0.87)		0.72(0.10–1.46)		1.20(0.50–1.90)		0.96(0.66–1.26)
Protein C (U/mL)	0.35(0.17–0.53)		0.42(0.20–0.64)		0.43(0.21–0.65)		0.54(0.28–0.80)		0.59(0.37–0.81)		0.96(0.64–1.28)
Protein S (U/mL)	0.36(0.12–0.60)		0.50(0.22–0.78)		0.63(0.33–0.93)		0.86(0.54–1.18)†		0.87(0.55–1.19)†		0.92(0.60–1.24)
TM (AU)°°	10.55(4.84–16.25)								7.26(3.96–10.56)		4.60(2.9–6.3)
TFPI (U/mL)§	0.7331†										0.8270

	Premature Infants (30–36 weeks' gestation)										
	Day 1		**Day 5**		**Day 30**		**Day 90**		**Day 180**		**Adult**
Inhibitor Levels	**M**	**(B)**	**M**	**(B)**	**M**	**(B)**	**M**	**(B)**	**M**	**(B)**	**M** **(B)**
AT (U/mL)	0.38(0.14–0.62)‡		0.56(0.30–0.82)		0.59(0.37–0.81)‡		0.83(0.45–1.21)‡		0.90(0.52–1.28)‡		1.05(0.79–1.31)
α_2M (U/mL)	1.10(0.56–1.82)‡		1.25(0.71–1.77)		1.38(0.72–2.04)		1.80(1.20–2.66)		2.09(1.10–3.21)		0.86(0.52–1.20)
C₁E-INH (U/mL)	0.65(0.31–0.99)		0.83(0.45–1.21)		0.74(0.40–1.24)‡		1.14(0.60–1.68)†		1.40(0.96–2.04)		1.01(0.71–1.31)
α_1AT (U/mL)	0.90(0.36–1.44)†		0.94(0.42–1.46)†		0.76(0.38–1.12)‡		0.81(0.49–1.13)†,‡		0.82(0.48–1.16)†		0.93(0.55–1.31)
HCII (U/mL)	0.32(0.10–0.60)‡		0.34(0.10–0.69)		0.43(0.15–0.71)		0.61(0.20–1.11)		0.89(0.45–1.40)†,‡		0.96(0.66–1.26)
Protein C (U/mL)	0.28(0.12–0.44)‡		0.31(0.11–0.51)		0.37(0.15–0.59)‡		0.45(0.23–0.67)‡		0.57(0.31–0.83)		0.96(0.64–1.28)
Protein S (U/mL)	0.26(0.14–0.38)‡		0.37(0.13–0.61)		0.56(0.22–0.90)		0.76(0.40–1.12)‡		0.82(0.44–1.20)		0.92(0.60–1.24)

° All values are expressed in units per milliliter (U/mL) where pooled plasma contains 1.0 U/mL. All values are given as a mean (M) followed by the lower and upper boundary encompassing 95% of the population (B). Between 40–75 samples were assayed for each value for the newborn. Some measurements were skewed due to a disproportionate number of high values. The lower limits that exclude the lower 2.5% of the population have been given (B).

AT, antithrombin; α_2-M, α_2-macroglobulin; C₁-INH, c₁esterase-inhibitor; α_1-AT, α_1-antitrypsin; HCII, heparin cofactor II; TM, thrombomodulin.

† Values that are indistinguishable from those of the adult.

‡ Values different from those of full-term infants.

§ Cord blood (Weissbach et al, 1994).

°° Data from Aurousseau et al, 1991.

From Andrew M, Paes B, Johnston M: Development of the hemostatic system in the neonate and young infant. Am J Pediatr Hematol Oncol 12:95, 1990.

in infants, requiring an exchange transfusion for hyperbilirubinemia, than in healthy adults (Schmidt et al, 1984). Reasons for the faster clearance of these proteins in newborns are incompletely understood but may be in part due to increased basal metabolic rate in newborns (Pencharz et al, 1977). Rapid clearance of coagulation proteins not only affects physiologic values but also influences replacement therapy strategies for sick newborns.

Endogenous Regulation of Thrombin. Endogenous activation of coagulation can be quantitated by activation peptides such as prothrombin fragment 1.2 (F1.2), FPA, and protein C activation peptide; or enzyme-inhibitor complexes such as thrombin-AT (TATs), thrombin-α_2M, protein C inhibitor, and protein C-α_1AT. There is considerable evidence that blood coagulation is activated at the time of birth. Plasma concentrations of FPA, TATs, and thrombin-α_2M complexes are increased at birth (Schmidt et al, 1989; Suarez et al, 1988; Suarez et al, 1988; Yuen et al, 1989). However, this process seems to be well controlled and self-limited. Indeed, activation of coagulation during the birth process does not result in significant consumption of circulating plasma coagulation proteins or clinical morbidity (Andrew, O'Brodovich, Mitchell, 1988; Kisker et al, 1981).

Fibrinolysis

Once a fibrin clot has formed in vivo, it is modified by the fibrinolytic system (Fig. 88–2). Activities of the fibrinolytic system are localized to the fibrin clot through specific lysine-binding sites. Plasminogen is converted to plasmin by several activators, of which tissue plasminogen activator (tPA) is secondarily important. Although plasminogen is also converted to plasmin by components of the contact system, this process has no physiologic importance. Analogous to thrombin, plasmin is the critical enzyme in fibrinolysis. Plasmin is a serine proteinase that cleaves fibrin in sequential steps, resulting in fibrin degradation products (FDPs) and the specific fibrin fragment, D-dimer.

The fibrinolytic system is regulated by inhibitors of plasmin and of the plasminogen activators. Plasmin is inhibited primarily by α_2M. However, when bound to the fibrin surface, plasmin is relatively protected from inhibition by α_2AP. The activators of plasminogen are inhibited by plasminogen activator inhibitors (PAIs), of which PAI-1 is the most important during infancy and childhood.

The Fibrinolytic System in Newborns

Plasma Concentrations. Plasma concentrations of components of the fibrinolytic system are age dependent (Table

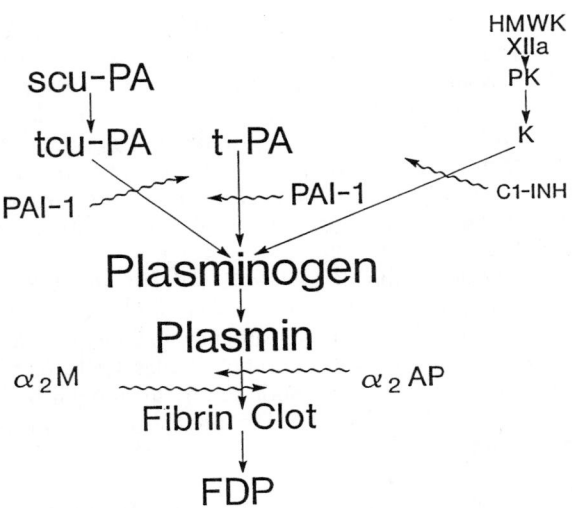

FIGURE 88–2. Physiology of fibrinolysis.

88–4). At birth, plasminogen levels are 50%, and α₂AP levels are 80% of adult values (Andrews, Paes, Johnston, 1990; Corrigan, 1988; Corrigan et al, 1989). In contrast, plasma concentrations of PAI-1 and tPA are significantly increased over adult values. The increased plasma levels of tPA and PAI-1 in newborns on day 1 of life are in marked contrast with values from cord blood, in which concentrations of these two proteins are significantly decreased com-

pared with adult values (Corrigan et al, 1989; Ginsberg, 1989). The discrepancy between newborn and cord plasma concentrations of tPA and PAI-1 can be explained by the enhanced release of tPA and PAI-1 from the endothelium shortly after birth. PAI-1 levels are detectable in cord blood but at significantly lower concentrations than for pregnant women (Lecander and Astedt, 1987). Histidine-rich glycoprotein (HRGP) levels in premature and full-term newborns are 7.0% and 14.0%, respectively, of adult values (Corrigan and Jeter, 1990). By 6 months of age, plasma concentrations of plasminogen and α₂AP are similar to adult values, whereas physiologic plasma concentrations of tPA are decreased and PAI-1 are increased (see Table 88–4).

Fetal Plasminogen. At birth, plasminogen is present in a "fetal" form characterized by increased amounts of mannose and sialic acid. Fetal plasmin may have mildly decreased enzymatic activity (Edelberg et al, 1990; Summaria, 1989) as well as decreased binding to cellular receptors for plasminogen (Edelberg et al, 1990; Summaria, 1989).

Activation of the Fibrinolytic System at Birth. Short whole blood clotting times, short euglobulin lysis times, and increased plasma concentrations of the Bβ15–42 fibrin-related peptides all suggest that the fibrinolytic system is activated at birth (Corrigan et al, 1989; Ekelund et al, 1970; Ginsberg, 1989; MarKarlan, 1967; Suarez et al, 1985). The clinical significance of an activated fibrinolytic system at birth is uncertain.

TABLE 88–4

Reference Values* for the Components of the Fibrinolytic System in Healthy Infants During the First Six Months of Life

	Full-Term Infant											
Fibrinolytic System	**Day 1** M (B)		**Day 5** M (B)		**Day 30** M (B)		**Day 90** M (B)		**Day 180** M (B)		**Adult** M (B)	
Plasminogen (U/mL)	1.95(1.25–2.65)		2.17(1.41–2.93)		1.98(1.26–2.70)		2.48(1.74–3.22)		3.01(2.21–3.81)		3.36(2.48–4.24)	
TPA (ng/mL)	9.60(5.00–18.9)		5.60(4.00–10.0)†		4.10(1.00–6.00)†		2.10(1.00–5.00)†		2.80(1.00–6.00)†		4.90(1.40–8.40)	
α₂AP (U/mL)	0.85(0.55–1.15)		1.00(0.70–1.30)†		1.00(0.76–1.24)†		1.08(0.76–1.40)†		1.11(0.83–1.39)†		1.02(0.68–1.36)	
PAI (U/mL)	6.40(2.00–15.1)		2.30(0.00–8.10)†		3.4(0.00–8.80)†		7.20(1.00–15.3)		8.10(6.00–13.0)		3.6(0.00–11.0)	

	Premature Infants											
Fibrinolytic System	**Day 1** M (B)		**Day 5** M (B)		**Day 30** M (B)		**Day 90** M (B)		**Day 180** M (B)		**Adult** M (B)	
Plasminogen (U/mL)	1.70(1.12–2.48)‡		1.91(1.21–2.61)‡		1.81(1.09–2.53)		2.38(1.58–3.18)		2.75(1.91–3.59)‡		3.36(2.48–4.24)	
TPA (ng/mL)	8.48(3.00–16.70)		3.97(2.00–6.93)†		4.13(2.00–7.79)†		3.31(2.00–5.07)†		3.48(2.00–5.85)†		4.96(1.46–8.46)	
α₂AP (U/mL)	0.78(0.40–1.16)		0.81(0.49–1.13)‡		0.89(0.55–1.23)‡		1.06(0.64–1.48)†		1.15(0.77–1.53)		1.02(0.68–1.36)	
PAI (U/mL)	5.40(0.00–12.2)†,‡		2.50(0.00–7.10)†		4.30(0.00–11.8)†		4.80(1.00–10.2)†,‡		4.90(1.00–10.2)†,‡		3.60(0.00–11.0)	
uPA (ng/mL)	0.18(0.08–0.28)§,°°										0.32(0.18–0.46)°°	
PAI-2 (ng/mL)	<1.6§										<1.6	

° For α₂AP, values are expressed as units per milliliter (U/mL) where pooled plasma contains 1.0 U/mL. Plasminogen units are those recommended by the Committee on Thrombolytic Agents. Values for TPA are given as nanograms per milliliter. Values for PAI are given as units per milliliter where 1 unit of PAI-1 activity is defined as the amount of PAI-1 that inhibits 1 international unit of human single-chain TPA. All values are given as a mean (M) followed by the lower and upper boundary encompassing 95% of the population (B).
† Values that are indistinguishable from those of the adult.
‡ Values that are different from those of the full-term infant.
§ Cord blood.
°°Data from Reverdiau-Moalic et al, 1991.
TPA, tissue plasminogen activator; α₂AP, α₂-antiplasmin; PAI, plasminogen activator inhibitor.
From Andrew M, Paes B, Johnston M: Development of the hemostatic system in the neonate and young infant. Am J Pediatr Hematol Oncol 12:95, 1990.

Regulation of Plasmin. The capacity to generate plasmin is reduced in plasma from newborns because plasminogen levels are 50% of adult values and α_2AP levels are 80% of adult values. The contribution of "fetal" plasminogen to impaired fibrinolysis is uncertain (Edelberg et al, 1990; Summaria, 1989). By 6 months of age, plasma concentrations of tPA plasma are decreased and PAI-1 are increased compared with adults, suggesting that the fibrinolytic system is suppressed (Andrew, Vegh, Johnston, 1992; Siegbahn and Ruusuvaara, 1988).

Platelets and the Vessel Wall

Platelets are disk-shaped cells produced by megakaryocytes in the bone marrow and released into the circulation. Platelet counts in newborns are similar to adults and range between 150,000 and 400,000 $\times$ 10^9/L, with mean volumes of 7 to 9 fL. The life span of platelets in healthy infants is likely similar to adults at approximately 7 to 10 days, at which time platelets are removed from the circulation by macrophages in the reticuloendothelial system (Castle et al, 1988). Platelet survival in thrombocytopenic infants is shorter than in adults, with the least thrombocytopenic infants having the longest survivals (Castle et al 1985a, 1985b; Elasas et al, 1967). Together these studies suggest that platelet survivals in newborns likely do not differ significantly from those in adults.

Platelet Structure. The outer surface of platelets contains several adhesive glycoproteins (GPs) that bind specific adhesive proteins to facilitate platelet-to-surface interactions (adhesion) and platelet-to-platelet interactions (aggregation). Under the glycocalyx there is a phospholipid bilayer that provides a procoagulant surface after platelets are activated and an internal membrane system that participates in platelet secretion of granular contents. Platelets contain two types of granules: dense bodies and α-granules. Dense bodies contain substances that promote platelet aggregation such as adenosine diphosphate (ADP), serotonin, and calcium. α-Granules contain several substances that have a wide variety of functions, including thrombospondin, an adhesive protein; growth factors such as platelet-derived growth factor (PDGF), tissue growth factor-beta (TGF-β), fibroblast growth factor (FGF); platelet factor 4 (PF4), a substance that interferes with heparin-AT interaction; several coagulation proteins; and β-thromboglobulin, a marker of platelet activation.

Platelet Function. Under normal circumstances, platelets circulate without adhering to vessel walls or to other cells. When the endothelial lining of blood vessels is damaged or removed, platelets adhere to subendothelial layers, undergo shape change, spread over the surface, and bind to each other. Adhesion initiates that secretion of platelet granule contents. These substances promote adhesion and formation of aggregates. Platelets also participate in coagulation by providing a lipoprotein surface on which the soluble coagulation factor complexes can form, resulting in the generation of thrombin and the formation of fibrin. As discussed earlier, thrombin itself is a potent stimulus of platelet aggregation.

The process of platelet adhesion is mediated by an integral membrane protein specific to the platelet membrane (glycoprotein Ib [GP Ib]). There are approximately 25,000 molecules of GP Ib per platelet, and they serve as binding sites for von Willebrand factor (vWF), an adhesive protein. vWF is secreted by endothelial cells and platelet and is present in the subendothelium and in plasma. Both the plasma concentrations of vWF and the proportion of high-molecular-weight multimers of vWF are important for adhesive function.

Following activation of platelets, GP IIb and GP IIIa come together on the platelet surface to form a 1-to-1 complex that forms a binding site for fibrinogen and, to a lesser extent, vWF and fibronectin. Platelet-to-platelet adherence or aggregation is mediated by fibrinogen bound to GP IIb/IIIa. GP IIb and GP IIIa are the most abundant platelet surface glycoproteins, with approximately 50,000 copies of each per platelet.

Occupation of platelet surface receptors by a variety of extracellular molecules (such as thrombin, collagen, and ADP) activates membrane-associated enzymes that, in turn, generate intracellular second messengers that promote platelet activation and secretion. Platelet secretion is a process whereby platelet granules form a cluster, fuse with the membranes of other granules or the open connected canalicular system, and promote platelet aggregation.

Platelet Function at Birth

Platelet function at birth has been assessed using cord platelets and, less frequently, platelets from newborns. Most studies show that cord platelets function differently from adult platelets. Electron microscopy studies show normal numbers and types of granules in cord platelets (Saving et al, 1991; Ts'ao, 1976). However, serotonin and ADP, which are stored in dense granules, are present at concentrations less than 50% of adult values (Corby and Zuck, 1976; Stuart, 1976).

Adhesion. The components required for platelet adhesion, GP Ib and vWF, are present at birth (Gruel et al, 1986). Both plasma concentrations and proportion of high-molecular-weight multimers are increased in newborns and may be responsible for enhanced cord platelet agglutination to low concentrations of ristocetin (Katz et al, 1989; Ts'ao et al, 1976; Weinstein et al, 1989). The multimeric forms appear similar to those released by endothelial cells, suggesting that mechanisms for processing the multimers may not be fully developed at birth (Hrodek, 1966).

Aggregation. Platelet GP IIb and IIIa are present on fetal platelet membranes from early gestation (Gruel et al, 1986; Israels et al, 1990). The capacity of cord platelets to aggregate following exposure to a variety of agonists has been variable, with some observations more consistent than others (Corby and O'Barr 1981a, 1981b, 1981c; Stuart et al, 1982). Cord platelet aggregation in response to eninephrine is markedly impaired owing to decreased numbers or occupation of α-adrenergic receptors (Alebouyeh, 1978; Corby and O'Barr, 1981; Jones et al, 1985; Stuart et al, 1984). Of the other agonists, decreased cord platelet aggregation to collagen is the most consistent defect (Hickman et al, 1979; Israels et al, 1987).

Activation and Secretion. Studies of activation pathways leading to release have not identified specific abnormalities in cord platelets (Israels et al, 1990). Inositol phosphate production and protein phosphorylation, as well as production of arachidonic acid and its metabolites (Stuart et al, 1982) are normal. In fact, cord platelets release more arachidonic acid than do adult platelets in response to stimulation by thrombin (Stuart, 1979). The latter may be due to platelet membranes made more reactive by low levels of vitamin E (Stuart and Oski, 1979). Agonist receptors, with the exception of the α-adrenergic receptor discussed previously, do not appear to be decreased in number (Israels et al, 1987). Despite a poor response to collagen stimulation, cord platelets have normal amounts of the collagen receptor GP Ib/IIa. Coupling of agonist receptors to phospholipases may be the site of this transient activation defect in response to collagen (Corby and O'Barr, 1981).

Platelets from Newborns. Recent studies, using whole blood flow cytometry, show that neonatal platelets are hyporeactive to thrombin, a combination of ADP and eninephrine, and a thromboxane A₂ analogue (Rajasekhar et al, 1994). Platelet aggregation studies show normal aggregation studies by 48 hours of age (Zandolfi et al, 1988).

Activation of Platelets During the Birth Process. Increased plasma levels of thromboxane B₂ β-thromboglobulin, PF4, and decreased granular content and eninephrine receptor availability all are consistent with activation of platelets during the birth process (Suarez et al, 1988). The mechanisms of activation are likely multifactorial.

The Vessel Wall

Studies in the last decade have established that the endothelium plays a complex role in hemostasis, preventing thrombotic complications under physiologic conditions and promoting fibrin formation when injured (Fig. 88–3). A review of these processes is beyond the scope of this chapter. The following describes some age-related features of endothelial cell anticoagulant properties.

Eicosanoids. One anticoagulant property of endothelial cell surfaces is mediated by lipoxygenase and cyclo-oxygenase metabolites of unsaturated fatty acids synthesized by the endothelium (Lagarde, 1988; Needleman et al, 1986). Prostacyclin (PG12) is a potent vasodilator that inhibits platelet aggregation and release and enhances fibrinolysis. PG12 regulates the extent of in vivo platelet plug formation in response to injury (Jacqz et al, 1985). Produced by the lipoxygenase pathway, 13-hydroxyoctadecadienoic acid (13-HODE) inhibits the adhesion of platelets to endothelial surfaces (Cairney et al, 1987; Croset and Lagarda, 1983). PG12 production by cord vessels exceeds that of adults (Jacqz et al, 1985).

Endothelial Cell Surface Proteoglycans. Endothelial cell surface heparan sulfate proteoglycans promote AT neu-

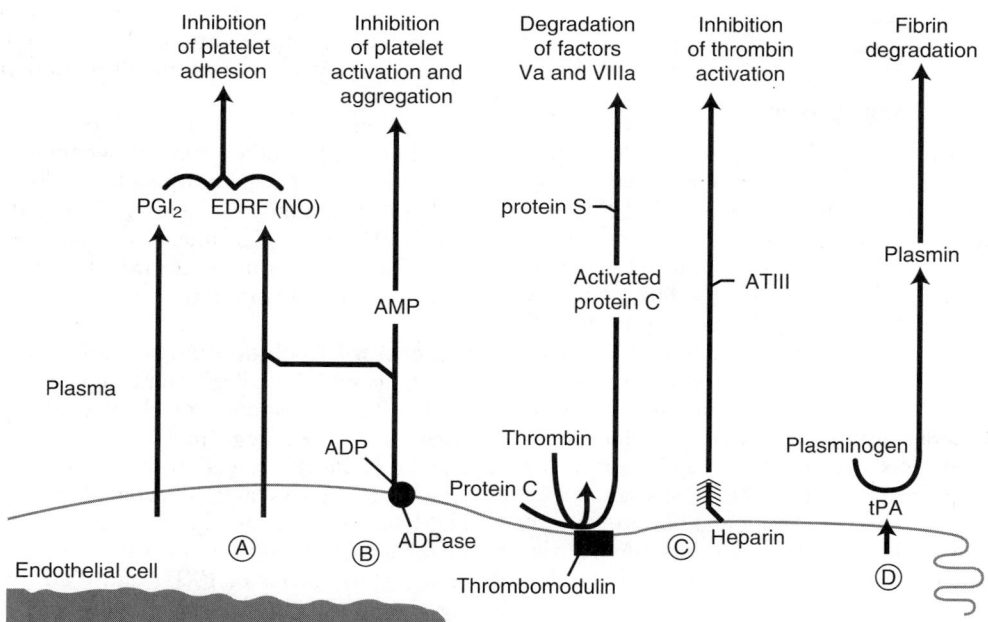

FIGURE 88–3. The vascular endothelium maintains blood fluidity in the absence of significant insult by the action of several molecules that are either on the surface of endothelial cells or released by them. Included are prostacyclin (PGI₂) and endothelium-dependent relaxing factor (EDRF), or nitric oxide (NO), which inhibit platelet adhesion **(A)**. Along with adenosine diphosphatase (ADPase), PGI₂ and EDRF (NO) also inhibit platelet activation and aggregation **(B)**. Thrombomodulin and heparin-like molecules inhibit coagulation **(C)**, and tissue-type plasminogen activator (t-PA) activates fibrinolysis **(D)**. At III, antithrombin III; ADP, adenosine diphosphate; AMP, adenosine monophosphate.

tralization of thrombin as well as other serine proteases (Xu et al, 1995). However, even in the presence of endothelium, $\alpha_2 M$ continues to be a more important inhibitor of thrombin in cord compared with adult plasma (Schmidt et al, 1989; Xu et al, 1995). Structurally, there is some evidence that vessel wall proteoglycan distribution differs in the young (Andrew, Mitchell, Paes, 1992; Kumar et al, 1967). Cord plasma glycosaminoglycan (GAG) composition in newborns also differs from that in adults, perhaps reflecting differences in the composition of the vessel wall (Andrew, Mitchell, Paes, 1992).

Nitric Oxide (NO): NO (endothelium-derived relaxing factor [EDRF]) modulates vascular tone in the fetal and postnatal lung and contributes to the normal decline in pulmonary vascular resistance at birth (Forestier et al, 1986). Like PG12, NO is a potent inhibitor of platelet activation and adhesion to the damaged vessel wall (Bodzenta-Lukaszyk et al, 1994).

Protein C/Protein S System. The endothelial cell receptor TM binds thrombin, which accelerates protein C activation to APC. APC in the presence of protein S proteolytically inactivates FVa and FVIIIa (see previous section). Although plasma concentrations of TM are increased in the young (Hurousseau et al, 1991), endothelial cell expression of TM in the young has not been measured.

Fibrinolysis. Endothelial cells produce many components of the fibrinolytic system, including tPA, PAI-1, and urokinase (UK). Endothelial cells also have binding sites for some components of the fibrinolytic system. The capacity of endothelial cells to release tPA and PAI-1 is reduced in the young.

Bleeding Time

Currently, the bleeding time is the best in vivo test of platelet interactions with the vessel wall. This is particularly true for newborns, in whom traditional platelet aggregation studies frequently are not feasible. Bleeding times in infants during the first week of life are significantly shorter than in adults (Andrew, Paes, Bowker, 1990; Andrew, 1991). Several mechanisms probably contribute to this enhanced platelet–vessel wall interaction, including increased plasma concentrations of vWF in newborns; enhanced function of vWF owing to increased amounts of high-molecular-weight, active multimers; large red blood cells; and high hematocrit levels (Aarts et al, 1983; Fernandez, 1985; Gerrard, 1989; Katz et al, 1989; Weinstein, 1989). The significance of mild platelet aggregation defects in cord platelets compared with adult platelets is uncertain when bleeding times in newborns are even shorter than in adults.

HEMORRHAGIC DISORDERS

All infants with clinically significant bleeding should be evaluated for a hemostatic deficit. Although acquired problems are more frequent, severe forms of congenital factor deficiencies often first present in early infancy and should be seriously considered in otherwise healthy infants (An-

drew and Brooker, 1995). Evaluation of any infant with hemorrhagic complications includes a careful history of family bleeding problems, outcome of previous pregnancies, maternal illnesses (especially infections), drug administration (maternal and neonatal), and documentation that VK was given at birth.

Simple observations on physical examination, such as localized versus diffuse bleeding and healthy or sick appearance of the infant, have tremendous importance for the classification of hemorrhagic disorders. Healthy infants frequently have petechiae over presenting parts secondary to venous congestion and the trauma of delivery. These petechiae are seen shortly after birth but gradually disappear and are not associated with bleeding. Infants with isolated platelet disorders generally appear healthy except for progressive petechiae, ecchymoses, and mucosal bleeding. Hemorrhages due to VK deficiency or inherited coagulation defects characteristically occur in apparently healthy children with large ecchymoses or localized bleeding (large cephalohematomas, umbilical cord bleeding, or gastrointestinal hemorrhage). Bleeding due to disseminated intravascular coagulation (DIC) or liver injury is generally seen in sick infants with diffuse bleeding from several sites.

Clinical Presentation. The clinical presentation of bleeding disorders differs in newborns compared with children or adults. Severe congenital factor deficiencies commonly present with bleeding from the umbilicus, from mucous membranes, following circumcision, from peripheral blood sampling sites, into the scalp forming large cephalohematomas, and into the skin. Hemarthrosis, a common presentation of severe congenital factor deficiencies in older children, rarely occurs in newborns. A small but important proportion of infants presents with an intracranial hemorrhage (ICH) as the first manifestation of their bleeding tendency.

In otherwise healthy infants, the most common causes of bleeding are thrombocytopenia secondary to transplacental passage of a maternal antiplatelet antibody, VK deficiency, and less commonly, a congenital coagulation factor deficiency. Although sick infants may have an underlying congenital deficit, acquired disorders such as DIC and liver failure are more common.

Laboratory Evaluation. The initial laboratory evaluation of infants with bleeding complications should include a PT, APTT, TCT, fibrinogen level, platelet count, and on rare occasion, a bleeding time. Abnormalities in these tests usually guide the selection of additional tests such as specific factor assays and paracoagulation tests. For a male child in whom hemophilia A or B is suspected, specific factor assays should be performed regardless of the APTT value. Deficiencies of FXIII and $\alpha_2 AP$ do not prolong the screening tests and must be measured directly if they are suspected. Differentiation of congenital and acquired deficiencies from physiologic values can be difficult for some coagulation proteins, a problem unique to newborns.

Management. The appropriate management of an infant with a hemorrhagic disorder is dependent on the current identification of the hemostatic defect. Options for replacement therapy consist of specific factor concentrates, fresh-frozen plasma (FFP), stored plasma, platelet concentrates, and cryoprecipitate. Other problems to consider are technical access, particularly if an exchange transfusion is planned, and the risk of graft-versus-host disease.

Congenital Factor Deficiencies

For most congenital coagulation factor deficiencies, both a severe and a milder form occur. Only the severe deficiencies usually present in the neonatal period. A MEDLINE search identified 62 publications describing 226 infants who bled from a congenital factor deficiency at birth (Table 88–5). These reports and information from older patients form the basis for the diagnosis and management guidelines for coagulation factor deficiencies in newborns.

Inheritance. Deficiencies of FXII, PK, and HMWK do not result in hemorrhagic complications and are not considered further. Most of the genetic coagulation disorders that present in newborns are the sex-linked defects, FVII (hemophilia A) and FIX deficiency (hemophilia B). Factors II, VII, V, and XI, are rare, autosomal inherited disorders, with consanguinity present in many families. Combined deficiencies of FII, FVII, FIX, and FX; or FV and FVIII are extremely rare but frequently present in the neonatal period (Mazzone et al, 1982; MacMillan and Roberts, 1966). Prenatal diagnosis of most congenital factor deficiencies is available at a molecular level (Smith, 1990).

Clinical Presentation. An otherwise healthy newborn with unexplained bleeding should be carefully investigated for a severe congenital coagulation factor deficiency (see Table 88–5). The most common sites of bleeding include circumcision, umbilical, ICH, scalp, and peripheral heelsticks. Massive bleeding may occur, resulting in concurrent DIC, which can mask the underlying factor deficiency (Rohyans et al, 1982). Full-term infants with unexplained ICH should be carefully evaluated for congenital or acquired hemostatic defects (Girolami et al, 1985; Cartwright et al, 1979; Chaplin et al, 1979; Gockos-Thocin et al, 1982; Gunn et al, 1985; Jackson and Blumhagen, 1983; Mackay et al, 1984; Palma et al, 1979; Scher et al, 1982; Serfontain, 1980). All severe congenital coagulation protein deficiencies can present with ICH at birth (Smith, 1990). The widespread use of ultrasonography during pregnancy has resulted in the detection of ICH in utero and has provided a safe modality for monitoring fetuses at risk. In utero factor replacement also has been accomplished in a few infants (Daffos et al, 1988).

Diagnosis. The diagnosis of a previously unexpected inherited coagulation protein deficiency is usually initiated by abnormal coagulation screening tests and completed by subsequent specific factor assays. Plasma concentrations of any coagulation protein must be interpreted in the context of age-specific physiologic values. Severe deficiencies of FV, FVIII, FIX, and FXIII result in levels less than 0.01 U/mL, which are easily distinguishable from physiologic values. In contrast, homozygous deficiencies of FII, FX, and FXI are defined by levels less than 0.20, 0.10, and 0.15 U/mL, respectively, which all overlap with physiologic

TABLE 88–5

Cases of Congenital Factor Deficiencies Presenting with Bleeding in Newborns*

Factor	n	ICH	Circ	Umbil	Hematoma	Punc Site	Ceph Hemat	Subgal	GI
Fibrinogen	7	0	2	5	1	—	—	—	—
II	1	0	—	—	—	—	—	—	1
V	4	2	—	1	1	—	—	—	—
VII	12	11	1	2	—	2	1	—	2
VIII	144	23	75	3	4	17	9	10	2
IX	27	3	16	2	3	3	1	1	—
vWf	4	1	—	1	2	1	—	—	—
X	5	4	—	—	—	1	1	—	2
XI	1	0	1	—	—	—	—	—	—
XIII	25	4	—	24	4	13	—	—	—
II,V,IX,X	1	0	—	—	—	—	—	—	—
V + VIII	1	0	—	—	—	—	—	—	—

° All sites of bleeding are included for each patient.

ICH, intracranial hemorrhage; Circ, circumcision; Umbil, umbilicus; Punc Site, puncture site; Ceph Hemat, cephalhematoma; Subgal, subgaleal; GI, gastrointestinal; vWf, von Willebrand factor.

levels. Although it seems probable that patients with severe factor deficiencies would have values outside the physiologic range, this has not been confirmed.

Treatment. The fundamental principle of treatment in the presence of active bleeding or a planned hemostatic challenge is to increase the plasma concentration of the deficient coagulation protein to a minimal hemostatic level. A minimal hemostatic level of a particular coagulation protein varies and is dependent on the protein and the nature of the hemostatic challenge. Table 88–6 provides minimal hemostatic levels and treatment options to achieve these levels.

ACQUIRED HEMOSTATIC DISORDERS
Disseminated Intravascular Coagulation

Historically, the term *DIC* has referred to diffuse fibrin deposition in the microvasculature (Balakrishnan et al,

1991). Subsequently, a relationship among fibrin deposition, clinical bleeding, and decreased concentrations of some coagulation factors was observed. Currently, the term *DIC* includes patients with in vivo activation of the coagulation and fibrinolytic systems as detected by sensitive assays of thrombin and plasmin generation (Balakrishnan et al, 1991).

Etiology. DIC is not a primary diagnosis but a secondary process related to a variety of primary disease states. Common etiologies in the neonatal period include asphyxia and shock (usually related to pathologic disorders involving the fetal-placental unit), infection, hypothermia, meconium aspiration, and disorders related to prematurity.

Clinical Presentation. Unlike bleeding due to VK deficiency or inherited factor deficiencies, DIC occurs in sick

---

TABLE 88–6

Coagulation Factor Proteins

Factor	Plasma Concentration	Half-Life	Minimum Hemostatic Value	Replacement Therapy
Fibrinogen	1.56–4.00 g/L	3–5 d	0.5–1.0 g/L	Plasma Cryo C
II	0.10 mg/mL	72 hr	0.4 U/mL	FIIC PCC Plasma
V	4–14 μg/mL	12–36 hr	0.25 U/mL	FFP Cryo
VII	300–500 ng/mL	3–7 hr	0.15 U/mL	FVIIC PCC Plasma
VIII	0.2 μg/mL	8–12 hr	0.30 U/mL	FVIIIC
IX	4 μg/mL	24 hr	0.10 U/mL	FIXC PCC
vWf	3–12 μg/mL	1–4 hr	0.25–0.50 U/mL	vWFC Cryo
X	4–10 μg/mL	24–56 hr	0.10 U/mL	PCC Plasma
XI	2–7 μg/mL	40–80 hr	0.20 U/mL	FXIC Plasma
XIII	A: 15 μg/mL B: 21 μg/mL	4–14 d	0.10 U/mL	FXIIIC Cryo Plasma
AT	0.30 mg/mL	17–26 hr	0.38–0.49	ATIIIC Plasma
Protein C	0.004 mg/mL	10 hr	0.38–0.49	Protein CC FFP
Protein S	25 μg/mL	24 hr	0.40–0.55	FFP

Cryo, cryoprecipitate; FFP, fresh frozen plasma; PCC, prothrombin complex concentrate; C, concentrate; AT, antithrombin.

infants, most commonly premature infants. The clinical spectrum of DIC is changing, reflecting the ever-improving perinatal care of sick infants. Intensity and duration of activation of the hemostatic system, degree of impaired blood flow, and liver function all influence the clinical severity of DIC (Haneberg, 1983; Hjort et al, 1964). In the past, infants who clinically manifested hemorrhagic or thrombotic complications from DIC frequently died. Currently, most infants with DIC survive, and for some, DIC is of little immediate clinical significance.

Diagnosis. The laboratory diagnosis of severe DIC is characterized by prolonged PT and APTT, depletion of certain coagulation factors (fibrinogen, FV, FVIII), increased FDPs, thrombocytopenia, and a microangiopathic hemolytic anemia. Pathologic decreases in fibrinogen FV and FVIII are readily identifiable because physiologic concentrations of these proteins at birth are similar to those of adult values. The availability of sensitive markers for endogenous thrombin and plasmin generation has complicated the diagnosis of DIC in newborns. For example, plasma concentration of TATs is increased in the first hours of postnatal life in healthy infants, probably reflecting activation of the coagulation system during birth (Suarez et al, 1984; Suarez et al, 1988; Yuen et al, 1989). Positive results for these sensitive paracoagulation tests indicate neither the presence of DIC nor the need to intervene. In practice, no single laboratory test can be used to confirm or exclude DIC.

Treatment. The cornerstone of management of DIC remains the successful treatment of the underlying problem. The decision to treat the hemostatic disorder is often difficult to make. In the absence of clinical manifestations, newborns probably do not require therapy for the hemostatic disorder itself. In the presence of clinically significant bleeding, therapeutic intervention with plasma products is indicated and often improves hemostasis. For infants between these two ends of the spectrum, treatment is dictated by the severity of the hemostatic impairment and the underlying problem. In general, the more pronounced the laboratory abnormalities, the greater the risk of bleeding or thrombotic complications. The argument that replacement therapy may "fuel the fire" is theoretical and not proven to occur.

Therapeutic interventions in infants with DIC include FFP, cryoprecipitate, factor concentrates (i.e., AT concentrates and prothrombin complex concentrates [PCCs]), anticoagulants, and exchange transfusions. FFP is extensively used because it contains all the coagulation proteins present in adult concentrations. Cryoprecipitate provides high concentrations of fibrinogen and FVIII, two proteins that are frequently depleted in DIC. Exchange transfusions are occasionally used in severe DIC, but their effects are transient unless the underlying problem resolves. PCCs have been used in newborns but are not generally recommended because of the potential thrombotic and infectious side effects (Andrew and Brooker, 1995).

Table 88–7 summarizes the clinical trials that used replacement therapy to correct the hemostatic defect in newborns with DIC (De Lemos et al, 1973; Gray et al, 1968; Gross et al, 1982; Hambleton and Appleyard, 1973; Turner,

1981; Waltt et al, 1973). Unfortunately, the timing and design of the available clinical studies do not permit strong recommendations to be made. Similarly, there are no clinical data supporting the use of heparin for most infants with DIC (Corrigan, 1974; Corrigan et al, 1977). In the absence of definitive clinical trials, reasonable goals are to maintain platelet counts above 50×10^9/L, fibrinogen concentrations over 1.0 g/L, and PT values at normal levels for postnatal age and GA.

Liver Disease

A MEDLINE search identified only 28 publications focused on coagulopathies of liver disease in newborns, and all were case series. The limited information available reflects the relative rarity of severe liver disease in newborns. The coagulopathies of liver disease in newborns are similar to those in adults and reflect the failure of hepatic synthetic functions superimposed on a physiologic immaturity, activation of the coagulation and fibrinolytic systems, poor clearance of activated coagulation factors, and loss of hemostatic proteins into ascitic fluid (Kelly and Summerfield, 1987). Some of the common pathologic causes of hepatic dysfunction in newborns are viral hepatitis, hypoxia, total parenteral nutrition, shock, and fetal hydrops.

Diagnosis. The laboratory diagnosis of hemostatic abnormalities due to liver failure includes prolongation of the PT, reflecting low plasma concentrations of FV, the VK-dependent proteins, and fibrinogen (di-Dattista et al, 1981; Dupuy et al, 1975; Hope et al, 1982; Mercier et al, 1976; Mindrum and Gloeck, 1959; Olivera et al, 1986). The secondary effects of liver disease on platelet number and function also occur in newborns (Rubin et al, 1977; von Breedin, 1962; Weston et al, 1977). The etiology of the thrombocytopenia is multifaceted and includes impaired platelet production, splenic sequestration, and accelerated clearance (Aster, 1966; Chesney et al, 1978; Lafer and Morrison, 1966; Osborn and Shanidi, 1973; Stein and Harker, 1982; Zinkham et al, 1967). Secondary VK deficiency occurs owing to impaired utilization (Blanchard et al, 1981) and impaired absorption. As a result, babies with cholestatic liver disease may develop VK deficiency and require parenteral treatment with VK.

Treatment. Patients with clinical bleeding may benefit temporarily from replacement of coagulation proteins with FFP, cryoprecipitate, and exchange transfusion. However, without recovery of hepatic function, replacement therapy is futile. VK should be administered to infants in whom cholestatic liver disease is suspected. PCCs containing FI, FVII, FIX, and FX should, in general, be avoided in newborns owing to the high risk of transmitting hepatitis and the risk of thrombotic disease (Goldsmith et al, 1992).

Periventricular-Intraventricular Hemorrhage

The most frequent form of ICH in premature infants is periventricular-intraventricular hemorrhage (PIVH) (Volpe, 1989). The natural history and immediate effects of specific therapeutic interventions can be accurately assessed by

TABLE 88–7

Clinical Trials Assessing the Benefits of Plasma Products

Author	n	Outcome		Comment
Beverley et al (1985)		**IVH**		
Treatment (FFP)	36	5 (14%)		No effect on the PT or APTT
Control	37	15 (41%)		
Gross et al (1982)		**Death**		
Treatment (ET)	11	4		No effect on the PT or fibrinogen level
Treatment (FFP)	11	5		
Control	11	3		
Turner (1981)		**Death**		
Treatment (FFP, Cryo, FIXC)	39	23		PT, APTT, and fibrinogen level improved in
Control	39	22		treatment group
Waltt et al (1973)		**Death**	**ICH**	
Treatment (FIXC)	40	19 (47%)	12	TT lower in control group on day 1
Control	40	16 (40%)	4°	
De Lemos et al (1973)		**Death**		
Treatment (ET)	20	4 (25%)		Prolonged APTT associated with a poorer outcome
Control	20	16 (80%)°		
Hambleton and Appleyard (1973)		**Death**	**ICH**	
Treatment (FFP)	33	9	2	Minor improvements on the PT and APTT
Control	33	10	3	
Gray et al (1968)		**Death**		
Treatment (FFP)	26	1 (4%)		TT lower in infants who died
Control	48	9 (19%)		

°A significant difference between groups of at least $P < 0.05$.

FFP, fresh frozen plasma; ET, exchange transfusion; C, concentrate; PT, prothrombin time; APTT, activated partial thromboplastin time; TT, thrombotest; Cryo, cryoprecipitate; ICH, intracranial hemorrhage; n, number.

ultrasound through the anterior fontanelle. The incidence of PIVH in premature infants is decreasing, likely reflecting improving neonatal care.

Antenatal VK. Table 88–8 summarizes the four clinical trials that assessed the effect of antenatal VK on plasma activities of VK-dependent coagulation proteins in premature infants (Kazzi et al, 1989; Morales et al, 1988; Pomerance et al, 1987; Thorp et al, 1994). Two reported a benefit and one did not (Kazzi et al, 1989; Morales et al, 1988; Pomerance et al, 1987; Thorp et al, 1994). The inconsistencies in results and methodologic problems prevent a recommendation for antenatal VK. This statement is not to be confused with the well-substantiated need for VK supplementation postnatally.

Coagulation Factor/Platelet Replacement Studies. Table 88–8 also summarizes the three clinical trials since 1980 that assessed coagulation factor and platelet replacement in newborns at risk for PIVH (Andrew, Caco, Vegh, 1991; Beverley et al, 1985; Shirahata, 1990). One trial assessed FFP because of the potential contribution of low plasma concentrations of many coagulation proteins at birth to PIVH. A position effect was reported but without a placebo control. It is possible that the observed beneficial effect was not the result of the increase in plasma concentrations of coagulation proteins (Beverley et al, 1985). A second trial assessed the effects of FXIII concentrates because

of the potential benefit of enhanced fibrin cross-linking (Shirahata et al, 1990). Although this study reported a significant effect, the analysis was performed on a small subset of infants that was not balanced. In addition, there is no strong biologic rationale because FXIII levels are well within the adult range at birth. A third trial assessed the effects of platelet concentrates administered to thrombocytopenic premature infants because of the association of thrombocytopenia and PIVH (Andrew, Caco, Vegh, 1991; Andrew, Caco, Vegh, 1993). No beneficial effect on PIVH was shown in this study, which was designed to detect a 25% effect or greater.

Antifibrinolytic Therapy. One trial assessed the effects of an antifibrinolytic agent, transexamic acid, because fibrinolytic activity is increased at birth and could contribute to PIVH (see Table 88–8) (Gilles et al, 1971; Hensey et al, 1984). No significant effect was demonstrated.

Recommendations. At this time, no firm recommendations can be made for any of the intervention modalities discussed because of a lack of consistent results and neurodevelopmental follow-up (Ment et al, 1988). Ongoing clinical studies are necessary to test potentially beneficial therapeutic agents within the context of the improving clinical care.

Respiratory Distress Syndrome

RDS, an acute lung disorder that primarily affects premature infants, is characterized by diffuse atelectasis, hyaline membrane formation, permeability edema, and right-to-left shunting of pulmonary blood flow (see Chapter 11).

Potential Role of Coagulation. One of the pathologic characteristics of RDS is fibrin deposition in both intra-alveolar and intravascular sites (Bachofen and Weibel, 1982; Gajl-Peczalska, 1964; Gitlen et al, 1964). Early studies suggested that decreased plasma concentrations of some coagulation proteins and inhibitors correlated with the severity of RDS (Damiano et al, 1990; Fukuda et al, 1987; Saldeen, 1982; Seeger et al, 1985). A recent study convincingly showed a direct correlation among in vivo markers of thrombin generation (TATs, F1.2), decreased levels of the major inhibitor of coagulation, AT, and severity of RDS. Other studies show that fibrin deposition within the lung likely contributes to the severity of lung disease (Damiano et al, 1990; Fukuda et al, 1987; Saldeen, 1982; Seeger et al, 1985). In a piglet model of neonatal acute lung injury, increasing plasma concentrations of AT by infusion of AT concentrates decreased the severity of the lung disease (Schmidt et al, 1993). These studies suggest that in vivo generation of thrombin is linked to fibrin deposition in the lung and this phenomenon may contribute to neonatal lung diseases.

Intervention Trials Influencing Hemostasis. Table 88–9 summarizes the four intervention studies directed at decreasing fibrin deposition in the lung by the use of plasminogen/plasmin heparin and AT concentrates (Ambrus et al, 1966; Ambrus et al, 1977; Markarian et al, 1971; Muntean and Rosseger, 1989). Plasminogen/plasmin infusions were tested in two trials (Ambrus et al, 1977; Muntean and Rosseger, 1989). A substantial decrease in the severity of RDS and mortality was demonstrated in both trials (Ambrus et al, 1977; Muntean and Rosseger, 1989). Although these results are compelling, the trials were performed in the 1960s and the results cannot be extrapolated to modern neonatal care. A third trial assessed the potential benefit of heparin therapy on the development of RDS and PIVH (Markarian et al, 1971). In the primary analyses, there was no difference in the number of deaths, incidence of RDS, or bleeding. A subanalysis, in which seven moribund infants treated with heparin and three moribund infants treated with saline were excluded, showed a positive effect on mortality (Markarian et al, 1971). A fourth trial compared AT concentrates to placebo in newborns with RDS. There was no difference in duration of ventilation, PIVH, or mortality (Muntean and Rosseger, 1989). At this time, neither fibrinolytic agents or anticoagulants can be recommended for the treatment of RDS. However, the biology of RDS and the results of early clinical trials support further investigation with antithrombotic agents in neonatal RDS.

Vitamin K Deficiency

The discovery of VK and its important role in hemostasis was intertwined with the role of VK in the treatment and subsequent prevention of hemorrhagic disease of the newborn (HDN). HDN consists of bleeding from multiple sites in otherwise healthy infants in the absence of trauma,

TABLE 88–8

PIVH Prevention Studies

Study	n	Weight (kg)	Dose 1 (mg/kg)	Dose 2 (mg/kg)	PIVH
Vitamin K					
Pomerance et al (1987)	53	1.5	10 mg	10 × 2	↓
Morales et al (1988)	100	1.5	10 mg	10 E 5 d	↓
Kazzi et al (1989)	98	2.5	10 mg	20 E d	⇄
Thorp et al (1994)	164	1.3	10 mg	10 × 1	↔
Blood Products					
Beverley et al (1985) (FFP)	73	1.5	10 mL	10 mL × 2	↓
Shirahata et al (1990) (FXIII-C)	21	—	100 U	none	↓
Andrew et al (1991) (platelet-C)	154	1.5	10 mL	10 mL × 1–3	⇄
Transexamic Acid					
Hensey et al (1984)	105	1.25	25 (IV)	25 × 20	⇄
Ethamsylate					
Morgan et al (1981)	73	1.5	12.5	12.5 × 16	↓
Benson et al (1986)	330	1.5	12.5	12.5 × 16	↓
Indomethacin					
Hanigan et al (1988)	111	1.3	0.4	0.4 × 3	↓
Ment et al (1988)	36	1.25	0.1	0.1 × 3	↓
Bandstra et al (1988)	199	1.3	0.2	0.1 × 2	↓
Bada et al (1989)	141	1.5	0.2	0.1 × 2	↓
Mahony et al (1985)	104	1.3	0.2	0.1 × 2	↓
Ment et al (1985)	48	1.25	0.6	0.1 × 8	↓
Rennie et al (1986)	50	1.75	0.2	0.2 × 2	⇄
Vincer et al (1987)	30	1.5	0.2	0.2 × 2	⇄

n, number; PIVH, periventricular-intraventricular hemorrhage; FFP, fresh frozen plasma; FXIII-C, factor XIII concentrate; platelet-C, platelet concentrate.

TABLE 88–9

Clinical Trials Assessing the Potential Benefits of Anticoagulant or Thrombolytic Therapy in Newborns with RDS

Author	n	Outcome		
		Death (%)	RDS (%)	ICH (%)
Markarian et al (1971)				
Heparin	39	17 (44)NS‡	26 (68.8)NS‡	40 mild°
				10 severe
Placebo	42	16 (38)	22 (53.3)	0 mild
				61 severe
Ambrus et al (1966)				
UK-plasmin	32	9 (28)†	—	7 (22)NS
Placebo	28	17 (61)		6 (21)
Ambrus et al (1977)				
Plasminogen C	251	6 (2)†	35 (14) mild NS	1 (0.4)NS‡
			19 (7) severe†	
Placebo	249	20 (8)	22 (9) mild	1 (0.4)
			31 (12) severe	
Muntean and Rosseger (1989)				
ATIII C	45	9 (20)NS‡	23 (51)NS‡	—
Control	53	8 (15)	28 (53)	—

°Patients who were diagnosed with ICH at autopsy.
†Significantly different than placebo/control group.
‡NS, not significantly different than placebo/control group.
  n, number; RDS, respiratory distress syndrome; ICH, intracranial hemorrhage; UK, urokinase; ATIIIC, antithrombin III concentrate; plasminogen C, plasminogen concentrate.

asphyxia, or infection on days 1 to 5 of life (Townsend, 1894). The link between VK deficiency and spontaneous hemorrhaging was first seen in chicks by Dam in 1929. The association between VK deficiency and HDN quickly followed with subsequent treatment of infants with HDN (Aballi and de Lamerens, 1962; Brinkhous et al, 1937; Bruchsaler, 1941; Dam et al, 1939). The original term *HDN* has been changed to *VK-dependent bleeding* (VKDB) because the original term *HDN* included many infants with bleeding from other causes.

Clinical Presentation. Infants are at greater risk for VKDB than are similarly affected adults because plasma concentrations of VK-dependent factors are physiologically decreased (Aballi and de Lamerens, 1962; Andrew, Paes, Johnston, 1990; Andrew, Paes, Milner, 1987, 1988; Kries et al, 1988; Lehmann, 1944). The clinical presentation of VKDB can be classified into three patterns (early, classic, late) based on the timing and type of complications (Table 88–10). The classic form of VKDB presents on days, 2 to 7 of life in breast-fed, healthy full-term infants. Etiologies include poor placental transfer of VK, marginal VK content in breast milk, inadequate milk intake, and a sterile gut. VKDB rarely occurs in formula-fed infants because formula is supplemented with VK (approximately 4 to 100 μg/L). The frequency of classic VKDB, without VK prophylaxis, depends on the population studied, the supplemental formula, and the frequency of breast feeding. In the absence of prophylactic VK, the frequency of VKDB ranges from 1.7% to 0.25%.

The early form of VKDB presents in the first 24 hours of life and is linked to maternal use of specific medications

that interfere with VK stores or function (Laosombat, 1988; Mountain et al, 1970; Srinivason et al, 1982). The late form of VKDB presents between weeks 2 and 8 of life and is linked with disorders that compromise the supply of VK (Sutor et al, 1995).

Laboratory Diagnosis. Laboratory tests used to detect VK deficiency include screening tests, factor assays, detection of decarboxylated forms of VK-dependent factors (protein induced by vitamin K antagonists [PIVKA]), and direct measurements of VK. Clinically, a prolonged PT is usually the first laboratory test to indicate that VK deficiency is present.

Forms of Vitamin K. VK exists in three forms: VK (phytonadione), which is present in leafy green vegetables; VK_2 (menaquinone), which is synthesized by intestinal bacterial flora; and VK_3 (menadione), a synthetic, water-soluble form. VK_3 is rarely used in newborns because in high doses it causes hemolytic anemia, resulting in jaundice and potential morbidity (Aballi and de Lamerens, 1962; Committee on Nutrition, 1961; Lucey and Dolan, 1959). Newborn stores of VK are low, as evidenced by low levels of VK in cord blood and livers of aborted fetuses (Greer et al, 1988; Hiraike, 1988a; 1988b; Shearer et al, 1982). Recent studies measuring placental transport of VK show that only about 10% of maternally administered VK reaches the fetus (von Kries and Hanawa, 1993).

Prophylactic Vitamin K. Most of the controversy concerning the prophylactic use of VK can be explained by the design of the trials and subsequent interpretations. There are two well-controlled studies that assessed the benefits of VK prophylaxis, using clinical bleeding as the outcome measure (Sutherland and Glueck, 1967; Vietti et al, 1960). Both trials showed a significantly positive result for prophylactic VK administration. In addition, numerous laboratory studies showed biochemical evidence of VK deficiency in infants who did not receive VK at birth (Greer et al, 1988; Hall and Pairaudeau, 1987; Hiraike et al, 1988a, 1988b; Shearer et al, 1982).

Further support for prophylactic VK comes from cohort studies reporting biochemical indices of VK deficiency at birth (Greer et al, 1988; Hall and Pairaudeau, 1987; Hiraike et al, 1988a, 1988b; Shearer et al, 1982). Population-based studies generally show that VKDB rarely occurs when VK prophylaxis is used, but it does occur when prophylactic VK is withdrawn. Finally, there are numerous case reports of infants with VKDB whom, for a variety of reasons, did not receive VK at birth (Behrmann, 1985; Binder, 1986; Lane et al, 1983).

Prophylactic Vitamin K Administration. Daily requirements of VK for newborns are approximately 1 to 5 μg/kg of body weight (van Kries and Hanawa, 1993). Recommendations for VK prophylaxis are similar in most countries (van Kries and Hanawa, 1993) and consist of a single dose of 0.5 to 1 mg intramuscularly or an oral dose of 2 to 4 mg

at birth, with subsequent dosing for breast-fed infants. Recent studies show that the oral route of administration of VK is as effective, less expensive, and less traumatic compared with intramuscular administration in preventing the classic presentation of VK deficiency (Hathaway et al, 1991; von Kries and Hanawa, 1993). However, oral VK_1 or VK_3 is not as effective as intramuscular VK in the prevention of late VK deficiency (see Table 88–10). Strategies to prevent late VK deficiency include repeated administration of oral VK (McNinch and Tripp, 1991; von Kries and Gobel, 1992) or continuous low-dose VK supplementation.

Certain risk groups require, in addition to general prophylaxis at birth, further VK prophylaxis (i.e., infants with α_1-antitrypsin deficiency, chronic diarrhea, cystic fibrosis, or celiac disease). Pregnant women receiving oral anticonvulsant therapy should receive about 5 mg of VK daily during the third trimester to prevent overt VK deficiency in their infants at birth.

In 1990, an unexpected association between childhood cancer and prophylactic VK was reported, based on a 1970 birth cohort (Butler et al, 1982). Subsequently, a case control study by the same group reported a significant association between intramuscular VK and cancer when compared with no VK or oral VK (Golding et al, 1992). However, two other large case control studies from 1993 (Ekelund et al, 1993; Pell et al, 1993) found no significant

TABLE 88–10

Forms of Vitamin K Deficiency Bleeding (VKDB) in Infancy

Early Form	Classic Form	Late Form
Age		
<24 hr	Days 2–7	0.5–6 mo
Causes and Risk Factors		
Medications during pregnancy		Marginal VK content in breast milk due to low VK intake and absorption
Anticonvulsants	Breast-feeding	Cystic fibrosis
Oral anticoagulants (rifampin, isoniazid)	Inadequate VK intake	Diarrhea
Antibiotics (rarely idiopathic or hereditary)		α_1AT deficiency
		Hepatitis
		Celiac disease
Localization in Order of Frequency		
ICH	ICH	ICH (>50%)
GI	GI	GI
Umbilicus	Umbilicus	Skin
Intraabdominal	ENT region	ENT region
Cephalhematoma	Injection sites	Injection sites
	Circumcision	Urogenital tract
		Intrathoracic
Frequency Without VK Prophylaxis		
Very rare	1.5%–1/10,000 births	4–10/10,000 births°
Prophylaxis		
	Adequate VK supply	Adequate VK supply
Discontinue or replace offending medications	Early and adequate breast-feeding	Adequate breast-feeding
Maternal VK prophylaxis	Formula	Formula
	VK prophylaxis	VK prophylaxis†

°More common in southeast Asia.

†Single intramuscular injection is better than single oral; repeated small doses are closer to physiologic conditions. Warning signs: neonatal icterus, poor feeding, failure to thrive, any form of bleeding.

ICH, intracranial bleed; GI, gastrointestinal bleed; ENT region, ear, nose, and throat region.

link between intramuscular VK and cancer. At this time, a strong recommendation can be made for the administration of prophylactic VK to newborns.

Treatment of Vitamin K Deficiency. An infant suspected of having VKDB should be treated immediately with VK pending laboratory confirmation. VK should not be given intramuscularly to infants with VKDB, because large hematomas may form at the site of the injection. The absorption of subcutaneous VK is rapid, and its effect is only slightly slower than systematically administered VK. Intravenous VK should be given slowly because it may induce an anaphylactoid reaction. Infants with major bleeding secondary to VK deficiency should also be treated with plasma products to rapidly increase levels of VK-dependent proteins. Plasma is the product of choice for treatment of a non–life-threatening hemorrhagic event, and PCCs should be considered for life-threatening bleeding.

Extracorporeal Membrane Oxygenation

Extracorporeal membrane oxygenation (ECMO) began in the 1960s and has been used to treat thousands of infants with a survival rate of approximately 60%. ECMO permits the transfer of oxygen into blood across a semipermeable membrane and is currently used for infants with life-threatening severe respiratory insufficiency. Underlying disorders include meconium aspiration syndrome, severe RDS, congenital diaphragmatic hernia, persistent pulmonary hypertension, and sepsis. Despite the widespread use of ECMO, few controlled trials assessing its efficacy have been published (Bartlett et al, 1985; Rosenburger and Lachin, 1993; Truog, 1992; Zreik et al, 1995). Clearly, more definitive trials are needed to validate the use of ECMO. The follow-up studies of the survivors of ECMO are most encouraging, with most infants having normal developmental follow-up.

Intracranial hemorrhage is the most important side effect and the leading cause of death in infants on ECMO. Etiologies for intracranial hemorrhage are multifactorial and include alterations in flow secondary to catheters, a consumptive coagulopathy, a hyperfibrinolytic state, anticoagulation with heparin, and thrombocytopenia (Plotz et al, 1993; Robinson et al, 1993). Heparin is used in full systemic doses, with a bolus of 100 to 150 U/kg followed by a continuous infusion of systemic heparin at 20 to 70 U/kg per hour. The ACT is used to monitor heparin therapy and is generally targeted to values two to three times baseline values (240 to 280 seconds). Although anticoagulation is required for ECMO, the optimal doses of heparin or potentially safer anticoagulants such as low-molecular-weight heparin (LMWH) have never been tested in patients receiving ECMO.

THROMBOTIC DISORDERS
Congenital Prethrombotic Disorders

Patients with single gene defects for recognized inherited prethrombotic disorders rarely present with their first thromboembolic event during infancy, unless there is another pathologic event that unmasks the defect. In contrast, patients who are homozygotes or double heterozygotes for

a congenital prethrombotic disorder usually present in the neonatal period.

Homozygous Prethrombotic Disorders

A MEDLINE search of the literature since 1980 identified 23 articles describing 40 patients with homozygous protein C deficiency and 1 patient with homozygous protein S deficiency. All affected newborns had undetectable levels of protein C (or protein S), whereas children with delayed presentation had detectable levels ranging between 0.05 and 0.20 U/mL.

Clinical Presentation. The classic clinical presentation of homozygous protein C/S deficiency consists of cerebral and ophthalmic damage that occurred in utero, purpura fulminans within hours or days of birth, and, on rare occasions, large-vessel thrombosis. Purpura fulminans is an acute, lethal syndrome of DIC with rapidly progressive hemorrhagic necrosis of the skin due to dermal vascular thrombosis (Adcock and Hicks, 1990; Adcock et al, 1990; Huletta and Headington, 1988). The skin lesions start as small ecchymotic sites that increase in a radial fashion, become purplish black with bullae, and then necrotic and gangrenous (Adcock et al, 1990; Adcock and Hicks, 1990). The lesions occur mainly on the extremities but can occur on the buttocks, abdomen, scrotum, and scalp. They also occur at pressure points, at sites of previous punctures, and at previously affected sites. Affected infants also have severe DIC with secondary hemorrhagic complications.

Diagnosis. The diagnosis of infants with homozygous protein C/S deficiency depends on the appropriate clinical picture, a protein C/S level that is usually undetectable, a heterozygous state in the parents and, ideally, the identification of the molecular defect. The presence of very low levels of protein C/S in the absence of clinical manifestations and family history cannot be considered diagnostic because physiologic plasma levels can be as low as 0.12 U/mL. Homozygous forms of AT or HCII deficiencies have not been confirmed in newborns, but one would anticipate that they would present with severe life-threatening thromboembolic complications.

Initial Treatment. The diagnosis of homozygous protein C/S deficiency is usually unanticipated and is made at the time of the clinical presentation. Although numerous forms of initial therapy have been used, 10 to 20 mL/kg of FFP every 6 to 12 hours is usually the form of therapy immediately available (Estelles et al, 1984). Plasma levels of protein C achieved with these doses of FFP vary from 15% to 32% at 30 minutes after the infusion and 4% to 10% at 12 hours (Marlar et al, 1989). The plasma level of protein S, which was entirely bound to C4b, was 23% at 2 hours and 14% at 24 hours, with an approximate half-life of 36 hours (Mahasandana et al, 1990). Doses of protein C concentrate have ranged from 20 to 60 U/kg. In one study a dose of 60 U/kg resulted in peak protein C levels above 0.60 U/mL (Dreytus et al, 1991). Replacement therapy should be continued until all of the clinical lesions resolve, which is usually 6 to 8 weeks. In addition to the clinical course, plasma D-dimer concentrations may be useful for monitoring the effectiveness of protein C replacement (Reverdiau-Moalic et al, 1991).

Long-Term Therapy. The modalities used for long-term management of infants with homozygous protein C/S deficiency include oral anticoagulation therapy, replacement therapy with protein C concentrate, and liver transplantation (Marlar et al, 1989). To avoid skin necrosis when oral anticoagulation therapy is initiated, replacement therapy should be continued until the INR is therapeutic. The therapeutic range for the INR can be individualized to some extent but is usually between 2.5 and 4.5. The risk with oral anticoagulation therapy includes bleeding with high INRs and recurrent purpuric lesions with low INRs. Frequent monitoring of INR values is required to avoid these complications. Bone development should also be monitored because the long-term effects of warfarin on bones is unknown in young infants.

Acquired Prothrombotic Disorders

Reviews of the literature (McDonald and Hathaway, 1983; Schmidt and Andrew, 1988; Schmidt and Zipursky, 1984) and an international registry of neonatal thrombotic disease have provided valuable information on the epidemiology of venous and arterial thrombotic disease in newborns. Symptomatic secondary thromboembolic complications occur more frequently in sick newborns than at any other age during childhood, with an incidence of approximately 2.4 per 1000 hospital admissions to the neonatal intensive care unit (NICU) (Schmidt and Andrew, 1995). Catheters are responsible for more than 80% of venous and 90% of arterial thrombotic complications. Catheters provide many of the requirements that initiate thrombus formation, such as a foreign surface, endothelial cell damage, impaired flow, and infusion of noxious substances (Schmidt and Andrew, 1995). Renal vein thrombosis is the most frequent form of non–catheter-related thrombosis. Other risk factors include increased blood viscosity, poor deformability of physiologically large red blood cells, polycythemia, dehydration, and activation of the coagulation and fibrinolytic systems secondary to a variety of medical problems. The following section discusses the epidemiology, diagnosis, and treatment of thromboembolic complications in newborns.

Venous Catheter–Related Thrombosis

Umbilical venous catheters (UCs) and other forms of central venous catheters (CVLs) are associated with a significant risk of thrombosis (Andrew, David, et al, 1994; David and Andrew, 1993). Based on autopsy studies, 20% to 65% of infants who die with UC in place have an associated thrombus. A MEDLINE search of the literature from 1966 to 1995 identified 60 references (most are case reports) to catheter-related thrombosis in infants. Short-term consequences of venous catheter thrombi include loss of access, pulmonary embolism (PE), superior vena cava syndrome, and organ impairment, if the catheter is improperly placed (i.e., hepatic vein thrombosis). Until recently, PE was rarely diagnosed in sick newborns because the clinical signs were easily confused with RDS. The use of ventilation lung scintigram in newborns has facilitated the diagnosis of PE

(O'Brodovich and Coates, 1984). Long-term sequelae of umbilical venous catheterization have not been rigorously studied, but they include portal hypertension, splenomegaly, gastric and esophageal varices, hypertension, and postphlebitic syndrome.

Diagnosis. The diagnosis of venous catheter thrombi is usually made with ultrasonography. However, the sensitivity and specificity of this diagnostic tool have never been compared with venography in newborns. Recent studies suggest that ultrasonography may be missing the presence and extent of venous catheter-related thrombosis in the small infant (Andrew, Marzinotto, 1995).

Arterial Catheter–Related Thrombosis

Seriously ill infants require indwelling arterial catheters, which incur a risk for thrombosis, regardless of the vessel and type of catheter (Ankola and Atakent, 1993). Catheter-related thrombosis not only occludes catheters, resulting in loss of patency, but may also obstruct major arterial vessels. In a retrospective examination of approximately 4000 infants who underwent umbilical artery catheterization, severe symptomatic vessel obstruction was observed in 1% of infants. Asymptomatic catheter-related thrombi occur more frequently, as evidenced by postmortem (3% to 59% of cases) and angiographic studies (10% to 90% of cases).

Diagnosis. For arterial thrombosis, contrast angiography is considered the reference test. Noninvasive techniques such as Doppler ultrasonography offer advantages, but their sensitivity and specificity are unknown. A review of 20 neonates with aortic thromboses treated in one institution revealed that ultrasonography failed to identify thrombi in four patients, three of whom had complete aortic obstruction (Vailas et al, 1986).

Sequelae. The sequelae of catheter-related thrombi can be immediate or long term. Acute symptoms reflect the location of the catheter and include renal hypertension, intestinal necrosis, and peripheral gangrene (Schmidt and Andrew, 1988). The long-term side effects of symptomatic and asymptomatic thrombosis of major arteries have not been studied but are probably significant (Schmidt and Andrew, 1988).

Prophylaxis with Heparin (Table 88–11). A low-dose, continuous heparin infusion (3 to 5 U per hour) is commonly used to maintain arterial catheter patency. The effectiveness of heparin was assessed in seven studies using three outcomes; patency, local thrombus, and ICH (Ankola and Atakent, 1993; Bosque and Weaver, 1986; David et al, 1981; Horgan et al, 1987; Jackson et al, 1987; Rajani et al, 1979). Patency, which is likely linked to the presence of a local thrombus, is prolonged by the use of low-dose heparin. Local thromboses were assessed by ultrasonography in two randomized studies. Unfortunately, the sample sizes were too small to draw conclusions. The evidence linking heparin to ICH in newborns is similarly weak. Thus, the magnitude of risk for ICH from heparin is uncertain (Lesko et al, 1986). Heparin is used in at least 75% of American

TABLE 88–11

Umbilical Artery Catheterization

Reference	Level	Intervention	Patient No.	Outcome Bleeding	Outcome Event (B or TE)
Jackson et al, 1987	II	HB-PU	61	†	13 TE
		PVC	64	†	23 TE
Horgan et al 1987	II	Heparin	59	†	16 TE
		No Heparin	52	†	18 TE
Rajani et al, 1979	I	Heparin	32	†	4 B‡
		Placebo	30	†	19 B
David et al, 1981	II	Heparin	26	0°	3 B‡
		No Heparin	26	0°	15 B
Bosque and Weaver, 1986	II	Heparin (C)	18	†	0 B‡
		Heparin (I)	19	†	8 B
Horgan et al, 1987	II	Heparin	59	†	2 B‡
		No Heparin	52	†	10 B
Ankola and Atakent, 1993	II	Heparin	15	4 ICH	2 B‡
		No Heparin	15	5 ICH	11 B

° No hemorrhage.
† Hemorrhage not reported.
‡ Indicates $P < 0.05$.
 B, blocked; TE, thromboembolic event; HB-PU, heparin-bonded polyurethane; PVC, polyvinylchloride; C, continuous; I, intermittent; ICH, intracranial hemorrhage.

nurseries to preserve arterial catheter patency (Schmidt and Andrew, 1988).

Renal Vein Thrombosis

Renal vein thrombosis (RVT) occurs primarily in newborns and young infants. The MEDLINE search identified 268 patients with RVT in 80 publications: 67 case reports and 13 case series. Of the 268 valuable cases, 79% presented within the first month, usually within the first week of life. Some infants developed RVT in utero. The incidence in males and females was similar, and the left and right side were equally affected. Bilateral RVT occurred in 24% of pediatric patients.

Clinical Presentation and Etiology. Presenting symptoms and clinical findings differ between neonates and older patients and are influenced by the extent and rapidity of thrombus formation. Neonates usually present with a flank mass, hematuria, proteinuria, thrombocytopenia, and nonfunction of the involved kidney. Clinical findings suggestive of acute inferior vena cava thrombosis include cold, cyanotic, and edematous lower extremities. RVT results from pathologic states characterized by reduced renal blood flow, increased blood viscosity, hyperosmolality, or hypercoagulability.

Coagulation Abnormalities. The most common coagulation abnormality is thrombocytopenia, which is usually mild, with average values of $100,000 \times 10^9/L$. Coagulation

screening tests may be prolonged and fibrin/fibrinogen degradation products increased. Infants with RVT should be evaluated for a congenital prethrombotic disorder (Rogers et al, 1989).

Diagnosis and Treatment. The diagnosis of RVT has changed from an autopsy finding to an antemortem diagnosis, which requires confirmation with an objective test. Ultrasonography is the radiographic test of choice because of ease of testing and sensitivity to an enlarged kidney. Treatment options include supportive care, anticoagulation, and thrombolytic therapy. In the 1990s, there is uniform agreement that aggressive supportive care is indicated. However, the use of anticoagulants and thrombolytic agents is controversial. One approach is to use supportive care to unilateral RVT in the absence of uremia and extension into the inferior vena cava. Heparin therapy should be considered for unilateral RVT that does extend into the inferior vena cava or bilateral RVT because of the risk of PE and complete renal failure. Thrombolytic therapy should be considered in the presence of bilateral RVT and pending renal failure. Thrombectomy, although a common therapeutic choice in the past, is rarely indicated.

Outcome. The outcome of RVT has changed from a frequently lethal complication to one in which more than 85% of children survive. Unfortunately, there are no recent studies assessing long-term morbidity, such as hypertension and renal atrophy.

Spontaneous Venous and Arterial Thrombosis

Spontaneous venous thromboses occur in the adrenal veins, inferior vena cava, portal vein, hepatic veins, and the venous system of the brain (Schmidt and Andrew, 1988; Schmidt and Zipursky, 1984). Spontaneous occlusion of arterial vessels in the absence of a catheter is unusual but can occur in ill infants. Similar to catheter-related thrombi, the clinical presentation reflects the vessel that is occluded. Complete occlusion of a vessel can lead to gangrene and loss of the affected limb or ischemic organ damage (Schmidt and Andrew, 1988; Schmidt and Zipursky, 1984). The presence of systemic hypertension in newborns is frequently related to renal artery thrombosis, even in the absence of a catheter.

Heparin Therapy in Newborns

The lack of consensus for prophylaxis and treatment of thromboembolic complications in newborns reflects the lack of controlled trials in this area. Recommendations for adult patients provide useful guidelines but may not reflect optimal therapy for newborns. Current therapeutic options include supportive care alone, anticoagulant therapy, thrombolytic therapy, and thrombectomy. For most infants who develop thrombotic complications, it is a catheter-related thrombus and is usually clinically silent. In most nurseries, catheters are not routinely screened for associated thrombosis; therefore, by exclusion, most infants with clinically silent thrombi receive supportive care alone. If the decision is made not to use anticoagulants to treat a catheter-related thrombus, the thrombus size should be carefully followed with an objective to determine if it is increasing in size. Anticoagulation should be instituted if the thrombus continues to extend or impair organ function.

Age-Dependent Features. Heparin's anticoagulant activities are mediated by catalysis of AT inhibition of thrombin and, secondarily, of other serine proteases. Although the dosing of heparin therapy in newborns will likely differ from adults, optimal dosing cannot be predicted. Some observations suggest that heparin requirements in newborns will be decreased compared with adults. For example, (1) the capacity of plasmas from healthy newborns to generate thrombin is both delayed and decreased compared with adults and similar to plasma from adults receiving therapeutic amounts of heparin (Andrew et al, 1987; Schmidt et al, 1988); (2) at heparin concentrations in the therapeutic range, the capacity of plasmas from healthy newborns to generate thrombin is barely measurable (Andrew et al, 1994); and (3) the amount of clot-bound thrombin is decreased in newborns owing to low plasma concentrations of prothrombin likely decreasing heparin requirements (Patel et al, 1995). Other observations suggest that heparin requirements will be increased compared with adults. For example, (1) the clearance of heparin is accelerated in newborns (Andrew et al, 1994; McDonald et al, 1981); (2) plasma concentrations of AT are decreased to levels frequently less than 0.40 Units/mL in premature infants, which may limit heparin's antithrombotic activities (Andrew et al, 1987; Andrew et al, 1990; Andrew et al, 1988); and (3) studies in a newborn piglet model of venous thrombosis have shown that low AT levels limit the anticoagulant and antithrombotic effectiveness of heparin (Schmidt et al, 1988; Shiozaki et al, 1993).

Indications, Therapeutic Range, and Dose. Indications for heparin therapy in newborns remain unclear. Although the benefits of heparin therapy in newborns are likely similar to those in adults, the relative risk of major bleeding may be increased. Infants with extending thrombotic complications, or with threatened organ or limb viability, may benefit from heparin therapy.

Therapeutic ranges reflect the optimal risk/benefit ratio of anticoagulant therapy with regard to recurrent thrombotic events and bleeding complications. In the absence of clinical trials in newborns, one approach is to use heparin in doses that achieve the lower therapeutic range for adults (Michelson et al, 1995; Schmidt and Andrew, 1992). Close monitoring of the thrombus with objective tests such as ultrasonography is recommended.

Average doses of heparin required in newborns to achieve adult therapeutic APTT values are bolus doses of 75 to 100 U/kg and average maintenance doses of 28 U/kg per hour (Andrew, Marzinotto, 1994). The duration of heparin therapy required for the treatment of thromboembolic complications is uncertain. One approach is to treat for 10 to 14 days with heparin alone (Michelson et al, 1995; Schmidt and Andrew, 1992). If there is subsequent extension of the thrombus in the absence of anticoagulation therapy, further treatment with heparin or oral anticoagulants therapy should be considered. In general, oral anticoagulants should be avoided whenever possible for newborns because of the risk of bleeding and the difficulties in monitoring. There are clear exceptions to this approach, such as homozygous protein C/S deficiency and recurrent thrombotic events.

Adverse Effects. There are two clinically important adverse effects of heparin therapy: major bleeding and, heparin-induced thrombocytopenia (HIT) (Mocan et al, 1991; Murdoch et al 1993; Spadone et al, 1992). In the absence of an alternative etiology, thrombocytopenic patients should be evaluated for HIT and treated with alternative therapy if anticoagulation is required (Hirsh et al, 1995).

Future. In the future, safer anticoagulant agents will be available for newborns (Hirsh and Levine, 1992; Schmidt and Andrew, 1988). For example, in adults LMWH has consistently been shown to be as efficacious and safer than heparin for the prevention and treatment of thrombotic complications. The advantages of LMWH include predictable bioavailability, minimal monitoring, ease of administration, less bleeding, and equal or increased efficacy. LMWHs are particularly helpful in patients, such as sick premature infants, who are vulnerable to bleeding complications. A pilot study has established doses per kilogram required to achieve adult therapeutic ranges (Massicotte et al, 1995).

Oral Anticoagulant Therapy in Newborns

Age-Dependent Features. Oral anticoagulants function by reducing plasma concentrations of the VK-dependent proteins. At birth, levels of the VK-dependent proteins are similar to those found in adults receiving therapeutic amounts of oral anticoagulants for deep venous thrombosis (DVT/PE). In addition, stores of VK are low and a small number of newborns have evidence of a functional VK deficiency state (Bovill et al, 1993). These features significantly increase the sensitivity of newborns to oral anticoagulants and, potentially, their risk of bleeding. Oral anticoagulant therapy should be avoided, when possible, during the first month of life. Unfortunately, a small number of infants require extended anticoagulation therapy; however, heparin cannot be used for extended periods because of the risk of osteopenia. LWMH is an option to be considered; however, studies in newborns are limited.

Indications, Therapeutic Range, and Dose. The optimal therapeutic INR range is unknown for newborns and almost certainly differs from that of adults. Recommendations for oral anticoagulation therapy in adults can be used as a guideline, with the goal of using the lowest effective dose, which can be individualized to some extent. Maintenance doses for therapeutic amounts of oral anticoagulants are age dependent, with infants having the highest requirements per unit of body weight (0.32 mg/kg).

Adverse Effects. Close monitoring of oral anticoagulation in newborns is required to prevent hemorrhagic and recurrent thrombotic complications. Unfortunately, infants have poor venous access as well as complicated medical problems. Weekly or biweekly measurements of the INR are required with frequent dose adjustments (Andrew, Marzinotto, 1994). Doses are affected by diet, medication, and intercurrent illnesses. Breast-fed infants are very sensitive to oral anticoagulants owing to low concentrations of VK in breast milk (Andrew 1992). Daily supplementation of breast-fed infants with small amounts of commercial formulas reduces their sensitivity to oral anticoagulants and their risk of sudden increases in INR values. In contrast with breast-fed infants, infants receiving commercial formulas or total parenteral nutrition are resistant to oral anticoagulants owing to VK supplementation (Haroon et al, 1982; Von Kries et al, 1985). Reducing or removing VK supplementation of total parenteral nutrition significantly reduces the dose requirements. Most infants requiring oral anticoagulants also require other medications on an intermittent and long-term basis. The effects of dosage changes and the introduction of new medications must be closely supervised. A whole blood monitor has been used with success in the monitoring of oral anticoagulants in infants (Massicotte et al, 1995). However, these infants were followed through a pediatric anticoagulation clinic with staff availability at all times.

Antiplatelet Agents in Newborns

Antiplatelet agents are rarely used in newborns for the purpose of antithrombotic therapy. The hyporeactivity of neonatal platelets and the paradoxically short bleeding time suggest that optimal use of antiplatelet agents differs in newborns compared with adults. Aspirin is the most commonly used antiplatelet agent. Empiric low doses of 1 to 5 mg/kg per day have been proposed as adjuvant therapy for

Blalock-Taussig shunts, some endovascular stents, and some cerebrovascular events (Hathaway, 1984).

Thrombolytic Therapy in Newborns

Age-Dependent Features. The activities of thrombolytic agents are dependent on the endogenous concentrations of plasminogen, which are physiologically decreased at birth (Andrew, Brooker, Paes, 1992). Low plasminogen levels result in an impaired capacity to generate plasmin (Corrigan et al, 1989) and a decreased capacity to thrombolyse fibrin clots (Andrew, Brooker, Paes, 1992). Increasing plasma concentrations of plasminogen with purified plasminogen resulted in fibrin clot lysis that was greater than for adult plasma, likely due to the decreased levels of $\alpha_2 AP$ in newborns' plasma. If an infant does not respond to thrombolytic therapy, replacement of plasminogen should be considered.

Indications, Therapeutic Range, and Dose. Infants who develop serious thrombotic complications, defined by organ or limb impairment, may benefit from thrombolytic therapy. The clinical objective is to remove the clot as quickly and safely as possible. The surgical removal of a clot in a major vessel in infants can be curative; however, it is technically difficult and poses a considerable life-threatening risk to infants who often are premature. In the absence of contraindications, the use of thrombolytic agents for these infants is a preferred approach.

There is no therapeutic range for thrombolytic agents. However, a variety of coagulation tests are used to monitor the activities of thrombolytic agents to ensure that a fibrinogen/fibrinolytic effect is present. These tests include fibrinogen concentrations, thrombin clotting time, fibrin/fibrinogen degradation products, and D-dimer. When thrombolytic therapy is used, it is advisable when possible, to correct other concurrent hemostatic problems such as thrombocytopenia and VK deficiency.

Thrombolytic therapy is used in low doses to restore catheter patency and in higher doses in children with extensive DVT or massive PE. Streptokinase (SK) should not be used to re-establish CVL patency because of the possibility of allergic reactions with repeated doses. For CVL patency, one commonly used low-dose protocol is to instill 2 or 3 mL of urokinase (UK) (5000 U/mL) for 2 to 4 hours (Kellam et al, 1987; Mirro et al, 1989; Morris et al, 1990; Winthrop and Wesson, 1984). Short infusions of low-dose UK have also been used if direct instillation of UK did not re-establish patency. One approach is to infuse UK at 150 U/kg per hour for 8 hours and reassess with objective tests.

A wide range of higher doses was used for systemic therapy with all three thrombolytic agents (Leaker et al, 1995). The most commonly used protocols are summarized in Table 88–12. The choice of agent reflected the decade and indication. In the 1970s and 1980s, SK was most commonly used for thrombotic complications of cardiac catheterization (92%), whereas tPA became the preferred agent during the 1990s (76%). In contrast, UK was the most commonly used agent for thromboembolism due to CVL (58%) and UC (27%).

Delivery of thrombolytic agent was agent specific. UK

TABLE 88-12

Thrombolytic Therapy for Pediatric Patients*

Low Dose for Blocked Catheters		
	Regimen	Monitoring
Instillation	UK (5000 U/mL) 1.5–3 mL/lumen 2–4 hr	None
Infusion	UK (150 U/kg/hr) per lumen 12–48 hr	Fibrinogen, TCT, PT, APTT

Systemic Thrombolytic Therapy†			
	Load	Maintenance	Monitoring
UK	4000 U/kg	4000 U/kg/hr	Fibrinogen, TCT, PT, APTT
SK	4000 U/kg (maximum 250,000 units)	2000 U/kg/hr	Same
TPA	None	0.5 mg/kg/hr for 6 hr	Same

* Values provided are starting suggestions; some patients may respond to longer or shorter courses of therapy.

† Start heparin therapy either during or immediately on completion of thrombolytic therapy. A loading dose of heparin may be omitted. The length of time for optimal maintenance is uncertain.

UK, urokinase; SK, streptokinase; TPA, tissue plasminogen activator; TCT, thrombin clotting time; PT, prothrombin time; APTT, partial thromboplastin time.

was usually administered locally using an indwelling catheter (61% of patients), whereas both tPA and SK were usually administered from a peripheral site (87% and 98% of patients, respectively). The duration of tPA therapy was 12 hours or less in 91% of patients compared with a minimum of 48 hours in 66% of patients treated with UK and a median of 24 hours for SK therapy in 78% of patients (Leaker et al 1995a, 1995b).

Efficacy and Adverse Effects. Resolution of thrombosis was difficult to assess accurately because objective testing was not uniformly applied or reported (69%). The literature and institutional study suggest that resolution was accomplished in more than 80% of patients with all three agents but with vastly different durations of therapy (Leaker et al, 1995a, 1995b). Bleeding at local sites was frequent and required transfusion in 54% of children (Leaker et al, 1995a, 1995b). However, severe bleeding, such as into the central nervous system, was rare (<1%) (Deeg et al, 1992). Treatment of mild bleeding secondary to thrombolytic therapy consists of local measures (pressure, topical thrombin preparations), and transfusion of packed red blood cells (PRBCs) is necessary. Treatment of major bleeding consists of stopping the thrombolytic therapy, plasma, and/or cryoprecipitate and consideration of an antifibrinolytic agent.

QUANTITATIVE PLATELET DISORDERS

Platelet counts in healthy infants and fetuses (18 to 30 weeks' GA) are similar to adults ($150 \times 10^9/L$) (Aballi and

de Lamerens, 1962; Andrew and Kelton, 1984; Beverley et al 1984; Forestier et al, 1986; Gill, 1983; Mehta et al, 1980; Pearson, 1978). Thrombocytopenia in newborns is defined as a platelet count less than $150 \times 10^9/L$ and requires investigation but not necessarily treatment. Mean volumes of newborn platelets are similar to adults, with values less than 10 fL (range of 7 to 9 fL) (Beverley et al, 1984; Castle et al, 1986; Mehta et al, 1980). Postnatally, mean platelet volumes increase slightly over the first 2 weeks of life, concomitant with an increase in platelet count (Arad et al, 1986; Kipper and Sieger, 1982).

Epidemiology

Thrombocytopenia is the most common hemostatic abnormality in NICUs. One prospective study (Andrew, 1987; Castle et al, 1986) and five retrospective reviews (Austin and Darlow, 1988; Gajl-Paczaloska, 1964; Mehta et al, 1980; Lupton et al, 1988; Samuels et al, 1987) provide the most reliable information on the epidemiology and clinical impact of thrombocytopenia in newborns. Nearly 25% of sick infants develop thrombocytopenia, which is trivial for some infants with a platelet count between 100 and 150 $\times 10^9/L$. However, in more than 50% of affected infants platelet counts fall below $100 \times 10^9/L$ and 20% of infants have platelet counts less than $50 \times 10^9/L$. The natural history of thrombocytopenia in sick newborns is remarkably consistent. It is present by day 2 of life in 75% of infants, reaches a nadir by day 4, and recovers to more than 150 $\times 10^9/L$ by day 10 of life in nearly 90% of infants. Although mild thrombocytopenia may not be clinically relevant, it is indicative of an underlying pathologic process. However, the clinical relevance of mild thrombocytopenia remains to be proved.

Pathogenesis

The pathogenesis of neonatal thrombocytopenia can be considered to be the result of decreased platelet production, increased platelet destruction, platelet pooling in an enlarged spleen, or a combination of these mechanisms. Determining the mechanism responsible for thrombocytopenia is important because the risk of bleeding and management is dependent on the mechanism. Increased platelet destruction is the mechanism responsible for thrombocytopenia in most infants (Castle et al, 1986; Castle et al, 1987). Splenic sequestration contributes to thrombocytopenia in some infants (Castle et al, 1987).

The evidence for increased platelet consumption consists of increased mean platelet volumes (MPVs), the presence of megakaryocytes in the bone marrow, and short platelet survivals. Although the MPV is similar to that of adults at birth, it increases by day 7 of life in both thrombocytopenic infants and sick nonthrombocytopenic infants. The increase in MPV parallels a decrease in platelet count, suggesting that increased consumption of platelets occurs in many sick infants. Similar numbers of megakaryocytes are present in bone marrow biopsies from thrombocytopenic infants and nonthrombocytopenic infants. Finally, the strongest evidence of platelet consumption comes from uniformly short platelet survivals in thrombocytopenic infants. Hypersplenism also contributed to thrombocytopenia in some infants.

Increased Platelet Destruction

Increased platelet destruction causing thrombocytopenia can be classified as nonimmune or immune events. For newborns, nonimmune causes of thrombocytopenia include DIC and exchange transfusion (Castle et al, 1986). Exchange transfusions and intrauterine transfusions cause thrombocytopenia by a dilutional effect, depending on the amount of blood transfused (Austin and Darlow, 1988; Stuart et al, 1987). After an exchange transfusion, platelet counts increase within 3 days and reach pre-exchange levels by about 7 days (Hathaway and Bonnar, 1978). Increased platelet-associated IgG (PAIgG) or complement causes immune thrombocytopenia. For reasons that are not clear, 50% of infants with platelet counts less than $100 \times 10^9/L$ have increased amounts of PAIgG on their platelets (Samuels et al, 1987; Tate et al, 1981). Underlying diseases for these infants include sepsis (Tate et al, 1981), preeclampsia (Podolsak, 1973), maternal idiopathic thrombocytopenic purpura, and neonatal alloimmune thrombocytopenia.

Disease States Associated with Platelet Consumption.
Table 88–13 delineates the many pathologic states associated with neonatal thrombocytopenia (Andrew and Kelton, 1984; Gill, 1983; Hathaway and Bonnar, 1978; Pearson and McIntosh, 1978). Thrombocytopenia secondary to acute and chronic asphyxia is likely the result of concurrent DIC (Castle et al, 1988). Mechanisms responsible for bacterial sepsis-induced thrombocytopenia include DIC, endothelial damage, platelet aggregation secondary to binding of bacterial products to platelet membrane, immune-mediated thrombocytopenia, and decreased production due to marrow infection (Patrick and Lazarchick, 1990; Tate et al, 1981; Weinblatt et al, 1987). Mechanisms responsible for thrombocytopenia due to viruses include loss of sialic acid from platelet membrane due to viral neuraminidase, intravascular platelet aggregation, and degeneration of megakaryocytes. Congenital rubella causes thrombocytopenia in 75% of affected infants with platelet counts ranging from 20 to $60 \times 10^9/L$ for the first 4 to 8 weeks of life. For premature infants, thrombocytopenia frequently complicates other disorders such as RDS, persistent pulmonary hypertension, necrotizing enterocolitis, preeclampsia, and hyperbilirubinemia treated with phototherapy (Ballin et al, 1987; Stuart et al, 1987). Persistent pulmonary hypertension in newborns may be due to intrapulmonary platelet aggregation and release of platelet-derived vasoactive substances such as thromboxane A_2 (Horgan et al, 1985). Infants with necrotizing enterocolitis are frequently thrombocytopenic with laboratory evidence of DIC. Hyperbilirubinemia and phototherapy are associated with mild thrombocytopenia and short platelet survivals (Castle et al, 1987).

Giant Hemangiomas.
Giant hemangiomas, or Kasabach-Merritt syndrome (Andrew, 1992; Shim, 1995), cause a local consumptive coagulopathy characterized by hypofibrinogenemia, elevated fibrinogen-FDPs, microangiopathic fragmentation of red blood cells, and thrombocytopenia. The thrombocytopenia is usually severe, with platelet

---

TABLE 88–13

Disease States Associated with Neonatal Thrombocytopenia

I. Increased destruction
  A. Immune mediated
      Maternal ITP
      Maternal SLE
      Maternal hyperthyroidism
      Maternal drugs
      Maternal preeclampsia
      Neonatal alloimmune thrombocytopenia
  B. Nonimmune—likely related to DIC
      Asphyxia
      Perinatal aspiration
      Necrotizing enterocolitis
      Hemangiomas
      Neonatal thrombosis
      Respiratory distress syndrome
  C. Unknown
      Hyperbilirubinemia
      Phototherapy
      Polycythemia
      Rh hemolytic disease
      Congenital thrombotic thrombocytopenic purpura
      Total parenteral nutrition
      Inborn error of metabolism
      Wiskott-Aldrich syndrome
      Multiple congenital anomalies
II. Hypersplenism
III. Decreased production of platelets
  A. Bone marrow replacement disorders
      Congenital leukemia
      Congenital leukemoid reactions
      Neuroblastoma
      Histiocytosis
      Osteopetrosis
  B. Bone marrow aplasia
      Thrombocytopenia absent radii
      Amegakaryocytic thrombocytopenia
      Fanconi's anemia
      Other marrow hypoplastic or aplastic disorders

ITP, idiopathic thrombocytopenic purpura; SLE, systemic lupus erythematosus; DIC, disseminated intravascular coagulation.

---

counts less than $50 \times 10^9/L$. Approximately 50% of affected infants experience systemic bleeding during the first month of life.

Drug-Induced Thrombocytopenia.
On rare occasion, transplacental passage of drugs and drug-dependent antibodies can result in both maternal and neonatal thrombocytopenia (Cariou et al, 1988; Corby and Schulman, 1971; Haslom et al, 1974; Levy and Garrettson, 1974; Ylikorkala et al, 1986). Agents implicated are quinine, hydralazine, tolbutamide, and thiazine diuretics. Recently, heparin has been implicated as a cause of thrombocytopenia (heparin-induced thrombocytopenia [HIT]). If HIT is suspected, heparin should be discontinued immediately, and alternative forms of anticoagulation therapy should be considered if necessary.

Other Associations.
Thrombocytopenia is associated with thromboembolic complications, polycythemic infants, he-

molytic anemia, hemolytic-uremic syndrome, and thrombotic thrombocytopenic purpura (TTP) (Murphy et al, 1987).

Decreased Platelet Production

Thrombocytopenia due to decreased platelet production accounts for less than 5% of thrombocytopenic infants (Table 88–14). Etiologies include congenital leukemia, leukemoid reactions in patients with Down syndrome, neuroblastoma, histiocytosis, some viral infections, osteoporosis, and disorders of bone marrow failure. Aplastic disorders include thrombocytopenia absent radius (TAR) syndrome, and amegakaryocytic thrombocytopenia (Hall et al, 1969; Hedberg and Lipton, 1988). Infants with aplastic disorders are at the greatest risk of serious bleeding in the first months of life. Neither splenectomy nor steroids are of benefit for infants with TAR syndrome (Hall et al, 1969; Hedberg and Lipton, 1988). Platelet transfusions are highly effective but should be reserved for symptomatic infants because prophylactic platelet transfusions could result in refractoriness owing to alloimmunization (Hedberg and Lipton, 1988). By several months of age, increased numbers of megakaryocytes usually appear in the bone marrow and platelet counts increase (Hedberg and Lipton, 1988). A functional platelet defect may be present in some children with TAR syndrome (Homans et al, 1988). Isolated amegakaryocytic thrombocytopenia may present with bleeding during the newborn period (Lecompte, 1988).

Hypersplenism

Splenic sequestration, demonstrated by decreased recovery of ^{111}In-oxine–labeled platelets, is a contributing cause of thrombocytopenia and is usually mild, with platelet counts ranging from 50 to 100 $\times$ 10^9/L (Castle et al, 1987).

Clinical Impact of Neonatal Thrombocytopenia

Newborns with consumptive thrombocytopenia are less likely to bleed than are infants with decreased production of platelets. If a platelet function defect is present in addition to thrombocytopenia, the bleeding risk is increased. Choosing a platelet count at which one should intervene, although simplistic, provides a guideline for therapy. Platelet counts less than 50 $\times$ 10^9/L place some otherwise healthy full-term newborns at risk for ICH (Hall et al, 1969; Hedberg and Lipton, 1988; Hegde, 1985). The importance of "moderate" thrombocytopenia (platelet counts between 50 and 100 $\times$ 10^9/L) in sick premature infants has been controversial. The bleeding time, which reflects platelet number and function, is prolonged in about 60% of premature infants with moderate thrombocytopenia and shortens when the platelet count increases above 100 $\times$ 10^9/L (Andrew, Castle, Saigal, 1987). However, maintaining a platelet count over 150 $\times$ 10^9/L with platelet concentrates did not have a beneficial effect on ICH, although it did reduce blood product requirements (Andrew et al, 1993).

Treatment

The management of thrombocytopenic infants depends in part on the underlying disorder. If the infant is bleeding, a trial of platelet concentrates (10 to 20 mL/kg) is indicated. The increased platelet count usually shortens the bleeding time and is frequently clinically effective (Andrew, 1987). Autoimmune and alloimmune thrombocytopenia do not respond to random donor platelet concentrates and require specific forms of therapy.

Alloimmune and Autoimmune Thrombocytopenia

Immune thrombocytopenia should always be suspected in otherwise healthy infants with isolated severe thrombocytopenia. An IgG antiplatelet autoantibody or alloantibody is produced in mothers and crosses the placenta, causing fetal thrombocytopenia. Since the antibody is not autologous, the thrombocytopenia persists only as long as the maternal IgG antibody remains in the infant's circulation. Normally, this would be several months, because the half-life of IgG is approximately 21 days. However, since the antibody binds to platelets, its life span is dependent on the life span of the sensitized platelets and, therefore, can be very short. Therefore, immune thrombocytopenic disorders of neonates are usually short lived but can cause serious bleeding, making the correct diagnosis and management of these disorders all the more important. The differentiation of autoimmune from alloimmune thrombocytopenia in neonates is critical, since the management and severity of these disorders are quite different.

Neonatal Alloimmune Thrombocytopenia

Neonatal alloimmune thrombocytopenia is similar to HDN and neonatal alloimmune neutropenia. All three disorders are caused by maternal IgG alloantibodies that cross the placenta into the fetal circulation, bind to specific cell antigens, and accelerate the removal of the cell type in question from the circulation. Mothers of infants with alloimmune thrombocytopenia have normal platelet counts and no bleeding history, although they may have previously delivered thrombocytopenic newborns. Maternal IgG allo-

TABLE 88–14

Investigations for Classifying Thrombocytopenia by Mechanism

Laboratory Parameter	Increased Platelet Destruction	Decreased Platelet Production
Platelet size	Increased	Normal
Platelet survival	Decreased	Normal
Platelet associated IgG	Often very increased	Usually normal or slightly increased
Bleeding time	Usually prolonged	Prolonged
Other cell lines	Usually normal	Often abnormal
Megakaryocytes	Normal or increased	Decreased
Other bone marrow Cell lines	Normal	Often decreased or abnormal

antibodies are directed against specific paternally derived antigens on the infant's platelets, which are absent from the mother's platelets. The most frequently implicated allo-antigen (in > 75% of cases) is the Pl[A1] (Zw[a]) antigen, which is present on the platelets of 98% of the general population. The second most common alloantigen is Br[a] (Zav[a] Hc[a]) (Karpatkin et al, 1986). Table 88–14 provides the platelet-specific antigen and phenotype frequency in European populations (Moake et al, 1994; Muira et al, 1984). ABO and HLA alloantibodies are infrequent causes of neonatal alloimmune thrombocytopenia (Moake et al, 1994). One potential explanation is that maternal HLA alloantibodies do not enter the fetal circulation in sufficient quantities because they are absorbed by foreign HLA antigens on the placenta (Muira, 1984).

The frequency of neonatal alloimmune thrombocytopenia is approximately 1:3000 to 5000 newborns (Berberich et al, 1974; Blanchette, 1988; Blanchette et al, 1990; Elias et al, 1988; Moake et al, 1994; Mueller-Eckhardt et al, 1989), which is considerably lower than the actual risk based on the frequency of the alloantigens. There is evidence that one or more immune response genes determine the formation of alloantibodies. For example, women possessing the HLA-DR3 alloantigen constitute 70% to 95% of affected patients, corresponding to a 10- to 30-fold increased risk of forming anti-Pl[A1] alloantibodies (De Waal et al, 1986; Mueller-Eckhardt et al, 1989; Reznikoff-Etrevont, 1988; Reznikoss-Etievant 1981). Alloimmunization against the Br[a] alloantigen is associated with Drw6 (Mueller-Eckhardt et al, 1989).

The clinical presentation of neonatal alloimmune thrombocytopenia is usually severe, isolated thrombocytopenia in a healthy, full-term infant. First-born infants are affected as often as subsequent infants. Minor bleeding in the form of petechiae, gastrointestinal tract hemorrhage, hematuria, or hemoptysis frequently occurs (Blanchette, 1988; Mueller-Eckhardt et al, 1989). Of great concern and serious morbidity is the occurrence of ICH in as many as 15% of infants (Blanchette, 1988; Mueller-Eckhardt et al, 1989). ICH may occur prenatally as well as postnatally. Hydrocephalus (Mueller-Eckhardt et al, 1989), porencephalic cysts (Burrows et al, 1988; Friedman and Aster, 1985; Herman et al, 1986; Lam and Shulman, 1985; Mueller-Eckhardt et al, 1989), and epilepsy are a few of the outcomes of ICHs. The severity of bleeding in infants with alloimmune thrombocytopenia may reflect not only the severe thrombocytopenia but also an additional platelet dysfunction caused by antiplatelet alloantibody impairing aggregation by binding to the GP IIb/IIIa.

The diagnosis of alloimmune thrombocytopenia is based on the clinical presentation and the presence of severe thrombocytopenia with a platelet count frequently less than 10×10^9/L. Confirmation by serologic testing follows; however, specific therapy should be instituted immediately. The serologic testing includes typing the mother to determine which platelet alloantigen she is missing and whether an antiplatelet alloantibody is present in her serum (McFarland et al, 1989; Mueller-Eckhardt et al, 1989; von dem Borne et al, 1981). Not infrequently, no alloantibodies can be detected in the maternal serum (Mueller-Eckhardt et al, 1989). Sometimes, testing maternal serum against paternal platelets detects the alloantibody. Platelet-associated IgG is elevated on the newborn's platelets (Kelton et al, 1980).

There are several possible treatments for managing a woman who has had a previously affected infant. First, there is a high probability that all subsequent infants will be affected. Because of the risk of ICH in utero, monitoring for the presence of ICH and therapeutic intervention begin prenatally. All potentially affected fetuses should be monitored by ultrasonography after approximately 20 weeks, with the objective of detecting evidence of ICH. In some centers, cordocentesis is performed to confirm the presence of thrombocytopenia as well as to provide a route for the regular administration of compatible platelets to treat affected fetuses (Daffos et al, 1984; Daffos et al, 1985; Kaplan et al, 1988; Nicolini et al, 1988). An alternative, less invasive approach is the intravenous administration of IgG (with or without dexamethasone) to the mother in the latter part of the pregnancy (Bussel et al, 1988; Davies et al, 1986; Tchernia et al, 1984). However, this approach is not effective for all fetuses (Mir et al, 1988). The relative safety and efficacy of these differing approaches require further clarification. Elective cesarean section is recommended at the time of fetal maturity to facilitate the postnatal management of the infant (Editorial, 1989). The necessity of cesarean section to prevent ICH has not been proved.

The cornerstone of management of affected infants is the transfusion of washed, irradiated maternal platelets (Adner et al, 1969). These platelets can be prepared before delivery if a planned cesarean section is the mode of delivery. Although matched platelets from an unrelated donor may also be used, maternal platelets are preferred because of their certain compatibility, availability, and safety. Most prepartum or postpartum mothers can easily tolerate the removal of 1 unit of whole blood and subsequent reinfusion of their red blood cells. Maternal platelets must be washed to remove maternal alloantibody and irradiated to prevent graft-versus-host disease caused by maternal lymphocytes (Martin et al, 1983). Frozen maternal platelets have also been used successfully (Liebermann, 1961). Random donor platelets should be used in an infant with significant hemorrhage while awaiting maternal platelets. The infusion of random donor platelets may transiently help the bleeding infant, and the lack of increase in platelet number confirms the diagnosis. Intravenous IgG may also be effective in raising the platelet count in affected infants in the absence of, or in addition to, maternal platelets (Blanchette, 1988; Elases et al, 1967; Mueller-Eckhardt et al, 1989; Sidiropoulos and Straume, 1984). Other forms of therapy that have been previously used include corticosteroids (Pearson et al, 1964) and exchange transfusions to remove maternal alloantibody. Such approaches are no longer indicated and probably are not effective (Katz et al, 1984; McIntosh et al, 1973; Pearson et al, 1964).

Autoimmune Neonatal Thrombocytopenia

Newborns with thrombocytopenia secondary to maternal autoimmune disorders present with a milder clinical course compared with that in newborns affected with alloimmune disorders. Usually the mother has ITP, but autoimmune platelet consumption can also be associated with other maternal disorders such as systemic lupus erythematous (SLE), lymphoproliferative disorders, and hyperthyroidism. Serologically, the antibody is directed against antigens common to maternal and neonatal platelets. The management of the fetus and infant of a mother with ITP is controversial. First, maternal ITP must be distinguished from the frequent occurrence of mild thrombocytopenia in healthy pregnant women at term. The latter appears to have no adverse effect on either the mothers or their infants and does not necessitate any specific treatment or delivery by cesarean section (Burrows and Kelton, 1988).

Based on case reports of ICH in infants affected by maternal ITP, recommendations for delivery by cesarean section (Jerrito et al, 1973) and prenatal platelet count monitoring have been made in hopes of lowering infant morbidity and mortality (Daffos et al, 1988). However, recent information from a large consecutive case study has drawn these recommendations into question (Burrows and Kelton, 1990). In the older reports, the lowest platelet count, not the cord platelet count, was used to support the recommendation of cesarean section for the fetus. The platelet count nadir for infants with thrombocytopenia secondary to maternal ITP occurs not at birth but several days subsequent to birth (Karpatkin et al, 1981; Kelton, 1983). Consequently, the decision for prenatal obstetric intervention must be made on the basis of the platelet count at the time of birth and the risk of ICH. The cord platelet count is rarely below 50×10^9/L. ICH rarely, if ever, occurs prenatally, and it is not clear that it is related to the birth process. In the infant, the true risk of ICH secondary to maternal ITP is unclear, because the older literature is biased by the inclusion of mothers with disorders other than ITP, such as SLE.

Based on recent consecutive patient cohort clinical studies, the following recommendations for management can be made. The pregnant mother should be treated according to her own platelet count and not the hemostatic risk to the fetus. There are no reliable predictors of severe thrombocytopenia in the infant except for the direct determination of the fetal platelet count by cordocentesis. However, this procedure has risks itself of fetal morbidity and mortality that appear similar to, or perhaps in excess of, the risk of serious bleeding in utero for maternal ITP (Moise et al, 1988). Fetal scalp sampling to determine fetal platelet counts has been advocated in the past (Ayromlooi, 1978; Scott et al, 1980); however, the low platelet count results in many unnecessary cesarean sections. The maternal platelet count itself does not predict which infants will be thrombocytopenic (Barbul et al, 1985). Some women who are "cured" of ITP by splenectomy can still deliver thrombocytopenic babies. Other women who are severely thrombocytopenic will not deliver thrombocytopenic infants. The predictive values of both elevated maternal PAIgG (Kelton et al, 1982) and serum platelet-bindable IgG (Cines et al, 1982; Mazzucconi et al, 1985) are too low to permit any role in the management of patients with ITP. Thus, there are no reliable predictors of severe thrombocytopenia in the infant. Most infants born to mothers with ITP do not have serious thrombocytopenia at birth. Therefore, prenatal treatment of mothers with corticosteroids or intravenous IgG would be rarely indicated for the treatment of the fetus (Blanchette et al, 1989; Davidson et al, 1987; Sacher and King, 1988; Wenske et al, 1983).

If the woman has had previous uncomplicated deliveries and the obstetrician anticipates no problems, spontaneous vaginal delivery is appropriate. Infants for whom a difficult procedure is anticipated can be delivered by cesarean section, but the evidence indicating that this approach is safer for the fetus is lacking. The percentage of infants with platelet counts less than 150×10^9/L ranges from 36% to 41% (Muira, 1984), and less than 50×10^9/L ranges from 10% to 58% (Muira, 1984). However, the frequency of cord platelet counts fewer than 150×10^9/L is only 18%, demonstrating that most infants are born with normal platelet counts (Burrows and Kelton, 1990). Infants born to mothers with ITP should be monitored closely, because the platelet count often falls postnatally. A platelet count of fewer than 50×10^9/L is a useful guide for institution of therapy.

Clinically, the infants are full term and very healthy, with either no clinical manifestations or mild clinical manifestations of thrombocytopenia in the form of petechiae. These infants do not have clinical or laboratory evidence of any other neonatal problems, such as DIC, hepatosplenomegaly, and dysmaturity. The diagnosis of autoimmune thrombocytopenia in newborns is made predominantly by the clinical presentation of mother and infant as well as the exclusion of other known causes of thrombocytopenia. In the past, case reports or case series have suggested that a combination of therapeutic maneuvers may be helpful. These interventions include irradiated platelet transfusion and corticosteroids (Karpatkin, 1984; Kryc and Corrigan, 1983; Sacher and King, 1988). More recently, intravenous IgG has been used after delivery (Ballin et al, 1988; Barton et al, 1987; Castaman et al, 1985; Chirico et al, 1983; Ciccimarra et al, 1984; Hanada and Ono, 1985; Hara et al, 1988; Le Gall et al, 1986; Newland et al, 1984; Ronconi et al, 1986; Stabile et al, 1986; Wenske et al, 1984) and is safe and effective, resulting in an 80% response rate in the infant when it is used alone or in combination with steroids. It is unclear whether the addition of steroids to intravenous IgG is beneficial. The 90% response rate is similar to the response rate of childhood ITP to intravenous IgG, and the response rate is faster than that due to corticosteroids alone (Bullin et al, 1988; Barton et al, 1987; Karpatkin, 1984). Clearly, prospective studies are required to confirm the high rate of response to intravenous IgG and the beneficial effects of intravenous IgG over other forms of therapy. We recommend the use of 1 g/kg, and if the infant is bleeding, irradiated platelet transfusions should also be given at doses of 10 to 20 mL/kg. A poor increment as well as a rapid fall in platelet number supports the diagnosis of autoimmune thrombocytopenia. If the infant does not respond and has evidence of bleeding, methyl prednisolone (3 mg/kg) may be substituted for prednisone, and intravenous IgG therapy is repeated.

Giant Hemangiomas

Giant hemangiomas, or Kasabach-Merritt syndrome (Fost and Esterly, 1968; Johnson et al, 1984; Orchard et al, 1989; Shim, 1995), cause a local consumptive coagulopathy characterized by hypofibrinogenemia, elevated fibrinogen/

fibrin degradation products, microangiopathic fragmentation of red blood cells, and thrombocytopenia (Larsen et al, 1987). The thrombocytopenia is usually severe, with platelet counts less than 50×10^9/L (Andrew, 1992). Approximately 50% of affected infants experience systemic bleeding during the first month of life (Andrew, 1992).

Thrombocytosis

Elevated platelet counts occur frequently in premature infants at approximately 4 to 6 weeks' postnatal age (Chan et al, 1989). There are no clinical manifestations of neonatal thrombocytosis, and therapeutic intervention is not indicated.

QUALITATIVE PLATELET DISORDERS

There is no evidence to suggest that the physiologic hyporeactivity of neonatal platelets in response to some agents contributes to bleeding. Pathologic impairment of platelet function may occur in some pathologic states in both mothers and infants. In mothers, conditions that have been implicated include some drugs, diabetes, diet, smoking, and ethanol. For infants, implicated conditions include some drugs, perinatal aspiration syndrome, hyperbilirubinemia, phototherapy, renal failure, and hepatic failure.

Aspirin

Salicylate crosses the placenta and can be detected in fetuses following maternal ingestion (Ylikorkala et al, 1986). Clearance of salicylate is slower in newborns than adults, potentially placing infants at risk for longer periods (Levy and Garrettson, 1974). However, in vitro studies have not demonstrated an additive effect of aspirin on newborn platelets (Stuart and Dusse, 1985; Ts'ao, 1977), and evidence linking maternal aspirin ingestion to clinically important bleeding in newborns is weak (Pomerance et al, 1987). There is little reason to have serious concerns about maternal ingestion of aspirin, but it is reasonable to advise mothers not to ingest aspirin, unless specifically indicated by their physician.

Indomethacin

Indomethacin is an antiplatelet agent used for nonsurgical closure of a patent ductus arteriosus in premature infants (Heymann et al, 1976). Indomethacin, like salicylate, has a longer half-life in newborns (21 to 24 hours) compared with adults (2 to 3 hours) and probably results from underdevelopment of hepatic drug metabolism, renal excretory function, or altered protein binding. Indomethacin inhibits platelet function in newborns, as evidenced by prolonged bleeding times. Randomized, controlled trials have provided conflicting conclusions on the effect of indomethacin on intraventricular hemorrhage in premature infants (Ment et al, 1988).

Maternal Diabetes

The reactivity of platelets from diabetic mothers and their infants is increased, with enhanced thromboxane B_2 pro-

duction, enhanced platelet aggregation (Kaapa et al, 1986; Shearer et al, 1982), and a lower threshold to many aggregating agents (Sagel et al, 1975). The enhanced platelet function in diabetes is associated with an increased synthesis of a prostaglandin E–like material that crosses the placenta and can affect the fetus (Halushka et al, 1977). The evidence linking enhanced platelet reactivity to thromboembolic complications in newborns is weak (Cowett and Schwartz, 1982; Oppenheimer and Esterly, 1965).

Diet

Alterations in the diet of mothers or infants during the postnatal period can affect newborn platelet function. Increasing the ratio of polyunsaturated to saturated fatty acids in the diet of mothers breast-feeding their infants results in an increased concentration of linoleic acid and enhanced thromboxane B_2 production (Kaapa et al, 1986). Infants receiving a diet deficient in essential fatty acids may have arachidonic acid depletion and platelet dysfunction (Dixon and Rosse, 1975; Friedman et al, 1976; Friedman et al, 1978). Vitamin E functions as an antioxidant and an inhibitor of platelet aggregation/release in humans. There are case reports of vitamin E–deficient infants with increased platelet aggregation that reversed following vitamin E supplementation (Khurshid et al, 1975; Lake et al, 1977).

Amniotic Fluid

Amniotic fluid contains procoagulant activity that enhances the generation of thromboxane A_2 by platelets (Levin et al, 1983; Segall et al, 1980; Stuart et al, 1987; Suzuki et al, 1976). Infants who develop a perinatal aspiration syndrome have pulmonary hypertension characterized by platelet thrombi in the pulmonary microcirculation. The exact mechanisms leading to persistent pulmonary hypertension in these infants are unknown, although alterations in prostaglandin synthesis have been suggested (Kaapa, 1987; Lake et al, 1977), in addition to thrombocytopenia, hypoxia, and acidosis (Levin et al, 1983; Mehta et al, 1980; Segall et al, 1980; Stuart et al, 1987; Suzuki et al, 1976).

Nitric Oxide

NO prevents adhesion of platelets to endothelial cells and inhibits aggregation of cord platelets induced by ADP, similar to results in adults (Bodzenta-LaRoszyk et al, 1994).

REFERENCES

Aarts PAMM, Bolhuis PA, Sakariassen KS, et al: Red blood cell size is important for adherence of blood platelets to artery subendothelium. Blood 62:214, 1983.

Adcock D, Brozna J, Marlar R: Proposed classification and pathologic mechanisms of purpura fulminans and skin necrosis. Semin Thromb Haemostas 16:333, 1990.

Adcock D, Hicks M: Dermatopathology of skin necrosis associated with purpura fulminans. Semin Thromb Haemostas 16:283, 1990.

Adner MM, Fisch GR, Starobin SG: Use of "compatible" platelet transfusions in treatment of congenital isoimmune thrombocytopenic purpura. N Engl J Med 280:244, 1969.

Ahlsten G, Ewald U, Kindahl H, Tuvemo T: Aggregation of and thromboxane B_2 synthesis in platelets from newborn infants of smoking and non-smoking mothers. Pros Leuk Med 19:167, 1985.

Ahlsten G, Ewald U, Tuvemo T: Maternal smoking reduces prostacyclin formation in human umbilical arteries: A study on strictly selected pregnancies. Acta Obstet Gynecol Scand 65:645, 1986.

Alebouyeh M, Lusher J, Ameri M, et al: The effect of 5-hydroxytryptamine and epinephrine on newborn platelets. Eur J Pediatr 128:163, 1978.

Ambrus C, Weintraub D, Ambrus J: Studies on hyaline membrane disease: III. Therapeutic trial of urokinase-activated human plasmin. Pediatrics 38:231, 1966.

Ambrus C, Choi T, Cunnanan E, et al: Prevention of hyaline membrane disease with plasminogen: A cooperative study. JAMA 237(17):1837, 1977.

Ambrus C, Jung O, Ambrus J, et al: The fibrinolysin system and its relationship to disease in the newborn. Am J Pediatr Hematol Oncol 1(3):251, 1979.

Andrew M: Platelets in newborns: Physiology and pathology. *In* Luban N (Ed): Transfusion Sciences. Elmsford, NY, Pergamon Press, 1991, p 207.

Andrew M: The hemostatic system in the infant. *In* Nathan D, Oski F (Eds): Hematology of Infancy and Childhood. Philadelphia, WB Saunders, 1992, p 115.

Andrew M, Brooker L: Blood component therapy in neonatal hemostatic disorders. Transf Med Rev 9(3):231, 1995.

Andrew M, Brooker L, Paes B, Weitz J: Fibrin clot lysis by thrombolytic agents is impaired in newborns due to a low plasminogen concentration. Thromb Haemostas 68(3):325, 1992.

Andrew M, Caco C, Vegh P, et al: Benefits of platelet transfusions in premature infants: A randomized, controlled trial [Abstract]. Thromb Haemostas 65(6):721, 1991.

Andrew M, Caco C, Vegh P, et al: A randomized controlled trial of platelet transfusions in thrombocytopenic premature infants. J Pediatr 123:285, 1993.

Andrew M, Castle V, Mitchell L, Paes B: A modified bleeding time in the infant. Am J Hematol 30:190, 1989.

Andrew M, Castle V, Saigal S, et al: Clinical impact of neonatal thrombocytopenia. J Pediatr 110:457, 1987.

Andrew M, Mitchell L, Berry L, et al: Fibrinogen has a rapid turnover in the healthy newborn lamb. Pediatr Res 23:249, 1988.

Andrew M, David M, Adams M, et al: Venous thromboembolic complications (VTE) in children: First analyses of the Canadian Registry of VTE. Blood 83(5):1251, 1994.

Andrew M, Marzinotto V, Blanchette, V, et al: Heparin therapy in pediatric patients: A prospective cohort study. Pediatr Res 35:78, 1994.

Andrew M, Marzinotto V, Brooker L, et al: Oral anticoagulant therapy in pediatric patients: A prospective study. Thromb Haemostas 71(3):265, 1994.

Andrew M, Marzinotto V, Pencharz P, et al: A cross-sectional study of catheter-related thrombosis in children receiving total parenteral nutrition at home. J Pediatr 126:358, 1995.

Andrew M, Mitchell L, Paes B, et al: An anticoagulant dermatan sulphate proteoglycan circulates in the pregnant women and her fetus. J Clin Invest 89:321, 1992.

Andrew M, Mitchell L, Vegh P, Ofosu F: Thrombin regulation in children differs from adults in the absence and presence of heparin. Thromb Haemostas 72(6):836, 1994.

Andrew M, O'Brodovich H, Mitchell L: The fetal lamb coagulation system during normal birth. Am J Hematol 28:116, 1988.

Andrew M, Ofosu F, Schmidt B, et al: Heparin clearance and ex vivo recovery in newborn piglets and adult pigs. Thromb Res 52:517, 1988.

Andrew M, Paes B, Bowker J, Vegh P: Evaluation of an automated bleeding time device in the newborn. Am J Hematol 35:275, 1990.

Andrew M, Paes B, Johnston M: Development of the hemostatic system in the neonate and young infant. Am J Pediatr Hematol Oncol 12:95, 1990.

Andrew M, Paes B, Milner R, et al: Development of the human coagulation system in the full-term infant. Blood 70(1):165, 1987.

Andrew M, Paes B, Milner R, et al: Development of the human coagulation system in the healthy premature infant. Blood 72:1651, 1988.

Andrew M, Schmidt B, Mitchell L, et al: Thrombin generation in newborn plasma is critically dependent on the concentration of prothrombin. Thromb Haemostas 63:27, 1990.

Andrew M, Vegh P, Johnston M, et al: Maturation of the hemostatic system during childhood. Blood 80(8):1998, 1992.

Ankola P, Atakent Y: Effect of adding heparin in very low concentration to the infusate to prolong the patency of umbilical artery catheters. Am J Perinatol 10(3):229, 1993.

Aster R: Pooling of platelets in the spleen: Role in the pathogenesis of "hypersplenic" thrombocytopenia. J Clin Invest 45:645, 1966.

Auberger K: Evaluation of a new protein C concentrate and comparison of protein C assays in a child with congenital protein C deficiency. Ann Hematol 64(3):146, 1992.

Auletta M, Headington J: Purpura fulminans: A cutaneous manifestation of severe protein C deficiency. Arch Dermatol 124:1387, 1988.

Aurousseau M, Amiral J, Boffa M: Level of plasma thrombomodulin in neonates and children [Abstract]. Thromb Haemostas 65(6):1232, 1991.

Austin N, Darlow BA: Transfusion-associated fall in platelet count in very-low-birthweight infants. Aust Paediatr J 24:354, 1988.

Ayromlooi J: A new approach to the management of immunologic thrombocytopenic purpura in pregnancy. Am J Obstet Gynecol 130:235, 1978.

Bada H, Korones S, Kolni H, et al: Partial plasma exchange transfusion improves cerebral hemodynamics in symptomatic neonatal polycytemia. Am J Med Sci 291:11, 1986.

Balakrishnan G, Brownlie J, Webber R, Gibson B: Enhanced thrombin generation in patients receiving intensive care. Arch Dis Child 66:1413, 1991.

Ballin A, Andrew M, Ling E, et al: High-dose intravenous gammaglobulin therapy for neonatal autoimmune thrombocytopenia. J Pediatr 112:789, 1988.

Ballin A, Koren G, Kohelet D, et al: Reduction of platelet counts induced by mechanical ventilation in newborn infants. J Pediatr 111:445, 1987.

Bandstra E, Montalvo BM, Goldberg RN: Prophylactic indomethacin for prevention of intraventricular hemorrhage in premature infants. Pediatrics 82(4):533, 1988.

Barbui T, Cortelazzo S, Viero P, et al: Idiopathic thrombocytopenic purpura and pregnancy: Maternal platelet count and antiplatelet antibodies do not predict the risk of neonatal thrombocytopenia. La Ric Clin Lab 15:139, 1985.

Barnard D, Simmons M, Hathaway W: Coagulation studies in extremely premature infants. Pediatr Res 13:1330, 1979.

Bartlett R, Roloff D, Cornell R, et al: Extracorporeal circulation in neonatal respiratory failure: A prospective randomized study. Pediatrics 76(4):479, 1985.

Barton JC, Saleh MN, Stedman CM, Lobuglio AT: Immune thrombocytopenia: Effects of maternal gammaglobulin infusion on maternal and fetal serum, platelet, and monocyte IgG [Case report]. Am J Med Sci 293:112, 1987.

Behrmann BA, Chan WK, Finer NN: Resurgence of hemorrhagic disease of the newborn: A report of three cases. Can Med Assoc J 133:884, 1985.

Ben-Tal O, Zivelin A, Seligsohn U: The relative frequency of hereditary thrombotic disorders among 107 patients and thrombophilia in Israel. Thromb Haemostas 61(1):50, 1989.

Berberich FR, Cuene SA, Chard RL, Hartmann JR: Thrombotic thrombocytopenic purpura. J Pediatr 84:503, 1974.

Benson JWT, Drayton MR, Hayward C, et al: Multicentre trial of ethamsylate for prevention of periventricular haemorrhage in very-low-birthweight infants. Lancet 2:1297, 1986.

Binder L: Hemorrhagic disease of the newborn: An unusual etiology of neonatal bleeding. Ann Emerg Med 15:935, 1986.

Blanchard RA, Furie BC, Jorgensen M, et al: Acquired vitamin K–dependent carboxylation deficiency in liver disease. N Engl J Med 305:242, 1981.

Blanchette V: Neonatal alloimmune thrombocytopenia: A clinical perspective. Curr Stud Hematol Blood Transfus 54:112, 1988.

Blanchette VS, Chen LC, Salomon de Friedberg Z, et al: Alloimmunization to the P1A1 platelet antigen: Results of a prospective study. Br J Haematol 74:209, 1990.

Blanchette VS, Sacher RA, Ballem PJ, et al: Commentary on the management of autoimmune thrombocytopenia during pregnancy and in the neonatal period. Blut 59:121, 1989.

Bleyer WA, Breckenridge RT: Studies on the detection of adverse drug reactions in the newborn: II. The effects of prenatal aspirin on newborn hemostasis. JAMA 213:2049, 1970.

Bodzenta-Lukaszyk A, Gabryelewicz A, Lukaszyk A, et al: Nitric oxide synthase inhibition and platelet function. Thromb Res 75(6):667, 1994.

Bosque E, Weaver L: Continuous versus intermittent heparin infusion of umbilical artery catheters in the newborn infant. J Pediatr 108:141, 1986.

Bovill E, Soll R, Lynch M, et al: Vitamin K_1 metabolism and the production of des-carboxy prothrombin and protein C in the term and premature neonate. Blood 81(1):77, 1993.

Brinkhous KM, Smith HP, Warner ED: Plasma prothrombin level in normal infancy and in hemorrhagic disease of the newborn [Abstract]. Am J Med Sci 193:475, 1937.

Brockmeier FK, Nordhagen R, Finne PH: Neonatal alloimmune thrombocytopenia. Acta Paediatr Scand 72:583, 1983.

Brown AK, Zeulzer WW, Burnett HH: Studies on the neonatal development of the glucoronide system. J Clin Invest 37:332, 1958.

Bruchsaler FS: Vitamin K and the prenatal and postnatal prevention of hemorrhagic disease in newborn infants. J Pediatr 18:317, 1941.

Burrows R, Caco C, Kelton J: Neonatal alloimmune thrombocytopenia: Spontaneous in utero intracranial hemorrhage. Am J Hematol 28:98, 1988.

Burrows RF, Kelton JG: Incidentally detected thrombocytopenia in healthy mothers and their infants. N Engl J Med 319:142, 1988.

Burrows R, Kelton J: Low fetal risks in pregnancies associated with idiopathic thrombocytopenic purpura do not justify obstetrical interventions. Am J Obstet Gynecol 163:1147, 1990.

Bussel J, Berkowitz R, McFarland J, et al: Antenatal treatment of neonatal alloimmune thrombocytopenia. N Engl J Med 319:1374, 1988.

Butler NR, Golding J, Haslam M, Stewart-Brown S: Recent findings of the 1970 Child Health and Education Study: Preliminary communication. J R Soc Med 75:781, 1982.

Cairney AEL, Andrew M, Greenberg M, et al: Wilms' tumor in three patients with Bloom syndrome. J Pediatr 111:414, 1987.

Cariou R, Toblem G, Belucci S, et al: Effect of lupus anticoagulant or antithrombogenic properties of endothelial cells: Inhibition of thrombomodulin-dependent protein C activation. Thromb Haemostas 60:54, 1988.

Cartwright GW, Culbertson K, Schreiner RL, Garg BP: Changes in clinical presentation of term infants with intracranial hemorrhage. Dev Med Child Neurol 21:730, 1979.

Casella J, Bontempo F, Markel H, et al: Successful treatment of homozygous protein C deficiency by hepatic transplantation. Lancet 1 (8583):435, 1988.

Castaman G, Rodeghiero F, Ronconi G, Dini E: Successful treatment of neonatal autoimmune thrombocytopenia with high-dose intravenous immunoglobulins [Letter]. Haematologica (Pavia) 70:276, 1985.

Casteels-Van Daele M, Jaeken J, Eggermont E, et al: More on the effects of antenatally administered aspirin on aggregation of platelets of neonates. J Pediatr 80:685, 1972.

Castle V, Andrew M, Kelton JG, et al: Frequency and mechanism of neonatal thrombocytopenia. J Pediatr 108:749, 1986.

Castle V, Coates G, Kelton J, Andrew M: ^{111}Indium oxine platelet survivals in the thrombocytopenic infant. Blood 70:652, 1987.

Castle V, Andrew M, Kelton J, et al: The clinical impact and etiologic factors of neonatal thrombocytopenia—a prospective one-year study. Pediatr Res 19:4, 1985.

Castle V, Coates G, Mitchell L, et al: Platelet survivals in the newborn: Effect of hypoxia [Abstract]. Blood 66:301, 1985.

Castle V, Coates G, Mitchell L, et al: The effect of hypoxia on platelet survival and site of sequestration in the newborn rabbit. Thromb Haemostas 59:45, 1988.

Chan KW, Kaikov Y, Wadsworth LD: Thrombocytosis in childhood: A survey of 94 patients. Pediatrics 84:1064, 1989.

Chaplin ER Jr, Goldstein GW, Norman D: Neonatal seizures, intracerebral hematoma, and subarachnoid hemorrhage in full-term infants. Pediatrics 63:812, 1979.

Chesney PJ, Taner A, Gilbert EM, Shahidi NT: Intranuclear inclusions in megakaryocytes in congenital cytomagalovirus infection. J Pediatr 92:957, 1978.

Chessells J, Wigglesworth J: Coagulation studies in preterm infants with respiratory distress and intracranial hemorrhage. Arch Dis Child 47:564, 1972.

Chirico G, Duse M, Ugazio A, Rondini G: High-dose intravenous gammaglobulin therapy for passive immune thrombocytopenia in the neonate. J Pediatr 103:654, 1983.

Ciccimarra F, De Curtis M, Paludetta R, et al: Treatment of neonatal passive immune thrombocytopenia [Letter]. J Pediatr 105:677, 1984.

Cines DB, Dusak B, Tomaski A, et al: Immune thrombocytopenic purpura and pregnancy. N Engl J Med 306:826, 1982.

Cohen JR: Idiopathic thrombocytopenic purpura in Hodgkin's disease. Cancer 41:743, 1978.

Committee on Nutrition: Vitamin K compounds and water-soluble analogues: Use in therapy and prophylaxis in pediatrics. Pediatrics 28:501, 1961.

Corby D, O'Barr T: Decreased alpha-adrenergic receptors in newborn platelets: Cause of abnormal response to epinephrine. Dev Pharmacol Ther 2:215, 1981.

Corby DG, O'Barr TP: Neonatal platelet function: A membrane-related phenomenon? Haemostasis 10:177, 1981.

Corby DG, O'Barr TP: Newborn platelet function. In Lusher JM, Barnhart MI (Eds): Acquired Bleeding Disorders in Children: Platelet Abnormalities and Laboratory Methods. New York, Masson Publishers, 1981, p 31.

Corby DG, Schulman I: The effects of antenatal drug administration on aggregation of platelets of newborn infants. J Pediatr 79:307, 1971.

Corby DG, Zuck TF: Newborn platelet dysfunction: A storage pool and release defect. Thromb Haemostas 36:200, 1976.

Corrazza MS, Davis RF, Merritt A, et al: Prolonged bleeding time in preterm infants receiving indomethacin for patent ductus arteriosus. J Pediatr 105:292, 1984.

Corrigan JJ: Heparin therapy in bacterial septicemia. J Pediatr 91:695, 1977.

Corrigan J: Normal hemostasis in fetus and newborn: Coagulation. In Polin R, Fox W (Eds): Fetal and Neonatal Physiology. Philadelphia, WB Saunders, 1992, p 1368.

Corrigan JJ, Jeter M: Histidine-rich glycoprotein and plasminogen plasma levels in term and preterm newborns. Am J Dis Child 144:825, 1990.

Corrigan JJ, Jordan C, Bennett BB, et al: Disseminated intravascular coagulation in septic shock: Report of three cases not treated with heparin. Am J Dis Child 126:629, 1974.

Cowett RM, Schwartz R: The infant of the diabetic mother. Pediatr Clin North Am 29:1213, 1982.

Cox AC, Rao GHR, Gerrard JM, White JG: The influence of vitamin E quinone on platelet structure, function, and biochemistry. Blood 55:907, 1980.

Croset M, Lagarde M: Stereospecific inhibition of PGH2-induced platelet aggregation by lipoxygenase products of icosaenoic acids. Biochem Biophys Res Commun 112:878, 1983.

Daffos F, Capella-Pavlovsky M, Forestier F: Fetal blood sampling during pregnancy with use of a needle guided by ultrasound: A study of 606 consecutive cases. Am J Obstet Gynecol 153:655, 1985.

Daffos F, Forestier F, Kaplan C, Cox W: Prenatal treatment of alloimmune thrombocytopenia [Letter]. Lancet 2:632, 1984.

Daffos F, Forestier F, Kaplan C, Cox W: Prenatal diagnosis and management of bleeding disorders with fetal blood sampling. Am J Obstet Gynecol 158(4):939, 1988.

Dam CPH: Cholesterinstoffwechsel in Huhnereierin und Huhnchen. Biochemischeschr Zeitschrift 215:475, 1929.

Dam H, Tage-Hansen E, Plum P: K-avitaminose hos spaede born som aarag til hemorrhagisk diathese. Ugesk Laeger 101:896, 1939.

Damiano V, Cherian P, Frankel F, et al: Intraluminal fibrosis induced unilaterally by lobar instillation of CdC122 into the rat lung. Am J Pathol 137(4):883, 1990.

David M, Andrew M: Venous thromboembolism complications in children: A critical review of the literature. J Pediatr 123(3):337, 1993.

David R, Merten D, Anderson J, Gross S: Prevention of umbilical artery catheter clots with heparinized infusates. Dev Pharmacol Ther 2(2):117, 1981.

Davidson BN, Rayburn WF, Bishop RC, et al: Immunoglobulin therapy for autoimmune thrombocytopenic purpura during pregnancy: A report of two cases. J Reprod Med 32:107, 1987.

Davies SV, Murray JA, Gee H, Giles HM: Transplacental effect of high-dose immunoglobulin in idiopathic thrombocytopenic purpura (ITP). Lancet 1:1098, 1986.

Davis RB, Leuschen MP, Boyd D, Goodlin RC: Evaluation of platelet function in pregnancy: Comparative studies in non-smokers and smokers. Thromb Haemostas 46:175, 1987.

De Lemos R, McLaughlin G, Koch H, Diserens H: Abnormal partial thromboplastin time and survival in respiratory distress syndrome: Effect of exchange transfusion [Abstract]. Pediatr Res 7:396, 1973.

De Swiet M: Maternal autoimmune disease and the fetus. Arch Dis Child 60:794, 1985.

De Waal LP, Van Dalen CM, Engelfriet CP, von dem Borne: Alloimmunization against the platelet-specific Zw^a antigen, resulting in neonatal thrombocytopenia or posttransfusion purpura, is associated with the supertypic DRw52 antigen including DR3 and DRw6. Human Immunol 17:45, 1986.

Deeg K, Wolfel D, Rupprecht T: Diagnosis of neonatal aortic thrombosis by colour-coded Doppler sonography. Pediatr Radiol 22(1):62, 1992.

Deguchi K, Tsukada T, Iwasaki E, et al: Late-onset homozygous protein C deficiency manifesting cerebral infarction as the first symptom at age 27. Intern Med 31(7):922, 1992.

Delorme M, Berry L, Mitchell L, et al: Isolation of anticoagulant dermatan sulphate proteoglycan from term human placenta [Abstract]. Blood 80(10):166a, 1991.

Delorme M, Saeed N, Sevcik A, et al: Plasma dermatan sulfate proteoglycan in a patient on chronic hemodialysis. Blood 82(11):3380, 1993.

di-Dattista C: Hereditary tyrosinemia in acute form. Pediatr Med Chir 3:101, 1981.

Dixon RH, Rosse WF: Platelet antibody in autoimmune thrombocytopenia. Br J Haematol 31:129, 1975.

Dreyfus M, Magny J, Bridey F, et al: Treatment of homozygous protein C deficiency and neonatal purpura fulminans with a purified protein C concentrate. N Engl J Med 325(22):1565, 1991.

Dupuy J, Frommel D, Alagille D, et al: Severe viral hepatitis B in infants. Lancet 1:191, 1975.

Edelberg JM, Enghild JJ, Pizzo SV, Gonzalez-Gronow M: Neonatal plasminogen displays altered cell surface binding and activation kinetics: Correlation with increased glycosylation of the protein. J Clin Invest 86:107, 1990.

Editorial: Management of alloimmune neonatal thrombocytopenia. Lancet 1:137, 1989.

Edson J, Blaese R, White J, Krivit W: Defibrination syndrome in an infant born after abruptio placentae. J Pediatr 72:342, 1968.

Ekelund H, Finnstrom O, Gunnarskog J, et al: Administration of vitamin K to newborn infants and childhood cancer. BMJ 307:89, 1993.

Ekelund H, Hedner U, Nilsson I: Fibrinolysis in newborns. Acta Paediatr Scand 59:33, 1970.

El Makhlouf A, Friedli B, Oberhansli, I, et al: Prosthetic heart valve replacement in children. J Thorac Cardiovasc Surg 93:80, 1987.

Elasas LJ, Whittemore R, Burrow GN: Maternal and neonatal Grave's disease. JAMA 200:250, 1967.

Elias M, Horowitz J, Tal I, et al: Thrombotic thrombocytopenic purpura and haemolytic uraemic syndrome in three siblings. Arch Dis Child 63:644, 1988.

Estelles A, Garcia-Plaza I, Dasi A, et al: Severe inherited protein C deficiency in a newborn infant. Thromb Haemostas 52(1):53, 1984.

Fernandez F, Gaudable C, Sie P, et al: Low hematocrit and prolonged bleeding time in uraemic patients: Effect of red cell transfusions [Abstract]. Br J Haematol 59:139, 1985.

Fetus and Newborn Committee: Canadian Pediatric Society: The use of vitamin K in the perinatal period. Can Med Assoc J 139:127, 1988.

Feusner JH: Normal and abnormal bleeding times in neonates and young children utilizing a fully standardized template technique. Am J Clin Pathol 74:73, 1980.

Feusner J, Slichter S, Harker L: Acquired haemostatic defects in the ill newborn. Br J Haematol 53:73, 1983.

Fischer A: Respective roles of ATIII and α_2M in thrombin inactivation. Thromb Haemostas 45:51, 1981.

Fost NC, Esterly NB: Successful treatment of juvenile hemangiomas with prednisone. J Pediatr 72:351, 1968.

Friedman JM, Aster RH: Neonatal alloimmune thrombocytopenic purpura and congenital porencephaly in two siblings associated with "new" maternal antiplatelet antibody. Blood 65:1412, 1985.

Friedman WF, Hirschklau MJ, Printz MP, et al: Pharmacologic closure of patent ductus arteriosus in the premature infant. N Engl J Med 295:526, 1976.

Friedman Z, Danon A, Stahlman MT, et al: Rapid onset of essential fatty acid deficiency in the newborn. Pediatrics 58:640, 1976.

Friedman Z, Lamberth ELJ, Stahlman MT: Platelet dysfunction in the neonate with essential fatty acid deficiency. J Pediatr 90:439, 1977.

Friedman Z, Seyberth H, Lamberth EL, Oates J: Decreased prostaglandin E turnover in infants with essential fatty acid deficiency. Pediatr Res 12:711, 1978.

Friedman Z, Whitman V, Maisels MJ, et al: Indomethacin disposition and indomethacin-induced platelet dysfunction in premature infants. J Clin Pharmacol 18:272, 1978.

Fujimura Y, Okubo Y, Sakai T, et al: Studies on precursor proteins PIVKA-II, -IX, and -X in the plasma of patients with "hemorrhagic disease of the newborn." Haemostasis 14:211, 1984.

Fukuda Y, Ishizaki M, Masuda Y, et al: The role of intraalveolar fibrosis in the process of pulmonary structural remodelling in patients with diffuse alveolar damage. Am J Pathol 126:171, 1987.

Galanakis DK, Mosesson MW: Evaluation of the role of in vivo proteolysis (fibrinogenolysis) in prolonging the thrombin time of human umbilical cord fibrinogen. Blood 48:109, 1976.

Galea P, Patrick MJ, Goel KM: Isoimmune neonatal thrombocytopenic purpura. Arch Dis Child 56:112, 1981.

Garrow D, Chisolm M, Radford M: Vitamin K and thrombotest values in full-term infants. Arch Dis Child 61:349, 1986.

Gerrard J, Docherty J, Israels S, et al: A reassessment of the bleeding time: Association of age, hematocrit, platelet function, von Willebrand factor, and bleeding time thromboxane B_2 with the length of the bleeding time. Clin Invest Med 12:165, 1989.

Gersony WM, Peckham GJ, Ellison RC, et al: Effects of indomethacin in premature infants with patent ductus arteriosus: Results of a national collaborative study. J Pediatr 102:895, 1983.

Gill EM: Thrombocytopenia in the newborn. Semin Perinatol 7:201, 1983.

Gladson C, Groncy P, Griffin J: Coumarin necrosis, neonatal purpura fulminans, and protein C deficiency. Arch Dermatol 123(12):1701a, 1987.

Golding J, Birmingham K, Greenwood R, Mott M: Intramuscular vitamin K and childhood cancer. BMJ 305:341, 1992.

Goldsmith J, Kasper C, Blatt P, et al: Coagulation factor IX: Successful surgical experience with a purified factor IX concentrate. Am J Hematol 40:210, 1992.

Gralnick HR, Gilvelber H, Abrams E: Dysfibrinogenemia associated with hepatoma: Increased carbohydrate content of the fibrinogen molecule. N Engl J Med 299:221, 1978.

Gray O, Ackerman A, Fraser A: Intracranial hemorrhage and clotting defects in low-birth-weight infants. Lancet 1:545, 1968.

Greer FR, Mummah-Schendel LL, Marshall S, Suttie JW: Vitamin K_1 (phylloquinone) and vitamin K_2 (menaquinone) status in newborns during the first week of life. Pediatrics 81:137, 1988.

Gross S, Filston H, Anderson J: Controlled study of treatment for disseminated intravascular coagulation in the neonate. J Pediatr 100:445, 1982.

Gruel Y, Boizard B, Daffos F, et al: Determinations of platelet antigens and glycoproteins in the human fetus. Blood 68:488, 1986.

Grundy C, Melissari E, Lindo, V, et al: Late-onset homozygous protein C deficiency. Lancet 338(8766):575, 1991.

Guckos-Thoeni U, Boltshauser E, Willi UV: Intraventricular hemorrhage in full-term neonates. Dev Med Child Neurol 24:704, 1982.

Guignard JP, Torrado A, Da Cunha O, et al: Glomerular filtration rate in the first three weeks of life. J Pediatr 87:268, 1975.

Gunn TR, Mok PM, Becroft DMO: Subdural hemorrhage in utero. Pediatrics 76:605, 1985.

Hall JG, Levin J, Kuhn JP, et al: Thrombocytopenia with absent radius. Medicine 48:411, 1969.

Hall MA, Pairaudeau P: The routine use of vitamin K in the newborn. Midwifery 3:170, 1987.

Halushka PU, Lurie D, Colwell JA: Increased synthesis of prostaglandins E–like material by platelets from patients with diabetes mellitus. N Engl J Med 297:1306, 1977.

Hambleton G, Appleyard W: Controlled trial of fresh frozen plasma in asphyxiated low-birthweight infants. Arch Dis Child 48:31, 1973.

Hamulyak K, de Boer-van den Berg MAG: The placental transport of [^{3}H] vitamin K_2 in rats. Br J Haematol 65:335, 1987.

Hamulyak K, Nieuwenhuizen W, Devillee PP, Hemker HC: Re-evaluation of some properties of fibrinogen purified from cord blood of normal newborns. Thromb Res 32:301, 1983.

Hanada H, Ono I: A neonate with passive ITP effectively treated with high-dose intravenous gammaglobulin. Rinsho Ketsueki 27:808, 1985.

Hanawa Y, Maki M, Murata B, et al: The second nation-wide survey in Japan of vitamin K deficiency in infants. Eur J Pediatr 147:472, 1988.

Haneberg B, Gutteberg TJ, Moe PJ, et al: Heparin for infants and children with meningococcal septicemia. NIPH Ann 6:43, 1983.

Hanigan WC, Kennedy G, Roemisch F, et al: Administration of indomethacin for the prevention of periventricular-intraventricular hemorrhage in high-risk neonates. J Pediatr 112:941, 1988.

Hara T, Kukita J, Yamashita H, et al: Intravenous gamma globulin for prolonged passive immune thrombocytopenia. Acta Paediatr Jpn 30:627, 1988.

Harada Y, Imai Y, Kurosawa H, et al: Ten-year follow-up after valve replacement with the St. Jude Medical prosthesis in children. J Thorac Cardiovasc Surg 100:175, 1990.

Haroon Y, Shearer MJ, Rahim S, et al: The content of phylloquinone (vitamin K_1) in human milk, cow's milk and infant formula foods determined by high-performance liquid chromatography. J Nutr 112:1105, 1982.

Hartman R, Manco-Johnson M, Rawlings J, et al: Homozygous protein C deficiency: Early treatment with warfarin. Am J Pediatr Hematol Oncol 11(4):395, 1989.

Haslam RR, Ekert H, Gillam GL: Hemorrhage in a neonate possibly due to maternal ingestion of salicylate. J Pediatr 84:556, 1974.

Hassan H, Leonardi C, Chelucci C, et al: Blood coagulation factors in human embryonic-fetal development: Preferential expression of the FVII/tissue factor pathway. Blood 76(6):1158, 1990.

Hathaway W, Mull M, Pechet G: Disseminated intravascular coagulation in the newborn. Pediatrics 43:233, 1969.

Hathaway W, Isarangkura P, Mahasandana C, et al: Comparison of oral and parenteral vitamin K prophylaxis for prevention of late hemorrhagic disease of the newborn. J Pediatr 119(3):461, 1991.

Hathaway W, Corrigan J: Report of scientific and standardization subcommittee on neonatal hemostasis. Thromb Haemostas 65(3):323, 1991.

Hathaway WE: Use of antiplatelet agents in pediatric hypercoagulable states. Am J Dis Child 138:301, 1984.

Hathaway WE: ICTH Subcommittee on Neonatal Hemostasis. Thrombos Haemostas 55:145, 1986.

Hathaway WE: New insights on vitamin K. Hematol Oncol Clin North Am 1:367, 1987.

Hathaway WE, Bonnar J: Hemostatic Disorders of the Pregnant Woman and Newborn Infant. New York, Elsevier, 1987.

Hedberg VA, Lipton JM: Thrombocytopenia with absent radii: A review of 100 cases. Am J Pediatr Hematol Oncol 10:51, 1988.

Hegde UM: Immune thrombocytopenia in pregnancy and the newborn. Br J Obstet Gynaecol 92:657, 1985.

Hensey OJ, Morgan MEI, Cooke RW: Tranexamic acid in the prevention of periventricular hemorrhage. Arch Dis Child 59:719, 1984.

Herman J, Jumbelic MI, Anconer RJ, Kickler TS: In utero cerebral haemorrhage in alloimmune thrombocytopenia. Am J Pediatr Hematol Oncol 8:312, 1986.

Herman J, Resnitzky P, Fink A: Association between thyrotoxicosis and thrombocytopenia: A case report and review of the literature. Isr J Med Sci 14:469, 1978.

Heymann MA, Rudolph AM, Silverman NH: Closure of the ductus arteriosus in premature infants by inhibition of prostaglandin synthesis. N Engl J Med 295:530, 1976.

Hickman RO, Buckner CD, Clift RA, et al: A modified right atrial catheter for access to the venous system in marrow transplant recipients. Surg Gynecol Obstet 148:871, 1979.

Hiraike H, Kimura M, Itokawa Y: Determination of K vitamins (phylloquinone and menaquinones) in umbilical cord plasma by a platinum-reduction column. J Chromotogr 430:143, 1988.

Hiraike H, Kimura M, Itokawa Y: Distribution of K vitamins (phylloquinone and menaquinones) in human placenta and maternal and umbilical cord plasma. Am J Obstet Gynecol 158:564, 1988.

Hirsh J, Dalen J, Warkentin T, et al: Heparin: Mechanism of action, pharmacokinetics, dosing considerations, monitoring, efficacy and safety. Chest 108(4):258S–275S, 1995.

Hirsh J, Levine M: Low-molecular-weight heparin. Blood 79:1, 1992.

Hjort PF, Rapaport SI, Jorgensen L: Purpura fulminans: Report of a case successfully treated with heparin and hydrocortisone: Review of 50 cases from the literature. Scand J Haematol 1:169, 1964.

Homans AC, Cohen JL, Mazur EM: Defective megakaryocytopoiesis in the syndrome of thrombocytopenia with absent radii. Br J Haematol 70:205, 1988.

Hope P, Hall M, Millward-Sadler G, Normand I: Alpha-1-antitripsin deficiency presenting as a bleeding diathesis in the newborn. Arch Dis Child 57(1):68, 1982.

Horgan M, Bartoletti A, Polonsky S, Peters J, Manning T, Lamont B: Effect of heparin infusates in umbilical arterial catheters on frequency of thrombotic complications. J Pediatr 111:774, 1987.

Horgan MJ, Carrasco NJM, Risemberg H: The relationship of thrombocytopenia to the onset of persistent pulmonary hypertension of the newborn in the meconium aspiration syndrome. NY State J Med 85:245, 1985.

Hrodek O: Blood platelets in the newborn: Their function in haemostasis and haemocoagulation. Acta Univ Carol Med Monogr 22:1966.

Israels S, Daniels M, McMillan E: Deficient collagen-induced activation in the newborn platelet. Pediatr Res 27:337, 1990.

Israels SJ, Gowen B, Gerrard JM: Contractile activity of neonatal platelets. Pediatr Res 21:293, 1987.

Jackson J, Truog W, Watchko J, et al: Efficacy of thromboresistant umbilical artery catheters in reducing aortic thrombosis and related complications. J Pediatr 110:102, 1987.

Jackson JC, Blumhagen JD: Congenital hydrocephalus due to prenatal hemorrhage. Pediatrics 72:344, 1983.

Jacqz EM, Barrow SE, Dollery CT: Prostacyclin concentrations in cord blood and in the newborn. Pediatrics 76:954, 1985.

Johnson DH, Vinson AM, Wirth FH: Management of hepatic hemangioendotheliomas of infancy by transarterial embolization: A report of two cases. Pediatrics 73:546, 1984.

Jones CR, McCabe R, Hamilton CA, Reid JL: Maternal and fetal platelet responses and adrenoreceptor binding characteristics. Thromb Haemostas 53:95, 1985.

Kaapa P: Immunoreactive thromboxane B_2 and 6-keto-prostaglandin F_1a in neonatal hyperbilirubinemia. Pros Leuk Med 17:97, 1985.

Kaapa P: Platelet thromboxane B_2 production in neonatal pulmonary hypertension. Arch Dis Child 62:195, 1987.

Kaapa P, Knip M, Viinikka L, Ylikorkala O: Increased platelet thromboxane B_2 production in newborn infants of diabetic mothers. Prost Leuk Med 21:299, 1986.

Kaapa P, Uhari M, Nikkari J, et al: Dietary fatty acid and platelet thromboxane production in puerperal women and their offspring. Am J Obstet Gynecol 155:146, 1986.

Kaden B, Rosse W, Hauch T: Immune thrombocytopenia in lymphoproliferative diseases. Blood 53:545, 1979.

Kaplan C, Daffos F, Forestier F, et al: Management of alloimmune thrombocytopenia: Antenatal diagnosis and in utero transfusion of maternal platelets. Blood 72:340, 1988.

Karim MAG, Clelland IA, Chapman IV, Walker CHM: B-thromboglobulin levels in plasma of jaundiced neonates exposed to phototherapy. J Perinat Med 3:141, 1981.

Karpatkin M: Corticosteroid therapy in thrombocytopenic infants of women with autoimmune thrombocytopenia. J Pediatr 105:623, 1984.

Karpatkin M, Blei F, Hurlet A, et al: Prothrombin expression in the adult and fetal rabbit liver. Pediatr Res 30:266, 1991.

Karpatkin M, Manucci PM, Mannuccio Manniuci P, et al: Low protein C in the neonatal period. Br J Haematol 62:137, 1986.

Karpatkin M, Porges RF, Karpatkin S: Platelet counts in infants of women with autoimmune thrombocytopenia: Effects of steroid administration to the mother. N Engl J Med 305:936, 1981.

Karpatkin S, Strick N, Karpatkin M, Siskind A: Cumulative experience in the detection of antiplatelet antibody in 234 patients with idiopathic thrombocytopenic purpura, systemic lupus erythematosus, and other clinical disorders. Am J Med 52:776, 1972.

Katz J, Hodder FS, Aster RS, et al: Neonatal isoimmune thrombocytopenia: The natural course and management and the detection of maternal antibody. Clin Pediatr 23:159, 1984.

Katz J, Moake J, McPherson P, et al: Relationship between human development and disappearance of unusually large von Willebrand factor multimers from plasma. Blood 73:1851, 1989.

Kellam B, Fraze D, Kanarek K: Clot lysis for thrombosed central venous catheters in pediatric patients. J Perinatol 7(3):242, 1987.

Kelly D, Summerfield J: Hemostasis in liver disease. Semin Liver Dis 7:182, 1987.

Kelton J: Management of the pregnant patient with idiopathic thrombocytopenic purpura. Ann Intern Med 99:796, 1983.

Kelton JG, Blanchette VS, Wilson WE, et al: Neonatal thrombocytopenia due to passive immunization: Prenatal diagnosis and distinction between maternal platelet alloantibodies and autoantibodies. N Engl J Med 302:1401, 1980.

Kelton JG, Inwood MJ, Barr RM, et al: The prenatal prediction of thrombocytopenia in infants of mothers with clinically diagnosed immune thrombocytopenia. Am J Obstet Gynecol 144:449, 1982.

Khurshid M, Lee TJ, Pealre IR, Bloom AL: Vitamin E deficiency and platelet functional defect in a jaundiced infant. BMJ 4:19, 1975.

Kisker C, Robillard J, Clarke W: Development of blood coagulation—a fetal lamb model. Pediatr Res 15:1045, 1981.

Kisker CT, Perlman S, Bohlken D, Wicklund D: Measurement of prothrombin mRNA during gestation and early neonatal development. J Lab Clin Med 112:407, 1988.

Kotohara K, Endo F: Effect of vitamin K administration of acarboxy prothrombin (PIVKA-II) levels in newborns. Lancet 2:243, 1985.

Kries RV, Shearer MJ, Gobel U: Vitamin K in infancy. Eur J Pediatr 147:106, 1988.

Kryc JJ, Corrigan JJ: Idiopathic thrombocytopenic purpura during pregnancy. A pediatric viewpoint. Am J Pediatr Hematol Oncol 5:21, 1983.

Kumar, V, Berenson G, Ruiz H, et al: Acid mucopolysaccharides of human aorta. I. Variations with maturation. J Atheroscler Res 7:573, 1967.

Lafer C, Morrison A: Thrombocytopenic purpura progressing to transient hypoplastic anemia in a newborn with rubella syndrome. Pediatrics 38:499, 1966.

Lagarde M: Metabolism of fatty acids by platelets and the functions of various metabolites in mediating platelet function. Prog Lipid Res 27:135, 1988.

Lake AM, Stuart MJ, Oski FA: Vitamin E deficiency and enhanced platelet function: Reversal following E supplementation. J Pediatr 90:722, 1977.

Lam AH, Shulman LA: Ultrasound in congenital haemorrhage secondary to isoimmune thrombocytopenia. Pediatr Radiol 15:8, 1985.

Landolfi R, De Cristofaro R, Ciabattoni G, et al: Placental-derived PGI_2 inhibits cord blood platelet function. Haematologica (Pavia) 73:207, 1988.

Lane PA, Hathaway WE, Githens JH, et al: Fatal intracranial hemorrhage in a normal infant secondary to vitamin K deficiency. Pediatrics 72:562, 1983.

Laosombat V: Hemorrhagic disease of the newborn after maternal anticonvulsant therapy: A case report and literature review. J Med Assoc Thailand 71:643, 1988.

Larsen EC, Zinkham WH, Eggleston JC, Zitelli BJ: Kasabach-Merritt syndrome: Therapeutic considerations. Pediatrics 79:971, 1987.

Le Gall E, Picaud J, Treguier C, et al: High-dose intravenous gammaglobulin therapy for autoimmune thrombocytopenia in two neonates. Arch Franc Pediatr 43:191, 1986.

Leaker M, Massicotte MP, Brooker L, Andrew M: Thrombolytic therapy in pediatric patients: A comprehensive review of the literature. Thromb Haemost 76:132, 1996.

Lecander I, Astedt B: Specific plasminogen activator inhibitor of placental type PAI 2 occurring in amniotic fluid and cord blood. J Lab Clin Med 110(5):602, 1987.

Lecompte T: Hereditary thrombocytopenias. Curr Stud Hematol Blood Transfus 55:162, 1988.

Lehmann J: Vitamin K as a prophylactic in 13,000 infants. Lancet 1:493, 1944.

Lesko S, Mitchell A, Epstein M, et al: Heparin use a risk factor for intraventricular hemorrhage in low-birth-weight infants. N Engl J Med 314:1156, 1986.

Levin DL, Weinberg AG, Perkin RM: Pulmonary microthrombi syndrome in newborn infants with unresponsive persistent pulmonary hypertension. J Pediatr 102:299, 1983.

Levy G, Garrettson LK: Kinetics of salicylate elimination by newborn infants of mothers who ingested aspirin before delivery. Pediatrics 53:201, 1974.

Liebermann J: The nature of the fibrinolytic enzyme defect in hyaline membrane disease. N Engl J Med 265:363, 1961.

Lucey JF, Dolan RG: Hyperbilirubinemia of newborn infants associated with the parenteral administration of a vitamin K analogue to the mothers. Pediatrics 23:553, 1959.

Lupton BA, Hill A, Whitfield MF, et al: Reduced platelet count as a risk factor for intraventricular haemorrhage. Am J Dis Child 142:1222, 1988.

Machlin LJ, Filipski R, Willis AL, et al: Influence of Vitamin E on platelet aggregation and thrombocythemia in the rat. Proc Soc Exp Biol Med 149:275, 1973.

Mackay RJ, Crespigny L, Laurence J, et al: Intraventricular hemorrhage in term neonates: Diagnosis by ultrasound. Aust Paediatr J 18:205, 1984.

Mahasandana C, Suvatte, V, Chuansumvita A, et al: Homozygous protein S deficiency in an infant with purpura fulminans. J Pediatr 117(5):750, 1990.

Mahony L, Caldwell R, Girod D, et al: Indomethacin therapy on the first day of life in infants with very low birthweight. J Pediatr 106:801, 1985.

Manco-Johnson M, Abshire TC, Jacobson LJ, Marlar RA: Severe neonatal protein C deficiency: Prevalence and thrombotic risk. J Pediatr 119:793, 1991.

Manco-Johnson M, Marlar R, Jacobson L, et al: Severe protein C deficiency in newborn infants. J Pediatr 113(2):359, 1988.

Mandelbrot L, Guillaumont M, Forestier F, et al: Placental transfer of vitamin K_1 and its implications in fetal haemostasis. Thromb Haemostas 60:39, 1988.

Markarian M, Lindley A, Jackson J, Bannon A: Coagulation factors in pregnant women and premature infants with and without the respiratory distress syndrome. Thromb Diath Haemorrh 17:585, 1967.

Markarian M, Luchenco LO, Rosenblut E: Hypercoagulability in premature infants with special reference to the respiratory distress syndrome and hemorrhage. II. The effect of heparin. Biol Neonate 17:98, 1971.

Marlar R, Adcock D, Madden R: Hereditary dysfunctional protein C molecules (type II): Assay characterization and proposed classification. Thromb Haemostas 63(3):375, 1990.

Marlar R, Montgomery R, Broekmans A: Report on the diagnosis and treatment of homozygous protein C deficiency. Report of the working party on homozygous protein C deficiency of the ISTH—Subcommittee on protein C and protein S. Thromb Haemostas 61(3):529, 1989.

Marlar R, Montgomery R, Broekmans A, and the Working Party: Diagnosis and treatment of homozygous protein C deficiency. J Pediatr 114:528, 1989.

Marlar R, Neumann A: Neonatal purpura fulminans due to homozygous protein C or protein S deficiencies. Semin Thromb Haemostas 16(4):299, 1990.

Marlar R, Sills R, Groncy P, et al: Protein C survival during replacement therapy in homozygous protein C deficiency. Am J Hematol 41:24, 1992.

Martin B, Robin H, Williams R, Ornelas W: Neonatal graft vs. host disease following transfusion of maternal platelets [Abstract]. Transfusion 23:417, 1983.

Martin-Bouyer G, Linh PD, Tuan LC: Epidemic of haemorrhagic disease in Vietnamese infants caused by warfarin-contaminated talcs. Lancet 1:230, 1983.

Massicotte P, Adams M, Marzinotto, V, et al: Low-molecular-weight heparin in pediatric patients with thrombotic disease: A dose-finding study. J Pediatr 128:313, 1996.

Massicotte P, Marzinotto, V, Vegh P, et al: Home monitoring of warfarin therapy in children with a whole blood prothrombin time monitor. J Pediatr 127:389, 1995.

Maurer HM, Haggins JC, Still WJS: Platelet injury during phototherapy. Am J Hematol 1:89, 1976.

Mazzone D, Fichera A, Pratico G, Sciacca F: Combined congenital deficiency of factor V and factor VIII. Acta Haematol 68:337, 1982.

Mazzucconi MG, Francesconi M, Fidani P, et al: Pregnancy, delivery, and detection of antiplatelet antibodies in women with idiopathic thrombocytopenic purpura. Haematologica (Pavia) 70:506, 1985.

McDonald M, Hathaway W: Neonatal haemorrhage and thrombosis. Semin Perinatol 7:213, 1983.

McDonald MM, Jacobson LJ, Hay WW, Hathaway WE: Heparin clearance in the newborn. Pediatr Res 15:1015, 1981.

McFarland JG, Frenzke M, Aster RH: Testing of maternal sera in pregnancies at risk for neonatal alloimmune thrombocytopenia. Transfusion 29:128, 1989.

McGrath L, Gonzalez-Lavin L, Edlredge W, et al: Thromboembolic and other events following valve replacement in a pediatric population treated with antiplatelet agents. Ann Thorac Surg 43:285, 1987.

McIntosh S, O'Brien RT, Schwarz SO, Pearson H: Neonatal isoimmune purpura: Response to platelet infusions. J Pediatr 82:1020, 1973.

McMillan C, Roberts H: Congenital combined deficiency of coagulation factors II, VII, IX, and X. N Engl J Med 274(23):1313, 1966.

McNinch A, Tripp J: Haemorrhagic disease of the newborn in the British Isles: Two-year prospective study. BMJ 303:1105, 1991.

Mehta P, Vasa R, Newman L, Karpatkin M: Thrombocytopenia in the high-risk infant. J Pediatr 97:791, 1980.

Mennuti M, Schwartz RH, Gill F: Obstetric management of isoimmune thrombocytopenia. Am J Obstet Gynecol 118:565, 1974.

Ment LR, Duncan CC, Ehrenkranz RA: Randomized indomethacin trial for prevention of intraventricular hemorrhage in very-low-birth-weight infants. J Pediatr 107:937, 1985.

Ment LR, Ehrenkranz RA, Duncan CC: Intraventricular hemorrhage of the preterm neonate: Prevention studies. Semin Perinatol 12:359, 1988.

Mercier J, Bourrillon A, Beaufils F, et al: Hereditary fructose intolerance with early onset. Arch Fr Pediatr 10:945, 1976.

Michelson AD, Bovill E, Andrew M: Antithrombotic therapy in children. Chest 108(4):506S, 1995.

Miletich J, Sherman L, Broze GJ: Absence of thrombosis in subjects with heterozygous protein C deficiency. N Engl J Med 317(16):991, 1987.

Mindrum G, Glueck H: Plasma prothrombin time in liver disease: Its clinical and prognostic significance. Ann Intern Med 50:1370, 1959.

Mir N, Samson D, House M, Kavan I: Failure of antenatal high-dose immunoglobulin to improve fetal platelet count in neonatal alloimmune thrombocytopenia. Vox Sang 55:188, 1988.

Mirro JJ, Rao BN, Stokes DC, et al: A prospective study of Hickman/Broviac catheters and implantable ports in pediatric oncology patients. J Clin Oncol 7:214, 1989.

Moake J, Chintagumpala M, Turner N, et al: Solvent/detergent-treated plasma suppresses shear-induced platelet aggregation and prevents episodes of thrombotic thrombocytopenic purpura. Blood 84:490, 1994.

Moalic P, Gruel Y, Body G, et al: Levels and plasma distribution of free and c₄b-BP-bound protein S in human fetuses and fullterm newborns. Thromb Res 49:471, 1988.

Mocan H, Beattie T, Murphy A: Renal venous thrombosis in infancy: long-term follow-up. Pediatr Nephrol 5:45, 1991.

Moise KJ, Carpenter RJ, Cotton DB, et al: Percutaneous umbilical cord blood sampling in the evaluation of fetal platelet counts in pregnant patients with autoimmune thrombocytopenia purpura. Obstet Gynecol 72:346, 1988.

Morales WJ, Angel JL, O'Brien WF, et al: The use of antenatal vitamin K in the prevention of early neonatal intraventricular hemorrhage. Am J Obstet Gynecol 159(3):774, 1988.

Morgan MEI, Ben JWT, Cooke RWI: Ethamsylate reduces the incidence of periventricular haemorrhage in very-low-birth-weight babies. Lancet 2:830, 1981.

Morris J, Occhionero M, Gauderer M, et al: Totally implantable vascular access devices in cystic fibrosis: A four-year experience with fifty-eight patients. J Pediatr 117(1):82, 1990.

Motohara K, Endo F, Matsuda I: Screening for late neonatal vitamin K deficiency by acarboxyprothrombin in dried blood spots. Arch Dis Child 62:370, 1987.

Motohara K, Kuroki Y, Kan H, et al: Detection of vitamin K deficiency by use of an enzyme-linked immunosorbent assay for circulating abnormal prothrombin. Pediatr Res 19:354, 1985.

Mountain KR, Hirsh J, Gallius AS: Neonatal coagulation defect due to anticonvulsant drug treatment in pregnancy. Lancet 1:265, 1970.

Mueller-Eckhardt C, Kiefel, V, Grubert A, et al: 348 cases of suspected neonatal alloimmune thrombocytopenia. Lancet 1:363, 1989.

Mueller-Eckhardt C, Kiefel V, Kroll H: HLA-DRw6, a new immune response marker for immunization against the platelet alloantigen Brᵃ. Vox Sang 57:90, 1989.

Muira M: Efficacy of several plasma components in a young boy with chronic thrombocytopenia and hemolytic anemia who responds repeatedly to normal plasma infusions. Am J Hematol 17:307, 1984.

Muira M, Koizumi S, Nakamura K, Ohno T, Tachinami T, Yamagami M, Taniguchi N, Kinoshita S, Abilgaard C: Efficacy of several plasma components in a young boy with chronic thrombocytopenia and hemolytic anemia who responds repeatedly to normal plasma infusions. Am J Hematol 17:307, 1984.

Muntean W, Rosseger H: Antithrombin III concentrate in preterm infants with IRDS: An open, controlled, randomized clinical trial [Abstract]. Thromb Haemostas 62:288, 1989.

Murdoch I, Beattie R, Silver D: Heparin-induced thrombocytopenia in children. Acta Paediatr 82:495, 1993.

Murphy WG, Moore JC, Kelton JG: Calcium-dependent cysteine protease activity in the sera of patients with thrombotic thrombocytopenic purpura. Blood 70:1683, 1987.

Nathan D, Snapper I: Simultaneous placental transfer of factors responsible for LE cell formation and thrombocytopenia. Am J Med 25:647, 1958.

Needleman P, Turk J, Jakschik B, et al: Arachidonic acid metabolism. Annu Rev Biochem 55:69, 1986.

Newland AC, Boots MA, Patterson KG: Intravenous IgG for autoimmune thrombocytopenia in pregnancy. N Engl J Med 310:261, 1984.

Nicolini U, Rodeck CH, Kochenour NK, et al: In utero platelet transfusion for alloimmune thrombocytopenia. [Letter]. Lancet 2:506, 1988.

O'Brodovich H, Coates J: Quantitative ventilation perfusion lung scans in infants and children: Utility of a submicronic radiolabelled aerosol to assess ventilation. J Pediatr 105:377, 1984.

Olson T, Levine R, Mazur E, et al: Megakaryocytes and megakaryocyte progenitors in human cord blood. Am J Pediatr Hematol Oncol 14(3):241, 1992.

Oppenheimer EH, Esterly JR: Thrombosis in the newborn: Comparison between infants of diabetic and non-diabetic mothers. J Pediatr 67:549, 1965.

Orchard PJ, Smith CMI, Woods WG, et al: Treatment of haemangioendotheliomas with alpha interferon. Lancet 2:565, 1989.

Osborn J, Shahidi N: Thrombocytopenia in murine cytomagalovirus infections. J Lab Clin Med 81:53, 1973.

Ostermann H, van de Loo J: Factors of the hemostatic system in diabetic patients: A survey of controlled studies. Haemostasis 16:386, 1986.

Ozkutlu S, Saraclar M, Atalay S, et al: Two-dimensional echocardiographic diagnosis of tricuspid valve noninfective endocarditis due to protein C deficiency (lesion mimicking tricuspid valve myxoma). Jpn Heart J 32(1):139, 1991.

Palma PA, Miner ME, et al: Intraventricular hemorrhage in the neonate at term. Am J Dis Child 133:941, 1979.

Palmisano PA, Cassady G: Salicylate exposure in the perinate. JAMA 209:556, 1969.

Patel P, Weitz J, Brooker L, et al: Decreased thrombin activity of fibrin clots prepared in cord plasma compared to adult plasma. Pediatr Res 39:826, 1996.

Patrick CH, Lazarchick J: The effect of bacteremia on automated platelet measurements in neonates. Am J Clin Pathol 93:391, 1990.

Pearson HA, McIntosh S: Neonatal thrombocytopenia. Clin Haematol 7:111, 1978.

Pearson HA, Shulman NR, Marder VJ, Cone TE: Isoimmune neonatal thrombocytopenic purpura: Clinical and therapeutic considerations. Blood 23:154, 1964.

Pell J, McIver B, Stuart P, et al: Comparison of anticoagulant control among patients attending general practice and a hospital anticoagulant clinic. Br J Gen Prac 43:152, 1993.

Pencharz P, Steffee W, Cochran W, et al: Protein metabolism in human neonates: Nitrogen-balance studies, estimated obligatory losses of nitrogen, and whole-body turnover of nitrogen. Clin Sci Molec Med 52:485, 1977.

Pescatore P, Horellou H, Conard J, et al: Problems of oral anticoagulation in an adult with homozygous protein C deficiency and late onset of thrombosis. Thromb Haemostas 69(4):311, 1993.

Peters C, Casella J, Marlar R, et al: Homozygous protein C deficiency: Observations on the nature of the molecular abnormality and the effectiveness of warfarin therapy. Pediatrics 81(2):272, 1988.

Peters M, Jansen E, ten Cate JW, et al: Neonatal antithrombin III. Br J Haematol 58:579, 1984.

Petrini P, Segnestam K, Ekelund H, Egberg N: Homozygous protein C deficiency in two siblings. Pediatr Hematol Oncol 7(2):165, 1990.

Plotz F, van Oeveren W, Bartlett R, Wildevuur C: Blood activation during neonatal extracorporeal life support. J Thorac Cardiovasc Surg 105(5):823, 1993.

Podolsak B: Thrombocytopoiesis in newborn infants after exchange blood transfusion. Zeitschrift fur Kinderheilkd 114:13, 1973.

Pomerance JJ, Teal JG, Gogdok JF, et al: Maternally administered antenatal vitamin K₁: Effect on neonatal prothrombin activity, partial thromboplastin time, and intraventricular hemorrhage. Obstet Gynecol 70:235, 1987.

Rajani K, Goetzman B, Wennberg R, Turner E, Abildgaard C: Effect of heparinization of fluids infused through an umbilical artery catheter on catheter patency and frequency of complications. Pediatrics 63:552, 1979.

Rajasekhar D, Kestin A, Bednarek F, et al: Neonatal platelets are less reactive than adult platelets to physiological agonists in whole blood. Thromb Haemost 72(6):957, 1994.

Rao S, Solymar L, Mardini M, et al: Anticoagulant therapy in children with prosthetic valves. Ann Thorac Surg 47:589, 1989.

Rappaport E, Speights V, Helbert B, et al: Protein C deficiency. South Med J 80(2):240, 1987.

Remuzzi G: Bleeding in renal failure. Lancet 1:1205, 1988.

Rennie JM, Doyle J, Cooke RWI: Early administration of indomethacin to preterm infants. Arch Dis Child 61:233, 1986.

Reverdiau-Moalic P, Gruel Y, Delahousse B, et al: Comparative study of the fibrinolytic system in human fetuses and in pregnant women. Thromb Res 61:489, 1991.

Reznikoff-Etievant MF, Dangu C, Lobet R, et al: HLA-B8 antigens and anti-PLᵃˡ allo-immunization. Tissue Antigens 18:66, 1981.

Reznikoff-Etievant MF, Kaplan C, Durieux I, et al: Alloimmune thrombocytopenias, definition of a group at risk: A prospective study. Curr Stud Hematol Blood Transfus 55:119, 1988.

Robinson T, Kickler T, Walker L, et al: Effect of extracorporeal membrane oxygenation on platelets in newborns. Crit Care Med 21(7):1029, 1993.

Rogers P, Silva M, Carter J, Wadsworth L: Renal vein thrombosis and response to therapy in a newborn due to protein C deficiency. Eur J Pediatr 149(2):124, 1989.

Rohyans J, Miser A, Miser J: Subgaleal hemorrhage in infants with hemophilia: Report of two cases and review of the literature. Pediatrics 70(2):306, 1982.

Roman J, Velasco F, Fernandez M, et al: Coagulation, fibrinolytic, and kallikrein systems in neonates with uncomplicated sepsis and septic shock. Haemostasis 23:142, 1993.

Ronconi GF, Castaman G, Fantuz E, Rodeghiero F: Treatment of passive-acquired immune thrombocytopenia of the newborn with high-dose intravenous gammaglobulin infusion. Pediatr Med Chir 7:567, 1986.

Rose SJ: Neonatal hemorrhage and vitamin K. Acta Haematol 74:121, 1985.

Rosenburger WF, Lachin JM: The use of response-adaptive designs in clinical trials. Contr Clin Trials 14:471, 1993.

Rubin M, Weston MJ, Bullock G, et al: Abnormal platelet function and ultrastructure in fulminant hepatic failure. Q J Med 46:339, 1977.

Rumack CM, Guggenheim MA, Rumack BH, et al: Neonatal intracranial hemorrhage and maternal use of aspirin. Obstet Gynecol 58:Suppl 525, 1981.

Runnebaum IB, Maurer SM, Daly L, Bonnar J: Inhibitors and activators of fibrinolysis during and after childbirth in maternal and cord blood. J Perinat Med 17:113, 1989.

Sacher R, King J: Intravenous gammaglobulin in pregnancy: A review. Obstet Gynecol Surv 44:25, 1988.

Sade R, Crawford FJ, Fyfe D, Stroud M: Valve protheses in children: A reassessment of anticoagulation. J Thorac Cardiovasc Surg 95(4):553, 1988.

Sagel J, Colwell JA, Crook L, Laimins M: Increased platelet aggregation in early diabetes mellitus. Ann Intern Med 82:733, 1975.

Saldeen T: Fibrin-derived peptides and pulmonary injury. Ann NY Acad Sci 384:319, 1982.

Samuels P, Main E, Tomaski A, et al: Abnormalities in platelet antiglobulin tests in preeclamptic mothers and their neonates. Am J Obstet Gynecol 157:109, 1987.

Saving K, Aldag J, Jennings D, et al: Electron microscopic characterization of neonatal platelet ultrastructure: Effects of sampling techniques. Thromb Res 61:65, 1991.

Scher MS, Wright FS, Lockman LA, Thompson TR: Intraventricular hemorrhage in the fullterm neonate. Arch Neurol 39:769, 1982.

Schmidt B, Andrew M: Neonatal thrombotic disease: Prevention, diagnosis, and therapy. J Pediatr 113:407, 1988.

Schmidt B, Andrew M: Report of Scientific and Standardization Subcommittee on Neonatal Hemostasis: Diagnosis and treatment of neonatal thrombosis. Thromb Haemostas 67(3):381, 1992.

Schmidt B, Andrew A: A prospective international registry of neonatal thrombotic diseases [Abstract]. Pediatr Res 35(4): Part 2:170a, 1994.

Schmidt B, Andrew M: Neonatal thrombosis: Report of a prospective Canadian and International registry. Pediatrics 96:939, 1995.

Schmidt B, Buchanan M, Ofosu F, et al: Antithrombotic properties of heparin in a neonatal piglet model of thrombin-induced thrombosis. Thromb Haemostas 60:289, 1988.

Schmidt B, Davis P, LaPointe H, et al: Efficacy of thrombin inhibition in a piglet model of neonatal acute lung injury [Abstract]. Thromb Haemostas 69(6):1020, 1993.

Schmidt B, Mitchell L, Ofosu F, Andrew M: Standard assays underestimate the concentration of heparin in neonatal plasma. J Lab Clin Med 112:641, 1988.

Schmidt B, Mitchell L, Ofosu F, Andrew M: Alpha-2-macroglobulin is an important progressive inhibitor of thrombin in neonatal and infant plasma. Thromb Haemostas 62:1074, 1989.

Schmidt B, Wais U, Pringsheim W, Kunzer W: Plasma elimination of antithrombin III is accelerated in term newborn infants. Eur J Pediatr 141:225, 1984.

Schmidt B, Zipursky A: Disseminated intravascular coagulation masking neonatal hemophilia. J Pediatr 109:886, 1986.

Schwarz HP, Muntean W, Watzke H, et al: Low total protein S antigen but high protein S activity due to decreased c_4b-binding protein in neonates. Blood 71:562, 1988.

Scott JR, Cruikshank DP, Kochenouri NK, et al: Fetal platelet counts in the obstetric management of immunologic purpura. Am J Obstet Gynecol 136:495, 1980.

Seeger W, Stohr G, Wolf H: Alteration of surfactant function due to protein leakage: Special interaction with fibrin monomer. J Appl Physiol 58:326, 1985.

Segall ML, Goetzman BW, Schick JB: Thrombocytopenia and pulmonary hypertension in the perinatal aspiration syndromes. J Pediatr 96:727, 1980.

Seguin JH, Topper H: Coagulation studies in very low-birthweight infants. Am J Perinatol 11(1):27, 1995.

Seip M: Systemic lupus erythematosus in pregnancy with haemolytic anemia, leukopenia, and thrombocytopenia in the mother and her newborn infant. Arch Dis Child 35:364, 1960.

Serfontein GL, Rom S, Stein S: Posterior fossa subdural hemorrhage in the newborn. Pediatrics 65:40, 1980.

Serra A, McNicholas K, Olivier HJ, et al: The choice of anticoagulation in pediatric patients with the St. Jude Medical valve prostheses. J Cardiovasc Surg 28:588, 1987.

Setzer ES, Webb IB, Wassenaar JW, et al: Platelet dysfunction and coagulopathy in intraventricular hemorrhage in the premature infant. J Pediatr 100:599, 1982.

Shah J, Mitchell L, Paes B, et al: Thrombin inhibition is impaired in plasma of sick neonates. Pediatr Res 31:391, 1992.

Shapiro AD, Jacobson LJ, Aramon ME, et al: Vitamin K deficiency in the newborn infant: Prevalence and perinatal risk factors. J Pediatr 109:675, 1986.

Shapiro ME, Riodvien R, Bauer KA, Salzman EW: Acute aortic thrombosis in antithrombin III deficiency. JAMA 245:1759, 1981.

Shearer MJ, Barkhan P, Rahim S, Stimmler L: Plasma vitamin K_1 in mothers and their newborn babies. Lancet 2:460, 1982.

Shim KT: Hemangiomas of infancy complicated by thrombocytopenia. Am J Surg 116:896, 1995.

Shinnar S, Molteni A, Gammon K, et al: Intraventricular hemorrhage in the premature infant: A changing outlook. N Engl J Med 306:1464, 1982.

Shiozaki A, Arai T, Izumi R, et al: Congenital antithrombin III deficient neonate treated with antithrombin III concentrates. Thromb Res 70:211, 1993.

Shirahata A, Nakamura T, Shimono M, et al: Blood coagulation findings and the efficacy of factor XIII concentrate in premature infants with intracranial hemorrhages. Thromb Res 57:755, 1990.

Shulman NR, Aster RH, Pearson HA, Hiller MC: Immunoreactions involving platelets: VI. Reactions of maternal isoantibodies responsible for neonatal purpura: Differentiation of a second platelet antigen system. J Clin Invest 41:1059, 1962.

Shulman NR, Marder VJ, Hiller MC, Collier EM: Platelet and leukocyte isoantigens and their antibodies: Serologic, physiologic, and clinical studies. Progress Haematol 4:222, 1964.

Sidiropoulos D, Straume B: The treatment of neonatal isoimmune thrombocytopenia with intravenous immunoglobulin (IgG iv). Blut 48:383, 1984.

Siegbahn A, Ruusuvaara L: Age dependence of blood fibrinolytic components and the effects of low-dose oral contraceptives on coagulation and fibrinolysis in teenagers. Thromb Haemostas 60(3):361, 1988.

Sitarz AL, Driscoll JMJ, Wolff JA: Management of isoimmune neonatal thrombocytopenia. Am J Obstet Gynecol 124:39, 1976.

Smith P: Congenital coagulation protein deficiencies in the perinatal period. Semin Perinatol 14(5):384, 1990.

Spadone D, Clark F, James E, et al: Heparin-induced thrombocytopenia in the newborn. J Vasc Surg 15:306, 1992.

Spevak P, Freed M, Castaneda A, et al: Valve replacement in children less than 5 years of age. J Am Cardiol 8:901, 1986.

Srinivasan G, Seeler RA, Tiruvury A, Pildes RS: Maternal anticonvulsant therapy and hemorrhagic disease of the newborn. Obstet Gynecol 59:250, 1982.

Stabile A, Pesaresi M, Sopo S, Segni G: Effective high-dose intravenous gamma globulin therapy for passive immune thrombocytopenia in the neonate. Eur J Pediatr 146:90, 1986.

Stein S, Harker L: Kinetic and functional studies of platelets, fibrinogen, and plasminogen in patients with hepatic cirrhosis. J Lab Clin Med 99:217, 1982.

Steiner M, Anastasi J: Vitamin E—an inhibitor of the platelet thromboxane production. J Pediatr 110:289, 1987.

Stewart S, Cianciotta D, Alexson C, Manning J: The long-term risk of warfarin sodium therapy and the incidence of thromboembolism in children after prosthetic cardiac valves. J Thorac Cardiovasc Surg 93:551, 1987.

Stuart M, Dusse J, Clark A, Walenga R: Differences in thromboxane production between neonatal and adult platelets in response to arachidonic acid and epinephrine. Pediatr Res 18:823, 1984.

Stuart MJ: Vitamin E deficiency: Its effect on platelet-vascular interaction in various pathologic states. Ann NY Acad Sci 393:277–288, 1982.

Stuart MJ: A storage pool deficiency in neonatal platelets [Abstract]. Thromb Haemostas 38:4, 1976.

Stuart MJ: Platelet function in the neonate. Am J Pediatr Hematol Oncol 1:227, 1979.

Stuart MJ, Elrad H, Graeber JE, et al: Increased synthesis of prostaglandin endoperoxides and platelet hyperfunction in infants of mothers with diabetes mellitus. J Lab Clin Med 94:12, 1979.

Stuart MJ, Gross SJ, Elrad H, Graeber JE: Effects of acetylsalicylic acid ingestion on maternal and neonatal hemostasis. N Engl J Med 307:909, 1982.

Stuart MJ, Oski FA: Vitamin E and platelet function. Am J Pediatr Hematol Oncol 1:77, 1979.

Stuart MJ, Sunderji SG, Allen JB. Decreased prostacyclin production in the infant of the diabetic mothers. J Lab Clin Med 98:412, 1981.

Stuart MJ, Wu J, Sunderji S, Cranley C: Effect of amniotic fluid on platelet thromboxane production. J Pediatr 110:289, 1987.

Suarez CR, Menendez CE, Walenga JM, Fareed J: Neonatal and maternal hemostasis. Value of molecular markers in the assessment of hemostatic status. Semin Thromb Haemostas 10:280, 1984.

Suarez CR, Gonzalez J, Menendez C, et al: Neonatal and maternal platelets: Activation at time of birth. Am J Hematol 29:18, 1988.

Suarez CR, Walenga J, Mangogna LC, Fareed J: Neonatal and maternal fibrinolysis: Activation at time of birth. Am J Haem 19:365, 1985.

Suen Y, Chang M, Lee S, Buzby J, Cairo M: Regulation of interleukin-11 protein and mRNA expression in neonatal and adult fibroblasts and endothelial cells. Blood 84(12):4125, 1994.

Summaria L: Comparison of human normal, full-term, fetal and adult plasminogen by physical and chemical analyses. Haemostasis 19:266, 1989.

Sutherland JM, Glueck HI: Hemorrhagic disease of the newborn: Breast feeding as a necessary factor in the pathogenesis. Am J Dis Child 113:524, 1967.

Sutor A: Thrombosis in the newborn and infants. In Poller L, Thomson J (Eds): Thrombosis and Its Management. Edinburgh, Churchill Livingstone, 1992, p 126.

Sutor A, Dagres N, Neiderhoff H: Late form of vitamin K deficiency bleeding in Germany. Klin Padiatr (Germany) 207:89, 1995.

Suzuki S, Wake N, Yoshiaki K: New neonatal problems of blood coagulation and fibrinolysis: II. Thromboplastic effect of amniotic fluid, and its relation to lung maturity. J Perinatal Med 4:221, 1976.

Tate DY, Carlton GT, Johnson D, et al: Immune thrombocytopenia in severe neonatal infections. J Pediatr 98:449, 1981.

Tchernia G, Dreyfus M, Laulrian Y, et al: Management of immune thrombocytopenia in pregnancy: Response to infusions of immunoglobulins. Am J Obstet Gynecol 148:225, 1984.

Territo M, Finklestein J, Oh W, et al: Management of autoimmune thrombocytopenia in pregnancy and in the neonate. Obstet Gynecol 41:579, 1973.

Thorp JA, Parriott J, Ferrette-Smith D, et al: Antepartum vitamin K and phenobarbital for preventing intraventricular hemorrhage in the premature newborn: A randomized, double-blind, placebo-controlled trial. Obstet Gynecol 83(1):70, 1994.

Townsend CW: The haemorrhagic disease of the newborn. Arch Pediatr 11:559, 1894.

Tripodi A, Franchi F, Krachmalnicoff A, Mannucci P: Asymptomatic homozygous protein C deficiency. Acta Haematol 83(3):152, 1990.

Truog R: Randomized, controlled trials: Lessons from ECMO. Clin Res 40:519, 1992.

Ts'ao C, Green D, Schultz K: Function and ultrastructure of platelets of neonates: Enhanced ristocetin aggregation of neonatal platelets. Br J Haematol 32:225, 1976.

Ts'ao CH: Comparable inhibition of PRP of neonates and adults by aspirin. Haemostasis 6:118, 1977.

Tuddenham E, Takase T, Thomas A, et al: Homozygous protein C deficiency with delayed onset of symptoms at 7 to 10 months. Thromb Res 53(5):475, 1989.

Turner T: Randomized sequential control trial to evaluate effect of purified factor II, VII, IX, and X concentrate, cryoprecipitate, and platelet concentrate in management of preterm low-birthweight and mature asphyxiated infants with coagulation defects. Arch Dis Child 51:810, 1981.

Vailas G, Brouillette R, Scott J, et al: Neonatal aortic thrombosis: Recent experience. J Pediatr 109:101, 1986.

Vermylen C, Levin N, Lanham J, et al: Decreased sensitivity to heparin in vitro in steroid-responsive nephrotic syndrome. Kidney Int 31:1396, 1987.

Vieira A, Ofosu F, Andrew M: Heparin sensitivity and resistance in the neonate: An explanation. Thromb Res 63(1):85, 1991.

Vietti TJ, Murphy TP, James JA, Pritchard JA: Observation on the prophylactic use of vitamin K in the newborn. J Pediatr 56:343, 1960.

Vincer M, Allen A, Evans J, et al: Early intravenous indomethacin prolongs respiratory support in very-low-birthweight infants. Acta Paediatr Scand 76:894, 1987.

Volpe J: Intraventricular hemorrhage in the premature infant—current concepts: I. Ann Neurol 25:3, 1989.

Von Breedin K: Hamorrhagische diathesen bei lebererkrankungen unter besonderer berucksichtigung der thrombocytenfunction. Acta Haematol 27:1, 1962.

Von Kries R, Gobel U: Vitamin K prophylaxis and late haemorrhagic disease of newborn (HDN). Acta Pediatr Scand 81:655, 1992.

Von Kries R, Hanawa Y: Neonatal Vitamin K prophylaxis: Report of Scientific and Standardization Subcommittee on Perinatal Haemostasis. Thromb Haemostas 69(3):293, 1993.

Von Kries R, Shearer MJ, McCarthy PT, et al: Vitamin K_1 content of maternal milk: Influence of the stage of lactation, lipid composition, and vitamin K_1 supplements given to the mother. Pediatr Res 22:513, 1987.

Von Kries R, Stannigel H, Gobel U: Anticoagulant therapy by continuous heparin-antithrombin III infusion in newborns with disseminated intravascular coagulation. Eur J Pediatr 114:191, 1985.

Von dem Borne A, van Leeuwen EF, Von Reisz LE, et al: Neonatal alloimmune thrombocytopenia: Detection and characterization of the responsible antibodies by the platelet immunofluorescent test. Blood 57:649, 1981.

Vukovich T, Auberger K, Weil J, et al: Replacement therapy for a homozygous protein C deficiency state using a concentrate of human protein C and S. Br J Haematol 70(4):435, 1988.

Waltt H, Kurz R, Mitterstieler G, et al: Intracranial haemorrhage in low-birth-weight infants and prophylactic administration of coagulation factor concentrates. Lancet 1:1284, 1973.

Warr T, Warn-Cramer B, Rao L, Rapaport S: Human plasma extrinsic pathway inhibitor activity: I. Standardization of assay and evaluation of physiologic variables. Blood 74:201, 1989.

Weinblatt ME, Scimeca PG, James-Herry AG, Pahwa S: Thrombocytopenia in an infant with AIDS. Am J Dis Child 141:15, 1987.

Weinstein M, Blanchard R, Moake J, et al: Fetal and neonatal Von Willebrand factor (vWF) is unusually large and similar to the vWF in patients with thrombotic thrombocytopenia purpura. Br J Haematol 72:68, 1989.

Weissbach G, Harenberg J, Wendisch J, et al: Tissue factor pathway inhibitor in infants and children. Thromb Res 73(6):441, 1994.

Wenske C, Gaedicke G, Heyes H: Idiopathic thrombocytopenic purpura in pregnancy and neonatal period. Blut 48:377, 1984.

Wenske C, Gaedicke G, Kuenzlen E, et al: Treatment of idiopathic thrombocytopenic purpura in pregnancy by high-dose intravenous immunoglobulin. Blut 46:347, 1983.

Weston M, Langley PG, Rubin MH, et al: Platelet function in fulminant hepatic failure and effect of charcoal haemoperfusion. Gut 18:897, 1977.

Whaun JM, Smith GR, Sochor V: Effect of prenatal drug administration on maternal and neonatal platelet aggregation and PF4 release. Haemostasis 9:226, 1980.

Widdershoven J, Kollee L, van Munster P, et al: Biochemical vitamin K deficiency in early infancy: diagnostic limitation of conventional coagulation tests. Helvetica Paediatrica Acta 41:195, 1986.

Widdershoven J, Lambert W, Motohara K, Monnens L, de Leenheer A, Matsuda I, Endo F: Plasma concentrations of vitamin K_1 and PIVKA-II in bottle-fed and breast-fed infants with and without vitamin K prophylaxis at birth. Eur J Pediatr 148:139, 1988.

Winthrop AL, Wesson DE: Urokinase in the treatment of occluded central venous catheters in children. J Pediatr Surg 19(5):536, 1984.

Witt I, Muller H, Kunter LJ: Evidence for the existence of fetal fibrinogen. Thromb Diath Haemorrh 22:101, 1969.

Woods A, Vargas J, Berri G, Kreutzer G, Meschengieser S, Lazzari MA: Antithrombotic therapy in children and adolescents. Thromb Res 42(3):289, 1986.

Xu L, Delorme M, Berry L, Ofosu F, Mitchell L, Paes B, Andrew M: Alpha-2-macroglobulin remains as important as ATIII for thrombin regulation in cord plasma in the presence of endothelial cell surfaces. Pediatr Res 37:1, 1995.

Yamamoto K, Matsushita T, Sugiura, I, et al: Homozygous protein C deficiency: Identification of a novel missuse mutation that causes impaired secretion of the mutant protein C. J Lab Clin Med 119(6):682, 1992.

Ylikorkala O, Halmesmaki E, Viinikka L: Effect of ethanol on thromboxane and prostacyclin synthesis by fetal platelets and umbilical artery. Life Sci 41:371, 1987.

Ylikorkala O, Makila UM, Kaapa P, Viinikka L: Maternal ingestion of acetyl-salicylic acid inhibits fetal and neonatal thromboxane in humans. Am J Obstet Gynecol 155:345, 1986.

Yuen PMP, Yin JA, Lao TTH: Fibrino-peptide A levels in maternal and newborn plasma. Eur J Obstet Gynecol 30:239, 1989.

Zinkham W, Medearis DN Jr, Osborn JE: Blood and bone marrow findings in congenital rubella. J Pediatr 71:512, 1967.

Zreik H, Bengur R, Meliones J, et al: Superior vena cava obstruction after extracorporeal membrane oxygenation. J Pediatr 127:314, 1995.

CHAPTER 89

Erythrocyte Disorders in Infancy

William C. Mentzer and Bertil E. Glader

NORMAL ERYTHROCYTE PHYSIOLOGY IN THE FETUS AND NEWBORN
Fetal Erythropoiesis

Fetal erythropoiesis occurs sequentially during embryonic development in three different sites: yolk sac, liver, and bone marrow. The growth factors and cytokines that regulate embryonic hematopoiesis in humans are not yet defined, but animal work suggests that they are different from those that regulate proliferation and differentiation of stem cells in later life (Zon, 1995). Yolk sac formation of red blood cells (RBCs) is maximal between the 2nd and 10th weeks of gestation. Myeloid, or bone marrow, production of RBCs begins around the 18th week, and by the 30th week of fetal life, bone marrow is the major erythropoietic organ. At birth, almost all RBCs are produced in the bone marrow, although a low level of hepatic erythropoiesis persists through the first few days of life. Sites of fetal erythropoiesis are occasionally reactivated in older patients with hematologic disorders such as myelofibrosis, aplastic anemia, and severe hemolytic anemia.

RBC production in extrauterine life is controlled in part by erythropoietin, a humoral erythropoietic stimulating factor (ESF) produced by the kidney. The role of erythropoietin in the developing fetus has not been completely defined. Current thoughts are that ESF does not influence yolk sac or hepatic erythropoiesis, but it may partially regulate myeloid RBC production (Finne and Halvorsen, 1972). ESF is detected in fetal blood and amniotic fluid during the last trimester of pregnancy. The concentration of this hormone increases directly with the period of gestation, and thus, erythropoietin levels in term newborns are significantly higher than in premature infants. This difference may reflect some degree of fetal hypoxia during late intrauterine life. Increased ESF titers also are seen in placental dysfunction, fetal anemia, and maternal hypoxia (Finne, 1966). Fetal RBC formation is not influenced by maternal erythropoietin, because transfusion-induced maternal polycythemia (decreased maternal ESF levels) has no effect on fetal erythropoiesis (Jacobson et al, 1959). Maternal nutritional status also is not a significant factor in the regulation of fetal erythropoiesis, because iron, folate, and vitamin B_{12} are trapped by the fetus irrespective of maternal stores. Most studies have demonstrated that women with severe iron deficiency bear children with normal total body hemoglobin content (Lanzkowsky, 1961).

Hemoglobin, hematocrit, and RBC count increase throughout fetal life (Table 89–1). Extremely large RBCs (mean corpuscular volume [MCV] of 180) with an increased hemoglobin content (mean corpuscular hemoglobin [MCH] of 60) are produced early in fetal life. The size and hemoglobin content of these cells decrease throughout gestation, but the mean corpuscular hemoglobin concentration (MCHC) does not change significantly. Even at birth, the MCV and MCH are greater than those seen in older children and adults. Many nucleated RBCs and reticulocytes are present early in gestation, and the percentage of these cells also decreases as the fetus ages.

Hemoglobin production increases markedly during the last trimester of pregnancy. The actual hemoglobin concentration increases, but, more important, body weight, blood volume, and total body hemoglobin triple in size during this period. Fetal iron accumulation parallels the increase in total body hemoglobin content. The neonatal iron endowment at birth, therefore, is directly related to total body hemoglobin content and length of gestation. Term infants have more iron than premature infants.

RBC Physiology at Birth

In utero, the Po_2 in blood delivered to the tissues is only one third to one fourth of the value in adults. This relative hypoxia may be responsible for the increased content of erythropoietin and signs of active erythropoiesis (nucleated RBCs, increased reticulocytes) seen in newborns at birth. When lungs become the source of oxygen, hemoglobin-O_2 saturation increases to 95% and erythropoiesis decreases. Within 72 hours after birth, erythropoietin is undetectable, nucleated RBCs disappear, and reticulocytes decrease to less than 1%.

The concentration of hemoglobin during the first few hours of life increases to values greater than those seen in cord blood. This is both a relative increase caused by a reduction in plasma volume (Gairdner et al, 1958) and an absolute increase caused by placental blood transfusion (Usher et al, 1963). The umbilical vein remains patent long after umbilical arteries have constricted, and thus transfusion of placental blood occurs when newborns are held at a level below the placenta. The placenta contains approximately 100 mL of fetal blood (30% of the infant's blood volume). Approximately 25% of placental blood enters the newborn within 15 seconds of birth, and by 1 minute, 50% is transfused. The time of cord clamping is thus a direct determinant of neonatal blood volume. The blood volume of term infants (mean of 85 mL/kg) varies considerably (50 to 100 mL/kg) because of different degrees of placental transfusion (Usher et al, 1963). These differences are readily apparent when the effects of early versus delayed cord clamping are compared at 72 hours of age: 82.3 mL/kg (early clamping) versus 92.6 mL/kg (delayed clamping). These changes are largely the result of differences in RBC mass (early clamping, 31 mL/kg; delayed clamping, 49 mL/kg). The blood volume of premature infants (89 to 105 mL/kg) is slightly greater than that of term infants, but in large part this is due to an increased plasma volume (Usher and Lind, 1965). The RBC mass of

TABLE 89–1

Mean Red Blood Cell (RBC) Values During Gestation

Age (Weeks)	Hb (g/dL)	Hematocrit (%)	RBC (10⁶/mm³)	Mean Corpuscular Volume (fl)	Mean Corpuscular Hb (pg)	Mean Corpuscular Hb Concentration (g/dL)	Nucleated RBCs (% of RBCs)	Reticulocytes (%)	Diameter (μ)
12	8.0–10.0	33	1.5	180	60	34	5.0–8.0	40	10.5
16	10.0	35	2.0	140	45	33	2.0–4.0	10–25	9.5
20	11.0	37	2.5	135	44	33	1.0	10–20	9.0
24	14.0	40	3.5	123	38	31	1.0	5–10	8.8
28	14.5	45	4.0	120	40	31	0.5	5–10	8.7
34	15.0	47	4.4	118	38	32	0.2	3–10	8.5

Hb, hemoglobin.
From Oski FA, Naiman JL: Hematologic Problems in the Newborn. 3rd ed. Philadelphia, WB Saunders, 1982.

premature infants, expressed as milliliters per kilogram, is the same as in term newborns.

Fetal and Neonatal Hemoglobin Function

A variety of hemoglobins are present during fetal and neonatal life (see Hemolysis due to Hemoglobin Disorders). Fetal hemoglobin is the major hemoglobin in utero, whereas hemoglobin A is the normal hemoglobin of extrauterine life. A single RBC may contain both hemoglobin F and hemoglobin A in varying proportions, depending on gestational and postnatal age. One major difference between hemoglobins A and F is related to oxygen transport.

The transport of oxygen to peripheral tissues is regulated by several factors, including blood oxygen capacity, cardiac output, and hemoglobin-oxygen affinity. (1) Oxygen capacity is a direct function of hemoglobin concentration (1 g hemoglobin combines with 1.34 mL oxygen). (2) Compensatory changes in cardiac output can maintain normal O_2 delivery under conditions in which oxygen capacity is significantly reduced. (3) The oxygen affinity of hemoglobin also influences oxygen delivery to tissues. Hemoglobin A is 95% saturated at arterial oxygen tensions (100 mm Hg), but this decreases to 70% to 75% saturation at a venous PO_2 of 40 mm Hg. The difference in O_2 content at arterial and venous oxygen tensions reflects the amount of oxygen that can be released. Changes in hemoglobin affinity for oxygen can influence O_2 delivery (Fig. 89–1). At any given PO_2, more oxygen is bound to hemoglobin when oxygen affinity is increased. Stated in physiologic terms, increased hemoglobin-oxygen affinity reduces oxygen delivery, whereas decreased hemoglobin-oxygen affinity increases oxygen release to peripheral tissues.

The oxygen affinity of hemoglobin A in solution is greater than that of hemoglobin F. Paradoxically, however, whole blood from normal children (hemoglobin A) has a lower oxygen affinity than neonatal blood (hemoglobin F) (Allen et al, 1953). This difference is related to an intermediate of RBC metabolism, 2,3-diphosphoglycerate (2,3-DPG). This organic phosphate compound interacts with hemoglobin A to decrease its affinity for oxygen and thereby enhance O_2 release. Fetal hemoglobin does not interact with 2,3-DPG to any significant extent (Bauer et al, 1968); consequently, cells containing hemoglobin F have a higher oxygen affinity than those containing hemoglobin A.

The increased oxygen affinity of fetal RBCs is advantageous for extracting oxygen from maternal blood within the placenta. A few months after birth, however, infant blood acquires the same oxygen affinity as that of older children (Fig. 89–2). The postnatal decrease in O_2 affinity is due to a reduction in hemoglobin F and an increase in hemoglobin A (which interacts with 2,3-DPG). Oxygen delivery (the difference in arterial and venous O_2 content) actually increases while oxygen capacity (hemoglobin concentration) decreases during the 1st week of life (Fig. 89–3). This enhanced delivery is largely a reflection of the decreased

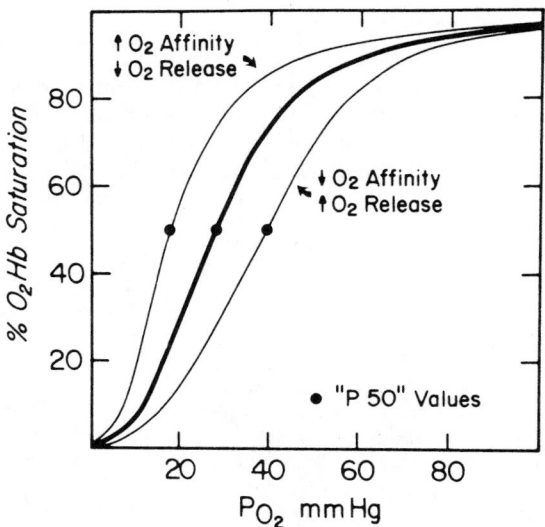

FIGURE 89–1. The oxygen dissociation curve of normal adult hemoglobin (dark line). The percent oxygen saturation (ordinate) is plotted for arterial oxygen tensions between 0 and 100 mm Hg (abscissa). As the curve shifts to the right, more oxygen is released at any given PO_2. Conversely, as the curve shifts to the left, more oxygen is retained on hemoglobin at any given PO_2. The "P 50" refers to that PO_2 in which hemoglobin is 50% saturated with oxygen. This term is useful in comparing the oxygen affinity of different hemoglobins. (From Oski FA, Delivoria-Papadopoulos M: The red cell, 2,3-diphosphoglycerate, and tissue oxygen release. J Pediatr 77:941, 1970.)

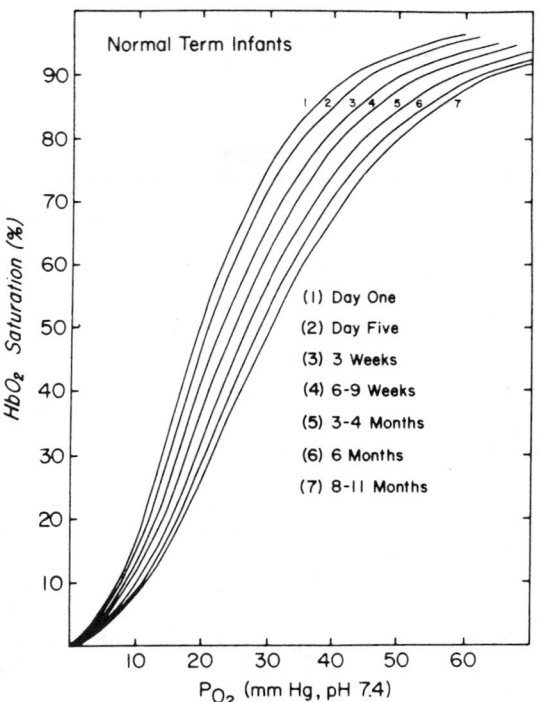

FIGURE 89–2. The oxygen affinity of blood from term infants at birth and at different postnatal ages. The gradual rightward shift of the oxygen saturation curve indicates increased oxygen release from hemoglobin as infants get older. This decreased oxygen affinity is due to a decrease in hemoglobin F and an increase in hemoglobin A. (From Oski FA, Delivoria-Papadopoulos M. The red cell, 2,3-diphosphoglycerate, and tissue oxygen release. J Pediatr 77:941, 1970.)

oxygen affinity of infant blood (Delivoria-Papadopoulos et al, 1971). The oxygen affinity of blood from premature infants is higher than that of term infants, and the normal postnatal changes (decrease in oxygen affinity, increase in

oxygen delivery) occur much more gradually in premature infants (see Fig. 89–3).

GENERAL APPROACH TO ANEMIC INFANTS
Medical History and Physical Examination

The cause of anemia frequently can be ascertained by medical history and physical examination. Particular importance is given to family history (anemia, cholelithiasis, unexplained jaundice, splenomegaly), maternal medical history (especially infections), and obstetric history (previous pregnancies, length of gestation, method and difficulty of delivery). The age at which anemia becomes manifest also is of diagnostic importance. Significant anemia at birth invariably is due to blood loss or alloimmune hemolysis. After 24 hours, internal hemorrhages and other causes of hemolysis become manifest. Anemia that appears several weeks after birth can be caused by a variety of conditions, including abnormalities in the synthesis of hemoglobin-beta chains, hypoplastic RBC disorders, and the physiologic anemia of infancy or prematurity.

Infants with anemia resulting from chronic blood loss may appear pale, without other evidence of clinical distress. Acute blood loss can produce hypovolemic shock and a clinical state similar to severe neonatal asphyxia. Newborns with hemolytic anemia frequently show a greater than expected degree of icterus. In addition, hemolysis often is associated with hepatosplenomegaly, and in cases resulting from congenital infection, other stigmata may be present.

Laboratory Evaluation of Anemia

A simple classification of neonatal anemia based on physical examination and simple laboratory tests is presented in Table 89–2. More esoteric RBC tests are described elsewhere (Alter, 1989).

FIGURE 89–3. Oxygen delivery in normal term and premature infants. Oxygen content (a function of total hemoglobin) is on the ordinate. Oxygen tension is on the abscissa. Oxygen delivery is measured by the difference in oxygen content at arterial (100 mm Hg) and venous (40 mm Hg) oxygen tensions. For both term and premature infants, oxygen delivery (shaded areas) increases with age. This occurs despite a decrease in oxygen content. (From Delivoria-Papadopoulos M, Roncevic NP, Oski FA: Postnatal changes in oxygen transport of term, premature, and sick infants: The role of red cell 2,3-diphosphoglycerate and adult hemoglobin. Pediatr Res 5:235, 1971.)

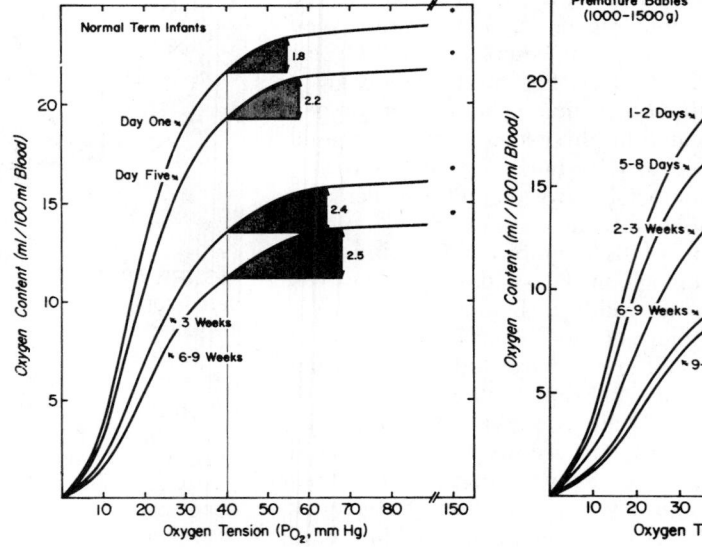

Differential Approach to Anemia in Newborn Period

Hemoglobin	Reticulocytes	Bilirubin	Coombs Test	Clinical Considerations
Decreased	Normal/decreased	Normal	Negative	Physiologic anemia of infancy and prematurity
				Hypoplastic anemia
Decreased	Normal/increased	Normal	Negative	Hemorrhagic anemia
Decreased	Normal/increased	Increased	Positive	Immune-mediated hemolysis
Decreased	Normal/increased	Increased	Negative	Acquired or hereditary RBC defects
				Enclosed hemorrhage with resorption of blood
				Coombs-negative ABO incompatibility

RBC Count, Hemoglobin, Hematocrit, and RBC Indices

RBC values during the neonatal period are more variable than at any other time of life. The diagnosis of anemia must therefore be made in terms of "normal" values appropriate for gestational and postnatal age. The mean cord blood hemoglobin of healthy term infants ranges between 14 and 20 g/100 mL (Table 89-3). Shortly after birth, however, hemoglobin concentration increases. This increase is both relative (owing to a reduction of plasma volume) and absolute (owing to placental RBC transfusion). Failure of hemoglobin to increase during the first few hours of life may be the initial sign of hemorrhagic anemia. RBC values at the end of the 1st week are virtually identical with those seen at birth. Anemia during the 1st week of life is thus defined as any hemoglobin value less than 14 g/100 mL. A significant hemoglobin decrease during this time, although within the normal range, is suggestive of hemorrhage or hemolysis. For example, 14.5 g hemoglobin at 7 days of age is abnormal for a term infant whose hemoglobin was 18.5 g at birth. A slight hemoglobin reduction normally occurs in premature infants during the 1st week of life. Beyond the 1st week, however, the hemoglobin concentration decreases in both term and premature infants (see Physiologic Anemia of Infancy and Prematurity).

The electronic equipment currently used for blood counts also gives statistical information regarding erythrocyte size (MCV) and hemoglobin content (MCH). The normal MCV (fl) in older children ranges from 75 to 90. MCVs of less than 75 are considered microcytic, whereas those over 100 indicate macrocytosis. Normal infant RBCs are large (MCV, 105 to 125), and not until 8 to 10 weeks of age does cell size approach that of older children. Neonatal microcytosis is defined as an MCV of less than 95 at birth. The RBC hemoglobin content of neonatal cells (MCH, 35 to 38) is greater than that seen in older children (MCH, 30 to 33). Neonatal hypochromia is defined as an MCH of less than 34. Hypochromia and microcytosis generally occur together, and invariably these abnormalities are due to hemoglobin production defects. Neonatal hypochromic microcytosis is seen with iron deficiency (chronic blood loss) and thalassemia disorders (alpha and gamma thalassemias).

The site at which blood is obtained is important, because higher hemoglobins and hematocrits occur in capillary blood compared with simultaneously obtained central venous samples (up to 20%). This difference can be minimized by warming an extremity to obtain "arterialized capillary blood" (Oh and Lind, 1966). In the face of acute hemorrhage, however, central venous samples must be obtained because of marked peripheral vasoconstriction.

Reticulocyte Count

The normal reticulocyte count of children and older infants is 1% to 2%. The reticulocyte count in term infants ranges

RBC Values in Term and Premature Infants During the 1st Week of Life

	Hgb (g/100 mL)	Hct (%)	Reticulocytes (%)	Nucleated RBCs (cells/1000 RBCs)
Term				
Cord blood	17.0	53.0	<7	<1.00
	(14–20)	(45–61)		
Day 1	18.4	58.0	<7	<0.40
Day 3	17.8	55.0	<3	<0.01
Day 7	17.0	54.0	<1	0
Premature (weighing less than 1500 g)				
Cord blood	16.0	49	<10	<3.00
	(13.0–18.5)			
Day 7	14.8	45	<3	<0.01

between 3% and 7% at birth, but this decreases to 1% to 3% by 4 days and to less than 1% by 7 days of age (see Table 89-3). In premature infants, reticulocyte values at birth are higher (6% to 10%) and may remain elevated for a longer period of time. Nucleated RBCs are seen in newborn infants, but they generally disappear by the 3rd day of life in term infants and in 7 to 10 days in premature infants. The persistence of reticulocytosis or nucleated RBCs suggests the possibility of hemorrhage or hemolysis. Hypoxia, in the absence of anemia, also can be associated with increased release of reticulocytes and nucleated RBCs.

Peripheral Blood Smear

Examination of the peripheral blood smear is an invaluable aid in the diagnosis of anemia. In particular, the smear is evaluated for alterations in the size and shape of RBCs as well as abnormalities in leukocytes and platelets. Erythrocytes of older children are approximately the size of a small lymphocyte nucleus, whereas those of newborns are slightly larger. RBC hemoglobinization (e.g., hypochromia) is estimated by observing the area of central pallor, which is one third the diameter of normal RBCs and more than one half the diameter of hypochromic cells. Spherocytes are detected by the complete absence of central pallor. The degree of reticulocytosis can be estimated, because these cells are larger and have a bluish coloration.

Coombs' Test

Most cases of neonatal hemolytic anemia are due to isoimmunization. The Coombs' test detects the presence of antibody on RBCs (direct Coombs') or in the plasma (indirect Coombs'). The direct Coombs' test also is known as the *direct antiglobulin test* (DAT). The clinician must search diligently to rule out an isoimmune disorder before embarking on a more wide-ranging (and expensive) work-up of hemolysis.

Blood Transfusions in the Treatment of Anemia

A hemoglobin of 14 g/100 mL corresponds to a RBC mass of 31 mL/kg. This implies that a transfusion of 2 mL RBC/kg increases the hemoglobin concentration by approximately 1 g/100 mL. Packed RBCs (hematocrit approximately 67%) contain 2 mL of RBC/3 mL packed RBC. Whole blood (hematocrit approximately 33%) contains 2 mL RBC/6 mL whole blood. Thus, the transfusion of 3 mL packed RBC/kg or 6 mL whole blood/kg increases hemoglobin concentration by approximately 1 g/100 mL.

Packed RBCs are the product of choice when transfusion is necessary for simple anemia, as occurs in hemolysis. If anemia is accompanied by hypovolemia from acute blood loss, volume expansion must be achieved promptly, using either whole blood or packed RBCs and a colloid such as 5% serum albumin or plasma protein fraction (infused separately). Because of the reduced availability of whole blood, owing to the demand for components, the usual choice is packed RBCs and colloid. The previously common practice of reconstituting RBCs with fresh-frozen

plasma to make "whole blood" is no longer acceptable because the increased donor exposure increases the risk of transmitting infectious disease. When packed RBCs need to be diluted to facilitate nonurgent transfusion, isotonic saline is the preferred diluent. If exchange transfusion is needed to treat hyperbilirubinemia, the capability of albumin to improve bilirubin binding and removal is ample reason to request whole blood. Although fresh blood less than 2 days old is ideal because there is a reduced risk of hyperkalemia, this is not usually available. An acceptable substitute is packed RBCs less than 4 to 5 days old. These packed RBCs provide adequate oxygen delivery; hyperkalemia can be prevented by washing the RBCs once in saline, then reconstituting with normal saline. Washing is not required for the usual small simple transfusions of packed RBCs, wherein the small volume of plasma negates any toxic effect of increased concentration of potassium in the plasma.

Blood currently available in most blood banks is anticoagulated with citrate-phosphate-dextrose (CPD) or CPD-adenine (CPDA-1), with shelf-lives of 21 or 35 days, respectively. Hematocrit usually ranges between 65 and 80% for packed RBCs. Near-normal 2,3-DPG levels are maintained for up to 12 to 14 days, which is advantageous when transfusing infants with acute hypoxia or those receiving large volumes of blood. Newer additive preparations in which most of the plasma is replaced by a solution containing saline, adenine, glucose (and, in some preparations, mannitol) support storage of RBCs up to 42 days. (Although these are the predominant RBCs available, the longer shelf-life is of no advantage for newborns, in whom fresher cells are preferred.) Hematocrits range from 55% to 65%, thus facilitating flow during infusion. Limited experience suggests that these preparations are well tolerated by newborns.

Preterm infants born weighing less than 1250 g are uniquely susceptible to potentially serious cytomegalovirus (CMV) infection from transfused blood, particularly if they lack immunity because their mothers are seronegative. This can be prevented by using blood products only from seronegative donors (Yeager et al, 1981). Because approximately 40% to 60% of adults are seropositive, this limits the availability of seronegative donors. Reserving seronegative blood for the minority of infants who are seronegative can reduce the demand for such donors. Alternatively, because CMV resides mainly in leukocytes, removal of such cells could prevent transmission of the virus. Frozen thawed, deglycerolized RBCs (Brady et al, 1984) and high-efficiency leukocyte depletion filters (Gilbert et al, 1989) have proved effective. Conventional saline-washed RBCs are not effective, presumably because they contain greater numbers of residual leukocytes (Demmler et al, 1986). A potential disadvantage of using CMV-seronegative blood in CMV-positive infants receiving large amounts of blood is dilution of infant's antibody level, resulting in increased susceptibility to nursery-acquired CMV infection.

Graft-versus-host (GVH) reaction rarely follows transfusion and occurs mainly in certain newborns at risk. For this to occur, viable lymphocytes in cellular blood products must be able to engraft and react against foreign antigens on tissues of the recipient. Infants at risk include those with congenital or acquired defects of cellular immunity, fetuses receiving intrauterine transfusion of RBCs or platelets, newborns receiving exchange transfusion following intrauterine transfusion (Naiman et al, 1969; Parkman et al, 1974), and infants receiving directed blood donations from first-degree relatives (whose genetic similarity may increase the likelihood of engraftment). Irradiation of RBCs, whole blood, platelets, and granulocytes with a minimum of 1500 rads has proved effective in preventing GVH reaction. Reports of GVH reaction after RBC transfusion in very premature infants without known risk factors (Enoki et al, 1985; Sanders et al, 1989) have prompted some workers to recommend irradiation of blood given to all infants with this condition. Logistics difficulties in providing routine irradiation preclude general endorsement of such recommendations.

HEMORRHAGIC ANEMIA

Anemia frequently follows fetal blood loss, bleeding from obstetric complications, and internal hemorrhages associated with birth trauma (Table 89–4). The clinical presentation of anemia depends on the magnitude and acuteness of blood loss.

Infants with anemia subsequent to moderate hemorrhage or chronic blood loss are generally asymptomatic. The only physical findings are pallor of the skin and mucous membranes. Laboratory studies can range from a mild normochromic-normocytic anemia (hemoglobin 9 to 12 g/100 mL) to a more severe hypochromic-microcytic anemia (hemoglobin 5 to 7 g/100 mL). The only therapy required for asymptomatic children is iron (2 mg elemental iron/kg, three times per day for 3 months). RBC replacement is indicated only if there is evidence of clinical distress (tachycardia, tachypnea, irritability, feeding difficulties). In most cases, increasing the hemoglobin to 10 to 12 g/100 mL removes all signs and symptoms associated with anemia. Because severely anemic infants are frequently in incipient heart failure, however, these children should be transfused

---

TABLE 89–4

Causes of Hemorrhagic Anemia in Newborns

Fetal hemorrhage
  Spontaneous fetomaternal hemorrhage
  Hemorrhage following amniocentesis
  Twin–twin transfusion
  Nuchal cord
Placental hemorrhage
  Placenta previa
  Abruptio placentae
  Multilobed placenta (vasa previa)
  Velamentous insertion of cord
  Placental incision during cesarean section
Umbilical cord bleeding
  Rupture of umbilical cord with precipitous delivery
  Rupture of short or entangled cord
Postpartum hemorrhage
  Bleeding from umbilicus
  Cephalhematomas, scalp hemorrhages
  Hepatic rupture, splenic rupture
  Retroperitoneal hemorrhages

TABLE 89–5

Comparative Clinical Findings in Neonatal Asphyxia and Acute Hemorrhage

	Neonatal Asphyxia	Acute Blood Loss
Heart rate	Decreased	Increased
Respiratory rate	Decreased	Increased
Intercostal retractions	Present	Absent
Skin color	Pallor with cyanosis	Pallor without cyanosis
Response to oxygen and assisted ventilation	Marked improvement	No significant change

---

very slowly (2 mL/kg per hour). If signs of congestive heart failure appear, a rapid-acting diuretic (furosemide, 1 mg/kg intravenously) should be given before proceeding with the transfusion. An alternative approach is to administer a partial exchange transfusion with packed RBCs to severely anemic infants. This increases the hemoglobin concentration without the danger of increasing blood volume and precipitating congestive heart failure.

A simple formula for the volume of RBCs needed in a partial exchange transfusion to correct severe anemia has been described by Nieburg and Stockman (1977): Packed RBC volume needed (mL) = body weight (kg) × 75 mL/kg × desired hemoglobin change/[22 g/dL − Hgb_w], where 75 mL/kg approximates the average blood volume and 22 g/dL represents the hemoglobin concentration of packed RBCs. The term Hgb_w is a reflection of the hemoglobin removed during the exchange transfusion, and this is approximated by (initial hemoglobin + desired hemoglobin)/2. For each infusion and withdrawal, syringe volumes up to 5% of the blood volume are well tolerated. For example, in the case of a 3-kg newborn with a hemoglobin of 3 g/dL that needs to be raised to a hemoglobin of 10 g/dL, approximately 100 mL of packed RBCs are needed for the procedure; syringe volumes of 15 mL can be used for each cycle of infusion and withdrawal of blood.

Infants who rapidly lose large volumes of blood appear to be in acute distress (pallor, tachycardia, tachypnea, weak pulses, hypotension, and shock). This presentation is distinct from that seen in neonatal respiratory asphyxia (slow respirations with intercostal retractions, bradycardia, and pallor with cyanosis) (Table 89–5). The clinical response to assisted ventilation and oxygen is also different: Infants with respiratory problems demonstrate a marked improvement, whereas there is little change in anemic newborns. Cyanosis is not a feature of severe anemia because the hemoglobin concentration is too low (clinical cyanosis indicates at least 5 g/100 mL of deoxygenated hemoglobin). The hemoglobin concentration immediately after an acute hemorrhage may be normal, because the initial response to acute volume depletion is vasoconstriction. A decreased hemoglobin may not be seen until the plasma volume has re-expanded several hours later. In view of these hemodynamic considerations, it is apparent that the diagnosis of acute hemorrhagic anemia is based largely on physical findings and evidence of blood loss. It is important to recognize these clinical features because immediate therapy is required. Treatment is directed at rapid expansion of the vascular space (20 mL fluid/kg). This is most quickly accomplished by rapid infusion of either isotonic saline or 5% albumin, followed by either type-specific, cross-matched whole blood, or packed RBCs resuspended with saline depending on availability. Fresh-frozen plasma, formerly used for reconstituting RBCs, is no longer acceptable because of the increased donor exposure with resultant increased risk of transfusion-transmissible infection. In infants in whom anemia and hypoxia are severe, non-cross-matched group O, Rh-negative RBCs are an acceptable alternative. Infants with hypovolemic shock caused by acute external blood loss usually show marked clinical improvement after this treatment. A poor response is seen in newborns with severe internal hemorrhage.

Fetal Hemorrhage

Fetomaternal Hemorrhage

Significant bleeding into the maternal circulation occurs in approximately 8% of all pregnancies and thus represents one of the most common forms of fetal bleeding. Small amounts of fetal blood are lost in most cases, but in 1% of pregnancies fetal blood loss may be as great as 40 mL (Cohen et al, 1964). Fetomaternal hemorrhage occasionally follows amniocentesis and placental injury (Zipursky et al, 1963), although anemia is seen only after unsuccessful amniocentesis or when there is evidence of a bloody tap (Woo Wang et al, 1967). For this reason, infants born to mothers who have had amniocentesis should be observed closely for signs of anemia. The effects of anemia resulting from fetomaternal hemorrhages are variable. Large acute hemorrhages can produce hypovolemic shock (Raye et al, 1970), whereas slower, more chronic blood loss results in hypochromic microcytic anemia resulting from iron deficiency (Pearson and Diamond, 1959). Some infants with severe chronic anemia (hemoglobin as low as 4 to 6 g/100 mL) may have minimal symptoms. An examination of the maternal blood smear for the presence of fetal cells (Kleihauer-Betke preparation) is necessary in any infant with suspected fetomaternal hemorrhage. This test is based on the principle that hemoglobin A is eluted from RBCs at an acid pH, whereas hemoglobin F is not affected by these conditions. Consequently, when alcohol-fixed and acid-treated RBCs are stained with eosin, those containing hemoglobin A are colorless, whereas those containing hemoglobin F (fetal RBCs) appear normally colored. Approximately 50 mL of fetal blood must be lost to produce significant neonatal anemia. This volume is greater than 1% of the maternal blood volume, and therefore fetal cells within the maternal circulation may be detected readily. This test is not valid when there is coexistence of maternal hemoglobinopathies with increased hemoglobin F levels. In addition, fetomaternal ABO incompatibility may cause rapid removal of fetal RBCs and thus obscure any significant hemorrhage. For this reason, it is important to examine maternal blood as soon as anemia from fetal hemorrhage is suspected. An unusual form of fetal blood loss is presumed to occur in infants born with a nuchal cord. In these cases, anemia is caused by compression of the umbilical vein, preventing placental blood from returning to the fetus (Shepherd et al, 1985).

Twin–Twin Transfusion

Transfusion of blood from one homozygous twin to another can result in anemia in the donor twin and polycythemia in the recipient. Significant hemorrhage is seen only in monochorionic monozygous twins (approximately 70% of all monozygous twins). In approximately 15% of these pregnancies, there is a twin–twin transfusion (Rausen et al, 1965). Bleeding occurs because of vascular anastomosis in monochorionic placentas. The anemic donor twin is usually smaller than the polycythemic recipient, with a greater than 20% difference in birth weight. Polyhydramnios is frequently seen in the recipient twin and oligohydramnios is seen in the donor. Twin–twin transfusions should be suspected when the hemoglobin concentration of identical twins differs by more than 5 g/100 mL; however, such a difference in hemoglobin concentration does not prove there has been a twin–twin transfusion. Recent studies indicate that this major hemoglobin difference can exist in some dichorionic twins, in whom there are no vascular anastamoses and therefore no possibility for twin–twin transfusion (Danskin and Neilson, 1989).

Placental Blood Loss

Placental bleeding during pregnancy is common, but in most cases hemorrhage is from the maternal aspect of the placenta. In placenta previa, however, the thin placenta overlying the cervical os frequently results in fetal blood loss. The vascular communications between multilobular placental lobes are also very fragile and are easily subjected to trauma during delivery. Vasa previa is the condition in which one of these connecting vessels overlies the cervical os and thus is prone to rupture during delivery. Abruptio placentae generally causes fetal anoxia and death, although some infants survive but can be severely anemic. Bleeding also follows inadvertent placental incision during cesarean sections (Montague and Krevans, 1966), and thus the placenta should be inspected for injury following all cesarean sections.

Umbilical Cord Bleeding

The normal umbilical cord is resistant to minor trauma and does not bleed. The umbilical cord of dysmature infants, however, is weak and liable to rupture and hemorrhage (Raye et al, 1970). In cases of precipitous delivery, a rapid increase in cord tension can rupture the fetal aspect of the cord and cause serious acute blood loss. Short or entangled umbilical cords and abnormalities of umbilical blood vessels (velamentous insertions into the placenta) are also liable to rupture and hemorrhage. Bleeding from injured umbilical cords is rapid but generally ceases after a short period of time, owing to arterial constriction. The umbilical cord should always be inspected for abnormalities or signs of injury, particularly after unattended, precipitous deliveries.

Hemorrhage After Delivery

Hemorrhagic anemia due to internal bleeding is occasionally associated with birth trauma. Characteristically, internal hemorrhages are asymptomatic during the first 24 to 48 hours of life, with signs and symptoms of anemia developing after this time. Cephalhematomas can be sufficiently large to cause anemia and hyperbilirubinemia, owing to the resorption of blood (Leonard and Anthony, 1961). Subgaleal hemorrhages are seen infrequently, sometimes after vacuum extraction used during delivery. These hemorrhages may be extensive because bleeding is not limited by periosteum. Adrenal and kidney hemorrhages occasionally follow difficult breech deliveries. Splenic rupture and hemorrhage occur most commonly in association with splenomegaly, as in erythroblastosis fetalis. Hepatic hemorrhages are generally subcapsular and may be asymptomatic. Rupture of the hepatic capsule results in hemoperitoneum and hypovolemic shock. Hepatic hemorrhages are suspected when a previously healthy infant goes into shock with clinical manifestations of an increasing right upper quadrant abdominal mass, shifting dullness on percussion, and evidence of free fluid on abdominal radiographs. In contrast to newborns with acute blood loss from fetomaternal or umbilical vessel bleeding, infants with hepatic hemorrhage generally demonstrate a poor clinical response to blood replacement.

HEMOLYTIC ANEMIA

RBCs from children and adults normally circulate for 100 to 120 days. Erythrocyte survival in newborns is somewhat shorter: 70 to 90 days in term infants, 50 to 80 days in premature infants (Pearson, 1967). Hemolytic anemia that further shortens RBC survival may arise for many reasons (Table 89–6). The precise mechanism of cell destruction is not always known, although membrane deformability is thought to be an important determinant (LaCelle, 1970). Erythrocytes are 7 to 8 μm wide, whereas the vascular diameter in some areas of the microcirculation may be less than 3 μm. Consequently, RBCs must deform their membranes and intracellular contents in order to pass through these narrow channels. This is no problem for normal RBCs. Abnormalities in RBC metabolism, hemo-

globin, or cell shape, however, all lead to decreased RBC membrane deformability. The consequence of this decreased membrane flexibility is RBC sequestration and removal by reticuloendothelial cells of the spleen and liver.

In older infants and children, the usual response to increased RBC destruction is enhanced erythropoiesis, and there may be little or no anemia if the rate of production matches the accelerated rate of destruction. In these cases of well-compensated hemolysis, the major manifestations are due to increased erythrocyte destruction (hyperbilirubinemia) and augmented erythropoiesis (reticulocytosis). During the early neonatal period, however, the increased oxygen-carrying capacity of blood (see Physiologic Anemia of Infancy) may blunt any compensatory erythropoietic activity in cases of mild hemolysis. Consequently, hyperbilirubinemia in excess of normal neonatal levels may be the only apparent manifestation of hemolysis. In most cases of significant hemolysis, however, some degree of reticulocytosis is usually present. The degree of hyperbilirubinemia and reticulocytosis must be interpreted in terms of values appropriate for gestational and postgestational age.

Immune Hemolysis

Placental transfer of maternal antibodies directed against fetal RBC antigens is the most common cause of neonatal hemolysis. This is a consequence of maternal sensitization to fetal RBC antigens inherited from the father. Hemolysis occurs only in the fetus. The spectrum of clinical problems ranges from minimal anemia and hyperbilirubinemia to severe anemia with hydrops fetalis. At one time, before effective prevention of Rh sensitization was available, hemolytic disease of the newborn was responsible for more than 10,000 deaths annually in the United States (Freda et al, 1975). Since the development of immunoprophylaxis against Rh D sensitization, the overall incidence of alloimmune hemolysis has decreased dramatically. Nevertheless, the majority of *serious* alloimmune hemolysis cases are still due to Rh D incompatibility, although ABO maternal-fetal incompatibility is much more common. A much smaller fraction of neonatal hemolytic disease is due to sensitization to Kell, Duffy, Kidd, and other Rh antigens.

Rh Hemolytic Disease (Erythroblastosis Fetalis)

The role of Rh antibody in classic erythroblastosis fetalis was first elucidated in 1941 by Levine and Katzin. There are several recognized Rh antigens, each of which is detected by specific antibodies. It is known that Rh blood-group antigens are determined by at least two homologous but distinct membrane-associated proteins. Two of these membrane proteins have separate isoforms (C and c; E and e), which are detected by specific antibodies (anti-C and anti-c; anti-E and anti-e). The most important of the membrane Rh proteins is the D antigen. Rh-positive RBC are those that possess this antigen. The symbol "d" (used to denote the absence of D, or Rh-negative) is not related to a specific antigen in that no anti-d serum has been identified. Rh proteins are encoded by two separate genes located on chromosome 1; they are designated Rh CcEe and Rh D (Mouro et al, 1993). The Rh CcEe gene encodes for both the C/c and E/e proteins. The Rh D gene encodes

---

TABLE 89–6

Causes of Hemolytic Anemia During the Newborn Period

Immune
　Isoimmune: Rh and ABO incompatibility
　Maternal immune disease: autoimmune hemolytic anemia, systemic lupus erythematosus
　Drug induced: penicillin
Acquired red blood cell (RBC) disorders
　Infection: cytomegalovirus toxoplasmosis, syphilis, bacterial sepsis
　Disseminated and localized intravascular coagulation, respiratory distress syndrome
Hereditary RBC disorders
　Membrane defects: hereditary spherocytosis, hereditary elliptocytosis
　Enzyme abnormalities: glucose-6-phosphate dehydrogenase pyruvate kinase
　Hemoglobinopathies: alpha-thalassemia syndromes, gamma/beta-thalassemia

for the Rh D proteins. The Rh-negative phenotype results from deletion of the Rh D gene on both chromosomes. In most cases, the Rh-negative phenotype also is associated with Rh c and Rh e (i.e., Rh cde). The frequency of Rh negativity varies in different racial groups. It is high in whites (15%), lower in blacks (5%), and virtually nonexistent in Asians. The Rh-positive phenotype may result from homozygosity (DD) or heterozygosity (Dd) for the D antigen. In Rh-positive whites, approximately 44% are homozygous (DD) and 56% are heterozygous (Dd). Knowledge of differences in Rh D genotype are important because approximately 25% of fetuses of couples with an Rh D–negative mother and an Rh D–positive father will be Rh D negative.

Current understanding of the natural history of Rh sensitization largely is derived from clinical experience gained before the immunologic prevention of neonatal hemolysis was readily available. The pathophysiology of alloimmune hemolysis resulting from Rh incompatibility includes the following: an Rh-negative mother, an Rh-positive fetus, leakage of fetal RBCs into maternal circulation, maternal sensitization to D antigen on fetal RBCs, production and transplacental passage of maternal anti-D antibodies into fetal circulation, attachment of maternal antibodies to Rh-positive fetal RBCs, and destruction of antibody-coated fetal RBCs. Historically, Rh hemolytic disease was rare (1%) during the first pregnancy involving an Rh-positive fetus; however, the likelihood of an infant being affected increased significantly with each subsequent pregnancy. Small volumes of fetal RBCs enter the maternal circulation throughout gestation, although the major fetomaternal bleeding responsible for sensitization occurs during delivery (Zipursky et al, 1963). Once sensitization has occurred, re-exposure to Rh D RBCs in subsequent pregnancies leads to an anamnestic response, with an increase in the maternal anti–Rh D antibody titer. Currently, significant hemolysis occurring in the first pregnancy indicates prior maternal exposure to Rh-positive RBCs, a consequence of fetal bleeding associated with a previous spontaneous or therapeutic abortion, ectopic pregnancy, or a variety of different prenatal procedures. On occasion the sensitization may be a consequence of an earlier transfusion in which Rh-positive RBCs were administered by mistake or in which some other blood product (e.g., platelets) containing Rh D RBCs was transfused.

The major factor responsible for the reduced death rate is the development of Rh immune globulin to prevent maternal sensitization. Important early observations were that fetomaternal RBC transfer (and thereby sensitization) primarily occurs during delivery and that the frequency of Rh immune hemolytic disease was much lower in ABO-incompatible pregnancies (maternal RBC type O, fetal RBC type A or B). The apparent beneficial effect of ABO incompatibility is due to the fact that maternal anti-A and anti-B antibodies recognize the corresponding A and B fetal RBCs, leading to their destruction before sensitization can occur. As a result of these early observations, it became standard practice for unsensitized Rh-negative mothers to receive a single intramuscular dose of Rh immune globulin (300 μg) within 72 hours of delivering of an Rh-positive infant (Freda et al, 1975). The results of this therapy were remarkable, with the virtual elimination of Rh D

sensitization as a major cause of hemolytic disease in newborns. The few treatment failures seen were attributed to fetomaternal bleeding of greater than 30 mL at delivery or bleeding that occurred antenatally. The current standard of practice is to administer Rh immune globulin to all unsensitized Rh-negative women at 28 weeks' gestation, with an additional second dose given at birth if the infant is Rh-positive. Moreover, the dose of Rh immune globulin should be increased proportionately when there is evidence of larger than normal fetomaternal bleeding at delivery. In suspicious cases (e.g., placental abruption, neonatal anemia), the volume of fetal hemorrhage can be quantified using the Kleihauer-Betke stain. Rh immune globulin also should be administered to unsensitized Rh-negative women after any event known to be associated with increased risk of fetomaternal hemorrhage (e.g., spontaneous or therapeutic abortion, amniocentesis, or chorionic villus biopsy). The risk of anti-Rh desensitization ranges from 0.6% to 5.4% when nonsensitized Rh-negative women undergo amniocentesis (Spinnato, 1992).

In pregnant Rh-negative women previously sensitized to Rh D, the transplacental passage of maternal anti-Rh D leads to a positive DAT on Rh D fetal RBCs. Depending on the amount of anti-D absorbed, varying degrees of fetal hemolysis occur, thereby leading to anemia, hepatosplenomegaly, and increased bilirubin formation. In utero, bilirubin is removed by transfer across the placenta into the maternal circulation; therefore, hyperbilirubinemia is not a problem until after delivery when levels may increase because of immaturity of hepatic conjugating enzymes. The major threat to the fetus is severe anemia leading to hydrops fetalis and intrauterine death. The clinical severity of neonatal hemolytic disease varies.

Mild hemolytic disease is most common, and affected infants have a positive DAT with minimal hemolysis, no significant anemia (cord blood hemoglobin greater than 14 g/dL), and minimal hyperbilirubinemia (cord blood bilirubin less than 4 mg/dL). Aside from early phototherapy, these newborns generally require no therapy unless the postnatal bilirubin increase is greater than expected. Infants who do not become sufficiently jaundiced to require exchange transfusion are at risk of development of severe anemia associated with a low reticulocyte count at 3 to 6 weeks of age; thus it is important to closely monitor hemoglobin levels after hospital discharge.

Moderate hemolytic disease is found in a smaller fraction of affected infants, and this is characterized by hemolysis, moderate anemia (cord blood hemoglobin less than 14 g/dL), and increased cord blood bilirubin levels (greater than 4 mg/dL). The peripheral blood may reveal numerous nucleated RBCs, decreased numbers of platelets, and occasionally a leukemoid reaction with large numbers of immature granulocytes. The cause of thrombocytopenia is not understood, but it is unlikely to be an immune reaction, because platelets lack Rh antigens. Similarly, the cause of the leukemoid reaction is not defined, although rarely it may be confused with congenital leukemia. Infants with Rh disease also may exhibit marked hepatosplenomegaly, a consequence of extramedullary hematopoiesis and sequestration of antibody-coated RBCs. The risk of development of bilirubin encephalopathy is high if these neonates do not receive treatment. Thus, early exchange transfusion with type-O Rh-negative fresh RBCs is usually necessary in conjunction with intensive phototherapy. This approach has been responsible for the favorable outcome of most infants with moderate alloimmune hemolysis. It is common for newborns treated who receive exchange transfusion to demonstrate a lower than normal hemoglobin measurement at the nadir of their "physiologic" anemia. Therefore, follow-up of hematocrits for at least 2 months is important. In part this may be due to persistence of some anti-D antibodies and destruction of the patient's own Rh D–positive RBCs. Also, this low hemoglobin measurement may reflect the decreased p50 and enhanced oxygen delivery of adult RBCs used for the exchange process, thereby blunting the expected erythropoietic response to hypoxia. Preliminary data suggest that the administration of recombinant human erythropoietin may minimize this late anemia of Rh hemolytic disease (Ovali et al, 1996; Scaradavou et al, 1993).

Severe hemolytic disease is seen in approximately 25% of affected infants, who are either stillborn or hydropic at birth. Understanding of hydrops fetalis, originally attributed to high-output cardiac failure secondary to severe anemia, is incomplete. Two other consequences of anemia also may contribute to the edema of hydrops. One of these is low colloid osmotic pressure resulting from hypoalbuminemia, a consequence of hepatic dysfunction. The second is a capillary leak syndrome secondary to tissue hypoxia. Management of seriously affected fetuses is directed at the prevention of severe anemia and death. To accomplish this, it first is necessary to identify those fetuses at risk. An increase in the maternal Rh D antibody titer in a previously sensitized Rh-negative woman is a good serologic measure of a fetus in potential jeopardy. Moreover, a previous history of neonatal hemolytic disease resulting from anti–Rh D suggests that the current fetus also may be at risk. In this regard it may be useful to know the fetal Rh blood type because this identifies those Rh-negative infants who are not at risk. In many cases this can be accomplished by direct Rh typing of fetal RBCs obtained via cordocentesis. Alternatively, molecular biologic techniques can be used to determine the Rh genotype in DNA obtained from amniocytes or chorionic villus samples (Bennett et al, 1993; Fisk et al, 1994). When the fetus is found to be Rh negative, no further maternal monitoring or fetal blood studies are necessary.

An increase in the maternal titer of IgG anti-D indicates maternal sensitization but does not accurately predict the potential severity of fetal hemolysis. A better correlation is obtained by spectrophotometric estimation of bile pigment in amniotic fluid as measured by the deviation in optical density (OD) at 450 nm (Fig. 89–4). Plotting the "delta OD 450 nm" against fetal age provides a good correlation with the severity of fetal hemolysis during the 3rd trimester, and the trend of two or more values is a more reliable predictor of severity of fetal disease (Liley, 1961). Fetuses with amniotic fluid delta OD values in zone 3 or increasing toward zone 3 are at greatest risk of intrauterine death from severe anemia and hydrops fetalis.

In earlier studies, at-risk fetuses older than 32 weeks' gestation with evidence of mature lung function were delivered early. However, for those fetuses less than 32 weeks' gestation with immature lung function, early delivery was

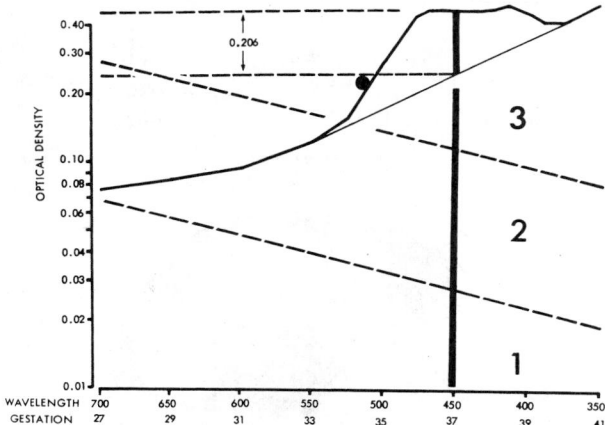

FIGURE 89–4. This composite graph depicts how spectrophotometric estimation of amniotic fluid bilirubin levels can be used as an indicator of fetal jeopardy from hemolytic disease. (1) The optical density of amniotic fluid (ordinate) is measured from 700 to 350 nm (abscissa—top). This absorption curve is depicted as the heavy solid line. (2) The contribution of bilirubin to this absorption is then calculated by subtracting the optical density of the projected baseline (fine solid line) from the measured optical density at 450 nm. In this case, the calculated value is 0.206. (3) This calculated contribution of bilirubin is then plotted as a function of gestational age (abscissa—bottom). In this particular patient, the gestational age of 34.5 weeks and the bilirubin absorption of 0.206 determine the point indicated by the solid dot. (4) The dashed lines demarcate three zones (1, 2, and 3): Zone 1 indicates an Rh negative infant or very mild hemolytic disease. Zone 2 indicates mild to moderate hemolytic disease. Zone 3 represents severe hemolytic disease with impending fetal death. Because the bilirubin concentration of amniotic fluid decreases with gestational age, the absolute optical density that places a fetus in zone 3 decreases as the length of gestation increases. In the case depicted here, an absorption of 0.206 at 34.5 weeks' gestation indicated this fetus was in zone 3 and thus seriously at risk. (From Bowman JM, Pollock JM: Amniotic fluid spectrophotometry and early delivery in the management of erythroblastosis fetalis. Pediatrics 35:815, 1965. Reproduced with permission from Pediatrics.)

not possible and fetal RBC transfusions were given. Initially, intrauterine RBC transfusions were administered through the peritoneal cavity, and this procedure ameliorated the anemia sufficiently to save many otherwise doomed fetuses (Liley, 1963). However, in some of these cases in which hydrops was already present, the success rate was much lower because RBC absorption from the peritoneal cavity (complicated by ascites) did not effectively reverse the effects of severe anemia and hypoxia.

In severely affected fetuses, hydrops may occur as early as 20 to 22 weeks' gestation. Moreover, in these instances, the Liley amniocentesis curves (which are derived from studies of fetuses after 27 weeks' gestation) do not accurately predict severe disease (Nicolaides et al, 1988). However, the development of high-resolution ultrasound has been a major advance that facilitates detection of early hydrops (ascites and edema) and enables direct percutaneous umbilical blood sampling (PUBS) (cordocentesis) for determination of red cell antigen typing and measurement of fetal hematocrit or hemoglobin levels (Fig. 89–5). Fetal

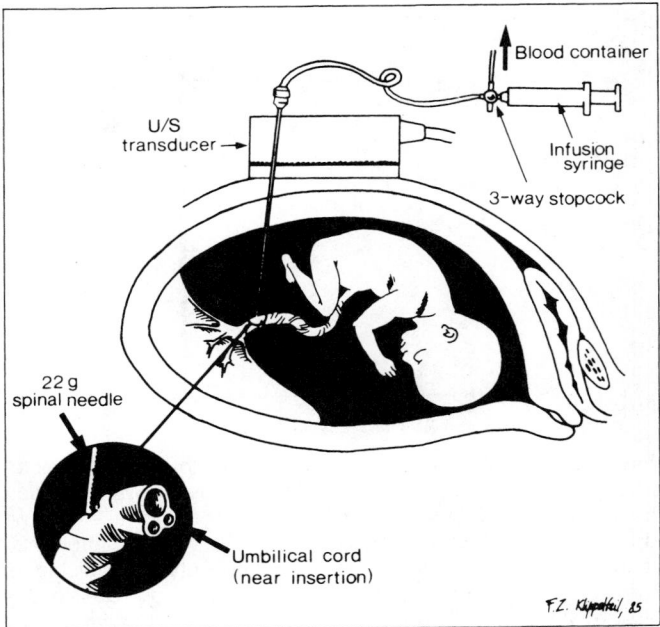

FIGURE 89–5. Diagrammatic view of in utero direct intravascular transfusion. U/S ultrasound. (From Grannum PA, Copel JA, Plaxe SC, et al: In utero exchange transfusion by direct intravascular injection in severe erythroblastosis fetalis. N Engl J Med 314:1431, 1986. Reprinted by permission of the New England Journal of Medicine.)

hydrops does not occur until hemoglobin concentration of the fetus decreases below approximately about 4 g/dL (or hematocrit below approximately 15%). However, the hemoglobin concentration of normal fetuses increases gradually during the latter part of pregnancy; thus the interpretation of hemoglobin values in affected fetuses must be compared with normal subjects for the state of gestation (Nicolaides et al, 1988). A reference range for normal fetuses and fetuses with varying degrees of hemolysis is seen in Figure 89–6. Expressing the degree of anemia as "hemoglobin deficit" (gram per deciliter below the normal mean hemoglobin value for age), three zones of severity have been defined:

- Zone I (mild): deficit less than 2 g/dL
- Zone II (moderate): deficit 2 to 7 g/dL
- Zone III (severe, hydropic): deficit 7 to 10 g/dL

The use of ultrasound, which allows fetal blood sampling through a 22-gauge spinal needle, has reduced the fetal trauma and morbidity of cordocentesis to less than 2% (Parer, 1988). Cordocentesis also has facilitated direct intravascular RBC transfusion to rapidly correct severe life-threatening anemia, with the rapid reversal of established hydrops in most cases (Grannum et al, 1988; Rodeck et al, 1984). Depending on the age of the fetus and severity of anemia, the desired volume of RBCs transfused generally is that which will achieve a post-transfusion hematocrit of approximately 35% to 45%. When RBC transfusion induces a reversal of hydrops, the serum albumin also increases, thus, supporting the role of anemia in the pathogenesis of the low albumin levels. Both simple transfusions and

intrauterine exchange transfusions have been performed in a number of fetuses (Grannum et al, 1986). Most perinatologists prefer simple RBC transfusion because of its shorter duration, aiming for a post-transfusion hematocrit no greater than 45% to avert circulatory overload (Weiner et al, 1991).

Hyperbilirubinemia (with elevation of the conjugated fraction) often develops in newborns who have received intrauterine RBC transfusions and they may require multiple exchange transfusions. This hyperbilirubinemia reflects the severity of hemolysis and its effects on the fetal liver. In some cases, anemia may be minimal or absent, and the DAT may be negative if the Rh-negative RBCs transfused prenatally still predominate. These infants may not require exchange transfusion. Neonatal exchange transfusion, amniocentesis, selective early induction of delivery, and intrauterine fetal blood transfusions all have contributed to the declining neonatal death rate from Rh incompatibility (Fig. 89–7).

ABO Incompatibility

Hemolysis associated with ABO incompatibility is similar to Rh hemolytic disease in that maternal anti-A or anti-B antibodies enter the fetal circulation and react with A or B antigens on the erythrocyte surface (Table 89–7). In type A and B individuals, naturally occurring anti-B and anti-A isoantibodies largely are IgM molecules that do not cross the placenta. In contrast, the alloantibodies present in type O individuals are predominantly IgG molecules (Abelson and Rawson, 1961). For this reason, ABO incompatibility is largely limited to type O mothers with type A or B fetuses. The presence of IgG anti-A or anti-B antibodies in type O mothers also explains why hemolysis caused by ABO incompatibility frequently occurs during the first

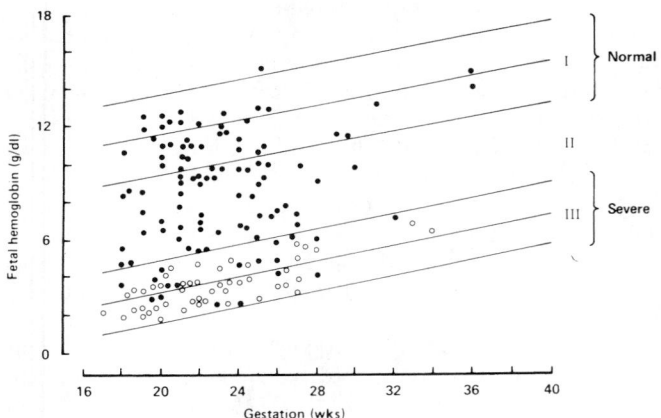

FIGURE 89–6. Fetal hemoglobin concentration of 48 hydropic (open circles) and 106 nonhydropic (solid circles) fetuses from red blood cell isoimmunized pregnancies at time of first fetal blood sampling. Values are plotted on the reference range of fetal hemoglobin for gestation. The individual 95% confidence intervals of the normal hemoglobin for gestation define zone I and the individual 95% confidence intervals of the hemoglobin for gestation define zone III. Zone II indicates moderate anemia. (From Nicolaides JH, Soothill PW, Clewell WH, et al: Fetal hemoglobin measurement in the assessment of red cell isoimmunization. Lancet 1:1073, 1988.)

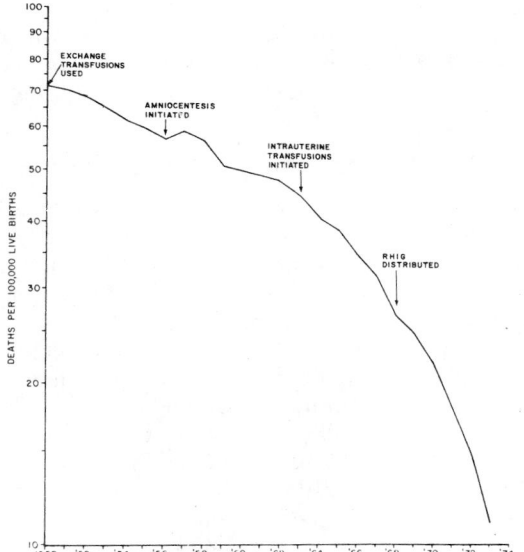

FIGURE 89–7. Infant death rates from hemolytic disease of the newborn, United States, 1950 to 1973. (From Centers for Disease Control: Rh Hemolytic Disease Surveillance Annual Report, June 1975.)

pregnancy without prior "sensitization." ABO incompatibility is present in approximately 12% of pregnancies, although evidence of fetal RBC sensitization (i.e., positive DAT) is found in only 3% of births, and less than 1% of live births are associated with significant hemolysis (Kaplan et al, 1976; Zipursky et al, 1963). The relative mildness of neonatal ABO hemolytic disease contrasts sharply with the findings in Rh incompatibility. In large part, this is because A and B antigens are present in many tissues besides RBCs; consequently, only a small fraction of anti-A or anti-B antibody that crosses the placenta actually binds to erythrocytes, the remainder being absorbed by other tissues and soluble A and B substances in plasma.

TABLE 89–7

Clinical and Laboratory Features of Immune Hemolysis Due to Rh Disease and ABO Incompatibility

	Rh Disease	ABO Incompatibility
Clinical Features		
Frequency	Unusual	Common
Pallor	Marked	Minimal
Jaundice	Marked	Minimal to moderate
Hydrops	Common	Rare
Hepatosplenomegaly	Marked	Minimal
Laboratory Features		
Blood type		
Mother	Rh(−)	O
Infant	Rh(+)	A or B
Anemia	Marked	Minimal
Direct Coombs' test	Positive	Frequently negative
Indirect Coombs' test	Positive	Usually positive
Hyperbilirubinemia	Marked	Variable
RBC morphology	Nucleated RBCs	Spherocytes

Although hemolytic disease resulting from ABO incompatibility is clinically milder than that from Rh disease, severe hemolysis occasionally occurs, and hydrops fetalis has been reported. In such cases it is essential to exclude other antibodies and other causes of hemolysis such as glucose-6-phosphate dehydrogenase (G6PD) deficiency or hereditary spherocytosis. In most cases, pallor and jaundice are minimal (see Table 89–7). Hepatosplenomegaly is uncommon. Laboratory features include minimal to moderate hyperbilirubinemia and, occasionally, some degree of anemia. The DAT (direct Coombs' test) frequently is negative, although the indirect antiglobulin test (neonatal serum plus adult A or B RBCs) more commonly is positive. This paradox is related to the fact that fetal RBCs, compared with adult erythrocytes, have less type-specific antigen on their surface (Voak and Williams, 1971). Heat-elution is the most sensitive test for anti-A or anti-B antibodies on infant red cells, but like the antiglobulin tests, it has poor predictive value for hemolysis. Studies of the subclass of the IgG anti-A and anti-B in maternal serum and on red cells of ABO-incompatible infants point to a possible explanation (Brouwers et al, 1988). The most common subclass is IgG2, which crosses the placenta but does not bind to Fc-receptors of phagocytic cells and therefore is incapable of causing cell lysis. This accounts for the frequent observation of positive indirect and direct antiglobulin tests with little or no hemolysis. On the other hand, IgG3 antibodies and to a lesser extent IgG1 antibodies, although present in lower concentrations on fetal RBCs, do bind to Fc-receptors and have strong lytic activity. This seems to account for cases of hemolysis associated with a negative or only weakly positive DAT.

The peripheral blood smear is characterized by marked spherocytosis, which is thought to be due to the reduced RBC surface area that results as antibody and membrane are removed by splenic macrophages. Autoimmune hemolytic anemia in older children is associated with antibodies directed against the Rh locus, and these cases also are characterized by spherocytosis. For unknown reasons, spherocytes are not a prominent feature of neonatal hemolysis resulting from Rh incompatibility.

Hemolysis in ABO incompatibility is usually mild, presenting with some degree of hyperbilirubinemia. Of major concern in the current managed health-care environment is that some infants with ABO incompatibility may be discharged home from medical establishments before significant clinical jaundice is evident. *It is critical that infants with ABO incompatibility be monitored closely for evolving jaundice and hyperbilirubinemia in the first few days of life.* In most cases hyperbilirubinemia is readily controlled by phototherapy (Osborn et al, 1984). When hyperbilirubinemia is not controlled by phototherapy, exchange transfusion is necessary using group O Rh-compatible RBCs. Tin-protoporphyrin, an inhibitor of heme catabolism to bilirubin, may help prevent hyperbilirubinemia in ABO-incompatible infants (Kappas et al, 1988). Additional follow-up at 2 to 3 weeks of age to check for anemia in these infants is essential.

Minor Blood Group Incompatibility

With the sharp decline of hemolytic disease caused by Rh incompatibility, the proportion of cases caused by Rh c, Rh

E, Kell, Duff, and Kidd incompatibility has increased from the previous estimates of 1% to 3%. The pathophysiology of these disorders is similar to that of Rh and ABO incompatibility. The infrequency of minor group incompatibility is primarily a reflection of the lower antigenicity of these RBC antigens. Diagnosis of minor group incompatibility is suggested by hemolytic anemia with a positive DAT in the absence of ABO or Rh incompatibility and with a negative maternal DAT. Definitive diagnosis requires identification of the specific antibody in neonatal serum or an eluate from neonatal RBCs. This is readily accomplished by testing maternal serum against a variety of known RBC antigens. With some antibodies such as Kell, antibody titer and amniocentesis findings may underestimate the severity of fetal hemolysis. Therefore, frequent ultrasound monitoring may be necessary, with fetal blood sampling being done in worrisome cases. Fetal blood sampling also is useful in determining whether the fetus of a heterozygous father has inherited the offending RBC antigen. This identifies those fetuses that need further serial evaluations.

Immune Hemolytic Anemia Due to Maternal Disease

Maternal autoimmune hemolytic anemia or lupus erythrematous during pregnancy may be associated with passive transfer of IgG antibody to the fetus. The diagnosis is suggested by the presence of neonatal hemolytic disease, a positive DAT, absence of Rh or ABO incompatibility, and antiglobulin-positive hemolysis in the mother. Treatment with prednisone in the mother may reduce both maternal hemolysis and neonatal morbidity. As in other cases of neonatal hemolysis, attempts are made to prevent hyperbilirubinemia and kernicterus.

Drug-Induced Immune Hemolysis

The classic example of drug-induced immune hemolysis is seen with penicillin and appears when an antibody is directed to a complex of penicillin bound to the RBC membrane. No hemolysis occurs in the absence of penicillin, even though antibody persists in the circulation. This type of drug-mediated immune hemolysis is seen rarely in newborn infants. Cephalosporin drugs also have been implicated to cause immune-mediated hemolysis by a similar mechanism. In all of these cases, the DAT may be positive only when the test is done in the presence of the drug in question. Moreover, hemolysis ceases once the drug is withdrawn.

Nonimmune Acquired Hemolytic Disease
Infection

Cytomegalic inclusion disease, toxoplasmosis, syphilis, and bacterial sepsis all can be associated with hemolytic anemia. In most of these conditions, some degree of thrombocytopenia also exists. Generally, there is hepatosplenomegaly. In cases of bacterial sepsis, both the direct and indirect bilirubin may be elevated. The mechanism of hemolysis is not clearly defined, but it may be related to RBC sequestration in the presence of marked reticuloendothelial hyperplasia associated with infection. Documentation of infec-

tion as the cause of hemolysis is made by the presence of other clinical and laboratory stigmata of neonatal infections. Hemolysis caused by infections may be exhibited early in the neonatal period, or it can be delayed for several weeks.

Disseminated Intravascular Coagulation

Disseminated intravascular coagulation is discussed in Chapter 88. The hemolytic component of this disorder is secondary to the deposition of fibrin within the vascular walls. When erythrocytes interact with fibrin, fragments of RBCs are broken off, producing fragile, deformed RBCs, or schistocytes. These cells are relatively rigid and thus incapable of normal deformation within the microcirculation. The hemolytic-uremic syndrome represents a localized form of intravascular coagulation that is characterized by thrombocytopenia, renal disease, and hemolytic anemia. Hemolysis is characterized by RBC fragmentation, presumably for the aforementioned reasons.

Hereditary RBC Disorders
Membrane Defects

The customary findings in RBC membrane disorders are the presence of dominant inheritance, abnormal RBC morphology (Fig. 89–8), and either increased or decreased osmotic fragility. Aside from hereditary spherocytosis, these disorders are uncommon.

Hereditary Spherocytosis

The hallmark of hereditary spherocytosis is the presence in the circulation of spherocytes, cells that have become spheroid because of a loss of membrane surface with no concomitant loss in volume. Inherited mutations in components of the membrane cytoskeleton (spectrin, ankyrin, or band 3) weaken the stability of the interactions between the cytoskeleton and the membrane lipid bilayer, promoting vesiculation and loss of bits of the bilayer, thus leading to progressive loss of membrane surface area (Palek and Jarolim, 1993). As the RBC becomes more spherical, it loses flexibility and becomes vulnerable to entrapment in the spleen, where metabolic depletion and attack by the reticuloendothelial system lead to hemolysis. Removal of the spleen allows hereditary spherocytes to have a near-normal life-span despite their cytoskeletal defects and abnormal shape.

The clinical manifestations of hereditary spherocytosis range from life-threatening anemia requiring regular RBC transfusions to fully compensated hemolysis marked by reticulocytosis but no anemia. Neonatal hemolysis or hyperbilirubinemia appears in approximately half of all affected infants (Stamey and Diamond, 1957). In most cases, other family members are affected in a pattern consistent with autosomal dominant inheritance. In 20% to 30% of cases, recessive inheritance is noted and only homozygotes express the clinical features of spherocytosis. Occasionally, the appearance of a new case of spherocytosis in a previously unaffected family is due to spontaneous mutation.

The diagnosis of spherocytosis is suspected when spherocytes are seen on the blood smear and the RBC osmotic

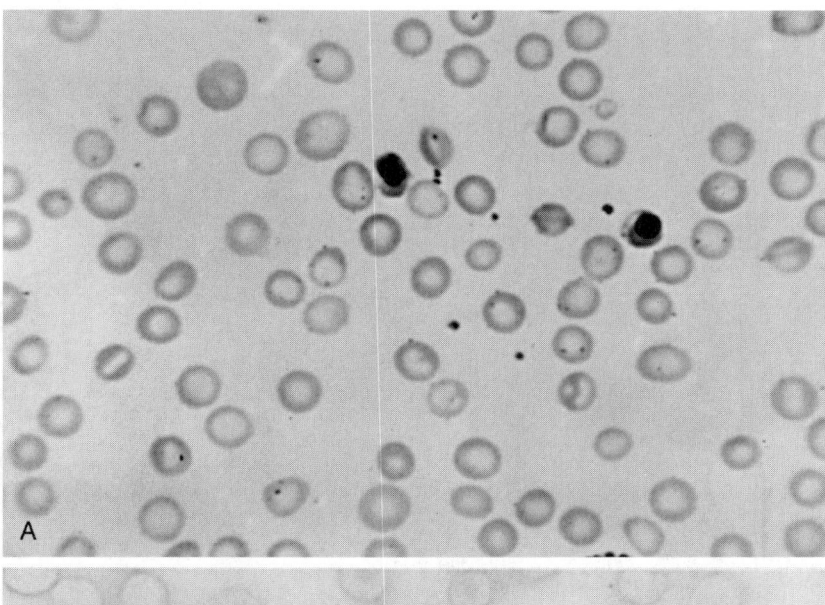

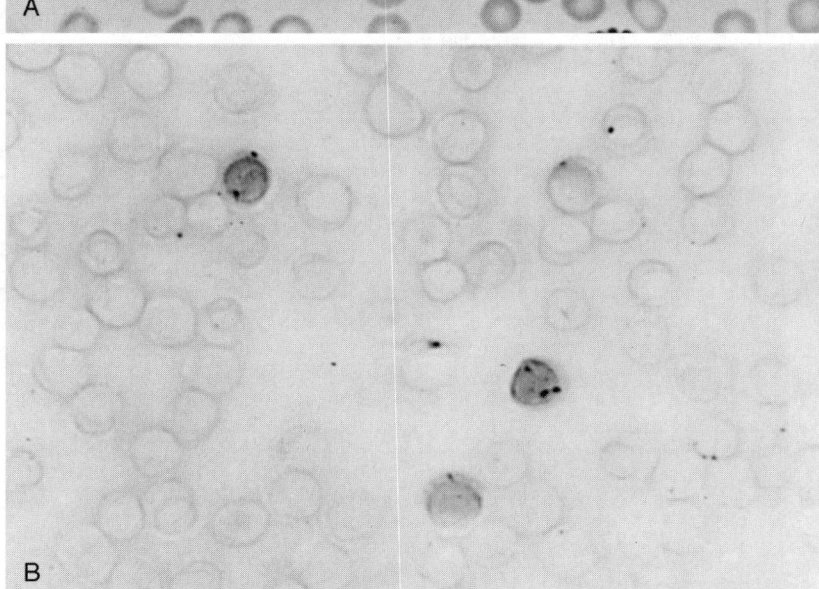

FIGURE 89–8. *A*, Hypochromic-microcytic red blood cells (RBCs) secondary to chronic fetal blood loss. *B*, Fetal RBCs in the maternal blood after a fetomaternal hemorrhage (acid-elution technique).

Illustration continued on following page

fragility is increased in a patient with laboratory evidence of hemolysis. In the newborn, morphologic assessment of the RBCs is sometimes difficult because even normal newborns may possess a minor population of spherocytes; conversely, in hereditary spherocytosis fewer spherocytes may be evident than will be the case later in life. Furthermore, interpretation of the osmotic fragility curve has to take into account the relative osmotic resistance of normal neonatal RBCs. If this is done by using newborns rather than adult normal controls, the fragile RBCs of infants who have hereditary spherocytosis can easily be identified (Shröter and Kahsnitz, 1983). Immune hemolysis, which also generates spherocytes, must always be ruled out in the work-up of a suspected case of hereditary spherocytosis. In the newborn, maternal antibody rather than autoantibody must be suspected if immune hemolysis is present. Spherocytes are commonly observed in ABO incompatibility, but not in Rh disease. Blood typing and a Coomb's test usually confirm a diagnosis of ABO incompatibility, but the Coombs' test may occasionally be negative and thus mis-leading. In this situation, evaluation of the family for other individuals affected with spherocytosis may point to a hereditary rather than an acquired cause. Sometimes it is necessary to wait until the infant age is 3 months or so to obtain a definitive laboratory diagnosis of hereditary spherocytosis, because, by this age, the confounding effects of maternal antibody and fetal RBCs are no longer present.

Treatment during the newborn period is directed toward management of hyperbilirubinemia, which is often present. Less commonly, RBC transfusions may be required for management of symptomatic anemia. Splenectomy is the definitive treatment for hereditary spherocytosis, but it is best deferred until the child is at least the age of 5 years because of the increased risk of overwhelming sepsis with encapsulated organisms such as *Haemophilus influenzae* or *Streptococcus pneumoniae* (Diamond, 1969) that occurs following splenectomy in infants and young children. Partial splenectomy may reduce the rate of hemolysis without increasing the risk of overwhelming infection (Tchernia et al, 1993).

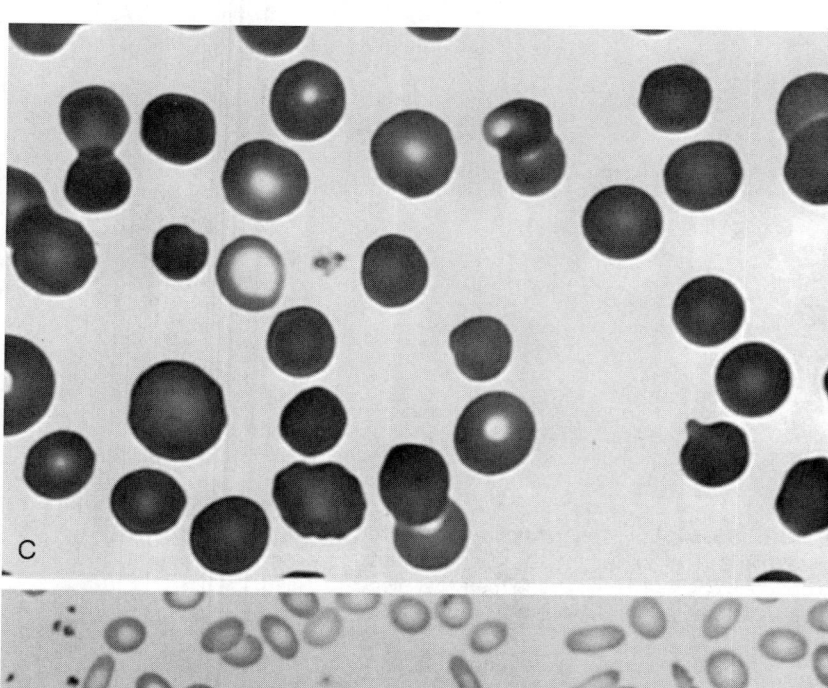

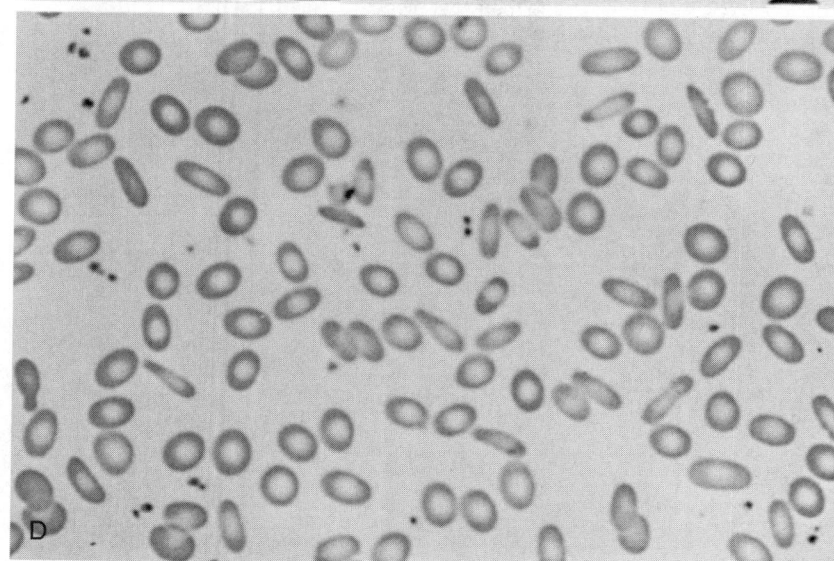

FIGURE 89–8 *Continued. C*, Hereditary spherocytosis. *D*, Hereditary elliptocytosis.

Hereditary Elliptocytosis

Hereditary elliptocytosis is a heterogeneous group of disorders that are caused by mutations of the RBC membrane cytoskeletal proteins (usually spectrin or protein 4.1) that weaken skeletal protein interactions and increase RBC mechanical fragility (Palek and Jarolim, 1993). Elliptocytes are evident on the blood smear, but in most instances hemolysis is absent. Some mutations weaken the cytoskeleton sufficiently to cause significant hemolysis accompanied by striking abnormalities in RBC morphology (hereditary pyropoikilocytosis). Asymptomatic elliptocytosis is inherited as an autosomal dominant trait, whereas individuals with hereditary pyropoikilocytosis inherit elliptocytosis from one parent and another, sometimes clinically silent, membrane protein mutation from the other parent. Transient poikilocytosis and hemolysis may occur during the newborn period in infants destined ultimately to have asymptomatic elliptocytosis (Austin and Desforges, 1969). RBC membrane mechanical fragility is strikingly abnormal in these infants, probably as a consequence of the destabilizing influence of large amounts of free intraerythrocytic 2,3-DPG, a by-product of the presence of fetal hemoglobin (Mentzer et al, 1987). As fetal hemoglobin levels decline postnatally in affected infants, membrane mechanical fragility improves, hemolysis disappears, and RBC morphology undergoes a transition from poikilocytosis to elliptocytosis. Without knowledge of the membrane protein mutations present in the infant and the infant's family, it is difficult to predict at birth who will have transient poikilocytosis with ultimate recovery and who is destined to have life-long pyropoikilocytosis with hemolysis.

RBC Enzyme Abnormalities

Hyperbilirubinemia, anemia, and even hydrops fetalis can be the result of inherited RBC enzymopathies. Except for G6PD deficiency (sex-linked) and adenosine deaminase excess (autosomal dominant), these disorders are autosomal recessive and heterozygotes are clinically normal. RBC morphology is usually normal and diagnosis requires assay

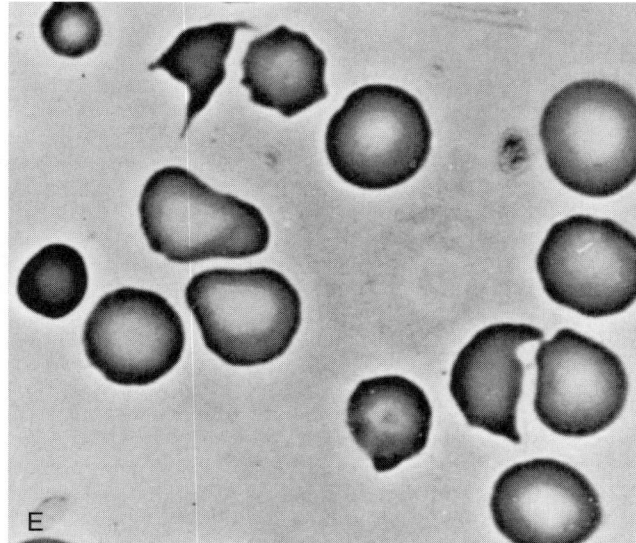

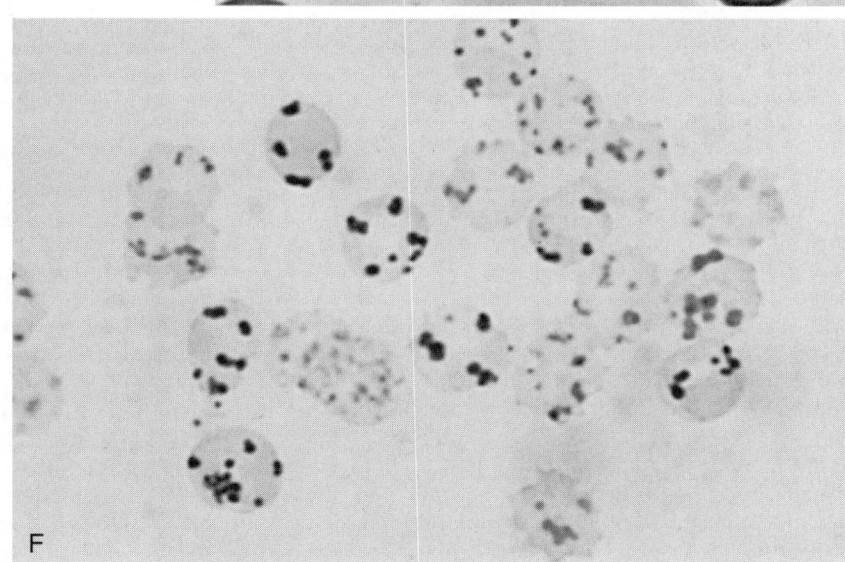

FIGURE 89-8 *Continued. E,* G6PD-deficient RBCs during acute hemolytic episode. *F,* Heinz bodies in patient with G6PD-deficient hemolysis (stained with supravital dye).

of the activity of the enzyme suspected to be abnormal. It is usually prudent to rule out common causes of hemolysis that are easily diagnosed before embarking on an expensive search for RBC enzymopathies, which, except for G6PD deficiency, are rare. Overviews of this group of disorders are available elsewhere (Luzzato L, 1997; Mentzer WC, 1997), and the special features of RBC enzymopathies in the newborn period have also been summarized (Matthay and Mentzer, 1981).

Glucose-6-Phosphate Dehydrogenase Deficiency

G6PD deficiency is a sex-linked disorder that affects millions of people throughout the world, particularly in Mediterranean countries, Africa, and China. Like sickle cell trait and thalassemia, G6PD deficiency is thought to have become common because it provides a measure of protection against malaria. In all but a few G6PD-deficient individuals, hemolysis and anemia are present only after exposure to medications that are potent oxidants or during

infections. Occasionally, hemolytic anemia is chronic rather than episodic and occurs even in the absence of obvious exposure to oxidant stress. Rarely, anemia may be so severe as to require regular RBC transfusions. The clinical heterogeneity of G6PD deficiency is due to the very large number of different mutations, usually single amino acid substitutions, that lead to altered enzyme function (Beutler and Yoshida, 1988; Miwa and Fujii, 1996). Normal RBCs contain abundant amounts of reduced glutathione (GSH), a sulfhydryl-containing tripeptide that serves as an intracellular antioxidant, neutralizing peroxides that form during metabolism or are introduced directly from the extracellular environment. Because of their enzyme deficiency, G6PD-deficient RBCs have a limited capacity to regenerate GSH from oxidized glutathione (Fig. 89-9). In the absence of GSH, RBCs are vulnerable to oxidant injury. The effects of oxidants on the RBC are multifocal. Denatured globin precipitates, termed Heinz bodies, bind to the cell membrane, unfavorably altering its structure and function. Membrane lipid peroxidation may contribute to

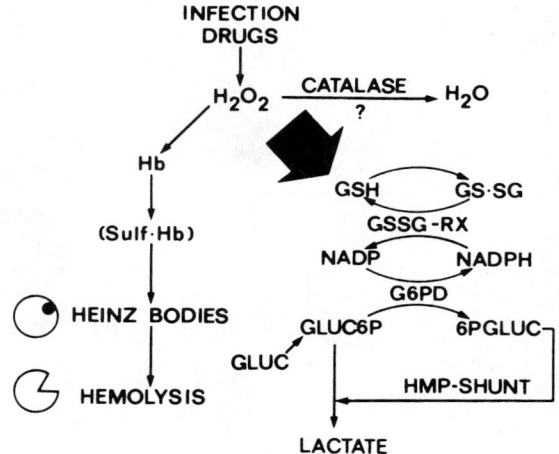

FIGURE 89–9. G6PD hemolysis—pathophysiology.

altered function. The activity of intracellular enzymes may decline. The ultimate result of these insults is hemolysis.

Race and sex are determinants of the severity of hemolysis in G6PD deficiency.

Race. The mutation G6PD A− that is responsible for nearly all of the G6PD deficiency seen in Africans (and is present in approximately 10% of American blacks) affects the stability of the enzyme, causing a gradual decline in activity during the life span of the RBC. Only in the oldest RBCs does enzyme activity reach low enough levels to create vulnerability to oxidant hemolysis. For this reason, hemolysis, if it occurs, is usually mild and self-limited. In contrast, in Asians and persons of Mediterranean descent, the common mutations causing G6PD deficiency alter enzyme activity in young and old RBCs alike. Hemolysis is usually more severe and can be fatal. In these ethnic groups, inheritance of an as yet unidentified factor renders G6PD-deficient individuals susceptible to severe and even fatal episodes of hemolysis following exposure to fava beans (favism). Favism is not seen in blacks.

Sex. The gene for G6PD is located on the X chromosome. All the RBCs of hemizygous G6PD-deficient males are affected by the enzyme deficiency. In contrast, a variable proportion of the RBCs of heterozygous G6PD-deficient females are enzyme deficient, depending on whether the process of random inactivation of the X chromosome that occurs early in embryonic development involves the chromosome carrying the normal or the mutant G6PD gene. When a large proportion of their RBCs are enzyme deficient, females exhibit an equivalent degree of hemolysis after exposure to oxidants as do their male counterparts. When a smaller proportion of cells are affected, hemolysis is milder or absent. For these reasons, hemolysis is more commonly seen in G6PD-deficient populations of male hemizygotes than female heterozygotes.

The diagnosis of G6PD deficiency is suggested by the appearance of a Coombs'-negative anemia in association with infection or the administration of drugs. Cells that appear as if a "bite" had been taken from them (due to splenic removal of Heinz bodies) are occasionally seen on the peripheral blood smear. Supravital stains of the peripheral blood with crystal violet may reveal Heinz bodies during hemolytic episodes. Although screening tests are available, definitive diagnosis requires assay of RBC G6PD activity or identification of a specific G6PD mutation by DNA analysis (Beutler, 1988; Miwa and Fujii, 1996). Measurement of enzyme activity may not reveal the deficiency in American blacks immediately after a hemolytic episode, because the population of deficient cells has been eliminated, or in transfused patients because of the presence of normal, enzyme-replete RBCs. Repeating the assay after at least 3 months ensures that any transfused cells are gone and that the population of deficient cells has been regenerated so that a more accurate determination of the presence of G6PD deficiency can be made.

Hemolysis resulting from G6PD deficiency is well documented in the newborn period (Valaes, 1994). Although the usual factors (drugs and infection) may be implicated, often there is no obvious cause for hemolysis. Premature (Eshaghpour et al, 1967) but not term black G6PD-deficient newborns (O'Flynn and Hsia, 1963) have more hyperbilirubinemia than normal infants. Severe hemolysis and hyperbilirubinemia can follow exposure to known hemolytic agents in black G6PD-deficient newborns (Brown, 1992) but can be seen even in the absence of exposure to such agents in Asian or white G6PD-deficient infants. These ethnic differences reflect the different G6PD mutations that are present in blacks, Asians, and whites. In one study from Greece (Doxiadis and Valaes, 1964), approximately 30% of all exchange transfusions done in the nursery were in G6PD-deficient infants who had no evidence of isoimmune hemolytic anemia. In Taiwan, the incidence of hyperbilirubinemia requiring phototherapy was higher in G6PD-deficient than in normal infant males, particularly if the nt 1376 mutation was present. Other mutations were associated with lesser degrees of hyperbilirubinemia and responded more favorably to phototherapy (Huang et al, 1996).

Therapy for neonatal hemolysis and hyperbilirubinemia resulting from G6PD deficiency includes (1) phototherapy or exchange transfusion to prevent kernicterus, (2) RBC transfusion for symptomatic anemia, (3) removal of potential oxidants that may be contributing to hemolysis, and (4) treatment of infections, using agents that do not themselves initiate hemolysis. Neonatal screening for G6PD deficiency has been very effective in reducing the incidence of favism later in life in Sardinia (Meloni et al, 1992) and other regions where this potentially fatal complication is common (Valaes, 1994). In the United States, where the most common G6PD mutation is the A− variant found in blacks (who are not susceptible to favism and in whom life-threatening hemolytic episodes are rare), neonatal screening has not been thought to be cost effective.

CASE STUDY 1

A male infant weighing 2722 g was born at 38 weeks' gestation to a 30-year-old Chinese, gravida 3, para 1, aborta 1 mother. Apgar score at birth was 1. Despite intensive resuscitative measures, the infant died after 2 hours, never having established spontaneous respirations. Autopsy disclosed hepatosplenomegaly, bile-filled canaliculi within the liver, bone marrow erythroid hyperplasia, and other evidence of severe intrauterine hemolysis. Hemoglobin was 9.8 g/100 mL, and the white blood cell count was 7200/µL. There was marked polychromatophilia (reticulocytosis), and numerous nucleated RBCs were seen in the peripheral smear. The infant's blood type was AB-positive, the mother's blood type was B-positive, and the Coombs' test (direct and indirect) was negative. Hemoglobin electrophoresis revealed 52% hemoglobin F, 45% hemoglobin A, and no hemoglobin Barts or hemoglobin H. RBC G6PD activity was decreased in the infant and in his mother. Four weeks before delivery, the mother had an upper respiratory infection and took ascorbic acid (250–500 mg/day) for a period of 2 weeks as treatment. On at least one occasion during the last month of pregnancy, she also ate fava beans (Mentzer and Collier, 1975).

Comment

As illustrated by this case, G6PD deficiency should be considered in the differential diagnosis not only of hyperbilirubinemia and hemolytic anemia but also of hydrops fetalis. The reason for the disastrous course in this infant is not known. Infection, ascorbic acid (an intracellular oxidant), or favism could have been responsible.

Pyruvate Kinase Deficiency

Pyruvate kinase (PK) is an autosomal recessive disorder that occurs in all ethnic groups. Although the most common of the Embden-Meyerhof glycolytic pathway defects, it is rare in comparison to G6PD deficiency. Approximately 350 cases, mostly in Northern Europeans, have been described (Mentzer, 1997). PK is one of the two key enzymatic steps that generate adenosine triphosphate (ATP) in RBCs. Impairment of ATP production is the central pathophysiologic abnormality in PK deficiency. Because nonerythroid tissues have alternative means of generating ATP, clinical abnormalities in PK deficiency are limited to RBCs. Thirty-three mutations of PK have been defined at the nucleic acid level and many more in terms of abnormalities of the PK protein (Mentzer, 1997). Reflecting this genetic diversity, the hemolytic anemia that characterizes PK deficiency varies considerably in severity from family to family. Approximately one third of PK-deficient individuals experience hyperbilirubinemia during the newborn period. Jaundice tends to appear early (on the 1st day of life), and may require exchange transfusion (Matthay and Mentzer, 1981). Death or kernicterus may occur. Severe intrauterine anemia and hydrops fetalis have been reported (Mentzer, 1997).

The diagnosis of PK deficiency should be considered in a jaundiced newborn with evidence of nonimmune hemolysis in the absence of infections or exposure to hemolytic agents. Hemoglobinopathies and membrane disorders should be ruled out by examination of the blood smear and other appropriate diagnostic tests before proceding to assay

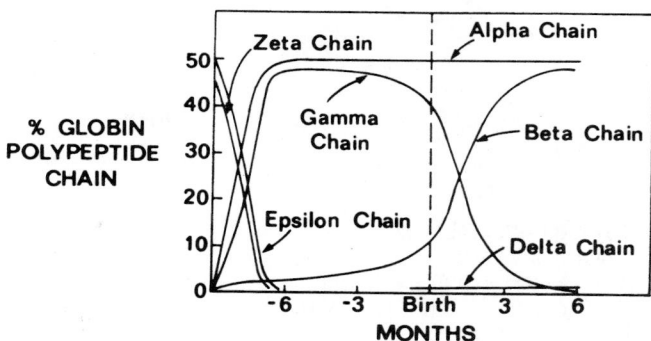

FIGURE 89–10. Fetal and neonatal hemoglobin production.

of RBC PK activity, which is the definitive test for the disorder. RBC morphology is basically normal in PK deficiency, although a few dense cells with irregular margins (echinocytes) are occasionally seen. PK heterozygotes are clinically and hematologically normal, but usually have roughly half the normal amount of RBC PK activity.

Treatment of hyperbilirubinemia by phototherapy and exchange transfusion if necessary is usually the only therapy necessary in the newborn period. RBC transfusions for anemia may occasionally be required. Splenectomy may reduce the rate of hemolysis but should be avoided in infancy and early childhood due to the high risk of infection after splenectomy.

Hemolysis due to Hemoglobin Disorders

To understand the hemoglobinopathies that are seen in the newborn, it is first necessary to review the normal developmental changes that occur in globin synthesis during fetal and neonatal life. In adults, the predominant hemoglobin tetramer (hemoglobin A) is composed of two alpha globin chains and two beta globin chains. In very young embryos, alpha chains are replaced by zeta chains and beta chains by epsilon chains. The transition from zeta to alpha globin chains is complete by the end of the 1st trimester. Epsilon chains disappear more slowly and are replaced first by gamma chains and then later by the beta chains of adult hemoglobin. By the time of birth, the transition from gamma to beta globin synthesis is well underway (Fig. 89–10). The various possible combinations of these different globin chains form a number of different hemoglobin tetramers that are characteristically found in embryonic, fetal, or postnatal life (Fig. 89–11). In contrast

	HEMOGLOBIN	GLOBIN POLYPEPTIDES	% IN CORD BLOOD
EMBRYONIC	GOWER-1	Zeta-2, Epsilon-2 ($\zeta_2\epsilon_2$)	0
	GOWER-2	Alpha-2, Epsilon-2 ($\alpha_2\epsilon_2$)	0
	PORTLAND	Zeta-2, Gamma-2 ($\zeta_2\gamma_2$)	0
FETAL	BARTS	Gamma-4 (γ_4)	<1%
	Hgb F	Alpha-2, Gamma-2 ($\alpha_2\gamma_2$)	60-85%
ADULT	Hgb A	Alpha-2, Beta-2 ($\alpha_2\beta_2$)	15-40%
	Hgb A₂	Alpha-2, Delta-2 ($\alpha_2\delta_2$)	<1%

FIGURE 89–11. Hemoglobin composition of cord blood.

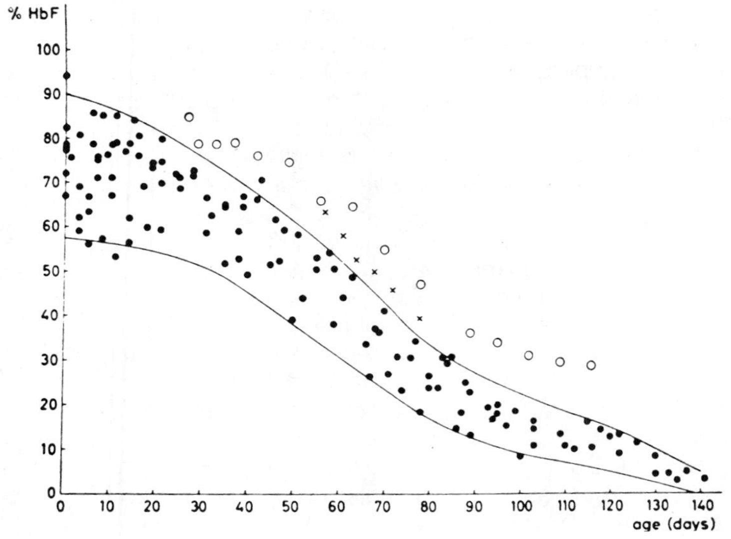

FIGURE 89–12. Decreasing concentration of fetal hemoglobin after birth. (Garby L, Sjöhn S, Vuille JC: Studies of erythro-kinetics in infancy. II. The relative rate of synthesis of haemoglobin F and haemoglobin A during the first months of life. Acta Paediatr 51:245, 1962.)

to globin, the heme moiety is unchanged in structure in embryonic, fetal, and postnatal hemoglobin molecules.

Fetal hemoglobin (alpha-2-gamma-2) is the major hemoglobin found in fetuses after the 1st trimester. Its replacement by adult hemoglobin (hemoglobin A) begins before birth, so that only approximately 60% to 90% of the hemoglobin found in the normal term infant is fetal hemoglobin (hemoglobin F). After birth, gamma chain synthesis declines rapidly as beta chain synthesis increases (see Fig. 89–10) so that most newly formed hemoglobin is hemoglobin A. As RBCs made before birth are replaced by cells made postnatally, the percentage of hemoglobin F declines rapidly, reaching a level of approximately 5% by 6 months of age (Fig. 89–12). Only trace amounts of the minor adult hemoglobin, hemoglobin A₂ (alpha-2-delta-2), and of the homotetramer of gamma globin chains, hemoglobin Barts, are present in cord blood. With postnatal maturation, the hemoglobin A₂ level increases gradually to the adult level of 2% to 3% while hemoglobin Barts quickly disappears.

Beta globin disorders such as sickle cell disease or beta thalassemia major do not become apparent clinically until several months of age, when the switch from hemoglobin F to hemoglobin A synthesis reveals the defect. In contrast, gamma globin mutations are most evident in fetal and neonatal life, then disappear by approximately 3 months of age as gamma globin synthesis is replaced by beta globin synthesis. Structural mutations of gamma globin may be associated with transient cyanosis during the newborn period if they form methemoglobin (see Methemoglobinemia) or are associated with low oxygen affinity (Kohli-Kumar et al, 1995). The alpha globin disorders are evident at all stages of development from fetal to adult.

Thalassemia Syndromes

The fundamental lesion in the thalassemias is absent or deficient synthesis of one or another of the normal globin chains, leading to a relative excess of the complementary or partner chain. For example, in alpha-thalassemia there

is diminished synthesis of alpha globin chains, leading to an excess of beta chains (or, in the fetus, of gamma chains). The opposite is true of beta-thalassemia, in which it is excess alpha globin chains that accumulate. Aggregates of free alpha chains or homotetramers of beta chains (hemoglobin H) or of gamma chains (hemoglobin Barts) form in the absence of more suitable partner globin chains, leading to RBC membrane damage and rapid hemolysis. In addition, the decrease in overall production of hemoglobin produces small RBCs (microcytosis) that are often filled with less than the normal amount of hemoglobin (hypochromia). Although in most instances, the globin chains produced by the thalassemic locus are normal in structure, there are mutations, termed thalassemic hemoglobinopathies, in which a structurally abnormal globin chain is found. In these cases, the instability of the hemoglobin tetramer formed from abnormal globin chains may also contribute to the hemolytic process.

Alpha-Thalassemia

Alpha-thalassemia is of particular importance to neonatologists because its clinical manifestations are present in utero and at birth. The more severe forms of alpha-thalassemia are found in Southeast Asians and less commonly in infants of Mediterranean origin. The molecular basis for alpha-thalassemia is usually deletion of one or more of the four alpha globin genes. Nondeletional forms of alpha-thalassemia are also known but are less common. A thalassemic hemoglobinopathy, hemoglobin Constant Spring, may also behave functionally as a mild form of alpha-thalassemia. Clinical severity is dictated by how many alpha globin genes are absent or nonfunctional. An infant can inherit 0, 1, or 2 alpha-thalassemia genes from each parent, giving rise to the following four clinical syndromes:

1. Silent carrier state. Deletion or nonfunction of a single alpha globin gene is not accompanied by any clinical or hematologic abnormalities.
2. Alpha-thalassemia trait. Deletion or nonfunction of two alpha globin genes, in *cis* or *trans*, is associated

with mild microcytic anemia, without hemolysis or reticulocytosis.

3. Hemoglobin H disease. When three of four alpha globin genes are deleted or nonfunctional, a moderate hemolytic anemia is found. The RBCs are hypochromic and microcytic and contain inclusions of hemoglobin Barts or hemoglobin H when appropriate staining is performed.

4. Homozygous alpha-thalassemia. Lack of all four alpha globin genes is associated with a severe intrauterine hemolytic anemia, hydrops fetalis, with massive hepatosplenomegaly, and, in most instances, fetal demise. The RBCs are very hypochromic, fragmented, and bizarre in shape. Erythroblastosis is present.

The diagnosis of the alpha-thalassemia syndromes is easily made during the newborn period by correlation of the clinical and hematologic appearance of the child with the amount of hemoglobin Barts (gamma$_4$) present in the RBCs (Table 89–8). The large amount of hemoglobin Barts found in the RBCs of homozygotes for alpha-thalassemia contributes to the clinical severity of the syndrome, because the markedly increased oxygen affinity of this hemoglobin makes it incapable of delivering oxygen to the tissues. DNA-based diagnostic tests are available for prenatal diagnosis, which is often carried out when a pregnancy at risk for a fetus with homozygous alpha-thalassemia is identified. The increased risk of eclampsia in mothers of such fetuses is an important justification for early identification and termination of the pregnancy.

No treatment is needed for the silent carrier state or for alpha-thalassemia trait, but studies to determine the thalassemia status of other family members, particularly those in their reproductive years, are recommended so that genetic counseling (and prenatal diagnosis if indicated) can be provided. Parents of infants who have hemoglobin H disease should be instructed to avoid oxidant agents that can cause hemolysis (the same list that is given to patients with G6PD deficiency). Although these infants are usually only mildly anemic, they may experience severe episodes of hemolysis during infections or exposure to oxidant agents. Fetuses with homozygous alpha-thalassemia who are not aborted are usually stillborn, but several have been born alive, resuscitated, and placed on chronic RBC transfusion programs (Beaudry et al, 1986; Bianchi et al, 1986). Experimental treatment of homozygous alpha-thalassemia in utero by means of hematopoietic stem cell transplantation is currently under evaluation.

Beta-Thalassemia

Like alpha-thalassemia, beta-thalassemia is found in regions of the world where malaria was formerly endemic: Southeastern Asia, India, Africa, and the Mediterranean basin. Although deletion of the beta globin locus is an occasional cause of beta-thalassemia, most cases are caused by point mutations that affect transcription, mRNA processing, or translation (Galanello, 1995; McDonagh and Nienhuis, 1993). Two general types of beta-thalassemia are recognized. In beta^0-thalassemia no beta globin at all is produced by the thalassemic locus, whereas in beta$^+$-thalassemia there is reduced but measurable output of beta globin. The severity of homozygous beta-thalassemia (or beta-thalassemia major) is greatest when two beta^0-thalassemia genes are inherited and usually much milder when two beta$^+$-thalassemia genes are inherited. Severe beta-thalassemia is associated with lifelong hemolytic anemia, dependence on regular RBC transfusions for survival, and the gradual development of transfusion-associated hemosiderosis. The clinical abnormalities of beta-thalassemia are not evident at birth, but first present only after 3 months of age, when beta globin normally becomes the dominant form of non-alpha globin synthesized. Although affected newborns appear clinically normal, the diagnosis of beta^0-thalassemia can be made at birth by detecting a complete absence of hemoglobin A, using hemoglobin electrophoresis or similar techniques. Definitive diagnosis of beta$^+$-thalassemia by these techniques, however, is not possible

TABLE 89–8

Alpha Thalassemia Syndromes

		Anemia	Hemolysis	α:β Chain Synthesis	Abnormal Hemoglobins	
					Cord Blood	Adult Blood
Normal	α/α α/α	None	None	0.95–1.10	0%–1% γ$_4$	—
Silent carrier	α/— α/α	None	None	0.85–0.95	1%–2% γ$_4$	—
Alpha-thalassemia trait	—/— α/α	Mild Hypochromic Microcytic	None	0.72–0.82	5%–6% γ$_4$	—
Hemoglobin "H" disease	—/— α/—	Moderate Hypochromic Microcytic	Moderate	0.30–0.52	20%–40% γ$_4$ 0–5% β$_4$	20%–40% β$_4$
Homozygous alpha-thalassemia ("hydrops")	—/— —/—	Severe Hypochromic Microcytic	Severe	0	70%–80% γ$_4$ 15%–20% β$_4$ 0–10% ζ$_2$γ$_2$	

in the newborn period, because the reduced amount of hemoglobin A produced overlaps the range for normal babies. Direct identification of beta-thalassemia mutations by DNA diagnostic techniques is increasingly available and does allow the identification at birth of all infants with beta-thalassemia major. These techniques, however, are more commonly used for prenatal diagnosis of beta-thalassemia syndromes. DNA can be obtained during midtrimester from fetal amniocytes (15 to 17 weeks) or during the 1st trimester from chorionic villi (9 to 11 weeks) and the assay completed within a few days, allowing families to make informed decisions regarding termination of pregnancy (Kazazian and Boehm, 1988). The implementation of a strategy of carrier detection, genetic counseling, and prenatal diagnosis in countries where beta-thalassemia is common has led to a striking reduction in the number of births of infants with beta-thalassemia major (Cao, 1996).

Hemoglobin E–Beta-Thalassemia

Hemoglobin E is a structurally abnormal hemoglobin that results from an amino acid substitution (lysine for glutamine) at the number 26 amino acid of beta globin, counting from the NH2 terminus. Because this mutation also adversely affects mRNA processing, there is reduced output of beta globin mRNA. Hemoglobin E is, therefore, an example of a thalassemic hemoglobinopathy. The thalassemic component of the condition is mild (a beta$^+$-thalassemia), so that hemoglobin E carriers are microcytic but not anemic. Even hemoglobin E homozygotes have little or no anemia. However, co-inheritance of hemoglobin E trait and beta^0-thalassemia trait can give rise to a transfusion-dependent form of beta-thalassemia major (Hurst, 1983). As with other types of beta-thalassemia major, clinical abnormalities are not seen until the infant is 3 to 6 months of age. However, the presence of hemoglobin E is easily detected at birth by hemoglobin electrophoresis or related techniques. Infants found to have hemoglobin E need careful follow-up to exclude the possibility of hemoglobin E beta-thalassemia. DNA-based detection of the hemoglobin E mutation is feasible (Embury, 1990) and has been applied to both prenatal and neonatal diagnosis.

Gamma-Thalassemia

Large deletions within the beta globin gene cluster may remove both gamma globin genes ($^A\gamma$ and $^G\gamma$) as well as the delta and beta globin genes. The resulting gamma-delta-beta-thalassemia is lethal in the homozygous state, but in the heterozygote produces a transient but moderately severe microcytic anemia in the newborn. Over the first few months of life, the anemia improves without specific therapy and eventually the hematologic picture is that of beta-thalassemia trait. At least eight different gamma-delta-beta deletions have been reported, all but one in families of European origin (McDonagh and Nienhuis, 1993).

CASE STUDY 2

A full-term 2300-g girl became jaundiced at 24 hours of age (total bilirubin 13.7 mg/dL). The hemoglobin was 10.4 gm/dL, hematocrit 32%, RBC count $3.8 \times 10^6/\mu$L, MCV 84 fl, and MCH 27 pg. The reticulocyte count was 26% and there were 400 nucleated RBC/100 WBC. Rh and ABO incompatibility was absent; the Coombs' test was negative. Iron and iron-binding capacity were normal, and there was no detectable RBC enzyme deficiency. The hemoglobin F level was 52% (normal is 60% to 85%). Hemoglobin Barts was not detected. An RBC transfusion was given and over the next few days nucleated RBCs disappeared, the reticulocyte count decreased, and the hematocrit remained stable. The mother was hematologically normal but the father had a mild hypochromic microcytic anemia that resembled beta-thalassemia trait. At several months of age, the infant had improved and had only a mild hypochromic microcytic anemia that clearly resulted from beta-thalassemia trait (Kan et al, 1972).

Comment

We frequently see newborns with severe hemolytic anemia that resolves or improves spontaneously over the first few months of life, suggesting that some unique property of the fetal RBC contributes to the severity of hemolysis. The presence of a hypochromic microcytic anemia not related to iron deficiency (which can occur with chronic fetal blood loss) suggests one of the thalassemia disorders. Either alpha- or gamma-thalassemia could produce this degree of anemia. The absence of hemoglobin Barts in the cord blood RBCs rules out alpha-thalassemia. Measurement of reticulocyte globin chain synthesis in vitro showed diminished production of both gamma and beta chains, consistent with a diagnosis of gamma-beta-thalassemia. The severe neonatal hemolytic anemia was due to accumulation of excess alpha globin chains, unable to form normal hemoglobin tetramers because of the lack of partner gamma or beta chains. As the infant matured and began to synthesize more beta chains, the globin chain imbalance lessened and hemolysis diminished. Eventually, the hematologic picture in the infant resembled that in her father, that is, classic beta-thalassemia trait.

Sickle Cell Disease

The sickling hemoglobinopathies are beta globin mutations that, like beta thalassemia, do not become clinically evident until several months of age. Sickle cell anemia, the most severe of the disorders, is the result of inheritance of two beta^S mutations (substitution of valine for glutamic acid at the sixth amino acid on the beta globin chain), one from each parent. Sickle-beta^0-thalassemia, phenotypically identical to sickle cell anemia, is caused by inheritance of one beta^S and one beta-thalassemia mutation. The third common form of sickle cell disease, hemoglobin S-C disease, is somewhat milder than sickle cell anemia or sickle-beta^0-thalassemia. It is the consequence of inheritance of one beta^S mutation and one beta^c mutation (the substitution of lysine for glutamic acid at the sixth amino acid on the beta globin chain). Although no clinical abnormalities are present at birth, early diagnosis is important, because two potentially fatal but largely preventable complications may occur during the 1st year of life. The first is the splenic sequestration crisis, an unpredictable pooling of large numbers of RBCs in the spleen, which leads to a rapid decrease in hematocrit and, in the most severe cases, cardiovascular collapse and death. The second is overwhelming septicemia, usually caused by *S. pneumoniae* or *H. influenzae*. The unusually high susceptibility to infection with encapsulated organisms such as *S. pneumoniae* is the consequence of functional asplenia, which commonly appears by 1 year of age in sickle cell anemia or sickle-beta⁰-thalassemia infants (but not until later in hemoglobin S-C disease). Prompt treatment of splenic sequestration with RBC transfusions is lifesaving so that parents are taught to recognize early manifestations such as splenic enlargement, lethargy, or pallor. Overwhelming sepsis can be prevented in most instances by early immunization with *H. influenzae* vaccine, beginning at 2 months of age, and by institution of daily prophylactic penicillin at a dose of 125 mg twice daily (Gaston et al, 1986). It is the need to institute these prophylactic measures within the first 1 to 2 months of life that provides a compelling rationale for the neonatal diagnosis of the sickling disorders. In many states, all newborns are screened for these disorders, whereas in others only high-risk ethnic groups are targeted. Usually a dried sample of blood on filter paper, collected at the same time as other screening tests for inherited metabolic disorders, is used, but cord blood is also satisfactory. Tests that quantitate the amount of hemoglobin S, such as high-performance liquid chromatography, thin-layer isoelectric focusing, or electrophoresis on both cellulose acetate (in an alkaline buffer) and citrate agar (in an acid buffer), are adequate, but sickle solubility tests or the sodium metabisulfate "sickle prep" are not, because sickle cell disease cannot be distinguished from sickle cell trait and the tests are not sensitive enough to detect reliably the small percentage of hemoglobin S present in the RBCs of the newborn. An excellent overview of issues related to newborn screening for sickle cell disease has been published by Wethers and colleagues (1989). Extensive experience with mandatory statewide screening for all infants has been accumulated in New York (Diaz-Barrios, 1989), California (Lorey et al, 1994), and elsewhere (Wethers et al, 1989).

Infants without a hemoglobinopathy born to mothers with sickle cell disease present more of a clinical problem during gestation and the neonatal period than infants who actually have sickle cell disease. Spontaneous abortion, intrauterine growth retardation (approximately 15%), stillbirth (6%), preterm labor and delivery, and perinatal mortality (approximately 15%) are all more frequent in the infants of mothers with sickle cell anemia (Koshy and Burd, 1995). These problems may be traced to abnormalities of the placenta such as small size, infarction, and an increased incidence of placenta previa and abruptio placentae, which appears to be the consequence of sickle vaso-occlusive events within the maternal side of the placental circulation. They are not caused by the presence of the sickle trait, beta-thalassemia trait, or hemoglobin C trait in the infant, because no hematologic disease is associated with the carrier state for these mutations, even in adult life when they

are fully expressed, except under conditions of extreme hypoxia.

One caveat regarding sickle trait blood is that blood from an adult donor who has sickle trait should not be used for exchange transfusions in the newborn, particularly if hypoxemia is present, because sickle trait RBCs in this setting may contribute to a fatal outcome (Veiga and Vaithianathan, 1963).

HYPOPLASTIC ANEMIA

The two major causes of pure RBC aplasia in children are Diamond-Blackfan anemia (DBA) and transient erythroblastopenia of childhood (TEC). Approximately 25% of DBA infants are anemic at birth. In contrast, TEC is a disease that is not seen before 1 to 2 months of age (Alter and Young, 1993), and, although it can present in the 1st year of life (Miller and Berman, 1994; Ware and Kinney, 1991) most children with this disorder are older infants or young children.

Diamond-Blackfan Syndrome

Also known as congenital hypoplastic anemia, Diamond-Blackfan syndrome is characterized by the absence of recognizable erythroid precursor cells in the bone marrow (Alter and Young, 1993). An as yet uncharacterized defect in erythroid progenitor cells appears to be responsible for the profound erythroid hypoplasia. Anemia is lifelong but the onset of the disease is variable. Approximately 10% of affected infants are severely anemic in the newborn period and pallor at birth or soon thereafter has been a feature of the disease in most cases (Alter and Young, 1993). Growth retardation, skeletal abnormalities, or other congenital anomalies are seen in almost one third of patients. The diagnosis of DBA is suggested by anemia and reticulocytopenia appearing in the first 6 months of life. Certain unusual features of the RBCs (macrocytosis, elevated fetal hemoglobin, increased adenosine deaminase activity) may assist in diagnosis. DBA can be cured by allogeneic bone marrow transplantation. Many patients achieve durable remissions from anemia when treated with corticosteroids. Those who do not require chronic RBC transfusions and are at risk of transfusion hemosiderosis. The incidence of leukemia is increased in older DBA patients, but the basis for this predisposition is unknown (Alter and Young, 1993; Glader, 1987).

Transient Erythroblastopenia of Childhood

TEC is an acquired hypoplastic anemia that usually appears several weeks after an acute viral infection (Wranne, 1970). Evidence of a humoral or cellular immune response directed against erythroid precursor cells has been obtained in many affected children. As in DBA, the hallmarks of the disorder are anemia and reticulocytopenia, with an absence of erythroid precursors in the bone marrow. The platelet count is sometimes increased and neutropenia may be present (Rogers et al, 1989). The abnormal RBC features seen in DBA are not seen in TEC. The natural history of TEC is one of spontaneous recovery over a period of several weeks, and because most children are recognized at the nadir of their anemia, evidence of recovery may already be present. RBC transfusion may be required to treat symptomatic anemia but steroid therapy is unnecessary and not effective. There are no long-term hematologic sequelae of TEC, and recurrences are rare.

PHYSIOLOGIC ANEMIA OF INFANCY AND PREMATURITY

At birth, the mean hemoglobin of term infants (17 g/100 mL) is slightly greater than in premature infants (16 g/100 mL). The hemoglobin concentration in term infants subsequently decreases to a plateau at which it remains throughout the 1st year of life (Table 89–9). Termed the *physiologic anemia of infancy*, this low (relative to adults) hemoglobin is a normal part of development and has no adverse clinical effects. A similar process (*anemia of prematurity*) occurs in premature infants, but the hemoglobin decreases more rapidly and reaches a lower nadir. After 1 year of age, there is little difference between the hemoglobin values of term and premature infants.

Physiologic Anemia of Infancy

With the onset of respirations at birth, considerably more oxygen is available for binding to hemoglobin and the hemoglobin–oxygen saturation increases from approximately 50% to 95% or more. Furthermore, the normal developmental switch from fetal to adult hemoglobin synthesis actively replaces high oxygen affinity fetal hemoglobin with lower oxygen affinity adult hemoglobin, which can deliver a greater fraction of hemoglobin-bound oxygen to the tissues. Therefore, immediately after birth the increase in blood oxygen content and tissue oxygen delivery downregulates erythropoietin production and, as a consequence, erythropoiesis is suppressed. In the absence of erythropoiesis, hemoglobin levels decrease because there is no replacement of aged RBCs as they are normally removed from the circulation. Iron from degraded RBCs is stored for future hemoglobin synthesis. The hemoglobin concentration continues to decrease until tissue oxygen needs are greater than oxygen delivery. Normally, this point is reached between 6 and 12 weeks of age when the hemoglobin concentration is 9.5 to 11 g/dL. As hypoxia is detected by renal or hepatic oxygen sensors, erythropoietin production increases and erythropoiesis resumes. The iron previously stored in reticuloendothelial tissues can then be used for hemoglobin synthesis. The supply of stored iron is sufficient for hemoglobin synthesis, even in the absence of dietary iron intake, until approximately 20 weeks of age. It is unnecessary to administer iron during this period, because it does not prevent the physiologic decrease in hemoglobin. Any iron administered is added to stores for future use. This physiologic hemoglobin decrease does not represent anemia in the true sense of the term; rather, it is a normal adjustment reflecting the presence of excess capability for oxygen delivery relative to tissue oxygen requirements. There is no hematologic problem, and no therapy is required.

Anemia of Prematurity

The physiologic anemia seen in preterm infants is more profound and occurs earlier (see Table 89–9). Because symptoms may occur, the anemia of prematurity is considered nonphysiologic. The cause of anemia is multifaceted. The lower hemoglobin may in part be a physiologic response to the lower oxygen consumption of premature infants compared with that of term infants, a consequence of their diminished metabolic oxygen needs (Mestyan et al, 1964). An important component in the first few weeks of life is blood loss as a result of sampling for the many laboratory tests necessary to stabilize the clinical status of these infants, particularly those with cardiorespiratory problems. The erythropoietic response to anemia is also suboptimal, a significant problem because demands on erthyropoiesis are heightened by the short survival of the RBCs of premature infants (approximately 40 to 60 days instead of 120 days as in adults) and the rapid expansion of the RBC mass that accompanies growth. The basis for suboptimal erythropoiesis in prematurity appears to be inadequate synthesis of erythropoietin in response to hypoxia. Figure 89–13 illustrates the magnitude of the deficiency, which, as shown by Stockman and colleagues (1984), is greatest in the smallest, least mature infants. Because the liver is the predominant source of erythropoietin during fetal life, it has been proposed that relative insensitivity of the hepatic oxygen sensor to hypoxia explains the blunted erythropoietin response seen in premature infants (Dallman, 1993). The spontaneous resolution

TABLE 89–9

Hemoglobin Changes During the 1st Year of Life

Week	Term	Premature (1.2–2.5 kg)	Premature (<1.2 kg)
0	17.0 (14.0–20.0)	16.4 (13.5–19.0)	16.0 (13.0–18.0)
1	18.8	16.0	14.8
3	15.9	13.5	13.4
6	12.7	10.7	9.7
10	11.4	9.8	8.5
20	12.0	10.4	9.0
50	12.0	11.5	11.0
Lowest hemoglobin (mean)	10.3 (9.5–11.0)	9.0 (8.0–10.0)	7.1 (6.5–9.0)
Time of nadir	6–12 weeks	5–10 weeks	4–8 weeks

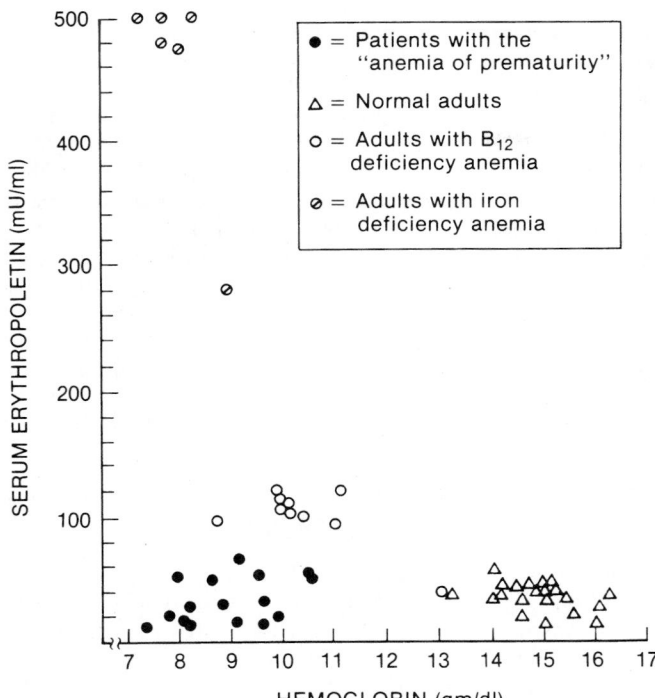

FIGURE 89–13. Hemoglobin levels and corresponding serum erythropoietin levels are shown. Values from each of the study subjects, normal adults, adults with vitamin B_{12} deficiency anemia, and adults with iron deficiency anemia also are shown. (From Ross MP, Christensen RD, Rothstein G, et al: A randomized trial to develop criteria for administering erythrocyte transfusions to anemic preterm infants from 1 to 3 months of age. J Perinatol 9:246, 1989. Reprinted by permission of Appleton & Lange, Inc.)

of the anemia that occurs by approximately 40 weeks' gestational age is in keeping with a developmental switch from the relatively insensitive hepatic oxygen sensor to the renal oxygen sensor, which is exquisitely sensitive to hypoxia, because by this time the predominant site of erythropoietin synthesis has shifted to the kidneys. The problem does not lie with altered sensitivity of erythroid progenitors to erythropoietin because this has been shown to be normal (Shannon et al, 1987).

The anemia of prematurity occurs even in nutritionally sufficient infants, but it may be heightened by deficiencies of folate, vitamin B_{12}, or vitamin E (Worthington-White et al, 1994). Premature infants are endowed at birth with significantly less vitamin E than term infants, and unless supplemental vitamin E is provided, this deficiency state persists for 2 to 3 months. Vitamin E is an antioxidant compound vital to the integrity of erythrocytes, and in its absence, these cells are susceptible to lipid peroxidation and membrane injury. One clinical consequence of vitamin E deficiency is that hemolytic anemia can occur in small premature infants (weighing less than 1500 g) at 6 to 10 weeks of age (Oski and Barness, 1967; Ritchie et al, 1968). This hemolytic anemia, which is characterized by reduced vitamin E levels and increased RBC peroxide hemolysis, rapidly disappears following vitamin E administration. A logical conclusion is that vitamin E deficiency might con-

tribute to the anemia of prematurity in a more general sense. In fact, premature infants given daily vitamin E (15 IU per day) had higher hemoglobin levels and lower reticulocyte levels than a control group not given the vitamin, as shown in Table 89–10 (Oski and Barness, 1967). A more recent study found no hematologic benefit to the administration of 25 IU of vitamin E daily to premature infants (Zipursky et al, 1987). Although it has become standard practice to administer vitamin E to all premature infants, the hemoglobin nadir in these babies is still lower than that in term newborns, indicating that anemia is largely caused by other factors such as erythropoietin deficiency.

Treatment of Anemia of Prematurity with Recombinant Human Erythropoietin

Because a relative deficiency of erythropoietin is present in the anemia of prematurity, a number of studies have evaluated the safety and efficacy of recombinant human erythropoietin (rH EPO) therapy in this setting. If adequate doses of rH EPO are used, reticulocytosis and a retardation in the development of anemia are regularly achieved (Gallagher and Ehrenkranz, 1993; Mentzer and Shannon, 1995). Several large multicenter trials have documented a modest but statistically significant reduction in the RBC transfusion requirements of treated infants compared with control subjects (Maier et al, 1994; Meyer et al, 1994; Shannon et al, 1995). Erythropoietin treatment may have a particularly important role to play in the management of infants whose parents refuse to allow blood transfusions on religious grounds (Davis et al, 1991). The optimal timing for initiation of rH EPO therapy and the optimal dose have yet to be determined. To achieve the best results, supplemental oral iron at a dose of at least 6 mg/kg per day needs to be administered. It may be possible to use parenteral iron supplements, particularly in young very-low-birth-weight infants who are not able to take oral iron (Heese et al, 1990). Adequate vitamin E supplementation is of particular importance if intramuscular iron is used (Graeber et al, 1977). Although concern was raised

TABLE 89–10

Effect of Supplemental Vitamin E on Anemia of Prematurity*

	Control	Vitamin E (15 IU/Day)
Birth weight	1176 ± 182 g	1278 ± 180 g
6–8 weeks of age		
Vitamin E (mg/100 mL)	0.22 ± 0.10	1.00 ± 0.25
H_2O_2 hemolysis (%)	66 ± 21	9 ± 9
Lowest hemoglobin (g/100 mL)	7.7 ± 1.5	9.2 ± 1.3
Highest reticulocytes (%)	6.7 ± 2.5	3.1 ± 0.7

* Premature infants were given prophylactic vitamin E (15 international units per day) and the vitamin E level, peroxide hemolysis, hemoglobin concentration, and reticulocyte count were measured after 6 to 8 weeks. These values were compared with those from a group of control infants not given vitamin E supplements.

Data from Oski FA, Barness LA: Vitamin E deficiency: A previously unrecognized cause of hemolytic anemia in the premature infant. J Pediatr 70:211, 1967.

over two rH EPO–treated infants in one study who subsequently died of sudden infant death syndrome (SIDS) (Emerson et al, 1993), SIDS has not been a feature of rH EPO treatment in other studies. Early concerns about rH EPO–induced neutropenia (Christensen et al, 1991) have, similarly, not been borne out (Shannon et al, 1995). Therefore, the current consensus is that use of this agent appears to be safe in premature infants. Very small premature infants (less than 1300 g birth weight) are those most likely to benefit from therapy (Strauss, 1994). There is disagreement regarding the cost-benefit relation of rH EPO therapy (Maier et al, 1994; Shireman et al, 1994; Wandstrat and Kaplan, 1995).

RBC Transfusion Therapy in Premature Infants

It has been estimated that of the approximately 38,000 infants born weighing less than 1500 g in the United States each year, 80% will receive multiple RBC transfusions (Strauss, 1991). Most transfusions given in the first several weeks of life are to replace phlebotomy losses required for laboratory monitoring during ventilator support and other intensive care measures. The mean blood loss resulting from phlebotomy during the 1st week of life in one group of 20 successive very ill premature infants admitted to the intensive care nursery was 38.9 mL, an impressive figure considering that the total blood volume of such infants is approximately 80 mL/kg body weight (Shannon, 1990). After the first few weeks of life, most transfusions are given to treat the symptoms of anemia of prematurity. The risks of allogeneic RBC transfusion in premature infants include exposure to viral infections, GVH disease, electrolyte and acid-base imbalances, exposure to plasticizers, hemolysis when T antigen activation of RBCs has occurred, and immunosuppression (Strauss, 1991).

Many strategies to reduce the need for allogeneic RBC transfusion in premature infants have been developed. Reducing phlebotomy losses by use of noninvasive monitoring techniques has been of only limited usefulness (Strauss, 1991). Donor exposures can be reduced by assigning a specified bag of adult donor blood to a sick neonate for multiple transfusions (Cook et al, 1993), particularly because it has been shown that blood stored for up to 35 days in citrate-phosphate-dextrose A1 is safe for use in this setting (Liu et al, 1994). Defining strict criteria for RBC transfusions can also reduce the number of donor exposures in routine nursery practice (Batton et al, 1992). Traditionally, RBC transfusions have been given to replace phlebotomy losses or in the presence of symptoms thought to reflect hypoxia (e.g., tachycardia, tachypnea, dyspnea, apneic spells, and poor feeding) (Oski and Naiman, 1982; Wardrop et al, 1978). However, studies to validate such practices have yielded conflicting results. Stockman and Clark (1984) showed a beneficial effect of transfusion on weight gain, but no benefit was found by Blank and coworkers (1984). Similarly, apneic spells were reduced in frequency following RBC transfusion in the studies of Joshi and associates (1987) and Ross and coworkers (1989) but not in those of Blank and colleagues (1984), Keyes and coworkers (1989), or Bifano and colleagues (1992). Lachance and colleagues (1994) measured oxygen consumption, myocardial function, resting energy expenditure, and other physiologic variables before and after RBC transfusions. They concluded that in asymptomatic anemic premature infants, oxygenation was well maintained without RBC transfusions when the hemoglobin level was 6.5 g/dL or more. Nelle and coworkers (1994) studied a similar group of asymptomatic anemic premature infants and found that RBC transfusion improved systemic oxygen transport as well as transport in the cerebral and gastrointestinal arteries. When clinical findings of hypoxia are absent or confusing, an elevated blood lactate level may predict a need for transfusion (Izraeli et al, 1993). At present, most intensive care nursery units have abandoned earlier practices of automatically replacing phlebotomy losses in favor of transfusing for clear-cut symptoms of hypoxia or for significant anemia unaccompanied by evidence of an adequate erythropoietic response.

POLYCYTHEMIA

Neonatal polycythemia is usually caused by one of two conditions: increased intrauterine erythropoiesis or fetal hypertransfusion (Table 89–11). Other causes seen in older children such as arterial hypoxemia (cyanotic heart disease, pulmonary disease), abnormal hemoglobins, or hypersecretion of erythropoietin by tumors are rare, and primary polycythemia or polycythemia vera is virtually nonexistent. In normal term infants, delayed clamping of the cord leading to an increased transfer of placental blood to the infant is the most common cause of polycythemia. In the setting of acute intrapartum hypoxia, increased placental transfusion may also account for the observed increase in fetal RBC mass, according to animal studies by Oh and

TABLE 89–11

Etiology of Neonatal Polycythemia

Active (Increased Intrauterine Erythropoiesis)	Passive (Secondary to Erythrocyte Transfusions)
Intrauterine hypoxia	Delayed cord clamping
Placental insufficiency	Intentional
Small-for-gestational-age infants	Unassisted delivery
Postmaturity	Maternofetal transfusion
Toxemia of pregnancy	Twin–twin transfusion
Drugs (propranolol)	
Severe maternal heart disease	
Maternal smoking	
Maternal diabetes	
Neonatal hyperthyroidism or hypothyroidism	
Congenital adrenal hyperplasia	
Chromosome abnormalities	
Trisomy 13	
Trisomy 18	
Trisomy 21 (Down syndrome)	
Hyperplastic visceromegaly (Beckwith syndrome)	
Decreased fetal erythrocyte deformability	

From Oski FA, Naiman JL: Hematologic Problems in the Newborn, 3rd ed. Philadelphia, WB Saunders, 1982.

coworkers (1975). Placental insufficiency and chronic intrauterine hypoxia, as seen typically in small for gestational age infants, most commonly underlie increased intrauterine erythropoiesis.

As the hematocrit increases, blood viscosity increases exponentially (Fig. 89–14). Blood flow is impaired by hyperviscosity at hematocrits of 60% or more. Oxygen transport, which is determined by both hemoglobin levels (i.e., oxygen binding capacity) and blood flow, is maximal in the normal hematocrit range. At low hematocrits, oxygen transport is limited by reduced oxygen binding capacity, whereas at higher hematocrits reduction in blood flow secondary to hyperviscosity may similarly limit oxygen transport. At any given hematocrit, expansion of the blood volume beyond the normal level (hypervolemia) distends the vasculature, decreases peripheral resistance, and increases blood flow and, ultimately, oxygen transport. These physiologic observations have implications for therapy of polycythemia.

Most polycythemic infants have no symptoms, particularly if the polycythemia becomes apparent only upon routine neonatal screening. Symptoms, when present, are usually attributable to hyperviscosity and poor tissue perfusion or to associated metabolic abnormalities such as hypoglycemia and hypocalcemia. Common early symptoms include plethora, cyanosis (resulting from peripheral stasis), lethargy, hypotonia, poor suck and feeding, and tremulousness. Serious complications include cardiorespiratory distress (with or without congestive failure), seizures, peripheral gangrene, necrotizing enterocolitis, renal failure (occasionally resulting from renal vein thrombosis), and priapism. Because the elevated RBC mass increases the catabolism of hemoglobin, hyperbilirubinemia is common and gall stones occasionally occur.

In the symptomatic infant, a venous hematocrit of 65% or more (or a hemoglobin greater than 22 g/dL) confirms the presence of polycythemia. In screening apparently healthy newborns for polycythemia, however, account must be taken of a number of physiologic variables that influence the hematocrit during the first 12 hours of life:

1. Time of cord clamping—immediate clamping (within 30 seconds) minimizes placental transfusion.
2. Age at sampling—values increase from birth to a peak at 2 hours, gradually decreasing to cord levels around 12 to 18 hours (Ramamurthy and Berlanga, 1987; Shohat et al, 1984).
3. Site of sampling—values from blood extracted by the heelstick method exceed those from venous blood (the difference can be minimized by prewarming the heel.
4. Method of hematocrit determination—spun values are higher than those obtained by electronic cell counter and show better correlation with blood viscosity (Villalta et al, 1989).

One way to standardize and simplify screening for polycythemia is as follows: At birth, clamp the cord at about 30 to 45 seconds; at 4 to 6 hours of age obtain a blood sample from a warmed heelstick and perform a spun hematocrit. If the result is greater than 70%, repeat the test on a venous sample. A venous hematocrit of 65% or more indicates polycythemia. By this approach, 1% to 5% of newborns are polycythemic; the range largely reflects differences in altitude at which the study population resides. Because the hematocrit is lower with increasing prematurity, polycythemia is less frequently seen in preterm infants than in term babies.

Following diagnosis, an attempt should be made to determine the cause of polycythemia (see Table 89–11). The condition is particularly common in infants of diabetic mothers or those with Down syndrome (Mentzer, 1978) and may also occur in the setting of maternal hypertension (Kurlat and Sola, 1992). However, no apparent cause is found in most cases. Studies to determine the effects of polycythemia are dictated by the clinical findings but should usually include serum bilirubin, glucose, calcium, blood urea nitrogen, and creatinine levels.

Treatment by isovolumetric partial exchange transfusion is recommended to reduce the RBC mass without inducing hypovolemia. A beneficial effect of isovolumetric hemodilution on skin capillary perfusion (Norman et al, 1992) and on skin vasomotor activity (Norman et al, 1993) has been documented in polycythemic infants. At the University of California at San Francisco, all symptomatic newborns whose venous hematocrit is greater than 60% and asymptomatic newborns whose hematocrit is greater than 65% undergo partial exchange transfusion, using either normal saline or 5% albuminated saline (Levy et al, 1990). Unlike fresh-frozen plasma, these products do not carry a risk of

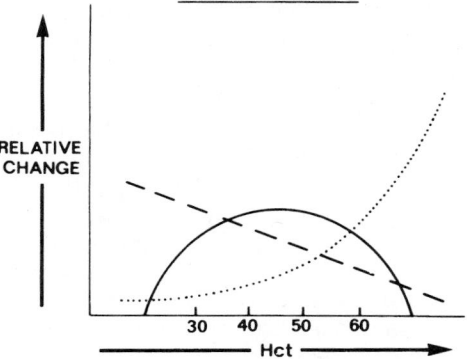
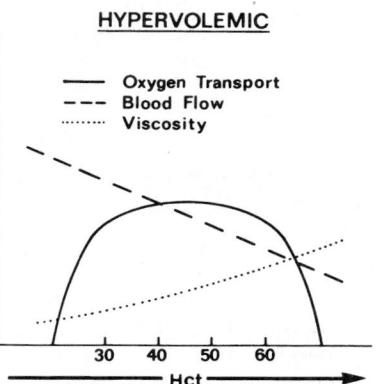

FIGURE 89–14. Effect of hematocrit on viscosity, blood flow, and oxygen transport.

transmitting viral infections. Furthermore, partial exchange transfusion with fresh-frozen plasma has been associated with the appearance of necrotizing enterocolitis (Black et al, 1985), whereas purified plasma protein derivatives such as albumin have not (Hein and Lathrop, 1987). Withdrawal of blood for a partial exchange transfusion is most easily done using an umbilical artery catheter. Any vessel may be used for blood withdrawal, and all but arterial lines can be used to infuse volume. An umbilical venous catheter inserted into the right atrium also provides acceptable access, but if correct placement cannot be achieved the catheter should be inserted just far enough into the vessel to allow blood to be withdrawn. Calculation of the total volume of blood to be exchanged for diluent uses the following formula (Oski and Naiman, 1982):

$$\text{Exchange volume} = \frac{\text{observed Hct} - \text{desired Hct} \times \text{BV (mL/kg)} \times \text{weight (kg)}}{\text{observed Hct}}$$

where blood volume (BV) is usually 100 mL/kg but in infants of diabetic mothers it may be lower (80 to 85 mL/kg).

EXAMPLE: A 3-kg dyspneic infant with an 80% hematocrit requires a partial exchange transfusion.

$$\text{Blood volume} = 3 \text{ kg} \times 100 \text{ mL/kg} = 300 \text{ mL}$$

$$\frac{\text{Observed Hct} - \text{desired Hct}}{\text{Observed Hct}} = \frac{80 - 55}{80} = 0.31$$

Therefore, volume of exchange = 300 mL × 0.31 = 93 mL.

Some neonatal programs have more stringent hematocrit thresholds (e.g., >70%) (Carmi et al, 1992; Levy et al, 1990) for partial exchange transfusion of asymptomatic polycythemic infants than that cited previously (>65%). Although asymptomatic infants have an increased risk of late, mild neuropsychologic handicaps, prospective studies have failed to demonstrate major benefit from partial exchange transfusion (Delaney-Black et al, 1989). Because coexisting hypoglycemia is an important determinant of adverse neurologic outcome, careful monitoring and maintenance of adequate glucose levels and hydration are important.

CASE STUDY 3

A gravida 2, para 1 white female delivered a 2950-g male infant after a normal pregnancy, labor, and delivery. At birth, the child had an Apgar score of 6. Physical examination revealed a cyanotic infant with a grade III/VI systolic heart murmur. The liver edge was palpable 2 cm below the right costal margin, and the spleen tip was palpable. Chest radiograph revealed a markedly enlarged heart with increased pulmonary vascular markings. The hemoglobin was 26 g/dL, and the hematocrit was 79%. There were no other hematologic abnormalities. The infant was partially exchanged with 5% albumin and the postexchange hematocrit was 62%. Subsequently, the infant's color improved, the heart murmur disappeared, and there were no remaining signs of congestive heart failure.

Comment

The clinical findings in this infant were initially suggestive of organic heart disease. Rapid disappearance of the cardiac abnormalities following recognition and treatment of polycythemia indicated that these abnormalities were the result of polycythemia-induced hyperviscosity. In older children with cyanotic heart disease, polycythemia is a physiologic response that allows adequate oxygen transport to occur in the presence of arterial hypoxemia. Phlebotomy in these children may produce an acute hypoxic insult and should be undertaken with caution if at all. In striking contrast, in the newborn period, infants with cyanotic heart disease are not polycythemic (Gatti et al, 1966). Therefore, phlebotomy should improve, not worsen, oxygen transport, as it did in Case Study 3.

METHEMOGLOBINEMIA

Methemoglobin is an oxidized derivative of hemoglobin in which heme iron is in the ferric (Fe^{3+}) or oxidized state rather than the ferrous (Fe^{2+}) or reduced state. Because methemoglobin is unable to bind (or release) oxygen, the presence of significant amounts of this respiratory pigment adversely affects blood oxygen binding capacity and transport. Normally, small amounts of methemoglobin are formed daily in vivo by the action of endogenous agents, which may include oxygen itself (auto-oxidation). However, any methemoglobin formed is rapidly reduced through the action of RBC NADH-methemoglobin reductase (also known as cytochrome b_5 reductase) so that in normal individuals levels of methemoglobin seldom exceed 1%. A second methemoglobin reductase, dependent on NADPH as cofactor, is also present in RBCs. Although this enzyme is not active under normal physiologic conditions, it is greatly activated by the presence of certain redox compounds such as methylene blue, forming the basis for treatment of methemoglobinemia by this agent.

Acquired methemoglobinemia occurs when normal individuals are exposed to chemicals such as aniline dyes that readily oxidize hemoglobin iron. Newborns are particularly susceptible because fetal hemoglobin is more readily oxidized to the ferric state than is hemoglobin A (Martin and Huisman, 1963) and because RBC NADH-methemoglobin reductase activity is low during the first few months of life (Bartos and Desforges, 1966). Merely marking the diapers of newborns with aniline dyes has caused methemoglobinemia. Drugs such as prilocaine, administered before birth to provide local anesthesia, can produce methemoglobinemia in both mother and infant (Climie et al, 1967). Perhaps the best known agent that may cause methemoglobinemia is nitrite, either present de novo in ingested material or converted from nitrates by the action of intestinal bacteria or by administering nitric oxide to term babies in high concentrations for treatment of persistent pulmonary hypertension (see Chapter 53). It is for the latter reason that well water (Comly, 1945) or foods (e.g., cabbage, spinach, beets, carrots) (Keating et al, 1973) with a high nitrate content can produce methemoglobinemia in infants. Accumulation of nitrate in the intestinal tract of infants with diarrhea and acidosis (Kay et al, 1990; Yano et al, 1982) or symptomatic dietary protein intolerance (Murray and Christie, 1993) is also thought to underlie the transient methemoglobinemia that occurs in these conditions.

Congenital methemoglobinemia is due to inherited disorders of hemoglobin structure or to a severe deficiency of NADH methemoglobin reductase activity. The seven inherited abnormalities of hemoglobin structure that give rise to methemoglobinemia, known collectively as the hemoglobin M disorders, are rare autosomal dominant defects caused by point mutations that alter a single amino acid in the structure of normal globin. The altered conformation that ensues favors the persistence of the ferric rather than the ferrous form of heme iron. The normal methemoglobin reductive capacity of the RBC cannot compensate for such instability of ferrous heme. Two of the mutations affect the a globin chain, three affect the beta globin chain, and two affect the gamma chain. Only the alpha and gamma globin chain mutations are associated with neonatal methemoglobinemia, because these are the globins that form hemoglobin F, the predominant hemoglobin found in neonatal RBCs. Neonatal methemoglobinemia is transient when produced by one of the two gamma chain mutations, hemoglobin FM-Osaka (Hayashi et al, 1980) or hemoglobin FM-Fort Ripley (Priest et al, 1989), because the normal developmental switch from fetal to adult hemoglobin eliminates all but a trace of the mutant hemoglobin. Hemoglobin M heterozygotes inheriting alpha or beta globin mutations appear cyanotic all their lives because of the increased methemoglobin levels present in their RBCs but they are otherwise asymptomatic. No therapy is needed (and none is possible). The homozygous state is incompatible with life. Diagnosis of the hemoglobin M disorders is by hemoglobin electrophoresis.

NADH-methemoglobin reductase deficiency is an uncommon autosomal recessive disorder. Heterozygotes are asymptomatic and do not have methemoglobinemia under normal circumstances. If challenged by drugs or chemicals that cause methemoglobinemia, however, patients become cyanotic and symptomatic at doses that have no effect in normal individuals. Homozygotes have lifelong methemoglobinemia at a level of 15% to 40% and are cyanotic but otherwise asymptomatic unless exposed to toxic agents. Diagnosis of NADH-methemoglobin reductase deficiency is by assay of the RBC enzyme activity, a procedure available only in specialized hematology laboratories.

The cardinal clinical manifestation of methemoglobinemia is cyanosis not resulting from cardiac or respiratory disease. Cyanosis present at birth suggests hereditary methemoglobinemia whereas that appearing suddenly in an otherwise asymptomatic infant is more consistent with acquired methemoglobinemia (Table 89–12). The blood is dark and, unlike deoxygenated venous blood, does not turn

---

TABLE 89–12

Approach to Infants with Cyanosis and Methemoglobinemia

Cyanosis associated with respiratory and cardiac findings
  Blood turns red when mixed with air
  Decreased arterial P_{O_2}
  Consider pulmonary, cardiac, or central nervous system disease
Cyanosis with or without respiratory and cardiac findings
  Blood turns red when mixed with air
  Normal arterial P_{O_2}
  Consider polycythemia syndromes
Cyanosis without respiratory or cardiac findings
  Blood remains dark after mixing with air
  Arterial P_{O_2} normal
  Consider methemoglobinemia syndromes:
  1. Rapid clearing of methemoglobin following methylene blue
    a. Consider toxic methemoglobinemia (look for environmental oxidants)
    b. Consider NADH-methemoglobin reductase deficiency (perform enzyme assay)
  2. Reappearance of methemoglobinemia after initial response to methylene blue
    a. Consider NADH-methemoglobin reductase deficiency
  3. No change in methemoglobin following methylene blue
    a. Consider hemoglobin M disorders (perform hemoglobin electrophoresis)
    b. Consider associated G6PD deficiency (perform enzyme assay)

---

red when exposed to air. Rapid screening for methemoglobinemia can be done by placing a drop of blood on filter paper and then waving the filter paper in air to allow the blood to dry. Deoxygenated normal hemoglobin turns red whereas methemoglobin remains brown. Methemoglobin levels of 10% or more can be detected (Harley and Celermajer, 1970). More accurate determination of methemoglobin levels is accomplished in the blood gas laboratory by co-oximetry or in the clinical laboratory using a spectrophotometer. Cyanosis is first clinically evident when methemoglobin levels reach approximately 10% (1.5 g/dL), but symptoms attributable to hypoxemia and diminished oxygen transport do not appear until levels increase to 30% to 40% of total hemoglobin. Death occurs at levels of 70% or greater. Methemoglobinemia is not associated with anemia, hemolysis, or other hematologic abnormalities.

In newborns, treatment with intravenous methylene blue (1 mg/kg as a 1% solution in normal saline) is indicated when methemoglobin levels are greater than 15% to 20%. The response to methylene blue is both therapeutic and diagnostic. Methemoglobin levels decrease rapidly, within 1 to 2 hours, if methemoglobinemia is caused by a toxic agent or by a deficiency of NADH-methemoglobin reductase. In contrast, the hemoglobin M disorders do not respond to methylene blue. Reappearance of methemoglobinemia after an initial response to methylene blue suggests a deficiency of NADH-methemoglobin reductase or the persistence of an occult oxidant. A poor response to methylene blue is also seen in G6PD-deficient individuals, not because G6PD deficiency is a cause of methemoglobin formation but because there is suboptimal generation of NADPH, a required cofactor in the reduction of methemoglobin by methylene blue in deficient individuals. In general, most infants with hereditary methemoglobinemia are asymptomatic and require no therapy. Older children are sometimes given daily administration of oral ascorbic acid or methylene blue to decrease cyanosis for cosmetic reasons. Methylene blue produces blue urine, but this is harmless.

REFERENCES

Normal Erythrocyte Physiology in the Fetus and Newborn

Allen DW, Wyman J, Smith GA.: The oxygen equilibrium of fetal and adult hemoglobin. J Biol Chem 203:81, 1953.

Bauer C, Ludwig I, Ludwig M: Different effects of 2,3-diphosphoglycerate and adenosine triphosphate on oxygen affinity of adult and fetal hemoglobin. Life Sci 7:1339, 1968.

Delivoria-Papadopoulos M, Roncevic NP, Oski FA: Postnatal changes in oxygen transport of term, premature, and sick infants: The role of red cell 2,3-diphosphoglycerate and adult hemoglobin. Pediatr Res 5:235, 1971.

Finne PH: Erythropoietin levels in cord blood as an indicator of intrauterine hypoxia. Acta Paediatr Scand 55:478, 1966.

Finne PH, Halvorsen S: Regulation of erythropoiesis in the fetus and newborn. Arch Dis Child 47:683, 1972.

Gairdner D, Marks J, Roscoe JD, et al: The fluid shift from the vascular compartment immediately after birth. Arch Dis Child 33:489, 1958.

Jacobson LO, Marks EK, Gaston EO: Studies on erythropoiesis. XII. The effect of transfusion-induced polycythemia in the mother on the fetus. Blood 14:644, 1959.

Lanzkowsky P: The influence of maternal iron deficiency on the haemoglobin of the infant. Arch Dis Child 36:205, 1961.

Oski FA, Delivoria-Papadopoulos M: The red cell, 2,3-diphosphoglycerate, and tissue oxygen release. J Pediatr 77:941, 1970.

Usher R, Lind J: Blood volume of the newborn premature infant. Acta Paediatr Scand 54:419, 1965.

Usher R, Shepard M, Lind J: The blood volume of the newborn infant and placental transfusion. Acta Paediatr Scand 52:497, 1963.

Zon LI: Developmental biology of hematopoiesis. Blood 86:2876, 1995.

General Approach to Anemic Infants

Alter BE: Methods in Haematology, Perinatal Haematology, Vol 21. Edinburgh, Churchill Livingstone, 1989.

Brady MT, Milam JD, Anderson DC, et al: Use of deglycerolized red blood cells to prevent posttransfusion infection with cytomegalovirus in neonates. J Infect Dis 150:334, 1984.

Demmler GJ, Brady MT, Bijou H, et al: Posttransfusion cytomegalovirus infection in neonates; role of saline-washed red blood cells. J Pediatr 108:762, 1986.

Enoki M, Goto R, Goto A, et al: Graft-versus-host reaction in an extremely premature infant after repeated blood transfusions. Acta Neonatol Jpn 21:696, 1985.

Gilbert GL, Hayes K, Hudson IL, et al: Prevention of transfusion-acquired cytomegalovirus infection in infants by blood filtration to remove leucocytes. Lancet 1:1228, 1989.

Naiman JL, Punnett HH, Lischner HW, et al: Possible graft-versus-host reaction after intrauterine transfusion for Rh erythroblastosis fetalis. N Engl J Med 281:697, 1969.

Oh W, Lind J: Venous and capillary hematocrit in newborn infants and placental transfusion. Acta Paediatr Scand 55:38, 1966.

Parkman R, Mosier D, Umansky I, et al: Graft-versus-host disease after intrauterine and exchange transfusions for hemolytic disease of the newborn. N Engl J Med 209:359, 1974.

Sanders MR, Graeber JE, Vogelsang G, et al: Post-transfusion graft versus host disease in a premature infant without known risk factors. Pediatr Res 25:272A, 1989.

Schwartz AD: Differential diagnosis of neonatal anemia. Paediatrician 3:107, 1974.

Yeager AS, Grumet FC, Hafleigh EB, et al: Prevention of transfusion-acquired cytomegalovirus infections in newborn infants. J Pediatr 98:281, 1981.

Hemorrhagic Anemia

Cohen F, Zuelzer WW, Gustafson DC, Evans MM: Mechanisms of isoimmunization. I. The transplacental passage of fetal erythrocytes in homo-specific pregnancies. Blood 23:621, 1964.

Danskin FH, Neilson JP: Twin-to-twin transfusion syndrome: What are appropriate diagnostic criteria? Am J Obstet Gynecol 161:365, 1989.

Leonard S, Anthony B: Giant cephalohematoma of newborn. Am J Dis Child 101:170, 1961.

Montague ACW, Krevans JR: Transplacental hemorrhage in cesarean section. Am J Obstet Gynecol 95:1115, 1966.

Nieburg PI, Stockman JA: Rapid correction of anemia with partial exchange transfusion. Am J Dis Child 131:60, 1977.

Oski FA, Naiman JL: Hematologic Problems in the Newborn. 3rd ed. Philadelphia. WB Saunders, 1982.

Pachman DJ: Massive hemorrhage in the scalp of the newborn infant. Hemorrhagic caput succedaneum. Pediatrics 29:907, 1962.

Pearson HA, Diamond LK: Fetomaternal transfusion. Am J Dis Child 97:267, 1959.

Philipsborn HF, Traisman HS, Greer D: Rupture of the spleen: A complication of erythroblastosis fetalis. N Engl J Med 252:159, 1955.

Rausen AR, Seki M, Strauss L: Twin transfusion syndrome. A review of 19 cases studied at one institution. J Pediatr 66:613, 1965.

Raye JR, Gutberlet RL, Stahlman M: Symptomatic posthemorrhagic anemia in the newborn. Pediatr Clin North Am 17:401, 1970.

Shepherd AJ, Richard J, Brown JP: Nuchal cord as a cause of neonatal anemia. Am J Dis Child 139:71, 1985.

Woo Wang MYF, McCutcheon E, Desforges JF. Fetomaternal hemorrhage from diagnostic transabdominal amniocentesis. Am J Obstet Gynecol 97:1123, 1967.

Zipursky A, Pollock J, Chown B, Israels LG: Transplacental fetal maternal hemorrhage after placental injury during delivery or amniocentesis. Lancet 2:493, 1963.

Hemolytic Anemia

Abelson NM, Rawson AJ: Studies of blood group antibodies. V. Fractionation of examples of anti-B, anti-A,B, anti-M, anti-P, anti-JK^a, anti-Le^a, anti-D, anti-CD, anti-K, anti-Fy^a, anti-S, and anti-Good. Transfusion 1:116, 1961.

Austin RF, Desforges JF: Hereditary elliptocytosis: An unusual presentation of hemolysis in the newborn associated with transient morphologic abnormalities. Pediatrics 44:196, 1969.

Bard H: The postnatal decline of hemoglobin F synthesis in normal full-term infants. J Clin Invest 55:395, 1975.

Beaudry MA, Ferguson DJ, Pearse K, et al: Survival of a hydropic infant with homozygous alpha-thalassemia-1. J Pediatr 108:713, 1986.

Bennett PR, Le Van Kim C, Colin Y, et al: Prenatal determination of fetal RhD type by DNA amplification. N Engl J Med 329:607, 1993.

Beutler E, Yoshida A: Genetic variation of glucose-6-phosphate dehydrogenase: A catalog and future prospects. Medicine 67:311, 1988.

Bianchi DW, Beyer EC, Stark AR, et al: Normal long-term survival with alpha-thalassemia. J Pediatr 108:716, 1986.

Boehm CD, Antonarakis SE, Phillips JA, et al: Prenatal diagnosis using DNA polymorphisms. N Engl J Med 308:1054, 1983.

Bowman JM: Rh erythroblastosis fetalis. Semin Hematol 12:110, 1975.

Brouwers HAA, Overbeeke MAM, van Ertbrugeen I, et al: What is the best predictor of the severity of ABO-haemolytic disease of the newborn? Lancet 2:641, 1988.

Brown AK: Hyperbilirubinemia in black infants: Role of glucose-6-phosphate dehydrogenase deficiency. Clin Pediatr 31:712, 1992.

Cao A, Galanello R, Rosatelli MC, et al: Clinical experience of management of thalassemia: The Sardinian experience. Semin Hematol 33:66, 1996.

Diamond LK: Splenectomy in childhood and the hazard of overwhelming infection. Pediatrics 43:886, 1969.

Diaz-Barrios V: New York's experience. Pediatrics (Suppl) 83:2, 1989.

Doxiadis SA, Valaes T: The clinical picture of glucose-6-phosphate dehydrogenase deficiency in early infancy. Arch Dis Child 39:545, 1964.

Embury SH, Kropp GL, Stanton TS: Detection of the hemoglobin E mutation using the color complementation assay: Application to complex genotyping. Blood 78:619, 1990.

Eshaghpour E, Oski FA, Williams M: The relationship of erythrocyte glucose-6-phosphate dehydrogenase deficiency to hyperbilirubinemia in Negro premature infants. J Pediatr 70:595, 1967.

Fisk NM, Bennett P, Warwick RM, et al: Clinical utility of fetal RhD typing in alloimmunized pregnancies by means of polymerase chain reaction on amniocytes or chorionic villi. Am J Obstet Gynecol 171:50, 1994.

Freda VJ, Gorman JG, Pollack W, Bowe E: Prevention of Rh hemolytic disease—10 years' clinical experience with Rh immune globulin. N Engl J Med 292:1014, 1975.

Galanello R: Molecular basis of thalassemia major. Int J Pediatr Hematol/Oncol 2:383, 1995.

Gaston MH, Vertier JI, Wood G, et al: Prophylaxis with oral penicillin in children with sickle cell anemia. N Engl J Med 314:1593, 1986.

Glader BE, Nathan DG: Haemolysis due to pyruvate kinase deficiency and other glycolytic enzymopathies. Clin Haematol 4:123, 1975.

Glader BE, Look K: Hematologic disorders in children in Southeast Asia. Pediatr Clin North Am 43:665, 1996.

Grannum PA, Copel JA, Moya FR, et al: The reversal of hydrops fetalis by intravascular transfusion in severe isoimmune fetal anemia. Am J Obstet Gynecol 158:914, 1988.

Grannum PA, Copel JA, Plaxe SC, et al: In utero exchange transfusion by direct intravascular injection in severe erythroblastosis fetalis. N Engl J Med 314:1431, 1986.

Huang CS, Hung KL, Huang MJ, et al: Neonatal jaundice and molecular mutations in glucose-6-phosphate dehydrogenase deficient newborn infants. Am J Hematol 51:19, 1996.

Hurst D, Tittle B, Kleman KM, et al: Anemia and hemoglobinopathies in Southeast Asian refugee children. J Pediatr 102:692, 1983.

Kan YW, Forget BG, Nathan DG: Gamma-beta thalassemia: A cause of hemolytic disease of the newborn. N Engl J Med 286:129, 1972.

Kaplan E, Herz F, Scheye E: ABO hemolytic disease of the newborn, without hyperbilirubinemia. Am J Hematol 1:279, 1976.

Kappas A, Drummond GS, Manola T, et al: Sn-protoporphyrin use in the management of hyperbilirubinemia in term infants with direct Coombs-positive ABO incompatibility. Pediatrics 81:485, 1988.

Kazazian HH, Boehm CD: Molecular basis and prenatal diagnosis of β-thalassemia. Blood 72:1107, 1988.

Kohli-Kumar M, Zwerdling T, Rucknagel DL: Hemoglobin F-Cincinnati, $\alpha_2{}^G\gamma_241(C7)$ Phe→Ser in a newborn with cyanosis. Am J Hematol 49:43, 1995.

Koshy M, Burd L: Obstetric and gynecologic issues. *In* Embury SH, Hebbel RP, Mohandas N, Steinberg MH (Eds): Sickle Cell Disease: Basic Principles and Clinical Practice. New York, Raven Press, 1995, p 689.

LaCelle PL: Alteration of membrane deformability in hemolytic anemias. Semin Hematol 7:355, 1970.

Levine P, Katzin EM, et al: Isoimmunization in pregnancy, its possible bearing on the etiology of erythroblastosis fetalis. JAMA 116:825, 1941.

Liley AW: Liquor amnii analysis in the management of pregnancy complicated by rhesus sensitization. Am J Obstet Gynecol 82:1359, 1961.

Liley AW: Intrauterine transfusion of fetus in hemolytic disease. BMJ 2:1107, 1963.

Lorey F, Cunningham G, Shafer F: Universal screening for hemoglobinopathies using high-performance liquid chromatography: Clinical results of 2.2 million screens. Eur J Hum Genet 2:262, 1994.

Luzzatto L: Glucose-6-phosphate dehydrogenase deficiency and hemolytic anemia. *In* Nathan DG, Oski FA (Eds): Hematology of Infancy and Childhood, 5th ed. Philadelphia, WB Saunders, 1997.

Lyon MF: Gene action in the X-chromosome of the mouse. Nature 190:372, 1961.

Matthay KK, Mentzer WC: Erythrocyte enzymopathies in the newborn. Clin Haematol 10:31, 1981.

McDonagh KT, Nienhuis AW: The thalassemias. *In* Nathan DG, Oski FA (Eds): Hematology of Infancy and Childhood, 4th ed. Philadelphia, WB Saunders, 1993, pp 783–880.

Meloni T, Forteleoni G, Meloni GF: Marked decline of favism after neonatal glucose-6-phosphate dehydrogenase screening and health education: The northern Sardinian experience. Acta Haematol 87:29, 1992.

Mentzer WC: Pyruvate kinase deficiency and disorders of glycolysis. *In* Nathan DG, Oski FA (Eds): Hematology of Infancy and Childhood, 5th ed. Philadelphia, WB Saunders, 1997.

Mentzer W, Glader BE: Disorders of erythrocyte metabolism. *In* Mentzer WC, Wagner GM (Eds): The Hereditary Hemolytic Anemias. Edinburgh, Churchill Livingstone, 1989, pp 267–318.

Mentzer WC Jr, Collier E: Hydrops fetalis associated with erythrocyte G-6-PD deficiency and maternal ingestion of fava beans and ascorbic acid. J Pediatr 86:565, 1975.

Mentzer WC, Iarocci TA, Mohandas N, et al: Modulation of erythrocyte membrane mechanical stability by 2,3-diphosphoglycerate in the neonatal poikilocytosis/elliptocytosis syndrome. J Clin Invest 79:943, 1987.

Miwa S, Fujii H: Molecular basis of erythroenzymopathies associated with hereditary hemolytic anemia: Tabulation of mutant enzymes. Am J Hematol 51:122, 1996.

Mouro I, Colin Y, Cherif-Zahar B, et al: Molecular genetic basis of the human rhesus blood group system. Nature Genet 5:62, 1993.

Nicolaides JH, Soothill PW, Clewell WH, et al: Fetal hemoglobin measurement in the assessment of red cell isoimmunization. Lancet 1:1073, 1988.

O'Flynn MED, Hsia DY: Serum bilirubin levels and glucose-6-phosphate dehydrogenase deficiency in newborn American Negroes. J Pediatr 63:160, 1963.

Orkin SH, Goff SC: The duplicated human alpha-globin genes: Their relative expression as measured by RNA analysis. Cell 24:345, 1981.

Osborn LM, Lenarsky C, Oakes RC, et al: Phototherapy in full-term infants with hemolytic disease secondary to ABO incompatibility. Pediatrics 74:371, 1984.

Ovali F, Samanci N, Dagoglu T, et al: Management of late anemia in rhesus hemolytic disease: Use of recombinant human erythropoietin (a pilot study). Pediatr Res 39:831, 1996.

Palek J, Jarolim P: Clinical expression and laboratory detection of red blood cell membrane protein mutations. Semin Hematol 30:249, 1993.

Parer JT: Severe Rh isoimmunization—Current methods of in utero diagnosis and treatment. Obstet Gynecol 158:1323, 1988.

Pearson HA: Life-span of the fetal red blood cell. J Pediatr 70:166, 1967.

Rodeck CH, Nicolaides KH, Warsof SL, et al: The management of severe rhesus isoimmunization by fetoscopic intravascular transfusions. Am J Obstet Gynecol 150:769, 1984.

Scaradavou A, Inglis S, Peterson P, et al: Suppression of erythropoiesis by intrauterine transfusions in hemolytic disease of the newborn: Use of erythropoietin to treat the late anemia. J Pediatr 123:279, 1993.

Schmaier AH, Maurer HM, Johnston CL, et al: Alpha thalassemia screening in neonates by means corpuscular volume and mean corpuscular hemoglobin determination. J Pediatr 83:794, 1973.

Schröter W, Kahsnitz E: Diagnosis of hereditary spherocytosis in newborn infants. J Pediatr 103:460, 1983.

Spinnato JA: Hemolytic disease of the fetus: A plea for restraint. Obstet Gynecol 80:873, 1992.

Stamatoyannopoulos G: Gamma-thalassemia. Lancet 2:192, 1971.

Stamey CC, Diamond LK: Congenital hemolytic anemia in the newborn. Am J Dis Child 94:616, 1957.

Tanaka KR, Paglia DE: Pyruvate kinase deficiency. Semin Hematol 8:367, 1971.

Tchernia G, Gauthier F, Mielot F, et al: Initial assessment of the beneficial effect of partial splenectomy in hereditary spherocytosis. Blood 81:2014, 1993.

Valaes T: Severe neonatal jaundice associated with glucose-6-phosphate dehydrogenase deficiency: Pathogenesis and global epidemiology. Acta Paediatr Suppl 394:58, 1994.

Valaes T, Karaklis A, Stravrakakis D, et al: Incidence and mechanism of neonatal jaundice related to glucose-6-phosphate dehydrogenase deficiency. Pediatr Res 3:448, 1969.

Valaes T, Petmezaki S, Henschke C, et al: Control of jaundice in preterm newborns by an inhibitor of bilirubin production: Studies with tin-mesoporphyrin. Pediatrics 93:1, 1994.

Veiga S, Vaithianathan T: Massive intravascular sickling after exchange transfusion with sickle cell trait blood. Transfusion 3:387, 1963.

Voak D, Williams MA: An explanation of the failure of the direct antiglobulin test to detect erythrocyte sensitization in ABO hemolytic disease of the newborn and observations on pinocytosis of IgG anti-A antibodies by infant (cord) red cells. Br J Haematol 20:9, 1971.

Weiner CP, Williamson RA, Wenstrom KD, et al: Management of fetal hemolytic disease by cordocentesis. Am J Obstet Gynecol 165:1302, 1991.

Wethers D, Pearson H, Gaston M: Newborn screening for sickle cell disease and other hemoglobinopathies. Pediatric (Suppl) 83:2, 1989.

Zipursky A, Pollock J, Chown B, et al: Transplacental fetal hemorrhage after placental injury during delivery or amniocentesis. Lancet 2:493, 1963.

Hypoplastic Anemia

Alter BP, Young NS: The bone marrow failure syndromes. *In* Nathan DG, Oski FA (Eds): Hematology of infancy and childhood. Philadelphia, WB Saunders, 1993.

Diamond LK, Blackfan KD: Hypoplastic anemia. Am J Dis Child 56:464, 1938.

Glader BE: Diagnosis and management of red cell aplasia in children. Hematol Oncol Clin North Am 1:431, 1987.

Miller R, Berman B: Transient erythroblastopenia of childhood in infants < 6 months of age. Am J Pediatr Hematol Oncol 16:246, 1994.

Rogers ZR, Bergstrom SK, Amylon MD, et al: Reduced neutrophil counts in children with transient erythroblastopenia of childhood. J Pediatr 15:746, 1989.

Wranne L: Transient erythroblastopenia in infancy and childhood. Scand J Haemotol 7:76, 1970.

Ware RE, Kinney TR: Transient erythroblastopenia in the first year of life. Am J Hematol 37:156, 1991.

Physiologic Anemia of Infancy and Prematurity

Batton DG, Goodrow D, Walker RH: Reducing neonatal transfusions. J Perinatol 12:152, 1992.

Bifano EM, Smith F, Borer J: Relationship between determinants of oxygen delivery and respiratory abnormalities in preterm infants with anemia. J Pediatr 120:292, 1992.

Blank JP, Sheagren TG, Vajara J, et al: The role of RBC transfusion in the premature infant. Am J Dis Child 138:831, 1984.

Brown MS, Berman ER, Luckey D: Prediction of the need for transfusion during anemia of prematurity. J Pediatr 116:773, 1990.

Christensen RD, Liechty KW, Koenig JM, et al: Administration of erythropoietin to newborn rats results in diminished neutrophil production. Blood 78:1241, 1991.

Cook S, Gunter J, Wissel M: Effective use of a strategy using assigned red cell units to limit donor exposure for neonatal patients. Transfusion 33:379, 1993.

Dallman PR: Anemia of prematurity: The prospects for avoiding blood transfusions with recombinant erythropoietin. Adv Pediatr 40:385, 1993.

Davis P, Herbert M, Davies DP, et al: Erythropoietin for anaemia in a preterm Jehovah's Witness baby. Early Hum Dev 1:279, 1991.

Emmerson AJB, Coles HJ, Stern CMM, et al: Double blind trial of recombinant human erythropoietin in preterm infants. Arch Dis Child 63:291, 1993.

Gallagher PG, Ehrenkranz RA: Erythropoietin therapy for anemia of prematurity. Clin Perinatol 20:169, 1993.

Graeber JE, Williams ML, Oski FA: The use of intramuscular vitamin E in the premature infant. J Pediatr 90:282, 1977.

Heese H De V, Smith S, Watermeyer S, et al: Prevention of iron deficiency in preterm neonates during infancy. S Afr Med J 77:339, 1990.

Izraeli S, Ben-Sira L, Harell D, et al: Lactic acid as a predictor for erythrocyte transfusion in healthy preterm infants with anemia of prematurity. J Pediatr 122:629, 1993.

Joshi A, Gerhardt T, Schandloff P, et al: Blood transfusion effect on the respiratory pattern of premature infants. Pediatrics 80:79, 1987.

Keyes WG, Donohue PK, Spivak JL, et al: Assessing the need for transfusion of premature infants and role of hematocrit, clinical signs and erythropoietin level. Pediatrics 84:412, 1989.

Lachance C, Chessex P, Fouron JC, et al: Myocardial, erythropoietic, and metabolic adaptations to anemia of prematurity. J Pediatr 125:278, 1994.

Liu EA, Mannino FL, Lane TA: Prospective, randomized trial of the safety and efficacy of a limited donor exposure transfusion program for premature neonates. J Pediatr 125:92, 1994.

Maier RF, Obladen M, Scigalla P, et al: The effect of epoetin beta (recombinant human erythropoietin) on the need for transfusion in very-low-birth-weight infants. N Engl J Med 330:1173, 1994.

Mentzer WC, Shannon KM: The use of recombinant human erythropoietin in preterm infants. Int J Pediatr Hematol Oncol 2:97, 1995.

Mestyan J, Fekete M, Bata G, et al: The basal metabolic rate of premature infants. Biol Neonatol 7:11, 1964.

Meyer MP, Meyer JH, Commerford A, et al: Recombinant human erythropoietin in the treatment of the anemia of prematurity: Results of a double-blind, placebo-controlled study. Pediatrics 93:918, 1994.

Nelle M, Höcker C, Zilow EP, et al: Effects of red cell transfusion on cardiac output and blood flow velocities in cerebral and gastrointestinal arteries in premature infants. Arch Dis Child 71:F45, 1994.

Oski FA, Barness LA: Vitamin E deficiency: A previously unrecognized

cause of hemolytic anemia in the premature infant. J Pediatr 70:211, 1967.

Ritchie JH, Fish MB, McMasters V, et al: Edema and hemolytic anemia in premature infants. N Engl J Med 279:1185, 1968.

Ross MP, Christensen RD, Rothstein G, et al: A randomized trial to develop criteria for administering erythrocyte transfusions to anemic preterm infants 1 to 3 months of age. J Perinatol 9:246, 1989.

Shannon KM: Anemia of prematurity: Progress and prospects. Am J Pediatr Hematol Oncol 12:14, 1990.

Shannon KM, Keith JF III, Mentzer WC, et al: Recombinant human erythropoietin stimulates erythropoiesis and reduces erythrocyte transfusions in very low birth weight preterm infants. Pediatrics 95:1, 1995.

Shannon KM, Naylor GS, Torkildson JC, et al: Circulating erythroid progenitors in the anemia of prematurity. N Engl J Med 317:728, 1987.

Shireman TI, Hilsenrath PE, Strauss RG, et al: Recombinant human erythropoietin vs transfusions in the treatment of anemia of prematurity. Arch Pediatr Adolesc Med 148:582, 1994.

Stockman JA, Clark DA: Weight gain: A response to transfusion in selected preterm infants. Am J Dis Child 138:828, 1984.

Stockman JA III, Graeber JE, Clark DA, et al: Anemia of prematurity: Determinants of the erythropoietin response. J Pediatr 105:786, 1984.

Strauss RG: Transfusion therapy in neonates. Am J Dis Child 145:904, 1991.

Strauss RG: Erythropoietin and neonatal anemia. N Engl J Med 330:1227, 1994.

Wandstrat TL, Kaplan B: Use of erythropoietin in premature neonates: Controversies and the future. Pediatrics 29:166, 1995.

Worthington-White DA, Behnke M, Gross S: Premature infants require additional folate and vitamin B_{12} to reduce the severity of the anemia of prematurity. Am J Clin Nutr 60:930, 1994.

Zipursky A, Brown EJ, Watts S, et al: Oral vitamin E supplementation for the prevention of anemia in premature infants: A controlled trial. Pediatrics 79:61, 1987.

Polycythemia

Black VD, Rumack CM, Lubchenko LO, et al: Gastrointestinal injury in polychemic term infants. Pediatrics 76:225, 1985.

Carmi D, Wolach B, Dolfin T, et al: Polycythemia of the preterm and full-term newborn infant: Relationship between hematocrit and gestational age, total blood solutes, reticulocyte count, and blood pH. Biol Neonate 61:173, 1992.

Delaney-Black V, Camp BW, Lubchenko LO, et al: Neonatal hyperviscosity association with lower achievement and IQ scores at school age. Pediatrics 83:662, 1989.

Gatti RA, Muster AJ, Cole RB, et al: Neonatal polycythemia with transient cyanosis and cardiorespiratory abnormalities. J Pediatr 69:1063, 1966.

Hein HA, Lathrop SS: Partial exchange transfusion in term, polycythemic neonates: Absence of association with severe gastrointestinal injury. Pediatrics 80:75, 1987.

Kurlat I, Sola A: Neonatal polycythemia in appropriately grown infants of hypertensive mothers. Acta Paediatr 81:662, 1992.

Levy I, Pmerlob P, Ashkenazi S, et al: Neonatal polycythaemia: Effort of partial dilutional exchange transfusion with human albumin on whole blood viscosity. Eur J Pediatr 149:354, 1990.

Mentzer WC: Polycythaemia and the hyperviscosity syndrome in newborn infants. Clin Haematol 7:63, 1978.

Norman M, Fagrell B, Herin P: Effects of neonatal polycythemia and hemodilution on capillary perfusion. J Pediatr 121:103, 1992.

Norman M, Fagrell B, Herin P: Skin microcirculation in neonatal polycythaemia and effects of haemodilution. Interaction between haematocrit, vasomotor activity and perfusion. Acta Paediatr 82:672, 1993.

Oh W, Omori K, Emmanouilides GC, Phelps DL: Placenta to lamb fetus transfusion in utero during acute hypoxia. Am J Obstet Gynecol 122:316, 1975.

Ramamurthy RS, Berlanga M: Postnatal alteration in hematocrit and viscosity in normal and polycythemic infants. J Pediatr 110:929, 1987.

Shohat M, Merlob P, Reisner SH: Neonatal polycythemia: Early diagnosis and incidence relating to time of sampling. Pediatrics 73:7, 1984.

Villalta IA, Pramanik AK, Diaz-Blanco J, et al: Diagnostic errors in neonatal polycythemia based on method of hematocrit determination. J Pediatr 115:460, 1989.

Methemoglobinemia

Bartos HR, Desforges JF: Erythrocyte DPNH dependent diaphorase levels in infants. Pediatrics 37:991, 1966.

Climie CR, McLean S, Starmer GA, Thomas J: Methaemoglobinaemia in mother and foetus following continuous epidermal analgesia with prilocaine. Br J Anaesthesiol 39:155, 1967.

Comly HR: Cyanosis in infants caused by nitrates in well water. JAMA 129:112, 1945.

Harley JD, Celermajer JM: Neonatal methaemoglobinaemia and the "red-brown" screening test. Lancet 2:1223, 1970.

Hayashi A, Fujita T, Fujimura M, et al: A new abnormal fetal hemoglobin, Hb FM-Osaka. Hemoglobin 4:447, 1980.

Kay MA, O'Brien W, Kessler B, et al: Transient organic-aciduria and methemoglobinemia with acute gastroenteritis. Pediatrics 85:589, 1990.

Keating JP, Lell ME, Strauss AW, et al: Infantile methemoglobinemia caused by carrot juice. N Engl J Med 288:824, 1973.

Martin H, Huisman THJ: Formation of ferrihaemoglobin of isolated human haemoglobin types by sodium nitrate. Nature 200:898, 1963.

Murray KF, Christie DL: Dietary protein intolerance in infants with transient methemoglobinemia and diarrhea. J Pediatr 122:90, 1993.

Priest JR, Watterson J, Jones RT, et al: Mutant fetal hemoglobin causing cyanosis in a newborn. Pediatrics 83:734, 1989.

Yano SS, Danish EH, Hsia YE: Transient methemoglobinemia with acidosis in infants. J Pediatr 100:415, 1982.

CHAPTER 90

Leukocyte Disorders in the Newborn*

Robert W. Sweetman, Joseph Rosenthal and Mitchell S. Cairo

A relatively small number of pluripotent hematopoietic stem cells, residing during early fetal life in the liver and spleen and later in the bone marrow, undergo proliferation and differentiation to give rise to large numbers of functionally diverse mature cells. The development of stem cells and progenitor cells into peripheral blood effector cells involves complex interactions between hematopoietic cells, cytokines, and the microenvironment at the site of hematopoiesis. An intact phagocyte system is critical to successful antimicrobial defense. Neutrophils and macrophages are responsible for the ingestion and killing of invading organisms. To function effectively, phagocytes must be present in an adequate number in the peripheral blood, respond to signals from invading pathogens, migrate to the site of infection, ingest the invading organism, and kill it by either oxygen-dependent or oxygen-independent mechanisms. Peripheral neutropenia and defective neutrophil functions are common findings during neonatal sepsis and are associated with poor prognosis (Siegel et al, 1981). Neonatal neutropenia may be caused by any one of a combination of defects in myelopoiesis involving production, maturation, or release. The pathophysiologic mechanisms responsible for neonatal neutropenia and defective neutrophil functions and the treatment of these conditions are discussed in this chapter.

FETAL AND NEONATAL HEMATOPOIESIS

The differentiation and maturation of progenitor cells into peripheral blood effector cells involves complex interactions between progenitor cells, the microenvironment at the site of hematopoiesis, and hematopoietic cytokines.

Stem Cells and Progenitor Cells

Till and McCulloch (1961) were the first to demonstrate that when bone marrow cells were transfused into lethally irradiated mice, separate colonies of hematopoietic cells could be identified in the spleen of the recipient. Each colony, containing neutrophils, monocytes, erythrocytes, megakaryocytes, eosinophils, and basophils, was derived from an individual cell, and many of the colonies contained cells that were capable of such colony formation when transplanted into a second irradiated animal. Such cells, which are capable of unlimited self-renewal, have been referred to as pluripotent stem cells. The hematopoietic stem cell is, therefore, a cell that is not committed to any particular hematopoietic lineage and has the capacity for proliferation as well as for differentiation into mature blood cells. The murine stem cell has been identified as Thy

$1.1^{lo}Lin-^{/lo}Sca-1^+$ (Uchida et al, 1992). The exact identity of the human hematopoietic stem cell is still under investigation. The earliest form of the committed myeloid progenitor cell is termed a colony-forming unit–granulocyte, erythrocyte, macrophage, and megakaryocyte (CFU-GEMM). CFU-GEMM are not true pluripotent cells because they have a limited self-renewal capacity. CFU-GEMM differentiate into more committed progenitor cells such as the granulocyte-macrophage colony-forming unit (CFU-GM) and the erythroid burst-forming unit (BFU-E). These are further differentiated to form committed and unilineage colony-forming units such as the granulocyte colony-forming unit (CFU-G), macrophage colony-forming unit (CFU-M), eosinophil colony-forming unit (CFU-E), and basophil colony-forming unit (CFU-B).

In human ontogeny, the process of maturation involves the orderly shift of hematopoiesis from extramedullary organs to the bone marrow (Nathan, 1989). Hematopoiesis is first observed by day 15 in blood islands formed by the yolk sac (Zon, 1995). Migliaccio and colleagues (1986) have identified pluripotent, erythroid, and granulocyte-macrophage progenitor cells in the yolk sac, liver, and blood from human embryos. The erythroid lineage is predominant during the yolk sac hematopoiesis. Yolk sac erythrocytes have distinctive morphologic and functional features. They are large nucleated cells, expressing the products of certain genes that are unique to this phase of development. Definitive cells that migrate to the fetal liver and subsequently to the fetal bone marrow are thought to originate either from the yolk sac or dorsal mesenteric hematopoietic cells (Zon, 1995). The transition of embryonal hematopoiesis from the yolk sac to the liver is associated with development of a differentiating program in proliferating stem cells as shown by their erythroid progeny, and therefore parallels changes of multiple parameters (e.g., morphology and globin expression) (Migliaccio et al, 1986). The combinations of gene expression that characterize fetal erythrocytes persist as hematopoiesis shifts from the liver to the bone marrow at the end of the second trimester of pregnancy. CFU-GM have been identified in fetal liver as early as 5 weeks' gestation. However, their number is low compared to the erythroid lineage. Ohls and coworkers (1995) examined the liver and bone marrow in midtrimester fetuses and compared them with bone marrows of adults and historic data of bone marrows from term neonates. They concluded that neutrophils were seen in the bone marrow of fetuses as early as 14 weeks' gestation but that they were limited in number. Myeloid cells (neutrophil progenitor cells) comprised less than 5% of nucleated marrow cells compared to 31% to 69% in term neonates and 25% to 52% in adults (Ohls et al, 1995).

Microenvironment

A group of supporting cells making up the microenvironment surrounding the hematopoietic cells are important for

*Supported in part by grants from the Pediatric Cancer Research Foundation, the CHOC Research and Education Foundation, and the Walden W. and Jean Young Shaw Foundation.

sustained hematopoiesis both *in vivo* and *ex vivo* (Gordon, 1993). The processes of intramedullar migration, adhesion, proliferation, and differentiation of hematopoietic cells are normally regulated by multiple cell types of several lineages, many derived from nonhematopoietic cells, arranged in a complex interactive nature in the medullary cavity (Torok-Storb, 1988). Stromal cells, fibroblasts, endothelial cells, macrophages, and adventitial reticulum cells interact with hematopoietic cells. The information required for these functions is transmitted by diffusable growth factors via cell junctions of the hematopoietic progenitor cells and the stromal cells.

Cytokines

The regulation of hematopoiesis is a complex biologic process involving multifactorial mechanisms. A relatively small and common set of pluripotent stem cells gives rise to large numbers of functionally diverse mature cells. Cell proliferation and differentiation is regulated and controlled by highly specific protein factors, affecting single- and multiple-lineage hematopoiesis. These growth promoting factors are named colony-stimulating factors (CSFs). CSFs are a group of glycoproteins with a molecular weight of 18 to 90 kD, defined by their abilities to support proliferation and differentiation of hematopoietic cells of various lineages (Fig. 90–1).

Although most CSFs possess similar and sometimes overlapping activities, no sequence homology or common secondary structure exists between any of the CSFs except for interleukin-6 (IL-6) and granulocyte colony-stimulating factor (G-CSF). Most factors are synthesized with a hydrophobic leader peptide that is proteolytically cleaved from the active molecule. The carbohydrate component is variable according to the tissue source, is not required for receptor binding or activation, and may play a role in protecting these proteins from degradation. Attempts to derive or synthesize small segments of the CSFs have failed to generate the biologic effects of the whole molecule, suggesting that a complex three-dimensional configuration of the molecule is essential for biologic activity.

Each growth factor is coded for by a single unique gene. A cluster of genes that encodes for granulocyte-macrophage CSF (GM-CSF), IL-3, IL-4, IL-5, and the receptor for macrophage CSF (M-CSF) are located on the long arm of chromosome 5 in humans. The full implication of this clustering remains to be determined.

The rate of hematopoiesis and specific lineage proliferation and differentiation is regulated by up-regulation of receptors induced by growth factors, and down-regulation by inhibitors such as interferons, macrophage-inhibiting protein 1-alpha, transforming growth factor-beta (TGF-β), and tumor necrosis factor (TNF) (Robinson et al, 1990). There are at least two classes of colony-stimulating growth factors that influence hematopoiesis and effector cell differentiation. Class I includes IL-1, IL-3, IL-6, IL-11, stem cell factor (Steel factor, SLF), and the recently identified ligand for FLT3/FLK2 receptor (Hannum et al, 1994). These factors affect the production of multilineage blood cell formation and regulate the proliferation of early committed progenitor cells. The Class II factors act on committed progenitor cells and have effects on the activation and function of mature effector cells. These are the GM-CSF, G-CSF, M-CSF, erythropoietin, and thrombopoietin. Two hematopoietic growth factors, G-CSF and GM-CSF, have been used in various clinical situations over the past decade.

Granulocyte Colony-Stimulating Factor

Human G-CSF was first purified to homogeneity from a medium conditioned by the bladder carcinoma cell line 5637 (Welte et al, 1987). The molecular weight of this glycoprotein is between 18 and 20 kD and the gene has been localized to chromosome 17 q11-21. It has been identified in the 15 to 17 chromosomal translocation commonly found in acute promyelocytic leukemia (Welte et al, 1987). G-CSF stimulates the proliferation of committed myeloid progenitor cells and has specific activity toward granulocyte colony formation with pure neutrophil colony proliferation. G-CSF has the capacity to induce differentiation of myelomonocytic leukemia cells (Souza et al, 1986). Additionally, G-CSF affects mature neutrophil effector function and primes neutrophils to increase expression of chemotactic receptors and to enhance bactericidal and phagocytic activity, superoxide generation, and antibody-dependent cellular cytotoxicity (Platzer et al, 1985; Souza et al, 1986). When used in addition to other cytokines or accessory cells, G-CSF appears to indirectly promote the formation of colonies derived from BFU-E and CFU (mix) (Simmers et al, 1987).

Clinical studies have shown that G-CSF therapy results in a dose-dependent increase in the circulating neutrophil count in children and adults with congenital and acquired neutropenia syndromes as well as chemotherapy-induced neutropenia (Bonilla et al, 1989; Hammond et al, 1989; Miller, 1994).

Granulocyte-Macrophage Colony-Stimulating Factor

GM-CSF was purified from a medium conditioned by the HTLV-II-infected T-lymphoblast cell line MO (Gasson et al, 1984). Characterization of the purified material showed that GM-CSF is a glycoprotein of 22 kD, and the gene is located on chromosome 5 q21-32 (Huebner et al, 1985). Potential physiologic sources for GM-CSF are T and B lymphocytes, macrophages, fibroblasts, endothelial cells, mesothelial cells, and osteoblasts (Gasson et al, 1984).

GM-CSF acts as a potent growth factor both *ex vivo* and *in vivo* by stimulating proliferation and maturation of myeloid progenitor cells, subsequently giving rise to neutrophilic and eosinophilic granulocytes and monocytes (Gasson et al, 1984). GM-CSF has direct and indirect effects on human neutrophils. Direct effects include inhibition of neutrophil migration, degranulation, changes in receptor expression, and changes in cytoskeleton and cell shape. Indirect actions enhance the ability of the neutrophil to respond to triggering stimuli. Among these effects are increased superoxide generation, Ca^{2+} fluxes, and production of inflammatory mediators such as leukotriene B_4.

Administration of GM-CSF in clinical trials results in an immediate and transient decrease in circulating neutrophils, eosinophils, and monocytes, followed by a recovery to baseline within 2 hours. A second phase follows, in

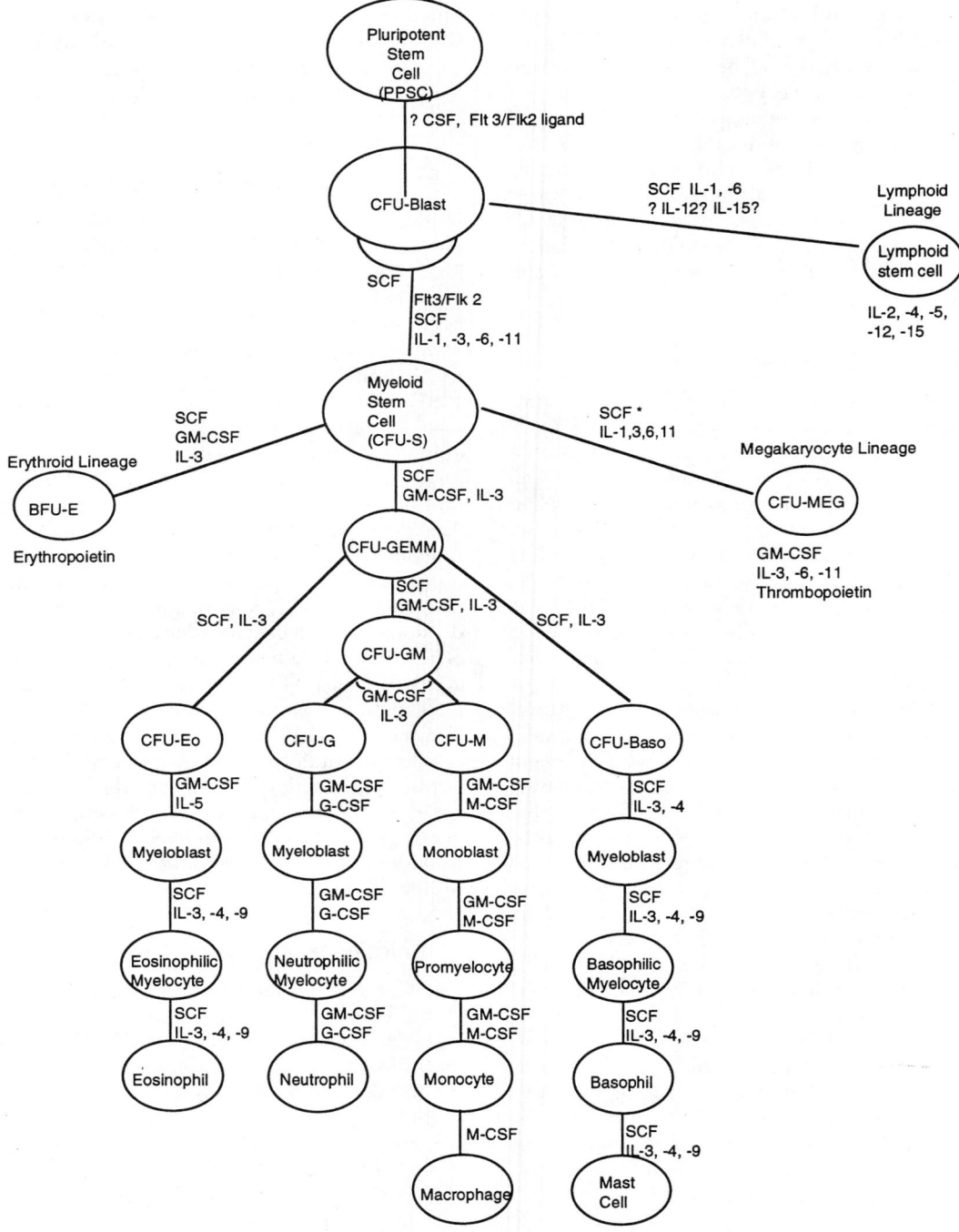

FIGURE 90–1. Colony-stimulating factors in hematopoiesis. SCF, stem cell factor; IL, interleukin; CFU-Blast, blast colony-forming unit; GM-CSF, granulocyte-macrophage colony-stimulating factor; CFU-GEMM, granulocyte, erythrocyte, macrophage and megakaryocyte colony-forming unit; CFU-GM, granulocyte-macrophage colony-forming unit; CFU-Eo, eosinophil colony-forming unit; CFU-G, granulocyte colony-forming unit; CFU-M, macrophage colony-forming unit; CFU-Baso, basophil colony-forming unit; CFU-MEG, megakaryocyte colony-forming unit; BFU-E, erythroid blast-forming unit; G-CSF, granulocyte colony-stimulating factor; M-CSF, macrophage colony-stimulating factor.

which the number of leukocytes increases with a marked shift to the left as a result of demargination from the bone marrow neutrophil storage pool (NSP) and increased myeloid production in the marrow.

GM-CSF has been investigated in numerous clinical situations. GM-CSF has been shown to induce a temporary increase in neutrophils and a decrease in infectious complications in adults and children with refractory aplastic anemia (Champlin et al, 1988; Guinan et al, 1990; Vadhan-Raj et al, 1989). Accelerated myeloid recovery after autologous bone marrow transplantation in patients with lymphoid malignancies was demonstrated by Nemunaitis and coworkers (1991). Gerhartz and colleagues (1993) established the efficacy of GM-CSF in patients with non-Hodgkin lymphoma receiving conventional-dose chemotherapy in terms of accelerated myeloid recovery, decreased infection rate, and length of hospitalization. GM-CSF has also been used in mobilizing hematopoietic cells in normal donors for allogeneic stem cell transplantation (Lane et al, 1995). Riikonen and associates (1994) reported an accelerated myeloid recovery and a reduction in hospitalization in oncology patients with febrile neutropenia when given GM-CSF.

The biologic activity of GM-CSF following myeloablative chemotherapy has been demonstrated in several nonrandomized studies and subsequently confirmed in randomized placebo-controlled studies. The results of these studies have been recently reviewed (Barge, 1993). Most studies have shown that GM-CSF was associated with an accelerated neutrophil recovery. In randomized, placebo-controlled studies, GM-CSF was associated with a significantly faster recovery of neutrophil counts by 3 to 13 days. A substantial increase in neutrophil and other myeloid cells, but without decrease in the number of opportunistic infections, has been demonstrated in patients with acquired immunodeficiency syndrome (AIDS) receiving zidovudine and GM-CSF (Groopman et al, 1987).

QUANTITATIVE AND QUALITATIVE DEFECTS IN THE NEONATAL PHAGOCYTE

The host response to infection involves a complex series of neutrophil responses including recognition, chemotaxis, adhesion, extravasation, activation, and phagocytosis. The average granulocyte has a half-life in the peripheral blood of approximately 7 hours. The body is therefore dependent on a continuing replenishment from the bone marrow. However, newborns and especially preterm infants have minimal granulocyte reserves compared with adults, predisposing them to neutropenia, especially in critically ill neonates. Additionally, neonates have other immunologic abnormalities that predispose them to an increased incidence of sepsis.

Quantitative Defects of Neonatal Neutrophils

Neonatal Neutropenia

Manroe and coworkers (1979) established reference values for absolute neutrophil counts in term and preterm infants during the first 28 days of life for both healthy infants and those with perinatal complications (Fig. 90–2). Mouzinho and associates (1994) studied serial white blood cells counts in healthy preterm very-low-birth-weight (VLBW) infants to investigate whether this subgroup of patients had different neutrophil counts compared to previous studies consisting mostly of term infants. They found that there was a wider range of the absolute total neutrophil count (ATN), mostly resulting from a downward shift of the lower boundary, especially during the first 60 hours of life. However,

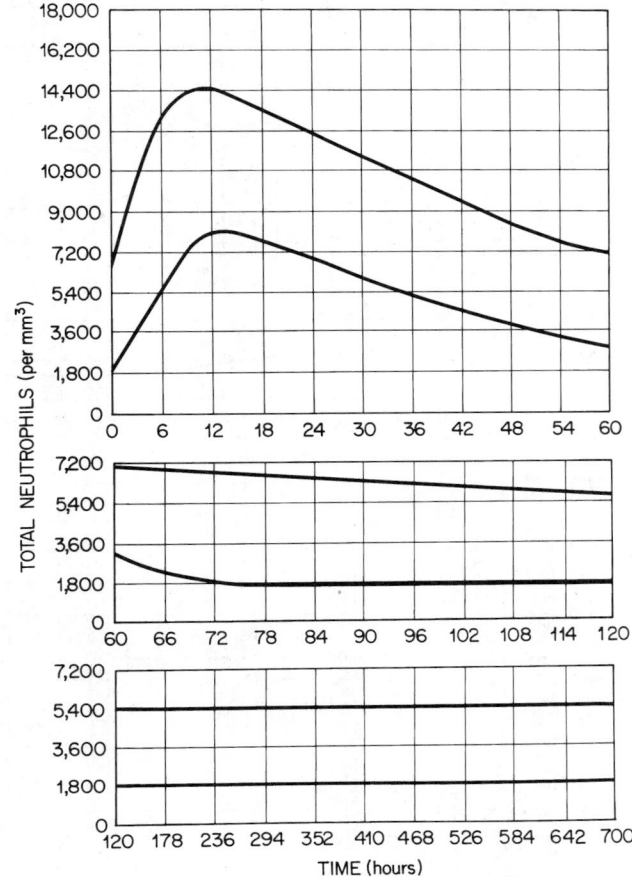

FIGURE 90–2. Reference values for neutrophilic cells in the newborn infant. (Adapted from Manroe BL, Weinberg AG, Rosenfeld CR, et al: The neonatal blood count in health and disease: I. Reference values for neutrophilic cells. J Pediatr 95(1):89–98, 1979.)

there was no difference in absolute total immature neutrophil counts or its ratio to total neutrophils (I:T) (Fig. 90–3). Similar findings were noted by Gessler and colleagues (1995) who studied, retrospectively, neutropenia in low-birth-weight infants and its relationship to maternal disease, sepsis, and antibiotic therapy. They noted that neutropenia during the 2nd week of life was most commonly related to antibiotic use.

Neutropenia may be caused by any one or a combination of defects in production, maturation, or release of neutrophils from the bone marrow to the peripheral blood. The pathophysiologic mechanisms responsible for neonatal neutropenia may be either exhaustion of myeloid committed progenitor cells or inadequate response of progenitor cells to proliferative or maturational signals. In a series of studies, Christensen and Rothstein (1984) documented significant differences in myeloid progenitor pools and cell kinetics in fetal and neonatal rats compared to adult rats (Table 90–1). In the newborn rat, the myeloid progenitor pool, consisting of CFU-GMs in the bone marrow, is only 25% of that of adult animals and requires 4 weeks of maturation to reach adult levels. Additionally, despite a lower number, the CFU-GM of the newborn rat is in a state of near-

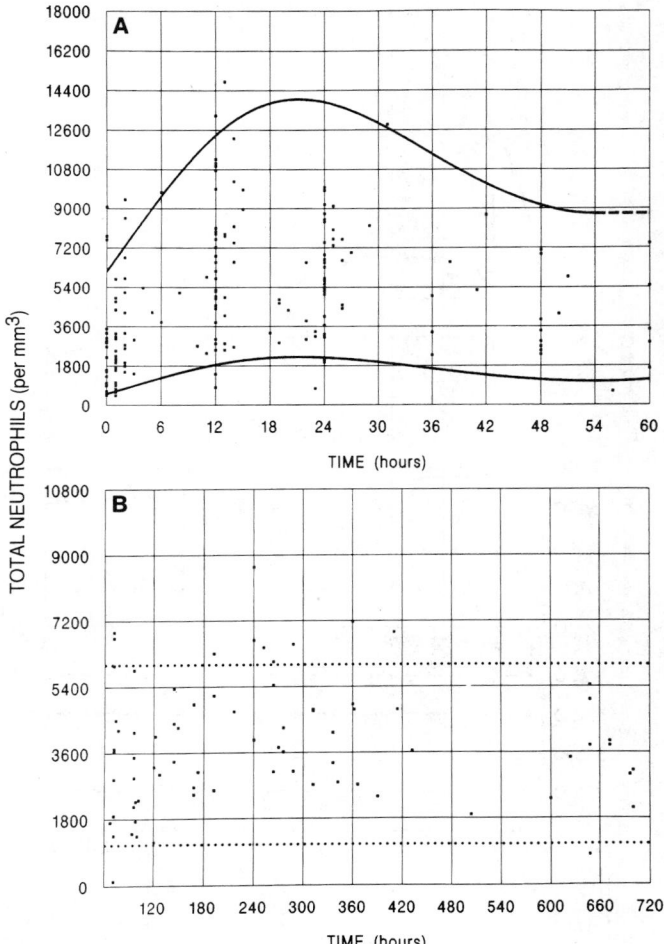

FIGURE 90–3. *A* and *B*, Total absolute neutrophil reference ranges for very-low-birth-weight neonates from birth to 60 hours *(A)* and 60 hours to 28 days *(B)*. (From Mouziaho A, et al: Pediatrics 1994(1):76–82, 1994. Reproduced by permission of Pediatrics, Copyright 1994.)

and mature neutrophils in the bone marrow. The NSP cells reach adult levels in the neonate rat at 4 weeks of age (Erdman et al, 1982). Following experimental sepsis with group B streptococcus (GBS), adult rats respond with a transient decrease in circulating neutrophil counts followed by significant neutrophilia associated with a twofold to threefold increase in the progenitor pool (CFU-Meg) and an increase in the proliferative rate to 75% of the maximal capacity (Christensen et al, 1982, 1983). In contrast, neonatal rats under the same conditions had a decrease by 50% of their progenitor pool and failed to increase their myeloid proliferative rate, which, as discussed previously, was already at near-maximal levels. Most importantly, during experimental sepsis, neonatal rats had further depletion of their already reduced NSP reserves by almost 80% compared to a decline of 33% in adult rats (Christensen et al, 1982, 1983; Christensen and Rothstein, 1984).

An additional immaturity in neonatal neutrophil kinetics that may further contribute to neonatal neutropenia is a defect in the regulation of release and migration of neutrophils from the bone marrow to the peripheral blood. A release of 10% of NSP has been documented in adult rats given subcutaneous inflammatory stimuli compared to 80% release in neonatal rats under the same conditions (Christensen and Rothstein, 1980). Similar incidences of neutropenia during neonatal sepsis have been documented in human neonates (Christensen et al, 1986; Christensen and Rothstein, 1980).

In summary, neutropenia in the neonate is thus likely to be a result of several factors:

■ Both the myeloid progenitor pool and the NSP in the newborn rat are only approximately 25% the size of those in adult animals and require 4 weeks of developmental maturation to reach adult values.

■ Despite a lower number of CFU-GM, the myeloid proliferative rate is near maximal capacity (75%) and cannot meet the increasing demands of sepsis.

■ There is a defect in regulation of release and mobilization of the neutrophil from the bone marrow reserves into the peripheral blood.

Severe Congenital Neutropenia (Kostmann Syndrome)

Kostmann syndrome is an autosomal recessive disorder that manifests within the first few months of life by severe, persistent neutropenia, with absolute neutrophil counts (ANCs) of less than 500 cells/μL and often less than 200 cells/μL. Bone marrow examination typically demonstrates a maturational arrest at the promyelocyte stage (Kostmann,

maximal proliferative capacity, the maximal rate of proliferation being 75% to 80%, whereas that of adult CFU-GM is only 25% (Christensen and Rothstein, 1984). Concomitantly with reduced numbers of myeloid progenitor cells (lower numbers of CFU-GM), and lower expansion capacity (already near maximal proliferative rate), the neonatal rat also possesses reduced numbers (25% of adult) of NSP cells, defined as the percentage of metamyelocytes, bands,

TABLE 90–1

Neutrophil Kinetics: Differences Between Adult and Neonatal Rats

	Adult Rat		Neonatal Rat	
	At Rest	**Stimulated**	**At Rest**	**Stimulated**
Proliferative pool (% CFU-GM)	100	×2–3 increase	10	Decrease
Proliferative rate (%)	25	75	80	80
Neutrophil storage pool (%)	100	Mild decrease	25	Significant decrease

1956). These children have recurrent infections especially of the skin and oral mucosa. G-CSF has been used with success in increasing the ANC and decreasing the number of infections (Bonilla et al, 1989; Daghistani et al, 1990; Welte et al, 1990). Bone marrow transplantation has also been used for those patients with a human leukocyte antigen (HLA)-identical unaffected sibling (Rappeport et al, 1980).

Alloimmune Neonatal Neutropenia

Alloimmune neonatal neutropenia occurs as a result of maternal sensitization and production of IgG to neutrophil antigens that are present on the infants' neutrophils, paternally acquired, which are not present on the maternal neutrophils. It is estimated to occur at a frequency of 3% of live births (Curnette, 1993). The most common antigens involved are NA1 and NA2. Peripheral blood counts show profound neutropenia and often demonstrate a monocytosis and eosinophilia (Cartron et al, 1991). The condition is self-limiting and typically lasts for 6 to 7 weeks during which time the neonate is susceptible to infections mostly cutaneous in nature but can be life-threatening and require intensive support. Kemp and Lubitz (1993) describe an infant with alloimmune neutropenia who experienced a delay in cord separation of 8 weeks. Therapeutic interventions that have been attempted include, in addition to antimicrobials, intravenous immune globulin (IVIG) infusions with mixed success as well as granulocyte infusions that lack the offending antigen. Gilmore and coworkers (1994) and Dale and associates (1993) have described the successful use of G-CSF in the treatment of infants, children, and adults with both congenital neutropenia and cyclic neutropenia with significant laboratory and clinical responses.

Maternal Hypertension–Associated Neutropenia

One of the most common and well-described causes of transient neonatal neutropenia is maternal hypertension. In a prospective study, Mouzinho and colleagues (1994) analyzed the incidence of neonatal neutropenia in relation to birth weight, gestational age, and severity of maternal hypertension. They concluded that the neonatal neutropenia was inversely related to the birth weight and gestational age and directly related to the severity of the preeclampsia. The incidence was nearly 80% among neonates less than 30 weeks' gestation and was statistically different from similar infants born of normotensive mothers. In most cases, the neutropenia resolves within 72 hours but there have been cases in which the neutropenia has persisted and G-CSF has been used to increase the neutrophil count (La Gamma et al, 1995).

Eosinophilia

Eosinophilia has frequently been observed in the newborn nursery with uncertain significance and cause. Many theories have been proposed, for example, it is a result of establishing a positive nitrogen balance or it is an antigen response to intravenous or nasogastric catheters or endotracheal tubes. Patel and associates (1994) retrospectively analyzed neonates with eosinophilia and matched control infants and found that sepsis developed in all infants with eosinophilia less than 26 weeks' gestation as it did in most infants more than 26 weeks' gestation. In most cases, the eosinophilia occurred after the onset of clinical symptoms of sepsis. The only other factor that was associated with eosinophilia, when compared to matched control groups, was mechanical ventilation.

Qualitative Defects of Neonatal Neutrophils

In addition to the quantitative defects in neonatal myelopoieses, numerous *in vitro* neutrophil functional defects have been documented. An effective antimicrobial defense depends on, in addition to a normal neutrophil count, normal neutrophil functions in three areas: chemotaxis, phagocytosis, and intracellular killing. Chemotaxis is the first step in the inflammatory response, consisting of a series of processes that start with stimuli from the invading microorganism followed by the directed migration of neutrophils to the site of invasion. Chemotactic defects in the neonatal neutrophil include abnormal motility of neutrophils derived from cord blood, decreased deformability, decreased generation of filamentous actin, defective adherence, decreased migration, and irreversible aggregation when exposed to chemotactic factors (Anderson et al, 1984, 1987, 1981, 1984; Krause et al, 1986; Mease et al, 1981; Miller, 1971).

The second phase of neutrophil activity is phagocytosis. The phagocytic activity of the neonatal neutrophil is not different from adult neutrophils when assayed in the presence of normal adult serum or plasma (Miller, 1979). However, when assayed under conditions of "stress" such as sepsis, the phagocytic activity of neonatal neutrophils is decreased compared with adult neutrophils (Forman et al, 1969; Matoth, 1952). Overall phagocytosis in newborns appears to be deficient only under severe conditions (Miller, 1979).

The final step of neutrophil activity is intracellular killing of the organism. The major bactericidal function of the neutrophil is carried out by an oxygen-dependent chain of reactions, also known as the neutrophil respiratory burst, in which toxic oxygen metabolites such as hydrogen peroxide, superoxide anion, and hydroxyl radicals are produced. Superoxide anion production in neutrophils obtained from neonates is comparable to that in adult cells, whereas hydroxyl radical production is decreased (Ambruso et al, 1984; Shigeoka et al, 1981). Direct bacterial killing tests measuring the actual killing capacity of neonatal neutrophils have shown decreased activity by neonatal granulocytes during overwhelming sepsis.

Leukocyte Adhesion Deficiency

Leukocyte adhesion deficiency (LAD) is a rare autosomal recessive disorder manifested by recurrent infections in the newborn period and is usually associated with delayed separation of the umbilical cord. Infections are usually associated with an accompanying neutrophilia but granulocytes fail to accumulate at the site of infection. Perirectal cellulitis or abscess, stomatitis, and gingivitis are frequent complications. The disorder is thought to be a deficiency of a family of surface membrane glycoproteins known as integrins, specifically the B$_2$ family. The responsible gene has been located on chromosome 21q22.3 (Corbi et al, 1988; Curnette, 1993). The diagnosis is made by flow cytometric analysis for the B$_2$ integrins. Screening for the genetic mutation is also possible via chorionic villus sampling or amniocentesis. The treatment has included granulocyte transfusions, G-CSF, and allogenic stem cell transplantation.

Myeloproliferative Disorders

Congenital or neonatal leukemia is extremely rare and occurs at an approximate incidence of 1 per 200,000 live births (Bader et al, 1979). Unlike other childhood acute leukemias occurring after the 1st year of life, most cases are of nonlymphocytic origin. The most common subtypes of acute nonlymphocytic leukemia (ANLI) found in the neonatal period are monocytic or myelomonocytic (M$_5$ or M$_4$). Leukemia cutis occurs in 25% to 30% of cases with congenital leukemia and appears as red, blue, or purple papules (Resnik et al, 1993). Infants with trisomy 21 have an increased incidence of neonatal leukemia. Infants born with an increased white blood cell count and organomegaly with or without other hematopoietic abnormalities must be evaluated for a myeloproliferative disorder in addition to other conditions that may present similarly, such as congenital or neonatal infections.

Infants with trisomy 21 may also exhibit a transient leukemoid or myeloproliferative disorder that may be indistinguishable from acute leukemia. Typically, this is of the myeloid line but lymphoid leukemoid reactions have been reported (Fernandez de Castro et al, 1990). The condition resolves, over a period of weeks to months, without the use of chemotherapy. This phenomenon has also been seen in phenotypically normal infants whose bone marrow blast cells exhibit a trisomy 21 but whose circulating nonleukemoid cells demonstrated a normal karyotype (Jiang et al, 1991; Jones et al, 1987). Cytogenetics are an extremely important part of the evaluation in a newborn infant suspected of having a malignant process. The most frequent chromosomal change found in neonatal leukemias, excluding trisomy 21, is 11q23 (Sansone and Negri, 1992). The presence of chromosomal changes other than trisomy 21 strongly favors acute leukemia. ANLL has been reported to develop in children with trisomy 21 who experience a leukemoid reaction that resolves within the neonatal period (Jiang et al, 1991; Wong et al, 1988). It may be helpful to follow serial peripheral chromosomes in this population to detect abnormal clonigenic activity.

MANAGEMENT OF NEUTROPENIA AND NEUTROPHIL DYSFUNCTION DURING NEONATAL SEPSIS
Granulocyte Transfusions

The rationale for granulocyte (neutrophil) transfusions from adult donors for treatment of overwhelming neonatal sepsis is to use a large number of normal adult cells to overcome the quantitative and qualitative defects that have been demonstrated during neonatal myelopoiesis and neu-

trophil dysfunction. Several studies have investigated the efficacy of granulocyte transfusions and were reviewed by Sweetman and Cairo (1995). Two studies demonstrated no advantage of neutrophil transfusions (buffy coats) in reversing the detrimental outcome of neonatal sepsis (Baley et al, 1987; Wheeler et al, 1987).

A recent trial of neutrophil transfusion has demonstrated a significant improvement in survival in neonates during bacterial sepsis (Cairo et al, 1992b). This prospective randomized trial compared granulocyte transfusions to supportive care with or without IVIG. In the group of neonates receiving granulocyte transfusions, there were 43 of 45 survivors (96%) compared to 20 of 30 survivors in the supportive care with or without IVIG ($P<0.002$) (Cairo et al, 1992b). The efficacy of granulocyte transfusion seems to be greater in the setting of neonatal sepsis than it is in adults. One possible explanation is that the average cells per harvest are 1 to 2 $\times$ 10^{10}, which represents approximately 10% of the daily adult granulocyte production, whereas it is 100% of the average daily production in the newborn. Although a number of questions remain to be answered regarding the future role of adult granulocyte transfusion in the treatment of neonatal sepsis, it seems that it has a beneficial effect by improving both total neutrophil number and neutrophil function, resulting in improved survival. With the apparent safety of administering G-CSF to normal donors before leukopheresis (Bensinger et al, 1993), the yield will increase and the benefits of granulocyte transfusion as an adjunctive therapy will likely also increase.

Hematopoietic Growth Factors in Neonatal Sepsis
Granulocyte Colony-Stimulating Factor

Significant differences between adults and newborns, especially preterm infants, have been reported in G-CSF serum levels, mRNA expression, and activity. Laver and colleagues (1990) have studied the plasma levels of G-CSF and GM-CSF and the frequency of CFU-GMs in the umbilical cord blood of normal term newborns. Plasma levels of G-CSF and GM-CSF at birth were significantly higher than adult levels. Cairo and associates (1993) compared circulating serum levels of stem cell factor (SCF) and G-CSF in preterm and term newborns with those of adults. There were no significant differences in SCF serum levels between preterm and term newborns and adults. In addition, there were no differences in G-CSF levels between third trimester maternal levels and matched term newborns. However, G-CSF levels were higher in preterm infants compared with term infants and adults. In contrast to these findings, English and coworkers (1992) reported that mean serum concentrations of G-CSF at birth were higher in infants older than 37 gestational weeks compared with newborns of 32 to 37 gestational weeks of age, and these differences resulted in higher neutrophil counts in term infants. Russell and colleagues (1994) have studied G-CSF levels at birth and their relationship with neutrophil count and various perinatal conditions. High G-CSF levels at birth were associated with infection and maternal pregnancy-induced hypertension (maternal PIH), but not with gestational age. Gessler and coworkers (1993) reported G-CSF serum levels at birth with respect to neutrophil count, infection, and gestational age. Serum concentrations of G-CSF in term and preterm neonates without infection reached peak levels within the first 7 hours of life (mean values: 261 pg/mL and 126 pg/mL in term and preterm infants, respectively). Levels decreased to normal adult range (<50 pg/mL) between 4 and 7 days of age, and were unchanged at 2 to 3 weeks of age. Peak G-CSF levels preceded peak neutrophil levels between 7 and 12 hours of life, similar to the interval noted between exogenous administration of recombinant G-CSF and neutrophilia seen in other clinical settings (Gabrilove, 1992; Lieschke et al, 1992; Stute et al, 1992). Term and preterm infants with signs of bacterial infection soon after birth had significantly higher levels of G-CSF compared with noninfected infants. Newborns born to mothers with maternal PIH tended to have lower, but not significantly different, G-CSF levels and neutrophil counts compared with healthy newborns. The lower G-CSF levels in offsprings of mothers with maternal PIH could explain, in part, the neutropenia reported in these infants (Koenig et al, 1989).

Cairo and associates (1992a) have shown that G-CSF production from stimulated adult mononuclear cells was higher than that from cord blood (P<0.007). Additionally, there were significantly more G-CSF mRNA transcripts from adult than from cord mononuclear cells. No differences were found in affinity, binding, and number of G-CSF receptors on cord and adult peripheral effector cells.

Cairo and colleagues have previously demonstrated that G-CSF, given to neonatal rats, induces neutrophilia similar to that seen in adult animals (Cairo et al, 1990b). Administration of G-CSF postnatally to newborn rats over a period of 7 days resulted in a profound peripheral neutrophilia within 24 hours and a sustained and increased response for the following 7 days. At the end of 7 days, an increase in bone marrow (BM) NSP without the depletion of early BM progenitor cells has been documented (Cairo et al, 1990). Iguchi and colleagues (1991) have investigated the effects of repetitive administration of G-CSF on the kinetics of neutrophil production in rats. Although G-CSF–treated rats showed a significant dose-dependent increase in total leukocyte and neutrophil counts compared with control animals, death rates after inoculation with GBS were not significantly different between the two groups (Iguchi et al, 1991). The effect of single-pulse rhG-CSF in the treatment and prophylaxis of experimental group B streptococcal sepsis has been evaluated in neonatal rats. Administration of a single intraperitoneal dose of G-CSF at the time of experimental GBS resulted in a synergistic effect on survival compared to animals given antibiotics alone (91% versus 28%, respectively) (P<0.001) (Cairo et al, 1990a). Another study demonstrated the efficacy of G-CSF prophylaxis in newborn rats over control animals which received no adjuvant prophylactic CSF therapy. In that study, newborn rats were given placebo or G-CSF for 7 days and then they were inoculated with experimental GBS, followed by treatment with or without antibiotics. Seventy-two hours after experimental GBS inoculation, there was still 100% survival in the rhG-CSF plus antibiotic-treated group as compared with survival of only 50%

in the placebo plus antibiotic group (P<0.001) (Cairo et al, 1990a).

A recent study has investigated the safety, pharmacokinetics, and biologic efficacy of administration of G-CSF to newborn infants with sepsis (Gillan et al, 1994). Forty-two newborn infants (gestational age 26–40 weeks) with presumed sepsis within the first 3 days of life were randomized to receive either placebo or varying doses of rhG-CSF. The growth factor was given for 3 days at doses of 1, 5, or 10 μg/kg every day or 5 or 10 μg/kg twice a day. The half-life of rhG-CSF was 4.4 ± 0.4 hours. Intravenous rhG-CSF was well tolerated at all gestational ages receiving treatment and was not associated with any recognized acute toxicity. RhG-CSF induced a significant increase in the ANC within 24 hours following doses of 5 and 10 μg/kg given either every 24 or divided every 12 hours. The increased neutrophil count was maintained for 96 hours, 48 hours after the last rhG-CSF dose. BM aspirates demonstrated a dose-dependent increase in the NSP following treatment with rhG-CSF. In addition, C3bi expression was significantly increased at 24 hours following 10 μg/kg of rhG-CSF given every 24 hours. The enhancement of neonatal neutrophil C3bi expression indicates that rhG-CSF may induce functional maturation in neonatal neutrophils.

A recent 2-year follow-up analysis in these patients has shown that rhG-CSF therapy for presumed neonatal sepsis was not associated with long-term hematologic, immunologic, or developmental adverse effects (Rosenthal et al, 1995).

Granulocyte-Monocyte Colony-Stimulating Factor

Bailie and coworkers (1994) have reported an inverse linear relationship between maternal GM-CSF levels and gestational age. In neonates, a quadratic association was found between GM-CSF and gestational age. Levels were not related to neutrophil count, perinatal complications, or the presence of infection. Cairo and colleagues (1989) investigated the affinity and quantity of rhGM-CSF receptors in neutrophils and GM-CSF production and GM-CSF mRNA expression from activated neonatal and adult T cells. Whereas the affinity and number of GM-CSF receptors were similar in neonatal and adult neutrophils, the GM-CSF production and GM-CSF mRNA expression were reduced in activated T cells derived from neonates compared to those from adults. English and colleagues (1992) assessed the ability of mononuclear and T cells from neonates and adults to produce GM-CSF after stimulation with concavalin A with and without phorbol myristase acetate. Neonatal mononuclear cells and T cells produce only 30% as much GM-CSF mRNA compared with adult cells.

Cairo and associates (1989, 1991b) have previously reported the effects of GM-CSF on neonatal neutrophils. In a study on the effect of GM-CSF on neonatal neutrophil function, GM-CSF was shown to enhance neonatal neutrophil oxidative metabolism, chemotaxis, bacterial killing, and induction of MO-1 expression with increased adherence and aggregation.

The modulating effects of a single pulse of GM-CSF on neonatal rat neutrophilia has been demonstrated by intraperitoneal administration of GM-CSF. Significant neutrophilia was induced within 6 hours of administration.

This early neutrophilia appears to be secondary to egress of bone marrow NSP cells. Additionally, GM-CSF induced an increase in marrow myeloid proliferation within 24 to 48 hours after intraperitoneal administration in the neonatal rat. Seven days of intraperitoneal administration of GM-CSF in neonatal rats resulted in a significant increase in peripheral neutrophilia, an increase in bone marrow NSP, and a slight increase in the newborn rat bone marrow CFU-GM proliferative rate (Cairo, 1989; Cairo et al, 1991b). Wheeler and Givner (1992) demonstrated that GM-CSF could improve outcome in neonatal sepsis. Newborn rats infected intraperitoneally with GBS were given GM-CSF 7 to 19 hours later. The mortality rate was 67% and 37% ($P = 0.003$), and peritoneal cultures were positive in 86% and 44% ($P = 0.017$) in the control and rhGM-CSF groups, respectively. Chemiluminescence was also significantly increased in the treated animals (Wheeler and Givner, 1992). Frenck and associates (1990) have demonstrated that GM-CSF significantly improved survival when given prophylactically. Administration of GM-CSF to neonatal rats 6 hours before a 90% lethal dose of *Staphylococcus aureus* resulted in 54% versus 10% survival in the control group ($P < 0.001$) (Frenck et al, 1990).

A recent phase I/II study has reported the feasibility, safety, and biological response of GM-CSF in VLBW neonates (Cairo et al, 1995). Twenty VLBW neonates (500–1500 g, ≤72 hours old) were randomized to receive either placebo (n = 5), rhGM-CSF 5 μg/kg once daily (n = 5), 5 μg/kg twice daily (n = 5), or 10 μg/kg once daily (n = 5), given via 2-hour intravenous infusion for 7 days. GM-CSF was well tolerated at all dose levels without grade III or IV toxicity. At doses of 5 μg/kg twice daily and 10 μg/kg once daily, a significant increase in the circulating neutrophil count (ANC) was noted within 48 hours of treatment, which continued for at least 24 hours after discontinuation of rhGM-CSF. There was a significant increase in the ANC on days 6 and 7 at all dose levels when the ANC was normalized for each patient's first count. By day 7, all tested doses of rhGM-CSF resulted in an increase in the absolute monocyte count compared with placebo-treated neonates. A significant increase in the bone marrow NSP was demonstrated at doses of 5 μg/kg twice daily and 10 μg/kg once daily. In addition, neutrophil C3bi receptor expression was significantly increased 24 hours after the first dose of rhGM-CSF, suggesting improved neutrophil function with GM-CSF versus placebo. These results suggest that prophylactic treatment with rhGM-CSF may reduce the risk of infections in high-risk VLBW neonates. A multicenter, randomized, prospective, double-blinded, placebo-controlled phase III trial is currently underway (Cairo et al, 1995).

SUMMARY

Fetal and neonatal granulopoiesis is in a dynamic continuum. With improved survival of preterm infants, understanding this process becomes of paramount importance. The development of mature, functional granulocytes involves complex interactions between the myeloid progenitor cells, the microenvironment, and cytokines. Understanding this process and the quantitative and qualitative defects of neonatal granulocytes will allow future clinicians

to modulate the myeloid lineages to accommodate for these deficiencies.

REFERENCES

Fetal and Neonatal Hematopoiesis

Barge AJ: A review of the efficacy and tolerability of recombinant haematopoietic growth factors in bone marrow transplantation. Bone Marrow Transplant 11(Suppl 2):1–11, 1993.

Bonilla MA, Gillio AP, Ruggeiro M, et al: Effects of recombinant human granulocyte colony-stimulating factor on neutropenia in patients with congenital agranulocytosis. N Engl J Med 320:1574–1580, 1989.

Champlin RE, Nimer SD, Ireland P, et al: Treatment of refractory aplastic anemia with recombinant human granulocyte-macrophage-colony stimulating factor. Blood 73:694–699, 1988.

Gasson JC, Weisbart RH, Kaufman SE, et al: Purified human granulocyte-macrophage colony stimulating factor: Direct action on neutrophils. Science 226:1339–1342, 1984.

Gerhartz HH, Engelhard M, Meusers P, et al: Randomized, double-blind, placebo-controlled, phase III study of recombinant human granulocyte-macrophage colony-stimulating factor as adjunct to induction treatment of high-grade malignant non-Hodgkin's lymphomas. Blood 82:2329–2339, 1993.

Gordon MY: Perspective: Physiological mechanisms in BMT and haemopoiesis—Revisited. Bone Marrow Transplant 11:193–197, 1993.

Groopman JE, Mitsuyasu RT, DeLeo MJ, et al: Effect of recombinant human granulocyte-macrophage colony-stimulating factor on myelopoiesis in the acquired immunodeficiency syndrome. N Engl J Med 317:593–598, 1987.

Guinan EC, Sieff CA, Oette DH, et al: A phase I/II trial of recombinant granulocyte-macrophage colony-stimulating factor for children with aplastic anemia. Blood 76:1077–1082, 1990.

Hammond WP, Price TH, Souza LM, et al: Treatment of cyclic neutropenia with granulocyte colony-stimulating factor. N Engl J Med 320:1306–1311, 1989.

Hannum C, Culpepper J, Campbell D, et al: Ligand for FLT3/FLK2 receptor tyrosine kinase regulates growth of haematopoietic stem cells and is encoded by variant RNAs. Nature 368:643–648, 1994.

Huebner K, Isobe M, Croce CM, et al: The human gene encoding GM-CSF is at 5q21-q32, the chromosome region deleted in the 5q-anomaly. Science 230:1282–1285, 1985.

Lane TA, Law P, Maruyama M, et al: Harvesting and enrichment of hematopoietic progenitor cells mobilized into the peripheral blood of normal donors by granulocyte-macrophage colony-stimulating factor (GM-CSF) or G-CSF: Potential role in allogeneic marrow transplantation. Blood 85:275–282, 1995.

Migliaccio G, Migliaccio AR, Petti S, et al: Human embryonic hemopoiesis. Kinetics of progenitors and precursors underlying the yolk sac–liver transition. J Clin Invest 78:51–60, 1986.

Miller LL: American Society of Clinical Oncology recommendations for the use of hematopoietic colony-stimulating factors: Evidence-based, clinical practice guidelines. J Clin Oncol 12(11):2471–2508, 1994.

Nathan DG: The beneficence of neonatal hematopoiesis. N Engl J Med 321:1190–1191, 1989.

Nemunaitis J, Rabinowe S, Singer J, et al: Recombinant granulocyte-macrophage colony-stimulating factor after autologous bone marrow transplantation for lymphoid cancer. N Engl J Med 324:1773–1778, 1991.

Ohls R, Li Y, Abdel-Mageed A, et al: Neutrophil pool sizes and granulocyte colony-stimulating factor production in human mid-trimester fetuses. Pediatr Res 37:806–811, 1995.

Platzer E, Welte K, Gabrilove JL, et al: Biological activities of human pluripotent hematopoietic colony-stimulating factor on normal and leukemic cells. J Exp Med 162:1788–1801, 1985.

Riikonen P, Saarinen UM, Makipernaa A, et al: Recombinant human granulocyte-macrophage colony-stimulating factor in the treatment of febrile neutropenia: A double blind placebo-controlled study in children. Pediatr Infect Dis J 13:197–202, 1994.

Robinson B, Quesenberry P: Hematopoietic growth factors: Overview and clinical applications, Part II. Am J Med Sci 300:237–244, 1990.

Siegel J, McCracken G: Sepsis neonatorum. N Engl J Med 304:642–647, 1981.

Simmers RN, Webber LM, Shannon MF, et al: Localization of the G-CSF gene on chromosome 17 proximal to the breakpoint in the t(15;17) in acute promyelocytic leukemia. Blood 70:330–332, 1987.

Souza LM, Boone TC, Gabrilove J, et al: Recombinant human granulocyte-colony-stimulating factor: Effects on normal and leukemic myeloid cells. Science 232:61–65, 1986.

Till J, McCulloch E: A direct measurement of the radiation sensitivity of normal mouse bone marrow cells. Radiat Res 14:213–222, 1961.

Torok-Storb B: Cellular interactions. Blood 72:373–385, 1988.

Uchida N, Weissman I: Searching for hematopoietic stem cells: Evidence that Thy-1.11o Lin-Sca-1+ cells are the only stem cells in C57BL/Ka-Thy-1.1 bone marrow. J Exp Med 175(1):175–184, 1992.

Vadhan-Raj S, Buescher S, Broxmeyer HE, et al: Stimulation of myelopoiesis in patients with aplastic anemia by recombinant human granulocyte-macrophage colony-stimulating factor (published erratum appears in N Engl J Med 320:329, 1989). N Engl J Med 319:1628–1634, 1989.

Welte K, Platzer E, Lu L, et al: Purification and biochemical characterization of human pluripotent hematopoietic colony-stimulating factor. Proc Natl Acad Sci U S A 82:1526–1530, 1987.

Zon L: Developmental biology of hematopoiesis. Blood 86:2876–2891, 1995.

Quantitative and Qualitative Defects in the Neonatal Phagocyte

Ambruso D, Bentwood B, Henson P: Oxidative metabolism of cord blood neutrophils: Relationship to content and degranulation of cytoplasmic granules. Pediatr Res 18:1148–1153, 1984.

Anderson DC, Freeman KL, Heerdt B, et al: Abnormal stimulated adherence of neonatal granulocytes: Impaired induction of surface Mac-1 by chemotactic factors or secretagogues. Blood 70:740–750, 1987.

Anderson DC, Hughes BJ, Smith CW: Abnormal mobility of neonatal polymorphonuclear leukocytes: Relationship to impaired redistribution of surface adhesion sites by chemotactic factor or colchicine. J Clin Invest 68:863–874, 1981.

Anderson DC, Hughes BJ, Wible LJ, et al: Impaired motility of neonatal PMN leukocytes: Relationship to abnormalities of cell orientation and assembly of microtubules in chemotactic gradients. J Leuko Biol 36:1–15, 1984.

Anderson DC, Pickering LK, Feigin RD: Leukocyte function in normal and infected neonates. J Pediatr 85:420, 1974.

Bader JL, Miller RW: US cancer incidence and mortality in the first year of life. Am J Dis Child 133:157–159, 1979.

Bonilla MA, Gillio AP, Ruggeiro M, et al: Effects of recombinant human granulocyte colony-stimulating factor on neutropenia in patients with congenital agranulocytosis. N Engl J Med 320:1574–1580, 1989.

Cartron J, Tchernia G, Celtron J, et al: Alloimmune neonatal neutropenia. Am J Pediatr Hematol Oncol 13:21–25, 1991.

Christensen RD, Harper TE, Rothstein G: Granulocyte-macrophage progenitor cells in term and preterm neonates. J Pediatr 109:1047–1051, 1986.

Christensen RD, Hill HR, Rothstein G: Granulocytic stem cell (CFU-C) proliferation in experimental group B streptococcal sepsis. Pediatr Res 17:278–280, 1983.

Christensen RD, Macfarlane JL, Taylor NL, et al: Blood and marrow neutrophils during experimental group B streptococcal infection: Quantification of the stem cell, proliferative, storage and circulating pools. Pediatr Res 16:549–553, 1982.

Christensen RD, Rothstein G: Efficiency of neutrophil migration in the neonate. Pediatr Res 14:1147, 1980a.

Christensen RD, Rothstein G: Exhaustion of mature marrow neutrophils in neonates with sepsis. J Pediatr 96:316, 1980b.

Christensen RD, Rothstein G: Pre and post-natal development of granulocyte stem cells (CFUc) in the rat. Pediatr Res 18:599–602, 1984.

Corbi AL, Larson RS, Kishimoto TK, et al: Chromosomal location of the genes encoding the leukocyte adhesion receptors LFA-1, MAC-1 and p150, 95. Identification of a gene cluster involved in cell adhesions. J Exp Med 167:1597–1607, 1988.

Curnette J: Disorders of granulocyte function and granulopoiesis. In Nathan DG, Oski FA (Eds): Hematology of Infancy and Childhood, 4th ed. Philadelphia, WB Saunders, 1993, pp 904–961.

Daghistani D, Jimenez J, Toledano S, et al: Congenital neutropenia: A case study. Am J Pediatr Hematol Oncol 12:210–214, 1990.

Dale DC, Bonilla MA, Davis MW, et al: A randomized controlled phase III trial of recombinant human granulocyte colony-stimulating factor

(filgrastim) for treatment of severe chronic neutropenia. Blood 81:2496–2502, 1993.

Erdman SH, Christensen RD, Bradley PP, et al: Supply and release of storage neutrophils: A developmental study. Biol Neonate 41:132–137, 1982.

Fernandez de Castro M, Salas S, Martinez A, et al: Transitory T-lymphoblastic leukemoid reaction in a neonate with Down syndrome. Am J Pediatr Hematol Oncol 12:71–73, 1990.

Forman ML, Stiehm ER: Impaired opsonic activity but normal phagocytosis in low-birth-weight infants. N Engl J Med 281:926–931, 1969.

Gessler P, Luders R, Konig S, et al: Neonatal neutropenia in low birthweight premature infants. Am J Perinatol 12:34–38, 1995.

Gilmore M, Stroncek D, Korones D: Treatment of alloimmune neonatal neutropenia with granulocyte colony-stimulating factor. J Pediatr 125:948–951, 1994.

Jiang CJ, Liang DC, Tien HF: Neonatal transient leukemoid proliferation followed by acute myeloid leukaemia in a phenotypically normal child. Br J Haematol 77:247–248, 1991.

Jones G, Weaver M, Laug W: Transient blastemia in phenotypically normal newborns. Am J Pediatr Hematol Oncol 9:153–157, 1987.

Kemp AS, Lubitz L: Delayed umbilical cord separation in alloimmune neutropenia. Arch Dis Child 68:52–53, 1993.

Kostmann R: Infantile genetic agranulocytosis. Acta Paediatr Scand Suppl 105:1, 1956.

Krause PJ, Herson VC, Boutin-Lebowitz J, et al: Polymorphonuclear leukocyte adherence and chemotaxis in stressed and healthy neonates. Pediatr Res 20:296–300, 1986.

La Gamma E, Alpan O, Kocherlakota P: Effect of granulocyte colony-stimulating factor on preeclampsia-associated neonatal neutropenia. J Pediatr 126:457–459, 1995.

Manroe BL, Weinberg AG, Rosenfeld CR, et al: The neonatal blood count in health and disease. J Pediatr 95:89–98, 1979.

Matoth Y: Phagocytic and ameboid activities of the leukocytes in the newborn infant. Pediatrics 9:748–754, 1952.

Mease AC, Burgess DP, Thomas PJ: Irreversible neutrophil aggregation: A mechanism of decreased newborn neutrophil chemotactic response. Am J Pathol 104:98–102, 1981.

Miller M: Chemotactic function in the human neonate: Humoral and cellular aspects. Pediatr Res 5:487–492, 1971.

Miller ME: Phagocyte function in the neonate: Selected aspects. Pediatrics 64:709–712, 1979.

Mouzinho A, Rosenfeld C, Sanchez P, et al: Revised reference ranges for circulating neutrophils in very-low-birth-weight neonates. Pediatr 94:76–82, 1994.

Patel L, Garvey B, Arnon S, et al: Eosinophilia in newborn infants. Acta Paediatr 83:797–801, 1994.

Rappeport JM, Parkman R, Newburger P, et al: Correction of infantile agranulocytosis (Kostmann's syndrome) by allogeneic bone marrow transplantation. Am J Med 68:605–609, 1980.

Resnik KS, Brod BB: Leukemia cutis in congenital leukemia. Analysis and review of the world literature with report of an additional case (Review). Arch Dermatol 129:1301–1306, 1993.

Sansone R, Negri D: Cytogenetic features of neonatal leukemias. Cancer Genet Cytogenet 63:56–61, 1992.

Shigeoka AO, Charette RP, Wyman ML, et al: Defective oxidative metabolic responses of neutrophils from stressed neonates. J Pediatr 98:392–398, 1981.

Welte K, Zeidler C, Reiter A, et al: Differential effects of granulocyte-macrophage colony-stimulating factor and granulocyte colony-stimulating factor in children with severe congenital neutropenia. Blood 75:1056–1063, 1990.

Wong K, Jones M, Srivastova A, et al: Transient myeloproliferative disorder in acute nonlymphoblastic leukemia in Down syndrome. J Pediatr 112:18–22, 1988.

Management of Neutropenia and Neutrophil Dysfunction During Neonatal Sepsis

Bailie KE, Irvine AE, Bridges JM, et al: Granulocyte and granulocyte-macrophage colony-stimulating factors in cord and maternal serum at delivery. Pediatr Res 35(2):164–168, 1994.

Baley J, Stork E, Warkentin P, et al: Buffy coat transfusions in neutropenic neonates with presumed sepsis: A prospective randomized trial. Pediatrics 80:712–720, 1987.

Bensinger WI, Price TH, Dale DC, et al: The effects of daily recombinant human granulocyte colony stimulating factor administration on normal granulocyte donors undergoing leukopheresis. Blood 81:1883–1888, 1993.

Cairo M: Host defense and new treatment strategies in neonatal sepsis—Introduction. Am J Pediatr Hematol Oncol 11(2):213–214, 1989.

Cairo MS, Christensen R, Sender LS, et al: Results of a phase I/II trial of recombinant human granulocyte-macrophage colony-stimulating factor in very low birthweight neonates: Significant induction of circulatory neutrophils, monocytes, platelets and bone marrow neutrophils. Blood 86:2509–2515, 1995.

Cairo MS, Gillan ER, Buzby JS, et al: Circulating Steel factor (SLF) and G-CSF levels in preterm and term newborn and adult peripheral blood. Am J Pediatr Hematol Oncol 15:311–315, 1993.

Cairo M, Mauss D, Kommareddy S, et al: Prophylactic or simultaneous administration of recombinant human granulocyte colony stimulating factor in the treatment of group B streptococcal sepsis in neonatal rats. Pediatr Res 27:612–616, 1990a.

Cairo M, Plunkett J, Mauss D, et al: Seven-day administration of recombinant human granulocyte colony stimulating factor to newborn rats: Modulation of neonatal neutrophilia, myelopoiesis, and group B streptococcus sepsis. Blood 76:1788–1794, 1990b.

Cairo M, Suen Y, Knoppel E, et al: Decreased G-CSF and IL-3 production and gene expression from mononuclear cells of newborn infants. Pediatr Res 31:574–578, 1992a.

Cairo MS, van de Ven C, Mauss D, et al: Modulation of neonatal rat myeloid kinetics resulting in peripheral neutrophilia by single pulse administration of Rh granulocyte-macrophage colony-stimulating factor and Rh granulocyte colony-stimulating factor. Biol Neonate 59:13–21, 1991b.

Cairo MS, van de Ven C, Toy C, et al: Recombinant human granulocyte-macrophage colony stimulating factor primes neonatal granulocytes for enhanced oxidative metabolism and chemotaxis. Pediatr Res 26(5):395–399, 1989.

Cairo MS, van de Ven C, Toy C, et al: GM-CSF primes and modulates neonatal PMN motility: Upregulation of C3bi (Mo1) expression with alteration in PMN adherence and aggregation. Am J Pediatr Hematol Oncol 13(3):249–257, 1991a.

Cairo MS, Worcester C, Rucker R, et al: Randomized trial of granulocyte transfusions versus intravenous immune globulin therapy for neonatal neutropenia and sepsis. J Pediatr 120:281–285, 1992b.

English K, Hammond W, Lewis D, et al: Decreased granulocyte-macrophage colony stimulating factor production by human neonatal blood mononuclear cells and T cells. Pediatr Res 31:211–216, 1992.

Frenck RW, Sarman G, Harper TE, et al: The ability of recombinant murine granulocyte-macrophage colony-stimulating factor to protect neonatal rats from septic death due to *Staphylococcus aureus.* J Infect Dis 162:109, 1990.

Gabrilove JL: Clinical applications of granulocyte colony stimulating factor (G-CSF). Growth Factors 6:187, 1992.

Gessler P, Kirchmann N, Kientsch-Engel R, et al: Serum concentrations of granulocyte-colony stimulating factor in healthy term and preterm neonates and in those with various diseases including bacterial infections. Blood 82:3177–3182, 1993.

Gillan ER, Christensen R, Suen Y, et al: A randomized, placebo-controlled trial of recombinant human granulocyte-colony stimulating factor administration in newborn infants with presumed sepsis: Significant induction of peripheral and bone marrow neutrophilia. Blood 84:1427–1433, 1994.

Iguchi K, Inoue S, Kumar A: Effect of recombinant human granulocyte colony-stimulating factor administration in normal and experimentally infected newborn rats. Exp Hematol 19(5):352–358, 1991.

Koenig JM, Christensen RD: Incidence, neutrophil kinetics, and natural history of neonatal neutropenia associated with maternal hypertension. N Engl J Med 321:557–562, 1989.

Laver J, Duncan E, Abboud M: High levels of granulocyte and granulocyte-macrophage colony-stimulating factors in cord blood of normal full-term neonates. J Pediatr 116:627–632, 1990.

Lieschke GJ, Burgess AW: Granulocyte colony-stimulating factor and granulocyte-macrophage colony-stimulating factor. N Engl J Med 327:28, 1992.

Rosenthal J, Healey T, Ellis R, et al: A two-year follow-up of neonates with presumed sepsis treated with recombinant human granulocyte colony-stimulating factor during the first week of life. J Pediatr 128:135–137, 1995.

Russell AR, Davies EG, McGuigan S, et al: Plasma granulocyte-colony stimulating factor concentrations (G-CSF) in the early neonatal period. Br J Haematol 86:642–644, 1994.

Stute N, Santana VM, Rodman JH, et al: Pharmacokinetics of subcutaneous recombinant human granulocyte colony-stimulating factor in children. Blood 79:2849–2854, 1992.

Sweetman R, Cairo MS: Blood component and immunotherapy in neonatal sepsis. Trans Med Rev 9:251–259, 1995.

Wheeler JG, Chauvenet AR, Johnson CA, et al: Buffy coat transfusions in neonates with sepsis and neutrophil storage pool depletion. Pediatrics 79:422–425, 1987.

Wheeler JG, Givner LB: Therapeutic use of recombinant human granulocyte-macrophage colony-stimulating factor in neonatal rats with type III group B streptococcal sepsis. J Infect Dis 165:938–941, 1992.

CHAPTER **91**

Renal Morphogenesis and Development of Renal Function

Jean-Pierre Guignard

RENAL MORPHOGENESIS

The fetal kidney develops from three successive mesodermic structures: the pronephros, the mesonephros, and the metanephros. Differentiation of the metanephros starts around the 5th week of gestation, and the first nephrons are formed by the 8th week. Nephrogenesis continues up to the 34th to 35th week, with the deep nephrons being formed first. From the completion of nephrogenesis around the 35th week until birth, the nephrons only grow in size. At birth, juxtamedullary nephrons are more mature than superficial nephrons. The total number of nephrons varies widely from 600,000 to 1.2 million per kidney. Fetal growth retardation reduces the number of nephrons, so that a positive correlation exists between birth weight and the final number of nephrons (Merlet-Bnichou et al, 1993).

The glomerular diameter approximates 110 μm at birth (280 μm in the adult), and the average proximal tubular length reaches 2 mm (20 mm in the adult). Postnatal growth is characterized by accelerated growth of the proximal tubular volume compared to the glomerular filtering area. The glomerular basement membrane, which behaves as a filtration barrier, is thinner in newborns (100 nm) as compared to adults (300 nm). The size of the apertures in the barrier limits the passage of compounds through the capillary wall. In addition, an electrostatic barrier, resulting from the presence of negatively charged glycosialoproteins in the glomerular capillary wall, further restricts the filtration of negatively charged molecules. The permeability of the glomerular basement membrane is greater in newborn than in more mature animals (Savin et al, 1985).

During the second half of gestation, the kidney weight increases proportionally to gestational age, body weight, and body surface area. The kidney and bladder can be visualized by ultrasonography from the 15th week of gestation, although the precise renal architecture is only clearly defined by the 20th week. Kidney size (Y), as measured by ultrasonography, increases proportionally to gestational age: Y (cm) = 16.19 + 0.61 gestational weeks (Jeanty et al, 1982). The ratio between the renal and the abdominal circumferences at the level of the umbilical vein remains constant during gestation, with its value varying from 0.27 to 0.30 (Grannum et al, 1980). At birth, renal volume approximates 10 mL, and it reaches 23 mL by the 3rd week of life. Each kidney weighs about 12.5 g (150 g in the adult) and has a length of about 4.5 cm (11.5 cm in

the adult) at birth. The surface of the kidney is lobulated and remains so for months after birth. Fetal bladder volume can also be assessed by ultrasonography. With a maximal capacity of 10 mL at the 32nd week, the bladder can contain up to 40 mL near term.

RENAL FUNCTION IN UTERO

The placenta is the major regulatory organ of the fetus, so that renal growth does not appear to be governed by functional requirements. Urine formation starts around the 10th to 12th week of gestation. Fetal urine is a major constituent of amniotic fluid, and its production increases with age. Mean hourly urine flow rate is high and approximates 5 mL at 20 weeks, 10 mL at 30 weeks, and 30 mL at 40 weeks of postconceptional age (Rabinovitz et al, 1989). Fetal oliguria with consequent oligohydramnios is associated with pulmonary hypoplasia.

The fetal urine is hypotonic throughout gestation, with sodium as the major osmotic component. The kidney actively reabsorbs electrolytes and solutes from the glomerular ultrafiltrate. Elevated concentrations of sodium (>100 mmol/L), chloride (>90 mmol/L), and osmolality (>210 mosm/L) in the urine of a dilated kidney have been considered as indicating poor renal postnatal prognosis (see Chapters 12 and 92). Sensitivity (40% to 80%) and specificity (<80%) of these parameters, however, are not ideal.

Fetal renal blood flow (RBF), as measured by Doppler ultrasonography, reaches 20 mL per minute at 25 weeks' gestation and 60 mL per minute near term (Veille et al, 1993). The low rate of RBF in the fetus is associated with an elevated renal vascular resistance. The fetus appears to be able to autoregulate RBF within modest limits (Robillard and Weitzman, 1980).

Fetal glomerular filtration rate (GFR) increases rapidly as the number and size of nephrons increase. When the full complement of nephrons is achieved, GFR increases in parallel with renal mass and hence with body weight and body surface area. From the 28th to the 35th week of gestation, GFR (measured by inulin clearance in 1- to 2-day-old newborns) increases proportionally to gestational age (GFR = −28.1 + 1.37 weeks gestation) then levels off up to the time of birth (Fig. 91–1) (Guignard and John, 1986).

Several vasoactive agents and hormones play a major role in modulating the fetal RBF and GFR, including the

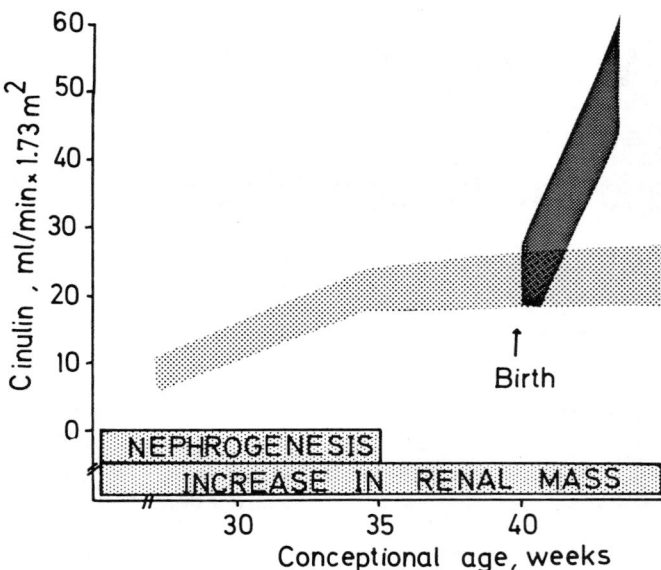

FIGURE 91–1. Maturation of glomerular filtration rate (C_{inulin}) in relation to conceptional age. (From Guignard JP: *In* Gruskin AB, Norman ME [Eds]: Pediatric Nephrology. The Hague, Martinus Nijhoff, 1981; with kind permission from Kluwer Academic Publishers.)

renin-angiotensin system, the catecholamines, the prostaglandins, the kallikrein-kinin system, and the atrial natriuretic peptide (Table 91–1). Interference with these systems can lead to severe renal dysfunction in the fetus. Clinical examples include fetal renal failure after administration to the mother of inhibitors of the angiotensin-converting enzyme or of prostaglandin synthesis (see Chapter 34). In the former situation, the decrease in the GFR probably results from the attenuated vasoconstriction of the efferent artery by angiotensin II inhibition, whereas reduced prostaglandin-dependent afferent vasodilation and the unopposed vasoconstrictive effects of angiotensin II and catecholamines may explain the drop in GFR observed in fetuses of mothers given indomethacin or nonsteroidal anti-inflammatory medications.

POSTNATAL MATURATION OF RENAL BLOOD FLOW

RBF is determined mainly by the mean arterial pressure and the resistance at the level of the renal glomerular arterioles. In the adult, physiologic intrinsic autoregulation

TABLE 91–1

Vasoactive Factors Modulating Renal Blood Flow and Glomerular Filtration Rate in the Immature Kidney

Adenosine	Nitric oxide
Angiotensin II	Norepinephrine
Atrial natriuretic peptide	Prostaglandin E_1
Bradykinin	Prostaglandin E_2
Epinephrine	Thromboxane A_2
Dopamine	Vasopressin
Endothelin	

maintains a constant RBF at perfusion pressures varying from 80 to 200 mm Hg. In children and adults, RBF approximates 20% to 25% of cardiac output, that is, 1200 mL/min × 1.73 m². The major part of the blood flow supplies the cortex, with medullary blood flow representing only 10% of the total RBF.

During fetal life, RBF is low, representing only 2% to 4% of the total cardiac output. This proportion increases after birth, from a value of 5% in the first 12 hours of life to 10% at the end of the 1st week. As a consequence, RBF increases rapidly from a value of 250 mL/min × 1.73 m² at 8 days of age to approximately 750 mL/min × 1.73 m² by 5 months of age. The postnatal maturation of RBF is associated with a striking decrease in renal vascular resistance and a marked increase in systemic blood pressure (see Chapter 95). The decrease in renal vascular resistance occurs along with a decrease in the resistance of both the afferent and efferent arterioles. Animal studies suggest that autoregulation of RBF is present in the immature kidney but is set at a lower range of blood pressure (Chevalier et al, 1987).

Several autocrine, paracrine, and endocrine factors regulate RBF, intrarenal hemodynamics, and GFR (see Table 91–1; Fig. 91–2) (Bailie, 1992; Guignard et al, 1991; Seri, 1995). Overactivation of the vasoconstrictive forces that regulate renal hemodynamics in the neonatal period may impair the maturation of RBF and induce renal hypoperfusion. Such an activation is seen during respiratory distress, hypoxemia and asphyxia, metabolic acidosis and hypercapnia, hyperthermia and hypothermia (Gillieron et al, 1995), and positive-pressure ventilation as well as in response to the administration of various medications (Guignard and John, 1986).

POSTNATAL MATURATION OF GLOMERULAR FILTRATION RATE
Determinants of Glomerular Filtration Rate

The rate of filtration is governed by the rate at which plasma flows into the glomerular capillaries, the balance of

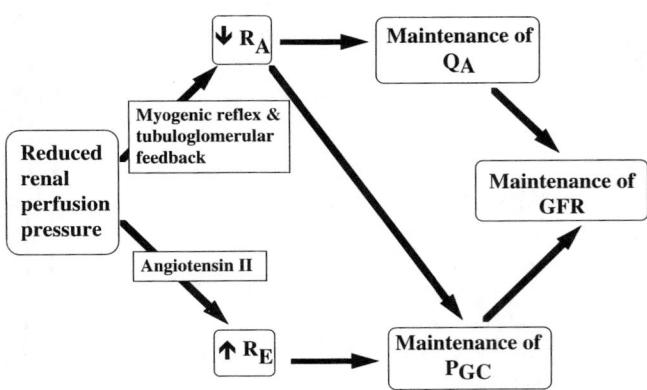

FIGURE 91–2. Mechanisms contributing to the autoregulation of renal blood flow and glomerular filtration rate (GFR). R_A, afferent arteriolar resistance; R_E, efferent arteriolar resistance; Q_A, glomerular plasma flow rate; P_{GC}, glomerular capillary hydraulic pressure). (From Badr KF, Ichikawa I: Prerenal failure: A deleterious shift from renal compensation to decompensation. N Engl J Med 319:623–629, 1988. Copyright © 1988 Massachusetts Medical Society. All rights reserved.)

Starling forces across the glomerular capillary walls, the permeability of the glomerular capillary wall to water and small solutes, and the total surface area of the capillaries. The ultrafiltration coefficient (K_f) represents the product of the permeability of the glomerular membrane and the glomerular filtering area. GFR is proportional to the Starling forces across the glomerular capillaries $\times$ the K_f:

$$GFR = K_f \times [P_{GC} - (P_{IT} + \pi_{GC})]$$

where P_{GC} is hydrostatic pressure in the glomerular capillary, P_{IT} is the proximal intratubular hydrostatic pressure, and π_{GC} is the oncotic pressure in the glomerular capillary. In adults, the average value of P_{GC} probably approximates 60 mm Hg, the proximal intratubular pressure 15 mm Hg, and the oncotic glomerular capillary pressure 27 mm Hg. Thus, the average net filtration pressure is close to 18 mm Hg. The relative state of vasoconstriction in the afferent and efferent arterioles plays a major role in regulating the intracapillary hydrostatic pressure. The factors modulating the state of vascular contraction are listed in Table 91–1.

During the early newborn period, the factors regulating GFR mature rapidly. Systemic blood pressure and mean transcapillary hydraulic pressure increase (see Chapter 34), followed by a parallel increase in GFR (Guignard and John, 1986). The plasma oncotic pressure also increases but at a lower rate than the transcapillary hydraulic pressure, so that the net ultrafiltration pressure increases. The low glomerular plasma flow rate present at birth is due to elevated afferent and efferent arteriolar resistances. A systemic increase in the ultrafiltration coefficient also occurs during maturation and may be attributed to an increase in both the hydraulic permeability and the glomerular capillary area.

In the fetus and newborn, the low systemic and hence the glomerular capillary hydrostatic pressure is the main factor limiting the rate of filtration. Vasoactive factors modulating the intraglomerular filtration pressure thus play a key role in maintaining filtration (Bailie, 1992; Guignard et al, 1991). The vasodilatory prostaglandins, the concentration of which is elevated during fetal life and early postnatal life, favor filtration by vasodilating the afferent arteriole. Angiotensin II also favors filtration by preferentially constricting the efferent arteriole. Minute-to-minute regulation of the contractile tone also depends on endothelium-released vasoactive factors such as nitric oxide and endothelin. Although endogenous endothelin behaves as a potent constrictor in the adult, it might vasodilate the afferent artery in the immature kidney (Semama et al, 1993). Atrial natriuretic peptide, the concentration of which is also elevated in early life, vasodilates the afferent artery (Robillard et al, 1992). Adenosine, a regulator of the tubuloglomerular feedback mechanism, is an efferent vasodilator. When acting in conjunction with elevated levels of angiotensin II, it also vasoconstricts the afferent arteriole (Gouyon and Guignard, 1989). Although the overactivation of adenosine plays a critical role in the pathogenesis of the hypoxemia-induced vasomotor insufficiency, the exact physiologic role of intrarenal adenosine in the fetus and newborn is still ill defined.

Assessment of Glomerular Filtration Rate

Inulin is the gold standard for measuring GFR in both the immature and the mature kidney. It is freely filtered, even by the preterm newborn with a gestational age as low as 27 weeks. The postnatal development of GFR has been assessed in premature newborns at different gestational ages and in term newborns. From a value of 20 mL/min $\times$ 1.73 m² at birth, GFR doubles in the first 2 weeks of life in term newborns (Fig. 91–3) (Guignard et al, 1975). GFR is lower in premature infants and develops at a lower velocity.

Creatinine, the most commonly used glomerular marker in mature subjects, is also frequently used to assess GFR in newborns. It presents, however, with several drawbacks. The concentration of creatinine is elevated after birth, the more so in the most immature infants (Fig. 91–4) (Bueva and Guignard, 1994; Van den Anker et al, 1995). The elevated creatinine concentration in the newborn has usually been considered as reflecting the maternal creatinine plasma concentration. Because of the back-diffusion of creatinine across leaky immature tubules, however, filtered creatinine is partly reabsorbed by the immature kidney. The reabsorption of creatinine by the premature infant probably accounts for the negative correlation between gestational age and the plasma creatinine during the first weeks of life (see Fig. 91–4) as well as for the finding that in very premature newborns creatinine clearance often underestimates inulin clearance (Coulthard and Ruddock, 1983). Despite these drawbacks, creatinine clearance correlates with inulin clearance (Stonestreet et al, 1979), and creatinine clearance studies in newborns have confirmed the rapid development of GFR in the first weeks of life and that GFR develops at a lower velocity in premature infants (Bueva and Guignard, 1994; Vanpee et al, 1992) (Fig. 91–5A). The differences in the GFR among infants with different gestational and postnatal age explain why the specific dosage recommendations are tailored to the given gestational and postnatal age for medications primarily eliminated via glomerular filtration (i.e., aminoglycosides).

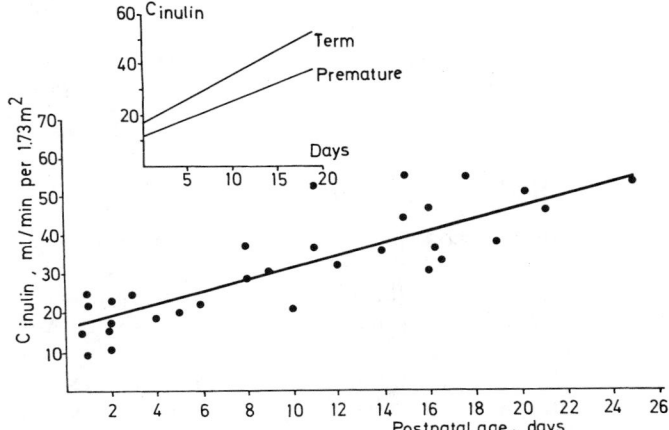

FIGURE 91–3. Maturation of glomerular filtration rate (C_{inulin}) in relation to postnatal age in term and preterm infants. (From Guignard JP: *In* Gruskin AB, Norman ME [Eds]: Pediatric Nephrology. The Hague, Martinus Nijhoff, 1981; with kind permission from Kluwer Academic Publishers.)

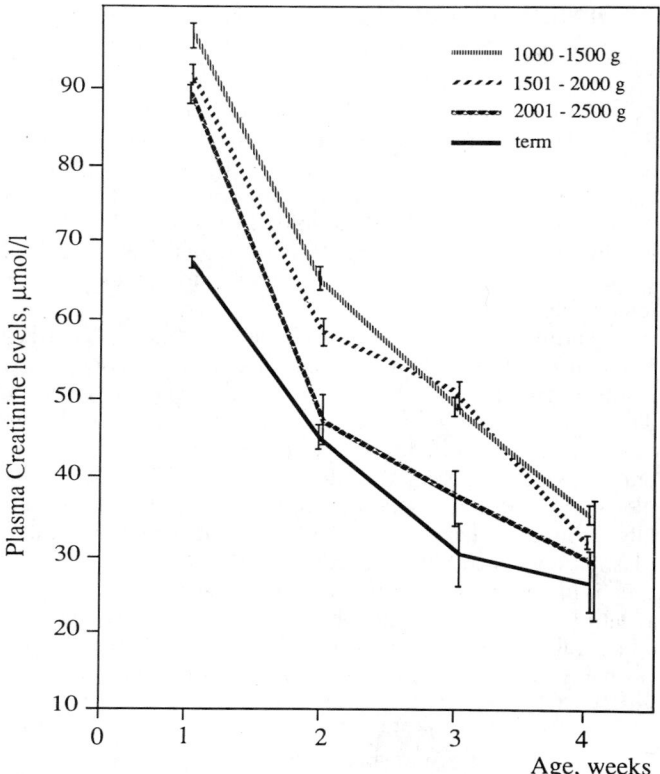

FIGURE 91–4. Plasma creatinine in term and low-birth-weight infants during the first 4 weeks of life. (From Bueva A, Guignard JP: Renal function in preterm neonates. Pediatr Res 36:572–577, 1994.)

REGULATION OF BODY FLUID TONICITY AND VOLUME

The kidney is responsible for maintaining the extracellular fluid volume (ECF) and osmolality constant despite large variations in salt and water intake. By modulating the renal conservation of water, the antidiuretic hormone (ADH) system plays a central role in the regulation of body fluid tonicity. Sodium chloride, the major osmotically active solute in ECF, determines its volume. The balance between the intake and the renal excretion of sodium thus regulates ECF volume (see Chapter 34).

Sodium and Water Reabsorption

Active sodium reabsorption occurs throughout the nephron, driven by a Na⁺,K⁺-ATPase localized to the basolateral membrane. Two thirds of the filtered Na⁺ load is reabsorbed in the proximal tubule via the Na⁺/glucose, Na⁺/amino acid, Na^+/PO_4^{-3}, and Na⁺/lactate symporters and by the Na⁺/H⁺ antiporter. Because water passively follows Na⁺ across the highly water-permeable proximal tubule, the osmolality of the proximal tubule fluid remains isotonic. Twenty percent of the sodium filtered load are reabsorbed in the ascending limb of the loop of Henle, which is impermeable to water. Accumulation of sodium chloride and recycling of urea into the medullary interstitium lead to the formation of a hyperosmotic medulla. The

thick ascending limb also reabsorbs calcium, magnesium, and potassium. The distal tubule and collecting duct reabsorb 10% of the filtered Na⁺ and Cl⁻ load. In the distal tubule, the continuing sodium chloride reabsorption in the absence of water reabsorption further decreases the osmolality of the tubular fluid, allowing the formation of a

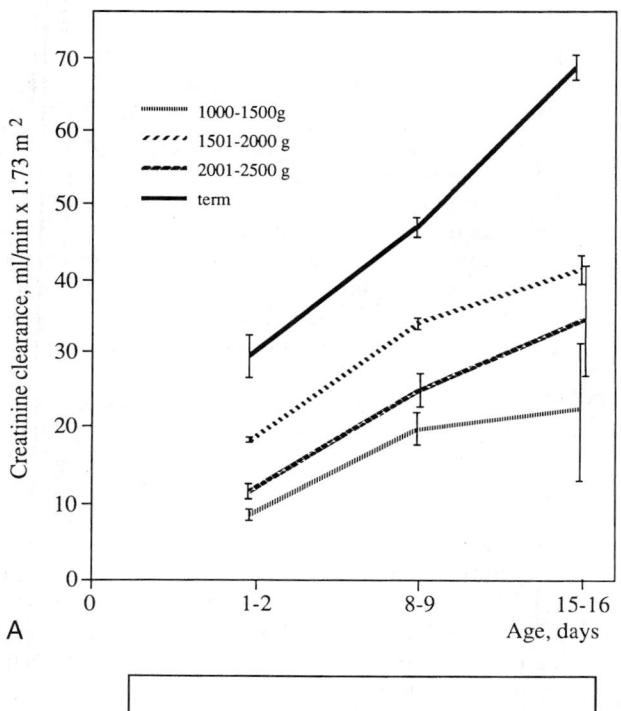

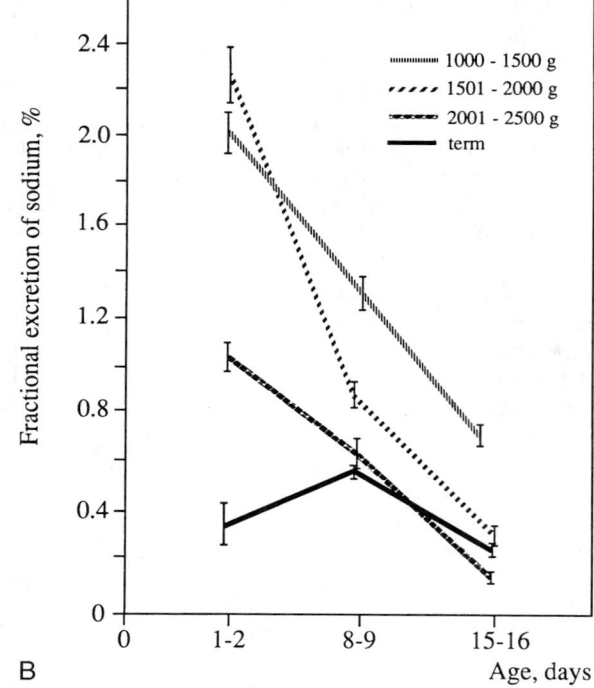

FIGURE 91–5. *A,* Creatinine clearance as a function of postnatal age in term and low-birth-weight infants. *B,* Fractional excretion of sodium as a function of postnatal age in term and low-birth-weight infants. (From Bueva A, Guignard JP: Renal function in preterm neonates. Pediatr Res 36:572–577, 1994.)

hypotonic urine. Excretion of solute-free water thus depends on Na^+ delivery to and reabsorption at the distal diluting site. The permeability of the collecting duct to water depends on the presence of ADH or arginine vasopressin (AVP). The release of AVP by the posterior pituitary is regulated by osmoreceptors located in the supraoptic nucleus of the hypothalamus. By binding to its cell membrane receptors and thus activating adenylate cyclase, AVP increases the intracellular levels of cyclic adenosine monophosphate (cAMP). This increase ultimately leads to phosphorylation of the water channels, which, in turn, results in insertion of these channels into the luminal membrane of the collecting duct cells, rendering the collecting duct permeable to water (see Chapter 34). In the absence of AVP, a large volume of hypotonic urine is excreted. In contrast, when elevated levels of AVP are present, water passively diffuses out of the collecting duct into the hyperosmotic interstitium, and a small volume of concentrated urine is excreted.

Water transport depends on the intact function of the aquaporin family of water channel proteins, specifically AQP2 (Lee et al, 1997). Patients who lack a functioning AQP2 have a severe form of nephrogenic diabetes insipidus, confirming that this protein is the vasopressin-regulated water channel in the collecting tubule (Deen et al, 1995; Lee et al, 1997).

During development, Na^+ reabsorption per unit of proximal convoluted tubule length increases threefold to fourfold (Celsi et al, 1986). The increase in active Na^+ reabsorption is associated with a threefold increase in Na^+,K^+-ATPase activity per millimeter of tubule length (Celsi et al, 1986) and with an increase in the number of cotransporters for glucose and bicarbonate reabsorption (Schwarz and Evan, 1983). The immature proximal tubule has a lower reflection coefficient for mannitol, indicating increased permeability of the proximal tubule to various solutes. The low capacity of the immature thick ascending limb of the loop of Henle to reabsorb Na^+ is associated with a low activity of the tubular Na^+,K^+-ATPase. As the consequence of the reduced Na^+ reabsorption in the loop of Henle, immature nephrons deliver a greater fraction of filtered Na^+ to the distal nephrons. The activity of the Na^+,K^+-ATPase also increases in this segment during development (Aperia et al, 1981). As a result of the maturational process, the fractional excretion of Na^+ decreases during development, from a value of 13% in the fetus to 3% in premature newborns less than 30 weeks of gestation and to 1% in term newborns (Fig. 91–5*B*) (Bueva and Guignard, 1994). Very-low-birth-weight infants may be at risk of negative sodium balance around the 2nd to 3rd week of life, when Na^+ retention is required for growth.

Body Fluid Tonicity

Although the volume of body fluids varies during growth, the tonicity of ECF is maintained constant by the kidneys, which excrete or retain appropriate amounts of water (see Chapter 34).

Excretion of Free Water

When the plasma osmolality decreases, the release of ADH also diminishes, leading to the excretion of dilute urine.

The newborn infant, preterm or term, is able to decrease urine osmolality to values as low as 40 mosm/L (Guignard et al, 1976). Because GFR is low in the newborn infant, the infant's ability to excrete large amounts of free water and consequently to cope with a hypotonic fluid load is limited leading to hyponatremia.

Hyponatremia may also occur in the syndrome of inappropriate secretion of ADH (SIADH), when the excretion of free water is impaired. This syndrome can occur in term as well as in preterm infants presenting with various cerebral injuries, pulmonary disorders, artificial ventilation, and drug toxicity (see Chapter 34).

Concentration of Urine

By comparison with adults who can concentrate urine up to 1400 mosm/L, the concentrating ability is limited in the newborn. The maximal urine osmolality achieved after dehydration or exogenous vasopressin administration (DDAVP 10 μg) remains below 430 and 630 mosm/L in 1- to 3-week-old and 4- to 6-week-old term infants. Osmolalities achieved by preterm newborns are slightly lower (Swenningsen and Aronson, 1974). The relative ineffectiveness of the concentrating ability of the newborn is related to several factors, including the low corticomedullary solute gradient associated with a limited accumulation of sodium chloride and urea in the medullary interstitium, the decreased formation of cAMP in response to ADH, the shortness of the loops of Henle, and the interference of prostaglandins with the vasopressin-stimulated cAMP synthesis (Joppich et al, 1979).

Extracellular Fluid Volume

Under normal conditions, plasma volume is closely related to ECF volume. Volume receptors distributed both on the venous (low-pressure receptors) and on the arterial side of the circulation sense the changes in plasma volume. Arterial sensors perceive the effective arterial volume. Atrial filling volume is monitored by stretch receptors, which mediate the release of the natriuretic peptide (Semmekrot and Guignard, 1991), promoting diuresis and natriuresis. Effective renal arterial volume is also sensed by baroreceptors located in the juxtamedullary apparatus of the kidney. A decrease in renal perfusion pressure activates the renin-angiotensin-aldosterone system (see Fig. 91–2). Angiotensin II, a potent renal and peripheral vasoconstrictor, then promotes sodium reabsorption, stimulates thirst, and favors the renal production of prostaglandins and bradykinin, hormones that play a role in sodium homeostasis. Aldosterone increases sodium reabsorption in the distal tubule promoting conservation of ECF volume. The neonatal period is characterized by the rapid physiologic constriction of the expanded ECF volume as well as by elevated levels of several hormonal systems participating in the regulation of sodium balance (see Chapter 34).

Although angiotensin II favors sodium retention by a direct action on the proximal tubule and by stimulating aldosterone secretion, the role of atrial natriuretic peptide in defending the plasma volume is still unclear. Elevated levels of atrial natriuretic peptide are present in the early postnatal period (Tulassay et al, 1987), but the relation to sodium homeostasis is still unclear (see Chapter 34). The same doubt applies to the relative importance of the kallikrein-kinin system and renal nerve activity in the defense of sodium homeostasis (see Chapter 34). The elevated levels of plasma renin activity, which are inversely correlated to gestational age, may be important for the maintenance and distribution of blood flow to various organs. The integrity of the renin-angiotensin system also appears crucial for the maintenance of RBF and GFR at low perfusion pressures (Guignard et al, 1991).

REGULATION OF ACID-BASE BALANCE

The kidney maintains acid-base balance by reclaiming the filtered bicarbonate and by excreting the daily production of fixed acids (see Chapter 34). Bicarbonate reabsorption occurs mainly in the proximal tubule. It is mediated by an active secretion of hydrogen ions and is closely linked to the tubular reabsorption of sodium. The excretion of fixed acids occurs mainly in the distal tubule, where secreted hydrogen ions are buffered by NH_3 and HPO_4^{-2} and excreted as NH_4^+ and $H_2PO_4^-$ (titratable acid). Free hydrogen ions determine the urine pH. The reabsorption of bicarbonate is increased by extracellular volume contraction, hypercapnia, hypokalemia, chloride deficiency, and aldosterone, and it is depressed by volume expansion, parathormone, and probably dopamine administration.

During fetal life, the placenta is responsible for the excretion of hydrogen ions. In experimental studies, the fetus responds to acid loading by increasing the excretion of NH_4^+ and titratable acid and by decreasing the urine pH. In human newborns, the threshold for bicarbonate reabsorption is reduced, leading to physiologic plasma bicarbonate concentrations as low as 16 to 20 mmol/L in the extremely immature infant and 19 to 21 mmol/L in term infants (Schwartz et al, 1979). The newborn infant is able to lower urine pH and increase both the excretion of NH_4^+ and titratable acidity in response to an acid load. Because of the tubular immaturity or relative unresponsiveness of the distal tubule to aldosterone, the response is somewhat blunted in the preterm infant. Proximal tubule immaturity or the relative expansion of the ECF volume at birth may account for the reduced bicarbonate threshold. Carbonic anhydrase, which accelerates bicarbonate reabsorption in the proximal tubule, is already present in the fetus and newborn and does not appear to be a limiting factor for bicarbonate reabsorption by the immature kidney (see Chapter 34).

The postnatal renal compensation for hypercapnia involves increased bicarbonate reabsorption and excretion of fixed acids to blunt a decrease in plasma pH. Whether this response, which has been found to be well developed in newborn animals (Heijden and Guignard, 1989), is mature in human newborns remains to be determined.

REGULATION OF POTASSIUM HOMEOSTASIS

Ninety-eight percent of the potassium in the body is intracellular, with a concentration close to 150 mmol/L. A high intracellular concentration of potassium is required for cell growth and division. Potassium homeostasis depends on an internal balance, which maintains a constant potassium concentration in the intracellular fluid and ECF space, and on an external balance, which requires that the potassium absorbed by the gastrointestinal tract in excess of the amount needed for growth be eventually excreted by the kidneys.

Potassium is actively reabsorbed in the proximal tubule and ascending limb of the loop of Henle, and the overall rate of excretion is determined by the function of the distal tubule and collecting duct. Plasma potassium concentration and aldosterone are the major physiologic regulators of potassium secretion. Hyperkalemia stimulates the Na^+, K^+-ATPase (see Chapter 34), increases the permeability of the luminal membrane to potassium, and stimulates the secretion of aldosterone by the adrenal cortex. Aldosterone, in turn, stimulates sodium reabsorption and enhances potassium secretion by stimulating the basolateral Na^+,K^+-ATPase leading to an elevation of the intracellular concentration of potassium and by increasing the permeability of the luminal membrane to potassium. Other factors favoring potassium secretion by the distal tubule and collecting duct include a rise in tubular flow rate, alkalosis, and an increase in the tubular fluid sodium concentration.

Potassium excretion remains low throughout gestation, and its concentration in fetal urine is below 3 mmol/L in healthy fetuses at 21 to 24 weeks of gestation (Golbus et al, 1985). The estimated daily rate of fetal accumulation of potassium lies between 0.6 and 0.8 mmol/kg (Wharton, 1987).

In healthy preterm infants with a positive potassium balance, potassium excretion remains stable during the 1st month of life, with mean values ranging from 1.29 to 1.48 mmol/kg per day (Guignard and John, 1986). The high sodium/potassium ratio present at birth decreases significantly with gestational and postnatal age (Sulyok et al, 1979), and it is thought to indicate the relative unresponsiveness of the distal tubule and collecting duct to aldosterone (Vanpee et al, 1988). In contrast with healthy premature infants, critically ill and stressed premature newborns may develop a negative potassium balance. In sick newborns, potassium losses can be exaggerated by the use of diuretics and volume expansion (see Chapter 34).

REGULATION OF CALCIUM, PHOSPHATE, AND MAGNESIUM HOMEOSTASIS

The kidney, in conjunction with the gastrointestinal tract and bone, plays a major role in maintaining calcium, phosphate, and magnesium homeostasis.

Regulation of Calcium Homeostasis

The total calcium concentration in plasma is maintained within narrow limits around 2.5 mmol/L. The distribution of calcium between the intracellular (bone) and extracellular compartment is mainly regulated by parathormone. Parathormone increases plasma calcium concentration by stimulating bone resorption, by activating the synthesis of $1,25(OH)_2$ vitamin D_3, and by increasing calcium reabsorption by the kidney. Normally 99% of the filtered calcium is reabsorbed by the nephron, mainly by the proximal tubule and the loop of Henle. In the proximal tubule and the thick ascending limb, calcium reabsorption is passive and closely linked to sodium reabsorption. By contrast, in the distal tubule and collecting duct, calcium reabsorption is active and independent of sodium transport, so that net calcium and sodium excretion do not always change in parallel. Parathormone is the main regulator of the renal excretion of calcium and it strongly stimulates calcium reabsorption in the distal tubule and collecting duct, resulting in a reduced calcium excretion. Volume expansion depresses both sodium and passive calcium reabsorption in the proximal tubule and thus increases calcium excretion. Calcium excretion is increased by acidosis and decreased by alkalosis. Finally, $1,25(OH)_2$ vitamin D_3 stimulates distal calcium reabsorption and thus decreases its excretion.

During the 26th to 36th weeks of gestation, the mean fetal accumulation of calcium is about 130 mg/kg per day (Forbes, 1976; Wharton, 1987). The calcium levels in fetal plasma are higher than the maternal levels. The fetal kidney is also able to produce $1,25(OH)_2$ vitamin D_3 effectively (Moore et al, 1985). During the neonatal period, the urinary calcium/creatinine ratio is higher in newborns than later in infancy (2.5 versus 0.7) (Matos et al, 1997). Loop diuretics are potent calciuric agents that may lead to neonatal nephrocalcinosis (see Chapter 34).

Regulation of Phosphate Homeostasis

Plasma phosphate approximates 2 mmol/L and is regulated by the kidney. In the urine, phosphate binds hydrogen ions and is eliminated as acid phosphate (a component of titratable acid). The phosphate released from the intracellular stores (mainly bone) is increased by parathormone and $1,25(OH)_2$ vitamin D_3. The proximal tubule reabsorbs approximately 80% of the filtered phosphate load, approximately 10% is reabsorbed by the distal tubule, and approximately 10% is excreted in the urine. Factors that increase the excretion of phosphate include parathormone, glucocorticoids, volume expansion, and acidosis. Parathormone is the main hormone regulating renal phosphate excretion, and it exerts this effect mainly by the inhibition of the Na^+/PO_4^{-3} cotransporter in the proximal tubule. Changes in dietary phosphate also modulate phosphate renal transport.

During the 26th to 36th weeks of gestation, the mean fetal accumulation of inorganic phosphate is close to 75 mg/kg per day (Wharton, 1987). At birth, 80% of the phosphorus is in bones (Royer, 1981). During early postnatal life, as a result of the efficient intestinal absorption and renal retention of phosphate, the newborn is in a positive phosphate balance and presents with elevated plasma concentrations of this anion (Brodehl et al, 1982; Key and Carpenter, 1990). Although fetuses and newborns appear to synthesize parathormone in response to hypocalcemia the phosphaturic response to parathormone is attenuated. This phenomenon may be due to a decreased sensitivity of the proximal tubule to the hormone and probably reflects homeostatic regulation at a time when phosphate retention is essential for growth. Growth hormone stimulates renal phosphate retention and increases the plasma concentration of phosphate.

Regulation of Magnesium Homeostasis

Magnesium is the second most abundant intracellular cation. It plays a major role in the regulation of protein synthesis and bone formation. The kidney maintains magnesium balance by excreting in the urine the amount of magnesium that is absorbed by the gastrointestinal tract in excess of the amount retained for growth. In normal conditions, approximately 3% of the magnesium filtered load is excreted in the urine. Magnesium is passively reabsorbed by the proximal tubule and the thick ascending limb. Regulation of magnesium excretion takes place in the thick ascending limb, where approximately 65% of the filtered load is reabsorbed. Factors that increase magnesium excretion include ECF volume expansion, acidosis, hypercalcemia, and hypermagnesemia. Parathormone decreases the excretion of magnesium.

During the 26th to 36th weeks of gestation, the mean fetal accumulation of magnesium approximates 3.5 mg/kg per day (Wharton, 1987). At birth, the serum magnesium concentration is close to 0.75 mmol/L and increases rapidly to 0.87 mmol/L during the first 3 days of life, at a time when the urinary excretion of magnesium is low (Chan et al, 1984). Magnesium excretion increases 10-fold during the 1st month of life to reach values close to 2 mg/kg per day (DeSanto et al, 1988). Serum magnesium level follows a circadian rhythm, being higher at night (DeSanto et al, 1988). Newborn hypomagnesemia is associated with intrauterine growth retardation. Newborn hypermagnesemia frequently occurs after maternal magnesium administration in the immediately before birth.

REFERENCES

Aperia A, Larsson L, Zetterström R: Hormonal induction of Na-K-ATPase in developing proximal tubular cells. Am J Physiol 241:F356, 1981.

Bailie MD: Development of the endocrine function of the kidney. Clin Perinatol 19:59, 1992.

Brodehl J, Gellissen K, Weber HP: Postnatal development of tubular phosphate reabsorption. Clin Nephrol 17:163, 1982.

Bueva A, Guignard JP: Renal function in preterm neonates. Pediatr Res 36:572, 1994.

Celsi G, Larsson L, Aperia A: Proximal tubular reabsorption and Na-K-ATPase activity on remnant kidney of young rats. Am J Physiol 251:F588, 1986.

Chan GM, Nordmeyer FR, Richter BE, et al: Comparison of serum total calcium, dialysable calcium and dialysable magnesium in well and sick newborns. Clin Physiol Biochem 2:154, 1984.

Chevalier RL, Carey RM, Kaiser DC: Endogenous prostaglandins modulate autoregulation of renal blood flow in young rats. Am J Physiol 253:F66, 1987.

Coulthard MG, Ruddock V: Validation of inulin as a marker for glomerular filtration in preterm babies. Kidney Int 23:407, 1983.

Deen PMT, Croes H, van Aubel R, et al: Water channels encoded by mutant aquaporin-2 genes in nephrogenic diabetes insipidus are impaired in their cellular routing. J Clin Invest 95:2291, 1995.

Delivoria-Papadopoulos M, Battaglia FC, Bruns PD, et al: Total, protein-bound, and ultrafilterable calcium in maternal and fetal plasma. Am J Physiol 21:363, 1967.

DeSanto NG, Dilorio B, Capasso G, et al: Circadian rhythm with acrophase at night for urinary excretion of calcium and magnesium in childhood: Population-based data of the Cimitile study in southern Italy. Miner Electrolyte Metab 14:235, 1988.

Forbes GB: Calcium accumulation by the human fetus. Pediatrics 57:976, 1976.

Gilliéron P, Thonney M, Cochat P, et al: Mild hypothermia or hyperthermia significantly affect renal function in immature rabbits. Pediatr Nephrol 9:C48, 1995.

Golbus MS, Filly RA, Callen PU, et al: Fetal urinary tract obstruction: Management and selection for treatment. Semin Perinatol 9:91, 1985.

Grannum P, Bracken M, Silverman R, et al: Assessment of kidney size in normal gestation by comparison of ratio of kidney circumference to abdominal circumference. Am J Obstet Gynecol 136:249, 1980.

Gouyon JB, Guignard JP: Adenosine in the immature kidney. Dev Pharmacol Ther 13:113, 1989.

Guignard JP: Renal function in the newborn infant. Pediatr Clin North Am 29:777, 1982.

Guignard JP, Torrado A, Da Cunha O, et al: Glomerular filtration rate in the first three weeks of life. J Pediatr 87:268, 1975.

Guignard JP, Torrado A, Mazouni SM, et al: Renal function in respiratory distress syndrome. J Pediatr 88:845, 1976.

Guignard JP, John EG: Renal function in the tiny, premature infant. Clin Perinatol 13:377, 1986.

Guignard JP, Gouyon JB, John EG: Vasoactive factors in the immature kidney. Pediatr Nephrol 5:443, 1991.

Heijden vd AJ, Guignard JP: Bicarbonate reabsorption by the kidney of the newborn rabbit. Am J Physiol 256:F29, 1989.

Jeanty P, Dramaix WM, Elkhazen N, et al: Measurement of fetal kidney growth on ultrasound. Radiology 144:159, 1982.

Joppich R, Kollmann D, Ingrich U, et al: Urinary cyclic AMP and renal concentrating capacity in infants. Eur J Pediatr 124:113, 1979.

Key LL, Carpenter TO: Metabolism of calcium, phosphorus and other divalent ions. *In* Ichikawa I (Ed): Pediatric Textbook of Fluids Electrolytes. Baltimore, Williams & Wilkins, 1990, p 98.

Lee MD, King LS, Agre P: The aquaporin family of water channel proteins in clinical medicine. Medicine 76:141, 1997.

Matos V, Van Melle G, Boulat O, et al: Urinary phosphate, calcium and magnesium to creatinine ratios in a healthy pediatric population. J Pediatr 131:252, 1997.

Merlet-Bnichou C, Leroy B, Gilbert T, et al: Retard de croissance intra-uterine et deficit en nephrons. Med Sci 9:777, 1993

Moore ES, Langmann CB, Favus MJ, et al: Role of fetal 1,25-dihydroxyvitamin D production in intrauterine phosphorus and calcium homeostasis. Pediatr Res 19:566, 1985.

Rabinovitz R, Peters MD, Vyas C, et al: Measurement of fetal urine production in normal pregnancy by real-time ultrasonography. Am J Obstet Gynecol 161:1264, 1989.

Robillard JE, Segar JL, Smith FG, et al: Regulation of sodium metabolism and extracellular fluid volume during development. Clin Perinatol 19:15, 1992.

Robillard JE, Weitzman RE: Developmental aspects of the fetal renal response to exogenous arginine vasopressin. Am J Physiol 238:F407, 1980.

Royer P: Growth and development of bony tissue. *In* Davis JA, Dobbing J (Eds): Scientific Foundations of Paediatrics. London, William Heinemann Medical Books Ltd, 1981, p 565.

Savin VJ, Beason-Griffin C, Richardson WP: Ultrafiltration coefficient of isolated glomeruli of rats aged 4 days to maturation. Kidney Int 28:926, 1985.

Schwarz GJ, Evan AP: Development of solute transport in rabbit proximal tubule: I. HCH_3^- and glucose absorption. Am J Physiol 245:F382, 1983.

Schwarz GJ, Haycock JB, Edelmann CM Jr, et al: Late metabolic acidosis: A reassessment of the definition. J Pediatr 95:102, 1979.

Semama DS, Thonney M, Guignard JP: Role of endogenous endothelin in renal hemodynamics of newborn rabbits. Pediatr Nephrol 7:886, 1993.

Semmekrot B, Guignard JP: Atrial natriuretic peptide during early human development. Biol Neonate 60:341, 1991.

Seri I: Cardiovascular, renal and endocrine actions of dopamine in newborns and children. J Pediatr 126:333, 1995.

Stonestreet BS, Bell EF, Oh W: Validity of endogenous creatinine clearance in low-birth-weight infants. Pediatr Res 13:1012, 1979.

Swenningsen NW, Aronson AS: Postnatal development of renal concentration capacity as estimated by DDAVP test in normal and asphyxiated neonates. Biol Neonate 25:230, 1974.

Sulyok E, Nemeth M, Tenyi I, et al: Postnatal development of renin-angiotensin aldosterone system (RAAS) in relation to electrolyte balance in premature infants. Pediatr Res 13:817, 1979.

Tulassay T, Seri I, Rascher W: Atrial natriuretic peptide and extracellular volume contraction after birth. Acta Paediatr Scand 76:444, 1987.

Van den Anker JN, De Groot R, Broerse HM, et al: Assessment of glomerular filtration rate in preterm infants by serum creatinine: Comparison with inulin clearance. Pediatrics 96:1156, 1995

Vanpee M, Blennow M, Linne T, et al: Renal function in very low birth weight infants: Normal maturity reached during early childhood. J Pediatr 121:784, 1992.

Vanpee M, Herin P, Zetterström R: Postnatal development of renal function in very low birth weight infants. Acta Paediatr Scand 77:191, 1988.

Veille JC, Hanson RA, Tatum K, et al: Quantitative assessment of human fetal renal blood flow. Am J Obstet Gynecol 169:1399, 1993.

Wharton BA: Calcium, phosphorus and magnesium. *In* Nutrition and Feeding of Preterm Infants. Oxford, Blackwell Scientific, 1987, p 111.

CHAPTER 92

Clinical Evaluation of Renal and Urinary Tract Disease

Istvan Seri and Jacquelyn Evans

PRENATAL EVALUATION OF RENAL AND URINARY TRACT DISEASE

Prenatal Diagnosis

Ultrasonography has become the most widely used and effective diagnostic tool in the prenatal evaluation of the fetal kidneys and urinary tract. Since the first report of the in utero ultrasound diagnosis of congenital renal disease in 1970 by Garett and colleagues, the prenatal diagnosis of most forms of congenital renal and urinary tract malformations has been reported. The detection rate of fetal congenital urologic abnormalities by ultrasonography is approximately 0.2% (Arger et al, 1986; Shackelford et al, 1992). As the incidence of renal and urinary tract malformations in the general population is close to 1%, approximately one in five cases is diagnosed prenatally by ultrasonography.

The most common indication for an ultrasound survey of the fetal genitourinary tract is the presence of oligohydramnios (Bruno et al, 1985). Another important indication is a positive family history for renal disease because fetal urinary tract abnormalities have been reported in 8% of pregnancies with a family history of renal anomalies (Reuss et al, 1987).

The fetal kidneys can be identified early in the second trimester (Patten et al, 1990). A more detailed view of the kidneys, however, is usually appreciated only from the 30th week of gestation. The normal ureter cannot be visualized by prenatal ultrasonography. The normal fetal bladder can be routinely identified by the 16th week of gestation, although it sometimes can be visualized as early as the 13th week (Patten et al, 1990).

Hydronephrosis is readily identifiable by prenatal ultrasonography and is most frequently due to ureteropelvic obstruction. Other causes of fetal hydronephrosis include bladder outlet or ureteral obstruction, polycystic kidney disease, multicystic dysplastic kidney disease, renal agenesis, congenital megaureter, duplication anomalies, reflux, and prune-belly syndrome. A mildly dilated (1 to 2 mm) renal pelvis has been reported in 41% of routine prenatal ultrasound examinations (Cohen and Haller, 1987). This is often a normal prenatal finding reflecting the functional dilation of the urinary tract secondary to high fetal urine flow rates.

Although prenatal ultrasonography has become standard for fetal evaluation, there are many potential pitfalls of this technique even in experienced hands. Because diagnostic error may occur in up to 30% of the cases (Colodny, 1987), appropriate postnatal studies should always confirm the prenatal diagnosis.

Fetal karyotype analysis and, in cases of certain types of obstructive uropathy, serial measurements of urine osmolality and electrolyte and protein excretion assist in the intrauterine diagnostic evaluation of fetuses with suspected renal and urinary tract anomalies (Johnson et al, 1994; Sullivan and Adzick, 1994). Detection of elevated amniotic fluid alpha-fetoprotein in conjunction with normal acetylcholinesterase activity suggests the intrauterine diagnosis of congenital nephrotic syndrome (Ghidini et al, 1994). Prenatal diagnosis of the autosomal dominant form of polycystic kidney disease using DNA probes has also become available.

Prenatal Management

In the fetus with severe obstructive uropathy, if the condition is bilateral or if there is a solitary kidney, the decrease in fetal urine output results in severe oligohydramnios or anhydramnios leading to pulmonary hypoplasia, the Potter sequence, and extremely high neonatal mortality. Early obstruction affects normal glomerular and tubular differentiation and, if untreated, leads to the development of irreversible renal dysplasia. Percutaneous vesicoamniotic shunt, bladder stent, and open bladder marsupialization encompass the choices of fetal intervention (Sullivan and Adzick, 1994). The goal of prenatal management is to relieve the obstruction during the most active period of nephrogenesis (i.e., between 20 and 32 weeks of gestation).

The integrated evaluation of the findings of prenatal ultrasound; fetal karyotyping; and fetal urine electrolyte, osmolality, and protein studies has been used to identify fetuses with bilateral obstructive uropathies who have not yet progressed to a stage of irreversible renal damage. Because only the third or fourth urine sample is predictive of long-term prognosis (Evans et al, 1991; Johnson et al, 1994), serial vesiconcenteses are recommended to be performed at 48- to 72-hour intervals. Fetuses whose third or fourth urine examination shows a sodium of less than 100 mg/dL, osmolality of less than 200 mOsm/L, total protein of less than 20 mg/dL, and beta$_2$-microglobulin of less than 4 mg/L are considered to be candidates for fetal surgery.

In addition to the predicted long-term renal outcome, other important factors influencing prenatal management of fetuses with obstructive uropathy include gestational age, lung maturity, and associated anomalies. If associated life-threatening anomalies or chromosome abnormalities are detected, the options are expectant management or termination of pregnancy. For the fetus with isolated obstructive uropathy and predicted irreversible renal dysplasia, in utero decompression is not recommended. In fetuses with isolated obstructive uropathy but predicted good long-term renal outcome, treatment depends on gestational age and lung maturity. If the fetus is less than 32 weeks of gestation, intrauterine decompression is advocated. If the fetus is 32 weeks or more of gestation, maternal steroid treatment and, once lung maturity is achieved, delivery of the fetus is recommended. Fetuses with immature lungs and isolated obstructive uropathy with normal or only mildly diminished amniotic fluid volume do not require active intervention in utero (Johnson et al, 1994).

POSTNATAL EVALUATION OF RENAL AND URINARY TRACT DISEASE
History

Renal disease in the newborn is more likely when there is a *family history* of renal disease, including urinary tract anomalies; renal agenesis; hereditary nephritis; polycystic kidney disease; medullary cystic disease; vesicoureteral reflux; and tubular disorders such as Fanconi syndrome, cystinuria, and nephrogenic diabetes insipidus. Appropriate screening of newborns for renal disease who have a positive family history of inherited diseases associated with renal anomalies is also indicated.

Prenatal and Perinatal History

A history of oligohydramnios or anhydramnios suggests the presence of bilateral renal agenesis, severe renal dysplasia, or obstructive uropathy. Polyhydramnios may occur with fetal nephrogenic diabetes insipidus. A difficult delivery secondary to increased abdominal girth may signal the presence of renal masses. A disproportionally large placenta should prompt the clinician to rule out congenital nephrotic syndrome in the newborn (Mahan et al, 1984). A history of perinatal asphyxia, acute hemorrhage, sepsis, hyaline membrane disease, antenatal or postnatal indomethacin therapy, and hypernatremic dehydration of the very-low-birth-weight newborn are conditions that should alert the clinician to the possibility of the development of postnatal acute renal failure.

Evaluation of Presenting Signs and Symptoms
Laboratory Tests and Methods of Evaluation of Renal Function
Urine Collection

Urine collection in the newborn is most commonly performed by the use of special collection bags. With the exemption of urine culture studies, this method provides an adequate sample for most of the routine tests. To document urinary tract infection, suprapubic bladder aspiration is recommended as the most reliable method. Bladder catheterization is mainly used in infants who fail to pass urine after the 1st day of life and in severely ill newborns who are paralyzed or heavily sedated.

Urinalysis

Analysis of the urine in the normal term newborn during the first few days of life shows a specific gravity of 1001 to 1021 with a corresponding osmolality of 50 to 800 mOsm/L. Maximal urine osmolality in preterm infants is less than in term newborns. The impaired concentrating capacity of the newborn kidney is the consequence of renal anatomic and functional immaturity, including the decreased hypertonicity of the renal medulla and the relative insensitivity of the immature collecting tubule to vasopressin (Roy et al, 1992).

Proteinuria

During the first few days of life, proteinuria can be detected in 76% of healthy newborns. Conditions affecting renal blood flow and tubular function, such as dehydration or perinatal asphyxia, frequently result in a usually transient but significant proteinuria. Proteinuria greater than 30 mg/dL in a concentrated urine persisting beyond the 1st week of life, however, suggests glomerular or tubular injury and requires further evaluation (Aviles et al, 1992). Persistent and massive proteinuria may indicate congenital nephrotic syndrome and necessitate renal biopsy.

Hematuria, Hemoglobinuria, and Myoglobinuria

Normal newborns do not have hematuria, hemoglobinuria, or myoglobinuria. Hematuria may occur in patients with perinatal asphyxia, acute renal failure, renal vein or artery thrombosis, congenital urinary malformations including autosomal recessive polycystic kidney disease and obstructive uropathies, coagulopathies, urinary tract infections, and trauma. Hematuria in a newborn with an umbilical arterial catheter in place should alert the clinician to the possibility of aortic and renal artery thrombosis. Finally, transient hematuria is a common finding in critically ill newborns. Hemoglobinuria and myoglobinuria may present in patients with intravascular hemolysis and rhabdomyolysis.

Uric Acid, Electrolyte, Glucose, and Amino Acid Excretion

As a result of increased uric acid production and fractional excretion, urinary excretion of uric acid is high during the 1st week in normal preterm and full-term infants, causing colored diaper stains and false-positive tests for proteinuria. Because the newborn's urine is dilute and not significantly acidic, however, uric acid precipitation and acute urate nephropathy are rare in the neonatal period. Because of the immaturity of their renal tubular transport processes, premature newborns also excrete more sodium, bicarbonate, phosphorus, glucose, and amino acids in the urine compared to full-term newborns (Jones and Chesney, 1992).

Sediment

The urinary sediment of the normal newborn contains fewer than 5 squamous epithelial cells, 0 to 2 red blood cells, and fewer than 5 white blood cells per high-power field. The most common cause of leukocyturia is urinary tract infection. The presence of casts in the sediment usually suggests an involvement of the upper urinary tract in the disease process. Red blood cell casts indicate glomerular injury, whereas white blood cell casts are present with infection or interstitial or tubular damage. Epithelial cell casts and granular casts may be seen in newborns with severe dehydration or may also represent interstitial or tubular injury. Hyaline casts are detected in cases of severe proteinuria or dehydration.

Serum Chemistry and Clearance Studies

Serum chemistry and clearance studies reflect the status of fluid and electrolyte balance and renal function. Mainly as a result of their excessive insensible water losses during the first few days of life (Sedin, 1995), very immature preterm infants cared for under radiant warmers require frequent serum electrolyte studies as well as close monitoring of the changes in their body weight and urine output to guide daily fluid administration (see Chapter 35).

An endogenous substance that can best be used to characterize glomerular function must have a constant turnover rate and be freely filtered and must not be reabsorbed; secreted; protein bound; or subject to synthesis, metabolism, or storage by the kidney. Although the turnover rate of creatinine is unknown in sick newborns and creatinine is not only filtered, but also secreted and reabsorbed by the immature kidney (Aviles et al, 1992; Bueva and Guignard, 1994), it is the endogenous substance that comes closest to fulfilling the above-mentioned requirements. In clinical practice, sequential determination rather than a single value of serum creatinine gives the most valuable information on glomerular filtration rate.

In term infants, serum creatinine is approximately 0.8 mg/dL at birth and remains between 0.7 to 0.9 mg/dL during the first 2 days of life (Bueva and Guignard, 1994; Feldman and Guignard, 1982). Thereafter serum creatinine gradually decreases to approximately 0.5 mg/dL by 1 week of age and to approximately 0.4 mg/dL by the end of the 1st month (Bueva and Guignard, 1994; Feldman and Guignard, 1982). During the first few days of life, serum creatinine levels are significantly higher in preterm than in term infants (0.8 to 1.8 mg/dL versus 0.7 to 0.9 mg/dL), with the highest levels observed in the most immature newborns (Bueva and Guignard, 1994; Stonestreet and Oh, 1978). This finding supports the notion that glomerular filtration rate is low in the preterm infant, who, immediately after birth, is unable to eliminate the excess creatinine transferred in utero from the mother (Aviles et al, 1992; Bueva and Guignard, 1994). By the 2nd week of life, however, serum creatinine begins to fall and drops below 0.6 mg/dL, even in the very-low-birth-weight infant (Bueva and Guignard, 1994).

In addition to serum creatinine, blood urea nitrogen (BUN) has been used widely in clinical practice to assess renal function. Because BUN is also influenced by the state of hydration, protein intake, and urinary flow rate, however, it is a much less reliable marker of renal function than serum creatinine.

Applying the concept of clearance measurements, the rate of sodium and water reabsorption may also be estimated in the different nephron segments (Aviles et al, 1992). Despite its limitations, this is the only way to assess sodium and water reabsorption along the nephron in the intact human kidney. The information obtained may then be used to detect changes in proximal and distal tubule sodium and water handling during development or disease. For a concise review on this subject, the reader is referred to the article by Avilles and colleagues (1992).

Physical Examination

Disorders of Micturition

Although many healthy newborn infants do not void until 12 to 24 hours of life, 92% to 100% of them pass urine by the end of the 1st day (Clark, 1977). The delay in voiding in the healthy newborn is mostly due to the labor and delivery–triggered cardiovascular and hormonal changes and their effects on renal function. Among others, a significant increase in vasopressin (Ramin et al, 1991) and catecholamine release (Lagerkrantz and Bistoletti, 1973; Mehandru et al, 1993) occurs during labor and delivery. These hormonal changes contribute to the decrease in the effective circulating plasma volume (Brace, 1992) and directly cause renal vasoconstriction and an augmentation of sodium and water reabsorption. If a normotensive newborn has not passed urine during the first 24 hours of life, the presence of hypovolemia or other causes of compensated shock or severe bilateral renal or urinary tract anomalies should be considered.

Abdominal Masses

Deep abdominal palpation can be most easily performed during the first 24 hours of life when abdominal tone is still somewhat decreased, and air does not completely fill the gastrointestinal tract. Thereafter, deep abdominal palpation is best done with the sucking reflex evoked because this reflex also induces abdominal muscle relaxation. Palpable abdominal masses are present in 0.2% to 0.6% of newborns (Museles et al, 1971; Perlman and Williams, 1976). Two thirds of these masses are of renal origin, and most of the remaining arise from the adrenal gland, the gastrointestinal tract, the female genitalia, or the liver. Hydronephrosis and dysplastic and polycystic kidney disease lead most frequently to palpable renal masses during the neonatal period. In the case of a midline abdominal mass, the presence of posterior urethral valves or a neurogenic bladder should always be considered. The discovered abdominal mass should then be further studied by ultrasonography, computed tomography (CT) scan, or magnetic resonance imaging (MRI) and, if appropriate, by renal cystourethrography, radionuclide scan, or intravenous pyelography.

Edema

Accumulation of fluid in the interstitial space occurs because of an imbalance in Starling forces and is a frequent finding in the preterm and term newborn. In the newborn with acute renal failure, *generalized edema* is most frequently due to a relative fluid overload in face of the markedly decreased glomerular filtration rate. In neonatal nephrotic syndrome, edema develops because increased urinary protein losses result in a marked drop in colloid osmotic pressure. In the edematous newborn with renal disease, additional hormonal factors may also contribute to the pathophysiology of edema formation. Such factors include the elevated activity of the renin-angiotensin-aldosterone system, increased bradykinin and prostaglandin production, high neonatal plasma prolactin levels, and attenuation of the renal effects of atrial natriuretic peptide.

Generalized edema in the neonatal period occurs most frequently, however, with conditions other than primary renal disease. Otherwise healthy premature newborns and full-term infants born to diabetic mothers may present with generalized edema owing to complex, hormone-regulated alterations in the dynamics of their physiologic fluid shift during early neonatal adaptation. Iatrogenic causes of edema formation frequently include volume overload, aggressive sodium supplementation during the period of early neonatal adaptation, and, in cases of late edema formation of the preterm newborn, maintenance of a high sodium intake after the infant converts from the sodium-losing to the sodium-retaining state (see also Chapter 35). Generalized edema is also a prominent clinical feature of congestive heart failure and of neonatal conditions characterized by generalized capillary leak, including hypoxia, hydrops, sepsis, and shock. Other, less common causes of generalized edema include severe anemia, liver failure, protein-losing enteropathy, congenital infections, syndrome of inappropriate secretion of antidiuretic hormone, congenital analbuminemia, vitamin E deficiency, hyperaldosteronism, and hereditary angioneurotic edema.

Characteristic congenital *localized edema* is present in newborns with gonadal dysgenesis and primary lymphedema (Milroy disease) (Greenlee et al, 1993). Localized edema in the sick newborn also occurs with impairment of venous return or lymphatic drainage as seen in the frequently catheter-related thromboses of major veins including the superior and inferior vena cava and the femoral and axillary veins. Iatrogenic and mostly benign occurrence is the localized limb edema associated with the use of restrictive boards to protect intravenous sites.

Ascites

Renal causes of intraperitoneal accumulation of fluid in the newborn include congenital urinary tract obstruction and nephrotic syndrome. The ascites in congenital urinary tract obstruction represents urine that has entered the peritoneal cavity after the rupture of the renal pelvis or one of the calyces. The ascitic fluid usually undergoes peritoneal dialysis and may lose most of the chemical characteristics of the urine. If the abdominal ultrasound study also demonstrates the presence of a thickened bladder, bladder outlet obstruction is the most likely diagnosis. The ascites in nephrotic syndrome has the character of an exudate. Nonrenal causes of ascites include bacterial or chemical peritonitis, congenital anomalies of the abdominal lymphatic system or biliary tree, malrotation, incomplete volvulus, ruptured ovarian cyst, and, extremely rarely, pancreatitis secondary to congenital pancreatic duct anomaly.

External Genitalia

In general, an association between anomalies of the external genitalia and the upper urinary tract is infrequent. In the male, however, abnormalities of mesonephric development may lead to unilateral or bilateral renal agenesis and lack of testicular development. In the female, such abnormalities may result in unilateral or bilateral renal agenesis and uterine abnormalities. Furthermore, newborns with bilateral cryptorchidism, unilateral cryptorchi-

dism and hypospadias, or penoscrotal or perineoscrotal hypospadias, who require thorough clinical and genetic evaluation for appropriate sex assignment, may also benefit from a renal ultrasound study to rule out possible renal or upper urinary tract anomalies (Laurance et al, 1976).

Hypertension

As discussed in detail in Chapter 99, renal vascular and parenchymal diseases as well as urinary tract anomalies may lead to the development of systemic hypertension. Therefore, the diagnostic work-up of neonatal hypertension should always include, but not be limited to, the evaluation of renal anatomy, function, and vascular integrity.

Evaluation of Renal and Urinary Tract Morphology

Ultrasonography

Ultrasonography has become the primary imaging technique in the postnatal evaluation of renal and urinary tract disorders in the newborn. Prenatal findings suggestive of urogenital anomalies should be followed up with a postnatal sonogram. The most common reasons for postnatal ultrasonographic assessment of the urinary tract are the prenatal finding of fetal hydronephrosis, the presence of urinary tract infection, and the detection of an abdominal mass in the newborn. Oligohydramnios in the absence of signs of placental dysfunction, unexplained tension pneumothorax in a nonventilated infant, failure to void, a poor urinary stream, the presence of a single umbilical artery, abnormal or low-set ears, perineal or anal anomalies, vertebral anomalies with or without VATER/VACTERL association, decreased abdominal wall musculature, unexplained elevation of serum creatinine, significant hematuria, proteinuria, and renal tubular acidosis are also indications for ultrasonographic evaluation of the urinary tract in the neonatal period. Finally, because prolonged administration of furosemide is associated with an increased incidence of nephrocalcinosis, screening ultrasound examinations are warranted in newborns on long-term diuretic treatment with furosemide in the presence of hematuria. Doppler ultrasound, a noninvasive method of detecting renal blood flow, is helpful in the evaluation of suspected renal arterial and venous thrombosis.

Voiding Cystourethrography

Voiding cystourethrography, an important complement to ultrasonography, can identify anatomic and functional abnormalities in lower urinary tract disorders. It is particularly important in the evaluation of urinary tract infection for the detection and assessment of vesicoureteral reflux.

Radionuclide cystography significantly decreases radiation exposure to the patient and has gained acceptance in the pediatric population, especially for the follow-up of vesicoureteral reflux in children. It has considerable technical limitations in the newborn, however, and it has not been widely used in this patient population.

Radionuclide Renal Imaging

Renal scintigraphy provides information about renal blood flow and function and is primarily used in the follow-up of infants with obstructive uropathy. It has all but replaced intravenous urography in the newborn, especially during the first 2 weeks of life, when the renal concentration of iodinated agents is limited. Although renal scintigraphy provides less anatomic detail than intravenous urography, it offers useful physiologic information with reasonable anatomic definition and less radiation exposure. It is also a reliable quantitative method of following renal function before and after surgery for obstructive uropathy.

Angiography

Because of advances in Doppler ultrasonography and radionuclide scintigraphy techniques, renal angiography has been used less frequently in the newborn. It provides accurate anatomic information of the renal arterial and venous circulation but is invasive and poses a significant radiation exposure to the newborn.

Renal Computed Tomography and Magnetic Resonance Imaging

Both CT and MRI provide high-resolution cross-sectional imaging. For most indications of neonatal renal imaging, however, CT and MRI do not offer a significant advantage over sonography or renal scintigraphy. CT and MRI also usually require sedation and immobilization. These techniques may play a role in neonatal uroimaging when findings of other techniques are inconclusive.

Renal Biopsy

Ultrasound-guided renal biopsy is performed in neonatal renal diseases if a tissue sample is required for the final diagnosis. Such conditions include but are not limited to Finnish-type nephrotic syndrome, nail-patella syndrome, autosomal recessive and autosomal dominant polycystic kidney disease, glomerulocystic kidney disease, and complex tubular functional abnormalities.

Acknowledgment

The authors thank Drs. Richard D. Bellah and Seth Schulman for their critical review of the manuscript.

REFERENCES

Arger PH, Coleman BG, Mintz MC, et al: Routine fetal genitourinary tract screening. Radiology 156:485, 1986.

Aviles DH, Fildes RD, Jose PA: Evaluation of renal function. Clin Perinatol 19:69, 1992.

Brace AB: Fluid distribution in the fetus and neonate. *In* Polin RA, Fox WW (Eds): Fetal and Neonatal Physiology. Philadelphia, WB Saunders, 1992, pp 1288–1298.

Bruno AN, Lavin JP, Nasrallah PF: Ultrasound experience with prenatal genitourinary abnormalities. Urology 26:196, 1985.

Bueva A, Guignard JP: Renal function in preterm neonates. Pediatr Res 36:572, 1994.

Clark DA: Times of first void and first stool in 500 newborns. Pediatrics 60:457, 1977.

Cohen HL, Haller JO: Diagnostic sonography of the fetal genitourinary tract. Urol Radiol 9:88, 1987.

Colodny AH: Antenatal diagnosis and management of urinary abnormalities. Pediatr Clin North Am 34:1365, 1987.

Crombleholme TM, Harrison MR, Longaker MT, Langer JC: Prenatal diagnosis and management of bilateral hydronephrosis. Pediatr Nephrol 2:334, 1988.

Evans MI, Sacks AJ, Johnson MP, et al: Sequential invasive assessment of fetal renal function and intrauterine treatment of fetal obstructive uropathies. Obstet Gynecol 77:545, 1991.

Feldman H, Guignard JP: Plasma creatinine in the first month of life. Arch Dis Child 57:123, 1982.

Garett WJ, Grunwald G, Robinson DE: Prenatal diagnosis of fetal polycystic kidney disease by ultrasound. Aust N Z J Obstet Gynaecol 10:7, 1970.

Ghidini A, Alvarez M, Silverberg G, et al: Congenital nephrosis in low-risk pregnancies. Prenat Diagn 14:599, 1994.

Greenlee R, Hoyme H, Witte M, et al: Developmental disorders of the lymphatic system. Lymphology 26:156, 1993.

Johnson MP, Bukowski TP, Reitleman C, et al: In utero surgical treatment of fetal obstructive uropathy: A new comprehensive approach to identify appropriate candidates for vesicoamniotic shunt therapy. Am J Obstet Gynecol 170:1770, 1994.

Jones DP, Chesney RW: Development of tubular function. Clin Perinatol 19:33, 1992.

Lagerkrantz H, Bistoletti P: Catecholamine release in the newborn infant at birth. Pediatr Res 11:889, 1973.

Laurance BM, Darby CW, Vanderschueren-Lodeweyck M: Two XX males diagnosed in childhood: Endocrine, renal, and laboratory findings. Arch Dis Child 51:144, 1976.

Mahan JD, Mauer SM, Sibley RK: Congenital nephrotic syndrome, evolution of medical management and results of renal transplantation. J Pediatr 105:549, 1984.

Mehandru PL, Assel BG, Nuamah IF, et al: Catecholamine response at birth in preterm newborns. Biol Neonate 64:82, 1993.

Museles M, Gaundry CL, Bason MW: Renal anomalies in the newborn found by deep palpation. Pediatrics 47:97, 1971.

Patten RM, Mack LA, Wang KY, Cyr DR: The fetal genitourinary tract. Radiol Clin North Am 28:115, 1990.

Perlman M, Williams J: Detection of renal anomalies by abdominal palpation in the newborn infant. BMJ 2:347, 1976.

Ramin SM, Porter JC, Gilstrap LC III, Rosenfeld CR: Stress hormones and acid base status of human fetuses at delivery. J Clin Endocrinol Metab 73:182, 1991.

Reuss A, Wladimiroff JW, Niermeijer MF: Antenatal diagnosis of renal tract anomalies by ultrasound. Pediatr Nephrol 1:546, 1987.

Roy DR, Layton HE, Jamison RL: Countercurrent mechanism and its regulation. *In* Seldin DW, Giebisch G (Eds): The Kidney: Physiology and Pathophysiology, 2nd ed. New York, Raven Press, 1992, pp 1649–1692.

Sedin G: Fluid management in the extremely preterm infant. *In* Hansen TN, McIntosh N (Eds): Current Topics in Neonatology. London, WB Saunders, 1995, pp 50–66.

Shackelford GD, Kees-Folts D, Cole BR: Imaging the urinary tract. Clin Perinatol 19:85, 1992.

Stonestreet BS, Oh W: Plasma creatinine levels in low birth weight infants during the first three months of life. Pediatrics 61:788, 1978.

Sullivan KM, Adzick NS: Fetal surgery. Clin Obstet Gynecol 37:355, 1994.

CHAPTER 93

Developmental Abnormalities of the Kidneys

Bernard S. Kaplan

The increasing use of prenatal ultrasonography, continuing improvements in ventilator and nutritional support, and progress in dialysis techniques for newborns and renal transplantation for young children have changed the natural history of cystic and dysplastic kidney diseases. To manage a newborn with a genetic or developmental disorder of the kidneys optimally, much information must be gathered from many sources and must be carefully evaluated. Clearly a team approach is needed. Errors occur with insufficient data, inadequate communication, and when the natural history of these conditions is not understood. Because newborns can be dialyzed and transplanted when they reach 8 to 10 kg, some of these problems impose enormous emotional and financial burdens on families. Therefore a precise diagnosis must be made before starting dialysis. The diagnosis depends on the evaluation of the prenatal history, results of fetal ultrasonography, family history, clinical examination, imaging studies of the infants and parents when indicated, laboratory studies (including DNA tests if available), and interpretation of pathology.

Several guiding principles are worth keeping in mind. Few genetic renal disorders are confined to the kidneys, and many syndromes have renal involvement. Therefore, ultrasonography of the kidneys and urinary tract should be done in all newborns with multiple defects. Also, ultrasonographic features can change over time. Variable expression of congenital renal defects may occur within and among kindreds; this is particularly true in autosomal recessive polycystic kidney disease. There are many classifications of cystic and dysplastic kidneys, but the one shown in Table 93–1 lists the conditions that can be seen in newborns.

ECTOPIC KIDNEY, HORSESHOE KIDNEY, AND CROSSED FUSED ECTOPIA

Ectopic kidney, horseshoe kidney, and crossed fused ectopia are abnormalities in the position of the kidney(s) that do not have important long-term effects unless associated with lower urinary tract anomalies, such as reflux or obstruction. In essence, these kidneys are at risk for the same problems as those in normal positions. Horseshoe kidney, however, does occur with increased frequency in Turner syndrome and other syndromes. A voiding cystourethrogram should be done to exclude the possibility of reflux, and a technetium 99m–labeled diethylenetriaminepentaacetic acid (DTPA) scan should be done if there is evidence on ultrasonography of an obstruction.

MULTICYSTIC KIDNEY

Multicystic kidney is the second most common cause of a flank mass in the newborn with a prevalence of 1 in 4300. Multicystic kidney is almost always a sporadic, nonsyndro-

mal, congenital anomaly. The diagnosis is made by in utero ultrasonography or by detection of an abdominal mass. Multicystic kidney is rarely the cause of symptoms in the newborn. Pathologic findings are ureteropelvic dysplasia or atresia, enlarged kidney, cysts of varying size that do not communicate, and no demonstrable pelvis or calyces (Fig. 93–1). Microscopic examination shows rudimentary lobes with no corticomedullary differentiation (Bernstein, 1991). Multicystic kidney must be differentiated from obstructive cystic renal dysplasia associated with hydronephrosis and other causes of obstructive uropathy by doing a DTPA scan. The multicystic kidney does not function. The contralateral kidney is usually normal, but in up to 50% of the cases it may be absent, hydronephrotic, ectopic, refluxing, and occasionally dysplastic (Atiyeh et al, 1992). There may be a spectrum, within and among kindreds, of calyceal diverticulum, pyelogenous cyst, ureteropelvic junction stenosis, infundibular stenosis, pelvic stenosis, and multicystic kidney (Kelalis and Malek, 1981). Most patients are followed by ultrasonography, and spontaneous involution often occurs without complications of infection, bleeding, or malignancy (Wacksman and Phipps, 1993).

RENAL ADYSPLASIA AND DYSPLASIA

The term *adysplasia* encompasses a spectrum of renal anomalies that include renal agenesis, hypoplasia, and dysplasia that occur in a patient (such as unilateral agenesis with contralateral dysplasia) or within a kindred (Buchta et al, 1973). Dysplastic kidneys can be unilateral or bilateral, often contain cysts, are disorganized, and may also contain ectopic cartilage and muscle. They may or may not function. The clinical picture depends on the severity of the renal anomaly, whether it is unilateral or bilateral, and the presence of associated anomalies (Fitch, 1977). The newborn may look normal or may have features of the oligohydramnios sequence, prune-belly syndrome, or malformation syndromes. If a vaginal or rectal atresia is associated with renal agenesis, this implies a more caudad developmental abnormality that encompasses the urorectal sinus. In these patients, the kidneys may be severely dysplastic, and the contralateral kidney may be absent. Adysplasia and dysplasia can be the result of a single gene disorder that may be autosomal recessive (Cole et al, 1976) or dominant (McPherson et al, 1987) or can occur by multifactorial inheritance (Holmes, 1989), in chromosomal disorders (Egli and Stalder, 1973), and as a consequence of in utero infections or exposure to toxins. Prenatal diagnosis by ultrasonography is possible, especially if there is oligohydramnios or associated anomalies such as limb defects.

Unilateral Renal Agenesis

Unilateral renal agenesis is usually an isolated (nonsyndromal), sporadic abnormality that is detected during prenatal

TABLE 93–1

Cystic and Dysplastic Kidneys in Newborns

Multicystic kidney
Renal adysplasia/dysplasia
  Isolated adysplasia/dysplasia°
  Adysplasia in regional defects
  Usually sporadic
    Prune-belly syndrome
    Posterior urethral valves†
    Genital anomalies and renal adysplasia/dysplasia
  Adysplasia/dysplasia in multiple congenital abnormalities
    syndrome
    Autosomal dominant
      Branchio-otorenal syndrome
      Ectodermal dysplasia, ectrodactyly, cleft lip/palate syndrome
      Radial ray aplasia and renal anomalies‡
    Autosomal recessive
      Fanconi pancytopenia syndrome
      Thrombocytopenia absent radius syndrome
      Radial ray aplasia and renal anomalies‡
      Fraser syndrome
      Fryns syndrome
    Usually sporadic
      VACTERL§
      Pallister-Hall syndrome
Cystic kidneys
  Autosomal recessive
    Autosomal recessive polycystic kidney disease

Meckel syndrome
Jeune syndrome
Renal-hepatic-pancreatic dysplasia
Glutaric aciduria Type II
Zellweger syndrome
Carbohydrate-deficient glycoprotein syndrome
  Autosomal dominant
    Autosomal dominant polycystic kidney disease: PKD1; PKD2
    Tuberous sclerosis
Glomerulocystic kidneys
  Isolated glomerulocystic kidneys
  Associated with other kidney diseases
  Autosomal dominant
    Familial hypoplastic glomerulocystic kidney
Dysgenetic kidneys
  Autosomal Recessive
    Congenital hypernephronic nephromegaly with tubular
      dysgenesis
Teratogens and renal abnormalities
  Anticonvulsants
  Cocaine
  Indomethacin
  Lead
  Phenacetin and salicylate
  Warfarin

° Occasionally recessive or dominant.
† Posterior urethral valves have been reported in sibs.
‡ Some kindreds with recessive, others with dominant inheritance.
§ Dominant inheritance has been reported.
From Kaplan BS, Kaplan P, Ruchelli E: Hereditary and congenital malformations of the kidneys. Perinat Clin North Am 19:197, 1992.

ultrasonography. Unilateral renal agenesis is an important finding if the solitary kidney is abnormal, is part of a syndrome, or is an expression of hereditary renal adysplasia (Moerman et al, 1994). The incidence is between 1 in 500 and 1 in 800 live births. If the solitary kidney is normal, there is little risk of chronic renal failure in adulthood.

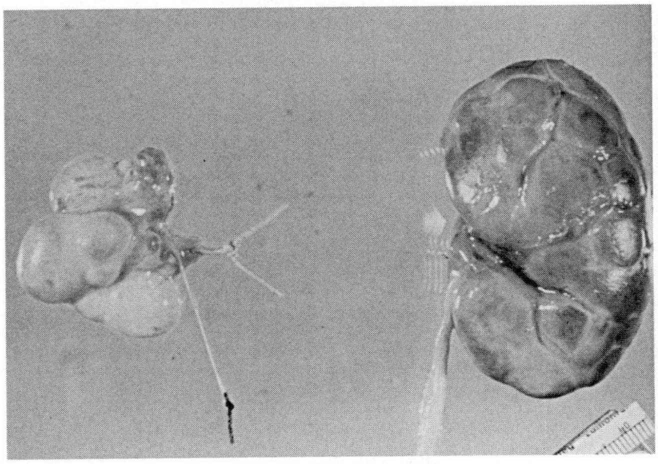

FIGURE 93–1. Multicystic kidney with atretic ureter (right). Large cysts with no normal renal tissue.

The newborn must be examined carefully for additional anomalies—cleft palate, preauricular pits, cardiac and vertebral defects, and müllerian duct aplasia (Tarry et al, 1986). A voiding cystourethrogram should be done to exclude reflux. No further evaluations are needed beyond 1 year of age, if at that time renal ultrasonography shows that the kidney is growing normally with appropriate compensatory hypertrophy.

Bilateral Renal Agenesis

Bilateral renal agenesis can occur as an isolated (nonsyndromal), sporadic abnormality detected during prenatal ultrasonography. It can also be a component of a syndrome such as the branchio-otorenal syndrome, or an expression of hereditary renal adysplasia. There can be variable expression within a family, and both autosomal recessive and dominant inheritance occur. The incidence is about 1 in 3000 births. Bilateral renal agenesis is an important cause of the oligohydramnios sequence (Potter syndrome), in which decreased amniotic fluid causes uterine compression of the fetus. This produces the characteristic Potter facies—wide-set eyes, a prominent skin fold that extends from medial canthus to cheek, a parrot-beak nose, pliable low-set ears, and receding chin. There are also lower limb deformations and, most importantly, a narrow, small chest with pulmonary hypoplasia. The infant is anuric and dies from pulmonary insufficiency. Bilateral renal agenesis is the most important cause of oligohydramnios, and the diagnosis can be confirmed by prenatal ultrasonography.

Isolated Dysplasia and Adysplasia

The incidence of isolated (nonsyndromal) bilateral renal dysplasia is about 15 per 100,000 newborns (Holmes, 1989). Modes of transmission are autosomal dominant inheritance with reduced penetrance and multifactorial inheritance. A parent and siblings may be unaffected, have unilateral dysplasia, or unilateral agenesis. Sporadic adysplasia may be caused by a new mutation or inheritance of the gene(s) from a nonmanifesting parent. First-degree relatives should be screened by ultrasonography to provide genetic counseling. The empiric risk of bilateral renal adysplasia for future sibs is 3.5% (Carter, 1970). The recurrence risk increases if two sibs are affected.

Dysplasia and Adysplasia in Regional Defects: Prune-Belly Syndrome and Posterior Urethral Valves

Renal adysplasia occurs in prune-belly syndrome and posterior urethral valves possibly as a result of obstructive uropathy (Bernstein, 1991). The renal pathology ranges from minor anomalies to severe dysplasia with and without cysts. The features of prune-belly syndrome are deficient abdominal wall muscles (Fig. 93–2), unilateral or bilateral undescended testes, and urinary tract abnormalities. Females are rarely affected but may have uterine or vaginal anomalies. Prune-belly syndrome is also associated with lower intestinal tract malrotation and atresias, lower limb deformations, and cardiovascular defects. Posterior urethral valves are characterized by urethral valves (either a flap

valve or a diaphragm in the prostatic urethra) and features of obstructive uropathy. The most frequent clinical presentation in the newborn of both conditions consists of features of the oligohydramnios sequence. A dilated prostatic urethra, megacystis, and megaureters can occur in both conditions. The survival of newborns with prune-belly syndrome or posterior urethral valves depends on the severity of pulmonary hypoplasia and the severity of renal dysplasia. Both conditions are *usually* isolated occurrences, although posterior urethral valves may occur in families and in malformation syndromes. Prenatal diagnosis and treatment are discussed in detail in Chapters 12, 16, and 92.

Dysplasia and Adysplasia with Multiple Congenital Anomalies

Branchio-Otorenal Syndrome

The spectrum of renal anomalies in branchio-otorenal syndrome ranges from unilateral dysplasia to bilateral agenesis. The kidneys may be even be normal (Fitch and Srolovitz, 1976). Renal function ranges from normal to severe reduction in glomerular filtration rate. Extrarenal manifestations are preauricular pits, branchial clefts, sensorineural deafness, and lacrimal duct atresia. The incidence is about 1 in 40,000. Inheritance is autosomal dominant with high penetrance and variable expression. The gene has been localized to chromosome 8q (Kumar et al, 1992). The prognosis depends on the severity of the renal disorder.

Acrorenal Syndromes

Radial and renal anomalies occur in ectodermal dysplasia–ectrodactyly–cleft lip plus palate syndrome (Rollnick and Hoo, 1988), VACTERL constellation of defects, Townes-Brock radial-ear-anal-renal syndrome (Kurnit et al, 1978),

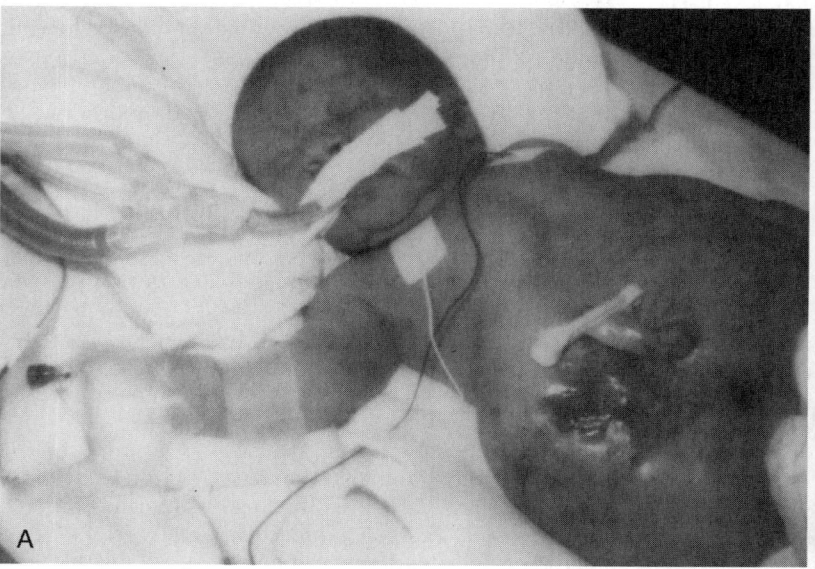 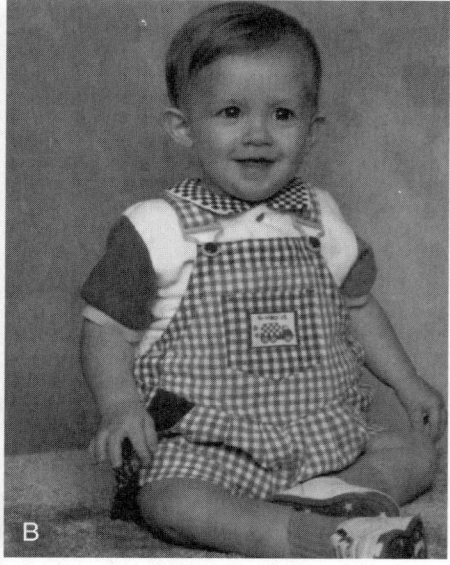

FIGURE 93–2. *A,* Newborn with prune-belly syndrome. The abdomen is protuberant, and the outlines of the intestines can be seen. The right ureter ruptured into the amniotic sac and thereby prevented the features of oligohydramnios sequence. *B,* The same patient at age 19 months.

Fanconi pancytopenia syndrome (Glanz and Fraser, 1982), thrombocytopenia absent radius syndrome (Fivush et al, 1990), Fraser syndrome (Boyd et al, 1988), Fitch-Fryns (Fryns) syndrome (Moerman et al, 1988), and Pallister-Hall congenital hypothalamic hamartoblastoma syndrome (Iafolla et al, 1989).

POLYCYSTIC KIDNEYS

To prevent confusion, the term *polycystic kidneys* should be applied only to autosomal recessive polycystic kidneys and autosomal dominant polycystic kidneys. In these conditions, there are many cysts in both kidneys, there is no evidence of renal dysplasia, and there is continuity of the lumen of the nephron from the uriniferous space to the urinary bladder. Patients with tuberous sclerosis can have cystic kidneys that appear identical by ultrasonography to autosomal dominant polycystic kidneys.

Autosomal Recessive Polycystic Kidney Disease

The incidence of autosomal recessive polycystic kidney disease is about 1 in 16,000 newborns, inheritance is autosomal recessive, there may be variable expression within a sibship (Kaplan, et al, 1988), and the gene has been assigned to chromosome 6p (Zerres et al, 1994). In the newborn, the kidneys are much more severely affected than the liver, whereas liver disease is more prominent when the disorder is diagnosed in older children. There are features of the oligohydramnios sequence if there is severe oliguria or anuria in utero. The abdomen is protuberant, and the kidneys are large and easily palpable. Hypertension is often severe, may be caused by volume expansion, and can be difficult to control. Peripheral renin activity and aldosterone excretion are reduced (Kaplan et al, 1989a). Hyponatremia is often induced iatrogenically as a result of inappropriate administration of free water and is not associated with increased urinary losses of sodium (Kaplan et al, 1989a). Furosemide or metolazone may correct hyponatremia, but additional sodium chloride may also be needed. The hypertension often responds to treatment with an angiotensin-converting enzyme inhibitor and a loop diuretic.

Renal sonography has superseded excretory urography and even histology as the preeminent diagnostic procedure. The sonographic appearances in the newborn are large kidneys, increased echogenicity of the parenchyma, loss of corticomedullary differentiation, and loss of central echo complex (Metreweli and Garel, 1980). The cortex is preserved, and the papillae are echogeneic. There may be macrocysts that are less than 2 cm in diameter. The liver is echodense, and biliary ducts are dilated. It is important to remember that renal ultrasonography does not always distinguish between autosomal recessive polycystic kidneys and autosomal dominant polycystic kidneys, between autosomal recessive polycystic kidneys and transient nephromegaly (Stapleton et al, 1981), or between autosomal recessive polycystic kidneys and glomerulocystic kidneys (Fitch and Stapleton, 1986). Kidney and liver biopsies are indicated in ambiguous cases.

At postmortem, the kidneys are enlarged, are spongy, and maintain their renal contours (Fig. 93–3A). The dilated collecting ducts are neatly arranged perpendicular to the surface of the kidney (Fig. 93–3B). There are no dysplastic elements. The liver is always involved; portal areas are expanded by increased numbers of dilated bile ductules surrounded by fibrous tissue. The dilated ductules may become cystic. The liver cells are normal.

Autosomal recessive polycystic kidneys can be diagnosed after 24 weeks' gestation by ultrasonographic demonstration of large hyperechogenic kidneys, oligohydramnios, and an empty bladder (Romero et al, 1984). Most infants who are symptomatic at birth die from respiratory or renal causes. Respiratory and renal function can improve in some cases, and a small number of patients who survive the neonatal period may maintain adequate renal function into adolescence. Bilateral nephrectomies have been done to improve ventilation (Sumfest et al, 1993). Seventy-five percent of those who survive to 1 year of age can live for more than 15 years (Kaplan et al, 1989a).

Autosomal Dominant Polycystic Kidney Disease

The incidence of autosomal dominant polycystic kidney disease in liveborns is 1 to 3 per 100,000. Although this is the second most common autosomal dominant mutation in humans with an estimated prevalence in the population of between 1 in 200 and 1 in 1000, autosomal dominant polycystic kidneys rarely present with clinical findings at birth (Fick et al, 1993). The inheritance is autosomal dominant with variable expression. At ages above 10 years, and especially over 30 years, a negative ultrasound examination provides reassurance for persons at 50% risk (Bear et al, 1992). Occasionally an infant may have symptoms before the parent. Prediction by DNA analysis complements ultrasonography for detection, is not age dependent, and may not be informative in every family. In about 85% of families, there is linkage with a gene, PKD1, on 16p13.3 (European Chromosome Polycystic Kidney Disease Consortium, 1994). A wide variety of haplotypes are represented on PKD1 chromosomes; this suggests that many different independent mutations gave rise to PKD1. In about 5% of families, linkage has been established between autosomal dominant polycystic kidneys and chromosome 4q13–q23 (PKD2) (Kimberling et al, 1993; Peters et al, 1993). These patients have the same clinical phenotypes as PKD1. Autosomal dominant polycystic kidney disease has been detected prenatally by ultrasonography (Sedman et al, 1987). Occasional patients have the oligohydramnios sequence, enlarged kidneys, and hematuria. Associated abnormalities reported in infants with autosomal dominant polycystic kidneys are endocardial fibroelastosis, an intracerebral vascular anomaly, pyloric stenosis, and hepatic fibrosis (Cobben et al, 1990). The demonstration of hepatic fibrosis in some patients can render differentiation between autosomal recessive polycystic kidneys and autosomal dominant polycystic kidneys difficult unless there is a positive family history of autosomal dominant polycystic kidneys. Ultrasonography and computed tomography scans are more sensitive methods for detecting the cysts than intravenous urography. Cysts may be seen in liver, pancreas, and spleen.

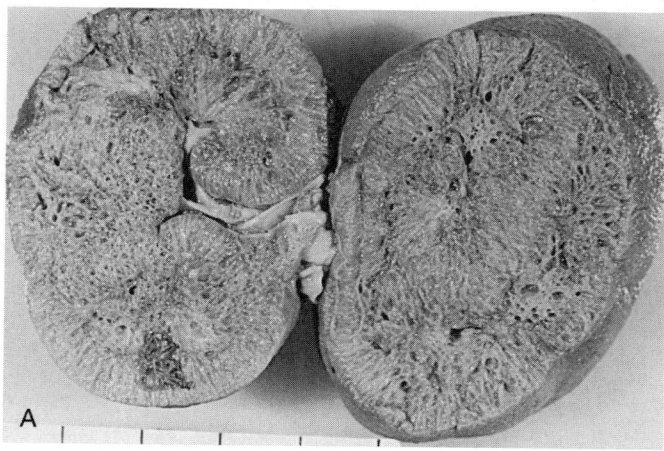 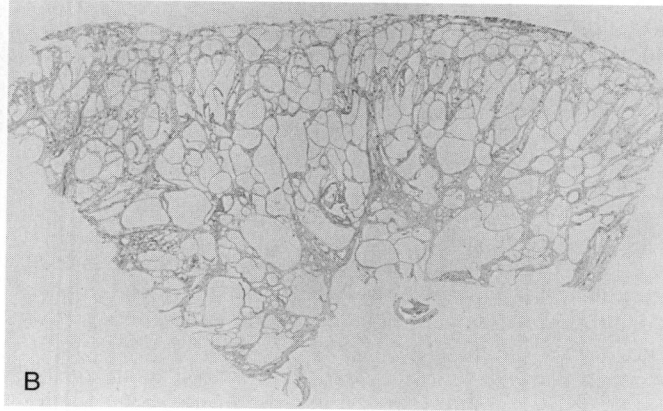

FIGURE 93–3. *A*, Large spongy kidneys (autosomal recessive kidneys). *B*, Photomicrograph of autosomal recessive kidneys with dilated tubules and paucity of glomeruli.

The kidneys are enlarged and lobular, and the calyces are stretched and distorted by cysts, which produce smooth or irregular indentations. Numerous cysts of various sizes are seen in the parenchyma of severely affected cases. At postmortem, the kidneys are large with numerous round protuberances on their surfaces (Fig. 93–4). Cysts are irregularly dispersed through the parenchyma and arise from many nephron segments.

About 50% of patients who present at birth die in the neonatal period or infancy from respiratory failure or sepsis (Freycon et al, 1982). Control of hypertension improves the prognosis, but renal failure eventually occurs in some survivors (Fick et al, 1993). Progressive loss of renal tubules by apoptosis is one mechanism of renal failure (Woo, 1995).

Tuberous Sclerosis

In tuberous sclerosis, there is a high spontaneous mutation rate with autosomal dominant inheritance, variable penetrance and expression, and localization to 16p (European Chromosome 16 Tuberous Sclerosis Consortium, 1993). Polycystic (Wentzl et al, 1970) and unilateral cystic disease

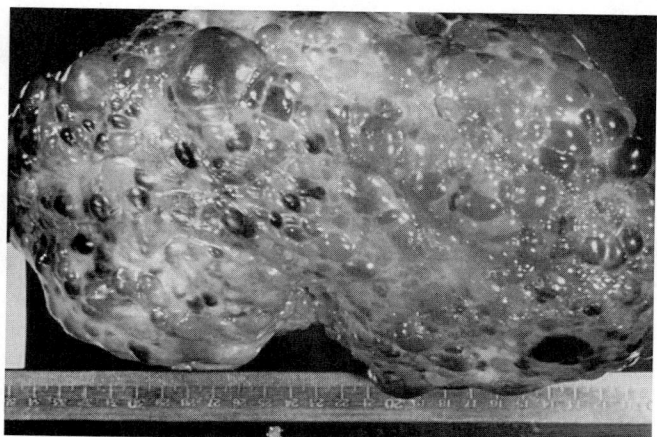

FIGURE 93–4. Autosomal dominant polycystic kidney. The kidney is large, and there are numerous cysts on the surface.

are occasionally found in newborns in whom a diagnosis of tuberous sclerosis is made later. Ash leaf depigmented nevi may be the only skin manifestation of the disease in infancy, and therefore infants with polycystic kidneys must be examined under ultraviolet light for the nevi. Seizures may occur in infancy. The parents must also be examined for stigmata of tuberous sclerosis. Renal cysts and polycystic disease in tuberous sclerosis are identical in their ultrasonographic, intravenous urographic, or computed tomographic appearances to simple cysts or autosomal dominant polycystic kidneys (Bernstein, 1993a). Some contain mural calcifications. Computed tomography studies may show fat-containing angiomyolipomas. These patients usually survive into adolescence and adulthood, although those with early-onset polycystic kidneys can progress to end-stage renal failure.

CYSTIC KIDNEYS WITH AUTOSOMAL RECESSIVE INHERITANCE
Meckel Syndrome

Inheritance in Meckel syndrome is autosomal recessive with variable expression within and between families (Fraser and Lytwyn, 1981). The features are postaxial polydactyly, microphthalmia, encephalocele, cystic kidneys, ambiguous genitalia, and hepatic fibrosis. Fifty percent have oligohydramnios. Goldston syndrome (cystic kidneys, hepatic fibrosis, Dandy-Walker malformation, autosomal recessive) may be part of the spectrum or a discrete entity (Glanz and Fraser, 1982). Histopathologic findings are spherical, cortical cysts that increase in size toward the medulla and are separated by interstitial stroma. Prenatal diagnosis is possible by ultrasonography and increased amniotic alpha-fetoprotein. The prognosis is dismal with death in the perinatal period.

Jeune Asphyxiating Thoracic Dystrophy Syndrome

Jeune asphyxiating thoracic dystrophy syndrome has autosomal recessive inheritance and variable expression. Respiratory distress, dysostoses, short ribs, small and long thoracic cage, small pelvis, trident acetabular margins, short and thick second and third phalanges, cone-shaped epiphyses, handle-bar clavicle, mesomelic shortening of limbs, renal cystic disease, and congenital hepatic fibrosis characterize the disorder (Donaldson et al, 1985). Three different morphologic lesions of the kidneys have been described: (1) dilated proximal and distal tubules and Bowman capsule with interstitial fibrosis, (2) cystic dysplasia and disorganized renal architecture, and (3) chronic tubulointerstitial disease resembling juvenile nephronophthisis. The differential diagnosis includes Ellis-van Creveld syndrome, Saldino-Noonan short rib–polydactyly syndrome (Type II), Majewski short rib–polydactyly syndrome, and Naumoff syndrome (Type III). Survivors develop metaphyseal dysplasia with short-limbed dwarfism. Treatment of renal failure may require dialysis and transplantation. Prenatal diagnosis by ultrasonography is possible by 18 weeks (Elejade et al, 1985).

Renal-Hepatic-Pancreatic Dysplasia (Ivemark Syndrome)

Inheritance of Ivemark syndrome is autosomal recessive. Patients may have the oligohydramnios sequence. The kidneys may be dysplastic with peripheral cortical cysts, primitive collecting ducts, glomerular cysts, and metaplastic cartilage (Bernstein et al, 1987). There is fibrosis of the liver and pancreas. Most patients die from respiratory insufficiency in the newborn period.

INBORN ERRORS OF METABOLISM

Several inborn errors of energy metabolism that manifest in the newborn period have morphologic and functional abnormalities of the kidneys. These are all rare conditions.

Glutaric Aciduria Type II (Multiple Acyl-CoA-Dehydrogenase Deficiencies)

In glutaric aciduria Type II, the deficiencies in mitochondrial enzymes (electron transfer flavoprotein or electron transfer ubiquinone oxidoreductase) are inherited as autosomal recessive traits. Clinical features are prematurity, hypotonia, hepatomegaly, nephromegaly, craniofacial anomalies, rocker bottom feet, anterior abdominal wall defects, and external genital anomalies. An odor of sweaty feet may be present. Within 24 hours, there is severe hypoglycemia but no ketosis, a metabolic acidosis with an increased anion gap, and mild hyperammonemia. Organic acids, including glutaric acid, ethylmalonic acid, isovaleric acid, and medium-chain dicarboxylics, are elevated in the urine, cerebrospinal fluid, and blood. Renal cystic dysplasia occurs in many cases (Wilson et al, 1989). Prenatal diagnosis may be possible by assaying the enzyme in amniocytes or elevated glutaric acid in amniotic fluid. Prenatal ultrasonography may show enlarged cystic kidneys. Treatment is unsuccessful, and death occurs in days to months.

Zellweger Cerebrohepatorenal Syndrome

The clinical features of Zellweger cerebrohepatorenal syndrome, an autosomal recessive condition, are similar to glutaric aciduria Type II (Patton et al, 1972). In addition, there may be nystagmus, cataracts (sometimes *oil droplets*), pigmentary retinopathy, optic disc pallor, and stippled epiphyses of patella and acetabulum. There is no abnormal odor. Kidneys are enlarged. All peroxisomal functions are abnormal: Plasma very-long-chain fatty acids, bile acids, pipecolic acid, phytanic acid, and urine dicarboxylic acids are elevated, and cholesterol and triglycerides levels are low. Cortical renal cysts, brain heterotopias, abnormal gyri, absent corpus callosum, and micronodular cirrhosis are seen at postmortem examination. Prenatal diagnosis is possible by enzyme assays in amniocytes or in chorionic villus cells. Most affected infants die by 6 months, but those with a milder form survive into their teens with deafness, retardation, and seizures.

Carbohydrate-Deficient Glycoprotein Syndrome

Multiple renal microcysts are found in the carbohydrate-deficient glycoprotein syndrome (Strom et al, 1993). There is multisystem involvement with olivopontocerebellar atrophy, retinitis pigmentosa, testicular atrophy, hypothyroidism, and immune deficiency. Several glycoproteins are deficient in their carbohydrate moieties. Inheritance is autosomal recessive, and the prognosis is variable.

HYPOPLASTIC KIDNEYS

Hypoplastic kidneys are small, have fewer calyces, and may be dysplastic. Simple hypoplasia, oligomeganephronia, and renal dysplasia are the types of small kidneys that are seen in newborns. In older children, small kidneys may also be the result of chronic pyelonephritis, chronic glomerulonephritis, renovascular accident, or nephronophthisis. In simple hypoplasia, the renal architecture is normal, but there are a decreased number of reniculi and small nephrons. Oligomeganephronic kidneys are small and have a decreased number of *enlarged* glomeruli (Royer et al, 1974). This is probably not a specific clinicopathologic entity.

GLOMERULOCYSTIC KIDNEYS

In the purest form of glomerulocystic kidney, there are dilated Bowman spaces, with few or no cysts in the tubule (Bernstein, 1993b). The rest of the renal architecture is normal. The kidneys may be large or small. The liver is normal. Most cases have occurred sporadically, but autosomal dominant inheritance has also been described (Kaplan et al, 1989b). Glomerular cysts are also seen in obstructive uropathy, in autosomal dominant polycystic kidneys, in association with malformations of other organs, in dysplastic kidneys, and in infants whose mothers received phenacetin or indomethacin during pregnancy. Glomerular cysts are often subcapsular and may contain more than one glomeruloid structure (Fig. 93–5).

DYSGENETIC KIDNEYS

Clinical features of congenital hypernephronic nephromegaly with tubular dysgenesis, a rare autosomal recessive condition, include late-onset oligohydramnios after 24

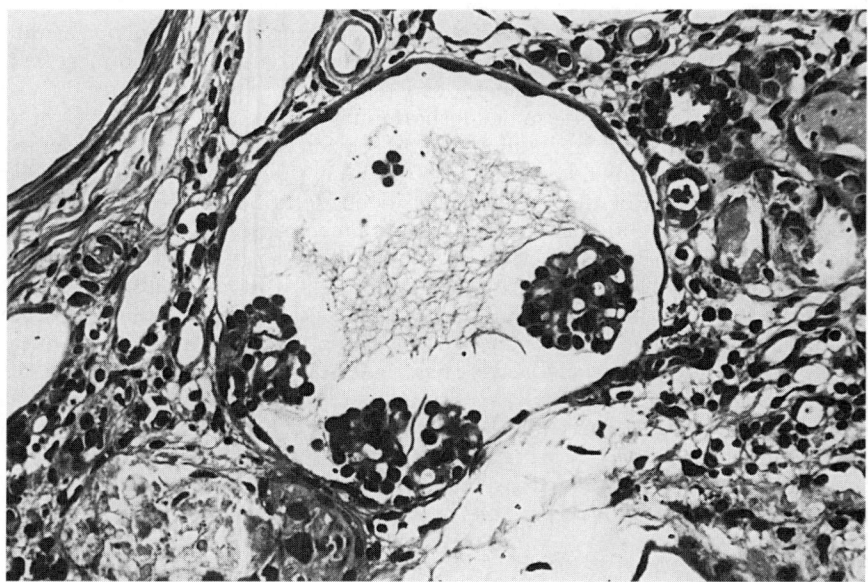

FIGURE 93–5. Glomerulocystic kidneys. Photomicrograph of glomerulus with three glomeruloid structures in a dilated Bowman capsule.

weeks of gestation and large nonfunctioning kidneys (Allanson et al, 1992). The calvaria may be underdeveloped with wide sutures. Similar calvarial anomalies occur in patients with the Finnish-type congenital nephrotic syndrome and in infants exposed in utero to angiotensin-converting enzyme inhibitors. The kidneys are enlarged symmetrically by ultrasonography, and the corticomedullary junction is poorly defined. There is an apparent increase in the number of glomeruli, and there are immature tubules without proximal convolutions. Prenatal diagnosis is not possible before 20 weeks. All the patients have died in the neonatal period.

IN UTERO EXPOSURE TO TERATOGENS

No convincing proof of a cause-and-effect relationship has been provided for associations of in utero exposure to teratogens. Urogenital anomalies are found occasionally in infants exposed in utero to valproic acid and other anticonvulsant agents (Ardinger et al, 1988). Maternal cocaine (and polydrug) use may produce genitourinary abnormalities (Chasnoff et al, 1988). Indomethacin may cause renal dysgenesis in fetal monkeys and possibly in humans exposed early in utero to prolonged high doses (Kaplan et al, 1994). Prenatal lead exposure is incriminated as a possible cause of the VACTERL association (Levine and Muenke, 1991). Glomerulocystic disease was reported in an infant exposed to phenacetin and salicylate in utero (Krous et al, 1977). Unilateral renal agenesis and abnormalities of position were noted in three infants exposed prenatally to warfarin (Hall, 1989).

REFERENCES

Allanson JE, Hunter AGW, Mettler GS, Jimenez C: A not uncommon autosomal recessive syndrome: A review. Am J Med Genet 43:811, 1992.

Ardinger HH, Atkin JF, Blackston RD, et al: Verification of the fetal valproate syndrome phenotype. Am J Med Genet 29:171, 1988.

Atiyeh B, Husmann D, Baum M: Contralateral renal abnormalities in multicystic-dysplastic kidney disease. J Pediatr 121:65, 1992.

Bear JC, McManamon P, Morgan J, et al: Age at clinical onset and at ultrasonographic detection of adult polycystic kidney disease: Data for genetic counselling. Am J Med Genet 18:45, 1984.

Bear JC, Parfrey PS, Morgan JM, et al: Autosomal dominant polycystic kidney disease: New information for genetic counselling. Am J Med Genet 43:548, 1992.

Bernstein J: The multicystic kidney and hereditary renal adysplasia. Am J Kidney Dis 17:495, 1991.

Bernstein J: Renal cystic disease in the tuberous sclerosis complex. Pediatr Nephrol 7:490, 1993a.

Bernstein J: Glomerulocystic kidney disease—nosological considerations. Pediatr Nephrol 7:464, 1993b.

Bernstein J, Chandra M, Cresswell J, et al: Renal-hepatic-pancreatic dysplasia: A syndrome reconsidered. Am J Med Genet 26:391, 1987.

Boyd PA, Keeling JW, Lindenbaum RH: Fraser syndrome (cryptophthalmos-syndactyly syndrome): A review of eleven cases with postmortem findings. Am J Med Genet 31:159, 1988.

Buchta RM, Visesku C, Gilbert EF, et al: Familial bilateral renal agenesis and hereditary renal adysplasia. Z Kinderheilk 115:111, 1973.

Carter CO: Genetics of polycystic disease of the kidney. Birth Defects 6:11, 1970.

Chasnoff IJ, Chisum GM, Kaplan WE: Maternal cocaine use and genitourinary tract malformations. Teratology 37:201, 1988.

Cobben JM, Breuning MH, Schoots C, et al: Congenital hepatic fibrosis in autosomal-dominant polycystic kidney disease. Kidney Int 38:880, 1990.

Cole BR, Kaufman RL, McAlister WH, et al: Bilateral renal dysplasia in three siblings: Report of a survivor. Clin Nephrol 5:83, 1976.

Donaldson MDC, Warner AA, Trompeter RS, et al: Familial juvenile nephronophthisis, Jeune's syndrome, and associated disorders. Arch Dis Child 60:426, 1985.

Egli F, Stalder G: Malformations of kidney and urinary tract in common chromosomal aberrations: I. Clinical studies, Humangenetik 18:1, 1973.

Elejade BR, de Elejade MM, Pansch D: Prenatal diagnosis of Jeune syndrome. Am J Med Genet 21:433, 1985.

European Chromosome 16 Tuberous Sclerosis Consortium: Identification and characterization of the tuberous sclerosis gene on chromosome 16. Cell 75:1305, 1993.

European Chromosome Polycystic Kidney Disease Consortium: The polycystic kidney disease 1 gene encodes a 14 kb transcript and lies within a duplicated region on chromosome 16. Cell 77:881, 1994.

Fick GM, Johnson AM, Strain JD, et al: Characteristics of very early onset autosomal dominant polycystic kidney disease. J Am Soc Nephrol 3:1863, 1993.

Fitch N: Heterogeneity of bilateral renal agenesis. Can Med Assoc J 116:381, 1977.

Fitch N, Srolovitz H: Severe renal dysgenesis produced by a dominant gene. Am J Dis Child 130:1536, 1976.

Fitch SJ, Stapleton FB: Ultrasonographic features of glomerulocystic disease in infancy: Similarity to infantile polycystic kidney disease. Pediatr Radiol 16:400, 1986.

Fivush B, McGrath S, Zinkham W: Thrombocytopenia absent radius syndrome associated with renal insufficiency. Clin Pediatr 29:182, 1990.

Fraser FC, Lytwyn A: Spectrum of anomalies in the Meckel syndrome, or: "Maybe there is a malformation syndrome with at least one constant anomaly." Am J Med Genet 9:63, 1981.

Freycon M-T, Boyer C, Lauras B, et al: Reins polykystiques a transmission dominante chez un nourrisson. Pediatrie 38:287, 1982.

Glanz A, Fraser FC: Spectrum of anomalies in Fanconi anemia. J Med Genet 19:412, 1982.

Hall BD: Warfarin embryopathy and urinary tract anomalies: Possible new association. Am J Med Genet 34:292, 1989.

Holmes LB: Prevalence, phenotypic heterogeneity and familial aspects of bilateral renal agenesis/dysgenesis. *In* Liss AR (Ed): Genetics of Kidney Disorders. New York, Alan R. Liss, 1989, pp 1–11.

Iafolla K, Fratkin JD, Spiegel PK, et al: Case report and delineation of the congenital hypothalamic hamartoblastoma syndrome (Pallister-Hall syndrome). Am J Med Genet 33:489, 1989.

Kaplan BS, Fay J, Dillon MJ, et al: Autosomal recessive polycystic kidney disease. Pediatr Nephrol 3:43, 1989a.

Kaplan BS, Kaplan P, de Chadarevian J-P, et al: Variable expression within a family of autosomal recessive polycystic kidney disease and congenital hepatic fibrosis. Am J Med Genet 29:639, 1988.

Kaplan BS, Kaplan P, Ruchelli E: Hereditary and congenital malformations of the kidneys. Perinat Clin North Am 19:197, 1992.

Kaplan BS, Pincott J, Gordon I, et al: Autosomal dominant hypoplastic glomerulocystic kidney disease. Am J Med Genet 34:569, 1989b.

Kaplan BS, Restaino I, Raval DS, et al: Renal failure in the newborn associated with in utero exposure to non-steroidal anti-inflammatory agents. Pediatr Nephrol 8:700, 1994.

Kelalis PP, Malek RS: Infundibular stenosis. J Urol 125:568, 1981.

Kimberling WJ, Kumar S, Gabow PA, et al: Autosomal dominant polycystic kidney disease: Localization of the second gene to chromosome 4q13–q23. Genomics 18:467, 1993.

Krous HF, Richie JP, Sellers B: Glomerulocystic kidney: A hypothesis of origin and pathogenesis. Arch Pathol Lab Med 101:462, 1977.

Kumar S, Kimberling WJ, Kenyon JB, et al: Autosomal dominant branchio-oto-renal syndrome—localization of a disease gene to chromosome 8q by linkage in a Dutch family. Hum Mol Genet 1:491, 1992.

Kurnit DM, Steele MW, Pinsky L, et al: Autosomal dominant transmission of a syndrome of anal, ear, renal and radial congenital malformations. J Pediatr 93:268, 1978.

Levine F, Muenke M: VACTERL association with high prenatal lead exposure. Pediatrics 87:390, 1991.

McPherson E, Carey J, Kramer A, et al: Dominantly inherited renal adysplasia. Am J Med Genet 26:863, 1987.

Metreweli C, Garel L: The echographic diagnosis of infantile renal polycystic disease. Ann Radiol 23:103, 1980.

Moerman P, Fryns J-P, Sastrowijoto SH, et al: Hereditary renal adysplasia: New observations and hypotheses. Pediatr Pathol 14:405, 1994.

Moerman P, Fryns J-P, Vandenberghe K, et al: The syndrome of diaphragmatic hernia, abnormal face and distal limb anomalies (Fryns syndrome): Further delineation of this multiple congenital anomaly (MCA) syndrome. Am J Med Genet 31:8054, 1988.

Patton RG, Christie DL, Smith DW, et al: Cerebro-hepato-renal syndrome of Zellweger. Am J Dis Child 124:840, 1972.

Peters DJM, Spruit L, Saris JJ, et al: Chromosome 4 localization of a second gene for autosomal dominant polycystic kidney disease. Nat Genet 5:359, 1993.

Rollnick BR, Hoo JJ: Genitourinary anomalies are a component manifestation in the ectodermal dysplasia, ectrodactyly, cleft lip/palate (EEC) syndrome. Am J Med Genet 29:131, 1988.

Romero R, Cullen M, Jeanty P, et al: The diagnosis of congenital renal anomalies with ultrasound: II. Infantile polycystic kidney disease. Am J Obstet Gynecol 150:259, 1984.

Royer P, Habib RN, Mathieu H, Broyer M: Pediatric Nephrology. Philadelphia, WB Saunders, 1974, p 9.

Sedman A, Bell P, Manco-Johnson M, et al: Autosomal dominant polycystic kidney disease in childhood: A longitudinal study. Kidney Int 31:1000–1005, 1987.

Stapleton FB, Hilton S, Wilcox J: Transient nephromegaly simulating infantile polycystic disease of the kidneys. Pediatrics 67:554, 1981.

Strom EH, Stromme P, Westvik J, et al: Renal cysts in the carbohydrate-deficient glycoprotein syndrome. Pediatr Nephrol 7:253, 1993.

Sumfest JM, Burns MW, Mitchell ME: Aggressive surgical and medical management of autosomal recessive polycystic kidney disease. Urology 42:309, 1993.

Tarry WF, Duckett JW, Stephens FD: The Mayer-Rokitansky syndrome: Pathogenesis, classification and management. J Urol 136:648, 1986.

Wacksman J, Phipps L: Report of the multicystic kidney registry: Preliminary findings. J Urol 150:1870, 1993.

Wentzl JE, Lagos JC, Albers DD: Tuberous sclerosis presenting as polycystic kidneys and seizures in an infant. J Pediatr 77:673, 1970.

Wilson GN, de Chadarevian J-P, Kaplan P, et al: Glutaric aciduria type II: Review of the phenotype and report of an unusual glomerulopathy. Am J Med Genet 32:395, 1989.

Woo D: Apoptosis and loss of renal tissue in polycystic kidney diseases. N Engl J Med 333:18, 1995.

Zerres K, Mucher G, Bachner L, et al: Mapping of the gene for autosomal recessive polycystic kidney disease (autosomal recessive polycystic kidneys) to chromosome 6p21-cen. Nat Genet 7:429, 1994.

CHAPTER 94

Developmental Abnormalities of the Genitourinary System

Stephen A. Zderic

This chapter covers the major urologic presentations associated with developmental abnormalities of the genitourinary system in the newborn that a neonatologist likely will encounter. The most frequent consultations from the neonatal intensive care unit (NICU) and the most common questions a urologist is asked serve as the basis for how much attention each particular topic is assigned. This chapter also aids the neonatologist to better use the urologic consultants.

PRENATAL DIAGNOSIS

The recent major advances in prenatal diagnosis have been made possible by our better understanding of the human development and the increased diagnostic accuracy of fetal ultrasound, amniocentesis, magnetic resonance imaging (MRI), and genetic testing (see Chapters 12 and 92). In addition, an increasing array of fetal interventions is rapidly moving from the laboratory stages of development to clinical applicability (Crombleholme, 1994). Therefore, the urologist is now able to prenatally identify and, in selected cases, manage fetuses with congenital abnormalities of the urinary tract, design a plan for further evaluation in the postnatal period, and establish a relationship with the family that has come to seek the prenatal consultation.

HYDRONEPHROSIS

The primary diagnosis made with prenatal sonography at present is hydronephrosis. The work-up of prenatally diagnosed hydronephrosis continues to evolve, and a brief outline of today's approach to its diagnosis and management is presented here. Many patients with prenatally diagnosed hydronephrosis have only transient dilations of the urinary tract that may reflect the increased distensibility of the fetal urinary tract and the massive fetal diuresis that produces large urinary volumes (Homsy et al, 1986). The decrease in urine output after delivery (see Chapters 34 and 91) may alone explain why many cases of prenatal renal and ureteral dilation resolve after birth. In addition, the ureter may contain small kinks or folds that resolve, producing normal morphology and function. Finally, the postnatal decrease in the distensibility of the urinary tract also contributes to the resolution of many cases of prenatal hydronephrosis.

For a newborn with hydronephrosis, the neonatal work-up is dictated by the newborn's gender and whether the hydronephrosis is unilateral or bilateral (Blyth et al, 1993). Bilateral hydronephrosis in a boy should lead one to consider posterior urethral valves and obtain both an ul-

trasound and a voiding cystourethrogram (VCUG) in the immediate neonatal period. In contrast, unilateral hydronephrosis in a male or bilateral hydronephrosis in a female can be managed by obtaining an ultrasound of the kidneys and bladder at 2 to 5 days of age. In these latter cases, obtaining an ultrasound earlier increases the likelihood that one may miss a significant hydronephrosis secondary to the relative intravascular volume depletion and transient oliguria of the immediate postnatal period (Djeter and Gibbons, 1989). If the ultrasound confirms the presence of hydronephrosis, the next phase of the work-up may take place at 3 to 5 weeks of age, when a VCUG and renal ^{99m}Tc-diethylenetriaminepenta-acetic acid (DTPA) scan may be performed. In the interim, it is absolutely essential that the infant be discharged home on antimicrobial prophylaxis, usually on amoxicillin (12.5 mg/kg once a day). The algorithm presented in Figure 94–1 is a reasonable approach to the management of neonatal hydronephrosis.

There is ample controversy, however, about the fine points and subtleties in the management that this algorithm cannot resolve. Since 20% of newborns with prenatal hydronephrosis have reflux, one could argue that all newborns with prenatally diagnosed hydronephrosis should also be studied with a VCUG or at least started on oral antibiotic prophylaxis, irrespective of the finding of their first ultra-

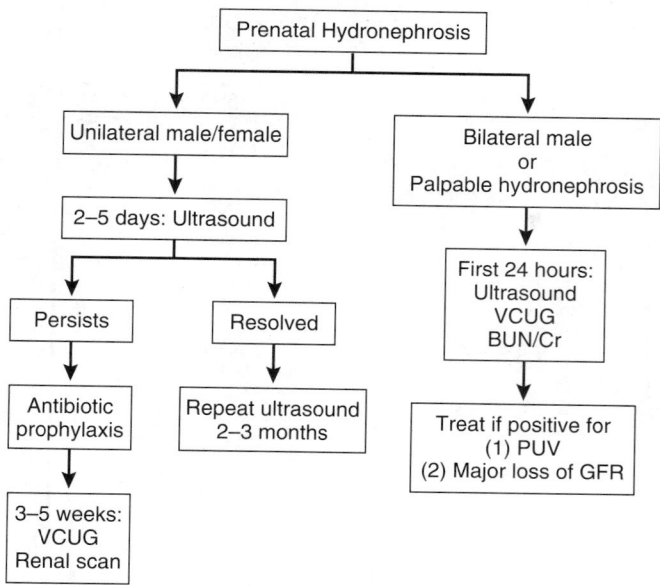

FIGURE 94–1. An approach to the initial management of prenatal hydronephrosis in the neonatal intensive care unit. PUV, posterior urethral valves; VCUG, voiding cystourethrogram; BUN, blood urea nitrogen; Cr, creatinine; GFR, glomerular filtration rate.

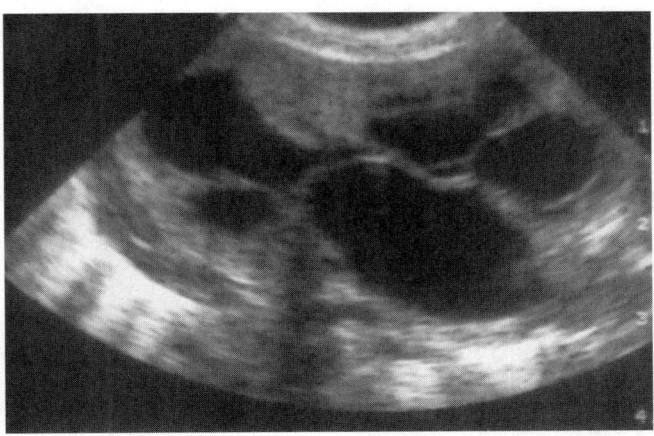

FIGURE 94–2. Ultrasound view demonstrates a classic partial ureteropelvic obstruction in which there is dilation of the renal pelvis and calyces. This image of anatomy alone says little about the severity of this obstruction, which must be ascertained by the use of a functional study such as a renal DTPA scan.

sound. Since antibiotic prophylaxis is cost effective in preventing urosepsis, it is the bias of this author to provide prophylaxis with antibiotics until the second ultrasound is obtained 2 to 3 months after birth, even if the initial postnatal ultrasound shows the resolution of the prenatal hydronephrosis. However, in the face of a significant urinary tract obstruction, oral antibiotics alone may not be effective in maintaining sterile urine.

OBSTRUCTIVE UROPATHY
Ureteropelvic Junction Obstruction

The diagnosis of a ureteropelvic junction (UPJ) obstruction is made by ultrasonography, which will reveal a dilated renal pelvis with or without caliectasis and no dilation of the ureter (Fig. 94–2). This is in marked contrast to the ureterovesical junction (UVJ) obstruction or megaureter, in which case the proximal ureter is dilated as well. The presence of a UPJ obstruction demonstrated by sonography is not predictive of the functional significance of the obstruction, and many infants with fairly impressive dilations of the renal pelvis in the neonatal period show partial or even complete resolution of their hydronephrosis with preservation of renal function. Thus, it is critical to ensure that additional imaging is obtained prior to any surgical repair. Although one study has found that any kidney with an anteroposterior diameter of greater than 2 cm has a greater chance of having functional compromise, many of these patients show stable renal function on close follow-up (Koff and Campbell, 1994; Ransley et al, 1990). In these cases, the use of DTPA renal scans has enabled the pediatric urologist to carefully select out those newborns in whom the aberrant anatomy has resulted in a loss of function as defined by a decreased glomerular filtration rate. However, it remains unclear at what level of functional impairment should intervention be considered (Allen, 1992). Some advocate intervention only if the differential function in the affected kidney falls below 35% (Cartwright, 1992), whereas others intervene only at 40%. Still

others rely heavily on a "well-tempered" diuretic renogram and the furosemide washout curves to define those patients who are obstructed (Conway et al, 1992). Finally, an intravenous pyelogram is favored by some to better define the anatomy prior to any planned surgical procedure. However, this procedure involves contrast agent exposure, repeat doses of ionizing radiation, and, in contrast with a renal radionuclide scan, does not quantify the function.

Therefore, in neonates in whom UPJ obstruction is diagnosed by sonography, a VCUG and a radionuclide renal scan should be performed to rule out possible reflux and to evaluate the renal function. If the radionuclide renal scan shows diminished renal function, surgical management is indicated. There is no preoperative test that will predict recovery of renal function following relief of obstructive uropathy. Therefore, one is left with the option of placing a temporary percutaneous nephrostomy or carrying out a primary repair. Figure 94–3 is illustrative of a patient with severe unilateral UPJ obstruction. Prenatal ultrasonography in this fetus revealed the presence of a unilateral hydronephrosis with no oligohydramnios and evidence of bladder emptying. On delivery, the newborn presented with a palpable flank mass, and a repeat ultrasound confirmed massive left-sided hydronephrosis with an anteroposterior diameter of greater than 2 cm. The VCUG showed no reflux, and the renal scan revealed that the left kidney had less than 10% function. Placing this neonate on antimicrobial prophylaxis would not have prevented an infection owing to the limited antibiotic delivery into the collecting system by the poorly functioning left kidney. At 1 week of life, a dismembered pyeloplasty was carried out, and the biopsy demonstrated normal glomeruli and distended tubules. The follow-up nephrostogram at 2 weeks after surgery revealed good urine flow into the bladder and that this kidney now supplied 40% of the total glomerular filtration rate. Although most of the UPJ obstructions that are this severe do not recover full function, this may be seen occasionally.

However, most newborns with UPJ obstruction have good renal function so as to allow for elective work-up at 3 to 6 weeks of life while the patient is maintained on antibiotic prophylaxis. At this point, these infants may be divided into three groups (Homsy et al, 1990). One third are obstructed and require immediate intervention, one third has a normal follow-up evaluation, and one third may be followed further with serial sonograms and renal scans. Of this last group, up to one third may ultimately require surgical correction.

In summary, the work-up of prenatally diagnosed hydronephrosis induced by UPJ obstruction (or by any other etiology) requires three key elements. The first element is the close and ongoing communication between the neonatologist and the pediatric urologist. The second element is the provision of antimicrobial prophylaxis during the follow-up period until the urinary tract is judged normal or surgical correction is carried out. Finally, by eliminating surgery that may prove to offer little benefit, expectant management is beneficial for the patient, his or her family, and society. However, this comes at the price of careful and close follow-up, which must be made clear to the family in no uncertain terms.

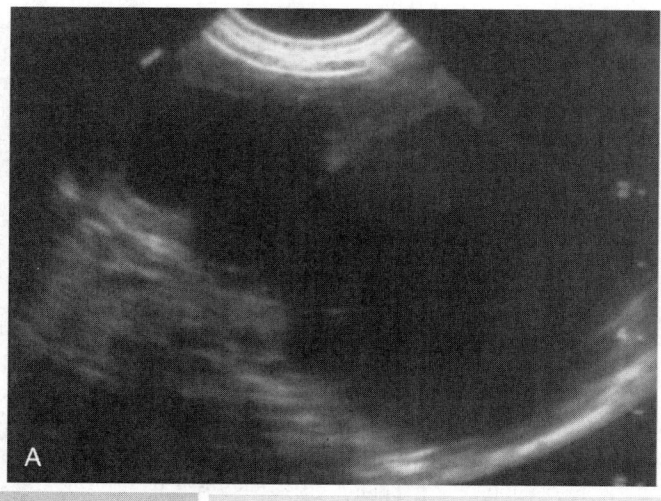

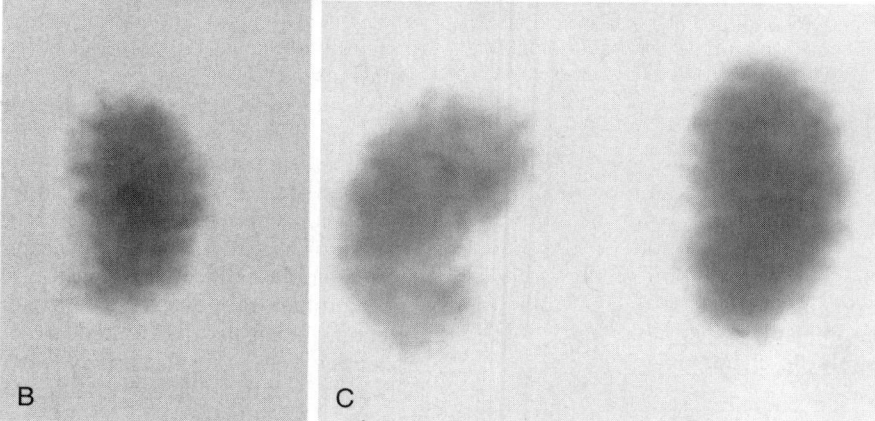

FIGURE 94–3. Ultrasound view *(A)* of a severe ureteropelvic junction obstruction shows a massive dilation of the renal pelvis and calyces with distortion of the renal parenchyma. A renal DTPA scan showed this kidney contributed under 5% of renal function *(B)*. Following a pyeloplasty in the neonatal period, functional recovery was seen in this kidney on follow-up DTPA renal scan *(C)*.

Ureterovesical Junction Obstruction (Megaureter)

Approximately 15% of the cases of prenatally diagnosed hydronephrosis prove to ultimately have a primary megaureter. In this instance, the ultrasound demonstrates not only marked pelviectasis and caliectasis but also significant ureteral dilation. The best ultrasound views to look for ureteral dilation are seen behind a distended bladder (Fig. 94–4A). In the newborn with megaureter, a VCUG is essential to exclude reflux. Some would argue that a refluxing primary megaureter should be repaired since an infection that develops in a partially obstructed system can be especially severe. However, recent data indicate that if the renal DTPA scan (Fig. 94–4B) reveals good renal function, these patients may be safely followed on antimicrobial prophylaxis instead. In a longitudinal study of the same cohort of patients, renal function was found to be well preserved, and in many instances the morphologic appearance was also substantially improved (Baskin et al, 1994). Unlike the UPJ obstructions, in which there is always a 20% to 30% risk of renal decompensation with need for subsequent surgery, primary megaureters seem to do better

with very few changes during the course of the management, with only about 10% of patients experiencing breakthrough urinary tract infections requiring reimplantation. The good results with conservative management occurred in a select group of patients with good renal function at the outset defined as a kidney contributing better than 35% to the overall glomerular filtration rate by radionuclide scan (Baskin et al, 1994). For kidneys whose split function fell below 35%, surgery to relieve obstructive uropathy remains the preferred mode of treatment.

Posterior Urethral Valves

The major obstructive uropathy that must be diagnosed early in the newborn period is posterior urethral valves. In fact, most cases are detected on prenatal sonography. It remains to be determined whether posterior urethral valves occur because of the failure of urethral alignment at a critical point in early development or whether there is an abnormal displacement of the mesonephric structures. However, there is little debate about the fact that posterior urethral valves present with a wide spectrum of findings. At the severe end of the spectrum is the neonate born with chronic renal insufficiency in whom prenatal sonography would have revealed severe oligohydramnios. If the obstruction is severe enough to result in oligohydramnios, these infants may also suffer from lung hypoplasia. In such cases, extracorporeal membrane oxygenation has been used in the NICU to get past the initial period of respiratory compromise, and long-term survivors have been reported. However, most of these infants require renal transplantation at some point in the future (Gibbons et al, 1993). At the other end of the spectrum is the child whose valve is of minimal functional significance and escapes prenatal detection only to present at age 6 or 7 years with a urinary tract infection or incontinence. In general, these children with late presentations have a good renal prognosis.

The prenatal diagnosis by ultrasound offers the pediatric urologist an opportunity to intervene before the obstructive uropathy is further compromised by the imposition of the additional burden of infection. As many as 30% of these patients may well require renal replacement therapy during their lifetime (Smith et al, 1996). Hence, it is imperative that in the newborn period every effort is made to optimize their renal function and maintain the urinary tract free of infection. The maternal obstetric history is extremely important in establishing the risk factors for the postnatal course. Obviously, the presence of oligohydramnios is a major warning sign for the possible development of respiratory and renal failure. Fetal surgery for obstructive uropathy either by percutaneous shunting or open procedures has not been shown to improve renal function (Coplen et al, 1996) but has been found to improve pulmonary function (see Chapters 12 and 92). The subset of patients with oligohydramnios are at increased risk of requiring urgent intervention and should be encouraged to deliver in tertiary

care settings. In situations where there is no oligohydramnios and the family elects to deliver closer to home, a plan for an appropriate postnatal evaluation is essential, as outlined earlier in this chapter. However, every male newborn with prenatal hydronephrosis does not have posterior urethral valves.

The postnatal evaluation of a child with suspected posterior urethral valves should begin with a renal and bladder ultrasound. The examination should first be performed without a catheter in the bladder so as to reveal the anatomy of the urinary tract in its distended form. There usually is bilateral hydroureteronephrosis. In severe cases, the renal parenchyma is of extremely poor quality, comprising a thin rim with a highly echogenic nature. When these findings are associated with a thick-walled bladder in a male infant, the diagnosis is almost certainly that of posterior urethral valves. Ultrasound examination of the bladder may also reveal a dilated posterior urethra (Fig. 94–5A). Thereafter, a catheter should be passed into the newborn's bladder and the sonographic views should be repeated to assess whether bladder decompression improves the morphology of the upper urinary tract at all.

In the event that an immediate urologic consultation is not available, there are several hints to passing a catheter under these circumstances. Generally speaking, an 8-French pediatric feeding tube will work well if it is adequately lubricated. However, in some cases, the posterior urethra is so severely distorted that the catheters curls up within it. Under these circumstances, it is best to try to pass an 8-French coudé-tipped catheter. The coudé-tipped catheter has a slightly curved tip at the end that allows it to slide through the posterior urethra. Should this not work, placing a small finger within the child's rectum allows

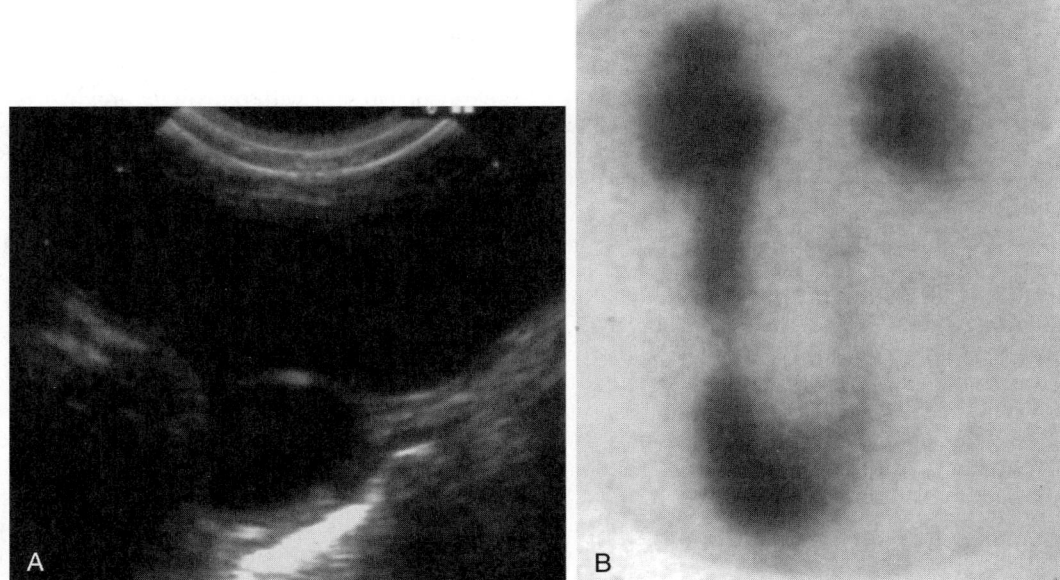

FIGURE 94–4. Ultrasound view of a primary megaureter shows a dilated ureter behind the urinary bladder; it is the bladder views that help distinguish a ureteropelvic junction obstruction from an obstruction at the ureterovesical junction *(A)*. Most megaureters have excellent renal function, which can be documented by DTPA renal scan *(B)*, and most may be followed conservatively with good outcomes.

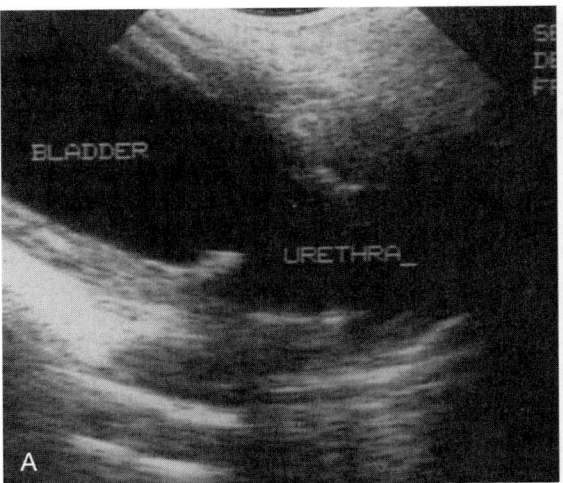

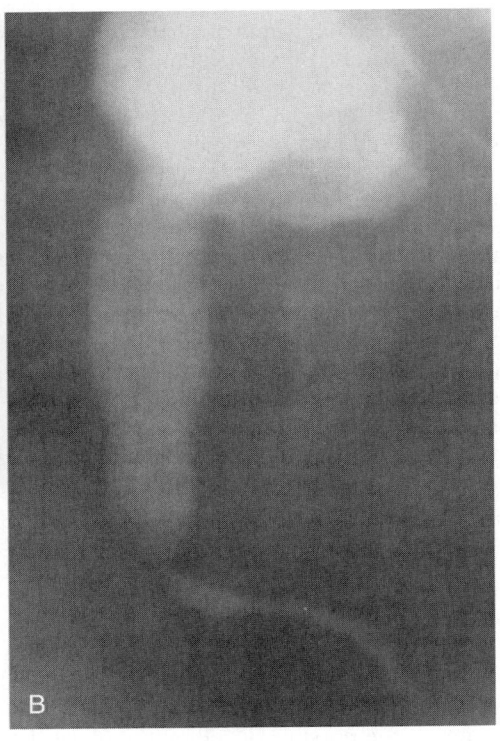

FIGURE 94–5. Ultrasound view of the bladder in a child with a posterior urethral valve demonstrates the classic thick-walled bladder and dilated posterior urethra that, in addition to hydronephrosis (not seen on this view), are characteristic of this diagnosis (A). A VCUG confirmed these findings of a dilated posterior urethra that terminates at the valve cusps (B).

one to deflect the catheter upward into the bladder. However, one must be extremely careful to avoid perforation of the urethra while trying to advance the catheter into the bladder.

In severe cases of posterior urethral valves, placing a catheter and achieving decompression may result in postobstructive diuresis. For this reason, newborns with posterior urethral valves who undergo decompression with placement of a catheter should remain in the NICU to closely monitor their fluid and electrolyte balance. Failure to keep up with the urinary electrolyte and free water losses can easily produce intravascular volume depletion, resulting in hypotension and a decreased renal blood flow that further aggravates the renal insufficiency. Once the newborn has been catheterized, antibiotics should be started and the overall medical condition should be optimized before any thought is given to further diagnostic steps and operative intervention.

A well-done VCUG remains the study of choice for making an accurate diagnosis of posterior urethral valves. This study is done in fluoroscopy usually via the catheter that was placed at the time of the bedside sonogram. It demonstrates a dilated posterior urethra and valve cusps at the distal aspect of the prostatic fossa (Fig. 94–5*B*). In severe cases, it also shows a heavily trabeculated bladder, a high-grade vesicoureteral reflux, or both. In a newborn who is critically ill, it is best to leave the catheter in place and wait until the patient's medical condition stabilizes to allow for transportation to the fluoroscopy suite for the VCUG to be carried out.

Once the VCUG has been reviewed, the pediatric urologist can plan for the initial surgical management. Most cases are managed with an endoscopic transurethral resection of the posterior urethral valve leaflets (Zderic, 1996).

However, in the preterm newborn, a vesicostomy may be the initial procedure of choice since forcing the smallest endoscope into a tiny urethra may produce a severe stricture that could become a source of long-term morbidity. Once the preterm newborn has gained weight, it is easy to close the vesicostomy and resect the valve. Since available information suggests an increased susceptibility to urinary tract infections in the uncircumcised male (Wiswell and Geschke, 1989), it is the preference of this author to also perform a circumcision at the time of the valve resection.

There is a subset of newborns with posterior urethral valves who present with only unilateral hydronephrosis and dysplasia. In most of these cases, the massive hydronephrosis and dysplasia are associated with a unilateral reflux that serves as a protective mechanism by acting as a pop-off valve to lower bladder pressure and spare the contralateral kidney. The vesicoureteral reflux with dysplasia (VURD) syndrome has been shown to correlate well with a good long-term renal outlook for these patients. A number of other pop-off mechanisms have also been described, and all are associated with an improved prognosis for long-term renal (Rittenberg et al, 1988) and bladder (Kaefer et al, 1995) function.

Discharge can be anticipated within several days after surgery once the fluid and electrolyte status is stable and the newborn has been demonstrated to void. It is important to caution the families that these infants have poor urinary concentrating ability and thus may have increased fluid requirements, making them susceptible to dehydration with even mild diarrhea or emesis. The initial follow-up should be performed within a month, and it consists of a follow-up physical examination, renal bladder ultrasound, and serum creatinine determination. This author prefers to maintain these infants on antibiotic prophylaxis even in the absence of reflux because they may be somewhat more susceptible to urinary tract infections owing to some degree of stasis in the distended collecting system and bladder. For the newborn with severe posterior urethral valves with evidence of chronic renal insufficiency, the teamwork in the NICU involving the urologists, nephrologists, neonatologists, and social workers plays a crucial role. The team members should meet the family to appropriately prepare them for the problems that lie ahead. In these cases, long-term follow-up care consists of visits to the urology and nephrology clinics as well as to the newborn follow-up clinic. For the family, the NICU is an ideal place to establish the relationship with each of these specialties in preparation for the future care of their son.

Ureterocele

A ureterocele is a cystic dilation of the distal ureter that protrudes into the urinary bladder and may extend past the bladder neck into the urethra. The embryologic basis for ureterocele formation has been postulated to be a prolonged existence of the Chwalla's membrane, which results in a temporary occlusion of the ureter and allows for the development of hydroureteronephrosis. Ureteroceles are mostly found in duplex systems, where they are always associated with the upper-pole renal parenchyma. The renal parenchyma seen in the upper pole of the duplex system is usually of poor quality and may even contain dysplastic elements. A ureterocele is, by definition, an obstructed system, and as such it must be dealt with on an urgent basis. Failure to do so may result in an infant who presents with urosepsis even if he or she has been maintained on antimicrobial prophylaxis.

On the renal and bladder ultrasound, the ureterocele originating from a duplex system is characteristically associated with the finding of hydronephrosis of the upper pole, a significant ureteral dilation down to the level of the bladder, and a cystic lesion within the lumen of the bladder close to the bladder base. A VCUG completes the workup and aids the urologist in assessing whether any reflux occurs into the ipsilateral or contralateral ureter(s). The surgical options that exist for the management of the newborn with a ureterocele include an endoscopic incision, upper-pole partial nephrectomy, and excision of the ureterocele with a combined reimplantation. However, one may first perform a cutaneous ureterostomy in the neonate and wait to carry out a definitive lower tract reconstruction in the older infant.

Ureteroceles may prolapse into the urethra; this type represents the most common form of bladder outlet obstruction in female neonates. In some patients, the ureterocele may prolapse completely outside the urethral meatus to produce a cystic bulge within the labia.

Ectopic Ureters

Much like ureteroceles, the possibility of urosepsis makes the early diagnosis of ectopic ureter of paramount importance. Most of these systems are detected with prenatal sonography that results in an immediate postnatal evaluation of the newborn. The physical examination in these patients usually is unremarkable. However, in a female with a suspected ectopic ureter, it is always imperative to check the vaginal introitus to look for urinary collections. If a ureter is ectopic to the urethra or vaginal vault, it will dribble urine on a continuous basis that often is apparent on physical examination (Fig. 94–6). Making the diagnosis of ectopic ureter early in life prevents urosepsis and simplifies the process of toilet training for a young female. An ectopic ureter often presents as the young female patient who "has never been dry a day in her life." Because of the embryology of ureteral bud migration from the metanephros, a male's ureter always enters above the external sphincter and therefore he will never be incontinent secondary to an ectopic ureter.

Similar to ureteroceles, most ectopic ureters also are found in duplex systems, where they always represent the upper-pole moiety. The ultrasound findings in ectopic ureter include a hydronephrosis usually in an upper pole of a duplex system, a dilated distal ureter that lies behind the bladder, and an extension of this dilated distal ureter past the bladder neck. However, contrary to that found in the case of a ureterocele, there is no cystic lesion seen with ectopic ureters within the bladder itself (Fig. 94–7). Ectopic ureters may present anywhere from the bladder neck to the distal urethra or vagina, so it is not surprising that there is a good deal of variety to the ultrasonographic findings. The VCUG is important in the evaluation of these patients, because in approximately 70% of the cases there is reflux into the ectopic ureter. However, this may not be apparent on the first void, and it may be necessary to

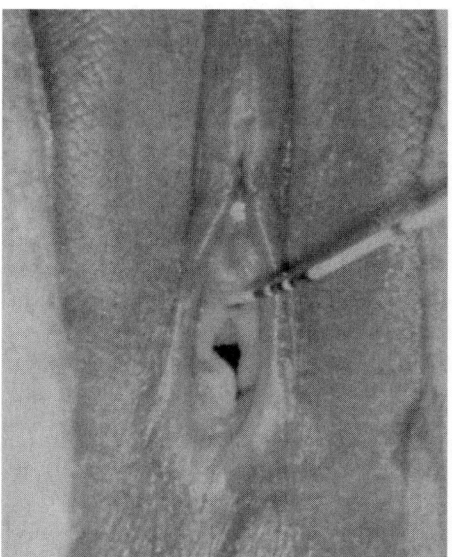

FIGURE 94–6. This is a classic finding in a female with an ectopic ureter which can present outside the confines of the external striated sphincter. In this case (at the time of surgery) the retrograde catheter has been passed into the ectopic ureter located at the 6 o'clock position just below the normal urethral meatus. This child presented at an older age due to unremitting urinary incontinence. This child might have also presented in the neonatal period with urosepsis; the incidence of such presentations has been diminished by prenatal sonography which leads to the use of antibiotic prophylaxis and earlier diagnosis and treatment.

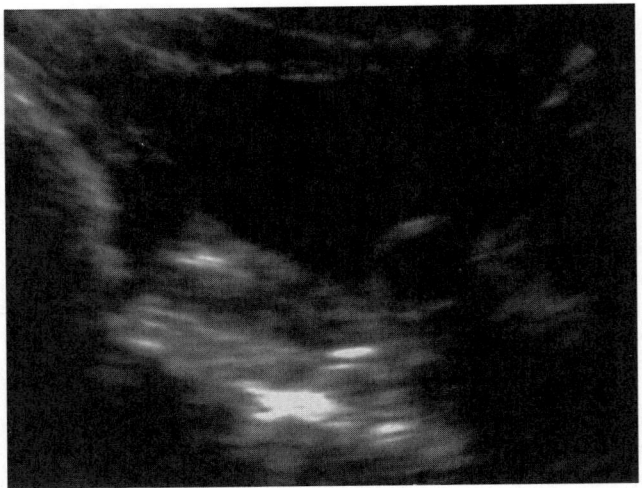

FIGURE 94–7. This ultrasound view of an ectopic ureter shows a dilated ureter behind the bladder which should arouse the suspicion of a diagnosis of ectopic ureter. This is especially true if the ureter cannot be shown on live time images to enter the bladder (doppler analysis can demonstrate ureteral jets of peristatic activity into the bladder). In such cases a VCUG is indicated. In addition careful observation of the perineum and vaginal introitus in a newborn female may reveal a continous dribbling of urine from the ectopic ureter (see Fig. 94–6).

cycle the bladder several times before such reflux may be demonstrated.

Surgical management of ectopic ureters includes an upper-pole partial nephrectomy (or a complete nephrectomy in a nonfunctioning kidney) with or without an excision of the distal stump, a temporizing cutaneous ureterostomy with delayed reimplantation and excision of the distal stump, and an immediate complete reconstruction with reimplantation and excision of the ectopic stump (Snyder, 1996). The benefit of the cutaneous ureterostomy is that it allows for a rapid decompression of the dilated ureter with a 30-minute procedure that does not preclude discharge within a 24-hour period following surgery. When the child is about 1 year of age, a ureteral reimplantation of the now much less dilated ureter and excision of the distal stump are performed.

SPINA BIFIDA

The child with spina bifida has many special needs, including an adequate urologic follow-up. The urologist's aims in managing a patient with spina bifida include to stabilize and maintain renal and upper urinary tract function, aid in achieving continence of urine and stool, and later in life provide sexual function counseling. The first and foremost goal is the preservation of the upper urinary tract and renal function, which is the focus of the initial assessment and management in the NICU. The evaluation and care of these patients requires a coordinated teamwork provided by the pediatric neurosurgeon, urologist, pediatricians, and physical therapists specialized in the care and follow-up of these patients (the spina bifida team), and the neonatologist. Following the neurosurgical repair of the dysraphism, the time spent in the NICU is an ideal point for the family

to meet the caregivers, especially the members of the spina bifida team, and begin the educational process.

The main threat to the renal function of the newborn with spina bifida may be traced to bladder function that is affected by the dysraphic state and the superimposed (and unavoidable) neurosurgical closure. This author begins the work-up by obtaining a renal bladder ultrasound within 1 week of closure to look for any evidence of hydronephrosis. If this sonogram is normal, the child is discharged home and a urodynamic assessment is carried out at 4 weeks of age. If the first ultrasound is abnormal, showing dilated upper tracts, a cystogram is obtained to rule out the possibility of vesicoureteral reflux. If reflux is present, the institution of prophylactic antibiotic treatment is mandatory and a urodynamic assessment prior to discharge is strongly recommended. The purpose of these urodynamic studies (Bauer, 1992) is to identify in advance the "hostile bladder," that is, the bladder whose poor function is compromising renal function.

Among the parameters of the urodynamic studies, the level of the leak point pressure may be of the greatest practical importance. Since up to 40% of children with an elevated leak point pressure above 40 cm H_2O may show signs of upper urinary tract deterioration, this finding dictates that some form of intervention is needed. Some pediatric urologists favor the immediate institution of clean intermittent catheterization in conjunction with antimicrobial prophylaxis and anticholinergic medications (Kasabian et al, 1992; Sutherland et al, 1995). Others advocate that such urodynamic data should be used to increase the frequency of screening ultrasounds to every 3 or 4 months to look for signs of hydronephrosis, and once these appear, institute some regimen of medical management. However, it is uniformly excepted that once upper tract changes are documented in the presence of an elevated leak point pressure, some intervention must be instituted. One option to consider other than medications and clean, intermittent catheterization is the surgical creation of a vesicostomy. This is tolerated well by the neonate and the parents, may be a more practical solution in families where both parents work, is associated with preservation of the upper urinary tract (Snyder et al, 1983), and can dramatically diminish admission rates for urosepsis (Zhylan et al, 1993). Newborns with low leak point pressures may be followed with serial ultrasound examinations every 6 to 12 months, with the realization that their chances for upper urinary tract decompensation are less than 10%.

IMPERFORATE ANUS

The diagnosis of imperforate anus prompts an immediate general surgical consultation and management. However, in the flurry of surgical preparation, it is worth remembering that these infants often have associated urologic findings (Rich et al, 1988). Up to 40% of those newborns with imperforate anus in whom the rectum ends in the supralevator position may have an associated lumbosacral finding such as spina bifida occulta and a tethered cord. This is an important subset of patients to identify, because their bladders are already at risk for voiding dysfunction even before any surgical procedure is performed.

The uroradiographic work-up for these patients should

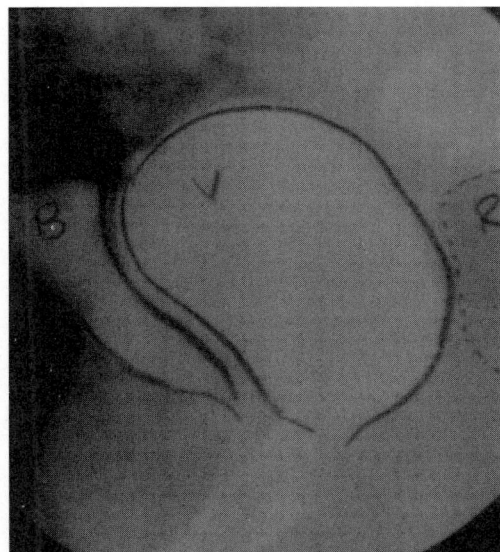

FIGURE 94–8. This child's genitogram is presented as an example of a cloacal anomaly. In this case the child had a normal rectum, but upon close exam had no distinct vaginal introitus or urethral meatus. Separation of the genitalia revealed one common opening to a urogenital sinus with a length of 3 centimeters. At that point the urethra branched anteriorly out to arrive at a functional bladder neck, and a dilated and distended vagina branched out posteriorly. This child presented with a palpable abdominal mass which represented a distended vagina filled with urine. B, bladder; V, vagina; R, rectum.

consist of a renal bladder ultrasound and a VCUG. The renal sonogram identifies patients with renal agenesis, anomalies of renal fusion, or occasional obstructive uropathy. The VCUG identifies those patients who reflux (almost 30%) so that antibiotic prophylaxis may be initiated. In addition, the VCUG may identify any signs of a colopros-tatic or colovaginal fistula and aid in the design of the subsequent anorectal reconstruction.

CLOACAL ANOMALIES

Cloacal anomalies of caudal differentiation present as a wide spectrum. One common variant has a completely "normal," although anteriorly placed, rectum and a urogenital sinus into which the vagina and urethra merge (Fig. 94–8). These female newborns may present with a pelvic mass that is cystic and posterior to the bladder on pelvic sonography. Close inspection of their genitalia reveals one common sinus that is narrow and offers a high resistance to urinary flow. As a consequence, the bladder empties into a vaginal vault that progressively expands, and in severe cases, it may even produce ureteral obstruction and hydronephrosis. The definitive diagnosis is made by a genitogram. In some affected neonates, there is a complete fusion, so that the urethra, vagina, and rectum empty into the perineum via one common channel. The embryology, anatomy, and complex management of these rare cases represent neonatal surgical emergencies in which management decisions are highly individualized (Pena, 1995).

Cloacal Exstrophy

The infant with cloacal exstrophy (Fig. 94–9A) presents with several obvious clinical features, including two bladder halves fully exposed on the abdomen (one on each side of the midline), an abdominal midline consisting of the entire wide-open cecal plate allowing for egress of stool, a protruding limb of prolapsed distal ileum, and an omphalocele of varying size. In addition to these obvious malformations, 50% of these children have associated spinal dysraphism of varying degrees (Fig. 94–9B). This infant represents a medical and social emergency (Canning et al, 1996). The risks of hypothermia, dehydration, and infection from the exposed viscera mandate immediate admission to the NICU.

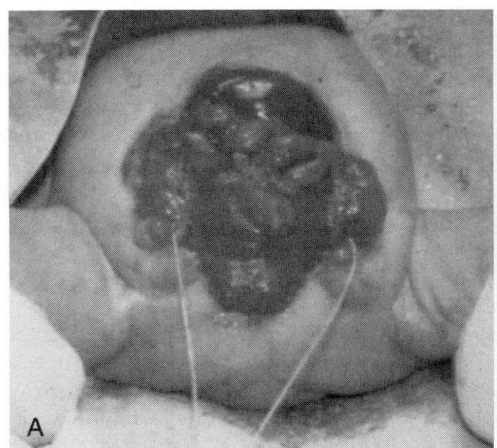
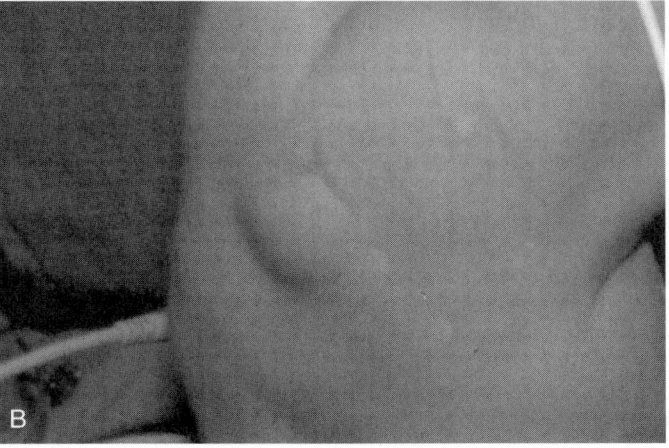

FIGURE 94–9. Cloacal exstrophy *(A)* presents with two bladder halves separated by an open cecal plate. Above this lies an omphalocele, which can be very large. To the right and left are rudimentary corporal bodies, which are almost always inadequate for phallic construction. The standard of care for these patients has been for assignment to the female gender. Fifty percent of these patients present with associated spinal anomalies such as spina bifida or a lipomeningocele *(B).*

All exposed viscera should be covered preferentially with Saran Wrap since gauze sponges tend to be abrasive and should be avoided. It is imperative that such infants are being cared for in a center experienced in the surgical management of cloacal exstrophy. The first stage of reconstruction should be undertaken as soon as the newborn's condition has stabilized. A central line is also placed because all these children will have some element of short bowel syndrome and will require hyperalimentation for varying periods postoperatively. The goals of the initial surgery are to tubularize the cecal plate and create a colostomy, followed by a reapproximation of the two bladder halves. The latter step is done in conjunction with the creation of a neo-urethra from adjacent skin flaps. These infants are left incontinent of urine until they reach the age of 5 to 7 years, when they undergo a second urologic reconstruction to create a competent bladder neck.

The social emergency of cloacal exstrophy arises because in half of these cases, the infant presents with testes and rudimentary corporal bodies. The ability to create a functional phallus in these cases is severely compromised by the hypoplastic corpora and the wide displaced pubic rami. Therefore, the widely accepted recommendation is that these infants be raised in a female gender. It is crucial that the neonatologists, urologists, and the nursing staff meet in advance so that the family does not receive mixed messages about their child's gender (see section on ambiguous genitalia).

Bladder Exstrophy

The patient with classic bladder exstrophy presents with a bladder plate that is protruding in the suprapubic area and extends to just below the umbilicus (Fig. 94–10). Bladder exstrophy is an isolated event not associated with other major congenital anomalies. In males, there is an associated epispadias because the urethra never develops. There is no formation of the bladder neck or trigone in both sexes, and as a consequence, there is no mechanism for urinary continence. The goals of the initial surgery are to create a neo-urethra out of adjacent skin flaps and tubularize the bladder plate (Canning et al, 1996). This should be carried out within the first 24 hours of life because the pelvic bones are most readily realigned during this period. For males, an epispadias repair is carried out at 2 years of age. Recently, a one-stage repair in the neonatal period, including primary bladder closure as well as epispadias repair, has been proposed. These infants are then left incontinent of urine until they reach the age of 5 to 7 years, when they undergo a second urologic reconstruction to create a competent bladder neck. Up to 50% of the patients may ultimately require clean, intermittent catheterization over their lifetime. Overall, newborns with bladder extrophy have an excellent prognosis and, with proper management, can lead nearly normal lives.

DISORDERS OF THE GENITALIA
The Undescended Testes

The presence of an undescended testis in the NICU is fairly common, considering that this diagnosis may be made

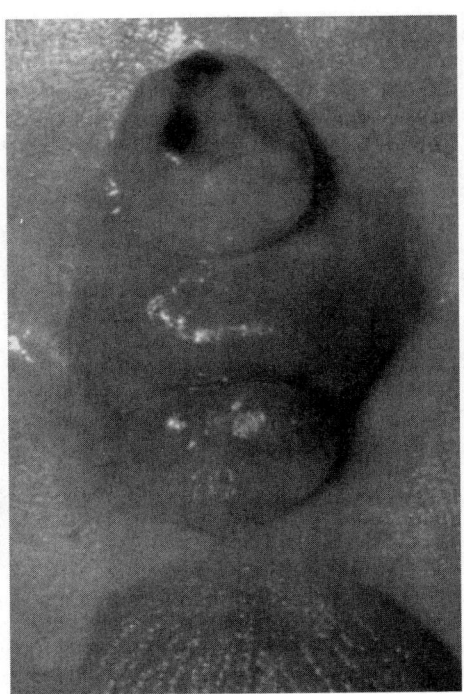

FIGURE 94–10. Classic exstrophy presents with exposed bladder mucosa that has prolapsed onto the abdomen beginning just below the umbilicus and extending on down to the pubis. Covering this mucosa with Saran Wrap and not cotton dressings prevents abrasions and inflammation that make the surgical closure more difficult. Primary surgical closure can be readily accomplished in the first 24 hours of life.

in up to 3% of all term males. However, most of the testes that are undescended in the neonatal period descend by 6 to 9 months of life, and the incidence of cryptorchidism is only 0.8% at the age of 18 years. Up to 30% of neonates may present with bilateral undescended testes. Since the presence of bilateral impalpable undescended testes in a newborn male must be considered as an intersex state until proven otherwise, it is especially important to note whether any gonadal tissue is palpable in these cases. Failure to follow this approach may delay the diagnosis of congenital adrenal hyperplasia, leaving these neonates with inadequate cortisol and mineralocorticoid function and thus susceptible to the development shock. Furthermore, if the diagnosis of congenital adrenal hyperplasia is delayed beyond the first few months of life, the subsequently necessary feminizing genitoplasty imposes an immense social burden on the family. For these reasons, an adequate diagnosis is both lifesaving and protective of the family's emotional needs (see section on ambiguous genitalia).

The infant with bilateral undescended testes and a normal phallus is usually referred to the pediatric urologist during the first few months of life and followed until 6 months of age. The infant with a unilateral undescended testis and a normal phallus may be referred for a urologic follow-up only at 6 months of age. If a testis is impalpable at this time, it will not descend on its own. The impalpable testis may be due to a true intra-abdominal gonad, a testis that is intermittently passing in and out of a large patent processus vaginalis, or a completely absent one secondary to an antenatal torsion. If testicular agenesis is present, the contralateral testis has usually undergone some degree of compensatory hypertrophy, with an increased volume noted by examination or by sonographic measurements (Huff et al, 1992). However, the measurement of volume alone does not preclude the need for exploration since there is an overlap in the distributions. At this point, if a testes is found, an orchiopexy may be safely performed.

The child who presents at age 6 months with an undescended testis high in the inguinal canal is also a candidate for surgical intervention since this is unlikely to descend on its own. However, if the testis is near the scrotum, a repeat examination is prudent. A retractile testis may also present at this point, in which case the testis may be pulled into the scrotal sack, but it only stays down if there is a gentle overstretch of the cremasteric muscle fibers. These infants should also be followed closely.

There are three major issues that should be addressed with families regarding cryptorchidism. First, the family should be reassured that, following orchiopexy, their son will have a normal-appearing scrotal sac, unless testicular atrophy is diagnosed. In these cases, as well as in cases of bilateral agenesis secondary to torsion, or in the rare infant with orchiectomy secondary to malignancy, testicular implants make a difference later in life. Although it is certainly possible to place such implants in infancy, the preference of this author is to wait until the child is older. These days the silicone testicular implants are being replaced by new saline implants. The second major issue concerns fertility. Recent series showed that 90% of men with unilateral cryptorchidism are fertile, and this is irrespective of the age of surgical correction (Lee et al, 1996). However, a previous study on males undergoing testicular biopsies on both testes revealed that as unilateral orchiopexy was deferred to the prepubertal years, the number of germ cells seen per tubule decline (Huff et al, 1989). For this reason the trend has been to carry out orchiopexy at least by the end of the first year of life if a testis is felt to be undescended. Long-term follow-up studies are underway to begin to determine the benefits of orchiopexy early in life. Finally, although the relative risk for testis cancer increases anywhere from 9- to 40-fold in cases of undescended testes, this observation must be tempered with the reality that testicular cancer is rare. Thus, the overall lifetime risk is low, even for the patient with abdominal undescended testes where the risk of testicular cancer is in the higher range.

Testicular Torsion

Torsion of the testes is a fairly rare event in the neonatal period (1 in 7000 live births). However, there is controversy as to its optimal management. The most important point in arriving at a management decision is the determination of what the scrotum looked like at birth. A newborn who presents in the delivery room with a painless, blue, and tense hemiscrotum most likely has had an antenatal torsion. In this type of torsion, the entire tunica vaginalis and spermatic vessels are twisted in such a way as to occlude the vascular pedicle and render the testes ischemic. This may often occur during the last trimester, and thus what one is seeing in the delivery room is a late presentation of

a process that has been ongoing for some time. In fact, if the antenatal torsion occurs early enough in gestation, all inflammation will have resolved, and the newborn presents with a contralateral solitary testis and an ipsilateral testis that is nonpalpable. In these cases, the surgeon finds blood vessels and a vas deferens that end blindly at a common point, where a small nubbin is occasionally found. On the other hand, the acute scrotum that develops after birth represents a surgical emergency, since the testis may be saved if the ischemia has not become complete or has not been long-lasting.

The controversy about management of torsion revolves around what to do for the infant who is born with the torsion. Past experience has shown that immediate exploration in the hours after birth does not produce testicular salvage, and this is well agreed on in the urologic literature. The unsettled issue is what to do about the contralateral side (Jerkins et al, 1983; Kaplan and Silber, 1989) since the initially normal testis may subsequently also undergo a torsion (Kay et al, 1980). For this reason some authors have advocated proceeding with an exploration to surgically tack down the normal testis and prevent a torsion in the remaining healthy gonad. Others, including the author, prefer to observe and follow closely and intervene only if the opposite side becomes symptomatic. This approach is also helpful in ruling out the extremely rare yolk sac tumors in these patients, since the serial examinations at 1-month intervals will confirm that the shrinking testicular "mass" is really a resolving torsion, which will ultimately be completely reabsorbed.

Hydrocele

A hydrocele is nothing more than a collection of fluid between the tunica vaginalis, which is the liner of the scrotal sac, and the tunica albuginea, which covers the surface of the testes. In the newborn, this fluid has its origin within the peritoneal cavity, which communicates with the scrotal sac via an evagination or extension of the peritoneum called a *patent processus vaginalis*. If the patency is small enough, it may actually function as a one-way valve, allowing fluid into, but not out of, the scrotum. This explains the slow and progressive increases in scrotal size that may be seen in some cases. In other cases with a large patency, the fluid may move in and out of the scrotum with ease such that when the consulting urologist arrives to examine the neonate, the swelling is gone. It is important to reassure families that these infants often improve over time, although the patency of the processus vaginalis persist in approximately 20% of men. It is also extremely important to distinguish a hydrocele from a testicular torsion. However, this is usually easy to do since, in the case of an hydrocele, one can palpate a nontender testis in a scrotum that transilluminates easily. Hydroceles often develop in neonates following the placement of ventriculoperitoneal shunts or peritoneal dialysis catheters. In these instances, even with unilateral presentation, both sides should be repaired since there is an approximately 30% chance that the contralateral side will also become symptomatic.

In general, overly aggressive therapy of the neonatal hydrocele should be avoided in the otherwise healthy newborn because many of these hydroceles will resolve on their own, and because the surgery always carries with it the attendant risk of damage to the vas deferens, testicular vessels, and possibly the development of testicular atrophy, especially in a small newborn (Scherer and Grosfeld, 1993).

Hypospadias

The diagnosis of hypospadias is readily made in more than 90% of the cases by a close examination of the genitalia. The examination reveals a urethral meatus that may open anywhere from the glans to the perineum, a foreskin that has not developed symmetrically, and, in severe cases, a marked tethering of the penis referred to as a *chordee penis*. The priority once the diagnosis of hypospadias is made is to make absolutely certain that the child is not circumcised. In hypospadias cases, the foreskin is crucial for use in the urethral reconstruction and correction of the chordee. Loss of this valuable foreskin may transform a simple hypospadias repair into an unnecessarily complex procedure with a higher complication rate.

However, up to 10% of newborns with hypospadias may have an intact foreskin, and the diagnosis is made only after the circumcision. These cases comprise the megameatus–intact prepuce variants. In these cases, an elective repair of the hypospadias is performed when the infant is 6 months old, and the cosmetic results in megameatus intact prepuce are outstanding, and the loss of foreskin does not in any way compromise the final surgical outcome.

On making the diagnosis of hypospadias, the examining physician must immediately check to see if both testes are palpable. For a newborn with a hypospadias and two testes that are properly placed in the scrotum, an outpatient evaluation with a urologist may be arranged within 1 week so as to allay parental concerns even though the reconstruction is deferred until 6 months of age. However, in severe hypospadias cases, urologic consultation in the NICU may help allay parental fears about gender assignment and long-term outcome. Completely elective outpatient surgery is believed to be safest after 6 months of age; only rarely is it necessary to repair a hypospadias in a younger infant.

The easiest and best cosmetic results are obtained in the simpler cases. However, even the most severe hypospadias may be reconstructed with good cosmetic results, although the likelihood increases that it may require more than one procedure. Half of all hypospadias are in the glanular position and readily amenable to a simple advancement technique, with success rates in the 98% range. Another 25% present in the midshaft region, and the use of a pedicled foreskin flap produces excellent cosmetic and functional results, with success rates in the 90% range. Even the 25% of cases comprising the most severe penoscrotal hypospadias may be reconstructed with good cosmetic and functional results, provided that circumcision was avoided in the neonatal period (Baskin and Duckett, 1996).

Finally, if a hypospadias is seen in conjunction with an undescended testis, the possibility of an intersex state exists (Rajfer and Walsh, 1976). This is particularly true if both testes are undescended and impalpable, in which case a diagnosis of congenital adrenal hyperplasia must be ruled out at once (see section on ambiguous genitalia). If there is a hypospadias present and one testis is impalpable, some

consideration must be given to the possibility of the diagnosis of mixed gonadal dysgenesis or androgen insensitivity syndromes (Borer et al, 1995), and an immediate urologic consultation is indicated.

Ambiguous Genitalia

The diagnosis and management of the neonate with ambiguous genitalia remain a medical and social emergency. The social component of this dilemma for a family cannot be emphasized enough. A complete discussion of genital ambiguity is beyond the scope of this section, and only the most salient features are discussed here. Whereas in the past this dilemma came as a total surprise in the delivery suite, recent advances in prenatal diagnosis have allowed for discussions about genital ambiguity to begin in advance. The increasing use of ultrasound in conjunction with amniocentesis has allowed for the in utero diagnosis of virilizing congenital adrenal hyperplasia or complete androgen resistance syndromes since, in these cases, the sonographic appearance of the genitalia will not match the karyotype obtained at amniocentesis. Still, one must be prepared to deal with the situation where no amniocentesis data are available, and none or only one early gestational maternal sonogram was performed.

The most common finding is the female newborn with congenital adrenal hyperplasia and varying severity in the clinical presentations of ambiguous genitalia. Findings on physical examination range from severe clitoromegaly to a fully developed phallus with no palpable gonads (Fig. 94–11A). As emphasized earlier, a phenotypic male with bilateral impalpable testes may be a severely virilized female owing to the overproduction of androgens. Often the older sibling has already been diagnosed with this condition and, in such a case, it is imperative to quickly ascertain if a karyotype was done during gestation. If this was not done or the results are not available, an ultrasound of the pelvis may be ordered to look behind the bladder for any müllerian remnants. This is a rare diagnosis, and most newborns with a well-formed penis and bilateral impalpable testes prove to be normal males. What one must not do is to defer consultation until a child is 6 months of age, only to then discover the true diagnosis. Once the diagnosis of virilizing congenital adrenal hyperplasia is established, appropriate hormonal replenishment must be initiated. A genitogram delineates the extent of surgery required. In the past, surgical reconstruction was deferred to when the child was 1 or 2 years of age, but there has been a trend with experienced surgeons to carry out feminizing genitoplasty in the first 3 months of life with good cosmetic results (Fig. 94–11B).

Another common presentation is the newborn with androgen insensitivity who presents as a phenotypic female despite an amniocentesis showing an XY karyotype. This situation arises because for virilization to occur, the androgens must first bind to their receptors in the cytosol. Mutations in this cytosolic receptor or at other points downstream then result in a phenotypic female who at subsequent laparotomy is found to have testes. Furthermore, since the testes have continued to produce müllerian inhibitory substance, these newborns have a missing uterus and the upper two thirds of the vaginal vault. There are

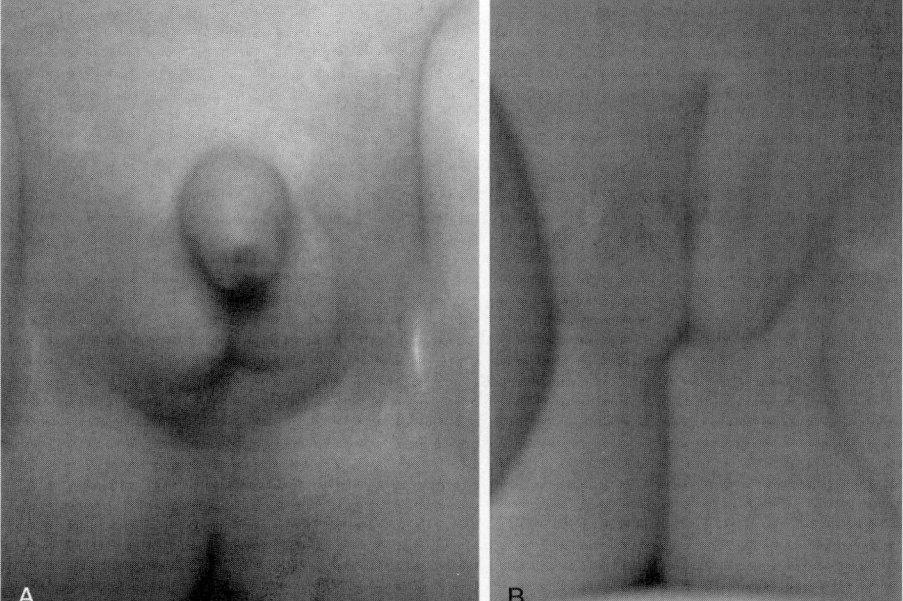

FIGURE 94–11. Congenital adrenal hyperplasia may present as a completely virilized female. The neonatologist must be suspicious of this diagnosis in any "male" with bilateral undescended testes. As shown in A, the degree of virilization can be striking, yet the absence of palpable testes led to immediate urologic consultation. An ultrasound demonstrated a uterus behind the bladder. In experienced hands, a feminizing genitoplasty may be carried out at 2 months (B).

no surgical management issues for these patients in the neonatal period.

Another presentation that must be considered in the neonatal period is the syndrome of mixed gonadal dysgenesis. These patients often present with a severe hypospadias and a unilateral undescended testis. Although many of these newborns may prove to be a straightforward combination of an undescended testis and a hypospadias, there also is a relatively high incidence of intersex disorders in this group of patients, with mixed gonadal dysgenesis being one of the more commonly made diagnoses (Rajfer and Walsh, 1976). These patients may have a normal XY or a mosaic karyotype. At exploratory laparotomy, a gonadal biopsy is performed and a testis will be found on one side and a primitive streak on the opposite side. On the side of the streak gonad, rudimentary müllerian structures may be seen, including a hypoplastic uterus. The streak gonads should be removed because of their malignant potential. The issue of gender is determined by the adequacy of the phallus; in patients where mixed gonadal dysgenesis is associated with small hypoplastic corporal bodies, a feminizing genitoplasty is the accepted management (Borer et al, 1995).

HERNIA

In cases where the patency is large enough, it is possible that intestine and other viscera (including the urinary bladder) may migrate into the scrotal sac. This is an easily reducible hernia without the urgency for repair (Scherer and Grosfeld, 1993). In contrast, a hernia that is difficult to reduce or incarcerated should prompt an elective repair. If the neck of the sac is so tight that the hernia cannot be reduced, the blood supply to the intestine will be compromised and this is classified as a strangulated hernia, which represents a surgical emergency.

CIRCUMCISION

Few topics arouse as much controversy, office visits, phone calls, and annoyance for families, neonatologists, pediatricians, and urologists as does the issue of routine circumcision in the newborn male. Circumcision has been practiced for centuries, and despite all-out efforts in the late 1970s and early 1980s to discourage it, families have continued to clamor for this procedure. It is a fact that, in the United States, around 80% of the male population is circumcised, and hence for many families, the concept that one could forgo this procedure is a surprise. It is reasonable to assume that the main reason most Americans seek routine circumcision is cosmetic. The other reason that families cite in their decision for circumcision is ease of maintaining hygiene. Superimposed on this are number of other arguments, including the "threat" of penile cancer and an "increased risk of sexually transmitted disease." It is true that for patients with poor hygiene, a nonretractile foreskin masks the onset of carcinoma of the penis. It is also true that this is a rare malignancy in the United States and a common malignancy in underdeveloped nations, where circumcision is not practiced. However, this fails to explain why in Europe, where the overwhelming majority of men are not circumcised, penile cancer is rare. The reasons relate to access to regular bathing, basic hygiene, and the ability to retract the foreskin when sexual activity begins. The etiology of carcinoma of the penis is polyfactorial, and as long as the foreskin may be retracted to allow for good hygiene, the threat of malignancy is in and of itself a nonindication for circumcision. Likewise, the threat of sexually transmitted diseases is of polyfactorial etiology, and circumcision will not eradicate this family of diseases. Educational efforts on behalf of diminished promiscuity, condom use, and basic hygiene will produce a greater benefit for society as a whole than circumcision alone.

All these rational arguments in favor of noncircumcision

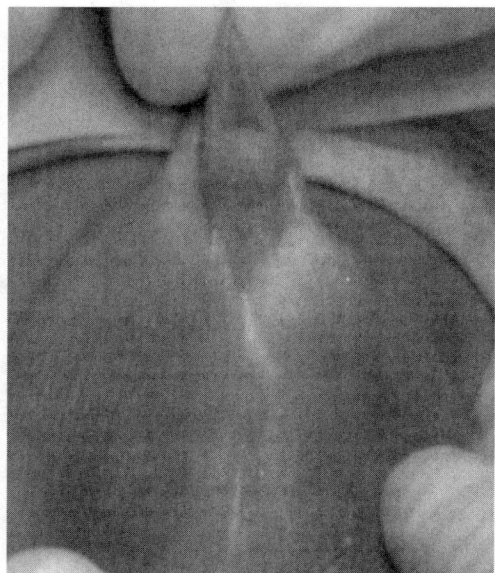

FIGURE 94–12. A severe hypospadias in which the urethral meatus is located at the penoscrotal junction. The foreskin is a well-developed hood located dorsally and is in the examiner's fingers. It is absolutely essential that it is preserved for use in this child's reconstruction. A circumcision should never be performed in any child with an obvious hypospadias or epispadias.

tend to fall short of their mark; most Americans still request routine circumcision. However, parents may also cite a significant study reported in several stages (Wiswell and Geschke, 1989; Wiswell and Hachey, 1993), in which a small medical benefit to circumcision was identified. These studies have demonstrated that the presence of the foreskin increases the chances of a urinary tract infection by about fourfold in the male during the first year of life, which implies that it is necessary to circumcise 99 newborns to gain a benefit for one. Although this is a small benefit, it is a real one. Long-term studies are underway to see if such

an effect carries over into adolescence. More important, based on the findings of these studies, circumcision is advocated for any newborn with an underlying congenital anomaly of the urinary tract such as reflux, posterior urethral valves, or megaureters, where the added burden of a urinary tract infection could have more serious consequences.

The use of regional anesthesia is preferred by some physicians: a circumferential block may be placed at the site where the clamp will be applied with 1% lidocaine (7 mg/kg body weight) and epinephrine (1:100,000 dilution). After the block is placed, the parent may hold and calm the newborn prior to placing the baby in the restraining device. With a successful block, a hemostat applied to the foreskin produces no signs of distress or altered heart rate, and the procedure can be performed without any discomfort to the patient. The three main techniques for circumcision include the use of the Plastibell, the Gomco clamp, or the Mogen clamp. The Plastibell is a plastic bell-shaped device that slips into the groove between the fully retracted foreskin and the coronal margin of the glans. The foreskin is then pulled forward over the Plastibell, and a suture is tied around the outside of the foreskin, thus compressing this skin against the plastic. The resulting skin necrosis in 3 to 5 days allows for the Plastibell and excess foreskin to fall away. This method works well, provided the suture is tight enough and does not slip. The disadvantage of this method is the resulting unsightly necrotic mass that does not slough away for several days. This author's preference is to use the Gomco clamp technique in which a metal bell-shaped device is fitted into the subcoronal groove. The foreskin is then pulled back over this bell, which is then inserted into a circular opening in a steel handle; this allows the foreskin to be crushed between the bell and the metal rim of the handle when the bell is tightened by use of a lever. The Mogen clamp is a guillotine device that has been used by Mohels in ritual circumcision as prescribed by the Jewish faith. Although there is the possibility of the inclusion of parts or potentially all of the glans, in the hands of an expert, the Mogen clamp produces an excellent cosmetic result.

FIGURE 94–13. About 10% of the hypospadias cases may be associated with an intact foreskin *(A)*, and are referred to as megameatus–intact prepuce (MIP) variants. In this case in an older child, the retracted foreskin demonstrates the hypospadias *(B)*, which may not always be possible in the neonate. Most of these children are diagnosed only after circumcision, but this is acceptable care. For these children reconstruction does not require the full foreskin, and beautiful results can be obtained.

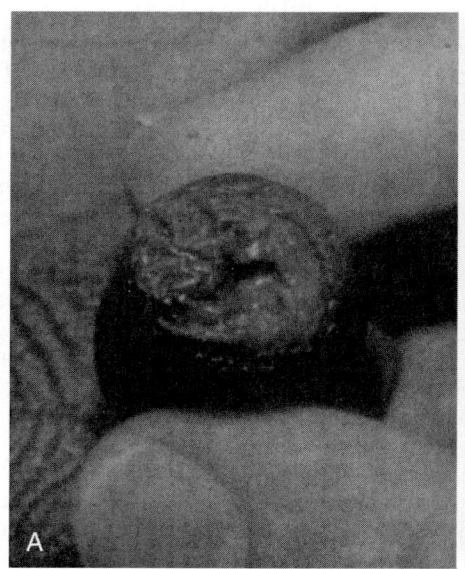
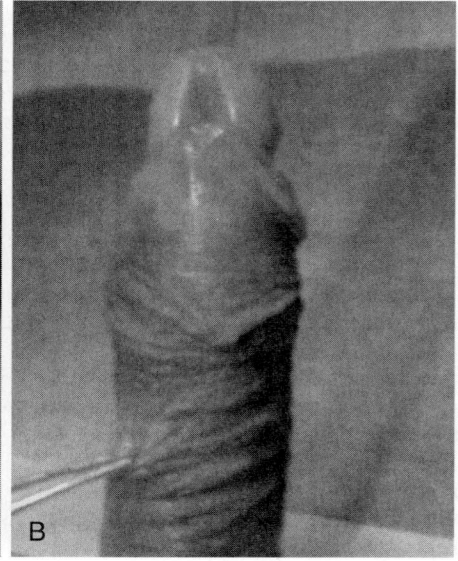

The leading contraindication to circumcision is a sick newborn with lung or heart disease. A premature newborn may also present a technical challenge owing to the smaller size, since the proper fit between infant and equipment is essential. In such instances, circumcision may be deferred until just prior to discharge from the NICU. In the newborn with a history of a complex medical course, this offers the physician a chance to carry out a circumcision with full monitoring of heart rate and pulse oximetry, which is not always available in an office-based setting.

As emphasized earlier, circumcision must never be performed in any child with a hypospadias or epispadias (Fig. 94–12) because the foreskin is essential to the urethral reconstruction. However, if one carried out a circumcision in a child with a completely normal fully circumferential foreskin (Fig. 94–13) and a hypospadias is then noted, this represents the megameatus–intact prepuce variant (5% to 10% of all hypospadias), as described in the section on hypospadias. This is no cause for alarm because in this case the foreskin is not needed for reconstruction, and the parents must be reassured that the standard of care has been rendered and the management of the child will not be altered. It is also important that this be diagnosed correctly as a megameatus–intact prepuce variant of hypospadias and not an injury of circumcision.

Besides injury to the glans and urethra (Baskin et al, 1996), complications of circumcision may include bleeding and, in rare instances, infection. In cases of prolonged and severe bleeding, coagulopathy should be suspected; hemophilia and von Willebrand disease may present in this manner. However, some bleeding after a routine circumcision may be seen in 10% to 20% of the cases. If blood has passed on to the diaper, and a repositioning of the pressure dressing fails to stop the bleeding, the frenulum should also be inspected since this is where most bleeding vessels are found. Although the physician experienced in circumcision should always consider technical factors first in the assessment of bleeding, as mentioned earlier, one should have a low threshold for obtaining coagulation studies.

REFERENCES

Allen TD: The swing of the pendulum. J Urol 148: 534, 1992.
Baskin LS, Zderic SA, Snyder HM, Duckett JW: Primary dilated megaureter: Long-term followup. J Urol 152:618, 1994.
Baskin LS, Duckett JW: Hypospadias. *In* Gillenwater J, Grayhack J, Howards S, Duckett J (Eds): Adult and Pediatric Urology, 3rd ed. Chicago, Year Book, 1996, pp 2549–2590.
Baskin LS, Canning DA, Snyder HM, Duckett JW: Treating complications of circumcision. Pediatr Emerg Care 12:62–68, 1996.
Bauer SB: Neurogenic vesical dysfunction in children. *In* Walsh PC, Retik AB, Stamey TA, Vaughan ED (Eds): Campbell's Urology, 6th ed. Philadelphia, WB Saunders, 1992, pp 1634–1637.
Blyth B, Snyder HM, Duckett JW: Antenatal diagnosis and subsequent management of hydronephrosis. J Urol 149:693–698, 1993.
Borer J, Nitti VW, Glassberg K: Mixed gonadal dysgenesis and dysgenetic male pseudohermaphroditism. J Urol 153:1267–1273, 1995.
Canning DA, Koo HP, Duckett JW: Anomalies of the bladder and cloaca. *In* Gillenwater J, Grayhack J, Howards S, Duckett J (Eds): Adult and Pediatric Urology, 3rd ed. Chicago, Year Book, 1996, pp 2445–2488.
Cartwright PC, Duckett JW, Keating MA, et al: Managing apparent ureteropelvic junction obstruction in the newborn. J Urol 148:1224, 1992.
Conway JJ, Maizels M: The "well-tempered" diuretic renogram: A standard method to examine the asymptomatic neonate with hydronephrosis or hydroureteronephrosis. J Nucl Med 33:2047–2051, 1993.
Coplen DE, Hare JV, Zderic SA, et al: A 10-year experience with antenatal intervention. J Urol 156:1142–1145, 1996.
Crombleholme TM: Invasive fetal therapy: Current status and future directions. Semin Perinatol 18: 385–396, 1994.
Djeter SW, Gibbons MD: The fate of infant kidneys with fetal hydronephrosis but initially normal postnatal sonography. J Urol 142:661–662, 1989.
Gibbons MD, Horan HA, Dejter SW, Keszler M: Extracorporeal membrane oxygenation: An adjunct in the management of the neonate with severe respiratory distress and congenital urinary tract anomalies. J Urol 150:434–437, 1993.
Homsy YL, Williot P, Danais S: Transitional neonatal hydronephrosis: Fact or fantasy. J Urol 136:339–341, 1986.
Homsy YL, Saad F, Laberge I, et al: Transitional hydronephrosis of the newborn and infant. J Urol 144:579–583, 1990.
Huff DS, Hadziselimovic F, Synder HM III, et al: Postnatal testicular maldevelopment in unilateral cryptorchidism. J Urol 142:546–548, 1989.
Huff DS, Snyder HM III, Hadziselimovic F, et al: An absent testis is associated with contralateral testicular hypertrophy. J Urol 148:627–628, 1992.
Jerkins GR, Noe HN, Hollabaugh RS, et al: Spermatic cord torsion in the neonate. J Urol 129:543–549, 1983.
Kaplan GW, Silber I: Neonatal torsion—to pex or not? *In* King LR (Ed): Urologic Surgery in Infants and Children. Philadelphia, WB Saunders, 1989, pp 386–395.
Kasabian NG, Bauer SB, Dyro FM, et al: The prophylactic value of clean intermittent catheterization in the treatment of infants and children with myelomeningocele and neurogenic bladder dysfunction. Am J Dis Child 146:840–844, 1992.
Kaefer M, Keating MA, Adams MC, Rink R: Posterior urethral valves, pressure pop-offs, and bladder function. J Urol 154:708–711, 1995.
Kay R, Strong DW, Tank ES: Bilateral spermatic cord torsion in the neonate. J Urol 123:293–294, 1980.
Koff SA, Campbell KD: Nonoperative management of unilateral neonatal hydronephrosis: Natural history of poorly functioning kidneys. J Urol 152:593–595, 1994.
Lee PA, O'Leary LA, Songer NJ, et al: Paternity after unilateral cryptorchidism: A controlled study. Pediatrics 98:676–679, 1996.
Pena A: Anorectal malformations. Semin Pediatr Surg 4:35–40, 1995.
Rajfer J, Walsh PC: The incidence of intersexuality in patients with hypospadias and cryptorchidism. J Urol 116:769–773, 1976.
Ransley PG, Dhillon HK, Gordon I, et al: The postnatal management of hydronephrosis diagnosed by prenatal ultrasound. J Urol 144: 584–589, 1990.
Rich MA, Brock WA, Pena A: Spectrum of genitourinary anomalies in patients with imperforate anus. Prd Surg Int 3:110–113, 1988.
Rittenberg MH, Hulbert WC, Snyder HM III, Duckett JW: Protective factors in posterior urethral valves. J Urol 140:993–996, 1988.
Scherer LR III, Grosfeld JL: Inguinal hernia and umbilical anomalies. Pediatr Clin North Am 40:1121–1131, 1993.
Smith GH, Canning DA, Schulman SL, et al: The long-term outcome of posterior urethral valves treated with primary valve ablation and observation. J Urol 155:1730–1734, 1996.
Snyder HM: Anomalies of the ureter. *In* Gillenwater J, Grayhack J, Howards S, Duckett J (Eds): Adult and Pediatric Urology, 3rd ed. Chicago, Year Book, 1996, pp 2197–2232.
Snyder HM, Kalichman MA, Charney E, et al: Vesicostomy for neurogenic bladder with spina bifida: A followup study. J Urol 130:724–727, 1983.
Sutherland RS, Mevorach RA, Baskin LS, Kogan BA: Spinal dysraphism in children: An overview and an approach to prevent complications. Urology 46:294–299, 1995.
Wiswell TE, Geschke DW: Risks from circumcision during the first month of life compared to those for uncircumcised boys. Pediatrics 83:1011–1015, 1989.
Wiswell TE, Hachey WE: Urinary tract infection and the uncircumcised state: An update. Clin Pediatr 32: 130, 1993.
Zderic S: The endoscopic management of urethral valves. *In* Smith AD, Badlani GH, Bagley, D, et al (Eds): Smith's Textbook of Endourology. St Louis, Quality Medical, 1996, pp 1323–1332.
Zhylan O, Zderic SA, Duckett JW, et al: Vesicostomy in the management of the myelomeningocele patient: An 18-year experience. J Urol 149:259A, 1993.

CHAPTER 95

Renal Insufficiency and Acute Renal Failure

Istvan Seri, Jacquelyn Evans and Tivadar Tulassay

DEFINITION AND INCIDENCE OF NEONATAL ACUTE RENAL FAILURE

Neonatal acute renal failure (ARF) is defined as the sudden, severe derangement of glomerular filtration and tubular function and is diagnosed when serum creatinine is greater than 1.5 mg/dL regardless of the rate of urine output. ARF should also be suspected in the newborn if serum creatinine fails to decline below maternal levels by at least the 5th to 7th days of life or is rising by 0.3 mg/dL per day (Karlowicz and Adelman, 1992).

Neonatal ARF has conventionally been subdivided into prerenal, intrarenal (intrinsic), and postrenal (obstructive) renal failure according to the primary site of the disorder. The overall incidence of neonatal ARF is approximately 20% of all neonatal intensive care unit admissions (Karlowicz and Adelman, 1992; Stapleton et al, 1987). Greater than 70% of these cases represent prerenal ARF with the rest being intrinsic or obstructive ARF. It is important to remember that the conventional classification of neonatal *obstructive* renal failure as ARF is incorrect; this disorder rather represents the acute onset of a chronic renal failure when separation from the placental circulation at birth occurs.

PATHOPHYSIOLOGY OF NEONATAL ACUTE RENAL FAILURE
Prerenal Acute Renal Failure

Prerenal ARF is the most common form of ARF in the newborn. The cause of prerenal ARF is renal hypoperfusion owing to systemic hypotension or to selective decreases in renal blood flow in response to tissue hypoxia without significant systemic hypotension. Under these circumstances, renal autoregulation fails to maintain renal blood flow (RBF) and glomerular filtration rate (GFR) in the physiologic range. Correction of the underlying condition immediately restores normal renal function unless renal hypoperfusion has been severe or prolonged so that renal parenchymal damage has already developed. When this occurs, prerenal ARF evolves into intrinsic ARF.

In prerenal ARF, despite the decrease in RBF, GFR is initially relatively preserved leading to enhanced tubular reabsorption of solutes and water. The increase in filtration fraction (GFR/RBF $\times$ 100) increases peritubular oncotic pressure resulting in enhanced proximal tubular sodium and water reabsorption (Feld et al, 1986). Furthermore, vasopressin and endothelin secretion as well as the activity of the renin-angiotensin-aldosterone system and the renal sympathetic nerves increases, leading to further enhancement of renal tubular solute and water absorption. The net result of these renal hemodynamic and hormonal changes is oliguria, decreased urinary sodium concentration, and increased urinary osmolality. In some newborns, however,

oliguria does not develop because of decreased pituitary release of, or renal responsiveness to, vasopressin (Dixon and Anderson, 1985) and because in these cases less significant alterations in the renal microcirculation may occur. Thus, the rate of urine output has a somewhat limited diagnostic value in newborns (see later). Urine output is an important prognostic factor, however, because morbidity and mortality of the nonoliguric ARF are decreased compared to the oliguric form even if the condition develops features of intrinsic renal failure (Chevalier et al, 1984; Karlowicz and Adelman, 1995).

Severe perinatal blood loss, perinatal asphyxia, respiratory distress syndrome, dehydration of the extremely immature preterm infant owing to increased transepidermal free water loss, necrotizing enterocolitis, hydrops, septic shock, and the use of certain pharmacologic agents (see later) are the most frequent conditions associated with absolute or relative decreases of intravascular volume or renal hypoperfusion (or both) resulting in the development of prerenal ARF in the newborn (Table 95–1). In addition, acute decreases in cardiac output during cardiac surgery or placement on extracorporeal membrane oxygenation may also lead to the development of prerenal ARF.

Intrinsic Acute Renal Failure

Approximately 6% to 8% of newborns admitted to neonatal intensive care units have intrinsic ARF with severe perinatal asphyxia being the most common cause (Stapleton et al, 1987). In contrast to in prerenal ARF, the renal functional abnormalities in intrinsic ARF are not immediately reversible. The severity of intrinsic ARF ranges from mild tubular dysfunction to acute tubular necrosis with or without oliguria and anuria and to renal infarction and corticomedullary necrosis with irreversible renal damage (see Chapter 99). It is of great clinical importance that untreated and sustained prerenal or obstructive ARF can eventually develop into intrinsic ARF. Conditions most commonly associated with the development of intrinsic ARF in the newborn are listed in Table 95–1.

The term *acute tubular necrosis* has been used interchangeably with ARF. Although extensive tubule injury is a frequent pathologic finding in ARF, acute tubular necrosis should be used only for cases of intrinsic ARF secondary to renal ischemia or nephrotoxic substances in which tubular necrosis is always one of the main mechanisms causing the renal failure (Kon and Ichikawa, 1984).

The course of intrinsic ARF may be subdivided into initiation, maintenance, and recovery phases. The initiation phase includes the original insult and the associated events. The sustained low GFR, tubular dysfunction, and azotemia represent the maintenance phase. The duration of the maintenance phase depends, at least in part, on the severity

TABLE 95–1

Causes of Acute Renal Failure in the Newborn*

Prerenal Acute Renal Failure	Intrinsic Acute Renal Failure	Obstructive Renal Failure
Loss of effective circulating blood volume	Acute tubular necrosis (long-lasting, severe renal ischemia,	Congenital malformations
Absolute loss	nephrotoxins)	Imperforate prepuce
Hemorrhage	Congenital malformations	Urethral stricture
Dehydration	Bilateral renal agenesis	PUV
Relative loss	Renal dysplasia	Urethral diverticulum
↑ Capillary leak (sepsis, NEC, RDS,	Polycystic kidneys	Primary VUR
asphyxia, ECMO)	Infections	Ureterocele
Renal hypoperfusion	Congenital infections (syphilis, toxoplasmosis)	Megaureter
All of the above	Pyelonephritis	UPJ obstruction
Congestive heart failure	Bacterial endocarditis	Extrinsic compression
Cardiac surgery	Renal vascular causes	Sacrococcygeal teratoma
Pharmacologic agents	Renal artery thrombosis	Hematocolpos
Indomethacin	Renal vein thrombosis	Intrinsic obstruction
Tolazoline	DIC	Renal calculi
ACE inhibitors	Nephrotoxins	Fungus balls
	Aminoglycosides	Neurogenic bladder
	Indomethacin	
	Amphotericin B	
	Methicillin	
	Radiocontrast dyes	
	Intrarenal obstruction	
	Uric acid nephropathy	
	Myoglobinuria	
	Hemoglobinuria	

° In many cases, a combination of several causative factors contributes to the development of acute renal failure. For instance, absolute hypovolemia, increased capillary leak–induced loss in effective circulating blood volume, hypotension, and reflex renal vasocontriction all result in renal hypoperfusion and ensuing renal injury in newborns with severe forms of shock.

ACE, angiotensin-converting enzyme; DIC, disseminated intravascular coagulation; ECMO, extracorporeal membrane oxygenation; RDS, respiratory distress syndrome; NEC, necrotizing enterocolitis; PUV, posterior urethral valve; UPJ, ureteropelvic junction; VUR, vesicoureteral reflux.

Modified from Karlowicz MG, Adelman RD: Acute renal failure in the neonate. Clin Perinatol 19:139, 1992.

and duration of the initial insult. The recovery phase is characterized by the gradual restoration of GFR and tubular functions. Recognition of the different phases of neonatal intrinsic ARF is helpful in the diagnosis, clinical management, and prognostication of the disorder.

Changes in renal hemodynamics brought about by the excessive production and release of vasoconstrictive hormones, including the renin-angiotensin system, epinephrine, norepinephrine, endothelin, adenosine, vasocontrictive prostaglandins, and vasopressin, play an important role in the development and maintenance of intrinsic renal failure (Karlowicz and Adelman, 1992). In addition, alterations in the function and ultrastructure of the nephron, including the decrease in the permeability and surface area of the glomerular capillary, intratubular obstruction to tubular flow by cellular debris, and tubular backleak, contribute to the impairment of renal function in intrinsic ARF. Finally, the deterioration of hemodynamic and tubular functions is associated with intracellular events, such as enhanced free radical injury with reperfusion of the kidneys and accumulation and sequestration of intracellular calcium in mitochondria resulting in phospholipase activation and the ensuing deterioration of mitochondrial structure and function. If the initiating insult is severe, sustained, or repeated, the intracellular events may lead to widespread epithelial cell death and irreversible tissue damage.

Ischemic-Hypoxic Injury

Despite being the best oxygenated organ, the kidney is susceptible to ischemic-hypoxic injury because of the redistribution of its blood flow under pathologic circumstances as well as because of the unique vascular supply of the renal medulla. The presentation and course of the renal damage depend on the severity and duration of the insult. Mild ischemia results in transient loss of renal concentrating capacity owing to the extreme sensitivity of the medullary thick ascending limb to tissue hypoxia (Brezis et al, 1984). This loss may be difficult to detect, however, in immature preterm newborns with the underlying and developmentally regulated immaturity of their renal concentrating capacity (see Chapter 92). More prolonged injury produces widespread tubular dysfunction with significant impairments in sodium and water reabsorption and decreases in GFR. This is the degree of severity of intrinsic ARF most frequently seen in full-term newborns with severe perinatal asphyxia who present most commonly with the nonoliguric form (Karlowicz and Adelman, 1995). Finally, as mentioned earlier, prolonged or repeated insults may result in the irreversible form of intrinsic ARF with oliguria and anuria and persistent tubular and glomerular damage.

The primary pathomechanism of ischemic-hypoxic intrinsic ARF is the damage to the renal tubular epithelium resulting in backleak of the glomerular filtrate and intraluminal obstruction with necrotic cellular debris (Kon and Ichikawa, 1984). The latter results in an elevation of the pericapillary hydrostatic pressure in the Bowman space leading to further decreases in GFR. The tubuloglomerular feedback mechanism may also be activated by the compensatory increases in the delivery of sodium and water to the distal parts of the nephron in the unobstructed tubules resulting in a further loss in GFR (Myers and Moran, 1986). In addition, abnormalities in the ultrastructure of the glomerulus and decreases in the total filtering surface area occur (Feld et al, 1986; Kon and Ichikawa, 1984). The cumulative effect of these changes in the most severe cases of intrinsic ARF is the complete cessation of glomerular filtration.

The use of some medications, including captopril or enalaprilat (Rasoulpour and Marinelli, 1992) (see Chapter 99) and tolazoline (Guignard and Gouyon, 1988), may also lead to the development of ischemic intrinsic ARF in the sick newborn. The angiotensin-converting enzyme inhibitors (captopril and enalaprilat) may induce unpredictable decreases in systemic blood pressure so that renal perfusion pressure drops below the autoregulatory range leading to tissue hypoperfusion with subsequent hypoxic-ischemic damage to the renal epithelium. Tolazoline, in addition to causing systemic hypotension, may also induce severe renal vasoconstriction, which further compromises renal perfusion (Guignard and Gouyon, 1988).

Nephrotoxic Injury

The predominant lesion in nephrotoxic ARF is the damage to the proximal tubule cells (Feld et al, 1986). In clinical practice, aminoglycoside administration to the newborn is one of the most common conditions in which such damage can occur. Aminoglycosides inhibit lysosomal phospholipases leading to tubule cell phospholipidosis and subsequent necrosis (Giuliano et al, 1984). Changes in the ultrastructure of the glomerulus also occur (Kon and Ichikawa, 1984). The immature kidney appears to be less susceptible to aminoglycoside toxicity than that of the adult (Pelayo et al, 1983). The clinician must also remember that aminoglycoside toxicity is usually *nonoliguric,* and therefore serial monitoring of serum creatinine values is necessary, especially during prolonged administration of these antibiotics, to detect their potential nephrotoxicity in the newborn. The mechanisms of aminoglycoside toxicity appear to be activated even when serum levels are in the accepted range for toxicity in the newborn (Adelman et al, 1987). The potential long-term consequences of this observation on neonatal renal function are unknown.

Combined Ischemic and Nephrotoxic Injury

Other medications, including amphotericin B and indomethacin, exert their renal side effects by causing both ischemic and direct nephrotoxic renal injury. Amphotericin B alters renal function by reducing RBF and GFR and by directly affecting tubular function resulting in renal tubular acidosis and increased urinary potassium excretion. Although these renal toxic effects are most often reversible, cases of fatal neonatal renal failure owing to amphotericin

B toxicity have also been reported (Baley et al, 1984). Serum creatinine and electrolytes should be closely monitored; the dosing interval should be prolonged if serum creatinine rises, and replacement therapy with potassium and bicarbonate should be provided if indicated.

Severe, although usually transient, nephrotoxicity can occur with indomethacin administration. The potentiation of the vasoconstrictive and sodium-retaining and water-retaining effects of angiotensin II, norepinephrine, and vasopressin by the indomethacin-induced inhibition of renal prostaglandin production is the mechanism of the renal actions of the drug. Because neonatal renal function is more dependent on local prostaglandin production than that of the euvolemic adult (especially when intravascular volume is decreased owing to fluid restriction and increased capillary leak in the preterm infant with patent ductus arteriosus), indomethacin administration is almost always associated with elevated serum creatinine concentrations, decreased urine output, and hyponatremia (Cifuentes et al, 1979). In addition, indomethacin may also exert a direct aldosterone-like effect on the distal tubule. Because the renal side effects of indomethacin are mostly transient, some clinicians prefer to wait until spontaneous recovery of renal function occurs while maintaining a restricted fluid intake without additional sodium supplementation. Alternatively, concomitant low-dose dopamine infusion may be used to aid in the recovery from the renal tubular side effects of indomethacin treatment (Seri, 1995). If severe oliguria and anuria develops in the preterm infant, however, furosemide administration may become necessary to prevent the persistence of the ARF caused by indomethacin (Yeh et al, 1982). Serum creatinine and electrolytes as well as urine output should be closely monitored in these newborns. If gentamicin or other nephrotoxic medications are being concomitantly administered, the dose interval of these medications should be prolonged when increases in serum creatinine occur.

A less common form of neonatal intrinsic ARF associated with hypoxia, perinatal asphyxia, or polycythemia is uric acid nephropathy (Karlowicz and Adelman, 1992; Stapleton, 1987). In such cases, precipitation of uric acid or monosodium urate crystals results in obstruction of the renal tubules causing intrinsic ARF. Because newborns normally excrete more uric acid, they may be prone to the development of uric acid nephropathy if severe and prolonged hyperuricemia develops (Stapleton, 1987). In addition, intrinsic ARF, partly as a result of intratubular obstruction, may develop with cases of rhabdomyolysis in severe perinatal asphyxia (Kojima et al, 1985) or with massive hemoglobinuria resulting from intravascular hemolysis. Finally, radiopaque contrast agents may also cause intrinsic ARF, especially in newborns who already have compromised renal function, such as those with congenital heart disease undergoing cardiac catheterization (Karlowicz and Adelman, 1992).

Obstructive Renal Failure

Obstructive renal failure can be caused by a variety of congenital malformations of the kidneys and the urinary collecting system (see Table 95–1; also see Chapters 93 and 94). Some of these newborns have reversible renal failure, whereas others have renal dysplasia with irreversible intrinsic renal failure at the time of diagnosis (see Chapters 93 and 94).

DIAGNOSIS OF NEONATAL ACUTE RENAL FAILURE

Despite its limitations, serum creatinine is the most widely used measure to evaluate glomerular filtration in the clinical setting and is more specific than blood urea nitrogen (BUN) (see Chapter 93). Because the production of BUN is increased by a high dietary protein intake, gastrointestinal bleeding, and hypercatabolic states, BUN levels are elevated out of proportion to changes in GFR under these conditions. Moreover, the renal excretion of urea is also influenced by tubular function, especially under conditions associated with changes in tubular water reabsorption. Therefore, as a general rule, if the BUN/serum creatinine ratio exceeds 20, increased urea production or increased renal urea reabsorption (or both) should be suspected (Feld et al, 1986).

The major goal in the initial evaluation of neonatal ARF is to diagnose prerenal ARF and obstructive renal failure promptly to prevent their transition to intrinsic ARF. The medical history of the pregnancy, the findings of prenatal tests and ultrasound studies, and the physical examination usually provide important clues as to urinary tract obstruction in the newborn presenting with oliguria and anuria in the immediate postnatal period. If obstruction is suspected, a renal and bladder ultrasound study should be performed without delay (see Chapter 92). In cases in which oliguria and elevated serum creatinine values are associated with hematuria or hypertension (or both), the possibility of renal vascular disease should also be considered (see Chapter 99).

The clinically most reliable diagnostic tool to differentiate prerenal ARF from intrinsic ARF is the provision of an appropriate fluid challenge, unless the newborn is suspected of having a urinary outlet obstruction or renal hypoperfusion secondary to congestive heart failure. Isotonic solution (usually normal saline) should be given in a dose of 20 mL/kg or more over a period of 30 minutes to 2 hours. If urine output remains less than 1 mL/kg per hour after 2 hours and there are no clinical signs of intravascular volume deficit, 1 to 2 mg/kg of furosemide should be administered. Alternatively, low-dose dopamine infusion may be used in addition to the volume challenge, especially if systemic blood pressure is labile or remains low after the volume challenge is completed. Low-dose dopamine improves renal perfusion, increases GFR, and increases renal sodium and free water excretion in the newborn (Seri, 1995). In addition, primarily along the proximal parts of the nephron, dopamine inhibits renal tubular Na^+,K^+-ATPase activity and decreases renal oxygen consumption when oxygen delivery is limited (Seri, 1995). The clinical importance of this effect of the drug, however, remains to be demonstrated in the newborn. Furthermore, because dopamine blunts the tubuloglomerular feedback and increases solute delivery to the distal parts of the nephron, oxygen consumption in the outer medulla may increase rather than decrease, at least in the euvolemic animal (Heyman et al, 1995). Under pathologic conditions, however, dopamine restores the diminished outer medullary

blood flow and ameliorates outer medullary hypoxia caused by indomethacin or by the inhibition of nitric oxide synthesis (Heyman et al, 1995). Therefore, the use of dopamine may be beneficial in the sick preterm and term infant with renal vasoconstriction caused by hypoxemia, acidosis, or indomethacin administration (Seri, 1995) (see earlier). Finally, although widely used in children and adults to diagnose prerenal ARF, the mannitol test is contraindicated in newborns with a predisposition to the development of intraventricular hemorrhage or periventricular leukomalacia because of the drug-induced sudden increase in serum osmolality.

In comparision to intrinsic ARF, prerenal ARF is associated with a low urinary sodium excretion, fractional excretion of sodium (FENa), and renal failure index and with high urine/plasma osmolar and creatinine ratios compared to intrinsic ARF (Table 95–2). Although these diagnostic indices are helpful in differentiating prerenal ARF from intrinsic ARF in older children and adults, there are important limitations to their use in the sick preterm and term newborn. Some newborns, especially immature preterm infants, with prerenal ARF have values overlapping those attributed to intrinsic ARF (Ellis and Arnold, 1982). Furthermore, FENa in preterm infants under 32 weeks of gestation with normal renal function is usually higher than 3%, and there are no data of FENa in these infants with intrinsic ARF. Finally, because of the developmentally regulated limitation of their concentrating capacity and the effects of low protein intake and urea excretion on urine osmolality (Feld et al, 1986), the urine/plasma creatinine ratio instead of the urine/plasma osmolal ratio should be used in newborns to evaluate their renal tubular reabsorptive capacity.

Laboratory tests to be followed in ARF include serum sodium, potassium, chloride, bicarbonate, calcium, phosphorus, magnesium, creatinine, uric acid, and glucose as well as BUN, blood gases, and a complete blood count with platelets. If urine is available, a urinalysis; urine culture; and a spot urine sample for sodium, creatinine, and osmolality should be obtained. Findings in a given spot urine sample may significantly differ from those of another one, and repeat analyses or a timed urine collection may become necessary in selected cases to aid in the differential diagnosis.

TREATMENT OF NEONATAL ACUTE RENAL FAILURE
Prerenal Acute Renal Failure

The approach of diagnosing prerenal ARF with the provision of fluid boluses and diuretic treatment (if appropriate) also serves as the initial management of the condition. Most newborns admitted to neonatal intensive care units with ARF have the prerenal form of ARF and respond to fluid therapy. If systemic hypotension develops despite adequate volume administration, early initiation of dopamine with the subsequent normalization of blood pressure ensures appropriate renal perfusion (Seri et al, 1993). Other management goals include the maintenance of normoxemia and normal pH to avoid the recurrence of renal vasoconstriction and to improve capillary integrity as well as the replacement of blood and free water losses as needed.

TABLE 95–2

Diagnostic Indices Suggestive of Prerenal or Intrinsic Renal Failure in the Newborn

	Prerenal Acute Renal Failure	Intrinsic Acute Renal Failure
Urine flow rate (mL/kg/h)	Variable	Variable
Urine osmolality (mOsm/L)	>400	≤400
Urine/plasma osmolar ratio	>1.3	≤1.0
Urine/plasma creatinine ratio	29.2 ± 1.6‡	9.7 ± 3.6‡
Urine [Na⁺] (mEq/L)	10–50	30–90
FENa (%)°	<3.0 (0.9 ± 0.6)‡	>3.0 (4.3 ± 2.2)‡
RFI°†	<3.0 (1.3 ± 0.8)‡	>3.0 (11.6 ± 9.6)‡
Response to fluid challenge (± furosemide)	Increased urine output	No effect on urine output

° Fractional excretion of sodium (FENa) = (Urine [Na⁺] / Serum [Na⁺]) / (Urine [Cr] / Serum [Cr]) × 100.
† Renal failure index (RFI) = Urine [Na⁺] / (Urine [Cr] / Serum [Cr]).
‡ Mean ± SD.
Table compiled from data in Feld et al, 1986; Karlowicz and Adelman, 1992; and Mathew et al, 1980.
See text for details.

Intrinsic Acute Renal Failure

Whenever possible, newborns presenting with conditions potentially associated with the development of intrinsic ARF should be monitored closely and, if available, preventive measures applied before the onset of renal injury. In established intrinsic ARF of the newborn, management centers around providing appropriate *supportive care* until renal function recovers (see later). Additional *nonspecific therapy* includes the use of furosemide (Fildes et al, 1986) and dopamine (Karlowicz and Adelman, 1992; Seri et al, 1993; Tulassay et al, 1983). Although there is no conclusive evidence that the attempt to provide selective renal vasodilation and diuresis improves renal function or prognosis in intrinsic ARF, patients who respond to diuretic management with an increase in urine output early in the course of renal failure are more likely to survive (Fildes et al, 1986). In addition, the use of these medications may aid in ensuring an appropriate fluid and electrolyte balance. If dopamine is used, it should be started early in the course of the disease and at low doses (1 to 4 μg/kg per minute) to avoid unnecessary increases in systemic blood pressure and possible renal vasoconstriction (Karlowicz and Adelman, 1992; Seri, 1995; Seri et al, 1993; Tulassay et al, 1983). The combined use of dopamine and furosemide may have a synergistic effect on inducing diuresis even in the preterm newborn (Tulassay and Seri, 1986). The potential toxicity of long-term and aggressive furosemide therapy, including ototoxicity, interstitial nephritis, osteopenia, nephrocalcinosis, hypotension, and persistence of patent ductus arteriosus, should be taken into consideration, especially in the preterm newborn (Karlowicz and Adelman, 1992) (see also Chapters 35 and 99).

There is no accepted *specific therapy* in the clinical practice for intrinsic ARF. Experimental findings suggest that early administration of adenosine triphosphate–magnesium chloride (ATP-MgCl₂) or thyroxine may decrease the extent of cellular damage in experimental intrinsic ARF (Karlowicz and Adelman, 1992). Both agents exert their protective effects mainly by improving the recovery of renal cellular ATP (Boydstun et al, 1995; Karlowicz and Adelman, 1992). Because of its serious hemodynamic side

effects, however, administration of ATP-MgCl₂ is probably contraindicated in sick newborns. With regard to thyroxine, there is only one noncontrolled clinical study in which the hormone was implicated in the recovery of renal function in eight children with ARF (Straub, 1976). The potential of thyroxine as well as adenine nucleotides and several growth factors to facilitate recovery of experimental ARF will likely by used in future clinical trials in an attempt to improve further recovery and survival of patients with intrinsic ARF (Wagener et al, 1995).

Supportive care includes prevention, early recognition, and aggressive management of complications of neonatal intrinsic ARF, including fluid overload, hypertension, electrolyte disturbances, nutritional deficiency, metabolic acidosis, and sepsis. Severe fluid restriction limiting intake to insensible and gastrointestinal and renal losses is required to avoid fluid overload with the development of pulmonary edema, congestive heart failure, hypertension, and hyponatremia. Fluid restriction also mandates the placement of a central venous line and the use of high glucose concentrations with little or no sodium and no potassium in the infusate.

Hypertension usually develops as a consequence of fluid overload or hyperreninemia resulting from the renal damage. The evaluation, diagnosis, and treatment of neonatal hypertension is described in Chapter 99 in detail.

Hyponatremia, hyperkalemia, hyperphosphatemia, and hypocalcemia frequently develop and require close monitoring and aggressive treatment when indicated. In cases of nonsymptomatic hyponatremia (serum sodium concentrations usually between 120 and 130 mEq/L), further restriction of free water intake is recommended. If hyponatremia at this level becomes symptomatic (lethargy, seizures) or serum sodium concentration falls below 120 mEq/L, 3% sodium chloride should be administered over 2 hours according to the following formula:

$$Na^+_{required} (mEq) = ([Na^+]_{desired} - [Na^+]_{actual}) \times \text{body weight (kg)} \times 0.8$$

Possible complications of hypertonic saline administration, especially if infused over less than 1 to 2 hours, include congestive heart failure, pulmonary edema, hypertension, intraventricular hemorrhage, and periventricular leukomalacia.

Signs of progressive hyperkalemia on the electrocardiogram, in order of severity, consist of tall peaked T waves, heart block with widened QRS complexes, arrhythmia, the development of sine waves, and finally cardiac arrest. If diuretics are ineffective and all potassium intake has been abolished (including that in medications), with serum potassium levels between 6 and 7 mEq/L and associated electrocardiographic changes or with serum potassium greater than 7 mEq/L in the absence of characteristic electrocardiogram changes, additional treatment is necessary. Under these conditions, management of hyperkalemia includes the administration of calcium gluconate, sodium bicarbonate, and insulin with glucose (Table 95–3). Although sodium polystyrene may also be administered, it must be remembered that it may take up to 6 hours until any effect is seen, and the exchange resin may be ineffective in preterm infants less than 29 weeks of gestation (Malone, 1991). Hyperkalemia unresponsive to medical management is one of the most common indications for peritoneal dialysis in the newborn with intrinsic ARF (Karlowicz and Adelman, 1992).

Hyperphosphatemia is common in ARF and should be treated with low phosphorus intake. Significant elevations in serum phosphate represent a risk of extraskeletal calcifications of the heart, blood vessels, and kidneys in the newborn, especially when the calcium-phosphorus product exceeds 70 (Lerner and Gruskin, 1990). Low phosphorus formulas should be provided for those newborns who tolerate feeding. Soy formulas should be avoided because of their high aluminum content. Although calcium carbonate may be used as a phosphate binding agent, severe hyperphosphatemia is best treated with peritoneal dialysis.

Although total calcium levels are frequently low in newborns with intrinsic ARF, ionized calcium is less commonly decreased because of concurrent hypoalbuminemia and metabolic acidosis. If ionized calcium is decreased and the newborn is symptomatic, 10 to 20 mg/kg of calcium gluconate should be infused over 10 to 20 minutes and repeated every 4 to 8 hours as necessary. The usual maintenance doses of elemental calcium (50 to 100 mg/kg per day) should also be provided in the form of calcium gluconate or calcium carbonate. If the newborn is being fed, dihydrotachysterol or calciferol may be administered to increase intestinal reabsorption of calcium.

Nutritional deficiency almost always develops in newborns with intrinsic ARF. The goal is to provide 100 kcal/kg with carbohydrates and fat, and 1 to 2 g/kg per day of high biologic value protein or an amino acid equivalent. Metabolic acidosis should usually be treated only when pH is less than 7.20, unless the newborn presents with associated pulmonary vascular reactivity and persistent pulmonary hypertension. The latter clinical scenario represents an extreme clinical challenge and may require the initiation of extracorporeal membrane oxygenation to treat both the pulmonary vascular and the renal disease. Finally, because sepsis is a common cause of death in newborns with intrinsic ARF, infection control must be rigorously observed, and when sepsis is suspected appropriate diagnostic steps should be taken and non-nephrotoxic antibiotic therapy administered. Because ARF alters the volume of distribution, protein binding, and renal excretion of many antibiotics, drug doses and dose intervals should frequently be adjusted. Furthermore, many hepatically metabolized antibiotics still require renal excretion of their potentially toxic metabolites.

When renal failure is prolonged beyond 1 to 2 weeks, supportive therapy is unsuccessful, or both, serious complications of intrinsic ARF develop. Such complications include severe fluid overload, electrolyte abnormalities (especially hyperkalemia or severe hyponatremia refractory to medical management), symptomatic uremia (tremors, vomiting, irritability), rapidly rising serum creatinine and BUN, and hypertension. When complications develop, dialysis should be initiated. Dialysis should be started when the newborn is still hemodynamically stable so that this treatment modality can affect morbidity and mortality from ARF. Peritoneal dialysis is preferred over hemodialysis in the newborn because it is similarly effective, probably safer, and technically less demanding. The peritoneal catheter may be placed either percutaneously or surgically. Relative contraindications to peritoneal dialysis include necrotizing enterocolitis; coagulopathy; hemodynamic instability; and the presence of an intra-abdominal foreign body, such as a ventriculoperitoneal shunt or a diaphragmatic patch.

Continuous arteriovenous hemofiltration uses the patient's cardiac output as the driving force for the hemofilter, which has a high ultrafiltration coefficient. The advantage of this technique is that it avoids rapid fluid shifts and the occurrence of hypotension by providing slow, continuous removal of an isotonic solute. It requires systemic heparinization, however, making the technique contraindicated in newborns at high risk for intracranial bleeding. Furthermore, clotting of the catheters occurs frequently, especially after prolonged use (Ronco et al, 1986).

TABLE 95–3

Medical Management of Hyperkalemia in the Newborn

Drug	Dose	Onset of Action	Duration of Action
Calcium gluconate (10%)	0.5–1.0 mL/kg (IV over 10 min)	1–5 min	15–60 min
Sodium bicarbonate (3.75% solution)	1.0–2.0 mEq/kg (IV over 10 min)	5–10 min	2–6 h
Insulin	1 IU/5 g glucose (IV bolus or continuous infusion)	15–30 min	4–6 h
Glucose	≤14 mg/kg/min (IV bolus or continuous infusion)	15–30 min	4–6 h
Sodium polystyrene sulfonate	1 g/kg dose every 6 h as needed (orally/rectally)	1–2 h°	4–6 h

° Onset of action may take up to 6 hours, and the drug may be ineffective in preterm infants <29 weeks of gestation (Malone, 1991).
See text for details.

Obstructive Renal Failure

Management of obstructive renal failure centers around the immediate relief of the obstruction, supportive medical care, and surgical correction of the underlying congenital malformation as described in detail in Chapter 94. Polyuria with electrolyte losses may occur following the relief of the obstruction, and close monitoring of serum electrolytes and appropriate fluid and electrolyte replacement therapy are necessary in the clinical care of such newborns.

CLINICAL COURSE OF NEONATAL ACUTE RENAL FAILURE

Derangement of glomerular and tubular function may last for up to 3 to 6 weeks in newborns with ARF. In the case of oliguric ARF, recovery is usually heralded by a gradual increase in the urine output over the course of several days and, in some cases, by the appearance of a polyuric phase. The free water and electrolyte losses associated with the polyuric phase of recovery mandate monitoring of serum electrolytes and appropriate replacement therapy with sodium, potassium, and free water if indicated. Serum creatinine and BUN usually start decreasing later in the course of polyuria.

OUTCOME OF NEONATAL ACUTE RENAL FAILURE

The mortality rate of newborns with ARF caused by congenital malformations or acquired diseases is around 50% for the oliguric form (Karlowicz and Adelman, 1992; Stapleton et al, 1987), whereas newborns with nonoliguric ARF have a much better prognosis (Chevalier et al, 1984; Karlowicz and Adelman, 1992). The long-term sequelae of neonatal ARF include reduced GFR in cases with excessive nephron losses and tubular dysfunction. GFR remains decreased in approximately 40% of newborns in both acquired oliguric (Stapleton et al, 1987) and nonoliguric (Chevalier et al, 1984) ARF. Newborns with the history of ARF secondary to congenital malformation have the worst long-term prognosis; close to 80% of such infants later develop chronic renal failure (Reimold et al, 1977).

With regard to renal tubular dysfunction, a permanent decrease in the concentrating capacity owing to injury to the epithelium of the thick ascending limb (see earlier) is the most frequent finding on follow-up. Other abnormalities include chronic hypertension; renal tubular acidosis; impaired renal growth; and, mostly in cases of renal cortical necrosis, nephrocalcinosis (Karlowicz and Adelman, 1992).

REFERENCES

Adelman RD, Wirth F, Rubio T: A controlled study of the nephrotoxicity of mezlocillin and gentamycin plus ampicillin in the newborn. J Pediatr 111:888, 1987.

Baley JE, Kliegman RM, Fanaroff AA: Disseminated fungal infections in very low birth weight infants: Therapeutic toxicity. Pediatrics 73:153, 1984.

Boydstun I, Najjar S, Kashgarian M, et al: Postischemic thyroxin stimulates renal mitochondrial adenine nucleotide translocator activity. Am J Physiol 268:E651, 1995.

Brezis M, Rosen S, Silva P, Epstein FH: Selective vulnerability of the medullary thick ascending limb to anoxia in the isolated perfused rat kidney. J Clin Invest 73:182, 1984.

Chevalier RL, Campbell F, Brenbridge AN: Prognostic factors in neonatal acute renal failure. Pediatrics 74:265, 1984.

Cifuentes RF, Olley PM, Balfe JW, et al: Indomethacin and renal function in premature infants with persistent patent ductus arteriosus. J Pediatr 95:583, 1979.

Dixon BS, Anderson RJ: Nonoliguric acute renal failure. Am J Kidney Dis 6:71, 1985.

Ellis EN, Arnold WC: Use of urinary indices in renal failure in the newborn. Am J Dis Child 136:615, 1982.

Feld LG, Springate JE, Fildes RD: Acute renal failure: I. Pathophysiology and diagnosis. J Pediatr 109:401, 1986.

Fildes RD, Springate JE, Feld LG: Acute renal failure: II. Management of suspected and established disease. J Pediatr 109:567, 1986.

Giuliano RA, Paulus GJ, Verpooten GA, et al: Recovery of cortical phospholipidosis and necrosis after acute gentamicin loading in rats. Kidney Int 26:838, 1984.

Guignard JP, Gouyon JB: Adverse effects of drugs on the immature kidney. Biol Neonate 53:243, 1988.

Heyman SN, Kaminski N, Brezis M: Dopamine increases renal medullary blood flow without improving regional hypoxia. Exp Nephrol 3:331, 1995.

Karlowicz MG, Adelman RD: Acute renal failure in the newborn. Clin Perinatol 19:139, 1992.

Karlowicz MG, Adelman RD: Nonoliguric and oliguric acute renal failure in asphyxiated term newborns. Pediatr Nephrol 9:718, 1995.

Keys TF, Kurtz SB, Jones JD, Muller SM: Renal toxicity during therapy with gentamycin and tobramycin. Mayo Clin Proc 56:556, 1981.

Kojima T, Kobayashi T, Matsuzaki S, et al: Effects of perinatal asphyxia and myoglobinuria on development of acute, neonatal renal failure. Arch Dis Child 60:908, 1985.

Kon V, Ichikawa I: Research seminar: Physiology of acute renal failure. J Pediatr 105:351, 1984.

Lerner GR, Gruskin AB: Acute renal failure. *In* Nelson NM (Ed): Current Therapy in Neonatal-Perinatal Medicine, 2nd ed. Toronto, BC Decker, 1990, pp 173–177.

Malone T: Glucose and insulin versus cation-exchange resin for the treatment of hyperkalemia in very low birth wieght infants. J Pediatr 118:121, 1991.

Mathew OP, Jones AS, James E, et al: Neonatal renal failure: Usefulness of diagnostic indices. Pediatrics 65:57, 1980.

Myers BD, Moran SM: Hemodynamically mediated acute renal failure. N Engl J Med 314:97, 1986.

Pelayo JC, Andrews PM, Coffey AK, et al: The influence of age on acute renal toxicity of uranyl nitrate in the dog. Pediatr Res 17:985, 1983.

Rasoulpour M, Marinelli KA: Systemic hypertension. Clin Perinatol 19:121, 1992.

Reimold EW, Don TD, Worthen HG: Renal failure during the first year of life. Pediatrics 59:987, 1977.

Ronco C, Brendolan A, Bragantini L, et al: Treatment of acute renal failure in newborns by continuous arteriovenous hemofiltration. Kidney Int 29:9008, 1986.

Seri I: Cardiovascular, renal, and endocrine actions of dopamine in newborns and children. J Pediatr 126:333, 1995.

Seri I, Rudas G, Bors ZS, et al: The effect of dopamine on renal function, cerebral blood flow and plasma catecholamine levels in sick preterm newborns. Pediatr Res 34:742, 1993.

Stapleton FB, Jones DP, Green RS: Acute renal failure in newborns: Incidence, etiology and outcome. Pediatr Nephrol 1:314, 1987.

Straub E: Effects of L-thyroxine in acute renal failure. Res Exp Med 168:81, 1976.

Tulassay T, Seri I: Interaction of dopamine and furosemide in acute oliguria of preterm infants with hyaline mebrane disease. Acta Paediatr Scand 75:420, 1986.

Tulassay T, Seri I, Machay T, et al: Effects of dopamine on renal functions in premature infants with respiratory distress syndrome. Int J Pediatr Nephrol 4:19, 1983.

Wagener OE, Lieske JC, Toback FG: Molecular and cell biology of acute renal failure: New therapeutic strategies. New Horiz 3:634, 1995.

Yeh TF, Wilks A, Singh J, et al: Furosemide prevents the renal side effects of indomethacin therapy in premature infants with patent ductus arteriosus. J Pediatr 101:433, 1982.

CHAPTER 96

Glomerulonephropathies and Disorders of Tubular Function

Bernard S. Kaplan

GLOMERULONEPHROPATHIES

Glomerulonephropathies generally present with the nephrotic syndrome or with a nephritic syndrome. The nephrotic syndrome is characterized by massive proteinuria, hypoalbuminemia, hyperlipidemia, and edema. Newborns may have transient proteinuria without apparent glomerular injury, and serum albumin levels can be in the nephrotic range in normal premature infants. Therefore, the diagnosis of nephrotic syndrome should be made only in patients with persistent, massive proteinuria; severe hypoalbuminemia; hyperlipidemia not caused by hyperalimentation; and edema that is not the result of fluid overload, capillary leak, or both. Nephritis (hematuria, red blood cell casts, oliguria or anuria, hypertension, and azotemia) is extremely uncommon in newborns.

The nephrotic syndrome can be inherited as an entity isolated to the kidneys (congenital nephrotic syndrome of the Finnish type (CNF) or as part of a defined malformation syndrome (Denys-Drash syndrome, Galloway-Mowat syndrome, nail-patella syndrome). The types of glomerular injury that may occur in newborns and infants with nephrotic syndrome can also be divided into primary glomerular conditions with nephrotic syndrome (e.g., CNF) and secondary glomerular conditions (e.g., congenital syphilis). The assignment of the locus for CNF to chromosome 19q12-q13.1 (Kestila et al, 1994) is a major advance in the classification of a group of conditions that can present with features of the nephrotic syndrome in the 1st year of life (Habib, 1993).

Only CNF and congenital syphilis *typically* present with nephrotic syndrome at birth. Diffuse mesangial sclerosis (DMS), Denys-Drash syndrome, and Galloway-Mowat syndrome rarely manifest in the neonatal period (Table 96–1). Minimal change nephrotic syndrome, focal segmental glomerulosclerosis, membranous glomerulonephritis, collagen type III glomerulopathy, mercury toxicity, and systemic lupus do not occur in newborns but occasionally present in infants. Renal vein thrombosis can be a consequence of the nephrotic syndrome but is never a cause of the syndrome. There is no convincing evidence that intrauterine infections with cytomegalovirus (Batisky et al, 1993), rubella (Beale et al, 1979), or toxoplasmosis (Shahin et al, 1974) are causes of neonatal nephrotic syndrome. Finally, there are reports of *unique* family syndromes in which congenital nephrotic syndrome occurred in association with other congenital anomalies, such as buphthalmos; reports of congenital glomerular injury that elude classification; and reports of spontaneous remission of apparent congenital nephrotic syndrome (Haws et al, 1992).

Congenital Nephrotic Syndrome, Finnish Type

CNF has also been called *infantile microcystic disease* because of the presence of dilated proximal renal tubules in many cases. Inheritance is autosomal recessive. The locus for CNF is assigned to 19q12-q13.1 (Kestila et al, 1994). It has not been determined whether all patients with apparent CNF have the same mutation(s) or whether there may be non-Finnish types of congenital nephrotic syndrome. There is intrafamilial and interfamilial variability in the severity and age of onset of the nephrotic syndrome. CNF occurs in all population groups, with the highest prevalence in Finland with an incidence of 12.2 per 100,000 newborns (Huttunen, 1976). The absence of a history of Finnish ancestry does not exclude the diagnosis. No biochemical abnormalities have been found to account for the proteinuria (Kestila et al, 1994). Proteinuria is

TABLE 96–1

Glomerulonephropathies and Renal Tubular Disorders in Newborns

Syndrome	Neonatal Onset	In Utero Diagnosis
Glomerulonephropathies		
Congenital nephrotic syndrome, Finnish type	Yes	Yes
Diffuse mesangial sclerosis	Rarely	No
Denys-Drash syndrome	No	No
Galloway-Mowat syndrome	Yes	Possibly
Congenital syphilis	Yes	Yes
Disorders of Renal Tubular Function		
Renal Fanconi syndrome		
Idiopathic	Yes	
Fructose intolerance	Yes°	Yes
Galactosemia	Yes°	Yes
Cystinosis	Not in proband	Yes
Cytochrome *c* oxidase deficiency	Yes	Unreliable
Proximal renal tubular acidosis	Yes	
Distal renal tubular acidosis	Yes	
Bartter syndrome	Yes	Yes
Pseudohypoaldosteronism		
Autosomal dominant	Yes	
Congenital X-linked nephrogenic diabetes insipidus	Yes	Yes

°If exposed to sucrose or fructose.

Time of Detection of Proteinuria and Onset of Edema and Abdominal Distention in Congenital Nephrotic Syndrome, Finnish Type

Time	Documentation of Proteinuria (%)	Onset of Edema and/or Abdominal Distention (%)
At birth	19	26
During 1st week	71	52
During 2nd month	100	100

Adapted from Huttunen N-P: Congenital nephrotic syndrome of Finnish type: Study of 75 patients. Arch Dis Child 51:344, 1976.

detected within the 1st week of life in 71% of cases and by 2 months in all affected infants (Table 96–2) (Huttunen, 1976). Proteinuria is highly selective, but the demonstration of this characteristic is not necessary to make the diagnosis. Early onset of hypertension and renal failure is uncommon. Infants are often premature and small for gestational age. Although there are no typical dysmorphic features, large anterior fontanels, limb deformations, and pyloric stenosis do occur (Sibley et al, 1986). Maternal serum and amniotic fluid alpha-fetoprotein levels are elevated (Seppala et al, 1976), and increased concentrations of albumin are detected in the amniotic fluid of some cases. The diagnosis may be made coincidentally by the finding of a low thyroxine level during screening for hypothyroidism (Finnegan et al, 1980). Most of these patients have a primary form of hypothyroidism characterized by low thyroxine and high thyroid-stimulating hormone levels caused by urinary losses of thyroxine and iodine (McLean et al, 1982). In CNF, the placenta is large with a mean placenta/neonatal weight ratio of 0.43 compared with a normal ratio of 0.18.

The kidneys are echodense and symmetrically enlarged on ultrasonography. The renal histopathologic findings are not pathognomonic. Proximal tubules are dilated in 74% of cases. The glomeruli initially appear normal by light microscopy. Ultrastructural studies show the effacement (*fusion*) of epithelial cell foot processes that is found in all patients with massive proteinuria regardless of the cause. Later in the course, there may be interstitial fibrosis, lymphocytic and plasma cell infiltration, periglomerular fibrosis, and progressive glomerular sclerosis (Habib, 1993). CNF must be differentiated from diffuse mesangial sclerosis, although the latter rarely presents in newborns.

The course is characterized by unremitting nephrotic syndrome complicated by failure to thrive, recurrent infections, and eventual chronic renal failure. Renal vein thrombosis may occur in utero and postpartum. Parents must be counseled that the inheritance is autosomal recessive. Treatment with corticosteroids and alkylating agents is futile. Aggressive feeding via nasogastric or gastrostomy tubes can ensure weight gain. Massive edema is treated with intravenous albumin and furosemide infusions if the patient is not volume depleted. Hypothyroidism is treated with thyroxine. Bilateral nephrectomies and dialysis are indicated if edema, volume depletion, and inanition cannot be controlled. Long-term peritoneal dialysis is difficult, but

feasible, in small infants. The results of living-related renal transplantation are encouraging, and CNF does not recur after transplantation (Mahan et al, 1984). A unique type of post-transplantation nephrosis resembling transplant glomerulopathy occurs in a quarter of the patients 1 to 33 months after transplantation (Laine et al, 1993). The response to treatment with prednisone and cyclophosphamide is poor (Laine et al, 1993).

Diffuse Mesangial Sclerosis

The nephrotic syndrome with DMS and chronic renal failure can be inherited as an autosomal recessive condition. DMS can also occur sporadically, and it can be seen as a component of the Denys-Drash syndrome (Habib, 1993). DMS has been reported in an 18-week fetus (Spear et al, 1991) and occasionally can present in the neonatal period (Scott and Rochefort, 1992). Maternal and fetal alpha-fetoprotein concentrations and placental size are usually normal (Scott and Rochefort, 1992). Most patients present between 3 and 6 months because of increasing edema, are hypertensive, and are in advanced renal failure. There are no dysmorphic features. The kidneys are enlarged and echodense by ultrasound examination. Early renal light microscopic findings are a fibrillar increase and expansion of mesangial matrix without an increase in mesangial cells. Podocytes are hypertrophied. The fully developed lesion consists of mesangial sclerosis, collapsed tufts, embedded mesangial cells, thick glomerular basement membranes, and tubulointerstitial lesions (Habib, 1993).

There is no specific treatment. Hypertension is treated with angiotensin-converting enzyme inhibitors but often requires several additional agents for optimal control. Treatment of DMS includes optimal calories, peritoneal dialysis, and transplantation. DMS does not recur after transplantation. It is important to determine whether there is a mutation in the WT1 gene on chromosome 11p to rule out Denys-Drash syndrome. If that cannot be done, renal ultrasound examinations may be warranted every few months.

Denys-Drash Syndrome

Early onset of nephrotic syndrome with DMS can also occur in the Denys-Drash syndrome. The syndrome consists of overlapping features of ambiguous genitalia, nephrotic syndrome with DMS (Habib, 1993), Wilms tumor, and a zinc finger mutation on chromosome 11p (Pelletier et al, 1991). Occasional patients present with nephrotic syndrome in the neonatal period (Gertner et al, 1980). Siblings are not affected. Most patients die by 4 years of age unless transplanted.

Galloway-Mowat Syndrome

The Galloway-Mowat syndrome is a rare condition (about 22 reported cases) that consists of abnormal central nervous system development and nephrotic syndrome (Cooperstone et al, 1993). Inheritance is autosomal recessive with variable expression in one family as shown in three siblings who had combinations of cataracts, anterior cleavage syndrome, microcephaly, diffuse sclerosis of white matter, and nephrotic syndrome (Cohen et al, 1994). Patients may be small for gestational age. Onset of nephrotic syndrome was between birth and 3 years in all cases and before 3 months of age in half of the reported cases. There are no consistent glomerular histopathologic changes. Basement membrane irregularities and dilated tubules are reported, but there is no pathognomonic abnormality (Cohen et al, 1994). Neurologic findings are microcephaly, wide sulci, abnormal gyral patterns, developmental retardation, and seizures (Roos et al, 1987). Large floppy ears, a receding forehead, and hiatal hernia occur in some cases (Cooperstone et al, 1993).

The prognosis is dismal with death before the age of 6 months in most cases. The nephrotic syndrome does not respond to steroids or cyclophosphamide. Renal transplantation is not encouraged because of the progressive nature of the neurologic disorder. Increased maternal serum and amniotic fluid alpha-fetoprotein assays and abnormal renal ultrasonographic findings may prove useful for prenatal diagnosis (Palm et al, 1986).

Congenital Syphilis

Congenital syphilis is the best characterized of the acquired causes of nephrotic syndrome in infants. Clinical features of nephrotic syndrome are more frequent than those of nephritis. The diagnosis must be suspected in an infant who has edema, proteinuria, and signs of congenital syphilis (McDonald et al, 1971). The renal histopathologic findings implicate an immune pathogenesis with subepithelial deposits that contain immunoglobulin G (IgG) and treponema antigen (O'Regan et al, 1976). Treatment with penicillin results in permanent remission of the glomerulopathy.

DISORDERS OF RENAL TUBULAR FUNCTION

A diagnosis of a renal tubular disorder cannot be made without an appreciation of normal renal maturation. Premature newborns (and even full-term newborns) can waste sodium and chloride and have variable combinations of aminoaciduria, glucosuria, phosphaturia, impaired potassium excretion, reduced reabsorptive capacity for sodium bicarbonate, and inability to concentrate the urine maximally. In healthy newborns, these are transient aberrations that tend to be isolated and that do not cause problems except for the low bicarbonate threshold in preterm infants. This can lead to mild metabolic acidosis during the first few months of life. Very-low-birth-weight newborns may have nonoliguric hyperkalemia, in part secondary to decreased Na^+,K^+-ATPase activity, which increases with maturation. Therefore, except in specific circumstances, it is not necessary to embark on a full-scale evaluation.

A renal tubular disorder may be suspected and confirmed in utero. A prenatal diagnosis that requires chorionic villus sampling or amniocentesis can be made only after the diagnosis of the condition in an older sibling. Postnatally the possibility of a tubular disorder may arise when abnormal blood gas and electrolyte results are obtained. The initial manifestations of a renal tubular disorder may not include all the findings associated with the disorder.

Three constellations of fluid and electrolyte imbalances should alert a neonatologist to the possibility of a disorder of renal tubular function. The combination of *metabolic acidosis, hyperkalemia, and hyponatremia* is seen in renal dysplasias, obstructive uropathy (especially if complicated by a urinary tract infection), and pseudohypoaldosteronism. Furthermore, congenital adrenal hyperplasia can present with these abnormalities. *Metabolic acidosis, hypokalemia, and hypophosphatemia* are the characteristic findings seen in patients with the renal tubular Fanconi syndrome. Finally, *metabolic alkalosis, hypokalemia, and hyponatremia* occur in Bartter syndrome.

Important clinical clues for the presence of a renal tubular disorder are poor feeding, unexplained vomiting, dehydration, failure to thrive, drowsiness, irritability, tetany, seizures, and unexplained icterus. Isolated proximal renal tubular acidosis (RTA) is uncommon. Large quantities of bicarbonate to correct a hyperchloremic metabolic acidosis is a clue to the diagnosis. Fructose intolerance and galactosemia must be considered in a jaundiced newborn who has Fanconi syndrome. Hypophosphatemia and renal phosphate wasting are manifestations of X-linked hypophosphatemic rickets, but it is uncommon for this to be diagnosed in a newborn. Hyperchloremic metabolic acidosis with a decrease in the unmeasured anion gap and in the absence of diarrhea raises the possibility of distal RTA. Distal RTA rarely presents in the neonatal period, however. Pseudohypoaldosteronism, Bartter syndrome, and renal adysplasias must be considered in newborns with severe hyponatremia and renal salt wasting. Infants with Bartter syndrome are hypokalemic, whereas those with renal adysplasia, pseudohypoaldosteronism, and the renal tubular hyperkalemia syndromes are hyperkalemic. Hematuria, renal calculi, and nephrocalcinosis with hypercalciuria can occur in newborns with and without prolonged use of furosemide (see Chapter 34).

Fanconi Syndrome of Proximal Tubular Dysfunction

Fanconi syndrome is characterized by generalized proximal renal tubular dysfunction with impaired net reabsorption of amino acids, bicarbonate, glucose, phosphate, urate, sodium, potassium, magnesium, calcium, and low-molecular-weight proteins. Renal excretion of these solutes and water is increased, and the serum concentrations of some are variably reduced. Hypophosphatemia results in vitamin D–resistant rickets, and bicarbonaturia causes a hyperchloremic metabolic acidosis. In newborns, the clinical manifestations of Fanconi syndrome may include polyuria, dehydration, metabolic acidosis, and glycosuria. These features are often asynchronous. Growth retardation and rickets mostly occur later in infancy.

Hereditary Fructose Intolerance

Hereditary fructose intolerance presents only in newborns fed sucrose or fructose in formula, antibiotics, fruit juices, or honey. The symptoms are poor feeding, vomiting, and failure to thrive (Gitzelman et al, 1989). The diagnosis can be made by molecular analysis of the aldolase-B gene in blood (Brooks and Tolan, 1993). Inheritance is autosomal recessive. Fructose-containing foods must be withdrawn from the diet as soon as the condition is suspected.

Galactosemia

Two of the three autosomal recessive inherited disorders of galactose metabolism (transferase and epimerase deficiency) manifest in newborns with signs of toxicity a few days after milk ingestion. Signs are vomiting, diarrhea, direct hyperbilirubinemia, hepatomegaly, ascites, and cataracts. There is an increased prevalence of *Escherichia coli* sepsis. In many countries and some states in the United States, newborn screening programs exist for early detection of galactosemia. The diagnosis is made by demonstrating increased concentrations of galactose (*reducing substances*) in blood and urine. The urine is positive only after ingestion of lactose or galactose. The diagnosis is confirmed by demonstrating deficient galactose-1-phosphate uridyl transferase in red blood cells. Milk and milk-containing products must be withdrawn completely from the diet.

Cytochrome *c* Oxidase Deficiency

A fatal infantile cytopathy involving brain, muscle, liver, and occasional renal tubular Fanconi syndrome is one of the *mitochondrial cytopathy* syndromes associated with defects in complex IV of the respiratory chain. Clinical features include neonatal onset of hypotonia; hyporeflexia; respiratory failure; elevated levels of lactic and pyruvic acids in blood, cerebrospinal fluid, or urine; and renal Fanconi syndrome (Biervliet et al, 1977). Cytochrome *c* oxidase activity and reducible cytochrome aa_3 activity are absent or reduced in liver, muscle, or kidney. Inheritance may be autosomal recessive. There is no treatment, prognosis is dismal, and most affected newborns die in infancy. Prenatal diagnosis is unreliable.

Cystinosis

The diagnosis of cystinosis is rarely made in a proband before 6 months of age. Affected individuals appear normal at birth and develop manifestations of the Fanconi syndrome after 6 months. The diagnosis must be considered, however, whenever there are features of Fanconi syndrome in a newborn. Inheritance is autosomal recessive. Cystinosis can be diagnosed in utero by cystine measurements in chorionic villi or amniocytes. Early and adequate treatment with cysteamine slows down the inexorable progression to end-stage renal failure (McSherry and Morris, 1978).

Renal Glycosuria

Isolated forms of renal glycosuria rarely present in the newborn and are benign. Intermittent or constant renal glycosuria can be detected in newborns who have the rare and possibly autosomal recessive condition of glucose and galactose malabsorption (Markello et al, 1993).

Distal Renal Tubular Acidosis

Infantile RTA (Lightwood syndrome) includes transient distal RTA, transient distal RTA with bicarbonate wasting, and transient proximal RTA (Igarashi et al, 1992). These patients have anorexia; failure to thrive; hypotonia; a persistently low serum bicarbonate; elevated serum chloride; inappropriately high urine pH; and, in some cases, nephrocalcinosis. Additional findings are decreased urinary excretion of titratable acid, NH_4^+, and citrate. Low doses of alkali (2 to 3 mEq/kg per day) are needed to maintain normal serum bicarbonate concentrations.

Type I distal RTA or classic distal RTA presents with the same findings as transient RTA. There are few reports of Type I distal RTA in newborns (McSherry and Morris, 1978). The diagnosis of distal RTA is made erroneously in infants with a hyperchloremic metabolic acidosis who have an *inappropriate* urine pH above 6 (Izraeli et al, 1990). "It is important to pHorget the urine pH" and exclude diarrhea, a more common explanation for these findings (Carlisle et al, 1991). Ammonium chloride loading should not be used to make the diagnosis in a newborn. The treatment of transient or permanent distal RTA is bicarbonate, citrate, or acetate. This treatment can be stopped after several months to challenge the diagnosis, or the infant can be allowed to outgrow the dose.

Hypokalemic Tubular Disorders

There are two forms of Bartter syndrome that occur in newborns. The *Proesmans type* of neonatal Bartter syndrome is characterized by the onset of polyuria in utero causing acute polyhydramnios and premature labor (Proesmans et al, 1985). Increased urinary excretion of prostaglandins also occurs, but this is thought to be secondary to the primary abnormality of chloride wasting. Amniotic fluid chloride concentrations are markedly elevated, but sodium and potassium levels are normal. This type of neonatal Bartter syndrome is a chronic, congenital tubular disorder, with hyperkaliuria; hypokalemia; hypochloremia; metabolic alkalosis; hyperaldosteronism; resistance to the pressor effect of angiotensin; juxtaglomerular apparatus hyperplasia; increased renal renin production; and, in some patients, hypercalciuria and nephrocalcinosis. There is no renomedullary cell hyperplasia. Inheritance is autosomal recessive. Similar features occur with prolonged use of loop diuretics and in the syndrome of congenital chloride diarrhea.

A congenital hypokalemic disorder described by Seyberth and colleagues (1985) has similar features to those of neonatal Bartter syndrome. These are polyhydramnios, premature labor, failure to thrive, febrile episodes, vomiting, diarrhea, polyuria, renal losses of electrolytes, hypercalciuria, nephrocalcinosis, and osteopenia. There is marked stimulation of renal and systemic prostaglandin E_2 production in the absence of a defect in the tubular reabsorption of chloride. In this abnormality, the basic defect may be primary hyperprostaglandism. Both types of hypokalemic tubular disorders are treated with indomethacin.

Renal Tubular Hyperkalemia Syndromes

The causes of renal tubular hyperkalemia in the newborn include marked prematurity, renal adysplasia, urinary tract obstruction, acute pyelonephritis, congenital adrenal hypoplasia, and pseudohypoaldosteronism. Renal tubular hyperkalemia is defined by hyperkalemia, inappropriately low urine potassium excretion, renal salt wasting, and metabolic acidosis. The serum creatinine concentration is often increased.

Pseudohypoaldosteronism

Type I or Renal Pseudohypoaldosteronism. This disorder usually manifests in early infancy with salt-wasting caused by diminished renal tubular responsiveness to aldosterone. This results in hyponatremia, hyperkalemia, markedly elevated plasma aldosterone, and hyperreninemia (Hanukoglu, 1991). Some patients die in infancy, whereas others may be asymptomatic. Treatment is sodium chloride supplementation for at least 2 years. Serum electrolyte concentrations become normal with increasing age, but aldosterone levels remain elevated. Mutation of genes encoding the subunits of the human amiloride-sensitive epithelial sodium channel on the short arm of chromosomes 16 and 12 may be responsible for this disorder (Strautnieks et al, 1996).

Multiple-Organ Pseudohypoaldosteronism. In some individuals, there is an impaired responsiveness to aldosterone in salivary and sweat glands, renal tubules, and colonic mucosal cells. These patients have a protracted course complicated with life-threatening episodes of salt wasting. Pseudohypoaldosteronism may be inherited as an autosomal dominant trait in some families and as an autosomal recessive trait in others.

Congenital X-Linked Nephrogenic Diabetes Insipidus

Congenital X-linked nephrogenic diabetes insipidus is a rare disorder with defective renal and extrarenal arginine-vasopressin V_2 receptor responses caused in part by mutations in the arginine-vasopressin V_2 receptor gene in Xq28 (Bichet et al, 1994). Vasopressin regulates water reabsorption primarily through water channels, and mutations in *AQP2* gene are also associated with severe nephrogenic diabetes insipidus (Deen et al, 1994). As a result, the kidneys cannot concentrate urine, and large quantities of hypotonic urine (50 to 100 mOsmol/kg water) are excreted. Affected newborns are irritable, feed poorly, do not gain weight, and have episodes of dehydration and fever. Serum concentrations of sodium, chloride, creatinine, and blood urea nitrogen are elevated. Serum levels of vasopressin are increased, and there is no response to exogenous vasopressin. Combined administration of indomethacin and hydrochlorothiazide or hydrochlorothiazide and amiloride is used, with varying degrees of success, to treat these patients.

REFERENCES

Batisky DL, Roy S III, Gaber LW: Congenital nephrosis and neonatal cytomegalovirus infection: A clinical association. Pediatr Nephrol 7:741, 1993.

Beale MG, Strayer DS, Kissane JM, Robson AM: Congenital glomerulosclerosis and nephrotic syndrome in two infants. Am J Dis Child 133:842, 1979.

Bichet DG, Birnbaumer M, Lonergan M, et al: Nature and recurrence of AVPR-2 mutations in X-linked nephrogenic diabetes insipidus. Am J Hum Genet 55:278, 1994.

Biervliet JPAM, Bruinvis L, Ketting D, et al: Hereditary mitochondrial myopathy with lactic aciemia, a De Toni-Fanconi-Debre syndrome, and a defective respiratory chain in voluntary striated muscle. Pediatr Res 11:1088, 1977.

Brooks CC, Tolan DR: Association of the widespread A 149 P hereditary fructose intolerance mutation with newly identified sequence polymorphisms in the aldolase gene. Am J Med Genet 52:835, 1993.

Carlisle EJF, Donnelly SM, Halperin ML: Renal tubular acidosis (RTA): Recognize the ammonium defect and pHorget the urine pH. Pediatr Nephrol 5:242, 1991.

Cohen AH, Turner MC: Kidney in Galloway-Mowat syndrome: Clinical spectrum with description of pathology. Kidney Int 45:1407, 1994.

Cooperstone B, Friedman A, Kaplan BS. The Galloway-Mowat syndrome of abnormal Gyral pattern and Glomerulopathy. Am J Med Genet 47:250, 1993.

Deen PMT, Verdijk MAJ, Knoers N, et al: Requirement of human renal water channel aquaporin-2 for vasopressin-dependent concentration of urine. Science 264:92, 1994.

Finnegan JT, Slosberg EJ, Postellon DC, Primack WA: Congenital nephrotic syndrome detected by hypothyroid screening. Acta Paediatr Scand 69:705, 1980.

Gertner JM, Kauschansky A, Giesker DW, et al: XY gonadal dysgenesis associated with the congenital nephrotic syndrome. Obstet Gynecol 55:665, 1980.

Gitzelman R, Steinmann B, van den Berghe G: Disorders of fructose metabolism. *In* Scriver C, Beaudet AL, Sly WS, Valle D (Eds): The Metabolic Basis of Inherited Disease, 6th ed. New York, McGraw-Hill, 1989, pp 399–424.

Habib R: Nephrotic syndrome in the 1st year of life. Pediatr Nephrol 7:347, 1993.

Hanukoglu A: Type I pseudohypoaldosteronism includes two clinically and genetically distinct entities with either renal or multiple organ defects. J Clin Endocrinol Metab 73:936, 1991.

Haws RM, Weinberg AG, Baum M: Spontaneous remission of congenital nephrotic syndrome: A case report and review of the literature. Pediatr Nephrol 6:82, 1992.

Heiman-Patterson TD, Bonilla E, DiMauro S, et al: Cytochrome-C-oxidase deficiency in a floppy infant. Neurology 32:898, 1982.

Huttunen N-P: Congenital nephrotic syndrome of Finnish type: Study of 75 patients. Arch Dis Child 51:344, 1976.

Igarashi T, Sekine Y, Kawato H, et al: Transient distal renal tubular acidosis with secondary hyperparathyroidism. Pediatr Nephrol 6:267, 1992.

Izraeli S, Rachmel A, Frishberg Y, et al: Transient renal acidification defect during acute infantile diarrhea: The role of urinary sodium. J Pediatr 117:711, 1990.

Kestila M, Mannikko C, Gyapay G, et al: Congenital nephrotic syndrome of the Finnish type maps to the long arm of chromosome 19. Am J Hum Genet 54:757, 1994.

Knoers N, Monnens LAH: Nephrogenic diabetes insipidus: Clinical symptoms, pathogenesis, genetics and treatment. Pediatr Nephrol 6:476, 1992.

Kozlowski PB, Sner JH, Nicastri AD, et al: Brain morphology in the Galloway syndrome. Clin Neuropathol 8:85, 1989.

Laine J, Jalanko H, Holthofer H, et al: Post-transplantation nephrosis in congenital nephrotic syndrome of the Finnish type. Kidney Int 44:867, 1993.

Levin B, Snodgrass GJ, Oberholzer VG, et al: Fructosemia: Observations on seven cases. Am J Med 45:826, 1968.

Mahan JD, Mauer SM, Sibley RK, Vernier RL: Congenital nephrotic syndrome: Evolution of medical management and results of renal transplantation. J Pediatr 105:549, 1984.

Markello TC, Bernardini IM, Gahl WA: Improved renal function with cystinosis treated with cysteamine. N Engl J Med 328:1157, 1993.

McLean RH, Kennedy TL, Ratzan SK, et al: Hypothyroidism in congenital nephrotic syndrome. J Pediatr 101:72, 1982.

McDonald R, Wiggelinkhuizen J, Kaschula ROC: The nephrotic syndrome in very young infants. Am J Dis Child 122:507, 1971.

McSherry E, Morris RC Jr: Attainment of normal stature with alkali therapy in infants and children with classic renal tubular acidosis. J Clin Invest 61:509, 1978.

O'Regan S, Fong JSC, de Chadarevian JP, et al: Treponemal antigens in congenital and aquired syphilitic nephritis. Ann Intern Med 85:325, 1976.

Palm L, Hagerstrand I, Kristoffersson U, et al: Nephrosis and disturbances of neuronal migration in male siblings—a new hereditary disorder? Arch Dis Child 61:545, 1986.

Pelletier J, Bruening W, Kashten CE, et al: Germline mutations in Wilms' tumor suppressor gene are associated with abnormal urogenital development in Denys-Drash syndrome. Cell 67:437, 1991.

Peral B, Ward CJ, San Millan JL, et al: Evidence of linkage disequilibrium in the Spanish polycystic kidney disease I population. Am J Hum Genet 54:899, 1994.

Proesmans W, Devlieger H, van Assche A, et al: Bartter syndrome in two siblings—antenatal and neonatal observations. Int J Pediatr Nephrol 6:63, 1985.

Roos RAC, Maaswinkel-Mooy PD, vd Loo EM, et al: Congenital microcephaly, infantile spasms, psychomotor retardation, and nephrotic syndrome in two sibs. Eur J Pediatr 146:532, 1987.

Scott RJ, Rochefort M: Fatal perinatal nephropathy with onset in intrauterine life. Arch Dis Child 67:1212, 1992.

Sedman A, Bell P, Manco-Johnson M, et al: Autosomal dominant polycystic kidney disease in childhood: A longitudinal study. Kidney Int 31:1000, 1987.

Seppala M, Rapola J, Huttunen N-P, et al: Congenital nephrotic syndrome: Prenatal diagnosis and genetic counselling by estimation of amniotic-fluid and maternal serum alpha-fetoprotein. Lancet 11:123, 1976.

Seyberth HW, Rascher W, Schweer H, et al: Congenital hypokalemia with hypercalciuria in preterm infants: A hyperprostaglanduric tubular syndrome different from Bartter syndrome. J Pediatr 107:694, 1985.

Shahin B, Papadopoulou ZL, Jenis EH: Congenital nephrotic syndrome associated with congenital toxoplasmosis. J Pediatr 85:366, 1974.

Sibley RK, Mahan JD, Vernier RL: Congenital and infantile nephrotic syndrome: A clinicopathologic study of 46 cases. Kidney Int 27:544, 1986.

Spear GS, Steinhaus KA, Quddusi A: Diffuse mesangial sclerosis in a fetus. Clin Nephrol 36:46, 1991.

Strautnieks SS, Thompson RJ, Gardiner RM, Chung E: A novel splice-site mutation in the gamma subunit of the epithelial sodium channel gene in three pseudohypoaldosteronism type 1 families. Nat Genet 13:248, 1996.

Torres VE: Genetics of renal cystic diseases. *In* Spitzer A, Avner ED (Eds): Inheritance of Kidney and Urinary Tract Diseases. Boston, Kluwer, 1990, pp 175–219.

Van den Heuvel LPW, Van den Born J, Jalanko H, et al: The glycosaminoglycan content of renal basement membranes in the congenital nephrotic syndrome of the Finnish type. Pediatr Nephrol 6:10, 1992.

CHAPTER 97

Infection of the Urinary Tract and Vesicoureteral Reflux

Stephen A. Zderic

The goal of this chapter is to provide an overview of the epidemiology, pathophysiology, diagnostic approaches, management, and follow-up radiographic evaluation of urinary tract infections in the newborn. Although a urinary tract infection may develop as the clinical presentation of congenital anomalies of the kidneys and the urinary tract as discussed in detail in Chapters 93 and 94, this chapter focuses on the diagnosis and management of vesicoureteral reflux. A major concept to stress at the outset is that reflux itself does not cause infections; studies have shown that many children may reflux without developing an infection. Instead, the susceptibility of the individual appears to play a major role in the etiology of neonatal urinary tract infections, especially in the absence of predisposing congenital anomalies.

URINARY TRACT INFECTIONS IN THE NEWBORN

Epidemiology

The incidence of urinary tract infection requiring hospitalization is approximately 0.5% during the first year of life (Wiswell and Hachey, 1993). Within the first several months, urinary tract infections are more common in boys. However, after the first 6 months of life, the incidence in girls increases steadily as that in boys declines (Shortliffe, 1992). For boys during the first year of life, an additional risk factor for urinary tract infection is the presence of the prepuce because noncircumcised male infants have an approximately 10-fold higher incidence of urinary tract infection during this period as compared with their circumcised counterparts (Wiswell and Geschke, 1989, Wiswell and Hachey, 1993; see also Chapter 94). For ages 1 to 3 years, the incidence of urinary tract infection in girls may be anywhere from 10- to 15-fold higher than in boys.

Pathophysiology

Urinary tract infections are polyfactorial in their etiology and clearly represent an altered balance between host and pathogen. Hematogenous spread of bacteria to the urinary tract occurs, but it is extremely rare. Most urinary tract infections start in the bladder and then ascend to produce pyelonephritis. This ascent of infected urine from the bladder to the kidney may take place via two major mechanisms: (1) the bacteria may be extremely virulent and produce pilli, which allow the bacteria to attach themselves to the ureter and migrate upstream or (2) the patient may reflux and shower the renal pelvis, which the allows for intrarenal reflux and seeding of the renal parenchyma (Fig. 97–1). Once bacteria are injected into the renal parenchyma under high pressure, areas of focal infection and inflammation develop (Fig. 97–2) and a series of complex

steps in the inflammatory cascade takes place (Roberts, 1992). If not interrupted by treatment, the ensuing inflammation can produce severe renal injury or scarring. Moreover, if repeated infectious insults continue without adequate therapy, the long-term result is significant renal scarring that, in its extreme, produces reflux nephropathy leading to end-stage renal disease.

Equally important in the pathogenesis are the individual characteristics of the patient or host. It is accepted that many patients are more susceptible to bacterial urinary tract infections because their bladder mucosa expresses cell surface proteins (receptors) that have a high affinity for the cell surface antigens on the bacterial cell wall. Some of these complex glycoproteins expressed by the bladder mucosa are mannose sensitive; thus, the receptor-ligand interaction between pathogen and host is based on the molecular recognition of mannose-6-phosphate (Schaeffer et al, 1984). The bladder mucosa itself is a dynamic component of the bladder wall, with a high-energy expenditure as

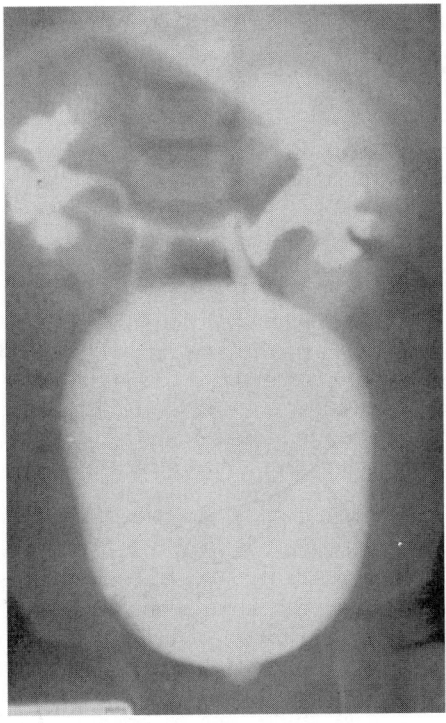

FIGURE 97–1. A VCUG showing a classic vesicoureteral reflux in a female neonate. The degree of filling required to produce voiding probable and the softer, thinner, and stretchier tissues of the neonate tend to make this reflux difficult to compare with a similar grade in an older child. Note that on the left side there is evidence of intrarenal reflux, in which contrast agent extravasates into the papillae and out into the cortex.

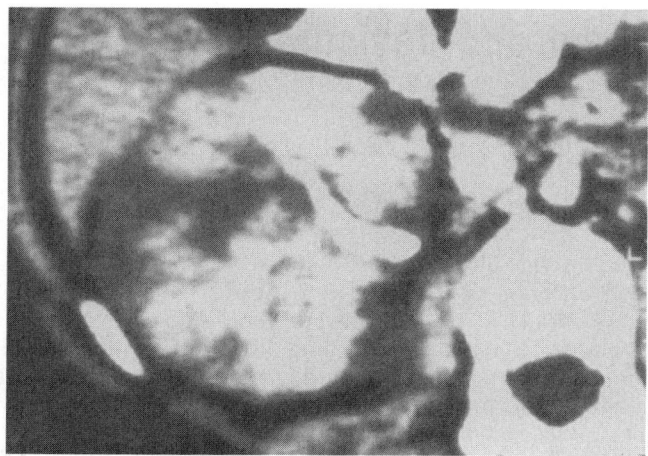

FIGURE 97–2. Computed tomography (CT) scan images of the right kidney in an infant with reflux and urosepsis demonstrating areas poor perfusion consistent with lobar nephronia or segmental pyelonephritis. Often fever persists despite 5 to 7 days of the appropriate antibiotic, which should prompt a search for any collections requiring drainage. In this case a CT scan was obtained to ensure that no abscess had developed.

reflected by the several-fold higher activity of its citrate synthetase compared with that of the bladder smooth muscle (Hypolite et al, 1993). When one considers the tremendous demands on the urothelium in terms of maintaining the osmotic gradient between urine (600 mOsm) and plasma (300 mOsm) this is hardly surprising.

To further complicate the pathophysiology of urinary tract infection, one must consider what happens when a urinary tract infection develops in something other than the normal urinary tract. It used to be extremely common for obstructive uropathies to present after urosepsis had developed. Fortunately, the increasing use of prenatal sonography makes these presentations less frequent. In the case of reflux, it is easy to understand why a simple case of cystitis can be transformed into pyelonephritis. However, even in the patient with a long-standing ureteropelvic junction (UPJ) obstruction and no evidence of reflux, urosepsis may develop. In this setting one has a dangerous combination of infected urine, stasis, and a warm environment with a near-ideal culture broth. Although infection was always an uncommon presentation of UPJ obstruction, it will become even more rare with the routine use of prenatal sonography.

If a severe infection has been established in a newborn or infant with a previously known obstructed urinary tract, the management may be altered by the use of temporary drainage by percutaneous nephrostomy. On the other hand, if a patient without a history of urinary tract obstruction and with acute pyelonephritis does not defervesce after 72 hours of antibiotic treatment, one must always suspect the possibility of an underlying obstruction. Under these circumstances an ultrasound is warranted and one may discover that infections have become established in primary megaureters, UPJ obstructions, ureteroceles, or ectopic ureters. Because the production of urine allows for some antibiotic to reach these bacteria, many of these infants can be managed medically if treated early on in their course. However, in advanced cases, or in patients with poor renal function, only temporary drainage procedures such as percutaneous nephrostomy may allow for the condition to stabilize (see Chapter 94).

Diagnosis

The diagnosis of a urinary tract infection in a newborn or young infant is not always straightforward, and a high index of suspicion is required because the symptoms are generalized. In one study of 100 infants with urinary tract infection, all patients were febrile above 38° C, 70% had fever above 39° C, 60% were irritable, 50% were feeding poorly, and 40% had vomiting or diarrhea (Ginsburg et al, 1982). Therefore, with the exception of newborns with suspected sepsis during the first few days of life, a urine specimen for analysis and culture must also be obtained in addition to the blood and cerebrospinal fluid (CSF) cultures, complete blood count, and CSF analysis in newborns and young infants presenting with these clinical symptoms.

Much has been said and written about the procurement of specimens by the techniques of clean catch, bags, catheterization, or suprapubic puncture. Clean-catch or bagged specimens are valid only if they are truly negative. It is intuitively obvious why these collection methods are susceptible to contamination in girls and especially so in uncircumcised males (Fig. 97–3). The composition of the preputial or vaginal flora is of little help in managing the febrile child; what matters most is the composition of the urine within the bladder itself. Another problem arises with the definition of what a negative urine culture means in clean-catch and bagged specimens. In many instances the reports state that such cultures are negative but only because the cutoff of 100,000 colony-forming units (CFU) per cubic centimeter is used to define a positive culture. Recent work suggests that 10,000 to 49,000 CFU/cm³ usually represent contamination, whereas counts in excess of 50,000 CFU/cm³ are more characteristic of a true positive culture in clean-catch and bagged specimens (Hoberman et al, 1994). However, there are significant overlaps, and numeric quantitation remains an inexact tool with such collection methods. Therefore, specimens obtained by the catheterization of the bladder or by a suprapubic tap should be used in patients with suspected urinary tract infection.

Although the gold standard for specimen collection for urine culture is the suprapubic aspirate, even urologists rarely use this method. A catheterized specimen is easy to obtain and provides accurate results especially if one discards the first 2 to 3 mL of urine, which may contain urethral contaminants. However, the suprapubic aspirate can also be safely performed in a newborn since the bladder is a pelvic organ. A 21-gauge needle may be inserted into the palpable bladder just above the pubic symphysis in the midline to collect a urine aspirate. Although, as mentioned earlier, this is a safe procedure in expert hands, complications may occur including bleeding, infection, or bowel perforation.

Most urologists and neonatologists would agree that in a febrile newborn or young infant presenting with urosepsis, either of the latter two methods is warranted and appropriate and that bagged urine specimens and clean-catch methods should not be used in these cases. First, the use

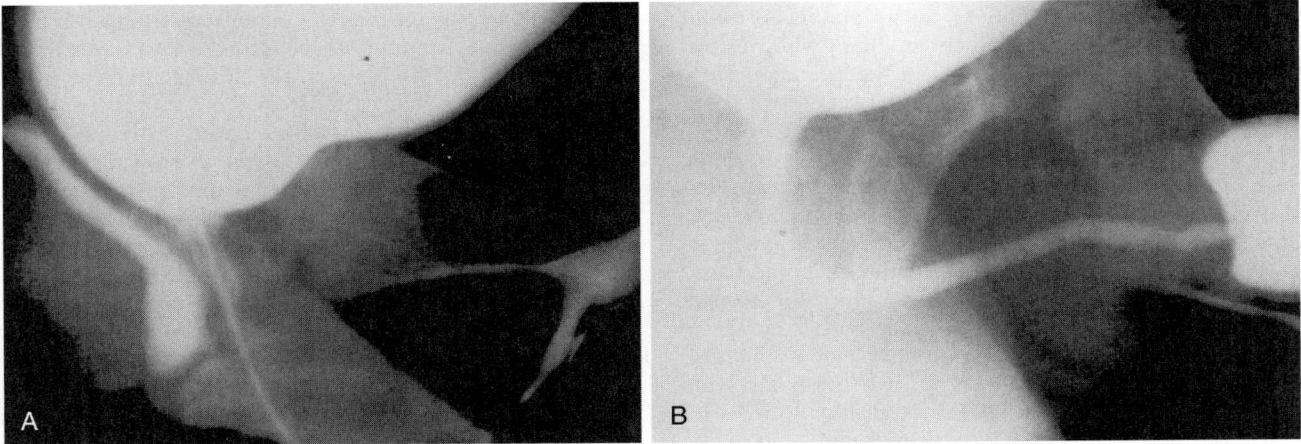

FIGURE 97–3. The errors inherent in bagged specimens are shown in these two VCUG images from a female *(A)* and uncircumcised male *(B)*. The contributions of vaginal and preputial flora to the specimens are obvious. When one also factors in how long it can take for such urine to be plated out in the laboratory, and that *Escherichia coli* have a doubling time for 20 minutes, the high incidence of false positives is easy to understand.

of bagged specimens and clean-catch methods increases the incidence of false-positive cultures so that more patients will be likely to undergo antibiotic therapy that is of no benefit. Of additional concern is the cost effectiveness of then ordering a renal bladder ultrasound and a voiding cystourethrogram (VCUG) based on a false-positive urine culture result. Information obtained from poorly collected specimen early on in the process leads to the well-described, expensive, and occasionally harmful cascade effect in clinical care (Mold et al, 1986).

Finally, an additional problem in establishing the accurate diagnosis arises in the newborn or infant who is on antimicrobial prophylaxis or has been medicated prior to the appearance of symptoms suggestive of infection. This point is illustrated by the case of a 2-year-old child with a fever of 40° C and a catheterized urine specimen that showed signs of white blood cells and nitrates, but in whom the culture remained negative. However, her renal ^{99m}Tc-dimercaptosuccinic acid (DMSA) scan (Fig. 97–4) showed the classic photopenic area consistent with pyelonephritis, and her VCUG demonstrated bilateral reflux. On questioning, the family reported having administered several doses of a leftover antibiotic.

Treatment

The infant with suspected urosepsis should be treated with broad-spectrum antibiotic coverage until the microbial sensitivity studies dictate a shift to the use of a single antibiotic. Ampicillin and gentamicin provide an excellent coverage for the most common pathogens that are likely to be present. The most likely pathogen is *Escherichia coli*,

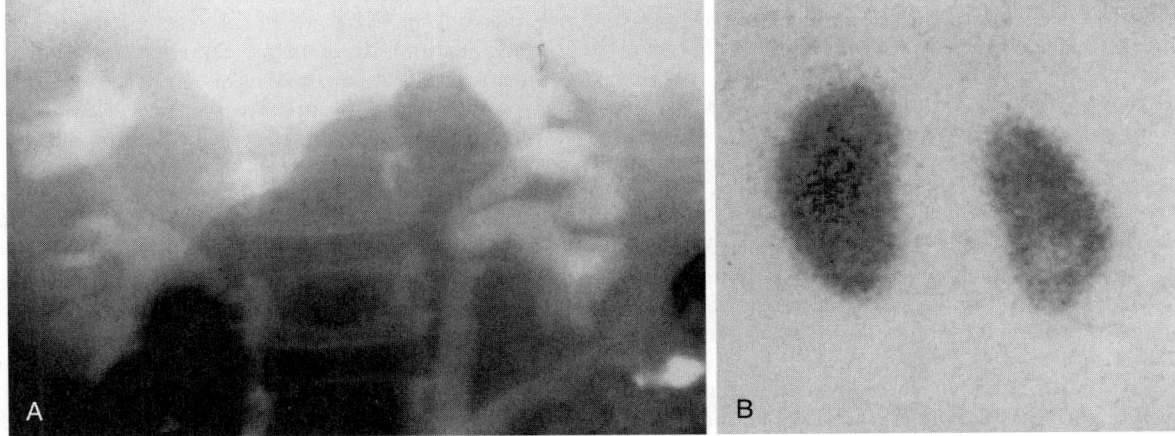

FIGURE 97–4. This VCUG demonstrates bilateral Grade III reflux in an infant who was not on antibiotic prophylaxis at the time of the study *(A)*. The urologist first learned of this patient when the child presented with a high fever and lethargy. A catheterized urine specimen was positive for white blood cells, red blood cells, and bacteria on urinalysis, yet the culture was negative. The family emphatically denied having given the child antibiotics, yet the DMSA scan was positive, with an obvious photopenic area showing evidence of pyelonephritis *(B)*.

but there is always a possibility of pseudomonas or other gram-negative bacteria, especially in an infant who was just discharged to home following a stay in the neonatal intensive care unit. The duration of intravenous antibiotic treatment for pyelonephritis is debated; certainly parenteral therapy avoids the concern of compliance issues. However, there is experimental evidence to suggest that reflux-associated pyelonephritis confirmed by DMSA scan can be successfully treated with only oral antibiotics (Risdon et al, 1994). Given the expense of hospitalization or home-based intravenous antibiotic therapy, the mandatory duration of parenteral therapy will continue to be debated. However, most would agree that combined parenteral and oral antibiotic therapy should be continued for 10 to 14 days, and this should then be followed up with a urine culture.

Once the acute infection has been treated, antibiotic prophylaxis should be instituted until the newborn or young infant is ready for radiographic imaging studies. The use of amoxicillin (12.5 mg/kg) in newborns or trimethoprim-sulfamethoxazole in infants is accepted for prophylaxis. The long-term use of low-dose, prophylactic trimethoprim-sulfamethoxazole treatment in urologic patients does not lead to shifts in the normal fecal flora (Stamey, 1980). In contrast, high doses of trimethoprim-sulfamethoxazole and especially of broad-spectrum antibiotics produce significant shifts in the fecal flora. This is extremely important, since the feces serve as the origin for more than 90% of the bacteria that colonize the perineum and vagina and ultimately produce a urinary tract infection.

The Radiographic Work-Up

Once a diagnosis of urinary tract infection has been established and treatment has begun, it is important to initiate a radiographic work-up to look for any underlying structural anomalies. It has been stated that up to 30% of infants and children with a urinary tract infection have an aberrant renal or urinary tract anatomic structure. The radiographic evaluation should consist of an ultrasound of the kidneys and the bladder followed by a carefully done VCUG (Lebowitz and Mandell, 1987). Most often, a 2- to 4-week period is allowed between infection and the radiographic imaging, but this interval is arbitrary. It is important to obtain a sterile urine specimen prior to the VCUG, and the patient should be maintained on antimicrobial prophylaxis until imaging rules out any urinary tract pathology. On sonography, kidney and bladder views are stressed because sometimes the kidneys alone are imaged and shown to be normal, and thus the work-up is terminated. In many of these cases, several infections later, a bladder ultrasound is performed showing a stone, ureterocele, or diverticulum (see Fig. 97–1). Even if a VCUG is done on the same day, a small ureterocele might be missed at fluoroscopy that would be seen on the bladder sonogram.

The VCUG must be done carefully and requires patience on the part of all concerned. The V stands for voiding, which is required to demonstrate 20% to 30% of the reflux cases that would be missed if the infant were anesthetized for a static cystogram. The policy of the author's institution is to obtain a classic fluoroscopic study first so as to define the anatomy and accurately grade the reflux if it is present. Some groups have advocated that

nuclear VCUG be used as the initial screening study. However, to define anatomy, the contrast VCUG remains the gold standard. As discussed in the next section, the cornerstone of accurate management of the reflux is the grading that is best provided by a well-executed study.

In recent years there has been a growing literature regarding the efficacy of DMSA scanning to identify patients with acute pyelonephritis. It is this author's bias that a well-collected urine specimen showing signs of infection in a febrile patient is adequate to establish this diagnosis. However, in cases where the index of suspicion for infection is high based on the clinical picture and a urinalysis (see Fig. 97–4), the DMSA scan is most helpful. Furthermore, this technique is useful in assessing the patient with abnormal anatomy secondary to extrophy or spina bifida whose chronic catheterization regimens result in chronic urinary tract colonization. This author has been extremely selective in the use of the DMSA scan but has been satisfied with the additional information it provides under the earlier described circumstances.

VESICOURETERAL REFLUX

The treatment of vesicoureteral reflux has continued to evolve over the past 40 years, creating a voluminous literature. Vesicoureteral reflux exists when urine flows from the bladder back toward the kidney, and this may occur during bladder filling and emptying (voiding). Using the contrast VCUG, it is possible to grade reflux from I through V (Fig. 97–5). Grading is valuable because it allows physicians to communicate the findings quickly and also provides information about the chances of spontaneous resolution. In the clinical practice, it is absolutely crucial that the consulting urologist personally reviews the films since many clues appear on the hard-copy views that may not make it to a typed report.

The etiology of reflux remains debated, but there is growing agreement that this condition is a syndrome. Some patients with reflux have a congenital malalignment of the ureter and bladder trigone and thus the normal flap valve to prevent reflux has not developed. This forms the basis for the anatomic or *primary reflux*. Many neonates with posterior urethral valves may be seen to have reflux, only to have the reflux disappear once the valves are resected. Reflux secondary to obstruction or neurogenic bladder is referred to as *secondary reflux*. This distinction is important: the rules for primary reflux resolution do not apply to the cases of reflux secondary to obstructing lesions. Of even greater significance for the neonatologist is the growing clinical evidence for elevated voiding pressures in infants with primary reflux (Sillen et al, 1992). Voiding pressure in infants with primary reflux is often threefold to fourfold higher than that seen in older children. Experimental evidence in rabbits suggests that voiding pressures are higher in the normal newborn bladder and diminish over time (Keating et al, 1990). Whether these diminishing voiding pressures reflect the increased capacity of the bladder, alterations in excitation coupling (Zderic et al, 1995), or both remains unclear. However, the neonatologist should remember that voiding pressures are elevated in the newborn with primary reflux and that these pressures diminish

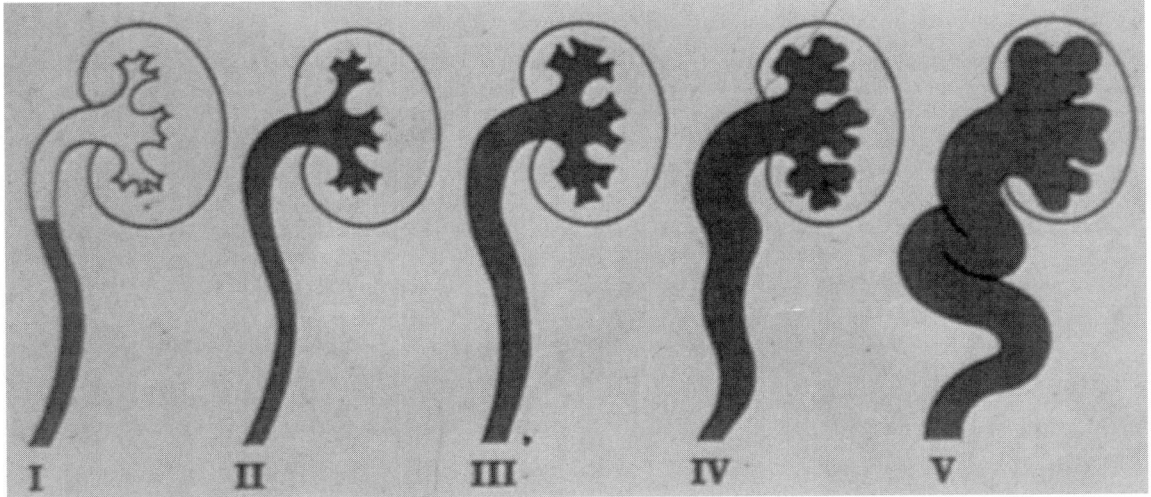

FIGURE 97–5. The international reflux grading scale is used to assign a prognosis for the spontaneous resolution of primary reflux. It also allows for effective communication between radiologists, urologists, and pediatricians. It may not be applied to assign a prognosis for any child with posterior valves or spina bifida.

over time. This has great bearing on how reflux resolution rates should be interpreted in the newborn.

An international reflux study was carried out over a decade and produced a comprehensive view of the natural history of primary reflux. The European data (Tamminen-Mobius et al, 1992) presented the outcomes of resolution of the disorder for unilateral and bilateral reflux for both randomized (Grades I to IV) and sideline follow-up of patients. Patients in the latter group declined randomization or were followed at the attending physicians' discretion. Randomized bilateral Grade III and IV primary reflux had a 30% and 10% chance, respectively, of resolving over a 4-year follow-up period. Children followed in the sideline arm had a better chance of resolving their reflux, which points out that many other intangibles enter into the decision-making process about when to intervene for reflux. The problem with this study for the neonatologist is that the average age of entry was 3.5 years. It is not possible to extrapolate these results to the newborn period, given the incredible differences in bladder function that have been documented clinically (Sillen et al, 1993) and experimentally (Keating et al, 1990; Zderic et al, 1995).

Outcomes for primary reflux resolution in newborns must be studied further. This should be made easier by the increased number of cases detected by prenatal sonography. Preliminary evidence in small series suggests that primary reflux detected in the first 6 months of life has a better chance for spontaneous resolution grade for grade than that diagnosed in the child presenting at 2 to 4 years of age. The recommendations one can make based on the available limited information about reflux management in the neonate also are affected by the mode of presentation and social circumstances (compliance issues). One can make an argument for a more aggressive surgical approach if a newborn presents with urosepsis and high-grade (Grade IV or V) primary reflux. In contrast, for a newborn with a diagnosis of Grade IV or V primary reflux made secondary to investigation for prenatally detected hydrone-

phrosis but without the presentation of urosepsis, expectant observation with antibiotic prophylaxis seems a reasonable alternative. Moreover, based on the findings of clinical and experimental physiology, it is the bias of this author that newborns with any grade of primary reflux should be placed on antimicrobial prophylaxis and followed conservatively for 1 year. The key to this approach is antibiotic prophylaxis, parent education, and close follow-up; therefore, an unstable social situation with noncompliance is a valid reason for surgical intervention. This is a controversial topic, and certainly for the higher grades of reflux, some urologists will continue to advocate operative intervention. With regard to reimplant surgery, it is absolutely crucial to understand that it only diminishes but does not eradicate the likelihood of pyelonephritis. A newborn or infant with innate susceptibility will still experience bladder infections despite the absence of primary reflux (Walker, 1994).

REFERENCES

Ginsberg CM, McCracken GH Jr: Urinary tract infections in young infants. Pediatrics 69:409–412, 1982.

Hoberman A, Wald ER, Reynolds EA, et al: Pyuria and bacteriuria in catheterized urine specimens obtained from young children with fever. J Pediatr 124:513–519, 1994.

Hypolite JA, Longhurst PA, Gong C, et al: Metabolic studies on rabbit bladder smooth muscle and mucosa. Mol Cell Biochem 125:35–42, 1993.

Keating MA, Duckett JW, Snyder HM, et al: Ontogeny of bladder function in the rabbit. J Urol 144:766–770, 1990.

Lebowitz L, Mandell J: Urinary tract infections in children: Putting radiology in its place. Radiology 165:1–9, 1987.

Mold JW, Stein HF: The cascade effect in the clinical care of patients. N Engl J Med 314:512–515, 1986.

Risdon RA, Godley ML, Parkhouse HF, et al: Renal pathology and the ^{99m}Tc-DMSA image during the evolution of the early pyelonephritic scar: An experimental study. J Urol 151(3):767–773, 1994.

Roberts JA: Vesicoureteral reflux and pyelonephritis in the monkey: A review. J Urol 148:1721–1724, 1992.

Schaeffer AW, Chmiel JS, Duncan JL, et al: Manose sensitive adherents of *E. coli* to epithelial cells from women with recurrent urinary tract infections. J Urol 131:906–910, 1984.

Shortliffe M: Urinary tract infections in infants and children. *In* Walsh PC, Retik AB, Stamey TA, Vaughan ED (Eds): Campbell's Urology, 6th ed. Philadelphia, WB Saunders, 1992, pp 1669–1686.

Sillen U, Hjalmas K, Aili M, et al: Pronounced detrusor hypercontractility in infants with gross bilateral reflux. J Urol 148:598–599, 1992.

Stamey TA: Pathogenesis and Treatment of Urinary Tract Infections. Baltimore, Williams & Wilkins, 1980.

Tamminen-Mobius T, Brunier E, Ebel KD, et al: Cessation of vesicoureteral reflux for 5 years in infants and children allocated to medical therapy. J Urol 148:1662–1666, 1992.

Walker RD: Vesicoureteral reflux update: Effect of prospective studies on current management. Urology 43:279–283, 1994.

Wiswell TE, Geschke DW: Risks from circumcision during the first month of life compared to those for uncircumcised boys. Pediatrics 83:1011–1015, 1989.

Wiswell TE, Hachey WE: Urinary tract infections and the uncircumcised state: An update. Clin Pediatr 1993 32:130–134, 1993.

Zderic SA, Gong C, Hypolite JA Levin RM: Developmental aspects of excitation contraction coupling in urinary bladder smooth muscle. Adv Exp Med Biol 385:105–116, 1995.

CHAPTER 98

Renal Vascular Disease in the Newborn

Tivadar Tulassay, Istvan Seri and Jacquelyn Evans

Neonatal hemostasis is characterized by a decrease in both the concentration and the function of the procoagulant and anticoagulant proteins. The balanced immaturity of the opposing hemostatic factors contributes to the low incidence of coagulation abnormalities in the healthy newborn. Under pathologic conditions, however, such as hypoxia, hypovolemia, hypotension, infection, and polycythemia, this delicate balance is easily compromised leading to an increased incidence of bleeding or thrombosis in the sick newborn. In addition to the pathologic conditions, the placement of an indwelling arterial or venous catheter resulting in endothelial injury appears to play a major role in thrombus formation in these patients. This notion is supported by the observation that 89% of all major vessel thromboses in the newborn are associated with catheter placement (Schmidt and Andrew, 1995).

The neonatal kidney is especially at high risk for thrombus formation. In addition to the use of umbilical arterial catheters, the low renal blood flow, the relatively small caliber of the renal vessels, and the enhanced renal vasoconstrictor and angioproliferative effects of endothelin and angiotensin II contribute to the increased risk of thrombogenesis in the neonatal kidney. The incidence of renovascular thrombosis in the newborn is unknown. In the past, renal venous thrombosis was more common. Since the introduction of umbilical arterial catheters in the routine care of the sick newborn, however, renal arterial thrombosis has become more frequent. Although renal vascular events usually present with the development of renal dysfunction, the function of other organs may also be affected, leading to the development of adrenal hemorrhage, congestive heart failure, systemic hypertension, inadequate perfusion of the lower extremities, and multiorgan failure.

RENAL ARTERIAL OBSTRUCTION
Etiology and Incidence

In the vast majority of the cases, renal arterial obstruction is the consequence of intra-arterial thrombus formation. Before the introduction of umbilical artery catheterization, only a few cases of renal artery thrombosis were reported, with shock, coagulopathy, and congestive heart failure being the principal causative factors (Adelman, 1988). The introduction of umbilical arterial catheterization in the early 1970s resulted in a significant increase in the incidence of neonatal aortic thrombosis. Because the presence of a catheter-related aortic thrombus is associated with an involvement of one or both of the renal arteries in 30% to 50% of the affected newborns, umbilical arterial catheter placement also increases the incidence of renal artery thrombosis (Schmidt and Andrew, 1995; Seibert et al, 1987). Ultrasonographic findings suggest that catheter-related asymptomatic aortic thrombi are present in 17% to

31% of newborns (Horgan et al, 1987; Oppenheimer et al, 1982), although the Doppler ultrasound technique may underestimate the real incidence (Schmidt and Andrew, 1995). The incidence of *severe symptomatic thrombosis* after umbilical arterial catheter placement is much less and is reported to be around 1% (O'Neill et al, 1981). Because the trauma to the vessel wall inflicted at the time of the placement of the catheter appears to play the most important role in aortic thrombus formation (Goetzman et al, 1975; Rasoulpour and Marinelli, 1992), the procedure should be done carefully to minimize endothelial injury and the attendant thrombus formation. Continuous infusion of low-dose heparin is also recommended. Although not shown directly to decrease the incidence of catheter-related thrombi, continuous low-dose heparinization prolongs the patency of umbilical arterial lines (Rajani et al, 1979) and may lower the incidence of thrombotic sequelae (Horgan et al, 1987).

In addition to the endothelial injury caused by catheter placement, several other risk factors for aortic and renal arterial thrombosis have been identified. Systemic infection; birth weight less than 1500 g; perinatal asphyxia; intrauterine cocaine exposure; maternal diabetes mellitus; maternal lupus; congenital heart disease; hypercoagulability; dehydration (especially hypernatremic dehydration); and infusion of calcium salts, hyperalimentation, or intravenous fat preparations through the umbilical arterial catheter are the most important additional risk factors for aortic and renal thrombosis in the newborn (Schmidt and Andrew, 1995; Seibert et al, 1987; Vailas et al, 1986). Although the incidence of aortic thrombus formation does not appear to be influenced by the type of catheter used (heparin bonded polyurethane or polyvinyl chloride) (Jackson et al, 1987), the level of catheter tip placement may be of importance; newborns with a high umbilical arterial catheter in place more frequently develop aortic and renal thrombosis (Seibert et al, 1987).

Finally, severe acquired or congenital protein C deficiency may also be associated with neonatal aortic thrombus formation even in the absence of umbilical catheter placement (Manco-Johnson et al, 1988). In cases of homozygous congenital protein C deficiency with associated thrombosis, the administration of supplemental protein C is necessary to correct the hypercoagulable prothrombotic condition in addition to the anticoagulant therapy (Dreyfus et al, 1991).

Clinical Presentation and Laboratory Findings

The symptoms of aortic and renal arterial thrombosis depend on the severity and extension of thrombus formation. Some infants may remain asymptomatic for a longer period of time, whereas others may show severe symptoms immediately after thrombus formation. Thrombosis of the abdominal aorta and the renal arteries should be suspected in newborns with a history of umbilical arterial catheterization who exhibit signs of congestive heart failure, hypertension, oliguria, renal failure, bowel ischemia or frank necrotizing enterocolitis (secondary to obstruction of the superior mesenteric artery), or decreased femoral pulses with lower limb ischemia (Schmidt and Andrew, 1995; Vailas at al, 1986). Aortic and renal thrombosis may be classified according to the severity of the clinical findings. *Minor thrombosis* presents with mildly decreased limb perfusion, hypertension, and hematuria; *moderate thrombosis* is present when decreased limb perfusion, hypertension, oliguria, and congestive heart failure occur; and *major thrombosis* is characterized by hypertension and signs of multiorgan failure. Laboratory findings associated with aortic thrombosis most frequently are thrombocytopenia, hypofibrinogenemia, elevated fibrin split products, variable prothrombin and thromboplastin times, conjugated hyperbilirubinemia, elevated blood urea nitrogen and serum creatinine, hyperreninemia, and hematuria.

Diagnosis

Although ultrasonography may fail to detect small intraarterial renal thrombi, especially in immature preterm infants (Schmidt and Andrew, 1995; Seibert et al, 1987; Vailas et al, 1986), the diagnosis of aortic and main renal artery thrombosis is most frequently made by real-time and Doppler ultrasonography (Schmidt and Andrew, 1995). Radionuclide imaging may also be useful in cases of suspected catheter-related renal artery thrombosis if the ultrasonographic findings are inconclusive (Molteni et al, 1993; Schmidt and Andrew, 1995). In cases in which intrathrombic fibrinolytic therapy or surgical intervention is considered, aortography through the umbilical arterial line should confirm the diagnosis (Richardson et al, 1988; Schmidt and Andrew, 1995).

Treatment

Prospective studies have shown that a large number of newborns with umbilical arterial catheters may develop asymptomatic aortic thrombosis (Oppenheimer et al, 1982; Seibert et al, 1987, 1991; Vailas et al, 1986). Because most of these thrombi resolve spontaneously, only supportive care, removal of the umbilical arterial catheter, and close ultrasonographic follow-up are recommended for the asymptomatic or the minimally symptomatic newborn (Schmidt and Andrew, 1995; Vailas et al, 1986). In more severe cases when fibrinolytic therapy is considered, the umbilical arterial line may be left in place (see later).

In the symptomatic patient with stable thrombosis of the aorta and renal arteries and only mild signs of organ dysfunction, supportive medical management consists of treatment of systemic hypertension and of the usually transient renal insufficiency and mild congestive heart failure. At present, heparin is the anticoagulant of choice in these newborns (Payne et al, 1989; Richardson et al, 1988; Schmidt and Andrew, 1995). Its initial loading dose is 75 to 100 IU/kg followed by 28 IU/kg per hour continuous infusion (Andrew et al, 1994). Laboratory monitoring to

avoid excessive heparinization and close follow-up of the clinical response by Doppler flow measurements and real-time ultrasonography are obligatory. Heparin has a large volume of distribution in newborns resulting in faster drug clearance (Schmidt and Andrew, 1995). Newborns at high risk for intracranial bleeding and those with established intracranial bleeding or with active bleeding elsewhere may not be candidates for systemic heparinization. The duration of heparin therapy depends on the clinical response measured by the improvement in organ function and should last for at least 7 days (Schmidt and Andrew, 1995). It is important to note that, in some newborns, a resistance to heparin therapy secondary to inherited or acquired antithrombin III deficiency may occur. In such cases, the administration of supplemental antithrombin III may be necessary to restore the effectiveness of heparin treatment. Finally, there is no evidence that long-term oral anticoagulation therapy is necessary after the resolution of neonatal aortic and renal thrombosis.

Medical management of cases with potential life-threatening complications of aortic or renal thrombosis includes systemic (Schmidt and Andrew, 1995) or intrathrombic (Schmidt and Andrew, 1995; Strife et al, 1988) application of fibrinolytic therapy and aggressive supportive care of organ dysfunction. Concomitant systemic heparinization is probably unnecessary and may increase the risk of intracranial bleeding. The intrathrombic infusion of the fibrinolytic agent reduces cumulative dose requirements and possibly the untoward systemic effects of fibrinolytic therapy. The fibrinolytic agents used in the clinical management of newborns with major thrombosis are streptokinase, urokinase, and tissue plasminogen activator (Schmidt and Andrew, 1995). These agents act by directly or indirectly converting plasminogen to plasmin, thus activating fibrinolysis. Streptokinase forms a protein complex with plasminogen, which, in turn, converts other plasminogen molecules to plasmin (Holden, 1990). The theoretical drawbacks of streptokinase application are depletion of the substrate and possible toxic reactions. Urokinase, a nonantigenic protein, directly converts plasminogen to plasmin in both the systemic circulation and the thrombus (Holden, 1990). At present, urokinase is the most frequently used fibrinolytic agent in newborns (Schmidt and Andrew, 1995). The suggested initial dose of systemic urokinase infusion is 4400 IU/kg over 20 minutes followed by 4400 IU/kg per hour of continuous infusion usually for 2 days. In cases of direct intrathrombic infusion, the cumulative dose should be decreased. Laboratory response includes a decrease in fibrinogen concentration and an increase in fibrin split products. In cases with a poor laboratory and clinical response, supplementation of plasminogen by the administration of fresh frozen plasma may be considered. Close ultrasonographic or angiographic follow-up is mandatory to evaluate the thrombolytic response. Tissue plasminogen activator is a fibrin-specific plasminogen activator that binds poorly to circulating plasminogen or fibrinogen (Haire, 1992). Thus, at least in theory, the use of this agent minimizes systemic proteolysis with maximal fibrinolytic activity on the surface of the thrombus. Although there are studies demonstrating the successful treatment of neonatal large vessel thrombosis with tissue plasminogen activator (Dillon et al, 1993), it is expensive, and no data have so far indicated the superiority of this agent over urokinase in the clinical setting (Schmidt and Andrew, 1995).

The major complication of fibrinolytic therapy is the occurrence of intracranial hemorrhage, especially in the sick preterm infant (Strife et al, 1988). Therefore, intrathrombic rather than systemic fibrinolytic therapy with radiologic imaging studies including serial head ultrasound examinations and laboratory monitoring of the appropriate coagulation parameters before, during, and after treatment constitute the suggested specific management of the newborn at high risk for intracranial bleeding who presents with a life-threatening aortic or renal arterial thrombosis. Although surgical thrombectomy has been successfully performed in newborns (Payne et al, 1989; Schmidt and Andrew, 1995), guidelines for the indication and timing of surgical management of neonatal aortic and renal thrombosis are not well established. Moreover, it must be emphasized that there is also no validated approach at present for the use of anticoagulant or fibrinolytic agents in newborns with aortic and renal thrombosis owing to the lack of scientific evidence concerning optimal management strategies. The above-described empiric approach to medical management summarizes the most recent recommendations based on the results of case reports, in the absence of well-designed controlled clinical studies.

Prognosis

Gestational and postnatal age; underlying pathologic conditions of the newborn; and the age, size, and location of the thrombus all have an impact on the outcome of neonatal aortic and renal arterial thrombosis. The overall mortality rate is around 20% (Schmidt and Andrew, 1995). Mortality rates with major aortic and renal arterial thrombosis, however, are higher (Vailas et al, 1986), whereas most newborns with minor or moderate thrombi recover.

The most frequent long-term morbidity in the affected newborn is renovascular hypertension. Although hypertension may persist for months or sometimes years, blood pressure eventually becomes normal, and the majority of the patients remain normotensive even after the antihypertensive treatment has been discontinued. It is not known, however, whether these children will have a higher incidence of hypertension or renal failure in adulthood. Chronic renal insufficiency develops less frequently during infancy and early childhood and is always the consequence of severe aortic and bilateral renal arterial thrombosis causing irreversible renal parenchymal damage.

RENAL VEIN OBSTRUCTION

Although renal vein thrombosis may occur at any age, newborns are particularly at risk for the development of this vascular event—60% to 75% of the patients with renal vein thrombosis are less than 1 month of age. Prenatally demonstrated renal vein thrombosis has also been reported, mainly in fetuses of diabetic mothers (Duncan et al, 1991; Sanders and Jaquier, 1989).

Incidence

Although autopsy findings indicate that the incidence of renal vein thrombosis is 1 in 40 to 1 in 300 in newborns who died (Arneil et al, 1973), the overall incidence of neonatal renal vein thrombosis is incompletely defined.

Etiology

The anatomy of the renal vasculature and the differences between the left and the right renal venous drainage determine the response of the renal venous system to injury. The drainage of the left adrenal vein into the left main renal vein explains why ipsilateral adrenal hemorrhage more frequently accompanies left-sided than right-sided renal vein thrombosis. The lack of venous collaterals in the right kidney is responsible for the more rapid and severe occurrence of clinical symptoms of venous thrombosis on this side. In the primary and most frequent form of renal vein thrombosis in the newborn, clotting starts in the small intrarenal veins when venous stasis occurs. As a result of the free anastomoses within the renal venous system, microthrombi spread distally and involve the renal cortex and medulla extending into larger veins (Arneil et al, 1973). In the secondary form of renal vein thrombosis, a thrombus in the inferior vena cava extends into the renal vein.

Decreases in renal blood flow and the occurrence of prethrombotic or hypercoagulable prothrombotic states are factors most frequently involved in the pathogenesis of renal vein thrombosis in the newborn. The normally low venous blood flow in the newborn may be further reduced by intravascular volume loss (bleeding or dehydration), hypoxia, infection, polycythemia, or cyanotic congenital heart disease. The ensuing venous stasis and hemoconcentration, especially when accompanied by disturbances in fluid and electrolyte homeostasis and acid-base balance, result in sludging and thrombosis in the small interlobular veins. The microthrombi in the small veins then spread distally involving the larger vessels. In thromboembolic states, subsequent renal vein involvement occurs with the proximal extension of the thrombus from the pelvicaliceal veins and from the inferior vena cava. In the newborn, renal vein thrombosis most frequently occurs after a central line placement through the femoral vein or if hemorrhagic shock develops. Finally, infants of diabetic mothers are at an especially high risk of renal vein thrombosis as a result of a combination of several risk factors, including their hypercoagulable state and relatively low extracellular water content as well as the often associated polycythemia, perinatal asphyxia, and respiratory distress.

Clinical Presentation and Laboratory Findings

The development of a unilateral or bilateral flank mass in association with a sudden deterioration of clinical status should raise the possibility of renal vein thrombosis in the newborn. Other clinical signs and laboratory findings consistent with renal vein thrombosis include oliguria or anuria, gross hematuria, thrombocytopenia, hemolytic anemia, metabolic acidosis, and azotemia. Prothrombin time and partial thromboplastin time may be prolonged because of consumption of coagulation factors. At the beginning, blood pressure is often low. Although hypertension may develop later in the course of the disease, the increase in blood pressure usually does not reach the level seen in cases of renal arterial thrombosis. Some newborns, however, whose early clinical symptoms are mild or overlooked may present with hypertension days or weeks after the development of the renal vein thrombosis.

Diagnosis

The diagnosis of renal vein thrombosis in the newborn is suspected based on the above-described clinical presentation and laboratory findings and confirmed by the results of real-time and Doppler ultrasonography (Schmidt and Andrew, 1995; Slovis et al, 1993). Sonography confirms the diagnosis with an approximately 92% accuracy (Ricci and Lloyd, 1990). The real-time ultrasonographic features are nonspecific and include renal enlargement and evidence of edema causing distortion of the renal architecture with an inhomogeneous appearance of the parenchyma and loss of corticomedullary differentiation. The findings of color Doppler sonography are more specific and make the diagnosis relatively easy once the thrombus has reached the larger renal veins. Among the survivors, characteristic calcification of intrarenal veins is detected in 60% of the cases (Slovis et al, 1993).

Renal vein thrombosis should always be differentiated from renal artery thrombosis. The latter occurs mostly in newborns with catheterization of the umbilical artery, it does not present with renal enlargement, and the subsequent systemic hypertension is usually more pronounced than that in renal vein thrombosis.

Treatment

Initial treatment is directed toward correcting the abnormalities in the fluid, electrolyte, and acid-base balance. The use of hypertonic infusions, nephrotoxic medications, and hyperosmolar radiographic contrast agents should be avoided. Diuretics are of limited value, and their use may further propagate hemoconcentration. If hemoconcentration cannot be corrected by infusion therapy, peritoneal dialysis may be indicated.

Although the correction of hemoconcentration and hyperviscosity in most patients prevents further propagation of the thrombus, intravenous heparin may be of some value in preventing extension of the thrombus (Ricci and Lloyd, 1990). Heparin treatment does not prevent the development of renal dysfunction (Mocan et al, 1991; Nuss et al, 1994). Successful thrombolytic therapy with urokinase infused through a lower extremity vein has also been reported (Duncan et al, 1991). Because active bleeding and the risk for intraventricular hemorrhage are the main contraindications of anticoagulant and thrombolytic therapy, their use is recommended mostly in the full-term newborn (see earlier).

The role of surgical intervention in the treatment of renal vein thrombosis has been extensively debated. Theoretically in the primary form of renal vein thrombosis, thrombectomy precludes extension of the thrombus into the vena cava or opposite kidney and prevents infections and the development of hypertension caused by renal ischemia. Because the smaller intrarenal veins are almost always occluded, however, extraction of thrombus from the main renal vein does not alleviate renal infarction in most cases of renal vein thrombosis. Moreover, an advantage of

early thrombectomy or nephrectomy has not been demonstrated, even with bilateral involvement (Ricci and Lloyd, 1990).

Prognosis

The survival rate of newborns with renal vein thrombosis has improved during the past decade and is around 80% to 95% (Ricci and Lloyd, 1990; Schmidt and Andrew, 1995). Most deaths are due to the underlying disease and not the renal vein thrombosis or the ensuing renal dysfunction. The extent of recovery of the involved kidney after renal vein thrombosis varies from a complete restoration of renal function to the development of a nonfunctioning shrunken kidney, partially fibrous kidney, renal hypertension, nephrotic syndrome, or chronic renal tubular dysfunction. Although follow-up data on survivors of neonatal renal vein thrombosis are limited, at a median follow-up period of 12 years in one study, glomerular filtration rate and urinary concentration remained within normal limits in two thirds and one half of 16 patients (Mocan et al, 1991). Because persistent renal imaging abnormalities were present in more than 80% of these patients (Mocan et al, 1991), however, the long-term outcome of renal function in patients with neonatal renal vein thrombosis remains uncertain, and continuing follow-up is absolutely necessary.

RENAL CORTICAL AND MEDULLARY NECROSIS

Renal cortical, renal medullary, and combined cortical and medullary necrosis are uncommon disorders in the newborn. They occur only in critically ill newborns who, in most of the cases, present with irreversible shock. Therefore, renal cortical and medullary necrosis is the manifestation of an end-organ insult to the kidney caused most frequently by extreme perinatal or postnatal stress, and it is seldom recognized while the newborn is alive.

Incidence and Etiology

Autopsy findings indicate that the incidence of renal cortical and medullary necrosis is around 5% in infants who die at less than 3 months of age (Lerner et al, 1992). Risk factors for the development of renal cortical and medullary necrosis include prematurity, congenital heart disease associated with low renal perfusion or poor tissue oxygenation, perinatal asphyxia, sepsis, bleeding diathesis or coagulopathy, and respiratory distress resulting in cardiovascular compromise. In addition, the use of contrast agents during cardiac catheterization also appears to be a risk factor.

Pathomechanism and Clinical Presentation

The clinical manifestations of renal cortical and medullary necrosis (hematuria, oliguria or anuria, and renal enlargement) are nonspecific and are present in several more common neonatal renal abnormalities. Because renal cortical and medullary necrosis occurs only in newborns with shock caused by a life-threatening condition, its recognition is often delayed or the diagnosis is never even considered.

It is unclear why some affected newborns preferentially develop medullary necrosis, whereas others present with cortical necrosis of the kidney. The severity of the intrarenal arteriolar vasoconstriction and the magnitude of the underlying resistance of the capillary bed in the renal cortex and medulla may have a major impact on the primary localization of the necrotic process.

Increased local production of vasodilator prostaglandins attenuate renal vasoconstriction under acute circulatory collapse (Gleason, 1987). Because inhibition of prostaglandin synthesis by indomethacin enhances renal ischemia under these circumstances, administration of the drug may contribute to the development of renal cortical and medullary necrosis in premature newborns with severely compromised cardiovascular status.

Hyperosmotic radiocontrast agents may also produce marked and protracted medullary vasoconstriction and hypoxia probably by affecting renal medullary prostaglandin synthesis (Gruskin et al, 1974; Nygren et al, 1988). Their use in newborns with congenital heart disease during cardiac catheterization may contribute to the development of renal cortical and medullary necrosis in this patient population. Whether the use of isosmotic contrast agents results in similar renal response is unknown.

Diagnosis, Management, and Prognosis

There are no specific clinical, laboratory, or imaging findings to aid in the diagnosis of neonatal renal cortical and medullary necrosis, and there is no specific therapy available. In all critically ill newborns with shock or thrombosis of the renal vessels, or after the administration of a hyperosmolar contrast agent during cardiac catheterization, the clinician should maintain a high degree of suspicion until the presence of a major renal insult can safely be ruled out. Differential diagnoses include all causes of neonatal acute renal failure, including bilateral renal arterial or renal vein thrombosis, autosomal recessive polycystic kidney disease, and bilaterally multicystic or hydronephrotic kidneys. During the acute phase, renal scintigraphy and magnetic resonance imaging may be of value in the diagnosis. The decreased ability of the critically ill newborn to tolerate transport in the acute phase of the disease, however, renders these studies impractical.

The prognosis of neonatal renal cortical and medullary necrosis depends on the underlying disease. Excretory urography in survivors shows characteristic bizarre-appearing dilated calices with variable amount of scarring. These morphologic changes are most frequently associated with reduced glomerular filtration rate, renal concentration defect, hypertension, and segmental hypoplasia. As in the cases of renal artery and vein thrombosis, the long-term effects of neonatal cortical and medullary necrosis on renal function remain to be determined.

ADRENAL HEMORRHAGE
Incidence

The incidence of detected neonatal adrenal hemorrhage ranges from 1.7 to 2.1 per 1000 births (Marino et al, 1990). Because adrenal bleeding may remain asymptomatic, the real occurrence is probably higher. In newborns who die, the incidence of adrenal hemorrhage is around 10%. In the majority of the cases, the bleeding locates to one side, and only 5% to 8% of adrenal hemorrhages are bilateral (Marino et al, 1990).

Pathomechanism

The fetal and neonatal adrenal glands are relatively large in size and are more vascularized than later in life, which may predispose them to bleeding. Risk factors associated with adrenal hemorrhage in the newborn include birth trauma, perinatal asphyxia, shock, infection, thrombosis of the inferior vena cava and left renal vein, and hemorrhagic disorders.

Clinical Presentation

Clinical symptoms are nonspecific and most frequently include unexplained jaundice, mild anemia, and presence of an abdominal mass. In the case of bilateral adrenal hemorrhage, hypoglycemia and hypotension may be the presenting findings. Rarely, neonatal adrenal hemorrhage presents with the clinical manifestation of a scrotal hematoma (Putnam, 1989). The simultaneous occurrence of adrenal bleeding and incomplete rotation of the colon leading to early duodenal obstruction has also been reported (Cheves et al, 1989). Finally, many affected infants remain completely asymptomatic.

Diagnosis

Suprarenal masses in the newborn that should be considered in the differential diagnosis of neonatal adrenal hemorrhage include abscesses; neuroblastoma; renal duplication; hydronephrosis; Wilms tumor; enteric duplications; and renal, pancreatic, hepatic, ovarian, and choledochal cysts. If adrenal hemorrhage is suspected, laboratory tests including a complete blood cell count, serum bilirubin, serum glucose, and urinary excretion of catecholamines and their metabolites aid in establishing the diagnosis. In typical cases, the diagnosis is confirmed by ultrasonography. Usually the whole gland is affected, but occasionally an uninvolved adrenal limb may be detected adjacent to the suprarenal mass. Because hemorrhage into the adrenal gland is usually followed by necrosis and later resolution with fibrosis and calcification, the evolution of these signs is characteristic on the sonographic follow-up examinations. Calcification of the adrenal gland is usually noted about 2 weeks after the hemorrhage. Despite the high resolution of ultrasound imaging, the use of magnetic resonance imaging, computed tomography, or radionuclide renal scan is sometimes necessary to differentiate between an atypical adrenal hemorrhage and neurobalstoma or a renal mass. Surgical exploration is seldom needed.

In utero adrenal bleeding of the fetus should be considered if a cystic mass in the suprarenal area is detected on prenatal ultrasonography (Marino et al, 1990). It is extremely difficult, however, to distinguish between fetal adrenal hemorrhage and cystic neuroblastoma without histologic examination. Because adrenal hemorrhage shows progressive changes within 2 weeks, whereas neuroblastoma usually remains unchanged during this time, a repeat prenatal ultrasound study may be helpful in establishing the diagnosis. A hemorrhage into an adrenal neuroblastoma may also cause progressive cystic changes on repeat ultrasonographic examinations making the prenatal differential diagnosis extremely difficult. In such cases, intrauterine evaluation of the suprarenal mass by magnetic resonance imaging may be informative.

The occurrence of benign hemorrhagic adrenocortical cysts has also been reported in Beckwith-Wiedemann syndrome, a condition also associated with a high incidence of adrenocortical carcinoma (McCauley et al, 1991). The differentiation of these benign hemorrhagic lesions of the adrenals from common adrenal hemorrhage may be difficult by imaging studies alone.

Outcome

In the majority of cases, the prognosis of neonatal adrenal hemorrhage is excellent. The disease is self-limiting and except for the rare bilateral cases requires no specific treatment.

HYPERTENSION IN THE NEWBORN

The first reported blood pressure measurement in the newborn was performed by the direct determination of the pressure in the umbilical artery in 1879 (Ribemont, 1879). Since then, the ever-increasing body of information on arterial blood pressure in the newborn has generated new and yet unanswered questions. For example, because the physiologic blood pressure range in the neonatal period, especially in the immature preterm infant, remains unknown, hypotension and hypertension cannot be adequately defined in this patient population.

Blood Pressure Measurement Techniques

The requirements for the techniques of blood pressure measurement include that the method should be simple, painless, and reliable with an acceptable risk/benefit ratio, and it should give information continuously or at least in frequent intervals without disturbing the newborn.

Invasive Measurement

The most widely used method of blood pressure measurement in the critically ill newborn is by means of an indwelling umbilical or peripheral artery catheter connected to a blood pressure transducer. Three sources of error are of importance when this method is used. First, if the catheter is too small in diameter, it underestimates the systolic pressure because of loss of higher frequencies. Second, the position of the catheter tip too close to the wall of the vessel or the presence of a clot at the tip of the catheter may result in dampening of the pressure waves and lead to an underestimation of the blood pressure. Finally, the presence of even small air bubbles in the system generates a resonant frequency, which then alters the measured systolic, diastolic, and, to a lesser extent, mean blood pressure

values (Weindling, 1989). The position of the umbilical arterial catheter tip in the aorta (high versus low) does not influence the measured value. Occasionally, both peripheral and umbilical arterial lines are placed and transduced in extremely labile, critically ill full-term newborns. In these cases, the peripheral arterial catheter may read higher systolic pressures than the umbilical line (Adelman, 1988).

Noninvasive Measurement

There are three noninvasive methods used in clinical practice. The traditional methods using auscultation, palpation, or the flush technique are insensitive, especially when the stroke volume is low. The Doppler ultrasound method is reliable for the measurement of systolic values, but it cannot accurately detect the diastolic pressure (Emery and Greenough, 1992). Automatic oscillometry method is the most commonly used noninvasive technique that provides an accurate, reproducible, and convenient estimate of blood pressure in most newborns, provided that the appropriate size cuff is used with a cuff width/arm circumference ratio of 0.44 to 0.55 (Low et al, 1995; Sonesson and Broberger, 1987). In very-low-birth-weight newborns, however, as well as in cases of extreme hypotension, some inaccuracy may occur (Rasoulpour and Marinelli, 1992).

Definition and Incidence

Despite the large body of information on blood pressure values in the neonatal period, there is no accurate definition of pathologic blood pressure values for the newborn and, in particular, for the very-low-birth-weight infant (see earlier). In the clinical practice, the infant's blood pressure and tissue perfusion are generally considered to be adequate as long as urine output and capillary refill are within normal limits in the absence of metabolic acidosis. Although this approach may be an appropriate clinical approximation for hypotension, it is not at all useful in cases of hypertension because there are no specific clinical or laboratory signs to indicate the level of systemic blood pressure elevation that has the potential of causing end-organ damage in the given newborn. In the pediatric population, hypertension is defined as the average systolic or diastolic blood pressure (or both) equal to or greater than the 95th percentile for age and sex when measured on at least three occasions. This definition, however, cannot be applied to neonatal hypertension because it presupposes an accurate definition of normal neonatal blood pressure (see earlier). Therefore, neonatal hypertension remains arbitrarily defined as the systolic blood pressure greater than 90 mm Hg and diastolic blood pressure greater than 60 mm Hg in the full-term newborn and systolic blood pressure greater than 80 mm Hg and diastolic blood pressure greater than 50 mm Hg in the preterm infant (Adelman, 1988). At present, this arbitrary definition is widely accepted and referred to in the literature. Based on these criteria, the reported incidence of neonatal hypertension ranges from 0.7% to 3.2% (Adelman, 1988; Rasoulpour and Marinelli, 1992). In the less than 1000 g extremely-low-birth-weight infant, however, even the arbitrary limits of hypertension are not agreed on (Spinazzola et al, 1991). Obviously, additional well-designed studies are needed to

TABLE 98–1

Blood Pressure in Healthy Term Newborns and Infants During the 1st Year of Life

Age	n	State	Systolic (mm Hg)	Diastolic (mm Hg)	Mean (mm Hg)
1 hour°	17		70	44	53
12 hour°	17		66	41	50
1st day†	46	Asleep	70 ± 9	42 ± 12	55 ± 11
		Awake	71 ± 9	43 ± 10	55 ± 9
3rd day†	46	Asleep	75 ± 11	48 ± 10	59 ± 9
		Awake	77 ± 12	49 ± 10	63 ± 13
6th day†	46	Asleep	76 ± 10	46 ± 12	58 ± 12
		Awake	76 ± 10	49 ± 11	62 ± 12
2nd week‡	566		78 ± 10	50 ± 9	
3rd week‡	77		79 ± 8	49 ± 8	
4 weeks‡	642		85 ± 10	46 ± 9	
6 weeks§	1131	Asleep	89 ± 11		
		Awake	96 ± 11		
6 months	525‡		92 ± 9	55 ± 9	
	858§		93 + 14		
12 months	427‡		95 ± 8	56 ± 8	
	1338§		94 + 11		

Table composed from data in Kitterman et al, 1969 (°, average values), Tan, 1987 (†), Zinner et al, 1985 (‡), and de Swiet et al, 1980 (§, mean values and 95th percentile).

follow the normal changes in neonatal blood pressure with time to provide more appropriate 95% confidence limits for use in the diagnosis of neonatal hypertension.

Factors directly associated with increases in blood pressure in the newborn include maternal smoking during pregnancy (Beratis et al, 1996); gestational and postnatal age (Georgieff et al, 1996; Rasoulpour and Marinelli, 1992; Spinazzola et al, 1991; Versmold et al, 1981); stress; agitation; application of topical mydriatics; crying; upright position; and, provided that the newborn is euvolemic, abdominal compression. Endotracheal suctioning results in a biphasic blood pressure response with an initial brief drop followed by a greater rise of longer duration (Perry et al, 1990).

Blood Pressure Standards

Table 98–1 describes the normal blood pressure values in healthy term newborns during the 1st year of life. Blood pressure increases with postnatal age by 1 to 2 mm Hg per day during the 1st week and by approximately 1 mm Hg per week during the first 6 weeks of life. Because blood pressure is affected by gestational age and birth weight, it is lower in premature infants than in full-term newborns (Emery and Greenough, 1992; Hegyi et al, 1994; Versmold et al, 1981; Weindling, 1989). Among premature infants, however, the limits of systolic and diastolic blood pressure appear to be less dependent of weight and gestational age if they do not require mechanical ventilation and have a stable cardiovascular status (Hegyi et al, 1994). Similar to that in the term infant, blood pressure in preterm newborns also increases with postnatal age (Table 98–2).

Etiology

Neonatal hypertension is associated with certain congenital malformations and acquired diseases (Table 98–3). The most common causes of hypertension seen in neonatal intensive care units are thrombosis of the renal artery owing to umbilical arterial catheterization, bronchopulmonary dysplasia, extracorporeal membrane oxygenation, and coarctation of the aorta (Rasoulpour and Marinelli, 1992; Seibert et al, 1991).

Clinical Signs

Approximately one third of patients with neonatal hypertension remain asymptomatic (Adelman, 1987). In those who develop clinical signs, the symptoms are rather nonspecific, and the presence or severity of the symptoms is not related to the magnitude of the blood pressure elevation. The clinical manifestation of neonatal hypertension

TABLE 98–2

Systolic Blood Pressure in Preterm Infants with Birth Weight <1500 g During the 1st Week of Life

Age (days)	n	Systolic Blood Pressure (mm Hg)	+2 SD (mm Hg)*
1	44	39.2 ± 7.6	54.4
2	37	45.3 ± 7.8	60.9
3	33	45.2 ± 7.8	60.8
4	27	46.0 ± 8.9	63.8
5	23	46.0 ± 8.7	63.4
6	22	47.5 ± 9.9	67.3
7	19	51.1 ± 9.9	70.9

*In children, +2 SD is considered as the upper normal limit (see text for details).

From Emery EF, Greenough A: Non-invasive blood pressure monitoring in preterm infants receiving intensive care. Eur J Pediatr 151:136, 1992. © 1992 Springer-Verlag.

TABLE 98–3

Causes of Neonatal Hypertension

Vascular

Renal artery thrombosis
Aortic thrombosis
Coarctation of the aorta
Hypoplastic aorta
Renal vein thrombosis
Thrombosis of the ductus arteriosus
Renal artery stenosis/intimal hyperplasia
Idiopathic arterial calcification

Renoparenchymal

Acute renal failure
Polycystic kidney disease
Renal cortical and medullary necrosis
Hypoplastic, dysplastic kidney
Acute renal infection
Pyelonephritis with scarring
Obstructive uropathy
Constrictive perirenal hematoma or urinoma
Congenital mesoblastic nephroma
Nephrolithiasis
Following pyeloplasty of a hydronephrotic kidney
Multicystic kidney

Endocrine

Pheochromocytoma
Neuroblastoma
Adrenal disorders (hyperplasia, hyperaldosteronism, carcinoma,
  hematoma)
Hyperthyroidism

Other

Drugs (corticosteroids, theophylline, pancuronium, intrauterine
  cocaine exposure, phenylephrine eye drops)
Extracorporeal membrane oxygenation
Bronchopulmonary dysplasia
Increased intracranial pressure/seizures
Fluid and electrolyte overload
Closure of an abdominal wall defect

---

includes signs of dysfunction of the cardiovascular system (congestive heart failure, decreased or unequal pulses, cardiomegaly, hepatomegaly, vasomotor instability), the respiratory system (tachypnea, cyanosis), the central nervous system (tremors, seizures, lethargy, coma, apnea, abnormal muscle tone, opisthotonus, asymmetric reflexes, facial palsy, hypertensive retinopathy, cerebral edema and hemorrhage), and the kidneys (dehydration, sodium wasting, oliguria or anuria, renal enlargement). In addition, nonspecific general symptoms of hypertension (abdominal distention, edema, fever, and failure to thrive) may also be encountered. Most infants develop hypertension during the first 2 weeks of life with a range of 1 to 45 days (Adelman, 1988). Approximately 50% of newborns with hypertension exhibit signs of hypertensive retinopathy, including a decreased ratio of the arterial to venous caliber, vascular tortuosity, and exudate formation (Skalina et al, 1983).

Evaluation of Neonatal Hypertension

After the thorough review of the history and the physical examination, appropriate laboratory and imaging studies should be performed according to the suspected cause. In the hypertensive newborn with an indwelling umbilical arterial catheter in place, a urinalysis and the evaluation of serum electrolytes, creatinine, and blood urea nitrogen should be followed by a real-time and Doppler ultrasonographic study of the kidneys, perirenal regions, renal arteries and veins, aorta, and inferior vena cava. Dynamic (technetium 99m-diethylenetriaminepenta-acetic acid) and static (technetium 99m-dimercaptosuccinic acid) renal radionuclide scans are additional valuable tests in newborns with suspected renovascular hypertension, providing information about renal blood flow and its intrarenal distribution as well as about renal function (see Chapter 92). An aortography through the umbilical arterial catheter is seldom indicated. Evaluation of the role of pain sensation or agitation in the cause of hypertension and four-extremity blood pressure measurements should also be part of the initial work-up. A more detailed cardiac evaluation, including an electrocardiogram, a chest radiograph, and an echocardiographic study, is necessary in cases in which a cardiac cause of the hypertension is suspected. In most newborns, the above-described work-up is sufficient for the diagnosis. If the patient's clinical or the laboratory findings indicate, however, further studies may be warranted to rule out other less frequent conditions associated with neonatal hypertension, including endocrine disorders or pheochromocytoma.

Treatment

As a result of inability to define neonatal hypertension accurately and the lack of information about the short-term and long-term side effects of antihypertensive medications in the newborn, firm clinical guidelines regarding the treatment of neonatal hypertension cannot be postulated. In asymptomatic newborns, with only mild to moderate elevation of blood pressure and without an identified cause, close observation and no aggressive antihypertensive treatment is recommended, unless clinical or echocardiographic evidence of hypertension develops. The definitive therapy of neonatal hypertension is to treat the primary cause whenever possible (e.g., removal of the umbilical catheter, discontinuation of an offending medication). In asymptomatic newborns with severe hypertension and in all symptomatic newborns even with only mild to moderate blood pressure elevation, treatment of the hypertension with antihypertensive agents is the presently accepted clinical practice (Table 98–4).

For mild hypertension with a component of fluid retention, diuretics including furosemide or a thiazide diuretic with or without spironolactone are recommended. In the long-term diuretic treatment of neonatal hypertension, thiazide diuretics are preferred over furosemide because long-term furosemide treatment is associated with potentially detrimental side effects, including severe electrolyte imbalance resulting in failure to thrive, calciuria, nephrocalcinosis, and osteopenia.

For the initial treatment of moderate to severe hypertension, the direct vascular smooth muscle relaxant hydralazine is used frequently. Hydralazine may also decrease pulmonary vascular resistance in infants with bronchopulmonary dysplasia. Hydralazine may be given alone or in

TABLE 98–4

Antihypertensive Agents Used in the Treatment of Hypertension in Newborns

Medications	Route	Dose	Comments
Diuretics			
Furosemide	IV, (oral)	1–2 mg/kg/dose (q 12–24 h)	Hyponatremia, hypokalemia, hypochloremia, hypercalciuria, nephrocalcinosis, osteopenia, ototoxicity
Chlorothiazide	Oral	5–50 mg/kg/d	Hyponatremia, hypokalemia, hypochloremia, calcium sparing
Spironolactone	Oral	1–3 mg/kg/d	Weak diuretic, hyperkalemia
Adrenergic Blockers			
β-adrenergic blockers			
Propranolol	Oral	0.5–2 mg/kg/d	Precipitation of heart failure, bronchospasm, hypoglycemia, ↓ renin release, recommended in combination with hydralazine
α₁/β-adrenergic blockers			
Labetalol	IV	0.5–1 mg/kg/h	Limited experience in neonatal hypertensive emergencies
Vasodilators			
Hydralazine°	IV	0.1–2 mg/kg/dose (q 6–12 h)	Reflex tachycardia, paroxysmal atrial tachycardia, emesis, diarrhea, positive ANA (SLE-like syndrome)
	Oral	0.25–1 mg/kg/dose (q 6–12 h)	
Diazoxide°	IV	1–3 mg/kg/dose	Hypotension, hyperglycemia, sodium and water retention
Nitroprusside°	IV	0.2–10 μg/kg/min	Thiocyanate and cyanide toxicity, methemoglobinemia; drug must be protected from light (↑ photochemical degradation)
Angiotensin-Converting Enzyme Inhibitors			
Captopril	Oral	10–50 μg/kg/dose (q 8–24 h) (may titrate to 0.5 mg/kg/dose)	Oliguria, renal failure, hyperkalemia, apnea, seizures, cough
Enalaprilat	IV	5–15 μg/kg/dose (q 8–24 h)	Oliguria, renal failure, hyperkalemia, cough
Calcium Channel Blockers			
Nifedipine	Oral, sublingual	0.25–0.5 mg/kg/dose	Limited experience

°Recommended in neonatal hypertensive emergencies.
SLE, systemic lupus erythematosus; ANA, antinuclear antibody.

combination with a beta blocker. Among the beta blockers, the nonselective beta blocker propranolol has been used most widely because it appears to increase the efficacy of hydralazine, while decreasing thiazide-induced tachycardia. Propranolol may precipitate heart failure, however, and cause hypoglycemia and bronchospasm.

The use of an angiotensin-converting enzyme inhibitor, primarily captopril, has become the treatment of choice in severe neonatal renovascular hypertension not responding to other medications. Mostly because of the higher postnatal renin levels and the immaturity of their renal function, newborns are extremely sensitive to the antihypertensive effects of captopril. When it was given at the originally recommended higher doses (0.3 mg/kg), unpredictable decreases in the systemic blood pressure occurred in some of the newborns resulting in renal failure (Rasoulpour and Marinelli, 1992) and neurologic complications (Perlman and Volpe, 1989). Therefore, captopril should be started at lower doses, and the dose should be titrated so that the lowest effective dose is administered long-term (see Table 98–4). The intravenous angiotensin-converting enzyme inhibitor enalaprilat has also been used successfully for the

treatment of severe neonatal renovascular hypertension (Mason et al, 1992).

Hypertensive emergencies in the newborn are usually managed with hydralazine, diazoxide, or sodium nitroprusside. To avoid a rapid and substantial drop in blood pressure and thus tissue perfusion, stepwise dose increases are recommended. Diazoxide, a direct arteriolar smooth muscle relaxant, must be given rapidly because it avidly binds to protein. Side effects of its repeated use include sodium and water retention and hyperglycemia. Sodium nitroprusside acts via the generation of nitric oxide, and thus its effect is dependent on the intact function of the endothelium. This photosensitive agent is an extremely potent vasodilator and must be administered in titrated continuous infusion while being shielded from light. Owing to its mechanism of action and metabolism, it may cause methemoglobinemia and cyanide toxicity. Because its administration to newborns at doses of 0.2 to 6 μg/kg per minute for up to 4 days has been found safe, routine monitoring of thiocyanate levels may not be necessary if the drug is administered in the aforementioned dose range and for a short period only (Benitz et al, 1985). The development of an unexplained metabolic acidosis with increased mixed venous oxygen content must prompt the discontinuation of the drug infusion and the measurement of plasma cyanide levels.

In hypertensive infants with stenosis of the renal artery, a balloon angioplasty or surgical reconstruction of the renal artery may be attempted. Only the poorly functioning, sclerotic, and shrunken kidney with established hypertension represents an indication for nephrectomy.

Prognosis

In the majority of cases of neonatal hypertension, systemic blood pressure can be adequately controlled by pharmacologic management and hypertension eventually resolves (Adelman, 1987; Rasoulpour and Marinelli, 1992). The long-term outcome, however, remains unclear. Newborns with hypertension of renovascular or renoparenchymal origin and those with persistent abnormalities of renal size and function, especially with concurrent bronchopulmonary dysplasia, require close and long-term follow-up because the scars and atrophic regions in the kidney carry the possibility of recurrence of hypertension as well as that of the development of renal insufficiency at a later age.

Acknowledgment

The authors thank Nathan Hagstrom, MD, and Rita Jew, PharmD, for their valuable help during the preparation of the manuscript.

REFERENCES

Adelman RD: Long term follow up of neonatal renovascular hypertension in the newborn. Pediatr Nephrol 1:35, 1987.

Adelman RD: The hypertensive newborn. Clin Perinatol 15:567, 1988.

Andrew M, Marzinotto V, Massicotte P, et al: Heparin therapy in pediatric patients: A prospective cohort study. Pediatr Res 35:78, 1994.

Arneil GC, MacDonald AM, Sweet EM: Renal venous thrombosis. Clin Nephrol 1:119, 1973.

Benitz WE, Malachowski N, Cohen RS, et al: Use of sodium nitroprusside in newborns: Efficacy and safety. J Pediatr 106:102, 1985.

Beratis NG, Panagoulias D, Varvarigou A: Increased blood pressure in newborns and infants whose mothers smoked during pregnancy. J Pediatr 128:806, 1996.

Cheves H, Bledsoe F, Rhea WG, Bomar W: Adrenal hemorrhage with incomplete rotation of the colon leading to early duodenal obstruction: Case report and review of the literature. J Pediatr Surg 24:300, 1989.

de Swiet M, Fayers P, Shinebourne EA: Systolic blood pressure in a population of infants in the first year of life: The Brompton study. Pediatrics 65:1028, 1980.

Dillon PW, Fox PS, Berg CJ, et al: Recombinant tissue plasminogen activator for neonatal and pediatric vascular thrombolytic therapy. J Pediatr Surg 28:1264, 1993.

Dreyfus M, Magny JF, Brifey F, et al: Treatment of homozygous protein C deficiency and neonatal purpura fulminans with purified protein C concentrate. N Engl J Med 325:1565, 1991.

Duncan BW, Adzick NS, Longaker MT, et al: In utero arterial embolism from renal vein thrombosis with successful postnatal thrombolytic therapy. J Pediatr Surg 26:741, 1991.

Emery EF, Greenough A: Non-invasive blood pressure monitoring in preterm infants receiving intensive care. Eur J Pediatr 151:136, 1992.

Georgieff MK, Mills MM, Gomez-Marin O, Sinaiko AR: Rate of change of blood pressure in premature and full term infants from birth to 4 months. Pediatr Nephrol 10:152, 1996.

Gleason CA: Prostaglandins and the developing kidney. Semin Perinatol 11:12, 1987.

Goetzman BW, Stadalnik RC, Bogren HG, et al: Thrombotic complica-

tions of umbilical artery catheters: A clinical and radiographic study. Pediatrics 56:374, 1975.

Gruskin AB, Auerbach VH, Black IF: Intrarenal blood flow in children with normal kidneys and congenital heart disease: Changes attributable to angiography. Pediatr Res 8:561, 1974.

Haire WD: Pharmacology of fibrinolysis. Chest 101:91S, 1992.

Hegyi T, Carbone MT, Anwar M, et al: Blood pressure ranges in premature infants: I. The first hours of life. J Pediatr 124:627, 1994.

Holden RW: Plasminogen activators: Pharmacology and therapy. Radiology 174:993, 1990.

Horgan MJ, Bartoletti A, Polansky S, et al: Effect of heparin infusates in umbilical arterial catheters on frequency of thrombotic complications. J Pediatr 111:774, 1987.

Jackson JC, Truog WE, Watchko JF, et al: Efficacy of thromboresistant umbilical artery catheters in reducing aortic thrombosis and related complications. J Pediatr 110:102, 1987.

Kitterman JA, Phibbs RH, Tooley WH: Aortic blood pressure in normal newborn infants during the first 12 hours of life. Pediatrics 44:959, 1969.

Lerner GR, Kurnetz R, Bernstein J, et al: Renal cortical and renal medullary necrosis in the first 3 months of life. Pediatr Nephrol 6:516, 1992.

Low JA, Panagiotopoulos C, Smith JT, et al: Validity of newborn oscillometric blood pressure. Clin Invest Med 18:163, 1995.

Manco-Johnson MJ, Marlar RA, Jacobson LJ, et al: Severe protein C deficiency in newborn infants. J Pediatr 113:359, 1988.

Marino J, Martinez-Urrutia MJ, Hawkins F, et al: Encysted adrenal hemorrhage: Prenatal diagnosis. Acta Paediatr Scand 79:230, 1990.

Mason T, Polak MJ, Pyles L, et al: Treatment of neonatal renovascular hypertension with intravenous enalapril. Am J Perinatol 9:254, 1992.

McCauley RG, Beckwith JB, Elias ER, et al: Benign hemorrhagic adrenocortical macrocysts in Beckwith-Wiedemann syndrome. AJR Am J Roentgenol 157:549, 1991.

Mocan H, Beattie TJ, Murphy AV: Renal venous thrombosis in infancy: Long-term follow-up. Pediatr Nephrol 5:45, 1991.

Mokrohisky ST, Levine RL, Blumhagen JD, et al: Low positioning of umbilical-artery catheters increases associated complications in newborn infants. N Engl J Med 299:561, 1978.

Molteni KH, George J, Messersmith R, et al: Intra-thrombic urokinase reverses neonatal renal artery thrombosis. Pediatr Nephrol 7:413, 1993.

Nuss R, Hays T, Manco-Johnson M: Efficacy and safety of heparin anticoagulation for neonatal renal vein thrombosis. Am J Pediatr Hematol Oncol 16:127, 1994.

Nygren A, Ulfendahl HR, Hansell P, Erikson U: Effects of intravenous contrast media on cortical and medullary blood flow in the rat kidney. Invest Radiol 23:753, 1988.

O'Neill JA Jr, Neblett WW III, Born ML: Management of major thromboembolic complications of umbilical artery catheters. J Pediatr Surg 16:972, 1981.

Oppenheimer DA, Carroll BA, Garth KE: Ultrasonic detection of complications following umbilical arterial catheterization in the newborn. Radiology 145:667, 1982.

Payne RM, Martin TC, Bower RJ, Canter CE: Management and follow-up of arterial thrombosis in the neonatal period. J Pediatr 114:853, 1989.

Perlman JM, Volpe JJ: Neurologic complications of captopril treatment of neonatal hypertension. Pediatrics 83:47, 1989.

Perry EH, Bada HS, Ray JD, et al: Blood pressure increases, birth weight-dependent stability boundary, and intraventricular hemorrhage. Pediatrics 85:727, 1990.

Putnam MH: Neonatal adrenal hemorrhage presenting as a right scrotal mass. JAMA 261:2958, 1989.

Rajani K, Goetzman BW, Wennberg RP, et al: Effect of heparinization of fluids infused through an umbilical artery catheter on catheter patency and frequency of complications. Pediatrics 63:552, 1979.

Rasoulpour M, Marinelli KA: Systemic hypertension. Clin Perinatol 19:121, 1992.

Ribemont A: Recherches sur la tension du sang dan les vaisseaux du foetus et du nouveau-n propos du moment on lon doit lier le cordon ombilical. Arch Tocol 6:577, 1879.

Ricci MA, Lloyd DA: Renal venous thrombosis in infants and children. Arch Surg 125:1195, 1990.

Richardson R, Applebaum H, Touran T, et al: Effective thrombolytic therapy of aortic thrombosis in the small premature infant. J Pediatr Surg 23:1198, 1988.

Sanders LD, Jaquier S: Ultrasound demonstration of prenatal renal vein thrombosis. Pediatr Radiol 19:133, 1989.

Schmidt B, Andrew M: Neonatal thrombosis: Report of a prospective Canadian and international registry. Pediatrics 96:939, 1995.

Seibert JJ, Taylor BJ, Williamson SL, et al: Sonographic detection of neonatal umbilical-artery thrombosis: Clinical correlation. Am J Roentgenol 148:965, 1987.

Seibert JJ, Northington FJ, Miers JF, Taylor BJ: Aortic thrombosis after umbilical artery catheterization in newborns: Prevalence of complications on long-term follow-up. Am J Roentgenol 156:567, 1991.

Skalina ME, Annable WL, Kliegman RM, Fanaroff AA: Hypertensive retinopathy in the newborn infant. J Pediatr 103:781, 1983.

Slovis TL, Bernstein J, Gruskin A: Hyperechoic kidneys in the newborn and young infant. Pediatr Nephrol 7:294, 1993.

Sonesson SE, Broberger U: Arterial blood pressure in the very low birthweight newborn: Evaluation of an automatic oscillometric technique. Acta Paediatr Scand 76:338, 1987.

Spinazzola RM, Harper RG, de Soler M, Lesser M: Blood pressure values in 500- to 750-gram birthweight infants in the first week of life. J Perinatol 11:147, 1991.

Strife JL, Ball WS Jr, Towbin R, et al: Arterial occlusions in newborns: Use of fibrinolytic therapy. Radiology 166:395, 1988.

Tan KL: Blood pressure in full-term healthy newborns. Clin Pediatr 26:21, 1987.

Vailas GN, Brouillette RT, Scott JP, et al: Neonatal aortic thrombosis: Recent experience. J Pediatr 109:101, 1986.

Versmold HT, Kitterman JA, Phibbs RH, et al: Aortic blood pressure during the first 12 hours of life in infants with birth weight 610 to 4,220 grams. Pediatrics 67:607, 1981.

Weindling AM: Blood pressure monitoring in the newborn. Arch Dis Child 64:444, 1989.

Zinner SH, Rosner B, Oh W, Kass EH: Significance of blood pressure in infancy: Familial aggregation and predictive effect on later blood pressure. Hypertension 7:411, 1985.

PART XV

ENDOCRINE DISORDERS

CHAPTER 99

Disorders of Calcium and Phosphorus Metabolism

Lewis P. Rubin

GENERAL CONSIDERATIONS

Calcium plays two important physiologic roles. Calcium salts in bone provide structural integrity. Regulation of calcium ions present in the cytosol and extracellular fluid (ECF) is essential for maintenance and control of numerous biologic processes, including cell–cell communication, cell aggregation, cell division, coagulation, neuromuscular excitability, membrane integrity and permeability, and enzymatic and secretory activities. This diversity of functions is made possible by the maintenance of a large electrochemical gradient between ECF Ca^{+2}, which is in the 1 mmol/L range, and resting intracellular (cytosolic) Ca^{+2}, which is about 0.1 μmol/L.

Significant alterations in serum calcium concentration occur frequently during the neonatal period. It is important to evaluate these alterations in light of the normal dynamic changes that take place during the extrauterine transition. After the first 2 to 3 extrauterine days, normal serum calcium concentrations vary only slightly with age and range between 8.8 and 10.6 mg/dL, with an average of 10 mg/dL. Serum or plasma calcium levels usually are reported as mg/dL (mg%) and may be converted to molar units by dividing by 4 (e.g., 10 mg/dL converts to 2.5 mmol/L).

Approximately 55% to 60% of the total plasma calcium is diffusible (or ultrafilterable) and the rest is protein-bound. Most diffusible calcium is ionized, but about 5% of total circulating calcium is complexed to plasma anions, such as phosphates, citrate, and bicarbonate. Ionized calcium (Ca^{+2}) is the only biologically available fraction of ECF calcium and is subject to precise metabolic control. Hypoalbuminemia leads to a decline in total serum calcium, but a proportionate increase in the ionized fraction usually maintains serum Ca^{+2} within the normal range. Acute alkalosis (e.g., hyperventilation or bicarbonate infusion) or rapid administration of citrate-buffered blood (e.g., during exchange transfusion, extracorporeal membrane oxygenation [ECMO], cardioplegia, or organ transplantation) acutely lowers serum Ca^{+2} by increasing albumin binding and citrate chelation of Ca^{+2}, respectively, but does not change total measured calcium. These conditions can produce transient clinical manifestations of hypocalcemia but will not affect total serum calcium concentration. Electrocardiogram Q-oTc intervals (Nelson et al, 1989) and algorithms for correcting serum total calcium for alterations in serum albumin concentration and/or pH or for calculating "free" calcium concentration have not proven to be reliable compared with actual measurement of Ca^{+2} using ion-selective electrodes (Zaloga et al, 1985). These caveats aside, for routine clinical purposes, measurement of total serum calcium often suffices.

Although the intestine has considerable calcium absorptive potential, renal tubular calcium reabsorption exceeds intestinal absorption by at least 40-fold. Renal calcium reabsorption occurs principally in the proximal tubule and is coupled with sodium reabsorption. Regulation of urinary calcium excretion is accomplished in the distal nephron and is subject to the action of calcitropic hormones.

More than 98% of total body calcium is in the skeleton as hydroxyapatite $[Ca_5(OH)(PO_4)_3]$; the remainder is contained in the ECF and soft tissues. A small fraction of skeletal calcium freely exchanges with the ECF and serves as an important buffer of circulating calcium. Consequently, decreased skeletal calcium is a hallmark of most chronic neonatal metabolic bone diseases.

The serum inorganic phosphate (Pi) concentration varies with age and is highest during infancy, then gradually declines to adulthood. Approximately 10% of inorganic phosphate in serum is noncovalently bound to protein, whereas 90% circulates as HPO_4^{-2} and HPO_4^{-1} ions or as complexes with sodium, calcium, or magnesium. About 80% to 85% of total body phosphorus is contained in the hydroxyapatite lattice of bone and contributes to mechanical support. The remainder is distributed in the ECF, largely in the form of inorganic ions or complexes, and in soft tissues as phosphate esters. Intracellular phosphate esters and phosphorylated intermediates regulate cell metabolism and gene expression (via kinase and phosphatase actions) as well as generate and transfer cellular energy (e.g., via adenosine triphosphate). Cytosolic and ECF phosphorus levels (approximately 0.1 mmol/L and 0.2 mmol/L, respectively), are less stringently regulated than are Ca^{+2} or Mg^{+2}.

The kidney is the principal regulatory organ for phosphorus homeostasis. This regulation is accomplished primarily through varying the threshold for phosphate reabsorption in the proximal tubule (the tubular maximum for Pi/glomerular filtration rate, or TmP/GFR). Hormones (parathyroid hormone [PTH], parathyroid-related protein [PTHrP], growth hormone) and dietary phosphate reset this theoretical threshold by regulating apical tubular Na-P cotransporters (Murer and Biber, 1995). Essentially, the TmP/GFR is the "set point" that defines the fasting serum phosphorus concentration; at lower serum phosphorus levels most of the filtered phosphorus is reabsorbed, and at higher levels most of the filtered phosphorus is excreted. A nomogram has been constructed so that TmP/GFR can be easily derived from the values of both fractional phosphorus reabsorption (TRP) and serum phosphorus concentration (Bijvoet, 1980).

The higher serum phosphate levels in infants (e.g., 4.5 to 9.3 mg/dL) compared to adults (3.0 to 4.5 mg/dL) reflect infants' higher rates of tubular phosphate resorption (Brodehl et al, 1982; Senterre and Salle, 1988). This adaptation permits avid tubular phosphate conservation despite the high ambient serum phosphate levels. Neonatal disorders of chronic hypophosphatemia and/or phosphorus depletion usually result from inadequate dietary supply (preterm infants) or intrinsic (e.g., familial hypophosphatemic rickets) or extrinsic (e.g., hyperparathyroidism) alterations in TmP/GFR. Similarly, chronic hyperphosphatemia usually implies either intrinsic (e.g., renal insufficiency) or extrinsic (e.g., hypoparathyroidism) abnormalities in TmP/GFR.

The homeostatic control of magnesium is less well characterized than that of calcium and phosphorus, but the same organ systems are involved: the intestine, bone, and kidneys (Ariceta et al, 1995).

In mammals, calcium and phosphate homeostasis is controlled by a parathyroid-renal hormonal axis involving PTH and 1,25-dihydroxyvitamin D [1,25(OH)$_2$D]. The influence of these two hormones on bone deposition, mobilization of mineral, and regulation of intestinal and renal absorption is outlined in Figure 99–1. Deficiency or excess of either hormone causes hypocalcemia and hypercalcemia, respectively.

PTH is a single-chain polypeptide consisting of 84 amino acids with a molecular weight of 9500. PTH is synthesized in the parathyroid glands, which are derived from the embryonic third and fourth pharyngeal pouches. Immunocytologic studies indicate the presence of immunoreactive PTH-containing cells in human fetal parathyroid glands at 10 weeks gestation (Leroyer-Alizon et al, 1981). The messenger RNA (mRNA) for PTH encodes the 84 amino acids of the mature peptide, an amino-terminal "pre" sequence of 25 amino acids and a basic "pro" hexapeptide, which is clipped intracellularly. Following secretion, the intact PTH molecule [PTH(1–84)] is subject to further metabolism and is rapidly cleared from the circulation with a half-life of less than 4 minutes. The amino-terminal portion (1–34) of the PTH molecule shows full biologic activity on the PTH receptor, whereas the carboxy-terminus has specific, albeit poorly understood, activities in osteoclasts and osteoclastic precursors (Kaji et al, 1994).

Secretion of PTH fragments by the parathyroid glands and prolonged clearance of carboxy-terminal PTH metabolites contribute to the considerable immunoheterogeneity of circulating PTH and account for numerous inconsistencies found in reports on PTH pathophysiology until the mid- to late 1980s. The current two-site immunoradiometric and immunochemiluminescent PTH assays are sufficiently sensitive and specific to detect physiologic levels of biologically active, intact PTH(1–84) and to distinguish hypoparathyroid from euparathyroid states (Nussbaum et al, 1987). The normal circulating levels of intact PTH range from approximately 10 to 60 pg/mL and the maximally stimulated and maximally suppressed levels are about 100 to 150 pg/mL and 5 to 10 pg/mL, respectively.

Parathyroid cells are exquisitely sensitive to changes in ambient Ca^{+2}. PTH secretory dynamics may be described as an inverse sigmoidal hysteretic relationship between serum [PTH] and Ca^{+2} with a parathyroid cell "set point" (the Ca^{+2} at which PTH secretion is half-maximal) of 1.2 to 1.25 mmol/L (Brown, 1983). This parathyroid "calciumstat" detects perturbations of blood Ca^{+2} of as little as 0.025 to 0.05 mmol/L and promptly adjusts PTH secretion (Grant et al, 1990). The molecular mechanism by which parathyroid cells "sense" these physiologic changes in ECF Ca^{+2} recently was determined. Parathyroid and renal tubular cells express a 7-transmembrane G protein-coupled Ca^{+2}-sensing receptor (CASR) that alters phosphatidylinositol turnover and intracellular calcium, ultimately effecting an increase in PTH secretion by the parathyroid gland and adjustment of calcium excretion by the kidney (Brown et al, 1995). As described later, gain-of-function (or activating) mutation in the CASR gene is responsible for neonatal primary hypercalcemia and familial hypocalciuric hypercalcemia, whereas loss-of-function mutations result in autosomal dominant neonatal hypocalcemia.

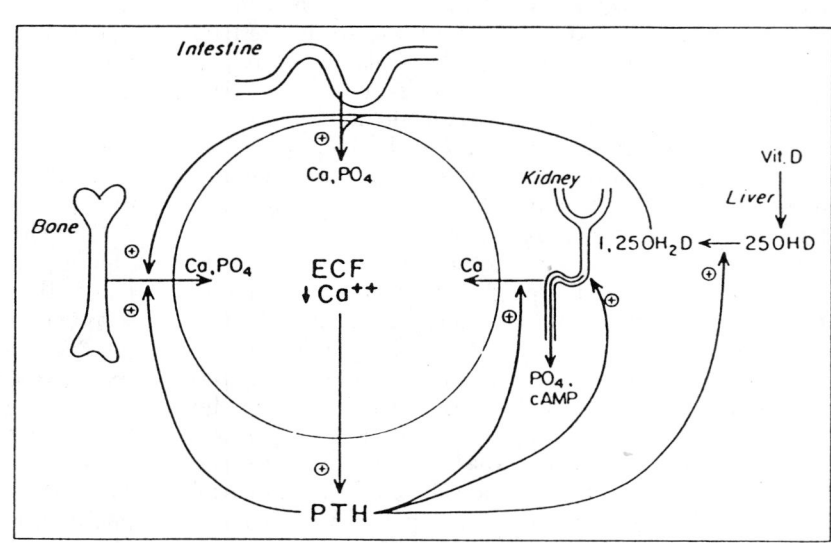

FIGURE 99–1. Hormonal regulation of calcium and phosphate by PTH and 1,25(OH)$_2$D. Decreased Ca^{+2} stimulates PTH and 1,25(OH)$_2$D secretion. Renal, gastrointestinal, and skeletal mechanisms increase Ca^{+2}, inhibiting PTH secretion and closing the negative feedback loop. PTH, parathyroid hormone; 1,25(OH)$_2$D, 1,25-dihydroxyvitamin D; 25(OH)D, 25-hydroxyvitamin D; Ca^{+2}, ionized calcium; PO$_4$, inorganic phosphate; ECF, extracellular fluid; cAMP, cyclic adenosine monophosphate.

PTH mobilizes calcium and phosphorus from bone, stimulates calcium reabsorption, inhibits phosphorus reabsorption from glomerular filtrate, and stimulates the renal synthesis of 1,25(OH)$_2$D, which participates with PTH in bone resorption and increases the efficiency of intestinal absorption of calcium and phosphorus. PTH reduces the renal TmP/GFR. Therefore, PTH secretion causes the serum calcium concentration to increase and the serum phosphorus concentration to be maintained or decrease.

A second member of the PTH family, PTHrP (Yasuda et al, 1989), has been discovered. PTHrP was first identified as the cause of humoral hypercalcemia of malignancy. As disclosed by molecular cloning, the amino acid sequence of PTHrP is homologous with the sequence of PTH only at the amino-terminus, where 8 of the first 13 amino acids in PTH and PTHrP are identical. Beyond this region, the sequences have little in common. PTHrP is a multifunctional molecule, like the neuropeptide pro-opiomelanocortin (the precursor of corticotropin, opiate molecules, and melanocyte-simulating hormones). The three PTHrP isoforms of 139, 141, and 173 amino acids (whose sequences are identical through amino acid 139) give rise to several secreted peptide fragments. PTHrP is widely expressed, especially in fetal tissues, and has important local functions in organogenesis and differentiation. The normal circulating level of PTHrP is considerably lower than the level of PTH, and it is doubtful that PTHrP has a major role in the day-to-day maintenance of calcium homeostasis. Two important exceptions are the fetus and lactating woman, where PTHrP appears to be an important calcitropic hormone.

The principal PTH receptor (PTH/PTHrP receptor) is a 7-transmembrane G protein-coupled receptor that belongs to a newly appreciated receptor subfamily that includes receptors for calcitonin, secretin, and corticotropin-releasing hormone. This versatile receptor mediates actions of two physiological ligands, PTH and PTHrP, in multiple tissues and signals through several-second messenger pathways (Juppner, 1994). The best characterized mediator of PTH's action is cyclic adenosine monophosphate (cAMP). A related receptor (designated PTHR2) has been identified that selectively recognizes PTH (Usdin et al, 1995). It is most abundantly expressed in the brain, pancreas, testis, and placenta and does not act via cAMP. The physiologic role of the PTHR2 in perinatal metabolism and in mineral or bone disorders remains to be determined.

Vitamin D is a secosteroid that is synthesized in the skin or is absorbed from the diet. Exposure to sunlight (290 to 320 nm) cleaves the B ring of 7-dehydrocholesterol (7-DHC or provitamin D), the immediate precursor of cholesterol, to form the sterol previtamin D. Previtamin D in the skin undergoes thermally-induced isomerization into biologically inert vitamin D. Vitamin D enters the circulation bound to vitamin D–binding protein and is transported to the liver, where the cytochrome P450-vitamin D-25-hydroxylase produces 25-hydroxyvitamin D [25(OH)D] (Dilworth et al, 1995). Provitamin D, or 25(OH)D, is the major circulating vitamin D metabolite. Its measurement, consequently, is a useful assessment of vitamin D stores. In proximal tubule cells, the cytochrome P450-mono-oxygenase, 25(OH)D-α-hydroxylase, metabolizes 25(OH)D to the biologically active hormone, 1,25(OH)$_2$D. The normal

circulating level of 25(OH)D is approximately 10 to 50 ng/mL. The normal circulating concentration of 1,25(OH)$_2$D ranges from 30 to 75 pg/mL, or about 1/1000 that of 25(OH)D.

Serum 25(OH)D levels are increased by exposure to sunlight and by ingestion of vitamin D and are decreased in vitamin D deficiency and in hepatobiliary disorders. Circulating 1,25(OH)$_2$D levels are increased by hyperparathyroidism and phosphate depletion and are reduced in hypoparathyroidism. 1,25(OH)$_2$D is biologically inactivated through a series of reactions beginning with 24-hydroxylation. 1,25(OH)$_2$D induces the 24-hydroxylase in vitamin D target cells, whereas hypocalcemia, through increased PTH levels, suppresses the enzyme. The 24-hydroxylase metabolizes 25(OH)D as well as 1,25(OH)$_2$D. When vitamin D is required, the kidney preferentially 24-hydroxylates the vitamin D prohormone, 25(OH)D, to 24,25(OH)$_2$D. In vitamin D–sufficient states, 25(OH)D-1α-hydroxylase is preferentially activated for the synthesis of circulating 1,25(OH)$_2$D.

The major biologic function of vitamin D is to maintain calcium homeostasis by increasing the intestinal absorption of dietary calcium and phosphorus. Although both minerals are absorbed along the entire length of the small intestine, most phosphate transport is located in the jejunum and ileum, whereas calcium absorption occurs principally in the duodenum. In bone, 1,25(OH)$_2$D stimulates osteoclast differentiation and bone resorption. Most identified biologic actions of 1,25(OH)$_2$D are mediated by binding to the vitamin D receptor (VDR), a member of the superfamily of trans-acting transcriptional regulatory factors that include the steroid and thyroid receptors.

The parathyroid-renal (PTH-1,25[OH]$_2$D) axis, reminiscent of the hypothalamic-pituitary-adrenal axis, is the principal means by which the organism responds to either a prolonged or a major hypocalcemic challenge. In this long-loop feedback system, 1,25(OH)$_2$D-mediated calcium absorption provides the ultimate feedback on PTH secretion. PTH secreted in response to hypocalcemia is the principal regulator of renal production of 1,25(OH)$_2$D that, in turn, decreases the expression of the PTH gene in parathyroid cells (Naveh-Many et al, 1990). Maximal adjustments to the rate of intestinal calcium absorption via the PTH-1,25(OH)$_2$D axis require 1 to 2 days to become fully operative so that 1,25(OH)$_2$D effects come into play only when the hypocalcemic stimulus is of a more chronic nature. In contrast, PTH regulates the minute-to-minute perturbations of ECF [Ca^{+2}].

Calcitonin, a peptide hormone synthesized by the parafollicular C cells of the thyroid, has an antihypercalcemic effect, that is, opposite to the actions of PTH. Human calcitonin is a 32-amino acid chain with a 1,7 disulfide bridge and a carboxy-terminal prolinamide. Alternative RNA splicing of the several transcripts of the single calcitonin gene is responsible for the production of different polypeptide products. Katacalcin is a 21-amino acid peptide that flanks calcitonin on its C-terminal in the large precursor polyprotein from which calcitonin is cleaved; like calcitonin, it may be involved in plasma calcium regulation and skeletal maintenance (Hillyard et al, 1983). A functionally related hormone, stanniocalcin, is synthesized in the nephron (Olsen et al, 1996). Currently, there is no compelling evidence that these calcium-lowering hormones, including calcitonin, are critical regulators of calcium homeostasis in the nonpregnant human adult. However, calcitonin may have important calcitropic functions in the pregnant and lactating woman, fetus, and neonate. Immunocytologic studies indicate the presence of immunoreactive calcitonin in the C cells of the human fetal thyroid gland as early as 14 weeks' gestation (Leroyer-Alizon et al, 1980). The C-cell population and the concentration of immunoreactive calcitonin in the thyroid gland of newborns are much greater than in older subjects, and serum concentrations of calcitonin in newborns are considerably higher than adult values. The primary stimulus for calcitonin secretion is a rise in the circulating calcium concentration. Calcitonin lowers serum calcium and phosphorus principally by inhibiting bone resorption.

PERINATAL MINERAL METABOLISM

During the past several years, molecular cloning techniques, improved immunoassay and bone densitometry techniques, and application of stable isotope methodology (Abrams et al, 1994; Ernst et al, 1995) have helped to elucidate many aspects of perinatal mineral metabolism. During human pregnancy, approximately 30 g of calcium and more than 16 g of phosphorus are transferred transplacentally from the maternal circulation to the growing fetus (Givens and Macy, 1933; Widdowsen and Dickerson, 1961), the bulk during the third trimester when fetal calcium accretion is approximately 150 mg/kg per day. This transplacental calcium pump is principally regulated by a mid-molecule PTHrP hormone (Kovacs et al, 1996) expressed by fetal parathyroid and placenta. In humans, the formidable demand on maternal calcium is met by a doubling of intestinal calcium absorption with a net increase of calcium accretion into bone (Heaney and Skillman, 1971).

Pregnancy constitutes a unique hormonal milieu that promotes a state of "physiologic absorptive hypercalciuria" (Gertner et al, 1986). Maternal total serum calcium declines slightly during pregnancy, reaching a nadir at the middle of the third trimester, and then increases slightly toward term (Pitkin et al, 1979). The maternal serum phosphorus and magnesium levels exhibit patterns similar to that of calcium during pregnancy. Maternal serum 25(OH)D varies with the season and vitamin D intake, whereas the transport protein for vitamin D metabolites (DBP) increases in maternal serum during pregnancy (Bouillon and van Assche, 1982). Serum $1,25(OH)_2D$ concentrations are increased in early pregnancy and rise through gestation (Kumar et al, 1979; Bikle et al, 1984; Paulson and DeLuca, 1986; Seely et al, 1997). The calculated free concentration of $1,25(OH)_2D$ also rises. For many years, it was believed that PTH levels also increased steadily through pregnancy. However, use of more accurate immunoassays indicates that PTH actually declines during the course of pregnancy (Davis et al, 1988; Saggese et al, 1991; Seely et al, 1997). PTHrP levels, in contrast, may be higher in pregnant than in nonpregnant women (Bertelloni et al, 1994). The role of circulating calcitonin in pregnancy is unclear (Stevenson et al, 1979; Bucht et al, 1986; Saggese et al, 1990).

Currently, it appears that maternal $1,25(OH)_2D$ drives enhanced intestinal mineral absorption while the interplay of calcitropic and progestational hormones protects the maternal skeleton from demineralization. Following parturition, $1,25(OH)_2D$ concentrations (Wilson et al, 1990) and calcium absorption rates (Kent et al, 1991) fall to prepartum levels. During the relatively low estrogen state of lactation, calcium becomes mobilized principally from bone stores (Sowers et al, 1993), possibly under the influence of PTHrP (Grill et al, 1992; Dobnig et al, 1995).

Toward the end of gestation, total and ionized calcium and phosphorus levels in fetal plasma are higher than maternal levels, and there is a state of "physiological fetal hypercalcemia" (Garel, 1987; Rubin et al, 1991). Fetal plasma PTH is low (Rubin et al, 1991), calcitonin levels are high (Hillman et al, 1977), and circulating PTHrP is detectable. There is a close correlation between maternal and fetal serum 25(OH)D levels, consistent with transplacental transfer of this metabolite (Bouillon and van Assche, 1982; Ron et al, 1984). Low levels may be found in infants born of mothers with low circulating levels of 25(OH)D resulting from poor dietary intake of vitamin D and lack of sunlight exposure. Fetal plasma $1,25(OH)_2D$ also is relatively low, despite robust renal 25(OH)D-1α-hydroxylase activity, whereas concentrations of $24,25(OH)_2D$ are high (Hollis and Pittard, 1984). In fact, the major function of the kidneys in fetal calcium homeostasis appears to be the production of $1,25(OH)_2D$ rather than renal tubular regulation of calcium excretion (Stewart et al, 1992). The high circulating concentrations of calcitonin may support this stimulated fetal 25(OH)D-1α-hydroxylase activity (Kawashima et al, 1986). In contrast, the relatively low circulating fetal $1,25(OH)_2D$ concentrations are a consequence of a several-fold enhancement of fetal clearance rate of $1,25(OH)_2D$ contributed by the placenta (Ross et al, 1989). Constitutively activated placental 24-hydroxylase activity (Rubin et al, 1993) preferentially hydroxylates maternally-derived 25(OH)D to $24,25(OH)_2D$, which appears to be an independent embryonic and fetal skeletal hormone. This placental capacity to metabolize 25(OH)D and $1,25(OH)_2D$ probably accounts for the enhanced clearance of fetal $1,25(OH)_2D$, limits access of placentally synthesized $1,25(OH)_2D$ to the fetal and maternal circulations, and, in effect, partitions the maternal and fetal vitamin D pools.

At birth, the placental transfer of calcium ceases abruptly, and human term newborn total calcium concentration and $[Ca^{+2}]$ decline from nearly 11 mg/dL and nearly 6 mg/dL, respectively, in umbilical cord blood to serum levels of 8 to 9 mg/dL and 5 mg/dL by 24 to 48 hours. In healthy term newborns, the nadir of $[Ca^{+2}]$ has ranged from 4.4 to 5.4 mg/dL (Loughead et al, 1988). Concomitant rises in PTH and $1,25(OH)_2D$ (Steichen et al, 1980) stabilize serum calcium and facilitate adaptation to extrauterine mineral and bone homeostasis. Serum calcitonin levels increase sharply during the first day and remain elevated compared to adults. Lactating mammary tissue expresses PTHrP under the control of prolactin and PTHrP is secreted into milk at concentrations 10,000-fold higher than its serum concentration (Budayr et al, 1989). The abundant amount of PTHrP ingested by the neonate may also be important for mineral regulation. By two weeks, serum calcium rises to the mean values observed in older children and adults (Specker et al, 1986). In preterm infants, calcium absorption from the intestine is nonsaturable and may be vitamin D independent (Bronner et al, 1992).

During the first week of life, urinary phosphate excretion is significantly higher in preterm than in term infants; after the first week, urinary phosphate excretion in premature infants approximates that of term infants, possibly due to accelerated postnatal renal maturation. Calcium excretion is low during the first week, when the newborn must compensate for the postpartum fall in serum calcium. After the first several days, calcium excretion increases with a magnitude inversely proportional to gestation. The high urinary calcium/creatinine ratio (UCa/Cr) of young infants then steadily declines with age (Sargent et al, 1993). However, in preterm breast-fed infants who are more than 2 weeks old, the UCa/Cr generally exceeds 2.0 (Karlen et al, 1985). These changes reflect the state of relative phosphate deficiency, resulting in an adaptively low urinary phosphate excretion and an inability to form bone minerals, and therefore, relatively high urinary calcium excretion.

CALCIUM METABOLISM IN THE NEWBORN
Neonatal Hypocalcemia

Neonatal hypocalcemia has been variously defined as a serum calcium level of less than 8 mg/dL, less than 7.5 mg/dL, or less than 7.5 mg/dL and as a Ca^{+2} level of less than 4.0 mg/dL. Under conditions of normal acid-base status and normalbuminemia, the serum calcium level and Ca^{+2} are linearly correlated, so that total serum calcium measurements remain useful as a screening test. However, because Ca^{+2} is the physiologically relevant fraction, in sick infants it is preferable directly to determine Ca^{+2} in freshly obtained blood samples. A precise definition of hypocalcemia, like hypoglycemia, in preterm infants is particularly difficult and is probably best defined with reference to Ca^{+2}.

A useful approach to the classification of neonatal hypocalcemia is by the time of onset. "Early" and "late" occurring hypocalcemias have different causes (Table 99–1), usually occur in different clinical settings, and prompt different strategies of evaluation and patient management.

Clinical Findings

Because Ca^{+2} is the coupling factor linking excitation and contraction in skeletal and cardiac muscle, increased neuromuscular excitability (tetany) is a cardinal feature of hypocalcemia; however, signs in neonates are variable and may not correlate with the magnitude of the depression in Ca^{+2}. Although some infants are severely affected, others with equally depressed serum calcium levels may be asymptomatic.

Increased neuromuscular irritability and seizures are the characteristic signs of neonatal tetany. Tetanic infants are jittery and hyperactive, and they frequently exhibit muscle jerking and twitching. Generalized or focal clonic seizures may occur at any time during the calcium derangement. Hyperacusis may be detected as a exaggerated response to environmental noises. Occasionally, respiratory or gastrointestinal signs, rather than neurologic findings, predominate. Laryngospasm with inspiratory stridor, at times severe

TABLE 99–1

Causes of Neonatal Hypocalcemia

Early-onset hypocalcemia (<48 hr of age)
  Prematurity
  Perinatal distress/asphyxia
  Infants of diabetic mothers
  Intrauterine growth restriction
Late-onset hypocalcemia (1st week of life)
  High phosphate load ± hypoparathyroidism or vitamin D deficiency
Neonatal hypoparathyroid syndromes
  Parathyroid agenesis
  DiGeorge syndrome (22q11.2 deletions, CATCH 22 syndrome)
  "Familial isolated hypoparathyroidism"
    PTH gene mutations
    Activating mutations of the Ca^{+2}-sensing receptor
  Neonatal hypoparathyroidism secondary to maternal hyperparathyroidism
  Kenny-Caffey syndrome
  Sanjad-Sakati syndrome ("Near Eastern neonatal hypoparathyroidism")
  Polyglandular autoimmune syndrome type I
PTH resistance (transient neonatal pseudohypoparathyroidism)
Hypomagnesemia ± distal renal tubular acidosis
Abnormal vitamin D [1,25(OH)$_2$D] production or action
  Vitamin D deficiency (secondary to relative maternal vitamin D deficiency)
  Acquired or inherited disorders of vitamin D metabolism
  Resistance to the actions of vitamin D
Hyperphosphatemia
  Excessive dietary phosphate
  Rhabdomyolysis-induced acute renal failure
  Advanced renal insufficiency
"Hungry bones syndrome" (skeletal mineralization significantly outpacing osteoclastic bone resorption)
Neonatal hypocalcemia associated with certain skeletal dysplasias
Other causes
  Bicarbonate therapy, metabolic or respiratory alkalosis
  Rapid transfusion or plasmapheresis with citrated blood
  Furosemide induced
  Phototherapy
  Lipid infusions
  Pancreatitis
  Pseudohypocalcemia (hypoalbuminemia)

enough to cause cyanosis or anoxia, or wheezing due to bronchospasm, may be the presenting manifestation of neonatal hypocalcemia. Vomiting, possibly related to pylorospasm, occurs relatively frequently in neonatal tetany, and in a few instances may cause hematemesis or melena. At times, the gastrointestinal signs are severe enough to mimic intestinal obstruction. Other signs that have been described in neonatal tetany include extensor hypertonia, apnea, tachycardia, tachypnea, and edema. Carpopedal spasm and Chvostek's sign are not as reliably elicited in newborns as in adults with tetany.

Early Neonatal Hypocalcemia

Hypocalcemia occurring during the first 3 days of life, usually between 24 and 48 hours postpartum, is termed "early neonatal hypocalcemia." It is a pathologic exaggeration of the normal decline in circulating calcium that is part of physiological transition to the extrauterine environment. Characteristically, early neonatal hypocalcemia is seen in one of four circumstances, namely, preterm infants, asphyxiated infants, infants of diabetic mothers, and infants with significant intrauterine growth restriction. Typically, in preterm infants, the postnatal decline in serum calcium level is steeper and occurs more rapidly than in term infants, the magnitude of the depression being inversely proportional to the gestation. Many low-birth-weight infants, and essentially all extremely low-birth-weight infants (ELBWs), exhibit total calcium levels of less than 7.0 mg/dL by day 2. However, the fall in Ca^{+2} is not proportionate to the fall in total calcium concentration and the ratio of ionized to total Ca is higher in these infants (Scott et al, 1979). The reason for the maintenance of Ca^{+2} is uncertain but is probably related to the low serum protein concentration and pH associated with prematurity. The sparing effect of the Ca^{+2} may, in part, explain the frequent lack of signs in preterm infants with low total calcium levels.

The neonatal parathyroid glands, regardless of degree of prematurity, appear capable of mounting an appropriate physiologic response to hypocalcemia. Hypocalcemia in extremely preterm newborns (Rubin et al, 1991) or infants undergoing cardiac bypass (Robertie et al, 1992) has been shown to provoke increases in intact PTH levels that are at least as great as those reported in adult subjects during citrate-induced hypocalcemia (Grant et al, 1990). Refractoriness to PTH action plays an uncertain role in early neonatal hypocalcemia. A several day delay in the phosphaturic and renal cAMP responses to PTH in preterm and term infants has inconsistently been reported, suggesting that there might be a maturational delay in response to PTH by the nephron. High renal sodium excretion in preterm infants also probably aggravates calciuric losses. The preterm infant's exaggerated rise in calcitonin (Romagnoli et al, 1987) may promote hypocalcemia. Currently, there is no convincing evidence that abnormalities in 25(OH)D metabolism play a pathogenic role in the hypocalcemia of preterm infants and, like fetuses, even extremely preterm newborns efficiently synthesize 1,25(OH)$_2$D if vitamin D stores are adequate (Hillman et al, 1985).

Early neonatal hypocalcemia and hyperphosphatemia are frequently observed in asphyxiated or severely stressed infants. The causes are probably multifactorial and may include, to varying degrees, renal insufficiency, tissue catabolism, and acidosis. The serum calcitonin response is augmented, and PTH levels are elevated. Hyperphosphatemia may induce relative PTH resistance in these infants (Tsang et al, 1974).

Infants of diabetic mothers (IDMs) also demonstrate an exaggerated postnatal drop in circulating calcium levels when compared to gestational age controls. The natural history usually is similar to that of early neonatal hypocalcemia in preterm infants, but hypocalcemia sometimes persists for several additional days. Maternal and neonatal hypomagnesemia (Mimouni et al, 1986) and low fetal PTH/PTHrP biological activity (Rubin et al, 1991) may be causative factors. The greater bone mass with relative undermineralization typical of macrosomic IDMs also may increase the neonatal demand for calcium, producing a more profound and prolonged decline in postnatal serum calcium

levels. Similar mechanisms may come into play in the transient hypocalcemia often observed in small-for-gestation (SGA) infants. Hypercalcitonemia, hypoparathyroidism, abnormalities in vitamin D metabolism and hyperphosphatemia all have been implicated, but none has been consistently found.

Historically, symptomatic neonatal hypocalcemia in IDMs has been associated with the severity of maternal diabetes (White classification) and inadequate glycemic control. Preterm IDMs that have sustained intrauterine growth restriction and asphyxia secondary to uteroplacental insufficiency invariably develop very low serum calcium levels. In recent years, improved metabolic control for pregnant diabetic women has markedly diminished the occurrence and severity of early neonatal hypocalcemia in IDMs (Demarini et al, 1994). In our experience, healthy IDMs that are able to begin milk feedings on the first day do not require serum calcium monitoring unless suggestive signs (e.g., jitteriness, stridor) occur.

Late Neonatal Hypocalcemia

Late neonatal hypocalcemia, or hypocalcemia occurring after 3 to 5 days of life, occurs more frequently in term than in preterm newborns and is not correlated with maternal diabetes, birth trauma, or asphyxia. Historically, it has been associated with cow's milk or cow's milk formula feedings, but occasionally does occur in breast-fed infants. The entity of "late infantile tetany" seen in infants fed whole cow's milk has become a rarity in the United States with adjustment of phosphorus content in humanized cow's milk and soy infant formulas. Human milk contains 150 mg/L of phosphorus as compared with over 500 mg/L in infant formulas prepared from cow's milk, whey, or soy protein. Therefore, a relatively low-phosphate "humanized" formula preparation is recommended for the first 2 weeks of life for full-term newborns who are not breast-fed, as well for any infant with hyperphosphatemic renal failure.

The hyperphosphatemia that is a prominent feature of late neonatal hypocalcemia may result from varying combinations of dietary phosphate load, immaturity of renal tubular phosphate excretion, transiently low levels of circulating PTH, hypomagnesemia, or marginal maternal vitamin D intake. The ingestion of a relatively high phosphate load coupled with a low GFR leads to an increase in serum phosphate levels and a reciprocal decline in serum calcium levels. However, the normal response to hypocalcemia is an increase in PTH secretion leading to an increase in both urinary excretion of phosphate and tubular resorption of calcium. It is relevant, therefore, that low circulating PTH levels have sometimes been observed in infants with late neonatal hypocalcemia. Serum calcium levels frequently increase when these infants are placed on a lower phosphate formula and calcium supplements. After several days to weeks, the serum PTH usually increases and the infants are able to tolerate higher dietary phosphate loads. The pathogenesis of this "transient hypoparathyroidism" in late neonatal hypocalcemia is poorly understood. Some of these infants have a persistent or recurrent inability to mount an adequate PTH response to a hypocalcemic challenge (Bainbridge et al, 1987) and, therefore, may have a forme fruste congenital hypoparathyroidism. In other affected infants, hypoparathyroidism may not be contributory (Venkataraman et al, 1985). Maternal vitamin D deficiency also is an important cause of late (and occasionally of an "early") neonatal hypocalcemia. It is investigated by assay of maternal and neonatal serum 25(OH)D levels. A role for maternal vitamin D deficiency role is also implicated by the increased occurrence of late neonatal hypocalcemia in winter (Cockburn et al, 1980) and the high incidence of enamel hypoplasia of incisor teeth reported in these infants, which indicates a defect in mineralization during the third trimester of pregnancy.

Low serum calcium and hyperphosphatemia after the first 1 to 2 days should prompt a thorough investigation for underlying cause(s). Hypocalcemia in this setting usually implies some primary or secondary dysregulation of the parathyroid-renal [PTH-1,25(OH)$_2$D] axis, hypomagnesemia, or renal insufficiency. The primary hormonal and end-organ disturbances that cause neonatal hypoglycemia syndromes are described below. In addition, the earlier observations of a universally favorable neurologic outcome in newborns with hypocalcemic or hypomagnesemic seizures (that may be valid for those who have a nutritional cause for the metabolic disturbance) may be less relevant to the current neonatal population in whom hypocalcemia or hypomagnesemia from dietary phosphate overload is seldom observed. In this group, neurologic prognosis may be more related to associated medical conditions (Lynch and Rust, 1994).

Hypocalcemia Caused by Hypoparathyroid Syndromes

The recognition of the importance of PTH deficiency presenting during the first weeks of life has grown with improved clinical laboratory techniques. Cytogenetic and molecular genetic diagnosis has provided the means to characterize several forms of congenital hypoparathyroidism. The biochemical hallmarks of hypoparathyroidism are hypocalcemia and hyperphosphatemia in the presence of normal renal function. Serum PTH concentrations are inappropriately low or undetectable. Individuals eventually diagnosed with a PTH resistance syndrome (pseudohypoparathyroidism) generally do not manifest hypocalcemia in the neonatal period. However, transient neonatal pseudohypoparathyroidism has been reported (Minagawa et al, 1995), which may explain some instances of late neonatal hypocalcemia.

Isolated absence of parathyroid gland development may be inherited in X-linked or autosomal recessive fashion. Congenital hypoparathyroidism also occurs as the DiGeorge syndrome (DGS), which comprises hypoparathyroid hypocalcemia, thymic hypoplasia with T cell incompetence, cardiac outflow tract defects, and dysmorphic facies. The DGS phenotype results from defects in cervical neural crest migration into the derivatives of the third and fourth pharyngeal (branchial) pouches. Currently, in at least 90% individuals with a clinical diagnosis of DGS, deletions (monosomy or partial monosomy) of chromosome region 22q11.2 are detectable by molecular dosage analysis and fluorescent in situ hybridization (FISH) using 22q11 probes or by high resolution banding studies (Driscoll et al, 1992; Wilson et al, 1992). The rare identification of other cytogenetic abnormalities suggests that the disturbance of neural crest migration presumed to underlie DGS may be caused by several distinct molecular defects. Frequently, DGS is sporadic and results from de novo 22 deletion. Numerous familial clusters also have been described in which the variable phenotype behaves as an autosomal dominant trait. In familial transmission, there appears to be a strong tendency for 22q11.2 deletions to be of maternal origin (Demczuk et al, 1996). In members of the same family, the 22q11 deletion often is associated with different sequelae, depending on whether endocrinologic, cardiac, or craniofacial and palatal abnormalities are the focus of attention: Shprintzen (or velocardiofacial) syndrome (Shprintzen, 1994); concotruncal anomaly face (or Takao) syndrome; or isolated cardiac outflow tract defects. Even transient congenital hypoparathyroidism in the absence of a DGS phenotype can be associated with the 22q11 deletion (Greig et al, 1996), and these infants should be evaluated and monitored for recurrence of hypocalcemia. Because of this heterogeneity, the mnemonic CATCH 22 (*C*ardiac defects, *A*bnormal facies, *T*hymic hypoplasia, *C*left palate and *H*ypocalcemia resulting from 22q11 deletion) has been proposed to encompass the various manifestations of a common genetic etiology (Wilson et al, 1993). A population study in northern England indicated a prevalence of DGS of at least 1 in 4000 live births (Burn et al, 1995).

DGS often presents in the first week of life with hypocalcemic tetany or seizures. Craniofacial features of the neonatal phenotype include microretrognathia, submucous cleft palate, low set and abnormal pinnae, telecanthus with short palpebral fissures, short philtrum, and a relatively small mouth. The presence of outflow tract or aortic arch abnormalities (especially, tetralogy of Fallot, type B interrupted aortic arch, truncus arteriosus, right aortic arch, and aberrant right subclavian artery), even in the absence of other DGS features, should prompt investigation with a standard karyotype to exclude major rearrangements and FISH using probes from within the deletion segment (Webber et al, 1996). Parents of an infant with DGS should be screened for carrier status. These infants require close anticipatory monitoring for the onset of hypocalcemia. Because of the potential for inducing graft-versus-host disease and until immunocompetence has been demonstrated, only irradiated blood products should be administered. Detection of a thymic shadow in a stressed newborn is very unreliable. The deficit in thymic function may be demonstrated by measuring the proportion of CD4 cells.

Normal PTH levels obtained when the infant is relatively normocalcemic do not exclude the diagnosis. It is interesting that these infants typically show resolution of hypoparathyroidism by early childhood, although parathyroid reserve may remain inadequate for defense against hypocalcemic stresses (Gidding et al, 1988; Greig et al, 1996).

The Kenny-Caffey syndrome is another congenital disorder featuring transient neonatal hypoparathyroidism and skeletal dysplasia with dwarfism, macrocephaly, delayed fontanel closure, dysmorphic facies, and cortical thickening of tubular bones (Fanconi et al, 1986; Franceschini et al, 1992). Congenital hypoparathyroidism in association with short stature, poor growth, characteristic facies, small hands and feet, and developmental delay (Sanjad-Sakati syndrome or "Near Eastern hypoparathyroidism") (Sanjad et al, 1991) is a distinct, probably autosomal recessive entity reported in Arab families from Saudi Arabia, Qatar, and Israel. Hypocalcemic seizures usually commence in the first 1 to 2 weeks of life. The polyglandular autoimmune syndrome type I (PGA I) is a triad of Addison's disease, hypoparathyroidism and chronic mucocutaneous candidiasis (Neufeld et al, 1980). These individuals also frequently develop chronic active hepatitis, malabsorption, juvenile-onset pernicious anemia, alopecia, and primary hypogonadism. When PGA I is diagnosed in early infancy, which is rare, it is the hypocalcemia (with or without candidiasis) that predominates.

Recently, forms of so-called "familial isolated hypoparathyroidism" with autosomal dominant, autosomal recessive, and X-linked inheritance patterns (Ahn et al, 1986) have been associated with allelic variants of the PTH or calcium-sensing receptor (CASR) genes. By definition, these infants have subnormal or undetectable serum levels of PTH with no demonstrable anatomic cause or developmental field defects, no evidence of candidiasis or autoimmune polyglandular failure, and no antiendocrine antibodies. Both autosomal dominant (Arnold et al, 1990) and autosomal recessive (Parkinson and Thakker, 1992) forms of familial isolated hypoparathyroidism have been related to mutations in the PTH gene. Activating missense mutations in the CASR gene produce a form of autosomal dominant hypocalcemia (Pollak et al, 1994; Baron et al, 1996); the set-point of the parathyroid cell is reset downward so that hypocalcemia does not elicit normal, compensatory PTH secretion. Occasionally, in infants with DGS, an autosomal dominant, apparently isolated hypoparathyroidism may dominate the clinical picture.

Neonatal Hypocalcemia Associated with Maternal Hypoparathyroidism

Hypocalcemia is commonly observed in infants born to hyperparathyroid mothers. These infants frequently manifest signs of increased neuromuscular irritability during the first 3 weeks of life but occasionally do so much later, as their limited PTH reserve and latent hypoparathyroidism emerge under stress or with time (Cuneo et al, 1996). The serum calcium levels range from 5.0 to 7.5 mg/dL and the serum phosphate levels are often greater than 8.0 mg/dL. Hypocalcemic signs may be exacerbated by feeding higher phosphate (cow's milk formula) diets. Indeed, there are reports of infants born to hyperparathyroid mothers who exhibited signs of hypocalcemia for the first time at 5 months of age (Friderichsen, 1938) and 1 year (Bruce and Strong, 1955), respectively, shortly after addition of cow's milk to the diet. In some instances, the symptoms of hypocalcemia are quite severe, and they may be resistant to antitetany therapy. There is eventual improvement with calcium therapy, which in some instances must be continued for several weeks.

In maternal hyperparathyroidism, the increased maternal serum calcium facilitates transplacental calcium transport to the fetus, producing fetal hypercalcemia beyond the physiologic, moderate elevations of serum calcium observed in the third trimester. As a result, fetal PTH secretion is suppressed more than it is in normal pregnancy and the suppressed parathyroids are not able to maintain nor-

mal serum calcium levels postpartum. Whether the maternal elevated PTH or a potentially suppressed expression of fetal PTHrP contribute to the pathophysiology is not known. The reason for the hypomagnesemia observed in some infants born to hyperparathyroid mothers also is uncertain but may be secondary to (1) maternal magnesium depletion, which could be a complication of hyperparathyroidism; (2) transient neonatal hypoparathyroidism; and (3) hyperphosphatemia, which may result from transient hypoparathyroidism or high dietary phosphate intake or both.

The mothers of affected infants are hypercalcemic and hypophosphatemic. They may also be asymptomatic, and hypocalcemic tetany occurring in the infant can lead to diagnosis of hyperparathyroidism in an asymptomatic mother. Maternal serum calcium values that are within the upper normal range can be falsely reassuring if the samples were obtained during the pregnancy, a time when serum calcium levels normally show a decline.

Neonatal Hypocalcemia Associated with Hypomagnesemia or Renal Tubular Acidosis

Hypomagnesemia may produce hypocalcemia by impairing parathyroid function. Hypomagnesemia interferes with PTH secretion (Anast et al, 1972; Rude et al, 1978) and it also blunts the end organ response to PTH (Rude et al, 1976). Depression of serum magnesium levels in newborns is either due to: (1) chronic congenital low serum magnesium levels or primary hypomagnesemia with secondary hypocalcemia, or (2) transient hypomagnesemia.

Primary familial hypomagnesemia with secondary hypocalcemia presents in infancy with persistent hypocalcemia and seizures that cannot by controlled with anticonvulsants and/or calcium gluconate. It is a rare, probably autosomal recessive disorder resulting from primary defects in intestinal and/or renal tubular transport of magnesium (Manz et al, 1978; Pronicka and Gruszczynska, 1991). The clinical spectrum includes polyuria, hyposthenuria, a moderate degree of metabolic acidosis with an inappropriately high urine pH and a positive urine anion gap, low citrate excretion, renal wasting of magnesium and calcium, secondary renal potassium wasting, nephrocalcinosis, muscle weakness, persistent tetany, seizures, and sometimes abnormal facies and sensorineural hearing loss. The partial distal acidification defect, which is probably a secondary effect of a medullary interstitial nephropathy, can be functionally distinguished from that present in primary distal renal tubular acidosis (RTA I) (Rodriguez-Soriano and Vallo, 1994). The serum magnesium is frequently less than 0.8 mg/dL (normal 1.6 to 2.8 mg/dL), and circulating levels of PTH are low despite the presence of hypocalcemia. The administration of magnesium to these infants leads to spontaneous parallel increases in serum PTH levels, serum calcium levels, and renal phosphate clearance.

Transient hypomagnesemia in newborns often occurs in association with hypocalcemia. Less commonly, the serum calcium level may be normal. In transient hypomagnesemia, the decrease in serum magnesium level typically is less severe (0.8 to 1.4 mg/dL) than it is in magnesium transport defects. In many infants with transient hypomagnesemia, the serum magnesium level increases spontaneously as the serum calcium level returns to normal following the administration of calcium supplements. However, in other cases the hypocalcemia responds poorly to calcium therapy, but when magnesium salts are given, both serum calcium and magnesium levels rise.

Phenocopies of transient hypomagnesemia (secondary renal magnesium wasting) can be caused by administration of loop diuretics, aminoglycosides, amphotericin B, urinary tract obstruction, or the diuretic phase of acute renal failure. The disorder also may be mistaken for a form of neonatal hypoparathyroidism because of the tetany and hypocalcemia, or as Bartter syndrome (hypokalemic alkalosis with hypercalciuria) because of secondary potassium wasting. An index of suspicion is raised when hypomagnesemia occurs in one of the situations listed previously. The diagnosis can be made by finding low serum magnesium levels with inappropriately high urinary magnesium excretion. A common laboratory feature of magnesium depletion, regardless of cause, is hypokalemia. Attempts to replete the potassium deficit with potassium therapy alone usually are not successful without simultaneous magnesium therapy.

The distal type of renal tubular acidosis (RTA I) is characterized by hypocalcemia, hypercalciuria, varying degrees of hypomagnesemia, hyperchloremia, low serum bicarbonate, and fixed urinary specific gravity and urinary pH (about 5.0). The mineral excretion defect leads to nephrocalcinosis and metabolic bone disease. RTA I sometimes presents during early infancy, when the hypocalcemia may precede the RTA. Lewis (1992) proposed that Tiny Tim in Dickens' *A Christmas Carol* had RTA I, which explains his growth failure, osteomalacia, pathologic fractures, and neuromuscular features.

Hypocalcemia Resulting from Vitamin D Disorders

In older children and adults, hypocalcemia as an isolated finding that results from disorders of vitamin D intake or metabolism is rare. Most individuals with abnormalities in either the production or the action of $1,25(OH)_2D$ chiefly show rickets or osteomalacia. In young infants, however, hypocalcemic tetany may manifest before the rachitic features become very conspicuous. Abnormalities in vitamin D metabolism can be divided into three broad categories: vitamin D deficiency, acquired or inherited disorders of vitamin D metabolism, and resistance to the actions of vitamin D.

As described previously, maternal vitamin D deficiency is the major risk for neonatal vitamin D deficiency presenting as hypocalcemia. Vitamin D deficiency is unusual in the United States because of the common practice of vitamin D supplementation of dairy products and other foods. However, it does occur in women in whom both sunlight exposure and dietary intake of vitamin D are inadequate. Recent immigrants from the Middle East or South Asia who continue to wear traditional dress *and* may have inadequate dietary vitamin D intake are particularly at high risk (Watney et al, 1971; Ahmed et al, 1995). Breast-fed infants of strictly vegetarian mothers are also susceptible to early onset hypocalcemic rickets (Bachrach et al, 1979). Neonatal rickets be prevented by daily supple-

mentation of 400 IU for infants and 800 IU for pregnant and lactating women.

Intestinal absorption of fat-soluble vitamin D requires a functioning pancreas, biliary system, and bowel mucosa. Consequently, pregnant women with malabsorption syndromes may be vitamin D deficient. Maternal anticonvulsant therapy (phenobarbital, diphenylhydantoin) during pregnancy, which increases hepatic catabolism of vitamin D, also can induce maternal and fetal vitamin D deficiency (Markestadt et al, 1984). Pregnant women who take anticonvulsants should receive vitamin D supplementation (800 to 1000 IU/day).

Other Causes of Neonatal Hypocalcemia

Various common therapeutic interventions are associated with hypocalcemia. Bicarbonate therapy, as well as any form of metabolic or respiratory alkalosis, decreases ionized calcium levels and bone resorption of calcium. Transfusion and plasmapheresis with citrated blood can form nonionized calcium complexes, thus decreasing Ca^{+2}. Furosemide therapy promotes calciuresis as well as nephrolithiasis. Phototherapy for hyperbilirubinemia may be associated with mild hypocalcemia. This effect has been attributed to decreased melatonin secretion, which potentiates glucocorticoid actions on bone metabolism. Lipid infusions may elevate serum-free fatty acid levels, which form insoluble complexes with calcium. Most of these effects are transient, and cessation of therapy is associated with a return to normal serum calcium levels. The major exception is aggressive furosemide therapy, which, when prolonged, may lead to bone demineralization and renal dysfunction (Downing et al, 1992). The addition of a thiazide diuretic may decrease these effects.

The systemic response to hyperphosphatemia is hypocalcemia. Clinical settings conducive to phosphate-induced neonatal hypocalcemia, in addition to excessive dietary phosphate, are rhabdomyolysis-induced acute renal failure and the hypocalcemia of advanced renal insufficiency. Pancreatitis can cause hypocalcemia and tetany through the action of pancreatic lipase on retroperitoneal and omental fat to release free fatty acids (FFAs) into the peritoneum. FFAs avidly chelate calcium and remove it from the ECF (Dettelbach et al, 1990). Pancreatitis also may release pancreatic calcium-lowering factors (Tomomura et al, 1995). Sepsis and septic shock cause hypocalcemia by unknown mechanisms. It is important to recognize that hypocalcemia also may be precipitated when the rate of skeletal mineralization significantly outpaces the rate of osteoclastic bone resorption. Examples of this type of hypocalcemia occur with overzealous vitamin D replacement in infants with rickets or hypoparathyroidism. Finally, certain skeletal dysplasia syndromes are associated with neonatal hypocalcemia, which may be severe (Peeden et al, 1992).

Treatment

The decision to treat the hypocalcemic infant depends on the severity of the hypocalcemia and the presence of clinical signs and symptoms. The morbidities associated with calcium treatment must be weighed against the potential benefits of treatment. Hypocalcemic preterm infants who have no symptoms and are not ill from any other cause probably do not need specific treatment. The early neonatal hypocalcemia should resolve by day 3. Many clinicians begin treatment in preterm newborns once serum calcium levels have dropped to 6.0 to 6.5 mg/dL and Ca^{+2} to 2.5 to 3.0 mg/dL. Another reasonable approach is to initiate prophylactic calcium infusions for all extremely premature ELBW newborns within the first 24 hours. There is no role for prophylaxis or treatment with pharmacologic doses of vitamin D. For newborns who exhibit cardiovascular compromise (e.g., severe respiratory distress, pulmonary hypertension, asphyxia, sepsis) or who require cardiotonic drugs or blood pressure support, a different therapeutic threshold is justified, and monitering blood $[Ca^{+2}]$ is particularly helpful, with the aim of preventing the onset of significant hypocalcemia.

The mainstay of treatment for neonatal hypocalcemia is intravenous administration of calcium salts. Calcium gluconate is preferred over calcium chloride (which, in sufficient doses, can produce hyperchloremic acidosis) or calcium lactate. A 10% solution of calcium gluconate contains 9.4 mg Ca/mL. A constant infusion of approximately 45 to 75 mg/kg per day usually produces a sustained increase in serum calcium level (7 to 8 mg/dL). Bolus infusions are hazardous and only transiently effective.

The risks associated with calcium infusions can be minimized by paying attention to detail. Rapid intravenous infusion of calcium can cause sudden elevation in serum calcium level, leading to bradyarrhythmias. Bolus infusion of calcium should be reserved for treatment of hypocalcemic tetany and seizures. Extravasation of calcium solutions into subcutaneous tissues may cause necrosis and subcutaneous calcifications. Therefore, scrupulous attention to peripheral intravenous catheter sites is particularly important when calcium-containing solutions are infused. Inadvertent intrahepatic injection of calcium through an umbilical venous catheter (due to failure to reach the inferior vena cava) can cause hepatic necrosis. Rapid intra-aortic infusion via the umbilical artery can cause arterial spasm and, at least experimentally, intestinal necrosis.

For emergency treatment of hypocalcemic crisis with seizures, tetany, or apnea, 1 to 2 mL/kg of a 10% solution of calcium gluconate should be administered over 5 to 10 min. The initial serum calcium level may be less than 5.0 mg/dL. Careful observation of the infant and the infusion site is essential, and the infusion should be discontinued if there is bradycardia, or when the desired clinical result is obtained. The intravenous dose of calcium gluconate necessary to stop convulsions is usually 1 to 3 mL/kg. Toxic reactions may be avoided if the maximum intravenous dose of calcium gluconate administered at any one time does not exceed 2 mL/kg; doses above 3 mL/kg should be administered with caution. If necessary, intravenous calcium therapy may be repeated 3 or 4 times in 24 hours to help control acute symptoms.

After acute symptoms have been controlled, calcium therapy should be continued as needed to maintain the serum calcium level above 7.0 mg/dL. In part, the level of serum calcium to be achieved depends on the level of serum total protein, particularly serum albumin. In hypoalbuminemic infants, lower levels of total serum calcium are normally present. In preterm and sick infants in whom the oral intake is limited, 5 to 8 mL/kg of 10% calcium gluconate (45 to 75 mg Ca/kg) may be infused with intravenous fluids over a 24-hour period. The lower dose range is preferred whenever there is hyperphosphatemia. If oral feedings are tolerated, 10% calcium gluconate may be given in the same daily dose divided into four to six feedings. Alternatively, Neo-Calglucon (calcium glubionate), which contains 23.6 mg Ca/mL, may be given in a dose of 2 mL/kg/day divided into feedings. Oral calcium gluconate is better tolerated by young infants because the high sugar content and osmolality of Neo-Calglucon may cause gastrointestinal irritation or diarrhea. Intravenous or oral calcium supplements are continued until the serum calcium level stabilizes.

In late neonatal tetany, dietary factors and hypoparathyroidism are important, and the goals of therapy are to reduce the phosphate load and to increase the calcium/phosphorus ratio of feedings to 4 to 1. This can be accomplished by the use of low phosphorus feedings such as human milk or Similac PM 60/40 Low Iron in conjunction with calcium supplements. These measures will inhibit intestinal absorption of phosphorus. Phosphate binders are generally not necessary. The serum calcium and phosphorus levels should be monitored once to twice weekly and the calcium supplements discontinued in a stepwise fashion after several weeks.

When hypomagnesemia contributes to (or causes) the hypocalcemia, administration of magnesium salts is indicated. Magnesium may be administered intramuscularly as a 50% solution of magnesium sulfate (50% $MgSO_4 \cdot 7H_2O$ contains 4 mEq/mL of magnesium). The suggested intramuscular or intravenous dose of 50% magnesium sulfate is 0.1 to 0.2 mL/kg. Intravenous infusions should be administered slowly with electrocardiographic monitoring to detect acute rhythm disturbances, which may include prolongation of atrioventricular conduction time and sinoatrial or atrioventricular block. The magnesium dose may be repeated every 12 to 24 hours, depending on clinical response and monitering of serum magnesium levels. Serum magnesium levels should be carefully monitored to guard against hypermagnesemia. Many infants with transient hypomagnesemia will respond sufficiently to 1 or 2 injections of magnesium. Infants with primary hypomagnesemia have permanent magnesium wasting and low serum magnesium levels and require lifelong treatment with magnesium supplements.

Infants with normal intestinal absorption who develop late hypocalcemia with vitamin D deficiency rickets usually respond within 4 weeks to 1000 to 2000 IU/day of oral vitamin D. These infants should receive at least 40 mg/kg per day of elemental calcium in order to prevent hypocalcemia because the unmineralized osteoid is able to mineralize when vitamin D is provided ("hungry bones" syndrome). In the various forms of persistent congenital hypoparathyroidism, long-term treatment with vitamin D or its therapeutic natural or synthetic metabolites is indicated.

Neonatal Hypercalcemia

Hypercalcemia usually is defined as a total serum calcium concentration greater than 11.0 mg/dL and a Ca^{+2} greater than 5.0 mg/dL. Neonatal hypercalcemia is found in association with several clinical entities (Table 99–2). It may be asymptomatic and discovered incidentally or may present dramatically (especially if serum calcium is 14.0 mg/dL or greater) and be life-threatening, requiring immediate intervention. The clinical findings include poor feeding, vomiting, constipation, hypotonia, lethargy, polyuria, hypertension, tachypnea, dyspnea, and seizures. Hypercalcemia causes polyuria and polydipsia by interfering with the action of vasopressin on the renal collecting ducts, resulting in dehydration. The central nervous manifestations result from direct neuronal effects of calcium as well as from hypertensive encephalopathy and cerebral ischemia. The hypertension is probably due to a direct vasoconstrictive effect of elevated ECF calcium as well as to increased activity of the renin-angiotensin system resulting from renal arteriolar constriction. Persistent hypercalcemia may produce extraskeletal calcification in kidney, skin, subcutaneous tissue, falx cerebri, arteries, myocardium, lung, or gastric mucosa. Nephrocalcinosis, nephrolithiasis, diffuse bone demineralization (and occasionally osteitis fibrosa) are well recognized hypercalcemic complications. In infants, the predominant manifestation of chronic, moderate elevations of serum calcium may be failure to thrive.

Normally, the parathyroid-renal axis prevents hypercalcemia via inhibition of PTH secretion and $1,25(OH)_2D$ synthesis, which reduces calcium absorption from the intestine, mobilization from bone, and reabsorption from the kidney. (The physiological role of calcitonin is not clear.) An elevated serum calcium, therefore, indicates that there is inappropriate calcium influx to the ECF from one or more of these pools. Because the kidney is the principal organ for stoichiometric calcium balance, hypercalcemia usually means that the capacity of the kidneys to excrete calcium has been exceeded. In fact, abnormalities in distal tubular resorption are involved in the pathogenesis of many hypercalcemic conditions (e.g., hyperparathyroidism) and renal impairment frequently accompanies many hypercalcemic syndromes.

Neonatal Hyperparathyroid Syndromes and Familial Hypocalciuric Hypercalcemia

Neonatal severe primary hyperparathyroidism (NSPHP) is an uncommon, life-threatening disorder. The parathyroid glands are refractory to regulation by $[Ca^{+2}]$, resulting in marked hypercalcemia, although milder clinical expression also occurs. These infants usually appear normal at birth but may have a narrow thorax, depressed sternum, or thoracolumbar kyphosis. Signs of hypercalcemia usually develop during the first days of life. Repeated serum calcium levels may range between 15 and 30 mg/dL, serum phosphorus concentration is frequently less than 3.5 mg/dL with significant hyperphosphaturia, and PTH levels are very elevated. Anemia, hepatomegaly, and splenomegaly have been reported. Skeletal radiographs reveal generalized demineralization, irregular metaphyses (subperiosteal bone resorption), and multiple pathologic fractures. Renal calcinosis is common. The bony findings may initially suggest a diagnosis of osteogenesis imperfecta (Bai et al, 1997).

Inheritance studies have long suggested a connection with a milder disease, familial hypocalciuric hypercalcemia (FHH), also called familial benign hypercalcemia (Marx et al, 1982), as well as a relationship of both to PTH-independent "resetting" of parathyroid Ca^{+2} sensing and renal calcium handling. The recent cloning of a parathyroid and renal Ca^{+2}-sensing receptor (CASR) clinches these relationships. Homozygosity for activating CASR mutations causes NSPHP, whereas heterozygosity at these loci results in FHH (Pollak et al, 1993; Pearce et al, 1995). Additionally, heterozygous (autosomal dominant) CASR mutations account for some cases of NSPHP (Pearce et al, 1995; Bai et al, 1997).

Newborns (and older children and adults) with FHH have mild (often asymptomatic) and intermittent hypercalcemia without hypercalciuria. In distinction to neonatal hyperparathyroidism, circulating levels of PTH, phosphorus and $1,25(OH)_2D$ tend to be normal. At least two other distinct genetic FHH entities have been described. Parents who have FHH are at risk for having an infant with NSPHP. Conversely, parents of an infant with hyperparathyroidism should receive screening with serum calcium and phosphorus levels and a urinary calcium/creatinine ratio. A UCa/Cr below 0.01 supports the diagnosis. Early diagnosis and subtotal parathyroidectomy have been necessary for survival in NSPHP.

Neonatal hyperparathyroidism occasionally occurs as part of the syndrome of multiple endocrine adenomatosis. There also have been reports of sporadic and familial forms of renal tubular acidosis with secondary hyperparathyroidism manifesting as hyperchloremia, hypercalcaemia, elevated serum PTH, and severe metabolic acidosis (Nishiyama et al, 1990; Savani et al, 1993). Serum calcium and PTH may promptly revert to normal values on initiation of

---

TABLE 99–2

Causes of Neonatal Hypercalcemia

Disorders of parathyroid function
  Neonatal severe primary hyperparathyroidism (homozygosity for activating Ca^{+2}-sensing receptor mutations)
  Familial hypercalcemic hypocalciuria (heterozygosity for activating Ca^{+2}-sensing receptor mutations)
  Neonatal hyperparathyroidism associated with multiple endocrine adenomatosis
  Renal tubular acidosis with secondary hyperparathyroidism
  Neonatal hyperparathyroidism secondary to maternal hypoparathyroidism
Williams syndrome (elastin gene locus deletions)
Idiopathic infantile hypercalcemia (Lightwood syndrome)
Phosphate depletion
Hypervitaminosis D
Subcutaneous fat necrosis
Blue diaper syndrome
Hypercalcemia associated with skeletal dysplasias
  Infantile hypophosphatasia
  Jansen metaphyseal chrondrodysplasia (activating mutations of the PTH/PTHrP receptor)
Other causes
  Tumor-associated hypercalcemia
  Congenital lactase deficiency
  Acute adrenal insufficiency
  Hypervitaminosis A
  Thyrotoxicosis

alkali therapy. Often, the acidification defect will be transient (Igarashi 1992). As the hyperparathyroidism and volume contraction are corrected, serum calcium normalizes.

Neonatal Hyperparathyroidism Associated with Maternal Hypoparathyroidism

Fetal and neonatal hyperparathyroidism may occur in infants born to mothers with poorly treated idiopathic or surgical hypoparathyroidism (Aceto et al, 1966; Loughead et al, 1990). Maternal hypocalcemia leading to impaired transplacental calcium transfer causes chronic stimulation of the fetal parathyroid glands. In contrast to infants with NSPHP, these newborns frequently have low birth weight, serum calcium levels that may be depressed or normal rather than elevated, and serum phosphorus levels that are normal to mildly elevated rather than depressed. The reasons for these differences in the biochemical findings between the two groups are unknown. In one infant delivered to a hypoparathyroid mother, there was radiographic evidence of rickets as well as hyperparathyroidism, and the serum 25(OH)D level was low (Saan et al, 1976). The authors concluded that the hyperparathyroidism induced a state of vitamin D deficiency, possibly by increasing the requirement for vitamin D, as has been reported in some adults with primary hyperparathyroidism. The mortality rate in infants born to poorly or untreated hypoparathyroid mothers has been high, especially for significantly intrauterine growth restricted newborns. In survivors, the skeletal abnormalities regress spontaneously, and bone radiographs normalize by 4 to 7 months. Correction of hypocalcemia in hypoparathyroid women during pregnancy with calcium and vitamin D supplements prevents the development of fetal hyperparathyroidism.

Williams Syndrome and Idiopathic Infantile Hypercalcemia

Williams syndrome (Williams et al, 1961; Beuren, 1972) is an autosomal dominant disorder that in full-blown form includes transient hypercalcemia in infancy, supravalvular aortic stenosis, multiple peripheral pulmonary arterial stenoses, "elfin" facies, mental and statural deficiency, and characteristic dental malformation (Grimm and Wesselhoeft, 1980). The typical facial features include supraorbital fullness with a broad forehead, short palpebral fissures with a medial flare to the eyebrows, a flat nasal bridge with a full tip and anteverted nostrils, occular hypertelorism, strabismus, stellate iris, malar hypoplasia with a wide mouth and a full lower lip, and hypoplastic teeth with malocclusion. Hallux valgus with a small curved fifth digit is common. Pectus excavatum and an umbilical or inguinal hernia are less commonly noted. Two thirds of newborns with Williams syndrome are small for gestational age, and many are born post-term. The frequency of Williams syndrome is estimated to be about 1 in 10,000 to 20,000. Recent evidence indicates that mutations in the elastin gene are responsible, at least in part, for this disorder. Moreover, Williams syndrome is a contiguous gene syndrome in which up to 2.5 Mb of genomic DNA distal to the elastin gene locus may be missing (Urban et al, 1996). Deletion of several specific genes in the Williams syndrome

region (7q11.23) appears to be pathogenetic for the distinct physiognomic and cognitive features. The extent of expression of the full Williams phenotype may be related to the size of the deletion. Currently, FISH for the detection of elastin deletions is a useful initial diagnostic assay for this disorder.

Although the hypercalcemia is often first diagnosed after the first month, Williams syndrome can present to clinical attention in the neonatal period (Shimizu et al, 1994). Heightened awareness of the syndrome may increase the frequency of neonatal diagnosis. The hypercalcemia rarely persists beyond several months and generally resolves spontaneously, but the hypercalciuria may persist. The pathogenesis of hypercalcemia in Williams syndrome remains unknown. Elevated serum calcium associated with normal or increased serum phosphorus levels and characteristic radiographic findings differentiate Williams syndrome from primary hyperparathyroidism. In some older infants, the serum calcium level is normal, but the presence of nephrocalcinosis and other soft tissue calcification suggests that hypercalcemia was previously present. Increased calcium absorption has been demonstrated, but enhanced vitamin D sensitivity or other disorders of specific calcitropic hormones have not been consistently found. A cautionary note is that many of these children were studied after resolution of their hypercalcemia. A low calcium diet usually controls the hypercalcemia.

In the early 1950s in England, Lightwood (1952) reported a series of infants with severe hypercalcemia. Findings consistent with hypervitaminosis D were found, including osteoporosis and dense bands of mineralization at the metaphyseal ends of long bones. Epidemiologic investigations have revealed that the majority of infants were born to mothers ingesting foods heavily fortified with vitamin D. Some infants were receiving 3000 to 4000 IU of vitamin D daily as part of a concerted effort to prevent nutritional deficiencies in infants subjected to the disruptions of wartime. With reduction of vitamin D supplementation, the incidence of infantile hypercalcemia declined dramatically. However, other instances have been described in which there is no known previous exposure to excessive maternal vitamin D intake, and the incidence of this "idiopathic" infantile hypercalcemia (IIH) has remained relatively fixed over time. IIH in the absence of Williams features is sometimes called Lightwood syndrome. Severely affected infants may have cardiac lesions and facial features similar to those seen in Williams syndrome. The distinction between the two syndromes remains problematic (Martin et al, 1984), and clarification probably awaits more extensive genetic analysis or definition of the mineral metabolic derangement(s). In contrast to Williams syndrome, serum calcium levels remain elevated for a prolonged period in severely affected infants with IIH. Therefore, in addition to dietary calcium restriction and avoidance of vitamin D, therapy has included the use of glucocorticoids to reduce gastrointestinal calcium absorption.

Neonatal Hypercalcemia Associated with Subcutaneous Fat Necrosis

Infantile hypercalcemia occurs in association with subcutaneous fat necrosis (Hicks et al, 1993). In afflicted infants, erythematous to violaceous, firm, subcutaneous nodules appear approximately 1 to 4 weeks after delivery, followed by an onset of signs and symptoms of hypercalcemia. Frequently, there is a history of difficult delivery, hypothermia, or asphyxia. The serum phosphorus and alkaline phosphatase levels are normal. Radiographs of the long bones are usually normal, although periosteal elevation has been described in one case, and findings similar to those in Williams syndrome were reported in another. Ectopic calcification may be present. Biopsy of the indurated plaques shows panniculitis with necrotic adipocytes and granulomatous infiltration. In experimental systems, stimulated macrophages can express 25(OH)D-1α-hydroxylase activity, and unregulated production of 1,25(OH)$_2$D by the granulomas in fat necrosis may cause the hypercalcemia (Finne et al, 1988; Kruse et al, 1993), in a manner analogous to the hypercalcemia encountered in sarcoidosis and other granulomatous diseases. Another potential mechanism is excess prostaglandin E release from the lesions (Veldhuis et al, 1979). Prostaglandins of the E series can stimulate osteoclastic bone resorption and have been linked to hypercalcemia and increased bone resorption associated with malignancy and chronic inflammation. The hypercalcemia associated with subcutaneous fat necrosis may persist for several days or weeks. Prognosis depends on the duration of the hypercalcemia. Treatment has consisted of glucocorticoids, volume expansion with saline, furosemide diuresis, and avoidance of excess dietary calcium and vitamin D.

Blue Diaper Syndrome

Blue diaper syndrome is a rare familial disease in which hypercalcemia and nephrocalcinosis are associated with a defect in the intestinal transport of tryptophan (Drummond et al, 1964). Bacterial degradation of tryptophan in the intestine leads to excessive indole production, which is converted to indican in the liver and causes indicanuria. Oxidation conjugation of two molecules of indican forms the water-insoluble dye indigo blue (indigotin), which causes a peculiar bluish discoloration of the diaper. The clinical course is characterized by failure to thrive, recurrent unexplained fever, infections, marked irritability, and constipation. The mechanism of the hypercalcemia is uncertain, although oral tryptophan loading in humans and experimental animals produces an increase in the serum calcium level. Treatment consists of glucocorticoid administration and a low calcium, low vitamin D diet.

Hypercalcemia Associated with Skeletal Dysplasias

Several skeletal dysplasia syndromes are associated with hypercalcemia. Their distinctive phenotypes guide appropriate diagnosis. Infantile hypophosphatasia is a deficiency of tissue-nonspecific alkaline phosphatase activity with onset in utero or in early postnatal life. Prominent features are craniosynostosis, severe skeletal abnormalities, and hypercalcemia. Mortality in the first year is common. Chlorthiazide therapy ameliorates the hypercalcemia, hypercalciuria and chronic bone demineralization (Barcia et al, 1997). Jansen syndrome presents in newborns with hypercalcemia and skeletal radiographs that mimic rachitic changes. This metaphyseal chrondrodysplasia is the result of an amino acid substitution mutation in the PTH/PTHrP receptor that activates the receptor in the absence of ligand (Schipani et al, 1996). PTH and PTHrP levels are low to undetectable. The functional consequences are chrondrodysplasia and hypercalcemia, which similar to that of primary hyperparathyroidism and hypercalcemia of malignancy.

Hypercalcemia Associated with Phosphate Depletion

Hypercalcemia occurs in phosphate depletion, which, in the neonatal period, is most commonly seen in very low-birth-weight infants who are fed unsupplemented human milk (Rowe et al, 1984). The low phosphate concentration in human milk leads to hypophosphatemia, which, in turn, leads to an increase in circulating 1,25(OH)$_2$D with an attendant increased intestinal absorption of calcium. In the presence of hypophosphatemia, only limited amounts of calcium can be deposited in bone and rickets with hypercalcemia and hypercalciuria results. We have observed extremely high serum calcium levels (greater than 15 mg/dL, with serum phosphorus less than 2.5 mg/dL and suppressed PTH) in ELBW infants in this setting. These infants respond to cautious phosphate replenishment. The condition is preventable by anticipatory monitoring of serum calcium and phosphorus levels. Hypophosphatemic bone disease is discussed later in the section on Osteopenia in Preterm Infants.

Other Causes of Neonatal Hypercalcemia

Unlike adults, in neonates tumor-associated hypercalcemia is extremely rare. Congenital lactase deficiency is associated with rapid onset of hypercalcemia, hypercalciuria and medullary nephrocalcinosis (Saarela et al, 1995). The calcium derangements are well managed by a lactose-free diet. Modest hypercalcemia may occur in acute adrenal insufficiency. The pathogenesis is uncertain, but there is evidence that total but not the ionized calcium concentration is increased.

Excessive supplementation with vitamin D is a common cause of hypercalcemia in newborns and infants. In preterm infants, prolonged feeding with premature formula (Nako et al, 1993) or mineral and vitamin D supplemented human milk fortifiers have led to mild to significant hypercalcemia. Infants respond to discontinuation of vitamin D supplements. These occurrences have prompted vitamin reformulation of these products. Hypervitaminosis D laboratory values typically show elevation of 25(OH)D but not of 1,25(OH)$_2$D. Serum PTH usually is suppressed by the hypercalcemia. Biochemical resolution may be protracted because of sterol deposition in fat stores. Hypervitaminosis A and thyrotoxicosis also accelerate bone turnover and can induce hypercalcemia.

Treatment

The first principle in the medical management of hypercalcemia is to increase the urinary excretion of calcium by maximizing glomerular filtration and the urinary excretion of sodium. In the normal kidney, sodium clearance and calcium clearance are very closely linked during water or osmotic diuresis. Infants with severe hypercalcemia are frequently dehydrated. Two thirds normal to isotonic saline containing 30 mEq of potassium chloride per liter may be infused intravenously at a rate to correct dehydration and maximize the GFR. After rehydration, furosemide in a dose of 1 mg/kg may be given intravenously at 6- to 8-hour intervals to inhibit tubular reabsorption of calcium as well as sodium and water. In situations in which severe hypercalcemia is associated with hypophosphatemia, oral or intravenous phosphorus may be given in a dose of 30 to 50 mg/kg per day of phosphorus as a phosphate salt. Unlike sodium, phosphate does not remove calcium from the body but causes a redistribution of calcium. The goal of phosphate therapy is to maintain serum phosphorus levels in a range of 3 to 5 mg/dL. The oral route for phosphate therapy is preferrable because serious immediate reactions have been reported with intravenous phosphate treatment. Therapy usually results in a significant reduction in serum calcium concentration over a 24- to 48-hour period. In more severe and resistant cases, cortisone, 10 mg/kg, or prednisone, 2 mg/kg, can be added to the therapeutic regimen. The hypocalcemic effects of glucocorticoids result from decreased intestinal absorption of calcium as well as increased renal excretion. Although effective in several types of hypercalcemic states, glucocorticoids are relatively ineffective in the treatment of hypercalcemia associated with primary hyperparathyroidism. There is little experience with use of calcitonin or bisphosphonates in infants. More definitive and specific therapy depends on the underlying cause of the hypercalcemia.

The mainstays of nonacute treatment of milder neonatal hypercalcemia are restriction of dietary calcium, elimination of vitamin D supplements, and limiting sunlight exposure.

Neonatal Disorders of Serum Magnesium

Neonatal hypomagnesemia is discussed in a preceding section, Neonatal Hypocalcemia Associated with Hypomagnesemia.

Magnesium sulfate is a mainstay of the management of preeclampsia. Magnesium given to the mother readily crosses the placenta and causes elevation of fetal magnesium levels and neuromuscular depression of the newborn. The hypermagnesemic newborn may exhibit varying degrees of flaccidity, unresponsiveness, respiratory insufficiency and apnea, ileus, and delayed passage of meconium. The signs may be mistaken for perinatal asphyxia. Occasionally, temporary endotracheal intubation and mechanical ventilation are required. Feedings should be deferred until normalization of bowel sounds. Prolonged fetal hypermagnesemia may be a risk factor for meconium obstructions. Aside from this latter sequela, the neonatal effects of hypermagnesemia appear to be transient and usually disappear within several hours. Because the newborn effectively excretes the magnesium load, serial monitoring of serum levels is not indicated. Infusion of calcium salts may antagonize some of the adverse effects of excess magnesium.

OSTEOPENIA IN PRETERM INFANTS

Osteopenia in the context of this discussion is defined as radiographic evidence of diminished bone density. Osteopenia is present in rickets, osteomalacia, and osteoporosis.

Rickets is a disorder of mineralization of the bone matrix, or osteoid, in growing bone; it involves both the growth plate (epiphysis) and newly formed trabecular and cortical bone. Radiographic features in rickets include osteopenia and characteristic findings at the cartilage-shaft junction of growing bones, including an increase in the width of the growth plate, cupping, and fraying. In rickets, the serum phosphorus or calcium level or both are characteristically depressed, and the serum alkaline phosphatase level is elevated. *Osteomalacia* is rickets that occurs in the presence of little or no linear growth, such as might occur in some preterm infants. Radiologically, osteomalacia is characterized by osteopenia but lacks the radiographic features of rickets at the cartilage-shaft junction. *Osteoporosis* is defined as a state of reduced bone mass per unit volume with a normal ratio of mineral to matrix. Unlike rickets and osteomalacia, in which the primary abnormality is a defect in mineralization, the primary abnormality in osteoporosis is either a decrease in matrix formation or an increase in matrix and mineral resorption. Osteoporosis may not be distinguishable from osteomalacia radiographically because both are characterized by an osteopenia without the rachitic changes at the cartilage-shaft junction. In contrast to patients with rickets and osteomalacia, patients with osteoporosis have normal serum concentrations of calcium, phosphorus, and alkaline phosphatase. In some disorders, histologic examination reveals evidence of both osteoporosis and osteomalacia.

Osteopenia with or without radiologic evidence of rickets at the cartilage-shaft junction is commonly observed between 3 and 12 weeks of age in preterm infants. The incidence and severity of this disorder increase with decreasing gestation and birth weight and are more common in infants with a complicated course. On the other hand, osteopenia usually is not a problem for the low-birth-weight, healthy preterm infant. In osteopenic VLBW babies, postnatal bone mineralization lags significantly behind expected intrauterine bone mineralization. Radiologic and biochemical monitoring suggests that the pathogenesis of this disorder is increased endosteal resorption rather than decreased bone formation, that is, it is a high turnover osteopenia (Beyers et al, 1994).

The clinical findings in preterm infants with osteopenia include a widened anterior fontanel, craniotabes (with the "ping pong ball" sign), bony expansion of the wrists, costochondral beading, and rib or long bone fractures (Dabezies et al, 1997). Respiratory distress (tachypnea) may occur secondary to demineralization and softening of the thoracic cage (Glasgow and Thomas, 1977). Long-term effects of osteopenia in preterm infants include delays in dental maturation (Seow, 1996) and linear growth.

Unlike nutritional rickets in term infants and older children, the osteopenia associated with prematurity is chiefly caused by deficiencies in dietary phosphate and calcium rather than by vitamin D deficiency. Eighty percent of bone mineralization in the fetus occurs during the third trimester when fetal calcium and phosphorus requirements are at least 100 to 120 mg/kg per day and 60 to 75 mg/kg per day, respectively (Ziegler et al, 1976). Diets that are particularly low in mineral content predispose preterm infants to osteopenia and rickets. The greatest risks for phosphate deficiency rickets result from feeding unsupplemented human milk (Sagy et al, 1980; Rowe et al, 1984) or milk formulas not designed for use in preterm infants, and from prolonged parenteral nutrition.

The pathogenesis of phosphate deficiency rickets differs from that of vitamin D and calcium deficiency in that neither hyperparathyroidism nor vitamin D deficiency is present. In contrast, the pathogenesis of calcium deficiency rickets is similar to that of vitamin D deficiency rickets in that the hypocalcemia causes hyperparathyroidism. The elevated PTH will increase bone resorption and enhance the renal conversion of 25(OH)D to 1,25(OH)$_2$D to increase intestinal calcium and phosphorus absorption. Individual preterm babies may exhibit predominantly phosphate depletion or a mixed phosphate and calcium deficiency; isolated calcium deficiency is rare (Kooh et al, 1977). The biochemical features will distinguish among these causes (see section on Hypercalcemia Associated with Phosphate Depletion). Commonly, there is dual mineral deficiency, and laboratory values may show a low, normal, or slightly elevated serum calcium and a low to low-normal phosphorus. In severe or complicated bone disease, serum 25(OH)D is a useful screen for establishing the sufficiency of vitamin D stores; levels less than 6 ng/mL indicate severe vitamin D deficiency. Serum alkaline phosphatase, which is a marker of osteoblastic bone formation, is frequently used to monitor skeletal metabolism in preterm infants. The magnitude of elevations in alkaline phosphatase (or osteocalcin) concentrations are not good predictors of the extent of the bone mineral deficits (Ryan et al, 1993; Pittard et al, 1992). The longitudinal assessment of bone mineral content by x-ray absorptiometry (Salle and Glorieux, 1993) is valuable but is not widely available.

Severe phosphate depletion and rickets may occur in rapidly growing preterm infants fed unsupplemented human milk that has a low phosphate content. Characteristically, these infants have hypophosphatemia, hypophosphaturia, hypercalcemia, hypercalciuria, normal or depressed serum PTH levels, normal 25(OH)D levels, and elevated serum 1,25(OH)$_2$D levels. The hypophosphatemia is the stimulus for the production of 1,25(OH)$_2$D, which, in turn, increases the intestinal absorption of calcium. However, in the presence of hypophosphatemia, only limited amounts of calcium can be deposited in bone, and hypercalcemia and hypercalciuria result. The hypercalcemia inhibits PTH secretion. This form of rickets does not respond to vitamin D therapy. In fact, vitamin D supplementation without correcting the underlying dietary phosphate deficit may aggravate the hypercalcemia and hypercalciuria by enhancing intestinal calcium absorption. The bone disease in these infants does respond to increased dietary phosphate, which is accomplished by adding a human milk supplement designed for preterm infants or switching to a preterm milk formula; both diets provide additional calcium as well as phosphorus. Addition of 20 to 25 mg/kg per day of potassium phosphate also will increase serum phosphorus levels. However, because phosphate repletion will permit bone mineralization, serum calcium may fall to subnormal levels (the "hungry bones" syndrome) unless supplemental calcium (e.g., 30 mg/kg per day) also is provided. Current recommended intakes of calcium and phosphorus

(Schanler and Rifka 1994; Atkinson, 1994) promote normalized bone growth and mineralization in preterm infants. For VLBW infants, it is important to maintain a mineral-enriched diet and laboratory monitoring for several weeks to months after hospital discharge.

Human milk has a low total antirachitic sterol activity of only 25 to 50 IU/L (Reeve et al, 1982), which may be insufficient for maintaining normal 25(OH)D levels in preterm infants. Therefore, if preterm infants are fed unsupplemented human milk they also should receive 400 to 600 IU daily of vitamin D. There is no apparent benefit for additional vitamin D intake for VLBW infants feeding high-calcium and high-phosphorus preterm infant formulas (Koo et al, 1995).

Additional, non-nutritional risk factors for osteopenia are lack of mobility (Moyer-Mileur et al, 1995) and therapy with dexamethasone (Kamitsuka et al, 1995), methylxanthines (Zanardo et al, 1995) or aminoglycosides (Giapros et al, 1995) in ill preterm infants, which increase urinary calcium excretion and the risk of serum mineral imbalance, nephrocalcinosis, and osteopenia. Copper deficiency is an unusual cause of osteopenia in preterm infants (Tanaka et al, 1980).

REFERENCES

Abrams SA, Schanler RJ, Yergey AL, et al: Compartmental analysis of calcium metabolism in very low-birth-weight infants. Pediatr Res 36:424, 1994.

Aceto T Jr, Batt RE, Bruck ES, et al: Intrauterine hyperparathyroidism: A complication of untreated maternal hypoparathyroidism. J Clin Endocrinol 26:487, 1966.

Ahmed I, Atiq M, Iqbal J, et al: Vitamin D deficiency rickets in breast-fed infants presenting as hypocalcemic seizures. Acta Paediatr 84:941, 1995.

Ahn TG, Antonarakis SE, Kronenberg HM, et al: Familial isolated hypoparathyroidism: A molecular genetic analysis of 8 families with 23 affected persons. Medicine 65:73, 1986.

Anast CS, Mohs JM, Kaplan SL, Burns TW: Evidence for parathyroid failure in magnesium deficiency. Science 177:606, 1972.

Ariceta G, Rodriguez-Soriano J, Vallo A: Magnesium homeostasis in premature and full-term neonates. Pediatr Nephrol 9:423, 1995.

Arnold A, Horst SA, Gardella TJ, et al: Mutation of the signal peptide-encoding region of the preproparathyroid hormone gene in familial isolated hypoparathyroidism. J Clin Invest 86:1084, 1990.

Atkinson SA: Calcium and phosphorus needs of premature infants. Nutrition 10:66, 1994.

Bachrach S, Fisher J, Parks J: An outbreak of vitamin D deficiency rickets in a susceptible population. Pediatrics 64:871, 1979.

Bai M, Pearce SHS, Kifor O, et al: In vivo and in vitro characterization of neonatal hyperparathyroidism resulting from a de novo, heterozygous mutation in the Ca(2+)-sensing receptor gene: Normal maternal calcium homeostasis as a cause of secondary hyperparathyroidism in familial benign hypocalciuric hypercalcemia. J Clin Invest 99:88, 1997.

Bainbridge R, Mughal Z, Mimouni F, Tsang RC: Transient congenital hypoparathyroidism: How transient is it? J Pediatr 114:866, 1987.

Barcia JP, Strife CF, Langman CB: Infantile hypophosphatasia: Treatment to control hypercalcemia, hypercalciuria, and chronic bone demineralization. J Pediatr 130:825, 1997.

Baron J, Winer KK, Yanovski JA, et al: Mutations in the Ca^{+2}-sensing receptor gene cause autosomal dominant and sporadic hypoparathyroidism. Hum Mol Genet 5:601, 1996.

Bertelloni S, Baroncelli GI, Pelletti A, et al: Parathyroid hormone-related protein in healthy pregnant women. Calcif Tissue Int 54:195, 1994.

Beuren AJ: Supravalvular aortic stenosis: A complex syndrome with and without mental retardation. Birth Defects Original Article Series 8:45, 1972.

Beyers N, Alheit B, Taljaard JF, et al: High turnover osteopenia in preterm babies. Bone 15:5, 1994.

Bijvoet OLM: Indices for the measurements of the renal handling of phosphate. *In* Massry SG, Fleisch H (Eds): Renal Handling of Phosphate. New York, Plenum Press, 1980, p 37.

Bikle DD, Gee E, Halloran B, et al: Free 1,25-dihydroxyvitamin D levels in serum from normal subjects, pregnant subjects and subjects with liver disease. J Clin Invest 74:1966, 1984.

Bouillon R, van Assche FA: Perinatal vitamin D metabolism. Dev Pharmacol Ther 4:1, 1982.

Brodehl J, Gellissen K, Weber HP: Postnatal development of tubular phosphate reabsorption. Clin Nephrol 17:163, 1982.

Bronner F, Salle BL, Putet G, et al: Net calcium absorption in premature infants: Results of 103 metabolic balance studies [published erratum appears in Am J Clin Nutr 57:451, 1993]. Am J Clin Nutr 56:1037, 1992.

Brown EM: Four-parameter model of the sigmoidal relationship between parathyroid hormone release and extracellular calcium concentration in normal and abnormal parathyroid tissue. J Clin Endocrinol Metab 56:572, 1983.

Brown EM, Pollak M, Seidman CE, et al: Calcium–ion-sensing cell-surface receptors. N Engl J Med 333:234, 1995.

Bruce J, Strong JA: Maternal hyperparathyroidism and parathyroid deficiency in child, with account of effect of parathyroidectomy on renal function and attempt to transplant part of tumor. Q J Med 24:307, 1955.

Bucht E, Telenius-Berg M, Lundell G, Sjoberg HE: Immunoextracted calcitonin in milk and plasma from totally thyroidectomized women: Evidence of monomeric calcitonin in plasma during pregnancy and lactation. Acta Endocrinol 113:529, 1986.

Budayr AA, Halloran BP, King JC, et al: High levels of a parathyroid hormone-like protein in milk. Proc Natl Acad Sci U S A 86:7183, 1989.

Burn J, Wilson DI, Cross I, et al: The clinical significance of 22q11 deletion. *In* Clark EB, Markwald RR, Takao A (Eds): Developmental Mechanisms of Heart Disease. Armonk, NY, Future Publishing, 1995, p 559.

Cockburn F, Belton NR, Purvis RJ, et al: Maternal vitamin D intake and mineral metabolism in mothers and their newborn infants. BMJ 288:11, 1980.

Cuneo BF, Langman CB, Ilbawi MN, et al: Latent hypoparathyroidism in children with conotruncal cardiac defects. Circulation 93:1702, 1996.

Dabezies EJ, Warren PD: Fractures in very low birth weight infants with rickets. Clin Orthopaed Rel Res 335:233, 1997.

Davis OK, Hawkins DS, Rubin LP, et al: Serum parathyroid hormone (PTH) in pregnant women determined by an immunoradiometric assay for intact PTH. J Clin Endocrinol Metab 67:850, 1988.

Demarini S, Mimouni F, Tsang RC, et al: Impact of metabolic control of diabetes during pregnancy on neonatal hypocalcemia: A randomized study. Obstet Gynecol 83:918, 1994.

Demczuk S, Levy A, Aubry M, et al: Excess of deletions of maternal origin in the DiGeorge/velo-cardio-facial syndromes: A study of 22 new patients and a review of the literature. Hum Genet 9:1996, 1996.

Dettelbach MA, Deftos LJ, Stewart AF: Intraperitoneal free fatty acids induce severe hypocalcemia in rats. J Bone Miner Res 5:1249, 1990.

Dilworth FJ, Scott I, Green A, et al: Different mechanisms of hydroxylation site selection by liver and kidney cytochrome P450 species (CYP27 and CYP24) involved in vitamin D metabolism. J Biol Chem 270:16766, 1995.

Dobnig H, Kainer F, Stepan V, et al: Elevated parathyroid hormone-related peptide levels after human gestation: Relationship to changes in bone and mineral metabolism. J Clin Endocrinol Metab 80:3699, 1995.

Downing GJ, Egelhoff JC, Daily DK, et al: Kidney function in very low-birth-weight infants with furosemide-related renal calcifications at ages 1 to 2 years. J Pediatr 120:599, 1992.

Driscoll DA, Budarf ML, Emanuel BS: A genetic etiology for DiGeorge syndrome: Consistent deletions and microdeletions of 22q11. Am J Hum Genet 50:924, 1992.

Drummond KN, Michael AF, Ulstrom RA, Good RA: The blue diaper syndrome: Familial hypercalcemia with nephrocalcinosis and indicanuria: A new familial disease, with definition of the metabolic abnormality. Am J Med 37:928, 1964.

Ernst JA, Cruse WK, Lemons JA: Metabolic balance studies in premature infants. Clin Perinatol 22:177, 1995.

Fanconi S, Fischer JA, Wieland P, et al: Kenny syndrome: Evidence for idiopathic hypoparathyroidism in two patients and for abnormal parathyroid hormone in one. J Pediatr 109:469, 1992.

Finne PH, Sanderud J, Aksnes L, et al: Hypercalcemia with increased and unregulated 1,25-dihydroxyvitamin D production in a neonate with subcutaneoud fat necrosis. J Pediatr 112:792, 1988.

Franceschini P, Testa A, Bogetti G, et al: Kenny-Caffey syndrome in two sibs born to consanguinous parents: Evidence for an autosomal recessive variant. Am J Med Genet 42:112, 1992.

Friderichsen C: Hypocalcemie bei einem Brustkind und Hypercalcemie bei der Mutter. Monatschr Kinderheilkd 75:146, 1938.

Garel JM: Hormonal control of calcium metabolism during the reproductive cycle. Physio Rev 67:1, 1987.

Gertner JM, Coustan DR, Kliger AS, et al: Pregnancy as a state of physiologic absorptive hypercalciuria. Am J Med 81:451, 1986.

Giapros VI, Andronikou S, Cholevas VI, Papadopoulou ZL: Renal function in premature infants during aminoglycoside therapy. Pediatr Nephrol 9:163, 1995.

Gidding SS, Minciotti AL, Langman CB: Unmasking of hypoparathyroidism in familial partial DiGeorge syndrome by challenge with disodium edetate. N Engl J Med 319:1589, 1988.

Givens MH, Macy IG: The chemical composition of the human fetus. J Biol Chem 102:7, 1933.

Glasgow JFT, Thomas PS: Rachitic respiratory distress in small preterm infants. Arch Dis Child 52:268, 1977.

Grant FD, Conlin PR, Brown EM: Rate and concentration dependence of parathyroid hormone dynamics during stepwise changes in serum ionized calcium in normal humans. J Clin Endocrinol Metab 71:370, 1990.

Greig F, Paul E, DiMartino-Nardi J, Saenger P: Transient congenital hypoparathyroidism: Resolution and recurrence in chromosome 22q11 deletion. J Pediatr 128:563, 1996.

Grill V, Hillary J, Ho PM, et al: Parathyroid hormone-related protein: A possible endocrine function in lactation. Clin Endocrinol 37:405, 1992.

Grimm T, Wesselhoeft H: Zur Genetik des Williams-Beuren-Syndroms und der isolierten Form der supravalvulaeren Aortenstenose (Untersuchungen von 128 Familien). Z Kardiol 69:168, 1980.

Heaney RP, Skillman TG: Calcium metabolism in normal human pregnancy. J Clin Endocrinol Metab 33:881, 1971.

Hicks MJ, Levy ML, Alexander J, Flaitz CM: Subcutaneous fat necrosis of the newborn and hypercalcemia: Case report and review of the literature. Pediatr Dermatol 10:271, 1993.

Hillman LS, Rojanasathit S, Slatopolsky E, et al: Serial measurements of serum calcium, magnesium, parathyroid hormone, calcitonin and 25-hydroxyvitamin D in premature and term infants during the first week of life. Pediatr Res 11:739, 1977.

Hillman LS, Salmons S, Dokoh S: Serum 1,25-dihydroxyvitamin D concentrations in premature infants: Preliminary results. Calcif Tissue Int 37:223, 1985.

Hillyard CJ, Myers C, Abeyasekera G, et al: Katacalcin: A new plasma calcium-lowering hormone. Lancet 1:846, 1983.

Hollis BW, Pittard WB: Evaluation of the total fetomaternal vitamin D relationships at term: Evidence for racial differences. J Clin Endocrinol Metab 59:652, 1984.

Igarashi T, Sekine Y, Kawato H, et al: Transient neonatal distal renal tubular acidosis with secondary hyperparathyroidism. Pediatr Nephrol 6:267, 1992.

Juppner H: Molecular cloning and characterization of a parathyroid hormone-parathyroid hormone-related peptide receptor: A member of an ancient family of G protein-coupled receptors. Curr Opin Nephrol Hypertens 3:371, 1994.

Kaji H, Sugimoto T, Kanatani M, et al: Carboxyl-terminal PTH fragments stimulate osteoclast-like cells formation and osteoclastic activity. Endocrinology 134:1897, 1994.

Kamitsuka MD, Williams MA, Nyberg DA, et al: Renal calcification: A complication of dexamethasone therapy in preterm infants with bronchopulmonary dysplasia. J Perinatol 15:359, 1995.

Karlen J, Aperia A, Zetterstrom R: Renal excretion of calcium and phosphate in preterm and term infants. J Pediatr 106:814, 1985.

Kawashima H, Torikai S, Kurokawa K: Localization of 25-hydroxyvitamin D3-1-hydroxylase and 24-hydroxylase along the rat nephron. Proc Natl Acad Sci U S A 78:1199, 1986.

Kent GN, Price RI, Gutteridge DH, et al: The efficiency of intestinal calcium absorption is increased in late pregnancy but not in established lactation. Calcif Tissue Int 48:293, 1991.

Koo WW, Krug-Wispe S, Neylan M, et al: Effect of three levels of vitamin D intake in preterm infants receiving high mineral-containing milk. J Pediatr Gastroenterol Nutr 21:182, 1995.

Kooh SW, Fraser D, Reilly BJ, et al: Rickets due to calcium deficiency. N Engl J Med 297:1264, 1977.

Kovacs CS, Lanske B, Hunzelman JL, et al: Parathyroid hormone–related peptide (PTHrP) regulates fetal–placental calcium transport through a receptor distinct from the PTH/PTHrP receptor. Proc Natl Acad Sci U S A 93:15233, 1996.

Kruse K, Irle U, Uhlig R: Elevated 1,25-dihydroxyvitamin D serum concentrations in infants with subcutaneous fat necrosis. J Pediatr 122:460, 1993.

Kumar R, Cohen WR, Silva P, et al: Elevated 1,25-dihydroxyvitamin D plasma levels in normal human pregnancy and lactation. J Clin Invest 63:342, 1979.

Leroyer-Alizon E, David L, Anast CS, et al: Immunocytological evidence for parathyroid hormone in human parathyroid glands. J Clin Endocrinol Metab 52:513, 1981.

Leroyer-Alizon E, David L, Dubois PM: Evidence for calcitonin in the thyroid gland of normal and anencephalic human fetuses: Immunocytological localization, radioimmunoassay, and gel filtration of thyroid extracts. J Clin Endocrinol Metab 50:316, 1980.

Lewis DW: What was wrong with Tiny Tim? Am J Dis Child 146:1403, 1992.

Lightwood RL: Idiopathic hypercalcemia with failure to thrive. Arch Dis Child 27:302, 1952.

Loughead JL, Mimouni F, Tsang RC: Serum ionized calcium concentrations in normal neonates. Am J Dis Child 142:516, 1988.

Loughead JL, Mughal Z, Mimouni F, et al: Spectrum and natural history of congenital hyperparathyroidism secondary to maternal hypocalcemia. Am J Perinatol 74:350, 1990.

Lynch BJ, Rust RS: Natural history and outcome of neonatal hypocalcemic and hypomagnesemic seizures. Pediatr Neurol 11:23, 1994.

Manz F, Scharer K, Janka P, Lombeck J: Renal magnesium wasting, incomplete tubular acidosis, hypercalciuria and nephrocalcinosis in siblings. Eur J Pediatr 128:67, 1978.

Markestadt T, Ulstein M, Strandjord RE, et al: Anticonvulsant drug therapy in human pregnancy: Effects of serum concentrations on vitamin D metabolites in maternal and cord blood. Am J Obstet Gynecol 150:254, 1984.

Martin NDT, Snodgrass GJAI, Cohen RD: Idiopathic infantile hypercalcemia—a continuing enigma. Arch Dis Child 59:605, 1984.

Marx SJ, Attie MF, Spiegel AM, et al: An association between neonatal severe primary hyperparathyroidism and familial hypocalciuric hypercalcemia in three kindreds. N Engl J Med 306:257, 1982.

Mimouni F, Tsang RC, Hertzberg VS, Miodovnik M: Polycythemia, hypomagnesemia and hypocalcemia in infants of diabetic mothers. Am J Dis Child 140:798, 1986.

Minagawa M, Yasuda T, Kobayashi Y, Niimi H: Transient pseudohypoparathyroidism of the neonate. Eur J Endocrinol 133:151, 1995.

Moyer-Mileur L, Luetkemeier M, Boomer LC, Chan GM: Effect of physical activity on bone mineralization in premature infants. J Pediatr 127:620, 1995.

Murer H, Biber J: Molecular mechanisms in renal phosphate reabsorption. Nephrol Dial Transplant 10:1501, 1995.

Nako Y, Fukushima N, Tomomasa T, et al: Hypervitaminosis D after prolonged feeding with a premature formula. Pediatrics 92:862, 1993.

Naveh-Many T, Silver J: Regulation of parathyroid hormone gene expression by hypocalcemia, hypercalcemia, and vitamin D in the rat. J Clin Invest 86:1313, 1990.

Nelson N, Illes L: The Q-oTc and Q-Tc interval and ionized calcium in newborns. Clin Physiol 9:39, 1989.

Neufeld M, Maclaren N, Blizzard R: Autoimmune polyglandular syndrome. Pediatr Ann 9:154, 1980.

Nishiyama S, Tomoeda S, Inoue F, et al: Self-limited neonatal familial hyperparathyroidism associated with hypercalciuria and renal tubular acidosis in three siblings. Pediatrics 86:421, 1990.

Nussbaum SR, Zabradnik R, Lavigne J, et al: Highly sensitive two-site immunoradiometric assay for parathyrin and its clinical utility in evaluating patients with hypercalcemia. Clin Chem 33:1364, 1987.

Olsen HS, Cepeda MA, Zhang QQ, et al: Human stanniocalcin: A possible hormonal regulator of mineral metabolism. Proc Natl Acad Sci U S A 93:1792, 1996.

Parkinson DB, Thakker RV: A donor splice site mutation in the parathyroid hormone gene is associated with autosomal recessive hypoparathyroidism. Nature Genet 1:149, 1992.

Paulson SK, DeLuca HF: Vitamin D metabolism during pregnancy. Bone 7:331, 1986.

Pearce SHS, Trump D, Wooding C, et al: Calcium-sensing receptor mutations in familial benign hypercalcemia and neonatal hyperparathyroidism. J Clin Invest 96:2683, 1995.

Peeden JN Jr, Rimoin DL, Lachman RS, et al: Spondylometaphyseal dysplasia, Sedaghatian type. Am J Med Genet 44:651, 1992.

Pitkin RM, Reynolds WA, Williams GA, et al: Calcium metabolism in normal pregnancy: A longitudinal study. Am J Obstet Gynecol 133:781, 1979.

Pittard WB 3d, Geddes KM, Hulsey TC, Hollis BW: Osteocalcin, skeletal alkaline phosphatase, and bone mineral content in very low-birth-weight infants: A longitudinal assessment. Pediatr Res 31:181, 1992.

Pollak M, Brown EM, Chou Y-HC, et al: Mutations in the human Ca^{+2}-sensing receptor gene cause familial hypocalciuric hypercalcemia and neonatal severe hyperparathyroidism. Cell 75:1297, 1993.

Pollak MR, Brown EM, Estep HL, et al: An autosomal dominant form of hypocalcemia caused by a mutation in the human Ca^{+2}-sensing receptor gene. Nature Genet 8:303, 1994.

Pronicka E, Gruszczynska B: Familial hypomagnesemia with secondary hypocalcemia—autosomal or X-linked inheritance? J Inherit Metab Dis 14:397, 1991.

Reeve LE, Chesney RW, DeLuca HF: Vitamin D of human milk: Identification of biologically active forms. Am J Clin Nutr 36:122, 1982.

Robertie PG, Butterworth JF 4th, Prielipp RC, et al: Parathyroid hormone in marked hypocalcemia in infants and young children undergoing repair of congenital heart disease. J Am Coll Cardiol 20:672, 1992.

Rodriguez-Soriano J, Vallo A: Pathophysiology of the renal acidification defect present in the syndrome of familial hypomagnesaemia-hypercalciuria. Pediatr Nephrol 8:431, 1994.

Romagnoli C, Zecca E, Tortorolo G, et al: Plasma thyrocalcitonin and parathyroid hormone concentrations in early neonatal hypocalcemia. Arch Dis Child 62:580, 1987.

Ron M, Levitz M, Chuba J, Dancis J: Transfer of 25-hydroxyvitamin D3 and 1,25-dihydroxyvitamin D3 across the perfused human placenta. Am J Obstet Gynecol 148:370, 1984.

Ross R, Halbert K, Tsang RC: Determination of the production and metabolic clearance rates of 1,25-dihydroxyvitamin D3 in the pregnant sheep and its chronically catheterized fetus by primed infusion technique. Pediatr Res 26:633, 1989.

Rowe JC, Rowe D, Horak E, et al: Hypophosphatemia and hypercalcemia in small premature infants fed human milk: Evidence for inadequate dietary phosphorus. J Pediatr 104:112, 1984.

Rubin LP, Posillico JT, Anast CS, Brown EM: Circulating levels of biologically active and immunoreactive intact parathyroid hormone in human newborns. Pediatr Res 29:201, 1991.

Rubin LP, Yeung B, Vouros P, et al: Evidence for human placental synthesis of 24,25-dihydroxyvitamin D3 and 23,25-dihydroxyvitamin D3. Pediatr Res 34:98, 1993.

Rude RH, Oldham SB, Singer FR: Functional hypoparathyroidism and parathyroid end-organ resistance in human magnesium deficiency. Clin Endocrinol 5:209, 1976.

Rude RH, Oldham SB, Sharp CF, Singer FR: Parathyroid hormone secretion in magnesium deficiency. J Clin Endocrinol Metab 47:800, 1978.

Ryan SW, Truscott J, Simpson M, James J: Phosphate, alkaline phosphatase and bone mineralization in preterm infants. Acta Paediatr 82:516, 1993.

Saan R, David L, Thomas A, et al: Congenital hyperparathyroidism and vitamin D deficiency secondary to maternal hyperparathyroidism. Acta Paediatr Scand 65:381, 1976.

Saarela T, Simila S, Koivisto M: Hypercalcemia and nephrocalcinosis in patients with congenital lactase deficiency. J Pediatr 127:920, 1995.

Saggese G, Baroncelli GI, Bertelloni S, et al: Intact parathyroid hormone levels during pregnancy, in healthy term neonates and in hypocalcemic preterm infants. Acta Paediatr Scand 80:36, 1991.

Saggese G, Bertelloni S, Baroncelli GI, et al: Evaluation of a peptide family encoded by the calcitonin gene in selected healthy pregnant women. Horm Res 34:240, 1990.

Sagy M, Birenbaum E, Balin A, et al: Phosphate-depletion syndrome in a premature infant fed human milk. J Pediatr 96:683, 1980.

Salle BL, Glorieux FH: Assessment of bone mineral content in infants: The new age. Acta Paediatr 82:709, 1993.

Sanjad SA, Sakati NA, Abu Osba YK, et al: A new syndrome of congenital hypoparathyroidism, seizure, growth failure and dysmorphic features. Arch Dis Child 66:193, 1991.

Sargent JD, Stukel TA, Kresel J, Klein RZ: Normal values for random urinary calcium to creatinine ratios in infancy. J Pediatr 123:393, 1993.

Savani RC, Mimouni F, Tsang RC: Maternal and neonatal hyperparathyroidism as a consequence of maternal renal tabular acidosis. Pediatrics 91:661, 1993.

Schanler RJ, Rifka M: Calcium, phosphorus and magnesium needs for the low-birth-weight infant. Acta Paediatr Suppl 405:111, 1994.

Schipani E, Langman CB, Parfitt AM, et al: Constitutively activated receptors for parathyroid hormone and parathyroid hormone–related peptide in Jansen's metaphyseal chondrodysplasia. N Engl J Med 335:736, 1996.

Scott SM, Ladenson JH, Aguanno JJ, Hillman LS: Ionized calcium in the sick neonate. Pediatr Res 13:505, 1979.

Seely EW, Brown EM, DeMaggio DM, et al: A prospective study of calciotropic hormones in pregnancy and postpartum: Reciprocal changes in serum intact parathyroid hormone and 1,25-dihydroxyvitamin D. Am J Obstet Gynecol 176:214, 1997.

Senterre J, Salle B: Renal aspects of calcium and phosphorus metabolism in preterm infants. Biol Neonate 53:220, 1988.

Seow WK: A study of the development of the permanent dentition in very-low-birthweight children. Pediatr Dent 18:379, 1996.

Shimizu H, Kodama S, Takeuchi A, et al: Idiopathic infantile hypercalcemia discovered in the newborn period. Acta Paediatr Jpn 36:720, 1994.

Shprintzen RJ: Velocardiofacial syndrome and DiGeorge sequence [letter] J Med Genet 31:423, 1994.

Sowers M, Corton G, Shapiro B, et al: Changes in bone density with lactation. JAMA 269:3130, 1993.

Specker BL, Lichtenstein P, Mimouni F, et al: Calcium-regulating hormones and minerals from birth to 18 months of age: A cross sectional study, II: Effects of sex, race, age, season and diet on serum minerals, parathyroid hormone, and calcitonin. Pediatrics 77:891, 1986.

Steichen JJ, Tsang RC, Gratton TL, et al: Vitamin D homeostasis in the perinatal period: 1,25(OH)2D in maternal, cord and neonatal blood. N Engl J Med 302:315, 1980.

Stevenson JC, Hillyard CJ, MacIntyre I: A physiological role for calcitonin: Protection of the maternal skeleton. Lancet ii:769, 1979.

Stewart CL, Devarajan P, Mulroney SE, et al: Transport of calcium and phosphorus. *In* Polin RA, Fox WW (Eds): Fetal and Neonatal Physiology. Philadelphia, WB Saunders, 1992, p 1223.

Tanaka Y, Hatano S, Nishi Y, Usui T: Nutritional copper deficiency in a Japanese infant on formula. J Pediatr 96:255, 1980.

Tomomura A, Tomomura M, Fukushige T, et al: Molecular cloning and expression of serum calcium-decreasing factor (caldecrin). J Biol Chem 270:30315, 1995.

Tsang RC, Chen I, Hayes W, et al: Neonatal hypocalcemia in infants with birth asphyxia. J Pediatr 64:428, 1974.

Urban Z, Helms C, Gerardo A, et al: 7q11.23 deletions in Williams syndrome arise as a consequence of unequal meiotic crossover [letter]. Am J Hum Genet 59:958, 1996.

Usdin TB, Gruber C, Bonner TI: Identification and functional expression of a receptor selectively recognizing parathyroid hormone, the PTH2 receptor. J Biol Chem 270:15455, 1995.

Veldhuis JD, Kulin HE, Demers CM, Lambert PW: Infantile hypercalcemia with subcutaneous fat necrosis: Endocrine studies. J Pediatr 95:460, 1979.

Venkataraman PS, Tsang R, Greer F, et al: Late infantile tetany and secondary hyperparathyroidism in infants fed humanized cow milk formula: Longitudinal follow-up. Am J Dis Child 139:664, 1985.

Watney PJ, Chance GW, Scott P, Thompson JM: Maternal factors in neonatal hypocalcemia: A study in three ethnic groups. BMJ 2:432, 1971.

Webber SA, Hatchwell E, Barber JCK, et al: Importance of microdeletions of chromosomal region 22q11 as a cause of selected malformations of the ventricular outflow tracts and aortic arch: A three-year prospective study. J Pediatr 129:26, 1996.

Widdowsen EM, Dickerson JWT: Chemical composition of the body. *In* Comar CL, Brunner F (Eds): Mineral Metabolism. Orlando, Academic Press, 1961.

Williams JC, Barratt-Boyes BG, Lowe JB: Supravalvular aortic stenosis. Circulation 24:1311, 1961.

Wilson DI, Burn J, Scambler P, Goodship J: DiGeorge syndrome, part of CATCH 22. J Med Genet 30:852, 1993.

Wilson DI, Cross IE, Goodship JA, et al: A prospective cytogenetic study of 36 cases of DiGeorge syndrome. Am J Hum Genet 51:957, 1992.

Wilson SG, Retallack RW, Kent JC, et al: Serum free 1,25-dihydroxyvitamin D and the free 1,25-dihydroxyvitamin D index during a longitudinal study of human pregnancy and lactation. Clin Endocrinol 32:613, 1990.

Yasuda T, Banville D, Hendy GN, Goltzman D: Characterization of the human parathyroid hormone-like peptide gene: Functional and evolutionary aspects. J Biol Chem 264:7720, 1989.

Zaloga GP, Chernow B, Cook D, et al: Assessment of calcium homeostasis in the critically ill patient—diagnostic pitfalls of the McLean Hastings nomogram. Ann Surg 202:587, 1985.

Zanardo V, Dani C, Trevisanuto D, et al: Methylxanthines increase renal calcium excretion in preterm infants. Biol Neonate 68:169, 1995.

Ziegler EE, O'Donnell AM, Nelson SE, Forman SJ: Body composition of the reference fetus. Growth 40:329, 1976.

CHAPTER 100

Disorders of the Adrenal Gland*

Daniel H. Polk

GENERAL CONSIDERATIONS

The mammalian adrenal gland is a dual endocrine organ, consisting of a cortex and medulla within a common capsule. The two glands have distinct embryologic origins and different functions. In the 5th week of fetal life, the primitive adrenal cortex is formed from cells of the coelomic mesoderm. During the 7th week, the cortex is invaded by ectodermal neural crest cells that aggregate to form a central cell mass, the adrenal medulla.

Adrenal cortical cells produce a variety of steroid hormones, and the medulla produces the catecholamines norepinephrine and epinephrine. Adrenal catecholamines are important for successful neonatal adaptation. The consequences of catecholamine excess are discussed in the section on neuroblastoma. This chapter focuses on development and function of the adrenal cortex.

Adrenal steroid production can be detected by the 9th week of gestation, and by the 12th week the adrenal glands are as large as the kidneys. The primitive, or fetal, zone of the adrenal cortex accounts for most of its bulk. This zone involutes slowly during the 3rd trimester and more rapidly after birth. There is no intrinsic difference between male and female adrenal function in utero, and the adrenal does not contribute to normal genital differentiation. The primary role of the fetal adrenal appears to be production of inactive steroid precursors, such as dehydroepiandrosterone sulfate, which the placenta can convert to estrogens.

During the second half of pregnancy, the permanent adrenal cortex emerges as a distinct anatomic structure and begins to synthesize the glucocorticoids and mineralocorticoids that are required for successful adaptation to extrauterine life (Fig. 100–1). Glucocorticoids, of which cortisol is the most important in humans, play a major role in carbohydrate metabolism. They promote gluconeogenesis and synthesis of liver glycogen and act to elevate blood glucose levels. Cortisol has enzyme-inducing capabilities that doubtless affect many organs and prepare the infant for postnatal life. This aspect of glucocorticoid action has been most completely delineated in the discussion of late fetal development (see Chapter 4).

Early evidence suggesting that human chorionic gonadotropin (hCG) is adrenocorticotropic in the fetus during the first half of pregnancy varies with reports failing to demonstrate such an effect (Walsh et al, 1979). In the second half of pregnancy, the growth and secretory activity of the adrenal depend on adrenocorticotropic hormone (ACTH).

The ACTH concentration is relatively high in fetal, neonatal, and maternal plasma (Simila et al, 1977; Winters et al, 1974). Winters and coworkers reported mean afternoon ACTH values of 43 ± 4 pg/mL in normal adults, 194 ±

29 pg/mL in maternal plasma during labor, 241 ± 33 pg/mL in cord blood before 34 weeks' gestation, 143 ± 7 pg/mL in cord blood at term, and 120 ± 8 pg/mL during the 1st week of life. Measurements of fetal and neonatal plasma ACTH levels reflect secretion of this hormone by the fetoplacental unit, because ACTH does not cross the placenta. There is evidence for placental as well as pituitary secretion of ACTH; pro-opiomelanocortin (POMC), the precursor peptide for ACTH, is demonstrable in placental extracts. Control of fetal ACTH production is uncharacterized. Large amounts of biologically active corticotropin-releasing hormone (CRH) are present in fetal and cord blood (Goland et al, 1988).

There is limited information regarding plasma cortisol concentrations during fetal life. In 1973, Beitins and coworkers reported a mean value of 2.1 ± 1.2 μg/dL in fetuses of 3 to 6 months' gestation as compared with a mean value of 6.3 ± 2.9 μg/dL in the cord blood of infants born at term by cesarean section. Although the human fetal plasma cortisol concentration may increase between midpregnancy and term, there is not the abrupt increase in late pregnancy that has been observed in some nonprimate animals. Cortisol crosses the placenta, but approximately 80% of maternal cortisol is converted to cortisone when it traverses the placenta (Campbell and Murphy, 1977). Cord arterial levels are higher than cord venous levels, indicating that a significant amount of circulating cord cortisol is of fetal origin. It has been estimated that near term, 50% to 75% of fetal plasma cortisol is derived from the fetal adrenal, and 25% to 50% originates from maternal cortisol that traverses the placenta (Beitins et al, 1973). The concentrations of corticosteroid-binding globulin (CBG), total cortisol, and unbound cortisol are lower in fetal than in maternal plasma (Ohrlander et al, 1976; Simmer et al, 1974).

Fetal plasma cortisol increases in association with a stress-induced increase in maternal plasma cortisol during labor (Ohrlander et al, 1976), and there is evidence to indicate that fetal plasma ACTH or cortisol is altered in response to fetal stress. Fetal plasma ACTH levels are elevated after labor and vaginal delivery when compared with elective cesarean section (Pohjavuori and Fyhrquist, 1983). Plasma levels of corticotropin-releasing factor (CRF) and arginine vasopressin (AVP), the primary hypothalamic peptides involved in stimulation of ACTH secretion, are also elevated at birth (Sasaki et al, 1984). The perinatal increase in ACTH is associated with fetal adrenal secretion of cortisol and pregnenolone (Arai and Yanaihara, 1977) as well as other POMC-derived peptides. In contrast to reports in other species, there is no evidence to support the concept that the human fetal adrenal cortex plays a role in the initiation of labor.

The plasma cortisol concentration decreases after birth, reaching a nadir at 24 to 36 hours of age, and then rapidly

---

*Revised from C. Anast, 5th edition.

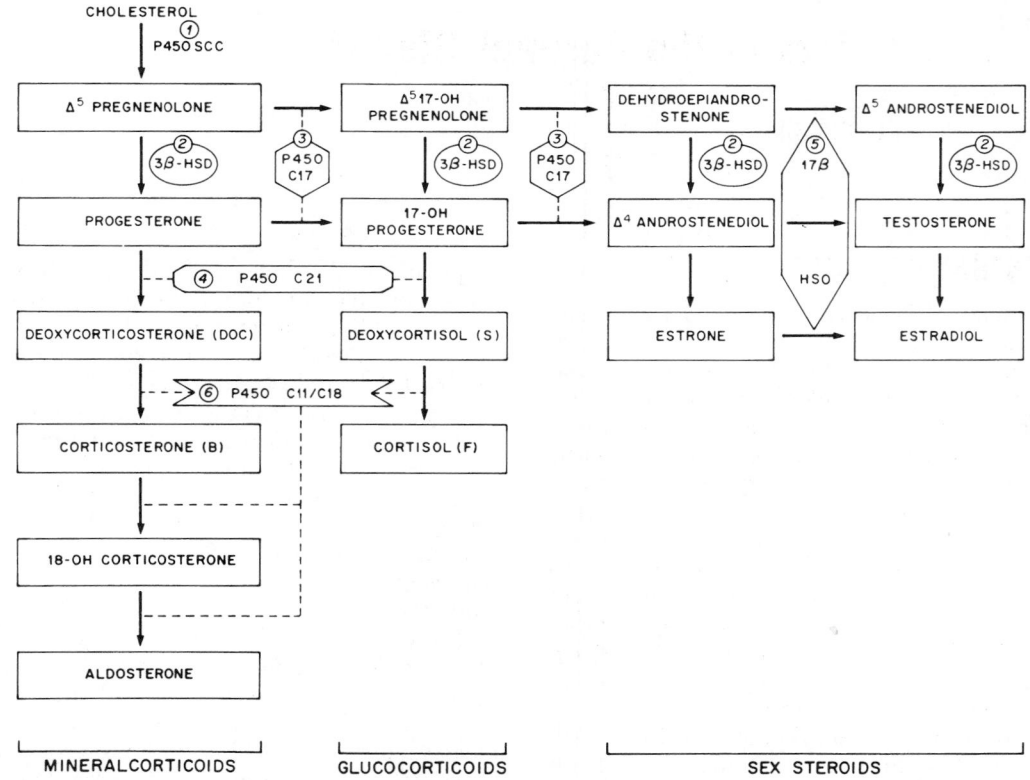

FIGURE 100–1. Steroid biosynthetic pathways: 1, P450 SCC, formerly termed *20,22-desmolase,* mediates side-chain cleavage and 20,22-hydroxylation of cholesterol. 2, 3β-hydroxysteroid dehydrogenase, a non-P450 enzyme. 3, P450 c17 mediates both 17-hydroxylation and 17,20-lyase activities. 4, P450 c21 mediates 21-hydroxylation. 5, 17β-hydroxysteroid oxidoreductase, a non-P450 enzyme. 6, P450 c11/c18 mediates three reactions: 11β-hydroxylation, 18-hydroxylation, and 18-methyl oxidation.

increases to levels that are equal to or greater than those later in infancy (Sperling, 1980). The response to exogenous ACTH is normal immediately after birth, but there is a smaller response in the initial days of life corresponding to the period of low plasma cortisol levels. After 5 days of life, there is a pronounced increase in serum cortisol in response to exogenous ACTH (Sperling, 1980). The age at which the circadian rhythm of ACTH and cortisol secretion becomes established is not known. The adult pattern of high morning and low nocturnal plasma 17-hydroxycorticosteroids does not appear to be present before 1 to 3 years of age (Franks, 1967).

ACTH contributes relatively little to the regulation of aldosterone synthesis. The main homeostatic mechanism involves release of renin from renal juxtaglomerular cells in response to diminished renal arteriolar pressure. Renin acts to increase angiotensin II, which in turn, increases aldosterone secretion and has a direct effect on vascular contractility. Increased intravascular pressure or volume acts to diminish renin production, thus closing the feedback loop. Low sodium and high potassium intakes also enhance aldosterone secretion, the latter by a mechanism that does not depend on the renin–angiotensin system.

The newborn is able to regulate aldosterone secretion in an appropriate manner. Kowarski and colleagues (1974) found that aldosterone levels in umbilical and newborn venous plasma were comparable to adult values. The levels

increased to values above the adult range between 11 days and 1 year of age.

The fetus does not depend on endogenous glucocorticoid or mineralocorticoid production. Its needs can be met by transplacental passage of maternal hormones, and deficiencies, per se, are not evident at delivery. However, the catastrophic consequences of defective organogenesis or of enzymatic errors soon become apparent. Glucocorticoid deficiency can result in hypoglycemia within hours of birth, and mineralocorticoid deficiency manifests as salt loss and adrenal crisis within days or weeks after birth. The differential diagnosis of neonatal adrenal insufficiency is presented in the following sections and summarized in Table 100–1.

ADRENAL HEMORRHAGE

The large adrenal glands of the newborn are vulnerable to mechanical trauma during labor and delivery. Focal hemorrhage at the junction of the fetal zone and the permanent cortex is a common finding in infants dying of other causes (Boyd, 1967). Minor bleeding into the adrenal cortex may not produce symptoms but may be associated with adrenal calcifications noted incidentally later in life. To result in adrenal insufficiency, hemorrhage must involve both adrenals and at least 90% of the adrenocortical tissue must be destroyed (Black and Williams, 1973). Massive adrenal hemorrhage is an uncommon but life-threatening event. Predisposing factors include large birth weight, prolonged or difficult labor, placental bleeding, and perinatal anoxia. Adrenal hemorrhage may occur in premature infants without obvious trauma. The adrenal may be a site of hemorrhage in infants with sepsis or with primary coagulopathies. In most published series, affected male infants outnumber females by 3 to 1.

The affected infant may show signs of hypovolemic shock, but commonly presents with pallor, apnea, and hypothermia accompanied by a falling hematocrit and jaundice. A large flank mass may be palpated, more commonly on the right side. In only 5% to 10% of cases the hemorrhage is bilateral. The condition must be differentiated from renal vein thrombosis. In both conditions, there may be azotemia, proteinuria, and hematuria, but in adrenal hemorrhage the hematuria is of a lesser degree. Intravenous pyelograms typically reveal no function on the affected side when a renal vein or artery has been thrombosed. Adrenal hemorrhage typically displaces the kidney downward and rotates it laterally, with flattening of the upper calyces.

Signs of adrenal insufficiency may be subtle and delayed. Even with extensive bilateral hemorrhage, functioning islands of zona glomerulosa cells are generally preserved. Hypoglycemia is a more common finding than is salt loss.

Immediate management is directed at blood and volume replacement. Indications for steroid replacement include bilateral hemorrhage, failure to respond to volume expansion, hypoglycemia, polyuria, hyponatremia, hyperkalemia, or anticipated general anesthesia.

Within 1 to 3 weeks after the hemorrhage, a thin zone of calcification appears at the periphery of the gland. As blood and necrotic adrenal tissue are resorbed, the area of calcification shrinks and assumes the shape and size of the original gland. Such calcification may persist for life. Adrenal function generally improves with resolution of the hemorrhage. ACTH stimulation with measurement of plasma or urinary corticoid responses is indicated after the acute

phase of the illness; late adrenal insufficiency has been reported.

TRANSIENT ADRENAL INSUFFICIENCY

In 1946, Jaudon described a series of 14 infants with dehydration, salt loss, and failure to gain weight. All responded to steroid replacement, and in each case it was eventually possible to discontinue treatment without a recurrence of symptoms. Other researchers have reported additional infants with an apparent delay in maturation of adrenal cortical function. Bongiovanni (1962) described a premature infant with marked hyponatremia and hyperkalemia and no detectable serum cortisol or urinary corticoids. The infant did well on cortisol replacement, and at age 6 months, following discontinuation of steroid treatment, he showed normal cortisol and aldosterone responses to ACTH. Kreines and DeVaux (1971) described a similar course in an infant born to a mother with Cushing syndrome resulting from an adrenal adenoma.

Rarely, transient adrenal insufficiency is observed in a newborn whose mother received glucocorticoids during pregnancy. The type of glucocorticoid administered to the mother may be important in this regard. Substantial amounts of cortisol and prednisolone are converted to less active metabolites during their traversal across the placenta as well as in the fetal circulation by both the placenta and other fetal tissues. Thus, when the mother is given cortisol or prednisolone, the fetal plasma concentration of these active steroids is only a small fraction of that in the mother (Dorr et al, 1986). However, following administration of dexamethasone to the mother, the concentrations in fetal and maternal plasma are similar (Charnvises et al, 1985).

The combination of hyponatremia, hyperkalemia, and polyuria may occur in acutely ill infants under a variety of other circumstances that do not involve adrenal insufficiency. Infants recovering from hypovolemic shock and acute tubular necrosis demonstrate these features, as do infants given furosemide without replacement of sodium. In doubtful cases, one may collect serum and urine specimens during a therapeutic trial of desoxycorticosterone acetate. This agent, given intramuscularly in a dosage of 0.5 mg/kg per day, provides a potent mineralocorticoid effect and does not inhibit pituitary ACTH or interfere with serum cortisol or urinary corticoid estimation. If steroid measurements do not support a diagnosis of adrenal insufficiency and if serum sodium levels do not increase and serum potassium levels decline in response to desoxycorticosterone acetate, then the medication may safely be discontinued.

ADRENAL HYPOPLASIA

In the absence of pituitary gland function, the adrenal glands fail to develop normally. The adrenal glands of anencephalic infants weigh less than 0.5 g at birth, as opposed to normal combined weights greater than 6 g. Arrested development of the adrenals has been attributed to a lack of trophic stimulation of ACTH. Pituitary hypoplasia can also occur in infants without major central nervous system malformations. In these infants, severe hypoglycemia can result in death within the first 48 hours of life.

TABLE 100–1

Causes of Neonatal Adrenal Insufficiency

Adrenal hemorrhage
Transient adrenal insufficiency
Congenital adrenal hypoplasia
    Primary: X-linked, autosomal recessive
    Secondary: Adrenocorticotropic hormone (ACTH) deficiency
Congenital adrenal hyperplasia
    21-hydroxylase deficiency (P450 C21)
    11-beta-hydroxylase deficiency (P450 C11/C18)
    17-hydroxylase deficiency (P450 C17)
    3-beta-hydroxysteroid dehydrogenase deficiency (3-HSD)
    20,22-desmolase deficiency (P450 SCC)
Isolated aldosterone deficiency
    18-hydroxylase deficiency (P450 C11/C18)
Pseudohypoaldosteronism
Congenital adrenal ACTH resistance
Neonatal adrenoleukodystrophy
Infantile glycerol kinase deficiency

Blizzard and Alberts (1956) described a male infant who had, in addition, microphallus and cryptorchidism. The association has been noted in several other cases and probably reflects a lack of trophic hormone stimulation of both adrenals and testes. Prompt glucocorticoid replacement is required.

Adrenal hypoplasia occurs in infants with anatomically and functionally intact pituitary glands (Pakravan et al, 1974; Roselli and Barbosa, 1965; Sperling et al, 1973). Isolated and familial forms, with either X-linked or autosomal recessive transmission, have been described. Early recognition, cortisol replacement, and prolonged survival have permitted studies of the mechanisms that underlie familial adrenal hypoplasia. The disease is manifested in infancy or early childhood by hyperpigmentation as a consequence of elevated ACTH levels and by hypoglycemia as a consequence of glucocorticoid deficiency. In contrast to congenital adrenal hyperplasia, familial adrenal hypoplasia has no associated excess of abnormal steroid metabolites. Mineralocorticoid production is generally unimpaired. A possible defect might involve the adrenal membrane receptor for ACTH (Migeon et al, 1968).

CONGENITAL ADRENAL HYPERPLASIA

Adrenal steroid biosynthesis requires a sequence of enzymatic reactions that are illustrated in Figure 100–1. Studies using techniques of molecular biology have demonstrated that the synthesis of cortisol and aldosterone requires only five apoenzymes, some having more than one function. Four of these enzyme systems belong to the cytochrome P450 family of oxidases. The two mitochondrial P450 enzymes are involved in the side-chain cleavage of cholesterol (P450 SCC, formerly 20,22-desmolase) and the hydroxylation of cholesterol carbons C11 and C18 (P450 C11/C18). There are two microsomal P450 enzymes: one having 17-hydroxylase and 17,20-desmolase activities (P450 C17) and one with 21-hydroxylase activity (P450 C21). The fifth enzyme, microsomal in location, has 3-beta-hydroxysteroid dehydrogenase and delta-5–3 ketosteroid isomerase activities (3β-HSD). In recent years, complementary DNA probes have been cloned, permitting gene mapping and sequencing of these particular protein products (Miller, 1988). The disease states in this category have several features in common. Each condition is inherited in an autosomal recessive manner. Thus, multiple sibling involvement is common, and recurrence risk in subsequent pregnancies is 25%. Each, with the exception of 18-hydroxysteroid dehydrogenase deficiency, involves hyperplasia of the adrenal cortex under the stimulus of elevated ACTH levels. In each case, the disorder may be managed well with appropriate steroid replacement.

Clinical manifestations of adrenal hyperplasia depend on the site and severity of the enzymatic block. With a block, precursors accumulate and are diverted into alternative metabolic pathways. Laboratory confirmation of a suspected defect involves measurement of these metabolites. The pathophysiology of all of these enzyme deficiencies is related to (1) the specific enzyme involved and severity of the defect, (2) the amount and type of precursor overproduction, (3) the impact of precursors on differentiation of the external genitalia, (4) the severity of glucocorticoid deficiency, and (5) the severity of mineralocorticoid deficiency. The defects listed in Table 100–1 are discussed in the following paragraphs.

Deficiency of 21-Hydroxylase

The 21-hydroxylase deficiency is the most common form of congenital adrenal hyperplasia as well as the most common cause of ambiguous genitalia. The incidence of 21-hydroxylase deficiency is estimated to be 1 in 15,000 in whites in the United States and Europe. However, the gene frequency varies in different ethnic groups, and a high incidence of the disorder (1 in 490) has been reported in the Yupik Eskimos of Alaska (Hirschfeld and Fleishman, 1969). The gene that codes for 21-hydroxylation is located on the short arm of chromosome 6 in proximity to the locus of the histocompatibility gene HLA-B and the loci for complement factors C4a and C4b (New et al, 1981). Knowledge of this genetic linkage has led to the use of human leukocyte antigen (HLA) typing in families with affected individuals for detection of heterozygotes as well as for the prenatal diagnosis of affected fetuses (Levine et al, 1980a; New et al, 1981; Pollack et al, 1981; Sherman et al, 1988). Newer techniques relying on demonstration of the specific gene defect have also been successful in the prenatal diagnosis of 21-hydroxylase deficiency (Wilson et al, 1995).

Hydroxylation at the C21 position is required for synthesis of glucocorticoids and mineralocorticoids. There are two clinical syndromes of congenital adrenal hyperplasia due to a 21-hydroxylation defect: simple virilization and virilization with salt wasting. In both forms, defective cortisol synthesis leads to increased secretion of ACTH, which, in turn, stimulates the adrenal to produce increased amounts of cortisol precursors, including androgens and androgen precursors. The plasma concentrations of 17-hydroxyprogesterone, androstenedione, and testosterone are elevated in affected patients, and the metabolites of these steroids result in increased urinary excretion of 17-ketosteroids and pregnanetriol. As a result of high levels of circulating fetal androgens, female newborns demonstrate varying degrees of virilization, ranging from mild to severe clitoral enlargement with complete labial fusion and a phallic urethra. Affected males are formed normally at birth. If the condition is untreated, both females and males show progressive virilization during infancy and early childhood with rapid linear growth and skeletal and somatic maturation. In addition to virilization, some infants show signs of salt wasting and aldosterone deficiency with failure to thrive, hyponatremia, hyperkalemia, and ultimately vascular collapse. Salt-losing crisis is uncommon before 6 days of age but occurs in approximately 50% of affected infants between 6 and 14 days of age. Patients with virilization and salt wasting are aldosterone deficient, as reflected by reduced circulating aldosterone levels and increased plasma renin activity. By contrast, patients with simple virilization have normal or elevated serum aldosterone levels and plasma renin activity in the baseline state that increase in response to sodium restriction. The reason for the increased circulating aldosterone in patients with simple virilization is uncertain.

The phenotype of 21-hydroxylase deficiency may encompass a variety of previously described abnormalities. Accumulated evidence suggests that classic congenital adrenal hyperplasia, "acquired or late onset" adrenal hyperplasia, and "cryptic" adrenal hyperplasia are all forms of 21-hydroxylase deficiency with a wide range of clinical abnormalities (Levine et al, 1980a; Lorenzen et al, 1980; New et al, 1981; Pollack et al, 1981).

Congenital adrenal hyperplasia should be suspected in all infants with ambiguous genitalia or a family history of either this condition or unexplained infant death and in all infants with vomiting, sluggish feeding, dehydration, or failure to thrive. The significant morbidity and mortality associated with this deficiency, especially in unrecognized males, has prompted screening by measurement of 17-hydroxyprogesterone (17-OHP) in filter paper blood spots.

The evaluation of an infant with ambiguous genitalia is outlined in Chapter 101. The steroidal biochemical findings in 21-hydroxylase deficiency include elevated urinary excretion of 17-ketosteroids and pregnanetriol and elevated plasma levels of 17-OHP and delta-4 androstenedione. The most useful test is the determination of plasma 17-OHP. The concentration of 17-OHP is normally elevated in umbilical cord blood with a mean value of 1700 ng/dL but rapidly decreases to 100 to 200 ng/dL after 24 hours of age (Grumbach and Conte, 1981). Although cord blood levels of 17-OHP may not be diagnostic of 21-hydroxylase deficiency, after 24 hours of age plasma 17-OHP and delta-4 androstenedione levels usually distinguish infants with 21-hydroxylase deficiency from normal infants. However, sick unaffected infants may have elevated 17-OHP and delta-4 androstenedione levels that confuse the diagnosis of 21-hydroxylase deficiency. In affected patients, the plasma 17-OHP levels usually range from 3000 to 40,000 ng/dL, depending on the age and severity of 21-hydroxylase deficiency (Grumbach and Conte, 1981). Borderline normal levels of plasma 17-OHP are rarely reported in patients with mild 21-hydroxylase deficiency or in heterozygotes. In these instances, the effect of ACTH administration on the increase of plasma 17-OHP and the ratio of 17-OHP to cortisol usually identifies affected infants (Levine et al, 1981). Cortisol levels may be normal in affected infants depending on the severity of the enzyme defect. In general, cortisol determinations are not useful in the diagnosis or management of this disease. In families with an affected member, HLA genotyping distinguishes between heterozygosity and a mild form of the disorder in a homozygous infant.

The urinary excretion of 17-ketosteroids and pregnanetriol has also been used in the diagnosis of 21-hydroxylase deficiency. During the first few days of life, the urinary 17-ketosteroids may be as high as 2 to 4 mg per 24 hours in normal infants, whereas urinary pregnanetriol may be normal in affected infants. After the early days of life, urinary 17-ketosteroid excretion values of greater than 2.5 mg per 24 hours and pregnanetriol values greater than 0.5 mg per 24 hours are diagnostic.

The combined use of HLA typing of amniotic fluid cells and the determination of 17-OHP and delta-4 androstenedione in amniotic fluid permits the definitive prenatal diagnosis of 21-hydroxylase deficiency. Amniotic fluid concentrations of 17-OHP and delta-4 androstenedione are elevated in affected fetuses between 14 and 20 weeks' gestation (Nagamani et al, 1978; Pang et al, 1980). HLA typing of amniotic fluid cells obtained from mothers who had a previously affected offspring permits identification of fetuses who are homozygous or heterozygous for 21-hydroxylase deficiency (Pollack et al, 1981). Newer techniques including allele-specific polymerase chain reaction can also be used. Various fetal treatment schemes have been used to block the influence of unchecked ACTH stimulation on adrenal steroid production in affected fetuses (David and Forest, 1984). Maternal administration of dexamethasone inhibits fetal ACTH overproduction especially early in pregnancy (1st trimester), which can significantly reduce virilization in affected females (Mercado et al, 1995).

In the infant with severe salt loss, initial treatment requires volume expansion with isotonic saline in 5% or 10% dextrose administered intravenously at a rate of 100 to 120 mL/kg per day with 25% of this amount given in the first 2 hours. Fifty mg/m² of hydrocortisone sodium succinate should be given as a bolus intravenously and another 50 to 100 mg/m² added to the infusion fluid over the first 24 hours. When hyponatremia and hyperkalemia are present, desoxycorticosterone acetate may be given intramuscularly in a dosage of 1 mg every 24 hours.

Chronic medical treatment of congenital adrenal hyperplasia requires the provision of sufficient cortisol to suppress adrenal androgen production and to protect against stress. The required dosage is generally in the range of 15 to 20 mg/m² of hydrocortisone per day, given in three divided oral doses. Cortisone acetate may be given intramuscularly every 3 days for long-term replacement. The dosage should be doubled or tripled during acute illnesses, and intramuscular cortisone acetate should be substituted in a dosage of 25 to 50 mg/m² per day during protracted vomiting or surgical stress. Inadequate dosage permits excessive production of androgens and excessively rapid growth and skeletal maturation. Overdosage produces slowing of growth and other features of the Cushing syndrome.

Infants with proven or suspected salt loss should also receive mineralocorticoid replacement and salt supplements (1 to 3 g/day orally). Fludrocortisone acetate (Florinef) in an oral dose of 0.025 to 0.1 mg/day is commonly used for mineralocorticoid replacement. During the first 2 years of life, some physicians prefer to implant one or two 125-mg desoxycorticosterone acetate pellets rather than prescribe Florinef. The pellets are absorbed slowly and last for 6 to 9 months. Suboptimal growth occurs with inadequate replacement, and excessive doses produce failure to thrive as well as hypertension.

Besides the evaluation of growth, skeletal maturation, and signs of virilization, adequacy of glucocorticoid therapy is assessed by monitoring urinary excretion of 17-ketosteroids and pregnanetriol and plasma levels of 17-OHP (Hughes and Winter, 1976). In this regard, plasma levels of 17-OHP have not been found more useful than urinary 17-ketosteroids (Grumbach and Conte, 1981). Indeed, there is uncertainty regarding the value of plasma 17-OHP measurements in assessing the quality of treatment (Frisch et al, 1981). Plasma levels of sodium and potassium and plasma renin activity are useful in evaluating the adequacy of mineralocorticoid therapy.

Surgical correction of mild to moderate clitoral enlargement is generally not required. Clitoral size tends to remain stable or even decrease as the child grows. When indicated, surgery may be performed at 4 to 12 months of age. The best age for correction of labial fusion is probably about 2 years. Some girls may require more complicated vaginoplasty at a later age. The prognosis for normal psychosexual development and reproductive function is excellent in boys and girls with 21-hydroxylase deficiency.

Deficiency of 11-Beta-Hydroxylase

Hydroxylation at the C11 position is required for cortisol and aldosterone synthesis. As originally reported by Eberlein and Bongiovanni (1956), deficiency of 11-beta-hydroxylase results in virilization of the female infant together with a variable degree of hypertension. There is accumulation of the immediate precursors 11-deoxycortisol (compound S) and desoxycorticosterone in the plasma and increased urinary excretion of their tetrahydro metabolites. Whereas compound S is biologically inert, desoxycorticosterone has mineralocorticoid effects and contributes to the hypertensive state. Neither compound is recognized by the hypothalamic-pituitary regulatory system, and an increase in ACTH secretion occurs (Levine et al, 1980b). Hydrocortisone replacement suppresses ACTH production and thereby prevents further virilization and relieves hypertension. Transient hyponatremia and hyperkalemia may occur after the initiation of glucocorticoid therapy as a result of inhibition of ACTH-stimulated desoxycorticosterone secretion before the inhibited renin-angiotensin-aldosterone system has had time to recover (Holcombe et al, 1980). Monitoring of treatment requires determination of urinary 17-ketosteroid or tetrahydro-S excretion.

The 11-beta-hydroxylase gene is located on chromosome 8 and thus is not linked to the HLA loci. The frequency of 11-beta-hydroxylase deficiency is rare, comprising less than 3% of the total cases of adrenal hyperplasia. In certain Middle Eastern populations, the two defects occur with equal frequency. The defect may be partial, and hypertension either may be absent or may not appear until late childhood or adulthood. Similarly, signs of virilization in the female may not appear until adolescence (Cathelineau et al, 1980).

Deficiency of 17-Hydroxylase

Hydroxylation at the C17 position is required for cortisol, androgen, and estrogen synthesis but is not involved in the synthesis of mineralocorticoids. Several different allelic gene defects for cytochrome P450 C17 have been associated with decreased activity of 17-hydroxylase. Biglieri and coworkers (1966) described four adult females with lack of secondary sexual development, hyperkalemic alkalosis, and hypertension who proved to have deficiency of this enzyme. They demonstrated excessive plasma levels of desoxycorticosterone and corticosterone and excessive excretion of their urinary metabolites. Aldosterone levels tended to be low, presumably owing to inhibition of the renin–angiotensin system. In affected XX females, both internal and external genitalia are normal. In males, impaired testosterone synthesis by the fetal testes results in either phenotypic female external genitalia or ambiguous genitalia, but the female müllerian duct derivatives are absent. Failure of pubertal development in females and defective virilization in males, as described by New and Suvannakul (1970), provide evidence that adrenal and gonadal 17-hydroxylase activities are under common genetic control. Cortisol replacement inhibits ACTH production and relieves hypertension. Exogenous androgens or estrogens are required at the age of puberty.

Deficiency of 3-Beta-Hydroxysteroid Dehydrogenase

Conversion of pregnenolone to progesterone requires oxidation at the 3 position and isomerization of a double bond from the delta-5 to the delta-4 position. The defect results in defective synthesis of cortisol, aldosterone, and potent androgens and estrogens. Bongiovanni (1962) originally described several infants with defects in this crucial enzyme complex. These infants had severe salt and water loss and, despite adequate steroid replacement, did not survive infancy. Urinary and plasma steroid metabolites are predominantly of the delta-5, beta-hydroxy configuration and include pregnanetriol and dihydroepiandrosterone. However, during the first few weeks of life, the delta-5, 3-beta-hydroxysteroids may be elevated in normal premature and full-term infants. It is therefore necessary to interpret the levels of these steroids in early infancy in relation to normal values for age. As a result of accumulation of dihydroepiandrosterone, a weak androgen, and defective conversion to the more potent androgens, androstenedione and testosterone, both males and females have partial virilization. Males have hypospadias and may have a bifid scrotum with or without cryptorchidism. Females have slight to moderate clitoral enlargement, which may be associated with labial fusion. Affected males have developed gynecomastia at puberty. Mild forms of 3-beta-hydroxysteroid dehydrogenase deficiency may not become clinically evident until adolescence (Parks et al, 1971; Rosenfield et al, 1980). In infancy, urinary 17-ketosteroids and pregnanetriol are elevated. The latter finding differentiates the defect from the more common deficiency of 21-hydroxylase. Both glucocorticoid and mineralocorticoid replacement are required throughout life.

Deficiency of 20,22-Desmolase

Conversion of cholesterol to pregnenolone is an essential step in the synthesis of mineralocorticoids, glucocorticoids, androgens, and estrogens. In rare instances, infants with a homozygous defect in P450 SCC activity have been described. They cannot synthesize any glucocorticoid, mineralocorticoid, or sex steroid. Defects in this early set of reactions lead to severe salt and water loss and hypoglycemia. Female infants have normal genitalia at birth but are incapable of producing estrogens at the time of puberty. Male infants with this defect usually have feminized external genitalia with a blind vaginal pouch but no müllerian duct derivatives. Little or no C21 or C19 steroids are detectable in plasma or urine. The adrenal glands and gonads are enlarged and filled with cholesterol and other lipids, hence, the name "lipoid adrenal hyperplasia." Most patients have died in infancy, but in a few (who perhaps have had less severe defects), steroid treatment has permitted prolonged survival.

ISOLATED ALDOSTERONE DEFICIENCIES
Deficiency of 18-Hydroxylase

The final steps in aldosterone synthesis involve hydroxylation and dehydrogenation at C18. Deficiency at this level results in aldosterone deficiency and salt loss without any alteration in the synthesis of cortisol or the sex steroids. Several authors have postulated that the transient salt wasting of infancy described by Jaudon (1946) might result from delayed maturation of these enzymes. Appropriate therapy consists of a mineralocorticoid and supplemental sodium chloride. Glucocorticoid replacement is not required.

PSEUDOHYPOALDOSTERONISM

Pseudohypoaldosteronism (end-organ unresponsiveness to aldosterone) is a salt-wasting disorder that results from renal tubular unresponsiveness to aldosterone (Proesmans et al, 1973). Characteristically, there is urinary sodium wasting, hyponatremia, hyperkalemia, vomiting, and dehydration in early infancy. Urinary 17-ketosteroids and plasma androgens are normal, whereas plasma aldosterone and renin concentrations are elevated. The infants do not respond to mineralocorticoid therapy, and treatment with supplemental sodium chloride is necessary.

CONGENITAL ADRENAL RESISTANCE TO ADRENOCORTICOTROPIN HORMONE

Infants affected by congenital adrenal resistance to ACTH have recurrent hypoglycemia and skin hyperpigmentation. Serum electrolytes are normal, and there are no manifestations of mineralocorticoid deficiency. These findings suggest glucocorticoid deficiency and ACTH excess. Plasma concentrations of cortisol are low, whereas those of aldosterone and corticosterone are normal or elevated. Urinary 17-ketosteroids are low, whereas urinary aldosterone levels are elevated. Plasma ACTH levels are strikingly elevated, and there is no response in plasma 17-hydroxysteroids, cortisol, or aldosterone levels to pharmacologic doses of ACTH. Aldosterone levels do increase in response to sodium restriction. These findings suggest adrenal resistance to ACTH with preservation of a normal mineralocorticoid response to the renin–angiotensin system. Accordingly, the adrenal glands of affected patients are small, with atrophy of the zona fasciculata and sparing of the zona glomerulosa. Treatment consists of appropriate glucocorticoid replacement.

NEONATAL ADRENOLEUKODYSTROPHY

There seems to be a neonatal form of adrenoleukodystrophy, a chronic X-linked disease of childhood that is inherited as an autosomal recessive trait and may present in the weeks following birth. Jaffe and coworkers (1982) have described infants with craniofacial and central nervous system abnormalities that are associated with progressive adrenal insufficiency. They postulated that the progressive adrenal defects might be secondary to the primary disorder of fatty acid metabolism with effects on receptor binding of ACTH.

INFANTILE GLYCEROL KINASE DEFICIENCY

Infantile glycerol kinase deficiency is an X-linked disease that presents in male infants as an acute salt-wasting crisis with blood steroid determinations that suggest adrenal hypoplasia (Kohlschutter et al, 1987). They are distinguished from the latter by elevated blood glycerol and creatinine kinase levels. The diagnosis may be delayed until the onset of developmental and myopathic symptoms. The diagnosis is confirmed by demonstrating the mitochondrial enzyme defect in biopsy material. These patients may actually represent a deletion in the X-chromosome for three closely linked gene loci (glycerol kinase, adrenal hypoplasia, and progressive muscular dystrophy).

ADRENAL OVERACTIVITY

Glucocorticoid excess results in hyperphagia, obesity, and impairment of linear growth, together with hypertension, osteoporosis, and polycythemia. The Cushing syndrome is extremely rare in infants except as a result of administration of glucocorticoids or ACTH. The cases that have been reported show a preponderance of adrenal tumors, both adenomas and carcinomas. There may be overproduction of androgens as well as glucocorticoids. There is no suppression of circulating corticoids with administration of dexamethasone. Surgical treatment involves extirpation with attendant glucocorticoid replacement to prevent acute adrenal insufficiency.

REFERENCES

Arai K, Yanaihara T: Steroid hormone changes in fetal blood during labor. Am J Obstet Gynecol 127:879, 1977.

Beitins IZ, Bayard F, Ances IG, et al: The metabolic clearance rate, blood production, interconversion and transplacental passage of cortisol and cortisone in pregnancy near term. Pediatr Res 7:509, 1973.

Biglieri EG, Herron MA, Brust N: 17-Hydroxylation deficiency in man. J Clin Invest 45:1946, 1966.

Black J, Williams DI: Natural history of adrenal haemorrhage in the newborn. Arch Dis Child 48:183, 1973.

Blizzard RM, Alberts M: Hypopituitarism, hypoadrenalism and hypogonadism in the newborn infant. J Pediatr 48:782, 1956.

Bongiovanni AM: Adrenogenital syndrome with deficiency of 3β-hydroxysteroid dehydrogenase. J Clin Invest 41:2086, 1962.

Bongiovanni AM: Disorders of adrenal steroid biogenesis. In Stanbury JB, Wyngaarden JB, Fredrickson DS (Eds): The Metabolic Basis of Inherited Disease. New York, McGraw-Hill, 1972, p 857.

Boyd JF: Disseminated fibrin thromboembolism among neonates dying within 48 hours of birth. Arch Dis Child 42:401, 1967.

Campbell AL, Murphy BEP: The maternal-fetal cortisol gradient during pregnancy and delivery. J Clin Endocrinol Metab 45:435, 1977.

Cathelineau G, Brerault J, Fiet J, et al: Adrenocortical 11β-hydroxylation defect in adult women with postmenarcheal onset of symptoms. J Clin Endocrinol Metab 51:287, 1980.

Charnvises S, de Fencl M, Osthanondh R, et al: Adrenal steroids in maternal and cord blood after dexamethasone administration at midterm. J Clin Endocrinol Metab 61:1220, 1985.

David M, Forest MG: Prenatal treatment of congenital adrenal hyperplasia resulting from 21-hydroxylase deficiency. J Pediatr 105:799, 1984.

Dorr HG, Versmold HT, Sippell WG, et al: Antenatal beta-methasone therapy: Effects on maternal, fetal and neonatal mineralocorticoids, glucocorticoids and progestins. J Pediatr 108:990, 1986.

Eberlein WR, Bongiovanni AM: Plasma and urinary corticosteroids in hypertensive form of congenital adrenal hyperplasia. J Biol Chem 223:85, 1956.

Franks RD: Diurnal variation of plasma 17-hydroxycorticosteroids in children. J Clin Endocrinol Metab 27:75, 1967.

Frisch H, Parth K, Schober E, et al: Circadian patterns of plasma cortisol, 17-hydroxyprogesterone, and testosterone in congenital adrenal hyperplasia. Arch Dis Child 56:208, 1981.

Goland RS, Wardlow SL, Blum M, et al: Biologically active corticotropin-releasing hormone in maternal and fetal plasma during pregnancy. Am J Obstet Gynecol 159:884, 1988.

Grumbach MM, Conte FA: Disorders of sex differentiation. *In* Williams RH (Ed): Textbook of Endocrinology. Philadelphia, WB Saunders, 1981, p 423.

Hirschfeld AJ, Fleishman JK: An unusually high incidence of salt-losing congenital adrenal hyperplasia in the Alaskan Eskimo. J Pediatr 75:492, 1969.

Holcombe JA, Keenan B, Nichols B, et al: Neonatal salt loss in the hypertensive form of congenital adrenal hyperplasia. Pediatrics 65:777, 1980.

Hughes IA, Winter JSD: The application of a serum 17-OH-progesterone radioimmunoassay to the diagnosis and management of congenital adrenal hyperplasia. J Pediatr 88:766, 1976.

Jaffe R, Cromline P, Hashida Y, et al: Neonatal adrenoleukodystrophy. Clinical, pathological and biochemical delineation of a syndrome affecting both males and females. Am J Physiol 198:100, 1982.

Jaudon JC: Addisons' disease in an infant. J Clin Endocrinol Metab 6:558, 1946.

Kohlschutter A, Willig HP, Schlamp D, et al: Infantile glycerol kinase deficiency—A condition requiring prompt identification. Eur J Pediatr 146:575, 1987.

Kowarski A, Katz H, Migeon CJ: Plasma aldosterone concentration in normal subjects from infancy to adulthood. J Clin Endocrinol Metab 38:498, 1974.

Kreines K, DeVaux WD: Neonatal adrenal insufficiency associated with maternal Cushing's syndrome. Pediatrics 47:516, 1971.

Levine LS, Dupont B, Lorenzen F, et al: Genetic and hormonal characterization of cryptic 21-hydroxylase deficiency. J Clin Endocrinol Metab 53:1193, 1981.

Levine LS, Dupont B, Lorenzen F, et al: Cryptic 21-hydroxylase deficiency in families of patients with classical congenital adrenal hyperplasia. J Clin Endocrinol Metab 51:1316, 1980a.

Levine LS, Rauh W, Gottediener K, et al: New studies of the 11β-hydroxylase and 18-hydroxylase enzymes in the hypertensive form of congenital adrenal hyperplasia. J Clin Endocrinol Metab 50:258, 1980b.

Lorenzen F, Pang S, New M, et al: Studies of the C-21 and C-19 steroids and HLA genotyping in siblings and parents of patients with congenital adrenal hyperplasia due to 21-hydroxylase deficiency. J Clin Endocrinol Metab 50:572, 1980.

Mercado AB, Wilson RC, Cheng KC, et al: Prenatal treatment and diagnosis of congenital adrenal hyperplasia owing to steroid 21 hydroxylase deficiency. J Clin Endocrinol Metab 80(7):2014, 1995.

Migeon CJ, Kenny FM, Kowarski A: The syndrome of congenital unresponsiveness to ACTH. Pediatr Res 2:501, 1968.

Miller WL: Molecular biology of steroid hormone synthesis. Endocrinol Rev 9:295, 1988.

Nagamani M, McDonough P, Ellegood J, et al: Maternal and amniotic fluid 17α-hydroxyprogesterone levels during pregnancy. Diagnosis of congenital adrenal hyperplasia in utero. Am J Obstet Gynecol 130:791, 1978.

New MI, Dupont B, Pang S, et al: An update of congenital adrenal hyperplasia. Recent Prog Horm Res 37:105, 1981.

New MI, Suvannakul L: Male pseudohermaphroditism due to 17α-hydroxylase deficiency. J Clin Invest 49:1930, 1970.

Ohrlander S, Genuser G, Encroth P: Plasma cortisol levels in the human fetus during parturition. Obstet Gynecol 48:381, 1976.

Pakravan P, Kenny FM, Depp R, et al: Familial congenital absence of adrenal glands: Evaluation of glucocorticoid, mineralocorticoid, and estrogen metabolism in the perinatal period. J Pediatr 84:74, 1974.

Pang S, Levine L, Cederquist M, et al: Amniotic fluid concentrations of Δ5 and Δ4 steroids in fetuses with congenital adrenal hyperplasia due to 21-hydroxylase deficiency and in anencephalic fetuses. J Clin Endocrinol Metab 51:223, 1980.

Parks GA, New MI, Bermudez JA, et al: A pubertal boy with the 3β-hydroxysteroid dehydrogenase defect. J Clin Invest 33:269, 1971.

Pohjavuori M, Fyhrquist F: Vasopressin, ACTH and neonatal haemodynamics. Acta Paediatr Scand Suppl 305:79, 1983.

Pollack MS, Levine LS, O'Neill GJ, et al: HLA linkage and B14, DR1, BfS haplotype association with the genes for late onset and cryptic 21-hydroxylase deficiency. Am J Hum Genet 33:540, 1981.

Proesmans W, Geussens H, Corbeel L, et al: Pseudohypoaldosteronism. Am J Dis Child 126:510, 1973.

Roselli A, Barbosa LT: Congenital hypoplasia of the adrenal glands: Report of 2 cases in sisters, with necropsy. Pediatrics 35:70, 1965.

Rosenfield RL, Rich B, Wolfsdorf J, et al: Pubertal presentation of congenital Δ5-3β-hydroxysteroid dehydrogenase deficiency. J Clin Endocrinol Metab 51:345, 1980.

Sasaki A, Liotta AS, Luckey MM, et al: Immunoreactive corticotropin-releasing factor is present in human maternal plasma during the third trimester of pregnancy. J Clin Endocrinol Metab 59:812, 1984.

Sherman SL, Aston CE, Morton NE, et al: A segregation and linkage study of classical and nonclassical 21-hydroxylase deficiency. Am J Hum Genet 42(6):830, 1988.

Simila S, Kauppila A, Ulikorkala O, et al: Adrenocorticotrophic hormone during the first day of life. Eur J Pediatr 124:173, 1977.

Simmer HH, Frankland MV, Greipel M: Unbound unconjugated cortisol in umbilical cord and corresponding maternal plasma. Gynecol Invest 5:199, 1974.

Sperling MA: Newborn adaptation: Adrenocortical hormones and ACTH. *In* Tulchinsky D, Ryan KJ (Eds): Maternal-Fetal Endocrinology. Philadelphia, WB Saunders, 1980, p 387.

Sperling MA, Wolfsen AR, Fisher DA: Congenital adrenal hypoplasia: An isolated defect of organogenesis. J Pediatr 82:44, 1973.

Walsh SW, Normal RL, Novy MJ: In utero regulation of rhesus monkey fetal adrenals: Effects of dexamethasone, adrenocorticotropin, thyrotropin releasing hormone, prolactin, human chorionic gonadotropin and melanocyte stimulating hormone in fetal and maternal plasma steroids. Endocrinology 104:1805, 1979.

Wilson RC, Wei JQ, Cheng KC, et al: Rapid deoxyribonucleic acid analysis by allele-specific polymerase chain reaction for detection of mutations in the steroid 21-hydroxylase gene. J Clin Endocrinol Metab 80(5):1635, 1995.

Winters AJ, Oliver S, Colston C, et al: Plasma ACTH levels in the human fetus and neonate as related to age and parturition. J Clin Endocrinol Metab 39:269, 1974.

CHAPTER 101

Abnormalities of Sexual Differentiation*

Daniel H. Polk

GENERAL CONSIDERATIONS

Anatomic differentiation of the external genitalia is usually complete in the human infant by birth, enabling the obstetrician and proud parents to proclaim "It's a girl" or "It's a boy." Permanent gender assignment is made instantaneously. Occasionally, genital differentiation is incomplete or ambiguous. The physician's reactions to this medical emergency have an immense impact on these children and their families. It is important to have a sound understanding of normal sexual development and to be able to initiate steps that will lead to appropriate gender assignment, diagnosis, and management.

Two principles emerge in the consideration of embryologic sexual differentiation. First, sexual organs at all three levels—gonads, internal duct structures, and external genitalia—develop from identical undifferentiated structures in the male and female fetus. Second, differentiation along female anatomic lines proceeds passively unless opposed by active male factors.

Male and female gonads develop from anlagen located on the urogenital ridge. Before 6 weeks of gestational age, testis and ovary are indistinguishable. In the fetus with a 46,XY chromosome constitution, definite testicular differentiation occurs rapidly over the ensuing weeks. By 12 weeks, both testicular testosterone concentration (Reyes et al, 1973) and the ability to convert pregnenolone to testosterone enzymatically (Siiteri and Wilson, 1974) are maximal. Peak concentrations of testosterone in the fetal circulation are reached at 16 weeks and are comparable to those of the adult male. Thereafter, the testosterone concentration decreases, and after 24 weeks, the concentration is in the early pubertal range (Kaplan and Grumbach, 1978). In contrast, ovarian differentiation occurs later in gestation and is not a prerequisite for normal female genital development. In the fetus with a 46,XX chromosome complement, oocytes appear at about the 12th week. Primordial follicles, containing oocytes surrounded by a layer of granulosa cells, are recognizable by the 12th week. The circulating estrogens in the fetus are primarily of placental origin, with little contribution from the fetal ovary. The ovary has no apparent role in sex differentiation of the female genital tract.

The advances in molecular biology have significantly contributed to current understanding of the genes controlling early sexual development. The testis-determining factor gene has been putatively mapped to the short arm of the 4 chromosome. Expression of this gene, called SR-4 (sex determining region 4) is required for testis determination of the pleuripotent gonadal anlagen (Berta et al, 1990; Koopman et al, 1990). The protein encoded by this locus contains a region termed the HMG which binds DNA,

resulting in a conformational change. Sex-reversing mutations in the SR-4 gene generally involve sequences within the HMG region. SR-4 expression, in turn, likely regulates expression of other important genes; evidence for regulation of antimüllerian factor has been proposed. Other regulators of SR-4 activity have also been suggested. These include steroidogenic factor 1 (SF-1) as well as products of the Wilms' tumor gene (WT-1) (Hsu et al, 1995; Ingraham et al, 1994). Finally, the genes involved in campomyelic dysplasia (SOX 9) and X-linked adrenal hypoplasia (DAX-1) have also been suggested to play roles in regulating gonadal development. However, precise mechanisms for their involvement remain to be described.

A schematic of fetal genital development is shown in Figure 101–1. At 7 weeks' gestation, the fetus has precursors of both male and female genital ducts. The müllerian ducts are anlagen of the fallopian tubes, uterus, and proximal vagina. Wolffian ducts are anlagen for the epididymis, vas deferens, seminal vesicles, and ejaculatory ducts of the male. The experiments of Josso (1972) have shown that the fetal testis produces a locally active macromolecular hormone that induces regression of the müllerian ducts. This action cannot be mimicked by androgens. However, high local concentrations of testosterone, produced by the fetal testis, are required for further development of the wolffian ducts. Genital duct development is nearly complete by 12 weeks of gestation.

Male and female external genitalia are identical during the 2nd month of pregnancy. Three structures are easily recognizable (see Fig. 101–1). These structures are the genital tubercle, the genital folds, and the genital swellings. Testosterone—more specifically, its active intracellular metabolite dihydrotestosterone (DHT)—is required for male differentiation. Without testosterone, the genital tubercle remains small and forms the clitoris, the genital folds remain separate and form the labia minora, and the genital swellings form the labia majora. Under the influence of DHT, the genital tubercle enlarges and forms the penis, the genital folds fuse to form a phallic urethra, and the genital swellings fuse to form the scrotum. Fusion is complete by the 12th week of gestation, but phallic enlargement continues to term.

Most of the known errors of human sexual differentiation can be provisionally explained by genetic or biochemical alterations in the aforementioned sequence of events. Conte and Grumbach (1989) have written excellent detailed reviews of this area. This discussion follows the classification scheme shown in Table 101–1. The first category entails disorders of gonadal differentiation, usually in association with abnormal number or structure of the X or Y chromosomes. The second category involves virilization of the female fetus; the third, undervirilization of the male fetus. The last category involves anatomic defects that,

---

*Revised from C. Anast, 5th edition.

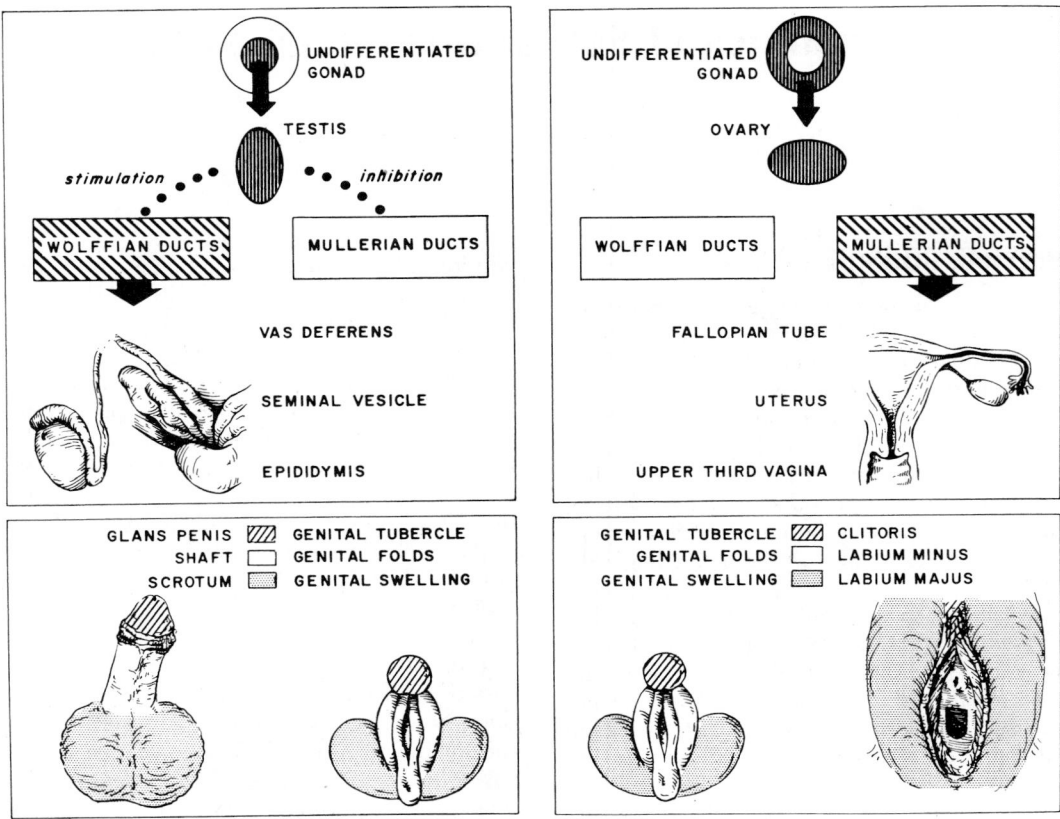

FIGURE 101–1. Outline of genital development. Note that gonadal development occurs from a common indifferent gonad, the internal genitalia develop from separate primordia present in both sexes, and the external genitalia develop in a continuous transformation of anlage common to both sexes. (From Fedeman DD: Disorders of sexual development. N Engl J Med 277:351, 1967. Reprinted by permission of the New England Journal of Medicine.)

in most cases, do not have a definite chromosomal or hormonal etiology.

DISORDERS OF GONADAL DIFFERENTIATION
Klinefelter Syndrome

Klinefelter syndrome is one of the most common sex chromosome anomalies, occurring in 1 in 1000 male births. The 47,XXY chromosome constitution arises during meiotic division in either parent or, less commonly, from mitotic nondisjunction in the zygote and is associated with advanced maternal age. Infants with 47,XXY karyotype as a group have lower birth weights than control subjects and have an increased incidence of major and minor congenital anomalies, especially clinodactyly. Although the testes may be noticeably small during infancy, there are seldom any genital abnormalities, and the diagnosis is seldom made during early childhood. Presenting features in older children and adolescents include low verbal intelligence quotient (I.Q.), behavioral disorders, poor gross motor control, eunuchoid habitus, gynecomastia, and variable virilization. Variants involving 46,XY/47,XXY individuals have been described. In addition 46,XX males occur with an incidence of 1 in 20,000 males. They share the endocrine manifesta-

tions of 47,XXY individuals but typically have normal stature. The biochemical basis for this defect is unknown but may involve Y chromosome translocations (Page et al, 1987b).

Turner Syndrome and Variants

Turner syndrome is defined as gonadal dysgenesis due to a missing or structurally defective X chromosome. The 45,X karyotype is associated with a high intrauterine mortality rate. Its frequency is 1 per 20 spontaneous abortuses but only 1 per 10,000 live newborn females. The incidence of 45,X karyotype is increased in the pregnancies of teenaged mothers. The condition should be suspected in female infants with webbing of the neck, edema of the extremities, or coarctation of the aorta. In most infants with gonadal dysgenesis, the external genitalia and internal duct structures are unequivocally female. Half the individuals with 45,X genotype also exhibit renal anomalies, some of which may not be suspected clinically (Shawker et al, 1987). More subtle findings include low birth weight for gestational age, ptosis, hypertelorism, micrognathia, hypertension, low-set or deformed ears, cubitus valgus, and dysplasia of fingernails and toenails. In the newborn, pleural effusions and ascites that clear spontaneously are not uncommon, and pericardial effusion has been reported. In other affected girls, somatic abnormalities are minimal and the condition is suspected because of short stature, failure of breast development, and primary amenorrhea at the age of puberty. A lack of feedback inhibition of hypothalamic-pituitary axis by the dysgenic ovary is reflected in elevated serum follicle-stimulating hormone (FSH) and luteinizing hormone (LH) levels in affected infants as early as 5 days of age (Conte et al, 1980).

Roughly 85% of the girls with gonadal dysgenesis have a 45,X karyotype. The remainder have either mosaicism or a structural abnormality of the X chromosome. Structural abnormalities include isochromosomes of either the short (XXpi) or long arm (XXqi), deletion of the short (XXp⁻) or long arm, or ring chromosomes. The diagnosis is thus confirmed by chromosome analysis and banding studies.

Suspicion and confirmation of gonadal dysgenesis in a newborn confers an unusual responsibility upon the physician. There is seldom any doubt about gender assignment, because these infants are females. However, their ovaries have in most instances regressed to vestigial streaks by the time of birth. Most of these girls are short and infertile as

TABLE 101–1

Classification of Abnormalities of Sexual Differentiation

I. Disorders of gonadal differentiation
  A. Klinefelter syndrome: 47,XXY and variants
  B. Turner syndrome (gonadal dysgenesis): 45,X and variants
  C. Pure gonadal dysgenesis: 46,XX
  D. True hermaphroditism
II. Virilization of the female fetus: 46,XX
  A. Due to maternal ingestion of drugs
  B. Due to maternal overproduction of androgens
  C. Due to congenital adrenal hyperplasia
    1. P450 C21 deficiency
    2. 3-Beta-hydroxysteroid dehydrogenase deficiency
    3. P450 C11/C18 deficiency
III. Undervirilization of the male fetus: 46,XY
  A. Anorchia, or vanishing testis syndrome
  B. Genetic defects in testosterone biosynthesis
    1. Defects common to cortisol and testosterone pathways
      a. 3-Beta-hydroxysteroid dehydrogenase deficiency
      b. P450 C17 deficiency
    2. Defects unique to androgen and estrogen synthesis
      a. 17, 20-Desmolase deficiency
      b. 17-Beta-hydroxysteroid oxidoreductase deficiency
  C. End-organ insensitivity to testosterone
    1. 5-Alpha-reductase deficiency
    2. Testicular feminization
    3. Partial testicular feminization
  D. Testicular unresponsiveness to human chorionic gonadotropin and luteinizing hormone
  E. Maternal ingestion of progestins and estrogens
IV. Anatomic abnormalities
  A. As isolated findings
    1. Hypospadias
    2. Cryptorchidism
    3. Persistence of müllerian structures
  B. Associated with other birth defects

adults. The parents should be told that their child will be shorter than average and probably infertile and will require hormone replacement at the age of puberty to foster a growth spurt, breast development, and menstrual cycles. However, even though streak gonads are the rule in 45,X gonadal dysgenesis, exceptions have been documented. Primary follicles have been observed in the ridges of some 45,X individuals in adolescence, and this correlates with the rare occurrence of menarche and a variable but attenuated period of regular menses. Moreover, conceptions have been documented in some women in whom extensive karyotypic studies revealed only 45,X cell line in multiple tissues (King et al, 1978; Kohn et al, 1980). Some fertile 45,X women may be unrecognized sex chromosome mosaics.

Mosaicism involving the Y chromosome is less common than classic Turner syndrome and produces a wider variety of phenotypes. Infants with 45,X/46,XY karyotypes commonly have ambiguous genitalia. Gender assignment should be in accordance with the expected potential for adult sexual function. Gonads in these individuals generally consist of bilateral dysgenic testis and a contralateral gonadal streak. Either or both gonads may have failed to produce müllerian-inhibiting substance, and there may be a uterus and unilateral or bilateral fallopian tubes. Depending on the extent and timing of intrauterine testosterone production, there may also be well-developed wolffian structures. Short stature and the somatic abnormalities of Turner syndrome are inconstant findings. Dysgenic gonads are predisposed to neoplasia and should be removed at an early age. Hormone replacement at the age of puberty must be concordant with the sex of rearing.

Pure Gonadal Dysgenesis

Pure gonadal dysgenesis is a term applied to phenotypic females with bilateral streak gonads who lack the somatic stigmata of Turner syndrome and who are of normal or tall stature. Karyotype may be either 46,XX or 46,XY. The internal and external genitalia of the 46,XX individuals with gonadal dysgenesis are normal female. The 46,XX patients seldom show clitoral enlargement, may show ovarian function at puberty, and are not prone to gonadal neoplasms. Familial cases are not uncommon in 46,XX gonadal dysgenesis, and transmission is consistent with an autosomal recessive trait. Deafness is an associated finding in some families with 46,XX gonadal dysgenesis (Simpson, 1976). Inheritance consistent with an X-linked or male-limited dominant trait has been observed. Usually, the external and internal genital tract is completely female. However, clitoral enlargement occurs, and affected siblings may have ambiguous external genitalia and development of the genital ducts. Both H-Y antigen–positive and H-Y antigen–negative forms have been described, findings that further reflect the genetic heterogeneity of this syndrome.

True Hermaphroditism

True hermaphroditism is a rare condition that requires the presence of both ovarian and testicular tissue in the same individual. The tissue may be present in the same or opposite gonads. In almost half of the cases there is an ovotestis on one side and an ovary or testis on the other. In one fifth of cases there are bilateral ovotestes, and in one third there is an ovary on one side and a testis on the other. The external genitalia are extremely variable, but roughly three fourths of patients have phallic enlargement, generally with hypospadias, and many have been raised as males. Cryptorchidism is common, and an inguinal hernia that may contain a gonad or uterus is present in about half of the cases. A uterus is usually present and often asymmetric. Genital ducts develop in accordance with the function of the ipsilateral gonad. Most patients with an ovotestis have predominantly female development of the genital ducts. Chromosomal findings are varied and do not correlate with gonadal histology or external genital appearance. Approximately 70% of patients with true hermaphroditism are X chromatin-positive. Van Niekerk (1981) reported that of 148 patients, 89 were 46,XX, 18 were 46,XY, 21 were XX/XY chimeras, and the remainder were sex chromosome mosaics. All patients with true hermaphroditism are H-Y antigen-positive. The presence of H-Y antigen in 46,XX true hermaphroditism supports the postulate that the structural gene for H-Y antigen is on an autosome and not the Y chromosome. Therefore, an autosomal mutation affecting the structural gene for H-Y antigen results in the differentiation of a testis or ovotestis in an XX individual (Fraccaro et al, 1979). However, until the sites of the putative regulatory genes that may affect the expression of H-Y are determined, the pathogenesis of true hermaphroditism in relationship to H-Y antigen remains uncertain.

At puberty, breast development is common, menses occurs in more than half the patients, and virilization occurs in a large number. Although spermatogenesis is rare, ovulation is not uncommon, and pregnancy and childbirth have occurred in several patients with an XX karyotype (Kim et al, 1979).

True hermaphroditism should be considered in any infant or child with ambiguous genitalia in whom an alternative explanation cannot be established from chromosomal, hormonal, and radiologic contrast studies. Diagnosis requires laparotomy and biopsy of gonads. Management involves surgical removal of gonads, internal duct structures, and features of the external genitalia that are incongruous with gender assignment.

VIRILIZATION OF THE FEMALE FETUS

Virilization of the female fetus is the most common category of disorders producing ambiguity of the external genitalia. As previously stated, in the absence of androgens, external female genitalia proceed to develop along female lines. Androgens, which may be derived from either maternal or fetal sources, can cause the external genitalia of otherwise normal 46,XX girls to virilize. In some cases, this process is so complete as to mimic the external genitalia of a cryptorchid male. Fusion of the genital folds or the genital swellings is a result of androgen exposure before the 12th gestational week. Clitoral enlargement can occur with androgen exposure at any time. Buccal smears are chromatin-positive, and karyotypes are 46,XX. Management of underlying pathologic processes and surgical correction of anatomic abnormalities are followed by normal

pubertal development and normal adult sexual and reproductive function.

Virilization by Maternal Ingestion of Drugs

Virilization of the female fetus has been attributed to testosterone, the 19-nortestosterone progestins, progesterone, and even, paradoxically, diethylstilbestrol. In each case, a fairly small proportion of exposed infants had clinically evident virilization. There was seldom evidence of virilization in the mother (Jones, 1981). It is not known which of these compounds act directly on the external genitalia and which act indirectly through altering androgen synthesis by the mother or fetus. It seems reasonable to speculate that differences in maternal, placental, or fetal metabolism of the synthetic steroids determine which infants are affected.

The incidence of this condition has diminished as the use of synthetic estrogens and progestins for management of threatened abortion has waned. However, the condition is still seen in offspring of women who unknowingly continue to take birth control pills following conception. Severity of virilization ranges from mild clitoral enlargement to complete labial fusion with a phallic urethra. The infant does not show progressive virilization or accelerated growth and skeletal maturation after birth. Even in the presence of a positive history of maternal hormone ingestion, it is mandatory to obtain a buccal smear or a chromosome analysis and a determination of 17-ketosteroids or 17-hydroxyprogesterone to exclude other possible diagnoses.

Virilization by Maternal Overproduction of Androgens

Severe disorders of maternal androgen production generally preclude pregnancy. However, artificial induction of ovulation in a virilized woman or development of a virilizing neoplasm during pregnancy can set the stage for virilization of a female infant. In most cases, the mother has clinical signs of virilization, such as hirsutism, acne, clitoromegaly, and deepening of the voice. Virilization has been observed in a female infant born to a mother with a virilizing form of congenital adrenal hyperplasia (Kai et al, 1979). The clinical features of the offspring of virilized mothers are identical with those described previously for girls whose mothers received sex hormones. Diagnosis requires demonstration of elevated urinary 17-ketosteroids or plasma testosterone in the mother as well as exclusion of alternative diagnoses in the infant.

Congenital Adrenal Hyperplasia

The category of diseases encompassed by congenital adrenal hyperplasia is discussed more fully in Chapter 100. Inherited enzymatic blocks in the synthesis of cortisol lead to overproduction of androgens and virilization of the female fetus. Defects in P450 C21, 3-beta-hydroxysteroid dehydrogenase, or P450 C11/C18 can each produce this result. Buccal smear is chromatin-positive, and urinary excretion of 17-ketosteroids remains above 2.5 mg per 24 hours. In infants with a defect in 21-hydroxylase, the plasma 17-hydroxyprogesterone level is elevated. Treatment with cortisol suppresses adrenal androgen production and prevents further virilization and excessively rapid growth and skeletal maturation. In infants with salt-losing forms of congenital adrenal hyperplasia, cortisol and mineralocorticoid replacement are lifesaving.

UNDERVIRILIZATION OF THE MALE FETUS

Complete male genital differentiation requires the presence of testes, the ability of testes to produce testosterone, and the ability of the genital anlagen to recognize and respond to testosterone. Defects can occur at each of these levels and result in genitalia that are either ambiguous or unambiguously female. The degree of virilization of 46,XX individuals can be remarkable, and that male sex assignment to infants born with bilateral cryptochordism may result in multiple surgical and medical interventions in what otherwise would have been a normal fertile female. The converse is also true, that is, that one should not hesitate to make an assignment of female gender to individuals with third-degree hypospadias and microphallus with bilateral anorchia despite the presence of a Y chromosome.

Anorchia

A spectrum of genital anomalies is observed in patients with a 46,XY karyotype resulting from cessation of testicular function during the critical stages of male sexual differentiation between 8 and 14 weeks' gestation. Deficiency of testicular function before 8 weeks' gestation results in female external and internal genitalia, whereas lack of testicular function beginning between 8 and 10 weeks' gestation results in ambiguous genitalia. Loss of testicular function after 14 weeks' gestation results in anorchia, or vanishing testes syndrome, in which there is normal male differentiation both internally and externally but no gonadal tissue. The diagnosis of anorchia is made in infants with apparent bilateral cryptorchidism, 46,XY karyotype, and elevated circulating gonadotropin levels, who fail to demonstrate a testosterone response to human chorionic gonadotropin administration (Lustig et al, 1987). As previously discussed, gender assignment in infants with this syndrome and ambiguous genitalia should be female, despite the presence of 46,XY karyotype.

Genetic Defects in Testosterone Biosynthesis

In several varieties of congenital adrenal hyperplasia, the enzymatic defect is shared by adrenal and gonadal tissues. The result is undervirilization of the affected male resulting from impairment of fetal testosterone production. Specific defects include 3-beta-hydroxysteroid dehydrogenase and 17-beta-hydroxylase deficiencies, discussed in Chapter 100. In these conditions, the enzyme deficiency impairs synthesis of cortisol as well as testosterone.

Defects may also occur in metabolic pathways unique to the synthesis of sex steroids. The 17,20-desmolase enzyme converts 17-alpha-hydroxypregnenolone to dehydroepiandrosterone and 17-alpha-hydroxyprogesterone to androstenedione. Deficiency leads to severe hypospadias, with

or without cryptorchidism, and an elevated urinary excretion of pregnenetriol and 11-ketopregnanetriol, suggesting elevated plasma levels of 17-alpha-hydroxyprogesterone and 17-alpha-hydroxypregnenolone. Occurrence in siblings and an "aunt" indicate X-linked recessive or male-limited autosomal dominant inheritance. In 1976, Goebelsman and coworkers reported a 46,XY phenotypic female with normal external genitalia, no müllerian structures, atrophic wolffian derivatives, abdominal testes, and biochemical findings suggestive of a defect in 17,20-desmolase activity.

The next step in testosterone synthesis involves 17-beta-hydroxysteroid oxidoreductase, which converts dehydroepiandrosterone to 5-androstenediol, androstenedione to testosterone, and estrone to estradiol. Deficiency results in ambiguous genitalia and elevated plasma androstenedione and estrone levels in postpubertal patients (Conte and Grumbach, 1989). Puberty in the patients reported by Saez and colleagues (1972) was characterized by virilization and gynecomastia. The latter finding was attributed to elevated concentrations of the estrogen estrone.

End-Organ Insensitivity to Testosterone

Deficiency of 5-Alpha-Reductase

The external genital anlagen of the fetus normally possess 5-alpha-reductase activity and can convert testosterone to the active metabolite dihydrotestosterone. This compound is required for complete male genital development, and a defect at this level may explain an autosomal recessive condition known as "pseudovaginal perineoscrotal hypospadias." An interesting variant of this condition, known as the "penis at twelve" syndrome, involves marked virilization and phallic growth at puberty. This condition presumably results from an incomplete block in reductase activity, which is overcome by increases in circulating testosterone which occur at puberty (Imperato-McGinley et al, 1984). Infants with 5-alpha-reductase deficiency have 46,XY karyotype, normally differentiated testes, male internal ducts, and ambiguous external genitalia. Bilateral inguinal or labial masses, representing testes, may prompt evaluation, but usually these patients present during puberty.

Testicular Feminization

Recognition of testosterone or DHT by target tissues requires the participation of a cytoplasmic receptor protein that binds the steroid, enters the nucleus, and interacts with nuclear chromatin. Genetic disorders in the rat and mouse involving receptor defects closely parallel the human condition of testicular feminization.

In the complete form of the disorder, 46,XY infants have unambiguously female external genitalia. Unless there are inguinal hernias containing testes, recognition may be delayed until puberty, when these girls show normal breast development but lack sexual hair and fail to menstruate. The vagina ends blindly, and the uterus and fallopian tubes are absent, reflecting the intrauterine production of and response to müllerian-inhibiting substance. The disorder is familial, with multiple sibling involvement and occurrence in maternal aunts suggesting X-linked recessive or male-limited autosomal dominant inheritance. The gender assignment is unquestionably female. Gonads should be removed because of a recognized incidence of malignant degeneration. Estrogen replacement at puberty enhances breast development but does not induce menses because there is no uterus.

Partial Testicular Feminization

Partial testicular feminization implies a partial defect in the biologic actions of testosterone with an attendant partial inhibition of male genital differentiation. Wilson and co-workers (1974) have suggested that many familial cases of microphallus, hypospadias, and gynecomastia with normal testosterone production at puberty fall in this category.

Studies of DHT binding by cultured fibroblasts from genital skin have shown two patterns in both the complete and partial forms of testicular feminization (Griffen and Wilson, 1980; Kaufman et al, 1979). In one, there are quantitatively reduced or absent (complete form) cytosol receptors for DHT and testosterone; in the other, cytosol binding and nuclear binding of DHT are normal. The latter presumably represents an as yet undefined postreceptor defect or subtle qualitative abnormality in the androgen receptor itself.

Testicular Unresponsiveness to Human Chorionic Gonadotropin and Luteinizing Hormone

Another form of male pseudohermaphroditism has been described in which there is Leydig cell hypoplasia or agenesis, apparently secondary to a deficiency or abnormality of the human chorionic gonadotropin (HCG)-LH receptor on the plasma membrane of the fetal and postnatal Leydig cell (David et al, 1984). The external genitalia in these 46,XY patients were female except for slight posterior labial fusion and clitoromegaly in one patient. Separate vaginal and urethral openings were present, but uterus and fallopian tubes were absent. Plasma LH levels were elevated, and plasma FSH levels were normal. Plasma testosterone levels were low and did not increase in response to HCG. It is thought that the resistance of undifferentiated embryonic and fetal Leydig cells to HCG results in fetal testicular deficiency with female or predominantly female differentiation of the external genitalia.

Maternal Ingestion of Progestins and Estrogens

Animal studies have suggested an antiandrogen effect of progestins on the male fetus. Maternal ingestion of progestins and estrogens has been implicated but not proved as a rare cause of male undervirilization in humans. Some studies have suggested an association between progestins and hypospadias (Aarskag, 1979); others have suggested that effects of maternal diethylstilbestrol ingestion during early pregnancy on male sexual differentiation are minimal (Leary et al, 1984). In vitro studies have demonstrated that progestins can inhibit 5-alpha-reductase activity (Voight and Hsia, 1973), which as discussed earlier, converts testosterone to dihydrotestosterone, the active metabolite that is required for complete male development.

ANATOMIC ABNORMALITIES
Isolated Findings

A complete discussion of hypospadias and cryptorchidism is presented in Chapter 94. Virilization of otherwise functional 46,XX girls may at times be so remarkable as to result in the inappropriate assignment of male sex. Any child who presents with bilateral cryptorchidism and hypospadias should be carefully evaluated at the time of birth for the existence of a more serious underlying defect.

Persistence of Müllerian Ducts

A fully developed uterus and fallopian tubes may be discovered incidental to surgery in phenotypic males with normal 46,XY karyotypes. The theoretical explanation of this finding is a failure of production or recognition of müllerian-inhibiting substance. The condition may be transmitted as an autosomal recessive trait, although X-linked recessive inheritance and genetic heterogeneity have not been excluded (Summitt, 1979). Treatment consists of removal of organs that are discordant with the patient's gender.

Anatomic Abnormalities in Association with Other Defects

Malformations of the external genitalia may be a part of a more complicated embryopathy. In females, genital abnormalities may be associated with imperforate anus, renal agenesis, congenital nephritis, and other congenital malformations of the lower intestine and genitourinary tract. Drash and coworkers (1970) have reported an association between degenerative renal disease, Wilms tumor, and ambiguity of the external genitalia in males. Rimoin and Schimke's monograph (1971) has an excellent discussion of associations between genital abnormalities and largely nonendocrine syndromes. In many instances, such infants have severe defects incompatible with life, but there is still the problem of assigning gender.

EVALUATION OF INFANTS WITH AMBIGUOUS GENITALIA

It is extremely important that the evaluation of a newborn with ambiguous genitalia be carried out immediately after birth. The flow chart in Figure 101–2 indicates studies that can be carried out to provide a provisional diagnosis and a firm gender assignment within the first 72 hours. The parents should be advised that their infant's genital development has not been completed by birth, that the baby is all girl or all boy and not a little of both, that tests will be done to determine the correct sex, and that announcement

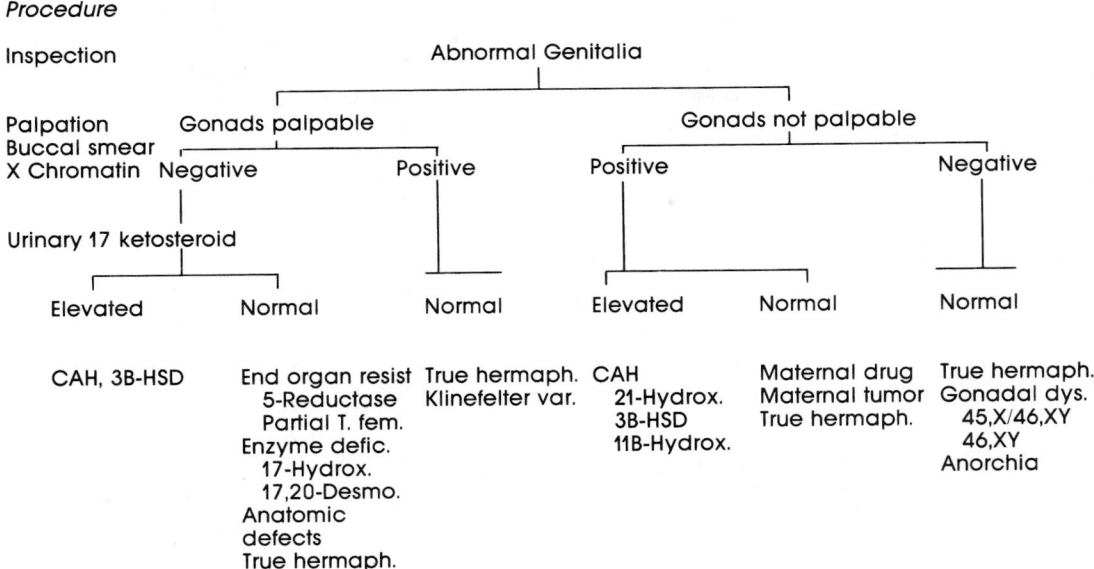

FIGURE 101–2. Investigation of the infant with ambiguous genitalia. Palpation of gonads is useful in that it usually is associated with an X chromatin-negative buccal smear and a 46,XY karyotype. However, testicular nondescent can occur in virtually all of the enzymatic deficiency syndromes. Infants with 21-hydroxylase deficiency have elevated plasma levels of 17-hydroxy-progesterone. CAH, congenital adrenal hyperplasia; 3B-HSD, 3β-hydroxysteroid dehydrogenase.

of the birth to friends and relatives should be delayed until the tests are returned.

Inspection of the external genitalia may reveal a phallic structure that is small for a male or large for a female. There is likely to be chordee with hypospadias. The genitalia swellings may be fused or open. A urologic surgeon should be involved early in the examination of the infant. If the phallic structure shows little potential for penile function, a female gender assignment should be made regardless of further findings. However, the converse is not true; the degree of phallic enlargement should not preclude a female gender assignment. Palpation of the labial-scrotal structures for gonads is extremely important, because these gonads are usually testes.

The buccal smear for determination of sex chromatin should be done on the 1st day of life. Although the number of positive chromatin bodies may be diminished in comparison to adult values, there should be no overlap of results between 46,XX females and 46,XY males. The chromatin-positive infant should be considered to have virilizing congenital adrenal hyperplasia until proved otherwise. Lymphocyte karyotyping should be done on the same indications as the buccal smear, but analysis takes weeks rather than hours. Techniques using actively dividing cells aspirated from bone marrow may shorten the time required for karyotyping.

Determination of 17-ketosteroid and pregnanetriol excretion can be accomplished in the first 72 hours. Infants with congenital adrenal hyperplasia resulting from a deficiency of 21-hydroxylase or 3-beta-hydroxysteroid dehydrogenase show an increase rather than a decrease in 17-ketosteroid excretion during the 1st week, with levels remaining above 2.5 mg per 24 hours. A striking increase in

plasma 17-hydroxyprogesterone is found in infants with defective 21-hydroxylation. Vomiting, dehydration, hyperkalemia, and hyponatremia are observed in salt-losing forms of 21-hydroxylase and 3-beta-hydroxysteroid dehydrogenase deficiencies.

Obtaining the history is extremely important. There should be a complete inquiry about all medications taken during pregnancy. Family history may reveal unexplained infant deaths among siblings of infants with salt-losing congenital adrenal hyperplasia. Infants with defects in testosterone synthesis or with partial testicular feminization commonly have hypogonadal maternal uncles or maternal "aunts" with primary amenorrhea.

By 72 hours, a definite gender assignment can be made in most cases. Chromatin-positive infants almost always are female. Those who do not have congenital adrenal hyperplasia, virilization from maternal drugs or tumor, or associated birth defects will probably require laparotomy and gonadal biopsy in later infancy. Chromatin-negative infants may have a male or female gender assignment, depending on phallic structure. They require karyotyping to exclude 45,X/46,XY mosaicism, further serum and urinary steroid measurement to define rare abnormalities of adrenal or gonadal steroid synthesis, and contrast studies of the genitourinary tract to search for müllerian duct structures. Laparotomy and gonadal biopsy can safely be deferred to a later age.

The pioneering studies of Money and colleagues (1955) have shown that karyotype, gonads, internal ducts, and hormones have very little to do with behavior and psychosexual inclinations. These features are chiefly influenced by gender assignment and home environment. If the parents are secure about their boy or girl, the gender role is firmly established in early infancy and can rarely be reversed. The physician's role is to be sure that the physical and hormonal state of the growing child is not seriously at odds with the gender assignment. In the girl with congenital adrenal hyperplasia, this involves glucocorticoid replacement, consideration of clitorectomy and vaginoplasty if needed in infancy, and continued follow-up after maturity. In the boy with hypospadias and deficient testosterone production, it means surgical repair of hypospadias and evaluation of the need for testosterone replacement at the age of puberty. The genetic male with a female gender assignment needs protection from confusing information about chromosomes and may require gonadectomy before puberty to prevent virilization.

PRENATAL DIAGNOSIS OF ABNORMALITIES OF SEXUAL DIFFERENTIATION

Amniocentesis, ultrasonography, and studies of maternal blood and urine provide tools for the prenatal diagnosis of abnormalities of sexual differentiation. Abnormalities of sex chromosome number and structure can be determined by karyotypic analysis of chromosomes from amniotic fluid obtained as early as 14 to 16 weeks' gestation and from chorionic villous biopsy specimens as early as 8 weeks' gestation. Human leukocyte antigen (HLA) typing of amniotic fluid cells may aid in the prenatal diagnosis of certain forms of congenital adrenal hypoplasia when HLA typing of previously affected family members is available. Moreover, elevated amniotic fluid levels of 17-hydroxyprogesterone and androstenedione are present in male and female fetuses with 21-hydroxylase deficiency (Pang et al, 1980). Similarly, a fetus affected with 11-beta-hydroxylase deficiency can be detected by measurement of 11-deoxycortisol in amniotic fluid or in maternal plasma and urine (Rosler et al, 1979; Schumert et al, 1980). Estriol concentrations in maternal plasma and urine reflect the functional integrity of the fetal adrenal and placenta; low levels are observed in disorders of fetal hypothalamic-pituitary-adrenal function (Davies, 1980). Fetal sexing is possible with ultrasonography after 28 weeks' gestation (LeLann, 1979).

REFERENCES

Aarskog D: Maternal progestins as a possible cause of hypospadias. N Engl J Med 300:75, 1979.

Berta P, Hawkins JR, Sinclair AH, et al: Genetic evidence equating SR4 and the testis-determining factor. Nature 348(6300):448, 1990.

Conte FA, Grumbach MM: Pathogenesis, classification, diagnosis and treatment of anomalies of sex. *In* DeGroot LJ (Ed): Endocrinology. Philadelphia, WB Saunders, 1989, p 810.

Conte FA, Grumbach MM, Kaplan SC, et al: Correlation of luteinizing hormone-releasing factor, induced luteinizing hormone, and follicle-stimulating hormone release from infancy to 19 years with the changing pattern of gonadotropin secretion in agonadal patients: Relation to restraint of puberty. J Clin Endocrinol Metab 50:163, 1980.

David R, Yoon DY, Landin L, et al: A syndrome of gonadotropin resistance possibly due to a luteinizing hormone receptor defect. J Clin Endocrinol Metab 59:156, 1984.

Davies J: The fetal adrenal. *In* Tulchinsky D, Ryan K (Eds): Maternal-Fetal Endocrinology. Philadelphia, WB Saunders, 1980.

Drash A, Sherman F, Hartmann WH, et al: A syndrome of pseudohermaphroditism, Wilms' tumor, hypertension, and degenerative renal disease. J Pediatr 76:585, 1970.

Fraccaro M, Tiepolo L, Zuffardi D, et al: Familial XX true hermaphroditism and the H-Y antigen. Hum Genet 48:45, 1979.

Goebelsmann U, Zachmann M, Darajan R, et al: Male pseudohermaphroditism consistent with 17,20-desmolase deficiency. Gynecol Invest 7:138, 1976.

Griffen JE, Wilson JD: The syndrome of androgen resistance. N Engl J Med 302:198, 1980.

Hsu SY, Kubo M, Chun Sy, et al: Wilms tumor protein WT1 as an ovarian transcription factor: Decreases in expression during follicle development and repression of inhibin-alpha gene promoter. Mol Endocrinol 9(10):1356, 1995.

Imperato-McGinley J, Peterson RE, Gautier T: Primary and secondary 5α-reductase deficiency. *In* Serio M, Mota M, Zanisc M, et al: (Eds): Sexual Differentiation: Basic and Clinical Aspects. New York, Raven Press, 1984, p 233.

Ingraham HA, Lala DS, Ikeda Y, et al: The nuclear receptor steroidogenic factor 1 acts at multiple levels of the reproductive axis. Genes Dev 8(19):2302, 1994.

Jones HW Jr: Nonadrenal female pseudohermaphroditism. *In* Josso N (Ed): Pediatric and Adolescent Endocrinology, Vol 8. Basel, Karger, 1981, p 65.

Josso N: Permeability of membranes to the müllerian-inhibiting substance synthesized by the human fetal testis in vitro: A clue to its biochemical nature. J Clin Endocrinol Metab 34:265, 1972.

Kai H, Nose O, Iida Y, et al: Female pseudohermaphroditism caused by maternal congenital adrenal hyperplasia. J Pediatr 95:418, 1979.

Kaplan NM: Male pseudohermaphroditism: Report of a case, with observations on pathogenesis. N Engl J Med 261:641, 1959.

Kaplan SL, Grumbach MM: Pituitary and placental gonadotropins and sex steroids in the human and sub-human primate fetus. Clin Endocrinol Metab 7:487, 1978.

Kaufman M, Pinsky L, Baird PA, et al: Complete androgen insensitivity with a normal amount of 5α-dihydrotestosterone–binding activity in labium majus skin fibroblasts. Am J Med Genet 4:401, 1979.

Kim MH, Gumpel JA, Graff P: Pregnancy in a true hermaphrodite ("es"). Obstet Gynecol 53(3 Suppl):40S, 1979.

King CR, Magenis E, Bennett S: Pregnancy and the Turner syndrome. Obstet Gynecol 52:617, 1978.

Kohn G, Yarkoni S, Cohen MM: Two conceptions in a 45,X woman. Am J Med Genet 5:339, 1980.

Koopman P, Munsterberg A, Capel B, et al: Expression of a candidate sex-determining gene during mouse testis differentiation. Nature 348(6300):450, 1990.

Leary FJ, Reseguie LJ, Kurland LT, et al: Males exposed in utero to diethylstilbestrol. JAMA 252:2984, 1984.

LeLann D: Diagnostic échographique antinatal du sexe masculin et féminin. Nouv Presse Med 8:2760, 1979.

Lustig RH, Conte FA, Kogan BA, et al: Ontogeny of gonadotropin secretion in congenital anorchia: Sexual dimorphisim versus syndrome of gonadal dysgenesis and diagnostic considerations. J Urol 138:587, 1987.

Money J, Hampson JG, Hampson JL: Hermaphroditism: Recommendations concerning assignment of sex, change of sex and psychologic management. Bull Johns Hopkins Hosp 96:253, 1955.

Page DC, Mosher R, Simpson EM, et al: The sex-determining region of the Y chromosome encodes a finger protein. Cell 51:1091, 1987a.

Page DC, Brown LG, de la Chapelle A: Exchange of terminal portions of X and Y chromosomal short arms in human XX males. Nature 328:437, 1987b.

Pang S, Levin LS, Cederquist LC, et al: Amniotic fluid concentrations of Δ^5 and Δ^4 steroids in fetuses with congenital adrenal hyperplasia due to 21-hydroxylase deficiency and in anencephalic fetuses. J Clin Endocrinol Metab 51:223, 1980.

Reyes FI, Winter JSD, Faiman C: Studies on human sexual development. I. Fetal gonadal and adrenal sex steroids. J Clin Endocrinol Metab 37:74, 1973.

Rimoin DL, Schimke RN: Genetic Disorders of the Endocrine Glands. S Louis, CV Mosby, 1971.

Rosler A, Leiberman E, Rosenmann A, et al: Prenatal diagnosis of 11β-hydroxylase deficiency congenital adrenal hyperplasia. J Clin Endocrinol Metab 49:546, 1979.

Saez JM, Morera AM, dePeretti E, et al: Further in vivo studies in male pseudohermaphroditism with gynecomastia due to a testicular 17-ketosteroid reductase defect (compared to a case of testicular feminization). J Clin Endocrinol Metab 34:598, 1972.

Schumert Z, Rosenmann A, Landau H, et al: 11-Deoxycortisol in amniotic fluid: Prenatal diagnosis of congenital adrenal hyperplasia due to 11β-hydroxylase deficiency. Clin Endocrinol 12:257, 1980.

Shawker TH, Garra BS, Loriaux DL, et al: Ultrasonography of Turner's syndrome. J Ultrasound Med 5:125, 1987.

Siiteri PK, Wilson JD: Testosterone formation and metabolism during male sexual differentiation in the human embryo. J Clin Endocrinol Metab 38:113, 1974.

Simpson JL: Disorders of Sexual Differentiation: Etiology and Clinical Delineation. New York, Academic Press, 1976.

Summitt RL: Genetic forms of hypogonadism in the male. *In* Steinberg AG, Bearn AG, Motulsky AG, et al (Eds): Progress in Medical Genetics, Vol 2. Philadelphia, WB Saunders, 1979.

van Niekerk WA: True hermaphroditism. *In* Josso N (Ed): Pediatric and Adolescent Endocrinology, Vol 8. Basel, Karger, 1981, p 80.

Voight W, Hsia SL: Further studies on testosterone 5α-reductase of human skin: Structural features of steroid inhibitors. J Biol Chem 248:4280, 1973.

Wilson JD, Harrod MJ, Goldstein JL, et al: Familial incomplete male pseudohermaphroditism, type I. Evidence for androgen resistance and variable clinical manifestations in a family with the Reifenstein syndrome. N Engl J Med 290:1097, 1974.

CHAPTER 102

Disorders of the Thyroid Gland

Daniel H. Polk and Delbert A. Fisher

EMBRYOGENESIS AND HISTOLOGIC DEVELOPMENT OF THE THYROID GLAND

The human thyroid gland is a derivative of the primitive buccopharyngeal cavity. It develops from contributions of two anlagen: (1) a midline thickening of the pharyngeal floor (median anlage) and (2) paired caudal extensions of the fourth pharyngobranchial pouch (lateral anlagen). All of these structures are discernible by day 16 or 17 of gestation; by the 24th day of gestation the median anlage has developed a thin flasklike diverticulum extending from the floor of the buccal cavity down to the fourth branchial arch. At 40 days of gestation, the median and lateral anlagen have fused, and by 50 days of gestation the buccal stalk has ruptured. During this period, the thyroid gland migrates caudally to its definitive location in the anterior neck, helped in part by its relationship with developing cardiac structures.

Developmental abnormalities of the thyroid gland usually represent defects in early morphogenesis resulting from aberrant thyroid tissue migration. The most common anomaly is the persistence of the thyroglossal duct. This is not usually associated with altered thyroid status in the newborn but may present in later life as an infected fistulous tract. Abnormalities of thyroid embryogenesis (thyroid dysgenesis) include agenesis or ectopic tissue in sublingual, cervical, mediastinal, or even intracardiac locations. Although ectopic thyroid tissue may manifest some function, these infants usually exhibit some degree of hypothyroidism. In addition, calcitonin deficiency is present in children with congenital hypothyroidism. However, hypoparathyroidism is not associated with thyroid dysgenesis, although the parathyroid glands may be ectopic in these children.

Thyroid Hormone Synthesis

Circulating plasma iodide enters the thyroid follicular cells and is combined with tyrosine through a series of enzymatically mediated reactions to form the active thyroid hormones 3,5,3′ triiodothyronine (T_3) and thyroxine (T_4). The steps in synthesis and release of thyroid hormones include (1) active transport of inorganic iodide from plasma to thyroid cell, (2) synthesis of tyrosine-rich thyroglobulin, which acts as the intermediate iodine acceptor, (3) organification of trapped iodide as iodotyrosines, (4) coupling of monoiodotyrosines (MIT) and diiodotyrosines (DIT) to form the iodothyronines, T_3 and T_4, with storage of iodotyrosines and iodothyronines in follicular colloid, (5) endocytosis and proteolysis of colloid thyroglobulin to release MIT, DIT, T_3, and T_4, and (6) deiodination of released iodotyrosines within the thyroid cell with reutilization of the iodine. These steps and their inhibitors are outlined in Table 102–1. Certain defects in these biochemical processes have been identified, clinically leading in most cases

to hypothyroidism. These are discussed in Congenital Hypothyroidism.

Fetal-Placental-Maternal Thyroid Interaction

The relative independence of the maternal and fetal hypothalamic-pituitary-thyroid hormone systems is suggested by several clinical observations. The placenta is impermeable to thyroid-stimulating hormone (TSH) and largely impermeable to the thyroid hormones. These data were recently reviewed by Roti (1988) and are summarized in Table 102–2. Direct evidence of placental transfer of thyroid hormones is provided by studies using various thyroid hormone analogues and tracers. Human studies have shown limited transfer from mother to fetus. Large doses of T_4 given to women produced only minor changes in cord serum concentrations of hormonal iodine. Supraphysiologic doses of T_3 chronically administered to pregnant women several weeks before delivery significantly increased maternal serum T_3 levels but only minimally lowered fetal T_4 values. Thus, it is clear that under physiologic conditions, placental transfer of thyroid hormones is limited. This limitation is due, at least in part, to the presence in placental tissue of an inner (tyrosyl) ring iodothyronine deiodinase, which converts T_4 to inactive reverse T_3 and converts T_3 to inactive diiodothyronine, or T_2. Of interest is recent data suggesting that the maternal compartment might significantly contribute to fetal thyroid hormone levels in the hypothyroid fetus (Vulsma et al, 1989). The physiologic significance of this observation is uncertain.

Maternal immunoglobulins of the IgG subclass are selectively transported across the placenta, particularly late in gestation. Hyperthyroidism or hypothyroidism has been reported in response to maternally derived TSH receptor-stimulating or TSH receptor-blocking antibodies. These syndromes are usually detected by either newborn screening or neonatal symptoms and signs (Matsurra et al, 1980;

TABLE 102–1

Biochemical Steps to Thyroid Hormone Synthesis

Step	Inhibitor
Iodide transport	CIO_4^- and SCN^-
Thyroglobulin synthesis	Protein synthesis inhibitors
Organification of iodide	PTU, MMI
MIT, DIT coupling	PTU, MMI
Thyroglobulin endocytosis and proteolysis	I^-, Li^-, colchicine, and cytochalasin B
Deiodination	Dinitrotyrosine

MIT, monoiodotyrosine; DIT, diiodotyrosine; PTU, propylthiouracil; MMI, methimizole.

TABLE 102–2

Placental Permeability for Substances Affecting Thyroid Function

Substance	Placental Permeability
I⁻	+ + + +
TRH	+ + +
Thiourylenes	+ + +
IgG antibodies	+ + +
T_3	0
T_4	+
TSH	0

TRH, thyrotropin-releasing hormone; TSH, thyroid-stimulating hormone.
Data from Roti E: Regulation of thyroid-stimulating hormone (TSH) secretion in the fetus and neonate. J Endocrinol Invest 11:145–150, 1988.

Zakarija and McKenzie, 1983). Thyroid scanning in affected infants reveals the presence of a normally situated thyroid gland; the clinical abnormalities wane with degradation of the maternal antibody. The half-life in newborn blood for the maternally derived IgG antibodies approximates 20 days.

The placenta is freely permeable to iodide, and the fetal thyroid is particularly sensitive to the inhibitory effects of iodine on thyroid function (Theodoropoulos et al, 1979). Relatively small amounts of maternal iodine exposure have been associated with transient neonatal hypothyroidism. The source may be radiopaque dyes used for radiographic procedures as well as maternal medications, including topically applied iodine washes, which may be absorbed across mucous membrane surfaces. This effect is more fully described in the section on congenital hypothyroidism.

The thioureylene antithyroid drugs cross the placenta and may compromise fetal and neonatal thyroid function (Marchant et al, 1977). The placenta also is permeable to selected synthetic thyroid hormone analogues such as 3',5'-dimethyl, 5-isopropyl thyronine (DIMIT). However, there is no current rationale for use of these analogues because of their low biological activity. Finally, the placenta is permeable to the hypothalamic peptide thyrotropin-releasing hormone (TRH). Both primate and human fetuses early in the 3rd trimester respond to pharmacologic doses of exogenous TRH with an increase in serum TSH. However, little endogenous TRH is normally detected in adult humans because of the presence of TRH-degrading enzyme systems in the blood. Although the sera of pregnant women contain somewhat lower levels of these enzymes than nonpregnant sera, the nearly immeasurable levels of TRH in the maternal circulation have little effect on fetal thyroid function.

In addition to producing TRH, the placenta produces thyrotropin-like activity. The alpha subunit of TSH is identical to that of human chorionic gonadotropin (hCG), and the beta subunit of hCG has structural homology with the beta subunit of TSH; thus, hCG has some TSH-like bioactivity. However, the biologic potency of hCG is only about 0.01% that of TSH, and hCG normally has little influence on fetal thyroid system development or function. Because of the hyperthyroidism sometimes seen in patients with choriocarcinoma, a unique chorionic thyrotropin has

been proposed, and a glycoprotein with thyrotropic activity has been isolated from human placenta. However, a structure has never been characterized, and it seems likely that this chorionic thyrotropin represents a variant form of hCG (Harada and Hershman, 1978).

In summary, placental permeability to maternal molecules might be a factor affecting fetal thyroid function as a result of maternal pathophysiologic states (acute iodide administration, autoimmune thyroid disease, or pharmacotherapy of thyrotoxicosis). However, the fetal pituitary-thyroid axis normally develops independently of the maternal thyroid axis influence. The placenta and selected fetal tissues may serve as sources of TRH or TSH, but the extent of this influence on fetal thyroid function is uncertain.

Control of Thyroid Hormone Production

The pattern of perinatal thyroid hormone secretion in the human is shown in Figure 102–1. Maturation of thyroid system control can be considered in three phases—hypothalamic, pituitary, and thyroidal. Changes in these systems are complex and superimposed on the increasing production and increasing serum concentration of serum thyroid hormone–binding globulin (TBG) as well as the changing pattern of fetal tissue iodothyronine deiodination during gestation. Maturation of these latter systems is described in the following section.

Although the fetal thyroid gland is able to concentrate iodide and synthesize thyroglobulin at 70 to 80 days of gestation, little thyroid hormone synthesis occurs until about 18 weeks' gestation. At this time, thyroid follicular cell iodine uptake increases, and T_4 becomes measurable in the serum. Both total and free T_4 concentrations then increase steadily until the final weeks of pregnancy (Fisher, 1985). This pattern differs from the development of serum T_3 levels in the fetus. The fetal serum T_3 concentration is low (<15 µg/dL) until 30 weeks of gestation and then increases slowly in two distinct phases, a prenatal and a postnatal phase. Prenatally, serum T_3 increases slowly after

Maturation of Thyroid Hormone Secretion in the Human Fetus

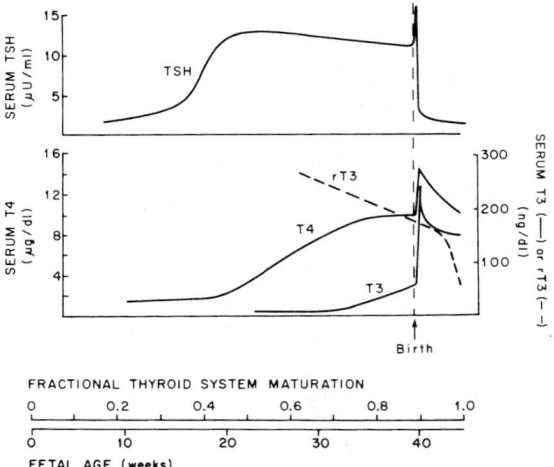

FIGURE 102–1. Patterns of circulating levels of thyroid-stimulating hormone (TSH), rT_3, T_4 and T_3 in the fetus and newborn.

30 weeks of gestation to reach a level of approximately 50 µg/dL in term cord serum (Fisher and Klein, 1981). Postnatally, both T_3 and T_4 serum concentrations increase fourfold to sixfold within the first few hours of life, peaking at 24 to 36 hours after birth. These levels then gradually decline to adult values over the first 4 to 5 weeks of life. The prenatal increase in serum T_3 seems to be largely due to progressive maturation of hepatic type I (phenolic) outer ring iodothyronine deiodinase activity and increasing hepatic conversion of T_4 to T_3, although other tissue sources of deiodinase, such as brown fat and the kidney, may be involved.

Fetal serum TSH increases rapidly from a low level at 18 weeks' gestation to a peak value at 24 to 28 weeks' gestation then gradually declines until term. At the time of parturition, partly in response to cold stress, there is an acute release of TSH resulting in an elevated level by 30 minutes of life. The level of circulating TSH remains modestly elevated for 2 to 3 days after birth. The increases in thyroid hormone that occur immediately after birth are not totally dependent on TSH and may represent other influences in the thyroid gland at the time of parturition. The high postnatal T_3 levels in the days following birth are due to both TSH stimulation of thyroidal T_3 secretion and further rapid maturation of tissue outer ring monodeiodinase activity.

Fetal thyroid gland function develops under the influence of a moderately elevated TSH level during the last half of gestation. The increase in serum T_4 that occurs during the last trimester is accompanied by a progressive decrease in serum TSH suggesting that changes in both thyroid follicular cell sensitivity to TSH and pituitary thyrotroph sensitivity to the negative feedback effect of thyroid hormones occur during this period. The pituitary gland contains a type II outer ring iodothyronine deiodinase, which converts T_4 to active T_3, which in turn modulates TSH production. In most circumstances, it is circulating T_4 that is most important in TSH control. Thus, even when the circulating T_3 level is low (as in midgestation), there may be significant negative feedback control (by T_4) of pituitary TSH secretion.

The ontogeny of TRH secretion and function in the fetus remain somewhat obscure. TRH immunoactivity is detectable in the hypothalamus by midgestation, increasing markedly in the third trimester after the peak in serum TSH activity is noted. The premature infant (before 30 to 32 weeks) is characterized by low levels of T_4 and free T_4, a normal or low level of TSH, and a normal or prolonged TSH response to TRH indicating a state of physiologic TRH deficiency. The full-term human fetus responds to pharmacologic maternal doses of TRH with a somewhat prolonged increase in TSH, suggesting a degree of relative hypothalamic (tertiary) hypothyroidism (Roti et al, 1981). Fetal sources of nonhypothalamic TRH (placenta and pancreas) probably contribute to the elevated circulating levels of fetal and cord blood TRH and presumably account for the high circulating TSH level characteristic of the midgestation fetus. However, the significance of ectopic TRH to the development of thyroid system control remains to be investigated.

In summary, the control of fetal thyroid hormone secretion can be characterized as a balance among increasing hypothalamic TRH secretion, increasing thyroid follicular cell sensitivity to TSH, and increasing pituitary sensitivity to thyroid hormone inhibition of TSH release. The fetus progresses from a state of both primary (thyroidal) and tertiary (hypothalamic) hypothyroidism in midgestation through a state of mild tertiary hypothyroidism during the final weeks of pregnancy and to fully mature thyroid function in the perinatal period.

Fetal Thyroid Hormone Metabolism

Although the thyroid gland is the sole source of T_4, most of the T_3 that circulates in the adult is derived from conversion of T_4 to T_3 via monodeiodination in peripheral tissues. Deiodination of the iodothyronines is the major route of metabolism, and monodeiodination may occur either at the outer (phenolic) ring or the inner (tyrosyl) ring of the iodothyronine molecule. Outer ring monodeiodination of T_4 produces T_3, the active form of thyroid hormone with greatest affinity for the nuclear thyroid hormone receptor. Inner ring monodeiodination of T_4 produces reverse T_3 (rT_3), an inactive metabolite. In mature humans, between 70% and 90% of circulating T_3 is derived from peripheral conversion of T_4, and 10% to 30% from direct glandular secretion. Nearly all the circulating rT_3 derives from peripheral conversion with only 2% to 3% coming directly from the thyroid gland. T_3 and rT_3 are progressively metabolized to diiodo, monoiodo, and noniodinated forms of thyronine, none of which possess biologic activity.

Two types of outer-ring iodothyronine monodeiodinases (5'MDI) have been described. Type I 5'MDI, predominantly expressed in the liver and kidney, is an enzyme inhibited by propylthiouracil, and its activity is stimulated by thyroid hormone. Type II 5'MDI, predominantly located in the brain, pituitary, and brown adipose tissues, is insensitive to propylthiouracil, and its activity is inhibited by thyroid hormone (Refetoff and Larsen, 1989). Type I 5'MDI activity in the liver and perhaps the kidney and muscles probably accounts for most of the peripheral deiodination of T_4; type II 5'MDI acts primarily to increase local intracellular levels of T_3 in the brain and pituitary and is important to brown adipose tissue function during the immediate postnatal period. The outer ring iodothyronine deiodinase also deiodinates reverse T_3 to diiodothyronine.

Both type I and type II 5'MDI are present in 3rd trimester fetuses (Polk et al, 1988b). Both deiodinase species are thyroid hormone responsive. However, hepatic type I 5'MDI activity becomes thyroid hormone responsive (e.g., activity decreases with hypothyroidism) only during the final weeks of gestation. Brain type II activity, in contrast, is responsive (increases with hypothyroidism) throughout the final trimester of gestation. Thus, type II deiodinase probably plays an important role to provide a source of intracellular T_3 to those tissues (such as the pituitary and in some species brown fat and the brain) dependent on T_3 during fetal life, whereas the ontogeny of the type I enzyme (to provide increased serum T_3 levels) increases only during the final weeks of gestation and during postnatal life.

An inner (tyrosyl) ring iodothyronine monodeiodinase (type III 5'MDI) has been characterized in most fetal tissues, including the placenta. This enzyme system catalyzes the conversion of T_4 to rT_3 and T_3 to diiodothyronine. Fetal thyroid hormone metabolism is characterized by a predominance of type III enzyme activity, particularly in the liver, kidney, and placenta, and this accounts in part for the increased circulating levels of rT_3 observed in the fetus. Placental type III deiodinase contributes to amniotic fluid rT_3 levels and presumably also contributes to circulating fetal rT_3. However, the persistence of high circulating rT_3 levels for several weeks in the newborn indicates that type III 5'MDI activities expressed in nonplacental tissues are also important to the maintenance of high circulating rT_3 levels.

Both T_3 and T_4 in blood are associated with various plasma proteins including TBG, thyroxine-binding prealbumin (TBPA), and albumin. TBG serves as the primary transport protein for both T_3 and T_4; 70% of the total T_4 and 40% to 60% of total T_3 are bound to TBG. The rest of the thyroid hormones are distributed almost equally between TBPA and albumin. The binding affinities of these proteins are such that adult free T_4 and T_3 concentrations are about 0.03% and 0.3% respectively, of the total hormone concentrations. TBG, TBPA, and albumin are produced by the liver, and production of these proteins increases progressively during the final half of gestation. Hepatic TBG production is stimulated by estrogen, and the increasing levels of estrogens during pregnancy account, at least in part, for the total plasma T_4 concentration, which increases progressively from midgestation until 34 to 35 weeks' gestation.

Thyroid System Effects and Adaptation to Extrauterine Life

In general, much of the fetal thyroid development is preparatory, providing for the relatively large amounts of thyroid hormones required for normal postnatal development. The production of active thyroid hormones is markedly increased in association with the events of parturition (see Fig. 102–1). During the first hours after birth, there are abrupt threefold to sixfold increases in circulating T_4 and T_3 levels, coincident with an increase in serum TSH concentrations. The initial increases in circulating thyroid hormone levels are due largely to increased hormone secretion from the thyroid gland. Substances other than TSH may also modulate the acute increases in circulating thyroid hormones at birth. A postnatal increase in serum catecholamine concentrations occurs at the time of parturition (Padbury et al, 1985), and the thyroid gland is adrenergically innervated. The cold-stimulated TSH surge is short-lived, and the decrease in TSH that follows during the 72 to 96 hours after birth is due to feedback inhibition by T_4 at either the hypothalamic or pituitary levels (or both). The serum TRH concentration is elevated in cord blood and declines in the days following birth. A clear increase in the serum TRH value coincident with the increase in TSH after parturition has not been reported, but the parallel increases in both TSH and prolactin levels in the early hours after birth support the view that the TSH surge is mediated by TRH (Roti, 1988). Thyroid hormone levels in the newborn gradually return to adult levels by about 1 month of age. The high level of circulating rT_3 characteris-

tic of the fetus persists following birth, gradually declining to the adult range by 4 to 6 weeks of age.

The metabolic significance of the neonatal thyroid hormone surge is not entirely clear. Physiologic processes known to be modulated by thyroid hormone in adults, such as thermogenesis and cardiovascular responses, clearly are important in the transition from intrauterine to extrauterine life, and it is tempting to link these transitional events with changes in thyroid hormone metabolism. Several studies using animal models have attempted to establish such a link and support the view that the level of thyroid function during the final weeks of gestation is more important than the neonatal increases in T_3 and T_4 for successful neonatal transition (Polk et al, 1988a). The situation in the human newborn may be somewhat different. Newborns with congenital thyroid agenesis have few if any signs or symptoms of thyroid hormone deficiency, and their postnatal environmental adaptation usually is not impaired. The precise timing of maturation of thyroid hormone effects on thermogenesis and cardiovascular function in the human newborn has not been defined.

In humans thyroid hormone nuclear receptors have been reported in fetal lung, brain, heart, and liver at 13 to 19 weeks' gestation by Gonzales and Ballard (1981) and Bernal and Pekonen (1984). The only thyroid hormone actions that have been characterized in the fetus are the effects of hypothyroidism on serum TSH and bone maturation. Most effects of thyroid hormone on perinatal developmental processes occur postnatally (Fig. 102–2).

In summary, thyroid hormones affect important postnatal processes including growth, thermogenesis, and development. The largely successful transition of athyrotic infants to extrauterine life speaks to the limited importance of fetal thyroid hormones in all but the final weeks of gestation. An exception to this may be the fetal brain, a major site of type II iodothyronine monodeiodinase activity in the fetus. The presence of this enzyme system in the brain early in development as well as its demonstrated response to fetal hypothyroidism in the rat and sheep suggests that intracellular conversion of T_4 to T_3 in the brain is important in these species for normal development

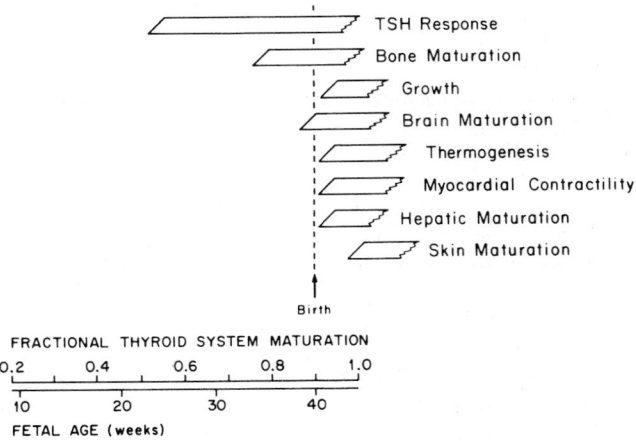

FIGURE 102–2. Onset of actions of thyroid hormone in the developing human. The left edge of the bar indicates the initiation of thyroid hormone responsiveness of the indicated parameter.

and differentiation of the central nervous system. The critical period for this effect is not known for the human fetus, but early treatment of congenital hypothyroidism in the newborn prevents mental retardation, suggesting that the period of thyroid dependency of the human brain extends into the postnatal period.

CONGENITAL HYPOTHYROIDISM

Congenital hypothyroidism has been recognized for centuries and its treatment known for decades, but only recently has the link between early treatment and the prevention of sequellae been proposed. With the emphasis being placed on early screening, many conditions that lead to the syndrome of congenital hypothyroidism have been recognized (Table 102–3). The importance of adequate neonatal screening in the management of newborn thyroid diseases must be emphasized. Before the advent of screening, less than one third of the infants found to ultimately have congenital hypothyroidism were given the diagnosis before 3 months of age, and only half by 6 months of age; irreversible brain damage developed in most of these infants (Jacobsen and Brandt, 1981).

Newborn screening programs for congenital hypothyroidism are designed to detect elevated serum TSH levels in blood samples collected on filter paper. Some programs measure TSH directly, and others measure TSH in samples with low or low-normal T_4 concentrations. In most programs in the United States, an initial T_4 measurement is conducted, and TSH is measured in samples with the lowest 10% of T_4 values. An elevated TSH level (>20 μIU/mL) suggests primary hypothyroidism. Most screening programs are just that, and some infants with hypothyroidism are missed in the screening process. Thus, no infant

TABLE 102–3

Thyroid Disorders and Their Approximate Prevalences in the Neonatal Period

Disorder	Incidence
Thyroid Dysgenesis	1:4,000
Agenesis	
Hypogenesis	
Ectopia	
Thyroid Dyshormonogenesis	1:30,000
TSH receptor defect	
Iodide trapping defect	
Organification defect	
Iodotyrosine deiodinase deficiency	
Defect in thyroglobulin	
Transient Hypothyroidism	1:40,000
Drug induced	
Maternal-antibody–induced	
Idiopathic	
Hypothalamic-Pituitary Hypothyroidism	1:100,000
Hypothalamic-pituitary anomaly	
Panhypopituitarism	
Isolated TSH deficiency	

TSH, thyroid-stimulating hormone.

TABLE 102–4

Clinical Signs and Symptoms of Congenital Hypothyroidism in Infancy

Age	Frequency (%)
0 to 7 Days	
Prolonged jaundice >3 days	73
Birth weight >4 kg	40
Poor feeding	40
Transient hypothermia	38
Large posterior fontanel (>5 mm)	32
1 to 4 Weeks	
Failure to gain weight	45
Constipation	35
Hypoactivity	33
1 to 3 Months	
Failure to thrive	90
Umbilical hernia	49
Macroglossia	43
Myxedema	40
Hoarse cry	30

who presents with signs or symptoms suggestive of thyroid dysfunction (Table 102–4) should be excluded from investigation on the basis of previous screening results. A determination of serum T_4 and TSH values is necessary in any infant with suspicious clinical or laboratory findings. With this as a background, the following is discussion of the major pathophysiologic states leading to congenital thyroid dysfunction (see Table 102–3).

Thyroid Dysgenesis

The term *thyroid dysgenesis* describes infants with ectopic or hypoplastic thyroid glands (or both) as well as those with total thyroid agenesis. Thyroid dysgenesis is the etiologic factor in most infants with permanent congenital hypothyroidism detected in newborn screening programs. Some thyroid tissue probably is present in two thirds of these infants, so that they represent a spectrum of severity of thyroid deficiency. A normal or near-normal circulating level of T_3 in the face of a low T_4 value suggests the presence of residual thyroid tissue, and this can be confirmed by a thyroid scan. A measurable level of serum thyroglobulin also indicates the presence of some thyroid tissue; athyrotic infants have no circulating thyroglobulin (Dammacco et al, 1985).

Thyroid dysgenesis occurs in 1:4000 live-born infants and is more prevalent in female than in male infants by a ratio of almost 2:1. Studies by Frasier and colleagues (1982) and Brown and coworkers (1981) suggest the disorder has been reported to be less common in black (1:32,000) than in white infants and may be more frequent (1:2000) in Hispanic infants. Although thyroid dysgenesis usually is sporadic, rare familial cases have been described, and the incidence is increased in infants with Down syndrome (Fort et al, 1984). Seasonal variations in incidence have been observed in Japan, Australia, and Canada. In isolated instances thyroid dysgenesis has occurred in association with maternal autoimmune thyroiditis. However, this may be coincidence; there usually is no correlation between thyroid dysgenesis and the presence of maternal autoimmune thyroiditis or circulating thyroid antimicrosomal or antithyroglobulin autoantibodies (Dussault et al, 1980). Immune globulins blocking TSH-stimulated thyroid cell growth in tissue culture have been reported in both maternal and newborn blood in about half of the cases of sporadic congenital hypothyroidism, but a role for such growth-blocking immune globulins in the pathogenesis of congenital hypothyroidism in vivo has not been established.

As discussed, most newborns with thyroid dysgenesis are asymptomatic, and few infants have signs of hypothyroidism during the early weeks of life. Most affected infants have low serum T₄ and high TSH concentrations in cord blood or in filter-paper blood spots collected at 2 to 5 days of age. Ten percent to 20% of hypothyroid infants have T_4 levels in the low-normal range with increased TSH values. These infants usually have ectopic functional thyroid tissue on scanning and significant levels of circulating thyroglobulin. Another 5% have a delayed elevation of serum TSH and are missed in the screening process unless a second screening test is done (LaFranchi et al, 1985). Again, thyroid function should be determined in any infant presenting with suspicious clinical signs or symptoms (see Table 102–4). Individuals with thyroid dysgenesis also show abnormalities of thyroidal C cells; calcitonin levels and responsiveness are reduced throughout infancy and childhood. Urinary calcium and hydroxyproline levels are increased, and there is a tendency toward osteopenia, but this seems of limited clinical significance (Kruse et al, 1987).

Hypothalamic-Pituitary Defects

Congenital hypothyroidism resulting from ineffective TSH stimulation of thyroid hormone secretion can result from a variety of abnormalities in TSH synthesis and metabolism. These include anomalous hypothalamic or pituitary development, isolated or familial deficiencies in TRH or TSH secretion, or TSH deficiency in association with other pituitary hormone deficiencies. Several TSH deficiency syndromes have been described: hypothalamic (tertiary) hypothyroidism with TRH deficiency or pituitary insensitivity (or both), isolated TSH deficiency, familial panhypopituitarism, congenital absence of the pituitary, and panhypopituitarism with absence of the sella turcica. The combined prevalence of these abnormalities associated with congenital hypothyroidism approximates 1:60,000 to 140,000 live births (Stanbury and Dumont, 1983).

Inborn Defects of Thyroid Hormone Production

Infants with inborn defects in thyroid metabolism account for nearly 10% of newborns with congenital nonendemic hypothyroidism (see Table 102–3). The defects in such patients include (1) a decreased thyroid response to TSH, (2) decreased thyroid iodide trapping, (3) defective organification of trapped iodide, (4) decreased capacity for deiodinating iodotyrosines, and (5) abnormalities in thyroglobulin synthesis, storage, or release. These disorders usually are transmitted as autosomal recessive traits (Lever et al,

1983). Except for the familial incidence and tendency for goiter to develop in affected individuals, the clinical manifestations of congenital hypothyroidism resulting from a biochemical defect are similar to those in infants with thyroid dysgenesis. Thyroid enlargement may be manifest at birth, but in many patients development of the goiter is delayed.

Transient Congenital Hypothyroidism

Congenital hypothyroidism may present as a transient defect persisting for a variable period after birth. Usually, transient neonatal hypothyroidism is caused by maternal ingestion of goitrogenic substances that reach the fetus via placental transfer. One frequently ingested goitrogenic drug is iodide prescribed in expectorants for the treatment of asthma or as treatment for maternal thyrotoxicosis. The mothers of these infants often have taken large doses of iodide for many years without development of large goiters and have been euthyroid during pregnancy. The fetal thyroid gland is unusually sensitive to iodide-induced hypothyroidism because of immaturity of the mechanisms that decrease thyroid iodide uptake in response to high plasma iodide levels. Urine iodine concentrations in affected infants usually exceed 1 mg/L.

Other substances that have been associated with neonatal goiter include thioureylene (antithyroid) drugs, sulfonamides, and hematinic preparations containing cobalt. Neonatal goiters resulting from antithyroid drug administration are uncommon unless large doses of the drugs are given to the mother (more than 150 mg per day propylthiouracil or equivalent near term). Amniotic injection of radiographic contrast agents used during amniofetography also can lead to transient congenital hypothyroidism.

Maternal-to-fetal transfer of TSH-receptor–blocking antibodies also can lead to transient perinatal hypothyroidism (Drexhage and Bottazzo, 1985). This condition is rare but has been reported in the newborns of women with either euthyroid or hypothyroid autoimmune thyroid disease. In these infants, TSH-receptor autoantibodies are detectable in maternal and cord blood. These antibodies can be measured either as TSH-binding–inhibiting immune globulins (TBII) or TSH (cAMP) blocking antibodies (TBA). The duration of the hypothyroid state in these newborns is correlated with the initial titer of blocking antibody and the duration of its presence in newborn blood. Transient congenital hypothyroidism must be differentiated from transient hyperthyrotropinemia (see the section on thyroid dysfunction in preterm infants).

Diagnosis and Management

Infants with congenital hypothyroidism are born with little or no clinical evidence of thyroid hormone deficiency. Thus, detection based on signs and symptoms usually is delayed 6 to 12 weeks or longer. Even though the emphasis in diagnosis of congenital hypothyroidism currently focuses on newborn screening, not all infants with congenital hypothyroidism are detected by these systems. Early clinical diagnosis must be based on a high index of suspicion regarding nonspecific symptoms and signs. These are outlined in Table 102–4 along with their relative frequency.

The diagnosis should be considered in any infant with prolonged jaundice, transient hypothermia, an enlarged (>1 cm) posterior fontanel, failure to feed properly, or respiratory distress with feeding.

The classic signs evolve during the first weeks after birth. There is a rapid reduction in growth rate after birth and a progressive accumulation of myxedema in the subcutaneous tissues and in the tongue. The thickened tongue becomes protuberant, and increasing difficulty in nursing and handling salivary secretions develops. The cry is hoarse because of myxedema of the vocal cords. There is marked muscular hypotonia, an umbilical hernia, constipation, bradycardia, and extremities that are cool to the touch and may exhibit pallor and circulatory mottling. The cardiac silhouette may be enlarged; the electrocardiogram shows low voltage and a prolonged conduction time. Some of the signs and symptoms are present by 6 to 12 weeks, especially lethargy, constipation, and the umbilical hernia. The cretinoid facies and growth retardation become progressively more obvious during the first several months of life.

As discussed previously, infants can escape detection by screening because of a delayed elevation in serum TSH or because of errors in sample collection or laboratory routine; it is estimated that 5% to 8% of affected infants might be missed. Infants with TSH deficiency are not detected since most newborn screening programs report only those infants with elevated TSH levels. Congenital primary hypothyroidism is associated with a low serum T_4 and a high TSH concentration in individual cord blood or neonatal blood samples. A cord serum T_4 of 6.0 μg/dL or less with a TSH in excess of 80 μIU/mL suggests hypothyroidism. At 3 to 5 days of age, a serum T_4 less than 7 μg/dL with a serum TSH in excess of 20 μIU/mL suggests hypothyroidism. However, 10% to 20% of infants with congenital hypothyroidism have T_4 values in the low-normal range (7 to 11 μg/dL). During the first 24 to 48 hours of life, serum TSH levels normally are elevated because of the neonatal TSH surge. Sampling infants during this time increases the number of false-positive results, but infants with congenital hypothyroidism are not usually missed.

The diagnosis of congenital hypothyroidism must be confirmed by measurement of serum T_4 and TSH concentrations in any infant with suspicious screening or neonatal sampling results. After 7 days of age a serum T_4 less than 6 μg/dL with a TSH more than 50 μIU/mL indicates primary hypothyroidism. A serum T_4 in the 6 to 11 μg/dL range with a TSH in the 20 to 50 μIU/mL range is suggestive, and repeat testing is necessary. Eight percent to 10% of infants with congenital hypothyroidism have screening TSH values less than 50 μIU/mL, and one in 12 to 24 hypothyroid infants (1:50,000 to 100,000 newborns) will have a screening TSH level less than 20 μIU/mL with a delayed postnatal increase to hypothyroid levels.

Hypothalamic-pituitary hypothyroidism is more difficult to diagnose. The disorder is characterized by a low serum T_4 concentration with a normal TSH value. In contrast, a low T_4 and TSH pattern most commonly reflects prematurity or a low TBG concentration. Measurement of a low serum TBG concentration or a normal free T_4 level identifies the low TBG patients. An infant with a low free T_4 concentration should be carefully examined for evidence of hypothyroidism, and other tests of pituitary function

should be conducted. A subnormal TSH response to TRH confirms a diagnosis of pituitary TSH deficiency. The TSH deficiency may be isolated or associated with other pituitary hormone deficiencies. If the peak level of TSH after TRH stimulation is normal or prolonged, hypothalamic TRH deficiency is likely.

The treatment of hypothyroidism relies on replacement with exogenous thyroid hormone. Sodium–L-thyroxine (Na T_4) is the drug of choice because of its uniform potency and reliable absorption. Appropriate doses of synthetic T_4 produce normal serum levels of T_3 via peripheral conversion. The best guide to adequacy of therapy is periodic measurement of circulating levels of T_4 and TSH; during the initial stages of treatment, a T_3 determination also may be of value. The history and physical examination are important in follow-up, but mild hypothyroidism or hyperthyroidism cannot always be excluded on clinical grounds. The usual starting dose of Na T_4 for hypothyroid infants is 10 to 15 μg/kg per day; we routinely begin treatment in term infants with a 50-μg T_4 tablet daily crushed and given orally in a small amount of liquid. Using Na T_4 for treatment, the goal of therapy is to maintain the serum T_4 in the upper normal range (10 to 16 μg/dL), which should result in normal serum T_3 levels (70 to 220 ng/dL).

Serum TSH levels may remain elevated in adequately treated patients. The thyroid hormone–pituitary feedback set-point seems to be altered in some infants with congenital hypothyroidism, and in such infants the serum TSH concentration remains elevated in the face of a normal or even elevated serum T_4 level (McCrossin et al, 1980).

Infants with presumably transient hypothyroidism resulting from maternal goitrogenic drugs need not be treated unless the low serum T_4 and elevated TSH levels persist beyond 2 weeks. Hyperthyroid mothers on antithyroid drugs may breast-feed their infants, because the concentration of drug in breast milk is very low. Infants with TSH-receptor–blocking antibody-induced hypothyroidism may require treatment for as long as 2 to 5 months.

Adequate dosage of thyroxine in the 1st year usually ranges between 25 and 50 μg daily. The growth rate should accelerate after initiation of therapy, and any growth deficit is commonly restored within a few months. Bone age is a sensitive index of thyroid deficiency, and delayed bone maturation suggests inadequate treatment even when other signs of hypothyroidism have ameliorated. Overtreatment can induce tachycardia, excessive nervousness, disturbed sleep patterns, and other findings suggesting thyrotoxicosis. Excessive thyroxine administered over a long period can produce premature synostosis of cranial sutures and undue advancement of bone age.

THYROID DYSFUNCTION SYNDROMES IN THE PREMATURE INFANT

Although the preterm infant is subject to the same pathophysiologic processes affecting the term infant, certain disorders of thyroid function are more common as a result of prematurity and are discussed in the following sections.

Transient Hypothyroxinemia

Serum T_4 concentrations increase progressively with gestational age (see Fig. 102–2). Most term infants have serum

T_4 concentrations above 6.5 μg/dL; only 2% to 3% have serum T_4 levels below this level. In contrast, some 50% of premature infants delivered before 30 weeks' gestation have serum T_4 values below 6.5 μg/dL (Hadeed et al, 1981). These preterm infants with hypothyroxinemia also have relatively low levels of free T_4. These levels are not as low as those in newborns with congenital hypothyroidism; rather, they are similar to the levels in adults. These relatively low free T_4 levels in premature infants are associated with normal or even low serum TSH values and normal TSH and T_4 responses to TRH, indicating responsive pituitary and thyroid glands. The hypothyroxinemia is transient, correcting spontaneously (in 4 to 8 weeks) with progressive maturation. The physiologic significance of these changes remains controversial. Previous studies have suggested that replacement therapy does not improve postnatal growth or subsequent development (Chowdrey et al, 1984). However, more recent studies have suggested that low T_4 values are associated with poorer neurologic outcome in preterm infants after attempting to adjust for other confounding variables (den Ouden et al, 1996; Reuss et al, 1996). These observations have led to studies examining the influence of thyroxine supplementation on these outcomes. In infants born before 30 weeks' gestation, exogenous thyroxine administration did not improve developmental outcome determined at 2 years of age (Van Wassenaer et al, 1997). Further studies involving more targeted populations of infants or relying on other dosing strategies are in progress.

Transient Primary Hypothyroidism

Transient hypothyroidism in the newborn, characterized by low serum T_4 and high TSH concentrations, is more common in Europe than in the United States; its prevalence varies geographically relative to iodine intake. In Belgium, it occurs in 20% of premature infants, with the incidence increasing as gestational age decreases (Delange et al, 1985). Cord blood T_4 and TSH values in these infants are usually in the normal range for premature infants. However, premature infants require higher iodine intake levels than term infants to maintain a positive iodine balance in the extrauterine environment, so in iodine-deficient geographic areas, neonatal iodine deficiency may develop in preterm infants. The primary hypothyroid state develops during the first weeks of extrauterine life and often is superimposed on the transient hypothyroxinemia characteristic of prematurity. Urinary iodine excretion and thyroid iodine content are low. The hypothyroidism is transient but may persist for 2 to 3 months so that treatment is recommended. Iodine treatment also corrects this transient primary hypothyroid state. The average time to recovery of function and discontinuation of treatment in Belgium was 50 days.

Premature infants also are particularly susceptible to transient, iodine-induced hypothyroidism (Delange et al, 1985). The mechanism by which the thyroid cell inhibits iodide transport in response to increased plasma iodide levels matures near term. Thus, either in utero or in the postnatal period, administration of iodine-containing drugs to the mother or amniotic injection of radiographic contrast agents for amniofetography has induced hypothyroidism. Premature infants are more susceptible, but iodide-induced hypothyroidism can also develop in term infants. The dose of iodine required approximates 50 to 100 μg/kg per day. Urine iodine levels in iodine-induced hypothyroid infants usually exceed 1 mg/L. The hypothyroidism, with or without goiter, is characterized by low serum total T_4 and free T_4 concentrations and high levels of TSH and urinary iodide. Treatment of these infants is indicated.

Transient Hyperthyrotropinemia

Idiopathic hyperthyrotropinemia is a rare disorder. The serum TSH concentration is increased, often markedly, but other thyroid function parameters are normal, and the infants are euthyroid. In Japan, Miyai and coworkers (1979) have reported an incidence of 1:15,000 to 20,000 newborns; the prevalence in Europe and the United States is not precisely known but is much lower. The serum TSH concentration may remain elevated for as long as 9 months before spontaneously normalizing. Affected infants do not require treatment, but prolonged follow-up is necessary to exclude the possibility of a permanent disorder, such as an ectopic thyroid gland, an inborn defect in thyroid hormonogenesis, or a thyroid hormone resistance syndrome. Transient hyperthyrotropinemia without hypothyroxinemia in the newborn also may occur in response to intrauterine antithyroid drug exposure, intrauterine iodine excess or deficiency, or a maternal TSH-receptor–blocking antibody and has been recorded as a TSH assay artifact. The mechanism of transient idiopathic hyperthyrotropinemia is not clear. Delayed maturation of thyroid responsiveness to TSH or of the iodothyronine feedback control of pituitary TSH secretion have been suggested.

Low T_3 Syndrome in Premature Infants

In the preterm infant the changes in thyroid function parameters during neonatal adaptation are qualitatively similar to those in term infants but are quantitatively obtunded (Fisher and Klein, 1981). The neonatal TSH surge and the neonatal T_4 and T_3 peak responses decrease with decreasing gestational age, and the transient low T_3 state that follows probably is related to the state of relative undernutrition in the neonatal period. Premature infants have an increased susceptibility to neonatal morbidity including birth trauma, acidosis, hypoxia, hypoglycemia, hypocalcemia, and infection all superimposed on feeding disorders and relative malnutrition. All of these factors tend to inhibit peripheral T_4 to T_3 conversion and aggravate the extent of the low T_3 state characteristic of prematurity. Serum T_3 values may remain low in these infants for 1 to 2 months.

Features of the low T_3 syndrome in premature infants include a low serum T_3 concentration secondary to a decreased rate of conversion of T_4 to T_3, variable but usually elevated serum rT_3 levels, and normal or low total serum T_4 concentrations. Free T_4 levels usually are in the range of values for healthy premature infants of matched gestational age and weight. TSH values are low in these infants. Treatment is not warranted.

The wide application of neonatal screening programs for congenital hypothyroidism has resulted in the identification of other causes of low values of T_3 and T_4 in the newborn. Although physiologically these individuals are euthyroid, a discussion of these syndromes is warranted due to their impact on reported values of T_3 and T_4 in the perinatal period.

DISORDERS OF THYROID HORMONE CARRIER PROTEINS

The major determinants of the levels of circulating thyroid hormones are the concentrations of thyroid-hormone–binding proteins. As discussed, TBG, TBPA, and albumin all participate as thyroid hormone carrier proteins. Abnormalities of serum albumin concentration have been described; the major categories are dysalbuminemia and analbuminemia. However, albumin usually binds only about 10% of the circulating T_4 and 30% to 50% of T_3, and the concentrations of TBG and TBPA are normal or increased in these disorders. Consequently, the levels of thyroid hormones in these patients usually are in the normal range (Hollander et al, 1985). No confirmed primary disorder of TBPA resulting in abnormal thyroid hormone levels has been described to date. Thus, the plasma protein disorders associated with abnormal serum T_4 levels include only the variations in TBG and the recently described hyperthyroxinemic state "familial dysalbuminemic hyperthyroxinemia."

Thyroxine-Binding Globulin Deficiency

The prevalence of TBG deficiency varies from 1:5000 to 12,000 newborns and is transmitted as an X-linked trait. Serum TBG levels are very low in affected males and approximately half of normal in carrier females. In about half the families, the TBG level shown by radioimmunoassay (RIA) is very low; in the other half, the defect is partial; serum T_4 levels vary similarly. Affected subjects are euthyroid with normal serum TSH responses to exogenous TRH. Treatment is not indicated.

There are many structural defects of the TBG molecule accounting for defective TBG-T_4 binding. Variants have been reported in Australian aborigines and American blacks as well as in other populations. These inherited defects seem not to be due to large fragment deletions, insertions, or rearrangements of DNA; consequently, polymorphism studies have not been helpful in detection or screening. A single amino acid substitution (asparagine for isoleucine) at position 96 of the TBG molecule accounts for the marked reduction of T_4-binding capacity of TBG-Gary (Takamatsu et al, 1987). Table 102–5 summarizes the reported properties of several variant TBG molecules investigated. Most patients with partial TBG deficiency demonstrated elevated levels of denatured TBG measured by RIA, and each manifested a defective molecule with reduced stability and decreased binding capacity. Patients with severe TBG deficiency have been postulated to have a defect in hepatic TBG synthesis, but the molecular mechanism remains obscure.

Thyroxine-Binding Globulin Excess

Subjects with increased levels of TBG have increased total serum T_4 concentrations with normal TSH levels. Serum

TABLE 102–5

Properties of Reported Abnormal Thyroxine-Binding Globulin Molecules*

	TBG Concentrations		T_4 Concentration	TBG Affinity
	Normal	**Denatured**		
Normal TBG	100	100	100	100
TBG-S	88	100	84	100
TBG-A	74	100	58	54
TBG-Quebec	16	260	41	70
TBG-Montreal	14	390	38	<3
TBG-Gary	1	1000	24	<5

° Values listed as percentage of values in normal subjects. Normal absolute values for the measured parameters are TBG RIA 1.1 to 2.1 mg/dL; TBG-denatured <2 to 8 μg/dL; T_4 5 to 12 μg/dL; TBG affinity constant for T_4, 0.7 to 1.35 × 10^{-10}/M^{-1}.

RIA, radioimmunoassay; TBG, thyroxine-binding globulin.

Adapted from Takamatsu J, Refetoff S, Charbonneau M, et al: Two new inherited defects of the thyroxine-binding globulin (TBG) molecule presenting as partial TBG deficiency. J Clin Invest 79:833–840, 1987.

T_3 concentrations are modestly increased. In these subjects, as in those with low TBG concentrations, TBG production rates and serum levels are correlated, suggesting that the mechanism for the high TBG concentrations is increased production, presumably by the liver. TBG levels are increased fourfold to fivefold in affected individuals. Early reports suggested a dominant mode of inheritance, but subsequent studies are compatible with an X-linked mode of inheritance.

Familial Dysalbuminemic Hyperthyroxinemia

Several groups of investigators have reported euthyroid subjects with increased serum T_4 concentrations but normal free T_4, total serum T_3, and TSH levels (Ruiz et al, 1982). There is increased binding of T_4 to albumin, and the albumin in these patients has an affinity for T_4 binding intermediate between TBG and TBPA. T_3 is less avidly bound, accounting for the preferential increase in serum T_4 concentration. Patients with the disorder are euthyroid with normal thyroid hormone production rates. The abnormal albumin seems to be transmitted as an autosomal dominant trait.

Diagnosis in these patients is confirmed by protein electrophoresis of serum containing labeled T_4. The fraction of T_4 label associated with TBG, TBPA, or albumin is measured, and the albumin-bound T_4 can be calculated and related to normal values. Measurements of TBG and TBPA concentrations also are useful. Antithyroid therapy is not necessary in these patients, but it is important to make the diagnosis to avoid a misdiagnosis of hyperthyroidism.

Finally, although the emphasis of neonatal thyroidology is on early detection and appropriate therapy of the hypothyroid state, hyperthyroid states do occur and are associated with significant morbidity.

Neonatal Thyrotoxicosis

Neonatal Graves disease is rare, probably because of the low incidence of thyrotoxicosis in pregnancy (1 to 2 cases per 1000 pregnancies) and the fact that the neonatal disease occurs only in about one of 70 cases of thyrotoxic pregnancy (Burrow, 1974). In most cases, the disease is due to transplacental passage of thyroid-stimulating antibody (TSA) from a mother with active or inactive Graves disease or Hashimoto thyroiditis. Thus, prediction of neonatal Graves disease from the maternal clinical status is not always possible. However, it is possible to predict the occurrence of Graves disease in newborns on the basis of maternal TSA titers. In a report by Zakarija and coworkers (1986), all women with TSA titers exceeding 500% of control values (measured by stimulation of cAMP in human thyroid slices) delivered thyrotoxic infants, whereas those with lower titers delivered euthyroid infants. In some infants, both TSH-receptor–stimulating and TSH-receptor–blocking antibodies are acquired from the mother, and the blocking antibodies have been reported to block the effect of the stimulating antibodies for 4 to 6 weeks so that late-onset neonatal Graves disease develops in a previously unrecognized infant (McKenzie and Zakarija 1978).

Graves disease in the newborn is manifested by irritability, flushing, tachycardia, hypertension, poor weight gain, thyroid enlargement, and exophthalmos. Thrombocytopenia, hepatosplenomegaly, jaundice, and hypoprothrombinemia also have been observed. Arrhythmias, cardiac failure, and death may occur if the thyrotoxicity is severe and the treatment is inadequate. Mortality rate approaches 25% in disease severe enough to be diagnosed. In some infants the onset of symptoms and signs may be delayed as long as 8 to 9 days. This is due to the postnatal depletion of transplacentally acquired blocking doses of maternal antithyroid drugs and to the abrupt increase in conversion of T_4 to active T_3 shortly after birth in the newborn. The diagnosis is confirmed by measuring high levels of T_4, free T_4, and T_3 in postnatal blood. Cord blood values may be normal or near normal whereas levels at 2 to 5 days may be markedly increased; the serum TSH is low. Neonatal Graves disease resolves spontaneously as maternal TSA in the newborn is degraded. The usual clinical course of neonatal Graves disease extends 3 to 12 weeks.

The treatment of hyperthyroidism in the newborn includes sedatives and digitalis as necessary. Iodide or antithyroid drugs are administered to decrease thyroid hormone secretion. These drugs have additive effects with regard to inhibition of hormone synthesis; in addition, iodide rapidly inhibits hormone release. Lugol solution (5% iodine and 10% potassium iodide; 126 mg of iodine per milliliter) is given in doses of one drop (about 8 mg) three times daily. Methimazole, carbimazole, or propylthiouracil are administered in doses of 0.5 to 1 mg, 0.5 to 1 mg, or 5 to 10 mg, respectively, per kilogram daily in divided doses at 8-hour intervals. A therapeutic response should be observed within 24 to 36 hours. If a satisfactory response is not observed, the dose of antithyroid drug and iodide can be increased by 50%. Corticosteroids in anti-inflammatory doses and propranolol (1 to 2 mg/kg per day) also may be helpful. Radiographic contrast agents (ipodate, 200 mg/kg per day) also may be useful in treatment either alone or in conjunction with antithyroid drug treatment.

REFERENCES

Bernal J, Pekonen F: Ontogenesis of nuclear 3,5,3′ triiodothyronine receptors in human fetal brain. Endocrinology 114:667–679, 1984.

Brown A, Fernhoff PM, Milner J, et al: Racial differences in the incidence of congenital hypothyroidism. J Pediatr 99:934–937, 1981.

Burrow GN: The Thyroid Gland in Pregnancy. Philadelphia, WB Saunders, 1974, pp 83–100.

Chowdry P, Scanlon JW, Auerbach R, et al: Results of a controlled double-blind study of thyroid replacement in very low birth weight premature infants with hypothyroxinemia. Pediatrics 73:301–304, 1984.

Dammacco F, Dammacco A, Cavallo T, et al: Serum thyroglobulin and thyroid ultrasound studies in infants with congenital hypothyroidism. J Pediatr 106:451–453, 1985.

Delange F, Bourdoux P, Ermans AM: Transient disorders of thyroid function and regulation in preterm infants. *In* Delange F, Fisher DA, Malvaux P (Eds): Pediatric Thyroidology. Basel, Karger, 1985, pp 369–393.

den Ouden AL, Kok JH, Verkerk RH, et al: The relation between neonatal thyroxine levels and neuro developmental outcome at age 5 and 9 years in a national cohort of very preterm and/or very low birth weight infant. Pediatr Res 39:142–145, 1996.

Drexhage HA, Bottazzo GF: The thyroid and autoimmunity. *In* Delange F, Fisher DA, Malvaux P (Eds): Pediatric Thyroidology. Basel, Karger, 1985, pp 90–105.

Dussault JH, Letarte J, Guyda H, et al: Lack of influence of thyroid antibodies on thyroid function in the newborn infant and on a mass screening program for congenital hypothyroidism. J Pediatr 96:385–387, 1980.

Fisher DA: Thyroid hormone and thyroglobulin synthesis and secretion. *In* Delange F, Fisher DA, Malvaux P (Eds): Pediatric Thyroidology. Basel, Karger, 1985, pp 44–56.

Fisher DA, Klein AH: Thyroid development and disorders of thyroid function in the newborn. N Engl J Med 304:702–708, 1981.

Fort P, Lifschitz F, Bellisario R, et al: Abnormalities of thyroid function in infants with Down syndrome. J Pediatr 104:545–549, 1984.

Frasier SD, Penny R, Synder R: Primary congenital hypothyroidism in Spanish-surnamed infants in Southern California. J Pediatr 101:315–317, 1982.

Gonzales LA, Ballard PL: Identification and characterization of nuclear 3,5,3′-triiodothyronine binding sites in fetal human lung. J Clin Endocrinol Metab 53:21–28, 1981.

Hadeed AJ, Asay LD, Klein AH, et al: Significance of transient hypothyroxinemia in premature infants with and without respiratory distress syndrome. Pediatr Res 68:494–497, 1981.

Harada A, Hershman JM: Extraction of human chorionic thyrotropin (hCT) from term placentas: Failure to recover thyrotropic activity. J Clin Endocrinol Metab 47:681–685, 1978.

Hollander CS, Bernstein G, Oppenheimer JH: Anomalies in thyroid hormone transport proteins. *In* Delange F, Fisher DA, Malvaux P (Eds): Pediatric Thyroidology. Basel, Karger, 1985, pp 394–406.

Jacobsen BB, Brandt NJ: Congenital hypothyroidism in Denmark. Arch Dis Child 56Z:134–136, 1981.

Kruse K, Suss A, Busse M, et al: Monomeric serum calcitonin and bone turnover during anticonvulsant treatment and in congenital hypothyroidism. J Pediatr 111:57–65, 1987.

LaFranchi SH, Hanna CE, Krainz PL, et al: Screening for congenital hypothyroidism with specimen collection at two time periods: Results of the Northwest Regional Screening Program. Pediatrics 76:734–740, 1985.

Lever EG, Medeiros-Neto GA, DeGroot LJ: Inherited disorders of thyroid metabolism. Endocr Rev 4:213–247, 1983.

Marchant B, Brownlie BEW, Hant DM, et al: The placental transfer of propylthiouracil, methimazole and carbimazole. J Clin Endocrinol Metab 45:1187–1193, 1977.

Matsurra N, Yamamoto Y, Nohara Y, et al: Familial neonatal transient hypothyroidism due to maternal TSH-binding inhibitor immunoglobulins. N Engl J Med 303:733–741, 1980.

McCrossin RB, Sheffield LJ, Robertson EF: Persisting abnormality in the pituitary-thyroid axis in congenital hypothyroidism. *In* Nagetaki S, Stockgit JHR (Eds): Thyroid Research VIII. Canberra, Australian Academy of Science, 1980, pp 37–40.

McKenzie JM, Zakarija M: Pathogenesis of neonatal Graves' disease. J Endocrinol Invest 2:183–187, 1978.

Miyai K, Amino N, Nishi K, et al: Transient infantile hyperthyrotropinemia. Arch Dis Child 54:965–967, 1979.

Padbury JF, Polk DH, Newnham JP, et al: Neonatal adaptation: Greater sympathoadrenal response in preterm than full-term fetal sheep at birth. Am J Physiol Endocrinol Metab 11:E443–E447, 1985.

Polk DH, Callegari CC, Newnham JP, et al: Effect of fetal thyroidectomy on newborn thermogenesis in lambs. Pediatr Res 21:453–457, 1988a.

Polk DH, Wu SY, Wright C, et al: Ontogeny of thyroid hormone effect on tissue 5′ monodeiodinase activity in fetal sheep. Am J Physiol Endocrinol Metab 17:E337–E341, 1988b.

Refetoff S, Larsen PR: Transport, cellular uptake and metabolism of thyroid hormone. *In* DeGroot LJ, et al (Eds): Endocrinology. Philadelphia. WB Saunders, 1989, pp 541–561.

Reuss ML, Paneth N, Pihto-Martin JA, et al: The relation of transient hypothyroxinemia in preterm infants to neurological development at two years of age. N Engl J Med 39:142–145, 1996.

Roti E, Gnudi A, Braverman LE, et al: Human cord blood concentrations of thyrotropin, thyroglobulin and iodothyronines after maternal administration of thyrotropin-releasing hormone. J Clin Endocrinol Metab 53:813–817, 1981.

Roti E: Regulation of thyroid-stimulating hormone (TSH) secretion in the fetus and neonate. J Endocrinol Invest 11:145–150, 1988.

Ruiz M, Rajatanavin R, Young RA, et al. Familial dysalbuminemic hyperthyroxinemia. N Engl J Med 306:635–639, 1982.

Stanbury JB, Dumont JE: Familial goiter and related disorders. *In* Stanbury JB, et al (Eds): The Metabolic Basis of Inherited Disease. New York, McGraw Hill, 1983, pp 231–269.

Takamatsu J, Refetoff S, Charbonneau M, et al: Two new inherited defects of the thyroxine-binding globulin (TBG) molecule presenting as partial TBG deficiency. J Clin Invest 79:833–840, 1987.

Theodoropoulos T, Bravermann LE, Vagenakis AG: Iodide-induced hypothyroidism: A potential hazard during perinatal life. Science 205:502–503, 1979.

Van Wassenaer AG, Kok JH, de Vijlder JJM, et al: Effects of thyroxine supplementation on neurologic development in infants born at less than 30 weeks gestation. N Engl J Med 336:21–26, 1997.

Vulsma T, Gons MN, de Vijlder JJM: Maternal-fetal transfer of thyroxine in congenital hypothyroidism due to a total organification defect or thyroid agenesis. N Engl J Med 321:13–16, 1989.

Zakarija M, McKenzie JM: Pregnancy-associated changes in the thyroid stimulating antibody of Graves' disease and the relationship to neonatal hyperthyroidism. J Clin Endocrinol Metab 57:1036–1039, 1983.

Zakarija M, McKenzie JM, and Hoffman WH: Prediction and therapy of intrauterine and late onset neonatal hyperthyroidism. J Clin Endocrinol Metab 62:368–374, 1986.

CHAPTER 103

Disorders of Carbohydrate Metabolism

Daniel H. Polk

DISORDERS OF CARBOHYDRATE METABOLISM

Even though abnormalities of carbohydrate metabolism represent a wide spectrum of pathophysiologic states (inborn errors of metabolism, abnormal endocrine responses, nonspecific hypermetabolic states), they are included in this section on perinatal endocrine function because of the critical integration that must occur among a variety of organs to achieve glucose homeostasis. This section outlines the major endocrine pathways that regulate glucose levels and the pathophysiologic states that affect neonatal glucose metabolism. Because of the impact that maternal diabetes mellitus plays in altering neonatal glucose homeostasis, a discussion of infants born to mothers whose pregnancies are complicated by diabetes is also included.

Patterns of Perinatal Glucagon, Insulin, and Somatostatin Secretion

The pancreas appears during the 4th week of gestation in the human fetus. Development of the islets of Langerhans is classically divided into primary and secondary transition phases. During primary transition, the various secretory products of the alpha cell (glucagon), beta cell (insulin), and D cell (somatostatin) are immunohistochemically demonstrable. Through the influence of as yet uncharacterized pancreatic mesenchymal differentiation factors, further differentiation of these cell lines occurs. The phase of secondary transition involves the organization of these various cell types into mature islets.

Even though the pancreatic insulin concentration is higher in the fetus than adult and blood levels are comparable, the regulation of insulin secretion between the two varies markedly. Acute changes in fetal plasma glucose are not associated with significant changes in the pattern of plasma insulin levels (Menon and Sperling, 1988). This lack of insulin response is most likely caused by defects in the cAMP generating system of the beta-cell; phosphodiesterase inhibitors seem to augment an insulin response. Insulin receptors are abundant in many fetal tissues, representing the largely anabolic role of insulin in the fetus. The chronic effect of hyperglycemia on fetal insulin secretion is well known. Hypertrophy and hyperplasia of pancreatic islets and increased pancreatic insulin content are classically described in infants born to mothers whose own glucose metabolism is impaired as a result of diabetes mellitus. These infants also have a more mature pattern of insulin secretion in utero (Oakley et al, 1972). It is likely this maturational effect is due to a variety of influences including amino acids, catecholamines, and poorly understood influences of the fetal hypothalamic-pituitary axis (Grasso et al, 1973; Sperling et al, 1980a; Van Assche et al, 1970). Thus, whereas insulin is readily demonstrable in the developing fetus, control of secretion and patterns of

receptor ontogeny suggest the largely trophic function of this hormone in the fetus.

Glucagon is detectable in the fetal pancreas between the 6th and 8th week of gestation in the human (Schaeffer et al, 1973). The human placenta is impermeable to glucagon, and fetal plasma glucagon levels increase steadily from about the 15th week of gestation until term (Adam et al, 1972; Sperling et al, 1977). The fetal glucagon response, like that of insulin, is also relatively insensitive to acute changes in fetal glucose concentrations (when compared to responses in the adult). Hyperglycemia does not suppress glucagon levels in fetal sheep, and chronic but not acute hypoglycemia modulates fetal glucagon levels in the rat (Fiser et al, 1974; Girard et al, 1974). Amino acids (particularly alanine and arginine) are potent secretagogues for fetal pancreatic glucagon, as are acetylcholine and epinephrine (Sperling et al, 1980a). Fetal glucagon responses are also impaired. Physiologic doses of glucagon do not result in fetal hepatic glucose production, probably because of a paucity of fetal hepatic glucagon receptors. Incomplete glucagon receptor linking to cAMP in the fetus has also been proposed (Menon and Sperling, 1988).

The role of somatostatin in the maintenance of fetal glucose homeostasis is not well documented. In adults, somatostatin infusion suppresses both insulin and glucagon secretion. This is accompanied by an initial decrease in plasma glucose concentrations (resulting from the initial glucagon deficiency), which then normalize. These observations have been extended to the newborn lamb (Menon and Sperling, 1988). The role for fetal somatostatin remains to be described.

FETAL GLUCOSE METABOLISM

In the basal nonstressed state, placental transport of glucose from mother to fetus meets all of the fetal glucose requirements. This observation is supported by several investigators. Using glucose tracer techniques, Kalhan and coworkers (1979) have shown that no net glucose production can be demonstrated in the human fetus at term. Hay and associates (1983) have used the Fick principle and glucose isotope dilution techniques to show that umbilical vein glucose uptake equals fetal glucose utilization. Finally, in fetal sheep, no gluconeogenesis is demonstrable under basal, nonstressed conditions (Sperling et al, 1980b). In all species studied, fetal glucose concentrations are related to, but lower than, maternal glucose concentrations. The rate of glucose utilization in the human fetus is uncertain; values of 6 to 10 mg/kg per minute have been described in studies of fetal sheep.

Glucose may not be the sole energy source for the fetus. Basal measurements of placental substrates and fetal oxygen consumption suggest that as much as 50% of the substrates used for fetal respiration are derived from lactate and amino acids (Battaglia and Meschia, 1978). This proportion may change in response to maternal starvation as well as during periods of fetal stress. In vivo measurements of oxygen consumption in various organs suggest that the majority of glucose is used to support fetal brain metabolism. The relative dependence of the fetus on maternal sources of glucose may be altered during fetal stress. Catecholamines, particularly epinephrine, are released in large quantities following a variety of physiologic states including fetal hypotension and hypoxia. Fetal epinephrine infusion at physiologic concentrations results in significant increases in fetal glucose and fatty acid levels resulting from stimulation of hepatic and adipocyte beta-adrenergic receptors. The substrate-mobilizing threshold for this catecholamine effect is much lower than the level of epinephrine required for fetal insulin or glucagon stimulation (Padbury et al, 1987).

Glucose Homeostasis at Parturition

At birth, a variety of events occur that permit the newborn to assume its own glucose homeostasis. In general, changes in circulatory insulin and glucagon levels as well as changes in their related receptors are accompanied by increases in enzyme activities essential for glycogenolysis and gluconeogenesis. Both serum glucagon and catecholamines increase threefold to fivefold in response to umbilical cord-cutting (Padbury et al, 1981; Sperling et al, 1980a). Circulating insulin levels usually decrease in the immediate newborn period and remain low for several days. The high epinephrine, high glucagon, and low insulin state may be related: epinephrine both stimulates pancreatic glucagon release and inhibits the release of insulin. The dependence of normal neonatal glucose homeostasis on adrenal epinephrine release has been demonstrated in adrenalectomized newborn sheep (Padbury et al, 1987). Thus, the depressed serum insulin and elevated glucagon and epinephrine levels (along with elevated serum growth hormone levels) at birth favor glycogenolysis, lipolysis, and gluconeogenesis. This is supported by observations in newborns. After a transient decrease immediately after birth, serum glucose levels increase, hepatic glycogen stores deplete, and plasma fatty acid concentrations reflecting lipolysis increase. Gluconeogenesis (predominantly from alanine), which is difficult to demonstrate in the fetus, becomes evident in the newborn.

Changes in various hormonal receptors also modulate these processes. Hepatic glucagon receptors increase in number and become functionally linked with cAMP responses (Ganguli et al, 1983). The functional significance of the decrease in insulin receptors that occurs during this time is unknown, but it parallels the decrease in postnatal serum insulin levels.

Neonatal glucose homeostasis also requires appropriate enzyme maturation and response in the newborn. The neonatal liver, in contrast to that of the fetus, is characterized by an increase in glycogen phosphorylase activity and a decrease in glycogen synthetase activity, consistent with the rapid depletion of hepatic glycogen seen during the newborn period. Phosphoenolpyruvate carboxykinase activity, which is the rate-limiting enzyme required for gluconeogenesis, also increases during the immediate postnatal period. This is likely a response to the changes in glucagon and insulin that occur during the immediate postnatal period (Girard, 1986; Granner et al, 1983). Gluconeogenesis provides about 10% of the glucose metabolized in the newborn during the hours following birth (Frazier et al, 1981). Thus, hormonal, receptor, and enzyme activities in the fetus provide for anabolism and substrate accretion, whereas those in the newborn period predominantly provide for the maintenance of glucose homeostasis in response to the abrupt interruption of maternal glucose supply. As can be inferred, many pathophysiologic states may impact this balance leading to hypoglycemia or hyperglycemia in the newborn.

HYPOGLYCEMIA
Definition and Diagnosis

In adults, brain metabolism accounts for nearly 80% of the total glucose comsumption. This value may be higher in newborns in whom the brain represents a proportionally larger tissue mass. Thus, glucose utilization is highest in the preterm infant when compared with term infant and adult values. The rate of glucose utilization in preterm infants is approximately 6 to 8 mg/kg per minute, whereas adult values range from 2 to 4 mg/kg per minute (Bier et al, 1977). That the brain is the primary site for glucose utilization and uses glucose as a primary energy source leads to the predominance of neurologic symptoms that accompany hypoglycemia (Table 103–1).

Blood glucose values in term and preterm infants after birth are shown in Figure 103–1. There is no consensus defining a blood glucose level diagnostic of hypoglycemia. Earlier data defining hypoglycemia as blood glucose levels of 30 mg/dL in term infants and 20 mg/dL in preterm infants relied on measurements in fasted infants and are probably not valid. Other concerns about the long-term effects of asymptomatic neonatal hypoglycemia, first raised by Pildes and coworkers (1974), have led to efforts to aggressively diagnose and treat this entity. There are limited data correlating the length of the hypoglycemic period with outcome or the relative risk of symptomatic versus asymptomatic hypoglycemia (Lucas et al, 1988). Because of these concerns and uncertainties, it seems prudent to aggressively screen infants at risk for hypoglycemia and treat those with values less than 40 mg/dL (Schwartz, 1997). In most nurseries, this consists of heelstick whole blood determinations of glucose using a commercially available indicator (Dextrostix or Chemstrip). Although useful, these methods have limitations. Various agents including fluoride, uric acid, bilirubin, acetaminophen, and isopropyl alcohol have been shown to interfere with these determinations. Additionally, low glucose values as reported by the

TABLE 103–1

Symptoms in Neonatal Hypoglycemia

Jitteriness	Apnea
Lethargy	Cyanosis
Feeding intolerance	Seizures

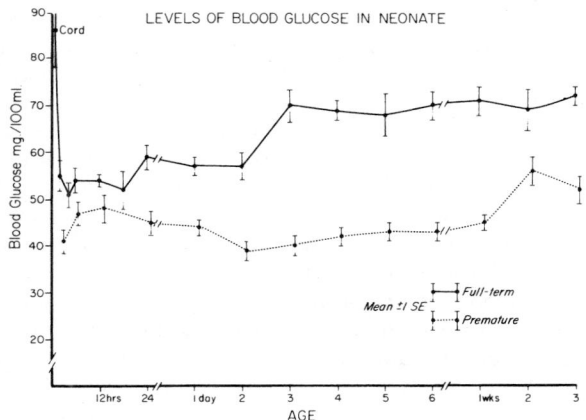

FIGURE 103–1. A total of 206 determinations of blood glucose levels was obtained in 179 full-sized infants (>2.5 kg), and a total of 442 determinations was made in 104 low-birth-weight infants (<2.5 kg) throughout the neonatal period. (From Cornblath M, Reisner S: N Engl J Med 273:378, 1965. Reprinted by permission of the New England Journal of Medicine.)

reagent strips tend to underestimate the degree of hypoglycemia present. Values close to those representing hypoglycemia (<40 mg/dL) or hyperglycemia (> 125 mg/dL) should be confirmed by actual laboratory chemical analysis. Initial therapies, especially in asymptomatic infants, should not be postponed in borderline cases, but continuation of therapy should be based on reliable laboratory glucose values. Because the onset and duration of hypoglycemia is variable in infants at risk, repeated routine screening of these infants should continue until the risk period for development of hypoglycemia has passed. Certain pathophysiologic states (infants of diabetic pregnancies or infants who are small for gestational age) may require screening over several days (Koh et al, 1988).

Conditions Associated with Neonatal Hypoglycemia

In general, hypoglycemia develops in newborns as a result of one or more of three basic mechanisms: (1) limited glycogen stores, (2) hyperinsulinism, or (3) diminished glucose production. Each of these categories is associated with several different disease states (Table 103–2). In addition, various other conditions are associated with hypoglycemia through unknown mechanisms.

Limited Glycogen Stores

Preterm Infants

Most hepatic glycogen accumulation occurs in the 3rd trimester of pregnancy. Prematurity is associated with decreased hepatic stores of glycogen and thus may predispose infants to hypoglycemia. Hypoglycemia develops in as many as 15% of preterm infants in the first hours of birth. As a variety of other conditions, associated with a risk of hypoglycemia (e.g., sepsis, feeding intolerance, and hypothermia), may develop, there may be additive effects on the duration and course of their hypoglycemia. The relatively

increased proportion of brain tissue in preterm infants may also contribute to increased glucose requirements. Because hypoglycemia is so prevalent in preterm infants, routine blood glucose screening while the infant is sick or until feedings are well established is critical. The onset of hypoglycemia after the immediate newborn period in an otherwise stable preterm infant should prompt an evaluation for other associated conditions (e.g., sepsis).

Perinatal Distress

Infants who are stressed in utero or intrapartum are at risk for hypoglycemia. Hypoxia and acidosis lead to increased catecholamine activity, which promotes hepatic glycogenolysis. Hypoxia also accelerates glucose utilization due to the effects of anaerobic metabolism. Roughly 18 times more glucose is required to produce comparable amounts of adenosine triphosphate (ATP) during anaerobic metabolism. There is evidence that neurologic outcome in stressed fetuses requiring resuscitation at birth is improved by early glucose administration (Dawes et al, 1963). However, others have reported detrimental effects of hyperglycemia in association with or following fetal/neonatal asphyxia. In the absence of better data, euglycemia is the goal.

Disorders of Glycogen Metabolism

Three disorders of glycogen metabolism may present with hypoglycemia in the newborn period. Glucose-6-phosphatase deficiency, amylo-1,6-glucosidase deficiency, and phosphorylase deficiency limit either glycogen metabolism or glucose release, resulting in excess glycogen stores, hepatomegaly, and hypoglycemia. Diagnosis of these disorders ultimately rests on laboratory analysis of biopsy material in children with characteristic phenotypes (cherubic face,

---

TABLE 103–2

Conditions Associated with Neonatal Hypoglycemia

Limited Glycogen Supply

Prematurity
Perinatal stress
Starvation
Glycogen storage disease

Hyperinsulinism

Infant of a diabetic mother
Beckwith-Wiedemann syndrome
Maternal drug therapy
Islet cell adenoma or nesidioblastosis
Erythroblastosis fetalis

Diminished Glucose Production

Small-for-gestation-age infants
Inborn errors of metabolism

Others

Hypothermia
Sepsis
Hypothalamic or hypopituitary disorders
Adrenal insufficiency
Polycythemia

truncal obesity, and hepatomegaly). These disorders are inherited primarily in an autosomal recessive manner.

Hyperinsulinism

Infant of a Diabetic Mother

A variety of disorders leading to neonatal hypoglycemia are the result of fetal or neonatal hyperinsulinism. The prototype for this condition is the infant of a diabetic mother. These children are at risk for neonatal hypoglycemia caused by the persistence of fetal hyperinsulinism in the face of an interrupted supply of maternal glucose. Other maternal metabolic substrates (amino acids and lipids) may also play a role in maintaining the fetal hyperinsulinemic state. The fetal hyperinsulinemic state is induced by these abnormal quantities and types of metabolic fuels transplacentally acquired, resulting in fetal pancreatic beta-cell hypertrophy. Hypoglycemia in affected infants frequently occurs 4 to 6 hours after birth, although the coexistence of other complications may impact this timing. These infants also manifest augmented pancreatic beta-cell sensitivity to glucose, which persists for several days after birth, and thus continue to be at risk for hypoglycemia during this time (Molsted-Peterson and Jorgensen, 1972).

The persistent fetal hyperinsulinemia leads to effects on all insulin-sensitive tissues, giving rise to the myriad of clinical signs and symptoms seen in these infants (Table 103–3). In addition to the disorders of carbohydrate metabolism, these infants are at significant risk for other types of perinatal morbidity. The observed increased incidence of respiratory distress in these infants is the result of many factors; the influences of glucose and insulin on surfactant and pulmonary function have been extensively studied. This work is outlined in Chapters 4 and 48. Affected infants may exhibit all of the manifestations of respiratory distress syndrome despite advanced gestational age or documented amniotic fluid lecithin-to-sphingomyelin ratios of more than 2:1.

The effects of chronic stimulation of insulin and insulin-like growth factor receptors in many fetal tissues including placenta, liver, heart, and adipose tissues may lead to large-for-gestational-age infants with their attendant difficulties during labor and delivery. The increased incidence of intra-partum fetal distress and third trimester fetal demise may result from placental dysfunction caused by abnormal substrate accretion and decreased diffusion capacity. Perinatal stress may have an additive effect on the degree of hypoglycemia via effects of catecholamines, glucocorticoids, and glycogen depletion. Plethora and hyperviscosity resulting from increased red blood cell mass may further compromise these infants who are at risk of development of venous thromboses. Erythropoietin levels are elevated in the infants of diabetic mothers, but the relative contributions of placental insufficiency, perinatal stress, and insulin to increased red blood cell mass are not well characterized. Hyperbilirubinemia may be present as a result of the increased red cell mass or secondary to placental or hepatic dysfunction. These infants may also manifest hypocalcemia—again, reflecting reduced placental function; hypoxia and perinatal stress probably also contribute to neonatal hypocalcemia in affected infants. A subgroup of infants born to diabetic mothers have marked hypertrophy of the cardiac septum and present with congestive heart failure. The increased incidence of other structural heart lesions may complicate the differential diagnosis of these infants; specific diagnosis is usually confirmed by cardiac ultrasound.

The observed increase in congenital malformations in infants of diabetic mothers led to the hypothesis that alterations in maternal glucose metabolism in the first weeks of pregnancy may cause defects in organogenesis. The work by Miller and coworkers (1981) correlated excess maternal glucose levels during the 1st trimester with an increased incidence of congenital malformations in their infants. Insulin does not seem to be teratogenic, but hyperglycemia, hyperketonemia, and hyperosmolality have all been shown to disrupt organogenesis in animal models. Increased attention to maternal glucose homeostasis later in pregnancy has dramatically improved perinatal mortality; the same may be true for early attention ameliorating associated congenital malformations (Reece et al, 1988). Transient hypoglycemia may also disrupt organogenesis as well as affect later fetal growth indices; both extremes of maternal hyperglycemia and hypoglycemia are therefore to be avoided (Buchanan et al, 1986).

In certain instances, the phenotype and clinical symptoms of hyperinsulinemic infants are so striking as to suggest the diagnosis of maternal diabetes mellitus. This diagnosis is supported by the finding of increased maternal levels of circulating glycosylated hemoglobin (Hgb A_1c). Although glucose homeostasis frequently returns toward normal in the days following delivery in women with gestational diabetes mellitus, Hgb A_1c levels remain elevated for weeks after delivery. Because of the impact of this condition on subsequent pregnancies, this diagnosis should be actively pursued in pregnancies complicated by inadequate prenatal care and large-for-gestational-age infants.

Mothers with severe long-standing diabetes associated with vasculopathy or retinopathy (White class F) may give birth to infants who are small for gestational age and prone to all the perinatal complications described. This condition is more fully described in Chapters 7 and 48.

Other Causes of Hyperinsulinism

In rare instances, primary abnormalities of pancreatic beta-cell development result in sustained neonatal hyperinsulinism and hypoglycemia. "Nesidioblastosis" is characterized by a proliferation of pancreatic beta cells. In addition, discrete islet-cell adenomas may mimic most of the features of nesidioblastosis. Because these abnormalities may be present during fetal development, affected infants may initially

TABLE 103–3

Associated Conditions in Infants of Diabetic Mothers

Congenital malformations	Hypocalcemia
Macrosomia	Hyperviscosity
Fetal distress	Hyperbilirubinemia
Sudden fetal demise	Respiratory distress
Hypoglycemia	Feeding difficulties

be indistinguishable from infants of diabetic mothers, but the persistence of prolonged hypoglycemia usually suggests the diagnosis. Inappropriately elevated blood insulin–to–glucose ratios (plasma insulin greater than 10 μIU/mL when plasma glucose is less than 40 mg/dL) or increased requirements (typically greater than 15 mg/kg per minute) frequently are present, although these findings are not specific for primary pancreatic beta-cell disorders. Medical management (steroids, diazoxide, or somatostatin) may ameliorate these conditions, but surgery may offer a definitive means of both diagnosis and treatment (Levitt Katz et al, 1997.

Beckwith-Wiedemann Syndrome

Infants with the syndrome of exopthalmos, macroglossia, and gigantism often have associated omphaloceles, macrosomia, and neonatal hypoglycemia. This condition is associated with pancreatic beta-cell hypertrophy and hyperinsulinism; the metabolic defect is unknown. Most cases of Beckwith-Wiedemann syndrome are sporadic, but there is some evidence that it may be inherited as an autosomal dominant trait (Engstrom et al, 1988). Early recognition and treatment of the attendant hypoglycemia is likely to improve the intellectual outcome of these infants.

Erythroblastosis Fetalis

Infants with erythroblastosis fetalis complicating Rh incompatibility may also manifest hypoglycemia secondary to hyperinsulinism. Pancreatic beta-cell hyperplasia is demonstrable, but the underlying biochemical defect is unknown. Although unrelated, infants undergoing exchange transfusion for any cause are at risk for hypoglycemia afterward because of the transient stimulation of endogenous insulin by the added dextrose in citrated stored blood products. The insulin response then leads to rebound hypoglycemia as the infused glucose is metabolized (Schiff et al, 1971). Heparinized blood contains no added glucose, but may lead to hypoglycemia owing to limited substrate availability during a double-volume exchange procedure.

Maternal Drug Effects on Neonatal Glucose Metabolism

Maternal chlorpropamide and benzothiazides increase fetal insulin secretion and predispose the newborn to hypoglycemia. The teratogenicity of chlorpropamide precludes most fetal exposure. Propranolol may also induce neonatal hypoglycemia via inhibition of catecholamine-induced glycogenolysis. Beta-sympathomimetics, commonly used in the prophylaxis of preterm labor, have been occasionally associated with neonatal hypoglycemia (Ogata, 1981). This may result from both direct effects on fetal insulin secretion as well as effects mediated via abnormal maternal glucose concentrations. Inappropriate intrapartum maternal glucose administration may also lead to transient fetal hyperinsulinism and attendant neonatal hypoglycemia. This is particularly important as a consequence of inappropriate fluid management in the treatment of epidural anesthesia-associated hypotension.

Diminished Glucose Production

Small for Gestational Age

Infants born small for gestational age not only have decreased glycogen stores but impaired gluconeogenesis. Elevated levels of gluconeogenic precursors (particularly alanine) have been reported in the blood of these infants. Defects in phosphoenolpyruvate carboxykinase activity (the rate-limiting enzyme for gluconeogenesis) have been suggested (Bussey et al, 1985). While insulin and glucagon secretion are similar in appropriate and small-for-gestational-age infants, the plasma amino acid response to glucagon may be altered in hypoglycemic small-for-gestational-age infants. Commonly, several days are required for these infants to maintain normal glucose homeostasis; thus, they remain at risk for hypoglycemia for an extended time after birth.

Inborn Errors of Metabolism

Rarely, aminoacidopathies (particularly those amino acids involved in gluconeogenesis) may be associated with neonatal hypoglycemia. The diagnosis rests on the demonstration of abnormal concentrations of amino acids in blood or urine samples.

Other Causes Associated with Neonatal Hypoglycemia

Hypothermia has been associated with hypoglycemia in part through the augmented effects of circulating catecholamines. The infants most likely at risk for hypothermia are those who are least able to support their own glucose requirements; thus, preterm stressed infants requiring resuscitation are at major risk for hypoglycemia. Infants exhibiting temperature instability should have their glucose status evaluated as well. Cortisol and growth hormone deficiencies are associated with hypoglycemia secondary to effects on hepatic glycogenolysis and gluconeogenesis. Polycythemia may lead to hypoglycemia as a direct result of increased glucose consumption by the red cell mass as well as secondary to effects on the intestinal absorption of substrates. Postprandial hypoglycemia has been noted in infants who are leucine-sensitive. This may be mediated by leucine effects on insulin secretion. Appropriate alteration of feeding schedules usually obviates these effects.

DIAGNOSIS AND TREATMENT OF NEONATAL HYPOGLYCEMIA

All infants at risk for development of neonatal hypoglycemia should be monitored, because anticipation and prevention are much more effective in the improvement of neonatal outcome than treatment. Blood glucose values less than 40 mg/dL should be verified and treated. Anticipation requires that screening continue for several days in infants of diabetic mothers and those born small for gestational age. Preterm infants should also be routinely monitored until feedings are well established.

The treatment of hypoglycemia depends on several factors. Infants who are asymptomatic with borderline glucose levels and capable of enteral feeds may receive either formula or 5% dextrose in water as an initial therapy.

Hypoglycemia may progress or persist in these infants, and they should continue to be closely monitored. Infants with symptomatic hypoglycemia should be given intravenous glucose solutions. I favor an initial bolus of 100 mg/kg of 10% dextrose in water solution (1 mL/kg). This is followed by a continuous infusion of 6 mg/kg per minute of 10% dextrose in water. This method is associated with a much lower incidence of rebound hyperglycemia or hypoglycemia than previous approaches based on 20% or 50% dextrose solutions (Lilien et al, 1980). The rate of infusion can be titrated to provide for normal blood glucose levels. The use of a peripheral vein for infusion is preferable to an umbilical vessel, particularly for prolonged infusions. Infusions of glucose into an umbilical artery have been associated with hyperinsulinism via direct pancreatic stimulation by the infused glucose.

In circumstances of extremely high glucose utilization associated with hyperinsulinism, corticosteroids, glucagon, diazoxide, and somatostatin have all been suggested as additional adjunctive therapy. Although successful, their use should be restricted to isolated cases or when in collaboration with endocrine consultants.

HYPERGLYCEMIA

Hyperglycemia, defined as a blood glucose greater than 125 mg/dL, is most commonly encountered in the very-low-birth-weight (< 1500 g) infant receiving intravenous glucose infusions. The glucose infusion rate may inadvertently exceed 6 to 8 mg/kg per minute as the fluids are advanced if the concentration of glucose is not adjusted accordingly. The osmotic diuresis and resultant dehydration can be marked in these cases; the resultant hyperosmolar state has been associated with intraventricular hemorrhage.

Sepsis and stress have also been associated with hyperglycemia in any infant. This is probably caused by multiple influences of catecholamines, cortisol, and acid-base status on the mobilization of glycogen, gluconeogenesis, and insulin responses. Endotoxins have been proposed to have direct effects on insulin actions in septic infants.

A transient state of neonatal diabetes mellitus has also been described. In approximately one third of the cases there is a positive family history of diabetes mellitus. Some of these infants are thought to have a deficiency in pancreatic beta-cell adenylcyclase activity, which improves with time (Haymond et al, 1989). The defect in the remaining infants is unknown. Many of these infants are small for gestational age and present with polyuria, glucosuria, and hyperglycemia. They may progress to severe dehydration, acidosis, and ketonemia. These infants require prompt attention to maintain their fluid and electrolyte balance and insulin therapy. The syndrome is usually self-limiting, and normal glucose homeostasis after the neonatal period is common. Rarely, hyperglycemia may be noted in infants receiving methylxanthines (theophylline). It is speculated that the increased levels of cAMP associated with this therapy activate hepatic glucose output.

Finally, several pitfalls in the diagnosis of neonatal hyperglycemia have been described. Glucose values of blood samples obtained from umbilical catheters concurrently used for glucose infusion are unreliable unless strict attention is paid to inadvertent glucose contamination. In cases of concern, heelstick blood may provide a more reasonable value.

Tests using Benedict solution (alkaline solution of cupric-citrate ions) for carbohydrate determination in urine are not glucose-specific and react with any reducing sugar (notably galactose). Thus, glycosuria can be inadvertently diagnosed and galactosemia missed unless specific glucose or galactose determinations are made. In the same manner, urine dipstick methods using glucose oxidase are specific for glucose as a substrate; galactose does not react with this agent.

REFERENCES

Adam PAJ, King KC, Schwartz R, et al: Human placental barrier to ^{125}I-glucagon early in gestation. J Clin Endocrinol Metab 34:772–775, 1972.

Battaglia FC, Meschia G: Principal substrates of fetal metabolism. Physiol Rev 58:499–531, 1978.

Bier DM, Leake RD, Haymond MW, et al: Measurement of "true" glucose production rates in infancy and childhood with 6,6-dideutero-glucose. Diabetes 26:1016–1023, 1977.

Buchanan T, Schweiner JK, Freinkel N: Embryotoxic effects of brief maternal insulin-hypoglycemia during organogenesis in the rat. J Clin Invest 78:643–649, 1986.

Bussey ME, Finley S, Ogata ES: Hypoglycemia in the newborn growth-retarded rat. Delayed phosphoenol pyruvate carboxylase induction despite increased glycogen availability. Pediatr Res 19:363–367, 1985.

Dawes GS, Jacobsen HN, Moh JC, et al: The treatment of asphyxiated mature foetal lambs and rhesus monkeys with intravenous glucose and sodium carbonate. J Physiol 169:167–184, 1963.

Engstrom W, Lindham S, Schofield P: Wiedmann-Beckwith syndrome. Eur J Pediatr 147:450–457, 1988.

Fiser RH, Erenberg A, Sperling MA, et al: Insulin-glucagon substrate interrelations in the fetal sheep. Pediatr Res 8:951–953, 1974.

Frazier TE, Karl IE, Hillman LS, et al: Direct measurement of gluconeogenesis from (2,3,[13]C2) alanine in the human newborn. Am J Physiol 240:E615–E621, 1981.

Ganguli S, Sinha MK, Sterman B, et al: Ontogeny of hepatic insulin and glucagon receptors and adenylate cyclase in the rabbit. Am J Physiol 244:E624–E631, 1983.

Girard J: Gluconeogenesis in late fetal and early neonatal life. Biol Neonate 50:237–258, 1986.

Girard JR, Kervan A, Soufflet E, et al: Factors affecting the secretion of insulin and glucagon by the rat fetus. Diabetes 23:310–314, 1974.

Granner D, Andreone T, Sabitie K, et al: Inhibition of transcription of the phosphoenol pyruvate carboxykinase gene by insulin. Nature 305:549–551, 1983.

Grasso S, Messina A, DiStefano G, et al: Insulin secretion in the premature infant: Response to glucose and amino acids. Diabetes 22:349–353, 1973.

Hay WW Jr, Sparks JW, Wilkening RB, et al: Fetal glucose uptake and utilization as functions of maternal glucose concentration. Am J Physiol 245:E347–E350, 1983.

Haymond MH, Pagliara AS, Bier DM: Endocrine and metabolic aspects of fuel homeostasis in the fetus and neonate. *In* DeGroot LJ, Besser GM, Cahill GF, et al. (Eds): Endocrinology. Philadelphia, WB Saunders, 1989, pp 2215–2241.

Kalhan SC, D'Angelo LJ, Savin SM, et al: Glucose production in pregnant women at term gestation. J Clin Invest 63:388–394, 1979.

Koh THHG, Aynsley-Green A, Tarbit M, et al: Neonatal hypoglycaemia: The controversy regarding definition. Arch Dis Child 63:1386, 1988.

Levitt Katz LE, Satin-Smith MS, Collett-Solberg P, et al: Insulin-like growth factor binding protein-1 levels in the diagnosis of hypoglycemia caused by hyperinsulinism. J Pediatr 131:193–199, 1997.

Lilien LD, Pildes R, Srinivasan G, et al: Treatment of neonatal hypoglycemia with minibolus and intravenous glucose infusion. J Pediatr 97:295–298, 1980.

Lucas A, Morley R, Cole JJ: Adverse neurodevelopmental outcome of moderate neonatal hyperglycaemia. BMJ 297:304, 1988.

Menon RK, Sperling MA: Carbohydrate metabolism. Semin Perinatol 12:157–162, 1988.

Miller E, Hare JW, Cloherty JP, et al: Elevated maternal hemoglobin A$_{1c}$ in early pregnancy and major congenital anomalies in infants of diabetic mothers. N Engl J Med 304:1331–1334, 1981.

Molsted-Peterson L, Jorgensen KR: Aspects of carbohydrate metabolism in newborn infants of diabetic mothers. III. Plasma insulin during intravenous glucose tolerance test. Acta Endocrinol 71:115–126, 1972.

Oakley NW, Beard RW, Turner RC: Effect of sustained maternal hyperglycemia on the fetus in normal and diabetic pregnancies. BMJ 1:466–473, 1972.

Ogata ES: Isoxysuprine infusion in the rat: Maternal fetal and neonatal glucose homeostasis. J Perinatol Med 9:293–301, 1981.

Padbury J, Roberman B, Oddie TH, et al: Fetal catecholamine release in response to labor and delivery. Obstet Gynecol 60:607–611, 1981.

Padbury J, Agata Y, Ludlow J, et al: Effect of fetal adrenalectomy on catecholamine release and physiologic adaptation at birth of sheep. J Clin Invest 80:1096–1103, 1987.

Pildes RS, Cornblath M, Warren I, et al: A prospective controlled study of neonatal hypoglycemia. Pediatrics 54:5–14, 1974.

Reece EA, Gabrielli S, Abdalla M: The prevention of diabetes-associated birth defects. Semin Perinatol 12:292–301, 1988.

Schaeffer LD, Wilder ML, Williams RH: Secretion and content of insulin and glucagon in human fetal pancreas slices in vitro. Proc Soc Exp Biol Med 143:314–318, 1973.

Schiff D, Aranda JV, Colle E, et al: Metabolic effects of exchange transfusions II. Delayed hypoglycemia following exchange transfusion with citrated blood. J Pediatr 79:589–593, 1971.

Schwartz RP: Neonatal hypoglycemia: How low is too low? J Pediatr 131:171–173, 1997.

Sperling MA, Christiansen RA, Artal R, et al: The nature and significance of amniotic fluid (AF) glucagon. Pediatr Res 11:412 (Abstract), 1977.

Sperling MA, Christiansen R, Ganguli S, et al: Adrenergic modulation of pancreatic hormone secretion in utero: Studies in fetal sheep. Pediatr Res 14:203–208, 1980a.

Sperling MA: Carbohydrate metabolism: Glucagon, insulin and somatostatin. *In* Tulchinsky D, Ryan K, (Eds): Maternal-Fetal Endocrinology. Philadelphia, WB Saunders, 1980b, pp 333–353.

Van Assche FA, Gepts W, DeGasparo M: The endocrine pancreas in anencephalics: A histological, histochemical and biological study. Biol Neonate 14:374–377, 1970.

PART XVI
NEOPLASIA

CHAPTER 104

Congenital Malignant Disorders

Katherine K. Matthay[*]

Neonatal malignancies differ in incidence, clinical behavior, and heritable features from the cancers seen in older children. Exposure to potential carcinogens or teratogens during the prenatal period may be related etiologically. Special consideration must also be given to treatment problems peculiar to the newborn age group, including differences in drug metabolism and pharmacokinetics from older children and the possible intolerance of rapidly growing and developing normal tissues to the inhibitory effects of antineoplastic chemotherapy and radiation. Late effects on reproductive capacity, intellectual development, and induction of secondary malignancy are also of heightened concern in treatment in the newborn. The epidemiology of neonatal malignancy is reviewed here, followed by disease-specific discussions of the most commonly encountered malignancies in the newborn. Other malignancies specific to individual organ systems are discussed elsewhere in this book.

EPIDEMIOLOGY
Incidence and Mortality

A study of death certificates by Fraumeni and Miller during the 5-year period ranging from 1960 to 1964 revealed that the death rate from malignant diseases in infants younger than 28 days of age was 6.25 per 1 million live births (Table 104–1). More than one half of cancer deaths in the neonatal period occurred in the 1st week of life, and more than one third occurred on the 1st day (Fraumeni and Miller, 1969).

Basing their report on the Third National Cancer Survey (1969–1971), Bader and Miller (1979) found the incidence of malignant neoplasms in the United States to be 183.4 per 1 million live births in infants younger than 1 year and 36.5 per 1 million live births in newborns younger than 29 days. The cancer incidence in those younger than 1 year was almost 3 1/2 times greater than mortality determined from death certificates from 1960 to 1969. When mortality of infants younger than age 1 year is used as an indicator of frequency, leukemia appears to be the most common cancer, followed by neuroblastoma, central nervous system tumors, and renal tumors. When ranked by incidence, neuroblastoma is most common, followed by leukemia, renal tumors, sarcomas, retinoblastomas, and central nervous system tumors. Because retinoblastoma is so often

cured, the incidence is 159 times greater than the mortality rate.

Among newborns, the incidence of neuroblastoma is more than 10 times greater than the mortality rate for this tumor, whereas the incidence of leukemia is less than 2 times greater than its mortality rate. Thus, a study of mortality rates differs markedly from one of incidence, because certain malignancies are rapidly fatal, others lead to death beyond the neonatal period, and a large number are curable or undergo spontaneous regression. Data from the Third National Cancer Study indicate that approximately 653 cancers are diagnosed annually in infants in the United States and that 130 of these cancers are found in newborns. A summary of incidence, mortality, and types of malignancies seen in the newborn and infant is shown in Table 104–2. Although there is no more recent national update of neonatal cancer incidence available, the relative frequency and incidence of childhood cancer has changed little in the period from 1973 to 1987. In the 0- to 4-year age group, there has been an overall increase of 0.3 per 100,000, whereas the incidence of leukemia in this age

TABLE 104–1

Mortality from Malignant Neoplasms in United States Children Younger than 5 Years as Compared with Those Younger than 28 Days of Age, 1960–1964

| Neoplasm | No. Deaths in Children Aged Younger than 5 Years | No. Deaths in Children Aged Younger than 28 Days | | |
		No.	Rate per 10^6 Live Births	Percent[°]
Leukemia	4592	44	2.11	1.0
Neuroblastoma	1049	27	1.30	2.6
Brain tumor	1035	7	0.34	0.7
Wilms tumor	696	9	0.43	1.3
Liver cancer, primary	196	10	0.48	5.1
Teratoma	111	9	0.43	8.1
Sarcoma, type specified	1940	12	0.58	1.2
Other		12	0.58	
TOTAL	9619	130	6.25	1.4

[°]Percentage of neonatal deaths among type-specific cancers in patients younger than 5 years of age (e.g., for leukemia = [44 × 100]/4592 = 1.0).

From Fraumeni JF, Miller RW: Cancer deaths in the newborn. Am J Dis Child 117:186, 1969. Copyright 1969, American Medical Association.

* Revised from the chapter originally written by Allan P. Schwartz.

1243

TABLE 104–2

Incidence and Mortality Rate of Malignant Tumors in U.S. Newborns and Infants

Tumor Type	Incidence				Mortality				Ratio (A/B)
	<29 Days		12 Mos.		<29 Days		12 Mos.		
	No.	Rate	No.	Rate° (A)	No.	Rate	No.	Rate° (B)	
Leukemia	5	4.7	34	31.8	101	2.6	807	20.8	1.5
Neuroblastoma	21	19.7	67	62.7	70	1.8	302	7.8	8.0
Central nervous system	1	0.9	15	14.0	12	0.3	257	6.6	2.1
Kidney	5	4.7	21	19.7	21	0.5	141	3.6	5.4
Reticuloendotheliosis	0	0	3	2.8	7	0.2	131	3.4	—
Sarcoma	4	3.7	19	17.8	29	0.7	129	3.3	5.4
Liver	0	0	8	7.5	15	0.4	99	2.6	2.9
Lymphoma	1	0.9	2	1.9	2	<0.1	60	1.5	1.3
Teratoma	0	0	3	2.8	11	0.3	28	0.7	4.0
Carcinoma	1	0.9	6	5.6	6	0.2	18	0.5	11.2
Germ cell, excluding teratoma	0	0	0	0	0	0	6	0.2	
Retinoblastoma	0	0	17	15.9	1	<0.1	4	0.1	159.0
Other	1	0.9	1	0.9	20	0.5	62	1.6	
TOTAL	39	36.4	196	183.4	295	7.6	2044	52.7	3.5

°Per one million live births per year.

From Bader JI, Miller RW: U.S. cancer incidence and mortality in the first year of life. Am J Dis Child 133:157, 1979. Copyright 1979, American Medical Association.

group has remained stable (Miller et al, 1994). A summary of five recently reported surveys from Los Angeles (Isaacs, 1985), Toronto (Campbell et al, 1987a), Memphis (Crom et al, 1989), Denmark (Borch et al, 1992), and our San Francisco experience is shown in Table 104–3. The relative frequencies of most types of malignancy are unchanged from those reported earlier (see Table 104–2), except for retinoblastoma, which is seen to occur more frequently than shown in Table 104–2, perhaps because of referral patterns at University of California–San Francisco and Hospital for Sick Children, Toronto.

PATHOGENESIS
Transplacental Tumor Passage and Twin-to-Twin Transmission

A few cases of malignant melanoma of the mother with spread to the fetus have been reported and reviewed (Anderson et al, 1989; Campbell et al, 1987b). The infant reported by Cavell (1963) recovered from the metastatic disease. Factors found to suggest an unfavorable fetal/infant outcome are maternal age younger than 30 years, primiparity, leg primary lesion, onset of disease more than

TABLE 104–3

Diagnoses in 221 Cases of Neonatal Malignancy

Center (Dates)	Neuroblastoma	Leukemia	Retinoblastoma	Sarcoma	Wilms	Central Nervous System	Other*
CHLA, Los Angeles† (1955–1982)	14	11	2	8	3	2	6
HSC, Toronto‡ (1922–1982)	48	8	17	12	4	9	4
SJCRH, Memphis§ (1962–1988)	19	6	3	0	2	0	4
UCSF, San Francisco°° (1942–1987)	11	4	9	2	5	1	7
DCR, Copenhagen†† (1943–1985)	20	12	2	11	4	8	11
TOTAL (No.)	112	41	33	33	18	20	32
TOTAL (%)	38.7%	14.2%	11.4%	11.4%	6.2%	6.9%	11.1%

°Includes 14 malignant germ cell tumors or teratomas, 5 hepatoblastomas, 2 melanomas, 1 blue nevus, 3 carcinomas, 2 histiocytoses, 2 reticulosarcomas, 2 schwannoma, and 1 unspecified.

†From Isaacs (1985)

‡From Campbell et al (1987a)

§From Crom et al (1989)

°°From Matthay (unpublished data). Courtesy of the Cancer Patient Data Program, Cancer Research Institute, and the Cancer Registry of UCSF, 1990.

††From Borch et al (1992)

CHLA, Children's Hospital of Los Angeles; HSC, Hospital for Sick Children; SJCRH, St. Jude's Children's Research Hospital; UCSF, University of California, San Francisco; DCR, Danish Cancer Registry, Copenhagen, Denmark.

3 years before pregnancy, metastatic status before pregnancy, birth at more than 36 weeks' gestation, and male sex. Maternal virilizing tumors have resulted in fetal virilization resulting from transplacental passage of androgens secreted by the neoplasm, but the tumors have not spread to the fetus (Haymond and Weldon, 1973). Multiple myeloma has been reported in a small number of pregnant women (Lergier et al, 1974). In two instances no abnormal myeloma protein was found in the infants, but a transient abnormal protein believed to be passively transferred from the mother was demonstrated in two others. None of the infants had evidence of disease.

Leukemia has not been found in newborns of women with this malignancy, although disease developed in two children of affected mothers at 5 and 9 months of age. In these instances, both mothers and children had acute lymphoblastic leukemia (Bernard et al, 1964; Cramblett et al, 1958). Although leukemia in mice can be transmitted to their offspring by viruses in breast milk, there is no evidence that leukemia is passed to the human infant in this manner. However, intrauterine transmission of leukemia between monozygotic twins has been documented by showing the monoclonal origin of the leukemia cells in the two individuals, using Southern blot and restriction fragment analysis of leukemia DNA (Mahmoud et al, 1995).

The development of choriocarcinoma in an infant as a complication of placental choriocarcinoma is rare. In at least four instances, both mother and infant have been affected. This represents tumor transmission from the fetus to the mother because the trophoblast, the site of origin, is composed of fetal rather than maternal tissue. In most of the recorded cases, there was either a recognized placental choriocarcinoma or absence of a primary site in the infants with disseminated malignancy. The characteristic presentation is of hematemesis or hemoptysis, anemia, hepatomegaly, and pulmonary metastasis in the infant. The diagnosis is established by the demonstration of an elevated urinary or plasma beta human chorionic gonadotropin (Belchis et al, 1993).

Environmental Factors

The review by Fraumeni and Miller (1969) showed no significant annual variation or aggregation of cases of neonatal cancers in the United States. A number of authors have reported that abdominal radiation to the mother during pregnancy increases the risk of the child in utero for subsequent development of leukemia, whereas others do not substantiate the existence of a relationship between prenatal x-ray exposure and childhood cancer. Children exposed prenatally to the atomic bombs in Hiroshima and Nagasaki have no significant excess of mortality from leukemia or other cancers. An epidemiologic study of 234 cases of childhood leukemia/lymphoma (McKinney et al, 1987) failed to reveal any significant association with prenatal x-ray exposure, maternal drug ingestion and smoking, or parental medical conditions or occupations. However, a more recent report by Yoshimoto and colleagues (1991) suggests that with longer follow-up, the relative risk of cancer in adult life after the intrauterine exposure is significantly increased. Another study from the Children's

Cancer Study Group shows an association of paternal x-ray exposure and infant leukemia (Shu et al, 1994).

A recent comprehensive review by Gold and Sever (1994) summarizes data on the studies of preconceptual and postconceptual parental exposures to chemicals, solvents, radiation, and electromagnetic field exposure as they relate to cancer incidence in offspring. Although many moderately significant correlations have been reported between prenatal exposures and various childhood cancers, the studies are often contradictory. Many possible mechanisms and factors must be considered in studies of the relationship of environmental factors to cancer pathogenesis in children. For example, preconception exposures could lead to genetic alterations transmitted to offspring by either parent. Also, a link to a particular exposure might really be a surrogate for another; thus, an occupation in the lumber and paper industry might reflect hydrocarbon exposure as well as wood dust. A paternal contribution to cancer initiated during gestation might be due to transmission of carcinogenic agents in spermatozoa or through contaminated clothing.

In 1977, Herbst and coworkers reported that large doses of diethylstilbestrol (DES) given to pregnant women were related to the development of adenocarcinoma of the vagina in their daughters of that pregnancy from 14 to 22 years later. A relationship between exposure in utero to DES and its close synthetic analogues during the first half of pregnancy and the later development of clear cell adenocarcinoma of both vagina and cervix is well established. According to the 1977 calculations of Herbst and colleagues, the risk of development of such tumors is 0.14 to 1.4 per 1000 DES-exposed females up until the age of 24 years. Melnick and coworkers (1987) reported the risk up to age 34 is 1 case per 1000. The tumors are rare in females younger than 14 years of age, but the frequency increases rapidly to a peak at age 17 to 22 years, after which there is a precipitous drop. In addition to neoplastic changes, several nonmalignant epithelial and structural alterations of the lower genital tract have been noted (Robboy et al, 1979), as have deformities of the endometrial cavity. Other authors have reported an increased risk of unfavorable outcome of pregnancy in daughters exposed to in utero DES. Detailed studies of males exposed in utero to DES showed increased frequencies of testicular hypoplasia, cryptorchidism, epididymal cysts, microphallus, increased abnormal spermatazoa forms, and lowered sperm counts. An estimated 30% of the males studied are probably infertile (Bibbo et al, 1977; Gill et al, 1979), and a few have been found to have seminomas (Conley et al, 1983).

A number of other agents known to cross the placenta may possibly be carcinogenic to the offspring. In utero exposure to phenytoin or possibly other antiepileptic drugs is associated with a syndrome in the newborn that includes hypoplasia of the midface, tapering of the fingers, and toes, and hypoplasia or aplasia of the nails. At least five children with this syndrome have been reported to have neuroblastoma (Ehrenbard and Chaganti, 1981; Jiminez et al, 1981), and one has been found to have an extrarenal Wilms tumor (Taylor et al, 1980). One young adult with a history of exposure in utero to phenytoin has developed a malignant mesenchymoma (Blattner et al, 1977).

The fetal alcohol syndrome, a disorder occurring in the

children of mothers who consume excessive amounts of alcohol, is characterized by developmental delay, growth deficiency, and multiple minor anomalies. One child with this syndrome has been reported with neuroblastoma (Kinney et al, 1980), a second with hepatoblastoma, and a third with adrenocortical carcinoma, but there is no evidence of increased incidence.

The association of neoplasms with other environmental agents has been inconclusive. Jick and associates (1981) noted an increase in pregnancies ending in spontaneous abortion and in congenital anomalies in live infants born to women presumed to have used vaginal spermicides near the time of conception. Two of the children were found to have neoplasms shortly after birth. A case-controlled study of neuroblastoma suggested increased risk associated with use in pregnancy of neurally active drugs, diuretics, and hair dyes and with alcohol consumption and sex hormone exposure (Kramer et al, 1987). Paternal exposure to electromagnetic fields has been suggested as a risk factor (Spitz and Johnson, 1985).

Agents implicated in childhood neoplasia following in utero exposure also often have teratogenic effects (Table 104–4). In the case of DES, the same organ appears to be at risk for both the oncogenic and teratogenic effects of the drug. Phenytoin exposure in the adult has been associated with the development of lymphomas, whereas phenytoin exposure in utero has been associated with neuroblastomas. Thus, an agent may have various teratogenic or oncogenic effects, depending on the susceptibility of the target organ at the time of exposure, prenatally or well into adulthood. The same toxic agent has been shown in animals to be teratogenic to the fetus in the second quarter of pregnancy and carcinogenic in the latter half of pregnancy (Napalkov, 1973).

Genetic Factors and Congenital Defects

Certain host factors seem to predispose a person to the development of neoplastic disease. There is an increased

TABLE 104–4

Drugs Associated with Teratogenic and Carcinogenic Disorders Following In Utero Exposure

Drug	Teratogenic Effects	Carcinogenic Effects
Diethylstilbestrol	Structural alterations on genital tract	Vaginal and cervical adenocarcinoma
Phenytoin	Fetal hydantoin syndrome	Neuroblastoma° Wilms tumor°
Alcohol	Fetal alcohol syndrome	Neuroblastoma° Hepatoblastoma° Adrenocortical carcinoma°
Vaginal spermicides	Limb reduction deformities° Chromosomal abnormalities° Hypospadias°	Medulloblastoma° Nesidioblastosis°
Phenobarbital	Microcephaly°	Brain tumors°

°Present data are only suggestive of an etiologic association.

incidence of leukemia in persons with Down syndrome, Fanconi aplastic anemia, and Bloom syndrome and of leukemia and lymphoreticular malignancies in persons born with immunodeficiency disorders such as ataxia-telangiectasia, Wiskott-Aldrich syndrome, and severe combined immunodeficiency. Down syndrome is more common than usual among siblings of children with leukemia. Both Down syndrome and leukemia occur more frequently among children of older mothers. Others have reported cytogenic variants of prezygotic origin in 4 of 25 non-Down syndrome children with acute leukemia and suggested that the aneuploid cell might be more susceptible to malignant change.

Although the risk of development of leukemia is increased slightly in a dizygotic twin or other sibling of a child who has the disease, the chance of leukemia developing is greatest in a monozygotic twin. If one monozygotic twin has leukemia, the co-twin has approximately a 25% chance of leukemia developing, usually within weeks or months of the diagnosis of the sibling. As discussed, this may be due to twin-to-twin transmission rather than to simultaneous development.

A small number of well-defined hereditary conditions are associated with an increased incidence of certain neoplasms: Von Hippel-Lindau syndrome (hemangioblastoma, pheochromocytoma, and renal cell carcinoma), Li-Fraumeni syndrome (sarcomas, breast cancer, central nervous system tumors, adrenocortical carcinomas, leukemia, melanoma, germ cell tumor, Wilms tumor), neurofibromatosis (central nervous system tumors, peripheral nerve tumors, rhabdomyosarcoma, leukemia, and juvenile chronic myelogenous leukemia), tuberous sclerosis; Gorlin syndrome (basal cell carcinomas, medulloblastomas, and ovarian fibromas), familial Wilms tumor, and retinoblastoma. Except for retinoblastoma, the neoplasms seldom present in the neonatal period, but the associated abnormalities may be recognized early and the family history alerts the clinician to the need for screening. In almost all of these neoplasms, the genetic defect has been identified. For example, NF-1 is located at 17q11.2 and produces a protein, neurofibromin, which acts as an "off" switch for the *ras* oncogene, resulting in dysregulation of cell growth when a mutation is present. In Li-Fraumeni syndrome, germ line mutations in a tumor suppressor gene, p53, have been demonstrated in some of these families in which members had sarcomas, breast cancer, brain tumors, and leukemia (Malkin et al, 1990).

An unexpectedly large number of childhood tumors occur in association with certain congenital defects. Children with Wilms tumor have an increased incidence of congenital aniridia. Aniridia is a rare anomaly, found in only 1 of 75,000 persons. It is about 1000 times more likely to occur in children with Wilms tumor (1 in 75). The association with a deletion in chromosome 11 has been described in at least 20 patients (Yunis and Ramsay, 1980). Most of these patients also have genitourinary abnormalities and mental retardation. From the clinical perspective, if an infant has aniridia, chromosome analysis should be undertaken. If a deletion of chromosome 11 is found, the child should be monitored for Wilms tumor with serial ultrasonographic studies of the kidneys. Wilms tumor develops in approximately half of these patients. Other problems associated with Wilms tumor include anomalies of the genitourinary tract and cardiac septal defects. Wilms tumor as well as several other childhood neoplasms are associated with the constellation of anomalies comprising the Beckwith-Wiedeman syndrome, typified by macroglossia, gigantism, and exophthalmos, but also includes visceromegaly, flame nevus, neonatal hypoglycemia, microcephaly, retardation, and hemihypertrophy (Sotelo-Avila et al, 1980). The associated neoplasms are seen in approximately 8% of infants with either the complete or partial syndrome and include Wilms tumor, adrenal cortical carcinoma, and hepatoblastoma, tumors of the same organs in which visceromegaly develops. Also reported are rhabdomyosarcoma, neuroblastoma, ganglioneuroma, and adenomas and hamartomas. These relationships among hemihypertrophy, visceral cytomegaly syndrome, hamartomas, and malignancy have been shown to be caused by specific chromosomal aberrations. The Beckwith-Wiedeman syndrome is linked with abnormalities of 11p15, where the insulin-like growth factor II gene and H19 tumor suppressor gene are located (Kubota et al, 1994). Three distinct nonoverlapping regions of chromosome 11p allelic loss have been identified in infantile tumors of adrenal and liver (Byrne et al, 1993).

CONGENITAL LEUKEMIA

Leukemia rarely occurs during the 1st month of life. Only 3% of all children with acute lymphoblastic leukemia are younger than 1 year of age; of 115 infants entered on Children's Cancer Study Group protocols, only two had congenital leukemia (Reaman et al, 1985). Most of the neonatal cases reported have acute nonlymphoblastic leukemia, in contrast to the predominance of acute lymphoblastic leukemia found in later childhood. In the Children's Cancer Study Group, 18% of all children undergoing treatment for acute nonlymphoblastic leukemia were infants (<1 year). No child born to a mother with leukemia has been found to have the disease during the neonatal period. Instances of familial neonatal leukemia are extremely rare. Campbell and coworkers (1962) described male and female siblings who died at 10 and 8 weeks of age, respectively, of myelogenous leukemia and a third female in the family who died at 4 weeks of age with a clinical course similar to that of her siblings, although a definite diagnosis was not made.

Congenital leukemia is occasionally associated with a number of congenital anomalies and with chromosomal disorders such as Down syndrome, trisomies D and E, and a number of nonspecific chromosomal abnormalities. Subtle cytogenetic abnormalities may occur more commonly than was previously believed in affected infants and their parents when studied with newer cytogenetic techniques (Pui, 1995).

Clinical Manifestations

The clinical signs of leukemia may be evident at birth, with hepatosplenomegaly, petechiae, and ecchymoses. Leukemic cell infiltration into the skin (leukemia cutis) results in nodular fibroma-like masses. These tumors are freely movable over the subcutaneous tissue and result in a blue or gray discoloration of the overlying skin (Fig. 104–1). Such cutaneous lesions are commonly found when the

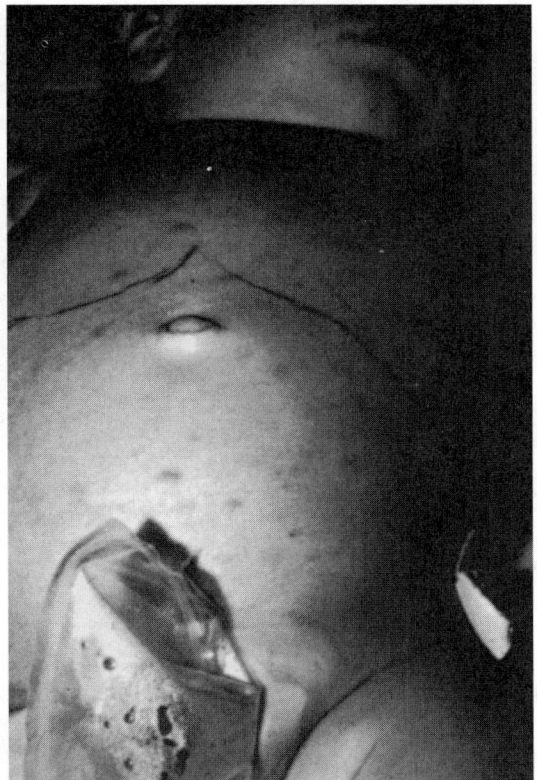

FIGURE 104–1. Leukemia cutis in a newborn infant.

disease appears at birth and have been noted in stillborn premature infants with leukemia. They may be the first clinical sign of the disease. At birth, many of the infants have respiratory distress from either leukemia infiltration in the lungs or atelectasis. Severe respiratory difficulty may develop soon after birth from pulmonary hemorrhage secondary to thrombocytopenia.

In those infants in whom signs of the disease develop within the 1st month but in whom no detectable signs of leukemia were noted at birth, the symptoms are often ill defined, with low-grade fever, diarrhea, hepatomegaly, and failure to gain weight. Hemorrhagic manifestations are often the first signs of the disease, and leukemia cutis is less common.

Hemoglobin levels are often normal at first, but they soon decline to low levels. Total white blood cell counts may be within normal limits or diminished, but leukocytosis is usually present. White blood cell counts of 150,000 to 250,000/mm³ or more are not unusual, and counts as high as 1.3 million/mm³ have been recorded. Leukocyte counts often increase progressively before death. There is usually a predominance of blast cells and immature granulocytes. Auer rods may be present in the blast cells (Fig. 104–2). These intracellular inclusions are composed of lysosomes and are considered to be pathognomonic of acute myelogenous leukemia.

Differential Diagnosis

A number of newborns reported in the earlier literature who were originally believed to have leukemia were later

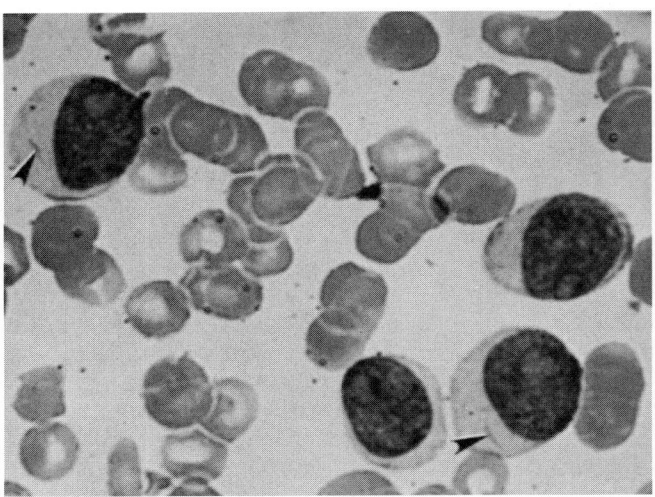

FIGURE 104–2. Malignant blast cells with Auer rods (arrowheads) present in cytoplasm diagnostic of acute myelogenous leukemia.

found to have other diseases. The predominance of myelogenous leukemia in this age group has contributed to the difficulty in differentiating the disorder from leukemoid reactions. Confusion with infections such as congenital syphilis, cytomegalovirus infection, toxoplasmosis, and bacterial septicemia may occur because of the leukocytosis, organomegaly, and thrombocytopenia that may accompany these diseases. The low platelet counts and leukemoid reactions reported in infants with congenital amegakaryocytic thrombocytopenia may also lead to an incorrect diagnosis of leukemia, but the absence of radii commonly seen in these children is a major clue to the correct diagnosis.

Severe erythroblastosis fetalis can mimic leukemia. Such infants usually have hepatosplenomegaly, large numbers of nucleated erythroblasts in the peripheral blood, and, occasionally, thrombocytopenia. Small infiltrates of extramedullary erythropoiesis may appear in the skin and superficially resemble leukemia cutis.

Infants with neonatal neuroblastoma often have hepatomegaly and may also have discolored tumor nodules in the subcutaneous tissue (see Figs. 104–4 and 104–6). Their blood cell counts are usually normal without circulating blasts, and specimens of bone marrow, if involved, reveal small clusters of neuroblastoma cells (see Fig. 104–5). Although these cells may resemble leukemia blast cells, their tendency to occur in clumps in an otherwise normal bone marrow distinguishes them from leukemic cells, which usually completely replace the normal bone marrow. In cases of complete bone marrow replacement, increased excretion of catecholamine metabolites and the presence of an abdominal mass or other primary lesion are clues to the diagnosis of neuroblastoma.

Congenital human immunodeficiency virus infection may also rarely be confused with leukemia. Clonal B-cell expansions in such patients may cause lymphadenopathy. One newborn reported by Voelkerding and coworkers (1988) presented with thrombocytopenia and had lymphocyte clusters in the bone marrow that were of B-cell lineage, clonal as defined by immune globulin gene arrange-

ment and positive for the common acute lymphocytic leukemia antigen. However, the patient was well and without evidence of lymphoproliferative disease a year later.

A marked but transient leukemoid reaction may occur in the newborn following in utero exposure to betamethasone (Anday and Harris, 1982). Lack of the usual clinical and laboratory findings of leukemia and a history of maternal drug exposure usually exclude the diagnosis of leukemia.

Pathology

Biopsy or autopsy shows heavy infiltration of many immature leukocytes into extrahematopoietic tissues. The bone marrow is hypercellular, with a marked predominance of the immature cells of the series affected, either myeloid or lymphoid. Cirrhosis of the liver has been noted at autopsy in several infants.

Cellular Morphology, Immunophenotype, and Chromosomes

Both acute lymphoblastic and acute nonlymphoblastic leukemia may be found in newborns. These diseases are differentiated on the basis of typical morphologic characteristics, such as the presence of granules or Auer rods and nuclear and cytoplasmic morphology and by cytochemical stains. Periodic acid–Schiff stain shows large aggregates of glycogen in the blast cells in acute lymphoblastic leukemia, whereas the pattern in acute nonlymphoblastic leukemia is finely granular and diffuse. Most acute lymphoblastic leukemia cells stain positively for terminal deoxynucleotidyl transferase, a DNA polymerase that catalyzes the polymerization of deoxynucleotides in thymocytes. This enzyme is present in 90% of acute lymphoblastic leukemia, but less than 5% of acute nonlymphoblastic leukemia. Activity can be measured by enzyme-linked immunosorbent assay, immunofluorescence, immunoperoxidase stain, and enzyme assay (Diamond and Matthay, 1988). Both types of leukemia are subclassified according to an international French-American-British classification (FAB) based on cell morphology and histochemistry and are divided into subtypes based on morphologic characteristics (Pui, 1995) (Table 104–5). The most common subtype by far in infantile and neonatal acute nonlymphoblastic leukemia is the monocytic variety (Odom and Gordon, 1984; van Wering and Kamps, 1986).

Immunophenotype determined using a panel of monoclonal antibodies against differentiation antigens and detected by fluorescence is helpful both in differentiating the lymphoid and nonlymphoid leukemias and in further subtyping (Poplack, 1993; Pui, 1993). The nonlymphoblastic leukemias react with antibodies to the CD13/CD33 antigens, present on cells of myeloid and monocytic lineage. The only exception is the M7 category, acute megakaryoblastic leukemia, seen in Down syndrome, which expresses the CD41/CD42 platelet glycoprotein. Most of the neonatal and infant acute lymphoblastic leukemia cells exhibit an early pre–B-cell phenotype, including Ia positivity, negativity for CD10 (common acute lymphoblastic leukemia antigen), unlike most childhood acute lymphoblastic leukemias, and positivity for CD19 and CD24 (early

TABLE 104–5

Morphologic and Immunophenotypic Classification of Childhood Acute Leukemia

FAB	Morphology		Antigen Expression[†]
ALL[°]			
L$_1$	Small cells, homogeneous Regular nuclei, scant cytoplasm Inconspicuous nucleoli	Pre B	HLA-DR, CD10, CD19, CD20, CD24
OR			
L$_2$	Large cells, heterogeneous, irregular or cleft nuclei May be multiple large nucleoli Moderate cytoplasm	OR T	CD2, CD5, CD7
L$_3$	Large cells, homogeneous Regular nuclear shape Prominent nucleoli Moderately abundant, deeply basophilic cytoplasm with vacuolation	B	HLA-DR, CD10, CD19, CD20, CD24, Slg +
ANLL			
M0	Minimal myeloid differentiation (MPO −)		CD13, CD33, CD34
M1	Poorly differentiated myeloblasts (MPO +)		CD13, CD33, CD34
M2	Myeloblastic with differentiation (MPO +)		CD13, CD33, CD34
M3	Promyelocytic (MPO +)		CD11b, CD13, CD33, CD34
M4	Myelomonoblastic (MPO +, NSE +)		CD11b, CD13, CD14, CD15, CD33, CD34
M5	Monoblastic (NSE +)		CD11b, CD13, CD14, CD15, CD33, CD34
M6	Erythroleukemic (MPO +, PAS +)		glycophorin A, CD34
M7	Megakaryoblastic (PPO +)		CD41, CD42, CD34, CD61

°L$_1$ or L$_2$ may show either pre-B or T antigens
†The indicated FAB type may express some or all of indicated antigens.
Slg, surface immune globulin; MPO, myeloperoxidase; NSE, nonspecific esterase; PPO, platelet peroxidase; ALL, acute lymphocytic leukemia; FAB, French-American-British.

B-cell markers) (Crist et al, 1986; Katz et al, 1988; Pui et al, 1987). The frequent rearrangements of the immune globulin heavy-chain gene, and occasionally the light-chain gene but almost never the T-cell receptor gene, may also be helpful in subclassification and understanding the biology of neonatal acute lymphoblastic leukemia (Felix et al, 1987; Ludwig et al, 1989). The acute leukemia surface antigen expression is shown in Table 104–5.

Chromosomal abnormalities in the leukemic cells have gained increasing importance in subclassification and prognosis of both acute lymphoblastic and acute nonlymphoblastic leukemia. A number of chromosomal translocations and deletions have been found to carry an unfavorable prognosis, such as the t(4;11), which is commonly present in infants with leukemia (Nagasaka et al, 1983). The most common chromosome involved in translocations in infantile acute lymphoblastic leukemia and acute nonlymphoblastic leukemia is the 11q23, found in at least 50% of infant leukemia and in a predominance of neonatal cases (Kaneko et al, 1988). The fact that 11q23 rearrangements are the most common clonal chromosomal abnormality in infant leukemias, coupled with the fact that this same rearrangement is seen in secondary acute nonlymphoblastic leukemia induced by epipodophyllotoxin therapy, suggests that intrauterine exposure to carcinogenesis is responsible for some cases of leukemia in infants. The gene that is disrupted by 11q23 translocations, designated HRX, MLL, ALL-1, or HTRX-1, has been cloned and characterized. It encodes a 431-kD protein that contains putative DNA-binding motifs. The 11q23 translocation can be detected in up to 80% of infants with acute lymphoblastic leukemia

by molecular analysis and is generally associated with an exceedingly poor prognosis (Chen et al, 1991; Heerema et al, 1994; Rubnitz et al, 1994). This rearrangement is the most common abnormality in monoblastic infant leukemia and is associated with hyperleukocytosis, coagulation abnormalities, and central nervous system dissemination.

Treatment and Prognosis

The course of congenital leukemia has usually been one of rapid deterioration and death from hemorrhage or infection. Although the length of survival has been significantly prolonged in children with leukemia, success has been limited in treatment in newborns. The infant with leukemia frequently presents with hyperleukocytosis (blast cell count in excess of 100,000/mm^3). This syndrome may result in sludging of blast cells in capillaries with resultant intracranial hemorrhage, respiratory distress, or problems from tumor lysis with hyperkalemia, hyperphosphatemia, hypocalcemia, hyperuricemia, and renal failure. These metabolic problems must be corrected before initiation of chemotherapy. In the infant, exchange transfusion is the easiest way to accomplish this and simultaneously lower the white blood cell count, which further decreases tumor lysis problems once chemotherapy is begun. Disseminated intravascular coagulation is another common complication seen in hyperleukocytosis and infantile leukemia, wherein monocytic subtypes are common. The monoblasts release procoagulants and cause consumptive coagulopathy, which may initially be exacerbated owing to further blast cell lysis with chemotherapy and require support with transfusion of platelets and fresh frozen plasma. Central nervous system involvement is common in infants with acute lymphoblastic leukemia and those with monocytic leukemia. Evaluation of cerebrospinal fluid and intrathecal prophylactic chemotherapy should be a routine part of treatment.

The current improved success of remission induction with treatment of acute nonlymphoblastic leukemia in infants younger than 1 year is similar to that in older children, using intensive combination chemotherapy regimens (Lampkin et al, 1984). The experience with newborns is limited, but between 1984 and 1989, 5 of 12 newborns with acute nonlymphoblastic leukemia sustained complete remissions with chemotherapy; all were in the myelomonocytic or monocytic category (Kaneko et al, 1988; Odom and Gordon, 1984). However, in acute lymphoblastic leukemia, the treatment outcome is significantly poorer in infants younger than 1 year at diagnosis (23% disease-free survival compared with 70% for older children) and may be even lower in newborns. Several studies of infant leukemia report only 10% to 20% survival for infants younger than 6 months of age at diagnosis compared with 40% for those older than 6 months (Chessells et al, 1994; Heerema et al, 1994). Fewer than 15% of newborns with acute lymphoblastic leukemia have remissions lasting more than a few months.

Although exchange transfusions may cause clinical improvement by rapidly decreasing an extremely high white blood cell count, the response is usually transient. The same chemotherapeutic agents used for older children with acute lymphoblastic leukemia may be used in infants, with the precaution that dosages may need to be altered to prevent undue toxicity. Furthermore, dosages should be calculated on the basis of body weight, rather than by the surface area calculation used in an older child. Infants have been shown to experience excessive neurotoxicity with vincristine, with hypotonia, a poor cry, inability to feed, and flaccid paralysis (Reaman et al, 1985). Radiation therapy, used for central nervous system leukemia, may also result in more marked neurotoxicity than in older children, and generally more intensive intrathecal chemotherapy or high-dose intravenous methotrexate is substituted. The relatively lower renal function and biliary excretion in newborns may also result in unexpected toxicity of certain drugs. Accordingly, many of the drugs commonly used in the treatment of infantile leukemias will require dosage modifications, including vincristine, anthracyclines, cyclophosphamide, epipodophyllotoxins (etoposide, teniposide), prednisone, cytarabine, 6-mercaptopurine, and methotrexate (Reaman, 1989). Spontaneous remissions, which occur in Down syndrome infants with leukemia, are rarely experienced by the normal child. Sansone (1989) reported an infant with myelomonocytic leukemia who relapsed after initial chemotherapy and then had a spontaneous remission persisting for more than 3 years at the time of the report.

LEUKEMIA WITH DOWN SYNDROME

An increased incidence of acute leukemia in children with Down syndrome (10- to 30-fold increased risk) is well recognized (Fong and Brodeur, 1987). A review of the world literature by Rosner and Lee (1972) revealed 227 children with both disorders; 31% had acute myeloblastic leukemia, and 69% had acute lymphoblastic leukemia.

Among 47 such infants with leukemia, 58% had myeloblastic leukemia and 42% had lymphoblastic leukemia. In infants younger than 3 years of age with Down syndrome and leukemia, the rare megakaryoblastic subtype (M7) predominates (Pui, 1995). Eighteen additional Down syndrome infants who had a transient disorder initially indistinguishable from acute myelogenous leukemia experienced complete clinical and hematologic recovery. In those with "transient leukemia" who died of other causes, no evidence of leukemia could be found at postmortem examination. The transient leukemoid reaction may result from a defect in the regulation of granulocyte multiplication and maturation, possibly related to the chromosomal abnormality. The same transient myeloproliferative disorder may be seen in trisomy 21 mosaicism (Seibel et al, 1984). It has even been reported in two normal infants in whom the trisomy was detected only in the leukemic cells (Ridgway et al, 1990). The increased incidence of neonatal polycythemia in Down syndrome patients observed by Weinberger and Oleinick (1970) has led these investigators to propose that the abnormality in the regulation of hematopoiesis is not limited to granulocyte production. Miller and Cosgriff (1983) found a hematologic abnormality in 28 of 81 newborns with Down syndrome (35%). The most common problem was polycythemia (21), the second most common, thrombocytopenia (7), and third was transient leukocytosis (2). However, a number of infants with transient leukemia have had recurrence of their disease leading to death, indicating that the disorders of marrow dysfunction and neonatal leukemia may not be separate entities but may be intimately related. Some infants with the transient myeloproliferative syndrome without Down syndrome have also been reported, and true leukemia has subsequently recurred (Brissette et al, 1994).

Attempts to differentiate the transient myeloproliferative disorder from a true leukemia have been made clinically, morphologically, through cell culture, and by chromosomal analysis. The self-limited transient myeloproliferative disorder is usually not associated with anemia, neutropenia, or thrombocytopenia, despite the presence of blast cells in the peripheral blood; the percentage of blast cells is greater in the blood than in the bone marrow; and the blast cells demonstrate trisomy 21 with no other cytogenetic abnormalities. Suda and coworkers (1987) showed that bone marrow blast cells cultured from such a patient resulted in colony formation with differentiation into normal basophils, neutrophils, eosinophils, macrophages, and erythrocytes. This differs from true acute nonlymphoblastic leukemia, in which in vitro colony formation is abnormal with lack of maturation. Hayashi and colleagues (1988) studied the chromosomes of 13 patients with Down syndrome and acute leukemia compared with 15 patients with Down syndrome and transient myeloproliferative disorder. Clonal chromosomal abnormalities were found in the cells of all patients with leukemia but not in the cells of those with the transient myeloproliferative disorder. However, Lazarus and coworkers (1981) reported one infant with transient myeloproliferative disorder whose cells demonstrated chromosomal abnormalities including −22,t(Xp;8q),t(21q;22q), which disappeared as the syndrome resolved spontaneously.

The high incidence of spontaneous remission of leukemia in infants with Down syndrome makes it difficult to interpret their response to antileukemic therapy. It may be most prudent to withhold the use of chemotherapeutic agents in this unusual group of newborns unless the clinical course is one of rapid deterioration.

NEUROBLASTOMA

Neuroblastoma is the most common malignant tumor in infants with approximately 20% of all cases occurring before age 6 months (Huddart et al, 1993) (see Tables 104–2 and 104–3). The neoplasm originates from neural crest cells that normally give rise to the adrenal medulla and sympathetic ganglia. In infants, the first clinical manifestations in more than half the cases usually result from the presence of metastatic disease rather than the primary tumor. Yet despite the occurrence of widespread disease, the prognosis in the newborn is remarkably good.

Clinical Manifestations

Neuroblastoma may present as a tumor mass anywhere that sympathetic neural tissue normally occurs. More than half of affected children have the primary tumor within the abdomen, arising in the adrenal medulla or a sympathetic ganglion. The tumor may arise in the posterior mediastinum, and because of bronchial obstruction the symptoms may be either increasing dyspnea or pulmonary infection. The neoplasm may also arise in the neck or pelvis. Involvement of the stellate ganglion may result in Horner syndrome, which includes sinking in of the eyeball, ptosis of the upper eyelid, slight elevation of the lower lid, constriction of the pupil, narrowing of the palpebral fissure, and anhidrosis (Fig. 104–3). The neoplasm arising from a paravertebral sympathetic ganglion has a tendency to grow into the intervertebral foramina, causing spinal cord compression and resultant paralysis. Careful periodic neurologic evaluation should be performed on the child with a neuroblastoma arising from this location, because the onset of cord compression may necessitate emergency neurosurgical intervention. The late diagnosis of this complication has resulted in permanent paraplegia (Matthay, 1994).

Metastatic lesions, especially of the skin and liver, are common presenting findings during the neonatal period.

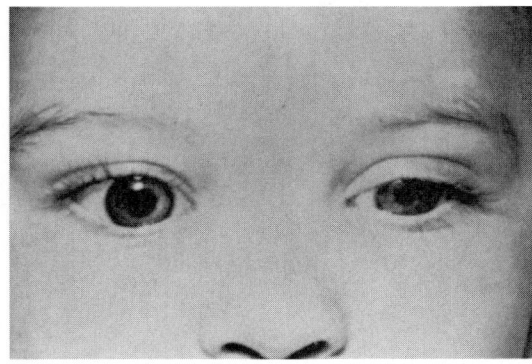

FIGURE 104–3. Horner syndrome in an infant with neuroblastoma arising from the left cervical sympathetic ganglion.

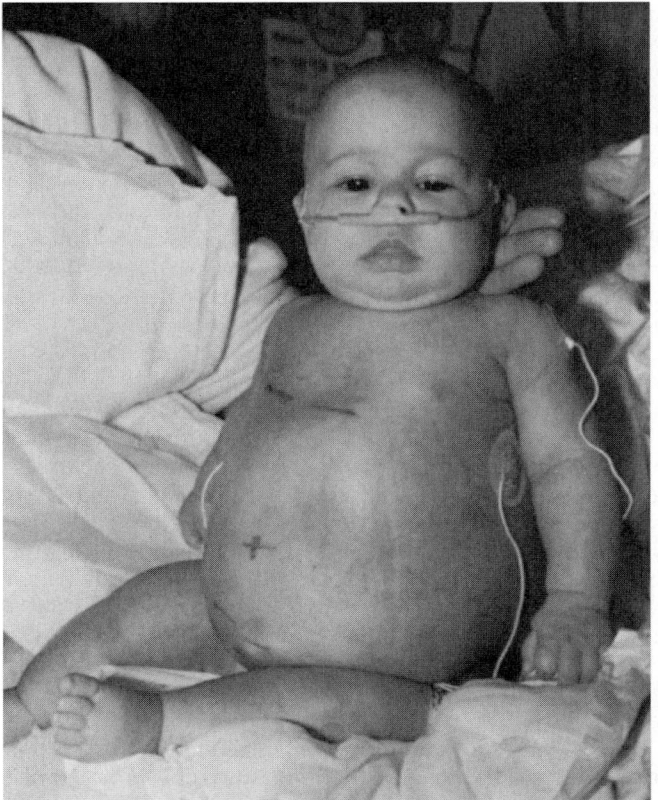

FIGURE 104–4. Stage 4S neuroblastoma causing abdominal distention and respiratory distress due to hepatic infiltration.

Often the primary site cannot be discovered. The skin nodules may first become erythematous for 2 or 3 minutes after palpation and then blanch, presumably owing to vasoconstriction from release of catecholamines from the tumor cells. This may be a diagnostic sign of subcutaneous neuroblastoma (see Fig. 104–7).

The liver often bears the brunt of metastatic dissemination, becoming studded with innumerable foci of tumor growth. The infant has a distended abdomen and respiratory distress (Fig. 104–4) from the rapidly growing hepatic neoplasm. Rarely, stippled calcifications occur in the liver metastases. The liver may be large enough at the time of birth to cause dystocia. The massive liver involvement common in newborns with disseminated neuroblastoma causing respiratory distress and coagulopathy is responsible for the higher mortality rate seen in newborns compared with older infants (Nickerson et al, 1985).

Neuroblastomas arising from sympathetic ganglia lower in the abdomen give rise to the clinical pictures consistent with their locations. Thus, presacral neuroblastomas may simulate presacral teratomas and be distinguished from them only by biopsy.

Unusual Presentations

Several children with neuroblastoma have been reported whose sole presenting symptom was persistent, intractable diarrhea. The children were believed to have had either cystic fibrosis or celiac syndrome before roentgenographic discoveries of calcified masses were made. Their symptoms dramatically abated following surgical removal of the tumors. It is thought that such symptoms are due to excessive excretion by the tumor of a vasoactive intestinal peptide (Swift et al, 1975).

The association of acute myoclonic encephalopathy and neuroblastoma has been described by numerous authors. This usually consists of rapid multidirectional eye movements (opsoclonus), myoclonus, and truncal ataxia in the absence of increased intracranial pressure. Removal of the tumor may not result in improvement in neurologic signs and symptoms. In general, the prognosis for survival of children with opsomyoclonus is excellent, although long-term neurologic deficits are common.

A report from the Netherlands suggests that there may be signs and symptoms in mothers whose fetuses have neuroblastoma. Vôute and coworkers (1970) reported six women who had sweating, pallor, headaches, palpitations, hypertension, and tingling in the feet and hands during the 8th and 9th months of pregnancy. All the children delivered were given the diagnosis of neuroblastoma shortly after birth or during the first few months of life. Because the mothers' symptoms disappeared postpartum, the authors proposed that they were caused by fetal catecholamines entering the maternal circulation.

Occasionally, a newborn with congenital neuroblastoma may be thought to have erythroblastosis. Severe jaundice with hepatosplenomegaly and an increase of nucleated red blood cells have been noted. Anders and coworkers (1973) described two newborns with congenital neuroblastoma that had metastasized to the liver and placenta who were throught to have hydrops fetalis. In one, the diagnosis was established by histologic examination of the placenta.

Familial neuroblastoma has been reported only rarely, with a review by Kushner et al (1986) citing 22 familial cases. However, two recent reports suggest that, in some such cases, a constitutional deletion of chromosome 1p36 may be present, the same site showing deletion or loss of heterozygosity in many neuroblastoma tumors (Biegel et al, 1993; Laureys et al, 1990).

Diagnosis

Neuroblastoma of the newborn most commonly manifests by enlargement of the liver alone (65%), followed by subcutaneous metastases (32%). These figures differ strikingly from those for older infants and children (Table 104–6). Metastases to lungs, bones, skull, and orbit are rare in the newborn, although clumps of tumor cells are often found if bone marrow aspiration specimens are carefully examined (Fig. 104–5). Otherwise, a localized primary tumor may be palpable or cause symptoms from spinal cord compression or Horner syndrome. Metastatic evaluation should include computed tomography or magnetic resonance imaging of the primary lesion, magnetic resonance imaging of the spine for paraspinal and posterior mediastinal lesions, bone scan, bone marrow aspirate and biopsy, and an ^{123}I or ^{131}I metaiodobenzylguanidine (MIBG) scan. MIBG is a norepinephrine analogue specifically taken up by neuroblastoma both in bone and soft tissue and provides a sensitive modality for disease localization (Feine et al, 1987;

TABLE 104–6

Incidence of Metastases in the Newborn with Neuroblastoma

Site	Number	Percentage	Percent
Liver	20	64.6	24.3
Subcutaneous	10	32.3	2.6
Marrow	3	9.7	
Lung	2	6.5	13.2
Spleen	2	6.5	2.0
Kidney	2	6.5	2.0
Pancreas	2	6.5	
Brain	2	6.5	15.8
Bone	1	3.2	47.4
Nodes	1	3.2	32.2
Pleura	1	3.2	
Myocardium	1	3.2	
Periadrenal	1	3.2	

From Schneider KM, Becker JM, Krasna IH: Neonatal neuroblastoma. Pediatrics 36:359, 1965.

Geatti et al, 1985). Immunocytologic staining of bone marrow with antineuroblastoma monoclonal antibodies can increase sensitivity of detection of bone marrow disease (Moss et al, 1985).

Biochemical Features

In 1957, Mason and colleagues reported an increased excretion of pressor amines in the urine of an infant with neuroblastoma. Subsequent studies in children with neuroblastoma have shown elevated levels of norepinephrine as well as its biochemical precursors and their metabolites in the urine, including dopa, dopamine, normetanephrine, homovanillic acid (HVA), and vanillylmandelic acid (VMA). As many as 95% of patients have an elevated urinary excretion of VMA or HVA or both. Currently, accurate VMA and HVA determinations can be made on random urine samples when normalized for creatinine concentration. In occasional cases, however, there is no elevation of catecholamines, necessitating a 24-hour urine collection. It is therefore important to measure urinary catecholamines in a child before surgical removal of a neuroblastoma or initiation of therapy to determine whether it is a catechola-

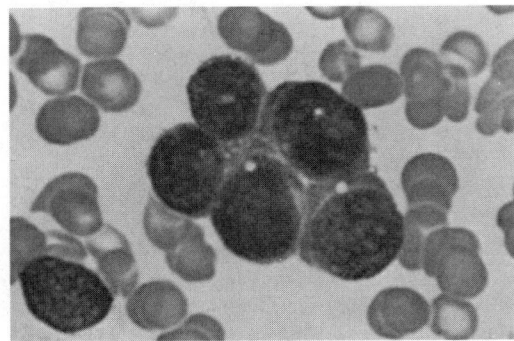

FIGURE 104–5. Clump of neuroblastoma cells found in bone marrow aspiration.

mine-producing tumor. This unique property of the neoplasm can be used not only as a diagnostic aid but also as a means of assessing the response to therapy or detecting the recurrence of tumor.

Urinary excretion of cystathionine is detectable in most patients with neuroblastoma but is also found in a number of other childhood neoplasms. Plasma carcinoembryonic antigen levels are also elevated in many cases, but this finding also is nonspecific. Serum lactic acid dehydrogenase levels increase with advanced disease, decrease with remission, and increase with recurrence. The degree of initial elevation may have prognostic significance in patients with advanced disease (Quinn et al, 1980). Other serum markers that are elevated in advanced disease include chromogranin, GD_2 ganglioside, neuron-specific enolase, and ferritin (Matthay, 1994).

Newborn Screening

Urinary catecholamine screening for neuroblastoma has been proposed by Woods and coworkers (1987) because the incidence of 8.7 per 1 million children per year is comparable to or higher than that of other congenital diseases for which screening is already in place, such as hypothyroidism, galactosemia, and phenylketonuria. The poor prognosis for advanced neuroblastoma in children older than 12 months of age at diagnosis compared to the favorable outcome for those diagnosed in infancy, raised the expectation that diagnosis at an earlier age might improve overall outcome. Rapid quantitative screening methods have been developed that have a high degree of sensitivity and specificity. Using such methods, researchers in Japan have demonstrated a dramatic improvement in the survival of infants detected on screening for neuroblastoma compared with those who were diagnosed clinically (Sawada et al, 1984). Studies have been conducted in North America as well as Japan with mass urinary screening at 3 weeks and 6 months to further determine the usefulness of this test (Lemieux et al, 1989). The results of most of these studies thus far underway or completed have shown a dramatic increase in the number of cases detected before 1 year of age, but no corresponding decrease in these same populations of cases after 1 year of age. In addition, most of the cases detected by mass screening have favorable biologic characteristics, suggesting that these are patients who would have had a good prognosis even if detected clinically (Goodman, 1991; Takeuchi et al, 1995; Woods et al, 1992). Many patients have been reported who had a negative screening result at 6 months, but who subsequently presented with advanced disease after 1 year of age (Kaneko et al, 1990; Nakagawara et al, 1991).

Pathology

The most primitive histologic subgroup of neuroblastoma is very cellular and is composed of small round cells with scant cytoplasm. The ganglioneuroma, its more benign counterpart, is composed of large, mature ganglion cells with abundant cytoplasm, whereas the ganglioneuroblastoma is intermediate in the degree of cellular differentiation. However, the histologic appearance of an individual tumor may show various degrees of cellular maturation.

Past attempts at correlation of prognosis with histologic grading have been contradictory. However, Shimada and coworkers (1984) have developed a system of histologic grading based on the amount of stroma, the degree of differentiation, and the nuclear morphology (mitosis and karyorrhexis). Using this classification, patients with a favorable prognosis can be separated from those who do not, although the classification is most helpful in patients with stage 1, 2, 3, and 4S, because most of the patients with stage 4 disease in this initial report had unfavorable histopathology. A study of patients with stage 3 and 4 disease from the Children's Cancer Study Group (Chatten et al, 1988) confirms the value of the Shimada classification for both these stages of disease with a highly significant difference in survival of patients with favorable versus unfavorable histopathology.

Prognosis

The outcome for patients with neuroblastoma has long been known to depend on the age at diagnosis and the stage of disease. However, these two variables alone do not define a homogeneous group with respect to outcome. Additional characteristics that have been correlated with prognosis include serum markers, N-*myc* oncogene amplification, chromosomal IP deletions, cellular DNA content, and histopathology.

Although different staging systems have been used for neuroblastoma, the system that is currently internationally accepted, which was modified from the original systems of Evans and St. Jude's is shown in Table 104-7 (Brodeur et al, 1993). Patients with stage 1 neuroblastoma have a 96% to 100% survival rate with surgery alone, as shown in cooperative studies reported by Evans and coworkers (1984). Similarly, for stage 2 neuroblastoma, surgery alone is sufficient to provide a 90% disease-free survival rate. Initial cooperative studies showed no benefit from the addition of chemotherapy to surgery with local irradiation for patients with stage 2 disease; subsequent review of 156 children with stage 2 neuroblastoma showed no significant benefit from the addition of radiation therapy to surgery alone, even in patients with microscopic or gross residual disease (Matthay et al, 1989). Infants with stage 3 and 4 disease have a poorer survival, even with aggressive chemotherapy, although the outcome, with better than 50% surviving overall, is far better than the 10% to 20% reported for older children.

Stage 4S comprises a unique group of patients with disseminated disease but a good prognosis, occurring exclusively in infants younger than 1 year old. This special group of children have remote spread of tumor involving the liver, skin, or bone marrow without roentgenographic evidence of skeletal metastases. The primary tumor may be unidentifiable or else no more extensive than defined by stage 1 or stage 2. Eighteen of 20 infants younger than the age of 1 year with stage 4S disease in the original observation by D'Angio and associates (1971) were cured of their disease. The 2-year survival rate of all of those with stage 4S disease is 80% as compared to 10% of all children with stage 4 disease, or the 50% to 70% in infants younger than 1 year with stage 4 disease (De Bernardi et al, 1992; Nickerson et al, 1985). Haas and colleagues (1988) re-

TABLE 104–7

International Staging System for Neuroblastoma

Stage	Definition
Stage 1	Localized tumor confined to the area of origin; complete gross excision, with or without microscopic residual disease; identifiable ipsilateral and contralateral lymph nodes negative microscopically. (Adherent nodes may be positive.)
Stage 2A	Localized tumor with incomplete gross excision; identifiable ipsilateral and contralateral lymph nodes negative microscopically.
Stage 2B	Localized tumor with complete or incomplete gross excision, with positive ipsilateral nonadherent regional lymph nodes; identifiable contralateral lymph nodes negative microscopically.
Stage 3	Unresectable tumor initiating across the midline with or without regional lymph node involvement; or, unilateral tumor with contralateral regional lymph node involvement; or, midline tumor with bilateral regional lymph node involvement; bilateral extension by infiltration.
Stage 4	Dissemination of tumor to distant lymph nodes, bone, bone marrow, and liver and/or other organs (except as defined in stage 4S).
Stage 4S	Localized primary tumor as defined for stage 1 or 2 with dissemination limited to liver, skin, and bone marrow in infant <1 year of age.

From Brodeur GM, Pritchard J, Berthold F, et al: Revisions of the international criteria for neuroblastoma diagnosis, staging and response to treatment. J Clin Oncol 11:1466, 1993.

viewed 212 infants with stage 4S neuroblastoma and found that only 13% died of disease progression whereas 12% died of therapy-related causes. Biologic differences have been demonstrated between stages 4S and 4 neuroblastoma, with lack of elevation of serum ferritin levels in stage 4S being compared with stage 4 (Hann et al, 1981). There is usually lack of N-*myc* oncogene amplification in stage 4S tumors compared with stage 4 tumors (Seeger et al, 1985).

Levels of several serum markers including ferritin, neuron-specific enolase, lactic dehydrogenase, GD$_2$ ganglioside, and chromogranin, have all been shown to be elevated in the serum of patients with advanced neuroblastoma. Analysis of these markers at diagnosis is helpful in distinguishing those patients with stage 3 and 4 disease who may have a more favorable survival prognosis and therefore require less intensive treatment. Hann and coworkers (1981) initially showed that ferritin levels were elevated in 15 of 17 children with stage 4 disease, but in none of 13 children with stage 4S disease. Subsequently, they demonstrated that ferritin was a prognostic factor independent of age and stage for children with stage 3 and 4 neuroblastoma: progression-free survival at 24 months of follow-up for patients with stage 3 tumor with normal ferritin levels was 76% versus 23% with elevated ferritin levels, whereas for stage 4 disease survival was 27% versus 3%,

respectively (Hann et al, 1985). Zeltzer and coworkers (1986) demonstrated similar findings for neuron-specific enolase, a cytoplasmic protein found in normal neural tissue and present in elevated quantities in the serum of patients with neuroblastoma. In patients with stage 3 and 4 neuroblastoma, only 5% survived who had neuron-specific enolase levels greater than 100 ng/mL, whereas 63% survived with neuron-specific enolase levels less than 100 ng/mL. Similar studies show improvement in survival for patients with lower lactate dehydrogenase (nonspecific marker) and for chromogranin A (Hsiao et al, 1990) and GD$_2$ ganglioside (Valentino et al, 1990), both shed by neuroblastoma into the circulation.

Amplification of the N-*myc* oncogene in primary neuroblastoma has also been shown to correlate with advanced stage disease and with rapid tumor progression regardless of stage (Brodeur et al, 1984; Seeger et al, 1985). Estimated progression-free survival was 68%, 30%, and 0%, respectively, for patients whose tumors had 1, 3 to 10, or more than 10 copies of the N-*myc* oncogene. Patients with stage 1 or 4S disease have N-*myc* amplification only rarely; when present, it has been associated with rapid disease progression in these usually favorable stages (Bourhis et al, 1991). Approximately 10% of patients with stage 2 disease have amplification; most of such patients to date have development of rapid disease progression and death within 2 years of diagnosis. Thus, N-*myc* amplification is a significant prognostic factor that is independent of stage. It will be most helpful in detecting the newborns with high-risk disease. In the most recent Children's Cancer Group study of stage 4 neuroblastoma in infants, the progression-free survival after 2 years is less than 10% in those with tumor N-*myc* amplification in contrast to 95% for those with single-copy tumors.

Total cellular DNA content may also predict response to therapy in infants with neuroblastoma (Look et al, 1991). Infants with hyperdiploid tumors had a significantly better response to therapy than did those with diploid tumors. Furthermore, hyperdiploidy correlated with stage 4S. Diploidy often correlates with tumor N-*myc* amplification, although, even in rare cases of hyperdiploidy with N-*myc* amplification, the N-*myc* amplification portends an unfavorable outcome, overriding the effect of hyperdiploidy. Other researchers confirmed the poor prognosis of patients with diploid (euploid) tumors and correlated tumor DNA with histologic grading and clinical stage (Gansler et al, 1986; Hayashi et al, 1989).

Tumor karyotype may also influence outcome in neuroblastoma: abnormalities of the short arm of chromosome 1 are more common in patients with metastatic disease but are rare in patients with stage 1, 2, and 4S disease (Christiansen and Lampert, 1988; Fong et al, 1989). Both allelic losses on chromosome 1 and additional material on chromosome 17q are unfavorable prognostic factors in neuroblastoma (Caron, 1995). It has recently been shown by multiple groups that expression of high-affinity nerve growth factor receptors (gp 140[trk-A]) is a favorable prognostic factor, which is highly predictive of a good outcome regardless of age. Infants whose tumor lacks gp 140[trk-A] expression have a 26% survival rate compared to an 87% in those in whom there is high expression (Nakagawara et al, 1993; Suzuki et al, 1993).

A number of children have experienced spontaneous tumor regression despite the presence of metastases, most commonly in infants with stage 4S disease. In other instances, malignant neuroblastomas have apparently undergone maturation into benign ganglioneuromas. The case (Haas et al, 1988) shown in Figure 104–6 is an example of spontaneous maturation and regression.

The diagnosis of neuroblastoma was made before the age of 6 months in 21 of 29 case reports collected by Everson and Cole (1966) in which spontaneous regression occurred. The remainder were diagnosed in patients between 6 and 24 months of age. This relationship of spontaneous regression to age has also been noted by Evans and coworkers (1971), who found that the majority of those with tumor regression were younger than 6 months of age and were usually those with stage 2 or stage 4S disease. Some patients with spontaneous regression of stage 4 disease have been reported (Sitarz et al, 1975). Patients with stage 1 disease, however, could not be evaluated because the tumor was usually completely resected. The mechanism of the spontaneous regression is uncertain, although in at least three cases, pathologic differentiation and maturation to ganglioneuroma have been documented.

Treatment

The unpredictable course of neuroblastoma, with its occasional spontaneous maturation or regression, not only makes the tumor unusual but also causes difficulty in evaluating therapy. The type and intensity of treatment can be based on the ability to define infants with relatively good, intermediate, and poor prognoses based on stage, pathology, ferritin level, and N-*myc* amplification. Patients who have localized disease (stage 1 or 2) without amplification of N-*myc* have a 90% to 100% survival with surgery alone, even if the tumor is not completely resected. Such patients should have surgical resection or partial resection, but they will probably not derive any additional benefit from postoperative radiation or chemotherapy. An exception to this rule would be in the case of spinal cord compression, in which prompt decompression either with osteoplastic laminotomy, limited chemotherapy, or local radiation therapy may be used to preserve function. The combination of extensive laminectomy with postoperative irradiation should be avoided, because later spinal deformity is almost inevitable in the infant. If a recurrence develops after local therapy in stage 2 neuroblastoma, such patients are almost always salvageable with further treatment (Matthay et al, 1989).

Patients with stage 4S disease have a highly favorable prognosis and may require minimal therapy. Because many patients undergo spontaneous regression without chemotherapy and the disease-free survival overall is 85% to 90%, therapy should be directed toward supportive care with minimal chemotherapy and surgery. The main cause of death is massive hepatic involvement resulting in respiratory insufficiency or compromise of renal or gastrointestinal function. In a review of 212 cases in the literature, 21

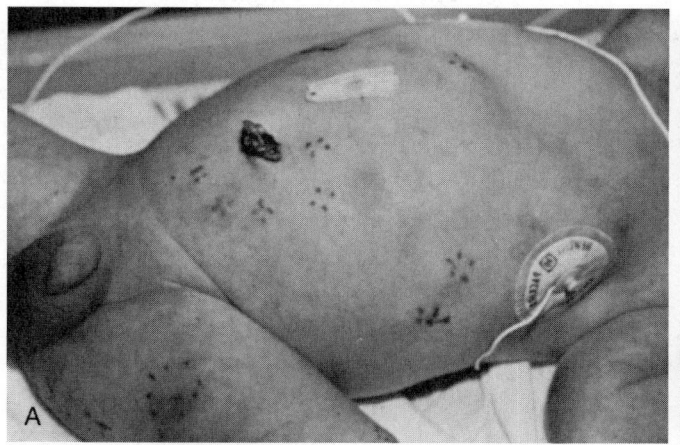

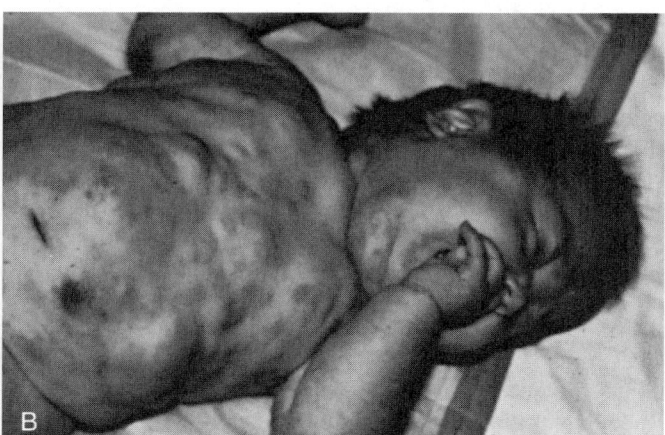

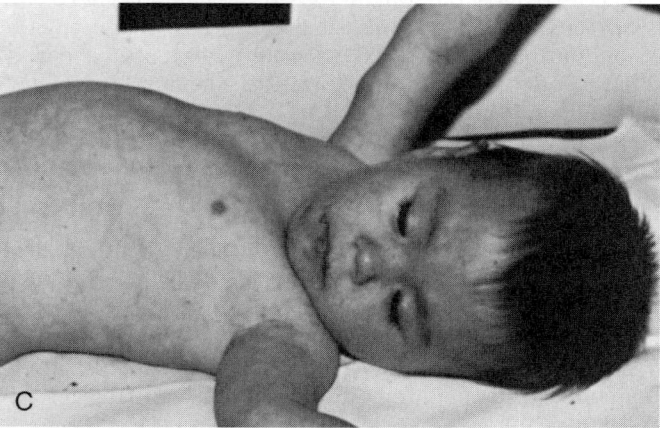

FIGURE 104–6. A newborn with Stage 4S neuroblastoma in whom progression was followed by spontaneous maturation and regression. *A*, birth; *B*, 3 months; *C*, 10 months.

patients died of local disease progression, 20 died of therapy-related causes, and only 7 died of progression to a stage 4 tumor. The hepatic tumor often regresses with low-dose radiation therapy at a dose of 450 cGy given in three fractions through across-table, opposed ports angled to avoid the kidneys, spine, and ovaries. Concomitant low-dose cyclophosphamide often hastens tumor regression. No benefit has been shown to result from resection of the primary tumor, despite anecdotal case reports. Nutritional and blood product support may also be necessary until the lesions begin to resolve. Only in the rare 3% of cases in which progression to a stage 4 lesion occurs is intensive antineoplastic treatment required.

Infants with the less favorable stages, 3 and 4, are usually treated with combination chemotherapy and local surgery and radiation therapy as necessary to eradicate residual disease. It is possible that the use of the newer prognostic factors, pathologic studies, N-*myc*, ferritin levels, and DNA ploidy may obviate the need for intensive therapy for patients with favorable stages. Active drugs that are most commonly used in treatment programs for advanced neuroblastoma include cisplatin, etoposide, doxorubicin, cyclophosphamide, vincristine, and ifosfamide. A few infants with a very unfavorable prognosis include patients with stage 4 disease with amplification of the N-*myc* oncogene; it is possible that for such patients, as in older children with neuroblastoma, standard chemotherapy regimens will be insufficient for cure. In these high-risk patients, myeloablative therapy followed by bone marrow infusion may offer additional benefit (Philip et al, 1991; Seeger et al, 1991).

MELANOTIC NEUROECTODERMAL TUMORS

Melanotic neuroectodermal tumors of infancy are uncommon neoplasms derived from cells of the neural crest. These melanin-containing tumors usually are diagnosed between 1 and 8 months of age and most commonly appear overlying the maxilla. With few exceptions, the tumor behaves in a benign manner (Cutler et al, 1981).

WILMS TUMOR

Wilms tumor, or nephroblastoma, the most common intra-abdominal tumor of childhood, but relatively rare in the neonatal period, occurs in 1 in 8000 children. In some children with aniridia, for instance, the risk is much higher. In contrast to neuroblastoma, this neoplasm, with optimal treatment, is associated with an increasing rate of cure that has been one of the dramatic success stories in the field of cancer therapy. The National Wilms Tumor Study, established in 1969, has helped in the rapid accumulation of information regarding the prognosis and treatment of this tumor, which results in death if untreated.

Clinical Manifestations

Most children with Wilms tumor have either an abdominal mass or an increase in abdominal size noted as the first clinical evidence of disease. This is often first discovered by a parent and brought to the attention of the physician.

The tumor lies deep in the flank, is attached to the kidney or is part of it, and is usually firm and smooth. It seldom extends beyond the midline, even though it may grow downward beyond the iliac crest. In 5% to 10% of all cases, tumors involve both kidneys. Gross hematuria is a rare presenting symptom, but microscopic hematuria is found in approximately one fourth of cases. However, hematuria in Wilms tumor is not a poor prognostic sign, as it is in adults with hypernephroma. Hypertension, occasionally noted in older infants and children, has not been observed in the newborn. The tumor may sometimes present with abdominal pain and be discovered at laparotomy, and occasionally acute hemorrhage into the tumor may result in a rapidly enlarging mass, usually associated with anemia and fever.

Wilms tumor is seldom diagnosed at birth or during the neonatal period, although several renal tumors have been so large as to have caused dystocia during delivery. Characteristics associated with an earlier presentation include bilaterality or associated aniridia or hypospadias (Pastore et al, 1988) and positive family history.

Rare cases of Wilms tumor associated with polycythemia have been reported. This finding is secondary to an increased production of erythropoietin by the neoplasm. The demonstration of elevated plasma erythropoietin levels in nonpolycythemic children with Wilms tumor studied preoperatively led to the suggestion that this test may be useful in the diagnosis and evaluation of response to therapy.

Differential Diagnosis

The other intra-abdominal tumor that may be easily confused with Wilms tumor is neuroblastoma. Although Wilms tumor distorts the kidney whereas neuroblastoma displaces it, preoperative distinction may be difficult when neuroblastoma arises within kidney substance. Less common intrarenal neoplasms that may be seen are rhabdoid tumor, mesoblastic nephroma, renal cell carcinoma, rhabdomyosarcoma, hemangiopericytoma, and lymphoma. Benign processes that may simulate Wilms tumor include multicystic kidneys, hematomas, and renal carbuncles.

Hereditary Associations and Congenital Anomalies

The association among Wilms tumor, hemihypertrophy, cardiac anomalies, congenital aniridia, hamartomas, and genitourinary defects and associated chromosomal changes has been discussed earlier in this chapter (see Genetic Factors and Congenital Defects). The finding of hemihypertrophy should alert the physician to observe the child for the possible development of Wilms tumor, adrenal cortical tumor, or hepatoma. Some of these patients may have incomplete forms of the Beckwith-Wiedemann syndrome (Sotelo-Avila et al, 1980). It is interesting that abnormalities of chromosome 11 are seen in tumor cells from Wilms tumor, rhabdomyosarcoma, and hepatoblastoma, all tumors associated with Beckwith-Wiedemann syndrome (Cowell and Pritchard, 1987). A number of cases of pseudohermaphroditism, nephron disorders (diffuse mesangial sclerosis), and Wilms tumor have also been reported (Gallo and

Chemes, 1987). Occasionally, certain members of a family may have the congenital anomaly and others may have the neoplasm. Meadows and coworkers (1974) reported one family in which a mother had congenital hemihypertrophy, three of the children had Wilms tumor, and a fourth had a urinary tract anomaly.

Aniridia is usually inherited in an autosomal dominant pattern with high penetrance and little variability of phenotypic expression. The child with aniridia who has Wilms tumor does not have this usual inheritance pattern but has sporadic congenital aniridia. Pilling (1975) reported 26 children with aniridia, 20 of whom had the sporadic type. Wilms tumor developed in 7 of the 20. It appears that the risk of development of Wilms tumor is higher if the sporadic aniridia is accompanied by a major genitourinary tract anomaly, severe mental retardation, or both. The Wilms tumor–aniridia syndrome, a combination of mental retardation, microcephaly, bilateral aniridia, anomalies of the pinna, Wilms tumor, and ambiguous genitalia, is associated with a small deletion of chromosome 11 (11p13-14.1). In some tumor tissues, the same section of DNA deleted from one chromosome may be duplicated on another. The behavior is compatible with a recessive oncogene. Although usually sporadic, this syndrome may occasionally be familial (Yunis and Ramsay, 1980). Rarely, affected persons may demonstrate all the findings except the Wilms tumor (Riccardi et al, 1978). There are two reports of aniridia in monozygous twins in which Wilms tumor developed in only one member of each pair (Maurer et al, 1979; Miller, 1979). Other congenital conditions that may predispose the patient to Wilms tumor include Turner syndrome and trisomy 18. There is also a variant mutation at 11p13 that results in Denys-Drash syndrome of Wilms tumor, genital anomalies, and nephropathy (Coppes et al, 1994). More recently, some familial and sporadic cases of Wilms tumor have also been shown to involve loss of heterozygosity at 16q (Newsham et al, 1995) and in rare cases, changes in chromosome 7 (Wilmore et al, 1994). Bloom syndrome, a rare autosomal recessive disease previously associated with a high risk of cancer, has been reported to predispose patients to Wilms tumor (Cairney et al, 1987). Reports of tumors occurring in siblings, identical twins, parent–child pairs, and cousins with no malformations indicate that hereditary factors at times may play a major role in the development of this neoplasm. Pedigrees showing a predisposition to Wilms tumor are rare, with only 1% of patients having affected siblings or parents, although such cases tend to occur earlier in infancy. The specific germ line abnormality has not yet been successfully localized, although a number of such cases have been examined for the candidate loci on 11p and 16q (Baird et al, 1994). However, heritability of the unilateral sporadic form of Wilms tumor was examined by Li and associates (1988) in 96 long-term survivors. No Wilms tumor developed in 179 offspring of these patients, confirming the low likelihood of heritability in the sporadic form.

Prognostic Factors

Several factors seem to influence the response to therapy and ultimate prognosis of the child with Wilms tumor: the histologic pattern, the age of the patient at the time of

TABLE 104–8

Clinicopathologic Staging of Wilms Tumor

Stage I:	Tumor limited to the kidney and completely resected.
Stage II:	Tumor extending beyond the kidney but completely resected. The tumor may have been biopsied, or there may have been local spillage.
Stage III:	Residual nonhematogenous tumor confined to the abdomen, including any of the following: lymph node involvement in the abdomen, diffuse peritoneal spillage or tumor growth that has penetrated the peritoneal surface, peritoneal implants, gross or microscopic extension beyond surgical margins, or unresectable because of infiltration into vital structures.
Stage IV:	Hematogenous metastases. Deposits beyond stage III (i.e., lung, liver, bone, and brain).
Stage V:	Bilateral renal involvement at diagnosis.

diagnosis, and the extent of disease. Tumors with better differentiation, showing glomeruloid and tubular formation, indicate a better chance for survival than do those with anaplastic and sarcomatous patterns. Patients younger than 2 years of age at diagnosis have fewer relapses, especially to distant sites, than do older children. Age, however, seems to be of little prognostic significance regarding mortality. Specimens weighing more than 250 g and positive regional lymph nodes, however, are often important predictors of both relapse and mortality.

The most common staging system in use is that devised by the National Wilms Tumor Study (Table 104–8). The clinical staging is an important factor in predicting survival; those with more extensive spread have a poorer prognosis. Therefore, adequate evaluation of the extent of tumor involvement is essential and should include computed tomography of the abdomen and chest to fully evaluate both kidneys, the inferior vena cava for tumor thrombus, and the liver and lungs, which are the most commonly involved areas of hematogenous spread (Fig. 104–7). Other commonly involved sites of metastatic spread are the retroperitoneum, peritoneum, mediastinum, and pleurae. If the histology shows a clear cell sarcoma, bone metastases may occur, so a bone scan should be included in the evaluation; rhabdoid tumors, which frequently metastasize to brain,

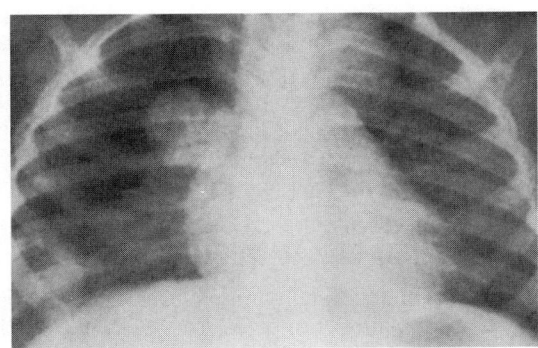

FIGURE 104–7. Pulmonary metastases of Wilms tumor.

necessitate computed tomography or magnetic resonance imaging of the brain.

Treatment and Prognosis

Before 1950, the two major modalities of therapy for Wilms tumor, surgical removal and radiation therapy, resulted in cure rates approaching 50%. The advantage of treatment with the chemotherapeutic agent dactinomycin was demonstrated in 1966 by Farber, who reported an 89% survival rate in children who had no evidence of metastatic disease at the time of diagnosis and who were followed up for at least 2 years, and a 53% survival rate in those presenting with evidence of metastatic disease. The drug therapy appeared to prevent clinical hematogenous metastases following surgical removal and radiation to the tumor bed by presumably destroying nondetectable, microscopic tumor foci, especially in the lungs. Vincristine also has striking activity against Wilms tumor and appears to be at least as effective as dactinomycin. Other single agents shown to have activity against this tumor include doxorubicin, cyclophosphamide, ifosfamide, and bleomycin.

Infants younger than 12 months of age have experienced undue toxicity to the liver, hematopoietic system, and lungs from the prescribed doses of dactinomycin, vincristine, and doxorubicin. On the earlier National Wilms Tumor Studies, 47% of infants had severe hematologic toxicity and there were toxic deaths in 6%. Dosages were subsequently reduced to 50% of the usual per kilogram dose given to older children, with a decrease in hematologic toxicity to 13% and elimination of toxic deaths. It is interesting that the dosage reduction did not compromise therapeutic effect as judged by the 2-year relapse-free survival figures (Morgan et al, 1988).

Results of the first two National Wilms Tumor Studies show that treatment with vincristine and dactinomycin is superior to treatment with either drug alone. Postoperative radiation therapy adds little benefit to those with totally excised tumors, and 6 months of therapy with two drugs appears to be as effective as 15 months of therapy in such patients. Patients with more advanced disease fared better following treatment with three drugs (dactinomycin, vincristine, doxorubicin) than with two (dactinomycin, vincristine). Patients with unfavorable histology had a significantly poorer prognosis than did those with favorable histology, as did those with positive nodes (D'Angio et al, 1981). Current treatment results from the third National Wilms Tumor Study (D'Angio et al, 1989) in children with Wilms tumor according to stage and histology are shown in Table 104–9. Thus, Wilms tumor, a neoplasm that is fatal if untreated, presently has a cure rate overall approaching 90%. The use of newer therapeutic agents may continue to improve these remarkably successful results. It has been suggested that infants with small, totally resected tumors may not need any more treatment than surgery.

OTHER RENAL NEOPLASMS

A number of neonatal renal tumors have been confused with the typical Wilms tumor in the past. Since these neoplasms have been recognized as separate entities, they are more commonly diagnosed during the neonatal period

TABLE 104–9

Treatment Results of the Third National Wilms Tumor Study According to Stage and Histology

Stage	Histology	No.	% Relapse-Free 2 Yr	% Relapse-Free 4 Yr	% Alive 4 Yr
I	Favorable	607	91.6	90.4	96.5
II	Favorable	278	90.4	88.1	92.3
III	Favorable	275	79.8	79.0	87.0
IV	Favorable	120	76.0	74.9	82.5
I–III	Unfavorable	130	69.7	64.8	68.4
IV	Unfavorable	29	55.6	55.6	55.3
All patients		1439	85.0	83.3	89.1

Data from D'Angio GI, Breslow N, Beckwith B, et al: Treatment of Wilms' tumor: Results of the Third National Wilms' Tumor Study. Cancer 64:349, 1989.

than is the classic nephroblastoma, which rarely occurs during the 1st month of life.

Rhabdoid Tumor of Kidney

Rhabdoid tumor of the kidney is an uncommon renal tumor of children that is one of the most lethal neoplasms of early neonatal life, with a mortality rate exceeding 80%. It has a predilection for males, with a male-to-female ratio of 1.5:1, and for infants, with median age at diagnosis of 11 months. Overall, rhabdoid tumors comprised 1.8% of all malignant childhood renal tumors entered on the National Wilms Tumor Study. Rhabdoid tumors frequently present simultaneously with embryonal primary tumors of the central nervous system, such as medulloblastoma (Bonnin et al, 1984). Originally believed to represent a "rhabdomyosarcomatoid" pattern of Wilms tumor, it subsequently was shown to lack any evidence of myoblastic differentiation or any morphologic or clinical linkage to Wilms tumor. Review of 111 cases by Weeks and coworkers and the National Wilms Tumor Study (1989) showed several findings suggesting that rhabdoid tumors may arise from cells involved in formation of the renal medulla but that they have no histogenic relationship to Wilms tumor. The prognosis is poor, particularly for infants with evidence of dissemination. The only patients who survived were those with completely resected disease and negative lymph nodes (50%), whereas all those with metastases died.

Mesoblastic Nephroma

The congenital mesoblastic nephroma, or fetal mesenchymal hamartoma, is clearly distinguishable from Wilms tumor by its benign nature. The involved kidney is usually greatly enlarged and distorted by the tumor, but, contrary to the findings with Wilms tumor, there is usually no lobulation, necrosis, hemorrhage, or discrete capsule between neoplasm and compressed kidney (Fig. 104–8). Although most cases present as an asymptomatic abdominal mass, the large size may cause problems. Polyhydramnios and premature labor occur with increased frequency in

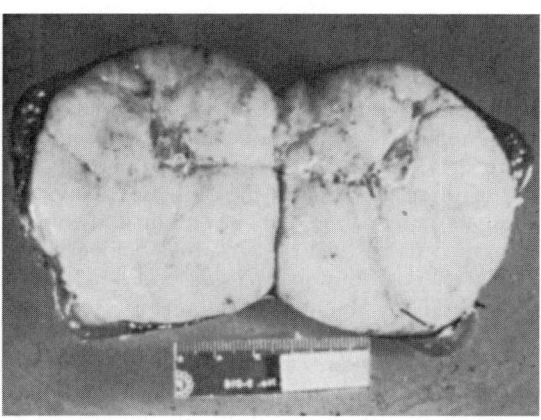

FIGURE 104–8. Congenital mesoblastic nephroma compressing and nearly totally replacing the kidney.

women whose infants have mesoblastic nephroma. The tumor may be diagnosed prenatally with ultrasonography, which helps to differentiate it from Wilms tumor because of its typical sonographic appearance of concentric echogenic and echo-poor ring pattern (Chan et al, 1987). Prenatal diagnosis may allow earlier treatment in symptomatic cases, such as that reported by Matsumura and colleagues (1993) in which compression of the aorta caused severe congestive heart failure in the fetus, necessitating emergency surgery. The histologic picture is of a preponderance of interlacing bundles of spindle-shaped cells within which dysplastic tubules and glomeruli are irregularly scattered. Extrarenal infiltration is common, especially into the perihilar connective tissues. Since that initial description, a cellular or atypical variant of congenital mesoblastic nephroma with focal hemorrhage, necrosis, hypercellularity, and a high mitotic index was described. The atypical variants usually present at a later age (mean 5.3 months) than the classic type (mean 16 days) (Pettinato et al, 1989). Despite pathologic variation, efforts to predict clinical behavior on this basis have failed. In the 16 cases of congenital mesoblastic nephroma reported by Pettinato and associates, all of the patients survived with surgery alone, despite frequent extension into psoas and perirenal fat and despite atypical histology in 10 tumors.

Most patients have been cured by nephrectomy alone, even in the presence of localized extrarenal extension. There is good evidence that more patients with mesoblastic nephroma have died as a result of aggressive chemotherapy and irradiation than from the tumor itself. Radical nephrectomy alone is the treatment of choice; however, in rare instances the tumor is unusually aggressive.

Persistent Renal Blastema and Nephroblastomatosis

Accumulations of immature renal tissue are not normally found beyond 36 weeks' gestation, the time at which nephrogenesis normally ceases. Nodular renal blastema is characterized by microscopic nests of primitive cells in the subcapsular renal cortex resembling the blastemal cells of Wilms tumor but lacking mitoses. Although benign, these nodules are believed to have the potential for neoplastic

transformation. They are found in one of every 200 to 400 postmortem examinations of infants younger than 4 months of age, but they are discovered in the kidneys of children older than 4 months of age only in cases of Wilms tumor. When nodular renal blastema becomes massive and confluent and replaces the cortex, it is referred to as "nephroblastomatosis" (Bove and McAdams, 1976). Kumar and associates (1978) reported the nodular renal blastema–nephroblastomatosis complex in 8 of 118 patients (6.8%) with Wilms tumor. Five of these eight patients had bilateral tumors. Children with this disorder may also have the congenital anomalies associated with Wilms tumor (Fig. 104–9). The fact that nodular renal blastema is rarely found in older children suggests that the majority of these lesions regress, a situation analogous to the course of neuroblastoma in situ. It is believed that those that persist give rise to Wilms tumor, whereas a small number progress to diffuse nephroblastomatosis. Complete progression of nodular renal blastema to nephroblastomatosis to Wilms tumor has been documented (Kulkarni et al, 1980). Children with massive bilateral involvement often respond to therapy used for Wilms tumor. Although persistent renal blastema is not a true malignancy, it probably has been confused with Wilms tumor in the past, and it appears in many instances to be a precursor of this malignancy.

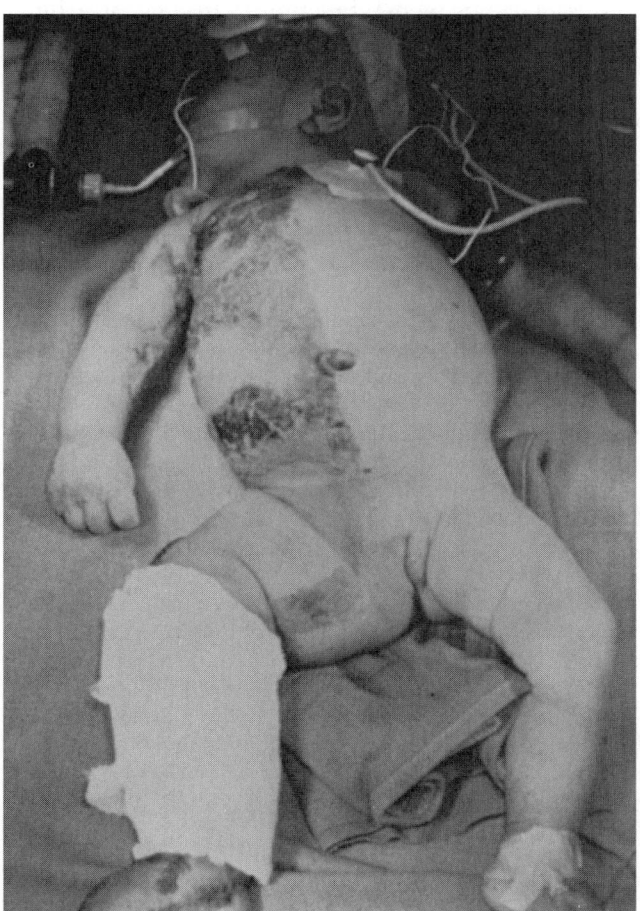

FIGURE 104–9. Congenital epidermal nevus in association with hemihypertrophy and nephroblastomatosis.

Cystic Partially Differentiated Nephroblastoma

A renal neoplasm in infants is known by a variety of names: polycystic nephroblastoma, benign multilocular cystic nephroma, well-differentiated polycystic Wilms tumor, and cystic partially differentiated nephroblastoma. It is a cystic encapsulated tumor occurring before 2 years of age. The cysts are lined by epithelium and show a mixture of partially differentiated and undifferentiated metanephrogenic blastema that differentiates this lesion from multilocular cysts of the kidney. The tumor appears to have a benign course, and nephrectomy is the treatment of choice (Joshi et al, 1977). These neoplasms probably represent a differentiated form of nephroblastoma.

RETINOBLASTOMA

Retinoblastoma is a malignant ocular tumor that arises in embryonic retinal cells. The incidence of retinoblastoma in the United States is approximately 1:18,000 live births. Bilateral involvement is observed in 20% to 35% of retinoblastomas; in as many as one fourth of these patients, the tumor is initially detected in only one eye.

Genetics

The gene for retinoblastoma, located on chromosome 13q14, has been cloned and belongs to a class of tumor suppressor genes whose function is to control cellular growth. When the gene is inactivated, either by a mutation or deletion, the block to cellular proliferation is removed, leading to tumor formation. Mutations at the retinoblastoma locus can be inherited in an autosomal dominant pattern or arise spontaneously. The Knudson "two hit" hypothesis postulates that the first gene change can occur in a germ cell (inherited cases) or in a retinoblast (in sporadic cases); only when the second gene change develops in a somatic target cell (retinoblast) already carrying a first hit will that cell be transformed. All patients with bilateral retinoblastoma have a new germinal mutation or an inherited one. Approximately 80% of unilateral retinoblastomas occur as a result of a somatic nonheritable mutation (Cowell and Pritchard, 1987). The germinal trait responsible for retinoblastoma is a dominant one with 80% to 96% penetrance. There are also a small number of patients (5% of retinoblastoma) born with a constitutional deletion of chromosome 13, 13q-, who have the associated anomalies of microencephaly, macrognathia, malformed ears and thumbs, hypertelorism, microphthalmia, ptosis, protruding upper incisors, short stature, cleft palate, developmental delay, and psychomotor retardation (Knudson et al, 1976). Children with the bilateral and hereditary form are diagnosed at an earlier age, because the chromosomal abnormality is present at birth, providing a greater susceptibility to tumorigenesis. It is possible, using DNA restriction-fragment length polymorphisms, to predict susceptibility to retinoblastoma (Cavenee et al, 1986; Wiggs et al, 1988).

Clinical Manifestations

Retinoblastoma commonly presents either with leukocoria or "cat's eye" on ocular examination or with strabismus caused by loss of vision in the affected eye. Multifocal retinal involvement is common, occurring in 84% of patients. Intraocular spread may fill the vitreous body by extension or seeding, whereas exophytic tumors arise from the outer retinal layer and cause retinal detachment. Extraocular spread is seen in less than 15% of patients, usually occurring by direct invasion of the optic nerve and eventually leading to subarachnoid involvement and intracranial spread. In such cases the cerebrospinal fluid may contain tumor cells. Rarely, tumors may spread by invasion of the orbit or by hematogenous dissemination to bones and bone marrow.

The diagnosis is made by ophthalmoscopic examination under anesthesia. Computed tomography or magnetic resonance imaging of the eye is useful to determine tumor extent and optic nerve involvement. A lumbar puncture for cerebrospinal fluid cytology should be obtained if there is optic nerve invasion; bone scan and bone marrow biopsy detect hematogenous spread. In general, repeated metastatic evaluations are not indicated for follow-up of this tumor because of the extreme rarity of extraocular dissemination. Only cases with extraocular involvement initially or with clinical findings compatible with spread require such evaluations. Tumors are then staged according to the Reese-Ellsworth classification based on the number and size of the lesions and whether they extend anterior to the ora serrata. In addition, any extraocular extension must be specified.

Treatment

Because extraocular spread and death from dissemination are rare, the main goal of treatment is local control and preservation of vision. Surgical enucleation is used only when there is no chance for useful vision, if glaucoma is present, or if conservative measures fail to control tumor. External beam radiation therapy, administered by experienced clinicians using careful positioning and general anesthesia, has been the standard treatment for cure of retinoblastoma. Doses range from 3500 to 5000 cGy given in three fractions per week. Occasionally, radioactive plaques are used for local recurrences. If local extension has occurred, the field must be enlarged to include the orbit or a craniospinal field for meningeal or brain involvement (Donaldson and Smith, 1989). Small tumors confined to the retina, occurring either before or after radiation therapy, can often be controlled with cryotherapy and photocoagulation. Because of the late effects of radiation on bony growth and second tumor induction, it is preferable to use aggressive cryotherapy and laser therapy when possible. Chemotherapy, including agents such as vincristine, doxorubicin, cyclophosphamide, cisplatin, and etoposide, has achieved responses and may be indicated in patients with disseminated disease. Thus far, no advantage has been demonstrated for the use of chemotherapy as adjuvant treatment given in addition to radiation therapy or enucleation.

The prognosis for children with unilateral retinoblastoma is excellent, with cure rates of 85% to 90% using conservative local treatment. However, patients with bilateral disease have a much lower long-term survival, not because of the retinoblastoma but because of a high predisposition to second malignancy, which may occur from 5 years up to the rest of the patient's life. Local extension also confers a poor prognosis, with survival rates being less than 40% with optic nerve invasion and less than 10% with orbital extension or distant dissemination.

HEPATIC MALIGNANCIES

Primary malignant tumors of the liver are uncommon in infants and children. The most common malignant neoplasm involving the liver in infancy is metastatic neuroblastoma. The two major histologic types of hepatomas are hepatoblastoma and hepatocellular carcinoma. Hepatoblastomas usually occur in infants and are rarely seen after 3 years of age. In the 129 cases reported by Exelby and coworkers (1975), almost half of the patients were 18 months of age or younger, 11 were younger than 6 weeks of age, and 3 were newborns. Hepatocellular carcinomas, however, appear to have a bimodal age distribution, occurring either in very young children younger than 4 years of age or in patients between the ages of 12 and 15 years. Both types of tumors occur more commonly in males. Hepatoblastoma occurs in association with Beckwith-Wiedemann syndrome and its variants. Hemihypertrophy occurs in 2% of hepatoblastoma patients.

Chromosome abnormalities in tumor tissue include loss of heterozygosity at 11p15.5, the Beckwith-Wiedemann locus, and, in non–Beckwith-Wiedemann syndrome patients, i(8q) and trisomy 20. There is also an increased risk of hepatoblastoma in familial adenomatosis polyposis coli, a gene which maps to chromosome 5q (Phillips et al, 1989).

The most common presenting symptoms of hepatic tumors are an upper abdominal mass and an enlarging abdomen. Anorexia, weight loss, and pain also frequently occur. Laboratory studies of liver function are rarely helpful in establishing a diagnosis and are usually normal. Alpha-fetoprotein, an alpha$_1$-globulin that occurs normally in the fetus and disappears in the first few weeks of life, is often present in the serum of the child with hepatic malignancy. A number of children with hepatoblastoma have elevated levels of the amino acid cystathionine in their urine. If present, cystathioninuria may allow differentiation among hepatoblastoma and a number of benign and malignant disorders, but elevated levels of cystathionine also occur in about 50% of patients with neuroblastoma.

Hepatic calcification is demonstrated in 10% of cases on the plain abdominal roentgenogram. Ultrasound is useful to distinguish cystic and solid masses from a diffusely enlarged liver. Computed tomography shows the extent of tumor involvement, anatomic landmarks, and operability, whereas magnetic resonance imaging most accurately shows adenopathy, tumor margins, and vessel involvement. Magnetic resonance imaging may often obviate the need for more invasive angiographic procedures preoperatively. If one lobe is free of malignancy and there is no evidence of distant metastatic disease, a lobectomy of the involved portion of the liver should be performed despite the high operative mortality rate. Surgery appears to be the best means for cure. Sixty percent of those with hepatoblastoma and 33% with hepatocellular carcinoma were cured if the tumor could be completely excised. The subgroup with pure "fetal" histology and complete resection have 100%

survival (Weinberg and Finegold, 1983). However, a number of cases have been reported since in which initially inoperable tumors could be removed and the patient cured by a second surgical procedure following reduction in tumor size by the use of chemotherapy and radiation therapy (Ortega et al, 1991). Chemotherapy after total gross tumor resection may increase survival rates (Wheatley and LaQuaglia, 1993). Three patients with unresectable disease, including one with pulmonary metastases, were rendered disease free with cisplatin and doxorubicin and remained in remission off treatment (Quinn et al, 1985). New approaches to initially unresectable tumors beyond chemotherapy include chemoembolization, and, in rare cases, liver transplantation.

In addition to hepatomas, a variety of rare liver tumors have been reported in infants. Angiosarcomas are believed to be the malignant form of infantile hemangioendotheliomas. One case occurred in a 20-month-old child following in utero exposure to arsenic (Falk et al, 1981), a toxin implicated in hepatic angiosarcomas in adults. Seventeen cases of hepatic teratomas have been reported in children, the majority occurring in females younger than 3 years of age. About one half of hepatic teratomas are malignant.

SACROCOCCYGEAL TERATOMAS

Teratomas are neoplasms that contain derivatives of more than one of the three primary germ layers of the embryo. Although these tumors are often benign, one or more of the germ layer derivatives may develop malignant characteristics. Teratomas arise in a wide variety of locations of the body but usually occur along the axial midline during early childhood. After puberty, teratomas most frequently occur in the gonads, particularly the ovary. A recent epidemiology study of malignant germ cell tumors in children by Shu and colleagues (1995) shows a correlation with prematurity, parental exposure to solvents and to plastic and resin fumes, maternal prenatal urinary tract infections, and higher birth weight.

The sacrococcygeal region is the most common site of teratomas in the 1st year of life, and the sacrococcygeal teratoma is the most common solid tumor in the newborn, although it is rarely malignant. Females are affected two to four times more frequently than males. The earliest detection of a teratoma may occur prenatally or at birth. Polyhydramnios, nonimmune fetal hydrops, and dystocia have all been described in association with germ cell tumors. Congenital anomalies are often present in association with sacrococcygeal teratomas, including genitourinary, hind gut, and lower vertebral malformations. Most tumors present as a mass protruding between the coccyx and rectum and may be quite large (Fig. 104–10). About 10% are found by rectal examination. Nearly all arise at the tip or inner surface of the coccyx and can be diagnosed early in life by the pediatrician who makes the rectal examination a routine part of the physical examination. An estimated 30 children per year are diagnosed in North America with sacrococcygeal teratomas before the age of 2 to 3 months.

Sacrococcygeal teratomas may be confused with meningomyeloceles, rectal abscesses, pelvic neuroblastomas, pilonidal cysts, and a variety of very rare neoplasms that may occur in that region. Most benign teratomas in this area

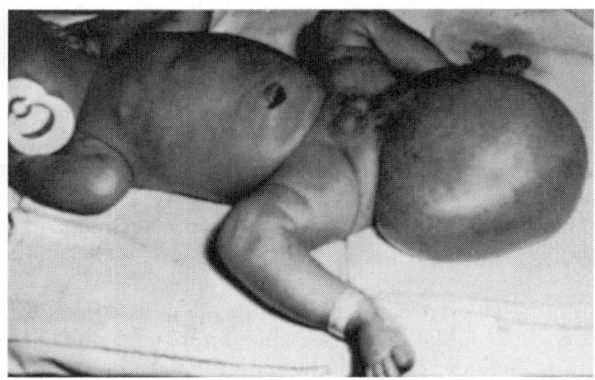

FIGURE 104–10. Large sacrococcygeal teratoma in a newborn girl.

produce no functional difficulties, even when marked intrapelvic extension is present. Thus, bowel or bladder dysfunction, painful defecation, and vascular or lymphatic obstruction suggest that the lesion is malignant.

Treatment of sacrococcygeal tumors is primarily surgical. They should be excised as soon as possible because small, undifferentiated foci may proliferate and become aggressive. They are attached to the coccyx, and therefore removal of the entire coccyx is a necessary part of the surgical procedure. Failure to remove the coccyx results in a 30% to 40% risk of local recurrence.

Sixty percent to 70% of sacrococcygeal teratomas in newborns are unequivocally benign, as determined by the presence of mature tissues. Embryonic or immature somatic tissues are present in 10% to 15% of cases, and the remaining tumors contain malignant elements as defined by the presence of an endodermal sinus tumor or highly undifferentiated neoplasm resembling neuroblastoma (Dehner, 1983). In general, the risk for malignancy is only present in the sacrococcygeal tumors, whereas those in the nasopharynx, neck, mediastinum, or retroperitoneum do not usually contain malignant germ cell elements. Local recurrence or metastasis of teratoma is rare but may occur when immature elements are present. In an early series reported by Gonzalez-Crussi and associates (1978), there were two of four recurrences in immature teratomas. However, there were no recurrences in eight infants with immature neuroepithelial or renal elements in a later series of 68 sacrococcygeal teratomas reported by Valdiserri and Yunis (1981). However, nine patients with endodermal sinus tumor in the same series all had metastases and all died. Hawkins and coworkers (1993) reported six children with the diagnosis of teratoma in the neonatal period who subsequently presented at a median age of 17 months with recurrent endodermal sinus tumor. Review of the initial disease identified small foci of yolk sac tumor in four patients. This illustrates the importance of careful pathologic examination of these neonatal teratomas with examination of multiple sections. Alpha-fetoprotein is usually markedly elevated in the serum of patients with endodermal sinus tumor and provides a useful marker of disease status. This must be interpreted with careful reference to normal values in infants, whose serum levels are normally high but decline with age in a predictable fashion (Blair et

al, 1987). In the series of 398 cases reported by Altman and associates (1974), 60% of the patients with malignant tumors died within 10 months of surgery, 21% were alive with residual disease, 11% were alive without apparent disease, and 9% were lost to follow-up. These findings contrast markedly to the mortality rate reported for children with benign lesions, which was approximately 5%.

A topographic classification for sacrococcygeal tumors appears valuable in predicting potential for metastatic behavior and survival (Fig. 104–11). An internal location predisposes the tumor to metastatic behavior, possibly because the delay in diagnosis is associated with a greater risk of malignant transformation. Therapy for children with malignant sacrococcygeal teratoma is far from optimal. Even those who have localized tumor that is grossly completely excised usually have recurrence. The tumor may respond to combination chemotherapy and radiation therapy in similar regimens to those used for germ cell tumors in general, and occasional cures, even in those patients with metastatic and unresectable disease, have been reported. The addition of regimens containing cisplatin, carboplatin, etoposide, and bleomycin to the therapy for disseminated germ cell tumors has improved the disease-free survival to more than 50% (Ablin et al, 1991; Marina et al, 1992; Nair et al, 1994). Some infants have died of the complications of the intensive therapy (Raney et al, 1981), and it is important to make appropriate dose modifications.

SARCOMAS

Soft tissue sarcomas are rarely seen in newborns, accounting for only 2% of all childhood sarcomas in a study of 357 patients in Germany (Koscielniak et al, 1989) and in the Intergroup Rhabdomyosarcoma Study (Ragab et al, 1986). Fibrosarcomas account for one fifth of these tumors in infants, a 10-fold excess compared with those in older children. The other subtypes seen are rhabdomyosarcoma (67%) and undifferentiated sarcoma (5%). The most common sites affected are the genitourinary tract and the extremities. However, any site may be affected, and rare cases of chest wall tumors (Shamberger et al, 1989) or pericardial tumors (Lazarus et al, 1989) have been reported. A case of Kaposi sarcoma has been reported in a 6-day-old infant with congenital human immunodeficiency virus infection (Gutierrez-Ortega et al, 1989). The prognosis in infantile sarcomas may be similar to that of older children, who have a 5-year overall survival rate of approximately 50%. The outlook is particularly favorable for infantile fibrosarcomas; five such patients survived in the series reported by Koscielniak and coworkers (1989). The majority of sarcomas are unresectable at diagnosis and therefore require combination chemotherapy and, occasionally, radiation. As in treatment of other infantile malignancies, it is necessary to decrease the doses by 50% to prevent excessive toxicity. The value of adjuvant therapy for fibrosarcomas is uncertain, because all those completely resected did well without further treatment. Radiation therapy for residual disease is problematic in the newborn, because of the possible deleterious effects on growth.

MELANOMA

Congenital malignant melanoma is exceedingly rare, with fewer than 30 cases reported in the medical literature.

TYPE I

Predominantly external
with minimal presacral
component

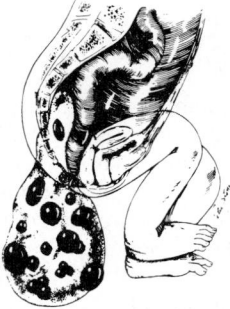

TYPE II

Presenting externally
but significant intrapelvic
extension

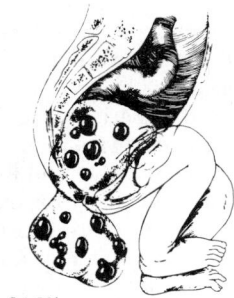

FIGURE 104–11. Location of sacrococcygeal teratoma in 398 patients. (From Altman RP, Randolph JG, Lilly JR: Sacrococcygeal teratoma: American Academy of Pediatrics Surgical Section Survey—1973. J Pediatr Surg 9:389, 1974. Reprinted by permission.)

Frequency 46.6%
Metastatic rate 0%
Mortality rate 11%

Frequency 34.6%
Metastatic rate 6%
Mortality rate 18%

TYPE III

Predominant mass
pelvic with extension
into abdomen

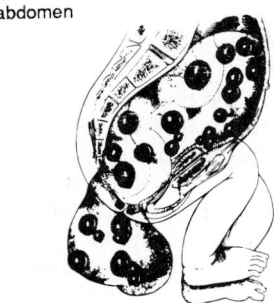

TYPE IV

Entirely presacral with
no external presentation

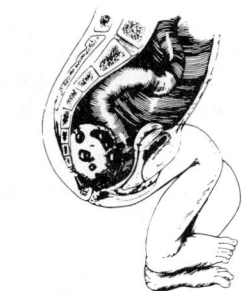

Frequency 8.8%
Metastatic rate 20%
Mortality rate 28%

Frequency 10%
Metastatic rate 8%
Mortality rate 21%

Although usually cutaneous, occasional cases arising in the eye have been described (Broadway et al, 1991). The tumor may be acquired transplacentally from the mother or may arise de novo. Those in the latter group may be associated with a congenital melanocytic nevus. Transplacentally acquired melanoma from an affected mother is usually evident at birth. The placenta may have a mottled brown-black discoloration. Malignant cells are evident on microscopic examination of the intervillous space and have been reported in cord blood. The tumor may involve any part of the body, may be manifest as an external mass or organ enlargement, or may involve the neural axis. Metastases usually develop in those with congenital de novo melanoma (seven of eight cases) during the 1st year of life (Prose et al, 1987). Before 1965, the outcome was uniformly poor for newborns with malignant melanoma, whether it was maternal in origin or de novo (Campbell et al, 1987b). However, in four of the seven cases in the literature since then the patients had a prolonged (5- to 18-year) survival even with metastases, suggesting that such lesions may have a more favorable prognosis in infancy than later childhood. Local excision is the currently accepted therapy, with chemotherapy if dissemination is present.

CENTRAL NERVOUS SYSTEM TUMORS

Central nervous system malignancies are a mixed group in newborns, which altogether comprise less than 5% of newborn cancers. Only 13% of all pediatric brain tumors occur before age 2 years, and only a few of these in the neonatal period. The usual presentation is with enlarging head circumference. Other clinical features may be protean, including irritability, listlessness, vomiting, and failure to thrive (Pollack, 1994). Supratentorial locations are more common than infratentorial, unlike the pattern in older children (Campbell et al, 1987a). Many types of brain tumors have been reported in newborns, including astrocytoma, peripheral neuroectodermal tumor, teratoma, medulloblastoma, ependymoma, choroid plexus papilloma, craniopharyngioma, myxofibrosarcoma, and vascular tumors (Dehner, 1983). The most common in a series of 103 neonatal brain tumors was teratoma (53%), usually occurring in the region of the pineal gland. Treatment for residual disease with radiation is again especially problematic in the newborn, whose brain development is likely to be more susceptible to radiation damage than that of an older child. For such patients in cases in which tumors are likely to be responsive to cytotoxic drugs, chemotherapy as a primary modality is preferable to radiation for local control in unresectable cases (Duffner et al, 1993).

HISTIOCYTOSES

The histiocytoses represent a spectrum of rare, poorly understood disorders of histiocytes ranging from benign to clearly malignant. These diseases have recently been classified by an international group, The Histiocyte Society, on the basis of pathology (Writing Group, 1987). The cytologically benign end of the spectrum (class I disease) comprises the childhood histiocytic syndromes, formerly called histiocytosis X (encompassing eosinophilic granuloma, Letterer-Siwe disease, and Hand-Schüller-Christian disease), currently known as Langerhans cell histiocytosis. It is postulated that an immunologic stimulus to a normal antigen-processing cell, the Langerhans cell, results in uncontrolled proliferation. Langerhans cells with cleaved nuclei and Birbeck granules are seen by electron microscopy; cell surface antigens include S-100 and CD-1, and multinucleated giant cells are sometimes seen. The class II histiocytoses include the familial erythrophagocytic lymphohistiocytosis and the infection-associated hemophagocytic syndrome. They are believed to be a secondary histiocytic reaction to an unknown antigenic stimulation or infectious agent, with erythrophagocytosis possibly reflecting foreign antigens adsorbed on erythrocytes or activation of macrophages by excess lymphokine production because of abnormal immunoregulation. The lesions are characterized by morphologically normal, reactive macrophages without Birbeck granules and with prominent erythrophagocytosis, and the process involves the entire reticuloendothelial system. The infiltrates are mixed lymphohistiocytic, unlike class I disease, in which either mixed histiocytic-eosinophilic or pure histiocytic infiltrates are seen. The class III histiocytoses are the truly malignant disorders of mononuclear phagocytes, including acute monocytic leukemia, malignant histiocytosis, and histiocytic lymphoma. These represent a local or disseminated clonal proliferation of neoplastic macrophages or their precursors.

Langerhans Cell Histiocytosis

Although traditionally Langerhans cell histiocytosis has been regarded as malignant, the high incidence of spontaneous remission and the histologic features, argue against this view. Studies have suggested that the disease has an immunologic basis. Most patients with Langerhans cell histiocytosis have a deficiency of circulating suppressor lymphocytes and an increased peripheral blood helper-suppressor cell ratio, suggesting immune dysregulation as the cause of the abnormal macrophage behavior. In some patients there is histologic evidence of an abnormal thymus.

Langerhans cell histiocytosis is occasionally seen in the newborn, generally in the disseminated (Letterer-Siwe) form or as an isolated spontaneously resolving cutaneous involvement, which has been called congenital self-healing reticulohistiocytosis or Hashimoto-Pritzker disease. The infant with Langerhans cell histiocytosis often presents with extensive hepatosplenomegaly, lymphadenopathy, and skin infiltration. Fever and jaundice are often present. Lytic

bone lesions eventually are seen, although they may not always be present at diagnosis in the infants. These lesions most typically involve the skull, ribs, pelvis, and scapula but may also be seen in the long bones and spine. Exophthalmos may result from a tumor mass in the orbit, and otitis media with drainage is often associated with destruction of the mastoid and petrous portion of the temporal bone. Pulmonary involvement may cause interstitial infiltrates and respiratory compromise. The disseminated form with multiple organ dysfunction has a poor prognosis, with less than 40% survival rate (Raney and D'Angio, 1989). In contrast, many infants have been described who present with isolated skin lesions of Langerhans cell histiocytosis that resolve over months to years without dissemination or any specific therapy (Kanitakis and colleagues, 1988). These infants present soon after birth with red-violaceous or brown, firm nodules scattered over the scalp and face, where they are more numerous, and also over the trunk and proximal part of the limbs. No systemic manifestations are present, and health is good. Sometimes the cutaneous form may present as an erythematous, scaly maculopapular rash on the scalp and intertriginous areas, which may include vesicular and crusted lesions. It is often confused with seborrhea, but the reddish-brown or purpuric papules are typical of histiocytosis. Histochemical and cell surface phenotype of the cutaneous self-healing and systemic disease appear to be indistinguishable.

Although Langerhans cell histiocytosis appears to respond to radiation and to many chemotherapeutic agents, including vincristine, vinblastine, prednisone, 6-mercaptopurine, chlorambucil, methotrexate, and cyclophosphamide, investigators have been unable to show any definitive improvement in cure rates using these modalities. The rarity of the disease combined with the high rate of self-healing has made prospective studies problematic. Langerhans cell histiocytosis responds locally to low-dose radiation therapy, 600 to 1000 cGy, which can be used for troublesome bone lesions that threaten well-being. For life-threatening disseminated histiocytosis with organ dysfunction, single-agent or combination chemotherapy has produced responses. In general, the minimal therapy that controls the disease is advised. For isolated skin lesions, topical corticosteroid preparations and expectant care only are recommended.

Familial Erythrophagocytic Lymphohistiocytosis

Like infants with Letterer-Siwe disease, infants with familial erythrophagocytic lymphocytosis also become ill within the first few months of life, with fever, anorexia, and wasting. However, this disease is differentiated by the presence of hemophagocytosis and a positive family history. This rare and fatal disease has an autosomal recessive pattern of inheritance, although a genetic marker is as yet unidentified. The proliferating histiocytes in familial erythrophagocytic lymphohistiocytosis have a phenotype similar to that of normal reactive sinusoidal histiocytes and lack the typical S-100 protein, CD-1, and Birbeck granules found in Langerhans cell histiocytosis (Wieczorek et al, 1986).

Patients present with fever, wasting, hepatosplenomegaly, and progressive pancytopenia. Central nervous system symptoms with seizures, disorientation, and coma with elevated cerebrospinal fluid protein levels and pleocytosis are common. Biopsy specimens of lesions found in the liver, spleen, lymph nodes, lungs, or bone marrow show marked erythrophagocytosis and a lymphohistiocytic infiltrate. The disease usually has a fulminant downhill course, with death in virtually all patients regardless of treatment. Etoposide and other antineoplastic drugs have induced temporary remission but have not changed the outcome. Plasmapheresis has also been tested with only temporary clinical improvement and correction of depressed cellular immune responses; bone marrow transplantation has also been used successfully in one patient (Ladisch and Jaffe, 1989).

Malignant Histiocytosis

Malignant histiocytosis has been reported occasionally in newborns (Ishii et al, 1987). It is characterized clinically by similar symptoms to familial erythrophagocytic lymphohistiocytosis, with fever, hepatosplenomegaly, lymphadenopathy, and pancytopenia. However, the family history is negative and pathologic examination shows malignant cells with large nuclei and prominent nucleoli that have histochemical features of histiocytes (stain positively with alphanaphthyl butyrate esterase). Erythrophagocytosis may be present but less prominent than in familial erythrophagocytic lymphohistiocytosis. The disease is more responsive to chemotherapy regimens containing cyclophosphamide, prednisone, doxorubicin, vincristine, etoposide, and cytarabine. Such regimens have been reported to produce 3-year disease-free survival in 40% to 50% of patients.

PRENATAL DIAGNOSIS AND TREATMENT OF MALIGNANCY

Prenatal diagnosis of malignant tumors has become increasingly common with the routine use of ultrasonography. Early diagnosis may allow earlier life-saving treatment or early procedures to preserve function. The most common lesions detected prenatally are teratoma and neuroblastoma. The prenatal detection of sacrococcygeal teratoma may result in a decision for early delivery and use of cesarean section to avoid dystocia and possible neurologic damage to the infant. Prenatal detection of sacrococcygeal teratoma may depend on the uterus being large for gestational dates, which is caused by rapid enlargement of tumor mass or by polyhydramnios. Less common are maternal preeclampsia, spotting, or weight gain. Untreated, the lesion may cause fetal death either through hemorrhage, preterm labor, or vascular "steal" with high-output failure and hydrops. In rare cases, fetal surgery has been performed to resect the large sacrococcygeal teratoma with hydrops, but maternal complications in one case and preterm labor in the other resulted in death of the fetus (Flake, 1993).

The management of the less common cervicofacial teratomas is even more complicated because of frequent respiratory compromise. In a review of 20 neonates from a Children's Cancer Group retrospective study (Azizkhan et al, 1995), a diagnostic prenatal ultrasound was performed in six patients. Two of these six survived only because

tracheostomies were performed at birth by pediatric surgeons present in the delivery room. Twenty percent of all the cases had malignant disease, and 35% had life-threatening airway obstruction. Four children were left with developmental delay, in part resulting from hypoxia. Diagnosis of intracranial teratoma with prenatal ultrasound has also been reported, although the usually fatal nature of these lesions and association with pulmonary hypoplasia may prevent amelioration of outcome for the fetus (Ng and Ong, 1993; Weyerts et al, 1993).

Prenatal detection of neuroblastoma, both localized and metastatic, has been achieved in many instances, usually in the 3rd trimester. The suprarenal mass may show areas of calcification and occasionally results in hydronephrosis, and it may metastasize in utero. The long-term prognosis in such cases, as in most cases of neonatal neuroblastoma, is excellent (Ho et al, 1993; Jennings et al, 1993). Because the abdominal tumors may occasionally cause fatal hemorrhage at birth, or may rarely result in catecholamine excess, preeclampsia, or hydrops fetalis, such prenatally detected tumors should be followed up carefully and early delivery performed if necessary.

It is also possible to detect retinoblastoma prenatally, which can allow earlier treatment and preservation of vision in families with a known hereditary predisposition (Pierro et al, 1993). A family history of tuberous sclerosis should alert clinicians to possible intracardiac tumors, which can also be detected prenatally, allowing decisions to be made about treatment or termination of pregnancy (Groves et al, 1992). Other tumors that have been detected prenatally include mesoblastic nephroma and brain tumors.

REFERENCES

Ablin AR, Krailo MD, Ramsay NK, et al: Results of treatment of malignant germ cell tumors in 93 children: A report from the Children's Cancer Study Group. J Clin Oncol 9:1782, 1991.

Allan RA, Wadsworth LD, Kalousek DK, Massing BG: Congenital erythroleukemia: A case report with morphological, immunophenotypic, and cytogenetic findings. Am J Hematol 31:114, 1989.

Allen JE: Teratomas in infants and children. *In* Holland JF, Frei E III (Eds): Cancer Medicine. Philadelphia, Lea & Febiger, 1973.

Altman RP, Randolph JG, Lilly JR: Sacrococcygeal teratomas: American Academy of Pediatrics Surgical Section Survey—1973. J Pediatr Surg 9:989, 1974.

Anday EK, Harris MC: Leukemoid reaction associated with antenatal dexamethasone administration. J Pediatr 101:614, 1982.

Anders D, Kindermann G, Pfeifer U: Metastasizing fetal neuroblastoma with involvement of the placenta simulating fetal erythroblastosis. J Pediatr 82:50, 1973.

Anderson JF, Kent S, Machin GA: Maternal malignant melanoma with placental metastasis: A case report with literature review. Pediatr Pathol 9:35, 1989.

Azizkhan RG, Haase GM, Applebaum H, et al: Diagnosis, management and outcome of cervicofacial teratomas in neonates: A Children's Cancer Group study. J Pediatr Surg 30:312, 1995.

Bader JL, Miller RW: U.S. cancer incidence and mortality in the first year of life. Am J Dis Child 133:157, 1979.

Baird PN, Pritchard J, Cowell JK: Molecular genetic analysis of chromosome 11p in familial Wilms tumour. Br J Cancer 69:1072, 1994.

Barnes AB, Colton T, Gundersen J, et al: Fertility and outcome of pregnancy in women exposed in utero to diethylstilbestrol. N Engl J Med 302:609, 1980.

Belchis DA, Mowry J, Davis JH: Infantile choriocarcinoma. Re-examination of a potentially curable entity. Cancer 72:2028, 1993.

Bell RJM: Fetal virilisation due to maternal Krukenberg tumour. Lancet 1:1162, 1977.

Bennett JM, Catovsky D, Daniel MT, et al: Proposals for the classification of the acute leukaemias: French-American-British (FAB) Co-operative Group. Br J Haematol 33:451, 1976.

Bernard J, Jacquillat C, Chavalet F, et al: Leucemie aigue d'une enfant de 5 mois née d'une mere atteinte de leucemie aigue au moment de l'accouchement. Nouv Rev Fr Hematol 4:140, 1964.

Bibbo M, Gill WB, Azizi F, et al: Follow-up study of male and female offspring of DES-exposed mothers. Obstet Gynecol 49:1, 1977.

Biegel JA, White PS, Marshall HN, et al: Constitutional 1p36 deletion in a child with neuroblastoma. Am J Hum Genet 52:176, 1993.

Blair JI, Carachi R, Gupta R, et al: Plasma α-fetoprotein reference ranges in infancy: Effect of prematurity. Arch Dis Child 62:362, 1987.

Blattner WA, Henson DE, Young RC, Fraumeni JF Jr: Malignant mesenchymoma and birth defects, prenatal exposure to phenytoin. JAMA 238:334, 1977.

Bonnin JM, Rubinstein LJ, Palmer NF, Beckwith JB: The association of embryonal tumors originating in the kidney and in the brain: A report of seven cases. Cancer 54:2137, 1984.

Borch K, Jacobsen T, Olsen JH, et al: Neonatal cancer in Denmark 1943–1985. Pediatr Hematol Oncol 9:209, 1992.

Bourhis J, Dominici C, McDowell H, et al: N-*myc* genomic content and DNA ploidy in stage IVS neuroblastoma. J Clin Oncol 9:1371, 1991.

Bove KE, McAdams AJ: The nephroblastomatosis complex and its relationship to Wilms' tumor: A clinicopathologic treatise. Perspect Pediatr Pathol 3:185, 1976.

Brissette MD, Duval-Arnould BJ, Gordon BG, Cotelingam JD: Acute megakaryoblastic leukemia following transient myeloproliferative disorder in a patient without Down syndrome. Am J Hematol 47:316, 1994.

Broadbent V, Pritchard J: Histiocytosis X—Current controversies. Arch Dis Child 60:605, 1985.

Broadway D, Lang S, Harper J, et al: Congenital malignant melanoma of the eye. Cancer 67:2642, 1991.

Brodeur GM, Azar C, Brother M, et al: Neuroblastoma: Effect of genetic factors on prognosis and treatment. Cancer 70:1685, 1992.

Brodeur GM, Pritchard J, Berthold F, et al: Revisions of the international criteria for neuroblastoma diagnosis, staging, and response to treatment. J Clin Oncol 11:1466, 1993.

Brodeur GM, Seeger RC, Schwab M, et al: Amplification of N-*myc* in untreated human neuroblastoma correlates with advanced disease stage. Science 224:1121, 1984.

Byrne JA, Simms LA, Little MH, et al: Three non-overlapping regions of chromosome arm 11p allele loss identified in infantile tumors of adrenal and liver. Genes Chrom Cancer 8:104, 1993.

Cairney AEL, Andrews M, Greenberg M, et al: Wilms tumor in three patients with Bloom syndrome. J Pediatr 111:414, 1987.

Campbell AN, Chan HSL, O'Brien A, et al: Malignant tumours in the neonate. Arch Dis Child 62:19, 1987a.

Campbell WA, Macafee AL, Wade WB: Familial neonatal leukaemia. Arch Dis Child 37:93, 1962.

Campbell WA, Storlazzi E, Vintzileos AM, et al: Fetal malignant melanoma: Ultrasound presentation and review of the literature. Obstet Gynecol 70:434, 1987b.

Caron H: Allelic loss of chromosome 1 and additional chromosome 17 material are both unfavourable prognostic markers in neuroblastoma. Med Pediatr Oncol 24:215, 1995.

Cavell B: Transplacental metastasis of malignant melanoma. Acta Paediatr Suppl 146:37, 1963.

Cavenee WK, Murphree AL, Shull MM, et al: Prediction of familial predisposition to retinoblastoma. N Engl J Med 314:1201, 1986.

Chan HSL, Cheng M-Y, Mancer K, et al: Congenital mesoblastic nephroma: A clinicoradiologic study of 17 cases representing the pathologic spectrum of the disease. J Pediatr 111:64, 1987.

Chatten J, Shimada H, Sather HN, et al: Prognostic value of histopathology in advanced neuroblastoma: A report from The Children's Cancer Study Group. Hum Pathol 19:1187, 1988.

Chen C-S, Medberry PS, Arthur DC, Kersey JH: Breakpoint clustering in t(4;11) (q21;q23) acute leukemia. Blood 78:2498, 1991.

Chessells JM, Eden OB, Bailey CC, et al: Acute lymphoblastic leukaemia in infancy: Experience in MRC UKALL trials: Report from the Medical Research Council Working Party on Childhood Leukemia. Leukemia 8:1275, 1994.

Christiansen H, Lampert F: Tumour karyotype discriminates between good and bad prognostic outcome in neuroblastoma. Br J Cancer 57:121, 1988.

Coldman AJ, Fryer CJH, Elwood JM, Sonley MJ: Neuroblastoma: Influ-

ence of age at diagnosis, stage, tumor site, and sex on prognosis. Cancer 46:1896, 1980.

Conley GR, Sant GR, Ucci AA, Mitcheson HD: Seminoma and epididymal cysts in a young man with known diethylstilbestrol exposure in utero. JAMA 249:1325, 1983.

Coppes MJ, Haber DA, Grundy PE: Genetic events in the development of Wilms' tumor. N Engl J Med 331:586, 1994.

Cowell J, Pritchard J: The molecular genetics of retinoblastoma and Wilms' tumor. Science 7:153, 1987.

Cramblett HG, Friedman JL, Najjar S: Leukemia in an infant born of a mother with leukemia. N Engl J Med 259:727, 1958.

Crist W, Pullen J, Boyett J, et al: Clinical and biological features predict a poor prognosis in acute lymphoid leukemias in infants: A Pediatric Oncology Group Study. Blood 67:135, 1986.

Crom DB, Williams JA, Green AA, et al: Malignancy in the neonate. Med Pediatr Oncol 17:101, 1989.

Cutler LS, Chaudry AP, Topazian R: Melanotic neuroectodermal tumor of infancy: An ultrastructural study, literature review, and reevaluation. Cancer 48:257, 1981.

D'Angio GJ, Breslow N, Beckwith B, et al: Treatment of Wilms' tumor: Results of the Third National Wilms' Tumor Study. Cancer 64:349, 1989.

D'Angio GJ, Evans A, Breslow N, et al: The treatment of Wilms' tumor: Results of the Second National Wilms' Tumor Study. Cancer 47:2302, 1981.

D'Angio GJ, Evans AE, Koop CE: Special pattern of widespread neuroblastoma with a favorable prognosis. Lancet 1:1046, 1971.

De Bernardi B, Pianca C, Boni L, et al: Disseminated neuroblastoma (stage IV and IV-S) in the first year of life. Cancer 70:1625, 1992.

Dehner LP: Neoplasms of the fetus and neonate. *In* Naeye RL, Kissane JM, Kaufman N (Eds): Perinatal Diseases. International Academy of Pathology Monograph No. 22. Baltimore, Williams & Wilkins, 1981, p 286.

Dehner LP: Gonadal and extragonadal germ cell neoplasia of childhood. Hum Pathol 14:493, 1983.

Diamond CA, Matthay KK: Childhood acute lymphoblastic leukemia. Pediatr Ann 17:156, 1988.

Donaldson S, Smith LM: Retinoblastoma: Biology, presentation, and current management. Oncology 3:45, 1989.

Dryja TP, Cavenee W, White R, et al: Homozygosity of chromosome 13 in retinoblastoma. N Engl J Med 310:550, 1984.

Duffner PK, Horowitz ME, Krischer JP, et al: Postoperative chemotherapy and delayed radiation in children less than three years of age with malignant brain tumors. N Engl J Med 328:1725, 1993.

Ehrenbard LT, Chaganti RSK: Cancer in the fetal hydantoin syndrome. Lancet 2:97, 1981.

Esseltine DW, De Leeuw NKM, Berry GR: Malignant histiocytosis. Cancer 52:1904, 1983.

Evans AE, D'Angio GJ, Randolph JR: A proposed staging for children with neuroblastoma: A report for The Children's Cancer Study Group. Cancer 27:374, 1971.

Evans AE, Brand W, De Lorimier A: Results in children with local and regional neuroblastoma managed with and without vincristine, cyclophosphamide, and imidazolecarboxamide. Am J Clin Oncol 6:3, 1984.

Evans AE, Land VJ, Newton WA, et al: Combination chemotherapy (vincristine, adriamycin, cyclophosphamide, and 5-fluorouracil) in the treatment of children with malignant hepatoma. Cancer 50:821, 1982.

Everson TC, Cole WH: Spontaneous Regression of Cancer: A Study and Abstract of Reports in the World Medical Literature and of Personal Communications Concerning Spontaneous Regression of Malignant Disease. Philadelphia, WB Saunders, 1966, pp 88–163.

Exelby PR, Filler RM, Grosfeld JL: Liver tumors in children in particular reference to hepatoblastoma and hepatocellular carcinoma: American Academy of Pediatrics Surgical Section Survey—1974. J Pediatr Surg 10:325, 1975.

Falk H, Herbert JT, Edmonds L, et al: Review of four cases of childhood hepatic angiosarcoma: Elevated environmental arsenic exposure in one case. Cancer 47:382, 1981.

Farber S: Chemotherapy in the treatment of leukemia and Wilms' tumor. JAMA 108:826, 1966.

Feine U, Muller-Schauenburg W, Treuner J, Klingebiel T: Metaiodobenzylguanidine (MIBG) labeled with $^{123}I/^{131}I$ in neuroblastoma diagnosis and follow-up treatment with a review of the diagnostic results of the International Workshop of Pediatric Oncology held in Rome, September 1986. Med Pediatr Oncol 15:181, 1987.

Felix CA, Reaman GH, Korsmeyer SJ, et al: Immunoglobulin and T cell regulator gene configuration in acute lymphoblastic leukemia of infancy. Blood 70:536, 1987.

Finklestein JZ: Neuroblastoma: The challenge and frustration. Hematol Oncol Clin North Am 1:675, 1987.

Flake AW: Fetal sacrococcygeal teratoma. Semin Pediatr Surg 2:113, 1993.

Flake AW, Harrison MR: Fetal surgery. Annu Rev Med 46:67, 1995.

Fong C, Brodeur GM: Down syndrome and leukemia: Epidemiology, genetics, cytogenetics and mechanisms of leukemogenesis. Cancer Genet Cytogenet 28:55, 1987.

Fong C, Dracopoli NC, White PS, et al: Loss of heterozygosity for the short arm of chromosome 1 in human neuroblastomas: Correlation with N-*myc* amplification. Proc Natl Acad Sci U S A 86:3753, 1989.

Fraumeni JF, Miller RW: Cancer deaths in the newborn. Am J Dis Child 117:186, 1969.

Gallo GE, Chemes HE: The association of Wilms' tumor, male pseudohermaphroditism and diffuse glomerular disease (Drash syndrome): Report of eight cases with clinical and morphologic findings and review of the literature. Pediatr Pathol 7:175, 1987.

Gansler T, Chatten J, Varello M, et al: Flow cytometric DNA analysis of neuroblastoma. Cancer 58:2453, 1986.

Geatti O, Shapiro B, Sisson JC, et al: Iodine-131 metaiodobenzylguanidine scintigraphy for the location of neuroblastoma: Preliminary experience in ten cases. J Nucl Med 26:736, 1985.

Gill WB, Schumacher GFB, Bibbo M, et al: Association of diethylstilbestrol exposure in utero with cryptorchidism, testicular hypoplasia, and semen abnormalities. J Urol 122:36, 1979.

Gold EB, Sever LE: Childhood cancers associated with parental occupational exposures. Occup Med 9:495, 1994.

Gonzalez-Crussi F, Winkler RF, Mirkin DL: Sacrococcygeal teratomas in infants and children. Arch Pathol Lab Med 102:420, 1978.

Goodman SN: Neuroblastoma screening data: An epidemiologic analysis. Am J Dis Child 145:1415, 1991.

Greenberger JS, Crocker AC, Vawter G, et al: Results of treatment of 127 patients with systemic histiocytosis (Letterer-Siwe syndrome, Schüller-Christian syndrome, and multifocal esoinpholic granuloma). Medicine 60:311, 1981.

Groves AMM, Fagg NLK, Cook AC, Allan LD: Cardiac tumours in intrauterine life. Arch Dis Child 67:1189, 1992.

Gutierrez-Ortega P, Hierro-Orozco S, Sanchez-Cisneros R, Montano LF: Kaposi's sarcoma in a 6-day-old infant with human immunodeficiency virus (letter). Arch Dermatol 125:432, 1989.

Haas D, Ablin AR, Miller C, et al: Complete pathologic maturation and regression of stage IVS neuroblastoma without treatment. Cancer 62:818, 1988.

Haicken BN, Miller DR: Simultaneous occurrence of congenital aniridia, hamartoma, and Wilms' tumor. J Pediatr 78:497, 1971.

Hann HL, Evans AE, Cohen IJ, Leitmeyer JE: Biological differences between neuroblastoma stages IV-S and IV: Measurement of serum ferritin and E-rosette inhibition in 30 children. N Engl J Med 305:425, 1981.

Hann HL, Evans AE, Siegel SE, et al: Prognostic importance of serum ferritin in patients with stages III and IV neuroblastoma: The Children's Cancer Study Group experience. Cancer Res 45:2843, 1985.

Hawkins E, Issacs H, Cushing B, Rogers P: Occult malignancy in neonatal sacrococcygeal teratomas. Am J Pediatr Hematol Oncol 15:406, 1993.

Hayashi Y, Eguchi M, Sugita K, et al: Cytogenetic findings and clinical features in acute leukemia and transient myeloproliferative disorder in Down syndrome. Blood 72:15, 1988.

Hayashi Y, Kanda N, Inaba T, et al: Cytogenetic findings and prognosis in neuroblastoma with emphasis on marker chromosome 1. Cancer 63:126, 1989.

Haymond MW, Weldon VV: Female pseudohermaphroditism secondary to a maternal virilizing tumor: Case report and review of the literature. J Pediatr 82:682, 1973.

Heerema NA, Arthur DC, Sather H, et al: Cytogenetic features of infants less than 12 months of age at diagnosis of acute lymphoblastic leukemia: Impact of the 11q23 breakpoint on outcome: A report of the Children's Cancer Study Group. Blood 83:2274, 1994.

Herbst AL, Cole P, Colton T, et al: Age-incidence and risk of diethylstilbestrol-related adenocarcinoma of the vagina and cervix. Am J Obstet Gynecol 128:43, 1977.

Ho PTC, Estroff JA, Kozakewich H, et al: Prenatal detection of neuroblastoma: A ten-year experience from the Dana-Farber Cancer Institute and Children's Hospital. Pediatrics 92:358, 1993.

Hsiao RJ, Seeger RC, Yu AL, O'Connor DT: Chromogranin A in children with neuroblastoma; serum concentration parallels disease stage and predicts survival. J Clin Invest 85:1555, 1990.

Huddart SN, Muir KR, Parkes S, et al: Neuroblastoma: A 32-year population-based study—Implications for screening. Med Pediatr Oncol 21:96, 1993.

Isaacs H Jr: Perinatal (congenital and neonatal) neoplasms: A report of 110 cases. Pediatr Pathol 3:165, 1985.

Ishii E, Hara T, Okamura J, et al: Malignant histiocytosis in infants: Surface marker analysis of malignant cells in two cases. Med Pediatr Oncol 15:102, 1987.

Jablon S, Kato H: Childhood cancer in relation to prenatal exposure to atomic-bomb radiation. Lancet 2:1000, 1970.

Jennings RW, LaQuaglia MP, Leong K, et al: Fetal neuroblastoma: Prenatal diagnosis and natural history. J Pediatr Surg 28:1168, 1993.

Jick H, Walker AM, Rothman KJ, et al: Vaginal spermicides and congenital disorders. JAMA 245:1329, 1981.

Jiminez JF, Brown RE, Seibert RW, et al: Melanotic neuroectodermal tumor of infancy and fetal hydantoin syndrome. Am J Pediatr Hematol Oncol 3:9, 1981.

Joshi VV, Banenee AK, Yadav K, Pathak IC: Cystic partially differentiated nephroblastoma. Cancer 40:789, 1977.

Kaneko Y, Kanda N, Maseki N, et al: Current urinary mass screening for catecholamine metabolites at 6 months of age may be detecting only a small portion of high-risk neuroblastomas: A chromosome and N-*myc* amplification study. J Clin Oncol 8:2005, 1990.

Kaneko Y, Shikano T, Maseki N, et al: Clinical characteristics of infant acute leukemia with or without 11q23 translocations. Leukemia 2:672, 1988.

Kanitakis J, Zambruno G, Schmitt D, et al: Congenital self-healing histiocytosis (Hashimoto-Pritzker). Cancer 61:508, 1988.

Katz F, Malcolm S, Gibbons B, et al: Cellular and molecular studies on infant null acute lymphoblastic leukemia. Blood 71:1438, 1988.

Kinney H, Faix R, Brazy J: The fetal alcohol syndrome and neuroblastoma. Pediatrics 66:130, 1980.

Knudson AF, Meadows AT, Nichols WW, Hill R: Chromosomal deletion in retinoblastoma. N Engl J Med 295:1120, 1976.

Kojima S, Mimaya J, Tonouchi T, et al: Identification of myeloid origin in undifferentiated congenital leukemia by in vitro marrow culture study. Am J Pediatr Hematol Oncol 11:337, 1989.

Koscielniak E, Harms D, Schmidt D, et al: Soft tissue sarcomas in infants younger than 1 year of age: A report of the German Soft Tissue Sarcoma Study Group (CSW-81). Med Pediatr Oncol 17:105, 1989.

Kramer S, Ward E, Meadows AT, Malone KE: Medical and drug risk factors associated with neuroblastoma: A case-control study. J Natl Cancer Inst 78:797, 1987.

Kretschmar CS, Frantz CN, Rosen EM, et al: Improved prognosis for infants with stage IV neuroblastoma. J Clin Oncol 2:799, 1984.

Kubota T, Saitoh S, Matsumoto T, et al: Excess functional copy of allele at chromosomal region 11p15 may cause Wiedemann-Beckwith (EMG) syndrome. Am J Med Genet 49:378, 1994.

Kulkarni R, Bailie MP, Bernstein J, Newton B: Progression of nephroblastomatosis to Wilms' tumor. J Pediatr 96:178, 1980.

Kumar APM, Pratt CB, Coburn TP, Johnson WW: Treatment strategy for nodular renal blastema and nephroblastomatosis associated with Wilms' tumor. J Pediatr Surg 13:281, 1978.

Kushner BH, Gilbert F, Helson L: Familial neuroblastoma: Case reports, literature review and etiologic considerations. Cancer 57:1887, 1986.

Ladisch S, Jaffe ES: The histiocytoses. *In* Pizzo PA, Poplack DG (Eds): Pediatric Oncology. Philadelphia, JB Lippincott, 1989, pp 491–504.

Lampkin B, Buckley J, Nesbit M, et al: Clinical and laboratory findings and responses to therapy in infants less than one year of age with acute non-lymphoblastic leukemia (ANLL). Proc Am Soc Clin Oncol 3:201, 1984.

Langer JC, Harrison MR, Schmidt KG, et al: Fetal hydrops and death from sacrococcygeal teratoma: Rationale for fetal surgery. Am J Obstet Gynecol 160:1145, 1989.

Laureys G, Speleman F, Opdenakker G, Leroy J: Constitutional translocation t(1;17)(p36; q12–21) in a patient with neuroblastoma. Genes Chromosomes Cancer 2:252, 1990.

Lazarus KH, D'Orsogna DE, Bloom KR, Rouse RG: Primary pericardial sarcoma in a neonate. Am J Pediatr Hematol Oncol 11:343, 1989.

Lazarus KH, Heerema NA, Palmer CG, Baehner RL: The myeloproliferative reaction in a child with Down syndrome: Cytological and chromosomal evidence for a transient leukemia. Am J Hematol 11:417, 1981.

Lemieux B, Auray-Blais C, Giguere R, Scriver CR: Neuroblastoma screening: The Canadian experience. Med Pediatr Oncol 17:279, 1989.

Lergier JE, Jiminez E, Maldonado N, Veray F: Normal pregnancy in multiple myeloma treated with cyclophosphamide. Cancer 34:1018, 1974.

Li FP, Williams WR, Gimbrere K, et al: Heritable fraction of unilateral Wilms tumor. Pediatrics 81:147, 1988.

Look AT, Hayes FA, Shuster JJ, et al: Clinical relevance of tumor cell ploidy and N-*myc* gene amplification in childhood neuroblastoma: A Pediatric Oncology Group study. J Clin Oncol 9:581, 1991.

Ludwig W-D, Bartram CR, Harbott J, et al: Phenotypic and genotypic heterogeneity in infant acute leukemia: I. Acute lymphoblastic leukemia. Leukemia 3:431, 1989.

Mahmoud HH, Ridge SA, Behm FG, et al: Intrauterine monoclonal origin of neonatal concordant acute lymphoblastic leukemia in monozygotic twins. Med Pediatr Oncol 24:77, 1995.

Malkin D: p53 and the Li-Fraumeni syndrome. Biochim Biophys Acta 1198:197, 1994.

Marina N, Fontanesi J, Kun L, et al: Treatment of childhood germ cell tumors. Review of the St. Jude experience from 1979 to 1988. Cancer 70:2568, 1992.

Martin ES, Griffith JF: Myoclonic encephalopathy and neuroblastoma. Am J Dis Child 122:257, 1971.

Mason GA, Hart-Mercer J, Miller EJ, et al: Adrenaline-secreting neuroblastoma in an infant. Lancet ii:322, 1957.

Matsumura M, Nishi T, Sasaki Y, et al: Prenatal diagnosis and treatment strategy for congenital mesoblastic nephroma. J Pediatr Surg 28:1607, 1993.

Matthay KK: Neuroblastoma. *In* Pochedly C (Ed): Neoplastic Diseases in Childhood. Switzerland, Harwood Academic Publishers, 1994, pp 735–778.

Matthay KK, Sather HN, Seeger RC, et al: Excellent outcome of stage II neuroblastoma is independent of residual disease and radiation therapy. J Clin Oncol 7:236, 1989.

Maurer HS, Pendergrass TW, Borges W, Honig GR: The role of genetic factor in the etiology of Wilms' tumor: Two pairs of monozygous twins with congenital abnormalities (aniridia; hemihypertrophy) and discordance for Wilms' tumor. Cancer 43:205, 1979.

McKinney PA, Cartwright RA, Saiu JMT, et al: The interregional epidemiological study of childhood cancer (IRESCC): A case control study of aetiological factors in leukaemia and lymphoma. Arch Dis Child 62:279, 1987.

Meadows AT, Lichtenfeld JL, Koop CE: Wilms' tumor in three children of a woman with congenital hemihypertrophy. N Engl J Med 291:23, 1974.

Melnick S, Cole P, Andersen D, Herbst A: Rates and risks of diethylstilbestrol-related clear-cell carcinoma of the vagina and cervix: An update. N Engl J Med 316:514, 1987.

Miller M, Cosgriff JM: Hematological abnormalities in newborn infants with Down syndrome. Am J Med Genet 16:173, 1983.

Miller RW: Persons at exceptionally high risk of leukemia. Cancer Res 27:2420, 1967.

Miller RW: Relation between cancer and congenital defects: An epidemiologic evaluation. J Natl Cancer Inst 40:1079, 1968.

Miller RW: Discordance for Wilms' tumor in MZ twins with aniridia. Childhood Cancer Etiol Newsletter No. 56, 1979.

Miller RW, Young JL, Novakovic B: Childhood cancer. Cancer 75:395, 1994.

Moe PG, Nellhaus G: Infantile polymyoclonia-opsoclonus syndrome and neural crest tumors. Neurology 20:756, 1970.

Morgan E, Baum E, Breslow N, et al: Chemotherapy-related toxicity in infants treated according to the Second National Wilms' Tumor Study. J Clin Oncol 6:51, 1988.

Moss TJ, Seeger RC, Kindler-Rohrbora A, et al: Immunohistologic detection and phenotyping of neuroblastoma cells in bone marrow using cytoplasmic neuron-specific enolase and cell surface antigens. *In* Evans AE, D'Angio GJ, Seeger RC (Eds): Advances in Neuroblastoma Research. New York, Alan R Liss, 1985, pp 367–378.

Murphree AL, Benedict WF: Retinoblastoma: Clues to human oncogenesis. Science 223:1028, 1984.

Nagasaka M, Maeda S, Maeda H, et al: Four cases of t(4:11) acute leukemia and its myelomonocytic nature in infants. Blood 61:1174, 1983.

Nair R, Pai SK, Saikia TK, et al: Malignant germ cell tumors in childhood. J Surg Oncol 56:186, 1994.

Nakagawara A, Arima-Nakagawara M, Scavarda NJ, et al: Association between high levels of expression of the TRK gene and favorable outcome in human neuroblastoma. N Engl J Med 328:847, 1993.

Nakagawara A, Zaizen Y, Ikeda K, et al: Different genomic and metabolic patterns between mass-screening positive and mass-screening negative later-presenting neuroblastoma. Cancer 68:2037, 1991.

Napalkov N: *In* Tomatis L, Mohr U, Davis W (Eds): Transplacental Carcinogenesis: International Agency for Research on Cancer Scientific Publication No. 4, 1973.

Nesbit MD Jr, O'Leary M, Dehner LP, Ramsay NKC: The immune system and the histiocytosis syndromes. Am J Pediatr Hematol Oncol 3:141, 1981.

Newsham I, Kindler-Röhrborn A, Daub D, Cavenee W: A constitutional BWS-related t(11;16) chromosome translocation occurring in the same region of chromosome 16 implicated in Wilms' tumors. Genes Chromosomes Cancer 12:1, 1995.

Ng HN, Ong CL: Two case reports of intracranial teratoma diagnosed antenatally. Ann Acad Med, Singapore 22:823, 1993.

Nickerson HJ, Nesbit ME, Grosfeld JL, et al: Comparison of stage IV and IV-S neuroblastoma in the first year of life. Med Pediatr Oncol 13:261, 1985.

Odom LF, Gordon EM: Acute monoblastic leukemia in infancy and early childhood: Successful treatment with an epipodophyllotoxin. Blood 64:875, 1984.

Olson JM, Hamilton A, Breslow NE: Non-11p constitutional chromosome abnormalities in Wilms' tumor patients. Med Pediatr Oncol 24:305, 1995.

Ortega JA, Krailo MD, Haas JE, et al: Effective treatment of unresectable or metastatic hepatoblastoma with cisplatin and continuous infusion doxorubicin chemotherapy: A report from the Children's Cancer Study Group. J Clin Oncol 9:2167, 1991.

Padilla RS, McConnell TS, Gribble JT, Smoot C: Malignant melanoma arising in a giant congenital melanocytic nevus. Cancer 62:2589, 1988.

Parkin DM, Stiller CA, Draper GJ, Bieber CA: The international incidence of childhood cancer. Int J Cancer 42:511, 1988.

Pastore G, Carli M, Lemerle J, et al: Epidemiological features of Wilms' tumor: Results of studies by the International Society of Paediatric Oncology (SIOP). Med Pediatr Oncol 16:7, 1988.

Pettinato G, Manivel JC, Wick MR, Dehner LP: Classical and cellular (atypical) congenital mesoblastic nephroma: A clinicopathologic, ultrastructural, immunohistochemical, and flow cytometric study. Hum Pathol 20:682, 1989.

Phillip T, Zucker JM, Bernard IL: Improved survival at 2 and 5 years in the LMCI unselected group of 72 children with stage IV neuroblastoma older than 1 year of age at diagnosis: Is cure possible in a small subgroup? J Clin Oncol 9:1037, 1991.

Phillips M, Dieks-Mireaux C, Kingston J, et al: Hepatoblastoma and polyposis coli (familial adenomatous polyposis). Med Pediatr Oncol 17:441, 1989.

Pierce MI: Leukemia in the newborn infant. J Pediatr 54:691, 1959.

Pierro L, Brancato R, Capoferri C: Prenatal detection and early diagnosis of hereditary retinoblastoma in a family. Ophthalmologica 207:106, 1993.

Pilling GP: Wilms' tumor in seven children with congenital aniridia. J Pediatr Surg 10:87, 1975.

Pollack IF: Brain tumors in children. N Engl J Med 331:1500, 1994.

Poplack DG: Acute lymphoblastic leukemia. *In* Pizzo PA, Poplack DG (Eds): Pediatric Oncology. Philadelphia, JB Lippincott, 1993, pp 431–481.

Posnick JC, Chen P, Zuker R, et al: Extensive malignant melanoma of the uvea in childhood: Resection and immediate reconstruction with microsurgical and craniofacial techniques. Ann Plastic Surg 31:265, 1993.

Prose NS, Laude TA, Heilman ER, Coren C: Congenital malignant melanoma. Pediatrics 79:967, 1987.

Pui C-H: Childhood leukemias. N Engl J Med 332:1618, 1995.

Pui C-H, Behm FG, Crist WM: Clinical and biologic relevance of immunologic marker studies in childhood acute lymphoblastic leukemia. Blood 82:343, 1993.

Pui C-H, Raimondi SC, Murphy SB, et al: An analysis of leukemic cell chromosomal features in infants. Blood 69:1289, 1987.

Quinn JJ, Altman AJ, Frantz CN: Serum lactic dehydrogenase, an indicator of tumor activity in neuroblastoma. J Pediatr 97:89, 1980.

Quinn JJ, Altman AJ, Robinson HT, et al: Adriamycin and cisplatin for hepatoblastoma. Cancer 56:1926, 1985.

Ragab AH, Heyn R, Tefft M, et al: Infants younger than one year of age with rhabdomyosarcoma. Cancer 58:2606, 1986.

Raney RB Jr, Chatten J, Littman P, et al: Treatment strategies for infants with malignant sacrococcygeal teratoma. J Pediatr Surg 16:573, 1981.

Raney RB Jr, D'Angio GJ: Langerhans cell histiocytosis (histiocytosis X): Experience at the Children's Hospital of Philadelphia, 1970–1984. Med Pediatr Oncol 17:20, 1989.

Reaman G: Special considerations for the infant with cancer. *In* Pizzo PA, Poplack DG (Eds): Pediatric Oncology. Philadelphia, JB Lippincott, 1989, pp 263–274.

Reaman G, Zeltzer P, Bleyer WA, et al: Acute lymphoblastic leukemia in infants less than one year of age: A cumulative experience of the Children's Cancer Study Group. J Clin Oncol 3:1513, 1985.

Reinberg Y, Anderson GF, Franciosi R, et al: Wilms tumor and the VATER association. J Urol 140:787, 1988.

Riccardi VM, Sujansky E, Smith AC, Francke U: Chromosomal imbalance in the aniridia-Wilms' tumor association: 11p interstitial deletion. Pediatrics 61:604, 1978.

Ridgway D, Benda GI, Magenis E, et al: Transient myeloproliferative disorder of the Down type in the normal newborn. Am J Dis Child 144:1117, 1990.

Robboy SJ, Kauffman RH, Prat J, et al: Pathologic findings in women enrolled in the National Cooperative Diethylstilbestrol Adenosis (DE-SAD) Project. Obstet Gynecol 53:309, 1979.

Rosner F, Lee SL: Down syndrome and acute leukemia: Myeloblastic or lymphoblastic? Report of forty-three cases and review of the literature. Am J Med 53:203, 1972.

Rubnitz JE, Link MP, Shuster JJ, et al: Frequency and prognostic significance of HRX rearrangements in infant acute lymphoblastic leukemia: A Pediatric Oncology Group study. Blood 84:570, 1994.

Sansone R, Haupt R, Stigini P, et al: Congenital leukemia: Persistent spontaneous regression in a patient with an acquired abnormal karyotype. Acta Haematol 81:48, 1989.

Sawada T, Kidowaki T, Sakamoto I, et al: Neuroblastoma: Mass screening for early detection and its prognosis. Cancer 53:2731, 1984.

Schneider KM, Becker JM, Krasna IH: Neonatal neuroblastoma. Pediatrics 36:359, 1965.

Schneiderman H, Wu AY-Y, Campbell WA, et al: Congenital melanoma with multiple prenatal metastases. Cancer 60:1371, 1987.

Schoeck VW, Peterson RDA, Good RA: Familial occurrence of Letterer-Siwe disease. Pediatrics 32:1055, 1963.

Schwartz AD, Dadash-Zadeh M, Lee H, Swaney JJ: Spontaneous regression of disseminated neuroblastoma. J Pediatr 85:760, 1974.

Seeger RC, Brodeur GM, Sather H, et al: Association of multiple copies of the N-*myc* oncogene with rapid progression of neuroblastomas. N Engl J Med 313:1111, 1985.

Seeger RC, Villablanca JG, Matthay KK, et al: Intensive chemoradiotherapy and autologous bone marrow transplantation for poor prognosis neuroblastoma. *In* Evans AE, D'Angio GJ, Knudson A, Seeger RC (Eds): Advances in Neuroblastoma Research 3. New York, Wylie/Liss, 1991, p 527.

Seibel NL, Sommer A, Miser J: Transient neonatal leukemoid reactions in mosaic trisomy 21. J Pediatr 104:251, 1984.

Shamberger RC, Holcombe EG, Weinstein HJ, et al: Chest wall tumors in infancy and childhood. Cancer 63:774, 1989.

Shimada H, Chatten J, Newton WA Jr, et al: Histopathologic prognostic factors in neuroblastic tumors: Definition of subtypes of ganglioneuroblastoma and an age-linked classification of neuroblastomas. J Natl Cancer Inst 73:405, 1984.

Shu X-O, Nesbit ME, Buckley JD, et al: An exploratory analysis of risk factors for childhood malignant germ-cell tumors: Report from the Children's Cancer Group (Canada, United States). Cancer Causes Control 6:187, 1995.

Shu X-O, Reaman GH, Lampkin B, et al: Association of paternal diagnostic x-ray exposure with risk of infant leukemia. Cancer Epidemiol Biomarkers Prev 3:645, 1994.

Sitarz AL, Santulli TV, Wigger HJ, Berdon WE: Complete maturation of neuroblastoma with bone metastases in documented stages. J Pediatr Surg 10:533, 1975.

Solis V, Pritchard J, Cowell JK: Cytogenetic changes in Wilms' tumors. Cancer Genet Cytogenet 34:223, 1988.

Sotelo-Avila C, Gonzalez-Crussi F, Fowler JW: Complete and incomplete forms of Beckwith-Wiedemann syndrome: Their oncogenic potential. J Pediatr 96:47, 1980.

Spitz M, Johnson CC: Neuroblastoma and paternal occupation: A case-control analysis. Am J Epidemiol 121:924, 1985.

Stark B, Hershko C, Rosen N, et al: Familial hemophagocytic lymphohistiocytosis (FHLH) in Israel: I. Description of 11 patients of Iranian-Iraqi origin and review of the literature. Cancer 54:2109, 1984.

Stark B, Vogel R, Cohen IJ, et al: Biologic and cytogenetic characteristics of leukemia in infants. Cancer 63:117, 1989.

Suda J, Eguchi M, Akiyama Y, et al: Differentiation of blast cells from a Down syndrome patient with transient myeloproliferative disorder. Blood 69:508, 1987.

Sullivan KM, Adzick NS: Fetal surgery. Clin Obstet Gynecol 37:355, 1994.

Suzuki T, Bogenmann E, Shimada H, et al: Lack of high-affinity nerve growth factor receptors in aggressive neuroblastomas. J Nat Cancer Inst 85:377, 1993.

Swift PGF, Bloom SR, Harris F: Watery diarrhea and ganglioneuroma with secretion of vasoactive intestinal peptide. Arch Dis Child 50:896, 1975.

Takaku A, Kodama N, Ohara H, Hori S: Brain tumor in newborn babies. Child's Brain 4:365, 1978.

Takeuchi LA, Hachitanda Y, Woods WG, et al: Screening for neuroblastoma in North America: Preliminary results of pathology review from the Quebec Project. Cancer 76:2361, 1995.

Taylor WF, Myers M, Taylor WR: Extrarenal Wilms' tumour in an infant exposed to intrauterine phenytoin. Lancet ii:481, 1980.

Touran T, Applebaum H, Frost DB, et al: Congenital metastatic cervical teratoma: Diagnostic and management considerations. J Pediatr Surg 24:21, 1989.

Valdiserri RO, Yunis EJ: Sacrococcygeal teratomas: A review of 68 cases. Cancer 48:217, 1981.

Valentino L, Moss T, Olson E, et al: Shed tumor gangliosides and progression of human neuroblastoma. Blood 75:1564, 1990.

van Wering ER, Kamps WA: Acute leukemia in infants: A unique pattern of acute nonlymphocytic leukemia. Am J Pediatr Hematol Oncol 8:220, 1986.

Voelkerding KV, Sandhaus LM, Belov L, et al: Clonal B-cell proliferation in an infant with congenital HIV infection and immune thrombocytopenia. Am J Clin Pathol 90:470, 1988.

Voûte PA Jr, Wadman SK, van Putten WJ: Congenital neuroblastoma: Symptoms in the mother during pregnancy. Clin Pediatr 9:206, 1970.

Weeks DA, Beckwith JB, Mierau GW, Luckey DW: Rhabdoid tumor of kidney. Am J Surg Pathol 13:439, 1989.

Weinberg AG, Finegold MJ: Primary hepatic tumors of childhood. Hum Pathol 14:512, 1983.

Weinberger MM, Oleinick A: Congenital marrow dysfunction in Down syndrome. J Pediatr 77:273, 1970.

Weyerts LK, Catanzarite V, Jones M, Mendoza A: Prenatal diagnosis of a giant intracranial teratoma associated with pulmonary hypoplasia. J Med Genet 30:880, 1993.

Wheatley JM, LaQuaglia MP: Management of hepatic epithelial malignancy in childhood and adolescence. Semin Surg Oncol 9:532, 1993.

Wieczorek R, Greco MA, McCarthy K, et al: Immunophenotypic, immunohistochemical, and ultrastructural demonstration of the relation to sinus histiocytes. Hum Pathol 17:55, 1986.

Wiggs J, Nordenskjold M, Yandell D, et al: Prediction of the risk of hereditary retinoblastoma, using DNA polymorphisms within the retinoblastoma gene. N Engl J Med 318:151, 1988.

Wilmore HP, White GFJ, Howell RT, Brown KW: Germline and somatic abnormalities of chromosome 7 in Wilms' tumor. Cancer Genet Cytogenet 77:93, 1994.

Woods WG, Lemieux B, Tuchman M: Neuroblastoma represents distinct clinical-biologic entities: A review and perspective from the Quebec Neuroblastoma Screening Project. Pediatrics 89:114, 1992.

Woods WG, Tuchman M: Neuroblastoma: The case for screening infants in North America. Pediatrics 79:869, 1987.

Woods W, Tuchman M, Bernstein M, et al: Screening for neuroblastoma in North America, 2 year results from the Quebec project. Am J Pediatr Hematol Oncol 14:313, 1992.

Writing Group of the Histiocyte Society: Histiocytosis syndromes in children. Lancet 1:208, 1987.

Yoshimoto Y, Kato H, Schull WJ: Cancer risk among in utero-exposed survivors. J Radiat Res (Suppl):231, 1991.

Yunis JJ, Ramsay NKC: Familial occurrence of the aniridia–Wilms' tumor syndrome with deletion 11p13-14.1. J Pediatr 96:1027, 1980.

Zeltzer PM, Marangos PJ, Evans AE, Schneider SL: Serum neuron-specific enolase in children with neuroblastoma. Cancer 57:1230, 1986.

PART XVII

DERMATOLOGIC CONDITIONS

CHAPTER 105

Newborn Skin: Basic Concepts

Elaine C. Siegfried and Nancy B. Esterly

SKIN DEVELOPMENT

Skin is the interface between an organism and its environment. It plays an important role in fluid balance and temperature regulation and provides a barrier against invading microbes and systemic absorption of topically applied agents. This chapter provides an overview of skin development. Emphasis has been placed on factors that influence the clinical management of premature infants and the prenatal diagnosis of heritable skin diseases.

The study of skin ontogenesis has been primarily organized based on the development of individual components: epidermis, basement membrane zone, dermis immigrant cells, and appendegeal structures. However, the initiation, differentiation, and growth of all of its components are intimately related. Prenatal skin biopsy for early diagnosis of severe genodermatoses is a useful procedure that depends on precise knowledge of the details of skin development (see Chapter 106). Disorders of keratinization, basement membrane integrity, melanocytes, and epidermal appendages have been detected as early as 16 weeks using this technique. In turn, fetal skin biopsy has helped to further clarify the details of epidermal development (Holbrook, 1991; Holbrook et al, 1993).

Epidermis

The epidermis consists of ectodermally derived, stratified squamous cells with localized proliferations that form the appendages: hair follicles, sebaceous glands, eccrine sweat glands, apocrine glands, and the nail matrix. Melanocytes immigrate into the epidermis from the neural crest and Langerhans' cells immigrate from mesoderm. The epidermis forms initially as a single layer of "indifferent ectoderm" and then differentiates into two layers of epidermal cells by 6 weeks. The outermost layer, called periderm, covers the basal layer stem cells. During the next 2 weeks, the basal cells give rise to an intermediate layer beneath the periderm. By 8 weeks epithelial cells are capable of expressing keratins, the major cytoskeletal proteins of the epidermis. K5 and K14 are the high-molecular-weight keratins primarily expressed by basal cells, whereas intermediate cells express K1 and K10 (Smack et al, 1994). Genetic abnormalities of these cytoskeletal components give rise to a spectrum of inherited scaling skin diseases that can now be detected by fetal skin biopsy or amniocentesis (see Chapter 106). The third month of gestation is an important period in skin development. Differentiation of the epider-

mis begins as two to three more layers of "intermediate cells" are added between the basal cells and periderm as coordinated maturation progresses within other strata of the skin. By 22 to 24 weeks, granular cells have formed beneath the periderm. Granular cells are named for their prominent organelles, the keratohyalin granules. These granules contain a high-molecular-weight protein called profillagrin, which plays a crucial role in terminal differentiation of keratinocytes in the stratum corneum. Cornified cells first appear within the pilosebaceous follicle as early as 15 weeks. Interfollicular keratinization follows at 24 to 26 weeks' gestation. At 28 weeks the stratum corneum consists of two to three cell layers. By 32 weeks there are more than 15 layers of corneocytes, equivalent to adult skin (Holbrook, 1991).

Basement Membrane Zone

Components of the basement membrane zone appear with the first epidermal cells at 35 days of gestation. Important components of the dermoepidermal junction, such as hemidesmosomes, anchoring filaments, and anchoring fibrils, are completely formed by 8 to 10 weeks. The epidermis and basement membrane are generally flat during fetal development. The undulating rete ridges that expand the surface area of the dermoepidermal junction do not appear until the third trimester and are not fully developed until 6 months after birth, coincident with accumulation of dermal matrix (Holbrook, 1991).

Dermis

A network of stellate mesodermal cells is present beneath the epidermis of a 1- to 2-month embryo. The primary matrix secreted by these cells is composed of glycosaminoglycans (GAG). Hyaluronic acid is the predominant GAG during the first trimester. Matrix proteins are also synthesized in the first trimester, including immature fibers resembling elastin and collagen types I, III, V, and VI. Types III and V collagen are increased in quantity compared with adult dermis. In the third month, the dermis is transformed from a cellular to a fibrous tissue, coincident with epidermal differentiation. During months 3 to 5, the size and quantity of the matrix proteins increase, and the composition of glycosaminoglycans changes. Immigrant cells, including Schwann cells, Merkel cells, melanoblasts, pericytes, and mast cells, are found in the dermis by the 5th month. The dermis continues to mature for approximately 6 months postnatally (Holbrook, 1991).

Human fetal skin wounds reportedly heal without scarring. This clinical observation, first made by surgeons pioneering antenatal diagnosis and treatment, has been followed by an explosion of experimental data elucidating the unique aspects of fetal wound healing (Dostal and Gamelli, 1993; Longacker and Adzick, 1991; Mast et al, 1992). Wound healing in the fetus differs from that of the adult by several factors, including tissue environment, inflammatory response, and components of the dermal extracellular matrix (Table 105–1). Wounds can cause scars in some human infants (Carthidge et al, 1990; Den Ouden et al, 1986), but prospective examination of sternotomy scars (Lista and Thompson, 1988) and bacille Calmette:Guérin (BCG) vaccinations (Sivarajah et al, 1990) in children found a direct correlation between increasing age and more prominent scarring.

Immigrant Cells

Melanocytes from the neural crest and mesenchymally derived Langerhans' cells migrate to the epidermis by the 8th week but do not develop their characteristic organelles until after 65 days estimated gestational age (EGA). Melanin production and transfer to adjacent keratinocytes occurs during the 4th to 5th month, but melanin production is relatively low, even at birth. The antigen-presenting function of Langerhans' cells has not been documented in utero (Holbrook, 1991).

Epidermal Appendages

Primordia of hair follicles, apocrine glands, eccrine sweat glands, and nails first appear at 10 to 12 weeks EGA. The pilosebaceous unit is formed, hair is keratinized, and sebum is synthesized as early as 16 to 18 weeks. Sebum production and secretion are greatly increased in the third trimester under the influence of fetal and maternal androgens. The number of lipid-filled sebocytes in amniotic fluid has been used to assess fetal maturity. Sebaceous lipids, squalane, and wax esters comprise the majority of vernix caseosa, especially in males. The vernix of female infants has a slightly higher proportion of cholesterol and cholesterol esters, lipids derived from keratinocytes (Holbrook, 1991; Nazzaro-Porro et al, 1979). Apocrine gland formation follows that of the sebaceous glands by 8 weeks. Apocrine secretion has been detected during the 3rd trimester but not in the neonatal period. The palmoplantar eccrine sweat ducts are the first portion of the apparatus to develop. By 22 weeks' EGA, they open to the surface and join the differentiated secretory cells of the eccrine sweat gland. Maturation of the eccrine apparatus elsewhere on the body follows at 24 to 26 weeks. Neither the morphology of the glandular coil cells nor eccrine gland function are fully developed in the premature infant, but the full complement of the sweat glands and hair follicles is completely formed in utero, making them more densely distributed in infant than adult skin. Nail primordia begin to form at 8 to 10 weeks. Nail plate formation is initiated at 17 weeks and is complete by the 5th month (Holbrook, 1991).

NEWBORN SKIN

The most clinically significant difference between the skin of premature and term infants is in the structure of the stratum corneum. Infants born before 32 weeks gestation have a very thin stratum corneum, which gives rise to a variety of problems (Rutter, 1988). The primary functions of the stratum corneum are conservation of body water and barrier protection. A premature stratum corneum does not effectively prevent transepidermal water loss, percutaneous absorption of exogenously applied compounds, or invasion of microbes. In the dry postnatal environment, the premature infant experiences excessive losses of body fluid and heat (Baumgart, 1982; Rutter and Hull, 1979). A variety of seemingly benign clinical interventions can dramatically increase these losses. Desiccated skin is even more easily injured, providing a portal of entry for invading microbes and increasing the risk of disseminated infection (Baumgart, 1982; Gunnar et al, 1985; Harper and Rutter, 1983; Rosen et al, 1995; Rutter, 1988). A premature infant's increased ratio of body surface area to body weight, diminished metabolic capacity, and decreased immune responses compound these problems.

Rates of transepidermal water loss (TEWL) are objective measures of stratum corneum integrity. TEWL has been well studied in premature infants, using the evaporimeter, a piece of equipment that provides direct measurements (Gunnar et al, 1985). During the first 4 weeks after birth, there is an exponential relationship between TEWL and gestational age in appropriate for gestational age (AGA) infants. TEWL is up to 15 times higher in 1-day-old infants born at 25 weeks gestation than in term neonates. In very-low-birth-weight infants, this can translate into a fluid loss of up to 30% of total body weight in 24 hours. As the stratum corneum develops, TEWL gradually decreases, but at 4 weeks postgestation TEWL from an

TABLE 105–1

Comparison of Fetal and Adult Wound Repair

Variable	Fetus (<24 wk)	Adult
Tissue environment	Amniotic fluid rich in growth factors and hyaluronic acid Relative hypoxemia Sterile	Air
Inflammatory infiltrate	Limited; neutrophils and lymphocytes predominate	Macrophages predominate
Extracellular matrix	Nonexcessive deposition of Types III and V collagen organized into a reticular pattern Increased amount of hyaluronic acid	Abundant Type I collagen deposited into disorganized bundles

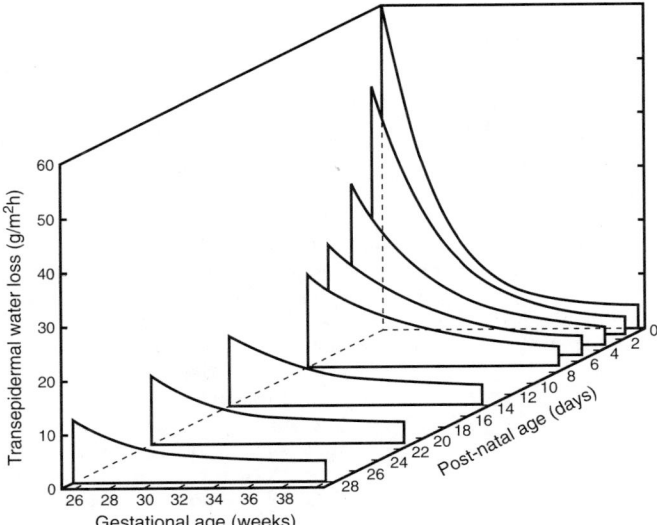

FIGURE 105–1. Transepidermal water loss in relation to gestational age at different postnatal ages in appropriate-for-gestational-age infants. (From Hammarlund K, Sedin G, Stromberg B: Transepidermal water loss in newborn infants: VIII. Relation to gestational age and postnatal age in appropriate and small for gestational age infants. Acta Paediatr Scand 72:721, 1983.)

infant born at 26 weeks is still twice that of a term infant (Fig. 105–1).

Loss of body water is accompanied by evaporative heat loss at a rate of 2.4 × 10 (Smack et al, 1994)[3] J/g (or 576 calories of body heat for every milliliter of water) (Hammarlund and Sedin, 1982). Evaporative losses are greatest in younger, more premature infants. Routine clinical interventions can exacerbate TEWL. Maintenance on an open radiant warmer bed in a nursery with low ambient humidity results in high evaporative loss of body water and heat (Le Blanc, 1991). Higher ambient temperatures are required to maintain normal body temperature under these conditions (Hammarlund and Sedin, 1982). Traditional efforts to minimize these losses have centered on intravascular fluid replacement and modification of the infant's hospital bed. These approaches have inherent problems. Evaporative losses originate as free water from the extracellular compartment. Replacement has been conventionally determined by calculation based on standardized maintenance fluid requirements and measured changes of body weight and extracellular electrolytes, which have a typical lag time of several hours. Replacement fluids given in the form of isotonic intravenous solutions may result in sodium and glucose overload. Enclosed isolettes with high ambient humidity carry a risk of colonization with pathogenic bacteria, although an increased incidence of infection has not been documented (Le Blanc, 1991). Shielding devices used on open radiant warmer beds limit access to infants. Furthermore, some materials used for shielding (glass, Plexiglas, Lucite, Perspex) absorb infrared energy, blocking overhead transmission of heat to the infant (Baumgart, 1990; Le Blanc, 1991). Pure polyethylene plastic wraps (e.g., Glad Wrap) are transparent to infrared heat, but plastic wrap made of more complex polymers may retain heat and have the potential to burn contacted skin (Le

Blanc, 1991). More recent data have focused on limiting skin injury and developing methods to improve the cutaneous barrier.

Clinically occult skin injury accompanies routine care. Skin stripping by removal of adhesive-backed products causes acute injury as well as the potential for secondary infection and significant scarring (Cartlidge et al, 1990). Removal of a piece of tape or an adhesive-backed electrode will markedly compromise the stratum corneum (Cartlidge and Rutter, 1987; Harper and Rutter, 1983), an observation that has been used in a positive way to facilitate transcutaneous monitoring of serum glucose in newborns (De Boer et al, 1994). We have observed several cases of full-thickness skin injury from presumed innocuous local application of pressure or thermal heat (Fig. 105–2). The precise causes of this type of wound are often difficult to identify and remain unreported. Ultraviolet light burns have occurred in association with white light phototherapy for jaundice, from relatively limited, inadvertent exposure to near-ultraviolet A (UVA) light, which is 1000 times less erythemogenic than ultraviolet B UVB (Siegfried et al, 1992). A Plexiglas safety shield, placed in front of daylight fluorescent bulbs, will filter out the UVA. However, white light phototherapy is also a source of infrared heat, and heat stress will exacerbate TEWL. In contrast, phototherapy delivered with blue light alone does not increase TEWL (Kjartansson et al, 1992).

Increased percutaneous absorption of topically applied compounds through an immature stratum corneum has been both advantageous and hazardous to neonates. This phenomenon was described in 1971 as "racoon facies," a visible periorbital ring of pallor from cutaneous vasoconstriction after the application of phenylephrine eyedrops (Rutter, 1987). This effect can be quantified and is directly proportional to measurements of TEWL. Both methods have been established as useful markers of stratum corneum integrity in infants (Plentin et al, 1992; Rutter, 1987). Transdermal delivery may be the optimal route of administration for theophylline (Cartwright et al, 1990; Rutter, 1987) and diamorphine (Barrett et al, 1993) in premature infants. Lidocaine applied topically to premature skin is probably much more effective than after application to mature skin (Barrett and Rutter, 1994). Even supplemental

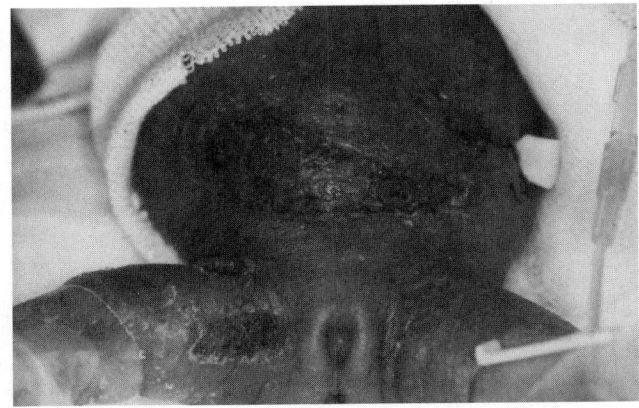

FIGURE 105–2. The cause of this full-thickness skin injury on a 26-week-old infant was innocuous enough to elude identification.

TABLE 105–2

Reported Hazards of Percutaneous Absorption in the Newborn

Compound	Reference	Product	Toxicity
Aniline	Rutter, 1987	Dye used as a laundry marker	Methemoglobinemia,[*] death
Mercury	Dinehart et al, 1988	Diaper rinses; teething powders	Rash, hypotonia
Phenolic compounds:			
Pentachlorophenol	West et al, 1981	Laundry disinfectant	Tachycardia, sweating, hepatomegaly, metabolic acidosis, death
Hexachlorophene		Topical antiseptic (pHisoHex)	Vacuolar encephalopathy, death
Resorcinol	West et al, 1981	Topical antiseptic	Methemoglobinemia[*]
Boric acid	Goldbloom and Goldbloom, 1953	Baby powder	Vomiting, diarrhea, erythroderma, seizures, death
Lindane	Rutter, 1987; West et al, 1981	Scabicide	Neurotoxicity
Salicylic acid	Abidel-Magid and El Awad Ahmed, 1994; West et al, 1981	Keratolytic emollient	Metabolic acidosis, salicylism
Isopropyl alcohol (under occlusion)	Rutter, 1987	Topical antiseptic	Cutaneous hemorrhagic necrosis
Silver sulfadiazine	Payne et al, 1992	Topical antibiotic (Silvadene)	Kernicterus (sulfa component), argyria (silver component)
Urea	Anonymous, 1987	Keratolytic emollient (Carmol)	Uremia
Povidine-iodine	Rutter, 1987; West et al, 1981	Topical antiseptic (Betadine)	Hypothyroidism, goiter
Neomycin	Rutter, 1987	Topical antibiotic	Neural deafness
Corticosteroids	Rutter, 1987; West et al, 1981	Topical anti-inflammatory (Lotrisone)	Skin atrophy, adrenal suppression
Benzocaine	Gelman et al, 1996	Mucosal anesthetic (teething products)	Methemoglobinemia[*]
Prilocaine	Frayling et al, 1990; Reynolds, 1996	Epidermal anesthetic (Emla)	Methemoglobinemia[*]

[*]Heritable glucose-6-phosphate deficiencies are associated with an increased susceptibility to methemoglobinemia, as are coadministration of several drugs, including sulfonamides, acetaminophen, nitroprusside, phenobarbital, and phenytoin.

oxygen has been administered percutaneously to very small preterm infants with poor pulmonary function (Cartlidge and Rutter, 1988a, 1988b).

In contradistinction, there have been numerous reports of percutaneous toxicity in infants caused by absorption of topically applied agents (Lane, 1987; Rutter, 1987). Published accounts serve to document the most severe cases of toxicity, often manifest as nursery epidemics of obvious clinical signs or deaths (Table 105–2). The potential for subclinical toxicities must be considered by everyone caring for small newborns (Table 105–3). When several topical therapeutic options are available, the one with the least potential for toxicity should be used. *Poisindex(R)* is an extensive, frequently-updated, computer-based reference source for the identification of potentially toxic compounds (Micromedex, 1995). The information from this data base

TABLE 105–3

Topically Applied Products that Should Be Used with Caution in the Newborn

Compound	Product	Concern
Triclosan	Lever 2000, liquid deodorant soaps	Risk of toxicities seen with other phenolic compounds
Propylene glycol (MacDonald et al, 1987)	Emollients, cleansing agents (Cetaphil lotion)	Excessive enteral and parenteral administration has caused hyperosmolality and seizures in infants
Benzethonium chloride	Skin cleansers	Poisoning by ingestion, carcinogenesis
Glycerin	Emollients, cleansing agents (Aquanil lotion)	Hyperosmolality, seizures
Ammonium lactate	Keratolytic emollient (Lac-Hydrin)	Possible lactic acidosis
Coal tar (van Shooten et al, 1994)	Shampoos, topical anti-inflammatory ointments	Excessive use of polycyclic aromatic hydrocarbons is associated with an increased risk of cancer

TABLE 105-4

Metabolic and Nutritional Disorders Presenting with Dermatitis

Disorder	Reference
Acrodermatitis enteropathica	Goskowics and Eichenfield, 1993
Biotin-dependent multiple carboxylase deficiency	Wolf and Heard, 1991
Prolidase deficiency	Bissonnette et al, 1993
Methylmalonic acidemia	Bodemer et al, 1994; de Raeve et al, 1994
Maple syrup urine disease	Giacoia and Berry, 1994
Propionic acidemia	Bodemar et al, 1994; de Raeve et al, 1994
Citrullinemia	Goldblum et al, 1986
Cystic fibrosis	Darmstadt et al, 1992
Gaucher's disease	Sherer et al 1993; Sidransky et al, 1992
Kwashiorkor	Goskowics and Eichenfield, 1993

and current published literature indicates a lower risk of percutaneous or systemic toxicity from chlorhexidine skin antisepsis than povidone-iodine.

The important role of nutrition in skin maturation and wound healing can be overlooked in small, sick infants who are maintained on varying amounts of complex parenteral fluids. Acquired deficiencies as well as those resulting from inborn errors of metabolism (Table 105–4) are associated with classic cutaneous findings. These include deficiencies of protein, essential fatty acids, zinc, biotin, and vitamins

A, C, and several B vitamins. Daily requirements for most of these nutrients are higher in premature than term infants (Table 105–5).

Attention to skin integrity will help control translocation of water through the skin of premature neonates. Appropriate hydration of keratinocytes is essential for normal skin maturation (Rawlings et al, 1994), an optimized barrier against exogenous assault, and maintenance of thermal, fluid, and electrolyte balance. A successful basic skin care regimen should also allow easy access and handling of infants. Therapeutic goals include minimizing postnatal trauma and providing an artificial barrier until the stratum corneum matures. Currently, there is no uniformly defined or accepted standard of care for the skin of premature infants. Formal clinical investigation has been limited. A few studies have verified the safety and efficacy of semiocclusive, adhesive-backed polyurethane membrane barriers in preventing fluid losses (Barak et al, 1989; Knauth et al, 1989; Mancini et al, 1994; Vernon et al, 1990). However, these dressings are not widely used because they are difficult to apply and thought to limit available area for surface monitors. Neonatal intensive care unit (NICU) staff often provide topical emollient therapy to infants in a random way. The risks and benefits of commercially available topical emollients have not been well defined. Concerns include the risk of systemic absorption and resulting toxicity, overgrowth of microbes, and secondary heat accumulation that could increase surface and core temperature.

There have been many studies of the mechanism of action and benefits of emollients on injured and diseased skin in adults. Petroleum wax–based ointment emollients (e.g., Vaseline petroleum jelly) act primarily by decreasing TEWL and accelerating barrier recovery (Ghadially and Elias, 1992). Some oils, such as safflower oil, contain essen-

TABLE 105-5

Nutritional Requirements and Cutaneous Signs of Deficiency

Nutrient	Infant's Daily Requirement Premature	Term	Cutaneous Signs
Protein (g/kg/day)	2.7–3.0	2.5–2.7	"Flaky paint" scaling, hypopigmentation, peripheral edema
Linoleic acid (g/kg/day)	1.2	0.3–0.8	Alopecia, erythema with coarse scaling, erosive intertriginous dermatitis, poor wound healing
Zinc (μg/kg/day)	400	100	Alopecia, acral and periorificial erosive, pustular dermatitis, poor wound healing
Biotin (μg/kg/day)	6.0	5.0 (not >20)	Alopecia, intertriginous and periorificial dermatitis, generalized scaling
Vitamin C (mg/kg/day)	25	20 (not >80)	Perifollicular hemorrhages, poor wound healing, friable gums
Vitamin A (μg/kg/day)	500	175 (not >700)	Generalized scaling
Riboflavin (mg/kg/day)	0.15	0.35° (not >1.4)	Intertriginous and periorificial dermatitis, mucositis
Pyridoxine (mg/kg/day)	0.18	0.25° (not >1.0)	Intertriginous and periorificial dermatitis, mucositis
Niacin (mg/kg/day)	6.8	4.25° (not >17)	Mucositis, symmetric hyperpigmented plaques at sun-exposed sites

°For full-term infants, the recommended doses of some water-soluble vitamins are probably high because toxicity has not been reported.

Adapted from Greene HL, Hambridge KM, Schanler R, Tsang RC: Guidelines for the use of vitamins, trace elements, calcium, magnesium, and phosphorus in infants and children receiving total parenteral nutrition: Report of the Subcommittee on Pediatric Parenteral Nutrient Requirements from the Committee on Clinical Practice Issues of the American Society for Clinical Nutrition 1–3. Am J Clin Nutr 48:1324, 1988; © Am J Clin Nutr American Society for Clinical Nutrition; and (2) Miller SJ: Nutritional deficiency and the skin. J Am Acad Dermatol 21:1, 1989. Used with permission.

tial fatty acids, which greatly influence cutaneous structure and function (Schurer et al, 1991; Ziboh and Chapkin, 1987). However, topical application of safflower oil does not prevent essential fatty acid deficiency in preterm infants (Lee et al, 1993). Oils, oil-and-water–based creams, and lotion emollients have greater tactile acceptance than greasy ointments. However, these preparations provide a less effective moisture barrier than ointment emollients (Lane and Drost, 1993). In addition, formulation of a cream or lotion emulsion requires the addition of several potentially irritating or toxic ingredients. Eucerin Creme is an emollient that has been studied for use in the nursery (Lane and Drost, 1993). It contains water, petrolatum, mineral oil, ceresin, lanolin alcohol, and methylchloroisothiazolinone/methylisothiazolinone (CMI/MI). Although susceptibility of premature infants to allergic contact sensitization is unknown, CMI/MI has been associated with allergic contact sensitization in up to 10% of exposed adults (Frosch et al, 1994). Aquaphor ointment contains essentially two ingredients: petrolatum in ointment—liquid (mineral oil) and solid (mineral wax) phases—and wool wax alcohol. A recent study documented that application every 12 hours reduced TEWL, improved skin integrity, did not alter skin flora, and was associated with a significant reduction of the incidence of sepsis. No adverse effects were reported (Nopper et al, 1994). Skin surface temperature was stable, and there was no evidence of hyperthermia or burns after application of the petroleum-based emollient used under infrared warmers, even for infants receiving concomitant white light phototherapy, confirming the results of a previous pilot study (Schwayder and Hetzel, 1989). Increased understanding of the mechanisms contributing to skin development may one day provide therapy to accelerate barrier maturation in very premature infants. Until that time, therapy should be directed toward providing a safe, temporary barrier and minimizing additional skin injury. Proposed recommendations for the care of premature skin are outlined in Table 105–6. A summary of dressing materials is outlined in Table 105–7.

DIFFERENTIAL DIAGNOSIS BY CUTANEOUS MORPHOLOGY

Diagnosis of skin disease is based on recognition of definitive morphology of the cutaneous examination. Dermatologists are trained to interpret the important features, including color, shape, texture, and distribution, while ignoring unimportant or misleading features. Skin disease is often categorized into morphologic groups based on the most prominent primary lesion. This helps formulate a differential diagnosis and direct further investigation. Important morphologic groups in neonatal dermatology are vesicles and pustules, erythroderma, collodion baby, nonblanching violaceous papules and plaques, pigmented lesions, vascular defects, and midline anomalies. Refer to subsequent chapters for more detailed information on specific disorders.

Vesicles and Pustules

Many conditions cause blisters and pustules in the newborn. Vesicles are, by definition, small intra- or subepidermal pockets of clear fluid. If the lesions are large (>1 cm),

---

TABLE 105–6

Proposed Guidelines for Basic Skin Care of the Newborn

1. *Use adhesives sparingly.*
   Place protective dressing (e.g., DuoDerm or Tegaderm) at sites of frequent taping (endotracheal tube and nasogastric tube placement).
   Use nonadhesive electrodes, and change them only when they become nonfunctional (Cartlidge and Rutter, 1987).
2. *Limit bathing.*
   Defer initial cleansing until body temperature has stabilized.
   Avoid cleansing agents for the first 2 weeks.
   Use warm water and moistened cotton pledgets in a humid environment.
   Surface cleansing is required no more than twice a week.
   If antimicrobial skin preparation is required, use short-contact chlorhexidine (except on the face)
3. *Be aware of the composition and quantity of all topically applied agents.*
   This includes antimicrobial cleansers, diaper wipes, adhesive removers, and perineal products.
   Dispense from single-use containers, if possible.
4. *Ensure adequate intake of protein, essential fatty acids, zinc, biotin, and vitamins A, D, and Bs.*
   Erosive periorificial dermatitis is a sign of nutritional deficiency.
5. *Apply a simple cream or ointment emollient every 8 hours* (Nopper et al, 1994).
6. *Guard against excessive thermal and ultraviolet exposure.*
   Use thermally controlled water for bathing.
   Avoid surface monitors with metal contacts.
   Use Plexiglas shielding over daylight fluorescent phototherapy.
7. *Protect sites of cutaneous injury with the appropriate occlusive dressing.*
   Use a film dressing on nonexudative sites (Barak et al, 1989; Knauth et al, 1989; Vernon et al, 1990).
   Use a hydrogel dressing on exudative wounds.
   Maintain appropriate hydration at the skin-dressing interface.
   Remove necrotic debris with each dressing change.

TABLE 105–7

Occlusive Dressing Materials

Class	Examples	Indications
Films		
Polyurethane ± adhesive backing	Tegaderm, Op-Site, Bioclusive, Omniderm	Superficial, nonexudative wounds, sites of friction
Microporous Teflon/silicone	Silon	
Hydrocolloids		
Hydrophilic colloidal particles in polyurethane foam	DuoDerm, Cutinova hydro, Restore	Exudative wounds, sites of friction
Hydrogels		
Cross-linked polyvinyl or other polymer; 80–99% water	Vigilon, Cutinova gel, Biofilm	Exudative wounds, fragile skin, sites of friction

Reprinted from Dermatologic Surgery, Kannon GA, Garrett AB: Moist wound healing with occlusive dressings, p 583. Copyright 1995, with permission from Elsevier Science Inc.

they are referred to as bullae. Pustules are filled with purulent fluid. Diseases in this category range from the totally innocuous and self-limited to the severe and life threatening.

A directed history, including family history of blistering diseases, and physical examination, including examination of the placenta, can focus the differential diagnosis. Small lesions in an otherwise healthy infant usually suggest a purely cutaneous process. Bullae and widespread involvement should prompt a more aggressive work-up.

The initial diagnostic work-up should include

Fluid aspirate taken from an intact pustule for Gram's stain, Wright's stain, and fungal, viral, and bacterial cultures.

Potassium hydroxide (KOH) preparation (or calcofluor white immunofluorescence), of the blister roof.

Scraping from the base of the blister for Tzanck smear.

Scraping from a carefully selected intact lesion, mounted in mineral oil, for scabies preparation.

Skin biopsy as indicated, depending on the morphology and extent of the lesions, and results of other evaluations.

Differential Diagnosis

Infections Localized to Skin

Candidiasis: KOH (or calcofluor white) preparation of the blister roof reveals pseudohyphae.

Bullous impetigo: Wright's stain reveals polymorphonuclear neutrophil leukocytes (PMNs); Gram's stain shows gram-positive cocci.

Gram-positive folliculitis: Wright's stain reveals PMNs; Gram's stain shows gram-positive cocci.

Pityrosporum folliculitis: Kott reveals short hyphae and spores.

Neonatal herpes: Tzanck smear reveals viral cytopathic changes.

Scabies: mineral oil preparation reveals mites, ova, and feces.

Transient Noninfectious Causes

Erythema toxicum neonatorum: Wright's stain shows eosinophils.

Neonatal pustular melanosis: Wright's stain shows keratinous debris with PMNs; the Gram's stain is negative.

Neonatal acne: close inspection reveals comedones.

Milia: Wright's stain shows keratinocytes only.

Miliaria crystallina: these tiny, superficial noninflammatory vesicles represent obstruction of the sweat duct.

Infantile acropustulosis: this pruritic condition mimics infantile scabies.

Eosinophilic pustular folliculitis.

Bullae and Extensive Blistering

The diseases in this category may be life threatening and may be impossible to distinguish from one another without skin biopsy. Appropriate therapy depends on correct diagnosis.

Staphylococcal scalded skin syndrome: skin biopsy reveals a split in the superficial epidermis. Culture of blister contents is negative; the locus of infection is nasopharyngeal, perianal, focus of impetigo, or abcess.

Congenital herpes simplex infection: skin, eye, or mouth lesions are presenting signs in one third of infants.

Toxic epidermal necrolysis: skin biopsy reveals a split at the dermoepidermal junction.

Bullous mastocytosis: stroking will produce a wheal and flare (Darier's sign).

Genetic disorders: these disorders have variable extent of severity and long-term sequelae. Early diagnosis and genetic counseling are important aspects of management (see Chapter 106).

Epidermolysis bullosa: blisters are most prominent at sites of friction. Familial forms are classified as simplex, junctional, and dystrophic, based on the skin cleavage plane. Electron microscopic analysis or immunofluorescence mapping, or both, are required for precise diagnosis.

Incontinentia pigmenti: vesicular skin lesions have a characteristic distribution along the lines of Blaschko. This striking pattern is seen with a variety of cutaneous abnormalities as a result of genetic mosaicism.

Additional information is summarized in Table 105–7 (Frieden, 1989).

Erythroderma

Generalized redness and scaling in infancy have an alarming appearance and are often clinically and histologically nonspecific. An infant's general state of well-being is an important clue to the extent of the disease. Definitive diagnosis may be possible only after a period of observation.

Careful history, family history, physical examination, and directed laboratory evaluation may help clarify the cause. The spectrum of disease includes common conditions limited to skin, infections, nutritional deficiencies, and immunologic disorders.

Infectious causes of erythroderma should always be considered first. The infant's skin should be carefully examined for more specific primary skin lesions. Laboratory evaluation should include complete blood count; KOH preparation (or calcofluor white immunofluorescence); Tzanck smear; and surveillance cultures of the nasopharynx, rectum, umbilicus, conjunctivae, urine, and blood. Consider syphilis serology and human immunodeficiency virus (HIV) studies in epidemiologically relevant locales. Begin empiric therapy, as needed.

The diagnostic evaluation should be more aggressive in any infant who is not thriving to search for metabolic or immunologic abnormalities. This should include dietary history, electrolytes, protein, albumin, alkaline phosphatase, microscopic examination of hair, and a sweat test. The results of these screening tests can suggest the need for further laboratory evaluation.

More directed laboratory evaluation includes blood smear for leukocyte vacuoles, HIV screen, plasma zinc, serum linoleic and arachidonic acids, amino acid profile, specific assays for biotinidase activity, antinuclear antibody (SS-A and SS-B titers), quantitative immunoglobulins, tests of cell-mediated immunity, skeletal survey, hair examination, and skin biopsy.

Differential Diagnosis

Systemic Infections Associated with Erythroderma
Candidiasis
Staphylococcal scalded skin syndrome
Syphilis
Acquired immunodeficiency syndrome (AIDS)

Primary Cutaneous Conditions
Atopic dermatitis: pruritus and involvement of the face and extensor extremities with marked sparing of the diaper area are helpful diagnostic clues.
Seborrheic dermatitis: the diaper area and skinfolds are often prominently involved.
Psoriasis: skin lesions are often sharply circumscribed, but scale may not be prominent.

Genodermatoses
The ichthyoses-associated abnormalities or skin biopsy help distinguish between the disorders in this category: lamellar ichthyosis, congenital nonbullous ichthyosiform erythroderma, epidermolytic hyperkeratosis, X-linked ichthyosis, multiple sulfatase deficiency, neutral lipid storage disease, Sjögren-Larsson syndrome, trichothiodystrophy, Netherton's syndrome, or X-linked dominant chondrodysplasia punctata.

Ectodermal Dysplasias. This is a group of disorders with abnormalities of the skin and its appendages. Excessive desquamation resembling postmaturity is a characteristic finding. The most well-recognized form is X-linked recessive hypohidrotic ectodermal dysplasia. Infants with this disorder have a decreased ability to sweat and a tendency toward hyperthermia.

Immunologic Disorders Associated with Erythroderma
A clinical syndrome of erythroderma, diarrhea, and failure to thrive in infancy was first described in 1908 by Leiner, in association with unsupplemented breast-feeding. Subsequently, similar signs have been reported in infants with increased susceptibility to infection. A defect in yeast opsonization was found in two infants with "Leiner's disease" in 1972. However, this defect, present in 5% of the general population, does not define the disease. Other patients had dramatic clinical improvement after infusion of fresh plasma or a purified preparation containing the fifth component of complement, C5. Consequently, Leiner's disease has been associated with C5 dysfunction. More recently, a variety of immunologic abnormalities have been reported in infants with similar clinical presentation under the name *syndrome of erythroderma, failure to thrive, and diarrhea in infancy* to avoid confusion (Glover et al, 1988). Other defined disorders in this category include the following:

Primary immunodeficiencies (severe combined immunodeficiency [SCID], Wiskott-Aldrich, hyperimmunoglobulin E syndrome, Omenn syndrome)
Secondary immunodeficiencies (AIDS, graft-versus-host disease)
Langerhans' cell histiocytosis
Neonatal lupus
Diffuse cutaneous mastocytosis

Metabolic and Nutritional Disorders Associated with Erythroderma
Patients in this group often present with erosive, periorificial dermatitis (see Table 105–5).

Other
Boric acid poisoning: This condition was reported with the use of boric acid baby powders. It can be clinically indistinguishable from staphylococcal scalded skin syndrome (Goldbloom and Goldbloom, 1953).

Collodion Baby

Collodion baby is a distinct subset of neonatal erythroderma that can be a clinical marker of a variety of underlying abnormalities. The phenotype includes parchment-like hyperkeratosis, pseudocontractures, ectropion, eclabium, absence of eyebrows, and sparse hair. These infants have defective cutaneous barrier function, with resultant losses of free water and thermal energy. They are extremely susceptible to hypothermia, hypernatremic dehydration, and percutaneous infection (see Chapter 106).

Nonblanching Violaceous Papules and Plaques

Nonblanching violaceous papules and plaques may be localized or disseminated. Infants with widespread lesions have been described as "blueberry muffin babies." The diseases in this category represent a variety of processes; most require aggressive evaluation and treatment.

Initial evaluation of a blueberry muffin infant should include complete blood count with white blood cell differential; platelet count; reticulocyte count; liver function tests; maternal and neonatal TORCH (*t*oxoplasmosis, *o*ther infections, *r*ubella, *c*ytomegalovirus infection, and *h*erpes simplex) titers; rapid plasma reagin (RPR); blood cultures for bacteria; urine, nasopharyngeal and rectal samples for viral cultures; and ophthalmologic examination.

Skin biopsy is necessary to distinguish between simple hemorrhage into the dermis (purpura) and other infiltrative conditions (e.g., dermal hematopoiesis, tumor) presenting in the neonatal period.

Differential Diagnosis

Purpura

Ecchymoses: this is traumatic purpura, usually secondary to labor and delivery.

Bland thrombosis: conditions in this category that can occur in the neonatal period include the following:

Embolization of foreign material. This has been reported in infants receiving extracorporeal membrane oxygenation (ECMO).

Purpura fulminans: neonatal purpura fulminans is most often associated with homozygous protein C or protein S deficiency (Marlar et al, 1989).

Cryoglobulinemia.

Infectious vasculitis: purpuric lesions represent infectious, inflammatory microemboli, most commonly associated with the following:

Gram-negative bacterial sepsis, including *E. coli, meningococcus,* and ecthyma gangrenosum *(Pseudomonas).*

Listeriosis

Aspergillosis

Thrombocytopenia: this usually presents with widely scattered petechiae.

Isoimmune thrombocytopenic purpura (ITP)

Maternal ITP

Disseminated intravascular coagulopathy

Dermal Hematopoiesis

This is the histology of the blueberry muffin skin lesions. Before 34 weeks' gestation, the skin serves as a hematopoietic center. It has yet to be shown whether blueberry muffin lesions are due to persistence or recurrence of the fetal potential.

Rubella
Cytomegalovirus
Syphilis
Other viral infections (e.g., coxsackievirus B2)
Twin transfusion syndrome
Rh hemolytic disease of the newborn

Malignancy

Congenital leukemia
Langerhans' cell histiocytosis
Neuroblastoma

Vascular Defects

It can be difficult to distinguish between the different forms of cutaneous vascular lesions presenting in the neonatal period. Nonvascular look-alikes also fall into this category but can be differentiated by skin biopsy (see Chapter 109).

Differential Diagnosis

Hemangioma

The most common tumor of infancy, this lesion usually becomes apparent during the first 2 to 4 weeks after birth and exhibits a characteristic rapid growth phase, peaking at 12 months, followed by slow involution over the next 5 to 10 years.

Vascular Malformation

This is a group of lesions, usually apparent at birth, that do not generally grow or involute. Some vascular malformations are associated with characteristic extracutaneous abnormalities.

Salmon patch
Nevus flammeus (port-wine stain)
Klippel-Trénaunay syndrome
Cobb syndrome
Arterial, lymph, venous, or mixed malformations
Cutis marmorata telangiectatica congenita

Lesions that Mimic Vascular Birthmarks

Pilomatrixoma
Giant juvenile xanthogranuloma
Langerhans' cell histiocytosis
Congenital myofibromatosis
Midline facial lesions (see Chapter 108)
  Dermoid
  Nasal glioma
  Encephalocele

Pigmented Lesions

It can be difficult to distinguish between the lesions in the pigmented lesion category without histopathologic examination. The majority of congenital pigmented lesions are isolated and benign, but it is important to recognize those that are syndrome associated or potentially life threatening. Both melanocytic and nonmelanocytic lesions are included in this category.

In general, skin biopsy of a congenital pigmented lesion can be postponed until after the neonatal period. The one exception is a nodular lesion suggestive of melanoma. (See Chapter 109 for additional details.)

Differential Diagnosis

Congenital nevocellular nevus
Café au lait macule
Nevus spilus (speckled lentiginous nevus)
Mongolian spot
Smooth muscle hamartoma
Plexiform neurofibroma

Nevus of Ota
Epidermal nevus
Urticaria pigmentosa, solitary mastocytoma
Lentigines

REFERENCES

Abidel-Magid EHM, El Awad Ahmed FR: Salicylate intoxication in an infant with ichthyosis transmitted through skin ointment. Pediatrics 94:939, 1994.

Anonymous: High plasma urea concentrations in collodion babies. Arch Dis Child 62:212, 1987.

Barak M, Hershkowitz S, Rod R, Dror S: The use of a synthetic skin covering as a protective layer in the daily care of low birth weight infants. Eur J Pediatr 148:665, 1989.

Barrett DA, Rutter N: Percutaneous lignocaine absorption in newborn infants. Arch Dis Child 71:F122, 1994.

Barrett DA, Rutter N, Davis SS: An in vitro study of diamorphine permeation through premature human neonatal skin. Pharm Res 10:583, 1993.

Baumgart S: Radiant energy and insensible water loss in the premature newborn infant nursed under a radiant warmer. Clin Perinatol 9:483, 1982.

Baumgart S: Radiant heat loss versus radiant heat gain in premature neonates under radiant warmers. Biol Neonate 57:10, 1990.

Bissonnette R, Friedmann D, Giroux JM, et al: Prolidase deficiency: A multisystemic hereditary disorder. J Am Acad Dermatol 29:818, 1993.

Bleacher J, Adolph V, Dillon P, Krummel T: Fetal tissue repair and wound healing. Dermatol Clin 11:677, 1993.

Bodemer C, de Prost Y, Bachollet B, et al: Cutaneous manifestations of methylmalonic and propionic acidaemia: A description based on 38 cases. Br J Dermatol 131:93, 1994.

Cartlidge PHT, Fox PE, Rutter N: The scars of newborn intensive care. In Early Human Development. Nottingham, Ireland, Elsevier Scientific, 1990: pp 1–10.

Cartlidge PH, Rutter N: Karaya gum electrocardiographic electrodes for preterm infants. Arch Dis Child 62:1281, 1987.

Cartlidge PH, Rutter N: Percutaneous oxygen delivery to the preterm infant. Lancet 1:315, 1988a.

Cartlidge PH, Rutter N: Percutaneous respiration in the newborn infant: Effect of ambient oxygen concentration on pulmonary oxygen uptake. Biol Neonate 54:68, 1988.

Cartwright RG, Cartlidge PH, Rutter N, et al: Transdermal delivery of theophylline to premature infants using a hydrogel disc system. Br J Clin Pharmacol 29:533, 1990.

Darmstadt GL, Schmidt CP, Wechsler DS, et al: Dermatitis as a presenting sign of cystic fibrosis. Arch Dermatol 128:1358, 1992.

De Boer J, Baarsma R, Okken A, et al: Application of transcutaneous microdialysis and continuous flow analysis for on-line glucose monitoring in the newborn infants. J Lab Clin Med 124:210, 1994.

De Raeve L, De Meirleir L, Ramet J, et al: Acrodermatitis enteropathica-like cutaneous lesions in organic aciduria. J Pediatr 124:416, 1994.

Den Ouden AL, Berger HM, Ruys JH: Scarring of the hands resulting from venipunctures in babies. Eur J Pediatr 145:58, 1986.

Dinehart SM, Dillard R, Raimer SS, et al: Cutaneous manifestations of acrodynia (pink disease). Arch Dermatol 124:107, 1988.

Dostal G, Gamelli R: Fetal wound healing. Surg Gynecol Obstet 176:299, 1993.

Frayling IM, Addison GM, Chattergee K, Meaklin G: Methaemoglobinaemia in children treated with prilocainelignocaine cream. BMJ 301:153, 1990.

Frieden I: Blisters and pustules in the newborn. Curr Probl Pediatr Nov:555, 1989.

Frosch PJ, Lahti A, Hannuksela M, et al: Chloromethylisothiazolone/methylisothiazolone (CMI/MI) use test with a shampoo on patch-test-positive subjects. Contact Derm 32:210, 1994.

Gelman CR, Rumack BH, Hess AJ: Benzocaine [Abstract]. Englewood, CO, Micromedex, Inc. (electronic version), 1996.

Ghadially R, Elias P: Effects of petrolatum on stratum corneum structure and function. J Am Acad Dermatol 26:387, 1992.

Giacoia GP, Berry GT: Acrodermatitis enteropathica-like syndrome secondary to isoleucine deficiency during treatment of maple syrup urine disease. Am J Dis Child 147:954, 1994.

Glover MT, Atherton DJ, Levinsky RJ: Syndrome of erythroderma, failure to thrive, and diarrhea in infancy: A manifestation of immunodeficiency. Pediatrics 81:66, 1988.

Goldbloom RB, Goldbloom A: Boric acid poisoning. J Pediatr 43:631, 1953.

Goldblum OM, Brusilow SW, Maldonado YA, Farmer ER: Neonatal citrullinemia associated with cutaneous manifestations and arginine deficiency. J Am Acad Dermatol 14:321, 1986.

Goskowics M, Eichenfield LF: Cutaneous findings of nutritional deficiencies in children. Curr Opin Pediatr 5:441, 1993.

Greene HL, Hambridge KM, Schanler R, Tsang RC: Guidelines for the use of vitamins, trace elements, calcium, magnesium, and phosphorus in infants and children receiving total parenteral nutrition: Report of the Subcommittee on Pediatric Parenteral Nutrient Requirements from the Committee on Clinical Practice Issues of the American Society for Clinical Nutrition 1–3. Am J Clin Nutr 48:1324, 1988.

Gunnar S, Hammarlund K, Nilsson GE, et al: Measurements of transepidermal water loss in newborn infants. Clin Perinatol 12:79, 1985.

Hammarlund K, Sedin G: Transepidermal water loss in newborn infants. Acta Pediatr Scand 71:191, 1982.

Harper VA, Rutter N: Barrier properties of the newborn infant's skin. J Pediatr 102:419, 1983.

Holbrook KA: Structure and function of the developing human skin. In Golsmith LA (Ed): Physiology, Biochemistry and Molecular Biology of the Skin. New York, 1991, pp 63–110.

Holbrook KA, Smith LT, Elias S: Prenatal diagnosis of genetic skin disease using fetal skin biopsy samples. Arch Dermatol 129:1437, 1993.

Kannon GA, Garrett AB: Moist wound healing with occlusive dressings. Dermatol Surg 21:583, 1995.

Kjartansson SK, Hammarlund K, Sedin G: Insensible water loss from the skin during phototherapy in term and preterm infants. Acta Pediatr 81:764, 1992.

Knauth A, Gordin M, McNeils W, Baumgart S: Semipermeable polyurethane membrane as an artificial skin for the premature neonate. J Pediatr 83:945, 1989.

Lane AT: Development and care of the premature infant's skin. Pediatr Dermatol 4:1, 1987.

Lane AT, Drost SS: Effects of repeated application of emollient cream to premature neonate's skin. Pediatrics 92:415, 1993.

LeBlanc MH: Thermoregulation: Incubators, radiant warmers, artificial skins, and body hoods. Clin Perinatol 18(3):403, 1991.

Lee EJ, Gibson RA, Simmer K: Transcutaneous application of oil and prevention of essential fatty acid deficiency in preterm infants. Arch Dis Child 68:27, 1993.

Lista FR, Thomson HG: The fate of sternotomy scars in children. Plast Reconstr Surg 81:35, 1988.

Longaker M, Adzick N: The biology of fetal wound healing: A review. Plast Reconstr Surg 87:788, 1991.

MacDonald MG, Getson PR, Glasgow AM, et al: Propylene glycol: Increased incidence of seizures in low birth weight infants. Pediatrics 79:622, 1987.

Mancini AJ, Sookdeo-Drost S, Madison KC, et al: Semipermeable dressings improve epidermal barrier function in premature infants. Pediatr Res 36(3):306, 1994.

Mast B, Diegelmann R, Krummel T, Cohen I: Scarless wound healing in the mammalian fetus. Surg Gynecol Obstet 174:441, 1992.

Micromedex: Poisindex(r) System. Englewood, CO, Micromedex, 1995.

Miller SJ: Nutritional deficiency and the skin. J Am Acad Dermatol 21:1, 1989.

Nazzaro-Porro M, Passi S, Bonifort L, Belsito F: Effects of aging on fatty acids in skin surface lipids. J Invest Dermatol 73:112, 1979.

Nopper AJ, Horli K, Sookdeo-Drost S, et al: Topical ointment therapy reduces the risk of nosocomial infection in premature infants. Paper presented at the Society of Pediatrics at Hilton Head, SC, June 1994.

Payne CM, Bladin C, Colchester AC, et al: Argyria from excessive use of topical silver sulphadiazine. Lancet 340:126, 1992.

Plantin P, Jouan N, Karangwa A, et al: Variations of the skin permeability in premature newborn infants: Value of the skin vasoconstriction test with neosynephrine. Arch Franc Pediatr 49:623, 1992.

Rawlings AV, Scott IR, Harding CR, Bowser PA: Stratum corneum moisturization at the molecular level. In Moshell AN (Ed): Progress in Dermatology. Evanston, Illinois, 1994: pp 1–12.

Report of the Working Party: Diagnosis and treatment of homozygous protein C deficiency. J Pediatr 114:528, 1989.

Reynolds JEF: Prilocaine hydrochloride [Abstract]. Englewood, CO, Micromedex, Inc. (electronic version), 1996.

Rosen JL, Atkins JT, Levy ML, et al: Invasive fungal dermatitis in the ≤1000-gram neonate. Pediatrics 95:682, 1995.

Rutter N: The immature skin. Br Med Bull 44:957, 1988.

Rutter N: Percutaneous drug absorption in the newborn: Hazards and uses. Clin Perinatol 14:911, 1987.

Rutter N, Hull D: Water loss from the skin of term and preterm babies. Arch Dis Child 54:858, 1979.

Schurer NY, Plewig G, Elias PM: Stratum corneum lipid function. Dermatologica 183:77, 1991.

Schwayder T, Hetzel F: Effects of emollients on skin temperature under infrared warmers. Paper presented at the 5th International Congress of Pediatric Dermatology, Milan, Italy, July 1989.

Sherer DM, Metlay LA, Sinkin RA, et al: Congenital ichthyosis with restrictive dermopathy and Gaucher disease: A new syndrome with associated prenatal diagnostic and pathology findings. Obstet Gynecol 81:842, 1993.

Sidransky E, Sherer DM, Ginns EI: Gaucher disease in the neonate: A distinct Gaucher phenotype is analogous to a model created by targeted disruption of the glucocerebrosidase gene. Pediatr Res 32:494, 1992.

Siegfried EC, Stone MS, Madison KC: Ultraviolet light burn: A cutaneous complication of visible light therapy for neonatal jaundice. Pediatr Dermatol 9:278, 1992.

Sivarajah N, Jegatheesan J, Gnananathan V: BCG vaccinations and development of a scar. Ceylon Med J 36:75, 1990.

Smack DP, Korge BP, James WD: Keratin and keratinization. J Am Acad Dermatol 30:85, 1994.

Van Shooten FJ, et al: Are coal-tar shampoos safe? Lancet 344:1505, 1994.

Vernon HJ, Lane AT, Wischerath LJ, et al: Semipermeable dressing and transepidermal water loss in premature infants. J Pediatr 86:357, 1990.

West DP, Worobec S, Solomon LM: Pharmacology and toxicology of infant skin. J Invest Dermatol 76:147, 1981.

Wolf B, Heard GS: Biotinidase deficiency. Adv Pediatr 38:1–21, 1991.

Ziboh VA, Chapkin RS: Biologic significance of polyunsaturated fatty acids in the skin. Arch Dermatol 123:1686, 1987.

CHAPTER 106

Congenital and Hereditary Disorders of the Skin

Elaine C. Siegfried and Nancy B. Esterly

The heritable disorders of skin (genodermatoses) feature diverse aberrations of color, texture, and structural integrity of the epidermis, epidermal appendages, and connective tissue. Some of these diseases are cutaneous only, others are associated with anomalies of multiple organ systems. Several genodermatoses can be diagnosed prenatally, by skin biopsy (Holbrook et al, 1993) (Table 106–1). This technique is being replaced gradually by molecular diagnostic methods as the genetic nature of these disorders is revealed. Understanding of the molecular basis of each disease will, in turn, facilitate the formulation of definitive therapy in the future (Francis, 1994).

GENODERMATOSES THAT REPRESENT MOSAICISM

A *genetic mosaic* is an organism composed of two or more genetically different populations of cells that originate from one zygote. When the skin is involved, unique patterning is seen, reflecting the cellular heterogeneity. Variations of this striking pattern were clinically described and mapped in 1901 by Alfred Blaschko. The distribution is known as Blaschko's lines. Blaschko's lines are distinct from dermatomes, skin tension lines, and lines of lymphatic drainage. The pattern is linear and whorled, and may be bilaterally symmetric, with a midline demarcation (Fig. 106–1). An anatomic equivalent has been described in the eyes and teeth (Bolognia et al, 1994). Several diseases are expressed in this fashion. The first to be recognized were X-linked disorders. Affected females are obligate heterozygotes, owing to the Lyon effect of X-inactivation. Examples include female carriers of the X-linked recessive disorder, hypohidrotic ectodermal dysplasia, and females with the X-linked dominant disorders, incontinentia pigmenti, chondrodysplasia punctata, CHILD syndrome (see later), and focal dermal hypoplasia. These conditions are seen almost exclusively in females, presumably because they are lethal in males. Autosomal mosaicism is not heritable unless the germ cells are affected (Happle, 1993).

The Ichthyoses

The *ichthyoses* are a diverse group of heritable and acquired skin disorders that share the primary problem of widespread scaly, dry skin. Several distinct types of ichthyosis have been described on the basis of their clinical and histologic features and their patterns of genetic transmission (Williams, 1983 and 1986), but the nosology is evolving as the molecular basis of these disorders is revealed. Several types of ichthyoses are primary disorders of cornification, with manifestations confined to the skin. Ichthyosiform syndromes have characteristic extracutaneous manifestations. More precise diagnostic criteria and better treatments are being recognized through collaborative research efforts, including genetic analysis. The National Registry for Ichthyosis and Related Disorders was created in 1995 to aid this effort. (For more information, call 800-595-1265.) The Foundation for Ichthyosis and Related Skin Types (FIRST) is a privately funded national organization providing information and support for families with these disorders; they may be contacted by mail at P.O. Box 669, Ardmore, Pennsylvania 19003; and by telephone, 800-545-3286.

Ichthyoses that Present in the Neonatal Period

Three ichthyosiform conditions have alarming presentations at birth. Two of these, the collodion baby and harlequin ichthyosis, have been historically described as distinct entities based on their striking and unique clinical appearance. Long-term survival of these infants, and more refined diagnostic studies, have identified these conditions as phenotypically distinct but genotypically heterogeneous. A third condition, epidermolytic hyperkeratosis (autosomal dominant bullous congenital ichthyosiform erythroderma), has an equally striking neonatal appearance. Another se-

---

TABLE 106–1

Genodermatoses Diagnosed Prenatally Using Fetal Skin Samples (Holbrook et al, 1993)

Epidermolysis bullosa (EB)
  Junctional EB
  Recessive dystrophic EB
  Dominant dystrophic EB
  EB simplex (general)
  EB simplex Dowling-Meara
  Unidentified forms of EB
Keratinization disorders
  Bullous congenital ichthyosiform erythroderma
  Nonbullous congenital ichthyosiform erythroderma/lamellar
    ichthyosis
  Harlequin ichthyosis
  Sjögren-Larsson syndrome
Pigment disorders
  Tyrosinase-negative oculocutaneous albinism
  Congenital nevus
  Incontinentia pigmenti
Disorders of epidermal appendages
  X-linked hypohidrotic ectodermal dysplasia
  Autosomal-recessive anhidrotic ectodermal dysplasia
Other disorders
  Tay's syndrome
  Chédiak-Higashi syndrome
  Griscelli disease
  Restrictive dermopathy

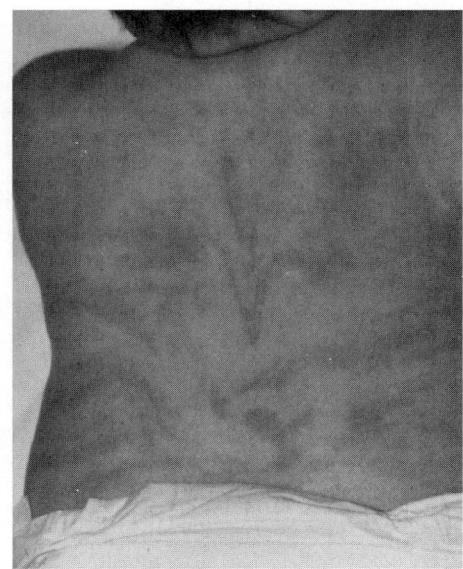

FIGURE 106–1. Blashchko's lines are a distinct linear and whorled pattern, to be distinguished from dermatomes or skin tension lines, characterized by midline demarcation with a central V. This pattern is the cutaneous clinical manifestation of a variety of mosiac genetic conditions.

vere category of infantile ichthyosis, congenital nonbullous ichthyosiform erythrodermal/lamellar ichthyosis, is a difficult diagnostic and management problem. Recognition of these conditions and appropriate management are vital to the survival of these infants.

Collodion Baby

Neonates affected with this uncommon condition have a pathognomonic appearance. With time, they usually express more specific features of one of the ichthyoses.

Clinical Findings. Collodion babies are often premature and small for gestational age (SGA). Their skin is parchment-like, shiny and thickened at birth, distorting their facial features with ectropion and eclabium, flattening the ears and causing pseudocontractures of the digits (Fig. 106–2). Histologic examination of the skin at this stage has been nonspecific, revealing a markedly thickened, compact stratum corneum. Nonetheless, these infants have a very ineffective barrier against transepidermal water loss and invasion of pathogenic microbes, with accompanying temperature instability.

Causes. Several genetically distinct outcomes have been reported for the collodion baby phenotype (see Table 106–1). Two thirds of these infants have nonbullous ichthyosiform erythroderma. Fifty percent of affected infants have no family history suggestive of ichthyosis (Pongprasit, 1993).

Diagnosis. Skin biopsy can be helpful, but is not likely to be specific until after the collodion appearance has resolved. Diagnostic studies should be carefully selected,

based on the evolution of the cutaneous findings, associated abnormalities, and family history (Table 106–2). Several outcomes have been reported, including complete healing without sequelae (Shwayder and Ott, 1991; Frenk, 1992). A prolonged period of observation may be required to determine the precise diagnosis and prognosis. As soon as a definite diagnosis has been made, genetic counseling should be provided.

Treatment. Complications include marked temperature instability, defective barrier function, increased insensible water loss predisposing to hypernatremic dehydration (Boyse et al, 1993), pneumonia secondary to aspiration of squamous material in the amniotic fluid, and cutaneous infections from gram-positive organisms and *Candida albicans*.

Treatment consists of aggressive supportive care. Infants must be placed in a highly humidified isolette. Fluid and electrolyte balance must be closely monitored. A high index of suspicion must be maintained for signs of cutaneous or systemic infection. But overzealous administration of antibiotics may lead to gram-negative infections and subsequent septicemia. Topical skin care should include application of a bland occlusive ointment emollient every 6 to 8 hours until the hyperkeratosis has resolved. Potentially toxic topical agents should be avoided, because of the increased risk of percutaneous absorption. Manual debridement is not indicated. The eyes should be protected with a bland lubricating ointment; aggressive surgical management of ectropion is almost never necessary. Systemic retinoids have not been useful (Waisman et al, 1989). With optimal supportive care, the thickened stratum corneum usually resolves in 2 to 4 weeks but can persist, especially in infants with lamellar ichthyosis.

Harlequin Ichthyosis

This rare congenital abnormality has a more striking appearance and a more grave prognosis than that of collodion baby. Most infants have been stillborn or died in infancy. Survival beyond infancy has only recently been possible. The harlequin phenotype is inherited as an autosomal recessive trait; several biochemical defects probably underlie the clinical condition.

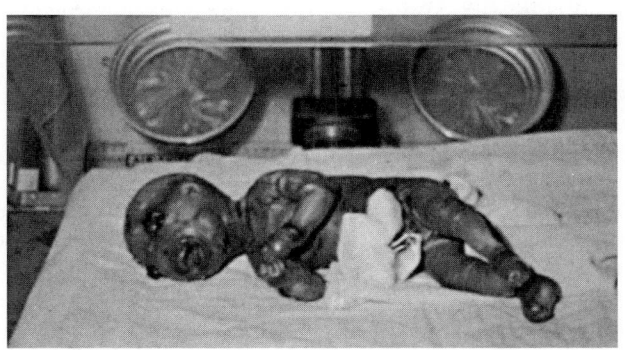

FIGURE 106–2. Harlequin fetus. (Courtesy of Dr. Marvin Cornblath.)

TABLE 106–2

Collodion Baby: Differential Diagnosis and Laboratory Evaluation

Diagnosis	Inheritance	Associated Abnormalities	Diagnostic Tests*
Nonbullous ichthyosiform erythroderma (>60%)	AR, AD		Histology is nonspecific; fetal skin biopsy is unreliable; the gene defect has not been identified
Lamellar ichthyosis	AR, AD	Persistent ectropion	Histology is nonspecific; fetal skin biopsy is unreliable; the gene defect has been identified
X-linked ichthyosis	X-linked recessive	Maternal failure to initiate labor; hypogonadism, undescended testis; corneal opacities (carrier females and affected males)	Histology is nonspecific; decreased serum cholesterol sulfate and steroid sulfatase activity; the gene defect has been mapped to Xp22.3
Netherton's syndrome	Sporadic	Ichthyosis linearis circumflexa, atopic diathesis, impaired cellular immunity	Histology in non-specific; microscopic examination of the hair shaft reveals pathognomonic trichorrhexis invagina
Gaucher's disease	AR	Hepatosplenomegaly, thrombocytopenia, neurologic abnormalities	Liver biopsy; beta glucocerebroside activity; the gene defect has been mapped to 1q21, and sequenced
Trichothiodystrophy (Tay's syndrome)	AR	Progeric facies, neurologic abnormalities, hypogonadism, cataracts, dental problems	Hair analyses: polarizing light microscopic examination reveals characteristic banding; there is decreased content of sulfer-rich matrix proteins
Sjögren-Larsson syndrome	AR	Spasticity, retardation, seizures	Pathognomonic retinal changes; fibroblast culture for fatty alcohol oxidoreductase activity
No detectable abnormality ("Lamellar exfoliation of the newborn")	AR, sporadic		Watchful waiting

*In the immediate neonatal period, skin biopsy may be nonspecific. Histologic evaluation may be postponed until after age 3–6 months.
AR, autosomal recessive; AD, autosomal dominant.
Data on diagnostic tests from Paller AS: Laboratory tests for ichthyosis. Dermatologic Clinics 12:99–107, 1994.

Clinical Findings. The clinical findings are unforgettable. The cutaneous scale is firm and plate-like, distorting and flattening the nose and ears. Skin rigidity also causes deep fissures, marked ectropion, eclabium, and pseudocontractures of all joints. Chemosis of the conjunctivae obscures the globes. The nails and hair are hypoplastic or absent (Fig. 106–3). Primary extracutaneous abnormalities are not prominent.

Diagnosis. The diagnosis is made by the pathognomonic appearance. The light microscopic findings always demonstrate compact hyperkeratosis. Additional light and electron microscopic abnormalities of the stratum corneum have not been identified consistently, supporting the theory that harlequin ichthyosis may represent a common phenotype for several different genetic errors of cornification (Hashimoto, et al, 1993).

Causes. The cause of harlequin ichthyosis is unknown. Although abnormalities of keratinization and epidermal lipid metabolism have been reported, few affected infants have been studied, and no single defect has been identified consistently (Dale and Kam, 1993).

Prognosis and Treatment. Treatment consists of supportive care in a humid, temperature-controlled environment and frequent application of topical emollients to skin and mucosal surfaces, as for collodion baby (Prasad et al, 1994). Nevertheless, infants given these therapies almost invariably succumb to their disease from sepsis, inability to feed, and inadequate ventilation. Survival beyond 6 weeks was extremely unusual prior to the use of oral retinoids. Recent reports have documented successful therapy of several affected infants using oral retinoids, with improved quality of life and survival well into childhood. Etretinate has been used most often, at doses of 1 mg/kg per day. Treated infants must be monitored for toxic effects. All survivors have had severe ichthyosis as an outcome; some have had intellectual impairment. Genetic counseling for the families of these infants is mandatory. Prenatal diagnosis may be made by fetal skin biopsy (Holbrook et al, 1993).

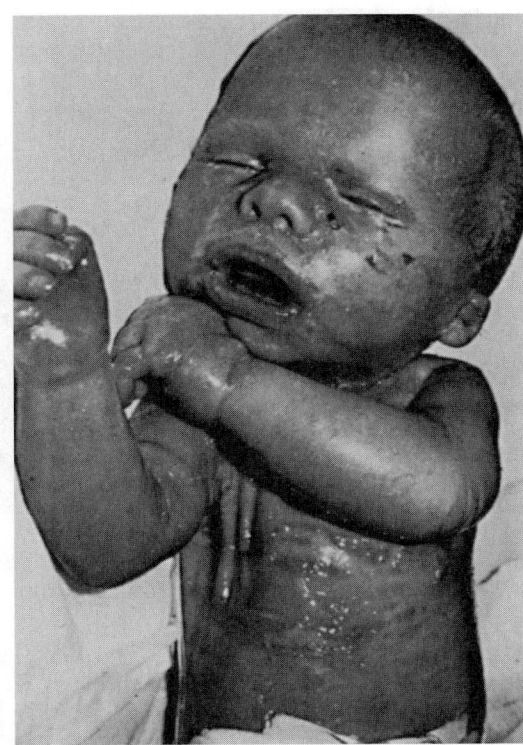

FIGURE 106–3. Collodion baby. Note the ectropion, eclabium, and areas of rupture in the membrane over the anterior thorax.

Epidermolytic Hyperkeratosis (Congenital Bullous Ichthyosiform Erythroderma)

Epidermolytic hyperkeratosis (EHK) is rare, with an estimated incidence of 1:250,000. Neonates with EHK are born with generalized erythroderma and blistering. Their clinical appearance shares cutaneous features of other infantile bullous disorders, especially epidermolysis bullosa (EB). Molecular defects responsible for EHK have recently been identified, proving a biochemical similarity between EHK, EB simplex, and other disorders of keratinization.

Clinical Findings. Infants may be born with generalized erythroderma and blistering. Hyperkeratosis may not be readily apparent. The neonatal course is complicated by temperature instability, susceptibility to hypernatremia, and sepsis, similar to that of the other severe neonatal ichthyoses. With time, the skin changes evolve to include characteristic ridged scales, accentuated in the flexural areas. Palms and soles are usually involved. Excessive bacterial colonization often causes a distressingly foul odor. There are no extracutaneous manifestations.

Diagnosis. There is significant clinical similarity to other bullous disorders of infancy, including epidermolysis bullosa, SSSS, and TEN. Precise diagnosis can be life-saving. Skin biopsy should be performed emergently, with examination of frozen sections. The histologic features of EHK are distinctive, showing intercellular edema, and coarse, clumped material in the upper, granular layers of the epidermis. Prenatal diagnosis is possible by fetal skin biopsy (Holbrook et al, 1993).

Causes. EHK is transmitted in an autosomal dominant fashion, with a high rate of spontaneous mutation. Ultrastructural analysis of skin from affected patients suggests an abnormality of keratin filaments in the suprabasal cells. Molecular analysis of affected families has identified genetic mutations in the genes that code for the synthesis of the keratin filaments that are preferentially expressed in the superficial epidermis, K1 (located within the type I keratin gene cluster at chromosome 17q) or K10 (located within the type II keratin gene cluster at chromosome 12q) (Francis 1994; Nirunsuksiri et al, 1995; Smack et al, 1994; Steijlen et al, 1994). The disorder can also be expressed in mosaic fashion as an epidermal nevus oriented along the lines of Blaschko (Paller et al, 1994). Prenatal studies for EHK may be indicated for offspring of parents with extensive epidermal nevi.

Prognosis and Treatment. Infants with widespread blistering should be managed with the same principles and techniques used for collodion babies. Attention to gentle handling will minimize further trauma. Application of a nonadhesive biooclusive dressing (e.g., hydrogel or foam; see Chapter 105, Table 105–7) will promote healing of denuded areas. Infants should be closely monitored for the development of secondary infection.

Nonbullous Congenital Ichthyosiform Erythroderma/Lamellar Ichthyosis

This category of infantile ichthyosiform skin disease, as distinct from the bullous variety (EHK), was initially characterized by its severity and autosomal recessive inheritance pattern. The term *nonbullous congenital ichthyosiform erythroderma* (CIE) generally refers to a milder clinical variant. Ultrastructural differences have been described in skin biopsy specimens. Recently, the phenotypically more severe lamellar ichthyosis has proved to be genetically distinct as well (Russell et al, 1995).

Clinical Findings. These conditions are characterized by congenital erythroderma and a variable degree of generalized scaling. Face, flexural sites, palms, and soles are also involved. The majority of collodion babies have these types of ichthyosis. In lamellar ichthyosis, the scales evolve to be thick, dark, and platelike (Fig. 106–4). Facial involvement causes chronic ectropion. Hair growth may be sparse, and nails may be dystrophic. Children with CIE have generalized erythema with finer, white scales. There is no associated ectropion. Secondary cutaneous infections with bacteria, yeast, and dermatophytes are common complications.

Diagnosis. Until recently, the diagnosis of these forms of ichthyosis has been based on clinical features alone. Skin biopsy is nonspecific; a normal granular layer is present. The differential diagnosis includes other causes of erythroderma and collodion baby (see Chapter 105). Prenatal diagnosis is possible for affected families (Holbrook et al, 1993). For patients without a previously defined family history, the appropriate laboratory assessment can be arranged through the National Registry for Ichthyosis and Related Disorders.

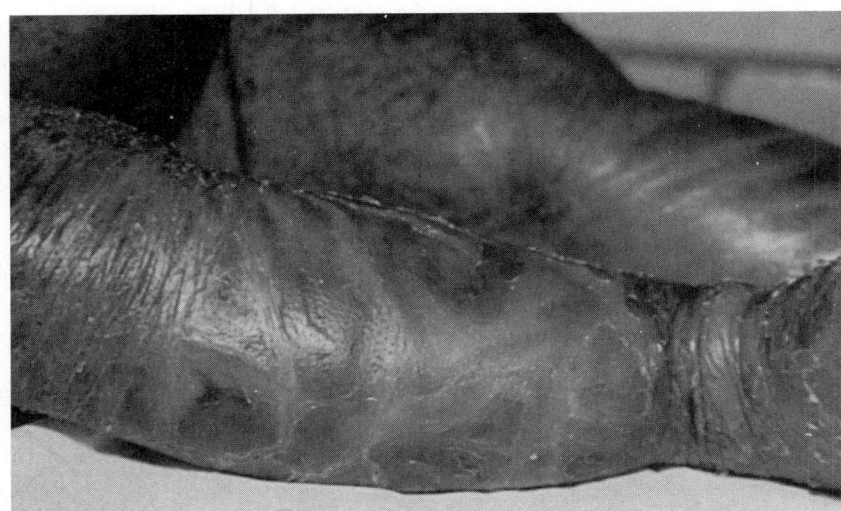

FIGURE 106–4. Large dark scales characteristic of lamellar ichthyosis on the leg of an affected infant.

Causes. The majority of cases are inherited in an autosomal recessive fashion, but an autosomal dominant form of lamellar ichthyosis has also been described. In 1995, a common locus of genetic mutations was identified in several families with recessive lamellar ichthyosis (Russell et al, 1995). The linked defects, located on chromosome 14, result in production of abnormal transglutaminase 1. This enzyme normally promotes cross-linking of intracellular proteins in the stratum corneum during terminal differentiation (Russell et al, 1994; Huber et al, 1995).

Prognosis and Treatment. The same management principles recommended for neonates presenting with the collodion baby phenotype can be applied to infants with erythroderma, although their neonatal course is marked by fewer complications. The mainstay of therapy for children with lamellar ichthyosis is the use of topical emollients and keratolytic agents. Successful treatment with topical calcipotriol has recently been described (Delfino et al, 1994; Russell and Young, 1994). Any topically applied agent will be transcutaneously absorbed to a much higher degree than through normal skin; dosing must be carefully monitored (Lucker, 1994; Abdel-Magid and el-Awad, 1994). Treatment with systemic retinoids has had variable success (Steijlen et al, 1994; Waisman et al, 1989).

Ichthyosiform Syndromes

Several syndromes presenting in the neonatal period have ichthyosis as a major feature.

Recessive X-linked Ichthyosis

Recessive X-linked ichthyosis (RXLI) is an uncommon condition, affecting 1 in 6000 males. Signs of the disorder are present at birth in one fifth of affected individuals; 85% develop skin changes by 3 months of age. The characteristic cutaneous finding is coarse brownish scaling most prominent on the neck and extensor extremities. The palms and soles are spared. Extracutaneous manifestations include hypogonadism and cryptorchidism, in up to 25% of affected males. Severely affected males can have short stature and mental retardation, a variant that has been referred to as Rud's syndrome. Characteristic corneal opacities are seen in affected males and heterozygote females but usually not until late childhood or adolescence. Carrier females experience failure to initiate or prolonged labor. Light microscopic and ultrastructural features of skin biopsy specimens are unremarkable. The pathogenesis of RXLI is aberrant production of the enzyme steroid sulfatase (a form of arylsulfatase C), with accumulation of cholesterol sulfate (Williams, 1986). The genetic abnormality has been localized to the distal short arm of the X chromosome (Xp22.3). Contiguous proximal genetic abnormalities produce the features of Kallman syndrome; distal abnormalities are identified in Conradi syndrome (Goldsmith, 1990).

Ichthyosis Linearis Circumflexa/Netherton's Syndrome

Netherton's syndrome is a rare, autosomal recessive condition. It often presents at birth, as ichthyosiform erythroderma, with flexural accentuation. The characteristic migratory, polycyclic lesions with a peripheral double-edged scale, referred to as ichthyosis linearis circumflexa, do not appear until after age 2. The syndrome is characterized by congenital ichthyosis, hair shaft defects (principally trichorrhexis invaginata), and atopic features (pruritus, hayfever, facial angioedema, and elevated IgE) but diagnosis may not be possible for several years (Judge et al, 1994). Generalized aminoaciduria and impaired cellular immunity have also been reported. This distinctive pattern of ichthyosis linearis circumflexa can also present as an isolated cutaneous condition.

Sjögren-Larsson Syndrome

This autosomal recessive disorder usually presents at birth with ichthyosiform erythroderma. The syndrome includes features that become evident only after the neonatal period: spastic diplegia, characteristic retinal lesions ("glistening dots"), and mental retardation. The diagnosis is supported by finding reduced or absent enzymatic activity of fatty alcohol oxidoreductase from cultured skin fibroblasts, amniocytes, or chorionic cells.

Chondroplasia Punctata Syndromes (Conradi and Conradi-Hünermann)

This loosely defined group of syndromes share distinctive skin and bony abnormalities that are present at birth but may disappear with time. The skin lesions consist of patterned hyperkeratosis along the lines of Blaschko. Orthopedic abnormalities (including asymmetric shortening of the long bones) prompt radiologic evaluation that reveals chondrodysplasia punctata, characteristic punctate calcifications of the epiphyses and cartilage. Abnormal facies and cataracts are associated features. Autosomal dominant, autosomal recessive, and X-linked dominant forms have been reported. The genetic abnormality associated with X-linked dominant Conradi syndrome may be contiguous with that of X-linked recessive ichthyosis.

CHILD Syndrome

This striking phenotype consists of *c*ongenital *h*emidysplasia, unilateral *i*chthyosiform erythroderma, and *l*imb *d*efects and is also known as unilateral congenital ichthyosiform erythroderma. This may represent a variant of X-linked dominant Conradi syndrome.

Keratitis, Ichthyosis, Deafness (KID) Syndrome

This rare, sporadic syndrome consists of congenital ichthyosiform erythroderma with characteristic pebbly palmoplantar thickening, abnormalities of nails, hair, and teeth, vascularizing keratitis, and sensorineural deafness. A few affected patients have died in infancy from overwhelming sepsis (Caceres-Rios et al, 1996).

Neutral Lipid Storage Disease (Chanarin-Dorfman Disease)

This autosomal recessive disorder consists of congenital ichthyosiform erythroderma, myopathy, neurosensory deafness, and cataracts. Vacuolated leukocytes, seen on peripheral smear, help establish the diagnosis (Judge et al, 1994).

Trichothiodystrophy

This is an autosomal recessive disorder that includes a spectrum of ectodermal abnormalities: congenital ichthyosis (sometimes presenting as collodion baby), brittle hair, and short stature (Kousseff, 1991). More severely affected patients have a constellation of findings that has been referred to as *Tay syndrome*. These include abnormal dentition, cataracts, nail dystrophy, progeric facies, photosensitivity with an increased incidence of skin cancers, and a wide variety of central nervous system (CNS) abnormalities. Diagnosis is supported by detection of characteristic alternating light and dark bands within the hair shaft on examination under polarizing microscopy. Further analysis of hair and nails reveals a decrease in the sulfur-rich proteins (Itin and Pittelkow, 1990).

Primary Cutaneous Ichthyoses

Primary cutaneous ichthyoses are a group of familial disorders that have no prominent extracutaneous manifestations. Lamellar ichthyosis, congenital nonbullous icthyosiform erythroderma, and EHK are also primary cutaneous ichthyoses.

Ichthyosis Vulgaris

This is the most common form of ichthyosis, with an estimated incidence of 1 in 250. It is inherited as an autosomal dominant trait. Onset is usually after the first 3 months of life. Scaling is most prominent on the extensor surfaces of the limbs. The palms and soles are also affected. Affected individuals often have coexisting keratosis pilaris and atopic dermatitis (Rabinowitz and Esterly, 1994). Skin biopsy distinguishes ichthyosis vulgaris from the other forms of ichthyosis by revealing small or absent keratohyalin granules. A major component of these granules, profillagrin, is reduced or undetectable in the skin of affected individuals (Nironsuksiri et al, 1995).

Erythrokeratodermia Variabilis

This type of ichthyosis is also very rare; it is inherited in an autosomal dominant fashion and can present in infancy. Affected individuals have transient migratory areas of discrete macular erythema as well as fixed hyperkeratotic plaques.

Prognosis and Treatment. It is important to distinguish between the various forms of ichthyosis so that the physician can offer a prognosis and appropriate genetic counseling to the family. The prognosis is related to the severity of the condition and the type of ichthyosis. The clinical signs and pedigree data sometimes provide sufficient information to make a diagnosis. Skin biopsy for light microscopy is diagnostic only for EHK and ichthyosis vulgaris. Other general screening laboratory tests are equally nonspecific. Unfortunately, a period of observation beyond the first 4 weeks of life is frequently needed, and laboratory confirmation of the correct diagnosis requires specialized studies (Holbrook et al, 1993).

Standard therapy begins with topical care designed to hydrate the stratum corneum. Frequent, brief tepid water baths should be immediately followed by liberal application of a bland ointment or cream emollient, such as petrolatum, Aquaphor, or Eucerin. Emollients containing keratolytics such as urea (10% to 25%), salicylic acid, propylene glycol, and alpha-hydroxy acids are also effective but are recommended only after infancy because of the risk of toxicity associated with increased percutaneous absorption. Irritating soaps and detergents should be avoided. Topical calcipotriol has been safe and effective as a short-term therapy in adults with a variety of ichthyoses (Kragballe et al, 1995).

Albinism

The term *oculocutaneous albinism* refers to a group of congenital disorders that are clinically manifest by absence of pigment of the skin, hair, and eyes, with associated photophobia and nystagmus. All races are affected; estimates of gene frequency vary depending on the population under consideration. As with many genetic disorders, the incidence of affected individuals is increased in certain racial isolates in which there is a high percentage of consanguineous marriages (Witkop et al, 1989).

Causes. All forms of oculocutaneous albinism but one are inherited in an autosomal recessive fashion. The characteristic pigmentary changes are due to a spectrum of biochemical defects that interfere with melanin synthesis or transport. Recent advances in the molecular biology of pigmentation have helped elucidate the pathogenesis of a subset of these disorders. Two types of oculocutaneous albinism have been mapped to specific chromosomal regions that code for regulatory proteins in the transport and synthesis of tyrosine, a precursor in the melanin synthesis pathway (Oetting and King, 1994).

Diagnosis. There are two main subtypes of oculocutaneous albinism, distinguished on the basis of subtle clinical differences and the presence or absence of tyrosinase activity. The tyrosinase-negative variant can be diagnosed prenatally by fetal skin biopsy (Holbrook et al, 1993). Several defects in the tyrosinase gene have been described (Tomita, 1994). Oculocutaneous albinism should be distinguished from simple ocular albinism, which has sex-linked, autosomal dominant and autosomal recessive forms.

Clinical Findings. Affected infants, regardless of their familial skin type, have a decrease in skin pigment. Hair and iris pigmentation can vary, depending on the genotype. Photophobia and nystagmus of variable degree are also type-specific. Visual acuity is almost always impaired. Patients with tyrosine-negative oculocutaneous albinism have the most severe form of visual impairment. Associated abnormalities may include hemorrhagic diathesis (Hermansky-Pudlak syndrome), small stature, and defective mentation. Deafness can occur in association with oculocutaneous albinism as well as with a number of other pigmentary disorders (Konigsmark, 1972).

Prognosis and Treatment. The most significant associated problems are visual impairment and the increased risk of sun-induced carcinogenesis. Treatment is supportive. Religious use of broad-spectrum sunblock with the highest available sun protection factor (SPF) is mandatory to protect against excessive exposure to sunlight. The safest approach for infants is zinc oxide ointment, sun-protective clothing (Sun Precautions, Seattle, WA; 1-800-882-7860), and sun avoidance. Individuals with tyrosinase-positive albinism accumulate pigment with increasing age, decreasing the risk of sun-induced complications. NOAH (National Organization for Albinism & Hypopigmentation) can provide additional information and support for affected families (1-800-473-2310).

Piebaldism

Piebaldism is an autosomal dominant congenital leukoderma, characterized by a white forelock. Histologic studies show an absence of melanocytes in the depigmented areas of skin and normal melanocytes in the uninvolved skin (Jimbow et al, 1975). The molecular basis of the disease has been identified as a defect of the c-kit proto-oncogene. This gene encodes the cell-surface receptor transmembrane tyrosine kinase for an embryonic growth factor. When c-kit function is reduced, the migration of melanocytes is curtailed during embryogenesis (Tomita, 1994).

Clinical Findings. A white forelock is present in 90% of cases. Other areas of the ventral skin may also be devoid of pigment, including the central forehead, chin, and trunk, with relative sparing of the dorsal surface. Eyebrows and midarm and midleg skin may also be depigmented. Within these areas, smaller normally pigmented or hyperpigmented patches may be evident (Fig. 106–5).

Diagnosis. The disorder is readily differentiated from albinism, in which the absence of pigment is uniform. Vitiligo may have a similar appearance, but it is not congenital and usually does not remain fixed. Occasional families may have associated defects such as sensorineural deafness and mental retardation (Telfer et al, 1971). Piebaldism is unrelated to Waardenburg syndrome, an unrelated autosomal dominant condition that features a white forelock, widened nasal bridge, and cochlear deafness.

Prognosis and Treatment. The leukoderma and white forelock remain constant throughout life. Cosmetic camouflage is a treatment option suitable for infants and children. Surgical options are evolving.

Aplasia Cutis Congenita

The congenital absence of skin is a cutaneous anomaly most often seen on the scalp but may involve the skin of the trunk and extremities.

Causes. Several distinct subtypes of aplasia cutis have been described based on the distribution, mode of inheritance, and associated abnormalities (Frieden, 1986). Most aplasia cutis congenita occur sporadically; autosomal dominant and autosomal recessive transmission have also been well documented (Sybert, 1985). Associated abnormalities include cleft lip and palate, limb anomalies, cutaneous organoid nevi, and epidermolysis bullosa. Aplasia cutis may overlie embryologic malformations such as meningomyelocele and spinal dysraphia, omphalocele, and gastroschesis (Frieden, 1986; Sybert, 1985). In addition, scalp defects are associated with specific teratogens (methimazole, intrauterine varicella, and herpes simplex) and malformation syndromes (trisomy 13, Johanson-Blizzard syndrome, amniotic band disruption complex, and the ectodermal dysplasias). Extensive aplasia cutis has been associated with elevated alpha-fetoprotein in maternal serum and amniotic fluid (Gerber et al, 1995).

The cause of aplasia cutis congenita is unknown. Basically, it is a phenotypic physical finding signifying disruption of the skin in utero attributable to any of numerous causes. The findings of a twin fetus papyraceous or a placental infarct have suggested vascular thrombosis as a cause in

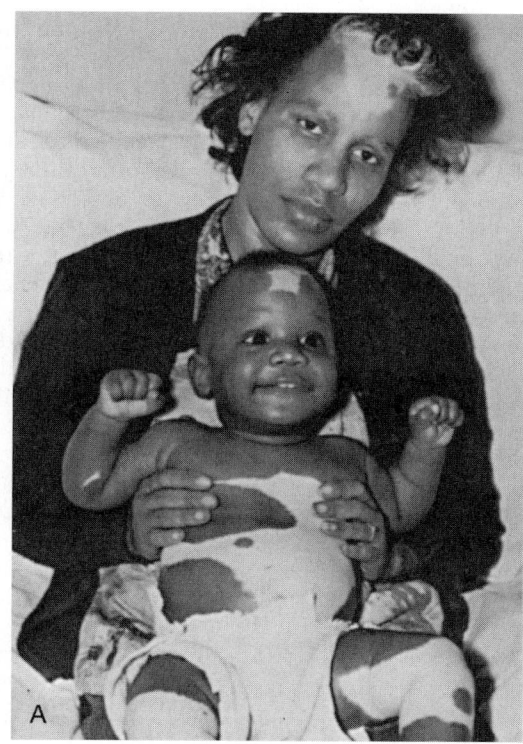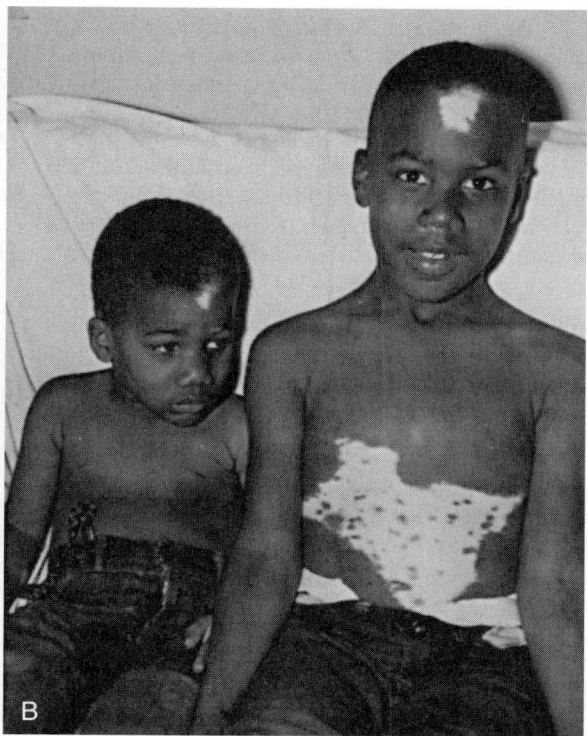

FIGURE 106–5. *A*, Mother and child with piebaldism. Both have patches on the forehead, although of different sizes and shapes. The areas of nonpigmentation on the infant's trunk and extremities are unusually extensive. *B*, Siblings with different degrees of piebaldism. (From Jahn HM, McIntire MS: Am J Dis Child 88:481, 1954. © American Medical Association.)

infants with lesions on the trunk and limbs (Levin et al, 1980).

Clinical Findings. The defect is usually along the midline of the scalp in the parietal or occipital areas. Lesions are sharply marginated and may present as ulcers, bullae, or scars. Lesions may be solitary or multiple, measuring up to several centimeters in diameter (Fig. 106–6). Up to 30% have underlying defects of the calvarium. Multiple defects, particularly those on the trunk and extremities, may be strikingly symmetric in distribution (Levin et al, 1980). Larger defects are often deeper and may extend to the dura or meninges. These may be complicated by meningitis, hemorrhage (which can be fatal), or venous thrombosis.

Histologic examination of tissue from the defect demonstrates an absent epidermis and a diminished number of appendageal structures and dermal elastic fibers or, in deeper lesions, the absence of all layers of the integument. There is no evidence of inflammation or pathogenic organisms.

Prognosis and Treatment. Cutaneous and bony lesions can heal spontaneously over a period of weeks to months. A hypertrophic or atrophic patch of alopecia remains. Patients with larger and deeper lesions must be observed for the possibility of a complicating meningitis. Prophylactic excision with repair should be considered in these cases. Lesions that fail to heal or produce cosmetically unacceptable scars can be excised with primary closure (Kosnik and Sayers, 1975).

Incontinentia Pigmenti

Incontinentia pigmenti (IP), also known as the Bloch-Sulzberger syndrome, is a disorder of the developing neuroectoderm, characterized by three distinctive, transient stages of cutaneous lesions and variable persistant abnormalities of the CNS, eyes, teeth, hair, and nails.

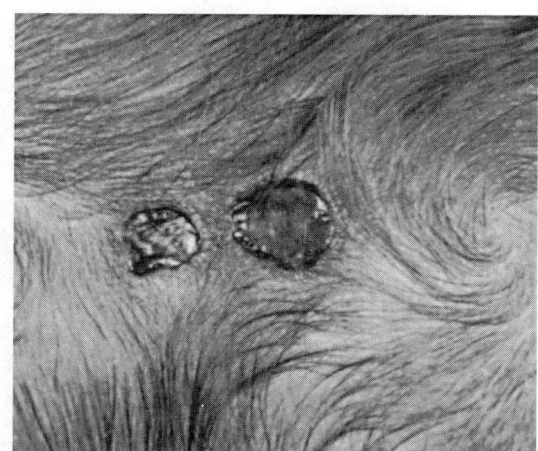

FIGURE 106–6. Two sharply marginated areas of absent skin on the scalp of a normal newborn male infant whose mother's labor and delivery were normal. The defects extended to the subcutaneous tissue and healed in 3 weeks with the formation of thin, white atrophic scars.

Causes. IP is inherited in an X-linked dominant fashion. Surviving females are mosaics, whereas most hemizygous males do not survive embryogenesis. Geneologic analyses have described a male-to-female ratio of 37:1. There is a high rate of spontaneous abortion of at-risk males (Emery et al, 1993). Two distinct gene loci have been identified. X/autosome translocations have suggested a locus on the short arm of X (Xp11.21), and linkage analysis has mapped the gene to Xq28 (Emery et al, 1993).

Clinical Findings. The diagnosis of IP is made by cutaneous examination. Most patients exhibit three stages of skin lesions that persist for variable periods (O'Brien and Feingold, 1985). The vesiculobullous phase presents at birth and generally lasts for several months. It is characterized by widespread inflammatory vesicular lesions on the scalp, trunk, and extremities in a whorled and linear distribution along the lines of Blaschko (Fig. 106–7A). The infant is otherwise well, although a peripheral eosinophilia as high as 50% may be associated. The vesicular phase evolves into a verrucous phase, in which warty lesions appear in roughly the same distribution as the blisters but are most pronounced on the hands and feet. The third stage is characterized by macular gray or brown pigmentation distributed along Blaschko's lines, independent of the sites of previous lesions (see Fig. 106–7B). The pigmentary lesions usually fade in later years and may disappear by adulthood. Rarely, the stage three pigmentary changes are present at birth, and the first two stages are never evident (Lerer et al, 1973). Fourth-stage lesions seen in some affected women consist of hypopigmented, atrophic, anhidrotic streaks, usually localized to the legs (Moss and Ince, 1987).

Eighty percent of affected individuals have extracutaneous involvement, including CNS aberrations (seizures, microcephaly, retardation, and spastic paralysis), patchy alopecia, defective dentition, ocular abnormalities, and less commonly, bony defects (Carney, 1976).

Diagnosis. Infants with IP usually present with blisters. The linear distribution of blisters is often so characteristic that it permits instant recognition of the disorder. But other causes of blisters must be considered in the differential diagnosis (see Chapter 105). Skin biopsy during the bullous phase will show intraepidermal vesicles filled with eosinophils. These features are not pathognomonic but help exclude more ominous causes of neonatal blistering.

Prognosis and Treatment. Treatment of the skin lesions is not necessary. Occasionally, vesicular lesions become extremely inflamed or secondarily infected. Patients should be monitored for the development of other anomalies, especially of the eyes, teeth, and CNS. Genetic counseling is indicated.

Cutis Laxa

Cutis laxa is a rare, heterogeneous group of genetic abnormalities of connective tissue with striking cutaneous features. Autosomal dominant, autosomal recessive, and X-linked forms have been described (Beighton, 1972; Byers

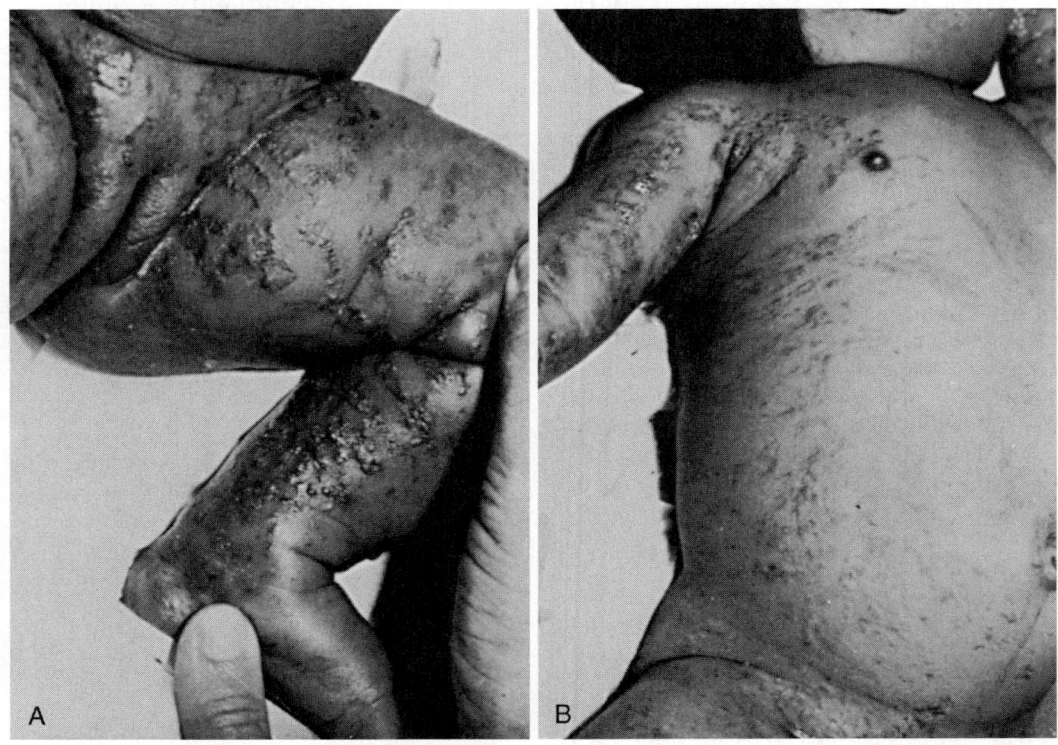

FIGURE 106–7. Incontinentia pigmenti. *A,* Inflammatory vesicular and crusted lesions on the legs. *B,* Whorled pigmentation developing on the trunk of a 1-month-old infant who still has inflammatory lesions on the limbs.

et al, 1980). Cutis laxa-like skin changes can also be found in other disorders (e.g., combined immunodeficiency disease and the Prader-Willi and Langer-Giedion syndromes).

Clinical Features. The skin of cutis laxa hangs in pendulous folds, producing a facies with hooked nose, everted nostrils, a long upper lip, sagging cheeks, and a prematurely aged appearance (Fig. 106–8). The infant may have a hoarse cry due to redundant laryngeal tissue. Individuals with the autosomal dominant form of cutis laxa suffer few ill effects, apart from their altered appearance, and enjoy good health and a normal life span. Pulmonary and cardiovascular manifestations are absent or minimal. In contrast, patients with the recessive form of the disorder are often seriously compromised and may die in childhood of pulmonary or cardiovascular complications. Systemic manifestations include diverticula of the gastrointestinal and urogenital tracts, rectal prolapse, multiple hernias, pulmonary emphysema, and cardiac disease (Mehregan et al, 1978). A few infants have been reported who manifested additional defects, such as skeletal anomalies, dislocation of the hips, and intrauterine growth retardation (Sakati et al, 1983).

Diagnosis. The clinical manifestations of cutis laxa can be attributed to abnormalities of elastin. Elastic fibers are diminished in the papillary and upper dermis, whereas those in the lower dermis undergo fragmentation and granular degeneration (Mehregan et al, 1978). Similar changes occur in the elastic tissue of affected viscera. Autosomal recessive cutis laxa has been associated with a deficiency of lysyl oxidase, a copper-dependant enzyme mapped to chromosome 5 (Khakoo et al, 1997). The X-linked form has been associated with abnormal intracellular copper metabolism, with a decrease in the activity of lysyl oxidase. This form of cutis laxa has also been classified as a subtype (Type IX) of Ehlers-Danlos syndrome. It is probably allelic to Menkes syndrome (see Fig. 106–8) (Goldsmith, 1990; Byers, 1994).

Treatment

Plastic surgery can improve the physical appearance of these patients (Thomas et al, 1993). The internal manifestations are not amenable to therapy.

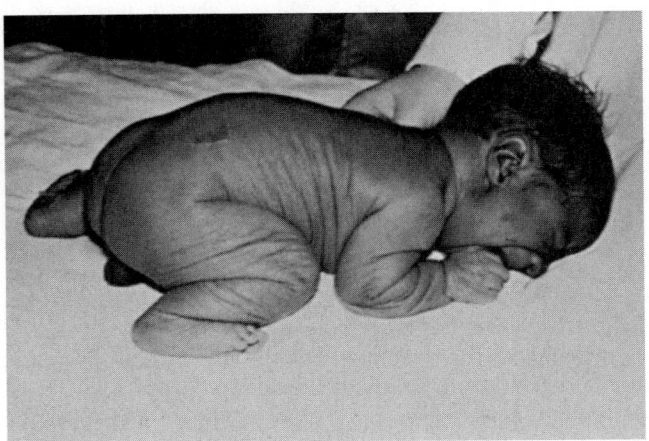

FIGURE 106–8. Newborn infant with clinical features of Menkes syndrome and cutis laxa.

Ehlers-Danlos Syndrome

The Ehlers-Danlos syndrome (EDS) is another heterogeneous group of inherited connective tissue disorders. In contrast to patients with cutis laxa, those with EDS have skin that is hyperextensible rather than loose; when stretched, the skin readily snaps back into place. Skin fragility is another feature, leading to easy bruising and bleeding, gaping wounds, and numerous cigarette-paper–like scars. Joint hypermobility is another major manifestation. Five types of EDS can be distinguished by associated clinically apparent abnormalities. Four additional subsets are defined on the basis of biochemical or molecular genetic studies. Individuals with type IV EDS can be easily distinguished from the other forms by their thin, translucent skin, marked bruising, and normal range of motion. It is especially important to identify this group because of its life-threatening complications (Byers, 1994).

Causes. More than 10 forms of EDS have been delineated on the basis of differences in clinical, genetic, and biochemical findings (Byers, 1994; Schachner and Hansen, 1988). All forms of EDS are believed to be due to defects in the biogenesis of collagen. Type IV EDS is characterized by a variety of defects in the synthesis of type III collagen, type VI by lysyl hydroxylase deficiency, type VII by procollagen N-proteinase deficiency, type IX by reduced activity of lysyl oxidase, and type X by a defect in fibronectin. These specific defects can be identified by culture of dermal fibroblasts from a skin biopsy.

Treatment. Recognition of the correct subtype is important for prognosis. EDS type IV is particularly important to identify because of the life-threatening association with arterial, bowel, and uterine rupture. There is no effective treatment for the various forms of EDS. These patients tolerate surgical procedures poorly because of difficulty in healing and frequent dehiscence of surgical wounds. Repair of cutaneous wounds may require the services of a plastic surgeon and progressive joint disease will require ongoing orthopedic care. The Ehlers-Danlos National Foundation can provide additional information and support for affected families: 6399 Wilshire Boulevard, Suite 510, Los Angeles, CA 90048; (213) 651-3038.

Epidermolysis Bullosa

Epidermolysis bullosa (EB) is a diverse group of diseases that is characterized by skin blistering. Classification is based on clinical characteristics, inheritance pattern, and the level of cleavage within the skin, as determined by skin biopsy. This prominent histologic feature defines three main groups: simplex (within the basal cells of the epidermis), junctional (within the lamina lucida of the basement membrane zone), and dystrophic (beneath the lamina densa of the basement membrane). At each level, there are several protein components that contribute to skin integrity. These molecules are all expressed in utero during the first trimester, allowing prenatal diagnosis by skin biopsy (Holbrook et al, 1993). Many patients have been described with clinical variants of these major forms, and more than 20 subtypes have been delineated (Fine et al,

1991; Fine et al, 1994). Research efforts have been greatly enhanced by DEBRA (Dystrophic Epidermolysis Bullosa Research Association of America, Inc.) and the National Epidermolysis Bullosa Registry (Fine et al, 1994). Identification of the molecular basis of a number of EB genotypes has not only facilitated prenatal and postnatal diagnosis but has also provided insight into the pathogenesis of blistering diseases, as well as the basic mechanisms of epithelial and basement membrane integrity.

Epidermolysis Bullosa Simplex

Epidermolysis bullosa simplex features blisters that arise within the basal layer of the epidermis. For this reason, the lesions of EB simplex do not scar. Two localized and seven generalized forms have been reported (Fine et al, 1991). The molecular defects of EB simplex have been localized to the keratin filaments, K14 (located on chromosome 17) and K5 (located on chromosome 12). These keratins are predominantly expressed in the basal cells of the epidermis. As a primary defect of keratin, this disorder is closely related to epidermolytic hyperkeratosis (Francis, 1994) (see the section on ichthyoses). The three most well-defined subtypes are described.

Generalized Epidermolysis Bullosa Simplex, Koebner Variant

This form of EB, inherited as an autosomal dominant trait, is present at birth or early in infancy. Bullae arise most frequently over pressure points, such as the elbows and knees as well as on the legs, feet, and hands. Mucous membrane involvement occurs primarily during infancy. The extensive erosions that sometimes result from the trauma of birth may be mistaken for aplasia cutis. Nails may be lost but almost always regrow. The prognosis is relatively good, and the propensity to blister may decrease with age.

Generalized Epidermolysis Bullosa, Dowling-Meara Variant

This autosomal dominant variant of EB simplex causes generalized, often extensive, blistering in the neonatal period and early years of life. Herpetiform grouping of the blisters is characteristic. Additional findings include nail dystrophy, palmoplantar keratoderma as a late feature, and improvement with age.

Localized Epidermolysis Bullosa, Weber-Cockayne Variant

The blisters in this disease are usually limited to the hands and feet, although they occasionally occur elsewhere on the body. This type of epidermolysis bullosa, which is inherited in an autosomal dominant fashion, usually does not occur during the neonatal period.

Junctional Epidermolysis Bullosa

Junctional EB is characterized by cleavage within the lamina lucida of the basement membrane zone. Four localized variants and three generalized variants have been described (Fine et al, 1991). Molecular defects have been recognized within several proteins that make up the anchoring filaments (e.g., kalinin, epiligrin, nicein, BM 600). Several subtypes of junctional EB are relatively localized and benign. The most severe form is described below.

Junctional Epidermolysis Bullosa, Herlitz Type

Autosomal recessive junctional EB, Herlitz type, has also been known as EB gravis or letalis because many of these patients die in infancy. Blistering is noted at birth. The most serious associated extracutaneous manifestation is gastric outlet obstruction, which should be assumed in an affected neonate born following polyhydramnios. Individuals with this form of junctional EB can, however, exhibit a spectrum of severity. Bullae and moist erosions occur on the scalp, in the perioral area, and over pressure points elsewhere on the body (Fig. 106–9A). Some of these erosions become the sites of vegetating granulomas, a pathognomonic finding. The hands and feet are relatively spared, and digital fusion, inevitable in the recessive dystrophic type of epidermolysis bullosa, does not occur. Nails are affected and may be lost permanently. Defective dentition is the rule, but mucous membrane erosions are inconspicuous and rarely cause problems. Laryngeal involvement can occur in childhood, manifested as hoarseness or stridor. These patients grow poorly, appear malnourished, and have chronic recalcitrant anemia. The anchoring filaments responsible for attachment of the basal cells to the basement membrane are reduced in number and abnormally structured, owing to a defect in the protein kalinin (Francis, 1994).

Dystrophic Epidermolysis Bullosa

Dystrophic EB is characterized by subepidermal blistering, below the level of the lamina densa of the basement membrane. The anchoring fibrils that link the lower part of the basement membrane to the papillary dermis are comprised of Type VII collagen. Mutations of the gene that codes for Type VII collagen have been identified in several forms of dystrophic EB. This group of diseases is clinically characterized by milia and scarring at sites of healed blisters. At least four localized and four generalized forms have been described. Of the generalized forms, two are autosomal recessive and two are dominant. All are present at birth (Fine et al, 1991). Prenatal diagnosis as early as 8 to 10 weeks is possible by molecular techniques for some families. Selected subtypes are described below.

Transient Bullous Dermolysis of the Newborn

This rare variant was first reported in 1985. Affected neonates present with alarming acral or generalized blistering that heals with scars. Histologic analyses have localized the abnormality to the precursors of the anchoring fibrils and lamina densa, components of the subepidermal zone (Hashimoto and Eng, 1992). Autosomal dominant and recessive forms have been described. This condition is unique among the subsets of EB because it spontaneously resolves within the first year of life.

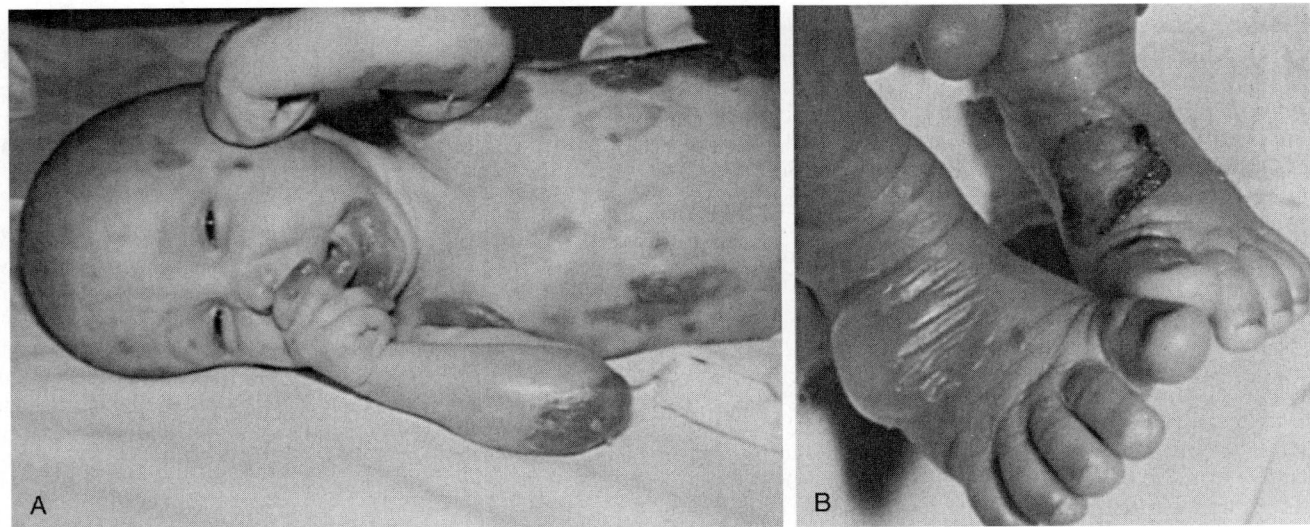

FIGURE 106–9. *A*, Multiple moist erosions characteristic of junctional epidermolysis bullosa. Note involvement of fingers and perioral skin. *B*, Large bullae on the feet of an infant with a scarring form of epidermolysis bullosa.

Recessive Dystrophic Epidermolysis Bullosa Gravis, Hallopeau-Siemens Variant

This variant is the more severe form of recessive dystrophic EB. Infants with Hallopeau-Siemens EB often have extensive denuded lesions at birth and during the neonatal period. Bullae may be hemorrhagic and occur on all surfaces, including the hands and feet; loss of the nails is usual. Over subsequent years the mobility of the fingers and toes becomes severely restricted, as fusion of digits, bone resorption, and the inevitable mitten-like deformity of the hands and feet ensue. Mucous membrane involvement may be severe, resulting in esophageal strictures and serious impairment of nutrition due to the restriction of oral intake. These bullae are subepidermal and always eventuate in scarring. Electron microscopy reveals diminished or absent anchoring fibrils associated with marked degeneration of Type VII collagen in the papillary portion of the dermis. Also evident is excess abnormal collagenase in fibroblast cultures.

Dominant Dystrophic Epidermolysis Bullosa

Most of the localized forms of dystrophic EB are autosomal dominantly inherited. The localized forms may cause blistering only in very specific areas and may become less pronounced with increasing age.

The two generalized forms of dominant dystrophic EB (Cockayne-Touraine and Pasini variants) tend to be less severe than recessive dystrophic EB. The bullae are subepidermal and heal with scarring, but the process may be relatively limited, involving mainly hands, feet (see Fig. 106–9*B*), and skin over bony protuberances or may be generalized, particularly in the Pasini variant. Nails may be lost. Milia are common and may appear in profusion in the soft, wrinkled scars; pigmentary changes are also usual. Mucous membrane lesions, if present, are mild, and general health may be unimpaired. The appearance of albo-papuloid lesions on the trunk during adolescence is a unique feature of the Pasini variant.

Diagnosis. Arriving at the correct diagnosis can be difficult, especially in the neonatal period. The differential diagnosis includes the spectrum of blisters and bullae outlined in Chapter 105. The distribution of blisters can be a clue. In EB, the earliest lesions occur on points of friction, such as the heels, wrists, knees, and sacrum. The fluid within the bullae is likely to be clear or hemorrhagic, rather than purulent. A careful family history for blistering diseases should be obtained. The most precise diagnostic tool is a carefully performed skin biopsy for immunofluorescence mapping and ultrastructural study. The sample for immunofluorescence should be obtained from normal or perilesional skin, excluding the palms or soles, and placed in Zeus's or Michel's transport medium. The ideal specimen for electron microscopy is a new spontaneous or induced blister preserved in glutaraldehyde (Fine et al, 1994). After the diagnosis of simplex, junctional, or dystrophic EB is made, further subclassification can be difficult during infancy, for subsets without a defined genotype. In these patients without relevant family history, distinguishing clinical features may take months or years to develop.

Treatment. To date, the mainstay of therapy for this group of disorders is supportive. The infant should be protected from frictional trauma; direct pressure is tolerated. Latex gloves can stick to the skin and should be lubricated with petrolatum. Bedding should be of a soft material. Dressing changes should be performed daily. Adequate premedication for pain control should be given. Bathing may have to be restricted to avoid excessive handling. Compresses with normal saline or Burow solution for eroded areas may be helpful in some instances. Tepid compresses should be used because warm temperatures increase the tendency to blister. Intact blisters should be lanced with an adequate incision to drain the fluid while maintaining the roof, as a "biologic dressing." Wounds should be covered with petrolatum-impregnated gauze. Topical antibiotics may promote healing, but content and quantity should be carefully monitored in young infants (see Chapter 105). Topical mupirocin is the antibiotic of choice at several EB centers; bacterial resistance has been reported in chronic users with EB. Commercially available nonadhesive dressings are simpler to use and more effective than plain gauze wraps. Exudry pads, secured with Surginet or Conforming Gauze, are recommended for draining wounds on the body. Omiderm (Doak Pharmaceuticals) is a nonadhesive, polyurethane dressing that provides an excellent barrier for moist wounds on the face and hands. Adhesive tape should never be applied because large areas of epidermis may be torn off with its removal. Dressing should be applied to blistered areas only to maximize the infant's tactile stimulation. For the newborn, environmental (isolette) temperature must be carefully monitored; overheating may result in extensive blistering. For patients with mucous membrane involvement, soft nipples, bulb syringes, and devices used for feeding infants with cleft palates should be used. Chronic serosanguinous drainage and gastrointestinal involvement often result in poor nutritional status. Iron-deficiency anemia is another common complication in infants with severe disease. Aggressive nutritional supplementation is routinely recommended. After discharge, cribs, high chairs, and infant seats should be well padded, and only soft toys offered for play (Gibbons, 1990).

Caregivers should be given anticipatory guidance about protective measures, wound care, and nutrition. Encourage contact with DEBRA. This privately funded organization is an excellent resource for affected families. DEBRA can provide practical information for day-to-day care and direct families to the appropriate regional center for specialized care: 141 Fifth Avenue, Suite 7-S, New York, NY 10010; (212) 995-2220.

To register newly diagnosed patients, contact the National EB Registry: c/o Jo-David Fine, MD, Principal Investigator, or Lorraine B. Jonnson, ScD, Coordinator; Department of Dermatology, University of North Carolina; Suite 3100, Thurston Building CB #7287; Chapel Hill, NC 27599; (919) 966-6383. The west coast registry is located at Stanford University Medical Center. Referrals may be arranged by contacting Dr. Lexie Nall: (415) 725-8839.

Neonatal Lupus Erythematosus

Neonatal lupus erythematosus (NLE) is an uncommon immune-mediated disease that results from transplacental transfer of maternal IgG antinuclear antibodies. It presents within the first 2 months of life. Infants manifest a spectrum of signs, including transient cutaneous lesions, thrombocytopenia, hepatitis, and/or congenital heart block; all have serologic evidence of lupus erythematosus during the first few months of life (Lee, 1993; Lee and Weston, 1984; Provost et al, 1987).

Causes. Neonatal lupus erythematosus is always marked by the presence of anti-Ro (SS-A), anti-La (SS-B), and/or anti-U_1RNP autoantibodies in mother and infant. With the exception of congenital heart block, most of the manifestations of neonatal lupus resolve with disappearance of maternal antibody, suggesting an important role for these antibodies in pathogenesis. An association with HLA-DR$_3$ in the mother but not the infant has also been documented (Lee and Weston, 1984). Ro-positive, HLA-DR$_2$ mothers, in contrast, produce unaffected infants (Provost et al, 1987).

Clinical Findings. Half of affected infants have skin lesions. These may be present with or without evidence of systemic disease (Hardy et al, 1979). Skin lesions are typically annular erythematous scaling plaques (Fig. 106–10), with a predilection for sun-exposed areas. These begin to resolve at about 6 months concurrent with the disappearance of maternal antibodies. Persistent telangiectatic matting in a characteristic distribution, involving the scalp, lips, and vulva, has also been described (Fig. 106–11) (Thornton et al, 1995).

Diagnosis. The skin lesions of NLE can be mistaken for several cutaneous disorders including syphilis, seborrheic dermatitis, dermatophytosis, atopic dermatitis, and psoriasis. Skin biopsy may demonstrate the histopathologic features of lupus. More reliable, however, is the detection of Ro (SS-A) and/or La (SS-B) antibody in serum from the infant and mother. The North American Collaborative Study of NLE is headed by Earl Silverman, MD. This is a prospective study of all aspects of the disease. Enrollment and serologic testing can be arranged at The Hospital for Sick Children, 555 University Avenue, Toronto, Ontario, Canada M5G 1X8; (416) 813–6249.

Prognosis and Treatment. Affected infants should be protected from sources of ultraviolet light (sunlight and daylight fluorescent bulbs) by application of a broad-spectrum sunscreen like titanium dioxide, zinc oxide, and sun-protective clothing (Sun Precautions, Seattle, Washington; 1-800-882-7860). Active skin lesions may be treated with a topical corticosteroid.

It is important to recognize that asymptomatic mothers are at risk for development of disorders associated with their abnormal serologies (e.g., Sjögren's syndrome, subacute cutaneous lupus, or systemic lupus erythematosus). There is a 25% risk of involvement for each subsequent

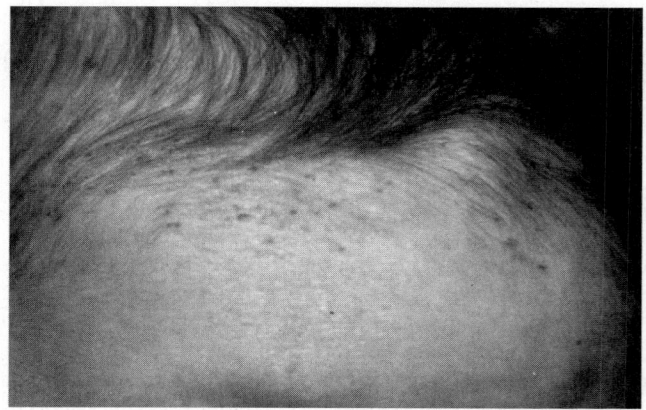

FIGURE 106–10. Newborn with cutaneous lesions of neonatal lupus erythematosus.

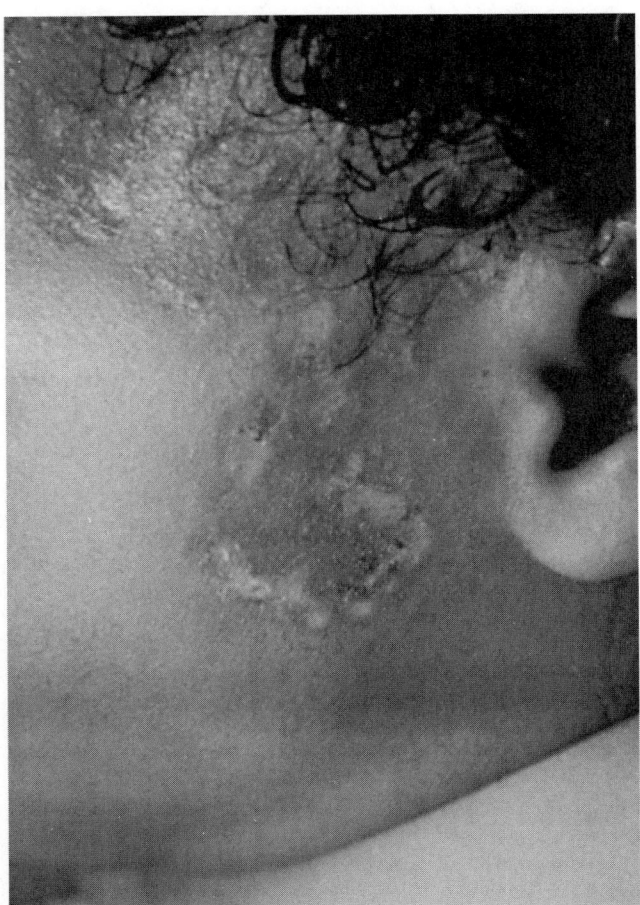

FIGURE 106–11. Telangiectatic matting of the scalp, lips, and groin is a recently recognized cutaneous marker of neonatal lupus.

pregnancy (Gawkrodger and Beveridge, 1984; McCune et al, 1987).

Ectodermal Dysplasias

The ectodermal dysplasias are a heterogeneous group of inherited disorders characterized by defects in the development of two or more structures of ectodermal origin. The major structures involved are hair follicles, nails, teeth, and sweat glands; sebaceous glands, conjunctivae, and/or the lens may also be affected. A formal classification system has been created for the EDs, based on the particular structures affected (Pinheiro and Freire-Maia, 1994). One hundred fifty-four syndromes have been included in this grouping. Several of these, such as incontinentia pigmenti and syndromes associated with ichthyosis, have not been traditionally regarded as ED. Many others have been reported rarely. The National Foundation for Ectodermal Dysplasias (NFED, 219 E. Main St., Mascouteh, Illinois 62258; [618] 566-2020) is a privately funded organization committed to locating affected families and providing them with information and support. The NFED also coordinates and funds research efforts.

Three of the more well-described types of ED are described.

Hypohidrotic Ectodermal Dysplasia

This X-linked recessive disorder was the first type of ED described, as Christ-Siemens-Touraine syndrome. It was previously referred to as "anhidrotic," but affected individuals may have a limited capacity to sweat, and the preferred descriptor is "hypohidrotic." This type of ED occurs in 1 in 100,000 male births and presents during the first year of life. The most serious problem is diminution of the sweating response due to rudimentary or absent eccrine sweat glands, which results in marked heat intolerance and episodes of hyperpyrexia, frequently misinterpreted as fever of unknown origin (Richards and Kaplan, 1969). If ED is not considered in the differential diagnosis, these infants may be subjected to numerous unnecessary hospitalizations and tests.

Clinical Features. Patients with hypohidrotic ectodermal dysplasia have several characteristic features that may be subtle in the newborn. One common neonatal sign is severe peeling or scaling skin. This skin change, which can be misconstrued as an indication of postmaturity, may provide a valuable clue to the diagnosis (Executive and Scientific Advisory Boards of the NFED, 1989). Thereafter, the skin may appear relatively pale and dry, with a prominent venous pattern over most of the body, but hyperpigmented and wrinkled in the periorbital area (Fig. 106–12).

The craniofacial characteristics of frontal bossing, depression of the central face, flattened nasal bridge, thick protruding lips, and prominent chin may not be readily apparent in the newborn. Likewise, the sparse, unruly, light-colored hair and scanty brows and lashes are also difficult to appreciate in the first few months. The changes in dentition cannot, of course, be detected until late infancy. Hypodontia with conical, poorly formed teeth is the rule; these changes can be identified on dental panoramic radiographs prior to eruption of the teeth. Atrophic rhinitis, diminished lacrimation, hoarseness, and hypoplastic or absent mucous glands in nasotracheobronchial passages are also frequent findings in these patients (Reed et al, 1970). If the diagnosis is in doubt, palmar skin biopsy may demon-

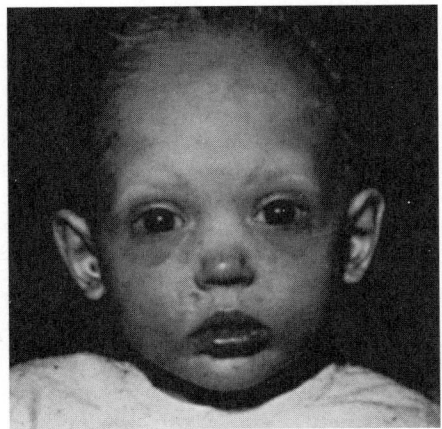

FIGURE 106–12. Female with fully expressed anhidrotic ectodermal dysplasia. Note the sparse, wispy hair, hyperpigmentation around the eyes, depressed nasal bridge, and protruding lips and ears.

strate absent or hypoplastic eccrine sweat glands. Techniques used to elicit sweating, such as pilocarpine iontophoresis or examination of the sweat pores on the palm with *O*-phthalaldehyde, can also be utilized to demonstrate the defect (Esterly et al, 1973). Atopic dermatitis occurs frequently in these children (Reed et al, 1970), as well as a decrease in T-cell function (Davis and Solomon, 1976).

This disorder is transmitted as an X-linked recessive trait. The gene has been localized to Xq11.21.1. First trimester prenatal diagnosis is possible (Zonana et al, 1990). All affected males fully express the disease, whereas carrier females have variable expression of the clinical signs. This expression can be explained by the inactivation of a random percentage of abnormal X chromosomes. In these females, hypohidrosis can be demonstrated in areas of skin marking the lines of Blaschko (see the section on mosaicism) (Bolognia et al, 1994; Crump and Danks, 1971; Esterly et al, 1973; Gorlin et al, 1970).

Once the diagnosis is made, it is important to educate parents so that these children are protected from overheating. Defective lacrimation can be palliated by the use of artificial tears. The nasal mucosa should be treated with saline drops or irrigation followed by application of petrolatum. Regular dental evaluations should be started early in life and dentures fitted to promote good nutrition, articulation, and normal appearance prior to starting school. Some of these children also choose a wig and reconstructive procedures later in life to improve facial configuration.

Hidrotic Ectodermal Dysplasia

Hidrotic ED, also known as Clouston syndrome, is an autosomal dominant condition. Affected individuals have characteristic abnormalities of skin, hair, and nails, whereas eccrine and sebaceous functions and dentition are normal. The phenotype is easily recognizable in early childhood, including thickened, conical nails and widening of the distal periungual area with cerebriform furrowing. The skin over the joints is often hyperpigmented. The degree of alopecia is variable. Neither the genetic locus nor molecular basis of the disorder has been discovered.

EEC Syndrome

The EEC syndrome is an autosomal dominant condition, featuring ectodermal dysplasia (including dental, ocular, nail, and hair defects), ectrodactyly (lobster-claw deformity of the hand), and cleft lip-palate. The cutaneous and appendageal anomalies include diffuse hypopigmentation affecting both skin and hair, scanty scalp hair and eyebrows, dystrophic nails, and small teeth with enamel hypoplasia. Sweating appears to be intact, and sweat glands are present on skin biopsy. The clefting of the lip is usually complete and bilateral, and the palate has a median cleft. Dry granulomatous lesions in the corners of the mouth are often secondarily infected with *Candida albicans*. Other findings include scarred lacrimal ducts, blepharitis and conjunctivitis, xerostomia, conductive hearing loss, and retardation. Neither the genetic abnormality nor the molecular defect have been identified.

REFERENCES

Abdel-Magid EH, el-Awad FR: Salicylate intoxication in an infant with ichthyosis transmitted through skin ointment—a case report. Pediatrics 94:939–940, 1994.

Beighton P: The dominant and recessive forms of cutis laxa. J Med Genet 9:216, 1972.

Bolognia JL, Orlow SJ, Glick SA: Lines of blaschko. J Am Acad Dermatol 31:157–190, 1994.

Briggaman RA: Hereditary epidermolysis bullosa with special emphasis on newly recognized syndromes and complications. Dermatol Clin 1:263, 1983.

Buyse L, Marks R, Wijeyesekera K, et al: Collodion baby dehydration: The danger of high transepidermal water loss. Br J Dermatol 129:86–88, 1993.

Byers PH: Ehlers-Danlos syndrome: Recent advances and current understanding of the clinical and genetic heterogeneity. J Inves Dermatol 103:47S–49S, 1994.

Byers PH, Siegel RC, Holbrook KA, et al: X-linked cutis laxa. N Engl J Med 303:61, 1980.

Caceres-Rios H, Tamayo-Sanchez L, Duran-McKinster C, Ruiz-Maldonado R: Keratitis, ichthyosis, and deafness (KID syndrome): Review of the literature and proposal of a new terminology. Pediatr Dermatol 13(2):105–113, 1996.

Carney RG Jr: Incontinentia pigment: A world statistical analysis. Arch Dermatol 112:535, 1976.

Clarke A, Sarfarazi M, Thomas NS, et al: X-linked hypohidrotic ectodermal dysplasia: DNA probe linkage analysis and gene localization. Hum Genet 75:378, 1987.

Cooper TW, Bauer EA: Epidermolysis bullosa: A review. Pediatr Dermatol 1:181, 1984.

Crump JA, Danks DM: Hypohidrotic ectodermal dysplasia. J Pediatr 78:466, 1971.

Dale BA, Kam E: Harlequin ichthyosis. Arch Dermatol 129:1471–1477, 1993.

Davis JR, Solomon LM: Cellular immunodeficiency in anhidrotic ectodermal dysplasia. Acta Derm Venereol 56:115, 1976.

Delfino M, Fabbrocini G, Sammarco EM, Santoianni P: Efficacy of calcipotriol versus lactic acid cream in the treatment of lamellar and x-linked ichthyoses. Journal of Dermatological Treatment 5:151–152, 1994.

Emery MM, Siegfried EC, Stone MS, et al: Incontinentia pigmenti: Transmission from father to daughter. J Am Acad Dermatol 29:368–372, 1993.

Esterly NB, Pashayan HM, West CE: Concurrent hypohidrotic ectodermal dysplasia and X-linked ichthyosis. Am J Dis Child 126:539, 1973.

Executive and Scientific Advisory Boards of the National Foundation for Ectodermal Dysplasia: Scaling skin in the newborn: A clue to the early diagnosis of X-linked hypohidrotic ectodermal dysplasia (Christ-Siemens-Touraine syndrome). J Pediatr 114:600, 1989.

Fine JD: Changing clinical and laboratory concepts in inherited epidermolysis bullosa. Arch Dermatol 124:523, 1988.

Fine JD: Epidermolysis bullosa: Clinical aspects, pathology, and recent advances in research. Internat J Dermatol 25:143, 1986.

Fine JD: Laboratory tests for epidermolysis bullosa. Dermatol Clin 12(1):123–132, 1994.

Fine JD, Bauer EA, Briggaman RA, et al: Revised clinical and laboratory criteria for subtypes of inherited epidermolysis bullosa. J Am Acad Dermatol 24(1):119–135, 1991.

Fine JD, Johnson LB, Suchindran CM: The national epidermolysis bullosa registry. J Invest Dermatol 102(6):54s–56s, 1994.

Fine JD, Johnson LB, Wright JT: Inherited blistering diseases of the skin. Pediatrician 18:175–187, 1991.

Francis JS: Genetic skin diseases. Curr Opin Pediatr 6(4):447–453, 1994.

Franco HL, Weston WL, Peebles C, et al: Autoantibodies directed against sicca syndrome antigens in the neonatal lupus syndrome. J Am Acad Dermatol 4:67, 1981.

Freire-Maia N, Pinheiro M: Ectodermal Dysplasias: A Clinical and Genetic Study. New York, Alan R. Liss, 1984.

Frenk E, de Techtermann F: Self-healing collodion baby: Evidence for autosomal recessive inheritance. Pediatr Dermatol 9(2):95–97, 1992.

Frieden IJ: Aplasia cutis congenita: A clinical review and proposal for classification. J Am Acad Dermatol 14:646, 1986.

Gawkrodger DJ, Beveridge GW: Neonatal lupus erythematosus in four successive siblings born to a mother with discoid lupus erythematosus. Br J Dermatol 111:683, 1984.

Gerber M, de Veciana M, Towers CV, Devore GR: Aplasia cutis congenita: A rare cause of elevated alpha-fetoprotein levels. Am J Obstet Gynecol 172(3):1040–1041, 1993.

Gibbons S: Care of epidermolysis bullosa patients: A nursing challenge. Dermatology Nursing 2(4):195–214, 1990.

Goldsmith LA: Look at the genes, see what's in the jeans. Arch Dermatol 126:585–586, 1990.

Gorlin RJ, Old T, Anderson VE: Hypohidrotic ectodermal dysplasia in females: A critical analysis and argument for genetic heterogeneity. Z Kinderheilkd 108:1, 1970.

Haber RM, Hanna W, Ramsay CA, et al: Hereditary epidermolysis bullosa. J Am Acad Dermatol 13:252, 1985.

Happle R: Mosaicism in human skin. Arch Dermatol 129:1460–1470, 1993.

Hardy JD, Solomon S, Barwell GS, et al: Congenital complete heart block in the newborn associated with maternal systemic lupus erythematosus and other connective tissue disorders. Arch Dis Child 54:7, 1979.

Hashimoto K, De Dobbeleer G, Kanzaki T: Electron microscopic studies of harlequin fetuses. Pediatric Dermatology 10(3):214–223, 1993.

Hashimoto K, Eng AM: Transient bullous dermolysis of the newborn. Journal of Cutaneous Pathology 19:496–501, 1992.

Holbrook KA, Smith LT, Elias S: Prenatal diagnosis of genetic skin disease using fetal skin biopsy samples. Arch Dermatol 129:1437–1454, 1993.

Huber N, Rettler I, Bernasconi K, et al: Mutations of keratinocyte transglutaminase in lamellar ichthyosis. Science 267:525–528, 1995.

Itin PH, Pittelkow MR: Trichothiodystrophy: Review of sulfur-deficient brittle hair syndromes and association with the ectodermal dysplasias. J Am Acad Dermatol 22:705–717, 1990.

Jimbow K, Fitzpatrick TB, Szabo G, et al: Congenital circumscribed hypomelanosis: A characterization based on electron microscopic study of tuberous sclerosis, nevus depigmentosus and piebaldism. J Invest Dermatol 64:50, 1975.

Judge MR, Atherton DJ, Salvayre R, et al: Neutral lipid storage disease: Case report and lipid studies. Br J Dermatol 130(4):507–510, 1994.

Judge MR, Morgan G, Harper JI: A clinical and immunological study of Netherton's syndrome. Br J Dermatol 131:615–621, 1994.

Khakoo A, Thomas R, Trompeter R, et al: Congenital cutis laxa and lysyl oxidase deficiency. Clin Genet 51:109–114, 1997.

King RA, Olds DP: Hairbulb tyrosinase activity in oculocutaneous albinism: Suggestions for pathway control and block location. Am J Med Genet 20:49, 1985.

Konigsmark B: Hereditary childhood hearing loss and integumentary system disease. J Pediatr 80:909, 1972.

Kosnik EJ, Sayers MP: Congenital scalp defects: Aplasia cutis congenita. J Neurosurg 42:32, 1975.

Kousseff BG: Collodion baby, sign of Tay syndrome. Pediatrics 87(4):571–574, 1991.

Kragballe K, Steijlen PM, Ibsen HH, et al: Efficacy, tolerability and safety of calcipotriol ointment in disorders of keratinization: Results of a randomized double-blind, vehicle-controlled, right/left comparative study. Arch Dermatol 31(5):556–560, 1995.

Lawlor F: Harlequin fetus progression to nonbullous ichthyosiform erythroderma. Pediatrics 82:870, 1988.

Lee LA: Neonatal lupus erythematosus. J Invest Dermatol 100(1):9–13, 1993.

Lee LA, Weston WL: New findings in neonatal lupus syndrome. Am J Dis Child 138:233, 1984.

Lerer RJ, Ehrenhranz RA, Campbell AGM: Pigmented lesions of incontinentia pigmenti in a neonate. J Pediatr 83:503, 1973.

Levin DL, Nolan KS, Esterly NB: Congenital absence of skin. J Am Acad Dermatol 2:203, 1980.

Lipson AH, Rogers M, Berry A: Collodion babies with Gaucher's disease—a further case. Arch Dis Child 66:667, 1991.

Lucker GPH: Effect of topical calcipotriol on congenital ichthyoses. Br J Dermatol 131:546–550, 1994.

McCune AB, Weston WL, Lee AA: Maternal and fetal outcome in neonatal lupus erythematosus. Ann Intern Med 106:518, 1987.

McKusick VA: Heritable Disorders of Connective Tissue. St. Louis, C. V. Mosby, 1972.

Mehregan AH, Lee SC, Nabai H: Cutis laxa (generalized elastolysis): A

report of four cases with autopsy findings. J Cutan Pathol 5:116, 1978.

Moss C, Ince P: Anhidrotic and achromians lesions in incontinentia pigmenti. Br J Dermatol 116:839, 1987.

Nirunsuksiri W, Presland RB, Brumbaugh SG, et al: Decreased profilaggrin expression in ichthyosis vulgaris is a result of selectively impaired posttranscriptional control. J Biol Chem 270(2):871–876, 1995.

O'Brien JE, Feingold M: Incontinentia pigmenti: A longitudinal study. Am J Dis Child 139:712, 1985.

Oetting WS, King RA: Molecular basis of oculocutaneous albinism. J Invest Dermatol 103(5 suppl):131S–136S, 1994.

Paller AS: Laboratory test for ichthyosis. Dermatol Clin 12(1):99–107, 1994.

Paller AS, Syder AJ, Yiu-Mo Chan BS, et al: Genetic and clinical mosaicism in a type of epidermal nevus. New Engl J Med 331:1408–1415, 1994.

Pinheiro M, Freire-Maia N: Ectodermal dysplasia: A clinical classification and a casual review. Am J Med Genet 53(2):153–162, 1994.

Pinnel SR, Krane SM, Kenzora J, et al: A new heritable disorder of connective tissue with hydroxylysine-deficient collagen. N Engl J Med 286:1013, 1972.

Pongprasit P: Collodion baby: The out-come of long-term follow-up. J Med Assoc Thail 76(1):17–22, 1993.

Prasad RS, Pejaver RK, Hassan A, et al: Management and follow-up of harlequin siblings. Br J Dermatol 130(5):650–653, 1994.

Pries C, Mittleman D, Miller M, et al: The EEC syndrome. Am J Dis Child 127:840, 1974.

Provost TT, Watson R, Gaither KK, et al: The neonatal lupus erythematosus syndrome. J Rheumatol 14(suppl 13):199, 1987.

Rabinowitz LG, Esterly NB: Atopic dermatitis and ichthyosis vulgaris. Pediatr Rev 15(6):220–226, 1994.

Reed WB, Lopez DA, Landing B: Clinical spectrum of anhidrotic ectodermal dysplasia. Arch Dermatol 102:134, 1970.

Richards W, Kaplan M: Anhidrotic ectodermal dysplasia: An unusual cause of hyperpyrexia in the newborn. Am J Dis Child 117:597, 1969.

Roberts LJ: Long-term survival of a harlequin fetus. J Am Acad Dermatol 21:335, 1989.

Rogers M, Scarf C: Harlequin baby treated with etretinate. Pediatr Dermatol 6:216, 1989.

Rosenfeld S, Smith ME: Ocular findings in incontinentia pigmenti. Ophthalmology 92:543, 1985.

Russell LJ, DiGiovanna JJ, Rogers R, et al: Mutations of the gene for transglutaminase 1 in autosomal recessive lamellar ichthyosis. Nat Genet 9(3):279–283, 1995.

Russell S, Young MJ: Hypercalcemia during treatment of psoriasis with calcipotriol. Br J Dermatol 130:795–796, 1994.

Sakati NO, Nyhan WL, Shear CS, et al: Syndrome of cutis laxa, ligamentous laxity, and delayed development. Pediatrics 72:850, 1983.

Schachner LA, Hansen RC (Eds): Pediatric Dermatology. New York, Churchill Livingstone, 1988.

Shwayder T, Ott F: All about ichthyosis. Pediatr Clin North Am 38(4):835–857, 1991.

Smack DP, Korge BP, James WD: Keratin and keratinization. J Am Acad Dermatol 30:85–102, 1994.

Solomon LM, Esterly NB: Neonatal Dermatology. Philadelphia, W. B. Saunders Company, 1973.

Solomon LM, Keuer EJ: The ectodermal dysplasias. Arch Dermatol 116:1295, 1980.

Steijlen PM, Kremer H, Fereydoun V, et al: Genetic linkage of the keratin type II gene cluster with ichthyosis bullosa of siemans and with autosomal dominant ichthyosis exfoliativa. J Invest Dermatol 103:282–285, 1994.

Steijlen PM, Van Dooren-Greebe RJ, Van de Kerkhof PC: Acitretin in the treatment of lamellar ichthyosis. Br J Dermatol 130(2):211–214, 1994.

Sybert VP: Aplasia cutis congenita: A report of 12 new families and a review of the literature. Pediatr Dermatol 3:1, 1985.

Telfer MA, Sugar A, Jaeger EA, et al: Dominant piebald trait (white forehead and leukoderma) with neurological impairment. Am J Hum Genet 23:383, 1971.

Thomas WO, Moses MH, Craver RD, Galen WK: Congenital cutis laxa: A case report and review of loose skin syndromes. Ann Plast Surg 30(3):252–256, 1993.

Thornton CM, Eichenfield LF, Shinall EA, et al: Cutaneous telangiectases in neonatal lupus erythematosus. J Am Acad Dermatol 33:19–25, 1995.

Tomita Y: The molecular genetics of albinism and piebaldism. Arch Dermatol 130:355–358, 1994.

Waisman Y, Rachmel A, Metzker A, et al: Failure of etretinate therapy in twins with severe congenital lamellar ichthyosis. Pediatric Dermatology 6(3):226–228, 1989.

Williams ML: A new look at the ichthyoses: Disorders of lipid metabolism. Pediatr Dermatol 3:476, 1986.

Williams ML: The ichthyoses—pathogenesis and prenatal diagnosis: A review of recent advances. Pediatr Dermatol 1:1, 1983.

Witkop CJ Jr, Quevedo WC Jr, Fitzpatrick TB, King RA: *In* Scriver CR, Beaudet AL, Sly WS, Volle D (Eds): The Metabolic Basis of Inherited Disease, 6th ed. New York, McGraw-Hill, 1989, p 2905.

Workshop Proceedings: Pathogenesis, clinical features and management of the nondermatologic complications of epidermolysis bullosa. Arch Dermatol 124:705, 1988.

Zonana J, Schinzel A, Upadhyaya M, et al: Prenatal diagnosis of X-linked hypohidrotic ectodermal dysplasia by linkage analysis. Am J Med Genet 35:132–135, 1990.

CHAPTER 107

Infections of the Skin

Elaine C. Siegfried and Nancy B. Esterly

As a group of potentially life-threatening and often easily treatable diseases, infections are often suspected first in a neonate with skin lesions. Recognition of characteristic morphologic features, aided by a few easily performed tests, will greatly enhance correct diagnosis and early initiation of appropriate therapy of the most common cutaneous infections (see Chapter 105). In this chapter, we confine our discussion to the most common pathogens causing neonatal infections that present with skin lesions: *Staphylococcus aureus*, *Streptococcus* spp, *Candida albicans*, and Herpes simplex.

STAPHYLOCOCCUS AUREUS

S. aureus is a ubiquitous organism. Colonization of the anterior nares and perineum are common, with frequent hand carriage (Dancer and Noble, 1991). This bacterial family is responsible for a variety of skin lesions. Infants become colonized with *S. aureus* during the first few weeks of life, following inoculation at the perineum or from handling. Cutaneous signs of *S. aureus* are mediated by local or circulating bacterial toxins that act directly on components of the epidermal keratinocytes, or as "superantigens" to stimulate exuberant immunologic responses (Tokura et al, 1994).

Bullous Impetigo

Impetigo is a group of superficial skin infections caused by group A streptococci or *S. aureus*, or both. Lesions caused by *S. aureus* are primarily vesicular and referred to as bullous impetigo. This form of impetigo can occur in nursery-based, epidemic patterns.

Clinical Findings. Impetigo is one of the most common neonatal skin infections. It occurs during the latter part of the 1st week or as late as the 2nd week of life, manifest as vesicles or pustules on an erythematous base most often seen in the periumbilical area, diaper area, or skin folds. Because the blisters are superficial, intact lesions are usually less than 1 cm in diameter. Larger lesions are flaccid and rupture so easily that they are usually seen as erosions, with a red moist base that develops a thin varnish-like crust (Fig. 107–1). These lesions heal rapidly without scarring. Lesions are usually not closely grouped, distinguishing them from the vesicles of herpes simplex infection.

Etiology. Bullous impetigo is caused by toxigenic strains of coagulase-positive hemolytic *S. aureus*. Most often, the organism can be classified as one of the group II phage types. The incubation period is 1 to 10 days. Skin lesions are the result of local production of an epidermolytic exotoxin that acts within the granular layer of the epidermis, producing superficial blisters.

Epidemiology. Individuals with skin lesions are highly infectious, but the disease can also be transmitted by asymptomatic carriers. The anterior nares of 30% of the general population are colonized with *S. aureus*, providing a reservoir for hand carriage and nosocomial spread (Kragballe et al, 1995; Doebbeling, 1994). Colonization of health care workers by methicillin-resistant strains poses a potentially serious problem.

Sporadic cases of impetigo are common, but many nursery epidemics have been reported and should be treated aggressively (Dave et al, 1994). Infected infants may not develop skin lesions until after discharge, so infection control surveillance should include all exposed patients. Overcrowding, insufficient nursery personnel, and inadequate hand washing contribute to nosocomial spread. Treatment of the umbilical cord with an antimicrobial agent has been shown to control epidemic *S. aureus* infections in the neonatal intensive care unit (NICU) (Haley et al, 1995). In the setting of an outbreak, nursery personnel should be surveyed for colonization of hands and nares. Application of mupirocin ointment to the anterior nares twice daily for five days will eliminate nasal carriage for up to 1 year (Doebbeling et al, 1994). Effective hand washing can prevent nosocomial spread; chlorhexidine is among the safest and most effective antimicrobial cleansers for hospital use (Doebbeling et al, 1992).

Diagnosis. The diagnosis is supported by the presence of gram-positive cocci in clusters on Gram stain of the contents from an intact pustule and confirmed by bacterial culture.

Treatment. Bullous impetigo is benign if treated early, but local proliferation with exotoxin production or dissemination can be life threatening. Treatment should be instituted promptly, and strict isolation maintained until the lesions

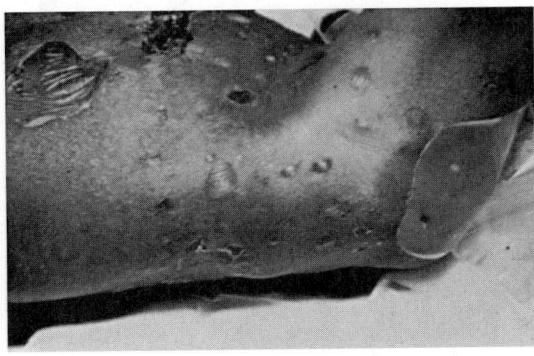

FIGURE 107–1. Bullous impetigo. Multiple intact and ruptured bullae on the abdomen, hip, and thigh of a newborn infant. No underlying erythema is present.

have resolved. Infants should be closely monitored, and a high index of suspicion maintained for evidence of systemic disease. Infants with periumbilical lesions are at risk for bacterial omphalitis. Extremely limited infections may be treated with topical mupirocin, but this form of therapy should be used with caution in neonates. Compresses with sterile water, normal saline, or Burow solution applied every few hours helps desiccate blisters. More extensive lesions require a systemically administered penicillinase-resistant antibiotic for 7 to 10 days. Sensitivities of the organism cultured should ultimately determine the choice of antibiotics.

Staphylococcal Scalded Skin Syndrome

Staphylococcal scalded skin syndrome (SSSS) occurs as a generalized manifestation of circulating *S. aureus* epidermolytic toxin. Affected infants are erythrodermic, a striking cutaneous finding that suggests a long differential diagnosis (see Chapter 105). Early diagnosis and treatment of SSSS can be life-saving.

Clinical Findings. Affected infants have abrupt onset of temperature instability and irritability with generalized skin tenderness and erythema that most often starts on the face and spreads rapidly. Erythema is often accentuated in skin folds. Facial edema, conjunctivitis, and crusting around the eyes, nose, and mouth give the infant a characteristic "sad mask" appearance. Flaccid bullae may develop, followed by widespread exfoliation (Fig. 107–2). Blistering is easily elicited by light stroking, a diagnostic feature called Nikolsky's sign. Widespread skin involvement can exacerbate fluid and electrolyte problems (Frieden, 1989).

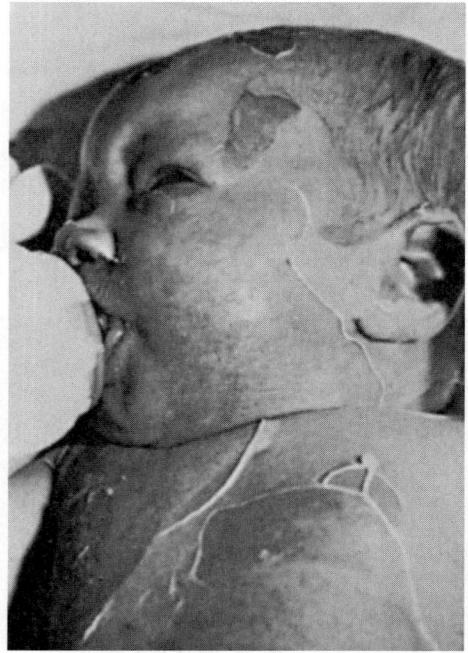

FIGURE 107–2. Staphylococcal scalded skin syndrome (Ritter disease). Intense erythema and peeling of large areas of epidermis are shown.

Etiology. The signs and symptoms of SSSS are the result of circulating epidermolytic toxin, produced from an often subclinical focus of *S. aureus* infection. Fresh skin lesions do not contain bacteria. Two distinct epidermolytic toxins have been identified in SSSS, produced by toxigenic strains of *S. aureus*, phage group I, II, or III. The toxins are thought to act primarily by disrupting proteins within the epidermal granular cells (Resnick, 1992), but superantigenic stimulation of cytokine production has also been demonstrated (Dave et al, 1994).

Diagnosis. If the diagnosis is in doubt, skin biopsy prepared for frozen section can be examined emergently. The presence of an intraepidermal, rather than full-thickness blister will distinguish SSSS from toxic epidermal necrolysis and allow rapid initiation of appropriate therapy. Other conditions can be ruled out by examination of permanent sections. If the clinical impression is strong, surveillance samples will define the primary focus of infection. Gram stains may be performed emergently; cultures will confirm the diagnosis. Common sites of primary infection are the nasopharynx, umbilicus, ocular conjunctivae, and in urine. Bullous lesions do not contain organisms. Blood cultures should be obtained because sepsis, although uncommon, may occur. Phage typing may be of interest in epidemics.

Treatment. Systemic administration of a penicillinase-resistant penicillin is the therapy of choice. Fluid and electrolyte replacement and measures for maintenance of normal body temperature may be required. Approximately 2 to 3 days after initiation of therapy, the denuded areas become dry, and a flaky desquamation ensues. Crusted and denuded areas may be treated with compresses of Burow or normal saline solution. Application of a bland ointment emollient may accelerate the return of the skin to normal during the flaky desquamative phase. Resolution occurs in another 3 to 5 days. Because the intraepidermal cleavage plane is at the level of the granular layer, scarring occurs only in instances of secondary complications (Frieden, 1989).

STREPTOCOCCUS SPECIES

Cutaneous streptococcal infections occur in the newborn but are less common than staphylococcal infections. Group A streptococci has been reported to cause disease of epidemic proportions (Dillon, 1966; Peter and Hazard, 1975) following the introduction of the organism into the nursery by maternal carriers or nursery personnel. The umbilicus is a frequent site of infection. Conjunctivitis, paronychia, vaginitis, and an erysipelas-like eruption have also been described (Dillon, 1966; Geil et al, 1970; Isenberg et al, 1984). Because sepsis and meningitis may result, infected infants should be treated promptly, and strict isolation should be instituted. As with staphylococcal infection, serious efforts should be made to identify the source of the organism. Several nursery outbreaks have been difficult to terminate because colonized infants may show little evidence of disease (Lehtonen et al, 1984). Isolation and treatment of infected infants, disinfection of the umbilical stump, the most likely reservoir of the organism, and penicillin prophylaxis for carriers and exposed infants have been the most effective measures. The infections respond readily to penicillin, which should be administered over a 10-day course.

Group B streptococci are now one of the most frequently encountered pathogens in the newborn nursery. Early-onset disease (during the 1st week of life), probably acquired in utero or during delivery, most commonly becomes manifest as septicemia with respiratory distress and shock. Late-onset disease (after the 1st week of life) is acquired postpartum and more often takes the form of meningitis. Patients with early-onset disease may harbor the organism on the skin; however, the presence of this agent on the skin is short lived as compared with other sites (Baker, 1977).

Skin infections caused by group B streptococcus are uncommon but have been documented (Belgaumkar, 1975; Hebert and Esterly, 1986; Howard and McCrackin, 1974). Vesiculopustular lesions, cellulitis, and small abscesses have all been noted. A 10-day course of procaine penicillin is considered the treatment of choice.

CANDIDA ALBICANS

C. albicans is a frequent pathogen of the female genital tract, especially during pregnancy. Infantile infection may be acquired in utero, during delivery, or postnatally.

Thrush

Clinical Findings. *C. albicans* colonizes the oral cavity and gastrointestinal tract of most neonates, peaking at 4 weeks of age (Russell and Lay, 1973). This peak corresponds to a peak incidence of thrush. The lesions are readily recognized as plaques of white, friable material on an erythematous base over the tongue, palate, buccal mucosa, and gingivae.

Diagnosis. Presumptive diagnoses are often made by physical examination, but microscopic examination of scrapings suspended in 10% potassium hydroxide for yeast and pseudohyphal forms is useful. The diagnosis may be confirmed by identification of the organism on culture.

Treatment. Nystatin is an antibiotic derived from *Streptomyces noursei* with activity against *Candida* but not dermatophytes. Oral lesions usually respond promptly to a course of nystatin suspension, 100,000 to 200,000 units, administered by mouth four times daily for 10 to 14 days. In refractory cases, an increased dosage of nystatin or systemic therapy may have to be instituted (Hebert and Esterly, 1986). Gentian (crystal) violet is a triphenylmethane antiseptic dye effective against *Candida* spp. In a 0.5% or 1% aqueous solution it has been a time-honored, safe, and effective treatment for thrush. Gentian violet is infamous for deep purple staining of the skin, which is transient. Prolonged use of gentian violet has been associated with nausea, vomiting, diarrhea, and mucosal ulceration. Carcinogenicity in mice has been reported (Rosenkranz and Carr, 1971).

Neonatal and Cutaneous Candidiasis

Neonatal candidiasis presents 3 to 7 days after birth with mucocutaneous lesions. Infection can be localized or generalized. The disease is rarely invasive in healthy full-term infants.

Clinical Findings. Localized cutaneous candidal infections are common in infants. Intertriginous areas, particularly the neck folds, axillae, and diaper area (Fig. 107–3A), are most frequently affected. Nails and periungual areas are also sites of predilection. Characteristic primary lesions are tiny vesicopustules that erode and merge, forming bright, erythematous, scaly plaques, often with a scalloped edge. "Satellite" pustules are commonly seen, but by no means are they pathognomonic for this condition.

Disseminated neonatal candidiasis can occur as a result of spread from an untreated localized site or by widespread inoculation during the process of birth (Fig. 107–3B). Generalized scaling is the dominant feature, but a careful

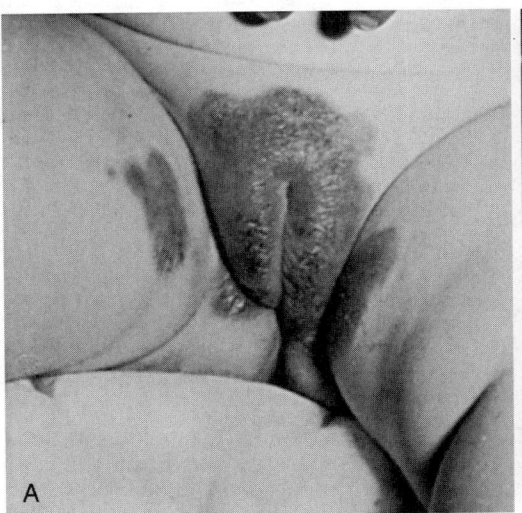
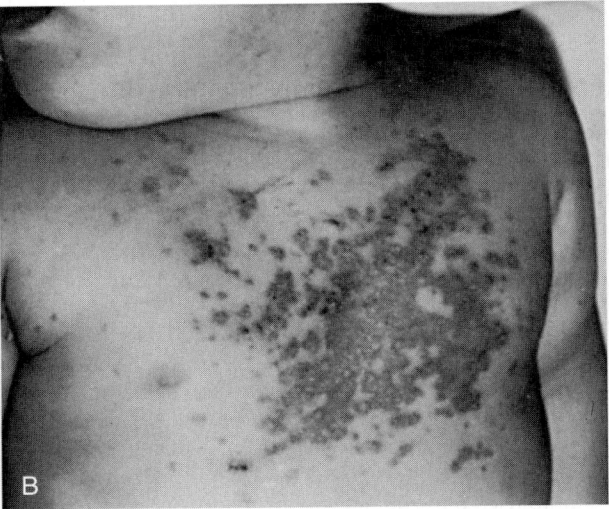

FIGURE 107–3. *A,* Sharply demarcated erythematous scaly candidal rash in the groin. *B,* Candidal eruption on the central chest of an infant.

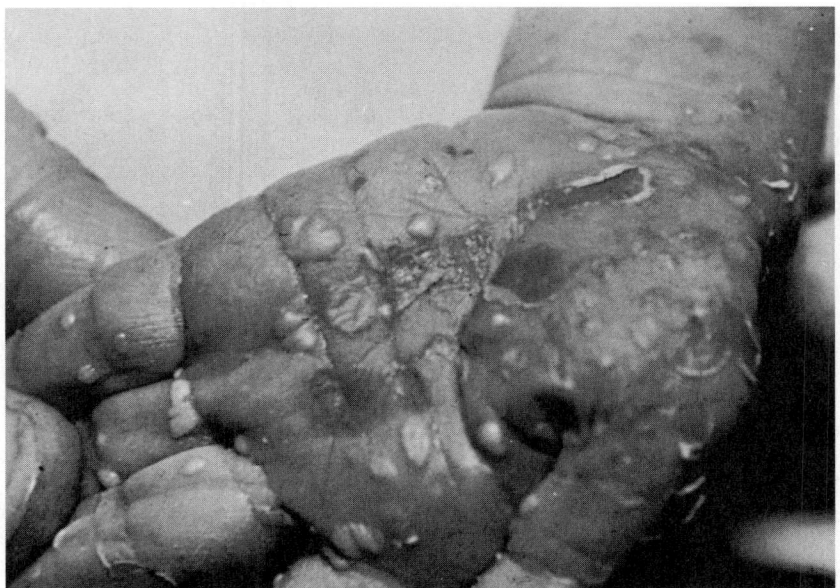

FIGURE 107–4. Congenital cutaneous candidiasis—pustular stage—in a 6-day-old infant. A maculopapular rash was present at birth. (Courtesy of P. J. Kozinn, N. Rudolf, A. A. Tariq, M. R. Reale, and P. K. Goldberg.)

search for primary vesicopustules and periungual or nail involvement are helpful diagnostic clues (Gibney and Siegfried, 1996).

Diagnosis. The differential diagnosis includes conditions that cause blisters and pustules (see Chapter 105). A potassium hydroxide preparation that reveals budding yeasts and pseudohyphal forms is the easiest and most cost-effective initial step in establishing the diagnosis. Calcofluor white stain and immunofluorescence microscopy is a more sensitive rapid technique. Cultures from an intact pustule, skin scrapings, or skin biopsy tissue also support the diagnosis.

Treatment. The eruption may resolve spontaneously or may become more widespread if left untreated. Localized cutaneous candidiasis in an otherwise healthy infant is most easily treated with a topical candidicidal agent, such as nystatin, one of the imidazoles (e.g., miconazole, clotrimazole, or ketoconazole), or ciclopirox olamine. Nystatin in an ointment vehicle may be the least irritating.

Congenital and Disseminated Candidiasis

Congenital candidiasis is assumed to result from ascending intrauterine infection. This form is usually seen in compromised, premature infants. Disseminated candidiasis can also be acquired during the neonatal period. Early recognition and appropriate therapy are life saving (Gibney and Siegfried, 1996).

Clinical Findings. Lesions of congenital candidiasis can be seen on the placenta and fetal membranes, including characteristic granulomas of the umbilical cord (Hebert and Esterly, 1986; Schirar et al, 1974). The cord lesions are multiple yellow-white papules, usually measuring 1 to 3 mm in diameter. The cutaneous eruption of congenital cutaneous candidiasis may be sparse or widespread and consists of papules and vesicopustules on an erythematous base. The face is relatively spared as are the oral mucous

membranes, and there is no predilection for the diaper area. Palmar and plantar pustules, paronychia, and nail dystrophy help distinguish this condition from more common, benign neonatal dermatoses (Fig. 107–4). Bullae and desquamation are usually late features (Fig. 107–5). Very low-birth-weight infants may present with a less specific, burn-like dermatitis.

Systemic involvement occurs via hematogenous or lymphatic spread, most frequently involving the kidney, central nervous system (CNS), and the skeletal system. Pneumonia may result from aspiration of infected amniotic fluid. Risk factors for congenital systemic infection include birth weight less than 1500 g, indwelling catheters, antibiotic therapy, steroid administration, and hyperalimentation. The clinician should have a lower threshold for parenteral therapy for infants with these risk factors (Johnson et al, 1984; Botas et al, 1995).

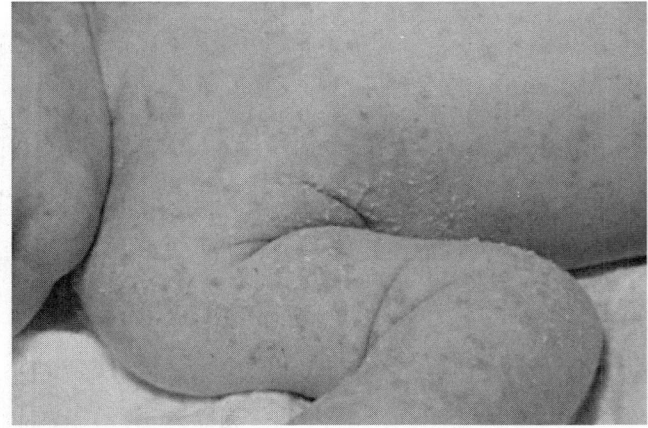

FIGURE 107–5. An 8-day-old infant with generalized erythematous, scaly eruption sparing only the face and scalp. Oral mucosa was not involved. Hyphae and budding yeasts were seen on potassium hydroxide preparation, and *Candida albicans* was cultured from the lesions. The infant's mother had candidal vaginitis during the pregnancy.

Etiology. Congenital candidiasis is presumed to invade as an ascending infection, crossing the fetal membrane and infecting surfaces that come in contact with amniotic fluid. Disease may be limited to chorioamnionitis and funisitis. Symptomatic vaginitis, chorioamnionitis, or ruptured membranes have no prognostic value for congenital disease (Gibney and Siegfried, 1996; Johnson et al, 1984).

Diagnosis. The differential diagnosis includes several other neonatal vesiculopustular eruptions that range from benign, self-limited cutaneous processes to rapidly progressive life-threatening disease (see Chapter 105). Early and correct diagnosis is essential. Organisms from skin are usually demonstrable on potassium hydroxide or calcofluor white preparations and cultures of scrapings from involved skin. Disseminated disease can be difficult to diagnose. Respiratory distress and infiltrates on chest radiograph will obscure evidence of *Candida* pneumonia because hyaline membrane disease often occurs in the same patient population. Ophthalmic examination, chest radiograph, blood, urine, and cerebrospinal fluid cultures may be helpful, but negative findings are not uncommon in disseminated candidiasis (Johnson et al, 1984). Histologic examination of the placenta and umbilical cord prepared with the appropriate stains may demonstrate fungal elements. Urinalysis positive for budding yeast or urine culture positive for *C. albicans* may be quickly dismissed as contaminant, but this is highly associated with systemic disease in infants at risk. The diagnosis of disseminated candidiasis can be expedited by a positive touch preparation of a punch biopsy specimen. Using this technique, one firmly imprints the dermal side of the specimen on a microscope slide and then looks for yeast after potassium hydroxide preparation or Gram's stain (Held et al, 1988).

Prognosis and Treatment. Systemic infection with *C. albicans* in premature infants is a serious infection with high morbidity and mortality (Johnson et al, 1984). Congenital or acquired candidiasis warrants parenteral antifungal therapy in the following situations, which increases the risk of disseminated disease: (1) evidence of respiratory distress or sepsis in the immediate neonatal period; (2) birth weight less than 1500 g; (3) treatment with broad spectrum antibiotics or corticosteroids; (4) extensive instrumentation during delivery or invasive procedures in the neonatal period; (5) positive systemic cultures; and (6) evidence of altered immune response. A critical factor for survival in systemic candidiasis is not extent of infection but the early initiation of antifungal therapy (Johnson et al, 1984; Botas et al, 1995). Healthy infants without visceral involvement respond rapidly to topical anticandidal agents (Gibney and Siegfried, 1996).

HERPES SIMPLEX

Early recognition and prompt initiation of therapy for neonatal herpes is critical. The consequences of delaying antiviral therapy can be devastating.

Clinical Findings. Onset of symptoms usually occurs at 1 to 2 weeks for most neonates, but congenital lesions have been reported (Salvadoret al, 1994). Only one third of infants present with cutaneous involvement (Frieden, 1989), although more than 80% develop typical skin lesions during the course of their disease (Overall, 1994). Characteristic skin lesions begin as isolated or grouped, tense vesicles on an erythematous base and evolve into pustules, crusts, or small erosions over several days. Forty percent of infected infants have disease limited to skin, eye, and mucosae (SEM disease). If treated early, these infants have an excellent prognosis; left untreated, 75% will progress (Arvin and Prober, 1992). Thirty-five percent have CNS disease, with a high incidence of developmental abnormalities. One fourth of infected infants present with disseminated disease (e.g., sepsis, liver dysfunction, coagulopathy, and respiratory distress). For this group, the prognosis is poor, with a 60% mortality rate and a 40% risk of long-term neurologic impairment in survivors (Arvin and Prober, 1992; Whitley, 1994).

Infants infected in utero have a distinctive clinical presentation. Skin lesions are almost always present at birth. These include widespread erosions and bullae, scars, and scalp lesions that resemble aplasia cutis. Other frequent findings include chorioretinitis, microcephaly, hydranencephaly, and microphthalmia (Arvin and Prober, 1992).

Etiology. The majority of cases of neonatal herpes simplex are the result of vertical transmission. Two thirds of cases are caused by HSV 2 and one third by HSV 1. The usual route of infection is via intrapartum contact with genital mucosa, but ascending infection accounts for 5% of cases of neonatal herpes. Infants who become infected in utero are more often premature or small for gestational age, with more widespread and severe disease (Arvin and Prober, 1992).

Epidemiology. The incidence of neonatal HSV is 1 in 500 to 1 in 7500 live births. One half of infected infants are born to mothers with primary infections. These women, who are usually without active lesions, have a 50% risk of transmitting disease to their newborn. One half of infants with neonatal herpes are born to mothers with recurrent genital herpes, generally HSV 2. Most of these women are also asymptomatic at the time of delivery, and may have no known history of genital herpes. In this group, the risk of transmitting infection is only 2.5%.

Diagnosis. A high index of suspicion is required. The differential diagnosis includes the causes of vesicles and pustules in the newborn outlined in Chapter 105. Tzanck smears, viral cultures, and direct fluorescent antibody detection are the most widely used tests to detect herpes infection. The diagnostic yield for each is variable, largely influenced by the age, quality, and handling of the specimen. Optimally, skin scrapings should be obtained from the base of a fresh vesicle. Other sites should be sampled as well, especially in infants suspected of having CNS or disseminated disease. Tzanck smear analysis is rapid and readily available but will reveal characteristic multinucleated giant cells in only 50% of HSV infections (Nahass et al, 1995). Immunofluorescence is 90% to 95% sensitive and specific but requires a specialized lab. Viral culture yields positive results for 80% of specimens by 24 hours, and 90% by 48 hours, under optimal conditions of handling and transport. Molecular diagnosis by polymerase chain reaction can detect HSV from specimens that would be suboptimal for the other methods (e.g., Tzanck smears, crusts, or paraffin-fixed biopsy specimens). Diagnostic polymerase chain reaction is now available at a limited number of centers but may be the easiest means of diagnosing HSV in the future (Nahass et al, 1995; Nahass et al, 1992).

Treatment. When diagnostic confirmation is delayed in suspected cases, presumptive therapy should be started. This therapy includes strict isolation and prompt administration of parenteral antiviral therapy. A 10-day course of acyclovir or vidarabine are equally effective in preventing severe disease in infants with SEM. Treatment is much less effective for infants with more widespread herpes infection (Arvin and Prober, 1992). Concomitant administration of immunoglobulin products may improve disease outcome for these infants (Whitley, 1994).

REFERENCES

Albert S, Baldwin R, Czekajewski S, et al: Bullous impetigo due to group II *Staphylococcus aureus*. Am J Dis Child 120:10, 1970.

Anthony BF, Giuliano DM, Oh W: Nursery outbreak of staphylococcal scalded skin syndrome. Am J Dis Child 124:41, 1972.

Arvin AM, Prober CG: Herpes simplex virus infections: The genital tract and the newborn. Pediatr Rev special edition:11–16, 1992.

Baker CJ: Summary of workshop on infections due to group B streptococcus. J Infect Dis 136:137, 1977.

Belgaumkar TK: Impetigo neonatorum congenita due to group B beta-hemolytic streptococcus infection. J Pediatr 86:982, 1975.

Botas CM, Kurlat I, Young SM, Sola A: Disseminated candidal infections and intravenous hydrocortisone in preterm infants. Pediatrics 95:883–887, 1995.

Curran JP, Al-Salihi FL: Neonatal staphylococcal scalded skin syndrome: Massive outbreak due to an unusual phage type. Pediatrics 66:285, 1980.

Dancer SJ, Noble WC: Nasal, axillary, and perineal carriage of Staphylococcus aureus among women: Identification of strains producing epidermolytic toxin. J Clin Pathol 44:681–684, 1991.

Dave J, Reith S, Nash JQ, et al: A double outbreak of exfoliative toxin-producing strains of staphylococcus aureus in a maternity unit. Epidemiology & Infection 112:103–114, 1994.

Dillon HC Jr: Group A Type 12 streptococcal infection in a newborn nursery. Am J Dis Child 112:177, 1966.

Doebbeling BN: Nasal and hand carriage of Staphylococcus aureus in healthcare workers. J Chemother 6:11–17, 1994.

Doebbeling BN, Reagan DR, Pfaller MA, et al: Long-term efficacy of intranasal ointment: A prospective cohort study of staphylococcus aureus carriage. Arch Intern Med 154:1505–1508, 1994.

Doebbeling BN, Stanley GL, Sheetz CT, et al: Comparative efficacy of alternative hand-washing agents in reducing nosocomial infections in intensive care units. New Engl J Med 327:88–93, 1992.

Elias PM, Fritsch P, Epstein EH Jr: Staphylococcal scalded skin syndrome. Clinical features, pathogenesis, and recent microbiological and biochemical developments. Arch Dermatol 113:207, 1977.

Elias PM, Mittermayer H, Tappeiner G, et al: Staphylococcal toxic epidermal necrolysis (TEN): The expanded mouse model. J Invest Dermatol 63:467, 1974.

Frieden I: Blisters and pustules in the newborn. Curr Probl Pediatr 555–615, 1989.

Gehlbach SH, Gutman LT, Wilfert CM, et al: Recurrence of skin disease in a nursery: Ineffectuality of hexachlorophene bathing. Pediatrics 55:422, 1975.

Geil CC, Castle WK, and Mortimer EA, Jr: Group A streptococcal infections in newborn nurseries. Pediatrics 46:489, 1970.

Gibney MD, Siegfried EC: Cutaneous congenital candidiasis: A case report. Pediatr Dermatol 2:359–363, 1996.

Guidelines for Perinatal Care: AAP Committee on the Fetus and New-born. ACOG Committee on Obstetrics: Maternal and Fetal Medicine, 2nd ed., 1988.

Haley RW, Cushion NB, Tenover FC, et al: Eradication of endemic methicillin-resistant Staphyloccus aureus indications from a neonatal intensive care unit. J Infect Dis 171:614–624, 1995.

Hebert AA, Esterly NB: Bacterial and candidal cutaneous infections in the neonate. Dermatol Clin 4:3, 1986.

Held JL, Berkowitz RK, Grossman ME: Use of touch preparation for rapid diagnosis of disseminated candidiasis. J Am Acad Dermatol 19:1063–1066, 1988.

Howard JB, McCrackin GH, Jr: The spectrum of group B streptococcal infections in infancy. Am J Dis Child 128:815, 1974.

Isenberg HD, Tucci V, Lipsitz P, et al: Clinical laboratory and epidemiological investigations of a *Streptococcus pyogenes* cluster epidemic in a newborn nursery. J Clin Microbiol 19:366, 1984.

Johnson DE, Thompson TR, Ferrieri P: Congenital candidiasis. Am J Dis Child 135:273, 1981.

Johnson DE, Thompson TR, Green TP, Ferrieri P: Systemic candidiasis in very low-birth-weight infants (<1,500 grams). Pediatrics 73:138–143, 1984.

Kam LA, Giacoia GP: Congenital cutaneous candidiasis. Am J Dis Child 129:1215, 1975.

Kragballe K, Steijlen PM, Ibsen HH, et al: Efficacy, tolerability and safety of calcipotriol ointment in disorders of keratinization: Results of a randomized double-blind, vehicle-controlled, right/left comparative study. Arch Dermatol 131:556–560, 1995.

Lehtonen OP, Ruuskanen O, Karo P, et al: Group-A streptococcal infection in the newborn. Lancet 2:1473, 1984.

Melish ME, Glasgow LA: Staphylococcal scalded skin syndrome—development of an experimental model. N Engl J Med 282:1114, 1970.

Melish ME, Glasgow LA: Staphylococcal scalded skin syndrome: The expanded clinical syndrome. J Pediatr 78:958, 1971.

Nahass GT, Goldstein BA, Zhu W, et al: Comparison of Tzanck smear, viral culture, and DNA diagnostic methods in detection of herpes simplex and varicella-zoster infection. JAMA 268:2541–2544, 1992.

Nahass GT, Mandel MJ, Cook S, et al: Detection of herpes simplex and varicella-zoster infection from cutaneous lesions in different clinical stages with the polymerase chain reaction. J Am Acad Dermatol 32:730–733, 1995.

Overall JC Jr: Herpes simplex virus infection of the fetus and the newborn. Pediatric Annals 23:131–136, 1994.

Overturf BD, Balfour G: Osteomyelitis and sepsis: Severe complications of fetal monitoring. Pediatrics 55:244, 1975.

Peter G, Hazard J: Neonatal group A streptococcal disease. J Pediatr 87:454, 1975.

Resnick SD: Staphylococcal toxin-mediated syndromes in childhood. Semin Dermatol 11:11–18, 1992.

Rosenkranz HS, Carr HS: Possible hazard in use of genitan violet. Br Med J 3:702–703, 1971.

Rubenstein AD, Mesher DM: Epidemic boric acid poisoning simulating staphylococcal toxic epidermal necrolysis of the newborn infant: Ritter's disease. J Pediatr 77:884, 1970.

Rudolph RI, Schwartz W, Leyden JJ: Treatment of staphylococcal toxic epidermal necrolysis. Arch Dermatol 110:559, 1974.

Rudolph N, Tariq AA, Reale MR, et al: Congenital cutaneous candidiasis. Arch Dermatol 113:1101, 1977.

Russell C, Lay KM: Natural history of Candida species and yeasts in the oral cavities of infants. Arch Oral Biol 18:957, 1973.

Salvador A, Meislich D, Tunnessen WW Jr: Picture of the month: Intra-uterine herpes simplex virus infection. Arch Pediatr Adoles Med 148:1311–1312, 1994.

Schirar A, Rendu C, Vielh JP, Gautray JP: Congenital mycosis (*Candida albicans*). Biol Neonate 24:273, 1974.

Sheagren JN: *Staphylococcus aureus*: The persistent pathogen (Parts I and II). N Engl J Med 310:1368, 1437, 1984.

Tokura Y, Yagi J, O'Malley M, et al: Superantigenic staphylococcal exotoxins induce T-cell proliferation in the presence of Langerhans cells or class II-bearing keratinocytes to produce T-cell activating cytokines. J Invest Dermatol 112:103–114, 1994.

Wagner MM, Rycheck RR, Yee RB, et al: Septic dermatitis of the neonatal scalp and maternal endomyometritis with intrapartum internal fetal monitoring. Pediatrics 74:81, 1984.

Whitley RJ: Neonatal herpes simplex virus infections: Is there a role for immunoglobulin in disease prevention and therapy? Pediatr Infect Dis 13:432–438, 1994.

CHAPTER 108

Common Newborn Dermatoses

Elaine C. Siegfried and Nancy B. Esterly

This chapter includes a group of cutaneous disorders that are unique to neonates. All have well-recognized clinical and/or histologic features. Most are asymptomatic and self-limited, so rigorous searches have not been made for precise pathogeneses or definitive therapies. These common neonatal dermatoses may be mistaken for more serious diseases, and serious diseases may be mistaken for common neonatal dermatoses. For this reason, verification of the correct diagnosis can obviate initiation of aggressive work-up and treatment. In other cases, it can be life saving. Differential diagnoses, based on clinical morphology, are outlined in Chapter 105.

ERYTHEMA TOXICUM NEONATORUM

Clinical Findings. Erythema toxicum is an inflammatory cutaneous disease of unknown origin that affects about half of all full-term newborns (Berg and Solomon, 1987). It occurs less frequently among preterm infants (Carr et al, 1966; Taylor and Bondurant, 1957). In the majority of infants, the lesions develop between 1 and 3 days of age but may occur as late as 3 weeks. No predilection of the disorder for race, sex, season, or geographic location has been reported.

Affected infants appear healthy. The basic skin lesion is a small (1 to 3 mm) papule that evolves into a pustule, with a prominent halo of erythema, that has been likened to a "flea bite." Individual lesions may persist only a few hours, but the eruption lasts for several days, and rarely, for several weeks. The number of lesions present may vary from a few to dozens. The trunk is the most frequent site of predilection, but the face and extremities may also be involved. Palms and soles are almost always spared. Several lesions may coalesce into plaques measuring several centimeters in diameter (Fig. 108–1).

Diagnosis. A Wright-stained smear of pustule contents reveals large numbers of eosinophils that supports the diagnosis. Skin biopsy may be necessary in clinically atypical cases. The histology consists of eosinophil-filled intraepidermal vesicles and a mixed intradermal inflammatory infiltrate that tends to localize around the superficial portion of the pilosebaceous follicle.

The differential diagnosis includes other benign, self-limited disorders such as transient neonatal pustular melanosis, miliaria, infantile acropustulosis, and eosinophilic pustular folliculitis, as well as infections such as bacterial folliculitis, bullous impetigo, candidiasis, herpes, and scabies. Urticaria pigmentosa and incontinentia pigmenti are more serious disorders that can be mistaken for erythema toxicum. The diagnostic work-up outlined in Chapter 105 can distinguish between these conditions.

Etiology. Erythema toxicum is a benign inflammatory disease of unknown cause. The eosinophilic infiltrate suggests that erythema toxicum is a hypersensitivity response, but studies attempting to incriminate chemical or microbiologic substances, acquired either transplacentally or vaginally from the mother, such as drugs, topical irritants, sebum, and milk, have failed to provide support for this hypothesis (Bassukas, 1992).

Treatment and Prognosis. Erythema toxicum is asymptomatic, resolves spontaneously, and requires no treatment. A prolonged course and recurrence are rare. Once the diagnosis is confirmed, anticipatory guidance and reassurance should be provided to parents.

TRANSIENT NEONATAL PUSTULAR MELANOSIS

Clinical Findings. This benign disorder is present at birth in 5% of black and 1% of white infants (Ramamurthy et al, 1976). Characteristic lesions are small, superficial pustules that rupture easily, leaving a collarette of fine scale and hyperpigmented macules (Fig. 108–2). The lesions may be profuse or sparse and can involve all body surfaces, including the palms, soles, and scalp (Fig. 108–3). The pustules last about 48 hours; the macules may persist for several months.

Diagnosis. Affected infants are otherwise well. A Wright-stained smear of pustule contents revealing keratinous debris and variable numbers of polymorphonuclear neutro-

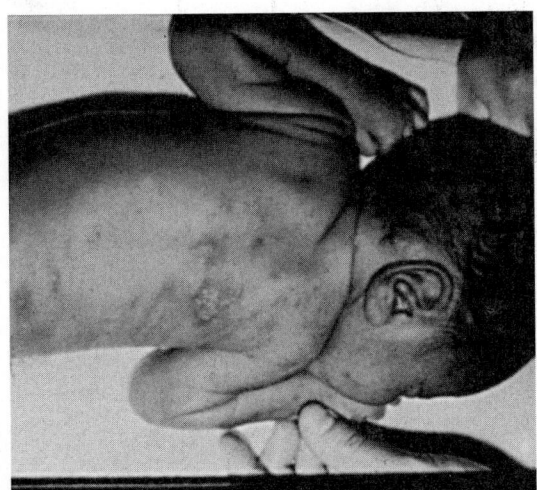

FIGURE 108–1. Florid lesions of erythema toxicum on the back of a newborn infant. The pustules are large and surrounded by an erythematous halo. Smears of the pustular contents showed only eosinophils.

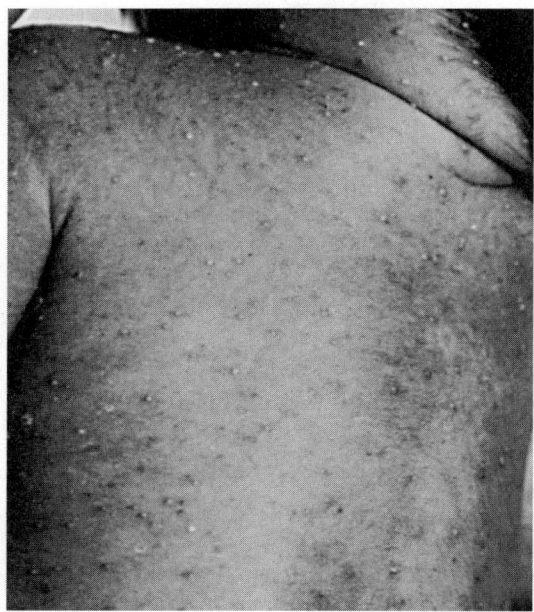

FIGURE 108–2. Numerous superficial pustules on the neck and back of a 1-day-old infant. A few pustules have ruptured, leaving a collarette of scale.

phils with few or no eosinophils supports the diagnosis. Gram's stain and bacterial cultures obtained from intact pustules uniformly fail to disclose the presence of organisms. The differential diagnosis includes the conditions listed for erythema toxicum.

Etiology. The cause of transient neonatal pustular melanosis is unknown. A prospective study reported that 17 infants with typical congenital lesions subsequently developed le-

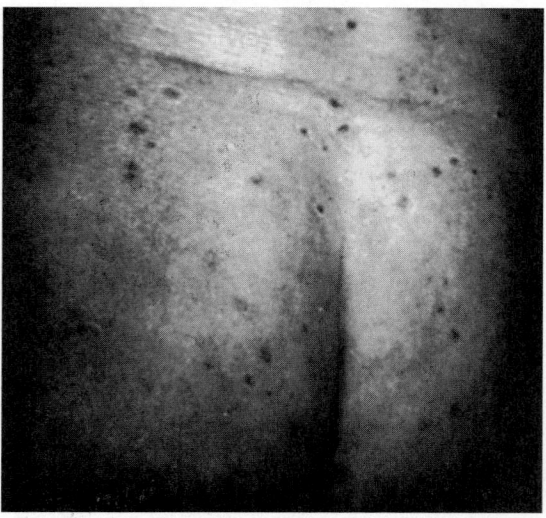

FIGURE 108–3. Transient neonatal pustular melanosis. Hyperpigmented macules on the lower back and buttocks, some of which are encircled by scale. (From Ramamurthy RS, Reveri M, Esterly NB, et al: Transient neonatal pustular melanosis. J Pediatr 88:831, 1976.)

sions of erythema toxicum, linking the two conditions (Ferrandiz et al, 1992).

Treatment. The disorder is asymptomatic and self limited. Once the diagnosis is confirmed, further therapy is not required.

MILIA, EPSTEIN PEARLS, AND SEBACEOUS HYPERPLASIA

Clinical Findings. Milia (single lesions are called *milium*) are found in 40% of full-term infants (Gordon, 1959). They are single or sparsely scattered 1- to 2-mm pearly lesions that occur on the face. The sites of predilection are the cheeks, forehead, and chin (Fig. 108–4). Large milia (larger than 2 mm) are found in infants with type I oral-facial-digital syndrome (Solomon et al, 1970). Rarely, milia may occur in unusual sites, such as on the arms, legs, or the foreskin.

Epstein pearls are the name given to milia that occur in the oral mucosa. These tiny cystic lesions occur in about 85% of newborn infants and are usually found on the palate, particularly along the midpalatine raphe and at the junction of the hard and soft palate. They are usually grouped, firm, and movable, and are an opaque white color.

Diagnosis. Histologically, a milium is an invagination of epidermal tissue, arising from the pilosebaceous apparatus of vellus hair, which forms a cyst filled with several layers of keratin-producing cells. The expressed contents of milial cysts resemble tiny white pearls and consist mostly of keratinocyte debris, a useful diagnostic feature.

Milia may be mistaken for sebaceous gland hyperplasia, which occurs in the same distribution. The papules of sebaceous gland hyperplasia are smaller (pinpoint), more yellow, and contain sebaceous lipids. Milia usually exfoliate spontaneously within a month. Epstein pearls are self limited but may take several months to resolve. Sebaceous hyperplasia also resolves spontaneously within the first few weeks of life.

MILIARIA

Clinical Findings. Miliaria neonatorum is a vesicular or pustular dermatitis arising from the eccrine duct. Four clinical variants have been described, their appearances

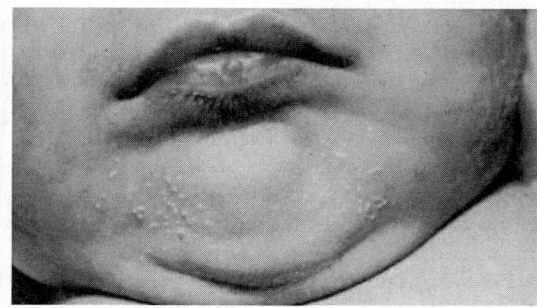

FIGURE 108–4. Numerous grouped milia on the chin of a newborn infant.

influenced by the site of obstruction within the duct. Miliaria crystallina (sudamina), are very superficial, clear, thin-walled, noninflammatory vesicles that rupture easily. The vesicle is localized within the stratum corneum. Miliaria rubra (prickly heat), are small, erythematous, grouped papules often localized to skin folds and areas covered by clothing. These lesions arise within the deeper levels of the epidermis and are accompanied by inflammation. The papules may become pustular if there is a prominent inflammatory component or secondary bacterial infection, a condition sometimes referred to as miliaria pustulosa. Miliaria profunda is a mildly inflammatory papular eruption that arises within the dermal portion of the eccrine duct.

Etiology. Miliaria is believed to be caused by sweat accumulation into obstructed eccrine ducts. Obstruction of the eccrine duct in adults has been reported to result from a variety of triggers including cutaneous injury, excessive hydration of the stratum corneum, or overgrowth of microbes (Fitzpatrick, 1990). Premature and even full-term neonates have a full complement of eccrine glands, distributed in greater density than after growth and increased skin surface area (Jordan and Blaney, 1982). Immature, incompletely canalized eccrine ducts could predispose the newborn to miliaria (Straka, et al, 1991). Overheating from excessive bundling and phototherapy probably contribute to its pathogenesis. The widespread availability of environmental temperature control has probably decreased the incidence of this condition.

Diagnosis. The differential diagnosis of miliaria includes the conditions listed above for erythema toxicum. Wright's stain of vesicle contents from miliaria crystallina will be cell-poor; that of miliaria rubra will usually reveal a majority of lymphocytes. If screening studies are nondiagnostic, a skin biopsy will be confirmatory (Fitzpatrick, 1990).

Treatment. Lesions rapidly resolve after the infant's environmental temperature is reduced. Application of occlusive emollients may exacerbate the eruption.

ACNE

Clinical Findings. The appearance of acne in infancy is similar to typical acne vulgaris of adolescence. The spectrum of lesions includes comedones, inflammatory papules, pustules, and rarely, cysts, generally limited to the face (Fig. 108–5). Comedones are an easily recognized, pathognomonic feature of acne.

The condition occurs in up to 20% of infants and is more common in boys. Acne occurs in a bimodal distribution during infancy. Early onset, *neonatal acne* occurs after 1 to 2 weeks of age and usually resolves spontaneously by 3 months. *Infantile acne* appears after 3 to 6 months and may persist for years.

Etiology. The pathophysiology of acne is similar at all ages. Important components are the increased size and activity of sebaceous glands, which are influenced by circulating levels of adrenal and gonadal androgens, of both endogenous and maternal origin. The role of *Propionibacterium acnes* in infantile acne has not been studied. This lipophilic,

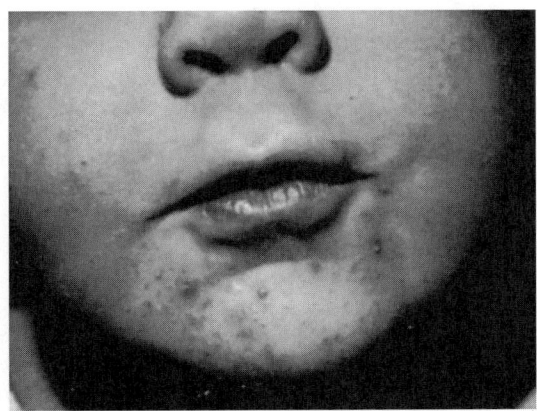

FIGURE 108–5. Papules, pustules, and comedones (diagnostic of acne) on the chin and cheeks of an infant male.

anaerobic gram-positive rod plays an important role in the pathogenesis of inflammatory lesions in adolescent acne. A family history of acne is common and affected infants have a higher risk of developing severe acne later in life (Hellier, 1954) suggesting a genetic predisposition (Forest et al, 1973).

Diagnosis. The differential diagnosis includes the papular and pustular disorders listed above, but the diagnosis of acne can almost always be made by clinical inspection. No other disorder features comedones. Infants with severe or persistent acne should be evaluated for androgenic endocrinopathy.

Treatment. Aggressive treatment of neonatal acne is rarely required. As initial therapy, topical 2% erythromycin or 2.5% to 5% benzoyl peroxide may be applied daily. Tretinoin and more potent benzoyl peroxides may be irritating. In more severe cases, a course of enteral erythromycin may be added, in divided doses of 30 to 50 mg/kg per day. Creams, ointments, and topical steroids may exacerbate the condition.

INFANTILE ECZEMA

The term *eczema* is derived from a Greek term meaning "to boil over." It refers to a clinical and histologic cutaneous phenotype characterized by erythema, edema, and scaling, often accompanied by crusting and, in severe cases, blistering. The histologic hallmark of acute eczema is epidermal intercellular edema (i.e., spongiosis). Epidermal thickening is present in chronic eczema. A mixed, perivascular inflammatory infiltrate is usually seen within the papillary dermis.

Different types of eczema can be defined by a spectrum of unifying clinical features. When a patient presents in infancy with widespread eczema, a precise diagnosis sometimes requires a period of observation. There are two common eczematous conditions that present in otherwise healthy infants: seborrheic dermatitis and atopic dermatitis. These diseases differ in pathogenesis, distribution of skin involvement, prognosis, and range of therapeutic options. Infants with widespread eczema who are not otherwise healthy, or those with prominent, erosive periorificial involvement should be evaluated for associated nutritional, metabolic, or immunologic abnormalities. A more extensive differential diagnosis is detailed under "Erythroderma" in Chapter 105.

Seborrheic Dermatitis

Clinical Findings. Infantile seborrheic dermatitis is characterized by greasy yellow scale on an erythematous base and minimal pruritus. Onset is usually within the first two months of life. The most common sites of involvement are the face, scalp, and diaper area. It may be localized or disseminated. Flexural areas such as the posterior auricular sulcus, neck, axillae, and inguinal folds can also be affected. Hypopigmentation is often striking in dark-skinned infants (Fig. 108–6). In severe cases, fissures may develop and become secondarily infected.

Causes. *Pityrosporum ovale* is a lipophilic yeast that is commonly present on normal skin, increasing in density during and after puberty. The mycelial form has been identified as a causative agent in tinea versicolor. For a century, the yeast form has been linked to adult seborrheic dermatitis. Therapeutic trials with yeast-inhibiting agents have supported a causal role (Straka, 1991). There is a higher incidence of seborrheic dermatitis in immunocompromised patients, especially those with AIDS (Prose, 1991). The association between *P. ovale* and infantile seborrheic dermatitis has been established more recently (Broberg and Faergemann, 1989; Ruiz-Maldonado et al, 1989). The pathogenesis of the disorder, the reason carriers remain asymptomatic and immunocompromised individuals can be more severely affected, remains unclear.

Treatment. Infantile seborrheic dermatitis spontaneously improves by the end of the first year of life. For infants with disfiguring or symptomatic disease, there are several therapeutic alternatives. Topical agents effective against *P. ovale* include topical ketoconazole, in a cream or shampoo base (Cutsem et al, 1990), shampoos containing 1% zinc pyrithione or 1% to 2.5% selenium sulfide, and propylene glycol (Faergemann, 1988). Propylene glycol is a hygroscopic preservative, with antimycotic activity against *P.*

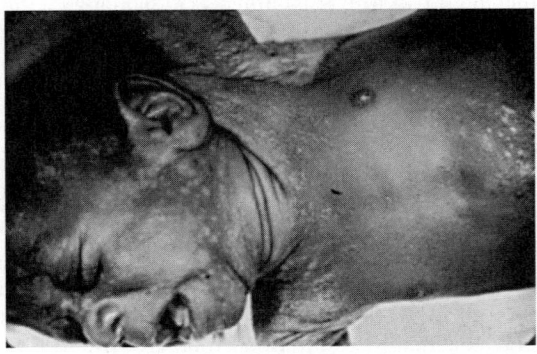

FIGURE 108–6. Infant with seborrheic eczema on the face and neck and in the axillae. Note the scaling and hypopigmentation. Temporary hypopigmentation is common in black infants with this disorder.

ovale, that has been widely used for over a century in foods and cosmetics. It is commercially available as a 1.5% soapless cleanser (Cetaphil lotion, Galderma Laboratories, Inc., Fort Worth, TX). The safety and efficacy for none of these products has been established in infants. But widespread availability and popular use has not produced reports of toxicity (see Chapter 105). Brief application with daily bathing is usually effective and limits excessive percutaneous absorbtion. Daily application of 0.5% to 1% hydrocortisone cream is another short-term alternative.

Atopic Dermatitis

Clinical Findings. Atopic dermatitis (AD) is a chronic, severely pruritic, familial disorder defined by a spectrum of defined cutaneous and extracutaneous manifestations (Hanifin, 1991; Paller, 1991). In 60% of cases, signs and symptoms begin in infancy; up to 10% of 1-year-old children are affected (Kay et al, 1994). The most easily recognized of the diagnostic criteria for atopic dermatitis may not be present until early childhood. These include onset of rash under the age of 2 years, flexural skin lesions, asthma or hay fever, and generalized dry skin (Williams et al, 1994). Atopic dermatitis and seborrheic dermatitis share clinical features, often making correct diagnosis difficult during the neonatal period. A common feature that may distinguish the two is involvement of the diaper area. This area is often dramatically spared in infants with atopic dermatitis and is primarily involved in infants with seborrheic dermatitis.

Etiology. Atopic disease has been clinically recognized since 1916; however, its pathogenesis remains elusive. Recent investigations of mechanisms and treatment of AD have focused on immune alterations. Blood eosinophilia, overproduction of IgE, and a diminished cell-mediated delayed-type hypersensitivity response are common features. Other, in vitro immune abnormalities have been described, including alterations in monocyte cAMP production, increased histamine release by basophils and mast cells, abnormal differentiation of antigen-presenting cells, increased serum levels of eosinophil cationic protein and interleukin-4, and diminished production of interferon gamma by circulating lymphocytes (Hanifin, 1991; Hanifin et al, 1993). These data support a hypothesis about the basic immune dysregulation causing AD. The theory assumes an imbalance of T-cell subsets, with inhibition of the cells that produce interferon gamma (Th1 T-cells) and a relative activation of the cells that produce interleukin-4 (Th2 T-cells). These assumed outcomes are believed to potentiate a vicious cycle of enhanced production of IgE, eosinophilia, mast cell proliferation, release of histamine by basophils and mast cells, and further expansion of Th2 cells (Hanifin, 1991; Hanifin et al, 1993).

Staphylococcus aureus plays an important role in the exacerbation of AD. Ninety percent of affected patients carry this microbe on their skin, and a course of antistaphylococcal antibiotics augments therapy during clinical flares. Staphylococcal exotoxins act as superantigens capable of stimulating a wide variety of T-cell responses (Leung et al, 1995).

Food and environmental allergens play a role in the

minority of patients (Hanifin, 1991). Prolonged breast-feeding and delayed exposure to diverse solid foods may protect against AD, especially in infants with a strong family of atopic disease (Zeiger, 1994).

Treatment. The goal of treatment is to control signs and symptoms. A definitive cure is not yet available, but spontaneous improvement occurs before puberty in 40% of patients (Hanifin, 1991). Maintenance therapy aims to hydrate the skin, reduce inflammation, control pruritus, and eliminate inciting factors. These goals are achieved with once-to-twice a day bathing with a mild antimicrobial cleanser, sparing application of topical corticosteroids, and liberal application of a bland ointment emollient. Addition of systemic antistaphylococcal antibiotics is sometimes necessary.

Infants with atopic dermatitis have a relative cutaneous anergy, and are at increased risk of cutaneous bacterial, yeast, fungal, and viral infections. A high index of suspicion for secondary infection must be maintained. Details of the diagnostic evaluation are outlined in Chapter 105.

Diaper Dermatitis

Etiology. Although diaper dermatitis was described over a century ago, and has been widely studied, the cause, true prevalence, and optimal treatment are still issues of debate. The majority of infants have episodes of diaper dermatitis, most commonly between 6 and 12 months of age (Jordan and Blaney, 1982). For decades, the condition was believed to be primarily due to the effects of ammonia. However, objective studies did not support this theory (Leyden et al, 1977). Many factors contribute to the pathogenesis of diaper dermatitis, but the nidus of the problem begins with occlusion, excessive hydration, friction, and maceration. Once skin barrier function has been compromised, irritants (urine, fecal lipases, proteases, bile salts) and microorganisms (urease-splitting bacteria, *S. aureus*, beta-hemolytic streptococcus, *Pseudomonas* spp, *Candida albicans*) exacerbate the problem. Exogenous irritants, such as soaps, commercial diaper wipes, and a myriad over-the-counter topical products, can perpetuate the process in susceptible infants.

Treatment. Clearly, the most important steps in preventing diaper dermatitis are maintaining skin barrier function and hygiene and preventing irritation. Traditionally, an effective but labor-intensive approach has been frequent diaper changes with gentle cleansing, thorough drying, and limited use of occlusive plastic or rubber diaper covers. This practice has been greatly simplified by the introduction of disposable diapers.

The first disposable diapers were marketed in 1963. For 20 years the absorbant core was composed primarily of cellulose fluff. During that time, several conflicting studies were done comparing the incidence of diaper dermatitis in infants using cloth versus disposable diapers (Jordan and Blaney, 1982). In the mid-1980s, a superabsorbant core material was developed, containing a cross-linked sodium polyacrylate. This material transforms and holds fluid within a gel, and has the capacity to absorb many times its own weight. Several studies have concluded that superabsorbant diapers are superior to cloth diapers in preventing

diaper dermatitis (Lane, 1990). In addition, superabsorbant diapers may prevent occult fecal contamination of clothing and fomites in daycare settings (Rory, 1991).

Routine use of topical preparations to prevent diaper dermatitis is not necessary for infants with normal skin. Some of these products have additional risks. Additives have the potential to cause contact sensitization or irritation. Powders applied vigorously enough to raise a cloud pose an aspiration hazard. This is especially true for talc, which can cause irritant pneumonitis. Talc (mainly hydrous magnesium silicate) may also cause granulomatous reactions when applied to wounds.

Appropriate treatment of diaper dermatitis begins with correct diagnosis of the underlying cause. Most infants develop acute diaper dermatitis as a result of the factors described previously. However, other primary pathologic processes must be considered for any infant with chronic, severe, or recurrent diaper rash. Primary cutaneous diseases that may present with diaper rash include allergic contact dermatitis, seborrheic dermatitis, psoriasis, and candidiasis. Several uncommon causes of diaper dermatitis such as histiocytosis, congenital syphilis, bullous pemphigoid, and staphylococcal scalded skin syndrome have serious implications (Lane, 1988).

Mild-to-moderate, common diaper dermatitis should be treated initially with traditional, frequent diaper changes, and/or leaving the area open. An interval change to superabsorbant diapers may be helpful for infants diapered with cloth. All potential irritants or sensitizers should be discontinued. Commercial diaper wipes are an often overlooked, common source of these. Washcloths, dampened paper towels, or mineral-oil soaked cotton balls are safe alternatives. Zinc oxide ointment or paste are inexpensive, bland, protective agents with antiseptic and astringent properties. Zinc may also play a role in wound healing (Maitra and Dorani, 1992; Okada et al, 1990; Rackett et al, 1993). Some caregivers may object to the difficulty in removing zinc oxide preparations. They should be reassured that it is not necessary to remove the salve. If a parent or clinician needs to remove zinc oxide to assess the skin, this can be easily accomplished with the help of mineral oil. If there is no objective evidence of candidiasis, a short course of a topical low-potency corticosteroid may be beneficial. A topical anticandidal agent should be used when potassium hydroxide preparation or culture suggests yeast infection. Combination products containing potent topical corticosteroids and antifungal agents are less effective than an antifungal used alone (Reynolds et al, 1991). Widespread use of one such product, combining a potent, fluoronated topical corticosteroid, 0.05% betamethasone diproprionate, with 1% clotrimazole (Lotrisone) applied under the occlusion of a diaper, has resulted in reports of skin atrophy, striae, and even adrenal suppression (Barkley, 1987). Clotrimazole and a similar product combining 0.1% triamcinolone acetonide and nystatin (Mycolog II) are contraindicated for diaper dermatitis.

HARLEQUIN COLOR CHANGE

Harlequin color change should not be confused with an entirely different disorder called *harlequin fetus.* Harlequin color change, first described in 1952, usually occurs during

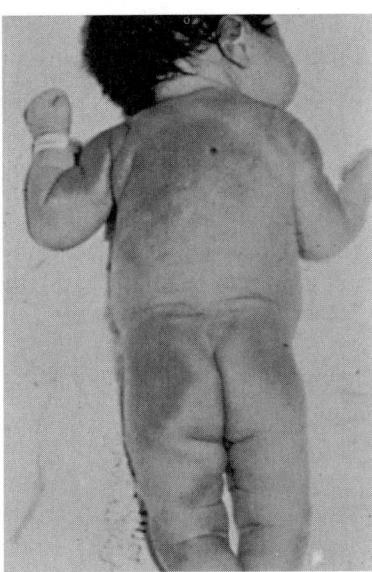

FIGURE 108–7. Rear view of newborn showing several large discolored areas of subcutaneous fat necrosis. They were irregular in size and shape, felt firm, and were not hot or tender.

the first 4 days of life (Mortensen and Stougard-Andresen, 1959). It is characterized by reddening of one half of the body and simultaneous blanching of the other half. A sharp, midline demarcation runs from the center of the forehead, down the face and trunk. Occasionally, the line of demarcation may be incomplete, sparing the face and genitalia. Turning the body from one side to the other accentuates blanching of the upper half and reddening of the lower half. There is no accompanying change in respiratory rate, pupillary reflexes, muscle tone, or response to external stimuli. The total duration of these episodes may range from a few minutes to several hours. Harlequin color change occurs most frequently in low-birth-weight infants but may be seen in up to 10% of term infants. The physiologic basis of the phenomenon has not been defined. It has no pathologic significance, requires no treatment, and can be expected to disappear no later than the third week of life.

SUBCUTANEOUS FAT NECROSIS

Clinical Findings. Subcutaneous fat necrosis affects full-term infants who have experienced perinatal distress. Lesions usually appear within the first 2 weeks of life. They may be single or multiple, poorly circumscribed, and are often tender nodules or plaques that are initially firm with a dusky reddish-purple hue. They are most often located in areas in which a fat pad is present: buttocks, back, arms, and thighs (Fig. 108–7). With time, subcutaneous calcification may develop and drain, with resultant scarring. The most serious association is hypercalcemia. Infants with hypercalcemia may be asymptomatic, so the incidence and time course has not been well documented (Cook and Stone, 1992). Symptoms include irritability, vomiting, poor feeding, and failure to thrive.

Causes. The development of subcutaneous fat necrosis has been related to ischemic injury from obstetric trauma,

intrauterine asphyxia (Chen et al, 1981), and hypothermia. Skin biopsy from a well-developed lesion will reveal a subcutaneous granulomatous infiltrate with multinucleated giant cells. Damaged lipocytes contain characteristic needle-shaped clefts. Soft-tissue necrosis and inflammation may stimulate local production of 1,25 dihydroxyvitamin D_3, resulting in hypercalcemia (Cook and Stone, 1992).

Treatment. In most infants, the process is self limited; resolution occurs over a period of weeks to months. Some recommend careful needle aspiration of fluctuant areas to reduce scarring (Hurwitz, 1985). Infants should be followed closely for the development of hypercalcemia for the first 6 weeks of life. Hypercalcemic infants should be treated initially with hydration and furosemide-induced diuresis. Restriction of oral calcium and vitamin D intake, and the administration of systemic corticosteroids may be necessary (Cook and Stone, 1992; Norwood-Galloway et al, 1987).

SCLEREMA NEONATORUM

The lesions of subcutaneous fat necrosis are histologically similar to those of sclerema neonatorum, raising unnecessary concern for stable, full-term infants with localized skin lesions. Sclerema neonatorum is a diffuse, systemic process with a grave prognosis (Fretzin and Arias, 1987).

Clinical Findings. Sclerema neonatorum occurs in debilitated or preterm neonates. It presents with widespread, stone-hard, nonpitting cutaneous induration. The skin appears pale and waxy, shaping the face in mask-like expression (Fig. 108–8); the joints are stiff. Associated metabolic

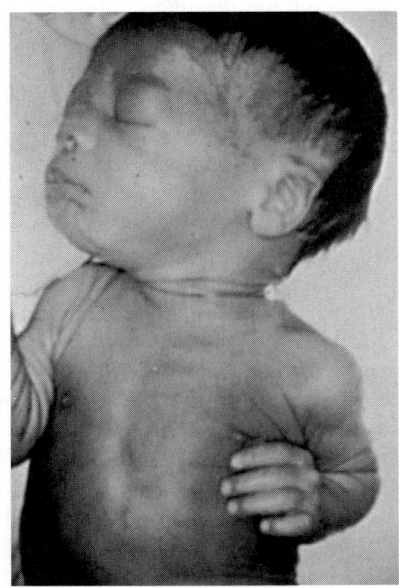

FIGURE 108–8. Sclerema neonatorum. Note the mask-like expression on the face, "pseudotrismus" of the partially immobilized mouth, and thickening of the skin over the face, arms, and hands. (From the Collection of the American Academy of Pediatrics. Reproduced with permission of the officers of the Academy.)

acidosis, hypoglycemia, hyperkalemia, hyponatremia, and azotemia may occur.

Etiology. The disorder has been associated with prematurity, low body weight, asphyxia, and hypothermia (Ji et al, 1993).

The histologic changes in sclerema are not specific. Fat necrosis with crystallization may be seen; thinning of the epidermis, dermal, and subcutaneous fibrosis with edema and thickening of the interlobular septa are more conspicuous features (Dasgupta et al, 1993).

The mechanism responsible for sclerema is unknown. Biochemical and crystalline changes in the subcutaneous fat of affected infants have suggested a decrease in the enzymatic desaturation of triglycerides (Horsefield and Yardley, 1965; Kellum et al, 1968).

Treatment. The treatment of sclerema neonatorum is supportive care. Corticosteroid therapy has not been effective in altering the 30% to 60% mortality rate (Levin et al, 1961).

REFERENCES

Barkley W: Strial and persistent tinea corporis related to prolonged use of betamethasone diproprionate. J Am Acad Dermatol 17:518–519, 1987.

Bassukas ID: Is erythema toxicum neonatorum a mild self-limited acute cutaneous graft–versus–host reaction from maternal-to-fetal lymphocyte transfer? Medical Hypotheses 38:334–338, 1992.

Berg FJ, Solomon LM: Erythema neonatorum toxicum. Arch Dis Child 62:327, 1987.

Bergbrant IM: Seborrhoeic dermatitis and pityrosporum ovale: Cultural, immunological and clinical studies. Acta Derm Venereol Suppl (Stockh); Suppl 167 (U1):7–36, 1991.

Broberg A, Faergemann J: Infantile seborrhoeic dermatitis and Pityrosporum ovale. Br J Dermatol 120:359–362, 1989.

Carr JA, Hodgeman JE, Freedman RJ, Levan NE: Relationship between toxic erythema and infant maturity. Am J Dis Child 112:129, 1966.

Chen TH, Shewmake SW, Hansen DD, Lacey HL: Subcutaneous fat necrosis of the newborn. Arch Dermatol 117:36, 1981.

Cook JS, Stone MS: Hypercalcemia in association with subcutaneous fat necrosis of the newborn: Studies of calcium-regulating hormones. Pediatrics 90:93–96, 1992.

Cutsem J, Gerven F, Fransen J, et al: The in vitro antifungal activity of ketoconazole, zinc pyrithione, and selenium sulfide against Pityrosporum and their efficacy as a shampoo in the treatment of experimental pityrosporosis in guinea pigs. J Am Acad Dermatol 22:993–998, 1990.

Dasgupta A, Ghosh RN, Pal RK, Mukherjee N: Sclerema neonatorum—histopathologic study. Indian Journal of Pathology & Microbiology 36:45–47, 1993.

Faergemann J: Propylene glycol in the treatment of seborrheic dermatitis of the scalp. Cutis 42:69–71, 1988.

Ferrandiz C, Coroleu W, Ribera M, et al: Sterile transient neonatal pustulosis is a precocious form of erythema toxicum neonatorum. Dermatology 185:18–22, 1992.

Fitzpatrick JE: Inflammatory reactions of the sweat unit. In Farmer ER, Hood AF (Eds): Pathology of the Skin. Norwalk, Appleton & Lange, 1990, pp 959–964.

Fitzpatrick R, Rapaport MS, Silva DG: Histiocytosis X. Arch Dermatol 117:253, 1981.

Forest MG, Cathiard AM, Bertrand GH: Evidence of testicular activity in early infancy. G Clin Endocrinol Metab 37:148, 1973.

Fretzin DF, Arias AM: Sclerema neonatorum and subcutaneous fat necrosis of the newborn. Pediatr Dermatol 4:112, 1987.

Gordon J: Miliary sebaceous cysts and blisters in the healthy newborn. Acta Obstet Gynaecol Scand 38:352, 1959.

Hanifin J: Atopic dermatitis in infants and children. Pediatr Clin North Am 38:763–789, 1991.

Hanifin J, Schneider L, Leung D, et al: Recombinant interferon gamma therapy for atopic dermatitis. J Am Acad Dermatol 28:189–197, 1993.

Hellier FF: Acneiform eruptions in infancy. Br J Dermatol 66:25, 1954.

Horsefield GJ, Yardley HJ: Sclerema neonatorum. J Invest Dermatol 44:326, 1965.

Hurwitz S: A visual guide to neonatal skin eruptions. Contemporary Pediatrics September, pp 82–92, 1985.

Ji XC, Zhu CY, Pang RY: Epidemiological study on hypothermia in newborns. Chinese Medical Journal 106:428–432, 1993.

Jordan W, Blaney T: Factors influencing infant diaper dermatitis. In Neonatal Skin: Predisposition, Structure and Function, vol 1. New York, Marcel Dekker Inc., 1982, pp 205–221.

Kay J, Gawkrodger DJ, Mortimer MJ, Jaron AG: The prevalence of childhood atopic eczema in a general population. J Am Acad Dermatol 30:35–39, 1994.

Kellum RE, Ray TL, Brown GR: Sclerema neonatorum: Report of case analysis of subcutaneous and epidermal-dermal lipids by chromatographic methods. Arch Dermatol 97:372, 1968.

Lane A: Diaper rash: Causes and cures. Patient Care 1988.

Lane A, Rehder P, Helm K: Evaluation of diapers containing absorbent gelling material with conventional disposable diapers in newborn infants. Am J Dis Child 144:315–318, 1990.

Leung DY, Travers JB, Norris DA: The role of superantigens in skin disease. J Invest Dermatol 105(suppl 1):37s–42s, 1995.

Levin SE, Milunsky A: Urea and electrolyte levels in the serum in sclerema neonatorum. J Pediatr 67:812, 1965.

Leyden J, Katz S, Stewart R, Kligman A: Urinary ammonia and ammonia-producing microorganisms in infants with and without diaper dermatitis. Arch Dermatol 113:1678–1680, 1977.

Maitra A, Dorani B: Role of zinc in post-injury wound healing. Arch Emerg Med 9:122–124, 1992.

Mortensen O, Stougard-Andresen P: Harlequin color change in the newborn. Acta Obstet Gynecol Scand 38:352, 1959.

Neligan GW, Strang LB: A "harlequin" colour change in the newborn. Lancet 2:1005, 1952.

Norwood-Galloway A, Lebwohl M, Phelps RG, et al: Subcutaneous fat necrosis of the newborn and hypercalcemia. J Am Acad Dermatol 16:435, 1987.

Okada A, Takagi Y, Nezu R, Lee S: Zinc in clinical surgery—a research review. Jpn J Surg 20:635–644, 1990.

Paller AS: Childhood atopic dermatitis: Update on therapy. Clin Case Dermatol 2:9–14, 1991.

Prose NS: Mucocutaneous disease in pediatric human immunodeficiency virus infection. Pediatr Clin North Am 38:977–990, 1991.

Rackett S, Rothe M, Grant-Kels J: Diet and dermatology—the role of dietary manipulation in the prevention and treatment of cutaneous disorders. J Am Acad Dermatol 29:447–461, 1993.

Ramamurthy RS, Reveri M, Esterly NB, et al: Transient neonatal pustular melanosis. J Pediatr 88:831, 1976.

Reynolds R, Boiko S, Lucky A: Exacerbation of tinea corporis during treatment with 1% clotrimazole/0.05% betamethasone diproprionate (Lotrisone). Am J Dis Child 145:1224–1225, 1991.

Rory V, Wun C, Morrow A, Pickering LK: The effect of diaper type and overclothing on fecal contamination in day-care centers. JAMA 265:1840–1844, 1991.

Ruiz-Maldonado R, Lopez-Matinez R, Chavarria E, et al: Pityrosporum ovale in infantile seborrheic dermatitis. Pediatr Dermatol 6:16–20, 1989.

Sharlin DN, Koblenzer P: Necrosis of subcutaneous fat with hypercalcemia: A puzzling and multifaceted disease. Clin Pediatr 9:290, 1970.

Straka BF, Cooper PH, Greer K: Congenital miliaria crystallina. Cutis 47:103–106, 1991.

Solomon LM, Esterly NB: Eczema in Neonatal Dermatology. Philadelphia, WB Saunders, 1973, p 125.

Solomon LM, Fretzin D, Pruzansky S: Pilosebaceous dysplasia in the oral-facial-digital syndrome. Arch Dermatol 102:596, 1970.

Solomon LM, Rostenberg A Jr: Atopic dermatitis and infantile eczema. In Samter M, Talmadge DW, Rose B, et al (Eds): Immunological Diseases, 3rd ed. Boston, Little, Brown, 1978, p 953.

Taylor WB, Bondurant CP: Erythema neonatorum allergicum. Arch Dermatol 76:591, 1957.

Williams HC, Burney PG, Pembroke AC, Hay RJ: The U.K. working party's diagnostic criteria for atopic dermatitis, III: Independent hospital validation. Br J Dermatol 131:406–416, 1994.

Zeiger RS: Dietary manipulations in infants and their mothers and the natural course of atopic disease. Pediatr Allergy Immunol 5 (suppl 6):26–28, 1994.

CHAPTER 109

Cutaneous Congenital Defects

Elaine C. Siegfried and Nancy B. Esterly

The spectrum of congenital cutaneous defects can be organized by tissue of origin or location within the skin. This spectrum is summarized in Table 109–1. However, in many cases the clinical appearance is not diagnostic for the specific condition or even the tissue type. An overview of differential diagnosis by clinical appearance is included in Chapter 105. This chapter includes information on the most common and clinically significant congenital cutaneous defects.

VASCULAR DEFECTS

Precise diagnosis and appropriate management of the cutaneous vascular defects have been confounded by tremen-

TABLE 109–1

Spectrum of Congenital Cutaneous Defects

Vascular Defects

Hemangiomas
Malformations: lymphatic, venous, arterial, capillary, mixed

Hypopigmented Lesions

Ash-leaf macules, confetti-like macules
Linear and whorled hypomelanosis
Nevus depigmentosis
Nevus anemicus
Hemangioma precursor

Melanin-Containing Lesions

Nevocellular nevi
Melanoma
Lentigines
Café-au-lait macules
Nevus spilus
Mongolian spots
Nevus of Ota and nevus of Ito

Tumors of Epithelial Origin

Epidermal (keratinocytic) nevi/sebaceous nevi-nevus unius lateris,
    nevus verrucosis, ichthyosis hystrix
Nevus comedonicus
Pilomatrixoma
Porokeratosis of Mibelli

Dermal Tumors

Connective tissue nevi: collagen, elastic tissue
Digital fibroma

Tumors of Extracutaneous Origin

Cutaneous mastocytosis: urticaria pigmentosa, solitary mastocytoma,
    diffuse cutaneous mastocytosis
Juvenile xanthogranuloma
Lipoma
Osteoma cutis
Nasal glioma
Dermoid cyst
Meningioma

dous confusion in nomenclature and poor understanding of the pathogenesis of the different conditions within this group. For example, the term *hemangioma* has been used indiscriminately to refer to lesions that differ considerably in morphology, behavior, and prognosis. A more meaningful classification system was proposed by Mulliken and Glowacki in 1982. This scheme separates vascular lesions of infants and children into two major categories: hemangiomas and malformations (Mulliken and Young, 1988). A hemangioma, by definition, is a benign tumor of vascular endothelium, characterized by a proliferative phase and an involutional phase (Fig. 109–1A). In contrast, a malformation is a developmental anomaly generated from a single or combination of vascular components: capillary, venous, arterial, or lymphatic. These two groups can be further differentiated by clinical, cellular, hematologic, radiologic, and skeletal characteristics (Table 109–2).

Hemangiomas

Hemangiomas are the most common tumors of infancy; mature lesions have been noted in 10% to 12% of 1-year old infants. They occur sporadically, most often as single lesions. For unclear reasons, hemangiomas are more common in premature infants. The male-to-female ratio in term infants is 1:3 (Esterly, 1995).

Clinical Findings. Typically, hemangiomas are not clinically apparent at birth but present within the first month of life as a faint blush or area of pallor, a change known as a *precursor lesion*. Most hemangiomas grow rapidly in the first 3 to 6 months; the rate and extent of growth is impossible to predict. The clinical appearance is dictated by the depth of the tumor. Superficial lesions are cherry red and sharply circumscribed. This type of hemangioma has been referred to as a "strawberry," "capillary," "plane," or "planotuberous" hemangioma. Lesions that are confined to the deep dermis and subcutis appear bluish and dome-shaped. This subset has been referred to as "cavernous" or "nodose." Most lesions have both superficial and deep components. The added descriptors have no functional or prognostic significance with one possible exception: The superficial component may herald residual change in skin texture, whereas the deep component may leave excess fibrofatty tissue. The growth phase usually slows after 6 months and ends by 12 months of age, followed by gradual involution. Flattening occurs by age 5 in half the cases, and by age 9 in an additional 40% (Esterly, 1995). Parents are frequently concerned about the risk of hemorrhage and should be reassured that this rarely occurs. However, several other complications are possible, and the more serious sequelae follow:

▮ Obstruction—A hemangioma that obstructs just one

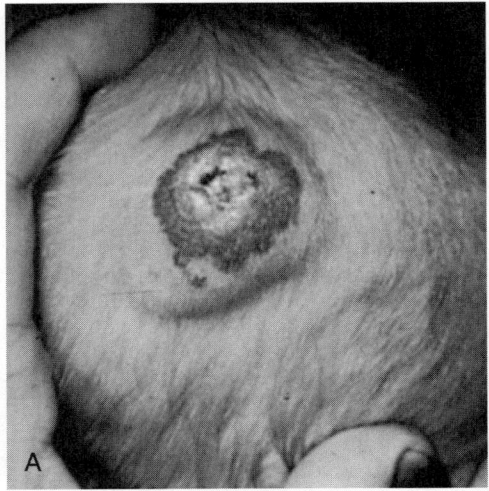

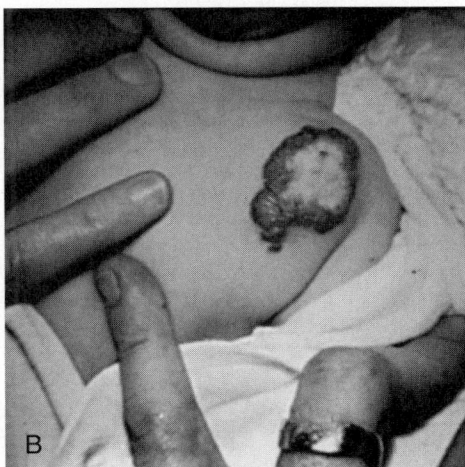

FIGURE 109–1. *A*, Hemangioma with small central ulceration on the scalp of an infant. *B*, Involuting hemangioma with central gray fibrotic area.

eye can pose a significant threat to visual development by limiting the visual field or compressing the globe. Obstruction of both external ear canals will impair development of hearing. Upper airway involvement may be marked by involvement of the beard area, and should be considered life-threatening.

■ Ulceration—This occurs in 5% of hemangiomas (Mulliken et al, 1995; Morelli et al, 1991; Morelli et al, 1994), most often in those located in areas of friction, (skin folds, diaper area), as well as in rapidly growing or involuting lesions. Ulcerated hemangiomas are painful and at risk for secondary infection.

■ Disfigurement—During the first year of life, the presence of a prominent hemangioma can elicit a disturbing amount of unwanted attention. Many parents require emotional support through this time. In addition to the transient disfigurement, lesions of the central face, and those with a significant superficial component, predispose to permanent scarring.

■ Kasabach-Merritt syndrome—This syndrome was originally described as a complication of infantile hemangioma, but may in fact be associated with a more

unusual vascular malformation (Enjolras et al, 1997). It consists of a rapidly expanding vascular tumor with primary platelet trapping and resultant consumptive coagulopathy. The mortality rate is 30% to 40%.

■ CNS anomalies—A giant facial hemangioma may be associated with defects of the posterior fossa (Reese et al, 1993).

■ Spinal dysraphism—A hemangioma over the sacrum may mark an underlying spinal cord abnormality (Tauafoghi et al, 1978; Albright et al, 1989).

■ Genitourinary abnormalities—Sacral hemangiomas may also be associated with imperforate anus, renal anomalies, or abnormalities of the external genitalia (Goldberg et al, 1986).

■ Visceral involvement—Diffuse neonatal hemangiomatosis presents as widely scattered small superficial hemangiomas. Infants with this pattern of cutaneous involvement may have a "benign" variant (i.e., lesions limited to skin). However, associated hemangiomatosis

TABLE 109–2

Characteristics of Vascular Birthmarks

Hemangioma	Malformation
Clinical	
Usually nothing seen at birth, 30 percent present as red macule	All present at birth; may not be evident
Rapid postnatal proliferation and slow involution	Commensurate growth; may expand as a result of trauma, sepsis, hormonal modulation
Female : male 3 : 1	Female : male 1 : 1
Cellular	
Plump endothelium, increased turnover	Flat endothelium, slow turnover
Increased mast cells	Normal mast cell count
Multilaminated basement membrane	Normal thin basement membrane
Capillary tubule formation in vitro	Poor endothelial growth in vitro
Hematologic	
Primary platelet trapping: thrombocytopenia (Kasabach-Merritt syndrome)	Primary stasis (venous); localized consumptive coagulopathy
Radiologic	
Angiographic findings; well-circumscribed, intense lobular-parenchymal staining with equatorial vessels	Angiographic findings: diffuse, no parenchyma Low-flow: phleboliths, ectatic channels High-flow: enlarged, tortuous arteries with arteriovenous shunting
Skeletal	
Infrequent "mass effect" on adjacent bone; hypertrophy rare	Low-flow: distortion, hypertrophy, or hypoplasia High-flow: destruction, distortion, or hypertrophy

From Mulliken JB, Young AE: Vascular Birthmarks, Hemangiomas and Malformations. Philadelphia, W. B. Saunders, 1988, p 35.

of the liver, GI tract, lungs and/or CNS, can be complicated by visceral hemorrhage or high-output cardiac decompensation, with a significant mortality rate. Congestive heart failure can also occur with a large, isolated cutaneous hemangioma (Mulliken et al, 1995).

Diagnosis. In most cases, a hemangioma can be diagnosed by its clinical appearance and pattern of evolution. A vascular lesion that is not obvious at birth, begins as a precursor noted during the first month of life, and exhibits rapid growth is undoubtedly a hemangioma. A lesion that deviates from this typical picture presents a diagnostic dilemma. The differential diagnosis includes atypical hemangioma, vascular malformation, or a nonvascular mimic. Doppler ultrasound is an easily performed test that may help to distinguish between a hemangioma and a high-flow malformation. Other imaging modalities, magnetic resonance imaging (MRI) or angiography, may be indicated for large or obstructive lesions (e.g., ocular or upper airway) to help define the extent of involvement or associated abnormalities (Esterly, 1995; Baker et al, 1993). Skin biopsy is diagnostic for nonvascular tumors that can mimic vascular birthmarks (e.g., pilomatrixoma, juvenile xanthogranuloma, Langerhans' cell histiocytosis, infantile myofibromatosis).

Pathogenesis. Hemangiomas in the proliferative phase are comprised of syncytial aggregates of endothelial cells. These cells, like mature endothelial cells, express alkaline phosphatase and factor VIII antigen, as well as Weibel-Palade bodies on electron microscopy, but [³H] labeling demonstrates active proliferation. Other histologic features that distinguish proliferating hemangiomas from malformations are the presence of multilaminate basement membranes bordering the endothelial syncytia, large numbers of mast cells (Esterly, 1995), and high expression of other immunohistochemical markers, including proliferating cell nuclear antigen, vascular endothelial growth factor, type IV collagenase, urokinase, and basic fibroblast growth factor (bFGF) (Takahashi et al, 1994). Elevated bFGF can be detected in urine from infants with hemangiomas, which may prove to be a useful diagnostic marker (Mulliken et al, 1995). Angiogenesis is a process that allows new blood vessel formation. It plays an important role in the growth of all vascular tumors, including hemangiomas. Identification of the basic processes that contribute to angiogenesis and effective angiogenesis inhibitors will provide insight into the pathogenesis and a more ideal therapy for hemangiomas (Mulliken, 1991; Morelli, 1993; O'Reilly et al, 1995).

Treatment. Eighty percent of hemangiomas are ultimately uncomplicated, and it is impossible to predict which ones will develop problems (Mulliken et al, 1995). For the majority of lesions, the initial treatment of choice is active nonintervention. During the phase of rapid proliferation, patients with uncomplicated hemangiomas should be examined at 2 to 4 week intervals for degree of growth and development of problems. During this phase, parents are often anxious and require ongoing, directed anticipatory guidance. A common concern is over the risk of significant hemorrhage. This is rare. Minor episodes of bleeding can

result from trauma and respond to short-term compression, like any superficial wound. Demonstration of before-and-after photographs of growing and involuted lesions in other children helps diminish concern. Local compression of accessible lesions (Mangus, 1973) may control growth and promote comfort. Coban dressing is a conveniently applied self-adhesive compressive wrap that easily provides compression (Kaplan and Palter, 1995).

Decades of aggressive therapy followed by suboptimal outcome from the 1940s through the 1960s was followed by a passive approach to the treatment of minimally complicated hemangiomas. The dogma has been to avoid treatment because children whose hemangiomas were allowed to involute spontaneously had less severe scarring than those subjected to cold steel or ionizing radiation. However, up to 20% of hemangiomas leave permanent skin changes that can be disfiguring (Enjolras and Mulliken, 1993). Psychological and social problems may result from facial or other visible deformities. Early intervention should be considered for lesions with a higher potential for complications. These include hemangiomas of the periorbital area, central face, skin folds, hands, and those with a pattern suggestive of visceral involvement (large or multiple lesions or "beard area"). Newer therapeutic approaches are aimed at minimizing growth or speeding slow resolution without the risk of additional scarring. In 1996, the benefits of newer approaches to therapy outweigh the risks in many cases. Early initiation of therapy, aimed at preventing growth, is easier and probably more effective than therapy that is delayed until maximal growth has been reached. Treatment options include pulsed dye laser, corticosteroids, and alpha-interferon, alone or in combination.

Several small uncontrolled studies have indicated that early treatment with yellow pulsed-dye laser can prevent growth of the superficial, but not the deep, component of proliferating hemangiomas. Later treatment of persistent hemangiomas may hasten, or ensure resolution (Ashinoff and Geronemus, 1991, 1993; Garden et al, 1992; Glassberg et al, 1989; Scheepers and Quaba, 1995; Sherwood and Tan, 1990; Waner et al, 1994; Wheeland, 1995). However, because the magnitude of growth, timing of involution, and degree of sequelae are variable and unpredictable, large, prospective, controlled studies are necessary to determine the laser's true efficacy and long-term effects.

Corticosteroids may be administered by topical application, intralesional injection or enteral/parenteral dosing. Each route utilizes corticosteroid preparations of different potency and duration of action. True comparative efficacy studies would be impossible. Experience is greatest with systemic administration, considered to be the optimal regimen by some experts; they recommend oral prednisone or prednisolone, 2 to 4 mg/kg per day as a single morning or divided dose (Esterly, 1995; Mulliken et al, 1995). Within 1 to 2 weeks, 30% of hemangiomas will show dramatic response; 40% will respond equivocally. In these patients, slowly tapering therapy is required through the proliferative phase. If no response is detected, the medication should be rapidly tapered after 2 weeks.

Intralesional injections may be preferred for well-localized hemangiomas, including those involving the eyelid. One-to-one mixtures of colloidal suspensions of triamcinolone and dexamethasone or betamethasone are used. Large doses are administered, in the range of 40 mg triamcinolone plus 6 mg of betamethasone in 2 mL of suspension (Kushner, 1979). Administration of this dose to a 5-kg infant is equivalent to 20 mg/kg of prednisone given as a single dose that may ultimately allow for a lower total systemic dose. Complications include cutaneous atrophy and skin necrosis.

The paucity of information on treatment of hemangiomas with topical steroids suggests that this route of administration has been ineffective. However, application of newer, more potent topical preparations may prove to be beneficial (Magana et al, 1994).

Recombinant interferon alfa-2a may be an effective therapy for life-threatening hemangiomas that are unresponsive to corticosteroids (Mulliken et al, 1995). Regression is not as dramatic as seen in corticosteroid-responsive lesions, making this form of therapy inadequate for vision-threatening hemangiomas; however, it is especially effective for Kasabach-Merritt syndrome. Interferon alpha-2a is administered as a subcutaneous injection, in the range of 3 million units/m² per day. Treatment must be continued for 6 to 10 months. Side effects include fevers up to 39° C, reversible elevations in liver transaminases, neutropenia, and anemia (Esterly, 1995; Mulliken et al, 1995).

Angiogenesis inhibitors offer promise for more predictably effective therapy in the future. Candidates include interleukin-12 (Voest et al, 1995) and AGM-1470 (a derivative of the fungal product fumagillin) (O'Reilly et al, 1995).

Ulceration is a therapeutic challenge that may be treated initially with the appropriate occlusive dressing. The choice of dressing and frequency of changes are dictated by the amount of exudate produced (see Table 105–7). Coban dressing is ideally suited to secure dressings over hemangiomas of the extremities (Kaplan and Paller, 1995). For sites that are difficult to dress, frequent, liberal application of zinc oxide paste is effective. To inspect the skin, zinc oxide is easily removed with mineral oil. Pain control should be prescribed. Alternating doses of acetaminophen and ibuprofen are usually sufficient, but overuse of the latter may increase the risk of bleeding and cause pain from GI upset that can be difficult to distinguish from the pain associated with ulceration. A high index of suspicion should be maintained for secondary infection, with a low threshold for either topical or systemic antibiotic therapy. If conservative therapy is unsuccessful, yellow light laser may relieve pain and speed reepithelialization (Morelli et al, 1991; Morelli et al, 1994; Achaver and Vanderkum, 1991). The ulcers will heal but will inevitably leave scars.

A hemangioma that interferes with the visual axis should be treated aggressively. Evaluation by an experienced pediatric ophthalmologist is recommended. A hemangioma that limits the visual field but does not distort the globe may be treated by patching the contralateral eye. More complicated lesions may be treated initially with corticosteriods: topical, enterally administered, or intralesional. The latter route of administration carries the risk of embolic occlusion of the retinal arteries. This tragic adverse effect can occur ipsilaterally, contralaterally, or bilaterally (Fig. 109–2) (Brown et al, 1972; Fost and Esterly, 1968; Zuniga et al, 1987). Surgical excision should be considered for vision-threatening hemangiomas that fail to respond to corticosteroids (Mulliken et al, 1995; Walker et al, 1994).

There is no uniformly successful therapy for seriously complicated or life-threatening hemangiomas. Reported treatment options include high-dose corticosteroids, aspirin, dipyridamole, interferon alpha, cold steel excision, sclerotherapy, arterial embolization, cyclophosphamide, and vincristine (Esterly, 1995; Mulliken et al, 1995; Payarols et al, 1995; Enjolras et al, 1990). All carry significant risks. The use of ionizing radiation is justified for alarming hemangiomas that have been unresponsive to other therapeutic modalities and are inoperable.

Vascular Malformations

Vascular malformations may be indistinguishable from hemangiomas by clinical and light microscopic examination; however, they are biologically distinct lesions.

Clinical Findings. Malformations are true structural anomalies, comprised of one or more types of vessels—capillaries, veins, arteries, and/or lymphatics. Unlike hemangiomas, they are always present at birth. They equally affect males and females. Growth is commensurate with the child, although they may expand as a result of local thrombosis or inflammation. Primary platelet trapping with consumptive coagulopathy (e.g., Kasabach-Merritt syndrome) does not occur. Local skeletal or soft tissue destruction or hypertrophy is common. Spontaneous resolution is not expected except in one specific malformation, the salmon patch. Vascular malformations occur either as isolated cutaneous defects or in association with a variety of well-defined syndromes. Variations include the following examples:

▌ Salmon patch (macular stain, nevus simplex)—The glabellar salmon patch, also known as "angel's kiss," is a bilaterally symmetric superficial capillary defect. It is the most common vascular malformation and the only one that almost always fades spontaneously. A similar lesion in the nuchal area, the "stork bite," is usually persistent. Large lesions may also involve the eyelids and alae nasi. Prominent glabellar salmon patches are associated with dysmorphic syndromes including Beckwith-Wiedemann syndrome and fetal alcohol syndrome (Burns et al, 1991).

▌ Nevus flammeus (port-wine stain)—This asymmetric postcapillary venule malformation occurs in 0.3% of neonates. The majority are isolated cutaneous lesions. At birth they are pink, macular, and blanchable. With time, most lesions darken; papulonodular surface change and ipsilateral soft tissue or even bony hypertrophy may occur. Facial nevus flammeus is a distribution that includes the forehead or upper eyelid and may be associated with buphthalmos or glaucoma. Emergent ophthalmologic examination is indicated for these infants. Sturge-Weber Syndrome (SWS) is a triad of facial nevus flammeus, leptomeningeal vascular malformation, and glaucoma that occurs sporadically. The classic finding of double-contoured (tramline) calcifications on skull film is not seen during infancy but develops during childhood. CNS lesions are most reliably detected by MRI after 6 months of age. SWS occurs in less than 30% of infants with facial

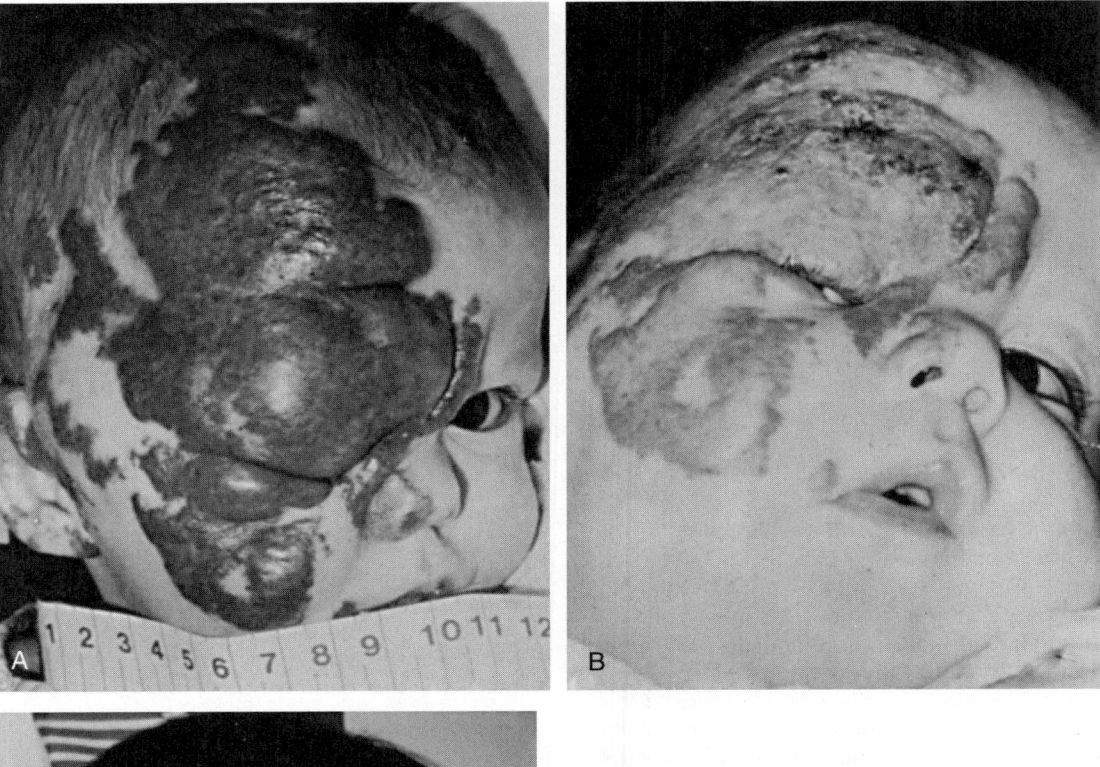

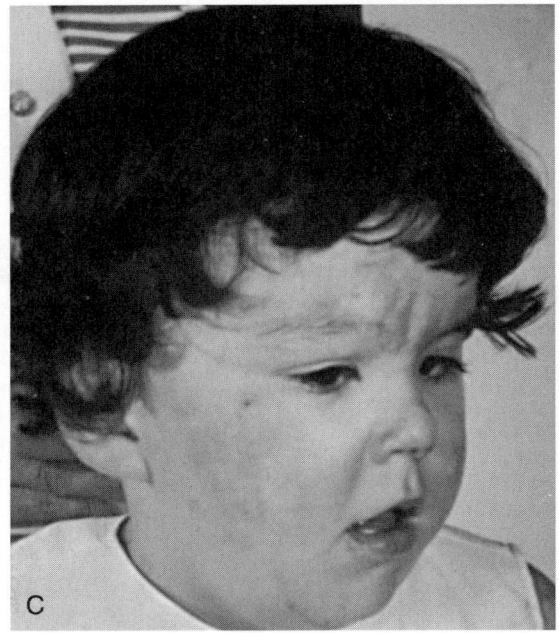

FIGURE 109–2. *A,* A flat hemangioma was noted at birth, and by 3 weeks of age had expanded, as shown. After 11 weeks of prednisone (20 mg per day), the lesion had regressed, as shown in *B. C,* Nearly complete regression is evident by age 4 years. She is a normally intelligent child whose only residual problem is strabismus.

port-wine stains; the risk is increased in infants with more extensive lesions (Tallman et al, 1991). The degree of CNS involvement is variable in SWS, ranging from subclinical lesions to intractable seizures and intellectual impairment. Two national organizations have been established to serve the needs of individuals and of families with an affected member: the National Vascular Malformations Foundation, Inc., 8320 Nightengale, Dearborn Heights, MI 48127; and The Sturge-Weber Foundation, P.O. Box 460931, Aurora, CO 80046.

▌ Arterial/lymph/venous malformation—This category includes a spectrum of isolated cutaneous vascular anomalies that have been given a variety of clinically descriptive names. These multifarious names do not offer insight into pathogenesis or natural history, and some experts advocate for a more simple classification, based on the type of anomalous vessel (Mulliken and Young, 1988). These include pure lymphangiomas (e.g., "cystic hygroma" and lymphangioma circumscriptum), arterial-venous malformations, and venous malformations. These lesions do not resolve spontaneously. Corticosteroid therapy is not beneficial. Complications are related to the flow rate and extent of the lesion. Localized thrombosis and phlebitis occur in low-flow lesions; high-flow lesions can cause significant bleeding, destructive interosseous changes, and high output cardiac failure (Mulliken and Young, 1988).

- Cutis marmorata telangiectatica congenita (CMTC)—This lesion is a distinct, reticulated capillary/venous malformation. CMTC can occur as a single isolated patch or involve an extensive area. With time, associated atrophy and ulceration may occur. The larger lesions may have ipsilateral hypertrophy or hypotrophy of the affected limb.
- Klippel-Trénaunay and Parkes Weber syndromes are clinically defined, sporadic conditions consisting of extensive nevus flammeus, most often occurring unilaterally on the lower extremity, associated with venous varicosities and progressive ipsilateral limb hypertrophy. Some authors differentiate Parkes-Weber syndrome, which also includes an A-V fistulae and its constellation of complications.
- Cobb syndrome is a sporadic condition consisting of a posterior truncal nevus flammeus overlying a vascular abnormality that involves the spinal cord.
- Bonnet-Dechaume-Blanc syndrome (also known as Wyburn-Mason syndrome)—This condition consists of a facial port-wine stain overlying a retinal and intracranial arteriovenous malformation. The retinal lesion appears as dilated, tortuous retinal vessels on routine ophthalmoscopy. Cranial bruit, mild proptosis, and conjunctival hyperemia may be present.
- Blue rubber bleb nevus syndrome—This autosomal dominant condition is characterized by venous malformations of the skin and GI tract associated with bleeding and iron deficiency anemia. Numerous lesions may be present at birth. They are blue macules or nodules that range in size from 1 mm to several centimeters, resembling the "blueberry muffin" lesions of congenital TORCH (*t*oxoplasmosis, *o*ther infections, *r*ubella, *c*ytomegalovirus, *h*erpes simplex) infection but easily compressible. They may be tender on palpation, or surmounted by droplets of sweat.
- Maffuci syndrome—This sporadic condition consists of mixed vascular malformations and characteristic enchondromas. Twenty-five percent of affected individuals have manifestations at birth or in early infancy.
- Bannayan-Riley-Ruvalcaba syndrome—The abnormalities included in this category are vascular malformations, macrocephaly, and lipomas. In combination with other features, separate conditions have been described: Bannayan-Zonana, Riley-Smith, and Ruvalcaba-Myhre-Smith. The usual inheritance pattern is autosomal dominant.
- Lymphedema—This term is used to describe diffuse soft tissue swelling characterized by firm, pitting edema. Lymphedema can occur in the setting of anomalous lymphatic drainage. Congenital variants have been reported. Females are affected more frequently than males. The lower limbs are the most common sites, but other sites may also be involved, and rarely, chylothorax or ascites may be present. Milroy disease is an autosomal dominant condition that presents with progressive lymphedema of the lower extremities. Lymphedema of the extremities occurs in Turner (XO) syndrome.

Treatment. Treatment for an uncomplicated capillary malformation is aimed at minimizing disfigurement. With time, these lesions thicken and develop irregular surface changes, often with friable nodules. In 1986, the yellow-light pulsed dye laser was FDA-approved for the treatment of nevus flammeus, as early as the neonatal period. The copper vapor laser and the argon-pumped tunable dye laser are also yellow light lasers. Most of the published data on laser treatment of port-wine stains in children is from studies utilizing the pulsed-dye laser. Children require an average of four to five pulsed-dye laser treatments for maximal lightening. The best results have been seen in children less than 4 years old. In this age group, 20% can expect 95% clearing (Goldman et al, 1993). Pulsed-dye laser therapy is less effective for facial port-wine stains that are close to midline or those on the extremities (Renfro and Geronemus, 1993; Garden and Bakus, 1993). Laser therapy can yield remarkable improvement for many port-wine stains, minimizing the emotional pain that accompanies facial disfigurement. Unfortunately, none of the currently available lasers is capable of permanently erasing port-wine stains in the majority of patients. The range of skin conditions that may benefit from yellow-light laser therapy is expanding rapidly to include a variety of skin lesions with vascular components.

HYPOPIGMENTED LESIONS

Localized areas of hypopigmentation on the skin of the newborn infant may be isolated phenomena, or they may be markers of extracutaneous abnormalities. The degree of hypopigmentation and distribution of the defect helps distinguish between the conditions.

Definition

A distinction must first be made between complete depigmentation and hypopigmentation. A depigmenting condition produces pure white lesions that are devoid of normal melanocytes. Even in fair-skinned infants, the lesions can be easily seen in ordinary daylight. This group includes tyrosinase-negative albinism and piebaldism (see Chapter 106) as well as vitiligo, which is rarely seen in infancy. A hypopigmented lesion is often subtly lighter in color than the surrounding skin. Histologic examination reveals a normal number of melanocytes. In fair-skinned children, these lesions may require Wood's light illumination to become obvious. The group includes anomalies with a deficient amount of either of the skin's pigments: melanin or hemoglobin. The ash-leaf macules and "confetti-like" lesions of tuberous sclerosis (Fig. 109–3), the linear and whorled patterning associated with hypomelanosis of Ito (Fig. 109–4A), and simple nevus depigmentosus are hypomelanotic lesions (Fig. 109–4B). Nevus anemicus and hemangioma precursors are areas of pallor that result from diminished superficial blood flow.

Ash-Leaf Macules

These are small oval areas of hypopigmentation, named for their similarity in size and shape to a European-mountain-

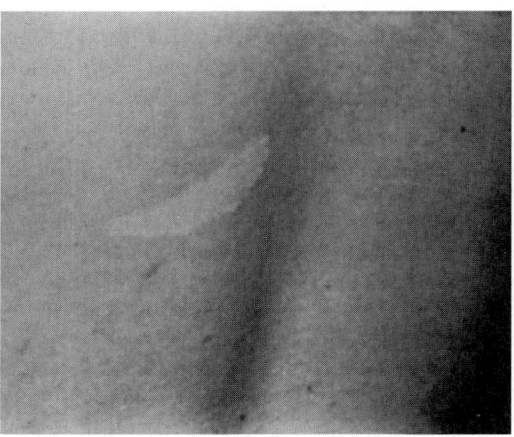

FIGURE 109–3. White ash-leaf macule on the back of a patient with tuberous sclerosis.

ash leaflet. They are one of the few congenital markers for infants with tuberous sclerosis. Tuberous sclerosis complex (TSC) is an autosomal dominant disorder with variable clinical manifestations characterized by the development of benign and malignant tumors in a variety of tissues: skin, central nervous system, and kidney. Serious complications of tuberous sclerosis include hamartomas of the lung and kidney and congenital rhabdomyomas of the heart. The diagnosis is currently made by meeting a set of diagnostic criteria, but the majority of manifestations are not present in infancy (Gomez, 1991; Janniger and Schwartz, 1993; Zvulunov and Esterly, 1995). Recently, abnormalities at two different genetic loci have been identified in kindreds with TS (Weinecke et al, 1995).

Hypomelanosis of Ito

The term *hypomelanosis of Ito* has been used as a diagnosis for a genetic disorder marked by a striking linear and whorled pattern of cutaneous pigment change oriented along the lines of Blaschko (see Chapter 106). Affected

individuals may have areas that are hyperpigmented or hypopigmented, or both. The pattern may be congenital or become apparent after birth. This condition is a form of genetic mosaicism. A subset of affected individuals has demonstrable karyotype abnormalities from affected sites. The majority of cases reported have extra cutaneous abnormalities (CNS, ocular, and skeletal) (Alvarez et al, 1993). Patterned pigment change confined to skin is probably a more common occurrence. For these individuals, the term *linear and whorled nevoid melanosis* may be more appropriate. Chromosomal analysis from separate tissues (e.g., blood and skin) is indicated for children with extensive skin lesions or evidence of extracutaneous involvement (Sybert, 1994).

MELANIN-CONTAINING LESIONS

Brown lesions usually represent an increased number of melanocytic cells or an excess of melanin. Brown coloration can also be associated with a thickened epidermis. It may be difficult to distinguish between the lesions in this category without histopathologic examination. The majority of congenital brown lesions are isolated and benign, but it is important to recognize those that are syndrome-associated or potentially life-threatening (see Chapter 105 for a differential diagnosis).

In general, skin biopsy of a congenital pigmented lesion can be postponed until after the neonatal period. The one exception is a nodular lesion suggestive of melanoma.

Nevocellular Nevi

This category includes congenital or acquired nevomelanocytic neoplasms. Nevomelanocytes are dendritic cells of neural crest origin. Nevocellular nevi have traditionally been categorized by the histologic position of the tumor nests within the skin. Junctional nevi are the most superficial, located at the junction between the epidermis and dermis. These lesions appear clinically as macules. Intradermal nevi are located deep to the dermoepidermal

FIGURE 109–4. Nevus depigmentosis is an isolated congenital skin lesion that presents as a hypomelanotic polygonal macule *(A)* or in a linear, Blaschko's distribution *(B)*.

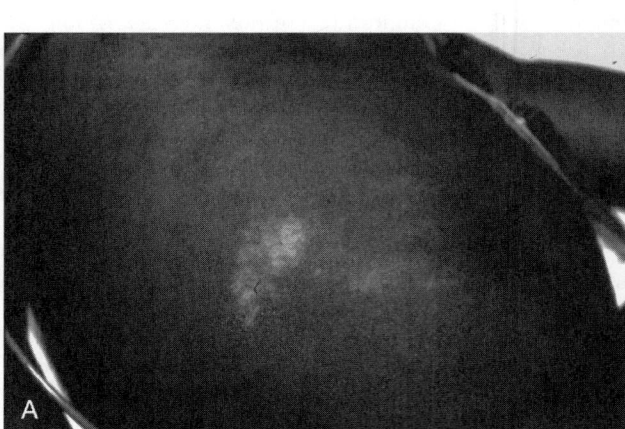

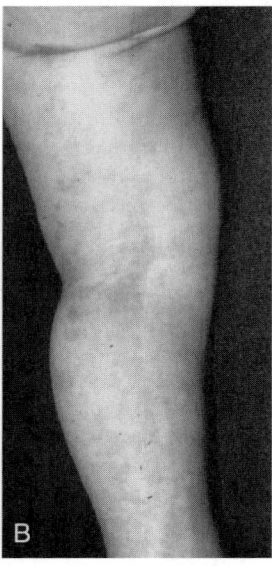

junction and are usually papular. "Blue" nevi are a variant located in the deep dermis, made up of cells that have elongated, neural features. Compound nevi have both junctional and dermal nests of nevomelanocytes.

Melanocytic nevi can be further divided into categories based on size: small (<1.5 cm), large (2 to 20 cm), and giant (>20 cm or 120 cm² surface area) (Zitelli et al, 1984); and time of onset: congenital, early-onset (<2 years), and acquired. Diagnostic histologic features have been described for congenital and acquired lesions, but these features may be found in both types.

Large, multiple, or congenital melanocytic nevi have been reported in association with several syndromes (Marghoob, Orlow, and Kopf, 1993) (Table 109–3).

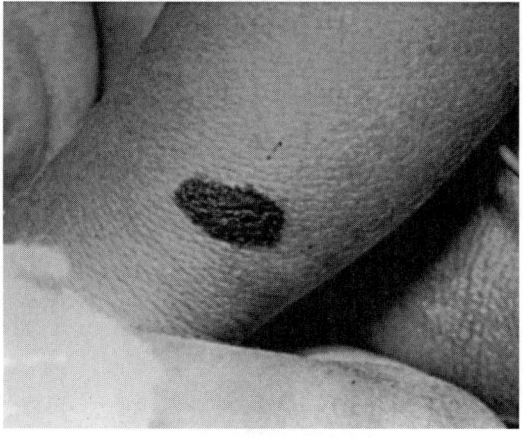

FIGURE 109–5. Dark brown irregular congenital nevus on the limb of an infant.

TABLE 109–3

Syndromes Associated with Melanocytic Nevi

Associated with:	Other Key Features
Congenital Nevi	
Carney syndrome (including LAMB and NAME syndromes)	Cardiac and cutaneous myxomas, endocrine abnormalities
Epidermal (linear sebaceous) nevus syndrome	Linear epidermal/sebaceous nevi, central nervous system and musculoskeletal defects
Neurocutaneous melanosis	Leptomeningeal melanocytosis and obstructive hydrocephalus
Neurofibromatosis type I	Cutaneous and plexiform neurofibromas, café-au-lait spots, Lisch nodules
Premature aging syndrome	Premature aging, short stature, bird-like facies, deafness
Occult spinal dysraphism/ tethered cord	Spinal cord abnormalities, lipomas, vascular malformations
Malformations associated with congenital melanocytic nevi	
Acquired Nevi	
Dysplastic nevus (atypical mole) syndrome	Increased incidence of cutaneous melanoma
Langer-Giedion syndrome	Distinctive facies, cone-shaped epiphyses, multiple exostoses
Congenital and/or Acquired Nevi	
EEC syndrome	Ectrodactyly, ectodermal dysplasia, cleft lip/palate, ocular abnormalities
Goeminne syndrome	Muscular torticollis, spontaneous keloids, genitourinary abnormalities
Kuskokwim syndrome	Skeletal abnormalities, joint contractures, muscle atrophy/ hypertrophy
Noonan's syndrome	Webbed neck, heart defects, multiple other anomalies
Turner's syndrome	Webbed neck, heart defects, multiple other anomalies, X-chromosome defect
Tricho-odonto-onychial dysplasia	Hypotrichosis, enamel defects, nail dystrophy

From Marghoob AA, Orlo SJ, Kopf AW: Syndromes associated with melanocytic nevi. J Am Acad Dermatol 29:373–388, 1993.

Congenital Nevocellular Nevi

Congenital nevocytic nevi are common and generally of little or no consequence. However, the infrequent but devastating association with malignant melanoma has made management a controversial issue.

Small congenital nevi measure less than 1.5 cm in diameter at birth (Fig. 109–5). Truely congenital lesions are present in 1% of white infants and 2% to 3% of black infants surveyed in the nursery (Osborn et al, 1987). There is a risk of malignancy associated with small nevi, but it may never be well defined. A distinct subset of melanocytic nevi in children, "early-onset nevi," has recently been recognized. These lesions are not necessarily congenital, appearing during the first 2 years of life. Early-onset nevi have been observed in 25% of children specifically examined for them. Twenty to fifty percent of melanomas arising in children and young adults may be associated with this type of nevus (Williams, 1993; Williams and Pennella, 1994). The frequency of congenital melanocytic nevi (CMN) is paradoxically increased in blacks, who have a much lower risk of melanoma (Shpall et al, 1994). The risk of melanoma in these very common pigmented skin lesions must be well below that of children with giant congenital nevi and possibly no higher than the 1% lifetime risk of malignant melanoma in the general white population. A decision about surgical removal of these lesions must be made on a case-by-case basis.

Large, giant or "garment" congenital nevi measure at least 20 cm or cover an entire body part (Fig. 109–6). These are rare, occurring in less than 1 in 20,000 neonates, and have a much greater potential for malignant degeneration. The cumulative risk of malignancy is estimated to be 2% to 15% over a lifetime, with a bimodal pattern of occurrence, either prior to age 3 or after puberty (Williams and Pennella, 1994; Kuflik and Janniger, 1994).

Conservative management of large congenital nevi by surveillance alone is complicated by the presence of features that strongly suggest melanoma. Most have an irregular surface appearance from birth and are variably thickened, hairy, verrucous, or nodular. Smaller, widely scattered "satellite lesions" are almost always present. Extracutaneous lesions have also been detected in several sites, includ-

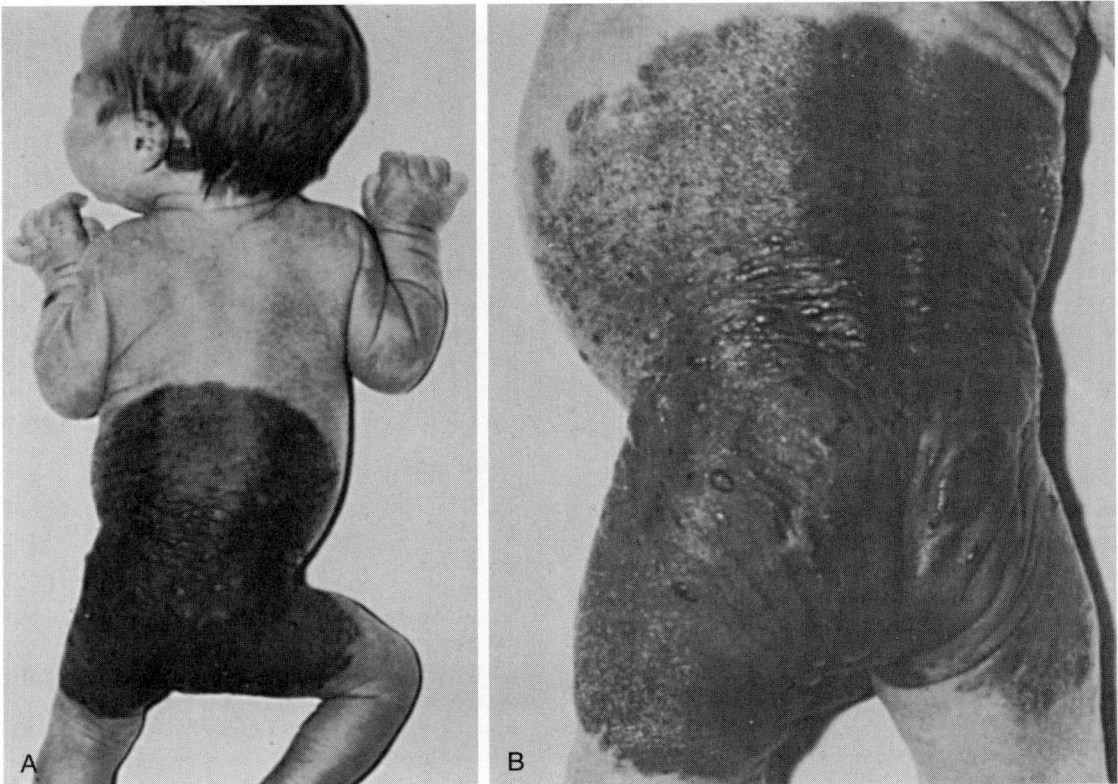

FIGURE 109–6. *A,* Newborn infant with large black nevus covering the "bathing trunk" area. The closer view *(B)* permits visualization of the nodular surface typical of giant nevi.

ing the meninges, lymph nodes, and placental villi. Often, these nevi have atypical histologic features as well. Children that develop malignant melanoma within a giant nevus have a very poor prognosis. However, many of the lesions with an alarming appearance from birth do not exhibit malignant behavior, have widespread metastases, or cause death. In fact, congenital melanoma is very rare and is associated with congenital nevi in less than 50% of reported cases (Williams and Pennella, 1994).

The management of CMN remains controversial, with equal numbers of advocates for and against prophylactic excision. Newly published data question the rationale for routine excision. But case reports of melanoma arising in smaller CMN, as early as 6 months of age, continue to dramatize the issue (Ozturkcan et al, 1994; DeFraeve et al, 1993; Ceballos et al, 1995).

The least controversial recommendation has been for surgical excision of large or multiple CMN during infancy (Casson and Colen, 1993). However, surgical removal is never an easy option. Multiple procedures are usually required, with the attendant high risks of significant morbidity sometimes yielding results that are more disfiguring than the birthmark (Figs. 109–7 and 109–8). Newer techniques performed in early childhood, such as tissue expansion (Vergnes et al, 1993) and partial thickness resection, (Sandsmark et al, 1993) may improve the aesthetic outcome. The efficacy of this approach in the prevention of malignancy has never been documented. A Congenital Nevocytic Nevus Registry was established at New York University Medical Center in 1978 to prospectively study

the natural history of giant CMN (Kopf et al, 1979; Gari et al, 1988). To participate by mail, contact the Skin and Cancer Unit, Department of Dermatology, NYU Medical Center, 550 First Ave, New York, NY 10016; call them at (212) 340-5260.

Families with an affected child may benefit from information provided by the "Nevus Network," a national sup-

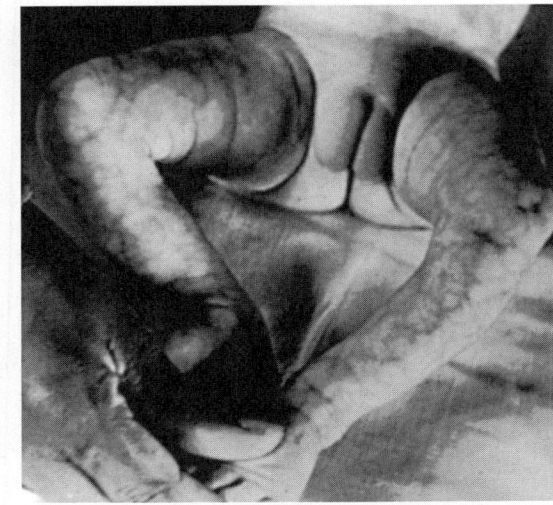

FIGURE 109–7. Cutis marmorata telangiectatica congenita. Note the striking network of dilated vessels most distinct over the extremities. (From Humphries JM. J Pediatr 40:486, 1952.)

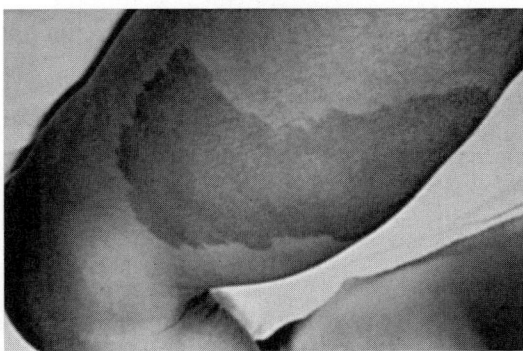

FIGURE 109–8. Large café-au-lait spot on the trunk of a newborn infant.

port group founded by Dr. Bari Joan Bett, a physician with a giant congenital nevus. To receive the newsletter, write c/o 1400 S. Joyce St. #C1201, Arlington, VA 22202, or call (703) 920-2349 or (405) 377-3403.

Neurocutaneous melanosis (NCM) is a congenital syndrome characterized by pigment cell tumors of the leptomeninges in patients with large or multiple (at least three) CMN of the head, neck, or posterior midline (Kadonaga and Frieden, 1991). Symptomatic NCM presents with signs or symptoms of increased intracranial pressure and has a poor prognosis (Sandsmark et al, 1994; Frieden et al, 1994). MRI can aid in the diagnosis of NCM (Barkovich et al, 1994). Although initial reports emphasized thickening of the leptomeninges, the most common MRI sign of NCM is actually T1 shortening in the parenchyma of the cerebellum or anterior temporal lobes (sometimes accompanied by T2 shortening). Radiologic identification of malignant degeneration is difficult. Roughly half of asymptomatic infants and children with giant CMN have evidence of NCM on MRI (Frieden et al, 1994), which suggests that numerous and extensive operations attempting to remove the cutaneous lesion may not be justified in these patients.

Other issues have been raised that challenge the interpretation of signs that have been accepted as ominous. The risk of melanoma in early infancy may have been overestimated by misinterpretation of the histology and extent of the lesions. Neither cellular atypia nor widespread involvement, including lymph nodes and placenta, prove malignancy (Carroll et al, 1994; Hara, 1993). Attempts to further define the risk of malignant degeneration in these lesions have not been insightful (Barnhill et al, 1994; Heimann et al, 1993).

Lentigines

Lentigines are small tan-to-dark brown macules that most commonly appear sporadically in adulthood. They are distinguished from other pigmented lesions by histologic examination that reveals elongated rete ridges, an increased number of singly dispersed melanocytes along the basal layer, and increased melanization of the basal keratinocytes. Multiple or congenital lentigines are features of several syndromes.

▪ Carney syndrome (including NAME and LAMB)—

These phenotypes share the features of *a*trial *m*yxoma and pigmented skin lesions. (NAME includes *n*evi and *e*phelides while LAMB includes *l*entigines and *b*lue nevi). Pigmented lesions are present at birth.

▪ LEOPARD syndrome—This is an autosomal dominant disorder that includes multiple *l*entigines, *e*lectrocardiogram defects, *o*cular hypertelorism, *p*ulmonic stenosis, *a*bnormal genitalia, growth *r*etardation, and sensorineural *d*eafness. Skin lesions do not appear until after the first year of life.

▪ Peutz-Jeghers syndrome—This autosomal dominant disorder includes mucocutaneous pigmented macules and intestinal polyposis. The pigmented lesions may be congenital and usually appear on the lips, buccal and gingival mucosa, and dorsae of the fingers and toes.

Café-au-Lait Macules

Café-au-lait macules (CALM) are light brown macules that vary in size from several millimeters to several centimeters. They cannot always be distinguished from nevocellular nevi on clinical grounds, but histologic features are diagnostic, showing increased melanin within the basal keratinocytes, without melanocyte proliferation. CALM are present in 2% of white and up to 12% of black infants. Large or multiple CALM in the neonatal period may be an isolated finding but should alert the physician to the possibility of an associated syndrome (see Table 109–4).

Neurofibromatosis

Neurofibromatosis (NF) is a group of variable multi-system disorders that include cutaneous neurofibromas and multiple CALM. A classification that includes eight subtypes has been defined (Riccardi, 1983). The great majority of patients with NF have subtype 1 (NF-1) or von Recklinghausen disease. NF-1 is a relatively common autosomal dominant disorder with a high rate of new mutation, occurring in 1 in 3500 people. The diagnosis has traditionally been made by fulfilling a set of diagnostic criteria; the presence of six or more CALM is the most common manifestation, occurring before age 6 in 99% of affected individuals (Zvulunov and Esterly, 1995). CALM may be present at birth but often arise and grow during childhood. Other diagnostic cutaneous findings are axillary or inguinal freckling (Crowe's sign) and neurofibromas, which may be present at birth. Diagnostic bony dysplasias (sphenoid wing dysplasia, pretibial pseudarthrosis) can also be detected at

---

TABLE 109–4

Syndromes that Feature Café au Lait Macules

Neurofibromatosis (NFI, II)	Turner syndrome
Albright syndrome	Noonan syndrome
Watson syndrome	Ataxia-telangiectasis
Ruvalcaba-Myhre-Smith syndrome	Tuberous sclerosis
Bloom syndrome	Basal-cell nevus syndrome
Russell-Silver syndrome	Hunter syndrome
	Gaucher syndrome

birth, in the minority of patients. Symptomatic central nervous system involvement (developmental delay, learning disabilities, seizures) occurs in about one third of patients with NF-1. The most ominous complication of NF-1 is the development of malignant tumors (neurosarcoma, pheochromocytoma, and juvenile chronic myelogenous leukemia) (Zvulunov and Esterly, 1995). The risk of leukemia is highest among children with both NF-1 and cutaneous juvenile xanthogranuloma (see later).

The genetic defects for NF-1 have been localized to chromosome 17q11;2. Most mutations occur on the paternally-derived chromosome. "Sporadic" cases may be the result of paternal transmission from a mosaic mutation of a fraction of spermatozoa from a clinically normal father (Lazaro et al, 1994). A portion of the NF-1 gene has homology with mammalian genes that encode for guanosine triphosphate-activating proteins (GAPs). GAPs function to regulate cell proliferation. Therefore, a functional mutation of the NF-1 gene would result in unsuppressed cellular proliferation (i.e., tumorigenesis). Prenatal diagnosis is now available for affected families by linkage analysis (Zvulunov and Esterly, 1995). Affected families may benefit from contact with the National Neurofibromatosis Foundation, 141 Fifth Avenue, Suite 7-S, New York, NY 10010; call at (800) 323-7938 or (212) 344-6633.

Type 2 neurofibromatosis (NF-2) is an autosomal dominant disorder with an incidence of about 1 in 40,000. It is characterized by bilateral acoustic neuromas. CALM are not as prominent or numerous as in NF-1, occurring in less than 40% of affected individuals. The gene defect has been localized to chromosome 22q11-q13 (Zvulunov and Esterly, 1995).

McCune-Albright Syndrome

McCune-Albright syndrome (MAS) is a sporadic disease characterized by polyostotic fibrous dysplasia, sexual precocity and other hyper functional endocrinopathies, and large café-au-lait spots (Schwindinger et al, 1992; Shenker et al, 1993). In contrast with the CAL seen in NF-1, the CAL in this syndrome may be unilateral with irregular borders, in a distribution that suggests the lines of Blashchko, and genetic mosaicism (Rieger et al, 1994) (see Chapter 106). Affected tissues from individuals with MAS have been found to harbor mutations of the gene that encodes the stimulatory G protein of adenylyl cyclase (Schwindinger et al, 1992; Shenker et al, 1993).

Nevus Spilus

Nevus spilus (speckled lentiginous nevus) is a hyperpigmented lesion that consists of focal proliferation of melanocytes along the basal layer of the epidermis (the dark spots) within a CAL. It may be disfiguring, but has no other associated abnormalities.

Blue-Gray Macule of Infancy (formerly mongolian spots)

More than 90% of black infants, 81% of Asians, and 10% of whites (Pratt, 1953) are born with mongolian spots.

These are brown, gray, or blue macules, most commonly located on the lumbosacral area, but they can occur anywhere. Mongolian spots may be single or multiple and vary in size from a few millimeters to several centimeters. They often fade within the first few years of life. Extensive lesions have been mistakenly attributed to abuse. Histologically, mongolian spots are collections of spindle-shaped melanocytes located deep in the dermis. Malignant change has never been reported.

Nevus of Ota/Ito

Nevus of Ota is a unilateral blue or grey discoloration involving the orbital and zygomatic area, including the sclera and fundus. It is a sporadic condition, but it occurs with the highest frequency in Asians, affecting up to 1% in Japan (Kopf and Weidman, 1962). The discoloration is detected at birth in 60% of cases. Glaucoma is a frequent complication. A similar lesion, located in the deltotrapezius area, is called nevus of Ito. Histologically, these lesions cannot be distinguished from mongolian spots. However, spontaneous resolution is not common, and association with malignant melanoma has been reported. Successful treatment has been achieved with Q-switched ruby and Q-switched YAG laser surgery.

TUMORS OF EPITHELIAL ORIGIN
Epidermal Nevus/Nevus Sebaceus

Epidermal nevus may present in the newborn period as a smooth hyperpigmented patch or rough, skin-colored plaque most often on the trunk or extremities, frequently oriented along the lines of Blashchko (see Chapter 106). With time, epidermal nevi may enlarge; most become verrucous. Nevus sebaceus has a yellow hue, occurs most often on the head, and may be nodular at birth and again after puberty, flattening during childhood. Up to 15% of sebaceous nevi develop a variety of neoplasms, both benign and malignant, including basal cell carcinoma. This rarely occurs before puberty.

Like other mosaic disorders, epidermal and sebaceous nevi are believed to be localized manifestations of somatic genetic mutations that would be lethal if fully expressed. A subset of patients with epidermal nevi are genetic mosaics of an autosomal dominant form of ichthyosis, called epidermolytic hyperkeratosis (or bullous ichthyosiform erythroderma). These individuals may be at risk for bearing children with total body involvement. The striking appearance of epidermal nevi has inspired descriptive nomenclature. *Nevus verrucosus* is a solitary plaque. *Nevus unius lateris* (Fig. 109–9) is an extensive linear lesion that is unilateral, following the lines of Blashchko. Both keratinocytic and sebaceous components may occur in the same patient, the former more commonly involving the trunk and extremities, and the latter more often involving the head and neck. The term *ichthyosis hystrix* refers to extensive, bilateral involvement with epidermal nevus.

Skin biopsy will rule out other conditions, distinguish between epidermal nevus and nevus sebaceus, and detect the diagnostic histologic features of epidermolytic hyperkeratosis. Small epidermal nevi do not require treatment.

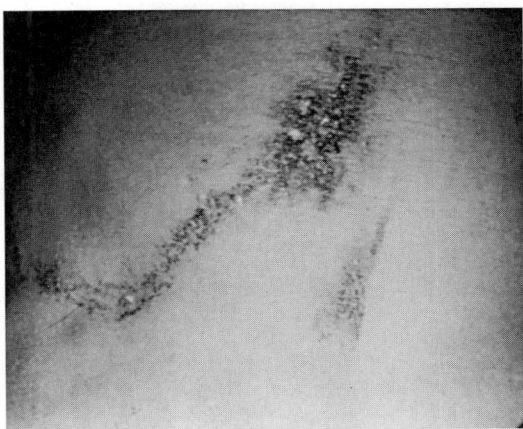

FIGURE 109–9. Linear hyperkeratotic epidermal nevus on the back and lateral thorax.

Nevus sebaceus carries a risk of malignant degeneration, and optimally is excised during early infancy or after childhood, using local anesthesia. There is no optimal therapy for larger lesions or those that are disfiguring. Full-thickness excision, including the subcutaneous tissue, is recommended to decrease the risk of recurrence. Laser therapy holds promise for the future. Topically applied keratolytic agents may be palliative. Genetic counseling about the risk for offspring of fully expressed disease should be considered for individuals with epidermal nevi that reveal the histologic features of epidermolytic hyperkeratosis.

Epidermal (linear sebaceous) Nevus Syndrome

In less than 10% of affected people, epidermal nevi and sebaceous nevi (especially those involving the head) are associated with a variety of extra cutaneous abnormalities, mainly ocular (33% of cases), neurologic (50%), and skeletal (70%), a condition referred to as *epidermal nevus syndrome.* Bony abnormalities include vertebral anomalies, kyphoscoliosis, limb shortening, and hemihypertrophy. CNS disorders include seizures, mental retardation, and hemiparesis; ocular abnormalities include eyelid/conjunctival nevus, coloboma, corneal opacity, and nystagmus. Malignancies also occur in this syndrome with a greater than expected frequency, including Wilms tumor, nephroblastoma, GI carcinomas, and rhabdomyosarcoma (Marghoob et al, 1993).

DERMAL TUMORS
Juvenile Xanthogranuloma

Juvenile xanthogranuloma (JXG) is a benign, self-healing, nonLangerhans' cell histiocytic tumor of infancy. JXG may be congenital; the majority of tumors present by 6 months of age (Nomland, 1959). Cutaneous lesions vary in color from red-brown to yellow. They occur most often on the upper half of the body (Fig. 109–10), may be solitary or multiple, and vary in size from several millimeters to several centimeters (see Fig. 109–4). JXG may also be localized to the eye or mucous membranes (De Raeve et al, 1994).

Skin biopsy is usually diagnostic, revealing characteristic foamy histiocytes and Touton giant cells within the dermis.

The vast majority of infants with JXG are otherwise healthy. Giant JXG can have an alarming appearance and may be confused with other types of histiocytic tumors (Magana et al, 1994). The most clinically significant associations are ocular JXG with its complications, and JXG, NF-1, and juvenile chronic granulocytic leukemia. Less than 0.5% of children with skin lesions have ocular involvement, but one half of children with ocular JXG have cutaneous lesions (Giacoia and Berry, 1994). Ocular tumors may present as unilateral glaucoma, uveitis, heterochromia iridis, or proptosis; ocular JXG is the most common cause of hyphema in infancy (Gaynes and Cohen, 1967; Zimmerman, 1965). The triple association of JXG, juvenile chronic granulocytic leukemia, and NF-1 has been reported in 24 cases. The appearance of JXG usually preceded the diagnosis of leukemia; the NF, marked by multiple CALM, was often missed (Sherer et al, 1993).

The majority of JXG are asymptomatic and self limited. Giant lesions have a similar prognosis (Magana et al, 1994). Ophthalmologic evaluation is indicated for children who present in the first two years of life with multiple lesions. Parents should be provided with anticipatory guidance about the ocular complications (Giacoia and Berry, 1994). JXG typically involute within 3 to 6 years (Hansen, 1992). Recurrence has been documented following surgical excision; this form of therapy is indicated only for lesions that are frequently traumatized or are more disfiguring than the resultant scar.

MASTOCYTOSIS

This group of disorders is characterized by increased numbers of tissue mast cells. The skin is the most common site of involvement, but the lymphoreticular system, GI tract, and bone marrow may also be affected. Symptoms result from the local or generalized effects following the release of histamine and other mast cell mediators. Pruritus, edema, blistering, and flushing are common. Abdominal

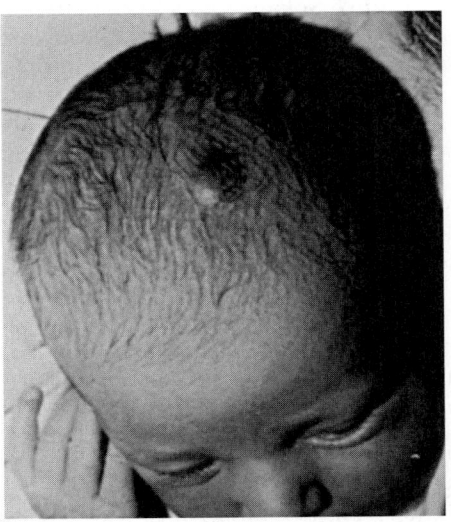

FIGURE 109–10. Solitary juvenile xanthogranuloma on the scalp, a typical site for these lesions.

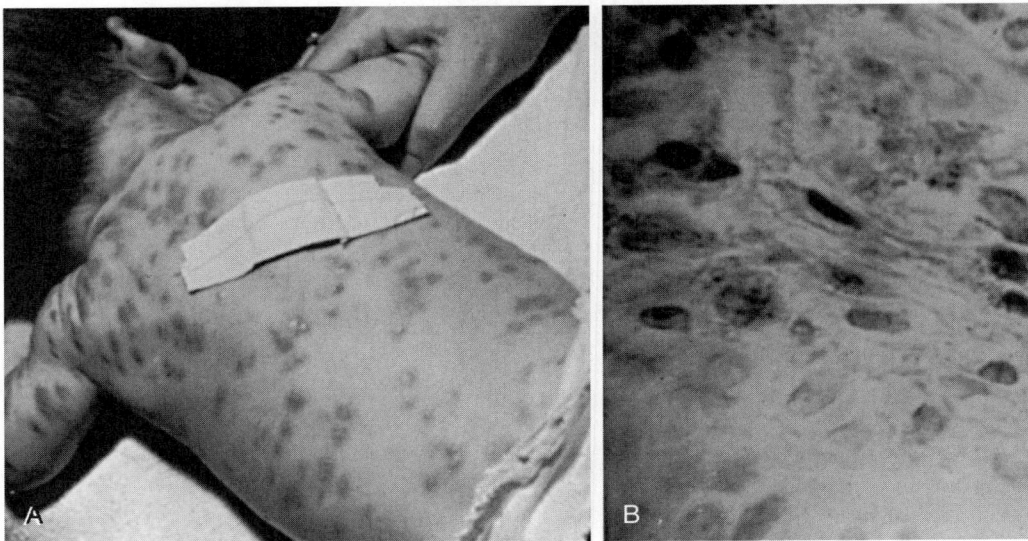

FIGURE 109–11. *A,* Deeply pigmented nodules and macules on the back of an infant with urticaria pigmentosa. A group of vesicles is visible just below the bandage that covers the biopsy site. *B,* Microscopic section from biopsy of patient stained with Giemsa. The mast cells can be identified as spindle-shaped cells containing granules that are located in the upper dermis.

pain, diarrhea, and vomiting are unusual. Hypotension is rare (Kettelhut and Metcalfe, 1991). If rubbed or traumatized, skin affected by mastocytosis will develop a diagnostic wheal ("Darier sign"). The site may blister or become hemorrhagic in a neonate.

Urticaria pigmentosa is the name given to the most common form of mastocytosis in infants, featuring multiple, small (1–3 cm) papules usually located on the trunk (Fig. 109–11). The disease may be congenital but usually presents within the first 6 months of life (Kettelhut and Metcalfe, 1991). A single, localized lesion is known as a solitary mastocytoma. These tumors can vary in size from a few to several centimeters. Diffuse cutaneous mastocytosis is an unusual condition that may present at birth with widespread blistering or diffuse thickening of the skin (Sagher and Evan-Paz, 1967; Solomon and Esterly, 1973).

The diagnosis may be confirmed by a skin biopsy, which reveals mast cell hyperplasia within the dermis. Plasma histamine levels are elevated in the majority of children with mastocytosis, sometimes to remarkably high levels. Further workup for evidence of systemic involvement should be limited to pediatric patients with extra cutaneous signs and symptoms, or those who require general anesthesia (Kettelhut and Metcalfe, 1991).

Caregivers should be educated to avoid exposing infants to factors that trigger mast cell degranulation, such as friction, pressure, temperature extremes, and substances that promote mast cell degranulation (aspirin, alcohol, narcotics, amphotericin B, or iodine-containing contrast media). If general anesthesia is required, perioperative administration of histamine-receptor blockers is recommended (Lerno et al, 1990).

For patients with limited skin involvement, application of potent topical corticosteroids may hasten involution of lesions. Symptomatic patients may be treated with a classical H1 antihistamine, such as hydroxyzine or cyproheptadine. An H_2-blocker, such as ranitidine, or oral disodium cromoglycate may be added in the presence of GI symptoms. Hypotension requires corticosteroids in addition to H_1 and H_2 antihistamines and intensive supportive care. Solitary mastocytomas usually involute by school age. Lesions of urticaria pigmentosa often resolve by puberty.

MIDLINE ANOMALIES

Congenital midline defects are a distinct group of diagnostically and therapeutically challenging conditions. These anomalies are located deep to the dermis, occurring at the cranial or caudal midline. Some of these lesions mark an underlying CNS problem or an intracranial connection. The differential diagnosis includes lesions that occasionally occur in the midline by serendipity; hemangiomas are the most common. Vascular malformations, hair tufts, dimples, and lipomas may also occur at the cranial or caudal midline and can mark a CNS or spinal malformation (Hayashi et al, 1984; Martinez-Lage et al, 1992). A midline mass in the nasal area may represent a dermoid cyst, encephalocele, or glioma (Paller et al, 1991). Occipital lesions include aplasia cutis congenita, encephalocele, and heterotopic brain tissue. The "hair collar sign" may mark ectopic neural tissue and CNS malformations (Commens et al, 1989; Drolet et al, 1995). Biopsy of a midline mass should not be performed unless an imaging study has been obtained to help clarify the nature of the lesion. If the possibility of an intracranial connection exists, referral to a neurosurgeon is indicated (Martinez-Lage et al, 1992).

REFERENCES

Achauer BM, Vander kam VM: Ulcerated anogenital hemangioma of infancy. Plast Reconstr Surg 87:861–868, 1991.

Albright AL, Gartner JC, Wiener ES: Lumbar cutaneous hemangiomas as indicators of tethered spinal cords. Pediatrics 83:977–980, 1989.

Alper J: Congenital nevi—the controversy rages on. Arch Dermatol 121:734, 1985.

Alper J, Holmes LB: The incidence of birthmarks in a cohort of 4,641 newborns. Pediatr Dermatol 1:58, 1983.

Alper J, Holmes LB, Mihm MC: Birthmarks with serious medical significance: Nevocellular nevi, sebaceous nevi, and multiple cafe-au-lait spots. J Pediatr 95:696, 1979.

Alvarez J, Peteiro C, Toribio J: Linear and whorled nevoid hypermelanosis. Pediatr Dermatol 10:156–158, 1993.

Amir T, Krikler R, Metzker A, et al: Strawberry hemangioma in preterm infants. Pediatr Dermatol 3:331, 1986.

Arons MS, Hurwitz S: Congenital nevocellular nevus: A review of the treatment controversy and a report of 46 cases. Plast Reconstr Surg 72:355, 1983.

Ashinoff R, Geronemus RG: Capillary hemangiomas and treatment with the flash lamp-pumped pulsed dye laser. Arch Dermatol 127:202–205, 1991.

Ashinoff R, Geronemus RG: Failure of the flashlamp-pumped pulsed dye laser to prevent progression to deep hemangioma. Pediatr Dermatol 10:77–80, 1993.

Baker LL, Dillon WP, Hieshima GB, et al: Hemangiomas and vascular malformations of the head and neck: MR characterization. Am J Neuroradiol 14:307–314, 1993.

Barkovich AJ, Frieden IJ, Williams ML: MR of neurocutaneous melanosis. Am J Neuroradiol 15:859–867, 1994.

Barksy SH, Rosen S, Geer DE, et al: The nature and evolution of port wine stains: A computer assisted study. J Invest Dermatol 74:154, 1980.

Barnhill RL, Aguiar M, Cohen C, et al: Congenital melanocytic nevi and DNA content: An analysis by flow and image cytometry. Cancer 74:2935–2943, 1994.

Berman B, Lim HWP: Concurrent cutaneous and hepatic hemangiomata in infancy: Report of a case and a review of the literature. J Cutan Surg Oncol 4:869, 1978.

Brown SH Jr, Neerhout RC, Fonkalsrud EW: Prednisone therapy in the management of large hemangiomas in infants and children. Surgery 71:168, 1972.

Browze NL, Whimster I, Stewart G, et al: The surgical management of lymphangioma circumscriptum. Br J Surg 73:535, 1986.

Burman D, Mansell PWQ, Warin RP: Miliary hemangiomata in the newborn. Arch Dis Child 42:193, 1967.

Burns AJ, Kaplan C, Mulliken JB: Is there an association between hemangioma and syndromes with dysmorphic features? Pediatrics 88:1257–1267, 1991.

Burrows DE, Mulliken JB, Fellows KE, et al: Childhood hemangiomas and vascular malformations: Angiographic differentiation. Am J Roentgenol 141:483, 1983.

Cainelli T, Marchesi L, Pasquali F, et al: Monozygotic twins discordant for cutaneous mastocytosis. Arch Dermatol 119:1021, 1983.

Carroll CB, Ceballos P, Perry AE, et al: Severe atypical medium-sized congenital nevus with widespread satellitosis and placental deposits in a neonate: The problem of congenital melanoma and its simulants. J Am Acad Dermatol 30:825–828, 1994.

Casson P, Colen S: Dysplastic and congenital nevi. Clin Plast Surg 20:105–111, 1993.

Cates CP, William ED, Ward-Booth RP, et al: Doppler ultrasound: A valuable diagnostic aid in a patient with facial hemangioma. Oral Surg 59:458, 1985.

Ceballos PI, Ruiz-Maldonado R, Mihm JMC: Melanoma in children. N Engl J Med 332:656–662, 1995.

Crocker AL: The histiocytosis syndromes. *In* Fitzpatrick TB, Eisen AA, Wolff K, et al (Eds): Dermatology in General Medicine, 2nd ed. New York, McGraw-Hill, 1979, p 1171.

Cohen PR, Zalar GL: Cutis marmorata telangiectatica congenita: Clinico-pathologic characteristics and differential diagnosis. Cutis 42:418, 1988.

Commens C, Rogers M, Kan A: Heterotrophic brain tissue presenting as bald cysts with a collar of hypertrophic hair. Arch Dermatol 125:1253–1256, 1989.

D'Armiento M, Reda E, Camagna A, et al: McCune-Albright syndrome: Evidence for autonomous multiendocrine hyperfunction. J Pediatr 102:585, 1983.

De Raeve L, Danau W, Debacker A, Otten J: Prepubertal melanoma in a medium-sized congenital nevus. Eur J Pediatr 152:734–736, 1993.

De Raeve L, De Meirleir L, Ramet J, et al: Acrodermatitis enteropathica-like cutaneous lesions in organic aciduria. J Pediatr 124:416–420, 1994.

Drolet BA, Clowry L, McTigue K, Esterly NB: The hair collar sign: Marker for cranial dysrahism. Pediatrics 96:309–313, 1995.

Eady PAJ, Sparrow GP, Grice K: Naevoid pigmentation with giant melanosomes: Two cases. Proc R Soc Med 68:759, 1975.

Elder DE: The blind men and the elephant—Different views of small congenital nevi. Arch Dermatol 121:1263, 1985.

Elder DE, Goldman LI, Goldman SC, et al: Dysplastic nevus syndrome. Cancer 46:1787, 1980.

Enjolras O, Mulliken JB: The current management of vascular birthmarks. Pediatr Dermatol 10:311–333, 1993.

Enjolras O, Riche MC, Merland JJ, Escande JP: Management of alarming hemangiomas in infancy: A review of 25 cases. Pediatrics 85:491–498, 1990.

Enjolras O, Wassef M, Mazoyer E, et al: Infants with Kasabach-Merritt syndrome do not have "true" hemangiomas. J Pediatr 130(4):631–640, 1997.

Esterly NB: Cutaneous hemangiomas, vascular stains and malformations, and associated syndromes. Curr Probl Dermatol 7:65–108, 1995.

Esterly NB: Kasabach-Merritt syndrome in infants. J Am Acad Dermatol 8:504, 1983.

Esterly NB, Margileth AM, Kahn G, et al: The management of disseminated eruptive hemangiomata in infants: Special symposium. Pediatr Dermatol 1:312, 1984.

Esterly NB, Sahihi T, Medenica M: Juvenile xanthogranuloma: An atypical case with study of ultrastructure. Arch Dermatol 105:99, 1972.

Fienman NL, Yakovac WC: Neurofibromatosis in childhood. J Pediatr 76:339, 1970.

Fretzin DF, Potter B: Blue rubber bleb nevus. Arch Intern Med 116:924, 1965.

Frieden IJ, Williams ML, Barkovich AJ: Giant congenital melanocytic nevi: Brain magnetic resonance findings in neurologically asymptomatic children. J Am Acad Dermatol 31:423–429, 1994.

Folkman J: How is blood vessel growth regulated in normal and neoplastic tissue? Cancer Res 46:467, 1986.

Fost NC, Esterly NB: Successful treatment of juvenile hemangiomas with prednisone. J Pediatr 72:351, 1968.

Fowler JF, Porsley W, Cotter PG: Familial urticaria pigmentosa. Arch Dermatol 122:80, 1986.

Garden J, Bakus A: Clinical efficacy of the pulsed dye laser in the treatment of vascular lesions. J Dermatol Surg Oncol 19:321–326, 1993.

Garden JM, Bakus AD, Paller AS: Treatment of cutaneous hemangiomas by the flashlamp-pumped pulsed dye laser: Prospective analysis. J Pediatr 120:555–560, 1992.

Gari LM, Rivers JK, Kopf AW: Melanomas arising in large congenital nevocytic nevi: A prospective study. Pediatr Dermatol 5:151–158, 1988.

Gaynes PM, Cohen GS: Juvenile xanthogranuloma of the orbit. Am J Ophthalmol 63:755, 1967.

Giacoia GP, Berry GT: Acrodermatitis enteropathica-like syndrome secondary to isoleucine deficiency during treatment of maple syrup urine disease. Am J Dis Child 147:954–956, 1994.

Glassberg E, Lask G, Rabinowitz LG, Tunnessen JWW: Capillary hemangiomas: Case study of a novel laser treatment and a review of therapeutic options. J Dermatol Surg Oncol 15:1214–1222, 1989.

Glovitzki P, Hallier CH, Telander RL, et al: Surgical implications of Klippel-Trenaunay syndrome. Ann Surg 192:353, 1983.

Goldman M, Fitzpatrick R, Ruiz-Esparza J: Treatment of port-wine stains (capillary malformation) with the flashlamp-pumped pulsed dye laser. J Pediatr 122:71–77, 1993.

Goldberg NS, Herbert AA, Esterly NB: Sacral hemangiomas and multiple congenital abnormalities. Arch Dermatol 122:684–687, 1986.

Golitz LE, Ruchkoff J, O'Meara P: Diffuse neonatal hemangiomatosis. Pediatr Dermatol 3:145, 1986.

Gomez MR: Phenotypes of the tuberous sclerosis complex with a revision of diagnostic criteria. Ann NY Acad Sciences 615:1–7, 1991.

Gordon L, Vujic I, Spicer KM: Visualization of cutaneous hemangiomas with Tc-99m tagged red cells. Clin Nucl Med 4:468, 1981.

Greene MH, Clark WH Jr, Tucker JH, et al: Managing the dysplastic naevus syndrome. Lancet 1:166, 1984.

Greeley PW, Middleton AG, Curtain JW: Incidence of malignancy in giant pigmented nevi. Plast Reconstr Surg 36:26, 1965.

Hansen RC: Dermatitis and nutritional deficiency. Arch Dermatol 128:1389–1390, 1992.

Hara K: Melanocytic lesions in lymph nodes associated with congenital nevus. Histopathology 23:445–451, 1993.

Harris LE, Stayura LA, Ramirez-Talavera PF, Anneger JF: Congenital and acquired abnormalities observed in liveborn and stillborn neonates. Mayo Clin Proc 50:85, 1975.

Hayashi T, Shyojima K, Honda E, Hasimoto T: Lipoma of corpus callosum associated with frontoethmoidal lipomeningocele: CT findings. J Comput Assist Tomogr 8:795–796, 1984.

Heimann P, Ogur G, Debusscher C, et al: Chromosomal findings in cultured melanocytes from a giant congenital nevus. Cancer Genet Cytogenet 68:74–77, 1993.

Hidano A, Nakajima S: Earliest features of the strawberry mark in the newborn. Br J Dermatol 87:138, 1972.

Hoffman HJ, Freeman A: Primary leptomeningeal melanoma in association with giant hairy nevi. Report of two cases. J Neurosurg 26:62, 1967.

Holden KR, Alexander R: Diffuse neonatal hemangiomatosis. Pediatrics 46:411, 1970.

Illig W, Weidner F, Hundeiker M, et al: Congenital nevi 10 cm precursors to melanoma: 52 cases, a review, and a new conception. Arch Dermatol 121:1274, 1985.

Janniger CK, Schwartz RA: Tuberous sclerosis: Recent advances for the clinician. Cutis 51:167–174, 1993.

Kadonaga JN, Frieden IJ: Neurocutaneous melanosis: Definition and review of the literature. J Am Acad Dermatol 5:747–755, 1991.

Kaplan M, Paller AS: Clinical pearl: Use of self-adhesive, compressive wraps in the treatment of limb hemangiomas. J Am Acad Dermatol 32:117–118, 1995.

Kettelhut BV, Metcalfe DD: Pediatric mastocytosis. J Invest Dermatol 96:15–18, 1991.

Kopf AW, Bart RS, Hennessey P: Congenital nevocytic nevi and malignant melanomas. J Am Acad Dermatol 1:123–130, 1979.

Kopf AW, Weidman AJ: Nevus of ota. Arch Dermatol 85:75–88, 1962.

Kuflik JH, Janniger CK: Congenital melanocytic nevi. Cutis 53:112–114, 1994.

Kushner BJ: Local steroid therapy in adnexal hemangioma. Ann Ophthalmol 11:1005–1009, 1979.

Lazaro C, Ravella A, Gaona A, et al: Neurofibromatosis type 1 due to germ-line mosaicism in a clinically normal father. New Engl J Med 331:1403–1407, 1994.

Lerno G, Slaats G, Coenen E, et al: Anaesthetic management of systemic mastocytosis. Br J Anaesthesia 65:254–257, 1990.

Lewis RA, Riccardi VM: Von Recklinghausen neurofibromatosis: Incidence of iris hamartoma. Ophthalmology 88:348, 1981.

Lund HA, Kraus JM: Melanotic tumors of the skin, Fascicle 3. *In* Atlas of Tumor Pathology. Washington, DC, Armed Forces Institute of Pathology, 1962.

Magana M, Vazquez R, Fernandez-Diez J, et al: Giant congenital juvenile xanthogranuloma. Pediatr Dermatol 11:227–230, 1994.

Mangus DJ: Continuous compression therapy of hemangiomas: Evaluation in two cases. Plast Reconstr Surg 49:490, 1973.

Marghoob AA, Orlow SJ, Kopf AW: Syndromes associated with melanocytic nevi. J Am Acad Dermatol 29:373–388, 1993.

Margileth AM: Developmental vascular abnormalities. Med Clin North Am 18:773, 1971.

Martinez-Lage J, Capel A, Costa T, et al: The child with a mass on its head: Diagnostic and surgical strategies. Child Nerv Syst 8:247–252, 1992.

Morelli JG: On the treatment of hemangiomas. Pediatr Dermatol 10:84, 1993.

Morelli JG, Tan OT, Weston WL: Treatment of ulcerated hemangiomas with pulsed tunable dye laser. Am J Dis Child 145:1062–1064, 1991.

Morelli JG, Tan OT, Yohn JJ, Weston WL: Treatment of ulcerated hemangiomas infancy. Arch Pediatr Adolesc Med 148:1104–1105, 1994.

Mulliken JB: A plea for a biologic approach to hemangiomas of infancy. Arch Dermatol 127:243–244, 1991.

Mulliken JB, Boon LM, Takahashi K, et al: Pharmacologic therapy for endangering hemangiomas. Curr Opin Dermatol 109–113, 1995.

Mulliken JB, Young AE: Vascular Birthmarks, Hemangiomas, and Malformations. Philadelphia, W. B. Saunders Company, 1988.

Mulliken JB, Glowacki J: Hemangiomas and vascular malformations in infants and children: A classification based on endothelial characteristics. Plast Reconstr Surg 69:421, 1982.

Mullins JF, Naylor D, Pedetski J: The Klippel-Trenaunay-Weber syndrome (nevus vasculosus osteohypertrophicus). Arch Dermatol 86:202, 1962.

Munkvad M: Blue rubber bleb nevus. Dermatologica 163:307, 1983.

National Institutes of Health Consensus Development Conference: Neurofibromatosis. Arch Neurol 45:575, 1988.

Nomland R: Nevoxanthoendothelioma, a benign xanthomatous disease of infants and children. J Invest Dermatol 22:207, 1959.

Oates CP, Williams ED, Ward-Booth RP, et al: Doppler ultrasound: A valuable diagnostic aid in a patient with a facial hemangioma. Oral Surg 59:958, 1985.

O'Reilly MS, Brem H, Folkman J: Treatment of murine hemangioendotheliomas with the angiogenesis inhibitor AGM-1470. J Pediatr Surg 30:325–329, 1995.

Osburn K, Schosser RH, Everett MA: Congenital pigmented and vascular lesions in newborn infants. J Am Acad Dermatol 16:788–792, 1987.

Ozturkcan S, Goze F, Atakan N, Icli F: Malignant melanoma in a child. J Am Acad Dermatol 30:493–494, 1994.

Paller AS: The Sturge-Weber syndrome. Pediatr Dermatol 4:300, 1987.

Paller AS, Pensler JM, Tomita T: Nasal midline masses in infants and children. Arch Dermatol 127:362–366, 1991.

Payarols JP, Masferrer JP, Bellvert CG: Treatment of life-threatening infantile hemangiomas with vincristine. New Engl J Med 333:69, 1995.

Peachy RDG, Lim CC, Whimster JW: Lymphangioma of skin: A review of 65 cases. Br J Dermatol 83:419, 1970.

Pinkus H, Mehregan AH: A Guide to Dermatohistopathology. New York, Appleton-Century-Crofts, Inc., 1969, pp 352–354.

Pratt AG: Birthmarks in infancy. Arch Dermatol 67:302, 1953.

Powell ST, Su WPD: Cutis marmorata telangiectasia congenita: Report of nine cases and review of the literature. Cutis 34:305, 1984.

Reed WB, Becker SW Sr, Becker SW Jr, Nickel WR: Giant pigmented nevi, melanoma and leptomeningeal melanocytosis. Arch Dermatol 91:100, 1965.

Reese V, Frieden IJ, Paller AS, et al: Association of facial hemangiomas with Dandy-Walker and other posterior fossa malformations. J Pediatr 122:379–384, 1993.

Renfro L, Geronemus RG: Anatomical differences of port-wine stains in response to treatment with the pulsed dye laser. Arch Dermatol 129:182–188, 1993.

Rhodes AR, Melski JW: Small congenital nevocellular nevi and the risk of cutaneous melanoma. J Pediatr 100:219, 1982.

Rhodes AR, Sober AJ, Day CL, et al: The malignant potential of small congenital nevocellular nevi: An estimate of association based on a histologic study of 234 primary cutaneous melanomas. J Am Acad Dermatol 6:620, 1982.

Riccardi VM: Early manifestations of neurofibromatosis: Diagnosis and management. Compr Ther 8:35, 1982.

Riccardi VM: Neurofibromatosis heterogeneity. J Am Acad Dermatol 8:518, 1983.

Riccardi VM: Von Recklinghausen neurofibromatosis. N Engl J Med 305:1617, 1981.

Riccardi VM, Eichner JE: Neurofibromatosis, Phenotype, Natural History and Pathogenesis. Baltimore, Johns Hopkins University Press, 1986.

Rieger E, Kofler R, Borkenstein M, et al: Melanotic macules following Blaschko's lines in McCune-Albright syndrome. Br J Dermatol 130:215–220, 1994.

Rodriguez-Erdmann F, Button L, Murray JE, Moloney M: Kasabach-Merritt syndrome: Coagulo-analytical observations. Am J Med Sci 261:9, 1971.

Rogers M, McCrossin I, Commens C: Epidermal nevi and the epidermal nevus syndrome: A review of 131 cases. J Am Acad Dermatol 20:476, 1989.

Sagher F, Evan-Paz Z: Mastocytosis and the Mast Cell. Chicago, Year Book Medical Publishers, 1967.

Saijo M, Munroe IR, Mancer K: Lymphangioma: Long-term follow-up study. Plast Reconstr Surg 56:642, 1975.

Sanchez NP, Rhodes AR, Mandell F, Mihm MC: Encephalocraniocutaneous lipomatosis: A new syndrome. Br J Dermatol 104:89, 1981.

Sandsmark M, Eskeland G, Ogaard AR, et al: Treatment of large congenital nevi: A review and report of six cases. Scand J Plast Reconstr Surg Hand Surg 27:223–232, 1993.

Sandsmark M, Eskeland G, Skullerud K, Abyholm F: Neurocutaneous melanosis: Case report and a brief review. Scand J Plast Reconstr Surg Hand Surg 28:151–154, 1994.

Scheepers JH, Quaba AA: Does the pulsed tunable dye laser have a role in the management of infantile hemangiomas? Observations based on 3 year's experience. Plast Reconstr Surg 95:305–412, 1995.

Schwindinger WF, Francomano CA, Levine MA: Identification of a mutation in the gene encoding the alpha subunit of the stimulatory G protein of adenylyl cyclase in McCune-Albright syndrome. Proc Natl Acad Sci 89:5152–5156, 1992.

Selmanowitz VJ, Orentreich N, Tiangco CC, Demis DJ: Uniovular twins discordant for cutaneous mastocytosis. Arch Dermatol 102:34, 1970.

Shenker A, Weinstein LS, Moran A, et al: Severe endocrine and nonendocrine manifestations of the McCune-Albright syndrome associated with activating mutations of stimulatory G protein GS. J Pediatr 123:509–518, 1993.

Sherer DM, Metlay LA, Sinkin RA, et al: Congenital ichthyosis with restrictive dermopathy and Gaucher disease: A new syndrome with associated prenatal diagnostic and pathology findings. Obstet Gynecol 81:842–844, 1993.

Sherwood KA, Tan OT: Treatment of capillary hemangioma with the flashlamp pumped-dye laser. J Am Acad Dermatol 22:136–137, 1990.

Shpall S, Frieden I, Chesney M, Newman T: Risk of malignant transformation of congenital melanocytic nevi in blacks. Pediatr Dermatol 11:204–208, 1994.

Smith JLS, Ingram RM: Juvenile oculodermal xanthogranuloma. Br J Ophthalmol 52:696, 1968.

Sober AJ: Solar exposure in the etiology of cutaneous melanoma. Photodermatology 4:23, 1987.

Solomon LM: Epidermal nevi: A study of 300 cases. In Fabrizi G, Serri F (Eds): Dermatologia Pediatrica. Transactions of a symposium on pediatric dermatology. Rome, Italy, CILAG SPA, 1985.

Solomon LM: The management of congenital melanocytic nevi. Arch Dermatol 116:1017, 1980.

Solomon LM, Esterly NB: Epidermal and other congenital organoid nevi. Curr Probl Pediatr 6:1, 1975.

Solomon LM, Esterly NB: Neonatal Dermatology. Philadelphia, W. B. Saunders Company, 1973.

Solomon LM, Fretzin DF, De Wald RL: The epidermal nevus syndrome. Arch Dermatol 97:273, 1968.

Swint RB, Klaus SW: Malignant degeneration of an epithelial nevus. Arch Dermatol 101:56, 1970.

Sybert VP: Hypomelanosis of Ito: A description, not a diagnosis. J Invest Dermatol 103:141s–143s, 1994.

Takahashi K, Mulliken JB, Kozakewich HP, et al: Cellular markers that distinguish the phases of hemangioma during infancy and childhood. J Clin Invest 93:2357–2364, 1994.

Tallman B, Tan OT, Morelli JG, et al: Location of port-wine stains and the likelihood of ophthalmic and/or central nervous system complications. Pediatrics 87:323–327, 1991.

Tan KL: Nevus flammeus of the nape, glabella, and eyelids. Clin Pediatr 11:112, 1972.

Tavafoghi V, Ghandchi A, Hambrick G, Udverhelyi G: Cutaneous signs of spinal dysraphism. Arch Dermatol 114:573–577, 1978.

Tsuchida T, Oksuka H, Riimura M, et al: Biochemical study of gangliosides in neurofibroma and neurofibrosarcomas of Recklinghausen's disease. J Dermatol (Tokyo) 11:129, 1984.

Vergnes P, Taieb A, Maleville J, et al: Repeated skin expansion for excision of congenital giant nevi in infancy and childhood. Plast Reconstr Surg 91:450–455, 1993.

Voest EE, Kenyon BM, O'Reilly MS, et al: Inhibition of angiogenesis in vivo by interleukin 12. J National Cancer Institute 87:581–586, 1995.

Wade TR, Kamino H, Ackerman AB: A histologic atlas of vascular lesions. J Dermatol Surg Oncol 4:845, 1978.

Walker RS, Custer PL, Nerad JA: Surgical excision of periorbital capillary hemangiomas. Ophthalmology 101:1333–1340, 1994.

Waner M, Suen JY, Dinehart S, Mallory SB: Laser photocoagulation of superficial proliferating hemangiomas. J Dermatol Surg Oncol 20:43–46, 1994.

Way BH, Hermana J, Gilbert EF, et al: Cutis marmorata telangiectatica congenita. J Cutan Pathol 1:10, 1974.

Wheeland RG: Advances in the surgical approach to pediatric dermatologic problems: The laser in vascular and pigmented pediatric lesions [abstract]. 53rd annual meeting of the American Academy of Dermatology. New Orleans, February 1995.

White CW, Sondheimer HM, Crouch EC, et al: Treatment of pulmonary hemangioma tests with recombinant interferon alfa-2a. N Engl J Med 320:1197, 1989.

Whitehouse D: Diagnostic value of the cafe-au-lait spot in children. Arch Dis Child 41:316, 1966.

Wienecke R, Konig A, DeClue JE: Identification of tuberin, the tuberous sclerosis-2 product: Tuberin possesses specific Rap1GAP activity. J Biol Chem 270:16409–16414, 1995.

Williams ML: Early onset nevi. Pediatr Dermatol 10:198, 1993.

Williams ML, Pennella R: Melanoma, melanocytic nevi, and other melanoma risk factors in children. J Pediatr 124:833–845, 1994.

Zimmerman LC: Ocular lesions of juvenile xanthogranuloma. Am J Ophthalmol 60:1011, 1965.

Zitelli GA, Grant MG, Abell E, et al: Histologic patterns of congenital nevocytic nevi and implications for treatment. J Am Acad Dermatol 11:402, 1984.

Zuniga S, Las Heras J, Benveviste S: Rhabdomyosarcoma arising in a congenital giant nevus associated with neurocutaneous melanosis in a neonate. J Pediatr Surg 22:1036–1038, 1987.

Zvulunov A, Esterly NB: Neurocutaneous syndromes associated with pigmentary skin lesions. J Am Acad Dermatol 32:915–935, 1995.

CHAPTER **110**

Retinopathy of Prematurity

Graham E. Quinn

Retinopathy of prematurity (ROP), recognized since the early 1940s (Terry, 1942), continues to be a cause of serious visual morbidity in very-low-birth-weight children, despite the fact that the condition had been declared "eliminated" in the 1960s and 1970s (Law, 1975). Rather than disappearing, this disorder of the developing retinal vasculature has been the focus of intense clinical and basic science research over the past 15 years. This time period has also been characterized by changes in terminology, classification, treatment options, and even the role of the ophthalmologist in the nursery. There is currently an internationally accepted classification of ROP (ICROP, 1984, 1987) and a treatment proven effective in a large, randomized multicenter trial, that is, cryotherapy for serious ROP as defined by the Cryotherapy for Retinopathy of Prematurity (CRYO-ROP) Cooperative Group (1990a, 1990b, 1993).

The original term of retrolental fibroplasia, indicating an end stage of fibrosis and scarring in the space behind the lens, no longer adequately describes the retinal vasoproliferative process seen in the eyes of premature infants. Therefore, retrolental fibroplasia has been replaced by the term, retinopathy of prematurity.

CLASSIFICATION

A unified classification system has allowed for major strides forward in clinical research and collaborative efforts among investigators. The impetus for the development of an international classification came at a Ross Laboratory–sponsored conference on ROP in December 1981 when a group of 23 ophthalmologists and ophthalmic pathologists from 11 countries formed a working group to develop a common classification of ROP. Before that time, several classifications were in common use (McCormick, 1977; Patz, 1972; Quinn et al, 1982; Reese et al, 1953; Schaffer et al, 1979) and each differed in emphasis, particularly in describing more severe retinopathy. Over the next few years, the group refined the protocol and put the developing system to use before recommending its broad use in the ophthalmic community. This effort resulted in the International Classification of Retinopathy of Prematurity (ICROP Committee, 1984). Further work by members of the committee as well as retinal specialists addressed the issue of late phases of retinopathy, including the characteristics of retinal detachment (ICROP Committee for Classification of Late Stages of ROP, 1987).

The basic premise of the classification is that more extensive and more posterior retinopathy is more serious

disease. The classification is based on four observations: (1) stage (or description in a 1 to 5 grading system) of the retinopathy occurring at the junction between the vascularized and unvascularized peripheral retina, (2) extent in 30-degree sectors of involvement of the retinopathy along the circumferential junction of the vascularized and unvascularized retina, (3) anterior-posterior location of the retinopathy within the retina, and (4) the presence or absence of plus disease, defined as engorged and tortuous posterior pole vessels.

The acute phases of retinopathy occur along the junction of vascularized and unvascularized peripheral retina and are divided into five stages. The working group agreed that an eye should be staged according to the worst disease observed in any area of the retina. Stage 1 ROP is a distinct white line or demarcation line between vascular and avascular retina, often with abnormal branching of vessels leading to it (Fig. 110–1). This was the earliest sign of ROP that the committee could agree on that would be clearly recognizable to ophthalmologists screening for ROP in the neonatal intensive care unit. The committee, however, recognized that earlier changes were observable, such as abnormal branching and equatorial turns of the vessels at the vascular-avascular junction. Stage 2 ROP consists of a heaping up of abnormal pink to salmon colored tissue in the region of the demarcation line that appeared to have depth when compared with the smooth surface of the retina. In stage 3 ROP, fine vessels appear along the surface of the ridge to just posterior to it and the fibrovascular proliferation invades the vitreous (Fig. 110–2). Stage 4 is a partial retinal detachment and is further subdivided into stage 4A for partial detachment not involving the macular region and stage 4B for partial detachment that involves the macula (Fig. 110–3). Stage 5 is a total retinal detachment, although this may be difficult to distinguish on clinical grounds if a partial detachment obscures the view of the retina.

Extent of retinal involvement along the vascular-avascular junction was determined in 30-degree segments along the circumference of this line. Therefore, up to 12 sectors of involvement were possible, even though the retinopathy of various stages may occur in the various sectors.

The major breakthrough that led to widespread use of the international classification was the adoption of a method to determine the anterior-posterior location of retinopathy. Because it was thought that more posterior disease was more ominous for the eye, being able to locate the retinopathy with certainty became important. Previous

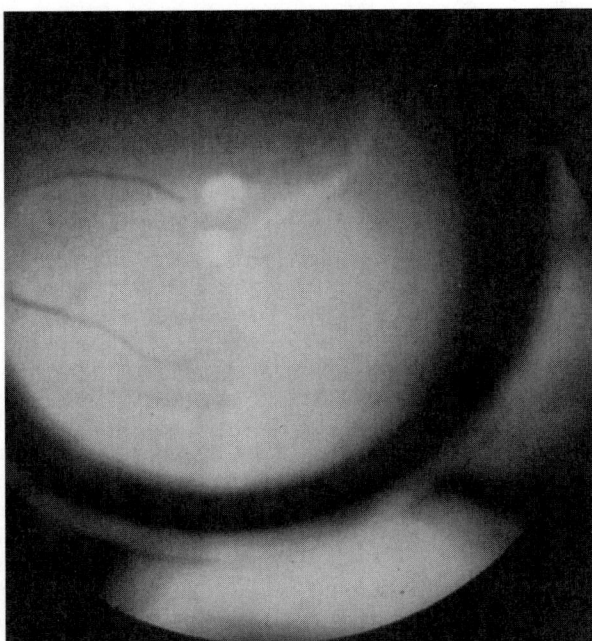

FIGURE 110–1. Stage 1 retinopathy of prematurity is defined as a thin white line (demarcation line) at the junction between the vascularized and avascular retina. (From the International Committee for the Classification of Retinopathy of Prematurity: Multicenter Trial of Cryotherapy: An international classification of retinopathy of prematurity. Arch Ophthalmol 102:1130–1134, 1984. Copyright 1984, American Medical Association.)

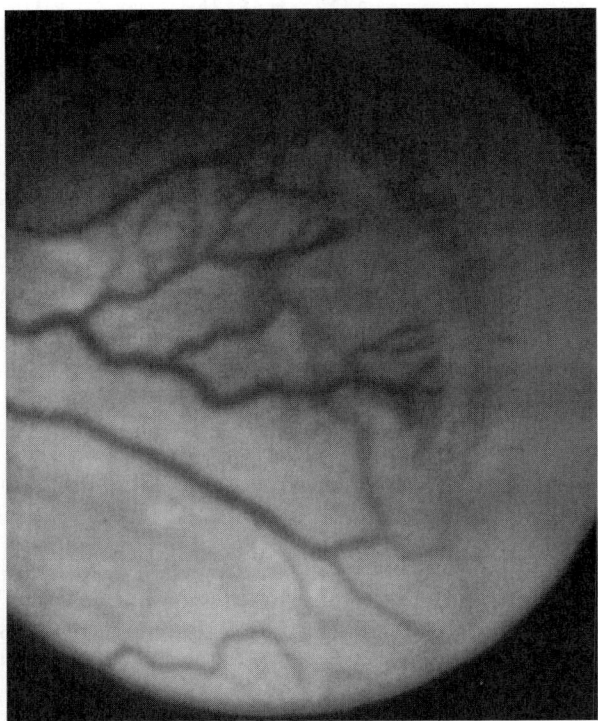

FIGURE 110–2. Stage 3 retinopathy of prematurity is characterized by the development of a ridgelike structure with width and volume that has developed fine new vessels extending into the vitreous. (From the International Committee for the Classification of Retinopathy of Prematurity: Multicenter Trial of Cryotherapy: An international classification of retinopathy of prematurity. Arch Ophthalmol 102:1130–1134, 1984. Copyright 1984, American Medical Association.)

classifications had used the traditional center of the eye as the macula and located disease in the peripheral retina in terms of distance from the macula. The committee, however, recommended using the optic nerve as the central reference point, taking into account that the retinal vessels emerge from the optic nerve and grow out over the retina in a centrifugal fashion. Three concentric areas of retina were described as potential "zones" of retinal involvement. As shown in Figure 110–4, the first area, zone 1, is the most posterior zone and is a circle centered on the optic nerve and with a radius of twice the distance from the optic nerve to the macula. Zone 2 is defined as that area outside zone 1 but within a circle defined by a radius of the distance from the optic nerve to the nasal ora serrata (where the peripheral retina ends just behind a flat area near the iris base). Zone 3 is that area of the retina that is peripheral to zones 1 and 2, and, as shown in the figure, is not present at the nasal meridian. Zone 3 enlarges in anterior-posterior extent toward the superior and inferior retina and reaches its broadest extent at the temporal meridian.

One final aspect of ocular findings included in the classification was the notation of the appearance of the posterior pole vessels. Abnormally dilated veins and tortuous arterioles in the posterior pole were thought to be ominous signs suggesting more serious and rapidly progressive ROP, and the presence of these findings was noted by appending a plus sign (+) to the stage designation. Abnormal posterior pole vessels are usually seen with iris vessel engorgement, poor dilation of the pupil, and vitreous haze.

The usual course of acute phase retinopathy is to regress

with few, if any, retinal sequelae. However, the long-term consequences for the child and family are extremely important because of the effect of retinal scarring on visual function (Birch and Spencer, 1991; Dobson et al, 1994) and because of the increased likelihood of later retinal problems such as retinal detachment (Tasman, 1979). Before the development of the international classification, most ophthalmologists had used the Reese classification (Reese et al, 1953) to describe long-term scarring or cicatricial phase of ROP. Unfortunately, that classification had tied increasingly severe retinal scarring with refractive error ranges and recognition acuity scores, and the unpredictable correlation of these three ocular findings had not sustained its continued use. Therefore, the ophthalmologists who developed the classifications in 1984 and 1987 recommended recording the retinal findings in terms of retinal location, posterior or peripheral, and whether the findings were more vascular or retinal (Table 110–1). The task of ordering the findings in terms of severity awaits more information about the impact of these findings on visual function and refractive error development. In the past decade, several investigators have added to knowledge of the effect of retinal residua of ROP on visual function (Birch and Spencer, 1991; Dobson et al, 1994; Gilbert et al, 1992; Mintz-Hittner et al, 1992; Reynolds et al, 1993), and that phase of the classification is near completion.

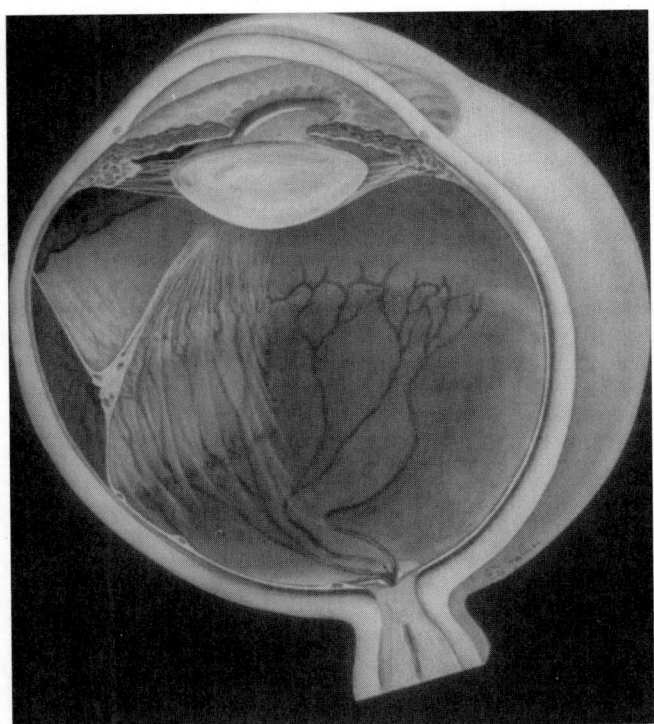

FIGURE 110–3. Stage 4A retinopathy of prematurity is defined as a partial retinal detachment that does not involve the fovea. (From the International Committee for the Classification of Retinopathy of Prematurity: An international classification of retinopathy of prematurity: II. The classification of retinal detachment. Arch Ophthalmol 105:906–912, 1987. Copyright 1987, American Medical Association.)

TABLE 110–1

Findings of Regressed Retinopathy of Prematurity

Location	Vascular	Retinal
Posterior	Tortuosity Straightening of vessels Decrease in angle of insertion of major temporal arcade	Pigmentary changes Macular ectopia Retinal fold Vitreoretinal interface changes Vitreous membranes Retinal detachment
Peripheral	Incomplete vascularization Abnormal branching Vascular arcades Telangiectasia	Pigmentary changes Vitreoretinal interface changes Retinal thinning Retinal folds Vitreous membranes

Adapted from ICROP Committee for Classification of Late Stages of ROP: An international classification of retinopathy of prematurity: II The classification of retinal detachment. Arch Ophthalmol 105:906–912, 1987. Copyright 1987, American Medical Association.

nopathy. The ability to document early acute phase retinopathy makes the direct comparison of acute phase disease incidence between reports from the 1940s, 1950s, and 1960s, with later reports virtually impossible. Any comparison of incidence must clearly distinguish between acute phase retinopathy and the long-term cicatricial forms.

At Pennsylvania Hospital in Philadelphia, the incidence of ROP has been documented using a classification for acute phases of ROP since the early 1970s. Over this period, the number of low-birth-weight infants who survive has increased, but it appears that the incidence of ROP has only decreased in the larger birth-weight infants. As shown in Table 110–2, a comparison of the incidence of ROP from the early 1970s to the early 1980s shows a decrease in the incidence of ROP in larger birth-weight infants. The survival rate and number of infants in whom ROP develops in 1972 to 1975 versus 1981 to 1982 is

INCIDENCE

The use of the indirect ophthalmoscope and the routine screening of premature infants in the intensive care units increased awareness of the early peripheral phases of reti-

FIGURE 110–4. Zones 1, 2, and 3 are identified for the right and left eyes. (From the International Committee for the Classification of Retinopathy of Prematurity: Multicenter Trial of Cryotherapy: An international classification of retinopathy of prematurity. Arch Ophthalmol 102:1130–1134, 1984. Copyright 1984, American Medical Association.)

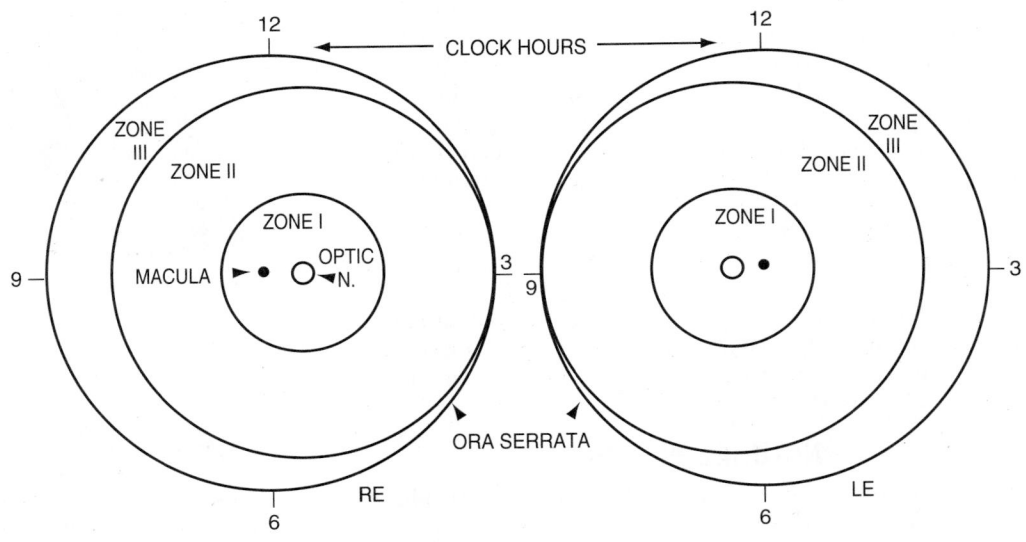

TABLE 110–2

Survival Rate and Number of Infants with Retinopathy of Prematurity

Birth Weight	Time Intervals	Survival Rate	No ROP	Yes ROP	*P* Value*
500–1000 g	1972–1975	15%	0	7	NS
	1981–1982	65%	11	36	
1001–1250 g	1972–1975	48%	5	15	<0.02
	1981–1982	95%	22	17	
1251–1500 g	1972–1975	75%	16	15	<0.01
	1981–1982	96%	42	6	
1501–2000 g	1972–1975	87%	74	14	<0.01
	1981–1982	99%	83	1	

*Comparing no ROP to yes ROP.

From Johnson LH, Quinn GE, Abbasi S, Bowen FW: Retinopathy of prematurity: Prevalence and treatment over a 20 year period at Pennsylvania Hospital. Doc Ophthalmol 74:213–222, 1990. Reprinted by permission of Kluwer Academic Publishers.

provided in Table 110–2, with the infants grouped in four birth-weight categories: 500 to 1000 g, 1001 to 1250 g, 1251 to 1500 g, and 1501 to 2000 g. The incidence of ROP cared for with the nutritional support regimen and neonatal care used at Pennsylvania Hospital has declined during this period in the larger birth-weight infants (Johnson, 1990).

Keith and Doyle (1995), in a report comparing incidence and severity of ROP for infants with birth weights of 500 to 999 g born between 1977 and 1992 in a perinatal center in Australia, documented that the incidence of ROP decreased significantly from 48% (68/141) in 1977 to 1984 to 36% (105/293) in 1985 to 1992. At the same time, survival rates increased from 34% (145/420) in 1977 to 1984 to 54% (312/581) in the 1985 to 1992 time period.

At this time, the report involving the largest number of serial eye examinations undertaken to document the incidence of acute phase ROP is from the CRYO-ROP study of infants with birth weights of less than 1251 g who were born during the 2-year period from 1986 to 1987 (Palmer et al, 1991). Eye examinations were undertaken from 4 to 6 weeks after birth in 4099 low-birth-weight infants to monitor the onset and course of the acute phase of ROP. The overall incidence of ROP observed was 65.8%, with the highest incidence (90%) being in the children with birth weights of less than 750 g, and lower incidences of 78% in the 751 to 1000 g birth-weight group and 47% in the largest 1000 to 1250 g birth-weight group. Stages 1, 2, or 3 ROP were the highest stage of ROP seen in 25%, 22%, and 18%, respectively, of the infants examined. As seen in Figure 110–5, the proportion of eyes in which more severe ROP develops is inversely related to the birth-weight group of the child. Also noted in the figure is the distribution of plus disease for the three birth-weight groups. The incidence of plus disease in the overall study population was 11%. There was no significant difference with race, gender, or single compared to multiple births (Palmer et al, 1991).

NATURAL HISTORY

In general, the natural course of ROP is an acute phase retinopathy to (1) develop in the weeks before term, (2)

reach a peak severity around term, and then, (3) begin to regress with remodeling of the retinal vasculature or with cicatrization that sometimes leads to retinal detachment. The following discussion addresses these three periods.

The vascularization of the peripheral retina in preterm infants proceeds in an orderly fashion from the optic nerve and reaching the ora serrata by about term due date. To determine whether this is an orderly process or a serendipitous event, investigators in the CRYO-ROP study examined the relation of vascularization of the retina in terms of postnatal age and postconceptional age (gestational age plus postnatal age) for infants with birth weights of less than 1251 g. There were 1400 infants in whom ROP did not develop during the neonatal period and who underwent serial eye examinations as part of the study (Palmer et al, 1991). In Figure 110–6, the cumulative proportion of eyes with vascularization into zone 3 is shown for three birth-weight groups: less than 750 g, 751 to 1000 g, and 1001 to 1250 g. Based on these figures, a pattern of orderly vascularization of the peripheral retina is clearly related to postconceptional age, regardless of birth-weight group. This pattern of close relation to postconceptional age is also seen in the disrupted process of abnormal vessel formation that characterizes the development of acute phase ROP. As shown in Table 110–3, the median onset of stage 1 ROP is at 34.3 weeks postception, stage 2 ROP at 35.4 weeks, and stage 3 at 36.6 weeks. The median age at onset of threshold ROP (defined in the CRYO-ROP study) is 36.9 weeks postconception, with a 5th percentile of 33.6 weeks and 95th percentile of 42 weeks.

The data from the CRYO-ROP study argue for a simple relation between postconceptional age (as an indicator of retinal development) and age at onset of ROP, at least for infants with birth weights of less than 1251 g. The situation is more complex than this and it is undoubtedly perturbed by perinatal events that result in various degrees of insults.

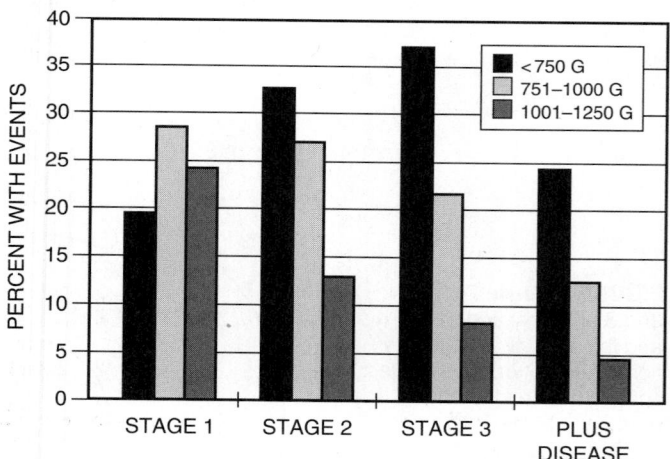

FIGURE 110–5. The percentage of eyes with stages 1, 2, and 3 retinopathy of prematurity is provided for three birth-weight groups: less than 750 g, 751 to 1000 g, and 1001 to 1250 g. In addition, the percentage of eyes that had evidence of plus disease is provided for the three birth-weight groups. (Data from Palmer EA, Flynn JT, Hardy RJ, et al: Incidence and early course of retinopathy of prematurity. Ophthalmology 98:1628–1640, 1991. Courtesy of Ophthalmology.)

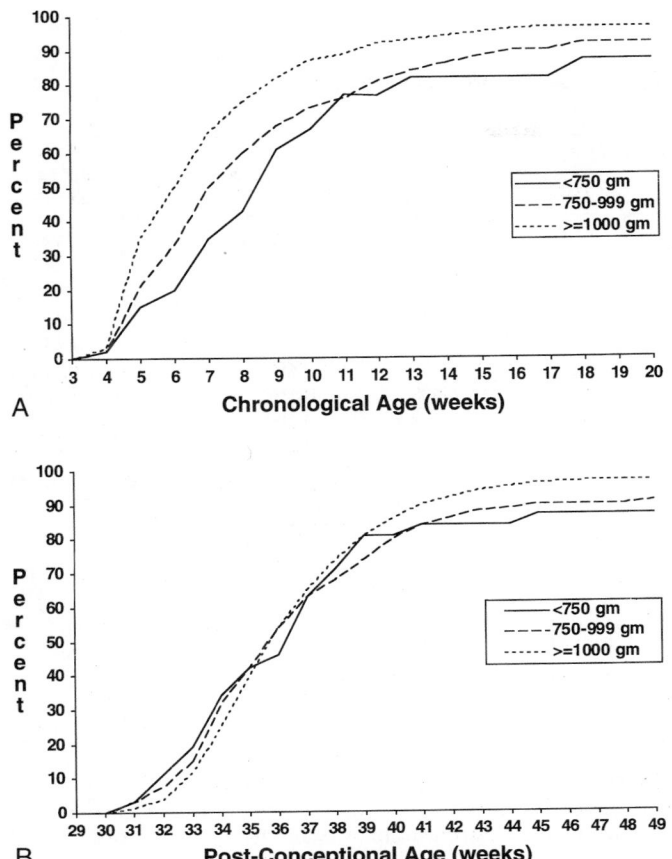

FIGURE 110–6. *A,* The cumulative proportion of eyes with retinal vascularized into zone 3 at various postnatal ages is presented by three birth-weight groups: less than 750 g, 751 to 1000 g, and 1001 to 1250 g. *B,* The cumulative proportion of eyes with retinal vascularized into zone 3 at various postconceptional ages is presented by three birth-weight groups: less than 750 g, 751 to 1000 g, and 1001 to 1250 g. (From Palmer EA, Flynn JT, Hardy RJ, et al: Incidence and early course of retinopathy of prematurity. Ophthalmology 98:1628–1640, 1991. Courtesy of Ophthalmology.)

Fielder and coworkers (1986) noted that ROP developed in infants with gestational ages of less than 28 weeks earlier than in later born infants (33.7 versus 35.7 weeks postconceptional age, respectively). Furthermore, in a report that included incidence data from larger birth-weight infants as well as those with birth weights of less than 1251 g, Quinn and colleagues (1992) showed that the onset of ROP becomes manifest later after birth, but earlier in infants who are born very early compared with later in gestation. This suggests an influence of perinatal events on the development of ROP and not just a strict postconceptional time course. Furthermore, the onset of ROP could be influenced by administration of vitamin E as prophylaxis of ROP, with ROP occurring later in the eyes of children who had received vitamin E (Quinn et al, 1990, 1992).

Most ROP regresses, but the natural history of regressing ROP is not well documented. Preslan and Butler (1994) reported that children in whom mild ROP developed in peripheral zone 2 or zone 3 had vascularization into zone 3 by around term and had completed vasculariza-

tion, and thus had complete regression, by 45 weeks' postconceptional age. Children in whom stage 3 ROP or ROP in zone 1 or posterior zone 2 developed had delay of retinal vascularization to an average of 51.7 to 55.4 weeks' postconceptional age. Therefore, more severe or more posterior ROP regresses more slowly and often lasts well into the time period after term due date (Preslan and Butler, 1994).

The incidence of long-term scarring resulting from ROP is less well documented, probably because of the difficulty of following up the premature infant on a long-term basis. The largest study reported is from the CRYO-ROP study and includes the ocular outcome at age 1 year of 5334 eyes of 2759 children with birth weights of less than 1251 g (Cryotherapy for Retinopathy of Prematurity Cooperative Group, 1994). These children had eye examinations at age 1 year and were among the 4099 children with acute phase data discussed previously. The outcome of eyes that underwent cryotherapy was not included in the report. The overall incidence of retinal residua involving the posterior pole was 3.7% (196 with macular heterotopia or worse among 5320 eyes; no data available on 14 eyes), with 113 eyes having extensive posterior pole scarring or detachment that was thought likely to cause significant visual handicap. Data in Table 110–4 suggest that more posterior disease and the greater the extent of stage 3-plus ROP, the more likely the outcome will be unfavorable (defined as grade III cicatricial or worse). For example the incidence of unfavorable outcomes in any ROP in zone 1 is 33.3%, whereas for ROP in zone 3 it is only 2.3%. Similarly unfavorable outcomes occur in 43.9% of eyes with 9 to 12 hours of stage 3-plus ROP in zone 2, compared with 8.8% for eyes with only 1 to 4 hours of stage 3-plus ROP in zone 2 (Cryotherapy for Retinopathy of Prematurity Cooperative Group, 1994).

Keith and Doyle (1995) reported that the occurrence of severe forms of ROP did not change significantly over the 1977 to 1992 period, but the trend was toward more children affected in a higher number of survivors (36/141[26%] in the earlier period versus 105/293 [36%] in the later period). Bilateral blindness from ROP was rare in Australia throughout the time period, affecting fewer than 1% in both periods.

TABLE 110–3

Onset of Various Stages of Retinopathy of Prematurity in Terms of Postconceptional Age in Weeks

	Median	5th Percentile	95th Percentile
Stage 1 ROP	34.3	°	39.1
Stage 2 ROP	35.4	32.0	40.7
Stage 3 ROP	36.6	32.6	42.9
ROP with plus disease	36.3	32.6	42.9
Threshold ROP	36.9	33.6	42.0

°Cannot be determined because 17% of infants had stage 1 retinopathy of prematurity (ROP) at the first eye examination.

Adapted from Palmer EA, Flynn JT, Hardy RJ, et al: Incidence and early course of retinopathy of prematurity. Ophthalmology 98:1628–1640, 1991. Courtesy of Ophthalmology.

TABLE 110–4

Anatomic Outcome (Reese Classification) Based on Zone and Stage of Most Severe Acute Phase Retinopathy of Prematurity*

Acute Phase Zone and Stage		Outcome at 1 Year (Cicatricial)†						Unfavorable Outcome (Grade III or Worse)	Total No. of Eyes‡
		<I	I	II	III	IV	V		
Zone 1	Any ROP	21	12	5	1	1	17	33.3%	58
Zone 2	St 3 +, 9–12 h	28	26	20	7	8	43	43.9%	134
	St 3 +, 5–8 h	38	19	12	3	0	17	22.5%	89
	St 3 +, 1–4 h	57	22	6	1	1	6	8.6%	94
	St 3, no plus	327	82	13	1	1	1	0.7%	425
	St 2	805	121	3	0	1	1	0.2%	935
	St 1	894	79	3	0	0	1	0.1%	977
Zone 3	Any ROP	575	40	1	0	0	1	0.2%	620
Other ROP		41	2	0	0	0	1	2.3%	44
No ROP		1826	128	0	0	0	0	0.0%	1958

*N = 5334 eyes.
†Based on Reese classification of cicatricial disease (Reese et al, 1953).
‡No data available on 14 eyes; therefore, 5320 total eyes in this table.
St, stage.
From Cryotherapy for Retinopathy of Prematurity Cooperative Group: The natural ocular outcome of premature birth and retinopathy: Status at 1 year. Arch Ophthalmol 112:903–912, 1994. Copyright 1994, American Medical Association.

DIFFERENTIAL DIAGNOSIS

Before the term due date, leukokoria caused by ROP is uncommon, because ROP does not usually progress to detachment by that time. Other causes of leukokoria in a young child include congenital nonattachment of the retina, persistent hyperplastic primary vitreous, retinal dysplasia, and retinoblastoma. In addition, vitreous hemorrhage from trauma or hematologic abnormalities should also be suspected. For an older child with peripheral retinal scarring, familial exudative vitreoretinopathy should be considered, as should Coats disease, myopic degeneration, trauma, and peripheral retinal uveitis (Palmer, 1984).

TREATMENT
Retinal Ablation

By the late 1960s and early 1970s, it was apparent that ROP was not a preventable condition in the neonatal nursery and attention was directed to surgical treatment of already established retinopathy. Two modalities were initially considered and attempted: laser photocoagulation and cryotherapy. Treatment was attempted in several countries including Japan, the United States, Switzerland, Israel, and Canada, with varying degrees of success (for review, see Fielder, 1992). The variable success rates likely resulted from (1) a lack of uniform indications for treatment including what stage of ROP should be treated and whether to treat in the presence of a retinal detachment, (2) variation in treatment techniques, such as treatment of the avascular region only or treatment of active retinopathy at the junction between the vascularized and avascular retina, and (3) techniques available for administration of the laser photocoagulation or cryotherapy. Relatively large series of 70 to 100 eyes reported by Nagata (1977) and Tagaki

(1978) gave treatment to between 20% and 30% of infants with birth weights of less than 1500 g and acknowledged that unnecessary treatment was being given to some children. Ben-Sira and coworkers (1980) reported a series of children with progressive ROP in whom treatment with cryotherapy had been confined to the avascular region of the retina, thus avoiding the fragile vessels of the acute phase ROP and the potential of hemorrhage. Eighty-three percent (15/18) of the eyes had little to no scarring of the posterior pole on follow-up examination. Tasman and colleagues (1985, 1986) subsequently reported a larger series that demonstrated that cryotherapy administered to eyes with severe acute phase retinopathy that had no evidence of retinal detachment led to significantly better outcomes than no treatment ($P < 0.001$).

Cryotherapy, rather than laser photocoagulation, emerged as the treatment modality of choice in the 1980s. This was largely based on the ease of administration of cryotherapy, because cryotherapy could be performed in the intensive care nursery with a neonatologist in attendance and using topical and subconjunctival anesthesia. Laser photocoagulation, on the other hand, required use of a cumbersome, nonportable instrument, usually required general anesthesia in the operating room, and was technically difficult in the sick, tiny premature infant.

Direct comparisons of the results obtained in the various small to medium size series of the 1970s and 1980s are not possible because no uniform classification system had yet been adopted. However, with the widespread use of ICROP, it was possible to address the important issue of at what stage to administer treatment in eyes likely to be blinded by acute phase ROP. Because the severe forms of ROP are relatively rare and no single center was likely to see enough serious retinopathy to achieve a convincingly sized clinical trial, a large, multicenter trial could be designed to determine the effect of cryotherapy on ROP.

Multicenter Trial of Cryotherapy

The multicenter trial of CRYO-ROP is a randomized study carried out at 23 centers in the United States and sponsored by the National Eye Institute that enrolled infants with birth weights of less than 1251 g who were born between January 1, 1986, and November 30, 1987. The study consisted of two arms. The first group was a cohort of 291 infants in whom threshold ROP (defined as zone 1 or 2 ROP, stage 3-plus with five contiguous or eight cumulative sectors of fibrovascular proliferation) developed in one or both eyes. When a child was found to have threshold ROP in both eyes at the same examination, one eye was randomly assigned to undergo cryotherapy within 72 hours of diagnosis and the fellow eye served as a control. When a child was found to have threshold ROP in only one eye and the fellow eye had less severe ROP or no ROP, the eye at threshold was randomly assigned to receive cryotherapy or no cryotherapy. Cryotherapy was applied to the avascular retina anterior to the edge of the ridge and effort was made not to involve the area of the active ROP. These children constituted the "randomized" group and were divided in some reports of the study into "symmetric" and "asymmetric" groups, indicating whether threshold ROP was diagnosed in both eyes at the same examination (symmetric) or as the worse ROP observed in only one eye (asymmetric). The mean birth weight for the randomized cohort was 800 g ($\pm$165 SD), mean gestational age was 26.3 weeks ($\pm$1.8 SD), and 82% had symmetric threshold ROP. Threshold ROP had developed at a mean postconceptional age of 37.7 weeks ($\pm$2.8 SD), with a range of 31.9 to 50.4 weeks (Cryotherapy for Retinopathy of Prematurity Cooperative Group, 1985, 1990a).

A second group of infants consisted of 4099 children who had been enrolled in 1 of the 23 study centers and who had serial eye examinations initiated during the neonatal period from 4 to 6 weeks after birth. In most of these children, there was no evidence of ROP, moderate or prethreshold ROP (prethreshold ROP defined as zone 1, any stage ROP, zone 2 with plus disease less than threshold criteria or, zone 2 with stage 3), or less than prethreshold ROP. Of this "natural history" group, threshold ROP developed in 218 children who were enrolled in the randomized portion of the study. The mean birth weight for the natural history cohort was 954 g ($\pm$185 SD) and mean gestational age 27.9 weeks ($\pm$2.2 SD) (Palmer et al, 1991).

Thus far, study examinations have been performed at 3 months after randomization or after term due date, and at ages 1 year, 2 years, 3 1/2 years, 4 1/2 years, and 5 1/2 years and are planned at ages 7 years, 8 years, 9 years, and 10 years. After the 2-year study examination, follow-up for the natural history cohort was limited to 5 of the 23 study centers (Portland, Philadelphia, Minneapolis, Columbus, and upstate New York [Buffalo, Rochester, Syracuse]) and, after the 5 1/2 year examination, follow-up was further limited to approximately 100 children at the Philadelphia center in whom ROP did not develop during the neonatal period.

At the 3-month study examination, the study measure used to determine the effect of cryotherapy was an anatomic one and was based on stereo fundus photographs of the posterior pole (Watzke et al, 1990). An "unfavorable"

outcome was defined as a posterior retinal fold involving the macula, a retinal detachment involving zone 1, or retrolental tissue obscuring the posterior pole.

The 3-month outcome report from the CRYO-ROP randomized trial documented a 98% follow-up rate with 273 of the eligible 279 infants returning for the examination (12 had died). Based on assessment by masked observers at the CRYO-ROP reading center in Portland, fundus photographs of 222 treated eyes and 216 control eyes could be assigned to the favorable or unfavorable categories. There was a 39.5% reduction of unfavorable outcome in treated eyes compared with control eyes ($\chi^2 = 25.4$, $P < 0.00001$). Among treated eyes, 31.1% had an unfavorable outcome and 51% of control eyes had an unfavorable outcome (Cryotherapy for Retinopathy Cooperative Group, 1990a). When more severe ROP residua are considered, there was a 44.4% reduction in the occurrence of total retinal detachment or total retrolental and a 53.6% reduction in the occurrence of posterior retinal fold in treated eyes compared with control eyes. In addition to the fundus photographs, an eye examination was performed at 3 months after randomization and the results were consistent with the anatomic outcomes on the fundus photographs. When demographic and disease-related characteristics were examined in relation to the outcome of children in whom symmetric threshold ROP developed, there were more unfavorable outcomes in smaller birth-weight infants compared with larger birth-weight infants, in threshold ROP in zone 1 compared with zone 2, and with 11 to 12 sectors of stage 3 ROP compared with 5 to 7 sectors of stage 3 (Table 110–5). In each case, the treated eyes had a lower likelihood of development of an unfavorable outcome.

Of particular importance in determining the cost-benefit

TABLE 110–5

Demographic and Disease Characteristics of Infants with Symmetric Threshold Retinopathy of Prematurity: Photographic Outcome at 3-Month Examination

	Treated Eyes		Control Eyes	
	N	**% Unfavorable**	**N**	**% Unfavorable**
Birth Weight				
<750 g	86	37.2%	84	58.3%
750–1000 g	86	25.6%	90	51.1%
1001–1250 g	28	32.1%	24	41.7%
Zone of ROP				
Zone 1, both eyes	18	77.8%	17	94.1%
Zone 2, both eyes	176	26.1%	175	48.6%
Sectors of Stage 3 ROP				
5–7	26	19.2%	27	40.7%
8–10	51	27.5%	52	44.2%
11–12	53	39.6%	47	74.5%

Adapted from Cryotherapy for Retinopathy of Prematurity Cooperative Group: Multicenter Trial of Cryotherapy for Retinopathy of Prematurity: Three-month outcome. Arch Ophthalmol 108:195–204, 1990. Copyright 1990, American Medical Association.

ratio of surgical intervention for threshold ROP, the cryo-therapy procedure itself was relatively free of serious complications. The most common ocular complications were subconjunctival hematoma (11.7%) and conjunctival laceration (5.3%), and the most common systemic complications were bradycardia (9.4%) and acquired or increased cyanosis (1.1%). Thus, the CRYO-ROP Cooperative Group concluded that administration of cryotherapy to eyes with threshold ROP was beneficial and the group recommended treatment of at least one eye of patients with symmetric threshold ROP. A recommendation for treatment of the fellow eye was not made, pending further follow-up.

By the time that the 1-year study examinations began, the CRYO-ROP Cooperative Group had included a quantitative assessment of visual acuity as an additional outcome variable to assess the benefit of cryotherapy administered at threshold ROP. Quantitative assessment of visual acuity had recently become feasible in a clinical setting by measuring grating acuity using the Teller Acuity Card (TAC) procedure (Dobson et al, 1990; McDonald et al, 1985). The procedure involves presenting a series of rectangular gray cards that have a patch of evenly spaced black and white stripes (gratings) on one end and a matched gray background on the other. The tester looks through a central peephole to determine which way the child is looking. The tester presents smaller (finer) and smaller gratings until the patch of stripes looks no different to the child than the gray background. The last stripes that the tester determines that the child can "see" is the threshold acuity (Dobson et al, 1990).

Assessment of grating acuity was conducted by one of four testers (P. Bartholomew [Portland], J. Evans [Philadelphia], L. Treub [Columbus], and A. Hamill [upstate New York]) who traveled to the 23 study centers to perform visual acuity testing on each child. The testers were masked to the treatment status of eyes tested and were trained in performing TAC testing in a standard manner (Dobson et al, 1990).

At 1 year after randomization, masked grading of fundus photographs and masked assessments of grating visual acuity were undertaken as outcome measures. Again, there was a high follow-up rate (94.%) with 246 patients returning for a study examination and only 14 failing to return (31 had died by the 1-year examination). Results of the 1-year anatomic outcome showed an overall reduction of 45.8% for unfavorable outcomes in treated eyes compared with control eyes ($\chi^2 = 26.4$, $P < 0.0001$). Among treated eyes, 25.7% had an unfavorable outcome whereas 47.4% of control eyes had an unfavorable outcome. Results of the 1-year grating acuity assessments showed an overall reduction of 37.8% for unfavorable outcomes in treated eyes compared with control eyes ($\chi^2 = 22.1$, $P < 0.0001$). Among treated eyes, 35.0% had an unfavorable outcome and 56.3% of control eyes had an unfavorable outcome (Cryotherapy for Retinopathy of Prematurity Cooperative Group, 1990b). Thus, a quantitative measure of visual acuity confirmed the benefit of administering cryotherapy to eyes with threshold ROP that had been documented with the fundus photographs of posterior pole residua of ROP. The CRYO-ROP Cooperative Group recognized the limited follow-up up to that time and emphasized clinical judgment in the decision about whether to treat both eyes.

In addition, when both anatomic and functional measures were considered, at least 25% of the eyes had poor outcomes despite the best treatment available. Because of these data, the CRYO-ROP Cooperative Group strongly urged "continued research . . . into prevention of prematurity and the prophylaxis and treatment of ROP."

The latest report of follow-up for the children in the randomized group is from the 3½-year study examination (Cryotherapy for Retinopathy of Prematurity Control Group, 1993). At that study examination, there were three outcome measures: (1) physician's clinical assessment of ROP residua based on an eye examination undertaken by study ophthalmologist, (2) grating acuity using the TAC procedure, and (3) recognition acuity testing using a crowded HOTV test. The latter method of testing letter recognition was used because the gold standard of acuity measure, Snellen acuity, was not reasonable to expect of many of the 3½-year-old children in the CRYO-ROP study. Two hundred and thirty-six (92.2%) of the children returned for the follow-up examination (236/256, 35 had died before the examination). The results at the 3½-year examination showed reductions of 19% in unfavorable outcomes using letter recognition ($P < 0.01$), of 20% in unfavorable outcomes using the TAC procedure ($P < 0.001$), and of 43% in unfavorable outcomes when considering the anatomic structure of the eye ($P < 0.0001$) (Cryotherapy for Retinopathy of Prematurity Cooperative Group, 1993).

As for the 3-month and 1-year study examinations, it was apparent that retinal status remained stable with an approximate reduction in unfavorable anatomic outcomes of 40%. However, the reduction in unfavorable grating acuity outcomes from 37.8% at the 1-year study examination compared with the 20% reduction observed at the 3½-year examination was worrisome. A possible explanation is seen when the data are looked at not as simply favorable or unfavorable, but rather when the data are divided into four categories: normal, below normal (defined as within one octave of normal range for age), poor, and blind. The "poor" and "blind" categories comprise the unfavorable outcomes. As shown in Table 110–6, the grating acuity results at 1 year had been essentially bimodal, with most of the eyes being in the normal category or the blind category. In contrast, the grating acuity data results at age 3½ years were more evenly distributed, with some of the eyes that had acuity in the normal range at age 1 year showing acuity in the below normal and poor range at age 3½ years. The reason for this apparent decreased benefit in older children who had cryotherapy for threshold ROP as infants is probably related to the fact that grating acuity improves with age. It is likely that acuity is not sufficiently developed in a 1-year-old child to detect the differences that were observed when the children were older and acuity was better developed (Cryotherapy for Retinopathy of Prematurity Cooperative Group, 1993). Despite the apparent lessened functional benefit at 3½ years, the benefit is still significant, with 50.8% (98/193) of eyes that underwent cryotherapy having an unfavorable outcome compared with 64.6% (124/192) for eyes that did not undergo cryotherapy ($P < 0.001$).

The first results of letter recognition acuity testing in children from the CRYO-ROP study support this interpretation of the grating acuity results. Recognition acuity re-

TABLE 110–6

Grating Acuity Results at 1-Year and 3½-Year Study Examinations*

		1 Year		3½ Year	
		Treated	Control	Treated	Control
Favorable	Normal	51 (31.9%)	80 (50.6%)	38 (20.3%)	35 (18.5%)
	Below normal	5 (3.1%)	9 (5.7%)	51 (27.3%)	30 (15.9%)
Unfavorable	Poor	8 (5%)	4 (2.5%)	41 (21.9%)	27 (14.3%)
	Blind	96 (60.0%)	65 (41.1%)	57 (30.5%)	97 (51.3%)
Total number of eyes that could be tested		160	158	187	189

*Grating acuity was tested in 178 children at the 1-year study examination and in 212 children at the 3½-year examination. At the 1-year examination, 1 treated and 4 control eyes were untestable. At the 3½-year examination, 6 treated and 3 control eyes could not be measured.

Data from Cryotherapy for Retinopathy of Prematurity Cooperative group (1990b, 1993).

sults using a crowded HOTV test could be obtained in approximately 3 of 4 of the children at the 3½-year study examination. This acuity task is more complex than performing grating acuity testing because it requires more cooperation and cognitive ability on this child's part. Nevertheless, a similar broad distribution of acuity results was also obtained. When these subcategories are combined into favorable (normal and below normal) and unfavorable (poor and blind) categories, there was a 19.0% reduction in unfavorable outcomes in treated eyes compared with control eyes ($P < 0.01$) (Cryotherapy for Retinopathy of Prematurity Cooperative Group, 1993).

The randomized subjects in the CRYO-ROP trial are participating in an extended follow-up with a final examination planned at age 10 years. Acuity testing using the ETDRS-Snellen chart, assessment of visual field extent measured using a double-arc perimeter, and color vision were measured as part of the 5½-year study examination; reports published in 1996 showed similar results (Cryotherapy for Retinopathy of Prematurity Cooperative Group, 1996). Other interim reports from the study may result from the findings at yearly examinations until age 10 years when Snellen acuity will again be tested, visual fields will be assessed using a kinetic perimetry technique in the Goldmann perimeter, and there will be further assessment of the long-term effect of cryotherapy on ROP residua and ocular status.

Laser Photocoagulation for Retinopathy of Prematurity

Over the past few years, laser photocoagulation for ROP has become feasible with the advent of a laser instrument mounted on an indirect ophthalmoscope, allowing easier administration of laser photocoagulation than was possible previously with floor-mounted instruments. The use of this modality in the treatment of threshold ROP continues to

be promising and outcomes after laser photocoagulation are similar to those obtained using cryotherapy at threshold ROP (Iverson et al, 1991; Landers et al, 1992; McNamara et al, 1992). The procedure appears to be less traumatic for the systemic and ocular condition of the infant. In addition, because the laser is applied directly to the retina and retina pigment epithelium and not transclerally as in cryotherapy, no conjunctival incision is needed (Brown et al, 1990; McNamara, 1993). It is unlikely that a single large trial comparing the results of cryotherapy and laser photocoagulation directly will be undertaken because the number of eyes needed to prove equality of outcomes is much larger than the CRYO-ROP study itself. However, the Laser ROP Study Group (1994) was formed to address this issue. As shown in Table 110–7, the group reported a meta-analysis on the results of four trials in which, at the diagnosis of threshold as defined in the CRYO-ROP study, one eye received cryotherapy and the fellow eye underwent laser photocoagulation (argon or diode). Two hundred and ninety-three eyes were reported from four studies (three randomized studies with 161 eyes and one nonrandomized study with 132 eyes). An odds ratio was calculated for each trial based on the proportion of unfavorable to favorable outcomes for laser and cryotherapy to determine equality of treatment (an odds ratio of 1 means equality in outcomes of laser and cryotherapy and an odds ratio of less than 1 means laser had greater success). For all four studies, the odds ratio was less than 1 (see Table 110–7). A combined estimate of the odds ratio for all trials is 0.44 (95% confidence intervals of 0.22 to 0.89), suggesting that laser is as effective as cryotherapy.

Laser photocoagulation may be of particular use in eyes with zone 1 ROP, because such eyes are difficult to treat with cryotherapy and the outcome of such eyes is still likely to be dismal despite timely administration of cryotherapy (see Table 110–5). Three of four eyes that received cryotherapy in the CRYO-ROP study had unfavorable structural outcomes at the 1-year study examination compared with more than 9 of 10 eyes that were not randomized to receive cryotherapy. In the intensive care nursery of the 1990s, it appears that laser photocoagulation for threshold ROP in zone 1 has a much better outcome than the historical control or treated eyes in the CRYO-ROP study that admitted infants from January 1986 to November 1987. Capone and colleagues (1993) reported favorable structural outcomes in 25 of 30 eyes (83%) with threshold ROP with at least one sector of zone 1 involvement. However, these results are not directly comparable with zone 1 eyes from the CRYO-ROP study because zone 1 threshold ROP in the CRYO-ROP trial was defined as having all ROP within zone 1. Still, such promising work is being explored in a randomized study (J. Vander, W. Tasman, personal communication).

Vitamin E

ROP is a consequence of oxidant radical injury to the developing retina and its vasculature. Because neither cryotherapy or laser photocoagulation are panaceas resulting in the eradication of poor vision from ROP, efforts need to be directed to the prevention of ROP or the prevention of the serious forms of ROP. The medical treatment of ROP,

TABLE 110–7

Comparison of Results of Treatment with Cryotherapy Versus Laser Photocoagulation in 293 Eyes

Clinical Trial	Cryotherapy		Laser Photocoagulation		Odds Ratio
	Favorable N (%)	Unfavorable N (%)	Favorable N (%)	Unfavorable N (%)	
McNamara et al (1991)	43 (81.1)	10 (18.9)	54 (85.7)	9 (14.3)	0.72
Iverson et al (1991)	5 (83.3)	1 (16.7)	6 (100)	0 (0)	0.28
Hunter and Repka (1992)	14 (93.3)	1 (6.7)	17 (94.4)	1 (5.6)	0.83
Unpublished data	50 (76.9)	15 (23.1)	64 (95.5)	3 (4.5)	0.18

From Laser ROP Study Group: Laser therapy for retinopathy of prematurity. Arch Ophthalmol 112:154–156, 1994. Copyright 1994, American Medical Association.

in addition to improvement of medical care, has largely centered on the use of antioxidants, in particular the naturally occurring antioxidant vitamin E. This fat-soluble compound is a potent free radical scavenger, and it has been used in trials of both prophylaxis of ROP and treatment of established disease.

The first trial of the efficacy of vitamin E in the prevention of blinding ROP was in 1949, and vitamin E prophylaxis in a small number of infants showed a beneficial effect (Owens and Owens, 1949). These data were not followed up until the early 1970s because of the clinical trials that showed a close correlation between oxygen administration and ROP and further problems with ROP were not expected after oxygen restriction (Patz, 1975). However, with the advent of neonatal intensive care units and increasingly specialized and sophisticated care, smaller, sicker infants survived in whom ROP developed. In the late 1970s and early 1980s, several clinical trials were undertaken to determine the effect of vitamin E on ROP. Comparison of the results of these trials is complicated because they predate the widespread use of a standard classification for ROP, they used somewhat different treatment regimens, and different forms of vitamin E were used. However, it is possible to identify eyes that would currently be graded as having stage 3-plus ROP using the ICROP standard. Table 110–8 compares the results of the trials of vitamin E prophylaxis in infants with birth weights of less than or equal to 1500 g, as summarized by Johnson and colleagues (1988). Using the end point of stage 3-plus ROP, it does appear that vitamin E prophylaxis significantly decreases the severity of ROP ($P < 0.02$). From these trials, it was also clear that there is a price to be paid for early administration of vitamin E, such as an increased incidence of necrotizing enterocolitis and sepsis in infants with birth weights of less than 1001 g (Johnson et al, 1985), thus increasing the risk-benefit ratio of ROP prophylaxis with vitamin E at pharmacologic serum levels.

However, because blindness from ROP still occurs despite the proven benefit of cryotherapy, Johnson and coworkers (1993) have continued to study the potential benefit of vitamin E in the prevention and treatment of ROP. On the basis of these data and on further studies, we

adopted a protocol in 1981 that included (1) maintenance of physiologic serum vitamin E levels from birth on (i.e., 1–2.3 mg/dL) and (2) pharmacologic vitamin E treatment, using a research protocol with informed parental consent, with target serum levels of 4 to 5 mg/dL in those children with threshold ROP. This protocol included cryotherapy or laser photocoagulation, when indicated by the retinal consultation, within 72 hours of the diagnosis of threshold ROP. From 1985 to 1991 at Pennsylvania Hospital, all 17 infants with threshold ROP received pharmacologic vitamin E treatment, in addition to cryotherapy in one (n = 10 patients) or both (n = 7 patients) eyes. When results of this small case series are compared with the results of the much larger CRYO-ROP study, the results suggest a benefit to using this protocol (Johnson et al, 1995).

Retinal Detachment Procedures

Over the past 15 years, the success rate for procedures that reattach total or partial retinal detachments caused by ROP has increased (Charles, 1986; Greven and Tasman, 1990; Hirose et al, 1981, 1993; Machemer, 1983; Tasman et al, 1987; Trese, 1984). The reason for using these procedures is that reattaching the retina may restore or preserve some degree of vision in eyes that are likely to be blind otherwise. For partial detachments, the procedure may include only a scleral buckling in which an external band is applied to the surface of the sclera to indent the sclera under the detached area and allow the detachment to settle down onto the retinal pigment epithelium. For complete retinal detachments, the surgical techniques include open sky or closed vitrectomy with removal of the lens and vitreous, releasing retinal traction and allowing the retina to settle down. Cryotherapy or scleral buckling procedures may also be added in some cases.

The level of vision that has been measured in eyes after vitrectomy procedures for total retinal detachment has been low and may be little different from the natural course of the disease. The largest report is based on acuity results of 129 eyes of 98 patients from the CRYO-ROP study (Quinn et al, 1991). Visual acuity was assessed at the 1-year study examination using the TAC procedure by one

TABLE 110-8

Comparison of Results of Vitamin E Prophylaxis of Retinopathy of Prematurity in Infants with Birth Weights of 1500 g or Less*

Clinical Trial	Placebo		Vitamin		95% Confidence Limits
	Total	No. with Stage 3+ ROP or Worse	Total	No. with Stage 3+ ROP or Worse	
Hittner et al, (1981)	51	5	50	0	−18.0 to −1.6
Finer et al, (1982)	114	5	111	3	−6.6 to +3.2
Puklin et al, (1982)	20	1	22	0	−14.6 to +4.6
Milner et al, (1981)	51	4	48	2	−12.9 to +5.6
Phelps et al, (1987)	99	5	97	5	−6.1 to +6.3
Johnson et al, (1989)	216	9	208	3	−5.9 to +0.3

*$\chi^2 = 5.78$ by Mantel-Haenszel technique for combining independent studies, $P < 0.02$.
From Johnson L, Abbasi S, Quinn GE, et al: Vitamin E and retinopathy of prematurity [Letter to the Editor]. Pediatrics 81:329–331, 1988. Reproduced with permission of PEDIATRICS.

of four testers who tested all children in the CRYO-ROP study. The testers were masked to status of the child's eyes. Two eyes of one infant had minimal pattern vision at the lowest level measurable using TAC procedure. In addition, none of the other eyes that had undergone vitrectomy and none of the eyes that did not undergo a procedure for total retinal detachment had evidence of pattern vision. The strengths of this report are that acuity was measured using a quantitative technique by masked observers who tested within a specified age range. However, the CRYO-ROP study was not designed to determine the effect on visual function of vitrectomy procedures performed for total retinal detachment. Instead, the decision about whether and when to perform the vitrectomy procedure was left to the individual physician caring for the child at one of the 23 centers that participated in the CRYO-ROP study. The study was also not designed to assess visual ability below pattern vision that might be useful in ambulation and spacial orientation.

Based on the dismal visual acuity results after vitrectomy procedures for total retinal detachment, it appears that efforts need to be concentrated on preventing retinal detachment and decreasing the number of eyes of children that reach the stage of total retinal detachment.

PROGNOSIS AND FOLLOW-UP REQUIREMENTS

ROP is not just an event that happens during the neonatal period and disappears without sequelae. It may lead to lifelong disabilities. Several recent reports have provided data that allow prediction during the neonatal period of the long-term morbidity for the individual child.

Schaffer and colleagues (1993) on behalf of the CRYO-ROP Cooperative Group reported on a series of ocular factors noted at the time of the ROP screening examinations in the nursery that allowed prediction of reaching threshold ROP or developing an unfavorable outcome. In this report, the data including ROP status and extent of vascularization were categorized according to the postconceptional age at the time of eye examination. As shown in Table 110–9, eyes with no ROP in which vascularization had only progressed into zone 1 before 35 weeks' gestation

were at high (about 1 in 3) risk for development of threshold ROP. Eyes in which vascularization had progressed into zone 2 were much less likely to go on to threshold ROP. Similarly, eyes that show evidence of plus disease in the earlier examination periods were much more likely to progress to threshold than eyes without plus disease. As expected, threshold ROP was more likely to develop in eyes of children with lower birth weights and shorter gestation as it was in eyes of children who were white, of multiple births, and born outside a study center nursery. The risk of development of an unfavorable structural outcome, as defined by the CRYO-ROP study, was increased with ROP occurring in zone 1, plus disease, severity of ROP, and extent of circumferential involvement. In addition, a faster rate of progression to both prethreshold and threshold ROP was found to be associated with unfavorable anatomic outcomes. These data give the ophthalmologist information to share with the family at the time of the examination about the likelihood of sight-threatening ROP developing.

The CRYO-ROP study has also provided data about the likelihood of abnormal visual function with various stages of ROP. In the 1994 report of the natural history subjects at age 1 year, eyes with ROP in zone 1 were more likely to have abnormal fixation (44%, 22/50) than eyes with ROP in zone 2 (8.2%, 183/2245) or zone 3 (3.3%, 18/546). Not all abnormal fixation in this population results from ROP residua, but the association is clear. Even when only zone 2 ROP is considered, there is a clear gradient for increasing severity of ROP and a higher likelihood of having abnormal fixation at 1 year.

Eyes in which ROP develops during the postnatal period are also at risk for numerous other ocular abnormalities, including myopia (Cats and Tan, 1989; Gallo et al, 1991; Gordon and Donzis, 1986; Nissenkorn et al, 1983; Page et al, 1993; Quinn et al, 1992; Snir et al, 1988), astigmatism (Kushner, 1982; Snir et al, 1988), anisometropia (Gallo et al, 1991; Reynolds, 1990; Schaffer et al, 1984; Snir et al, 1988), and strabismus (Gallo et al, 1991; Kushner, 1982; Page et al, 1993; Robinson and O'Keefe, 1993; Snir et al, 1988). The prevalence and degree of myopia appears to increase with the severity of acute phase retinopathy (Laws et al, 1992; Quinn et al, 1992). Quinn and coworkers

TABLE 110–9

Percentage of Eyes that Ultimately Reached Threshold ROP for Each Zone and Stage of ROP

		Postconceptional Age at Examination: Percent that Reach Threshold (No. Eye Examinations)				
		≤32 wks	33–34 wks	35–36 wks	37–38 wks	39–40 wks
Zone 2	Incomplete vessels	9.3% (1991)	5.5% (2166)	2.8% (1161)	1.4% (588)	2.4% (206)
	Stage 1°	7.5% (358)	6.5% (1138)	4.5% (1186)	1.5% (742)	1.4% (365)
	Stage 2°	3.9% (129)	5.5% (494)	4.4% (816)	2.3% (786)	1.2% (481)
	Stage 3°	NC (9)	15.7% (83)	13.2% (205)	8.5% (283)	2.2% (267)
	Stage 1 +	NC (2)	83.3% (12)	41.7% (12)	NC (6)	NC (4)
	Stage 2 +	NC (2)	44.0% (25)	33.9% (59)	25.0% (24)	16.7% (36)
	Stage 3 +	NC (2)	76.7% (30)	60.7% (61)	34.5% (87)	31.4% (51)
Zone 1	Incomplete vessels	32.8% (122)	37.0% (46)	6.7% (15)	35.7% (14)	NC (0)
	Stage 1	18.2% (11)	33.3% (27)	NC (8)	NC (3)	NC (0)
	All other ROP	NC (4)	NC (7)	NC (18)	NC (7)	NC (5)

°No eyes with plus disease included in these categories.
NC, number too small to calculate meaningful value.
Adapted from Schaffer DB, Palmer EA, Plotsky DF, et al: Prognostic factors in the natural course of retinopathy of prematurity. Ophthalmology 100:230–237, 1993; Courtesy of Ophthalmology.

(1992), reporting on behalf of the CRYO-ROP Cooperative Group, noted that 69.1% of eyes with stage 3-plus ROP in zone 2 or any ROP in zone 1 were myopic at the 1-year examination, compared with only 18.3% of eyes with mild ROP (stage 1 or 2 in zone 2 or any ROP in zone 3). High myopia of more than 5 diopters developed in 34.5% of eyes with severe ROP, compared with only 1.6% for eyes with mild ROP. In addition, eyes with ROP residua in the posterior pole were much more likely to have high myopia (Quinn et al, 1992). Astigmatism and anisometropia are also more common with more severe acute phase ROP, as was the presence of strabismus at 6 months (Laws et al, 1992) and at age 1 year (Cryotherapy for Retinopathy of Prematurity Cooperative Group, 1994).

PREVENTION AND NEW APPROACHES

It does not appear that ROP can be prevented in the neonatal intensive care nursery. Therefore, attention must be directed toward (1) detecting and treating ROP that is likely to lead to visual handicap, (2) developing strategies that make already established disease less severe or prevent its progression, and (3) decreasing the physiologic instabilities that increase susceptibility to ROP.

The CRYO-ROP study has provided data that indicate the postconceptional ages when ROP is most likely to develop in children with birth weights of less than 1251 g and therefore when ROP screening examinations are most likely to detect sight-threatening ROP. For these low-birth-weight infants, it appears that first screening examinations should take place around 31 to 32 weeks' postconceptional age and should continue on an every other week basis until prethreshold ROP develops, less severe ROP begins to regress, or vascularization has proceded well into zone 3. When prethreshold ROP develops, more frequent examinations are indicated (Palmer et al, 1991; Schaffer et al, 1993). Such a screening schedule is likely to detect threshold ROP at a time when it is still treatable.

Medical or surgical treatment may provide a sensible route to prevent progression of already established ROP. Besides examining the administration of vitamin E as discussed previously in this chapter, an attempt is underway to examine the effect of increased oxygen administration for children with already established prethreshold ROP to determine whether the progression to threshold severity can be halted. The rationale for the Supplemental Treatment with Oxygen of Prethreshold ROP (STOP-ROP) trial is that the florid vasoproliferation seen in severe acute phase ROP is, at least in part, caused by relative hypoxia, and supplemental oxygen may decrease new vessel formation (Szewczyk, 1953; Phelps, in press). Furthermore, from use in human subjects but based on the same rationale, is the use of an antivasoproliferative substance to decrease abnormal new vessel formation in severe acute phase ROP. It appears that molecules such as vascular endothelial growth factor (VEGF) are potent angiogenic factors whose production is increased by hyperoxia and may be involved with retinal neovascularization in humans. Drugs that prevent the formation or action of VEGF might prevent the active vasoproliferation of severe acute ROP (Aiello et al, 1994; D'Amore, 1994; Pierce et al, 1995).

In addition to decreasing insults to the developing retina by decreasing episodes of sepsis, hypoxia, hyperoxia, and other illness-related factors in the premature baby, a series of studies have been undertaken to determine whether reducing oxidant radical formation caused by light will decrease the incidence of ROP. Feasibility studies are underway, using patches over the infants' eyes until 31 weeks' postconceptional age, to determine whether a multicentered trial can be done to answer this question (James Reynolds and Rand Spencer, personal communication).

In conclusion, the data summarized in this chapter indicate that ROP, although it may be diagnosed during the neonatal period, is associated with considerable risk of ocular morbidity. Strabismus, myopia, astigmatism, and anisometropia are likely to develop in infants with ROP, and the children must be followed up for years to prevent the development of irreversible visual function abnormalities.

REFERENCES

Aiello LP, Avery RL, Arrigg PG, et al: Vascular endothelial growth factor in ocular fluid of patients with diabetic retinopathy and other retinal disorders. N Engl J Med 331:1480–1487, 1994.

Ben-Sira I, Nissenkorn I, Grunwald E, Yassur Y: Treatment of acute phase retinopathy of prematurity. Br J Ophthalmol 64:758–762, 1980.

Birch EE, Spencer R: Visual outcome in infants with cicatricial retinopathy of prematurity. Invest Ophthalmol Vis Sci 32:410–415, 1991.

Brown GC, Tasman WS, Naidoff M, et al: Systemic complications associated with retinal cryoablation for retinopathy of prematurity. Ophthalmology 97(7):855–858, 1990.

Capone A, Diaz-Rohena R, Sternberg P, et al: Diode-laser photocoagulation for zone 1 threshold retinopathy of prematurity. Am J Ophthalmol 116:444–450, 1993.

Cats BP, Tan KEWP: Prematures with and without regressed retinopathy of prematurity: Comparison of long-term (6–10 years) ophthalmological morbidity. J Pediatr Ophthalmol Strabismus 26:271–275, 1989.

Charles S: Vitrectomy with ciliary body entry for retrolental fibroplasia. In McPherson AR, Hittner HM, Kretzer FL (Eds): Retinopathy of Prematurity. Philadelphia, Decker, 1986, pp 225–243.

Multicenter Trial of Cryotherapy for Retinopathy of Prematurity Cooperative Group: Manual of Procedures. Springfield, VA, National Technical Information Service, US Department of Commerce, PB 88–163530, 1985.

Cryotherapy for Retinopathy of Prematurity Cooperative Group: Multicenter Trial of Cryotherapy for Retinopathy of Prematurity: Three-month outcome. Arch Ophthalmol 108:195–204, 1990a.

Cryotherapy for Retinopathy of Prematurity Cooperative Group: Multicenter Trial of Cryotherapy for Retinopathy of Prematurity: One year outcome—Structure and Function. Arch Ophthalmol 108:1408–1416, 1990b.

Cryotherapy for Retinopathy of Prematurity Cooperative Group: Multicenter Trial of Cryotherapy for Retinopathy of Prematurity: 3½-year outcome—Structure and function. Arch Ophthalmol 111:339–344, 1993.

Cryotherapy for Retinopathy of Prematurity Cooperative Group: The natural ocular outcome of premature birth and retinopathy: Status at 1 year. Arch Ophthalmol 112:903–912, 1994.

Cryotherapy for Retinopathy of Prematurity Cooperative Group: Multicenter Trial of Cryotherapy: Snellen visual acuity and structural outcome at 5½ years after randomization. Arch Ophthalmol 114:417–424, 1996.

D'Amore P: Mechanisms of retinal and choroidal neovascularization. Invest Ophthalmol Vis Sci 35:3974–3979, 1994.

Dobson V, Quinn G, Biglan A, et al: Acuity card assessment of visual function in the Cryotherapy for Retinopathy of Prematurity trial. Invest Ophthalmol 31:1702–1708, 1990.

Dobson V, Quinn GE, Flynn JT, et al: Multicenter trial of cryotherapy for retinopathy of prematurity—3-1/2 year outcome: Structure and function. Arch Ophthalmol 111:339–344, 1993.

Dobson V, Quinn GE, Summers CG, et al: Effect of acute-phase retinopathy of prematurity on grating acuity development in the very-low-birth-weight infant. Invest Ophthalmol Vis Sci 35:4236–4244, 1994.

Dobson V, Quinn GE, Tung B, et al: Comparison of monocular recognition and resolution acuities in eyes with and without residua of retinopathy of prematurity. Invest Ophthalmol Vis Sci 36:692–702, 1995.

Fielder AR, Ng YK, Levene MI: Retinopathy of prematurity: Age at onset. Arch Dis Child 61:774–778, 1986.

Fielder AR: Cryotherapy of retinopathy of prematurity. In Davidson SI, Jay B (Eds): Recent Advances in Ophthalmology, No. 8. Edinburgh, Churchill Livingston, 1992, pp 129–148.

Finer NN, Schindler RF, Grant G, et al: Effect of intramuscular vitamin E on frequency and severity of retrolental fibroplasia: A controlled clinical trial. Lancet 1:1087–1091, 1982.

Gallo JE, Holmstrom G, Kugelberg U, et al: Regressed retinopathy of prematurity and its sequelae in children age 5–10 years. Br J Ophthalmol 75:527–531, 1991.

Gibson DL, Sheps SB, Schecter MT, et al: Retinopathy of prematurity: A new epidemic? Pediatrics 83:486–492, 1989.

Gibson DL, Sheps SG, Uh SH, et al: Retinopathy of prematurity-induced blindness: Birth weight–specific survival and the new epidemic. Pediatrics 86:405–412, 1990.

Gilbert W, Dobson V, Quinn G, et al: The correlation of visual function with posterior retinal structure in severe retinopathy of prematurity. Arch Ophthalmol 110:625–631, 1992.

Gordon RA, Donzis PB: Myopia associated with retinopathy of prematurity. Ophthalmol 93:1593–1598, 1986.

Greven C, Tasman W: Scleral buckling in stages 4B and 5 retinopathy of prematurity. Ophthalmology 97:817–820, 1990.

Hirose T, Schepens CL, Lopansri C: Subtotal open-sky vitrectomy for severe retinal detachment as a late complication of ocular trauma. Ophthalmology 88:1–9, 1981.

Hirose T, Katsumi O, Mehta MC, Schepens CL: Vision in stage 5 retinopathy of prematurity after retinal reattachment by open-sky vitrectomy. Arch Ophthalmol 111:345–349, 1993.

Hittner HM, Godio, Rudolph AJ, et al: Retrolental fibroplasia: Efficacy of vitamin E in a double-blind clinical study of preterm infants. N Engl J Med 305:1365–1371, 1981.

Hunter DG, Repka MX: Diode laser photocoagulation for threshold retinopathy of prematurity: A randomized study. Ophthalmology 100:238–244, 1992.

International Committee for the Classification of Retinopathy of Prematurity: Multicenter Trial of Cryotherapy: An international classification of retinopathy of prematurity. Arch Ophthalmol 102:1130–1134, 1984.

International Committee for the Classification of Retinopathy of Prematurity: An international classification of retinopathy of prematurity. II. The classification of retinal detachment. Arch Ophthalmol 105:906–912, 1987.

Iverson DA, Trese MT, Orgel IK, Williams GA: Laser photocoagulation for threshold retinopathy of prematurity. Arch Ophthalmol 109:1342–1343, 1991.

Johnson L, Abbasi S, Quinn GE, et al: Vitamin E and retinopathy of prematurity. Letter to the Editor. Pediatrics 81:329–331, 1988.

Johnson L, Quinn G, Abbasi S, et al: Effect of sustained pharmacologic vitamin E levels on incidence and severity of retinopathy of prematurity: A controlled clinical trial. J Pediatr 114:827–838, 1989.

Johnson LH, Quinn GE, Abbasi S, Bowen FW: Retinopathy of prematurity: Prevalence and treatment over a 20 year period at Pennsylvania Hospital. Doc Ophthalmol 74:213–222, 1990.

Johnson LH, Quinn GE, Abbasi S: Vitamin E and ROP—The continuous challenge. In Klaus MH, Fanaroff AA (Eds): The Yearbook of Neonatal and Perinatal Medicine. St Louis, CV Mosby, 1993, pp xv–xxiv.

Johnson L, Quinn GE, Abbasi S, et al: Severe retinopathy of prematurity in ≤1250g birth weight infants: Incidence and outcome of treatment using pharmacologic serum levels of vitamin E in addition to cryotherapy. 1985–1991. J Pediatr 127:632–639, 1995.

Keith CG, Doyle LW: Retinopathy of prematurity in extremely low birth weight infants. Pediatr 95:42–45, 1995.

Kushner BJ: Strabismus and amblyopia associated with regressed retinopathy of prematurity. Arch Ophthalmol 100:256–261, 1982.

Landers MB III, Toth CA, Semple HC, Morsse LS: Treatment of retinopathy of prematurity with argon laser photocoagulation. Arch Ophthalmol 110:429–431, 1992.

Laser ROP Study Group: Laser therapy for retinopathy of prematurity. Letter to the Editor. Arch Ophthalmol 112:154–156, 1994.

Law FW: The history and traditions of Moorfields Eye Hospital, Vol II. London, HK Lewis, 1975, p 203.

Laws D, Shaw DE, Robinson J, et al: Retinopathy of prematurity: A prospective study. Review at six months. Eye 6:477–483, 1992.

Machemer R: Closed vitrectomy for severe retrolental fibroplasia in the infant. Ophthalmology 90:436–441, 1983.

McCormick A: The retinopathy of prematurity in the newborn. Curr Probl Pediatr 7:1, 1977.

McDonald M, Dobson V, Sebris SL, et al: The acuity card procedure: A rapid test of infant acuity. Invest Ophthalmol Vis Sci 26:1158–1162, 1985.

McNamara JA, Tasman W, Brown GC, Federman JL: Laser photocoagulation for stage 3+ retinopathy of prematurity. Ophthalmology 98:576–580, 1991.

McNamara JA, Tasman W, Vander JF, Brown GC: Diode laser photocoagulation for retinopathy of prematurity: Preliminary results. Arch Ophthalmol 110:1714–1716, 1992.

McNamara JA: Laser treatment for retinopathy of prematurity. Curr Opin Ophthalmol 4:76–80, 1993.

Milner RA, Watts JL, Paes B, Zipursky A: RLF in 1500 gram neonates: Part of a randomized clinical trial of the effectiveness of vitamin E. *In* Retinopathy of Prematurity Conferences Syllabus, Vol 2. Washington, DC, Dec 4–6, 1981, pp 703–716.

Mintz-Hittner HA, Prager TC, Kretzer FL: Visual acuity correlates with severity of retinopathy of prematurity in untreated infants weighing 750 g or less at birth. Arch Ophthalmol 110:1087–1091, 1992.

Nagata M: Treatment of acute proliferative retrolental fibroplasia with xenon-arc photocoagulation. Jpn J Ophthalmol 21:436–459, 1977.

Nissenkorn I, Yassur Y, Mashowski D, et al: Myopia in premature infants with and without retinopathy of prematurity. Br J Ophthalmol 67:170–173, 1983.

Owens WC, Owens EU: Retrolental fibroplasia in premature infants. II. Studies on the prophylaxis of the disease: The use of alpha-tocopheryl acetate. Am J Ophthalmol 32:1631–1637, 1949.

Page JM, Schneeweiss S, Whyte HEA, Harvey P: Ocular sequelae in premature infants. Pediatrics 92:787–780, 1993.

Palmer EA: Module 12: Retinopathy of prematurity. Focal Points 1984: Clinical modules for ophthalmologists, San Francisco, 1984, American Academy of Ophthalmology.

Palmer EA, Flynn JT, Hardy RJ, et al: Incidence and early course of retinopathy of prematurity. Ophthalmology 98:1628–1640, 1991.

Patz A: Retrolental fibroplasia. Surv Ophthalmol 14:1–15, 1972.

Patz A: The role of oxygen in retrolental fibroplasia. Graefes Arch Klin Exp Ophthalmol 102:77–85, 1975.

Phelps DL, Rosenbaum AL, Isenberg SJ, et al: Tocopherol efficacy and safety for preventing retinopathy of prematurity: A randomized, controlled, double-masked trial. Pediatrics 79:489–500, 1987.

Phelps DL, Palmer EA, Wood NE on behalf of the Executive Committee, STOP-Trial: Supplemental therapeutic oxygen for prethreshold ROP. *In* Shapiro M, Miller M (Eds): Retinopathy of Prematurity. New York, Kugler, in press.

Pierce EA, Avery RL, Foley ED, et al: Vascular endothelial growth factor/vascular permeability factor expression in a mouse model of retinal neovascularization. Proc Natl Acad Sci USA 92:905–909, 1995.

Preslan MW, Butler J: Regression pattern in retinopathy of prematurity. J Pediatr Ophthalmol Strabismus 31:172–176, 1994.

Puklin JE, Simon RM, Ehrenkranz RA: Influence on retrolental fibroplasia on intramuscular vitamin E administration during respiratory distress syndrome. Ophthalmology 89:96–102, 1982.

Quinn GE, Schaffer DB, Johnson L: A revised classification of retinopathy of prematurity. Am J Ophthalmol 94:744–749, 1982.

Quinn GE, Johnson L, Otis C, et al: Incidence, severity and time course of ROP in a randomized clinical trial of vitamin E prophylaxis. Doc Ophthalmologica 74:223–228, 1990.

Quinn G, Dobson V, Barr C, et al: Visual acuity in infants after vitrectomy for severe retinopathy of prematurity (ROP). Ophthalmol 98:5–13, 1991.

Quinn GE, Johnson L, Abbasi S: Onset of retinopathy of prematurity as related to postnatal and postconceptional age. Br J Ophthalmol 76:284–288, 1992.

Quinn GE, Dobson V, Repka MX, et al: Development of myopia in infants with birth weights less than 1251g. Ophthalmology 99:329–340, 1992.

Reese AB, King MJ, Owens WC: A classification of retrolental fibroplasia. Am J Ophthalmol 36:133–135, 1953.

Reynolds JD: Anisometropic amblyopia in severe posterior retinopathy of prematurity. Binoc Vis Q 5:153–158, 1990.

Reynolds J, Dobson V, Quinn GE, et al: Prediction of visual function in eyes with mild to moderate posterior pole residua of ROP. Arch Ophthalmol 111:1050–1056, 1993.

Robinson R, O'Keefe M: Follow-up on premature infants with and without retinopathy of prematurity. Br J Ophthalmol 77:91–94, 1993.

Schaffer DB, Quinn GE, Johnson L: Sequelae of arrested mild retinopathy of prematurity. Arch Ophthalmol 102:373–376, 1984.

Schaffer DB, Johnson L, Quinn GE, Boggs TR: A classification of retrolental fibroplasia to evaluate vitamin E therapy. Ophthalmology 86:1749–1760, 1979.

Schaffer DB, Palmer EA, Plotsky DF, et al: Prognostic factors in the natural course of retinopathy of prematurity. Ophthalmology 100:230–237, 1993.

Snir M, Nissenkorn I, Sherf I, et al: Visual acuity, strabismus and amblyopia in premature babies with and without retinopathy of prematurity. Ann Ophthalmol 20:256–258, 1988.

Szewczyk TS: Retrolental fibroplasia and related ocular diseases classification, etiology, and prophylaxis. Am J Ophthalmol 36:1333–1361, 1953.

Tagaki I: Treatment of acute retrolental fibroplasia. Ophthalmol Jpn 82:323–330, 1978.

Tasman W: Late complications of retrolental fibroplasia. Trans Am Acad Ophthalmol Otolaryngol 86:1724–1740, 1979.

Tasman W: Management of retinopathy of prematurity. Ophthalmology 92:995–999, 1985.

Tasman W, Brown GC, Schaffer DB, et al: Cryotherapy for active retinopathy of prematurity. Ophthalmol 93:580–583, 1986.

Tasman W, Borrone RN, Bolling J: Open sky vitrectomy for total retinal detachment in retinopathy of prematurity. Ophthalmology 94:449–452, 1987.

Terry TL: Extreme prematurity and fibroplastic overgrowth of the persistent vascular sheath behind the crystalling lens. Am J Ophthalmol 25:203–204, 1942.

Trese MT: Surgical results of stage V retrolental fibroplasia and time of repair. Ophthalmology 91:461–466, 1984.

Watzke RC, Robertson JE, Palmer EA, et al: Photographic grading in the retinopathy of prematurity trial. Arch Ophthalmol 108:950–955, 1990.

APPENDIX 1

DRUGS

Robert Levin

Pharmacopeia for the Newborn Period

ABBREVIATIONS:

ET—endotracheal	**PR**—by rectum
IM—intramuscularly	**SC**—subcutaneously
IT—intrathecally or intratracheally	**TOP**—topical
IV—intravenously	
PO—by mouth	

Drug	Route and Dose	Adverse Effects and Cautions
Acetazolamide	IV, PO: 5 mg/kg/dose q 6–8 h; increase as needed to 25 mg/kg/dose (*temporarily effective*), max dose 55 mg/kg/day	Hyperchloremic metabolic acidosis, hypokalemia, drowsiness, paresthesias
Acyclovir	PO, IV: 5–10 mg/kg/dose q 8 h, infuse over 1 h	Transient renal dysfunction; lengthen dose interval with renal failure
Albumin, 5%	IV: 0.5–1 gm/kg slowly	Hypovolemia, heart failure; monitor blood pressure
Albuterol	Aerosol: 0.5–1 mg/dose q 2–6 h PO: 0.1–0.3 mg/kg/dose q 6–8 h	Tachycardia, arrhythmias, tremor, irritability
Amikacin	IM, IV: Postnatal age 0–4 weeks, <1200 gm: 7.5 mg/kg/dose q 18–24 h ≤1 week, 1200–2000 gm: 7.5 mg/kg/dose q 12–18 h; and >2000 gm 10 mg/kg/dose q 12 h >1 week, 1200–2000 gm: 7.5 mg/kg/dose q 8–12 h; and >2000 gm 10 mg/kg/dose q 8 h	Nephrotoxicity; ototoxicity; blood level monitoring recommended (desirable levels: peak = 10–25 μg/ml; trough = 3–5 μg/ml)
Aminophylline	See Theophylline	
Amphotericin B	IV: 0.25–1 mg/kg/dose/day; on day 1 0.25 mg/kg/dose, diluted and infused over 4–6 h (*do not use filters with pore size <1 μm*); increase dose as tolerated; total dosage 30–35 mg/kg over 6 wk	Nephrotoxicity; fever; flushing; anemia; hypotension; hyposthenuria; hypokalemia; protect bottle and tubing from light with foil
Ampicillin	IM, IV: newborns <7 days = 25–50 mg/kg/dose q 8–12 h; >7 days old = 25–50 mg/kg/dose q 6–8 h Highest dose for meningitis Maintain q 12 h for 4 weeks for <1200 gm	
Amrinone	Initial: 0.75 mg/kg over 2–3 min; maintenance 3–5 μg/kg/min	Fluid balance; electrolytes; renal function
Ascorbic acid	See Vitamin C (ascorbic acid)	
Atropine	IV, IM, ET, SC: 0.01–0.03 mg/kg, repeat q 4–6 h prn	Hyperthermia, tachycardia, urinary retention
Bacitracin	Top: as ointment (500 units/gm), q 4–8 h	
Beractant	IT: *for prophylactic treatment:* Give 4 ml/kg as soon as possible; may repeat at 6-h intervals to a maximum of 4 doses in 48 hours IT: *for rescue treatment:* Give 4 ml/kg as soon as respiratory distress syndrome diagnosed; may repeat at 6-h intervals to a maximum of 4 doses in 48 h	May give additional doses if infant still has respiratory distress, or is intubated and needs >30% FiO₂ to keep PaO₂ ≤80 torr. Administer each dose as 4 doses of 1 ml/kg each, giving each dose over 2–3 seconds and turning newborn to a different position after each dose
Bethanechol	PO: 0.1–0.2 mg/kg/dose q 6–8 h or 3 mg/m²/dose q 8 h 20 min before feeding	Diarrhea, jitteriness, tremors, sleeplessness, bronchoconstriction, increased tracheobronchial secretions
Caffeine	PO, IV: loading dose = 10 mg/kg; maintenance dose = 2.5 mg/kg/dose q 24 h (*doses are for the nonsalt form of drug—caffeine base*).	Restlessness, emesis, tachycardia; therapeutic plasma concentration = 5–20 μg/ml free base
Calcium chloride 10% (27 mg elemental CA²⁺/ml)	IV: 0.35–0.70 ml (9–19 mg Ca²⁺)/kg/dose for acute hypocalcemia	Bradycardia if injected too quickly; necrosis from extravascular leakage
Calcium glubionate 6.47% (23 mg elemental Ca²⁺/ml)	PO: treatment = 500–1000 mg/kg/day q 3–4 h; supplement = 150 mg/kg/day q 3–4 h	High osmotic load of syrup may cause diarrhea
Calcium gluconate 10% (9.3 mg elemental Ca²⁺/ml)	IV: 1–2 ml (9–19 mg Ca²⁺)/kg/dose for acute hypocalcemia PO: 3–9 ml/kg/day in 2–4 divided doses (30–80 mg/Ca²⁺/kg/day) for chronic use	Bradycardia if injected too quickly; necrosis from extravascular leakage; gastric necrosis and calcification if it is too concentrated; diarrhea may potentiate digitalis effect
Calcium lactate 13% (130 mg elemental Ca²⁺/gm powder)	PO: 0.5 gm/kg/day in divided doses q 6–8 h	See Calcium gluconate; gastrointestinal irritation
Captopril	PO: 0.05–0.1 mg/kg/dose q 6–24 h; increase dose up to 0.5 mg/kg/dose to control blood pressure	High initial doses may cause hypotension and renal insufficiency

Drug	Route and Dose	Adverse Effects and Cautions
Cefotaxime	IV: 25–50 mg/kg/dose <7 days = q 12 h; >7 days = q 8 h	Adjust dose for renal impairment
Cefuroxime	IV, IM: 25 mg/kg/dose; <7 days q 12 h; >7 days q 8 h	
Cephalothin	IV, IM: 20 mg/kg/dose; preterm <7 days q 12 h (till 4 wk for <1200 gm) >7 days q 8 h; term <7 days q 8 h; >7 days q 6 h	
Chloral hydrate	PO, PR: sedative = 10–30 mg/kg/day divided q 6–8 h; hypnotic = 50 mg/kg as single dose	Gastric irritation; caution with hepatic, renal, cardiac, or pulmonary disease. Provides *no* analgesia
Chloramphenicol	IV, PO: loading dose = 20 mg/kg; maintenance = 5 mg/kg/dose q 6 h; maintenance doses vary 2.5–12.5 mg/kg/dose q 6 h; 25 mg/kg q 24 h for 4 wk for <1200 gm	Hematologic and blood level monitoring mandatory (usual therapeutic level 10–25 μg/ml). Cardiac toxicity, "gray baby" syndrome, dose-related bone marrow suppression, idiosyncratic aplastic anemia
Chlorothiazide	PO: 5–15 mg/kg/dose q 12–24 h	Hypokalemia; hyponatremia decreases calcium excretion; hyperglycemia
Chlorpromazine	PO, IM, IV: 0.2–0.5 mg/kg/dose prn withdrawal symptoms	Extrapyramidal symptoms; potentiates hypnotics and narcotics; hypotension
Cimetidine	PO, IV: 2.5–5 mg/kg/dose q 6 h according to gastric pH ≥5	Decreases drug clearance by hepatic cytochrome P450
Clindamycin	PO, IV: 5 mg/kg/dose preterm <1 wk = q 12 h, preterm >1 week or term <1 wk = q 8 h, term >1 wk = q 6 h, maintain q 12 h till 4 wk for <1200 gm	Pseudomembranous colitis is rare in newborns. Limited experience in newborns. Hepatic metabolism
Colfosceril palmitate	IT: *for prophylactic treatment:* Give 5 ml/kg as soon as possible; may repeat second and third doses 12 and 24 h later to those infants remaining on ventilators IT: *for rescue treatment:* Give 5 ml/kg as soon as respiratory distress syndrome diagnosed; may repeat second dose 12 h later	Administer each dose as 2 doses of 2.5 ml/kg each, giving each dose over 1–2 min; and turning newborn 45 degrees for 30 seconds to the right after the first dose and then similarly to the left after the second dose
Corticotropin	IM, IV, SC: 3–5 units/kg/day in 4 divided doses, usual maximum of 30 units/day	Hypertension, immunosuppression, electrolyte imbalance, cataracts, growth retardation, gastrointestinal ulcers or dysfunction
Cortisone Acetate	PO: 0.5–2 mg/kg/day, divided q 6 h	Treatment of more than 7–10 days requires gradual dosage reduction to avoid adrenal insufficiency. Immunosuppression, hyperglycemia, growth delay, leukocytosis, gastric irritation
Desoxycorticosterone acetate (DOCA) see Fludrocortisone		
Dexamethasone	IM, IV: bronchopulmonary dysplasia—0.25 mg/kg/dose q 8–12 h for 3–7 days	See Cortisone
Diazepam	PO, IV, IM: sedative = 0.02–0.3 mg/kg/dose q 6–8 h; seizure = 0.1–0.2 mg/kg/dose slow IV push	Diluted injection may precipitate; IM absorption is poor; respiratory depression, hypotension
Dicloxacillin	4–8 mg/kg/dose (PO) q 6 h	

Digoxin	IV: Acute digitalization°
	Prematures Loading dose (TDD)†
	  <1.5 kg 10–20 μg/kg
	  1.5–2.5 kg 20 μg/kg
	Term newborns 30 μg/kg
	Infants (1–12 mo) 35 μg/kg
	Maintenance dose: 1/8 TDD q 12 h
	  Begin 12 h after last digitalization dose
		Risk of arrhythmias is increased during digitalization. IV formulation is twice as concentrated as oral. Conduction defects, emesis, ventricular arrhythmias

Diphenhydramine	PO: 5 mg/kg/day q 6 h	Somnolence
Diphenylhydantoin	See Phenytoin	
Diphtheria antitoxin	IM, IV: 20,000–50,000 units/day for 2–3 successive days	Hypersensitivity reaction
Dobutamine	IV: 2–15 μg/kg/min by continuous infusion and titrate to desired effect	Tachycardia, hypotension
Dopamine	IV: 2–20 μg/kg/min by continuous infusion and titrate to desired effect	Extravasation may lead to necrosis. (Phentolamine is an antidote.) High dose may constrict renal arteries
Edrophonium	Tensilon test for myasthenia gravis SC, IM: 0.2–0.5 mg/kg; IV: preliminary test dose = 0.04 mg slow push, test dose = 0.16 mg/kg (1 min later)	Cardiac arrhythmia, diarrhea, tracheal secretions may require atropine antagonism
Epinephrine	Resuscitation: IV, ET—1:10,000: 0.05–0.1 ml/kg q 10–15 min Hypotension: 0.01–0.1 μg/kg/min by continuous infusion and titrate to desired effect	Tachycardia, arrhythmia

Drug	Route and Dose	Adverse Effects and Cautions
Erythromycin	PO, IV: 10 mg/kg/dose, <7 days = q 12 h, >7 days = q 8 h Eye prophylaxis at birth: ophthalmic ointment 0.5% in each eye	IV administration is painful. May affect theophylline serum levels
Ethacrynic acid	IV: 0.5–1.0 mg/kg/dose q 12–24 h	Ototoxicity with aminoglycosides: hypokalemia and hyponatremia
Exosurf	See Colfosceril palmitate	
Fentanyl	IV, IM: 1–2 μg/kg/dose, q 4–6 h prn	50–100 times the potency of morphine. Muscle rigidity ("stiff man" syndrome) may occur
Fibrinogen	IV: 50 mg/kg: repeated prn as determined by clotting time	
Flucytosine	PO: 20–40 mg/kg q 6 h	Monitor levels. Effective antifungal concentration: 35–70 μg/ml. Bone marrow dysfunction: >100 μg/ml. Renal dysfunction decreases clearance
Fludrocortisone	PO: 0.025–0.2 mg/day	Mineralocorticoid replacement where 0.1 mg of fludrocortisone is equivalent to DOCA 1 mg
Folic acid	PO: 50 μg/day for preterm newborns after feeding is established for maintenance; 500 μg/day for therapy	
Furosemide	IM, IV; 0.5–2 mg/kg/dose q 12–24 h PO: 1–2 mg/kg/dose q 12–24 h Bioavailability reduced by cor pulmonale	Hypokalemia, hyponatremia, hypochloremia; half-life prolonged in premature newborns
Gentamicin	IM, IV: postnatal age ≤7 days age: <1000 gm and <28 weeks 2.5 mg/kg/dose q 24 h; <1500 gm and <34 wk 2.5 mg/kg/dose q 18 h; >1500 gm and >34 wk 2.5 mg/kg/dose q 12 h >7–28 days age: <1200 gm 2.5 mg/kg/dose q 18–24 h; >28 days > 1200 gm 2.5 mg/kg/dose q 8 h	Blood level monitoring indicated for efficacy; toxicity is rare in newborn (desirable levels: trough <2 μg/ml to avoid toxicity; peak 5-10 μg/ml)
Gentian violet	Top (skin): as 1–2% aqueous solution, bid Top (oral): as 1% aqueous solution, bid	Stains skin
Glucagon	IM, IV: 30–100 μg/kg; may be repeated after 6–12 h; infant of diabetic mother may require 300 μg/kg	Maximum dose 1 mg; higher doses possibly toxic
Heparin	IV: Initial dose–50 units/kg; maintenance dose–100 units/kg q 4 h or 20–25 units/kg/h continuous infusion. Titrate doses to 1½–2 times baseline whole blood clotting time or activated partial thromboplastin time	Intractable bleeding (reversible with protamine); heparin half-life; prematures < term < adults
Hydralazine	PO, IM, IV: 0.15 mg/kg every 6 h; increase as needed in 0.1 mg/kg increments up to 4 mg/kg/day	Tachycardia, lupus-like reactions
Hydrochlorothiazide	PO: 2.0–2.5 mg/kg/day q 12 h	Hypercalcemia, hypokalemia, hyperglycemia
Hydrocortisone	PO, IM, IV: adrenal crisis, 3–10 mg/kg/day; PO: physiologic replacement, 1 mg/kg/day or 15–25 mg/m²/day	See Cortisone
Immunoglobulin intravenous, human	IV: 400–750 mg/kg/dose infused over 2–6 h	Studies in newborns are preliminary. Necrotizing enterocolitis, volume overload
Indomethacin	PO, IV: 0.1–0.2 mg/kg/dose q 12–24 h	Transient renal dysfunction, decreased platelet aggregation
Insulin (Regular)	IV: hyperglycemia infusion dose, 0.01–0.1 units/kg/h; SC; intermittent dose, 0.1–0.2 units/kg q 6–12 h	
Iron	PO: 2–6 mg/kg/day elemental iron	
Isoniazid	PO: 10 mg/kg/day, single dose or divided q 12 h	Newborns do not require pyridoxine supplement. Follow liver function test
Isoproterenol	IV: 0.05–0.5 μg/kg/min by infusion	Arrhythmias, systemic vasodilation, tachycardia, hypotension, hypoglycemia
Kanamycin	IM, IV: 7.5–10 mg/kg/dose; <7 days = q 12 h; >7 days = q 8 h	Nephrotoxicity, ototoxicity. Monitoring of blood levels useful (optimal serum peak concentrations 15–25 μg/ml)
Kayexalate	See Sodium polystyrene sulfonate (Kayexalate)	
Levothyroxine	PO: starting dose 8–10 μg/kg/day (round off to nearest 12.5, 25.0, or 37.5 μg to coincide with pill size). Increase by 12.5–25 μg/24 h every 2 weeks to desired effect; max 500 μg/day	Adjust dosage on 3–6 wk schedule by clinical response and T4. Optimal T_4 range 8–11 μg/dl
Lidocaine	IV: 1 mg/kg infused over 5–10 min; may be repeated q 10 min 5 times, prn; infusion dose 10–50 μg/kg/min or 1 mg/kg/h	Monitoring of blood levels useful (therapeutic range 1–6 μg/ml plasma); dilute for ET administration
Lorazepam	IV: 0.05–0.1 mg/kg infused over 2–5 min	Limited data in newborns, preparations may contain benzyl alcohol. Dilute
Magnesium sulfate	IM, IV: 25–50 mg/kg q 4–6 for 3–4 doses prn; use 50% solution IM; 1% solution IV	Hypotension, central nervous system depression; monitor serum concentration; calcium gluconate should be available as an antidote

Drug	Route and Dose	Adverse Effects and Cautions
Medium-chain triglyceride (MCT)	PO: 1–8 ml/24 h divided in feedings (7.7 cal/ml)	
Meperidine	IV, IM: 0.5 mg/kg/dose q 4 h prn PO: 0.5–1 mg/kg/dose q 4 h	Respiratory depression reversible with naloxone; underdosage increases pain perception
Methyldopa	IV, PO: 2–3 mg/kg q 6–8 h; increased as needed at 2-day intervals; maximum dosage 12–15 mg/kg/dose	Sedation, fever, false-positive Coombs' test, hemolysis; sudden withdrawal of methyldopa may cause rebound hypertension
Methylene blue	IV: 0.1–0.2 mg/kg of 1% solution for methemoglobinemia, infused slowly	
Methylprednisolone	IV, IM: 0.1–0.4 mg/kg/dose, q 6 h	Hydrocortisone preferred for physiologic replacement
Metoclopramide	PO, IV: 0.1–0.2 mg/kg/dose q 6–8 h or prior to each feeding	Dystonic reactions, irritability, diarrhea, decreases glomerular filtration rate in adults
Mezlocillin	75 mg/kg/dose <7 days q 12 h; >7 days q 8 h; maintain q 12 h for 4 wk for <1200 gm	Urinary retention
Midazolam	IV, IM: 0.07–0.20 mg/kg/dose q 2–4 h prn for sedation	Limited experience in newborns. Respiratory depression, apnea
Morphine sulfate	IV, IM, SC: 0.05–0.1 mg/kg/dose q 2–6 h prn	Respiratory depression reversible with naloxone
Mycostatin	PO: 100,000–200,000 units q 6 h Topical: as 2% ointment (in petrolatum 95% polyethylene 5%) 3–4 times daily	
Nafcillin	IV, IM: 25 mg/kg/dose, newborns 0–7 days = q 12 h, infants >7 days = q 6–8 h; double dosage for meningitis; maintain q 12 h for 4 wk for <1200 gm	Agranulocytosis; granulocytopenia; hepatic dysfunction; may require dosage adjustment
Naloxone	IV, IM, SC: 0.1 mg/kg/dose; may be repeated as necessary; delivery room, minimum = 0.5 mg for term newborn	Onset of action may be delayed 15+ min after IM or SC administration. Narcotic effects may outlast naloxone antagonism; dilute for ET administration
Neomycin	PO: 10–25 mg/kg/dose q 6 h Topical: 0.5% ointment, 3–4 times daily	Renal toxicity and ototoxicity if absorbed
Neostigmine	IM: Test for myasthenia gravis—0.1 mg/kg PO: Treatment for myasthenia gravis = 0.33 mg/kg/day q 3–6 h	Cardiac arrhythmia (atropine should be kept available)
Nitroprusside	IV: begin in dose of 0.5 μg/kg/min and vary as needed up to 8 μg/kg/min to control blood pressure	Profound hypotension possible; requires arterial line to monitor blood pressure; thiocyanate toxicity with long-term use or renal insufficiency
Oxacillin	IV, IM: 25 mg/kg/dose Preterm <4 wk old <1200 gm q 12 h; 1200–2000 gm q 12 h for <7 days old; 1200–2000 gm q 8 h for 7 days old; Term 25–40 mg/kg/dose <7 days old, q 12 h; >7 days old, q 6 h	Sterile abscess formation, nephrotoxicity; monitor liver enzymes and complete blood count
Pancreatin	PO: 2000 units of lipase with each feeding PR and into colostomy: 0.3–0.5 gm in sufficient liquid (for meconium ileus)	
Pancuronium	IV: 0.03–0.1 mg/kg/dose q 1–4 h prn; titrate to age and effect desired	Ensure adequate oxygenation and ventilation. Tachycardia, bradycardia, hypotension, hypertension. Potentiated by acidosis, hypothermia, neuromuscular disease
Paraldehyde	PR: 0.3 ml/kg q 4–6 h	Reserve for refractory status epilepticus. Local irritation, pulmonary edema, hemorrhage. Hepatic dysfunction decreases clearance. Avoid IM if possible. Do not give by arterial catheter. Avoid plastic containers
Penicillin G	IV, IM: sepsis 25,000–50,000 units/kg/dose, meningitis 75,000–100,000 units/kg/dose, q 8–12 h; <7 days and q 6–8 h; >7 days; *Use higher doses for group B* Streptococcus *infections* Maintain q 12 h for 4 wk for <1200 gm	Use for susceptible organisms such as streptococci; syphilis
Pentobarbital	PO, IM, IV: 2–6 mg/kg prn	Blood level monitoring helpful (sedative level 0.5–3 μg/ml). Higher doses may depress respirations. Monitor blood pressure
Phenobarbital	IV, IM, PO: anticonvulsant loading dose—15–20 mg/kg, may repeat 10 mg/kg/dose twice for status epilepticus; maintenance dose: 3–5 mg/kg/day q 12–24 h, begin 12–24 h after load dose: Sedation: 2–3 mg/kg q 8–12 h prn	Blood level monitoring helpful (therapeutic range 15–40 μg/ml). Half-life 40–200 h in infants, prolonged by asphyxia
Phentolamine	SC: dilute to 0.5 mg/ml, inject 0.2 ml at 5 sites around dopamine infiltration; max 2.5 mg total dose	
Phenytoin	IV: loading dose, 15–20 mg/kg, infused <0.5 mg/kg/min PO, IV: maintenance, 4–8 mg/kg/dose q 24 h; higher doses q 8 h >7 days. Flush IV with saline before/after dose	Therapeutic blood level monitoring indicated (desirable level 10–20 μg/ml). Infant clearance may be high

Drug	Route and Dose	Adverse Effects and Cautions
Phosphate, sodium, or potassium	PO: 1–3 mmol/kg/day in divided doses or supplement formula phosphorus intake to 75 mg/kg/day; diluted solution contains 3.3 mg phosphorus/ml; 1 packet of potassium PO_4 contains 250 mg (8 mmol) of phosphorus	Large amounts may cause catharsis; increase gradually to full supplementation
Piperacillin	IM, IV: 50–100 mg/kg/dose—preterm <7 days q 12 h, preterm >7 days q 8 h, term <7 days q 8 h, term >7 days q 6 h	
Pitressin	See Vasopressin	
Plasma	IV: 5–10 ml/kg; repeated prn	Volume overload, viral infection risk
Prednisone	PO: 0.5–2 mg/kg/day, q 6 h	See Cortisone
Procainamide	IV: 1.5–2.5 mg/kg infused over 10–30 min; may be repeated in 30 min if needed PO: 40–60 mg/kg/day q 4–6 h	Asystole, myocardial depression, anorexia, vomiting, nausea. Blood level monitoring helpful (therapeutic range: procainamide, 3–10 µg/ml; N-acetyl procainamide, 5–30 µg/ml)
Propranolol	IV: 0.01 mg/kg initial dose and 0.01–0.15 mg/kg infused over 10 min; may be repeated in 10 min and then q 6–8 h to max of 0.15 mg/kg/dose PO: 0.05–2 mg/kg q 6 h	Relatively contraindicated in low-output congestive heart failure and patients with bronchospasm
Propylthiouracil	PO: 2–4 mg/kg q 8 h. Increase to max of 10 mg/kg/dose. Onset of action may be delayed days to weeks	
Prostaglandin E_1, alprostodil	IV: 0.05–0.1 µg/kg/min. Often, dose may be reduced by ½ after initial response. Intra-arterial infusion offers no advantage	Apnea, seizures, fever, disseminated intravascular coagulation, diarrhea, cutaneous vasodilatation, decreased platelet aggregation, cortical bone proliferation during prolonged infusion
Protamine sulfate	IV: 1 mg for each 100 units of heparin in previous 30 min; 0.5–0.75 for 30–60 min; and 0.25–0.375 for heparin given >2 h before	Excessive doses induce coagulopathy
Pyridoxine	See Vitamin B_6	
Quinidine gluconate	PO, IM: 2–10 mg/kg/dose q 2–6 h until desired effect or toxicity occurs IV route not recommended in neonates	Check electrocardiogram before each dose; discontinue if QRS interval increases 50% or more. Maintain level of 2–6 µg/ml. Nausea, vomiting, diarrhea, fever, atrioventricular block
Ranitidine	PO, IV: 1–2 mg/kg q 8–12 h	H_2 antagonist minimally studied in newborns. Minimal inhibition of hepatic P450 enzymes
Ribavirin	6 g nebulized in hood with a solution of 20 mg/ml 12–18 h/day for 3–7 days	May precipitate in endotracheal tube; avoid exposure of pregnant staff; possible teratogenic effects
Silver nitrate (1% solution)	Prophylaxis: 1 or 2 drops each eye	Chemical conjunctivitis
Sodium bicarbonate (0.5 mEq/ml)	IV: 1–2 mEq/kg/dose infused slowly only if infant ventilated adequately	Intravascular hemolysis may be associated with rapid infusion
Sodium polystyrene sulfonate (Kayexalate)	PO, PR: 1 gm/kg; approximately q 6 h	Usually administered as a solution with 20% sorbitol to prevent intestinal obstruction; 20% sorbitol solution may injure intestinal mucosa of very-low-birth-weight newborns; may decrease serum calcium or magnesium
Spironolactone	PO: 1–3 mg/kg/day q 8–24 h	Contraindicated with hyperkalemia; onset of action delayed; drowsiness; nausea; vomiting; diarrhea; androgenic effects in females; gynecomastia in males
Streptomycin	IM: 10–20 mg/kg/day q 24 h	Nephrotoxicity, ototoxicity. Use in newborns as part of triple therapy for tuberculosis
Sulfisoxazole	PO, IV: 25 mg/kg q 6 h. Aggressive therapy is used only in full-term neonates >2 weeks old	In prematures or in presence of jaundice, may lead to kernicterus
Survanta	See Beractant	
Tetanus immune globulin	IM: 250–500 units/dose	Optimal dosage not established for newborns
Theophylline	PO, IV: loading dose: 5–6 mg/kg; maintenance dose: 1–2.5 mg/kg/dose q 6–12 h; aminophylline (IV) dose = theophylline (IV) dose × 1.25	Blood level monitoring indicated (therapeutic range: apnea, 7–12 µg/ml; bronchospasm, 10–20 µg/ml). Tachycardia at 15–20 µg/ml, seizures >40 µg/ml. Avoid rectal dosing owing to variable absorption. Clearance decreased by asphyxia and prematurity
Thiamine	See Vitamin B_1	
Ticarcillin	IM, IV: 75 mg/kg/dose <7 days q 12 h, >7 days q 8 h; maintain q 12 h for 4 wk for <1200 gm	Contains 5.2 mEq Na$^+$/gm; may inhibit platelet function
Tobramycin	See Gentamicin dosing guidelines	
Tolazoline	IV loading dose: 0.5–1 mg/kg over 10 min; maintenance dose 0.2–2 mg/kg/h	Hypotension; gastrointestinal and pulmonary bleeding; renal dysfunction. Accumulates with oliguria; no antidote
Vancomycin	PO: 10 mg/kg, q 6 h IV: postnatal age ≤7 days: <1200 gm 15 mg/kg/day q 24 h; 1200–2000 gm 15 mg/kg/day q 12–18 h; >2000 gm 30 mg/kg/day q 12 h; >7 days: <1200 gm 15 mg/kg/day q 24 h; 1200–2000 gm 15 mg/kg/day q 8–12 h; >2000 gm 45 mg/kg/day q 8 h Cerebrospinal fluid: 5–10 mg/day (cerebrospinal fluid trough <20 µg/ml)	Nephrotoxicity; ototoxicity. (Therapeutic levels: peak = 25–40 µg/ml; trough = 5–10 µg/ml). Rapid infusion may cause cutaneous vasodilatation and shock

Drug	Route and Dose	Adverse Effects and Cautions
Vasopressin	IM, SC: 2.5–10 U 2–4 times daily	20 units/ml aqueous injection
Vecuronium	IV: 0.08–0.1 mg/kg/dose, repeat prn at 0.03–0.15 mg/kg/dose q 1–2 h	Neuromuscular blockade potentiated by calcium channel blockers such as verapamil
Verapamil	IV: 0.1–0.2 mg/kg infused over 2 min; if response is inadequate, repeat in 30 min PO: 2–5 mg/kg/day in 3 divided doses	Monitor electrocardiogram during infusion. Bradycardia, atrioventricular block, asystole. Contraindicated in patients with 2nd or 3rd degree atrioventricular block during treatment with beta blockers
Vitamin A (oleovitamin A)	PO: preventive, 600–1500 units/day	
Vitamin B₁ (thiamine)	PO: preventive, 0.5–1 mg q day; PO: therapeutic, 5–10 mg q 6–8 h	
Vitamin B₆ (pyridoxine)	PO: preventive, 100 μg/l of ingested formula; therapeutic for deficiency, 2–5 mg/day q 6 h; test dose for pyridone dependency seizures, 50–100 mg IV	
Vitamin C (ascorbic acid)	IM, IV, PO: preventive, 25–50 mg/day (term infants); 100 mg/day (premature infants)	
Vitamin D₂ (ergocalciferol)	PO: preventive, 400–1000 IU/day (premature infants), 40–100 IU/day (term infants)	
Vitamin E (d-alpha tocopherol)	PO: prevention of hemolysis—25–50 IU/day (1 IU = 1 mg)	Some preparations are hyperosmolar
Vitamin K₁ (phytonadione)	SC, IM: preventive, 0.5–1.0 mg, single dose; therapeutic, 1–2 mg/kg/dose q 6–12 h according to prothrombin time	With thrombocytopenia, slow IV infusion at same dose. Anaphylaxis observed with rapid injection IV

°PO dose increased 20%.
†TDD (loading dose): 1/2, 1/4, 1/4 dose q 8 h.

References

1. Bhatt DR, Furman GI, Wirtschafter DD, and Reber DJ: Neonatal Drug Formulary, 1987–1988. Coving, CA, California Perinatal Association, 1988.
2. Bhatt DR, Reber DJ, Wirtschafter DD, et al: Neonatal Drug Formulary, 4th Ed. Los Angeles, NDF, 1997.
3. Levin RH: Drug disposition in neonates, infants, and children. *In* Rudolph AM (Ed): Rudolph's Pediatrics, 20th Ed. Appleton & Lange, 1996.
4. Taketomo CK, Hodding JH, Kraus DM: Pediatric Dosage Handbook, 3rd Ed. Lexi-Comp, 1996–1997.
5. Threlkeld DS (Ed): Facts and Comparisons. St. Louis, Facts and Comparisons, 1997.

THE TRANSFER OF DRUGS AND OTHER CHEMICALS INTO HUMAN MILK

Committee on Drugs

This statement was first published in 1983, with a revision published in 1989. Information about the transfer of drugs and chemicals into human milk continues to become available. This current statement is intended to revise the lists of agents transferred into human milk and describe their possible effects on the infant or on lactation, if known (Tables 1 through 7). The fact that a pharmacologic or chemical agent does not appear on the lists is not meant to imply that it is not transferred into human milk or that it does not have an effect on the infant; it only indicates that there were no reports found in the literature. These tables should assist the physician in counseling a nursing mother regarding breast-feeding when the mother has a condition for which a drug is medically indicated.

The following question and options should be considered when prescribing drug therapy to lactating women. (1) Is the drug therapy really necessary? Consultation between the pediatrician and the mother's physician can be most useful. (2) Use the safest drug, for example, acetaminophen rather than aspirin for analgesia. (3) If there is a possibility that a drug may present a risk to the infant, consideration should be given to measurement of blood concentrations in the nursing infant. (4) Drug exposure to the nursing infant may be minimized by having the mother take the medication just after she has breast-fed the infant and/or just before the infant is due to have a lengthy sleep period.

Data have been obtained from a search of the medical literature. Because methodologies used to quantitate drugs in milk continue to improve, this current information will require continuous updating. Drugs cited in Tables 1 through 7 are listed in alphabetical order by generic name; brand names are listed in Tables 8 and 9 in accordance with the current *Physicians Desk Reference, AMA Drug Evaluation,* and the *USAN and the USP Dictionary of Drug Names.*

Physicians who encounter adverse effects in infants fed drug-contaminated human milk are urged to document these effects in a communication to the American Academy of Pediatrics Committee on Drugs and to the Food and Drug Administration. This communication should include the generic and brand name of the drug, the maternal dose and mode of administration, the concentration of the drug in milk and maternal and infant blood in relation to the time of ingestion, the method used for laboratory identification, the age of the infant, and the adverse effect. Such reports may significantly increase the pediatric community's fund of knowledge regarding drug transfer into human milk and the potential or actual risk to the infant.

Reference: Shardern JL: Chemically Induced Birth Defects, 2nd ed. New York, Marcel Dekker, 1993.

The recommendations in this policy statement do not indicate an exclusive course of treatment or serve as a standard of medical care. Variations, taking into account individual circumstances, may be appropriate.

Adapted from PEDIATRICS 93:137–148, 1994, including Tables 1 through 9. Used with permission of the American Academy of Pediatrics.

TABLE 1

Drugs that Are Contraindicated During Breast-Feeding

Drug	Reason for Concern, Reported Sign or Symptom in Infant, or Effect on Lactation
Bromocriptine	Suppresses lactation; may be hazardous to the mother
Cocaine	Cocaine intoxication
Cyclophosphamide	Possible immune suppression; unknown effect on growth or association with carcinogenesis; neutropenia
Cyclosporine	Possible immune suppression; unknown effect on growth or association with carcinogenesis
Doxorubicin°	Possible immune suppression; unknown effect on growth or association with carcinogenesis
Ergotamine	Vomiting, diarrhea, convulsions (doses used in migraine medications)
Lithium	One-third to one-half therapeutic blood concentration in infants
Methotrexate	Possible immune suppression; unknown effect on growth or association with carcinogenesis; neutropenia
Phencyclidine (PCP)	Potent hallucinogen
Phenindione	Anticoagulant: increased prothrombin and partial thromboplastin time in one infant; not used in United States

°Drug is concentrated in human milk.

TABLE 2

Drugs of Abuse: Contraindicated During Breast-Feeding*

Drug Reference	Reported Effect or Reasons for Concern
Amphetamine†	Irritability, poor sleeping pattern
Cocaine	Cocaine intoxication
Heroin	Tremors, restlessness, vomiting, poor feeding
Marijuana	Only one report in literature; no effect mentioned
Nicotine (smoking)	Shock, vomiting, diarrhea, rapid heart rate, restlessness; decreased milk production
Phencyclidine	Potent hallucinogen

°The Committee on Drugs strongly believes that nursing mothers should not ingest any compounds listed in Table 2. Not only are they hazardous to the nursing infant, but they are also detrimental to the physical and emotional health of the mother. This list is obviously not complete; no drug of abuse should be ingested by nursing mothers even though adverse reports are not in the literature.

†Drug is concentrated in human milk.

TABLE 3

Radioactive Compounds that Require Temporary Cessation of Breast-Feeding*

Drug	Recommended Time for Cessation of Breast-Feeding
Copper 64 (^{64}Cu)	Radioactivity in milk present at 50 h
Gallium 67 (^{67}Ga)	Radioactivity in milk present for 2 wk
Indium 111 (^{111}In)	Very small amount present at 20 h
Iodine 123 (^{123}I)	Radioactivity in milk present up to 36 h
Iodine 125 (^{125}I)	Radioactivity in milk present for 12 d
Iodine 131 (^{131}I)	Radioactivity in milk present 2–14 d, depending on study
Radioactive sodium	Radioactivity in milk present 96 h
Technetium-99m (^{99m}Tc), ^{99m}Rc macroaggregates, ^{99m}Tc O4	Radioactivity in milk present 15 h to 3 d

°Consult nuclear medicine physician before performing diagnostic study so that radionuclide that has shortest excretion time in breast milk can be used. Before study, the mother should pump her breast and store enough milk in freezer for feeding the infant; after study, the mother should pump her breast to maintain milk production but discard all milk pumped for the required time that radioactivity is present in milk. Milk samples can be screened by radiology departments for radioactivity before resumption of nursing.

TABLE 4

Drugs Whose Effect on Nursing Infants Is Unknown But May Be of Concern

Psychotropic drugs, the compounds listed under antianxiety, antidepressant, and antipsychotic categories, are of special concern when given to nursing mothers for long periods. Although there are no case reports of adverse effects in breast-feeding infants, these drugs do appear in human milk and thus could conceivably alter short-term and long-term central nervous system function.

Drug	Reported or Possible Effect
Antianxiety	
Diazepam	None
Lorazepam	None
Midazolam	—
Perphenazine	None
Prazepam°	None
Quazepam	None
Temazepam	—
Antidepressants	
Amitriptyline	None
Amoxapine	None
Desipramine	None
Dothiepin	None
Doxepin	None
Fluoxetine	—
Fluvoxamine	—
Imipramine	None
Trazodone	None
Antipsychotic	
Chlorpromazine	Galactorrhea in adult; drowsiness and lethargy in infant
Chlorprothixene	None
Haloperidol	None
Mesoridazine	None
Chloramphenicol	Possible idiosyncratic bone marrow suppression
Metoclopramide°	None described; dopaminergic blocking agent
Metronidazole	In vitro mutagen; may discontinue breast-feeding 12–24 h to allow excretion of dose when single-dose therapy given to mother
Tinidazole	See metronidazole

°Drug is concentrated in human milk.

TABLE 5

Drugs that Have Been Associated with Significant Effects on Some Nursing Infants and Should Be Given to Nursing Mothers with Caution*

Drug	Reported Effect
5-Aminosalicylic acid	Diarrhea (1 case)
Aspirin (salicylates)	Metabolic acidosis (1 case)
Clemastine	Drowsiness, irritability, refusal to feed, high-pitched cry, neck stiffness (1 case)
Phenobarbital	Sedation; infantile spasms after weaning from milk containing phenobarbital, methemoglobinemia (1 case)
Primidone	Sedation, feeding problems
Sulfasalazine (salicylazosulfapyridine)	Bloody diarrhea (1 case)

°Measure blood concentration in the infant when possible.

TABLE 6

Maternal Medication Usually Compatible with Breast-Feeding*

Drug	Reported Sign or Symptom in Infant or Effect on Lactation	Drug	Reported Sign or Symptom in Infant or Effect on Lactation
Acebutolol	None	Digoxin	None
Acetaminophen	None	Diltiazem	None
Acetazolamide	None	Dipyrone	None
Acitretin	—	Disopyramide	None
Acyclovir†	None	Domperidone	None
Alcohol (ethanol)	With large amounts drowsiness, diaphoresis, deep sleep, weakness, decrease in linear growth, abnormal weight gain; maternal ingestion of 1 g/kg daily decreases milk ejection reflex	Dyphylline†	None
		Enalapril	—
		Erythromycin†	None
		Estradiol	Withdrawal, vaginal bleeding
		Ethambutol	None
Allopurinol	—	Ethanol (cf. alcohol)	—
Amoxicillin	None	Ethosuximide	None, drug appears in infant serum
Antimony	—	Fentanyl	—
Atenolol	None	Flecainide	—
Atropine	None	Flufenamic acid	None
Azapropazone (apazone)	—	Fluorescein	—
Aztreonam	None	Folic acid	None
B₁ (thiamin)	None	Gold salts	None
B₆ (pyridoxine)	None	Halothane	None
B₁₂	None	Hydralazine	None
Baclofen	None	Hydrochlorothiazide	—
Barbiturate	See Table 5	Hydroxychoroquine†	None
Bendroflumethiazide	Suppresses lactation	Ibuprofen	None
Bishydroxycoumarin (dicumarol)	None	Indomethacin	Seizure (1 case)
Bromide	Rash, weakness, absence of cry with maternal intake of 5.4 g/d	Iodides	May affect thyroid activity; see miscellaneous iodine
Butorphanol	None	Iodine (providone-iodine/vaginal douche)	Elevated iodine levels in breast milk, odor of iodine on infant's skin
Caffeine	Irritability, poor sleeping pattern, excreted slowly; no effect with usual amount of caffeine beverages	Iodine	Goiter; see miscellaneous, iodine
		Iopanoic acid	None
Captopril	None	Isoniazid	None; acetyl metabolite also secreted; ? hepatotoxic
Carbamazepine	None	K₁ (vitamin)	None
Carbimazole	Goiter	Kanamycin	None
Cascara	None	Ketorolac	—
Cefadroxil	None	Labetalol	None
Cefazolin	None	Levonorgestrel	—
Cefotaxime	None	Lidocaine	None
Cefoxitin	None	Loperamide	—
Cefprozil	—	Magnesium sulfate	None
Ceftazidime	None	Medroxyprogesterone	None
Ceftriaxone	None	Mefenamic acid	None
Chloral hydrate	Sleepiness	Methadone	None if mother receiving ≤20 mg/24 h
Chloroform	None	Methimazole (active metabolite of carbimazole)	None
Chloroquine	None		
Chlorothiazide	None		
Chlorthalidone	Excreted slowly	Methocarbamol	
Cimetidine†	None	Methyldopa	None
Cisapride	None	Methyprylon	None
Cisplatin	Not found in milk	Metoprolol†	None
Clindamycin	None	Metrizamide	Drowsiness
Clogestone	None	Mexiletine	None
Clomipramine	—	Minoxidil	None
Codeine	None	Morphine	None; infant may have significant blood concentration
Colchicine		Moxalactam	None
Contraceptive pill with estrogen/progesterone	Rare breast enlargement; decrease in milk production and protein content (not confirmed in several studies)	Nadolol†	None
		Nalidixic acid	Hemolysis in infant with glucose-6-phosphate dehydrogenase (G-6-PD) deficiency
Cycloserine	None		
D (Vitamin)	None; follow up infant's serum calcium level if mother receives pharmacological doses	Naproxen	—
		Nefopam	None
Danthron	Increased bowel activity	Nifedipine	—
Dapsone	None; sulfonamide detected in infant's urine	Nitrofurantoin	Hemolysis in infant with G-6-PD deficiency
Dexbrompheniramine maleate with d-isoephedrine	Crying, poor sleeping patterns, irritability		

Table continued on following page

TABLE 6

Maternal Medication Usually Compatible with Breast-Feeding* *Continued*

Drug	Reported Sign or Symptom in Infant or Effect on Lactation	Drug	Reported Sign or Symptom in Infant or Effect on Lactation
Norethynodrel	None	Sulfapyridine	Caution in infant with jaundice or G-6-PD deficiency, and ill, stressed, or premature infant; appears in infant's milk
Norsteroids	None		
Noscapine	None		
Oxprenolol	None		
Phenylbutazone	None	Sulfisoxazole	Caution in infant with jaundice or G-6-PD deficiency, and ill, stressed, or premature infant; appears in infant's milk
Phenytoin	Methemoglobinemia (1 case)		
Piroxicam	None		
Prednisone	None		
Procainamide	None	Suprofen	None
Progesterone	None	Terbutaline	None
Propoxyphene	None	Tetracycline	None; negligible absorption by infant
Propranolol	None	Theophylline	Irritability
Propylthiouracil	None	Thiopental	None
Pseudoephedrine†	None	Thiouracil	None mentioned; drug not used in United States
Pyridostigmine	None		
Pyrimethamine	None	Ticarcillin	None
Quinidine	None	Timolol	None
Quinine	None	Tolbutamide	None
Riboflavin	None	Tolmetin	Possible jaundice
Rifampin	None	Trimethoprim/ sulfamethoxazole	None
Scopolamine	—		
Secobarbital	None	Triprolidine	None
Senna	None	Valproic acid	None
Sotalol	—	Verapamil	None
Spironolactone	None	Warfarin	None
Streptomycin	None	Zolpidem	None
Sulbactam	None		

*Drugs listed have been reported in the literature as having the effects listed or no effect. The word "none" means that no observable change was seen in the nursing infant while the mother was ingesting the compound. It is emphasized that most of the literature citations concern single case reports or small series of infants.

†Drug is concentrated in human milk.

TABLE 7

Food and Environmental Agents: Effect on Breast-Feeding

Agent	Reported Sign or Symptom in Infant or Effect on Lactation
Aflatoxin	None
Aspartame	Caution if mother or infant has phenylketonuria
Bromide (photographic laboratory)	Potential absorption and bromide transfer into milk; see Table 6
Cadmium	None reported
Chlordane	None reported
Chocolate (theobromine)	Irritability or increased bowel activity if excess amounts (16 oz/d) consumed by mother
DDT, benzenehexachlorides, dieldrin, aldrin, hepatachlorepoxide	None
Fava beans	Hemolysis in patient with glucose-6-phosphate dehydrogenase (G-6-PD) deficiency
Fluorides	None
Hexachlorobenzene	Skin rash, diarrhea, vomiting, dark urine, neurotoxicity, death
Hexachlorophene	None; possible contamination of milk from nipple washing
Lead	Possible neurotoxicity
Methyl mercury, mercury	May affect neurodevelopment
Monosodium glutamate	None
Polychlorinated biphenyls and polybrominated biphenyls	Lack of endurance, hypotonia, sullen expressionless facies
Tetrachlorethylene-cleaning fluid (perchloroethylene)	Obstructive jaundice, dark urine
Vegetarian diet	Signs of B_{12} deficiency

TABLE 8

Generic Drugs and Corresponding Trade Names*†

Generic	Trade	Generic	Trade
acebutolol	Sectral	flecainide	Tambocor
acetaminophen	Tylenol, Anacin-3, Panadol, Tempra, Phenaphen	flufenamic acid	Arlef (foreign)
		fluoxetine	Prozac
acetazolamide	Diamox	fluvoxamine	—
acitretin	Soriatane	gold sodium thiomalate	Myochrysine
acyclovir	Zovirax	haloperidol	Haldol
allopurinol	Zyloprim	hydralazine	Apresoline
aminosalicylic acid	Rowasa	hydrochlorothiazide	HydroDIURIL
amitriptyline	Elavil, Endep	hydroxychloroquine	Plaquenil
amoxapine	Asendin	ibuprofen	Advil, Motrin
amoxicillin	Amoxil	imipramine	Tofranil, Janimine
amphetamine (dextroamphetamine)	Dexedrine	indomethacin	Indocin
		iopanoic acid	Telepaque
aspartame	NutraSweet	isoniazid	INH
atenolol	Tenormin	kanamycin	Kantrex
azapropazone (apazone)	Not available in US	ketorolac	Toradol
aztreonam	Azactam	labetalol	Normodyne, Trandate
baclofen	Lioresal	levonorgestrel	as Levlen, as Nordette, as Norplant, as Tri-Levlen, as Triphasil
bendroflumethiazide	Naturetin		
bishydroxycoumarin	Dicumarol	lidocaine	Xylocaine
bromocriptine	Parlodel	loperamide	Imodium
butorphanol	Stadol	lorazepam	Ativan
captopril	Capoten	medroxyprogesterone	Provera, Depo-Provera
carbamazepine	Tegretol	mefenamic acid	Ponstel
carbimazole	Neo-mercazole (foreign)	mesoridazine	Serentil
cefadroxil	Duricef	methadone	Dolophine
cefazolin	Ancef, Kefzol	methimazole	Tapazole
cefotaxime	Claforan	methocarbamol	Robaxin
cefprozil	Cefzil	methotrexate (amethopterin)	Folex, Rheumatrex
ceftazidime	Fortaz	methyprylon	Noludar
ceftriaxone	Rocephin	metoclopramide	Reglan
chloramphenicol	Chloromycetin	metoprolol	Lopressor
chloroquine	Aralen	metrizamide	Amipaque
chlorothiazide	Diuril, Chlotride (foreign)	metronidazole	Flagyl, Protostat
chlorpromazine	Thorazine	mexiletine	Mexitil
chlorprothixene	Taractan	midazolam	Versed
chlorthalidone	Hygroton, as Combipres	minoxidil	Loniten, Rogaine
cimetidine	Tagamet	monosodium glutamate	MSG, Accent
cisapride	Benzamide (foreign)	moxalactam	Moxam
cisplatin	Platinol	nadolol	Corgard
clemastine	Tavegil (foreign), Tavist	nalidixic acid	NegGram
clindamycin	Cleocin	naproxen	Naprosyn
clomipramine	Anafranil	nefopam	Acupan (unavailable in US)
colchicine	(Generic only)	nifedipine	Procardia
cyclophosphamide	Cytoxan	nitrofurantoin	Furadantin, Macrodantin
cycloserine	Seromycin	[³H]Norethynodrel	as Enovid
danthron	Dorbane, Istizin	noscapine	Tusscapine
dapsone	(Generic only)	oxprenolol	Trasicor (foreign)
desipramine	Norpramin, Pertofrane	perphenazine	Trilafon, as Etrafon, as Triavil
dexbrompheniramine maleate with *d*-isoephedrine	as Disophrol, as Drixoral	phenindione	Hedulin, Indon (unavailable in US)
		phenylbutazone	Azolid, Butazolidin
dextroamphetamine	Dexedrine	phenytoin	Dilantin
diazepam	Valium	piroxicam	Feldene
digoxin	Lanoxin, Lanoxicaps	prazepam	Centrax
diltiazem	Cardizem	prednisolone	Delta-Cortef, Meti-Derm, Prelone
dipyrone	Diprofarn, Novaldin (unavailable in US)	prednisone	Deltasone, Meticorten, Sterapred
disopyramide	Norpace	primidone	Mysoline
domperidone	Motilium (unavailable in US)	procainamide	Pronestyl
dothiepin	Prothiaden (unavailable in US)	propoxyphene	Darvon, Dolene, SK65
doxepin	Sinequan	propranolol	Inderal
doxorubicin	Adriamycin	propylthiouracil	(Generic only)
dyphylline	Dilor	pseudoephedrine	as Actifed, Novafed, as Sudafed
enalapril	Vasotec	pyridostigmin	Mestinon
ergotamine tartrate with caffeine	as Cafergot	pyrimethamine	Daraprim
		quazepam	Dormalin
estradiol	Estrace	quinine	as Quinamm
ethambutol	Myambutol	rifampin	Rifadin, Rimactane
ethosuximide	Zarontin	secobarbital	Seconal
fentanyl	Sublimaze	senna	Senokot

Table continued on following page

TABLE 8

Generic Drugs and Corresponding Trade Names*† *Continued*

Generic	Trade	Generic	Trade
sotalol	(Investigational)	ticarcillin	as Timentin
spironolactone	Aldactone	timolol	Blocadren, Timoptic
sulbactam	as Unasyn	tinidazole	Fasigyn, Simplotan (unavailable in US)
sulfasalazine (salicylazosulfapyridine)	Azulfidine	tolbutamide	Orinase
		tolmetin	Tolectin
sulfisoxazole	Gantrisin	trazodone	Desyrel
suprofen	Suprol	trimethoprim with sulfamethoxazole	Bactrim, Septra
temazepam	Restoril		
terbutaline	Bricanyl, Brethine	triprolidine	Actidil, as Actifed
tetracycline	Achromycin	valproic acid	Depakene
theophylline	Bronkodyl, Elixophyllin, Slo-Phyllin, Theo-Dur	verapamil	Calan
		warfarin	Coumadin, Panwarfin
thiopental	Pentothal	zolpidem	Ambien
thiouracil	Thiouracil (no longer marketed in US)		

*For convenience, one or more examples of the trade name are given.

†Inclusion of drug names in Table 8 does not constitute an endorsement by the American Academy of Pediatrics of the products listed. Names are included for informational purposes only.

TABLE 9

Trade Names and Generic Equivalents*

Trade	Generic	Trade	Generic
Accent	monosodium glutamate	Corgard	nadolol
Achromycin	tetracycline	Coumadin	warfarin
Actidil	triprolidine	Cytoxan	cyclophosphamide
as Actifed	triprolidine	Daraprim	pyrimethamine
as Actifed	pseudoephedrine	Darvon	propoxyphene
Acupan (unavailable in US)	nefopam	Delta-Cortef	prednisolone
Adriamycin	doxorubicin	Deltasone	prednisone
Advil	ibuprofen	Depakene	valproic acid
Aldactone	spironolactone	Depo-Provera	medroxyprogesterone
Ambien	zolpidem	Desyrel	trazodone
Amipaque	metrizamide	Dexedrine	dextroamphetamine
Amoxil	amoxicillin	Diamox	acetazolamide
Anacin-3	acetamethophan	Dicumarol	bishydroxycoumarin
Anafranil	clomipramine	Dilantin	phenytoin
Ancef	cefazolin	Dilor	dyphylline
Apresoline	hydralazine	Diprofarn (foreign)	dipyrone
Aralen	chloroquine	as Disophrol	dexbrompheniramine maleate
Arlef (foreign)	flufenamic acid	Diuril	chlorothiazide
Asendin	amoxapine	Dolene	propoxyphene
Ativan	lorazepam	Dolophine	methadone
Azactam	aztreonam	Dorbane	danthron
Azolid	phenylbutazone	Dormalin	quazepam
Azulfidine	sulfasalazine	as Drixoral	dexbrompheniramine maleate
Bactrim	trimethoprim with sulfamethoxazole	Duricef	cefadroxil
Benzamide (foreign)	cisapride	Elavil	amitriptyline
Blocadren	timolol	Elixophyllin	theophylline
Brethine	terbutaline	Endep	amitriptyline
Bricanyl	terbutaline	Enovid	[³H]Norethynodrel
Bronkodyl	theophylline	Estrace	estradiol
Butazolidin	phenylbutazone	as Etrafon	perphenazine
as Cafergot	ergotamine tartrate with caffeine	Fasigyn	tinidazole
Calan	verapamil	Feldene	piroxicam
Capoten	captopril	Flagyl	metronidazole
Cardizem	dilitiazem	Folex	methotrexate (amethopterin)
Cefzil	cefprozil	Fortaz	ceftazidime
Centrax	prazepam	Furadantin	nitrofurantoin
Chloromycetin	chloramphenicol	Gantrisin	sulfisoxazole
Chlotride (foreign)	cholothiazide	Haldol	haloperidol
Claforan	cefotaxime	Hedulin	phenindione
Cleocin	clindamycin	HydroDIURIL	hydrochlorothiazide
as Combipres	chlorthalidone	Hygroton	chlorthalidone

*

TABLE 9

Trade Names and Generic Equivalents* *Continued*

Trade	Generic	Trade	Generic
Imodium	loperamide	Restoril	temazepam
Inderal	propranolol	Rheumatrex	methotrexate
Indocin	indomethacin	Rifadin	rifampin
Indon	phenindione	Rifamycin	rifampin
INH	isoniazid	Rimactane	rifampin
Istizin	danthron	Robaxin	methocarbamal
Janimine	imipramine	Rocephin	ceftriaxone
Kantrex	kanamycin	Rogaine	minoxidil
Kefzol	cefazolin	Rowasa	mesalamine
Lanoxicaps	digoxin	Seconal	secobarbital
Lanoxin	digoxin	Sectral	acebutolol
as Levlen	levonorgestrel	Senokot	senna
Lioresal	baclofen	Septra	trimethoprim with sulfamethoxazole
Loniten	minoxidil	Serentil	mesoridazine
Lopressor	metoprolol	Seromycin	cycloserine
Macrodantin	nitrofurantoin	Simplotan (unavailable in US)	tinidazole
Mestinon	pyridostigmine		
Meticorten	prednisone	Sinequan	doxepin
Meti-Derm	prednisolone	SK65	propoxyphene
Mexitil	mexiletine	Slo-Phyllin	theophylline
Motilium	domperidone	Soriatane	acitretin
Motrin	ibuprofen	Sotalol	sotalol
Moxam	moxalactam	Stadol	butorphanol
MSG	monosodium glutamate	Sterapred	prednisone
Myambutol	ethambutol	Sublimaze	fentanyl
Myochrysine	gold sodium thiomalate	as Sudafed	pseudoephedrine
Mysoline	primidone	Suprol	suprofen
Naprosyn	naproxen	Tagamet	cimetidine
Naturetin	bendroflumethiazide	Tambocor	flecainide
NegGram	nalidixic acid	Tapazole	methimazole
Neo-mercazole (foreign)	carbimazole	Taractan	chlorprothixene
Noludar	methyprylon	Tavegil (foreign)	clemastine
as Nordette	levonorgestrel	Tavist	clemastine
Normodyne	labetalol	Tegretol	carbamazepine
Norpace	disopyramide	Telepaque	iopanoic acid
as Norplant	levonorgestrel	Tempra	acetomethophan
Norpramin	desipramine	Tenormin	atenolol
Novafed	pseudoephedrine	Theo-Dur	theophylline
Novaldin (unavailable in US)	dipyrone	Thiouracil (no longer marketed in US)	thiouracil
Nutrasweet	aspartame	Thorazine	chlorpromazine
Orinase	tolbutamide	as Timentin	ticarcillin
Parlodel	bromocriptine	Timoptic	timolol
Panadol	acetomethophan	Tofranil	imipramine
Panwarfin	warfarin	Tolectin	tolmetin
Pentothal	thiopental	Toradol	ketorolac
Pertofrane	desipramine	Trandate	labetalol
Phenaphen	acetomethophan	Trasicor (foreign)	oxprenolol
Plaquenil	hydroxycholoroquine	Triavil	perphenazine
Platinol	cisplatin	Trilafon	perphenazine
Ponstel	mefenamic acid	as Tri-Levlen	levonorgestrel
Prelone	prednisolone	as Triphasil	levonorgestrel
Procardia	nifedipine	Tusscapine (foreign)	noscapine
Pronestyl	procainamide	Tylenol	acetaminophen
Propacil	propylthiouracil	as Unasyn	sulbactam
Prothiaden (unavailable in US)	dothiepin	Valium	diazepam
		Vasotec	enalapril
Protostat	metronidazole	Versed	midazolam
Provera	medroxyprogesterone	Xylocaine	lidocaine
Prozac	fluoxetine	Zarontin	ethosuximide
as Quinamm	quinine	Zovirax	acyclovir
Quine	quinine	Zyloprim	allopurinol
Reglan	metoclopramide		

*Inclusion of drug names in Table 9 does not constitute an endorsement by the American Academy of Pediatrics of the products listed. Names are included for informational purposes only.

APPENDIX 2
SELECTED FORMULAS

Amounts Are Expressed per Liter

	Similac Natural Care Human Milk Fortifier (24 Cal/oz)	Similac Natural Care Preterm Milk in 1:1 Ratio	Preterm Human Milk	Enfamil Human Milk Fortifier	Enfamil HMF Plus Preterm Milk	Casec Protein Supplement	ProMod Protein Supplement	Moducal	Polycose Glucose Polymers	MCTaid	Enfamil w/Iron (20 Cal/oz)	Enfamil Premature Formula w/Iron (20 Cal/oz)	Enfamil Premature Formula w/Iron (24 Cal/oz)	ProSobee
Energy (cal)	806	737	660	140	800						676	676	812	676
Protein (g)	21.8	18.9	16.2	7	23	—			0	0	14.5	20	24	20
% of Total Calories			9.8	20	11.5	100%	100%			0	8.6	12	12	12
Source	Cow's milk plus whey	Human milk, cow's milk plus whey	Human milk	Cow's milk whey: casein 60-40	Human milk, cow's milk	Cow's milk	Whey protein concentrate				Reduced minerals whey, nonfat milk	Whey protein conc, nonfat milk	Whey protein conc, nonfat milk	Soy protein isolate, L-methionine
Amino Acids (mg)														
Histidine	440	455	419	140	559						280	390	470	400
Isoleucine	1300	1180	1056	439	1495						880	1160	1390	800
Leucine	2290	2060	1838	752	2590						1510	1940	2300	1310
Lysine	1870	1500	1129	501	1630						1010	1510	1810	1040
Tryptophan	310	320	328	112	440						220	310	380	210
Phenylalanine	910	855	801	284	1085						570	760	920	850
Tyrosine	820	840	856	329	1185						650	900	1080	590
Threonine	1360	1100	837	381	1218						770	1100	1320	550
Valine	1350	1220	1092	448	1540						900	1220	1460	800
Methionine	555	440	328	142	470						280	450	540	310
Cystine	340	325	309	86	395						173	220	260	156
Fat (g)	44.1	39.5	35	0	35	0		0	0	—	36	35	41	37
% of Total Calories	47.0		48	0	39	0			0	100%	48	44	44	48
Sources	MCT, soy, coconut oils	Human milk; MCT, soy, coconut oils	Human milk		Human milk			Corn starch		100% MCT	Palm olein, soy, coconut, high oleic sunflower	MCT, soy, coconut	MCT, soy, coconut	Palm, soy, coconut, high oleic sunflower
Fatty Acids														
Polyunsaturated (g)			6	0	6						6.8	8.8	10.3	7.1
Saturated (incl. medium chain) (g)			14.7	0	14.7						15.3	22.4	26.2	15.7
Monounsaturated (g)			13.4	0	13.4						13.7	3.9	4.6	14.1
Linoleic Acid (mg)	5645	5650	5650	0	5650						6200	7700	9000	6400
α-Linolenic Acid (mg)			375	0	375						600	1100	1300	700
E:PUFA Ratio	2.5		0.65		8.3						2	4.9	4.9	2
Carbohydrate (g)	86.1	79.5	73	27	100	0		—		0	73	75	90	68
% of Total Calories	42		44	80	50	0		100%	100%	0	43	44	44	40
Source	Hydrolyzed cornstarch, lactose	Lactose, hydrolyzed cornstarch	Human milk	Corn syrup, cow's milk	Human milk, corn syrup, cow's milk			Glucose polymers	Glucose polymers		Lactose	Corn syrup solids, lactose	Corn syrup solids, lactose	Corn syrup solids
Minerals														
Calcium (mg)	1705	478	250	900	1150						530	1120	1340	710
Phosphorus (mg)	853	499	150	450	600						360	560	670	560
Magnesium (mg)	97	65	33	10	43						54	46	55	74
Iron (mg)	3.0	2.0	0.9	0	0.9						12.2	12.2	14.6	12.2
Zinc (mg)	12.2	8.0	3.7	7.1	10.8						6.8	10.1	12.2	8.1
Manganese (μg)	97	50.3	3.6	47.4	51						101	43	51	169
Copper (μg)	2030	1205	380	620	1000						510	850	1010	510
Iodine (μg)	44	113.5	178	0	178						68	169	200	101

Nutrient	For lactose, sucrose, galactose, and cow's milk protein-intolerant infants	Growing ELBW infants	Growing LBW infants	Normal full-term infants					Human milk fortifier
Sodium (mg)	240	320	260	183	350	70	280	314.5	344
Potassium (mg)	810	840	700	730	660	160	500	774	1047
Chloride (mg)	540	690	570	430	760	180	580	619	658
Calcium-phosphorus ratio					2		2	2	2
Selenium (µg)	18.9	14.6	12.2	18.9	16	None added	16	°	°
Chromium (µg)	None added	3.2	2.7	None added	0.3	None added	0.3	None added	None added
Molybdenum (µg)	None added	2	1.7	None added	1.5	None added	1.5	None added	None added
Nonprotein nitrogen (cal/g)									206
Vitamins									
Vitamin A (IU)	2000	10100	8500	2000	10000	9500	480	5280	10081
Vitamin D (IU)	410	2200	1830	410	2200	2100	80	650	1218
Vitamin E (IU)	13.5	51	43	13.5	50	46	3.9	18.2	32.5
Vitamin K (µg)	54	65	54	54	64	44	20	59	97
Thiamine (vitamin B1) (µg)	540	1620	1350	540	1600	1510	89	1060	2030
Riboflavin (vitamin B2) (µg)	610	2400	2000	950	2400	2100	270	2650	5030
Vitamin B6 (µg)	410	1220	1010	410	1200	1140	62	1046	2030
Vitamin B12 (µg)	2	2	1.7	2	2	1.8	0.2	2.4	4.5
Niacin (µg)	6800	32000	27000	6800	32000	30000	2100	21350	40600
Folic Acid (folacin) (µg)	108	280	240	108	280	250	31	165	300
Pantothenic acid (µg)	3400	9700	8100	3400	9600	7300	2300	8865	15428
Biotin (µg)	20	32	27	20	32	27	5.4	152.7	300
Vitamin C (ascorbic acid) (mg)	81	162	135	81	160	116	44	172	300
Choline (mg)	81	97	81	81	89	None added	89	85	81
Inositol (mg)	115	138	115	41	450	None added	450	248	45
Carnitine (mg)	13.5	16.2	13.5	13.5	7	None added	7		
Nucleotides (mg)									
AMP (mg)	None added	None added	None added	26	26	None added	26	26	None added
CMP (mg)	None added	None added	None added	5	5	None added	5	5	None added
GMP (mg)	None added	None added	None added	11	11	None added	11	11	None added
UMP (mg)	None added	None added	None added	4	4	None added	4	4	None added
Other Nutrients									
Cholesterol (mg)	0	7.4	6.1	7.1	150	None added	150		
Taurine (mg)	41	49	41	41	41	None added	41	48	54
Water (g)	910	880	900	910	910	None added	910	898	885
Osmotic Characteristics									
Renal Solute Load (mOsm) Term	179	210	175	132	200	66	137	126.7	147.2
Premature								187.6	233.4
Osmolality (Osm/kg water)	200	310	260	300	425	120	300		280
Osmolarity (mOsm/L)	182	270	230	270	375	100	270		250
Indications	For lactose, sucrose, galactose, and cow's milk protein-intolerant infants	Growing ELBW infants	Growing LBW infants	Normal full-term infants					Human milk fortifier

Amounts Are Expressed per Liter *Continued*

	Nutramigen	Pregestimil Liquid (20 Cal/oz)	Pregestimil Powder (20 Cal/oz)	Pregestimil Liquid (24 Cal/oz)	Alimentum	Similac w/Iron 20 (improved)	Similac Special Care 24 w/ or w/o Iron	Similac PM 60/40 20 (from powder)	Isomil 20	Human Milk (mature)	Similac NeoCare (22 Cal/oz)
Energy (cal)	676	676	676	812	676	676	806	676	676	680	744
Protein (g)	19	19	19	23	18.9	14.0	21.8	14.9	18.2	10.2	19.3
% of Total Calories	11.4	11.4	11.4	11.4	11.2	8.3	10.8	8.8	10.8	6.0	10.0
Source	Casein hydrolysate, amino acids	Casein hydrolysate, amino acids	Casein hydrolysate, amino acids	Casein hydrolysate, amino acids	Casein hydrolysate, amino acid	Cow's milk and whey	Cow's milk and whey	Whey and caseinate	Soy protein isolate, L-methionine		Cow's milk and whey
Amino Acids (mg)											
Histidine	570	570	570	690	520	310	460	335			490
Isoleucine	1140	1140	1140	1380	1090	740	1210	905			1130
Leucine	1940	1940	1940	2300	1720	1370	2270	1580			2020
Lysine	1630	1630	1630	2000	1690	1220	1850	1310			1570
Tryptophan	300	300	300	370	310	210	370	265			305
Phenylalanine	910	910	910	1110	860	610	810	600			910
Tyrosine	420	420	420	510	400	570	770	560			740
Threonine	930	930	930	1130	880	750	1330	960			1120
Valine	1430	1430	1430	1730	1410	790	1280	940			1160
Methionine	590	590	590	710	520	370	550	400			520
Cystine	300	300	300	370	300	220	410	300			360
Fat (g)	34	38	38	45	37.2	36.5	43.5	38.0	37.2	38.8	40.9
% of Total Calories	45	48	48	48	49.5	48.6	48.6	50.4	49.5	51.3	49.0
Sources	Palm olein, soy, coconut, high oleic sunflower	MCT, soy, high oleic safflower	MCT, corn, soy, high oleic safflower	MCT, soy, high oleic safflower	MCT, safflower, soy oils	High-oleic safflower, coconut, and soy oils	MCT, soy, coconut oils	Corn, coconut, soy oils	High-oleic safflower, coconut, and soy oils		Soy, high-oleic safflower, MCT, and coconut oils
Fatty Acids											
Polyunsaturated (g)	6.4	8.6	8.1	10.2							
Saturated (incl. medium chain) (g)	14.6	23.3	23.1	27.7							
Monounsaturated (g)	12.9	6.2	6.8	7.4							
Linoleic Acid (mg)	5800	7600	7600	9000	10,811	6757	5645	8784	6757	3973	5580
α-Linolenic Acid (mg)	600	1000	500	1200							
E:PUFA Ratio	2.1	3	3.2	3	1.1	1.1	2.5	1.0	1.0	0.5	
Carbohydrate (g)	74	69	69	83	68.9	73.0	85.5	68.9	68.2	72.1	76.6
% of Total Calories	44	41	41	41	40.8	43.2	42.4	40.8	40.4	42.4	41.0
Source	Corn syrup solids, modified corn starch, glucose polymers	Corn syrup solids, modified corn starch	Corn syrup solids, dextrose, modified corn starch	Corn syrup solids, modified corn starch	Sucrose, modified tapioca starch	Lactose	Hydrolyzed corn starch, lactose	Lactose	Corn syrup, sucrose	Lactose	Corn syrup solids, lactose
Minerals											
Calcium (mg)	640	780	640	930	709	527	1452	380	709	279	781
Phosphorus (mg)	430	510	430	610	507	284	726	190	507	143	461
Magnesium (mg)	74	81	74	97	50.7	40.5	96.8	40.7	50.7	34.7	67
Iron (mg)	12.2	12.7	12.7	15.3	12.2	12.2	3.2 or 14.5	1.5	12.2	0.0	13.4
Zinc (mg)	6.8	7.4	6.4	8.9	5.1	5.1	12.1	5.1	5.1	1.2	8.9
Manganese (μg)	169	200	210	240	202.7	33.8	96.8	33.8	168.9	6.8	74.6
Copper (μg)	510	740	640	890	507	608	2016	608	507	252	896
Iodine (μg)	101	74	47	89	101	41	48	41	101	110	112

	1	2	3	4	5	6	7	8	9	10	11
Sodium (mg)	320	320	260	380	297	162	347	162	297	177	246
Potassium (mg)	740	74	740	890	797	709	1040	581	730	524	1060
Chloride (mg)	580	580	580	700	541	439	653	399	419	422	560
Calcium:phosphorus ratio					1.4	1.9	2.0	2.0	1.4	2.0	1.7
Selenium (µg)	18.9	18.9	18.9	23	20	15	°	°	14	°	°
Chromium (µg)	None added	None added	None added	None added	None added	None added	None added	None added	None added	None added	None added
Molybdenum (µg)	None added	None added	None added	None added	None added	None added	None added	None added	None added	None added	None added
Nonprotein calorie to nitrogen ratio					198	277	206	259	206	392	215
Vitamins											
Vitamin A (IU)	2000	2600	2600	3100	2027	2027	10081	2035	2027	2231	3422
Vitamin D (IU)	410	430	510	510	405	405	1210	407	405	20	595
Vitamin E (IU)	13.5	26	26	31	20.3	20.3	32.3	17.0	20.3	3.4	26.8
Vitamin K (µg)	54	127	127	153	101.4	54.1	96.8	54.3	74.3	2.0	82
Thiamine (vitamin B1) (µg)	540	540	530	650	405	676	2016	678	405	211	1637
Riboflavin (vitamin B2) (µg)	610	610	640	730	608	1014	5000	1017	608	347	1116
Vitamin B6 (µg)	410	410	430	490	405	405	2016	407	405	204	744
Vitamin B12 (µg)	2	2	2.1	2.4	2.70	1.69	4.03	2.03	2.70	0.68	3.0
Niacin (µg)	6800	6500	8500	8100	9122	7095	40323	7122	9122	1503	14508
Folic Acid (folacin) (µg)	108	108	106	130	101.4	101.4	298.4	101.7	101.4	50.3	186
Pantothenic acid (µg)	3400	3400	3200	4100	5068	3041	15323	3052	5068	1803	5952
Biotin (µg)	20	20	53	24	30.4	29.7	298.4	30.5	30.4	4.1	67.0
Vitamin C (ascorbic acid) (mg)	81	81	79	97	60.8	60.8	298.4	61.0	60.8	40.8	112
Choline (mg)	81	81	90	97	54.1	108.1	80.6	81.4	54.1	89.8	119
Inositol (mg)	115	115	32	138	33.8	31.8	44.4	162.8	33.8	149.0	45
Carnitine (mg)	13.5	13.5	13.5	16.2	10.8	11.5	47.6	11.5	10.8		44.0
Nucleotides (mg)											
AMP (mg)	None added	None added	None added	None added	None added	72	None added	None added	None added		None added
CMP (mg)	None added	None added	None added	None added	None added	11	None added	None added	None added		None added
GMP (mg)	None added	None added	None added	None added	None added	30	None added	None added	None added		None added
UMP (mg)	None added	None added	None added	None added	None added	15	None added	None added	None added		None added
Other Nutrients											
Cholesterol (mg)	2.2	2.2	2.2	2.7	None added	16	None added	None added	None added		None added
Taurine (mg)	41	41	41	49	45.3	45.4	54.0	45.4	45.3	40.1	50.0
Water (g)	910	900	910	880	899	899	879	905	899	878	888
Osmotic Characteristics											
Renal Solute Load (mOsm) — Term	172	174	169	210	124.3	93.5	147.2	93.0	116.4	73.8	130.8
Premature					185.8	133.8	226.4	129.4	176.8	99.5	192.0
Osmolality (Osm/kg water)	320	280	320	320	350	270	270	250	220	255	290
Osmolarity (mOsm/L)	290	250	290	280	330	270	270	220	220		260
Indications	For infants intolerant of cow's milk formulas	For fat-intolerant infants, those post NEC, small preemies with feeding intolerance			Hypoallergenic	Normal full-term infants	Growing LBW premature infants	Low mineral content	Lactose-free soy formula		For conditions such as prematurity

°Data not available.

Data courtesy of Mead Johnson Company and Ross Products Division, Abbott Laboratories.

Estimated Daily Requirements of Premature Infants*†: Growth and Nongrowth

	Body Weight Intervals (g)								
	750–1000	1000–1250	1250–1500	1500–1750	1750–2000	2000–2250	2250–2500	2500–2750	2750–3000
Energy									
Growth (kcal)	21	46	68	79	93	104	114	111	108
Nongrowth (kcal)	71	94	117	133	156	180	204	215	239
Total (kal/kg)	105	124	127	130	133	133	134	124	121
Protein									
Growth (g)	1.78	3.45	4.44	4.79	4.85	4.90	4.68	4.27	3.77
Nongrowth (g)	0.87	1.12	1.37	1.62	1.87	2.12	2.37	2.62	2.87
Total (g/kg)‡	3.02	4.06	4.22	3.94	3.58	3.30	2.96	2.62	2.30
Sodium									
Growth (mEq)	0.95	1.68	2.10	2.21	2.21	2.21	2.10	1.89	1.57
Nongrowth (mEq)	0.18	0.23	0.28	0.34	0.39	0.44	0.49	0.55	0.60
Total (mEq/kg)	1.29	1.69	1.73	1.56	1.38	1.24	1.09	0.92	0.75
Potassium									
Growth (mEq)	0.31	0.73	1.05	1.15	1.26	1.36	1.36	1.36	1.15
Nongrowth (mEq)	0.20	0.26	0.32	0.38	0.43	0.49	0.55	0.61	0.66
Total (mEq/kg)	0.58	0.88	0.99	0.94	0.90	0.87	0.80	0.75	0.63
Calcium									
Growth (mg)	148	317	442	530	592	632	660	627	592
Nongrowth (mg)	—	—	—	—	—	—	—	—	—
Total (mg/kg)	169	282	321	326	316	300	278	239	206
Phosphorus									
Growth (mg)	49	110	148	172	188	197	202	194	177
Nongrowth (mg)	12	27	37	43	47	49	50	49	44
Total (mg/kg)	70	121	135	132	125	116	106	93	77
Magnesium									
Growth (mg)	9.0	18.5	25.5	30.0	33.5	35.5	37.0	35.5	32.5
Nongrowth (mg)	—	—	—	—	—	—	—	—	—
Total (mg/kg)	10.3	16.4	18.6	18.5	17.8	16.7	15.6	13.5	11.3

*Assuming extent of intestinal absorption as follows: energy: 75% absorption for infants weighing 750–1500 g, 80% for those weighing 1500–2500 g, and 85% for those weighing more than 2500 g; protein: 75% absorption at 750–1250 g, 77% at 1250–1500 g, 80% at 1500–2250 g, 83% at 2250–2500 g, and 85% above 2500 g; sodium and potassium, 95% absorption throughout; calcium, 40%, phosphorus, 80%, magnesium, 20% throughout.

†See also chapter on nutrition.

‡Based on arithmetic mean weight for the weight interval. (Data of O'Donnell AM, Ziegler EE, Fomon SJ. Reproduced with permission of Dr. Fomon.)

APPENDIX **3**
ILLUSTRATIVE FORMS AND NORMAL VALUES

Neuromuscular Maturity

	-1	0	1	2	3	4	5
Posture							
Square Window (wrist)	>90°	90°	60°	45°	30°	0°	
Arm Recoil		180°	140°-180°	110°-140°	90-110°	<90°	
Popliteal Angle	180°	160°	140°	120°	100°	90°	<90°
Scarf Sign							
Heel to Ear							

Physical Maturity

Skin	sticky friable transparent	gelatinous red, translucent	smooth pink, visible veins	superficial peeling &/or rash. few veins	cracking pale areas rare veins	parchment deep cracking no vessels	leathery cracked wrinkled
Lanugo	none	sparse	abundant	thinning	bald areas	mostly bald	
Plantar Surface	heel-toe 40-50mm:-1 <40mm:-2	>50mm no crease	faint red marks	anterior transverse crease only	creases ant. 2/3	creases over entire sole	
Breast	imperceptible	barely perceptible	flat areola no bud	stippled areola 1-2mm bud	raised areola 3-4mm bud	full areola 5-10mm bud	
Eye/Ear	lids fused loosely:-1 tightly:-2	lids open pinna flat stays folded	sl. curved pinna; soft; slow recoil	well-curved pinna; soft but ready recoil	formed &firm instant recoil	thick cartilage ear stiff	
Genitals male	scrotum flat, smooth	scrotum empty faint rugae	testes in upper canal rare rugae	testes descending few rugae	testes down good rugae	testes pendulous deep rugae	
Genitals female	clitoris prominent labia flat	prominent clitoris small labia minora	prominent clitoris enlarging minora	majora & minora equally prominent	majora large minora small	majora cover clitoris & minora	

Maturity Rating

score	weeks
-10	20
-5	22
0	24
5	26
10	28
15	30
20	32
25	34
30	36
35	38
40	40
45	42
50	44

Expanded New Ballard Score includes extremely premature infants and has been refined to improve accuracy in more mature infants. (From Ballard JL, Khoury JC, Wedig K, et al: New Ballard Score, expanded to include extremely premature infants. J Pediatr 119:417–423, 1991.)

Correlations Between Gestation Length and Embryonic and Fetal Bodily Dimensions

Week of Gestation	Crown-Rump Length (cm)	Weight (cm)	Biparietal Diameter (cm)
6	0.5		
7	0.8	0.07	
8	1.5	0.22	
9	2.5	0.88	
10	3.5	3.5	
11	4.6	6.0	
12	5.7	11.0	
13	6.8	19.0	
14	8.1	33.0	
15	9.4	55.0	
16	10.7	80.0	
17	12.1	120.0	3.7
18	13.6	170.0	4.0
19	15.3	253.0	4.4
20	16.4	316.0	4.8
21	17.5	385.0	5.2
22	18.6	460.0	5.5
23	19.7	542.0	5.75
24	20.8	630.0	5.95
25	21.8	723.0	6.1
26	22.8	823.0	6.2
27	23.8	930.0	6.35
28	24.7	1045.0	6.5
29	25.6	1174.0	6.65
30	26.5	1323.0	6.85
31	27.4	1492.0	7.1
32	28.3	1680.0	7.3
33	29.3	1876.0	7.6
34	30.2	2074.0	7.8
35	31.1	2274.0	8.1
36	32.1	2478.0	8.35
37	33.1	2690.0	8.6
38	34.1	2914.0	8.9
39	35.1	3150.0	9.2
40	36.2	3405.0	9.55
41		3600.0	9.8
42		3650.0	9.85
		3750.0	10.0
		3900.0	10.2
		4000.0	10.3
		4200.0	10.6

Data based on the study of Bartolucci L: Am J Obstet Gynecol 122:439, 1975. Courtesy of Iffy L, et al: Pediatrics 56:173, 1975.

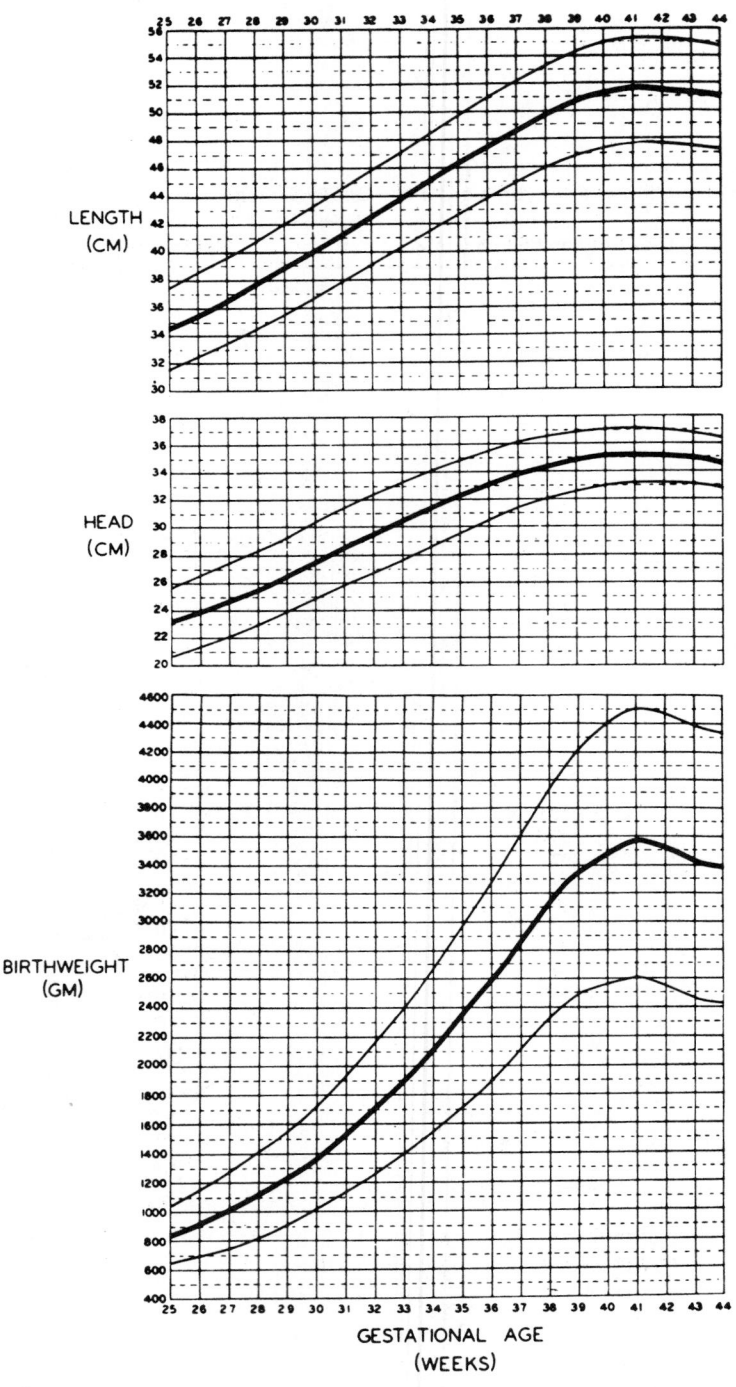

Intrauterine growth curves. (From Usher R, McLean F: J Pediatr 74:901, 1969.)

Longitudinal Head Circumference of 450 Infants; Single-Point Measurements From National Center for Health Statistics (NCHS) Norm

| | Mean ± SD Birth Weight (g) | | | | | | | | NCHS Norms | |
Corrected Age	501–750 (635 ± 61) n = 14	751–1000 (893 ± 53) n = 40	1001–1250 (1138 ± 76) n = 68	1251–1500 (1377 ± 70) n = 84	1501–1750 (1633 ± 73) n = 72	1751–2000 (1876 ± 70) n = 72	2001–2250 (2109 ± 68) n = 60	2251–2500 (2368 ± 93) n = 40	Boys	Girls
Birth	22.3 ± 0.9	23.9 ± 0.8	25.4 ± 0.8	27.5 ± 0.9	28.2 ± 1.0	29.4 ± 0.8	30.7 ± 0.7	31.7 ± 0.8	34.6 ± 0.8	34.1 ± 0.6
40 wk	31.3 ± 1.3	33.8 ± 1.4	34.7 ± 1.9	34.7 ± 1.3	36.9 ± 0.6	35.7 ± 1.2	36.1 ± 1.9	35.0 ± 1.2	34.6 ± 0.8	34.1 ± 0.6
1 mo	34.3 ± 1.0	34.7 ± 1.2	36.4 ± 1.5	36.7 ± 2.3	35.1 ± 1.4	38.0 ± 1.8	37.0 ± 1.9	36.7 ± 0.2	37.3 ± 0.7	36.5 ± 0.6
3 mo	39.5 ± 1.3	39.3 ± 1.7	40.7 ± 1.9	40.4 ± 2.2	40.7 ± 2.4	40.8 ± 1.1	39.7 ± 0.5	40.7 ± 1.2	40.6 ± 0.8	39.5 ± 0.7
6 mo	40.3 ± 0.9	41.6 ± 1.4	41.3 ± 1.5	43.6 ± 1.2	42.6 ± 1.6	43.9 ± 0.8	44.1 ± 1.8	43.0 ± 1.5	43.7 ± 0.7	42.4 ± 0.7
9 mo	42.1 ± 0.9	43.8 ± 1.0	43.9 ± 1.5	44.7 ± 0.8	45.3 ± 2.5	44.3 ± 0.9	45.7 ± 2.0	46.7 ± 1.5	45.8 ± 0.7	44.4 ± 0.7
12 mo	43.7 ± 2.3	45.0 ± 1.9	44.5 ± 1.7	46.3 ± 2.4	45.0 ± 1.6	46.7 ± 1.6	46.4 ± 0.6	45.2 ± 0.4	47.1 ± 0.7	45.6 ± 0.7
15 mo	45.9 ± 1.8	45.3 ± 1.7	45.9 ± 1.5	47.2 ± 1.1	47.9 ± 1.8	47.7 ± 1.4	47.0 ± 0.1	47.5 ± 0.9	NA°	NA°
18 mo	45.9 ± 1.3	45.8 ± 1.3	47.0 ± 1.1	47.4 ± 1.0	47.0 ± 1.5	47.9 ± 1.7	47.2 ± 0.5	47.4 ± 0.7	48.3 ± 0.7	47.1 ± 0.7

°NA indicates not available.

From Sheth RD, Mullett MD, Bodensteiner JB, Hobbs GR: Longitudinal head growth in developmentally normal. Arch Pediatr Adolesc Med 149:1360, 1995. Copyright 1995, American Medical Association.

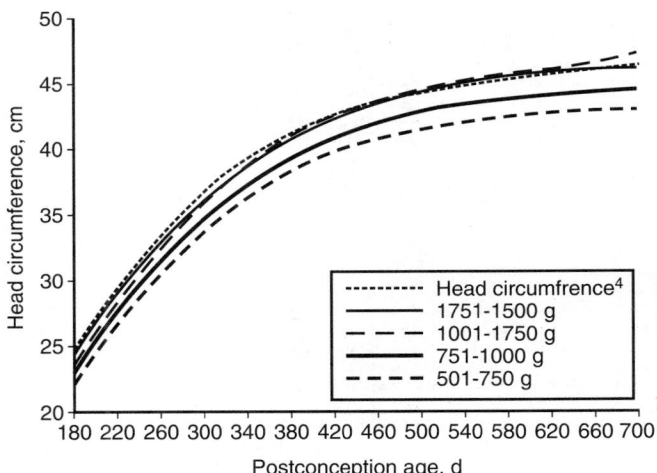

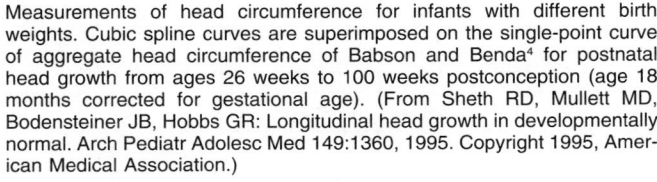

Measurements of head circumference for infants with different birth weights. Cubic spline curves are superimposed on the single-point curve of aggregate head circumference of Babson and Benda[4] for postnatal head growth from ages 26 weeks to 100 weeks postconception (age 18 months corrected for gestational age). (From Sheth RD, Mullett MD, Bodensteiner JB, Hobbs GR: Longitudinal head growth in developmentally normal. Arch Pediatr Adolesc Med 149:1360, 1995. Copyright 1995, American Medical Association.)

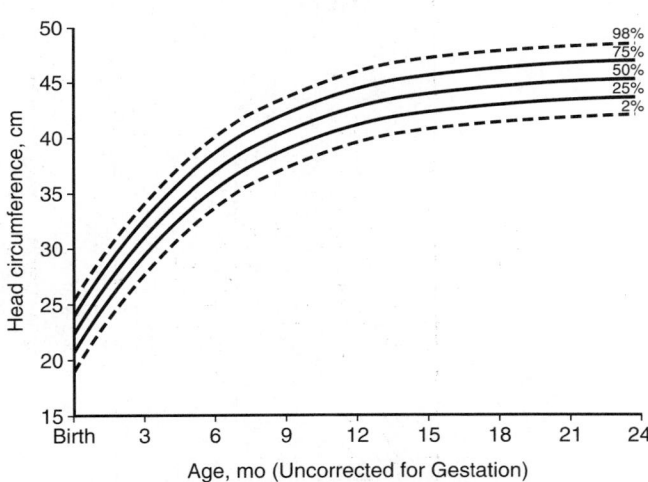

Percentile grid for growth of longitudinal head circumference for infants with a birth weight of 501 to 1000 g plotted from birth to age 24 months (actual age). (From Sheth RD, Mullett MD, Bodensteiner JB, Hobbs GR: Longitudinal head growth in developmentally normal. Arch Pediatr Adolesc Med 149:1360, 1995. Copyright 1995, American Medical Association.)

IHDP Growth Percentiles:
VLBW Premature Girls[1,2]
(≤1500 g BW, ≤37 wk GA)

Name_____

Record #_____

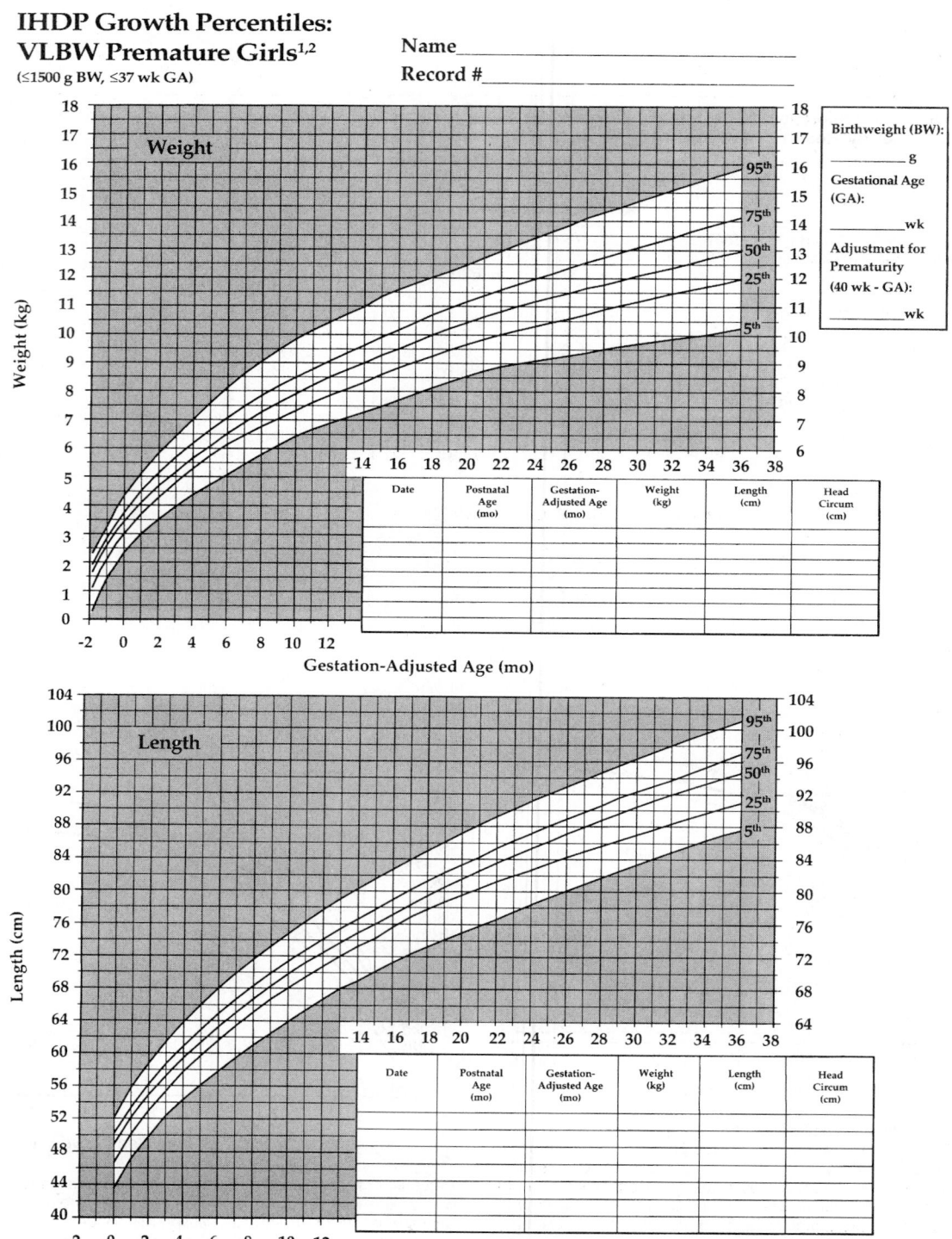

Birthweight (BW):

_____ g

Gestational Age (GA):

_____ wk

Adjustment for Prematurity (40 wk - GA):

_____ wk

IHDP Growth Percentiles: VLBW Premature Girls[1,2]

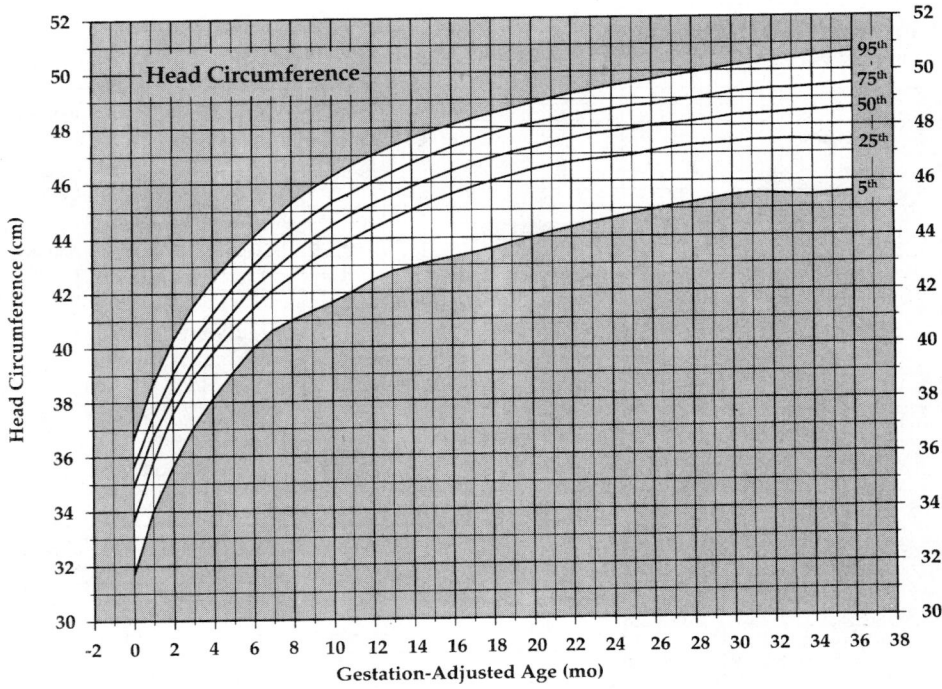

Growth of very-low-birth-weight (VLBW, ≤1500 g) and low-birth-weight (LBW, 1501 to 2500 g) premature (≤37 weeks, GA) infants differ from that of normal-birth-weight term infants during infancy and early childhood. Because these infants may not catch up to term infants in growth during the early years, their growth should be compared to that of premature infants of similar birth weight.

The growth percentiles presented here are based on a large sample of infants enrolled in the Infant Health and Development Program (IHDP).[1,2] Some infants most likely to experience growth problems from biologic or environmental causes, premature infants with birth weight greater than 2500 g, and small-for-gestational-age term infants were excluded.[1] Study infants, however, are probably typical of premature infants who receive modern neonatal intensive care.

References

1. The Infant Health and Development Program: Enhancing the outcomes of low-birth-weight, premature infants. *JAMA* 1990;263(22):3035–3042.
2. Casey PH, Kraemer HC, Bernbaum J, et al: Growth status and growth rates of a varied sample of low birth weight, preterm infants: A longitudinal cohort from birth to three years of age. *J Pediatr* 1991;119:599–605.

IHDP studies were supported by grants from the Robert Wood Johnson Foundation, Pew Charitable Trusts, and the Bureau of Maternal and Child Health, US Department of Health and Human Services. These graphs were prepared by SS Guo and AF Roche, Wright State University, Yellow Springs, Ohio. IHDP, its sponsors, and the investigators do not endorse specific products.

Courtesy of Ross Products Division, Abbott Laboratories, Columbus, OH.

Instructions for Use

1. Measure and record weight, length, and head circumference.
2. Calculate gestation-adjusted age by subtracting Adjustment for Prematurity in weeks from postnatal age in weeks. Adjustment for Prematurity equals 40 weeks minus GA. For example, at 12 wk postnatal age, an infant born at 30 wk GA would be 2 wk (0.5 mo) gestation-adjusted age.

IHDP Growth Percentiles:
LBW Premature Girls[1,2]
(1501 to 2500 g BW, ≤37 wk GA)

Name_____

Record #_____

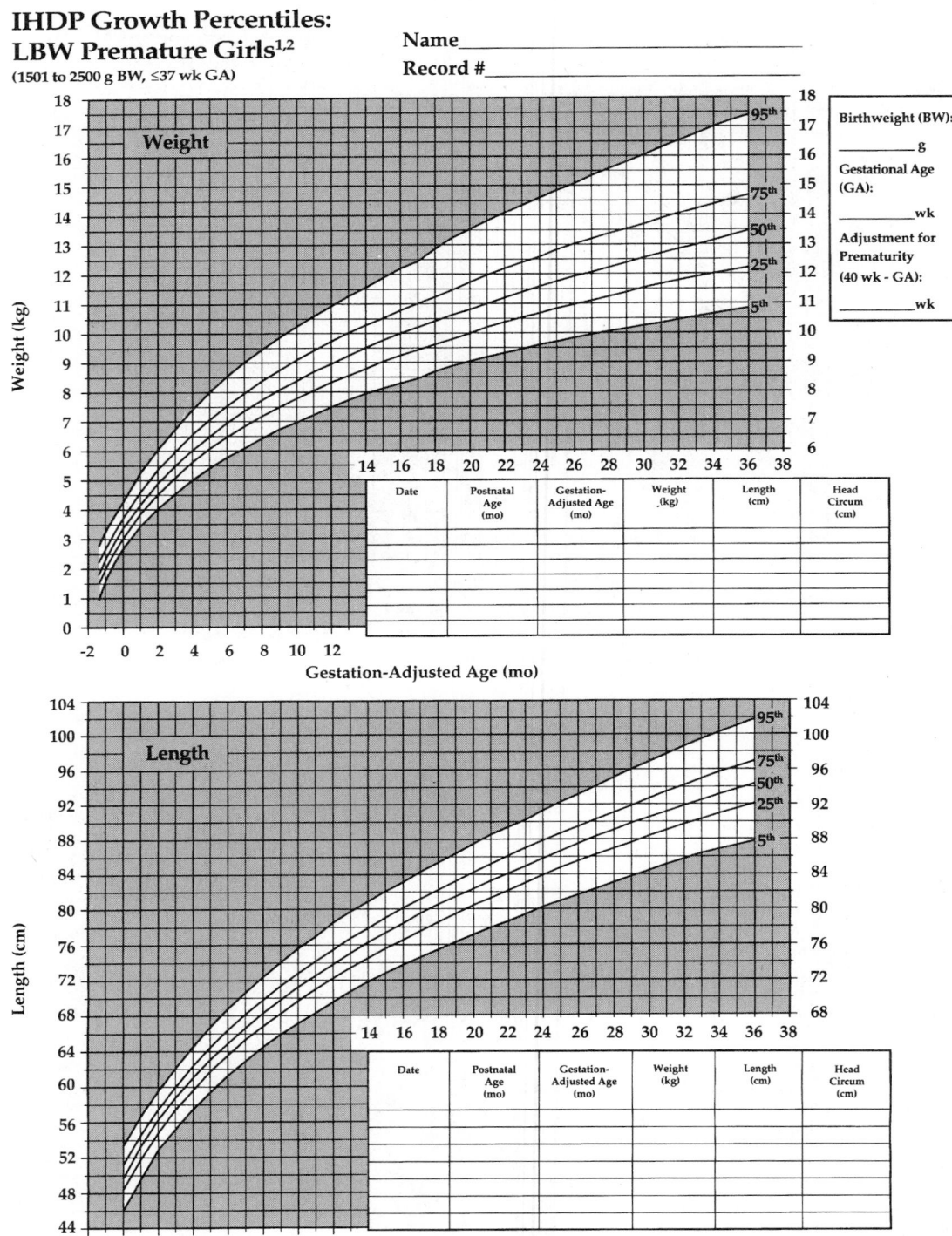

Birthweight (BW):

_____ g

Gestational Age (GA):

_____ wk

Adjustment for Prematurity (40 wk - GA):

_____ wk

Date	Postnatal Age (mo)	Gestation-Adjusted Age (mo)	Weight (kg)	Length (cm)	Head Circum (cm)

Date	Postnatal Age (mo)	Gestation-Adjusted Age (mo)	Weight (kg)	Length (cm)	Head Circum (cm)

IHDP Growth Percentiles: LBW Premature Girls[1,2]

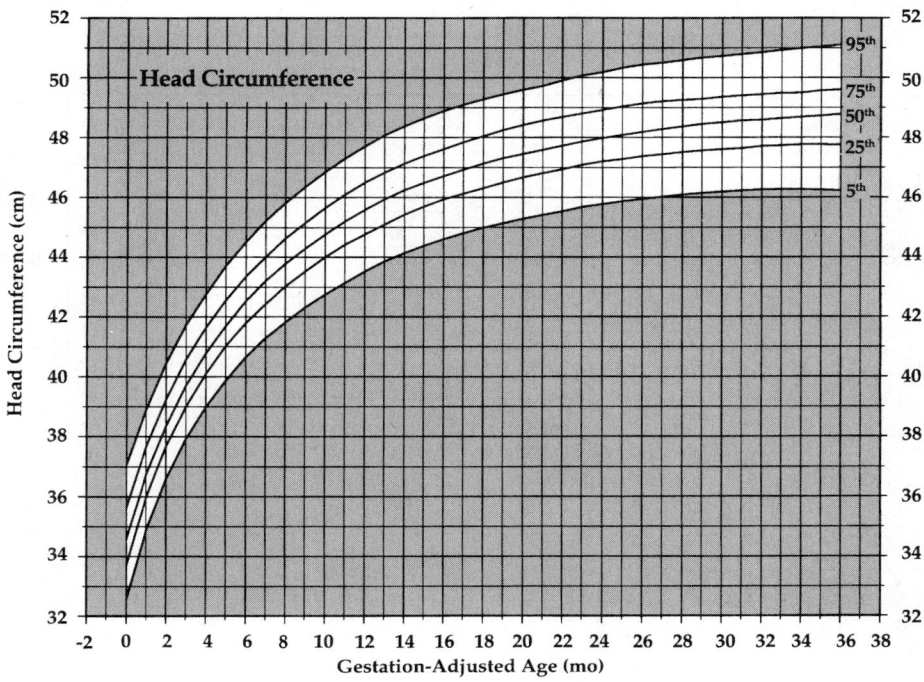

Growth of very-low-birth-weight (VLBW, ≤1500 g) and low-birth-weight (LBW, 1501 to 2500 g) premature (≤37 weeks, GA) infants differ from that of normal-birth-weight term infants during infancy and early childhood. Because these infants may not catch up to term infants in growth during the early years, their growth should be compared to that of premature infants of similar birth weight.

The growth percentiles presented here are based on a large sample of infants enrolled in the Infant Health and Development Program (IHDP).[1,2] Some infants most likely to experience growth problems from biologic or environmental causes, premature infants with birth weight greater than 2500 g, and small-for-gestational-age term infants were excluded.[1] Study infants, however, are probably typical of premature infants who receive modern neonatal intensive care.

Instructions for Use

1. Measure and record weight, length, and head circumference.
2. Calculate gestation-adjusted age by subtracting Adjustment for Prematurity in weeks from postnatal age in weeks. Adjustment for Prematurity equals 40 weeks minus GA. For example, at 12 wk postnatal age, an infant born at 30 wk GA would be 2 wk (0.5 mo) gestation-adjusted age.

References

1. The Infant Health and Development Program: Enhancing the outcomes of low-birth-weight, premature infants. *JAMA* 1990;263(22):3035–3042.
2. Casey PH, Kraemer HC, Bernbaum J, et al: Growth status and growth rates of a varied sample of low birth weight, preterm infants: A longitudinal cohort from birth to three years of age. *J Pediatr* 1991;119:599–605.

IHDP studies were supported by grants from the Robert Wood Johnson Foundation, Pew Charitable Trusts, and the Bureau of Maternal and Child Health, US Department of Health and Human Services. These graphs were prepared by SS Guo and AF Roche, Wright State University, Yellow Springs, Ohio. IHDP, its sponsors, and the investigators do not endorse specific products.

Courtesy of Ross Products Division, Abbott Laboratories, Columbus, OH.

IHDP Growth Percentiles: VLBW Premature Boys[1,2]
(≤1500 g BW, ≤37 wk GA)

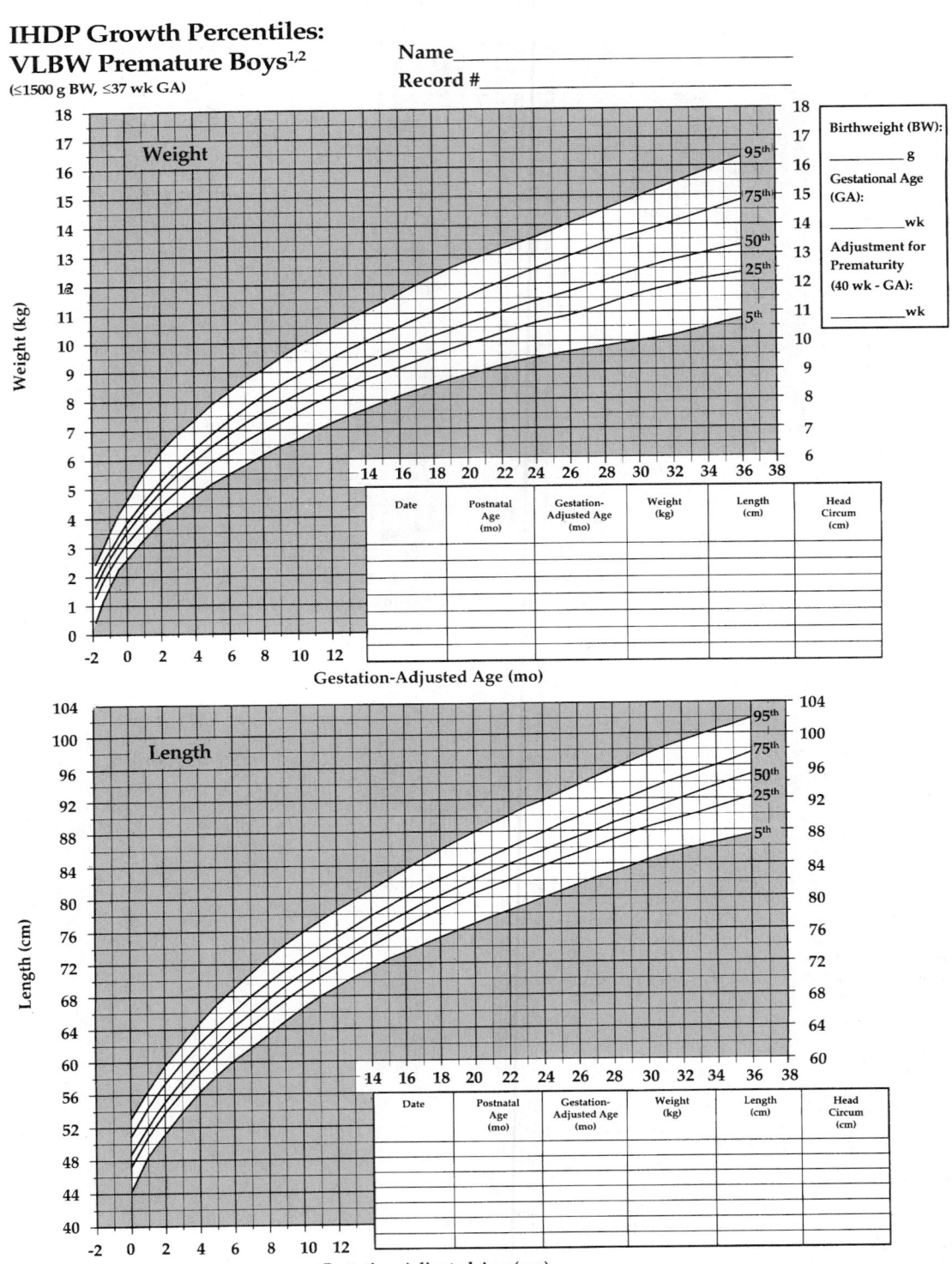

Name_____

Record #_____

Birthweight (BW):

_____ g

Gestational Age (GA):

_____ wk

Adjustment for Prematurity (40 wk - GA):

_____ wk

Date	Postnatal Age (mo)	Gestation-Adjusted Age (mo)	Weight (kg)	Length (cm)	Head Circum (cm)

Date	Postnatal Age (mo)	Gestation-Adjusted Age (mo)	Weight (kg)	Length (cm)	Head Circum (cm)

IHDP Growth Percentiles: VLBW Premature Boys[1,2]

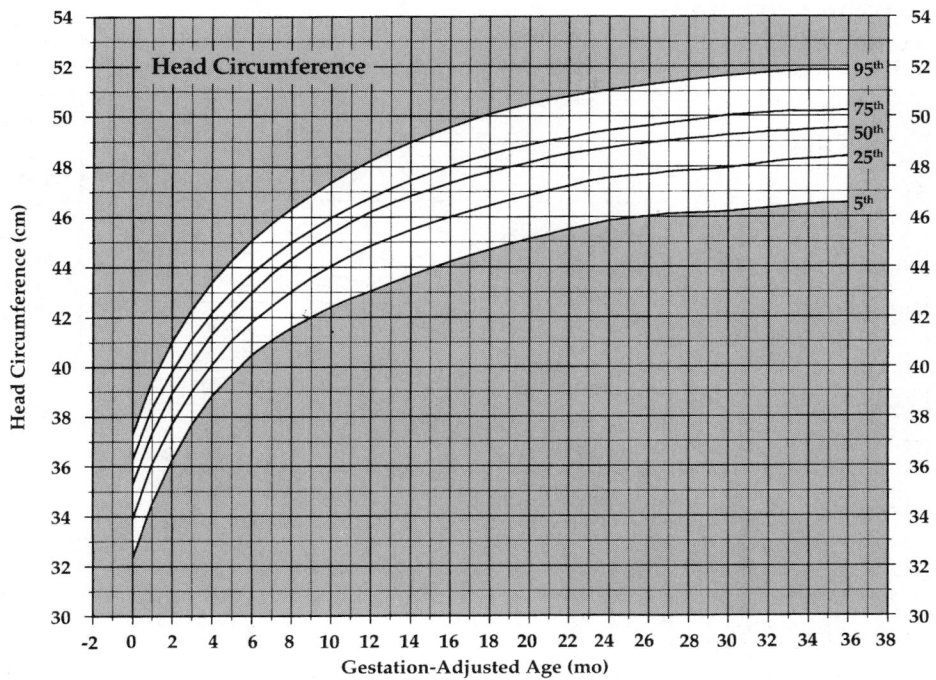

Growth of very-low-birth-weight (VLBW, ≤1500 g) and low-birth-weight (LBW, 1501 to 2500 g) premature (≤37 weeks, GA) infants differ from that of normal-birth-weight term infants during infancy and early childhood. Because these infants may not catch up to term infants in growth during the early years, their growth should be compared to that of premature infants of similar birth weight.

The growth percentiles presented here are based on a large sample of infants enrolled in the Infant Health and Development Program (IHDP).[1,2] Some infants most likely to experience growth problems from biologic or environmental causes, premature infants with birth weight greater than 2500 g, and small-for-gestational-age term infants were excluded.[1] Study infants, however, are probably typical of premature infants who receive modern neonatal intensive care.

Instructions for Use

1. Measure and record weight, length, and head circumference.
2. Calculate gestation-adjusted age by subtracting Adjustment for Prematurity in weeks from postnatal age in weeks. Adjustment for Prematurity equals 40 weeks minus GA. For example, at 12 wk postnatal age, an infant born at 30 wk GA would be 2 wk (0.5 mo) gestation-adjusted age.

References

1. The Infant Health and Development Program: Enhancing the outcomes of low-birth-weight, premature infants. *JAMA* 1990;263(22):3035–3042.
2. Casey PH, Kraemer HC, Bernbaum J, et al: Growth status and growth rates of a varied sample of low birth weight, preterm infants: A longitudinal cohort from birth to three years of age. *J Pediatr* 1991;119:599–605.

IHDP studies were supported by grants from the Robert Wood Johnson Foundation, Pew Charitable Trusts, and the Bureau of Maternal and Child Health, US Department of Health and Human Services. These graphs were prepared by SS Guo and AF Roche, Wright State University, Yellow Springs, Ohio. IHDP, its sponsors, and the investigators do not endorse specific products.

Courtesy of Ross Products Division, Abbott Laboratories, Columbus, OH.

IHDP Growth Percentiles:
LBW Premature Boys[1,2]
(1501 to 2500 g BW, ≤37 wk GA)

Name_____

Record #_____

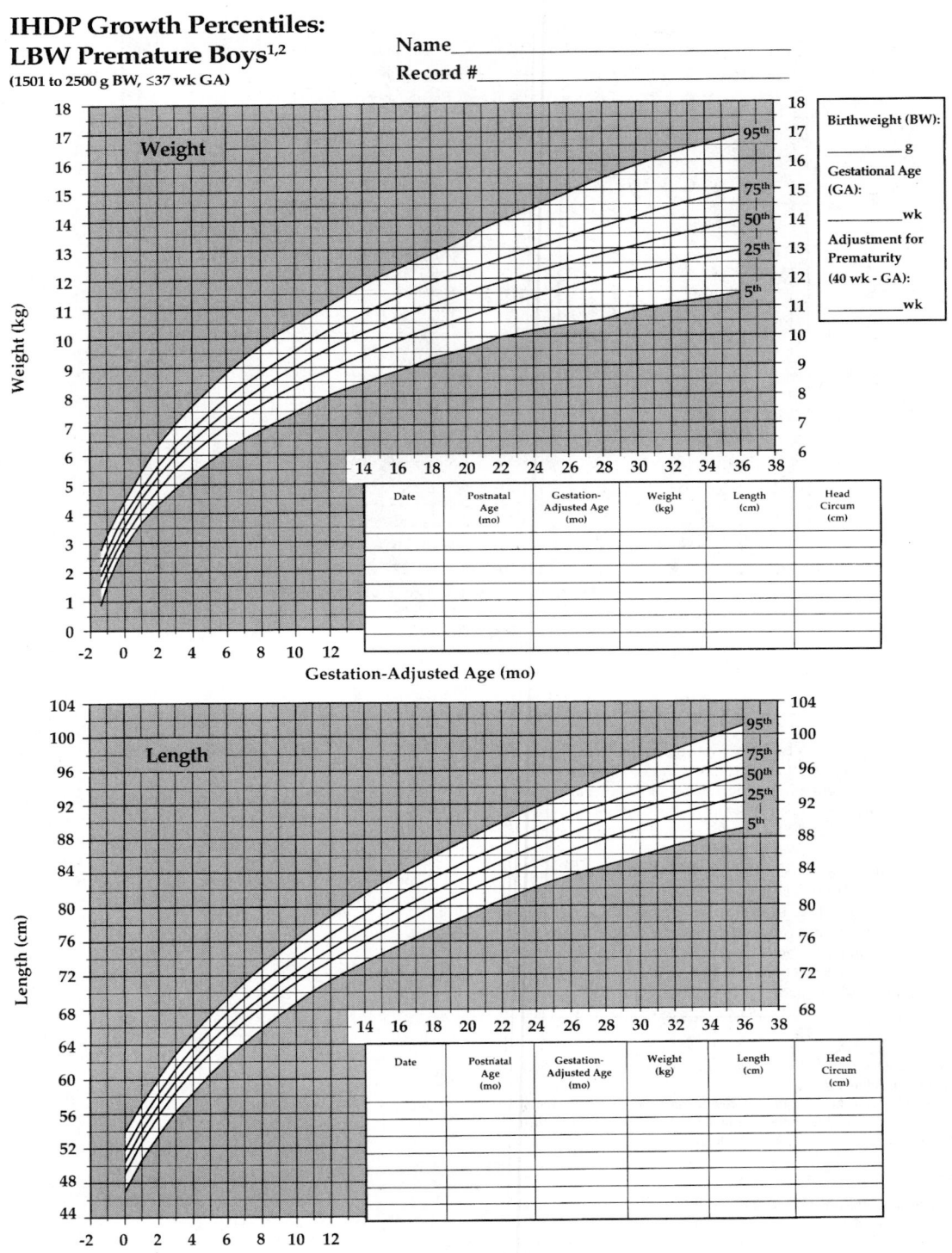

Birthweight (BW):

_____ g

Gestational Age (GA):

_____ wk

Adjustment for Prematurity (40 wk - GA):

_____ wk

Weight

Date	Postnatal Age (mo)	Gestation- Adjusted Age (mo)	Weight (kg)	Length (cm)	Head Circum (cm)

Gestation-Adjusted Age (mo)

Length

Date	Postnatal Age (mo)	Gestation- Adjusted Age (mo)	Weight (kg)	Length (cm)	Head Circum (cm)

Gestation-Adjusted Age (mo)

IHDP Growth Percentiles: LBW Premature Boys[1,2]

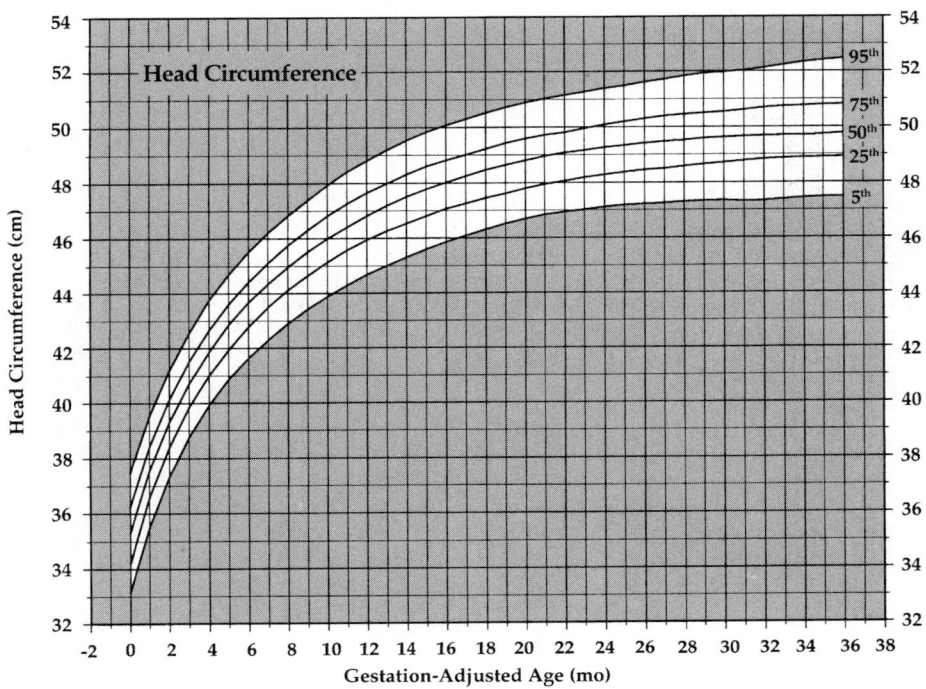

Growth of very-low-birth-weight (VLBW, ≤1500 g) and low-birth-weight (LBW, 1501 to 2500 g) premature (≤37 weeks, GA) infants differ from that of normal-birth-weight term infants during infancy and early childhood. Because these infants may not catch up to term infants in growth during the early years, their growth should be compared to that of premature infants of similar birth weight.

The growth percentiles presented here are based on a large sample of infants enrolled in the Infant Health and Development Program (IHDP).[1,2] Some infants most likely to experience growth problems from biologic or environmental causes, premature infants with birth weight greater than 2500 g, and small-for-gestational-age term infants were excluded.[1] Study infants, however, are probably typical of premature infants who receive modern neonatal intensive care.

References

1. The Infant Health and Development Program: Enhancing the outcomes of low-birth-weight, premature infants. *JAMA* 1990;263(22):3035–3042.
2. Casey PH, Kraemer HC, Bernbaum J, et al: Growth status and growth rates of a varied sample of low birth weight, preterm infants: A longitudinal cohort from birth to three years of age. *J Pediatr* 1991;119:599–605.

IHDP studies were supported by grants from the Robert Wood Johnson Foundation, Pew Charitable Trusts, and the Bureau of Maternal and Child Health, US Department of Health and Human Services. These graphs were prepared by SS Guo and AF Roche, Wright State University, Yellow Springs, Ohio. IHDP, its sponsors, and the investigators do not endorse specific products.
Courtesy of Ross Products Division, Abbott Laboratories, Columbus, OH.

Instructions for Use

1. Measure and record weight, length, and head circumference.
2. Calculate gestation-adjusted age by subtracting Adjustment for Prematurity in weeks from postnatal age in weeks. Adjustment for Prematurity equals 40 weeks minus GA. For example, at 12 wk postnatal age, an infant born at 30 wk GA would be 2 wk (0.5 mo) gestation-adjusted age.

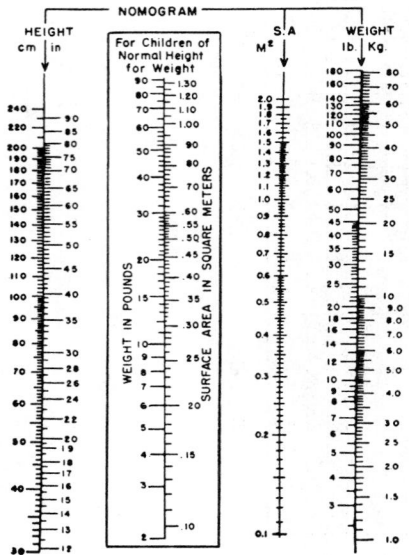

The West nomogram for the estimation of body surface area. The surface area is indicated where a straight line connecting height and weight intersects the surface area column. If the patient is roughly of average size, the surface area can also be estimated from the weight alone (enclosed area). (From Shirkey HC: Drug therapy. *In* Vaughan VC III, McKay RJ [Eds]: Nelson Textbook of Pediatrics, 10th ed. Philadelphia, WB Saunders, 1975.)

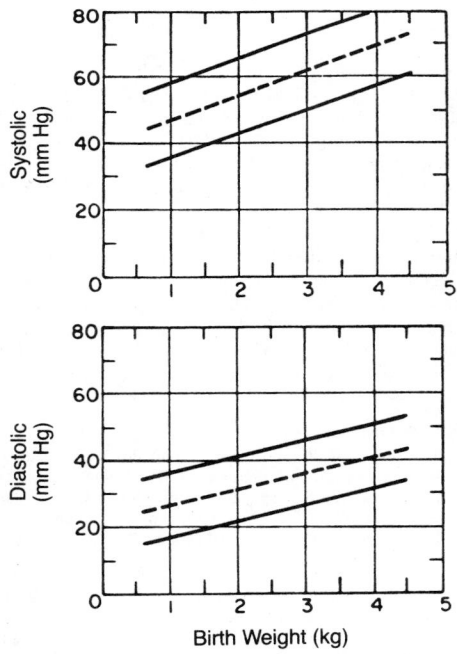

Linear regressions (broken lines) and 95% confidence limits (solid lines) of systolic (top) and diastolic (bottom) aortic blood pressures on birth weight in 61 healthy newborn infants during the first 12 hours after birth. For systolic pressure, $y = 7.13x + 40.45$; $r = 0.79$. For diastolic pressure, $y = 4.81x + 22.18$; $r = 0.71$. For both, $n = 413$ and $P < 0.001$. (From Versmold HT et al: Pediatrics 67:607, 1981. Reproduced by permission of Pediatrics © 1981.)

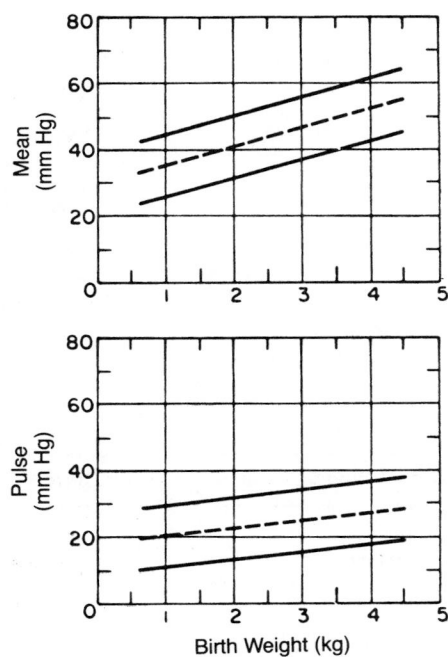

Linear regressions (broken lines) and 95% confidence limits (solid lines) of mean pressures (top) and pulse pressures (systolic-diastolic pressure amplitudes) (bottom) on birth weight in 61 healthy newborn infants during the first 12 hours after birth. For mean pressure, $y = 5.16x + 29.80$; $n = 443$; $r = 0.80$. For pulse pressure, $y = 2.31x + 18.27$; $n = 413$; $r = 0.45$. For both, $P < 0.001$. (From Versmold HT, et al: Pediatrics 67:607, 1981. Reproduced with permission of Pediatrics © 1981.)

Average Blood Pressure, Heart Rate, Hemoglobin, and Weight During First Week of Life

			Day						
			1	2	3	4	5	6	7
Systolic pressure	Awake	Mean	67.9	71.9	74.3	77.5	74.2	76.8	76.2
		(2 SD)	(30.8)	(33.6)	(31.4)	(37.0)	(29.2)	(31.0)	(29.6)
	Asleep	Mean	65.0	72.0	77.0	71.0	74.8	76.9	73.7
		(2 SD)	(27.2)	(33.0)	(31.4)	(41.2)	(27.2)	(33.8)	(27.0)
Diastolic pressure	Awake	Mean	43.5	48.3	49.3	52.5	49.0	51.8	47.6
		(2 SD)	(28.8)	(30.2)	(31.6)	(31.8)	(28.6)	(30.0)	(27.2)
	Asleep	Mean	41.4	48.9	52.7	50.7	49.3	53.0	46.7
		(2 SD)	(24.6)	(31.0)	(32.0)	(28.2)	(26.8)	(33.0)	(25.4)
Mean arterial pressure	Awake	Mean	57.7	59.6	63.7	65.0	61.9	63.5	63.5
		(2 SD)	(31.8)	(29.6)	(30.2)	(35.4)	(31.6)	(30.8)	(28.4)
	Asleep	Mean	55.8	60.9	64.8	62.6	61.7	64.4	61.0
		(2 SD)	(27.2)	(31.0)	(34.2)	(30.0)	(28.2)	(33.6)	(28.4)
Heart rate	Awake	Mean	169.2	164.6	167.2	173.2	169.2	172.9	170.9
		(2 SD)	(63.2)	(78.4)	(64.4)	(66.8)	(50.2)	(57.2)	(60.8)
	Asleep	Mean	177.5	173.1	169.1	176.4	166.3	173.1	168.9
		(2 SD)	(67.8)	(77.2)	(61.0)	(69.6)	(56.0)	(54.2)	(74.2)
PVC (%)		Mean	61.0		53.7				50.8
		(2 SD)	(18.2)		(21.2)				(16.8)
Hemoglobin (g/dL)		Mean	20.2		17.9				17.0
		(2 SD)	(6.0)		(7.0)				(5.2)
Wt (g)		Mean	1221.8		1171.1				1155.2
		(2 SD)	(342.8)		(314.0)				(382.8)

Right upper arm morning blood pressure, heart rate, packed volume of cells (PVC), hemoglobin (Hb), and weight in the first week of life for infants under 34 weeks' gestation and under 1500 g birth weight.

From Tan KL: J Pediatr 112:266, 1988.

Colloid Osmotic Pressure (mm Hg) in Infants' Blood

Term, vaginal delivery	19.5 ± 2.1 (SD)
Term, cesarean section	16.1 ± 2.0
Term, vaginal (sick)	19.5 ± 3.1
(sepsis, asphyxia, heart failure, abdominal surgery)	
Preterm (700–1980 g)	12.5 ± 2.5
(hyaline membrane disease, asphyxia, necrotizing enterocolitis, etc.)	

Data from Sola A, Gregory GA: Crit Care Med 9:568, 1981.

Normal Blood Chemistry Values in Term Infants

Determination	Sample Source	Cord	Age 1–12 hr	Age 12–24 hr	Age 24–48 hr	Age 48–72 hr
Sodium, mEq/L°	Capillary	147 (126–166)	143 (124–156)	145 (132–159)	148 (134–160)	149 (139–162)
Potassium, mEq/L		7.8 (5.6–12)	6.4 (5.3–7.3)	6.3 (5.3–8.9)	6.0 (5.2–7.3)	5.9 (5.0–7.7)
Chloride, mEq/L		103 (98–110)	100.7 (90–111)	103 (87–114)	102 (92–114)	103 (93–112)
Calcium, mg/100 mL		9.3 (8.2–11.1)	8.4 (7.3–9.2)	7.8 (6.9–9.4)	8.0 (6.1–9.9)	7.9 (5.9–9.7)
Phosphorus, mg/100 mL		5.6 (3.7–8.1)	6.1 (3.5–8.6)	5.7 (2.9–8.1)	5.9 (3.0–8.7)	5.8 (2.8–7.6)
Blood urea nitrogen, mg/100 mL		29 (21–40)	27 (8–34)	33 (9–63)	32 (13–77)	31 (15–68)
Total protein, gm/100 mL		6.1 (4.8–7.3)	6.6 (5.6–8.5)	6.6 (5.8–8.2)	6.9 (5.9–8.2)	7.2 (6.0–8.5)
Blood sugar, mg/100 mL		73 (45–96)	63 (40–97)	63 (42–104)	56 (30–91)	59 (40–90)
Lactic acid, mg/100 mL		19.5 (11–30)	14.6 (11–24)	14.0 (10–23)	14.3 (9–22)	13.5 (7–21)
Lactate, mm/L†		2.0–3.0	2.0			

°Acharya and Payne: Arch Dis Child 40:430, 1968.
†Daniel, Adamsons, and James: Pediatrics 37:942, 1966.

Serum Electrolyte Values in Preterm Infants

Constituent	Age 1 Week Mean	SD	Range	Age 3 Weeks Mean	SD	Range	Age 5 Weeks Mean	SD	Range	Age 7 Weeks Mean	SD	Range
Na (mEq/L)	139.6	± 3.2	133–146	136.3	± 2.9	129–142	136.8	± 2.5	133–148	137.2	± 1.8	133–142
K (mEq/L)	5.6	± 0.5	4.6–6.7	5.8	± 0.6	4.5–7.1	5.5	± 0.6	4.5–6.6	5.7	± 0.5	4.6–7.1
Cl (mEq/L)	108.2	± 3.7	100–117	108.3	± 3.9	102–116	107.0	± 3.5	100–115	107.0	± 3.3	101–115
CO_2 (mM/L)	20.3	± 2.8	13.8–27.1	18.4	± 3.5	12.4–26.2	20.4	± 3.4	12.5–26.1	20.6	± 3.1	13.7–26.9
Ca (mg/dL)	9.2	± 1.1	6.1–11.6	9.6	± 0.5	8.1–11.0	9.4	± 0.5	8.6–10.5	9.5	± 0.7	8.6–10.8
P (mg/dL)	7.6	± 1.1	5.4–10.9	7.5	± 0.7	6.2–8.7	7.0	± 0.6	5.6–7.9	6.8	± 0.8	4.2–8.2
BUN (mg/dL)	9.3	± 5.2	3.1–25.5	13.3	± 7.8	2.1–31.4	13.3	± 7.1	2.0–26.5	13.4	± 6.7	2.5–30.5

From Klaus MH, Fanaroff AA: Care of the High-Risk Neonate. 3rd ed. Philadelphia, WB Saunders, 1988. Adapted from Thomas J, Reichelderfer T: Clin Chem 14:272, 1968.

Thyroid Function in Full-Term and Preterm Infants

Serum Thyroxine (T₄) Concentration in Premature and Term Infants

	Estimated Gestational Age (wk)				
	30–31	32–33	34–35	36–37	Term
Cord					
Mean	6.5°	7.5	6.7†	7.5	8.2
SD	1.0	2.1	1.2	2.8	1.8
n	3	8	18	17	37
12–72 hr					
Mean	11.5‡	12.3‡	12.4‡	15.5†	19.0
SD	2.1	3.2	3.1	2.6	2.1
n	12	18	17	15	6
3–10 days					
Mean	7.7‡	8.5‡	10.0‡	12.7†	15.9
SD	1.8	1.9	2.4	2.5	3.0
n	7	8	9	9	29
11–20 days					
Mean	7.5†	8.3‡	10.5	11.2	12.2
SD	1.8	1.6	1.8	2.9	2.0
n	5	11	9	9	8
21–45 days					
Mean	7.8‡	8.0‡	9.3†	11.4	12.1
SD	1.5	1.7	1.3	4.2	1.5
n	11	17	13	5	5
46–90 days		(30–73 weeks)			
Mean		9.6			10.2
SD		1.7			1.9
n		16			17

°*P*<0.05 ⎫
†*P*<0.005 ⎬ for the comparison of premature vs. term infants (*t*-test)
‡*P*<0.001 ⎭

From Cuestas RA: J Pediatr 92:963, 1982.

Serum Free Thyroxine (T₄) Index in Premature and Term Infants

	Estimated Gestational Age (wk)				
	30–31	32–33	34–35	36–37	Term
Cord					
Mean			5.6	5.6	5.9
SD			1.3	2.0	1.1
n			12	10	14
12–72 hr					
Mean	13.1°	12.9°	15.5†	17.1	19.7
SD	2.4	2.7	3.0	3.5	3.5
n	12	14	14	14	6
3–10 days					
Mean	8.3°	9.0°	12.0‡	15.1	16.2
SD	1.9	1.8	2.3	0.7	3.2
n	6	9	5	4	11
11–20 days					
Mean	8.0§	9.1‡	11.8	11.3	12.1
SD	1.6	1.9	2.7	1.9	2.0
n	5	8	8	4	8
21–45 days					
Mean	8.4§	9.0‡	10.9		11.1
SD	1.4	1.6	2.8		1.4
n	11	17	5		5
46–90 days		30–35 weeks			
Mean		9.4			9.7
SD		1.4			1.5
n		13			10

°*P* 0.001 ⎫
†*P* 0.025 ⎬ for the comparison of premature vs. term infants (*t*-test)
‡*P* 0.01 ⎪
§*P* 0.005 ⎭

From Cuestas RA: J Pediatr 92:963, 1982.

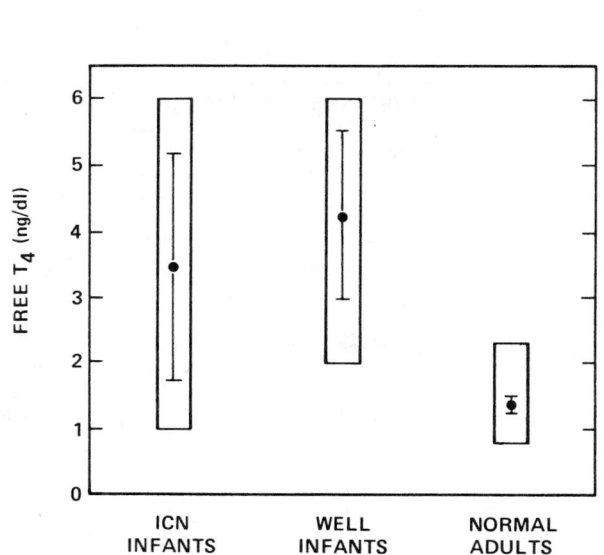

Free thyroxine (T₄) levels in sick intensive care nursery [ICN] infants, healthy term infants, and normal adults. The center • represents the mean ± SD. (From Wilson DM, et al: J Pediatr 101:113, 1982.)

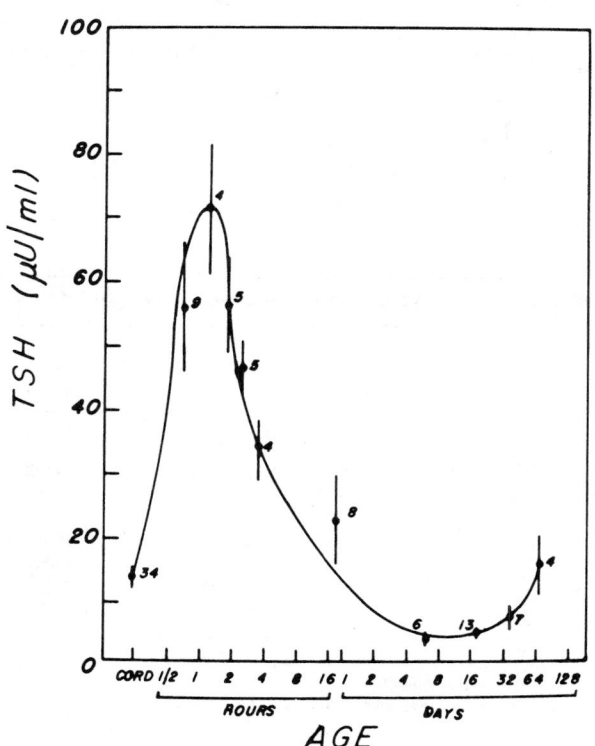

Thyroid-stimulating hormone (TSH) levels in healthy preterm infants. Mean, standard error of the mean, and sample size are shown. (From Cuestas RA: J Pediatr 92:963, 1982.)

Normal Values for Cerebrospinal Fluid

	Term Babies
Color	Clear or xanthochromic
White cell count	6–8 (range 0–34)
Protein	45 mg/100 mL (range 30–102)

Data from Samson: Ergebn d inn Med u Kinderh 41:553, 1931; Otilia: Acta Paed 35:Suppl 8, 1948; Bauer, et al: J Pediatr 66:1017, 1965; Wolf and Hoepffner: World Neurol 2:871, 1961; and Widell: Acta Paed 47:Suppl 115, 1958.

Cerebrospinal Fluid Values in Very-Low-Birth-Weight Infants on Basis of Birth Weight

	Group 1 (≤1000 g) (n = 38*)		Group 2 (1001–1500 g) (n = 33*)		P
	Mean ± SD	Range	Mean ± SD	Range	
Birth weight (g)	763 ± 115	550–980	1278 ± 152	1020–1500	
Gestational age (wk)	26 ± 1.3	24–28	29 ± 1.4	27–33	
Leukocytes/mm³	4 ± 3	0–14	6 ± 9	0–44	NS
Erythrocytes/mm³	1027 ± 3270	0–19,050	786 ± 1879	0–9750	
PMNs (%)	6 ± 15	0–66	9 ± 17	0–60	NS
MN leukocytes (%)	86 ± 30	34–100	85 ± 28	13–100	
Glucose (mg/dL)	61 ± 34	29–217	59 ± 21	31–109	NS
Protein (mg/dL)	150 ± 56	95–370	132 ± 43	45–227	NS

NS, not significant (P > 0.05); MN, mononuclear; PMN, polymorphonuclear leukocytes.
*Number of cerebrospinal fluid specimens.
From Rodriguez AF, Kaplan SL, Mason EO: Cerebrospinal fluid values and the very LBW infant. J Pediatr 116:971, 1990.

Cerebrospinal Fluid Values in Very-Low-Birth-Weight Infants, by Chronologic Age: Group 1 (Birth Weight ≤1000 g)

	Postnatal Age (Days)					
	0–7 (6 Infants; n = 6*)		8–28 (12 Infants; n = 17)		29–84 (10 Infants; n = 15)	
	Mean ± SD	Range	Mean ± SD	Range	Mean ± SD	Range
Birth weight (g)	822 ± 116	630–980	752 ± 112	550–970	750 ± 120	550–907
Gestational age at birth (wk)	26 ± 1.2	24–27	26 ± 1.5	24–28	26 ± 1.0	24–27
Leukocytes/mm³	3 ± 3	1–8	4 ± 4	0–14	4 ± 3	0–11
Erythrocytes/mm³	335 ± 709	0–1780	1465 ± 4062	0–19,050	808 ± 1843	0–6850
PMNs (%)	11 ± 20	0–50	8 ± 17	0–66	2 ± 9	0–36
Glucose (mg/dL)	70 ± 17	41–89	68 ± 48	33–217	49 ± 22	29–90
Protein (mg/dL)	162 ± 37	115–222	159 ± 77	95–370	137 ± 61	76–260

*Number of cerebrospinal fluid specimens.
PMN, polymorphonuclear leukocyte.
From Rodriguez AF, Kaplan SL, Mason EO: Cerebrospinal fluid values and the very LBW infant. J Pediatr 116:971, 1990.

Cerebrospinal Fluid Values in Very-Low-Birth-Weight Infants, by Chronologic Age: Group 2 (Birth Weight ≥1001 to 1500 g)

	Postnatal Age (Days)					
	0–7 (8 Infants; $n = 8°$)		8–28 (11 Infants; $n = 14$)		29–84 (6 Infants; $n = 11$)	
	Mean ± SD	*Range*	*Mean ± SD*	*Range*	*Mean ± SD*	*Range*
Birth weight (g)	1428 ± 107	1180–1500	1245 ± 162	1020–1480	1211 ± 86	1080–1300
Gestational age at birth (wk)	31 ± 1.5	28–33	29 ± 1.2	27–31	29 ± 0.7	27–29
Leukocytes/mm³	4 ± 4	1–10	7 ± 11	0–44	8 ± 8	0–23
Erythrocytes/mm³	407 ± 853	0–2450	1101 ± 2643	0–9750	661 ± 1198	0–3800
PMNs (%)	4 ± 10	0–28	10 ± 19	0–60	11 ± 19	0–48
Glucose (mg/dL)	74 ± 19†	50–96	59 ± 23	39–109	47 ± 13	31–76
Protein (mg/dL)	136 ± 35	85–176	137 ± 46	54–227	122 ± 47	45–187

°Number of cerebrospinal fluid specimens.
†$P = 0.004$. Infants up to 7 days of age had significantly higher value compared with those older than 29 days.
From Rodriguez AF, Kaplan SL, Mason EO: Cerebrospinal fluid values and the very LBW infant. J Pediatr 116:971, 1990.

Cerebrospinal Fluid (CSF) Analysis from Previous Studies in Premature Infants with Birth Weight ≤2500 g

Author	No. of Infants	Postnatal Age	Mean CSF Cells/mm³ (Range)	Mean Protein (mg/dL) (Range)
Samson	NR	Up to 1 mo	4	55
Otila	46	Up to 1 mo	10	101
Wolf and Hoepffner	22	1–3 days	2 (0–13)	105 (50–180)
Gyllenswärd and Malmström	36	1–40 days	7 (1–37)	115 (55–292)
Sarff et al	30	1–6 days	9 (0–29)	115 (65–150)

NR, Not recorded.
From Rodriguez AF, Kaplan SL, Mason EO: Cerebrospinal fluid values and the very LBW infant. J Pediatr 116:971, 1990.

TERM NEWBORN

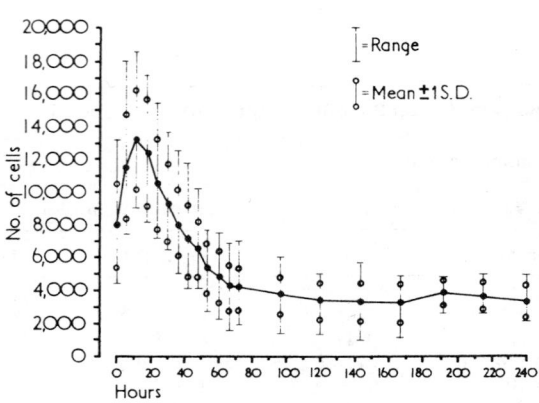

Means, ranges, and means ± 1 SD of neutrophils of 15 full-term healthy babies during the first 10 days of life. (Data from Xanthou M: Arch Dis Child 45:242, 1970.)

PREMATURES

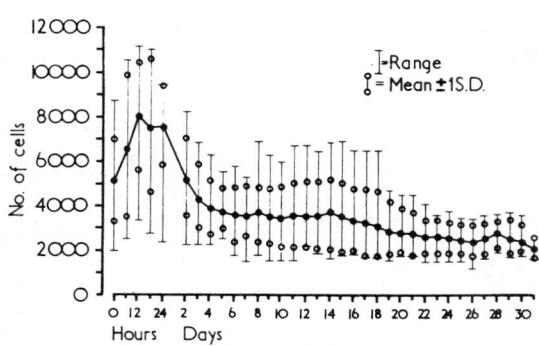

Means, ranges, and means ± 1 SD of neutrophils of 14 healthy babies during the first month of life (13 premature + 1 small for dates). (Data from Xanthou M: Arch Dis Child 45:242, 1970.)

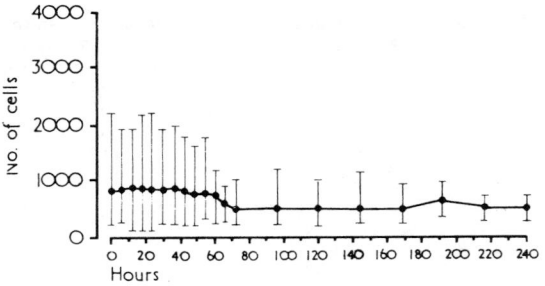

Means and ranges of the eosinophils of full-term babies during the first 10 days of life. (Data from Xanthou M: Arch Dis Child 45:242, 1970.)

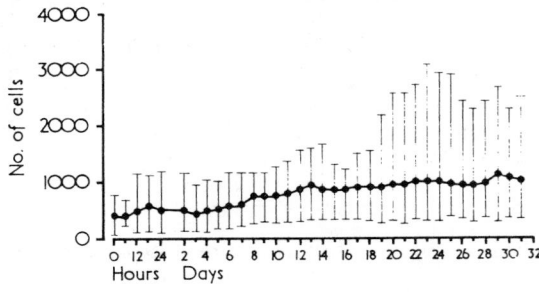

Means and ranges of eosinophils of low-birth-weight babies during the first month of life. (Data from Xanthou M: Arch Dis Child 45:242, 1970.)

TERM NEWBORN

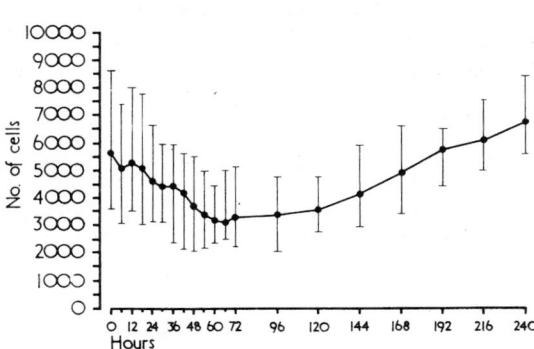

Means and ranges of lymphocytes of full-term babies during the first 10 days of life. (Data from Xanthou M: Arch Dis Child 45:242, 1970.)

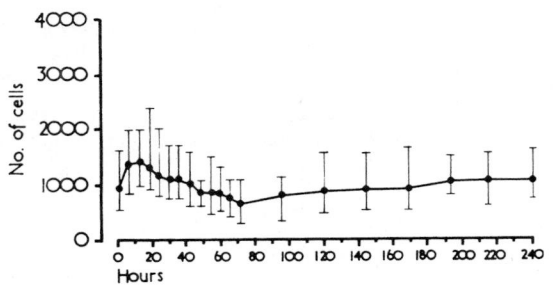

Means and ranges of the monocytes of healthy full-term babies during the first 10 days of life. (Data from Xanthou M: Arch Dis Child 45:242, 1970.)

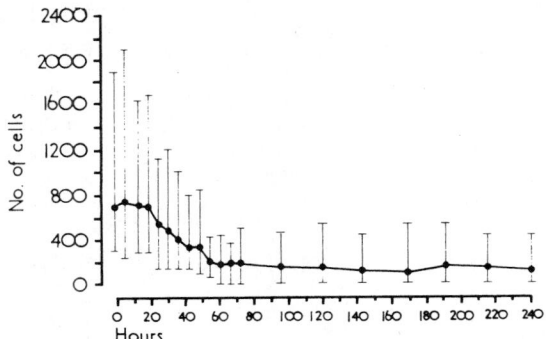

Means and ranges of metamyelocytes of full-term babies during the first 10 days of life. (Data from Xanthou M: Arch Dis Child 45:242, 1970.)

PREMATURES

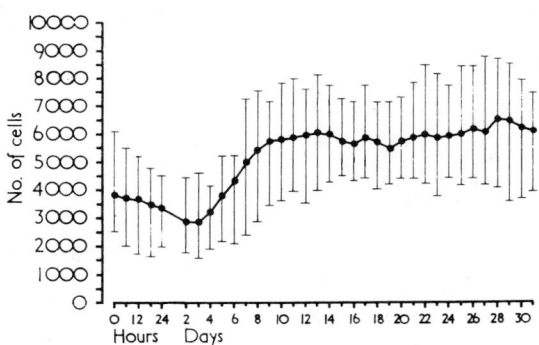

Means and ranges of lymphocytes of low-birth-weight babies during the first month of life. (Data from Xanthou M: Arch Dis Child 45:242, 1970.)

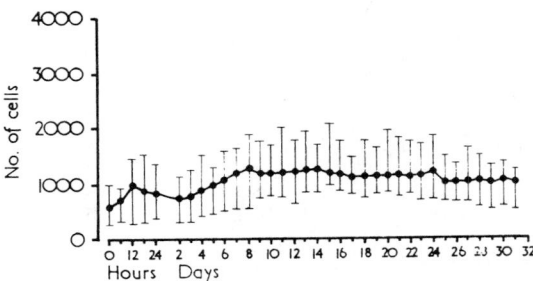

Means and ranges of monocytes of low-birth-weight babies during the first month of life. (Data from Xanthou M: Arch Dis Child 45:242, 1970.)

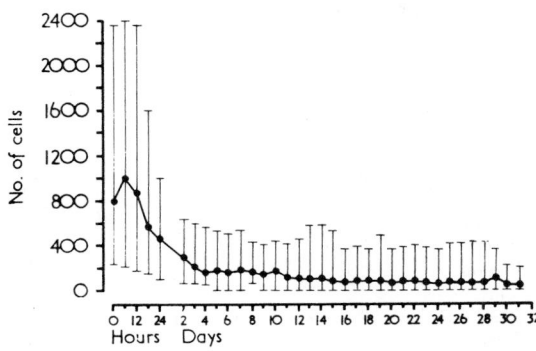

Means and ranges of metamyelocytes of 14 healthy babies during the first month of life. (Data from Xanthou M: Arch Dis Child 45:242, 1970.)

Nucleated Red Blood Cells in Normal Infants and Infants of Diabetic Mothers

Variables	Control Infants (*n* = 102)	Infants of Diabetic Mothers	
		No Perinatal Asphyxia (*n* = 54)	Perinatal Asphyxia (*n* = 25)
Gestational age (weeks)	39.5 ± 1.5	38.0 ± 1.0°	37.9 ± 1.2°
Birth weight (kg)	3.3 ± 0.3	3.5 ± 0.6°	3.6 ± 0.6°
Leukocyte count†	27.3 ± 9.2	17.1 ± 5.1°	16.8 ± 6.1°
NRBCs (absolute count)	0.4 ± 1.3	1.4 ± 3.1°	1.8 ± 2.3°
NRBCs/100 leukocytes	1.7 ± 6.2	8.3 ± 17.8°	13.0 ± 18.9°

°Significantly different from control infant values (*P* at least <0.05).
†Data are expressed as × 10⁹/L
NRBC, nucleated red blood cell
Adapted from Green DW, Mimouni F: J Pediatr 116:129, 1990.

Blood Gases: Representative Values in Normal Infants at Term

	Umbilical Vein	Arterial Blood					Reference
		30 min	1–4 hr	12–24 hr	24–48 hr	96 hr	
pH	7.33	—	7.30	7.30	7.39	7.39	
PCO_2, mm Hg	43	—	39	33	34	36	Reardon et al (1960)
HCO_3, mEq/L	21.6	—	18.8	19.5	20	21.4	Oliver et al (1961)
PO_2, mm Hg	28 ± 8	—	62 ± 13.8	68	63–87		Nelson et al (1962, 1963)
O_2 saturation			95%	94%	94%	96%	
Crying vital capacity, mL (for 3-kg infant)	77 range (56–110)				92 (69–128)	100	Sutherland and Ratcliff (1961)
Functional residual capacity mL/kg	22 ± 8	25 ± 8	21 ± 1	28 ± 7		39 ± 9	Klaus et al (1962)
Lung compliance mL/cm H_2O/kg	1.5 ± 0.05			2.0 ± 0.4		1.7	Cook et al (1957)
Lung compliance/FRC, mL/cm H_2O/mL		0.04 ± 0.10		0.053 ± 0.009		0.065	Chu et al (1964) Cook et al (1957)
Right-to-left shunt, percentage cardiac output		22% (range 11–29%)		24% (17–32%)			Prod'hom et al (1964)

		Comment	Reference
Respiratory frequency	34/min (range 20–60)	1–2 days 1–11 days	Cook et al (1995) Cross (1949)
Resistances, cm H_2O/L/sec	29, 26 18 ± 6/3	Total lung resistance Airway resistance	Cook et al (1949), Swyer et al (1960), Polgar (1962)
Flow rates, mL/sec	48–37 161–106	Max insp, max exp rest crying	Swyer et al (1957), Long and Hull (1961)
Ventilation, mL/kg/min	200		Cook et al (1955), Nelson et al (1962)
Dead space, mL	4.4–9.2	Term infants	Nelson et al (1962), Cook et al (1955), Strang (1961)
Alveolar ventilation, mL/kg/min	120–145	First 3 days of life	Nelson et al (1962)
O_2 consumption, mL/kg/min	6.2	At neutral temperature	Oliver ad Karlberg (1963)
CO_2 production, mL/kg/min	5.1	At neutral temperature	Oliver and Karlberg (1963)
Alveolar-arterial O_2 differences, mm Hg	28 ± 10, room air 311 ± 70, 100% O_2	Age 7 hr to 42 days Age 6–58 hr, 3 infants	Nelson et al (1963)
Arterial-alveolar CO_2 differences, mm Hg	1.8 ± 3.8	Age 3–74 hr	Nelson et al (1963)

From Avery ME, Normand C: Anesthesiology 26:510, 1965.

Body Composition of the Reference Fetus

Gestational Age (wk)	Body Weight (g)	Water (g)	Protein (g)	Lipid (g)	Other (g)	Water (g)	Protein (g)	Ca (mg)	P (mg)	Mg (mg)	Na (mEq)	K (mEq)	Cl (mEq)
		per 100-g Body Weight				per 100-g Fat-Free Weight							
24	690	88.6	8.8	0.1	2.5	88.6	8.8	621	387	17.8	9.9	4.0	7.0
25	770	87.8	9.0	0.7	2.5	88.4	9.1	615	385	17.6	9.8	4.0	7.0
26	880	86.8	9.2	1.5	2.5	88.1	9.4	611	384	17.5	9.7	4.1	7.0
27	1010	85.7	9.4	2.4	2.5	87.8	9.7	609	383	17.4	9.5	4.1	6.9
28	1160	84.6	9.6	3.3	2.4	87.5	10.0	610	385	17.4	9.4	4.2	6.9
29	1318	83.6	9.9	4.1	2.4	87.2	10.3	613	387	17.4	9.3	4.2	6.8
30	1480	82.6	10.1	4.9	2.4	86.8	10.6	619	392	17.4	9.2	4.3	6.8
31	1650	81.7	10.3	5.6	2.4	86.5	10.9	628	398	17.6	9.1	4.3	6.7
32	1830	80.7	10.6	6.3	2.4	86.1	11.3	640	406	17.8	9.1	4.3	6.6
33	2020	79.8	10.8	6.9	2.5	85.8	11.6	656	416	18.0	9.0	4.4	6.5
34	2230	79.0	11.0	7.5	2.5	85.4	11.9	675	428	18.3	8.9	4.4	6.4
35	2450	78.1	11.2	8.1	2.6	85.0	12.2	699	443	18.6	8.9	4.5	6.3
36	2690	77.3	11.4	8.7	2.6	84.6	12.5	726	460	19.0	8.8	4.5	6.1
37	2940	76.4	11.6	9.3	2.7	84.3	12.8	758	479	19.5	8.8	4.5	6.0
38	3160	75.6	11.8	9.9	2.7	83.9	13.1	795	501	20.0	8.8	4.5	5.9
39	3330	74.8	11.9	10.5	2.8	83.6	13.3	836	525	20.5	8.7	4.6	5.8
40	3450	74.0	12.0	11.2	2.8	83.3	13.5	882	551	21.1	8.7	4.6	5.7

Data from Ziegler, EE, et al: University of Iowa, Iowa City, 1975.

Plasma Immunoglobulin Concentrations in Premature Infants (25–28 weeks' gestation)

Age (mo)	n	IgG* (mg/dL)	IgM* (mg/dL)	IgA* (mg/dL)
0.25	18	251 (114–552)†	7.6 (1.3–43.3)	1.2 (0.07–20.8)
0.5	14	202 (91–446)	14.1 (3.5–56.1)	3.1 (0.09–10.7)
1.0	10	158 (57–437)	12.7 (3.0–53.3)	4.5 (0.65–30.9)
1.5	14	134 (59–307)	16.2 (4.4–59.2)	4.3 (0.9–20.9)
2.0	12	89 (58–136)	16 (5.3–48.9)	4.1 (1.5–11.1)
3	13	60 (23–156)	13.8 (5.3–36.1)	3 (0.6–15.6)
4	10	82 (32–210)	22.2 (11.2–43.9)	6.8 (1–47.8)
6	11	159 (56–455)	41.3 (8.3–205)	9.7 (3–31.2)
8–10	6	273 (94–794)	41.8 (31.1–56.1)	9.5 (0.9–98.6)

*Geometric mean.
†The normal ranges in parentheses were determined by taking the antilog of (mean logarithm ± 2 SD of the logarithms).
From Ballow M, et al: Pediatr Res 20:899, 1986.

Plasma Immunoglobulin Concentrations in Premature Infants (29–32 weeks' gestation)

Age (mo)	n	IgG* (mg/dL)	IgM* (mg/dL)	IgA* (mg/dL)
0.25	42	368 (186–728)†	9.1 (2.1–39.4)	0.6 (0.04–1)
0.5	35	275 (119–637)	13.9 (4.7–41)	0.9 (0.01–7.5)
1	26	209 (97–452)	14.4 (6.3–33)	1.9 (0.3–12)
1.5	22	156 (69–352)	15.4 (5.5–43.2)	2.2 (0.7–6.5)
2	11	123 (64–237)	15.2 (4.9–46.7)	3 (1.1–8.3)
3	14	104 (41–268)	16.3 (7.1–37.2)	3.6 (0.8–15.4)
4	21	128 (39–425)	26.5 (7.7–91.2)	9.8 (2.5–39.3)
6	21	179 (51–634)	29.3 (10.5–81.5)	12.3 (2.7–57.1)
8–10	16	280 (140–561)	34.7 (17–70.8)	20.9 (8.3–53)

*Geometric mean.
†The normal ranges in parentheses were determined by taking the antilog of (mean logarithm ± 2 SD of the logarithms).
From Ballow M, et al: Pediatr Res 20:899, 1986.

Temperature Equivalents

Celsius	Fahrenheit	Celsius	Fahrenheit
34.0	93.2	38.6	101.4
34.2	93.6	38.8	101.8
34.4	93.9	39.0	102.2
34.6	94.3	39.2	102.5
34.8	94.6	39.4	102.9
35.0	95.0	39.6	103.2
35.2	95.4	39.8	103.6
35.4	95.7	40.0	104.0
35.6	96.1	40.2	104.3
35.8	96.4	40.4	104.7
36.0	96.8	40.6	105.1
36.2	97.1	40.8	105.4
36.4	97.5	41.0	105.8
36.6	97.8	41.2	106.1
36.8	98.2	41.4	106.5
37.0	98.6	41.6	106.8
37.2	98.9	41.8	107.2
37.4	99.3	42.0	107.6
37.6	99.6	42.2	108.0
37.8	100.0	42.4	108.3
38.0	100.4	42.6	108.7
38.2	100.7	42.8	109.0
38.4	101.1	43.0	109.4

To convert Celsius to Fahrenheit:

$$9/5 \times \text{Temperature} + 32$$

Example: To convert 40° Celsius to Fahrenheit

$$9/5 \times 40 = 72 + 32 = 104° \text{ Fahrenheit}$$

To convert Fahrenheit to Celsius:

$$(\text{Temperature} - 32) \times 5/9$$

Example: To convert 98.6° Fahrenheit to Celsius

$$98.6 - 32 = 66.6 \times 5/9 = 37° \text{ Celsius}$$

Conversion of Pounds and Ounces to Grams

Ounces	1 lb	2 lb	3 lb	4 lb	5 lb	6 lb	7 lb	8 lb
				Grams				
0	454	907	1361	1814	2268	2722	3175	3629
1	482	936	1389	1843	2296	2750	3204	3657
2	510	964	1418	1871	2325	2778	3232	3686
3	539	992	1446	1899	2353	2807	3260	3714
4	567	1021	1474	1928	2381	2835	3289	3742
5	595	1049	1503	1956	2410	2863	3317	3771
6	624	1077	1531	1985	2438	2892	3345	3799
7	652	1106	1559	2013	2466	2920	3374	3827
8	680	1134	1588	2041	2495	2948	3402	3856
9	709	1162	1616	2070	2523	2977	3430	3884
10	737	1191	1644	2098	2552	3005	3459	3912
11	765	1219	1673	2126	2580	3033	3487	3941
12	794	1247	1701	2155	2608	3062	3515	3969
13	822	1276	1729	2183	2637	3090	3544	3997
14	851	1304	1758	2211	2665	3119	3572	4026
15	879	1332	1786	2240	2693	3147	3600	4054

Conversion of Inches to Centimeters

Inches	cm	Inches	cm	Inches	cm
10	25.40	15	38.10	20	50.80
10½	26.67	15½	39.37	20½	52.07
11	27.94	16	40.64	21	53.34
11½	29.21	16½	41.91	21½	54.61
12	30.48	17	43.18	22	55.88
12½	31.75	17½	44.45	22½	57.15
13	33.02	18	45.72	23	58.42
13½	34.29	18½	46.99	23½	56.69
14	35.56	19	48.26	24	60.96
14½	36.83	19½	49.53		

APPENDIX 4
COMMUNITY AND AGENCY RESOURCES

REPRESENTATIVE INTERNET WEB SITES—RESOURCES FOR PHYSICIANS AND PARENTS[4]

Food and Drug Administration
http://www.fda.gov
This site has information regarding the latest drugs and devices.

National Institutes of Health
http://www.nih.gov
This site is the gateway to a vast variety of basic and clinical research endeavors, including those supported by the National Institutes of Child Health and Human Development and the National Institute of Heart, Lung, and Blood.

World Health Organization
http://www.who.ch
WHO data and e-mail of those involved with epidemiology and infectious diseases throughout the world.

Division of Birth Defects and Developmental Disabilities, CDC
http://www.cdc.gov/nceh/programs/infants/brthdfct/prevent/bd-prev.htm

Food and Drug Administration
http://vm.cfsan.fda.gov/~dms/wh-folic.html

March of Dimes Birth Defects Foundation
http://www.modimes.org

Spina Bifida Association of America
http://www.infohiway.com/spinabifida

Dermatology Online Atlas
http://www.rrze.uni-erlangen.de/docs/FAU/fakultaet/med/kli/derma/bilddb/db.hm
This site has excellent pictures of a variety of dermatologic conditions.

Cedars Sinai Medical Center in Los Angeles
http://www.csmc.edu/neonatology/neo.links.html
This site is one of the best maintained neonatology sites with multiple linkages to other sites of interest to those caring for infants.

Johns Hopkins and Marshall University Departments of Pediatrics
http://www.med.jhu.edu/peds/neonatology/poi2.html
This is an excellent site with information on infants and children for parents and caregivers.

Academy of Pediatrics
http://www.aap.org

Online Mendelian Inheritance in Man (OMIN), National Center for Medical Genetics, Johns Hopkins University
http://www3.ncbi.nlm.nib.gov/Omim/symbol.html

Pediatrics Information Index from the University of Alabama
http://www.uab.edu/pedinfo

REFERENCES

1. De Ville KA: Internet list servers and pediatrics: Newly emerging legal and clinical practice issues: II. Pediatrics 98(3, Pt 1):453–454, 1996.
2. Elliott SJ, Elliott RG: Internet list servers and pediatrics: Newly emerging legal and clinical practice issues: I. Pediatrics 97(3):399–400, 1996.
3. Roberts JR, Spooner A: Pediatric Internet resources: Creation and growth of the PEDINFO index. Arch Pediatr Adolesc Med 151:592–597, 1997.
4. Sikorski R, Peters R: Internet anatomy 101: Accessing information on the World Wide Web. JAMA 277(2):171–172, 1997.
5. Sikorski R, Peters R: Medical literature made easy: Querying databases on the Internet. JAMA 26:277(12):959–960, 1997.

Recommended Childhood Immunization Schedule
United States, January - December 1998

Vaccines[1] are listed under the routinely recommended ages. ⬚Bars⬚ *indicate range of acceptable ages for immunization. Catch-up immunization should be done during any visit when feasible. Shaded* ⬭ovals⬭ *indicate vaccines to be assessed and given if necessary during the early adolescent visit.*

Age ▶ Vaccine ▼	Birth	1 mo	2 mos	4 mos	6 mos	12 mos	15 mos	18 mos	4-6 yrs	11-12 yrs	14-16 yrs
Hepatitis B[2,3]	Hep B-1										
			Hep B-2		Hep B-3					Hep B	
Diphtheria, Tetanus, Pertussis[4]			DTaP or DTP	DTaP or DTP	DTaP or DTP		DTaP or DTP[4]		DTaP or DTP	Td	
***H influenzae* type b**[5]			Hib	Hib	Hib	Hib					
Polio[6]			Polio[6]	Polio	Polio[6]				Polio		
Measles, Mumps, Rubella[7]						MMR			MMR[7]	MMR	
Varicella[8]						Var				Var	

Approved by the Advisory Committee on Immunization Practices (ACIP), the American Academy of Pediatrics (AAP), and the American Academy of Family Physicians (AAFP).

[1] This schedule indicates the recommended age for routine administration of currently licensed childhood vaccines. Some combination vaccines are available and may be used whenever administration of all components of the vaccine is indicated. Providers should consult the manufacturers' package inserts for detailed recommendations.

[2] *Infants born to HBsAg-negative mothers* should receive 2.5 µg of Merck vaccine (Recombivax HB) or 10 µg of SmithKline Beecham (SB) vaccine (Engerix-B). The 2nd dose should be administered at least 1 mo after the 1st dose. The 3rd dose should be given at least 2 mos after the second, but not before 6 mos of age.
Infants born to HBsAg-positive mothers should receive 0.5 mL of hepatitis B immune globulin (HBIG) within 12 hrs of birth, and either 5 µg of Merck vaccine (Recombivax HB) or 10 µg of SB vaccine (Engerix-B) at a separate site. The 2nd dose is recommended at 1-2 mos of age and the 3rd dose at 6 mos of age.
Infants born to mothers whose HBsAg status is unknown should receive either 5 µg of Merck vaccine (Recombivax HB) or 10 µg of SB vaccine (Engerix-B) within 12 hrs of birth. The 2nd dose of vaccine is recommended at 1 mo of age and the 3rd dose at 6 mos of age. Blood should be drawn at the time of delivery to determine the mother's HBsAg status; if it is positive, the infant should receive HBIG as soon as possible (no later than 1 wk of age). The dosage and timing of subsequent vaccine doses should be based upon the mother's HBsAg status.

[3] Children and adolescents who have not been vaccinated against hepatitis B in infancy may begin the series during any visit. Those who have not previously received 3 doses of hepatitis B vaccine should initiate or complete the series during the 11 to 12-year-old visit, and unvaccinated older adolescents should be vaccinated whenever possible. The 2nd dose should be administered at least 1 mo after the 1st dose, and the 3rd dose should be administered at least 4 mos after the 1st dose and at least 2 mos after the 2nd dose.

[4] DTaP (diphtheria and tetanus toxoids and acellular pertussis vaccine) is the preferred vaccine for all doses in the vaccination series, including completion of the series in children who have received 1 or more doses of whole-cell DTP vaccine. Whole-cell DTP is an acceptable alternative to DTaP. The 4th dose (DTP or DTaP) may be administered as early as 12 mos of age, provided 6 mos have elapsed since the 3rd dose and if the child is unlikely to return at age 15-18 mos. Td (tetanus and diphtheria toxoids) is recommended at 11-12 years of age if at least 5 years have elapsed since the last dose of DTP, DTaP or DT. Subsequent routine Td boosters are recommended every 10 years.

[5] Three *H influenzae* type b (Hib) conjugate vaccines are licensed for infant use. If PRP-OMP (PedvaxHIB [Merck]) is administered at 2 and 4 mos of age, a dose at 6 mos is not required.

[6] Two poliovirus vaccines are currently licensed in the US: inactivated poliovirus vaccine (IPV) and oral poliovirus vaccine (OPV). The following schedules are all acceptable to the ACIP, the AAP, and the AAFP. Parents and providers may choose among these options.
    1)   2 doses of IPV followed by 2 doses of OPV.
    2)   4 doses of IPV.
    3)   4 doses of OPV.
The ACIP recommends 2 doses of IPV at 2 and 4 mos of age followed by 2 doses of OPV at 12-18 mos and 4-6 years of age. IPV is the only poliovirus vaccine recommended for immunocompromised persons and their household contacts.

[7] The 2nd dose of MMR is recommended routinely at 4-6 yrs of age but may be administered during any visit, provided at least 1 mo has elapsed since receipt of the 1st dose and that both doses are administered beginning at or after 12 mos of age. Those who have not previously received the second dose should complete the schedule no later than the 11 to 12-year visit.

[8] Susceptible children may receive varicella vaccine (Var) at any visit after the first birthday, and those who lack a reliable history of chickenpox should be immunized during the 11-12-year-old visit. Susceptible children 13 years of age or older should receive 2 doses, at least 1 month apart.

INDEX

Note: Page numbers in *italics* refer to illustrations; page numbers followed by t refer to tables.

ISBN 0-7216-5751-6